MW01156745

T

U

V

W

PFENNINGER & FOWLER'S

Procedures for Primary Care

THIRD EDITION

Edited by

John L. Pfenninger, MD
President and Director, Medical Procedures Center, PC
Private Practice
Midland, Michigan
Senior Consultant and Founder
National Procedures Institute
Austin, Texas
Clinical Professor
Michigan State University College of Human Medicine
East Lansing, Michigan

Grant C. Fowler, MD
Professor and Vice Chair
Department of Family and Community Medicine
University of Texas Medical School at Houston
Houston, Texas

ELSEVIER
MOSBY

ELSEVIER
MOSBY

1600 John F. Kennedy Blvd
Ste. 1800
Philadelphia, PA 19103-2899

PFENNINGER & FOWLER'S PROCEDURES FOR PRIMARY CARE IBSN: 978-0-323-05267-2
THIRD EDITION

Notices

Knowledge and best practice in this field are constantly changing. As new research and experience broaden our understanding, changes in research methods, professional practices, or medical treatment may become necessary.

Practitioners and researchers must always rely on their own experience and knowledge in evaluating and using any information, methods, compounds, or experiments described herein. In using such information or methods they should be mindful of their own safety and the safety of others, including parties for whom they have a professional responsibility.

With respect to any drug or pharmaceutical products identified, readers are advised to check the most current information provided (i) on procedures featured or (ii) by the manufacturer of each product to be administered, to verify the recommended dose or formula, the method and duration of administration, and contraindications. It is the responsibility of practitioners, relying on their own experience and knowledge of their patients, to make diagnoses, to determine dosages and the best treatment for each individual patient, and to take all appropriate safety precautions.

To the fullest extent of the law, neither the Publisher nor the authors, contributors, or editors, assume any liability for any injury and/or damage to persons or property as a matter of products liability, negligence or otherwise, or from any use or operation of any methods, products, instructions, or ideas contained in the material herein.

Library of Congress Cataloging-in-Publication Data

Pfenninger and Fowler's procedures for primary care / edited by John L. Pfenninger, Grant C. Fowler.—3rd ed.
p. ; cm.
Other title: Procedures for primary care
Includes bibliographical references and index.
ISBN 978-0-323-05267-2
1. Primary care (Medicine) 2. Surgery, minor. I. Pfenninger, John L. II. Fowler, Grant C. III. Title: Procedures for primary care.
[DNLM: 1. Primary Health Care—methods. 2. Diagnostic Techniques and Procedures. 3. Surgical Procedures, Operative—methods. W 84.61 P528 2010]
RC48.P76 2010
616–dc22

2010008159

Acquisitions Editor: Kate Dimock
Developmental Editor: Julie Mirra
Publishing Services Manager: Pat Joiner-Myers
Project Manager: Joy Moore
Design Direction: Ellen Zanolle
Marketing Manager: Tracie Pasker

Printed in China

Last digit is the print number: 9 8 7 6 5 4

The first edition of this text was dedicated to my family. Grandma Rose helped awaken my curiosity in medicine and my parents supported it. My wife Kay and my children, Stacey, Matthew, and Dana provided the encouragement that was needed to persist and complete the book itself.

The second edition was dedicated to all my colleagues in family practice here in Midland who were so gracious in covering call for me during my travels and while writing.

As this third edition is published, medicine is in turmoil. We are trying to find direction. Our care is being driven by evidence-based medicine. A cost-effective approach to provide that care is of paramount importance. Finding a way to enable care for all and determining methods to support the aging population have gained center stage importance. With this in mind, this third edition is dedicated then to my two grandsons, Daniel and Ryan Maura. They are the future. They and their generation will need to pull and mold the best of the past to create a new world of healthcare to address these issues. It is for them that we strive to do our best. It will take their best to allow us to continue to provide the highest quality of medical care in the world.

John L. Pfenninger, MD

As they should be, the first and second editions were dedicated to our families, friends, and colleagues. They both inspired and tolerated us through this process, again and again. Likewise, this edition is dedicated to them.

This edition is also dedicated to primary care clinicians everywhere who have endured practicing in our current healthcare system; all of us know what that means and it has not always been nurturing and supportive. As we continue to endure, adapt, and persevere, this book is dedicated to those who continue to do the right thing, what's best for our patients, their families, our profession, and the healthcare system. Even though future healthcare systems are likely to be more complicated, new technologies and procedures will evolve that can keep it fun and exciting. And my prediction persists that patient outcomes and satisfaction as well as healthcare systems will be enhanced when as many procedures as possible are provided by primary care clinicians.

Grant C. Fowler, MD

CONTRIBUTORS

Suraj Achar, MD
Associate Clinical Professor, Associate Director of Sports Medicine, University of California–San Diego, San Diego, CA

Christopher F. Adams, MD, MBA
Fellow of Sports Medicine, University of Missouri–Kansas City, Kansas City, MO

Olasunkanmi W. Adeyinka, MD
Assistant Professor, Department of Family and Community Medicine, University of Texas Medical School at Houston; Medical Director, UT Physicians–Family Medicine, Houston, TX

Scott Akin, MD
Medical Staff, Contra Costa Regional Medical Center, Martinez, CA

Haneef Alibhai, MD, CM, CCFP, FCFP
Medical Director, MD Cosmetic & Laser Clinic, Abbotsford, Vancouver, BC, Canada

Philip J. Aliotta, MD, MSHA, FACS, CPI
Chief of Urology, Sisters of Charity Hospitals; Attending, Department of Urology, School of Biomedical Sciences and Medicine, SUNY–Buffalo; Attending and Director of Pelvic Floor Disorders and Neurogenic Bladder, Jacobs Neurologic Institute, Buffalo General Hosptial, Buffalo, NY; Instructor of Urology, New York Osteopathic Medicine, New York, NY; Instructor of Urology Lake Erie College of Osteopathic Medicine, Erie, PA

Michael A. Altman, MD
Associate Professor, Department of Family and Community Medicine, University of Texas Medical School at Houston, Houston, TX

Gerald A. Amundsen, MD
Faculty, Great Plains Family Medicine Residency, Oklahoma City; Physician, Mustang Family Practice, Mustang, OK

John J. Andazola, MD
Program Director, The Southern New Mexico Family Medicine Residency Program, Las Cruces, NM

Fatih Arikan, DDS, PhD
Associate Professor, Department of Periodontology, Ege University School of Dentistry, Bornova, Izmir, Turkey

K.M.R. Arnold, MD
Assistant Clinical Professor, Department of Family Medicine, University of Indiana, Indianapolis, IN

Darrin Ashbrooks, MD
Department of Family Medicine, University of Arkansas for Medical Science AHEC–Southwest, Texarkana, AR; Department of Sports Medicine, University of Kansas City–Missouri School of Medicine, Kansas City, MO

Barry Auster, MD
Clinical Instuctor of Dermatology, Michigan State University, East Lansing; Chair of Dermatology, Sinai-Grace, Detroit; Department of Dermatology, William Beaumont Hospital, Royal Oak, MI

Dennis E. Babel, PhD, HCLD (ABB)
Laboratory Director, Mycology Consultants Laboratory, Holland, MI

Thad J. Barkdull, MD, FAAFP, CAQSM
Clinical Assistant Professor, Department of Family Medicine, John A. Burns School of Medicine, University of Hawaii; Director of Sports Medicine, Family Medicine Residency, Tripler Army Medical Center, Honolulu, HI

Andy S. Barnett, MD
Clinical Instructor, Department of Family Medicine, University of Washington and Madigan Army Medical Center, Tacoma; Staff Physician, Department of Emergency Medicine, Jefferson General Hospital, Port Townsend, WA

Rebecca Beach, MD
Residency Faculty, Mercy Health System Family Medicine Residency; Family Physician, Mercy Clinic South, Janesville, WI; Clinical Assistant Professor, University of Wisconsin–Madison, Madison, WI

Jennifer Bell, MD
Clinical Instructor, Departments of Family and Preventive Medicine, University of Utah, Salt Lake City, UT

J. Michael Berry, MD
Associate Clinical Professor of Medicine, Division of Hematology–Oncology, University of California–San Francisco; Associate Director of HPV–Related Clinical Studies, UCSF Helen Diller Family Comprehensive Cancer Center, San Francisco, CA

Christopher J. Bigelow, MD
Ophthalmologist, MidMichigan Medical Center, Midland, MI

Lee I. Blecher, MD
Assistant Clinical Professor of Family Medicine, Virginia Commonwealth University School of Medicine; Fairfax Family Medicine, Fairfax, VA

David T. Bortel, MD, ABOS
Staff Orthopedic Surgeon–Joint Replacements, MidMichigan Medical Center, Midland, MI

David B. Bosscher, DO, FAAFP
Staff, Allegan General Hospital, Allegan, MI

Jamie Broomfield, MD
Associate Professor, University of Wyoming Family Medicine Residency Program at Cheyenne, Cheyenne, WY

Gregory L. Brotzman, MD
Professor of Family and Community Medicine, Medical College of Wisconsin, Milwaukee, WI

Mary Beth Brown, PT, ATC, PhD
Postdoctoral Fellow, Pulmonary and Critical Care, Department of Medicine, Indiana University School of Medicine, Indianapolis, IN

Gregory A. Buford, MD, FACS
Board Certified Plastic Surgeon; Fellowship Trained Cosmetic Surgeon; Founder and Medical Director, Beauty by Buford, Englewood, CO

Richard Castillo, DO, OD
Clinical Professor, College of Optometry, Northeastern State University; Ophthalmologist, Tahlequah City Hospital, Tahlequah, OK

Jonathan Chan, DO
Associate Physician, Department of Family Medicine, Kaiser Permanente, Southern California Permanente Medical Group, San Diego, CA

Marisha Chilcott, MD
Staff Physician, Contra Costa Regional Medical Center, Martinez, CA; Santa Rosa Memorial Hospital, Santa Rosa, CA

Beth A. Choby, MD, FAAFP
Assistant Professor, Department of Family Medicine, University of Tennessee–Chattanooga, Chattanooga, TN

Ashley Christiani, MD
Adjunct Clinical Professor, University of California–San Francisco School of Medicine, San Francisco; Adjunct Clinical Professor, College of Osteopathic Medicine, Touro University; Senior Physician, The Permanente Medical Group–Kaiser Vallejo Hospital, Vallejo, CA

Wendy C. Coates, MD
Professor of Medicine and Chair of Acute Care College, UCLA Geffen School of Medicine, Los Angeles; Director of Medical Education, Department of Emergency Medicine, Harbor–UCLA Medical Center, Torrance, CA

Andrew S. Coco, MD, MS
Assistant Clinical Professor of Family Medicine, Temple University Medical School, Philadelphia; Associate Director, Family Medicine Residency, Lancaster General Hospital; Medical Director, Louise von Hess Medical Research Institute at Lancaster General Hospital, Lancaster, PA

Gregory Costello, MD
Medical Director, RejuviSkin Medical Spa, Verona, NJ

Kevin Crawford, RN, PA, FNP
Owner/Director, Arizona Laser Skin Solutions, Tempe, AZ

Jacob Curtis, DO
Adjunct Assistant Professor of Primary Care, Department of Family Medicine, A.T. Sill University of Health Sciences, Kirksville, MI; Family Physician, Department of Family Medicine, Franklin County Medical Center, Preston, ID; Adjunct Assistant Professor of Primary Care, Department of Family Medicine, Touro University, Nevada College of Osteopathic Medicine, Las Vegas, NV

Paul W. Davis, MD
Associate Clinical Professor of Family Medicine, University of Washington School of Medicine, Seattle, WA; Director of GI Endoscopy, Kanakanak Hospital, Bristol Bay Area Health Corporation, Dilliningham, AK

Jeffrey R. Dell, MD, FACOG, FACS
Director, Urogynecology and Reconstructive Pelvic Surgery, Institute for Female Pelvic Medicine, Knoxville, TN

Daniel J. Derksen, MD
Professor, Department of Family and Community Medicine, University of New Mexico School of Medicine, Albuquerque, NM

Carlos A. Dumas, MD
Staff Physician, UT Physicians, Family Practice, Houston, TX

Scott W. Eathorne, MD
Medical Director, Providence Athletic Medicine, Providence Hospital, Southfield, MI

John Eckhold, MD
Staff Physician, Department of Orthopedics, MidMichigan Medical Center, Midland, MI

Steven H. Eisinger, MD, FACOG
Clincal Professor of Family Medicine and Obsetrics and Gynecology, University of Rochester School of Medicine and Dentistry, Rochester, NY

William Ellert, MD, MSN
Clinical Associate Professor, University of Arizona College of Medicine; Chief Medical Officer, Phoenix Baptist Hospital, Phoenix, AZ

Mel Elson, AB, MD
Director, Longevity Institute, LLC; CEO, Global Cosmeceutical Innovations, LLC, Nashville, TN

William Jackson Epperson, MD, MBA
Director, Inlet Medical Associates, PA, Murrells Inlet, SC

Joe Esherick, MD, FAAFP
Clinical Assistant Professor of Family Medicine, UCLA School of Medicine, Los Angeles; Associate Director of Inpatient Medical Services, Ventura County Medical Center, Ventura, CA; Instructor of Hospitalist Procedures Course, National Procedures Institute, Midland, MI

Azadeh Esmaeili, MD
Health Science Center, SUNY–Stony Brook, Stony Brook, NY

Linda Fanelli, RNC, RDMS
Registered Diagnostic Medical Sonographer, Covenant Medical Center, Saginaw, MI

Steven Fettinger, MD, FACOG, FACS
Associate Clinical Professor, College of Human Medicine and Behavioral Sciences, Michigan State University, East Lansing; Attending Physician at Covenant Medical Center and St. Mary's Medical Center, Saginaw, MI

Jeremy Fish, MD
Assistant Clinical Professor, Department of Community and Family Medicine, University of California–Davis; Residency Director, Contra Costa Family Medicine Residency Program, Martinez, CA

David Flinders, MD
Adjunct Assistant Professor, University of Utah College of Medicine, Salt Lake City; Assistant Residency Director, Utah Valley Family Medicine Residency, Provo, UT

Stuart Forman, MD
Attending Physician; Medical Director, Critical Care Unit, Contra Costa Regional Medical Center, Martinez, CA

Grant C. Fowler, MD
Professor and Vice Chair, Department of Family and Community Medicine, University of Texas Medical School at Houston, Houston, TX

Dan B. French, MD
Cleveland Clinic, Cleveland, OH

Roberta E. Gebhard, DO
Assistant Clinical Professor, SUNY–Buffalo, Buffalo, NY

Jeffrey A. German, MD
Associate Professor of Clinical Family Medicine, Louisiana State University Health Sciences Center, Shreveport, LA

Vincent C. Giampapa, MD, FACS
Assistant Clinical Professor, Department of Plastic and Reconstructive Surgery, University of Medicine and Dentistry of New Jersey, Newark; Attending Physician, Department of Plastic Surgery, Hackensack University Medical Center, Hackensack, NJ

Rebecca H. Gladu, MD
Clinical Associate Professor of Family Medicine, Baylor College of Medicine, Houston; Associate Director, San Jacinto Methodist Family Medicine Residency, Baytown, TX

Emily Godfrey, MD, MPH
Assistant Professor of Family Medicine and of Community Health Sciences, University of Illinois–Chicago College of Medicine and School of Public Health; Stroger Hospital of Cook County, Chicago, IL

Mitchel P. Goldman, MD
Volunteer Clinical Professor of Dermatology/Medicine, University of California–San Diego, San Diego, CA

Dolores M. Gomez, MD
Assistant Director, Advanced Hospital Training Fellowship for Family Physicians, Maricopa Integrated Health Systems, Phoenix, AZ

Jennifer L. Good, MD
Associate Director, Altoona Family Physicians Family Medicine Residency, Altoona; Clinical Assistant Professor of Family and Community Medicine, Milton S. Hershey Medical School, Penn State University, Hershey, PA

Ian M. Gralnek MD, MSHS, FASGE
Associate Professor of Medicine, Rappaport Faculty of Medicine, Technion-Israel Institute of Technology; Chief, Hospital-wide Ambulatory Care Services; Senior Physician, Department of Gastroenterology; Rambam Health Care Campus, Haifa, Israel

Lee A. Green, MD, MPH
Professor of Family Medicine, University of Michigan, Ann Arbor, MI

Maury J. Greenberg, MD, CAPT, MC, USPHS
Adjunct Associate Professor of Family Medicine, Uniformed Services University of the Health Sciences, Bethesda, MD; Clinical Associate Professor of Family Medicine, Stony Brook University School of Medicine, Stony Brook, NY

Peter W. Grigg, MD
Colorado Springs, CO

Stephen A. Grochmal, MD
Associate Clinical Professor, Division of Minimally Invasive Surgery; Adjunct Faculty, Department of Obstetrics and Gynecology, Howard University College of Medicine, Washington, DC; Medical Director, Center for Minimally Invasive Gynecologic Surgery and Cosmetic Gynecology, Paramus, NJ

Mark S. Grubb, MD
Associate Clinical Professor of Pediatrics, University of Washington, Seattle; Clinical Staff, Good Samaritan Hospital, Puyallup, WA

Sylvana Guidotti, MD, FACEP
Director of Emergency Department, Ventura County Medical Center, Ventura, CA

Ali Gürkan, DDS, PhD
Assistant Professor, Department of Periodontology, Ege University School of Dentistry, Bornova, Izmir, Turkey

Patrick J. Haddad, JD
Member, Kerr, Russell and Weber, PLC, Detroit, MI

Kim Haglund, MD
Staff Physician, Departments of Family Medicine and Surgery, Contra Costa Regional Medical Center, Martinez, CA

Basil M. Hantash, MD, PhD
Chair, Elixir Institute for Regenerative Medicine, San Jose, CA

Michael B. Harper, MD
Professor of Family Medicine, Louisiana State University Health Sciences Center, Shreveport, LA

George D. Harris, MD
Professor of Medicine, Department of Community and Family Medicine; Assistant Dean, Year 1 and 2 Medicine, University of Missouri–Kansas City School of Medicine; Medical Staff, Truman Medical Center–Lakewood, Kansas City, MO

Andrew Thomas Haynes, MD
Private practice, Bossier, LA

John Harlan Haynes III, MD, MSc, CPE
Assistant Professor, Department of Family and Community Medicine, University of Texas Southwestern Medical Center, Dallas; Department of Family Medicine, John Peter Smith Hospital, Fort Worth; Adjunct Assistant Professor, Department of Medical Education, University of North Texas Health Science Center–Fort Worth; Senior Vice President and Medical Director, JPS Health Network, Fort Worth, TX

Yves Hébert, MD
President, Canadian Association of Aesthetic Medicine, Vancouver, British Columbia, Canada

Harold H. Hedges III, MD
Associate Clinical Professor, Department of Community and Family Medicine, University of Arkansas School of Medicine; Staff, Arkansas Baptist and St. Vincent Hospitals, Little Rock, AR

Scott T. Henderson, MD
Program Director, Mercy Family Medicine Residency, Mercy Medical Center–North Iowa, Mason City, IA

John Hill, DO
Professor of Family Medicine and Sports Medicine; Director of Primary Care Sports Medicine, University of Colorado Health Sciences Center, Denver, CO

Terrance S. Hines, MD
Clinical Assistant Professor, Department of Family and Community Medicine, Texas A&M University System Health Science Center College of Medicine, Round Rock; Senior Staff Physician, Department of Family and Community Medicine, Scott & White Healthcare, Cedar Park West Clinic, Taylor, TX

John R. Holman, MD, MPH
Officer in Charge, Naval Branch Clinic, Bridgeport, CA

Thomas E. Howard, MD
Clinical Instructor, Department of Family Practice, University of Minnesota–Duluth School of Medicine, Duluth; Staff, Department of Family Practice and Emergency Medicine, Deer River Health Care Center, Deer River, MN

Karl S. Hubach, MD, RVT
Inlet Vein Specialists, PC, Murrells Inlet, SC

Eric M. Hughes, MD
Physician, Austin Regional Clinic, Austin, TX

James L. Jackson, MD, FACS
MidMichigan Medical Center–Midland, Midland, MI

Marjon B. Jahromi, DDS
Assistant Professor, Department of Dental Anesthesiology, Loma Linda University School of Dentristry; Attending Anesthesiologist, Special Care Dentistry Clinic, Loma Linda University, Loma Linda, CA

David James, MD, FCFP(EM)
Clinical Associate Professor, SUNY–Buffalo School of Medicine and Biomedical Sciences; Director, Emergency Department, Millard Fillmore Gates Circle Hospital, Attending Physician, Emergency Department, Valeida Health System, Buffalo, NY; Attending Physician, Emergency Department, Niagara Health System, Welland, Ontario, Canada

Robert E. James, MD
Urologist, Sutter Pacific Medical Foundation; Sutter Medical Group of the Redwoods; Sutter Medical Center of Santa Rosa; Santa Rosa, CA

Raymond F. Jarris, Jr., MD
Medical Director, Emergency Department; Assistant Chief, Emergency Medicine, Swedish Medical Center/Ballard, Seattle, WA

Naomi Jay, RN, PhD
Nurse Practioner, Dysplasia Clinic, University of California–San Francisco, San Francisco, CA

Robert L. Kalb, MD
Associate Professor, Medical College of Ohio; St. Anne Hospital, Toledo, OH

Bernard Katz, MD
Co-Chief Executive Officer, Santa Monica Bay Physicians Health Services, Inc., Santa Monica, CA

Barbara F. Kelly, MD
Associate Professor, Department of Family Medicine, University of Colorado–Denver; Medical Director, A.F. Williams Family Medicine Center, Denver, CO

Morteza Khodaee, MD, MPH
Assistant Professor, Department of Family Medicine, University of Colorado–Denver School of Medicine, Denver, CO

Yong Sik Kim, MD, PhD
Assistant Professor, Baylor College of Medicine; Green Health Clinic, Houston, TX

Thomas A. Kintanar, MD
Clinical Associate Professor, Department of Medicine, Indiana University School of Medicine; Director of Medical Education, St. Joseph Hospital, Fort Wayne, IN

Karyn B. Kolman, MD
Faculty, Maricopa Medical Center, Phoenix, AZ

Donna A. Landen, MD
Assistant Professor, Department of Family and Community Medicine, University of Alabama–Birmingham, Birmingham, AL

Dennis LaRavia, MD, FAAFP
Medical Director, Rayburn Correctional Center, Angie, LA; Director, Occupational Health, Temple-Inland Paper Co., Bogalusa, LA

Mark Lavallee, MD, CSCS, FACSM
Assistant Clinical Professor, Indiana University–South Bend School of Medicine; Co-Director, South Bend Sports Medicine Fellowship; Head Team Physician at Indiana University–South Bend and Holy Cross College, South Bend, IN; Co-Chair, Sports Medicine Committee USA Weightlifing, Colorado Springs, CO

Lawrence Leeman, MD, MPH
Associate Professor of Family and Community Medicine and Obstetrics and Gynecology, University of New Mexico School of Medicine; Director of Family Medicine, Maternal and Child Health; Co-Medical Director, Mother-Baby Unit, University of New Mexico Hospital, Albuquerque, NM

Ruth Lesnewki, MD
Medical Director, Department of Family Medicine, East 13th Street Family Practice, New York, NY

Madeline R. Lewis, DO, MS
Associate Director, Memorial Hospital Family Medicine Residency; Clinic Director, E.B. Warner Family Medicine Clinic, South Bend, IN

Mark Lewis, MD

Sandy T. Liu, BS
Medical Student, George Washington University School of Medicine, Washington, DC

Benjamin Mailloux, MD
Private practice; Waldo County General Hospital, Belfast, ME

Ashfaq A. Marghoob, MD
Associate Professor, SUNY–Stony Brook, Stony Brook, NY; Associate Member, Memorial Sloan Kettering Cancer Center, Hauppauge, NY

Gregory A. Marolf, MD
Assistant Clinical Director, Sports Medicine Fellowship, Bayfront Medical Center Family Practice Residency; Physician, Bayfront Convenient Care Clinics, St. Petersburg, FL

Coral D. Matus, MD
Associate Director, The Toledo Hospital Family Medicine Residency Program, Toledo, OH

William L. McDaniel, Jr., MD
Retired Clinical Associate Professor of Community Science Program, Department of Family Practice, Mercer University School of Medicine, Macon; Staff Physician, Department of Family Practice, Hamilton Medical Center, Dalton, GA (Whitfield)

Michael McHenry, MA, PA-C
Physician Assistant, Family Medicine Associates, Midland, MI

Greta McLaren, MD
Assistant Professor, University of Colorado Health Sciences Center; Medical Director, RenewSkin Clinic, Denver, CO

James W. McNabb, MD
Adjunct Associate Professor, Department of Family Medicine; Distinguished Teaching Professor of Medical Acupuncture, University of North Carolina School of Medicine, Chapel Hill; Family Physician, Full Circle Family Medicine of Piedmont HealthCare, Mooresville, NC

John M. McShane, MD
Assistant Clinical Professor, Departmet of Family Medicine, Jefferson Medical College, Philadelphia; President, McShane Sports Medicine, Villanova, PA

Thomas H. Mitchell, RRT
Director Cardiorespiratory Services, Truman Medical Center Lakewood, Kansas City, MO

Harris Mones, DO
Associate Professor, University of Osteopathic Medicine and Health Sciences, Des Moines, IA; Adjunct Clinical Associate Professor, Lake Erie College of Osteopathic Medicine, Bradenton; Associate Professor, NOVA Southeastern College of Osteopathic Medicine, Ft. Lauderdale; Director of Medicial Education, Westchester General Hospital, Miami, FL

Rolf O. Montalvo, MD
Assistant Professor and Residency Program Director, Department of Family and Community Medicine, University of Texas Medical School at Houston; Staff Physician, Department of Family and Community Medicine, Memorial Hermann Hospital Texas Medical Center and Lyndon B. Johnson General Hospital Houston, TX

Carlos A. Moreno, MD, MSPH
Professor and Chair, Department of Family and Community Medicine, University of Texas Medical School at Houston; Chief of Family Medicine, Memorial Hermann Hospital–TMC, Houston, TX

Mark Needham, MD
Co-Chief Executive Officer, Santa Monica Bay Physicians Health Services, Inc., Santa Monica, CA

Gary R. Newkirk, MD
Clinical Professor of Family Medicine, University of Washington School of Medicine; Residency Director, Family Medicine Spokane Residencies, Spokane, WA

Mary Jane Newkirk, MS, CCC-SLP
Speech-Language Pathologist, Spokane Public Schools, Spokane, WA

Jerry Ninia, MD, RVT, FACOG, FACS
Clinical Associate Professor, SUNY–Stony Brook School of Medicine, Stony Brook, NY; Director of Obstetrics and Gynecology, St. Charles Hosptial, Port Jefferson, NY

John O'Brien, MD
Associate Professor, Department of Family Medicine, Univeristy of Michigan Medical School, Ann Arbor, MI

Theodore O'Connell, MD
Clinical Instructor, David Geffen School of Medicine at UCLA, Los Angeles; Residency Program Director, Kaiser Permanente Woodland Hills, Woodland Hills, CA

Francis G. O'Connor, MD, MPH
Medical Director, Consortium for Health and Military Performance, Military and Emergency Medicine, Uniformed Services University of the Health Sciences, Bethesda, MD

Kathleen M. O'Hanlon, MD
Professor, Department of Family and Community Health, Marshall University School of Medicine, Huntington, WV

Carol Osborn, MD
Adjunct Professor, Deptartment of Family Practice Medicine, University of Utah Health Sciences Center; Staff Physician, Department of Family Practice Intermountain Healthcare, Salt Lake City, UT

Lori Oswald, PA-C
Physician Assistant, Medical Procedures Center, Midland, MI

Gary Page, MD
Medical Officer, Parker Indian Hospital, Parker, AZ

James R. Palleschi MD
Urologist, Sutter Medical Network; Sutter Pacific Medical Foundation; Sutter Medical Group of the Redwoods; Sutter Medical Center of Santa Rosa, Santa Rosa, CA

Scott A. Paluska, MD, FACSM
Clinical Associate Professor, University of Illinois–Urbana; Medical Director, OAK Orthopedics, Urbana, IL

Helen A. Pass, MD
Assistant Professor of Clinical Surgery, Columbia University College of Physicians and Surgeons, New York, NY

Dale A. Patterson, MD, FAAFP
Program Director, Memorial Hospital Family Medicine Residency, South Bend, IN

Mike Petrizzi, MD
Clinical Professor, Department of Family Medicine, Virginia Commonwealth University/Medical College of Virginia, Richmond; Medical Director, Hanover Family Physicians, Mechanicsville, VA

John L. Pfenninger, MD, FAAFP
President and Director, Medical Procedures Center, PC; Private practice, Midland, MI; Senior Consultant and Founder, National Procedures Institute, Austin, TX; Clinical Professor, Michigan State University College of Human Medicine, East Lansing, MI

Madelyn Pollock, MD
Medical Director, Executive Health Resources, Inc., Newtown Square, PA

John Bartels Pope, MD
Professor of Clinical Family Medicine, Louisiana State University Health Sciences Center, Shreveport, LA

Linda Prine, MD
Associate Clinical Professor of Family Medicine, Albert Einstein College of Medicine; Faculty, Beth Israel Residency in Urban Family Practice, New York, NY

Kalyanakrishnan Ramakrishnan, MD, FRCS
Professor, Department of Family and Preventative Medicine, University of Oklahoma Health Sciences Center, Oklahoma City, OK

Oscar Ramirez, MD, FACS
Clincal Faculty at Cleveland Clinic–Florida; Private practice, Sanctuary Plastic Surgery, Boca Raton, FL

Renae Rasmussen CRNA, APRN, CL
Anesthesia section, Bigfork Valley Hospital, Bigfork, MN

Stephen D. Ratcliffe, MD, MSPH
Program Director, Lancaster General Hospital Family Medicine Residency, Lancaster, PA

Duren Michael Ready, MD
Assistant Professor, Departments of Family and Community Medicine and Medical Humanities, Texas A&M University Health Science Center College of Medicine; Director, Headache Clinic, Department of Neurology, Scott and White Memorial Hospital and Clinic, Temple, TX

Bal Reddy, MD
Assistant Professor of Clinical Family Medicine, Predoctoral Director, Department of Family and Community Medicine, The University of Texas Medical School at Houston; UT Physicians–Family Medicine Center, Houston, TX

Sumana Reddy, MD, FAAFP
Founder, Acacia Family Medical Group, Salinas; District Director, California Academy of Family Physicians, San Francisco, CA

Peter L. Reynolds, MD
Assistant Professor, Saint Louis University Family Medicine Residency Program, Belleville, IL

Ronald D. Reynolds, MD, FAAFP
Professor of Family Medicine, University of Cincinnati College of Medicine, Cincinnati; Medical Leader, HealthSource–New Richmond Family Practice, New Richmond, OH

Terry Reynolds, BS, RDCS
School of Cardiac Ultrasound, Arizona Heart Foundation, Phoenix, AZ

David Roden, MD
Attending Otolayrngologist, MidMichigan Medical Center, Midland, MI

J.R. MacMillan Rodney, MD
Surgical Resident, Cornell University Medical College, New York, NY

Wm. MacMillan Rodney, MD
Adjunct Professor of Family Medicine, Meharry Medical College, Nashville; Professor and Chair, Medicos para la Familia, Intl., Memphis, TN

Montiel T. Rosenthal, MD
Associate Clinical Professor, Department of Family and Community Medicine, University of Cincinnati College of Medicine; Director, Prenatal Clinic, The Christ Hospital; Director, Family Medicine, Cincinnati Children's Hospital Medical Center; Attending Physcian, Good Samaritan Hospital, Cincinnati, OH

Steven E. Roskos, MD
Associate Professor, Department of Family Medicine, College of Human Medicine, Michigan State University, East Lansing, MI

Scott F. Ross, MD
Family Practicioner, Department of Family Medicine, MidMichigan Medical Center, Midland, MI

Matt D. Roth, MD
Family and Sports Medicine, Promedica Physician Group, Maumee OH

Terry S. Ruhl, MD
Associate Program Director, Altoona Family Physicians Residency, Altoona; Clinical Assistant Professor, Department of Family and Community Medicine, Penn State College of Medicine, Hershey, PA

Edmund S. Sabanegh, Jr., MD
Associate Professor and Chair, Department of Urology, The Cleveland Clinic Lerner College of Medicine, Case Western Reserve University; Director, Center for Male Infertility, Cleveland Clinic Foundation, Cleveland, OH

Robert Salinas, MD
Associate Professor, Department of Family and Preventive Medicine, University of Oklahoma Health Sciences Center, Oklahoma City, OK

Scott Savage, DO, FACEP, FSCP, FACHE, FAPWCA, CCHP, CHCQM
Associate Professor of Aerospace Medicine, University of Texas Medical Branch, Galveston, TX; Associate Clinical Professor of Emergency Medicine, Boonshaft School of Medicine, Wright State University, Dayton, OH; Space Flight Surgeon, NASA/Wyle/UTMB, Johnson Space Center, Houston, TX

Alon Scope, MD
Visiting Investigator, Dermatology Service, Memorial Sloan-Kettering Cancer Center, New York, NY

Todd M. Sheperd
Clinical Assistant Professor, Department of Family Medicine, Michigan State University College of Human Medicine, East Lansing; Medical Director, Acute Rehabilitation Unit Northern Michigan Regional Hospital; Attending Physician, Bayside Family Medicine, Petoskey, MI

James R. Shepich, MD, FACS
Staff Surgeon, MidMichigan Medical Center, Midland, MI

Julie M. Sicilia, MD
Clinical Assistant Professor, University of Washington, Seattle WA; Clinical Assistant Professor, Providence Alaska Family Medicine Residency, Anchorage, AK

Victor S. Sierpina, MD
W.D. and Laura Nell Nicholson Family Professor of Integrative Medicine; Professor, Family Medicine; Distinguished Teaching Professor of Medical Acupuncture, University of Texas Medical Branch, Galveston, TX

Larry Skoczylas, DDS, MS
Oral and Maxillofacial Surgeon, Midland Oral and Maxillofacial Surgery, PC, Midland, MI

Eric Skye, MD
Clinical Assistant Professor and Associate Chair for Educational Programs, Department of Family Medicine, University of Michigan, Ann Arbor, MI

Wendy L. Smeltzer, MD, CCFP, FCFP
Medical Director, Medical Esthetics, Sante Wellness Group; President and Medical Director, Medique Skincare Ltd., Calgary, Alberta, Canada

Al Smith MD
Smith & Robinson Family Medicine; ICAEL Accredited Echocardiography Lab, Raymondville, TX

Eric A. Smith, MD
Associate Staff, Wooster Community Hosptial, Wooster, OH

Farin W. Smith, MD
Clinical Assistant Professor, University of Alabama–Birmingham; Staff, Trauma Surgery and Surgical Critical Care, Huntsville Hospital System, Huntsville, AL

Jeffrey V. Smith, MD, JD
Staff Physician, Departments of Family Medicine and Surgery, Contra Costa Regional Medical Center, Martinez, CA

Gary L. Snyder, MD, RVT, DPM
Medical Director, Apollo International Institute of Medical Sciences, Big Lake, MN

Michael Stampar, DO
Assistant Clinical Professor, Department of Surgery, Michigan State University, East Lansing, MI; Owner, Spago Day Spa, Salon, and Medispa, Punta Gorda, FL

Sandra M. Sulik, MD, MS
Associate Professor Depart of Family Medicine, State University of New York Health Science Center/St. Joseph's Family Medicine Residency, Syracuse, NY

James A. Surrell, MD, FACSm FASCRS
Associate Clinical Professor of Surgery, College of Human Medicine, Michigan State University, East Lansing; Medical Director, Digestive Health Institute, Marquette General Health System, Marquette, MI

Michelle E. Szczepanik, MD
Resident, Dewitt Army Community Hospital, Ft. Belvoir, VA

Robert S. Tan, MD
Clinical Associate Professor, Department of Family and Community Medicine, University of Texas Medical School at Houston; Associate Professor, Department of Internal Medicine, Baylor College of Medicine; Staff, Michael E. DeBakey VA Medical Center, Extended Care Director, OPAL Medical Clinic, Houston, TX

Sheila Thomas, MD
Primary Care Family Practice Physician, UT Family Practice, University of Tennessee, Memphis, TN

Thomas N. Told, DO, FACOFPdist
Assistant Dean for Clinical Education, and Chief of Division of Rural and Wilderness Medicine, College of Osteopathic Medicine, Rocky Vista University, Parker CO; Kirksville College of Osteopathic Medicine, A.T. Still University, Kirksville, MO

Michael L. Tuggy, MD
Clinical Associate Faculty, University of Washington School of Medicine; Director, Swedish Family Medicine–First Hill Residency, Seattle, WA

Cathy Uecker, RN
Registered Nurse, Grand Rapids, MI

Hakan Usal, MD
Surgeon, Department of Plastic Surgery, Usal Cosmetic Surgery Center, Hackensack; Attending Physician, Department of Plastic Surgery, Hackensack University Medical Center, Hackensack; Staff, Department of Plastic Surgery, Valley Hospital, Ridgewood, NJ; Staff, Department of Plastic Surgery, Staten Island University Hospital, Staten Island, NY

Richard P. Usatine, MD
Professor, Departments of Family and Community Medicine and Dermatology and Cutaneous Surgery; Assistant Director, Medical Humanities Education, University of Texas Health Science Center–San Antonio; Medical Director, Skin Clinic, University Health System, San Antonio, TX

Peter Valenzuela, MD, MBA
Assistant Professor and Assistant Dean for Clinical Affairs, Texas Tech University Health Sciences Center at the Permian Basin, Odessa, TX

Renier van Aardt, MB, ChB, CCFP
Medical Director, Vitality Medi-Spa, Halifax; Medical Director, Laser Plus Medi-Spa, Truro, Nova Scotia, Canada

Deepa A. Vasudevan, MD
Assistant Professor, Department of Family and Community Medicine, University of Texas Medical School at Houston, Houston, TX

Roger K. Waage, MD
Associate Professor, University of Minnesota Medical School–Duluth; Program Director, Duluth Family Medicine Residency, Duluth, MN

Matti Waterman, MD
Clinical Lecturer, Rappaport Faculty of Medicine, Technion-Israel Institute of Technology; Senior Physician, Department of Gastroenterology and Department of Medicine, Rambam Health Care Campus, Haifa, Israel; Clinical Fellow, Advanced Fellowship in Inflammatory Bowel Disease, Department of Medicine, Division of Gastroenterology, Mount Sinai Hospital, Toronto, Ontario, Canada

Lydia A. Watson, MD, FACOG
Staff Physician, Department of Obstetrics and Gynecology, MidMichigan Medical Center, Midland, MI

David G. Weismiller, MD, ScM
Professor of Family Medicine, The Brody School of Medicine at East Carolina University; Associate Provost, East Carolina University, Greenville, NC

Stephen J. Wetmore, MD, CCFP, FCFP
Professor, Department of Family Medicine, Schulich School of Medicine and Dentistry, The University of Western Ontario, London, Ontario, Canada

Russell D. White, MD
Professor of Medicine, Director, Sports Medicine Fellowship Program, Medical Director, Sports Medicine Center, Department of Community and Family Medicine, University of Missouri–Kansas City School of Medicine; Truman Medical Center–Lakewood, Kansas City, MO

Carman H. Whiting, MD
Assistant Professor, Department of Family and Community Medicine, University of Texas Medical School at Houston, Houston, TX

Thad Wilkins, MD
Associate Professor, Department of Family Medicine, Medical College of Georgia, Augusta, GA

Verneeta L. Williams, MD
Associate Director, Riverside Family Medicine Residency, Newport News, VA

Charles L. Wilson, MD
Clinical Associate Professor, Department of Family Medicine, University of Washington School of Medicine; Private Practice, The Vasectomy Clinic, Seattle, WA

Thomas C. Wright, Jr., MD
Professor of Pathology, Columbia University, New York, NY

Gary Yen, MD
Lecturer, Department of Family Medicine, University of Michigan, Ann Arbor, MI

George G. Zainea, MD
Staff Surgeon, Department of Colon and Rectal Surgery, MidMichigan Physicians Group, Midland, MI

Michael Zeringue, MD
Physician, Sports Medicine and Interventional Pain Management Physician, Ponchartrain Bone and Joint, Metairie, LA

Edward M. Zimmerman, MD, PC
Las Vegas Laser & Lipo, Las Vegas, NV

Edward G. Zurad, MD
Clinical Professor, The Commonwealth Medical College, Scranton; Clinical Associate Professor, Temple University, Philadelphia; Medical Director, Procter & Gamble Paper Products, Mehoophany, PA

PREFACE

The face of medicine has changed drastically since the first edition of this text was published in 1994. The intervening 16 years have seen a revolution in computers and technology. New procedures have been introduced. Electronic medical records are being rapidly adopted. The government has just passed a new healthcare reform bill. Medicine has become more regulated and much more of a business. The vision of the family physician "who can provide a breadth and continuity of commonly needed healthcare services for adults and children; who can deliver babies, manage simple fractures, counsel single parents, go to the hospital, maintain an office, and, when all else fails, comfort the dying; ... who provides healthcare from the nursery to the nursing home, without taking the patient to the poorhouse along the way," as defined by Dr. Rodney in the forward to the first edition, becomes more elusive.*

This indeed is a time of change. Rapid change. Warp speed change. A time of excitement and confusion. A time of bewilderment and futuristic goals. A time for huge potential growth.

The primary care clinician stands at the threshold of this change. Measuring quality has been implemented. The Family Medical Home has been introduced and is being incorporated into routine care by many. It is now the focus of hope to manage healthcare delivery in the future.

In all this change and turmoil, we must be careful to recall that the care of the patient remains the primary goal of the medical system. The goal is not to meet some time constraint for an office visit or hospital stay, or to follow some protocol or clinical guideline, or to meet the budget. Rather, the goal of our care is the health of our patients and their families. That goal gives us our purpose and is the reason we became physicians, clinicians, and healers.

Having primary care providers perform procedures still makes sense in the new order of healthcare. It can be a part of the proposed Family Medical Home. Many of these procedures can be performed in the office, which reduces cost. They can be offered by clinicians who know their patients, which the patients appreciate. Performing procedures in the office reduces the time needed to complete referrals to other specialists and reduces delay in the diagnosis and treatment of many conditions. It also makes it easier to document that necessary procedures were actually performed and that patients were not lost in the system. If healthcare reimbursement becomes more "bundled," it will make sense for the primary care clinician to provide even more procedural care. Performing procedures is also rewarding for practitioners and can enhance their enjoyment of the practice of medicine. That said, the quality of the procedures performed can and must meet or surpass the highest of standards. This text helps meet that goal.

We appreciate the feedback we have received on the first two editions. New features in this edition include colored photos and two complete new sections: Aesthetic Medicine and Hospitalist Procedures. Adding these sections reflects some of the changes in medicine. The patient's desire to look younger and healthier has been coupled with advancements in technology to accomplish just that. Hospitalist care has become the norm and is more focused and complicated; yet the associated procedures are not out of the range of primary care clinicians. Family physicians and other primary care clinicians, because of their breadth and depth of training, can step up to these new areas of healthcare and bring these procedures to their patients.

Times change. The experts, academics, and politicians move on. New technology and procedures are invented. *But the need for that healer and caregiver who really does care will never change.* The fear and trepidation that a patient often experiences can only be alleviated by the touch, the words, and the expertise of the caring clinician. In our search for the knowledge and expertise to perform the procedures presented in this text, we should never forget that, first and foremost, we are people who treat patients and their families, not just their symptoms. We learn and gain the skills to perform the procedures reviewed in this text to aid healing. Procedures are not goals unto themselves; rather, they are included in our expertise as another way to help people feel better and be healthier.

John L. Pfenninger, MD
Grant C. Fowler, MD

*Pfenninger JL, Fowler GC: Procedures for Primary Care Physicians. Mosby, 1994.

PREFACE TO THE FIRST EDITION

The inspiration for this text came from busy primary care physicians across the country. Medicine in the 1990s is changing rapidly. The high cost of hospital care, emergency room visits, and even the expenses of freestanding day surgery centers have created a forceful impetus for physicians to perform previous hospital-based procedures and surgeries in the office. Fast-paced lifestyles have added performance pressure: the patient's time is at a premium. No longer will they accept referrals for simple procedures or the subsequent inconvenience. Patients expect their physician to perform most routine procedures. In certain areas of the country, competition for patients has increased, resulting in the need for physicians to master certain procedural skills to enhance their status and desirability. Overwhelmed with paperwork and other responsibilities, primary care physicians have little time to spend preparing for or performing a procedure (much less orienting their staff), and yet some procedures in the office are becoming more complex. Thus, among other things, physicians are pressured from patients, healthcare plans, greater competition, paperwork, and their own staff. It was at the urge and cry of these pressured physicians for a concise, and yet all-encompassing, reference for procedures that this book was created.

Coupled with these pressures, there has been a parallel explosion in new technology. There has also been a clarification and refinement in techniques and indications for older technology. Safer medications and monitoring units are also available to facilitate performing procedures in the office. However, few primary care physicians have the time to stay up-to-date with the changes in technology. New technology or new applications of old technology allow definitive care for conditions in a simpler fashion with less risk and expense than ever before. Radio-frequency loop cervical conization, which is now done in the office setting, has, or will soon, replace the majority of in-hospital cervical conizations. This procedure may cost as little as 20% of in-hospital costs. Fiberoptic diagnoses allow for a more comprehensive evaluation and earlier diagnosis of cancer. More importantly, these diagnoses can now be made by the same physician who cares for the patient most of the time. These technological advances save lives, add to the quality of life, are cost effective, and decrease liability.

Interestingly, there is a wide variety of procedures currently being performed by primary care physicians. However, there are large individual and geographic variations. These variations will no doubt diminish with the advent of managed care. It is well known that it is very cost effective to keep procedures in the hands of primary care physicians, yet there is no comprehensive text detailing the performance of these procedures. With our first attempt, this text is not yet perfect. We relied on authors from all over the country and more than 80 authors contributed. There is a wide range of style and practicality. The intent of the text is to give direction and to serve as a resource and brief review for a particular procedure—not to be all-inclusive in a single text.

The chapters in this book in no way intend to make the reader an expert at any procedure. It is a rare procedure that can be safely "learned from the book." The majority of procedures will be mastered by attending courses that are then followed by a preceptor arrangement. The text merely combines and lists those procedures that primary care physicians perform, sometimes on a daily basis. The text may also serve as a review for physicians and staff on those procedures that are not performed on a day-to-day basis.

Procedures for Primary Care Physicians is not a static document. It will grow and change with time. The chapters will be refined and the contents revised to be more concise and direct. This can only happen through feedback from the readers. Suggestions from you, the reader, would be most appreciated. Submissions of new, or even alternatives, to current chapters are most welcome.

As the title states, this text is directed to primary care physicians—family and general practitioners, emergency physicians, pediatricians, obstetricians, internists, house officers, medical students, military medics, paramedics, nurse practitioners, and all other "primary care providers." It is hoped that the contents will enhance the performance of procedures, improve patient care and satisfaction, and lead to greater physician self-fulfillment.

John L. Pfenninger, MD
Grant C. Fowler, MD

ACKNOWLEDGMENTS

We would like to give special thanks to Julie Mirra at Elsevier for persisting with us through this edition. Despite an incredible number of necessary communications to authors and editors, she kept us on track. Without her steadfast and unwavering support, we might still be working on this project!

We would also like to acknowledge the support of Rolla Couchman, with his good humor, Druanne Martin with her continuous, nurturing support, and Kate Dimock, our final connection at Elsevier. Delores Meloni also assisted us. Thanks to Adrianne Brigido who helped us get the project going and to others at Elsevier who also helped.

Nancy Lombardi did a tremendous job. Her attention to detail was amazing as she even corrected some errors that were present in the first and second editions. Her expertise was very much appreciated.

Thanks from Jack Pfenninger to the MidMichigan Medical Center medical librarians, Pat Wolfgram and Jill VanBuskirk, for their help in researching references, and to Kay Pfenninger for her many hours of scanning slides and overall editing support. Thanks, too, to my office staff who accepted all of my excuses for not completing office tasks on time while I worked on the book! They include Maggie Maurer, Linda Headley, Mary Dansa, Annette Reihl, June Waterman, Peggy Wisneski, and Deana Hegyi.

Grant Fowler would also like to acknowledge Margaret Zambrano and Carolyn Love for their outstanding administrative support of this and similar projects over the years.

ACKNOWLEDGMENTS TO THE FIRST EDITION

The number of people to be thanked in a text of this magnitude is too great to allow mention of them all. Each, in his or her own way, has added greatly to its value. The special people who provided their support and encouragement include: Grant Fowler, MD, for giving large blocks of his time and expertise—without his assistance, the text would be nowhere near completion; Len Scarpinato, DO, for his editorial assistance; Barbara Apgar, MD, for the moral support needed when the "going got rough;" Don DeWitt, MD, for encouraging the vision; Pat Wolfgram, the hospital librarian, for retrieving the voluminous number of reference articles; Joan Haddix, Joi Henton, and Shirley Marsh, for their typing assistance; and Beth Moe, Denise Willard, and Linda Hallman for their secretarial skills. To Ted Huff, I give my sincere thanks for developing educational diagrams out of what were sometimes mere scratchings of the pen. A sincere thanks goes to Cindy Trickel of Carlisle Publishers Services, who provided invaluable editorial guidance in converting thoughts into words.

A special thanks also goes to all the family physicians in Midland, Michigan. They not only provided after-hours coverage for me, but also provided the encouragement to continue on through many personal crises. My office staff and nurses also deserve my gratitude.

Each and every author of this book also deserves special recognition. There were many refusals to assist in this project because of over-commitment and lack of belief in the project. For those authors who did contribute, it meant extra sacrifice and dedication. They participated in a dream that has now come to fruition.

To all of these, a sincere thank you.

John L. Pfenninger, MD

A special thanks to the residents, faculty, and staff of the Hermann/LBJ Family Practice Program and the Department of Family Practice and Community Medicine at the University of Texas Houston Health Science Center–Medical School for their contributions, patience, and encouragement—without which this book might not have happened.

Grant C. Fowler, MD

FOREWORD

There are two sides to the complete primary care physician. One side is the compassionate listener, a person who can heal with words. The other side is the talented caregiver who can provide and apply medical science, including necessary or desired procedures for patients. People need people for good health, and those who have a complete primary care physician who knows them and treats them are among the luckiest people in the world. The complete primary care physician is a precious resource that has been endangered but is making a comeback.

Pfenninger and Fowler's *Procedures for Primary Care* is the bible for the laying on of hands in primary care practice. The first edition in 1994 sold over 40,000 copies and became a fixture in the library of every residency program. It is the one book that is worn and well-used. The second edition in 2003 had 82 new chapters and cemented the book as a must-have in every primary care office. The third edition expands this classic text to an amazing 234 chapters with two new sections, Aesthetic Medicine and Hospitalist Procedures.

The scope of primary care is expanding. After years of decline because of "turf wars" with specialists, health systems are appreciating more than ever that having multitalented primary care physicians is the key to efficient and high-quality healthcare delivery. Comprehensiveness is now back in style for primary care with the Patient-Centered Medical Home as the provider and coordinator of all healthcare services. This is not the "gatekeeping" of managed care but rather a "place" where patients share an information system with their personal physician and have all their services coordinated. The more the primary care physician team can do, the better for everyone.

I am fortunate to be "walking the talk" of the Patient-Centered Medical Home model. In 2009, I was asked to develop a new primary care practice network in a heavily doctored area of southern California. Building off the practice of one physician, we will have 9 offices and 26 physicians in early 2011. We are starting residency programs in family medicine and internal medicine. All practices qualify as advanced medical homes. We have established a variety of "procedure clinics" among our group, performing a wide variety of dermatologic procedures and aesthetics. We have expertise among us in sports medicine. We are developing our own hospitalist service. While no primary care physician will do all the procedures described in this book, among us we will do almost all of them. We will train a new generation of primary care physicians in as many procedures as time and interest allows. *Procedures for Primary Care* is our indispensable guide.

There is a renaissance underway in primary care. The internet and information technology change how we do most everything, and primary care is no exception. Patients now have access to a world of information for free, including healthcare and their medical records. Primary care physicians have become "information managers" for patients and access to communication online has become continuous. In this new world of information, communication, and continuous care, what patients need and want is shared decision making. For patients, an "I can do that for you" from their primary care physician is usually a welcome relief. The world of specialists is often confusing and usually very expensive. Good primary care exudes value, the combination of quality and efficiency, so needed and welcomed in healthcare today.

Knowledge is power and knowledge is abundantly available in *Procedures for Primary Care*. Jack Pfenninger and Grant Fowler have assembled a phenomenal group of talented authors who all "walk the talk" of their chapters. Need to remove a fishhook? Need to remove a ring from a swollen finger? Remove isolated hairs for good? Apply an Unna boot? Repair an earlobe? This book has procedures for them all, of course, and these examples are only a small slice of what is here. If you want to venture into Botox treatment or provide stress echocardiograms, this book will tell you how. We often go to workshops to learn new procedures, but what is helpful to keep doing them is a handy reference to remind us of all the elements of the procedure.

Patient safety requires that we have a checklist for each procedure and not just rely on what we and our staff remember at the time. This book has all the checklists. I imagine a thousand times a day physicians and office staffs somewhere are reviewing a chapter in this book before going into the treatment room. Copies of these checklists should become part of your office procedure manual.

I am certain that this will not be the last edition of *Procedures for Primary Care*. This resource is simply too valuable not to have, and access to it needs to be in print in every office. With this edition, the patient education sheets have been moved online to make downloading and printing easier and more convenient. I imagine synergy with the internet will grow over time as it has with other classic textbooks. For now, having a readily available copy of *Procedures for Primary Care* will be at the top of your office resources. Use it often to keep your quality of care high and your scope of practice broad for the benefit of your patients.

Joseph E. Scherger, MD, MPH
Vice President, Primary Care
Eisenhower Medical Center
Rancho Mirage, CA
Clinical Professor of Family Medicine
University of California, San Diego
University of Southern California

FOREWORD TO THE SECOND EDITION

As a comprehensive guide to performing medical and surgical procedures in the office, hospital, or emergency department, *Pfenninger and Fowler's Procedures for Primary Care* might be considered an antidote to the evils that originated from Pandora's box. According to Greek mythology, Pandora (whose name means "rich in gifts") found a buried box and impulsively removed its lid. Out of the box, scattering in every direction, came disease, death, and all the other evils that afflict humankind. Like Eve in the Christian scriptures, Pandora introduced mortality into our world. However, her box also contained an antidote—hope—and she closed the lid just in time to prevent this quality from escaping.

In combating the myriad diseases that Pandora supposedly unleashed, primary care clinicians have long been powerful agents for hope and healing. Because of advances in treatment options, including minimally invasive outpatient surgical techniques, many procedures that previously would have necessitated hospitalization or consultation now can be performed by primary care clinicians in the office, hospital, or emergency room. This arrangement allows continuity of care, hopefully provides excellent patient education, and, by moving some procedures out of the hospital, may offer significant economic advantages. However, as their role expands, these clinicians must continue to use sound judgment and keep the patient's welfare as the uppermost priority. They should avoid procedures beyond their expertise; they should avoid procedures that might necessitate repetition; and they should avoid procedures that might cause them medicolegal problems.

Like Pandora, *Pfenninger and Fowler's Procedures for Primary Care* is rich in gifts, but these are of the life-affirming kind. More than 200 chapters provide up-to-date information for a continually evolving specialty. The book includes practical, step-by-step instructions for performing an extensive array of medical and surgical procedures, as illustrated by line drawings and clear photographs. It also covers indications and contraindications, equipment and suppliers, complications, billing codes, and other practical topics. In the literature for primary care clinicians, few other books cover such a wide range of topics. Indeed, I know of no other volume that is likely to be more useful to its intended audience.

Some readers may wonder why this foreword is being written by a cardiovascular surgeon and not by a primary care clinician. Perhaps they will allow heart disease to serve as an example for many other diseases. Primary care clinicians are at the leading edge of the battle against many diseases—not only in treatment but also in prevention. Regarding heart disease, their advice is often the deciding factor in convincing patients to make positive changes with respect to fat intake, physical activity, cigarette smoking, and other lifestyle factors. An example from the recent literature supports this premise: in a study involving patients with coronary artery disease at Creighton University, recommendations from primary care clinicians concerning the assessment of lipid profiles and use of statin therapy significantly reduced the number of adverse cardiovascular outcomes. As the average age of the population continues to increase and congestive heart failure becomes increasingly prevalent, primary care clinicians can be expected to play an even greater role in diagnosing and treating this disorder. If primary care clinicians can do this with heart disease, it is my hope that they can use their abilities in many other areas of medicine.

The book also contains patient education handouts. When primary care clinicians perform a procedure, they must know the disease well. In so doing, they also have a golden opportunity to teach some prevention principles. I hope that they will never miss the opportunity to treat the whole patient and potentially change the course of the disease by educating the patient before, during, and after performing the procedure.

In conclusion, I congratulate Drs. Pfenninger and Fowler on producing such an excellent volume. It should help improve the quality of care in many aspects of medical practice, and I highly recommend it for every primary care clinician and trainee. There are some who consider me a pioneer in heart disease; I hope that this book encourages medical pioneers everywhere to prevent and treat early the diseases that Pandora supposedly released.

Denton A. Cooley, MD
Surgeon-in-Chief, Texas Heart Institute
Clinical Professor of Surgery
University of Texas Medical School at Houston
Houston, TX

FOREWORD TO THE FIRST EDITION

In 1930, more than 80% of the physicians in the United States were general family doctors, providing comprehensive health care at a reasonable cost. By 1980, the self-reported percentage of family doctors in the United States was 15%. Along with this trend of dwindling numbers has been a gradual decline of diagnostic and therapeutic skills held by those physicians who do practice general family medicine.

One definition of a generalist physician (formerly a general practitioner) is a family physician who can provide a breadth and continuity of commonly needed healthcare services. These physicians care for children, deliver babies, manage simple fractures, counsel single parents, go to the hospital, maintain an office, and, when all else fails, comfort the dying. Their goal is to provide health care from the nursery to the nursing home, without taking the patient to the poor house along the way

Today, of the 625,000 physicians in the United States, fewer than 10% comprehensively wield the clinical skills needed to provide such care. The headlong rush to subspecialize in medicine has left family physicians in the minority. Still, they are an important minority whose number is now growing in response to the projected needs of the twenty-first century American healthcare system.

Since 1983, a group of family physicians, supported by the American Academy of Family Physicians (AAFP), has constructed a series of demonstration projects to propagate diagnostic and therapeutic skills in family medicine. Many of the procedural pioneers in family practice have quietly and unselfishly contributed their professional energies to the resuscitation of full-service family practice within a medical education system gone far, far astray. This book stands as a contribution to that effort. Although some may view the teaching and learning of clinical skills as "proceduralism," the skills that are depicted in this book represent the desire of physicians to remain clinically excellent. No amount of psychosocial expertise can overcome the credibility lost when a physician cannot perform basic clinical services on behalf of his or her patient.

Recently a prominent dean of a well-known medical school asked me why the residency programs at my institution, the University of Tennessee, persisted in reaching a comprehensive set of procedural clinical skills when, in his opinion, managed care organizations and health maintenance organizations would effectively amputate these skills from the day-to-day practice of family physicians. I disagree with this vision of the future, but it is true that some family physicians voluntarily relinquish many of the clinical skills described in this book. It is my hope that the skills described in its pages will become required curriculum, not only for residents, but, particularly, for faculty. One of the major challenges for the success of this book (and the specialty of family practice) is the development of accountability in a healthcare system that has become overly fragmented, costly, and inaccessible.

Are these skills needed? During the past 20 years, family physicians have been manipulated, exploited, and oppressed in a variety of ways that makes study of their actual needs very complex. For example, a lack of reported interest in obstetrical care cannot be used to justify the tremendous void that exists in women's healthcare as provided by family physicians. Residents are not likely to acquire clinical skills that family physician faculty members cannot themselves demonstrate in their positions as role models. A lack of procedural skill among family practice faculty and practitioners is particularly troubling in rural and underserved communities. These communities cannot afford platoons of various subspecialized physicians.

Although excellent healthcare is available from a combination of obstetricians, pediatricians, and internists, a well-trained, comprehensive-care family physician should be able to deliver continuing healthcare unrestricted by age, sex, organ system, and pregnancy. The physician should be skilled in many of the procedures described here to screen for, prevent, and treat common disease entities. If family practice simply becomes synonymous with "generic primary care," there will be very little need for many of the skills described in this book. My compliments to the editors and the authors for executing a labor of love in an outstanding fashion. They have chosen the road less traveled.

Wm. MacMillian Rodney, MD, FAAFP, FACEP
Meharry/Vanderbilt Professor and Chair Department of Family and Community Medicine Professor Surgery/Emergency Medicine Meharry Medical College Nashville, TN

CONTENTS

Online Assets

Patient Education Handouts, Patient Consent Forms, Sample Operative Reports, and other miscellaneous forms and handouts are available at www.expertconsult.com.

Supplier information can be found in Appendix D, which is on page 1629 in print and online at www.expertconsult.com.

SECTION I

Anesthesia

Section Editor: THEODORE O'CONNELL

CHAPTER 1

Bier Block

Peter W. Grigg

Intravenous (IV) regional anesthesia, also known as a *Bier block*, is a useful method of providing operative anesthesia to wide areas of the distal portion of an extremity. When executed with proper technique, the Bier block is a safe alternative to local or hematoma infiltration, and provides anesthesia superior to these other methods. At the same time, it has the advantage of being technically simpler to perform than other regional alternatives (e.g., axillary or brachial plexus block).

Indications

Although the technique of IV regional anesthesia has been used on the lower extremity, it is most often used in applications involving the upper extremity. Bier blocks are useful for (1) surgery of the wrist, hand, and fingers (e.g., carpal tunnel release, foreign body removal, laceration repair, incision and drainage, and tendon release and repair); and (2) reduction of fractures or dislocation below the elbow. Bier blocks are also used in the treatment of complex regional pain syndromes.

Contraindications

Documented sensitivity to local anesthesia is an absolute contraindication. Relative contraindications include the following:

- Injuries to the proximal extremity that would be adversely affected by application of a tourniquet (e.g., crush injury)
- Conditions predisposing to arterial thrombosis (e.g., Raynaud's phenomenon, homozygous sickle cell disease)
- Fractures about and above the elbow
- Infection at or near the intended IV cannula insertion site
- Preexisting cardiac disorders affected by IV local anesthetic (e.g., untreated third-degree heart block)
- Difficulty in maintaining arterial occlusion with a tourniquet (e.g., inadequate cuff size in a massively obese patient)

Equipment

- Standard monitoring equipment (cardiac monitor, pulse oximeter, continuous blood pressure monitor)
- Standard Advanced Cardiac Life Support (ACLS) airway supplies and drugs, as well as drugs used for sedation (e.g., midazolam [Versed], fentanyl, and propofol [Diprivan])
- Double-cuff automatic pneumatic tourniquet that can individually or simultaneously inflate or deflate both cuffs to preset pressures (as an alternative, ordinary blood pressure cuffs can be used if the dimensions of the arm can accommodate two appropriately sized cuffs between the axilla and the elbow without overlap)
- Lidocaine (without epinephrine), 1 mL/kg of 0.5% solution for upper extremity blocks, 2 mL/kg of the 0.25% solution for lower extremity blocks
- Two IV catheters, a 22-gauge line for the operative side and a 20-gauge line for the arm on the nonoperative side, which can be used for sedation and administration of emergency drugs if needed
- Sterile skin preparation solution (e.g., povidone-iodine)
- Tape
- Elastic bandage of sufficient size to wrap the entire extremity distal to the tourniquet

Although the risk of serious adverse reaction is very small when the procedure is followed correctly, it should be conducted only in facilities capable of managing serious local anesthetic toxicities (see the Complications section, later).

American Society of Anesthesiologists standards require an anesthesiologist (or a similarly qualified practitioner other than the surgeon) to manage the patient during a Bier block. This person should not be the operating surgeon because the surgeon is busy doing the procedure and cannot effectively manage complications of the local anesthetic.

Preprocedure Patient Preparation

Advise the patient that 95% of patients experience good or complete anesthesia with a Bier block; the remainder require additional analgesics or sedatives. Explain the risks, alternatives, and potential complications to the patient and answer any questions. Note that anesthesia will resolve in 30 minutes or less after tourniquet release. See patient education and patient consent forms available online.

Technique

1. Perform a focused history and physical examination to ensure the patient is a candidate for a Bier block. Note NPO status, medical problems, medication allergies, and Mallampati airway classification (see Chapter 2, Procedural Sedation and Analgesia).
2. Attach the cardiac monitor and pulse oximeter. Place the blood pressure cuff on the nonoperative side and note the patient's blood pressure.
3. Place two IV lines—one on the operative side, and one on the nonoperative side. On the operative side, attach the syringe with lidocaine and tape in place.
4. An ACLS-trained practitioner should administer the sedation and monitor the patient as previously noted. An IV tranquilizer such as midazolam (Versed) 2 to 4 mg IV often is given for comfort, although sedation is not required.
5. Test the pneumatic tourniquet or blood pressure cuffs for accuracy and maintenance of pressure and then place them on the proximal portion of the extremity.
6. Have an assistant elevate the extremity above the heart while you wrap the elastic bandage around it, wrapping from distal to proximal (from fingers or toes up to the distal cuff). Be careful not to dislodge the needle or catheter.
7. Rapidly inflate the proximal cuff to 50 to 100 mm Hg above the systolic blood pressure for upper extremity blocks and twice the

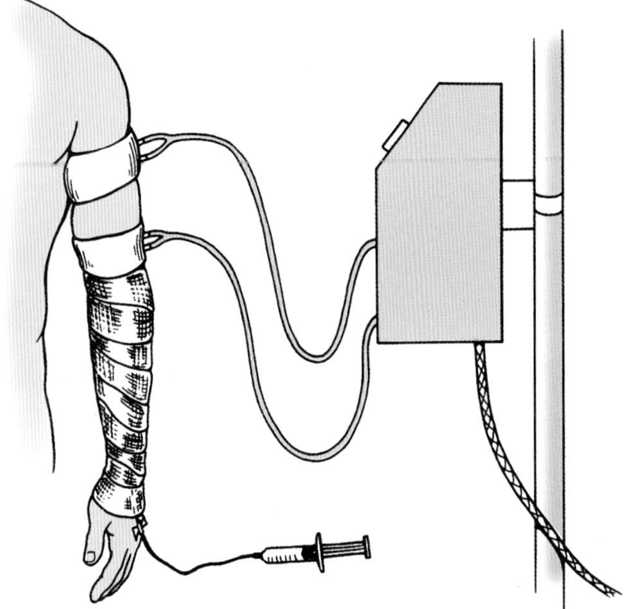

Figure 1-1 Bier block procedure, before removal of elastic bandage and injection of lidocaine, showing inflation of proximal cuff.

systolic blood pressure for lower extremity blocks. Assign an assistant to be responsible for continuously monitoring the maintenance of cuff pressure throughout the remainder of the procedure (Fig. 1-1).

8. Lower the extremity, remove the elastic bandage, and check the distal pulses. If no pulse is palpable and the extremity is blanched, inject the appropriate dose of lidocaine.
9. After approximately 10 to 15 minutes, check the adequacy of anesthesia by gently manipulating the operative site. Additional time may be required to achieve full effect.
10. After the initial 10 to 15 minutes, inflate the distal cuff to the same pressure as the proximal cuff, and then deflate the proximal cuff. This use of two cuffs reduces the pain associated with the occlusive tourniquet by allowing infusion of the anesthetic under the proximal cuff before it is inflated.
11. When anesthesia is deemed adequate, the IV line on the operative side may be removed. The limb is then prepared, and the operation may proceed up to a maximum inflation time of 2 hours. Periodically monitor the blood pressure on the contralateral side to ensure proper tourniquet pressure. The tourniquet may remain inflated during the process of taking intraoperative plain films.
12. At the completion of the procedure, but no sooner than 20 minutes after lidocaine injection (to permit diffusion of some of the lidocaine out of the vascular system), deflate and remove the cuffs. Some physicians recommend cycles of deflation and inflation, but this has no advantage in lowering systemic plasma lidocaine levels.
13. Observe the patient for 10 to 15 minutes for signs of toxicity or adverse reaction.

Complications

See Chapter 5, Local and Topical Anesthetic Complications.

- Complications arise from the lidocaine and the equipment used to produce the block. Minor adverse reactions to the lidocaine (e.g., dizziness, tinnitus, bradycardia) occur in fewer than 2% of patients after cuff deflation.
- Allergic reactions are very rare. Anaphylaxis is treated with oxygen therapy, IV fluid, epinephrine, antihistamines, and steroids.
- Seizures and cardiovascular collapse occur almost exclusively when the lidocaine is injected with the cuffs deflated—because of operator error or equipment malfunction—and are rare. Seizures may be self-limited and treated with airway management, IV benzodiazepines, barbiturates, or propofol.
- Dysrhythmias are treated according to ACLS algorithms.
- Hypotension may require IV fluids or vasopressors.
- Ecchymosis and subcutaneous hemorrhage can occur underneath the cuff site and can be minimized by placing padding (web roll) on the arm.
- Engorgement of the extremity can occur when arterial inflow of blood continues but venous drainage is restricted by the tourniquet. A fully functional tourniquet and checking for an absent pulse minimize this problem.
- Hematoma formation can occur at sites of unsuccessful IV attempts. Apply pressure for 3 minutes before applying elastic bandage. Apply pressure over the IV site when the functioning catheter is removed.

CPT/Billing Code

01995 Regional IV administration of local anesthetic agent (upper or lower extremity)

Acknowledgment

The editors wish to recognize the many contributions by Robert Williams, MD, MPH, to this chapter in the previous edition of this text.

Suppliers

(See online list for contact information.)

Double-cuff pneumatic tourniquet
Thomas Medical, Inc.
VBM Medical, Inc.
Zimmer, Inc.

Online Resources

LipidRescue.org
The New York School of Regional Anesthesia: 2010 World Anesthesia Conference. http://www.nysora.com.

Bibliography

American Society of Anesthesiologists Task Force on Sedation and Analgesia by Non-Anesthesiologists: Practice guidelines. Anesthesiology 96:1004–1017, 2002.
Bannister M: Bier's block. Anaesthesia 52:713, 1997.
Blasier RD, White R: Intravenous regional anesthesia for management of children's extremity fractures in the emergency department. Pediatr Emerg Care 12:404, 1996.
Bolte RG, Stevens PM, Scott SM, Schunk JE: Mini-dose Bier block intravenous regional anesthesia in the emergency department treatment of upper-extremity injuries. J Pediatr Orthop 14:534, 1994.
Brown EM, McGriff JT, Malinowski RW: Intravenous regional anesthesia (Bier block): Review of 20 years' experience. Can J Anaesth 36:307, 1989.
Farrell RG, Swanson SL, Walter JR: Safe and effective IV regional anesthesia for use in the emergency department. Ann Emerg Med 14:288, 1985.
Henderson CL, Warriner CB, McEwen JA, Merrick PM: A North American survey of intravenous regional anesthesia. Anesth Analg 85:858–863, 1997.

Lowen R, Taylor J: Bier's block: The experience of Australian emergency departments. Med J Aust 160:108, 1994.
Moore N, Kirton C, Bane J: Lipid emulsion to treat overdose of local anesthetic. Anaethesia 61:107–109, 2006.
Moore N, Kirton C, Bane J: Lipid emulsion to treat overdose of local anaesthetic [author reply]. Anaesthesia 61:607, 2006.
Salo M, Kanto J, Jalonen J, Laurikainen E: Plasma lidocaine concentrations after different methods of releasing the tourniquet during intravenous regional anaesthesia. Ann Clin Res 11:164, 1979.
Soltesz EG, van Pelt F, Byrne JG: Emergent cardiopulmonary bypass for bupivacaine cardiotoxicity. J Cardiothorac Vasc Anesth 17:357, 2003.
Tetzlaff JE: The pharmacology of local anesthetics. Anesthesiol Clin North Am 18:217, 2000.

CHAPTER 2

PROCEDURAL SEDATION AND ANALGESIA

Sylvana Guidotti

Procedural sedation and analgesia (PSA) is the clinical practice of using pharmacologic agents to achieve a measurable level of sedation, while performing typically painful or anxiety-provoking procedures. The term *conscious sedation* is no longer used because it describes neither the intent nor the outcome of the process. PSA allows the nonanesthesiologist to perform selected procedures in a safe and controlled setting.

The Joint Commission on Accreditation of Healthcare Organizations (JCAHO) has produced sedation guidelines to describe and define the spectrum of PSA. More important, the American Society of Anesthesiologists (ASA) and the American College of Emergency Physicians (ACEP) have published guidelines for PSA by nonanesthesiologists and emergency physicians, respectively. As defined by the ASA, PSA is a continuum from minimal sedation/analgesia to general anesthesia.

Minimal sedation occurs when the patient continues to respond normally to verbal commands without cardiopulmonary functions being affected. *Moderate sedation* is a state of depressed consciousness where the patient responds appropriately to verbal command with or without light tactile stimuli. *Dissociative sedation* should be considered a form of moderate sedation that occurs when a dissociative pharmacologic agent produces a trancelike state. The result is analgesia and amnesia while protective airway reflexes and cardiovascular stability are maintained. *Deep sedation* causes a depression of consciousness in which the patient is not easily arousable but responds purposefully with repeated or painful stimuli. At this level, the patient may require assistance in maintaining airway and ventilation. *General anesthesia* is at the end of the spectrum; consciousness is lost and the patient is unarousable to any stimuli. The patient requires ventilatory assistance, and cardiovascular function may be affected or impaired.

For coding purposes, the American Medical Association CPT coding manual describes "moderate (conscious) sedation" as a drug-induced depression of consciousness during which patients respond purposefully to verbal commands, either alone or accompanied by light tactile stimulation. No interventions are required to maintain a patent airway, and spontaneous ventilation is adequate. Cardiovascular function is maintained. It does not include minimal sedation (anxiolysis), deep sedation, or monitored anesthesia care (Table 2-1).

PSA comprises three components. First there is the *process of sedation*, which requires a thorough knowledge of the agents being administered. Next is the *intended procedure* to be performed. Finally, there are the *unpredictable side effects and untoward reactions* to the sedating medications, which can occur during or in the recovery phase of the procedure.

The physician should be familiar with all of the appropriate monitoring and rescue equipment. A suitably trained provider should assist with the sedation. All individuals who participate in the care of the patient undergoing PSA must demonstrate ongoing clinical competency and be privileged for the procedure if they will be performing it in a hospital setting.

INDICATIONS

As nonanesthesiologist physicians become more comfortable with PSA, the roster of appropriate procedures where these agents are beneficial continues to expand. The list includes, but is not limited to, the following:

- Anal procedures
- Biopsy procedures
- Bone marrow aspiration or biopsy
- Bronchoscopy
- Cardioversion (electrical or chemical)
- Dental/oral surgical procedures
- Endometrial biopsy
- Essure contraceptive placement
- Fracture reductions/care
- Gastrointestinal endoscopy
- Hysterosalpingography
- Lumbar puncture
- Magnetic resonance imaging/computed tomography scans/invasive radiographic procedures
- Office dilation and curettage/vacuum aspiration
- Orthopedic procedures
- Phlebectomy
- Plastic/cosmetic/laser procedures
- Wound repair/care, including burns; large excisions

PSA can be used in conjunction with and as a supplement to digital blocks, hematoma blocks, or regional nerve blocks as well as topical anesthetic agents. These modalities may obviate the need for deeper levels of sedation. Other distractions for the patient such as music or videos are useful adjuncts.

CONTRAINDICATIONS

Elective procedures on pregnant patients should be deferred until after delivery. Patients with severe unstable systemic disease and patients with potentially unstable airways should be directed to a higher level of care. The ASA classification of systemic disease is designed to guide the physician as to which patients are appropriate candidates for PSA (Table 2-2).

Class II patients include those with well-controlled hypertension, controlled non–insulin-dependent diabetes, and minimal cardiac or respiratory disease. Class III patients include those with insulin-dependent diabetes mellitus, poorly controlled hypertension, significant cardiac or respiratory disease, and significant renal

TABLE 2-1 Operational Definitions and Characterizations of Levels of Sedation–Analgesia

Sedation Score	Level of Sedation	Level of Consciousness	Response: Verbal	Response: Tactile	Response: Patency	Ventilation, Oxygenation
0	None	Fully aware of self and surroundings	P	P	P	P
1	"Minimal"	Mostly aware of self and surroundings, but sedate	P–L	P	P	P
2	"Moderate"	Slightly aware of self and surroundings, usually somnolent, arouses easily with stimuli	L–A	P–L	P–L*	P–L*
3	"Deep"†	Not aware of self or surroundings, little arousal with stimuli	A	L (to pain)	L–A	L
4	General anesthesia	Unconscious, no arousal with painful stimuli	A	A (to pain)	L–A	L–A

A, absent, inadequate; L, limited, partial, mildly abnormal; P, present, adequate, or normal.
*May need to supplement oxygen to maintain SaO_2.
†Deep sedation may be indistinguishable from general anesthesia and carries all the same risks.

or hepatic disease. Based on individual experience and skill in providing sedation, practitioners may decide to limit the amount of patient risk they are willing to accept, using the ASA guidelines.

In general, the nonanesthesiologist physician who provides PSA in the private office setting should do so on patients with class II status or less. For hospital-based procedures outside of the operating room, PSA may be performed on patients up to and including class III status.

The ASA has set forth *preprocedure fasting guidelines* for scheduled elective cases. However, in separate recommendations for PSA, the ASA states, "The literature does not provide sufficient evidence to test the hypothesis that preprocedure fasting results in a decreased incidence of adverse outcomes in patients undergoing either moderate or deep sedation." The current guidelines are the result of consensus, rather than being evidence based, with respect to the risk of aspiration. *The recommendations are 6 hours for solids, cow's milk, and infant formula; 4 hours for breast milk; and 2 hours for clear liquids.* ACEP recognizes that there are certain emergent situations in which the benefits of PSA at any sedation depth outweigh the potential risks. In all other circumstances, it would be best to strictly adhere to the fasting guidelines. Thus, if a patient has not followed the aforementioned fasting guidelines, it would be best to postpone the procedure or just not use significant PSA.

Equipment

- A single unit with blood pressure and electrocardiographic measurements, variable-pitch beep pulse oximeter, and recording device is the ideal monitor for PSA. Individual units are acceptable but require repeated manual recordings of the readings on the patient's chart.
- Angiocatheter for intravenous (IV) access (at least 20 gauge), IV solution, and stand.
- Oxygen source.
- Medications for sedation and analgesia.
- Reversal medications.
- Diphenhydramine and epinephrine to be used in the event of severe allergic reactions.
- Crash cart or Banyan kit with equipment and medications for basic and advanced cardiac life support (ACLS; see Chapter 220, Anaphylaxis).
- Suction device.
- Defibrillator (Fig. 2-1).

Although it is not a requirement for class I patients, the *application of oxygen* by nasal cannula should be used for every patient undergoing PSA because each patient has a unique and unpredictable response to the medications. *Capnometry* is another, more sensitive measurement of ventilatory status and is being used as part of PSA monitoring. As a measure of exhaled carbon dioxide, end-tidal CO_2 may detect hypoventilation before the development of oxygen desaturation.

Personnel

At least two providers must be involved in PSA. The physician who is performing the procedure is also ordering the medications. The assistant is typically a registered nurse who has fulfilled all of the requirements to administer PSA drugs, monitor the patient during the procedure and recovery phase, and participate in any needed resuscitations.

There should be a well-defined response for any cardiopulmonary emergency that results from PSA. Most hospitals have organized a "code team" to respond to such situations. In the nonhospital setting, the physician should be able to manage the emergency until emergency medical services personnel arrive for transport to a hospital.

Preprocedure Patient Assessment

Every patient who undergoes PSA should have a *complete history and physical examination* before the procedure. Included in the

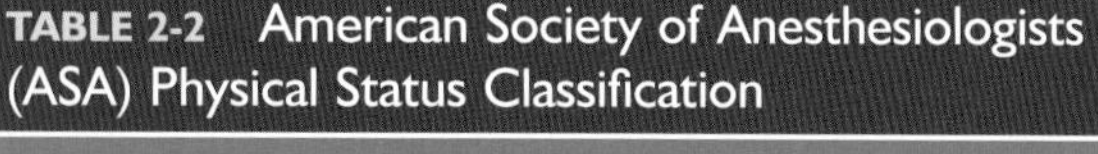
TABLE 2-2 American Society of Anesthesiologists (ASA) Physical Status Classification

ASA Classification	Sedation Risk
Class I: Normal healthy patient	Minimal
Class II: Mild systemic disease without physical limitation	Low
Class III: Severe systemic disease with functional limitations	Intermediate
Class IV: Severe systemic disease that is a constant threat to life	High
Class V: Moribund patient who may not survive without procedure	Extremely high

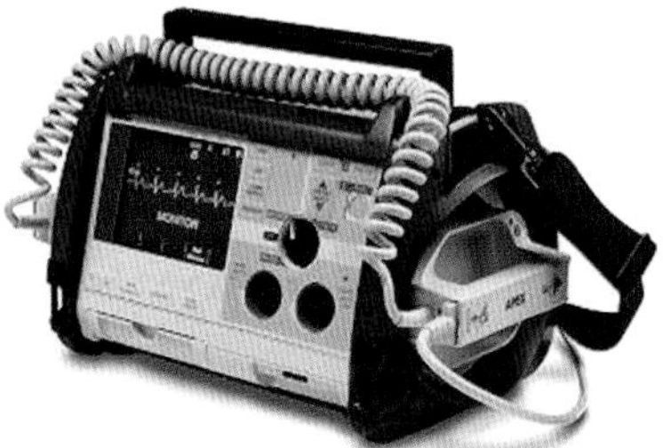

Figure 2-1 Defibrillator. (Courtesy of Zoll Medical Corp., Chelmsford, Mass.)

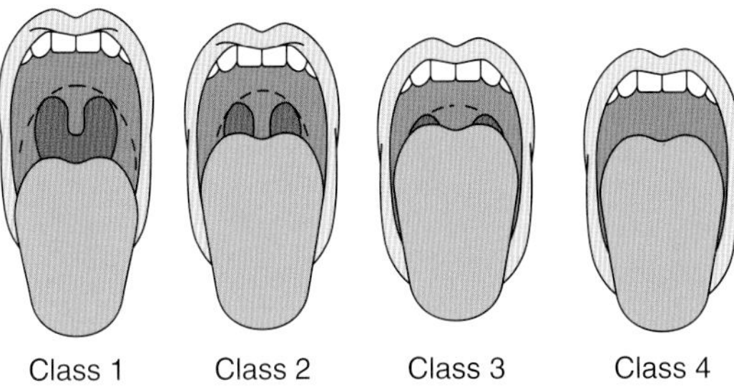

Figure 2-2 The Mallampati classification relates tongue size to pharyngeal size. It is based on the pharyngeal structures that are visible. Class 1: Visualization of the soft palate, fauces, uvula, anterior and posterior pillars. Class 2: Visualization of the soft palate, fauces, and uvula. Class 3: Visualization of the soft palate and the base of the uvula. Class 4: Soft palate not visible at all. (Modified from Mallampati SR, Gatt SP, Gugino LD, et al: A clinical sign to predict difficult tracheal intubation: A prospective study. Can J Anaesth 32:429–434, 1985.)

documentation are pertinent medical history, current medications, allergies (problems with sedative or analgesics), and review of systems (snoring or obstructive sleep apnea). The physical examination should focus on assessment of airway and cardiovascular system. Anatomic variants (macroglossia, micrognathia) and presence of a beard, dentures, or a short, arthritic neck should be noted. Direct evaluation of the patient's open mouth using the *Mallampati classification* measures how much the tongue obscures the uvula and soft palate (Fig. 2-2 and Table 2-3). Obtain and document an *informed consent* from the patient for both PSA and the procedure. Explain the sedation process, potential for failure, adverse effects, as well as alternatives to the procedure and the consequences of not providing sedation.

Preprocedure Patient Preparation

- Reconfirm the initial assessment and the patient's ASA classification.
- Document the fasting time.
- Check a pregnancy test on age-appropriate women.
- Make certain there is an adult to escort the patient home.
- Ask the patient to void, dress in a gown, and recline on the procedure bed.
- The IV line should be secured and functioning.
- Blood pressure cuff, cardiac monitor, and pulse oximeter should be applied and baseline vitals, including room air SaO_2, documented.
- Emergency resuscitation equipment and medications should be functional and at the ready.
- A PSA monitoring flow sheet is used to record preprocedure, intraprocedure, and postprocedure data. Document start and completion times, medications and dosages administered, as well as the level of sedation achieved throughout the procedure (see flow sheets online at www.expertconsult.com).
- The practice of premedicating the patient with histamine type 2 blockers or proton pump inhibitors is no longer recommended because of the lack of evidence with regard to the efficacy of these drugs to diminish gastric acid secretion and subsequent risk of aspiration.
- Before sedating the patient, physician and assistant must take a "*time out*" to once again identify the patient, the intended procedure, and the site. Once the procedure has started, the patient should be encouraged to tell the operator about any unusual discomfort, shortness of breath, chest pressure, or itching.

TABLE 2-3 Mallampati Classification*

Class I	Full view of soft palate, fauces, uvula, pillars, tonsils
Class II	Visible hard and soft palate, fauces, upper portion of tonsils, and uvula
Class III	Visible hard and soft palate, base of uvula
Class IV	Only hard palate is visible

*See also Figure 2-2.

Technique

1. Position the patient as comfortably as possible for the procedure, using warm blankets and placing pillows under the head or knees.
2. Use the single dose of medication that will provide a maximum level of sedation required to perform the procedure. Multiple small doses create discomfort for the patient and may culminate in oversedation. For painful procedures, begin IV administrations with a short-acting narcotic. For painless but anxiety-producing procedures, there should be more emphasis on anxiolysis. Maintain verbal contact with the patient. Observe the patient for slurred speech, droopy eyelids, and calm affect. The patient should stir to verbal commands and be able to follow them. Remember that the effects should start within several minutes but may not peak for up to 7 minutes.
3. Begin the procedure once the patient has achieved the desired depth of sedation.
4. If the patient is not sedated adequately after a modest dose of narcotic, administer a small dose of a short-acting benzodiazepine and continue to observe for effects. Recall the synergistic efforts of these drugs.
5. Record vital signs every 5 minutes. The assistant should remain at the patient's bedside throughout the procedure to observe the response to sedation and to respond to any monitor alarms. The patient must be monitored continually for head position, level of consciousness, airway patency, and adequacy of respiration and oxygenation. Observation of ventilation is essential, especially when using supplemental oxygen, which will delay the detection of apnea by pulse oximetry.
6. Naloxone and flumazenil should be at the bedside in the event any reversal is required.
7. The depth of sedation should be assessed at frequent intervals during the procedure. *If the sedation is too light* the patient may express displeasure or experience discomfort, as well as develop tachycardia or hypertension. *If sedation is too deep* the patient may develop periods of apnea; the oxygen saturation (SaO_2) will decrease and trigger the monitor alarm. Also, if side-stream end-tidal CO_2 is used, the earliest sign of respiratory compromise would be a steady rise of the end-tidal CO_2 above 40 mm Hg. Finally, the patient's Aldrete score (see flow sheet online at www.expertconsult.com) will decrease if sedation is too deep. If at any time during the procedure there is a change in or deterioration of the patient's condition, either suspend or abort the procedure, assess the patient, and commence any resuscitation.

Medications

There are several medications in the armamentarium of PSA. The physician must understand the pharmacology of these drugs and the appropriate settings in which to use them.

A short-acting analgesic should be used at the onset. Fentanyl has a very good safety profile with a rapid onset and short duration of action. It does not cause the extent of cardiorespiratory depression that is typical of other opioids. However, its side effects are magnified with benzodiazepines (Table 2-4).

If anxiolysis is the goal of PSA, fentanyl combined with *midazolam* provides a minimal level of sedation that is ideal for such procedures as cardioversion, endoscopy, lumbar puncture, and certain wound repairs. *When moderate sedation* is desired for particularly painful procedures, fentanyl can be used with *etomidate* to create relaxation

TABLE 2-4 Commonly Used Medications for Procedural Sedation and Analgesia

Medication	Class	Description	Initial IV Dose	Repeat Dose	Minimum Interval
Etomidate (Amidate)	Sedative-hypnotic	Rapid onset Short duration	0.1 mg/kg	0.1 mg/kg	5 min
Fentanyl (Sublimaze)	Opiate	Short acting	1 µgm/kg, up to 100 µg	25 50 µg	5 min
Flumazenil (Romazicon)	Benzodiazepine antagonist	Reversal agent for benzodiazepine	0.2 mg	0.2 mg, up to 1 mg total	1 min
Midazolam (Versed)	Benzodiazepine	Short acting Sedation/amnesia	1–2 mg	0.5–1 mg, up to 5 mg	5 min
Methohexital (Brevital)	Ultra–short-acting barbiturate	Nonanalgesic amnesia	0.75–1 mg/kg	0.5 mg/kg	2 min
Naloxone (Narcan)	Opiate antagonist	Reversal agent for opiate	0.2–0.4 mg	0.2 mg	2–3 min
Propofol (Diprivan)	Sedative-hypnotic	Rapid onset	1 mg/kg	0.5 mg/kg	3–5 min
Atropine	Anticholinergic Antiarrhythmic	Treatment of symptomatic bradycardia; decrease secretions	0.4 mg	0.4 mg, 3 mg max	3–5 min
Diphenhydramine (Benadryl)	Antihistamine Anticholinergic	Treats anaphylaxis; sedative; antiemetic	25 mg	25 mg	5–10 min
Metoclopramide (Reglan)	Central and peripheral dopamine antagonist	Antiemetric	10 mg	—	—
Ondansetron (Zofran)	Serotonin (5-HT_3) receptor antagonist	Antiemetic	4 mg	4 mg, 16 mg max	5–10 min

for closed reductions of joint dislocations or fractures. *Propofol* can be used for moderate or deep sedation. It has no analgesic properties and should be used with fentanyl. It is safest to deliver propofol as a continuous infusion that can be discontinued if any adverse reaction occurs. At low doses, *methohexital* produces a state of unconsciousness while preserving protective airway reflexes. It is purely an amnestic agent, and careful use with opioids is advised. Hypotension and histamine release are significant side effects.

Ketamine is a dissociative agent that has a long history of use for pediatric PSA. The data supporting the use of ketamine in adults are very few owing to the increased incidence of hallucinations during emergence from the drug.

COMPLICATIONS

Several factors are associated with adverse outcomes during PSA. In addition to the known effects of the drugs themselves, there are patient factors, inadequate preprocedural evaluation, drug–drug interactions, drug dosing errors, and inconsistent monitoring and observation.

Respiratory depression is the most common and profound adverse effect. All of the drugs used inhibit respiratory drive to some degree. The synergistic effects that occur when the drugs are combined can magnify the inhibition of the respiratory system. Should the SaO_2 fall below 90%, the procedure should be suspended and the patient evaluated. In addition, *chest wall and glottic rigidity are catastrophic side effects of fentanyl* that can occur when a high dose of the drug is injected rapidly. Under these circumstances the patient may require paralysis and mechanical ventilation until the symptoms resolve.

Sympathetic output from the central nervous system is similarly suppressed by all of the PSA drugs and can result in *bradycardia* and *hypotension*. Furthermore, there is a preponderance of patients who take β-adrenergic blockers and calcium channel blockers, which increase the risk for *dysrhythmias* and cardiovascular collapse during PSA. *Atropine 0.4 mg* IV push is used to treat symptomatic bradycardia (i.e., bradycardia associated with hypotension or heart block).

Nausea and vomiting are usually due to opioids. Preventing unwanted gastrointestinal side effects is important when the patient's sensorium is depressed because emesis could lead to aspiration. Noxious gastrointestinal symptoms also make for an unpleasant experience for the patient. *Zofran 4 to 8 mg* IV is an excellent antiemetic.

Should the patient experience any *itching* or if *urticaria* becomes apparent *(allergic reactions)*, *diphenhydramine 25 mg* IV should be administered. Auscultate the lungs for wheezing and check vital signs. Inhaled bronchodilators, IV corticosteroids, and subcutaneous epinephrine are appropriate for the management of allergic reactions and anaphylaxis.

In rare instances, *paradoxical reactions* to benzodiazepines can occur. Malignant hyperthermia must also be kept in mind as a potential complication.

POSTPROCEDURE RECOVERY AND PATIENT EDUCATION

Recovery should occur in a place where there is adequate cardiopulmonary monitoring and trained personnel for direct observation because the patient continues to be at risk for development of drug-related complications. If reversal agents are administered, continuous observation is required until sufficient time has elapsed for the last dose to wear off, thus avoiding resedation. The *Aldrete score* uses five criteria to determine a level at which it is safe to discharge the patient. The parameters include a measure of blood pressure and SaO_2 and an evaluation of the patient's mental status, airway patency, and motor function. (See flow sheet online at www.expertconsult.com.)

The patient's escort should be given both verbal and written instructions that include postprocedure activities, diet, and medications. Give the patient the following advice:

- Do not drive a car or operate hazardous equipment until the next day.
- Do not make important decisions or sign legal documents for 24 hours.
- Do not take medications, unless your physician has prescribed them specifically, for the next 24 hours.
- Avoid alcohol, sedatives, and other depressant drugs for 24 hours.
- Notify your health care provider of pain, severe nausea, difficulty breathing, difficulty voiding, bleeding, or other new symptoms.

PATIENT EDUCATION GUIDES

See patient education and consent forms and PSA monitoring flow sheets online at www.expertconsult.com.

CPT/Billing Codes

See the CPT definition for moderate sedation discussed earlier.

36000 Introduction of needle or intracatheter, vein
90760 IV therapy 1 hour
90774 IV injection (use in conjunction with J codes for drugs)
94760 Noninvasive ear or pulse oximetry for oxygen saturation
94761 Noninvasive single interpretation
97761 Noninvasive, multiple interpretations
99144 Sedation services provided by the same physician performing the diagnostic or therapeutic service that the sedation supports requiring the presence of an independent observer including monitoring of cardiorespiratory function (pulse oximetry, ECG, and blood pressure), age 5 years or older, first 30 minutes. When providing moderate sedation, the following services are included and *not* reported separately:

- Assessment of the patient (not included in intraservice time)
- Establishment of IV access and fluids to maintain patency, when performed
- Administration of agent(s)
- Maintenance of sedation
- Monitoring of SaO_2, heart rate, and blood pressure
- Recovery (not included in intraservice time)

Intraservice time starts with the administration of the sedation agent(s), requires continuous face-to-face attendance, and ends at the conclusion of personal contact by the physician providing the sedation.

99145 Each additional 15 minutes of intraservice time
99147 Moderate sedation services provided by a physician other than professional performing the procedure, first 30 minutes, age 5 years or older
99150 Each additional 15 minutes

Suppliers

(See contact information online at www.expertconsult.com.)

Banyan kits
Banyan International Corp.
Capnometry monitors
Nellcor Corp.
Heartstream semiautomatic defibrillator
Philips Medical Systems
Vital signs monitors
Welch Allyn

Bibliography

Bahn EL, Holt KR: Procedural sedation and analgesia: A review and new concepts. Emerg Med Clin North Am 23:509–517, 2005.

Frank LR, Strote J, Hauff SR, et al: Propofol by infusion protocol for ED procedural sedation. Am J Emerg Med 24:599–602, 2006.

Goodwin SA, Caro DA, Wolf SJ, et al: Clinical policy: Procedural sedation and analgesia in the emergency department. Ann Emerg Med 45:177–196, 2005.

Green SM, Roback MG, Miner JR, et al: Fasting and emergency department procedural sedation and analgesia: A consensus-based clinical practice advisory. Ann Emerg Med 49:454–467, 2007.

Joint Commission on Accreditation of Healthcare Organizations: 2001 sedation and anesthesia care standards. Available at www.jointcommission.org.

Miller MA, Levy P, Patel MM: Procedural sedation and analgesia in the emergency department: What are the risks? Emerg Med Clin North Am 23:551–572, 2005.

Practice guidelines for sedation and analgesia by non-anesthesiologists: An updated report by the American Society of Anesthesiologists Task Force on Sedation and Analgesia by Non-anesthesiologists. Anesthesiology 96:1004–1017, 2002.

CHAPTER 3

EPIDURAL ANESTHESIA AND ANALGESIA

Peter W. Grigg

Epidural anesthesia (i.e., complete relief of pain and significant motor block) and analgesia (i.e., the relief of pain only, with as little motor block as possible) can be accomplished by injecting opiates, local anesthetics, or a combination of these medications into the epidural space. An epidural is an extremely versatile procedure; it may be used to enhance the birthing experience or to provide anesthesia or analgesia during or after surgical procedures. For prolonged analgesia, a catheter may be left in the epidural space for several days to allow additional medication to be injected by repeated bolus, patient-controlled epidural anesthesia (PCEA) pump, or controlled continuous infusion.

From an anesthetic perspective, the *level* of anesthesia refers to an anatomic level or segment of effect (e.g., up to the level of the umbilicus [T10] or the level of the xiphoid [T8]), whereas *depth* refers to the amount of sensation or motor activity remaining. Depth of blockade is determined by choice of drugs and concentrations. Segmental level of anesthesia or analgesia can be controlled by the level of the injection, the volume of solution injected, as well as other factors (see the note after the Technique section), and the depth can be increased or decreased as the clinical situation dictates. Such control is one of the advantages of epidural anesthesia over other forms of regional anesthesia.

Clinicians administering epidural anesthesia must have a good understanding of not only the relevant anatomy and needle placement techniques, but the pharmacology and physiology involved. The clinician must be familiar and experienced with the diagnosis and management of possible complications. A review of and familiarity with the updated American Society of Anesthesiologists (ASA) Practice Guidelines for Obstetric Anesthesia (2007) and the ASA Difficult Airway Algorithm are highly recommended for medical professionals providing epidural services to obstetric patients. Epidural anesthesia or analgesia should be performed only in a hospital, surgery center, or facility where equipment and adequately trained personnel are available to manage any and all possible complications. The equipment available should be comparable with that of a hospital operating room.

EDITOR'S NOTE: Although there is general agreement that epidural anesthesia is safe and is the most effective method of pain relief in labor, there has been some controversy regarding possible side effects. Meta-analyses attempting to determine whether epidurals increase the risk for cesarean section are conflicting, but the majority of current evidence suggests they do not. However, there is consensus among studies that epidurals prolong labor—the first stage of labor by 12 minutes and the second stage of labor by 42 minutes. There is also consensus that epidurals increase the need for assisted delivery and the likelihood of maternal fever. (The cause of epidural-associated maternal fever is unknown.) Fetal heart rate changes are also common with epidurals during labor. Although the cause of heart rate changes is not known, one theory suggests reduced uterine blood flow from maternal hypotension as the mechanism. Intravenous (IV) fluid preloading (volume expansion) may help reduce the risk of maternal hypotension. However, IV fluid preloading must be performed cautiously or slowly in patients with pregnancy-induced hypertension.

ANATOMIC CONSIDERATIONS

The spinal canal contains the spinal cord, its coverings (i.e., pia mater, arachnoid mater, dura mater), and cerebrospinal fluid. The pia mater is closely attached or adherent to the spinal cord. The dura mater is the separate, toughest, and outermost covering of the spinal cord. The arachnoid membrane is a delicate membrane interposed between the dura mater and the pia mater. It is separated from the pia mater by the subarachnoid space, which contains the cerebrospinal fluid.

The epidural space is a potential space, external to the dura mater and located between the dura mater and the ligamentum flavum (connective tissue covering the vertebrae; Fig. 3-1). Although the epidural space is a potential space, it is filled with spongy connective tissue, fat, and blood vessels. This allows for solutions injected into the space to flow freely in all directions and to bathe the nerve roots as they exit the spinal canal.

PHYSIOLOGIC CONSIDERATIONS

When an epidural is used in labor and delivery, it is important to remember that visceral pain from uterine contractions is partly conducted through the sympathetic nervous system. Impulses travel through the inferior, middle, and superior hypogastric plexuses to the sympathetic chain. This chain then connects to the spinal cord through the 10th, 11th, and 12th thoracic nerves. Any effective analgesic solution must spread cephalad enough to affect these levels.

INDICATIONS

- As an alternative to general or spinal anesthesia for selected surgical procedures
- Requested by patient or suggested by clinician (e.g., to avoid maternal fatigue) for labor and delivery
- Postoperative analgesia

NOTE: Epidural analgesia should not be withheld on the basis of achieving an arbitrary cervical dilation.

NOTE: Continuous epidural analgesia is being used more and more for obstetrics and postoperative analgesia; however, spinal anesthesia is still the most commonly used regional technique for surgical procedures.

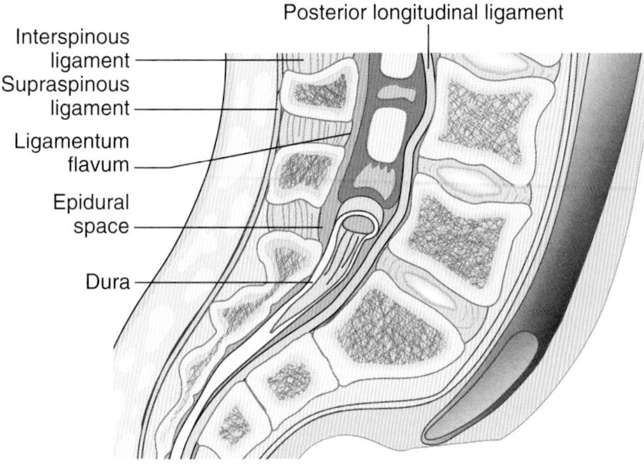

Figure 3-1 Anatomy of the vertebral column and its contents in the lower lumbar and upper sacral regions. (Redrawn from Moore DC: Regional Block, 4th ed. Springfield, Ill, Charles C Thomas, 1979.)

CONTRAINDICATIONS

- Patient declines
- Localized infection at the puncture site
- Severe, uncorrected hypovolemia
- Blood dyscrasias; coagulopathy; prolonged international normalized ratio (INR), prothrombin time (PT), or activated partial thromboplastin time (APTT); thrombocytopenia
- Anticoagulant therapy (e.g., heparin, warfarin, enoxaparin [Lovenox], fondaparinux [Arixtra], clopidogrel [Plavix])
- Allergy to specific epidural agents
- Spinal abnormalities, including scoliosis and other structural abnormalities
- Active systemic infection
- Lack of proper resuscitative equipment, skills, or trained staff
- Preexisting neurologic diseases (amyotrophic lateral sclerosis [ALS], other degenerative nerve diseases, polio)
- Preoperative headache (relative)
- Aortic stenosis
- Anemia

EQUIPMENT

- Disposable sterile gloves
- Equipment for the clinician to observe universal blood and body fluid precautions
- Disposable epidural tray containing the following:
  1. Appropriate prep solutions, swabs, and sterile 4 × 4 gauze pads
  2. Disposable drapes
  3. Epidural catheter, threading assist guide, and syringe adapter attachment
  4. Syringes
     a. Plastic Luer-Lok (3 mL) for local infiltration of lidocaine 1%
     b. Plastic syringe (20 mL) for administration of epidural agent
     c. Glass Luer-Lok procedural syringe (5 mL) filled with saline for loss-of-resistance technique (Fig. 3-2)
  5. Needles
     a. Skin puncture needle (18 gauge)
     b. Tuohy epidural needle (18 gauge) or other epidural needle
     c. Filter needle (19 gauge) for drawing solutions into the syringes
     d. Skin wheal needle (25 or 27 gauge)
  6. Filter (0.2 μm) and filter straw (4 inch)
  7. Medications
     a. Lidocaine 1% (5-mL vial) for local infiltration
     b. Sodium chloride 0.9% injectable (10-mL ampule)
     c. Test dose lidocaine 1.5% injectable, with epinephrine 1:200,000 (5-mL vial)
     d. Epinephrine injectable 1:1000 (1-mL vial)
- Epidural medications (Table 3-1)
- Patient-monitoring equipment (e.g., automated blood pressure [BP] device, continuous electrocardiogram [ECG] monitor, pulse oximeter, fetal monitor [if used for obstetrics])
- Emergency and resuscitative equipment (e.g., suction, Ambu-bag, oxygen, defibrillator) as well as an anesthesia machine
- Emergency and other drugs not included in the epidural kit:
  1. Ephedrine 5% (1 mL) for use if hypotension develops (usual dose to treat hypotension is 10 mg [0.2 mL] IV)
  2. Phenylephrine (Neo-Synephrine)
  3. Atropine
  4. Diphenhydramine (Benadryl)
  5. Metoclopramide (Reglan), ranitidine (Zantac), and Bicitra (a nonparticulate antacid; the generic is sodium citrate and citric acid solution 3 g/2 g per 30 mL)
  6. Diazepam or midazolam

NOTE: A 1% solution equals 10 mg/mL.

Epidural Agents: Local Anesthetics

The two most commonly used local anesthetics for epidural anesthesia are lidocaine and bupivacaine (see Table 3-1). Lidocaine has a rapid onset (5–15 minutes) and lasts 1 to 2 hours, whereas bupivacaine has a slower onset of action (10–20 minutes) and a longer duration of action, lasting 2 to 4 hours. In general, increasing the concentration of the drug while maintaining the same volume decreases the latency (time to onset of anesthesia). The addition of epinephrine to lidocaine (available premixed 1:200,000 with lidocaine) or to 0.25% (or less) bupivacaine appears to increase the duration of action.

Bupivacaine is widely used for both obstetric and surgical epidural anesthesia and analgesia. Bupivacaine 0.25% provides adequate sensory analgesia with minimal motor blockade for 1 to 3 hours, and it is well suited for both obstetric and postoperative analgesia (Table 3-2). When used at 0.5% concentration, bupivacaine produces significant motor blockade. Because of toxicity at higher levels, bupivacaine 0.75% is not recommended for use in obstetrics.

Levobupivacaine (Chirocaine) is a newer agent that is similar to bupivacaine in duration and action but with less central nervous system (CNS) and cardiac toxicity. Another agent, ropivacaine (Naropin), has less cardiotoxicity than bupivacaine but more than lidocaine. In addition, ropivacaine has a significantly higher threshold for CNS toxicity than bupivacaine. In studies, 15 to 30 mL ropivacaine 0.5% provided epidural anesthesia comparable to bupivacaine 0.5% for cesarean section; however, the duration of motor blockade was shorter with ropivacaine.

When lumbar epidural anesthesia is used for surgical procedures, initial volumes of 10 to 20 mL are recommended in adult patients, depending on the concentration of anesthetic and the desired level of anesthesia. Sensory levels are then checked and the dose adjusted accordingly. Additional incremental doses are administered through the epidural catheter as needed. Lower initial volumes (6 to 10 mL) are usually adequate for analgesia in the obstetric patient.

NOTE: The clinician should always use preservative-free local anesthetics and narcotic agents specifically formulated for spinal or epidural anesthesia.

Epidural Agents: Opiates

Anesthetic agents tend to cause motor blockade. Although they do not cause motor blockade, epidural opioids alone are not as effective as dilute concentrations of local anesthetics for anesthesia or analgesia. However, when opiates are used in combination with local

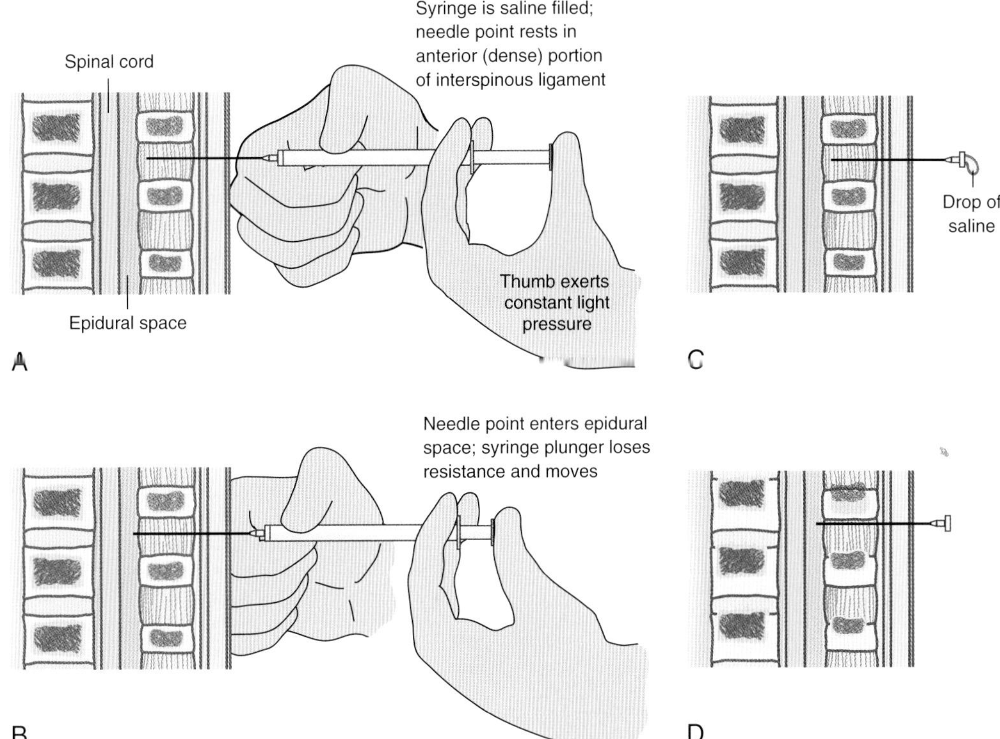

Figure 3-2 Loss-of-resistance and hanging-drop methods of ascertaining when the point of the needle rests in the epidural space. **A,** Needle rests in interspinous ligament. **B,** Syringe plunger loses resistance when needle enters epidural space. **C,** Saline-filled syringe has been removed, leaving a hanging drop. **D,** Hanging drop disappears when needle enters epidural space. (Redrawn from Moore DC: Regional Block, 4th ed. Springfield, Ill, Charles C Thomas, 1979.)

TABLE 3-1 Local Anesthetics Commonly Used for Epidural Anesthesia

Agent	Concentration (%)	Dose (mL)	Dose (mg)	Onset (min)	Duration (hr)	Sensory Block	Motor Block
Lidocaine	2	10–20	100–400	5–15	1–2	Good	Good
Bupivacaine	0.5	10–20	50–100	10–20	2–4	Good	Good
Levobupivacaine	0.5	10–20	50–150	10–15	4–6	Good	Good
Ropivacaine	0.5	15–30	75–150	15–30	2–4	Good	Good
Ropivacaine	0.75	15–25	113–188	10–20	3–5	Good	Excellent

TABLE 3-2 Local Anesthetics Commonly Used for Epidural Analgesia

Agent	Concentration (%)	Dose (mL)	Dose (mg)	Onset (min)	Duration (hr)	Sensory Block	Motor Block
Lidocaine	1	10–20	100–200	5–15	1–2	Good	Good
Bupivacaine	0.125–0.25	10–20	25–50	15–20	1–3	Good	Minimal
Chirocaine	0.125–0.25	10–20	25–50	15–20	1–2	Good	Minimal
Ropivacaine	0.2	10–20	20–40	10–15	0.5–1.5	Good	Minimal

TABLE 3-3 Concentrations of Bupivacaine with or without Opioids for Labor Analgesia (Bolus Injection)

Bupivacaine Concentration (%)*	Dose (mL)	Opioid	Result
0.5	5–10	None	Both sensory and motor blockade
0.25	10–15	None	Sensory and partial motor blockade
0.125	10–15	Fentanyl 1–3 μg/mL	Sensory and minimal motor blockade
0.06	10–15	Sufentanil 0.5 μg/mL	Analgesia and no motor blockade

*The higher concentrations are being used less frequently for labor analgesia. The trend is for use of higher-volume lower local concentrations.

anesthetic agents, they allow for a reduction in the necessary concentration of the anesthetic agents, thereby minimizing motor blockade. This makes epidural opioids particularly useful in situations where motor blockade is undesirable (e.g., labor, control of postoperative pain). Table 3-3 shows doses and effects of combining bupivacaine and opioids for control of labor pain.

Preprocedure Patient Preparation

A focused history (general maternal health, anesthesia problems, drug allergy, relevant obstetric issues, current medications, and NPO status) and physical examination should be performed with special attention to the airway, blood pressure, heart, lungs, and back for anatomic deformities or skin infection. Expert witnesses in medical liability cases often note a lack of preblock examination by the anesthesiologist. Laboratory studies are obtained on an individualized basis and should include a coagulation profile if indicated.

The patient should be informed of the available anesthesia and analgesia options. A fact sheet can be given to the patient to read before surgery or before the procedure is performed (see the sample patient education form available at www.expertconsult.com) or, for obstetric patients, before the onset of labor. For obstetric care, patients should be informed that any anesthetic procedure is optional and that there are associated risks. Preferably, the fact sheet is given to the patient as a part of the prenatal care. Desired anesthesia or analgesia should be included in the patient's birth plan.

Shortly before performing an epidural, the clinician should answer any questions, review the options again with the patient, including the benefits and specific risks, and obtain signed informed consent. Follow local NPO guidelines (usually nothing to eat or drink 8 hours before the scheduled procedure). Early and ongoing communication between the obstetrician or surgeon and the anesthesiologist is vital, particularly when significant anesthetic, obstetric, or surgical risk factors have been identified.

Technique

1. Consider giving nonparticulate antacids, H_2 blocker, and metoclopramide 30 minutes before an epidural if a cesarean delivery or postpartum tubal ligation is being performed.
2. Informed consent and permission forms should be signed and in order.
3. Establish IV access with a 20-gauge or larger catheter and give a bolus of 500 to 1000 mL of IV fluids. The patient should be well hydrated before the procedure to minimize the risk of hypotension.

   NOTE: Administer the IV fluids slowly in patients with pregnancy-induced hypertension.
4. Secure the continuous BP, ECG, and pulse oximetry monitors on the patient and record the initial values. Cycle the BP monitor to observe carefully for hypotension by measuring the BP every 2.5 minutes. Vital signs should be recorded on the anesthesia chart at least every 5 minutes. All medications, doses, routes, and times administered must be noted on the record. For obstetric patients, fetal monitoring should be used.
5. Open the disposable epidural kit and mix the appropriate solutions. Use the filtered needle to draw the solutions that will be administered epidurally. All epidural medications must be preservative free.
6. Place the patient in either the sitting or the lateral position, with the back and neck flexed and the spine straight and not rotated. An assistant should stand in front of the patient during the procedure, helping the patient to remain in that position.
7. Locate the appropriate interspace. Perform the sterile prep and drape the area.
8. A midline approach through the L2 to L3, L3 to L4, or L4 to L5 interspace is most commonly used for epidural anesthesia. Administer local anesthesia (lidocaine 1%) to the interspace area by first making a skin wheal, then injecting into the deeper tissues at the angle the epidural needle will follow.
9. Preliminarily puncture just the skin with an 18-gauge needle to allow for later easy passage of the epidural needle.
10. Pass the Tuohy epidural needle through the skin, angling it appropriately to pass directly toward the spinal canal, until it has firmly passed into the interspinous ligament. Using either the loss-of-resistance technique (with air or saline) or the hanging-drop method (see Fig. 3-2), the needle is now advanced into the epidural space.

    NOTE: The proper angle to direct the tip depends on which interspace is used. The proper angle is almost perpendicular at the L4 to L5 interspace (90 degrees), although it decreases to about 70 degrees at the L2 to L3 interspace. The proper location is usually just below the inferior border of the spinous processes. For epidural anesthesia, insertion angle and location are identical to those used for saddle block anesthesia; however, the depth of insertion is unique to each procedure.
11. Single-shot epidural injections may be used for surgical procedures of short duration. If a longer-duration procedure is anticipated or if postoperative pain relief is desired, place an epidural catheter. Catheter placement must be performed very carefully because improper placement can cause life-threatening complications (e.g., intravascular injection, or total spinal anesthesia if in the subarachnoid space). Rotate the needle so that the catheter will pass either cephalad or caudad as it exits the needle. Note the markings toward the hub of the epidural catheter that are usually 1 cm apart after the first mark. In most cases, the first mark is the same distance from the tip of the catheter as the needle is long. In other words, when inserting the catheter, after the first mark has passed into the needle hub, for every centimeter mark further that the catheter is advanced, the tip advances a centimeter into the spinal canal.
12. Place the tip of the catheter through the hub of the Tuohy epidural needle and advance it slowly through the needle and into the epidural space. A slight resistance is usually encountered as the catheter tip passes through the needle into the epidural space. Advance the catheter 5 cm into the epidural space. The needle is then slowly withdrawn over the catheter, and the catheter secured at the puncture site and along the back with tape. Tape the catheter in place after the patent sits up because the epidural catheter moves when changing from the flexed to straight up position, and may otherwise come out of the epidural space.

    NOTE: The clinician should *never* attempt to withdraw the catheter while the needle is in place. The catheter may shear off, leaving the distal segment in the epidural space. Never readvance the needle after the catheter is in place, for the same reason.

13. Secure the catheter hub so that it is easily accessible for injections from the head of the operating table. Fasten the syringe adapter filter to the proximal end of the catheter. Tape the hub to the epidural tubing and to the patient's gown to prevent dislodging with movement.
14. Administer the test dose through the catheter or through the needle hub if not using a catheter. The test dose is performed to detect either intravascular or subdural placement of the catheter or needle. Begin by aspirating to check for the presence of blood or cerebrospinal fluid. If either is present, the needle has been inserted improperly and must be corrected. Next, administer 2 to 4 mL of 1.5% lidocaine with 1 : 200,000 epinephrine. If the needle is intravascular, a noticeable increase in heart rate, BP, or both will usually be detected within 3 minutes after the injection. The patient may note tinnitus. Sensory and motor function of the lower extremities will be affected after 5 minutes if the catheter or needle is in the subdural space. If intravascular placement is detected, remove the catheter and repeat the procedure at a different interspace. If the catheter is intrathecal, then options exist: (1) remove and replace the catheter at a different interspace or (2) use as a continuous spinal catheter.
15. After the test dose has confirmed proper placement, the patient is ready for the epidural injection. Aspirate to check for the presence of blood or cerebrospinal fluid before each injection or before placing the patient on an infusion pump or PCEA pump. (Use of infusion pumps or PCEA pumps is beyond the scope of this chapter. Please refer to standard anesthesia textbooks for this information.) Check and record the level of analgesia after the injection. A relatively sharp object (e.g., a toothpick) can be used to do this. Do not use a needle.
16. Some anesthesiologists do a combined spinal/epidural technique, but this is not described here.

    NOTE: The factors affecting the level of epidural analgesia include the level of the epidural injection; the volume and concentration of anesthetic solution used; the rate of injection; the addition of a vasoconstrictor; patient age, height, and physical condition; and the position of the patient.

Complications

- Hypotension
  - It is the most common cardiovascular complication of epidural anesthesia.
  - It is caused by widespread sympathetic block.
  - Hypovolemic patients are more susceptible to hypotension.
  - The clinician should treat significant hypotension with positioning, IV fluids, and an IV vasopressor if needed.

  NOTE: Significant bradycardia may be treated with atropine.

- Subarachnoid injection: Injection of large volumes of anesthetic solution into the subdural or subarachnoid space may result in a high or total spinal block, with respiratory arrest, severe hypotension, and possibly cardiac arrest. These conditions must be recognized and treated immediately.
- Postspinal headache: Subdural puncture, always a risk when performing epidural anesthesia, carries a high risk for spinal headache, particularly in younger and pregnant patients. For severe or persistent headache, a blood patch may be necessary.
- Toxicity from anesthetic agents
  - See Chapter 5, Local and Topical Anesthetic Complications.
  - Accidental injection of local anesthetic into the bloodstream or anesthetic overdose may lead to systemic toxic reactions, including (1) *CNS toxicity* (which begins with numbness of tongue, lightheadedness, dizziness, tinnitus, blurred vision, disorientation, drowsiness, muscle twitching, and tremors, possibly progressing to convulsions); and (2) *cardiovascular toxicity* (initially a mild increase in BP and heart rate is observed, followed by hypotension). The clinician should treat initial hypotension with ephedrine. In severe cases the patient may experience an irreversible state of cardiovascular depression.

  NOTE: For CNS toxicity, treat convulsions by (1) maintaining a patent airway and assisted or controlled ventilation; and (2) administering IV thiopental (Sodium Pentothal), midazolam, or diazepam. Intubation may be required.

  - Local tissue toxicity is also possible (but it is rare when preservative-free anesthetic solutions are used).
- Respiratory complications, which can be caused by paralysis of intercostal muscles, and hypoxia or hypercarbia can occur, especially in patients with underlying respiratory disease (e.g., chronic obstructive pulmonary disease).
- Neurologic damage: Postepidural neurologic sequelae are due to (1) trauma; (2) anterior spinal artery syndrome (i.e., a syndrome resulting from damage or thrombosis of the anterior spinal artery caused by trauma from the epidural needle), which is almost always avoided by using a midline approach when inserting the needle; and (3) epidural hematoma.

  NOTE: Because of decreased peripheral sensation, the patient is at increased risk of lower extremity injury as long as the epidural is in place. Risk of neural injury in the operating room can be kept to a minimum through careful patient positioning. After surgery, patients must be followed closely to detect potentially treatable sources of neurologic injury, including expanding spinal hematoma or epidural abscess, constrictive dressings, improperly applied casts, and increased pressure on neurologically vulnerable sites. A neurologist or a neurosurgeon should evaluate new neurologic deficits promptly to formally document the patient's evolving neurologic status, arrange further testing or intervention, and provide long-term follow-up.

- Catheter complications
  - Epidural catheters may be inadvertently inserted into a blood vessel or into the subarachnoid space. The test dose is used to avoid this possibility and to prevent placing a large dose of anesthetic into either the circulation or the subarachnoid space. Epidural catheters can also migrate into blood vessels and the subarachnoid space, so watch for complications that may occur shortly after insertion.
  - The distal portion of the catheter may break off in the epidural space. This may occur if an attempt is made to withdraw the catheter through the epidural needle. It may also occur if the needle is readvanced after the catheter is deployed. If the catheter will not advance through the needle, remove the needle and catheter together and repeat the procedure at another interspace.

CPT/Billing Codes

62273 Injection, lumbar epidural, of blood or patch
62278 Injection of diagnostic or therapeutic anesthetic or antispasmodic substance (including narcotics); epidural, lumbar or caudal, single
62279 Injection of diagnostic or therapeutic anesthetic or antispasmodic substance (including narcotics); epidural, lumbar or caudal, continuous
62311 Epidural, lumbar, single
62319 Epidural, lumbar, continuous

ICD-9-CM Diagnostic Codes

For ICD-9-CM codes for other surgical procedures, see the appropriate chapter.

V22.2 Pregnant state, NOS
650 Spontaneous vaginal deliveries

A fifth digit (represented by the * symbol in the following codes) is used to denote the current episode of care for codes 640 to 648 and 651 to 669. Following are the digits used and the episodes of care they represent:

0 = Unspecified
1 = Delivered with or without mention of antepartum condition
2 = Delivered with mention of postpartum complication
3 = Antepartum condition or complication
4 = Postpartum condition or complication
644.2* Premature labor with delivery (less than 37 weeks)
652.2* Breech presentation
653.5* Unusually large fetus causing disproportion
660.4* Shoulder dystocia

The following are codes related to deliveries with forceps or vacuum:

659.7* Abnormality in fetal heart rate or fetal distress
662.2* Prolonged second stage of labor

The following are codes related to episiotomy, episiotomy repair, and repair of low vaginal lacerations:

664.0* First-degree perineal laceration
664.1* Second-degree perineal laceration
664.2* Third-degree perineal laceration
664.3* Fourth-degree perineal laceration
664.4* Unspecified perineal laceration

The following are codes that relate to pain:

719.4 Joint pain
724.5 Back pain
729.5 Limb or leg pain

NOTE: More specific locations will usually be reimbursed at higher levels.

307.80 Psychogenic pain, site unspecified
307.89 Psychogenic pain, other (This code can be used to indicate pain in most areas.)

Acknowledgment

The editors wish to recognize the many contributions by Thomas H. Corbett, MD, MPH, to this chapter in the previous editions of this text.

Suppliers

(See contact information online at www.expertconsult.com.)

Anesthesia and critical care pharmaceuticals
Baxter Healthcare Corp.
Becton, Dickinson and Co.
Rusch, Inc.
Sims Portex, Inc.
Disposable trays, infusion pumps, etc.
B. Braun Medical, Inc.
Epidural and saddle block needles
Kendall Company

Patient Education Guides

See the patient education form available at www.expertconsult.com.

BIBLIOGRAPHY

American College of Obstetricians and Gynecologists Committee on Obstetric Practice: ACOG committee opinion. No. 339: Analgesia and cesarean section delivery rates. Obstet Gynecol 107:1487–1488, 2006.
American College of Obstetricians and Gynecologists Committee on Obstetric Practice: ACOG committee opinion. No. 443: Optimal goals for anesthesia care in obstetrics. Obstet Gynecol 113:1197–1199, 2009.
American Society of Anesthesiologists Task Force on Management of the Difficult Airway: Practice guidelines for management of the difficult airway: An updated report by the American Society of Anesthesiologists Task Force on Management of the Difficult Airway. Anesthesiology 98:1269–1277, 2003.
American Society of Anesthesiologists Task Force on Obstetric Anesthesia: Practice guidelines for obstetric anesthesia: An updated report by the American Society of Anesthesiologists Task Force on Obstetric Anesthesia. Anesthesiology 106:843–863, 2007.
Echt M, Begneaud W, Montgomery D: Effect of epidural analgesia on the primary cesarean section and forceps delivery rates. J Reprod Med 45: 557–561, 2000.
Hawkins JL: Revised practice guidelines for obstetric anesthesia. ASA Newsletter 71:1, 2007.
Hofmeyr GJ: Prophylactic intravenous preloading for regional analgesia in labour. Cochrane Database Syst Rev:CD000175, 2000.
Horlocker TT: Complications of spinal and epidural anesthesia. Anesthesiol Clin North America 18:461–485, 2000.
McClellan KJ, Faulds D: Ropivacaine: An update of its use in regional anesthesia. Drugs 60:1065–1093, 2000.
Thorp JA: Epidural analgesia during labor. Clin Obstet Gynecol 42:785–801, 1999.

CHAPTER 4

LOCAL ANESTHESIA

Gerald A. Amundsen

The administration of local anesthesia is an extremely important practice in most clinical settings. Most wounds, traumatic and surgical, require some form of anesthesia before repair in order to maintain patient comfort and satisfaction. Over 100 million wounds are repaired in the United States each year, so it is imperative that most clinicians be well accustomed to the medications and techniques used to administer the medications.

The underlying action of local anesthetics is to prevent the generation and conduction of nerve impulses at the molecular level. The overall effect of an anesthetic is to reduce pain associated with trauma or procedures, and this effect is significantly affected by factors such as blood supply, the size of the area to be anesthetized, and the location of the wound in terms of nerve ending size and density. The fingers, toes, genitals, perianal area, and nose are especially sensitive. Patient factors such as infection, anxiety, and chronic disease (e.g., diabetes, peripheral vascular disease, obesity) also affect the success of the anesthetic. To achieve successful anesthesia, the clinician must be able to make decisions and react based on all of these factors. (Also see Chapter 10, Topical Anesthesia.)

INDICATIONS

- To relieve pain from a procedure (incision) or trauma (laceration/fracture)
- Diagnostic nerve blocks to isolate pathology

See Tables 4-1 and 4-2 for a selection of local anesthetics and their characteristics, and Box 4-1 for selection criteria for local anesthetics.

RELATIVE CONTRAINDICATIONS

- "Known" sensitivity to amide anesthetic medications (lidocaine, mepivacaine, bupivacaine) has never been reported and so is a relative contraindication. The older ester anesthetics (procaine, tetracaine) are more likely to cause true allergic reactions. Fortunately, there is no cross-reactivity between the classes, so the individual with known sensitivity to the ester anesthetics is not likely to experience a similar reaction with the amide group. The **parabens preservatives** used to prolong shelf life in multidose vials of amide anesthetics may induce sensitivity reactions similar to those of the ester group. Parabens are most likely the cause of the "allergy" ascribed to the amides. However, the incidence of parabens allergy is also quite low. If there is a concern about an allergy, use single-dose vials of the amide anesthetics that lack preservative and are inexpensive.
- History of central nervous system (CNS) symptoms (e.g., seizure, tremor, tinnitus) associated with anesthetic toxicity.
- History of cardiovascular reactions (e.g., hypotension, bradyarrhythmia) associated with previous anesthetic use.
- Epinephrine, frequently used in local anesthetics to prolong the action as well as to decrease the blood flow, may cause a variety of reactions either directly, in association with other medications the patient uses, or as a result of other existing comorbidities.
  - Epinephrine generally should also be avoided, because of vasoconstrictive properties, in the distal extremities (i.e., fingers, toes, penis, nose, earlobes), in contaminated wounds, or when the viability of a skin flap is in question.
  - Patients with known peripheral vascular disease may have an exaggerated vasoconstrictor response to epinephrine. Extreme care should be taken if local anesthetics with vasoconstrictors are used in patients with diabetes, hypertension, arteriosclerosis, thyrotoxicosis, heart block, or cerebral vascular disease.
  - If a skin flap has marginal viability or if blood flow to a flap is compromised, epinephrine should not be used.
  - If a wound is contaminated, epinephrine may increase the likelihood of infection because of the diminished blood flow.
  - Do not use epinephrine in patient taking monoamine oxidase inhibitors.

EQUIPMENT

Supplies necessary for the local administration of anesthetic are typically inexpensive and readily accessible.

- Anesthetic agents of choice (see Table 4-1 and Box 4-1)
- 18-gauge needle to draw up solution
- 25- to 30-gauge needles of various lengths
- Syringes (1–10 mL)
- Antiseptic (alcohol, povidone-iodine, chlorhexidine) to clean the vial top and the clinical area
- Sodium bicarbonate 7.5% (Neutra-Caine) or sodium bicarbonate 7% to 10% for buffering the anesthetic if desired to reduce the pain of injection (see later discussion)

EDITORS' NOTES: (1) In equipping the office, it is unnecessary to store every type of anesthetic at every concentration, and it is also unnecessary to stock the office with every size and length of needle. It is more practical and economical for the physician to be familiar with the equipment of choice and to stock the office according to preference. Typically, a long- and short-acting anesthetic with and without epinephrine and a few sizes of needle should suffice for most offices. (2) Melman and Siegel (1999) have shown that it is perfectly acceptable **to draw up buffered anesthetic solutions in syringes up to 14 days before use.** When stored at room temperature, there is no increased bacterial contamination or growth, and the anesthetic still functions. We used to pull up our syringes at the beginning of the day and then discard them at the end of the day, but there is no need to do this. We now fill numerous 1-mL syringes, date them, and continue to use them throughout the week. It is much more efficient for the nurse to pull up multiple syringes than to do just one at a time. It is not efficient for the physician to spend time pulling up anesthetic into the syringe! (3) Advanced Meditech International (AMI) has designed **a small anesthetic bottle holder that mounts on the wall** (VE-11 Handzfree Anesthetic Bottle

TABLE 4-1 Local Anesthetic Agents

Type	Name	Concentration (%)	Onset	Duration*	Maximum Adult Dose
Amino esters	Procaine (Novocain)	2	Slow	15–30 min plain 30–90 min w/epi	600 mg
	Tetracaine (Pontocaine)	0.25	Slow	120–240 min plain 240–480 min w/epi	100 mg plain 200 mg w/epi
	Chloroprocaine (Nesacaine)	2	Fast	15–30 min plain 30–90 min w/epi	800 mg plain 1000 mg w/epi
Amino amides†	Lidocaine (Xylocaine)	0.5–2	Fast	30–120 min plain 60–400 min w/epi	300 mg plain 500 mg w/epi
	Etidocaine (Duranest)	0.5	Fast	120–240 min plain	300 mg plain 400 mg w/epi
	Mepivacaine (Carbocaine)	1	Moderate	30–120 min plain 60–400 min w/epi	300 mg plain 500 mg w/epi
	Bupivacaine (Marcaine)	0.25	Slow	120–240 min plain 240–480 min w/epi	175 mg plain 225 mg w/epi

w/epi, with epinephrine.
*Duration of action for adults and older children; prolonged duration of action in neonates and young children possible.
†No known allergic reaction to the amides. If allergic reaction apparent with use, consider parabens preservatives as the cause. Use single-dose vials of anesthetics to avoid parabens.

TABLE 4-2 Maximum Dosages of Commonly Used Injectable Local Anesthetics

Anesthetic	Concentration (%)	Maximum Adult Dose
Lidocaine (Xylocaine)	1	4.5 mg/kg not to exceed 300 mg (30 mL in adult)
Lidocaine (Xylocaine) with epinephrine	1	7 mg/kg not to exceed 500 mg (50 mL in adult)
Bupivacaine (Marcaine) with epinephrine	0.25	3 mg/kg not to exceed 175 mg (50 mL per average adult)
Bupivacaine (Marcaine)	0.25	3 mg/kg not to exceed 225 mg

From McEvoy GK (ed): AHFS Drug Information. Bethesda, Md, American Society of Health-System Pharmacists, 1999.

Box 4-1. Selection of Local Anesthetics and Effects

Lidocaine (Xylocaine) without Epinephrine (1% to 2%)

Can cause vasodilation
Can last 30 to 60 minutes depending on site or vascularity
Use in contaminated wounds
Use in fingers, nose, penis, toes, earlobes
Use if vascular disease is present or if patient is immunocompromised
Use if there are cerebrovascular or cardiovascular risks
Use for nerve block

Lidocaine (Xylocaine) with Epinephrine (1% to 2%)

Causes vasoconstriction
Has longer duration
Use in highly vascular areas to improve visualization of field
Use in clean wounds
In general, do not use on fingers, nose, penis, toes, and earlobes

Bupivacaine (Marcaine)

For longer duration
For nerve blocks

Holder; Fig. 4-1). The cost is around $40, but in our office it is indispensable. It holds the anesthetic where it is readily available and makes filling syringes an easy task. It also allows the entire staff to see how much anesthetic is left in the bottle. There is nothing more frustrating than pulling out the drawer with the anesthetic solution and finding that the bottle is empty!

Options for Allergic Patients

- Use a cooling agent (e.g., ice cube, ethyl chloride).
- For small lesions, use no anesthetic.
- Use single-dose vials instead of multidose vials to avoid the parabens preservatives.
- Use bacteriostatic saline alone.
- Substitute an amide for an ester (if offending agent can be identified).
- Use diphenhydramine (Benadryl). Inject 10 to 50 mg in the usual fashion (50 mg/mL diphenhydramine mixed with 4 mL of normal saline).

Preprocedure Patient Preparation

Patients should be made aware of the anesthesia plan (local, digital block, nerve block, topical) and the potential discomfort they may briefly experience. A standard consent form is used for whatever procedure is to be performed. The risks include allergic reaction to the anesthetic, infection, bleeding, damage to the area resulting in ischemia (if epinephrine or other vasoconstrictors are used), and systematic absorption of the local anesthetic.

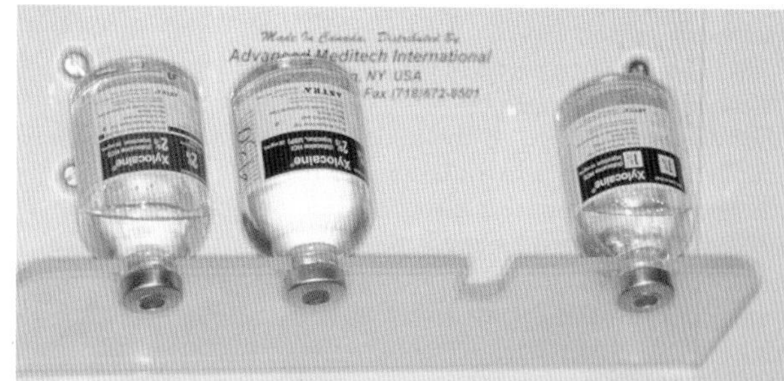

Figure 4-1 Anesthetic bottle holder. (Courtesy of Advanced Meditech International, Inc.; VE-11 Handzfree Anesthetic Bottle Holder.)

General Techniques

1. The top of the vial is wiped with alcohol, and the desired volume of anesthetic is withdrawn using an 18-gauge needle. Typically, 5 to 10 mL should suffice for most procedures, although less than 1 mL is usually enough for simple shave or punch biopsy procedures.
2. Discard the 18-gauge needle and replace it with an appropriately sized needle for the location and type of procedure. For most office procedures, a 27- or 30-gauge needle with a length of 1 or 1.5 inches is appropriate.
3. The local injection may be intradermal (creating a wheal) or subcutaneous (deep to the skin), depending on the intended procedure. Advance the needle to the desired location and draw back on the plunger before injecting to avoid systemic effects associated with injecting directly into a vessel. If there is blood return on aspiration, reposition the needle, aspirate again, and inject if there was no blood return during aspiration.
4. Before any digital or other block, a review of the related anatomy is recommended. In the case of digital blocks, it is important to remember the location and number of nerves supplying each digit (Fig. 4-2). (See Chapter 8, Peripheral Nerve Blocks and Field Blocks.)

Common Errors

- Injection while advancing the needle can result in systemic complications from introduction of the anesthetic directly into the vascular system. Inject only while withdrawing the needle.
- Inadequate anesthesia may be the result of failure to wait for the agent to work effectively. Allow time for the drug to diffuse and achieve the desired effect (4–5 minutes). If the injection is intradermal (causing a wheal), it will have a more rapid onset. If deeper (subcutaneous), it will take longer to achieve its effect.
- Injection directly into an area of infection will not achieve good anesthesia and may contribute to spread of the infection. Do not inject into an area of infection. Rather, inject around the area in a field block pattern (Fig. 4-3), and do not use epinephrine in areas near infection.
- Although there is no proof that injection directly into a suspected cancer will spread the cancer along the needle track, injection into or through a suspected cancer should be avoided if possible.
- Injection of too much anesthetic may distort a lesion in a way that inhibits the accuracy and completeness of the excision or destruction. It may also mask a lesion and make it difficult to palpate and find if it is below the skin. Use a field block (see Fig. 4-3) to avoid the lesion while achieving anesthesia.

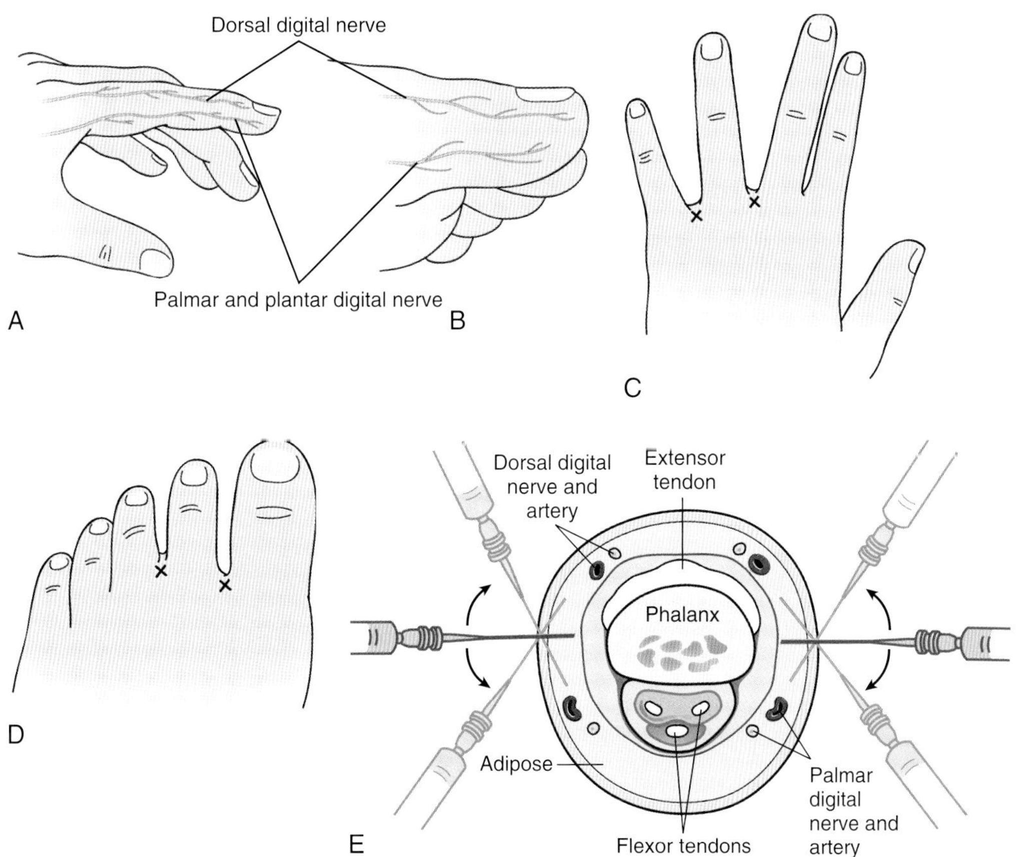

Figure 4-2 The anatomy of a digital block. In the finger (**A**) and toe (**B**), there are four nerves to block in order to obtain a successful digital block. A dorsal and palmar branch on each side of the digit needs to be blocked. If the proper sites of infiltration are chosen (**C,** finger, or **D,** toe), the four nerves should be well anesthetized. First, the web space on both sides of each digit is injected. Insert the needle parallel to the digits, directed toward the hand or foot. Insert 1 to 2 cm and inject 1 to 2 mL of anesthetic. Repeat on the other side. After the web space is infiltrated, insert the needle perpendicular to the base of the digit on each side of the digit. Insert until the needle touches bone. Withdraw a few millimeters and inject 1 mL of anesthetic (red needle and syringe). It is also helpful to then perform a "ring block" (**E**). Inject from the midline on top to the midline on the bottom from both sides to complete a "ring" around the entire digit (gray needle and syringe). A digital block may take several minutes to take effect because there is so much accessory innervation. In the case of a severely inflamed paronychia, or an ingrown toenail in which the nail must be partially or entirely removed, additional local anesthetic may still be necessary just proximal to the site of inflammation to eliminate pain and to allow the removal. It is best to avoid vasoconstrictor agents in local anesthetics for digital blocks. In addition, care should be taken to avoid systemic injection. See Figure 8-2 for more anatomic details.

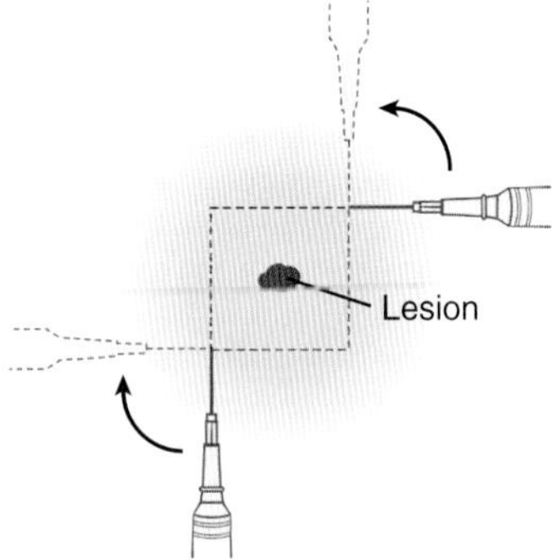

Figure 4-3 Field block. Inject at 90-degree angles on both sides of the skin lesion to be excised. Usually only two injection sites are necessary. After injecting in one direction, withdraw the needle, rotate it 90 degrees, and inject again. This avoids distortion of the central area around the lesion to be excised.

- Inappropriate administration of anesthetic creates increased pain and anxiety for the patient. Methods for reducing the pain of injection are discussed in Box 4-2.
- For adverse reactions and concerns about toxic doses, see Chapter 5, Local and Topical Anesthetic Complications.

Reduction of Pain of Injection

Sodium Bicarbonate

Injection of local anesthetics can cause pain, which is related to the size of the needle, the rapidity of injection, and the temperature of the anesthetic solution. The acidity of the solution (pH 4.05 to 6.49) also causes a significant burning sensation. This short-lived pain can be reduced by using a small needle, pinching up the skin, injecting slowly, warming the solution (room temperature), and adding 1 mL of sodium bicarbonate solution (7%–10%) to 9 mL of anesthetic. Patients, especially children, will note remarkable improvement in comfort. Infiltration with unbuffered solution has been found to be 2.8 to 5.7 times more painful than infiltration with buffered counterparts. There has been no significant difference detected in the time of onset or duration of anesthesia or in the surface area of skin anesthetized. Occasionally, the addition of bicarbonate can make the solution cloudy, but there are no known adverse effects from this. Other tips to reduce pain with injections are outlined in Box 4-2.

Box 4-2. Tips to Reduce Pain with Injections

Use warm solution (room temperature).
Use a small needle (30 gauge if possible).
Inject slowly.
Inject subcutaneously into the adipose tissue (vs. intradermally, which creates a wheal). It will take longer for subcutaneous injection to take effect but will be less painful.
Warn the patient that the most sensitive areas are fingers, toes, genitals, nose, and perianal area.
Use sodium bicarbonate.
Pinch up and "shake" the skin while the injection is being given.
Use a topical anesthetic (see Chapter 8, Peripheral Nerve Blocks and Field Blocks) before injection.
Use a topical refrigerant to cool the area before injection (e.g., MediFrig, ethyl chloride, Fluori-Methane [15% dichlorodifluoromethane, 85% trichloromonofluoromethane]).

Previously it was indicated that the buffered solution be discarded after 24 hours. Buffered lidocaine is stable for at least 1 week at room temperature. Refrigeration may nearly double that time. Warming the buffered solution to above room temperature may also decrease the discomfort of injection (see Box 4-2).

Topical Anesthetics

Certain clinical situations favor the use of a topical anesthetic (see Chapter 10, Topical Anesthesia). Examples include combative children too large for the papoose board and too young to reason with, and patients with nosebleeds, eye injuries, corneal abrasions, or lesions on mucous membranes that need to be treated with painful modalities, such as liquid nitrogen or electrosurgery. Mucous membranes (i.e., nose, mouth, throat, esophagus, anus, and genitourinary tract) can be anesthetized successfully with many of the local anesthetics by direct topical application. Care must be taken to avoid excess systemic absorption of the topical anesthetic near mucous membranes (see Chapter 5, Local and Topical Anesthetic Complications). On many occasions, the application of topical anesthetic before injection may allow for more accurate administration of injectable anesthetic.

Complications

Complications of anesthetic administration are listed here, and adverse effects of the drugs themselves are discussed in detail in Chapter 5, Local and Topical Anesthetic Complications. With proper administration, anesthetic complications are quite rare.

- Sensitivity reactions (with esters or multidose vials)
- CNS toxicity: seizure, tinnitus, visual disturbances, altered mental status (if an excess dose is given)
- Cardiovascular toxicity: arrhythmias, bradycardia, hypotension, congestive heart failure exacerbation
- Marked, prolonged vasoconstriction in digit if epinephrine was used (consider rubbing in nitroglycerin ointment for vasodilation)
- Methemoglobinemia
- Infection
- Bleeding
- Tissue/nerve trauma

Postprocedure Management and Concerns

Patients should be instructed to watch for redness, pus, swelling, streaking, or increased pain, all of which can be indicative of infection or local sensitivity. When a long-acting agent like bupivacaine is used, warn the patient to exercise caution with activity because the long-acting effect will mask pain and allow enough activity to sustain further injury.

CPT/Billing Code

Administration of local anesthetic is included in the CPT code for individual procedures, and no extra charge can be generated. When anesthetic is administered as part of a joint injection, the CPT code for the joint injection is used. Injection of an anesthetic for diagnostic purposes or a therapeutic nerve block can be billed under a CPT code.

64450 Introduction/injection of anesthetic (nerve block), diagnostic or therapeutic

Acknowledgment

The editors wish to recognize the many contributions by Daniel Derksen, MD, to this chapter in the previous edition of this text.

SUPPLIERS

(See contact information online at www.expertconsult.com.)

Advanced Meditech International, Inc. (AMI)
Delasco
MD, Inc.

Most medical suppliers can provide syringes and needles as well as anesthetics.

BIBLIOGRAPHY

Achar S, Kundu S: Principles of office anesthesia. Part 1. Infiltrative anesthesia. Am Fam Physician 66:91–94, 2002.

Denkler K: A comprehensive review of epinephrine in the finger: To do or not to do. Plast Reconstr Surg 108:114–124, 2001.

Denkler K: Dupuytren's fasciectomies in 60 consecutive digits using lidocaine with epinephrine and no tourniquet. Plast Reconstr Surg 115: 802–810, 2005.

Ernst AA, Marvez-Valls E, Nick TG, Wahle M: Comparison trial of four injectable anesthetics for laceration repair. Acad Emerg Med 3:228–233, 1996.

Fitzcharles-Bowe C, Denkler K, Lalonde D: Finger injection with high-dose (1:1000) epinephrine: Does it cause finger necrosis and should it be treated? Hand (NY) 2:5–11, 2007.

Holmes HS: Options for painless local anesthesia. Postgrad Med J 89:71–72, 1991.

Krunic AL, Wang LC, Soltani K, et al: Digital anesthesia with epinephrine: An old myth revisited. J Am Acad Dermatol 51:755–759, 2004.

Lalonde D, Bell M, Benoit P, et al: A multicenter prospective study of 3,110 consecutive cases of elective epinephrine use in the fingers and hand: The Dalhousie Project clinical phase. J Hand Surg Am 30:1061–1067, 2005.

Melman D, Siegel DM: Prefilled syringes: Safe and effective. Dermatol Surg 25:492–493, 1999.

Moy RL, Pfenninger JL: Taking the sting out of local anesthesia. Patient Care March 15:61–73, 2000.

Radovic P, Smith RG, Shumway D: Revisiting epinephrine in foot surgery. J Am Podiatr Med Assoc 93:157–160, 2003.

Scarfone RJ, Jasani M, Gracely EJ: Pain of local anesthetics: Rate of administration and buffering. Ann Emerg Med 31:36–40, 1998.

Soriano TT, Lask GP, Dinehart SM: Anesthesia and analgesia. In Robinson JK, Hanke CW, Sengelmann RD, Siegel DM (eds): Surgery of the Skin: Procedural Dermatology. Philadelphia, Mosby, 2005, pp 39–58.

Tetzlaff JE: The pharmacology of local anesthetics. Anesthesiol Clin North Am 18:217–233, 2000.

Thomson CJ, Lalonde DH, Denkler KA, Feicht AJ: A critical look at the evidence for and against elective epinephrine use in the finger. Plast Reconstr Surg 119:260–266, 2007.

Tuggy M, Garcia J: Procedures Consult. Available at www.proceduresconsult.com.

Usatine RP, May RL: Anesthesia in Skin Surgery: A Practical Guide. St. Louis, Mosby, 1998.

CHAPTER 5

LOCAL AND TOPICAL ANESTHETIC COMPLICATIONS

William L. McDaniel, Jr. • Raymond F. Jarris, Jr.

Many in-office surgical procedures require the use of local or topical anesthetics. *Topical* anesthetics are used more frequently in children for dermatologic procedures and in persons having nasopharyngoscopy and esophagogastroduodenoscopy (EGD). Various mixtures of potent topical medications are also being used more frequently, often under occlusion, to cover large surface areas for many aesthetic procedures. This markedly increases the risk for toxic levels to accumulate.

The primary care physician must have an understanding of the types of complications that may be encountered when using these anesthetics and must be equipped to diagnose and deal with them. For maximum recommended dosages, see Chapter 4, Local Anesthesia.

ALLERGIC REACTIONS

- Low incidence (<1%).
- Older agents such as procaine and tetracaine (esters) are more likely to cause allergic reactions because they are derivatives of para-aminobenzoic acid, a known allergen.
- *There are no reported allergic reactions to lidocaine (an amide) or any other amides.*
- In known or suspected local anesthetic allergy, avoid *multidose vials* of an amide such as lidocaine. Many contain methylparaben preservatives, which have a structure similar to para-aminobenzoic acid.
- True allergic reactions may vary from mild to life-threatening with anaphylaxis and circulatory collapse. In cases of anaphylaxis
  - Plasma losses may equal 35% of circulating blood volume within minutes.
  - Rapid replacement of volume with colloid and administration of epinephrine are indicated (see Chapter 220, Anaphylaxis).
  - If epinephrine fails, norepinephrine infusion may be lifesaving.

ALTERNATIVES TO OBTAIN PAIN RELIEF IN ALLERGIC PATIENTS

- Use *single-dose* vials of lidocaine, which lack preservative.
- Substitute an amide anesthetic for an ester.
- A small local anesthetic effect can be obtained by injecting sterile normal saline into tissue.
- Small lesions (e.g., skin tags) may not require an anesthetic for removal/treatment.
- Dilute 50 mg of diphenhydramine (1 mL from a 50 mg/mL vial) with 4 mL sterile normal saline. Inject 1 to 5 m (10 mg to 50 mg) of this dilute diphenhydramine locally for anesthetic effect.
- Use ice cubes, ethyl chloride spray (Frigiderm), liquid nitrogen (sparingly) to obtain topical anesthesia.
- Hypnosis.

EFFECTS OF EPINEPHRINE IN LOCAL ANESTHETICS

It has long been an admonition to students, residents, and practicing clinicians that epinephrine should never be used in areas of the body supplied by the fine terminal end arterioles such as the fingers and toes, penis, and nose. Theoretically, the epinephrine could cause prolonged spasm leading to ischemia and even necrosis of the tissue. This effect would be potentially magnified if the vessels were already diseased and narrowed, as occurs in smokers and patients with diabetes, peripheral vascular disease, and similar conditions. Hence, in the past, it was literally seen as substandard care to use epinephrine in these areas, especially when there was potential vascular disease or diminished blood supply.

In 2000, a series of articles began appearing in the literature to refute this "theoretical" adverse effect (see Bibliography). A paper by Denkler published in 2001 reviewed the literature from 1880 through 2000. The conclusion was: "An extensive literature review failed to provide consistent evidence that our current preparations of local anesthesia with epinephrine cause digital necrosis, although not all complications are necessarily reported. However, as with all techniques, caution is necessary to balance the risks of this technique...."

Digits can withstand prolonged periods of ischemia. Successful reimplantations have been reported 42 hours after traumatic amputations.

The usual concentration of epinephrine in local anesthetics is 1 : 100,000. Studies have been conducted using concentrations of 1 : 1000 with virtually no adverse consequences.

A multicenter prospective study of 3110 consecutive cases of elective epinephrine use in the fingers and hands (concentration ≤1 : 100,000) found that "the true incidence of finger infarction in elective low-dose-epinephrine injection into the hand and finger is likely to be remote, particularly with the possible rescue with phentolamine. Phentolamine was not required to reverse the vasoconstriction in any patients" (Lalonde et al, 2005).

"Phentolamine rescue" or reversal of epinephrine is not discussed in this text. Nitroglycerin ointment has also been suggested to reverse any apparent ischemia, however rare (or even possible) this event is.

It would seem acceptable then to use local anesthetics with epinephrine to control bleeding for optimal wound repair and also to prolong needed anesthesia in areas supplied by end arteries. It would appear that an age-old caveat has been disproven. The prudent physician would still observe at-risk patients closely and use epinephrine sparingly.

Overdose Reactions

Central Nervous System Toxicity

Local anesthetics reach the central nervous system after slow absorption or by direct intravenous (IV) injection. An inadvertent direct IV injection may create a transient high local central nervous system level of anesthetic, which can cause *seizures*. Most seizures created in this way terminate within minutes, provided the administration of the drug has stopped.

A warning of less serious central nervous system effects may include circumoral numbness, lightheadedness, tinnitus, visual disturbance, muscular twitching, and irrational behavior.

If high serum levels persist, grand mal seizures, apnea, unconsciousness, and death may occur. An alert patient, in most cases, tells the physician before a seizure develops. This would be absent in the case of rapid inadvertent IV injection.

Acidosis and hypercarbia increase the likelihood of central nervous system toxicity. Pulse oximetry monitoring during the procedure may be an invaluable tool to alert the clinician to some of the effects of toxicity.

With serious central nervous system toxicity, stop the offending agent and begin oxygen and support ventilation if needed. Alert patients can be asked to hyperventilate, which lowers the PCO_2 level and raises the seizure threshold. This may temporarily alleviate twitching. Seizures can usually be stopped with IV midazolam (Versed), diazepam (Valium), or lorazepam (Ativan). Lorazepam and diazepam are inconsistently absorbed by the intramuscular (IM) route. Midazolam may be used IM if an IV line is not available. Flumazenil (Romazicon) should be available as an antagonist for benzodiazepines in case of respiratory depression from the drugs.

Cardiovascular Toxicity

Cardiovascular toxicity can occur with any of the local anesthetic drugs. Local anesthetics prolong conduction through the Purkinje fibers and heart muscle. *Prolongation of PR interval* and *widening of the QRS* may be observed. Higher concentrations decrease heart muscle contractility. *Hypotension, respiratory depression*, and *bradycardia* are observed with lidocaine.

If cardiovascular toxic effects are suspected, discontinue or *remove the agent* when possible. *Basic cardiopulmonary resuscitation is the cornerstone* of immediate management. Advanced cardiac life support (ACLS) protocols should be initiated as necessary for serious rhythm disturbances. Various studies indicate the cardiotoxicity of bupivacaine is more severe and difficult to treat than that associated with lidocaine. Cardiology and anesthesiology consults should be obtained as soon as available.

Catecholamine Reactions

Catecholamine reactions are rarely associated with administered epinephrine but may be produced as a result of anxiety associated with the administration of a local anesthetic or the initiation of the procedure, or as a result of the initial injury that is being treated. Symptoms may include *tachycardia, palpitations, hypertension, apprehension, tremulousness, diaphoresis, tachypnea, pallor, and, on occasion, anginal chest pain*. Caution is recommended for patients who have hyperthyroidism, hypertension, or atherosclerotic cardiovascular disease, although these conditions do not contraindicate the judicious use of epinephrine-containing anesthetics. *Patients taking monoamine oxidase inhibitors should not receive epinephrine-containing anesthetics*. The treatment includes stopping further drug administration, observation of the patient, and administration of alpha- or beta-adrenergic antagonists or benzodiazepine agents, if necessary.

Vasovagal Reactions

A marked vasovagal reaction may occur if the patient experiences anxiety when an event, such as the sight or sensation of a needle insertion, causes a loss of sympathetic tone and an increased vagal tone. The resulting hypotension and bradycardia may lead to lightheadedness or syncope. If this occurs, the patient should be placed in the supine position with the legs elevated. Ammonia inhalant ("smelling salts") can be tried initially. A 0.3-mL ampule can be crushed and waved in front of the patient's nose. Should this not be effective, give 0.5 mL of atropine (1 mg/mL) IM. This may also be required for significant bradycardia. Practitioners need to be observant and aware that vasovagal syncope can occur even 10 to 15 minutes after a procedure/injection. This has been reported after immunizations also, and such reactions to the Gardasil vaccine have gained significant press.

EDITOR'S NOTE: I now include the questions, "How well do you tolerate pain?" (choices: well, okay, poorly) and "Do you have a tendency to faint with needles?" (choices: yes, no) on my intake forms and also on specific procedure questionnaires. If patients answer that they tolerate pain poorly or have a tendency to faint, we routinely give atropine before the surgery/procedure.

Methemoglobinemia

Methemoglobinemia is a rare but serious complication of topical and local anesthetic agents. It should be clinically suspected and diagnosed if topical or local anesthetics were given. Early diagnosis and treatment can prevent the serious complications of brain damage and death. One must be especially cautious now because, as noted, topical anesthesia is being used more frequently for aesthetic procedures.

The best way to illustrate the point is with a case history. A 27-year-old white man underwent outpatient EGD and developed unexplained cyanosis. During his recovery phase the nurse noted cyanosis, which did not resolve on high-flow oxygen. Vital signs and arterial blood gases were within the normal range. Diagnoses such as pulmonary thromboembolic phenomenon and allergic reactions to meperidine (Demerol) or diazepam (Valium) were considered.

An astute respiratory technician noted that the arterial blood drawn for the arterial blood gases was brown. The diagnosis of methemoglobinemia was suspected and confirmed by discovering a methemoglobin level of 14% (Fig. 5-1).

The patient involved had received Cetacaine spray (a combination of benzocaine, aminobenzoate, and tetracaine) four or five

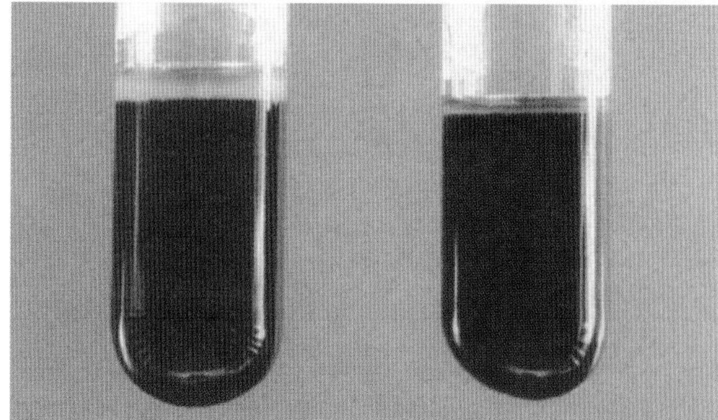

Figure 5-1 Normal arterial blood versus methemoglobinemia. Compare arterial whole blood with 1% methemoglobin *(left)* with arterial whole blood with 72% methemoglobin *(right)*. Note the characteristic chocolate-brown color of the sample with an elevated methemoglobin level. (From DeBaun MR, Vichinsky E: Hemoglobinopathies. In Kliegman [ed]: Nelson Textbook of Pediatrics, 18th ed. Philadelphia, Saunders, 2007, Fig. 462-6.)

times before the EGD procedure. The endoscopist had requested that the patient swallow the material each time. This spray contains about 14% benzocaine, which was the culprit in this case. The 2007 *Physicians' Desk Reference* lists methemoglobinemia as a rare adverse effect of Cetacaine spray and cautions that care should be used not to exceed a 2-second spray.

Normal hemoglobin contains iron in the ferrous (+2) state. Methemoglobin contains iron that has been oxidized to the abnormal ferric (+3) state. Normal levels of methemoglobin range up to 3%.

Prevent methemoglobinemia by avoiding overdose of benzocaine, prilocaine, and lidocaine. Prilocaine and lidocaine in a eutectic mixture of 2.5% each (EMLA) is considered safe when used as recommended. EMLA is applied topically and is often used in infants and children. One case of methemoglobinemia has been reported with its use over large areas for a long period of time. It is more likely to occur if used under occlusion for large areas for extended times.

Other drugs that can cause methemoglobinemia include sulfonamides, phenytoin (Dilantin), amyl nitrate, dapsone, sodium nitroprusside, quinolones, and nitroglycerin.

The following signs are noted at the various methemoglobin levels:

- Up to 15%: graying of skin
- 15% to 20%: cyanosis becomes apparent and the blood has a chocolate-brown color
- 20% to 50%: weakness, dizziness
- 50% to 70%: arrhythmias, acidosis, convulsions, and coma may occur
- Over 70%: death and cerebral anoxia may occur

Nitrates, foods, and contaminated well water may predispose to methemoglobinemia and may lower the threshold for local anesthetics.

Treatment varies with the level of methemoglobin present and the condition of the patient. Urgent administration of methylene blue is indicated for symptomatic hypoxia as evidenced by arrhythmias, angina, respiratory distress, seizures, coma, or methemoglobin levels greater than 30%. Methylene blue 1% administered IV slowly over 5 minutes should result in improvement. Adults and children are administered 1 to 2 mg/kg (0.1 to 0.2 mL/kg of 1% solution) or 25 to 50 mg/kg^2. A second dose can be repeated after an hour if the response was inadequate. Do not exceed 7 mg/kg.

Hyperbaric oxygen therapy may help by increasing the amount of dissolved oxygen in the blood. Consider exchange transfusions in the most severely affected patients. This may require a tertiary center.

Successful treatment will be unavailable unless the astute clinician considers the diagnosis of methemoglobinemia (Box 5-1).

Box 5-1. Factors Suggesting Acquired Methemoglobinemia

A local anesthetic agent was used.
A larger-than-usual dose was needed.
Environmental predisposition present (nitrates) or other predisposing drugs such as sulfonamides, phenytoin (Dilantin), amyl nitrate, dapsone, sodium nitroprusside, quinolones, nitroglycerin, and methamphetamines.
Cyanosis does not respond to usual O_2.
Arterial blood appears chocolate-brown (usually 15% to 20% levels of methemoglobin present).
Infants and the elderly seem more susceptible to development of methemoglobinemia.

BIBLIOGRAPHY

Cetacaine. In Physicians' Desk Reference. Oradell, NJ, Medical Economics, 2001.

Denkler K: A comprehensive review of epinephrine in the finger: To do or not to do. Plast Reconstr Surg 108:114–124, 2001.

Denkler K: Dupuytren's fasciectomies in 60 consecutive digits using lidocaine with epinephrine and no tourniquet. Plast Reconstr Surg 115: 802–810, 2005.

Fitzcharles-Bowe C, Denkler K, Lalonde D: Finger injections with high-dose (1 : 1000) epinephrine: Does it cause finger necrosis and should it be treated? Hand (NY) 2:5–11, 2007.

Greenberg MJ: Diagnosing acquired methemoglobinemia can be confusing at best. EMS News, January 8, 1995.

Krunic AL, Wang LC, Soltani K, et al: Digital anesthesia with epinephrine: An old myth revisited. J Am Acad Dermatol 51:755–759, 2004.

Lalonde D, Bell M, Sparkes G, et al: A multicenter prospective study of 3110 consecutive cases of elective epinephrine use in the fingers and hand: The Dalhousie Project clinical phase. J Hand Surg Am 30:1061–1067, 2005.

Lee JJ, Rubin AP: EMLA cream and its current uses. Br J Hosp Med 50: 463–466, 1993.

Marx JA, Hockberger RS, Walls RM (eds): Rosen's Emergency Medicine: Concepts and Clinical Practice, 6th ed. St. Louis, Mosby, 2004.

McCaughey W: Adverse effects of local anaesthetics. Drug Safety 7:178–189, 1992.

Radovic P, Smith RG, Shumway D: Revisiting epinephrine in foot surgery. J Am Podiatr Med Assoc 93:157–160, 2003.

Roberts JR, Hedges JR (eds): Clinical Procedures in Emergency Medicine, 4th ed. Philadelphia, Saunders, 2004.

Rodriguez LF, Smolik LM, Zbehlik AJ: Benzocaine-induced methemoglobinemia: Report of a severe reaction and review of the literature. Ann Pharmacother 28:643–649, 1994.

Smith C: Pharmacology of local anaesthetic agents. Br J Hosp Med 52: 455–460, 1994.

Thomson CJ, Lalonde DH, Denkler KA, Feicht AJ: A critical look at the evidence for and against elective epinephrine use in the finger. Plast Reconstr Surg 119:260–266, 2007.

CHAPTER 6

Nitrous Oxide Sedation

Marjon B. Jahromi

Nitrous oxide (N_2O) sedation was first used as an anesthetic agent in 1844 and can be considered a safe alternative to intravenous (IV) sedation. Nitrous oxide sedation has a long history of safety in the medical and dental community. It is now used by approximately 95% of pediatric dentists and is growing in popularity in general dental and medical offices. Most U.S.-trained dentists will become proficient in N_2O sedation as part of their undergraduate dental training. It is not necessary to have extensive experience with IV sedation to be able to perform N_2O sedation safely. Gaining experience with N_2O sedation can be achieved by observing an experienced practitioner and performing the sedation under supervision. Alternatively, continuing education courses are available. Practitioners who are not familiar with the technique are encouraged to participate.

Nitrous oxide is a relatively insoluble drug and is a rapidly effective sedative with an onset of effects within 2 to 3 minutes of administration and peak effects within 5 minutes. Dosing can be adjusted easily and rapidly to increase or decrease depth of sedation during the procedure. Recovery time is short because elimination through the lungs occurs as rapidly as absorption. N_2O is not metabolized in the body to any significant extent and therefore can be used safely on most patients. Patients remain conscious and protective reflexes are intact so there is minimal risk of aspiration or oversedation. In addition, N_2O does not cause respiratory depression, making it safer than fentanyl, midazolam, or chloral hydrate. Technically, it is easier to perform than IV sedation because there is no need to gain venous access. Nitrous oxide is administered through a face mask or nasal hood that is simply placed on the patient's face.

Indications

- Anxious and apprehensive patients undergoing minor office surgical or dental procedures
- Patients needing increased pain reaction threshold
- Patients who are unable to tolerate other sedatives

Contraindications

- Pregnancy (first trimester)
- Airway obstruction and severe asthmatic conditions
- Severe psychiatric disorders (N_2O can cause dreaming and hallucinations)
- Pulmonary hypertension
- Pneumothorax
- Severe cardiac disease
- Hyperthyroidism
- Sickle cell anemia
- Chronic bronchitis/emphysema
- Bowel obstruction

Nitrous oxide should *not* be used to replace local anesthesia but rather as an adjunct to local anesthesia. Nitrous oxide sedation is not a good option to control defiant or erratic behavior.

Advantages

- Rapid onset; monitoring time during recovery is brief.
- Good analgesic and amnestic (limited) properties.
- Unlike IV sedation, when nitrous oxide is used alone, a driver is not needed once the patient has recovered. Patients should be monitored for approximately 30 minutes after the use of N_2O to ensure return to baseline functional status before discharge.
- Patients may resume all normal activities after discharge and are not limited in their activities.

Limitations

- Lack of potency
- Expense of equipment
- Training required to become proficient

Equipment

- Inhalation sedation machine (Fig. 6-1)
- Breathing circuit
- Reservoir bag
- Scavenging system
- Nasal hood or facial mask
- Oxygen and N_2O supply (N_2O is stored in compressed form as a liquid in cylinders)
- Pulse oximeter
- Oral pharyngeal airway available

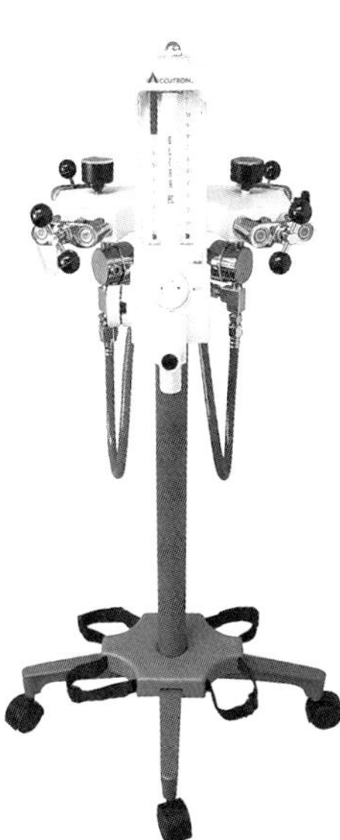

Figure 6-1 Accutron 4-Cylinder Portable Manifold. (Courtesy of Accutron, Inc., Phoenix, Ariz.)

- Emergency cart with appropriate drugs (consider the Banyan kit; see Chapter 220, Anaphylaxis)

Presedation Assessment and Concerns

Figure 6-2 shows an anesthesia evaluation form that can be used before and after the procedure.

- A complete medical history should be obtained from the patient. Relevant information includes a history of cardiac or respiratory disease, medications, allergies, prior surgeries and complications from anesthesia, history of tobacco use, and history of substance abuse.
- The oropharynx should be thoroughly evaluated for any abnormalities or evidence of obstruction. A history of sleep apnea may indicate airway abnormalities such as narrow airways and tonsillar hypertrophy. Obesity, especially involving the face and neck, may lead to difficulties in spontaneous ventilation under sedation.
- Nitrous oxide will potentiate drugs that depress the respiratory system.
- The procedure and all possible sensations should be described to the patient in advance. Nitrous oxide can produce a feeling of euphoria, dreaminess, and detachment. It can also cause numbness and tingling of the extremities. It may cause nausea, confusion, and sexual hallucinations in higher doses.

Preprocedure Patient Preparation

- An experienced assistant trained in Basic Life Support (BLS) should always be present.
- Patients do not need to fast if nitrous oxide is the sole anesthetic agent. However, if an oral sedative is to be used in combination with nitrous oxide, confirm that the patient has fasted for at least 6 hours for solid foods and nonclear liquids and at least 6 hours for clear liquids.
- Perform a full check of the inhalation sedation machine to ensure that it is safe to use and that it has an adequate supply of gases for completion of the procedure. Nitrous oxide is a compressed liquid at room temperature with a pressure of 745 pounds per square inch. A full E cylinder of N_2O will have 1590 mL of gas. The pressure indicator in a N_2O tank will show a constant pressure until only about 20% (400 mL) of N_2O is left in the cylinder. This is very different from oxygen, which is a nonliquified gas. The pressure indicator in an oxygen tank will indicate a proportional decrease in pressure as the volume of the gas is depleted. Therefore, the pressure indicator of a N_2O tank cannot be used to estimate the amount of gas remaining in the cylinder.
- The scavenging system should also be checked for proper functioning. It is below the standard of care to operate a N_2O unit without a scavenging apparatus.
- The health care practitioner should have all the necessary equipment and be prepared to handle all medical emergencies in the event the patient should reach a deeper level of sedation than initially planned. Although not required, a pretracheal stethoscope is an excellent method to monitor the patient's respirations and heart sounds. This may prevent the patient from becoming oversedated and losing consciousness. The conventional or newer wireless pretracheal stethoscope can be easily obtained by any health care practitioner (Figs. 6-3 and 6-4).

Documentation

- Informed consent should be obtained for both the planned procedure and the N_2O sedation. All written and verbal instructions, including consent with risks, benefits, alternatives, and contraindications, should be documented.
- The patient's vital signs, including blood pressure, heart rate, and oxygen saturation by pulse oximetry, should be recorded at regular intervals throughout the procedure and during recovery.
- Any standardized anesthesia form can be used for documentation (Fig. 6-5). Alternatively, vitals, level of sedation, and concentration of N_2O being administered can simply be recorded at 5-minute intervals (also see Chapter 2, Procedural Sedation [Sedation and Analgesia]).

Technique

1. Always have a BLS-trained assistant present.
2. Begin the inhalation sedation session with a full check of the inhalation sedation machine to ensure that it is safe to use and that it has an adequate supply of gases to allow the procedure to be completed. Also check the scavenging system for proper functioning.
3. Once the presedation check has been completed, position the patient properly for the procedure to be performed. Obtain and record baseline vital signs, including continuous pulse oximetry. A *pretracheal stethoscope* may also be placed at the lower end of the trachea and midline to the neck for additional monitoring of respirations.
4. Place a nasal hood or facial mask on the patient's face. The nasal hood should fit snugly around the patient's nose to minimize any leakage of gas. Nasal hoods come in a variety of sizes and may be scented for optimal patient comfort. Most nasal hoods manufactured now are also latex free.
5. Introduce 100% oxygen only. The initial gas flow rate should be set to 6 L/min. The patient should be instructed to take deep breaths through his or her nose. Adjust the flow rate so that the reservoir bag can be seen moving during each breath without completely emptying. If the reservoir bag completely empties, the flow rate should be increased until about two thirds of the bag empties with each patient breath.
6. Once the flow rate has been adjusted to the proper level, introduce the N_2O. Patient tolerance and N_2O requirement vary significantly for each person. It is important to titrate the dose slowly to prevent oversedation. Oversedation should be avoided because it can result in unpleasant feelings for the patient. Initially, 10% N_2O is introduced and the patient is allowed to breathe this mixture for 1 minute. The O_2 level should also be adjusted to maintain the constant flow rate that was previously established. Some inhalation sedation machines will also automatically decrease the O_2 flow as the N_2O flow is increased.
7. If this dose provides adequate sedation, the operative or dental procedure can begin. Signs of adequate sedation include a reduction in anxiety, increased relaxation, slowing of the blink reflex, decreased response to painful stimuli, and general decrease in movements.
8. If this level of sedation is not sufficient, provide an additional 10% N_2O and allow the patient to breathe the mixture for 1 minute before reassessment. This cycle can be repeated to a maximum mixture of 70% N_2O:30% O_2. Document the level and length of N_2O administered in the patient's medical chart.

   NOTE: Minimum dose is 10% N_2O:90% O_2. Maximum concentration is 70% N_2O:30% O_2. Average maintenance dose is typically between 20% N_2O:80% O_2 and 40% N_2O:60% O_2. Almost all ambulatory N_2O/O_2 delivery systems have an oxygen fail-safe mechanism that prevents N_2O from being administered unless there is adequate O_2 flowing to the system. Therefore, it is not possible to administer 100% N_2O.

9. Immediately reduce the N_2O concentration with the first sign of oversedation. *Signs of oversedation* include agitation, sweating, nausea, vomiting, lack of cooperation, diaphoresis, inability to keep eyes open, decreased response to questions, and loss of consciousness. The patient is also at risk for silent aspiration if vomit reaches the epiglottis. Patients may also complain of unpleasant feelings such as intense tingling or detachment from

Patient: ______________________________
Operating Surgeon: ______________________ Procedure: ______________________
Age: __________ Height: __________ Weight: __________ Pre-Op B/P: __________

MEDICAL HISTORY:

____
____
____

ANESTHETIC HISTORY:
Personal: ______________________________
Family: ______________________________

REVIEW OF SYSTEMS:

Heart:	CP DOE Orthopnea HTN CHF Dysrhythmias	______________
Pulmonary:	COPD Asthma URI Bronchitis Pneumonia	______________
Endocrine:	DM Thyroid Obesity Steroid use	______________
GI:	PUD Reflux HH	______________
Liver:	Hepatitis Cirrhosis	______________
Mus. Skel.:	Fractures MH	______________
CNS:	Seizures CVA Paralysis HA TIA	______________
GU:	CRF Infections Pregnant	______________
Hemo:	Coagulopathy Sickle Cell	______________
Habits:	Smoking EtOH Drugs	______________

MEDICATIONS: ______________________________

ALLERGIES: ______________________________

PHYSICAL EVALUATION:
Heart: ______________________________
Pulmonary: ______________________________
Airway: Classification 1 2 3 4 Head and Neck: _____ FBO: _____ Loose/Missing teeth _________

HOSPITALIZATIONS: ______________________________
____

ASA CLASSIFICATION: 1 2 3 4 5 E **NPO:** ______________________

ANESTHESIA PLAN: General Anesthesia Monitored Anesthesia Care Nitrous Oxide

PRE-OPERATIVE MEDICATIONS: ______________________________

CONSENT (Risks/Benefits/Alternatives discussed, Questions answered, Accepts risks) ______________

______________ ______________________
Date / Time Signature

DISCHARGE SUMMARY: ☐ VSS ☐ Alert/Awake ☐ Ambulatory ☐ IV removed intact ☐ Post-op instructions given to

____

Post-op transport provided by: Room Air SpO_2: %

____
____

POST-DISCHARGE NOTE:

____
____
____
____

ANESTHESIA EVALUATION

Figure 6-2 Anesthesia evaluation form used both before and after the procedure to document discharge status.

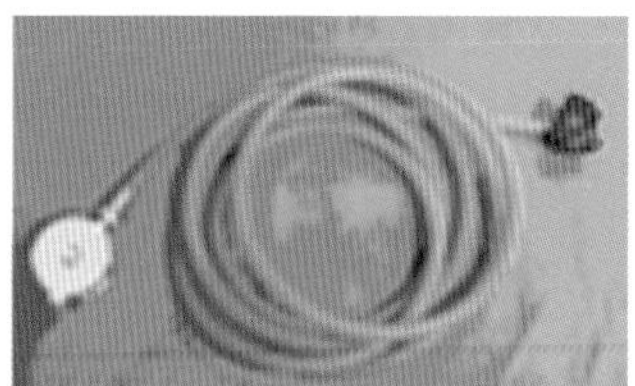

Figure 6-3 Conventional pretracheal stethoscope. (Author's own stethoscope. Chest piece from Hull Anesthesia, Inc. Earpiece and cord from Westone.)

reality. It is imperative that the health care provider constantly assess the level of sedation because changes in patient comfort may occur rapidly.

10. With lengthy administration (>30 minutes), reduce the N_2O concentration. The duration of exposure to an anesthetic can have an effect on recovery time. Accumulation of anesthetic in tissues such as muscle, skin, and fat increases with continuous inhalation and can delay recovery time. This is especially true of the more soluble anesthetics, but it can also occur to some degree with low-solubility anesthetics.
11. Once the procedure is complete, the N_2O can be reduced and the patient returned to breathing 100% O_2 for 3 to 5 minutes. This should be achieved by reducing the inspired concentration of N_2O by 20% per minute until it is reduced to zero.

Complications

- Oversedation or prolonged administration can lead to agitation, sweating, nausea, vomiting, feelings of detachment, confusion, hallucinations, and unconsciousness.
- Nitrous oxide can cause myocardial and respiratory depression in high doses (>70%).
- *Chronic* effects of N_2O exposure can include bone marrow suppression, mainly through inhibiting enzymes that depend on vitamin B_{12}. As a result, myelin formation and DNA synthesis may be affected. Megaloblastic anemia, pernicious anemia, peripheral neuropathies, and an increased incidence of miscarriages can also occur as a result of chronic N_2O use. Central nervous system degeneration is common among those who abuse N_2O. Scavenging of waste gases is therefore crucial to protect office staff. The National Institute for Occupational Safety and Health (NIOSH) recommends limiting the room concentration of N_2O to 25 ppm.

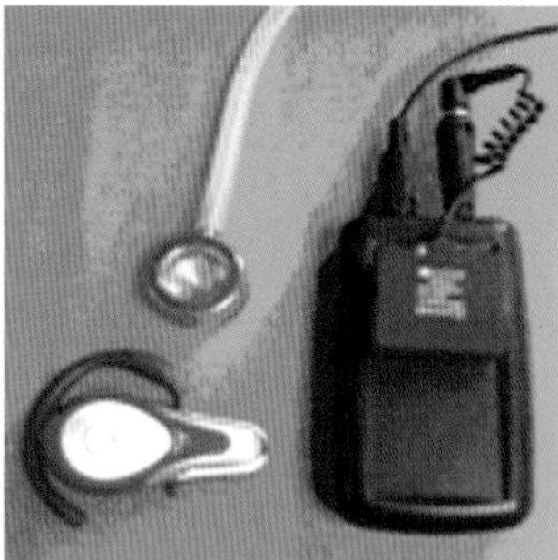

Figure 6-4 Wireless pretracheal stethoscope. (Courtesy of Sedation Resource, Inc., Lone Oak, Tex.)

Postprocedure Management and Concerns

- Monitoring of vital signs along with pulse oximetry should be continued during recovery.
- The patient should breathe 100% O_2 for 3 to 5 minutes after the procedure to prevent diffusion hypoxia.
- Diffusion hypoxia is a condition caused by the rapid release of N_2O from the blood. Because N_2O is insoluble, it leaves the bloodstream rapidly once the inspired concentration is reduced. If the inspired concentration of N_2O is high, then a large amount of gas will quickly emerge from solution into the alveoli, displacing O_2. This mechanism requires large volumes of N_2O to be released from the alveoli, which usually occurs during the first 5 minutes of recovery. Room air does not have an O_2 concentration high enough to compensate for the high N_2O concentration released from the alveoli after the procedure. Thus, hypoxia can occur if supplemental O_2 is not given and if the patient is not allowed to breathe 100% O_2 for 3 to 5 minutes after the discontinuation of N_2O sedation.
- Symptoms of diffusion hypoxia include disorientation, nausea, and severe headache.
- All written and verbal instructions that were given should be documented.
- Postoperative instructions are more relevant to the actual procedure that was performed; therefore there are no specific postoperative instructions for N_2O sedation.
- The patient should be alert and oriented before discharge. If nitrous oxide was the only sedation used, the patient may drive himself or herself home. However, if an oral sedative was used in combination with nitrous oxide, a driver is required to take the patient home.

CPT/Billing Codes

99141 Sedation with or without analgesia (conscious sedation); intravenous, intramuscular or inhalation.

NOTE: 94760–94762 may not be reported in addition to 99141.

Acknowledgment

The editors wish to recognize the many contributions by Jessica Y. Hackman, DMD, and Thomas A. Bzoskie, MD, to this chapter in the previous edition of this text.

Suppliers

(Full contact information available online at www.expertconsult.com.)

Nitrous oxide machines and supplies
Accutron, Inc.
Henry Schein Dental
Pretracheal stethoscopes
Hull Anesthesia, Inc.
Sedation Resource, Inc.
Westone

M F	Age	Ht	Wt	BP	SpO_2	ASA 1 2 3 4 5 E	NPO

MEDICAL HISTORY:

MEDICATIONS:

ALLERGIES:

PRE-OP MEDICATIONS:

☐ Unable to obtain baseline vital signs, patient is uncooperative

Time:

SpO_2
ECG
Temperature

☐ GA
☐ MAC
☐ Supine
☐

MONITORS
☐ Precordial
☐ Pulse Oximeter
☐ NIBP
☐ ECG
☐ Respirations
☐ Temperature
☐
☐

IV
☐ Hand
☐ Arm
☐ ACF
☐ Foot
☐ R ☐ L
☐ 20 ☐ 22 ☐ 24

200
150
100
50

Notes Anes X Surg O

Oxygen
Total

AIRWAY
☐ Nasal Cannula
☐ Nasopharyngeal
☐ Orotracheal Tube
☐ Nasotracheal Tube
☐ L M A
☐ R ☐ L
20 22 24 26

NOTES: ☐ Equipment checked ☐ Patient examined ☐ NPO verified ☐ Consent obtained

ANESTHESIA TIME
Anes end:
Anes start:
Anes total:

Procedure: Date:
Location:
Surgeon:
Anesthesiologist:

Patient Identification:

Figure 6-5 Anesthesia record.

BIBLIOGRAPHY

Clark MS, Brunick AL: Handbook of Nitrous Oxide and Oxygen Sedation, 3rd ed. St. Louis, Mosby, 2008.

Dorsch JA, Dorsch SE: Understanding Anesthesia Equipment, 5th ed. Philadelphia, Lippincott Williams & Wilkins, 2008.

Katzung BG: Basic and Clinical Pharmacology, 7th ed. New York, Appleton & Lange, 1998.

Meechan JG, Robb ND, Seymour RA: Pain and Anxiety Control for the Conscious Dental Patient. Oxford, Oxford University Press, 1998.

Miller RD, Cucchiara RF, Miller ED: Miller's Anesthesia, 2 Volumes, 6th ed. St. Louis, Elsevier Health Sciences, 2004.

Morgan GE, Mikhail MS: Clinical Anesthesiology, 4th ed. New York, Appleton & Lange, 2005.

Trojan J, Saunders B, Woloshynowych M, et al: Immediate recovery of psychomotor function after patient administered nitrous oxide/oxygen inhalation for colonoscopy. Endoscopy 29:17–22, 1997.

Wiener-Kronish JP, Gropper MA: Conscious Sedation. Philadelphia, Hanley & Belfus, 2001.

CHAPTER 7

Pediatric Sedation and Analgesia

Paul W. Davis

Over the past decade, various professional medical societies and hospital associations have readdressed the challenging issue of sedation and pain control in children with the goal of developing multidisciplinary guidelines for what constitutes acceptable and satisfactory care. These societies have included the American Academy of Pediatrics (AAP), the American Society of Anesthesiologists (ASA), and the Joint Commission for Accreditation of Healthcare Organizations (formerly, JCAHO). Their recommendations not only rely heavily on expert opinion and consensus but openly advise that all pediatric sedation be performed under the direction of pediatric subspecialists. We respectfully disagree with the assertion that only pediatricians and anesthesiologists can safely and effectively administer these medications.

The administration of medications for analgesia and moderate or deep sedation was previously termed *conscious sedation*. Because these medications actually do alter a patient's level of consciousness and perception of pain, however, the phrase is inaccurate and is now rarely used.

Historical Perspective on Undertreatment of Pain

Historically, the management of pain and anxiety in the pediatric population outside of the operating room has been inadequate. Indeed, several studies have suggested that inattention to painful conditions may be more prevalent for pediatric procedural care delivered outside of children's hospitals. Nevertheless, any physician who has performed even minor procedures for infants and children appreciates the value of being able to safely and predictably sedate them. Aside from the psychological shock and trauma imposed on infants and children because of a limited understanding of the purpose for a procedure, developmental responses to pain vary by age and can thwart the most well-meaning clinician's efforts to complete a needed procedure.

At least six factors have been identified as contributing to the undertreatment of pain and anxiety in the pediatric population: (1) lack of familiarity with the use of sedative agents; (2) the erroneous conception that newborns and infants do not feel pain; (3) the incorrect belief that children have a very short-term recollection of painful events; (4) the fear of adverse effects of sedatives and analgesics; (5) the fear of masking the symptoms and signs of progressive injury or complications of treatment; and (6) the overarching underestimation of pediatric pain because of the young patient's inability to describe or quantify it.

Developmental Differences in the Perception of Pain

Although the physiologic response to pain is similar in adults and children, recent studies involving young children and fetuses suggest that they may actually experience a heightened perception of pain. A child's perception of pain and clinical reaction to painful stimuli are influenced by several factors, including age, cognitive level, past experiences, extent of control over the situation, parental responses, and perceived cause and expected duration of the painful experience.

The plan for treatment should account for the differences in the pain response at different stages of development:

- *Less than 6 months*—Anticipatory fear is not present and the infant reflects the level of anxiety of the parent. Withdrawal, facial grimacing, thrashing, and brief crying are typical expressions of pain.
- *6 to 18 months*—Anticipatory reactions begin to appear in response to fear of a suspected painful experience (e.g., withdrawal of a limb at the sight of a needle).
- *18 to 24 months*—Children begin to use words like "boo boo" and "hurt" in response to expected painful stimuli.
- *3 years*—Children are still unable to understand the reason for pain but are able to localize pain and identify its cause. They are more capable of reliably assessing the pain they feel. Their tolerance for a painful procedure is improved by allowing them some sense of control over certain aspects of the situation (e.g., when it will be performed or how they are positioned).
- *5 to 7 years*—Continued improvements in understanding of purpose and necessity of painful stimuli occur at this age with consequent improved cooperation.
- *8 to 12 years*—Comprehension of the whole process continues to grow with improved understanding/localization of internal pain.
- *Adolescence*—Children are adept at qualifying and quantifying pain and they develop coping strategies similar to those of adults that help to diminish the perception of pain.

This chapter addresses the current breadth of effective pharmacologic and nonpharmacologic methods to alleviate both pain and anxiety in the pediatric patient before surgical operations and other procedures.

Nonpharmacologic Techniques

Needlesticks represent the most common source for iatrogenic procedural pain worldwide. From simple immunizations to venipuncture for laboratory studies to anesthetic injection before dermatologic procedures, laceration repair, and orthopedic reductions, needle pain is ubiquitous. In addition, more and more children are undergoing nonmedical procedures like body piercings and tattooing (or removal of tattoos).

Untreated pain in the pediatric population has been studied extensively and does have long-term emotional and medical outcomes that are lifelong. Children now receive more than 20 needlesticks for immunizations before they are 2 years of age and many develop needle phobia because only 1 in 9 is done with any kind of pain control. Adolescents subsequently avoid needed medical treatment, 16% to 75% of adults surveyed refuse to donate blood, patients with human immunodeficiency virus infection delay needed blood tests and continue to infect sexual partners, and geriatric patients refuse influenza and pneumococcal vaccines owing to fear of needle pain.

Physicians who perform neonatal elective circumcisions know first-hand the benefits associated with the oral administration of "sugar water." The analgesic effect and safety of sucrose for procedural pain both with and without the use of a pacifier (non-nutritive sucking) in neonates have been clearly demonstrated. Effectiveness in older patients is less clear, but it is easy to administer and there are no known adverse effects. Aspiration has not been a reported complication. The influence of age, intercurrent illness, type of procedure, and location of procedure is unclear at this time.

The simplest and most common nonpharmacologic method used with children is *voluntary and external distraction*. Giving the child and parent *verbal reassurance* by providing them with information about the procedure before it is started may help allay anxiety but might also make it worse. *Hypnosis* has been used to help direct children's focus away from the procedure. Young patients can be taught to *repeat positive statements* to themselves to distract them and relieve anxiety. These behavioral and cognitive approaches represent useful adjuncts that are frequently overlooked because of perceived time constraints in a busy office or emergency department. *Distraction techniques* include counting or saying the "ABCs," music and videotapes, bubble blowing, spinning pinwheels, using party blowers, playing "I Spy" games, and the use of "medical play" as employed by child life programs. *Behavioral treatments* include the techniques of desensitization (the gradual, increasing exposure to a procedure over time), positive reinforcement (rewards and positive statements during or after a procedure), and relaxation technique (the use of breathing, imagery, and self-hypnosis to decrease anxiety). Although all of these techniques have been shown to be very effective, they need props, take time, and require trained personnel.

The dorsal column of the spinal cord forms a common final pathway for several kinds of afferent neurologic stimuli, including pain, position, temperature sensation, and vibration. By applying the "gate theory" and stimulating nerve fibers with either cold or vibration, the sensation of sharp pain can be decreased or eliminated by interfering with its transmission because of the other impulses. The use of cold water or ice and the application of vibrating massagers represent effective ways of ameliorating pain. Cold sprays (e.g., Painease; Gebauer, Cleveland) have been widely used but the research into their efficacy in children has been equivocal at best. A device that uses vibration is currently under investigation (Buzzy; MMJ Labs, Atlanta). Pediatric dentists frequently use tactile vibration using their opposite hand in the delivery of oral anesthesia, with great success.

Topical Analgesics for Children

Also see Chapter 10, Topical Anesthesia.

Ease of administration with minimal trauma for the child and parent would make these the medications of choice for a large variety of procedures. The reality has never lived up to the promise, however.

The topical agent most commonly used for laceration repair in children is LET (a combination of lidocaine, epinephrine, and tetracaine) with an onset of action of 20 minutes. EMLA cream is a eutectic mixture of lidocaine and prilocaine but often requires application approximately 1 hour before the procedure, limiting its usefulness. LMX 4 is a nonprescription 4% liposomal lidocaine preparation that is also effective as a topical anesthetic agent.

Recently, Zingo (Anesiva, Inc., South San Francisco) has been approved by the U.S. Food and Drug Administration (FDA) for use on intact skin to provide topical local analgesia before venipuncture or peripheral intravenous cannulation in children 3 to 18 years of age. This needle-free product has a novel delivery system using pressurized gas jets that deliver lidocaine hydrochloride monohydrate, 0.5 mg, directly through the epidermis and into the dermis. Zingo comes as a ready-to-use, sterile, single-use, disposable, needle-free delivery system. The product consists of a drug reservoir cassette filled with 0.5 mg lidocaine powder (particle size of 40 μm), a pressurized helium gas cylinder, and a safety interlock. The safety interlock prevents premature triggering of the device. Once Zingo is pressed against the skin, the interlock is released, allowing the button to be depressed to deliver the anesthetic. Triggering the device results in a sound not unlike the popping of a balloon. Because the price of this single-use product is between $20 and $25, its use can increase the cost of venipuncture considerably. Although use can be repeated, if necessary, at a different site (a frequent requirement when attempting to place an intravenous catheter in dehydrated children), repeated use at the same site is not recommended and the clinician needs to pay heed to the total dosage of anesthetic administered to avoid toxicity.

Zingo provides local dermal analgesia within 1 to 3 minutes of application and analgesia diminishes within 10 minutes of treatment. Most adverse reactions were application site–related and included bruising, burning, pain, contusion, and hemorrhage. These occurred in 4% of pediatric patients. The most common systemic adverse reactions were nausea (2%) and vomiting (1%). Erythema, edema, pruritus, and petechiae occurred in approximately half of all patients and were brief and self-limited.

Pharmacologic Agents for Sedation and Analgesia

The ideal pediatric agent for procedural sedation would have certain characteristics. First, it would be both 100% safe as well as completely effective for the full range of desired properties—amnesia, analgesia, anxiolysis, motor control, and sedation. It would have rapid onset, fast recovery, a predictable duration of action, and would be completely reversible. In addition, it would be easy to titrate and painless to inject, provide choices for administration route, and be easy to administer. Finally, such an ideal agent would be entirely free of adverse effects and complications.

Needless to say, this ideal pediatric sedative agent has yet to be discovered. A wide range of approved short-acting agents are currently available for use as sedative–hypnotics or analgesics in infants and children. Each of these agents offers advantages in select situations and for specific patients. Procedures that are not painful but require patients to cease moving can be performed with sedation alone. Painful procedures, however, require both sedation and analgesia.

The American College of Emergency Physicians has developed an evidence-based clinical policy for the use of pharmacologic agents for sedation and analgesia in children. This policy focuses on etomidate, fentanyl/midazolam, ketamine, methohexital, pentobarbital, and propofol. The specific uses, recommendations, and cautions for both these and other agents are addressed in the following section. Specific indications and contraindications are addressed individually for each medication. The important characteristics of selected agents are summarized in Table 7-1 for easy reference.

Sedative–Hypnotic Agents

These medications provide anxiolysis, control of movement, sedation, and often amnesia for the painful event, but do not provide analgesia.

"Lytic Cocktail"

This time-honored mixture is addressed briefly here for historical reasons and because many older primary care physicians have used this regimen extensively in the past with great success. The "lytic

TABLE 7-1 Summary of Important Characteristics of Selected Agents

Characteristic	Chloral Hydrate	Fentanyl	Ketamine
Dose and route	Oral and rectal: 25–100 mg/kg up to 1 g/dose infants and 2 g/dose older children	IV: 0.5–2 μg/kg/dose Titrate q3min to desired effect Suggested max: 3 μg/kg	IV: 0.25–2 mg/kg; start with 0.25–0.5 mg/kg and titrate to effect q3–5min (suggested max: 2 mg/kg). Combine with atropine 0.01–0.02 mg/kg IV IM: 1–4 mg/kg (suggested max: 4 mg/kg). Combine with atropine 0.02 mg/kg IM Oral: 4–6 mg/kg (suggested max: 6 mg/kg). Combine with atropine 0.02–0.03 mg/kg Rectal: Same as oral
Onset of action/ time to peak effect	Onset 15–30 min Peak effect 30–60 min	Onset 1 min Peak effect 2–3 min	IV: onset <1 min, peak several minutes IM: Onset 2–5 min, peak 20 min (dose dependent) Oral and rectal: Onset >5 min, peak 30 min (dose dependent)
Duration of action	60 min—residual sedation may last longer in neonates and toddlers	30–45 min	IV: 15 min IM: 30–120 min Oral and rectal: Onset >5 min, peak 30 min (dose dependent)
Adverse reactions	Respiratory depression Airway obstruction	Respiratory depression Bradycardia Dysphoria Delirium Nausea Vomiting Pruritus Urinary retention Smooth muscle spasm Hypotension Allergic reaction Chest wall/glottic rigidity	Laryngospasm Rare respiratory depression Decreased response to hypercarbia Stimulation of salivary and tracheobronchial secretions Mild to moderate increase in blood pressure, heart rate, and cardiac output Emergence phenomena (hallucinations, nightmares, severe agitation) Paradoxical hypotension Skeletal muscle hypotonicity Rigidity Mild disequilibrium Random movements of head or extremities Elevated intracranial and intraocular pressure Nystagmus Vomiting Transient erythematous rash Loss of protective reflexes/aspiration Allergic reaction
Drug Interactions	Coadministration of other sedatives or narcotics increases risk of respiratory complications Can alter warfarin metabolism	Coadministration of other respiratory depressants like benzodiazepines increases the risk of respiratory depression	Half-life may be prolonged if given with other agents metabolized in the liver Coadministration with benzodiazepines or opiates may decrease the occurrence of hallucinations but may also prolong recovery
Contraindications	Repeated dosing in neonates Patients with significant liver or renal disease Patients with cardiac arrhythmias Patients with porphyria	Known allergy or prior serious adverse event	Presence of URI increases risk of laryngospasm to 9% Presence of potential head injury Known increased intracranial pressure Open globe injury Hypertensive disease Coronary artery disease Psychosis Prior adverse reaction to ketamine
Comments	Dose should be decreased in high-risk or debilitated patients Most effective in children under 4 yrs of age	Slow infusions and lower doses decrease the risk of chest wall rigidity Chest wall and glottic rigidity can be reversed with succinylcholine or naloxone Dose should be decreased in high-risk or debilitated patients Respiratory depressant effects may last longer than opioid effects Use with caution in patients at risk for cholelithiasis Delayed clearance in patients with hepatic disease	Causes dissociative reaction (a "trance-like" state) Provides amnesia, analgesia, immobilization, and sedation All-or-none sedation—no sedation continuum Especially useful for young children (lower incidence of emergence phenomena)
Antagonist	None	Naloxone—IV/IM/SQ at 10–100 mcg/kg Adolescent dose: 0.1–0.8 mg Titrate slowly to patient response waiting 2–3 min between doses	None

BP, blood pressure; CHF, congestive heart failure; CI, contraindicated; CNS, central nervous system; CO, cardiac output; HR, heart rate; IM, intramuscular; IV, intravenous; Min, minutes; Mo, months; Sec, seconds; SQ, subcutaneous; SVR, systemic vascular resistance; URI, upper respiratory infection; Yr, years.

cocktail" consists of chlorpromazine (Thorazine), promethazine (Phenergan), and meperidine (Demerol) and is given intramuscularly according to the weight of the child: chlorpromazine, 0.5 mg/kg; promethazine, 0.5 mg/kg; and meperidine, 0.7 mg/kg. It is *not recommended* because (1) the physician must deal with the side effects of three medications instead of one (polypharmacy); and (2) its effect can be erratic and unpredictable.

Benzodiazepines (Midazolam)

Benzodiazepines provide sedation, anxiolysis, and amnesia, but do not provide analgesia. There are several reasons why midazolam (Versed) is the most commonly used agent in this category and the *clear drug of choice for pediatric procedures requiring merely sedation and anxiolysis*. Midazolam has a rapid onset of action, short duration of action, and rapid recovery time. Although patients may not appear sedated when it is used as a single agent, they become more relaxed and cooperative, and there is the frequent (but not universal) benefit of a marked amnestic response for the event. Controversy exists as to whether this marked amnestic response actually blocks "intrinsic memory"—that is, although patients may not consciously recall the painful incident, the traumatic event is still recorded in the brain at the subconscious level. For this reason, it is advisable to coadminister an appropriate analgesic agent for painful procedures.

Midazolam offers great flexibility in route of delivery because it can be administered by the *oral, intranasal, sublingual, rectal, intramuscular (IM), or intravenous (IV) route*. Its efficacy is well established. When used as a single agent (i.e., not combined with an opiate, ketamine, or droperidol), however, it is inferior to other regimens or single agents, and patients may appear to be wide awake.

Recommended dosages vary depending on route of administration. *Oral* midazolam is given at doses of 0.5 to 1 mg/kg and results in the onset of mellowness at 15 to 30 minutes. *Intranasal* midazolam at recommended dosages of 0.3 to 0.5 mg/kg has a more rapid onset of action at 5 to 15 minutes, duration of action of 15 to 20 minutes, and some effects lingering for up to several hours. The solution is drawn up into a tuberculin syringe, the needle removed, and the drug then instilled into the child's nares with the child supine or the headed tilted back. Recommended *rectal doses* of midazolam are 0.45 to 1 mg/kg, with efficacy reported variably from 62% to 93% for laceration repair. Agitation (reported in up to 17%) has been the major drawback of this route of administration. The recommended *IV dose* of midazolam is 0.05 to 0.1 mg/kg and the *IM dose* is 0.05 to 0.15 mg/kg; time to peak effect is 3 to 5 minutes for the IV route and variable for the IM route. Duration of action is 2 to 4 hours.

Adverse effects are uncommon and include the atypical effects of paradoxical agitation and euphoria after administration or an emergence reaction when given IV (1.4%) or orally (6%). Hypotension and respiratory depression are rare but can occur, especially if a narcotic agent is coadministered. The antagonist flumazenil (Romazicon) at a dose of 0.002 to 0.02 mg/kg IV can be given to reverse the effects of midazolam, but patients will require a longer period of observation in recovery (2 hours is commonly recommended) because this agent may have a shorter duration of action than the benzodiazepine, with consequent recurrence of sedation or respiratory depression.

Chloral Hydrate

Not very many years ago, chloral hydrate was considered the mainstay of safe, effective pediatric sedation. Although it has a wide margin of safety, chloral hydrate is *primarily used to sedate children younger than 3 years of age for diagnostic imaging* because its effects on older children are unreliable. It can be administered *orally or rectally* at a dose of 25 to 100 mg/kg up to 1 g/dose for infants and 2 g/dose for older children. Chloral hydrate has an unpleasant smell and taste, making it difficult to entice a child to take much of it orally. Peak action occurs at 60 minutes, making it much less useful than other agents in the emergency setting. Its duration of action is quite variable, with sedation lasting from 1 to 4 hours after administration.

Adverse effects include prolonged sedation, paradoxical agitation, and coma, but airway obstruction and respiratory depression can occur and there is no consistent dose below which complications do not occur; deaths have been reported. In one published series, adverse events were reported in 33% of children who received chloral hydrate either alone or in combination with other sedatives. This relatively high rate of complications contrasts markedly with the widespread perception of its safety. There is no reversal agent for chloral hydrate and its use is contraindicated in patients with cardiac, hepatic, and renal disease as well as porphyria. In addition, its sedative effects can be difficult to predict. In the past, this agent was frequently used in unmonitored settings. In light of the difficulty in predicting its sedative effects and the attendant risks with its use, it is imperative that procedural sedation protocols for monitoring patients during and after administration of this agent be strictly followed.

Barbiturates (Methohexital, Thiopental, and Pentobarbital)

Barbiturates are *primarily used for sedating children younger than 3 years of age* to perform diagnostic imaging. They are relatively safe but are contraindicated in patients with porphyria. Major side effects include respiratory depression with apnea and hypotension, both of which are more common when barbiturates are used in combination with opiates or benzodiazepines.

Methohexital (Brevital) is an ultra–short-acting agent with an onset of action of 30 to 60 seconds and duration of effect of 5 to 10 minutes. It can be administered intravenously at a dose of 1 to 1.5 mg/kg to children 3 to 12 years of age. It is contraindicated in children with temporal lobe epilepsy because it can cause seizures in this subgroup.

Thiopental (Pentothal) is also a short-acting barbiturate with an onset of action of 30 to 60 seconds but a slightly longer duration of effect of 15 minutes. It *is generally given rectally* to children at a dosage of 5 to 10 mg/kg and has the notable side effect of decreasing intracranial pressure. It is therefore particularly useful in patients for whom increased intracranial pressure is a concern.

Pentobarbital (Nembutal) is a very useful barbiturate sedative for longer radiologic procedures like magnetic resonance imaging and positron emission tomography scans. It has an onset of action of 3 to 5 minutes when given IV and a duration of effect of 30 to 45 minutes. For children and infants more than 6 months of age, it can be given intravenously at a dosage of 1 to 3 mg/kg and titrated every 3 to 5 minutes to a maximum dosage of 100 mg, or intramuscularly at a dosage of 2 to 6 mg/kg to a maximum dosage of 100 mg.

Etomidate

Etomidate is an ultra–short-acting imidazole (nonbarbiturate) hypnotic agent with no analgesic properties. Although studies have been published supporting its safety and efficacy in children, the FDA does not currently recommend its use in children younger than 10 years of age.

Its consideration as a potential sedative for children stems from its use in the emergency department for both adults and children as an induction agent in rapid-sequence intubation. After the administration of the *recommended dose* of 0.3 mg/kg IV, etomidate has a rapid onset of action of 5 to 30 seconds and a duration effect of only 5 to 15 minutes. It has the major advantage of decreasing intracranial pressure, like thiopental, and not adversely affecting hemodynamic stability. Reported *adverse effects* include myoclonus (22% of children receiving it in one study) and oxygen desaturation. When given with fentanyl for analgesia, its safety and efficacy compare favorably with midazolam and fentanyl. Compared with pentobarbital for pediatric sedation before diagnostic imaging, etomidate provided a shorter duration of sedation, greater overall efficacy, fewer failures, and fewer adverse effects.

Propofol

Propofol is a nonopioid, nonbarbiturate sedative–hypnotic agent that produces deep sedation almost immediately after IV administration (the one arm–brain circulation time is approximately 40 seconds). It has no analgesic properties but does produce a modest amnestic effect (although weaker than that of midazolam) and is affectionately known as "oil of amnesia," although this term would be more aptly applied to midazolam. Propofol has been used extensively by anesthesiologists and pediatric intensivists as either an induction agent for general anesthesia or as a sedative in the pediatric intensive care unit for patients requiring mechanical ventilation or other uncomfortable procedures. It acts as a direct muscle relaxant and has both antiemetic and euphoric properties. It has no adverse effects on hepatic or renal function. Propofol does not increase either the intraocular pressure or intracranial pressure. When given in conjunction with an opioid analgesic agent, it provides very effective analgesia and sedation for painful procedures. It also has the benefit of an extremely short recovery time of 5 to 15 minutes. Even if deep sedation inadvertently drifts into general anesthesia, with the attendant need for assisted ventilation, the patient is likely to awaken within a few minutes after cessation of the IV infusion. Nevertheless, controversy remains intense regarding the use of propofol outside of the operating room or intensive care unit, or by nonanesthesiologists.

The *recommended induction dosage* for children 3 to 16 years of age is 2.5 to 3.5 mg/kg, administered IV over 20 to 30 seconds. A lower dosage should be administered in children with an ASA classification of III or IV. Intravenous infusion should follow using a rate of 200 to 300 μg/kg/minute for children 2 months to 16 years of age, decreasing the dose to 125 to 150 μg/kg/min after the infusion has been running 30 minutes or longer. Higher infusion rates may be required for children younger than 5 years of age.

Adverse effects noted with propofol include apnea, hypotension, bacterial contamination of the lipid emulsion, and pain at the site of injection (must be administered with lidocaine). Propofol decreases the systemic vascular resistance by an estimated 15% and cardiac output by more than 10%. Hypotension has been reported to occur between 17% and 92% of the time. Respiratory depression results in decreased tidal volume and unpredictable apnea. Oxygen desaturation has been reported in 5% of cases and simple airway interventions were required in 3% of patients; increased oxygen concentration sufficed for almost all other patients. The need for endotracheal intubation has been reported in only 0.03% of patients. *It is difficult to titrate this drug because of both its potency and its rapid onset of action and time to peak effect.* Indeed, this may be the root cause for the frequency with which this agent results in a deeper level of sedation than intended.

In several observational studies, propofol sedation has been reported to be both safe and effective when performed by trained emergency department personnel as long as established practice guidelines and hospital protocols are followed strictly. Because it is considered a general anesthetic agent, a second qualified and credentialed provider (i.e., not the physician performing the procedure) should be present to administer and monitor the patient throughout the procedure until the patient is fully awake. The patient should be carefully monitored with pulse oximetry as well as capnography and physical monitoring of spontaneous respiratory effort.

Propofol is relatively *contraindicated* in patients with a known allergy to eggs or soybeans because current formulations of propofol contain soybean oil, egg lecithin, and egg yolk phospholipids. The generic form contains sulfites, so the brand name Diprivan must be used for sulfite-allergic patients.

Propofol can be coadministered with opioid analgesics or midazolam, but the initiating and maintenance dosage of propofol will likely need to be decreased. The likelihood of sedation events and complications is increased with the coadministration of narcotics. Adverse events are also more likely when propofol is used for sedation in patients with an ASA classification of III or higher.

Other Agents

Ketamine

Ketamine is a phencyclidine derivative and is unique among the sedative–hypnotic and analgesic agents in that it is a "dissociative sedative." It actually produces a trancelike state and provides amnesia, analgesia, immobilization, and sedation. It is therefore an ideal agent for use in young children, often being used as a single agent, resulting in an enhanced safety profile. Unlike other tranquilizers, there is no "sedation continuum" (i.e., the sedative effect is either present or absent). *Ketamine is often used in young children for brief, painful procedures like fracture reduction and laceration repair.*

Not only is ketamine very effective when used according to practice guidelines, it is very safe. Patients almost always retain protective airway reflexes, intact upper airway muscular tone, and spontaneous breathing. It can be *administered orally* (4 to 6 mg/kg), *rectally* (4 to 6 mg/kg), *IM* (1 to 4 mg/kg), or *IV* (0.25 to 2 mg/kg). IV doses can be titrated to effect every 3 to 5 minutes starting with 0.25 to 0.5 mg/kg. *Onset of action* is less than 1 minute with IV use, with maximal effect noted at approximately 3 to 4 minutes. Onset of action is 2 to 5 minutes with IM use, with maximal effect noted at 20 minutes. Oral and rectal use results in an even slower onset of action, with peak effect at 30 minutes. With IV use the duration of effect is short, 15 minutes, but recovery times are much longer (30 to 120 minutes) and less predictable for oral, IM, and rectal use.

Side effects of ketamine include both vomiting and increased salivation. The latter can be controlled by preadministration of either atropine or glycopyrrolate. Laryngospasm occurs very rarely and can be managed by positive-pressure bag-mask ventilation. Ketamine is most known for the frequent occurrence of unpleasant hallucinations and nightmares as well as severe agitation during emergence from sedation. These emergence phenomena are much more common in patients older than 15 years of age and extremely rare in younger children. Coadministration of midazolam has been proposed to minimize this adverse effect, but to date there are no convincing large studies to support this. Although midazolam also decreases the incidence of vomiting with ketamine, it also results in a four- to fivefold increase in the incidence of oxygen desaturation. Still, ketamine with midazolam has been associated with fewer adverse events compared with ketamine combined with fentanyl or propofol, especially in children younger than 10 years of age.

Unfortunately, ketamine has *many contraindications*, including age less than 3 months, airway instability, cardiovascular or pulmonary diseases including bronchospasm, glaucoma or eye injury, increased intracranial pressure or head injury, porphyria, thyroid disease, and psychosis.

Nitrous Oxide

Also see Chapter 6, Nitrous Oxide Sedation.

Inhaled nitrous oxide provides amnesia, mild analgesia, anxiolysis, and sedation when mixed in a 1 : 1 ratio with oxygen and administered through a demand-valve mask. This system requires patient cooperation, so this method of sedation is generally reserved for children older than 4 years of age.

At the concentrations usually used for sedation and analgesia, nitrous oxide use preserves protective airway reflexes, normal blood pressure and pulse, and spontaneous respirations. It has an excellent safety profile, and *adverse effects* are typically mild, including nausea, vomiting, and occasional dysphoria. It can be used alone or in combination with other sedatives and analgesics and it has a proven track record of efficacy for a variety of painful procedures. *Contraindications* include pregnancy, vomiting, and the presence of known or presumed "trapped air" (e.g., bowel obstruction, pneumothorax, perforated viscus, or middle ear infection).

Opioid Analgesics (Fentanyl)

Opioids (narcotic agents) are widely used and well-established analgesics. Although morphine is the prototype drug in this class, and meperidine also has been used extensively in the past, fentanyl has rapidly become the opioid agent of choice for children requiring potent analgesia during procedural sedation. Fentanyl is a synthetic opioid that has 75 to 125 times the potency of morphine and a *very rapid IV onset of action* (2 to 3 minutes) with a relatively short duration of action (30 to 60 minutes). It is administered in an initial IV dose of 0.5 to 1 μg/kg and its pharmacokinetics permit smooth and safe titration either alone or in combination with midazolam at intervals of approximately 3 minutes until the desired effect is achieved.

Fentanyl has additional *advantages* over the longer-acting narcotic agents. It lacks the histamine release characteristic of morphine and the buildup of very–long-acting metabolites occasionally seen with meperidine (the so-called serotonin surge syndrome). It is also effective when administered *intranasally* or *by nebulizer*.

Adverse effects of fentanyl include hypoxemia and respiratory depression. Chest wall and glottic rigidity are uncommon but serious complications and have been reported in neonates receiving a single dose of fentanyl of between 3 and 5 μg/kg. In fact, *fentanyl has the highest reported complication rate of any agent used for procedural analgesia and sedation*. However, fentanyl is rarely used as a single agent so it is likely that much of the excess risk is due to polypharmacy. The practicing physician needs always to remain vigilant when using opioid–sedative combinations, especially when three or more medications have been administered.

The antagonist naloxone is an effective reversal agent for fentanyl. It is administered IV at a dose of 0.1 mg/kg for children 0 to 5 years of age and 2 mg/kg for children older than 5 years of age. The dose can be repeated. Its onset of action is 1 to 2 minutes, with a duration of effect of 20 to 40 minutes, resulting in complete reversal as a single dose most of the time when used with fentanyl. Incidentally, when used to reverse the effects of meperidine, naloxone can result in normeperidine-induced seizures. *If glottic or chest wall rigidity occurs, a neuromuscular blocking agent such as succinylcholine, rocuronium, or vecuronium may need to be administered to achieve an oral or endotracheal airway, along with bag-mask positive-pressure ventilation.*

If any significant sedation and anesthesia is going to be used other than basic anxiolytics (what was formerly called "conscious sedation"), strict adherence to safety and established guidelines is imperative (also see Chapter 2, Procedural Sedation and Analgesia).

Equipment

The equipment required for pediatric sedation and analgesia comprises everything that is needed to effectively and safely monitor the patient through induction, maintenance, and recovery from the effects of the medications used. In addition, equipment needs to be readily at hand to manage any complication that may arise from the unintended escalation of sedation level to either deep sedation or general anesthesia. A list of basic essential equipment appears in Box 7-1.

Box 7-1. Equipment Needs and Considerations for Pediatric Procedural Sedation

- Oxygen with a system that is capable of administering at least 90% O_2 at 10 L/min for 60 minutes
- Bag-mask system for positive-pressure ventilation
- Laryngoscope with appropriately sized blades and endotracheal tubes
- Suction catheters and apparatus
- Emergency cart with appropriate medications and Breslow tape
- Defibrillator
- Pulse oximeter
- Electrocardiograph monitor
- Noninvasive blood pressure apparatus
- Emergency antagonists, including naloxone and flumazenil
- IV start kit and appropriately sized IV catheters
- 500-mL bags of normal saline and Ringer's lactate
- Telephone or radio for summoning assistance in an emergency
- End-tidal CO_2 monitor (when available)
- Equipment for administering blood and blood components need to be readily available if transfusion becomes necessary
- Intraosseous catheter kit should be immediately available if IV access is lost and a standard IV line cannot be started

The majority of this equipment is available in the Banyan Kit (a "crash cart in a suitcase"), available commercially.

Presedation Evaluation

Box 7-2 summarizes a comprehensive and accepted set of required components for the safe administration of procedural sedation in the pediatric patient. This sedation model was developed at the Children's Hospital of Wisconsin. Pediatric sedation does not relieve the physician of the need to explain the anticipated procedure to both the child (when their cognitive level warrants) and the parent or guardian. Informed consent for both the sedation and the procedure should be obtained and documented in the medical record. An example of a procedural sedation informed consent form is available online at www.expertconsult.com.

A focused history and physical assessment should be performed before administering any sedative or analgesic agent. This evaluation can be performed any time within 30 days of an intended procedure, depending on institutional requirements and standards. However, the patient must be reassessed immediately before

Box 7-2. Components of the Children's Hospital of Wisconsin Sedation Model

Monitoring and personnel requirements
NPO guidelines
Presedation evaluation
Focused present and past history
Focused physical examination
Vital signs
GRA (graded risk assessment) documentation
Assignment of ASA physical status score
Generation of sedation plan
Informed parental consent
Equipment and monitoring standards based on actual level of sedation
Quantitative sedation scoring
Time-based recording of vital signs, oxyhemoglobin saturation, and sedation level
Recovery and discharge criteria
Standardized record

Essential components of the Children's Hospital of Wisconsin structured sedation program, adapted from American Society of Anesthesiologists (ASA) and American Academy of Pediatrics (AAP) guidelines. Each of these components is specifically prompted on a uniform sedation documentation record.

TABLE 7-2 Airway Assessment

Physical Characteristic	Specific Concerns
Body habitus	Obese vs. thin Size and length of neck
Presence of micrognathia (see Fig. 7-1)	Receding mandible Size of mandible in relation to face
Dentition status	Protruding incisors (buck teeth) Poor dental condition; caries Loose teeth or crowns Distance between upper and lower teeth, associated with the presence of high-arched palate
Joint mobility	Mobility of the head at the atlanto-occipital joint (see Fig. 7-2) Mobility of the mandible at the temporomandibular joint Mallampati classification (see Chapter 2, Procedural Sedation and Analgesia, Fig. 2-2)
Thyromental distance (>6 cm, three fingerbreadths)	By measuring the thyromental distance, the anatomic proximity of the glottis to the mandible and base of the tongue can be gauged
Intraoral concerns	Status of tonsils, intraoral tissues, torus palatinus, tumors, trauma Redundant tissue Presence of neonatal teeth Intra-oral, lingual, or labial body ornaments
Nasal concerns	Body ornaments: studs and rings Patient may require a nasal airway rather than oral

initiating procedural sedation to ensure his or her suitability for sedation as well as to reconfirm the appropriateness of the planned sedation regimen. The sedation plan and choice of sedative/analgesic agent(s) should be clearly documented on the presedation evaluation form.

The history should include allergies, use of medications or illicit drugs, diseases, operations, hospitalizations, previous exposure to sedation or general anesthesia, untoward reactions to anesthetic agents in the past, relevant family history, and the time and content of the last oral intake. The physical examination should include auscultation of the heart and lungs as well as a careful assessment of the airway (Table 7-2 and Figs. 7-1 and 7-2). Special attention should be given to identifying anatomic or clinical conditions that might interfere with endotracheal intubation and resuscitation should they become necessary. These conditions are summarized in Box 7-3.

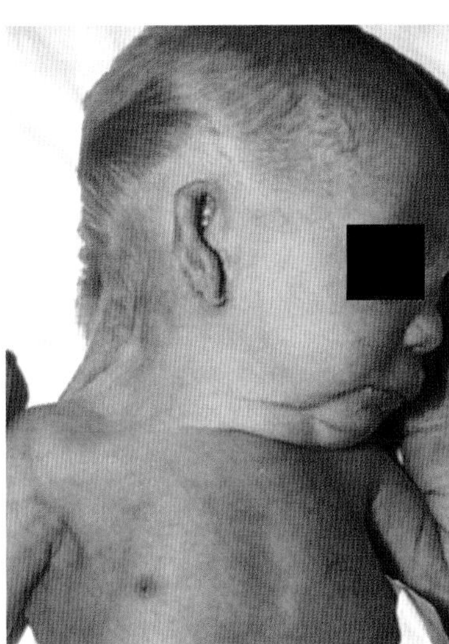

Figure 7-1 Micrognathia.

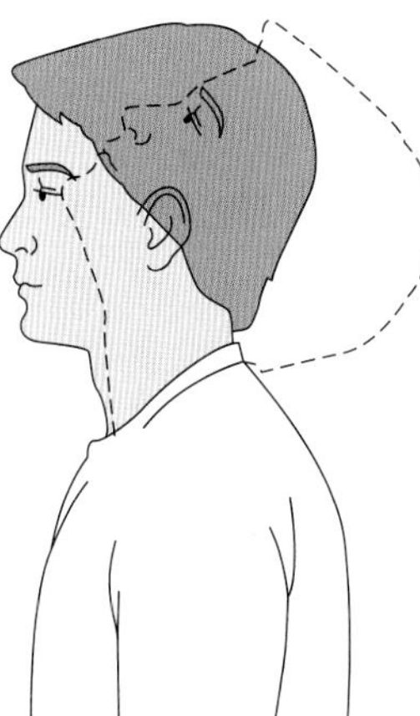

Figure 7-2 Mobility of the head at the atlanto-occipital joint.

Pediatric patients need to be assigned an ASA Physical Status Classification before performing any emergency or elective procedure. This classification is summarized in Chapter 2, Procedural Sedation and Analgesia, Table 2-2.

A pediatric patient's suitability for mild, moderate, or deep sedation outside of the operating room can range from excellent to very poor in each of the ASA classes, but is generally expected to be good for classes I and II. Formal published recommendations suggest that an anesthesiologist or subspecialist should be consulted for patients with ASA classes of III and IV to assist with airway abnormalities and management as well as other special needs. At the least, in clinical settings where such assistance is unavailable, a second trained and experienced physician should be consulted whose entire focus is the management of sedation throughout the procedure. For elective procedures, transfer to a larger facility where such help is available should be seriously considered.

Fasting before Sedation

There is limited evidence to support an optimum duration of fasting before sedation to reduce the risk of aspiration. The ASA guidelines, which are based on expert opinion and consensus, recommend a minimum fasting period of 2 hours for clear fluids, 4 hours for breast

Box 7-3. Sedation Graded Risk Assessment Tool—Sedation Risk Factors*

Snoring, stridor, or sleep apnea
Craniofacial malformation
History of airway difficulty
Vomiting, bowel obstruction
Gastroesophageal reflux
Pneumonia or oxygen requirement
Reactive airways disease
Hypovolemia, cardiac disease
Sepsis
Altered mental status
History of sedation failure
Inadequate NPO time
No identified risk factors

*Medical conditions and patient characteristics with known potential for increasing the risk of procedural sedation are specifically prompted on the sedation record.

TABLE 7-3 Fasting Guidelines before Procedural Sedation

Age	Milk/Solid	Clear Liquid/Breast Milk
Children <6 mo	4 hr	2 hr
Children >6 mo	6 hr	2 hr
Other children and adults	6 hr	6 hr

If food or fluids are ingested within these time periods

- The procedure may be delayed
- The case may be referred to a licensed anesthesia provider to help protect the airway.
- In emergent and urgent situations, the increased risk of aspiration must be weighed against the benefits of the procedure. The lightest effective sedation should be used.

milk, and 6 hours for formula, nonhuman milk, and solids. For children with normal airways and no clinical predisposition to aspiration, a systematic review of randomized trials failed to find any benefit for fasting from fluids for more than 6 hours compared with 2 hours. In addition, no statistically significant differences in intraoperative gastric volumes and pH were noted. According to an expert panel who published their findings in *Annals of Emergency Medicine* in 2007, the following considerations related to the risk of aspiration should dictate the planned depth and length of procedural sedation in the emergency department:

- Possibility of a difficult airway
- Conditions predisposing to esophageal reflux, including elevated intracranial pressure, gastritis, bowel obstruction, or ileus
- Age less than 6 months
- Severe systemic disease with functional limitation (ASA) class ≥3)
- Timing and nature of last oral intake
- Urgency of procedure

See Table 7-3 for a useful summary of accepted fasting guidelines before sedation.

Personnel

Physicians who administer procedural sedation must fully understand the pharmacology of the medications they use. They must also have the breadth of clinical experience and judgment to select a regimen that is appropriate for both the patient and the intended procedure. Because altered consciousness represents a continuum and not discrete "quantum" levels, clinicians should have the requisite training and current skill to deal effectively with complications arising from the patient drifting to the next deeper level of sedation than that intended.

Two trained and credentialed individuals are required when a patient is significantly sedated for a procedure, one to perform the procedure and the second to administer and monitor the sedation. Ideally, both individuals would be physicians, and this choice is probably prudent if deep sedation is planned (at the least, the second individual should be a licensed nurse anesthetist). In practice, the second individual is either a nurse or trained assistant (certified medical assistant, certified nursing assistant, or respiratory therapist). He or she monitors the patient and documents vital signs, level of consciousness, timing and dose of medication administration, and any complications. If the assistant is not a physician trained in sedation management, it is imperative that the physician in charge of the procedure be able to stop the procedure at any time to manage complications arising from sedation and analgesia.

Monitoring

Documentation of any procedure should be scrupulous and complete and include a description of the level of responsiveness of the patient, otherwise known as the sedation score (see Chapter 2, Procedural Sedation and Analgesia, Table 2-1). Document the issues discussed in obtaining informed consent in the patient record. Some medicolegal experts also recommend asking a parent or guardian to sign a form listing each procedure that the physician might perform. With regard to pediatric sedation, the physician should document how well the patient tolerated the method used. If side effects are noted or complications encountered, full documentation—including a careful record of all measures and medications used in dealing with them—must be given in the sedation report in the patient's medical record. A time-based record of heart rate (electrocardiographic monitor or pulse oximeter), oxygen saturation (pulse oximeter), end-tidal CO_2 (if used), as well as nursing assessments and monitoring must be made until the patient is fully recovered. For patients with an underlying illness or for whom deep sedation is planned, these measurements along with vital signs should be taken and recorded at least every 5 minutes.

The nurse should record all medications given (dose, route of administration, and time given), as well as fluids, blood loss, and any unusual events or complications. Supplemental oxygen should be administered prophylactically in all cases. IV access is strongly encouraged during pediatric sedation and analgesia, although it is not absolutely necessary for lighter levels of sedation or when sedative agents are administered by oral, nasal, rectal, or intramuscular routes. However, in these cases, equipment and skilled personnel capable of immediately establishing vascular access need to be present.

Recovery and Discharge Criteria

Monitoring must be continued by trained personnel until the infant or child has met pre-established criteria for safe discharge. These criteria include the following:

- Airway patency and stable cardiovascular function
- Easy arousability with intact protective reflexes
- Ability to talk (if age appropriate)
- Ability to sit up without assistance (if age appropriate)
- Adequate level of hydration

Disabled patients as well as young children and infants should be observed until they return to the same level of responsiveness noted before sedation. Numerous scoring systems have been published. Table 7-4 outlines the Aldrete Recovery Scale, a common system used at many health care institutions throughout the United States. As most of my residents and nurses have heard me chant, "When they meet the Aldrete, the patient's all ready."

TABLE 7-4 Aldrete Recovery Score*

Activity	Voluntary movement of all limbs to command—2 points Voluntary movement of two extremities to command—1 point Unable to move—0 points Apneic—0 points
Respiration	Breathe deeply and cough—2 points Dyspnea, hypoventilation—1 point
Circulation	BP ±20 mm Hg of preanesthesia level—2 points BP ±20–50 mm Hg of preanesthesia level—1 point BP >50 mm Hg of preanesthesia level—0 point
Consciousness	Fully awake—2 points Arousable—1 point Unresponsive—0 points
Color	Pink—2 points Pale, blotchy—1 point Cyanotic—0 points

BP, blood pressure.

*Total score must be greater than 8 at the conclusion of the monitoring.

Postsedation Concerns

Available evidence suggests that infants and children who have not experienced an adverse event during sedation can be safely discharged after 30 minutes of observation and monitoring.

What about the risk of adverse events occurring after discharge? In a large, well-designed, prospective study of 1341 pediatric sedation events occurring in the emergency department setting, adverse reactions were noted in 14% of patients and potentially life-threatening events occurred in 12%. Only 8% of all adverse events occurred after the procedure. Every child who experienced a post-procedure event had a similar adverse effect earlier in the sedation. All serious, potentially life-threatening events occurred within 25 minutes of the last sedative/analgesic dose. Parents or guardians should nevertheless be advised that minor side effects may occur after discharge from the recovery area and that full recovery after moderate or deep sedation may be prolonged. Discharge instructions should include the telephone number of a trained staff member to field any parental questions or concerns.

Patient Education Guides

See the sample patient and parent education handout available online at www.expertconsult.com.

CPT/Billing Codes

99143 Moderate sedation services provided by the same physician performing the diagnostic or therapeutic service that the sedation supports, requiring the presence of an independent trained observer to assist in the monitoring of the patient's level of consciousness and physiologic status in patients younger than 5 years of age, first 30 minutes intra-service time

99144 Patients age 5 years or older, first 30 minutes intra-service time

99145 Each additional 15 minutes intra-service time. (List separately in addition to code for primary service)

NOTE: This code list does not include simple or minimal office sedation techniques (anxiolysis).

BIBLIOGRAPHY

American Academy of Pediatrics Committee on Drugs: Guidelines for monitoring and management of pediatric patients during and after sedation for diagnostic and therapeutic procedures. Pediatrics 89:1110–1115, 1992.

Baxter AL: Topical anesthetics in children. MedscapeCME, 2008. Available at http://cme.medscape.com/viewarticle/570327.

Blike GT, Cravero JP: Pride, prejudice, and pediatric sedation: A multispecialty evaluation of the state of the art. Report from a Dartmouth summit on pediatric sedation. National Patient Safety Foundation, 2001. Available at www.npsf.org/pdf/r/PediatricSedation.pdf.

Borland M, Jacobs I, King B, O'Brien D: A randomized controlled trial comparing intranasal fentanyl to intravenous morphine for managing acute pain in children in the emergency department. Ann Emerg Med 14:335–340, 2007.

Brady M, Kinn S, O'Rourke K, et al: Preoperative fasting for preventing perioperative complications in children. Cochrane Database Syst Rev 2:CD005285, 2005.

Carr DB, Goudas LC: Acute pain. Lancet 353:2051–2058, 1999.

Chen E, Joseph MH, Zeltzer LK: Behavioral and cognitive interventions in the treatment of pain in children. Pediatr Clin North Am 47:513–525, 2000.

Cohen LL, MacLaren JE, Fortson BL, et al: Randomized clinical trial of distraction for infant immunization pain. Pain 125:165–171, 2006.

Coté CJ, Wilson S: Guidelines for monitoring and management of pediatric patients during and after sedation for diagnostic and therapeutic procedures: An update. Pediatrics 118:2587–2602, 2006.

Dartmouth Pediatric Sedation Project. Available at http://an.hitchcock.org/PediSedation. Accessed January 3, 2010.

Green SM, Krauss B: Clinical practice guideline for emergency department ketamine dissociative sedation in children. Ann Emerg Med 44:460–471, 2004.

Green SM, Roback MG, Miner JR, et al: Fasting and emergency department procedural sedation and analgesia: A consensus-based clinical practice advisory. Ann Emerg Med 49:454–461, 2007.

Hsu DC: Procedural sedation and analgesia in children. May 31, 2008. Available at www.uptodate.com.

Joseph MH, Brill J, Zeltzer LK: Pediatric pain relief in trauma. Pediatr Rev 20:75–83, 1999.

Krauss B, Zurakowski D: Sedation patterns in pediatric and general community hospital emergency departments. Pediatr Emerg Care 14:99–103, 1998.

Mace SE, Barata IA, Cravero JP, et al: Clinical policy: Evidence-based approach to pharmacologic agents used in pediatric sedation and analgesia in the emergency department. Ann Emerg Med 44:342–377, 2004.

Migita RT, Klein EJ, Garrison MM: Sedation and analgesia for pediatric fracture reduction in the emergency department: A systematic review. Arch Pediatr Adolesc Med 160:46–51, 2006.

Miner JR, Kletti C, Herold M, et al: Randomized clinical trial of nebulized fentanyl citrate versus i.v. fentanyl citrate in children presenting to the emergency department with acute pain. Acad Emerg Med 14:895–898, 2007.

Newman DH, Azer MM, Pitetti RD, Singh S: When is a patient safe for discharge after procedural sedation? The timing of adverse effect events in 1367 pediatric procedural sedations. Ann Emerg Med 42:627–635, 2003.

Practice guidelines for preoperative fasting and the use of pharmacologic agents to reduce the risk of pulmonary aspiration: Application to healthy patients undergoing elective procedures. A report by the American Society of Anesthesiologists Task Force on Preoperative Fasting. Anesthesiology 90:896–905, 1999.

Proudfoot J: Analgesia, anesthesia, and conscious sedation. Emerg Med Clin North Am 13:357–370, 1995.

Sacchetti A, Schafermayer R, Geradi M, et al., Pediatric Committee of American College of Emergency Physicians: Pediatric analgesia and sedation. Ann Emerg Med 23:237–250, 1994.

Selbst SM, Clark M: Analgesic use in the emergency department. Ann Emerg Med 19:1010–1013, 1990.

Sinha M, Christopher NC, Fenn R, Reeves L: Evaluation of nonpharmacologic methods of pain and anxiety management for laceration repair in the pediatric emergency department. Pediatrics 117:1162–1168, 2006.

Weaver CS, Hauter WE, Brizendine MS, Cordell WH: Emergency department procedural sedation with propofol: Is it safe? J Emerg Med 33:355–361, 2007.

CHAPTER 8

Peripheral Nerve Blocks and Field Blocks

Morteza Khodaee • Barbara F. Kelly

Many ambulatory procedures lend themselves well to local anesthesia with a field block or a peripheral nerve block. A *field block* is a method of providing anesthesia to a relatively small area by injecting a "wall" of anesthetic solution across the path of the nerves supplying the operative field (Fig. 8-1). Instead of the injection being made directly into the area of the procedure, it is made into the soft tissue some distance away, where the nerves are situated. Advantages include longer duration of anesthesia and no distortion of the operative field.

A *nerve block* is the infiltration of a local anesthetic near the nerve branch supplying sensation to a particular area. Blocking a nerve provides longer duration of anesthesia than that obtained with local cutaneous infiltration. Knowledge of the anatomy of peripheral nerves and a scrupulous sterile technique are important for successful peripheral nerve blocks. Use of this technique may reduce the amount of anesthetic needed, reduce distortion of tissues, and allow palpation of pathology to be excised.

Ultrasonography-guided nerve blocks may increase block quality parameters and decrease the potential complications (see Chapter 185, Musculoskeletal Ultrasonography).

In some sites (e.g., the breast) a nerve block cannot be obtained, and thus the field block is the only reasonable alternative. However, where possible, the nerve block may be the procedure of choice.

Also see Chapter 9, Oral and Facial Anesthesia.

Indications

- When local anesthetic at the site of incision may be ineffective (e.g., with infected tissue the pH is lower)
- When the edema from the local anesthetic injection would distort anatomic landmarks and make approximation and repair difficult
- To preserve palpation of the deep tissue to be excised
- When repairs or excisions are quite large and prohibit the use of large amounts of anesthetic
- For fracture and dislocation care
- For nail removal

Contraindications

Absolute Contraindications

- If it would require injecting through infected tissue
- Presence of septicemia
- Profound bleeding tendencies
- History of allergy to local anesthetics (see Chapter 4, Local Anesthesia, and Chapter 5, Local and Topical Anesthetic Complications)

Relative Contraindications

- Any neurologic damage existing before the procedure. Document findings before injection.
- In general, epinephrine-containing solutions should not be used in the fingers, toes, penis, nose, or ear, nor should epinephrine be used in areas with poor vascular supply. Use caution in patients with diabetes, peripheral vascular disease, or other conditions affecting vascular supply.

Equipment

- Sterile field and agent for sterile preparation of skin
- Local anesthetic agent (see Chapter 4, Local Anesthesia), usually 2% lidocaine without epinephrine
- 18-gauge needle to draw up solution
- 25- to 30-gauge needle for injection (1 to 10 mL)
- Appropriate-size syringe
- Gloves

Preprocedure Patient Preparation

There are few complications with field and nerve blocks. The benefits of the blocks versus the alternatives (e.g., general anesthesia, no anesthesia, and Bier block) may be explained. Depending on the agent used, the duration of anesthesia may be prolonged, and the patient should be informed of the expected length of action. In rare instances a nerve could be traumatized, but long-term consequences are rare. Any precautionary advice, such as avoidance of heat or cold after the procedure, should be given to the patient. The possibility of paresthesia during the injection should be explained.

Technique

Field Block

The technique of administering a field block is similar to the technique discussed for local anesthetics (see Chapter 4, Local Anesthesia). In this instance, however, the area to be incised is spared from the injection. Rather, the area around the site is injected (see Fig. 8-1). Repeat injections are made until the entire border of the field has been infiltrated. Allowing 5 to 10 minutes for the block to take effect improves the resulting anesthesia.

Nerve Block

1. Before beginning any peripheral nerve block, perform a neurologic examination of the area to be anesthetized and document

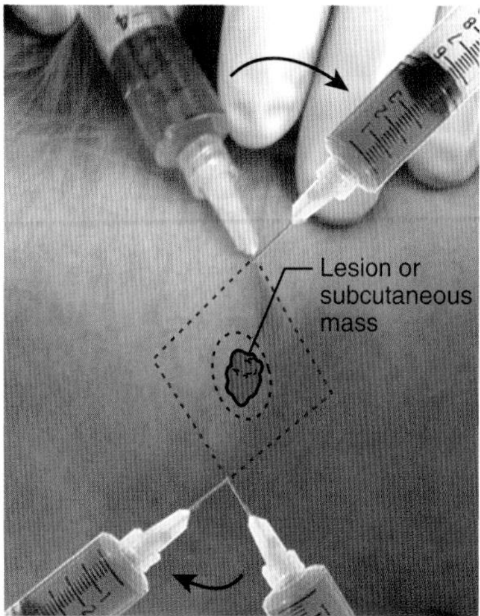

Figure 8-1 Field block technique. This method of injecting around the lesion prevents distortion of the anatomy and allows any deeper central lesion to remain palpable. The *red lines* indicate the path of the needle (four separate insertions). The *black line* indicates the incision line.

the results in the medical record. If any neurologic defect is present, include a description of it in the document of informed consent for the procedure, and have the patient sign a statement agreeing that the defect was present before the administration of the anesthetic.

2. Identify the appropriate nerve(s) and anatomic sites to accomplish the block.
3. Carefully clean and prepare the skin over the injection site in a sterile fashion.
4. Draw up the anesthetic. Usually a 25- to 30-gauge needle can be used to inject the anesthetic. The amount of anesthetic used varies depending on the location of the nerve.
5. Insert the needle into the site, withdrawing the plunger slightly to test for intravascular placement of the needle and moving the needle if necessary to avoid intravascular injection. If the patient experiences paresthesia, withdraw the needle slightly because it is probably within the nerve. *The goal is to inject perineurally*, not into the nerve itself. If no paresthesia is noted at the expected site, confirm that there is no potential for intravascular injection and slowly inject the anesthetic. If the proper site has been identified, often as little as 1 or 2 mL will provide an excellent anesthetic field.
6. Allow 5 to 15 minutes for the block to take effect. Confirm anesthesia to pinprick before making an incision.

Common Nerve Blocks

Also see Chapter 9, Oral and Facial Anesthesia.

1. **Digital block of finger or toe and nail anesthesia** (Fig. 8-2): Use 4 to 6 mL of 1% to 2% lidocaine *without* epinephrine for each finger, and 6 to 8 mL of the same for toes. Insert the 25- to 30-gauge, ½-inch needle fully into the skin at the base of the finger or toe into the web space and inject 1 mL (see Fig. 8-2B). Repeat this on the other side unless it is the first or fifth digit. Then insert the needle perpendicular to the bone at the base of the digit, touch the bone, and pull back a little (see Fig. 8-2B and D). Inject 1 mL into the lateral aspect, then 1 mL across the dorsal and another 1 mL under the ventral surfaces in the subcutaneous space. Repeat this on the contralateral side of the digit. Alternatively, the needle can be inserted dorsally, then ventrally (see Fig. 8-2E). The dorsal digital nerves in both

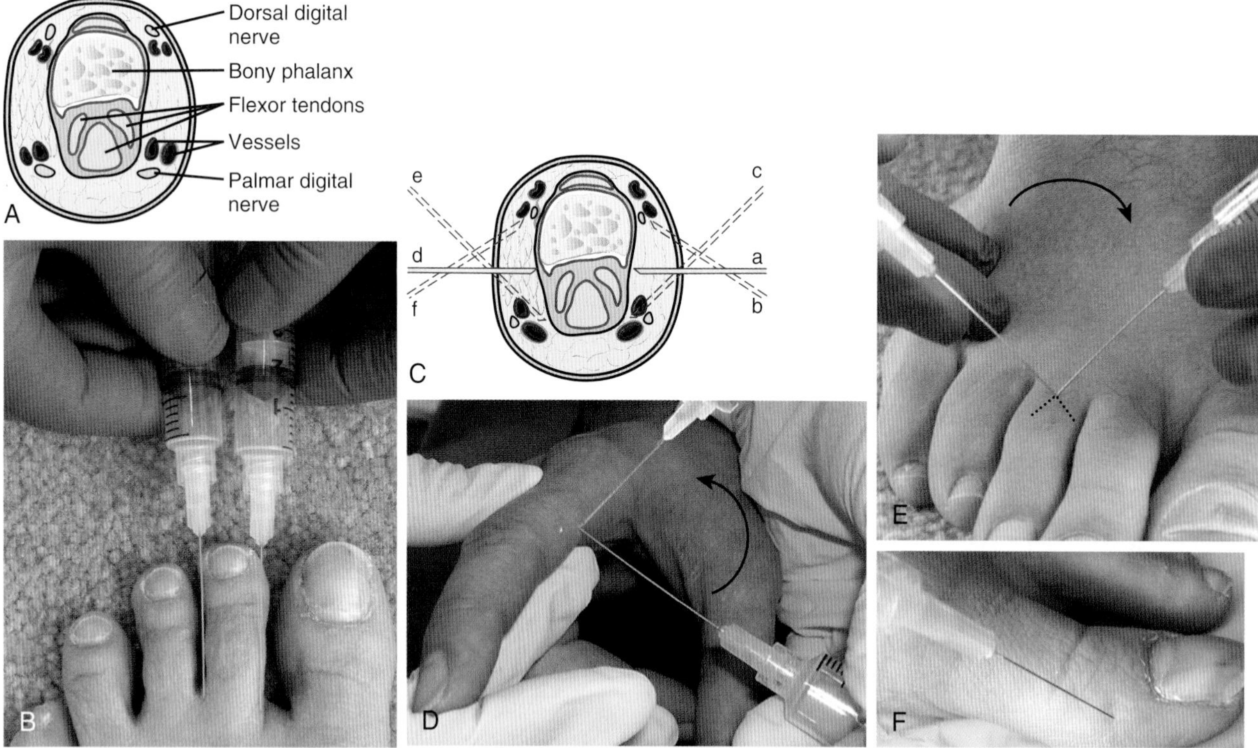

Figure 8-2 Anatomy and injection technique for digital nerve block. **A,** The four digital nerves. The bone is used as a landmark to find the proper plane of the dorsal digital nerve. **B,** Site of injection in web space. When removing a toenail, an additional 1 mL of anesthetic can be placed just proximal to the nail. **C** and **D,** Digital nerve block of the finger. The sites of the nerves are injected bilaterally. Insert the needle and, after touching bone, withdraw slightly and then inject 0.5 mL of anesthetic. **E,** Digital nerve block of the toe, showing an alternative method of injection from the dorsal aspect. This is followed by a ventral injection in the same manner. **F,** Nail wing block.

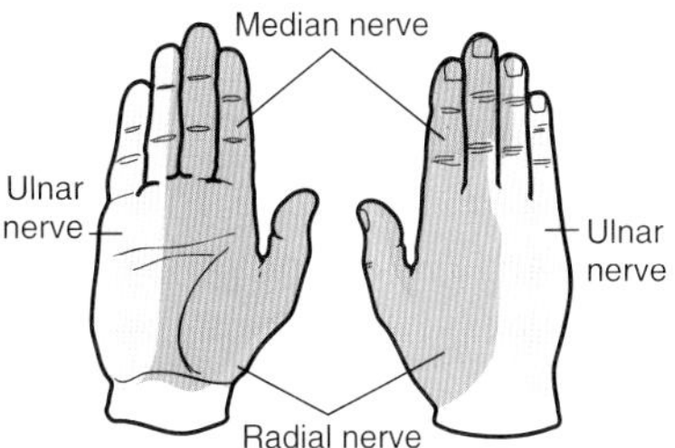

Figure 8-3 Distribution of cutaneous sensation of the hand by the radial, ulnar, and median nerves.

instances lie close to bone. As the bone is touched with the needle tip, withdraw 1 or 2 mm and inject the solution.

Nail anesthesia can be achieved by a *wing block* as well (see Fig. 8-2F). The injection site is 5 to 8 mm proximal and lateral to the corner of the nail. Direct the needle distally at a 45-degree angle, advance until bone is reached, and pull back slightly to avoid injecting the periosteum. Slowly inject 0.3 to 0.5 mL of anesthetic. This will blanch both the proximal and the lateral nail folds in a "winglike" pattern. To obtain full lateral anesthesia, a second injection of 0.3 to 0.5 mL into the entire length of the lateral nail fold should be performed in addition to the wing block to obtain anesthesia for the lateral half of the nail. A similar procedure can then be carried out on the other side of the toe if full nail anesthesia is needed.

2. **Median nerve block:** The median nerve supplies sensation to the palmar aspect of the thumb and index and middle fingers. In addition, the radial half of the palm is supplied by the median nerve (Fig. 8-3). A nerve block may be indicated for extensive lacerations and incisions in these areas. The median nerve lies between the flexor carpi radialis and the palmaris longus (Fig. 8-4A). With slight flexion of the wrist and simultaneous flexion of the middle finger only at the metacarpophalangeal joint, the palmaris longus stands out (Fig. 8-4B). The injection should be made at the flexor crease of the wrist just radial to the palmaris longus. Use 3 to 5 mL of 1% lidocaine *without* epinephrine (Fig. 8-4B and C).
3. **Ulnar nerve block:** The ulnar nerve innervates the dorsal and palmar aspects on the ulnar side of the hand (fifth finger and ulnar side of the fourth finger; see Fig. 8-3). The ulnar nerve divides to dorsal and palmar branches 4 to 5 cm proximal to the wrist. Therefore, the easiest way to obtain an ulnar block is to inject the ulnar nerve at the elbow where the nerve lies only 0.5 cm below the skin, between the medial epicondyle and the olecranon (Fig. 8-5A). Each branch can also be blocked separately at the wrist (Fig. 8-5B). The risk of nerve compression and postprocedure paresthesia is higher at the elbow. For all nerve blocks, it is best not to inject directly into the nerve but around it; 2 to 3 mL of 1% lidocaine should be sufficient here.
4. **Radial nerve block:** The radial nerve innervates the dorsum of the thumb, the index and middle fingers, and the radial portion of the dorsum of the hand (see Fig. 8-3). Because of multiple divisions of the radial nerve, 10 mL of anesthetic is often required to obtain good results. Inject 3 mL of solution along the lateral border of the radial artery two fingerbreadths above the wrist. Then lay a superficial ring of solution from this point extending dorsally over the border of the wrist and into the anatomic snuffbox area created by the tendons of the abductor pollicis longus and extensor pollicis brevis muscles. The nerve is in the superficial fascia just deep to the skin (Fig. 8-6).
5. **Facial nerve blocks** (also see Chapter 9, Oral and Facial Anesthesia):
   - **Supraorbital and supratrochlear nerve blocks (forehead block):** The supraorbital and supratrochlear nerves innervate the forehead and anterior scalp. The nerves exit at the supraorbital ridge. To ensure that both nerves have been injected, infiltrate just above the bone beneath the entire medial two thirds of the eyebrow (Fig. 8-7A).
   - **Infraorbital nerve block:** Palpate a notch in the infraorbital rim. The infraorbital nerve exits just beneath this small notch. Infiltrate through the skin directly over the infraorbital area, or use an intraoral technique. The latter approach requires a 1½-inch needle, ideally 27 gauge. Introduce the needle at the gingival–buccal margin over the maxillary canine tooth. Advance it under the skin until the infraorbital foramen is reached. Use approximately 2 mL of anesthetic. This block is used especially to repair upper lip lacerations so that the

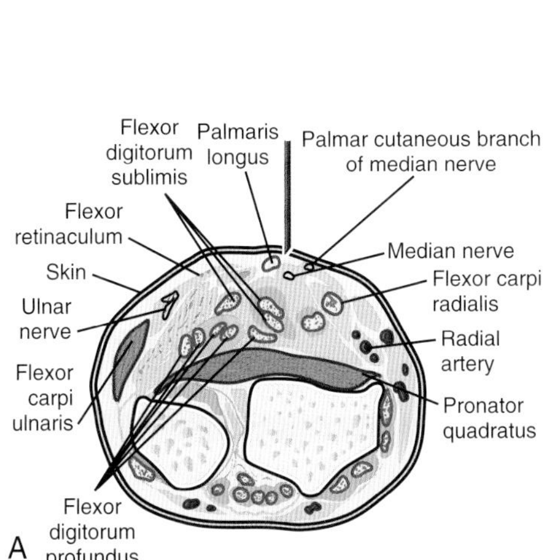

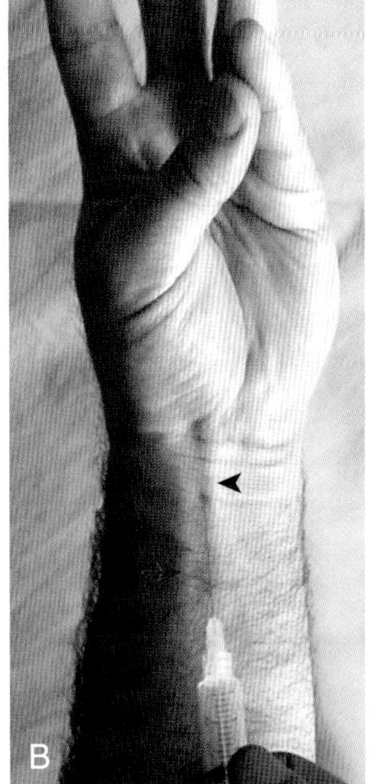

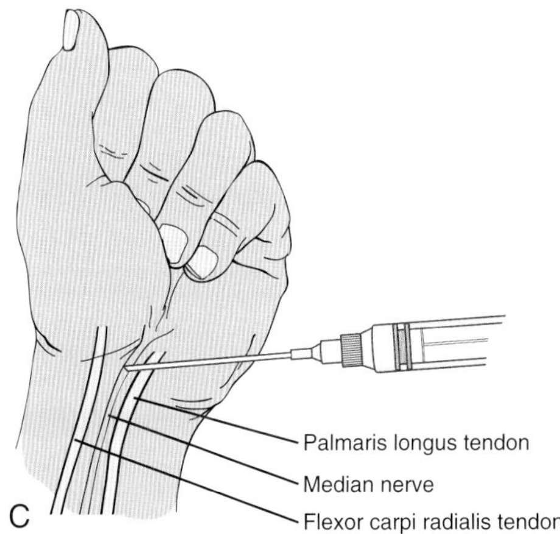

Figure 8-4 Median nerve block. **A,** Cross-sectional anatomy of the wrist (left wrist, palm up). **B,** Site of injection between flexor carpi radialis tendon (*arrow*) and palmaris longus tendon (*arrowhead*). **C,** Location of injection. (**A** and **C,** Adapted from Trott A: Wounds and Lacerations: Emergency Care and Closure, 3rd ed. St. Louis, Mosby, 1997.)

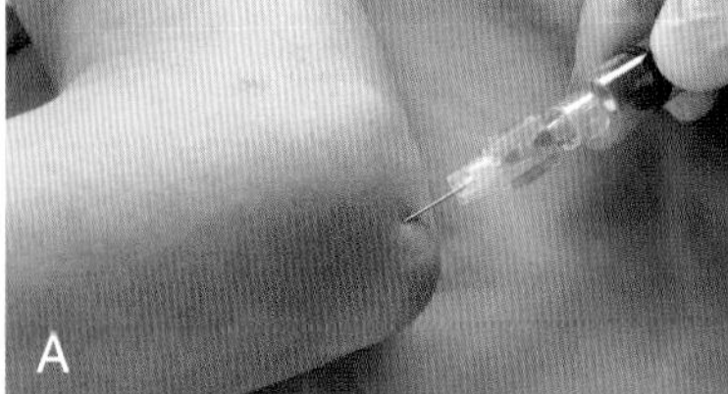

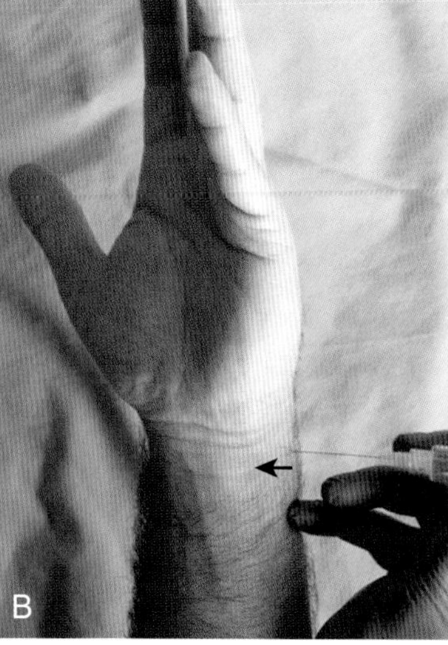

Figure 8-5 **A,** Site of an ulnar nerve block. **B,** Site of injection at wrist for palmar branch deep between the flexor carpi ulnaris tendon and ulnar artery (*arrow*), and for dorsal branch subcutaneously distal to the ulnar styloid process (needle).

vermilion border can be approximated appropriately. It can also be used for lacerations of the lower lateral nose and the lower eyelid (Fig. 8-7B and C).

- **Mental nerve block:** The mental nerve innervates the lower half of the lip. To avoid distortion that is inevitable with local injection around the vermilion border, inject the mental nerve. In adults the nerve exits the mandible just inferior to the second mandibular bicuspid, midway between the upper and lower edges of the mandible, and 2.5 cm from the midline of the jaw. As with the infraorbital nerve injection, introduce the needle at the gingival–buccal margin inferior to the second bicuspid. Another option is a transcutaneous approach 1.5 cm posterior and lateral to the mental foramen, which can be palpated through the skin. After aspiration, inject 2 mL of anesthetic (Fig. 8-7D and E).
- **Lip block:** The *upper lip* can also be blocked by injection of 5 to 10 mL of anesthetic along two lines in the direction of the nasal alae (Fig. 8-7F). An option for blocking the *lower lip* is to insert the needle at the midpoint of the chin, aiming toward the angle of the mouth (Fig. 8-7G).

6. **Ear block:** Because of complex innervations of the ear, it is impossible to infiltrate a solitary nerve. In addition, it is difficult to infiltrate *over* the cartilage because the skin here is so thin. A complete block of the auricle can be obtained by infiltrating completely around the ear with approximately 10 mL of 1% lidocaine *without* epinephrine (Fig. 8-8). This block will not numb the concha or the ear canal.
7. **Foot block:** Foot blocks are indicated not so much to prevent distortion but rather to limit discomfort. The sole of the foot is exquisitely sensitive to injection, and it is often subject to puncture wounds, lacerations, and foreign bodies. Nerve blocks can actually be more comfortable than direct infiltration and are discussed in detail in the following.
   - **Posterior ankle block:** The sural nerve (Su) runs behind the fibula and lateral malleolus to supply the lateral aspect of the heel and foot. The tibial nerve (LP, MP, MC) is found between the Achilles tendon and the medial malleolus, and its course is along the posterior tibial artery. The tibial nerve supplies the medial portion of the sole and the medial side of the foot (Fig. 8-9). To block the sural nerve, insert the needle lateral to the Achilles tendon 1 to 2 cm proximal to the level of the distal tip of the lateral malleolus. To ensure that the entire nerve is infiltrated, introduce the needle several times in a fan-shaped motion, directing it to the posterior medial aspect of the fibula (Fig. 8-10).

     To obtain a tibial nerve block, identify the posterior tibial pulsation. Pass the needle medial to the Achilles tendon toward the posterior tibial artery behind the medial malleolus. Infiltration is around the artery, and careful aspiration must be carried out to prevent intra-arterial injection (Fig. 8-11).
   - **Anterior ankle block:** The superficial peroneal nerve (SP) supplies the majority of the dorsal foot. It can be blocked by inserting the needle subcutaneously at the superior and medial aspect of the medial malleolus (Fig. 8-12).

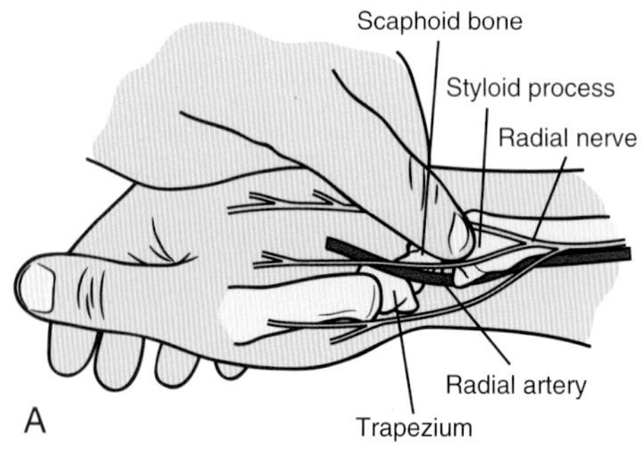

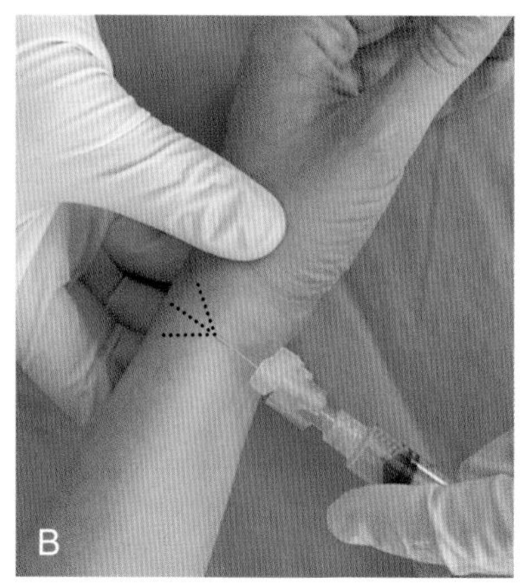

Figure 8-6 Radial nerve block. **A,** Identification of radial artery, the radial styloid, and the anatomic snuffbox. **B,** Begin on the ventral surface 2 cm above the wrist, just lateral to the radial artery. Extend over the dorsum of the wrist; *dotted lines* show subcutaneous injection of anesthetic. (**A,** Adapted from Rosen P, Chan TC, Vilke GM, Sternbach G: Atlas of Emergency Procedures. St. Louis, Mosby, 2001.)

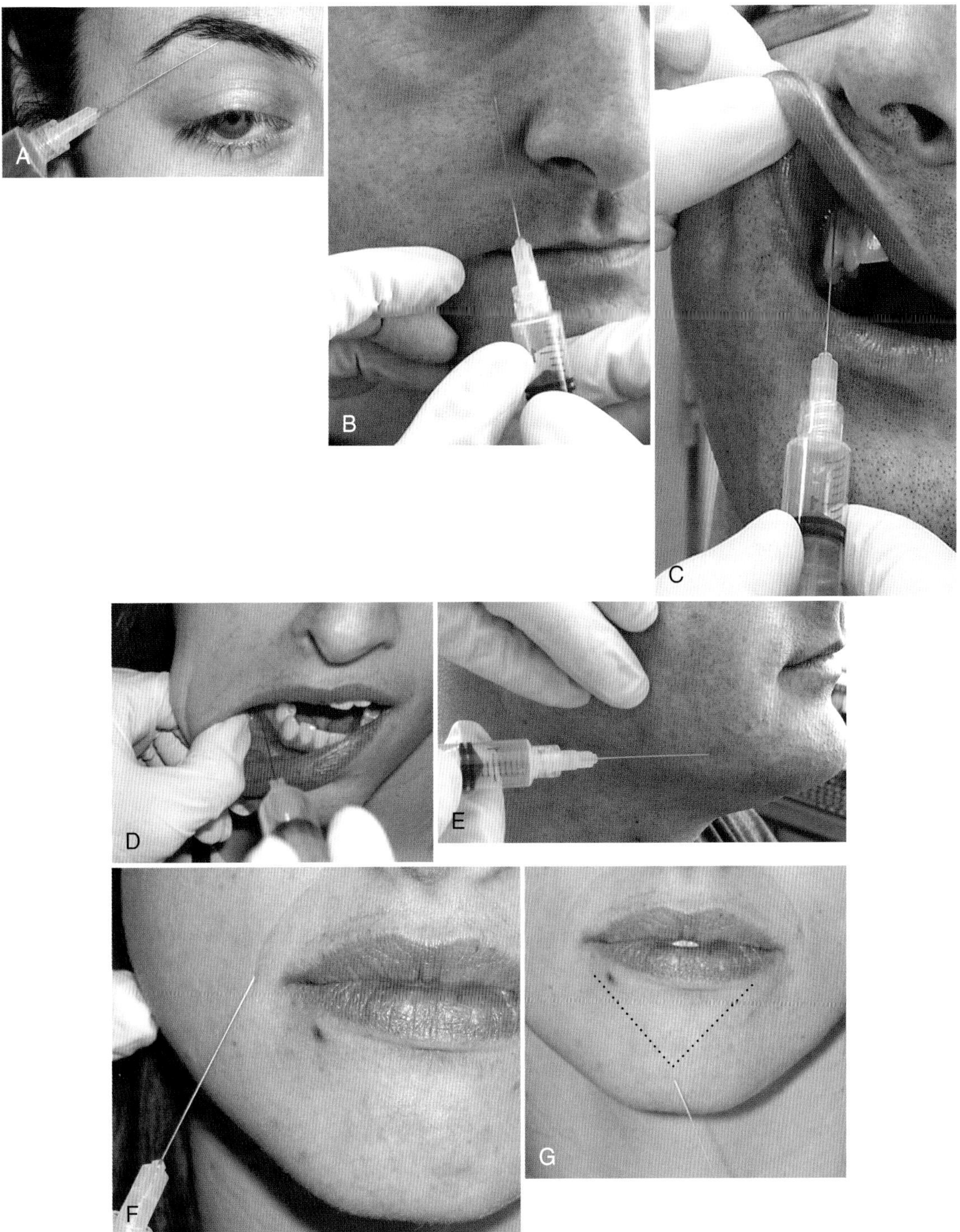

Figure 8-7 Locations of various nerves of the face and methods to obtain a nerve block. **A,** Technique for deposition of anesthetic to accomplish a supratrochlear and supraorbital (forehead) nerve block. **B,** Transcutaneous infraorbital nerve block. **C,** Intraoral technique to anesthetize the infraorbital nerve. **D,** Intraoral technique to anesthetize the mental nerve. **E,** Transcutaneous mental nerve block. **F,** Upper lip block. **G,** Lower lip block; *dotted lines* show subcutaneous injection of anesthetic. Also see Chapter 9, Oral and Facial Anesthesia.

8. **Other regional nerve blocks:** Other regional nerve blocks are dealt with in other chapters: oral-facial and nose (Chapter 9, Oral and Facial Anesthesia), penile (Chapter 117, Adult Circumcision), paracervical (Chapter 173, Paracervical Block), pudendal nerve (Chapter 174, Pudendal Anesthesia). Also see Chapter 4, Local Anesthesia, and Chapter 5, Local and Topical Anesthetic Complications.

CPT/Billing Code

64450 Introduction/injection of anesthetic agent (nerve block), diagnostic or therapeutic

Be sure to document both the diagnostic and procedural code for the local anesthesia. The CPT system allows separate billing for local anesthetic if it is administered by a physician different than

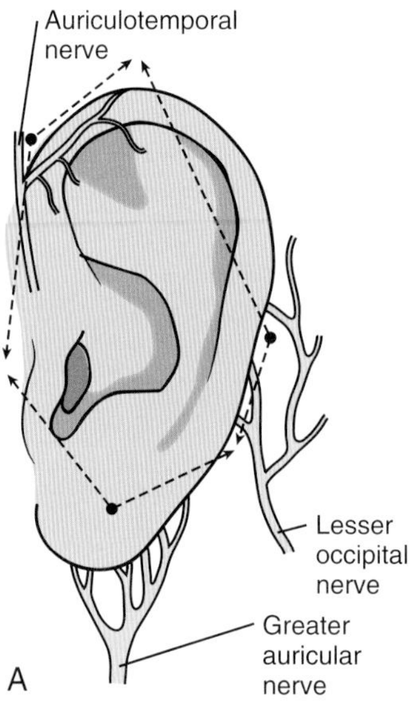

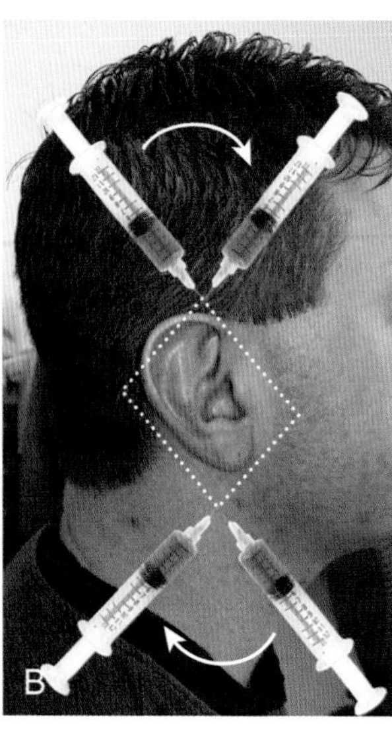

Figure 8-8 **A,** Ear block. *Dots* show insertion sites of needles; *arrows* show direction of needles injecting anesthetic. **B,** Alternative technique to achieve field anesthesia of the ear; *dotted lines* show subcutaneous injection of anesthetic. (**A,** Modified from Robinson JK: Atlas of Cutaneous Surgery. Philadelphia, WB Saunders, 1996. **B,** Adapted from Trott A: Wounds and Lacerations: Emergency Care and Closure, 3rd ed. St. Louis, Mosby, 1997.)

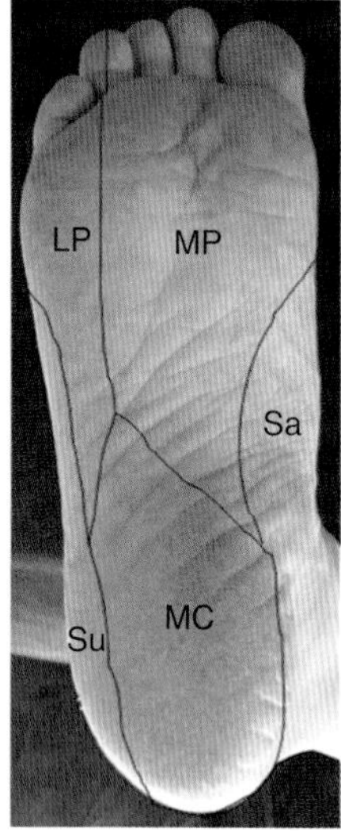

Figure 8-9 Distribution of sensory innervation to the foot. LP, lateral plantar branch of tibial nerve; MC, medial calcaneal branches of tibial nerve; MP, medial plantar branch of tibial nerve; Sa, saphenous nerve; Su, sural nerve.

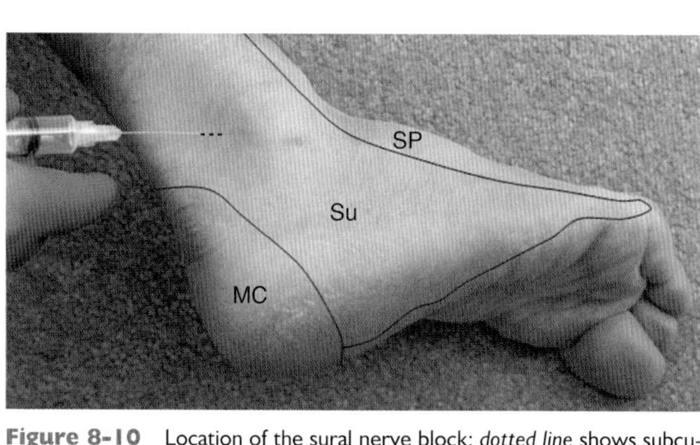

Figure 8-10 Location of the sural nerve block; *dotted line* shows subcutaneous injection of anesthetic. MC, medial calcaneal branches of tibial nerve; SP, superficial peroneal nerve; Su, sural nerve.

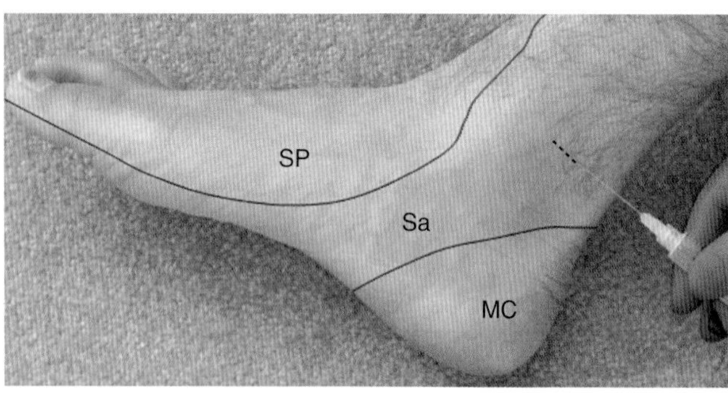

Figure 8-11 Location of the tibial nerve block; *dotted line* shows subcutaneous injection of anesthetic. MC, medial calcaneal branches of tibial nerve; SP, superficial peroneal nerve; Su, sural nerve.

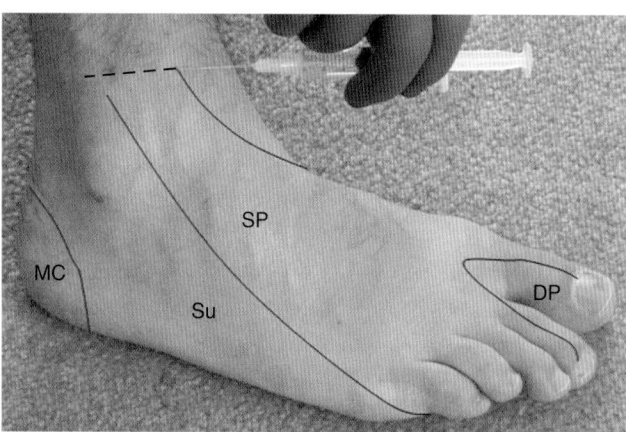

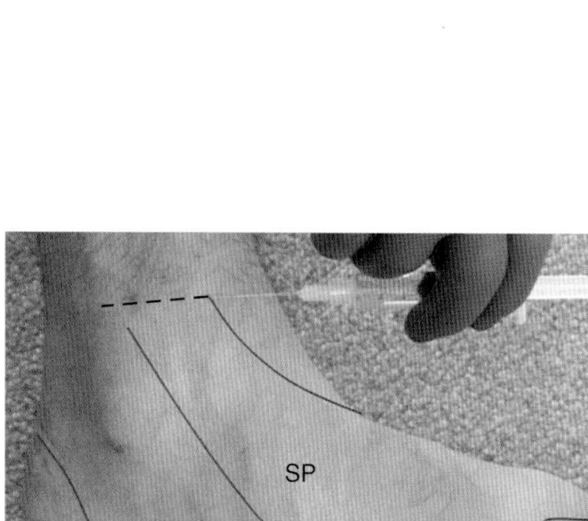

Figure 8-12 Location of the superficial peroneal nerve block; *dotted line* shows subcutaneous injection of anesthetic. DP, deep peroneal nerve; MC, medial calcaneal branches of tibial nerve; SP, superficial peroneal nerve; Su, sural nerve.

the surgeon, but the CPT code includes local anesthesia for the surgical procedure in most cases. A code for the instrument tray is allowed if the procedure requires more than basic instruments. If the nerve blocks are performed for diagnostic reasons, they can be billed separately.

ICD-9-CM Diagnostic Codes

ICD-9-CM codes are variable depending on the diagnosis.

Additional Resources

See the patient education and patient consent forms available at www.expertconsult.com.

Acknowledgment

The editors wish to recognize the contributions by Julie Graves Moy, MD, MPH, to this chapter in the previous two editions of this text.

ONLINE RESOURCES

American Society of Anesthesiologists: http://www.asahq.org/patientEducation/officebased.htm.
Society for Ambulatory Anesthesia: http://www.sambahq.org.

BIBLIOGRAPHY

Hadžić A, Volka JD: Peripheral Nerve Blocks: Principles and Practice. New York, McGraw-Hill, 2004.
Hahn MB, McQuillan PM, Sheplock GJ (eds): Regional Anesthesia. St. Louis, Mosby, 1996.
Krunic AL, Wang LC, Soltani K, et al: Digital anesthesia with epinephrine: An old myth revisited. J Am Acad Dermatol 51:755–759, 2004.
Meier G, Buettner J: Peripheral Regional Anesthesia: An Atlas of Anatomy and Techniques. Stuttgart, Thieme Medical Publishers, 2007.
Mulroy MF: Regional Anesthesia: An Illustrated Procedural Guide. Boston, Little, Brown, 1989.
Richert B: Basic nail surgery. Dermatol Clin 24:313–322, 2006.
Roberts JR, Hedges JR (eds): Clinical Procedures in Emergency Medicine, 4th ed. Philadelphia, Saunders, 2004.
Salam GA: Regional anesthesia for office procedures: Part I. Head and neck surgeries. Am Fam Physician 69:585–590, 2004.
Salam GA: Regional anesthesia for office procedures: Part II. Extremity and inguinal area surgeries. Am Fam Physician 69:896–900, 2004.
Simon RR, Brenner BE: Anesthesia and Regional Blocks in Emergency Procedures and Techniques, 3rd ed. Baltimore, Williams & Wilkins, 1994. **EDITOR'S NOTE:** This is an excellent resource.
Trott A: Wounds and Lacerations: Emergency Care and Closure, 3rd ed. St. Louis, Mosby, 1997.

CHAPTER 9

Oral and Facial Anesthesia

Larry Skoczylas

The ability to perform site-specific oral and facial regional nerve blocks is an important adjunct to almost any medical practice. Physicians are often the first practitioners to evaluate facial pain. This pain may be due to trauma, localized swelling and infection, or even facial neuralgias and tics. Properly infiltrated local anesthetic can eliminate discomfort when closing wounds, can provide pain control to a patient with a tooth abscess until he or she can be treated, or can be used as a diagnostic test to see if a suspected neuralgia is due to a peripheral or a central source. If peripheral, pain should be eliminated by the anesthesia. If central, the pain may persist.

This discussion involves both intraoral and extraoral anesthetic techniques. Therefore, an understanding of regional anatomy is crucial to properly perform these infiltrations and nerve blocks. The sensory innervation of the face and oral cavity is primarily from the trigeminal nerve (fifth cranial nerve). This nerve is divided into ophthalmic (V_1), maxillary (V_2), and mandibular branches (V_3; Figs. 9-1 and 9-2).

The *ophthalmic division* is purely sensory and supplies the eyeball, conjunctiva, lacrimal gland, parts of the mucous membrane of the nose, paranasal sinuses, and the skin of the forehead, eyes, and nose. When this nerve is paralyzed, the ocular conjunctiva becomes insensitive to touch. Sensory anesthesia of V_1 is usually obtained by local infiltration with a supraperiosteal extraoral block.

The *maxillary division*, like the ophthalmic division, is purely sensory. It supplies innervation to the skin of the middle portion of the face, lower eyelid, side of the nose, upper lip, maxillary teeth, and periodontal tissues. In addition, this nerve is sensory to the mucous membrane of the nasopharynx, maxillary sinus, tonsils, and hard and soft palate. This nerve can be blocked by both intraoral and extraoral injection.

The *mandibular division* has a large sensory as well as a small motor component. Blockage of the motor division can lead to decreased muscle function of the masseter, temporalis, pterygoid, mylohyoid, digastric, and soft palate elevators. Sensory innervation is to the temporal region and ear, cheek, lower lip and chin, parotid gland, temporomandibular joint, and mastoid area. Orally, the mandibular teeth and periosteal tissues, bone of the mandible, anterior two thirds of the tongue, and all intraoral mucosa are affected. The majority of anesthetic given for the mandibular division is intraoral, although some extraoral blocks may be indicated.

Indications

- Whenever anesthesia is desired in a fairly large anatomic area
- To limit the amount of medication given
- For laceration repair or lesion removal
- Around infection sites for incision and drainage
- To limit distortion of tissues and allow a better repair
- To anesthetize periosteum before more painful subperiosteal procedures such as tooth removal
- As a diagnostic block to determine the cause or site of pain
- To control pain

Contraindications

- History of allergy or reaction to local anesthetics (or bisulfite/parabens preservatives)
- Risk of hematoma (e.g., in patients with hemophilia or anticoagulant use); trauma to vascular bundles can increase risk of bleeding and hematoma *(relative contraindication)*
- Uncooperative patients (e.g., pediatric patients or patients with mental retardation may require sedation before local anesthetic; *relative contraindication*)

Complications

See Chapter 5, Local and Topical Anesthetic Complications.

- *Syncope:* Most common untoward reaction to anesthetic injections, often resulting from pain during the injection. A semisupine or supine position and slow injection technique are recommended.
- *Broken needle:* Very rare, but it is best to always leave some needle showing and not to "bury" to the hub when injecting.
- *Hematoma:* Rare, often resulting from torn capillaries or vessels that are punctured during injection.
- *Persistent paresthesia:* Occurs after the anesthetic should have worn off. Indicates damage to the nerve from physical or local chemical trauma. Can be temporary or permanent.
- *Ischemic ulcer:* Usually resulting from vasoconstrictor use in relatively *avascular* tissue (e.g., subperiosteally in the hard palate). Skin is very vascular, and ischemia is extremely rare when local anesthetic with epinephrine of a low concentration (1/100,000 or 1/200,000) is used.
- *Blanching:* Occurs at the site of injection because of pressure of anesthetic and vasoconstriction. If remote from the injection site, then it is probably due to inadvertent intravascular injection. No treatment is needed.
- *Tachycardia:* Can occur from pain of injection, but it is most likely due to intravascular injection or rapid absorption of local anesthetic with epinephrine.
- *Paralysis:* Results from inadvertent anesthesia of facial nerve (seventh cranial nerve). It is usually temporary. If longer-acting anesthetics such as bupivacaine are used and the patient cannot close the eyelid, the lid can be taped down (to avoid dryness of the eye) until the anesthetic wears off.
- *Visual disturbance:* Rare, probably due to vascular spasm or intra-arterial injection. Normal vision usually returns in about 30 minutes.
- *Overdosage:* Seizures and cardiac arrhythmias.

Equipment

- 10-mL syringe with Luer-Lok hub (for aspiration)
- 1- or 1½-inch (25- to 30-gauge) needle
- Local anesthetic, such as 2% lidocaine with or without 1 : 100,000 epinephrine, or 0.5% bupivacaine with or without 1 : 200,000 epinephrine

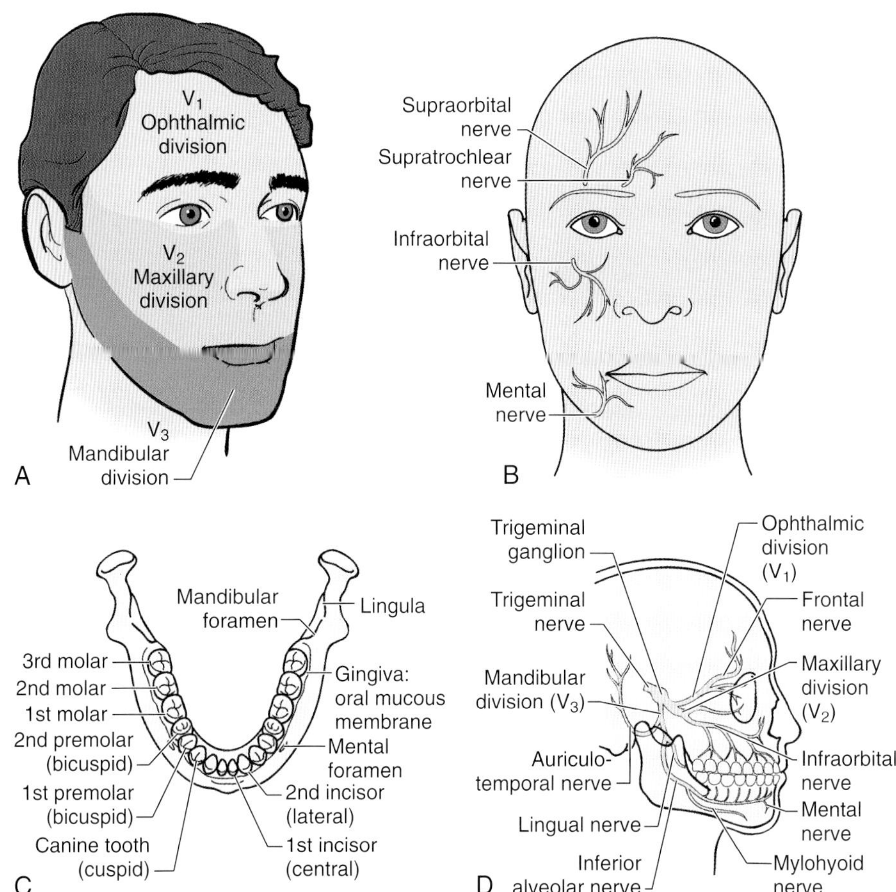

Figure 9-1 Sensory innervation of the face and oral cavity is primarily from the trigeminal nerve. **A,** The trigeminal nerve is divided into three branches: the ophthalmic branch (V_1), the maxillary branch (V_2), and the mandibular branch (V_3). **B,** Sensory distribution of the terminal branches of the trigeminal nerve: the supratrochlear nerve, supraorbital nerve, infraorbital nerve, and mental nerve. **C,** Anatomy of the mandibular arch and the lower teeth. **D,** Distribution of the trigeminal nerve. (**D,** Modified from Roberts JR, Hedges JR: Clinical Procedures in Emergency Medicine, 2nd ed. Philadelphia, WB Saunders, 1991.)

- Mepivacaine (pK_a 7.6; may give better anesthesia in infected tissue, which usually has an acidic environment [pK_a <7.5])
- Dental aspirating syringe (a good alternative; would need specific anesthetic carpules and needles for this system)

General Technique

1. Anesthetic solution is usually deposited just above the bone around the nerve trunks in the submucosa or subcutaneous tissue, where the nerves exit from the bone itself (e.g., supraorbital, infraorbital, or mental nerves). This technique is known as a *supraperiosteal injection*. It may be approached from either an intraoral or extraoral route, depending on the nerve block desired.
2. If going through facial skin, clean the skin with alcohol. If giving local anesthetic to repair traumatic lacerations, clean thoroughly with normal saline. Tent or support the tissue and slowly infiltrate (for 30–60 seconds) into the area to be addressed. Identify landmarks before infiltration; they can become "ballooned" and hard to appreciate after local anesthetic is given.

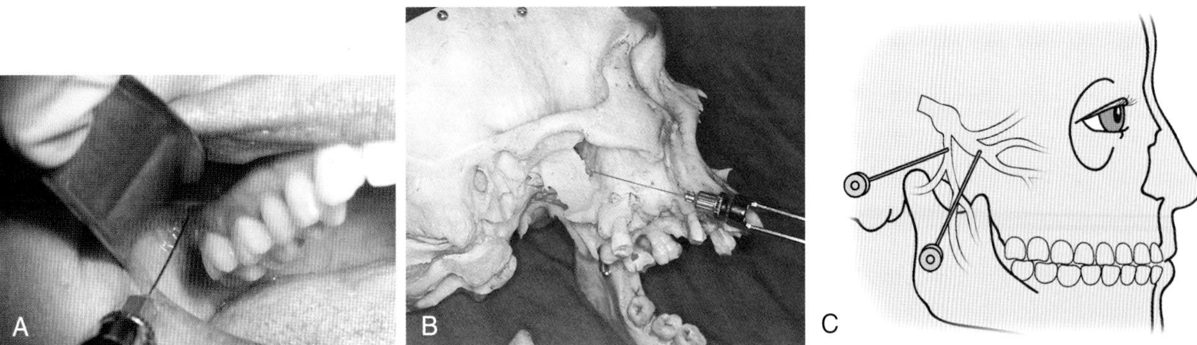

Figure 9-2 Maxillary nerve block. **A,** View with patient. **B,** Angle of needle to obtain intraoral maxillary (V_2) block. **C,** Location of needles for extraoral block (not described). Note that needle is not placed directly into the nerve.

3. If going through the oral mucosa, tissues are rarely scrubbed before injection. Cleaning any obvious debris in a trauma site with normal saline is indicated before closure. Lift up and tent lips or cheek. The target of the injection should be the procedure site.

INTRAORAL APPROACHES

Maxillary (V_2) Intraoral Nerve Block

See Figures 9-1 and 9-2.

Indications

- Anesthesia of the entire hemimaxilla for trauma repair or pathologic surgery
- For diagnostic blocks of the second division of the trigeminal nerve to evaluate neuralgias and tics
- To aid in anesthetizing infected sites or areas of tooth removal

Advantage

Decreases the amount of anesthetic solution used and the number of injection sites needed for maxillary anesthesia.

Technique

1. Place patient in a semisupine position. Partially open the patient's mouth and pull mandible toward side of injection (mandible to right for upper right injection).
2. Pull taut and retract cheek with index finger to gain visibility.
3. Aim for the area posterior and lateral to back of upper jaw (pterygopalatine fossa area). The area of insertion is the height of the mucobuccal fold above the distal aspect of the upper wisdom tooth area (lateral to the approximate junction of the hard and soft palate). Orient the bevel of the needle toward the bone.
4. Advance the needle slowly in the superomedial direction to a depth of about 30 mm (if necessary, measure on the needle beforehand to get an idea of the length).
5. No resistance should be felt. If resistance is noted, the angle of the needle toward the midline is too great.
6. Aspirate and deposit the local anesthetic (2 to 3 mL): continue to aspirate intermittently throughout the course of injection.

Mandibular (V_3) Intraoral Inferior Alveolar Nerve Block

See Figures 9-1 and 9-3.

Indications

- For anesthesia of entire hemimandible; can be achieved bilaterally if anesthesia of entire mandible or anterior mandible is needed
- For fracture repair, bone biopsy, removal of teeth, or pain control resulting from tooth infection or swelling

Disadvantages

- Not 100% successful (80% to 85%).
- Blind technique (by palpating landmarks). Intraoral swelling can make palpation of landmarks difficult.
- Intraoral landmarks are different in children than in adults. The lingula (a small bony bump) of the inner ramus of the mandible (where the nerve enters the jaw) is at a lower level in children.

Technique

1. Place the patient in a semisupine position and instruct him or her to keep the mouth open.
2. The target site is the lingula, a small bony bump about halfway back on the inner ramus of the mandible, where the inferior alveolar nerve enters the jaw.
3. Place the *thumb* of the noninjecting hand over the pterygomandibular raphe (the band of tissue in the posterior cheek between the upper and lower wisdom teeth). Use the thumb to pull the tissue laterally until the *deepest* depression in the anterior border of the ramus is felt. This creates a tense area for needle penetration.
4. Gently grasp the posterior border of the mandible with the middle finger of the noninjecting hand, as high superiorly as the ear allows. The line between the thumb and finger establishes the vertical height of the target area on the inner aspect of the ramus. The lingula should always be on or just below this line (and will always be below this line in children).
5. The anteroposterior position of the nerve (the target site) is located midway between the thumb and middle finger. The line of needle insertion is an oblique angle estimated by placing the barrel of the syringe over the bicuspid teeth (or mid-mandibular body region) of the opposite side.
6. The needle is inserted to the target site until bone is gently contacted. Depth of penetration is 1 to 2 cm. Always leave part of the needle showing to identify direction. Correct length should be about one half to three fourths of a 1½-inch needle.
7. If bone is contacted before half the length of the needle is inserted, the angle of penetration is usually too anterior. If no bone is contacted, the angle is too parallel to the inner aspect of the ramus of the mandible. In these instances it is best to withdraw the needle and start again.
8. Aspirate and slowly inject over 60 seconds. Continue to aspirate intermittently while injecting.

Akinosi Intraoral Closed Mouth Mandibular (V_3) Block

See Figure 9-4.

Indications

- For mandibular V_3 anesthesia
- When the patient is unable to open his or her mouth because of pain, swelling, trismus, or infection

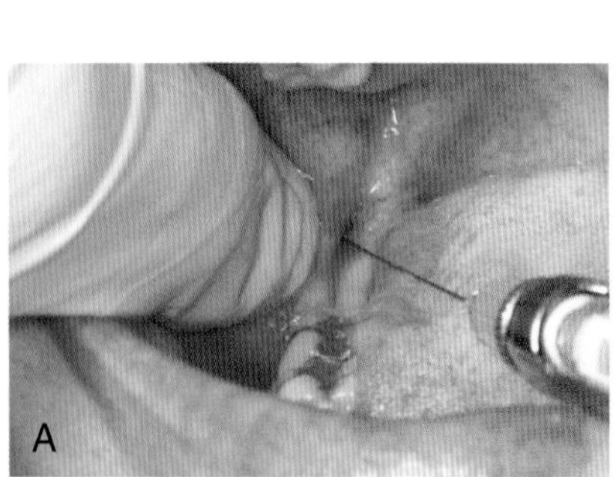

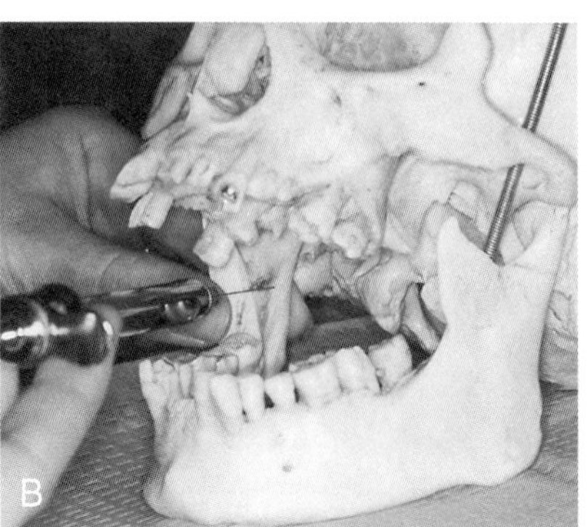

Figure 9-3 Site of intraoral mandibular (V_3) inferior alveolar block. **A,** Patient; **B,** skull.

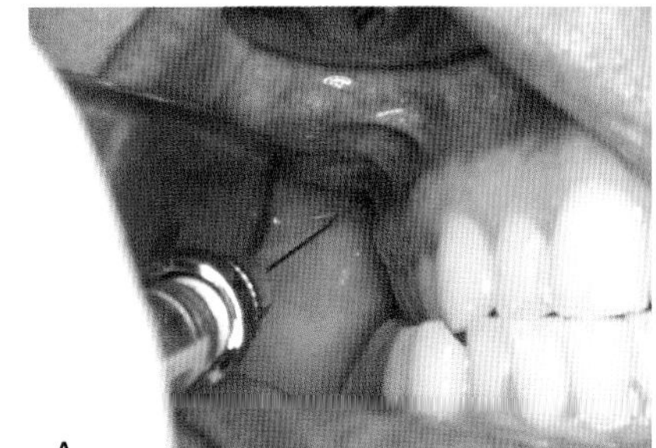

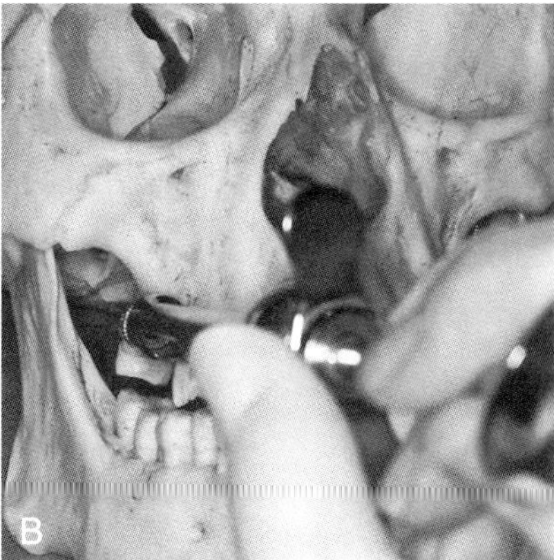

Figure 9-4 Position of needle for closed-mouth Akinosi intraoral mandibular (V_3) block. **A,** Patient; **B,** skull.

- For an uncooperative patient
- When conventional mandibular block has failed

Technique

1. Place the patient in the same position as that for the V_3 block.
2. Place the noninjecting finger (the thumb may be too big) at the greatest depression of the anterior ramus, as previously described for the V_3 block.
3. Identify the maxillary tuberosity—essentially a rounded area of bone just past the upper wisdom tooth area intraorally, which is the end of the maxillary bone.
4. Hold the barrel of the syringe parallel to the plane of the upper teeth, with the bevel of the needle toward the midline of the upper jaw.
5. The needle is inserted at the gingival (gum) level, about 0.5 cm superior to the tooth–gum interface.
6. Advance the needle between your finger and the maxillary tuberosity about 25 mm into the tissue, directing the needle slightly laterally to stay parallel to the plane of the upper teeth.
7. Aspirate and inject 2 to 3 mL of local anesthetic slowly over 60 seconds. Motor nerve paralysis of the masseter and lateral pterygoid muscles often occurs and can help decrease trismus. There can also be a facial nerve palsy if injection is through the sigmoid notch of the mandibular ramus and into the parotid gland. Maintaining the correct depth of penetration will help decrease this complication.

EXTRAORAL APPROACHES

Extraoral Block of Infraorbital Nerve

See Figures 9-1 and 9-5.

Indications

- To anesthetize the upper face, lips, or nose for trauma repair or excision
- To provide local anesthetic effect when infection intraorally causes too much pain to tolerate intraoral injection
- For diagnostic nerve block for neuralgias or tics

This is an easy block to administer, whether the intraoral or extraoral approach is used. It is also frequently used because it avoids the distortion created by direct local injection when lip repair and fine approximation are needed to avoid unsightly scars.

Disadvantage

The technique is performed by blind palpation of infraorbital foramen.

Technique

1. Palpate the infraorbital foramen just below the lowest level of the infraorbital rim, on a line between the pupil and the corner of the mouth.
2. Approach the infraorbital nerve from 1 cm below the bony rim and slightly medial to the palpated foramen. It is *not* necessary to enter the infraorbital foramen.
3. Slowly deposit 1 to 3 mL of local anesthetic. Paresthesia of the upper lip is sometimes (but not always) noted when the nerve is touched by the needle before injection.
4. For an intraoral approach, use the same anatomic landmarks, and approach the nerve through the mucobuccal fold over the maxillary second bicuspid, aiming at the infraorbital foramen. A long needle will be needed.

Maxillary Extraoral Block of Supraorbital and Supratrochlear Nerves

See Figures 9-6 and 9-7.

Indications

- To anesthetize the forehead (supraorbital nerve lateral, supratrochlear nerve medial)
- Use with infraorbital block to anesthetize periorbital tissues

Technique

1. Palpate the supraorbital foramen, which lies just superior to the supraorbital notch. This lies on a vertical line with the pupil when the eye is focused forward.
2. Insert the needle just above the notch and inject 2 to 4 mL of anesthetic. You do *not* need to be injecting directly into the foramen to block the supraorbital nerve.
3. The supratrochlear nerve can be blocked by redirecting the needle to 1 cm below and medial to the supraorbital foramen, staying on the bony rim, and injecting another 2 mL.

Mandibular Extraoral Mental Nerve Block

See Figures 9-1 and 9-8.

Indications

- To anesthetize the lower lip and chin area for trauma repair or excision
- To provide local anesthetic effect when infection intraorally causes too much pain to tolerate intraoral injection
- For diagnostic nerve blocks for lower face neuralgias and tics

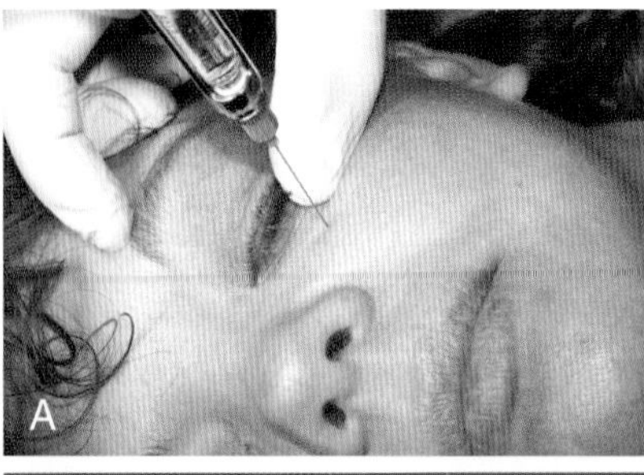

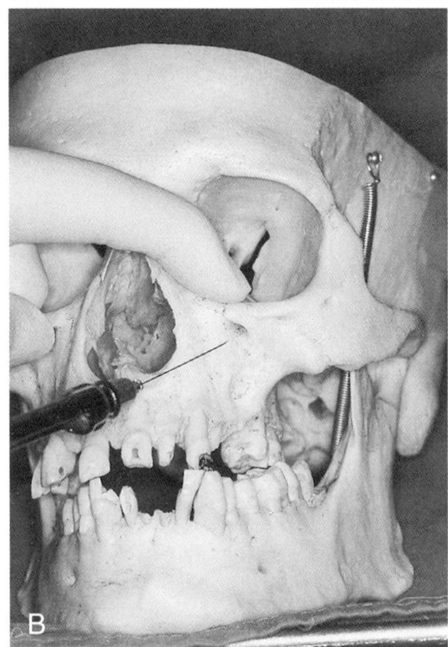

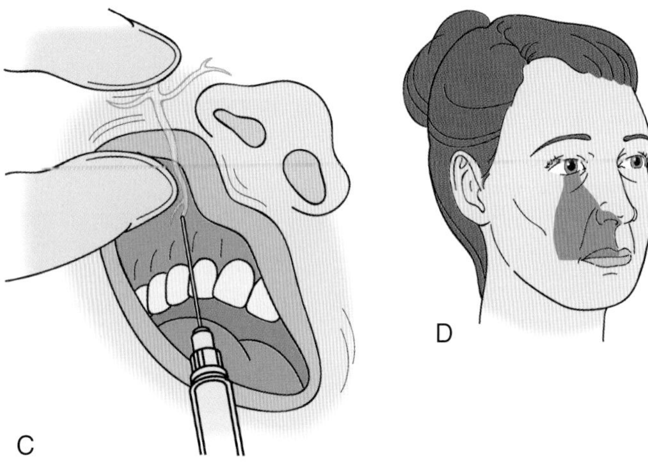

Figure 9-5 Infraorbital nerve block. **A,** View of patient receiving extraoral infraorbital nerve block. **B,** Proper location for an extraoral infraorbital nerve block. **C,** Intraoral infraorbital nerve block (see text). **D,** Area of anesthesia obtained with infraorbital blocks. (**C** and **D,** From Rosen P, Chan TC, Vilke GM, Sternbach G [eds]: Atlas of Emergency Procedures. St. Louis, Mosby, 2001.)

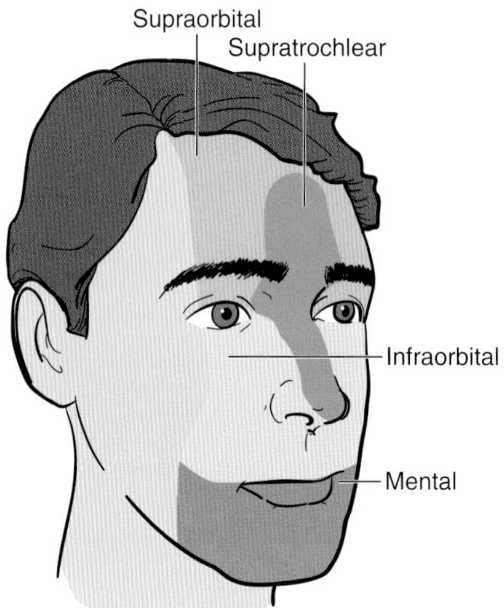

Figure 9-6 Sensory distribution of the terminal branches of the trigeminal nerve.

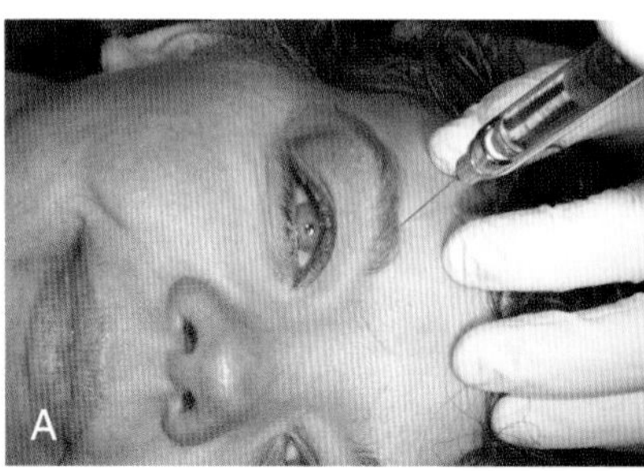

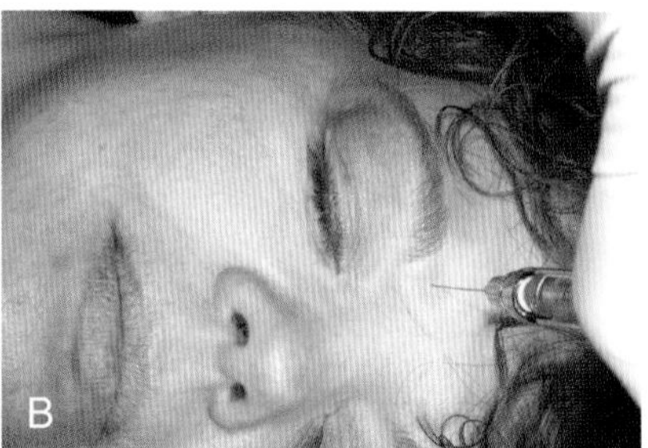

Figure 9-7 **A,** Supraorbital nerve block. **B,** Supratrochlear nerve block.

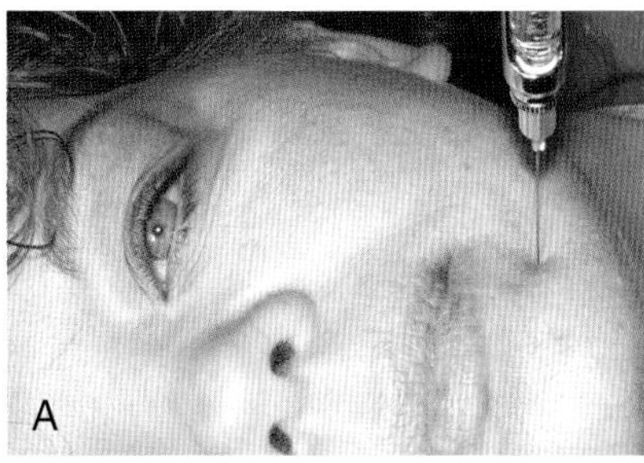

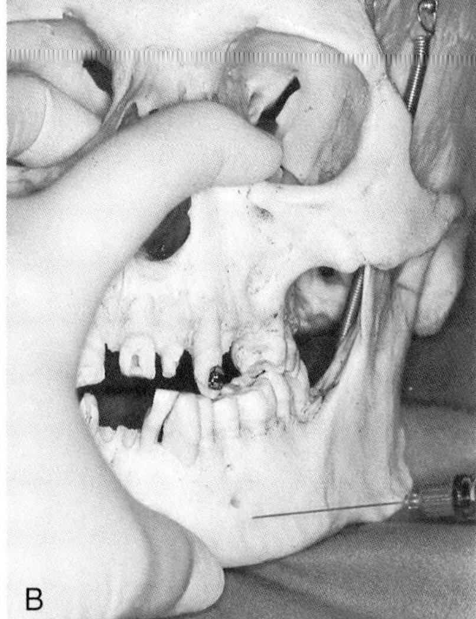

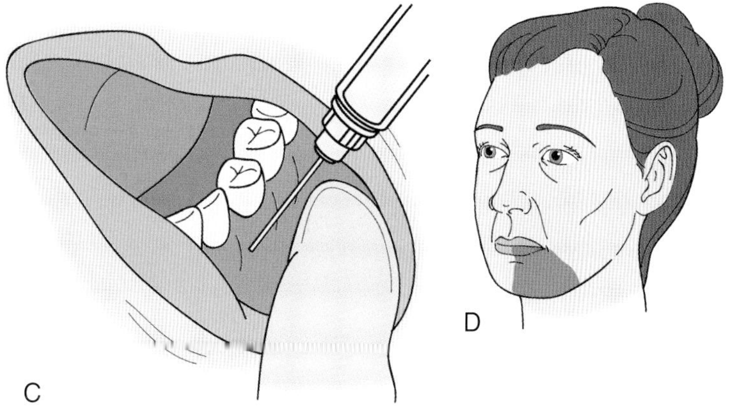

Figure 9-8 Mental nerve block. **A,** View of patient receiving extraoral mental nerve block. **B,** Site of extraoral mental nerve block. **C,** Intraoral approach. **D,** Area of anesthesia obtained with mental nerve block. (**C** and **D,** From Rosen P, Chan TC, Vilke GM, Sternbach G [eds]: Atlas of Emergency Procedures. St. Louis, Mosby, 2001.)

Disadvantage

The technique is performed by blind approximation of the mental nerve position in the mandible.

Technique

1. Approach the mandible extraorally from a position below the bicuspid teeth. The mental nerve foramen is located in the middle of the lower jaw on a line exactly vertically down from the previously described infraorbital nerve foramen. (This area can also be approached vertically from the inferior border of the mandible.)
2. Enter the skin with the needle perpendicular to the bone. Advance the needle until bone is touched, then back off 2 to 3 mm. It is *not* necessary to enter the mental foramen.
3. Deposit 1 to 3 mL of local anesthetic. Paresthesia of the lower lip is sometimes (but not always) noted when the nerve is touched by the needle.
4. The mental nerve can also be approached intraorally. The needle is inserted in front of the teeth at the junction of the gum and lip mucosa at the level of the premolar/molar teeth (fifth tooth from the midline). Direct the needle inferiorly just above bone for approximately 1 cm and inject 2 to 3 mL of anesthetic.

Nose: Skin and Nasal Mucosa

See Figure 9-9.

Indications

- For paranasal biopsy, or repair of bony or soft tissue nasal trauma (anesthesia for elective rhinoplasty is quite specific and will not be covered)
- Often used in conjunction with extraoral infraorbital nerve block for nasal procedures

Disadvantage

It can be painful to administer in the awake patient.

Technique

1. Apply topical spray anesthetic to each nostril.

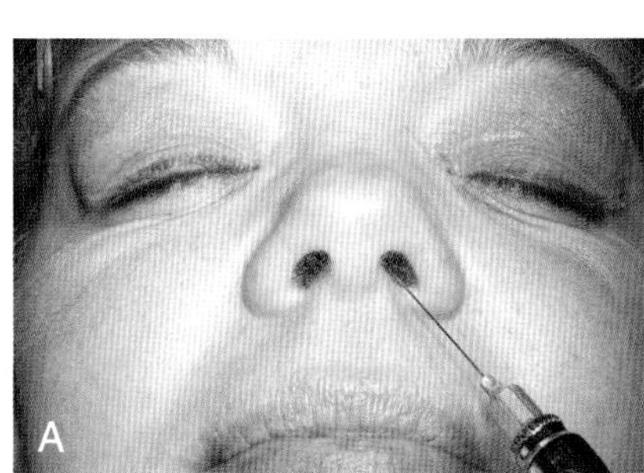

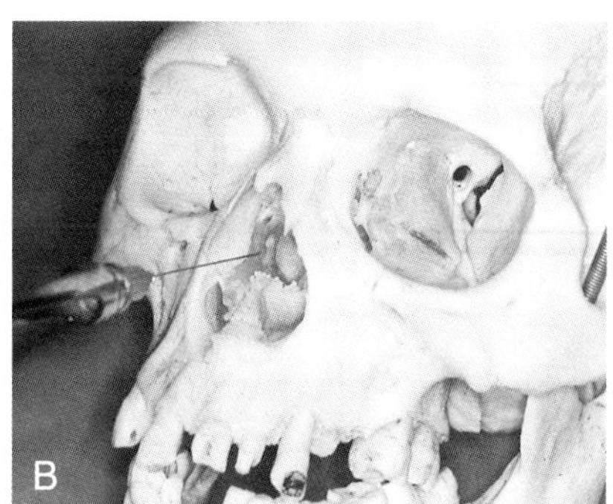

Figure 9-9 **A,** View of patient receiving nasal septal anesthesia. **B,** Proper location for administering nasal septal anesthesia.

2. Cotton-tipped applicators with 4% cocaine solution are used to paint the nasal mucosa. Leave in place for 5 minutes. This may be contraindicated in patients with cardiac disease.
3. Perform bilateral infraorbital nerve blocks, extraoral technique (see earlier).
4. Infiltrate the skin along the base of the nares, and continue as subcutaneous infiltration up the nasal-facial crease.
5. Inject the septal mucosa with local anesthetic containing vasoconstrictor to help decrease bleeding, especially in nasal or septal fractures. Use 1½-inch needle and inject from posterior to anterior. Now inject subperiosteally between the nasal bones and the tissue, and along the lateral nasal region.

CPT/Billing Code

64400 Injection, anesthetic agent; trigeminal nerve, any division or branch

BIBLIOGRAPHY

Allen GD: Dental Anesthesia and Analgesia (Local and General). Baltimore, Williams & Wilkins, 1984.

Bramhall J: Regional anesthesia for aesthetic surgery. In Kaminer MS, Dover JS, Arndt KA (eds): Atlas of Cosmetic Surgery. Philadelphia, WB Saunders, 2002, pp 73–94.

Budac S, Suresh S: Emergent facial lacerations repair in children. Anesth Analg 102:1091–1092, 2006.

Eaton JS, Grekin RC: Regional anesthesia of the face. Dermatol Surg 27:1006–1009, 2001.

Edlich EF, Rodeheaver GT, Thacker JG: Local and regional anesthesia for wound repair. In Tintinalli JE, Krome RL, Ruiz E (eds): Emergency Medicine: A Comprehensive Study Guide, 4th ed. New York, McGraw-Hill, 1996.

Hahn MB: Distributions of the trigeminal nerve. In Hahn MB, McQuillan PM, Sheplock GJ (eds): Regional Anesthesia: An Atlas of Anatomy and Techniques. St. Louis, Mosby, 1996, pp 45–52.

Hanke CW: The tumescent facial block. Dermatol Surg 27:1003–1005, 2001.

Higgenbotham E, Vissers RJ: Local and regional anesthesia. In Tintinalli JE, Krome RL (eds): Emergency Medicine: A Comprehensive Study Guide, 6th ed. New York, McGraw-Hill, 2004.

Katz J: Atlas of Regional Anesthesia. Norwalk, Conn, Appleton-Century-Crofts, 1985.

Kretzschmar JL, Peters JE: Nerve blocks for regional anesthesia of the face. Am Fam Physician 55:1701–1704, 1997.

Malamed SF: Handbook of Local Anesthesia. St. Louis, Mosby, 1990.

Malamed SF: Nerve injury caused by mandibular block analgesia. Int J Oral Maxillofac Surg 35:876–877, 2006.

Mulroy MF: Peripheral nerve blockade. In Barash PG, Cullen BF, Stoelting RK (eds): Clinical Anesthesia, 5th ed. Philadelphia, Lippincott Williams & Wilkins, 2006.

Pascal J, Charier D, Perret D, et al: Peripheral blocks of trigeminal nerve for facial soft-tissue surgery. Eur J Anaesthesiol 22:480–482, 2005.

Reichman EF, Tolsar DR: Regional nerve blocks (regional anesthesia). In Reichman EF, Simon PR (eds): Emergency Medicine Procedures. New York, McGraw-Hill, 2004, pp 939–983.

Roberts GJ, Rosenbaum NL: Color Atlas of Dental Anesthesia and Sedation. Alesbury, United Kingdom, Hazell Books, 1991.

Salam GA: Regional anesthesia for office procedures. Am Fam Physician 69:585–590, 2004.

Schimek F, Fahle M: Techniques of facial nerve block. Br J Ophthalmol 79:166–173, 1995.

Simpson S: Regional nerve blocks. Aust Fam Physician 30:565–568, 2001.

Smith DW, Peterson MR, DeBerard SC: Regional anesthesia. J Postgrad Med 106:69–73, 77–78, 1999.

Soriano TT, Lask GP, Dinehart SM: Anesthesia and analgesia. In Robinson JK, Hanke DW, Sengelmann RD, Siegel DM (eds): Surgery of the Skin: Procedural Dermatology. Philadelphia, Mosby, 2005, pp 39–58.

CHAPTER 10

Topical Anesthesia

Suraj Achar • Jonathan Chan

Topical anesthesia offers patients an alternative to local injectable anesthetics. The ideal topical anesthetic should provide 100% anesthesia with rapid onset of action, have prolonged duration, and have no local or systemic side effects. To date, the perfect topical agent has not been developed. New formulations have improved efficacy and application options. (Also see Chapter 4, Local Anesthesia; Chapter 229, Transcutaneous Electrical Nerve Stimulation, Phonophoresis, and Iontophoresis; and Chapter 5, Local and Topical Anesthetic Complications.)

There are many benefits and some drawbacks of topical anesthetics compared with local injectable anesthetics. First, application of topical anesthetics is painless. In addition, topical anesthetics do not distort wound margins in laceration repairs. One drawback is the extra time required to achieve effective anesthetic effect.

Although the first topical anesthetics were developed in the latter half of the 19th century with the first uses of topical cocaine, safer and more effective agents have more recently become available. The use of TAC (tetracaine, adrenalin, cocaine), one of the first topical anesthetic creams to be developed, is no longer supported by the literature. LET/LAT (lidocaine, epinephrine/adrenalin, tetracaine) solution-gel has been found to be equally efficacious as TAC. LET eliminates cocaine (thus lessening the risk for toxicity and seizures), avoids documentation issues, and lowers the cost.

EMLA (eutectic mixture of local anesthetics), which was approved by the U.S. Food and Drug Administration (FDA) in 1992, is now commonly used. A *eutectic mixture* is one in which the melting point of the mixture is lower than that of the individual components; in the case of EMLA, the components (lidocaine and prilocaine) remain liquid at room temperature. LMX 4 (4% liposomal lidocaine) and LMX 5 (5% liposomal lidocaine) are liposomal agents that are available over the counter. LMX 4 and LMX 5 were formerly called ELA-Max. Liposomes are synthetic biologic membranes composed of an aqueous core surrounded by a lipid layer. This delivery system allows medications to penetrate the stratum corneum more readily because they resemble cell membranes, thus strengthening the onset of action while controlling release of the action drug for a longer duration of action.

More recently, the S-Caine Patch has been developed. This 1:1 eutectic mixture of 70 mg lidocaine and 70 mg tetracaine base has a disposable, oxygen-activated heating element. The heat is maintained at 39° C to 41° C for a 2-hour period. Heat has been shown to enhance the delivery of topical creams.

Categories of topical anesthetics can be divided into those applied on intact skin, nonintact skin, and mucous membranes. This categorization is important because a topical anesthetic (e.g., lidocaine) applied to the mucous membrane may result in blood levels comparable with those achieved with parenteral administration (Table 10-1). Available topical anesthetics for intact skin are EMLA/EMLA Disc, LMX 4, LMX 5, and iontophoretic preparations. Also, with the development of many new aesthetic procedures, many clinicians now have various mixtures compounded (see later, as well as Chapter 59, Skin Peels).

In addition to creams and ointments, cooling can also be used to provide brief, temporary anesthesia (e.g., ethyl chloride spray or ice cubes).

Indications

Intact Skin

LMX 4/LMX 5

- FDA: temporary relief of pain associated with minor cuts, abrasions, minor burns, skin irritation, and insect bites.
- Literature-supported uses: venipuncture, venous cannulation, arterial puncture, suture removal, shave biopsy, punch biopsy, chemical peels, curettage of molluscum contagiosum, cryotherapy of venereal warts, intracutaneous allergy testing, epilation, débridement of otitis media with an intact tympanic membrane, removal of an embedded foreign body, circumcision at more than a 37-week gestation, skin grafting, débridement of ulcers, lumbar puncture.
- Adjunct to: vasectomy, dermabrasion, laser resurfacing, postsurgical discomfort.
- Nonsurgical uses: postherpetic neuralgia, meralgia paresthetica.
- Used for intact skin. Efficacy is similar to EMLA, but LMX 4 is less expensive than EMLA.

EMLA

FDA: for use on intact skin for local anesthesia.

Lidoderm Patch

FDA: relief of pain associated with postherpetic neuralgia.

BLT Triple Anesthetic Gel (20% Benzocaine, 6% Lidocaine, 4% Tetracaine)

- Used for intact skin.
- Percentages may vary.
- This is usually compounded.

S-Caine Patch/S-Caine Peel

- Used for intact skin.
- Approved for children 3 years of age or older.

Nonintact Skin

Topicaine (4% or 5% Lidocaine Gel)

- Minor skin cuts or abrasions.
- Available over the counter.

TABLE 10-1 Summary of Topical Anesthetics

Agents	Concentration	Status	Maximum Dose or Area*	Onset of Action	Duration	Pregnancy Category†
Intact Skin						
EMLA cream or anesthetic disc	2.5% lidocaine/2.5% prilocaine	Rx	20 g/200 cm^2 for 7–12 yr of age and >20 kg (A) and (C)	60–120 min	180 min	B
LMX 4/5	4% lidocaine plus vitamin E, propylene glycol, benzyl alcohol, lecithum, cholesterol, carborner-940, triethanolamine, polysorbate 80	OTC	100 cm^2 (A)	‡	‡	B
Amethocaine gel	4% tetracaine	Europe	50 mg (A)	40 min	240 min	C
Lidocaine acid mantle (Novartis)	30%–40% lidocaine	Rx		20 min	30–60 min	
Patch (Lidoderm)	5% lidocaine	Rx	420 cm^2 (three patches)		12 hr max duration of patch time	B (patch not studied in pregnancy)
S-Caine Patch/Peel	Lidocaine 70 mg, tetracaine 70 mg	Rx	One patch	30 min	Patch time	
BLT gel	20% benzocaine, 6% lidocaine, 4% tetracaine			15 min	60 min	C
Ethyl chloride spray	Skin refrigerant	OTC		<1 min	Transient	
Topicaine	4%–5% lidocaine	OTC	600 cm^2 (A), 100 cm^2 (C >10 kg)	Rapid	30–60 min	
Nonintact Skin						
LET/LAT	4% lidocaine/1 : 2000 epinephrine/1% tetracaine	Compounded				
Mucous Membrane						
Xylocaine		Rx	300 mg (A)/100 mg (C)	2–5 min	15–45 min	B
Viscous solution	2% lidocaine			1–2 min	15–20 min	
Liquid	5% lidocaine			2 min		
Ointment	2.5%, 5% lidocaine					
Benzocaine						
Cetacaine						
spray	14% benzocaine	Rx				
liquid	2% tetracaine	Rx				
gel						
ointment						
Hurricaine						
liquid	20% benzocaine	OTC		<5 min	15–45 min	C
gel						
spray						
Cocaine solution	4% and 10%	C-II§	200 mg (A)	1–5 min	30–60 min	C
Ophthalmic						
Alcaine solution	0.5% proparacaine	Rx		20 sec	15–20 min	C
Pontocaine solution	0.5% tetracaine	Rx	50 mg (A)	20 sec	15–20 min	C

EMLA, eutectic mixture of local anesthetics; LAT, lidocaine, adrenalin, tetracaine; LET, lidocaine, epinephrine, tetracaine; OTC, over the counter; Rx, prescription; TAC, tetracaine, adrenalin, cocaine.

*A, Adults; C, children.

†Pregnancy category B: Animal studies have not shown a fetal risk but there are no controlled studies in pregnant women. Pregnancy category C: Animal studies are not available. Safety for use during pregnancy has not been established. Use only when potential benefits outweigh potential hazards to the fetus.

‡No clinical studies.

§C-II: Controlled substances schedule II drug (Controlled Substances Act of 1970). Cocaine must be stored in a locked cabinet; and separate written records must be maintained for a period of 2 years after the drug is dispensed.

Adapted from Huang W, Vidimos A: Topical anesthetics in dermatology. J Am Acad Dermatol 43:286–298, 2000.

LET/LAT (Lidocaine, Epinephrine/Adrenalin, Tetracaine)

- Scalp and facial lacerations.
- Does not work on intact skin.

Mucous Membranes

Lidocaine (Xylocaine), Benzocaine

- Painful, irritated, inflamed mucous membranes: anesthesia before minor surgical procedure and esophagogastroduodenoscopy.
- 2% viscous lidocaine for aphthous ulcers and mucositis in immunosuppressed patients.

Ophthalmic Preparations

Removal of foreign bodies, short eyelid procedures (e.g., chalazion removal), and placement of eye shields.

Mechanical Methods

Thermal: Ice/Ethyl Chloride Spray

Skin tag clipping, incision and drainage of simple abscess, and injections (blood draws, skin grafting, sports injuries).

For Aesthetic Procedures

Many noninvasive aesthetic procedures (e.g., deep skin peels, facial resurfacing) require some type of topical anesthetic. Oral analgesic medications and anxiolytics can also be beneficial. Everyone seems to have his or her own favorite compounded preparation. With the rapid growth of procedures in this field, few studies have been published to compare the various combinations and their efficacy.

BLT (Benzocaine, Lidocaine, Tetracaine)

BLT is a favorite compounded mixture. The percentages may vary (e.g., 20%, 7%, 7%, or 20%, 6%, 4%). With most BLT preparations, it takes 45 to 60 minutes to obtain good effect.

Quadri-Caine

Quadri-Caine (Scripts Pharmacy, St. Joseph, Mich) is a compounded topical anesthetic that has a more rapid onset (10 to 15 minutes). Standard Quadri-Caine consists of 10% lidocaine, 5% tetracaine, 5% prilocaine, and 1% bupivacaine in an emollient cream plus a penetration enhancer. Quadri-Caine VC contains the vasoconstrictor phenylephrine.

Quadri-Caine, as with most of these potent compounded preparations, should be used only under the direction of physicians experienced in the use of high-potency topical anesthetics. It is unknown what amounts of the topical anesthetics in Quadri-Caine reach the systemic circulation. The amount to apply must be determined on a case-by-case basis. It is recommended that not more than 3 g of Quadri-Caine be applied in 24 hours.

Quadri-Caine is not for resale. It must be purchased by a medical office or clinic for use during a patient visit or may be ordered by prescription specifically for individual patient use.

Quadri-Caine and Quadri-Caine VC are registered trademarks and, as compounded products, have not undergone FDA review.

NOTE: Compounded products are not produced under the same standards as FDA-approved products. The levels of lidocaine may vary dramatically, and toxicity studies using moderate or large amounts of compounded products have not been performed.

CONTRAINDICATIONS

Many preparations contain preservatives that can cause allergic reactions. If a patient develops an allergic dermatitis while using a topical anesthetic, he or she may not be allergic to the active drug itself, but rather to other components in the cream or ointment. An allergy to lidocaine is extremely rare, if it occurs at all.

LET/LAT

Sensitivity to tetracaine, epinephrine, or lidocaine

EMLA

- Advanced liver disease (hepatic metabolism)
- Methemoglobinemia risk

LMX 4/LMX 5

- Sensitivity to lidocaine.
- Avoid mucous membranes: absorption increases toxicity risks.
- Efficacy diminishes as the skin thickness (lack of absorption) and vascularity (rapid clearance) increases. Essentially ineffective on the palms and soles even if occluded for hours.

Lidoderm 5% Patch

- Sensitivity to lidocaine (rare); denuded skin; mucous membranes.
- Do not use more than 12 hours out of 24-hour period to avoid toxicity. Do not use with methemoglobinemia-inducing agents on infants younger than 12 months of age (Box 10-1).
- Use with caution in infants younger than 3 months of age (maximum dose of 1 g for 1-hour application if term).

BLT Triple Anesthetic Gel

- Allergy to p-aminobenzoic acid (PABA), hair dyes, and sulfonamides
- Sensitivity to benzocaine, lidocaine, or tetracaine

S-Caine Patch/S-Caine Peel

Sensitivity to lidocaine or tetracaine

Topicaine (4% to 5% Lidocaine Gel)

Sensitivity to lidocaine

Box 10-1. Agents Associated with Methemoglobinemia*

Acetaminophen	Nitroprusside
Acetanilid	Pamaquine
Aniline dyes	Para-aminosalicylic acid
Benzocaine	Phenacetin
Chloroquine	Phenobarbital
Dapsone	Phenytoin
Naphthalene	Primaquine
Nitrates and nitrites	Quinine
Nitrofurantoin	Sulfonamides
Nitroglycerin	

*Use with caution with eutectic mixture of local anesthetics (EMLA).

From Huang W, Vidimos A: Topical anesthetics in dermatology. J Am Acad Dermatol 43:286–298, 2000.

Thermal: Ice/Ethyl Chloride Spray

- Raynaud's phenomenon, cryoglobulinemia
- Not effective for skin biopsy, alters specimen

Lidocaine (Xylocaine), Benzocaine (Mucous Membranes)

- Sensitivity to Xylocaine or benzocaine

Ophthalmic Preparations

- Not to be used to control pain over long term
- Inhibits healing and, because no sensation, may lead to inadvertent trauma
- May also eliminate blinking, leading to drying of cornea

TECHNIQUE

NOTE: Precautions must be taken to avoid high blood levels of anesthetics. This is especially true with the use of compounded products or FDA-approved products used under occlusion. Part of the confusion that providers face relates to the need to use occlusion with EMLA because of its poor penetration through the stratum corneum. With LMX 4/LMX 5, occlusion is not needed because the liposomes appear to enhance absorption. However, physicians may accidently or purposely use these newer agents under occlusion. Small doses of these drugs have been shown to be safe when used with occlusion, but large doses (>60 g) may be toxic.

LET/LAT

Apply 1.5 to 3.0 mL of LET to a soaked gauze and wipe in and over a facial or scalp laceration. Avoid mucous membranes and end-arteriolar parts of the body such as the digits. Contact with wound should be a minimum of 10 minutes and a maximum of 30 minutes. Watch for blanching, which correlates with anesthesia. Onset of action is 15 to 30 minutes.

EMLA/EMLA Disc

EMLA cream is a eutectic mixture of 2.5% lidocaine and 2.5% prilocaine. A eutectic mixture is one that melts at a lower temperature than does any of its ingredients. Therefore, both anesthetics exist in a liquid form.

Remove oil from skin with an alcohol or acetone swab. Consider thinning the stratum corneum through tape stripping of superficial cells. Apply the disc or 1 to 2 g per 10 cm^2 of the cream. Cover with an occlusive dressing (Tegaderm, OpSite, or Band-Aid) for 60 minutes for a 3-mm depth. Every additional 30 minutes provide 1 mm of more depth; a 2-hour maximum time is equivalent to 5 mm. Cream should still be visible when the dressing is removed. If it is not visible, an inadequate amount was used (Table 10-2).

TABLE 10-2 Recommended Maximum Dose and Application Area of Eutectic Mixture of Local Anesthetics

Age	Body Weight (kg)	Maximum Total Dose and Time	Maximum Application Area (cm^2)
1–3 mo	<5	1 g (1 hr)	10
4–12 mo	>5	2 g (4 hr)	20
1–6 yr	>10	10 g (4 hr)	100
7–12 yr	>20	20 g (4 hr)	200

Adapted from Huang W, Vidimos A: Topical anesthetics in dermatology. J Am Acad Dermatol 43:286–298, 2000.

LMX 4/LMX 5

Apply for 15 to 40 minutes without occlusion. A transient erythema may develop, but no serious side effects have been observed. In children weighing less than 20 kg, apply cream to an area no larger than 100 cm^2 to prevent systemic toxicity.

Lidoderm 5% Patch

Apply up to three patches at one time to cover the most painful area (e.g., postherpetic neuralgia) for a maximum of 12 hours in a 24-hour period. Patches may be cut to smaller sizes for smaller lesions or impaired elimination (e.g., hepatic disease).

BLT Triple Anesthetic Gel

Apply to intact skin for 10 to 30 minutes. Recent studies note that BLT provides effective analgesia after 15 minutes of application.

S-Caine Patch/S-Caine Peel

Apply S-Caine Patch and use disposable heating element as instructed. Time to effect is 20 to 30 minutes.

Apply S-Caine Peel to area. The cream dries on exposure to air and becomes flexible and is peeled off skin after 20 to 30 minutes. The advantage of this flexible membrane is delivery of topical anesthetic to contoured areas of the body. Do not leave on longer than 30 minutes.

Topicaine

Apply a moderately thick layer (about 1/8 inch) to affected area. Best anesthetic results occur in 20 minutes to 1 hour.

Lidocaine (Xylocaine), Benzocaine (Mucous Membranes)

Wolfe and colleagues reported in 2000 that atomized lidocaine 4% solution decreased the discomfort of nasogastric tube placement. The combination of 1.5 mL atomized lidocaine applied intranasally plus 3.0 mL applied oropharyngeally plus 5 mL 2% lidocaine jelly applied intranasally is superior to jelly alone. Caution should be used because of impaired swallowing after use. Patients should expectorate excess anesthetic to avoid systemic absorption and toxicity. Plasma levels are similar to those obtained with intravenous injection. For viscous solution, do not exceed 1 tablespoon (15 mL) every 3 hours or 1 teaspoon (5 mL) of 5% liquid in an adult (see Chapter 4, Local Anesthesia, and Chapter 5, Local and Topical Anesthetic Complications, for maximum doses). Ingestion of food should be avoided for at least 1 hour after oral use to prevent aspiration.

Thermal: Ice/Ethyl Chloride Spray

For skin tag clipping hold ice in direct contact for 10 seconds and clip skin tag immediately.

For skin tag clipping or draining an abscess spray the vaporized coolant for 1 to 2 seconds until the dermis turns white and immediately clip the tag or incise and drain the abscess. Use caution because overapplication causes blistering.

Ophthalmic Use

Apply one or two drops in the eye. The effects of the anesthetic are rapid (30 seconds) and persist up to 15 minutes. An additional drop can be placed every 5 to 10 minutes for a total of 7 to 10 drops.

Conclusion

Topical anesthetics may offer a painless alternative to painful injectable anesthetics. Since the advent of TAC, there have been numerous advances. EMLA cream and over-the-counter LMX are now available. Moreover, advances in delivery modes, including heat in S-Caine Patch and flexible membranes in S-Caine Peel, allow the provider to tailor topical anesthetics to specific clinical situations.

Acknowledgment

The editors wish to recognize the contributions by William Dery, MD, to this chapter in the previous edition of this text.

Supplier

(See contact information online at www.expertconsult.com.)

Quadri-Caine
Scripts Pharmacy

BIBLIOGRAPHY

Crystal CS, Blankenship RB: Local anesthetics and peripheral nerve blocks in the emergency department. Emerg Med Clin North Am 23:477–502, 2005.

Crystal CS, McArthur TJ, Harrison B: Anesthetic and procedural sedation techniques for wound management. Emerg Med Clin North Am 25:41–71, 2007.

Eidelman A, Weiss JM, Enu IK, et al: Comparative efficacy and costs of various topical anesthetics for repair of dermal lacerations: A systematic review of randomized, controlled trials. J Clin Anesth 17:106–116, 2005.

Eidelman A, Weiss JM, Lau J, Carr DB: Topical anesthetics for dermal instrumentation: A systematic review of randomized, controlled trials. Ann Emerg Med 46:343–351, 2005.

Ernst AA, Marvez E, Nick TG, et al: Lidocaine adrenaline tetracaine gel versus tetracaine adrenaline cocaine gel for topical anesthesia in linear scalp and facial lacerations in children aged 5 to 17 years. Pediatrics 95:255–258, 1995.

Huang W, Vidimos A: Topical anesthetics in dermatology. J Am Acad Dermatol 43:286–298, 2000.

Kundu S, Achar S. Principles of office anesthesia: Part II. Topical anesthesia. Am Fam Physician 66:99–102, 2002.

Lander J, Brady-Fryer B, Metcalfe JB, et al: Comparison of the ring block, dorsal penile nerve block, and topical anesthesia for neonatal circumcision: A randomized controlled trial. JAMA 278:2157–2162, 1997.

Lener EV, Bucalo BD, Kist DA, Moy RL: Topical anesthetic agents in dermatologic surgery: A review. Dermatol Surg 23:673–683, 1997.

Moy RL, Pfenninger JL: Taking the sting out of local anesthesia. Pat Care March 15:61, 2000.

Nestor MS: Safety of occluded 4% liposomal lidocaine cream. J Drugs Dermatol 5:618–620, 2006.

Package Insert: EMLA, Westborough, Mass, Astra USA.

Package Insert: Iontocaine, North Chicago, Ill, Abbott Laboratories.

Topicaine Topical Anesthetic Gel. Available at http://www.esbalabs.com/top4.htm. Accessed September 9, 2008.

Wolfe TR, Fosnocht DE, Linscott MS: Atomized lidocaine as topical anesthesia for nasogastric tube placement: A randomized, double blind, placebo-controlled trial. Ann Emerg Med 35:421–425, 2000.

SECTION 2

Dermatology

Section Editor: THEODORE O'CONNELL

CHAPTER 11

ACNE THERAPY: SURGICAL AND PHYSICAL APPROACHES

Michael A. Altman

Acne is the most common skin disease of childhood and adolescence and is estimated to affect 80% of individuals between 11 and 30 years of age and up to 95% of all adolescents. It is a disease of the pilosebaceous unit. Acne involves increased sebum production, obstruction of the pilosebaceous glands with keratinization of the canal, bacterial proliferation, and inflammation. Many topical and systemic medications have been developed to treat acne. When these medications fail to control the disease, or when significant lesions develop, several procedures may be used to intervene. This chapter focuses on the procedures a primary care physician might consider in the office treatment of acne.

COMEDO REMOVAL

The removal of open comedones (blackheads, noninflamed plugged pores) enhances the patient's appearance while preventing the development of inflamed acne lesions and cysts (with their complications). Instruments such as the round loop (or oval loop) extractor (Fig. 11-1) or the Schamberg extractor effectively extract the plug by allowing uniform, smooth pressure to encircle the pore (Fig. 11-2). Downward pressure allows the comedo or pus to exit through the hole in the extractor. Extractors can be obtained from any medical supply provider, and some are even sold over the counter.

Open comedones that offer resistance can be loosened with one of two techniques:

1. Application of tretinoin (Retin-A), a topical keratolytic, for 1 month before comedo extraction.
2. Use of a no. 11 blade, tip of a needle, or the pointed end of a comedo extractor to stretch the walls or slightly incise the pore opening. The physician should insert the scalpel point 1 mm into the comedo, following the angle of the follicle opening, and angle the tip to bring the plug upward through the enlarged pore opening.

If there is still resistance, the comedo extractor should be held in the other hand and lateral pressure applied with the blunted end to the base of the lesion as the blade lifts the plug through the center of the extractor. A large amount of sebaceous material may be found beneath the plug and should be removed.

ACNE SURGERY FOR PUSTULES AND CYSTS

The surgical drainage of acne pustules and cysts, when performed correctly, speeds resolution of the lesions, prevents subdermal rupture, and enhances cosmetic appearance. Closed comedones can also be opened to prevent their progression to inflammatory lesions.

Enter the head of a white pustule with a small (25-gauge) needle, with the tip (tiny nick) of a no. 11 blade, or the pointed end of the comedo extractor. Drain the pustule with lateral pressure or with the assistance of an extractor. Superficial cysts that have thin roofs and easily palpated fluid can be drained by making a small incision less than 4 mm long. Some physicians advocate that the base of a drained superficial cyst be gently curetted to dislodge any necrotic debris. Nodules and large cysts may best be treated by intralesional corticosteroid injection.

INTRALESIONAL CORTICOSTEROID INJECTION

Individual nodular or cystic acne lesions often dramatically decrease in size after intralesional injection of a corticosteroid. It is reassuring to patients to know that a fast, relatively painless procedure is available when lesions arise. Patients with severe acne often require repeated injections every 2 to 3 weeks. Multiple cysts can be treated in one session.

The steroid preparation triamcinolone acetonide 10 mg/mL (e.g., Kenalog-10) is a preferred agent and should be diluted to about 2.5 mg/mL with saline or local anesthetic (e.g., 1% lidocaine). Saline is the preferred diluent because injections of local anesthetics are painful. Triamcinolone acetonide is particularly useful in that it is insoluble and therefore can remain deposited for months at the injection site, achieving its desired local effect without risk for adrenal suppression.

When preparing for an injection, shake the steroid vial to disperse the suspension. First draw the saline into a tuberculin syringe, followed by an appropriate amount of triamcinolone. (If lidocaine is the diluent, use only single-dose vials to prevent precipitation of the steroid.) An air bubble can be aspirated into the syringe to mix the two. Then insert a 30-gauge needle through the thinnest portion of the cyst roof and deliver 0.05 to 0.3 mL of the resulting 2.5-mg/mL triamcinolone acetonide mixture. Limit the maximum volume to 0.2 mL per lesion to reduce the risk of skin atrophy. The injection usually blanches the cyst.

Inject directly into the cyst, not the skin. Skin atrophy can follow injections if the steroid is deposited into the skin below the cyst or if the steroid concentration is too high. One session of injections should not exceed a total of 10 to 20 mg of triamcinolone, to avoid systemic effects. It may be necessary to repeat intralesional injections at 2-week intervals, not to exceed three total sessions.

Fluctuant lesions can be aspirated first with a large-bore needle attached to a 1- or 3-mL syringe before steroid injection. Skin atrophy remains unlikely, but the patient should be forewarned that atrophy still may occur independent of the injection because of

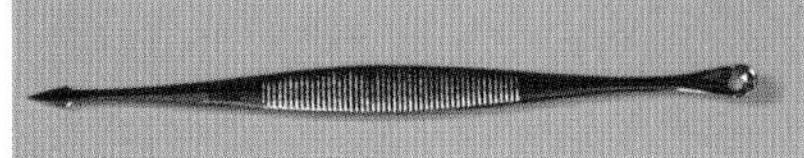

Figure 11-1 Comedo extractor. Note pointed end and cupped end with central opening.

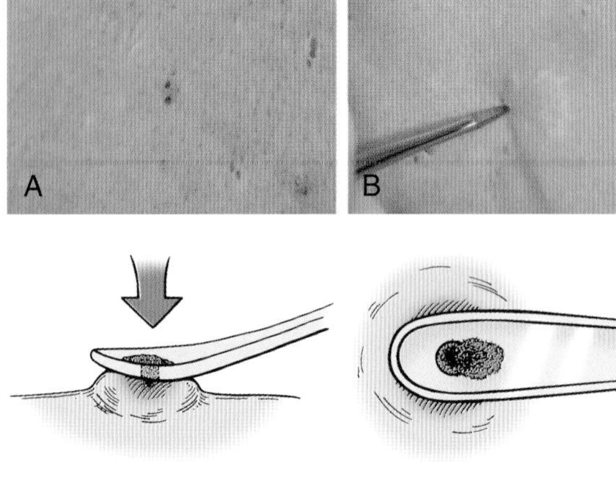

Figure 11-2 Use of comedo extractor to express cystic contents. **A,** Comedo. **B,** Incising over comedo to enlarge opening using sharp end of extractor. **C,** Applying pressure over comedo to express contents through central opening of extractor. **D,** Graphic representation of **C**.

underlying inflammation involving the collagen bed. Secondary bacterial infections do not occur. Avoid injecting the periorbital and perinasal areas because steroid crystals inadvertently injected into vessels may drain into the cerebral venous sinuses or central retinal artery. Finally, counsel patients that skin depression may occur, but in most cases it is temporary and gradually resolves in 4 to 6 months.

Cryotherapy

Cryotherapy has been found to be effective against pustular acne but not against comedonal or papular acne. It is most effective against superficial cystic lesions and least effective against deeper lesions. Any softening effect on scars is usually temporary. Application is painful and burning discomfort may last up to 4 hours. In current dermatology, it has fallen out of general use for acne management.

Other Current Approaches

Photodynamic therapy (see Chapter 60, Photodynamic Therapy), microdermabrasion (see Chapter 58, Microdermabrasion and Dermalinfusion), and chemical peels (see Chapter 59, Skin Peels) can also be used to control acne by physical techniques.

Scar Revision

1. A variety of procedures can be used to remove or revise acne scars. Deep, "ice-pick" scars can be excised using a punch biopsy and immediately replacing the scar plug with a full-thickness punch graft of normal skin. This procedure is relegated to early scar revision now that laser skin resurfacing is available.
2. Another technique, punch-graft elevation, uses a punch just slightly larger than the pitted scar. A cylindrical incision is made into the dermis, allowing the core to "pop out" above the skin surface. A Steri-Strip secures this skin core just above the surrounding skin. Dermabrasion of the remaining treatment site may be required at a later date. Results are unpredictable.
3. Collagen injections can be used to smooth the skin surface, but are a temporary solution (see Chapter 57, Tissue Filler).
4. Dermabrasion involves the use of a high-speed hand drill with a diamond-studded steel sander under local anesthesia to smooth out scars. Microdermabrasion (see Chapter 58, Microdermabrasion and Dermalinfusion) can also be used. It is less aggressive and there is little recovery time, but many (six to eight) visits may be needed. It is best reserved for more superficial scars.
5. The latest carbon dioxide laser methods use a fractionated column of light to smooth the skin (e.g., Active FX and Fraxel). This affords less "down time" because it is less aggressive than previous laser treatments. At the same time, it can smooth the skin more effectively and with fewer treatments than microdermabrasion or chemical peels.
6. Scar revisions should not be performed for 6 months to 1 year after use of oral isotretinoin.

Complications

Complications include adverse pigmentary changes, deeper and longer scars, and increased skin sensitivity to sunlight.

CPT/Billing Codes

10040	Acne surgery, opening of multiple cysts, comedones, or pustules
10060	Incision and drainage of abscess
11900	Intralesional injection of up to 7 lesions
11901	Intralesional injection of more than 7 lesions
15780–87	Dermabrasion
15790–91	Chemical peel
17340	Cryotherapy (CO_2 slush)
17360	Chemical exfoliation for acne

ICD-9-CM Diagnostic Codes

695.3	Acne rosacea
706.1	Acne

Bibliography

Berson DS, Chalkner DK: Current concepts in the treatment of acne: Report from a clinical round table. Cutis 72(Suppl):5–13, 2003.

Briden ME: Alpha-hydroxyacid chemical peeling agents: Case studies and rationale for safe and effective use. Cutis 73(2 Suppl):18–24, 2004.

Brody HJ: Complications of chemical resurfacing. Dermatol Clin 19: 427–438, 2001.

Gold MH: Dermabrasion in dermatology. Am J Clin Dermatol 4:467–471, 2003.

Habif TP: Clinical Dermatology: A Color Guide to Diagnosis and Therapy, 4th ed. St. Louis, Mosby, 2004.

Nguyen QH, Kim YA, Schwartz RA: Management of acne vulgaris. Am Fam Physician 50:89–96, 1994.

Taub AF, Procedural treatments for acne vulgaris. Dermatol Surg 33:1005–1026, 2007.

CHAPTER 12

APPROACH TO VARIOUS SKIN LESIONS

John L. Pfenninger

This chapter provides guidelines for the diagnosis and treatment of common skin lesions. Table 12-1 can be used as a guide for proper biopsy and treatment techniques. The specifics of performing the procedures are reviewed elsewhere in this textbook. These guidelines are not intended to be all-inclusive, but they do provide a framework for the approach to common skin lesions.

All excised skin lesions are best sent to the pathologist for definitive diagnosis. With selected lesions, such as skin tags or sebaceous cysts, many physicians will rely on their clinical judgment and avoid the added laboratory expense. However, in today's litigious society, the physician must be absolutely certain of the diagnosis when deciding not to send tissue to the pathologist for evaluation. Numerous benign lesions can be placed in a single formalin container (e.g., skin tags, obviously benign nevi) to cover the legal aspects and yet conserve costs. The fee to process each bottle (regardless of the number of samples in it) is approximately $160 to $200 for the routine dermatologic lesion.

ANGIOMA (HEMANGIOMA)

If the angiomas are small, use a ball electrode to cauterize them lightly. If larger than 2 mm, local anesthesia may be needed. Tissue should be wiped away and the process repeated until no vessel is seen (Fig. 12-1). Focal cryotherapy or sclerotherapy will also work. If the angiomas are large, a superficial shave excision or curettement followed by light cautery of the base works best.

ACROCHORDON (SKIN TAG)

Although many physicians prefer to use electrosurgery or cryotherapy to remove acrochordons, the most direct and simple approach is to elevate the tag with pickups and excise it with sharp tissue scissors at the level of the surrounding skin (Fig. 12-2). If it has a broad base, a local anesthetic may be required. Monsel's solution (ferric subsulfate) or aluminum chloride may be used for hemostasis. It is essential to have good-quality scissors so the lesion is cut, not "pinched."

If the tag is small enough, a ball electrode can be used to lightly and quickly cauterize the tag. It is then simply "wiped away," similar to the treatment of a small angioma (see earlier).

Cryocautery can be effective, but it is difficult to limit the freeze solely to the tag. A unique method with liquid nitrogen is to use the Styrofoam cup method, dipping the flat pickups in the liquid, and then grasping the tag with the cooled metal. The tag usually necroses off. The tag should be frozen twice in the same visit. Special thickened metal forceps are available from Brymill Cryogenic Systems (Ellington, Conn) that stay colder longer and can be used to treat multiple lesions without having to dip into the liquid nitrogen repeatedly (Fig. 12-3).

ACTINIC KERATOSES

Actinic keratoses (Fig. 12-4) are sun-induced, premalignant lesions. Single lesions can be shaved, cauterized, or, most commonly, treated with *cryotherapy*. When multiple lesions are present, they can be treated with 5-fluorouracil (5-FU, Efudex), masoprocol (Actinex) cream, imiquimod (Aldara) cream, or photodynamic therapy with δ-aminolevulinic acid (Levulan) in conjunction with light therapy (e.g., blue light, intense pulsed light [IPL]). *Lesions that do not resolve require surgical sampling for histology*. They are then frequently squamous cell carcinomas (SCCs; see treatment methods, later). The risk that actinic keratoses will progress to SCC is probably less than 1% in early lesions, and as high as 10% to 20% for persistent hypertrophic lesions. The patient should be counseled that both 5-FU and masoprocol cause significant erythema and tenderness in the areas treated. For 5-FU and masoprocol, the medication is applied twice a day for 3 to 4 weeks to the face and three to four times per day on the arms. (See patient education form online at www.expertconsult.com. The manufacturer will also provide a patient education videotape.) Treatment with imiquimod is significantly more expensive, with less efficacy (Table 12-2). Steroid creams may be used to reduce the inflammatory response. Alternatively, daily application of retinoic acid (Retin-A) 0.025% or 0.05% may resolve early lesions and prevent new ones. Protection from the sun is essential.

BASAL CELL CARCINOMA

Basal cell carcinomas (BCCs) characteristically have small, centrally ulcerated depressions and raised, pearly borders (*nodular-cystic type*; (Fig. 12-5A and B). However, their actual appearance can vary markedly from the classic description. *Sclerosing* (or morpheaform; Fig. 12-5C) BCCs may manifest as flat lesions with nondescript borders. Others are nonhealing ulcerations that never do become elevated. Some are *pigmented* (Fig. 12-5D) and may be confused with seborrheic keratoses (SKs), nevi, or even melanomas. They may appear erythematous and bleed easily, mimicking a pyogenic granuloma. *Superficial* (Fig. 12-5E) BCCs commonly occur on the back and are flat and scaly. They may look like an SCC, actinic keratoses, eczema, or even tinea. A biopsy should be taken of all nonhealing, changing, or enlarging skin lesions. Once a diagnosis is made, proper treatment can be planned. Chronic sun exposure, chronic irritation, and the human papillomavirus appear to be the most common causative factors.

When a biopsy is taken of a suspected BCC, almost any area of the lesion is appropriate for sampling. If the lesion is ulcerated, it is best to sample the nonulcerated portion because the ulcer may show only necrotic changes if enough depth is not included in the sample. Normal skin from the margin is *not* needed in the specimen.

TABLE 12-1 Surgical Diagnosis and Management of Common Skin Lesions

Lesion	Procedure							
	Punch Biopsy	Shave Biopsy	Shave Removal	Fusiform Excision	Incisional Biopsy	Curettement Alone	Cautery/ Curettement (ED & C)	Cryotherapy
Acrochordon (skin tags)		X[a]	X[a]					X
Actinic keratosis	X	X	X[a]	X[l]	X	X	X[a]	X[a]
Angioma, cherry		X	X			X	X[a]	X
Angioma, spider								
Bowen's disease (SCC in situ)	X	X	X	X[am]	X		X[a] if <1 cm	X[a] if <1 cm
Cancer, basal cell	X	X		X	X		X[a]	X
Cancer, squamous cell	X			X[a]	X		X	
Condylomata acuminata[c]	X	X	X	X[d]		X	X	X
Dermatofibroma	X	X	X[a]	X[a]	X			
Hemangioma, cherry		X	X			X	X[a]	X
Keratoacanthoma	X	X		X[a]	X		X[a]	X
Lentigo	X	X	X		X			X[a]
Lentigo maligna	X			X[a]	X			
Lipomas				X				
Melanoma	X			X[am]	X			
Milia	X	X	X			X[a]		
Molluscum contagiosum	X[d]	X	X			X[a]		X
Mucocele				X				X
Neurofibroma	X	X	X[f]	X	X		X[g]	
Nevi, acquired	X	X	X[h]	X	X			
Nevi, atypical	X	X	X[ai]	X[a]	X			
Nevi, giant congenital	X			X	X			
Paronychia								
Pyogenic granuloma	X	X	X	X			X[a]	X
Rashes	X	X						
Sebaceous cysts				X				
Sebaceous hyperplasia	X	X	X			X	X[a]	X
Seborrheic keratosis	X	X	X[a]	X[d]	X	X	X	X[a]
Telangiectases								
Warts	X	X	X		X[d]		X[a]	X[a]
Warts, planar	X	X	X			X[a]	X	X
Warts, plantar	X	X					X	X[a]
Xanthelasma		X	X	X				

IPL, Intense pulsed light; SCC, squamous cell carcinoma.
[a]**Procedure of choice.**
[b]Face only; legs require sclerotherapy or laser. Extremely fine veins may require IPL or laser.
[c]Imiquimod (Aldara), podofilox (Condylox), interferon; see Chapter 155, Treatment of Noncervical Condylomata Acuminata.
[d]Used only if cancer is a possibility or nature of lesion unknown.
[e]Not approved by the Food and Drug Administration.
[f]Followed by cautery and curettement.
[g]Preceded by shave removal.
[h]Use only if certain that lesion is not a melanoma.
[i]If used here, must be sure to use deep, saucer-shaped shave and that entire lesion removed in initial sample (*do not* use if suspect melanoma).
[j]*Candida* antigen; bleomycin, imiquimod (Aldara), see Chapter 42, Wart (Verruca) Treatment.
[k]Retin-A.
[l]Generally not indicated unless large, recurrent, or severely dysplastic.
[m]See Table 12-3.
[n]Radiation generally reserved for large, unresectable or recurrent lesions.
[o]Levulan plus IPL/light therapy.
[p]IPL, scleropathy.

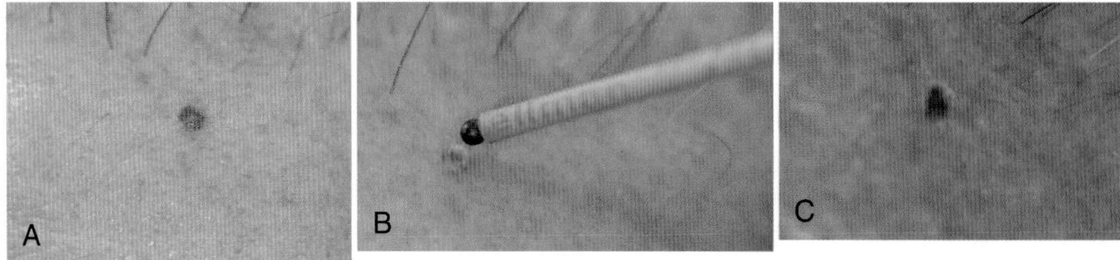

Figure 12-1 **A,** Hemangioma. **B,** Cautery of hemangioma. **C,** Hemangioma after cautery.

Surgical Diagnosis and Management of Common Skin Lesions—cont.

Electrosurgery (Radiofrequency)	85% Trichloroacetic Acid	Laser Ablation	Radiation	Fluorouracil 5% (Efudex) or Masoprocol 10% (Actinex)	Incision and Drainage	Other
X						
X	X	X		X[ac]		X[cok]
X[a]		X				
X[b]		X				X[p]
		X				
		X	X[n]	X[c]		
		X	X[n]	X		
X	X	X		X[e]		X[c]
		X				
X[a]		X				
		X		X		
X	X	X				X[ap]
						X[a] (see text)
						X
X					X[a]	
X	X					X[j]
X						
X[g]						
X[g]						
		X[h]				
					X[a]	X
X		X				
						X
					X[a]	X
X						
X		X				X
X[b]		X				X[p]
X	X	X				X[aj]
X	X	X				X[ak]
X	X	X				X[aj]
X		X				X

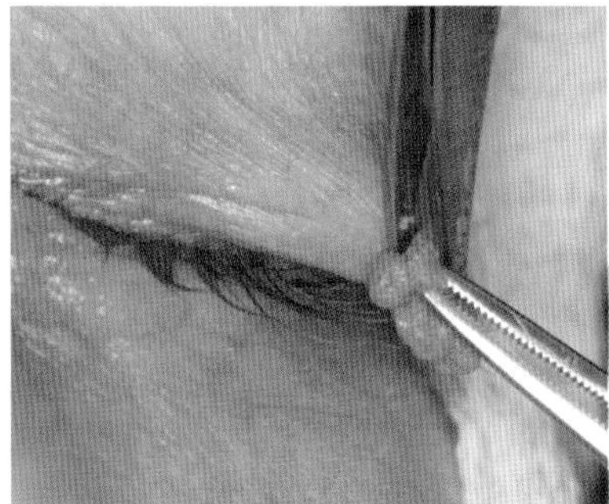

Figure 12-2 Acrochordon removal with sharp tissue scissors.

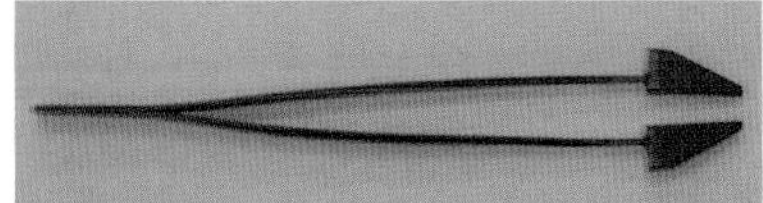

Figure 12-3 Special cryosurgical forceps (Brymill Cryogenic Systems) with extra mass at tips to allow freezing of multiple lesions before needing recooling. No anesthesia is needed.

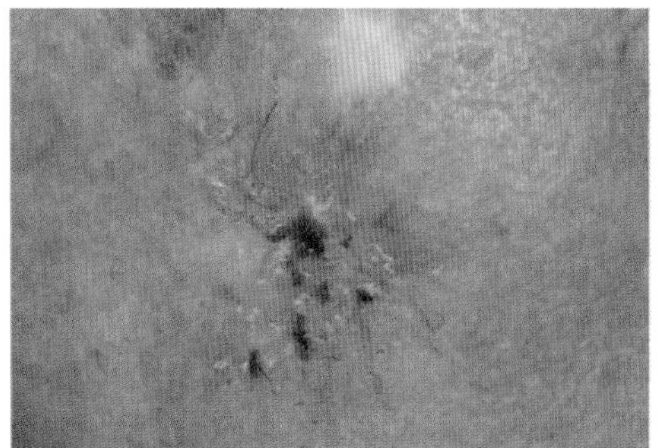

Figure 12-4 Advanced actinic keratosis of the right cheek.

TABLE 12-2 Comparison of Costs for Topical Treatment of Actinic Keratoses

Agent and Preparation	Treatment Regimen	Cost of One Treatment
δ-Aminolevulinic acid (Levulan), 20% sol	+ Blue light or intense pulsed light	$108.02+
Diclofenac (Solaraze), 3% gel	Twice daily for 60–90 days	$105.00
5-Fluorouracil (generic), 2% solution	Twice daily for 2–4 wk	$51.40
5-Fluorouracil (generic), 5% solution	Same	$74.50
5-Fluorouracil (Efudex)		
5% cream	Same	$102.25
2% solution	Same	$69.70
5% solution	Same	$102.90
5-Fluorouracil (Fluoroplex), 1% cream	Twice daily for 2–6 wk	$80.40
5-Fluorouracil (Carac), 0.5% cream	Once daily (max. 4 wk)	$98.10
Imiquimod (Aldara), 5% cream	Twice weekly for 16 wk	$518.76

Prices have increased significantly since 2004. The cost to the patient for one tube of Efudex 5% cream (40 g) on March 17, 2009 was $342.00, while the generic was $257.00 (Rite-Aid, Midland, Mich.)

From Imiquimod (Aldara) for actinic keratoses. Med Lett Drugs Ther 46:42–44, 2004.

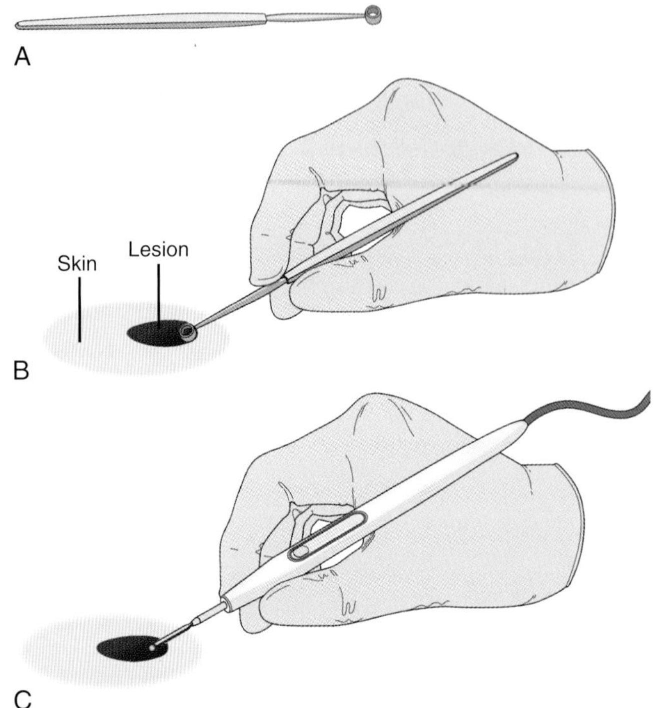

Figure 12-6 Electrodesiccation and curettage for a basal cell carcinoma. Sequence is repeated a total of three times. **A,** Dermal curette (available as disposable and reusable). Generally, for cancers, the reusable curettes are used because they are not as sharp and are less likely to penetrate the dermis. **B,** Lesion is curetted away. This tissue is sent to pathology for histologic diagnosis. **C,** Cautery of curetted area.

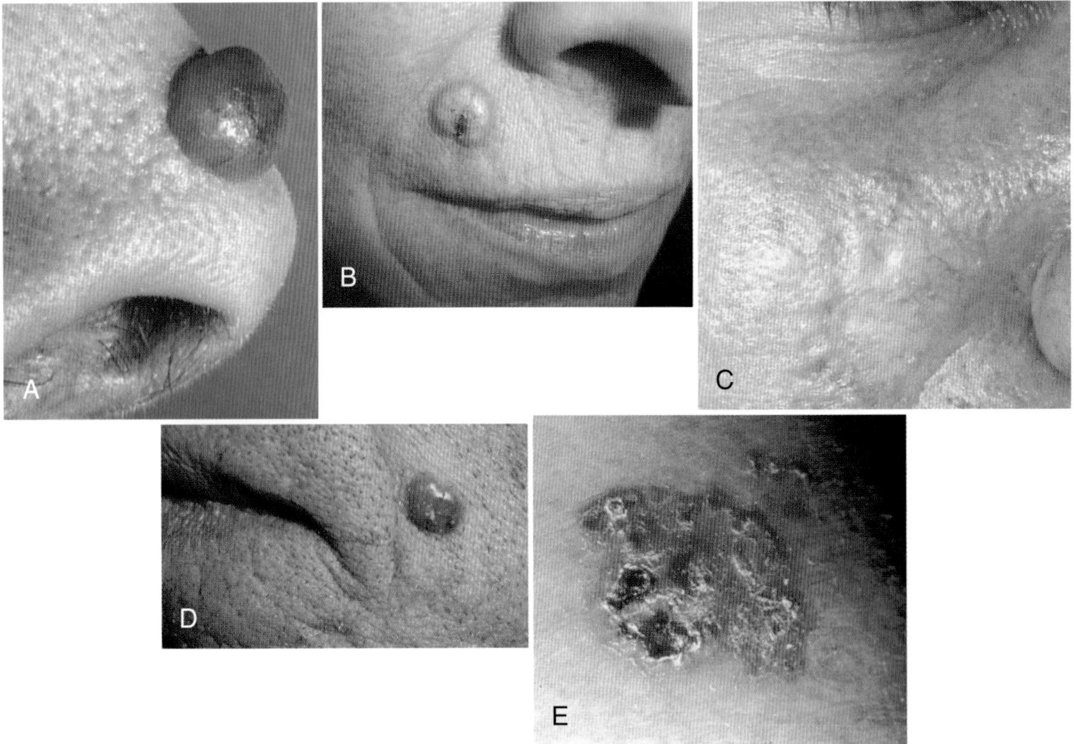

Figure 12-5 Basal cell carcinoma. **A,** Nodular; **B,** nodular ulcerative; **C,** morpheaform; **D,** pigmented; **E,** superficial.

The treatment of BCCs is rather straightforward. No one dies from BCCs unless there is long-term total neglect, and they almost never metastasize, so failure of treatment will generally lead only to recurrence, which then may need referral or more aggressive treatment. They can be difficult to treat, with higher recurrence rates in the nasolabial folds and the preauricular areas. The inner canthal area can be an especially difficult area to excise and treat because of tear duct involvement. Careful follow-up is needed to detect early recurrences. Any lesion that is less than 5 to 6 mm in any location generally has an excellent response to almost any treatment modality.

There are many approaches to the treatment of BCCs. *Radiation therapy* is rarely used, but it may be necessary when the lesions are located in areas such as the lid margins, and in large lesions found on elderly patients. It is usually not recommended for sclerotic/morpheaform types, around the tear ducts where there can be scarring, or in young people when there can be long-term sequelae from the radiation.

BCCs usually involve the upper portions of the skin and, again, very rarely metastasize. Deaths are extremely rare and reportable. For the majority of lesions that are smaller than 1 cm, treatment with *cautery and curettement (electrodesiccation and curettage [ED&C])* is a rapid and effective solution. Cure rates approach 95% to 98%, and scarring is usually minimal (Figs. 12-6 and 12-7). The technique is as follows:

1. After local anesthesia, scoop out the lesion with a large reusable dermal curette. The disposable units are too sharp for this procedure. Scrape the base of the lesion until a gritty feeling is encountered. Usually, it is rather easy to determine when all of the soft necrotic tissue is removed. If the lesion has not been previously sampled, send this first curettement to pathology. (Do not include tissue that is obtained after the cautery; see Fig. 12-7B.)
2. Then fulgurate or cauterize the entire base with a ball electrode to destroy remaining cells and control bleeding.
3. After the first cauterization, again vigorously curette the site to remove any of the char. Scrape until "grittiness" is palpable once again.
4. Perform fulguration or cauterization a second time, as before.
5. Carry out the third and final curettement with a smaller dermal curette that more easily enters any tiny crevices in the wound site. Be careful not to penetrate too deeply and pass through the entire dermis. If this should happen, a small window of fatty tissue will be visible in the bottom of the wound, and formal excision is indicated because the tumor most likely went deep into the subcutaneous tissue.
6. After the third curettement, fulgurate or cauterize the lesion for the final time. Place some topical astringent, a small amount of antibiotic ointment, and a dressing. Although the wound appears significantly ulcerated at this point, the long-term cosmetic results of this procedure are excellent if patients follow *moist healing* practices (see the sample patient education form available online at www.expertconsult.com).

Encourage the patient to *gently* wash the area three or four times a day with soap and water to prevent an eschar from forming. Immediately after washing, have the patient apply an antibiotic ointment to keep the area moist. The ointment can be applied six or eight times a day, not so much to prevent infection but to aid the reepithelialization of the wound. Petroleum jelly may work as well. Allow the wound to be open unless it is under clothing. Cover it at night if necessary to keep it moist.

Lesions in younger patients, larger-sized (>1 cm) lesions, lesions in more aggressive locations (nasolabial folds, preauricular areas, eyelids), sclerosing-type BCC lesions, recurrent lesions, and lesions with ill-defined margins may require *complete excision* to enable the pathologist to examine the margins. Remove 3 to 4 mm of normal skin around all edges (Table 12-3). Margins can be marked to aid in the histologic evaluation. Some physicians believe that excision is more cosmetically acceptable than cautery and curettement. An advantage of ED&C over cryotherapy is that the necrotic lesion can be "felt" with the curette, so the surgeon knows how far and deep to proceed with the scraping. If properly cared for, most lesions treated with ED&C will only have some mild depigmentation after 4 to 6 months. Although *cryotherapy* reportedly is very successful, the surgeon cannot often "feel" or see the margins of the tumor. All the various clinical factors should be weighed when selecting the method for lesion removal.

Laser therapy can be used to ablate the lesions. *Topical 5-FU* and *imiquimod* have been approved to treat superficial BCCs. *Cryotherapy* has excellent results for lesions less than 1 cm wide. A good freeze 5 mm past the lesion is required, followed by thawing, then a repeat freeze (see Chapter 14, Cryosurgery). It is critical to note the thaw time. Cure rates of 98% are reported (see caveat previously).

Follow-up 3 months after treatment to ensure success of treatment is recommended. The patient must be followed closely because

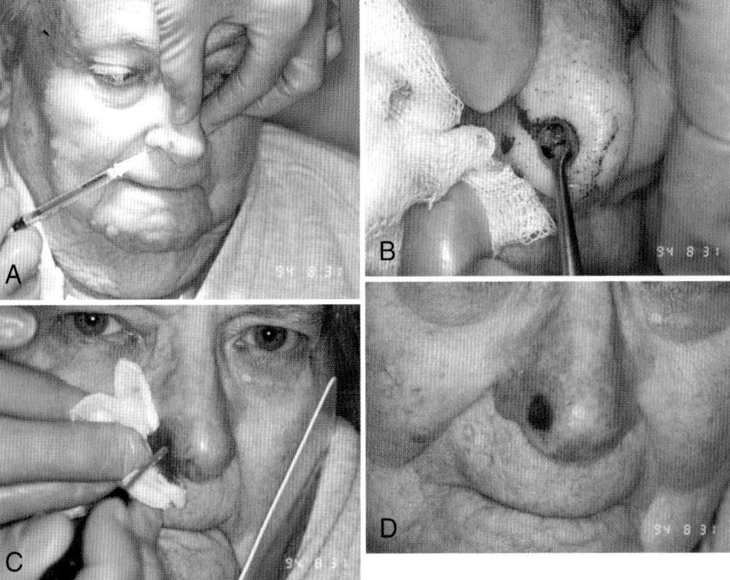

Figure 12-7 **A,** Basal cell carcinoma of right nose. **B,** After administration of local anesthetic, the lesion is curetted. **C,** Cautery of the base with a ball electrode. Repeat curettement and cautery for a total of three times. **D,** Appearance of wound after completion of treatment. (Courtesy of The Medical Procedures Center P.C., Midland, Mich.)

TABLE 12-3 Excisional Margins of Normal Tissue for Various Skin Lesions

Lesion	Margins
Atypical nevi	
Atypical or mild dysplasia	Be certain margins are clear (shave acceptable)
Moderate dysplasia	2–3 mm
Severe dysplasia	3 mm
Actinic keratoses	2–3 mm
Bowen's disease (squamous cell carcinoma in situ)	3 mm
Basal cell carcinoma	
Superficial	3 mm
Nodular/ulcerative	3 mm
Morpheaform (sclerotic, "aggressive")	5 mm
Squamous cell carcinoma	5 mm
Lentigo maligna (Hutchinson's freckle)	3 mm
Lentigo maligna melanoma	As for melanoma, below
Melanoma	
In situ	5 mm
Invasive to 1 mm (no ulceration, low mitotic count)	1 cm
>1 mm depth of invasion or ulcerated, increased mitotic count	Refer

30% of patients will develop new BCCs somewhere within 3 years (Table 12-4).

Mohs chemosurgery is not indicated for routine treatment of BCCs. Consider it for recurrent, morpheaform-type, or very large lesions. It may also be used for larger lesions in high-risk sites. The cost does not justify routine use because cure rates are so good with the other methods discussed here.

Squamous Cell Carcinoma

Squamous cell carcinoma (Fig. 12-8) often appears as a diffuse, nonhealing, crusted lesion. It frequently occurs at the base of an actinic keratosis or cutaneous lesion. The lesions may be multifocal in origin and, as with actinic lesions, are due to solar damage. SCCs are more aggressive than BCCs and can metastasize. Because the margins of these lesions are often not very clear, many clinicians prefer to excise all invasive SCCs. If 5-FU (Efudex) or masoprocol (Actinex) creams or cryotherapy are used to treat diffuse actinic changes, any post-treatment residual lesions (after 6 to 8 weeks) should be removed for biopsy to rule out SCC. *When a biopsy is performed* on a suspected SCC, try to include portions of the central area. A deep punch biopsy into subcutaneous fat is preferred by many pathologists, but a deep saucer-type shave is adequate, with definitive therapy after pathology results. Early or small lesions can be treated with cautery and curettement (see Figs. 12-6 and 12-7) or with cryotherapy, with excellent results (see earlier). If the lesion

TABLE 12-4 Follow-up of Various Skin Cancers after Treatment (Nonmetastatic)

Cancer	Follow-up
Basal cell carcinoma	3 mo
Squamous cell carcinoma	3 mo, 6 mo–1 yr
Melanoma	Every 4–6 mo (2–3 times) first year Every 6 mo (2 times) second year Every 1 yr lifetime (First-degree family members should be examined and counseled. Stress sun avoidance/protection.)

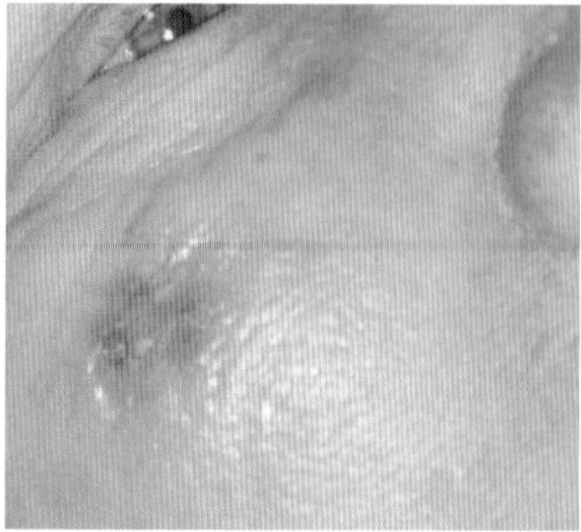

Figure 12-8 Squamous cell carcinoma.

is excised, remove at least 5 mm of normal tissue to be sure all margins are clear (see Table 12-3).

SCC in situ (Bowen's disease) is a severely dysplastic lesion that has not yet invaded beyond the epidermis. This lesion should be treated similarly to SCC, although excision is rarely needed.

Lesions (especially the more invasive ones) should be reevaluated in 3 and 6 months to document cure. Evaluation of the lymph nodes draining the area is also prudent (see Table 12-4).

Coding for skin cancer treatment is complicated. The biller must know the size, location, and method of removal to bill correctly.

Condylomata Acuminata

Many therapeutic interventions are available to treat condylomata acuminata. See Chapter 155, Treatment of Noncervical Condylomata Acuminata.

Dermatofibroma

Dermatofibromas (Fig. 12-9) often occur on the anterior surface of the lower leg. The etiology is unknown, but dermatofibromas may represent a fibrous reaction to trauma, viral infection, or insect bites. They are often confused with verrucae or nevi. Dermatofibromas do not progress to cancers, and once the diagnosis of dermatofibroma is confirmed, the physician often can merely observe the lesion. However, until the lesion is sampled, only an educated guess is possible. Many BCCs of the lower extremities mimic dermatofibromas. A rapidly growing lesion could be a dermatofibrosarcoma. Dermatofibromas are generally deep-seated and require excision if complete removal is desired. Cryotherapy can be attempted but dermatofibromas are generally quite cryoresistant. Because the lesions are often on the legs and are cut while shaving, the most judicious approach is to shave the lesion flat, which provides tissue for confirmatory diagnosis

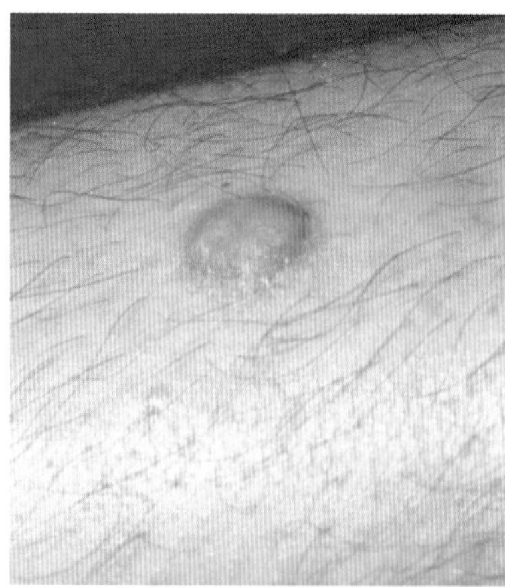

Figure 12-9 Dermatofibroma.

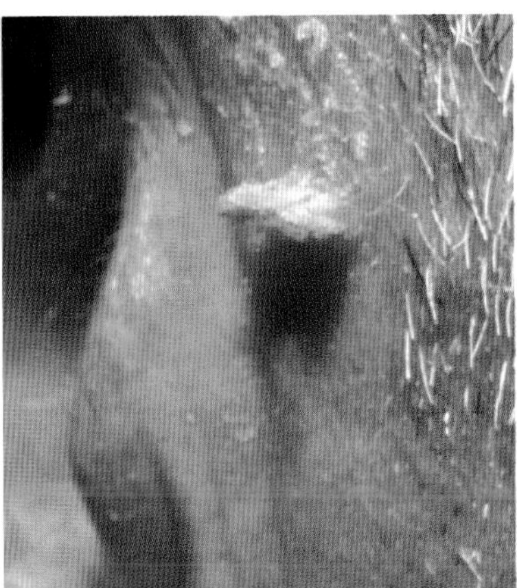

Figure 12-10 Cutaneous horn.

and reduces the likelihood of further trauma. A pigmented spot may remain, but at least it will be flat. If final results are not satisfactory, it can still be excised or cryotherapy can then be attempted.

Cutaneous Horn

A cutaneous horn (Fig. 12-10) is a type of actinic keratosis. Use caution to rule out an early SCC at the base. Usually a deep saucer-type shave is performed, followed by cautery. Tissue should be sent to pathology for verification.

Keratoacanthoma

Keratoacanthoma (Fig. 12-11) is a common, "benign" epithelial tumor found in elderly patients. This lesion may have a viral etiology. Keratoacanthoma often is confused with SCC, but it is a distinct entity and often considered an "SCC variant" because it cannot be differentiated histologically from SCC. *The history of rapid growth is critical* for the pathologist to make the proper diagnosis.

The lesion begins as a dome-shaped papule that continues to enlarge rapidly. A fully developed tumor is a round, dome-shaped mass with a central keratin-filled crater often 1 to 2 cm in size. The lesion may stop growing after 6 weeks, and then it may slowly regress over the next 12 months. These lesions often occur on the dorsum of the hands, ears, and neck. Clinically they often appear to be BCCs, but if curettement is attempted they are much more sclerotic and fibrous, unlike the classic BCC.

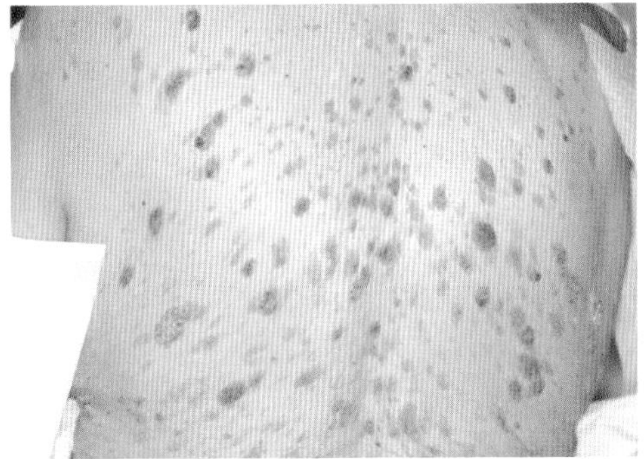

Figure 12-12 Seborrheic keratoses.

Because these lesions grow rapidly, most physicians do not advocate simple observation. Cryotherapy (small lesions only), a deep saucer-type shave, ED&C (×3), or conventional excision with 3- to 5-mm free margins provides acceptable treatment. Keratoacanthomas can recur, and patients should be followed closely during and after treatment. The major differential diagnoses for the clinician include BCC and SCC. Because of the rapid growth and high numbers of mitotic cells, even pathologists experience difficulty and often will report that they "cannot rule out SCC" at the base. Subsequently, the therapeutic approach is essentially the same as for an SCC.

Seborrheic Keratoses

Seborrheic keratoses (Fig. 12-12) are benign, hyperkeratinized, superficial epidermal lesions that occur commonly with aging. Their size ranges from 2 mm to 3 cm. They have no malignant potential. The typical lesion has the appearance that it can be easily lifted off with a fingernail. Patients often say that they have removed the lesion or rubbed it off with a towel, only to have it recur. SKs are occasionally confused with BCCs, SCCs, nevi, and verrucous lesions. Pathology reports often use the term *verruciform keratosis*.

Most SKs can be easily removed, after anesthesia, with the *radiofrequency* (electrosurgery) *shave* technique. Alternatively, *shave excision with mild curetting* of the base can be performed. Hemostasis can be accomplished with Monsel's solution or aluminum chloride. Minimal scarring should result because the lesion is so superficial.

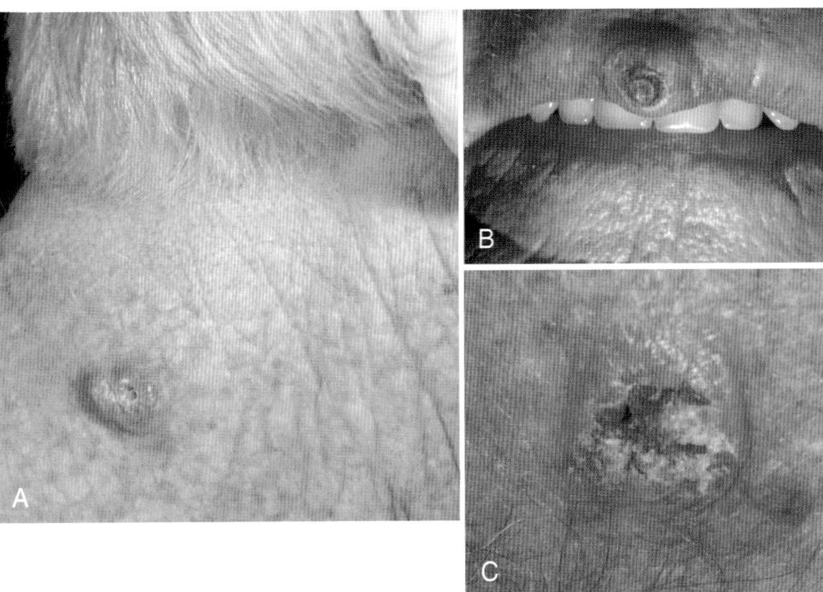

Figure 12-11 **A–C,** Keratoacanthomas.

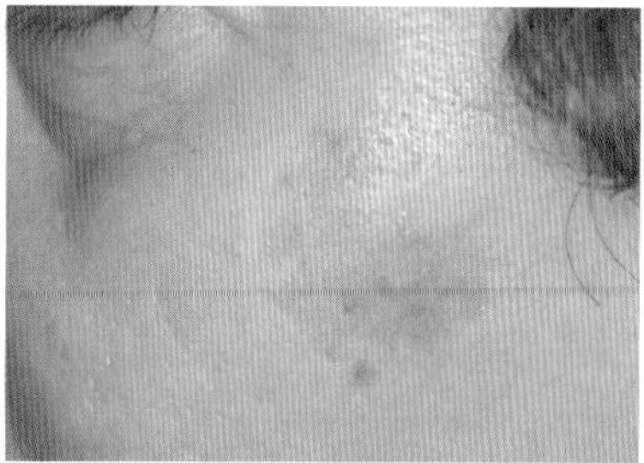

Figure 12-13 Lentigo.

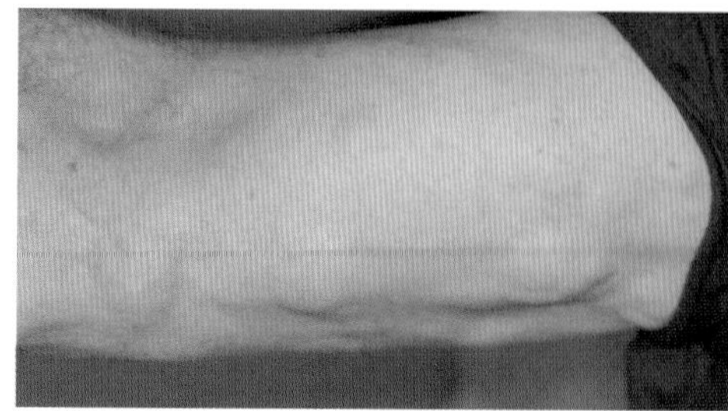

Figure 12-14 Arm with multiple lipomas.

Cryotherapy is the most frequently used method. No anesthesia is needed, but this treatment may cause a little more discomfort. Liquid nitrogen is the quickest approach, especially if multiple lesions are present (use the spray thermos applicators). After treatment, a blister may form or the lesion may just dry up and fall off. It is essential that the clinician be absolutely sure of the diagnosis if cryotherapy is to be used. Any lesions that persist need to be sampled. If many SKs occur all at once, consider an internal malignancy (Leser-Trélat sign).

Medicare does not reimburse for removal of SKs unless they are markedly irritated or pruritic, bleeding, or rapidly growing, or if the diagnosis is uncertain.

Lentigo

Lentigos (Fig. 12-13), or liver spots, are common, brownish or tan macules that occur on the sun-exposed areas of the face, shoulders, arms, and hands. They are often called "senior freckles." Lentigos increase in number during childhood and adult life and occasionally they fade spontaneously. Biopsy of lesions with irregular borders or dark pigmentation should be performed to rule out lentigo maligna melanoma. *Cryotherapy* is the treatment of choice. Although bleaching and depigmenting creams may be tried, they will need to be used lifelong. *Superficial ablation techniques* with laser, radiofrequency, or trichloroacetic acid also may work. The latest, most effective approach is to use IPL, but the technology is expensive (see Chapter 53, Fractional Laser Skin Resurfacing).

Lentigo Maligna (Melanoma in Situ)

Lentigo maligna is a sun-associated precursor of lentigo maligna melanoma, a type of invasive melanoma. These lesions can grow to be several centimeters in diameter and usually occur on the face. They are slow-growing macules with irregular borders and pigmentation. These lesions often are confused with "liver spots" (lentigos), which are smaller, have a homogeneous color, and appear mainly over the dorsa of the hands and forearms. The estimated lifetime risk of transformation from lentigo maligna to melanoma is only 4.7%, and some physicians prefer close observation as the treatment of choice. Unless absolutely sure of the diagnosis, a biopsy should be done. Removal is probably best done with complete surgical excision.

Lipomas

Lipomas (Fig. 12-14) present as a palpable mass under the skin. Most lesions are nontender, move freely, and have a soft, irregular consistency. The differential is usually a sebaceous cyst. Cysts have pores; lipomas do not. Cysts are more tense. Lipomas usually do not progress to malignancy, but rapidly growing or changing lesions should be removed to rule out liposarcoma. Removal also may be necessary when lipomas occur in areas of pressure or when they cause pain or discomfort. Lesions on the lower extremities have a higher likelihood of malignant degeneration. Lesions up to 3 cm are removed by making a 1- to 2-cm incision through the dermis after injecting as little as 1 mL of 2% lidocaine with epinephrine. Sterile preparation and draping are not needed. The clinician should make the incision in line with the skin lines and use hemostats or curved tissue scissors to dissect the lesion from the surrounding adhering tissue. Pressure on the base of the lesion often will extrude the lipoma through the small incision (Fig. 12-15). Some lipomas are encapsulated, but more often the margins are obscure. It may be difficult to determine whether all of the lesion has been removed because the fat involved looks just like normal fat. It is best to remove any loosely adhering fatty tissue in the cavity. Bleeding is minimal. Closure usually can be obtained with Steri-Strips or tissue glue, followed by a pressure dressing. Once the diagnosis of lipoma has been made in one area, other similar lesions do not necessarily require removal unless they are symptomatic. (Lesions that are larger than 3 to 4 cm may require formal excision with sterile technique and suture closure.)

There are special CPT codes for removal of these lesions under "Excision of Benign Tumors." The code is independent of the method used for removal (see Appendix G, Neoplasms, Skin: ICD-9 Codes).

Melanoma

The major caveat regarding melanomas (Fig. 12-16) is that the *depth of the lesion is very important in determining appropriate definitive treatment.* Primary care physicians should not feel uncomfortable about performing a biopsy of any lesion with characteristics that may be consistent with a melanoma. A biopsy does not spread the lesion or limit life expectancy in any way. On the contrary, early diagnosis may save the patient's life. The mnemonic *A, B, C, D, E, F, G* can be used as an aid for remembering the clinical features of malignant melanoma:

Asymmetry
Border irregularity
Color variegation
Diameter more than 6 mm
Elevation above skin surface
Feeling different (including pruritus); "F" also is a reminder to check family history
Growth or change

Because it is so important to determine the depth of the lesion, *never* perform a shave biopsy or shave removal *if melanoma is a serious consideration* (see Chapter 32, Skin Biopsy). *When choosing a site for punch or incisional biopsy* within a pigmented lesion, choose the area that is most nodular or atypical (darkest in color, inflamed, or irregular). The majority of pigmented lesions removed are atypical nevi. *Saucer-type shaves are acceptable for biopsy and removal if the clinical impression is that melanoma is unlikely.* The point is, all atypical nevi cannot be excised with suture closure. It is too time consuming and costly. If there is a strong clinical suspicion for melanoma, do a punch biopsy, which provides depth and the information needed for further treatment. However, if the working diagnosis is an atypical nevus, a shave biopsy is adequate. To save lives, atypical lesions need to be sampled, and shave excisions are the most expedient. Some

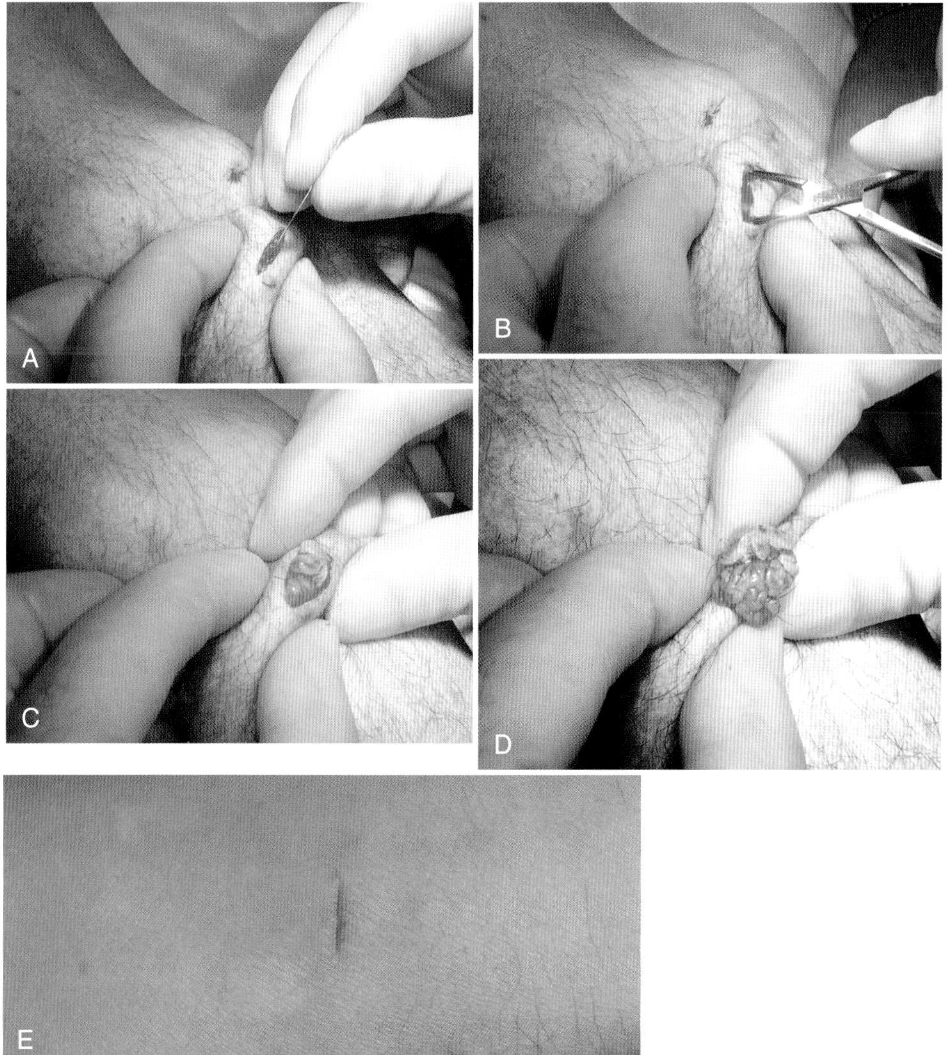

Figure 12-15 Simple technique for removing lipomas. **A,** After local anesthesia is administered, incise and drain the lipoma. **B,** Lysing adhesions with hemostat. **C,** Expressing the lipoma. **D,** Completing removal. Wound is closed with Steri-Strips and pressure dressing applied. **E,** Appearance 1 week after removal of lipoma using this technique.

unsuspected melanomas may be transected, but at least they will be diagnosed and further care can be initiated.

Recent National Institutes of Health (NIH) guidelines indicate that with lesions that invade less than 1 mm, 1-cm clear excisional margins around the lesion should be adequate for treatment. An extensive work-up for metastases is not indicated for the minimal-depth lesions (Table 12-5).

Molluscum Contagiosum

The lesions of molluscum contagiosum (Fig. 12-17) are small, 2- to 3-mm, papular, wartlike excrescences with central umbilication. They are painless and rarely cause pruritus. They usually appear as a crop of multiple lesions in young children, or later in adolescents and young adults as they become sexually active.

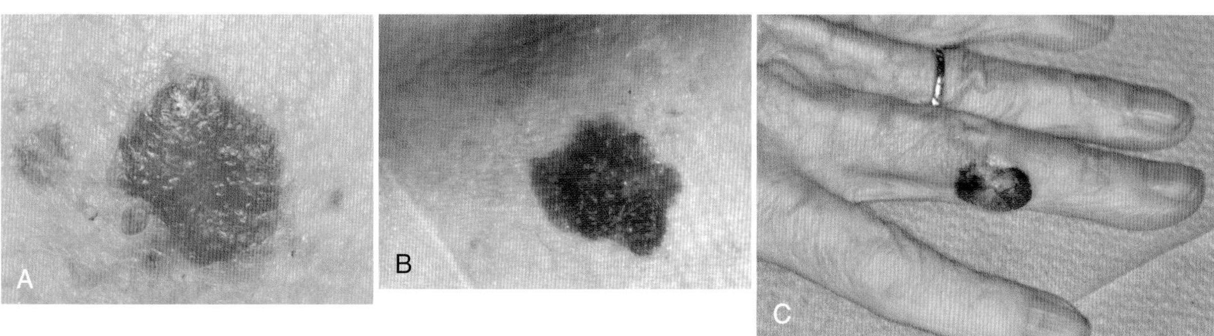

Figure 12-16 **A–C,** Melanomas.

TABLE 12-5 Treatment of Suspect Pigmented Lesions and Melanomas

Stage	Recommended Treatment	Survival
Suspect pigmented lesion	Punch, incisional, or excisional biopsy down to subcutaneous fat	Not affected by biopsy procedure
Suspected positive lymph node with melanoma	Fine-needle aspiration biopsy or excision	Not affected by biopsy procedure
Early melanoma		
Melanoma in situ (limited to epidermis)	Excision with margin of 0.5 cm normal skin and layer of subcutaneous tissue No further radiographs or laboratory work indicated	Not affected
Depth <1 mm	Excision with margin of 1 cm normal skin and subcutaneous tissue down to fascia No further radiographs or laboratory work indicated unless lesion is ulcerated or has high mitotic count	95% (8 yr)
Intermediate melanoma		
Depth 1–4 mm	After diagnostic biopsy, wide-margin excision and adjunctive therapy should be considered (refer)	Poor
High-risk melanoma		
Depth >4 mm	After diagnostic biopsy, wide-margin excision and adjunctive therapy should be considered (refer)	Poor

Modified from NIH Consensus Conference: Diagnosis and treatment of early melanoma. JAMA 268:1314–1319, 1992.

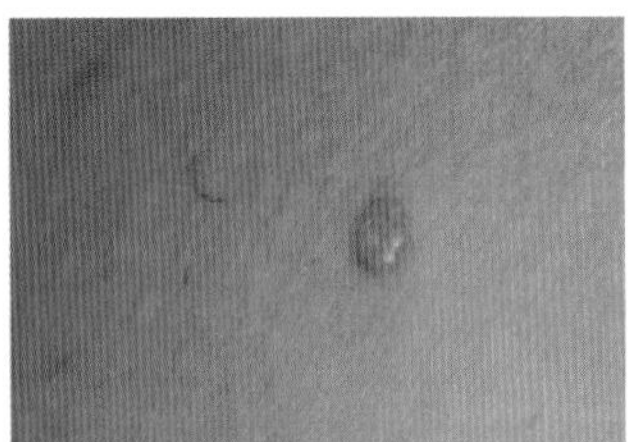

Figure 12-17 Molluscum contagiosum.

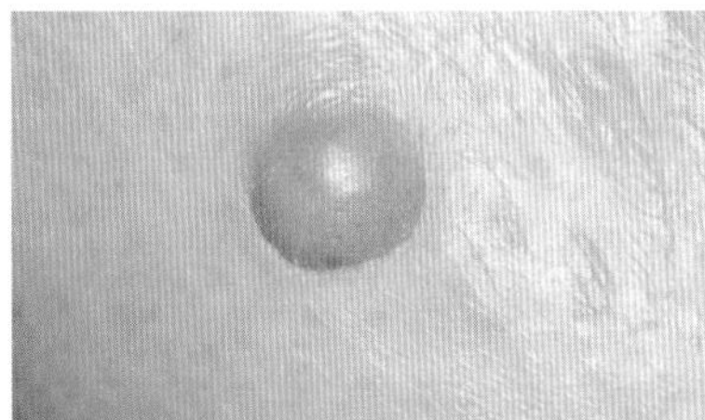

Figure 12-18 Neurofibroma.

Expectant observation is certainly acceptable because the lesions will spontaneously resolve (3 to 18 months), but many patients desire to have these viral lesions removed. Table 12-1 describes the treatments that are possible. Curettement with a small disposable (sharp) dermal curette or cryotherapy is the treatment of choice. Treatment rarely requires anesthesia, but topicals can be tried (see Chapter 10, Topical Anesthesia).

NEUROFIBROMAS

Neurofibromas (Fig. 12-18) are soft, nodular lesions that often appear to be minimally pigmented nevi. When a shave excision is performed, however, a soft, jelly-like material is seen at the base. This is the pathognomonic sign of a neurofibroma. The soft tissue is curetted and the base cauterized. A significant cavity may exist, but with moist healing techniques the results are excellent. These lesions do not have to be removed unless symptomatic or if a diagnosis is needed. Excision with suture closure is needed for the larger lesions. Free margins of 1 mm are adequate.

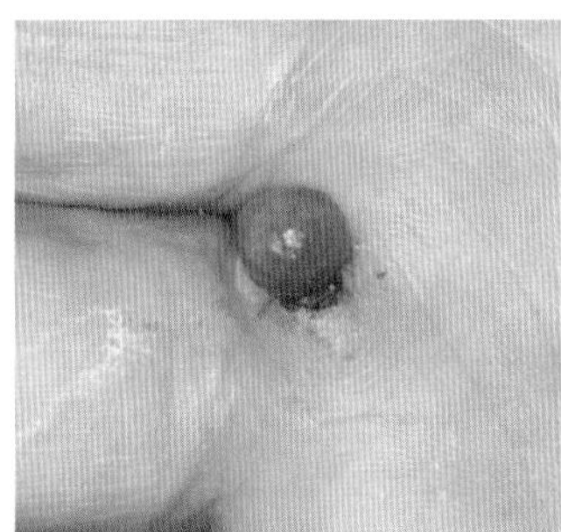

Figure 12-19 Pyogenic granuloma.

PYOGENIC GRANULOMAS

Pyogenic granulomas (Fig. 12-19) are small, rapidly growing, nodular, friable, vascular lesions that often bleed when touched. They occur at sites of trauma or previous surgery. Because of their vascular nature, pyogenic granulomas are best treated with curettement followed by cautery of the base. These lesions will recur if any tissue remains, and some physicians advocate complete excision. They can be confused with BCCs.

ACQUIRED NEVI ("MOLES")

Acquired nevi are benign, melanocytic nevi that are absent at birth and first appear in early childhood. The lesions become more numerous until middle age, and the majority of white adults have several acquired nevi. Lesions are generally found on sun-exposed areas because the sun induces their growth.

Common acquired nevi follow a predictable developmental progression (Fig. 12-20). The earliest lesions are junctional nevi (see Fig. 12-20A), with the nevus cells at the junction between the dermis and epidermis. By late adolescence, the growths develop into compound nevi (see Fig. 12-20B), with nevus cells in both the dermis and epidermis. Compound nevi may develop hairs. By late adulthood, the lesions regress into intradermal nevi and appear nonpigmented (see Fig. 12-20C).

If the lesions lose their pigment, they may turn pink or flesh-colored. At all stages, common benign acquired nevi have smooth, distinct, symmetric borders. Patients with large numbers of acquired nevi should be monitored closely because they are at higher risk for developing melanoma.

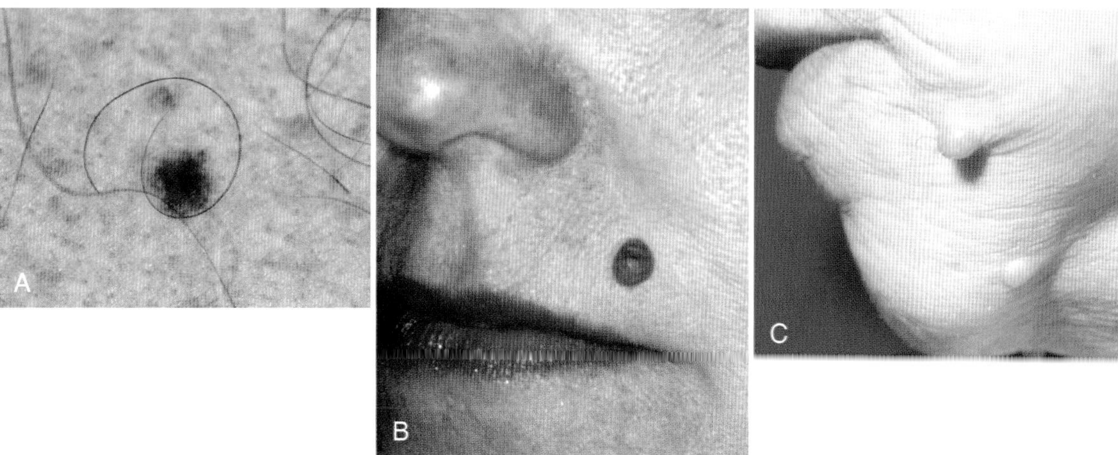

Figure 12-20 **A,** Junctional nevus. **B,** Compound nevus. **C,** Intradermal nevus.

Raised or pedunculated benign nevi can best be excised with a shave removal technique (optimized with the radiofrequency technique; see Chapter 30, Radiofrequency Surgery [Modern Electrosurgery]). There should be no suspicion whatsoever of melanoma if a shave technique is used. If malignancy is even a remote possibility, either a full-thickness biopsy of the lesion should be performed before removal, or the lesion should be treated by complete excision rather than shave removal. Treatment of melanomas is based solely on the depth of the lesion (see previous discussion). Superficial nevi usually do not recur, but the deeper compound nevi often do recur unless the full depth of the lesion is excised. It is difficult to determine when the entire lesion has been removed using a shave technique. The deeper dermal lesions are generally flat, whereas the superficial epidermal lesions are raised or pedunculated.

A *halo nevus* (Fig. 12-21) is an acquired nevus that develops a white halo around it. This is a sign that the immune system is activating against the mole, and it will soon disappear. It is the only change in a nevus that does not need a biopsy.

Dysplastic Nevi

Dysplastic nevi (Fig. 12-22; a histologic diagnosis), or atypical moles (a clinical diagnosis but now also used synonymously with "dysplastic" by many pathologists), are acquired nevi that become dysplastic (precancerous) over time. The lesions are usually larger than common acquired nevi (>5 mm) and may have irregular margins, variable pigmentation, and irregular surface contours. Because the risk for melanoma is increased in patients with atypical moles and because melanoma can develop from an atypical lesion, some physicians advocate full excision of suspect lesions. Shave excisions, if done, must be deep and saucer shaped to ensure the entire depth of the lesion is removed. Once the technique of the shave excision is mastered, six to eight nevi can be shaved off in a single 15-minute visit. Using the radiofrequency smoothing technique and moist healing minimizes scarring. Patients can have so many atypical nevi that it precludes excising all of them. These patients need to be followed closely, as do their family members. Sun protection is a must.

Should the pathologist report that the "margins are positive" in an atypical or dysplastic nevus, it behooves the surgeon to remove more tissue to ensure that the entire lesion has indeed been removed. Whether this removal is through another shave or a frank excision with suture closure depends on the exact pathology.

Congenital Nevi

The approach to congenital nevi is based on three factors: size, color, and family history. Congenital nevi *larger than 20 cm²* often extend over large portions of the body. The lesions grow proportionally with the anatomic site, their surfaces may be irregular, and they may contain coarse hairs. Their management is very controversial because excision is difficult and deforming. The lifetime risk of these nevi developing into melanoma is 5% to 20%; therefore, some physicians advocate early removal and grafting. Others advocate close monitoring. Melanoma can develop at any site in the lesion, and biopsies of the most irregular portions of the lesions may not detect malignant change. Efforts to completely eradicate these lesions must be tempered by the potential for treatment-induced scarring and disfigurement. A 1996 study by De Raeve and colleagues suggests that vigorous curettement in the first weeks of life may be the best alternative.

Lesions between 1.5 and 20 cm² are easier to excise, and this has been generally recommended. Lesions *less than 1.5 cm²* are the easiest to excise but also have the lowest malignant potential. Certainly, those that are located in areas that are difficult to observe (e.g., scalp, buttocks) should be removed. Shave excisions usually are not adequate because congenital nevi are deep lesions.

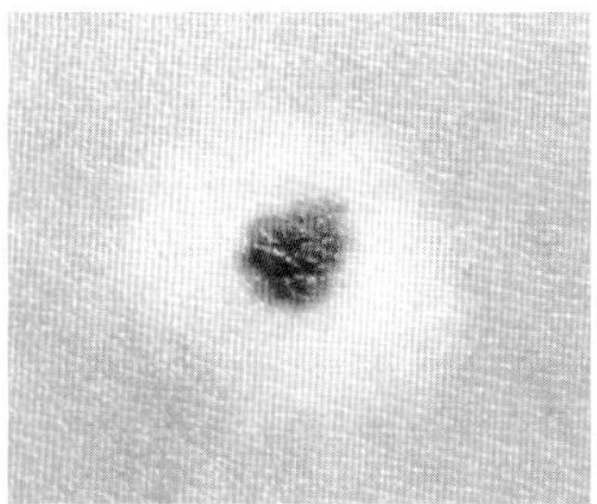

Figure 12-21 Halo nevus.

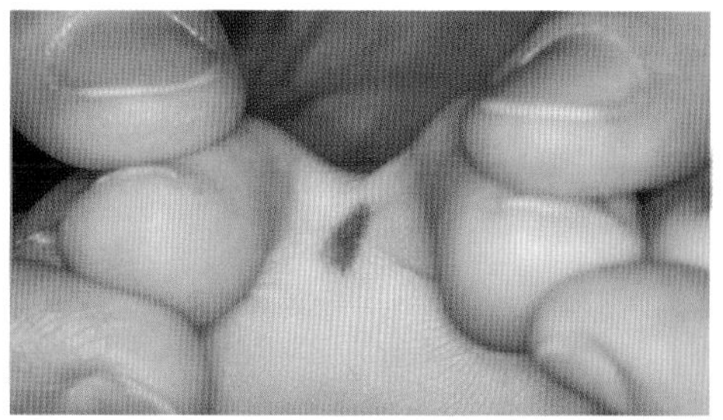

Figure 12-22 Dysplastic nevus.

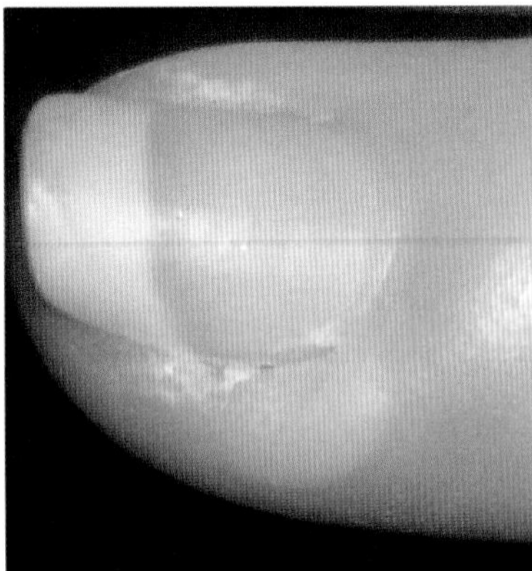

Figure 12-23 Paronychia.

Another factor to consider is the degree of pigmentation. *Very light moles* are less likely to degenerate into a cancer, do so later (after age 20 years), and allow early detection of changes. *Dark, almost black, lesions* are more likely to transform into a melanoma, do so earlier (teenage years), and are difficult to monitor, making their removal more appropriate.

The *latest recommendations suggest* observation for all congenital nevi, as with other nevi, unless changes are observed. The clinician will need to help the patient and the family sort through the various recommendations and decide on a course that is acceptable to all, including the local prevailing medical opinion.

PARONYCHIA

Paronychia (Fig. 12-23) is an infection of the distal phalanx along the proximal and lateral edges of the nail. Paronychia produces signs of local infection, including redness, tenderness, and swelling. Mild paronychia can be treated with soaks and topical antibiotics. More significant infections may develop into abscesses. As with all abscesses, it is best to incise and drain (I&D) them once a loculated area of purulence can be identified. A digital block may be needed, depending on size. The incision technique is illustrated in Figure 12-24. Occasionally packing may be used to keep the abscess from reaccumulating, but usually these abscesses are so small that it cannot be accomplished. Topical antibiotics (e.g., mupirocin [Bactroban]) may be beneficial, but unless there is marked cellulitis or the patient is immunocompromised, systemic antibiotics are rarely indicated. Chronic paronychia may be secondary to fungal infection.

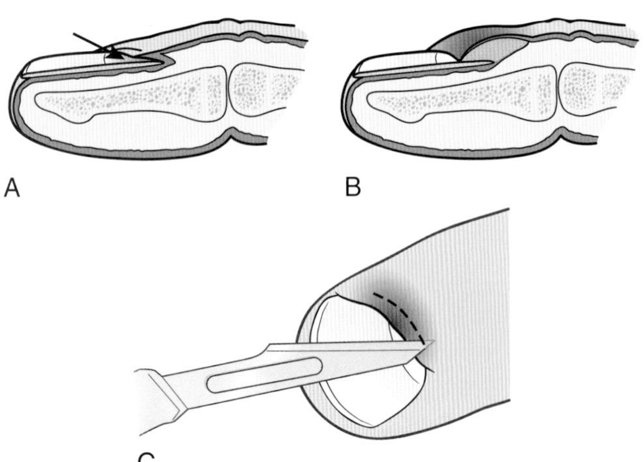

Figure 12-24 Separation of the cuticle from the nail *(arrow)* (**A**) can lead to a paronychia (**B**). In acute paronychia, drain any pus and consider a culture. A simple nick (**C**) through the most translucent area of the abscess is usually all that is required.

RASHES (EXANTHEMS, DERMATOSES)

In many cases, biopsy of a "rash" or ill-defined dermatologic lesion is not very helpful. Unless the clinical diagnosis is fairly clear, the primary care physician may be wise to obtain a dermatology consultation. Biopsies of these lesions may be indicated for clarification of a fairly discrete differential diagnosis (as with inflammatory dermatoses) or for ruling out a cutaneous neoplasm.

When multiple sites are involved, the following *simple guidelines* may be followed for selecting a lesion for a biopsy specimen: It is best to *select those areas that have the primary inflammatory changes* but are free from secondary changes such as crusting, fissuring, erosion, ulceration, and infection. *Choose sites where the scars will not be obvious* and where hypertrophic scarring is generally not a problem.

If the primary lesion is a *macule*, select a "fresh" lesion that is more abnormal in color. Generally, perform a punch biopsy, advancing the punch into the subcutaneous fat. *Papules* should be removed completely, if possible. Select a mature lesion without secondary changes. If the lesion is a *plaque*, the biopsy specimen should consist of the thickest area through the full depth into the subcutaneous fat. The same technique is used for *nodular* lesions and *suspected neoplastic* lesions. Alternatively, a fine-needle aspiration biopsy could be performed. For *vesicles and bullae, choose an intact lesion* whenever possible. Rupturing a sac makes histologic interpretation more difficult. *Sample these lesions at the margin where the blister roof is attached to the remainder of the specimen, and include normal skin.* This is virtually the only time normal skin is helpful in a biopsy to make a diagnosis (vesicular bullous disease). (See Chapter 32, Skin Bropsy.)

SEBACEOUS HYPERPLASIA (ADENOSUM SEBACEUM)

Adenosum sebaceum, or senile sebaceous gland hyperplasia, is characterized by small growths composed of enlarged sebaceous glands (Fig. 12-25A). These very small, 2- to 5-mm lesions can mimic early BCC. If numerous lesions are present in the temporal and forehead areas, they are very *unlikely* to be cancerous; BCCs are more often solitary. Treatment consists of removal of the elevated portions of the papule with shave, sharp curettement, or electrosurgical technique. Often the lesion is deep seated, and, unless curetted, it will not be entirely removed. Unlike a soft necrotic cancer, these lesions are very dense and fibrotic. Biopsy is indicated if the nature of the lesion is uncertain. However, treatment can usually be carried out on the basis of the clinical diagnosis. Cryotherapy also works well for smaller lesions.

SEBACEOUS CYSTS

The *epidermal cyst*, or *sebaceous cyst*, is a round, tense, keratinizing cyst that is freely mobile and very superficial (Fig. 12-25B and C). When located in the scalp, they are called *trichilemmal cysts* (*wens*, *pilar cysts*). Most patients present with a slowly growing lesion that on physical examination is subcutaneous, smooth, and nontender. A history of drainage or inflammation with purulent discharge may or may not be present, but it does help solidify the diagnosis. A small central punctum (pore) or opening helps differentiate it from a lipoma.

Note the following three precautions:

1. Lesions in the preauricular areas should be examined closely because parotid tumors (both adenomas and adenocarcinomas) can present as apparent "cysts." If there is any question, obtain a needle biopsy or computed tomography scan before attempting removal.

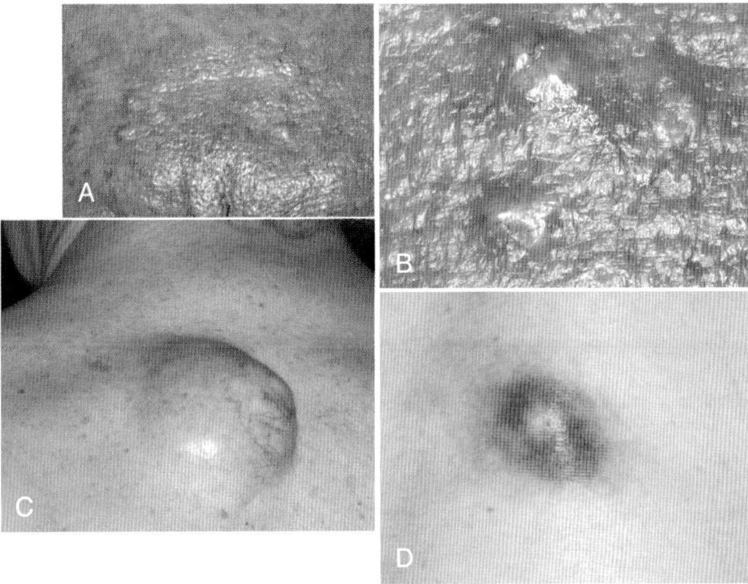

Figure 12-25 **A,** Sebaceous gland hyperplasia on the forehead of a 52-year-old male. Usually lesions are multiple and popular. **B,** When larger, or on close inspection, sebaceous gland hyperplasia can resemble basal cell carcinoma (BCC). However, BCCs are rarely multiple like this. **C,** Sebaceous cyst. **D,** Inflamed sebaceous cyst.

2. *"Cysts,"* especially *in infants* (but also in *children*) have a higher likelihood of being dermoids (also known as *fusion plane cysts*), which may have fistulous connections with deeper spaces. Fortunately, cysts in the most common location of the lateral third of the eyebrow can be easily removed. But all others, including on the nasal bridge, the scalp, the neck, and the postauricular areas, may have intracranial connections. Consider magnetic resonance imaging first to exclude a contiguous tract. If present, removal will require a neurosurgical consult. Seventy percent of dermoid cysts will appear by 5 years of age and are more worrisome if they contain hair or capillary changes.
3. *"Everything is what it is until it ain't!"* The majority of sebaceous cysts are easy to differentiate. However, they have been misdiagnosed, with the underlying pathologic process being metastatic melanoma or other cancer. The only way to be sure of the diagnosis is to remove them.

Many believe asymptomatic lesions can be watched. The down side to this strategy is that they can grow, making removal more difficult. Or, they can become infected. If the patient asks for removal because of irritative symptoms or growth, the lesion should be removed. Once the characteristic sebaceous material and smell are observed, they *do not* need to be sent to pathology.

In the past, a surgeon's adeptness was often judged by whether he or she could remove the lesion intact without rupturing the capsule. This requires sterile technique and a fairly generous incision over the area with judicious removal of the *entire* sac, to decrease the likelihood of any recurrence. The cavity is then irrigated and closed with sutures.

Another, simpler technique is preferred by patient and physician alike where the skin is thinner (e.g., face); it does not work well with thick skin (e.g., back). Maintaining an intact sac during removal is no longer thought to be required. After anesthesia, a small, 5- to 6-mm incision is made directly into the cyst using a no. 11 blade. Some prefer to use a 3- or 4-mm sharp dermal punch. All contents are expressed using external pressure. Frequently (especially in scalp cysts, where the sac is thick and firm), this external pressure will not only extrude the sebaceous material of the cyst but the sac itself (Fig. 12-26). (Do not use the punch method on the scalp because of the thickness of the sac.) If the sac is not produced, then curved hemostats are inserted into the wound and repeated attempts are made to grasp the sac and gently tug it out in its entirety. A 3- to 4-mm dermal curette can also be inserted into the cavity to curette away any possible residual sac. No suture closure is indicated, so sterile technique (e.g., draping) is not indicated. If blood accumulates or the wound gets infected (both very rare), the patient just expresses it. Should some of the sac be left behind and the cyst reform, then formal excision with suture closure will be required.

This simple method of cyst treatment is usually successful unless the cyst is quite large (>2 cm), it has been infected previously, a previous attempt at removal has been made (causing surrounding scarring), or it is deep in the skin tissue. Wens, large and small (0.5–4 cm), are almost always treated successfully with the minimal incision technique, even with prior infection. The sacs are much thicker—almost like ping-pong balls! Three to four wens can readily be removed in a 15-minute visit (Fig. 12-27). Up to 95% of all sebaceous cysts can be treated with this simple method, without recurrence.

A variation on the technique just described is to insert two large iodine crystals (iodine crystals USP) into the sac after expression of the contents. The sac for some reason contracts around the crystals in 48 to 72 hours; the clinician then easily expresses the entire complex through the incision. This technique can also be used if it appears that the entire sac has not been removed using the simple technique described previously.

For those cysts in which the aforementioned method is not recommended (as noted), excision is necessary. Perform a field block with local anesthesia. Using a scalpel, make a small fusiform incision in the direction of the skin lines over the top of the cyst that includes the punctum. The length should be just less than the size of the cyst. Be careful to incise lightly because the skin is often very thin. Dissect deeply first into the adipose tissue at the two ends of the incision, being careful not to rupture the sac. A curved Metzenbaum scissors works well. Use an Allis clamp to grasp the wedge of skin (still attached) over the cyst. Apply only light pressure because the skin separates easily. This traction, however, will lift up the cyst below. Continue dissection until the cyst is free. Should the cyst rupture, one can proceed with the dissection, or express the entire contents, then continue to dissect the sac out. Be sure to remove the entire sac or the cyst is more likely to recur. Irrigate the cavity with saline and then close, usually with an intermediate closure technique.

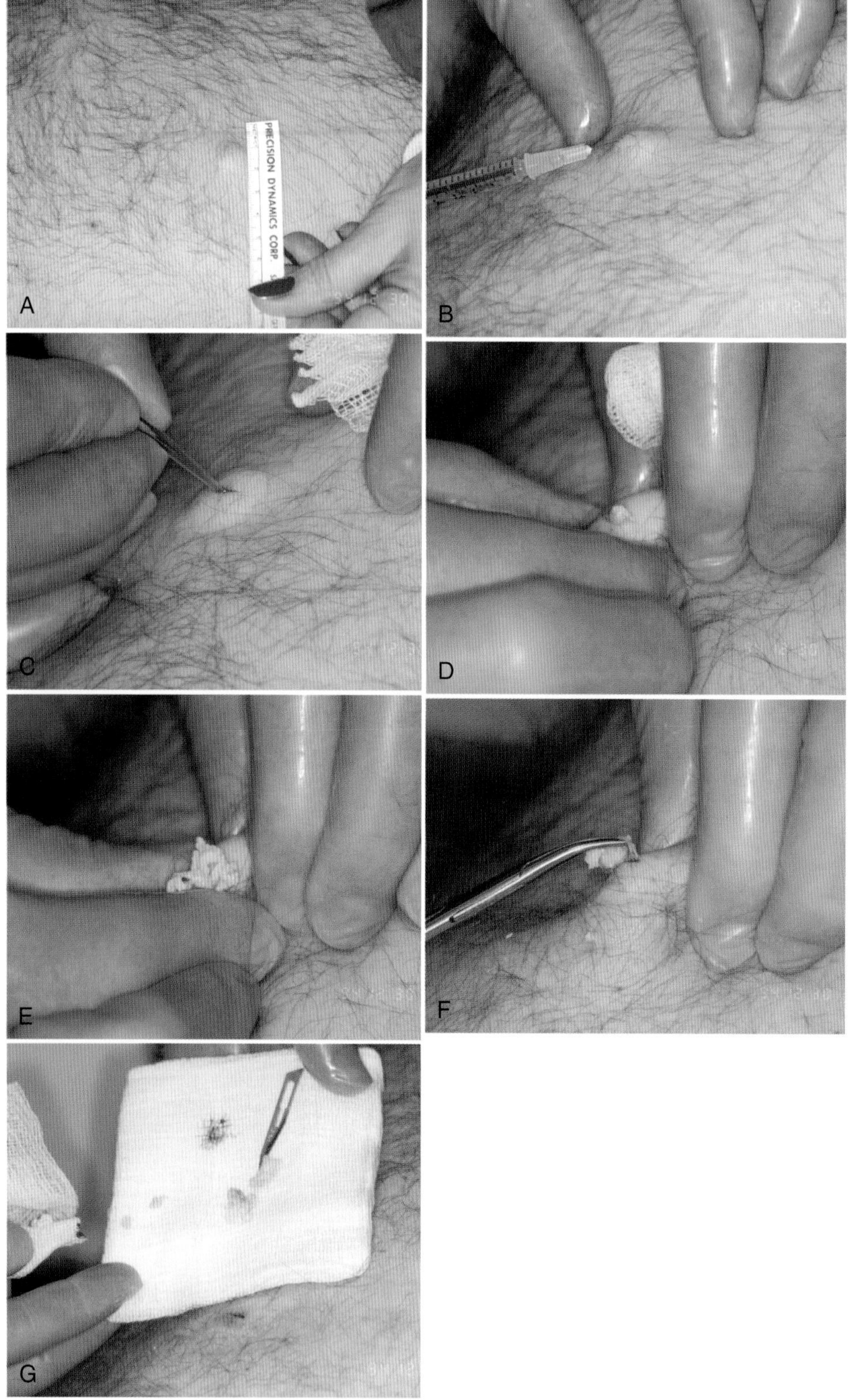

Figure 12-26 **A,** Sebaceous cyst (1.5 to 2 cm). **B,** Inject 1 mL of local anesthetic over the top of the cyst to form a wheal. **C,** Incise with a no. 11 blade directly into the cyst. **D,** Express the contents of the cyst. **E,** Sebaceous material. **F,** Grasp the sac with hemostats and tease it free with gentle pressure and a rocking motion. **G,** Sebaceous material and appearance of wound after removal. No closure is needed for a small incision. (Courtesy of The Medical Procedures Center, P.C., Midland, Mich.)

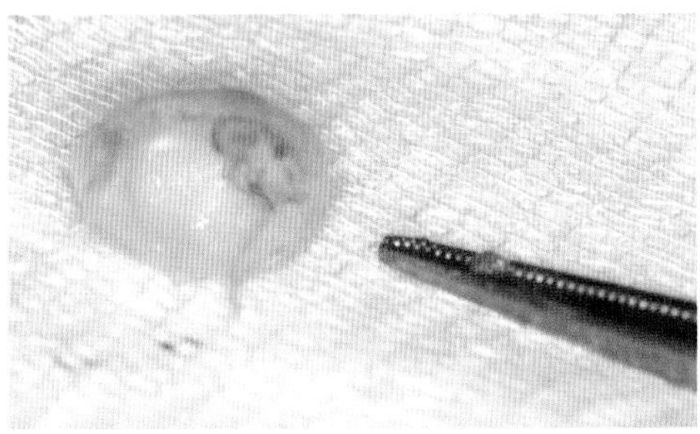

Figure 12-27 Typical sac from a trichilemmal (pilar) cyst, or wen.

If *infected*, sebaceous cysts pose a bigger problem. *The treatment for an abscess is to I&D it!* Antibiotics are costly and often there is not really an infection; rather, the cyst has ruptured, causing an inflammatory response. Treatment is the same: I&D. Formal excision is ill advised because infection is likely to occur if sutures are placed.

Technique

See Chapter 20, Incision and Drainage of an Abscess.

1. Prep with alcohol. Inject 2 mL of 2% lidocaine with epinephrine over the top of the lesion.
2. Use a no. 11 blade to incise the lesion. Be careful because the contents are often under pressure and come "flying out." All sebaceous material must be removed.
3. Insert hemostats to break up any pockets. Try to remove the sac as noted previously, but it is usually too friable. Use a reusable dermal curette and curette the inside, which may remove the sac.
4. Place ¼-inch iodoform gauze into the wound. Leave a small tail on the outside.
5. Cover with ointment so the dressing does not stick. Change the dressings two to three times per day. Change the gauze in 1 week and replace with clean gauze. Remove the new gauze in 3 weeks and let the wound heal.

Usually the cyst will not recur but rather scar down. If it recurs, formal excision is necessary, but not until the infection has resolved. No antibiotics are necessary after an I&D.

Telangiectases

Small *cherry hemangiomas*, a type of telangiectasia, are benign, small, red vascular lesions that do not require treatment. If irritated or bleeding, they can be lightly cauterized and wiped off with a gauze. (See earlier discussion.) Malignancy is not a consideration. *Spider veins*, another type of telangiectasia, are best treated with sclerotherapy if on the legs. Radiosurgery with a 30-gauge needle works extremely well on the face for isolated lesions, but works poorly in the lower extremities (see Chapter 30, Radiofrequency Surgery [Modern Electrosurgery]). Spider veins in the leg can produce significant pain and paresthesias if left untreated (see Chapter 92, Sclerotherapy). When the veins are very fine and dense such as with rosacea, IPL works extremely well.

Warts (Verruca Vulgaris and Plantaris)

The recurrence rates associated with all treatments of common warts are 30% or higher. Most over-the-counter and prescription preparations are acidic, caustic solutions. In time, 60% of warts resolve spontaneously. Vitamins enhance the immune system and may aid wart resolution. Numerous treatment methods are used and noted in Table 12-1 (see Chapter 42, Wart [Verruca] Treatment). *Candida* antigen injections are efficacious, cost effective, and the least traumatic of the alternatives, with virtually no residual scarring.

Plantar warts are treated with methods similar to those used with common warts. Physicians should avoid surgical excisions on the bottom of the feet because the scar tissue often remains painful after healing. A patient may suffer with the irritated scar, which produces an effect not unlike a pebble in a shoe. Soaking followed by paring of callous tissue will improve the efficacy of any treatment. Cryotherapy is effective and does not result in scarring. Treatment with *Candida* antigen has become the first-line approach in all but the simplest cases of verruca.

Warts (Condyloma Acuminata)

See Chapter 155, Treatment of Noncervical Condylomata Acuminata.

Wens

See the previous section on sebaceous cysts.

Xanthelasma

Xanthelasma, the most common form of xanthoma, is a yellow-white plaque on the eyelids. The diagnosis of xanthelasma can be made clinically. The goal of all treatments is to stay very superficial. Light fulguration or cauterization is often sufficient. With radiofrequency loop ablation, it is easier to control depth. Use the large loop at pure cutting level 2 (20 watts) and lightly vaporize the lesions until no residual white material exists. Often, if small, an incision can be made with an 18-gauge needle and the lesion can be expressed. Surgically removing the abnormal tissue with a curvilinear elliptical excision provides excellent results when repaired using a 6-0 suture. Because of the nature of the lesion, recurrences are common.

CPT/Billing Codes

10060	I&D cyst/abscess, simple
10061	I&D cyst/abscess, complex or multiple
11200	Skin tag removal by excision or destruction: 1-15
11201	Each additional 10 or portion thereof

NOTE: If the sac is removed or gauze is placed, this is considered "complex."

Coding and billing of lesion removal and destruction are very complex. There are excision codes with simple and intermediate closures. Shave excisions are another whole section in the CPT code book. Destruction of lesions depends on whether they are benign or malignant, their size, and where they are located. For genital and anal lesions, it also depends on how they are "destroyed." It is of the utmost importance that the clinician differentiates the methods for the treatment of these lesions when coding and billing. Clinicians should consider obtaining the current year's edition of *The NPI Reimbursement Manual for Office Procedures* (Pfenninger JL, editor, The National Procedures Institute, www.npinstitute.com). This manual not only lists appropriate procedure codes but provides a comparison and suggested fee for each procedure code commonly used for all procedures by primary care clinicians, not just dermatologists. A videotape/DVD discussing coding and billing is also available from the same source.

Additional Resources

Multiple patient education forms for different diagnoses and conditions are available at www.expertconsult.com.

Multiple videotapes/DVDs are available from the National Procedures Institute depicting treatment techniques for the methods and approaches discussed in this chapter. www.npinstitute.com (phone 1-866-NPI-CME1).

BIBLIOGRAPHY

American Cancer Society and National Comprehensive Cancer Network: Melanoma: Treatment guidelines for patients (Part 1). Dermatol Nurs 17:119–131, 2005.

American Cancer Society and National Comprehensive Cancer Network: Melanoma: Treatment guidelines for patients (Part 2). Dermatol Nurs 17:191–198, 2005.

American Society of Plastic Surgeons: Evidence-Based Clinical Practice Guidelines: Treatment of Cutaneous Melanoma. Arlington Heights, Ill: American Society of Plastic Surgeons, 2007.

Bialy TL, Whalen J, Veledar E, et al: Mohs micrographic surgery vs traditional surgical excision: A cost comparison analysis. Arch Dermatol 140:736–742, 2004.

Bowen GM, White GL Jr, Gerwels JW: Mohs micrographic surgery. Am Fam Physician 72:845–848, 2005.

Cohen PR, Schulze KE, Nelson BR: Cutaneous carcinoma with mixed histology: A potential etiology for skin cancer recurrence and an indication for Mohs microscopically controlled surgical excision. South Med J 98:740–747, 2005.

Coit DG, Andtbacka R, Bichakjian CK, et al: Melanoma. J Natl Compr Canc Netw 7:250–275, 2009.

Cook J, Salasche S: Mohs surgery: An informed view. Plast Reconstr Surg 115:945–946, 2005.

Cook J, Zitelli JA: Mohs micrographic surgery: A cost analysis. J Am Acad Dermatol 39(Pt 1):698–703, 1998.

Dandurand M, Petit T, Martel P, Guillot B, for ANAES: Management of basal cell carcinoma in adults: Clinical practice guidelines. Eur J Dermatol 16:394–401, 2006.

De Raeve LE, De Coninck AL, Dierickx PR, Roseeuw DI: Neonatal curettage of giant congenital melanocytic nevi. Arch Dermatol 132:20–22, 1996.

Dummer R, Hauschild A, Jost L, for the ESMO Guidelines Working Group: Cutaneous malignant melanoma: ESMO clinical recommendations for diagnosis, treatment, and follow-up. Ann Oncol 19(Suppl 2):ii86–ii88, 2008.

Dummer R, Panizzon R, Bloch PH, Burg G, for the Task Force on Skin Cancer: Updated Swiss guidelines for the treatment and follow-up of cutaneous melanoma. Dermatology 210:39–44, 2005.

Essers BA, Dirksen CD, Nieman FH, et al: Cost-effectiveness of Mohs micrographic surgery vs. surgical excision for basal cell carcinoma of the face. Arch Dermatol 142:187–194, 2006.

Folberg R, Salomao D, Grossniklaus HE, et al, for the Association of Directors of Anatomic and Surgical Pathology: Recommendations for the reporting of tissues removed as part of the surgical treatment of common malignancies of the eye and its adnexa. Hum Pathol 34:114–118, 2003.

Fraser MC, Goldstein AM, Tucker MA: Genetic testing for inherited predisposition to melanoma: Has the time come? J Drugs Dermatol 3:93–95, 2004.

Gillard M, Wang TS, Johnson TM: Nonmelanoma cuntaneous malignancies. In Chang AE, Ganz PA, Hayes DF, et al (eds): Oncology: An Evidence-Based Approach. New York, Springer, 2006.

Guidelines of care for cutaneous squamous cell carcinoma: Committee on Guidelines of Care. Task Force on Cutaneous Squamous Cell Carcinoma. J Am Acad Dermatol 28:628–631, 1993.

Guidelines of care for malignant melanomas: Committee on Guidelines of Care: Task Force on Malignant Melanoma. J Am Acad Dermatol 28:638–641, 1993.

Habif TP: Clinical Dermatology, 4th ed. St. Louis, Mosby, 2004.

Hatzis GP, Finn R: Using botox to treat a Mohs defect repair complicated by a parotid fistula. J Oral Maxillofac Surg 65:2357–2360, 2007.

Huang CL, Marghoob AA, Halpern AC: Management of dysplastic nevi and melanomas. In Robinson JK, Hanke DW, Sengelmann RD, Siegel DM (eds): Surgery of the Skin: Procedural Dermatology. Philadelphia, Mosby, 2005.

Jost LM, Jelic S, Purkalne G., et al, for the ESMO Guidelines Task Force: ESMO minimum clinical recommendations for diagnosis, treatment and follow-up of cutaneous malignant melanoma. Ann Oncol 16(Suppl 1):66–68, 2005.

Klin B, Ashkenazi M: Sebaceous cyst excision with minimal surgery. Am Fam Physician 41:1746–1748, 1990.

Krant JJ, Carucci JA: Benign subcutaneous lesions. In Robinson JK, Hanke DW, Sengelmann RD, Siegel DM (eds): Surgery of the Skin: Procedural Dermatology. Philadelphia, Mosby, 2005.

Krengel S, Hauschild A, Schäfer T: Melanoma risk in congenital melanocytic nevi: A systematic review. Br J Dermatol 155:1–8, 2006.

Kuflik AS, Janniger CK: Basal cell carcinoma. Am Fam Physician 48: 1273–1276, 1993.

Kurban RS, Kurban AL: Skin disorders of aging: Diagnosis and treatment. Geriatrics 48:30–42, 1993.

Lask G, Moy1 ED: Principles and Techniques of Cutaneous Surgery. New York, McGraw-Hill, 1996.

Leibovitch I, Huilgol SC, Selva D, et al: Basosquamous carcinoma: Treatment with Mohs micrographic surgery. Cancer 104:170–175, 2005.

Miller SJ: The National Comprehensive Cancer Network (NCCN) guidelines of care for nonmelanoma skin cancers. Dermatol Surg 26:289–292, 2000.

Miller SJ, Alam M, Andersen J, et al, for the National Comprehensive Cancer Network: Basal cell and squamous cell skin cancers. J Natl Compr Canc Netw 5:506–529, 2007.

Motley R, Kersey P, Lawrence C: Multiprofessional guidelines for the management of the patient with primary cutaneous squamous cell carcinoma. Br J Dermatol 146:18–25, 2002.

Nag S, Quivey JM, Earle JD, et al: The American Brachytherapy Society recommendations for brachytherapy of uveal melanomas. Int J Radiat Oncol Biol Phys 56:544–555, 2003.

Nguyen TH: Mohs bashing out of hand. Plast Reconstr Surg 115:361–362, 2005.

NIH Consensus Conference: Diagnosis and treatment of early melanoma. JAMA 268:1314–1319, 1992.

Otley CC: Cost-effectiveness of Mohs micrographic surgery vs. surgical excision for basal cell carcinoma of the face. Arch Dermatol 142:1235, author reply 1235–1236, 2006.

Otley CC: Mohs' micrographic surgery for basal-cell carcinoma of the face. Lancet 365:1226–1227, author reply 1227, 2005.

Pfenninger JL: The NPI Reimbursement Manual for Office Procedures. Midland, Mich, The National Procedures Institute, 2010.

Redondo P, Marquina M, Pretel M, et al: Methyl-ALA-induced fluorescence in photodynamic diagnosis of basal cell carcinoma prior to Mohs micrographic surgery. Arch Dermatol 144:115–117, 2008.

Rigopoulos D, Larios G, Gregoriou S, Alevizos A: Acute and chronic paronychia. Am Fam Physician 77:339–346, 2008.

Roenigk RK, Roenigk HH: Dermatologic Surgery: Principles and Practice, 2nd ed. New York, Marcel Dekker, 1996.

Shindel AW, Mann MW, Lev RY, et al: Mohs micrographic surgery for penile cancer: Management and long-term followup. J Urol 178: 1980–1985, 2007. [See comment in Nat Clin Pract Urol 5:364–365, 2008.]

Shuster S: Mohs' micrographic surgery for basal-cell carcinoma of the face. Lancet 365:1227–1228, 2005.

Stacano JJ, Juma A, Dhital SK, McGeorge DD: Excision margin for cutaneous squamous cell carcinoma: Is it standardized? Eur J Plast Surg 27: 135–139, 2004.

Stern RS, Boudreaux C, Arndt K: Diagnostic accuracy and appropriateness of care for seborrheic keratoses. JAMA 265:74–77, 1989.

Sterry W, for the European Dermatology Forum Guideline Committee: Guidelines: The management of basal cell carcinoma. Eur J Dermatol 16:467–475, 2006.

Stulberg DL, Crandell B, Fawcett RS: Diagnosis and treatment of basal cell and squamous cell carcinomas. Am Fam Physician 70:1481–1488, 2004.

Telfer NR, Colver GB, Morton CA, for the British Association of Dermatologists: Guidelines for the management of basal cell carcinoma. Br J Dermatol 159:35–48, 2008.

Tran KT, Wright NA, Cockrell CJ: Biopsy of the pigmented lesion: When and how. J Am Acad Dermatol 59:852–871, 2008.

Tromberg J, Bauer B, Benvenuto-Andrade C, Marghoob AA: Congenital melanocytic nevi needing treatment. Dermatol Ther 18:136–150, 2005.

Usatine RP: The Color Atlas of Family Medicine. New York, McGraw-Hill, 2009.

Usatine RP, Pfenninger JL, Stulberg DL, Small R: Dermatologic and Cosmetic Procedures in Office Practice. Philadelphia, Elsevier, 2010.

Whitaker DK, Sinclair W, for the Melanoma Advisory Board: Guideline on the management of melanoma. S Afr Med J 94(Pt 3):699–708, 2004.

CHAPTER 13

Burn Treatment

Roberta E. Gebhard

One million people seek medical advice for burns each year in the United States. Burn injuries can cause both severe psychological and physical disability. Early resuscitation and aggressive surgical intervention of burn injuries can reduce mortality and limit long-term morbidity.

Burn Complications Requiring Resuscitation

Inherent to burn injuries are a number of potential complications. Burn research has shown that the causes of early mortality are not the burns themselves, but complications related to hypoxia, hypoventilation, and circulation disorders, including hypovolemia and hypothermia. Complications requiring early resuscitation are as follows:

- Airway injury (airway edema from thermal or chemical burns)
- Inhalation injury/hypoxia
  - Chemical fumes are the most common cause of pneumonitis/pulmonary edema.
  - Smoke or other particulate material causes pneumonitis.
  - Carbon monoxide poisoning is common with fires in enclosed spaces.
- Hypothermia from loss of skin integrity and evaporative losses
- Hypovolemia or shock resulting from intravascular-to-extravascular fluid shifts and pain-vasoconstriction
- Cardiac asystole and arrhythmias (especially with high-voltage burns)

Resuscitation for Early Burn Complications

Advanced Burn Life Support (ABLS) courses are available both in traditional and online formats that help focus resuscitation efforts to the most critical patient needs by using a simple-to-remember alphabetic mnemonic: A = Airway, B = Breathing, C = Circulation, D = Disability, E = Exposure, F = Fluids (see the "Online Resources" section at the end of the chapter).

A = Airway

Airway management is the crucial first step in resuscitating a severe burn victim. Early endotracheal intubation is recommended when an injured airway is first diagnosed. Although airway edema normally stays above the vocal cords, delayed intubation can be much more difficult or traumatic. The manifestations of airway injury are often subtle and may not appear for 24 hours. A history of the victim being confined in a burning building (or closed space) or of having impaired mentation is suggestive of acute inhalational injury. With this history, a search for clinical evidence of inhalation injury should be undertaken carefully. Clinical clues to acute inhalation injury include facial burns, singed eyebrow or nasal hairs, oropharyngeal carbon deposits, acute inflammation, and carbonaceous sputum. If hoarseness, a brassy cough, or stridor develops, immediately intubate the patient. Intubation is also required before transport if transportation time will be prolonged. Airway injuries indicate major burn severity.

B = Breathing

Evaluate the patient for spontaneous respirations. Check for stridor, wheezing, or rales and administer 100% O_2 as soon as it is available. Carbon monoxide (CO) poisoning should be assumed if the burn victim was trapped in an enclosed space.

C = Circulation

Rapid shifts in intravascular fluid occur in burns of greater than 20% to 25% total body surface area (TBSA). Hypovolemia resulting from capillary leak and evaporative losses should be anticipated and corrected (see "F = Fluids" section). High-voltage burns can cause cardiac arrest. Lower-voltage injuries may cause delayed arrhythmias. After removing the electrical source with a nonconducting piece of equipment or turning off the power source, begin basic life support in the pulseless victim. Advanced cardiac life support measures should be initiated as soon as appropriate equipment is available.

D = Disability

Remember to stabilize the cervical spine to prevent further disability. High-voltage injuries can cause tetanic muscle contractions severe enough to fracture the cervical spine, lumbar spine, or limbs. Jumps from burning buildings can also cause fractures.

E = Exposure

- Expose the patient by removing any nonadherent clothing, especially chemically contaminated or smoldering clothing, constricting clothing, and jewelry.
- Examine for associated injuries. Document these injuries and address them after the patient is stabilized.
- Brush away residual dry chemicals. Irrigate liquid residual chemicals copiously with water. Alkalis may require forceful irrigation (such as a shower) for up to an hour.
- Cover the patient with a clean, dry blanket to prevent hypothermia.

F = Fluids

Aggressive fluid resuscitation is required in patients with burns covering more than 25% TBSA to prevent hypovolemia and shock resulting from capillary leak and evaporative losses.

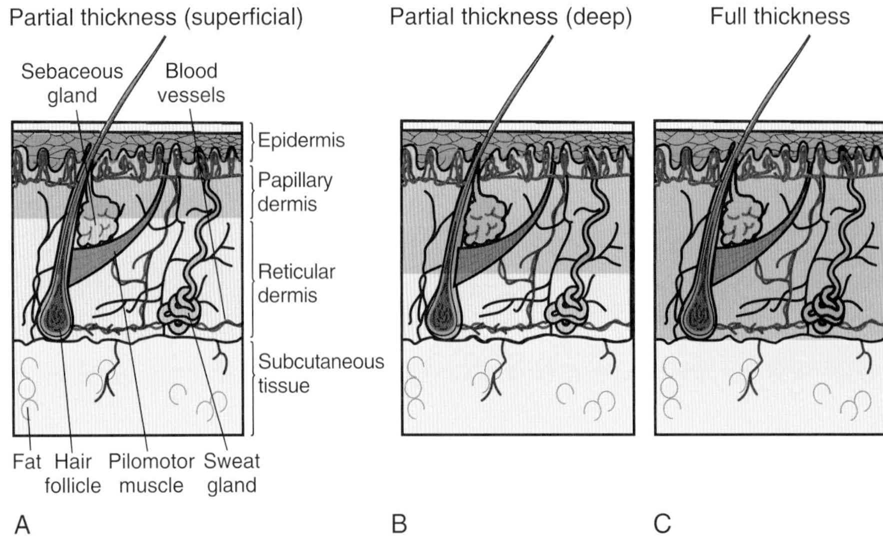

Figure 13-1 **A,** Superficial partial-thickness burn. **B,** Deep partial-thickness burn. **C,** Full-thickness burn. *Coral background area* denotes depth of burn injuries. (Reproduced from Edlich RF, Bailey TL, Bill TJ: Thermal burns. In Marx JA, Walls R, Hockberger R [eds]: Rosen's Emergency Medicine: Concepts and Clinical Practice, 5th ed. Philadelphia, Mosby, 2002, pp 802–813.)

Intravenous Access

Insert two large-bore intravenous (IV) lines, avoiding burned skin if possible. Central venous access may be needed.

Parkland Formula

The most widely used formula for fluid resuscitation is the Parkland Formula, although there is some controversy that it may underestimate the initial need for fluid (see Holm and colleagues, 2004). The greatest intravascular-to-extravascular fluid shifts occur in the first 8 hours. Significant but slower fluid shifts continue for the next 16 hours. All fluid resuscitation formulas are designed to replace the intravascular volume as it is lost, most rapidly in the first 8 hours, then the next 16 hours.

- *First 24 hours:* lactated Ringer's 4 mL/kg/percent burn (first half given in first 8 hours, second half given in next 16 hours). Time is measured from the onset time of burn.
- *Second 24 hours:* colloid 0.5 mL/kg/percent burn + 2000 mL of 5% dextrose in water (given over second 24 hours).
- *Example:* 70-kg adult with 50% TBSA partial- and full-thickness burns requires 14 L of lactated Ringer's over the first 24 hours (4 mL × 70 kg × 50% burn = 14,000 mL/24 hr). Seven liters is given in the first 8 hours (875 mL/hr) and 7 L given in the next 16 hours (437.5 mL/hr).
- Evaluation of fluid resuscitation efforts is best gauged by *urine output* (see "Inpatient Management for the Primary Provider" section).

Estimating Burn Severity

Burn depth, size, and locations on the body must be assessed to determine the burn severity.

Burn Depth

Figure 13-1 shows the skin in cross-section with the layers involved with superficial partial-thickness, deep partial-thickness, and full-thickness burns.

Superficial burns are erythematous without blister formation and involve only the epidermis; pain is localized (Fig. 13-2). *Superficial partial-thickness* burns are painful, warm, and moist with blister formation; they involve the epidermis and superficial papillary dermis (Fig. 13-3). With *deep partial-thickness* burns the skin is mottled, waxy, and white in appearance, with ruptured blisters. Pain sensation is absent, but pressure sensation is intact (Fig. 13-4). *Full-thickness* burns involve both the epidermis and dermis, have a white to gray, leathery appearance, and do not blanch with pressure. There is only sensation to deep pressure; there is no pain because pain receptors in the dermis are destroyed (Fig. 13-5).

Burn depth terminology no longer includes the use of "first-, second-, and third-degree burns." Note that superficial and superficial partial-thickness burns have minimal to no risk of scarring, are painful, and heal spontaneously by 3 weeks. Deep partial-thickness and full-thickness burns have a higher risk of scarring, decreased sensation, and delayed healing of greater than 3 weeks. *Fourth-degree burn* is the term still used to depict the most severe burns, extending through both the epidermis and the dermis and into the fascia and muscle. Fourth-degree burns are life-threatening and may never heal if they are present over more than 2% of TBSA (see later).

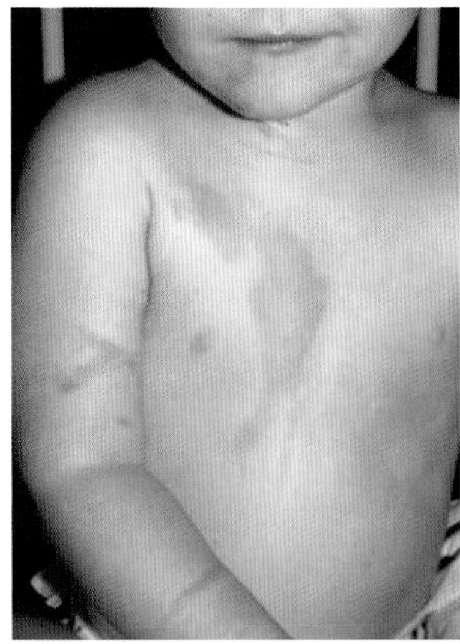

Figure 13-2 Superficial burns are erythematous without blister formation, involve only the epidermis, and are characterized by localized pain.

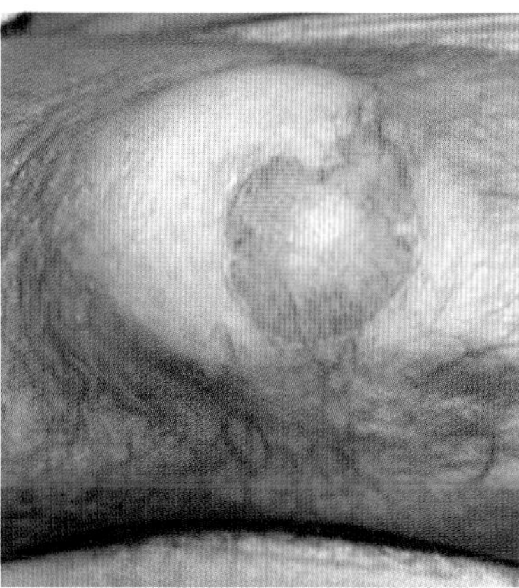

Figure 13-3 Superficial partial-thickness burns are painful, warm, and moist with blister formation, and involve the epidermis and superficial papillary dermis.

Initial estimates of the depth of the burn are crucial to timely triage. The final depth of injury cannot always be predicted at the initial evaluation; therefore, sequential evaluations may be needed to revise the depth of the burn over the days and weeks after the injury. See Figure 13-6 for treatment recommendations based on wound depth assessment.

Burn Size: Percentage of Total Body Surface Area

Burn size is an important determinant of burn healing. Healing occurs from fibroblasts migrating in from the burn margins and the oil glands and hair follicles (skin appendages). The skin appendages penetrate deep into the dermis and, except for full-thickness burns, are spared from destruction.

The adult body surface area can be divided into percentages of nine and multiples or fractions of nine: the "Rule of Nines" (Fig. 13-7). *Infants have a greater proportion of TBSA on the head and neck and less on the legs. The posterior torso, including buttocks, still equals 18%, with each buttock equaling 2.5%. Palms are 1.25%.*

Burn Locations

The determination of whether a particular burn injury should be treated as an ambulatory case, a local hospital admission, or a direct admission to a regional burn center depends on burn involvement in some highly critical areas.

The American Burn Association (ABA) has set up criteria for referral to a burn center for treatment (Box 13-1). The ABA's grading system recommends disposition to a burn center for these critical conditions because of the significantly increased risk of morbidity.

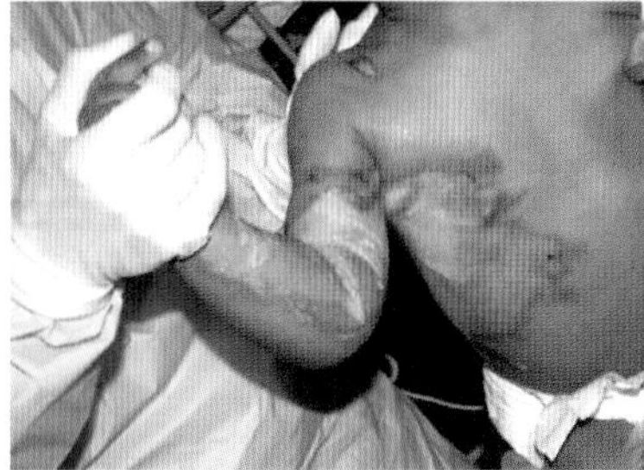

Figure 13-4 With deep partial-thickness burns the skin is mottled, waxy, and white in appearance, with ruptured blisters.

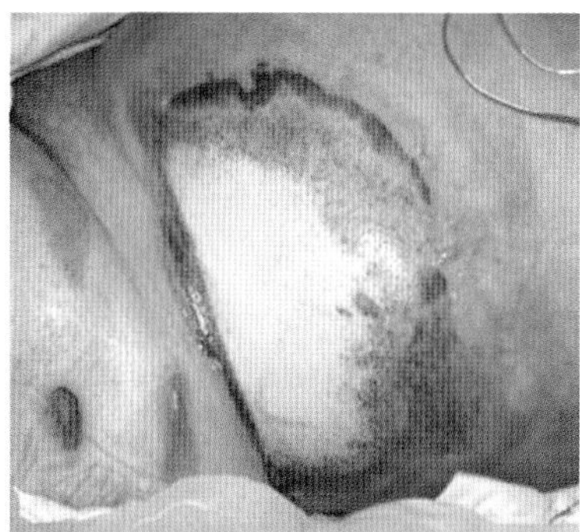

Figure 13-5 Full-thickness burns involve both the epidermis and dermis, have a white to gray, leathery appearance, and do not blanch with pressure.

Certain burn locations or other potential injuries lead to automatic classification as *moderate burn severity*. Fractures in association with burns increase the severity index.

Disposition of Patient Based on Burn Severity: American Burn Association Guidelines

The ABA guidelines for disposition of burn patients are based on burn severity, which is based on depth, size, and location of the burn (see Box 13-1).

- Minor burns: outpatient management
  - Involve less than 10% TBSA in adults, less than 5% TBSA in children and elderly
  - Less than 2% TBSA full-thickness burns
  - Do not involve face, hands, feet, genitalia, or respiratory tract
  - Are not circumferential
  - No associated injuries or comorbidities
- Moderate burns: hospitalization
- Major burns: burn center

Complications Encountered during Burn Management

Additional complications are encountered during the treatment of burns, whether in the hospital or as an outpatient. Any life-threatening complications encountered during the resuscitation phase of burn care require continued attention after the patient is stabilized and disposition has been determined. Burn centers offer expertise in wound management and vigilance in late complications. Other complications that must be prevented if possible and addressed if they occur despite all preventive efforts include the following:

- Airway injury
  - Hypoxia
  - Airway edema
  - CO poisoning: PO_2 levels on blood gases may be normal even in the presence of CO poisoning. Carboxyhemoglobin (CO-Hgb) levels should be measured. The presence of 100% O_2 provides appropriate supplementation and reduces CO levels. (The $T_{1/2}$ of CO-Hgb converting back to hemoglobin is reduced from 250 minutes on room air to 40 minutes on 100% O_2.) Severe cases of CO poisoning should receive hyperbaric oxygen therapy, which can be life-saving. See Figure 13-8 for an algorithm on using the hyperbaric chamber for CO poisoning.
  - CO poisoning symptoms are related to the percentage of CO-Hgb: CO-Hgb levels less than 20% are usually asymptomatic. At CO-Hgb levels of 20% to 30%, headache and nausea

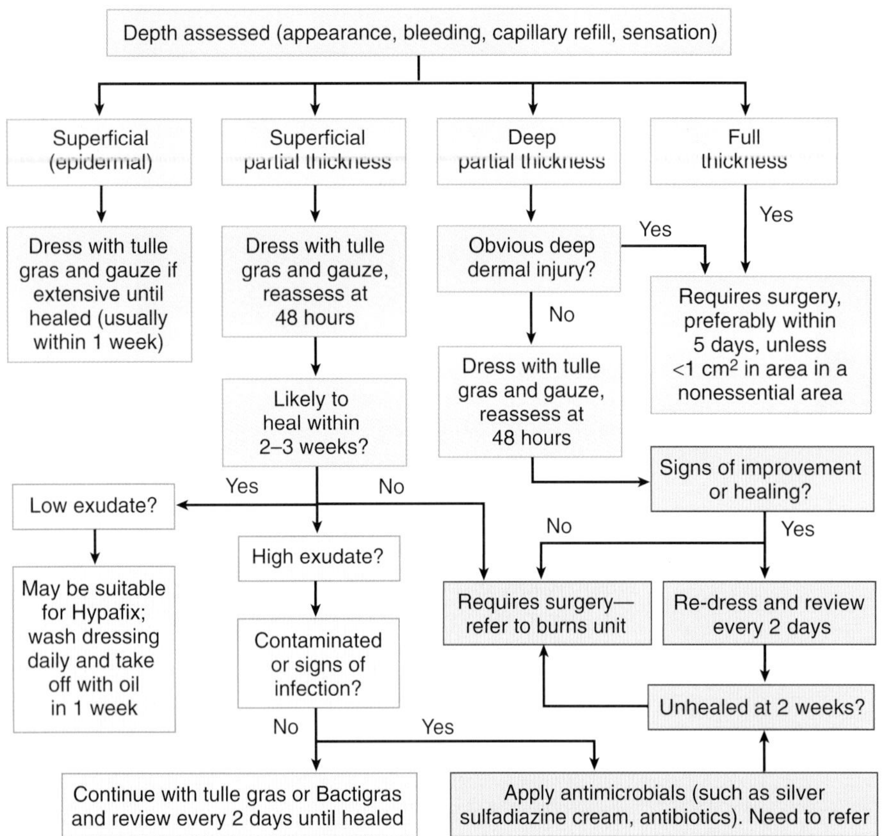

Figure 13-6 Algorithm for assessing depth of burn wounds and suggested treatment.

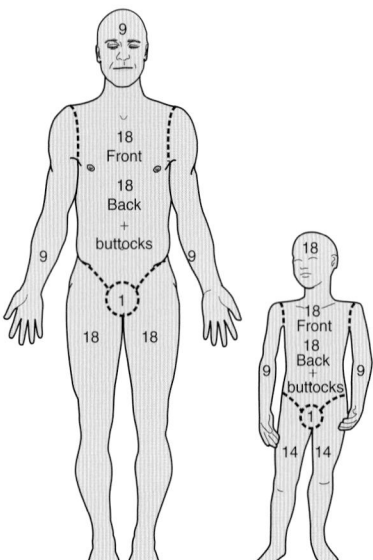

Figure 13-7 Rule of nines. (Modified from Krisanda TJ, Bethel CA: Burn care procedures. In Roberts JR, Hedges JR [eds]: Clinical Procedures in Emergency Medicine, 3rd ed. Philadelphia, WB Saunders, 1998.)

Box 13-1. Burn Center Referral Criteria

A burn center may treat adults, children, or both. Burn injuries that should be referred to a burn center include the following:

- Partial-thickness burns of greater than 10% of the total body surface area.
- Burns that involve the face, hands, feet, genitalia, perineum, or major joints.
- Third-degree burns in any age group.
- Electrical burns, including lightning injury.
- Chemical burns.
- Inhalation injury.
- Burn injury in patients with preexisting medical disorders that could complicate management, prolong recovery, or affect mortality.
- Any patients with burns and concomitant trauma (such as fractures) in which the burn injury poses the greatest risk of morbidity or mortality. In such cases, if the trauma poses the greater immediate risk, the patient's condition may be stabilized initially in a trauma center before transfer to a burn center. Physician judgment will be necessary in such situations and should be in concert with the regional medical control plan and triage protocols.
- Burned children in hospitals without qualified personnel or equipment for the care of children.
- Burn injury in patients who will require special social, emotional, or rehabilitative intervention.

Excerpted from Committee on Trauma, American College of Surgeons: Guidelines for the operation of burn centers. In Resources for Optimal Care of the Injured Patient 2006. Rockford, Ill, American College of Surgeons, 2006, pp 79–86.

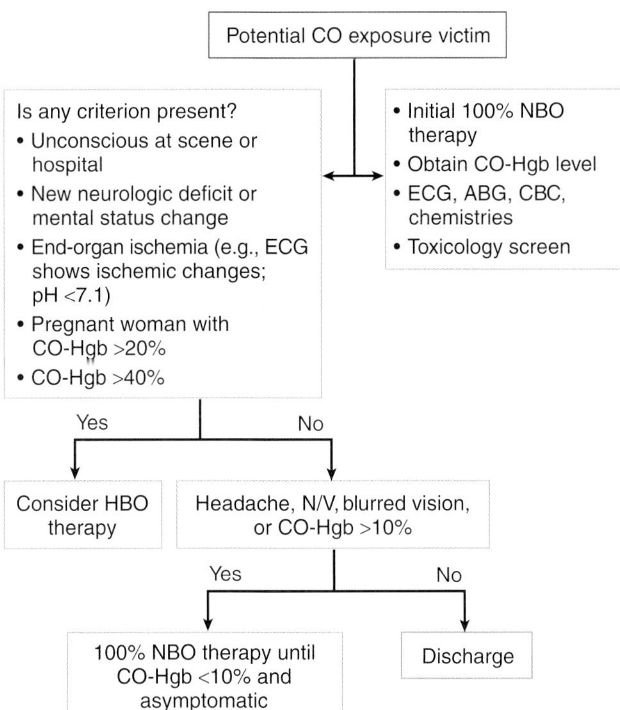

Figure 13-8 Algorithm for using normobaric oxygen (NBO) and hyperbaric oxygen (HBO) after carbon monoxide exposure. ABG, arterial blood gas; CBC, complete blood count; CO-Hgb, carboxyhemoglobin; ECG, electrocardiogram; N/V, nausea/vomiting. (Adapted from O'Brien C, Manaker S: Carbon monoxide and smoke inhalation. In Lanken PN, Hanson CW III, Manaker S [eds]: The Intensive Care Unit Manual. Philadelphia, WB Saunders, 2001.)

occur. At CO-Hgb levels of 30% to 40%, confusion occurs, and coma ensues when CO-Hgb levels reach between 40% and 60%. Levels over 60% cause death.

- Cardiac arrhythmias: Can occur for up to 3 days after high-voltage injury
- Pain
- Infection
  - Bacterial
  - Tetanus
  - Smoke inhalation/pneumonitis
  - Pneumonia
- Hypothermia
- Intravascular-to-extravascular fluid shifts
  - Hypovolemia/shock
  - Edema
  - Compartment syndrome
- Hypertrophic scars/contractures
  - Loss of function of hands, feet, eyes, joints, genitalia
  - Permanent disfigurement (Fig. 13-9)

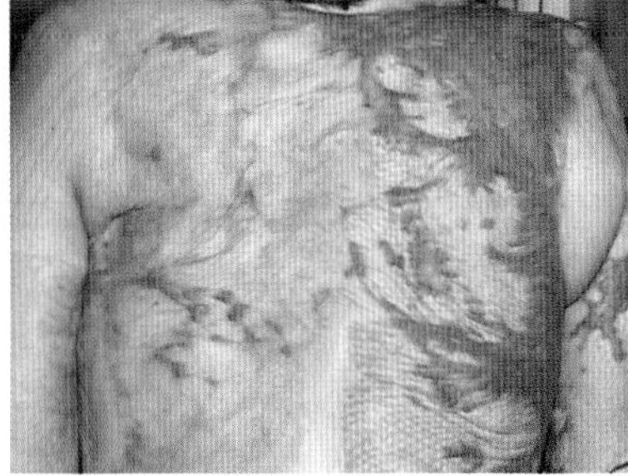

Figure 13-9 Permanent disfigurement.

- Pigmentary changes
  - Hypopigmentation for 6 to 24 months
  - Hyperpigmentation if not protected from ultraviolet damage
- Sensory dysfunction (sensory nerve damage)
  - Hyperesthesias
  - Pruritus
- Xerosis (damaged sweat glands)
- Psychological
  - Depression
  - Anxiety disorders
- Carcinoma (nonmelanoma skin cancers) in burn scars

Inpatient Management for the Primary Provider

According to the ABA's grading system for burn severity and disposition of patients, moderate and major burn injuries require hospitalization either locally or in a burn center. The primary provider may be the admitting provider for moderate and even severe burns if stabilization is needed before transfer to a burn center. The ABA's website (www.ameriburn.org) has search capability to assist in locating burn centers throughout the United States. Inpatient management of patients with moderate burn severity should include consideration of the following:

- History of burn injury
  - When? Initial time of burn important for fluid resuscitation.
  - How? Fire, steam, chemical, electrical, hot material?
  - Where? Enclosed space (inhalation injury)?
- Medical history
  - Medical problems: diabetes and chronic steroid use increase risk of infection. Cardiopulmonary disease decreases physical reserves. Other medical problems will need to be addressed.
  - Medications: steroid use, blood thinners, diabetic medications, and so forth.
  - Allergies: sulfa allergy (use bacitracin ointment).
  - Last tetanus: boost if not received in last 12 months.
- Airway: suspected airway injury may need intubation if oropharyngeal edema develops during the 12 to 24 hours after injury. Observe for raspy cough, hoarseness, or stridor.
- Breathing: monitor for hypoxia.
  - CO poisoning: 100% O_2 or hyperbaric oxygen therapy (see Fig. 13-8).
  - Pneumonitis or pulmonary edema: ventilation with high O_2 and positive end-expiratory pressure may be needed.
  - Pneumonia: treat with appropriate systemic antibiotics.
- Circulation
  - Monitor urine output for adequate rehydration.
  - Monitor for cardiac arrhythmias with telemetry. Patients with high-voltage (>440 V) injuries can develop ventricular arrhythmias up to 3 days after the injury. The most common electrocardiographic (ECG) finding of cardiac injury after electrical burn is nonspecific ST segment–T-wave abnormalities. These patients should be admitted to the telemetry unit for cardiac monitoring until the ECG normalizes. Treat with appropriate antiarrhythmics.
  - Monitor for compartment syndrome for circumferential wounds or if excessive rehydration.
    - Clinical diagnostic signs: delayed capillary refill, distal anesthesia, increasing limb pain, and decreased or absent distal pulses. Clinical signs are only 60% sensitive (they miss 40% of true compartment syndromes).
    - Measure direct compartment pressures (see Chapter 188, Compartment Syndrome Evaluation).
    - Obtain surgical consultation for escharotomy of affected limb, including across joints. Rarely needed for circumferential burns of trunk.
    - Fasciotomy will be necessary if escharotomy is not effective.

- Disability: obtain an x-ray skeletal survey for high-voltage burn or other suspected bone injury. Tetanic convulsion can cause fracture of cervical spine, lumbar spine, or limbs. A cross-table lateral view of the cervical spine should be obtained before removal of full cervical spine precautions. Monitor the level of consciousness; mental alertness confirms adequate circulation.
- Exposure: Avoid hypothermia, which can increase peripheral vasoconstriction. Evaporative fluid loss and loss of barrier to infection result from partial- and full-thickness burns. Consider early excision of eschar and skin grafting or artificial covering.
- Fluids: Continue rehydration per urine output. For adults, adequate urine output is 0.5 mL/kg/hr; for children, 1.0 mL/kg/hr is needed. A Foley catheter is required. Excessive fluid administration can lead to increased edema, increased rate of compartment syndrome, and unnecessary fasciotomies. Higher urine output and osmotic diuretics are normally required for high-voltage burns to prevent acute renal failure from rhabdomyolysis.
- Requirements decrease as the capillary leakage decreases over 2 to 7 days.
  - Admission weight and daily patient weights are required. Increased insensible losses through open wounds make patient weight invaluable.
  - Inputs and outputs: hourly fluid input and output are required to monitor the massive amounts of fluid used for resuscitation.
- Give tetanus prophylaxis for burns deeper than superficial partial thickness (if time since last tetanus booster is >12 months).
- Early nutrition first 12 to 24 hours, enteral if possible: Burn injuries are associated with an increased metabolism from 1.3× to 2× baseline. Enteral feedings decrease gastrointestinal ulceration. Parenteral feedings may be required but significantly increase the risk of sepsis at IV sites. Catheters should be replaced every 48 to 72 hours.
- Infection: Common sources of infection in burn patients include the burn wounds, pneumonia, IV line sepsis, and urinary tract sepsis from indwelling catheters. Burn wound infections usually require full-thickness biopsy and tissue culture to differentiate bacterial colonization from bacterial tissue invasion. Systemic antibiotics are required. Excision of infected burn tissue and grafting are often required. Culturing of central line catheter tips on replacement is recommended. Worsening pulmonary status should prompt a chest radiographic examination.
- Pain: Baseline pain medication with augmentation of pain relief by rescue medications is recommended. Some authorities recommend treatment of baseline pain with methadone and augmentation with morphine before dressing changes or activities such as physical therapy.

WOUND CARE

Burn Débridement

- Devitalized tissue removal is important to prevent bacterial colonization. Mild soaps such as chlorhexidine are recommended. Avoid povidone–iodine (Betadine), alcohol, and hydrogen peroxide, which inhibit fibroblasts as well as bacteria, delaying the healing process.
- Remove ruptured blisters, those blisters prone to break (e.g., over joints), and those with cloudy fluid that could be infected.
- Removal of small intact blisters is controversial. Some authorities recommend débridement of all blisters, whereas others recommend leaving them undisturbed as a natural sterile barrier to infection.

NOTE: Delayed blister resolution longer than 2 weeks may indicate deep partial-thickness burn. Consider consultation for excision and skin grafting.

- Removal of adherent tar or clothing can be facilitated by application of petroleum jelly or bacitracin ointment for softening and removal during washing at dressing changes. Whirlpool baths are well tolerated for wound débridement.

Dressings

- Standard dressings are changed twice a day. After dressing removal, the wounds are washed, inspected for healing or onset of infection, patted dry, treated with topical antibiotics, and covered with Telfa (Smith & Nephew, London), a nonadherent dressing, and gauze or stockinet. Tulle gras dressings are gauze impregnated with paraffin, and Bactigras (Smith & Nephew) is a tulle gras with 0.5% chlorhexidine acetate. Both can be used as an alternative to Telfa. Hypafix (Smith & Nephew) is an adhesive retention tape that is air and moisture permeable and completely covers the entire dressing to reduce contamination.
- Consider Unna paste dressings. Advocates cite benefits such as decreased scarring, discomfort, and cost without increased infection rate. Dressings are changed every 3 to 7 days. Concerns include delayed detection of infection and overlooking of early scarring or other complications because of infrequent wound observation.

Topical Antibiotics

Topical antibiotics are used to decrease bacterial colonization of open blisters and deep burns. Their use significantly decreases wound infections. No single agents can be used in all cases. Several choices include the following:

- *Silver sulfadiazine (Silvadene 1% cream)*. Silver sulfadiazine has intermediate eschar penetration and a broad spectrum of antibacterial and anticandidal activity. It is easy to apply but should not be used on the face because of staining or in patients with sulfa allergy or glucose-6-phosphate dehydrogenase (G6PD) deficiency. Silver sulfadiazine should not be used in pregnant women, newborns, and breast-feeding women of children 2 months of age or younger owing to risk of sulfonamide kernicterus if it is absorbed through the skin.
- *Mafenide acetate (Sulfamylon 8.5% cream)*. Mafenide acetate has excellent eschar penetration and has the best antibacterial spectrum. It should be used on ears for prevention of chondritis. Some authorities recommend it on all full-thickness burns. Mafenide is painful after it is applied and expensive. Sleep disturbance is fairly common after evening application. It is a carbonic anhydrase inhibitor; metabolic alkalosis may occur.
- *Bacitracin zinc ointment 1%*. Bacitracin is best used for facial burns, around mucous membranes, in patients with sulfa allergy, and for loosening adherent tar or clothing before removal. Advocates note that it is inexpensive, readily available without prescription, and often effective. Bacitracin does not have good eschar penetration, has a narrower spectrum of antibacterial action, and can cause topical sensitization. It has no activity against *Candida albicans*. Controlled trials are needed comparing bacitracin with silver sulfadiazine.
- *Combination*. Some authorities recommend Sulfamylon for morning dressing change and Silvadene for the evening dressing change. The latter is considered painless with less sleep disturbance.
- *Alternatives to topical antibiotics*. Biologic dressings such as pigskin or allografts; biosynthetic dressings such as Integra, Alloderm (LifeCell Corporation, Branchburg, NJ), Epicel (Genzyme, Cambridge, Mass), TransCyte and Biobrane (Smith & Nephew); and Xeroform (Smith & Nephew), a bismuth-impregnated petroleum gauze, produce faster healing and lower infection rates, but need to be placed within 6 hours of injury. Their use is limited by lack of availability at the point of entry to the health care system, high cost, and difficulty of use.

Excision and Skin Grafting

- Benefits of excision of the eschar and skin grafting include prevention of hypertrophic scarring and contractures as well as protection of deep tissues such as muscles and tendons (see Chapter 33, Skin Grafting). Decreases in evaporative fluid loss, pain, and susceptibility to infection are noted. Reduced time for rehabilitation and reduced time in hospital are also significant.
- A negative aspect of early excision and grafting is significant blood loss in a critically ill patient. Decreased blood loss occurs if excision is performed one day and grafting the following day.
- Options for skin grafting with the patient's own skin (autograft) include full-thickness versus split-thickness grafts as well as sheet grafts versus mesh grafts.
- Other grafting materials include allografts (cadaver), xenografts (usually porcine), cultured skin cells, and dermal substitutes such as collagen and bilayer substitutes (both dermal and epidermal components). See also the previous discussion of alternatives to topical antibiotics.

Prevention of Contractures and Hypertrophic Scarring

- Early consultation with a burn specialist or surgeon with burn experience is recommended. Hypertrophic scarring and contractures are best prevented and, once started, are more difficult to treat.
- Hypertrophic scarring can occur up to 2 years after the burn injury.
- There is an increased risk of contracture in deep partial-thickness burns and full-thickness burns, black patients, and at extremes of age range, both young and old.
- Late excision (after 2 weeks) of eschar and skin grafting for deep partial-thickness or full-thickness burns masked by blisters should be done. Nonresorption of blister by 2 weeks is a diagnostic clue.
- Early involvement with physical therapy and occupational therapy decreases contractures. Active range of motion (ROM) and stretching are superior to passive ROM in decreasing the risk of contracture. Avoid splinting of extremity burns if at all possible.
- Pressure dressings decrease hypertrophic scarring, even if initiated as late as 12 months after the burn injury, but early pressure dressing use is superior.
- Silicone sheeting like ReJuveness or Scar Fx (Scar Heal) can reduce hypertrophic scarring if used up to 12 years after the injury.

Ambulatory Management for the Primary Provider

Management of the majority of the 1 million burns per year in the United States occurs in an ambulatory setting. The primary provider is well equipped to manage the initial and follow-up burn care for minor burns. Minor burns involve less than 10% TBSA of adults, less than 5% TBSA of young and old patients, and less than 2% TBSA full-thickness burn; they do not involve the face, hands, feet, genitalia, or respiratory tract. They are not circumferential. These patients do not have significant associated injuries or comorbidities that predispose to infection.

Initial Ambulatory Visit

- Evaluation of burn severity and inclusion of only minor burns.
- Tetanus prophylaxis, if indicated.
- Burn débridement. (Give field block or regional anesthesia for discomfort; remove devitalized tissue, ruptured blisters, and blisters likely to rupture.*)
- Wound washed with mild soap and warm water. (This is a clean but not sterile procedure.*) Skin disinfectants are no longer recommended because they are thought to delay wound healing.
- Wound dressing changes twice a day.*
- Early referral for excision of eschar and skin grafting as outpatient, if indicated.†
- Pain control: nonsteroidal anti-inflammatory drugs or acetaminophen recommended for baseline pain. (Prescribe oral narcotic pain relievers [e.g., acetaminophen with codeine] for before-dressing changes, for breakthrough pain, and at bedtime for pain during sleep.)
- Avoidance of splinting and encouragement of active ROM and stretching.
- Full-thickness burns less than 3 cm in diameter in a nonfunctional, noncosmetic area with normal-thickness skin may be allowed to heal by contracture.
- Patient teaching guide (see the patient education form available online at www.expertconsult.com).
- Follow-up appointment scheduled for the day after the burn injury.

Second Ambulatory Visit

- During the dressing change, reevaluation of burn severity (location, size, and depth), evaluation of pain control, and possible further wound débridement.
- Teaching wound care and dressing changes at this visit.
- Teaching patient to observe for infection, scarring, or other complication.
- Patient referral to physical or occupational therapy for burns involving the hands, feet, or joints.

Subsequent Visits

- Follow-up weekly until the wound is epithelialized. Continue daily follow-up if compliance of patient or communication with provider is not optimal.
- Epithelialized wounds no longer need antibiotic ointments or dressings, but they do need daily sunblock (SPF 15 or higher) for 6 to 24 months to prevent hyperpigmentation. Once repigmentation is complete and the wound no longer blanches from red-pink to white with pressure, additional sunblock is not needed.
- Subsequent follow-up for at least 6 months and reevaluation every 4 to 6 weeks to check for hypertrophic scarring, which can occur up to 2 years after the burn.
- Hypoallergenic, unscented moisturizing creams (cocoa butter, mineral oil, or Vaseline Intensive Care lotion) for pruritus and xerosis. Antihistamines such as diphenhydramine or hydroxyzine pamoate.
- Patient education handout for home care. (See the patient education form available online at www.expertconsult.com.)

Considerations for Referral to Burn Specialist or Surgeon

- Black people, who have increased risk of hypertrophic scars (if not healed at 10 days)
- Children and elderly (if not healed at 2 weeks)
- Adults (if not healed at 3 weeks)
- Wound infection
- Early hypertrophic scarring

*The "Inpatient Management for Primary Provider" section of this chapter includes more extensive discussion of this topic.

†See the "Considerations for Referral to Burn Specialist or Surgeon" section.

PREVENTION

- Encourage installation of smoke detectors on each floor of domestic dwellings, particularly at prenatal visits or well-child visits.
- Encourage parents to teach their children about the proper fire safety precautions, fire escapes, and the hazards of matches and fireworks.
- Encourage families to know and practice fire escape routes. Purchase rope escape ladders for bedrooms on the second floor.
- Advise smokers to quit smoking and not to smoke in bed.

CONCLUSION

Burns are a common problem, most of which can be managed in an ambulatory setting. An understanding of burn depth, high-risk burn locations, and how to estimate the burned percentage of TBSA is necessary for appropriate patient disposition. Understanding the potential complications and management principles for burn injuries permits early and appropriate medical and surgical therapy. Helping patients to understand how to care for their burn injuries and what complications to look for will further decrease the complication rates. For slowly healing wounds, surgical referral for excision and skin grafting can reduce healing time, contractures, and infection. Encourage good prevention practices.

PATIENT EDUCATION GUIDES

See the sample patient education form available online at www.expertconsult.com.

CPT/BILLING CODES

16000	Burns, initial, superficial, when no more than local treatment required
16020	Burns, dressings and/or debridement of partial thickness, initial or subsequent, small (less than 5% TBSA)
16025	Burns, dressings and/or débridement, medium
16030	Burns, dressings and/or débridement, large
16035	Burns, escharotomy, initial incision
16036	Burns, escharotomy, each additional incision

See Chapter 33, Skin Grafting, for procedural coding for skin grafts or skin substitutes.

ICD-9-CM DIAGNOSTIC CODES

940.X	Burn, unspecified
940–947.X	Burns by specific site. Fourth digit of the code (0 to 5) indicates depth or severity.
948.XX	Burns classified according to extent of body surface involved. Fourth digit of the code indicates percentage of TBSA involved (0 = <10%, 1 = 10% to 19%, and so on up to 9 = 90% or more involved). Fifth digit of the code indicates percentage of TBSA involved in full-thickness burns.

ACKNOWLEDGMENT

The editors wish to recognize the contributions by J. Fintan Copper, MD, and Timothy J. Downs, MD, FAAFP, to this chapter in the previous edition of this book.

SUPPLIERS

(See contact information online at www.expertconsult.com.)

Genzyme Biosurgery
Integra LifeSciences Corp.
Kendall Customer Service c/o Covidien
LifeCell Corporation
ReJuveness, LLC
ScarHeal, Inc.
Smith & Nephew, Inc.

ONLINE RESOURCES

Advanced Burn Life Support course online. Available at www.aba.sitelms.org.

American Burn Association (listing regional burn centers by state). Available at www.ameriburn.org.

BIBLIOGRAPHY

Baxter CR: Management of burn wounds. Dermatol Clin 11:709–714, 1993.

Cameron JL (ed): Current Surgical Therapy, 6th ed. St. Louis, Mosby, 1998.

Clardy PF, Manaker S: Carbon monoxide poisoning. In Rose BD (ed): UpToDate. Waltham, Mass, UpToDate, 2008. Available at www.uptodate.com/home/index.html.

Holm C, Mayr M, Tegeler J, et al: A clinical randomized study on the effects of invasive monitoring on burn shock resuscitation. Burns 30:798–807, 2004.

Johnson KR: Sunburn. In Rose BD (ed): UpToDate. Waltham, Mass, UpToDate, 2008. Available at www.uptodate.com/home/index.html.

Lewis DP: Burns: Initial management and outpatient follow-up. Fam Pract Recert 23:19, 2001.

Monafo WW: Initial management of burns. N Engl J Med 335:1581–1586, 1996.

Morgan ED, Bledsoe SC, Barker J: Ambulatory management of burns. Am Fam Physician 62:2015–2026, 2000.

Morgan ED, Miser WF: Treatment of minor thermal burns. In Rose BD (ed): UpToDate. Waltham, Mass, UpToDate, 2008. Available at www.uptodate.com/home/index.html.

Papini R: ABC of burns: Management of burn injuries of various depths. BMJ 329:158–160, 2004.

Rice PL: Emergency care of moderate and severe thermal burns in adults. In Rose BD (ed): UpToDate. Waltham, Mass, UpToDate, 2008. Available at www.uptodate.com/home/index.html.

CHAPTER 14

CRYOSURGERY

James W. McNabb • John L. Pfenninger

Cryosurgery is the deliberate destruction of diseased tissue by freezing in a controlled manner. It is important that all primary care physicians master the art and technique of cryosurgery. The procedure is often a better alternative than surgical excision, especially when convenience, healing, disability during healing, infectious disease risk (human immunodeficiency virus, hepatitis), discomfort, and scar formation are considered. (See also Chapter 138, Cryotherapy of the Cervix.)

GENERAL CONSIDERATIONS

- Lesions treated with cryosurgery usually heal with minimal or no scar formation. Even if inadvertent excessive freezing is done, scarring is rarely significant.
- Complete healing may take more than 6 to 8 weeks in extreme cases, but the results are usually excellent. Selective destruction of cells occurs during the freeze. However, the collagen and fibroelastic structural framework is preserved, so the epithelial cells grow back in an organized fashion within the preserved matrix.
- The procedure is safe, simple, and easy to learn. It usually takes less time than conventional surgery.
- Patients may prefer to avoid injections of local anesthetic, which is usually possible with cryosurgery.
- A burning sensation is experienced with the initial freeze and again on thawing. Explain to patients that the freezing will feel like an ice cube stuck to the skin. This often reassures them enough to cope with the minimal amount of pain experienced. However, young children often will not accept the procedure without crying. Their fear of the unknown increases when the unpleasant cold sensation starts. They have difficulty trusting that the burning feeling will actually improve in a very short time instead of continually getting worse. In children and in some adults, a local anesthetic will be helpful, especially when freezing multiple or large lesions and when attempting a deep freeze for malignant lesions.
- Other than keeping the lesions clean and protected, patients can essentially ignore the cryotreated lesion between treatments. They appreciate the omission of suture insertion and removal. Patients also welcome being able to bathe and swim while the lesion is healing.
- Secondary infection usually is not a significant problem. Even with overfreezing and with cryosensitive patients who overreact with excessive tissue destruction, infection occurs rarely. Excessive freezing may result in wound weeping for longer than 1 to 2 weeks, but infection should not be expected unless the area receives poor skin care.
- Occasionally, a profuse watery discharge may persist more than 3 to 4 days after treatment. Débridement of the wound often alleviates the discharge.
- Two concerns exist regarding cryosurgery and use of the nitrous oxide closed system. The first is the spread of infectious agents by the equipment. Cryoprobes must be cleaned and sterilized between procedures using Cidex or an autoclave. Second, there can be adverse health effects from prolonged exposure to nitrous oxide at high levels—far higher than will ever be experienced using nitrous oxide closed systems for cryosurgery for mere minutes at a time. Air hunger, dizziness, confusion, headaches, nausea, vomiting, and loss of consciousness or death may occur if nitrous oxide is present in quantities sufficient to dilute the oxygen concentration in the air. This overexposure creates an altered (euphoric or excited) mental state. Long-term exposure to nitrous oxide has been associated with neuropathy, increased rates of spontaneous abortion, and congenital anomalies in offspring. Federal regulations require nitrous oxide gas to be vented outside of the examination/treatment room. This can be accomplished by simply extending the exhaust tube on the unit out a window or by installing vents in an outside wall. The likelihood of a patient receiving enough exposure to do harm is very small and has not yet been reported. In practice, considering the minimal amounts of nitrous oxide used, few practitioners "vent" the rooms. Carbon dioxide (which is an agent nearly as cold) can be substituted for nitrous oxide, if a closed system is desired.

ADVANTAGES OF CRYOTHERAPY (CRYOSURGERY)

- Local anesthesia is optional, so needles can usually be avoided.
- Freezing usually produces only minimal pain.
- Final healing is cosmetically excellent, with minimal or no scarring.
- Minimal physician time is required, and the procedure is easy to learn.
- Preoperative skin preparation is not required.
- Multiple lesions can be treated quickly in one office visit.
- Postoperative infection is rare.
- No complicated postprocedure care is needed.
- No significant disruption of postprocedure activity is required.
- The procedure is ideal for patients with light-complexioned skin.
- The procedure is inexpensive and cost effective.
- A wide variety of lesions can be treated without significant exposure to blood-borne pathogens.
- Units are portable and can be taken to nursing home facilities when needed.
- Units are relatively inexpensive with low start-up costs.
- Units take up little space in the office.

DISADVANTAGES OF CRYOSURGERY

- Use is limited in patients with darker skin because of pigment changes. Even with brief partial-thickness freeze technique, some melanocytes are destroyed and the healed cryolesion may be slightly lighter in color than the surrounding skin, even in fair-skinned individuals.
- Cryosurgery is not recommended in areas of hair growth, such as around the eyebrows and eyelashes, and on scalps with thin hair, because even brief freezing tends to destroy hair follicles.

- Healed cryolesions may not tan sufficiently, often are more susceptible to sunburn, and may require added sunscreen protection.
- Tissue is not available for histopathologic diagnosis, so certainty of complete removal is lacking.
- There is the possibility of exposure to nitrous oxide gas if closed units are used (see earlier).

Agents Used for Cryosurgery

There are three basic methods of cryosurgery (Table 14-1).

1. Closed systems (freezing is carried out with a cooled probe as opposed to the application of the agent itself)
   - Nitrous oxide
   - Carbon dioxide
   - CryoPen
2. Liquid nitrogen
   - Thermos bottle/spray unit (Brymill; Wallach)
   - Cotton-tipped applicators and Styrofoam cup
3. Aerosol canister
   - Tetrafluoroethane (Verruca-Freeze, Medi-Frig)
   - Ether/propane (Histofreezer)

Nitrous oxide is quite unstable, and once it is released into the probe, it immediately breaks down to molecular nitrogen and oxygen. The physical characteristics of the nitrous oxide gas enable the cryotip's temperature to be easily lowered to its boiling point of −89° C. With *carbon dioxide*, the tip is not as cold, and it will take slightly longer to achieve a quality freeze (−78.5° C).

Nitrous oxide comes in a closed gas cylinder (blue tank, versus brown for carbon dioxide and green for oxygen). The hand-held cryogun, which is connected to the tank with tubing, is structured differently from the liquid nitrogen guns. It is designed to allow a controlled, rapid expansion of nitrous oxide gas within the cryoprobe tip, lowering its temperature to −89° C. The storage tanks preserve nitrous oxide virtually "forever" by keeping the gas under pressure with no port for evaporation (except for cryogun activation). The tanks are moved from storage to use on small carts. The cryoprobes (tips) come in numerous shapes and sizes to match the lesion to be treated. The rounded, pointed, and slanted flat tips are popular for dermatologic applications (Fig. 14-1). The hemorrhoid tip is rarely, if ever, used for hemorrhoids, but its shape allows use for multiple dermatologic lesions. The flat and slightly conical 19- and 25-mm tips that are used for cryosurgery of the cervix can also be used for dermatologic applications.

Because nitrous oxide does not achieve a probe temperature as low as liquid nitrogen (−89° C versus −196° C), it is significantly slower at freezing tissue. This is especially important when treating multiple lesions. Both nitrous oxide and liquid nitrogen are effective for treating malignancies. Overlapping treatment areas for larger lesions using large probes ensures efficacy. Nitrous oxide units have an active defrost mode that rapidly frees the cryotip from frozen tissue.

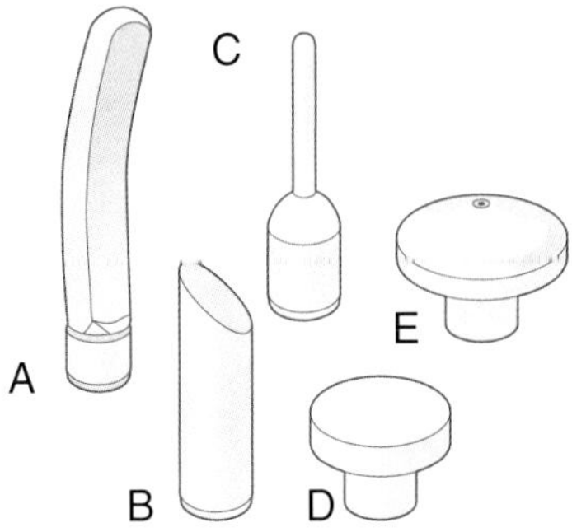

Figure 14-1 Sample of varying shapes of cryoprobe tips. Most come in variable sizes. **A,** Hemorrhoid tip. **B,** Slanted flat tip. **C,** Pointed tip. **D,** Flat cervical tip. **E,** Slight conical cervical tip.

CryoPen is a closed, self-contained refrigerant system. It uses an internal cryogen that is cooled in a free-standing unit to −95° C. It eliminates the handling of cryogen gases and liquids. CryoPen reusable tips are available in 3-, 5-, 7-, and 10-mm sizes. These are applied directly to the lesion and maintained in place until the clinical end point has been reached.

Liquid nitrogen is the coldest cryogen, effecting a rapid, deep freeze (boiling point −196° C). A large storage container (Dewar) is needed. Newer Dewars can store the liquid nitrogen for up to 1 year. Liquid nitrogen is relatively inexpensive, but if not used it will evaporate. Liquid nitrogen may be applied to the lesion directly using cotton-tipped applicators or sprayed using a thermos-type unit (Brymill CRY-AC and CRY-AC-3 [Brymill Cryogenic Systems, Ellington, Conn], or Wallach UltraFreeze [Wallach Surgical Devices, Orange, Conn]). The various apertures of the spray tips allow a variable amount of gas to cover a lesion, allowing control over the extent of freezing. A reusable plastic shield is available to limit gas spread. These spray units allow efficient and rapid treatment of multiple lesions in a single office visit. Additional probes are available that allow the thermos to be used as a closed system, but there is no active defrost. Subsequently, the tip may "stick" to the tissue for a significant length of time before it thaws and detaches.

Canister refrigerants are the least expensive agents used for cryosurgery. They come prepackaged in small hand-held canisters the

TABLE 14-1 Cryogenic Agents

	Agents				
Characteristics	**Liquid Nitrogen**	**N_2O**	**CO_2**	**Tetrafluoroethane**	**Ether/Propane**
Boiling point	−196° C	−89° C	−78.5° C	−47° C	−25° C
Effective treatment temperature	−196° C	−89° C	−78.5° C	−70° C	−55° C
Use	Thermos-type guns Cotton-tip applicator Stored in large Dewars	Cylinders with applicator gun (cryoprobe)	Cylinders with applicator gun (cryoprobe) Dry ice slush	Aerosol canister	Aerosol canister
Method/system	Open/closed	Closed	Closed/open	Open (spray/cones, buds)	Open (buds)
Shelf life	1 yr max. with best Dewars	Indefinite	Indefinite	5 yr	5 yr +
Flammable	No	No	No	No	Yes
Trade name	Cryogun (Brymill Cryogenic Systems) UltraFreeze (Wallach)	—	—	Verruca-Freeze (CryoSurgery) Medi-Frig (Ellman International)	Histofreezer (OraSure Technologies)
Indications	All	All	All	Superficial only (no cancers)	Superficial only (no cancers)

size of a soda can, making them portable for use in nursing homes, satellite clinics, and multiple examination rooms. They have a very long shelf life. Unfortunately, they do not achieve tissue temperatures low enough to treat very many lesions. These agents are *not* indicated for malignancies, deep lesions, or large lesions. *Trifluoroethane/pentafluoroethane/tetrafluoroethane* (Verruca-Freeze [CryoSurgery, Nashville, Tenn; Medi-Frig [Ellman International, Oceanside, NY]) is a nonflammable compressed gas that freezes tissue on vaporization (boiling point −47° C). *Dimethyl ether/propane/isobutane* (Histofreezer [OraSure Technologies, Bethlehem, Penn]) also comes in a canister but is not as cold (−25° C) and is flammable.

Over-the-counter skin refrigerants were approved for use by the U.S. Food and Drug Administration in 2003. Several products are available, including Dr. Scholl's Freeze Away, Wartner Plantar Wart Removal System, and Compound W Freeze Off. The first two products contain dimethyl ether and propane. Wartner's product also adds isobutane to these. Although the manufacturers state that temperatures as low as −57° C are achieved on skin application, such low temperatures were not realized in a recent study. There is significant concern regarding their ability to create local tissue necrosis because of their inability to reach low temperatures rapidly enough to achieve clinical effect. In contrast to other physician-applied options, these over-the-counter products are also dangerous because they are extremely flammable.

Tissue Effects: Principles for Treatment

It is important to recognize that at −2.2° C, cells begin to freeze. At −5° C, cells will supercool, but they recover. Tissue destruction begins only when the temperature is between −10° C and −20° C. A deeper freeze with temperatures between −40° C and −50° C ensures that malignant cells are completely destroyed.

The size of the ice ball that forms around the lesion provides a good estimate of the depth of the freeze. The *lethal zone* (tissue temperature less than −20° C) is 2 to 3 mm *inside* the outer margin of the ice ball (Fig. 14-2). This is especially crucial to remember in cases of premalignant or malignant lesions, which are deeper in the skin. *The size of the ice ball beyond the lesion is the most important criterion in determining how long to freeze.* Factors requiring prolonged freeze time include low tank pressure, increased tissue vascularity, excessive overlying keratin (needs to be removed or moistened), and poor tip-to-lesion contact. The use of different systems (e.g., nitrous oxide, liquid nitrogen, carbon dioxide, canister gases) dramatically affects the rapidity and depth of freeze. Likewise, the method of applying liquid nitrogen (with the cotton-tipped applicator or in a spray fashion) affects freezing parameters. Once an ice ball of the desired size has been obtained, it is just as important to observe *the time it takes for the area to thaw from the outer edge of the ice ball to the lesion edge* ("*halo thaw time*") and *the time for all the tissue to thaw* (*total thaw time*; Box 14-1). A brief freeze can turn tissue white, providing the ice ball desired; however, if it remains frozen only momentarily, it will have little effect.

Freeze times should be adjusted according to patient sensitivity, type and size of the lesion, presence of malignancy, and lesion vascularity. Table 14-2 shows the variations with nitrous oxide alone,

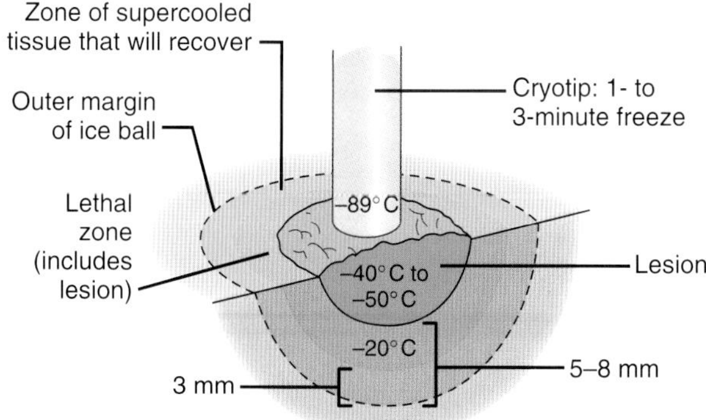

Figure 14-2 Nitrous oxide full-thickness destruction freeze technique (malignant lesions). Note that the outer supercooled area will recover. Monitoring thaw times for both malignant and benign lesions is extremely important (see Box 14-1).

Box 14-1. Freezing Guidelines for Skin

Benign Lesions
- Ice ball 2 mm beyond lesion borders.
- Correlate with thaw times (see below).
- Consider double freeze for difficult and/or premalignant lesions.

Malignant and Most Premalignant Lesions
- Ice ball 5 mm beyond lesion borders.
- Double freeze (freeze, thaw, refreeze, using same parameters).

Freeze Time
- Variable, depending on cryogen, pressure applied, size of lesion, type of lesion, size of nozzle/tip, expertise of operator.
- Second freeze is faster.

Halo Thaw Time
- 1 min (benign).
- 2–4 min (malignant).

Total Thaw Time
- 2–3 min (benign).
- 3–5 min (malignant).

Liquid Nitrogen
- Small swab (small lesions) and large swab (large lesions).
  - 10-sec freeze.
  - Total thaw time: 60 sec (superficial lesions).
- Spray: as noted above for other applications.

See text for details and for specific lesions.

TABLE 14-2 Freeze Time Guidelines for Nitrous Oxide Technique

Tissue	Lesion	Freeze Time*
Skin	Full-thickness, benign	1–1.5 min
	Full-thickness, malignant	1.5–3 min†
	Plantar warts (after débridement)	40 sec
	Condylomata	20–45 sec
	Verrucae	1–1.5 min
	Vascular lesions (with pressure)	1–1.5 min
	Seborrheic keratoses (2-mm margin)	30 sec†
	Actinic keratoses (3-mm margin)	1–1.5 min†
	Basal cell cancer (3- to 5-mm margin)	1.5 min†
Vascular	Hemorrhoids	
	Cryoligation	2 min
	Cryo without ligation	2–3 min†
Cervix	Cervicitis	3 min
	Cervical intraepithelial neoplasia I, II, III	3 min†
	Cervical intraepithelial neoplasia I, II (alternative method)	5 min

*Freeze times are approximate guidelines and should be adjusted to the size of the ice ball and the thaw time, which are far more important than the freeze time alone. Because nitrous oxide is slower and more controlled, freeze times are more reliable than with liquid nitrogen.
†Freeze-thaw-refreeze.

TABLE 14-3 Freeze Time Guidelines for Liquid Nitrogen Open-Spray Technique

Lesion	Common Freeze Time in Seconds
Actinic keratoses	5–15
Cherry angioma	5–10
Condylomata	5–10
Keloids	20–30
Lentigines	5–10
Molluscum contagiosum	5–10
Mucocele	10–30
Papilloma	5–10
Prurigo nodularis	10–30
Sebaceous hyperplasia	5–10
Seborrheic keratoses	10
Skin tags	5–10
Common warts	10–20

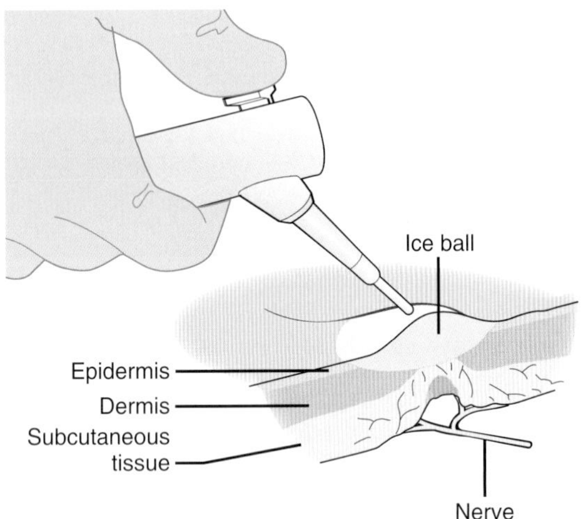

Figure 14-3 With nitrous oxide, once the cryotip is frozen to the skin, the probe can be retracted to avoid freezing nontarget underlying structures.

and Table 14-3 shows those with liquid nitrogen. Age, vascular flow, amount of pigment, depth of lesion, amount of keratin, location on the body, and cell type of the lesion all affect the amount of freezing required to destroy pathologic tissue. Adjust your freeze times accordingly. Applying pressure to the lesion with the fixed probes will increase the depth of freeze. Vascular lesions will require longer freezing times, and pressure from the probe should be applied to squeeze as much blood as possible out of the lesion before freezing. Any active bleeding from a prior shave or curettement will need to be controlled first.

For *benign lesions*, a single freeze/thaw cycle is sufficient. The ice ball should extend 2 to 3 mm beyond most lesion margins. Resistant lesions such as warts often require a freeze/thaw/freeze cycle. Complete thaw times should be 2 to 3 minutes for larger lesions.

For *malignant or premalignant lesions*, a freeze/thaw/freeze cycle is recommended. The ice ball should extend 5 mm beyond the lesion margin each time the tissue is frozen. The second freeze is usually quicker and less painful.

Dry, keratinized tissue will not freeze easily and insulates the lesion underneath from freezing. Remove as much keratin as possible before freezing, especially when using nitrous oxide, carbon dioxide, or the canister agents.

With the nitrous oxide cryotips, once the tip is "frozen" and fixed to the skin, the probe can be pulled back, tenting up the skin, to reduce the depth of freeze, thereby sparing deeper critical structures (such as nerves) from exposure to freezing (Fig. 14-3).

Bandages are not necessary unless the lesion is continually irritated (i.e., by clothing), develops a large blister, or develops a serous discharge.

Post-Treatment Physiologic Effects

Erythema and hyperemia are immediate responses to effective freezing. Edema and exudation (blister formation) peak within 24 to 48 hours and usually subside after 72 hours (Fig. 14-4). Blood may accumulate under the blister, making it appear black (Fig. 14-5). The extracellular collagen structures are more resistant to freezing than the cells themselves. Crust formation begins, and this crust will slowly contract over the next several days. Reepithelialization occurs from the outer margin inward. Fibroblasts lay down minimal new collagen along the preserved, well-formed collagen matrix, resulting in a lack of scar formation. If the collagen matrix has been destroyed by excessive cryoinjury, fibroblasts will produce collagen randomly, leading to scar formation (Fig. 14-6). Cartilage (e.g., in the ear) is preserved.

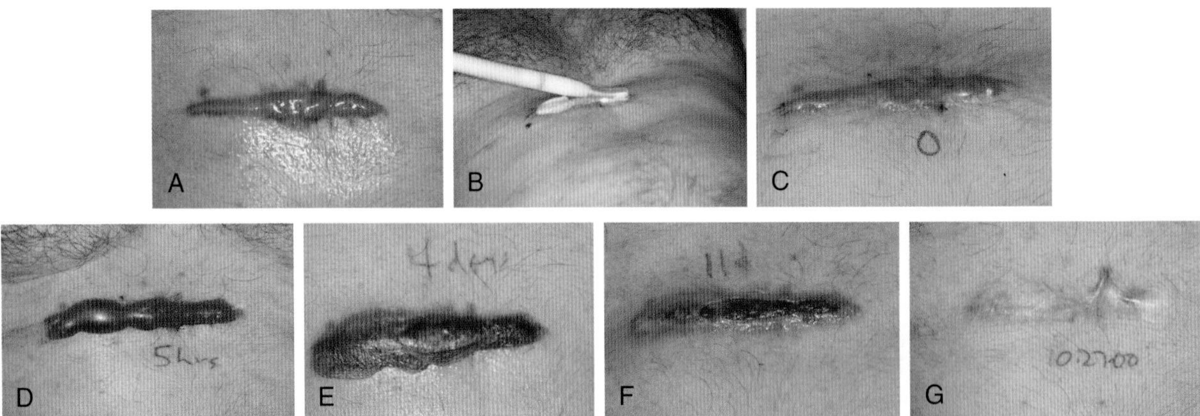

Figure 14-4 **A,** A 10-cm hypertrophic scar over upper abdomen. **B,** Application of nitrous oxide probe. **C,** Appearance immediately after thawing. **D,** Blister formation at 5 hours. **E,** Ruptured blister at 4 days. **F,** Appearance at 11 days. **G,** Final appearance after a second cryotherapy treatment several months later; the small residual scar resolved after the third focal treatment.

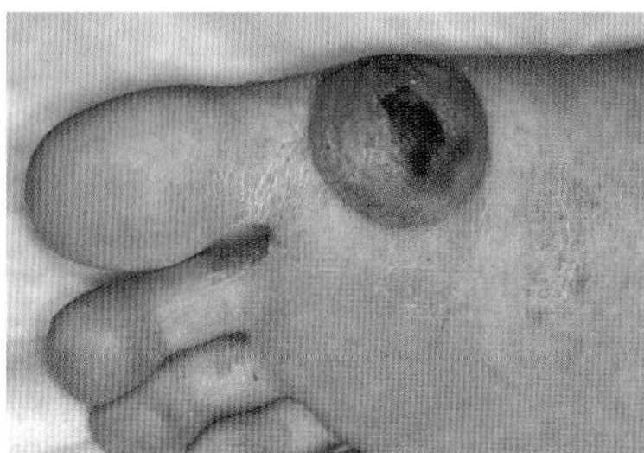

Figure 14-5 Appearance of a hemorrhagic bulb after cryotherapy of a plantar wart.

If the patient or physician desires, the treated lesion can be surgically débrided in 24 to 48 hours. During this time, the dermis and epidermis separate, lifting the lesion to the top of the blister. Removal of the prepared lesion with iris scissors is painless. After 72 hours, however, the lesion may stick like a graft and may bleed on attempts at removal. If completely left alone, the lesion will eventually slough spontaneously. (Surgical débridement 1 or 2 days after freezing effectively removes the lesion and satisfies some patients sooner. However, many patients are quite happy to avoid the early return visit and are willing to wait to see how much of the lesion sloughs before returning for another treatment.) A disadvantage of this technique is that a second office visit is needed for the 24- to 48-hour débridement procedure, and the serous discharge without the intact blister can be quite copious depending on the size of the lesion.

The healed cryolesion is soft, with minimal to no scarring. This allows erections if penile lesions have been frozen. Pigment is often decreased, and hair and sweat glands may be destroyed in the area of freezing. It is best to caution the patient *in advance* that although the area that was frozen is unlikely to develop much of a scar, the skin is often lighter. The inflammatory response may result in the development of a transient halo of hyperpigmentation. This will usually clear completely over several months.

Indications

- Actinic keratoses (full-thickness freeze)
- Angiomas or hemangiomas, including congenital strawberry hemangiomas (more difficult)
- Basal cell carcinoma (full-thickness destructive double-freeze)
- Bowen's disease (squamous cell carcinoma in situ)
- Cervical intraepithelial neoplasia (CIN, dysplasia), "cryoconization" (see Chapter 138, Cryotherapy of the Cervix)
- Chondrodermatitis helicis nodularis
- Condylomata acuminata
- Dermatofibromas (difficult)
- Freckles (lentigines)
- Granulation tissue
- Hemorrhoids (rarely done)
- Hypertrophic scars (often multiple treatments over time)
- Keloids (as for hypertrophic scars)
- Lentigos
- Molluscum contagiosum
- Mucocele
- Myxoid cysts
- Papular nevi (full-thickness freeze)
- Pyogenic granuloma
- Squamous cell carcinoma (full-thickness destructive double-freeze)
- Seborrheic keratoses (procedure of choice)
- Skin tags and polyps
- Verrucae (including plantar)
- Xanthoma

Contraindications

Absolute Contraindications

- Proven excessive reaction to cryosurgery
- Patient nonacceptance of the possibility of skin pigment changes
- Malignant melanoma
- Areas of end-stage compromised circulation
- Lesions in which identification of tissue pathology is required
- Sclerosing (morpheaform) or recurrent basal cell or squamous cell carcinoma

Relative Contraindications

- Basal cell or squamous cell carcinomas more than 1 cm in diameter
- Any condition with high levels of cryoglobulins (most are noted in this list)
- Immunoproliferative neoplasms (e.g., myeloma, lymphoma)
- Macroglobulinemia
- Active severe collagen vascular diseases
- Severe active ulcerative colitis
- Acute poststreptococcal glomerulonephritis (almost 100% of these patients have high levels of cryoglobulins)
- Active subacute bacterial endocarditis, syphilis, Epstein-Barr virus infection, cytomegalovirus infection
- Chronic severe hepatitis B
- High-dose steroid therapy

NOTE: The majority of patients with the preceding conditions are likely to have an exaggerated response to cryosurgery because they have high levels of circulating cryoglobulins. If cryosurgery is appropriate or necessary for any of these patients, be sure to obtain informed consent and perform a pretest in the axilla or thigh area before treating a more prominent or cosmetically sensitive area. Proceed with caution and greatly shorten the freezing times until the response can be predicted. You may be able to freeze lesions effectively and safely with a much shorter freeze time. With overfreezing, the risk of tissue slough and marked hypopigmentation increases. Therefore, start slowly and advise patients that extra visits and treatment sessions may be necessary. A conservative approach is best in light of their clinical situation.

Lesions Difficult to Treat with Cryosurgery

- Dermatofibroma (these lesions require a longer freeze time)
- Hidradenitis
- Flat nevi (must be absolutely sure the lesion in not a melanoma)
- Squamous cell cancer (usually reserved for practitioners who treat this cancer often)
- Most vascular lesions (especially if extensive)

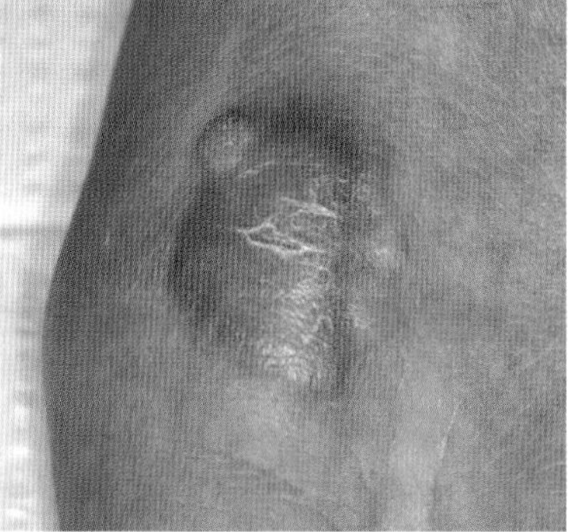

Figure 14-6 Excessive scarring (rare) after cryosurgery of verrucous lesion over first metatarsophalangeal joint of the large toe on the left foot.

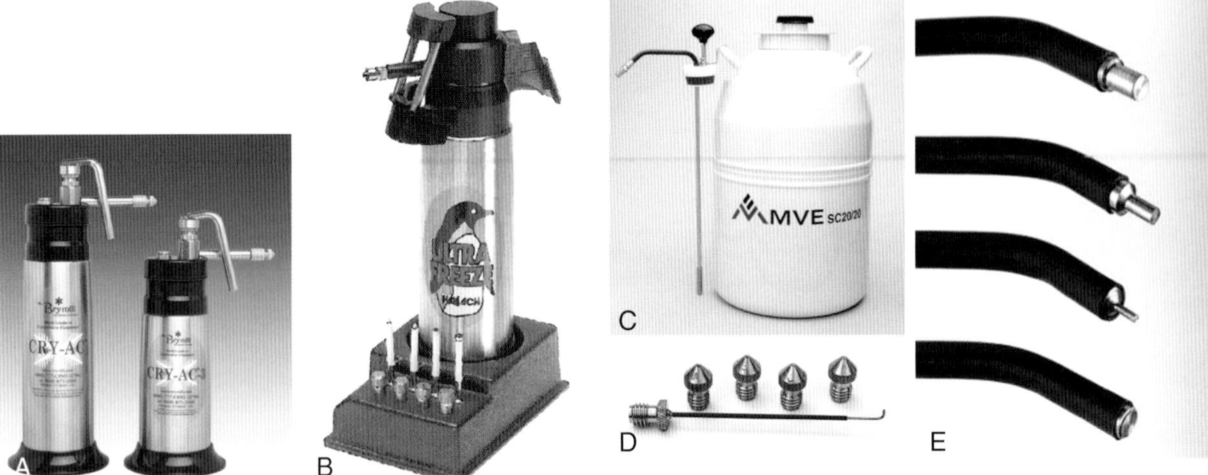

Figure 14-7 **A,** Brymill CRY-AC cryoguns are refillable with liquid nitrogen. **B,** Wallach UltraFreeze Cryosurgical System. **C,** Liquid nitrogen Dewar. **D,** Brymill open-spray aperture tips (openings of tip vary in size, with "A" the largest). **E,** Brymill closed miniprobes. (**A** and **C–E,** Courtesy of Brymill Cryogenic Systems, Ellington, Conn. **B,** Courtesy of Wallach Surgical Devices, Orange, Conn.)

Areas Not Recommended for Cryosurgery

- Areas where hair loss is critical to the patient
- Areas where pigment changes are critical to the patient
- Feet, ankles, and lower legs, when circulation is in question (especially patients with diabetes or peripheral vascular disease)
- Over superficial cutaneous nerves (unless adequate skin traction to pull the skin away from the nerve is possible, usually with nitrous oxide technique)
- Basal cell cancers in the nasolabial fold, in preauricular areas, and on lips (often more extensive and tend to recur)
- Any cancer that has not had histologic confirmation
- Periorbital area (may induce immediate and severe swelling)
- Port wine stain (use laser)

Equipment

Liquid Nitrogen

- Cryogen spray unit (Fig. 14-7A and B)
- Storage Dewar (Fig. 14-7 C)
- Assorted various-sized nozzles (Fig. 14-7D and E)
- Protective plastic shield with assorted opening sizes (Fig. 14-8)
- Styrofoam cups (if thermos canister is not available)
- Cotton-tipped applicators (small and large)
- Metal pickups (optional; Fig. 14-9)

Nitrous Oxide

- 20-lb tank (the "short, fat, blue one"; Fig. 14-10A)
- Mobile storage cart (see Fig. 14-10A)
- Cryoprobe regulator with gun (Fig. 14-10B)
- Cryoprobe tip assortment (Fig. 14-11)
- K-Y Jelly or cryogen gel; do not use anything that is not water soluble (e.g., petrolatum)

Canister Gas Refrigerants

- Can of Verruca-Freeze (Fig. 14-12A) or Medi-Frig (Fig. 14-12B) with various sizes of plastic limiting cones and buds (see Fig. 14-12A and C)
- Can of Histofreezer with applicators

CryoPen

- CryoPen base unit (Fig. 14-13)
- CryoPen reusable tips (3-, 5-, 7-, and 10-mm sizes)

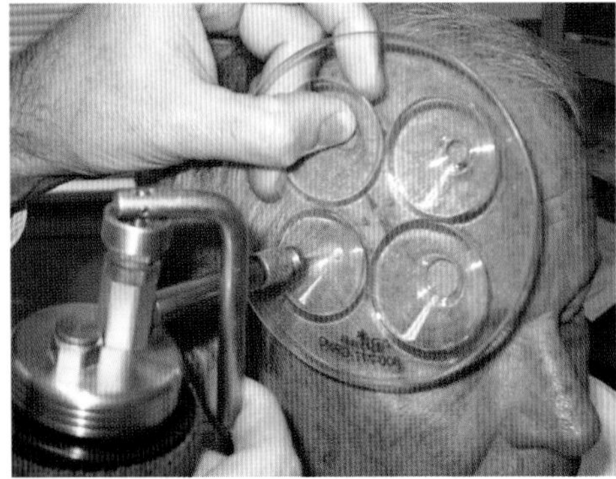

Figure 14-8 Protective shield (Brymill) with various-sized orifices, which limits the spread of open-spray liquid nitrogen and protects surrounding skin.

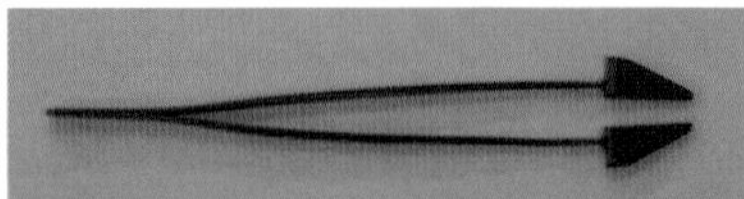

Figure 14-9 Special cryosurgical forceps (Brymill) with extra mass at tips to allow freezing of multiple lesions before recooling. No anesthesia is needed.

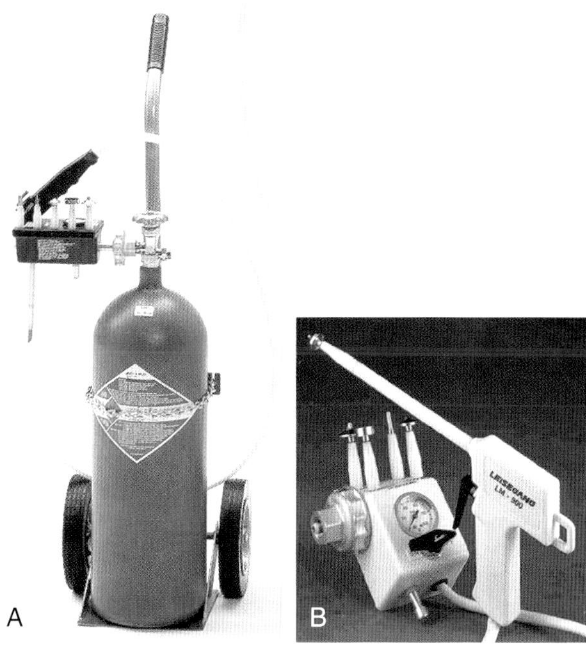

Figure 14-10 **A,** Nitrous oxide cryosurgical unit. Handpiece is placed in holder and connected to a 20-lb tank. **B,** Leisegang cryosurgical hand gun.

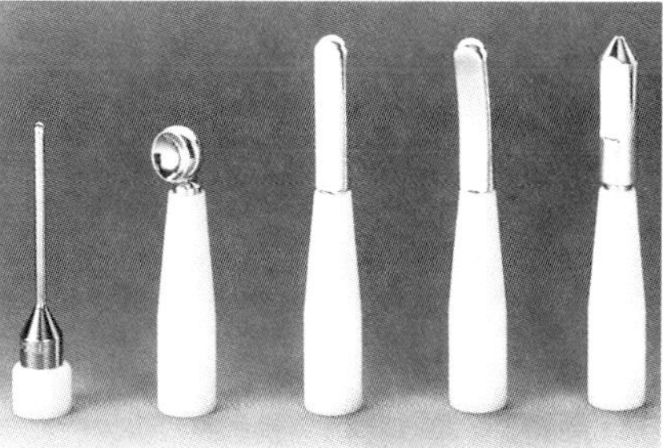

Figure 14-11 Various cryosurgical tips for treatment of a variety of dermatologic lesions with nitrous oxide. *Left to right:* Fine point, small cup, round tip, hemorrhoid tip, and slightly coned tip. (Also see Chapter 138, Cryotherapy of the Cervix.)

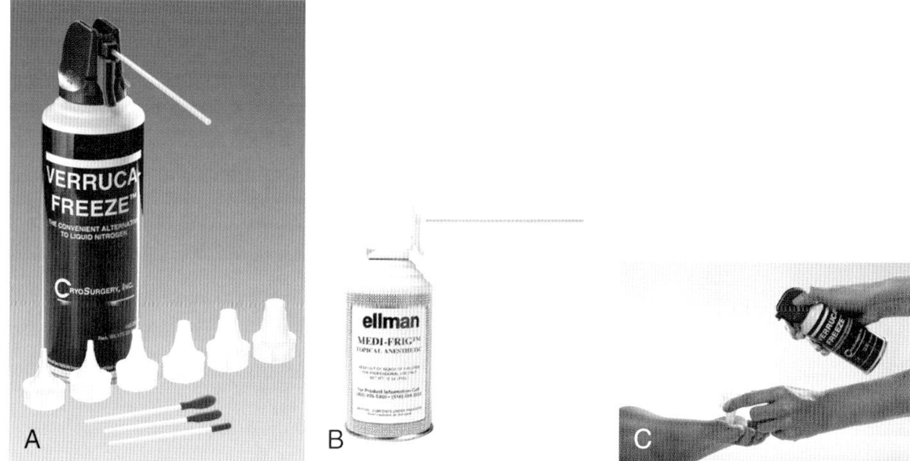

Figure 14-12 **A,** Self-contained Verruca-Freeze unit with various sizes of specula. **B,** Medi-Frig. **C,** Application of Verruca-Freeze using a transparent limiting cone. (**B,** Courtesy of Ellman International, Inc, Oceanside, NY.)

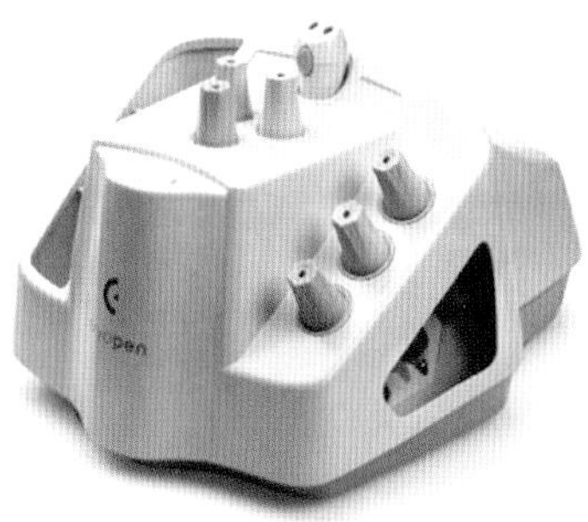

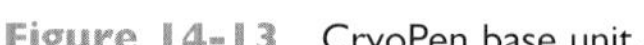

Figure 14-13 CryoPen base unit.

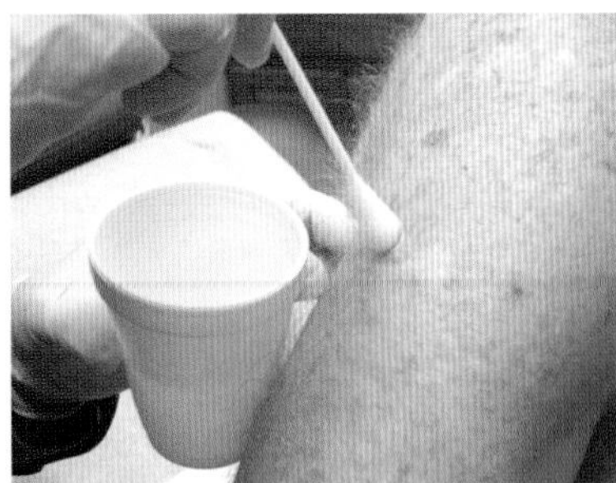

Figure 14-14 Liquid nitrogen applied directly to a skin lesion using the dipstick technique.

PREPROCEDURE PATIENT PREPARATION

Before the procedure, the patient should be advised of the basic technique, the expected sensation during treatment, and the possible complications. The advantages of and rationale for using cryosurgery also should be reviewed with the patient.

For all methods listed, consider local anesthesia for patient comfort and the ability to freeze long enough to obtain the desired effect. The need for anesthesia will depend on the size of the lesion, number of lesions, patient age, and other factors.

TECHNIQUE

Liquid Nitrogen

Cup/Cotton-Tipped Applicator or Metal Pickups Technique

1. Dispense a small amount of liquid nitrogen into a Styrofoam cup to prevent contaminating the primary source of liquid nitrogen.
2. Choose the size of the cotton-tipped applicator to match lesion.
3. Dip a clean cotton-tipped applicator into the cup and then touch the lesion with the applicator.
4. Keep the applicator cold by dipping it into the cup every several seconds and reapplying to the lesion to obtain the desired size of ice ball (Fig. 14-14). Do not place a cotton-tipped applicator that has touched the patient, or the treatment cup supply, into the primary source of liquid nitrogen because contamination can occur. Likewise, do not return any unused liquid into the Dewar. Viruses often are not killed by the cold and may be spread to others if contamination of the source occurs.
5. The size of the applicator and amount of pressure applied affect rapidity and depth of freeze.
6. Freezing times are markedly shortened with liquid nitrogen. The cotton-tipped applicator/cup method is not as fast as the cryogun, but it is still significantly faster than nitrous oxide and can be used readily for small lesions, if benign or premalignant (e.g., actinic keratosis).
7. A variant of the foregoing method can be used for pedunculated lesions such as skin tags. Metal needle drivers or metal pickups are dipped into the cup of liquid nitrogen. The lesions are then grasped. This technique limits the spread of the freeze and is very effective (Fig. 14-15).

Spray Technique Using a Cryogen Spray Gun: Brymill CRY-AC or Wallach UltraFreeze

The timed-spot freeze technique allows standardization of liquid nitrogen delivery.

1. *Select the nozzle size.* The "C" tip is the one chosen most commonly for use with the Brymill; this size is a starting point. Although the "D" has a smaller opening, the "B" tip has a larger orifice and can treat large lesions faster. The "A" tip is larger still (Fig. 14-7D).
2. *Position the nozzle* of the spray gun perpendicular to the lesion, 1 to 1.5 cm from the skin surface and aimed at the center of the target lesion (Fig. 14-16A). A tangential spray can be used to create a slower, more controlled freeze.
3. *Spray the lesion.* The spray gun trigger is depressed and liquid nitrogen is sprayed until an ice ball encompasses the lesion and the desired margin (see Box 14-1). The spray needs to be maintained in either a continuous or intermittent fashion to keep the target field frozen for an adequate time. This time may vary from 5 to 30 seconds. Spraying intermittently will keep the ice ball smaller. If more than one freeze/thaw cycle is required for lesion destruction, complete thawing should be allowed before the next cycle is started (usually 2 to 3 minutes; see Table 14-3).
4. *Little movement of the gun is needed* unless the lesion is large (>2 cm). Usually it is a direct spray technique as described previously. For large lesions, overlapping direct sprays can be

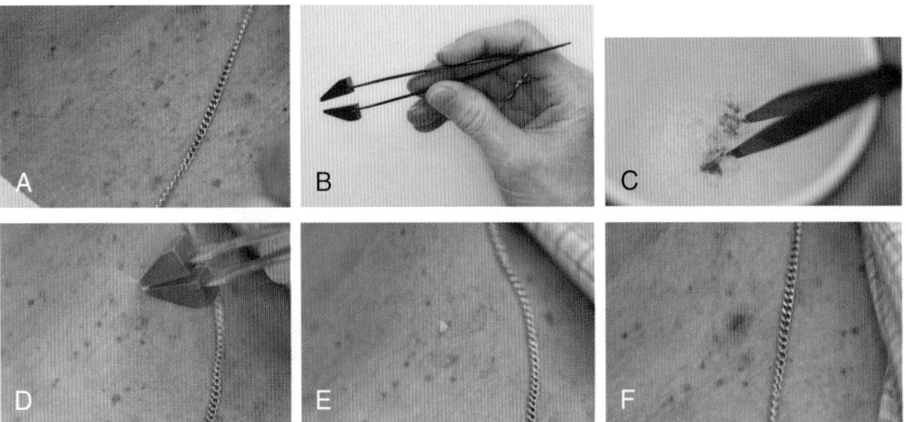

Figure 14-15 The treatment of a skin tag using cryosurgical forceps. **A,** Skin tag. **B,** Forceps. **C,** Forceps in Styrofoam cup with liquid nitrogen. **D,** Grasping the skin tag for a few seconds. **E,** Frozen tag. **F,** Appearance of tag 10 minutes after freezing.

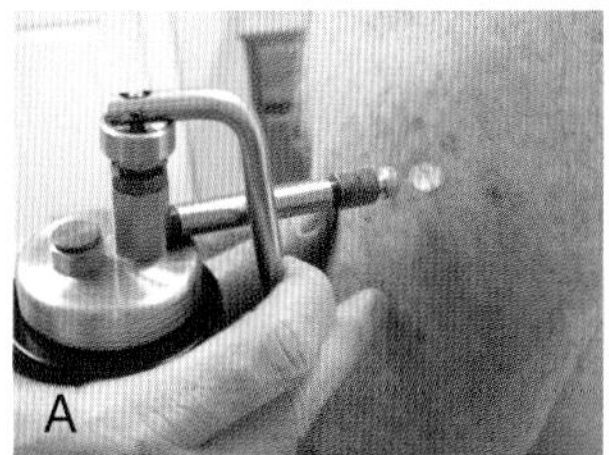

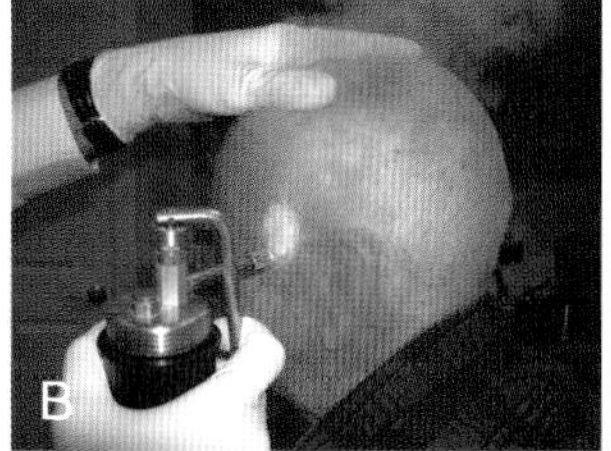

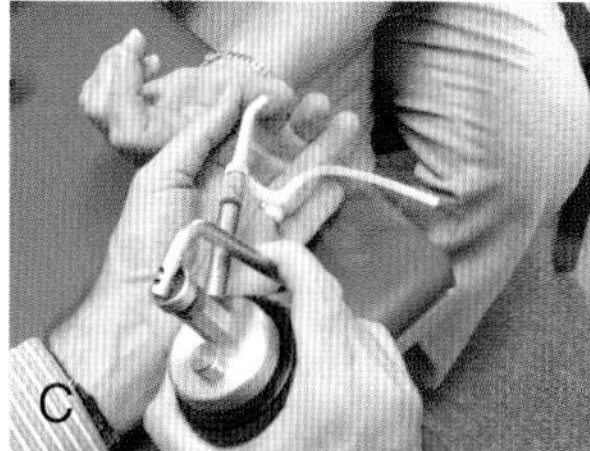

Figure 14-16 **A,** Perpendicular spray technique using liquid nitrogen in a cryogun. **B,** Open spray using a spiral pattern to cover a large area. **C,** Cryosurgery of a wart using the Brymill CRY-AC with a closed probe.

performed, or the lesion can be covered in a paintbrush or enlarging spiral pattern (Fig. 14-16B).

5. *Using a limiting cone* or plastic plate shield with variable-sized openings (see Fig. 14-8) is recommended for most smaller lesions because it focuses the spray onto the area desired and limits destruction of normal tissue. It is also helpful around critical areas like the eyes to limit the spread of the spray. Hold it tight against the skin to prevent leakage. Select the cone size to give the desired size of ice ball. The ice ball will still usually spread 1 to 2 mm beyond the size of the opening. Use freezing guidelines (see Box 14-1) for desired effect.

Liquid nitrogen spray techniques achieve desired freezing levels 8 to 10 times faster than nitrous oxide.

Contact Probes

Small, solid tips much like the nitrous oxide tips also can be used with the thermos guns, but the diameters are only 2 to 4 mm (Fig. 14-7E).

1. Select the appropriate size and apply the probe tip directly to the skin or lesion (see Fig. 14-16C).
2. Obtain the rim of ice ball size desired.
3. Allow to thaw.

The advantage of these tips is that the ice ball is well controlled and forms much faster than with nitrous oxide. They can also be used in areas such as around the eyes where it is necessary to avoid a wider spray. The disadvantage of using these probes is that the thawing is passive and can take a long time. Although large tips have been designed to apply to the cervix for dysplasia, studies proving adequacy are not available.

CryoPen Closed System

1. Select the appropriate size reusable tip to match the lesion.
2. Apply the CryoPen tip directly to the lesion.
3. The size of the tip and amount of pressure applied affect rapidity and depth of freeze.
4. Obtain the rim of ice ball size desired.
5. Allow to thaw.
6. Repeat the freeze if indicated.

The advantage of these tips is that the ice ball is well controlled. They can also be used in sensitive areas such as around the eyes where it is necessary to avoid cryogen spray.

Nitrous Oxide or Carbon Dioxide Closed System

1. *Débride* any keratin you can beforehand (e.g., plantar wart). This is usually done using a blade and shaving away any callus.
2. *Place a thin layer of water-soluble gel* on the lesion to hydrate the lesion and to enhance even contact with the cryoprobe. If the lesion is dry, soaking it well with a wet 4 × 4 gauze pad before application of the gel will enhance the effectiveness of the freeze, especially if it is a large lesion.
3. *Select a probe* with a size and shape that correspond to the lesion size (Fig. 14-17).
4. Hold the handpiece ("gun") with trigger in one hand, and *guide the probe tip* to a point over the site of freezing (see Fig. 14-17).
5. *Place the tip on the lesion and activate the gun*. The tip will stick to the skin within 3 to 5 seconds.

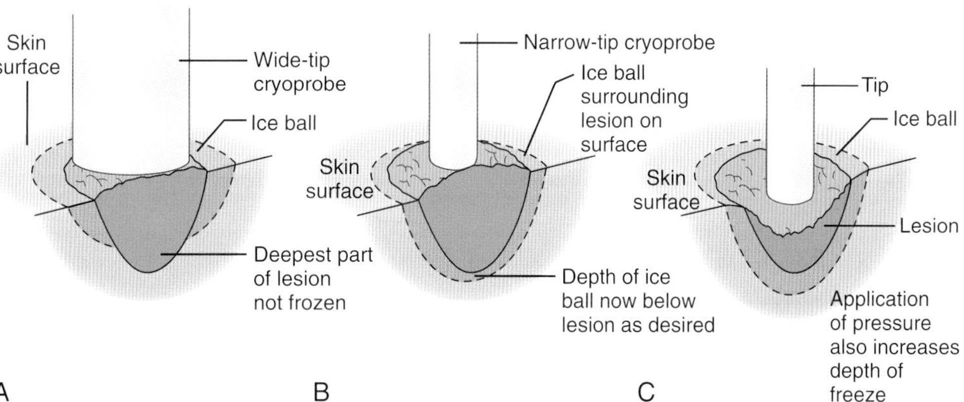

Figure 14-17 Cryosurgery of a deep but narrow lesion. **A,** If a wide cryoprobe tip is used, the deepest part of the lesion will not be frozen even though a 3- to 5-mm margin of ice ball is obtained. **B,** To ensure that the entire lesion is frozen, a tip smaller than the lesion may be used, thereby limiting the rapid lateral spread of the ice ball. **C,** Alternatively, the cryoprobe tip may be pressed down until the top of the lesion is below the skin surface. The cold will penetrate deeper before too much normal tissue is frozen by lateral spread.

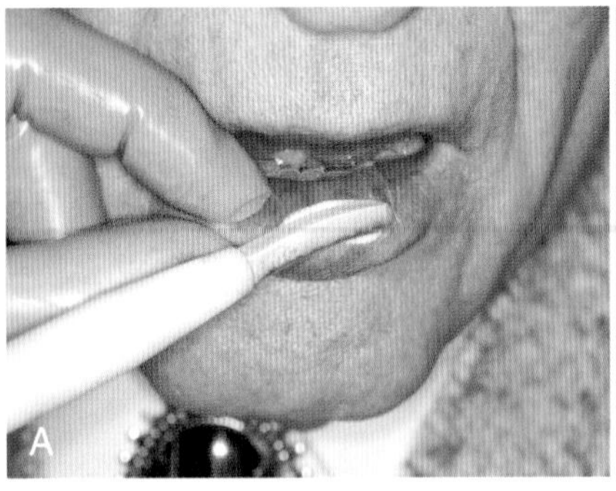

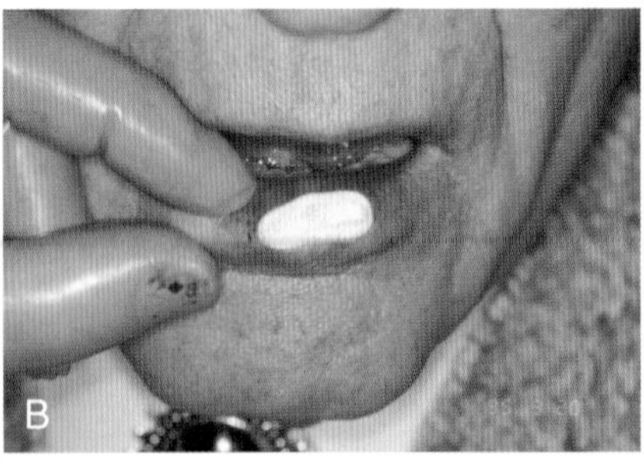

Figure 14-18 Cryosurgery of a lip lesion using a nitrous oxide closed system with a "hemorrhoid tip." **A,** Freezing the lesion. **B,** Appearance immediately after removing the tip.

6. *Freeze until desired ice ball is obtained* (Fig. 14-18A).
7. *Thaw.* This will be an active process. Some units will thaw automatically when the freeze trigger or button is released, whereas others require that a second button be pushed. *The gas from the tank to the handpiece must be turned on for this to occur!* The tip will "release" from the skin within seconds. The frozen skin will then thaw passively (Fig. 14-18B).

Cryogen Canister: Verruca-Freeze/Medi-Frig or Histofreezer

See Figure 14-12.

1. *Select a limiting cone size* that will completely encompass the lesion (which must be benign) plus 2 mm of normal tissue.
2. *Hold the cone securely* against the skin to prevent leakage (essential! see Figs. 14-12C and 14-17A).
3. Dispense enough liquid from the canister to *fill the cone to the line (approximately ⅛ to ¼ inch)*. Avoid splattering; use a gentle spray.
4. *Allow the fluid to evaporate* (30 to 60 seconds).
5. *Remove* the cone.
6. *Repeat*, if indicated.

Alternatively, the buds can be frozen and then applied to the lesions much like the cotton-tipped applicators with liquid nitrogen.

Technique for Specific Lesions

Keratin Removal

Lesions with dense keratin coverings (e.g., plantar warts) are very resistant to cryosurgery (especially to nitrous oxide and canister gases). The patient can help prepare a plantar wart with 2 weeks of salicylic acid application: After bathing and cleaning the area, the patient should apply a 17% solution (Compound W) to the wart(s). A piece of Mediplast (40% salicylic acid) or Trans-Ver-Sal, cut just a little larger than the wart, can also be used. This is left in place 24 hours until the next day's application. (If the pad migrates significantly during the day, it may be used at night only.) After 2 weeks, a soft white layer of keratin can be peeled away, revealing the base or root of the plantar wart lesion. Freezing time for the lesion should be shortened once the keratin layer and outer epidermis have been removed.

Alternatively, in lesions with significant keratin, a no. 10 or no. 15 scalpel blade can be used to shave off the keratin in thin layers until the first red punctate vasculature is seen (verruca). Stop débridement at this point (punctate bleeding) to minimize bleeding.

Actinic Keratoses

Usually actinic keratoses are quite superficial. If they are numerous, liquid nitrogen is much quicker to use than nitrous oxide. Anesthesia is rarely needed. Because these lesions are premalignant, however, a full-thickness freeze is suggested. Whichever technique is used, be sure to obtain at least a 3-mm ice ball. It may be best to freeze a second time. Moisten the lesion first (with K-Y Jelly) if nitrous oxide is used.

Nonmelanoma Skin Cancers

This technique is used for treating malignant lesions such as *basal cell carcinomas* less than 1 cm. Be sure to confirm the diagnosis by obtaining a biopsy specimen before treatment. Many physicians do not use cryosurgery on malignancies other than basal cell carcinomas, although studies would support treating smaller (<1 cm) squamous cell carcinomas also. Malignant cells are more cryoresistant, and destruction requires temperatures of −40° C to −50° C. Only liquid nitrogen or nitrous oxide may be used to treat malignancies. The canister cryogens do not achieve low enough tissue temperatures for effective treatment of these lesions. If cryosurgery is the chosen method of destruction for basal cell carcinoma, the probe can be applied directly to the lesion. Alternatively, shave off (debulk) most of the lesion and freeze the now thinned-out residual. Follow the steps outlined previously for the technique used, but continue the freeze until the ice ball is 5 mm beyond the margins of the lesion (see Fig. 14-2). When freezing is complete, allow the lesion to slowly completely thaw and repeat the freezing process a second time. Because a malignancy is being treated, it is wise to document the extent of the freeze and the thaw time. Freeze time will vary depending on the cryogen being used, but the thaw times should be the same—halo thaw time about 2 minutes with complete thaw time 3 to 5 minutes, depending on size (see Box 14-1).

Full-Thickness Freeze Technique for Anatomically Large or Irregular Skin Lesions

Some lesions are too large to be completely frozen by a cryoprobe in a single freeze. Some examples are Bowen's disease, keloids, vascular lesions, or mosaic warts. In such cases, note the central location of the cryoprobe. This spot will be the lateral margin of the cryoprobe placement (nitrous oxide) for the next adjacent freeze (after thawing occurs). This allows for the 50% overlap that is desired. Freezing of extremely large lesions can begin on one side, and then the opposite side can be frozen while the first is thawing. Progressing from opposite sides to the center will save time and still allow for a 40% to 50% freeze overlap.

Using liquid nitrogen, overlapping direct sprays can be performed or the lesion can be covered in a paintbrush or enlarging spiral pattern. It is important that a good freeze be obtained over the entire lesion.

Hypertrophic Scars and Keloids

Cryosurgery can be used in two different ways to treat scars. It can be used alone or before injection of steroids. The hyperemia and edema that immediately follow freezing and thawing soften the hypertrophic scar or keloid and allow easy penetration by a needle and a more even distribution of intralesional steroid. Cryosurgery alone, without steroids, will reduce the size of large keloids, but numerous treatments may be needed and more vigorous freezing is needed if steroids are not used (also see Chapter 38, Hypertrophic Scars and Keloids).

Use the following technique for nitrous oxide (see Fig. 14-4):

1. Select a cryotip slightly narrower than the scar. You do *not* want the ice ball to extend more than 1 mm beyond the scar.
2. Apply a thin coat of water-soluble gel to the scar only. (Do not cover any of the surrounding skin.)
3. Moisten and warm the cryotip in warm water. Freeze until the ice ball progresses just to the edge of the scar, usually for 20 seconds to 1 minute, occasionally longer if necessary.
4. If steroids will be used, wait approximately 10 to 15 minutes for mild tissue swelling, then proceed with intralesional injection using triamcinolone diacetate (Aristocort) or triamcinolone acetonide (Kenalog 10 mg/mL) with a small 30-gauge needle. Use very dilute solutions (0.1 mL diluted with 0.3 mL of a parabens-free 1% lidocaine *without* epinephrine) and a sufficient volume to infiltrate the entire scar. (Increase the concentration on successive visits as necessary, depending on response.)
5. For large scars, four to five treatments may be necessary at 6- to 8-week intervals to achieve optimal success.

Liquid nitrogen can also be used. It is quicker and very efficacious, but it may be more difficult to limit the size of the freeze with smaller lesions.

Treatment may produce a copious discharge during the first few postoperative days.

Condylomata Acuminata

See also Chapter 155, Treatment of Noncervical Condylomata Acuminata.

1. Penile, perianal, and vulvar areas are sensitive. Individual lesions and small groups of condylomata can be frozen without anesthetic. Topical anesthetics can also be applied before freezing. In some situations, 20% topical benzocaine (Hurricaine), 5% lidocaine, EMLA cream, or ELA-Max may be appropriate. Topical applications may require 30 to 60 minutes to achieve maximum effectiveness. ELA-Max is now available over the counter. Large or multiple lesions may require injections of local anesthetic.
2. Find all the lesions. For women, examine the genitalia and the cervix with a colposcope to look for very small lesions, particularly in the vaginal introitus, on the vaginal side walls, the vulva, and the rectum. Women with external condylomata have a high incidence of cervical dysplasia, and colposcopy may be indicated. (See Chapter 137, Colposcopic Examination, and Chapter 138, Cryotherapy of the Cervix.)
3. If nitrous oxide is used, moisten the skin lesions with a water-soluble gel. Touch the lesion(s) with an appropriately sized probe. Activate the nitrous oxide–powered tip, and effect adherence after 3 to 5 seconds. Then apply gentle traction. Do not pull too hard or you may tear the tissue being treated or the surrounding skin. Freeze for approximately 20 to 45 seconds. Judge actual freezing time by the size of the lesion and the ice ball, which should extend 2 mm beyond the margin of the lesion(s) (Fig. 14-19). Within minutes after freezing, the condylomata darken and then will turn black; they should slough within a few days. If they do not turn dark, refreezing may be necessary.
4. Liquid nitrogen in either form (spray, cotton-tipped applicator, or metal pickups) is quicker for treating multiple lesions. Needle drivers dipped into a cup of liquid nitrogen will also work.
5. A combination of electrosurgery (radiofrequency surgery) and cryosurgery may speed the treatment of extensive perianal, vulvar, or penile lesions. The cryosurgery component will allow preservation of the elastic tissue matrix and expandability of the anal canal, penis, and vulva after healing. The electrosurgery component is used for tissue débridement, making sure not to cut too deep. Then, the base of each lesion is frozen for 20 to 30 seconds. This technique can be used for treatment of large areas of condylomata often seen on the genitalia.

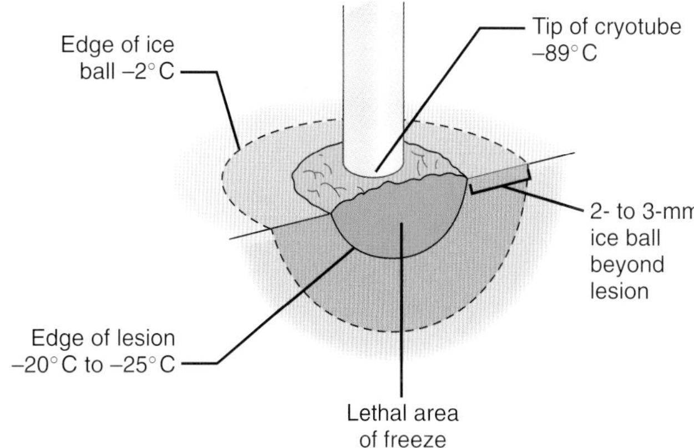

Figure 14-19 Treatment of benign lesions. To ensure that all of the tissue of the lesion reaches the –20° C to –25° C necessary for destruction, the outer edge of the frozen area (the ice ball) should extend at least 2 to 3 mm in all directions beyond the lesion.

Molluscum Contagiosum

Freezing is often an excellent, nearly painless treatment for molluscum contagiosum. Advise your patients, particularly children, to protect the healing crust to decrease the chance of scar formation.

1. If using nitrous oxide, prepare each lesion with a small amount of water-soluble gel. Freeze each lesion for 30 seconds to 1 minute. Use very fine-tipped probes to avoid freezing normal skin.
2. With liquid nitrogen, only brief freezes of several seconds are necessary.
3. Advise the patient and parent that the lesions should fall completely off within 2 weeks or less. If they do not, the patient should return soon for retreatment to prevent their spread.

Vascular Lesions (Hemangiomas and Strawberry Hemangiomas)

As with malignant lesions, vascular lesions are more cryoresistant, and a freeze/thaw/refreeze technique is recommended (Fig. 14-20). Nitrous oxide may be the preferred method both to control the extent of the freeze and to be able to compress the lesion to remove the blood, although liquid nitrogen can also be used.

1. Moisten and warm the cryotip in warm water, and apply water-soluble gel to the lesion.
2. Make contact with the probe on the hemangioma and *exert firm pressure* to squeeze the blood out of the vascular channels.
3. Activate the cryogun, and hold pressure against the lesion throughout the freeze. Begin timing when the ice ball becomes visible. For larger lesions, freeze for 1½ minutes or until the ice ball extends out 3 mm. Allow 5 to 7 minutes for thawing, and then repeat the freeze.

Skin Verrucae

Liquid nitrogen spray is the most effective and most rapid. Use a freeze/thaw/refreeze technique and obtain a 1- to 2-mm margin for each treated wart. Repeat the treatments every 1 to 3 weeks based on response. Débride any necrotic tissue before the next freeze.

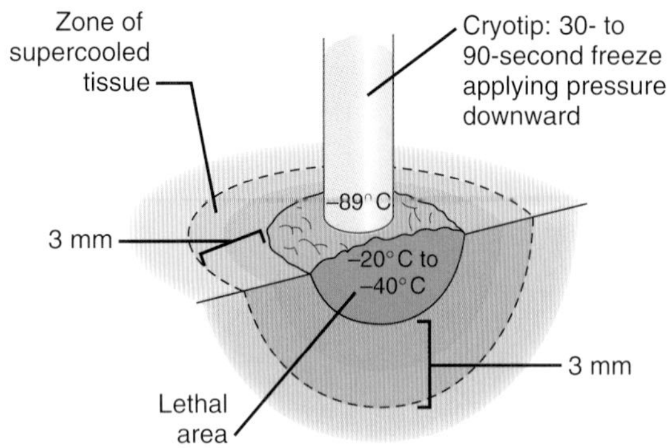

Figure 14-20 Full-thickness destructive freeze of vascular lesion. Pressure is applied to the tip to express as much blood as possible.

Seborrheic Keratoses

Seborrheic keratoses are usually quite superficial. However, they frequently demonstrate a thick raised component. They are quickly treated using liquid nitrogen because débridement, anesthesia, and soaking are usually not required. For nitrous oxide, the raised lesions may need to be débrided or hydrated before cryosurgery can be effective. Because the procedure takes longer, anesthesia using 1% lidocaine may be needed with nitrous oxide, especially in larger lesions. A 2-mm ice ball margin is sufficient for treatment (Fig. 14-21).

Cryotherapy for Cervical Intraepithelial Neoplasia

See Chapter 138, Cryotherapy of the Cervix.

Complications and Shortcomings

- Pigment cells and hair cells may be destroyed by cryosurgery.
- Hypertrophic scars, verrucae, and vascular lesions are quite resistant to treatment and may recur, requiring several treatments.
- Areas of poor circulation may be susceptible to *prolonged ulcer formation*, especially in elderly diabetic patients (e.g., anterior tibial compartment).

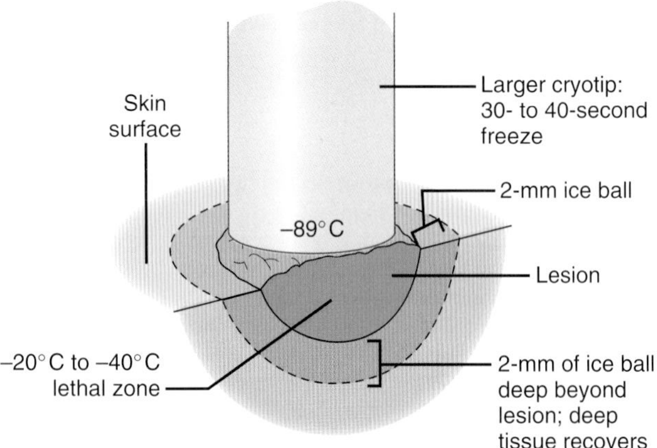

Figure 14-21 Nitrous oxide partial-thickness freeze used for removal of superficial lesions (e.g., seborrheic keratoses). Cryotip should cover or nearly cover entire lesion to limit depth of freeze. Halo thaw time should be approximately 30 to 45 seconds for all methods.

- Tissue pathology *documentation* and verification of *adequate destruction* of malignant lesions is *not possible* with cryosurgery. Pretreatment biopsy is recommended for all lesions suspect for malignancy. A presumed "benign lesion" may indeed be malignant and thus insufficiently treated with cryosurgery alone. So, if there is doubt concerning a possible melanoma or squamous cell cancer, biopsy is recommended first.
- Cryosurgery in the periorbital area may cause *excessive swelling*, in which the eyelid may be shut for several hours or days. However, cryosurgery of small, well-localized lesions on the eyelids is usually well tolerated. Be conservative on the freeze time until the individual patient's reaction is documented.
- *Peripheral neuropathy* (the ulnar nerve at the elbow or peripheral nerves on the lateral aspect of the digits) can result when areas adjacent to nerves are frozen. The nerve sheath is cryoresistant, but the nerve tissue is more susceptible to damage. This side effect can be minimized (if using a closed nitrous oxide or carbon dioxide system) by pulling the skin outward and away from the nerve, once good contact is achieved. If the nerve is affected, recovery occurs within 4 to 6 weeks, although 3 to 6 months may occasionally be required. Sensory nerves are more likely to be affected.
- In general, the skin of *infants and the elderly*, as well as previously damaged skin, is more susceptible to necrosis and blistering than normal skin. Thin skin can be a result of sun exposure, radiation, and chronic topical steroid application. Reduce freeze times until the reaction of a damaged area is known.
- One of the most common lesions treated with cryosurgery is active keratosis. Should any lesion not totally resolve after treatment, especially if it persists after a second cryosurgery session, it should be sampled. These resistant lesions are frequently found to be squamous cell carcinomas.

Postprocedure Patient Education

The patient should be informed of the anticipated healing time and results, as well as the need to call the office should there be an overreaction to freezing. If the blister enlarges more than 5 to 6 mm beyond the lesion, it might be best to open it. The basic instructions would be the same as those given with a second-degree burn. If the skin from the blister peels off, use moist healing techniques. Document that the patient was told of permanent pigment changes, possible nerve involvement, and hair loss. Placing a copy of the handout that was given to the patient in the chart provides excellent medical-legal documentation as well as an excellent medical reference for staff and physician alike. *See patient education and patient consent forms available online.*

Common Errors

The most common errors encountered in cryosurgery relate to undertreating the lesion. This usually occurs because of failure to ensure adequate ice ball formation in and around the lesion. Lack of consistent contact of the freezing tip with the lesion or failure to follow proper technique when using the liquid nitrogen spray leads to clinical failure. Inadequate freeze often occurs in plantar warts because of the insulating effect of keratin. Unless this is removed before treatment, cryosurgery is less likely to be effective. Selection of cryogen agent is important especially when treating malignancy. A canister refrigerant cannot achieve cold enough temperatures to treat malignancy effectively. Conversely, overfreezing lesions may lead to local side effects, especially hypopigmentation.

CPT/Billing Codes

Cryosurgery is billed out as "destruction of lesions." Certain areas require specific codes.

Destruction (Cryocautery, Electrocautery, Laser, Chemical, or Curettement)

Benign Lesions

(Site and size not needed, except for locations noted following)

11200 Skin tags, 1 to 15 lesions
11201 Skin tags, each additional 10 lesions or portion thereof
17000 Destruction of *premalignant* lesions (actinic keratosis); first lesion
17003 Second through 14 premalignant lesions, each (used in conjunction with 17000) (charge for each additional lesion treated)
17004 Destruction of *premalignant* lesions, 15 or more lesions (do not report 17004 in conjunction with 17000-17003)
17110 Benign other than skin tags 15 or less
17110 Destruction of benign lesions other than skin tags or cutaneous vascular lesions up to 14 lesions
30117 Destruction of intranasal lesion
46614 Anal, with anoscopy
46916 Anal (perianal), benign lesion, simple destruction, cryo
46924 Anal (perianal), benign lesion, extensive destruction
46934 Anal, internal hemorrhoid
46937 Anal, benign rectal tumor
54056 Genitals (male), penis, cryotherapy, simple destruction
54065 Genitals (male), penis, cryotherapy, extensive destruction
56501 Genitals (female), perineum, simple destruction
56501 Genitals (female), vulva/introitus, simple destruction
56515 Genitals (female), vulva/introitus, extensive destruction
57061 Genitals (female), vagina, simple destruction
57065 Genitals (female), vagina, extensive destruction
57511 Cervix
67850 Eyelid, lid margin
68135 Eyelid, conjunctiva

Malignant Lesions

See codes 17260 to 17286 as follows.

NOTE: All of these codes have a 10-day global fee surgical period. Destruction by any method, with or without curettement, includes local anesthesia and ablation, and usually does not require closure. Sizes listed describe *lesion* diameter, not the width of the skin area destroyed.

17260 Trunk, arm, or leg (TAL): <0.5 cm
17261 TAL: 0.6–1.0 cm
17262 TAL: 1.1–2.0 cm
17263 TAL: 2.1–3.0 cm
17264 TAL: 3.1–4.0 cm
17266 TAL: >4.0 cm
17270 Scalp, neck, hand, foot, or genitalia (SNHFG): <0.5 cm
17271 SNHFG: 0.6–1.0 cm
17272 SNHFG: 1.1–2.0 cm
17273 SNHFG: 2.1–3.0 cm
17274 SNHFG: 3.1–4.0 cm
17276 SNHFG: >4.0 cm
17280 Face, eyelid, ear, nose, lip, or mucous membrane (Face mm): <0.5 cm
17281 Face mm: 0.6–1.0 cm
17282 Face mm: 1.1–2.0 cm
17283 Face mm: 2.1–3.0 cm
17284 Face mm: 3.1–4.0 cm
17286 Face mm: >4.0 cm

ICD-9-CM Diagnostic Codes

See ICD-9-CM Code Book under "neoplasm, skin." Then identify anatomic site and whether lesion is benign, malignant (primary or secondary), carcinoma in situ, or uncertain.

Patient Education Guides

See patient education and patient consent forms available online at www.expertconsult.com.

Acknowledgment

The editors wish to recognize the many contributions by John E. Hocutt, Jr., MD, to this chapter in the previous edition of this text.

Suppliers

(See online list for contact information.)

Liquid nitrogen
Brymill Cryogenic Systems
CryoPen LLC
CryoSurgery, Inc.
Ellman International
OraSure Technologies
Wallach Surgical Devices, Inc.

Nitrous oxide units
CooperSurgical

BIBLIOGRAPHY

American Academy of Dermatology Committee on Guidelines of Care: Guidelines of care for cryosurgery. J Am Acad Dermatol 31:648–653, 1994.

Andrews MD: Cryosurgery for common skin conditions. Am Fam Physician 69:2365–2372, 2004.

Bacelieri R, Johnson SM: Cutaneous warts: An evidence-based approach to therapy. Am Fam Physician 72:647–652, 2005.

Bowen GM, White GL Jr, Gerwels JW: Mohs micrographic surgery. Am Fam Physician 72:845–848, 2005.

Burkhart CG, Pchalek I, Adlerb M, Burkhart CN: An in vitro study comparing temperatures of over-the-counter wart preparations with liquid nitrogen. J Am Acad Dermatol 57:1019–1020, 2007.

Castro-Ron G, Pasquali P: Cryosurgery. In Robinson JK, Hanke DW, Sengelmann RD, Siegel DM (eds): Surgery of the Skin: Procedural Dermatology. Philadelphia, Mosby, 2005, pp 191–202.

Cohen PR, Schulze KE, Nelson BR: Cutaneous carcinoma with mixed histology: A potential etiology for skin cancer recurrence and an indication for Mohs microscopically controlled surgical excision. South Med J 98:740–747, 2005.

Cook J, Salasche S: Mohs surgery: An informed view. Plast Reconstr Surg 115:945–946, 2005.

Dandurand M, Petit T, Martel P, Guillot B, for ANAES: Management of basal cell carcinoma in adults: Clinical practice guidelines. Eur J Dermatol 16:394–401, 2006.

Essers BA, Dirksen CD, Nieman FH, et al: Cost-effectiveness of Mohs micrographic surgery vs. surgical excision for basal cell carcinoma of the face. Arch Dermatol 142:187–194, 2006.

Habif TP: Clinical Dermatology: A Color Guide to Diagnosis and Therapy, 4th ed. St. Louis, Mosby, 2004.

Hatzis GP, Finn R: Using botox to treat a Mohs defect repair complicated by a parotid fistula. J Oral Maxillofac Surg 65:2357–2360, 2007.

Jackson A, Colver G, Dawber RPR: Cutaneous Cryosurgery: Principles and Clinical Practice, 3rd ed. London, Informa Healthcare, 2005.

Kuwahara RT: Cryotherapy. eMedicine, updated November 26, 2007. Available at http://www.emedicine.com/derm/topic553.htm.

Leibovitch I, Huilgol SC, Selva D, et al: Basosquamous carcinoma: Treatment with Mohs micrographic surgery. Cancer 104:170–175, 2005.

Miller SJ: The National Comprehensive Cancer Network (NCCN) guidelines of care for nonmelanoma skin cancers. Dermatol Surg 26:289–292, 2000.

Miller SJ, Alam M, Andersen J, et al, for the National Comprehensive Cancer Network: Basal cell and squamous cell skin cancers. J Natl Compr Canc Netw 5:506–529, 2007.

Nguyen TH: Mohs bashing out of hand. Plast Reconstr Surg 115:361–362, 2005.

Otley CC: Cost-effectiveness of Mohs micrographic surgery vs. surgical excision for basal cell carcinoma of the face. Arch Dermatol 142:1235, author reply 1235–1236, 2006.

Otley CC: Mohs' micrographic surgery for basal-cell carcinoma of the face. Lancet 365:1226–1227, author reply 1227, 2005.

Redondo P, Marquina M, Pretel M, et al: Methyl-ALA-induced fluorescence in photodynamic diagnosis of basal cell carcinoma prior to Mohs micrographic surgery. Arch Dermatol 144:115–117, 2008.

Shindel AW, Mann MW, Lev RY, et al: Mohs micrographic surgery for penile cancer: Management and long-term followup. J Urol 178:1980–1985, 2007. [See comment in Nat Clin Pract Urol 5:364–365, 2008.]

Shuster S: Mohs' micrographic surgery for basal-cell carcinoma of the face. Lancet 365:1227–1228, 2005.

Sterry W, for the European Dermatology Forum Guideline Committee: Guidelines: The management of basal cell carcinoma. Eur J Dermatol 16:467–475, 2006.

Stulberg DL, Crandell B, Fawcett RS: Diagnosis and treatment of basal cell and squamous cell carcinomas. Am Fam Physician 70:1481–1488, 2004.

Telfer NR, Colver GB, Morton CA, for the British Association of Dermatologists: Guidelines for the management of basal cell carcinoma. Br J Dermatol 159:35–48, 2008.

Tuggy M, Garcia J: Procedures Consult. Available at www.proceduresconsult.com.

Usatine RP, Tobinick EL: Cryosurgical techniques. In Usatine RP, Moy RL, Tobinick EL, Siegel DM (eds): Skin Surgery: A Practical Guide. St. Louis, Mosby, 1998, pp 137–164.

CHAPTER 15

DERMOSCOPY

Ashfaq A. Marghoob • Azadeh Esmaeili • Alon Scope

Skin cancer, the most common malignancy in the United States, is associated with significant morbidity and mortality. Fortunately, early detection of skin cancer, through visual examination of the entire cutaneous surface, can have a positive impact on patient outcomes. Because dermoscopy can assist clinicians in correctly identifying cutaneous malignancies, it has been well received by physicians engaged in skin cancer screening efforts.

Dermoscopy is a technique that requires the use of hand-held magnification devices known as *dermoscopes* (or *dermatoscopes*). These instruments illuminate the skin and, by exploiting the optical properties of the skin, allow the physician to visualize subsurface colors and structures. Dermoscopes are designed to reduce the amount of light reflected off the skin surface, thereby allowing clinicians to appreciate the appearance of the subsurface anatomic structures of the epidermis and papillary dermis that are otherwise not discernible to the unaided eye. Two types of dermoscopes are available, one using standard light-emitting diode (LED) illumination (i.e., *nonpolarized dermoscopy*) and the other using cross-polarized light (*polarized dermoscopy*; Fig. 15-1). To reduce skin surface light reflection, *nonpolarized dermoscopy* requires direct skin contact in the presence of a liquid interface (e.g., mineral oil or alcohol) between the dermoscope and the skin. *Polarized dermoscopy*, however, does not require an immersion liquid because one of the inherent properties of cross-polarized light is to filter out light reflected from the skin surface, allowing only light reflected from deeper layers of the skin to reach the observer's retina. Polarized and nonpolarized dermoscopy provide complementary information. For example, polarized dermoscopy is the preferred method for visualizing blood vessels because it does not require direct skin contact. The ability to see dermoscopic structures without direct skin contact eliminates the effect of contact pressure–induced blanching of the blood vessel. Nonpolarized dermoscopy, on the other hand, is better for visualizing structures within the superficial layers of the epidermis, such as milia cysts, which are important structures that enable observers to correctly identify seborreic keratoses. With these scopes, clinicians can now appreciate morphologic alterations in skin lesions as dermoscopic structures of different shapes and colors (Table 15-1). Because most dermoscopic colors and structures have been correlated with histopathologic findings, dermoscopy can be considered a form of bedside in vivo gross tissue inspection that can help to predict tissue pathology.

The overall clinical diagnostic accuracy for malignant melanoma (MM), without the added benefit of dermoscopy, for experienced dermatologists is only about 60%. Dermoscopy enhances the diagnostic accuracy for MM and helps triage those lesions requiring a biopsy. In a large meta-analysis of dermoscopy studies, Bafounta and colleagues revealed that dermoscopy significantly increased diagnostic accuracy (by 49%) compared with unaided examination, with mean sensitivity increasing by 19% and mean specificity by 6%. The increase in specificity with dermoscopy translates into a reduction in the excision of benign lesions. This is consistent with a retrospective analysis that showed a significant reduction in the benign–malignant ratio of excised melanocytic lesions from 18:1 in the predermoscopy era to 4:1 after dermoscopy was implemented by trained clinicians. The benefit of using dermoscopy greatly depends on experience, and reliance on dermoscopy by untrained or less experienced examiners was found to be no better than clinical inspection alone. However, studies indicate that participation in short dermoscopy training courses improves confidence and diagnostic performance of nonexperts when evaluating lesions by dermoscopy. The benefits provided by the use of dermoscopy are presented in Box 15-1.

EVALUATION TECHNIQUE: TWO-STEP DERMOSCOPY ALGORITHM

The two-step dermoscopy algorithm forms the foundation for the dermoscopic evaluation of skin lesions (Fig. 15-2).

The ***first step in performing dermoscopy*** *requires that the observer classify the lesion under investigation as either a growth of melanocytic or nonmelanocytic origin.* On nonglabrous skin, the presence of a pigment network, aggregated globules, streaks, or homogeneous blue pigmentation identifies the lesion as melanocytic (Figs. 15-3 through

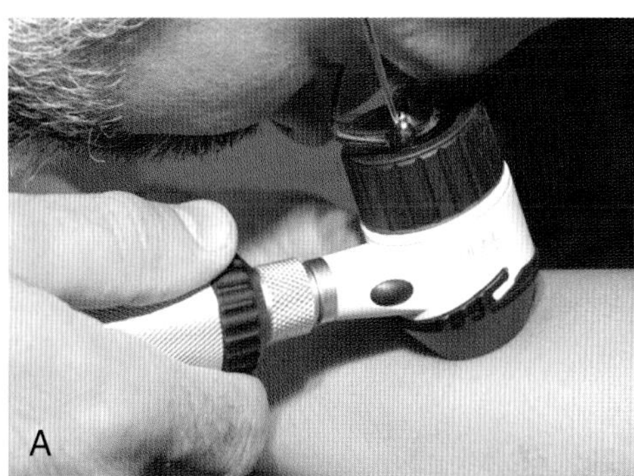

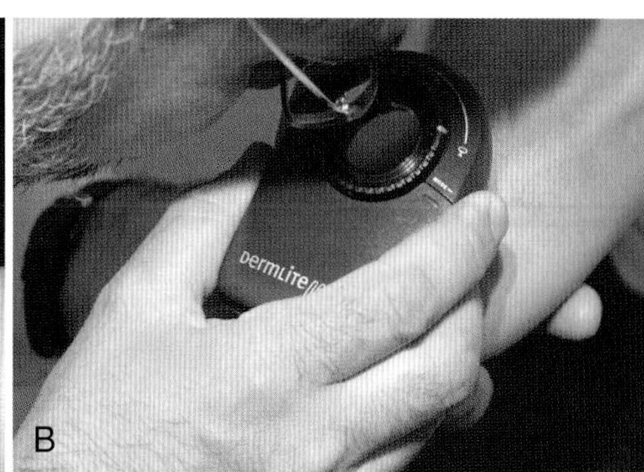

Figure 15-1 Physician examining a pigmented skin lesion under contact nonpolarized dermoscopy (**A**) and non-contact polarized dermoscopy (**B**).

TABLE 15-1 Dermoscopic Structures and Their Histopathologic Correlations

Dermoscopic Structures	Definition	Histopathologic Correlation
Pigment network (reticulation)	Gridlike network consisting of pigmented "lines" and hypopigmented "holes."	Melanin in keratinocytes or melanocytes along the epidermal rete ridges.
Pseudonetwork	In facial lesions, diffuse pigmentation interrupted by nonpigmented follicular openings, appearing similar to a network.	Pigment in the epidermis or dermis interrupted by follicular and adnexal openings of the face.
Structureless (homogeneous) areas	Areas devoid of dermoscopic structures and without regression. These areas can be pigmented or nonpigmented. If the area is uniformly dark, it is referred to as a "blotch" (see below).	Lack of melanin or presence of melanin in all layers of the skin.
Dots	Small, round structures less than 0.1 mm in diameter that may be black, brown, gray, or bluish.	Aggregates of melanocytes or melanin granules. Black dots represent pigment in the upper epidermis or stratum corneum. Brown dots represent pigment at the dermoepidermal junction. Gray-blue dots represent pigment in the papillary dermis.
Peppering	Tiny, blue-gray granules.	Melanin deposited as intracellular (mostly within melanophages) or extracellular particles in the upper dermis
Globules	Round to oval structures that may be brown, black, or red with diameters greater than 0.1 mm.	Nests of melanocytes in the dermis and dermal–epidermal junction.
Streaks (pseudopods, radial streaming)	Radially arranged projections of dark pigment (brown to black) at the periphery of the lesion.	Confluent junctional nests of melanocytes.
Blotches	Dark brown to black, usually homogeneous areas of pigment that obscure underlying structures.	Aggregates of melanin in the stratum corneum, epidermis, and upper dermis.
Regression areas	White, scarlike depigmentation (lighter than the surrounding skin, shiny white under polarized dermoscopy) often combined with or adjacent to blue-gray areas or peppering.	Scarlike changes: thickened fibrotic papillary dermis, dilated blood vessels, sparse lymphocytic infiltrates, and variable numbers of melanophages.
Blue-white veil	Irregular, confluent blue pigmentation with an overlying white "ground-glass" haze.	Aggregation of heavily pigmented cells (usually melanoma cells or melanophages) with compact orthokeratosis of the stratum corneum and acanthosis (thickened epidermis).
Vascular pattern	See Table 15-5 for vascular terminology.	Tumor neoangiogenesis and dilated blood vessels in the papillary dermis ("vascular blush").
Milia-like cysts	Round whitish or yellowish structures that shine brightly (like "stars in the sky") under nonpolarized dermoscopy.	Horn pseudocysts.
Comedo-like openings	"Blackhead"-like plugs on the surface of the lesion.	Concave clefts in the surface of the epidermis, often filled with keratin.
Fingerprint-like structures	Thin, light brown, parallel running lines.	Probably represent thin, elongated, pigmented epidermal rete ridges.
Ridges and fissures	Cerebriform surface resulting in gyri (ridges) and sulci (fissures). Confluence of adjacent comedo-like openings will create a fissure.	Wedge-shaped clefts of the surface of the epidermis, often filled with keratin (fissures).
"Moth-eaten" border	Concave invaginations of the lesion border.	Not available.
Leaf-like areas	Brown to gray-blue, discrete bulbous structures resembling a leaf pattern.	Large, complex nodules of pigmented basal cell carcinoma in the upper dermis.
Spoke-wheel–like structures	Well-circumscribed brown to gray-blue-brown radial projections meeting at a darker brown central hub.	Nests of basal cell carcinoma radiating from the follicular epithelium.
Large blue-gray ovoid nests	Large, well-circumscribed areas, larger than globules.	Large nests of basal cell tumor in the dermis.
Multiple blue-gray globules	Round well-circumscribed structures that, in the absence of a pigment network, suggest basal-cell carcinoma.	Small nests of basal cell tumor in the dermis.
Lacunae	Red, maroon, or black lagoons.	Dilated vascular spaces.
Parallel patterns	On acral areas, parallel rows of pigmentation following the furrows (nevi) or ridges (melanoma) of the dermoglyphics.	Pigmented melanocytes in the furrows (crista limitans) or ridges (crista intermedia) of acral skin.

Box 15-1. Benefits of Dermoscopy

- Allows the observer to formulate a logical differential diagnosis
- Differentiates melanocytic from nonmelanocytic skin lesions
- Differentiates benign from malignant skin lesions
- Provides earlier diagnosis of melanoma
- Improves diagnostic accuracy
- Increases the confidence in diagnosis
- Avoids unnecessary biopsies
- Helps isolate suspicious foci within a large lesion
- Helps define lesion borders for presurgical margin mapping
- Aids in monitoring patients with multiple nevi
- Helps reassure patients

15-6). In addition, a pseudonetwork pattern can be seen in melanocytic lesions on facial skin (Fig. 15-7). On the other hand, melanocytic lesions on the palms and soles are recognized primarily by the presence of a parallel pigment pattern (Fig. 15-8; see Table 15-1). If, however, the lesion does not manifest any of the aforementioned melanocytic criteria, the observer seeks to identify specific criteria that can identify the lesion as a nonmelanocytic lesion (see Fig. 15-2) such as basal cell carcinoma (Figs. 15-9 through 15-11), squamous cell carcinoma (Fig. 15-12), he mangioma (Fig. 15-13), seborrheic keratoses (Figs. 15-14 and 15-15), or dermatofibroma (Fig. 15-16). In addition, a group of lesions exists that is termed "structureless" in that they do not manifest any melanocytic or nonmelanocytic lesion structures. Because it is not uncommon to encounter amelanotic and hypomelanotic MMs that are structureless, all such lesions should be viewed with extreme suspicion, especially if the

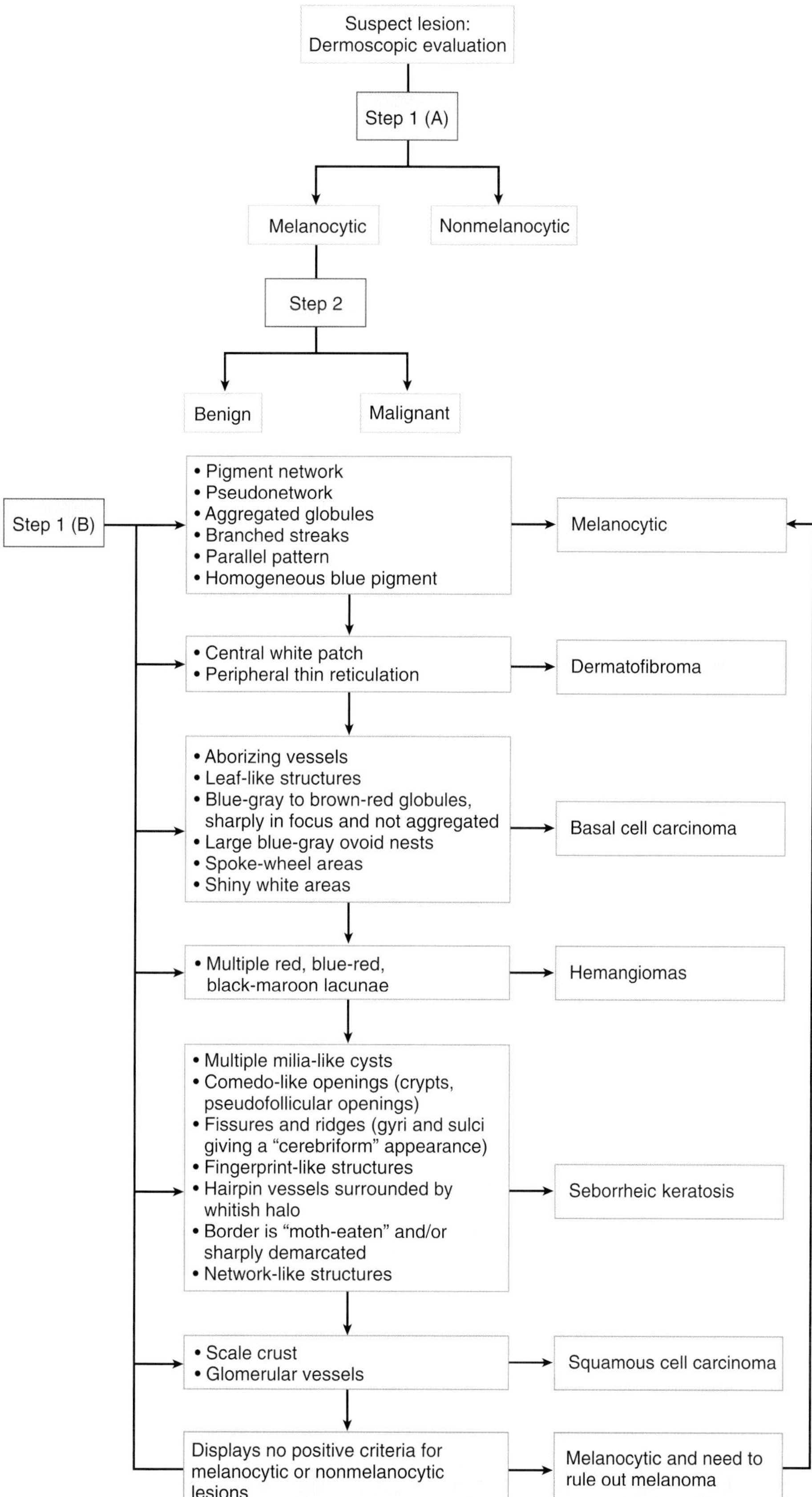

Figure 15-2 The two-step algorithm for the evaluation of the pigmented lesions. In the first step, the observer must decide whether the lesion is of melanocytic or nonmelanocytic origin (Step 1 [A]), using a stepwise evaluation of dermoscopic features (Step 1 [B]). In the second step, the observer differentiates between benign melanocytic nevi and melanoma using pattern analysis or one of the score-based algorithms mentioned in the text (e.g., ABCD rule, Menzies method, seven-point checklist).

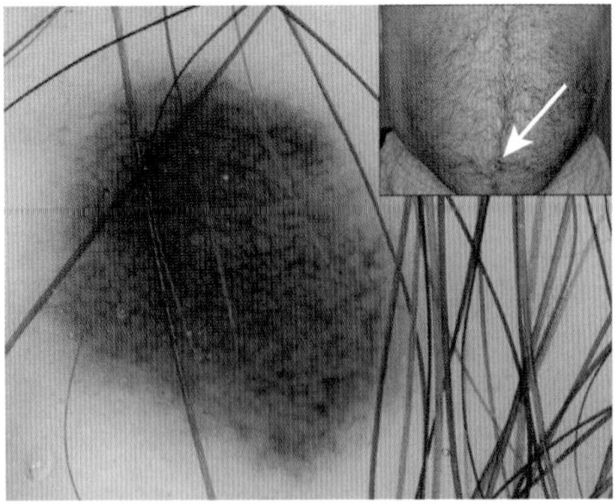

Figure 15-3 This abdominal pigmented lesion is larger and darker than the patient's other moles *(inset, arrow)* and thus can be considered an "ugly duckling" that requires close-up examination. On dermoscopy, there is a pigmented network, and thus the lesion is melanocytic in origin. The lesion displays a regular network thinning out at the periphery, which is a benign nevus pattern.

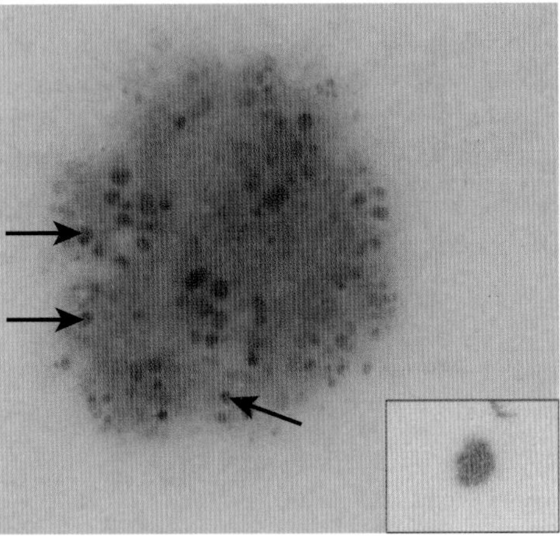

Figure 15-4 Pigmented lesion featuring aggregated globules *(arrows)* with an overall symmetric distribution, which is a benign nevus pattern.

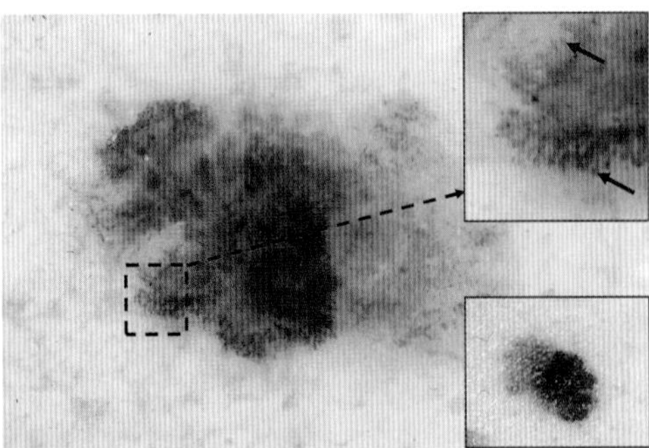

Figure 15-5 This lesion is clinically suspect by the ABCD criteria for melanoma *(inset)*. On dermoscopy, the lesion does not display any of the benign nevus patterns and has peripheral streaks shaped like pseudopods *(dotted box and corresponding inset)*. The streaks are focally placed; their presence indicates that the lesion is melanocytic and raises concern for melanoma. This was a 0.4-mm melanoma.

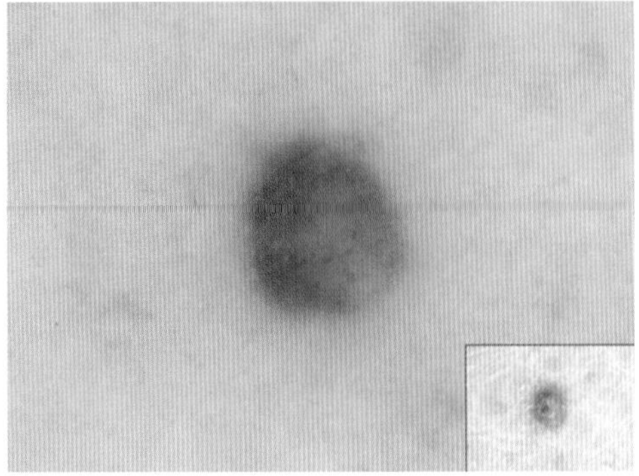

Figure 15-6 Blue nevus showing homogeneous steel-blue pigmentation (one of the benign nevus patterns: the homogeneous pattern).

lesion manifests linear irregular or dotted blood vessels, both commonly seen in MM (Fig. 15-17).

The ***second step*** *in the two-step dermoscopy algorithm pertains only to lesions that are deemed to be of melanocytic origin*, which include both lesions with melanocytic-specific features (Table 15-2) and those that are structureless. *The objective during this second-tier evaluation process is to differentiate benign nevi from* MM. Toward this goal, a number of algorithms have been created. Novices in dermoscopy may find one of the score-based algorithms useful in assessing melanocytic lesions (Box 15-2, Tables 15-3 and 15-4, and Figs. 15-18 and 15-19). However, once experience in dermoscopy is attained, most dermoscopists rely on pattern analysis to differentiate between nevi and MM.

Although pattern analysis requires experience; a *simplified form* of pattern analysis can be taught to novices in dermoscopy (Box 15-3). Fortunately, most benign nevi tend to manifest one of nine benign global patterns, all of which are characterized by symmetry of dermoscopic colors and structures. Hence, knowing these benign global patterns can prevent the excision of many atypical moles, most of which will reveal one of these benign patterns. Any lesion that deviates from one of these global benign patterns needs to be viewed with caution.

The nine benign global dermoscopic patterns include (1) diffuse reticular network, (2) patchy reticular network, (3) peripheral reticular network with central hypopigmentation, (4) peripheral reticular network with central hyperpigmentation, (5) peripheral reticular network with central globules, (6) globular pattern, (7) peripheral globules with central reticular network or starburst, (8) homogeneous pattern, and (9) symmetric multicomponent pattern (Figs. 15-20 and 15-21; see Box 15-3). Based on the aforementioned

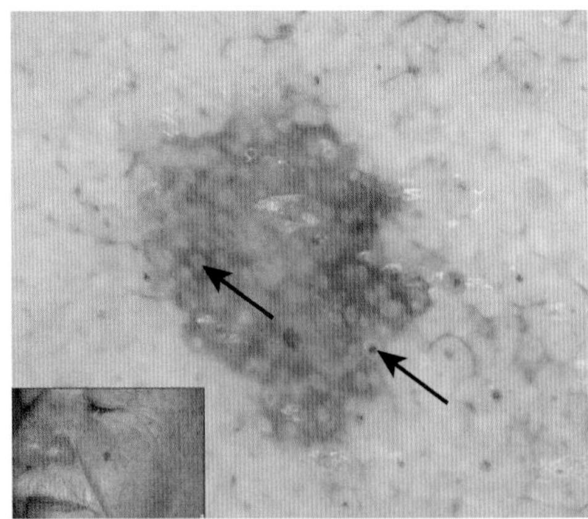

Figure 15-7 Pigmented lesion on the face featuring a pseudonetwork pattern, produced by pigmentation surrounding adnexal openings such as hair follicles *(arrows)*.

Text continued on p. 115

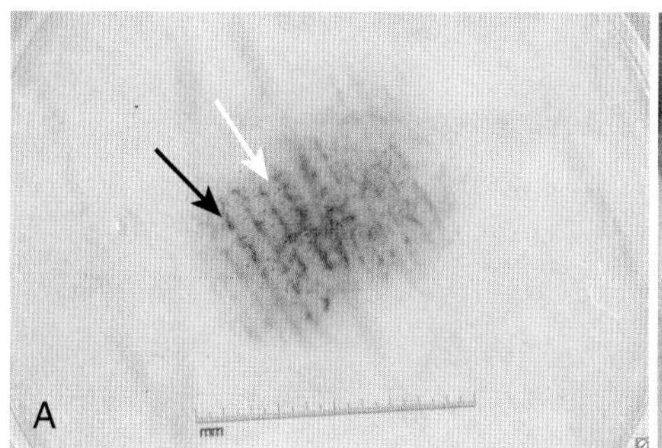

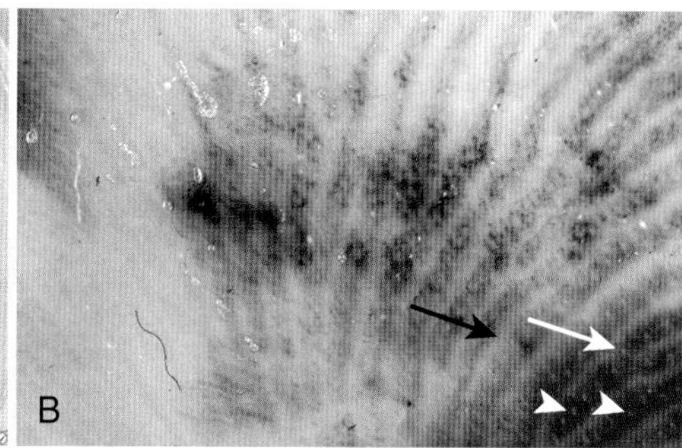

Figure 15-8 **A,** Acral nevus exhibiting a parallel furrow pattern, where pigmentation is seen in the furrows *(black arrow)* but does not involve the ridges *(white arrow)*. **B,** Acral melanoma displaying the opposite pattern, with the pigmentation on the ridges *(white arrow)* but not in the furrows *(black arrow)*. To help distinguish ridges from furrows, one can look for the sweat gland openings, which are always located on the ridges *(white arrowheads)*.

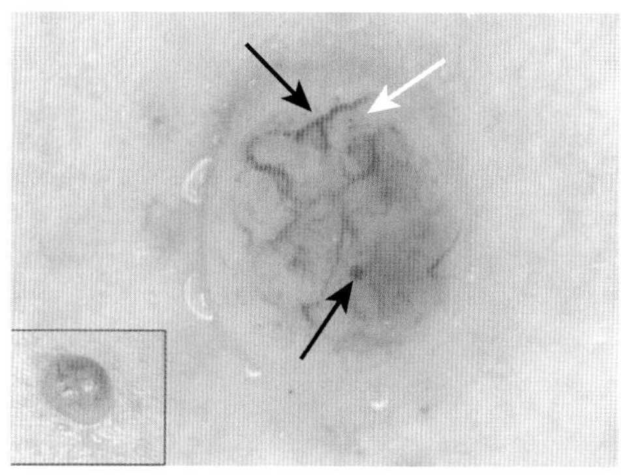

Figure 15-9 Pigmented nodular basal cell carcinoma featuring arborizing telangiectases *(black arrow, top)*, ovoid nest *(black arrow, bottom)*, and multiple blue-gray globules *(white arrow)*.

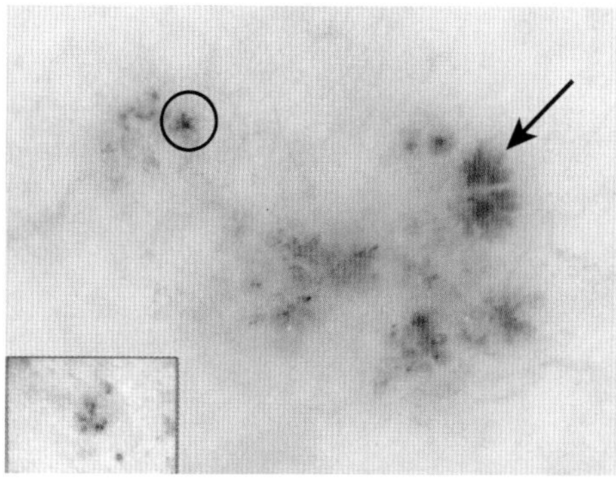

Figure 15-10 Pigmented basal cell carcinoma showing spoke-wheel–like structures *(circle)* and leaflike areas *(arrow)*. Both of these structures are 100% specific for the diagnosis of basal cell carcinoma.

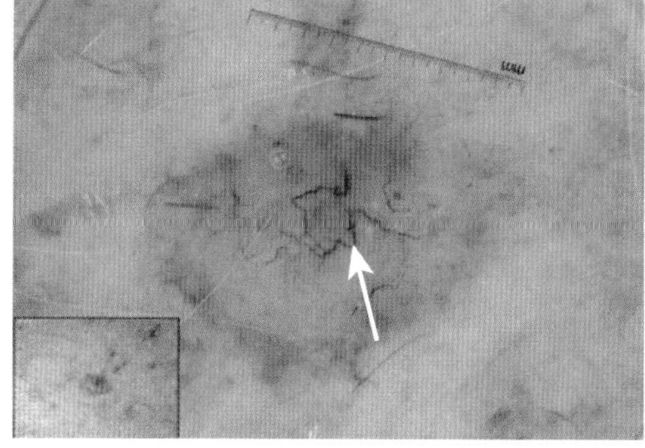

Figure 15-11 Nonpigmented basal cell carcinoma featuring arborizing telangiectases *(arrow)*.

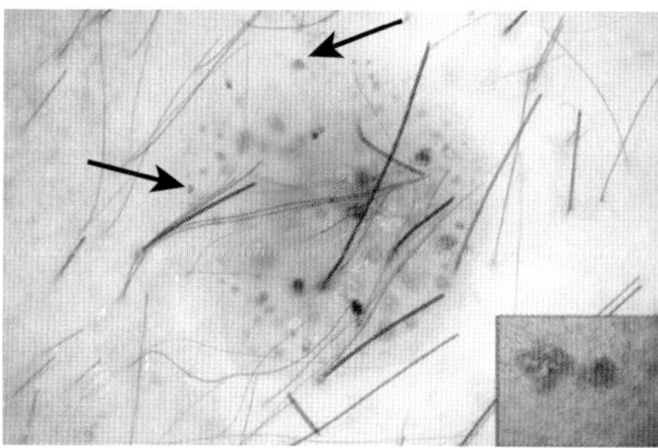

Figure 15-12 This keratotic lesion *(inset)* reveals clusters of glomeruloid vessels *(arrows)*, suggestive of the diagnosis of squamous cell carcinoma.

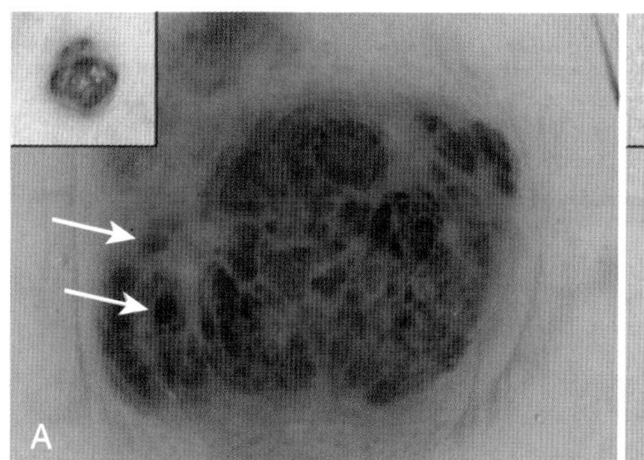

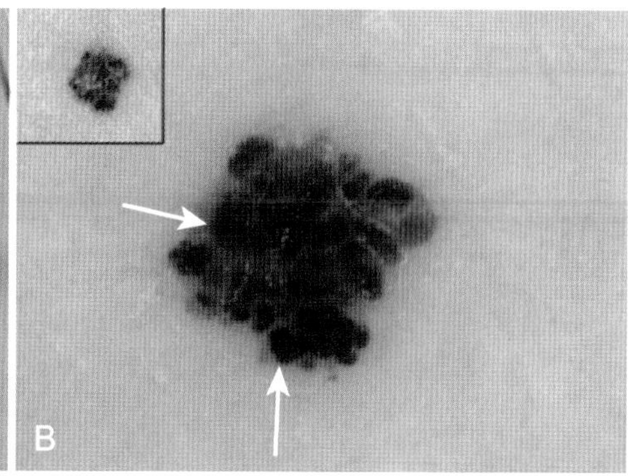

Figure 15-13 **A,** Hemangioma showing multiple lacunae of variable size, with a spectrum of colors from red to blue *(arrows)*. **B,** Cherry hemangioma showing multiple bright to dark red lacunae *(arrows)*.

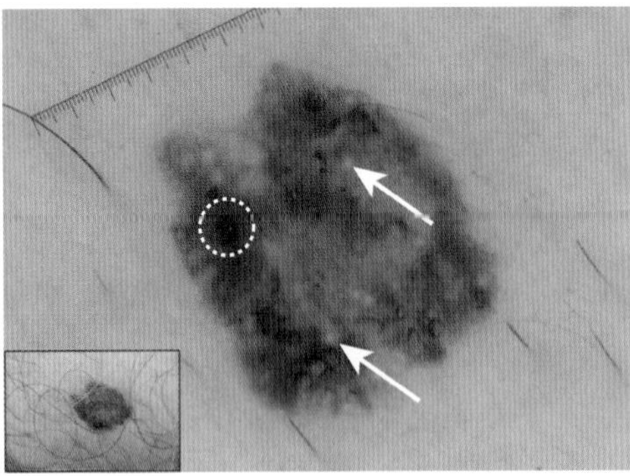

Figure 15-14 Seborrheic keratosis featuring sharp borders, comedo-like openings *(dotted circle)*, and multiple milia-like cysts *(arrows)*.

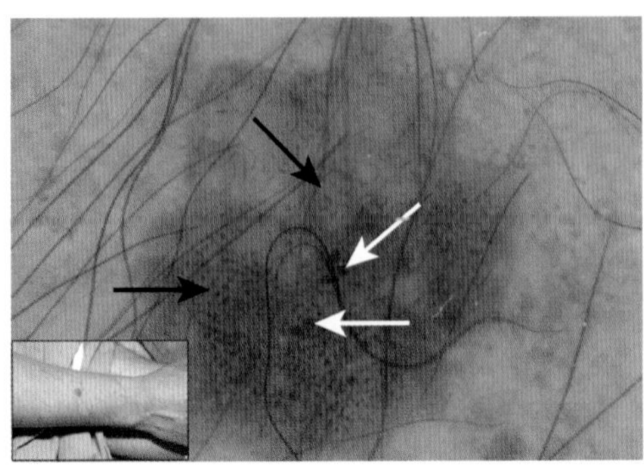

Figure 15-15 Seborrheic keratosis featuring a cerebriform pattern. The ridges (gyri, *black arrows*) are the raised portion of the lesion, and the fissures (sulci, *white arrows*) are crypts filled with keratin.

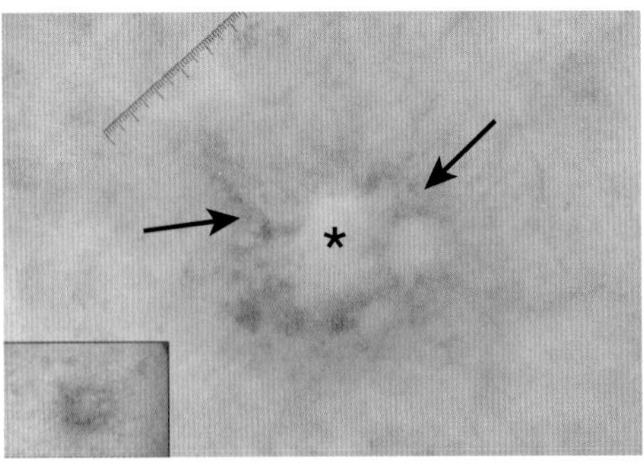

Figure 15-16 Dermatofibroma featuring a central depigmented scarlike area *(asterisk)* with surrounding peripheral network *(arrows)*.

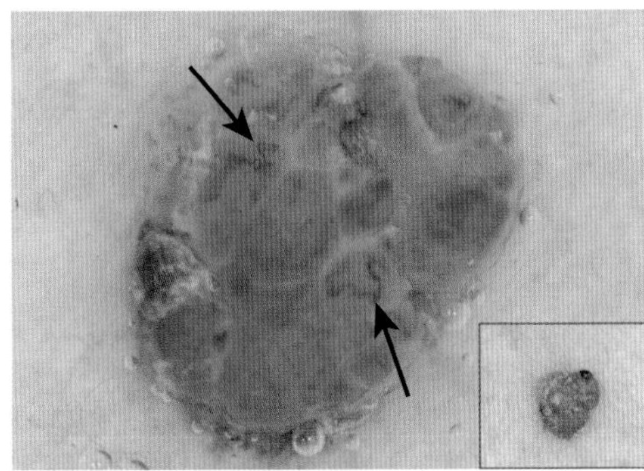

Figure 15-17 This nodule is amelanotic and lacks specific melanocytic or nonmelanocytic criteria of the two-step algorithm of dermoscopy. Thus, by default, one needs to consider melanoma in the differential diagnosis. Indeed, this lesion features atypical hairpin vessels *(arrows)*, a clue to the correct diagnosis. This proved to be a nodular melanoma.

TABLE 15-2 Dermoscopic Criteria for Melanocytic Lesions

Dermoscopic Criterion	Definition
Benign Nevi	
Reticular pattern	Pigment network of relative uniform thickness and color with holes of relative uniform size. Small brown or black dots can often be seen overlying the network or within the center of the lesion.
Globular pattern (includes cobblestone pattern)	Numerous, round-to-oval to angulated structures with various shades of brown. The globules are of uniform size, shape, and color and are distributed symmetrically.
Homogeneous pattern	Diffuse brown, gray-blue to blue-white pigmentation.
Starburst pattern	Finger-like projections seen at the edge of the lesion. The pigmented streaks are distributed symmetrically along the entire perimeter of the lesion in a radial arrangement.
Pseudonetwork pattern (face)	Pigmented lesion on facial skin with interruption of the pigment due to the presence of follicular and adnexal openings. This results in a network-like appearance.
Parallel furrow pattern (palms & soles)	Pigment located along the furrows of the palms and soles.
Melanoma	
Multicomponent pattern	Presence of three or more of the aforementioned patterns.
Atypical pigment network	Black, brown, or gray network with irregular-sized holes and thickened network lines. The network is often broken up, creating branched streaklike structures within the lesion.
Irregular dots/globules	Black, brown, round-to-oval structures distributed asymmetrically, not overlying the lines of a network, and often located toward the periphery of the lesion.
Irregular streaks	Finger-like projections seen at the edge of the lesion but distributed asymmetrically and focally along the perimeter of the melanoma.
Blotches	Black, brown, blue, or gray structureless areas distributed asymmetrically and not involving the entire lesion in a homogeneous manner.
Vascular structures	Dotted vessels, linear irregular vessels, thick and tortuous vessels, or erythema.
Annular-granular structures and pseudonetwork (Face)	Multiple blue-gray dots surrounding the follicular ostia, creating an annular-granular pattern. Once the pigment becomes confluent a pseudonetwork-like pattern emerges, which creates rhomboidal-like structures.
Parallel-ridge pattern (palms/soles)	Pigmentation aligned along the ridges on the palms and soles. This openings of the sweat ducts are located on the ridegs.

Box 15-2. Menzies Method

Negative Features (Neither Feature Found)

Symmetry of pattern (Assess only the colors and structures within the lesion. The symmetry/asymmetry of the contour/silhouette of the lesion is not a factor in this evaluation method.)

Presence of only a single color

Positive Features (At Least One Feature Found)

Blue-white veil
Pseudopods
Scarlike depigmentation
Multiple (5–6) colors
Broadened network
Multiple brown dots
Radial streaming
Peripheral black dots/globules
Multiple blue-gray dots ("peppering")

For melanoma to be diagnosed, the lesion must have neither of the two morphologic negative features and at least one of the nine positive features.

TABLE 15-3 ABCD Rule of Dermoscopy

Components of the ABCD Rule	Description	Score
Asymmetry	In 0, 1, or 2 perpendicular axes; assess not only contour, but also colors and structure	0–2
Border	Abrupt cut-off of pigment pattern at the periphery in 0 to 8 segments	0–8
Colors	Presence of up to 6 colors (white, red, light brown, dark brown, blue-gray, black)	1–6
Dermoscopic structures	Presence of network, structureless (homogeneous) areas, branched streaks, dots and globules	1–5

Calculation of Total Dermoscopy Score

A distinction between benign and malignant melanocytic lesions can often be made using the following formula: [(A score × 1.3) + (B score × 0.1) + (C score × 0.5) + (D score × 0.5)].

Interpretation of total score: <4.75, benign nevi; 4.75–5.45, suspicious for melanoma; >5.45, melanoma.

TABLE 15-4 Seven-Point Checklist

Criteria	Score
Major Criteria	
Atypical pigment network	2
Blue-white veil	2
Atypical vascular pattern	2
Minor Criteria	
Irregular streaks	1
Irregular dots/globules	1
Irregular blotches	1
Regression structures	1
Seven-Point Total Score	
Nonmelanoma	<3
Melanoma	≥3

By simple addition of the individual scores, one can differentiate between many benign nevi and melanoma. A minimum total score of 3 is required for the diagnosis of melanoma, whereas a total score of less than 3 indicative of a benign nevus.

Box 15-3. Revised Pattern Analysis

Nine Benign Nevus–Specific Patterns (All Exhibit Symmetry of Structure, Color, and Pattern)

1. Diffuse reticular network
2. Patchy reticular network
3. Peripheral reticular network with central hypopigmentation
4. Peripheral reticular network with central hyperpigmentation
5. Peripheral reticular network with central globules
6. Globular pattern
7. Peripheral globules with central reticular network or starburst
8. Homogeneous pattern
9. Symmetric multicomponent pattern

Nine Melanoma-Specific Structures

1. Atypical network
2. Streaks
3. Atypical dots or globules
4. Negative pigment network
5. Off-center pigmented blotch
6. Blue-white veil overlying flat areas
7. Blue-white veil overlying raised areas
8. Atypical vascular structures
9. Brown peripheral structureless area

Any lesion that does not conform to one of the benign nevus patterns or exhibits at least one of the melanoma-specific structures listed here should raise suspicion for melanoma. Thus, most melanomas will display asymmetry of structure, color, and pattern.

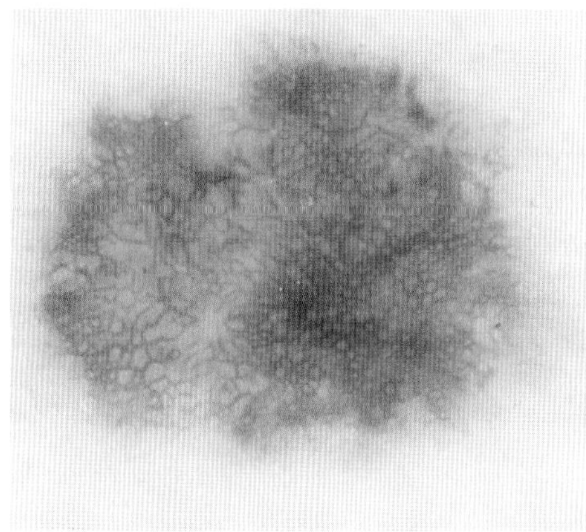

Figure 15-18 Lesion evaluation using various dermoscopic algorithms. The seven-point checklist of dermoscopy identifies only atypical network (two points). The total score is 2, denoting a benign lesion (i.e., nevus). Evaluation using the Menzies method also leads to the conclusion that this is a nevus because the lesion shows a single color and overall symmetry of structure and pattern. Lesion evaluation using the ABCD rule indicates a total score of 3.3 (A = 1.3 for asymmetry in one axis [comparing right and left halves of the lesion], B = 0 because the lesion gradually fades into the periphery, C = 1 for the color brown, and D = 1 for the presence of network). This score is within the benign range of the ABCD method.

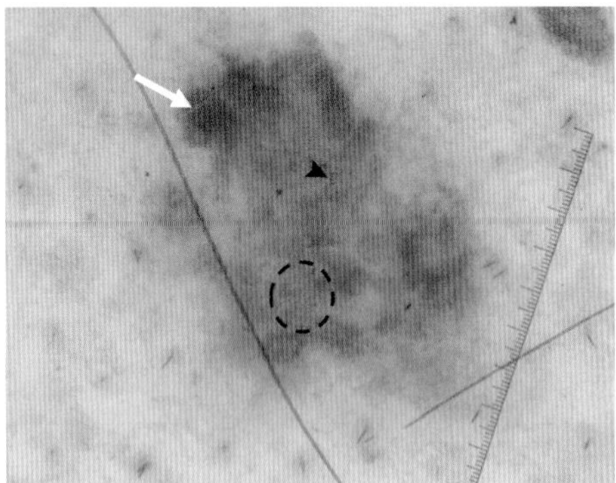

Figure 15-19 Lesion evaluation using various dermoscopic algorithms. By the seven-point checklist of dermoscopy the lesion displays an irregular blotch (*arrow*, one point), irregular dots/globules (*arrowhead*, one point), and regression structures with bluish peppering (*dotted circle*, one point). The total score is 3, denoting a melanoma. Evaluating the same lesion by the Menzies method also leads to the same conclusion because the lesion has more than one color and has asymmetry of structure and pattern. It also has blue-gray peppering *(dotted circle)*. Thus, this lesion is a melanoma. Lesion evaluation using the ABCD indicates a total score of 6.6 (A = 2.6 for two-axis asymmetry, B = 0 because the lesion fades gradually into the periphery, C = 2 for the presence of four colors [light and dark brown, blue-gray, and red], and D = 2 for the presence of network, structureless areas, and dots and globules). The lesion has dermoscopic features consistent with melanoma.

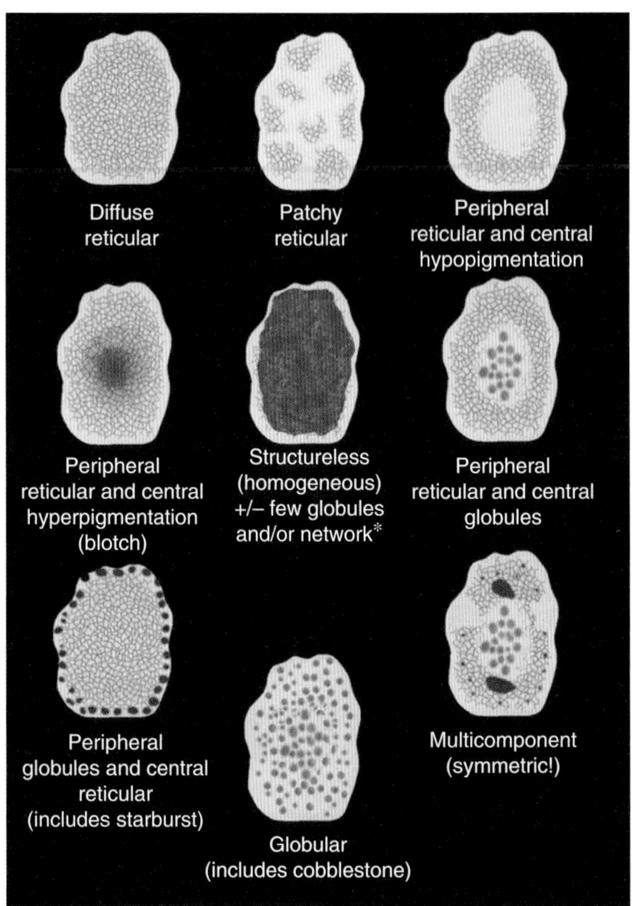

Figure 15-20 The nine benign global dermoscopic patterns of nevi. *"Structureless" refers to a hyper- or hypopigmented blotch.

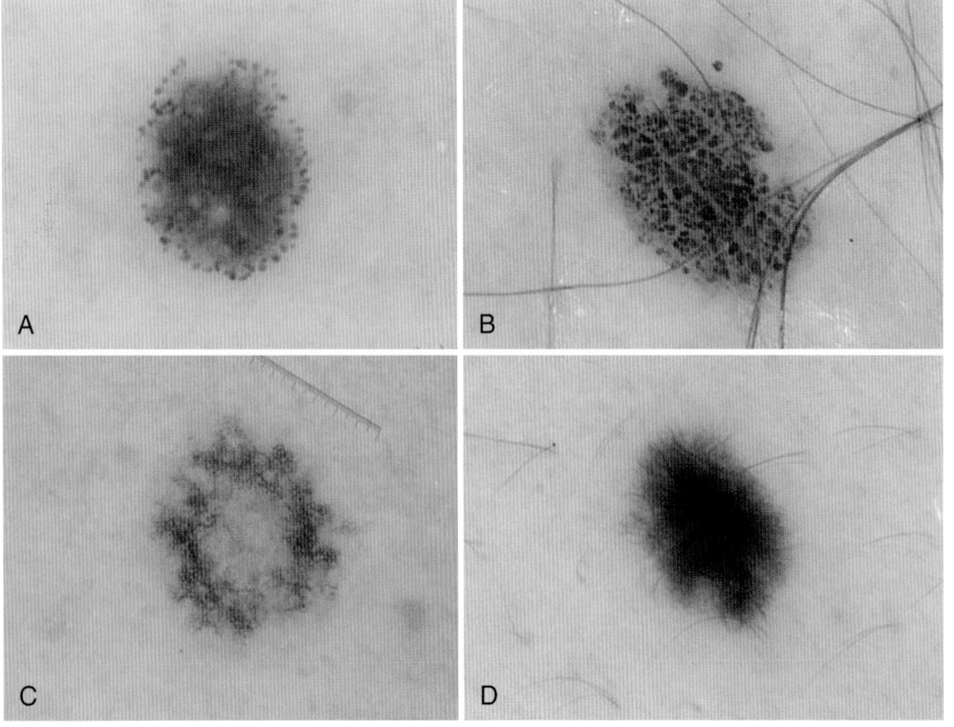

Figure 15-21 Examples of benign global dermoscopic patterns. **A,** Peripheral globules and central reticular. **B,** Globular pattern. This variant is called the "cobblestone" pattern because the globules are large and angulated, arranged almost back to back. **C,** Peripheral reticular and central hypopigmentation. **D,** Peripheral reticular and central hyperpigmentation.

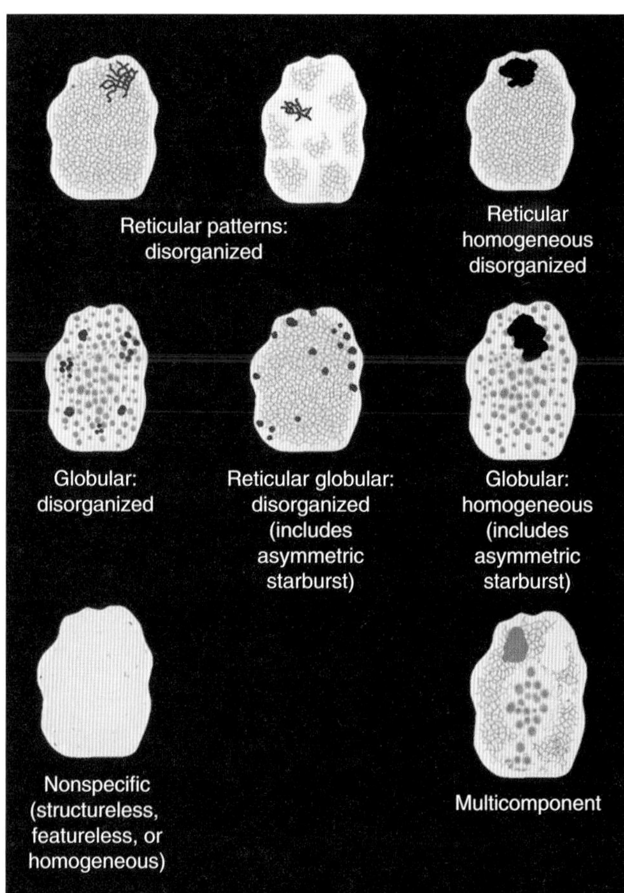

Figure 15-22 Global dermoscopic patterns commonly seen in melanoma. Specific (local) dermoscopic structures that should raise suspicion for malignancy include atypical network; streaks; atypical dots or globules; negative pigment network; off-center pigmented blotch; blue-white veil overlying flat areas; blue-white veil overlying raised areas; atypical vascular structures; and brown peripheral structureless area.

features common to benign nevi, it stands to reason that most melanocytic nevi will be symmetric, uniform, display less than three colors, and have an organized architecture.

In contrast, MM often exhibits a pattern that deviates from the aforementioned benign patterns, manifests asymmetry of dermoscopic colors and structures, and displays a disordered dermoscopic architecture. *Most MMs also contain at least one of the following nine specific dermoscopic structures*: (1) atypical network, (2) peripheral streaks, (3) atypical dots or globules, (4) negative pigment network, (5) off-center pigmented blotch, (6) blue-white veil overlying flat areas, (7) blue-white veil overlying raised areas, (8) atypical vascular structures, and (9) brown peripheral structureless area (Figs. 15-22 and 15-23; see Box 15-3).

Although most MMs display at least some degree of asymmetry of pattern, color, and structure, there exists a subset of early MMs that are structureless. Fortunately, most of these early MMs can be correctly identified based on observing their growth dynamics or by visualizing the presence of an increased vasculature.

Neoangiogenesis, resulting in an increased blood volume, is required for MM survival and growth. These neoangiogenic blood vessels can often be visualized under dermoscopy, and their presence can help correctly identify many MMs. Studies have shown that the specific morphology of the blood vessels observed under dermoscopy is correlated to specific tumors (Table 15-5). The most common vessel morphologies exhibited by MM are linear-irregular and dotted vessels (Fig. 15-24). Hence, the presence of such vessels in

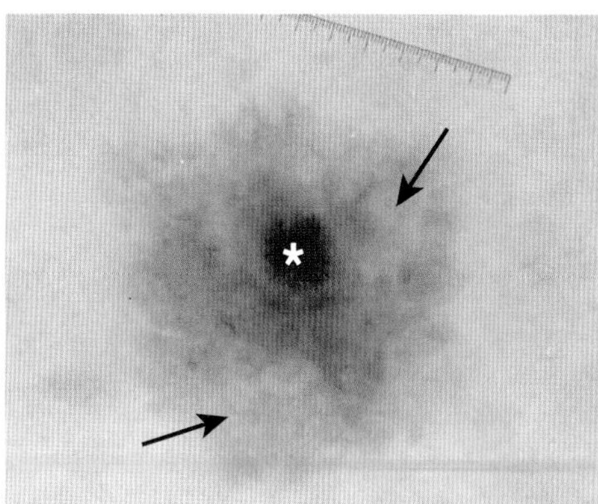

Figure 15-23 Although this lesion has symmetry of structure and pattern, it does not conform to one of the nine benign patterns. In addition, it has peripheral brown structureless areas *(arrows)* and an atypical network in the center *(asterisk)*. This was an in situ melanoma.

TABLE 15-5 Vascular Structures with Associated Tumors

Primary Vessel Morphology	Disease Entity
Arborizing vessels	Basal cell carcinoma
Comma vessels	Intradermal nevus Congenital melanocytic nevus
Corkscrew vessels	Nodular melanoma Cutaneous melanoma metastasis Desmoplastic melanoma
Dotted and globular vessels	Melanoma Spitz nevus Dysplastic nevus Squamous cell carcinoma
Glomerular vessels	Squamous cell carcinoma
Hairpin vessels	Keratoacanthoma Melanoma Irritated seborrheic keratosis Squamous cell carcinoma Spitz nevus
Linear irregular vessels	Melanoma Spitz nevus
Milky red area/globule	Melanoma
Polymorphous vessels	Melanoma

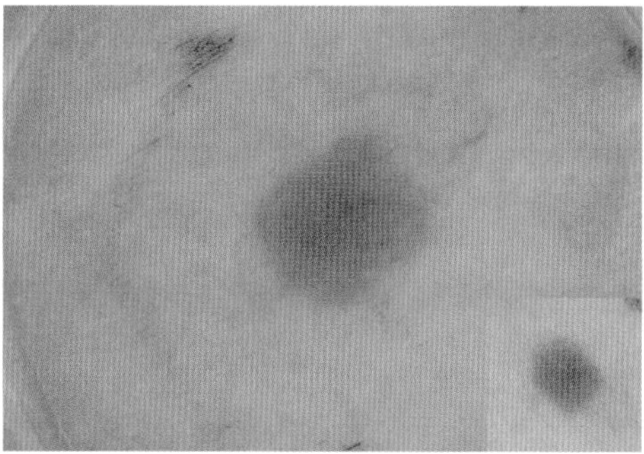

Figure 15-24 Invasive melanoma (0.45 mm in Breslow depth) lacking any pigmented dermoscopic features, and showing only dotted vessels throughout the lesion.

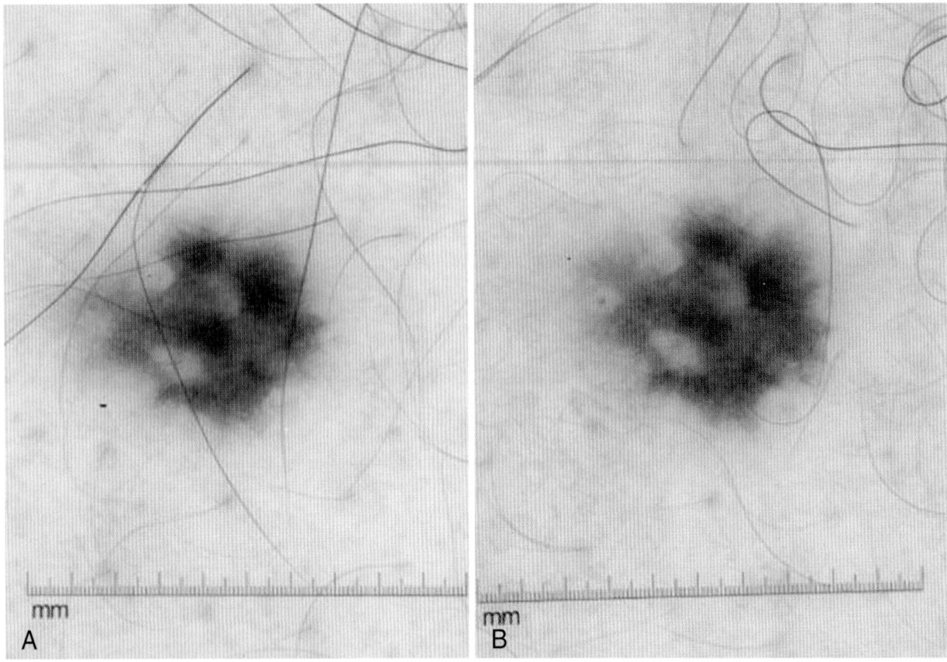

Figure 15-25 Side-by side comparison of sequential dermoscopic images at baseline (**A**) and 9-month follow-up (**B**). No dermoscopic changes are seen on follow-up examination; therefore, the lesion is considered biologically benign.

a hypopigmented or amelanotic lesion is an important clue to the diagnosis of MM.

Malignancies, being biologically active, are growing lesions, whereas benign nevi are usually in a state of senescence. This fact can be used by clinicians to help isolate early MMs that have not yet developed any of the MM-specific dermoscopic structures mentioned previously (i.e., structureless MM) from among many benign nevi. The acquisition of sequential dermoscopic images provides physicians with the ability to monitor lesions for change. This ability to compare baseline and follow-up dermoscopic images of the same lesion over time increases the specificity of MM diagnosis while at the same time maintaining a high sensitivity, which translates into the appropriate removal of MMs with a concomitant reduction in the unnecessary removal of benign lesions (Figs. 15-25 and 15-26).

Sequential imaging is usually restricted to patients with multiple atypical nevi because it is often more practical to simply remove a single atypical mole on a patient with few to no additional nevi than it is to follow them. For individuals possessing many nevi, the removal of all of their atypical moles would be impractical. In such patients, sequential dermoscopic imaging appears to be a reasonable management strategy. The principle is that if a lesion is found to be stable, the patient can be reassured that the lesion is biologically indolent at that moment in time and thus can be followed routinely.

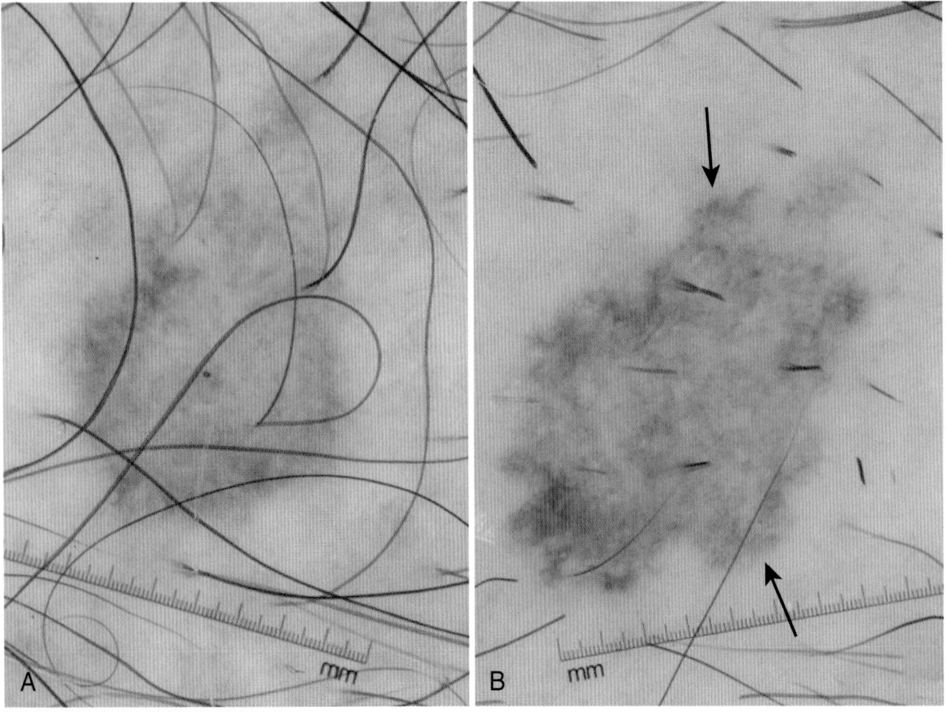

Figure 15-26 Dermoscopic follow-up using side-by side comparison of sequential dermoscopic images at baseline (**A**) and 4-month follow-up (**B**). At follow-up, radial growth of the lesion can be appreciated (**B,** *arrows*). This lesion, which otherwise does not display melanoma-specific dermoscopic features, proved to be an invasive melanoma 0.3 mm in Breslow depth.

Short-Term Mole Monitoring

The most timely method, short of performing a biopsy, for correctly segregating benign lesions from MM is by sequential "short-term" dermoscopic imaging (see Figs. 15-25 and 15-26). Menzies and colleagues (2001) introduced the concept of short-term mole monitoring, which involves sequential reexamination of the same lesion over a 3- to 4-month period. Short-term dermoscopic monitoring is aimed at increasing the specificity of evaluation of equivocal melanocytic lesions. It is used to evaluate melanocytic lesions that lack dermoscopic features of MM, yet appear somewhat atypical to the examiner or have a history of change. In this setting, any morphologic change observed during the 3-month monitoring period warrants an excision. The exceptions to this rule are when one observes an overall increase or decrease in pigmentation without accompanying architectural change or the loss or appearance of milia-like cysts.

The majority (81%) of the lesions followed up in the study by Menzies and colleagues did not change and thus were "spared" from undergoing unnecessary removal. Of the lesions that did reveal change, 11% were found to be MM, all of which proved to be histologically thin tumors, and none revealed any of the MM-specific dermoscopic structures mentioned previously. The specificity for the diagnosis of MM by means of short-term digital monitoring of dermoscopically equivocal lesions was reported to be 83%. In another study, Kittler and associates (2006) followed suspect lesions lacking MM-specific features at baseline for over 8 months. After follow-up of 1.5 to 4.5 months, only 38.2% of the MMs showed specific dermoscopic features for MM. This value increased to 55% after 4.5 to 8.0 months and to 64.9% after more than 8.0 months (Fig. 15-27). The observed changes in MM lesions included asymmetric enlargement, focal changes in pigmentation and structure, regression features, and change in color. Insignificant change observed in lesions after at least 6 months of follow-up included a darker or lighter overall appearance, change in the number or distribution of brown globules, and disappearance of parts of the pigment network. The conclusion of the study was that MM-specific dermoscopic criteria in structureless MMs become readily apparent as the length of follow-up increases. However, MMs that lack any specific features can in fact be detected by the short-term monitoring process. Thus, MMs lacking MM-specific dermoscopic features can now be detected based on observing their dynamic evolution over time.

Dermoscopy in the Primary Care Office

Approximately 40% of office visits to physicians in the United States are to a primary care physician (PCP), and although most patients with MM had at least one primary care visit in the year before diagnosis, only 20% report receiving a skin cancer examination. Compared with MM detection by the patient or family, MM detected by physicians is more likely to be thinner. PCPs, therefore, are in a unique position to perform skin cancer screening. Studies indicate that training PCPs to screen for MM using dermoscopy leads to increased diagnostic sensitivity without a significant decrease in specificity. Argenziano and colleagues (2006) introduced the three-point checklist for the purpose of improving sensitivity in skin cancer (i.e., MM and basal cell carcinoma) screening by PCPs (Table 15-6 and Figs. 15-28 through 15-30). The three-point checklist was meant to serve as a triage tool to help PCPs in deciding on referrals of pigmented lesions to dermatologists. The study indicated that dermoscopy allows PCPs to perform 25.1% better triage of skin lesions suggestive of skin cancer compared with naked-eye examination alone ($P = .002$).

In another study among general practitioners, sensitivity for MM diagnosis improved significantly from a clinical baseline pretest of 54% to a post-training dermoscopy diagnosis of 76%. In addition, dermoscopy education created an increased awareness of the clinical appearance of MM among PCPs and improved naked-eye diagnosis of MM. PCPs are encouraged to be formally trained in dermoscopy

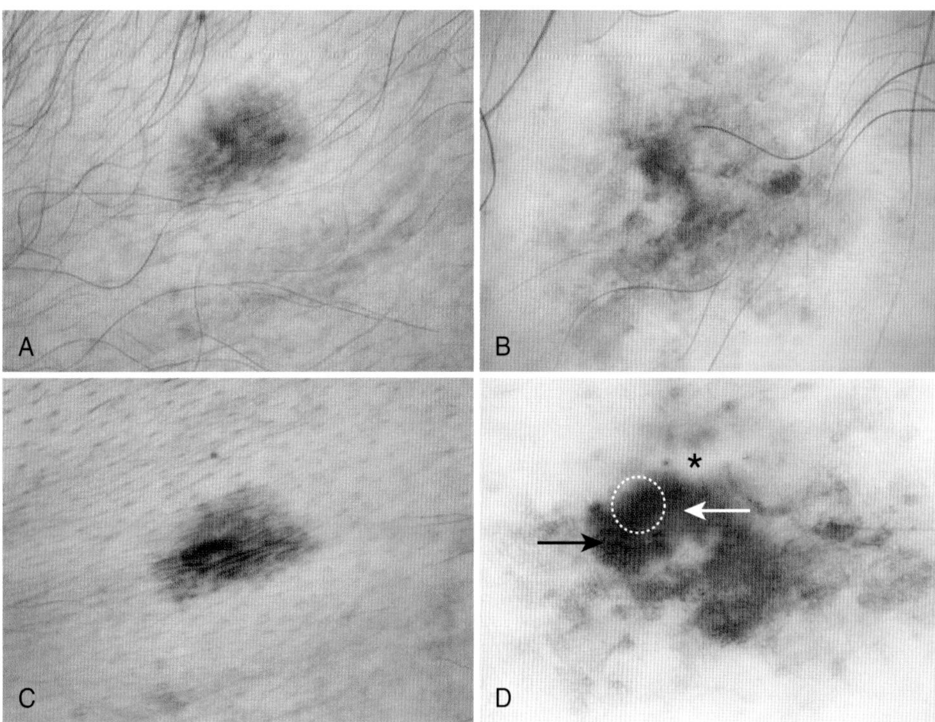

Figure 15-27 With long-term follow-up, malignant lesions will increasingly show melanoma-specific dermoscopic structures. This lesion was clinically inconspicuous (**A**) and dermoscopically showed only a reticular–homogenous pattern (**B**). However, at 2-year follow-up (**C**), the lesion was clinically more suspect, with asymmetry and multiple colors (brown, black, and pink). On dermoscopy at the 2-year follow-up (**D**), the lesion showed an atypical network *(black arrow)*, multiple dots *(dotted circle)*, and bluish-gray *(white arrow)* and white scar-like *(asterisk)* areas suggestive of regression. This was a melanoma 1.8 mm in Breslow depth.

TABLE 15-6 The Three-Point Checklist

Three-Point Checklist	Definition
Asymmetry	Asymmetrical distribution of colors and dermoscopic structures.
Atypical network	Pigmented network with irregular holes and thick line. Streaks are considered part of an atypical network.
Blue-white structures	Any type of blue or white color, including white scarlike depigmentation, blue-whitish veil and blue pepper-like granules (regression structures).

The presence of more than one criterion suggests a suspicious lesion.

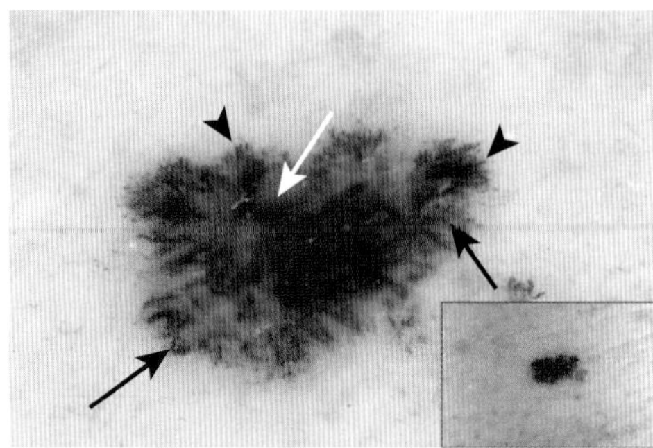

Figure 15-30 Evaluating this pigmented lesion using the three-point checklist indicates asymmetric distribution of dermoscopic structures, atypical network *(black arrows)*, and blue-white structures *(white arrow)*. The total score is 3. This lesion was a melanoma 0.3 mm in Breslow depth. Of note, the lesion also displays multiple peripheral streaks *(black arrowheads)*, which are considered to be part of the atypical network.

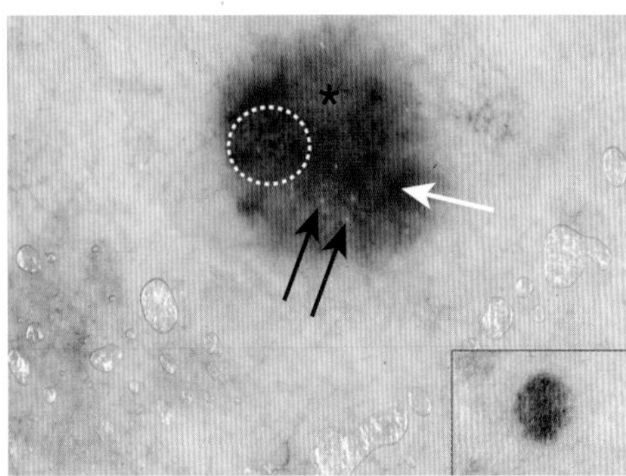

Figure 15-28 This lesion appears clinically symmetric *(inset)*. However, dermoscopic evaluation reveals asymmetric distribution of the dermoscopic structures: aggregated globules in the top left quadrant *(dotted circle)*, blue-white structures *(asterisk)*, blotches *(white arrow)*, and milia-like cysts *(black arrows)*. By the three-point checklist the lesion gets a score of 2 for the dermoscopic asymmetry and blue-white structures, denoting a suspect lesion. This lesion was a melanoma 0.5 mm in Breslow depth.

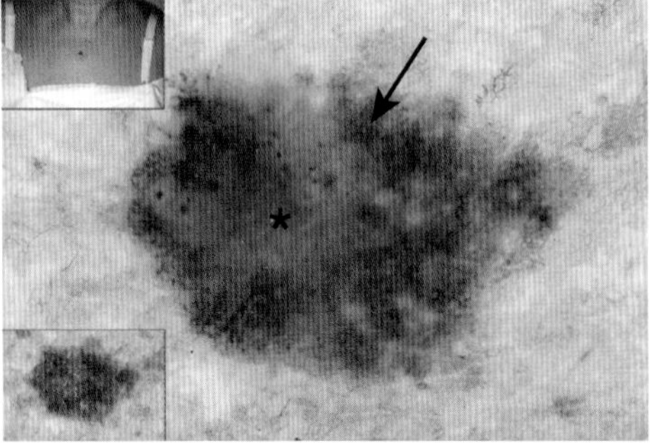

Figure 15-29 This lesion is an "ugly duckling" that stands out as different on the patient's chest *(top inset)* and shows clinical asymmetry and multiple colors *(bottom inset)*. Evaluating this pigmented lesion using the three-point checklist indicates asymmetric distribution of dermoscopic structures, atypical network *(arrow)*, and blue-white structures *(asterisk)*, for a total score of 3. This lesion was a melanoma 0.5 mm in Breslow depth.

for the clinical assessment of skin tumors, including MM. Australia and New Zealand have successfully implemented a wide network of skin cancer screening by PCPs. In a study assessing New Zealand general practitioners' diagnosis and management of skin cancer, the participating physicians were shown to have a high level of expertise in making the correct diagnosis and in deciding whether or not to biopsy the lesion.

It is important to acknowledge that dermoscopy constitutes only one portion of a thorough history and physical examination. We caution against *solely* relying on the dermoscopic findings while dismissing other clinical cues. For example, a lesion that appears different (either by clinical or dermoscopic examination) relative to its neighboring lesions, known as the *ugly duckling sign*, should raise suspicion in the observer even in the absence of definitive dermoscopic features of MM. The final decision-making process should always evaluate the dermoscopic findings in light of the patient's personal and family history, as well as other clinical parameters of the lesion such as symptoms of pain, bleeding, or itching.

In summary, there is compelling evidence that dermoscopy improves MM diagnosis at an earlier, curable stage while avoiding excessive scarring from removal of benign lesions. As a first-level screening tool, dermoscopy may improve the PCP's ability to detect skin cancer.

SUPPLIERS

(See contact information online at www.expertconsult.com.)

Dermatoscope
Heine USA
DermoGenius
BIOCAM GmbH
EpiScope
Welch Allyn
3Gen
Makers of dermlites

ONLINE RESOURCES

Dermoscopy [educational website]. Available at http://www.dermoscopy.org/; dermoscopy tutorial available at http://www.dermoscopy.org/atlas/base.htm.

International Society of Dermoscopy: Online discussion forum. Available at http://www.dermoscopy-ids.org/discussion/ [registration required].

Miami Medical: Episcope. Available at http://www.miami-med.com/episcope.htm. Accessed March 26, 2008.

BIBLIOGRAPHY

Argenziano G, Puig S, Zalaudek I, et al: Dermoscopy improves accuracy of primary care physicians to triage lesions suggestive of skin cancer. J Clin Oncol 24:1877–1882, 2006.

Argenziano G, Soyer HP, Chimenti S, et al: Dermoscopy of pigmented skin lesions: Results of a consensus meeting via the Internet. J Am Acad Dermatol 48:679–693, 2003.

Argenziano G, Zalaudek I, Corona R, et al: Vascular structures in skin tumors. Arch Dermatol 140:1485–1489, 2004.

Bafounta ML, Beauchet A, Aegerter P, Saiag P: Is dermoscopy useful for the diagnosis of melanoma? Results of a meta-analysis using techniques adapted to the evaluation of diagnostic tests. Arch Dermatol 137: 1343–1350, 2001.

Benvenuto-Andrade C, Dusza S, Hay J, et al: Level of confidence in diagnosis: Clinical examination versus dermoscopy examination. Dermatol Surg 32:738–744, 2006.

Benvenuto-Andrade C, Marghoob A: Ten reasons why dermoscopy is beneficial for the evaluation of skin lesions. Exp Rev Dermatol 1:369–374, 2006.

Binder M, Kittler H, Steiner A: Reevaluation of the ABCD rule for epiluminescence microscopy. J Am Acad Dermatol 40:171–176, 1999.

Bono A, Maurichi A, Moglia D, et al: Clinical and dermatoscopic diagnosis of early amelanotic melanoma. Melanoma Res 11:491–494, 2001.

Brochez L, Verhaeghe E, Bleyen L, Naeyaert JM: Diagnostic ability of general practitioners and dermatologists in discriminating pigmented skin lesions. J Am Acad Dermatol 44:979–986, 2001.

Carli P, de Giorgi V, Chiarugi A, et al: Addition of dermoscopy to conventional naked-eye examination in melanoma screening: A randomized study. J Am Acad Dermatol 50:683–689, 2004.

Carli P, De Giorgi V, Crocetti E, et al: Improvement of malignant/benign ratio in excised melanocytic lesions in the "dermoscopy era": A retrospective study 1997–2001. Br J Dermatol 150:687–692, 2004.

Chen SC, Pennie ML, Kolm P, et al: Diagnosing and managing cutaneous pigmented lesions: Primary care physicians versus dermatologists. J Gen Intern Med 21:678–682, 2006.

Cyr PR: Atypical moles. Am Fam Physician 78:735–740, 2008.

Epstein DS, Lange JR, Gruber SB, et al: Is physician detection associated with thinner melanomas? JAMA 281:640–643, 1999.

Fox FN: Dermoscopy: An invaluable tool for evaluating skin lesions. Am Fam Physician 78:704–706, 2008.

Gachon J, Beaulieu P, Sei JF, et al: First prospective study of the recognition process of melanoma in dermatological practice. Arch Dermatol 141:434–438, 2005.

Geller AC, Koh HK, Miller DR, et al: Use of health services before the diagnosis of melanoma: Implications for early detection and screening. J Gen Intern Med 7:154–157, 1992.

Haenssle HA, Krueger U, Vente C, et al: Results from an observational trial: Digital epiluminescence microscopy follow-up of atypical nevi increases the sensitivity and the chance of success of conventional dermoscopy in detecting melanoma. J Invest Dermatol 126:980–985, 2006.

Hennings JS, Dusza SW, Wang SQ, et al: The CASH (color, architecture, symmetry, and homogeneity) algorithm for dermoscopy. J Am Acad Dermatol 56:45–52, 2007.

Johr R, Soyer HP, Argenziano G, et al: Dermoscopy: The Essentials. St. Louis, Mosby, 2004.

Kittler H, Guitera P, Riedl E, et al: Identification of clinically featureless incipient melanoma using sequential dermoscopy imaging. Arch Dermatol 142:1113–1119, 2006.

Kittler H, Pehamberger H, Wolff K, Binder M: Follow-up of melanocytic skin lesions with digital epiluminescence microscopy: Patterns of modifications observed in early melanoma, atypical nevi, and common nevi. J Am Acad Dermatol 43:467–476, 2000.

Kittler H, Pehamberger H, Wolff K, Binder M: Diagnostic accuracy of dermoscopy. Lancet Oncol 3:159–165, 2002.

Malvehy J, Puig S, Braun RP, et al: Handbook of Dermoscopy. New York, Taylor & Francis, 2006.

Marghoob AA, Braun RP, Kopf AW: Atlas of Dermoscopy. New York, Taylor & Francis, 2005.

Marghoob AA, Korzenko AJ, Changchien L, et al: The beauty and the beast sign in dermoscopy. Dermatol Surg 33:1–4, 2007.

McGee R, Elwook M, Adam H, et al: The recognition and management of melanoma and other skin lesions by general practitioners in New Zealand. N Z Med J 107:287–290, 1994.

Menzies SW, Gutenev A, Avramidis M, et al: Short-term digital surface microscopic monitoring of atypical or changing melanocytic lesions. Arch Dermatol 137:1583–1589, 2001.

Menzies SW, Zalaudek I: Why perform dermoscopy? The evidence for its role in the routine management of pigmented skin lesions. Arch Dermatol 142:1211–1212, 2006.

Pagnanelli G, Soyer HP, Argenziano G, et al: Diagnosis of pigmented skin lesions by dermoscopy: Web-based training improves diagnostic performance of non-experts. Br J Dermatol 148:698–702, 2003.

Scope A, Benvenuto-Andrade C, Agero AC, et al: Correlation of dermoscopic structures of melanocytic lesions to reflectance confocal microscopy. Arch Dermatol 143:176–185, 2007.

Usatine RP (ed): Appendix: Dermoscopy. In Usatine RP (ed): The Color Atlas of Family Medicine, New York, McGraw-Hill, 2009.

Wang SQ, Scope A, Marghoob AA: Dermoscopic patterns of melanoma. G Ital Dermatol Venereol 142:99–108, 2007.

Westerhoff K, McCarthy WH, Menzies SW: Increase in the sensitivity for melanoma diagnosis by primary care physicians using skin surface microscopy. Br J Dermatol 143:1016–1020, 2000.

CHAPTER 16

Fishhook Removal

John Harlan Haynes III • Terrance S. Hines

Fishhook injuries are relatively common. Confidence in their management is paramount to successful outcomes. The method used to remove a fishhook depends on the anatomic location of the injury and the conditions under which the removal is to take place. The first and least harmful method described is the *string-yank* method, which may be used without anesthesia by anglers on the water. It is best used on the more resilient skin surfaces with underlying bone and muscle. For more embedded hooks, or for hooks in flaccid areas such as the earlobe, the needle cover *"barb-sheath"* or the *pull-through* technique may be more applicable. Local anesthesia with 1% lidocaine is well received by the anxious patient in an emergency setting. If the shank has already been clipped by a well-meaning first-aider, a strong needle driver or hemostat may be clamped over the exposed shank tip to facilitate removal.

Occasionally, radiographs may help in determining the type of fishhook and depth of penetration. Before a fishhook is removed, be sure to assess the proximity of the hook to underlying neurovascular or tendon structures and the potential for damage.

Indication

A fishhook embedded in subcutaneous tissue (most commonly, fingers and feet).

Contraindications

- Penetration into the eye with scleral perforation (dictates ophthalmology referral)
- Deeply embedded hooks in or near the neck, genitalia, arteries, or the wrist, or possible penetration of gastrointestinal mucosa

Angler's String-Yank Method

Equipment

- Silk suture (0 or larger diameter), umbilical tape, or ordinary string, 2 to 3 feet in length
- 2 to 3 mL of 1% lidocaine in syringe with a 30-gauge needle
- Protective eyewear

Technique

1. Cleanse the skin with an iodinated soap or similar antiseptic solution.
2. Inject 2 to 3 mL of 1% local anesthetic around the hook.
3. Tie the midpoint of the string or suture around the curve of the fishhook. Securely wrap the other ends several times around your index and middle finger (Fig. 16-1A).
4. Place the involved extremity on a flat surface to provide stabilization. Depress the shank of the hook against the skin with the index finger of your nondominant free hand until it meets resistance. The shaft of the hook is then lifted approximately parallel to the underlying skin by grasping the eye with the thumb and middle fingers (Fig. 16-1B). This maneuver disengages the barb from the subcutaneous tissue.
5. With the shank depressed and the barb disengaged, grasp the string 12 inches from the hook and firmly and quickly jerk the string, with follow-through, in one forceful move parallel to the shank (Fig. 16-1C). Sudden and forceful pulling on the suture is necessary to prevent failure of the technique. Bystanders should stand clear from the flight path, and protective eyewear should be worn. This method is effective and produces no additional wounds.

Needle Cover or "Barb-Sheath" Method

Equipment

- 0.5 mL lidocaine 1% in a syringe with a 30-gauge needle
- 18-gauge needle
- Protective eyewear

Technique

1. After local anesthesia is injected, introduce the 18-gauge needle through the entrance track along the inside curvature of the hook, parallel to the shank, with the bevel toward the inside of the curve so that the needle opening can engage the barb (Fig. 16-2A and B).
2. Advance the hook slightly to dislodge the barb from the tissue. Gently pull and twist the hook so that the barb is firmly sheathed by the lumen of the 18-gauge needle.
3. Back the hook and needle out together as a unit (Fig. 16-2C).

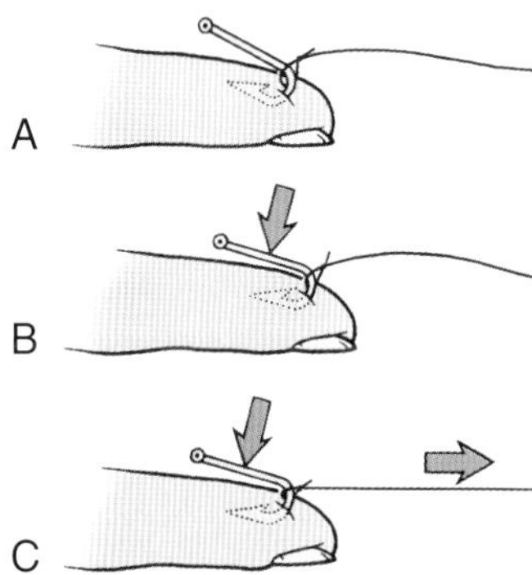

Figure 16-1 **A–C,** Angler's string-yank method of fishhook removal. See text for details.

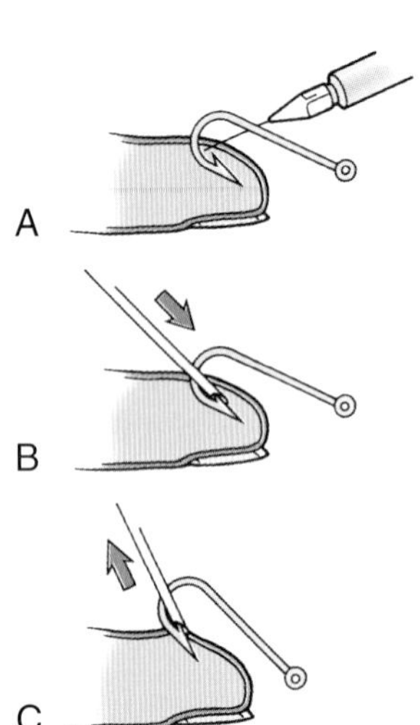

Figure 16-2 **A–C,** Removal of a fishhook with anesthetic when the hook is large and not too deep in the skin. See text for details.

TRADITIONAL PULL-THROUGH METHOD

Equipment

- 0.5 mL lidocaine 1% in syringe with a 27-gauge needle
- Wire clipper
- Protective eyewear

Technique

1. Provide local anesthesia over the point of the hook (Fig. 16-3A).
2. Force the point through the anesthetized skin (Fig. 16-3B).
3. When the barb tip is fully exposed, clip it off (Fig. 16-3C).
4. Back the hook out along the direction of entry (Fig. 16-3D).
5. Alternatively, if the shank has multiple barbs, clip off the eye of the hook and pull on the sharp end of the hook until the entire hook is removed (Fig. 16-4).

POSTPROCEDURE CARE

- Explore the wound for possible foreign bodies and débrid it.
- Administer tetanus toxoid if more than 5 years has elapsed since its last administration.
- Prophylactic antibiotic therapy may be considered for persons who are immunosuppressed or have diabetes or peripheral vascular disease. Prophylactic antibiotics may also be used for deeper or contaminated wounds. Coverage should include normal skin flora (*Staphylococcus aureus* and *Staphylococcus pyogenes*) as well as potential water-borne pathogens (*Aeromonas* species, *Edwardsiella tarda*, *Erysipelothrix rhusiopathiae*, *Vibrio vulnificus*, and *Mycobacterium marinum*). Empiric coverage for soft tissue infections after water exposure includes either a first-generation cephalosporin *or* clindamycin *plus* levofloxacin *plus* either metronidazole (sewage- or soil- contaminated wound, not necessary if clindamycin given) *or* doxycycline (coverage of *Vibrio* species if seawater exposure).
- Dress the wound with a sterile adhesive bandage and antibiotic ointment.
- Wash the area well with soap and water four to six times a day for 2 days.
- Warn the patient of the possibility of infection.

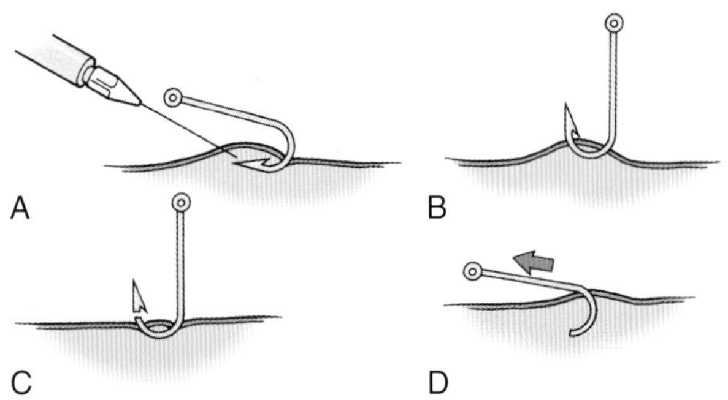

Figure 16-3 **A–D,** Traditional pull-through method for removing a small fishhook. See text for details.

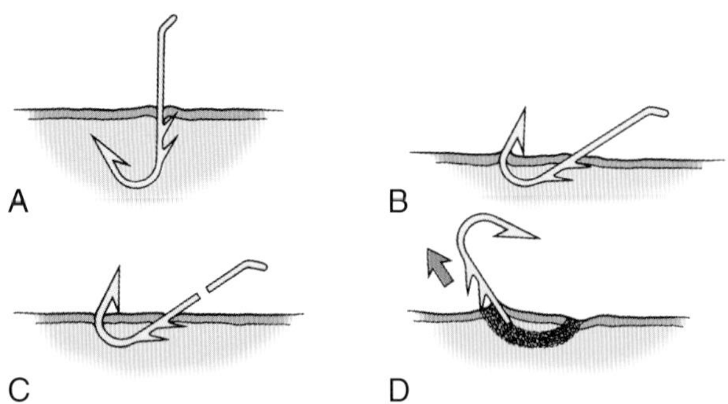

Figure 16-4 Removal of a barbed fishhook. **A,** The hook embedded in soft tissue. **B,** Twist the hook forward until the sharp end is visible. **C,** Cut off the eye of the hook. **D,** Pull on the sharp end to remove.

CPT/BILLING CODES

10120 Removal of subcutaneous foreign body, simple
10121 Incisional removal, foreign body, complex

Removal of foreign body from the following

20520 Muscle or tendon sheath, simple
23330 Shoulder subcutaneous
24200 Upper arm/elbow subcutaneous
27086 Pelvis/hip subcutaneous
28190 Foot subcutaneous
67938 Embedded eyelid

ICD-9-CM DIAGNOSTIC CODES

Foreign body in the following

729.6 Soft tissue
919.6 Superficial without major open wound
930.1 Eyelid
931 Auricle
931 Ear
932 Nose
932 Nostril
935 Mouth
955.4 Musculocutaneous

BIBLIOGRAPHY

American Academy of Orthopedic Surgeons: Fishhook removal. In Snider RK (ed): Essentials of Musculoskeletal Care. Rosemont, Ill, American Academy of Orthopedic Surgeons, 1997.

Baddour LM: Soft tissue infections following water exposure. Available at www.uptodate.com.

Bothner J: Fish-hook removal techniques. Available at www.uptodate.com.

Gammons M, Jackson E: Fishhook removal. Am Fam Physician 63: 2231–2236, 2001.

Halaas GW: Management of foreign bodies in the skin. Am Fam Physician 76:683–688, 2007.

Raveenthiran V: Soft palatal injury resulting from an unusual fishhook in a child. J Trauma 62:1060, 2007.

CHAPTER 17

FLAPS AND PLASTIES

Dennis LaRavia

Appropriate wound closure after excision is essential in achieving a cosmetically pleasing result. Although many elliptical defects can be repaired with a basic side-to-side closure, large or complex defects may require more advanced techniques. Several techniques for wound closure and scar revision are described in this chapter, including advancement and rotation flaps, V-Y plasties, M-plasties, and the management of dog-ears. The specific flaps and plastic surgery closures described are chosen for their utility, reliability, and predictability of aesthetic result.

INDICATIONS

- A soft tissue defect is so large that a simple primary closure is not possible. If an elliptical defect may not be pinched together easily between the fingers with minimal tension, a simple side-to-side closure will likely be insufficient.
- There is excessive skin tension with simple closure techniques, and simple closure would yield a poor cosmetic result.
- Surgical skin remodeling techniques, or "plasties," may be indicated when dealing with dog-ears, complex wounds, or other defects that would cause an undesirable scar.

CONTRAINDICATIONS (ALL RELATIVE)

When performed correctly, the closure techniques described in this chapter generally achieve good results. However, certain risk factors may lead to poor outcomes. Relative contraindications to complex skin closures and flaps include the following.

- Diabetes
- Impaired wound healing history
- Vascular compromise to region
- Keloid or hypertrophic scar formation history
- Prior radiation to region
- Coagulopathy (intrinsic or induced through anticoagulants such as warfarin)
- Wound location on lower extremity, especially the feet (due to slow healing)

Good healing can still be accomplished in most cases if the operator is careful to engage in appropriate communication with the patient to ensure compliance, provides the correct closure technique, and limits platelet aggregation inhibitors (i.e., aspirin, other nonsteroidal anti-inflammatory drugs, and clopidogrel) for 5 days before surgery if possible. If the patient cannot stop these agents, the surgery can still be performed, but the patient should expect more intraoperative bleeding and increased likelihood of postoperative oozing and ecchymoses in the operative area. Patients on warfarin can also have extensive plastic procedures with advanced flaps and closures but should expect slower healing and more prolonged bruising in the operative area. The current recommendation is that warfarin not be stopped for cutaneous surgery because there is a significant risk of stroke. However, depending on the size of the lesion, the procedures described in this chapter can be quite extensive and involved. Consider "bridge therapy" for those patients who need anticoagulation (see Appendix H, Pearls of Practice).

It is particularly important to ask the patient about any history of abnormal scarring, keloids, or poor healing. Certain areas of the body are especially prone to hypertrophic scar and keloid formation, such as the chest, earlobes, and shoulders (Fig. 17-1). Black skin and children's skin also tend to scar more. Any patient at high risk for keloid formation should receive thorough preoperative counseling before proceeding with any skin surgery. These patients should be followed closely after surgery because early keloid development may be curtailed by the judicious use of steroid injections and silicone gel sheeting. As a general rule, the physician should avoid the temptation to excise keloids unless special attention is paid to preparation of the area before surgery using intralesional steroids, and the patient agrees contractually to long-term (1 to 2 years) surveillance and follow-up treatment if needed (see Chapter 38, Hypertrophic Scars and Keloids, for details). Conservative methods should generally be tried before reexcision, which potentially could just lead to more scars.

EQUIPMENT

Most skin excisions and closures can be performed with fairly simple equipment (as shown in the following list). Electrocautery and suction are not always necessary but are strongly recommended for meticulous control of bleeding. Adequate hemostasis is critical in preventing hematomas, wound dehiscence, and infection. Typical equipment should include the following:

- Topical antiseptic wash: povidone–iodine (Betadine) or chlorhexidine gluconate (Hibiclens)
- 5-mL syringe with needles (16 to 20 gauge to draw up anesthetic and 27 to 30 gauge for tissue injection)
- Injectable local anesthetic: 1% to 2% lidocaine with epinephrine for most areas; previously epinephrine has been avoided in fingers, toes, and genitals. However, newer findings would indicate that it is safe.

A 1 : 1 mixture of 1% lidocaine with 1% lidocaine with epinephrine works well in major revisions or flaps on the nose to minimize the excessive bleeding that often occurs without epinephrine. Epinephrine is not used, however, in an elderly woman with Raynaud's disease or poor nasal/facial circulation. It is always helpful to have the vasoconstrictive effect of epinephrine, but if flap viability is going to be a concern, it is best to limit or eliminate its use.

- Sterile drape
- Sterile gloves
- Sterile gauze pads
- Telfa pad and Tegaderm for wound dressing
- Skin-marking pen (Fine-tipped pens are available and suggested when more cosmetic repairs are important.)
- Nylon suture (4-0, 5-0, or 6-0, depending on location)

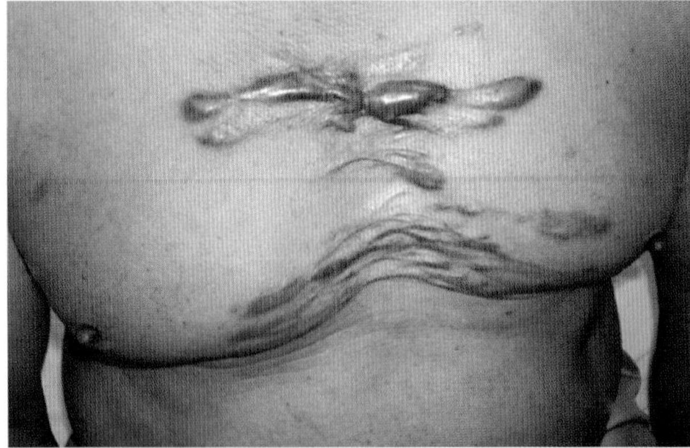

Figure 17-1 Keloid.

- 4-0, 5-0, or 6-0 absorbable suture such as Vicryl or Dexon if deep sutures are indicated
- Adson forceps
- Needle holder (smooth)
- No. 15 scalpel
- Suture scissors
- Two skin hooks
- Scissors, Metzenbaum, curved, 5 to 5½ inches
- Hemostats, curved, mosquito, 2 inches
- Hemostats, straight, small, 2 inches
- Good lighting

Strongly Recommended Equipment

- Electrocautery unit
- Suction device
- Crash cart including defibrillator, oxygen, and intubation equipment on site for emergencies (see Chapter 220, Anaphylaxis)

Preprocedure Patient Preparation

History and Physical

During the preoperative history, topics of discussion should include the following:

- Medications, including herbal supplements, that the patient has taken in the past 6 weeks
- Allergies or adverse reactions to medications including iodine and local anesthetics, suture material, bandages, and latex
- Past surgical history and any history of keloid formation, hypertrophic scars, or poor wound healing
- Past medical history, including cardiac disease, diabetes, human immunodeficiency virus infection, hepatitis, bleeding disorders, immunosuppression
- Whether the patient has a pacemaker or other implanted electronic device that may preclude the use of electrocautery
- Whether the patient has a history of valvular disease, rheumatic fever, joint replacement, or other indication for antibiotic prophylaxis
- The status of any anticoagulants and when the last dose was taken
- Pregnancy (in reproductive-age women)

Informed Consent

Before the procedure, the patient must give informed consent to undergo surgery. This includes a full description of the risks, benefits, and alternatives to the procedure. The patient must have the opportunity to ask questions regarding the procedure and have the answers provided to his or her satisfaction to constitute informed consent.

Informed consent to photography is also recommended to allow a pictorial history. Either still or movie photography can be used.

Risks

The risks of the procedure to be discussed with the patient include, but are not limited to, the following:

- Suboptimal result, including the possibility of a worse scar after wound healing
- Infection
- Wound dehiscence
- Hypertrophic scar, keloid formation, or other poor scar result
- Swelling or bruising of the tissue
- Bleeding
- Pain
- Damage to nerves
- An allergic reaction to sutures, dressing, anesthetic, or other medications
- Recurrence of lesion and possible need for further surgery

Benefits

Benefits of the procedure may include, but are not limited to, the following:

- Improved cosmetic result
- Improved wound healing
- Improved overall results compared with conventional side-to-side closure
- Removal of potentially dangerous lesion such as squamous cell carcinoma, basal cell carcinoma, or melanoma

Alternatives

Alternatives to the cosmetic surgical closures listed previously may include the following:

- Leaving the wound open to heal by secondary intention
- Side-to-side closure
- Performance of a skin graft
- Referral to a plastic surgeon

Antibiotic Prophylaxis

See Chapter 222, Prevention and Treatment of Wound Infections.

Surgical antibiotic prophylaxis should be used more liberally when flaps and plasties are performed because the blood supply is often compromised with these closures, increasing the risk of infection. Antibiotic prophylaxis should be strongly considered in the following cases:

- The surgical site involves an extremity or ear, and when it is difficult to keep the area clean such as the axilla, the perineum, genitalia, and other intertriginous areas (e.g., under the breasts)
- Diabetes or immunosuppression
- The wound is dirty, has been open more than 1 hour, or aseptic technique was not ideal
- Patient follow-up is difficult, or the patient is otherwise at increased risk of infection
- History of previously infected wounds for no apparent reason
- Male patients 6 to 16 years of age

Preoperative Medications and Anesthesia

The decision on whether to use sedation should be based on personal philosophy, patient desire, and the availability of proper monitoring. When performed correctly, most minor surgical procedures can be completed with minimal discomfort to the patient.

However, some sedation may be indicated in anxious patients when the procedure is extensive or if significant discomfort is anticipated (see Chapter 2, Procedural Sedation and Analgesia).

The use of local anesthetic warrants discussion. Lidocaine with epinephrine is preferable to lidocaine alone for nearly all cutaneous procedures. See the discussion regarding the use of epinephrine in the digits and end artery areas in Chapter 4, Local Anesthesia. In the doses administered in local anesthesia, epinephrine is generally safe and its vasoconstrictive properties are important in controlling bleeding and potentiating analgesia. Because epinephrine takes 7 to 10 minutes to achieve full effect, it is advisable to anesthetize the surgical site before preparing and draping the patient. The addition of 1 mL of sodium bicarbonate to every 9 mL of lidocaine with epinephrine helps neutralize the acidity of the solution and thus decreases the pain with injection. The addition of sodium bicarbonate to plain lidocaine does not benefit to the same extent because plain lidocaine is not as acidified. *Bupivacaine (Marcaine) precipitates at a neutral pH and should never be used with sodium bicarbonate.* When the longer-acting properties of bupivacaine are desired, it may be helpful to anesthetize the region using lidocaine with epinephrine (buffered with sodium bicarbonate) before injecting bupivacaine.

Additional techniques to minimize discomfort include the use of topical anesthetics, cryoanesthesia (e.g., topical ethyl chloride), slow injections, and initiation of the anesthesia injection on the subdermal plane. It is advisable to draw up all injectable medications in advance and to keep scalpels, needles, and syringes out of the patient's view, particularly when working with pediatric patients.

Preparation of Skin and Hair

Hair removal at the surgical site may be accomplished by shaving or by cutting the hair with scissors (to minimize microabrasions that may increase the risk of infection). On the scalp, ointment can be used to spread the hair away from the operative site and to minimize the need to cut the hair. The skin is prepared with a povidone–iodine (Betadine) or chlorhexidine (Hibiclens) solution with gentle scrubbing. Note that Betadine must be allowed to dry before it is considered effective, and Hibiclens should be avoided on the face because it is extremely toxic to the eye. Skin markings may be made before or after preparing the patient. An overzealous scrub or an alcohol wipe, however, may remove preoperative markings, and a pen used before the skin preparation is no longer sterile.

Drapes

Sterile drapes should be used with any skin procedures that require suturing to protect the suture material from becoming contaminated and introducing bacteria into the tissue. Fenestrated drapes that have adhesive around the opening to affix the hole securely over the surgical site are especially helpful. However, you may need to extend the aperture or design your own by cutting a hole in a sterile surgical drape. Sterile technique is particularly important with flaps and plasties because blood supply may be compromised, predisposing the wound to infection.

Technique

Also see Chapters 22 through 25, which cover various types of laceration and incision repair.

Tissue excision should be completed before committing to any particular flap or closure method. It is best to cut the shape of the defect, as well as the flap design, on a cotton towel before cutting the skin. This helps to prevent the common pitfall of creating flaps that are too short. The practitioner need not be limited to the following techniques. Some wounds may even heal best through secondary intention.

It is often preferable to convert a nonelliptical defect, such as a large punch biopsy site, to an ellipse along skin tension lines before closure. On occasion, a nonelliptical defect such as a triangle or rectangle may lend itself to a flap closure by advancement or rotation. Regardless of the shape of the defect, the base must be on an even plane in the subcutaneous tissue to allow for a good result.

The key to good wound closure is to provide optimal alignment of the skin edges under minimal tension. High-quality wound closures are best accomplished by adequate *undermining* of tissue, the use of Burow's triangles, the appropriate use of corner sutures, and selection of the proper plastic closure for the defect or lesion to be removed. The desired effect is to produce an excellent skin closure with little or no tension. By performing a *layered closure*, tension forces that tend to pull the skin apart can be diverted to the deep structures, limiting scarring on the visible surface area. All *buried sutures*, if necessary, should have the knot inverted (placed away from the skin side). Most skin sutures should be removed within 7 days to prevent the formation of "railroad track" scars. Exceptions are back and anterior tibial areas, which may require removal of sutures at 14 to 19 days because of the slow healing of those areas.

Flaps are composed of skin and subcutaneous tissue cut from the donor site and moved a small distance to a recipient site without removing it from its vascular supply. Local skin flaps consist of rotation flaps that pivot into place and advancement flaps that move laterally. *Rotation flaps* maintain a base of intact skin, whereas some *advancement flaps* are completely incised, with blood being supplied only from the subcutaneous tissues. Because flaps carry their own blood supply, it is important to avoid damaging the subdermal vascular plexus or cutting potential nutrient vessels. Flaps created with parallel incisions are at increased risk for necrosis because of limited blood supply, but they are sometimes unavoidable. Figure 17-2 illustrates the proper level for undermining the flap tissue.

Tissue handling techniques are important for flap success. It is crucial to handle skin gently with minimal trauma. Lifting the skin with skin hooks is preferable to manipulation with forceps or pickups. Use skin forceps primarily for avascular structures and grasping needles, not for grasping the skin. Skin forceps are capable of exerting forces of greater than 400 pounds per square inch, which will bruise the repaired area and increase the likelihood of skin infection with a poor healing response. If grasping the skin is absolutely necessary, grasp the deep dermis only and avoid the fragile epidermis. Skin forceps without teeth are preferable.

Elliptical Excisions

The elliptical excision technique is appropriate for the vast majority of lesions requiring tissue removal, and it generally facilitates wound closure. Length and width ratios should be greater than 3 : 1, and

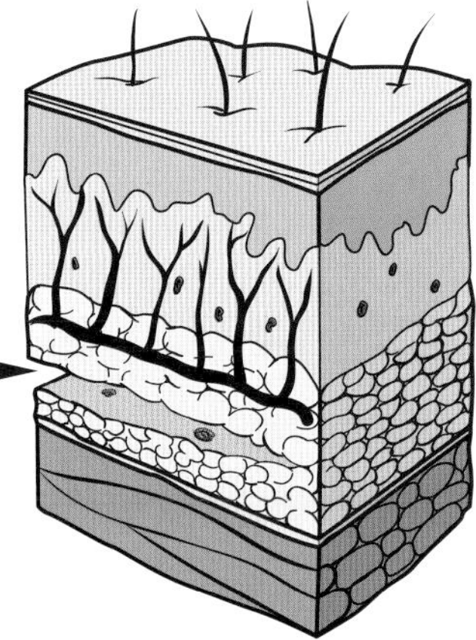

Figure 17-2 Skin flap *(arrowhead)*, with proper level of undermining in subcutaneous adipose layer. This can be performed with a blade or sharp tissue scissors. It is important to maintain integrity of vessels and not create a flap that is too thin.

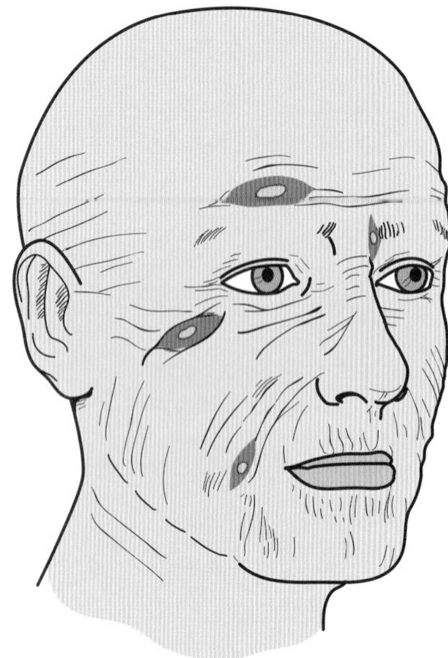

Figure 17-3 It is essential to place elliptical excisions in relaxed skin tension lines.

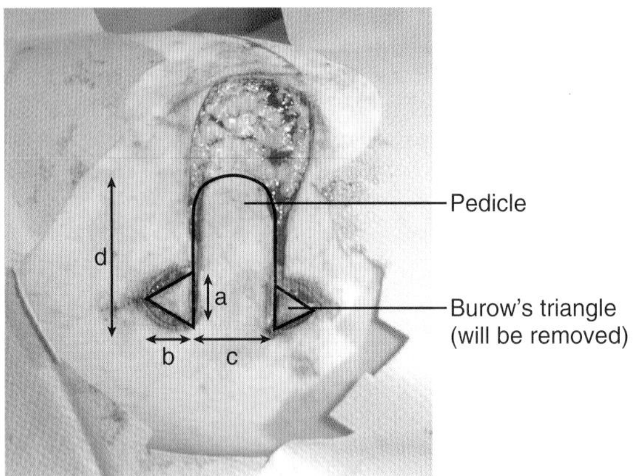

Figure 17-4 Burow's triangle: a, base of Burow's triangle; b, height of triangle; c, base of pedicle; d, length of pedicle. In planning Burow's triangle, the height (b) should equal half the base of its pedicle (c). The base of the triangle (a) should be one-third the length of the pedicle (d).

the terminal angles should be less than 30 degrees to avoid dog-ears. The long axis of the ellipse should run along wrinkle lines or, in younger patients, relaxed skin tension lines (Fig. 17-3; see Chapter 21, Incisions: Planning the Direction of the Incision).

If the closure is tight, gentle undermining may create more laxity. With flaps and plasties, some undermining will almost always be necessary. *Undermining* should be performed subdermally (between the skin and subcutaneous adipose tissue) to avoid injury to the vascular plexus (see Fig. 17-2 and Chapter 22, Laceration and Incision Repair). It is critical that the surgeon understands and uses undermining.

Description of Burow's Triangle

When side-to-side closure is difficult owing to skin tension, a variety of flaps can be used to close the defect, depending on skin availability and anatomic location. Simple elliptical closures usually have their best results in removal of small defects. Larger defects are almost always closed with a better result and a much lower likelihood of dehiscence with advanced closures and flaps.

In addition to undermining, another concept that must be mastered is the *Burow's triangle*. Corner sutures (three-point or half-buried mattress sutures) should be used in closing the Burow's triangles and in attaching the free end of the pedicle to the defect site. The Burow's triangles' height should be approximately half the width of the pedicle, and their base should be approximately one-third the length of the pedicle (Fig. 17-4).

Single Advancement Flap

This flap is a viable consideration *for defect closures on the trunk and thighs* (Fig. 17-5). Advancement flaps are conceptually simple but have limited application because of the parallel incisions required, as well as the increased skin tension created. The single-pedicle advancement flap, with or without Burow's triangles, may be useful in highly vascular, elastic areas. All advancement flaps are moved laterally without any rotation. In planning the flap, remember that *the length of a simple advancement flap should be two to three times the length of the defect to be closed*, depending on skin laxity. *On the face*, flaps should not exceed a 3 : 1 length/width ratio. As with the planning of all flaps, it may be helpful to cut the defect as well as the planned flap design on a surgical drape or other material before cutting skin.

1. Use a skin-marking pen to draw the desired flap on the patient's skin. In the case of a single advancement flap, it may be preferable cosmetically, although not necessarily, to round the advancing edge, creating a U-shaped closure, depending on the defect

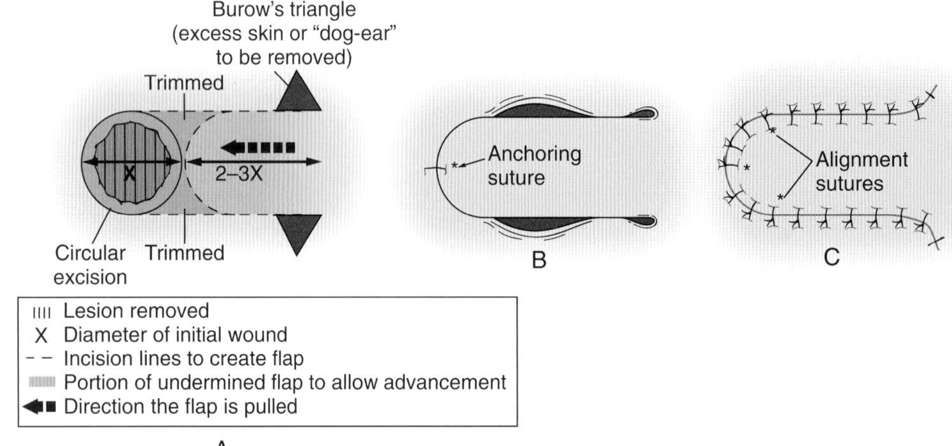

Figure 17-5 **A–C,** Single advancement flap. See text for details. *, Anchoring suture.

to be closed. At times, a rectangular end may be appropriate. Remember to make the base of the pedicle long and wide enough to avoid tension in the closure of the wound.
2. Undermine the intended flap at the level shown in Figure 17-2, and pull the flap into place.
3. Burow's triangles should be used to facilitate easy tissue movement and a closure with little or no tension. Burow's triangles should be placed at the pivot end of the pedicle on either side. This action greatly assists the operator in closing the wound.
4. Using the skin hook, advance the flap and place an anchoring suture. If the pedicle is rectangular rather than rounded, then corner sutures are critical to good position and healing (see Fig. 17-5B).
5. Place the next sutures as shown in Figure 17-5C to ensure proper alignment of the flap, then complete the closure.

Double Advancement Flap

Consider using double advancement flaps where *large defects are encountered on the trunk and the thighs*. If a double advancement flap is to be used (advancing a flap from two sides), the length of each flap should generally be one to two times the length of the defect.

1. Excise lesions with appropriate margins.
2. Draw out the anticipated repair with the skin-marking pen and create the incisions as shown. Trim the excess tissue to create a square defect (Fig. 17-6A).
3. Undermine areas to be advanced.
4. Place a Burow's triangle on both sides on both pedicles, similar to the single advancement flap. These Burow's triangles should be the following dimensions: the base should be one-third the length of the pedicles, and the height should be one-half the width of the pedicles.
5. Advance the opposing flaps toward each other and place the anchoring (tension-bearing) suture subcutaneously (Fig. 17-6B).
6. Use double corner sutures (three-point/half-buried mattress) at sites where the flaps meet each other and adjacent to normal skin (Fig. 17-6C).
7. Place corner sutures where the Burow's triangles were removed (Fig 17-6D).
8. Close the remainder of the wound site with simple interrupted sutures (Fig. 17-6E).

V-Y Plasty or Island Advancement Flap

These closures are satisfactory *for areas with excellent subcutaneous blood supply*. The V-Y plasty or flap is an advancement flap that may be *used in closing a circular defect*. The technique should be limited to skin that is highly mobile. The technique may be useful when a vital structure prevents the standard elliptical excision or when an elliptical excision is too large to be closed without excessive tension (Figs. 17-7 and 17-8). There is a reasonable likelihood of loss of part of these flaps if the procedure is not done in a meticulous fashion. For larger lesions, the V-Y flap may be advanced from both sides as a *double V-Y advancement* flap. The *disadvantage* of the V-Y flap is that the entire perimeter of the triangle is incised, which severely reduces the blood supply to only the vessels coming up from beneath the flap and thus limits the distance the flap can travel.

Use of the V-Y flap to close a circular defect is demonstrated as follows (see Fig. 17-7):

1. Excise the defect (Fig. 17-7A and B).
2. Plan a triangle with a base approximately the diameter of the circular defect and an apical angle of 30 to 45 degrees (Fig. 17-7C).
3. Incise the triangle and undermine laterally to allow eventual closure of the sides. *Do not* undermine under the flap itself because the blood supply to the "island" is provided by the subcutaneous vessels (Fig. 17-7D).
4. Trim the angles at the base of the triangle to fill the defect (Fig. 17-7E).
5. Using skin hooks, advance the flap into the defect and suture the top together (Fig. 17-7F).
6. Close the remainder of the incisions with simple interrupted sutures to create a Y-shaped scar (Fig. 17-7G).

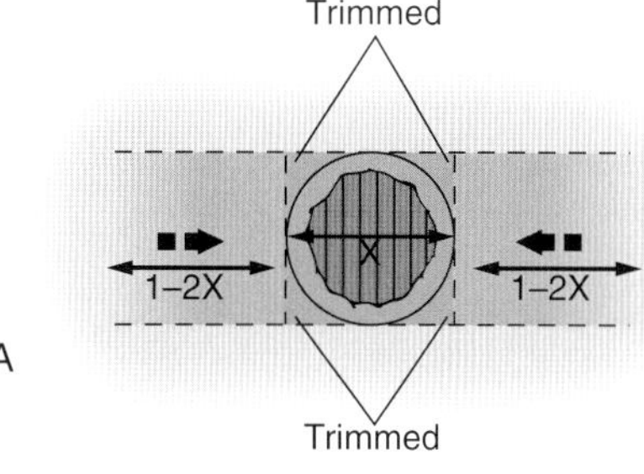

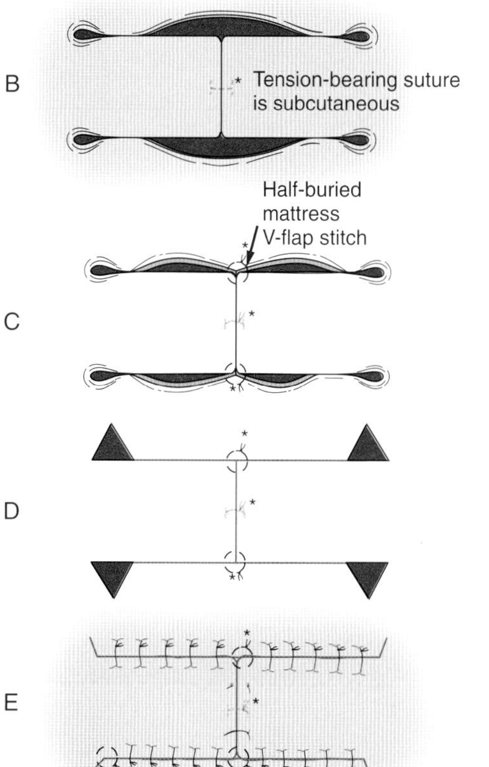

Figure 17-6 **A–E,** Double advancement flap. See text for details. *, Anchoring sutures. For further information, see Chapter 22, Laceration and Incision Repair.

Another method of creating a V-Y repair to close a wound under tension is as follows:

1. Create an elliptical excision large enough to remove the lesion (Fig. 17-7H).
2. A V-shaped incision is made, then undermined to reduce skin tension (Fig. 17-7I).

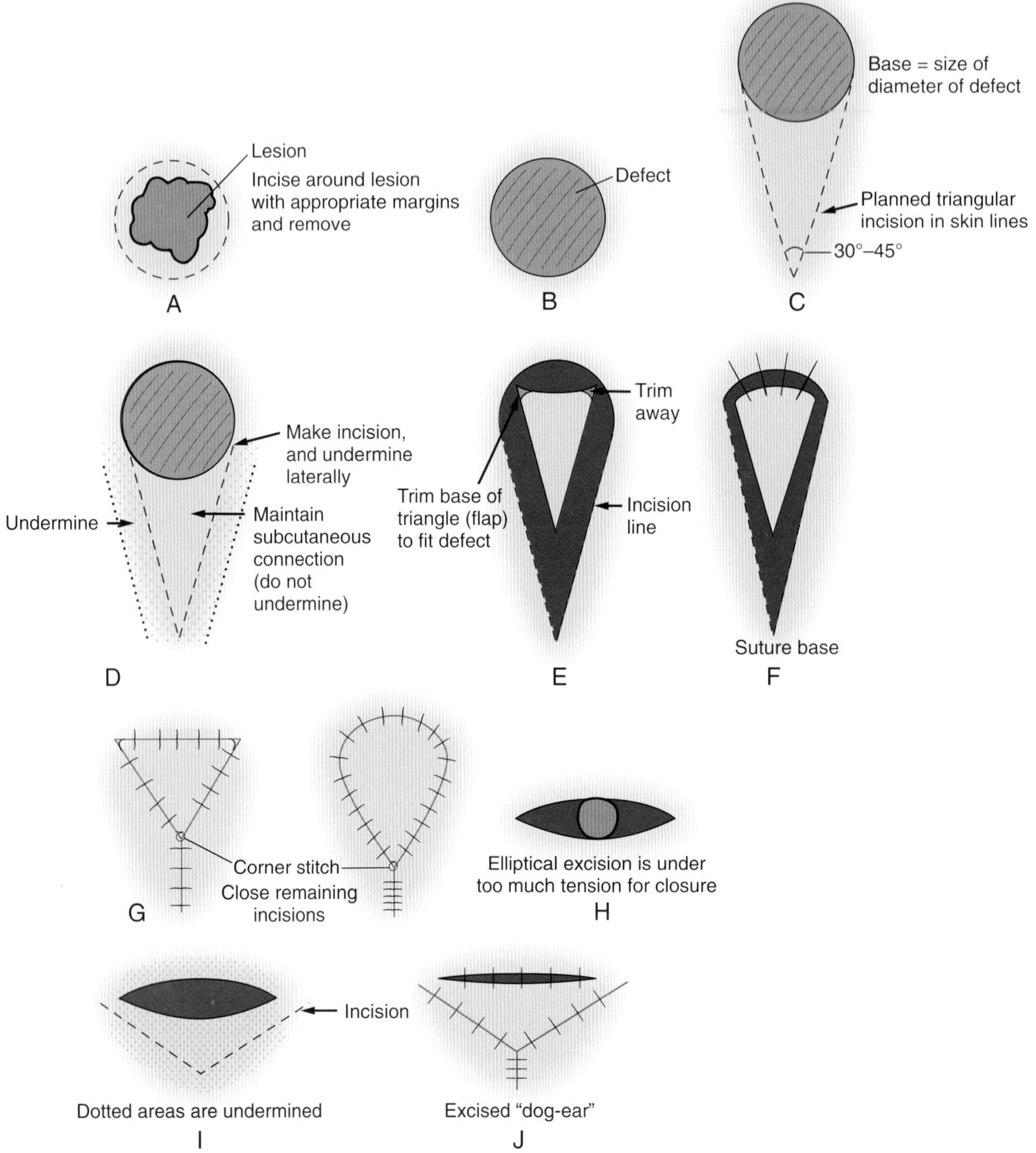

Figure 17-7 **A–J,** V-Y flap. See text for details.

3. Close the ellipse first. When the V is closed, there will be a dog-ear that will need to be excised. Closing this area will form the vertical portion of the Y (Fig. 17-7J).

The *double V-Y advancement flap* is performed in the same manner but with mirror-image triangular flaps that are advanced toward each other. This technique may be helpful for larger lesions.

1. Mark an elliptical area around the lesion. Excise only the abnormality in a circular fashion (Fig. 17-9A).
2. *Incise* the triangular flaps that were marked out previously. *Undermine laterally only*, not under the "triangles." Using skin hooks, gently advance the two flaps toward each other and place the anchoring suture (Fig. 17-9B).
3. Place the next sutures as shown to provide good alignment, followed by corner sutures. The closure may then be completed with subcutaneous or simple interrupted sutures (Fig. 17-9C).

Rotation Advancement Flap

The design of a rotation flap should be planned only after the original tissue has been excised completely. The flap length should be generous (usually an *arc length of four to five times the base of the defect to be closed*) to allow adequate tissue movement. The *advantages* of a rotation flap include the provision of good blood supply by avoiding parallel incisions, the ability to undermine the mobilized tissue if needed, and the ability to create a contralateral flap if more tissue is needed. The major *disadvantage* is that the final result may not blend into natural skin lines. *This closure allows the coverage of large defects if used correctly.* Some tissues like the face rotate easily. The scalp also closes satisfactorily with this approach. This is an effective closure in the neck region and most other areas where loose skin can be moved to an adjacent area requiring a defect to be closed.

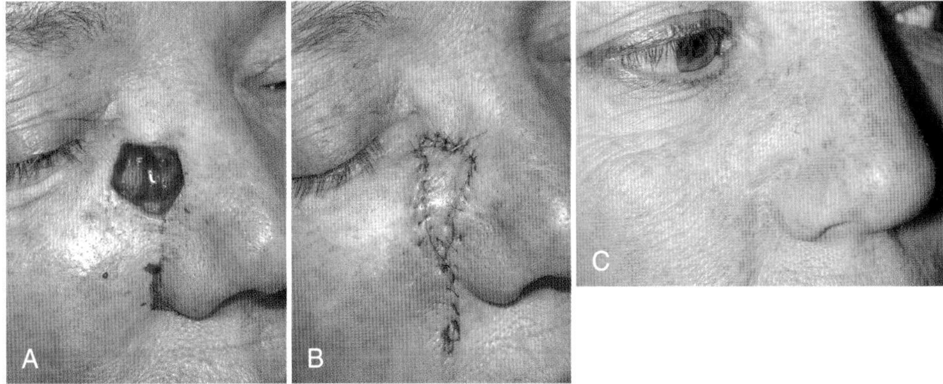

Figure 17-8 Island pedicle flap technique. **A,** Island pedicle repair of perinasal cheek defect. The flap can be advanced a great distance on a nasalis muscular swinging pedicle, which provides reliable blood supply. **B,** Note that although the flap was undersized, the surrounding tissues were undermined, and the flap was inset at the time of repair. **C,** There is slight flap elevation, a trapdoor deformity, at 6 months. (From Robinson JK, Hanke CW, Siegel DM, Sengelmann RD [eds]: Surgery of the Skin: Procedural Dermatology. Philadelphia, Mosby, 2005.)

1. The illustrated lesion lends itself to an excision that may be trimmed to create a triangular defect (Fig. 17-10A).
2. Draw the desired arc down to the "pivot point," according to the aforementioned guidelines (i.e., flap edge four to five times the length of the base of the triangular defect). Be sure to allow recruitment of sufficient tissue. Again, it may be helpful to cut the defect in a surgical drape, along with the proposed repair flap design, before incising the skin and committing to a particular repair (Fig. 17-10B). It is always helpful to first carefully draw the arc, lesion defect expected, and the Burow's triangle before any incisions are made. Excise the tissue to be removed.
3. Undermine the flap and surrounding tissue with curved Metzenbaum scissors or a blade (Fig. 17-10C). Make the Burow's triangle on the opposite side of the arc and at the other end of the arc. The Burow's triangle allows you to easily move the tissue of the flap into place (Fig. 17-10D).
4. Rotate the flap into place to fill the defect. The first suture is a corner suture reapproximating the skin at the corner of the Burow's

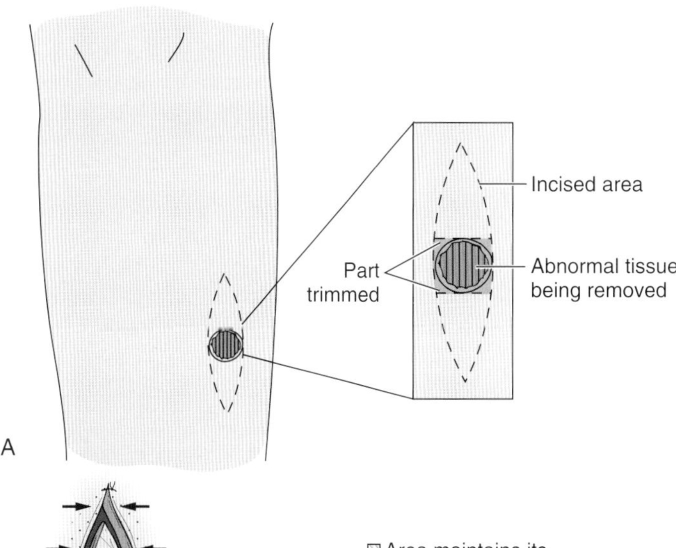

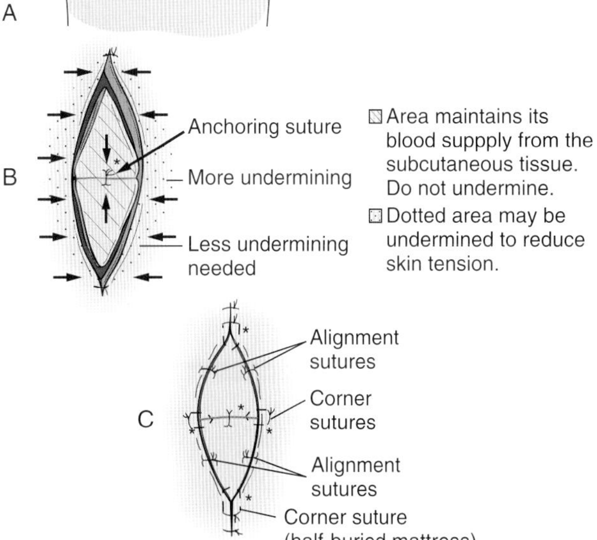

Figure 17-9 **A–C,** Double V-Y advancement flap. *, Anchoring sutures. See text for details.

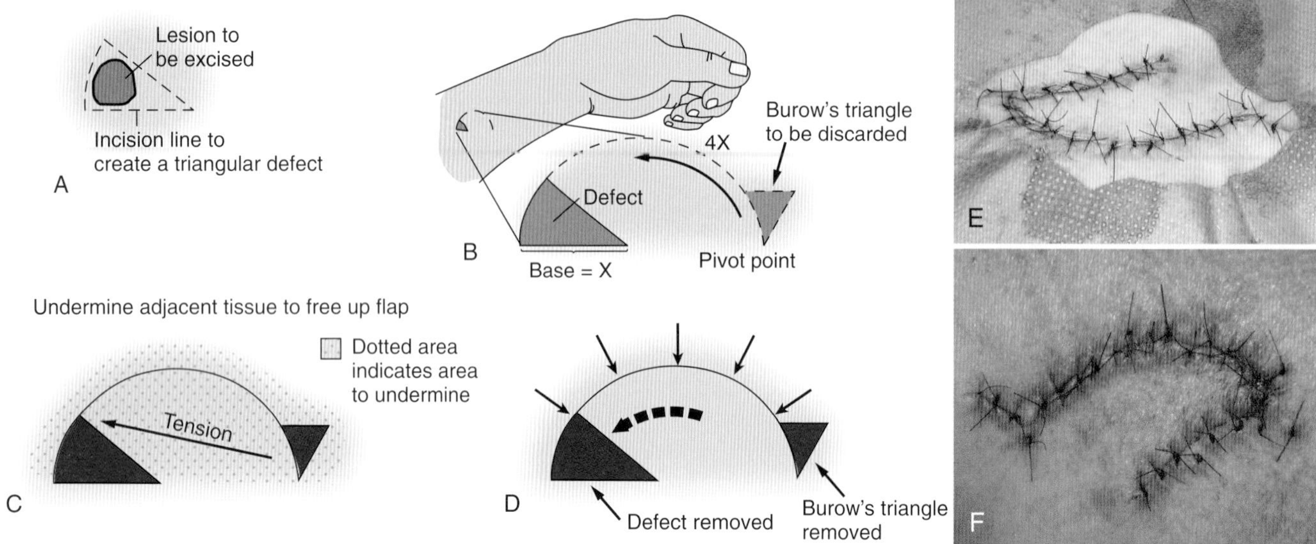

Figure 17-10 **A–F,** Rotation flap. See text for details.

triangle, and the second suture is the corner suture to connect the mobile end of the rotation flap to the other corner (Fig. 17-10E).

5. Suture the rest of the skin edges into place with simple interrupted sutures (Fig. 17-10F).

Z-Plasty

The *best sites in which to use this closure are over flexor and extensor joints of the hand and the sacral area, where pilonidal cysts occur.* The Z-plasty is a particularly useful technique *for scar revision to redirect a scar into skin tension lines (making it less visible) or to release scar contractures.* Scar contracture is apt to occur when a laceration is perpendicular to skin creases, as in the case of a vertical laceration on the finger (Fig. 17-11A). Healing often contracts the scar, pulling the finger into a flexed position. Redirection of the scar can release skin tension. The *major drawback* to the technique is that the length of the scar is increased.

1. Excise the linear scar or lesion in a narrow ellipse along its axis (Fig. 17-11B).

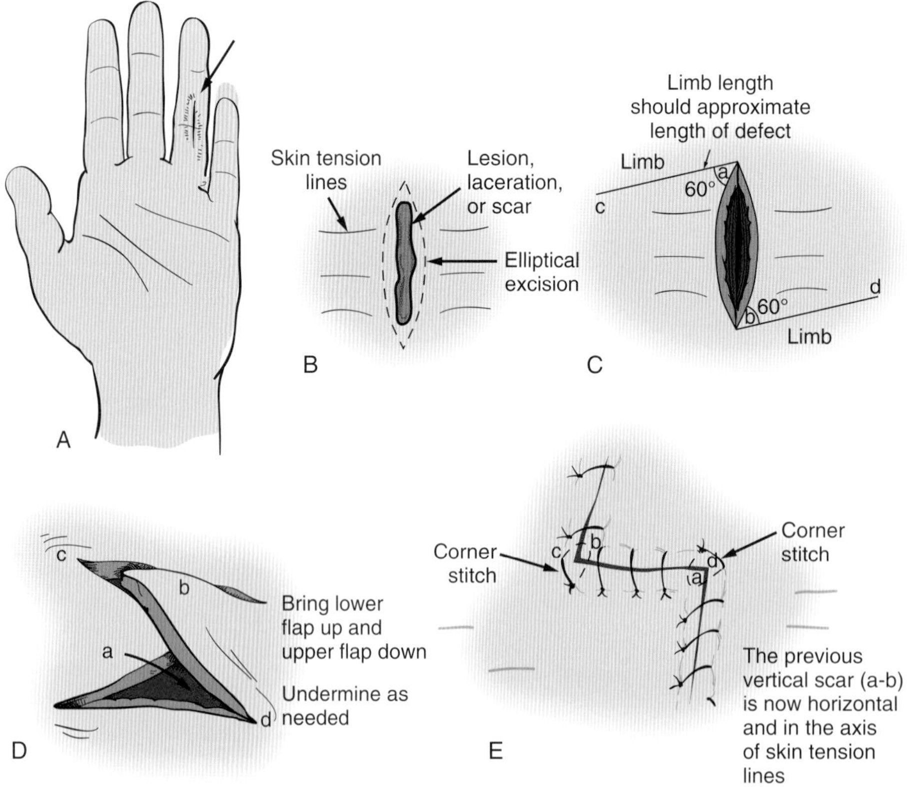

Figure 17-11 **A–E,** Z-plasty. See text for details.

2. Create the limbs of the "Z" at 60-degree angles from this axis. The length of each limb should equal the length of the defect (Fig. 17-11C).
3. Using skin hooks, advance the two triangles as shown, by crossing them over one another (Fig. 17-11D). Undermine the flaps as needed.
4. Place a "corner stitch" (half-buried mattress) at each of the flap tips, as shown in Figure 17-11E. Then complete the wound closure with simple interrupted sutures. The new scar will now lie within the axis of the skin tension lines.

M-Plasty

This is an excellent closure *when there is a paucity of skin for rotation or advancement flaps* and can be used on the face, scalp, neck, trunk, and extremities. It is truly a closure suitable for all areas and produces excellent results when the rules are followed. The design of this repair should be based on Langerhans' tension lines so the final closure is parallel with Langerhans' lines. The blood supply is excellent, and it is rare to lose any portion of the flap because of inadequate blood supply. The repair usually blends into the skin lines very well with time.

1. The lesion should lend itself to a linear-type closure. The outline of the lesion to be removed should fit into the center of the M-plasty drawing (Fig. 17-12A and B). The length/width ratio should be at least 3:1, with the length measured at the internal points of the Burow's triangles and the width being the total width of the excision (lesion plus margins). This is an extremely important measurement.
2. The base of each Burow's triangle should be approximately the same as the depth (height) to allow ideal closure. There certainly is room for variance and still get a good closure, but these guidelines are the best.
3. After the M-plasty is drawn on the skin, allowing adequate margins, the entire lesion and excess skin are removed (Fig. 17-12C).
4. The next step is to carefully undermine the surrounding tissue at the same depth as the lesion removed. The area to be undermined is usually about 10 mms, but it needs to be approximately equal to half of the width of the skin excised, with the undermining to be extended around the entire perimeter, including beneath the Burow's triangles at each end of the M-plasty.
5. The first suture placed is an anchor suture in the middle of the repair to bring the edges together (Fig. 17-12D). If the wound does not come together easily, then the undermining was inadequate or the 3:1 ratio was not upheld.
6. The second and third sutures to be placed are placed midway between the anchor (middle) suture and either end of the wound to be closed (Fig. 17-12E).
7. The fourth and fifth sutures to be placed are modified corner/subcuticular sutures placed near the end of the wound from each side into the subcuticular portion of the skin, then connecting the tip of each Burow's triangle (through the subcuticular tissue), then out through the subcuticular tissue on the other side and out the skin opposite the entry point on the opposite side of the wound. The suture through the skin should be placed about 2 to 3 mm central to the point of the Burow's triangle to allow a gentle pull of the triangle toward the center of the wound (Fig. 17-12F).
8. The other sutures needed are simply interrupted sutures to produce the appropriate closure.
9. When the sutures are removed, it is best to leave the anchor suture as the last one to be removed if the sutures are removed sequentially (not at the same time).

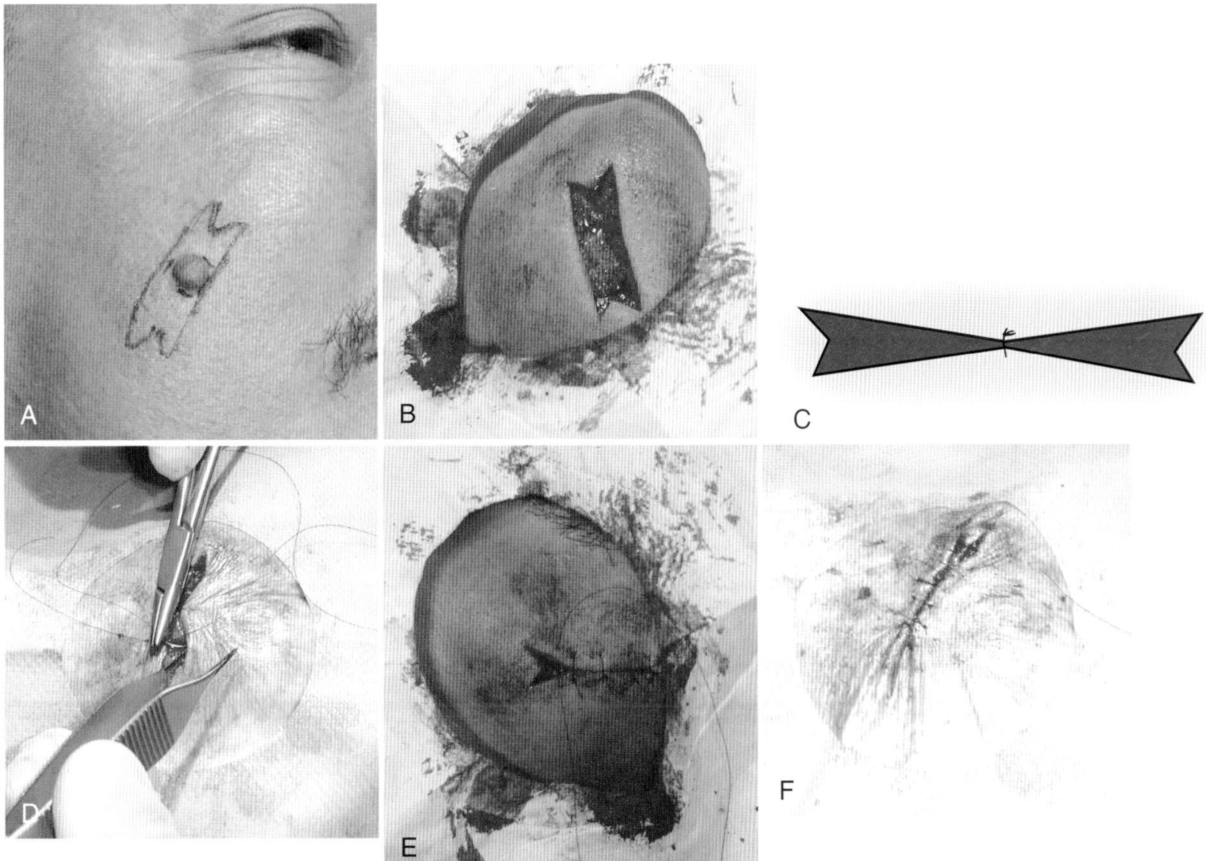

Figure 17-12 **A–F,** M-Plasty. See text for details.

Dog-Ears

Dog-ears are caused by excess skin left at the end of the suture line. They commonly occur when skin edges are rotated or pulled, when interrupted sutures are not placed evenly, or when one side of a wound is longer than the other. Dog-ears can be avoided by (1) closing the ends of an elliptical defect first and distributing the "extra skin" throughout the wound, (2) keeping ellipse incision angles 30 degrees or less, and (3) maintaining 3:1 length/width ratios or using advanced closures. The best technique for repair is demonstrated in Figure 17-13. *In this repair, the wound will be lengthened and excess tissue must be removed.*

It is easy with this technique to judge the amount of tissue that must be removed.

1. Excess tissue on one side of the wound closure creates a dog-ear (Fig. 17-13A).
2. At the apex of the wound, incise the tissue at a 150-degree angle to the wound. The length depends on the amount of excess tissue (Fig. 17-13B). Make the cut on the side of the wound where the excess tissue exists, making sure that you gently pull the excess tissue toward the wound along the long axis of the wound.
3. Using the skin hook, pull the apex of the dog-ear over the extended incision line and excise the excess tissue with a blade or tissue scissors (Fig. 17-13C). This action makes the repair close nicely using the Burow's triangle approach.
4. Close as shown using a corner suture and then interrupted sutures (Fig. 17-13D).

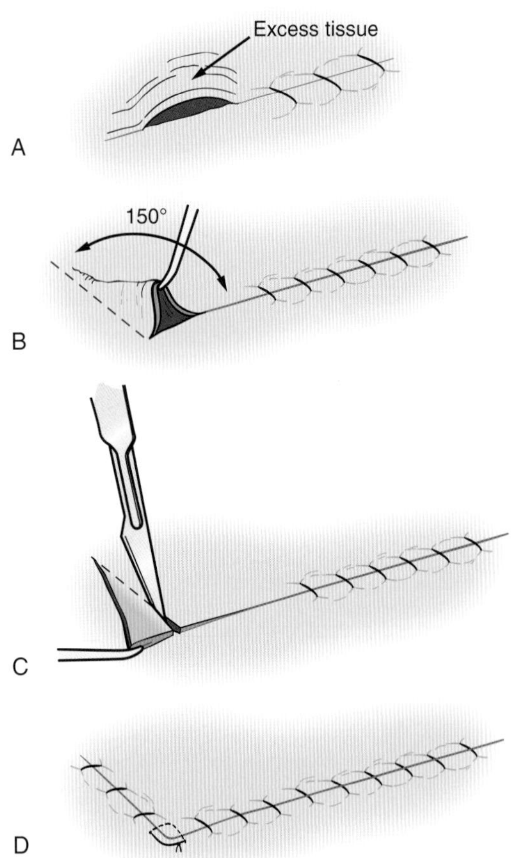

Figure 17-13 **A–D,** Dog-ear repair. See text for details.

Potential Complications of Advanced Closures and Flaps

Acute (within 2 Weeks)

- Bleeding
- Bruising
- Swelling
- Hematoma
- Pain
- Infection
- Wound dehiscence

Chronic or Permanent

- Scarring/contractures
- "Railroad tracks" from delayed suture removal
- Hypertrophic scars
- Keloid
- Hyperpigmentation
- Hypopigmentation
- Nerve damage
- Ectropion and entropion of eyelid
- Disruption of vermilion border of upper lip
- Skin atrophy
- Hair loss
- Recurrence of excised lesion

Additional Considerations

In the excision of potentially malignant lesions, tumor-free margins must always be obtained before committing to any flap closure. If a later pathology report indicates incomplete excision of a malignant lesion, the appropriate area around the previous closure area will need to be resected. If this involves a flap technique, there may already be significant skin tension or little skin may be available for further repairs. The patient requiring more extensive repairs or grafting may be left with a large defect. But usually, with a correct surgical approach, reexcision to accomplish a cure based on pathology should be possible.

Postprocedure Patient Education

Proper postoperative care is more critical with skin flaps and plasties than with simple closures. For the first 24 hours after surgery, the patient must rest and avoid exertion. Instruct the patient to refrain from bending, heavy lifting, and exercising until the sutures are removed. The wound should be kept clean and covered with a thin coat of antibiotic ointment particularly for first 24 hours. The patient should refrain from alcohol and aspirin-containing medicines for at least the first 24 hours after surgery. The wound should be dressed with a small piece of Telfa covered by Tegaderm or roll dressing, depending on the site, so a good seal develops over the wound. If subcuticular sutures are used, Steri-Strips are placed, followed by the Telfa and Tegaderm dressing. A thick outer dressing of 4 × 4 gauze or other bandage is then placed to provide a pressure dressing that limits bleeding and swelling. Ice on the area for 2 to 4 hours helps relieve pain, swelling, and bleeding.

After 24 hours the thick outer bandage may be removed. Most wounds heal faster and are less likely to develop secondary infection if left open. Each day the wound should be carefully checked to make sure there is no crust or blood accumulation. If there is blood or crust accumulation, this should be removed with gentle washing using soap and water. The wound should have a very thin layer of antibiotic ointment applied before bedtime. The exceptions to these guidelines are hand and foot wounds in boys or men who will continue to work and play. These selected patients should continue to have a wound covering at least during the daytime after the first 24 hours to keep the wound from getting wet or contaminated. If the wound dressing gets wet or contaminated, it should be replaced with a new dressing of antibiotic and Tegaderm or roll dressing. After 24 hours it is acceptable to shower and wash the wound. The area should not be scrubbed. If the wound bleeds at any time, the patient should apply firm pressure for 15 minutes and a new dressing should be placed over the wound. Instruct the patient to call the office or go to the emergency department if the wound bleeds significantly despite 15 minutes of firm pressure, if any signs of infection (e.g., purulence, redness, increased pain, swelling, or fever) are noted, or if there is any breakdown in wound or suture integrity.

In the case of surgery on the face, instruct the patient to sleep with his or her head slightly elevated for the first two nights after the procedure and to avoid sleeping on the same side as the wound. The patient should also avoid bending down (head below the heart) for the first 48 hours after the surgery. Arrange for office follow-up based on personal discretion, depending on the complexity of the procedure, the cleanliness of the wound, and patient factors. Sutures on the face are usually taken out within 4 to 7 days, depending on the size, position, and tension of the closure. If deep, buried sutures are used, skin sutures may be removed sooner than if no buried sutures are used. Sutures on the neck are generally left in place for 6 to 8 days depending on the size and tension of the closure. On the trunk, groin, and extremities, sutures are left in longer, usually 10 to 21 days, depending on the speed of healing. Usually the slowest areas to heal are the anterior tibial areas and the posterior trunk. Sutures on the scalp are usually removed in 7 to 10 days.

Conclusion

Achievement of a durable repair with a good cosmetic result after skin surgery is important. To obtain predictable, good-quality outcomes, focus on simplicity. An ellipse excision with primary closure is best used for small lesions. Other, larger defects, skin cancers that require wider excision, and any area that is likely to dehisce is usually much better served with a plastic/flap repair if done correctly. When wounds are difficult to close, flaps, skin grafts, and healing by secondary intention are always options, and usually better options for optimal long-term results.

It is prudent to remember the keys to excellent repairs in plastic closures: (1) proper width-to-length ratio of excision, (2) corner sutures placed appropriately, (3) undermining done carefully with Metzenbaum scissors, and (4) use of Burow's triangles to extend and move tissue. Observance of these four parameters will provide optimal outcomes.

Patient Education Guides

See the patient education and consent forms available online at www.expertconsult.com.

CPT/Billing Codes

Excision or repair by adjacent tissue transfer or rearrangement, including Z-plasty, V-Y plasty, rotation flap, and advancement flaps:

14000 Trunk <10 sq cm
14001 Trunk 10–30 sq cm
14020 Scalp, arms, legs <10 sq cm
14021 Scalp, arms, legs 10–30 sq cm
14040 Forehead, chin, cheek, mouth, neck, axilla, genitalia, hands, feet <10 sq cm
14041 Forehead, chin, cheek, mouth, neck, axilla, genitalia, hands, feet 10–30 sq cm
14060 Eyelids, nose, ears, lips <10 sq cm
14061 Eyelids, nose, ears, lips 10–30 sq cm
14300 Any area, unusual, or complicated repair, more than 30 sq cm
14350 Filleted finger or toe flap, including preparation of recipient site

NOTE: These codes generally apply to full-thickness excision and repair by adjacent tissue mobilization. For reporting laceration repairs, the procedure must be created by the surgeon and not by the incidental shape of the laceration. Refer to the CPT book for further description.

ICD-9-CM Diagnostic Codes

See Appendix G, Neoplasm, Skin: ICD-9 Codes.

Acknowledgment

The editors wish to recognize the many contributions by Ashley K. Christiani, MD, and Mats Hagstrom, MD, to this chapter in the previous two editions of this text.

Suppliers

(See contact information online at www.expertconsult.com.)

Acuderm, Inc.
Delasco Dermatologic Lab and Supply Co.
Miltex Instrument Company, Inc.
Moore Medical Corp.
SSR Surgical Instruments

VIDEOTAPES AND DVDS

Coding and Billing

Pfenninger JL: Billing/coding for dermatologic procedures. Creative Health Communications, 2005. Available at www.creativehealthcommunications.com.

Procedure Technique

Pfenninger JL: Common office dermatologic procedures, 2005. Creative Health Communications, 2005. Available at www.creativehealthcommunications.com.

Pfenninger JL: Excision and common wound repairs: Patient cases. Creative Health Communications, 2005. Available at www.creativehealthcommunications.com.

Pfenninger JL. Suturing and excision techniques. Exercises on pig's feet biopsy. Creative Health Communications, 2005. Available at www.creativehealthcommunications.com.

Thomsen TW, Barclay DA, Setnick GS: Videos in clinical medicine: Basic laceration repair. N Engl J Med 355:e18–e22, 2006.

Tuggy M, Garcia J: Procedures Consult. Available at www.proceduresconsult.com, and as an application at www.apple.com/iTunes.

BIBLIOGRAPHY

Arndt KA, Dover JS, Alam M: Procedures in Cosmetic Dermatology Series: Scar Revision. Philadelphia, Saunders, 2006.

Aston SJ, Beasley RW, Thorne CHM (eds): Grabb and Smith's Plastic Surgery, 5th ed. Philadelphia, Lippincott-Raven, 1997.

Brown JS: Minor Surgery: A Text and Atlas, 4th ed. London, Edward Arnold, 2001.

Denkler K: A comprehensive review of epinephrine in the finger: To do or not to do. Plast Reconstr Surg 108:114–124, 2000.

Fewkes JL, Pollack S, Cheney MC: Illustrated Atlas of Cutaneous Surgery. Philadelphia, Gower Medical, 1991.

Georgiade GS, Riefkohl R, Levin LS (eds): Plastic, Maxillofacial and Reconstructive Surgery, 3rd ed. Baltimore, Williams & Wilkins, 1997.

Grossman JA: Minor Injuries and Repair. New York, Gower Medical, 1993.

Hass AF, Grekin RC: Antibiotic prophylaxis in dermatologic surgery. J Am Acad Dermatol 32:155–176, 1995.

Jackson EA: The V-Y plasty in the treatment of fingertip amputations. Am Fam Physician 64:455–458, 2001.

Radovic P, Smith RG, Shumway D: Revisiting epinephrine in foot surgery. J Am Podiatr Med Assoc 93:157–160, 2003.

Robinson JK, Arndt KA, LeBoit PE, Wintroub BU: Atlas of Cutaneous Surgery. Philadelphia, WB Saunders, 1996.

Robinson JK, Hanke CW, Sengelmann RD, Siegel DM (eds): Surgery of the Skin: Procedural Dermatology. Philadelphia, Mosby, 2005.

Thomson CJ, Lalonde DH, Denkler K, Feicht AJ: A critical look at the evidence for and against elective epinephrine use in the finger. Plast Reconstr Surg 119:260–266, 2007.

Usatine RP, Moy RL (eds): Skin Surgery: A Practical Guide, 2nd ed. Philadelphia, Mosby, 2010.

CHAPTER 18

Foreign Body Removal from Skin and Soft Tissue

Grant C. Fowler

Patients frequently seek care from a primary care clinician for a foreign body in the skin or soft tissue. In fact, foreign bodies are present in 3% of wounds. In certain situations, removal may cause more trauma than leaving the object in place; hence, the patient may require only information or reassurance. However, the presence of a foreign body increases the risk of infection in most wounds, even if only slightly. A foreign body can also cause pain. Fortunately, removal is often accomplished with minimal trauma, usually resulting in considerable appreciation by the patient.

A foreign body should be suspected in all wounds caused by a high-velocity missile or a sharp, fragile object. Objects that splinter, shatter, or break in the process of causing a wound often leave remnants behind. For example, a piece of glass that caused a wound by breaking on impact with the skin is more likely to leave shards in the wound than a piece of glass that was previously broken.

All wounds should be probed manually for the presence of a foreign body. Up to 38% of embedded objects are missed on the initial assessment; consequently, the most common error in the management of soft tissue foreign bodies is the failure to detect their presence. Failure to diagnose soft tissue foreign bodies and manage them correctly is a common cause of malpractice litigation in both emergency and family medicine. With the techniques discussed in this chapter, attempts at removal may be simplified and the results optimized.

Indications

- Known foreign body in skin, subcutaneous, or soft tissue
- Pain or persistent inflammation from a foreign body
- Foreign body with toxic, infectious, or allergic potential
- Impairment of neurovascular or mechanical function due to a foreign body
- Foreign body near a fractured bone or open joint
- Foreign body causing a cosmetic deformity

NOTE: A general guideline is if one end of the foreign body can be palpated by hand or an instrument, it can be removed. Another is that removal may be more difficult than expected, even if the foreign body is large, palpable, and apparently superficial on radiographs; therefore adequate time should be set aside to evaluate, explore, plan, and pursue removal. However, some experts say spend no more than 15 to 20 minutes exploring; clinicians thereby avoid causing excessive damage by probing for too long "looking for a needle in a haystack." Yet another guideline is if a patient complains of a foreign body sensation, the clinician should assume that there is one, even if the radiographs are negative. One study found that a foreign body sensation in a patient was 43% sensitive and 83% specific for the presence of glass.

Contraindications

- Lack of knowledge of anatomic structures surrounding the foreign body
- Proximity of foreign body to a vital structure such as a nerve or artery
- An uncooperative patient who cannot be sedated (see Chapter 7, Pediatric Sedation and Analgesia) or anesthetized (see Chapter 4, Local Anesthesia)

NOTE: Consider referral for a foreign body in the soft tissues of the face or the deep spaces of the hands or feet, or for broken glass if there are multiple shards. Also, deeply imbedded objects, those in joints, and those impairing neurovascular or mechanical function may best be removed by a surgeon while the patient is under general anesthesia.

Equipment

- Blunt-tipped, stiff (but bendable), sterile metal probe
- Small, sharp-tipped dissecting scissors
- Sterile tweezers (splinter forceps are very helpful)
- Adson pickup forceps with teeth (an Allis clamp may also be helpful)
- Two mosquito hemostats
- Bright light that can be directed or focused (use of a headlamp allows both hands to be free for the procedure)
- Clear plastic tape
- Skin-marking pen or pencil
- Paper clips, BBs, or 27-gauge needles used for local anesthetic can be used as markers
- Scalpel (no. 11 or 15)
- Suture, if necessary for closure
- Local or topical anesthetic materials (see Chapter 4, Local Anesthesia, and Chapter 10, Topical Anesthesia)
- Irrigant, such as saline
- Syringe for irrigation (5 mL for small wounds, 10 to 30 mL for larger wounds) with optional 18-gauge needle
- Magnifying glass or loupes
- Povidone-iodine solution (Betadine)
- Powerful magnet for ferromagnetic objects
- Sterile adhesive bandage
- Liquid soap
- Blood pressure cuff to use as tourniquet and elastic (Ace) bandage *(optional)*
- Hair removal (depilatory) wax *(optional)*
- Skin hook *(optional)*
- 3-mm skin punch for biopsy *(optional)*
- 1-0 or 2-0 nylon suture, without needle, to use as probe *(optional)*
- Hemoclips, hemoclip applicator, and silk sutures *(optional)*

Preprocedure Patient Preparation

Patients should be aware that in some situations removal may be too complicated, unsuccessful, or impossible. The clinician should also explain that it is safe for certain objects to be left in the skin permanently. For example, wounds containing a small metal fleck in a nonvital area will often heal with no problems. Even lead and other metal objects are sometimes safe to let "rest" in the skin indefinitely. Their removal, especially if deeply embedded, may cause more trauma than leaving the object in place, especially if the patient is not experiencing symptoms and has no signs of infection. The body tends to wall off nonporous materials and smooth objects such as bullets, glass, metal, and even shrapnel; therefore, if deeply embedded they are often better left alone. However, heavily contaminated foreign bodies should be removed as soon as possible. Hair or marine foreign bodies, such as sea urchin spines, may cause granuloma formation, so they should usually be removed. Similarly, objects made of wood, vegetable fiber, or other organic materials, which are likely to cause an inflammatory reaction or infection, usually have to be removed. The same is true for any object with toxic or allergic potential.

Patients should also be aware that it may be necessary to leave the object in the tissue until it forms a cyst or localizes (i.e., edema subsides). Although it may take days, weeks, or even decades, certain objects will eventually work their way to the surface and can then be removed. If an infection develops, it will be treated with an antibiotic. If a small pocket of fluid develops, it may help with later removal. Inform the patient that if removal is attempted, certain techniques may be used to locate and remove the foreign body, including taking radiographs.

If removal is attempted, the patient should be informed that there is a chance that the object will not be able to be removed or may be only partially removed. Even with what appears to be a simple extraction (e.g., splinter), the clinician may want to be cautious about telling the patient that it was removed entirely; perhaps a better explanation is that all of the visible object was removed but that there is always the chance that small fragments may still be present that are currently undetectable. With removal, there will be minor trauma and possibly scarring (from the original wound, an incision, or from sutures), and there is a possibility of damage to vital structures surrounding the object such as a nerve, artery, vein, or tendon. Such trauma may be associated with discomfort during the procedure or some bleeding during or after the procedure. There is also risk of infection after the procedure. In certain situations, minimal or no anesthesia will be used at first in order to localize or grasp the object. A patient's intact sensation is usually much more accurate than probing blindly under anesthetized skin when attempting to locate an object, especially if the skin were to be distorted from an injection of the local anesthetic. For small or difficult-to-locate objects, the patient's intact sensation may be the only way to find the object. As soon as the object is grasped, stabilized, or removed, the discomfort is usually decreased or eliminated. After the object is grasped, local anesthetic may then be used to minimize any discomfort.

The patient should be aware that glass objects, especially small ones, may be difficult to visualize on radiographs and that there may be multiple shards. For various reasons, glass is probably the most difficult object to remove. If the clinician is not certain that all of the foreign object(s) has been removed, referral may be required.

If the decision is made to attempt to remove the object(s), the patient should be aware that the procedure may be time consuming, although usually not more than 15 to 20 minutes will be spent exploring to keep tissue damage to a minimum. He or she should be in a comfortable position that can be maintained for this amount of time. The patient should also be aware of the importance of remaining immobile during the procedure.

Technique

1. Before removal, obtain as much history as possible regarding the foreign body. Knowledge of the material and method of injury may help determine which technique to use and whether a diagnostic study such as a radiograph would be helpful. Knowledge of the angle of entry (e.g., whether tangential or perpendicular to the skin surface) may be helpful for localization. Information regarding the speed and force of entry may also be helpful.
2. Most superficially embedded, visible objects can be magnified and removed from soft tissue with a sterile needle and tweezers. For very fine splinters in the skin surface (e.g., cactus spurs, glass slivers), spreading liquid soap lightly over the skin will often enhance visualization. Alternatively, they can be removed by applying clear plastic tape or hair removal wax to the skin and then peeling it off.
3. Good judgment should be used when removing foreign objects in cosmetically sensitive areas. For example, the risk of tattooing from an object left in place (e.g., graphite from pencil or asphalt, tar, or gravel from road) must be weighed against the risk of a scar from removal.
4. Toothpicks and splinters usually enter tangentially, and their tract can usually be envisioned based on the history. Occasionally, instead of using forceps or making an incision, a hypodermic needle can be inserted perpendicular to the splinter to "spear" the splinter. The hypodermic is then used as a lever to ease the splinter out through the entry wound. Because wood splinters must be removed entirely to avoid local inflammation, instead of merely pulling the splinter out, many experts incise the entire tract of the splinter to remove it. They then irrigate the wound to ensure removal of any and all fragments. Although this may seem excessive, and creates a laceration where only a puncture wound existed, small pieces of the splinter may otherwise remain in the skin. This is especially important for splinters derived from cedar or California redwood because of the pliable and reactive nature of the wood.
5. If the object is not visible because it is below the skin, consider the use of radiographs or other imaging techniques for localization and documentation.
   - *Radiographs* are 98% sensitive for detecting radiopaque materials such as metal, gravel, pencil graphite, or teeth. Sand, mammalian bone, and certain fish bones (e.g., haddock, cod, grey mullet, sole, red snapper) are also usually radiopaque. Some plastics produce at least a slight shadow on x-ray films. Painted wood can also sometimes be seen on x-ray films. Although leaded glass is radiopaque, which improves its visibility on radiographs, the majority of glass is nonleaded. However, in one cadaver study, radiographs were 90% sensitive for detecting nonleaded glass, with a false-positive rate of only 10%. (It should be noted that a diameter of less than 1.5 mm was associated with risk of failed detection.) Radiographs are also helpful if the glass shattered near the skin surface to make sure there are not multiple shards. Routine lateral and anteroposterior views may suffice. By ordering "soft tissue" x-rays, slightly underpenetrated films are provided, which enhances visibility and localization efforts. (With digitized images, the contrast and brightness can be adjusted to produce the same effect.) If the object is positioned parallel to the central ray of the x-ray beam, it increases the likelihood of detection. Oblique and tangential views may also be helpful if the object is obscured by underlying bone.
   - *High-frequency ultrasonography* is available in most emergency departments as an alternative for localizing nonradiopaque objects (see Chapter 185, Musculoskeletal Ultrasonography, and Chapter 225, Emergency Department, Hospitalist, and Office Ultrasonography [Clinical Ultrasonography]). Most

authors have reported a greater than 90% sensitivity for detection of objects larger than 4 to 5 mm. Although ultrasonography has the benefit of avoiding radiation, it has the limitation of being operator dependent. Small objects perpendicular to the skin surface may also be difficult to visualize. The 7.5- to 10-MHz probe is better for shallow depths (<5 mm), whereas the 5-MHz probe should be used for deeper searching.

Xeroradiography (technology used in xeromammograms), although recommended in the past, has fallen out of favor because it has rarely been found to offer an advantage over plain radiographs. It also requires a much higher dose of radiation compared with plain radiographs and is not as readily available.

Fluoroscopy has received more attention lately as a diagnostic and therapeutic tool in the emergency department. Compared with plain radiographs, bedside fluoroscopy usually requires less irradiation and is faster, more convenient, and less expensive. For objects that must be removed, needle localization under fluoroscopy may remain the final option.

Computed tomography (CT) scanning is useful not only for further characterizing foreign objects seen on plain radiographs, but also for diagnosing possible complications such as an abscess. CT is often useful for visualizing nonradiopaque objects made of plastic or wood. Consequently, CT has evolved as the procedure of choice for excluding foreign objects if the plain radiograph is negative. With the development of spiral/helical CT scanning (i.e., real-time scanning), and its increased availability in emergency departments, the time required to visualize an image has been greatly reduced.

Magnetic resonance imaging (MRI) in comparison studies is the most accurate method of detecting foreign bodies such as thorns or those made of wood or plastic. MRI is also useful for detecting complications due to a foreign body such as an abscess or bony involvement. However, MRI is limited when scanning gravel or ferrometallic foreign bodies because they produce streaking that usually obscures visualization. And because CT scanning can also usually detect foreign bodies made of wood or plastic, and abscesses, MRI is rarely used because of the additional time it takes to obtain the images as well as the additional expense incurred.

6. Attempt to localize the object before incising the skin. Although the object may not be visible, there may be a discoloration beneath the skin. Any externally visible entry wound should be measured and the exact size and location recorded. Examine the wound entrance to determine the angle of penetration and possibly the depth of penetration. Palpate the object, determine the exact orientation and approximate depth (Fig. 18-1A), and measure and record it. For larger metal objects, a powerful magnet may pull the object to the surface and tent the skin. If the skin tents, mark the outline of the object with the skin-marking pen. Glass is the most common foreign body, yet it is one of the more difficult substances to remove because it is transparent and slippery, and the size and outline of the pieces are unpredictable. If glass is suspected, to avoid cutting yourself do not probe with your finger. An unknown number of shards may be involved, and if there is uncertainty about whether all of the shards have been removed, referral should be considered.

NOTE: Probing a wound with a gloved finger is not recommended for *any* possibly sharp foreign object because it may result in a puncture wound to the clinician and spread of a body fluid– or blood-borne infection.

7. If the object is not visible at the entrance wound, after palpation for orientation and depth, prepare the skin with povidone-iodine and carefully use a sterile probe or mosquito hemostat to

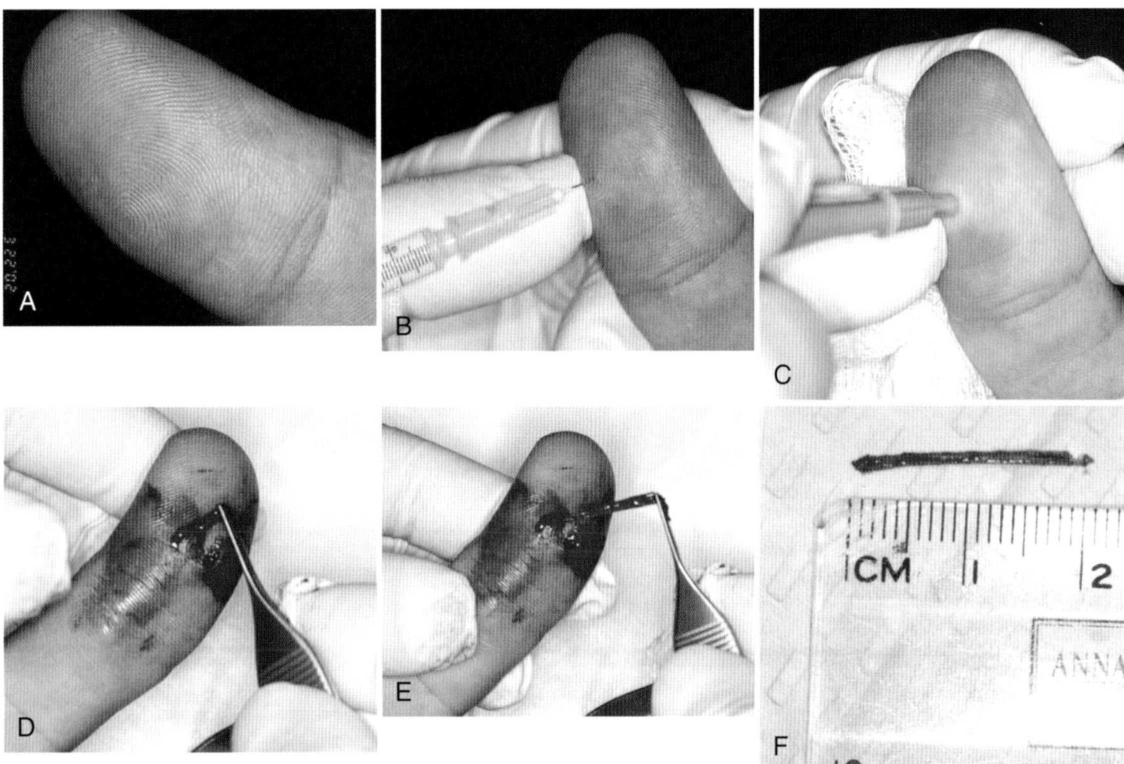

Figure 18-1 Patient reports sensation of sliver in palmar surface of distal phalanx. **A,** A fullness is palpable, but no real foreign body is detected. **B,** Lidocaine 2% 0.5 mL without epinephrine is injected. **C,** A 3-mm disposable skin punch is used. It is inserted until a gritty sensation is appreciated. **D,** Fine pickups without teeth are inserted and grasp the foreign body. **E,** A long wooden sliver is removed. **F,** The sliver.

enter the wound. Gently follow the apparent tract of the wound to locate the nearest edge. Use small, light, deliberate probing motions, gradually fanning in all directions, until contact is made with the object. This may be felt or heard as a clicking sound when the probe contacts the foreign body. (For metallic objects, a magnetic probe can be used in the same manner and the object will usually cause a click when it comes into contact with the magnet, and can then be pulled out of the wound.) Avoid excessive or unnecessary blind probing that may conceal the foreign body further with blood and edema, or push it deeper into the tissue. For small objects, before using local anesthetic, attempt to use the patient's sensation as a guide; it may be more accurate than using a probe. In this situation, avoidance of local anesthetic not only minimizes local skin distortion but limits the tissue destruction that may occur by cutting or exploring blindly under anesthesia. After the object is removed, if the patient has not been anesthetized and the symptoms have completely resolved, this is somewhat reassuring that everything was removed. If the patient continues to have a foreign body sensation, there may have been more than one foreign body and exploration may need to be continued.

8. If the object is not palpable, an attempt can be made to follow the tract of the wound with a probe. However, because of the nature of the tissue, following the tract may be more difficult in muscle or fat. That said, the clinician must avoid probing only superficially because the subcutaneous tissue can reapproximate and give the appearance of a superficial wound. If necessary, the wound edges should be extended with a scalpel for direct visualization if there is concern regarding a retained foreign body. If the bottom of the wound is less than 5 mm deep and visible, there is a 96% chance that a foreign body has been ruled out.
9. After the object is located, fixate the probe in the clinician's nondominant hand. Rest this hand on a firm surface. Administer or inject local anesthetic with the dominant hand (Fig. 18-1B). Occasionally, the injection of anesthetic beyond the foreign body or on each side of the entry wound will force the foreign body out. After excluding the presence of a neurovascular bundle, tendon, or other important structure, without moving the probe, cut down along the probe with a no. 11 or 15 scalpel blade until the foreign body is reached. Do not remove the probe. Reach into the incision and remove the foreign body with a pair of Adson forceps. Alternatively, if the entrance tract is fairly long, and if the foreign body is very superficial and easily palpable beneath the skin, it may be advantageous to simply cut down through the skin directly over the object to remove it without the use of a probe. The object should be stabilized between the fingers of the clinician's nondominant hand while the incision is being made.

   NOTE: An inadequate incision is a common source of frustration when attempting to remove a foreign object, so the clinician should usually plan a slightly larger-than-necessary incision when making it. Bleeding into the field, which may obscure the entrance wound or the object, can be another source of frustration. If the object is in the soft tissue of an extremity and the arterial circulation is otherwise intact, it is safe to inflate a proximal blood pressure cuff to greater than systolic arterial pressure for up to 2 hours to minimize bleeding. (Although this may cause some mild patient discomfort, patients usually tolerate it well.) The extremity can be elevated for a minute or an elastic (Ace) bandage can be wrapped tightly around the extremity, from distal to proximal, before inflating the blood pressure cuff to minimize venous backflow into the field. The elastic bandage can be removed as soon as the blood pressure cuff is inflated.

10. For a wound less than 48 hours old, one technique that has been found to have a 92% success rate uses nylon suture as a probe. The clinician grasps a 1-0 or 2-0 nylon suture (with no needle) between his or her thumb and index finger, then pushes it into the entrance wound while gently rotating it so that it follows the foreign body tract. Experienced clinicians report that the foreign body is easily felt when the suture contacts it. The suture is then left in the tract and the wound opened down to the foreign body by cutting alongside the suture with a scalpel.
11. If an edge of the object is somewhat superficial and easily located with a probe, and the entrance wound is large, simply enlarging the entrance wound slightly with mosquito forceps may provide the clinician enough room for a firm grasp on the object with the forceps. The object can then be removed. If the object has been in place for long enough to form a cyst, occasionally the cyst wall will need to be incised. This may be performed by the use of very small, deliberate strokes with the scalpel while the object is held by one set of mosquito forceps. The other set of mosquito forceps can then be used to bluntly dissect down to the object by spreading anything that was incised with the scalpel. If the object is visible after incision of the cyst wall, it should be grasped through the incision with the second set of forceps. The first set of forceps can then be relaxed and the object removed. If the object is not visible, which is often the case when a foreign body has been in place for a long time, constant traction on the object with the first set of forceps may cause one end of the cyst to tent. Incise through this tent with the scalpel until the object is freed.

    NOTE: Do not blindly grab something in a wound with a hemostat. Blind grasping can cause damage to a vital anatomic structure.

12. Another option for the not yet visible but readily palpable object is to perform a punch biopsy (Fig. 18-1C through F; see Chapter 32, Skin Biopsy). As the punch biopsy is being performed, a hard "click" may reveal the position of the foreign body, thereby both localizing the foreign body and avoiding the need to make a larger incision. After the biopsy is performed, tease apart the core of tissue removed and identify the foreign body. If the foreign body cannot be found in the tissue, probe the wound to make sure the foreign body is not still beneath the biopsy site. If the punch biopsy missed the foreign body (because of an angled entry wound, it may be lateral to the biopsy site), undermine the subcutaneous fat all around the site using dissecting scissors. After undermining, if pressure is applied from various locations around the site toward the center of the biopsy site, it may force the foreign body into the biopsy site. Foreign bodies located in subcutaneous fat are highly mobile, so lateral pressure can move them a considerable distance. If the foreign body is beneath the biopsy site, the decision can be made whether to deepen the site with the punch or to cut down with a no. 11 scalpel. Neither procedure should be performed if the object is located close to an underlying vital structure (e.g., nerve, artery, significant vein).
13. If a skin punch is not available, a simple elliptical excision of a block of skin overlying the foreign body can be performed in the same manner. Limit the incision to just the skin, and while applying upward traction on the ellipse with forceps (or an Allis clamp) and with the subcutaneous fat still attached beneath, probe the subcutaneous fat lateral to and beneath the incision for the foreign object. If the object is not found with probing, use the dissecting scissors to undermine the subcutaneous fat in the same directions, attempting to come into contact with the object. If the object is not found with undermining, the probe can be used again under the ellipse or directed laterally. If the object is still not located, apply pressure to the skin lateral to the incision, attempting to force the object into view.
14. If the object is neither palpable through the skin nor able to be located by probing through the entry wound (yet is visible on

x-ray films), paper clips or BBs may be used for localization with a radiograph. Bend the paper clips into various shapes and tape them to the skin with clear plastic tape, or tape the BBs over the skin above and beside the approximate location of the object. With lateral and anteroposterior radiographs taken at precisely 90 degrees, the location of the foreign body can be predicted by measuring the distance from the paper clips or BBs on the film. Transfer this measurement to the skin with a marking pen. Next, remove the tape and clips, apply povidone-iodine and local anesthetic, incise the skin in the correct location to the depth measured on the x-ray film, and remove the object. A punch biopsy may also be used in this manner if the measurements from the x-ray film are very accurate; however, if there is any error in the measurement, an incision may need to be made to expand the search for the object.

NOTE: It is very important to have true lateral and anteroposterior views in order to use radiographic measurements for localization before incision; otherwise any variance in the angle of the x-ray beam to the film will cause significant distortion of the apparent location of the foreign body. This is especially true for small metal flakes.

15. For deeply embedded objects, after injecting local anesthetic, two 27-gauge needles can be inserted at a 45-degree angle to the skin and directed toward the object from either side. Radiographs can then be used for localization, and an incision made down to the tip of the needle closest to the object. Needles used in such a manner are especially helpful when fluoroscopy is available; when the extremity is rotated under fluoroscopy, the needles provide a three-dimensional effect useful for localizing, planning the overlying incision, and removing the object.
16. Localizing even a superficial foreign body can be difficult after the procedure has begun because of distortion by local anesthetic, edema, and tissue retraction. It can be especially difficult to localize deeply embedded foreign bodies owing to these conditions. One reported technique for localizing radiopaque foreign bodies uses hemoclips with silk sutures tied to them. After the clinician dissects down to where he or she thinks the foreign body is located, two or three hemoclips can be placed into the depths of the wound. On subsequent radiographs, the hemoclip located closest to the foreign body should be verified. This one should be left in place and the others removed. The incision and dissection pathway should then follow the silk suture down to the foreign body.
17. After removal of the foreign body, the wound should be irrigated with any remaining anesthetic. This irrigation should be followed by sterile saline pulsated from a syringe. Irrigation is helpful for removing any small fragments or debris that may be remaining. A jetted irrigation can be performed by attaching an 18-gauge needle to the syringe.
18. If a significant incision was made or a punch biopsy performed, reapproximate the skin with suture. Cover the wound with a sterile adhesive bandage and give the patient postprocedure instructions.
19. For a splinter under a nail, either a "V" can be cut in the distal nail to allow it to be reached and grasped, or a portion or all of the nail can be removed under a local block (see Chapter 28, Nail Plate, Nail Bed, and Nail Matrix Biopsy, and Chapter 29, Ingrown Toenails, for similar situations). Alternatively, a 27-gauge needle can be bent at its tip to form a hook, inserted under the nail, and used to hook the splinter and drag it out. If the entire splinter cannot be removed, at least the part of the nail covering any possible splinter fragments should be removed to allow for irrigation. Otherwise, because the subungual area is very close to the distal phalanx, any remaining fragments may increase the risk of infection and subsequent rapid spread to osteomyelitis.
20. Tetanus prophylaxis should be provided if appropriate.

Complications

- Trauma to local vital structures, such as nerves, arteries, veins, or tendons.
- Infection or bleeding.
- Scarring from the original wound, or from the incision and sutures that were necessary to locate the object and close the wound.
- Failure to remove the object, partially or completely. Again, for those objects that must be removed, needle localization under fluoroscopy may remain the final option. The patient should be informed if there was failure to remove the object, and this should be documented as well as any agreed-on plan for follow-up or removal.

Postprocedure Patient Education

After removal, a dull ache or stretching sensation in the area is normal for up to a day, especially if sutures were placed. Instruct the patient to watch for signs of infection. Itching is a normal sign of healing. The patient should follow up with the clinician in 2 days to check for infection (earlier if there are significant signs) and again in the appropriate number of days (7 days in most cases) for suture removal if sutures were placed. A topical antibiotic may be applied, and the dressing should remain over the wound for 48 hours. It should be changed if it gets wet during that time. After the first 48 hours, a dressing should be applied only if the wound continues to drain or if it could get dirty. After the first 48 hours, the wound may be washed with soap and water.

CPT/Billing Codes

NOTE: As with all coding, the reimbursement is usually greater if there is a more descriptive code that includes the location, depth, and complexity (e.g., 23330 is approximately twice the RVUs as 10120, whereas 28192 is approximately four times that of 10120).

10120 Incision and removal of foreign body, subcutaneous tissues; simple
10121 Incision and removal of foreign body, subcutaneous tissues; complicated

For codes 20100 through 20103, exploration is defined as exploration and enlargement of the wound; extension of dissection (to determine penetration); débridement; removal of foreign body(s); or ligation or coagulation of minor subcutaneous and/or muscular blood vessel(s) of the subcutaneous tissue, muscle fascia, and/or muscle not requiring thoracotomy or laparotomy.

20100 Exploration of penetrating wound (separate procedure); neck
20101 Exploration of penetrating wound (separate procedure); chest
20102 Exploration of penetrating wound (separate procedure); abdomen/flank/back
20103 Exploration of penetrating wound (separate procedure); extremity
20520 Removal of foreign body in muscle or tendon sheath; simple
20525 Removal of foreign body in muscle or tendon sheath; deep or complicated
23330 Removal of foreign body, shoulder, subcutaneous tissue
24200 Removal of foreign body, upper arm or elbow area; subcutaneous tissue
24201 Removal of foreign body, upper arm or elbow area; deep (subfascial or intramuscular)
27086 Removal of foreign body, pelvis or hip; subcutaneous tissue
28190 Removal of foreign body, foot; subcutaneous tissue
28192 Removal of foreign body, foot; deep
28193 Removal of foreign body, foot; complicated

ICD-9-CM Diagnostic Codes

709.4 Foreign body granuloma of skin or subcutaneous tissue
729.6 Residual foreign body in subcutaneous or soft tissue
876.1 Foreign body back through open wound
879.3 Foreign body abdominal wall (anterior) through open wound
879.5 Foreign body abdominal wall (lateral) through open wound
880.13 Foreign body arm (upper) through open wound
882.1 Foreign body hand through open wound
884.1 Foreign body multiple arm through open wound
891.1 Foreign body calf, knee, leg through open wound
910.6 Foreign body face, neck or scalp superficial
910.7 Foreign body face, neck or scalp superficial infected
911.6 Foreign body abdominal wall, back, breast, buttock, chest, flank, groin, interscapular region, labia, penis, trunk, vagina or vulva superficial
911.7 Foreign body abdominal wall, back, breast, buttock, chest, flank, groin, interscapular region, labia, penis, trunk, vagina or vulva superficial infected
912.6 Foreign body arm, axilla superficial
912.7 Foreign body arm, axilla superficial infected
913.6 Foreign body forearm superficial
913.7 Foreign body forearm superficial infected
914.6 Foreign body hand superficial
914.7 Foreign body hand superficial infected
915.6 Foreign body finger superficial
915.7 Foreign body finger superficial infected
916.6 Foreign body calf, hip, knee or leg superficial
916.7 Foreign body calf, hip, knee or leg superficial infected
917.6 Foreign body foot or toe superficial
917.7 Foreign body foot or toe infected
919.6 Foreign body site NOS superficial
919.7 Foreign body site NOS superficial infected

BIBLIOGRAPHY

Buttaravoli P: Minor Emergencies: Splinters to Fractures, 2nd ed. St. Louis, Mosby, 2007.

Chan C, Salam GA: Splinter removal. Am Fam Physician 67:2557–2562, 2003.

Friedman EM, Munter DW, Richards JR, et al: When and how to retrieve foreign bodies. Patient Care 15:186, 1997.

Gutman SJ: Subcutaneous foreign body identification and removal. In Reichman EF, Simon RR (eds): Emergency Medicine Procedures. New York, McGraw-Hill, 2003, pp 762–771.

Lammers RL: Soft tissue foreign bodies. In Tintinalli JE, Kelen GD, Stapczynski JS (eds): Emergency Medicine: A Comprehensive Study Guide, 6th ed. New York, McGraw-Hill, 2004, pp 317–324.

Murtagh J: Removal of foreign bodies. In Murtagh J: Practice Tips, 4th ed. Sydney, Australia, McGraw-Hill, 2004, pp 113–127.

Thomas SH, Brown DFM: Foreign bodies. In Marx JA, Hockberger RS, Walls RM (eds): Rosen's Emergency Medicine, 6th ed. St. Louis, Mosby, 2006, pp 878–879.

CHAPTER 19

Fungal Studies: Collection Procedures and Tests

Dennis E. Babel

Diagnostic Methods

The three basic methods used to diagnose fungal infections are direct microscopy (e.g., potassium hydroxide [KOH] method), fungal culture, and biopsy with histopathology.

Direct Microscopy

Early diagnosis of cutaneous mycoses can be made in the physician's office by direct microscopy of infected tissue or lesion exudate. A number of different clearing solutions can be applied to collected material to assist in direct microscopy. These agents help distribute the specimen so the clinician can more readily visualize any fungal structure. These solutions include simple saline, potassium or sodium hydroxide in various formulas and preparations, and various coloring agents.

Fungal Culture

The ultimate identification of fungal pathogens requires their isolation on fungal culture medium. This isolation can take place in the physician's office using fungal media such as Sabouraud's dextrose agar with cycloheximide (to inhibit fungal contaminants) and chloramphenicol (to inhibit bacterial contaminants). These are commercially available as Mycosel agar (BBL Microbiology Systems, Becton Dickinson Co., Cockeysville, Md), Mycobiotic agar (Difco Laboratories, Detroit, Mich), and Dermatophyte Test Medium (DTM), a presumptive color-change medium (Hardy Diagnostics, Santa Maria, Calif). Of the three listed, only DTM is a color-change medium for purposes of this chapter. Inoculation of an appropriate patient specimen on these agars should allow the growth only of the true causative fungal organism.

Biopsy and Histopathology

Biopsy specimens obtained from fungal lesions can reveal the in vivo morphology of the infectious agent as well as the host response to this invasive presence. The appropriately stained histopathology section can provide the clinician with proof of the presence of a fungal pathogen, clues to its identity, the extent of infection, and the patient's ability to respond to this invasion. Although this procedure might be considered the gold standard for the diagnosis of human mycoses, it is an invasive procedure, is somewhat costly, and is seldom required for the identification of cutaneous mycoses. A 3-mm punch biopsy is usually sufficient. The pathologist must be alerted if a fungal infection is considered in the differential.

Equipment

This list includes materials for collecting and examining specimens for cutaneous mycoses as described in the text. Not every item is needed for each collection method.

- Alcohol swabs
- 3 × 3 gauze squares
- Scalpel blade (no. 15)
- Toothbrush
- Cotton-tipped applicator
- Disposable biopsy punch (3 mm)
- Glass microscope slide (1 × 3 in)
- Coverglass (22 × 22 mm)
- 20% KOH with dimethyl sulfoxide solution
- Chlorazol black E solution
- Microscope with 10× and 40× objectives
- Fungal culture media in tubes, vials, or Petri dishes (see "Fungal Culture" section, earlier)

Cutaneous Mycoses Specimen Collection (for KOH Preparations and Fungal Cultures)

Hair

The most common mycoses of the hair are tinea capitis and tinea barbae (Fig. 19-1).

- Clean the area of alopecia thoroughly with alcohol to remove foreign debris and minimize bacterial contamination. This will not affect the viability of the fungi in any manner (Fig. 19-2).
- Collect a specimen with a scalpel, glass slide edge, new toothbrush, 3 × 3 gauze square, or cotton-tipped applicator (Fig. 19-3).
- Appropriate specimen could include black dots (hair stubs) or scalp scale from the area of alopecia. (Long hairs and hair clippings are unacceptable because they are seldom actually infected and are frequently contaminated with bacteria.)

Skin

Fungal infections of the skin include tinea corporis, tinea cruris, tinea pedis, tinea manuum, and candidiasis (Fig. 19-4).

- For annular or serpiginous lesions of the skin, clean the advancing lesional edge with alcohol and obtain the scaling epithelium (avoid collecting scale from the center or oldest portion of the

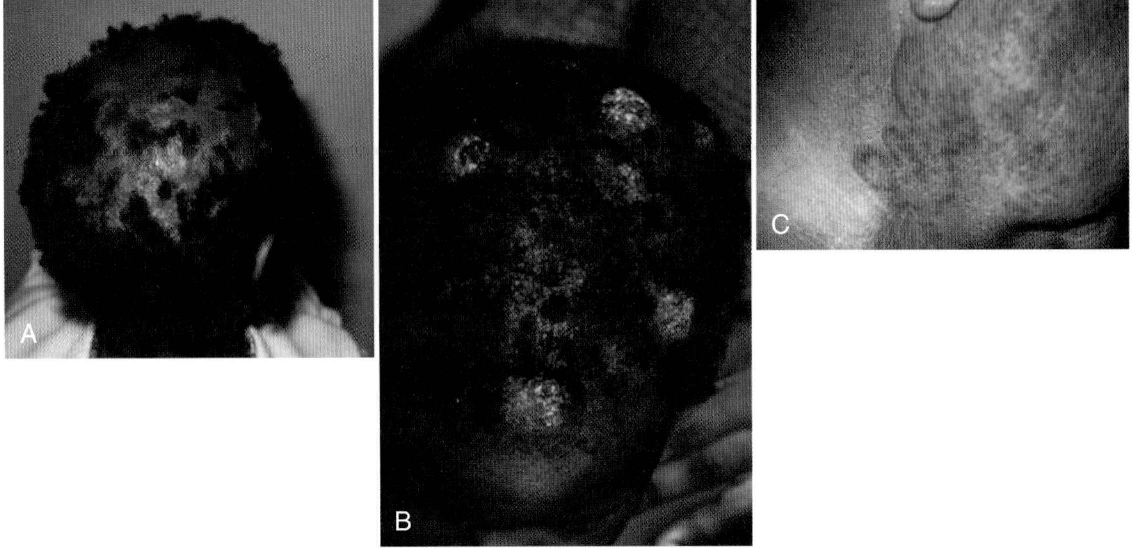

Figure 19-1 **A,** Black dot tinea capitis. **B,** Tinea capitis with kerion. **C,** Tinea barbae.

lesion because it is unlikely that the fungal pathogen is still present in that "healed" area). Scrape over the area firmly with the side of a scalpel blade to prevent bleeding. Loosened epithelial debris may be scraped directly onto a glass microscope slide for KOH examination and directly onto the fungal media surface for culture.

- For intertriginous mycoses, once again clean and collect material from the dry scaling edge. (Avoid any central, moist, macerated material because it is usually devoid of any viable fungi and is frequently contaminated with bacteria.)
- For vesicular mycoses of the skin, collect a portion of the vesicle roof by removing with a sterile scissors or scalpel blade. (Vesicular fluid and epithelium from the vesicle base are usually devoid of any fungi.)

Nail

Fungal infection of the nail (onychomycosis) is usually due to dermatophytes (tinea unguium) or *Candida* (Fig. 19-5).

- For *distal* subungual onychomycosis, trim back the nail to the leading edge of infection (edge closest to the proximal nail fold) and discard. Collect keratinaceous debris from beneath the remaining trimmed nail plate edge.
- For *proximal* subungual onychomycosis, reverse this process and collect material from the active edge closest to the distal end.
- For *white superficial onychomycosis*, clean and collect material by simply scraping the surface area of involvement.

NOTE: Less-than-ideal specimens are nail clippings and whole-removed nail plate because the true fungal reservoir is actually the nail bed (the exception being nail plate surface material from white superficial onychomycosis).

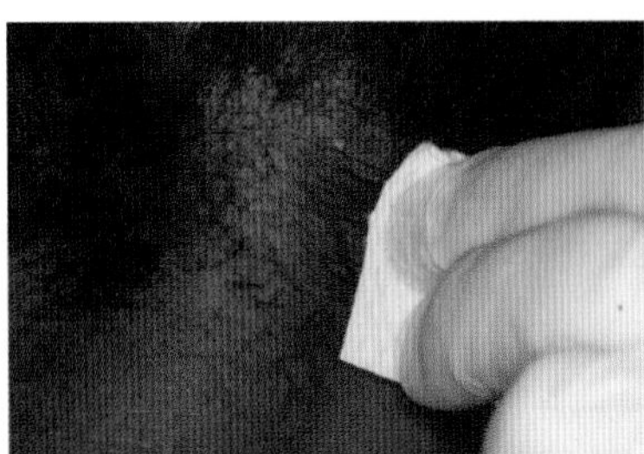

Figure 19-2 Clean area with alcohol wipe.

Technique for KOH Preparation

See Figure 19-6A.

1. Place appropriate specimen (collected as previously described) on a clean glass microscope slide.
2. Add one drop of 20% KOH with dimethyl sulfoxide solution.*
3. Add one drop of chlorazol black E solution.*
4. Place a coverglass on top of the slide preparation and press down to eliminate air bubbles.
5. Blot excess solution from the finished slide preparation.
6. Place the preparation on the microscope stage and examine it with the *low-power* (10×) objective.
7. To enhance contrast, reduce the microscope illumination by lowering the condenser until epithelial cells are clearly visible.
8. *Screen* the slide preparation under low power (10×) for the presence of fungal structures, such as hyphae or yeast.
9. Examine suspect structures with the 40× setting (high-power dry objective) to confirm the presence of fungi (an oil immersion objective is *not* needed).
10. The observation of hyphae or budding yeast and pseudohyphae constitutes a "positive" KOH preparation for fungus.

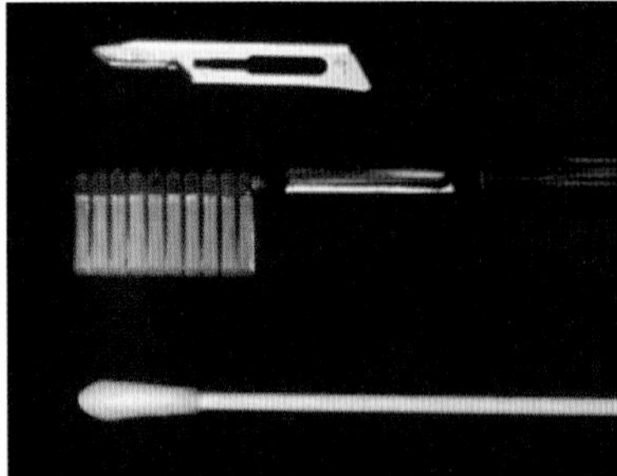

Figure 19-3 Tinea collection tools.

*These solutions are commercially available (see the "Suppliers" section).

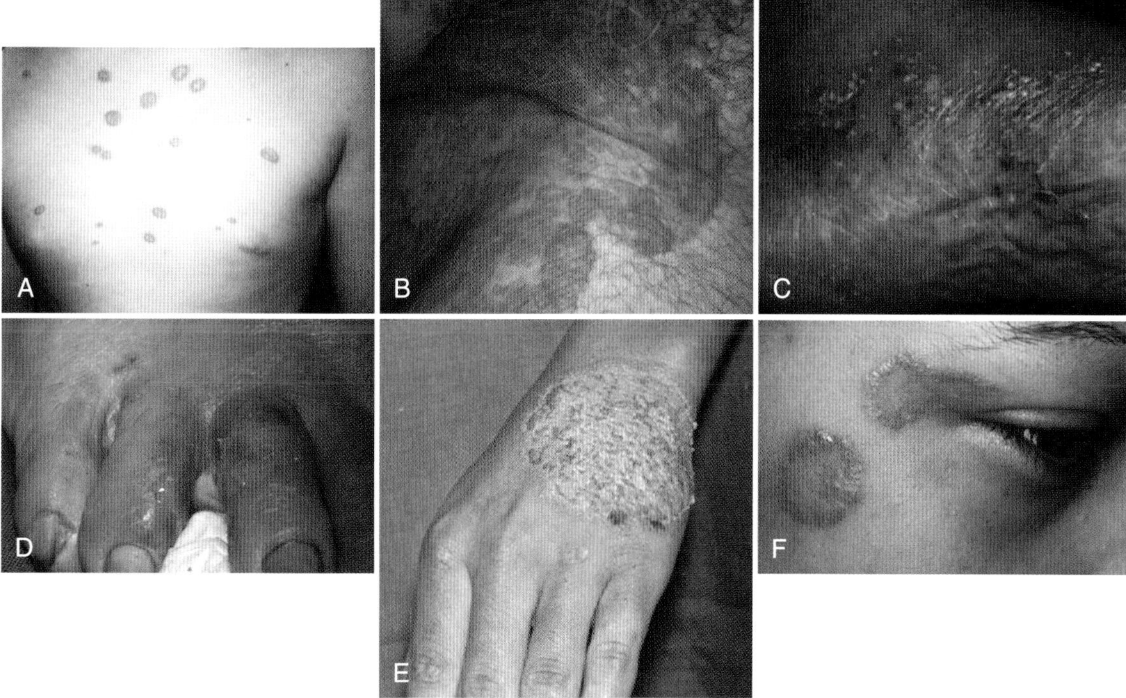

Figure 19-4 **A,** Tinea corporis (annular). **B,** Tinea cruris (serpiginous). **C,** Tinea pedis (vesicular). **D,** Tinea pedis (interdigital). **E,** Tinea manuum. **F,** Tinea faciei.

Positive KOH

1. *Dermatophyte (mold) causing tinea.* Look for hyaline, septate filaments with diameters at least four times the diameter of an epithelial cell wall. This diameter should be very consistent (5 to 7 μm). This filament is linear and may course across a number of keratinocytes and occasionally branch (Fig. 19-6B–F).
2. *Candida (yeast).* Look for round to oval budding cells as well as "stretched out" budding cells (pseudohyphae; Fig. 19-6G).
3. Malassezia furfur *(pityriasis versicolor).* Look for short, hyaline, septate hyphae as well as round, clustered yeast cells ("spaghetti and meatballs"; see Fig. 19-6F).

Common Errors in KOH Examinations

- Not collecting specimen from the leading edge of infection.
- Not thoroughly cleaning the sample site with alcohol before sampling.

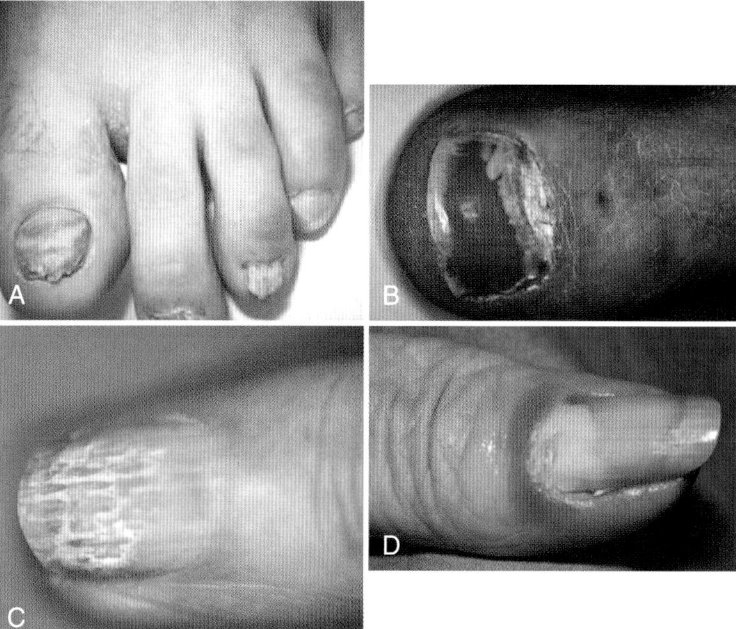

Figure 19-5 **A,** Distal subungual onychomycosis. **B,** Proximal subungual onychomycosis. **C,** White superficial onychomycosis. **D,** Candidal onychomycosis/paronychia.

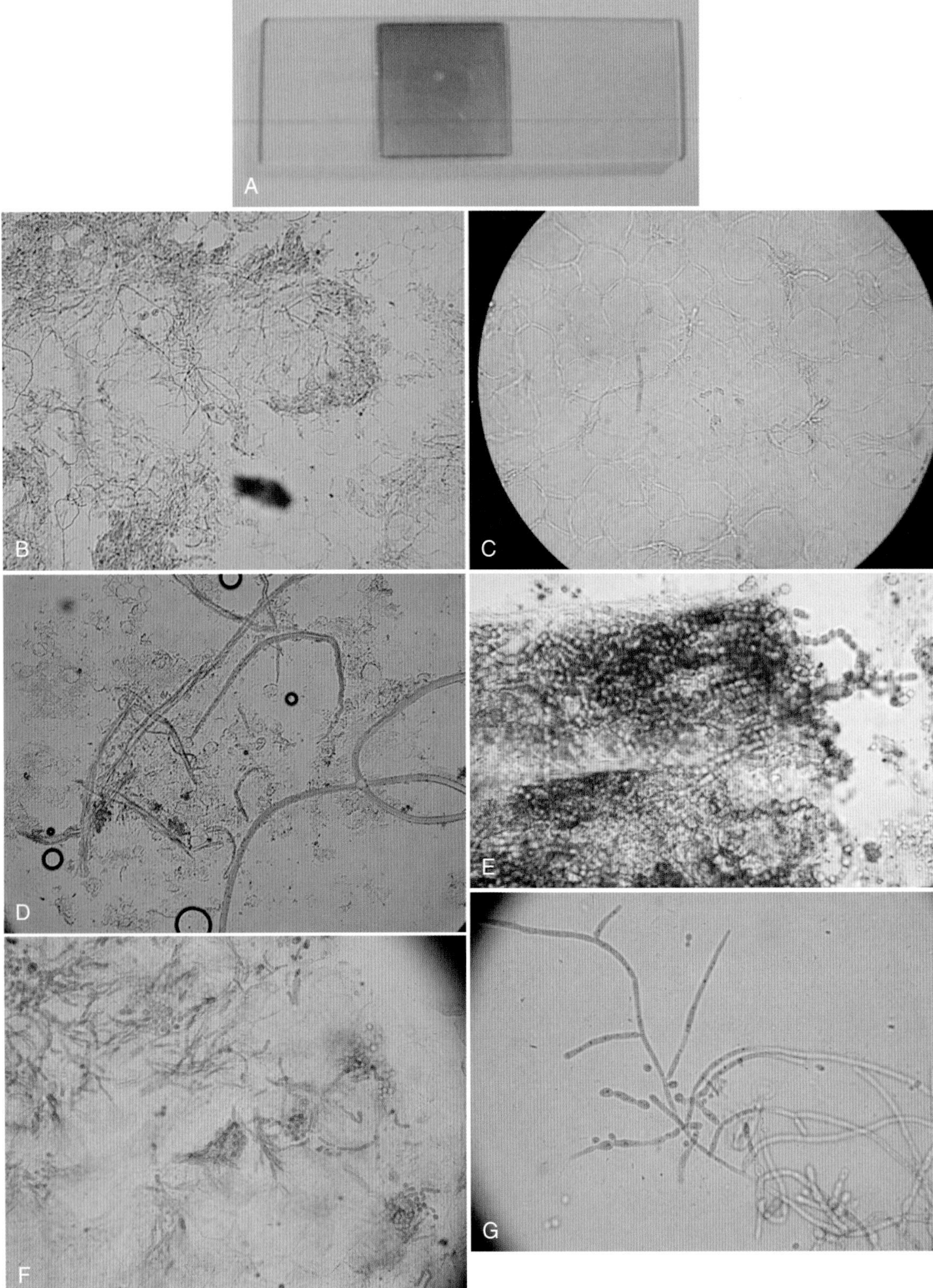

Figure 19-6 **A,** Glass slide KOH preparation. **B,** Positive KOH for hyphae (low power). **C,** Positive KOH for hyphae (high power). **D,** False-positive KOH preparation with foreign debris. **E,** Positive KOH for tinea capitis. **F,** Positive KOH for tinea versicolor ("spaghetti and meatballs"). **G,** Positive KOH for candidiasis.

- Not reducing the microscope light by racking down the microscope condenser to maximize contrast.
- Mistaking foreign matter (e.g., sock fibers, dirt, pollen) for fungal structures microscopically.
- Heating a KOH slide preparation to speed up the clearing process to the point where the chemical precipitates out. (Heating a slide preparation should not be necessary if using 20% KOH with dimethyl sulfoxide.)

Technique for a Fungal Culture (Office Procedure)

The greatest recovery of mycotic pathogens by fungal culture can be achieved through the inoculation of lesion material directly onto fungal media by the examining physician (Fig. 19-7). (Alternatively, the patient specimen that will be sent to an outside laboratory for inoculation should be packaged carefully and delivered in a timely fashion.)

1. The patient specimen should be gently pressed onto the agar surface. Minimize "stabbing" and avoid "slashing" the agar because these techniques may lead to a premature drying out of the culture system.
2. Fungal cultures from most cutaneous specimens should be incubated at room temperature (22° C to 27° C) in a draft-free location and out of direct sunlight.
3. Presumptive pathogen media such as DTM, which rely on a color change from orange to red when a fungal pathogen is present, should be observed for the first 10 days. The development of a red agar color after this period should be considered a false-positive result.

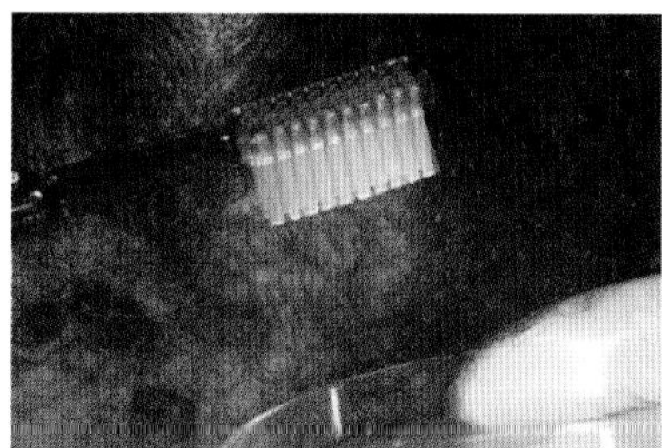

Figure 19-7 Fungal culture inoculation from tinea capitis with toothbrush.

Technique for Biopsy for the Identification of Cutaneous Mycoses

Biopsy specimens can be obtained for both the fungal culture and the histopathologic confirmation of the organism's presence in vivo.

1. A 3-mm punch biopsy obtained from the lesional edge is usually sufficient for both purposes (see Chapter 32, Skin Biopsy).
2. The biopsy material should be divided longitudinally into two equal parts.
3. One biopsy portion should be placed into *formalin* and sent to the pathology laboratory with a request for "fungal stains."
4. The second biopsy portion should be placed in *sterile saline* and sent to the microbiology laboratory for "fungal culture."

Suppliers

(See contact information online at www.expertconsult.com.)

Fungal culture isolation media
#X30—Mycobiotic agar, plastic Hardy flask
#X15—DTM (Dermatophyte Test Medium), plastic Hardy flask
Hardy Diagnostics
Instrument for trimming nail plate
#21-626 Ruskin double action forceps, 6″, straight
Miltex, Inc.
KOH solutions for micro preps
20% KOH with DMSO; chlorazol black E fungal stain
Dermatology Lab & Supply, Inc. (Delasco)

Bibliography

Aly R, Beutner KR, Malbach H (eds): Cutaneous Infection and Therapy. New York, Marcel Dekker, 1997.
Babel DE: Fungi. In Lesher J (ed): Manual of Cutaneous Microbiology for the Office Laboratory. Pearl River, NY, Parthenon Publishing, 2000.
Babel DE, Rogers AL: Dermatophytes: Their contribution to infectious disease in North America. Clin Microbiol Rev 5:81–85, 1983.
Babel DE, Rogers AL, Beneke ES: Dermatophytosis of the scalp: Incidence, immune response, and epidemiology. Mycopathologia 109:69–73, 1990.
Belsey RE, Skeels MR, Baer DM, Koneman EW: Basic Office Microbiology. Oradell, NJ, Medical Economics, 1990.
Daniel CR III, Elewski BE: The diagnosis of nail fungus revisited. Arch Dermatol 136:1162–1164, 2000.
Sauer GC, Hall JC (eds): Manual of Skin Diseases, 7th ed. Philadelphia, Lippincott-Raven, 1996.
Usatine RP: The Color Atlas of Family Medicine. New York, McGraw-Hill, 2009.

CHAPTER 20

Incision and Drainage of an Abscess

Daniel J. Derksen

An abscess is a localized infection characterized by a collection of pus surrounded by inflamed tissue. When a sweat gland or hair follicle infection forms an abscess, it is called a *furuncle*, or *boil*. If multiple follicles are involved with abscesses, it is referred to as a *carbuncle*. *Paronychia* is an abscess that involves the nail. A *felon* is an abscess in the tuft of soft tissue in the distal phalanx of the finger. A *hordeolum* is an abscess on the eyelid margin, whereas a *chalazion* is a chronic abscess of the eyelid itself in the meibomian glands beneath the tarsal plate (see Chapter 65, Chalazion and Hordeolum). *Hidradenitis suppurativa* is a chronic condition in the axilla and groin with recurrent abscess formation. *Pilonidal abscesses* are discussed in Chapter 109, Pilonidal Cyst and Abscess: Current Management; *perianal abscesses* in Chapter 107, Perianal Abscess Incision and Drainage; and *Bartholin's abscesses* in Chapter 131, Bartholin's Cyst and Abscess: Word Catheter Insertion, Marsupialization. For *olecranon* and *prepatellar* bursitis, see Chapter 192, Joint and Soft Tissue Aspiration and Injection (Arthrocentesis).

Most often, *Staphylococcus aureus* is the causative agent in abscesses, but some abscesses are due to *Streptococcus* species or a combination of microorganisms, including gram-negative and anaerobic bacteria. Perianal abscesses are usually caused by a mix of aerobic and anaerobic enteric organisms. Abscesses can occur in any location, but they are commonly found on the extremities, buttocks, and breast or in hair follicles.

A small abscess may respond to warm compresses or antibiotics and drain spontaneously. As the abscess enlarges, the inflammation, collection of pus, and walling off of the abscess cavity render such conservative treatments ineffectual. *The treatment of choice for an abscess is incision and drainage (I&D)*, and if this treatment is done properly, antibiotics are usually unnecessary. (See precautions for the facial triangle in "Contraindications," later.) In a nonlactating woman, a *breast abscess* that is not subareolar is rare. If an abscess occurs away from the areola, it should prompt a biopsy in addition to I&D and raise the clinician's suspicion of a malignant tumor.

Patients with diabetes, debilitating disease, or compromised immunity should be observed closely after I&D of an abscess. Although usually not necessary, consider a culture obtained by aspiration or swab of the abscess cavity because the abscess may have been caused by unusual organisms in these compromised patients. The infection may also warrant the administration of antibiotics that cover *Staphylococcus* infection.

If an abscess recurs after incision and drainage, methicillin-resistant *S. aureus* (MRSA) should be considered, a culture and sensitivity obtained, and the patient treated with appropriate antibiotics based on these results. Community-associated *S. aureus* is most often sensitive to clindamycin, trimethoprim/sulfamethoxazole, doxycycline, and rifampin. The frequency of MRSA skin and soft tissue infections has increased dramatically, and it is now the most common pathogen for these infections when patients present to the emergency department. Resistance changes rapidly and differs regionally. Initial treatment remains I&D, although some recommend treatment with one or more oral antibiotics based on culture and sensitivity.

Indications

A localized collection of pus that is tender and not spontaneously resolving. If the lesion is not "pointing" and localized, a trial of antibiotics may be indicated. However, antibiotics are usually inadequate once a collection of pus is present.

Contraindications

Small, nonfluctuant facial furuncles without surrounding cellulitis should not be incised or drained if located within the triangle formed by the bridge of the nose and the corners of the mouth. These infections should be treated with antibiotics, with coverage for MRSA, and warm compresses because there is a risk of septic phlebitis with intracranial extension after I&D of a furuncle in this area. However, if the lesion is large and fluctuant, drainage is recommended, regardless of the site. In most instances, drainage alone is adequate, but in this area antibiotics are also recommended.

Equipment

- Local anesthetic (1% to 2% lidocaine), sodium bicarbonate 7.5%, or diphenhydramine (Benadryl) 50 mg/mL
- Syringe with 25- to 30-gauge needle, usually ½ to 1 inch, because only the skin over the abscess is anesthetized
- Possibly a cryosurgery unit or ethyl chloride for anesthesia (to avoid a needle poke)
- Alcohol or povidone-iodine (Betadine) wipe
- 4 × 4–inch gauze
- No. 11 blade
- Curved hemostats
- Possibly iodoform gauze (¼- to ½-inch width, and up to 24 inches long depending on abscess size)
- Possibly culture materials
- Bandage scissors
- Dressing of choice

Technique

Protective eyewear should be worn.

1. Prepare the abscess area with povidone-iodine or alcohol.
2. Administer a field block with local anesthetic (see Chapter 8, Peripheral Nerve Blocks and Field Blocks) to allow an adequate

incision to be made. Avoid infiltration of the abscess cavity; rather, concentrate on anesthetizing the perimeter of the tissue around the abscess. Local anesthetics usually work poorly in the acidic milieu of an abscess. More anesthetic than usual may be needed to relieve pain. Alternatively, diphenhydramine 10 to 25 mg can be injected into the area for anesthesia. Dilute a 50-mg (1-mL) vial in a syringe with 4 mL of normal saline (Fig. 20-1A and B). Cryocautery can also be used to freeze the roof of the abscess. This can be performed with a nitrous oxide unit, liquid nitrogen, or ethyl chloride. The incision is then made through the cooled skin, which is now anesthetized.

EDITOR'S NOTE: Nearly always, lidocaine will be adequate, but larger volumes may be needed.

3. Make a sufficiently wide incision with a pointed no. 11 blade to allow drainage of the abscess cavity and to prevent premature closure of the incision. If a large abscess is present, a 1-cm incision is usually large enough. Make the incision in the skin lines. Recurrence of the abscess is most often due to an inadequate incision and premature closure of the incision (Fig. 20-1C and D). Purulent material can "squirt out," especially if digital pressure is applied. Protective glasses and other precautions are suggested.
4. If a culture is obtained, it should be from the abscess cavity and not from the superficial skin over the abscess. Alternatively, the abscess cavity can be aspirated with a large-bore (18-gauge) needle before the incision is made. The aspirated contents can then be sent for the appropriate cultures in more complicated cases. This is rarely helpful in routine superficial abscesses.
5. Apply external pressure to express all pus (Fig. 20-1E). The abscess cavity should also be thoroughly explored with a sterile cotton-tipped applicator or with hemostats. Attempts should be made to break down any walled-off pockets or possible septa (Fig. 20-1F). If the lesion began as a cyst (e.g., sebaceous cyst), a small reusable dermal curette can be used to curette the cavity in the hope of removing all of the sac (Fig. 20-1G). Disposable curettes are often too sharp and may cause excessive damage. A residual sac can lead to a recurrent cyst. The cavity can be packed with

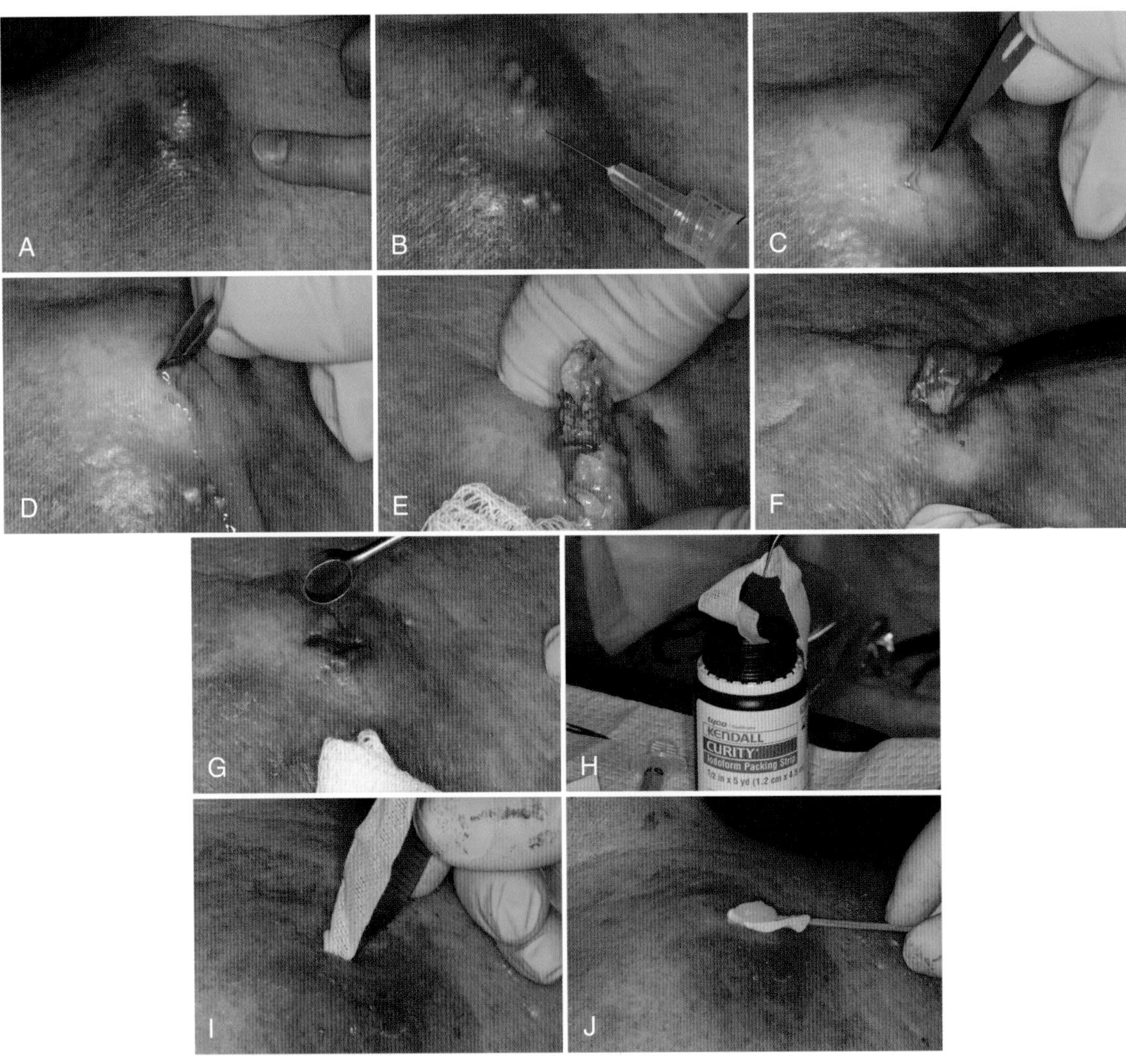

Figure 20-1 **A,** Large sebaceous cyst abscess of the back. **B,** Injecting local anesthetic (2% lidocaine with epinephrine). May augment with field block if desired. **C,** Incising abscess with no. 11 blade. **D,** Purulent material is released from the lesion. **E,** Apply digital pressure to evacuate contents of the infected cyst. **F,** In the case of sebaceous cyst abscesses, the sac can often be grasped and removed using hemostats. It may be so necrotic in some lesions that it fragments, making removal more difficult. **G,** In cases where total removal of the cyst sac is uncertain, a reusable dermal curette can be used to scrape the cavity and remove any residual sac. **H,** Iodoform gauze (¼- or ½-inch, depending on size of cavity) is used to pack the wound open. Premature closure will lead to recurrence of the abscess. Suturing the wound closed is contraindicated. **I,** Insert the gauze using pickups without teeth. **J,** Apply antibiotic ointment over the tail of the iodoform gauze to prevent the outer dressing from sticking to it.

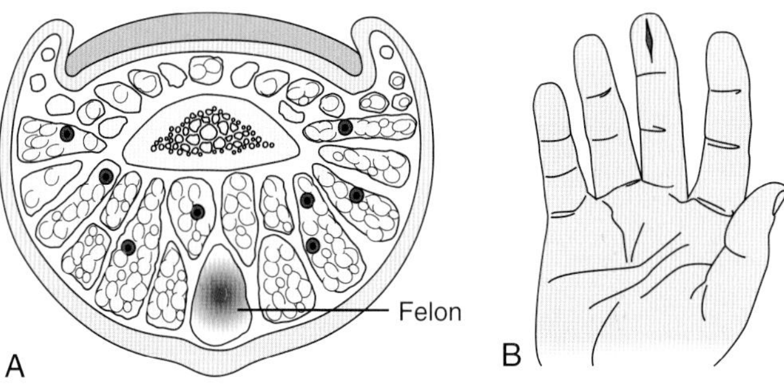

Figure 20-2 **A,** Anatomic cross-section of the distal phalanx, showing the numerous fascial septa and a felon. **B,** Incision of a felon. Incision should be in the longitudinal digital midline and should not cross a flexor crease.

a Penrose drain or with packing material, preferably iodoform gauze. The length and width depend on abscess size. A small "tail" of gauze should be left protruding from the wound for drainage. Apply an ointment over the wound to prevent the gauze from sticking to the overlying dressing and being inadvertently removed when the dressing is changed (Fig. 20-1H through J).
6. Depending on the location and the size of the abscess, the gauze can be removed slowly over several weeks. Slowly advancing the packing will ensure that the wound does not close off too soon, and decreases the recurrence rate. The packing material can be changed daily, but it is painful and there is no real advantage to changing it. There may be some advantage to changing it after 5 to 7 days to reduce purulence and recheck the wound. For larger abscess cavities, leave the "wick" in for 4 weeks so that the abscess scars down from the inside. The patient can advance the drain every few days and cut off 2 inches at a time.
7. A sterile dressing can be applied over the area to collect discharge. This should be changed several times daily. Healing should progress from the inside out; that is, epithelialization of the abscess cavity should occur before healing of the incision site to minimize the chance of recurrence.
8. In patients with hidradenitis, I&D may traumatize the area and cause more long-term abscesses. However, the pain is usually so severe and acute with an abscess that I&D is necessary. Most patients with hidradenitis require long-term antibiotics, similar to patients with chronic acne. Some patients may require resection of all axillary or groin tissue involved.
9. A felon is an abscess in the distal tuft of the phalanx (Fig. 20-2A). A digital block serves best to anesthetize the area. Prepare with alcohol or povidone-iodine. Incise the abscess in the midline parallel with the digit (Fig. 20-2B). The large bilateral incisions of the past are now generally avoided. A small wick of iodoform gauze can be placed in the cavity for 24 hours. Many physicians use antibiotics in patients with felons to cover for *S. aureus*.

Usually I&D is sufficient to resolve an abscess. If cellulitis is present or the patient is at high risk for infection, an antibiotic can be used. It should cover *S. aureus*.

Complications

If the packing is tight in the abscess cavity, the pain can be sufficient to warrant use of acetaminophen or nonsteroidal anti-inflammatory drugs. Narcotics are rarely needed. I&D alone may provide sufficient pain relief from a tense abscess such that no pain medication is needed. Complications include the following:

- Recurrence
- Scar or keloid
- A failure to resolve, causing a cellulitis, or the progression to septicemia
- Formation of a fistula
- Osteomyelitis

An abscess in the palmar aspect of the hand can extend from superficial to deep tissue through the palmar fascia. Deep infection is suspected when the simple I&D fails to reduce the erythema, pain, pus, or swelling. More extensive surgical débridement, hospitalization, and intravenous antibiotics may be necessary in a patient with a deep palmar abscess, which is a surgical emergency.

A recurrent paronychia may require removal of the nail to resolve the infection (see Chapter 29, Ingrown Toenails, and Chapter 12, Approach to Various Skin Lesions). Also, consider treatment for *Candida* infection in fingernail cases.

Postprocedure Patient Preparation

Some patients can be taught to change their own packing, replace the dressings, and advance the drain. Other patients may require a family member or home nurse visits or may have to return to the office to have this done. Patients should be instructed to watch for signs of recurrence of the abscess and for evidence of further infection such as cellulitis, and to notify the clinician immediately if any of the following occur:

- Recollection of pus in the abscess
- Fever and chills
- Increased pain or redness
- Red streaks near the abscess
- Increased swelling in the area

Generally, bathing and frequent changes of the overlying dressing are encouraged.

CPT/Billing Codes

Incision and drainage CPT codes vary by complexity and site.

10040	Acne surgery
10060	I&D one abscess
10061	I&D multiple/complex abscess
10080	I&D pilonidal cyst, simple
10081	I&D complicated pilonidal cyst
10140	I&D hematoma
10160	Aspirate abscess/cyst
10180	I&D complex/postoperative infection
19020	I&D deep abscess
21501	I&D deep, neck
23030	I&D deep, shoulder
23930	I&D deep, arm/elbow
23931	I&D infected olecranon bursa
25028	I&D deep, forearm
26010	I&D simple, abscess finger
26011	I&D complex, finger (felon)
26990	I&D deep, hip area
26991	I&D infected bursa, hip area
27301	I&D deep abscess/bursa knee
27603	I&D deep, leg/ankle
28001	I&D bursa, foot
28002	I&D deep, foot
30000	I&D drainage abscess or hematoma, nasal, internal approach
30020	I&D nasal septum (abscess hematoma)
40800	I&D vestibule mouth
40801	I&D complicated, mouth
41000	I&D lingual
41005	I&D sublingual (superficial)

41006 I&D sublingual, deep
41800 I&D gums
45005 I&D submucosal rect abscess
46040 I&D perirectal abscess
46050 I&D superficial perianal abscess
46083 I&D hemorrhoid, external
54015 I&D deep, penis
54700 I&D epididymis
55000 Aspirate hydrocele
55100 I&D scrotal wall abscess
56405 I&D vulva
56420 I&D Bartholin's abscess
67700 I&D eyelid abscess
69000 I&D abscess pinna
69005 I&D abscess, pinna, complicated
69020 I&D ear canal abscess

ICD-9-CM Diagnostic Codes

For ICD-9-CM diagnostic codes, look under "abscess" for specific site.

BIBLIOGRAPHY

Bamberger DM, Boyd SE: Management of *Staphylococcus aureus* infections. Am Fam Physician 72:2474–2481, 2005.

Bobrow BJ, Pollack CV Jr, Gamble S, Seligson RA: Incision and drainage of cutaneous abscesses is not associated with bacteremia in afebrile adults. Ann Emerg Med 29:404–408, 1997.

Brooks I, Frazier EH: The aerobic and anaerobic bacteriology of perirectal abscesses. J Clin Microbiol 35:2974–2976, 1997.

Hankin A, Everett WW: Are antibiotics necessary after incision and drainage of a cutaneous abscess? Ann Emerg Med 50:49–51, 2007.

Moran GJ, Krishnadasan A, Gorwitz RJ, et al: Methicillin-resistant *S. aureus* infections among patients in the emergency department. N Engl J Med 355:666–674, 2006.

Nagle D, Rolandelli RH: Primary care office management of perianal and anal disease. Prim Care 23:609–620, 1996.

Squires JA, Fish FS III: Incision, draining and exteriorization techniques. In Robinson JK, Hanke DW, Sengelmann RD, Siegel DM (eds): Surgery of the Skin: Procedural Dermatology. Philadelphia, Mosby, 2005, pp 213–225.

Tuggy M, Garcia J: Procedures Consult. Available at www.proceduresconsult.com.

Usatine RP: Incision and drainage. In Usatine RP, Moy RL, Tobinick EL, Siegel DM (eds): Skin Surgery: A Practical Guide. St. Louis, Mosby, 1998, pp 200–210.

Usatine RP: The Color Atlas of Family Medicine. New York, McGraw-Hill, 2009.

CHAPTER 21

Incisions: Planning the Direction of the Incision

Julie M. Sicilia

Although generally considered minor procedures, skin incisions are invasive. They cause permanent changes in skin architecture and carry the potential for deleterious patient outcomes in terms of cosmesis and function. Skin incisions must be made with careful, thoughtful consideration and advance planning.

Several general issues should be addressed before deciding to perform an incision:

- Overall health status of the patient, including assessment of risk for:
  - Significant bleeding (bleeding dyscrasias, medications including herbs)
  - Potential for delayed wound healing (e.g., smoking, collagen vascular disease, diabetes, obesity, immunosuppression, steroid use, malnutrition, and peripheral vascular disease)
  - Allergy to any substance being used in conjunction with the procedure, including latex and the parabens preservatives in multiple-dose vials of anesthetics
- Need for antibiotic prophylaxis (e.g., dirty wounds, bites, infection, puncture, immunosuppression, diabetes)
- Ability of the patient or caregivers to properly care for the surgical wound postoperatively
- Expected benefits versus risks of the procedure

The physician must obtain an informed consent and ensure that the patient knows the basic complications of pain, bleeding, infection, recurrence, scarring, and distortion of the anatomy. The physician must always consider the patient as a whole being and not simply focus on "the lesion." Many pitfalls are avoidable if this is kept in mind.

Technical factors to be considered include the following:

- Avoidance of damage to any underlying vital structures
- Proper orientation of incision lines
- Correct design and size of the excision
- Avoidance of significant anatomic distortion

Avoiding Damage to Underlying Structures

Simple full-thickness skin excisions performed with care usually do not pose a threat to underlying structures. The plane of removal should be at the junction of the adipose tissue and the dermis (Fig. 21-1). Nonetheless, familiarity with the anatomy of the proposed surgical site in regard to underlying nerves, vessels, tendons, bursae, and bony structures is essential. Of special concern are two nerves that lie superficially within the subdermal fat layer: the temporal branch of the facial nerve and the spinal accessory nerve (Figs. 21-2 and 21-3). Injury to the temporal branch of the facial nerve may cause inability to wrinkle the forehead and drooping of the eyebrow on the affected side. Damage to the spinal accessory nerve can lead to loss of use of the trapezius muscle. When performing excisions in these regions, physicians should consider less invasive alternative methods for treating the particular lesion, if possible. If an incisional approach must be used, the patient should be advised of the potential complications.

Orientation of the Incision

Skin incisions and excisions must take into account static and dynamic skin tension to minimize scarring and maximize function. Langer's lines of minimal skin tension, in general, lie perpendicular to the long axis of underlying musculature and can usually be demonstrated by pinching together a local area of skin or by having the patient contract the muscles under that area. On the face, wrinkles form along these lines as a result of repeated contraction of the facial musculature. ***Linear incisions*** (e.g., for removal of underlying lesions such as lipomas or for incision and drainage) should be oriented parallel to wrinkle lines when possible (parallel to the lines of minimal skin tension). With an ***elliptical excision***, in which a section of overlying skin is removed, the long axis of the ellipse should lie parallel to the lines of minimal skin tension. Standard depictions of Langer's lines (Fig. 21-4) assist in planning incisions, but lines of minimal tension must be evaluated on each patient individually before a procedure. For the face, the patient's simulating various facial expressions will aid in demonstrating natural wrinkle lines. It should also be noted that for certain elliptical excisions (especially on the face), the long axis of the excision may need to curve or angle instead of lying entirely in a straight line (Fig. 21-5). Planning incisions along lines of minimal tension decreases the forces on the wound that tend to pull it apart, thereby reducing scar potential. Certain areas, especially the deltoid and sternum, are invariably prone to experiencing transverse traction, with a subsequent wider scar and a higher propensity for keloid formation. Children also have an increased tendency to develop hypertrophic or keloid scars.

When lines of minimal tension are not apparent, even after the patient performs maneuvers to accentuate them, it may be helpful to first perform a circular excision, undermine the wound circumferentially, and then allow natural skin tension to orient the wound, usually into a more oval shape. At that point the resulting oval can be converted to an ellipse and the wound closed (Fig. 21-6).

Incisions across joint surfaces should be made transversely (or obliquely if necessary). Perpendicular lacerations or incisions across joint space lines have a tendency to contract, thus limiting range of motion. Chapter 17, Flaps and Plasties, includes a review of Z-plasty, an example of a situation in which a laceration extending across a joint is converted to a transverse wound to maximize joint function and minimize contracture.

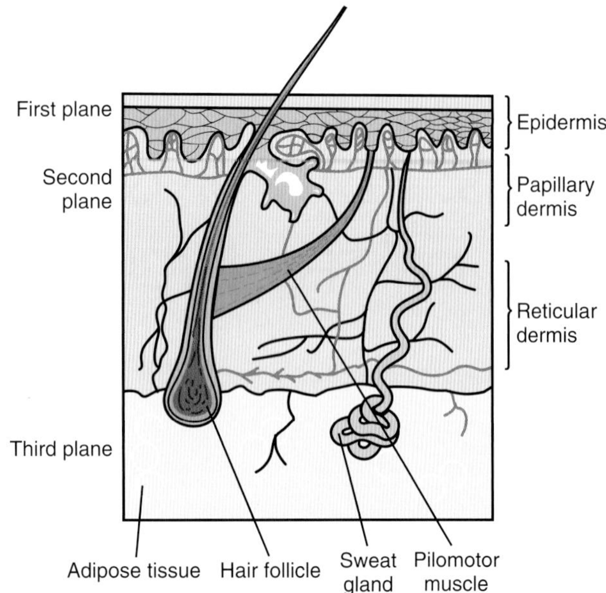

Figure 21-1 Skin anatomy.

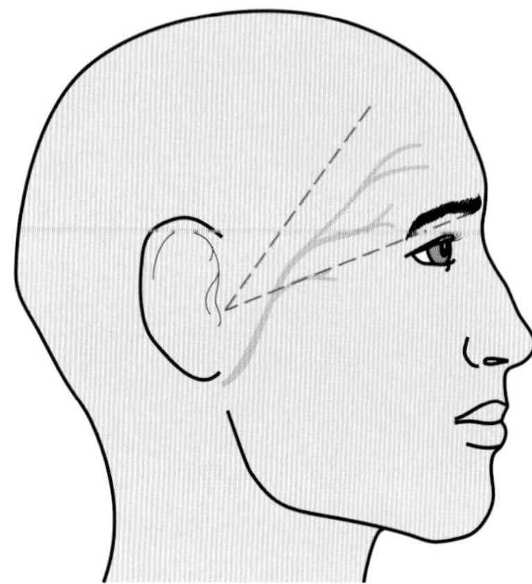

Figure 21-2 Temporal branch of facial nerve. The nerve lies superficially within a triangle created by a line extending from the tragus to the upper forehead wrinkle area and a line extending from the tragus to the lateral aspect of the eyebrow.

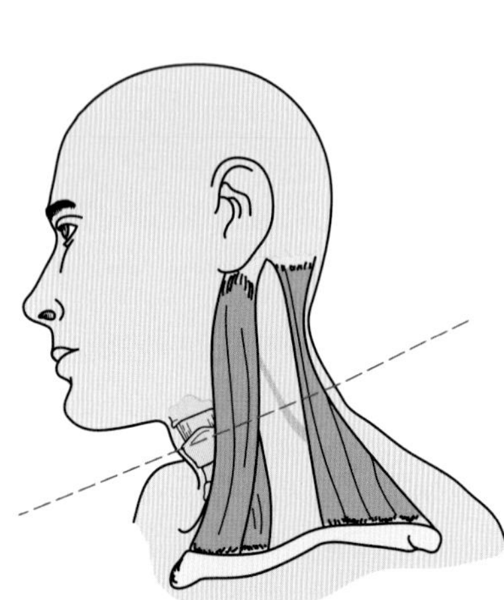

Figure 21-3 Spinal accessory nerve. The nerve lies superficially within the posterior triangle of the neck at the level of the notch in the superior thyroid cartilage.

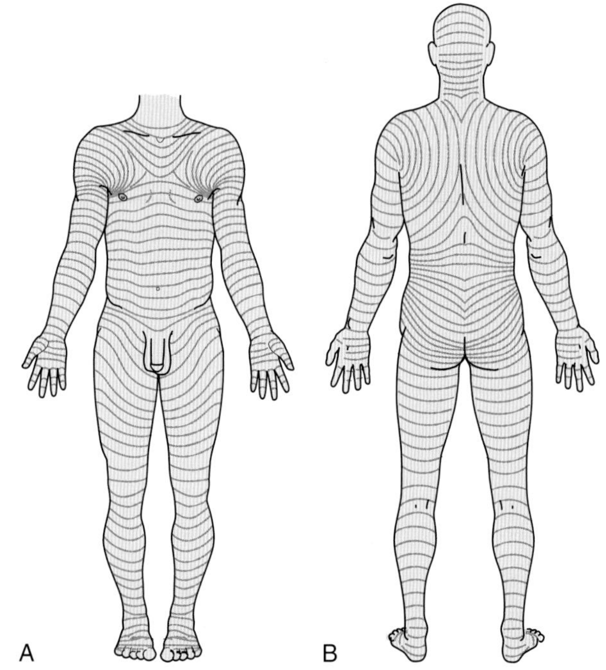

Figure 21-4 Lines of minimal skin tension. **A,** Anterior body. **B,** Posterior view.

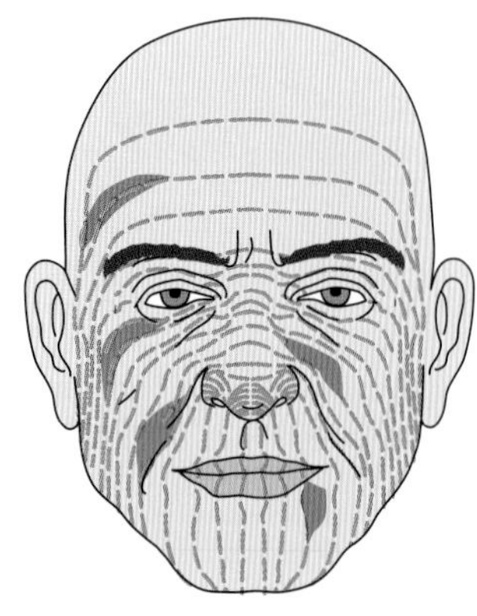

Figure 21-5 Skin tension lines on the face and proper excision shapes.

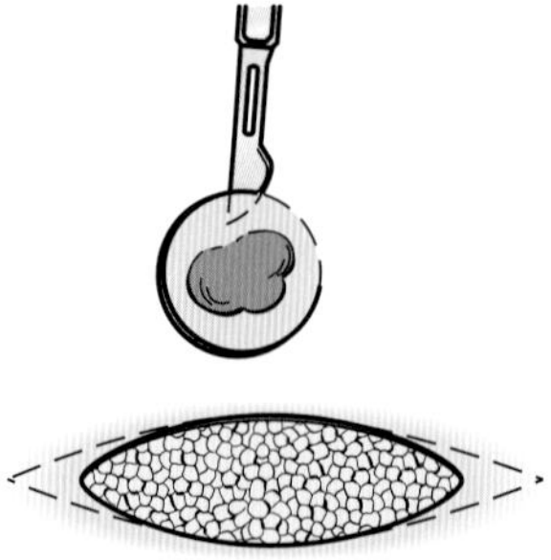

Figure 21-6 **A,** Creating a circular wound, with conversion to an ellipse. **B,** Creating an ellipse.

Design and Size of the Excision

Surgical marking pens should be used freely in designing incisions. Planning, measuring, and marking are essential steps toward an optimal result. The majority of skin excisions are elliptical in shape. The wound should be three times as long as it is wide (Fig. 21-7). A wound that is not long enough will create dog ears when repaired. Because alcohol will remove most marking pen inks, first use an alcohol wipe and anesthetize the wound, then mark and measure the planned excision, and finally anesthetize the surgical site. Next, prepare the site with povidone-iodine (Betadine), which will not remove the ink, and then drape the patient.

When incising with the scalpel, a no. 15 blade is used and should be held perpendicular to the skin or angled up to 15 degrees with the cutting edge angled away from the lesion (Fig. 21-8A and B). Remember that slight eversion during the repair is desirable (Fig. 21-8C). Slanting the blade in the opposite direction makes this difficult to accomplish. Remember to "build pyramids, not dig ditches"—when incising, the top of the blade should tilt slightly over the lesion, not away from it (Fig. 21-8D). Angling the blade more than 15 degrees creates a very thin "slice" of tissue on the remaining skin, which may necrose and lead to more scar formation.

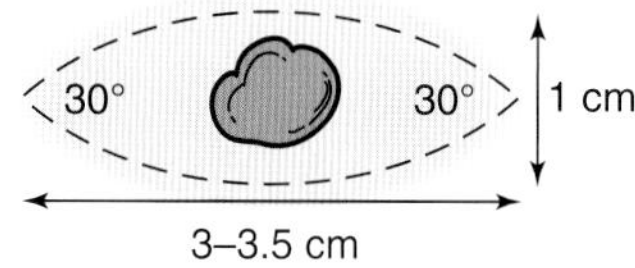

Figure 21-7 Creating an ellipse (proper dimensions).

Margins of normal tissue that should be removed vary depending on whether a lesion is benign or malignant, and, if malignant, the margins vary depending on the type of cancer (see Chapter 12, Approach to Various Skin Lesions). For benign lesions, the incision can be placed close to the lesion with only 1 or 2 mm of normal tissue excised. For *melanomas*, a 5-mm margin is needed if in situ, and a 1-cm margin is needed for any *invasive melanoma less than 1 mm*. If *greater than 1 mm* deep, consider referral.

For *basal cell carcinomas*, remove a 3- to 5-mm rim of normal tissue, and for squamous cell carcinomas, at least a 5-mm band of normal tissue around the lesion.

After the ellipse is made down to adipose, the tissue specimen is freed by cutting with the scalpel in the plane between dermis and adipose tissue. Using Adson pickups with teeth, grasp the end of the ellipse and dissect from one end to center. Then grasp the other end and do the same. This technique avoids the tendency to travel too deep within the excision (Fig. 21-9).

Avoiding Distortion of Surface Anatomy

The physician should always attempt to estimate the change in surface anatomy that results from an excision. Pinching together the two sides of a planned ellipse assists in demonstrating whether a defect can be closed in a direct side-to-side fashion and if significant distortion of surrounding tissue will occur. The presternal, scalp, and pretibial regions can be potentially quite difficult to close after a skin excision, as can wider excisions in any location. Excisions necessitating removal of a significant amount of tissue on the forehead, upper lip, and around the eyes often cause distortion of facial appearance (Fig. 21-10). Proper planning creates excellent cosmetic results (Fig. 21-11).

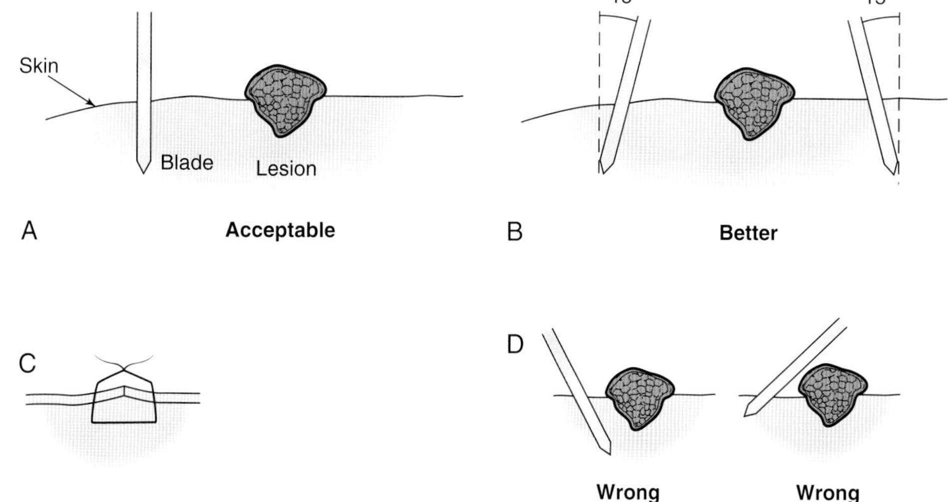

Figure 21-8 The proper angle of the scalpel when creating an ellipse. **A,** Acceptable angle. **B,** Better angle. **C,** Proper shapes of suture and skin margins on completion of closure. **D,** Wrong angles (see text).

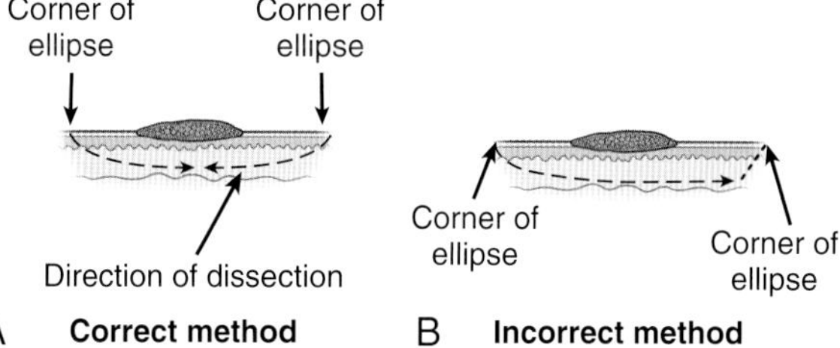

Figure 21-9 Method of dissecting tissue free after the ellipse is incised. **A,** Going from each end to the center. **B,** Going from one end to the opposite end (incorrect) leads to too deep of a dissection at the terminal end.

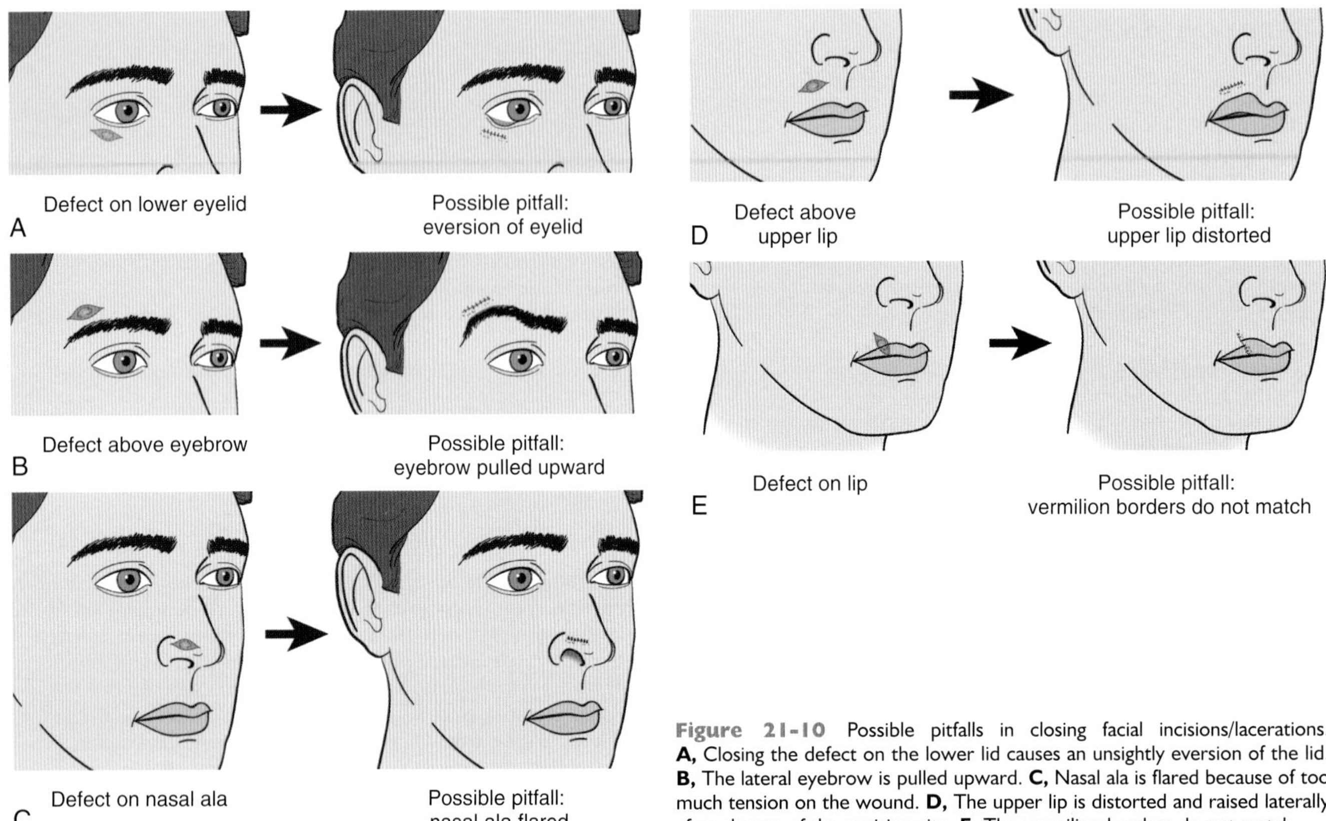

Figure 21-10 Possible pitfalls in closing facial incisions/lacerations. **A,** Closing the defect on the lower lid causes an unsightly eversion of the lid. **B,** The lateral eyebrow is pulled upward. **C,** Nasal ala is flared because of too much tension on the wound. **D,** The upper lip is distorted and raised laterally after closure of the excision site. **E,** The vermilion borders do not match.

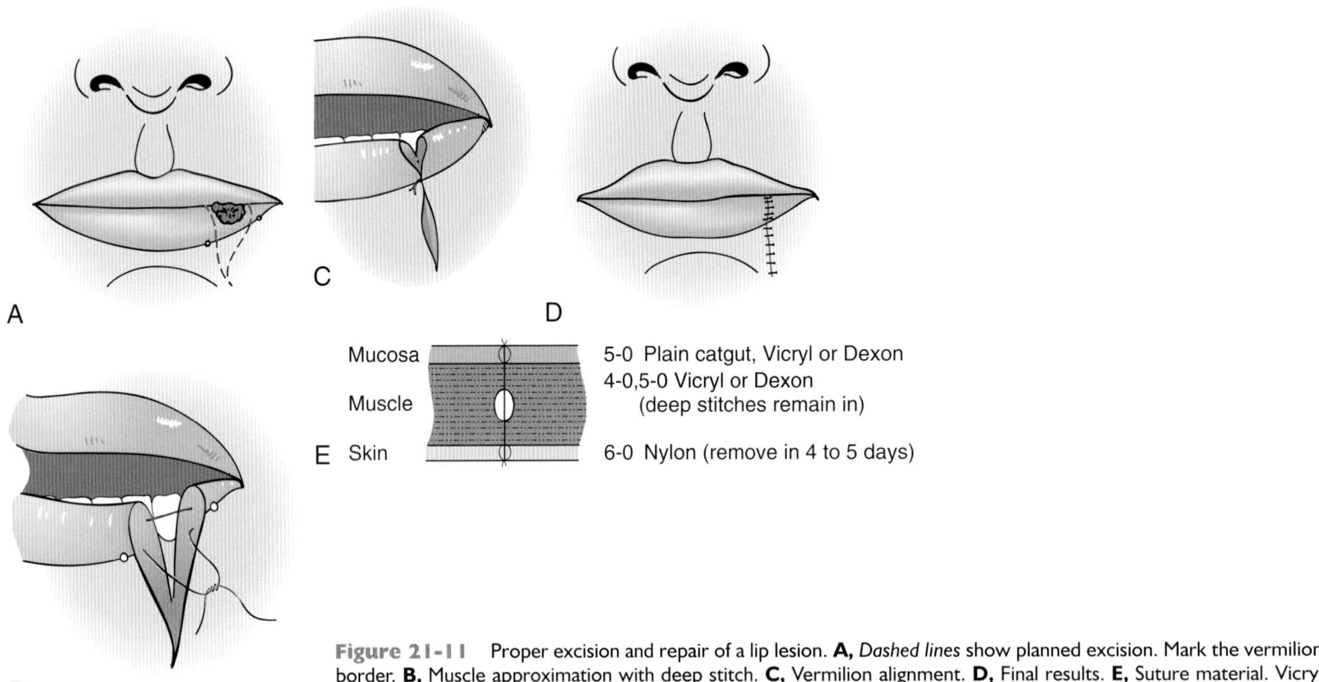

Figure 21-11 Proper excision and repair of a lip lesion. **A,** *Dashed lines* show planned excision. Mark the vermilion border. **B,** Muscle approximation with deep stitch. **C,** Vermilion alignment. **D,** Final results. **E,** Suture material. Vicryl or Dexon inside the mouth will need to be removed. Catgut will absorb in 3 to 4 days.

ACKNOWLEDGMENT

The editors wish to recognize the many contributions by Stephen K. Toadvine, MD, to this chapter in the previous edition of this text.

BIBLIOGRAPHY

Becker J, Stucchi AF (eds): Essentials of Surgery. Philadelphia, Saunders, 2005.

Moy RL, Usatine RP: Elliptical excision. In Usatine RP, Moy RL, Tobinick EL, Siegel DM (eds): Skin Surgery: A Practical Guide. St. Louis, Mosby, 1998, pp 120–136.

Salasche S, Orengo IF, Siegle RJ: Dermatologic Surgery Tips and Techniques. St. Louis, Mosby, 2007.

Trott A: Wounds and Lacerations: Emergency Care and Closure. St. Louis, Mosby, 1997.

Woods LK, Dellinger P: Current guidelines for antibiotic wound prophylaxis of surgery wounds. Am Fam Physician 57:2731–2740, 1998.

CHAPTER 22

Laceration and Incision Repair

Richard P. Usatine • Wendy C. Coates

Lacerations are a commonly seen problem in physicians' offices, urgent care centers, and hospital emergency departments. Lacerations can be repaired with sutures, wound closure tapes, staples (see Chapter 34, Skin Stapling), or tissue adhesive (see Chapter 37, Tissue Glues).

The goals of laceration and incision repair are as follows:

- Achieve hemostasis
- Prevent infection
- Preserve function
- Restore appearance
- Minimize patient discomfort

In repairing skin, it is helpful to understand the three phases of wound healing, which are listed in Box 22-1. Nonabsorbable skin sutures or staples are used to give the wound strength during the first two phases. After the nonabsorbable skin sutures are removed, wound closure tapes or previously placed deep absorbable sutures play an important role in the final phases of wound healing.

Indications

- Lacerations that are open and less than 12 hours old (<24 hours old on the face)
- Some bite wounds in cosmetically important areas (close follow-up recommended)
- Repair of sites where a lesion has been surgically removed

Contraindications

- Wounds more than 12 hours old (>24 hours old on the face)
- Animal and human bite wounds (exceptions: facial wounds, dog bite wounds)
- Puncture wounds

Equipment

- Surgical sterile preparation (Betadine, Hibiclens); alcohol swabs (not to be used inside the wound)
- Ruler in centimeters
- Irrigation device for contaminated wounds: 30-mL syringe with 18-gauge angiocatheter or commercially manufactured splash shield device (Fig. 22-1) and sterile saline
- Appropriate anesthetic, usually 1% or 2% lidocaine with or without epinephrine (see Chapter 4, Local Anesthesia)
- 1- to 10-mL syringe
- 27-gauge, 1¼-inch needle (small-gauge needles are preferred to administer anesthesia)
- Sterile drapes; fenestrated drape (applied over the lesion)
- 4 × 4 gauze sponges; sterile cotton applicators are useful for hemostasis
- Sterile pack containing 4½-inch needle holder; curved or straight iris scissors; one mosquito hemostat; suture scissors; Adson forceps with teeth; skin hook *(optional)*
- No. 15 blade for excisions with blade handle (single disposable unit also available)
- Appropriate suture (see Chapter 24, Laceration and Incision Repair: Suture Selection)
- Allis forceps for removal of deeper masses *(optional)*
- Skin marking pen (for excision, if wound revision is needed)
- Electrosurgical unit should be available for electrocoagulation
- Specimen jar (when lesions are being excised)
- Sterile gloves
- Protective mask with plastic shield for eyes or other types of personal protective equipment

Preprocedure Patient Preparation

The patient should be informed of the nature of his or her laceration. If the laceration is in a cosmetically important area, consider offering the option of a plastic surgeon for the repair. Advise the patient about the risks of pain, bleeding, dehiscence, infection, and scarring. In the case of lesion removal, warn that it is not always possible to be sure that the entire lesion is removed, so it could recur. Inform the patient that most repairs cause some permanent scarring, although attempts will be made to optimize the appearance. Patients should apply sunscreen to the area for at least 6 months after repair to minimize scarring. Warn the patient of the risks of hyperpigmentation or hypopigmentation, hypertrophic scars, keloids, nerve damage, alopecia, and distortion of the original anatomy. It is advisable to have the patient sign a consent form (see the consent form available online at www.expertconsult.com).

Initial Assessment

The initial evaluation *before anesthesia* should include a history of how the wound was sustained, factors that might impair healing, tetanus immunization history, and an assessment of peripheral neurovascular status.

For *elective excisions*, see Chapter 21, Incisions: Planning the Direction of the Incision, to plan the direction of the incision. If a traumatic laceration is to be repaired, see Table 22-1 for essentials of wound assessment. The clinician should consider the possibility of domestic violence in patients with traumatic wounds, especially if lacerations appear on the face or if multiple injuries of varying ages are noted.

In general, *antibiotics* are not needed for either wound or subacute bacterial endocarditis (SBE) prophylaxis for cutaneous procedures.

Box 22-1. Three Phases of Wound Healing

Phase 1 (Initial Lag Phase, Days 0–5)

No gain in wound strength

Phase 2 (Fibroplasia Phase, Days 5–14)

Rapid increase in wound strength occurs
At 2 weeks, the wound has achieved only 7% of its final strength

Phase 3 (Final Maturation Phase, Day 14 until Healing Is Complete)

Further connective tissue remodeling
Up to 80% of normal skin strength

For SBE prophylaxis guidelines, see Chapter 221, Antibiotic Prophylaxis. Consideration should be given to coverage for *Staphylococcus aureus* and methicillin-resistant *S. aureus* (MRSA) infection in several situations (Box 22-2).

The following are major goals for prescribing antibiotics before or after skin surgery:

- Prevention of a new wound infection
- Prevention of the spread of an existing local infection
- Treatment of an existing infection
- Prevention of bacterial endocarditis

The clinical decision-making process of whether or not to use antibiotics before or after skin surgery is complex. The physician must consider host factors, the anatomic location of the surgery, the sources that might contaminate the wound, and method of wound injury. Because this topic concerns wound repair after multiple types of trauma and elective procedures, the full complexity of the decision-making process is beyond the scope of this chapter. Box 22-2 lists the multiple factors to be considered when making a decision about antibiotic prophylaxis for skin procedures. See Chapter 222, Prevention and Treatment of Wound Infections.

The recommendations of the American Heart Association (AHA) for the *prevention of bacterial endocarditis* were last published in 2007. Endocarditis prophylaxis is not needed for incision or biopsy of surgically scrubbed skin. The 2007 guidelines state that antibiotic prophylaxis is recommended for procedures on infected skin and skin structures for patients with underlying cardiac conditions associated with the highest risk of adverse outcome from infective endocarditis. For individuals at highest risk for endocarditis (see Chapter 221, Antibiotic Prophylaxis) who undergo a surgical procedure that involves infected skin or skin structures, it is reasonable that the therapeutic regimen administered for treatment of the infection contain an agent active against staphylococci and beta-hemolytic streptococci, such as an antistaphylococcal penicillin or a cephalosporin. Vancomycin or clindamycin may be administered to patients unable to tolerate a beta-lactam antibiotic or who are known or suspected to have an infection caused by MRSA.

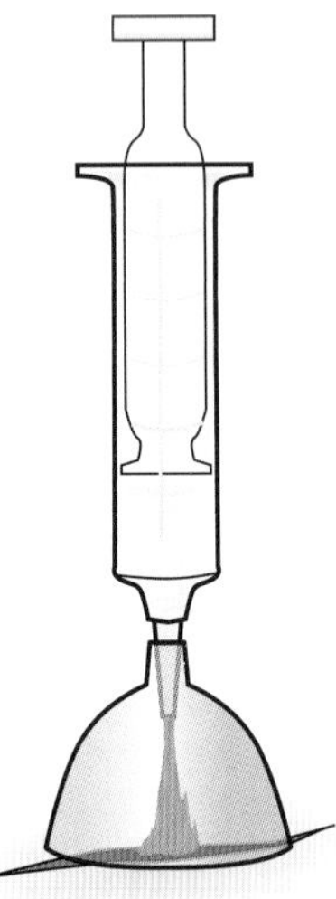

Figure 22-1 Irrigation of a dirty wound using a syringe and plastic shield.

TABLE 22-1 Essentials of Wound Assessment

Parameters	Factors to Consider
Mechanism of injury	Sharp vs. blunt trauma, bite
Dirty vs. clean	Outdoors vs. kitchen sink
Time since injury	Suture up to 12 hr; 24 hr on face
Foreign body	Explore and obtain radiograph for metal or glass
Functional examination	Neurovascular, muscular, tendons
Need for prophylactic antibiotics	If needed, give as soon as possible and cover *Staphylococcus aureus;* irrigate well

Cummings and Del Beccaro (1995) performed a meta-analysis of randomized studies on the use of antibiotics to prevent infection of simple wounds. They concluded that there is no evidence in published trials that prophylactic antibiotics offer protection against infection of nonbite wounds in patients treated in emergency departments. Cummings (1994) also performed a meta-analysis of randomized trials for antibiotics to prevent infection in patients with dog-bite wounds and found that prophylactic antibiotics reduce the incidence of infection in these patients.

Box 22-2. Possible Antibiotic Prophylaxis Situations or When to Consider Antibiotic Prophylaxis

Coexisting Conditions

Diabetes mellitus
Peripheral vascular disease
Elderly
Immunocompromised
Previous radiation to the site
Malnutrition (e.g., alcoholism, chemotherapy)
History of previous infection or slow healing
Chronic steroid use
Obesity

Locations

Increased bacteria
Axilla, mouth, anogenital areas
End-arterial locations (fingers, toes) with diseases of vascular compromise
Over joint spaces where there is a possibility of entering joint (e.g., metacarpophalangeal joints)

Contamination

Dirty wounds, especially those sustained at farms, meat-packing plants, etc.
Less than optimal sterile technique (should be rare)
Deep puncture wounds
Bites (especially human and cat bites)
Presence of a retained foreign body

Method of Wound Injury

Crush injury (10-fold increase in infection) with devitalized skin
Penetrating injury

Antibiotics have a role in the treatment of many established skin infections. However, *most skin abscesses are better treated with incision and drainage* rather than with antibiotics. For skin procedures, there is not a consensus on whether to give an antibiotic and the appropriate timing for its administration. Recommendations for timing before the procedure vary from 1 hour (which is typical timing for bacterial endocarditis prophylaxis) to within 30 minutes of the procedure. Although a single second dose 6 hours later was the standard in the past, it is no longer currently recommended for bacterial endocarditis prophylaxis but may be advocated for further treatment of the infection.

Controversy exists over which *bite injuries* should be treated with prophylactic antibiotics. Cat- and dog-bite injuries carry the risk of infection with *Pasteurella multocida*, and human-bite injuries carry the risk of infection with *Eikenella corrodens* and *S. aureus*. Based on the microbiology of these wounds, amoxicillin/clavulanate provides good prophylactic coverage for the bacteria affecting most bite injuries. Alternatives include second-generation cephalosporins or clindamycin with a fluoroquinolone.

The *best method for prevention of wound infections* is to clean and irrigate traumatic wounds well, rather than relying on prophylactic antibiotics. The physician needs to weigh the benefits and the risks of antibiotic use based on the individual patient and the circumstances of the wound repair or skin surgery. The factors listed in Box 22-2 and the references at the end of this chapter should provide guidance for the physician making decisions about antibiotic prophylaxis for skin surgery.

Local Anesthesia

In traumatic wounds, neurovascular integrity should be assessed *before* administration of anesthesia. The wound should then be fully anesthetized to allow for painless examination of the tissue damage, thorough irrigation, and adequate closure. Many wounds can be adequately anesthetized with 1% or 2% lidocaine. Consider using lidocaine with epinephrine to provide increased hemostasis if there are no contraindications to epinephrine in the patient, the location of the wound, or the wound itself. (See Chapter 4, Local Anesthesia, and Chapter 8, Peripheral Nerve Blocks and Field Blocks.) Topical anesthetics are effective for wounds that do not involve mucosal surfaces. A combination of lidocaine, epinephrine, and tetracaine (LET) applied with a saturated cotton ball or as a gel formulation directly into the wound provides adequate anesthesia for many wounds.

Perform the following to minimize the pain of injecting local anesthetic:

- Use a small-gauge needle (27 gauge or smaller)
- Inject slowly
- Inject directly into the dermis through the open wound (not through intact skin)
- Warm anesthetic to body temperature *(optional)*
- Buffer the anesthetic with sodium bicarbonate (10 mL to 1 mL) *(optional)*

Wound Preparation

After the initial assessment and administration of local or regional anesthetic, and antibiotics if indicated, wounds should be inspected thoroughly for foreign bodies, deep tissue layer damage, and injury to nerve, vessel, or tendon. A radiograph should be obtained to look for retained glass or metal in wounds sustained with broken glass or metal. Complex wounds or those in cosmetically important areas should be closed by a practitioner with the appropriate expertise.

Cleansing

After the wound is anesthetized, cleansing of a traumatic wound should be performed by irrigation with normal saline at approximately 15 psi of pressure. This can be accomplished by attaching an 18-gauge angiocatheter or a commercially available splash shield to a 30-mL syringe (see Fig. 22-1). At least 200 mL of irrigation is recommended. Moscati and associates (2007) performed a multicenter comparison of *tap water versus sterile saline* for wound irrigation showing equivalent rates of wound infection in immunocompetent patients. The tap water group irrigated their own wounds under the water tap for a minimum of 2 minutes after they had the wound anesthetized. Higher-risk wounds were excluded from the study, suggesting that tap water is a reasonable cleansing alternative only in low-risk lacerations. Chemical compounds such as hexachlorophene (pHisoHex), chlorhexidine gluconate (Hibiclens), or povidone–iodine (Betadine) should not be used inside wounds but may be applied to external, intact skin if desired. Greasy contaminants can be removed with any petroleum-based product, such as bacitracin ointment. To prevent a "road rash" tattoo, wrap petrolatum gauze around the fingers and wipe off the asphalt and other foreign material embedded in the skin after anesthesia.

For elective excisions, irrigation before closure is not generally needed. If there was a ruptured cyst or if the excisional area was open a considerable time, or if there was concern about contamination, irrigation with 10 mL of saline two or three times may be performed.

Débridement

After the cleansing process, wounds should be examined for devitalized tissue that needs removal or débridement. This débridement may convert a jagged, contaminated wound into a clean surgical one and can be accomplished with a scalpel or sharp tissue scissors (Fig. 22-2). Preserve as much tissue as possible in case future scar revision is necessary. After débridement, wound edges should be held together to see if they are under any tension. Wounds under significant tension are best repaired by a two-layer closure. In dirty wounds, however, this may increase the incidence of infection.

Undermining

Undermining can significantly reduce skin tension when there is a gap to be closed (Fig. 22-3). Undermining may increase the risk of infection and thus should be avoided in dirty wounds. Extreme care is also needed when undermining around vital structures. Approximately one third to one half of the undermined tissue is freed up to be brought into the defect. Undermine bilaterally as far back as the wound is wide.

TECHNIQUE

Ideally, four principles should be incorporated in the process of closing any wound:

1. *Control all bleeding before closure.* This can be accomplished by applying direct pressure for at least 5 minutes, adding epinephrine to the local anesthetic when appropriate, using electrocoagulation, or tying off bleeders with absorbable sutures.
2. *Eliminate "dead space"* where tissue fluid and blood can accumulate (Fig. 22-4).

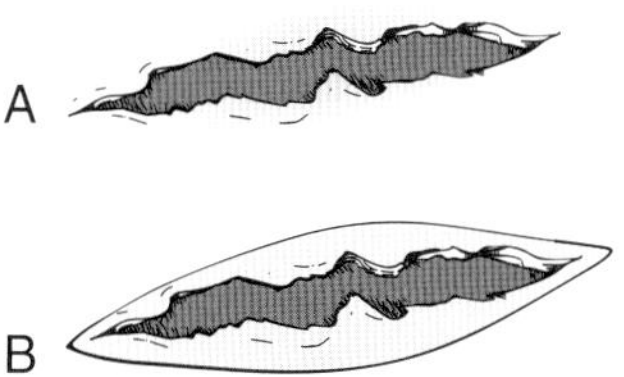

Figure 22-2 Débridement. **A,** Irregular jagged wound. **B,** Excise a jagged wound or crush injury to create a more readily reparable wound.

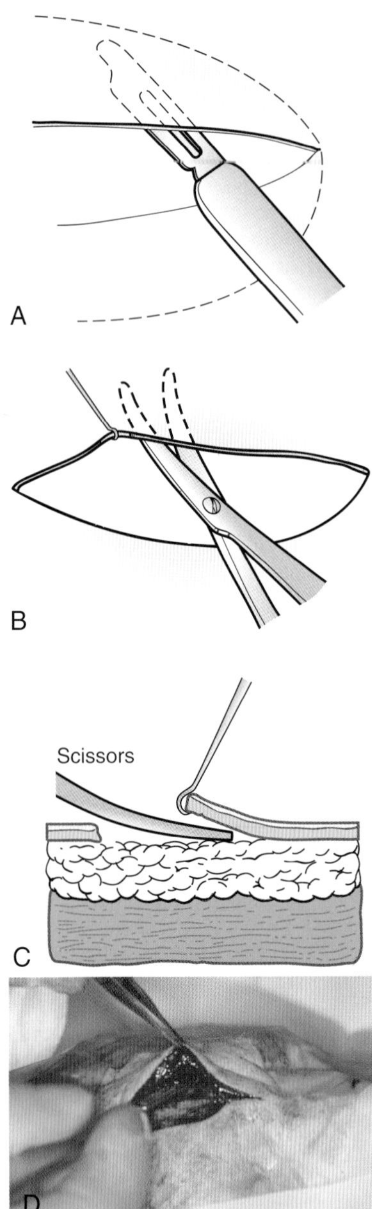

Figure 22-3 When skin margins approximate with tension, this can be relieved by undermining the margins through the use of a blade (**A**) or scissors (**B** and **C**). The usual plane is at the dermal–adipose junction. Undermine twice as far back as the wound is wide, if possible. The proper level of undermining to mobilize the skin is shown (**D**). (**D,** Courtesy of The Medical Procedures Center, PC, Midland, Mich, John L. Pfenninger, MD.)

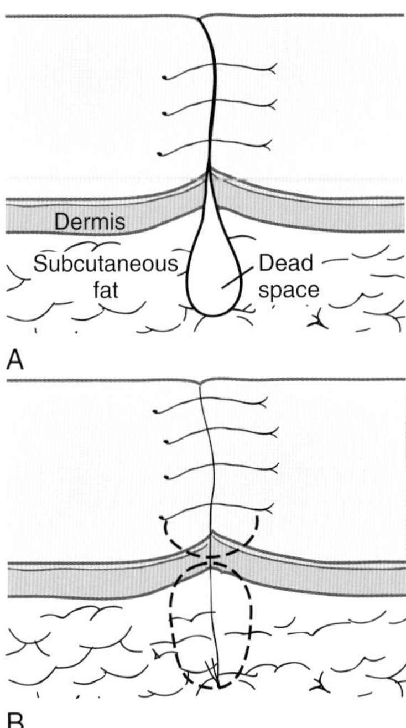

Figure 22-4 Closing the dead space. **A,** Improper closure with dead space not closed. **B,** Proper closure with dead space closed by deep sutures.

3. *Accurately approximate tissue layers* to each other. Scars are most visible when shadows are created by depressed or elevated tissue. Also be sure that anatomic areas match on each side in critical areas such as the vermilion border of the lip.
4. *Approximate the wound with minimal skin tension*. If there will be significant tension, undermining and deep inverted buried sutures are used to decrease the tension on the skin margin. Ideally, when the repair is completed the wound will be tented up slightly.

Lacerations and incisions are approximated using a variety of techniques:

- *Simple interrupted suture* (Fig. 22-5). On completion, the skin margins should be slightly everted (Fig. 22-6). The needle should enter the skin surface at a 90-degree angle (Fig. 22-7). The stitch should be as wide as it is deep. The suture on both sides of the wound should be of equal distance from the wound margin and of equal depth. The final shape should appear like an Erlenmeyer flask (Fig. 22-8). As a general rule, these sutures need to be no closer than 2 mm in a fine plastic closure and can be substantially farther apart in other types of closures. The distance between sutures should equal half the total distance of the sutures across

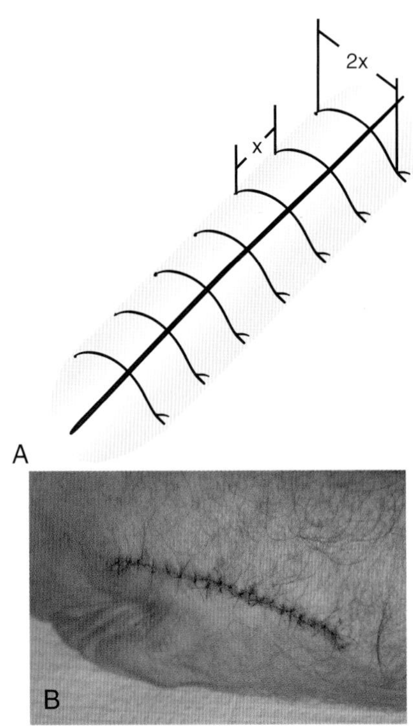

Figure 22-5 Simple interrupted suture. **A,** Proper spacing. **B,** Interrupted sutures after excision of a basal cell carcinoma of the elbow. (**B,** Courtesy of The Medical Procedures Center, PC, Midland, Mich, John L. Pfenninger, MD.)

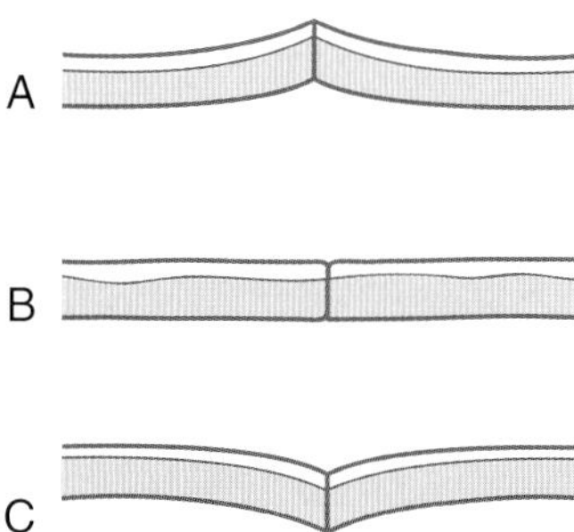

Figure 22-6 Wound margin appearance after closure. **A,** Proper eversion of the skin edges on closure ("build pyramids, not ditches"). **B,** Acceptable, but not optimal, closure. **C,** Improper closure because healing will lead to further contraction and scar depression.

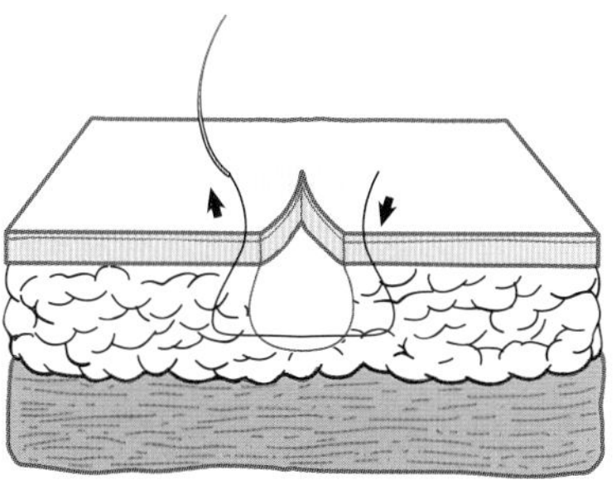

Figure 22-8 Use the Erlenmeyer flask–shaped pathway to promote eversion of skin edges. (Revised from Moy R: Suturing techniques. In Usatine RP, Moy RL, Tobinick EL, Siegel DM [eds]: Skin Surgery: A Practical Guide. St. Louis, Mosby, 1998, pp 88–100.)

the incision. Avoid tying the *knots* too tight. The knots should be lined up on one side of the wound. The finer the suture, the closer the stitches need to be. See Chapter 23, Laceration and Incision Repair: Needle Selection, and Chapter 24, Laceration and Incision Repair: Suture Selection, for needle and suture selection, respectively. See Chapter 25, Laceration and Incision Repair: Suture Tying, for tying techniques.

- *Simple running stitch* (Fig. 22-9). The *advantages* of the simple running stitch in sterile wounds under little or no tension are that it is quick and distributes tension evenly and provides excellent cosmetic results. Because there is an increased risk of contamination in traumatic lacerations, the simple running stitch is less desirable in these wounds. In case of infection, the entire wound closure would need to be removed. If there is significant gaping of the wound, interrupted suture methods should be used. The relative *disadvantage* is that the entire stitch must be removed at once; with interrupted techniques, some sutures may be removed early for better cosmesis whereas a few remaining ones can be left for prevention of dehiscence and removed at a later date. This stitch is ideal in the scalp and is the one generally used for episiotomy repairs.
- *Deep suture with inverted knot or "buried stitch"* (Fig. 22-10). Deeper wounds or wounds under tension are best closed by providing structural support and not relying solely on nonabsorbable superficial sutures. Well-placed, deep absorbable sutures can do much to aid in closing a wound, removing tension from the superficial skin sutures, and decreasing scarring by providing increased wound support long after the epidermal sutures have been removed. The inverted knot technique places the bulk of the knot as far below the skin margins as possible to avoid suture spitting (migration of deep sutures to the skin surface). It also keeps the ends of the cut suture from protruding through the wound margin. To start the stitch, begin at the bottom of the wound (in the undermined area if undermining was used) and come up usually just below the epidermal–dermal junction (remember, "Bottoms up!") to start. Go straight across the incision; enter at the same level at the opposite side; then go down to the base at the same depth as the contralateral side and tie. Care should be taken to achieve symmetry of depth and width on both sides of the laceration. After the appropriate number of deep inverted sutures is placed to approximate the skin margins, the surface (skin) is then fully closed with the closure of choice (nonabsorbable suture, wound closure tapes, or tissue adhesive).
- *Vertical mattress suture* (Fig. 22-11). This suture promotes eversion of the skin edges. It is useful when the natural tendency of loose skin is to create inversion of the wound margins, which is to be avoided. A good example is the loose, flabby skin under the triceps muscle and thin skin in older people. The stitch is also appropriate when the skin is very thin and interrupted sutures have a tendency to pull through.

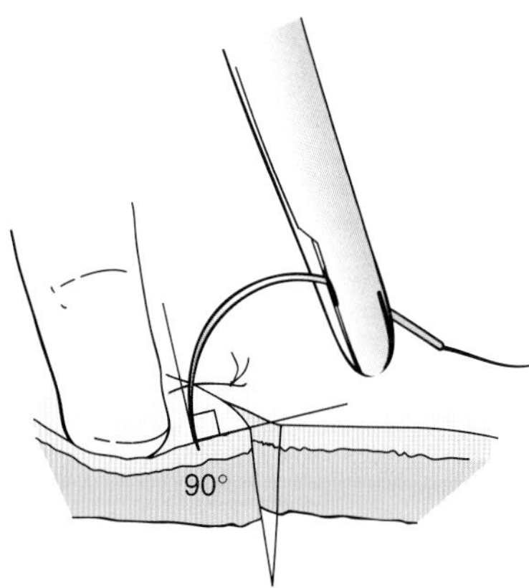

Figure 22-7 Needle should enter the skin surface at a 90-degree angle. (Revised from Moy R: Suturing techniques. In Usatine RP, Moy RL, Tobinick EL, Siegel DM [eds]: Skin Surgery: A Practical Guide. St. Louis, Mosby, 1998, pp 88–100.)

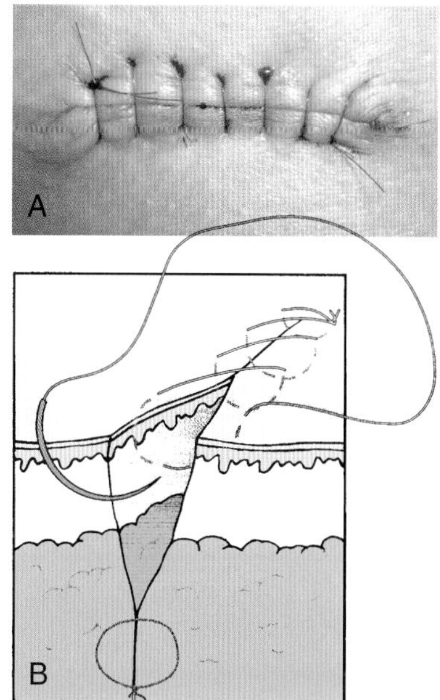

Figure 22-9 Running stitch. **A,** This is a good stitch to use if there is no tension on the wound or after deep stitches were already placed with good approximation of the wound edges. **B,** Always keep the depth of the suture placement the same on each side. (**A,** Courtesy of Richard P. Usatine, MD, San Antonio, Tex; **B,** From Moy R: Suturing techniques. In Usatine RP, Moy RL, Tobinick EL, Siegel DM [eds]: Skin Surgery: A Practical Guide. St. Louis, Mosby, 1998, pp 88–100.)

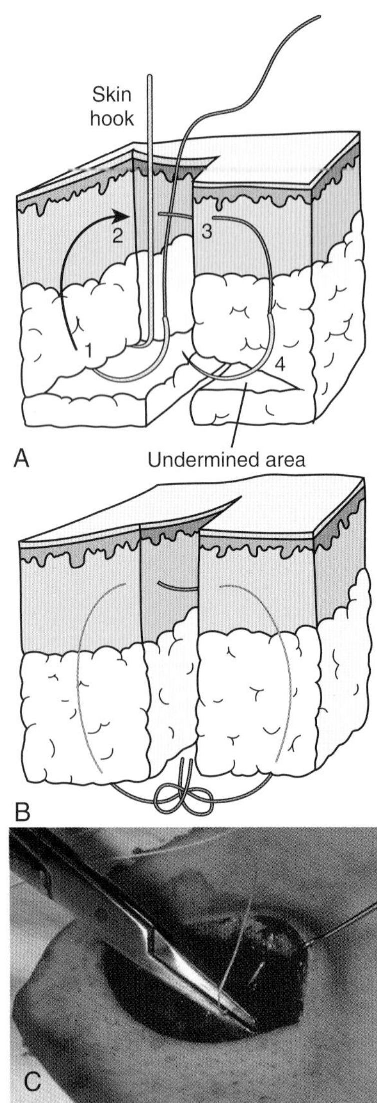

Figure 22-10 Deep stitch with absorbable suture material. **A,** Needle should enter deep in the skin below the dermis where the undermining was accomplished (1) and exit in the upper dermis (2). The needle enters in the upper dermis (3) and exits below the dermis where the undermining was accomplished (4). **B,** The deep inverted buried stitch is tied at the bottom of the wound to avoid having the knot stick out of the incision. **C,** Placing the deep stitch. (From Moy R: Suturing techniques. In Usatine RP, Moy RL, Tobinick EL, and Siegel DM [eds]: Skin Surgery: A Practical Guide, St Louis, Mosby, 1998, pp 88–100.)

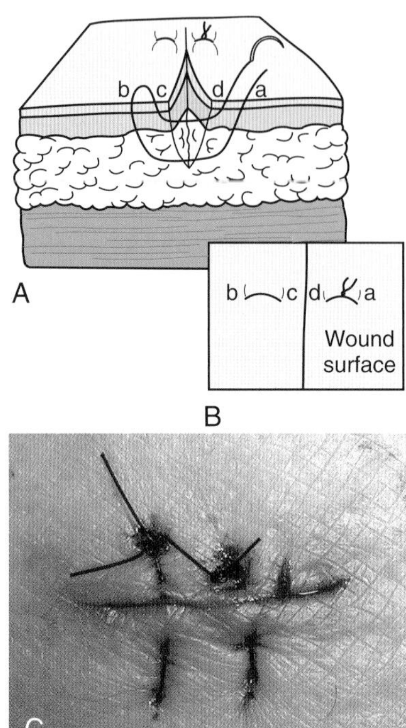

Figure 22-11 Vertical mattress suture. **A,** Cross-section. **B,** Overhead view. Begin at a, and go under skin to b. Come out, go in at c, and exit at d. **C,** Photograph of two vertical mattress sutures used to obtain wound eversion. (Courtesy of Richard P. Usatine, MD, San Antonio, Tex.)

- *Horizontal mattress suture* (Fig. 22-12). This suture is helpful in wounds under a moderate amount of tension and also promotes wound edge eversion. It is especially useful on palms or soles and in patients who are poor candidates for deep sutures because of susceptibility to wound infections.
- *Subcuticular running suture* (Fig. 22-13). This suture is used to close linear wounds that are not under much tension; it yields an excellent cosmetic result. The two ends can be tied over the wound, or a knot can be placed at each end to prevent slippage. The ends of the suture do not necessarily need to be tied; taping under slight tension preserves approximation. Usually a polypropylene-coated nylon works best. Steri-Strips, tapes, or tissue glue can be used to supplement this type of stitch. Special care must be taken to avoid pressure on the wound because this stitch separates easily. Applying Tegaderm or similar protective sheets provides added protection and strength.
- *Three-point or half-buried mattress suture, also known as the "corner stitch"*(Fig. 22-14). This suture technique is designed to permit closure of the acute corner tip of a laceration or of certain incisional techniques (e.g., Burow's triangle) without impairing blood flow to the tip. It is an intradermal stitch in which the needle is inserted initially into the intact skin on the nonflap portion of the wound and passed through the skin at the mid-dermis level; at the same level, the suture is then passed transversely through the tip of the flap, returned on the opposite side of the wound, and brought through the skin, paralleling the point of entrance. The suture is tied by drawing the tip snugly into place in good approximation. Care should be taken not to have the knot tied over the point of the flap (caused by having the needle insertion starting too far laterally). This same approach can be used in closing a stellate laceration, drawing the tips together in a purse-string fashion. Repair of a "T" laceration also uses this technique (Fig. 22-15).
- Repair of a *dog ear* or management of excess tissue can be performed as shown in Figure 22-16 (see Chapter 17, Flaps and Plasties). Figure 22-17 reviews the steps in the repair of a *C-flap* laceration.

NOTE: In one study, otherwise healthy children with facial lacerations were randomized to repair using fast-absorbing catgut or nylon suture (Luck and colleagues, 2008). There were no significant differences in the rates of infection, wound dehiscence, keloid formation, and parental satisfaction between the absorbable catgut and the nylon suture. Fast-absorbing catgut suture is not as easy to work with as nylon but does have the advantage of not requiring suture removal in children who may be very fearful of the suture removal process.

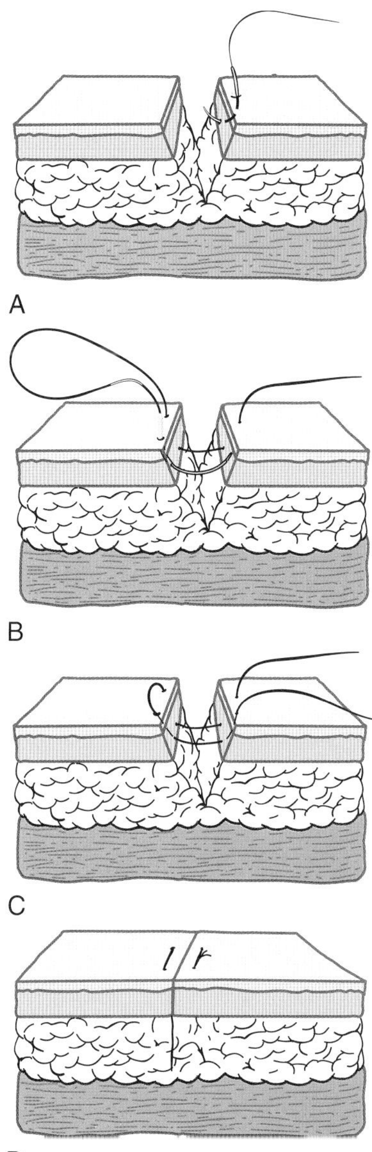

Figure 22-12 Horizontal mattress suture. **A,** Needle is passed 0.5 to 1 cm away from wound edge deeply into the wound. **B,** Needle is passed through the opposite side and reenters the wound parallel to the initial suture. **C,** Reenter the skin perpendicularly to provide some eversion of the wound edges. Enter and exit both the wound and skin at the same depth; otherwise, "buckling" and irregularities occur in the wound margin. **D,** Suture is then tied as shown.

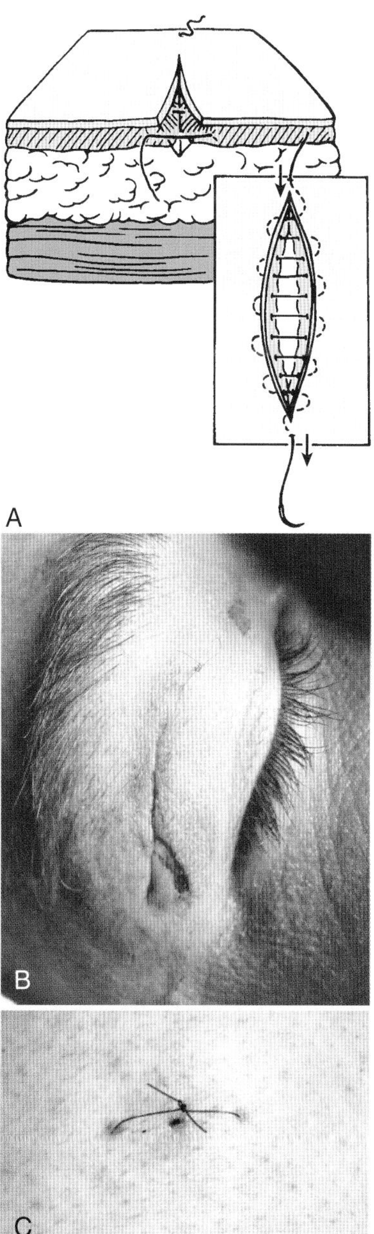

Figure 22-13 Subcuticular running suture. **A,** Graphic depiction. **B,** Prolene was used to repair this eyebrow laceration. The ends are knotted to prevent slippage. **C,** Appearance before removal after repair of a cheek excision. The ends are tied together to prevent slippage. (**B,** Courtesy of Joe Deng, MD, Loma Linda, Calif; **C,** Courtesy of The Medical Procedures Center, PC, Midland, Mich, John L. Pfenninger, MD.)

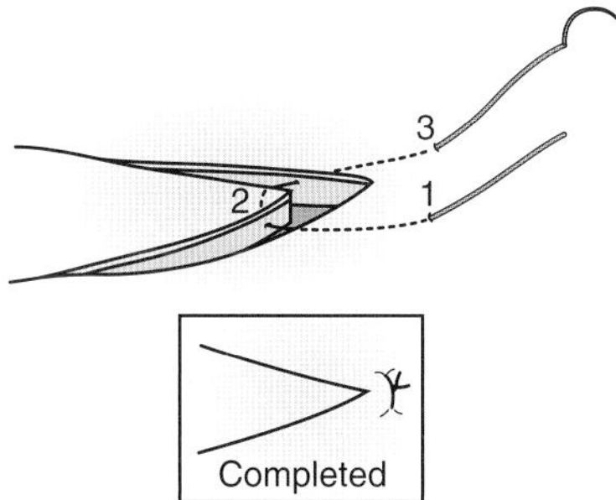

Figure 22-14 Three-point or half-buried mattress suture to repair a V-flap laceration.

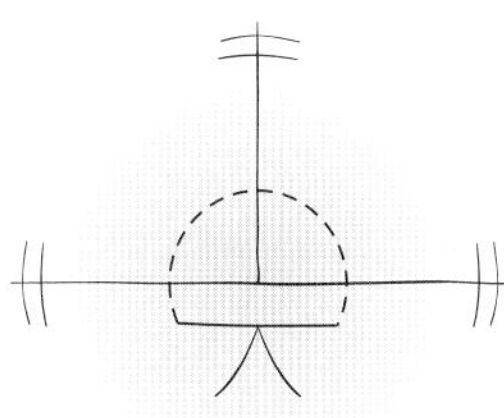

Figure 22-15 T-laceration repair using half-buried mattress suture technique.

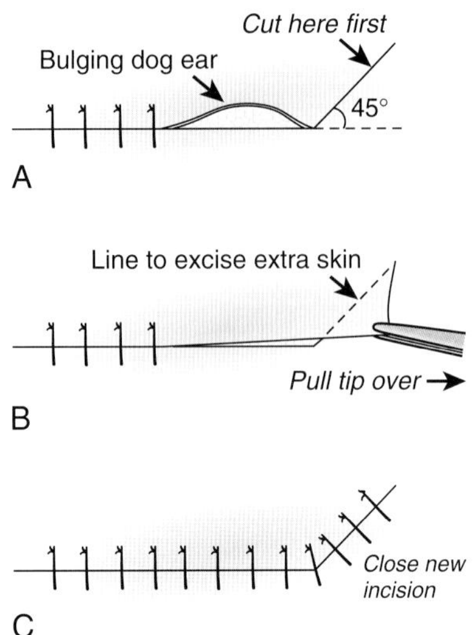

Figure 22-16 Dog-ear repair. **A,** Note site of initial incision of bulging dog ear. **B,** Pull the tip over and excise. **C,** Close the new incision for skin to lie flat.

Wound Closure Tapes and Strips

Wound closure tapes (Fig. 22-18) may be used alone for small, superficial wounds (especially in young children). When these tapes suffice to close a wound, they are easily placed without physical or psychological trauma to the patient. Wounds closed with tape are more resistant to infection than are sutured wounds. Tape cannot provide adequate skin edge eversion or deep tissue approximation when used alone. Thus tape is most commonly used as an adjunct to sutures or staples. Tape can help reinforce wounds closed subcuticularly or with conventional suturing techniques. Adhesion is enhanced by the application of a sticky substance to the skin surface. Traditionally, tincture of benzoin has been used for this purpose, but a preparation containing gum mastic (Mastisol) has been shown to provide stronger adhesion. Wound closure tapes are especially helpful after suture removal to prevent dehiscence and may be left on until they fall off. Patients may shower with them on after the initial 24 hours.

The proper method of applying the strips is to apply benzoin or Mastisol over the entire area, then place the strips in a parallel fashion without overlapping and without "tacking" strips (see Fig. 22-18).

Tissue Adhesive

Tissue adhesives may be used to close certain wounds that are not under significant tension and are not at risk for infection (see Chapter 37, Tissue Glues).

Delayed Primary Closure (Tertiary Intention)

Primary closure is defined by the use of sutures, tapes, or adhesives to close the wound at the time of initial surgery or evaluation. Healing by *secondary intention* occurs when no attempt is made to close the wound and the wound granulates in on its own. This method is used after a simple shave biopsy, in grossly contaminated or infected wounds, or in wounds that present far too late to consider closure. Delayed primary closure is healing by *tertiary intention*.

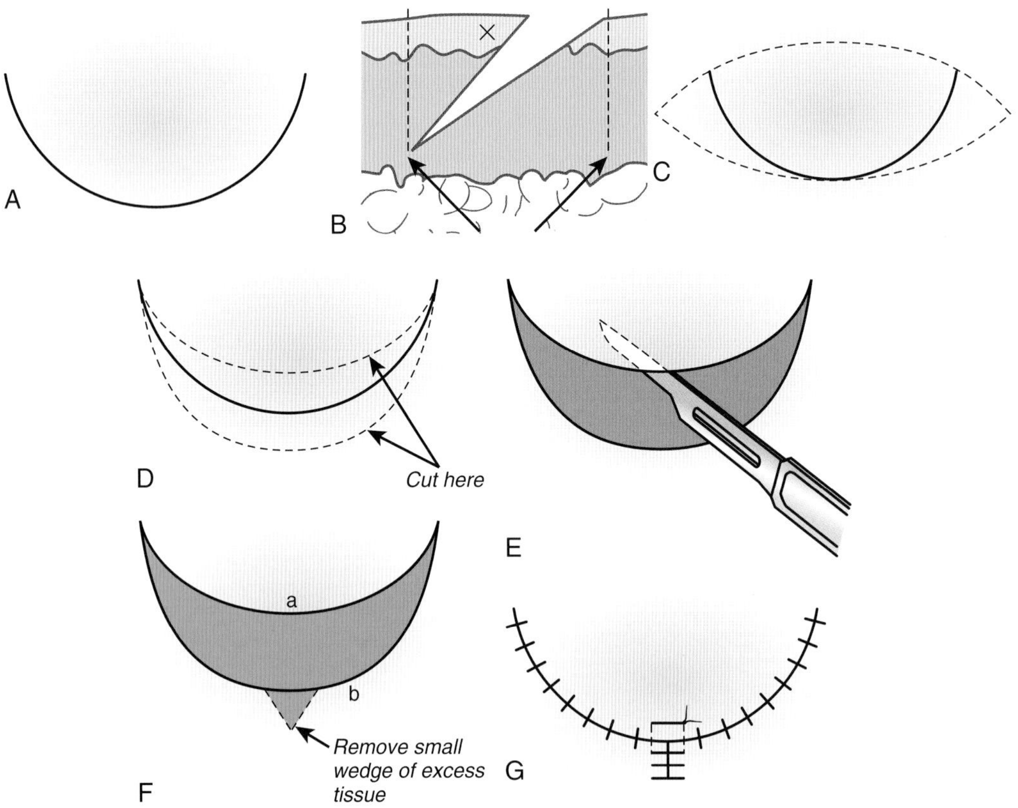

Figure 22-17 C-flap repair. **A,** Laceration. **B,** The problem: The point X is often very thin and may necrose. Even if it does not, contracture will occur after healing and the slim margin along the X will be depressed, causing a more visible scar. **C,** If small enough, convert the wound to an ellipse for easier repair. **D,** Alternatively, excise the angled margins of skin to obtain "square" borders. **E,** Undermine. **F,** Close with interrupted sutures. Because side a is smaller than side b, a small wedge of tissue may need to be removed. **G,** Complete closure.

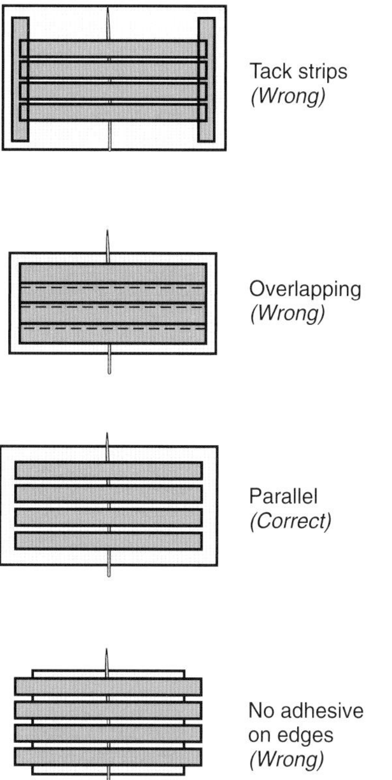

Figure 22-18 The red rectangles illustrate where Mastisol was applied to the skin.

Box 22-3. Pearls of Suturing

Use 27- to 30-gauge needle for anesthesia; slow injection; warm solution.
Use 1% to 2% lidocaine (epinephrine is helpful to achieve hemostasis). Avoid epinephrine or use with extreme care in fingers, toes, nose, ears, and penis. Do not use epinephrine in digital blocks.
Make elliptical excision at least three times as long as wide.
Follow Langer's lines.
Undermine. Undermine. Undermine. Double the width of the wound on each side.
Eliminate all dead space.
Use deep inverted buried absorbable sutures to reduce skin tension ("bottoms up").
Evert skin edges slightly ("build pyramids, not ditches"). Inversion of wound edges results in 300% increase in time for epithelial bridging.
Place interrupted sutures half as far apart as they are across. The more tension, the more sutures needed. Follow the Erlenmeyer flask shape. The finer the suture, the more sutures needed, but the less scarring.
Edema occurs after closure. Only approximate tissues; do not strangulate.
Begin gentle washing of wound after 12 to 24 hours; if Steri-Strips or tissue glues are not used, apply an ointment to keep the wound moist to speed healing.
Apply Steri-Strips after suture removal.

Delayed primary closure is used for wounds that are greater than 12 hours old (24 hours for facial lacerations) but would safely benefit from closure in a few days. Repairing them immediately could increase the chance of infection. After anesthetizing, evaluating, and irrigating the wound, insert a small piece of petrolatum gauze between the wound edges and place the patient on an antibiotic, such as cephalexin, for 5 days. On the third day, the patient should return for definitive repair. The wound is then anesthetized, reirrigated, and closed primarily with nonabsorbable sutures (i.e., no deep sutures because they increase the chance of infection).

See Box 22-3 for a summary of key points for suture repair (also included in Appendix H, Pearls of Practice).

Possible Complications of Laceration Repair

The following complications may occur within the first 2 weeks*:

- Infection
- Pain
- Bleeding
- Dehiscence
- Hematoma
- Bruising and swelling
- Suture spitting

Prolonged or permanent complications may include the following:

- Scarring
- Hypertrophic scars
- Keloid formation
- Hyperpigmentation
- Hypopigmentation
- Nerve damage
- Imperfect cosmetic alignment (e.g., the vermilion border)
- Suture spitting
- Recurrence of an incompletely excised lesion

*Adapted from Usatine RP, Moy RL, Tobinick EL, Siegel DM (eds): Skin Surgery: A Practical Guide. St. Louis, Mosby, 1998.

Postprocedure Patient Education

Most wounds are best protected with some sort of dressing during the first 24 to 48 hours after closure. Continued slight oozing of blood might be expected. For hemostasis, a pressure dressing should be applied. This could be folded gauze over a sterile ointment with tape over it or a nonstick type of gauze dressing covered with gauze and tape. Trade names for nonstick dressings include Xeroform, Adaptic, and Telfa. For the extremities, the use of a self-adherent wrap like Coban, CoFlex, and others provides a good pressure dressing to hold things in place. If on the lower extremities, elevation helps for 24 hours. Ice over the area for a few hours will reduce pain, swelling, and bleeding. It is not usually necessary to keep a wound completely dry after 24 hours. Therefore, patients may shower after 24 hours and redress the wound after gently drying it. Moist healing (application of some type of ointment after gentle washing twice daily) aids in quicker healing. Although it has been traditional to use antibiotic ointments for dressings postsurgically, Smack and colleagues (1996) determined that clean wounds heal just as well when white petrolatum is applied. Neomycin and bacitracin are frequent contact allergens. Alternatively, Tegaderm or Opsite (transparent, self-adherent, plastic wrap–type dressings that "breathe out" but do not let anything in) can be applied and left in place until the sutures are removed (Fig. 22-19). If bleeding occurs, the patient can replace the dressing after 24 to 48 hours because it is available over-the-counter. In addition to providing the optimal moist healing environment, these dressings provide added support to the sutured closure.

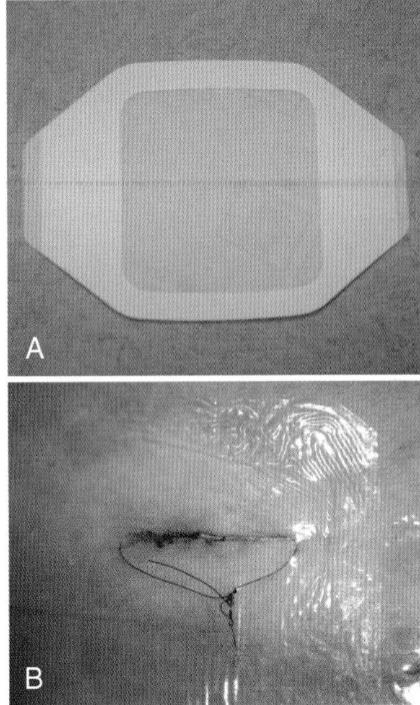

Figure 22-19 Tegaderm. **A,** The Tegaderm film patch. **B,** The film applied to a newly sutured wound. It is left in place until the subcuticular suture is removed, providing moist healing and support to the wound edges. (Courtesy of The Medical Procedures Center, PC, Midland, Mich, John L. Pfenninger, MD.)

Pull
Cut here
A Correct
Pull
Cut here
B Incorrect
C Correct
D Incorrect

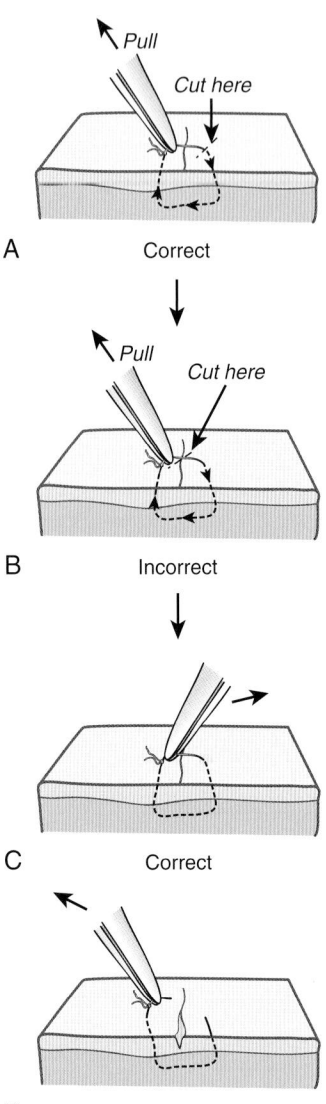

Figure 22-20 Suture removal. **A,** Cut where the suture enters the skin. **B,** Cutting suture near knot leaves length of suture that is "dirty" and pulled into the tissue. **C,** Pull the forceps over the wound, which approximates wound edges. **D,** Pulling suture out this way tends to pull wound edges apart. Also, note dirty length of suture being pulled through wound.

TABLE 22-2 Timing for Suture Removal

Anatomic Area	Days until Removal	External Suture Size	Buried Absorbable Suture Size
Face	4–5	5-0 or 6-0	5-0
Scalp	10–14	4-0, staples	3-0
Upper body	7–10	4-0	4-0
Hand	7–10	4-0 or 5-0	4-0
Lower body	10–14	4-0	3-0
Over joint (splint recommended)	14–21	4-0	3-0

Adapted from Coates WC: Lacerations to the face. In Tintinalli JE, Kelen GD, Stapczynski JS (eds): Emergency Medicine: A Comprehensive Study Guide, 6th ed. New York, McGraw-Hill, 2004, pp 298–304.

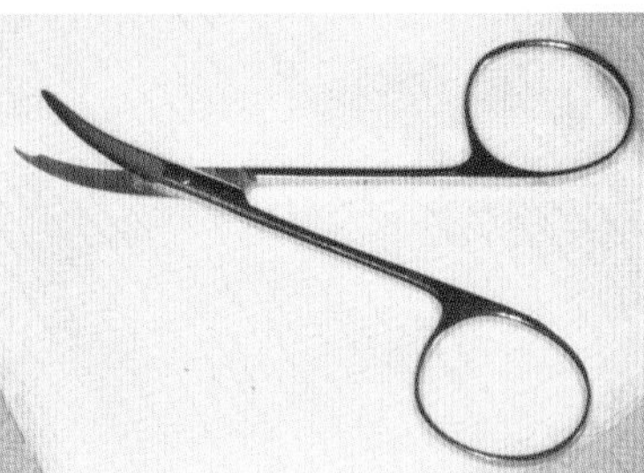

Figure 22-21 Suture removal scissors. (Courtesy of The Medical Procedures Center, PC, Midland, Mich, John L. Pfenninger, MD.)

Suggestions for the timing for skin suture removal are listed in Table 22-2. See Figure 22-20 for proper suture removal techniques. Using suture scissors makes removal much easier (Fig. 22-21). Because scarring increases the longer the sutures remain in place, consider removing them a few days early and applying a tissue adhesive (see Chapter 37, Tissue Glues). Early removal is possible only if there is little to no tension on the wound. Even when sutures are removed at the usual times, tissue glues help keep the wound edges opposed. The high cost of tissue glues is one barrier to this approach. IsoDent (Ellman Corp., Hewlett, NY) is markedly less expensive and works as well as the more common glues. Adhesive strips or another self-adherent transparent dressing can also be used.

Wounds on the face or scalp may be dressed with a thin layer of antibiotic ointment or petrolatum in lieu of a mechanical dressing. It is best to cover these wounds at night to avoid drying. Instruct patients to return if there are signs of wound infection, including erythema, pus, lymphangitis, or fever. A routine wound check is unnecessary for patients who understand the importance of monitoring wounds for signs of infection. An instructional handout can be given (see the patient education form available online at www.expertconsult.com).

Concurrent Treatment

Tetanus Prophylaxis

Table 22-3 is based on the current Centers for Disease Control and Prevention recommendations for tetanus prophylaxis in wound management.

Analgesic Medication

Analgesic medication may need to be administered for a few days depending on the extent of the trauma, the pain threshold of the patient, and the concerns of the family. For most patients, over-the-counter medications are sufficient, but in selected patients prescription narcotics may be indicated. If antibiotics are needed, refer to earlier discussion under Initial Assessment.

TABLE 22-3 Centers for Disease Control and Prevention Recommendations for Tetanus Prophylaxis in Wound Management

	Clean, Minor Wounds		All Other Wounds*	
Vaccination history	Td†	TIG	Td	TIG
Unknown or less than three doses	Yes	No	Yes	Yes
Three or more doses‡	No§	No	No‖	No

TIG, tetanus immune globulin.

*Such as, but not limited to, wounds contaminated with dirt, feces, soil, and saliva; puncture wounds; avulsions; and wounds resulting from missiles, crushing, burns, and frostbite.

†For children younger than 7 years of age, DTaP or DTP (DT, if pertussis vaccine is contraindicated) is preferred to tetanus toxoid alone. For patients older than 7 years of age, Td is preferred to tetanus toxoid alone.

‡If only three doses of fluid toxoid have been received, a fourth dose of toxoid, preferably an absorbed toxoid, should be given.

§Yes, if more than 10 years since last dose.

‖Yes, if more than 5 years since last dose. (More frequent boosters are not needed and can accentuate side effects.)

From Diphtheria, tetanus, and pertussis: Recommendations for vaccine use and other preventive measures: Recommendations of the Immunization Practices Advisory Committee (ACIP). MMWR Recomm Rep 40(RR-10):1–28, 1991.

Conclusion

In the treatment of lacerations, careful inspection, adequate irrigation, skilled closure, and appropriate wound care can produce the best functional and cosmetic results. The principles and steps covered in this chapter show how lacerations can be repaired with maximal skill and minimal discomfort to the patient. More advanced skills and knowledge can be developed through experience and by reading Chapter 17, Flaps and Plasties, and the sources listed in the bibliography.

Patient Education Guides

See the patient education and consent forms available online at www.expertconsult.com.

CPT/Billing Codes and ICD-9-CM Diagnostic Codes

Coding and billing become very complex for laceration repair and excisions. Important factors to list for billing personnel are as follows:

- Location
- Size of lesion
- Length of closure or excision
- Simple or intermediate repair (intermediate includes either undermining or placement of deep buried sutures)
- Benign or malignant status
- Whether a true skin lesion or subcutaneous tumor or deep tumor (e.g., lipoma) was excised
- Method of removal (shave, excision, destruction)

With an excision, when charging for the size of the lesion, also include the width of the margins. For example, if a basal cell carcinoma that has a diameter of 1 cm is being excised, there should be 0.3 cm free margins. The size charged for the excision would be 1.6 cm. Suture removal is included in the initial charge if the original sutures were placed by the same group of physicians. Suture removal can be billed if performed by an unassociated physician or group. Anesthetic, materials, and supplies are customarily also included in the reimbursement fees. If a lesion is excised and repaired in a simple fashion (no undermining, deep sutures, flaps, or plasties), the fee for excision then includes local anesthesia, repair, any interval care for 10 days, and suture removal. If an intermediate repair is done with an excision, two codes should be charged (the excision and the repair).

For CPT/billing codes, see Table 22-4. For ICD-9-CM diagnostic codes, see Appendix G. For specific skin lesion sites, and to code out lacerations, go to the ICD-9 manual and look under wounds for the specific site: Wound, open (by cutting or piercing instrument) (by firearms) (cut) (dissection) (incised) (laceration) (penetration) (perforating) (puncture) (with initial hemorrhage, not internal). (Laceration ICD codes are too extensive to list in detail here.) For fracture with open wound, see Fracture.

TABLE 22-4 CPT/Billing Codes

Benign Skin Excision

11200	Tags, up to/including 15 lesions
11201	Tags, each additional 10 lesions
11400	TAL <0.6 cm
11401	TAL 0.6–1.0 cm
11402	TAL 1.1–2.0 cm
11403	TAL 2.1–3.0 cm
11404	TAL 3.1–4.0 cm
11406	TAL >4.0 cm
11420	SNHFG <0.6 cm
11421	SNHFG 0.60–1.0 cm
11422	SNHFG 1.1–2.0 cm
11423	SNHFG 2.1–3.0 cm
11424	SNHFG 3.1–4.0 cm
11426	SNHFG >4.0 cm
11440	Face <0.6 cm
11441	Face 0.6–1.0 cm
11442	Face 1.1–2.0 cm
11443	Face 2.1–3.0 cm
11444	Face 3.1–4.0 cm
11446	Face >4.0 cm

Malignant Skin Excision

11600	TAL <0.6 cm
11601	TAL 0.6–1.0 cm
11602	TAL 1.1–2.0 cm
11603	TAL 2.1–3.0 cm
11604	TAL 3.1–4.0 cm
11606	TAL >4.0 cm
11620	SNHFG <0.6 cm
11621	SNHFG 0.6–1.0 cm
11622	SNHFG 1.1–2.0 cm
11623	SNHFG 2.1–3.0 cm
11624	SNHFG 3.1–4.0 cm
11626	SNHFG >4.0 cm
11640	Face <0.6 cm
11641	Face 0.6–1.0 cm
11642	Face 1.1–2.0 cm
11643	Face 2.1–3.0 cm
11644	Face 3.1–4.0 cm
11646	Face >4.0 cm

Simple Skin Repairs

12001	SNAGTE <2.6 cm
12002	SNAGTE 2.6–7.5 cm
12004	SNAGTE 7.6–12.5 cm
12005	SNAGTE 12.6–20.0 cm
12006	SNAGTE 20.1–30.0 cm
12007	SNAGTE >30.0 cm
12011	FEENLMM <2.6 cm
12013	FEENLMM 2.6–5.0 cm
12014	FEENLMM 5.1–7.5 cm
12015	FEENLMM 7.6–12.5 cm
12016	FEENLMM 12.6–20.0 cm
12017	FEENLMM 20.1–30.0 cm
12018	FEENLMM >30.0 cm
12020	Superficial wound dehiscence

Intermediate Skin Repairs

12031	SATAL <2.6 cm
12032	SATAL 2.6–7.5 cm
12034	SATAL 7.6–12.5 cm
12035	SATAL 12.6–20.0 cm
12036	SATAL 20.1–30.0 cm
12037	SATAL >30.0 cm
12041	NHFG < 2.6 cm
12042	NHFG 2.6–7.5 cm
12044	NHFG 7.6–12.5 cm
12045	NHFG 12.6–20.0 cm
12046	NHFG 20.1–30.0 cm
12047	NHFG >30.0 cm
12051	FEENLMM <2.6 cm
12052	FEENLMM 2.6–5.0 cm
12053	FEENLMM 5.1–7.5 cm
12054	FEENLMM 7.6–12.5 cm
12055	FEENLMM 12.6–20.0 cm
12056	FEENLMM 20.1–30.0 cm
12057	FEENLMM >30.0 cm

Benign Tumor Excisions (e.g., lipoma)

21550	Biopsy, soft tissue, neck/thorax
21555	Neck/thorax SQ*
21556	Neck/thorax deep*†
21930	Back/flank*
22900	Abdominal wall deep*†
23075	Shoulder SQ
23076	Shoulder deep*†
24075	Upper arm/elbow SQ*
24076	Upper arm/elbow deep*†
25075	Forearm/wrist SQ*
25076	Forearm/wrist deep*†
26115	Hand/finger SQ*
26116	Hand/finger deep*†
27047	Pelvis/hip SQ*
27048	Pelvis/hip deep*
27327	Thigh/knee SQ*
27328	Thigh/knee deep*†
27618	Leg/ankle SQ*
27619	Leg/ankle deep*†
28043	Foot SQ*
28045	Foot deep*
38500	Excision and/or biopsy, lymph node, superficial
41825	Gum/alveolar, no repair
41826	Gum/alveolar, simple rep

Face:	Face, ear, eyelid, nose, lip, or mucous membrane
FEENLMM:	Face, ear, eyelid, nose, lip, or mucous membrane
NHFG:	Neck, hand, foot, or external genitalia
SATAL:	Scalp, axilla, trunk, arm, or leg
SNAGTE:	Scalp, neck, axilla, genitalia, trunk, or extremity
SNHFG:	Scalp, neck, hand, foot, or genitalia
SQ:	Subcutaneous
TAL:	Trunk, arm, or leg

Codes in **bold** have a 10-day global fee surgical period.
The sizes listed in codes 11400 to 11646 describe lesion diameter, not the length of the skin excised.
*90-Day global fee surgical period.
†Deep excision includes subfascial or intramuscular lesions.

SUPPLIERS

(See contact information online at www.expertconsult.com.)

Zerowet splash shields and Klenzalac wound irrigation systems

IsoDent

Opsite

Tegaderm

Zerowet

VIDEOTAPES AND DVDS

Coding and Billing

Pfenninger JL: Billing/coding for dermatologic procedures. Creative Health Communication, 2005. Available at www.creativehealthcommunications.com.

Procedure Technique

Pfenninger JL: Excision and common wound repairs: Patient cases. Creative Health Communication, 2005. Available at www.creativehealthcommunications.com.

Pfenninger JL: Suturing and excision techniques: Exercises on pig's feet biopsy. Creative Health Communication, 2005. Available at www.creativehealthcommunications.com.

Pfenninger JL: Common office dermatologic procedures, 2005. Creative Health Communication, 2005. Available at www.creativehealthcommunications.com.

Thomsen TW, Barclay DA, Setnick GS: Videos in clinical medicine: Basic laceration repair. N Engl J Med 355:e18–e22, 2006.

BIBLIOGRAPHY

Coates WC: Lacerations to the face and scalp. In Tintinalli J, Kelen GD, Stapczynski JS (eds): Emergency Medicine: A Comprehensive Study Guide, 6th ed. New York, McGraw-Hill, 2004, pp 298–304.

Cummings P: Antibiotics to prevent infection in patients with dog bite wounds: A meta-analysis of randomized trials. Ann Emerg Med 23:535–540, 1994.

Cummings P, Del Beccaro MA: Antibiotics to prevent infection of simple wounds: A meta-analysis of randomized studies. Am J Emerg Med 13:396–400, 1995.

DeBoard RH, Rondeau DF, Kang CS, et al: Principles of basic wound evaluation and management in the emergency department. Emerg Med Clin North Am 25:23–39, 2007.

Fincher EF, Gladstone HB, Moy RL: Layered closures, complex closures with suspension sutures and plication of SMAS. In Robinson JK, Hanke CW, Sengelmann RD, Siegel DM (eds): Surgery of the Skin: Procedural Dermatology. Philadelphia, Mosby, 2005, pp 273–290.

Haas AF, Grekin RC: Antibiotic prophylaxis in dermatologic surgery. J Am Acad Dermatol 32:155–176, 1995.

Houck CS, Sethna NF: Transdermal anesthesia with local anesthetics in children: Review, update, and future direction. Expert Rev Neurother 5:625–634, 2005.

Jose RM, Vidyadharan J, Bragg TW, et al: Mammalian bite wounds: Is primary repair safe? Plast Reconstr Surg 119:1967–1968, 2007.

Katz KH, Desciak EB, Maloney ME: The optimal application of surgical adhesive tape strips. Dermatol Surg 25:686–688, 1999.

Kundu S, Achar S: Principles of office anesthesia: Part II. Topical anesthesia. Am Fam Physician 66:99–102, 2002.

Le BT, Dierks EJ, Ueeck BA, et al: Maxillofacial injuries associated with domestic violence. J Oral Maxillofac Surg 59:1277–1283, 2001.

Lloyd JD, Marque MJ 3rd, Kacprowicz RF: Closure techniques. Emerg Med Clin North Am 25:73–81, 2007.

Luck RP, Flood R, Eyal D, et al: Cosmetic outcomes of absorbable versus nonabsorbable sutures in pediatric facial lacerations. Pediatr Emerg Care 24:137–142, 2008.

Moscati RM, Mayrose J, Reardon RF, et al: A multicenter comparison of tap water versus sterile saline for wound irrigation. Acad Emerg Med 14:404–409, 2007.

Reichman EF, Simon RR: Emergency Medicine Procedures. New York, McGraw-Hill, 2004.

Robinson JK, Hanke CW, Sengelmann RD, Siegel DM: Surgery of the Skin: Procedural Dermatology. Philadelphia, Mosby, 2005.

Smack DP, Harrington AC, Dunn C, et al: Infection and allergy incidence in ambulatory surgery patients using white petrolatum vs bacitracin ointment: A randomized controlled trial. JAMA 276:972–977, 1996.

Usatine RP, Moy RL, Tobinick EL, Siegel DM (eds): Skin Surgery: A Practical Guide. St. Louis, Mosby, 1998.

Weitzul S, Taylor RS: Suturing technique and other closure materials. In Robinson JK, Hanke CW, Sengelmann RD, Siegel DM (eds): Surgery of the Skin: Procedural Dermatology. Philadelphia, Mosby, 2005, pp 225–244.

Wilson W, Taubert KA, Gewitz M, et al: Prevention of infective endocarditis: Guidelines from the American Heart Association. A guideline from the American Heart Association Rheumatic Fever, Endocarditis, and Kawasaki Disease Committee, Council on Cardiovascular Disease in the Young, and the Council on Clinical Cardiology, Council on Cardiovascular Surgery and Anesthesia, and the Quality of Care and Outcomes Research Interdisciplinary Working Group. Circulation 116:1736–1754, 2007.

Woods RK, Dellinger EP: Current guidelines for antibiotic prophylaxis of surgical wounds. Am Fam Physician 57:2731–2740, 1998.

Laceration and Incision Repair: Needle Selection

William Jackson Epperson

A large variety of needle types have been developed for specific surgical needs. The needle facilitates the appropriate placement of suture. Inappropriate needle selection can damage the tissues, causing poor results and delayed healing. For example, a tapered needle with a round shaft is needed in suturing bowel, where prevention of leakage is imperative. A cutting needle would never be appropriate in the reanastomosis of bowels or blood vessels.

Most needles are made of noncorrosive stainless steel. Through a process of heating the metal, maximum strength and ductility (the ability to bend under pressure without breaking) are achieved. Each needle type is sharpened to a varying degree depending on its use. Also, to assist with passage through tissues, most needles receive a thin coat of silicone or other lubricant.

Needle Design

The surgical needle is composed of a *swaged eye* or *shank*, a body, and a *point* (Fig. 23-1). There are *three types of needles*: the closed eye, the French (split or spring) eye, and the swaged eye. Both closed-eye and French-eye needles must be threaded (Fig. 23-2). Since the 1960s, needles have been almost exclusively swaged because threaded needles have many undesirable characteristics. The swaged portion of the needle is now commonly referred to as the *shank*. Within the shank the metal is literally molded around the suture, which alleviates most needle-to-suture attachment problems and prevents the repeated use of a dull, nonlubricated, or contaminated needle, problems associated with threaded needles.

Many terms have been developed by suture manufacturers to categorize their products for different purposes and to denote their size. Unfortunately, there is no standard nomenclature. On thick skin, "for skin" (FS) needles are acceptable, and most have a reverse cutting edge. On cosmetic areas, *plastic (P), plastic skin (PS), premium (PRE), or precision cosmetic (PC)* needles may offer some minor advantages for the surgeon, but at a significantly greater cost. These initial designations for the needles are the common nomenclature used by Ethicon, Inc. (Somerville, NJ) as marketing terms for their needles. Ethicon, Inc. manufactures over 80% of the needles used in North America. Other manufacturers include USSDG (Norwalk, Conn) and Surgical Specialties Corporation (e.g., LOOK, Sharpoint; Reading, Penn), who use somewhat similar needle description nomenclature.

Generally, a larger needle is used for deeply buried sutures, whereas a smaller needle can be used to close a thin layer of skin. Location of closure is also important. For instance, facial closures are often done with a P-3 needle, whereas other areas with thicker skin require an FS-2 or FS-3 needle. It is important to review the descriptions of the needle on the outside of the suture package, and often a picture of the needle will aid in proper needle selection.

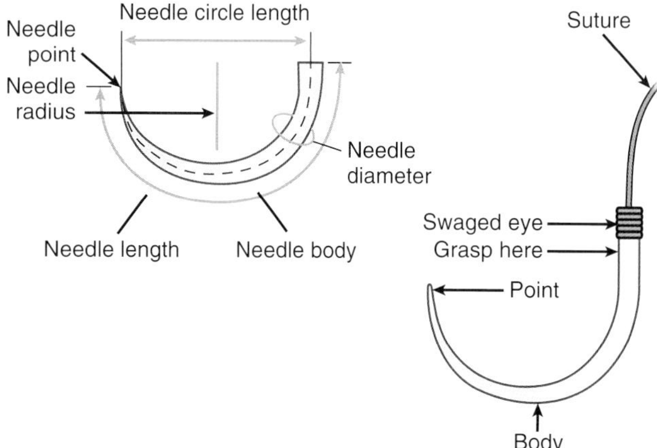

Figure 23-1 Anatomy of a surgical needle.

Needles should be handled only with needle holders. A proper-sized, high-quality needle holder is needed for suturing; no other instrument is acceptable for this task. This is one instrument that is worth investing in because it can make the suturing experience satisfying or totally frustrating. In general, gold-handled instruments are of superior quality. The needle should be grasped by the needle holder at a position about one needle holder's width past the curved center of the needle. Only one click of needle holder pressure should be applied to hold the needle in place. If the needle slips it may be that the needle holder is old and no longer will hold the needle, or the suturing attempt being made is not commensurate with the needle size and technique being applied.

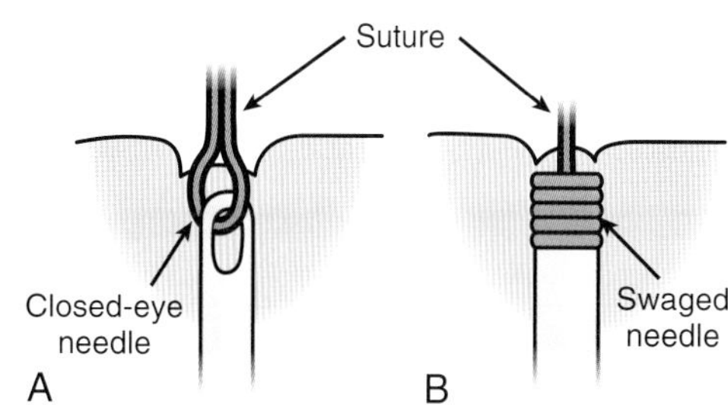

Figure 23-2 **A,** Tissue disruption can be caused by the double-suture strand with a closed-eyed needle. **B,** Tissue disruption is minimized by a single-suture strand swaged to needle.

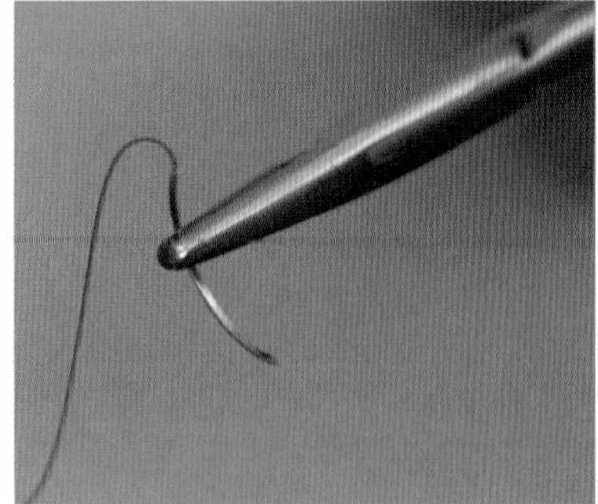

Figure 23-3 Needle holder with needle in place.

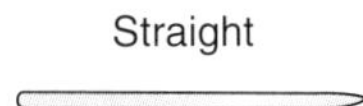

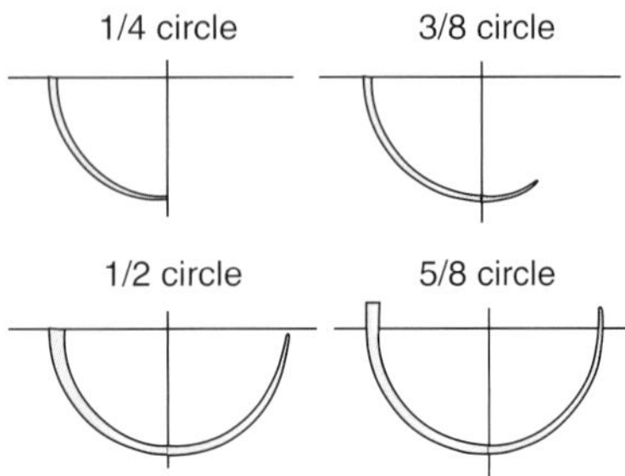

Figure 23-4 Needle body shapes.

A hemostat or other grasping instrument is not an acceptable substitute for a needle holder when suturing. The needle will easily roll out of position because it requires a flat surface to maintain its operative position. All grasping of the needle with any instrument causes a weakening of the metal with risk of breakage. This is less of a concern when a proper-sized needle holder is used with prudent application of force in achieving desired surgical results.

The needle should be grasped below the shank portion, but beyond the mid-body region (Fig. 23-3). The swaged metal must be sufficiently soft to crimp firmly around the suture and lock it in place. Therefore, if the needle is grasped by the needle holder at the shank, it can easily bend and weaken. The body of the needle is firm, not malleable, and less likely to bend. The tip of the needle holder should just cover the needle, and the handle should be closed only to the first or second ratchet. During needle placement the force must be advanced in the direction of the curvature of the needle. The wrist must be everted and supinated as the needle goes through tissue to avoid undue pressure and bending.

The *body of the needle* is important for both strength and grasping by the needle holder. Various shapes of the body are important for added strength as well as for matching the flow of the needle through the tissues as directed by the point. A flattened body with concave or convex surfaces helps to reduce unwanted needle rotation when suturing. The shape of the body of the needle allows for a variety of uses (Fig. 23-4). In general, a 3/8-inch curvature is adequate for most cutaneous procedures (Fig. 23-5).

Needle points are the most important needle consideration. The basic types of needle points include *cutting*, *tapered*, and *blunt* (Fig. 23-6). The *blunt-point* needle is used for friable parenchymal tissue such as liver and kidney. This point allows for dissection through tissues, avoiding the trauma of a cutting needle.

The two opposing edges of a *cutting needle* allow for easier passage through tough tissues. This makes cutting needles ideal for suturing skin with its dense supporting structures. However, these cutting edges have their drawbacks when it comes to tendons and oral mucous membranes, which are easily damaged by overcutting.

The *conventional cutting* needle has a cutting edge on its inside or concave curvature. The inside cutting in the direction of force is a negative characteristic of this needle. The suture force tends to concentrate at the apex of the triangle, and the tissues outside of the desired suture channel are cut. For this reason, a conventional

Ethicon

Precision point needles

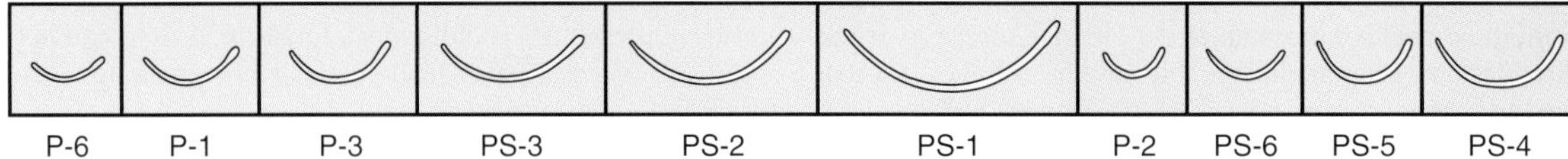

Precision cosmetic needles

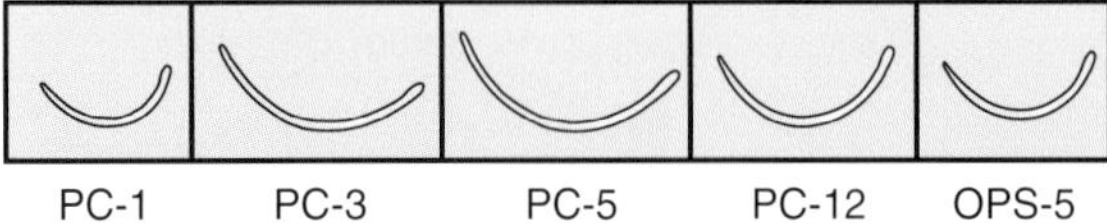

Davis & Geck

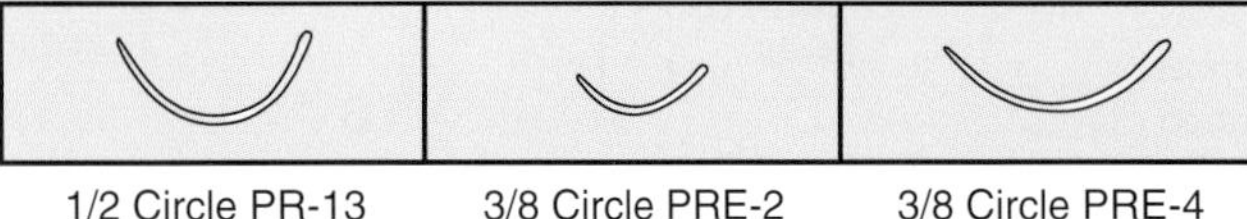

Figure 23-5 Ethicon and Davis & Geck (Kendall) needle nomenclature for facial closures (actual sizes).

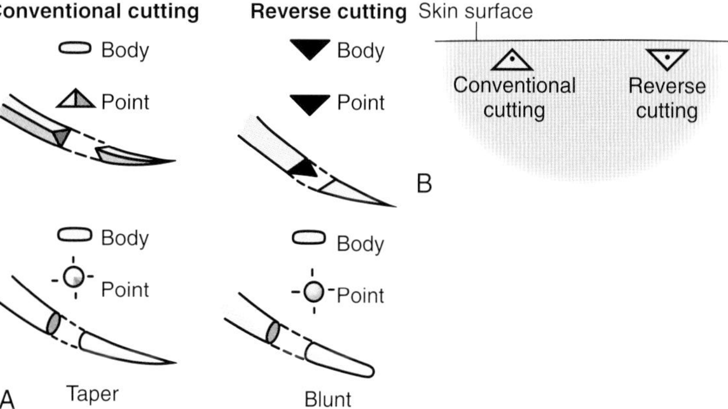

Figure 23-6 **A,** Needle points and body shapes. **B,** In conventional cutting needles the pressure is concentrated on the apex of the triangle, and the needle thereby has a tendency to tear through tissue. In reverse cutting, the advantage of piercing through tissue still exists, but the pressure from the suture is distributed over the whole base so unwanted tearing is reduced. *Black dot* indicates suture.

cutting needle is rarely used compared with the reverse cutting needle (see Fig. 23-6).

The *reverse cutting* needle has its cutting edge on the outer curvature of the needle. This provides a flat surface along the inner edge, thereby reducing the incidence of sutures pulling through tissues into the margin of the wound. Unless specified otherwise, a "cutting needle" now refers to a *reverse cutting design*.

Tapered cut or *round* needles have an oval body to reduce twisting in the needle holder. These points are useful in less dense tissues that require small holes and minimal tissue injury, such as fascia or bowel.

Complications

When inappropriately small suture needles are chosen, there is a high risk of needle bending or breaking. A lost needle tip can be a serious, time-consuming intraoperative problem. Other causes of needle breakage include an unexpected encounter with bone or scar tissue, inappropriate angle of penetration, or the use of a reshaped needle that was bent during usage.

The loss of the whole needle in tissues can be avoided by using good judgment in matching tissue bites to needle length. Avoid firm grasping of the suture material near the shank with the needle holder or forceps because it can weaken or cut the suture material, leaving an unattached needle. This free needle becomes a great risk to the surgeon for needlestick injury as well as an opportunity for complications in the patient.

The shank is the thinnest metal portion of the needle, and this thin metal is, of course, the weakest portion of the needle. Care must be taken never to apply force or attempt to use the needle holder on the shank when suturing. When a needle bends during suturing, the act of straightening it further weakens the metal. The surgeon must remain aware of this potential cause for complications.

In addition, multiple needle passes through tissues and associated frequent re-arming of the needle holder wears away the needle lubricant coating, which increases the force required for subsequent needle passes.

Conclusion

Often an ordinary suturing procedure becomes more difficult than expected. This difficulty can be ameliorated by reassessing the appropriateness of the instruments being used. Needle selection is often a key factor in facilitating the ease of the operation and ensuring ultimate good surgical results.

Suppliers

(See contact information online at www.expertconsult.com.)

Ethicon, Inc.
USSDG Sutures (now Syneture)
Most medical supply firms carry any suture material needed.

BIBLIOGRAPHY

Ethicon, Inc.: Wound Closure Manual. Somerville, NJ, Ethicon, Inc., 1985.

Goldwasser MS, Bailey JS (eds): Diagnosis and Management of Skin Cancer. Oral Maxillofac Surg Clin 17:133–240, 2005.

Moy RL: Suture material. In Usatine R, Moy R, Tobinick E, Siegel D (eds): Skin Surgery: A Practical Guide. St. Louis, Mosby, 1998, pp 77–87.

Moy RL, Waldman B, Hein DW: A review of sutures and suturing techniques. J Dermatol Surg Oncol 18:785–795, 1992.

Robinson JK, Hanke CW, Sengelmann RD, Siegel DM (eds): Surgery of the Skin: Procedural Dermatology. Philadelphia, Mosby, 2005.

Rohrer TE, Cook JL, Nguyen TH: Flaps and Grafts in Dermatologic Surgery. Philadelphia, Mosby, 2007.

Schwartz SI, Shires GT, Spencer FC, Storer EH (eds): Principles of Surgery, 7th ed. New York, McGraw-Hill, 1999.

Tier WC: Considerations in the choice of surgical needles. Surg Gynecol Obstet 149:84, 1979.

Way LW (ed): Current Surgical Diagnosis and Treatment, 9th ed. Norwalk, Conn, Appleton & Lange, 1991.

Weitzul S, Taylor RS: Suturing technique and other closure materials. In Robinson JK, Hanke DW, Sengelmann RD, Siegel DM (eds): Surgery of the Skin: Procedural Dermatology. Philadelphia, Mosby, 2005, pp 225–244.

CHAPTER 24

Laceration and Incision Repair: Suture Selection

William Jackson Epperson

Numerous suture types have been developed for specific tissue properties in the body. The qualities most important for suture include flexibility, strength, secure knotting, and a low propensity to contribute to inflammation or infection. The goal of suturing is to maintain the approximation of tissue securely until healing allows for tissue strength to be maintained alone.

The two main categories of suture are *absorbable* and *nonabsorbable*. All types of suture are foreign to the body; therefore the degree to which the body reacts against the suture is an important consideration in suture choice.

Suture size is indicated by the use of a "0," with the more "0"s designating smaller sutures (e.g., 4-0 is smaller than 3-0). Suture materials are standardized by specific regulations, which ensure tensile strength consistency.

Absorbable suture is a sterile strand of synthetic polymer or mammalian-derived collagen. The rate of absorption and duration of tensile strength are important considerations. For example, the suture may lose effective strength long before it has been absorbed. Various coatings and materials have been developed to prolong the tensile strength retention of absorbable sutures. These coatings also aid in the passage of suture through tissues by decreasing friction.

The *natural absorbable suture (mammalian collagen or gut sutures)* are derived mainly from the submucosa of sheep intestine, the serosa of cattle intestine, or the flexor tendons of cattle. They are available in plain or chromic (coated with chromic salts to help delay absorption). Tensile strength is determined by the percentage of collagen in the gut suture. Any collagen materials in the gut suture can cause severe tissue reactions, so purity of the protein is very important. Rare true suture allergy can be caused by foreign collagens or chromic salts in "gut" suture.

Common *synthetic absorbable* suture materials include polyglactic acid (Vicryl), polyglycolic acid (Dexon), and polydioxanone (PDS). These materials have the desirable property of extended time of tensile strength (Fig. 24-1).

Nonabsorbable suture is used for skin and for long-term internal placement such as in cardiovascular, orthopedic, and plastic surgery. Many raw materials are used, including silk, cotton, stainless steel, nylon, polyester, and polypropylene (Table 24-1). Table 24-2 reviews the various features of each of these sutures. All suture materials except stainless steel will lose at least some tensile strength if left in the body for long enough periods.

Nonabsorbable sutures are removed from the skin when no longer needed. In vascular and orthopedic applications there is often a need for more permanent materials that retain their tensile strength. Tendon repair requires prolonged healing time, so sutures need long-term tensile strength to give adequate time for self-repair. Vascular grafts must have the support of suture for an indefinite period. The anastomosis of a graft and a blood vessel is never secured by the fibroblast and collagen of the body alone.

Braided suture adds strength and helps to secure the knotting but is more likely to leak fluid, which is called *capillarity*. This quality increases the likelihood of harboring bacteria and subsequent infections. *Monofilament* is better to use in the presence of infection, but its knots are less dependable. Tissue reaction is important in delicate tissues in which scar and tissue formation may be a problem, which is why gut suture may not be a good choice for use on the face.

Other suture characteristics are also important. *Tensile strength* is the force necessary for a suture to break divided by its cross-sectional area. Tensile strength can be altered by twisting, braiding, increased age, heating, and moisture. Suture coatings reduce friction when passing through tissues. Braided suture has more friction than monofilaments. Coatings used include silicone, Teflon (DuPont; Wilmington, Del), and wax. Polyglactic suture has also been coated with triclosan, which is an antibacterial agent that may reduce the incidence of staphylococcal infections. *Memory* describes the characteristics of a suture material in returning to its original shape after bending. Increased memory is found in nylon and polypropylene, and their knots are more likely to untie spontaneously.

Sutures are foreign to tissues and all induce inflammatory responses. The larger stranded and multistranded sutures, in general, cause more tissue reactions than thin or monofilament sutures. Synthetic sutures of nylon and polypropylene cause less reaction than silk or surgical gut. The dissolution of absorbable sutures is accomplished by the homeostatic immune response. In general, less immunogenic suture materials are small diameter, synthetic, monofilament, and nonabsorbable. A greater immunologic response comes from suture materials that are larger diameter, natural fiber, multifilament, and absorbable.

Knots are an important consideration in terms of whether they remain tied and do not cause a significant reduction in the tensile strength of the suture material. The knot is the weakest part of the completed suture ligature. Proper knotting technique requires application of the square knot or a double loop followed by a square knot tie. Often knots are accomplished as half hitches that are weak and do not remain secure. The more friction the suture has, the less likely it is to incur slippage and loss of knot integrity. Braided suture knots rarely slip, whereas monofilament often comes untied in the absence of proper knotting technique. For proper tying techniques, see Chapter 25, Laceration and Incision Repair: Suture Tying.

Choosing a Suture

Each surgeon has his or her own choice of suture based on training and individual preferences. Choosing the appropriate suture characteristics in relation to the various applications will facilitate the operation and lead to an acceptable result. Table 24-3 generalizes some recommendations for sutures commonly used in an office

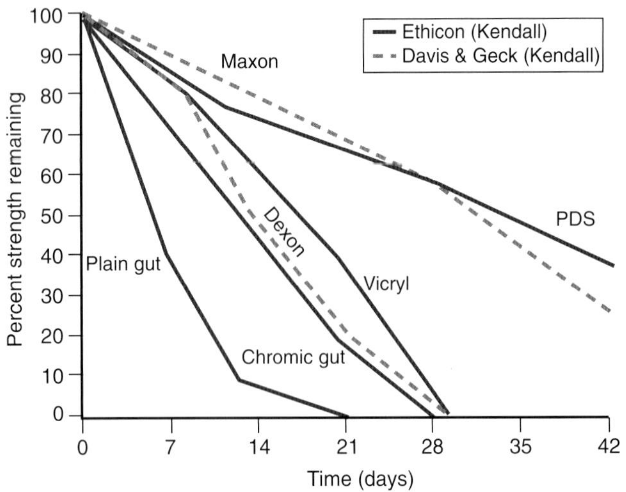

Figure 24-1 In vivo strength retention of absorbable sutures.

TABLE 24-1 Nonabsorbable Sutures

Material	Type	Tensile Strength	Tissue Reaction	Cost
Silk	Braided	Poor	High	Low
Nylon (Ethilon, Dermalon)	Mono	Good	Minimal	Low
Polypropylene (Prolene, Surgipro)	Mono	Excellent	Minimal	High
Uncoated braided polyester (Dacron, Mersilene)	Braided	Good	Moderate	High
Coated braded polyester (Ti-cron, Ethibond)	Braided	Good	Moderate	High
Polybutester (Novafil)	Mono	Good	Minimal	Moderate

TABLE 24-2 Common Suture Materials

Suture	Types	Makeup	Usage	Tissue Reaction	Absorption Time or Rate (total)	Tensile Strength Retention
Absorbable Sutures						
Gut	Plain multifilament twisted	Mammalian collagen	Superficial vessels and quick-healing subcutaneous tissues	High	70 days	7–10 days
Gut	Chromic multifilament twisted	Mammalian collagen	Versatile; also good in the presence of infection; do not use on skin because of reaction	Moderate	90 days	10–21 days
Polyglycolic acid (Dexon)*	Mono	Synthetic polymer	Buried sutures; good tensile and knot strength	Mild	40% in 7 days	20% in 15 days, 5% in 28 days
Polydioxanone (PDS)†	Mono	Polyester polymer	Versatile; body cavity closure; bowel; buried skin suture where more strength and longer retention needed	Mild	210 days	70% in 14 days, 50% in 28 days
Polyglactic acid (Vicryl)†	Braided	Coated polymer	Subcutaneous skin; buried sutures	Mild	60–90 days	60% in 14 days, 30% in 21 days
Polyglyconate (Maxon)	Mono	Polyester	Smoother knot and excellent first-throw holding; buried	Mild	180–210 days	80% in 14 days, 60% in 28 days
Nonabsorbable Sutures						
Cotton	Twisted fibers	Cotton fiber	Ligating, some skin but generally too reactive	Minimal	Nearly permanent, encapsulated in the body	50% in 6 mo, 30% in 2 yr
Silk	Braided	Silkworm-spun fiber	Ligating, some skin but rarely used	Moderate	2 yr	Gone in 1 yr
Steel	Mono	Alloy Fe-Ni-Cr	Tendons, sternum, abdominal wall	Low	Never; encapsulated in the body	Indefinite
Nylon (Ethilon, Dermalon)	Mono	Synthetic polymer	Skin	Very low	20% per year	Loses 20% per year
Polyester (Mersilene)	Braided	Polyester	Cardiovascular, general, and plastic surgery	Minimal	Nearly permanent; encapsulated in the body	Nearly indefinite
Polypropylene (Prolene)†	Mono	Synthetic polymer	Skin, vascular, plastic surgery—very "slippery" so needs extra knots; "stronger" than nylon	Minimal	Considered permanent; encapsulated in the body	Nearly indefinite

*Dexon Plus has a synthetic coating to facilitate knot tying and passage through tissue.
†Prolene, Ethilon, Ethibond, and PDS are registered trademarks of Ethicon, Inc. (Somerville, NJ).

TABLE 24-3 Common Sutures for Cutaneous Surgery

Area of Body	Skin (Interrupted)	Skin (Running Subcuticular)	Buried
Face	5-0 or 6-0 nylon	4-0 or 5-0 polypropylene	4-0, 5-0, or 6-0 synthetic absorbable or 6-0 clear nylon
Extremities, trunk	4-0 or 5-0 nylon	3-0 or 4-0 polypropylene or 3-0 or 4-0 synthetic absorbable (rarely used on extremities)	3-0 or 4-0 synthetic absorbable; occasionally 4-0 polypropylene if quite deep

setting. In general, the smaller the suture, the lower the tensile strength; thus, more sutures will be needed, but the cosmetic result will be better. Physicians vary greatly in their preferences, and no one suture is satisfactory for all situations. Nylon is a good, all-around, inexpensive material for surface skin suturing. It is not quite as strong or slippery as polypropylene, but it ties easier and takes fewer knots. Polypropylene is stronger and glides through tissue easily, but requires at least three, if not four, knots and still may not remain tight. Polypropylene works well for running subcuticular stitches, and often, because it is stronger, a smaller size can be used for interrupted closures.

Complications

Suture breakage can be a time-wasting inconvenience for the surgeon and present significant problems for wound healing. The direct application of inappropriate force to suture material may result in suture breakage, as may irregular surgical angles, rapid suture decomposition by infection, difficult-to-access surgical sites, and postoperative patient mobility. Complications may be reduced by applying an increased number of ligatures and by using suture diameter that is commensurate to the forces most likely to be experienced in the surgical situation. Of course, almost all applications of suture can reduce tissue blood supply, and proper surgical technique reduces the incidence of this complication. Running loops of suture in an effort to accomplish quicker wound closure increases the risk of wound dehiscence in the event of suture breakage. Interrupted suture ligatures greatly reduce this complication, but are extremely time consuming compared with running ligatures.

The tensile strength of the suture can be reduced by actions that cause fragmentation or splitting of the suture fibers, also known as *frays*. Common causes include friction caused by tying, especially with tension applied during long knot rundowns. Also, scar tissue, bone, or foreign material may damage suture within tissues, whereas retractors, forceps, clamps, and needle holders can cause damage to suture within the surgical field.

Tips

When purchasing your supply of office sutures, consider the following:

1. Nylon is most commonly used and least expensive for interrupted sutures in the skin (3-0 through 6-0).
2. For running subcuticular sutures, nylon will work, but only for shorter lengths. It is not very slippery and may break on removal. Polypropylene (Prolene) is "more slippery" and stronger.
3. For deep inverted sutures, generally use polyglactic acid (Vicryl) or polyglycolic acid (Dexon). Vicryl lasts a little longer.
   - If longer retention and greater strength are desired, consider polydioxanone (PDS II).
   - If a permanent deep suture is preferred, consider clear nylon.

Patient Education Guide

See the patient education form on care of sutures online at www.expertconsult.com.

Suppliers

(See contact information online at www.expertconsult.com.)

Most medical supply firms carry any suture material needed.

Ethicon Inc.
USSDG Sutures (now called Syneture after U.S. Surgical acquired Davis & Geck, a subsidiary of TYCO Healthcare)

Bibliography

Flippin AL, Cebrun H, Reichman EF: Basic wound closure techniques. In Reichman EF, Simon RR (eds): Emergency Medicine Procedures. New York, McGraw-Hill, 2004, pp 710–735.

Forsch RT: Essentials of skin laceration repair. Am Fam Physician 78: 945–951, 2008.

Goldwasser MS, Bailey JS (eds): Diagnosis and Management of Skin Cancer. Oral Maxillofac Surg Clin 17:133–240, 2005.

Moy RL: Suture material. In Usatine R, Moy R, Tobinick E, Siegel D (eds): Skin Surgery: A Practical Guide. St. Louis, Mosby, 1998, pp 77–87.

Moy RL, Waldman B, Hein DW: A review of sutures and suturing techniques. J Dermatol Surg Oncol 18:785–795, 1992.

Robinson JK, Hanke CW, Sengelmann RD, Siegel DM (eds): Surgery of the Skin: Procedural Dermatology. Philadelphia, Mosby, 2005.

Rohrer TE, Cook JL, Nguyen TH: Flaps and Grafts in Dermatologic Surgery. Philadelphia, Saunders, 2007.

Schwartz SI, Shires GT, Spencer FC, Storer EH (eds): Principles of Surgery, 7th ed. New York, McGraw-Hill, 1999.

Tier WC: Considerations in the choice of surgical needles. Surg Gynecol Obstet 149:84, 1979.

Way LW: Current Surgical Diagnosis and Treatment, 9th ed. Norwalk, Conn, Appleton & Lange, 1991.

Weitzul S, Taylor RS. Suturing technique and other closure materials. In Robinson JK, Hanke CW, Sengelmann RD, Siegel DM (eds): Surgery of the Skin: Procedural Dermatology. Philadelphia, Mosby, 2005, pp 225–244.

Wound Closure Manual. Somerville, NJ, Ethicon, 1985.

CHAPTER 25

Laceration and Incision Repair: Suture Tying

Ronald D. Reynolds

The knot is the weakest point of any suture. Even when properly tied, the knot is less than half the strength of the suture material that it is tied in and will always be the point at which a suture fails. Knots will slip apart if not correctly constructed. If excessive tension is applied, even to a properly tied suture loop, it will break at the knot because of internal shearing forces.

It is incumbent on the physician to know what suture material and size to use for each type of tissue that is to be approximated (see Chapter 24, Laceration and Incision Repair: Suture Selection). Once a suture is placed, it must be tied in an appropriate manner—not too tight or too loose and with a knot that will not fail before the tissue has healed. The knot must not be excessively large because inflammation and infection are directly correlated with knot volume in tissue.

General Principles of Knot Tying

A few generalities can be made about all knot tying. The suture material must always be treated with respect. Grasping the suture with an instrument will weaken it and thus should be avoided, except when holding a tail that will be cut away after an instrument tie. Shearing forces created by sawing two strands upon one another will weaken the strands. The first throw of a knot should just approximate the tissue, but subsequent throws must be tied firmly for knot security. Ideally, knots should be tied with equal tension on both strands. Tension should be applied parallel to the loop being closed and along the axis of the knot being tightened. Excessive throws do not add to knot security; they only add time and bulk.

Knot Mechanics

Suture knots are at the mercy of a number of factors. If the knot is tied in a *monofilament* material such as gut, nylon, polypropylene (Prolene), or polydioxanone (PDS), the *coefficient of friction* within the knot will be low, leading to a tendency to slip. These materials also have *memory*, a tendency to maintain the shape in which they were manufactured, giving a straightening tendency that can lead to untying. The *pliability*, or ability to form a tight loop, of nylon is higher than that of the other monofilament materials. Braided *multifilament* suture materials such as silk, polyester (Mersilene, Ethibond), polyglactin (Vicryl), and polyglycolic acid (Dexon) have a higher coefficient of friction and less memory, making them easier to tie and less prone to slippage. The absorbability of a suture does not have a direct influence on its tying characteristics.

When knots are tied, great care must be taken as to the details. The *square knot* (Fig. 25-1A) is the prototype suture knot because it is easy to tie, is strong, and does not loosen easily. Each twisting layer of the knot is called a *throw*. A square knot is constructed of one helical twist for the first throw, followed by one helical twist in the opposite direction for the second throw. If both helices are in the same direction, a *granny knot* (Fig. 25-1B) results. Granny knots slip much more easily than square knots and therefore should be avoided when tying sutures.

After a helix for a knot throw is made with two suture strands, it must be kept in a helical configuration as the knot is tightened. If too much tension is applied to one strand, that strand will straighten and a *half hitch* (Fig. 25-1C) in the other strand will result. As is obvious by its appearance, half hitches will slip on the straightened member of the suture and, therefore, are also to be avoided. It is unfortunately common for a physician who thinks that square knots are being laid down to instead make a series of slipping half hitches (Fig. 25-1D). This is due to too much tension being applied to one strand during the tightening phase of tying.

If there is excess tension on wound edges when a square knot is being tied, the first throw of the knot may loosen before the second throw is placed and allow the edges to gape apart. The *surgeon's knot* (Fig. 25-1E) is an adaptation of the square knot with two helical twists in the first throw. This additional twist increases the friction within the first throw and helps to hold it tight while the second throw is made. It is almost always used, but, whenever a surgeon's knot seems necessary, the clinician should always be sure that the deep space has been closed with a deep suture if possible to approximate wound edges and take tension off the skin closure.

Choosing a Suture Tying Technique

All physicians learn knot tying skills during medical school and become familiar with one-handed and two-handed ties, as well as instrument ties. There are some important points to consider when you decide which of these tying techniques to use.

Most procedures performed by primary care physicians are office procedures done on the skin. Physicians cannot afford to waste excess suture material just for the sake of knot tying. Studies of the economics of suture tying show that at least two to four times as many sutures can be constructed in a given length of suture material with an *instrument tie* than with a *hand tie*. Although instrument tying is slightly slower than hand tying, it is much more economical and is the preferred technique for all skin procedures.

If a hand tie is to be done, the preferred method is the two-handed tie. Although the one-handed tie may be slightly faster than a two-handed tie, it is difficult to do well. One-handed ties are prone to creating a series of half hitches, because it is common to keep too much tension on one strand during tying. Also, because most wounds are sutured with the needle movement directed toward the physician and it is this closest strand (with its needle attached) that is primarily manipulated during a one-handed tie, there is a possibility of needlestick injury during a one-handed tie. Therefore one-handed tying is not covered in this chapter.

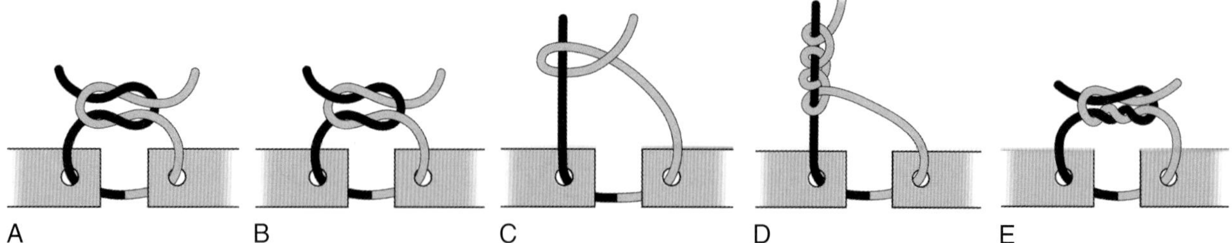

Figure 25-1 Suture knots. **A,** Square knot. **B,** Granny knot. **C,** Half hitch. **D,** Series of "square" half hitches. **E,** Surgeon's knot. (Redrawn from Zimmer CA, Thacker JG, Powell DM, et al: Influence of knot configuration and tying technique on the mechanical performance of sutures. J Emerg Med 9:107–113, 1991.)

How Tight to Tie the Loop

To appropriately approximate tissue, sutures must bring wound edges into apposition, but not place excessive force on the tissues ("approximate but don't strangulate"). If a suture loop is tied too loosely, a gap persists and the wound will not heal by primary intention but, instead, must heal by secondary intention from deeper within the defect. If tied too tightly, a suture loop will strangulate the tissue within, creating ischemia and poor wound healing. A too-tight skin suture will cut into the skin surface across the wound, creating a permanent "railroad track" scar.

Whether incised by accidental laceration or by an intentional surgical wound, all tissue will swell somewhat from the inflammation that is attendant in the healing process. Some allowance must be made for this anticipated swelling when tying each suture. It is the tension of the first throw, and maintenance of this tension while the second throw locks it in place that is critical. Additional throws beyond these do not change the tension within the original loop.

As tension is applied to the first throw of a knot, the tissue edges should just barely touch together. If the edges are bunched together initially, subsequent swelling will make the loop too tight. With skin sutures, two subtle indications of excess loop tension include (1) a puckering effect of each suture that makes the wound mound up slightly between each loop, and (2) a pale color of the skin underneath the suture. *It is far better to remove and replace an improperly tied suture than to leave it and hope for the best.*

How Many Throws to Place

How many additional throws to place on top of the basic square or surgeon's knot for knot security is a slippery question. Suture manufacturers will only say "additional throws as indicated by the surgical circumstance and the experience of the surgeon." (Believe me, they won't give a real answer, even when pressed. I've tried. Medicolegal concerns keep them from committing themselves.)

For a knot to be secure, additional throws are needed beyond the basic two throws. Without added throws, the knot will slip loose when tension is applied to the loop. Any loosely tied knot will slip, so all throws past the first must be tied quite firmly, but without excessive force that will damage the integrity of the suture material.

Placing more throws than needed will unnecessarily add operative time and increase the bulk of the knot, without adding strength to the knot. Extra throws in a skin suture knot add operative time but have no consequence for the tissue because they are not buried. If the knot is buried, as in a subcuticular suture, additional bulk adds to the tissue reaction and can increase the infection risk. It is therefore necessary to know the minimum number of throws to tie a secure knot in a variety of suture materials.

As a general rule, studies have shown that when 3- to 4-mm tails are left, monofilament materials need a total of four firm square throws to be secure, and braided materials need three. Obviously, if the knot is not tied squarely (made of alternating throws with helices in different directions), is tied loosely, or consists of half hitches rather than square throws, even the recommended number of throws will not suffice.

There are two exceptions to this general rule. First, nylon is pliable enough that it holds with three firm square throws. Second, when the suture is cut on the knot and no tails are left, one additional throw is required for knot security.

Techniques

Instrument Tie

An instrument tie uses the needle holder to form the twists in each throw. Directions are for a right-handed physician. Left-handed physicians can reverse the handedness in the directions and look at the figure in a mirror.

1. Place the suture moving toward yourself, and pull it through until just 2 to 3 cm of the tail is left outside the entry hole. Drop the needle beside the wound to minimize needlestick risk. Pick up the long end of the suture with your left thumb and index finger about 8 cm from its exit, and hold it above the wound.
2. Create the first throw by making a single twist (for a square knot) or double twist (for a surgeon's knot) around the tip of the needle holder with the long strand. To do this, the needle holder is held closed, but not locked, facing toward the left. The instrument tip approaches the long strand moving toward the physician. Both it and the long strand are moved in a clockwise motion to wrap the strand around the tip (Fig. 25-2A), with care taken not to pull the suture through the wound. Grasp the short end with the very tip of the needle holder. Pull the short end through the loops around the needle holder's tip (Fig. 25-2B). Keep even tension on both strands as you pull the short strand toward you with the needle holder and the long strand away from you with your left hand (Fig. 25-2C). The sutures should maintain a helical configuration all the way down to the wound. Apply enough tension to just appose the wound. Release the short end.
3. The second throw is created by reversing the rotation of the long strand around the needle holder tip. While still holding the long strand in the left hand, bring it toward you while moving the needle holder away from yourself. As the needle holder tip touches the long strand, wrap counterclockwise around it (Fig. 25-2D). Again grasp the short end in the needle holder tips (Fig. 25-2E), and pull the short strand away from yourself while pulling the long strand toward you (Fig. 25-2F). Carefully pull the throw down square to lock the knot. As you tighten this critical second throw, don't pull hard enough to disturb the first throw—this might loosen the careful apposition.
4. Additional throws must be made, with the number depending on the suture material and circumstances. Repeat the cycle of clockwise–counterclockwise throws, being careful to lay each throw down with opposite rotation to the last throw. Tie each throw square (not half-hitched) with firm and even tension on both ends as the knot is snugged tight. When the knot is

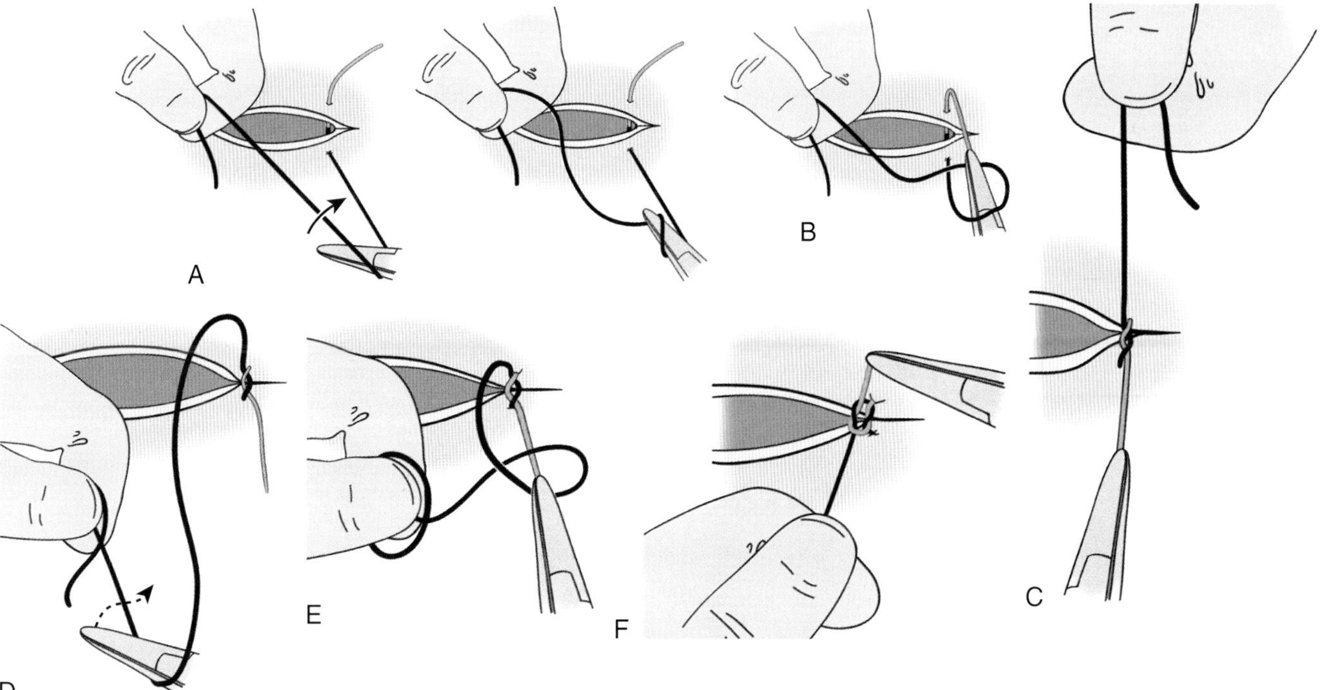

Figure 25-2 Instrument tie. **A,** The first clockwise wrap around the needle holder tip. **B,** Grasping the tail. **C,** Tensioning the first throw. **D,** Counter-clockwise wrap for the second throw. **E,** Grasping the tail. **F,** Tensioning the second throw.

completed, excess material is cut away, either on the knot if it is to be buried or leaving 3- to 4-mm tails if it is a skin suture.

Two-Handed Tie

This version of the two-handed tie presumes that the suture to be tied has been sewn toward you, with the needle on your side of the wound. Following this sequence prevents you from having to cross your hands over the top of the wound, a motion that blocks your vision of the knot being formed.

1. The two-handed tie starts like the instrument tie with the suture being placed in the tissue and being pulled through, but leaving about 10 cm of the tail outside the wound. Grasp the tail in your right hand and the long end in your left hand. Palms are up when initially grasping the strands, which are held between the last three fingers and the palm. To start the knot, grasp the short end between your right index finger and thumb. Use the back of your left thumb to hold the long end as shown. Lay the short end across the side of your left thumb to form a loop (Fig. 25-3A).
2. Drop your left index finger to contact the pad of your left thumb and hold the loop open. Maintaining the pinch, drop the loop off your thumb and move down to pinch the short end (Fig. 25-3B), leaving your left index finger inside the loop. Push the free end up through the loop with the left thumb by extending your left wrist (Fig. 25-3C). Release the free end from your right hand and regrasp it as it is pulled through the loop. This same maneuver can be redone to make the second twist needed for a surgeon's knot. Draw down the first throw and tighten evenly by bringing your left hand away from and your right hand toward yourself (Fig. 25-3D).
3. The second square throw is created by reversing these maneuvers. As you draw the long end back toward yourself with your left hand, use your left index finger to begin to create a loop. Reach under the short end with your left thumb (Fig. 25-3E), and push your thumb up to hold the side of the loop. Bring your left thumb and index finger together inside the loop (Fig. 25-3F). Lift the short end in your right hand, and place it in the pinch of your left thumb and index finger. Push the short end down through the loop with your left index finger, release it from the right hand, and then regrasp. The second throw is then brought down by bringing the right hand away and the left hand toward you (Fig. 25-3G). Be careful not to disturb the first throw as this critical second throw is tightened.
4. Additional throws are added as needed by alternating the same process of the first and second throws. Alternating the helix of the throws will keep the knot square. When the knot is completed, excess material is cut away, either on the knot if it is to be buried or leaving 3- to 4-mm tails if it is a skin suture.

Half Blood Knot

It is useful to know one additional knot for tying suture—the half blood knot. Fishermen use this slipping knot to tie lures onto the end of fishing line. It is a very strong knot, retaining almost all of the strength of the suture material. The half blood knot is the best knot for securing the beginning of a running suture, particularly with monofilament material. General surgeons commonly use it to secure the beginning of a running suture in the linea alba when closing the abdomen, but it also works well to start a running cuticular or subcuticular suture.

After the suture is placed in the tissue, the tail is passed around the working strand of the suture. Four twists of the tail around itself are made. More than four twists do not add to the strength of the knot. The tail is then passed up through the first loop, parallel to the working strand (Fig. 25-4). The knot is tightened by pulling on the tail with a needle holder, then is slipped down to secure the tissue. The working end continues on to construct a running suture line.

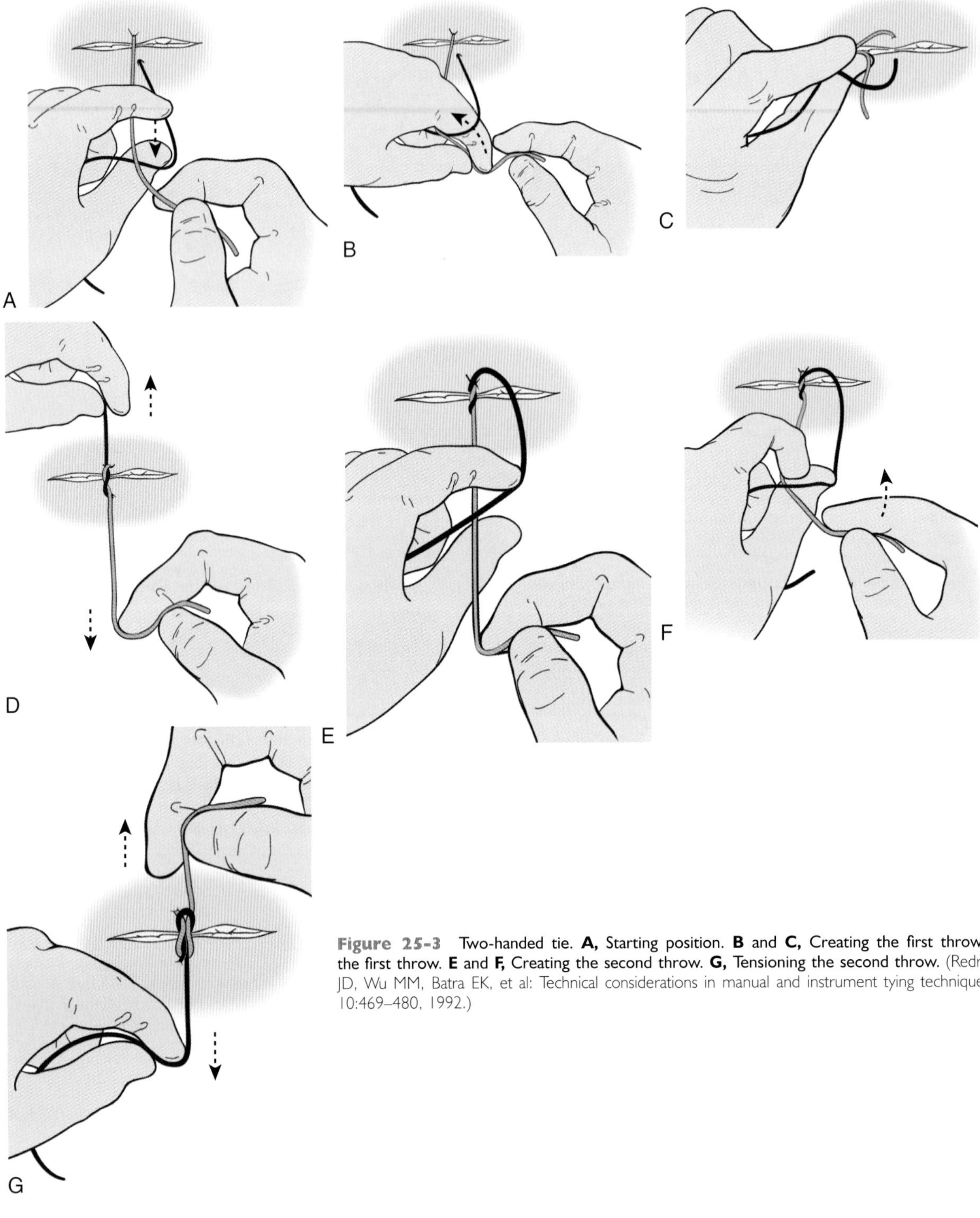

Figure 25-3 Two-handed tie. **A,** Starting position. **B** and **C,** Creating the first throw. **D,** Tensioning the first throw. **E** and **F,** Creating the second throw. **G,** Tensioning the second throw. (Redrawn from James JD, Wu MM, Batra EK, et al: Technical considerations in manual and instrument tying techniques. J Emerg Med 10:469–480, 1992.)

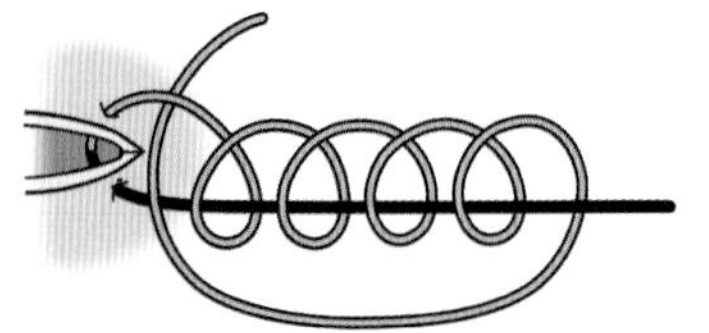

Figure 25-4 Half blood knot. The tail is passed around the long strand, then loops four times around itself, then the tail is put through the first loop.

COMMON ERRORS

- If the first throw of a knot slips loose before the second throw can be tied, additional measures are needed:
  - A double helix can be used as the first throw, creating the *surgeon's knot.*
  - An absorbable deeper suture can be placed to take tension off of the closure.
  - The extra hands of an assistant can hold the wound edges together as the suture loop is being tied.
  - A helper stitch can be placed and later removed. A horizontal mattress suture is placed in the middle of the wound to bring the skin edges partway together. Once the wound is completely closed, this "helper" stitch is often loose and can then be removed.
- A series of half hitches is tied rather than locking square knots. To prevent this, the surgeon must apply even tension to both strands as the knot is tightened, rather than hold one strand taut and tighten the other.
- The knot is tied too loosely. This may be caused by two different problems. First, the first throw must be tied tightly enough to just appose the wound edge. Second, the surgeon should not pull tension on either strand as the second throw is tied because this often loosens the first throw.
- The knot is tied too tightly. As each knot throw is constructed, attention must be given to not strangulating the tissue because this can lead to tissue ischemia and necrosis. The common result of too tight a suture loop is a "railroad track" appearance of the scar when the sutures are removed. It is best to remove and replace an improperly tied suture.

CONCLUSION

Suture tying is an art that develops with experience. Close attention to detail is necessary when approximating tissue. The goal is to bring tissue edges into apposition without causing strangulation inside the loop as postoperative swelling develops. The instrument tie is preferred for skin sutures. If a hand tie is to be done, the two-handed technique is preferred. The physician must tie firm, square throws by using even tension on each end and must know how many throws to place with each type of suture material to ensure knot security.

PATIENT EDUCATION GUIDE

See the patient education form on suture care online at www.expertconsult.com.

SUPPLIER

A useful *Knot Tying Manual* and "knot tying board" are available free of charge from Ethicon, Inc. (see contact information online at www.expertconsult.com).

ONLINE RESOURCES

Half Blood Knot

http://dorkingas.co.uk/Knots/Half%20Blood%20Knot/half_blood_knot.htm

Instrument Tie

http://www.bumc.bu.edu/Dept/Content.aspx?DepartmentID=69&PageID=5263
http://www.youtube.com/watch?v=0Ye3oYU_6A8

Two-Handed Tie

http://www.bumc.bu.edu/Dept/Content.aspx?DepartmentID=69&PageID=5262
http://www.youtube.com/watch?v=XHk_191uYP4&NR=1

BIBLIOGRAPHY

Behm T, Unger JB, Ivy JJ, Mukherjee D: Flat square knots: Are 3 throws enough? Am J Obstet Gynecol 197:172.e1–172.e3, 2007.

Ethicon, Inc.: Knot Tying Manual. Somerville, NJ, Ethicon, Inc., 1996.

Fong ED, Bartlett AS, Malak S, Anderson IA: Tensile strength of surgical knots in abdominal wound closure. Aust N Z J Surg 78:164–166, 2008.

Kim JC, Lee YK, Lim BS, et al: Comparison of tensile and knot security properties of surgical sutures. J Mater Sci Mater Med 18:2363–2369, 2007.

Scott DJ, Goova MT, Tesfay ST: A cost-effective proficiency-based knot-tying and suturing curriculum for residency programs. J Surg Res 141:7–15, 2007.

CHAPTER 26

Mucocele Removal

Andy S. Barnett

Oral mucous cysts (mucoceles) form as a result of obstruction or trauma involving the ducts of minor salivary glands. Mucoceles are the most common benign soft tissue mass of the oral cavity. Mucoceles occur most frequently in the mucosa of the lower lip. They appear as soft, nontender, compressible lesions with a pink or bluish tinge. Typical size ranges from a few millimeters up to 1 cm, but can be much larger. Superficial mucoceles may rupture and not recur, but larger lesions usually remain persistent or recurrent unless treated adequately.

Anatomy

Because most labial mucoceles occur as a result of mild trauma, location adjacent to the lower lip incisors is most common. Lesions on the lower lip can occur in any layer of tissue from the upper mucosa to beneath the submucosa and usually involve minor salivary glands without the involvement of significant neurovascular structures.

Indications

- Growth, pain
- Lesions refractory to superficial treatment (e.g., simple puncture or topical cryotherapy)
- Uncertain of clinical nature and biopsy is indicated
- Cosmetic concerns

Contraindications

- Atypical location (e.g., gingival or sublingual)
- Atypical gross appearance when perhaps just a biopsy is indicated
- Pulsating mass (consider an arterial aneurysm) *(relative)*

Equipment

- Lidocaine 2% with 1 : 100,000 epinephrine
- 1- to 3-mL syringe with a ½- to 1-inch, 27- or 30-gauge needle
- Scalpel with no. 11 blade and possibly a no. 15 blade
- Cryocautery or electrocautery unit

Precautions

Depending on location, consider a proximal duct stone or tumor occluding the duct. Be sure to include any unusual or palpable/thickened tissue in the specimen. Lesions that are atypical in appearance or location should be sent for pathologic evaluation to exclude carcinoma.

Preprocedure Patient Preparation

See the sample patient education handout titled "Mucocele Treatment" online at www.expertconsult.com.

Procedure

Small Lesions or Initial Treatment

An injection of lidocaine with epinephrine is given *under* the mucocele to produce anesthesia and to minimize bleeding by inducing vasoconstriction. The injection will often elevate the lesion, making it easier to see. Injecting in or above the lesion may have just the opposite effect.

With a no. 11 blade, a small stab wound is made in the cyst laterally, and the seromucinous contents are expressed. A freeze of the lesion (see Chapter 14, Cryosurgery) is performed to produce a 2- to 3-mm rim of ice around the lesion. As an alternative to cryotherapy, electrocautery may be used to lightly desiccate the lesion after incision and drainage. The ball cautery tip can be inserted directly into the cavity.

Larger Lesions

Because the tissue is so pliable it is often difficult to stabilize the lip. Consider using a large chalazion clamp, which also effectively controls bleeding.

Option 1

For larger lesions, recurrence is less likely if the roof is shaved off with a no. 15 blade before proceeding to cryotherapy or electrodesiccation (Fig. 26-1). Compress the area firmly between the fingers to reduce bleeding. If cryotherapy is chosen, hemostasis should be obtained before the freeze. A chemical coagulant, such as Monsel's solution, is useful here. The wound is allowed to heal by secondary intent, which takes 5 to 7 days. Caution the patient not to "bite" on the areas, which is tempting to do.

Option 2

Alternatively, after anesthesia, use a radiofrequency loop (cutting 20 W and coagulate 30 W or, if a single "cut and coag" setting available, about level 3 or 4) to remove the top of the lesion. Be careful not to go too deeply. Mucinous material appearing much like saliva will often come out of the cyst. A deeper wall of the cyst is usually evident at this point. Generally, a ball electrode is used to destroy the base, or cryotherapy can be considered.

Recurrent Lesions

Recurrent lesions may be retreated as described previously, but with a more aggressive approach. Persistently recurrent lesions or cysts located more deeply in the submucosa may need to be completely excised or marsupialized with interrupted fine absorbable sutures around the margins of the lesion (Fig. 26-2).

A micromarsupialization technique (Fig. 26-3) has recently been described that involves the placement of a 4-0 silk suture through the widest diameter of the dome of the lesion without involvement of the base. A surgical knot is made and the suture is left in place

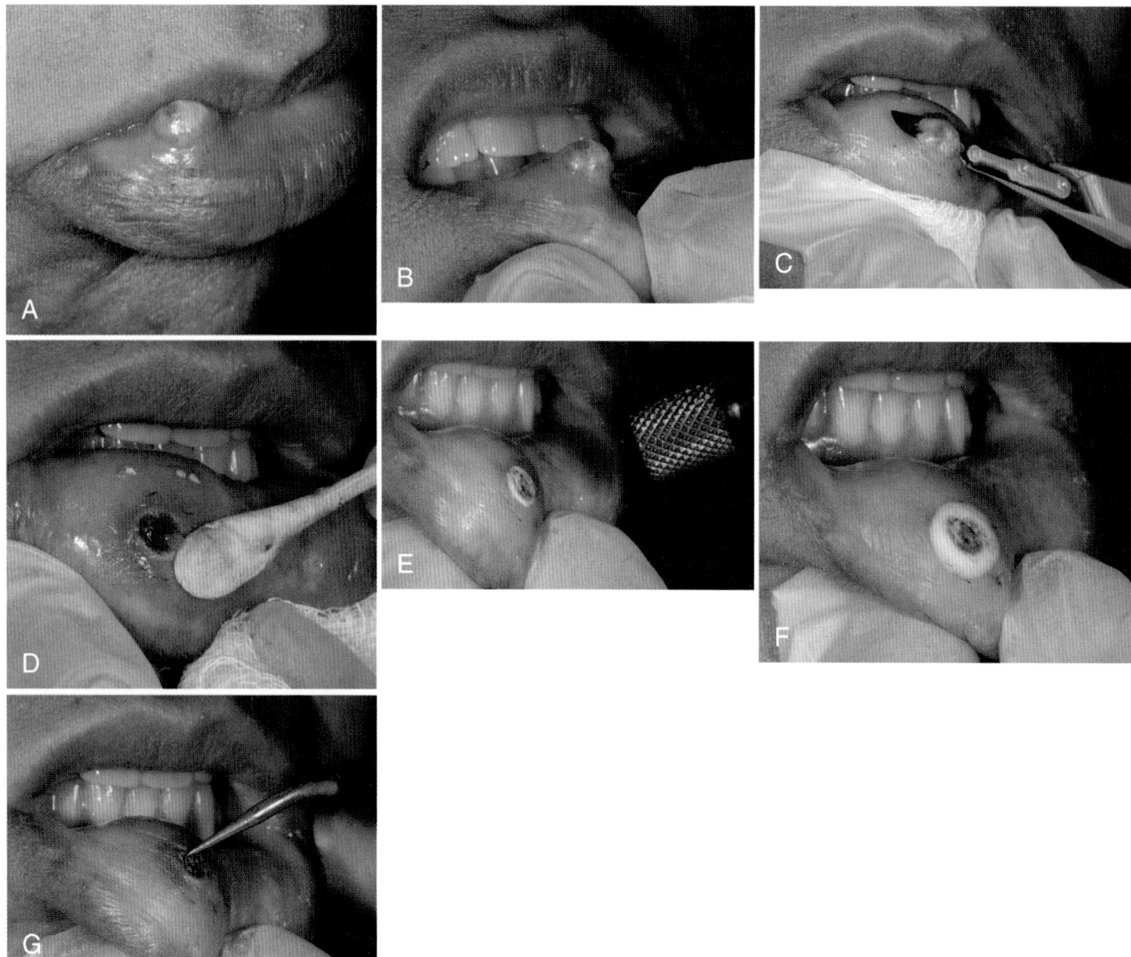

Figure 26-1 Mucocele removal. **A,** Large mucocele on the lip that recurred after previous incision, drainage, and cryosurgery. **B,** The lip is stabilized for administration of local anesthesia with lidocaine and epinephrine. **C,** The protruding tip of the mucocele is shaved off with a no. 15 blade. **D,** Preliminary hemostasis is achieved with Monsel's solution. **E,** Liquid nitrogen is sprayed to destroy the underlying lesion. **F,** Cryospray is continued until a 2-mm halo of normal tissue is frozen around the affected area. **G,** Electrosurgery is used to achieve final hemostasis after cryosurgery. (From Usatine RP, Moy RL, Tobinick EL, Siegel DM [eds]: Skin Surgery: A Practical Guide. St. Louis, Mosby, 1998.)

for 7 days. Patients must return to have the suture replaced if it is lost during this 7-day period.

Sample Operative Report

Procedure: Mucocele excision (or destruction)
Indication: Lower lip mucocele, refractory to simple cryotherapy
Consent: A consent form was signed and witnessed after a discussion with the patient/guardian of the *risks* (including but not limited to pain, bleeding, infection, scar formation, slow healing, recurrence of lesion, and failure to diagnose more serious pathology), *benefits* (treatment of lesion), and *alternatives* (including but not limited to simple aspiration, topical cryotherapy, and watchful waiting).
Technique: The mucosa surrounding the lesion was cleansed with Betadine and then anesthetized with lidocaine 1% with epinephrine 1:100,000 through a 30-gauge needle, using a total volume of 3 mL. Anesthesia was confirmed and then the lesion was unroofed around the margins of the dome with a sterile no. 15 blade. The removed portion was sent to pathology for histologic evaluation. Hemostasis was achieved with application of Monsel's solution. The base of the lesion was frozen with a 2-mm rim of normal tissue included for 5 seconds. Final hemostasis was achieved with brief application of electrocautery to any visible areas of bleeding. Antibiotic ointment was applied to the lesion.
Complications: None
Estimated blood loss: Less than 5 mL
Follow-up: If needed for any signs or symptoms of infection or recurrence of lesion and pending the pathology report.

Complications

Postoperative complications are very rare because of the forgiving nature of oral mucosal tissue.

- A minimal amount of postoperative *bleeding* can be controlled with direct pressure and should resolve within hours.
- Any *infection* should be treated with antibiotics to cover typical oral pathogens.
- *Pain* can be treated with over-the-counter (OTC) medications.
- If the biopsy specimen indicates *atypical, dysplastic,* or *neoplastic tissue,* conservative reexcision or referral should be considered based on the findings.
- *Recurrence* is the most common complication and can be dealt with using a more aggressive approach, as noted previously, or with referral.

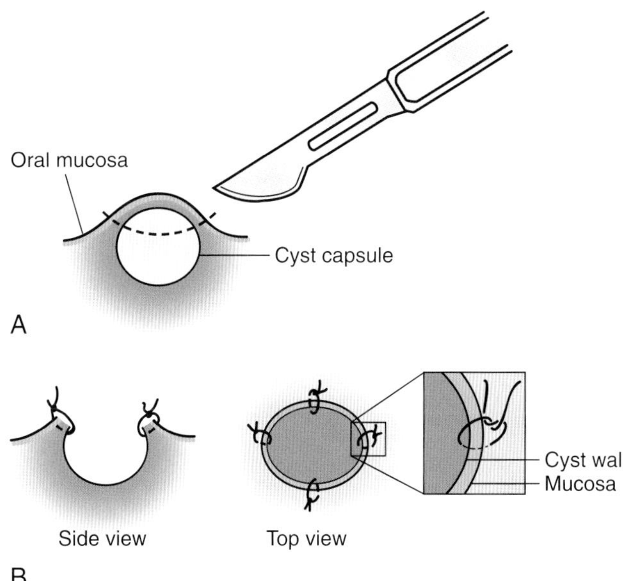

Figure 26-2 Marsupialization technique to allow continued drainage and promote epithelialization of mucocele cyst. **A,** Unroof the cyst with a no. 15 blade. **B,** Simple interrupted sutures (4-0 or 5-0 absorbable such as plain or chromic catgut, which dissolves quickly) are placed circumferentially through the cyst and oral mucosa.

- *Perforation/"button hole"* is a rare complication if the excision (especially with a radiofrequency loop) goes too deep. Often the wound can be left to heal on its own. If it is gaping open, a subcuticular closure may be necessary to limit scarring. Alternatively, an absorbable suture on the mucosal side may close the exterior wound nicely.

Postprocedure Management

Frequent topical application of antibiotic ointment may speed healing and prevent irritation of the healing mucosa by the adjacent teeth. Healing, even in delayed cases, should be complete within 2 weeks. Incomplete mucosal healing is suspect for more serious underlying pathologic process that requires excisional biopsy. Swelling is to be expected. Pain can generally be controlled with OTC medications.

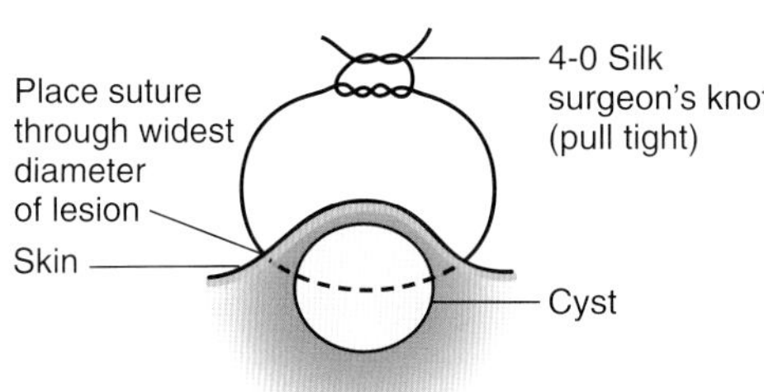

Figure 26-3 Micromarsupialization technique. Remove after 7 days.

Patient Education Guides

See the sample patient education forms online at www.expertconsult.com.

CPT/Billing Codes

40490 Biopsy of lip
40510 Excision of lip; transverse wedge excision with primary closure
  40520 with V-excision and primary direct linear closure
40808 Biopsy, vestibule of the mouth
40810 Excision/destruction, lesion of mucosa and submucosa (e.g., mucocele), vestibule of mouth, without repair
  40812 with simple repair
  40814 with complex repair
40820 Destruction of lesion or scar of vestibule of mouth by physical methods (e.g., laser, thermal, cryo, chemical)

ICD-9-CM Diagnostic Code

527.6 Oral mucocele

Lip Lesion (Upper and Lower)

173.0 Primary cancer
216.0 Benign
232.0 Carcinoma in situ
238.2 Uncertain behavior

Acknowledgment

The editors wish to recognize the many contributions by Stephen K. Toadvine, MD, MPH, to this chapter in the previous edition of this text.

Online Resource

Flaitz CM, Hicks MJ: Mucocele and ranula. Updated July 15, 2009. Available at www.emedicine.com.

Bibliography

Allen CM, Blozia GG: Oral mucosal lesions. In Cummings CW, Harker LA, Krause CJ, et al (eds): Otolaryngology: Head and Neck Surgery, 3rd ed. St. Louis, Mosby, 1998.
Baurmash HD: Mucoceles and ranulas. J Oral Maxillofac Surg 61:369–378, 2003.
Delbem AC, Cunha RF, Vieira AE, Ribeiro LL: Treatment of mucus retention phenomena in children by the micro-marsupialization technique: Case reports. Pediatr Dent 22:155–158, 2000.
Gill D: Two simple treatments for lower lip mucocoeles. Australas J Dermatol 37:220, 1996.
López-Jornet P: Labial mucocele: A study of eighteen cases. Internet J Dent Sci 3(2), 2006.
Usatine RP, Moy RL, Tobinick EL, Siegel DM (eds): Skin Surgery: A Practical Guide. St. Louis, Mosby, 1998.

CHAPTER 27

Nail Bed Repair

John Eckhold

The fingernail is a highly evolved structure designed to enhance the functions of the distal finger. The fingernail functions to (1) protect the distal phalanx, (2) enhance fine touch and fine digital movements, (3) facilitate scratching and grooming, and (4) provide aesthetic and cosmetic considerations.

Any disruption of the normal anatomy distal to the tendinous insertions of the extensor and deep flexor tendons on the finger or the thumb may adversely influence the growth, configuration, quality, and function of the nail plate unit. Sometimes a crushing injury with no penetration of the nail may cause more disfigurement than a sharp penetration, which may extend through the nail to the underlying phalanx. A good primary repair of the injured nail bed yields a high percentage of good results. Meanwhile, the results of excessively delayed repairs and revisions of faulty repairs have a much poorer prognosis. A severely deformed fingernail can be a source of embarrassment or functional impairment.

Consideration for repair includes (1) a thorough anatomic knowledge of the structure to be restored; (2) availability of all the sterile equipment required (including excellent lighting and magnification); (3) the ability to counsel the patient on what to expect over the 6 to 12 months of follow-up that will be required to see the final nail growth; and (4) the ability to recognize those injuries that may exceed the physician's training and experience, requiring referral to a hand surgeon.

Informing the patient *before* any repair effort that the resultant fingernail may be deformed or absent in spite of your best efforts spares the physician and the patient much grief in the end. Preoperative (close-up) photographs provide documentation of the severity of the injury. Patients sometimes forget what the physician had to start with and instead recall only how wonderful the fingernail looked before the injury, expecting the physician to replicate the preinjury status.

Anatomy

The nail unit is composed of four distinct epithelial structures: the *proximal nail fold*, the *germinal matrix*, the *sterile matrix*, and the *hyponychium* (Fig. 27-1). The *lateral nail folds* (Fig. 27-2) are adjacent normal epidermal folds that border the nail unit laterally. The proximal nail fits into a grove of tissue termed the *proximal nail fold*. The skin over the dorsum of the nail fold is the *nail wall*. The *eponychium* is the thin membrane extending from the nail wall onto the dorsum of the nail. The *lunula* is the curved, white opacity in the nail, just distal to the eponychium. It is the indicator of the junction between the germinal and sterile matrix. The *germinal matrix* is the most important component of the nail unit because it is responsible for the formation of the nail plate. A detailed anatomic understanding of the perionychial components of the nail area is required for consideration of nail repairs. The components are as follows:

1. *Nail plate (nail)*. Formation begins in the germinal matrix under the proximal nail fold. It is made up of desiccated, keratinized, squamous cells. Note how the nail plate fits into the groove of the proximal nail fold (see Fig. 27-1).
2. *Nail bed*. This lies under the nail plate, beginning at the proximal edge of the nail matrix and continuing until the hyponychium. It is very vascular and thus appears pink. The space between the nail bed and underlying bony structure is very thin (1 to 3 mm) without any subcutaneous tissue. The nail bed consists of the following:
    - The *eponychium*, which is the dorsal roof of the proximal fold and serves as protection for the underlying germinal matrix and provides a thin layer of cells producing the shiny dorsal nail surface
    - The *germinal matrix*, where nail production begins and which extends distally just beyond the eponychium to end at the distal border of the lunula
    - The *sterile matrix*, described by some observers as the "road bed" for the advancing nail, and which adds squamous cells to thicken the nail and enhance its adherence to the nail bed

    NOTE: The sterile matrix is the distal portion of the nail bed, beyond the germinal matrix. The germinal matrix serves as the nail origin; the sterile matrix only adds to the nail thickness.
3. *Hyponychium*. The distal site where the nail separates from the nail matrix. This area allows the nail to become independent of the nail matrix.
4. *Paronychium*. Consists of the lateral nail folds and adjacent cutaneous portions of the lateral nail borders.
5. *Lateral nail folds*. Epithelium bordering the nail laterally.
6. *Cuticle*. The translucent vein of tissue that extends out to the surface of the nail where it emerges from beneath the proximal nail fold. It acts as a barrier or seal to protect the nail unit from external irritants and seals the proximal nail fold to the nail.

Physiology

Nail formation occurs in three layers. The *dorsal* layer arises from the dorsal roof of the nail fold, the *intermediate* layer from the ventral floor and the lateral walls of the proximal nail, and the *ventral* layer from the sterile matrix of the nail bed. The ventral layer provides adherence and enhances the nail thickness to compensate for wearing away on the dorsal surface. The nail grows distally as a result of the force of the pressure placed on the growing cell mass beneath the proximal nail fold. The resultant nail advances distally, hugging the underlying nail bed. Any distortion of these anatomic templates (e.g., proximal nail fold, nail matrix contour and composition) can lead to a deformed and unattractive nail.

Full-length fingernail growth takes 4 to 6 months and is frequently suspended completely for 3 weeks after an acute traumatic event. Fingernails reportedly grow four times as rapidly as toenails. Peak nail growth rate occurs at about 30 years of age.

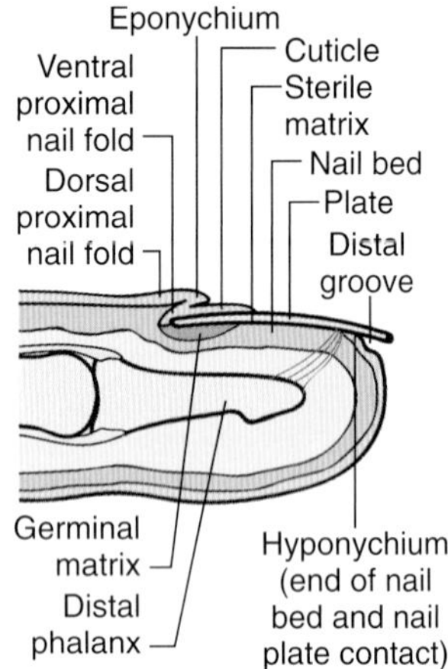

Figure 27-1 Sagittal view of the nail and distal phalanx.

Fractures

An x-ray examination must be performed on any crush, impact, or penetrating injury for possible involvement of the distal phalanx to avoid missing a fracture that may deform the nail bed if left unreduced or unstable. Fractures when accompanied by bleeding from under or around the nail plate, including a drained subungual hematoma, automatically become open fractures and must be treated with the appropriate caution and care. Fractures may require reduction and internal fixation before nail bed repair. Proximal nail bed injuries or avulsions in children are often open Salter epiphyseal fractures of the distal phalanx and should be treated appropriately.

Subungual Hematoma

See Chapter 35, Subungual Hematoma Evacuation.

The nail bed is a highly vascular area subject to bleeding with either sharp or nonpenetrating blunt trauma. To release the painful smaller hematoma, first cleanse the finger with povidone–iodine solution for several minutes (no anesthesia is required if the nail plate does not need to be removed). Use of a heated (red-hot) paper clip, drill, or microcautery releases the underlying pressure with minimal discomfort. The heated tip passes through the nail with minimal pressure and is cooled by the hematoma, thus not causing injury to the nail bed. The hole should be at least 2 mm in diameter to allow drainage to continue and not seal up when clot forms. If the nail is to be removed to inspect and possibly repair the nail bed, do not place the hole in the nail until the location of the repair site is known. After nail bed repair the vent hole should *not* overlay the repair site directly in order to achieve maximal contouring effect from the replaced nail plate.

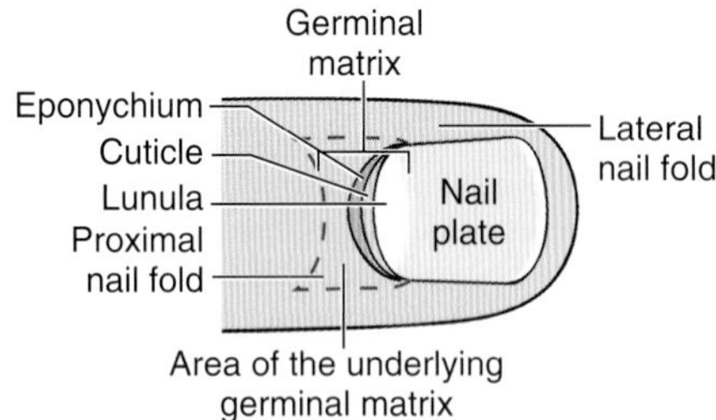

Figure 27-2 Dorsal view of the nail. The sterile matrix underlies the nail plate distal to the lunula (proximal to the lunula is the germinal matrix) under the nail plate.

If the trauma produces a large hematoma suspected of causing a significant nail bed injury, the nail should be removed to facilitate meticulous magnified inspection and careful repair of the nail bed. The prerequisites for inspection include (1) good anesthesia, (2) good light and magnification, (3) essential sterile equipment, (4) sterile saline for irrigation, and (5) adequate retraction assistance to carefully investigate the area deep to the proximal and lateral nail folds.

Equipment

- Surgical loupes or appropriate magnification providing 2.5× magnification or greater
- Freer septum elevator
- Kutz periosteal elevator
- Small periosteal Key elevator
- English nail splitter
- Small bone rongeur
- Small bone reduction forceps or clamps
- Single- and double-pronged skin hooks
- No. 11 or 15 surgical blade and handles
- Small cuticle scissors
- Needle holders
- Suture scissors
- ⅜-inch Penrose drain
- Small hemostats (2)
- 6-0 and 7-0 absorbable suture (gut or white Vicryl)
- Silicone sheeting (0.020-in thick)
- Petrolatum gauze
- Antibiotic ointment (e.g., Neosporin)
- Small syringe and 30-gauge needle
- Lidocaine 1% to 2% plain (generally no epinephrine in the fingers; however, see the discussions in Chapter 4, Local Anesthesia, and Chapter 5, Local and Topical Anesthetic Complications)
- Adson pickups, with and without teeth
- Finger dressing material, small metal splints, and arm sling for postoperative elevation

Nail Plate Avulsion (Surgical)

The nail must be removed when there is a large subungual hematoma or when the nail bed injury/laceration is directly visualized or strongly suspected (e.g., there is avulsion of the distal nail from the hyponychium or proximally from the eponychium; see the editor's note after the Bibliography). Verify at this time if there is (1) displaced, unstable phalangeal fracture (requiring fixation); (2) large nail bed avulsion (with missing tissue requiring nail bed grafts); or (3) significant distal amputation of tissue (requiring some type of graft for closure). Consider early referral of the injury if it exceeds personal training, experience, and comfort level.

Exploration of the nail bed can be completed under general anesthesia, scalene block, axillary block, Bier block, or digital block (see Chapter 1, Bier Block, and Chapter 8, Peripheral Nerve Blocks and Field Blocks). The first four can be used with an arm tourniquet and additional sedation as required for longer procedures in which multiple digits are involved. Uncooperative adults and restless children may be managed better with the use of a more formal type of anesthetic setting. Practitioners prefer to save the patients any additional anesthetic charges if possible, but their desire to economize should not compromise the examination or repair in any way when the patient is being uncooperative and moving about during a delicate repair under magnification.

After anesthesia the surgical field is prepared and draped in the usual manner to ensure sterility of the surgical field. At this time, if no other form of tourniquet is in use, a digital tourniquet can be established by use of a sterile ⅜-inch Penrose drain placed smoothly around the finger and secured with a small hemostat to occlude flow

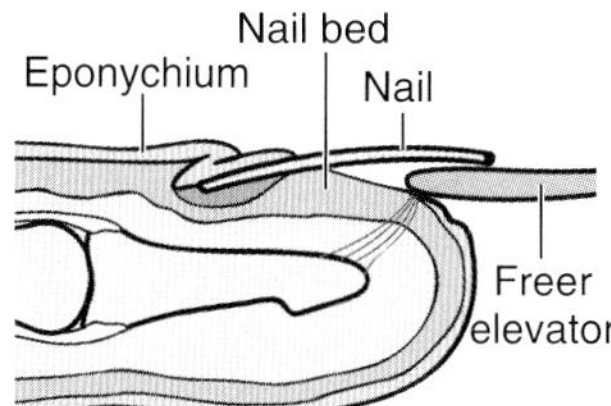

Figure 27-3 Freer elevator placed under the nail. The nail bed is made up of the germinal matrix proximal to the lunula and the sterile matrix distally.

through the digital vessels. Depending on the site of the injury and personal preferences, there are two techniques to remove the nail and visualize the nail bed.

Distal Technique

The Freer elevator is placed under the free edge of the nail (Fig. 27-3) and advanced proximally, following the plane of cleavage between the nail plate and the nail bed. Substantial resistance is encountered along the nail bed until the germinal matrix is reached, where the progress becomes easier. Be careful to avoid advancing the elevator excessively into the proximal nail groove. Now gently work the elevator medially and laterally to free up the last of the soft tissue attachments deep to the nail plate. Place the elevator under the cuticle (on the dorsum of the nail; Fig. 27-4) and dissect under the ventral portion of the proximal nail fold. Continue the dissection laterally on both sides to release any remaining soft tissue attachment while a hemostat is used to apply gentle distal traction, pulling distally. (The goal is to free the nail from any residual soft tissue attachments while not digging too deeply into either the proximal or lateral folds and not worsening any existing trauma.)

Proximal Technique

The proximal approach is often used when a distal cleavage plane cannot be identified because trauma or other pathology (such as onychomycosis) exists. The Freer elevator is placed under the cuticle and advanced to the proximal nail fold and worked to free the proximal and lateral gutters while avoiding damage to the cells in the depth of the folds. Proximal relaxing incisions (Fig. 27-5) facilitate exposure. Advance the elevator to locate the proximal edge of the nail plate. The skin hooks are now used to hold the eponychium folded proximally while the elevator comes over the top, then directed distally just deep to the nail plate as it dissects the plane between the nail plate and the nail bed. Keep the plane of the elevator turned so that the blade conforms as well as possible to the exact curvature of the nail plate in all areas.

General Considerations for Repair

When the nail is removed (by the trauma or the surgeon), carefully cleanse the area and examine it with magnification. Make an

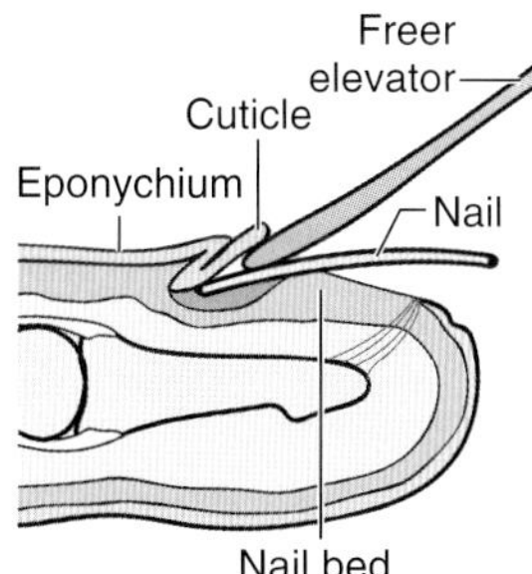

Figure 27-4 Freer elevator placed under the cuticle.

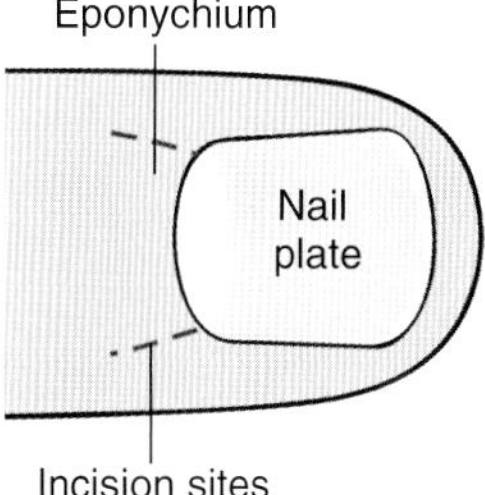

Figure 27-5 Proximal relaxing incisions are used to facilitate exposure.

adequate record of the status of the entire nail bed, the proximal and lateral nail folds, and the hyponychium. Record these findings as part of the operative findings of the distal phalanx.

Carefully scrape any residual nail bed tissue off the nail undersurface, and place the nail in sterile saline to soak while the nail bed is examined. With the tourniquet inflated, cleanse and lavage the nail bed. With excellent light and magnification, the defects can be identified and any gross irregularities trimmed while leaving all the tissue that can be repaired and contoured.

The best sutures for nail bed repair are absorbable 6-0 or 7-0 chromic or Vicryl. (Zook and colleagues [1980] have recommended 7-0 chromic on a micropoint spatula, double-armed, GS-9, ophthalmic needle [Ethicon, Somerville, NJ].) Either a 5-0 or 6-0 monofilament suture is used to repair lacerations or incisions in the skin.

Sometimes the germinal matrix and nail bed may be avulsed from their proximal origin below the proximal fold. When this occurs, use of a monofilament (5-0 or 6-0) horizontal mattress suture (Fig. 27-6) restores the anatomy.

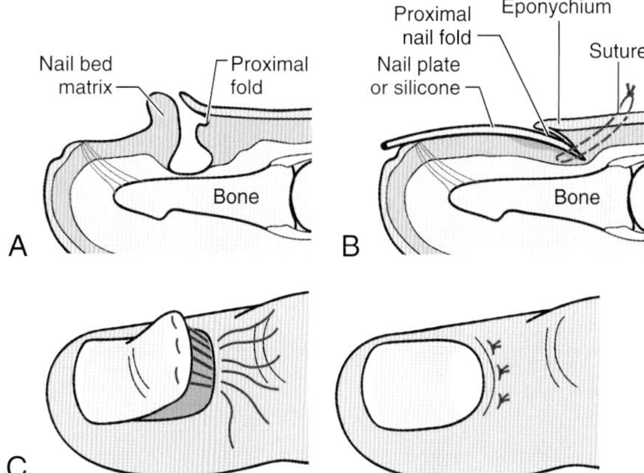

Figure 27-6 Proximal nail bed avulsion. The nail plate has been removed. The *nail bed* consists of the germinal and the sterile matrix. The *matrix* extends from a point just distal to the insertion of the extensor tendon to the end of the fingernail attachment. The *germinal matrix*, which produces most of the nail, begins just 3 to 5 mm proximal and deep to the *eponychium* and extends distally to the lunula. The *lunula* is the white portion of the germinal matrix just beyond the *cuticle*. It marks the end of that portion of the germinal matrix that produces the fingernail. The *sterile matrix* begins proximally at the distal edge of the lunula and extends distally to the *hyponychium*. It also plays some role in production of the nail. The *eponychium* is the flap or tuft of skin that covers over the proximal nail. **A,** Nail bed has been avulsed from its normal location and displaced dorsally. **B,** Horizontal mattress suture through the nail wall is used to anchor the nail bed into proper site for healing. Proximal nail fold must be held open (with fingernail or substitute) to prevent scarring down and closure of nail fold. The nail plate or silicone sheet has been placed and anchored (with suture) to hold the proximal nail fold open. **C,** Appearance of wound after suturing. Sutures are removed from the nail in 3 weeks. The replaced nail or silicone sheet will dislodge in 1 to 3 months. (**C,** From Chudnofsky CR, Sebastian S: Special wounds: Nail bed, plantar puncture, and cartilage. Emerg Med Clin North Am 10:808–822, 1992.)

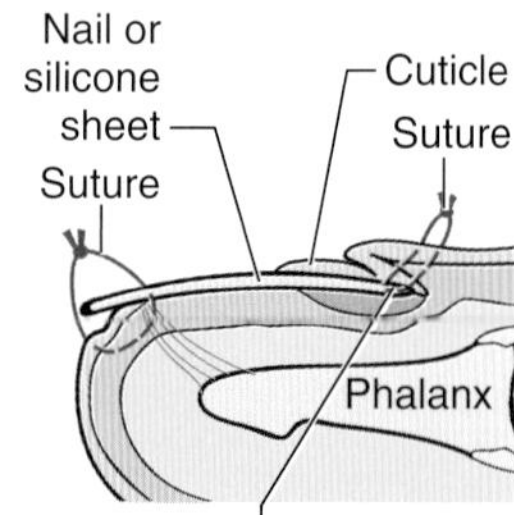

Figure 27-7 Replacement of the nail or substitute. The nail fold is held open to prevent it from scarring down when the nail bed has been avulsed or severely damaged. The nail itself or a silicone sheet is anchored by the horizontal mattress suture.

After repair of the nail bed, replace the nail. The nail serves as a stent to keep the nail folds open and to approximate the edges of the repair. The nail is well stabilized by the placement of a 5-0 or 6-0 monofilament suture through the nail into the fingertip area.

If the nail is not available or is damaged too badly to use as a stent, alternative materials may be used to provide contouring and protection to the nail bed. Materials such as medical-grade silicone sheeting (0.020 inch), petrolatum gauze, or Xeroform can be shaped to approximate the original nail (Fig. 27-7). They must be placed carefully so that they occupy the space of the proximal and lateral nail folds to prevent them from permanently scarring down. These stents must be anchored by a 6-0 monofilament or similar suture through the proximal portion of the nail folds to ensure their position. These stents will (1) protect the nail bed while healing, (2) maintain the contour of the nail bed and subsequent nail plate, and (3) prevent adherence of the proximal nail fold to the matrix.

Avoid making the postoperative dressing too tight. Instruct the patient to elevate the hand at all times. If nonadherent gauze is used as a stent on the nail bed to hold open the nail folds, the sutures may be removed at 7 to 10 days and gauze will subsequently peel off on its own. If the nail plate has been replaced, it will usually come off in about 3 weeks. Explain to the patient that the fingernail will require 6 to 12 months to grow out and to allow its final status to be determined. Trim the advancing rough edges to prevent accidental snags.

Classification of Nail Bed Injuries

The *type I* nail bed injury (Fig. 27-8A) is a small hematoma (<30% of visible nail) with no major matrix injury. Any injury that produces a subungual hematoma can be classified as a type I injury, including superficial lacerations of the nail bed.

The *type II* injury (Fig. 27-8B) is a large hematoma (>30% of visible nail) with a likely matrix injury (e.g., a severe crushing injury). These injuries have a poor prognosis because the fragments are much more difficult to reassemble anatomically and the viability of this tissue is severely reduced compared with that of simple or stellate lacerations. The need for radiographs to visualize fracture patterns and stability is increasingly important in these more complex injuries. The same general techniques as described previously are used, but more time is spent informing the patient of the poor prognosis and of the likely need for further surgery and possible partial or complete loss of the nail.

A *type III* nail bed injury (Fig. 27-8C) with or without a hematoma has a phalangeal fracture (distal phalangeal fracture–nail bed lacerations). These fractures may be nondisplaced or displaced and, more important, stable or unstable.

A *type IV* nail bed injury has extensive matrix fragmentation, but the bone is intact. The proximal nail plate may or may not be avulsed from the proximal nail fold (Fig. 27-8D).

A *type V* nail bed injury, involving matrix avulsion, can be categorized as follows:

- Avulsed segment available for repair (Fig. 27-8E)
- Small avulsion (less than 2 mm width)
- Large avulsion that requires a split- or full-thickness graft from adjacent finger or toe donor site

Treatment Guidelines

Type I injuries often go untreated or may benefit from decompression if throbbing pain occurs when the hematoma is small.

Type II injuries involve nail removal and suture repair of the nail matrix. Replace the nail plate as a template into the proximal and lateral nail folds, and anchor with 5-0 nylon sutures through the

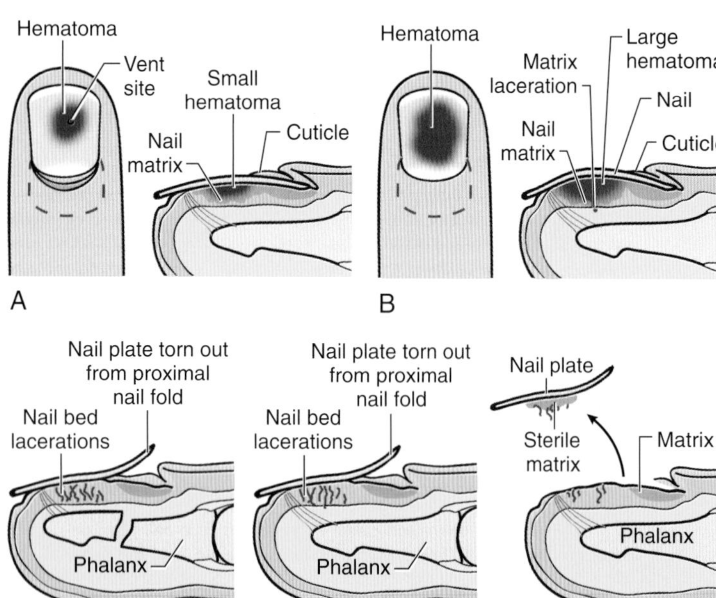

Figure 27-8 **A,** Type I nail bed injury: small hematoma. **B,** Type II nail bed injury: large hematoma (>30%) with likely matrix injury. **C,** Type III nail bed injury with phalangeal fracture. **D,** Type IV nail bed injury: extensive matrix injury with intact phalanx. **E,** Type V nail bed injury with matrix avulsion. This particular matrix avulsion shows an avulsed segment available for repair.

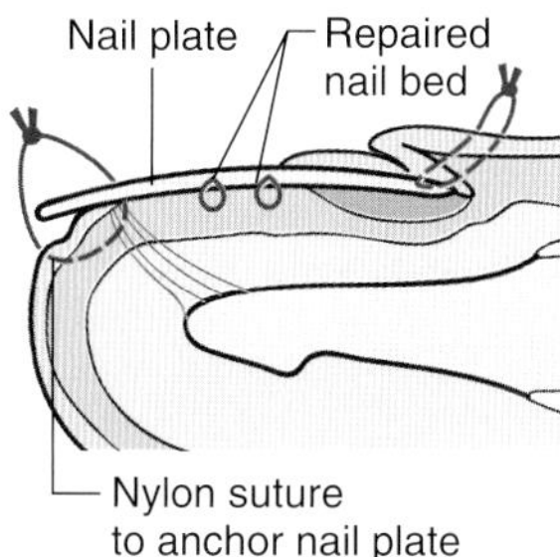

Figure 27-9 Repair of type II injury with nail reattached. The nail bed is repaired and the nail plate or substitute is anchored proximally and distally.

distal nail and hyponychium to prevent accidental removal (Fig. 27-9).

A careful search of the nail fragments should be undertaken to find segments of nail bed that can then be removed carefully with a small elevator and reattached to the nail bed as a free graft to reapproximate the original undamaged nail bed. Again, the intact nail plate or the silicone sheet is used to contour and protect the nail bed during the healing stage.

With *type III* injuries, remove the nail. Stabilize unstable or displaced fractures with small K-wires. Repair the viable matrix with absorbable suture and replace the nail for splinting (Fig. 27-10). If the nail is unavailable or unusable, create a template from sterile silicone sheeting (0.020 inch) and secure in the place of the nail plate.

If the fracture is nondisplaced at the time of the x-ray examination but is so unstable when examined surgically that it cannot be trusted to remain in anatomic position, it must be stabilized with K-wire fixation. Any inadvertent displacement of the dorsal phalangeal cortex during the healing leads to nail bed irregularities and resultant deformed fingernails. The previous principles of repair apply, and serial radiographs are required to verify position of bone fragments and to observe for indication of osteomyelitis. *As in other open fractures, prophylactic antibiotics are required until indication of proper wound healing is demonstrated.*

With *type IV* injuries, remove the nail and carefully repair the epithelial fragments. This may involve trimming some severely traumatized fragments with very minimal débridement because the nail plate will hold the fragments down into a vascular bed and contour them to heal with the nail bed.

With *type V* injuries, perform the following:

- With an available avulsed segment, carefully remove it from the nail plate and reattach to the nail bed with a 6-0 or 7-0 absorbable suture.
- Small avulsions (<2 mm wide) may be closed primarily if the nail bed can be undermined with a small elevator and the tissue closed without tension through the use of a 6-0 or 7-0 absorbable suture.
- Larger avulsions require split- or full-thickness grafts from adjacent fingers or toes (see Shepard, 1990a and 1990b).

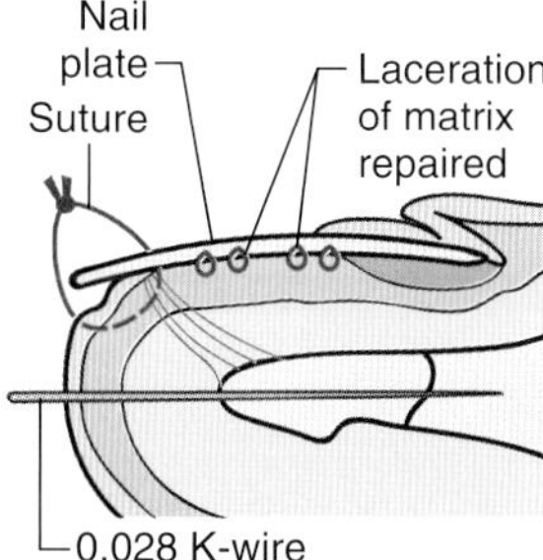

Figure 27-10 Repair of type III injury. The unstable fracture is stabilized, the matrix repaired, and the nail plate secured by nylon suture.

As mentioned previously, with an avulsed nail bed, look carefully for remnants of the nail bed on large pieces of the nail plate that may accompany the patient. Ask family members or coworkers to look for any amputated fingertips, which may provide needed tissue for the nail bed reconstruction. Sometimes a fingernail and part of the nail bed may still be inside a glove that was worn at the time of injury. If an adjacent finger was amputated or is otherwise irreparable, it may serve as a donor for a full- or partial-thickness nail bed graft for the defect in question. A small defect may be repaired with a small split-thickness graft from an undamaged segment of the involved nail. In larger defects a split-thickness graft from the sterile matrix (do not include the germinal matrix) of the great toe can be used. After removal of the great toenail, use a sterile surgical blade with a thick graft sawing motion to shave approximately 0.014 inch from the nail bed (it is preferable to cut too thin than too thick). Carefully sew the graft in place with fine absorbable sutures, reapply the nail or other template, and secure in place when properly positioned to maintain the proximal and lateral folds in an open position.

In general, consider perioperative antibiotic use for type III, IV, and V injuries, including distal amputations. Verify that tetanus status is up to date because many of these wounds are grossly contaminated.

Late Reconstruction of the Nail Matrix

Delayed reconstruction efforts are frequently associated with disappointment for the patient and the physician. Patients must know up front that odds of a major improvement after surgery are very guarded, and it is possible for the nail to look even worse regardless of best efforts and surgical technique.

- *Nail ridges* can result from either a scar below the nail bed or a fracture healing with a prominence on the dorsal phalangeal surface. Correction requires smoothing of the healed bone surface and removal of the scar tissue. The defect created by the scar removal must be closed either by undermining and direct approximation or by grafting, as mentioned previously.
- *Split nails* can result from a ridge or longitudinal scar in the germinal or sterile matrix. Resection of the scar in the sterile matrix and use of a free graft, if primary closure is impossible, may be helpful. Use of the proximal eponychial incisions to visualize and graft the germinal matrix may provide some improvement. Some authors advocate use of the second toe as a donor rather than the great toe to avoid cosmetic alteration of the larger great toenail. Use a germinal matrix graft of similar size and shape to fill the resected scar site, as a free graft.
- *Nonadherence* of the nail is caused from scars in the sterile matrix. Resection of the scar and replacement with a free split- or full-thickness matrix graft provides the best results.

CPT/Billing Codes

11760 Repair of nail bed
11762 Reconstruction of nail bed with graft

ICD-9-CM Diagnostic Codes

883.0 Wound, open, nail, finger(s), thumb
883.1 Complicated
893.0 Wound, open, nail, toe(s)
893.1 Complicated

ACKNOWLEDGMENT

The editors wish to recognize the contributions by Douglas R. Jackson, MD, to this chapter in the previous two editions of this book.

BIBLIOGRAPHY

Denkler K: A comprehensive review of epinephrine in the finger: To do or not to do. Plast Reconstr Surg 108:114–124, 2001.

Denkler K: Dupuytren's fasciectomies in 60 consecutive digits using lidocaine with epinephrine and no tourniquet. Plast Reconstr Surg 115: 802–810, 2005.

Fitzcharles-Bowe C, Denkler K, Lalonde D: Finger injections with high-dose (1 : 1000) epinephrine: Does it cause finger necrosis and should it be treated? Hand (NY) 2:5–11, 2007.

Fleckman P, Christopher A: Surgical anatomy of the nail unit. Dermatol Surg 27:257–260, 2001.

Hanke E, Lawry M: Nail surgery. In Robinson JK, Hanke DW, Sengelmann RD, Siegel DM (eds): Surgery of the Skin: Procedural Dermatology. Philadelphia, Mosby, 2005, pp 719–742.

Krunic AL, Wang LC, Soltani K, et al: Digital anesthesia with epinephrine: An old myth revisited. J Am Acad Dermatol 51:755–759, 2004.

Lalonde D, Bell M, Sparkes G, et al: A multicenter prospective study of 3110 consecutive cases of elective epinephrine use in the fingers and hand: The Dalhousie Project clinical phase. J Hand Surg Am 30:1061–1067, 2005.

Moossavi M, Scher RK: Complications of nail surgery: A review of the literature. Dermatol Surg 27:225–228, 2001.

Radovic P, Smith RG, Shumway D: Revisiting epinephrine in foot surgery. J Am Podiatr Med Assoc 93:157–160, 2003.

Reardon CM, McArthur PA, Survana SK, Brotherston TM: The surface anatomy of the germinal matrix of the nail bed in the finger. J Hand Surg Br 24:531–533, 1999.

Rich P: Nail biopsy: Indications and methods. Dermatol Surg 27:229–234, 2001.

Scher RK, Daniel CR III (eds): Nails: Therapy, Diagnosis, Surgery. Philadelphia, WB Saunders, 1990.

Shepard GH: Management of acute nail bed avulsions. Hand Clin 6:39–56, 1990a.

Shepard GH: Nail grafts for reconstruction. Hand Clin 6:79–102, 1990b.

Thomson CJ, Lalonde DH, Denkler KA, Feicht AJ: A critical look at the evidence for and against elective epinephrine use in the finger. Plast Reconstr Surg 119:260–266, 2007.

Van Beek AL, Kassan MA, Adson MH, Dale V: Management of acute fingernail injuries. Hand Clin 6:23–35, 1990.

Zook EG, Van Beek AL, Russell RC, Beatty ME: Anatomy and physiology of the perionychium: A review of the literature and anatomic study. J Hand Surg 5:528–536, 1980.

EDITOR'S NOTE: There is some controversy regarding the necessity to remove the nail regardless of the hematoma size. Traditional teaching recommended removal. The study by Roser and Gellman (1999) and others questions this practice. Consult the following sources:

Fieg EL: Letter to the editor. Am Fam Physician 65:1997, 2002.

Lammes RL, Trott AT: Methods of wound closure. In Roberts JR, Hedges JR (eds): Clinical Procedures in Emergency Medicine, 2nd ed. Philadelphia, WB Saunders, 1998.

Roser SE, Gellman H: Comparison of nail bed repair versus nail trephination for subungual hematomas in children. J Hand Surg Am 24:1166–1170, 1999.

Selbst SM, Magdy A: Minor trauma: Lacerations. In Fleisher GR, Ludwig S (eds): Textbook of Pediatric Emergency Medicine, 4th ed. Philadelphia, Lippincott Williams & Wilkins, 2001, p 1493.

Wang QC, Johnson BA: Fingertip injuries. Am Fam Physician 63:1961–1966, 2001.

CHAPTER 28

NAIL PLATE, NAIL BED, AND NAIL MATRIX BIOPSY

Steven E. Roskos

Nail biopsy is a simple procedure that can be used to diagnose tumors, inflammatory diseases, and infections of the nail. *Nail plate* biopsy is the simplest of the nail biopsies and is useful for diagnosing proximal subungual onychomycosis as well as distinguishing melanoma from other types of nail pigmentation. *Nail bed* biopsy is helpful in diagnosing many disorders, including psoriasis, lichen planus, squamous cell carcinoma, melanoma, and subungual epidermoid inclusions. *Nail matrix* biopsy is used to distinguish between benign pigmented streaks (longitudinal melanonychia) and melanoma.

The presence of melanocytes in the germinal tissue of the nail matrix makes this a possible site for development of melanoma. Primary subungual melanomas frequently appear as pigmented bands or streaks in the nail plate, and they account for up to 3.5% of all cutaneous malignant melanomas (15% to 20% in blacks). Distinction between the numerous benign causes of pigmented streaks (trauma, malnutrition, and normal occurrence in many blacks and Asians) and malignant lesions is frequently difficult. Biopsy is often recommended to confirm the diagnosis.

ANATOMY

The *nail plate* is the hard, translucent structure composed of keratinized squamous cells, commonly called the "nail" itself. The *nail bed* refers to the softer tissue beneath the nail that provides germinal tissue for the nail plate and to which the nail plate is attached (Fig. 28-1). The nail matrix lies beneath the proximal nail fold and synthesizes 90% of the nail plate.

INDICATIONS

- Thickened, distorted nail plate with a negative evaluation for fungal infection (potassium hydroxide [KOH] scraping, culture)
- Longitudinal pigmented linear streak in the nail plate suspect for malignancy
- Tumor of the nail bed
- Subungual hyperkeratosis
- Diagnosis of disorders such as psoriasis and lichen planus

CONTRAINDICATIONS

- Allergy or sensitivity to local anesthetics (see Chapter 4, Local Anesthesia)
- Bleeding diathesis or uncontrolled anticoagulation therapy (no need to stop warfarin, aspirin, or clopidogrel)

EQUIPMENT

- Antiseptic (chlorhexidine, povidone–iodine, or alcohol)
- Sterile gloves
- 3-mm disposable skin biopsy punch
- Local anesthetic (e.g., 1% or 2% lidocaine) *without* epinephrine
- 27-gauge needle (for toes) or 30-gauge needle (for fingers)
- Sterile scissors with straight blades (or a narrow Locke periosteal elevator)
- Sterile rubber band, small Penrose drain, or Ellman disposable digit tourniquet
- Two sterile, straight hemostats
- 5-0 or 6-0 nylon suture
- Needle driver
- No. 15 scalpel (for nail matrix biopsy)
- Fine sterile scissors with curved blades (for nail matrix biopsy)
- Steri-Strips (for nail matrix biopsy)
- Tissue forceps (for nail matrix biopsy)
- Xeroform gauze
- Sterile gauze and tubular gauze dressing
- Antibiotic ointment (Bacitracin or Polysporin)
- Adhesive bandage or an adhesive wrap like Coban or Co-Flex tape
- Suture scissors
- Sterile specimen container filled with 10% formalin (for histology)
- Sterile specimen container without formalin (for fungal culture)

PRECAUTIONS

When sampling the nail matrix, be careful not to damage the proximal matrix. Most linear melanomas (95%) originate from the distal matrix. Biopsies of the distal nail matrix are very unlikely to produce permanent scarring because this part of the matrix produces the ventral portion of the nail plate. Biopsies of the proximal nail matrix will usually cause a permanent nail plate abnormality in the form of a longitudinal fissure. For pigmented streaks less than 3 mm wide, punch biopsy as described in this chapter is an adequate technique. Larger lesions require more extensive excision and are more likely to cause nail deformity.

PREPROCEDURE PATIENT EDUCATION

It is important to explain to the patient what information you hope to gain from the biopsy and how it will affect treatment decisions. Explain that a biopsy is not guaranteed to produce an accurate diagnosis. Describe the procedure in detail, including the anesthesia. Make sure the patient understands the risks, which include bleeding, distortion of the nail during regrowth, infection, onycholysis (separation of nail from nail bed), permanent nail abnormality, and scarring. The patient should be given an opportunity to read the patient education handout and the consent form before signing it (see patient education and patient consent forms online at www.expertconsult.com).

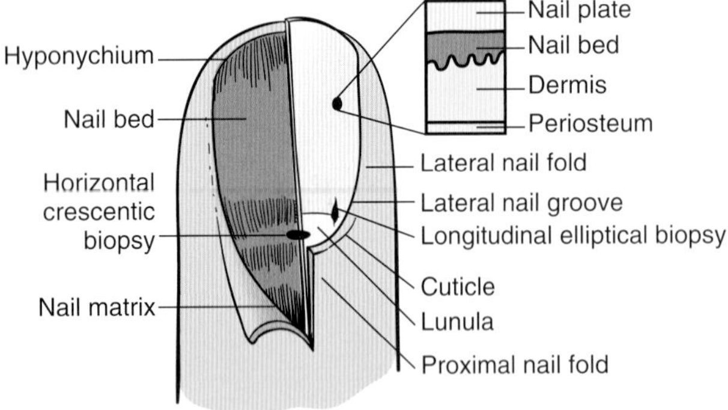

Figure 28-1 Anatomy of the nail, dorsal view. Also shows possible shapes for obtaining a nail biopsy.

TECHNIQUE

Nail Plate (Nail) Biopsy

1. Soak the affected digit and nail in warm water for 10 minutes to soften the nail plate.
2. With steady pressure, hold the punch perpendicular to the nail; rotation of the punch will produce a round biopsy specimen without pain. No anesthetic is required.
3. Elevate the biopsy sample and lyse the underlying nail bed tissue with the scissors or scalpel.
4. Place the specimen in a sterile container if it is being sent for fungal culture, or a formalin-filled container if it is being sent for histology or periodic-acid Schiff (PAS) staining.

Nail Bed Biopsy

1. Soak the digit in warm water for 10 minutes to soften the nail plate.
2. Prepare the patient's hand with antiseptic.
3. Perform a distal wing block or a digital block using 2% lidocaine without epinephrine (Fig. 28-2; see Chapter 8, Peripheral Nerve Blocks and Field Blocks).
4. Apply a tourniquet to decrease bleeding at the site and allow easier removal of specimen.
5. Partially remove the nail plate according to the procedure outlined in Chapter 29, Ingrown Toenails.
6. When the affected nail bed has been exposed, use a 3- or 4-mm punch to obtain the biopsy specimen as close as possible to the proximal origin of the pigmentation. However, there is a higher chance of a deformed nail if the biopsy is obtained from the root portion of the nail under the proximal nail fold. The biopsy specimen should be 2 to 3 mm in thickness. Alternatively, small elliptical excisions can be made (see Fig. 28-1 and Chapter 32, Skin Biopsy).
7. Close the biopsy site with one or two 5-0 or 6-0 nylon sutures oriented along the longitudinal plane.
8. Remove the tourniquet.
9. Apply a dressing of antibiotic ointment and sterile gauze.

Nail Matrix Biopsy

1. Soak the digit in warm water for 10 minutes to soften the nail plate.
2. Prepare the patient's hand with antiseptic.
3. Perform a digital block using lidocaine without epinephrine (see Fig. 28-2).
4. Apply a tourniquet to decrease bleeding at the site and allow easier removal of specimen.
5. Make two lateral incisions in the proximal nail fold at an angle of 45 degrees using a no. 15 scalpel (Fig. 28-3).
6. Use a periosteal elevator to detach the proximal nail fold from the nail plate. This should expose the entire nail plate and allow you to visualize the origin of the pigmented streak (longitudinal melanonychia). The nail plate can be left in place (Fig. 28-4) or reflected (see Fig. 28-3).
7. Place a 3-mm punch against and perpendicular to the nail plate directly over the origin of the pigmented streak (see Fig. 28-4A).
8. Rotate the punch between the thumb and forefinger.
9. After scoring the nail, check to be sure the origin of the band is entirely encompassed by the punch.
10. Reapply the punch and continue to rotate until you contact bone.
11. Gently lyse adhesions to the bone using fine curved scissors (see Fig. 28-4B).
12. Gently remove the specimen using the scissors or tissue forceps and place the whole specimen, including nail plate (which may be stuck inside the punch), in the formalin-filled specimen container. *Be careful not to crush the specimen.*

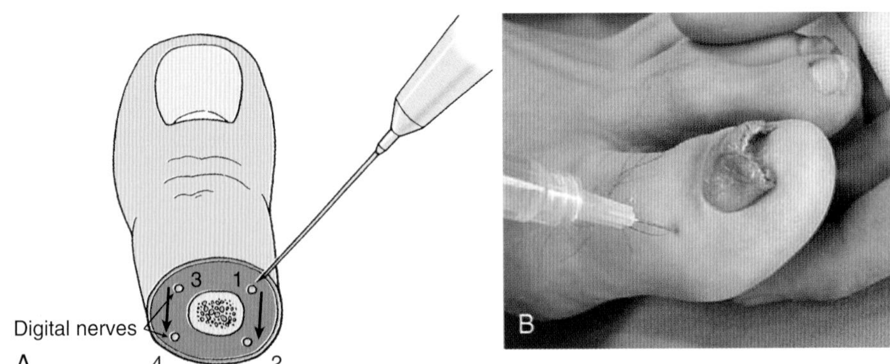

Figure 28-2 **A,** Ring block technique for digital nerve block. 1, Raise a wheal at the dorsal surface of the base of the digit. 2, Direct the needle toward the plantar surface, delivering 1 mL of anesthetic to the extensor and 1 mL to the plantar branches of the digital nerve. 3, Perform a second puncture at the corresponding site of the other side. 4, Advance the needle in the plantar direction to allow delivery of 1 mL of anesthetic to each branch of the digital nerve. A minimum of 4 mL of anesthetic is used. Also see Chapter 8, Peripheral Nerve Blocks and Field Blocks. **B,** Administering a distal wing block. Insert needle 5 to 8 mm proximal and lateral to the junction of the proximal nail fold and lateral nail fold. Inject anesthetic until it progresses as far as possible down the nail fold toward the tip of the digit, distending and blanching the lateral nail fold. This has the appearance of a "wing." Repeat on the other side of the nail. If necessary, inject at other already anesthetized areas around the nail until the entire digital tip is swollen and white. (**B,** From Richert B: Basic nail surgery. Dermatol Clin 24:313–322, 2006.)

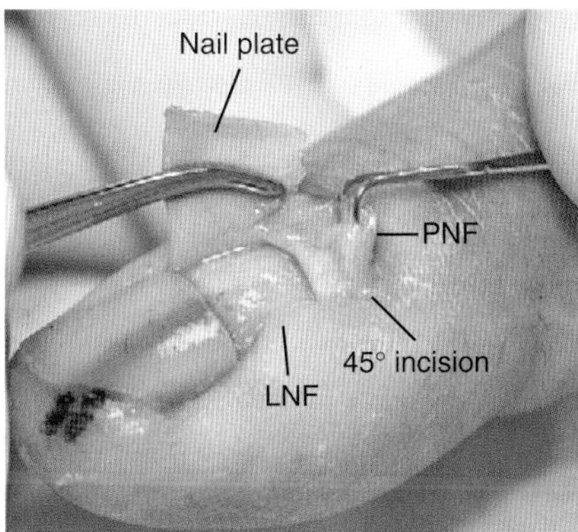

Figure 28-3 Proximal nail fold (PNF) is reflected (with skin hook) and proximal nail plate is partially avulsed and reflected (with hemostat), exposing the nail matrix. The nail plate can be reattached with nylon sutures to the lateral nail fold (LNF). (From Jellinek N: Nail matrix biopsy of longitudinal melanonychia: Diagnostic algorithm including the matrix shave biopsy. J Am Acad Dermatol 56:803–810, 2007.)

13. Apply Steri-Strips to the two lateral incisions and the defect in the nail plate.
14. Remove the tourniquet.
15. Dress the site as described in the next section.

The possible shapes and types of biopsies are summarized in Figure 28-5.

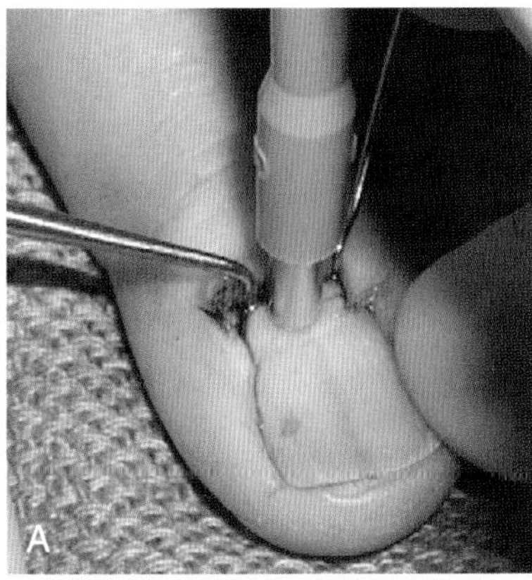

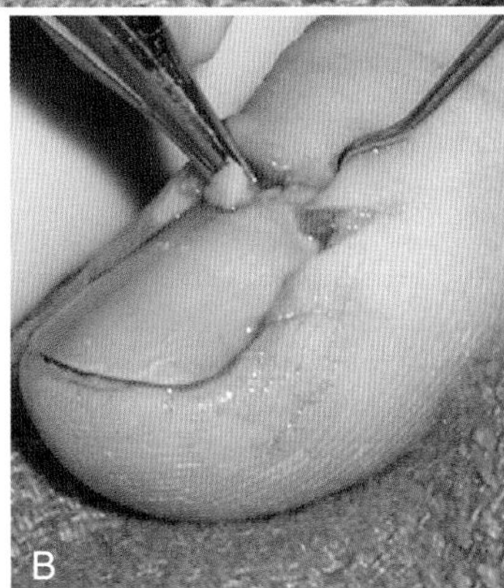

Figure 28-4 **A,** Nail matrix biopsy with nail plate in place. The proximal nail fold is reflected (with skin hooks, optional) while punch is held perpendicular to nail plate over origin of linear pigmentation (nail plate has not been reflected in this figure). Scarring is more likely to occur if the germinal matrix is sampled. **B,** Removing punch sample. Gently lyse adhesions to the bone using fine curved scissors, held nearly perpendicular to the nail plate. (From Jellinek N: Nail matrix biopsy of longitudinal melanonychia: Diagnostic algorithm including the matrix shave biopsy. J Am Acad Dermatol 56:803–810, 2007.)

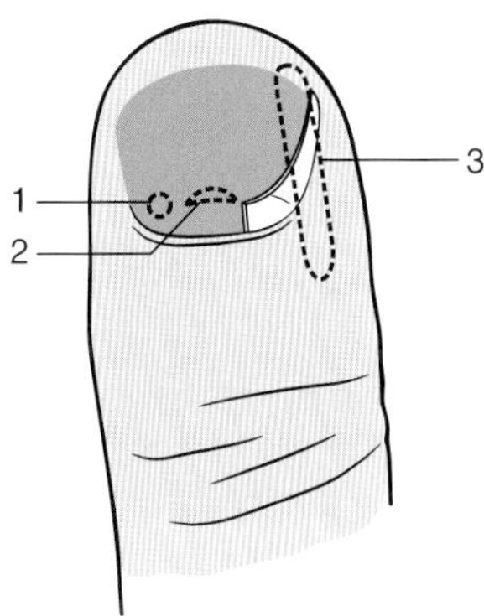

Figure 28-5 Alternative biopsy techniques. 1, Punch biopsy of nail matrix; 2, transverse biopsy of nail matrix, used for longitudinal pigmented streaks between 3 and 6 mm; 3, longitudinal nail biopsy for lateral nail pigmentation. (From Braun RP, Baran R, Le Gal FA, et al: Diagnosis and management of nail pigmentation. J Am Acad Dermatol 56:835–847, 2007.)

Postprocedure Management

1. Apply topical astringent (e.g., Monsel's solution), remove the tourniquet, and control bleeding with pressure.
2. Place a bulky dressing of gauze over the surgical site (except for the nail plate biopsy, where a simple adhesive bandage may be applied over antibiotic ointment). Use multiple 2 × 2 gauze pads, folded in half and wrapped over the nail transversely and longitudinally. Secure these with significant pressure and tape or adhesive dressing.
3. Observe the patient for 10 to 15 minutes. If blood soaks through the bandage, apply pressure to the lateral digital arteries and remove the bandage. Apply a clean, dry gauze pressure dressing while holding pressure on the arteries.

Postprocedure Patient Education

The patient should keep the limb elevated until the next day to decrease throbbing. Acetaminophen or ibuprofen may be used for pain. If the patient experiences increasing pain several hours after the procedure, the dressing may be acting as a tourniquet and should be removed. Otherwise, the patient should leave the dressing in place for 24 to 48 hours, after which he or she may remove the dressing, wash the wound with a 1 : 1 mixture of hydrogen peroxide and tap water or simple soap and water, and apply a large adhesive bandage over a gauze and antibiotic ointment. The patient should repeat this procedure two to three times daily until the area has healed.

Nail Biopsy Encounter Form

See Encounter Form, Nail Biopsy, online at www.expertconsult.com.

Complications

- Bleeding
- Infection
- Distortion of nail with regrowth and permanent nail abnormality (the greatest concern if the germinal matrix is sampled)
- Onycholysis (separation of the nail plate from the nail bed)
- Scarring

CPT/Billing Codes

11730 Avulsion of nail plate, partial or single
11732 Avulsion, each additional
11755 Biopsy nail unit, any method
11765 Wedge excision of skin of nail fold (e.g., for ingrown toenail)

ICD-9-CM Diagnostic Codes

110.1 Dermatophytosis of nail
117.9 Other and unspecified mycoses
172.6 Malignant melanoma of skin, upper limb, including shoulder
172.7 Malignant melanoma of skin, lower limb, including hip
173.6 Other malignant neoplasm of skin, upper limb, including shoulder
173.7 Other malignant neoplasm of skin, lower limb, including hip
216.6 Benign neoplasm of skin, upper limb, including shoulder
216.7 Benign neoplasm of skin, lower limb, including hip
239.2 Neoplasm of unspecified nature of bone, soft tissue, and skin
703.8 Other specified diseases of nail (besides ingrowing nail); includes dystrophia unguium, hypertrophy of nail, koilonychia, leukonychia (punctata) (striata), onychauxis, onychogryphosis, onycholysis
703.9 Unspecified disease of nail

ONLINE RESOURCES

Onumah N, Scher RK: Nail surgery. eMedicine. Available at http://www.emedicine.com/derm/topic818.htm.

Sinni-McKeehen B, Rich P: Fungal nail infections: Treating from head to toe. Medscape. Available at http://medscape.com/viewarticle/470942_19.

See patient education and patient consent forms available online at www.expertconsult.com.

BIBLIOGRAPHY

André J, Lateur N: Pigmented nail disorders. Dermatol Clin 24:329–339, 2006.

Braun RP, Baran R, Le Gal FA, et al: Diagnosis and management of nail pigmentations. J Am Acad Dermatol 56:835–847, 2007.

Denkler K: A comprehensive review of epinephrine in the finger. To do or not to do. Plast Reconstr Surg 108:114–124, 2001.

Denkler K: Dupuytren's fasciectomies in 60 consecutive digits using lidocaine with epinephrine and no tourniquet. Plast Reconstr Surg 115: 802–810, 2005.

Fitzcharles-Bowe C, Denkler K, Lalonde D: Finger injection with high-dose (1:1000) epinephrine: Does it cause finger necrosis and should it be treated? Hand (NY) 2:5–11, 2007.

Jellinek N: Nail matrix biopsy of longitudinal melanonychia: Diagnostic algorithm including the matrix shave biopsy. J Am Acad Dermatol 56:803–810, 2007.

Jellinek NJ: Nail surgery: Practical tips and treatment options. Dermatol Ther 20:68–74, 2007.

Krunic AL, Wang LC, Soltani K, et al: Digital anesthesia with epinephrine: An old myth revisited. J Am Acad Dermatol 51:755–759, 2004.

Lalonde D, Bell M, Benoit P, et al: A multicenter prospective study of 3,110 consecutive cases of elective epinephrine use in the fingers and hand: The Dalhousie Project clinical phase. J Hand Surg Am 30:1061–1067, 2005.

Radovic P, Smith RG, Shumway D: Revisiting epinephrine in foot surgery. J Am Podiatr Med Assoc 93:157–160, 2003.

Richert B: Basic nail surgery. Dermatol Clin 24:313–322, 2006.

Thomson CJ, Lalonde DH, Denkler KA, Feicht AJ: A critical look at the evidence for and against elective epinephrine use in the finger. Plast Reconstr Surg 119:260–266, 2007.

Usatine RP: The Color Atlas of Family Medicine. New York, McGraw-Hill, 2009.

CHAPTER 29

Ingrown Toenails

Madelyn Pollock

Ingrown toenails usually present with pain, redness, swelling, and sometimes discharge. It is not uncommon for patients to have attempted self-remedies. Often, the irritation is long-standing enough to cause granulation tissue to form. The great toe is virtually the only toe involved, and either the medial or lateral border of the nail may be affected.

Figure 29-1 is an algorithm for the suggested treatment of an ingrown toenail.

Removal of the toenail, either partial or total, remains the definitive treatment for bothersome ingrown nails. For recurrent episodes, ablation of the germinal matrix tissue can be used to prevent regrowth of the nail. Permanent destruction can be effected using chemicals or radiofrequency energy.

Anatomy

Figure 29-2 illustrates the nail bed anatomy.

Indications

- Onychocryptosis (ingrown nail)
- Onychomycosis (fungal infection of the nail) with significant pain; without medical treatment, however, the fungus will recur
- Chronic, recurrent paronychia (inflammation of the nail fold)
- Onychogryposis (deformed, curved nail)

For a first occurrence, it is reasonable to remove only the offending portion of the nail and allow regrowth while educating the patient to correct all offending practices such as overtrimming nails and wearing tight-fitting shoes. If an ingrown nail recurs, permanent ablation of the portion of nail matrix causing the problem is indicated.

Contraindications

- Allergy to local anesthetics (see Chapter 5, Local and Topical Anesthetic Complications).
- Bleeding diathesis.
- Diabetes mellitus and peripheral vascular disease are relative contraindications and should be considered on a case-by-case basis.
- Pregnant patients should not have phenol ablation.

Equipment and Supplies

- 5- or 10-mL syringe with long (1½-inch) needle (25 or 27 gauge).
- Local anesthetic generally *without* epinephrine (e.g., 2% lidocaine with or without sodium bicarbonate buffer to decrease the sting; see Chapter 4, Local Anesthesia). Recent research does not confirm the previous concerns that epinephrine might cause excess vasoconstriction in the digits. However, with patients at high risk, such as those with long-standing diabetes or severe peripheral vascular disease, it might be best to avoid it.
- Narrow Locke periosteal elevator (nail elevator; Fig. 29-3).
- Sterile scissors with straight blades (or an English nail splitter [Fig. 29-4] or miniblade with wedge tip).
- Wide rubber band, small Penrose drain, donut digital tourniquet (Ellman Corp.; Fig. 29-5), or a portable blood pressure cuff (tourniquets are optional but very helpful).
- Two straight hemostats.
- Silver nitrate sticks for cautery of granulation tissue (optional). Best to curette this tissue off with a reusable dermal curette.
- Alcohol swabs.
- Povidone–iodine (Betadine) solution.

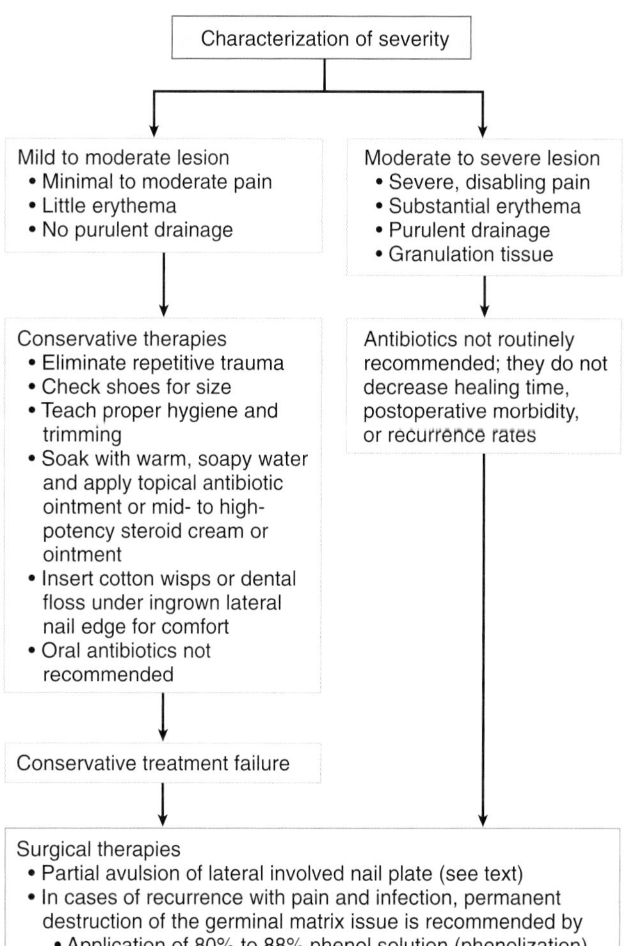

Figure 29-1 Algorithm for a suggested approach to the patient with an ingrown toenail. (Modified from Heidelbaugh JJ, Lee H: Management of the ingrown toenail. Am Fam Physician 79:303–308, 2009.)

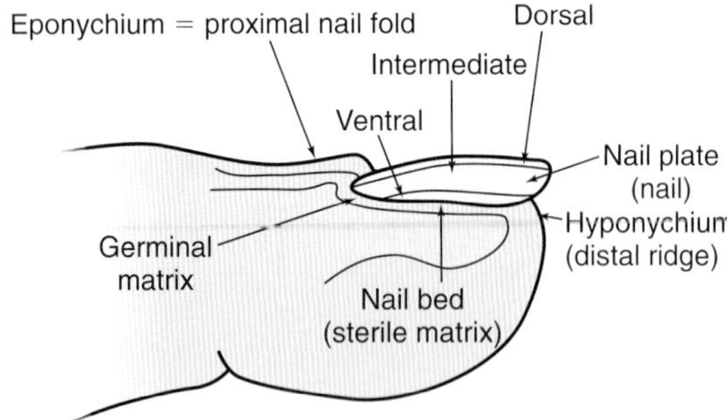

Figure 29-2 Nail bed anatomy and terminology. Also see more details in Chapter 27, Nail Bed Repair.

- Monsel's solution to control any possible bleeding after the tourniquet is removed.
- Sterile gauze and tubular gauze dressing.
- Antibiotic ointment (Polysporin or Bacitracin).
- Phenol solution (88%) and isopropyl alcohol for permanent ablation of the nail, if desired.
- As an alternative to phenol, the Ellman Surgitron (radiofrequency unit) with specially designed, Teflon-insulated matrix ablation tips (less inflammation and excellent results; see Chapter 30, Radiofrequency Surgery [Modern Electrosurgery]).

Preprocedure Patient Education and Consent

See the patient education form online at www.expertconsult.com.

A *signed* consent is not mandatory but the patient must be well informed of the procedures and the intended outcome. A patient education handout that explains the nature of ingrown nails is helpful. Before beginning the procedure, be sure the patient understands that providing anesthesia is uncomfortable, but after that there should be no pain. There is no guarantee that removing the portion of ingrown nail will resolve the problem, but generally it will if the nails are cared for properly afterward. The major benefit to removing the toenail (or a portion of it) is pain relief, with the secondary benefit of allowing the body to heal the inflamed area.

PROCEDURE

NOTE: Nonsterile gloves may be used in this procedure.

Removal of Partial or Full Nail

1. With the patient in the supine position, *prepare* the toe with Betadine. If the patient has significant discomfort, anesthesia (step 2) can precede this step for patient comfort.

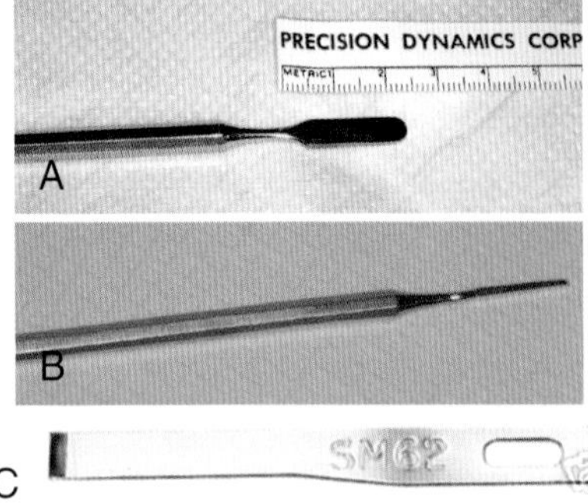

Figure 29-3 Locke periosteal elevator. **A,** Front view. **B,** Side view. **C,** Miniblade with wedge tip. (Courtesy of John L. Pfenninger, MD, The Medical Procedures Center, PC, Midland, Mich.)

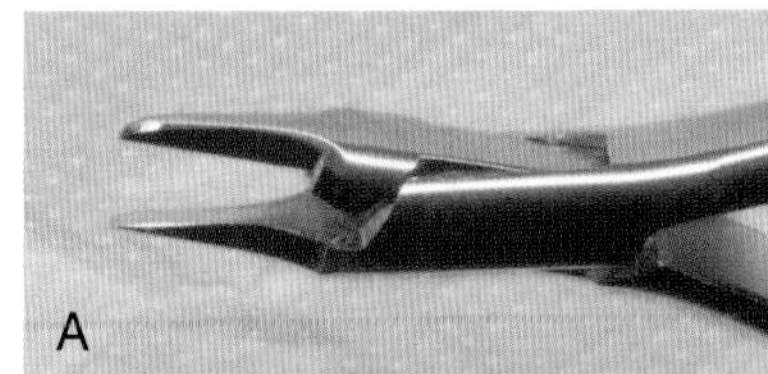

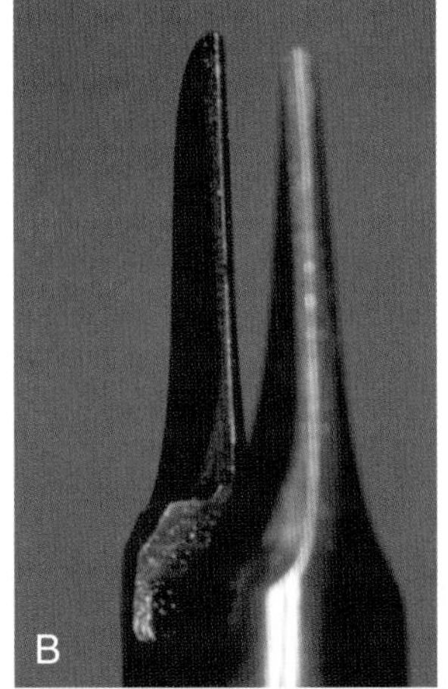

Figure 29-4 Nail splitter. **A,** Flat jaw on bottom. **B,** Beveled jaw on top. (Courtesy of John L. Pfenninger, MD, The Medical Procedures Center, PC, Midland, Mich.)

2. *Administer a digital block* as described in Chapter 8, Peripheral Nerve Blocks and Field Blocks.
3. *Apply a tourniquet* if desired. Options include the following:
   - Use a straight hemostat to firmly secure a wide rubber band or Penrose drain around the base of the toe.
   - Apply a blood pressure cuff at the calf so it will not affect the operative field. To use this method, place the cuff around the calf, elevate the foot to about a 45-degree angle at the hip, and, after 1 to 2 minutes of elevation, raise the cuff pressure to above systolic, lock the cuff it so it stays inflated, and then lower the foot to the operative field. Maintain the pressure until the procedure is completed.
   - The Ellman donut tourniquets (see Fig. 29-5) are disposable and come in various sizes. After the procedure, simply cut them with scissors to remove them.
4. Identify the portion of the nail to be removed, which is at least 20% to 25% of the nail.
5. When anesthesia is achieved (5 to 10 minutes), *loosen and lift the nail to be removed* from the nail bed by using the flat, rounded blade of the scissors, a single jaw of a straight hemostat, or a narrow periosteal elevator. The elevator works best to decrease the likelihood of injury to the nail bed (see Fig. 29-3). Introduce

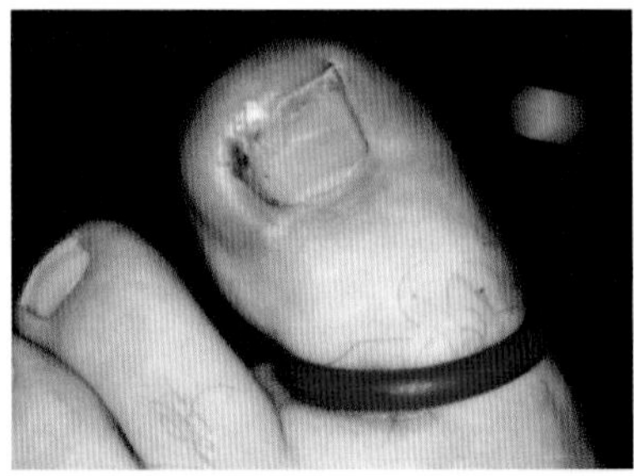

Figure 29-5 The Ellman digital tourniquet. (Courtesy of John L. Pfenninger, MD, The Medical Procedures Center, PC, Midland, Mich.)

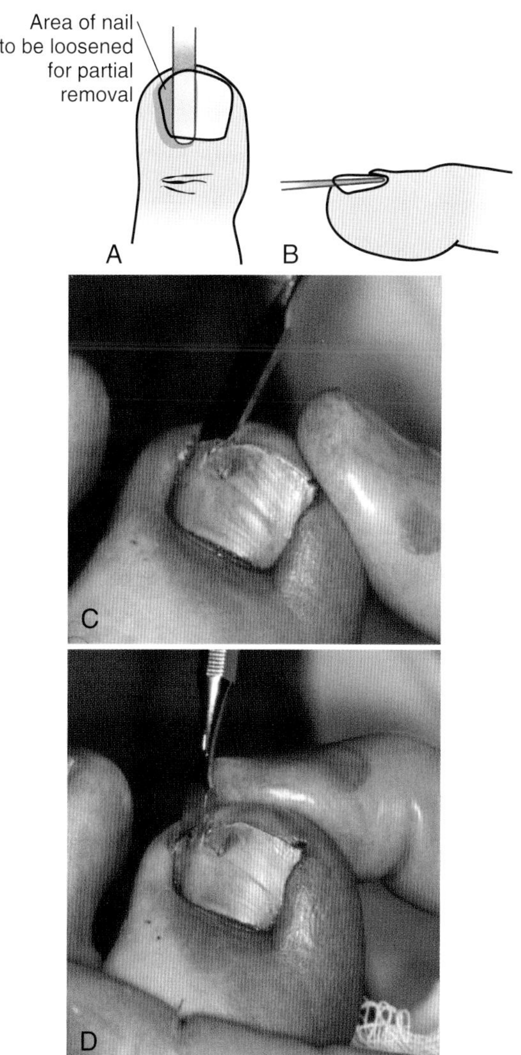

Figure 29-6 **A,** Periosteal elevator advanced all the way under the proximal nail fold. **B,** Lateral view. Advance with upward pressure on the nail with forward motion until more pressure is felt under the nail fold. **C,** Inserting the elevator. **D,** The instrument has been fully inserted, freeing up the lateral portion of the nail from the nail bed. (**C** and **D,** Courtesy of John L. Pfenninger, MD, The Medical Procedures Center, PC, Midland, Mich.)

and advance the instrument with continued upward pressure against the nail plate and away from the nail bed to minimize injury and bleeding (Fig. 29-6). It is important to completely free the proximal nail at its base under the nail fold to allow removal and to expose the germinal tissue of the nail bed. Push forward gently—the elevator moves easily when under the nail. Resistance will be felt when the proximal end of the nail plate has been loosened sufficiently. Release the entire nail plate in this fashion if the entire nail is to be removed.

6. For a partial nail removal, scissors or a nail splitter (see Fig. 29-4) should be used to *completely split the nail 5 to 6 mm in from the lateral or medial margin in a longitudinal direction* (Fig. 29-7). A miniblade with a wedge at the tip also works well. Include the base of the nail. This requires introducing your cutting instrument beneath the proximal nail fold. Take care to protect the nail fold from damage when making this part of the incision.
7. *Grasp that portion of the nail to be removed lengthwise with a straight hemostat and remove it,* using a steady pulling motion with a simultaneous upward twist of the hand toward the affected side (Fig. 29-8). This twisting action ensures that the nail will be rolled out from beneath the affected nail margin instead of rolling over it. *If the entire nail is to be removed,* the nail may be removed in two halves or in its entirety after a thorough loosening and lifting of the nail. In removing the entire nail, the forceps should apply lift and distal traction on the nail as it separates from the nail bed. Indications for total removal include onychomycosis that can cause painful pincer nails or perhaps having both the medial and lateral aspects of the nail ingrown (Fig. 29-9).
8. *Remove all granulation tissue* by grasping with hemostats and pulling. Light curettage with a reusable dermal curette (not as sharp as the disposables) removes any residual tissue from the nail groove. Without a tourniquet there will be significant bleeding during this portion of the procedure, especially if there is significant granulation tissue. Application of silver nitrate or Monsel's solution to the exposed nail bed will control bleeding and, with silver nitrate, discourage persistence of granulation tissue.
9. *If ablation is to be performed,* complete that portion at this step before the tourniquet is removed and the wound dressed (see later discussion).
10. *Remove any tourniquet* used.
11. Observe the area for hemostasis, using pressure as necessary. When hemostasis is obtained, *dress with antibiotic ointment, nonadherent gauze pad, and tube gauze* (Fig. 29-10).

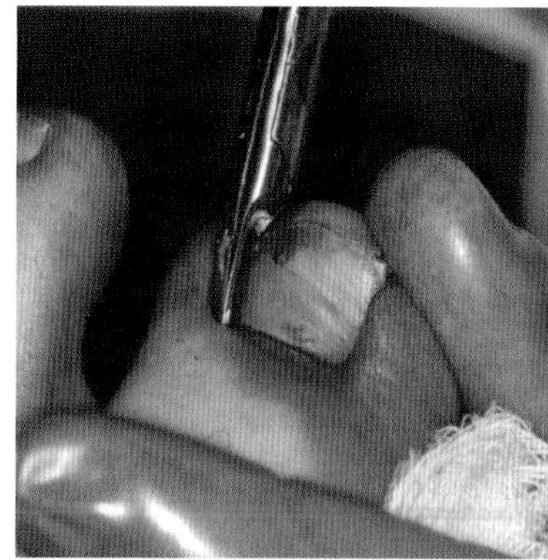

Figure 29-7 Using the nail splitter to "cut" through the nail. Flat jaw is down, beveled side is up. (Courtesy of John L. Pfenninger, MD, The Medical Procedures Center, PC, Midland, Mich.)

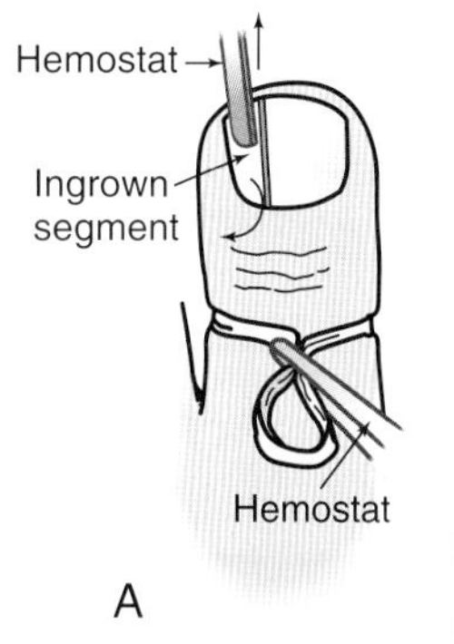

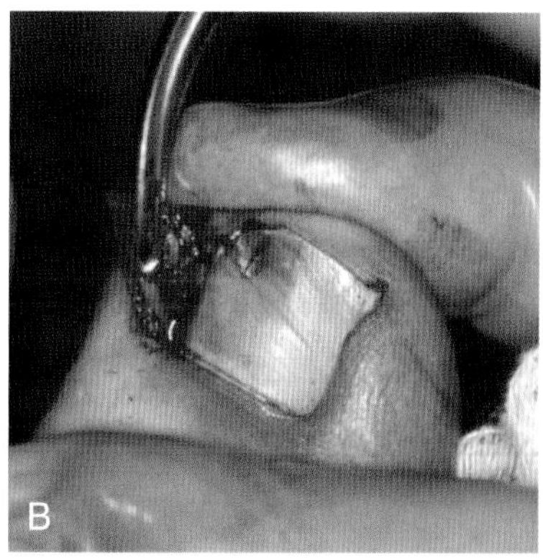

Figure 29-8 Technique for nail removal after nail has been elevated and split. **A** and **B,** Grasp that portion of the nail to be removed lengthwise with a straight hemostat, and remove it using a steady pulling motion with a simultaneous upward twist of the hand toward the affected side. (**B,** Courtesy of John L. Pfenninger, MD, The Medical Procedures Center, PC, Midland, Mich.)

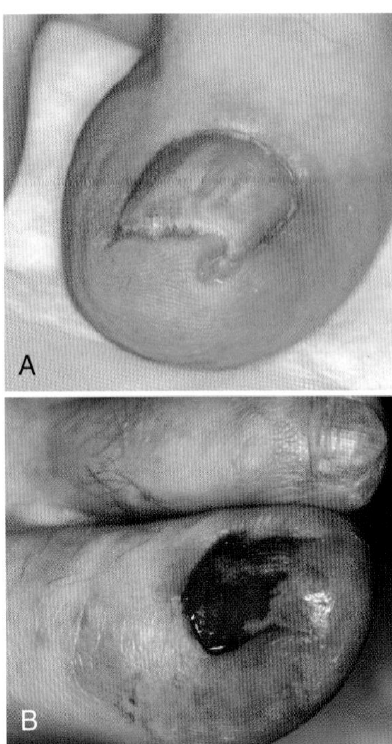

Figure 29-9 Complete removal of the toenail. **A,** Onychomycosis. **B,** Appearance after the nail has been removed. (Courtesy of John L. Pfenninger, MD, The Medical Procedures Center, PC, Midland, Mich.)

Nail Bed Ablation (Matrixectomy)

If recurrent regrowth of the toenail with resulting pain or infection occurs, permanent ablation of the germinal tissue is recommended (matrixectomy).

Phenol Chemical Method

1. Remove total or partial nail as described previously. The area must be dry and not bleeding. Remove all granulation tissue.
2. Sponge the exposed nail bed dry with cotton swabs and then cauterize the germinal tissue, including that under the nail fold, by application of phenol on a cotton swab to the nail bed tissues (Fig. 29-11). It is important to achieve good hemostasis before this step so that the tissue is dry. *Use caution to avoid phenol contact with normal skin.* A skin hook can be helpful in elevating the skin fold from the nail matrix. Hold the phenol-dampened cotton swab in place for 3 minutes. Three separate 60-second applications with drying of the surface in between is also reported to be effective. The tissue will pale or "gray" at the area of application.

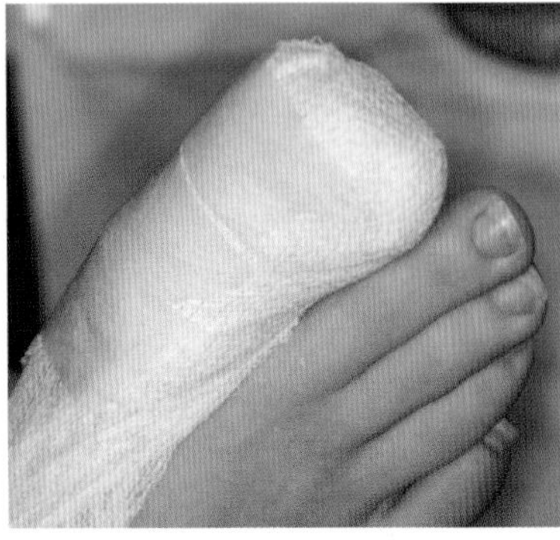

Figure 29-10 A compression dressing is applied after most toenail procedures. (Courtesy of John L. Pfenninger, MD, The Medical Procedures Center, PC, Midland, Mich.)

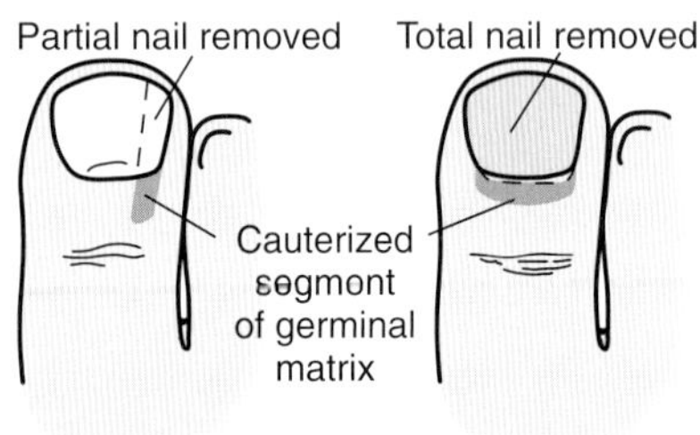

Figure 29-11 Area of nail bed to be cauterized in partial *(left)* and total permanent nail removal (matrixectomy) *(right)*.

3. After 3 minutes, drip 70% isopropyl alcohol into the nail groove and swab the area to neutralize the phenol.

Radiofrequency Method

See Chapter 30, Radiofrequency Surgery (Modern Electrosurgery).

The radiofrequency method of ablation is quick and easy. Although formal studies have not been performed, it is thought that radiofrequency causes markedly less pain, swelling, and discharge than other methods. It is difficult to control liquid agents, and they tend to destroy more tissue than desired.

1. Remove whole or partial nail as described previously.
2. Place antenna lead under the heel of foot.
3. Turn unit to "Hemo-part rect" (hemostasis/coagulation setting) and set the power at 2 to 3.
4. Insert wide or narrow insulated matrixectomy tip over nail matrix, under the eponychium as far as it will go, insulated side up (Fig. 29-12). These electrodes are insulated with Teflon on one surface to prevent damage to the undersurface of the

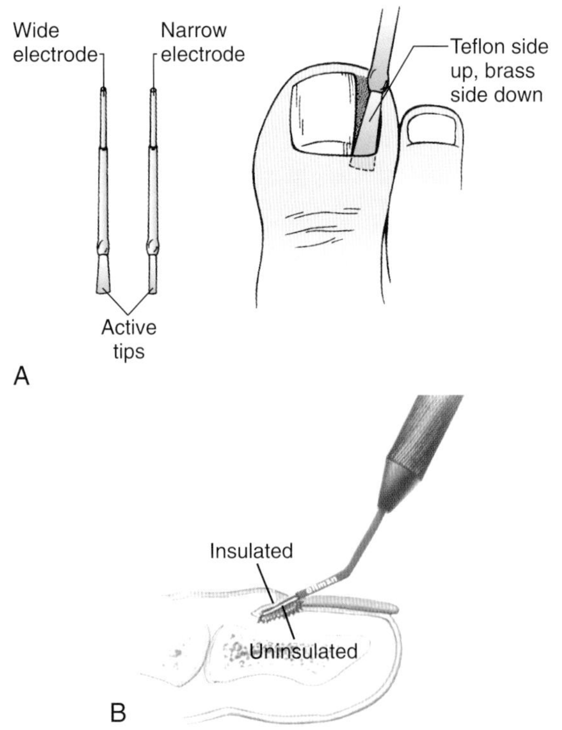

Figure 29-12 Application of nail matrixectomy electrode with Teflon-coated side up: top (**A**) and lateral (**B**) views. The lateral 25% of the nail has been removed.

proximal nail fold while ablating the nail matrix with the uninsulated surface beneath. A slight upward pressure should be exerted against the undersurface of the nail fold to ensure that no pressure is exerted on the underlying matrix. The field must be free of blood. For proper effect, there should be a slight gap between electrode and matrix.

5. Apply power and slowly withdraw the electrode pulling distally. Contact should last for only 1 to 2 seconds, and a sizzling sound should be heard. This step can be repeated once or twice over the same area after a 15-second cooling period. If the entire nail matrix is to be ablated, multiple applications are necessary with side-to-side placements of the electrode; slight overlapping should not be a problem. *Caution:* two to three passes (maximum) over the same tissue area are sufficient. *Avoid overtreatment.* The matrix is very thin and bone lies immediately beneath it. Overtreatment can cause burns with prolonged healing times of up to 6 to 8 weeks. It is often easier to use the narrower electrode because the power level can be set lower and it affords better control. Side-by-side applications may then be needed even for partial nail removal.

Other Methods

Sodium hydroxide (10% solution) and CO_2 laser are also described in the literature for use in matrixectomy. Sodium hydroxide is applied similarly to phenol and is thought by some to decrease postoperative drainage and speed healing compared with the phenol method. It is not as commonly used in the United States as phenol. The CO_2 laser requires special equipment and training and is usually operated by dermatologists or podiatrists.

When either partial or complete ablation is accomplished apply antibiotic ointment to the nail bed, cover with a sterile gauze pressure dressing, remove the tourniquet, and wrap with a tubular gauze dressing. Coban, CoFlex, and other similar self-adherent dressings provide a comfortable pressure wrap that holds the dressing in place.

Sample Operative Report

Informed consent obtained: Yes______ No______
Site (circle one): Left Right Medial Lateral great toe
Anesthesia: Digital block ______% Lidocaine without epi ____mL
Tourniquet used: Yes______ No______
Nail removal (circle one): Complete Partial
Granulation tissue removed: Yes______ No______ Cautery Y Chem/elect N
Ablation performed: No______ Yes______ (Phenol radioablation [tip ______ wide ______ narrow, setting ______])
Other____
Hemostasis was obtained.
The wound was dressed with antibiotic ointment and covered with a sterile dressing. The patient was given oral and written instructions in postoperative management. The patient tolerated the procedure without complications.

Common Errors

- Inadequate anesthesia resulting in patient discomfort. Ensure full anesthesia before starting procedure. Anesthetizing the toe generally requires 6 to 10 mL of lidocaine.
- Prolonged use of tourniquet resulting in ischemia. This can be avoided by foregoing use of the tourniquet in patients with possible decreased circulation and limiting the time under tourniquet pressure for all cases.
- Laceration of nail bed during lifting or splitting of the nail. This can result in difficult-to-control bleeding at the nail edge and scarring, leading to deformity of the nail when it grows back. Position any cutting instrument used such that the nail bed is protected during the incision. Use of the miniblade (also called *Beaver* or *wedge blade*), which has no sharp edge on the portion of the blade facing the nail bed, can help.
- Retained portion of nail results in persistent pain after procedure. Avoid this by careful examination of the nail fold and the removed portion of the nail after the procedure. A feathery edge of nail where it abuts the nail growth plate demonstrates that all the nail was removed. If necessary, explore the area and remove retained fragments.

Complications

- Infections (treat with soaking and appropriate antibiotics)
- Bleeding (generally controlled with pressure)
- Regrowth of nail and return of symptoms (regrowth rate after phenol cauterization is 4% to 25%; for radiofrequency, <5%)
- Excessive tissue destruction with radiofrequency unit, leading to prolonged healing time and possible osteomyelitis

Postprocedure Patient Education and Management

The foot should be rested and preferably elevated during the first 12 to 24 hours. Because phenol ablates the nerve endings of the nail plate, pain should be absent when it is used. There is minimal pain with the radiofrequency unit. Nonsteroidal anti-inflammatory drugs or acetaminophen may be taken for discomfort.

The dressing should be changed in 12 to 24 hours, at which point ambulation can be encouraged; however, vigorous exercise should be avoided for 1 week. The toe should be washed with soap and water at least twice daily (depending on soiling) until healed. Topical antibiotic ointment should be applied and the area kept clean until healed. Tell the patient to expect a sterile exudate from the nail bed for several weeks. Explaining that the wound will "heal like a burn" can help patients understand that the exudate is not an indication of infection. Emphasize proper nail hygiene to prevent further recurrences (Fig. 29-13).

CPT/Billing Codes

11730 Nail removal, partial or complete
11732 Avulsion each additional nail
11750 Permanent nail removal (matrixectomy), partial or complete

ICD-9-CM Diagnostic Codes

110.1 Onychomycosis
703.0 Ingrown toenail
703.8 Onychogryphosis

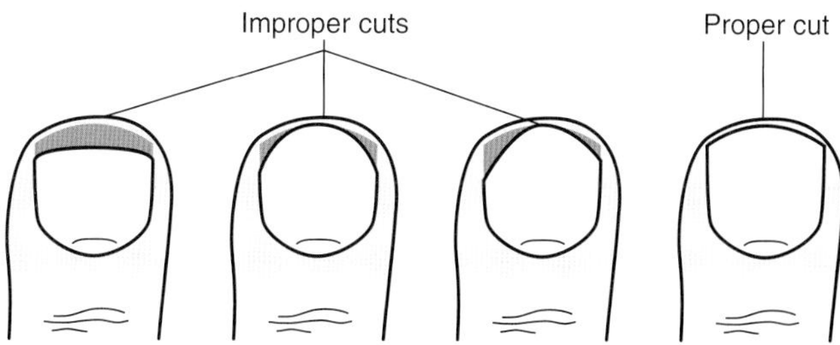

Figure 29-13 Examples of improper and proper nail care. Trim the nail flat and straight across and not too short. (Redrawn from Heidelbaugh JJ, Lee H: Management of the ingrown toenail. Am Fam Physician 79:303–308, 2009.)

Acknowledgment

The editors wish to recognize the many contributions by James F. Peggs, MD, to this chapter in the previous edition of this text.

Suppliers

(See contact information online at www.expertconsult.com.)

Toe tourniquets and Surgitron radiofrequency unit (see Chapter 30, Radiofrequency Surgery [Modern Electrosurgery])
Ellman

Other equipment can be obtained from most medical suppliers, such as Miltex and Delasco.

Bibliography

Bos AMC, van Tilburg MW, van Sorge AA, Klinkenbijl JH: Randomized clinical trial of surgical technique and local antibiotics for ingrowing toenail. Br J Surg 94:292–296, 2007.

Daniel CR III, Iorizzo M, Tosti A, Piraccini BM: Ingrown toenails. Cutis 78:407–408, 2006.

DeLauro NM, DeLauro TM: Onychocryptosis. Clin Podiatr Med Surg 21:616–630, 2004.

Denkler K: Dupuytren's fasciectomies in 60 consecutive digits using lidocaine with epinephrine and no tourniquet. Plast Reconstr Surg 115: 802–810, 2005.

Freiberg A, Dougherty S: A review of management of ingrown toenails and onychogryposis. Can Fam Physician 34:2675–2681, 1988.

Heidelbaugh JJ, Hobart L: Management of ingrown toenail. Am Fam Physician 79:303–308, 2009.

Hettinger DF, Valinsky MS, Nuccio G, Lim R: Nail matrixectomies using radio wave technique. J Am Podiatr Med Assoc 81:317–321, 1991.

Hill GJ: Outpatient Surgery, 2nd ed. Philadelphia, WB Saunders, 1980.

Ikard RW: Onychocryptosis. J Am Coll Surg 187:96–102, 1998.

Krunic AL, Wang LC, Soltani K, et al: Digital anesthesia with epinephrine: An old myth revisited. J Am Acad Dermatol 51:755–759, 2004.

Radovic P, Smith RG, Shumway D: Revisiting epinephrine in foot surgery. J Am Podiatr Med Assoc 93:157–160, 2003.

Reynolds J: Practical foot techniques [instructional video]. Austin, Tex, National Procedures Institute, 1989. Available at www.npinstitute.com.

Reyzelman AM, Trombello KA, Vayser DJ, et al: Are antibiotics necessary in the treatment of locally infected ingrown toenails? Arch Fam Med 9:930–932, 2000.

Robb JE, Murray WR: Phenol cauterization in the management of ingrowing toenails. Scott Med J 27:236–239, 1982.

Rounding C, Bloomfield S: Surgical treatments for ingrowing toenails. Cochrane Database Syst Rev 2:CD001541, 2005.

Thompson C, Lalonde D, Denkler K, Feicht A: A critical look at the evidence for and against elective epinephrine use in the finger. Plast Reconstr Surg 119:260–266, 2007.

Usatine R: Nail procedures. In Usatine RP, Pfenninger JL, Stulberg DL, Small R (eds): Dermatologic and Cosmetic Procedures in Office Practice. Philadelphia, Saunders, 2011, Chapter 18 (in press).

Yang KC, Li YT: Treatment of recurrent ingrown great toenail associated with granulation tissue by partial nail avulsion followed by matricectomy with sharpulse carbon dioxide laser. Dermatol Surg 28:419–421, 2003.

Zuber T, Pfenninger J: Management of ingrown toenails. Am Fam Physician 52:181–190, 1995.

Radiofrequency Surgery (Modern Electrosurgery)

John L. Pfenninger

Radiofrequency (RF) surgery—modern electrosurgery—has become a versatile tool for the primary care physician in dermatologic, surgical, and gynecologic applications. It is both time and cost effective, and it provides efficacious treatment for a multitude of lesions. Appropriate selection of waveform and current intensity allows excision (cutting), cutting and coagulation (blend), pure coagulation (hemostasis), or fulguration. Tissue either can be removed delicately with excellent cosmetic results or can be totally ablated. The electrosurgical unit (ESU) can be used for treatment of both benign and malignant lesions.

This chapter is based on the Ellman Surgitron (Ellman International, Inc., Hewlett, NY), a portable generator that creates high-frequency current of 3.8 to 4.0 MHz, which is comparable to the radiowave frequency for broadcasting (Figs. 30-1 and 30-2). ESU wave frequency for different brand models can vary from 500,000 to 4 million cycles (4.0 MHz) per second. All units can be used with a multitude of electrode tips for a large variety of applications. With the advent of the loop electrosurgical excision procedure (LEEP) in the 1990s, many companies introduced units into the market. Unless otherwise noted, discussion here will be in reference to the Ellman Surgitron because it is widely adapted to many dermatologic procedures. The reader can generalize the discussion to most other units quite readily.

There is a choice of three waveform outputs plus a fulguration current (four modes). By changing waveforms, practitioners obtain different effects. The settings of the Ellman unit are described as *filtered fully rectified*, *fully rectified*, and *partially rectified*. These correspond with a *pure cutting* effect (90% cutting, 10% coagulation),

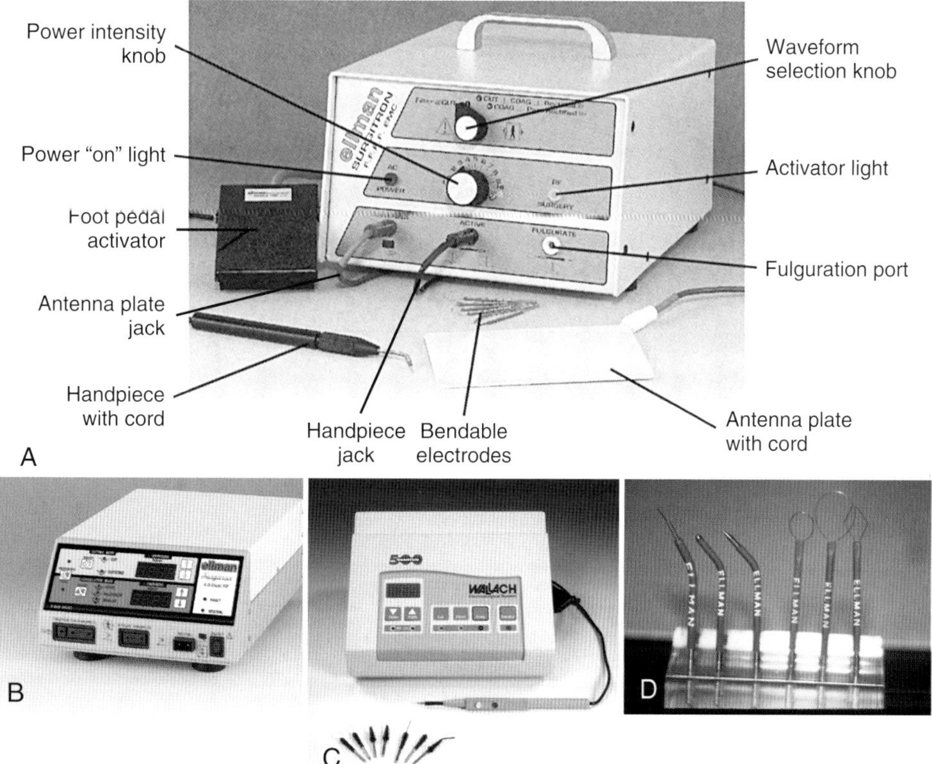

Figure 30-1 **A,** Ellman Surgitron radiofrequency unit with foot pedal, antenna plate, and hand wand tip holder. A variety of electrode tips are lying above the white antenna plate. **B,** Ellman Dual Frequency IEC II. **C,** The Wallach Q500 electrosurgical unit with finger control handpiece and a variety of electrodes. **D,** Typical electrodes (Ellman) for skin electrosurgery (*left to right*): vari-tip cutting wire; ball electrode and pointed electrode for cautery or fulguration; small and large loops; diamond-shaped electrode. (**A, B,** and **D,** Courtesy of Ellman International, Inc., Hewlett, NY. **C,** Courtesy of Bruno Ratensberger.)

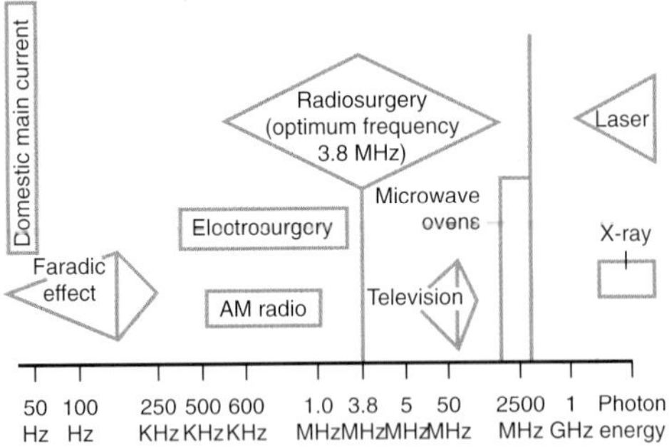

Figure 30-2 Comparison of uses and effects of various electrical frequencies. (Courtesy of Ellman International, Inc., Hewlett, NY.)

a *blended* current to allow 50% cut and 50% coagulation, and a 90% *coagulation* (hemostasis) effect, respectively. A separate outlet also provides a spark-gap fulgurating current (referred to as *hyfrecation*) for very superficial cautery (Fig. 30-3).

Advantages of using RF technique include rapidity of treatment, a nearly bloodless field, minimal postoperative pain, and rapid healing. Local anesthetic is used except in rare instances. Because the frequency is so high, the current from this unit passes through the body without causing painful muscle contractions or nerve stimulation (Faraday effects). Radiosurgery using the *cutting wave* cuts without pressure, needing only a feather-like touch, and thus minimizes tissue damage. The tissue damage that does occur is very superficial and comparable with that of proper laser use. This is in contrast to true cautery, which causes damage similar to third-degree burns. In addition, radiosurgery avoids the risk of electrical burns to the patient. Instead of a ground plate, an *antenna* is used to focus the "radio waves." In contrast to other electrical units, this antenna does not have to be in contact with a patient's skin; instead, it only needs to be under the patient near the operating field. (Most ESUs with lower-frequency output, however, do require true grounding pads or plates, so the manufacturer's recommendations must be followed.)

The high-frequency energy of this unit is concentrated at the tip of each electrode. During each procedure, the electrode itself remains cold; however, the highly concentrated electrical energy creates molecular energy inside each cell it contacts, thereby creating intracellular heat and actually vaporizing the cell, much as a laser does. The *amount of heat generated* depends on the amount of *time* the tip is in contact with the tissue, the *size* of the electrode, the *power setting*, the *type of waveform* selected, and the wave *frequency*. Higher frequency means less contact time, finer wire, less power, a more "cutting" waveform, and less tissue damage.

High-frequency electrosurgery is now replacing many laser applications because of the minimal tissue damage, low cost of equipment, minimal maintenance, ease of treatment, and excellent long-term results. It has replaced most laser applications for the gynecologic treatment of dysplasia (conization) and condylomata. It is now also being used for blepharoplasties, radioassisted uvulopalatoplasty (RAUP) for snoring, spinal procedures, skin tightening (dual-frequency unit), and many more applications.

Mode or function	Waveform	Configuration
Electrocoagulation Hemostasis Cautery	Partially rectified	
Blend Cut and coag	Fully rectified	
Cutting Electrosection	Fully filtered and fully rectified	
Fulguration Electrodesiccation	Markedly damped	

Figure 30-3 Common terminology for various modes, waveform characterization, and waveform configuration for the outputs of the radiofrequency unit.

Box 30-1. Common Uses of and Lesions Treated with Radiofrequency Surgery

Actinic keratoses
Basal cell cancers
Blepharoplasties
Cauterization of "bleeders"
Cervical biopsies
Cervical conizations (LLETZ, LEEP)*
Chalazions
Condylomata
Curettement and cautery (e.g., warts)
Electroepilation
Excisions
Hair transplants
Hemangiomas
Hemorrhoid tags
Incisions
Mucosal lesions
Nail plate ablation†
Nevi (benign)
Pyogenic granulomas
Radioassisted uvulopalatoplasties (RAUP)
Rhinophyma
Sebaceous gland hyperplasia
Seborrheic keratoses
Shave removals
Skin tags
Skin tightening (Radiage)
Squamous cell carcinomas
Syringomas
Telangiectases (spider veins) face (not recommended for legs)
Verrucae
Xanthelasma

*See Chapter 149, Loop Electrosurgical Excision Procedure for Treating Cervical Intraepithelial Neoplasia.
†See Chapter 29, Ingrown Toenails.

INDICATIONS

Radiofrequency surgery can be used for a variety of skin and mucosal lesions. It is especially helpful when good cosmetic results are essential. It is also very helpful in well-perfused areas like mucosa and the anal area because the "cut and coag" setting can be used to control the bleeding. Common uses and lesions treated are listed in Box 30-1.

CONTRAINDICATIONS

- *Cardiac pacemakers* (relative contraindication): Do not work near the heart and place the antenna (or grounding) plate well away from the heart. Use the least power possible. Activate the handpiece intermittently rather than continuously. The cutting mode is the most risky, so avoid it if possible. Use another form of treatment if it is an option. The pacers are purportedly "shielded" and the current in the ESUs should not affect them, but all things are not perfect! Therefore caution is needed. Asystole and tachycardia are potential adverse outcomes.
- *Uncooperative patient.*

Equipment

- Alcohol wipe
- Local anesthetic (e.g., 2% lidocaine with or without epinephrine)
- 1-mL syringe with 30-gauge needle
- ESU
- Electrode tips (depending on procedure performed): reusable or disposable
- No. 15 scalpel blade
- Antenna (or grounding) plate
- Handpiece for tips (unit can be finger-activated from this handpiece if desired)
- Foot pedal to activate handpiece (or use handpiece as above); foot pedal preferred for delicate surgeries
- Smoke evacuator (human immunodeficiency virus [HIV] and human papillomavirus [HPV] have been found in smoke plume)
- Room air purifier or exhaust fan (removes residual odor)
- Moveable cart to hold the ESU, smoker evacuator, tips, and all equipment for the procedures
- Mask
- Nonsterile gloves
- Aluminum chloride for topical control of bleeders (or Monsel's solution if face is not involved)
- Antibiotic ointment
- Band-Aid
- Patient education handout on moist healing (which is essential to obtain optimal results). (See the sample patient education handout available online at www.expertconsult.com.)
- For LEEP supplies, see Chapter 149, Loop Electrosurgical Excision Procedure for Treating Cervical Intraepithelial Neoplasia.

The *most common tips* used for removal of skin lesions are the large and small loops. The ball electrode is used frequently for coagulation and for ablation of lesions. Special tips are available for matrixectomy (see later discussion and Chapter 29, Ingrown Toenails) and skin tightening (see Chapter 52, Nonablative Radiowave Skin Tightening with the Ellman S5 Surgitron [The Pelleve Procedure]).

Disposable tips are convenient but can be costly. *Reusable tips* must be free of carbon buildup and shiny to obtain best results. After cleaning and sterilizing, and before repeat use, the tip must be examined. If it is not shiny, the carbon can be removed in several ways:

- Use a 2 × 2-inch piece of fine sandpaper and, using the index finger to support the back side of the loop, rub it over the sandpaper. Turn it over and do the reverse side. Be sure to clean the entire wire loop.
- Purchase the cleaning "blocks" available.
- Place the units in an ultrasonic cleaner.
- Use a moistened piece of 4 × 4 gauze, insert the tip into the folded material, and activate it on the cutting setting, level 5.

When complete, the wire should be shiny (like new). One of the most *common reasons for poor cutting and "stalls"* during RF surgery is "dirty" (carbon-covered) reusable loops, which is avoided if disposable tips are used.

Most ESUs have digital readouts for *wattage* (power intensity). The Ellman simply has an intensity dial labeled 1 to 10. Each unit roughly corresponds to 10 W. For skin surgery a setting of 2 to 4 (20 to 40 W) is usually needed. (*As a "default," remember "pure cutting on level 2."*)

Use of a *smoke evacuator* is essential. Not only have HPV and HIV been found in smoke plume (no infections have been documented), but the smell of burning flesh is very offensive and the examination room and office can smell for hours afterward.

The dual-frequency unit (Ellman Surgitron DF IEC II; see Fig. 30-1B) is being used with increasing frequency for plastic surgery and neurosurgery applications. Its coagulation potential is much better and it can coagulate in a "wet" (bloody) field using the bipolar modality. This is achieved through the dual frequencies of 4 MHz for cutting but 1.7 MHz for bipolar coagulation. This unit will not interfere with any nearby electronics or electrical circuits. Other benefits include a higher frequency (4.0 vs. 3.8 million cycles per second) than the original equipment. There is still minimal thermal damage when cutting. It meets national safety codes for operating room use, and it is more user friendly because there is a two-pedal foot switch for cutting or coagulation and a three-button finger switch (for each modality). It has a memory for the most recent settings when turned off, digital power settings, and an audible sound when activated. This unit is significantly more expensive, and whether the benefits warrant the extra cost for the average practitioner remains to be seen. The dual-frequency unit with the special electrodes must be used for skin-tightening procedures. Those considering offering aesthetic procedures in their practice may want to consider this unit.

Technique

Proper technique is accomplished when the loop electrodes pass through the tissue smoothly, like cutting through soft butter. Generally, a motion of 5 to 8 mm/sec is appropriate. *If there is excess sparking and smoke*, the power setting is too high. *If the flow is not smooth*, the operator is going too fast, the power setting is too low, the skin is too dry or hyperkeratotic, or the electrode is dirty (debris or carbon buildup). It is important to remember that the least tissue damage occurs with the pure cutting setting. Coagulation causes the most tissue destruction. If cosmetic results are desirable, judicious use of the coagulation setting and using as little power (watts) as possible is important.

The most common use for the RF unit in primary care is removal of elevated skin lesions such as nevi and seborrheic lesions. Commonly, when using a blade to shave off a benign nevus, two things result: bleeding and an irregular surface. As the surgeon tries to smooth out the "highs" in the base of the wound, blood obscures the area. Then, as the blade is used to shave off these highs, too much tissue is removed, leaving "dips." The "lows" (too much tissue removed) and the "highs" (too little) result in adverse outcomes with undesirable scarring. Using the RF technique, both bleeding and an uneven wound base can be avoided. In addition, any focal areas of undesirable residual tissue are removed and the edges can be smoothed for a more pleasing cosmetic result. Because the tissue left behind has minimal thermal damage, healing is quick and scarring is minimized.

The most successful technique for removing lesions appears to be first to "debulk" the majority of the lesion with a no. 15 blade in a shave fashion (see Chapter 32, Skin Biopsy). Then, use the loop electrode on a pure cutting setting of 2 (20 W) to smooth out or vaporize the base of the wound. Pinch the skin around the area to control bleeding, activate the loop, and very superficially pass the tip over/through the tissue, gradually going down until the lesion is smoothed out adequately (Fig. 30-4). This "smoothing out" of the base provides an excellent outcome with rapid healing. The "cutting" setting has 10% coagulation so bleeding is nicely controlled. The tissue is literally vaporized cell layer by cell layer. Healing results are excellent. Another advantage with the method described is that the tissue sent to pathology has no burn artifact.

Some advocate the removal of lesions primarily with the loop only (as opposed to using the blade). *Extreme caution is needed!* The loop cuts so quickly that it often goes too deep. Even in experienced hands too much tissue may be removed unless the process is very slow and meticulous with only a small amount of tissue removed each time. *Do not try to remove all of the lesion with the first pass!* The only time the "layered" or "feathering" removal technique is recommended is for larger condylomata (Fig. 30-5).

Another advantage of shaving the lesion first with a blade is that a good specimen is available for pathology. If the loop is used, there

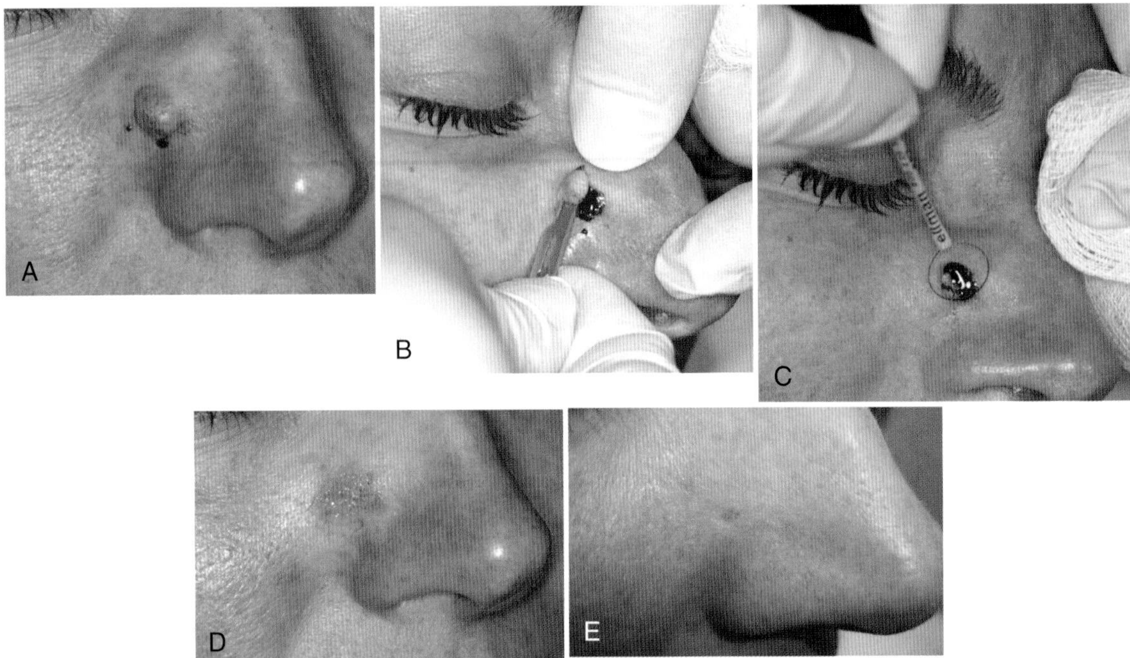

Figure 30-4 Preferred technique for removal of raised lesions with a broad base. **A,** Nasal nevus after infiltration with lidocaine. **B,** Shave the lesion with a no. 15 blade. Remove most of the lesion, being careful not to go too deep. **C,** Smooth out the base and control bleeding with a large loop electrode (cutting, 2). "Sculpt" the final result. Proceed very superficially and literally remove a few cell layers at a time to blend the edges. **D,** Appearance on completion of removal. **E,** Appearance 2 years after removal. (Courtesy of The Medical Procedures Center PC, Midland, Mich.)

will always be some coagulation artifact, albeit minimum. If total vaporization or the coagulation technique is used, minimal (if any) tissue can be sent. It is best that all pigmented lesions be sent for histology because this is a very litigious area of medicine, and the less "artifact" on a specimen the better.

The Ellman unit does have a "fulguration port." This setting provides a very intense but superficial burn/coagulation. It can be used in place of the coagulation mode in many instances, but in general it has little benefit over the coagulation setting and is rarely used.

Novices are most concerned about the proper choice of settings when beginning electrosurgery. *Here are some pointers:*

- For removal of tissue, use pure cutting mode.
- For cutting the skin, or for the shave technique noted previously, usually an intensity of 2 (≤20 W) is sufficient. For removing large areas (e.g., cervical conization) or if the skin is hyperkeratotic, the intensity will need to be increased, but rarely over 4 (40 W) for the skin and 6 for the cervix. *Remember the "default" setting:* cutting, level 2. The larger and drier the tissue, the higher the power will need to be.
- When tissue destruction (matrixectomy, epilation, telangiectases) or bleeding control is needed, turn to the coagulation mode. Most applications will require a level of 3 (30 W). When small areas are treated *without anesthesia* (epilation, telangiectases of the face), reduce the power level to 1.
- Use the cut/coagulation mode when bleeding is likely (e.g., inner lip, buccal mucosa) or where scarring is not so much of an issue (external hemorrhoidal tags). The setting will need to be a little higher (3, or 30 W).
- For removal of cervical tissue, the goal is to limit tissue artifact so the pathologist can readily read the specimen and discern if the entire lesion was removed. Use a *pure cutting mode*; although scarring is not a concern, bleeding still is. Amazingly, however, there is generally very little bleeding, even with pure cutting, and the pathologist will be able to read to the margins of the excision because the cutting mode leaves little burn artifact. (See Chapter 149, Loop Electrosurgical Excision Procedure for Treating Cervical Intraepithelial Neoplasia.)
- All electrosurgery will be accomplished easier at lower power (therefore causing less tissue destruction) *if the tissue is moist and*

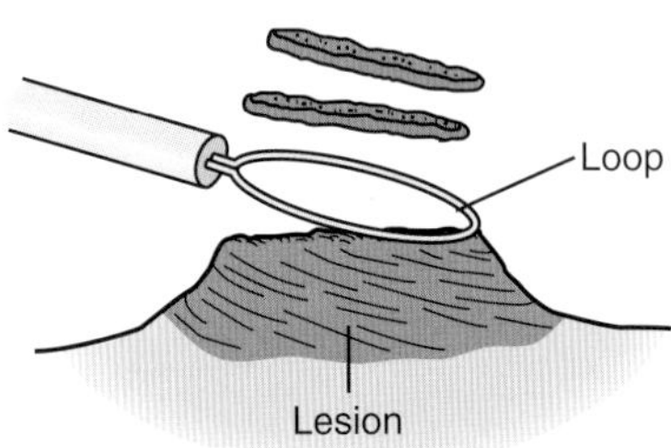

Figure 30-5 "Feathering" technique for lesion removal. Rather than removing the entire lesion in one pass, it is removed a small amount at a time. This avoids removing too much and going too deep, causing scarring.

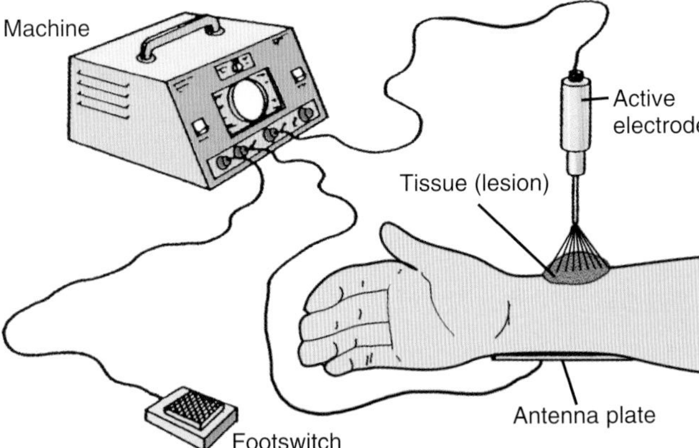

Figure 30-6 Diagrammatic illustration of radiosurgery showing the distribution of energy and the appropriate placement of the antenna plate near the lesion. (Courtesy of Ellman International, Inc., Hewlett, NY.)

TABLE 30-1 Proper Electrode Tips and Power Settings

Procedure	Mode	Power (Ellman/Watts)	Electrode
Condylomata	Cutting	2/20	Large or small round loop
Ear piercing	Cutting or cut/coag	2/20	Narrow, pointed tip
Electrodesiccation and curettage	Coag	3/25–30	Ball
Epilation	Coag	1/10	Vari-tip, 33-gauge needle on hub adaptors, or insulated needle
Epistaxis	Coag	3/30	Ball electrode
Hemorrhoid tags	Cut/coag	3/25–30	Large loop or vari-tip
Hemostasis, skin	Coag	2–3/20–30	Ball electrode
Incisions	Cutting	2–3/20–30	Vari-tip, fine needle, blade
LEEP	Cutting	4/35–40	Long, special LEEP electrodes
LEEP	Coag base/hemostasis	6/40–60	Long, special LEEP ball
Matrixectomy	Coag	2–3/20–30	Special insulated matrixectomy electrodes, raise up on the eponychium, do not overcoagulate
Rhinophyma	Cutting	2/20	Large loop or rounded surgical blade (no. 10A)
Shave excision/smoothing	Cutting	2/20	Large or small loop
Skin tags/small condylomata	Coag	3/25–30	Pickups with ball electrode, bipolar pickups
Telangiectases	Coag	1/10	Vari-tip, 33-gauge needle on hub adapters, or insulated needle
Undermining	Cutting or cut/coag	2–3/20–30	Vari-tip, blade
Vasectomy (cauterizing vas ends)	Coag	3/30	Narrow, pointed tip
Verruca	Cutting	3/25–30	Large loop, special cutting curette
Verruca	Coag	3/30	Ball electrode
Xanthelasma	Cutting	2/20–25	Large loop

LEEP, loop electrosurgical excision procedure.

hyperkeratotic material has been removed. Use a moistened 4 × 4 gauze pad and wipe it across the tissue after each pass or two.

- Most lesions will have to be anesthetized before removal with the RF unit.
- In general, place the antenna plate or grounding pad as close to the lesion as possible to limit the spread of the current and increase the intensity at the desired site (Fig. 30-6).
- The proper electrode tips and power settings are summarized in Table 30-1.
- Be sure to *hold the handpiece like a pencil*, and place the fifth finger on the patient for stabilization. If the patient jumps or moves, your hand thus moves with him or her. Otherwise, the patient may experience a significant laceration or burn.

Specific Approaches for Various Lesions

There are a multitude of applications possible with the variety of tips available (Fig. 30-7; see Fig. 30-1D). There are loop and straight-wire electrodes for excising, incising, or shaping tissue; ball electrodes for coagulation; and pointed rod electrodes for fulguration and desiccation. More specific electrodes are available for nail matrixectomies and LEEP of the cervix. *The tips are changed in the handpiece much like the bits are changed in an ordinary drill.* Most treatments are accomplished with simple local anesthesia, regional field blocks, or digital blocks. Radiosurgery is relatively atraumatic when correctly applied; consequently, the risks of scar tissue formation are minimal compared with those associated with scalpel surgery.

For the majority of cases, the handpiece is inserted into the color-coordinated "handpiece" port on the unit to enable the selection of various output modes. (If inserted into the "fulguration port," that will be the only output.)

Biopsies or excisions of lesions may be accomplished with the standard ellipse technique using the *vari-tip electrode* (Fig. 30-8) or a scalpel blade inserted into a *chuck adapter* (Fig. 30-9). The vari-tip has a fine wire that can be pulled out at variable distances to cut from 1 to 2 mm up to 1.5 cm deep. The unit is set at cutting mode. The proper power is usually between 2 and 3. The thickness and dryness of skin may cause some variation in the latter setting. Remove any hyperkeratinized tissue first, and be sure the skin is

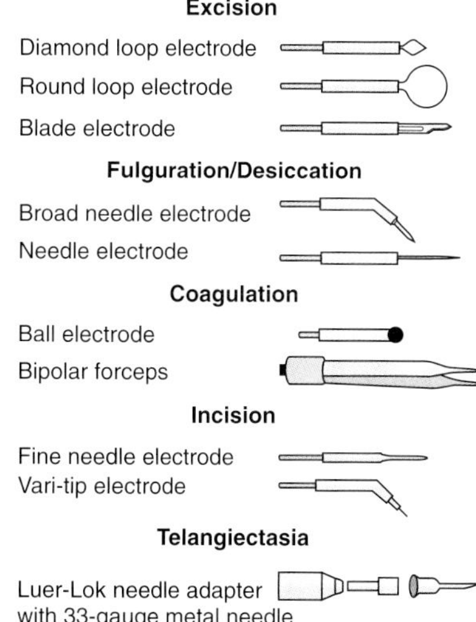

Figure 30-7 Multiple electrode tips available for the Ellman Surgitron radiofrequency unit.

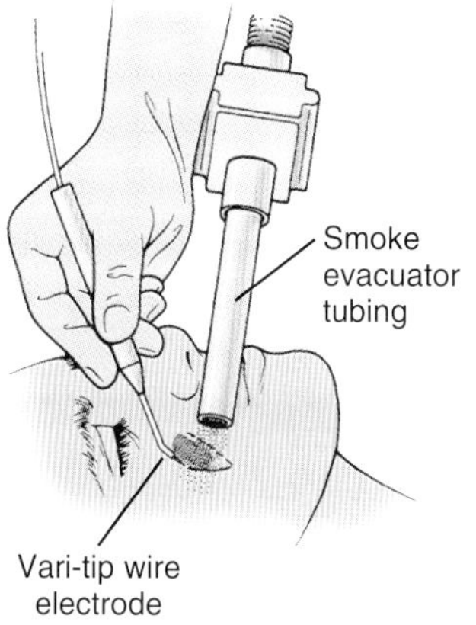

Figure 30-8 Use of the vari-tip wire electrode to carry out an elliptical excision.

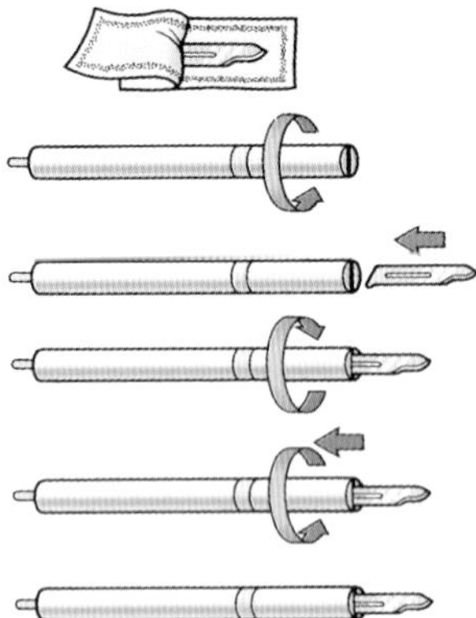

Figure 30-9 Technique of inserting scalpel blade into handle for radiofrequency surgery. Most surgery is carried out with the loop electrodes or vari-tip wire. The scalpel is used most frequently for "bloodless" undermining.

moist. In addition to incising and excising, these two electrodes are often used to undermine skin because bleeding will be controlled if the cut/coag (blend) mode is used. The cutting is very fast so be careful not to excise too deeply.

If the lesion to be removed is large and elevated, a biopsy specimen may be obtained by simply using the loop electrodes to remove the sample (Fig. 30-10). (See previously discussed precautions.) However, with smaller, flatter lesions, using the loop to obtain a shave biopsy specimen may cause sufficient artifact in the tissue specimen and obscure pathology. For smaller lesions, then, use a regular scalpel blade (without current) to obtain a shave biopsy specimen. Then use the loop electrode to smooth out the base and control bleeding. Remember, when obtaining a biopsy sample for suspected melanoma, the depth of lesion penetration is *very important*. Do *not* perform a shave biopsy of a pigmented lesion unless you are certain it is not a melanoma (see Chapter 32, Skin Biopsy).

Basal cell cancers are often best treated using a combination of curettement and cautery (or fulguration). A *ball electrode* is used in the handpiece with coagulation mode and the power set at approximately 3 to 4. After curetting the lesion, the base of the wound is cauterized. Cautery and curettement are usually carried out three times on the same visit. The tissue from the first curettement is sent for histology to confirm the clinical diagnosis (see Chapter 12, Approach to Various Skin Lesions, and Chapter 32, Skin Biopsy). Lesions less than 1 cm have a cure rate greater than 98%.

Condylomata acuminata may be excised using a loop electrode with the unit set at *cutting* (most commonly) or at *cut/coag* and power set at approximately 2 to 3. For larger lesions, "debulk" them with the initial pass, then successively remove more tissue, and finally feather out the edges with a very light touch. Be very careful not to go too deep and remove too much tissue with the first pass! Using a colposcope for magnification during the removal is very helpful. (Alternatively, any residual after the initial pass may be removed with coagulation of the bases of the wound.) *Small warts* on all parts of the body may be destroyed easily using a ball electrode with the unit set at coagulation and a power setting just strong enough to "cook" the lesions (1 to 2). The smaller lesions can also be grasped with metal pickups and the electrode applied to the pickups while lifting the lesion. Apply enough current so that the lesion can be wiped off with moist gauze after coagulating it.

Xanthelasma may be treated easily using a large loop in the cutting mode set at level 2. Use very superficial passes over the lesion until all white material is removed. Use ophthalmic ointment to keep the wound moist until it is healed. No suture closure is required.

Fibroepithelial skin tags may be removed simply, usually without anesthesia, with the loop electrode on the cut (or cut/coag) mode and power setting at slightly less than 2 (Fig. 30-11). They can also be treated like small condylomata, as noted previously. Larger lesions will require anesthesia.

Hemorrhoidal tags can be removed similarly to skin tags. Be careful that the local anesthesia does not distort the base of the tag, which can create a false sense that more tissue has to be removed. This could leave a larger wound than needed. The cut/coag mode at level 3 to 4 works best. Usually the wound is left open.

Seborrheic keratoses are successfully treated using the technique described previously for shave excisions. Remember, the lesion is very superficial, so deep removal is not necessary. This will minimize scarring. Use a blade to shave off the bulk of the lesion and follow it with a large loop, cutting mode, and setting of 2, using the feathering technique.

Sebaceous cysts may be uncovered for intact removal or extraction of the capsule by using a small ellipse around the central pore. The cutting mode is selected and the power dial is set at no more than 2. The length and depth of the ellipse obviously depend on the size of the cyst and thickness of the skin. The vari-tip electrode is set at skin thickness (estimate). With an Allis clamp, put slight traction on the ellipsed area over the cyst wall itself. The lesion is then bluntly dissected from surrounding deep tissue and removed.

Telangiectases (face only) are effectively treated with the electrocoagulation technique. Use the coagulation (hemostasis) mode with the power set at 1, and a fine needle. A hypodermic needle adaptor is available for the handpiece; a short 33-gauge hypodermic needle with a metal hub is then attached to the adaptor for this procedure (see Fig. 30-7). Insulated needles can also be purchased from the manufacturer (Fig. 30-12). The special needles are insulated and active only at the very tip. Generally, topical anesthetic is used (see Chapter 10, Topical Anesthesia). Treatment lasts a fraction of a second. The unit is activated before touching the telangiectases. Vessels should be penetrated minimally at approximately 1- to 2-mm intervals. Begin distally and work proximally. (Doing the opposite—proximal to distal—causes the vessels to go into spasm, making them hard to locate.) Facial lesions respond the

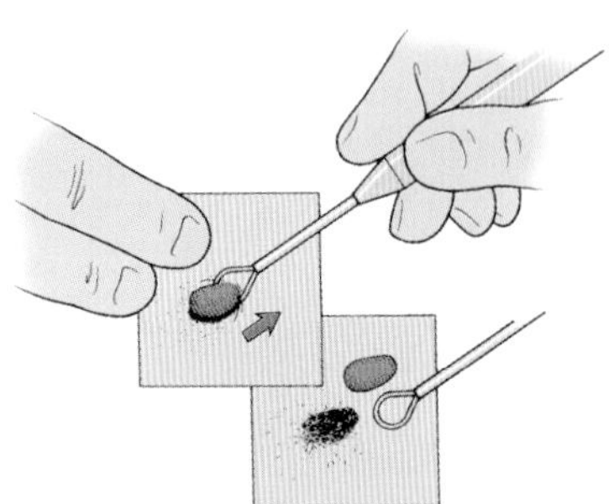

Figure 30-10 Another technique for removing a raised skin lesion with a broad base. Care must be taken not to excise too much tissue.

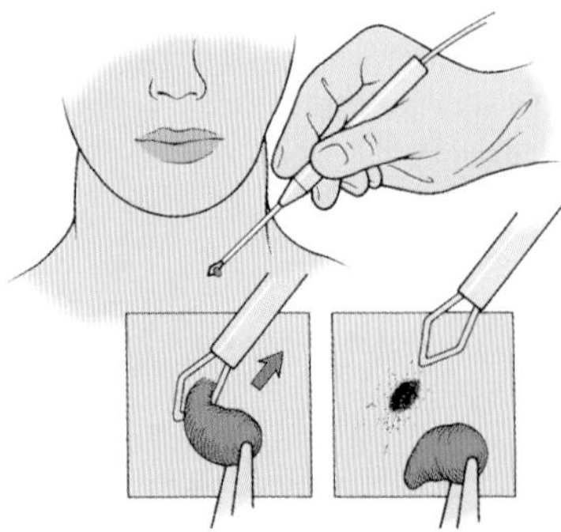

Figure 30-11 Technique for removing a lesion with a pedunculated base.

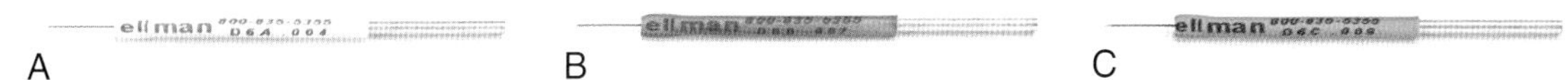

Figure 30-12 Insulated needles available for treatment of telangiectasia. **A**, #D6-A, .004; **B**, #D6-B, .007; **C**, #D6-C, .009. (Courtesy of Ellman International, Inc., Hewlett, NY.)

best, whereas spider veins on the lower extremity do not resolve well. There is often prolonged pigmentation and recurrence with leg veins. Sclerotherapy is the procedure of choice for the lower extremities (see Chapter 92, Sclerotherapy). *Spider angiomas* anywhere can be treated with the fine needle. Occasionally all that is needed is coagulation of one central vessel. *Cherry hemangiomas* are best treated using light ball electrode desiccation, then wiped away.

Epilation of isolated hairs deploys a similar technique and needle. Choose the coag setting at level 1, grasp the hair with pickups, and slide the needle down the shaft. Activate the electrode; as the hair follicle is "cooked," the hair comes out easily. Trichiasis is treated in this fashion too. For large areas of unwanted hair, use the modern techniques of removal (see Chapter 48, Laser and Pulsed-Light Devices: Hair Removal).

Actinic keratoses are very dry and, unless small, are best treated with cryosurgery or shave technique. If the electrodesiccation technique is used, however, those lesions that do not respond appropriately should be studied further to rule out neoplastic changes. If there is any doubt, obtain a shave biopsy sample before treatment.

Plantar warts are treated in a multitude of ways (see Chapter 42, Wart [Verruca] Treatment). When other methods fail (e.g., *Candida* antigen injections, topicals, cryotherapy, bleomycin), the wart may have to be removed with curettement and coagulation. Perform this carefully because scarring on the bottom of the feet can cause painful nodules. Some residual scarring is the norm rather than the exception. After anesthesia, curette the lesion and follow with ball electrode coagulation. Curette again to ensure all wart tissue has been removed. Do not penetrate the dermis; warts are epithelial. Alternatively, a loop can be used to excise the lesion, but it frequently goes too deep (see precautions discussed previously). The electrified curette works very well, but it too can go too deep, too fast, and too easily. Be careful and go slow.

For ingrown toenail surgery, where ablation of part or all of the growth center is desired, the matrixectomy electrodes perform superbly (Fig. 30-13; see Chapter 29, Ingrown Toenails).

Ear piercing: Use the thin, pointed electrode at the cutting or cut/coag setting, 2 to 3, or 25 to 30 W. Identify the sites bilaterally and mark them. Stabilize the earlobe and then advance the tip through the anesthetized tissue. Remove the tip and insert the earring stud.

Cervical dysplasia: For those trained in colposcopy and treatment of cervical intraepithelial neoplasia (CIN), this unit can be adapted to the LLETZ (large loop excision of the transformation zone) procedure with a special set of electrodes designed for this purpose (Fig. 30-14). This office procedure allows a "tailored" cervical conization (see Chapter 149, Loop Electrosurgical Excision Procedure for Treating Cervical Intraepithelial Neoplasia).

Rhinophyma: Extra tissue is removed using the large round electrode and sculpting the nose back to the original form (Fig. 30-15). Use pure cutting, level 2. Keep the tissue moist by continually wiping with a moist gauze pad.

Skin tightening (Radiage): The basic concept in skin tightening is to heat collagen, which then contracts during the healing process. No anesthesia is necessary. Special tips are used for this procedure (Fig. 30-16; see Chapter 52, Nonablative Radiowave Skin Tightening with the Ellman S5 Surgitron [The Pelleve Procedure]). The 10-mm "Radiage Wand" works for most areas, with the 5-mm one for areas around the eyes, where it is hard to maneuver.

For this procedure, the dual-frequency Ellman unit must be used. The cut/coag mode is preferred by some, although others use pure cutting, which also appears to create adequate heat. Long-term effects remain to be seen. Good immediate improvement can be seen in some patients, but contraction and, thus, tightening will continue for up to 3 months.

Typical power levels for the face are 16 to 20 W, with less for the neck (14 to 15 W) and much less for the eyelids (4 to 7 W) when done with the 5-mm tip.

Circular motions are recommended by the manufacturer, but a sweeping motion also works well. Most patients experience a pleasant sensation of warmth throughout the treatment of a given area until just before it is time to move the tip. At this point, it goes from feeling comfortable to very hot in a matter of 2 to 3 seconds. When the tip becomes too hot, move on to a new area. The excessive heat dissipates and patients are again comfortable in 2 to 3 seconds. Patients do not seem to mind this as long as the reason for it is explained to them at the beginning of the treatment.

Do not lift the wand off the skin with the handpiece activated. It will cause a small electrical shock that is uncomfortable for the patient.

Forty-five minutes is the typical treatment time for the face, including eyelids (use plastic eye shields). This does not include setup or cleanup time.

Ninety days is the expected time for revision and new collagen formation to be complete. Repeat treatment, if needed, may take place any time after that.

When using the eye shields, coat the inside with ointment-type eye lubricant to protect the corneal epithelium. Drops are not adequate. Erythromycin ophthalmic ointment works, but may cause

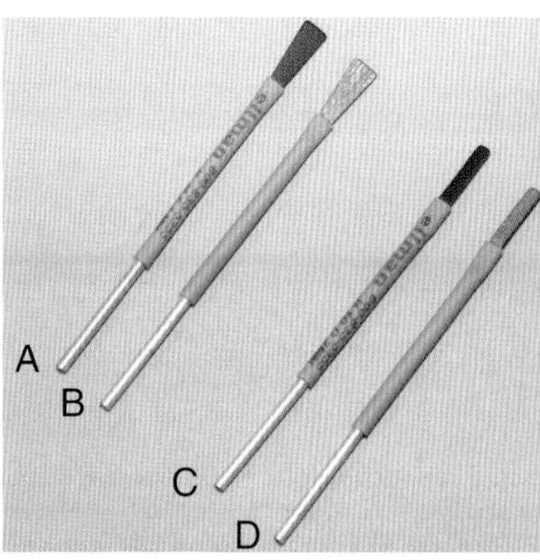

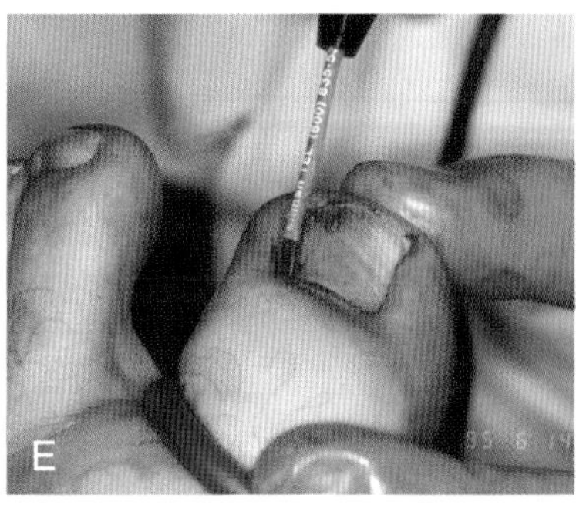

Figure 30-13 Toenail matrixectomy electrodes. **A,** Wide blade, coated Teflon side up. **B,** Wide blade, brass uncoated side up. **C,** Narrow blade, coated Teflon side up. **D,** Narrow blade, brass uncoated side up. The brass (active) side goes down, facing the matrix. The Teflon (coated, protective side) faces and lifts up against the eponychium as it is slowly withdrawn. **E,** Proper application of the matrixectomy electrode into the nail groove.

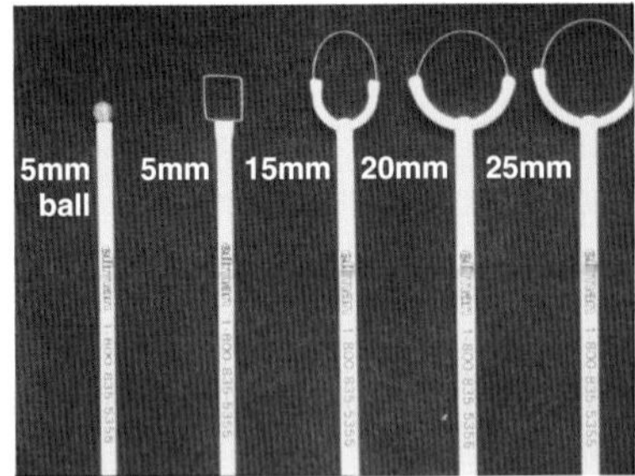

Figure 30-14 LLETZ (large loop excision of the transformation zone) electrodes used to perform office cervical conizations. (Courtesy of Ellman International, Inc., Hewlett, NY.)

allergic reactions. Consider "overnight" eye lubricants, such as GenTeal PM. Most of these seem to contain petrolatum (like LacriLube). The vision may be blurry for ½ hour or so after removal. This does not seem to be a problem if one treats the eyes first and then immediately removes the eye shields, giving time for the lubricant to dissipate during the remainder of the treatment (see Chapter 52, Nonablative Radiowave Skin Tightening with the Ellman S5 Surgitron [The Pelleve Procedure]).

Other lesions: These include tattoos, sebaceous hyperplasia, eccrine hidrocystomas, milia, verrucae plana, verrucae vulgaris, venous lakes, and trichoepitheliomas. For those performing laparoscopy, radiosurgical techniques can be used for endometriosis, pelvic inflammatory disease, myomectomy, and, in skilled hands, ectopic pregnancy. The vari-tip has also been used for blepharoplasties. The larger, pointed tips can be used for body piercing. Uvuloplasties are quite simple using excision or ablation techniques.

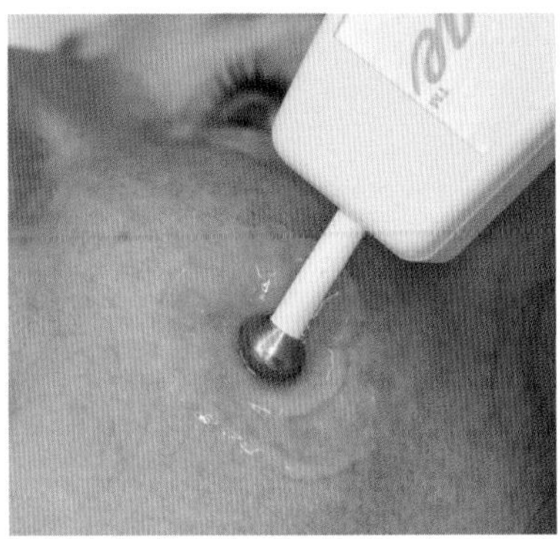

Figure 30-16 Technique for skin tightening (Radiage) using the special handpiece and tip.

Warning: As with laser, vaporization of viral particles (HPV and HIV) in the smoke plume that accompanies destruction or excision of tissues with these techniques has been documented. Those present in the room should wear protective masks, and a smoke evacuation system is mandatory (Fig. 30-17). The suction should be no further than 2 cm from the operative site. Proper vacuums have a viral filter as well as a charcoal filter to limit the offensive odor. Compact portable units are available from the same manufacturers who supply the ESUs.

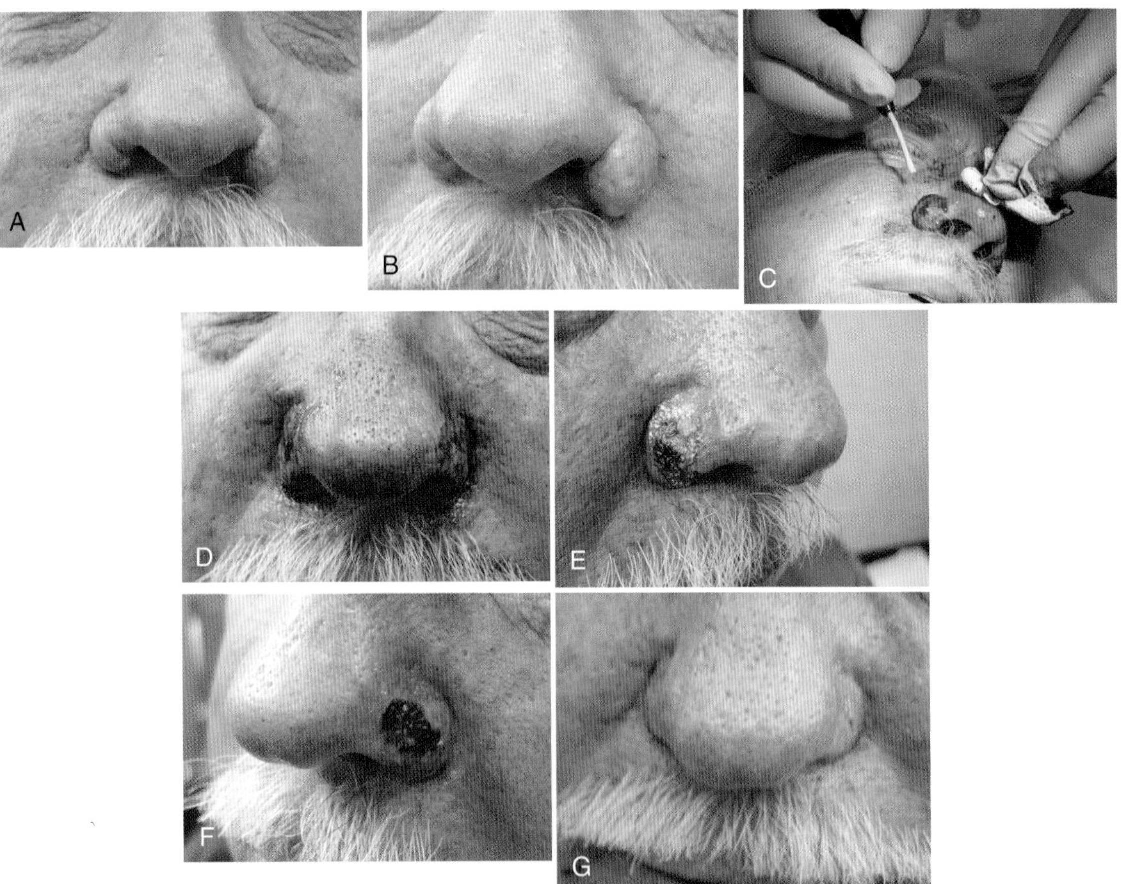

Figure 30-15 Use of radiofrequency loop to treat rhinophyma. **A,** Preoperative appearance. **B,** Preoperative appearance of left naris. **C,** Using the loop to remove tissue after a nasal block with lidocaine. **D,** Immediate postoperative appearance. **E,** Two weeks postoperative appearance, right naris. **F,** Two weeks postoperative appearance, left naris. **G,** One month postoperative appearance.

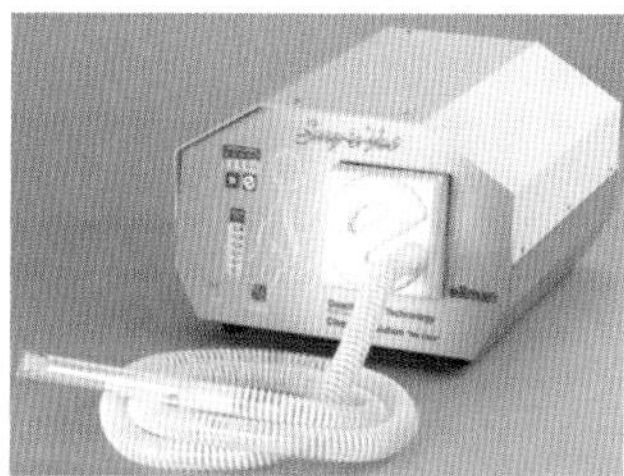

Figure 30-17 Smoke evacuator with both viral and charcoal filters. (Courtesy of Ellman International, Inc., Hewlett, NY.)

Some physicians have created their own vacuum exhaust systems leading to the exterior of the building or installed bathroom-type exhaust fans in the room.

Modern electrosurgery (RF) techniques are easily mastered and are best accomplished by attending a workshop on radiosurgery or by following the instructions given in Pollack's *Electrosurgery of the Skin*. These instructions can be practiced at home on a piece of beefsteak. Simplicity, economy, and versatility are unique to this instrument. The lesions that can be removed are myriad, depending on the practitioner's scope of practice and versatility.

Key Points

- If the ESU is adjusted to the *correct settings*, the tissue will cut like soft butter.
- If the power is too low, the stroke too fast, the skin too dry, or the electrodes not totally clean, the *electrode will stick or catch*.
- If the power is *too high*, there will be excessive sparking and smoke. The principle is to *minimize* the lateral heat. Less tissue damage occurs with the finer the tip, the less energy used, the less time the electrode stays in one spot, the more moist the tissue, use of a cutting mode, and use of a higher-frequency unit:

$$H = \frac{T \times I \times W \times S \times R}{F}$$

  where heat (H) depends on time (T), intensity of current (I), waveform (W), area of surface contact or electrode size (S), and resistance of tissue (R) divided by frequency (F).
- Once the lesion has been removed, any remaining bleeding can be controlled with topical astringents. Monsel's solution or aluminum chloride works best (see Chapter 40, Topical Hemostatic Agents).

Complications

- Broken wire causing laceration (discard worn tips).
- Too deep an excision, causing excessive scarring and trauma to undesired tissue.
- Destruction of tissue for pathologic review, caused by improper technique.
- Handpiece in wrong port or unit in wrong mode to obtain desired effect.
- Pacemaker dysfunction.
- Inadvertent burns, on either the patient or operator, resulting from unintended activation of handpiece.
- Poor healing.
- Pain, bleeding, and infection (extremely rare).
- Scarring (usually very minimal, but could result in a depression, hypopigmentation, or hyperpigmentation).
- Incomplete removal of a lesion.
- Recurrence of the lesion.
- Inadvertent shaving of a pigmented lesion that turns out to be a melanoma.
- Spreading infection between patients.
- Explosion of colonic gas (methane) from exposure to a spark (if the patient is asleep, a moist gauze should be placed in the anus to reduce the chance of a burn if performing a procedure in that area).
- Sparks can cause explosions should alcohol or other flammable agents be nearby.

Although some of these complications can be avoided, they still do occur on occasion. Removing a lesion on someone who is on aspirin or anticoagulant therapy may be accompanied by increased bleeding, necessitating heavier use of the coagulation waveform. But *do not* discontinue warfarin, aspirin, or clopidogrel. Another complication that may be seen in diabetic patients or older patients with thin, poorly perfused skin is slow or delayed healing. In this case, patients can often be instructed in self-care of the wound, with periodic inspections by the physician. Performing any procedures with these techniques on the lower extremities of diabetic patients can certainly be fraught with problems related to healing delay and possibly secondary infection. Scarring must also be considered a complication; however, once proper technique is established, a scar by this method of treatment is often less pronounced than those produced by other surgical and excisional techniques. Excising too deeply increases the likelihood of scars.

Postprocedure Patient Care

Several approaches are acceptable in the postprocedure care of these lesions. In general, the areas that were treated should be washed lightly four times per day with mild soap and water. The patient can use a washcloth for light débridement to prevent eschar formation. A topical antibiotic ointment is then applied as frequently as necessary to keep the lesion moist (even Vaseline will work). A dressing is not needed except at bedtime (or if under clothing) to ensure that the area stays moist (see the patient education handout online). Moist healing and prevention of eschar (scab) formation are essential to decrease the likelihood of scarring.

Moist healing can also occur when the lesion is simply covered with a small piece of synthetic material (e.g., Op-Site, Tegaderm) or the new Johnson & Johnson over-the-counter product called "Advanced Healing" (see Chapter 44, Wound Dressings). Leave these coverings in place for 1 week, provided there is not an excessive accumulation of serum. If serum does accumulate, the dressing should be changed. Usually, after 7 days, the wound can be left open to continue its healing process without any covering, unless it is in an area that may be irritated by clothing. This method is not practical in hair-bearing sites or if multiple lesions are removed.

CPT/Billing Codes

Billing codes for RF surgery are diverse depending on what was done. There is no special reimbursement if RF is used. Codes vary with the lesion size, benign or malignant characteristics, location, and type of removal. Some lesions would be billed out as true "excision." Others would be billed as "shave excision," and still others would be termed "destruction" or "biopsy." The reader is advised to consult the most recent CPT coding manuals and other sections of this text.

Acknowledgment

The author would like to thank J. Drlik, MD, for his contribution to the section on skin tightening (Radiage).

Suppliers

(See contact information online at www.expertconsult.com.)

Ellman International, Inc.
Wallach Surgical Devices, Inc.

For other suppliers, see Chapter 149, Loop Electrosurgical Excision Procedure for Treating Cervical Intraepithelial Neoplasia.

ONLINE RESOURCES

See patient education and patient consent forms available online at www.expertconsult.com.

Learning Tapes

Pfenninger JL: The Basics of Radiofrequency Surgery: A Guide for Clinicians (DVD). Creative Health Communications, 2005. Available through The National Procedures Institute at www.npinstitute.com.

BIBLIOGRAPHY

Brown JS: Electrocautery. In Minor Surgery: A Text and Atlas, 4th ed. New York, Oxford University Press, 2000.

Chiarello S: Controlled radio-vaporization of tumor tissue utilizing 4.0 MHz radiofrequency cutting current through a patented radiofrequency blade. Dermatol Surg 27:157, 2001.

El-Gamal HM, Dufresne RG, Saddler K: Electrosurgery, pacemakers and ICDs: A survey of precautions and complications experienced by cutaneous surgeons. Dermatol Surg 27:385–390, 2001.

Hainer BL: Fundamentals of electrosurgery. J Fam Pract 4:419–426, 1991.

Hainer BL, Usatine RB: Electrosurgery for the skin. Am Fam Physician 66:1259–1266, 2002.

Kannon GA: Moist wound healing with occlusive dressings: A clinical review. Dermatol Surg 21:583–590, 1995.

O'Grady KF, Easty AC: Electrosurgery smoke: Hazards and protection. J Clin Eng 21:149–155, 1996.

Pfenninger JL: Electrosurgery. In Usatine RP, Pfenninger JL, Stulberg DL, Small R (eds): Dermatologic and Cosmetic Procedures in Office Practice. Philadelphia, Saunders, 2011.

Pollack SV: Electrosurgery of the Skin. New York, Churchill Livingstone, 1991.

EDITOR'S NOTE: This is a comprehensive, concise, small text that provides a thorough practical review of radiosurgery.

Rex J, Ribera M, Bielsa I, et al: Surgical management of rhinophyma: Report of eight patients treated with electrosection. Dermatol Surg 28:347–349, 2002.

Soon SL, Washington CV Jr: Electrosurgery, electrocoagulation, electrofulguration, electrodesiccation, electrosection, electrocautery. In Robinson JK, Hanke DW, Sengelmann RD, Siegel DM (eds): Surgery of the Skin: Procedural Dermatology. Philadelphia, Mosby, 2005, pp 177–190.

Tuggy M, Garcia J: Procedures Consult. Available at www.proceduresconsult.com.

Usatine RP: Electrosurgery. In Usatine RP, Moy RC (eds): Skin Surgery: A Practical Guide. St. Louis, Mosby, 1998, pp 165–199.

Wedman J, Miljeteig H: Treatment of simple snoring using radio waves for ablation of uvula and soft palate: A day-case surgery procedure. Laryngoscope 112:1256–1259, 2002.

CHAPTER 31

Ring Removal from an Edematous Finger

John Harlan Haynes III • Andrew Thomas Haynes • Terrance S. Hines

Soft tissue swelling of a finger occurs with trauma, fluid retention, weight gain, arthritis, allergic reaction, infection, or iatrogenic infusion infiltration. When the finger is constricted by circumferential banding, such as with ring jewelry, venous outflow from the finger may be restricted, which can lead to nerve damage, ischemia, and digital gangrene if the ring is not removed promptly.

The involved finger should be evaluated initially for any lacerations or neurovascular compromise. This can be accomplished by testing for sensory deficits through the use of two-point discrimination to the distal fingertip and assessment of distal digital pulses with a Doppler flowmeter. In the absence of any signs of neurovascular compromise, ring-sparing techniques may be attempted initially; however, if signs of compromise are present, ring cutting is indicated. Embedded bands should be evaluated radiographically for bony involvement necessitating removal in the operating room.

Removal of a constricting ring is often described as a two-step process: (1) exsanguination of the finger and (2) removal of the ring. If a tourniquet is used to accomplish the first step, a maximum of 2 hours is recommended, although up to 4 hours has been reported. If ring removal is not accomplished by a trial of elevation, lubrication, application of ice for 5 minutes, application of a proximal blood pressure cuff, and circular traction, the clinician may use the various techniques for intact removal of a constricting band (e.g., string-wrap method or glove method). Alternatively, division of a constricting ring may be necessary using a variety of tools (e.g., conventional hand-operated or motorized circular saw, Steinmann pin cutter, wire or bolt cutters, or other commercially available cutting device). However, this damages jewelry and could injure the patient. Care should be taken to avoid implantation of metal filings, which may lead to foreign body granuloma and synovitis if the ring is cut. Rings removed by cutting are often repairable by a jeweler. After ring removal by any of these methods, a neurovascular examination should be performed as mentioned earlier. If any deficits in sensation or vascular flow are noted, prompt consultation with a hand specialist is required.

Indications

Acute or chronic finger edema with proximal band constriction

Relative Contraindications

- Open wound or fracture
- Deeply embedded ring erosion
- Lack of patient cooperation

String-Wrap Method

Equipment

- Between 2 and 3 yards of string, braided suture of 0 gauge or larger, or umbilical tape—preferably on a spool
- Adhesive tape
- Small hemostat
- 1.5 mL of 1% lidocaine *without* epinephrine *(optional)*
- 5-mL syringe with 27-gauge needle for digital nerve block *(optional)*
- Lubricating K-Y Jelly, mineral oil, vegetable oil, or the like

Technique

1. Some patients may require a digital block in case the pain increases from the compression and unwinding. If needed, 0.5 to 0.75 mL of 1% lidocaine is infiltrated deep into the neurovascular bundle on the proximal volar aspect of the affected finger bilaterally.
2. Lightly lubricate the finger near the ring. Pass the hemostat from distal to proximal under the ring, grasp the end of the string, and thread it beneath the ring, pulling several inches of string through (Fig. 31-1A). Tape the proximal end to the hand (Fig. 31-1B).
3. Wrap the string circumferentially around the finger, beginning just adjacent to the ring margin. Care should be taken to not wrap the string so tight as to obstruct arterial flow. Wind the string in a smooth single layer going distally, using moderate tension until it encompasses the point of greatest swelling (Fig. 31-1C).
4. Untape the proximal end of the string and pull distally toward the fingertip. Maintain tension along the long axis of the finger, moving the ring distally as the string unwinds beneath it. Force the ring over that portion of the finger that has been compressed by the wrap (Fig. 31-1D). Once past the area of largest diameter, usually the proximal interphalangeal joint, the ring will slide off easily.
5. Variations, including wrapping proximally to distally as well as vice versa, have been described. A number of devices have been used for this "sequential compression," including suture, thread, or floss; thicker umbilical tape, ribbon gauze, or tape; or more elastic items such as an intravenous tourniquet, rubber band, or Penrose drain.

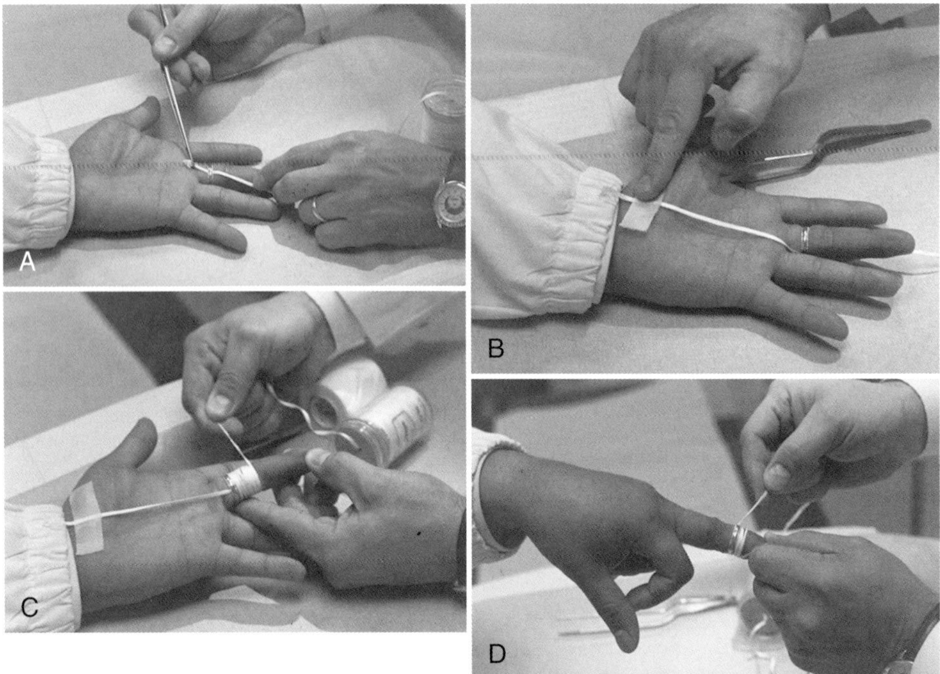

Figure 31-1 **A–D,** String-wrap method of removing ring from a swollen finger. See text for details.

Circular Saw or Steinmann Pin Cutter Method

Equipment

- Hand-held circular-blade ring cutter (e.g., Beaver) or Steinmann pin cutter with a McDonald elevator
- Large hemostats (e.g., Kelly clamps)
- 20-mL syringe filled with saline and 20-gauge Intracath sheath

Technique

1. Begin by draping the patient and providing eye protection to all persons in the work area. Slip the small hook of the ring cutter or elevator under the ring on the palmar surface to serve as a guide and barrier (Fig. 31-2). If elevation of this section is necessary for application of the ring cutter, the ring may be bent outward by using pliers with the jaws placed at 90 degrees from the cutting site.
2. Firmly grip the saw handle, and, using a 180-degree twisting motion, grind through the ring. Using the pin cutter, cut through the ring, over the elevator. This process generates heat and may be interrupted every 30 seconds to allow ring cooling to prevent further injury to the patient. Irrigation is helpful, but careful drying is necessary if electric tools are being used. Because sparks may be produced, flammable items (e.g., rubbing alcohol) must be removed.
3. The cut ends of the ring may be spread using hemostats with steady opposing force. If the ring must be cut in two places, sharp edges should be protected with a gauze covering.
4. Rinse the area with high-pressure saline to ensure evacuation of all metal filings.
5. Alternatives include the Moody GEM II motorized ring cutter, Dremel MultiPro+ cutting tool, fire department extrication tools, and carbide dental drills.
6. In cases of titanium or tungsten alloy bands causing constriction, we recommend the use of a high-speed Dremel tool with an abrasive carbide cutting wheel. A variable-speed Dremel tool and one-inch carbide cutting wheel are available at most hardware supply stores. The medial and lateral sides of the finger must be supported with malleable ribbons and the finger should be protected by a stainless steel ring support under the ring. A bulb syringe with sterile water is used to keep the ring as cool as possible while cutting. It may be necessary to consult a team member from maintenance or plant operations who is experienced in using a Dremel tool.

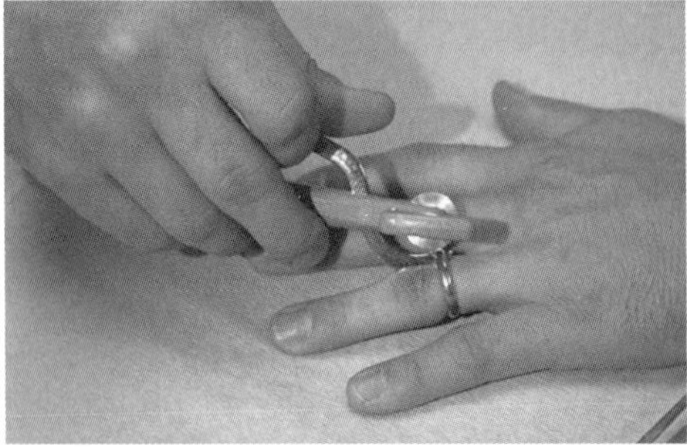

Figure 31-2 Hook of the ring cutter serves as a guide and barrier.

Surgical Glove Method

Discussion

- Not universally recommended
- Can be used in the presence of fractures or soft tissue injury
- Causes minimal additional pain

Technique

1. Cut one finger from a surgical glove (Fig. 31-3).
2. Place on involved finger.
3. Slip proximal end under ring using hemostats (Fig. 31-4A).
4. K-Y Jelly may be used to lubricate.
5. Pull proximal end back over ring (Fig. 31-4B).
6. Continue to pull and twist on the retroverted glove to advance ring distally (Fig. 31-4C).

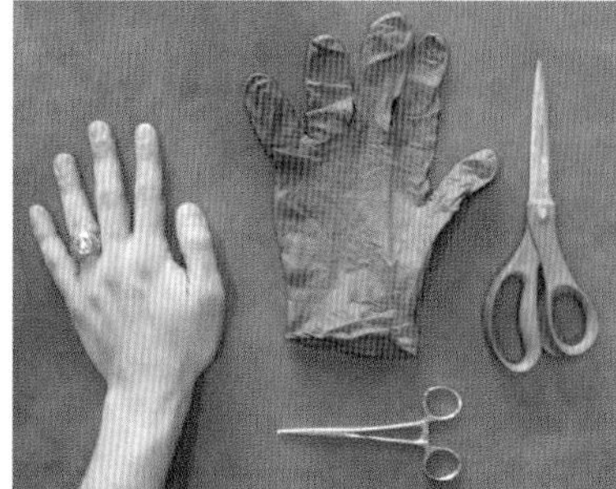

Figure 31-3 Materials needed for ring removal from an edematous finger using the surgical glove method: surgical glove, hemostat, scissors. One finger is cut from the glove and the tip is removed to form a "sleeve."

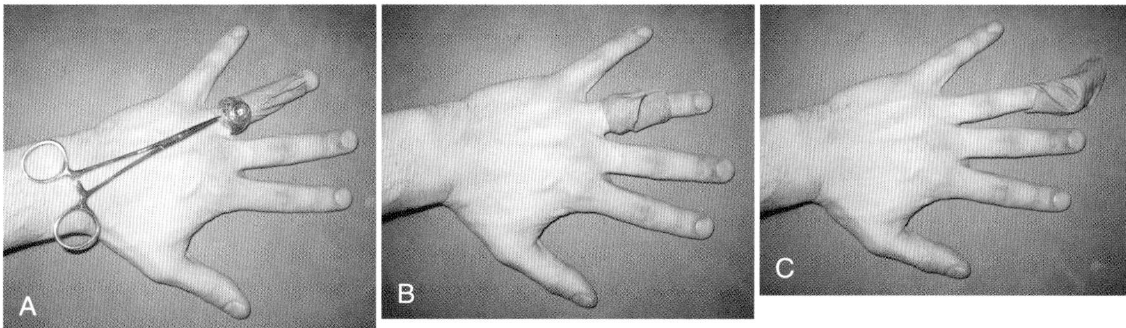

Figure 31-4 **A,** The rubber sleeve is pulled under the ring. **B** and **C,** The sleeve is pulled over the ring, removing it from the finger.

7. A variant of this technique involves using a Penrose drain. In the event of a failed removal, the drain may act as insulation against electrical burns should electrocautery be required during surgery.

Postprocedure Patient Care

- Consider appropriate tetanus prophylaxis.
- Consider antibiotics in cases of contaminated wounds, patients with diabetes, patients with comorbidities, or the immunocompromised.

CPT/Billing Codes

Ring removal is considered part of the standard evaluation and management (E&M) otherwise provided to the patient. However, if the ring removal were provided in the setting of a finger fracture, an appropriate CPT code (open, closed, manipulated) may be used if definitive treatment is provided. If definitive treatment is referred to another physician, coding for supplies and splinting may be used.

0 There is no specific code for removal of a ring. Use the appropriate E&M code.

BIBLIOGRAPHY

Belliappa PPL: A technique for removal of a tight ring. J Hand Surg [Br] 14:127, 1989.

Chiu TF, Chu SJ, Chen SG, et al: Use of a Penrose drain to remove an entrapped ring from a finger under emergent conditions. Am J Emerg Med 25:722–723, 2007.

Cresap C: Removal of a hardened steel ring from an extremely swollen finger. Am J Emerg Med 13:318–320, 1995.

Fasano FJ Jr, Hansen RH: Foreign body granuloma and synovitis of the finger: A hazard of ring removal by the sawing technique. J Hand Surg [Am] 12:621, 1987.

Fuchs SM: Ring removal. In Henretig FM, King C (eds): Textbook of Pediatric Emergency Procedures. Baltimore, Williams & Wilkins, 1997.

Inoue S, Akazawa S, Fukuda H, Shimizu R: Another simple method for ring removal. Anesthesiology 83:1133, 1995.

McElfresh EC, Peterson-Elijah RC: Removal of a tight ring by the rubber band. J Hand Surg [Br] 16:225, 1991.

Paterson P, Khanna A: A novel method of ring removal from a swollen finger [letter]. Br J Plast Surg 54:182, 2001.

Peckler B, Hsu C: Tourniquet syndrome: A review of constricting band removal. J Emerg Med 20:253–262, 2001.

Ruddy RM: Illustrated techniques of pediatric emergency procedures. In Fleisher GR, Ludwig S, Henretig FM (eds): Textbook of Pediatric Emergency Medicine, 5th ed. Philadelphia, Lippincott, Williams & Wilkins, 2006, p 1861.

Rudnitsky GS, Barnett RC: Soft tissue foreign body removal. In Roberts JR, Hedges JR (eds): Clinical Procedures of Emergency Medicine, 3rd ed. Philadelphia, WB Saunders, 1998.

Thilagarajah M: An improved method of ring removal. J Hand Surg [Br] 24:118–119, 1999.

Tintinalli JE, Ruiz E, Krome RL: Emergency Medicine: A Comprehensive Study Guide. New York, McGraw-Hill, 1996.

Tuggy M, Garcia J: Procedures Consult. Available at www.proceduresconsult.com.

CHAPTER 32

Skin Biopsy

John L. Pfenninger

Examination and appropriate history suffice to establish most dermatologic diagnoses. At times, however, biopsies are necessary. A skin biopsy is typically performed to make or confirm a diagnosis and to guide definitive treatment. In many instances, a biopsy serves as the means of both diagnosis and treatment if it removes the entire lesion. Needle aspiration biopsy (see Chapter 226, Fine-Needle Aspiration Cytology and Biopsy) is usually reserved for deeper lesions but at times can also be used to diagnose skin lesions.

Skin biopsies are generally quick, simple, and cost effective. Diagnoses obtained by biopsy also serve to build a physician's experience and skill in dermatologic diagnosis by providing feedback and confirming the clinical diagnosis, perhaps reducing the need for future biopsies of similar lesions.

To enable the pathologist to provide the most information possible, provide a good history with each specimen submitted. Include aspects of the "seven Ds":

1. *Demographics* (e.g., patient's age, history of travel, location of lesion)
2. *Diseases* (other diseases the patient has [e.g., lupus])
3. *Duration* (how long it has been present)
4. *Drugs* applied to the lesion or taken by the patient that could be the cause or change the appearance of the lesion (e.g., topical or oral steroids)
5. *Description* (e.g., papular, vesicular, hyperkeratotic)
6. *Diameter*
7. *Diagnosis* suspected

Skin biopsies are either partial or full thickness. Partial-thickness biopsies include shave excision and curettage. Full-thickness biopsies include standard excisional and incisional biopsies and the punch biopsy. Punch biopsies take only 5 to 7 minutes to complete; excisional or incisional types take longer. All of these may readily be incorporated in a primary care setting and can be performed when the patient first presents.

Priorities to be kept in mind when performing skin biopsies are (1) maintaining patient comfort and safety, (2) obtaining an appropriate tissue sample for pathologic diagnosis, and (3) producing the best cosmetic (least scarring) and functional result possible. Although written consent forms are usually not necessary for a skin biopsy, it is still important that patients understand the nature of the procedure, why it is being performed, and the possible complications.

Indications

- To obtain a tissue sample for diagnosis by histopathology, electron microscopy, or immunofluorescence testing
- To perform an excision for curative or cosmetic purposes
- To obtain a deep culture (bacterial or fungal) while avoiding superficial contamination of wounds (e.g., decubitus ulcers)

NOTE: Lyme disease can be confirmed through cultures of biopsy material.

In general, the main reasons to do a skin biopsy are to rule out cancer and to determine the disease process present. If the physician's answer to the question "What is it?" is "I don't know," that may be an indication for biopsy (not necessarily referral). The next question should be, "Could this be a melanoma?" If the answer is "yes," then a full-thickness biopsy (punch, incision, or excision) is indicated.

Contraindications

- Significant coagulopathy (warfarin, clopidogrel, and aspirin do not need to be stopped).
- Preparations, anesthetics, preservatives, or other materials to which the patient is allergic.
- Partial-thickness biopsies are discouraged if not contraindicated if melanoma is suspected (must "biopsy for depth").

A biopsy does *not* spread or activate the disease, distort a future diagnosis of a melanoma, or compromise future care (unless possibly if a melanoma is shaved and transected). The only potential error that can be made in sampling a lesion is to shave a melanoma and not include the entire depth. If the entire lesion is removed so its depth can be assessed, there is no consequence. However, if when performing a shave biopsy/removal, part of the lesion is left behind, thereby making it impossible to determine prebiopsy thickness, it could compromise appropriate care. Melanoma treatment and prognosis are based on depth of the neoplasm. Thus, if there is a true consideration for melanoma, it is best to perform "biopsy for depth," which means a punch or excision. The fear that any pigmented lesion "could be" a melanoma should not deter a clinician from doing a biopsy. In practice, the majority of atypical nevi are removed using a shave technique. It is impractical to remove every such nevus with a full-thickness frank excision using suture closure. It is far better to shave and transect a melanoma than to ignore a lesion and miss the melanoma. The point is to sample suspect lesions, or to refer the patient for biopsy and definitive care.

Equipment

- Nonsterile gloves (sterile if sutures are to be placed)
- Alcohol wipes
- Local anesthetic (0.5 to 1.0 mL of 1% to 2% lidocaine with or without epinephrine)
- Hemostatic agents (see Chapter 40, Topical Hemostatic Agents)
- Antibiotic ointment
- Adhesive bandage
- Specimen container, usually containing formalin

NOTE: Tissue for culture may need to be placed in saline, whereas immunofluorescent studies may require that the tissue be placed in dry ice. Check with the pathologist to determine the proper handling of tissue for the diagnosis of Lyme disease.

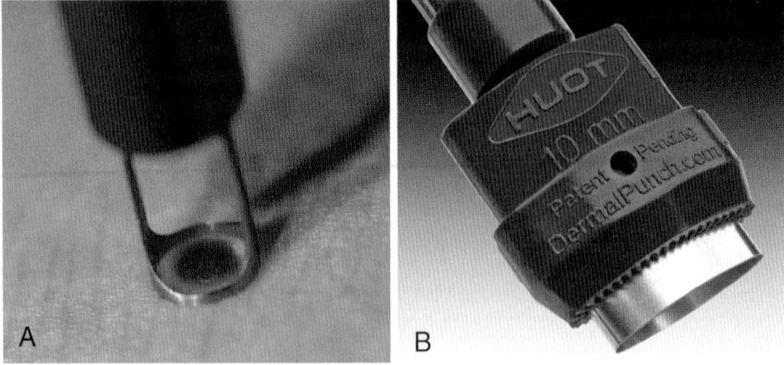

Figure 32-1 Biopsy punch tools. **A**, The VisiPunch. **B,** The Elliptiscalpel. (Courtesy of Huot Instruments, Menomonee Falls, Wisc.)

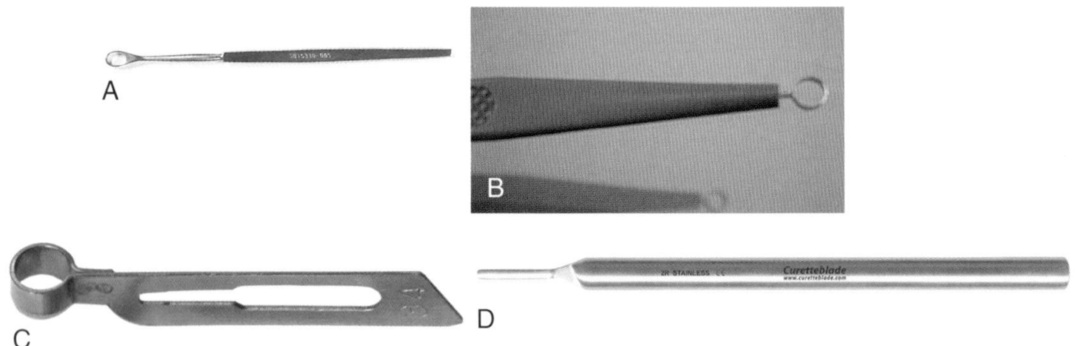

Figure 32-2 **A,** Fox dermal curette (reusable). **B,** Disposable curette. **C,** Disposable curette blade. **D,** Curette blade with smooth handle.

For Punch Biopsy

- A 2-, 3-, or 4-mm punch biopsy tool; disposable biopsy punches are convenient and inexpensive, and it is not necessary to clean, sterilize, or sharpen them. The 2-mm punch is used only for areas where scarring is to be avoided because such a small amount of tissue may lead to a missed diagnosis, or the tissue can become inappropriately crushed. Biopsies over 4 mm in size will leave more scarring and, if sutured, may leave a "dog-ear effect." Newer disposable punches (VisiPunch, Huot Instruments, Menomonee Falls, Wisc; Fig. 32-1A) allow better visualization of the tissue being sampled, whereas other types (the Elliptiscalpel, Huot Instruments; Fig. 32-1B) can remove larger lesions by performing an elliptical excision.
- Pickups.
- Sharp fine tissue scissors.
- Suture kit or Steri-Strips (only if the biopsy site is 4 mm or larger).

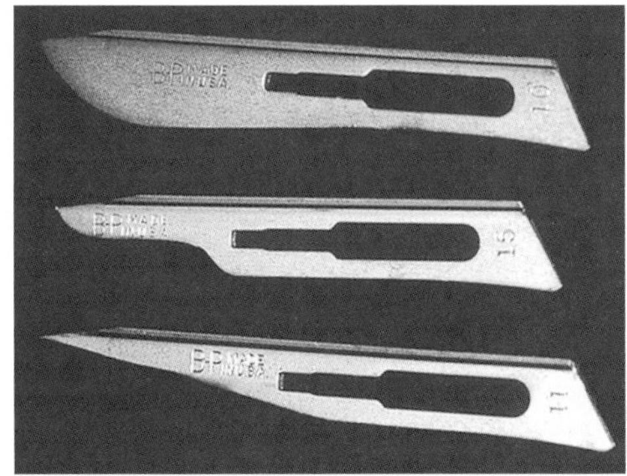

Figure 32-3 No. 10, 15, and 11 scalpel blades used for shave excisions.

For Curettage

A dermal curette (Fig. 32-2) is used. *Disposable* curettes are recommended for nonmalignant lesions. Disposables are very sharp and will cut into the skin quite readily so must be used with caution. They do have a tendency to bend if a lesion is fibrotic (e.g., verruca). *Reusable* curettes do not bend but are not as sharp and often are inadequate for benign lesions where tissue adhesion is good. Neoplastic tissue (e.g., basal cell carcinomas, squamous cell carcinomas), on the other hand, is necrotic and easily curetted. When used for this purpose, reusable curettes are also less likely to cut into the normal skin structures. The curette blade (see Fig. 32-2C and D) is interesting and has some excellent features. The curette is disposable, so it is sharp and fits on a scalpel handle. It also does not bend, so when curetting fibrotic tissue, like verrucae, it maintains its shape and curetting function. Curettes of 2, 3, 4, 5, and 6 mm should be available. The size used depends on the size of the lesion.

For Shave Excisions

A single-edge flexible razor blade or scalpel blade (no. 10 or 15) is used (Fig. 32-3). A scalpel handle is not needed; not only does it take time to insert and remove the blade on the handle, but medical personnel can be injured during the process. The blade itself or a radiofrequency unit may be used to smooth out the surface after the shave excision. (See Chapter 30, Radiofrequency Surgery [Modern Electrosurgery], to review the technique.) Sharp tissue scissors (Metzenbaum) can also be used to perform the "shave" by clipping off elevated lesions.

TABLE 32-1 Selection of Biopsy Site Based on Lesion Type

Lesion Suspected	Where to Biopsy
Basal cell carcinoma	Raised, nonulcerated area
Squamous cell carcinoma	Central, thickened area
Melanoma	Darkest, raised portion
Vesiculobullous disease	Fresh lesion at the margin; include some normal tissue (see Fig. 32-4)
Rashes	Primary lesion without secondary excoriation or infection

Normal tissue is not needed in most instances (only with vesiculobullous lesions).
A biopsy does not spread cancer.
In sampling a suspected melanoma, go for depth (i.e., a punch instead of a shave).
Most chronic dermatitis is nonspecific on biopsy. A dermatologic consult may be indicated and be more beneficial.

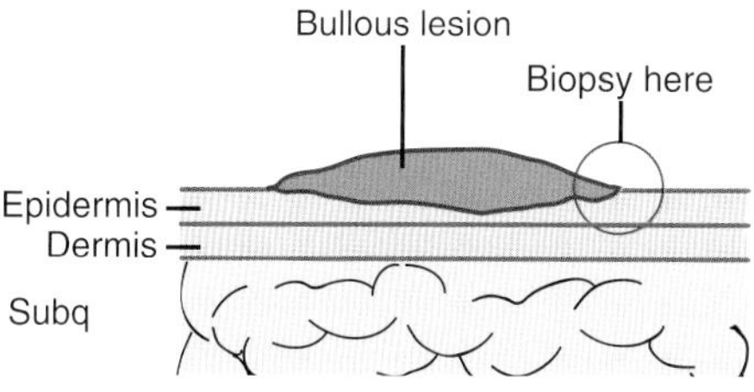

Figure 32-4 Obtaining a skin biopsy when a vesicle or bulla is present. Normal tissue should be included in the specimen. "Fresh" lesions that have not ruptured and are not crusted should be chosen.

For Incisions and Excisions

- Minor surgical or laceration tray with scalpel, skin hooks, pickups, tissue scissors, and suture (see Chapter 21, Incisions: Planning the Direction of the Incision; Chapter 22, Laceration and Incision Repair; and Chapter 24, Laceration and Incision Repair: Suture Selection)
- Radiofrequency unit if desired (see Chapter 30, Radiofrequency Surgery [Modern Electrosurgery])

TECHNIQUE

Choosing a Biopsy Site

Although any skin area can be sampled, being selective improves final outcome. See Table 32-1 for recommendations specific to particular lesions and Table 32-2 for anatomic sites.

It is *not necessary to include normal tissue* in the sample, except when sampling a vesiculobullous lesion. It is then necessary to sample (usually a punch) right at the margin where the epidermis is being lifted from the underlying tissue (Fig. 32-4). If the lesion is small, a deep shave removing the entire lesion is also acceptable.

TABLE 32-2 Site-Specific Biopsy Guidelines

Location	Comments
Breast	Punch or shave
Cervix	Mini-Townsend or baby Tischler forceps (see Chapter 137, Colposcopic Examination)
Eyelid	Sharp tissue scissors for shave removal
Gingiva	Shave; consider radiofrequency unit to limit bleeding if lesion is elevated
Intra-anal	Cervical biopsy forceps or flexible sigmoidoscopy biopsy forceps
Lip	Punch (bloody; heals quickly) or shave
Muscle	See Chapter 228, Muscle Biopsy
Nail bed	Remove portion of nail; use small punch (see Chapter 27, Nail Bed Repair)
Penis	Thin skin; use shave technique; stay superficial; scissors or sharp curette works best
Perianal	Sharp tissue scissors
Pinna	Shave; superficial punch; curette
Tongue	Punch; bloody; use suture; curette
Trunk	Any method
Vagina	Cervical biopsy forceps
Vulva	Hair-bearing area: use punch for depth Non–hair-bearing area: shave biopsy (see Chapter 159, Vulvar Biopsy)

When there are multiple lesions that could be sampled, **avoid** the following areas:

- Cosmetically important areas
- Upper chest and deltoid regions, where hypertrophic scarring is more common
- Fingers, toes, and areas overlying joints
- Regions in which secondary infection (e.g., axillae and groin) or delayed healing (e.g., pretibial) is common
- Areas that compromise underlying structures, including superficial nerves and vessels
- Old lesions (choose well-developed but "fresh" lesions free of excoriation or excessive inflammation)
- Ulcerated lesions (if the only available lesion is ulcerated, include a border of the lesion in the specimen)
- Areas of poor circulation

Punch Biopsy

The punch biopsy instrument is used to obtain a full-thickness cylindrical specimen. Punch biopsy is a good choice for complete removal of small lesions (<5 mm) or whenever there is doubt as to the diagnosis or optimal treatment for a particular lesion. It is strongly recommended when melanoma is a significant consideration because it provides information on the depth of the lesion. The whole lesion does not have to be removed at the time of biopsy, and a biopsy does not change the natural history of the lesion's progression in any way.

1. Prepare the selected site with alcohol. Sterile technique should be followed if sutures are intended; otherwise, nonsterile gloves can be used. Biopsies of 2 or 3 mm do not need to be closed with sutures. A 4-mm biopsy on the face may need to be sutured, and a 5-mm biopsy nearly always requires suturing.
2. Place a ring of anesthesia around the lesion (field block) or deep to the lesion.
3. Choose the appropriate-sized punch unit (2 to 5 mm). Remember that 2-mm biopsies may not provide adequate tissue for diagnosis and are somewhat difficult to handle. To minimize scarring, stretch the skin on both sides of the planned biopsy site away from the site, perpendicular to the lines of minimal skin tension, using the thumb and index finger of the nondominant hand (Fig. 32-5). Then push the unit vertically into the skin and rotate it back and forth to cut through the skin to the subcutaneous fat (Fig. 32-6A). A decrease in resistance should be felt at the point where the dermis is completely penetrated (much like doing a lumbar puncture).
4. Withdraw the punch. Push down with the fingers on each side of the biopsy. If the "plug" goes down with the skin, the biopsy has not gone deep enough. If the plug pops up instead of going down, then the adipose tissue has been entered and the tissue has been freed adequately. Gently grasp the specimen with forceps or a skin hook. Lift the specimen and free it by cutting the subcutaneous base with sharp tissue scissors (Fig. 32-6B and

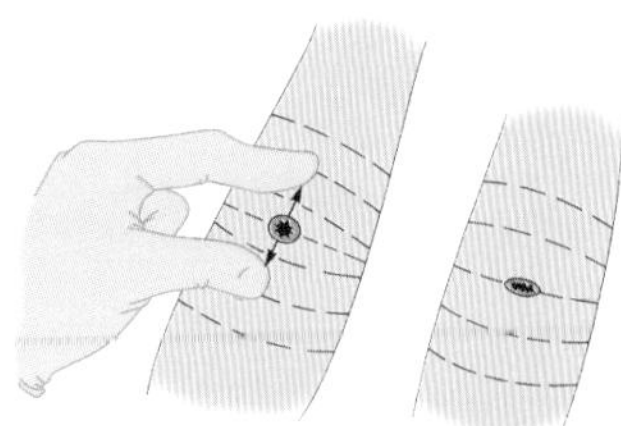

Figure 32-5 Proper stretching of skin tension lines before punch biopsy (arm). On release, the tendency of the skin is to make the circular biopsy become more elliptical and thus more cosmetically pleasing when healed.

C; Fig. 32-7). Apply pressure for hemostasis. Avoid chemical astringents in punch sites if the wound is to be closed with sutures, Steri-Strips, or glues; otherwise, apply Monsel's solution, aluminum chloride, or Gelfoam to control the bleeding. (Biopsies 3 mm or less rarely, if ever, need closure.) Rarely, electrocautery will be needed to control bleeds. A small pressure dressing with a folded 2 × 2 gauze under a Band-Aid is usually sufficient (Fig. 32-8).

5. Large punch instruments (>5 mm) are available, but closure of these wounds may require conversion of the circular defect into an ellipse because closure would otherwise cause "dog ears." Alternatively, consider using the Elliptiscalpel.
6. Use of absorbable sutures provides the same outcome cosmetically as does the use of nonabsorbable sutures, but they are more costly. With punch biopsies of 4 mm or less, outcomes are the same regardless of whether a suture is placed.

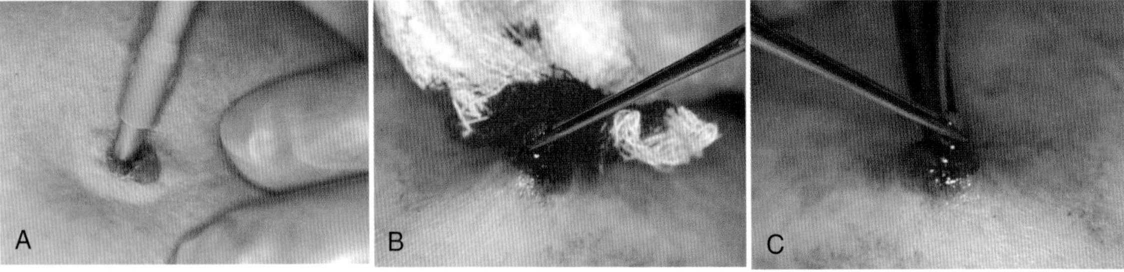

Figure 32-6 **A,** Applying the punch for a skin biopsy. **B,** Excising the tissue freed by the punch. **C,** Typical cylinder of tissue obtained from a 3-mm punch. (Courtesy of The Medical Procedures Center, PC, Midland, Mich.)

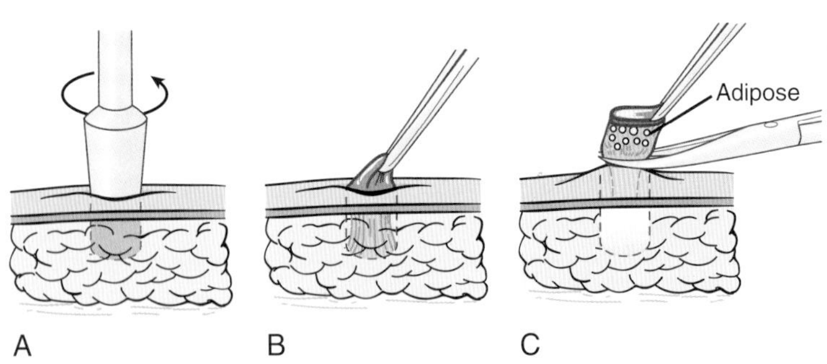

Figure 32-7 Graphic representation of the punch biopsy technique. **A,** Twisting the punch with gentle pressure. **B,** Picking up the loosened piece. **C,** Cutting with scissors or a blade.

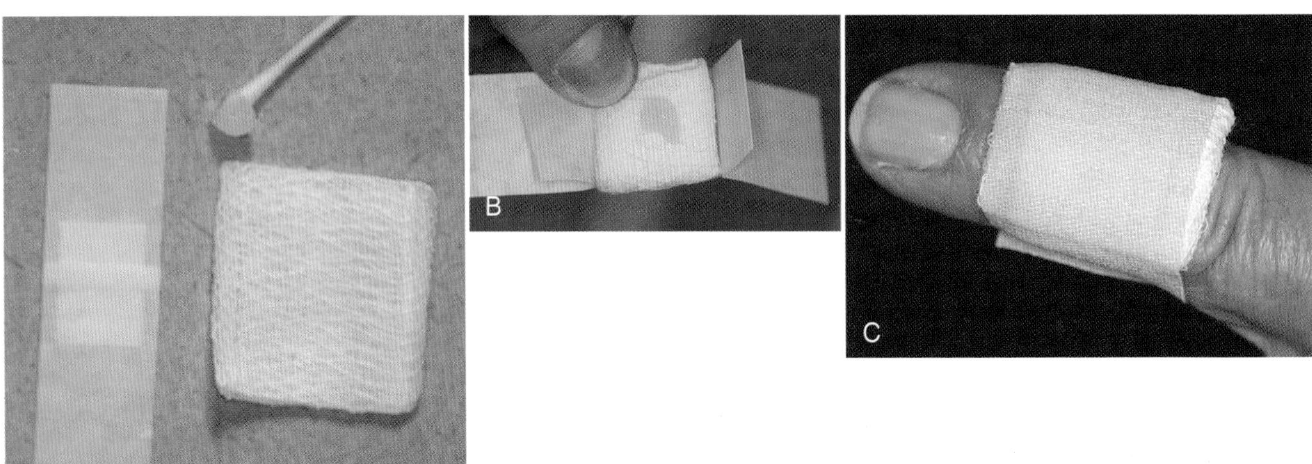

Figure 32-8 The pressure dressing for a biopsy. **A,** Components: gauze pad, antibiotic ointment, and Band-Aid. **B,** Gauze pad with antibiotic ointment. **C,** Pressure dressing on finger.

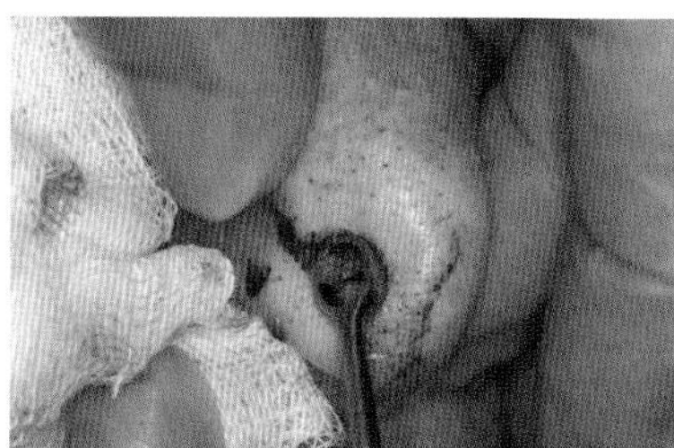

Figure 32-9 Skin biopsy performed using a reusable curette to obtain a sample. (Courtesy of The Medical Procedures Center, PC, Midland, Mich.)

Curettage

Curettage is a partial-thickness technique and is particularly well suited for biopsy removal of basal cell carcinomas and hyperkeratotic epidermal lesions such as warts, molluscum contagiosum, seborrheic keratoses, and actinic keratoses (see Chapter 12, Approach to Various Skin Lesions). A potential disadvantage of curettage in terms of obtaining a laboratory specimen is that, usually, multiple fragments of specimen are produced and the presence of disease-free margins cannot be determined. The physician performing the procedure decides if the removal is adequate. Many times, the initial curettement will reveal necrotic tissue consistent with a neoplasm such as a basal cell carcinoma. If it is elected to proceed with treatment at that time, only the first curettement specimen is sent to pathology.

NOTE: With benign lesions, it is clinically apparent when the abnormal tissue has been removed. For treatment (not just biopsy) of malignant lesions, continue curettement until there is a "gritty" tissue sensation, which is then followed by cautery. This process of curettement followed by cautery is done three times to ensure complete removal of any foci of *neoplastic* tissue (e.g., basal cell carcinoma, advanced actinic keratosis, or squamous cell carcinoma).

1. Prepare the area with alcohol and obtain an anesthetic wheal. Use the curette to scrape away or scoop out the lesion, typically in multiple fragments. Send the curetted tissue to pathology. (Remember to use disposable instruments for more fibrotic lesions and reusable curettes for necrotic tissue; see earlier discussion.)
2. Continue the curettage until only normal tissue remains at the margins. Usually, this is the upper aspect of the dermis, which feels "gritty" or "sandy" under the curette and demonstrates punctate surface bleeding. Use hemostasis as needed with topical hemostatic agents or light ball cautery. Carcinomas and severely dysplastic lesions generally feel soft and scrape out easily. Remember, when using curettage to treat a carcinoma, repeat a process of curettage and cautery three times (Fig. 32-9; see Chapter 12, Approach to Various Skin Lesions).
3. If, in the case of cancer, curettage (or shave excision) produces a full-thickness skin wound and adipose tissue is entered, this indicates that the tumor has probably invaded below the dermis. Set up a sterile field, excise the area, and close the wound with suture.

Shave Biopsy

Shave biopsy is used frequently and is best suited to remove the protruding portion of a raised skin lesion when a full-thickness sample is not required. Flat lesions such as nevi also can be removed/sampled using this technique, but rather than shaving flat across the surface, a saucer-shaped incision is made to go deeper in the center to remove the lesion.

Shave excisions should not be performed if a melanoma is suspected because they may interfere with the pathologist's ability to grade the depth of invasion. A melanoma is treated based on the depth of invasion, and a difference of 0.1 mm or even 0.01 mm could be the difference between little further treatment and a radical resection. Lesions most amenable to shave excision include compound or intradermal nevi, skin tags, seborrheic keratoses, actinic keratoses, lentigines, and small basal cell carcinomas.

Advantages of shave excision include minimal time requirement, simple equipment, lack of need for suturing, and generally excellent cosmetic results. Also, the pathologist can determine if the entire lesion has been removed.

1. Prepare the area with alcohol and use clean technique; sterile gloves are not necessary. Reserve full sterile setup for full-thickness skin excisions that will be sutured. Instill a local anesthetic within the dermis underneath the lesion to elevate the lesion slightly, facilitating removal.
2. Excise the lesion by shaving with a slightly bowed, flexible, single-edge razor blade or with a scalpel blade kept parallel to the skin (Fig. 32-10). The resulting defect should be essentially level,

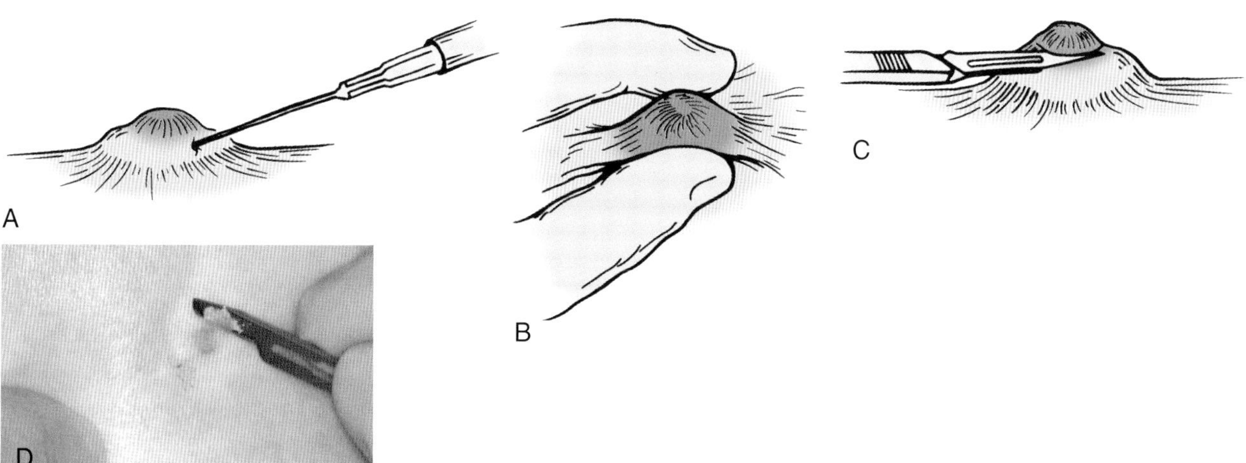

Figure 32-10 One technique of shave biopsy. **A,** Inject a local anesthetic to elevate the lesion. **B,** Roll the skin between the thumb and forefinger to create a flat cutting surface and a tamponade effect on the surrounding blood vessels. **C,** Holding a no. 15 blade parallel to the skin or at a slight downward angle, shave the lesion flush with or slightly below the surrounding skin. **D,** Shave technique using a no. 15 blade. *No scalpel handle is necessary.* (**A–C,** Courtesy of The Medical Procedures Center, PC, Midland, Mich.)

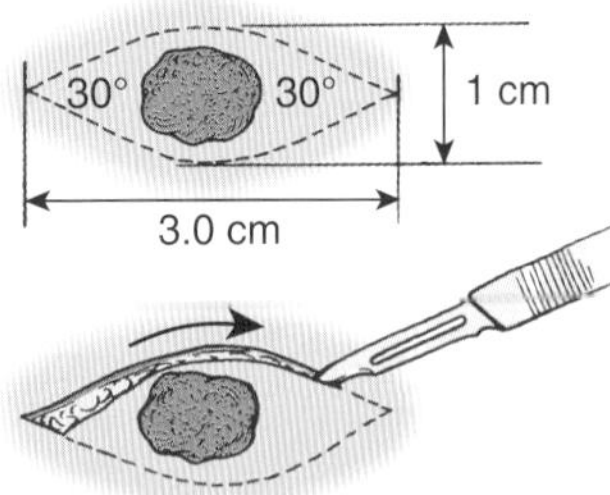

Figure 32-11 Elliptical excision biopsy technique. See text for details.

or minimally depressed, in relation to the surrounding skin. The greater the depth of the shave into the dermis, the more likely there will be resultant scarring. Apply simple pressure, pinpoint electrodesiccation, radiofrequency loop smoothing (pure cutting level 2/20 watts), or topical agents such as aluminum chloride or Monsel's solution to achieve hemostasis. Topical applications theoretically may inhibit healing. Monsel's solution and silver nitrate carry the risk of temporary staining.

3. Shave excision can also be performed using a radiofrequency loop. Heat artifact may occur at the margins of the excision, hindering histopathologic evaluation, or in the case of a very thin lesion, obliterating the lesion entirely. Also, because of the ease of cutting with the radiofrequency unit, the novice user may inadvertently go too deep with the loop, causing excessive and unnecessary scarring. Many practitioners perform a shave biopsy with a scalpel blade then use a radiofrequency loop to "feather out" the edges of the defect created to complete the procedure (see Chapter 30, Radiofrequency Surgery [Modern Electrosurgery]).
4. Sharp tissue scissors can be used, especially for pedunculated lesions, to effectively shave off the abnormality.
5. A variation of the shave biopsy is the **saucer excision.** With this technique, the central aspect of the biopsy, instead of being flat, is more depressed than the periphery. This technique might be used for actinic lesions, nevi, or dermatofibromas. In cases of suspected dysplastic nevi (but not a melanoma), one may cautiously perform a "deep saucer shave" because it allows histopathologic review of the tissue to ensure everything has been removed. Be sure, however, not to partially transect a melanoma; this is a very fine line. When in doubt, perform a deep punch biopsy first to confirm the nature of the lesion.

Excisional or Incisional Biopsy

An **excisional biopsy** is used to remove an entire lesion in a manner that obtains a full-thickness specimen of skin. It generally refers to traditional frank excision with suture closure. Diagnosis and treatment can be carried out at the same time. Excisional biopsy can be used for removal of malignant, or suspected malignant, skin lesions where margins can be assessed. The problem with this approach is that the recommendations for "clear margins" vary depending on the lesion involved (e.g., 1 to 2 mm for benign lesions, 3 mm for a basal cell carcinoma, 5 mm for a squamous cell carcinoma, 10 mm for invasive melanoma <1 mm deep), and this is often unknown until the histology report is obtained. Doing a primary excision for a biopsy may lead to an excessive and unnecessarily large excision, or may require repeat surgery so that more tissue can be removed. An **incisional biopsy** removes only a portion of a larger lesion, and residual abnormal tissue remains. In general, a single punch biopsy (or more, if the lesion is very large) would be quicker and more acceptable when the diagnosis is uncertain. Then, once the diagnosis is known, appropriate treatment may be addressed.

1. In performing an excision, use sterile technique. Establish anesthesia, preferably in a field block pattern. Use a surgical marking pen to outline the planned margins of excision, and orient the long axis of the excision parallel to the lines of minimal skin tension (see Chapters 22, Laceration and Incision Repair, through Chapter 25, Laceration and Incision Repair: Suture Tying). Form the planned excision in the shape of an ellipse with a length that measures three times its width. The corners of the ellipse should subtend approximately 30 degrees (Fig. 32-11). See Chapter 12, Approach to Various Skin Lesions, for a discussion of appropriate margins for various lesions.
2. With the scalpel, make the initial incision along the outlined excision, then free up one corner of the ellipse, excising the full thickness of skin. Excise from one end to the center, then from the opposite end to the center, obtaining a specimen of uniform thickness. (A common error is to perform only a partial-thickness excision in the corners or lateral aspects of the wound.)
3. After the specimen is freed, undermine the edges on each side of the wound to a distance measuring the width of the original wound (Fig. 32-12). Undermine between the dermis and subcutaneous tissue with a scalpel blade, tissue scissors, or a radiofrequency unit using a vari-tip or fine needle with the unit set on the cut and coagulation setting.
4. A simple single-layer closure suffices for wounds with minimal tension. Otherwise, absorbable subcutaneous sutures (e.g., Dexon, Vicryl, PDS II) placed with an inverted knot can be used to reduce tension on the skin edges before final closure is completed (Fig. 32-13; see also Chapter 22, Laceration and Incision Repair).

NOTE: The following topics can be found in their respective chapters: planning the excisional site (Chapter 22, Laceration and Incision Repair), choosing and administering the anesthetic (Chapter 4, Local Anesthesia), selecting the suture (Chapter 24, Laceration and Incision Repair: Suture Selection), performing proper closures (Chapter 25, Laceration and Incision Repair: Suture Tying), and choosing dressings (Chapter 44, Wound Dressing).

Complications

- *Pain:* Generally insignificant.
- *Infection:* If the patient washes the area three to four times per day with soap and water and applies ointment (antibiotic or otherwise) to keep it moist, there is rarely an infection.

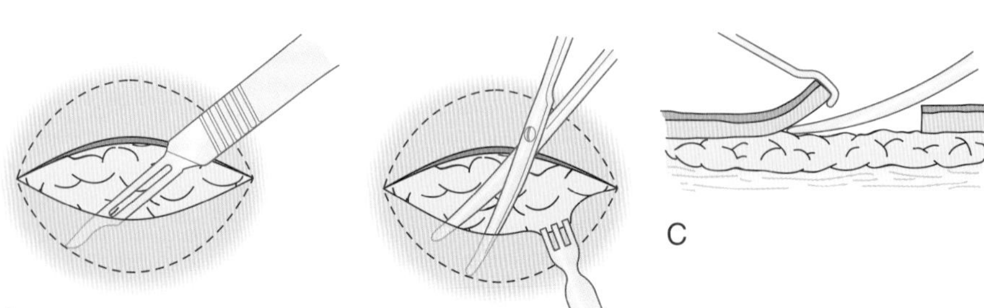

Figure 32-12 Subcutaneous undermining to release tension on wound margins with scalpel (**A**) and scissors (**B**). Proper level for undermining within subcutaneous fat (**C**).

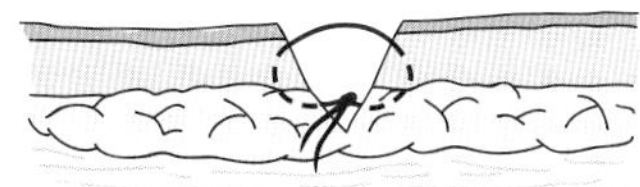

Figure 32-13 Deep inverted absorbable sutures to close dead space after excision.

- *Excessive bleeding:* Almost nonexistent.
- *Scarring:* Always a possibility. With punch biopsies, there may be an "acne-like" pockmark. Obviously, excision and incision leave a line and possibly suture tracks. All methods can leave hypopigmentation. Some topical hemostatic agents (Monsel's solution and especially silver nitrate) can leave prolonged hyperpigmentation.
- *Missing the correct diagnosis:* A lesion may be sent for biopsy, but unless it is totally removed, the most significant area could be missed. (Likewise, the practitioner could unknowingly shave and transect through a melanoma; therefore, if there is any doubt, perform the biopsy for depth.)
- *Allergic reactions:* To topical antibiotics, the anesthetic, dressings, and other agents (usually indicated by redness and itching).
- *Recurrence:* Even if it was thought that the entire lesion was removed, both benign and malignant lesions can recur.

Postprocedure Patient Education

Shave excisions and curettage require moist healing, as described for radiofrequency shave excisions in Chapter 30, Radiofrequency Surgery (Modern Electrosurgery). Care for sutured full-thickness wounds is like that for primary clean lacerations and incisions described in Chapter 22, Laceration and Incision Repair.

CPT/Billing Codes

11100	Skin biopsy, one lesion
11101	Biopsy, each additional lesion
11755	Biopsy nail unit
30100	Biopsy intranasal
38500	Biopsy/excision lymph node, superficial
38505	Biopsy lymph node, by needle
41100	Tongue, anterior two thirds
41105	Tongue, posterior one third
45100	Biopsy anorectal wall
54100	Biopsy penis, cutaneous
54105	Biopsy penis, deep
56605	Biopsy lesion, vulva or perineum
56606	Vulva, each additional
57100	Biopsy vagina, simple
57105	Biopsy vagina, extensive
57500	Biopsy cervix
67810	Biopsy eyelid
68100	Biopsy of conjunctiva
69100	Biopsy pinna
69105	Biopsy ear canal

ICD-9-CM Diagnostic Codes

See Appendix G for a listing of ICD-9-CM codes for the skin.

Suppliers

(See contact information online at www.expertconsult.com.)

Disposable and reusable punches and curettes

Acuderm, Inc.
CooperSurgical, Inc.
Curetteblade, Inc.
Delasco
Huot Instruments LLC (Wittenberg VisiPunch and ElliptiPunch)
Miltex

Any office medical supplier should be able to supply the basic instruments needed for skin biopsy.

Additional Resources

See information on moist healing in Chapter 30, Radiofrequency Surgery (Modern Electrosurgery).

See patient education and patient consent forms available online at www.expertconsult.com.

Bibliography

Achar S: Principles of skin biopsies for the family physician. Am Fam Physician 54:2411–2418, 1996.

American Cancer Society and National Comprehensive Cancer Network: Melanoma: Treatment guidelines for patients (Pt 1). Dermatol Nurs 17:119–131, 2005.

American Cancer Society and National Comprehensive Cancer Network: Melanoma: Treatment guidelines for patients (Pt 2). Dermatol Nurs 17:191–198, 2005.

Bergfield WF, Pfenninger JL, Weinstock MA: Skin biopsy: Selecting an optimal technique. Patient Care March 30:11, 2001.

Boyd AS, Neldner KH: How to submit a specimen for cutaneous pathology analyses: Using the "5 D's" to get the most from biopsies. Arch Fam Med 6:64–66, 1997.

Coit DG, Andtbacka R, Bichakjian CK, et al: Melanoma. J Natl Compr Canc Netw 7:250–275, 2009.

Dummer R, Hauschild A, Jost L, for the ESMO Guidelines Working Group: Cutaneous malignant melanoma: ESMO clinical recommendations for diagnosis, treatment and follow-up. Ann Oncol 19(Suppl 2):86–88, 2008.

Gabel EA, Jimenez GP, Eaglstein WH, et al: Performance of nylon and an absorbable suture material (Polyglactin 910) in the closure of punch biopsy sites. Dermatol Surg 26:750–752, 2000.

Garbe C, Hauschild A, Volkenandt M, et al: Evidence-based and interdisciplinary consensus-based German guidelines: Systemic medical treatment of melanoma in the adjuvant and palliative setting. Melanoma Res 18:152–160, 2008.

Garbe C, Hauschild A, Volkenandt M, et al: Evidence and interdisciplinary consensus-based German guidelines: Surgical treatment and radiotherapy of melanoma. Melanoma Res 18:61–67, 2008.

Harvey DT, Fensje NA: The razor blade biopsy technique. Dermatol Surg 21:345–347, 1995.

Jost LM, Jelic S, Purkalne G, et al, for the ESMO Guidelines Task Force: ESMO minimum clinical recommendations for diagnosis, treatment and follow-up of cutaneous malignant melanoma. Ann Oncol 16(Suppl 1):66–68, 2005.

Moy RL, Lee A, Zalka A: Commonly used suturing techniques in skin surgery. Am Fam Physician 44:1625–1634, 1991.

Oppenheim EB: Failure to biopsy skin lesions prompts litigation. Medical Malpractice Prevention Ap 1990.

Pfenninger JL: Billing/Coding for Dermatologic Procedures (DVD). Creative Health Communications, 2004. Available through The National Procedures Institute at www.npinstitute.com.

Pfenninger JL: Common Office Dermatologic Procedures (DVD). Creative Health Communications, 2004. Available through The National Procedures Institute at www.npinstitute.com.

Pfenninger JL: How to Perform Skin Biopsies: A Guide for Clinicians (DVD). Creative Health Communications, 2005. Available through The National Procedures Institute at www.npinstitute.com.

Saiag P, Bosquet L, Guillot B, et al: Management of adult patients with cutaneous melanoma without distant metastasis. 2005 update of the French Standards, Options and Recommendations guidelines. Summary report. Eur J Dermatol 17:325–331, 2007.

Salasche SJ, Grabski WJ: Transverse sectioning of a pigmented lesion. Dermatol Surg 23:578–582, 1997.

Schanbacher CF, Bennett RG: Postoperative stroke after stopping warfarin for cutaneous surgery. Dermatol Surg 26:785–789, 2000.

Siegel MS, Usatine RP: The punch biopsy. In Usatine RP, Moy RL, Tobinick EL, Siegel DM (eds): Skin Surgery: A Practical Guide. St. Louis, Mosby, 1998, pp 101–119.

Siegel MS, Usatine RP: The shave biopsy. In Usatine RP, Moy RL, Tobinick EL, Siegel DM (eds): Skin Surgery: A Practical Guide. St. Louis, Mosby, 1998, pp 55–76.

Tobinick EL, Usatine RP: Choosing the type of biopsy. In Usatine RP, Moy RL, Tobinick EL, Siegel DM (eds): Skin Surgery: A Practical Guide. St. Louis, Mosby, 1998, pp 40–54.

Tran KT, Wright NA, Cockerell CJ: Biopsy of the pigmented lesion: When and how. J Am Acad Dermatol 59:852–871, 2008.

Usatine RP, Moy RL, Tobinick EL, Siegel DM: Elliptical excision. In Usatine RP, Moy RL, Tobinick EL, Siegel DM (eds): Skin Surgery: A Practical Guide. St. Louis, Mosby, 1998, pp 120–136.

CHAPTER 33

SKIN GRAFTING

Thomas N. Told

PINCH (PATCH) GRAFTING

Pinch grafting (also known as *patch grafting*; first described in 1872) is a method of treating leg ulcers by grafting small pieces of full-thickness skin, usually harvested from the patient's medial thigh, to the ulcer site. With pinch grafting, leg ulcer healing rates of 20% to 50% can be anticipated, depending on the cause of the ulcer. Pinch grafting should be considered as an adjunct to conservative therapy and a therapeutic alternative for the inpatient or ambulatory management of leg ulcers. (Chapter 41, Unna Paste Boot: Treatment of Venous Stasis Ulcers and Other Disorders, describes another method for treating lower extremity venous ulcers using the Unna boot.) Pinch grafting requires no special training and no specialized equipment or supplies, but it does require a prolonged period of leg elevation and bed rest after the procedure.

Indications

Pinch grafting can be used to treat any *leg ulcer* or any other small, slow-healing ulcer of the trunk or extremities. Success rates for pinch grafting are highest for arterial ulcers (50%) and lowest for venous ulcers (20% to 40%). Compared with patients treated with conservative therapy, patients treated with pinch grafting have a shorter time to healing (reepithelialization) and a longer time until ulcer recurrence.

Contraindications

- Allergy to anesthetic or antiseptic agents
- Skin infection at potential donor sites
- Lack of granulation base in ulcer *(relative contraindication)*
- Patient unwillingness or inability to comply with postprocedure instructions

Equipment

- Syringe and needle for anesthetic injection
- 1% or 2% lidocaine *without* epinephrine
- Antiseptic agent for donor site preparation (e.g., povidone–iodine)
- Sterile drape for donor site
- Sterile gloves
- Tissue forceps with teeth
- Scalpel with no. 15 blade
- Ruler
- Dressings for grafted ulcer (options include petrolatum [Vaseline]–impregnated gauze; saline-soaked fine-mesh gauze; Adaptic [Johnson & Johnson, New Brunswick, NJ] nonadhering dressing; Xeroform gauze [Kendall, Mansfield, Mass]; or Biobrane [Smith & Nephew, Hull, United Kingdom])
- Two layers of dry gauze and a light pressure dressing
- Telfa pad (Kendall) to transport grafts
- Vaseline gauze, Telfa pad, or Adaptic or Xeroform gauze for dressing the donor site (there is also a dissolving Vaseline gauze that works well)

Preprocedure Patient Preparation

The patient must be willing and able to comply with postprocedure activity restrictions. The leg ulcer(s) must be clean and must have a granulation base. The ulcer base can be débrided with wet-to-dry saline gauze dressings for 3 to 4 days before the procedure. The relative risks and benefits of pinch grafting should be explained to the patient. All supplies and equipment should be gathered at bedside or in the examination–treatment room. The ulcers should be measured to provide an estimate of the number of grafts needed. The donor site (the proximal medial thigh is preferred) and the skin around the ulcer(s) should be prepared in a sterile manner. Pinch grafting should be performed under sterile conditions.

Technique

1. Prepare and drape both donor sites and ulcer(s).
2. Measure the ulcer(s).
3. *Inject local anesthetic* (without epinephrine) into the donor site to form wheals of 5 to 10 mm in diameter (the number of wheals should equal the number of grafts needed; Fig. 33-1).
4. Grasp the anesthetized skin with the tissue forceps and *remove full-thickness skin pieces* 3 to 5 mm in diameter, avoiding subcutaneous fat (Fig. 33-2). Trim off any fat that may be adherent.
5. Store the graft pieces on a Telfa pad moistened with normal saline.
6. *Place the skin pieces on the leg ulcer*. Leave 2- to 5-mm spaces between grafts as well as between grafts and the ulcer edge to allow drainage of wound secretions (Fig. 33-3).
7. *Dress the ulcer and grafts* with fine-mesh, petrolatum-impregnated gauze (e.g., Adaptic or Xeroform) to cover the whole ulcer, followed by an occlusive dressing with 4 × 4 gauze pads and a compressive dressing.
8. *Dress the donor site* with fine-mesh, petrolatum-impregnated gauze (e.g., Adaptic or Xeroform) followed by dry gauze in at least two layers and light compression with an Ace wrap or Coban (3M, St. Paul, Minn).
9. See later for postoperative care.

Substitutes for Autographs

The mathematics of skin loss is very precise; the body cannot afford to lose too much skin surface area before it is fatally compromised. In some cases there may not be adequate skin to harvest or the patient's skin condition may be too poor to supply autografts to cover defects. In these cases substitutes are available to cover defects and allow protection and healing.

Early *skin substitutes* such as Biobrane, which is a collagen-impregnated fabric that imparts a framework for fibroblasts to adhere

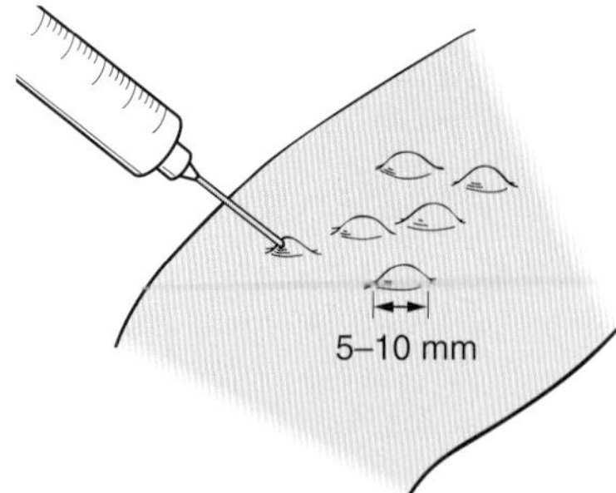

Figure 33-1 Local anesthetic (without epinephrine) is injected into the donor site, forming wheals 5 to 10 mm in diameter.

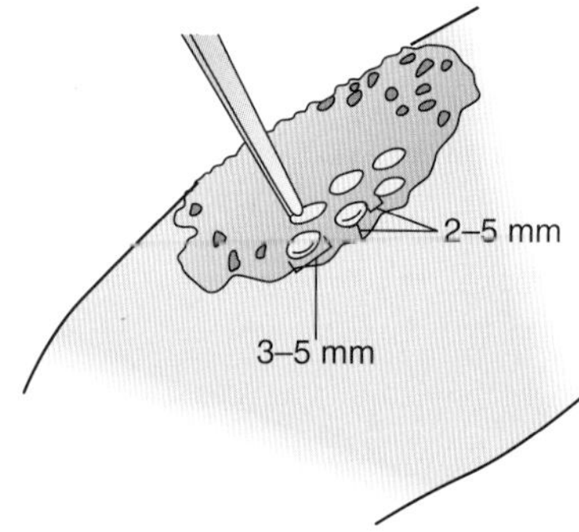

Figure 33-3 Skin pieces are placed on the leg ulcer, with 2- to 5-mm spaces left between grafts as well as between grafts and the ulcer edge to allow drainage of wound secretions.

to on the wound surface and thus accelerate the healing process, have been available for years. Unlike Telfa dressings, where the slick, shiny side of the dressing touches the wound to prevent adherence, with Biobrane the rough, collagen-bearing fabric side is placed next to the wound and left there until it falls off weeks later. With deep second-degree skin loss this is all that may be needed to stimulate healing.

Heterografts such as pig skin may be used to temporarily stabilize and débride large areas of skin loss that may need temporary coverage until autografting can take place with the patient's own skin.

Synthetic skin has undergone remarkable development from the early days of culturing fibroblasts from the foreskins of circumcised infants, to today's modern techniques of growing customized skin using stem cell technology. Currently, the major problem with these grafts is their lack of durability and short life span.

Allografting with banked cadaver skin is the mainstay of burn centers today. It is used for covering large, full-thickness areas of skin loss. There is a good supply of this material, but the potential to spread serious tissue-borne diseases always must be kept in mind and could limit general use.

Most of these materials are supplied in sheets, as a mesh, and are ready to be applied using the basic techniques for grafting previously covered. Before using them one must be familiar with all the supplier's recommendations for use.

Complications

- The most common complication is *graft failure*.
- *Infections* at the donor site or the ulcer are rarely reported.
- *Deep venous thrombosis* (DVT) is a possible complication of this procedure because of immobilization.
- *Bleeding* at the donor site occurs frequently but is almost always minor and easily controlled with local pressure.
- *Cosmetic outcome should be considered because grafts heal with a permanent studded appearance to the wound*, so they work best on smaller lesions in less cosmetically sensitive areas such as legs and ankles.

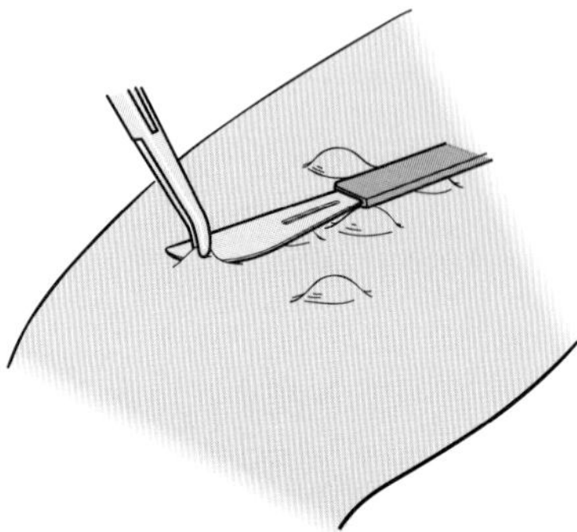

Figure 33-2 Anesthetized skin is grasped with the tissue forceps. Full-thickness pieces of skin 3 to 5 mm in diameter are removed.

Postprocedure Patient Education and Care

- Give the patient a handout on postoperative care. (See the sample patient education form online at www.expertconsult.com.)
- Patients must be placed on *bed rest*, with toilet privileges, with the grafted leg elevated for 7 days.
- The *donor site dressing* can be removed and replaced two to three times a day as needed. Wash gently with soap and water. Cover with petrolatum or antibiotic ointment, followed by the dressing.
- *At 7 days* after the procedure, the petrolatum *gauze covering the ulcer is removed* (if wound secretions are profuse, the compresses covering the petrolatum gauze are changed daily). After the petrolatum gauze is removed, a nonadhering dressing is applied and held in place with an elastic bandage. This dressing may be made by impregnating a stockinette with petrolatum ointment, or a commercially prepared product such as Adaptic or Xeroform gauze (bismuth tribromophenate) may be used.
- *At 7 days* after the procedure, the patient is allowed to *ambulate*.
- *At 14 days* after the procedure, the *stockinette is removed* and the ulcer dressed with gauze as needed.
- Some authorities recommend that low–molecular-weight heparin, or other *DVT prophylaxis*, be given to patients at high risk of venous thrombosis for 7 to 10 days after pinch grafting.
- *Prophylactic antibiotics* have generally not been used but could be considered in high-risk situations. If topical antibiotics are used, it is best to avoid those products containing neomycin owing to the high rate of allergic reactions.

Conclusion

Pinch grafting is a simple therapeutic procedure that may hasten and improve the healing of leg ulcers. The technique is relatively simple, can be performed at the bedside, and requires no special equipment or supplies. This procedure does require a prolonged period of postgraft ambulation restriction. Patients should know about and be prepared for this restricted ambulation. Clinicians should consider pinch grafting as an adjunct to conservative therapy for treatment of leg ulcers, especially when other therapies like the Unna boot have failed. Unna boots do not make a good outer covering dressing for skin grafts because they tend to apply too much compression for optimum vascularization of the new graft.

Full-Thickness and Split-Thickness Skin Grafts

Every primary care physician who manages wounds will encounter full-thickness skin loss that cannot be closed by conventional suturing methods. One of the best ways to solve these full-thickness skin loss problems is through the use of skin grafting techniques. The cutaneous surgeon possessing the basic skills of skin closure can easily master this most useful procedure. Donor skin reduces the size of the defect and speeds healing time. A properly selected and applied graft creates a minimal donor site defect and contributes to good function and cosmetic results.

Indications

- *Full-thickness abrasions and burns* where skin loss creates defects 1 cm or more in width between viable skin edges
- *Full-thickness skin loss on areas that have tight skin that cannot be advanced or undermined* (e.g., tip of the nose, fingers, and toes)
- *Large areas of skin loss* that need to be minimized for better function
- To provide essential covering for *defects that cannot be closed* (e.g., large skin excision sites, full-thickness skin flap donor sites, tendons, cartilage, and bone)
- Areas of skin loss *where excessive scarring of secondary granulation tissue may impair function* or create adverse cosmetic results

Contraindications

- Infection at the donor site
- Infection at the recipient site
- Excessive bleeding at the recipient site
- Contamination of the recipient site with imbedded foreign material
- Excessive edema at the recipient site
- Inadequate blood supply to sustain a graft

NOTE: Defects that are smaller than the size of a dime (1 cm in diameter) will heal well on their own without the need for grafting. If wounds are contaminated with foreign material or are infected, a delay of the grafting procedure will allow for the recipient site to establish granulation tissue that will better support the graft.

Skin Graft Types

Skin grafts are divided into two categories: *split thickness* and *full thickness* (Fig. 33-4):

Full-thickness grafts consist of the epidermis and the entire dermis. Full-thickness grafts are harvested by sharp dissection with a scalpel, and the thickness of the graft is determined by the region of the body where the donor skin originates.

Split-thickness grafts consist of the epidermis and a variable depth of dermis. *Split-thickness grafts* take only a part of the dermis, leaving the rest of the dermis at the donor site to regenerate. There are *three grades* of a split-thickness graft: *thin (0.005 to 0.010 inch)*, *medium*, and *thick*. The thickness is varied by the downward pressure the surgeon exerts on the dermatome handle, or by a steeper angle applied to the cutting blade. Mechanical dermatomes are available that have an adjustable gate, or a preset thickness setting, that will determine graft thickness (Fig. 33-5).

Whether the surgeon uses a free-hand shave technique or a preset dermatome, it takes practice to produce skin grafts of appropriate thickness.

NOTE: The tendency of the novice operator is to produce thicker split-thickness grafts than intended, even with the mechanical dermatome set on the thinnest settings.

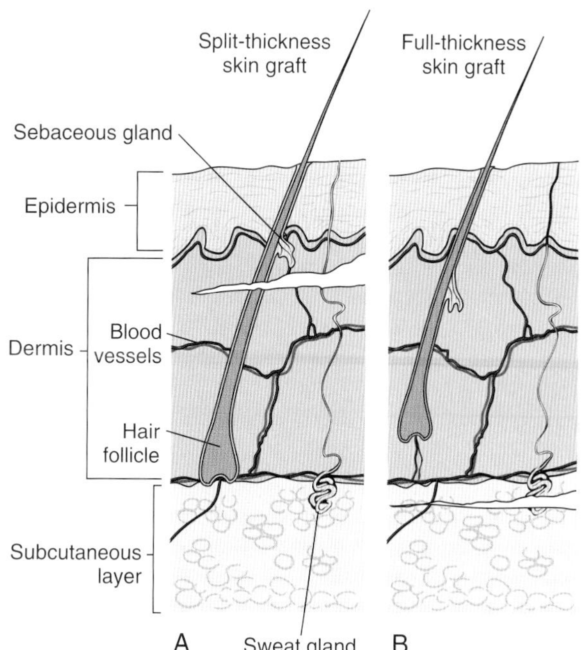

Figure 33-4 Free skin grafts are divided into two main types: split-thickness (**A**) and full-thickness (**B**).

Split-Thickness Grafts

ADVANTAGES

- Split-thickness grafts *can be "meshed"* and made to cover large areas of skin loss. In this technique, small slits are cut in the graft similar to the holes in a pie crust, allowing the sides of the graft to be stretched by an expansion ratio of 1 to 1½ times (Fig. 33-6).
- Thicker grafts can be placed in a *mechanical mesh maker* (Fig. 33-7) to form a uniform mesh pattern that covers large areas of skin loss from full-thickness burns. Extensive meshing promotes drainage of blood and serum from under the graft and improves success of donor skin revascularization.
- Very thin grafts (0.010 to 0.015 inch) vascularize quickly and heal much more rapidly.
- Split-thickness grafts tend to contract as they heal, thus drawing down the size of the original defect.
- Donor sites heal more rapidly.
- Grafts require less blood supply to survive and may be the best choice for sites where vascularization is less than optimal.

The thickness of the graft can vary to satisfy the need for wear, appearance, hair growth, and speed of healing. Thin grafts heal rapidly but are not as cosmetically pleasing. Grafts thicker than 0.015 inch look better and resist wear better but heal more slowly.

DISADVANTAGES

- Split-thickness skin grafts are not as resistant to trauma and *can be injured easily* in areas of friction and wear.
- They are *less like normal skin* in color, texture, suppleness, and hair growth. The mesh pattern is permanent and is not used in cosmetically sensitive areas such as the face or anterior neck.
- Meshing or "pie crusting" causes *additional scarring* and skin hypertrophy.
- Split-thickness grafts do not germinate over bone without periosteum, or cartilage without perichondrium.
- A dermatome must be used; for large grafts, an operating suite is necessary.
- Free-hand technique produces only postage stamp–sized grafts.
- These grafts *do not work well over joints* because they are more likely to cause contracture and restriction of the joint.

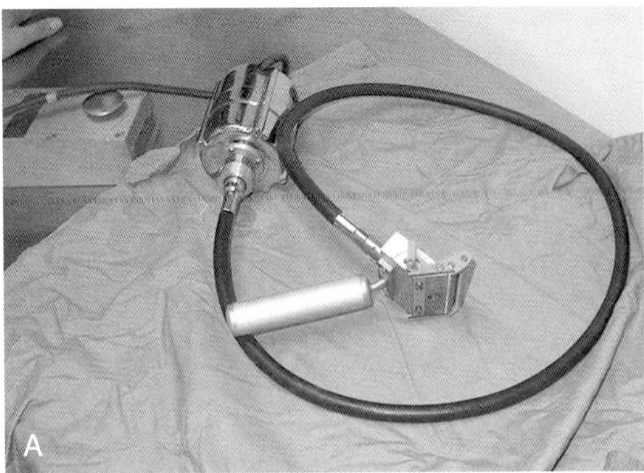

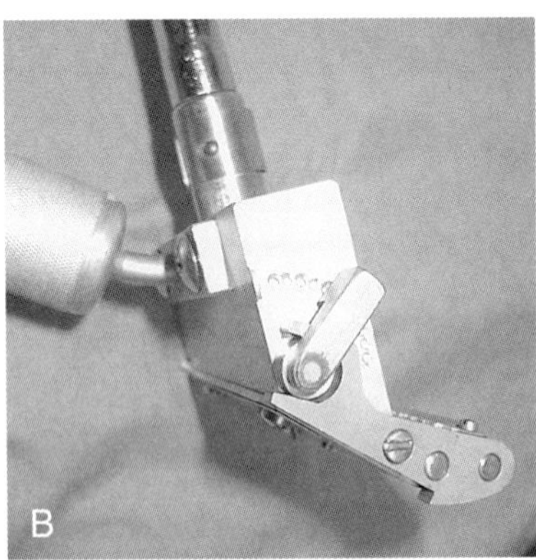

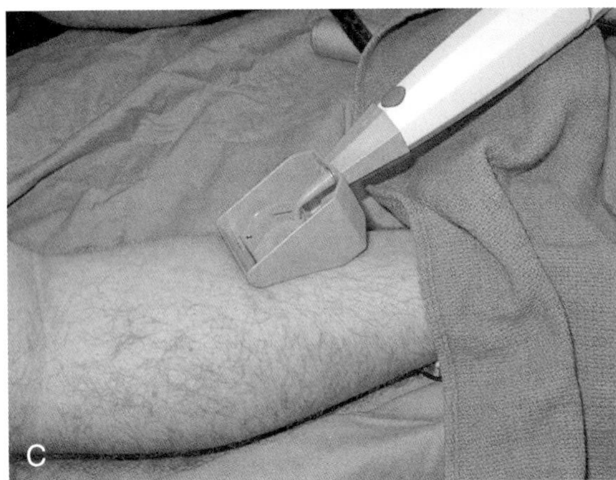

Figure 33-5 **A,** Adjustable-thickness motorized dermatome. **B,** Adjustment lever on the motorized dermatome that cams the blade up or down to control the thickness of the skin graft. **C,** Duval battery-powered dermatome with disposable, fixed-depth and fixed-width, detachable head.

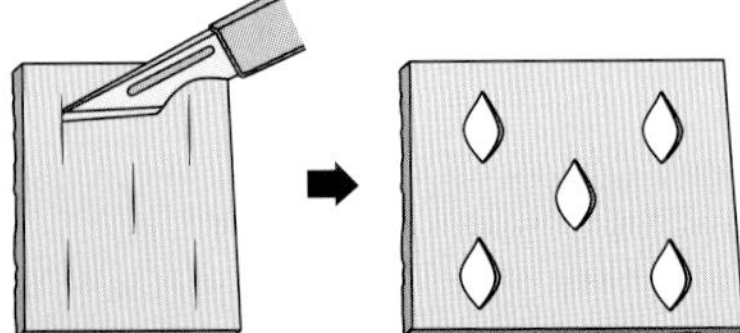

Figure 33-6 Split-thickness grafts can be expanded by "pie crusting" or cutting small slits in places that need expansion. This can expand a graft by 50% over the original size.

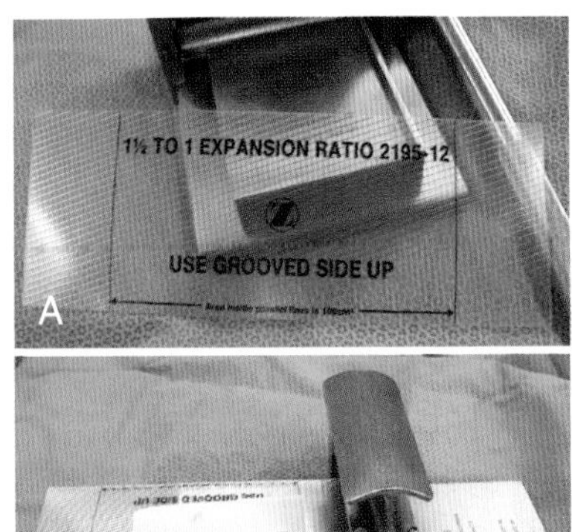

Figure 33-7 **A,** The skin graft is placed on the disposable clear plastic template with the dermis side resting on the grooves of the template. **B,** The handle is turned clockwise, rolling the graft through the press. A uniform meshed graft emerges on the opposite side. Meshing allows a 2-inch-wide graft to expand to cover a defect of 3 inches (1 : 1.5 ratio) and facilitates drainage of blood and fluids that may accumulate under the graft.

Full-Thickness Grafts

ADVANTAGES

- Full-thickness grafts *match* normal skin contours, color, and texture *better* than any other form of graft and are more aesthetically pleasing over time.
- They undergo *less postoperative contracture* and will not influence the size of the defect.
- Thick grafts *resist friction and wear better* than the thinner grafts.
- Full-thickness grafts can be used to cover bone without periosteum and cartilage without perichondrium.

DISADVANTAGES

- Full-thickness grafts cannot be used to cover large areas without carrying their own blood supply.
- Large full-thickness donor sites must be covered with split-thickness grafts to heal.
- Full-thickness grafts need a good supply of blood at the recipient site to survive.
- Thick grafts do not contract in total diameter with healing like split-thickness grafts do.
- Full-thickness grafts take the longest time of any graft to vascularize.
- The size of the donor site is determined by the defect size, and the graft cannot be meshed to expand its surface coverage.

Equipment

- Dermatome
  - Adjustable type with thickness settings, flexible shaft, and external power (see Figs. 33-5A and B)
  - Battery-powered, disposable-head type (see Fig. 33-5C)
- Sterile tongue blade
- 5 to 10 mL sterile mineral oil
- Petrolatum-impregnated gauze, Tegaderm (3M), or fine-mesh gauze
- Minor surgical tray
- 5-0 suture (polyethylene or Vicryl)
- Skin stapler if sutures are not used
- Steri-Strips
- Kerlix roll
- Ace wrap, Coban, or elastic stockinette
- No. 10 or larger blade or a razor blade
- Two Adson tissue forceps

- 5-inch Halsey needle holder
- 4-inch curved iris scissors
- 6-0 or 5-0 nylon sutures (monofilament, not braided)

Donor Sites

Full-Thickness Grafts

See Figure 33-8.

- Postauricular area
- Supraclavicular area
- Suprapalpebral area
- Antecubital area
- Volar wrist area
- Lower abdominal area
- Inguinal area

Split-Thickness Grafts

See Figure 33-9.

- Posterior lateral thigh
- Superior buttocks
- Anterior abdomen
- Anterior thigh
- Inner surface of the upper arm for hairless skin
- Flexor surface of the forearm

NOTE: Facial defects should be repaired with full-thickness grafts because these grafts cause less cosmetic disruption. Never use skin for the face from areas below the clavicle because these grafts do not match in color or texture and they contain hair follicles, resulting in lifelong deformity.

Techniques

Full-Thickness Grafts

1. Make sure no active folliculitis or cellulitis exists close to the donor site.
2. Prepare the skin for surgery using aseptic technique.
3. Drape the donor site.

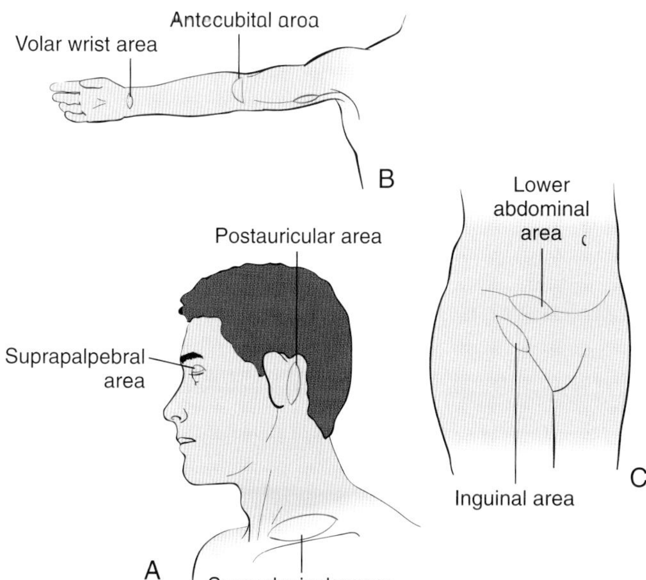

Figure 33-8 Potential harvest areas for full-thickness grafts. **A,** Head. **B,** Arm. **C,** Lower abdomen and inguinal areas. Do not use grafts from areas shown in (**B**) and (**C**) to graft the face, head, and neck (**A**). The color will never match and a permanent defect will remain.

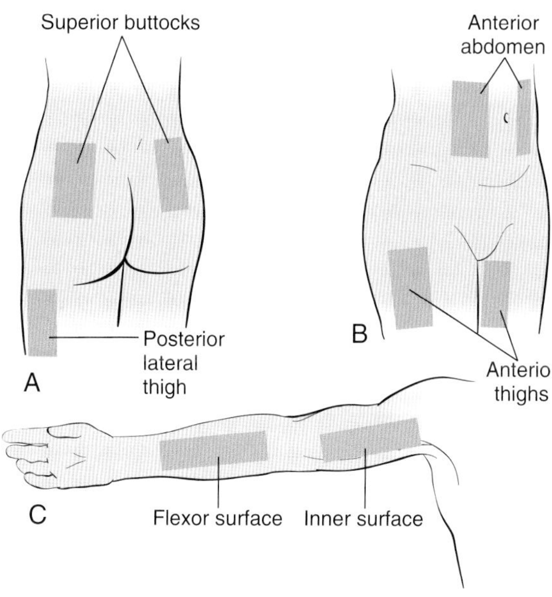

Figure 33-9 Potential harvest areas for split-thickness grafts. **A,** Posterior buttocks and lateral thigh. **B,** Anterior abdomen and thighs. **C,** Hairless areas of the arm.

4. Infiltrate the skin to be transferred with lidocaine without epinephrine for anesthesia.
5. Remove a fusiform piece of skin large enough to cover the defect without creating tension (Fig. 33-10A and B).
6. Remove as much subcutaneous fat as possible without buttonholing the graft (Fig. 33-10C and D).
7. Place the graft dermis side down on a saline-soaked gauze pad until ready for transfer.
8. Trim the graft to fit the defect.
9. Suture the graft into the defect, taking care to notice the skin lines and skin edges (Fig. 33-11A).
10. Use polyethylene suture, staples, or Steri-Strips.
11. Care must be taken to use the suture size and technique that will result in the least damage to the edges of the skin graft (small premium needles [size P-3] and suture 5-0 or less). Excessive bleeding at the edges will allow blood to flow under the new graft and prevent adherence of the graft.
12. A stent dressing best secures the graft (Fig. 33-11B).
13. Close the donor site in the usual fashion with sutures or staples. If the donor site cannot be closed without excess tension, a split-thickness graft can be used to cover it.

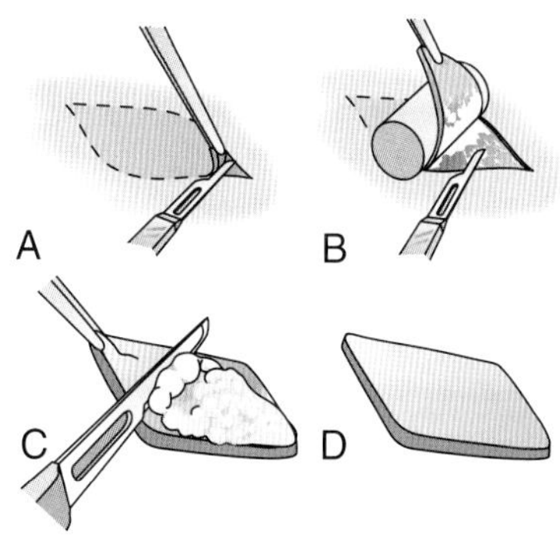

Figure 33-10 Full-thickness grafts should have all the subcutaneous fat removed before being placed on the graft site. **A,** Excising the graft. **B,** Using a small cotton roll to aid in keeping the graft flat. **C,** Removing the subcutaneous fat from donor skin. **D,** Graft skin ready to be applied.

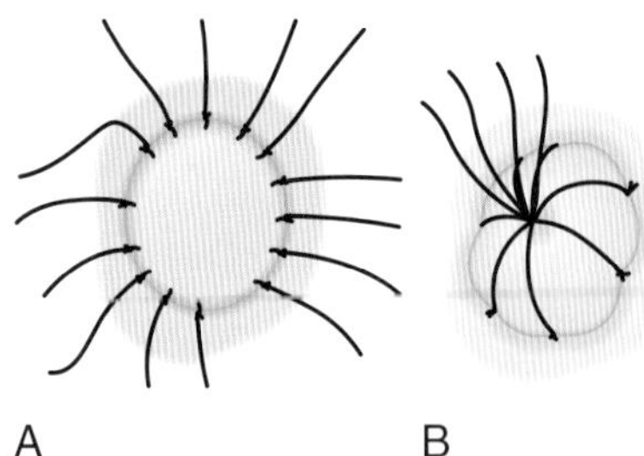

Figure 33-11 Grafts can be secured best by using a stent. Suture tails are left long at the time of attachment of the graft (**A**), then tied over the dressing (**B**) to provide pressure and anchor the graft in place. An initial layer of nonadherent material is applied, or the graft may be lubricated with antibiotic ointment to prevent the gauze stent from sticking.

14. Place a nonadherent dressing on the donor site and treat as a laceration.

Split-Thickness Grafts

HARVESTING TECHNIQUES: DERMATOME

1. Make sure no active infection or atrophic skin diseases exist on or near the donor or recipient site.
2. Prepare and drape the area with surgical scrub and drapes.
3. Ready the dermatome by *setting the desired thickness* on the gauge. *Usually the best intermediate setting is the thickness of a scalpel blade*. Thin grafts should transmit light like frosted glass. *Disposable dermatome heads* will produce thin grafts; the operator simply needs to decide on the blade width because various heads have various widths.
4. *Anesthetize* the skin to be harvested with local or regional anesthesia for small grafts. General anesthesia can be used when the areas to be grafted are large.
5. *Place a thin film of sterile mineral oil* on the skin that will be run through the dermatome. This lubricates the surfaces and helps maintain a uniform thickness.
6. Have an assistant use the sterile tongue blade to *depress the skin in front of the dermatome* and *provide countertraction to straighten out any wrinkles in the skin*.
7. *Start the dermatome* and approach the skin at a fairly steep angle until the blade catches the skin and begins cutting. When this happens, flatten the angle so the undersurface of the dermatome is aligned perfectly parallel with the skin surface. Downward pressure on the handle will place the blade deeper in the dermis and produce a thicker graft (Fig. 33-12).
8. The split-thickness graft will bunch up behind the blade and an assistant will need to *grasp the leading edges of the graft* and gently lift them straight up (the way a thin slice of cheese is lifted from a cheese cutter to keep it from bunching up). The total length of the graft can be determined easily as it is lifted off the blade.

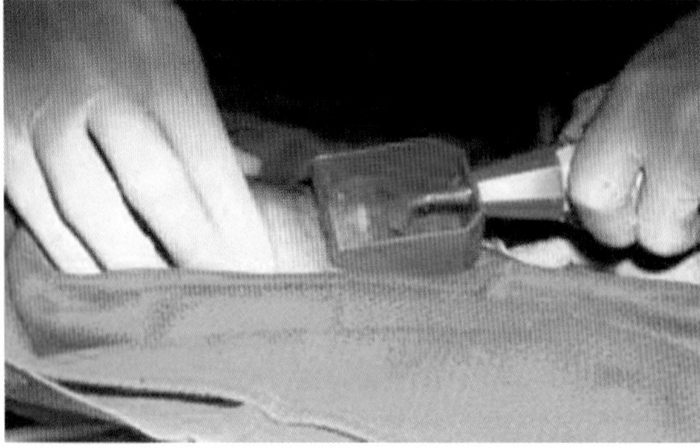

Figure 33-12 Battery-powered dermatome at the correct cutting angle.

9. *When the desired graft length is reached*, release downward pressure on the dermatome handle and point the blade in a steep upward angle, severing the graft.
10. Spread the graft out carefully, with the dermis side down, on saline-soaked gauze. In the case of extremely thin grafts, the skin can be floated on the surface of sterile saline in a basin before being transferred to the recipient site.

    NOTE: The *shiny side is always the dermis side (vs. epidermis) and must go next to the vascular surface* of the recipient site; otherwise it would be like laying grass sod upside down.

11. The donor site is dressed with Tegaderm or Adaptic, or Biobrane, or Xeroform gauze, or fine-mess gauze, which is left in place until it falls off in about 2 weeks. A gauze wrap and an Ace bandage can further protect the wound and reduce scar hypertrophy.

HARVESTING TECHNIQUES: FREE-HAND. This technique is well suited to the outpatient setting or emergency department, where small areas of skin loss elude conventional closure and require grafting.

1. A half-dollar–sized (3 × 3 cm) area on the forearm or thigh is infiltrated with 2% plain lidocaine without epinephrine, prepared with antiseptic solution, and draped for surgery (Fig. 33-13A).

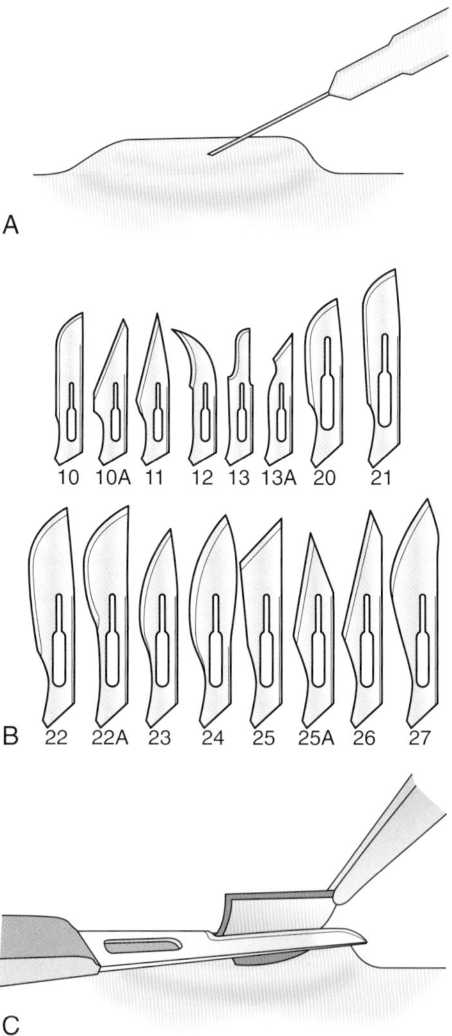

Figure 33-13 Free-hand split-thickness graft. **A,** Infiltration with local anesthesia will slightly raise the skin, making cutting easier. **B,** Scalpel blades of various sizes. **C,** The large scalpel blade is held at a shallow angle to the skin, and the graft is shaved off to a desired length.

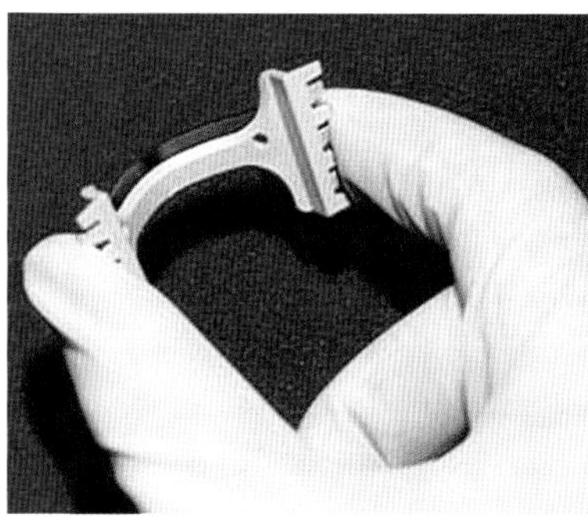

Figure 33-14 The Derma-blade is bent in a U-shape between the thumb and forefinger in preparation for harvesting a free-hand split-thickness graft. Widening the distance between the thumb and forefinger will widen the strip of skin being harvested. T-shaped gripping bars at each end of the blade improve control. (Courtesy of American Safety Razor, Cedar Knolls, NJ.)

2. Using a scalpel blade with a long straight cutting edge, like the no. 20, 21, or no. 22 in a scalpel handle (Fig. 33-13B), shave the skin at the desired thickness with a gentle slicing motion (Fig. 33-13C). A thin, standard double-edged razor blade or a specially prepared razor blade called a Derma-blade (American Safety Razor; Cedar Knolls, NJ) can also be used (Fig. 33-14). Both blades are straight when not in use, and are grasped between the thumb and index finger and gently bent into a U-shaped arc. The closer the thumb and index finger are drawn together the narrower the strip of skin will become. The Derma-blade is more expensive than a standard double-edged razor blade, but it has the advantage of being completely sterile and much safer to use. The graft is taken by applying light downward pressure on the blade and moving it side to side in smooth oscillating strokes. The greater the downward pressure on the blade the thicker the graft.
3. Widths up to 2 cm can be removed up to the length needed.
4. The skin can be transferred directly to the defect and sutured in place like any other split-thickness graft.

Recipient Site Preparation and Graft Stabilization

1. In the case of full-thickness grafts, *meticulous hemostasis* is the key to graft survival. *Bipolar* cautery (as opposed to the monopolar cautery generally used) is the best way to achieve homeostasis with very little thermal damage.
2. The full-thickness *graft must be tailored precisely to the defect* at the time of placement, whereas split-thickness grafts may overlap the margins.
3. The survival of split-thickness grafts depends on the growth of capillary beds into the raw undersurface of the graft. This may take several weeks of preparation to allow granulation tissue to develop. Try to use natural methods of débridement and capillary bed enhancement because enzymatic débriding agents will attack the graft as well.

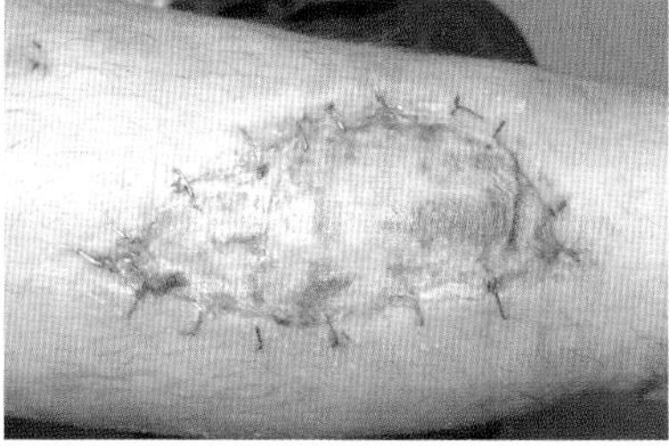

Figure 33-15 Split-thickness skin graft 10 days after surgery.

4. The graft must *not move* during the period of revascularization. The graft can be secured with a 6-0 or 5-0 monofilament suture. One tail of the suture is intentionally left twice as long as the diameter of the defect so a stent dressing can be tied over the graft (see Fig. 33-11). The dressing will stay in place for 7 to 10 days. Avoid the temptation to look under the dressing during the healing processes.
5. *Use as few sutures as necessary*. Simple interrupted suture with monofilament material is the best tolerated. Do not put too much tension on the graft or the sutures. If more stabilization is needed, Steri-Strips can be used. Some surgeons report good success with Steri-Strips alone. *Dermabond*, a commercial dermal adhesive, can stabilize fragile grafts; however, care must be taken not to allow the adhesive to flow between the graft and recipient site, which will prevent adherence.
6. In the case of large split-thickness grafts, skin staples can be used. This is a more rapid method of attachment and is relatively atraumatic (Fig. 33-15).
7. *Large skin grafts may require a "pie crust" maneuver to vent bubbles or blood* from under the graft itself. Small holes can be cut in the graft with fine scissors or a scalpel to let out the fluid (see Fig. 33-6).
8. *Cover the graft* with nonadherent material like Adaptic, Biobrane, Xeroform gauze, or Telfa. Make sure the new graft stays moist and out of the ambient air for extended periods. Cover the nonadherent material with saline-moistened gauze and at least two layers of protective gauze wrap and a light compressive dressing of Ace wrap or Coban.

   The dressings are not changed for the first 24 to 48 hours after graft placement unless soiled or bloody; then, for the next two daily outer dressing changes moistened gauze is replaced over the nonadherent dressing. It is best not to disturb the nonadherent dressing in direct contact with the graft to prevent movement of the new graft.
9. The graft *must be protected from trauma* and from loss of contact with the vascular bed. Some cutaneous surgeons prefer to roll a cotton-tipped applicator over the surface of the new graft, rolling from the middle of the newly applied skin to the outside. This expresses unwanted blood, fluids, or air bubbles that will lift the healing graft away from the recipient bed.

Common Errors

- *Placing the wrong surface of the graft against the donor site*. Care must be taken at all times to ensure that the graft is not turned over in transferring it from the donor site to the recipient site. Split-thickness grafts are the most susceptible to this mistake.
- *Allowing split-thickness grafts to dry out between harvesting and placement*. The graft should be kept in moist gauze or a small basin of saline. Blot, do not rub, the surfaces of the graft.
- *Causing excessive bleeding to the donor site before graft placement*. Excessive débridement or wiping of the site with antiseptic-saturated gauze may cause bleeding that will lift the graft from the surface after placement and encourage infection.
- *Not removing large air bubbles*. Air bubbles can become trapped under the graft during the placement process and before application of the dressing. Care must be taken to remove such bubbles or fluid pockets.
- *Not removing all the fat and subcutaneous tissue from the dermal side of a full-thickness skin graft*. The dermal side of a full-thickness graft should be free of any material that will block the migration of vascular elements into the skin graft.
- *Allowing edema or venous stasis to occur in the grafted extremity*. Edema and vascular congestion will cause the buildup of fluid under the graft and lift it away from the recipient site.
- *Attempting to remove an adherent covering in direct contact with the graft in less than 7 days*. Dressing edges can be trimmed when they spontaneously lift away from the surgical site, but the dressing should never be pulled off.

- *Loose-fitting dressings*. Loose dressings will cause excessive shear forces on the skin graft during the 7- to 14-day healing process. Movement of the graft will impede healing and adherence.

Complications

The major complication of skin grafting is *infection at the donor site* (causing it to become a full-thickness defect) and *loss of the graft at the recipient site* (causing another full-thickness defect). The use of prophylactic antibiotics cannot make up for poor planning and bad surgical technique; therefore, it is important to approach full-thickness skin loss with proper preparation.

Postprocedure Patient Education and Guides

See the sample patient education form online at www.expertconsult.com.

CPT/Billing Codes

15100 Split graft, trunk, arms, legs, first 100 cm^2
15120 Split graft, face, scalp, eyelids, mouth, neck, ears, orbits, genitalia, hands, feet, first 100 cm^2
15200 Full-thickness graft, including direct closure of the donor site, trunk, 20 cm^2 or less
15220 Full-thickness graft, including closure of the donor site, including scalp, arms, legs, 20 cm^2 or less
15240 Full-thickness graft, including donor site closure, forehead, cheeks, chin, mouth, neck, axilla, genitalia, hands and feet, 20 cm^2 or less
15260 Full-thickness, free, including closure of the donor site, nose, ears, eyelids, and/or lips, 20 cm^2 or less

ICD-9-CM Diagnostic Codes

Split-Thickness Grafts

707.0 Ulcers
709.2 Scar
879.0 to 881.2 Wounds
942.32 to 945.59 Burns

Full-Thickness Grafts

707.8 Ulcers
709.2 Scar
876.0 to 876.1 and 879.0 to 879.5 Open wounds
942.31 to 944.58 Burns

Acknowledgment

The author and editors wish to recognize the contributions of Paul M. Paulman, MD, to the section on Pinch (Patch) Grafting in the previous edition of this text.

Suppliers

(See contact information online at www.expertconsult.com.)

Adjustable dermatomes
Zimmer, Inc.
Medical and surgical supplies
Bergen Brunswig Medical Corp.
Surgical instruments
Miltex Instrument Co.

Bibliography

Adams DC, Ramsey ML: Grafts in dermatologic surgery: Review and update on full- and split-thickness skin grafts, free cartilage grafts, and composite grafts. Dermatol Surg 31:1055–1067, 2005.
Andreassi A, Bilenchi R, Biagioli M, D'Aniello C: Classification and pathophysiology of skin grafts. Clin Dermatol 23:332–337, 2005.
Christensen DR, Arpey CJ, Whitaker DC: Skin grafting. In Robinson JK, Hanke DW, Sengelmann RD, Siegel DM (eds): Surgery of the Skin: Procedural Dermatology. Philadelphia, Mosby, 2005, pp 365–380.
Collins L, Seraj S: Diagnosis and treatment of venous ulcers. Am Fam Physician 81:989–996, 2010.
Doherty GM (ed): Current Diagnosis & Treatment: Surgery, 13th ed. New York, McGraw-Hill, 2010.
Haas AF, Glogau RG: Composite graft. In Robinson JK, Arndt KA, LeBoit PE, Wintroub BU (eds): Atlas of Cutaneous Surgery. Philadelphia, WB Saunders, 1996, pp 165–168.
Hjerppe A, Sand M, Huhtala H, Vaalasti A: Pinch grafting of chronic leg ulcers. J Wound Care 119:37–40, 2010.
Kontos AP, Qian Z, Urato NS, et al: The use of a flexible razor blade in skin graft harvesting. Dermatol Surg 35:120–123, 2009.
Leffell DJ: Split-thickness skin grafts. In Robinson JK, Arndt KA, LeBoit PE, Wintroub BU (eds): Atlas of Cutaneous Surgery. Philadelphia, WB Saunders, 1996, pp 149–156.
Ogawa R, Hyakusoku H, Ono S: Useful tips for successful skin grafting. J Nippon Med Sch 74:386–392, 2007.
Oien RF, Hakansson A, Hansen BU: Leg ulcers in patients with rheumatoid arthritis: A prospective study of aetiology, wound healing and pain reduction after pinch grafting. Rheumatology 40:816–820, 2001.
Oien RF, Hansen BU, Hakansson A: Pinch graft skin transplantation for leg ulcers in primary care. J Wound Care 9:217–220, 2000.
Orgill DP: Excision and skin grafting of thermal burns. N Engl J Med 360:893–901, 2009.
Phillips TJ: Current approaches to venous ulcers and compression. Dermatol Surg 27:611–621, 2001.
Roenigk RK, Zalla MJ: Full-thickness skin grafts. In Robinson JK, Arndt KA, LeBoit PE, Wintroub BU (eds): Atlas of Cutaneous Surgery. Philadelphia, WB Saunders, 1996, pp 157–164.
Schwartz S (ed): Principles of Surgery, 9th ed. New York, McGraw-Hill, 2010.

CHAPTER 34

Skin Stapling

David James

In certain body areas, when performed with care, skin stapling provides a rapid and simple alternative to other methods of skin closure and wound repair. Clinical experience with stapling now spans decades, and improved equipment, such as absorbable staples, is being introduced constantly. A variety of staplers with specific features for the purpose to which they are being applied are available. For example, staplers designed for small lacerations may hold only 5 fine staples, whereas staplers for general-purpose closure may hold up to 35 heavier-gauge staples.

Advantages

The final result of a stapled wound depends directly on its location, the condition of the wound being stapled, and operator experience. The best cosmetic results are seen in clean, uninfected linear wounds of the scalp, torso, and proximal extremities that have some degree of a subcutaneous fat "bed" and that are not under undue tension. Poorer results occur when the wound is macerated, ragged, infected, under tension, or placed directly over a bony prominence with thinner skin.

Numerous studies have supported stapling as an acceptable alternative to suture closure, and in some studies a lower rate of infection after closure has been found with stapling. Staples are generally well accepted by patients, and, in most cases, it is a much faster procedure than suturing. Well-placed staples evert the wound edges optimally and place less tension on wound edges than sutures. Surgical stainless steel staples are less "reactive" than sutures and potentially result in less postclosure inflammation and infection. Staple ends do not completely meet in the deeper tissues, thus resulting in less tissue constriction; this may also promote a lower infection rate.

Disadvantages

Stapling has the potential to provide a result inferior to suturing. Staples certainly do leave larger puncture scars proportional to the time they remain in the wound, and the cost–benefit ratio of using a stapling device in smaller wounds is not advantageous. Recycling of the used devices are also problematic because most are made of plastic and are for single-use only.

Indications

- To secure skin grafts or repair wounds whose edges are easily approximated and not under undue tension
- Long, linear wounds of the scalp, proximal extremities, or the torso where cosmesis is not a concern

Contraindications

- Facial or neck tissue, or in areas where there is an inadequate subcutaneous base
- Over small mobile joints of the hand and foot, soles and palms, or any other location where the staples may interfere with function of a body part
- In wounds that are macerated or infected, or over areas of large tissue loss, unless the subcutaneous tissues may be easily approximated after undermining and use of buried deeper sutures to help approximate the skin edges

Equipment

- Skin hooks or two pairs of fine Adson forceps
- Skin stapler with appropriate-gauge staples (heavier gauge for longer wounds over thicker tissue, lighter gauge for smaller wounds)
- Sterile surgical skin preparation solution, sterile drapes, gloves for the operators
- Local anesthetic appropriate for the area to be repaired
- Suture kit with appropriate sutures on standby, in case deeper sutures need to be inserted to take tension off the skin edges
- Staple remover (usually given to patient if another practitioner will be removing the staples)

Preprocedure Patient Preparation

Community standards or facility type will dictate the nature and extent of any consent forms involved. In all cases, the patient should be informed about the procedure to close the wound, the intent to use staples, the relative advantages and disadvantages of staple use in his or her particular wound, how to care for the repaired wound, and when to return for recheck and/or suture removal.

Technique

1. The help of an assistant to hold the skin edges together for the stapler operator is often useful during the procedure (Fig. 34-1).
2. Prepare and drape the wound in the usual fashion.
3. Don sterile gloves.
4. Anesthetize the area to be repaired with injectable lidocaine 1% or 2% with or without epinephrine. Topical anesthetics (e.g., a solution of lidocaine, epinephrine, and tetracaine) may be used as an alternative to injectable anesthetics.
5. If there is tissue loss or if the wound is gaping, undermine the edges of the wound and close the deeper layers with buried absorbable sutures. The skin edges should be well approximated and under no tension before stapling is performed.
6. Have assistant (if present) pick up the skin edges of the wound in front of the stapler with the skin hooks/forceps, and gently hold them together and slightly elevate them.
7. Start at one end of the wound, pointing the stapler toward the opposite end. Position the stapler guide (usually an arrow) over the laceration and press the stapler gently down onto the skin.

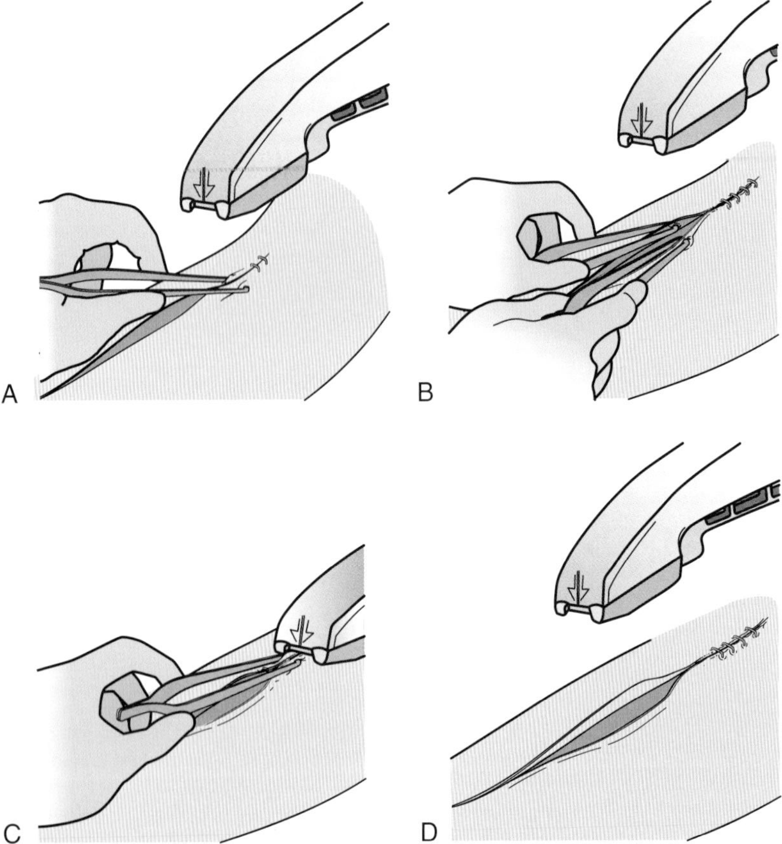

Figure 34-1 Use of a skin stapler. Approximate skin edges so they are slightly everted with one forceps (**A**) or two forceps (**B**). Position the instrument lightly over the everted skin edges, aligning the stapler arrow with the incision (**C**). Pressing down on the instrument too heavily may make staple removal difficult. Squeeze the trigger quickly and firmly until the trigger motion is halted (**D**). Release the trigger and back the instrument off the staple.

Squeeze the trigger, placing one staple. *Do not release the trigger*, but pull up gently on the stapler. This will pull up the wound edges.

8. Release the stapler trigger and remove the stapler.
9. Replace the guide over the laceration, and repeat step 6.
10. Alternate step 7, followed by step 6, until the end of the wound is reached. If there is a "dog-ear" of excess tissue, excise with forceps and iris scissors and place final staples.
11. The distance between staples depends on the operator and his or her experience, but the wound margins should be approximated without gaps when complete. Some clinicians prefer to start closing at the middle of a wound, lessening the chance of dog-ears.
12. A lone operator can approximate the skin edges with a single forceps by pulling the skin edges together before placing a staple, or by placing the thumb and forefinger of the non-operating hand along the edges of the skin to pull them together.
13. After stapling is complete, reclean the wound and place an appropriate dressing.
14. Arrangements for follow-up and staple removal should be made. In general, staples should remain in place for 8 to 10 days. Stapled scalps may be washed after staple placement if necessary.
15. Removal of staples is best accomplished by a staple remover that bends the staple arms up and out of the skin (Fig. 34-2). A hemostat may also be used to pry up each staple arm.

Complications

Complications, although rarely reported, include dehiscence, poor cosmesis, infection, and hematoma. These are similar to the complications seen with a sutured wound.

Postprocedure Patient Education

See the sample patient education handout online at www.expertconsult.com.

CPT/Billing Codes

Coding is the same as for suture repairs; see Chapter 22, Laceration and Incision Repair.

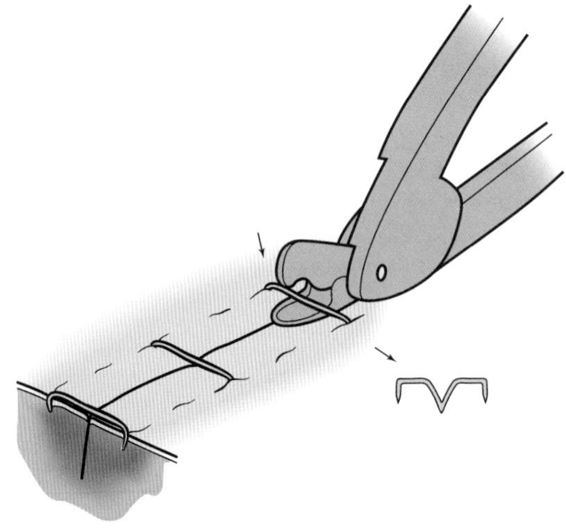

Figure 34-2 Use of a staple remover.

Acknowledgment

The editors wish to recognize the many contributions by J. Mark Wiedemann, MD, MS, to this chapter in a previous edition of this text.

Suppliers

(See contact information online at www.expertconsult.com.)

Minogue Medical
Most medical suppliers (e.g., Miltex, Delasco)
3M
Weck Closure Systems

BIBLIOGRAPHY

Brickman K, Lambert R: Evaluation of skin stapling for wound closure in the emergency department. Ann Emerg Med 18:1122–1125, 2009.

Dos Santos LR, Freitas CA, Hojaij FC, et al: Prospective study using skin staplers in head and neck surgery. Am J Surg 170:451–452, 1995.

James D: Repair of lacerations. In James D (ed): A Field Guide to Urgent and Ambulatory Procedures. Philadelphia, Lippincott Williams & Wilkins, 2001, pp 202–212.

Kanegaye JT, Vance CW, Chan L, Schonfeld N: Comparison of skin stapling devices and standard sutures for pediatric scalp lacerations: A randomized study of cost and time benefits. J Pediatr 130:808–813, 1997.

Orlinsky M, Goldberg RM, Chan L, et al: Cost analysis of stapling versus suturing for skin closures. Am J Emerg Med 13:77–81, 1995.

CHAPTER 35

Subungual Hematoma Evacuation

Rebecca Beach

Injuries to the nail bed and fingertip are the most common injuries to the upper extremity. Most common among these is a subungual hematoma, which results from a direct blow to the fingernail or a squeezing-type injury to the distal finger, causing bleeding into the space between the nail bed and the fingernail itself. Intense pain can result from the pressure generated by such a hematoma. Evacuation of the hematoma can produce significant relief and can be performed safely in the outpatient setting. Toenails can be treated in the same fashion. Evacuation of a hematoma may or may not prevent the eventual spontaneous avulsion of the nail that results from some hematomas. Patients should be made aware of this possibility. Radiographs may be necessary and, if a fracture is documented, antibiotics may be indicated because this would then essentially be an open fracture.

Indication

A visible, painful hematoma beneath the involved nail (Fig. 35-1) requires treatment.

Contraindications

- Crushed or fractured nail bed or fracture of distal phalanx.
- Hematomas involving greater than 50% of the nail *may* indicate laceration of the underlying nail bed. (Removal of the nail and repair of the laceration is recommended by some experts to avoid a post-traumatic nail deformity. Others recommend leaving the nail in place as a splint. The patient should be warned that the nail *may* be deformed unless the nail bed is examined and treated.)

Equipment

- Alcohol lamp or Bunsen burner (or cigarette lighter), metal paperclip, and forceps or hemostat
- *Or* battery-operated cautery unit
- *Or* 18-gauge needle or no. 11 scalpel
- *Or* automatic drill device (Dremel tool, dental burr, or PathFormer device)
- *Or* radiofrequency or electrocautery unit with needle or pointed electrode

Technique

1. Wash the digit as thoroughly as possible with an antibacterial soap to decrease the possibility of contamination of the hematoma and subsequent infection.
2. Consider a digital block with lidocaine without epinephrine because any pressure on the area can be painful.
3. Create a hole in the nail directly over the center of the hematoma to allow decompression.
   - *Paperclip method.* Partially straighten a metal paperclip, grasp it with the forceps, and heat it over the alcohol lamp, Bunsen burner, or lighter. Place the heated clip firmly on the nail, allowing it to melt the tissue for a few seconds until the nail is completely perforated (Fig. 35-2).
   - *Cautery method.* In similar fashion, apply battery cautery tip to the nail and create a hole in the nail bed (Fig. 35-3). Some electrocautery units may work, but there is often too much keratin in the nail for it to be effective.
   - *Drill method.* Twist a large-bore needle or scalpel between your fingers gently in one place to create a 1- to 2-mm hole over the central area of the hematoma. A 2-mm, sharp, disposable punch biopsy unit can also be tried. Alternatively, a drill device (Dremel tool, dental burr, or PathFormer device) may be used. The only drawback to this method is that any pressure on the nail can cause pain, so proceed gently.

In the first two procedures mentioned, the heated tip is cooled by the hematoma on perforation of the nail, thereby preventing injury to the nail bed. This effect is maximal in the center of the hematoma, where the distance between nail and tissue is greatest. Similarly, with the drill technique, the tip of any drill/needle/scalpel will not touch sensitive tissue if it is placed in the center of the hematoma. The hole created in the nail should be of sufficient size so as not to close off within a few hours (adequate size is 1 to 2 mm). Elevation of the finger, cool compresses, and a simple bandage are recommended during the first 12 hours. Use of antibiotic ointment can serve dual purposes—to moisturize (minimizing blood clotting so that the hematoma will drain maximally and prevent blood from adhering to the bandage) and to minimize infection. Because patient anxiety can be severe, passing the needle through the fibers of a 4 × 4 gauze so that the patient cannot visualize it may make the drilling procedure more tolerable for a child.

Complications

- Infection of the remaining hematoma
- Pain
- Inadvertently lacerating the nail bed
- Not recognizing a fracture beneath the hematoma

Cautions

- Neither the drill method nor the two heat methods by themselves should be painful, but the hematoma itself may be exquisitely tender, so the digit should be grasped gently, proximal to the injury.

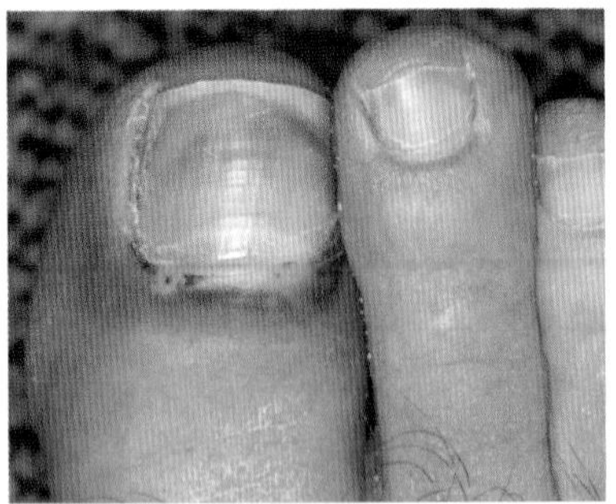

Figure 35-1 Subungual hematoma.

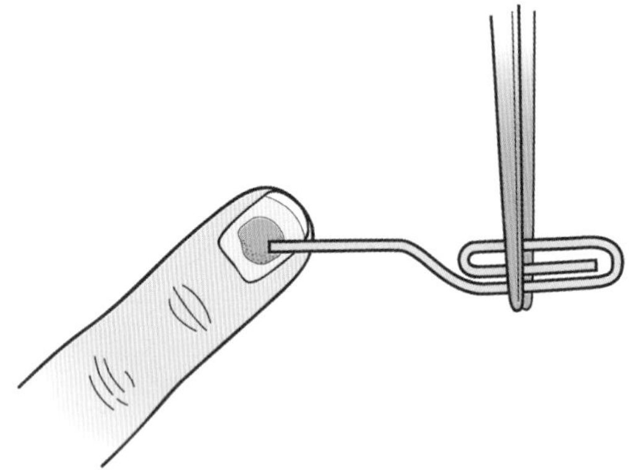

Figure 35-2 Heated paperclip is placed directly over the hematoma to create a perforation of the nail.

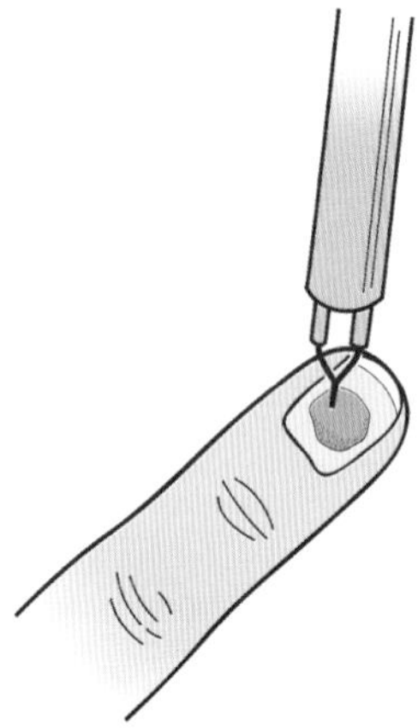

Figure 35-3 Cautery unit may be used to perforate the nail and evacuate the subungual hematoma.

- Either a local anesthetic or ethyl chloride may be used before these methods, if desired, to decrease pain. However, ethyl chloride is flammable and should not be used during or immediately before the cautery method or very close to the flame of the paperclip method. Holding the area in ice water is safer. Consider a digital block.
- Artificial acrylic nails may also be flammable.

CPT/Billing Code

11740 Subungual hematoma evacuation

ICD-9-CM Diagnostic Codes

959.5 Injury fingernail
923.3 Contusion finger(s) (nail) (subungual)

Acknowledgment

The editors wish to recognize the contributions by James F. Peggs, MD, to this chapter in the previous two editions of this text.

Suppliers

(See contact information online at www.expertconsult.com.)

AMI Battery Cautery
Delasco Dermatological Supplies
Hyfrecator Plus
Path Scientific, LLC
Surgitron and Battery Unit
Ellman International, Inc.

ONLINE RESOURCES

See patient education and patient consent forms available online at www.expertconsult.com.

BIBLIOGRAPHY

Salter SA, Ciocon DH, Gowrishankar TR, Kimball AB: Controlled nail trephination for subungual hematoma evacuation. Am J Emerg Med 24:875–877, 2006.
Simon RR, Wolgin M: Subungual hematoma: Association with occult laceration requiring repair. Am J Emerg Med 5:302–304, 1986.
Usatine RP: The Color Atlas of Family Medicine. New York, McGraw-Hill, 2009.
Van Beek AL, Kassan MA, Adson MH, Dale V: Management of acute fingernail injuries. Hand Clin 6:23–35, 1990.
Zook EG: Nail bed injuries. Hand Clin 1:701–716, 1985.

CHAPTER 36

Tick Removal and Prevention of Infection

David James

Persons frequenting outdoor areas may be exposed to ticks. Ticks often lurk in tall grasses or in overhead branches, and will attach themselves to persons passing by them in search of a blood meal. Although most tick bites are harmless, ticks may be the vectors of several significant diseases. Because it is impossible to identify in the field whether a tick carries an infectious disease, it is good medical practice to remove all ticks found on human skin promptly. Ticks feed slowly, and several hours of attachment are thought to be required for transmission of tick-borne illnesses.

Diseases Transmitted by Ticks

Ticks have eight legs and are members of the class Arachnida. Ticks belonging to the families Argasidae (soft ticks) and Ixodidae (hard ticks) are able to act as disease vectors to humans. The ixodid ticks *Dermacentor* and *Ixodes* are most likely to be encountered by humans in North America, and they can transmit microorganisms hematogenously during all phases of their development. See Box 36-1 for a list of tick-borne diseases.

Ticks have powerful mouthparts to break the skin of their hosts and enable a blood meal. The saliva of the tick has anticoagulant properties to keep blood flowing. Pathogens in the gut of the tick migrate to the tick's salivary glands, and thus are transmitted parenterally to the host during feeding. *Generally, a tick must be attached for longer than 8 hours for successful transmission of disease.*

Two of the tick-borne diseases bear special mention. *Tick-bite paralysis* is a serious illness that presents as an ascending neuromuscular paralysis, similar to Guillain-Barré syndrome. The paralysis is caused by envenomation of the host with a salivary neurotoxin secreted in the saliva of certain gravid *Dermacentor* ticks. Resolution of the paralysis occurs after removal of the often-overlooked tick.

Lyme disease is a fairly common illness affecting the cardiovascular, musculoskeletal, neurologic, and dermatologic systems. It is often seen in children and adults who spend time outdoors. Lyme disease is caused by the spirochete *Borrelia burgdorferi*, and is transmitted to humans by the bite of the hard *Ixodes* tick. White-footed mice and white-tailed deer are the major reservoirs for *B. burgdorferi*. This disease is becoming prevalent throughout northeastern North America, and is worth including in the differential diagnosis of unusual rashes, fevers, myalgias, and arthralgias. It is best diagnosed by enzyme-linked immunosorbent assay (ELISA) testing of serum for specific antibodies to *B. burgdorferi*. A Lyme disease preventative vaccine is now commercially available (LYMErix), and may be appropriate for those individuals living in high-prevalence locations who spend a great deal of time outdoors. Treatment of Lyme disease is discussed in the section on Complications and Disease Prevention. See Table 36-1 for a synopsis of presenting features of other tick-borne diseases.

Recently, the tick *Amblyomma americanum* has been associated with an erythema migrans–like rash in patients from the southeastern United States. This condition has been termed *southern tick-associated rash illness (STARI)*. It is distinct from Lyme disease because it is not caused by the spirochete *B. burgdorferi*, and some cases have been identified with a novel spirochete, *Borrelia longestari*. Treatment is with antibiotics, as listed in the section on Complications and Disease Prevention.

Hard ticks are best removed mechanically. Care must be taken to remove the tick's mouthparts, which will be firmly embedded in the host. The head and mouthparts may separate from the tick's body if not removed properly, thus increasing risk of disease transmission. A punch biopsy of the tissue surrounding the mouthparts may then be necessary. *Home remedies*, such as the placement of oil on the tick to smother it or burning the tick with a hot match or cigarette, are not recommended. Both techniques have the potential to cause the tick to regurgitate its blood meal and cause significant inoculation of disease pathogens.

Equipment

- Blunt curved forceps or tweezers
- Rubber gloves
- Povidone–iodine scrub and solution
- Normal saline specimen container or culture medium *(optional)*
- Gauze and bandage

In addition, for difficult removal or retained mouthparts:

- Punch biopsy equipment for 3- to 6-mm punch as appropriate
- Iris scissors
- Lidocaine 0.5 mL in syringe with 30-gauge needle
- Aluminum chloride solution 6.25% on a cotton-tipped swab *(optional)*
- 5-0 nylon suture and needle driver *(optional)*

Box 36-1. Tick-borne Diseases

Babesiosis
Human granulocytic and monocytic ehrlichiosis
Lyme disease
Q fever
Rocky Mountain spotted fever
Tick fever
Tick-bite paralysis
Tularemia
Typhus

TABLE 36-1 Common Tick-Borne Diseases and Their Management

	Lyme Disease	Ehrlichiosis	Rocky Mountain Spotted Fever	Tularemia
Pathogens	*Borrelia burgdorferi*	*Ehrlichia chaffeensis* *Ehrlichia ewingii*	*Rickettsia rickettsii*	*Francisella tularensis*
Geographic distribution in continental United States	Northeast and upper Midwest	South, Southeast, and Midwest	Southeast, Atlantic Coast states, Midwest	South and Midwest
Presenting symptoms	Erythema migrans, fatigue, myalgias, arthralgias, headache, fever, chills, neuropathies	Fever, chills, headache, myalgias	Macular rash, fever, myalgias, vomiting, fatigue, headache	Fever, chills, headache, cough, diarrhea, fatigue, vomiting, sore throat; contact with mice is a risk factor
Initial laboratory findings	Nonspecific; convalescent serology positive at 4–6 wk for antibodies to *Borrelia*	Leukopenia, thrombocytopenia, elevated liver aminotransferases; confirmatory convalescent serology at 1–2 wk	Leukopenia, thrombocytopenia, elevated liver aminotransferases, hyponatremia; confirmatory convalescent serology at 7–10 days	White blood cell count often normal, elevated erythrocyte sedimentation rate; confirmatory convalescent serology at 2 wk
Treatment	Doxycycline, tetracycline, amoxicillin-clavulanate, levofloxacin, erythromycin	Doxycycline, chloramphenicol, rifampin	Tetracycline, doxycycline, chloramphenicol	Streptomycin, gentamicin, tetracycline, chloramphenicol, fluoroquinolones

Technique

1. Gently paint the surrounding area with povidone–iodine solution.
2. With blunt forceps, tweezers, or gloved fingers, grasp the tick as close to the skin surface as possible and pull upward and perpendicular with steady, even pressure (Fig. 36-1).
3. *Do not* twist or jerk the tick because this may break off mouthparts.
4. *Never squeeze*, crush, or puncture the body of the tick because its fluids may contain infectious agents.
5. The tick may be sent for microscopic analysis of the *Borrelia* spirochete or cultured for other organisms.
6. Disinfect the bite site with povidone–iodine scrub or antibacterial soap.

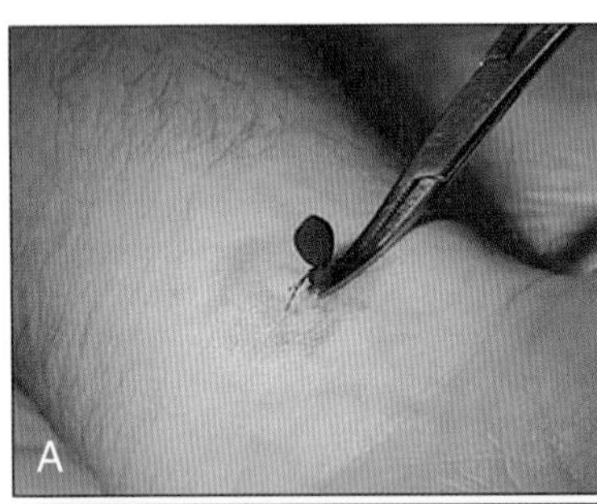

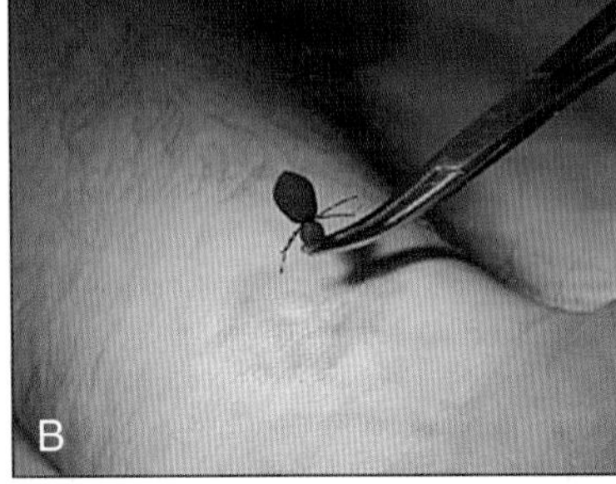

Figure 36-1 Technique of tick removal. **A,** Apply the instrument perpendicular to the skin, encompassing the tick. **B,** Pull upward with a steady, even pressure.

In cases of a particularly tenacious tick, retained mouthparts, or high-risk endemic areas, perform the following technique:

1. Disinfect the area with antibacterial soap. Infiltrate the area beneath the bite with lidocaine.
2. Apply the punch biopsy instrument perpendicular to the skin so that it encompasses the tick. Stretch the skin on each side of the lesion. Advance the biopsy punch downward with moderate pressure, using a clockwise–counterclockwise twisting motion. Penetration through the epidermis and dermis is confirmed with a marked decrease in resistance (see Chapter 32, Skin Biopsy).
3. Remove the punch. Lift the biopsy specimen with forceps and cut the pedicle with iris scissors. Submit the tissue for histologic study.
4. Disinfect the area again and apply pressure with gauze. If adequate hemostasis is not accomplished, cauterize with aluminum chloride solution or close with suture. Apply bandage.

Complications and Disease Prevention

Local complications of tick removal may include transient *bleeding* or *cellulitis*. Bleeding is managed by locally applied pressure, whereas cellulitis is prevented by attention to area cleanliness and follow-up care.

As Lyme disease is becoming more prevalent throughout North America, *prophylactic antibiotics* after a tick bite seem a reasonable approach to infection prevention. After tick removal, a 10-day course of antibiotics is recommended. Choices include doxycycline 100 mg orally twice daily or tetracycline 500 mg orally four times a day (for adults, and children 10 years of age and older); amoxicillin-clavulanate 400 to 875 mg orally twice daily; levofloxacin 500 mg orally daily; or erythromycin 125 to 500 mg orally four times a day.

Patient Education Guides

See patient education handouts available online at www.expertconsult.com.

CPT/Billing Codes

10120 Removal of superficial foreign body, skin
10121 Incisional removal of foreign body, complex

ICD-9-CM Diagnostic Codes

919.4 Injury, superficial, insect bite, without infection
919.5 Injury, superficial, insect bite, with infection (or see specific site, 910.4 to 919.4 without infection or 910.5 to 919.5 with infection)

Acknowledgment

The author wishes to recognize John Harlan Haynes III, MD, for contributions to this chapter in the previous edition of the text.

Bibliography

Gayle A, Ringdahl E: Tick-borne disease. Am Fam Physician 64:461–466, 2001.

Goodman JL: Ehrlichiosis: Ticks, dogs, and doxycycline. N Engl J Med 341:195–197, 1999.

James DM: Tick removal. In James DM (ed): Field Guide to Urgent and Ambulatory Care Procedures. Philadelphia, Lippincott Williams & Wilkins, 2001, pp 225–226.

Needham G: Evaluation of five popular methods for tick removal. Pediatrics 75:997–1002, 1985.

Tibbles C, Edlow J: Does this patient have erythema migrans? JAMA 297:2617–2627, 2007.

CHAPTER 37

TISSUE GLUES

Rebecca Beach

Cyanoacrylates have been in widespread use outside of the United States for years, and the U.S. Food and Drug Administration (FDA) approved their use for repair of incisions and lacerations in 1998. The agents combine cyanoacrylates and formaldehyde. Some have added plasticizers for extra strength and flexibility. Dermabond (2-octylcyanoacrylate; Ethicon Corp., Norwood, Mass) is available in small, single-use, glass vacuum vials, and it forms a polymeric bond across apposed tissue edges on contact with moisture or air. There are several newer brands, including SurgiSeal (Adhezion Biomedical, Wyomissing, Penn) and LiquiBand (MedLogic Global, Ltd., Plymouth, United Kingdom). Over-the-counter cyanoacrylates such as Super Glue and Crazy Glue are somewhat weaker and are not FDA approved for this indication but are used by many patients at home. The latter preparations have more difficulty binding to a moist surface. Cosmesis with tissue glues is comparable or superior to sutures, and there is much greater acceptance, especially with children. The products have antimicrobial properties and negligible tissue toxicity and are easily applied. They significantly decrease wound repair time.

INDICATIONS

- Nonmucosal laceration or incision repairs
- Facial, scalp, torso, or extremity wounds
- After deep suture placement if skin tension is minimal
- Wounds less than 8 cm (gap <0.5 cm)
- As an alternative to 5-0 or smaller suture
- Removal of foreign bodies in ear or nose (physicians can apply a small drop of glue on the wooden end of cotton swab, touch the object for 30 seconds, and remove)
- Repair of lacerated nails or nail beds
- Because there is more scarring the longer sutures are left in, consider removing any sutures a few days ahead of schedule after the wound has sealed over and applying a tissue glue to keep the wound edges together

CONTRAINDICATIONS

- Mucosal lesions
- Significant wound margin tension
- Noncompliant patient
- Heavily contaminated wounds requiring débridement
- Human or animal bite or scratch wounds
- Puncture wounds
- Stellate, jagged, or crush wounds
- Wounds on axillae, perineum, or feet
- Hand or joint lacerations (in which repetitive movement or washing can weaken bond)

ADVANTAGES

- Faster than suturing or stapling
- Less painful
- Less need for painful injectable anesthetic
- As effective as suturing in appropriately selected patients
- A lower infection rate compared with staples and sutures (according to some studies)
- No need for suture removal
- Low cost
- Reduces risk of needlestick injury
- Hair apposition technique allows treatment of scalp wounds without shaving, with less pain, and much more quickly than traditional techniques

DISADVANTAGES

- Bond reaches strength equivalent to naturally healed tissue at 7 days after repair.
- Early dehiscence is the most common complaint. Wound strength on the first day is significantly less than with suture.
- Glue is very liquid, and inadvertent spillage or excessive application can cause adherence to gloves or other tissues as well as pain from heat of exothermic reaction.
- Dermabond, LiquiBand, and SurgiSeal are available as single-use applicators at typically double or triple the cost of a single pack of nylon suture.

EQUIPMENT

- Dermabond single-use vials (Fig. 37-1A) or alternative brands. May find information on specific brands and their applicators at corporate websites: www.liquiband.com, www.adhezion.com (for SurgiSeal).
- Gloves.
- Single-use tissue approximators (Bionix Development Corp., Toledo, Ohio), gauze, or forceps (see Fig. 37-3A) *(optional)*.
- Super Glue remover *(optional)*. Acetone (nail polish remover) is the active ingredient.

PREPROCEDURE PATIENT PREPARATION

Obtain verbal informed consent for the procedure. Explain that the wound will be cleansed and prepared, possibly involving analgesia. Some children may need to be restrained. Explain the procedure and warn the patient there may be a slight sensation of heat or stinging.

TECHNIQUE

See Figure 37-2.

1. Meticulous wound preparation is essential and may require topical or infiltrated anesthetics. Good hemostasis must be achieved before application.
2. The patient should be positioned so that the fluid glue does not run off the wound to other areas.

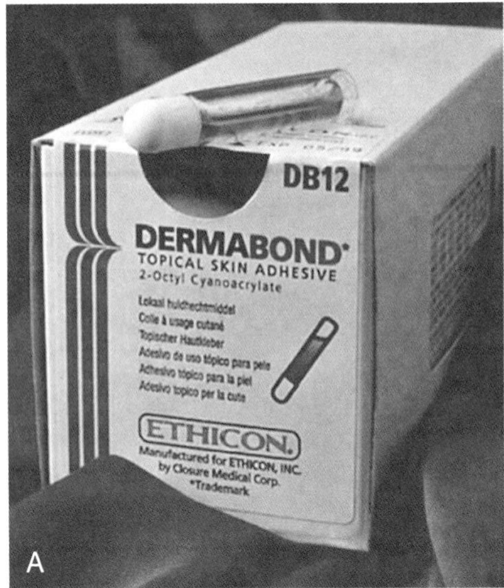

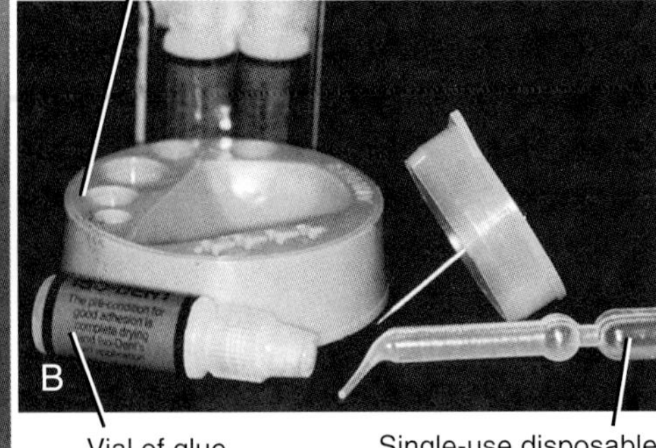

Figure 37-1 **A,** Dermabond single-use vials. **B,** Ellman IsoDent System. (**A,** Courtesy of Ethicon, Inc., Norwood, Mass. **B,** Courtesy of Ellman International, Inc., Hewlett, NY.)

3. The edges of the laceration are manually apposed. Clean, not sterile, gloves are acceptable for use, provided the wound is not inadvertently contaminated. For better traction, gauze, forceps, or disposable plastic tissue approximators may be used (Fig. 37-3).
4. The vial is crushed to start the flow of glue, and the glue touched to the wound edges. Dermabond and LiquiBand both have "chisel-tip" applicators, which purportedly improve accuracy. SurgiSeal has a sponge-tipped applicator.
5. The glue is gently painted over the wound. Care should be taken to keep the glue from entering into the wound, which can impair healing and precipitate a foreign body reaction. If there is doubt that the tissue edges can be reapproximated completely and evenly, suturing or stapling should be considered.
6. Apply only a few drops at a time. Heat is produced proportionately to the amount of adhesive applied and can be exquisitely painful. By the time the patient is feeling heat, it may be too late to wipe off the excess. Err on the side of caution.
7. The glue should be applied in an ovoid area (the wound being central) for best adhesive strength.
8. The manufacturer recommends a minimum of three separate coats. Each layer should be allowed to dry. The first will dry in about 2½ minutes. The surface, when dry, looks slightly rougher and more undulant than when it is wet. Subsequent layers dry more rapidly. Excess adhesive must be wiped off within 10 seconds.
9. Steri-Strips, applied after drying, can help prevent wound dehiscence.
10. Hair apposition technique (HAT) for scalp lesions:
    - Twist together one or two hairs from each side of scalp laceration.
    - Apply a few drops of glue to the hairs.
    - Repeat every few millimeters along the laceration until it is completely approximated.
    - Caution patient not to wash hair for 2 days or vigorously brush or comb around the area of the laceration.

Postprocedure Patient Education

The adhesive is water resistant, and further dressing is not needed. The patient may wet the area but should pat it dry. Soaking is not recommended. *Antibiotic ointment should be avoided* because it will weaken the bond and dissolve the glue. A bandage may be appropriate for active people, children, or those inclined to pick or pull at the wound. The adhesive spontaneously sloughs in 5 to 14 days.

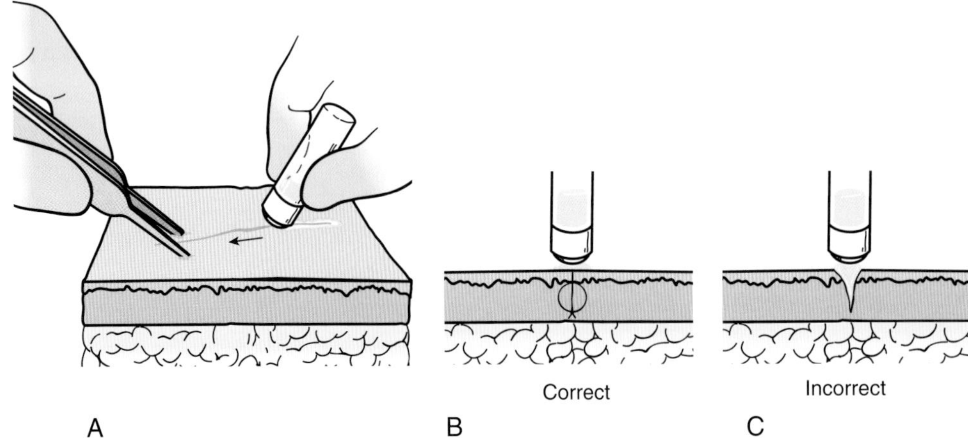

Figure 37-2 **A,** Approximate margins and apply glue. **B,** Correct application. **C,** Incorrect application into the wound itself.

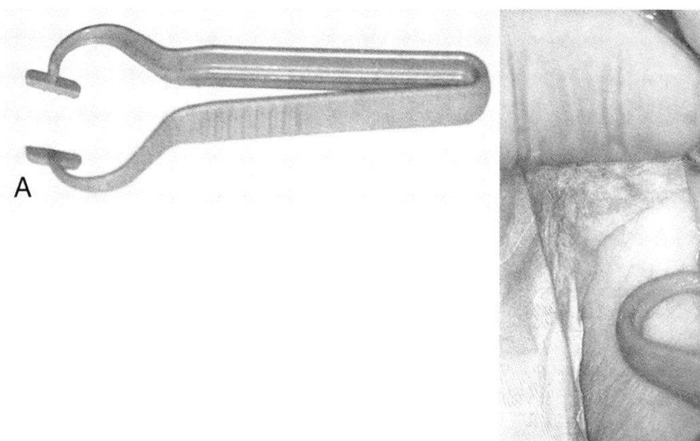

Figure 37-3 **A,** Plastic tissue approximators for the application of tissue glue. **B,** Application of tissue glue with the aid of plastic approximators.

Infections are unusual but can be detected early because the wound is visible and purulent exudate normally "unroofs" the adhesive. In these cases, the adhesive should be gently removed and standard wound infection treatment, possibly including systemic antibiotics, implemented. Reclosure with cyanoacrylate is not recommended.

Complications

- Early wound dehiscence.
- If the practitioner's instruments, gauze, or gloves accidentally adhere to the wound or patient, pressure is placed adjacent to the area and the object is "rolled off" in a way that does not place traction on the repair.
- Adhesive that inadvertently binds the eyelids should be covered with generous amounts of ophthalmic antibiotic ointment and not pried open. The bond usually weakens and separates—if not immediately, then in 1 or 2 days. Cyanoacrylates are not harmful to the eye and are used routinely in ophthalmologic practice. Appropriate placement of gauze during repairs can prevent spillage into the eyes.
- Petroleum jelly, antibiotic ointment, or a commercially available Super Glue remover can be used on dried runoff areas.
- Adhesive may insinuate itself between wound edges, resulting in unacceptable healing.

Patient Education Guides

See the sample patient education handout available online at www.expertconsult.com.

Cost

Updated in 2010, Dermabond is about $21 per *single-use* vial and comes in boxes of 12. Applying tissue glues conserves physician time, which is also a factor. Many institutions and offices are also now allowing other assistants to apply the adhesive.

CPT/Billing Codes

See Chapter 22, Laceration and Incision Repair, Table 22-4, for wound closure codes. The same codes are used whether the repair is performed with suture or with tissue glue.

ICD-9-CM Diagnostic Codes

ICD-9 codes for wound or laceration vary by location, degree, depth, and tendon involvement. See also Chapter 22, Laceration and Incision Repair.

Acknowledgment

The editors wish to recognize the contributions of J. Mark Wiedemanm, MD, and John L. Pfenninger, MD, to this chapter in the previous edition of this text.

Suppliers

(See contact information online at www.expertconsult.com.)

Dermabond
Ethicon, Inc.
LiquiBand
MedLogic Global, Ltd.
SurgiSeal
Adhezion Biomedical
Wound closure forceps
Bionix Development Corp.

BIBLIOGRAPHY

Bruns TB, Worthington JM: Using tissue adhesive for wound repair: A practical guide to Dermabond. Am Fam Physician 61:1383–1388, 2000.

Hock MO, Ooi SB, Saw SM, Lim SH: A randomized controlled trial comparing the hair apposition technique with tissue glue to standard suturing in scalp lacerations (HAT Study). Ann Emerg Med 40:19–26, 2002.

Pfenninger JL: Use of tissue glues (cyanoacrylate tissue adhesives). In Rakel R (ed): Saunders Manual of Medical Practice. Philadelphia, WB Saunders, 2000.

Quinn J, Wells G, Sutcliffe T, et al: A randomized trial comparing octylcyanoacrylate tissue adhesive and sutures in the management of lacerations. JAMA 277:1527–1530, 1997.

Simon HK, McLario DJ, Bruns TB, et al: Long-term appearance of lacerations repaired using a tissue adhesive. Pediatrics 99:193–195, 1997.

Singer AJ, Hollander JE, Valentine SM, et al: Prospective, randomized, controlled trial of tissue adhesive (2-octylcyanoacrylate) vs. standard wound closure techniques for laceration repair. Stony Brook Octylcyanoacrylate Study Group. Acad Emerg Med 5:94–99, 1998.

CHAPTER 38

HYPERTROPHIC SCARS AND KELOIDS

Harris Mones • Dennis LaRavia

The skin of predisposed individuals may respond to injury or surgery by developing excessive growths known as *hypertrophic scars* or keloids. *Hypertrophic scars* are self-limited growths that enlarge within the boundaries of a wound and then often regress over time. Many hypertrophic scars spontaneously involute within 2 years. *Keloids* are benign, hard, fibrous proliferations of collagen that expand, either slowly or rapidly, beyond the original size and shape of a wound. They tend to persist and often invade surrounding tissue. They may become painful or pruritic as well as unsightly.

Hypertrophic scars and keloids represent abnormalities in the synthesis and degradation of collagen and extracellular matrix components. Hypertrophic scars have a 3-fold increase in collagen synthesis enzymes compared with normal scars, whereas keloids may exhibit 20 times the normal levels. Hypertrophic scars can occur at any site of skin injury. Those following surgical incisions usually remain linear. Burns frequently produce unsightly, pink, hypertrophic scars that may contract. The scars may itch, but generally they do not produce the pain and hyperesthesia seen with keloids.

The most important risk factor for keloid formation is a wound healing by secondary intention. This is especially true if wound healing time is greater than 3 weeks. Although most cases of keloids are sporadic, some cases are familial. In familial cases the mode of inheritance is unknown.

The incidence of keloids in dark-skinned individuals is 15 to 20 times that found in light-skinned people, and is higher in Asians. Overall, there is an equal incidence of lesions in males and females, although young females have a higher incidence than young males. Hypertrophic scars and keloids are found only in humans, occur in 5% to 15% of wounds, and are rarely seen in people older than 65 years of age. Keloids appear frequently in anatomic sites that are subject to motion, that overlie bony prominences, or are areas of increased skin tension or recurrent stretch, such as the shoulders, upper back, and presternal areas. Keloids may develop on the face and scalp after acne, or on the earlobe after ear piercing. They are seen more frequently in wounds that cross skin lines. Children and pregnant women are more likely to experience both hypertrophic scars and keloids.

This chapter focuses on office techniques used in the treatment of hypertrophic scars and keloids. Because of the natural regression of hypertrophic scars, therapy for these lesions is usually limited to topical application or injection of steroids and compression. Keloids are considered by some clinicians to be low-grade, benign, cutaneous tumors, and radiation therapy has been advocated. This therapy is not reviewed here. The malignancy potential of radiation in the treatment of a benign disease as well as its expense make radiation therapy a last resort. No single therapy for keloids has proven experimentally superior. Location, size, and duration are factors in choosing the most appropriate therapy. Cryotherapy, corticosteroid injection, surgical excision, pressure therapy, and irradiation—or a combination of these modalities—may be chosen for the treatment of keloids.

PREVENTION

The most important thing to consider in the management of keloid scar formation is prevention. Before surgical procedures are performed, a thorough history of abnormal scar formation or a family history of keloid scar formation should be obtained from the patient. If a history of keloid formation is obtained, all nonessential surgery should be avoided, especially at sites that are at high risk. In circumstances where surgery cannot be avoided, all attempts must be made to minimize skin tension and secondary infection. Antibiotics, meticulous sterile technique, and, rarely, perioperative steroid injections (mixed with lidocaine) are helpful in prevention as well.

CRYOTHERAPY

Tissue destruction techniques used for treating keloids can incite further keloid formation. Cryotherapy, however, has been used with good results in 65% to 75% of cases. Both liquid nitrogen and nitrous oxide methods can be efficacious (see Chapter 14, Cryosurgery, Fig. 14-4). The more recent the keloid, the better the response to cryotherapy. A 10- to 15-second freeze with *liquid nitrogen* (−189° C) is usually required for keloids on most sites other than the mid-sternal region (small scars will take less time). Freezing for more than 10 to 15 seconds with liquid nitrogen can produce persistent post-treatment hypopigmentation. A 30- to 45-second freeze is usually adequate for most keloids when *nitrous oxide* (−89° C) is used. A better guide for any modality is to continue the freeze until 1 to 2 mm of normal tissue is involved and the complete *thaw time* is 1.5 to 2 minutes. During each treatment visit, the entire lesion must be treated with two to three freeze/thaw cycles.

After cryotherapy (see Chapter 14, Cryosurgery, Fig. 14-4), tissue edema will develop in 20 to 60 minutes. Within hours a significant bulla (blister) will appear. A rather copious serous discharge may follow. A moist environment (semiocclusive dressing) will aid healing. In southern and temperate climate areas, particularly during the summer months, occlusive therapy may prolong healing and increases the likelihood of secondary infection. Depending on the size of the lesion, five to eight treatments may be needed at 6-week intervals. Start conservatively and increase the freeze times if there are no untoward adverse effects.

Cryotherapy can also be used to soften hard keloids immediately before injection of steroids. Edema of the skin allows better dispersal of the steroid and minimizes its deposition into the subcutaneous or surrounding normal tissue. Cryotherapy before injection (liquid nitrogen spray for 3- to 5-second burst[s]) may also improve keloid regression, allows for lower injection pressures, and decreases the pain associated with injections. Allow 20 to 60 minutes for the edema to develop before proceeding with the injection.

Corticosteroid Injections

Once a scar is palpable, topical corticosteroids, even under occlusion (e.g., flurandrenolide [Cordran] tape), are rarely beneficial. Raised hypertrophic scars and keloids, however, may be softened and flattened by intralesional corticosteroid therapy. Corticosteroids represent effective monotherapy for some hypertrophic scars and small keloids, and they are frequently used as the initial therapy for large keloids.

Early, small, or narrow lesions are initially treated with intralesional injection every 4 to 6 weeks. Early keloids are softer and more responsive to injection than older, inactive lesions. Avoid injecting into surrounding normal skin to prevent perilesional subcutaneous atrophy and telangiectasis formation. When a lesion flattens to nearly the level of the skin surface, allow more time to pass before injecting again and decrease the concentration of the injections. Overaggressive therapy can lead to hypopigmentation and a depression resulting from the atrophy.

Injections are frequently performed with a 27- or 30-gauge needle on a Luer-Lok syringe. Locked syringes help to prevent needle disengagement when injecting under pressure. Consider using cryotherapy immediately beforehand (see the previous section) to ease injection and spread of the steroid.

Many steroid regimens have been developed, and there is considerable variation in guidelines and recommendations for dosages and drugs. No clear advantage has been shown for any one type of corticosteroid. Triamcinolone acetonide 10 mg/mL (Kenalog-10) is a popular choice because of its 4- to 6-week duration of action. Although undiluted steroid can be used for unresponsive or dense lesions, it is more prudent to dilute the triamcinolone 1:3 with physiologic saline or 1% lidocaine (single-dose vials) to create a 2.5 mg/mL solution. This dilute concentration limits postinjection hypopigmentation and atrophy. Injecting only lidocaine around the lesion using a 27- to 31-gauge needle before steroid injection improves patient comfort. Once the individual patient response is known, the concentration of triamcinolone acetonide can be increased to a dilution of 1:2 or 1:1 with lidocaine if necessary for future injections to increase the effect. If little effect is seen even without dilution, triamcinolone 40 mg/kg can be used and diluted as indicated. **A common error is to be too aggressive.** Go slowly to avoid the complication of atrophy. Hyaluronidase can be added to the solution to help disperse the steroid.

Administer the corticosteroid as the needle passes through the lesion. Keep the bevel of the needle pointed down. The scar may blanch temporarily with the injection. Try to keep the injection within the confines of the lesion to prevent side effects in the adjacent tissue. Firm lesions may limit the amount of medication that can be administered. The total amount will vary significantly depending on the size of the lesion. Keloids over 1 to 1.5 cm in diameter generally do not resolve as quickly or completely as smaller keloids. When the lesion is too dense to inject, consider treating with cryotherapy first, as previously discussed.

Another method of injecting steroids is to use the MadaJet Injector (see Pearl no. 8 in Appendix H, Pearls of Practice). The same concentration is used. The spring-loaded "gun" fires (dispenses) the solution, which is under pressure, into the lesion. No needles are involved, and there is less pain. Injections may again need to be repeated every 4 to 6 weeks to gain maximum benefit. The same dilutions are used.

Systemic effects from the corticosteroids are rare, but are possible with repeated injections of higher concentrations. Local effects include hypopigmentation, hyperpigmentation, perilesional atrophy, perilymphatic linear atrophy, and local telangiectasia. These effects often improve over time. This therapy is generally considered safe and effective.

Surgical Excision

Therapy of keloids limited to traditional surgical excision with primary closure leads to a recurrence rate of greater than 50%. Mixing corticosteroids with the local anesthetic at the time of surgical removal provides superior results. In treating recalcitrant keloids over 1 to 1.5 cm, the best surgical results have been obtained using intralesional corticosteroid injections of triamcinolone (diluted to 2.5 to 5.0 mg/mL) into the immediate subcutaneous interface of the keloid and normal deep skin structures. The steroid injections can be administered 3 months and 6 weeks before scheduled surgical excision and again on the day of skin surgery immediately before the procedure. Follow-up at 4 and 8 weeks after surgery is important to detect any recurrence, which can be aborted with further injections. For smaller lesions, many clinicians will just inject at the time of surgery.

Proper surgical technique during the excision reduces the recurrence of keloids. Because tissue trauma may incite excessive growth, the wound bed and surrounding tissues must be handled gently. Avoid the use of instruments that crush tissue as well as overly aggressive cautery. Superpulse carbon dioxide lasers allow precise excision and cautery and cause minimal thermal damage to surrounding tissue. This makes them useful in excising some keloids, despite their relative expense. Radiofrequency surgery has similar results (see Chapter 30, Radiofrequency Surgery [Modern Electrosurgery]).

When an excision is performed, close the skin under minimal tension. Consider gentle undermining to decrease wound tension. Some surgeons avoid subcuticular absorbable sutures, which may increase tissue reaction. Skin closure should be accomplished with a very fine nonabsorbable suture material, such as 6-0 nylon. Topical adhesives ("tissue glues" such as Dermabond or IsoDent) and wound closure strips help close the wound with the least possible trauma and reduce tension on wound edges. They may also reduce the total number of sutures needed.

Some surgeons advocate removal of every vestige of a keloid; however, wide excision of normal skin around keloids does not reduce the rate of recurrence. Other surgeons advocate leaving a rim of incompletely excised keloid in place to serve as a barrier to further keloid growth. It is unclear whether this technique provides significant benefit over standard excisions.

Local advancement flaps can be used to limit the wound tension after excision. Figure 38-1 shows a low-tension flap created after the

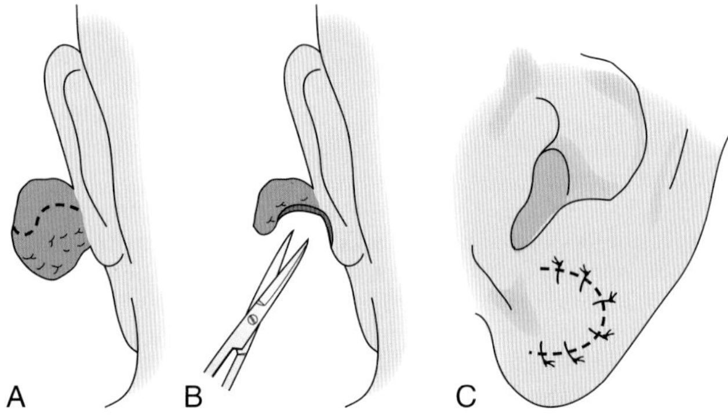

Figure 38-1 Resection of a keloid on an earlobe. The skin overlying a keloid can be used to create a low-tension wound closure. **A,** Half the skin is selected for the flap. **B,** The skin is sharply dissected from the underlying keloid, and the subcutaneous keloid is totally excised. **C,** The wound is closed with simple, interrupted, nonabsorbable 6-0 nylon suture.

removal of a globular earlobe keloid. Although some practitioners advocate skin grafting to provide low-tension skin closure, large donor site keloids can also develop. Advanced closure techniques such as rotation advancement or M-plasty to cover large areas of keloid removal may be indicated to minimize tension on skin edge closure.

Evidence suggests using Silastic–silicone preparations (e.g., Mederma, ReJuveness, Biodermis, Mepiform, Kelokote) immediately after surgery may reduce the occurrence of keloids in those prone to excessive scarring.

A final surgical method of removing keloids is radiofrequency surgery. The large loop is used on a pure cutting setting. After anesthesia (with a dilute steroid included) the keloid is shaved off, followed by radiofrequency surgery/smoothing (Fig. 38-2).

Before attempting surgical excision of keloids, counsel the patient well. Patients with current or previous hypertrophic scars or keloids are more likely to form these types of scars after most surgical procedures, including dermabrasion. However, sculpting hypertrophic scars with traditional dermabrasion or carbon dioxide laser is usually beneficial and generally does not lead to recurrence of hypertrophic scars. It is more common in cases that are complicated by other factors, such as previous isotretinoin therapy, infection, or patient noncompliance with postoperative therapy. A detailed informed consent is useful in creating appropriate patient expectations. Photographs can be helpful before the procedure, immediately after the procedure, 3 months after the procedure, and 1 year after the procedure.

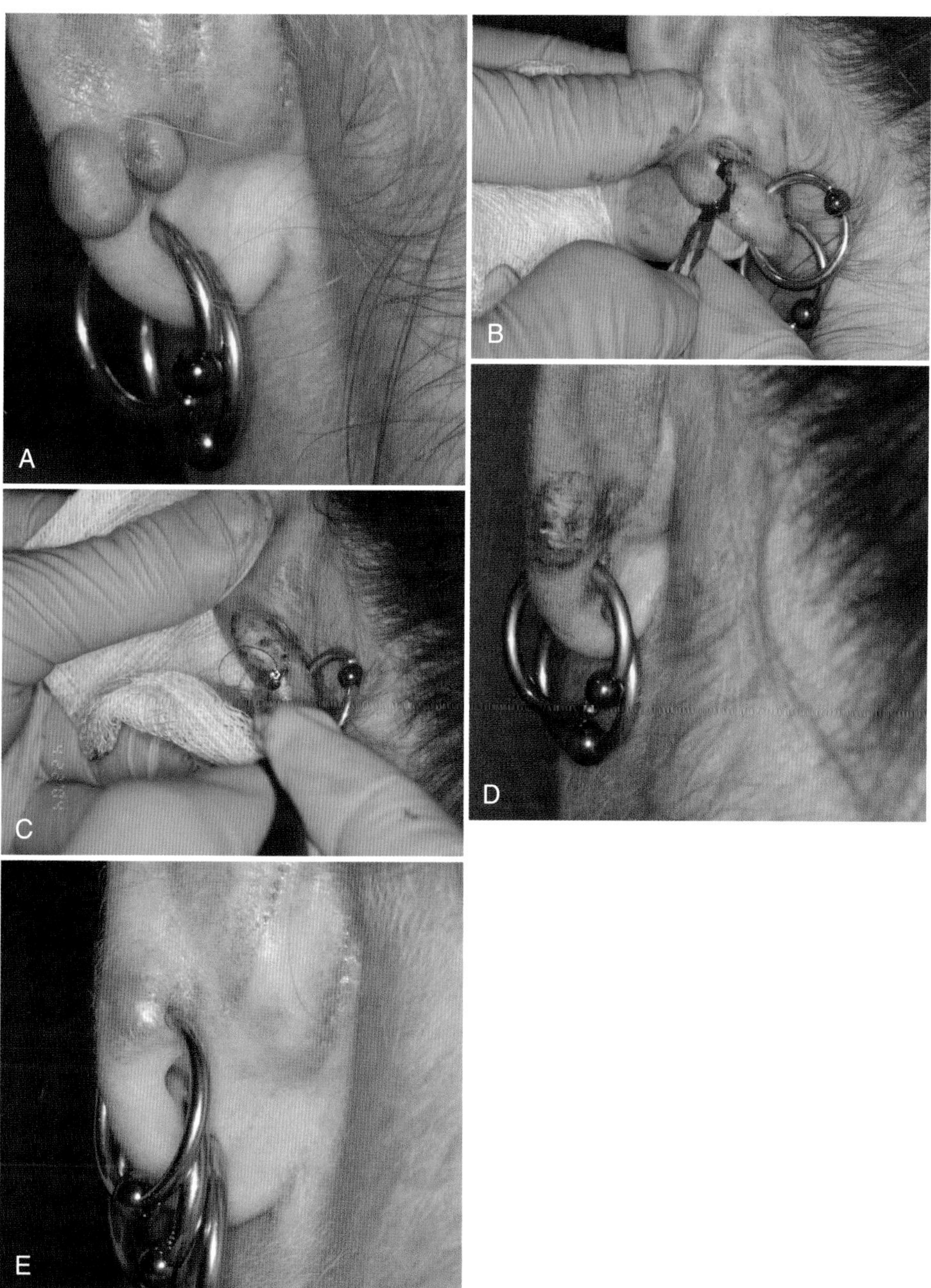

Figure 38-2 Removal of earlobe keloid using radiofrequency technique. **A,** Keloid. **B,** Shave removal of lesion after local anesthesia, including low-dose steroid. **C,** Radiofrequency smoothing of wound base, using pure cutting setting. **D,** Appearance of wound on completion of procedure. **E,** Appearance 1 month later. Unfortunately, patient has repierced the area!

Postoperative results vary widely, and patients must understand that keloids may recur regardless of the treatment methods used. Warn patients that pigment variations may take several months after surgery to resolve. Sunscreens are essential. Patients should be seen at monthly intervals to identify any recurrence, and steroid injections or silicone treatments should be initiated or reintroduced early before the lesion becomes mature and large. It is recommended that patients should agree to surveillance of the wound closure site at least every 3 months for 1 to 2 years to ensure early intervention with postoperative intralesional corticosteroid injection if there is evidence of return of the keloid.

Pressure Therapy

Pressure applied to burn sites can prevent hypertrophic scar formation or induce regression of early hypertrophic scars. Similarly, pressure dressings and garments after keloid surgery reduce their rate of recurrence. Pressure bandaging is used until the scar is no longer red; however, patient compliance may be poor when months or years of therapy are required. Many physicians prefer to use postoperative injections to ensure adequate therapy. However, when wounds are large or numerous, fitted pressure garments may be the best alternative.

After earlobe keloid excision, a pressure earring can be worn as soon as the skin sutures are removed (usually 5 to 7 days). A spring-loaded, light-pressure earring prevents the complication of skin necrosis. Hypoallergenic pressure earrings with a self-adjusting clasp are available from Padgett Instruments (Kansas City, Mo; 1-800-842-1029) and many other medical supply companies. These earrings cost about $40 and are available in a variety of styles and colors that encourage prolonged use. A less expensive alternative is to use large, flat, back-clip earrings lined with Silastic sheeting cut to fit inside them. Silastic sheeting alone has been therapeutic in reducing keloids and hypertrophic scars but is best combined with repetitive intralesional steroid injections and compression to hold it in place.

Light Therapy (Laser and Others)

Continuous-wave carbon dioxide laser used in the cutting mode has been shown to be effective for some refractory keloids. All possible keloid tissue is excised with the laser, and the wound is allowed to heal by secondary intention or is closed with minimal tension, as noted previously. Concurrent intralesional steroids, compression dressings, or silicone treatments may be helpful. Depending on the size, depth, and location of the wound, as well as the patient's health, healing may take as long as 3 months. Transient hypertrophic scars develop in up to 30% of cases; unfortunately, as with other treatments, recurrence rates are high. Superpulse carbon dioxide laser may prove to be better, but long-term studies are pending. Flashlamp-pumped pulsed-dye lasers (585 nm) and intense pulsed-light lasers (e.g., PhotoDerm) are used to treat relatively flat hypertrophic scars and keloids. The advantage of using lasers relates to the precision with which the light energy can be delivered to the target rather than the surrounding tissue and the absorption of specific wavelengths of light by the vascular components of the target. Multiple sessions are required and cost may be a factor for some patients, but results are frequently impressive.

Alternative Methods

Some investigators inject *hyaluronidase* with steroids after cryotherapy, with improved results. Others have applied Imiquimod 5% cream (Aldara) postoperatively to help prevent keloid recurrence after surgical excision. The cream is applied postoperatively on alternate nights for eight weeks. Although their mechanism of action is unknown, *topical silicone gel* and *silicone sheeting* are used with success. The gel's impermeability to water is thought to minimize evaporation and provides a semiocclusive dressing that accelerates healing and shortens the inflammatory phase. Topical Silastic gels and Mederma gel (a vegetable oil extract) have proved to be beneficial in reducing both volume and redness of lesions. The silicone sheets (e.g., Mederma, ReJuveness, Biodermis, Mepiform, Kelokote) must be worn 12 to 24 hours per day for 3 months or more. They are applied under tape or a pressure garment. The sheet is 3.5 mm thick and is applied over the scar only. It is held in place with paper tape and removed and washed daily. Its effect is unrelated to pressure. Perioperative injection with *interferon* has been used. One study of 12 patients showed a recurrence rate of less than 10% after traditional excision, interferon injection, and follow-up of nearly 15 months. Intralesional *bleomycin* has also been tried with some success. *5-Fluorouracil* 50 mg/mL mixed with triamcinolone 1 mg/mL injected one to three times weekly into hypertrophic scars may be efficacious in decreasing scar tissue. Verapamil, cyclosporine, D-penicillamine, relaxin, topical mitomycin C, Cordran tape, and tacrolimus are other options that have been studied.

Conclusion

Stepwise treatment as well as combination of modalities may prove to be the most effective manner to treat keloids. If initial topical (or injected, high-potency) steroids and compression do not resolve the lesion, cryotherapy may soften the lesion and allow improved injectability. Next, excision or careful vaporization of the bulk of a lesion with carbon dioxide superpulse laser may be indicated. If resection is attempted, careful, low-tension closure with minimal sutures or healing by secondary intention is recommended. Excision followed by several sessions of 500- to 600-nm pulsed light or laser or low-dose radiation is also an option. Application of topical gels and pressure dressings combined with various modalities seems to produce acceptable results even with difficult lesions.

CPT/Billing Codes

There are no specific codes for treatment or excision of hypertrophic scars or keloids.

11900 Intralesional injection up to and including 7
11901 Intralesional injection more than 7

Also include the J code and amount for substance used.

ICD-9-CM Diagnostic Code

701.4 Keloid or scar

Acknowledgment

The editors wish to recognize the many contributions by Edward M. Zimmerman, MD, to this chapter in the previous edition of this text.

Suppliers

(See contact information online at www.expertconsult.com.)

MadaJet injector
Delasco Dermatologic Lab and Supply Co.
Mederma gel
Merz Pharmaceuticals
Mepiform (self-adherent silicone dressing)
Byron Medical
PhotoDerm and lasers of all wavelengths
Lumenis (formerly ESC Medical Systems)
Pressure earrings
Padgett Instruments, Inc.

ReJuveness silicone sheets
ReJuveness, Inc.
Silastic gel sheeting and topical products
Biodermis
Silastic topical gel (Kelokote)
Allied Biomedical Corp.

ONLINE RESOURCES

See patient education and patient consent forms available online at www.expertconsult.com (link to Cryosurgery form).

For updated references, search "keloid treatment" at www.elibrary.com.

BIBLIOGRAPHY

Alster TS, Williams CM: Treatment of keloid sternotomy scars with 585 nm flashlamp-pumped pulsed-dye laser. Lancet 345:1198–1200, 1995.

Berman B, Bieley HC: Keloids. J Am Acad Dermatol 33:117–123, 1995.

Berman B, Bieley HC: Adjunct therapy to surgical management of keloids. Dermatol Surg 22:126–130, 1996.

Chuangsuwanich A, Gunjittisomram S: The efficacy of 5% Imiquinod cream in the prevention of recurrence of excised keloids. J Med Assoc Thai 90:1363–1367, 2007.

Coleman WP, Hanke CW, Alt TH, Asken S: Cosmetic Surgery of the Skin, 2nd ed. St. Louis, Mosby, 1997.

de Oliveira GV, Nunes TA, Magna LA, et al: Silicone versus nonsilicone gel dressings: A controlled trial. Dermatol Surg 27:721–726, 2001.

English RS, Shenefelt PD: Keloids and hypertropic scars. Dermatol Surg 25:631–638, 1999.

España A, Solano T, Quintanilla E: Bleomycin in the treatment of keloids and hypertropic scars by multiple needle punctures. Dermatol Surg 27: 23–27, 2001.

Fitzpatrick RE: Treatment of inflamed hypertrophic scars using intralesional 5-FU. Dermatol Surg 25:224–232, 1999.

Fitzpatrick TB, Wolff K, Johnson RA: Color Atlas and Synopsis of Clinical Dermatology, 3rd ed. New York, McGraw-Hill, 1997.

Gold MH: Topical silicone gel sheeting in the treatment of hypertrophic scars and keloids. J Dermatol Surg Oncol 19:912–916, 1993.

Gold MH, Foster TD, Adair MA, et al: Prevention of hypertrophic scars and keloids by the prophylactic use of topical silicone gel sheets following a surgical procedure in an office setting. Dermatol Surg 27:641–644, 2001.

Habif TP: Clinical Dermatology, 4th ed. St. Louis, Mosby, 2004.

Juckett G, Hartman-Adams H: Management of keloids and hypertophic scars. Am Fam Physician 80:253–260, 2009.

Kantor GR, Wheeland RG, Bailin PL, et al: Treatment of earlobe keloids with carbon dioxide laser excision: A report of 16 cases. J Dermatol Surg Oncol 11:1063–1067, 1985.

Marneros A, Noris JEC, Olsen BR, Reichenberger E: Clinical genetics of familial keloids. Arch Dermatol 137:1429–1434, 2001.

Murray JC: Keloids and hypertrophic scars. Clin Dermatol 12:27–37, 1994.

Nemeth AJ: Keloids and hypertrophic scars. J Dermatol Surg Oncol 19: 738–746, 1993.

Niessen FB, Spauwen PH, Schalkwijk J, Kon M: On the nature of hypertrophic scars and keloids: A review. Plast Reconstr Surg 104:1435–1458, 1999.

Rusciani L, Rossi G, Bono R: Use of cryotherapy in the treatment of keloids. J Dermatol Surg Oncol 19:529–534, 1993.

Stucker FJ, Shaw GY: An approach to management of keloids. Arch Otolaryngol Head Neck Surg 118:63–67, 1992.

Usatine RP: The Color Atlas of Family Medicine. New York, McGraw-Hill, 2009.

CHAPTER 39

EPILATION OF ISOLATED HAIRS (INCLUDING TRICHIASIS)

Kathleen M. O'Hanlon

The method used to permanently remove problem hairs, such as misdirected eyelashes or ingrown hairs, depends on the anatomic location of the hair and the condition of the surrounding skin. The simplest approach, typically used by electrologists, applies electrical current to cause follicular destruction. In radiofrequency surgery, household current is converted to a frequency of 3.9 MHz, resulting in heating and vaporization of water in the tissue and subsequent destruction of the hair root. This process results in minimal lateral heat transfer, allowing for selective ablation of lash follicles without the side effects on the lid previously experienced with electrocautery (see Complications). In the presence of inflammatory disease with ingrown hairs, a more comprehensive skin care program should be used first to decrease the density of papules and pustules. For removal of large areas of hair, new laser applications have been developed. The units are expensive but time saving and effective (see Chapter 48, Lasers and Pulsed-Light Devices: Hair Removal).

PHYSIOLOGY

Hair is formed by the replication of cells in hair follicles. The growth phase (anagen) commences with germinal papillae descending into the dermis. This is followed by cellular proliferation (catagen), during which a bulb and a hair are formed. Once growth has ceased, the follicle shrinks and enters into the resting phase (telogen). The duration of each phase of the cycle depends on the type and location of the hair. Short hairs, such as human eyelashes, spend the majority of their time in the telogen phase, during which the germinal cells reside near the base of the follicle. Hair ablative procedures therefore need to apply heat energy (electrolysis or radiosurgery) specifically to the base of these follicles.

Trichiasis

Abnormal eyelashes may be congenital or may result from trauma, infections, diseases such as Stevens-Johnson syndrome, chronic disease, and allergies, medication use, or even the aging process. *Cilia inversum* is a rare finding in which a lash originates in the tarsal conjunctiva instead of anterior to the tarsal plate. *Cilia incarnata*, an anomaly akin to ingrown hair, develops when a lash is trapped beneath the skin near the lid margin. In *distichiasis*, lashes grow from the meibomian gland orifices posterior to the normal lashes. True trichiasis, an acquired condition in which one or more lashes is misdirected posteriorly toward the conjunctiva or cornea, may pose a range of problems, from irritation to corneal abrasion or ulceration. Localized hairs may be suitable for tweezing, followed by permanent ablation if they recur. On the upper lid, the eyelash bulb has been determined to be about 2.4 mm below the surface of the lid margin, and the lower lid follicles are about 1.4 mm deep. Lanugo hairs or widespread trichiasis may require more specialized surgical procedures and should be referred to an ophthalmologist.

Ingrown Hairs

Ingrown hairs, *pili incarnati*, originate from a variety of causes. Razor-shaved hair ends have very sharp tips that may curve back toward the skin surface and reenter the epidermis a short distance from the mouth of the follicle (common in black people or people with curly hair). Double-edged razors, in which the hair is pulled out of the follicle by the first razor and cut by the second razor, leave the resultant hair tip recoiled in the follicle below the surface of the skin. The curved hair may then grow into the follicular wall. As the hair tips pierce the epidermis or penetrate the dermis, a foreign body inflammatory reaction ensues. Usually the ingrown hairs are completely buried, but they may have an identifiable recurving loop. In treating such hairs, the unattached end of the hair must be exposed above the surface of the skin using sharp forceps. Impacted hairs, which cannot be freed, should be left in place until a subsequent visit.

INDICATIONS

- Trichiasis
- Ingrown hairs (e.g., pseudofolliculitis barbae and other related disorders)

RELATIVE CONTRAINDICATIONS

- History of recurrent herpes (premedicate before epilation)
- Inflammatory skin condition (controlled)
- "Demand" cardiac pacemaker (radiofrequency wave can cause pacemaker malfunction, resulting in palpitations or even asystole)

ABSOLUTE CONTRAINDICATION

Active herpetic outbreak

EQUIPMENT

- Radiosurgery unit (Surgitron; Ellman International, Hewlett, NY).
- Ellman's "insulated needle electrode" (catalog no. D6) or flexible probes (fine wires or 33-gauge needles) may be necessary for the curvaceous ingrown hairs (Fig. 39-1).
- Small tweezers.
- Alcohol wipe.
- Loupes or magnification lamp (*optional—but very helpful*).
- Topical anesthetic (*optional*; e.g., EMLA, ELA-Max, Hurricaine Gel; see Chapter 10, Topical Anesthesia).

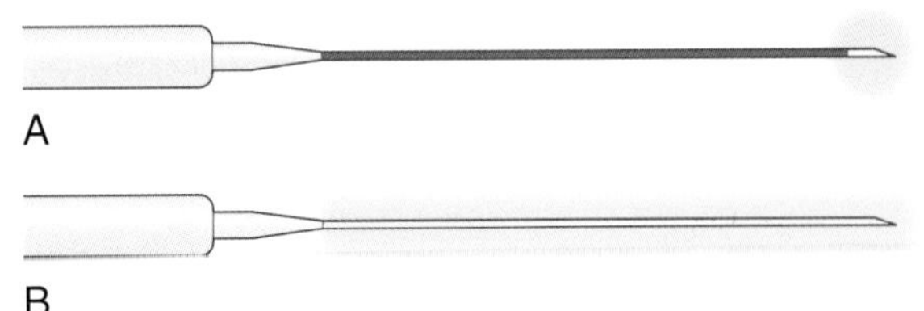

Figure 39-1 Two common needles used for epilation. **A,** Coated with only the tip active. **B,** Uncoated with entire needle active. (Courtesy of Ellman International, Hewlett, NY.)

Precautions

- Excess insertion depth of epilation needle can cause unnecessary scarring.
- Power set too high can result in lid or corneal side effects, including scarring.
- In the case of the ingrown hair, the shaft should be pulled gently to indicate the direction of the follicle, and a preferably *flexible* probe should be inserted for epilation. Probes that do not conform to the curvature of the hair may not reach the hair root. Although rare, incomplete electrolysis may create an ingrown hair if a distorted follicle is sealed off by the current.

Preprocedure Patient Education and Forms

See patient education, encounter, and consent forms online at www.expertconsult.com.

Procedure

See Figure 39-2.

- Prepare area with alcohol.
- Apply topical anesthetic *(optional)*.
- Set the Ellman Surgitron to 10 W or less (level 1) in the coagulation mode.
- Place the insulated needle electrode into the handpiece. Alternatively, use the 33-gauge needle and a needle hub adapter.

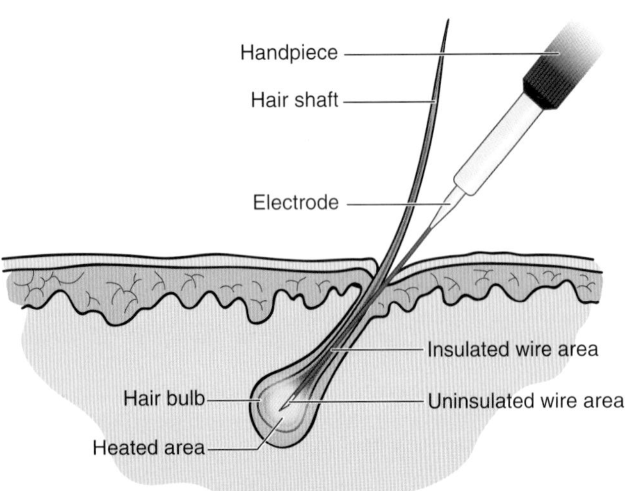

Figure 39-2 Using a fine needle electrode for epilation. (Courtesy of Ellman International, Hewlett, NY.)

- Identify the exposed end of the hair and, pulling the shaft gently with tweezers, insert the needle into the follicle until resistance is met, and activate the unit.
- Remove the hair with tweezers. It should come out easily.

Sample Operative Report

See sample operative report online at www.expertconsult.com.

Common Errors

- Inadequate penetration depth, resulting in unsuccessful permanent ablation
- Excessive cautery to the tissue

Complications

Although extremely rare, the following are potential complications:

- Recurrence of hair growth ("permanent" ablation is not 100% effective)
- Eyelid complications, including cellulitis, hypopigmentation or hyperpigmentation, lid deformities (e.g., notching, scarring—much more likely with *electrocautery*, which is not recommended by the author)
- Cicatricial conjunctival disease due to heat damage (also more likely with *electrocautery*)
- Potential hazard to the globe (due to close proximity)
- Activation of herpes zoster

Postprocedure Management

Antibiotic (eye) ointment for 3 to 5 days or until localized pits have granulated.

Postprocedure Patient Education

See patient education form online at www.expertconsult.com.

CPT/Billing Codes

17380	Electrolysis epilation; each ½ hour
67820	Correction of trichiasis; epilation by forceps only
67825	Correction of trichiasis epilation by electrosurgery, cryosurgery, or laser

ICD-9-CM Diagnostic Codes

374.00	Entropion
374.05	Trichiasis w/o entropion
374.54	Hypertrichosis of eyelid
704.1	Hirsutism/hypertrichosis (excessive growth of hair)
704.2	Trichiasis

Patient Education Guides

See patient education and consent forms and sample operative and encounter forms online at www.expertconsult.com.

Bibliography

Bartley GB: An experimental study to compare methods of eyelash ablation. Ophthalmology 94:1286–1289, 1987.

Crutchfield CE: The causes and treatment of pseudofolliculitis barbae. Cutis 61:351–356, 1998.

Elder MJ: Anatomy and physiology of eyelash follicles: Relevance to lash ablation procedures. Ophthal Plast Reconstr Surg 13:21–25, 1997.

Hurwitz JJ: Experimental treatment of eyelashes with high-frequency radio wave electrosurgery. Can J Ophthalmol 28:62–64, 1993.

Kezirian GM: Treatment of localized trichiasis with radiosurgery. Ophthal Plast Reconstr Surg 9:260–266, 1993.

CHAPTER 40

Topical Hemostatic Agents

Dale A. Patterson • Matt D. Roth

In medical training there is a cynical phrase quoted to novice medical students on a surgery rotation: "All bleeding stops eventually." Although this is true, the lesson to learn is that usually the best amount of bleeding is the least amount of bleeding. Effective, rapid hemostasis is the goal of physicians performing cutaneous surgery. This chapter covers the most useful methods of achieving topical hemostasis (Table 40-1).

The various methods range from physical techniques, such as simple pressure with an index finger and gauze pad, to chemical, electrical, and even laser techniques. The method used depends on the specifics of the surgery being performed, the experience of the office surgeon, and the availability of the agents or equipment.

Each method has its own benefits and drawbacks, and the astute clinician will match the method that best fits the needs of the particular patient. The older chemical agents (the so-called vasoconstrictive, vaso-occlusive, or denaturing agents) produce an eschar and actually cause some tissue damage. Newer, so-called physiologic agents facilitate the clotting mechanism but can be exorbitantly expensive (e.g., $30 or more for a single pack of Gelfoam). It is therefore important for the physician or health care provider to be familiar and accomplished with multiple methods to ensure the most positive outcome.

Indications

- For the treatment of
  - Bleeding after cutaneous surgery such as a shave biopsy
  - Abrasions or denuded skin
  - The nail bed after removal of either partial or full nail
  - Cuts or open wounds that cannot or will not be primarily closed
- To cauterize excess granulation tissue

Contraindications

Absolute

- Profuse bleeding. Topical agents will not control briskly bleeding vessels.
- Allergy to the hemostatic agent used.

Relative

- Large, deep wounds that require primary surgical closure with suture (use mechanical methods only).
- Cardiac pacemaker may preclude use of electrosurgery (e.g., Bovie, Hyfrecator).

NOTE: *Cautery* technically refers to a hot wire (most often, a battery-powered unit). This method is generally safe for patients with a pacemaker. On the other hand, *electrocautery* (e.g., Bovie, Hyfrecator, Ellman Surgitron) produces a low-amperage current (causing electrofulguration, electrodesiccation, or electrocoagulation) that may pose a risk to pacemaker users. Most new pacemakers are shielded. Use of these electrosurgical units should not be a problem, but other safe alternatives exist. See Chapter 30, Radiofrequency Surgery (Modern Electrosurgery), for details of electrosurgical principles.

Equipment and Supplies

Hemostatic Agents

See Figure 40-1 for a depiction of several common hemostatic agents.

Vaso-occlusive Denaturing Agents

Most commonly used

- Ferric subsulfate solution (20%; Monsel's solution)
- Aluminum chloride (30% solution; Drysol)
- Silver nitrate sticks or 20% to 50% solution
- Hydrophilic polymer and potassium salt (QR powder)

Not recommended

- Trichloroacetic acid (50% to 85% solution)
- Zinc chloride paste
- Phenol 50% solution
- Hydrogen peroxide 3% solution

Agents Producing a Physical Meshwork

- Absorbable gelatin sponge (Gelfoam)
- Oxidized cellulose (Surgicel)
- Microfibrillar collagen (Avitene)
- Cyanoacrylates (Dermabond, IsoDent; see Chapter 37, Tissue Glues)

Physiologic Hemostatic Agents

- Epinephrine, or lidocaine with epinephrine
- Thrombin (Thrombostat)
- Fibrin sealant
- Cocaine hydrochloride solution

Combination Products

- Flowable bovine collagen and bovine platelets (CoStasis)
- Flowable bovine gelatin matrix and bovine thrombin (FloSeal)

Agents for Traumatic Injuries

- QuikClot (granular zeolite powder)
- HemCon (Chitosan dressing)
- ChitoFlex (Chitosan dressing)

Mechanical Methods

- Electrocautery ("hot-wire," battery-operated unit)
- Electrosurgery (e.g., Bovie, Hyfrecator, Ellman Surgitron)

TABLE 40-1 Topical Hemostatic Agents

Generic/Product Name	Effectiveness	Difficulty of Preparation/ Application	Undesired Tissue Destruction	Chance of Pigment Stain (Usually Temporary)	Cost
Vaso-occlusive/Denaturing Agents					
Recommended					
Ferric subsulfate solution (20%; Monsel's solution)	+++	++	+	++	$$
QR powder (Quick Relief)	+++	+	–	–	$$
Aluminum chloride (30%)	++	++	+	–	$$
Silver nitrate sticks	+++	+	++	++++	$$
Not recommended					
Trichloroacetic acid (50%–85%)	++	+++	+++	–	$$
Zinc chloride paste	++	++	+	–	$$
Phenol 50%	++	++	+++	–	$$
Hydrogen peroxide	+	+	+	–	$
Agents Producing a Physical Meshwork					
Absorbable gelatin sponge (Gelfoam)	+++	++	–	–	$$$$
Oxidized cellulose (Surgicel)	++++	+++	–	–	$$$$
Microfibrillar collagen (Avitene)	+++++	+++++	–	–	$$$$$
Physiologic Hemostatic Agents					
Cocaine hydrochloride	+++	++++	–	–	$$$
Epinephrine	+++	+	–	–	$
Thrombin (Thrombostat)	+++++	++++	–	–	$$$$$
Fibrin sealant	+++++	++++	–	–	$$$$
Combination Agents					
CoStasis, FloSeal	+++++	+++++	–	–	$$$$$

Agents rated from
+ Mildly effective to +++++ Highly effective
+ Easy to prepare/apply to +++++ Difficult to prepare/apply
+ Minimal damage to +++++ Significant destruction
+ Low pigment stain to +++++ High chance of pigment stain
$ Low cost to $$$$$ High cost
– Indicates no effect.

- Laser (carbon dioxide)
- Shaw scalpel (a teflon-coated scalpel blade with a heating element)
- Application of ice
- Pressure dressings

PREPROCEDURE PATIENT EDUCATION

Discuss the procedure, including the rare but possible risks of further bleeding, infection, nerve damage, and scarring. Determine if the patient is known to be allergic to any of the agents. If using silver nitrate or Monsel's solution, inform the patient of the possibility of pigmentary change ("tattooing"), which is usually temporary but still requires discretion when being used in exposed areas such as the face.

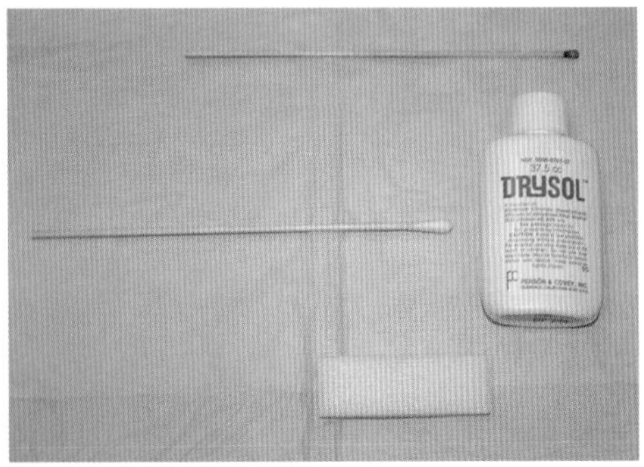

Figure 40-1 Common hemostatic agents. From top to bottom: silver nitrate stick, aluminum hydroxide with applicator, and absorbable Gelfoam.

PROCEDURE

Please see the corresponding chapter for the initial procedure being performed. *Topical hemostatic agents* are not a substitute for meticulous surgical technique, and many *cannot* be used inside a wound to be sutured. When topical hemostatic agents are required, ensure the patient is positioned on the examination or procedure table to provide adequate access to the wound.

Vaso-occlusive Denaturing Agents

These agents are applied topically and are *not* used if a wound is to be closed surgically. To maximize the coagulation effect, these agents should be applied as close to the source of bleeding as possible, and the wound should be sponged free of excess blood just before their application.

Ferric Subsulfate Solution (20%; Monsel's Solution)

First described by Leon Monsel in 1856, this liquid is perhaps the most commonly used topical hemostatic agent (Fig. 40-2). The solution is dark brown, almost black. If the bottle is left open, evaporation results in a pasty solution that, because it is more concentrated, is more effective. Do not let it become too thick, however. If it crystallizes, it can be reconstituted with water. Keep the container covered once the desired consistency is obtained. Hemostasis is effective with only rare staining, which can last up to 3 months. Application of Monsel's solution to a relatively dry wound bed (achieved by stretching and blotting the skin) controls oozing effectively.

Monsel's solution is applied with a cotton-tipped swab after drying and stretching the skin with the other hand. The swab is applied with light pressure. The low pH and the subsulfate group denature protein and occlude blood vessels. The practitioner cannot

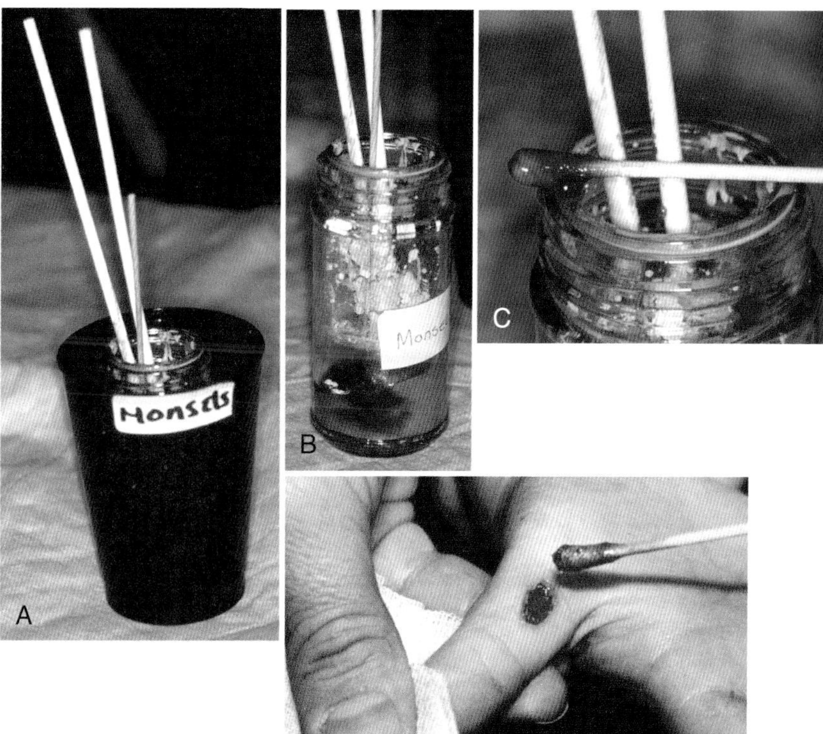

Figure 40-2 Topical astringent. **A,** Monsel's solution in open bottle, which allows it to thicken. **B,** Inner bottle. **C,** Cotton-tipped applicator used to apply thickened solution. Do not reinsert into bottle/container. **D,** Applying Monsel's with cotton-tipped applicator.

use too much. Once in contact with blood, the black, coagulated mixture can be wiped away. Monsel's works particularly well after cervical biopsies, loop electrosurgical excision procedures, and anorectal biopsies. It is also commonly used after shave excision and punch biopsies except in very fair-skinned individuals.

Monsel's solution is inexpensive, easily applied, easily stored, and readily available. However, there is a rare risk of "tattooing," so some physicians do not recommend it for the face, especially on light skin (Fig. 40-3). In clinical practice there is often a compromise in which Monsel's, given its superior hemostatic properties, is still used for the face and on patients with a very light complexion. (Aluminum chloride is nonstaining and should be tried first in these cases.) The tattooing can last several months. Monsel's may also cause temporary artifactual changes in skin and cervical biopsies, confounding the histologic evaluation of reexcisions for a few weeks thereafter. It also stains clothing. Stains on laboratory coats can be removed with dilute hydrochloric acid, such as that often found in toilet bowl cleaners, or by using Iron-Out. Monsel's stains need to be treated before washing in hot water or drying with heat because each seems to set the stain permanently.

Aluminum Chloride (30%)

Aluminum chloride is usually applied topically to a wound as a 30% solution (e.g., Drysol, Lumicaine) on a swab with light pressure (Fig. 40-4). It is colorless and forms a thin coagulum over the wound. Although not as effective as Monsel's solution, it does not cause tattooing. This solution is commonly used after surgical shave biopsies.

Silver Nitrate

Silver nitrate is available as a 20% to 50% solution and as a solid on a wooden stick. The sticks are more convenient and consequently more popular. The silver nitrate on the end is activated when the tip is placed on a moist wound bed. Silver ions cause proteins to precipitate, which occludes blood vessels. The eschar that forms in the wound bed prevents deeper tissue penetration

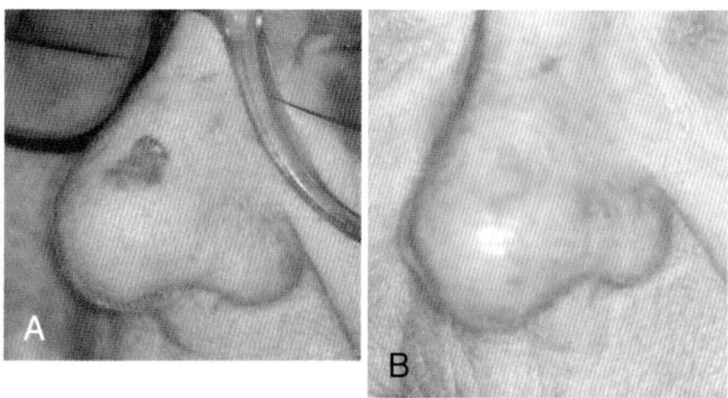

Figure 40-3 Monsel's staining. **A,** Three weeks after initial use. **B,** Spontaneous resolution after 6 to 8 weeks.

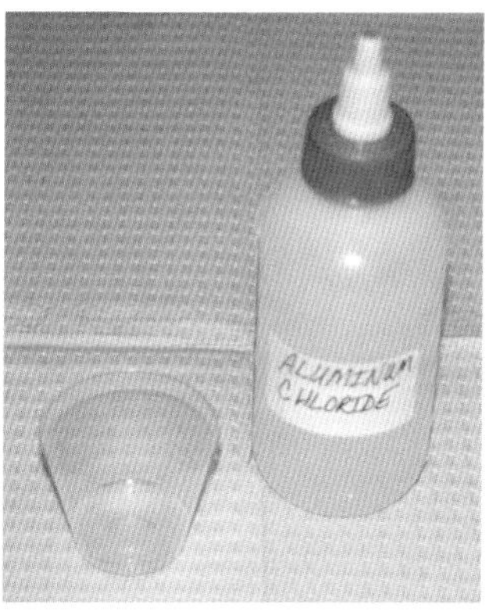

Figure 40-4 Aluminum chloride (clear solution).

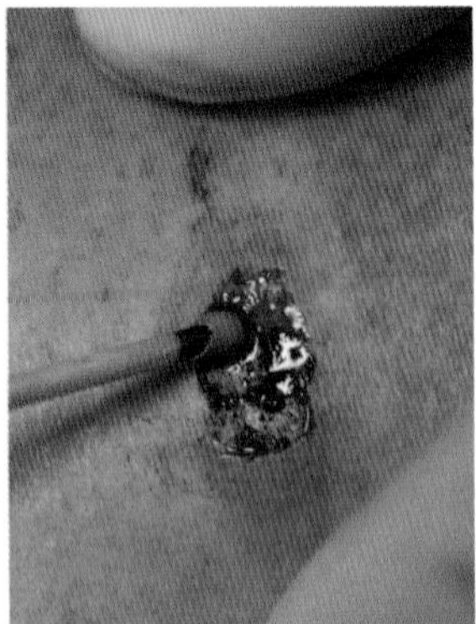

Figure 40-5 Shave biopsy partially cauterized by silver nitrate stick.

by the hemostatic agent. Silver salts stain the tissue black because of the deposition of reduced silver. Although most of the stain disappears spontaneously within a few weeks, there is a modest possibility of permanently tattooing the treated site. Care must be used with silver nitrate to avoid damaging normal tissue surrounding a wound. Because of these concerns, silver nitrate is most often restricted to cauterization of excess granulation tissue or for use in nonvisible areas (e.g., cervix, rectum). Figure 40-5 shows silver nitrate hemostasis of a shave biopsy.

Trichloroacetic Acid (50% to 85%)

Trichloroacetic acid is a topically applied agent that also forms an eschar at the wound bed. When it touches the tissue, the acid also causes superficial tissue destruction, and subsequently is *rarely used* for hemostatic purposes and is *not* recommended. Without anesthesia it can be painful, so application should be precise and rapid.

QR Powder (Hydrophilic Polymers and Potassium Salt)

This product is available over-the-counter and for professionals (Fig. 40-6). Blood must be present for it to work. The product is supplied in an individual-use packet with a cost of about $2 per packet. A thin coating of the powder is applied to the wound and pressure held for 15 to 60 seconds. Pressure is applied until bleeding stops (see Fig. 40-6D and E). If bleeding recurs, another application of the product can be made, even by the patient at home. The eschar should be left in place until it naturally "falls off." It is safe to wash and bathe the area 1 hour after application of the product. QR powder is not biologically derived and is not known to cause allergic reactions, tattooing, or discoloration of the skin. It can be used on any wound left to heal by secondary intention and has been successfully used to stop bleeding from the nose, abrasions, punctures, and minor surgical procedures. It should not be used below the surface of the skin on sutured wounds and is for topical/external use only. It does not cause pain or any pigment changes.

Other Agents

Zinc chloride paste is an effective hemostatic agent that was used in the original fixed-tissue Mohs' micrographic surgery, and it is still occasionally used today. *Phenol 50%* is effective, but the severe caustic effects on normal tissue may enlarge a wound. For this reason, it may be useful in nail removal for achieving hemostasis while providing destruction of the nail matrix. *Hydrogen peroxide* is readily available and is a weak hemostatic agent. It has obvious germicidal action, is inexpensive, and is easy to apply. Hydrogen peroxide is commonly applied directly to the wound in saturated gauze with direct pressure. It too causes some degree of tissue destruction and is rarely used for hemostasis alone.

Agents Producing a Physical Meshwork

Surgical wound closure is acceptable after use of most of the following agents.

Absorbable Gelatin Sponge (Gelfoam)

Gelatin powder is applied dry to the wound bed with light pressure. Absorbable gelatin sponges are manufactured in various forms from purified gelatin solution. Gelatin sponges can be applied dry or moistened with saline or thrombin. Absorbable gelatin holds blood

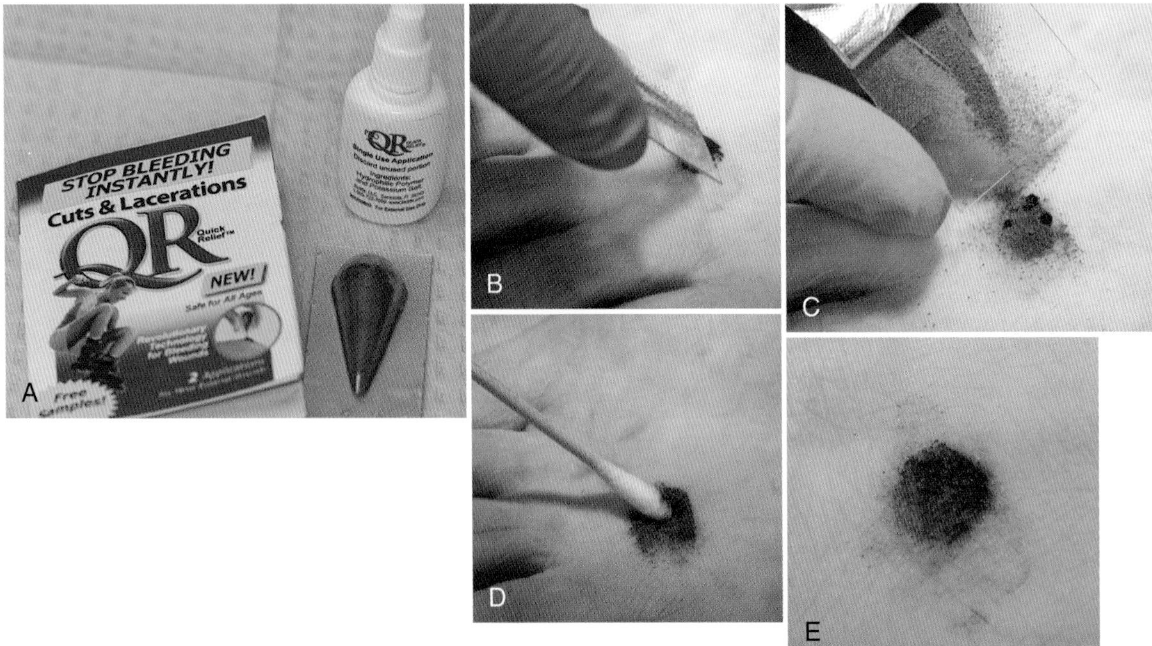

Figure 40-6 QR ("Quick Release") powder. **A,** Available in packets *(lower right)* or bottle dispensers. **B,** QR in use: applying from packet to shave excision. **C,** Appearance on wound before applying pressure. **D,** Applying pressure with a cotton-tipped applicator. **E,** Final appearance; hemostasis is obtained. A dressing is applied without antibiotic ointment.

and provides a matrix for clot formation and granulation tissue to form. The sponges are costly for a private office but are convenient and easy to handle. The gelatin powder can be difficult to handle and may be less effective than other meshwork agents.

Potential side effects include excessive granuloma formation and fibrosis. Care should be taken if these sponges are used near tendons because they have been known to cause excessive fibrosis especially in these areas.

Oxidized Cellulose (Surgicel)

Oxidized cellulose consists of absorbable fibers prepared from cellulose. Woven strips or sheets of cellulose can be cut and held with firm pressure on the wound bed. Oxidized cellulose provides a meshwork for coagulation and causes local vasoconstriction. This preparation is moderately priced, easy to handle, and mildly bactericidal.

Foreign body reaction is possible if excessive amounts of cellulose are left in a wound. Cellulose should not be used under grafts or flaps because it separates the graft from the blood supply. Some experts believe that the removal of oxidized cellulose after obtaining hemostasis frequently produces rebleeding.

Microfibrillar Collagen (Avitene)

Microfibrillar collagen is prepared by mechanically breaking down bovine collagen into fibrils. It is available in a fibrous (granular) form or a web form. The fibrous form is applied directly to the wound and held in place. The highly effective collagen products aggregate platelets on their surface. Collagen matrix applied to skin biopsy sites produces fewer infections, faster healing, and better cosmetic results than Monsel's solution.

Microfibrillar collagen adheres to wet gloves or surfaces, and it must be applied with dry instruments. Although the collagen is eventually absorbed, *it cannot be used at skin closure sites because it impedes the healing of wound edges*. The high cost and difficulty in handling make this agent impractical for most office dermatologic surgery.

Cyanoacrylates (Dermabond, IsoDent)

Tissue glues can seal wound edges and halt bleeding. See Chapter 37, Tissue Glues.

Physiologic Hemostatic Agents

Epinephrine

Epinephrine is a potent activator of adrenergic receptors, and the activation of α-adrenergic receptors produces vasoconstriction in the skin. Epinephrine is available in local anesthetics such as lidocaine with epinephrine or as adrenaline chloride solutions. Epinephrine is inexpensive and readily available, and it does not harm normal tissue at the base of the wound. It can be applied topically to control bleeding (e.g., the nose) or injected into a bleeding site (e.g., cervical biopsy). Effects are temporary (about 2 hours). Control of the bleeding, however, allows electrocoagulation or application of other topical agents if necessary.

Complications are quite rare. The precaution is always to avoid its use in end-arterial areas (i.e., finger, nose, penis, toes) for fear of causing distal necrosis. This rarely occurs. However, caution is advised in the vascular-compromised patient. Rebound vasodilation can potentially cause delayed bleeding. Cardiac arrhythmias and neurologic symptoms have been reported with the use of epinephrine in dermatologic procedures.

Thrombin (Thrombostat)

Thrombin is a potent physiologic clotting agent produced by the activation of bovine prothrombin. This freeze-dried powder either can be mixed with isotonic saline and sponged or sprayed on the wound bed or can be applied directly as powder. The wound should be sponged free of excess blood before thrombin is applied. For superficial surgery or plastic surgery involving flaps, dilute solutions of 100 units/mL may be effective.

Thrombin does not injure tissue or produce residue on the tissue bed. Once the solution is prepared, it must be used within 6 hours. Thrombin is expensive, prohibiting the routine use of this agent for office procedures.

Fibrin Sealant

Fibrin sealant is produced by making two components of human clotting factors immediately before application. Fibrin clot forms in about 30 seconds; the sealant can be applied with a special spraying device that mixes the components as they are delivered into the wound. Fibrin glue is one of the most effective agents available for hemostasis. The cost, the risk associated with the use of human blood products, and the cumbersome administration make this therapy undesirable for routine dermatologic surgery.

Cocaine Hydrochloride

Cocaine hydrochloride is useful as a powerful vasoconstrictor, but the potential for abuse, the cost, and the need for locked storage make its use problematic.

Combination Products

Combination products, such as CoStasis and FloSeal, use both meshwork and hemostatic agents in surgical procedures when conventional methods of hemostasis are unsuccessful. They are impractical for office procedures owing to their cost and limited applicability in routine procedures. A combination of a hydrophilic polymer and a potassium iron oxyacid salt, PRO QR powder, has more recently become available and is gaining popularity in office and emergency department settings.

Agents for Traumatic Injuries

QuikClot (Granular Zeolite Powder)

QuikClot has been approved by the U.S. Food and Drug Administration for the treatment of external hemorrhage. Much of the experience in the use of QuikClot has been in military applications. When applied to a wound, the granular zeolite powder attracts water and dries the wound in an exothermic reaction. This drying effect increases the rate at which red blood cells aggregate and decreases blood loss. The product has been shown to reduce hemorrhage from major traumatic wounds and has been used by the military in Iraq and Afghanistan. QuikClot is supplied in various forms, including sponges, bandages, granular packets, and nasal applicators. Each of these forms is applied directly to an external bleeding wound and combined with pressure to stop hemorrhage. The original product caused a significant temperature elevation in the surrounding tissue, but a reformulated product has been released that decreases the amount of heat released during application.

HemCon and ChitoFlex (Chitosan Dressings)

Chitosan is a mucoadhesive, biodegradable polysaccharide derived from shellfish. HemCon and ChitoFlex supply chitosan in ready-to-apply bandages. When exposed to blood, the bandages become extremely adherent and facilitate clotting. The molecule is also positively charged and may attract negatively charged erythrocytes, further enhancing clot formation. HemCon bandages are larger and supplied in various sizes to treat external wounds. ChitoFlex bandages are more flexible and compact, facilitating the treatment of penetrating trauma tracts. Both are latex free and have no known complications or contraindications. They can be left in place for up to 48 hours and should be removed with water or saline for definitive wound treatment.

Mechanical Methods

- *Cautery (electrosurgical or battery-operated unit):* For hemostasis, use the coagulation or fulguration settings and set at a very low power. Gently "tap" the area, being careful to avoid excessive tissue damage. Larger vessels (>3 mm) should be tied off rather than coagulated.
- *Laser (carbon dioxide):* Rarely used for this purpose.
- *Shaw scalpel* (a teflon-coated scalpel blade with a heating element).
- *Ice packs:* Cause vasoconstriction and reduce bleeding and swelling.
- *Pressure dressings* (see Chapter 32, Skin Biopsy, Fig. 32-8, for an example).

Common Errors

- Using agents capable of producing "tattooing" (Monsel's or silver nitrate) in a visible area on a light-skinned person. Choose an agent that does not have this risk.
- Overcauterizing an area of bleeding, leading to more tissue destruction than necessary. Use only the minimal amount of chemical, electric, or thermal cautery to stop the active bleeding.
- Using ferric subsulfate, aluminum chloride, or silver nitrate inside a wound that needs to be sutured closed.

Complications

- Rebound bleeding
- Infection
- Nerve damage
- Scarring or tattooing
- Swelling
- Excessive tissue damage

Postprocedure Patient Information

Instruct the patient on the following:

- Keep the area clean and moist, but avoid maceration. Any ointment, including those with antibiotics, aids healing.
- Change the dressing at least two to three times a day (preferably four) and wash gently with soap and water.
- Follow-up as directed; do so sooner if there is an increase in redness, swelling, pain, fever, night sweats or chills, or other signs of infection such as purulent drainage.
- Avoid cleansing with hydrogen peroxide because it kills fibroblasts.

Conclusion

Hemostatic agents are useful during cutaneous surgery or when faced with an open wound that cannot be primarily closed with sutures. Topical hemostatic agents are not a substitute for meticulous surgical technique, and many cannot be used inside a wound to be sutured. Physical measures such as direct pressure, cold application, or suture ligatures should also be considered when trying to control bleeding. The various agents have benefits and limitations. It is important to become familiar with several, such as Monsel's solution, aluminum chloride, absorbable gelatin sponge (Gelfoam), and oxidized cellulose (Surgicel).

Billing and Coding

Application of topical hemostatics is included in the wound care charge and should not be "unbundled." If a patient presents with a condition requiring topical hemostasis, the appropriate level of service should be billed. ICD-9-CM codes are indicated for the particular lesion or presenting concern being addressed.

Acknowledgment

The editors wish to recognize the many contributions by Jerry W. Hizon, MD, and Lee A. Kaplan, MD, to this chapter in the previous edition of this text.

Suppliers

(See contact information online at www.expertconsult.com.)

Nearly every medical supplier (such as Delasco) can provide the routine and common hemostatic agents. For the newer agents, consult the following:

HemCon Medical Technologies, Inc.
Z-Medica Corporation

BIBLIOGRAPHY

Gabay M: Absorbable hemostatic agents. Am J Health Syst Pharm 63: 1244–1253, 2006.

Guttman C: Pearls of wisdom: Dermatologist Susan H. Weinkle, M.D. Dermatol Surg 34:96, 2008.

Ho J, Hruza G: Hydrophilic polymers with potassium salt and microporous polysaccharides for use as hemostatic agents. Dermatol Surg 33: 1430–1433, 2007.

Kircik L: Comparative efficacy of topical hemostatic powder vs. foam sterile compressed sponge in second intention healing after Mohs micrographic surgery: Pilot study. Presented at the American College of Mohs Surgery Annual Meeting, Vancouver, British Columbia, Canada, May 3, 2008.

Kuwahara RT, Ammonette RA: A novel method to remove Monsel's stain. Dermatol Surg 26:507, 2000.

Mabry R, McManus JG: Prehospital advances in the management of severe penetrating trauma. Crit Care Med 36(Suppl):S258–S266, 2008.

Palm MD, Altman JS: Topical hemostatic agents: A review. Dermatol Surg 34:431–445, 2008.

Spitzer M, Chernys AE: Monsel's solution-induced artifact in the uterine cervix. Am J Obstet Gynecol 175:1204–1207, 1996.

Take 5: Surgical Pearls: QR powder to control bleeding. Practical Dermatology 5:64, 2008.

Wang DS, Chu LF, Olson SE, et al: Comparative evaluation of noninvasive compression adjuncts for hemostasis in percutaneous arterial, venous and arteriovenous dialysis access procedures. J Vasc Interv Radiol 19:72–79, 2008.

CHAPTER 41

Unna Paste Boot: Treatment of Venous Stasis Ulcers and Other Disorders

Paul W. Davis

Background

Venous stasis leg ulcers are the most common type of ulcers on the lower extremities. They most often occur on the medial aspect of the ankle and can be either partial or full thickness. Their shape is usually irregular and there is often associated edema, skin hyperpigmentation, induration, and thickening of the dermis and epidermis. Plaquelike lesions, called *lipodermatosclerosis*, are frequently observed. Erythema may be present, especially when the feet are dependent. This remarkable redness can frequently cause the clinician to suspect the presence of cellulitis. These ulcers are often painful and are accompanied by a significant amount of exudative drainage, again suggesting cellulitis.

Leg ulcers affect an estimated 500,000 to 1 million people in the United States. One percent of people in industrialized countries will suffer from a leg ulcer at some point in their lives and the vast majority of these are secondary to venous problems. Venous leg ulcers are the end result of chronic venous insufficiency (CVI), which leads to venous hypertension, inadequate venous blood return, and increased capillary pressure in the lower extremities. Chronic and recurrent venous obstruction, progressive valvular damage, and impairment of the calf muscle pump are the root causes of CVI.

A variety of hypotheses have been proposed to explain the pathophysiology of venous ulceration. One theory is that *sluggish venous flow leads to the adherence of leukocytes to the capillary walls*, resulting in obstruction of the local capillaries and the migration of additional leukocytes into the surrounding subcutaneous tissue. Proteolytic enzymes and toxic metabolites are released, increasing capillary permeability and destruction. Local ischemia, tissue necrosis, and ulceration are the final result. The *fibrin cuff theory* suggests that increasing venous hypertension causes fibrinogen molecules to leak out of the damaged capillary endothelial cells, polymerizing to fibrin and forming thick deposits around the remaining capillaries. Thus, "fibrin cuffs" form, posing a barrier to diffusion of oxygen and nutrients throughout the tissues of the lower extremities and leading to fibrosis, necrosis, and ulceration.

The *trap hypothesis* incorporates the theories described previously and further suggests the extravasation of erythrocytes from the capillary bed. These "trapped" red blood cells are broken down in the tissues and release hemoglobin, which is metabolized to hemosiderin. This hemosiderin is responsible for the brown hyperpigmentation, often referred to as *brawny edema*, characteristic of the advanced stages of CVI. The associated thin, glistening skin and induration of brawny edema result from the associated fibrin cuffs and fibrosis. Already prone to ischemia and tissue necrosis, the involved areas develop venous stasis dermatitis and attendant intense pruritus, resulting in scratching, skin breakdown, and ulceration.

Introduction

Surgical repair is not the standard or first-line treatment for venous stasis ulcers. The application of a firm compression garment to the involved lower leg has been used for thousands of years, and for more than 300 years, compression in one form or another has been the mainstay of treatment for venous stasis leg ulcers and CVI. As early as the 1600s, a rigid lace-up stocking was used, but it was not until the mid-1800s that elastic bandages were invented and used for treating this condition. Multiple forms of compression therapy are available today, including hosiery, bandages, boot systems, orthotics, pneumatic pumps, and various combinations of these.

The exact mode of action of compression is not fully understood, but the theory is that pressure applied to the calf muscle raises interstitial pressure, reduces venous insufficiency, lowers superficial venous hypertension, and facilitates venous return by supporting the calf muscle pump. Additional proposed benefits associated with compression therapy include the softening of lipodermatosclerosis, reduction of venous reflux, increase of arterial flow to the ulcer site, improvement in the microcirculation, increased oxygenation to the wound site, and stimulation of fibrinolysis. In short, continuous compression decreases venous congestion, lowering retained volume in the lower extremities and facilitating a favorable wound healing environment.

This chapter considers only one frequently used type of compression therapy, the Unna boot. It is important to understand that other compression systems are commercially available and effective for the treatment of venous stasis ulcers. Although the Unna boot is favored in the United States, the multilayered elastic compression bandage or wrap is more popular in the United Kingdom. Short stretch bandages are widely used throughout the remainder of Europe, as well as Australia. Which type of compression is the most effective remains unclear from a review of the most current evidence-based literature (see Bibliography). What is clear is that compression is more effective than no compression, high compression is more effective than low compression, and multilayered systems are more effective than single-layer systems.

The Unna paste boot is used primarily when a semi-immobilizing, soft-pressure or gradient-pressure dressing over a joint, extremity, or even the scalp is needed. It is commonly available in a 3- or 4-inch roll or bandage that is impregnated with a calamine–gelatin–zinc oxide compound (Fig. 41-1). Unna paste dressings are soothing and antipruritic and require less frequent dressing changes than

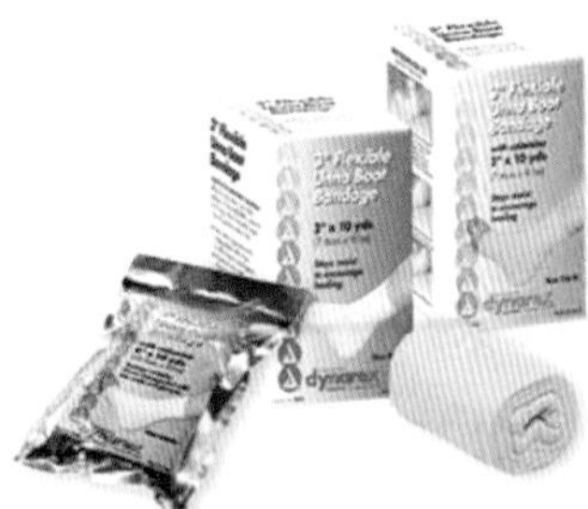

Figure 41-1 Examples of commercial Unna paste boot materials. (Courtesy of Dynarex Corporation, Orangeburg, NY.)

conventional dressings. When dressing changes can be scheduled from 3 to 11 days, instead of one to three times per day, savings in health care cost and patient convenience can be realized.

Indications

- Phlebitis and thrombophlebitis of the lower extremity
- Venous stasis ulcers
- Postphlebitic syndrome
- Lymphedema
- Split- and full-thickness skin graft sites
- Split- and full-thickness skin graft donor sites
- Acute and chronic tendonitis
- Acute ankle sprains without fracture

Use of the Unna paste dressing has varied over the years. With the advent of air cushion or foam splints, its use for ankle sprains has diminished. Unna paste dressings continue as a therapeutic mainstay for chronic venous disease with or without venous stasis ulcers. Without some type of dressing, healing-associated pruritus can lead to scratching and subsequent enlargement of the ulcers. The Unna boot can be used as a symmetric gradient-pressure dressing for venous stasis ulcers to help reduce venous hypertension, control edema, and counteract delayed venous return. As such, the Unna boot is a proven, effective part of overall therapy. Débridement should be carried out before application, if indicated, and then the ulcer should be covered with a permeable dressing, such as Tegaderm (pouched or regular).

Recent studies have advocated Unna paste dressings over split- or full-thickness skin grafting of burns on extremities. The advantages of using the Unna paste dressing compared with conventional dressing changes two to three times per day include earlier hospital discharge, patient comfort (because of fewer painful dressing changes), and higher graft acceptance rate (nearly 100% in some studies, probably because of less graft disturbance during critical microcirculation formation).

Unna paste dressings have been used over skin graft donor sites on the scalp. Use on scalp donor sites led to a significant reduction in a complication called *concrete scalp* (thick exudative crusting over the hair-bearing scalp, which tends to scar).

When pediatric patients excoriated their lower extremity skin grafts because of pruritus, the Unna paste dressings allowed healing and higher percentage skin graft acceptance. Parents spent less time changing the dressings (15 minutes vs. 3.5 hours per week), and the children had fewer play- and sleep-time disturbances compared with conventional three-times-per-day dressing changes and use of antihistamines.

When Unna paste dressings were used over skin-grafted, molten metal burns of the lower extremity, the benefits included early ambulation and earlier hospital discharge and return to work (44 vs. 84 days).

In acute and chronic tendonitis, the Unna boot acts as a soft immobilizer.

Contraindications

- Acute sprains with fractures
- Significant arterial insufficiency when used with compression covering
- Venous stasis ulcers that are infected and need débridement and cleaning (e.g., ulcers with heavy exudate and crusted ulcers with associated cellulitis)
- Active superficial phlebitis if infection is a major concern
- Sensitivity to any of the dressing components

Acute fractures can continue to swell. Because the gauze in the Unna paste dressing is nondistensible, pressure sores or compartment syndrome may occur if there is marked swelling after application.

Circulatory compromise and necrosis have been reported when a compression dressing is used in the presence of arterial insufficiency. Use a hand-held Doppler and blood pressure cuff to compare the ankle and brachial pressures. The ratio of the systolic pressure at the posterior tibial or dorsalis pedis artery divided by the brachial artery pressure should be equal to or greater than 1. If the ratio is 0.7 or less, significant arterial insufficiency is present and compression is contraindicated. If infection is a concern, use of a dressing that is not changed for 3 to 11 days may mask progressive infection and postpone appropriate treatment.

Technique

1. Cleanse the skin with slightly warm water or saline. If the skin is dry, petroleum jelly can be used as a moisturizer. Avoid topical antibiotics, povidone, and hexachlorophene, which can be topically sensitizing and cause a contact dermatitis. Topical steroids can be applied after washing if dermatitis is present.
2. For venous stasis ulcers, débride the ulcer. Hydrocolloid dressings such as DuoDerm can aid in healing. Some experts recommend extending the DuoDerm 1 inch past the edge of the ulcer. It is normal for these moist dressings to develop an anaerobic odor that does not necessarily indicate an infection. Alternatively, the ulcer can be covered with a permeable dressing like Tegaderm.
3. A smooth, snug layer of Kling or Kerlix can be used as an underwrap if desired. This may prevent chafing of the skin as the Unna paste dries.
4. For the lower extremity, keep the ankle at a right angle. Start wrapping at the metatarsal heads and roll proximally with a 50% overlap. It is important to avoid ridges, which can cause discomfort (Fig. 41-2).
5. Cover the heel completely. Alternate a horizontal wrap to cover the Achilles tendon with an oblique turn to cover the posterior aspect of the heel. Cut the dressing and start another wrap around the heel. Wrap snugly and cut the dressing frequently during the wrap. Avoid applying the edge of the dressing on the joint line, instead crossing the ankle with the full width of the

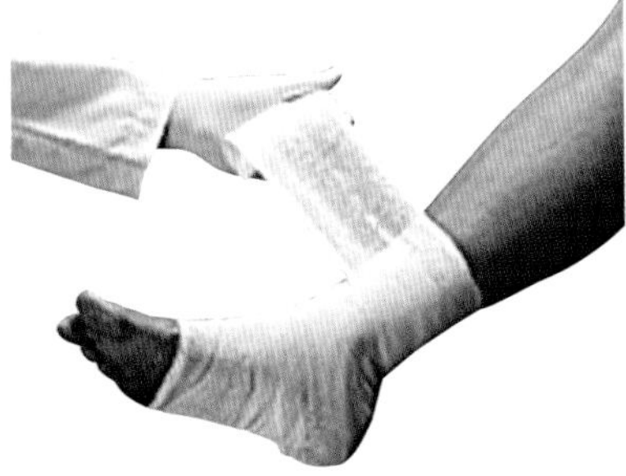

Figure 41-2 **Application of first layer of Unna paste boot with zinc oxide–impregnated gauze.** (Courtesy of Dynarex Corporation, Orangeburg, NY.)

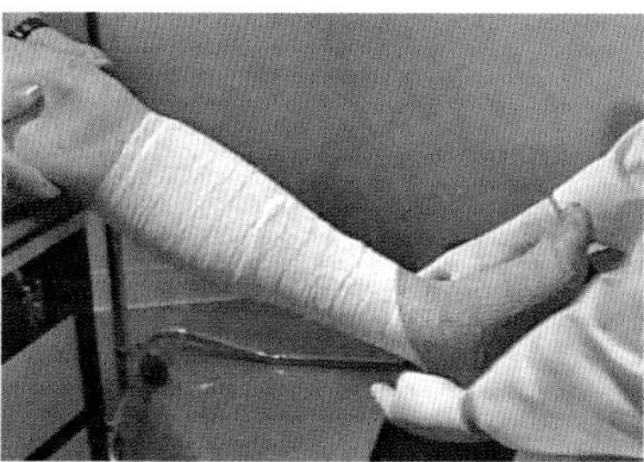

Figure 41-3 Application of second layer of Unna paste boot with Ace, Coban, Kling, or gauze wrap. (Courtesy of Dynarex Corporation, Orangeburg, NY.)

wrap. This helps prevent constriction bands and their tourniquet effect. *Do not reverse directions* as with plaster casting material; wrap only in one direction (clockwise or counterclockwise) to prevent ridges.

6. Wrap the Unna paste dressing in three layers and proceed all the way to the tibial tuberosity.
7. Several options for covering the Unna paste dressing include elastic bandage, Coban, Kling, or stockinette. Both the elastic bandage and Coban dressing help with needed compression (Fig. 41-3).
8. The final boot will consist of two or three distinct layers in addition to the specialized wound dressing if a venous leg ulcer is present (Fig. 41-4).
9. For wounds that are moist and draining, the dressing may need to be changed more frequently, as often as every 3 days. If moist discharge is minimal, the dressing can be changed about every 7 days and up to 11 days for patients on protracted therapeutic regimens. For patients with new applications of the Unna boot, it is wise to examine the patient and change the dressings more frequently to ensure that there are no complications.
10. The Unna "cap" for a skin graft donor site on the scalp is applied with an initial layer of Aquaphor gauze followed with an Unna paste dressing. Excellent results with no "concrete scalp" complications were achieved with dressing changes every 3 days in one small study.

Complications

- Occasional contact dermatitis
- Neurovascular compromise if dressing is applied too tightly or in the presence of arterial insufficiency
- Masking of cellulitis developing in a stasis ulcer under the dressing

Postprocedure Patient Education

- The dressing must be kept dry.
- Patients should cover the entire dressing with a plastic bag or other impermeable covering to bathe.
- Remove the boot with a pair of large bandage scissors. Lifting the bandage away from the skin and applying a thin film of petroleum jelly on the scissors can prevent discomfort or inadvertent injury during removal.
- Cleanse and dry the skin thoroughly. When the boot is used for stasis ulcers, inspect the area carefully for the presence of infection and débride again if necessary before applying a second boot. Venous stasis ulcers can take 2 to 3 months or more to heal.
- For best results, the patient must comply with all other aspects of medical therapy.
- As the swelling subsides in sprains, the compression advantage will be lost. Instruct the patient to return in 2 or 3 days or when the Unna paste dressing becomes loose or develops wrinkles because these can cause pressure sores. A second boot will need to be applied, or more appropriate therapy, such as an inflated splint, must be used.
- Teach the patient to check for signs of impaired circulation and to report any paresthesia, discoloration, or worsening discomfort promptly.

CPT/Billing Code

29580 Unna paste boot application

(When the code 29580 is used with the modifier -22, the procedure applies to the application of a multilayered, sustained, graduated high-compression bandage system, *not* to the standard three-layer Unna boot application.)

ICD-9-CM Diagnostic Codes

451.0 Phlebitis or thrombophlebitis, superficial vessels of lower extremities
451.1 Phlebitis or thrombophlebitis, of deep vessels of lower extremities
451.11 Phlebitis or thrombophlebitis, femoral vein (deep) (superficial)
451.19 Phlebitis or thrombophlebitis, other
Femoropopliteal vein, popliteal vein, tibial vein
451.2 Phlebitis or thrombophlebitis of lower extremities, unspecified
454.0 Varicose veins of the lower extremities with ulcer
454.1 Varicose veins of the lower extremities with inflammation (stasis dermatitis)
454.2 Varicose veins of the lower extremities with ulcer and inflammation
457.0 Noninfectious disorders of lymphatic channels
457.1 Lymphedema, acquired
459.1 Postphlebitic syndrome
459.11 Postphlebitic syndrome with ulcer
459.12 Postphlebitic syndrome with inflammation
459.13 Postphlebitic syndrome with ulcer and inflammation

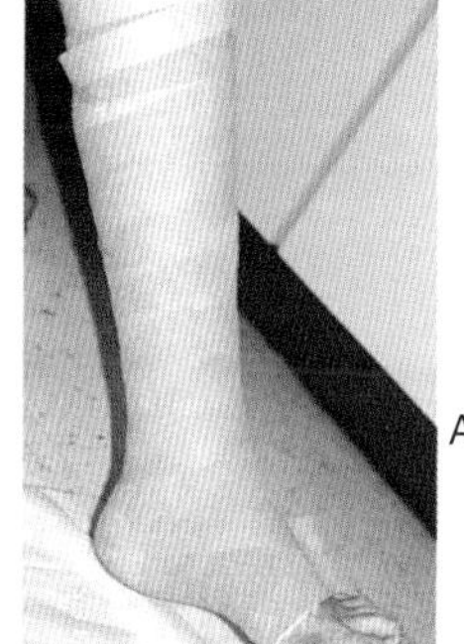

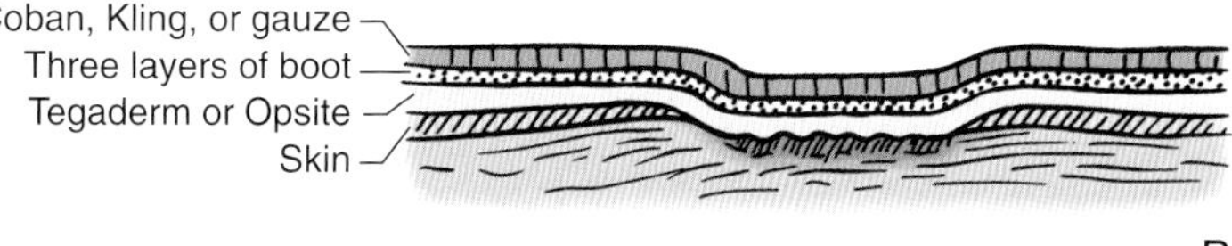

Figure 41-4 **A,** Unna paste boot, completed application. **B,** The layers of a completed boot application.

707.0	Decubitus ulcers
707.06	Decubitus ulcers, ankle
707.07	Decubitus ulcers, heel
707.09	Decubitus ulcers, other site
707.10	Ulcer of lower limb, unspecified
707.11	Ulcer of thigh
707.12	Decubitus ulcers, calf
707.13	Ulcer of ankle
707.14	Ulcer of heel and midfoot, or plantar surface of midfoot
782.3	Edema, legs
825.25	Metatarsal fractures

Some Medicare Carriers (MC) and Fiscal Intermediaries (FI) specify the diagnoses that support medical necessity for CPT 29580. One MC in Arkansas will cover Unna boots only for ulcers of the lower extremity (454.0, 454.2, 707.06, 707.07, 707.12, 707.13, and 707.14). Other MCs and FIs will accept a wider set of ICD-9-CM codes, so it is advisable to consult their written Articles and Local Coverage Decisions to ascertain what codes are covered in a specific locale.

SUPPLIERS

(See contact information online at www.expertconsult.com.)

Unna Paste Boot dressing is a trade name, and more than 25 companies make these dressings. Check with your local medical supply company or contact one of the following:

Aquaphor gauze
Beiersdorf

Dome-Paste medicated bandage (4-inch × 10-yard)
Miles, Inc. (Pharmaceutical Division)

Medicopaste bandage
Graham-Field, Inc.

Unna's Boot Elastic Paste Bandage
Surgical Supply Service

Unna-Flex bandage
ConvaTec (division of Bristol-Myers Squibb)

BIBLIOGRAPHY

Barone CM, Mastropieri CJ, Peebles R, Mitra A: Evaluation of the Unna boot for lower-extremity autograft burn wounds excoriated by pruritus in pediatric patients. J Burn Care Rehabil 14:348–349, 1993.

Carter YM, Summer GJ, Engrav LH, et al: Incidence of the concrete scalp deformity associated with deep scalp donor sites and management with the Unna cap. J Burn Care Rehabil 20:141–144, 1999.

Charles CA, Falabella AF, Fernandez-Obregon AC: Leg ulcer management. In Robinson JK, Hanke DW, Sengelmann RD, Siegel DM (eds): Surgery of the Skin: Procedural Dermatology. Philadelphia, Mosby, 2005, pp 743–766.

Collins L, Seraj S: Diagnosis and treatment of venous ulcers. Am Fam Physician 81:989–996.

Cullum N, Nelson EA, Fletcher AW, Sheldon TA: Compression for venous leg ulcers. Cochrane Database Syst Rev Issue 2, 2001.

Davis J, Gray M: Is the Unna's boot bandage as effective as a four-layer wrap for managing venous leg ulcers? J Wound Ostomy Continence Nurs 32:152–156, 2005.

Grube BJ, Heimbach DM, Engrav LH: Molten metal burns to the lower extremity. J Burn Care Rehabil 8:403–405, 1987.

O'Donoghue JM, O'Sullivan ST, Beausang ES, et al: Calcium alginate dressings promote healing of split skin graft donor sites. Acta Chir Plast 39:53–55, 1997.

Palfreyman SJ, Nelson EA, Lochiel R, Michaels JA: Dressings for healing venous leg ulcers. Cochrane Database Syst Rev Issue 3, 2006.

Phillips TJ: Current approaches to venous ulcers and compression. Dermatol Surg 27:611–621, 2001.

Sanford S, Gore D: Unna's boot dressings facilitate outpatient skin grafting of hands. J Burn Care Rehabil 17:323–326, 1996.

Schaum KD: Unna boots versus multilayered, sustained, graduated high compression bandage systems. Ostomy Wound Manage 51:28, 30, 2005.

Summer GJ, Hansen FL, Costa BA, et al: The Unna "cap" as a scalp donor site dressing. J Burn Care Rehabil 20:183–188, 1999; discussion 182.

Wells NJ, Boyle JC, Snelling CF, et al: Lower extremity burns and Unna paste: Can we decrease health care costs without compromising patient care? Can J Surg 38:533–536, 1995.

CHAPTER 42

WART (VERRUCA) TREATMENT*

Lori Oswald • John L. Pfenninger

Warts are a disease of antiquity. They have no regard for class or social status. They do not discriminate by race or color. There is an equal political distribution between Republicans and Democrats. They are annoying, sometimes disfiguring and painful, and to the angst of patient and physician, they frequently recur. With ardent attempts to rid the pest by heating, freezing, burning, cutting and electrifying, treatment has induced as much anxiety as the disease itself. But the physician persists.

William C. Everts, DO

Verrucae vulgaris (warts) are caused by the human papillomavirus (HPV). There are over 100 individual types and they are identified by numbers. *Common warts* are caused by types 1, 2, 4, 7, 27, 29, and 57; *flat (planar) warts*, by types 3, 10, 28, and 49; and *plantar warts*, by types 1, 2, and 4. Another series of HPV cause cervical dysplasia and condylomata. Most verruca vulgaris lesions form after a latent period of weeks to several months. The peak incidence occurs in late childhood and adolescence.

HPV causes numerous epithelial cancers. Cervical dysplasia and cervical cancer are the most commonly recognized types. However, 31% of squamous cell carcinomas and 36% of basal cell carcinomas of the skin contain HPV in nonimmunosuppressed patients. In immunosuppressed patients, 65% of squamous cell carcinomas and 60% of basal cell carcinomas contain HPV. As a result, treatment becomes more than just a cosmetic issue.

Warts have the following various presentations:

- Flat (planar)
- Filiform (small, fine, elongated lesions)
- Mosaic (a cluster of warts that fuse together)
- Verruca vulgaris, including periungual ("common wart")
- Plantar
- Genital/anal wart (condylomata acuminata)
- Laryngeal papillomatosis

DIFFERENTIAL DIAGNOSIS

- Actinic keratosis
- Seborrheic keratosis
- Nevus
- Molluscum contagiosum
- Callus
- Corn
- Nonspecific papule
- Cutaneous dysplasia

It can be difficult to differentiate the true nature of a plantar lesion. Hypertrophic callus buildup makes identification confusing. The tell-tale sign of a plantar wart is that, as the callus is pared away, the practitioner sees small, punctate sites of bleeding. This is nearly pathognomonic for HPV disease. Biopsies can be obtained when the diagnosis remains unclear.

*For the treatment of genital warts (condyloma), see Chapter 155, Treatment of Noncervical Condylomata Acuminata.

INDICATIONS FOR TREATMENT

- Pain
- Bleeding
- Recurrent trauma
- Lack of spontaneous resolution
- Psychosocial sequelae
- Employment repercussions (e.g., waitress)
- Rapid growth or multiplication
- Concerns regarding transmission
- Persistence as a possible cause of malignancy

A large number of verrucae do not resolve spontaneously. A longitudinal study concluded that only 40% of patients cleared their warts over a 2-year follow-up. HPV can remain dormant for long periods, then suddenly grow rapidly or multiply. With any treatment, the role of the immune system should not be underestimated. Induced inflammation from whatever treatment modality is used may finally trigger the immune system to recognize and then resolve the virus.

The virus itself is never totally eliminated. Rather, the immune system merely keeps it in remission, much like herpes. The virus can recur with any immunosuppressed state at any time during the patient's life. The goal of treatment is to eradicate active disease, not to eliminate the virus itself.

CONTRAINDICATIONS

- Lack of compliance
- Cellulitis
- Allergy to treatment modality
- Ambiguous diagnosis
- Bleomycin in the very young (relative)

TREATMENT

See Box 42-1 and Figure 42-1.

General

Transmission of HPV occurs by direct person-to-person contact or, possibly (and rarely), from fomites. The patient may also cause autoinoculation of verruca vulgaris by scratching, shaving, or traumatizing the skin. It is important to *enhance the immune system* as much as possible during the treatment of all wart manifestations. Smoking is known to increase the growth potential and the persistence of warts on the cervix. Smoking reduces the cells of Langerhans in the skin in general and subsequently decreases all immunity.

Box 42-1. Modalities for Treating Warts (Verruca Vulgaris)

General guidelines (maintaining healthy immune system)
- Eating a diet high in fruits and vegetables
- Taking vitamins with folic acid (may supplement folic acid up to 1 mg)
- Avoiding smoking and secondhand smoke
- Avoiding any immunosuppression when possible

Expectant observation

Hypnosis

Chemicals: topical
- Over-the-counter medication (usually an acid preparation)
- Topical salicylic acid 17%–40%
- Formalin
- Cantharidin (Cantharone) 0.7% collodion solution
- Trichloroacetic acid
- Bichloracetic acid
- Tretinoin (Retin-A 0.05% solution, or 0.025%, 0.05%, or 0.1% cream)
- 5-Fluorouracil (Efudex, Fluoroplex) 5% cream
- Imiquimod (Aldara)
- Podofilox (Condylox)
- Silver nitrate

Chemicals: oral
- Cimetidine (Tagamet) 20–40 mg/kg/day (especially in pediatric patients)
- Zinc sulfate 10 mg/kg to maximum of 600 mg/day (three divided doses, 2 mo maximum)

Chemicals: injection
- *Candida* antigen (Candin) 1:500 solution or generic 1:1000 solution
- Bleomycin (Blenoxane) 15-U vial
- Interferon

Mechanical
- Tape occlusion
- Cryotherapy
  - Liquid nitrogen (−196° C)
  - Nitrous oxide (−89° C)
  - Carbon dioxide (−78° C)
  - Tetrafluoroethane (−47° C/−70° C): MediFrig, Verruca Freeze
  - Dimethyl ether/propane (−29° C/−55° C): Histofreezer, Compound-W, Wartner, Dr. Scholl's

Electrodesiccation and curettage

Electrocautery (ball electrode)

Laser

Infrared coagulator (IRC)

Radiofrequency loop removal

Excision (discouraged)

Also see Chapter 155, Treatment of Noncervical Condylomata Acuminata.

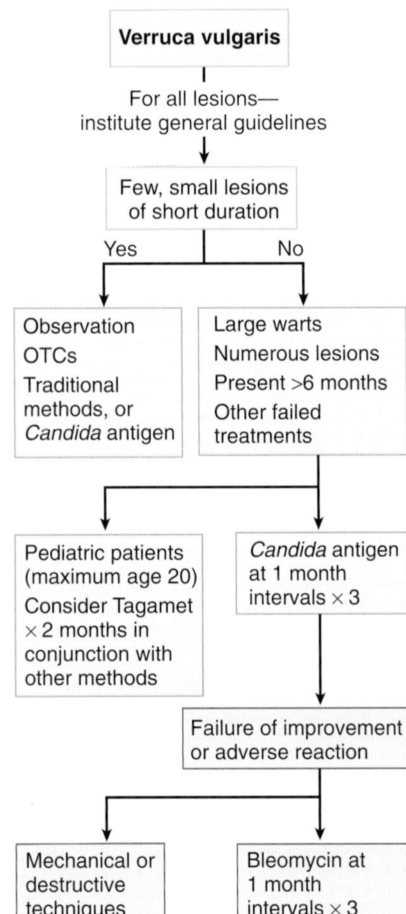

Figure 42-1 Selection of modalities for treating verrucae. At each visit, reinforce general guidelines. At times, especially with extensive lesions, bleomycin and *Candida* antigen can be injected at the same visit (use separate syringes). *Candida* and bleomycin may need to be used more than three times. As long as progress is being made, there is no need to change treatment. OTC, over the counter.

The patient must be advised to *stop smoking* (if applicable). *Illicit drugs* have been known to suppress the immune system and they, too, should be avoided. On the other hand, various *vitamins* (e.g., folic acid) have been shown to play a beneficial role in suppressing HPV. Subsequently, consider using a good multivitamin with minerals to maximize immune system capabilities. The patient should also be instructed to eat a *diet* that includes five helpings of fruits and vegetables a day to optimize immune function. Medications such as *steroids* that suppress immunity should be limited, if at all possible.

Treatment of verrucae in patients who are pregnant, have had organ transplants, are immunosuppressed as a result of diseases such as acquired immunodeficiency syndrome, or are taking immunosuppressants of any sort is difficult. Patients should be made aware that the success rate in such cases is poor.

Research into the efficacy of various treatments for warts is difficult. Some studies have shown that even hypnosis can resolve warts. Many folktales carry the belief that banana peels, raw potatoes, cerumen, spider webs, and other items resolve warts. Spontaneous resolution is always possible and often occurs for no apparent reason.

Many physicians recommend *expectant observation*. An old maxim states that "wart" patients should not be referred to a physician friend for treatment because it will generally make the physician look bad! Anyone who has treated warts can become frustrated in dealing with them. Not only can they persist, but they may indeed multiply. Frequently, treatment of a single wart with a modality such as cryotherapy or cautery will result in a ring of warts around the area that was frozen or burned. The simple common wart has indeed humbled the best clinicians. Subsequently, many again recommend simple observation.

Warts have no "roots" and are completely epidermal lesions. Treatment ideally should not cause scarring. There is no communication between warts—no "mother wart!" However, treatment of a single wart or some of the warts can lead to resolution of all the warts because of immune activation. Obtaining patient compliance for any regimen is often difficult, and home remedies frequently fail owing to lack of consistency in applying the treatment. It is not uncommon for a physician to have to treat a lesion(s) four or more times to resolve it.

Chemicals: Over-the-Counter Medications

Numerous over-the-counter (OTC) medications, usually mild acids in liquid form, are available for the treatment of warts. These include Compound-W, Mediplast, Trans-Ver-Sal, Occlusal, Duofilm, Premier, Salactic Film, Sal-Plant gel, Tinamed, Wart Off, and Duoplant. Forty percent salicylic acid treatments (Compound-W maximum-strength pads, Dr. Scholl's clear-away maximum-strength pads and invisible strips) may also be used and applied every 48 hours. (See also the discussion of "Tape Occlusion" in the section on "Mechanical Methods.")

Method: Pare away callus after soaking lesions in warm water. Hydrating the keratin allows better penetration of the liquid or agent being applied. Apply medication as directed by supplier and occlude the area. Repeat every other day, being sure to remove the dead tissue with paring or with a pumice stone. Treatment is nonscarring and generally effective but requires compulsive persistence with daily treatments, often for 4 to 6 weeks.

Chemicals: Physician Applied

Bichloracetic or Trichloroacetic Acid (50% to 85%)

These are potent chemicals and should not be provided for home treatment.

Method: Prepare the lesion as described for OTC medications. Apply the acid, being careful to avoid normal skin. If the lesion is raised and convoluted, work the acid into the lesion with a toothpick. Cover. Repeat weekly until the wart has resolved.

Cantharidin (Cantharone, Verr-Canth)

Cantharidin causes blistering at the dermoepidermal junction.

Method: Apply the chemical directly on the wart and cover it with tape for 48 hours. Evaluate the patient weekly and remove any residual blister, then reapply the cantharidin. Repeat until the wart has resolved.

Silver Nitrate

Method: Silver nitrate is available on the ends of sticks. Apply after paring as for OTC medications. Repeat weekly. Unfortunately, this method can leave a dark chemical "tattoo" that usually resolves but may last for months or years.

Prescription Creams

Tretinoin Cream (Retin A)

Method: Cream or solution at a concentration of 0.025%, 0.05%, or 0.1% is rubbed in thoroughly at bedtime. This is frequently used with diffuse flat warts on the legs or face, so it is rubbed over the entire area. The application may be repeated daily. The goal is to have a mild erythema with fine scaling. It is not uncommon to take months to resolve the warts. It can be used in combination with 5-fluorouracil or imiquimod.

5-Fluorouracil (Efudex, Fluoroplex)

5-Fluorouracil (5-FU) is a second-line treatment for truly resistant warts, and it has not been approved by the U.S. Food and Drug Administration (FDA) for this indication.

Method: A 2% solution or 5% cream is applied similarly to tretinoin cream. It is important to rub in thoroughly. 5-FU can also be used for condylomata (see Chapter 155, Treatment of Noncervical Condylomata Acuminata). 5-FU can cause significant inflammation in intertriginous areas and in areas with actinic skin change.

Imiquimod (Aldara)

Imiquimod is not a caustic agent but rather an immune enhancer. It is supplied in boxes of 12 or 24 packets. It is not approved by the FDA for verrucae (only for condylomata in those 12 years of age and older), but is frequently used as the sole treatment or as an adjunct in combination with other treatment therapies. It is essential to pare down the callus (especially on a plantar wart) and to rub in the imiquimod thoroughly. For verruca, it is applied *daily*, usually in the evening before sleep, and removed after 8 hours. It is not necessary to discard a packet if only a portion is used.

Podofilox (Condylox) Liquid

Refer to Chapter 155, Treatment of Noncervical Condylomata Acuminata.

Chemicals: Oral

Oral Cimetidine (Tagamet)

Method: Although controlled studies in children included small numbers, cimetidine appears to resolve verruca in some cases with dosages of 20 to 40 mg/kg/day for 2 months maximum. It can be used in addition to other caustic modalities to accentuate efforts. One study showed that adults with recalcitrant warts could be treated successfully with doses of 30 to 40 mg/kg (maximum dose of 3.5 g/day).

Oral Zinc

Zinc sulfate taken orally at 10 mg/kg/day to a maximum of 600 mg in three divided doses has been reported to result in complete resolution of resistant warts in 60.9% after 1 month and in 86.9% after 2 months. However, patients generally become nauseated and 20% experienced vomiting, which limits its overall acceptance.

Chemicals: Injected

Candida *Antigen*

EDITOR'S NOTE: After OTC topicals, this method is my absolute first choice to treat all but the simplest verrucae. I have not tried it on condylomata. It can be used on single large warts, on mosaics, or to treat patients with 80 to 100 lesions! I have used it for 18 years now, and results are excellent with few adverse reactions and no scarring. Multiple studies confirm its effectiveness.

Candida antigen is used for verruca vulgaris (nongenital HPV; Fig. 42-2). It has not been studied on condylomata acuminata. Although *Candida* antigen has been approved for over 40 years as the control

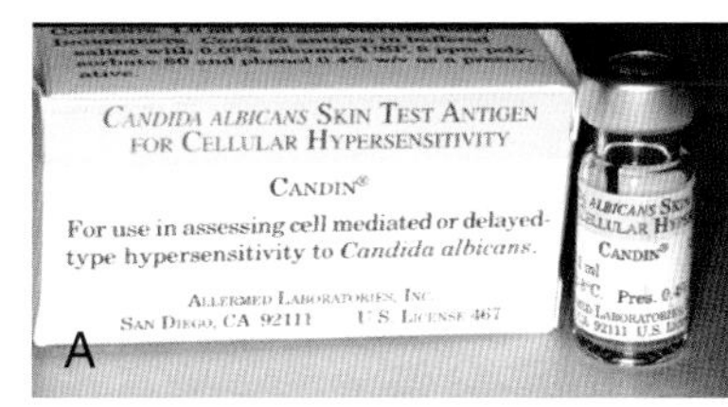

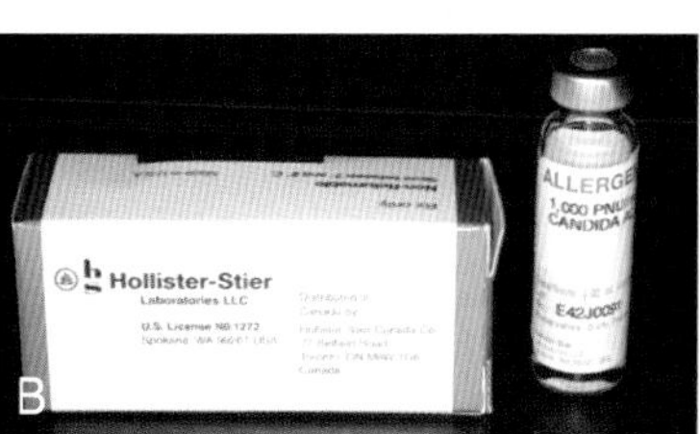

Figure 42-2 *Candida* antigen preparations: proprietary (**A**) and generic (**B**) (Hollister-Stier).

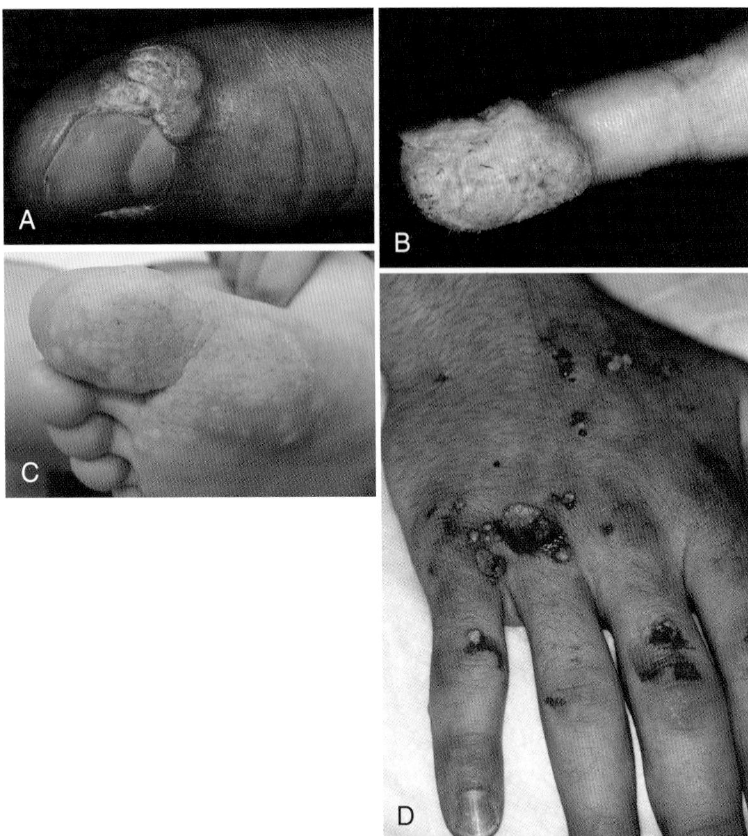

Figure 42-3 Examples of verrucae that are difficult to treat, but are well suited to *Candida* antigen injections: Periungual (**A**); large finger lesion (**B**); mosaic, toe and plantar aspect of metatarsal head (**C**); multiple lesions on the hand of a patient who had both hands affected (postinjection) (**D**).

for tuberculosis testing, it does not have FDA approval for treating verrucae. Its use is nevertheless covered by malpractice policies even when treating warts. *Candida* antigen can be especially helpful for large, extensive lesions, multiple lesions, and periungual lesions where other modalities would cause too much trauma (Fig. 42-3).

The concept is that nearly everyone has antibodies to *Candida*. When the antigens are injected into an area, there is an immediate immune response (redness, some swelling, occasionally mild pruritus). The increased immune activity in the area leads to recognition of the foreign material of the verruca, and an immune response ensues against that antigen as well. The body is then "sensitized" to the wart and eliminates all such lesions.

Pfenninger Protocol

- *Candida* antigen is available as Candin (1:500) and as a generic (1:1000). *Caution:* Some allergy desensitization extracts may be in concentrations as high as 1:50, which can cause excessive reactions.
- Mix 1:1 Candin and lidocaine 1% or 2% without epinephrine, or 1 part generic antigen with 4 parts lidocaine. (In spite of its lower concentration, the generic preparation appears to cause more reaction and thus needs greater dilution.)
- Topical anesthetic may be applied 15 minutes before injection.
- Inject 0.1 to 0.3 mL per wart (depending on size), using a 30-gauge needle and 1-mL Luer-Lok syringe. The Luer-Lok (screw-on) connection is important because it often takes considerable pressure to inject the solution into the wart/skin. This can cause a needle that is just pressed on to come off, spraying fluid everywhere.
- Try for an *intradermal* or *intralesional* injection to create an immune response. If the solution goes in easily, it is in too deep. Create a bleb if possible. Wear protective glasses because the material often "squirts" out through a verruca pore (Fig. 42-4).
- Limit the *total amount* to 1 mL at any one visit. If there are numerous warts, this may mean injecting only minute amounts into each one. Even if all the warts are not injected individually, the immune response may generalize and all warts may disappear.
- Repeat injection in 1 month if residual tissue remains.
- If the injections have not worked after three attempts 1 month apart, then they probably will not be successful. However, when warts are extensive, there are not many other options. As long as there is some progress, results have been obtained even after five or six monthly injection sessions.
- Expect 65% to 75% effectiveness with the first injection. Of the remainder, approximately 50% respond with each succeeding injection.
- Expect pruritus, drying of the lesion, and peeling of dead tissue. The lesion may turn black, regress spontaneously without any outward signs, or become erythematous (localized).
- *Adverse reactions* include rash (allergy), adenopathy, and persistence of the lesion, all very rare.

The *advantages* of the *Candida* antigen injection are that if the immune system can be activated to recognize the foreign tissue, all lesions will resolve. Allergic reactions are extremely rare. There is usually none of the scarring, hyperpigmentation, or hypopigmentation that can occur more commonly after some of the other modalities of treatment. There is no "downtime"; patients can exercise, play sports, go back to work, and do whatever they want immediately after treatment. There is minimal pain. The pain at the time of injection can be reduced through the use of the MadaJet to inject the solution (see Appendix H, Pearls of Practice). However, expensive solution is lost just to prime the "gun." The real advantage to using *Candida* antigen is that, unlike many of the other modalities, the immune system is induced into responding and resolving the lesion(s). Recurrences are rare, and efficacy is 80% to 85% after

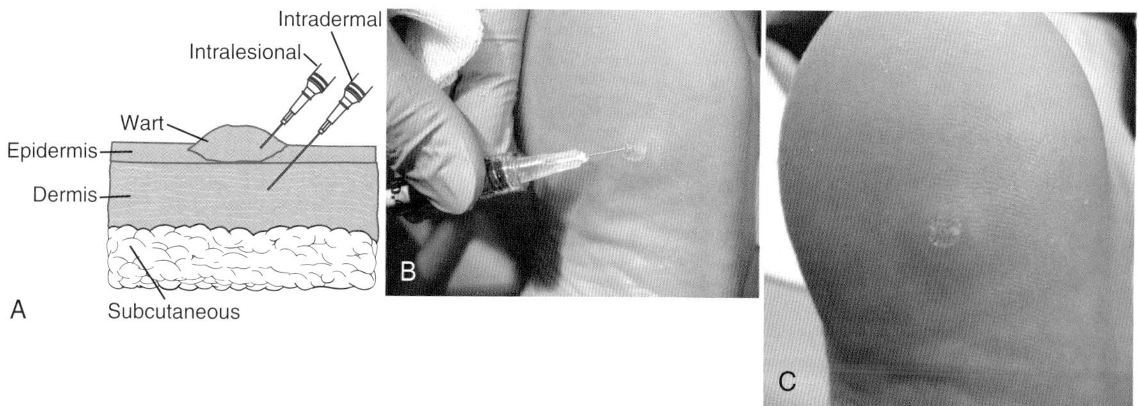

Figure 42-4 Injecting *Candida* antigen for the treatment of warts. **A,** Intralesional injection and intradermal injection. If injected into the subcutaneous tissue, the level is too deep. **B,** Injecting a heel lesion. **C,** Appearance postinjection.

three treatments at monthly intervals. It can be used in combination with almost all of the other treatment modalities to effect a synergy between the agents.

Proprietary *Candida* antigen is expensive, but a generic form is available. Practitioners often supply the antigen for the first visit, but write a prescription for the patient to bring the antigen in at subsequent visits. Outpatient hospital pharmacies usually carry it, but any pharmacy can order it. This markedly reduces costs for the clinician's office. Insurance companies generally do not reimburse the physician as there is no J code, but they will commonly pay for the patient's prescription. Note on the prescription, "Bring to the next office visit, for treatment of warts." Some insurance companies will not pay if it is being used for diagnostic purposes.

The most critical aspect of treatment is to inject the solution into the lesion itself or intradermally just below it. Do not go below the dermis. The injection should be difficult; if the solution goes in easily, the placement is too deep.

For a more complete review of the entire procedure, go to www.altoonafp.org/wartstudy.

Bleomycin

When all other methods fail, intralesional bleomycin can be considered. Pregnancy must be excluded before bleomycin injection is performed.

Method: A 15-U vial of bleomycin sulfate (Blenoxane; Bristol-Myers Squibb, Princeton, NJ) is diluted with 5 mL of bacteriostatic water or 0.9% sodium chloride to form a 3-U/mL solution. When stored at 4° C, the solution can be used for up to 4 months. Mix one part of this solution with five parts of 1% lidocaine without epinephrine (i.e., 0.1 mL of bleomycin with 0.5 mL of lidocaine). This provides 0.6 mL of solution with 0.5 U bleomycin/mL. Use a 30-gauge needle. Inject directly into the wart as follows:

Wart Size	Amount of Solution (0.5 U Bleomycin/mL)
Less than 5 mm	0.1 to 0.2 mL
5 to 10 mm	0.2 to 0.4 mL
Greater than 10 mm	Up to 1 mL
Multiple warts	Up to 3 mL (1.5 U)/visit

Warts will initially appear hemorrhagic, then clear (48% to 92%; Fig. 42-5). Repeat injection can be performed in 2 to 4 weeks. Three to four treatments may also be required for resistant lesions. Alternatively, the drug can be "dropped" onto the wart and "pricked" into the lesion using a Monolet needle. If tolerated well, the concentration of bleomycin can be gradually increased to 1 : 3 (bleomycin 0.5 U/mL to lidocaine).

Bleomycin is expensive. One vial will treat many patients. Patients can be given a prescription, which allows them to bring the drug to the office and saves office expense. It is also quite painful. The main mode of action of bleomycin is the inhibition of DNA synthesis, with some evidence of RNA inhibition. When injected locally it causes vascular microthrombosis; therefore, the patient may develop a hemorrhagic blister and may want it drained if the blister becomes uncomfortable. There have been very rare reports of Raynaud's phenomenon occurring after intralesional injection of bleomycin.

EDITOR'S NOTE: We have used bleomycin extensively for 10 years, treating five or six patients per week in a referral clinic. We have never seen Raynaud's phenomenon as a complication when using bleomycin as described.

Interferon

Alfa interferon is approved by the FDA for treatment of condylomata in patients older than 18 years of age. Two preparations are available:

- Alferon N injection (interferon alfa-n3): 1-mL vial, 0.05 mL/wart injected two to three times per week for up to 8 weeks
- Intron-A (interferon alfa-2b): 10 million IU/vial, 0.1 mL (reconstituted) per wart three times per week for 3 weeks

Some practitioners use interferon for verrucae as well. It is expensive and can often be followed by flulike symptoms for 24 hours. Subsequently, its use is quite limited. For more details on interferon use, see Chapter 155, Treatment of Noncervical Condylomata Acuminata.

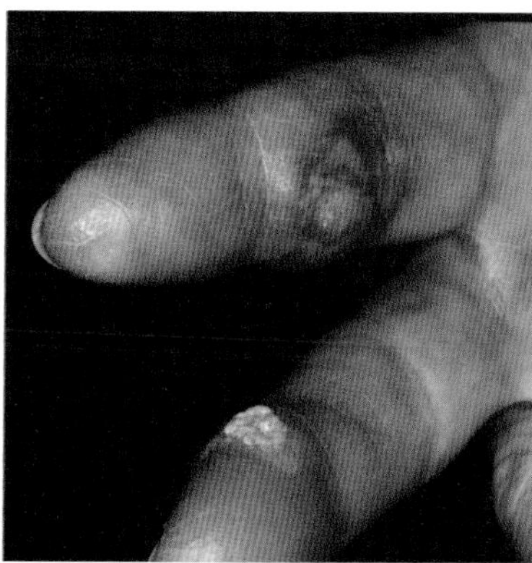

Figure 42-5 Bleomycin response 3 days after injection.

MECHANICAL METHODS

Tape Occlusion (Patient Applied)

For young children or for those who are afraid of needles, tape occlusion can be tried. However, in contrast to initial reports, recent studies have shown treatment with tape to be only 16% to 21% effective. The wart is simply covered with tape (usually duct tape) for a week. Tape is removed for 12 hours and then reapplied. The patient is seen 1 week later and macerated tissue is removed. The cycle is repeated until the wart(s) resolves, usually in 4 to 6 weeks. Obviously, this method is useful only if there are a limited number of lesions and if there is patient compliance. One of the major difficulties is keeping the tape in place.

Cryotherapy (Over-the-Counter and Physician Applied)

Cryotherapy is a destructive treatment of the skin because the cold by itself does not kill HPV. The real advantage to cryotherapy is that there is little disability and usually no scarring. The patient may initially experience localized erythema and edema, followed by blister formation. Some persistent hypopigmentation may occur. Cryotherapy with liquid nitrogen is usually performed using a thermos bottle spray unit or cotton-tipped applicators (Fig. 42-6). OTC "freeze treatments" are also available. They contain dimethyl ether and propane, but they are not as effective because they do not reach as cold a temperature as liquid nitrogen (−196° C). Examples of these products are Compound W-Freeze Off, Wartner-Freezing Wart Remover, and Dr. Scholl's Freeze Away (also makes a combination kit with salicylic acid). See Chapter 14, Cryosurgery, for further details.

Electrodesiccation and Curettage or Electrocautery

Warts can be treated readily with electrocautery. Small ones can be touched with the battery-powered "hot wires" and wiped away. Similarly, electrical units can be placed on fulguration or coagulation settings and the warts coagulated with the ball tips. It helps to have them moistened first. Smaller lesions can be grasped with metal pickups and the current transferred to the wart by touching the cautery tip to the forceps.

All lesions need to be anesthetized. Keratin (such as in plantar warts) must be pared away because it has little moisture and does not coagulate readily. That is why many practitioners curette the wart first and then coagulate the base. Bleeding from the curettage is controlled with digital pressure.

The major complication from electrodestruction is scarring, which occurs to some degree in all areas treated this way except for the very small superficial lesions. The provider must be especially careful on the plantar surface of the feet not to create a hypertrophic scar. This can become a persistently painful area analogous to walking on a stone in a shoe.

The greatest advantage of using curettage before electrocautery is that the abnormal tissue will usually separate from normal skin, defining what is abnormal from the normal tissue. A sharp disposable curette is needed; reusable curettes are often too dull. Unfortunately, the disposable curettes frequently bend. The Curetteblade (see Chapter 32, Skin Biopsy) is sharp and strong, so it does not bend. Cautery is then applied, and repeat light curettage is performed. This limits excessive removal of normal tissue and scarring. Alternatively, large warts can be shaved off to debulk them before cautery, but this will leave a significant amount of wart tissue behind and make cautery more difficult.

Primary excision using radiofrequency loop removal (see Chapter 30, Radiofrequency Surgery [Modern Electrosurgery]) is to be discouraged because the loop cuts so rapidly that it is easy to over-excise the lesion and leave a large pit and subsequent scarring. Tendons, nerves, and periosteal tissue can be injured inadvertently even by the experienced practitioner. It is critical to be familiar with the relevant anatomy when using any of the electrocautery techniques.

Of all methods, the electrocautery technique is one of the most effective. However, it has the disadvantages of prolonged healing with an open sore, scarring, and pain.

Laser Method

The laser method is expensive but offers the advantage of precise control of depth and removal of "just the right amount" of tissue. When properly used, results are excellent and scarring is minimal. Combining pulsed-dye laser with the application of salicylic acid has been shown to decrease the number of laser treatments needed.

Infrared Coagulation (Redfield)

One of the more recent treatments for warts—another method of destruction—is the use of the infrared coagulator. It is quick and effective. Much of the research has been done on condylomata. The probe is placed on the wart for 0.75 to 1 second, and the trigger is pulled. Local anesthesia is necessary. Blistering followed by sloughing and then superficial ulceration can be expected. Scarring is possible. See Chapter 106, Office Treatment of Hemorrhoids, for discussion on the use of the infrared coagulator.

Excision

Many pedunculated and filiform warts can be grasped with pickups and quickly excised with sharp tissue scissors, a curette, or a blade (shave excision). Consider using *Candida* antigen with lidocaine mixed per the Pfenninger protocol as the local anesthetic before excision to promote resolution of the wart. This is treating the wart with two different modes. After removal, cauterize the base lightly, not only to control the bleeding but to destroy any residual wart tissue. It is only in the extremely rare case of an isolated wart or two that has resisted everything that full-thickness skin excision with suture placement is necessary. This is especially discouraged on the

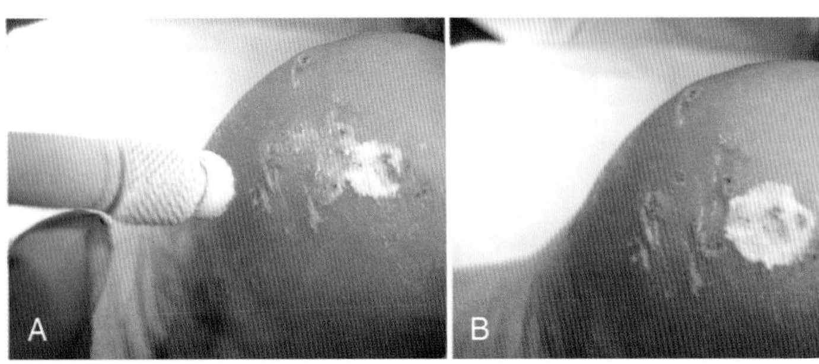

Figure 42-6 Treating a plantar wart with liquid nitrogen. **A,** Freezing the wart. **B,** Appearance after cryotherapy.

TABLE 42-1 Treatments of Choice Listed in Order of Preference

	Primary	Secondary
Filiform wart	STS excision	Electrocautery, cryotherapy, curettement
Flat warts (planar)	*Candida* antigen	Tretinoin, 5-FU, cryotherapy
Verruca		
Single or few, small	Cryocautery/*Candida* antigen	Electrocautery
Multiple	*Candida* antigen	Cryocautery
Mosaic	*Candida* antigen	Cryocautery
Plantar	*Candida* antigen	Cryocautery
Periungual	*Candida* antigen	Cryocautery
Resistant to *Candida* × 3	Bleomycin injection (off-label)	Cryocautery, electrocautery, IRC
Condylomata*	85% TCA	Radiofrequency loop excision, IRC, cryotherapy, imiquimod
Urethral meatus*	5-FU	STS excision; electrocautery
Vaginal*		
Few	85% TCA	Electrocautery, nitrous oxide cyrotherapy
Multiple	Imiquimod, 5-FU (both off-label)	Laser
Anal, vulvar*	85% TCA	Imiquimod, radiofrequency excision, cryocautery, IRC
Rectal*	85% TCA	Cryocautery, electrocautery, imiquimod, radiofrequency excision
Laryngeal papillomatosis	Laser	Mumps or *candida* antigen (injection; off-label)

*Also see Chapter 155, Treatment of Noncervical Condylomata Acuminata.
5-FU, 5-Fluorouracil; IRC, infrared coagulator; STS, sharp tissue scissor; TCA, trichloroacetic acid.

plantar surface of the feet because painful scarring can be a significant complication.

Table 42-1 shows the optimal methods of treating various wart presentations. OTC medications are often tried first. Treatments also can be combined to improve outcomes.

Combination Therapy for Resistant Warts

- *Candida* antigen solution for treatment and anesthesia followed by cryotherapy.
- Imiquimod (Aldara) cream or 5-FU cream can be used in addition to most therapies (especially *Candida* antigen injection). If mechanical methods are used, it will be necessary to allow some healing before applying the cream. The creams may be used immediately after paring away the hyperkeratotic tissue on plantar warts, however, and will be more efficacious if the callus is removed.
- Oral cimetidine (Tagamet) can be added to any regimen.
- For extensive lesions (e.g., entire planter surfaces) *Candida* antigen injections can be used for some lesions along with bleomycin for other lesions.
- Always reinforce a good diet and folic acid supplements with any treatment. Zinc can also be considered alone or in addition to any treatment modality, but is poorly tolerated.

Further Treatment Options

Because of the quest for the most efficacious treatment, multiple other treatments have been tried, including the following. Only limited studies have been done to determine their effectiveness:

- Zinc sulfate orally at 10 mg/kg daily, up to 600 mg/day in three divided doses (61% with complete clearing)
- Garlic extracts topically
- Cidofovir (compounded with Vanicream base to make 1–3% formulation)

Complications

- Allergic reactions
- Infection
- Blistering
- Scarring
- Persistence of lesion
- Pain
- Bleeding
- Traumatic seeding and increase in number of warts

CPT/Billing Codes

Intralesional injection
11900 Up to and including 7
11901 Over 7

For injections there is also generally a charge for the medication used, but there is no J code for *Candida* antigen. The provider is advised to provide a prescription to be taken to the pharmacy by the patient (see text).

The J code for bleomycin is J 9040. However, it may be advisable to give the patient a prescription to be filled, as is done with *Candida*.

Destruction (electrocautery, cryotherapy, laser, chemicals, and curettement)
17110 Benign lesions (e.g., flat warts) destruction, any method, up to 14
17111 15 or more

ICD-9-CM Diagnostic Codes

07810 Verruca vulgaris (all presentations)
07811 Condyloma acuminata

Patient Education Guides

See patient education and patient consent forms available online at www.expertconsult.com.

Suppliers

(See contact information online at www.expertconsult.com.)

***Candida* antigen (Candin)**
Allermed Laboratories
***Candida* antigen (generic)**
Antigen Laboratories, Inc.
Hollister-Stier Labs
MadaJet
MADA Medical Products

For cryotherapy, radiofrequency, and electrocautery units, see the appropriate chapters mentioned throughout this chapter. For the infrared coagulator, see Chapter 106, Office Treatment of Hemorrhoids.

ONLINE RESOURCE

http://www.cochrane.org/reviews/em/aboo1781.html.

BIBLIOGRAPHY

Al-Gurairi FT, Al-Waiz M, Sharquie KE: Oral zinc sulphate in the treatment of recalcitrant viral warts: Randomized placebo-controlled clinical trial. Br J Dermatol 146:423–431, 2002.

Amer M, Diab N, Ramadan A, et al: Therapeutic evaluation for intralesional injection of bleomycin sulfate in 143 resistant warts. J Am Acad Dermatol 18:1313–1316, 1988.

Brodell R, Marchese Johnson S: Warts, Diagnosis and Management: An Evidence-Based Approach. London, Martin Dunitz, Taylor and Francis Group, 2003.

Burkhart CG, Pchalek I, Adler M, et al: An in vitro study comparing temperatures of over-the-counter wart preparations with liquid nitrogen. J Am Acad Dermatol 57:1019–1020, 2007.

Cha S, Johnson L, Natkunam Y, Brown J: Treatment of verruca vulgaris with topical cidofovir in an immunocompromised patient: A case report and review of the literature. Transplant Infect Dis 7:158–161, 2005.

Cordro AA, Guglielmi HA, Woscoff A: The common wart: Intralesional treatment with bleomycin sulfate. Cutis 26:319–322, 1980.

Davis M, Gostout B, McGovern R, et al: Large plantar wart caused by human papillomavirus-66 and resolution by topical cidofovir therapy. J Am Acad Dermatol 43:340–343, 2000.

Epstein E: Immunotherapy of warts with masoprocol cream. Cutis 59: 287–289, 1997.

Eriksen K: Treatment of the common wart by induced allergic inflammation. Dermatologica 160:161–166, 1980.

Fleischer AB Jr, Feldman SR, McConnell RC: The most common dermatologic problems identified by family physicians, 1990–1994. Fam Med 29:648–652, 1997.

Focht D III, Spicer C, Fairchok M: The efficacy of duct tape vs. cryotherapy in the treatment of verruca vulgaris (the common wart). Arch Pediatr Adolesc Med 156:971–974, 2002.

Gibbs S, Harvey I: Topical treatments for cutaneous warts. Cochrane Database Syst Rev 2006, Issue 2, CD001781.

Glass A, Solomon B: Cimetidine therapy for recalcitrant warts in adults. Arch Dermatol 132:680–682, 1996.

Habif TP: Warts, herpes simplex and other viral infections. In Habif TF (ed): Clinical Dermatology, 4th ed. St. Louis, Mosby, 2004, pp 381–388.

Haen M, Spigt M, Caro JT, et al: Efficacy of duct tape vs. placebo in the treatment of verruca vulgaris (warts) in primary school children. Arch Pediatr Adolesc Med 160:1126–1129, 2006.

Haller KH: *Candida* antigen injection proves effective treatment for warts. Am Fam Physician 61:478, 2000.

Johnson SM, Roberson PK, Horn TD: Intralesional injection of mumps or *Candida* skin test antigens: A novel immunotherapy for warts. Arch Dermatol 137:451–455, 2001.

Lipke M: An armamentarium of wart treatments. Clin Med Res 4:273–293, 2006.

AUTHOR'S NOTE: Extremely valuable and comprehensive review. Highly recommended reading.

Marchese-Johnson S, Kincannon JM, Horn TD: A novel treatment for warts: Immunotherapy using mumps and *Candida* antigen. Presented at the Scientific Poster Discussion Session, 58th Annual Meeting of the American Academy of Dermatology, San Francisco, March 13, 2000.

Marchese-Johnson S, Roberson PK, Horn TD: Intralesional injection of mumps or *Candida* skin test antigens: A novel immunotherapy for warts. Arch Dermatol 137:451–455, 2001.

Miller OM, Brodell RT: Human papillomavirus infection: Treatment options for warts. Am Fam Physician 53:135–143, 1996.

Munn SE, Higgins E, Marshall M, Clement M: A new method of intralesional bleomycin therapy in the treatment of recalcitrant warts. Br J Dermatol 135:969–971, 1996.

Muzio G, Massone C, Rebora A: Treatment of non-genital warts with topical imiquimod 5% cream. Eur J Dermatol 12:347–349, 2002.

Naylor MF, Neldner KH, Yarbrough GK, et al: Contact immunotherapy of resistant warts. J Am Acad Dermatol 19:679–683, 1988.

Phillips RC, Ruhl TS, Pfenninger JL, Garber MR: Treatment of warts with *Candida* antigen injection. Arch Dermatol 136:1274–1275, 2000.

Price N: Bleomycin treatment for verrucae. Skinmed 6:166–171, 2007.

Shamanin V, zur Hausen H, Lavergne D, et al: Human papillomavirus infections in nonmelanoma skin cancers from renal transplant recipients and nonimmunosuppressed patients. J Natl Cancer Inst 88:802–811, 1996.

Signore R, Gillis K: *Candida albicans* intralesional injection immunotherapy of warts: A novel therapeutic approach. Presented at the Scientific Poster Discussion Session, 58th Annual Meeting of the American Academy of Dermatology, San Francisco, March 13, 2000.

Sollitto RJ, Pizzano DM: Bleomycin sulfate in the treatment of mosaic plantar verrucae: A follow-up study. J Foot Ankle Surg 35:169–172, 1996.

Sontheimer D, Brown M: Are oral agents effective for the treatment of verruca vulgaris? J Fam Pract 55:353–354, 2006.

Stulberg D, Hutchison A: Molluscum contagiosum and warts. Am Fam Physician 67:1233–1240, 2003.

Thomas K, Koegh-Brown M, Chalmers J, et al: Effectiveness and cost-effectiveness of salicylic acid and cryotherapy for cutaneous warts: An economic decision model. Health Technol Assess 10:iii, ix–87, 2006.

Tosti A, Piraccini BM: The nail unit: Surgical and non-surgical approaches. Dermatol Surg 27:235–239, 2001.

Trozak D, Tennenhouse D, Russell J: Dermatology Skills for Primary Care: An Illustrated Guide. Totowa, NJ, Humana Press, 2006.

Tuggy M, Garcia J: Procedures Consult. Available at www.proceduresconsult.com.

Usatine RP, Moy RL, Tobinick EL, Siegel DM (eds): Skin Surgery: A Practical Guide. St. Louis, Mosby, 1998.

Vanhooteghem O, Richert B, de la Brassinne M: Raynaud phenomenon after treatment of verruca vulgaris of the sole with intralesional injection of bleomycin. Pediatr Dermatol 18:249–251, 2001.

Wenner R, Askari S, Cham P, et al: Duct tape for the treatment of common warts in adults. Arch Dermatol 143:309–313, 2007.

CHAPTER 43

Wood's Light Examination

Roberta E. Gebhard

The Wood's lamp ("black light") produces ultraviolet rays with a wavelength of 365 nm and above by projecting a beam of light through a filter of glass containing nickel oxide. Invisible light in the long-wave ultraviolet range and visible blue-white light are created. The fluorescence produced as the light hits objects varies in color depending on qualities of the surface itself. Characteristic appearances have been described for several dermatologic conditions. The Wood's light examination provides a quick, inexpensive, and useful adjunct in their diagnosis (Fig. 43-1).

Diagnostic uses for the examination include the following:

- Tinea capitis
- Erythrasma
- Vitiligo, albinism, tuberous sclerosis, and other pigmentary conditions
- *Pseudomonas* infections
- Porphyria cutanea tarda
- Tinea versicolor
- Detection of some chemicals that are applied to the skin or taken systemically
- Adjunct in finding corneal abrasions or herpetic corneal lesion
- Identification of ejaculate in rape/sexual assault

Indications

- Any dermatitis in body folds such as the inguinal, perianal, interdigital, axillary, or inframammary areas (e.g., erythrasma, *Pseudomonas* infections)
- Patches of scalp scaling and partial hair loss, especially when the hairs are broken or shorter than normal (tinea capitis)
- Pigmentary conditions
- Blisters or punctate erosions on the exposed portions of the hands and forearms, with follow-up urine examination (porphyria cutanea tarda)
- Patches of scaling and altered pigmentation of the skin (tinea versicolor)

Technique

Let the light warm for a few minutes. From a distance of approximately 8 inches, focus the Wood's light on the area of interest. Darken the room to improve visualization of the resultant fluorescence. Observe and record findings carefully. It is crucial to observe the specific color of fluorescence, not simply its presence. Soaps, lotions, cosmetics, urine, other chemicals, and fragments of scaling skin may themselves yield fluorescence. In addition, *patients should not bathe 24 hours before the examination*. Otherwise the examination may show little or no fluorescence.

Common Findings

- *Tinea capitis*: The majority of cases in the United States are caused by *Trichophyton tonsurans*, which does *not* fluoresce. *Trichophyton verrucosum* does not fluoresce either. Hair (but not the skin of the scalp) may fluoresce yellow-green if infected with *Microsporum canis* or *Microsporum audouinii*, or a pale white-green in the rare event of *Trichophyton schoenleinii* infection. In these cases, sensitivity may be relatively low. Sensitivity of approximately 50% has been reported for M. *canis* (Kefalidou and colleagues, 1997). Fluorescence of affected hair should be sought, particularly in the follicular portion of the hair. Potentially infected, broken-off hair may be plucked and the subepidermal portion then viewed under the Wood's lamp (Fig. 43-2).
- *Tinea corpora*: Fungal infections of the skin do not fluoresce, except for tinea versicolor (usually a golden yellow).
- *Erythrasma*: This produces a brilliant coral-red fluorescence. Erythrasma, frequently confused with tinea, is not fungal in origin but is caused by *Corynebacterium minutissimum*. Treatment is with erythromycin (Fig. 43-3).
- Pseudomonas *infection*: This fluoresces aqua-green or white-green. Wood's light examination can be used to screen burned patients because infection fluoresces before it becomes clinically apparent. *Pseudomonas* can also be found in ear discharge, intertrigo pedis, and secondary pseudomonal infection of the scrotum.
- *Vitiligo*: Wood's light accentuates hypopigmented areas and is particularly useful for examining patients with fair complexions.
- *Tuberous sclerosis*: Wood's light is helpful in highlighting characteristic hypopigmented skin lesions exhibiting the shape of a mountain ash leaf.
- *Tinea versicolor*: This produces a pale yellow-gold fluorescence. In this case, Wood's light helps to differentiate skin lesions such as vitiligo.
- *Porphyria cutanea tarda*: Urine fluoresces a bright pink-orange. This may be accentuated by acidifying the urine, adding an equal volume of 1.5 N HCl (Fig. 43-4).
- *Tetracycline*: In patients taking tetracycline systemically, some inflammatory lesions (including acne papules) may exhibit a yellow fluorescence under the Wood's lamp. This fluorescence may also be observed in dried or concentrated urine containing the drug.
- *Fluorescein*: The dye is used topically by moistening a small strip of impregnated paper (available commercially) and allowing a drop to fall in the conjunctival sac. Any areas of denudation (e.g., trauma, herpes) on the cornea then fluoresce when viewed through the Wood's lamp (Fig. 43-5).
- *Miscellaneous*: Many cosmetics, topical medications, industrial chemicals, and even urine may be detected on the skin by their fluorescence. For this reason, the Wood's lamp is most useful for identifying areas for collection of samples for further forensic study in cases of suspected sexual abuse, rather than as proof of assault.

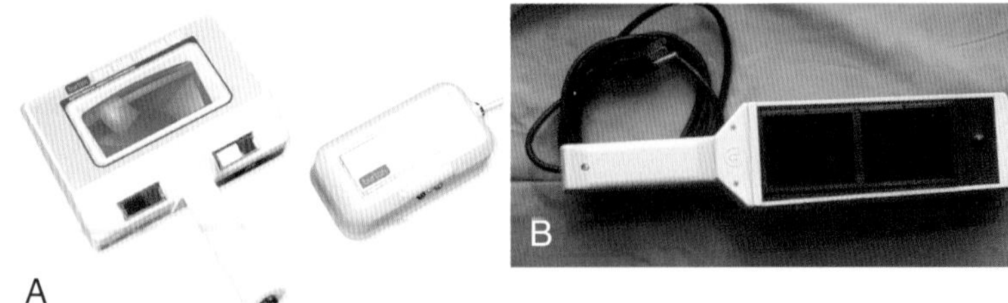

Figure 43-1 **A** and **B,** Examples of Wood's lamps (ultraviolet light). (**B,** Courtesy of Dennis Babel, PhD.)

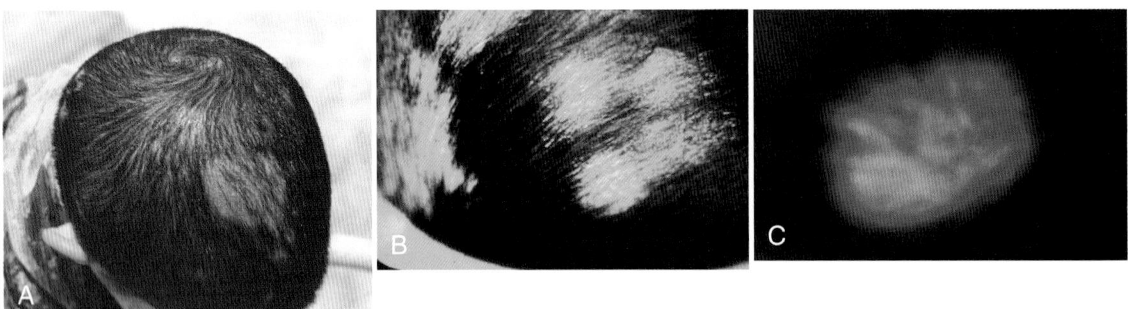

Figure 43-2 **A,** Clinical picture of nonfluorescent (black dot) tinea capitis. This is the most common presentation seen in North America. **B** and **C,** Wood's light–positive (fluorescent) tinea capitis. This fluorescence is caused by the fungal metabolite pteridine. (Courtesy of Dennis Babel, PhD.)

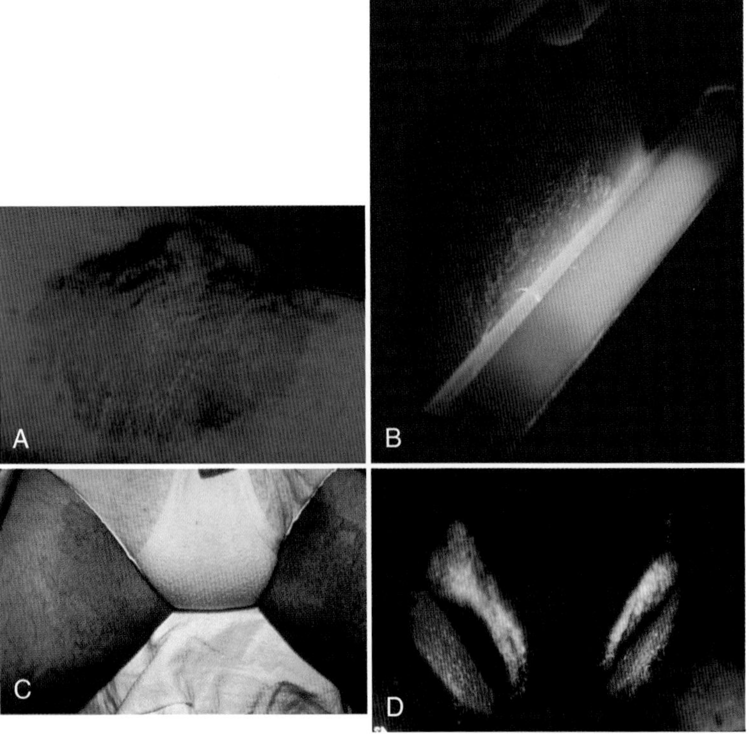

Figure 43-3 **A** and **B,** Erythrasma under Wood's light. **C,** Crural erythrasma caused by the bacterium *Corynebacterium minutissimum*. **D,** Wood's light–positive crural erythrasma. (**A,** From McPhee SJ, Papadakis MA, Tierney LM: Current Medical Diagnosis and Treatment 2008. New York, McGraw-Hill, 2008. **B,** Courtesy of Richard P. Usatine, MD, Florida State University, Tallahassee, Fla. **C** and **D,** Courtesy of Dennis Babel, PhD.)

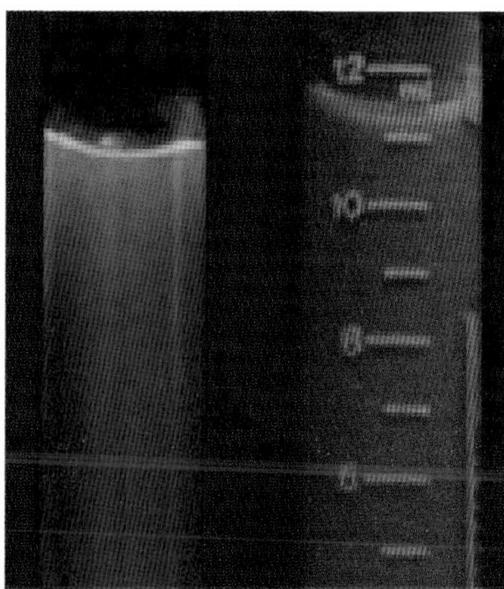

Figure 43-4 Urine fluoresces a bright pink-orange in porphyria cutanea tarda under Wood's light. (From Wolff K, Johnson RA, Suurmond D: Fitzpatrick's Color Atlas and Synopsis of Clinical Dermatology, 5th ed. New York, McGraw-Hill, 2005.)

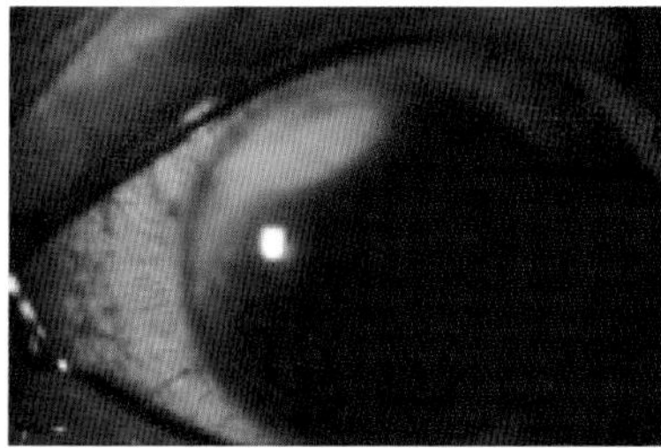

Figure 43-5 Corneal abrasion with fluorescein fluorescing under Wood's light. (From Knoop KJ, Stack LB, Storrow AB, Thurman RJ: Atlas of Emergency Medicine, 2nd ed. New York, McGraw-Hill, 2002.)

PRECAUTIONS

- Not all tinea fluoresces.
- Patients washing before the examination may yield a false-negative result.
- Do not confuse a pathologic process with other substances, such as lint, sulfur-laden scales of skin, serum exudate, ointment, deodorants, soaps, or tetracycline.

CPT/BILLING CODES

Use standard "Evaluation and Management" codes.

ICD-9-CM DIAGNOSTIC CODES

039.0	Erythrasma
110.0	Tinea capitis
110.0	Tinea barbae
110.0	Tinea tonsurans
110.2	Tinea manuum
110.3	Tinea cruris
110.4	Tinea pedis
110.5	Tinea corporis
111.0	Tinea versicolor
277.1	Porphyria cutanea tarda
709.01	Vitiligo

ACKNOWLEDGMENT

The author and editors wish to recognize the contributions of Stephen K. Toadvine, MD, MPH, to this chapter in the previous edition of this text.

SUPPLIER

(See contact information online at www.expertconsult.com.)

Burton Medical Products

BIBLIOGRAPHY

Bechtel K, Bennet BL: Evaluation of sexual abuse in children and adolescents. In Rose BD (ed): UpToDate. Waltham, Mass, UpToDate, 2008. Available at www.uptodate.com.

Chuh AA, Wong WC, Wong SY, Lee A: Procedures in primary care dermatology. Aust Fam Physician 34:347–349, 2005.

Habif TP: Clinical Dermatology: A Color Guide to Diagnosis and Therapy, 4th ed. St. Louis, Mosby, 2004.

Kefalidou S, Odia S, Gruseck E, et al: Wood's light in *Microsporum canis* positive patients. Mycoses 40:461–463, 1997.

Wolff K, Johnson RA, Suurmond R: Fitzpatrick's Color Atlas and Synopsis of Clinical Dermatology, 5th ed. New York, McGraw-Hill, 2005.

CHAPTER 44

Wound Dressing

Marisha Chilcott

Wound management is an often overlooked and undervalued aspect of patient care. Nonetheless, wounds are a source of significant patient, family, and clinician distress, causing readmission, long-term morbidity, and avoidable mortality. This brief overview of wound care and dressing selection intends to demystify basic wound management and improve patient outcomes.

There are three basic tenets to wound management:

1. To get rid of the "ick" (i.e., slough, pus, and necrotic debris)
2. To promote healthy tissue growth
3. To achieve wound closure

The *key steps* in attaining these goals are *first to prepare the wound bed and then to manage the progressive development of the healing tissue*. Selection of appropriate dressings is critical to succeed in these simple endeavors, and there is no single recipe that will work for all wounds. Dressing selection is determined by the individual wound itself, the available materials, and the psyche and physical health of the patient. For example, a wound in the perineum requires very different considerations than a wound on the scalp or back. A lower extremity wound in the exact same location is very different if the patient is diabetic, has peripheral vascular disease, or is an otherwise well patient with Hansen's disease (with neuropathy).

In addition to the *general wound types* most frequently encountered (e.g., *pressure ulcers, venous stasis ulcers, nonhealing infected surgical wounds*), the clinician will occasionally have to address the recalcitrant and *fungating malignant wound* of neoplasia. These wounds may need to be addressed somewhat differently because their management objective may not be actual healing. Rather, the objective may be to maintain quality of life for the patient who must live with the open wound for the remainder of his or her life. Thus, management of odor and appearance is of greater import than achieving resolution of the wound site.

Wounds with toxins, such as those produced by *brown recluse spider bites* or *infiltrated chemotherapeutic* agents, are also treated differently in that they require aggressive, usually wide surgical débridement to remove the offending agent and limit ongoing damage to tissue.

The range of dressing choices includes a variety of materials, forms, and structures. Their individual characteristics are governed by their principal purpose, be that absorption, bacterial growth inhibition, pain relief, débridement, occlusion, compression, or simple protection. Effective management of the stages of wound healing requires an understanding of the processes and the roles potentially played by the dressings available.

Wounds 101

The word *wound* is defined as a break in the epithelial integrity of skin with disruption of possibly deeper tissues, including dermis, fascia, muscle, and bone. Wounds then divide neatly into acute versus chronic, and clean versus infected. The ideal wound, from the standpoint of speed of healing, cosmesis, and function, is clean and acute. An example is the classic surgical wound created in a sterile environment and approximated to maximize the probability of primary closure. The most challenging wound, from either a patient's point of view or a clinician's management perspective, is infected and chronic. These can be decubitus sacral ulcers exposed to feces, foot injuries on the diabetic patient with severe tinea pedis and onychomycosis, abdominal wounds that have dehisced secondary to infected seromas, or any of a number of unfortunate breakdowns in integumentary integrity.

Clean or sterile acute wounds can heal by either primary or secondary intention and are relatively straightforward to manage. The fundamentals of that process are the basis for all wound care. In fact, *the goal of the management of the chronic infected wound* is to modify its conditions to approximate a clean acute wound so as to follow the same uneventful healing process.

Healing of acute wounds involves a cascade of overlapping processes that includes first *hemostasis*, then *inflammation*, followed by *proliferation*, and culminating with *remodeling*. Chronic wounds become chronic when they get stuck in the stage of inflammatory processes because of infection, poor circulation, inadequate enervation, repeated trauma, or some combination of those conditions. The role of dressing selection and wound care management comes down to ameliorating those conditions that impair the progression from inflammation to proliferation.

Wound types can be generally be categorized by their cause, their depth, and their appearance. Causes are almost always multifactorial, but the underlying pathologic process that predisposes a particular patient toward wound development is relevant in the overall care of the wound and the person who hosts it.

Depth is both a physical measurement (in millimeters to centimeters) and a characterization of penetration through the skin and underlying tissues. It is generally divided into *surface, partial thickness*, and *full thickness*.

A *categorization for pressure ulcers* was developed in 1975 by J. D. Shea, then refined and promoted as a tool to promote clear communication between clinicians in 1989 by the National Pressure Ulcer Advisory Panel (NPUAP). In 1997 and 2007, the NPUAP updated their pressure ulcer staging system to reflect the growing understanding of the multifactorial nature of wound development. The following *NPUAP definitions* are directed specifically at pressure ulcers and do not apply to wounds from other causes (e.g., venous insufficiency, diabetic foot wounds):

Pressure ulcer: A localized injury to the skin and/or underlying tissue, usually over a bony prominence, as a result of pressure, or pressure in combination with shear and/or friction.

Stage I: *Intact skin* with nonblanching redness of a localized area, usually over a bony prominence. Darkly pigmented skin may not have visible blanching; its color may differ from the surrounding area. *Note:* The area may be painful, firm, soft, warm, or cooler compared with adjacent tissues and may be difficult to detect in individuals with dark skin tones.

Stage II: *Partial-thickness loss of dermis* presenting as a shallow open ulcer with a red-pink wound bed, without slough. May also present as an intact or open/ruptured serum-filled blister. *Note:*

Presents as a shiny or dry shallow ulcer without slough or bruising. (Bruising may indicate deep tissue injury; see later discussion.) This stage should *not* be used to describe skin tears, tape burns, perineal dermatitis, maceration, or denudement.

Stage III: *Full-thickness* tissue loss. Subcutaneous fat may be visible but bone, tendon, or muscle is *not* exposed. Slough may be present but does not obscure the depth of tissue loss. *May* include undermining and tunneling. *Note:* The actual measured depth of the stage III pressure ulcer varies by anatomic location. The bridge of the nose, ear, occiput, and malleolus do not have subcutaneous tissue, and stage III ulcers can be quite shallow. In contrast, extremely deep stage III pressure ulcers can develop in areas of significant adiposity. The key feature is that bone/tendon is neither visible nor palpable.

Stage IV: *Full-thickness tissue loss with exposed bone, tendon, or muscle.* Slough or eschar may be present on some parts of the wound bed. Often includes undermining and tunneling. *Note:* As with stage III ulcers, the actual depth varies by anatomic location. Areas without significant subcutaneous tissue (e.g., nose, ear, malleolus) can have very shallow stage IV ulcers, with bone/tendon that is either visible or palpable.

Unstageable: Ulcers with full-thickness tissue disruption but with the base of the wound covered by slough and/or eschar are not stageable until the base of the wound is exposed.

Types or Healing Stages of Wounds

Acute wounds heal in a relatively orderly and well-organized fashion, with "coordinated actions of both resident and migratory cell populations within the extracellular matrix environment leading to repair of injured tissues." In contrast to this, some wounds fail to heal in a timely and orderly manner, resulting in chronic nonhealing wounds. As mentioned earlier, the usual stages of healing are hemostasis, inflammation, proliferation, and epithelialization.

Chronic wounds are those that fail to progress through the normal stages of healing. Although the most common place for a chronic wound to get "stuck" is in the inflammatory stage, a wound that is exposed to repeated trauma (because of a patient who "picks") can also be functionally chronic. The biologic foundations for the variety of reasons a wound becomes chronic are complex, but the facts that wounds have stages of evolution and that clinical interventions play a role in their development are the obvious motivations behind wound care and dressing selections (Table 44-1).

Wound Bed Preparation

A *clean acute wound* has, by definition, a prepared wound bed. That is, the injured tissue is disrupted but not necrotic or burdened by foreign bodies or bacterial load. It is ready to start healing and *needs dressings that simply protect it and keep it on its natural course* by preventing it from becoming infected, necrotic, or otherwise healing impaired. This is described further later.

Whether acute or chronic, *a dirty wound* has a wound bed that will not heal well because the inflammatory cascade is upregulated and proliferation of the various cell lines that make up the new tissue (basal cells, fibroblasts, myofibroblasts, and epithelial cells) is inhibited. Thus, the first step in the care of a dirty wound is to *prepare its bed.*

Wound bed preparation means creating an optimal environment for healing with a well-vascularized foundation that is stable and has minimal exudate. This preparation requires *reducing the bacterial load, removing necrotic tissue, and optimizing host systemic factors.* Bacterial load reduction is achieved through both appropriate systemic antibiotics and selection of a dressing that is bactericidal or at least bacteriostatic.

Dakin's solution and *acetic acid solutions* have been used for more than a century to decontaminate wounds. There is now clear clinical evidence that *these solutions are toxic to fibroblasts and impair healing.* However, this does not mean that they do not have a role. Both are extremely effective at reducing the bacterial burden of a wound infected with gram-negative organisms, particularly *Pseudomonas.* Although there is an element of toxicity to polymorphonuclear neutrophils and fibroblasts that slows healing, infection and colonization probably impair healing even more significantly. The judicious course of practice is to make staged use of these solutions as part of 1 to 2 days of wet-to-dry dressing management before converting to a more long-term, tissue-promoting (but less bactericidal) dressing choice.

Virtually all *necrotic tissue requires removal* to develop a healthy wound bed. The notable exception to this rule is the case of dry necrosis without infection. These cases occur under relatively special circumstances of severe frostbite, ischemic injury, and rare other circumstances. Such completely dry necrotic tissue can be *allowed to autoamputate*; however, if the dry necrosis is actually an eschar overlying wet necrosis, intervention is necessary. If there is any indication of infection (i.e., wet necrosis), aggressive débridement is a prerequisite to wound bed preparation and healing.

Débridement can be achieved through progressive dressing changes using a hydrogel and mechanical removal with gauze, surgical/sharp débridement, use of a vacuum device, or, if tolerable, larval therapy (i.e., medical maggots; see Chapter 45, Maggot Treatment for Chronic Ulcers). Under the appropriate conditions, larval therapy is the safest, fastest, and most efficacious method of wound débridement.

As implied earlier, wound bed preparation involves more than simply the local management of the wound. It also requires a perspective that includes the individual patient who harbors the wound. This means thinking about the patient as a whole person and recognizing that the greater milieu of the patient's health state is hugely influential on the outcome of the healing process. *Glycemic optimization* and *nutritional support* are often at the foundation of this multidisciplinary approach. A nutritional consult can aid tight glycemic control and suggest if supplementation of key minerals (e.g., *zinc*) and vitamins (e.g., *vitamins A, C, and E*) can benefit. Note that although supplementation with zinc in patients with deficiency enhances collagen formation, supplementation with zinc in patients who are *not* deficient can paradoxically cause copper deficiency. Copper deficiency in turn weakens scar tissue through decreased tensile strength. Also, vitamin stores and intake can vary widely depending on individual patient circumstances. Thus, a formal nutrition consult to assess a patient's current and impending status should guide supplementation, rather than wholesale recommendations for general replenishment. *Occupational therapy* consultation may aid with appropriate bed/chair fitting and selection. In addition, edema should be minimized through compression and elevation, and immunosuppressive drugs such as steroids avoided.

TABLE 44-1 Chronic Wound Characteristics and Descriptions

Wound Characteristic	Features
Necrotic	Devitalized epidermis Blackened in color Dry and retracted
Sloughy	Containing a layer of viscous, adherent slough Yellow in color Wet Potentially malodorous
Granulating	Significant amounts of highly vascularized granulation tissue Beefy red or deep pink in color
Epithelializing	Evidence of pink margin Isolated pink islands on the surface

TABLE 44-2 Examples of Antimicrobial Dressings

Silver-Based Dressings	Iodine-Based Dressings	Other Antimicrobials
Acticoat (Smith & Nephew, St. Petersburg, Fla) Silvadene Cream (Monarch Pharmaceuticals, Bristol, Tenn) Actisorb Silver 2000 (Johnson & Johnson, New Brunswick, NJ) Aquacel Ag (ConvaTec, Princeton, NJ)	Iodosorb (Smith & Nephew) Iodoflex (Smith & Nephew)	Metronidazole (Metrotop Gel; Pharmacia & Upjohn, Bridgewater, NJ) Bacitracin zinc and polymixin B sulfate (Polysporin; Johnson & Johnson) Neomycin sulfate, polymixin B sulfate, and bacitracin (Neosporin; Johnson & Johnson) Mupirocin (Bactroban; GlaxoSmithKline, London)

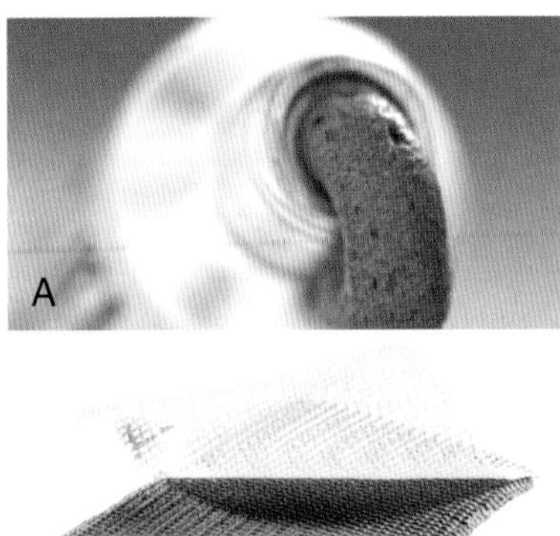

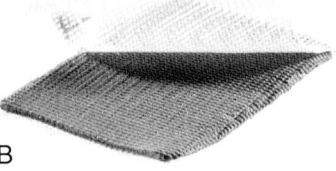

Figure 44-2 Iodine-containing products. **A,** Iodosorb cream. **B,** Iodoflex mesh. (Courtesy of Smith & Nephew, St. Petersburg, Fla.)

DRESSINGS BY DESIGN

The general objective of all dressings is to promote rapid and cosmetically acceptable healing with minimal patient discomfort. Within this greater expectation, however, dressing types vary greatly in their material composition and primary application. Absorption, infection prevention, infection amelioration, débridement, pain management, and protection are different dressing purposes.

The following describes various dressing types and their characteristics. Each description is followed by a table that includes brand name dressings in each category (where applicable). This section is by no means meant to be an endorsement of any specific product, nor does it claim to be an exhaustive list of products currently available. Nonetheless, it is often difficult for the clinician to recognize based on name or product labeling just what category a given product might fit into. Many health care organizations do not stock the entire line of a given supplier's products, and how to mix and match what is available at an institution to address the progressive dressing needs of a given wound can be very confusing. The purpose of the tables is to provide a basis for this sort of cross-reference.

Dressing Types and Characteristics

Antimicrobial

Antimicrobial dressings are used for locally infected or colonized wounds to reduce the microbiologic load (Table 44-2). Solutions of *acetic acid* or *dilute bleach (Dakin's solution)* have been used for years for this purpose but except in specific and judicious applications should be replaced with the less host-toxic options now available. Dressings made with *silver*, in ionic or nanocrystalline form, have been demonstrated to be very effective antimicrobials with bactericidal rather than just bacteriostatic qualities. Silver dressings include both silver-infused creams and meshes (Figs. 44-1 and 44-2).

Iodine is an excellent bacteria eradicator, but in some forms it has been clearly demonstrated to delay healing. *Povidone–iodine (Betadine)* in particular has been implicated as more toxic than others for overall healing in spite of its efficacy against bacterial infection and colonization. It remains an extremely effective preoperative skin preparation agent but should not be used directly in open wounds. There are, however, other iodine-based dressings that are indicated for wound care (see Fig. 44-2). For patients with thyroid disease, caution needs to be maintained and thyroid function monitored because it has been demonstrated that there is systemic uptake of iodine through dressings.

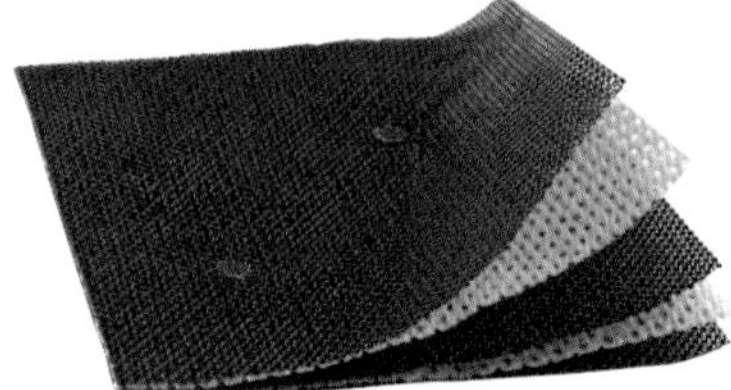

Figure 44-1 Acticoat, a silver-impregnated antimicrobial barrier dressing. (Courtesy of Smith & Nephew, St. Petersburg, Fla.)

Other *antibiotic ointments and creams* are useful in that they create a barrier to prevent new infection and can reduce the risk of cross-colonization with other wounds or uninfected tissues. Ointments or creams can be used directly on or over a wound and be subsequently covered with a dry gauze or bandage to form a basic antibacterial dressing.

Low-Adherent and Nonadherent

Low-adherent and nonadherent dressings are designed to reduce their adherence to the wound bed and either permit (*hydrophilic*) or prevent (*hydrophobic*) drainage of fluid from the wound (Table 44-3). The hydrophobic low-adherent and nonadherent dressings thus are also a form of occlusive dressing. The hydrophilic dressings are designed to be used with an overlying absorptive dressing that is in turn usually occlusive (e.g., a foam or gel dressing). Most of these are in the form of tulles, textiles, or multilayered or perforated plastic films.

Semipermeable

Semipermeable films consist of *transparent polyurethane sheets* that are coated with hypoallergenic acrylic adhesives. They promote a moist environment by occluding the wound, adhere to the healthy skin

TABLE 44-3 Low-Adherent and Nonadherent Dressings

Hydrophilic	Hydrophobic
Adaptic (Johnson & Johnson, New Brunswick, NJ) Xeroflo (Kendall, Ltd.) Mepitel (Mölnlycke Health Care, Norcross, Ga) Tegapore (3M, St. Paul, Minn) N-Terface (Winfield Labs, Richardson, Tex) Fine-mesh gauze or chiffon (not a brand, but a type of cloth)	Vaseline Gauze (Kendall, Ltd., Mansfield, Mass) Xeroform (Kendall, Ltd.) Telfa (Kendall, Ltd.) Scarlet Red Ointment Dressing (Kendall, Ltd.)

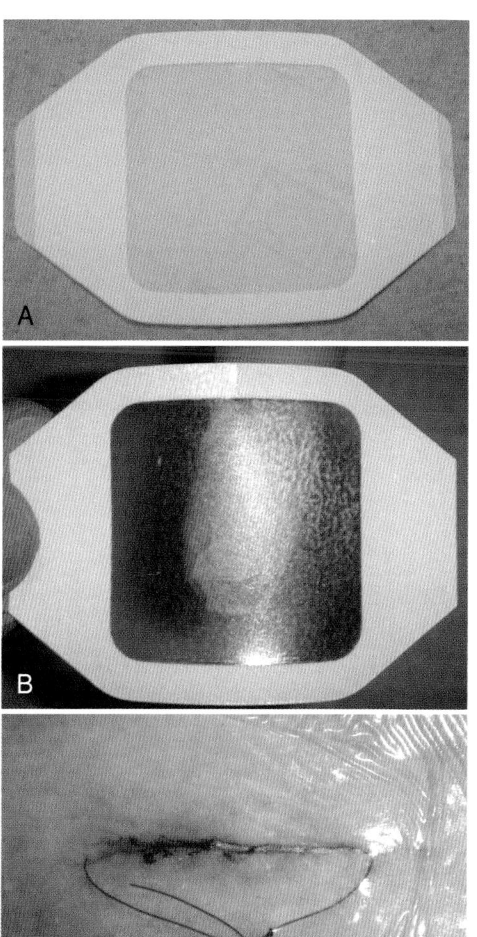

Figure 44-3 Tegaderm, a hydrophobic low-adherent dressing. **A,** The dressing with the protective backing in place. **B,** The protective backing has been removed, leaving a transparent window for proper application. **C,** Tegaderm placed over a recently closed excision (subcuticular running closure). The dressing provides not only moist healing/protection but support to the wound margins. (Courtesy of John L. Pfenninger, MD, The Medical Procedures Center, PC, Midland, Mich.)

(but not wound), and allow visualization of the wound and surroundings skin (Fig. 44-3). However, because they are just a film over the wound, they do not provide any padding, nor do they address the amount of exudate an infected wound often produces (Box 44-1). Thus they are most suitable for *flat, shallow wounds with low exudates*, or for use as a *secondary dressing* (i.e., in lieu of tape covering dry gauze to create an occlusive dressing). These dressings are often used over sutured wounds not only to provide protection and moist healing, but to decrease the tension on wound margins. Care is minimal because these covered wounds can become wet (e.g., bathing) without consequence.

Box 44-1. Examples of Semipermeable Film Dressings

Bioclusive (Johnson & Johnson, New Brunswick, NJ)
CarraFilm (Carrington, Irvine, Tex)
Mefilm (Mölnlycke Health Care, Norcross, Ga)
OpSite Flexigrid & OpSite Plus (Smith & Nephew, St. Petersburg, Fla)
Tegaderm (3M, St. Paul, Minn)

Box 44-2. Examples of Hydrocolloid Dressings

Comfeel (Coloplast, Humlebaek, Denmark)
Cutinova (Smith & Nephew, St. Petersburg, Fla)
DuoDerm (ConvaTec, Princeton NJ)
Hydrocol (Dow Hickam, Sugar Land, Tex)
NuDerm (Johnson & Johnson, New Brunswick, NJ)
Tegasorb (3M, St. Paul, Minn)

Hydrocolloids

Hydrocolloids are a class of nonbiologic occlusive dressings that contain a hydrocolloid matrix composed of carboxymethylcellulose, gelatin, elastomers, and pectin on an adhesive sheet or wafer, or as a paste or powder. Although their forms vary by brand and type, the hydrocolloid dressings have in common that they form a gel on contact with wound exudates (Box 44-2). Although there is little clinical evidence based on randomized, controlled trials to guide dressing choices generally, it has been fairly well established that hydrocolloids are more effective than either paraffin gauze or wet-to-dry gauze dressings.

Hydrogels are a matrix of insoluble polymers, usually sodium carboxymethylcellulose, modified starch, or sodium alginate, that are partially hydrogenated and able to simultaneously donate water molecules to the wound surface (maintaining moistness) and absorb some wound exudates. *They are the standard for management of sloughing or necrotic wounds*. They promote wound débridement by rehydration of nonviable tissue, thus encouraging autolysis (Fig. 44-4). All hydrogels may be left in place for multiple days but require a secondary dressing overlying them. For very dry wounds, the secondary dressing should be occlusive, such as a semipermeable film (Box 44-3).

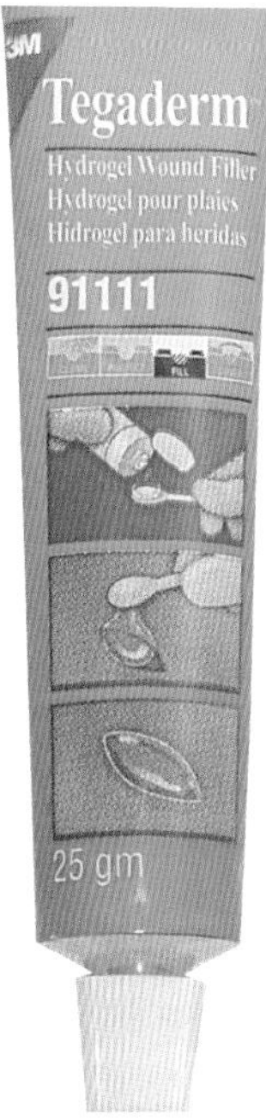

Figure 44-4 Tegaderm Hydrogel. (Courtesy of 3M, St. Paul, Minn.)

Box 44-3. Examples of Hydrogel Dressings

GranuGel (ConvaTec, Princeton, NJ)
Intrasite (Smith & Nephew, St. Petersburg, Fla)
Nu-Gel (Johnson & Johnson, New Brunswick, NJ)
Purilon (Coloplast, Humlebaek, Denmark)
Tegagel (3M, St. Paul, Minn)
Vigilon (Bard, Murray Hill, NJ)

Alginates

Alginates are made of the calcium and sodium salts of alginic acid, found in a class of brown seaweed (Phaeophyceae). Commercially produced alginates are either 100% calcium alginate or a combination of calcium with sodium alginate at a ratio of 80:20 (Box 44-4). The alginates, like the hydrocolloids, react on contact with the wound exudate to form a gel. Typically, they can absorb 15 to 20 times their weight of fluid and are *excellent choices for highly exudative wounds*. They should *not* be used in wounds with little exudate because they will dry out the wound surface, adhere to it, and cause pain on removal. With respect to removal, alginates need to be *changed daily* and to have a secondary dressing overlying them (i.e., gauze or film; Fig. 44-5). Those with higher concentrations of mannuronic acid (e.g., Kaltostat) can be washed off with saline, whereas those higher in guluronic acid (e.g., Sorbsan) will retain their structure and can be removed as a single piece.

Foam Dressings

Foam dressings are manufactured from either a polyurethane or silicone foam and are available as sheets (with and without integrated adhesives) or cavity-filling chips. Foam dressings are *excellent for absorbing large amounts of exudates, provide a level of protection in the form of padding, and are generally occlusive*, thus not requiring additional overlying dressing. Furthermore, under most circumstances, they may be left in place for 2 to 3 days at a time, reducing the cost and discomfort of frequent dressing changes (Table 44-4 and Fig. 44-6).

Vacuum Dressings

A *vacuum dressing* is a mechanical device that uses a reticulated foam dressing cut to the shape of the individual wound and then covered by an occlusive drape through which a sealed vacuum tube is placed. The tube is connected to a pump, which provides 50 to 125 mm Hg of negative pressure to the wound environment (Figs. 44-7 and 44-8). The technology is available through KCI Medical (San Antonio, Tex). The KCI V.A.C. device has been demonstrated to enhance local blood flow, diminish edema, limit bacterial proliferation, and accelerate granulation tissue formation. It has excellent capacity to remove drainage and exudates and acts as an effective débridement tool. Indications for using a KCI V.A.C. include chronic open wounds, dehisced incisions, meshed grafts, and flaps, as well as either chronic or acute traumatic wounds. Contraindications to its use are fistulas to organs or internal cavities, necrotic tissue in eschar, untreated osteomyelitis, and malignancy in the wound.

Box 44-4. Examples of Alginate Dressings

Algiderm (Bard, Murray Hill, NJ)
Algosteril (Johnson & Johnson, New Brunswick, NJ)
Kaltostat (ConvaTec, Princeton, NJ)
SeaSorb (Coloplast, Humlebaek, Denmark)
Sorbsan NA and Sorbsan SA (Dow Hickam, Sugar Land, Tex)
Tegagen (3M, St. Paul, Minn)

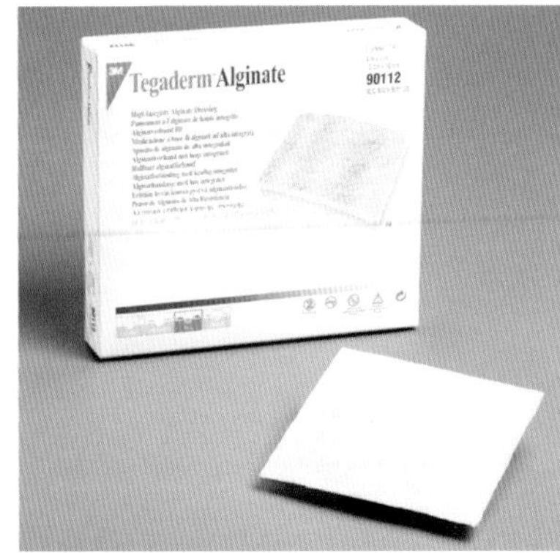

Figure 44-5 Tegaderm Alginate. (Courtesy of 3M, St. Paul, Minn.)

General Recommendations

Among the review articles and other published works on wound management from the past 15 years, there is a consensus statement by experts published in 2007 (Vaneau and colleagues, 2007). A steering committee selected a panel of 27 experts who had no declared conflicts of interest; they worked first from questionnaires, then discussion, followed by working-group peer review. Their recommendations are given here regarding the application of specific dressing types for specific wound stages:

- *Acute wounds, epithelialization stage* (i.e., postoperative): Low-adherent dressings
- *Epithelialization stage*: Hydrocolloid and low-adherent dressings
- *Débridement stage*: Hydrogels
- *Granulation stage*: Foam and low-adherent dressings
- *Hemorrhagic wounds*: Alginates (effective both for absorption of exudates and hemostasis)
- *Malodorous wounds*: Activated charcoal; metronidazole gel (good for anaerobic bacteria)

It should be noted, however, that a paucity of published evidence based on actual trials limits these recommendations. In particular, firm conclusions could be drawn on only three types of dressings (hydrocolloid, alginate, and foam dressings), and the committee made no comment one way or the other on either surgical/sharp

TABLE 44-4 Foam Dressings

Foam Adhesive Sheets	Foam Non-Adhesive Sheets	Foam Cavity Fillers
Allevyn Adhesive* (available in different shapes and sizes) Allevyn Lite Island Allevyn Thin and Allevyn Plus Adhesive Biatain Adhesive (Coloplast, Humlebaek, Denmark) Lyofoam Extra Adhesive (Seton Healthcare Group) Tielle and Tielle Lite (Johnson & Johnson, New Brunswick, NJ)	Allevyn Allevyn Lite Lyofoam and Lyofoam Extra (Seton Healthcare Group, Oldham, UK)	Allevyn Cavity Allevyn Plus Cavity Cavi-Care

*All Allevyn products and Cavi-Care are by Smith & Nephew (St. Petersburg, Fla).

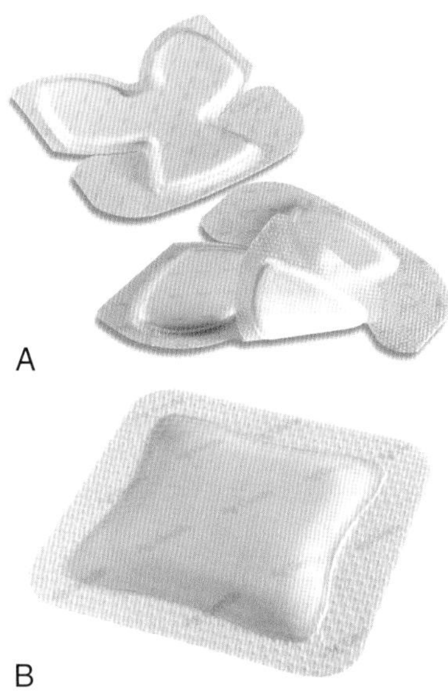

Figure 44-6 **A** and **B,** Allevyn Adhesive foam dressing in two shapes. (Courtesy of Smith & Nephew, St. Petersburg, Fla.)

débridement techniques or larval therapy (maggots) as methodologies for removal of necrotic tissue from wounds.

Other criteria that were agreed on as useful for individual clinicians' decision making but for which there was insufficient evidence to make specific recommendations included the following:

- Pain or discomfort on application and removal
- Management of exudates
- General dressing tolerance (e.g., ability of caregiver/nursing staff and patient to accept larval therapy)

Dressings for Specific Wound Types

Table 44-5 and Box 44-5 present general recommendations for types of dressings based on wound types and the healing objective of the dressing.

Other Considerations in Wound Management and Dressing Application

One of the most common problems in wound management is failure to protect the surrounding healthy skin or tissue and resultant expansion of the wound area. Although much of this discussion has focused on dressing choices that take the clinician away from traditional *wet to dry* gauze dressings, these outdated techniques nonetheless remain one of the most common choices (familiarity and lack of knowledge about other choices being the most likely reasons for this). A *common error* made by many nurses, physicians, and other caregivers who change dressings is that of allowing wet material to macerate dry, intact skin. This can be a problem with any dressing that either does not keep up with absorption of exudates or is oversized and sits on intact skin. For areas that are constantly exposed to moisture, a layer of *hydrophobic ointment* or *thick cream* (e.g., zinc oxide, A&E ointment, or Desitin cream) can prevent maceration and further breakdown of the skin.

Of additional concern, the dry, intact skin surrounding a wound is exposed to the adhesives of the binding layer of the dressing (i.e.,

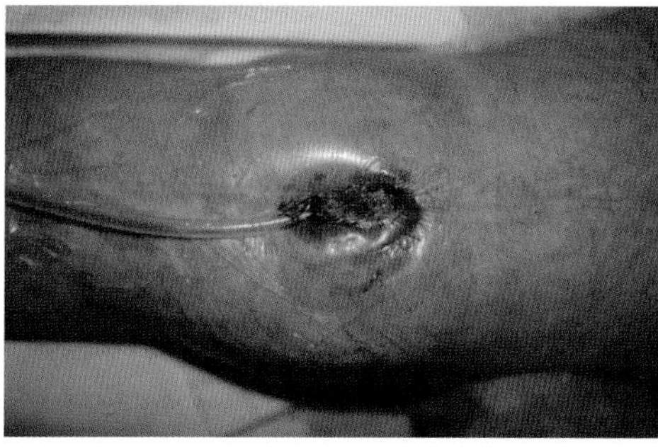

Figure 44-7 V.A.C. dressing in place in knee wound.

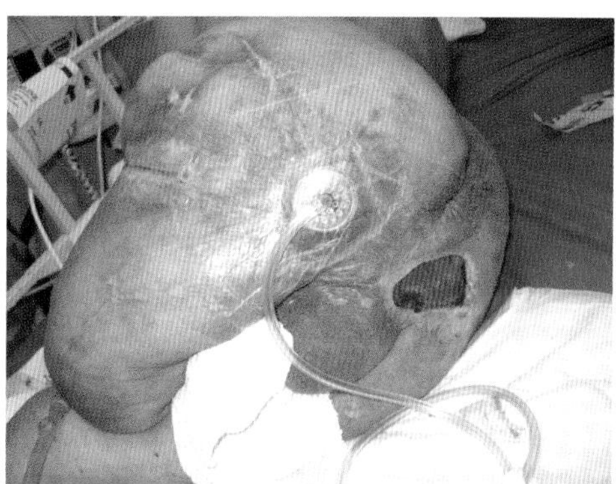

Figure 44-8 V.A.C. dressing in sacral wound, with adjacent wound before second dressing has been placed.

TABLE 44-5 Dressing Recommendations Based on Wound Type and Dressing Objectives

Wound Type	Dressing Objective	Dressing Recommendation
Incisional/Surgical wounds	Protect wound from contamination Immobilize wound edges Compression	Benzoin + Steri-Strips Antibacterial ointment Low-adherent dressing Semipermeable film
Skin tears	Protect wound from contamination Immobilize wound edges	Antibacterial ointment Low-adherent dressing Semipermeable film
Partial-thickness wounds or donor sites	Facilitate epithelialization Absorb exudate Protect wound from contamination	Low-adherent dressing + overlying absorptive layer (foam or gauze) Antibiotic cream/ointment + gauze or foam Occlusive dressing with absorptive property (hydrocolloid sheets or foam dressing)
Full-thickness wounds (pressure wounds, surgical site dehiscence, third-degree burns)	Maintain moisture Absorb exudate Débridement	Hydrogels Alginates Foam dressings KCI V.A.C. dressing
Any wound with heavy load of necrotic tissue	Absorb exudate Débridement	Larval therapy/dressing KCI V.A.C. dressing
Malignant wound	Maintain moisture Absorb exudate Odor control	Foam dressings for absorption Metronidazole gel Activated charcoal (Actisorb Plus or Lyofoam C)

Box 44-5. Factors Influencing Dressing Selection

Wound Depth
- Superficial
- Full thickness
- Cavity

Wound Description
- Necrotic
- Sloughing
- Granulating
- Epithelializing

Wound Characteristics
- Dry
- Moist
- Heavily exudative

Bacterial Profile
- Sterile
- Colonized
- Infected
- Infected and potential source of serious cross-infection

plastic or paper tapes, Coban, clear occlusive dressing), which can cause skin tears and irritation such as blisters and rash. Care should be taken to protect intact skin by using a skin protectant, either a thin liquid applied and dried or even a thin film dressing (e.g., Tegaderm or Op-Site), on areas of intact skin that are repeatedly exposed to adhesives and the mechanical irritation of their repeated removal and reapplication.

In addition to the general wound types most frequently encountered (e.g., pressure ulcers, venous stasis ulcers, nonhealing infected surgical wounds), the clinician will occasionally have to address the recalcitrant and fungating *malignant wound of neoplasia.* These wounds may need to be addressed somewhat differently because their management objective may not be actual healing. Rather, the objective may be to maintain quality of life for the patient, who must live with the open wound for the remainder of his or her life. Thus, *management of odor* and *appearance* is of greater import than achieving resolution of the wound site. Activated charcoal can reduce unpleasant odors and is found in dressings such as ActiSorb and Lyofoam Plus.

Wounds containing toxins, such as those produced by brown recluse spider bites or infiltrated chemotherapeutic agents, are also treated differently in that they require aggressive, usually wide surgical débridement to remove the offending agent and limit ongoing damage to tissue.

Summary and Resource References

Wound management is a challenging element of patient care that requires a multidisciplinary approach for optimization of the final outcome. It is incumbent on the clinician(s) to be willing to change course as the wound's character evolves. Dressing selection is a vital and dynamic, but not singular, element of the total wound care. No amount of dressing expertise can overcome the deleterious effects of ignoring the patient's condition as a whole—medical, metabolic, social, and emotional states are crucial for healing in the global sense.

CPT/Billing Codes

Procedures 16000 to 16030 refer to local treatment of burned surface only.

11000	Eczema/infected skin—first 10%
11001	Eczema/infected skin—each additional 10%
11040	Débridement partial-thickness skin
11041	Débridement full-thickness skin
11042	Débridement skin and subcutaneous tissue
11043	Débridement skin, subcutaneous tissue, and muscle
11044	Débridement skin, muscle, bone
15852	Dressing change (for other than burns) under anesthesia (other than local)
16000	Initial treatment, first-degree burn, when no more than local treatment is required
16010	Dressing/débridement, initial or subsequent, under anesthesia, small
16015	Under anesthesia, medium or large, or with major débridement
16020	Without anesthesia, office or hospital, small
16025	Without anesthesia, medium (e.g., whole face or whole extremity)
16030	Without anesthesia, large (e.g., more than one extremity)

Online Resources

Dressings.org: Available at www.dressings.org.
KCI: V.A.C. Therapy. Available at www.kci1.com/KCI1/vactherapy.
Monarch Labs: Available at www.monarchlabs.com.
World Wide Wounds: Available at www.worldwidewounds.com.

Bibliography

Black J, Baharestani MM, Cuddigan J, et al: National Pressure Ulcer Advisory Panel's updated pressure ulcer staging system. Dermatol Nurs 19:343–349, 2007.

Bluestein D, Javaheri A: Pressure ulcers. Am Fam Physician 78:1186–1196, 2008.

Chaby G, Senet P, Vaneau M, et al: Dressings for acute and chronic wounds: A systematic review. Arch Dermatol 143:1297–1304, 2007.

Enoch S, Price P: Cellular, molecular and biochemical differences in the pathophysiology of healing between acute wounds, chronic wounds and wounds in the aged. August 2004. Available at http://www.worldwidewounds.com/2004/august/Enoch/Pathophysiology-Of-Healing.html.

Kramer SA: Effect of povidone-iodine on wound healing: A review. J Vasc Nurs 17:17–23, 1999.

Leveriza-Oh M, Phillips TJ: Dressings and postoperative care. In Robinson JK, Hanke CW, Siegel DM, Sengelmann RD (eds): Surgery of the Skin: Procedural Dermatology. Philadelphia, Mosby, 2005, pp 117–136.

Morykwas MJ, Argenta LC, Shelton-Brown EI, McGuirt W: Vacuum-assisted closure: Method for wound control and treatment: Animal studies and basic foundation. Ann Plast Surg 38:553–562, 1997.

Piacquadio D, Nelson DB: Alginates: A "new" dressing alternative. J Dermatol Surg Oncol 18:990–998, 1992.

Reddy M, Gill SS, Kalkar SW, et al: Treatment of pressure ulcers. JAMA 300:2647–2662, 2008.

Sanchez R: Wound dressing. In Pfenninger JP, Fowler GC (eds): Procedures for Primary Care, 2nd ed. Philadelphia, Mosby, 2003, pp 295–304.

Stahl-Bayliss CM, Grandy RP, Fitzmartin RD, et al: The comparative efficacy and safety of 5% povidone-iodine for topical antisepsis. Ostomy Wound Manage 31:40–49, 1990.

Thomas S: A structured approach to the selection of dressings. July 1997. Available at www.worldwidewounds.com/1997/july/Thomas-Guide/Dress-Select.html.

Thomas S: MRSA and the use of silver dressings: Overcoming bacterial resistance. November 2004. Available at www.worldwidewounds.com/2004/november/Thomas/Introducing-Silver-Dressings.html.

Vaneau M, Chaby G, Guillot B, et al: Consensus panel recommendations for chronic and acute wound dressings. Arch Dermatol 143:1291–1294, 2007.

CHAPTER 45

Maggot Treatment for Chronic Ulcers

Kim Haglund • Marisha Chilcott

Pressure ulcers and other types of chronic wounds are commonly encountered by primary care providers, especially those who provide care for nursing home residents. Getting such wounds to heal can be a daunting task and requires attention not only to optimal wound dressings but to pressure relief measures, nutrition, and hygiene. The first step toward wound healing is to remove necrotic tissue from the wound and create a clean wound base. Necrotic tissue removal may be accomplished by surgical débridement, either in the operating room or at the bedside; chemical débridement with products that soften or liquefy dry necrotic tissue; or mechanical débridement, such as traditional "wet-to-dry" gauze dressings that pull adherent necrotic tissue from the wound bed when the gauze packing is removed. Although all of these methods have a role in chronic wound management, they all have some disadvantages. Each method can cause damage to adjacent viable tissue and can be uncomfortable for the patient. Surgical débridement in the operating room also exposes the patient, who may have multiple comorbidities, to the risks of anesthesia. Maggot débridement, on the other hand, has the advantages of not harming viable tissue, débriding accurately and completely even in areas of undermining or tunneling, and, in our experience, being very well tolerated in terms of patient comfort.

Indications

- Maggot therapy is indicated for débridement of soft tissue wounds with any type of devitalized tissue in the wound area, including dry eschar, densely adherent fibrinous exudates, or purulent exudates.
- Maggot therapy works well for pressure ulcers, venous stasis ulcers, neuropathic foot ulcers, and nonhealing traumatic or surgical wounds.

Relative and Absolute Contraindications

- Maggot therapy does not work very well for ischemic wounds because the maggots may débride tissue from the wound edges that, although not visibly necrotic, is not really viable owing to very poor perfusion, thereby enlarging the wound area. Such wounds should be treated first with revascularization; once good perfusion is restored, maggots may be used if needed.
- Wounds such as fistulas that communicate with internal organs or body cavities should never be treated with maggots.
- Wounds that are manifestations of an acute life- or limb-threatening infection.
- Allergy to brewer's yeast or soy protein (both used to grow the larvae).
- Allergy to the blowfly larvae.
- Bleeding from the wound bed is common during maggot débridement and, in patients on anticoagulation or with a coagulopathy, may be severe enough to require stopping therapy. Caution should be exercised when deciding whether to use maggot therapy for a patient on anticoagulation or with a coagulopathy.

Equipment and Supplies

To make a maggot dressing, you will need the following:

- Medical-grade maggots. In the United States, order from Monarch Labs (the only U.S. supplier of maggots for medical use; Fig. 45-1). Vial cost for 250 to 500 larvae is approximately $90 (2008 fee), with overnight shipping $39 to $47 additional. They should be used within 24 hours of receipt.
- "Cage" material, either Dacron chiffon (order from Monarch) or other small-pore fabric. We have used cut-up Ted hose with good results when Dacron was unavailable. Monarch will also provide custom-cut pieces of Dacron if you need a bigger piece. The Monarch website states that nylon stockings can be used, but you must select stockings with a weave that is tight enough to prevent the maggots from escaping when they are still small.
- Hydrocolloid dressing to protect skin around wound (not essential).
- Protective skin prep solution.
- Adhesive solution (e.g., benzoin).
- Saline solution.
- Dry gauze.
- Tape.
- Cotton-tipped applicators.
- Two plastic (red, biohazard) trash bags for disposal.
- Ethyl chloride.

Preprocedure Patient Education

Maggot therapy is not well known to the general public or even to many nurses or physicians. Thus, when instituting maggot treatment, it is important for the provider to demystify the procedure and remove the "yuck" factor as much as possible. Try to stress to patients that maggots work like tiny, flexible, and mobile surgical instruments to remove dead or infected tissue from tight corners or tunnels under the skin where human hands and instruments cannot reach. For patients who may be living in a long-term care facility, let the family know when and why maggot therapy is planned because they may misinterpret maggots in the wound as a sign of neglect. See the patient education form available online at www.expertconsult.com.

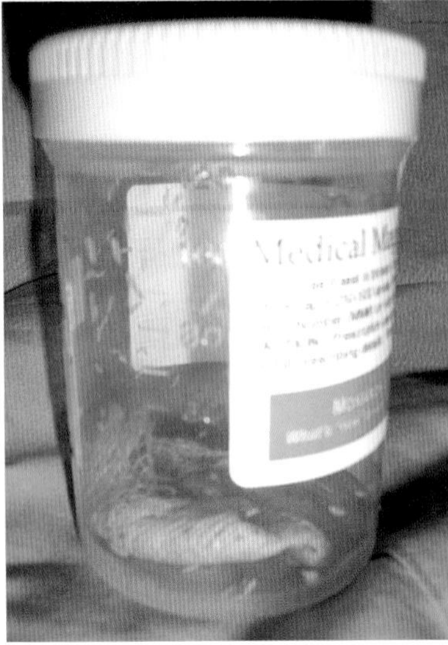

Figure 45-1 Vial of medical-grade maggots.

TECHNIQUE

Application of Maggots

1. Before starting, check the viability of the maggots—you should be able to see them crawling along the walls of the vial. If none are moving, make sure the vial is warm (room temperature at least). If still no movement after warming, contact Monarch Labs for a replacement.
2. Apply protective skin prep solution to intact skin around wound.
3. Cut a donut of hydrocolloid dressing to fit around the wound. (This step is not strictly necessary, but does protect vulnerable skin and allows the application of potentially irritating adhesive to the dressing rather than directly to skin.) The hole needs to match the wound in size and shape, leaving 2 to 3 cm of hydrocolloid margin around the wound (Fig. 45-2).
4. Apply the hydrocolloid donut to the skin, making sure it sticks securely and has no wrinkles.
5. Apply a layer of adhesive (benzoin works well) to the top surface of the hydrocolloid. If hydrocolloid is not being used, apply the adhesive to the prepared skin.

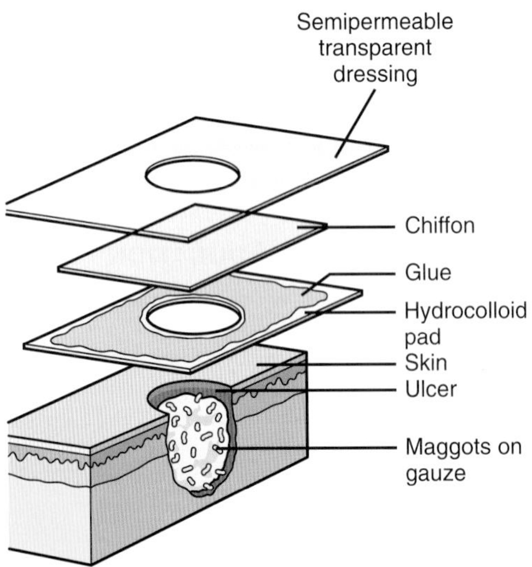

Figure 45-2 Cut a hole in the dressing to match the size of the wound. Typical layering of materials when using maggot therapy.

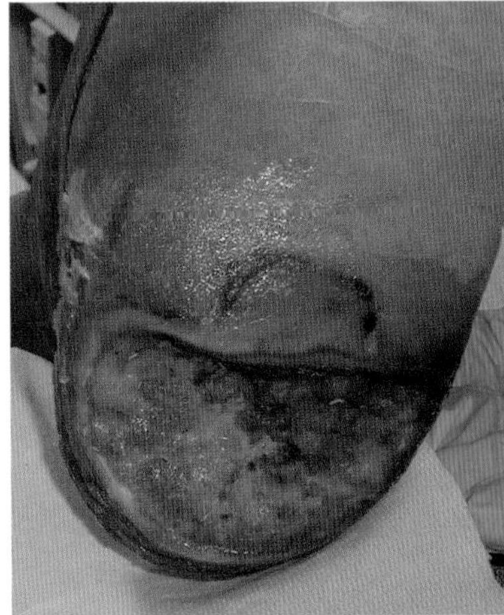

Figure 45-3 Ulcer prepared for medical maggot treatment.

6. With an open plastic trash bag tucked under the body part to which the maggots are being applied (to catch "runaways" and make cleanup easy), open the vial of maggots and gently use cotton-tipped applicators to nudge them into the wound bed. The recommended dose of maggots is five to eight maggots per square centimeter of wound area. For wounds larger than 5 × 5 cm, simply use the whole vial. The piece of damp gauze that comes in the vial may be used to gently wipe the maggots from the sides of the vial (many more will already be burrowed into the gauze itself) and then apply them to the wound. The gauze is then placed in the wound bed. The maggots tend to collect on the underside of the vial lid and in the crevice of the lid, so bang the vial against a hard surface before beginning to knock them to the bottom of the vial. If you are having trouble getting them out, an easy way is to pour a little saline in the vial, swirl, and pour out onto a gauze pad. Then put the damp gauze and maggots into the wound.
7. Once the maggots are in place, apply a little damp, loosely fluffed gauze to cover them and keep the wound bed moist.
8. Apply the Dacron or other fabric "cage" over the wound, sticking it to the prepared hydrocolloid while being careful to avoid wrinkles. Wrinkles create tunnels through which maggots can escape. The edges of the fabric can be taped to the skin or hydrocolloid for an extra measure of security.
9. Put a few squares of dry gauze on top of the fabric cage to absorb drainage, then secure with tape. Do not use too thick a pad of dry gauze or the maggots will be smothered. This dry dressing should be changed as often as needed, usually a few times a day. Although there may be substantial drainage, avoid the temptation to use an abdominal pad or other occlusive absorbent material because you will find that the maggots do not tolerate the lack of oxygen (Figs. 45-3 and 45-4).
10. When the maggots are secured in place, the patient may lie on the wound without concern for killing the maggots.
11. Put all maggot-related trash in plastic bag, double-bag, and dispose. You cannot save maggots for future use if you do not use them all.
12. Remove maggots (see next section) in 2 to 3 days and reapply new maggots with a fresh "cage" and dressings if débridement is incomplete.

Removal of Maggots

1. Place a biohazard plastic bag under the body part to be débrided.
2. Remove the dry gauze, fabric cage, and damp gauze from the wound bed and place in the trash bag. The damp gauze will have lots of maggots crawling in it. They should be much bigger than

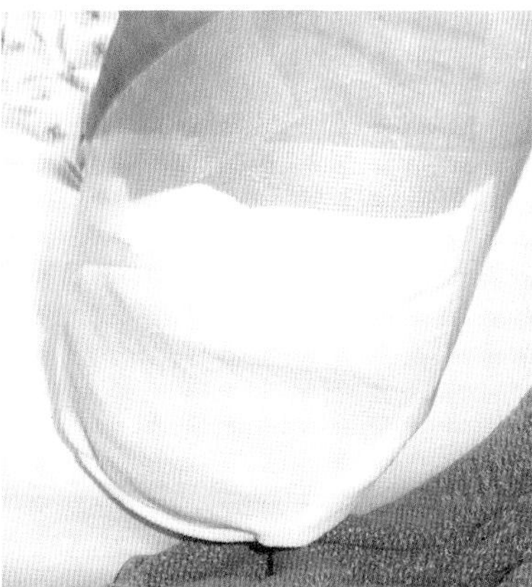

Figure 45-4 Ulcer dressed with medical maggots in place.

when applied—at least the size of grains of cooked rice—but there may seem to be many fewer because some may have died.

3. If there is any undermining or tunneling of the skin, maggots likely are in these spaces. Probe into tunnels with cotton-tipped applicators, wipe the wound with gauze, or flood the wound with saline to flush them out.
4. If you think there may be maggots left behind, apply a damp gauze dressing to the wound bed, cover with a fabric cage, and secure as for a regular maggot dressing. The maggots will stop eating when they are full and will migrate out of the wound and into the gauze. There is no danger of them eating healthy tissue even if all the necrotic tissue has been removed—they will simply migrate out of the wound and "hide" in the gauze. Change the gauze three or four times a day for a day or two and all the maggots should be gone.
5. Even if you are sure all the maggots appear to be gone, damp-to-dry gauze dressing changes should be made three to four times daily for 1 to 2 days between cycles of maggot therapy. This helps remove any material that has been liquefied by the maggots but not consumed.
6. Reapply a new vial of maggots 1 to 2 days after removal of the first set. Most wounds require only two or three cycles of maggot treatment. Very large wounds may need up to five or six treatments.
7. The hydrocolloid donut may be left in place for up to 1 week through multiple cycles as long as it is still adhering well and the skin beneath does not appear macerated.
8. If maggots are escaping from the trash bag while you are trying to remove them from the wound bed, they can be sprayed with ethyl chloride to slow them down.

Once the maggots have débrided all of the necrotic tissue and a clean wound bed is present, the wound will heal by secondary intention. The débrided wound may be left open or may be covered with a usual dressing to maintain a clean, moist wound environment

Once maggots have died, they should be removed. Otherwise, they may trigger an allergic response or become a catalyst for further infection.

Common Difficulties

- Escaped maggots due to wrinkles in cage material or tape.
  Resolution: Make sure the material is flat when laid down on the adhesive and take care with taping. Multiple pieces of flat tape are better than a few pieces with wrinkles or folds.
- Dead maggots when dressing removed.
  Resolution: Make sure the gauze dressing over the maggots is not too occlusive or too dry. Maggots need plenty of oxygen and a moist environment.
- Maggots escaping through the cage despite it being adequately secured around the edges.
  We have only had this problem when using nylon stockings to cover leg wounds, never with the Dacron chiffon pieces supplied by Monarch. Use the Dacron or a tightly woven stretch fabric (TED hose works) rather than ordinary pantyhose.

Complications

The most serious potential complication is *bleeding*. Although most wounds will have mild oozing from a healthy granulating base once the maggots have débrided off necrotic tissue, rarely will there be such heavy bleeding that maggot therapy will have to be abandoned. If the wound includes necrotic tissue through which blood vessels course, maggot débridement may also cause significant bleeding by débriding away the vessel wall. If this happens, the bleeding vessel will need to be controlled with a figure-of-eight stitch, or cautery if the vessel is small enough.

Maggots can also cause *pain or discomfort*. This usually occurs at 24 to 36 hours into therapy and increases as larvae grow larger. If analgesics do not help, remove the dressing, which generally affords immediate relief. Do not apply local anesthetics.

Billing and Coding

Medicare/Medicaid and most insurance companies will cover maggot therapy. If a patient is uninsured or his or her insurance does not cover maggots, there is a Patient Assistance Grant program offered through BTER Foundation (BioTherapeutics Education and Research Foundation) that will cover the cost of the maggots. See the BTER website or the Monarch Labs website for more information.

CPT/Billing Codes

ABC code for Maggots (EAACT) or HCPCS misc code A9270.

97597 For wounds 20 cm^2 or less
97598 For wounds greater than 20 cm^2

ICD-9 Diagnostic Codes

707.00 For decubitus ulcer (and gangrene) with following locations
- 707.01 Elbow
- 707.02 Upper back, shoulder blades
- 707.03 Lower back, sacrum
- 707.04 Hip
- 707.05 Buttock
- 707.06 Ankle
- 707.07 Heel
- 707.09 Head, other sites

879.8 Wound, skin, complicated NEC

If reimbursement is denied, appeal. The BTER Foundation will assist with appeals as well as provide Patient Assistance Grants.

Patient Education Guides

See patient education forms available online at www.expertconsult.com.

Suppliers

BioTherapeutics Education and Research (BTER) Foundation
Monarch Labs

ONLINE RESOURCES

BTER Foundation at http://www.bterfoundation.org.
Monarch Labs at http://www.monarchlabs.com.

BIBLIOGRAPHY

Courtenay M, Church JC, Ryan TJ: Larva therapy in wound management. J R Soc Med 93:72–74, 2000.

Jukema GN, Menon AG, Bernards AT, et al: Amputation-sparing treatment by nature: "Surgical" maggots revisited. Clin Infect Dis 35:1566–1571, 2002.

Sherman RA: Maggot debridement in modern medicine. Infect Med 15: 651–656, 1998.

Sherman RA: Maggot therapy for treating diabetic foot ulcers unresponsive to conventional therapy. Diabetes Care 26:446–451, 2003.

Sherman RA, Sherman J, Gilead L, et al: Maggot debridement therapy in outpatients. Arch Phys Med Rehabil 82:1226–1229, 2001.

SECTION 3

Aesthetic Medicine

Section Editor: HANEEF ALIBHAI

CHAPTER 46

Introduction to Aesthetic Medicine

Haneef Alibhai

As our world continues to evolve, investment in health and wellness is now, more than ever, a top priority for people living longer, healthier, and more active lives. With this comes an ever-growing demand for various surgical and nonsurgical cosmetic medical procedures to enhance one's appearance and overall wellness.

In 2008, over 10 million cosmetic medical procedures were performed in the United States. Eighty-three percent of these procedures were nonsurgical (American Society of Aesthetic Plastic Surgeons). Since 1997, surgical procedures increased by 80% and nonsurgical procedures increased by 233%. Ninety-two percent of the procedures were preformed on women. The top five nonsurgical cosmetic procedures in 2008 were botulinum toxin (Botox) injections (2,464,123 procedures), laser hair removal (1,280,964 procedures), hyaluronic acid dermal filler treatments (1,262,848 procedures), chemical peels (591,808 procedures), and laser skin resurfacing (570,880 procedures). The most popular procedure among people younger than 35 years of age was laser hair removal, whereas the most popular procedure among people older than 35 years was botulinum toxin injections. In 2008, Americans spent almost $11.8 billion on cosmetic procedures.

Aging Population

Currently, baby boomers—born between 1946 and 1964—are the most powerful consumers in the world of aesthetic and cosmetic treatments, with more each year spending millions on cosmetic and aesthetic procedures. In the United States, baby boomers now make up 51% of the total population, with 12,000 people turning 50 every day (one every 8 seconds). This trend will continue, with the number of Americans older than 55 years growing by 60% in the next 20 years.

Facial Aging Process

As we age, our skin matures (chronologic aging). This is generally accelerated because of a process known as *photo-aging*. Photo-aging refers to premature aging from sun exposure, smoking, and genetic predisposition. *Healthy skin* is defined as skin that is smooth, firm, glowing, clear of blemishes and vascular lesions, and plump with natural moisture. *Unhealthy skin* is defined as skin that is uneven, blotchy with pigmentation, poor in tone and elasticity (thin), leathery, dull, and covered with age spots, telangiectases, fine lines, and wrinkles. These unwelcome changes are brought about by the pull of gravity and the cumulative damage to DNA, collagen, and cell membranes by free radicals produced from normal cellular metabolism, environmental elements, and sun exposure. (Also see the discussion of aging skin in Chapter 59, Skin Peels.)

For centuries, we have strived to slow down the aging process in an attempt to look and feel younger. The facial rejuvenation process aims to achieve the following goals.

- Reverse sun damage and reduce the signs of aging (vascular and pigmented lesions)
- Renew and retrain skin cells to appear younger and function more effectively to maintain youthful appearance (smooth skin)
- Relax overactive muscles that cause wrinkles
- Replace lost volume
- Tighten sagging and loose skin
- Stimulate dermal collagen production

During the past decade, much progress has been made in the field of noninvasive facial rejuvenation. The list of noninvasive facial rejuvenation techniques has grown considerably in response to the aging baby boomer's demand for procedures that combine safety, efficacy, predictability, and, of course, minimal downtime. The following noninvasive facial rejuvenation techniques are the most widely performed and sought-after procedures:

- Cosmeceutical skin care
- Microdermabrasion and dermal infusion
- Chemical peels
- Photofacial rejuvenation (intense pulsed light, or IPL)
- Laser/IPL treatment of hair, veins, pigmented lesions, acne, and tattoos
- Ablative laser resurfacing (carbon dioxide, erbium:yttrium-aluminum garnet)
- Light-based therapies (e.g., radiofrequency [RF], light-emitting diode [LED] photomodulation, infrared [IR] devices, fractional resurfacing)
- Nonablative/fractional skin resurfacing
- Nonablative/fractional skin tightening (RF, IR)
- Ablative/fractional skin resurfacing
- Photodynamic therapy (PDT)
- Sclerotherapy
- Botulinum toxin injections
- Dermal filler treatments

Even more recently, cosmetic physicians have begun combining rejuvenation techniques in an attempt to provide better and longer-lasting results. Depending on the patient's concerns and goals, most facial rejuvenation procedures can be performed in concert to provide patients with excellent, long-lasting results. Indeed, when combined, these procedures offer far superior results compared with the results from any single procedure.

Without question, aesthetic medicine is the most exciting and rapidly growing field of medicine today. Given this staggering growth, it is more important than ever for providers to constantly seek education opportunities to keep up to date with recent advances in technology and new procedures in aesthetic medicine. This section of the text provides an overview of the most popular and sought-after cosmetic rejuvenation procedures available today. Those who want to enter the field of aesthetic medicine are strongly encouraged to undergo intensive hands-on clinical training with an experienced aesthetic physician.

Initial Cosmetic and Aesthetic Assessment Visit

Regardless of the reason for the initial visit, it is essential that a full evaluation be made of the *overall health status*. The general health history questionnaire can be used for an overview, but specific questions should then be asked about the skin (Fig. 46-1). It is important to determine exactly what it is the patient is concerned about because another procedure may be more appropriate than what the patient has requested.

For light-based therapies, determining the Fitzpatrick skin type (see Chapter 48, Lasers and Pulsed-Light Devices: Hair Removal, section on "Fitzpatrick Skin Types and Treatment Implications" and Fig. 48-7) is important because the amount of energy needed will vary depending on the skin type.

It is also important to determine if there has been recent use (within 6 months) of isotretinoin (Accutane) because it markedly increases the skin's sensitivity to light and many other products.

If the patient has a history of *herpes simplex*, it may be wise to use antiviral prophylaxis to prevent an outbreak if generalized facial procedures like ablative laser resurfacing or more aggressive peels are to be performed (e.g., valacyclovir [Valtrex] 2 g immediately, followed by 2 g 12 hours later).

Understanding what the patient has used for skin care and what is available to improve the appearance of the skin is very helpful (see Chapter 47, Cosmeceuticals and Skin Care).

Effective *topical anesthetics* are beneficial for many procedures. Care must be taken that they be used appropriately, especially if applied under occlusion, because side effects can be significant (see Chapter 5, Local and Topical Anesthetic Complications, and Chapter 10, Topical Anesthesia). In some instances, an *anxiolytic* (e.g., diazepam [Valium] 10 mg 30 minutes before the procedure) will make the experience easier (e.g., ablative laser resurfacing).

This initial visit not only allows a comprehensive evaluation of the patient, it allows the provider to assess the patient's psychological makeup. An honest discussion of findings is essential. Conditions such as body dysmorphic syndrome should be recognized and dealt with in a straightforward fashion lest the patient be harmed further. The main objective of the initial consultation is to educate the patient on the various nonsurgical cosmetic procedures that are available. The discussion focuses on the procedures deemed to be most appropriate for the patient. Based on the patient's concerns, timeline, goals, and budget, a customized treatment plan will be developed (Fig. 46-2). It is imperative that realistic expectations be set when discussing outcomes. Experience over the years has proved that it is best to be honest with patients and to "under-promise and over-deliver."

Before and After Photographs*

Obtaining before and after photographs can be very beneficial in an aesthetic practice and is strongly recommended. Photographs document the appearance before an intervention for both the patient and the provider. Patients frequently "forget" their initial appearance and see only what remains to be done. Having a "before" photograph can document the changes. Physicians can also use the photographs to gauge what interventions have had the most impact over time.

General Tips

- Ideally, all photographs should be taken in a designated room using a blue background.
  - Lighting, distance, background, and views taken should be duplicated for both the before and the after photographs.
  - Additional background options: dark solid wall color, posterboard, felt, blue window shade mounted on the back of a door.
- Limited or no jewelry for both before and after photographs.
- Hair pulled away from the face.
- Views should be consistent: full face/oblique/profile/close-up of treatment area.

"Before" Tips

- The "before" photograph should be taken during the initial consultation, before any treatment.
- If face has not been cleansed, use a makeup remover wipe to remove the majority of makeup.

"After" Tips

- "After" photographs should be as similar as possible to the "before" photograph.
  If no makeup is worn in the "before" (recommended), the "after" also should be taken without makeup.
- "After" photographs should be taken at predetermined time frames.
  Example: 7 to 10 days postpeel, and again at 3, 6, 9, and 12 months.

Preparing for the Photograph

- Take a *photograph of the name* on the chart before taking a photograph of the patient.
- *Adequate lighting:* If the picture is taken with a digital camera, the photograph should *not* have a yellow hue.
- *For dermal filler photographs, turn the flash off:* When using a digital camera, the flash washes out folds.
- *Date stamp:* Turned on for recording the date the photograph is taken.
- *Stool* with no back.
  - Patient should be sitting up straight and not leaning back against anything.
  - Position stool approximately 1 foot from the wall; check viewfinder for shadows.
  - Pull hair back away from the face and remove all or large jewelry.

Taking the Photo

- Head position
  - The *ala-tragus line should be parallel to the floor* (the ala-tragus line is an imaginary line that runs from the nostril to the cartilaginous projection in the middle of the ear).
  - Another way to check head position is to be sure the occlusal (biting) surface of the teeth is parallel to the floor.

Full-Face Photo

- Have the patient sit up straight.
- Head position: straight, ear not tipped toward either shoulder.
- Hair away from jaw line.
- Eyes open and focused straight ahead, not looking up or down.
- For "blinkers"—keep the eyes closed until you have the view in focus, then open eyes.

Additional Checks

- Ala-tragus line or occlusal surface parallel to the floor.
- Chin not tipped too far up or down.
- Lips in a neutral position—not smiling or frowning.
- Head should take up entire frame—do not crop off hair or chin.

*This section contains contributions by Cathy Uecker.

AESTHETIC SERVICES PATIENT PROFILE

Name: ______________________ DOB: _________ Age: _________ Gender: M/F

Have you completed our medical history form? Yes_____ No_____
Are you pregnant? Yes_____ No_____
Do you wear contact lenses? Yes_____ No_____
Have you had any skin cancers? Yes_____ No_____ Abnormal moles removed? Yes_____ No_____
Precancerous skin changes (actinic keratoses)? Yes_____ No_____
Do you currently have a sunburn/windburn/red face? Yes_____ Why?__________________ No_____
Are you in the habit of going to tanning booths? Yes_____ No_____ Last visit?__________
Please circle what best describes how your skin reacts to the sun (Fitzpatrick Classification):

- I Always burns, never tans—light white skin
- II Always burns, sometimes tans—light white skin
- III Sometimes bums, always tans—medium white skin
- IV Rarely burns, always tans—dark/olive white and Asian skin
- V Moderately pigmented—light brown skin
- VI Black skin—medium to dark brown, African and African-American skin

Do you currently get facial waxing/electrolysis/use depilatories? Yes_____ No_____
Are you currently using Biore/snore strips? Yes_____ No_____
Are you currently using Retin-A/Renova/Differin? Yes_____ No_____ What Strength? __________
For how long? _____ How frequently? _____ Where applied? _______________
Are you now or have you ever used Accutane? Yes_____ No_____ How long? _____ When? _____
Have you ever had microdermabrasion? Yes_____ No_____ When? _____ Where? _____
Do you have regular dermal filler injections? Yes_____ No_____
Do you have regular Botox injections? Yes_____ No_____
Have you ever had a chemical peel? Yes_____ No_____ Within the last 14 days? Yes_____ No_____
What kind? ____________________ Describe your reaction: ____________________
Have you recently had facial surgery? Yes_____ No_____ Describe: ______________ When? ________
Have you recently had laser resurfacing? Yes_____ No_____ When? _____ What Kind? __________________
What type of work do you do? __________________ Airline travel? Yes_____ How often? _____ No_____
Do you participate in vigorous aerobic activity or sports? Yes_____ No_____ What type? _______________
Do you smoke? Yes_____ No_____
Do you develop cold sores/fever blisters? Yes_____ No_____ Last breakout? ____________
Are you allergic/sensitive to (check all that apply) milk_____ apples_____ citrus_____ grapes_____
aloe vera_____ aspirin_____ perfumes_____ latex_____ hydroquinone_____
Other allergies? If so, what? _________________________
Are you sensitive to alcohol-based products? Yes_____ No_____
Please list all medications you take especially thyroid supplements, hormone replacement therapy, birth control pills, Accutane, Coumadin: ____
How would you describe your skin? (check all that apply) Thick_____ Thin_____ Sagging_____ Firm_____
Normal_____ Dry_____ Oily_____ Acne_____ Blackheads_____ Milia_____ Cysts_____ Breakouts_____
Acne scarred_____ Large pores_____ Small pores_____ Rosacea_____ Eczema_____ Freckled_____
Sun-damaged_____ Uneven/blotchy_____ Mature_____ Wrinkled_____ Patchy dryness on_______________
Sallow_____ Melasma_____ Perfume-stained_____ Hypopigmented_____ Hyper-pigmented_____ Psoriasis_____
Dehydrated (lacking moisture)_____ Telangiectasia (broken surface blood vessels)_____
Do you have a tendency to scar? Yes_____ No_____ Form keloids? Yes_____ No_____
Do you consider your skin sensitive_____ resilient_____ not sure_____
Eye color: Blue_____ Green_____ Hazel_____ Gray_____ Lt Brown_____ Med Brown_____ Dk Brown_____
Hair color: Blonde_____ Red_____ Lt Brown_____ Med Brown_____ Dk Brown_____ Black_____ Gray/Silver/White_____
Skin tone: Pale/Whlte_____ Light_____ Medium_____ Reddish_____ Freckled_____ Lt Olive_____ Med Ollve_____
Dark Olive_____ Lt Brown_____ Med Brown_____ Dk Brown_____ Soft Black_____ Black_____
What is your hereditary makeup (what nationality)? ____
Are you using glycolic/AHA home care products? Yes_____ No_____ If so, which one(s)?____________________
How does your skin react to them? _________________________
Have you ever used any products that caused a bad reaction? Yes_____ No_____ Describe ______________________
What is your daily home care regimen? ______________________
What are the cosmetic improvements you would like to see in your skin? ________________________
____

Patient/Client Signature: ______________________________ Date: _____________
Treatment recommendations: ____
____
____
____
Patch test: _________ Date _________ Solution _________ Test area _________ Result _________
Physician/Aesthetician Signature ______________________________ Date: _________

Figure 46-1 Aesthetic Services Patient Profile form.

CUSTOMIZED AESTHETIC TREATMENT PLAN

Name of Patient: ______________________________ M _____ F _____ Date of Birth: ______________

Date first evaluated: ________________ Date photos taken: ________________

SUBJECTIVE: Patient's initial concerns:
1. ____________________
2. ____________________
3. ____________________
4. ____________________

PAST MEDICAL HISTORY: Reviewed. See medical history form. Initial ______
PERTINENT FACTS:

Previous skin cancer:	Y ___	N ___	Previous actinics:	Y ___	N ___	Sun exposure:	Y ___	N ___
Cold sores:	Y ___	N ___	Tanning booth use:	Y ___	N ___	Scar easily:	Y ___	N ___
Heal poorly:	Y ___	N ___						

PREVIOUS TREATMENTS: Y ___ N ___ What _____________ When _____________ Where _____________
AESTHETIC QUESTIONNAIRE FORM: Reviewed. Initial ______
SKIN TYPE: I II III IV V

OBJECTIVE:
____
____
____

ASSESSMENT:
1. ____________________
2. ____________________
3. ____________________
4. ____________________

TREATMENT PLAN:

Botox:	1st Area: _________	Price: $ ________	Date Sch'd: ________	Date Tx: _________	Date Tx: _________
	2nd Area: _________	Price: $ ________	Date Sch'd: ________	Date Tx: _________	Date Tx: _________
	3rd Area: _________	Price: $ ________	Date Sch'd: ________	Date Tx: _________	Date Tx: _________
Cosmoderm:	Area: _________	Price: $ ________	Date Sch'd: ________	Date Tx: _________	Date Tx: _________
Juvederm:	Area: _________	Price: $ ________	Date Sch'd: ________	Date Tx: _________	Date Tx: _________

LIGHT SHEER/HAIR REMOVAL:

	Area: _________	Price: $ ________	Date Sch'd: ________	Date Tx: _________	Date Tx: _________
	Area: _________	Price: $ ________	Date Sch'd: ________	Date Tx: _________	Date Tx: _________
IPL:	1st Area: _________	Price: $ ________	Date Sch'd: ________	Date Tx: _________	Date Tx: _________
	2nd Area: _________	Price: $ ________	Date Sch'd: ________	Date Tx: _________	Date Tx: _________
Radiage:	Area: _________	Price: $ ________	Date Sch'd: ________	Date Tx: _________	Date Tx: _________
Active FX:	Area: _________	Price: $ ________	Date Sch'd: ________	Date Tx: _________	Date Tx: _________
Microdermabrasion:	_________	Price: $ ________	Date Sch'd: ________	Date Tx: _________	Date Tx: _________
Chemical Peel:	_________	Price: $ ________	Date Sch'd: ________	Date Tx: _________	Date Tx: _________

Skin Care Products: ______________________________ Price: $ ____________________
Skin Care Samples: ______________________________

Customized Plan Notes:
____
____
____

PROVIDER SIGNATURE:
______________________________ Date: ____________________

Figure 46-2 Customized Aesthetic Treatment Plan form.

Oblique View and Profile Views

- Repeat aforementioned positioning checks.
- Rotate the stool, not just the person's head.

PATIENT EDUCATION AND CONSENT

Probably more than in any other area of medicine, the time must be taken to evaluate the patient's condition and wishes. A frank discussion of risks, benefits, possible complications, alternative therapies, and expected outcomes is essential. It is important not to "oversell" a procedure (see consent forms online at www.expertconsult.com). Educational handouts explaining the procedure; before, during, and after photographs from previous patients; and written postprocedure instructions can be very helpful. The majority of the procedures in this section are elective, and it is essential that patients have realistic expectations of what can be accomplished.

Aesthetic medicine can be a very enjoyable and rewarding area in which to practice. The key to success is combination therapy because no single procedure will address all of the concerns that may bring a patient to a cosmetic clinic. Physicians must therefore be well trained and seek continuing education as this field continues to grow so rapidly. Ultimately, honest communication, patient education, outstanding customer service, and ethical care are the cornerstones of success in aesthetic medicine.

BIBLIOGRAPHY

Alam M, Dover JS, Nguyen TH: Procedures in Cosmetic Dermatology Series: Treatment of Leg Veins. Philadelphia, Saunders, 2006.

Arndt KA, Dover JS, Alam M: Procedures in Cosmetic Dermatology Series: Scar Revision. Philadelphia, Saunders, 2006.

Carruthers A, Carruthers J: Procedures in Cosmetic Dermatology Series: Botulinum Toxin, 2nd ed. Philadelphia, Saunders, 2005.

Carruthers A, Carruthers J: Procedures in Cosmetic Dermatology Series: Soft Tissue Augmentation. Philadelphia, Saunders, 2005.

Donofrio LM: Evaluation and management of the aging face. In Robinson JK, Hanke DW, Sengelmann RD, Siegel DM (eds): Surgery of the Skin: Procedural Dermatology. Philadelphia, Mosby, 2005, pp 425–436.

Draelos ZD: Procedures in Cosmetic Dermatology Series: Cosmeceuticals. Philadelphia, Saunders, 2005.

Glaser DA, Layman J: Psychosocial issues and the cosmetic surgery patient. In Robinson JK, Hanke DW, Sengelmann RD, Siegel DM (eds): Surgery of the Skin: Procedural Dermatology. Philadelphia, Mosby, 2005, pp 413–424.

Goldberg D: Procedures in Cosmetic Dermatology Series: Lasers and Lights, vol. 1: Vascular/Pigmentation/Scars/Medical Applications. Philadelphia, Saunders, 2005.

Goldberg D: Procedures in Cosmetic Dermatology Series: Lasers and Lights: vol. 2: Rejuvenation/Resurfacing/Treatment of Ethnic Skin/Treatment of Cellulite. Philadelphia, Saunders, 2005.

Goldman MP: Procedures in Cosmetic Dermatology Series: Photodynamic Therapy. Philadelphia, Saunders, 2005.

Haber RS, Stough D, Alam M: Procedures in Cosmetic Dermatology Series: Hair Transplantation. Philadelphia, Saunders, 2005.

Hanke CW, Sattler G, Dover JS: Procedures in Cosmetic Dermatology Series: Liposuction. Philadelphia, Saunders, 2006.

Moy RL, Dover JS: Procedures in Cosmetic Dermatology Series: Advanced Face Lifting. Philadelphia, Saunders, 2006.

Moy RL, Fincher EF: Procedures in Cosmetic Dermatology Series: Blepharoplasty. Philadelphia, Saunders, 2006.

Rubin MG, Dover JS, Alam M: Procedures in Cosmetic Dermatology Series: Chemical Peels. Philadelphia, Saunders, 2006.

Usatine RP: The Color Atlas of Family Medicine. New York, McGraw-Hill, 2009.

CHAPTER 47

COSMECEUTICALS AND SKIN CARE

Wendy L. Smeltzer

Products applied to the skin can range from purely cosmetic products to prescription drugs, but many fall somewhere in between and are commonly referred to as *cosmeceutical agents*. The term *cosmeceutical* is widely used in the skin care industry but is still not recognized by many regulatory bodies such as the U.S. Food and Drug Administration (FDA). However, cosmeceuticals are a reality, as evidenced by the widespread use of this term and a growing number of textbooks and symposia in the medical aesthetics field on this subject. The share of the skin care market comprising cosmeceuticals continues to grow and is the fastest-growing segment of skin care products in the marketplace.

DEFINITIONS

The term *cosmeceutical* was coined by Dr. Albert M. Kligman in the 1970s to focus on the ill-defined territory that falls between cosmetic products and therapeutic medications (drugs). Historically, topical skin care products have been divided into either cosmetics or drugs as defined by the Food, Drug and Cosmetic Act of 1938. A *cosmetic* is defined as "an article intended to be rubbed, poured, sprinkled, sprayed on, introduced into or otherwise applied to the human body or any part thereof for cleansing, beautifying, promoting attractiveness or altering appearance." The definition of a *drug* is "an article intended to affect the structure or any function of the body or articles intended for use in the diagnosis, cure, mitigation, treatment or prevention of disease in man." At a fundamental level, cosmetics alter the appearance of the skin, whereas drugs alter the structure and function of the skin.

Cosmetics do not require premarketing clearance, and it is up to the manufacturer to ensure that the ingredients and amounts used are not subject to drug regulations and that the product is safe when used as intended. On the other hand, drugs are subject to extensive premarketing research to prove their efficacy and safety. According to regulators, the intended use of a product can also determine its classification. Thus it is not only the ingredients in a skin care product but the claims in labeling and advertising that can affect its classification as a cosmetic or drug. Cosmeceuticals bridge the gap between cosmetics and drugs and refer to products that achieve cosmetic results by means of some degree of physiologic action. Other terms for cosmeceuticals are *performance cosmetics*, *active cosmetics*, *functional cosmetics*, and *dermoceuticals*.

COSMECEUTICAL CLASSES

Categories of cosmeceuticals, some of which overlap, include the following:

- Retinoids
- Exfoliants
- Vitamins
- Antioxidants
- Peptides
- Growth factors
- Skin-lightening agents
- Others

Retinoids

The *retinoids* are compounds that have the basic core structure of vitamin A and its derivatives. *All-trans retinoic acid* is the active form of vitamin A in the skin. It works by interacting with nuclear receptor proteins to form complexes that interact with DNA sequences to affect transcription and regulation of gene expression for skin keratinocyte growth and differentiation. This causes increased cell turnover in the epidermis. All-trans retinoic acid is quite irritating to the skin and has teratogenic effects. Derivatives such as *retinol* are commonly used in skin care products because they are have a lower irritation profile and fewer safety concerns. Once applied to the skin, retinol converts to retinaldehyde and then all-trans retinoic acid. The science and benefits of retinoids are well documented, with proven results in *reducing photodamage and fine lines of the skin as well as efficacy against acne and psoriasis*.

Exfoliants

The two key exfoliant cosmeceuticals are *alpha hydroxy acids (AHAs)* and *beta hydroxy acids (BHAs)*. The difference in their chemical structures leads to significant differences in their mechanisms of action, although both cause superficial skin cells to desquamate at an increased rate. This results in a smoothing of skin texture and reduction in photodamage.

Alpha Hydroxy Acids

The most widely used AHA in skin care products is *glycolic acid* because of its excellent penetration into the epidermis due to its small molecular size. However, *lactic acid* and other larger AHAs are found increasingly in skin care products. There are many studies on the science and effectiveness of AHAs since the introduction of these products in 1974 by Van Scott and Yu. The AHAs cause desquamation of skin cells in the epidermis by reducing cellular cohesion between keratinocytes. It is postulated that AHAs bind calcium, which decreases local calcium ion concentrations from cell adhesion molecules, thus disrupting intercellular adhesion and increasing exfoliation. There are also some stimulating effects on the dermis, including increased synthesis of collagen and glycosaminoglycans, which also results in a moisturizing effect.

AHAs are very *effective in the treatment of photodamaged skin as well as dry skin, seborrheic dermatitis, acne, and keratoses*. Concentrations up to 10% are used in home care products, whereas higher concentrations are used in professional treatments.

Beta Hydroxy Acids

Salicylic acid is the only BHA used extensively in skin care products. It has proven keratolytic effects and affects only the stratum corneum. It decreases cohesion between the corneocytes by denaturing glycoproteins and disrupting desmosomal attachments. *It has been used to treat hyperkeratotic conditions such as corns, warts, seborrheic dermatitis, psoriasis, and dandruff.* Because salicylic acid is lipophilic, it is *also very useful in the treatment of acne, and in treatment of photoaging and dyschromia.* Concentrations of 0.5% to 2% are commonly used in home care products. The concentration is usually limited by the amount of irritation it causes.

Amino Acid Filaggrins

These are amino acids found naturally in skin that foster moisture retention. However, they are used topically as a mild chemical peel to reduce wrinkles and improve skin texture, although more peer-reviewed research is required to define their optimal use.

Vitamins

Vitamin C

Vitamin C is a valuable topical cosmeceutical in skin care with significant data supporting its biologic activity and benefits to the skin. Vitamin C is *useful in treating photoaging* because it has an antioxidant effect *as well as a skin-lightening* effect through tyrosinase inhibition. It is also an essential cofactor for collagen production in the skin and has proven effects on *wrinkle reduction*. In addition, vitamin C is helpful in treating *acne* because of its anti-inflammatory properties due to deactivation of some factors responsible for the production of certain proinflammatory cytokines. The active form of vitamin C is *L-ascorbic acid*, which is a challenge to incorporate in topical products because of stability and absorption issues. It oxidizes easily, which leads to loss of potency, and it has poor skin penetration. Enhanced delivery systems and use of more stable derivatives such as *magnesium ascorbyl phosphate* make the use of topical vitamin C a mainstay in skin rejuvenation treatments.

Vitamins B and E

Vitamin B_3 (niacinamide) is used topically in skin care because it is well absorbed and well tolerated. The mechanism of action is not well elucidated, but it is a precursor to enzyme cofactors important in many cellular metabolic functions. There is some evidence that it improves the skin barrier function, which *reduces skin redness and irritation*. It may also *reduce hyperpigmentation and improve skin texture and wrinkle depth*.

Vitamin E (i.e., the *tocopherols*) is an anti-oxidant that is a well-documented free radical scavenger. In topical application to skin, there is good evidence that is it *photoprotective, helping prevent damage from ultraviolet (UV) radiation*. There is some controversy about its use in wound healing and scar prevention, and it may have some benefit in treatment of photodamaged skin.

Vitamin K

Vitamin K is a potent agent that increases coagulation of blood. When applied to the skin topically, there is some evidence that it *may reduce bruising*. There are studies showing reduced purpura after pulsed-dye laser treatments, but more research is required.

Antioxidants

Antioxidants protect the skin from free radical damage due to oxidant stress generated by sunlight and pollutants. The mechanism of action is the scavenging of singlet oxygen and reactive oxygen species. Many antioxidants have proved effective when taken orally, but not all are effective topically. The challenge is to get sufficient skin absorption of the correct form of the antioxidant agent with enough activity to achieve the desired effect. In addition to the following agents, some of the vitamins reviewed earlier are also antioxidants.

Ubiquinone

Ubiquinone, or *coenzyme Q10*, has been proven to absorb after topical application to skin. There are some studies to support improvement in photoaging of skin as well as decreased stratum corneum cell size due to a lessening of the slowdown of cell division that occurs with intrinsic aging.

Alpha Lipoic Acid

Alpha lipoic acid is a potent antioxidant that penetrates into the dermis of skin. There is some evidence that it may reduce both intrinsic and extrinsic aging of the skin due to free radical damage, as well as decreasing UV-B–induced erythema. Further investigation and peer-reviewed studies are still required.

Idebenone

This newer antioxidant is a synthetic version of ubiquinone. Some initial studies indicate effectiveness in treatment of photodamaged skin, but more studies are required.

Peptides

Peptides are short chains of amino acid sequences that make up larger proteins. There are three key cosmeceutical peptides that are useful topical agents for antiaging skin treatments, all with very different mechanisms of action. The cost and delivery mechanisms for these ingredients are challenging. There are limited peer-reviewed studies on these products, and research is ongoing.

Argireline

Argireline (acetyl hexapeptide-3; Lipotec, Barcelona) is a hexapeptide that inhibits neurotransmitter release. It therefore can theoretically reduce muscle movement. It may *decrease skin wrinkles* when delivered to targeted facial muscles, such as fine lines around the eyes and lips. It does not penetrate into deep facial muscles and is not a substitute for botulinum toxin in the treatment of dynamic wrinkles.

Matrixyl

Matrixyl (palmitoyl pentapeptide-3), a pentapeptide fragment of dermal collagen, acts as a feedback stimulator to increase collagen synthesis. It is nonirritating to skin and preserves the barrier function of skin. It is useful in the *reduction of wrinkle depth in the treatment of aging skin*.

Copper Peptide

Copper is a trace element necessary for wound healing and enzymatic processes that enhance collagen production and antioxidant activities. A tripeptide carrier may help deliver elements such as copper into the skin. The major effect of this peptide is as a delivery system rather than its own biologic activity.

Growth Factors

Growth factors are regulatory proteins that act as chemical messengers between and within cells. Hundreds of growth factors have now been identified, with many of them acting synergistically in wound healing and tissue regeneration, although their mechanisms of action are still poorly understood. Growth factors can be extracted from plants, cultured epidermal cells, placental cells, and human fibroblasts for use in cosmeceuticals. Some studies show improvement in photodamaged skin, which is similar to a chronic wound. There is also controversy about whether these molecules are too large to be absorbed, as well as theoretical concerns about their potential to contribute to hypertrophic scarring or cancerous growth. Growth factors used in skin care products include *kinetin*, a plant growth factor, and *human growth factor (HGF)*.

Skin-Lightening Agents

Unwanted pigmentation in the skin may be treated with a variety of cosmeceutical agents. However, only pigments in the epidermis will respond to topical agents; the deeper dermal pigments will not. Some of the aforementioned cosmeceuticals will decrease pigmentation, such as vitamins C and B_3, retinoids, and the AHAs and BHAs. Other agents also are useful as topical products to lighten pigmentation.

Hydroquinone

Hydroquinone (HQ) has been the standard in treatment of hyperpigmentation for many years. Its main mechanism of action is through inhibition of tyrosinase, an enzyme necessary for the production of melanin, but it may also alter the formation of melanosomes and selectively damage melanosomes and melanocytes. Although very effective, it commonly causes skin irritation and may have a cytotoxic effect on melanocytes. Concern over cytotoxicity has resulted in the banning of HQ from use in skin products in some countries.

Others

Kojic acid is a naturally occurring derivative from a fungus that acts as a tyrosinase inhibitor. At the 2% to 4% concentration used in skin products, it is mildly irritating and a possible allergen.

Azelaic acid, another effective skin-lightening agent, is isolated from *Pityrosporum ovale* and also inhibits tyrosinase. It is safe, although it may require a higher concentration (20%), which can cause contact dermatitis.

Other tyrosinase inhibitors, such as *arbutin* from bearberry fruit, *paper mulberry* extract from mulberry leaves, *aloesin* from aloe vera, and *glabridin* from licorice extract, may also be used as skin-lightening agents.

Other Cosmeceutical Agents

Dehydroepiandrosterone

Dehydroepiandrosterone (DHEA) is an adrenal steroid, levels of which naturally decline with age. There is some evidence that topically applied DHEA may increase collagen synthesis and decrease collagen breakdown, although more studies are needed.

Dimethylaminoethanol

Dimethylaminoethanol (DMAE) is a precursor of choline that increases neurotransmitter release and muscle tone. When applied topically, it may increase muscle tone, which may cause skin tightening for skin rejuvenation. Given that other cosmeceutical peptides designed for skin rejuvenation act by doing the reverse—relaxing muscle tone to smooth out wrinkles—one can see the potential for consumer confusion and the need for more research and clinical studies.

Sunscreens

Although sunscreens technically are not cosmeceutical agents, no discussion of skin care products is complete without reviewing sunscreens. Sunscreens are regulated by the FDA as over-the-counter (OTC) drugs and require a drug identification number (DIN). The use of a broad-spectrum sunscreen with minimum SPF 30 is important in any skin care regimen to prevent photoaging as well as skin cancers. Although in the past there has been a focus on damage caused by UV-B radiation (290 to 320 nm), we now know that UV-A radiation (320 to 400 nm) is also significant in both carcinogenesis and photodamage. UV-A has been called "the silent killer" because erythema does not occur with exposure, as it does with UV-B radiation. The SPF number listed on sunscreen labels refers to its "sun protection factor." This is the dose of UV radiation required to produce one MED (minimal erythema dose) on protected skin after application of 2 mg/cm^2 of product, divided by the UV radiation needed to produce one MED on unprotected skin. Because erythema is produced by UV-B radiation only, the SPF rating refers to its ability to protect from UV-B and *not* UV-A. There is no standard measure of UV-A protection. It is therefore important to choose a sunscreen that provides broad-spectrum protection and lists both UV-B (an SPF rating) and UV-A radiation (no current rating available) on its label.

TABLE 47-1 Common Chemical Sunscreen Agents

UV-A Filters	UV-B Filters	UV-A + UV-B Filters
Avobenzone (Parsol 1789) Encamsule (Mexoryl SX) Methyl anthranilate	Para-aminobenzoic acid (PABA) Cinoxate Homosalate Octyl methoxycinnamate (octinoxate; Eusolex 2292) Octyl salicylate (octisalate)	Dioxybenzone Drometrizole trisiloxane (Mexoryl XL) Octocrylene Oxybenzone (Eusolex 4360) Sulisobenzone

Sunscreens can be categorized as either physical or chemical sunscreens. Physical sunscreen agents work by physically blocking the penetration of UV radiation into the skin by reflecting or scattering light. The most common physical sunscreen agents are titanium dioxide and zinc oxide. Both of these block UV-A and UV-B radiation and are well tolerated on the skin, with a low risk of irritation. Chemical sunscreen agents work by absorbing the harmful UV rays and transforming them to harmless longer-wave radiation.

PABA (para-aminobenzoic acid) was one of the first chemical sunscreen agents available. It absorbs UV-B radiation but causes significant skin sensitivities, so it has generally been replaced by newer agents. Table 47-1 lists some of the common chemical sunscreen agents and their primary filtering actions.

Another factor to consider with sunscreens is their water resistance classification. For sunscreens to be labeled "water resistant," they must maintain their SPF level after 40 minutes of water immersion. "Very water resistant" sunscreens (formerly called "waterproof") maintain their SPF level after 80 minutes of water immersion.

Cosmetic Skin Care Products

In addition to the various cosmeceutical agents and sunscreens, it is important also to understand the use of cosmetic skin care products. Adults use an average of seven skin care products daily and billions of dollars are spent annually in the United States on skin cleansers and moisturizers; thus, it behooves the physician to have some understanding of skin care basics. The stratum corneum plays a key role in the use of cosmetic skin care products. The general appearance of the skin depends on the status of the stratum corneum. When it has adequate moisture, the stratum corneum is soft, pliant, and smooth and reflects light. The skin will then have a "radiance" or "glow." When the stratum corneum does not have adequate moisture, the skin will be rough and may have scaling or cracks. This roughness scatters light and the skin then has a dull appearance. Skin care involves cleansing the skin and ensuring adequate moisture content in the stratum corneum by preserving the integrity of the epidermal barrier. *Skin care regimens involve the daily use of cleansers, toners, and moisturizers.*

Cleansers

The basic function of a cleanser is to cleanse the skin. There is a hydrolipid film covering the surface of the skin that becomes soiled through contact with dirt and pollutants as well as by secretions from sebaceous and sweat glands. Shed corneocytes, decomposition products from the cornification process, as well as microorganisms also may contaminate this hydrolipid film. The challenge for cleansers is to remove this soil and not strip the hydrolipid film in the process, which would impair the epidermal barrier. There are two *major categories of cleansers: soap/detergents and emulsion cleaning agents*.

Soaps and detergents contain surfactant agents that increase the affinity of dissimilar phases for each other. This allows oil and water to mix. These are foaming cleansers and generally remove oil from skin, and thus are best as cleansers for oily skin. Soaps are the alkali salt of a fatty acid and leave an alkaline residue on the skin. This raises the pH of the skin, which increases *Propionibacteria* counts and can exacerbate acne. There are very few true soaps remaining in the marketplace; most have been replaced by synthetic detergents. Common detergent agents found in skin cleansers are sodium and ammonium lauryl sulfate, sodium laureth sulfate, cocamidopropyl betaine, and lauramphocarboxyglycinate.

Emulsion cleaning agents are oil-in-water emulsions or water-in-oil emulsions. They are usually cleansing milks or cleansing creams. They are less drying generally than detergents and can leave a residue of oil on the skin. These cleansers are better suited to drier skin types.

Toners

Toners are leave-on products applied to the skin after cleansing. They are designed to freshen and tone the skin and prepare the skin for the application of a moisturizer. When soaps were commonly used as cleansers, toners also served to remove the alkali residue and restore the acid mantle of the skin. In addition, toners are used to remove surface oil and debris and can be a delivery vehicle for other agents applied to the skin. Many toners have astringent agents such as witch hazel, ethanol, citrus extracts, and potassium alum as their key components. These are best for oily skin types. Alternatively, toners may have humectant agents such as propylene glycol, butylene glycol, and sorbitol, which may increase the moisture content of dry skin.

Moisturizers

Moisturizers are products applied to the skin that promote and restore the epidermal barrier function and thus increase the water content of the stratum corneum. We lose approximately 500 mL of water daily through our skin (i.e., transepidermal water loss). Moisturizers are designed to maintain the water content of skin between 10% and 30%. Skin moisturizers are classified as *occlusive agents, humectant agents, and emollient agents*. *Occlusive agents* act as an enhanced skin barrier by adding a hydrophobic film to the surface of the skin. This further impairs evaporation and conserves the moisture content of the stratum corneum. Common occlusive agents include *petrolatum, mineral oil, paraffin, silicone, fats, and wax*. *Humectant agents* attract water into the stratum corneum. This water usually is drawn from the dermis, but humectants can also attract water from the environment if the ambient humidity is over 70%. It is important to note that humectants can increase transepidermal water loss if the epidermal barrier is not intact. Humectant ingredients commonly found in skin moisturizers are *glycerin, hyaluronic acid, urea, propylene glycol, gelatin, honey, and sorbitol*. *Emollient agents* are substances that fill in the cracks and crevices in the stratum corneum. They are usually also barrier agents and include substances such as *mineral oil, lanolin, ceramides, silicone, fatty esters, and fatty alcohols*.

Most moisturizers are formulated as *creams*, which are water-in-oil emulsions, or as *lotions*, which are oil-in-water emulsions and are lighter than the cream formulations. The heaviness of the moisturizer depends on this formulation as well as the amount and characteristics of the occlusive agents. Night creams are examples of moisturizers designed as heavier creams, whereas a light, nongreasy moisturizer may be a lotion containing a weaker occlusive agent with the addition of humectant agents.

Choosing a Skin Care Regimen

Proper skin cleansing and moisturizing must work in harmony to maintain epidermal barrier integrity and adequate hydration of the stratum corneum. Before choosing a skin care regimen, it is important to consider the skin condition. Note the status of the stratum corneum and the epidermal barrier and determine whether the skin is oily or dry and whether it appears dehydrated. Sensitivities should be considered. The presence of acne lesions, dyschromias, and other signs of photodamage should be noted. The environment should also be considered because humidity, temperature, wind, and pollutants are factors affecting skin care choices.

There are as many individual skin care regimens as there are products to choose from. It is impossible to give a standard skin care regimen or list all brands of skin care products on the market. The following is this author's approach and may provide some general guidance.

For oily skin types, choose a foaming cleanser with an astringent toner and lighter moisturizer with less occlusive and more humectant properties. *For drier skin types*, a cleansing milk or cream is preferable with a humectant toner and heavier moisturizer with increased occlusive and emollient effect.

The choice then to add cosmeceutical agents to the basic regimen depends on the desired structural changes for the skin conditions present.

For acne-prone skin, the use of lotions for moisturizing is preferable to creams. AHAs and BHAs are very beneficial in exfoliating the skin and unblocking sebaceous glands. Retinols may also be useful, as well as the anti-inflammatory action of vitamin C serums.

For hyperpigmentation, products containing hydroquinone have been the mainstay of treatment. Other lightening agents such as kojic acid and azelaic acid are beneficial, as is vitamin C serum. Exfoliating agents such as retinol should be used, and daily use of sunscreen is important.

The largest demand for skin care advice is in the realm of *skin rejuvenation and the treatment of photodamage and aging of the skin*. In addition to the basic skin care regimen of appropriate cleansing and moisturizing, products with active cosmeceutical ingredients are beneficial, along with a sunscreen to prevent further damage. The daily use of a medical exfoliant such as retinol and an AHA is an important step in any skin rejuvenation regimen, along with the topical application of vitamin C serum. The use of a peptide cream with Argireline and Matrixyl may also be beneficial. A broad-spectrum sunscreen with minimum SPF 30 should be used daily. Although this is one suggested approach to skin rejuvenation, there are many other cosmeceutical ingredients and regimens that may be useful.

The Challenge of Cosmeceuticals

Cosmeceuticals represent the next new frontier in aesthetic medicine and the fastest-growing segment of the skin care industry. They are the driving force in the field of skin care research. However, there are very few peer-reviewed clinical trials for most of these products and there is little incentive to conduct extensive scientific research and studies. There is the concern that if research proves efficacy then the product would no longer be considered a cosmeceutical, but would be classified as a drug and be subject to the rigorous governmental approval processes. The dilemma for skin care companies is that physicians require scientific proof of efficacy, yet this proof would then remove the newly developed product from the market and subject it to scrutiny as a new drug. The current confusion in the marketplace about cosmeceuticals and the issue of hope versus hype versus fact is likely to remain until new regulations are in place.

BIBLIOGRAPHY

Draelos Z: Cutaneous exfoliation. Cosmet Dermatol 10:51–57, 2000.

Draelos Z: Procedures in Cosmetic Dermatology Series: Cosmeceuticals. Philadelphia, Saunders, 2005.

Draelos Z, Thaman L (eds): Cosmetic Formulation of Skin Care Products. New York, Taylor & Francis, 2006, pp 167–215.

Farris P: Cosmeceuticals: A review of the science behind the claims. Cosmet Dermatol 16:59–70, 2003.

Geffken C: What's in a name? Global Cosmetic Industry (GCI) 5:28–30, 2004.

Kligman D: Cosmeceuticals. Dermatol Clin 18:609–615, 2000.

O'Rourke K: Cosmetic pharmaceuticals in dermatology. Curr Probl Dermatol 12:291–293, 2000.

Small R: Skin care products. In Usatine R (ed): Dermatologic and Cosmetic Procedures in Office Practice. Philadelphia, Elsevier Saunders, 2010.

CHAPTER 48

LASERS AND PULSED-LIGHT DEVICES: HAIR REMOVAL

Barry Auster • Gary Page

Photoepilation (laser hair removal) is one of a variety of methods for the removal of unwanted hair. Others include electroepilation, mechanical epilation, depilatories, and waxing. Laser hair removal has rapidly evolved over the past 10 years and there are now numerous U.S. Food and Drug Administration (FDA)–approved laser or intense pulsed-light (IPL) devices available for hair removal. The current technologies evolved from the clinical observation of hair reduction in laser-treated congenital (pigmented) hairy nevi. The potential market for laser hair removal is tremendous.

PRINCIPLES FOR PHOTOEPILATION WITH LASERS

Light energy emitted from a monochromatic laser (a single wavelength of light) or an IPL source (produces a broad spectrum of light using filters to block unwanted wavelengths) is absorbed by a pigmented object (in this case, hair) and is converted into heat energy. This heat energy destroys the hair follicle, causing a long-term reduction in hair growth. This process of transforming light to heat energy and destroying targeted pigmented tissue is called *selective photothermolysis*.

The concept of selective photothermolysis was first presented by Anderson and Parrish in 1983. This is the process by which thermal damage is confined to the particular target tissue. It is based on two important concepts. The first is that *chromophores* (e.g., hair, blood vessels, melanosomes/pigment) are objects that preferentially absorb light of specific wavelengths (Fig. 48-1). The second is *thermal relaxation time* (TRT), which is defined as the time required for an object to cool to 50% of the temperature resulting from laser exposure. When the target tissue absorbs the laser light, energy is changed to heat, which causes thermal tissue damage and heat transference to the surrounding tissues. For lasers, *pulse width* is the duration (in milliseconds [msec]) that the light energy is applied. A laser with a pulse width less than the TRT of the target conducts very little heat to the surrounding tissues. Consequently, it is possible to confine the laser's destructive effect to a specific area of tissue based on the chromophore content and the rapidity at which the light energy is applied (Fig. 48-2).

Lasers are *monochromatic*, which means the light is of a single wavelength or color. Each type of laser has a different wavelength and each chromophore absorbs the specific light energy in that laser wavelength, converting it to thermal energy. Melanin is the target chromophore for photoepilation. Hemoglobin, another chromophore, is targeted to destroy vascular lesions. Water and collagen are also chromophores. Each chromophore has a spectral absorption pattern that determines the wavelengths of light that are most absorbed and converted to thermal energy. It is important to match the wavelength of the laser with the specific chromophore for targeted destruction and to avoid damage to adjacent tissues. *The amount of energy needed to destroy the hair follicle is usually close to the energy level at which skin damage occurs. Determining the treatment energy level for a particular patient without causing excessive surrounding tissue damage is the most clinically demanding task.* Certain types of lasers are then chosen because they are more effective at destroying hair follicles without causing excessive surrounding damage, which could lead to burns or scarring.

The lasers used for epilation fall into four categories: alexandrite (755 nm), neodymium-doped yttrium aluminum garnet (Nd:YAG; 1064 nm), ruby (694 nm), and diode (810 nm).

Treatment tip or spot sizes vary from 2 to 15 mm, and pulse widths vary from 10 to 100 msec. In addition, the repetition rate can vary from 1 to 10 or more pulses per second (hertz). Faster repetition rates improve efficiency in treating larger areas such as the back or legs. The size of the area being affected by each burst of energy (spot size) is variable from machine to machine and from laser tip to laser tip. In general, the larger the spot size, the greater the depth of light penetration at the same energy level. Lasers and IPL machines most often measure the energy level delivered to the skin in joules per square centimeter (J/cm^2), also known as *fluence* (Fig. 48-3A).

Intense pulsed-light (Fig. 48-3B and C) devices are flashlamp devices that emit light over the entire visual spectrum and hence are not monochromatic like lasers. Specificity for different hair colors and skin types may be achieved with various cut-off filters and fluence settings. Recently, IPL devices have increased in popularity because of their versatility and cost effectiveness. With one device and multiple handpieces/filters, physicians can treat most conditions. With regard to photoepilation, IPL devices are now equally as efficacious as lasers. In addition, a hybrid device (Syneron) uses a combination of IPL followed by radiofrequency. It is based on the principle of electrical impedance, whereby electrical energy flows preferentially to a warmer target. This device reportedly has some beneficial effects for gray and white hairs.

The ideal patient for photoepilation is someone with light skin and dark hair, so that all the generated thermal energy is focused on the melanin chromophore of the hair. Light hair is very difficult to treat because it is not differentiated from the surrounding light skin. Studies are ongoing using a melanin dye (Melamax; Creative Technologies, Chesapeake, VA) that is driven into the hair root by an ultrasound device. Preliminary data showed modest improvement in the effect of hair removal lasers on white or blonde hair. The effect was greater on vellus than terminal hairs. Similarly, it is very difficult in most instances to treat black hair on black skin. When patients are tanned, care must be taken lest the skin itself be burned during the treatments.

Cooling during treatment is important. IPL devices contact the skin and use a combination of a chilled gel and a chilled sapphire tip. The latter is a vast improvement over glass tips, which cracked frequently from the stress of temperature changes. Some devices

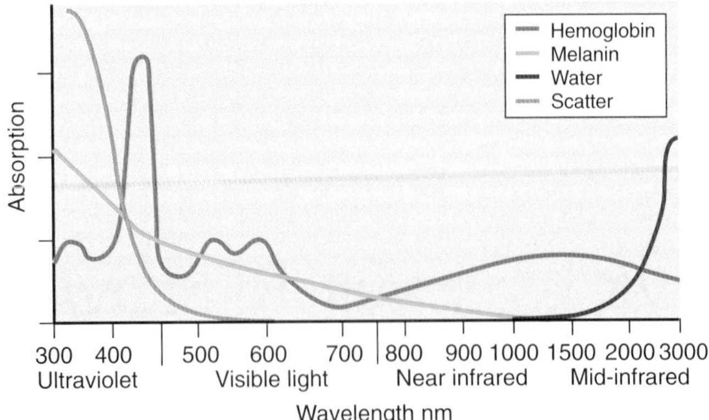

Figure 48-1 Relative absorption of light by biologic tissues. By selecting specific wavelengths of light, a selective effect on biologic tissue is achieved. Whenever light hits tissue, it can be transmitted, scattered, reflected, or absorbed, depending on the type of tissue and the selected wavelength(s) (color) of the light. However, light *absorption* and subsequent tissue heating must take place to achieve any biologic effect, and a given wavelength of light may be strongly absorbed by one type of tissue and be transmitted or scattered by another. Different tissues have different absorption characteristics depending on their specific components (i.e., skin is composed of cells, hair follicles, pigment, blood vessels, sweat glands). The main absorbing targets, or chromophores, of tissues are (1) hemoglobin in blood; (2) melanin in skin, hair, and moles; and (3) water (present in all biologic tissue).

(e.g., LightSheer Diode Laser; Lumenis, Santa Clara, Calif) use a cold-water chamber to cool tissue. Dynamic cooling devices use a chlorofluorocarbon, U.S. Environmental Protection Agency–approved refrigerant spray. This is available only on lasers produced by Candela (Wayland, Mass), which has proprietary rights to the technology. A final alternative chilling method is using cold air blown on the site being treated (Zimmer MedizinSystems Corp., Irvine, Calif).

The FDA has recently approved a home-use laser (TRIA Beauty, Dublin, Calif) for hair removal. This is a diode laser and costs approximately $600. Preliminary data, although limited, show beneficial results.

Hair Growth Phases and Treatment Implications

Hair follicles have been difficult to treat with lasers. There is a wide variation in depth at different anatomic sites, with the deepest follicular bulbs at 5 mm. This is beyond the range of penetration of

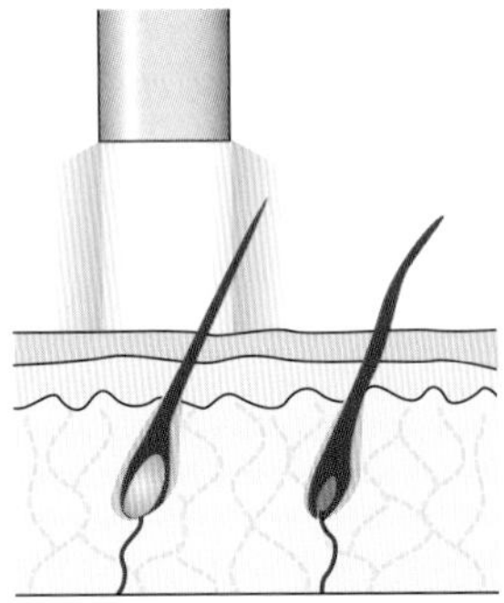

Figure 48-2 Three principles of selective photothermolysis: (1) Penetrating wavelength of light should be absorbed selectively by target tissue; (2) pulse duration should match thermal relaxation time of target tissue; and (3) sufficient fluence (J/cm^2) should be applied to damage target tissue. (Redrawn from a presentation by Brian Zelicksen, MD, American Society for Laser Medicine and Surgery Meeting, April 2002.)

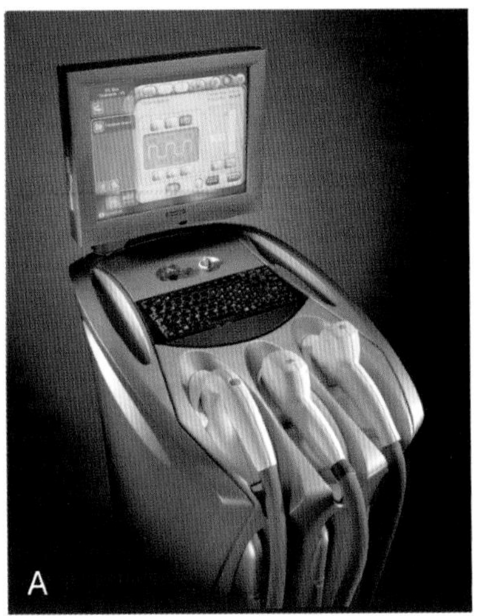

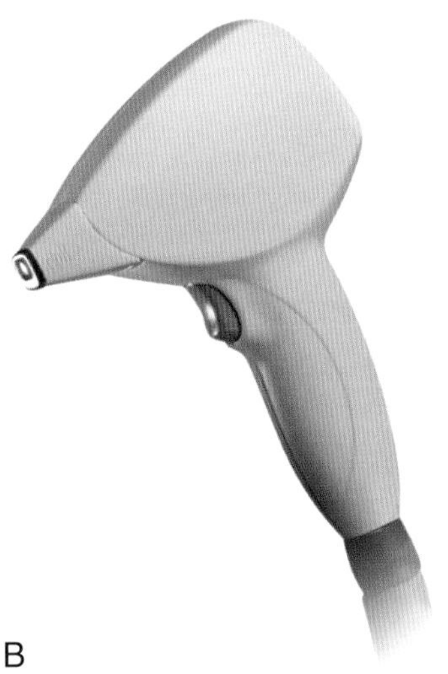

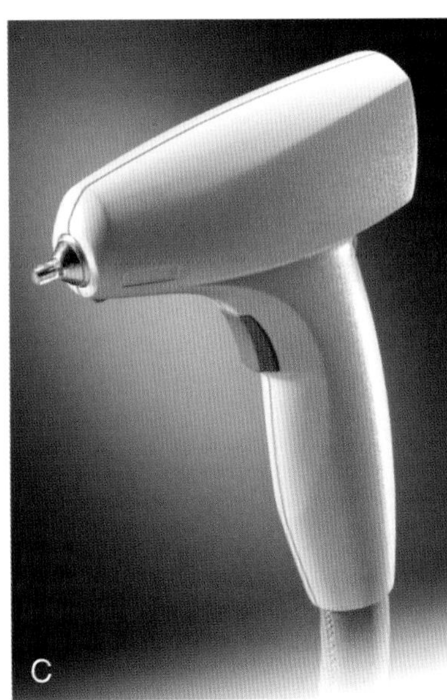

Figure 48-3 Intense pulsed-light and laser system. **A,** Lumenis One. **B,** LightSheer handpiece. **C,** Multi-Spot Nd:YAG handpiece. (Courtesy of Lumenis, Santa Clara, Calif.)

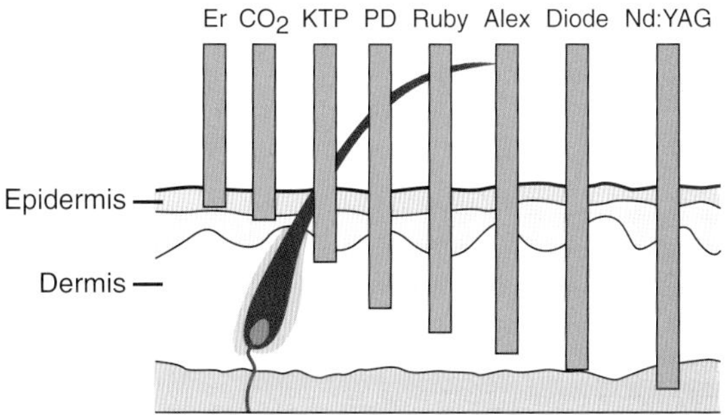

Figure 48-4 Depth of penetration of various cutaneous lasers. Alex, alexandrite; Er, erbium; KTP, potassium titanyl phosphate; PD, pulsed dye.

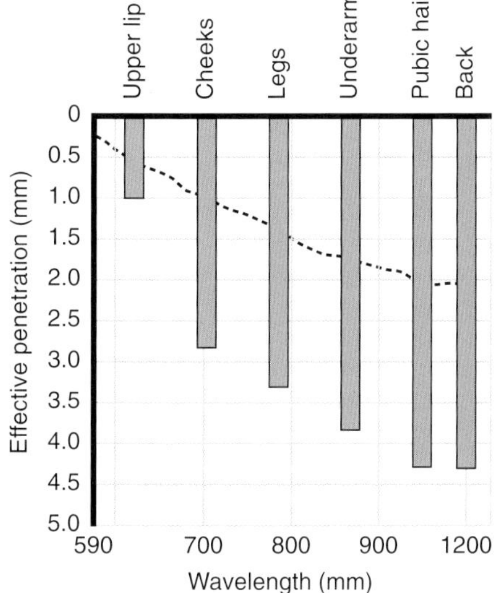

Figure 48-5 Depth of hair follicles in different body locations. *Dotted line* indicates penetration depth of light frequency.

most lasers (Figs. 48-4 and 48-5). Whereas upper lip hair follicles range from 1 to 2.5 mm in depth, pubic and axillary hairs may lay as deep as 5 mm. In addition, most authorities agree that *only the anagen phase* of follicular growth is responsive to laser-induced thermal energy damage. The percentage of follicles in the anagen phase at any one anatomic site varies from 30% on the trunk to as high as 80% on the scalp. Therefore, to understand laser hair removal more fully, a knowledge of hair anatomy and development is necessary.

Hair is composed of keratinous fibers that grow from follicles over the entire body surface except the palms and soles. The number of follicles is finite at birth. Growth involves three stages (Fig. 48-6). *Anagen* is the active growth phase of the hair follicle, during which the hair contains abundant melanin. *Catagen* is a period of regression when cell division terminates in the long part of the follicle and the lower part of the follicle begins to involute. The final, resting phase is called *telogen*, during which the old hair is emitted and shed before the development of a new hair begins. During telogen there is very little or no melanin in the *follicle* and hence laser treatments will have very little to no effect. The length of these three individual phases of hair growth varies widely with anatomic site (Table 48-1). Because of this, patients must be advised that 100% hair reduction may be impossible because of the relative unresponsiveness of the telogen follicle to laser photoepilation. Hairs, particularly on the trunk, may remain in telogen for longer than 3 months. Therefore, patients need to be advised that follow-up treatments may be needed up to 1 year after initiation of therapy to allow for conversion of telogen hairs to anagen.

Hairs are of two types: *terminal hairs* are thick, long, and pigmented with melanin and found throughout the body surface, whereas *vellus hairs* are thin, short, and depigmented.

Figure 48-6 demonstrates the structure and life cycle of a typical hair. The hair itself grows from the bulb, which consists of the hair matrix and the dermal papilla. The *papilla* is an area of highly vascularized connective tissue that provides the nutrients for the rapidly dividing cells of the matrix. During periods of active growth, matrix cells divide every 24 to 72 hours and migrate upward to become keratinized and packed into layers that compose the *hair shaft*.

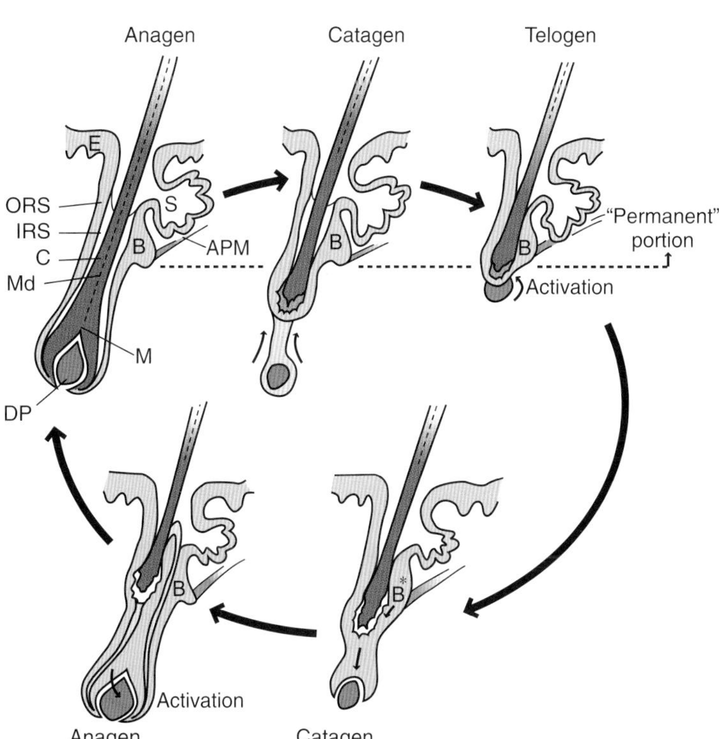

Figure 48-6 The different phases of the hair cycle: anagen, catagen, and telogen. Labeled structures include arrector pili muscle (APM), bulge (B), cortex (C), dermal papilla (DP), epidermis (E), inner root sheath (IRS), matrix (M), medulla (Md), outer root sheath (ORS), and sebaceous gland (S). B and B* denote quiescent and activated bulge cells, respectively. Follicular structures above the *dotted line* form the permanent portion of the follicle; keratinocytes below the bulge degenerate during catagen and telogen. (Redrawn from Cotsarelis G, Sun TT, Lavker RM: Label-retaining cells reside in the bulge area of pilosebaceous unit: Implications for follicular stem cells, hair cycle, and skin carcinogenesis. Cell 61:1329–1337, 1990.)

TABLE 48-1 Hair Depth and Hair Cycle

Body Area	Telogen Hair (%)	Anagen Hair (%)	Telogen Duration	Follicles Density (1/cm^2)	Follicle Depth (mm)
Scalp	13	85	3–4 mo	350	3–5
Beard	30	70	10 wk	500	2–4
Upper lip	35	65	6 wk	500	1–2.5
Axillae	70	30	3 mo	65	3.5–4.5
Trunk	70	30	12 wk	70	2–4.5
Pubic area	70	30	12 wk	70	3.5–4.5
Arms	80	20	18 wk	80	2.5–4
Legs and thighs	80	20	24 wk	60	2.5–4
Breasts	70	30	12 wk	65	3–4.5

The "bulge," which is a protrusion near the attachment of the arrector pili muscle, has recently been determined to consist of stem cells important in hair regeneration. The bulge is generally located 1 to 1.5 mm below the cutaneous surface. As mentioned previously, hairs grow in recurrent cycles (see Table 48-1). Therefore, the target of laser thermolysis is twofold: the bulge and the papilla.

Fitzpatrick Skin Types and Treatment Implications

As the thermolytic hair removal technique has developed, it has become clear that proper patient selection is critical for success. The two preeminent factors in patient selection are skin type and hair color (Fig. 48-7). Skin types are based on the Fitzpatrick classification system:

Type I Always burns, never tans
Type II Always burns, sometimes tans
Type III Sometimes burns, always tans
Type IV Rarely burns, always tans
Type V Moderately pigmented
Type VI Black skin

Fitzpatrick grouped patients into the six different skin types based on the amount of pigmentation found in the skin. Skin type I has the least pigment and type VI has the most. The lower skin types are most sensitive to ultraviolet (UV) radiation ("sunburn") and to development of solar damage such as pigmentation, skin thinning, actinic changes, and skin cancer. More freckles are also found in skin types I and II and fewer in type III and above. The higher the skin type, the more melanin is present in the epidermis and the more resistant the skin is to sunburn. Hair removal treatment is easier in patients who are most sensitive to UV radiation because they have less melanin *in their skin* to absorb the therapeutic light. More light energy passes through to the hair follicles itself and there is less risk of photothermal damage to the skin.

In general, skin types I and II are most easily treated. Types III, IV, and V are more difficult to treat. Skin type VI may be treated only in rare circumstances. Because of increased epidermal melanin, there is a higher risk of thermal damage to the skin in types V and VI, which may cause scarring or pigmentary alterations such as hypopigmentation or postinflammatory hyperpigmentation. Only a few devices (Nd:YAG and diode lasers) have received FDA approval to treat type VI skin. Extreme care must be taken in treating type V and VI skin types, particularly if the hairs are fine or light. Permanent dyspigmentation may occur if such patients are overtreated.

Indications

- Hypertrichosis
- Hirsutism
- Cosmetic (e.g., bikini lines)
- Pseudofolliculitis barbae

Hypertrichosis, excessive vellus or lanugo hair, may be localized or generalized and may occur in both men and women. It is not related to excess testosterone.

Hirsutism involves development of coarse terminal hair (e.g., on the face) in children or women resulting from increased levels of male hormone. In women, the most common clinical causes are congenital adrenal hyperplasia and polycystic ovaries. If a woman demonstrates symptomatology of these disorders (e.g., irregular menses, infertility, obesity, acne), then *appropriate laboratory testing should be performed*. These tests should be carried out under fasting conditions and include *insulin level, glucose, luteinizing hormone, follicle-stimulating hormone, prolactin, dehydroepiandrosterone (DHEA), and free testosterone*. If a woman does demonstrate androgen excess, referral to an endocrinologist is appropriate. Spironolactone, a competitive inhibitor of DHEA binding, may be used supplementally and also is effective in women with hypertrichosis without androgen excess.

Pseudofolliculitis barbae resulting from ingrown hairs is improved dramatically by photoepilation. By reducing the number of hairs, the severe infection may be significantly diminished and the patient's symptoms markedly improved. Although there may be some pigment changes, they may improve over time and the risks may be outweighed by the benefit to the patient's quality of life. Unwanted permanent hair loss may also occur because of treatment.

Contraindications

Absolute

- History of keloids
- Isotretinoin (Accutane) use in past 6 months

Relative

- Herpes simplex (active; use antiviral drugs if there is a history starting the day before and continuing for 5 days afterward)
- Photosensitizing medications (e.g., St. John's wort, tetracycline, thiazides, captopril)
- Recent plucking, waxing, or electrolysis
- Pregnancy (a general precaution; no adverse effects are known)
- White hair
- Recently tanned skin (relative, because degree of tan is important, and only a change in the parameters for treatment may be required; patients with a tan should know that treatments must be more conservative and therefore may not show the optimal benefit)

Individuals with a history of herpes simplex should be treated prophylactically with antiviral drugs before and during treatment. Individuals who have been on isotretinoin within 6 months tend to have adverse healing and susceptibility to hypertrophic scarring. In addition, patients on photosensitizing medications or supplements may be treated, but treatment settings should be conservative. Because the hair itself is the major chromophore for the laser, patients should be advised to *avoid* waxing, electrolysis, plucking, depilatories, or shaving immediately before treatment because the resulting inflammatory process generally involves more pigmented changes, which will absorb the light energy. In female patients who have plucked hair on a daily basis, the latter requirement may present a difficult conundrum because an effective treatment requires approximately 1 mm of hair protruding above the skin surface. Between treatments, patients are allowed to continue their own hair removal methods, with shaving being the preferred method.

Safety Issues

Physicians who use lasers for hair removal should be acutely aware of the potential for ocular damage. All of the devices may cause blindness. The importance of eye protection for both the practitioner (or technician) and the patient is paramount and cannot be overstressed. Laser goggles should be labeled with the wavelength they block. When working around the orbit, metallic, totally occlusive goggles are preferred (Oculo-Plastik, Inc., Montreal, Quebec); in some cases a corneal shield inserted under the lids is best. The laser or IPL handpiece must be carefully guarded, and those using it must ensure that it is pointed away from the eyes at all times. Some office practices designate one of the clinical personnel as the "laser safety officer" in charge of ensuring that eye protection is worn by all in the treatment rooms and that warning signs are posted outside the door when the laser is in operation. The warning sign should be taken down when the laser is not in use or the sign will soon be ignored.

Factors Influencing Type of Equipment Used

- Reliability
- Purchase price
- Technical support
- Training provided
- Cost of maintenance contract
- Space needed in office for storage
- Disposable materials cost
- Ease of operation
- Warranty period
- Length of time the particular company representative has been "in the business"

Purchasing a hair removal device is a challenging task. It is important to determine the reliability of the unit, the available warranty, and exchange and support contracts, including costs, because these units are mechanically complicated and do break down. The cost of a service contract should be considered part of the acquisition cost. Even more important is the educational support and training provided by the company for current and future staff members. All units have a learning curve, and training seminars with on-site education on an ongoing basis are crucial for safety and efficacy of treatments. Appropriate technical support is also an important consideration, as are anticipated upgrades. Repairs must be guaranteed on a timely basis. Finally, it is prudent to have frank discussions with physicians who currently use and have experience with the equipment being considered.

Equipment

- 4 × 4 gauze pads.
- Hair clippers.
- Alcohol to cleanse the skin.
- Cooling gel or Zimmer Chiller (depends on device used).
- Topical anesthetic. EMLA (eutectic mixture of local anesthetics) cream is preferable because of its vasoconstrictive effect, which reduces the competing chromophore of hemoglobin. Many offices use topical anesthetics prepared by specialty pharmacies that contain much higher concentrations of lidocaine. Recently, the FDA has begun to look into these formulations because they have not been tested for safety. Operators should be aware that these agents may be absorbed percutaneously with resultant neurologic and cardiac effects. There have been several deaths reported from overuse of these agents topically. Care should be taken to apply limited quantities and to avoid occluding them if large areas are involved. (See Chapter 5, Local and Topical Anesthesia Complications, and Chapter 10, Topical Anesthesia.)
- Protective laser eyewear (goggles and metal eyepieces).
- Laser/IPL equipment.
- Cooling pack/ice for post-treatment care.
- Smoke evacuator or a room exhaust fan to remove the smell of burning hair.
- For offices that have not previously used lasers there are certain U.S. Occupational Safety and Health Administration (OSHA) requirements for the treatment room. There should be no mirrors, or any present must be covered with paper. If the room is on the first floor it should have no windows or they should be covered with blackout shades. If the door to the room has a window it should also be covered. The door also should have a sign on the outside that says "Laser in Use." Although uncommon, OSHA inspections may result in fines in the tens of thousands of dollars if infractions are discovered.

Preprocedure Patient Preparation

The patient should fill out the aesthetics questionnaire form (see Chapter 46, Introduction to Aesthetic Medicine, Fig. 46-1) and be supplied with educational materials before the visit with the clinician (see patient education and consent forms online at www.expertconsult.com). The patient must not tan for 4 weeks prior and should not pluck any hair for at least 5 days prior.

It is extremely important to know the medical history, including use of medications and tanning history, and to determine Fitzpatrick skin type. The power settings for the full treatment are determined at this time and recorded. During the initial visit, many practices perform test patches with the settings that will be used. This is particularly important in types V and VI skin. For the darker skin types, adverse reactions such as edema and crusting may become evident up to 2 days after treatment. Some practitioners will treat the ideal patient (Fitzpatrick type I or II with dark brown or black hair) at this initial appointment, but will observe the effect of the test spots on other skin types before initiating the full treatment.

A useful adjunct for patients who have a combination of coarse and fine hairs is topical eflornithine (Vaniqa; SkinMedica, Inc., Carlsbad, Calif). This product inhibits hair growth. It is useful for vellus hairs and does not affect the treatment of terminal hairs. It can be used to improve the overall appearance at completion of the treatment process and can be started immediately after the consultation session. However, hair growth tends to recur once the medication is stopped.

Procedure and Technique of Hair Removal

1. The patient's skin type is determined on the Fitzpatrick skin type scale (see Fig. 48-7).
2. Proper settings are selected (individualized with each unit). Each company will provide training with its particular unit. The settings are too variable to list individually here.
3. The hair is clipped to a 1-mm length.
4. The skin is wiped with alcohol.
5. Various topical anesthetics may be used before treatment.

Skin Typing

For successful hair removal, it is necessary to determine the correct typing of your skin. Your doctor will consider your skin type when planning your treatment program.

Skin type is categorized by the Fitzpatrick skin type scale, which ranges from Type I (fair) to Type VI (black). The main factors that influence skin type are genetic disposition and reaction to sun exposure and tanning habits.

Skin type is determined genetically and is one of the many aspects of overall appearance. Genetics also determines the eye color, hair color, and the way skin pigments react to light. The way your skin reacts to sun exposure is important in correctly assessing your skin type. Sunbathing or artificial tanning (e.g., tanning creams) affects the evaluation of your skin color.

Please take a few minutes and fill out this questionnaire to help us determine your skin type and treat you properly.

Genetic Disposition

	0	1	2	3	4	Score
What color are your eyes?	Light blue, gray, green	Blue, gray, green	Blue	Dark brown	Brownish black	
What is the natural color of your hair?	Sandy red	Blonde	Chestnut/dark blonde	Dark brown	Black	
What color is your skin (unexposed areas)?	Reddish	Very pale	Pale with beige tint	Light brown	Dark brown	
Do you have freckles on unexposed areas?	Many	Several	Few	Incidental	None	
					Genetic Disposition Total	

Reaction to Sun Exposure

	0	1	2	3	4	Score
What happens when you stay too long in the sun?	Painful redness, blistering, peeling	Blistering followed by peeling	Burns sometimes followed by peeling	Rare burns	Never had burns	
To what degree do you turn brown?	Hardly or not at all	Light tan	Reasonable tan	Tan very easy	Turn dark brown quickly	
Do you turn brown with several hours of sun exposure?	Never	Seldom	Sometimes	Often	Always	
How does your face react to the sun?	Very sensitive	Sensitive	Normal	Very resistant	Never had a problem	
					Reaction to Sun Exposure Total	

Figure 48-7 Sample form to determine skin type. (Courtesy of John L. Pfenninger, MD, The Medical Procedures Center, PC, Midland, Mich.)

6. The cooling gel is applied; most lasers and IPL devices have integrated cooling systems.
7. Eye protection is provided to the practitioner and the patient.
8. Photoepilation is performed.
9. Observe for the proper tissue reaction (see later discussion).
10. Ice packs or chilled aloe gel are applied.
11. Follow-up sessions are scheduled.

At the treatment session, hairs are clipped to a 1-mm length because if long hairs are left on the skin surface there is a risk that they will act as a heat sink and singe the underlying epidermis. Protective goggles are placed on the patient, laser operator, and anyone else present in the room. Proximity of the spot treatments varies from one device to another, but in general they should either be abutted or slightly overlapped (10% to 20%). *Observation of clinical response during the treatment is essential.* If either obvious burning of the skin or no effect to hairs or follicles is noted, energy fluences should be adjusted accordingly. The *ideal cutaneous response* is discrete perifollicular erythema and edema without coalescence into solid erythema. Observe for shearing or fracture of about 20% to 30% of the hairs during the treatment session and note the "sulfur" smell of thermally damaged hair. Patients should be advised that additional hairs will fall out over the ensuing 2 to 3 weeks (Figs. 48-8 through 48-10).

Tanning Habits

	1	2	3	4	5	Score
When did you last expose your body to sun (or artificial sunlamp/tanning cream)?	More than 3 months ago	2–3 months ago	1–2 months ago	Less than a month ago	Less than 2 weeks ago	
Did you expose the area to be treated to the sun?	Never	Hardly ever	Sometimes	Often	Always	
					Tanning Habits Total	

Add up the total scores for each of the three sections for your Skin Type Score. This will give you a better evaluation of your skin type.

Summary

Genetic Disposition Total	
Reaction to Sun Exposure Total	
Tanning Habits Total	
Skin Type Score	

Your Fitzpatrick Skin Type

Skin Type Score	Fitzpatrick Skin Type
0–7	I
8–16	II
17–24	III
25–30	IV
Over 30	V–VI

Note: This questionnaire is intended as a guideline for skin typing. Final evaluation of skin type should be determined by your doctor.

Figure 48-7, cont.

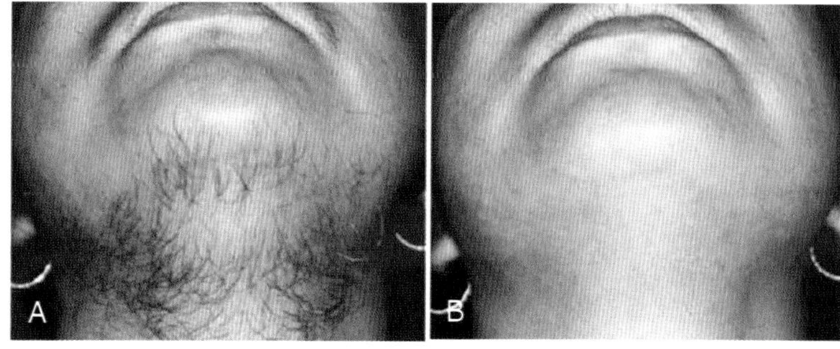

Figure 48-8 Before (**A**) and after (**B**) laser treatment for neck and face. (Courtesy of Nimish Patel, MD, The Laser Center, Ahmedabad, India.)

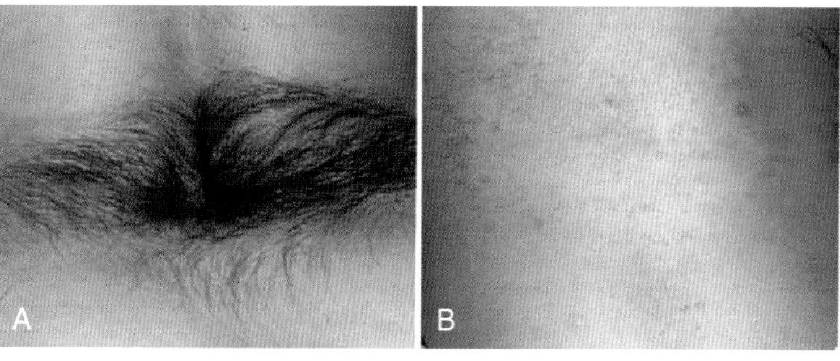

Figure 48-9 Before (**A**) and after (**B**) laser treatment for lower back. (Courtesy of Nimish Patel, MD, The Laser Center, Ahmedabad, India.)

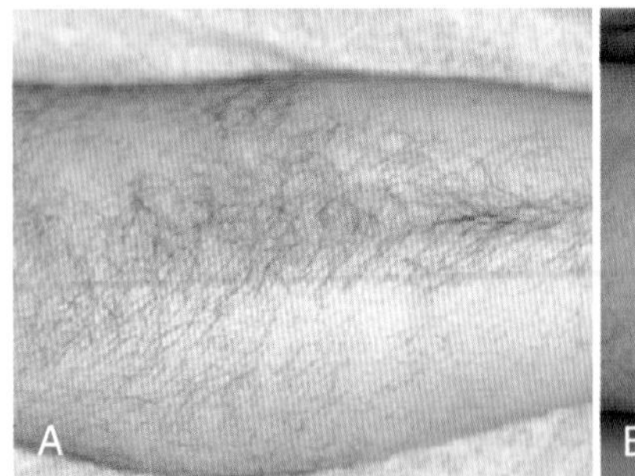

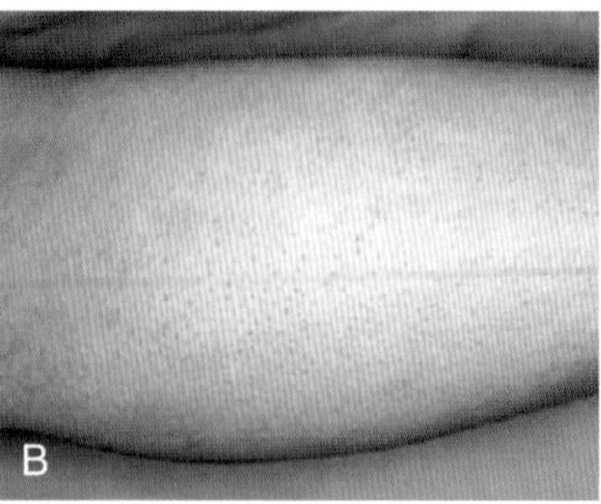

Figure 48-10 Before (**A**) and after (**B**) laser treatment for arm. (Courtesy of Valeria B. Campos, MD, Christine C. Dierickx, MD, and R. Rox Anderson, MD, Wellman Laboratories of Photomedicine, Harvard Medical School, Boston.)

Complications

- *Anesthesia complications*: Topical anesthetic creams may be used before treatment, but *caution should be used* because some deaths have been attributed to toxicity of anesthetics applied under occlusion over large areas.
- *Discomfort* associated with photoepilation is generally mild and transient and has been described as similar to a large rubber band snapping against the skin when the light pulse is triggered. *If the patient reports severe pain during the treatment, this should be considered as an indication of excessive energy with the potential for significant thermal injury.* Power should be immediately lowered and ice applied if the treated sites appear bright red or edematous.
- Ocular burns and blindness.
- Second-degree burns.
- *Hypopigmentation* is a difficult problem to treat but it usually improves on its own over a period of months to years.
- *Postinflammatory hyperpigmentation* may be treated with prescription as well as over-the-counter bleaching creams, light chemical peeling, or even pigment-specific lasers. Over-the-counter bleaching agents contain 2% hydroquinone and are modestly effective for this problem. Prescription agents containing 4% hydroquinone combined with tretinoin and fluocinolone (e.g., Tri-Luma Cream; Galderma Laboratories, Ft. Worth, Tex) are far more effective.
- *Scarring*: Hypertrophic scarring or keloids should be treated with currently acceptable modalities, which include intralesional steroid injections, silicone gel sheathing, and pulsed-dye laser treatments.
- Lack of satisfactory response with regrowth.
- *Stimulation of hair growth (rare)*: This is a rare event but does occur more commonly in dark, type III or IV skin types. This may be due to a biostimulatory rather than destructive effect. If it occurs, treatment with an alternative, longer-wavelength laser should be attempted.

Postprocedure Patient Education

The patient should be given the following instructions and advice:

- Do not pick at any skin peeling that may occur.
- Plucking residual hair is acceptable after treatment.
- Soothing gel, lotion, or cool packs may provide comfort.
- Makeup can be applied after 2 hours.
- Erythema may last for several hours.
- Sunscreen (SPF ≥ 30) should be used between sessions.
- Multiple treatments will be required at all anatomic sites, but the number varies.
- Treatment intervals will be every 3 to 4 weeks or longer depending on the site for five to six treatment sessions, then every 3 months for a year.

Cool compresses can be applied for 2 to 3 hours after treatment but are usually not needed after this time. On occasion, patients experience blistering that causes crusting. This usually does not occur until the following day. If it does occur, the patient can apply warm compresses and a topical antibiotic ointment. Future treatments will require that the settings be adjusted.

Conclusion

Photoepilation is a well-developed technology in the cosmetic medical field. Compared with electrolysis, treatments are more rapid, more comfortable, and more effective. The key to a successful laser hair removal practice is correct selection of patients for whom the treatment would be effective. Patients with dark skin types and light hair are poor candidates. Providing appropriate expectations for the patients before the onset of treatment is crucial. As our understanding and experience with this technology improve in the future, improved treatment responses as well as more acceptable home-use devices are likely to be seen.

CPT/Billing Code

17380 Electrolysis, epilation, each half-hour

ICD-9-CM Diagnostic Codes

704.1 Hirsutism, hypertrichosis
704.8 Pseudofolliculitis barbae
704.9 Disease of hair and follicle, NOS

Charges

A wide variation in charges for photoepilation exists between practices and within a practice. Variables that determine pricing include local competition, cost of equipment, size of the area being treated, and the duration of the treatment. Larger treatment areas require more provider or technician time and cause more "wear and tear" on the equipment. The majority of hair removal is considered to be cosmetic and thus patients need to pay out-of-pocket at the time of service. It is important that they understand this and sign an agreement beforehand stating the fees are known to them.

Suppliers

(See contact information online at www.expertconsult.com.)

Equipment
Candela Corp.
Cynosure, Inc.
Lumenis, Inc.
Palomar Medical Technologies, Inc.
Zimmer MedizinSystems, Inc.
Patient education materials
MJD Patient Communications

BIBLIOGRAPHY

Anderson RR, Parrish JA: Selective photothermolysis: Precise microsurgery by selective absorption of pulsed radiation. Science 220:524–527, 1983.

Babilas P, Schreml S, Szeimies RM, Landthaler M: Intense pulsed light (IPL): A review. Lasers Surg Med 42:93–104, 2010.

Draelos ZD: Hair removal techniques. In Merli GJ (ed): The Clinics Atlas of Office Procedures: Basic Cosmetic Procedures. Philadelphia, WB Saunders, 2000, pp 142–149.

Eremia S, Li C, Newman N: Laser hair removal with alexandrite versus diode laser using four treatment sessions: 1-Year results. Dermatol Surg 27:925–929, 2001.

Eremia S, Li CY, Umar SH, Newman N: Laser hair removal: Long-term results with a 755 nm alexandrite laser. Dermatol Surg 27:920–924, 2001.

Goldberg D: Procedures in Cosmetic Dermatology Series: Lasers and Lights, Volume 1: Vascular/Pigmentation/Scars/Medical Applications. Philadelphia, Saunders, 2005.

Goldberg D: Procedures in Cosmetic Dermatology Series: Lasers and Lights: Volume 2: Rejuvenation/Resurfacing/Treatment of Ethnic Skin/Treatment of Cellulite. Philadelphia, Saunders, 2005.

Goldberg DJ, Arndt KA: Is a medical degree necessary to perform laser and surgical procedures? Dermatol Surg 26:85–86, 2000.

Grossman MC, Dierickx C, Farinelli W, et al: Damage to hair follicles by normal-mode ruby laser pulses. J Am Acad Dermatol 35:889–894, 1996.

Orf RJ, Dierickx C: Laser hair removal. In Kaminer MS, Dover JS, Arndt KA (eds): Atlas of Cosmetic Surgery. Philadelphia, Saunders, 2002.

Page GW: Is there a doctor in the spa? Bodyworks 12:10, 2006.

Ross EV, Cooke LM, Timko AL, et al: Treatment of pseudofolliculitis barbae in skin types IV, V, and VI with a long-pulsed neodymium:yttrium aluminum garnet laser. J Am Acad Dermatol 47:263–270, 2002.

Sadick NS, Shaoul J: Hair removal using a combination of conducted radiofrequency and optical energies: An 18-month follow up. J Cosmet Laser Ther 6:21–26, 2004.

Small R: Hair removal with lasers. In Usatine RP, Pfenninger JL, Stulberg DL, Small R (eds): Dermatologic and Cosmetic Procedures in Office Practice. Philadelphia, Saunders, 2011, Chapter 26.

Sun TT, Cotsarelis G, Lavker RM: Hair follicular stem cells: The bulge-activation hypothesis. J Invest Dermatol 96(Suppl 5):77S–78S, 1991.

Tanzi EL, Alster TS: Long-pulsed 1064nm Nd:YAG laser-assisted hair removal in all skin types. Dermatol Surg 30:13–17, 2004.

Tope WD, Hordinsky M: A hair's breadth closer [editorial]. Arch Dermatol 134:867, 1998.

Wagner RF, Tomich JM, Grande DJ: Electrolysis and thermolysis for permanent hair removal. J Am Acad Dermatol 12:441–449, 1985.

Willey A, Torrontegui J, Azpiazu J, Landa N: Hair stimulation following laser and intense pulsed light photo-epilation: Review of 543 cases and ways to manage it. Lasers Surg Med 39:297–301, 2007.

CHAPTER 49

Lasers and Pulsed-Light Devices: Photofacial Rejuvenation*

Renier van Aardt

In 1983, Anderson and Parrish described the concept of selective *photothermolysis*. Their article simply stated that the matching of a specific wavelength and pulse duration of light can obtain selected effects on a targeted tissue with minimal changes to surrounding structures.

This was a breakthrough in the application of light and laser technology for the purpose of skin rejuvenation. Dr. Patrick Bitter is credited for developing the treatment and for coining the word *photofacial*, referring to the cosmetic improvement of facial skin using nonablative light-based technology.

Lasers have a relatively short history in medical use. In 1964, the Nd:YAG (neodymium-doped yttrium-aluminum garnet) laser and CO_2 (carbon dioxide) laser were developed at Bell Laboratories. Researchers found that a CO_2 laser beam could cut tissue like a scalpel, but with minimal blood loss. The surgical uses of this laser were investigated extensively from 1967 to 1970 by pioneers such as Thomas Polanyi and Geza Jako, and by the early 1970s use of the CO_2 laser in ear/nose/throat and gynecologic surgery had become well established but was limited to academic and teaching hospitals.

The single most significant advance in the use of medical lasers was the concept of *"pulsing"* the laser beam, which allowed for the aforementioned selective photothermolysis. The first lasers to fully exploit this principle were the pulsed-dye lasers introduced in the late 1980s for the treatment of port wine stains and strawberry birthmarks in children and, soon afterward, the first Q-switched lasers for the treatment of tattoos.

Another major advance was the introduction of scanning devices in the early 1990s, enabling precision computerized control of laser beams. Scanned, pulsed lasers revolutionized the practice of plastic and cosmetic dermatologic surgery by making safe, consistent laser resurfacing possible.

In recent years, the main focus of dermatologic laser research and development has been on laser hair removal, photorejuvenation, and the treatment of vascular lesions, including leg veins, using lasers and intense pulsed light (IPL). The thrust of current research is directed toward *nonablative laser resurfacing* (e.g., laser skin toning, photofacial), *fractionated ablative resurfacing, plasma resurfacing,* and *improved photodynamic therapy* (for treatment of sun damage and skin cancer and for hair removal).

The treatment known as *photofacial rejuvenation* stems from the inherent human desire to be socially acceptable and to appear young and attractive. Social pressure demands a flawless skin; when obvious blemishes are present, the individual can suffer significant psychological trauma. Patients seek treatments that will improve facial blemishes such as pigmented lesions, vascular lesions, scars, texture, rhytids, and tone without downtime and preferably without risk.

Skin deterioration is the result of a number of external and internal factors. The most common *external factor* is ultraviolet (UV) light from prolonged sun exposure as well as the popular use of tanning beds. The effects of UV light are cumulative over a person's lifetime and can result in *telangiectases, matting, poikiloderma, broken capillaries, actinic keratoses, skin cancer, seborrheic keratoses, solar lentigines, progression of chloasma and melasma, textural deterioration, accelerated skin atrophy, redundant skin, and the formation of rhytids*. These findings are more likely in patients with lighter skin types (Fitzpatrick types I, II, and III) who have less natural defense against UV light, resulting in more severe sun damage. Patients with sun-damaged skin are usually good candidates for IPL photorejuvenation, although expectations should be realistic and focused on the improvement of chromophores (pigmented spots) rather than rhytids. Mild to moderate rhytids can be improved with fractional, plasma, and ablative technologies, as outlined in the next section.

Internal factors that cause the skin to lose its youthful appearance include acne, rosacea, chronic illness, endocrine diseases, skin diseases, drug abuse, smoking, and congenital skin lesions.

It is therefore essential for any person desiring attractive skin in later life to practice healthy lifestyle habits, including sun avoidance and regular use of topical sun protection products, not smoking, and consuming a healthy diet and ample water. The degree of improvement of lesions will vary depending on the origin and characteristics of the lesion and the chosen treatment modality and parameters.

Indications

Type I Photorejuvenation (Intense Pulsed Light and Fractional Laser)

- Mild to moderately photoaged skin
- Benign vascular lesions (telangiectases, flushing, symptoms of rosacea)
- Dyschromia
- Erythema after laser resurfacing
- Pigmentary sun damage
- Mottled pigmentation
- Hyperpigmentation
- Lentigines

Type II Photorejuvenation (Fractional and Ablative Lasers)

- Dermal and epidermal structural changes
- Rhytids
- Elastotic changes
- Collagenous and connective tissue changes
- Large pores

*Photofacial is defined as facial skin treatment using light-based technology.

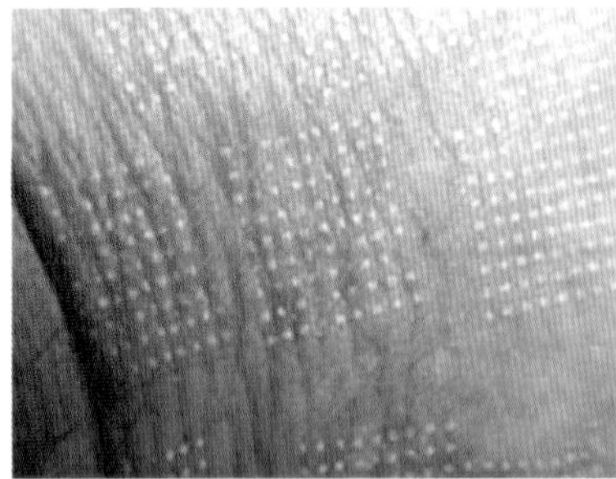

Figure 49-1 Appearance of the skin after application of the fractional laser, showing the typical areas of ablation (dots) and the spared areas in between that allow a much more rapid healing time. The treatment causes macroscopic erythema and edema that typically resolve within 24 hours. The beneficial effects of collagen contraction and skin tightening may continue for 4 to 6 months.

TREATMENT TYPES

Photofacial treatment can be categorized into two main types: *ablative* and *nonablative*. Ablative treatment vaporizes tissue at very high temperatures, whereas nonablative treatment uses gentler heat that may denature protein in certain targets but is insufficient to vaporize tissue. Photofacial treatments can be subdivided further into those that produce downtime versus those that have little or no downtime. Nonablative technologies typically do not produce significant downtime, whereas ablative treatment at a reasonable depth of treatment does. The exception is *fractional ablative therapy*, where tiny islands of tissue known as *microscopic treatment zones* (MTZs) are destroyed. The areas of normal tissue between the treated areas allow for a much more rapid healing time and little, if any, downtime (Fig. 49-1). The treatment causes macroscopic erythema and edema that typically resolves within 24 to 72 hours. The success of both ablative and nonablative laser treatments still depends on the skill of the operator. Figure 49-2 shows the pattern and depth of various treatments.

Ablative Laser

The two most commonly used ablative lasers are the CO_2 laser and the erbium laser. The CO_2 laser was the first to be used for ablative skin resurfacing and tends to create coagulation and significant bulk heating of the skin, and therefore carries a higher risk of complications such as hypopigmentation and permanent scarring. In skilled hands it remains the most effective way to achieve the best results in skin rejuvenation. CO_2 lasers emit light in the near-infrared region at 10,600 nm. They target intracellular water, which heats cells instantly to more than 100° C, resulting in vaporization and removal of a surface layer of cells, coagulation necrosis of cells and denaturing of extracellular proteins in a subjacent residual layer, and nonfatal damage to cells in a still deeper zone. The entire epidermis and a variable thickness of dermis are removed, with a resultant smoother skin due to heat-induced shrinkage of deeper collagen. Patients must accept post-treatment edema, burning, and crusting and an average of 4.5 months of post-treatment erythema. Traditional ablative therapy carries the risk of pigmentary changes, acne flares, herpes simplex virus infection, scars, milia formation, and dermatitis.

Erbium (Er:YAG) lasers are solid-state lasers whose lasing medium is erbium-doped yttrium aluminum garnet ($Er:Y_3Al_5O_{12}$). The erbium laser has become a more popular resurfacing modality than the CO_2 laser because of its precision and lower degree of bulk heating. It also targets intracellular water at 2940 nm, but it is considerably less ablative than the CO_2 laser. The ablation is more superficial and wounds heal more quickly, but it is less effective at equal fluence and with a similar number of passes compared with the CO_2 laser. To achieve an effective thermal damage effect to improve solar elastosis and rhytids, a longer pulse duration is required when using the erbium laser. A combination of erbium and CO_2 lasers may be used as an alternative to the CO_2 laser alone.

Nonablative Laser

Nonablative lasers can be used to selectively injure the dermis or a target in the skin while protecting the epidermis by cooling during treatment, such as the Nd:YAG laser used for collagen remodeling

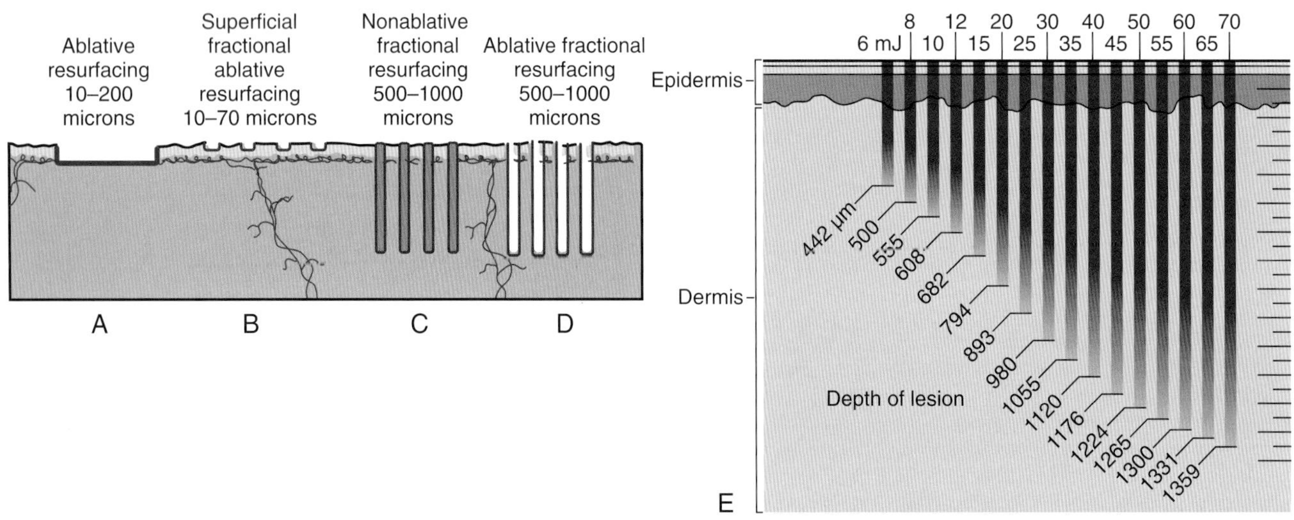

Figure 49-2 Diagram illustrating the difference between ablative and fractional resurfacing. **A,** Superficial layer of tissue is completely vaporized. **B,** Columns of tissue have been vaporized, leaving areas of normal tissue in between, which speeds healing. **C,** Nonablative fractional resurfacing, showing heated (injured) tissue that remains in the microchannels. **D,** Ablative fractional treatment with the tissue in the microchannels vaporized. Ablative and nonablative fractional laser treatments can essentially penetrate to the same depth; however, ablative laser vaporizes tissue, whereas nonablative laser leaves a plug of necrotic debris. **E,** Human skin and depth of penetration of the Fraxel laser with corresponding energy settings. (**E,** Courtesy of Reliant Technologies, Inc., Mountain View, Calif.)

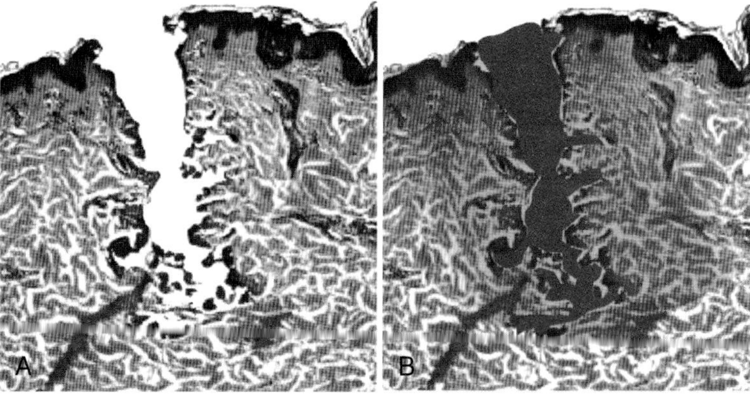

Figure 49-3 **A,** Ablative fractional laser treatment, immediately after treatment. Treatment depth up to 1500 μm. With fully ablated microchannels, necrotic tissue is completely vaporized, with the following results: (1) no residual heating, (2) more comfortable procedure, and (3) faster healing time. **B,** Nonablative fractional treatment, immediately after treatment. Treatment depth up to 1500 μm. Necrotic debris stays in the tissue, with the following results: (1) wide and deep zone of thermal necrosis, (2) more painful procedure, and (3) longer recovery time.

of the dermis or the treatment of leg, truncal, and facial veins. Like ablative lasers, nonablative lasers emit coherent light at wavelengths absorbed by water. This approach has less predictable efficacy compared with ablative laser techniques.

Fractional Therapies

Fractional photothermolysis using the erbium laser has been developed to overcome the disadvantages of conventional ablative and nonablative laser therapies. It produces columns of thermal damage or ablation called *foci*, or MTZs, ranging between 50 and 150 μm in diameter and located at specific depths from 0 to 550 μm (Fig. 49-3). Treatment time for each pulse (exposure duration) ranges between 3 and 30 milliseconds. The density of treatment corresponds to the inter-MTZ space and is adjustable. Because the MTZs are surrounded by uninjured tissue, keratinocytes have a shorter migration path and healing is much quicker (Fig. 49-4). The technique coagulates both the epidermis and dermis without affecting the stratum corneum, which acts as a natural bandage that protects the tiny wounds as they heal. To improve solar elastosis, scars, and rhytids, a course of treatments, typically three to five, is spaced at least 2 weeks apart. The treatments have fewer and less severe side effects than traditional, nonfractional ablative resurfacing and, with the exception of deep rhytids, the results in terms of skin tone, texture, dyschromia, and scars are essentially equivalent. More aggressive CO_2 laser fractional treatment vaporizes tiny columns of tissue entirely and may require fewer treatments than erbium devices, but it causes more downtime because of erythema and even crusting that can last a few days, with a possible higher incidence of postinflammatory hyperpigmentation. The ratio of risk to benefit always must be considered when choosing the appropriate device for the condition to be treated.

Fractional light therapy can be nonablative, using IPL or laser, or ablative with the CO_2 and erbium laser, with varying degrees of coagulation. Compared with a chemical peel, dermabrasion, or other forms of laser treatment, fractional laser allows the surgeon to customize the surgery more safely, not only to each patient but to each area of the face.

The newer photofacial resurfacing devices include the following:

- Matrix RF (radiofrequency device; Syneron, Inc., Irvine, Calif)
- Erbium (Er:YAG) fractional lasers
  - Lux2940 (Palomar Medical Technologies, Inc., Burlington, Mass)
  - Sciton Profractional (Sciton, Inc., Palo Alto, Calif; Fig. 49-5)
- CO_2 fractional lasers
  - Smartxide DOT (Deka Laser, Florence, Italy)
  - Fraxel re:pair (Solta Medical, Inc., Hayward, Calif)
  - Pixel CO_2 (Alma Lasers, Ltd., Caesarea, Israel)
  - SmartSkin CO_2 (Cynosure, Inc., Westford, Mass)
- Harmony^{XL} (pixel laser; multimodality skin rejuvenation; Alma Lasers, Ltd.; see Fig. 49-5)

The types of dermatologic lasers are listed in Box 49-1.

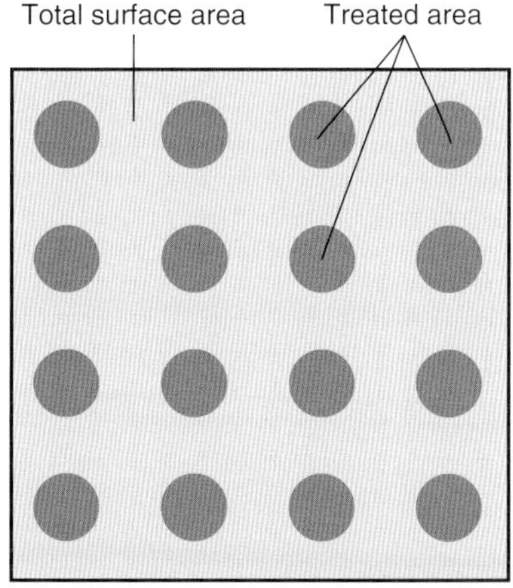

Figure 49-4 Fractionated columns of light versus the traditional laser. With fractional applications, the treated areas are affected by focal columns of light, leaving "dots" of destroyed tissue within the total surface area. In traditional laser ablation, the entire surface area (i.e., the box) would be orange, denoting the affected/ablated area.

Plasma Resurfacing

Skin resurfacing can also be accomplished with a plasma-based device (Rhytec Portrait PSR3; Rhytec, Inc., Waltham, Mass) instead of a laser, although its superiority to laser-based devices remains an open question. Nitrogen plasma energy is delivered to the skin to stimulate skin remodeling while creating a coagulated barrier out of the skin's outer layers that mitigates infection. Studies are lacking to assess its efficacy compared with traditional devices.

Intense Pulsed Light

Intense pulsed-light technology has been increasingly competitive with lasers since the mid-1990s, and owing to enhanced engineering and favorable pricing versus many lasers, IPL devices have proliferated in the skin rejuvenation market. These devices are quickly gaining acceptance in medical offices and spas; although the technology was initially decried as "the poor man's laser" and dismissed as having too many side effects and too little efficacy, the newest generation of devices have proved so popular that even "old guard" companies are adding IPL to their product offerings.

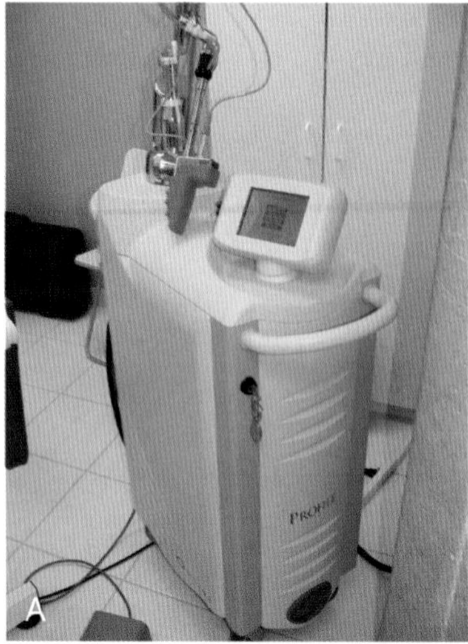

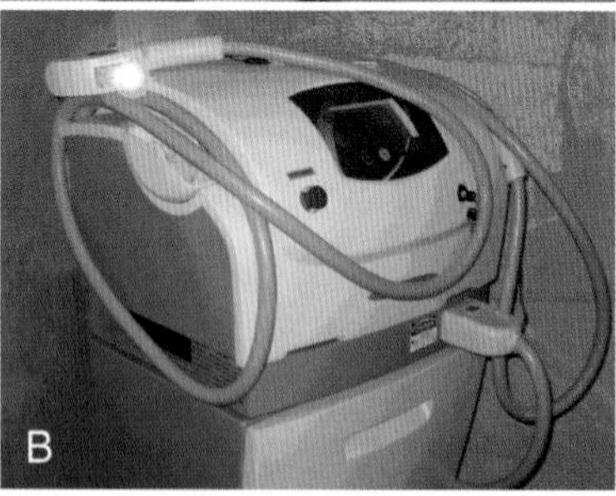

Figure 49-5 Sciton Profractional laser (**A**) and an Alma Harmony intense pulsed-light device (**B**).

Intense pulsed light has both *advantages and disadvantages* compared with lasers. Lasers are useful because they permit exquisite control of where and how much one heats the skin. Lasers allow for smaller handpieces, whereas IPL treatment heads house the flashlamp, cooling apparatus, and high-voltage wires, resulting in a bulkier and heavier handpiece. Like lasers, IPL devices are becoming smaller, more efficient, more powerful, and less expensive. Lasers are more intricate than IPL and therefore more vulnerable to breakdown, resulting in higher purchase costs and more expensive maintenance. Because laser is collimated light, it is less eye-safe than IPL. Collimated light is light whose rays are nearly parallel, and therefore spreads slowly as it propagates. A laser beam delivers more focused energy to the target than IPL and hence is potentially more harmful to the retina. It is imperative, however, to use protective eyewear when operating or undergoing treatment with any light-based device.

Because the *three main chromophores* in skin (hemoglobin, water, and melanin) have broad absorption peaks, monochromacity is not a prerequisite for selective heating, making IPL an adequate substitution for or, in some instances, even preferable to lasers. When treating sun damage, the targets consist of brown pigmentation (solar lentigines), redness (enlarged capillaries), and water and collagen (textural deterioration). Wavelengths between 515 and 600 nm are optimally absorbed by oxyhemoglobin and melanin, making this spectrum ideal for selective photothermolysis in treating the typical patient with sun-damaged skin (i.e., pigmented areas and redness). IPL devices use flashlamps, computer-controlled power supplies, and bandpass filters to generate light pulses of prescribed duration, intensity, and spectral distribution (see Chapter 48, Lasers and Pulsed-Light Devices: Hair Removal, Fig. 48-1). Flashlamps are high-intensity gas-discharge lamps filled with xenon gas that produce bright light when an electrical current passes through the gas. Electrical energy stored in capacitor banks is converted into optical energy, pulsing the lamps and covering the entire spectrum of light between UV and infrared.

To ensure an even flow of energy, most modern IPL systems use partial-discharge technology. Mirrors surround the xenon flashlamp

Box 49-1. Lasers Used in Dermatology

1. *CO_2 laser*: The light from these lasers is absorbed by water in the skin; hence, they are used for skin resurfacing, removal of benign skin tumors such as warts, xanthelasma, mucous cysts, cherry angiomas, and leukoplakia, and for surgical cutting.
2. *Nd:YAG laser*: The active medium is a neodymium-doped yttrium aluminum garnet, producing laser light at a wavelength of 1064 nm. Nd:YAG lasers have slight absorption in melanin and hemoglobin and are used for hair removal, vein treatments, photorejuvenation, acne treatments, and laser skin surgery.
3. *Q-switched Nd:YAG laser*: These lasers have strong absorption in dark tattoo inks, and hence are used in tattoo removal.
4. *Er:YAG laser*: The active medium is an erbium-doped yttrium aluminum garnet, producing laser light at a wavelength of 2940 nm. It is absorbed by water in the skin and is used for skin resurfacing, photorejuvenation, and removal of skin growths.
5. *Ruby laser*: A synthetic ruby crystal (chromium-doped aluminum oxide) is the gain medium, producing laser light at a wavelength of 694 nm. Ruby laser light has very strong absorption in melanin and black and dark blue ink pigments. These lasers are especially useful in tattoo removal, hair removal, and removal of pigmented (dark) skin lesions.
6. *KTP, or potassium titanyl phosphate, laser*: This frequency-doubled Nd:YAG laser with a 532-nm wavelength and absorption by hemoglobin and melanin is used to remove vascular and pigmented skin lesions.
7. *Alexandrite laser*: This Q-switched laser with a 755-nm wavelength is used to remove blue, black, and green tattoos and epidermal and dermal pigmentations (e.g., melasma).
8. *Diode laser*: These lasers have varying wavelengths, depending on the color of the target. The absorbing chromophores are melanin and hemoglobin. Diode lasers are used for hair removal, dilated vein treatments, and photorejuvenation.
9. *Dye laser*: These lasers contain organic compounds in solution (often rhodamine) as the active medium and have wavelength activity between 400 to 800 nm. The target chromophores are hemoglobin and melanin. Dye lasers are useful in treating vascular lesions and for nonablative skin rejuvenation.
10. *Excimer laser*: Compounds of xenon, krypton, and argon are the active media. These lasers target proteins and water and have wavelengths of 190 to 350 nm. They are useful in the treatment of psoriasis and vitiligo.
11. *Fractional lasers*: These lasers produce microscopic treatment zones and target specific depths in the dermis. These are especially useful for treatment of acne scars, wrinkles, sun damage, and melasma. CO_2 and erbium laser wavelengths are commonly used, and the target chromophore is water.

and the lamp is cooled by water circulating around a quartz envelope, filtering out most of the harmful far-UV output of the lamp. The light output is directed toward the distal end of the handpiece, and a sapphire or quartz block couples the light output to the skin. The normal, unfiltered output of a xenon lamp is between 370 and 1800 nm. Most IPL devices use dichromic filters to transmit a desired range of wavelengths. In other words, they use filters to select the wavelength of light desired to treat the particular entity (e.g., pigment, vessels, collagen). By adjusting the fluence, number of pulses, pulse duration, and the cut-off filter, and considering the patient's particular skin type, various skin targets can be selectively heated to achieve the desired clinical outcome. Most IPL devices have different spot sizes to choose from, facilitating adequate treatment over small or large surface areas.

Intense Pulsed-Light Photofacial Treatment

See Figures 49-6 through 49-8.

The majority of photofacial treatments are performed with IPL devices, and IPL has become a popular treatment in physician offices and spas. IPL is indicated for the treatment of mild to moderate photodamage (type I photorejuvenation).

Indications

- Solar lentigines
- Chloasma
- Melasma
- Postinflammatory hyperpigmentation
- Actinic lesions
- Telangiectases
- Spider angiomas
- Broken capillaries
- Diffuse erythema and poikiloderma

Skin texture and pore size may also improve from the stimulation of fibroblasts, resulting in collagen production and tightening. The final result of a series of photofacial treatments may only be evident a few months later because skin remodeling is a gradual process. Collagen may continue to contract for up to 3 months after treatment.

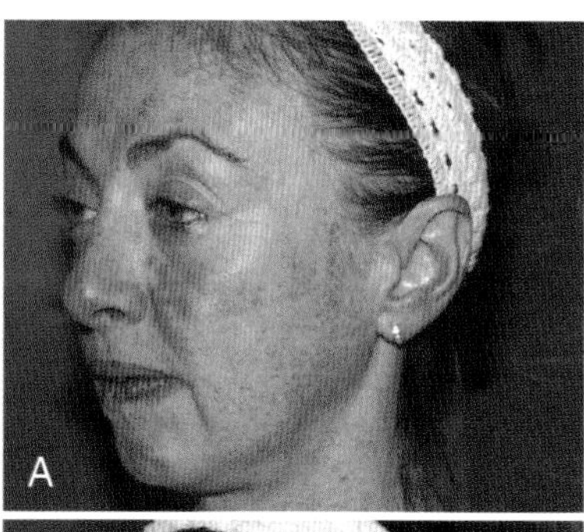

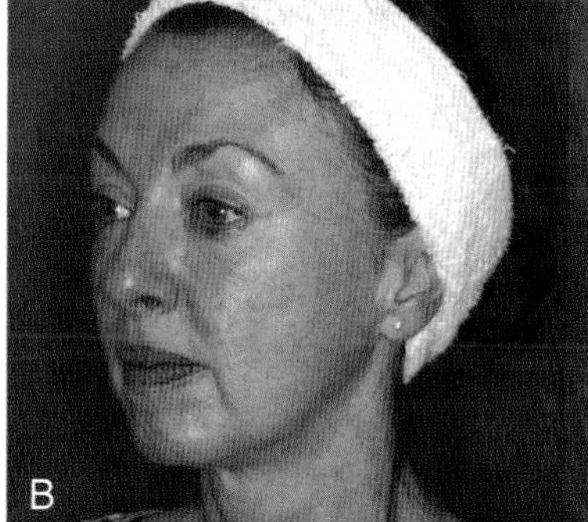

Figure 49-6 Before (**A**) and 1 month after (**B**) a series of five intense pulsed-light treatments with the Vasculight (Lumenis). Improvements in erythema and pigmentation are noted.

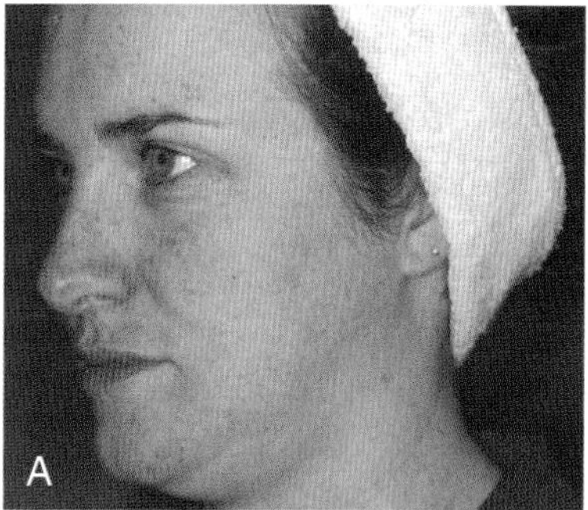

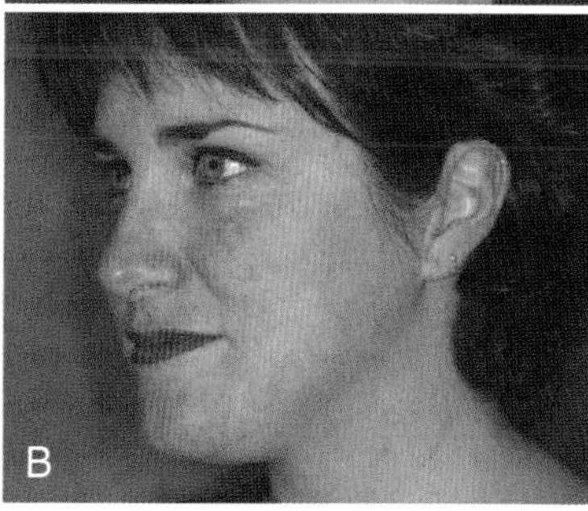

Figure 49-7 Before (**A**) and 2 weeks after (**B**) a single intense pulsed-light treatment with the Vasculight (Lumenis), showing improvement in dyschromia.

Contraindications

- *Patients with darker skin types, such as Fitzpatrick types V and VI,* are naturally protected from most UV damage and are generally not good candidates for photorejuvenation, with the possible exception of mild to moderate fractional laser resurfacing to address scars and melasma. They are also much more likely to suffer side effects from light-based treatments because of the high absorption of light by melanin. Practitioners should exercise particular caution because these patients are also more likely to develop keloid scars and hyperpigmentation or hypopigmentation if they sustain a burn wound from overly aggressive treatment.
- A generalized active inflammatory or infectious process of the skin.
- A history of herpes simplex without receiving antiviral prophylaxis (some procedures).
- *Photosensitizing medications*: If a patient is on Accutane, at least 6 months should pass after a course is completed before laser or IPL is used in order to avoid irreversible skin discoloration.
- *Suntan*: Patients should wait for a tan to fade before treatments commence to avoid burning the epidermis and risking hypopigmentation, which may take months or longer to heal.

Preprocedure Patient Education

See patient information and consent form online at www.expertconsult.com. In general, IPL treatments should be performed in a series of three to six treatments 2 to 4 weeks apart.

A medical history and clinical examination are required before treatments can commence. The skin should be carefully examined to rule out skin lesions such as actinic keratoses, basal cell carcinoma, squamous cell carcinoma, and melanoma, and such lesions should be treated appropriately before beginning light-based therapies.

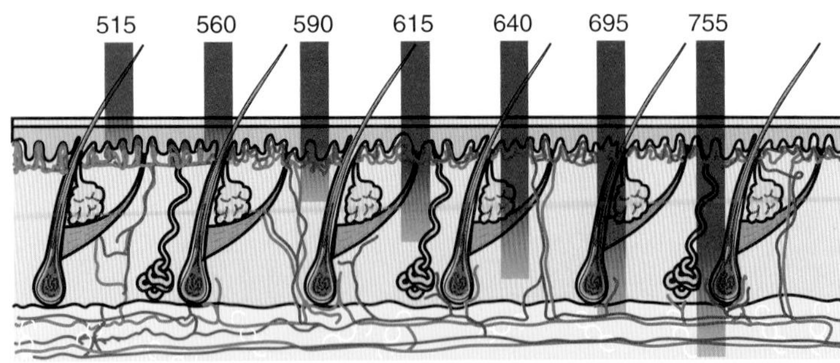

Figure 49-8 Depth of penetration of various cut-off filters used in intense pulsed-light devices for nonablative selective photothermolysis. A wavelength of 515 to 590 nm targets melanin and vascular structures and is used mainly for skin rejuvenation; 640 to 695 nm is used mainly for hair removal; and 755 nm is used for skin tightening. Besides wavelength, fluence and spot size also determine the depth of penetration.

Technique

The patient is placed in a comfortable reclined or supine position; good ambient lighting is needed. The skin must be cleansed and all makeup and skin cream removed before the procedure. Eye protection must be supplied for the patient and can consist of snug fitting metal eye shields or disposable stick-on eye protectors specifically designed for IPL use. The technician must wear appropriate IPL eye protection, and the use of gloves is recommended. Most IPL devices require the application of cool or chilled, clear ultrasound gel to provide a consistent light path and cooling to the skin. Devices that have handpieces with built-in cooling of the light guide require a thin layer of gel; if built-in cooling is absent, a thicker layer of cold gel serves to cool and protect the epidermis. Each manufacturer has specific recommendations for gel use and application related to its particular device design.

The spot size of IPL light guides varies, but the average size is about 2 inches × ¾ inch, whereas laser spot sizes are usually smaller. The handpiece and light guide must be properly cleaned and disinfected, using a medical-grade chemosterilant/high-level disinfectant such as hydrogen peroxide 7%, between treatments. The starting fluence for the first treatment is generally modest and is usually increased with each consecutive treatment. It is good practice to perform two or three "test pulses" in the preauricular area and monitor the treated area for 2 or more minutes to ensure that the chosen energy level does not cause excessive redness, swelling, ecchymosis, or blistering. It should be sufficient to cause end-point pigment darkening and capillary contraction or color changes. Manufacturers will provide suggested treatment settings related to their particular device.

The face is treated in sections that typically consist of each cheek area, from preauricular to midface, with the midface consisting of the nose, upper lip, chin area, and forehead. Care must be taken not to pass over the vermillion of the lips and not to treat closer than ½ inch from the eyebrows and hairline. Because most IPL wavelengths have a strong affinity for melanin and may cause a permanent reduction in darker hair, patients must be made aware of this fact, especially men, who may not want their beard hair decreased by treatment.

It is important to note that the midface is more sensitive than other areas of the face; the patient should be informed of this and that despite the eye protection, they will see bright flashes of light that will not be harmful to their eyesight. Depending on the device, the parameters, and the protocol, one or more passes may be made of the face or certain areas using the same or different cut-off filters. When the treatment has been completed, the gel must be removed, the skin gently cleansed, and a soothing aloe-based gel or protective moisturizing cream applied. The treatments are repeated every 2 to 3 weeks, with a total of three to six treatments being typical. Herpes simplex prophylaxis should be prescribed when laser or IPL devices are used in treating the perioral region for patients with a past history of herpes simplex type 1 infection. Valacyclovir 2 g 1 hour before the procedure and 2 g 12 hours after the first dose is effective.

Maintenance IPL treatments can be performed every 3 to 4 months, choosing parameters based on any skin pigmentary changes in the interim. Other areas of the body can be treated, including the neck, décolleté area, arms, hands, back, and legs. The fee for the procedure is calculated by either area or the number of pulses used.

Postprocedure Patient Education

Patients must be instructed to avoid sun exposure and use a good-quality, UVA/UVB broad-spectrum sunscreen (SPF 15 to 30) daily. If a patient has acquired a tan between treatments, any further treatments should be postponed until the tan has faded. Appropriate skin care is beneficial for patients undergoing a series of photofacial treatments. Exfoliation of the stratum corneum with microdermabrasion or gentle chemical peels can assist in removing surface pigmentation between IPL treatments, and using a daily moisturizer can treat dry skin caused by increased skin turnover after IPL treatment. Patients should also be made aware that maintenance treatments will be required every 3 to 4 months to avoid a gradual return to baseline. Patients should be educated regarding the dangers of UV light exposure and the continued use of a sunscreen because this information will help them prolong the beneficial effects of their photofacial treatments.

Complications

Surface cooling of the skin is extremely important with IPL to avoid side effects such as burns that can lead to pain, blisters, infection, scars, and hyperpigmentation, especially on darker skin types. Newer IPL devices have built-in contact cooling, allowing the light guide to be placed directly on the skin, achieving effective cooling and precisely duplicable results with each pulse. Other cooling methods include cold ultrasound gel, cold air devices, and cryogen spray.

Common Errors

- Single, aggressive treatments can yield impressive results, especially for superficial pigmentation; however, this approach is painful, the risk of short-term side effects is higher, and most patients desire a no-downtime treatment with an acceptable comfort level. Achieving a no-downtime treatment regimen requires starting treatments at a modest fluence and incrementally increasing the energy in subsequent treatments toward a target level.
- Care must be taken not to use too much pressure when treating capillaries because excessive pressure will result in blanching, and the target will be lost and not effectively treated.
- Some IPL devices rely on the use of cold ultrasound gel to be placed on the skin for cooling and "drifting" the light guide in the gel just above the skin surface. Although the technique is effective, the skill and experience of the operator are important in achieving consistent results.

Adjunctive Treatments

5-Aminolevulinic Acid (Levulan)

An adjunctive treatment that complements IPL extremely well is the use of the photosensitizing agent 5-aminolevulinic acid (Levulan, DUSA Pharmaceuticals, Inc., Wilmington, Del) to broaden the overall benefits and improve the end results achieved with photofacial treatments. The treatment is known as *photodynamic therapy* (also see Chapter 60, Photodynamic Therapy). 5-Aminolevulinic acid is approved for the treatment of actinic keratoses. It is used in the treatment of nonmelanoma skin cancer and of systemic cancers. It is also applied "off-label" with excellent results for the treatment of acne. Levulan is prepared by breaking chambers in a vial. It is then applied directly to skin that has been prepared with microdermabrasion, or by acetone or alcohol scrub, to break down the skin's lipid barrier. The material is allowed to be absorbed over time, which increases the effectiveness of light therapy. The interval between application and the start of IPL treatment is referred to as the *incubation time*.

When combined with IPL, short incubation times between 15 minutes and 1 hour can be used with good clinical response. Improved reduction of brown and red pigments, textural improvement, and pore minimization can be expected with this approach. Patients *must* avoid any sunlight or bright indoor light exposure to the treated skin for 24 hours after treatment to minimize erythema and avoid burns. Some erythema, flaking, swelling, or peeling can be expected with 5-aminolevulinic acid treatment.

Retinoids

Topical retinoids (i.e., tretinoin and isotretinoin) are another adjunctive treatment that has been shown to improve the outcome of IPL treatments. Patients should be motivated and prepared for possible erythema and dry, flaking skin with the use of topical retinoids. Patients should start using retinoids at least 2 weeks before commencing IPL, discontinue application 2 days before IPL, and resume use a day after treatment. Because retinoids are photosensitizing, increased flushing and some downtime may occur when they are used in conjunction with IPL to treat sun damage. For this reason, retinoids are reserved for more severe sun damage. Microdermabrasion is never used when a patient is using retinoids because of increased skin fragility and should be considered only after the retinoid has been discontinued for at least 1 month. Waxing should also be avoided when retinoids are being used. Retinoids alone have beneficial effects on sun-damaged skin, improving texture and dyschromia with consistent use, and may be used over the long term to reduce the frequency of maintenance IPL treatments.

Nonfacial Treatments

Other body areas can be treated with IPL with equal efficacy, including the neck, chest, arms, and legs. Fluences should be lowered when treating the neck and décolleté areas and always adapted to the particular skin area color. With years of sun damage, more exposed areas my have increased background melanin than less exposed areas and should be treated accordingly.

Conclusion

Photofacial treatments have become an accepted method of improving the appearance of the skin, especially photodamaged and aging skin. Many modalities are available, and it is up to the practitioner to decide on the most appropriate treatment to address the patient's concerns. In some cases, combination treatments may be required. The patient's expectations, budget, and clinical concerns must be considered when deciding on the appropriate treatment method. IPL has become the most common and popular treatment option for photodamaged skin because of its good safety profile, minimal downtime, low cost, and excellent results.

When IPL is used for the appropriate candidate, results can be dramatic and very pleasing for the patient as well as rewarding for the practitioner. The technology has seen significant advances in recent years, overcoming many of the initial barriers and objections to its use to such an extent that in some cases it is now preferred over laser treatment. For the cosmetic dermatology practitioner, IPL is a modality to combine with other, traditional laser devices to satisfy the demands of patients and allow for a comprehensive armamentarium of light-based skin treatment devices to be available to address various skin concerns.

Patient Education Guides

See the patient information and consent forms online at www.expertconsult.com.

J Code

J7308 5-Aminolevulinic acid (Levulan)

CPT/Billing Codes

Insurance providers do not reimburse for cosmetic procedures. However, they will reimburse for some of the following treatments:

17106 Destruction of cutaneous vascular proliferative lesions (e.g., laser) <10 cm^2
17107 Destruction of cutaneous vascular proliferative lesions 10 to 50 cm^2
17108 Destruction of cutaneous vascular proliferative lesions >50 cm^2
17110 Destruction of benign lesions, up to 14
17111 Destruction of benign lesions, >14
96567 Photodynamic therapy by external application of light to destroy malignant and/or nonmalignant lesions of the skin and adjacent mucosa (e.g., lip) by activation of photosensitive drug(s), each phototherapy session

ICD-9-CM Diagnostic Codes

448.1 Capillary angiomas
448.1 Facial telangiectases
448.1 Spider angiomas
692.74 Chronic skin damage/solar elastosis
695.3 Rosacea
701.4 Keloid
701.8 Other specified hypertrophic and atrophic skin conditions
701.8 Rhytids, face (wrinkles, lines)
702.0 Actinic (solar)/senile keratoses
702.11 Keratosis, seborrheic inflamed
702.19 Keratosis, seborrheic
701.8 Facial telangiectases
706.1 Acne vulgaris
709.00 Dyschromia skin (pigment disorder)
709.09 Chloasma
709.09 Lentigines
709.09 Melanosis
709.09 Melasma
709.09 Poikiloderma
709.2 Skin firbrosis/scar; cicatrix (excludes keloid)

Suppliers

(See contact information online at www.expertconsult.com.)

Selected IPL manufacturers

Aesthera Corp.
Alma Lasers, Ltd.
Cynosure, Inc.

Lumenis
Palomar Medical Technologies, Inc.
Sciton, Inc.
Syneron, Inc.

AUTHOR'S NOTE: Many different manufacturers produce IPL devices today, some of which are inexpensive and of low power, often purchased by spas and salons. High-quality equipment, supported by reputable clinical studies, ensures high-quality treatment, the best results, and high-quality support by the manufacturer. Proper research, discussion with peers, and attendance at national and international laser conferences, such as the ASLMS (American Society of Laser Medicine and Surgery), are strongly recommended before any purchase is made.

ONLINE RESOURCE

American Board of Laser Surgery: Available at www.americanboardoflasersurgery.org.

BIBLIOGRAPHY

Alster TS, Tanzi EL, Welch EC: Photorejuvenation of a facial skin with topical 20% 5-aminolevulinic acid and intense pulsed light treatment: A split-face comparison study. J Drugs Dermatol 4:35–38, 2005.

Anderson RR, Parrish JA: Selective photothermolysis: Precise microsurgery by selective absorption of pulsed radiation. Science 220:524–527, 1983.

Bjerring P, Christiansen K, Troilius A, Dierickx C: Facial photo rejuvenation using two different intense pulsed light wavelength bands. Lasers Surg Med 34:120–126, 2004.

Geronemus R: Fractional photothermolysis: Current and future applications. Lasers Surg Med 38:169–176, 2006.

Goldberg D: Procedures in Cosmetic Dermatology Series: Lasers and Lights, Volume 1: Vascular/Pigmentation/Scars/Medical Applications. Philadelphia, Saunders, 2005.

Goldberg D: Procedures in Cosmetic Dermatology Series: Lasers and Lights: Volume 2: Rejuvenation/Resurfacing/Treatment of Ethnic Skin/Treatment of Cellulite. Philadelphia, Saunders, 2005.

Goldman M: Clinical pearl: Observations on the use of fractionated CO_2 laser resurfacing. J Drugs Dermatol 8:82–86, 2009.

Ross EV: Laser versus intense pulsed light: Competing technologies in dermatology. Lasers Surg Med 38:261–272, 2006.

Saluja R, Khoury J, Detweiler S, Goldman M: Histologic and clinical response to varying density settings with a fractionality scanned carbon dioxide laser. J Drugs Dermatol 8:17–20, 2009.

Small R: Ablative lasers. In Usatine RP, Pfenninger JL, Stulberg DL, Small R (eds): Dermatologic and Cosmetic Procedures in Office Practice. Philadelphia, Saunders, 2011, Chapter 29 (in press).

Small R: Non-ablative lasers. In Usatine RP, Pfenninger JL, Stulberg DL, Small R (eds): Dermatologic and Cosmetic Procedures in Office Practice. Philadelphia, Saunders, 2011, Chapter 28 (in press).

Small R: Photorejuvenation with lasers. In Usatine RP, Pfenninger JL, Stulberg DL, Small R (eds): Dermatologic and Cosmetic Procedures in Office Practice. Philadelphia, Saunders, 2011, Chapter 27 (in press).

Tan KL, Kurniawati C, Gold M: Low risk of postinflammatory hyperpigmentation in skin types 4 and 5 after treatment with fractional CO_2 laser device. J Drugs Dermatol 7:774–777, 2008.

Waibel J, Beer K: Ablative fractional laser resurfacing for the treatment of a third-degree burn. J Drugs Dermatol 8:294–297, 2009.

CHAPTER 50

LASERS AND PULSED-LIGHT DEVICES: ACNE

Renier van Aardt

Acne vulgaris is a common chronic disease affecting the pilosebaceous follicle of the face, neck, back, chest, and other areas of the body. It affects 40 million American adolescents and 25 million adults. At least 50% of adults admit to having suffered with some degree of acne in their lifetime. In the past, people have treated it many different ways, with everything from handfuls of vervain (a flowering herb) to bloodletting (India). Even arsenic and x-rays were used with little benefit and considerable risk because people were willing to try anything for even minor improvements. Given the prevalence and number of patients who suffer from refractory acne, alternatives to existing treatments are constantly sought. Acne vulgaris is a disease that not only causes physical blemishes but has major psychological effects on its sufferers, including social withdrawal, clinical depression, and suicide. In recent years, the use of laser- and light-based devices has had a significant impact on our ability to manage acne.

CLINICAL APPEARANCE AND GRADING

Acne has been classified from grade 1 to grade 4 depending on its severity. Variations include minor blackheads and whiteheads and clogged pores (grade 1) that can become infected and inflamed (grade 2), leading to large red papules and pustules (grade 3) and cysts and nodules (grade 4). Lesions are often "popped" or picked by the patient. With the larger lesions, scarring is often the result. The usual type of depressed scarring can last throughout a person's life, and can become an extremely noticeable facial imperfection. Scars can be erythematous, irregular, textured lesions, enlarged pores, or deep icepick and cratered lesions. Treatment is primarily directed at reducing inflammation and preventing scars. However, light-based technologies also make scar reduction and skin remodeling possible to improve appearance.

INTERNAL CAUSES

There are many contributing factors to the severity of acne, but no clear single cause has been identified. Acne develops as the patient progresses through puberty and the sebaceous glands grow and increase their sebum secretion. Acne is more prevalent and severe in males because of the increased production of *testosterone* during puberty. Adult-onset acne in women may be attributed to cyclical variations in sex hormones, with an increase in androgenic hormone levels resulting in an increase in sebum production. This increase in sebum, coupled with the keratinization of the hair follicle, causes occlusion of the ducts and in turn the formation of comedones.

There is a correlation between the *depth of the hair follicle* and the size of the lesion. The deeper the follicle, the deeper the occlusion, which in turn results in a larger lesion.

The bacterium *Propionibacterium acnes* causes inflammation either because of an immune system reaction, inflammatory enzymes from the bacteria, or a combination of the two. *P. acnes* is a normal colonizer of the sebaceous follicles; it is a gram-positive, microaerophilic bacterium that, as part of its normal metabolic and reproductive processes, produces and accumulates endogenous porphyrins, namely protoporphyrin, uroporphyrin, and coproporphyrin III. Porphyrins can be visualized using a Wood's lamp or digital fluorescence photography because they absorb light energy at the near-ultraviolet and blue-light spectrum. This unique attribute of the bacterium lends to the therapeutic effects of some light-based treatments.

EXTERNAL CAUSES

External factors vary from patient to patient, but there are several factors that can affect the severity of acne. *Diet* will affect each patient individually, and although dairy products seem to cause problems in women, no other real universal dietary factors have been identified. *Thick makeup*, *hair spray*, *greasy hair gels*, and *hats*, *sweat bands*, or *athletic helmets* are all external factors that contribute to the severity of acne because of the combination of mechanical or chemical irritation, oil gland occlusion, and bacterial colonization. In some work environments, exposure to industrial products like cutting oils may produce acne. In addition, *inadequate cleansing* contributes to the development of acne. In all cases, the external factors aggravate acne, but are not the root cause of the disease.

Patients should be advised not to rub, scratch, pick, or squeeze their skin because *mechanical irritation* can aggravate acne and lead to scarring. Careful and controlled extraction of comedones by a trained aesthetician or nurse after steaming and appropriate skin preparation may be beneficial. Some *drugs* can cause or worsen acne, including iodides, bromides, and oral or injected steroids. A proper skin care regime is helpful to minimize the severity of acne by removing impurities and irritants.

TREATMENT OPTIONS

Because the pathogenesis of acne involves four factors (hypercornification of the pilosebaceous duct, increased sebum production, colonization by *P. acnes*, and the development of inflammation), a stepwise and systematic approach to treatment is best. Because acne is a chronic disease, its treatment is an ongoing process that requires educating the patient as well as patience on the part of both the patient and the clinician, to allow each step in the treatment process to take effect. Treatments aimed at clearance of *P. acnes* alone generally provide short-lived improvement; therefore, combination therapy is recommended (Table 50-1).

The first universal step is appropriate skin care. *Cleansing* the skin seems to help all patients, if only slightly, but acne is not directly

TABLE 50-1 Treatment Options in Acne Management

Acne Grade 1	Acne Grade 2	Acne Grade 3	Acne Grade 4	Rosacea Acne
Gentle skin care and extraction of comedones Topical retinoids Exfoliation: peels and/or microdermabrasion	Gentle skin care and extraction of comedones Blue light Topical retinoids Benzoyl peroxide Topical antibiotics Exfoliation: peels (salicylic/glycolic) and/or microdermabrasion Photodynamic therapy	Gentle skin care Blue light and red light Topical retinoids Benzoyl peroxide Systemic and/or topical antibiotics Hormonal therapy Exfoliation: peels (salicylic/glycolic) and/or microdermabrasion IPL and photodynamic therapy	Gentle skin care Blue light and red light Systemic antibiotics Hormonal therapy IPL (not with tretinoin) and photodynamic therapy Systemic isotretinoin	Gentle anti-inflammatory skin care Topical antibiotics and/or systemic tetracyclines Glycolic acid peels IPL and photodynamic therapy Avoid triggers

IPL, intense pulsed light.

caused by dirt. Cleansers have an antibacterial effect and may reduce bacterial colony counts. Toners may be helpful in restoring the pH balance of the skin after cleansing to an acidic state. Using gentle exfoliation such as *microdermabrasion* or *glycolic facials* may be helpful to remove excessive keratin from the epidermis and open pores, allowing sebum to drain freely. Overscrubbing is not recommended because the skin becomes dry, damaged, and inflamed and as a result can become less receptive to topical products. Abrasive home scrubs are therefore not recommended for acne-prone skin. A *gentle cleanser* is all that is necessary to cleanse the skin properly. *Moisturizers* that are noncomedogenic are helpful to prevent skin dehydration and to counteract the drying effect of many other active ingredients, such as benzoyl peroxide. The most commonly used cleansers are available over-the-counter and include Clearasil and PHisoderm, but aesthetic physicians' offices and spas also have a variety of excellent brands available to their clientele.

As with many other cosmetic treatments, combination therapy is the best approach to treating acne, which brings us to the *second step of treatment*. Using topical products, such as *topical retinoids*, maximizes the effect that an intense pulsed-light (IPL) treatment will have on the acne. Retinoids are comedolytic and act on the keratinization of the hair follicle. They are therefore beneficial for acne grades 1 and 2 where comedones predominate. Differin (adapalene) is the least irritating, but others, such as Retin-A (tretinoin) or Tazorac (tazarotene), may also be used. There are many over-the-counter retinoid creams on the market, but these do not usually deliver consistent levels of retinoid to the dermis.

Retinoids result in a decrease in sebaceous duct occlusion, preventing oil from accumulating in the sebaceous glands and creating a favorable habitat for bacterial colonization. Inflammatory acne, on the other hand, responds better to *topical antibiotics and photodynamic therapy* (PDT; Fig. 50-1). Preparations that combine antibiotics like clindamycin with benzoyl peroxide are available for better efficacy than single antibiotics alone. In addition, *blue light* (415-nm wavelength) has excellent antibacterial properties against porphyrin-producing bacteria because porphyrins release singlet oxygen when activated by this wavelength of light. Singlet oxygen is toxic to the bacteria (see Chapter 60, Photodynamic Therapy).

Hormonal therapy is a useful adjunct in the treatment of acne in female patients. The onset of acne is triggered by the increased production of androgens. Oral contraceptives inhibit ovulation, thereby preventing androgen production by the ovaries. Lower serum androgen levels reduce sebum secretion, which consequentially exerts an antiacne effect. The mean reduction in total facial acne lesions with the use of drospirenone and cyproterone acetate (components of birth control pills) has been shown to be 62% and 59%, respectively. Other contraceptives with antiacne effects include norgestimate and levonorgestrel.

Oral antibiotics and isotretinoin (Accutane) constitute the next level of traditional therapy. However, the availability of lasers, IPL devices, and PDT now provides excellent treatment options that avoid possible systemic side effects, leaving oral treatment as an alternative for severe and unusually refractive cases. *Intralesional steroids* are infrequently used and are more appropriate for early nodular lesions; they should not be a standard treatment for acne. Newer *devices that extract comedones* in the course of IPL treatment are excellent for grades 2 and 3 acne. Gently extracting large comedones and draining superficial cysts may be helpful when providing full-face treatments such as IPL and PDT. Strong pressure should never be applied to avoid spreading infection. *Oral antibiotics* such as minocycline are very effective in treating acute flare-ups of papulopustular acne. Oral antibiotics also reduce the severity of acne in conjunction with or before the initiation of light-based therapy. Combining tetracyclines with light therapy is a relative contraindication because the skin is more photosensitive, but in my experience the increased post-treatment erythema is worth the benefit. Patients need to be informed of the possible side effects.

Rosacea

Although rosacea is a different disease from acne vulgaris, it warrants discussion here because of the many similarities between the two, including an inflammatory component and small papules and pustules. When treating rosacea, skin care should be restricted to mild, hypoallergenic products. Prescription metronidazole preparations such as Rosasol and Metrogel are effective at controlling the

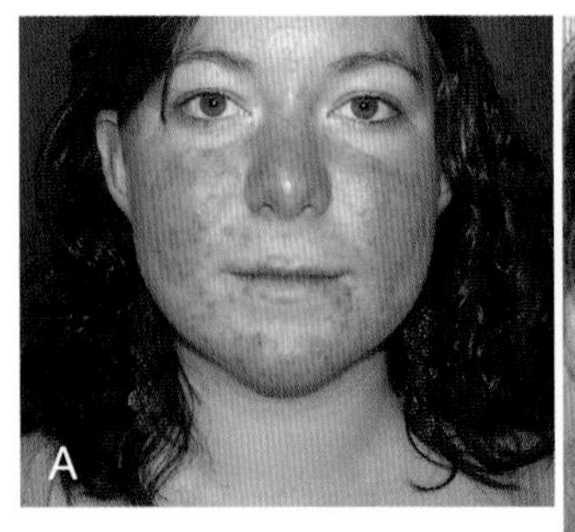

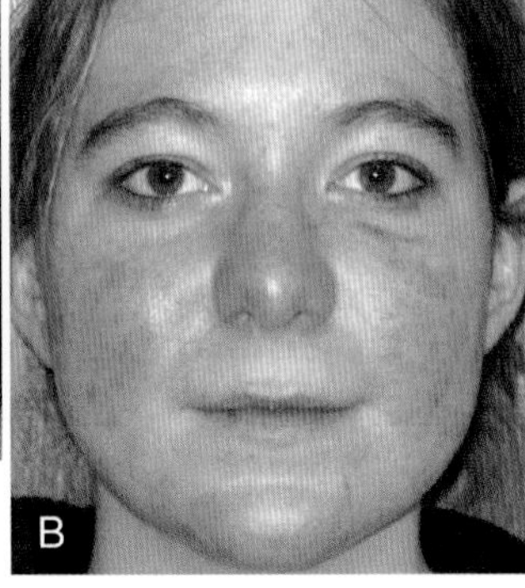

Figure 50-1 Treatment of inflammatory acne with scars. Five intense pulsed-light treatments were performed with the Vasculight (Lumenis, Yokneam, Israel) SR handpiece combined with three photodynamic therapy treatments with incubation periods lasting 30 to 90 minutes. **A,** Before treatment. **B,** After treatment.

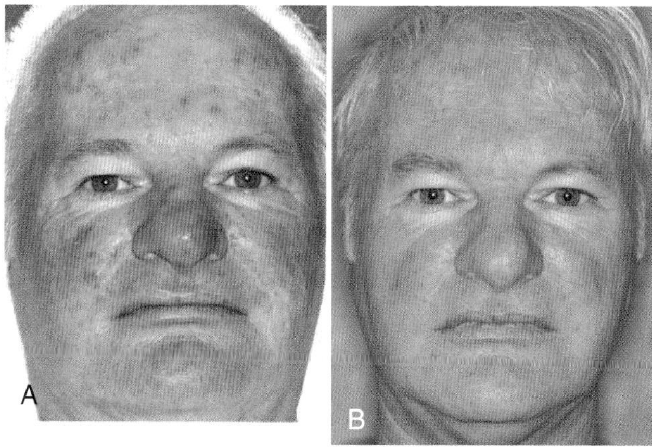

Figure 50-2 Treatment of refractory rosacea acne with five intense pulsed-light treatments with the Vasculight and three photodynamic therapy treatments with incubation periods of 60 to 120 minutes. **A,** Before treatment. **B,** After treatment.

disease activity, and IPL and PDT treatments can be highly effective in reversing erythema, telangiectasia, and the activity of the disease (Fig. 50-2).

Blue Light and Red Light Therapy

Approximately 70% of patients report improvement of their acne after sunlight exposure. In vivo studies, however, have provided insufficient evidence to justify the use of ultraviolet A and B as antiacne treatment, especially given their potential carcinogenicity. Because the strongest porphyrin photoexcitation band that produces singlet oxygen lies between 407 and 420 nm, irradiation of *P. acnes* with blue light leads to predictable bacterial destruction. Studies have shown a mean acne lesion reduction of 64% for papulopustular acne in a treatment course of two 15-minute sessions per week over 5 weeks. Various devices are available, such as the Clearlight, the Blu-U, and 410-nm IPL devices. The treatments are painless and have no side effects (Fig. 50-3).

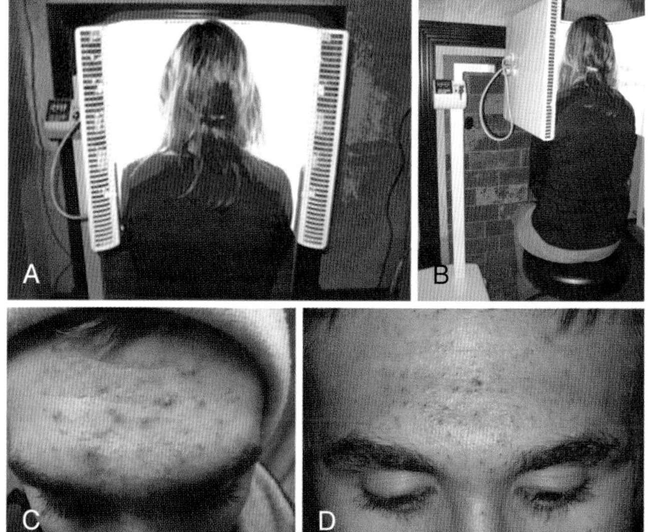

Figure 50-3 Blue light sessions combined with extractions and skin care (**A** and **B**). Before (**C**) and after (**D**) a 6-week course of twice-weekly treatments.

Although *blue light* has the strongest porphyrin photoexcitation ability, it is limited by its depth of penetration in skin. *Red light*, although a less effective photoexciting wavelength, has an increased depth of penetration in human skin and may also induce anti-inflammatory effects by stimulating cytokine release from macrophages. Improvements as high as 76% have been achieved in combined blue and red light studies, perhaps because of a synergistic effect of these wavelengths.

Photodynamic Therapy

Photodynamic therapy (see also Chapter 60, Photodynamic Therapy) refers to the topical application of D-aminolevulinic acid (ALA; e.g., Levulan) to the skin, which, when preferentially absorbed by pilosebaceous units, is metabolized through the heme synthesis pathway to produce protoporphyrin IX. PDT has been widely used for the treatment of a variety of skin diseases, including nonmelanoma skin cancer, actinic keratoses, warts, psoriasis, cutaneous T-cell lymphoma, and acne vulgaris.

When protoporphyrin IX is photoactivated by the appropriate wavelengths of light (intense pulsed light [IPL], pulse light, or blue light), singlet oxygen and free radicals are produced with cytotoxic effects. Not only is *P. acnes* destroyed, but the pilosebaceous unit is damaged or destroyed. ALA application time, also referred to as the incubation period, can vary between 15 and 120 minutes. Red light, blue light, IPL, diode laser, pulsed dye laser, and light-emitting diode (LED) sources have all been shown to be effective in activating protoporphyrin IX. Studies have shown a decrease in acne lesion counts that persists from 10 to 20 months after one to four treatments. Typically, three treatments are performed at 2- to 4-week intervals to achieve a remission of this duration. PDT results in a temporary reduction in skin oiliness, improvement in acne severity, and a cosmetic improvement of the skin with textural improvement and a reduction in sun damage and pore size. Cosmetic improvement of the skin is maximized when IPL parameters for skin rejuvenation are used at a moderate fluence. Possible side effects include initial burning discomfort, self-limiting crusting, erythema, mild edema, and hyperpigmentation. The side effects are reduced with short incubation periods and are self-limiting. Patients must stay out of the sun and bright rooms for a minimum of 24 hours after ALA is applied.

Intense Pulsed-Light Therapy

Intense pulsed light is a broadband light source that uses multiple wavelengths typically produced by a xenon flash-lamp, coupled with light filters to select specific bands of wavelengths to treat certain conditions. With acne, wavelengths are used that are highly absorbed into the sebum, the bacteria that are in the lesions, and the sebaceous glands (400 to 600 nm). These systems, such as the ClearTouch or Palomar Starlux with the LuxV handpiece, can be used on all skin types. The Lume 1 (Lumenis) is faster and can be used on all but the darkest skin types). Caution must be exercised when treating darker skin types because these wavelengths have an extremely high melanin absorption coefficient, so the risk of burning is high without proper settings, effective epidermal cooling, and testing. The broad range of emitted wavelengths covers the peak absorption of endogenous porphyrins produced by *P. acnes*, as well as that of hemoglobin in blood vessels close to the inflamed acne lesions, leading to both antibacterial and anti-inflammatory effects (Fig. 50-4).

Patients must be protected from any possible sun exposure before treatment because increased skin pigment (tanning) will increase the risk of epidermal burning from the artificial light sources. A very small amount of sun exposure can alter the pigment of the skin, restricting the technician's ability to treat at optimal settings. Self-tanning creams are also contraindicated because any darkening of the skin that increases absorption of light energy where it is not

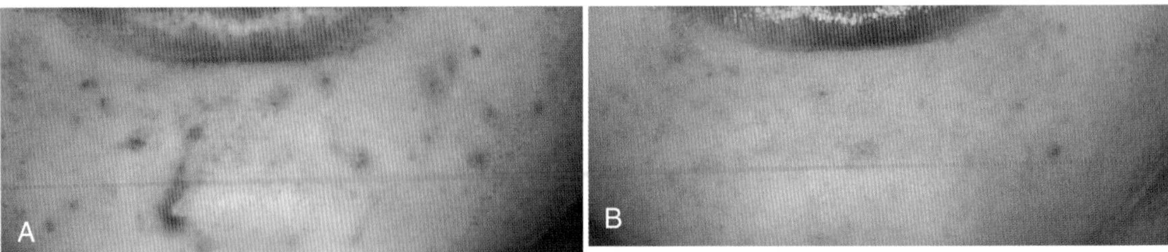

Figure 50-4 Treatment of recalcitrant acne on the chin. The patient received 2 weeks of twice-weekly treatments with the LuxV handpiece (Palomar Medical Technologies, Burlington, Mass). **A,** Before treatment. **B,** After treatment.

desired will restrict the amount of power that can be safely used. Areas of higher melanin concentration and areas of more sensitive skin should be evaluated and treated accordingly. Pretreatment of the skin with topical hydroquinone 4% twice a day for 2 to 4 weeks for patients with Fitzpatrick skin type 4 or higher will reduce the incidence of hyperpigmentation after laser and IPL treatments.

Treatment with light-based technology incorporates the ability to tailor both the pulse duration and the fluence energy used. Contact cooling before, during, and after the light pulse is also important. Tailoring *pulse duration* means altering the duration of light being emitted from the flash-lamp in milliseconds. The *delay* between pulses allows some cooling of surrounding tissue while target chromophores absorb additional energy with the second, shorter pulse. Cooling of the epidermis allows the user to deliver a larger amount of energy to the target and also reach deeper into the skin, while protecting the superficial layers of the skin. Some additional cooling may be necessary after treatment, both for comfort and to prevent blistering (e.g., ice pads). Using these principles, the initial treatment settings are often 100-msec pulse duration with fluences of 10 to 14 J/cm^2, followed by a second pass using a 20-msec pulse with fluences of 8 to 12 J/cm^2. Subsequent treatments will have the same pulse durations, but with increasing fluence. The first pulse penetrates deeper and allows for a longer heating time to affect the cysts and glands, whereas the second pass attacks the more superficial lesions. Most patients notice improvement with five to six treatments. If the fluence is not increased throughout the course of the treatments, results may not meet expectations. The treatment will cause some discomfort, and some redness is to be expected, but it typically clears within hours.

Treatments should be conducted at 2- to 3-week intervals for *teenagers* because their flare-ups seem to occur within this time frame, whereas *adults* respond better to monthly treatments. When treatment intervals are too short, flare-ups may occur; however, too long of an interval between treatments will also diminish the cumulative effect of treatments and the ultimate outcome.

With regard to *complications*, as stated earlier, there is a large amount of melanin absorption at these wavelengths, and therefore patients should be advised that permanent hair reduction may occur in the treated areas. Men are required to shave before treatment on the face, and some pain is to be expected in these areas. There can be lateral spread of the effect owing to diffusion of light in the skin, so if trying to avoid a hairline or eyebrow, stay at least 2 cm away from it to ensure that no thermal damage to the hair bulb or stem cells occurs.

"Major" complications include superficial blisters and burns. These are ultimately caused by overtreatment, too much sun exposure, or patients not following post-treatment instructions. Most burns and blisters can be treated with a class I steroid (clobetasol cream), and blisters can be treated with antibiotic/healing creams. Most burns resolve spontaneously within 2 months; however, hypopigmentation can still be seen after 8 to 12 months on some darker-skinned patients.

After treatment, in addition to immediate cooling with a cold pack, patients are told to limit sun exposure, use a noncomedogenic moisturizer that includes a sunscreen, and avoid external heating factors that could create an adverse reaction. Most patients are able to continue their combination oral or topical therapies during the treatment course, including tetracycline antibiotics. Combination therapy increases the treatment success rate. Some erythema secondary to the thermal damage is to be expected. This can be treated by short-term use of an over-the-counter hydrocortisone cream, which will not affect the treatment or cause further breakouts. LEDs such as the Gentlewaves (590-nm wavelength) can be used because LEDs are proven to aid the body in the thermal healing response.

Laser Therapy

Lasers with wavelengths used to treat vascular lesions and superficial pigmented lesions can also be used to treat acne. These wavelengths also act through photoactivation of bacterial porphyrins as well as potentially causing nonspecific thermal injury to sebaceous glands. Devices such as the Aura, a potassium titanyl phosphate (KTP) laser, and the NLite System, a pulsed dye laser, have been shown to provide a reduction in acne severity. Studies with as few as one treatment to biweekly treatments for 2 weeks reduced acne by 39% to 50%. Results were found to be more effective in combination with topical therapy than with lasers alone.

Infrared lasers have recently become one of the most effective available acne treatments because of their depth of penetration into the dermis. Experience with isotretinoin use has shown shrinkage of sebaceous glands and marked reduction of sebum production during treatment. Although sebum production returns to normal after cessation of treatment, many patients remain clear of acne, leading to the hypothesis that a temporary effect on sebaceous glands may be adequate to induce long-term acne clearance. With infrared lasers, the target chromophore is water, which is the dominant chromophore in sebaceous glands. The laser produces an injury zone in the dermal layer where sebaceous glands are located and in theory causes enough injury to arrest overproduction of sebum, thereby eliminating acne.

Both 1450-nm and 1540-nm lasers have been studied in trials. Initial biopsies confirmed thermal coagulation of the sebaceous gland, but biopsies at 2 and 6 months revealed no long-term alteration of the skin. Studies combining pulsed dye laser with infrared laser show synergistic effects, suggesting that infrared laser may have clinical use as a primary or adjunctive acne treatment in patients requiring an alternative to more traditional methods of treatment. Side effects are transient and local, including erythema and discomfort during treatment, without any delayed adverse effects.

Radiofrequency

Although radiofrequency is not a light-based technology, it has a similar effect on the sebaceous unit as laser by producing thermal injury to the dermis, including the sebaceous gland. The ThermaCool system has been studied and shows encouraging results in reducing acne and improving acne scarring, although the study size was small with limited follow-up, underscoring the need for larger studies with longer follow-up.

Conclusion

A proper history and physical examination with accurate diagnosis are imperative before treatment of acne commences. A stepwise approach and establishing realistic expectations are important. Patients need to understand the chronic nature of the disease and the possibility that acne will be refractory to treatment. Combination therapy remains the best approach in the treatment of acne.

Comedonal acne is best managed with skin care that includes appropriate exfoliation and topical retinoids. If multiple lesions are inflamed and infected, benzoyl peroxide and topical or oral antibiotics must be prescribed along with skin care to reduce the infection. Blue light, IPL, and PDT can be added for more severe cases.

Nodulocystic acne is unlikely to respond to topical therapy and, if the severity warrants, is best treated with oral antibiotics and PDT in combination with IPL and blue light or isotretinoin (Accutane). Unfortunately, recent continued negative publicity and its correlation with depression and suicide, as well as documented birth defects, may lead to Accutane's eventual recall from the U.S. market by the Food and Drug Administration.

The use of light-based technology has greatly increased the treatment success rate for acne. It may be considered after oral and topical therapy failure in patients with inflammatory acne without scarring, or in conjunction with current therapies as part of a first-line of therapy in patients presenting with both active acne and acne scars. However, cost, discomfort, erythema, multiple office visits, and complications are potential downsides to laser and other light-based therapies.

These newer treatments provide an attractive alternative for noncompliant patients and are free of complications such as antibiotic resistance and teratogenic side effect profiles. With continued technological advances in the ability to selectively target *P. acnes* and sebaceous glands, a new frontier of acne treatment is evolving, providing patients with safer and more effective treatment choices for one of the most prevalent and distressing skin conditions.

CPT/Billing Codes

10040 Acne surgery
10060 I&D one abscess
I&D multiple abscesses
11900 Intralesional injection ≥7
11901 Intralesional injection >7
96567 Photodynamic therapy

ICD-9-CM Diagnostic Codes

6953 Rosacea
7061 Acne

Suppliers

(See contact information online at www.expertconsult.com.)

Blue-U (blue light)
Clarion Medical Technologies, Inc.
Candela Smoothbeam diode laser
Northern Optotronics, Inc.
Intense pulsed-light devices
Clarion Medical Technologies, Inc.
NexGen Lasers, Inc.
Palomar Medical Technologies, Inc.
Isolaz Deep Pore Laser Therapy
SkinRx Distribution
Levulan
Clarion Medical Technologies, Inc.
Radiofrequency devices
NexGen Lasers, Inc.
Solta Medical

BIBLIOGRAPHY

Alexiades-Armenakas M: Long-pulsed dye laser-mediated photodynamic therapy combined with topical therapy for mild to severe comedonal, inflammatory, or cystic acne. J Drugs Dermatol 5:45–55, 2006.

Calderhead RG: The photobiological basics behind light-emitting diode (LED) phototherapy. Laser Ther 16:97–108, 2007.

Gold MH, Bradshaw VL, Boring MM, et al: The use of novel intense pulsed light and heat source and ALA-PDT in the treatment of moderate to severe inflammatory acne vulgaris. J Drugs Dermatol 3(Suppl):S15–S19, 2004.

Gold MH, Rao J, Goldman MP, et al: A multicenter clinical evaluation of the treatment of mild to moderate inflammatory acne vulgaris of the face with visible blue light in comparison to topical 1% clindamycin antibiotic solution. J Drugs Dermatol 4:64–70, 2005.

Goldberg D: Procedures in Cosmetic Dermatology Series: Lasers and Lights, Volume 1: Vascular/Pigmentation/Scars/Medical Applications. Philadelphia, Saunders, 2005.

Goldberg D: Procedures in Cosmetic Dermatology Series: Lasers and Lights, Volume 2: Rejuvenation/Resurfacing/Treatment of Ethnic Skin/Treatment of Cellulite. Philadelphia, Saunders, 2005.

Goldberg DJ, Russell BA: Combination blue (415 nm) and red (633 nm) LED phototherapy in the treatment of mild to severe acne vulgaris. J Cosmet Laser Ther 8:71–75, 2006.

Hongcharu W, Taylor CR, Chang Y, et al: Topical ALA-photodynamic therapy for the treatment of acne vulgaris. J Invest Dermatol 115:183–192, 2000.

Pregerson DB: Primary care procedures: Trephination of subungual hematoma. Consultant 48:241–244, 2008.

Taub AF: Photodynamic therapy for the treatment of acne: A pilot study. J Drugs Dermatol 3(Suppl):S10–S14, 2004.

Tzung T-Y, Wu K-H, Huang M-L: Blue light phototherapy in the treatment of acne. Photodermatol Photoimmunol Photomed 20:266–269, 2004.

Usatine RP: The Color Atlas of Family Medicine. New York, McGraw-Hill, 2009.

CHAPTER 51

Lasers and Pulsed-Light Devices: Skin Tightening

Gregory Costello

Advances in aesthetic and anti-aging medicine have led to treatments that were not available just a few decades ago. A multitude of options other than surgical intervention are now available to the patient who wishes to improve his or her appearance. The trend in aesthetic medicine has increasingly shifted from the concept of painful, long surgical recovery to multiple "minimal down time" procedures with little to no pain. This is especially true regarding the topic of skin tightening.

In the past, the concept of skin versus muscle laxity was irrelevant in terms of treatment because in either case the only treatment was surgical. However, with the advent of novel technologies that cause contraction, synthesis, and remodeling of collagen, "loose skin" can be addressed through noninvasive means. Laxity below the eyes, lowering of the brows, prominence of nasolabial folds, and formation of "jowls," among a multitude of other skin laxity issues, can be easily improved without painful surgery, long recovery times, or the risk of anesthesia.

Some types of sagging were and are still treated with surgery, such as an abdominoplasty (Fig. 51-1). This procedure is painful and requires general anesthesia. In addition, the procedure is costly, requires significant down time for recovery, and often leaves an unsightly scar.

This chapter focuses on the latest technologies developed specifically for tightening lax and sagging skin, which in turn reduces wrinkles and improves skin surface irregularities (Figs. 51-2 and 51-3). The latest technologies include intense pulsed light (IPL), radiofrequency (RF), and laser modalities to achieve a similar goal of dermal heating to produce changes in skins. (Also see Chapter 52, Nonablative Radiowave Skin Tightening with the Ellman S5 Surgitron [The Pelleve Procedure].) Most of these modalities show some immediate short-term results owing to temporary protein contraction; however, because of the stimulation of collagen formation, maximum results, which are also longer lasting, require up to 8 months to complete the remodeling process.

Skin Structure and Breakdown

As we age, our skin's structure deteriorates as a result of sun exposure, dietary habits, and natural processes. As the collagen in the skin breaks down, the skin's tightness and general elasticity decreases, causing a sagging or loose appearance. This tissue breakdown occurs at a depth of 3 to 5 mm in the dermis.

Treatment Evolution

The new technology that has evolved from older treatments involves passing certain types of light or current through the top layers of skin, leaving them undamaged but affecting a specific target deeper in the dermis, which in turn stimulates the production of "good" collagen. These treatments are mostly quite noninvasive and, in most cases, involve very little pain. They do involve multiple treatments, and the results are noticeable over time.

Light-Based Technology

In recent years, many systems have been developed using light to target the condition of loose skin. These systems use various wavelengths and different types of technology. In principle, light penetrates deep into the skin where it is absorbed by water and converted to heat energy. The thermal conversion then stimulates fibroblasts to produce new collagen. Some of the original systems, such as the CoolTouch (Roseville, Calif) system, used the 1320-nm neodymium-doped yttrium–aluminum garnet (Nd-YAG) wavelength. The 1440-nm Nd-YAG wavelength has also been used, but the results have been only slightly better than those with the 1320-nm systems. Good results have also been achieved with the use of IPL technology to deliver specified wavelength bands for a more efficient heating process. IPL technology uses several wavelengths banded together by light cut-off filters to specifically target certain chromophores in the skin. In the case of skin tightening, the target chromophore is water. Accordingly, for the treatments to be effective, the system must use wavelengths that are well absorbed by water.

Infrared Light

Infrared laser technology can be used to target water as a chromophore for photothermolysis. There are many examples of infrared technologies, both ablative and nonablative, that can be used to promote collagen growth in the dermis. The Cutera (Brisbane, Calif) 1064-nm Nd-YAG laser targets microvasculature to produce subdermal heating using high peak energies delivered through microsecond pulses. This gentle heating of the skin causes type I collagen formation, resulting in improvement in skin firmness and texture. Type I collagen is the most abundant type of collagen in the body and is found in blood vessels, multiple organs, tendons, and bone, as well as in skin. The proportion of type I collagen increases when tissue repair or healing occurs.

There are other wavelengths in the infrared spectrum that are surface ablative and promote collagen growth by means of deep dermal heating. Use of these lasers improves surface defects in the skin (e.g., roughness, sun damage, rhytids) as well as promotes collagen growth. The 2790-nm yttrium–scandium–gallium garnet (YSSG) laser (Pearl Laser; Cutera) uses water as a chromophore, causing vaporization of approximately 10 to 30 μm of epidermal tissue and coagulation of an additional 20 to 60 μm of tissue. Below this layer of coagulation, the tissue is heated. It is in this heated subcoagulation region where collagen stimulation occurs. The coagulated tissue acts as an occlusive dressing that quickly peels off, leaving behind a layer of skin where the collagen remodeling occurs.

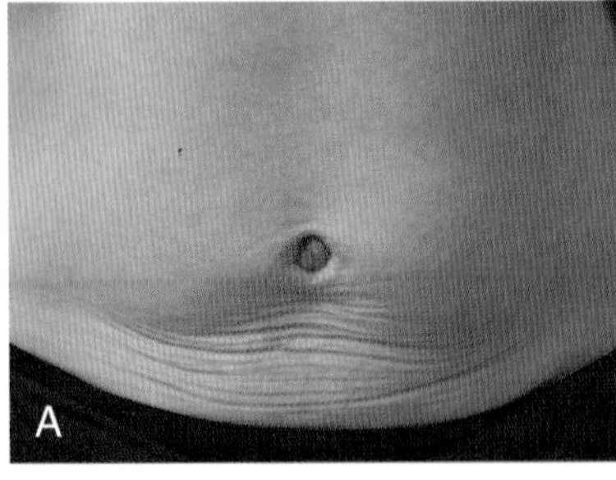

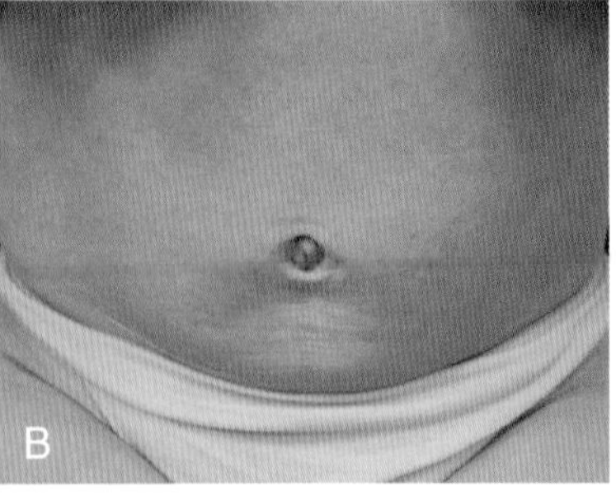

Figure 51-1 **A,** Preoperative photograph showing laxity of the abdominal skin. **B,** Same patient 3 months after treatment. (Courtesy of Palomar Medical Technologies, Inc., Burlington, Mass.)

The most widely used parameters for this treatment are between 1.0 and 3.5 J/cm^2, with a pulse width of 0.3 to 0.5 msec. Maximal dermal heating occurs with a higher pulse width with this procedure.

Fractionated Infrared Light

The use of *fractional light delivery* with infrared light allows for a higher fluence, resulting in a deeper thermal effect and thus deeper tightening. The idea of fractional energy delivery, which has been made popular recently by the Reliant Fraxel (Solta Medical, Hayward, Calif) and Palomar Lux IR (Palomar Medical Technologies, Burlington, Mass) systems, involves controlled thermal damage. The concept centers on the principle of using microlenses to focus light to create a significant amount of thermal damage in one column while leaving the surrounding tissue relatively undamaged. This stimulates the skin's normal healing response, including fibroblast activity that promotes new collagen production. In the case of the Palomar Lux IR fractional system, fractional delivery is combined with optimum wavelength selection to allow for deep thermal injury with minimal pain and risk. Cooling is absolutely necessary because these wavelengths are all very highly absorbed by water, and at the fluencies that are being used a burn is likely without proper cooling. This system is equipped with contact sensors, which allow the system to fire only if proper contact is achieved. This ensures that the skin is adequately cooled.

Intense Pulsed Light

Intense pulsed-light technology, in the infrared wavelengths, uses a spectrum of wavelengths to achieve collagen production through fibroblast stimulation. The Cutera Titan XL uses flash lamp technology in the 1100- to 1800-nm wavelengths, where water is the dominant chromophore. The challenge in IPL technology has always been to provide enough energy to the desired target without causing thermal damage to the surface tissue. The Titan XL overcomes this risk through a cycle of cooling before and after the delivery of energy to the desired target. The treatment area is covered with a thin layer of gel and the 3 × 1-cm IPL handpiece crystal is placed directly in contact with the skin. One second of cooling is followed by the delivery of heat at the selected fluence, followed by 2 more seconds of cooling. Both the cooling and delivery of energy take place through the contact crystal and are preprogrammed to occur automatically without having to lift the handpiece from contact with the skin. This automated cycle allows for the delivery of high amounts of energy deep into the skin while protecting the surface from visible damage.

RADIOFREQUENCY

Radiofrequency, unlike light-based technologies that operate based on absorption coefficients, is based on passing an RF current deep into the skin that is designed to denature collagen deeper in the skin while leaving the top layer undamaged. This causes immediate tightening and thermal damage, which stimulates new collagen growth. The thermal effect is generated by the tissue's natural resistance to the movement of ions within an RF field.

The ThermaCool TC system from Thermage (Solta Medical) is an example of a monopolar RF technology. This system uses a capacitive coupling membrane to couple the RF to the skin. A grounding plate is attached to the patient to dissipate the current, and the RF generator is then turned on. This type of delivery allows for deep penetration by the RF and, as a result, much better heating than that obtained with RF bipolar electrodes. Monopolar delivery of RF causes excellent volumetric tissue heating. Monopolar RF treatments are moderately painful and do pose a risk for scarring and burns when not operated correctly.

Another approach to skin tightening using RF technology is the addition of IPL. The ReFirme ST from Syneron (Irvine, Calif) uses pulses of infrared light in the 700- to 2000-nm wavelength range simultaneously with bipolar RF. The pulse of infrared light uses melanin and hemoglobin as chromophores, thus heating the dermis. The heating effect creates a path of optimal electrical conductivity or lower impedence. Because electricity prefers the path of lowest impedence, the electrical bipolar RF energy is concentrated at the target site preheated by the optical energy. Contact cooling at the treatment site minimizes electrical conduction to the epidermis and allows most of the energy to penetrate into deeper parts of the dermis.

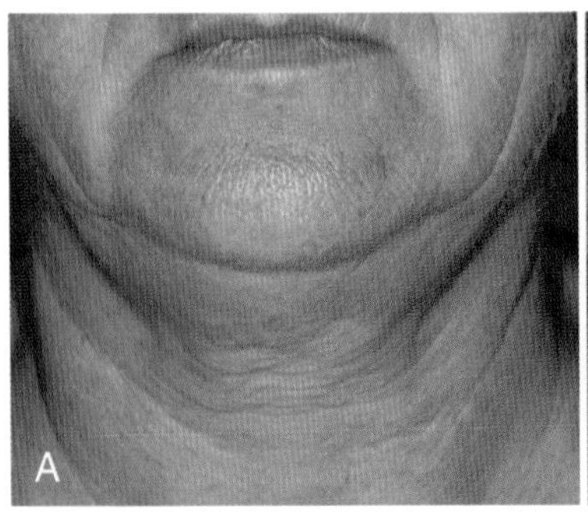

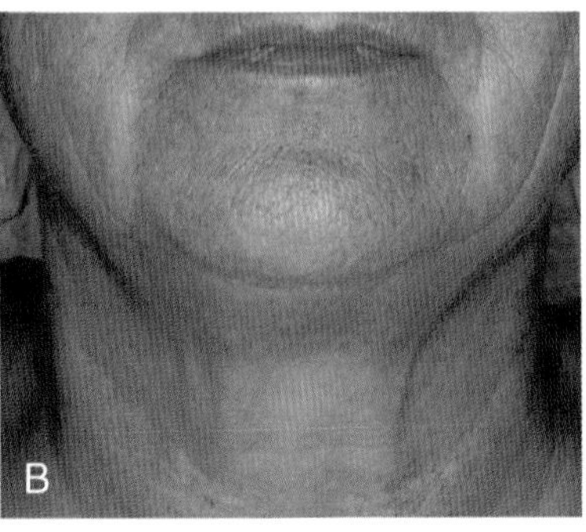

Figure 51-2 **A,** Preoperative frontal photograph showing sagging of the neck skin. **B,** Same patient 2 months after treatment. (Courtesy of Khalil A. Khatri, MD, Skin and Laser Surgery Center of New England, Nashua, NH, and Palomar Medical Technologies, Inc., Burlington, Mass.)

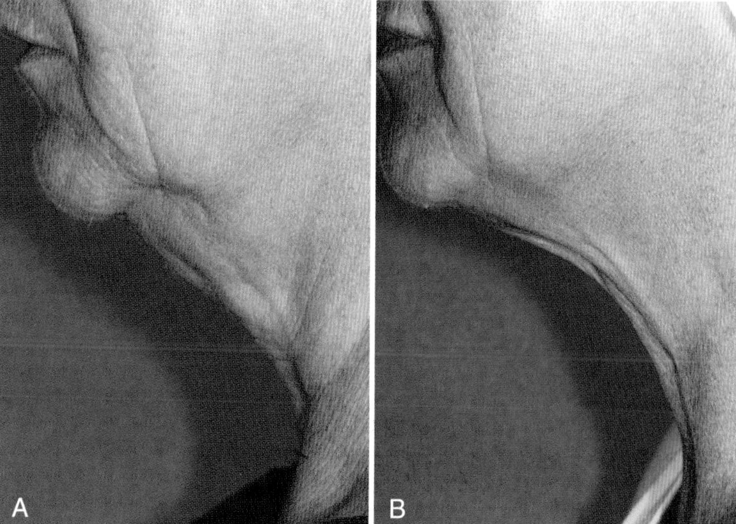

Figure 51-3 **A,** Preoperative photograph taken from the side showing laxity of the neck skin. **B,** Same patient 1 month after treatment. (Courtesy of Khalil A. Khatri, MD, Skin and Laser Surgery Center of New England, Nashua, NH, and Palomar Medical Technologies, Inc., Burlington, Mass.)

TIPS AND COMMON ERRORS

- Choose the right patient for best results. These systems are designed only to tighten skin, so muscle laxity and excessive fat will not improve in appearance.
- Be cautious with darker skin types (types 3 to 6) in any system that uses melanin as a chromophore.

CONCLUSION

As with most aesthetic procedures, patient selection is of the highest priority to maximize patient satisfaction. The aforementioned procedures work best in patients with mild to moderate skin laxity. The procedures will produce a subtle tightening of the loose or sagging skin but are not intended for correction of muscle laxity or severe skin laxity, or excess skin in overweight patients. Physicians must fully explain to patients what they should expect and what not to expect from their treatments to attain the highest patient satisfaction from any skin tightening device.

SUPPLIERS

(See contact information online at www.expertconsult.com.)

Cutera World Headquarters
Palomar Medical Technologies, Inc.
Syneron Medical LTD.
Thermage, Inc.

ONLINE RESOURCE

American Board of Laser Surgery. Available at www.americanboardoflasersurgery.org.

BIBLIOGRAPHY

Anderson RR, Parrish JA: Selective photothermolysis: Precise microsurgery by selective absorption of pulsed radiation. Science 220:524–527, 1983.

Dierickx CC: The role of deep heating for noninvasive skin rejuvenation. Lasers Surg Med 38:799–807, 2006.

Goldberg D: Procedures in Cosmetic Dermatology Series: Lasers and Lights, Volume 1: Vascular/Pigmentation/Scars/Medical Applications. Philadelphia, Saunders, 2005.

Goldberg D: Procedures in Cosmetic Dermatology Series: Lasers and Lights, Volume 2: Rejuvenation/Resurfacing/Treatment of Ethnic Skin/Treatment of Cellulite. Philadelphia, Saunders, 2005.

Goldberg DJ: Histologic changes after treatment with intense pulsed light. J Cutan Laser Ther 2:53–56, 2000.

Goldman M: Clinical pearl: Observations on the use of fractionated CO2 laser resurfacing. J Drugs Dermatol 8:82–86, 2009.

Kauvar A, Hruza G (eds): Principles and Practices in Cutaneous Laser Surgery. Boca Raton, Fla, Taylor and Francis, 2005.

Moy RL, Dover JS: Procedures in Cosmetic Dermatology Series: Advanced Face Lifting. Philadelphia, Saunders, 2006.

Sadick N: Combination radiofrequency and light energies: Electro-optical synergy technology in aesthetic medicine. Dermatol Surg 31:1211–1217, 2005.

Saluja R, Khoury J, Detwiler S, Goldman M: Histologic and clinical response to varying density settings with a fractionality scanned carbon dioxide laser. J Drugs Dermatol 8:17–20, 2009.

Schmults CD, Phelps R, Goldberg DJ: Nonablative facial remodeling: Erythema reduction and histologic evidence of new collagen formation using a 300-microsecond 1064-nm Nd:YAG laser. Arch Dermatol 140:1373–1376, 2004.

Small R: Combination cosmetic treatments. In Usatine RP, Pfenninger JL, Stulberg DL, Small R (eds): Dermatologic and Cosmetic Procedures in Office Practice. Philadelphia, Saunders, 2011.

Small R: Photorejuvenation with lasers. In Usatine RP, Pfenninger JL, Stulberg DL, Small R (eds): Dermatologic and Cosmetic Procedures in Office Practice. Philadelphia, Saunders, 2011.

Tan KL, Kurniawati C, Gold M: Low risk of postinflammatory hyperpigmentation in skin types 4 and 5 after treatment with fractional CO2 laser device. J Drugs Dermatol 7:774–777, 2008.

Waibel J, Beer K: Ablative fractional laser resurfacing for the treatment of a third degree burn. J Drugs Dermatol 8:294–297, 2009.

CHAPTER 52

Nonablative Radiowave Skin Tightening with the Ellman S5 Surgitron (The Pelleve Procedure)

Michael Stampar

The demand for procedures to rejuvenate aging skin has never been greater, and the baby boomer market demands results without downtime. Nonablative monopolar radiofrequency energy (NMRFE) has been shown to contract skin in both a horizontal and vertical axis through "volumetric" heating of the dermis and subdermis. This radiofrequency (RF) energy is conducted/passed through from the dome-shaped active handpiece touching the skin, directly to a passive antenna plate placed behind the body part. Heat is generated at the dermal–subdermal junction, where fat provides the highest resistance to the flow of electrons. This increased impedance causes heating of adjacent deep dermal type one and three collagen fibrils and causes contraction of skin in a horizontal plane. Further deeper heating, with conduction through vertical connective tissue bands, running through fat from the deep dermis to the underlying fascia, has been shown to be the mechanism responsible for vertical contraction, or a "shrink-wrap" effect with NMRFE. Many different RF devices have become available, but primary care providers interested in providing antiaging procedures require technology that offers reliable results, with little to no risk of true complications, at a reasonable cost, and with a predictable range of efficacy.

The Ellman Dual Frequency S5 Surgitron device (Fig. 52-1) is unique because of the very high frequency (4 MHz, or 4 million cycles per second) it produces as compared with other RF devices. Earlier monopolar versions have been available for over 20 years as a source of RF energy for office surgery, with diverse applications in many specialties (see Chapter 30, Radiofrequency Surgery [Modern Electrosurgery]). More recently, dome-shaped, hand-held, alloy electrode treatment tips have been developed. They are to be used only with the S5 Surgitron device, to allow continuous, gradual, volumetric dermal and subdermal heating. These smooth-edged domes use low energy levels and allow constant visual, tactile, and patient-generated feedback to ensure safety.

The efficacy of thermally induced skin contraction appears to be temperature dependant and based on the number of repeat passes required to induce collagen denaturation and restructuring in any given patient. This gradually progressive heat-generating technique allows thermal injury to occur in both deep and more superficial levels of the dermis. Controlled thermal injury causes three-dimensional skin contraction with immediate as well as delayed improvement in wrinkles, texture, and pore size. Horizontal dermal contraction provides lift and tightening, whereas vertical contraction firms the skin by making the subdermal fat layer more compact. Patients seeking dermal fillers have had enough dermal thinning to allow collapse and creasing. Volume replacement is aided by firming the subdermal "compartment" where the volumizing products are deposited. By treating not only to the point of visible contraction, but to an end point of no further observable contraction, a demonstrable result can be achieved in almost every case in a single treatment session.

The degree of improvement depends on the "skin age" more than chronologic age. The more reversibly bound collagen fibrils remaining the better, and more rapid, the immediate result. When properly used, the dome-shaped handpieces allow the physician to deliver each patient's therapeutic dose painlessly, without significant safety concerns. Favorable results have been seen in patients ranging from a 19-year-old fashion model with early fine forehead lines, to an 81-year-old with coarse neck creases. Skin in other areas of the body also has responded when heated thoroughly. The safety, reliability, and low treatment cost make skin tightening with the Ellman Dual Frequency unit (Ellman International, Inc., Oceanside, NY) a reasonable treatment modality for the primary care physician providing antiaging services. At this time, the Pelleve procedure has received FDA clearance for the treatment of moderate-to-fine facial wrinkles and folds in types I to IV skin. Neck and body use mentioned in this chapter represent "off-label" use, as does treating types V and VI skin in the United States. There are no such restrictions outside the United States.

Anatomy

The pertinent anatomy for skin tightening includes the location of the collagen bundles and vertical fibrous connective tissue bands. The greatest densities of bundles of collagen fibrils are in the deep dermis just superficial to the dermal–subdermal junction, but they are present throughout the dermis. The decrease in density of these bundles with photodamage and aging leads to dermal softening, allowing lines and creases to form. Thermal denaturation of collagen occurs at a temperature of 65° C, which causes a breakdown of covalent bonds and restructured contraction of the helical fibrils; cooling appears to cause more rapid skin contraction. The inflammatory response and subsequent repair of the thermal injury bring fibroblasts that lay down new collagen, further improving the appearance of the skin by reversing, to some degree, the aging process of the skin. The more superficially the dermis is injured by vertical penetration of the accumulating heat energy, the greater the effect on fine lines and texture.

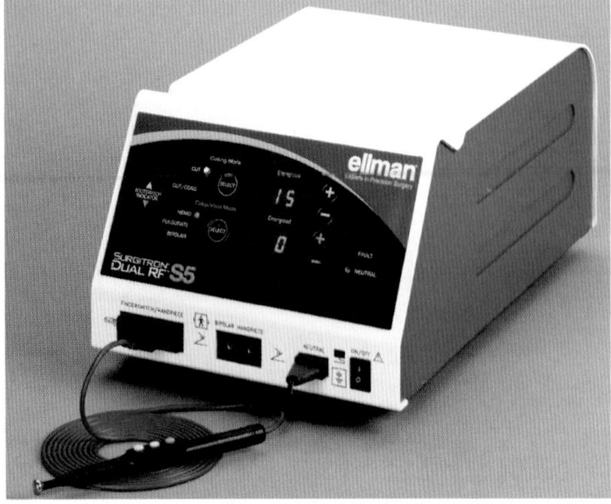

Figure 52-1 The Ellman Dual Frequency electrosurgical unit used for the Pelleve skin tightening procedure.

The vertical fibrous septa provide the path of least resistance for further energy flow to the passive electrode. The energy flows down these bands to their fascial origin, resulting in vertical contraction of the fibrous septa surrounding fat compartments that remain cool (Fig. 52-2).

Indications

Radiofrequency-generated thermal skin tightening with the Pelleve procedure is indicated in anyone showing signs of photodamaged or aging skin. Skin laxity—ranging from early softening of contours causing a vague, tired appearance to overt sagging—can benefit from the restoration of dermal collagen integrity. Ptotic brows and jawline, double chins, and an overall "melting" appearance of the skin on the face can be improved.

Significant improvement has been seen in these areas:

- Softened jaw contours (jowling)
- Flattened brow arch with or without forehead creasing
- Nasolabial and melolabial folds
- Crow's feet
- Excess upper lid skin
- Forehead and glabellar creasing and softening
- Double chin
- Neck softening and creasing
- Perioral lip lines
- Large pores and thick skin on the nose and chin
- Aged loose skin in the face, neck, arms, and abdomen (off-label)
- Dermal-filler patients (off-label)

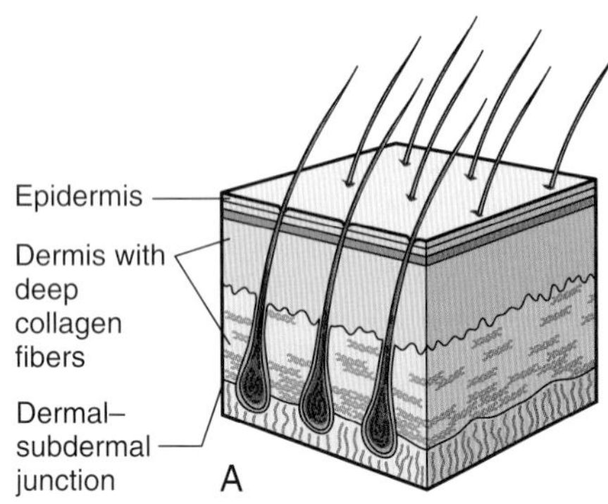

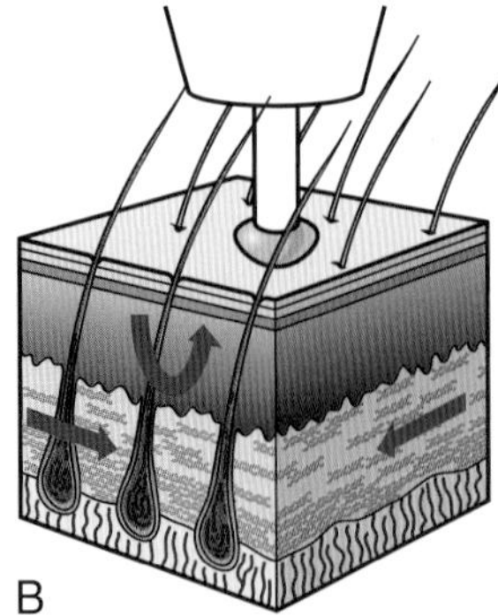

Figure 52-2 **A,** Diagram of actinically damaged or aged skin. **B,** Application of the S5 Surgitron probe. *Straight arrows* show horizontal saturation of deep collagen. *Curved arrow* shows heat rising more superficially to affect wrinkles.

Contraindications and Relative Contraindications

Currently in the United States the Pelleve procedure is cleared for use in patients with types I to IV skin. Despite the general acceptance that RF energy is "color blind," no patients with type V or VI skin were included in the study population. When combining RF skin tightening with botulinum toxin (Botox) or fillers, tighten first, then inject. Successful skin tightening will alter the amount of filler needed in glabellar and perioral lines and folds, so filling after skin tightening is advised. On the other hand, studies have shown no detrimental effects of heating with RF energy over all commonly used dermal fillers. Avoid heating over areas injected with Botox within 7 days to allow proper tissue penetration.

Contraindications include the following:

- The presence of any topical, local, regional, or general anesthetic that can alter the patient's perception of heat on the skin. Patients need to provide feedback on heat sensation to avoid burns and overheating.
- Pacemakers and implanted defibrillators (the "shielding" built into new devices decreases the risk, but patients should be cleared by a cardiologist familiar with the specific device before proceeding).
- Open skin lesions in the treatment area.
- Any neuropathy that alters pain sensation to the areas being treated.

NOTE: The use of anticoagulation is not a contraindication.

Equipment and Supplies

- Ellman Dual Frequency 4.0 radiofrequency generator with antenna plate (other, lower-frequency units, and coagulation- or hyfrecation-only units will not work safely!)
- Dome-shaped skin tightening handpieces: 5 mm for eyelids, 10 mm for face, 15 mm for face and neck (off-label)
- Pelleve cooling gel (ultrasound gels also work well, but others may coagulate or allow burns)
- Reusable soft gel cool packs
- Eye shields for direct eyelid treatment and anesthetic ophthalmic drops
- Nonsterile 4 × 4 gauze pads
- Elastic headband

NOTE: *Do not use any topical anesthetic on the skin!*

Preprocedure Care

- Ask patients to arrive with no makeup or remove makeup on arrival.
- Tell patients not to take pain medications or sedatives and avoid anti-inflammatory medicines for 1 week before and 4 weeks after

the procedure, if possible, to avoid blunting the inflammatory response to the treatment.

PROCEDURE

Photos are vital and should be taken. Take them with the patient standing in five positions and with appropriately lit close-ups of wrinkles in the forehead, periorbital, cheek, or lip areas. The lighting, positioning, and framing should be standardized for your camera and facility to ensure reliable comparisons of before and after photographs. Asymmetry between the two sides of the face or brow position, orbital height, or cheek volume should be reviewed with the patient in the mirror before starting the procedure. A headband can be used to keep dispersion gel out of the patient's hair, and also adds consistency to photographs.

The Pelleve procedure is performed with the patient placed in the *supine position* on a treatment table that allows the operator to sit at the head. Adequate lighting should be provided to allow close observation of changes in skin redness and texture as the treatment progresses. The passive electrode pad is placed against the skin of the upper back for face and neck treatments or, when treating other areas, directly under the treatment area. The *pure cut* waveform is used for the most efficient delivery of the RF energy. For facial applications, the 10-mm tip is used. When treating on or around the eyelids, *eye shields* provided with the device should be carefully inserted after topical anesthetic drops are instilled (see Chapter 10, Topical Anesthesia). *Dispertion gel* can be applied directly to the skin, or the dome-shaped electrode can be dipped into a reservoir of the gel, and is spread with the continuous *random circular* or *linear movement* of the tip on the treatment area. Failure to cover all areas with a layer of gel can result in rapid excessive heat delivery and burns. The dispertion gel provides smooth gliding over the skin and keeps the epidermis cooler than the dermis, where the therapeutic heating occurs. To provide the treatment safely and painlessly, contact of the treatment electrode with the skin through the dispertion gel *must* be established *before* activating the electrode.

Prior to activating the electrode on facial skin, "patient tuning" can be done on the back of the hand to determine the approximate heat threshold for each patient. Because of variability in local and total body impedance between patients, all treatments should be started with continuous movement at a power level of *20 watts* on *pure cutting mode* and increased a few watts at a time to find an effective but comfortable working level. Comfortable treatment levels will vary over the face and neck, with lower levels on the thinner skin of the forehead and periorbital area and higher levels in the cheek and neck areas.

The power setting should be adjusted based on patient feedback to allow a gradual, progressive warming from a "3 to 4" to a "7 to 8" on a scale where "10" would cause the patient to pull away. To optimize treatment time and patient comfort, a proper level of energy will require 10 to 15 seconds of continuous random-pattern contact to reach the heat perception level of 7 to 8 over an *area* of 6 to 10 cm^2.

Treatment level and heat perception can be adjusted by changing the power level of the pure cut mode or by changing the speed of movement or amount of area covered between passes. Initially the provider may completely depend on the patient's feedback to decide when to move to the next treatment area. But, with experience, observed color and texture changes will indicate that the tissue temperature is near threshold before the patient needs to alert you to increased heat sensation. A dialogue should be maintained between the operator and patient to develop an understanding of the patient's heat tolerance and variations in heat perception in all treatment areas. Handheld infrared temperature guns can be used to spot-monitor the temperature to help avoid undertreating easily reddened skin and to monitor progress.

Slower, more concentrated movements in an area will often result in "jumping" from a 5 to 9 on the heat perception scale, whereas rapid movements over a large area may seem never to achieve that threshold temperature to allow collagen remodeling. A compromise between these two extremes should be reached.

Passes over sensitive areas such as the orbital rim under the brow are incorporated into other periocular passes over crow's feet and the temple because all these areas require a lower treatment energy than the thicker cheek and forehead skin. Avoid heating directly over the brow hairs, as this may cause a spark gap or tattooed brows to change color.

So, in addition to patient feedback, control of the treatment level also requires observing the skin for redness, visible smoothing, and contraction. A *"pass"* is counted each time an *area* is taken from warm to almost too warm on "threshhold temperature," when visible contraction is seen or the patient repeats "that's hot." Circular or linear motions can be made (Fig. 52-3). If the patient repeatedly reports the sensation is too warm too quickly, the power setting should be turned down on the unit. Passes should be repeated until no further contraction or smoothing occurs with continued energy delivery. This end point must be reached for a demonstrable result. In general, when addressing wrinkles directly, the operator will return to the previously treated area for additional passes after going over the next one or two adjacent areas to allow some gel pack cooling between passes. When performed properly at appropriate energy settings, the procedure should be essentially painless.

In contrast to other devices that are limited by pulses to be delivered, *continuous confluent energy should be applied to all facial skin*, hairline to hairline laterally, and to the clavicle inferiorly when treating the neck (off-label in the United States). By extending the facial treatment to the firm, adherent skin of the scalp and over the sternocleidomastoid muscle in the neck, the contraction achieved after several passes has an anchor point for pulling the skin taut rather than simply contracting concentrically. In the midface, more energy should be delivered laterally and across the jawline, where maximal horizontal contraction and tightening will occur relative to the medial cheek fat pad areas, where vertical contraction will firm and smooth the skin. Excessive malar flattening should be avoided. All forehead and neck areas are treated evenly to the therapeutic end point of definitive visible firming, contraction, or smoothing. It will take several passes over an area to get to a point that the skin can be seen to contract, firm, or smooth with each additional application of heat, followed by a cold pack. In a split-face, one-month study of four consecutive patients, the author demonstrated greater midface contraction when heating and cooling, versus just heating, was used

The time it takes to treat adjacent areas to tolerance allows enough cooling time to then *return to the initial area for added passes*. If discomfort occurs immediately, decrease the energy level or terminate the treatment for that area. The skin will progress to a point of no further contraction in two to five additional passes after seeing contraction after the first pass. Typically, one pass in each area per decade of age is required for maximal contraction and smoothing.

A full face and neck procedure takes approximately 40 to 60 minutes, depending on the skin condition and size of the patient.

At the point of completion for an anatomic area, *cold gel packs* are applied with gentle pressure in the desired direction of contraction to rapidly chill the freshly denatured collagen bundles, primarily in the midface, where three-dimensional contraction provides lift. The theory behind this is that rapid cooling will force tighter contraction of covalent bonding of the collagen helices, similar to setting a molten mold.

NOTE: *Care should be taken not to activate the electrode treatment tip before skin contact is established and not to lose contact while energy is being delivered*. Disrupting the contact between the treatment electrode and the dispertion gel while the electrode is active will cause a spark gap to occur, which causes an "electric shock"-type feeling. This can happen if the patient pulls away, the operator pulls away, a dry area is touched, or thicker hair is crossed. This typically startles the subject but has not been observed to cause any significant

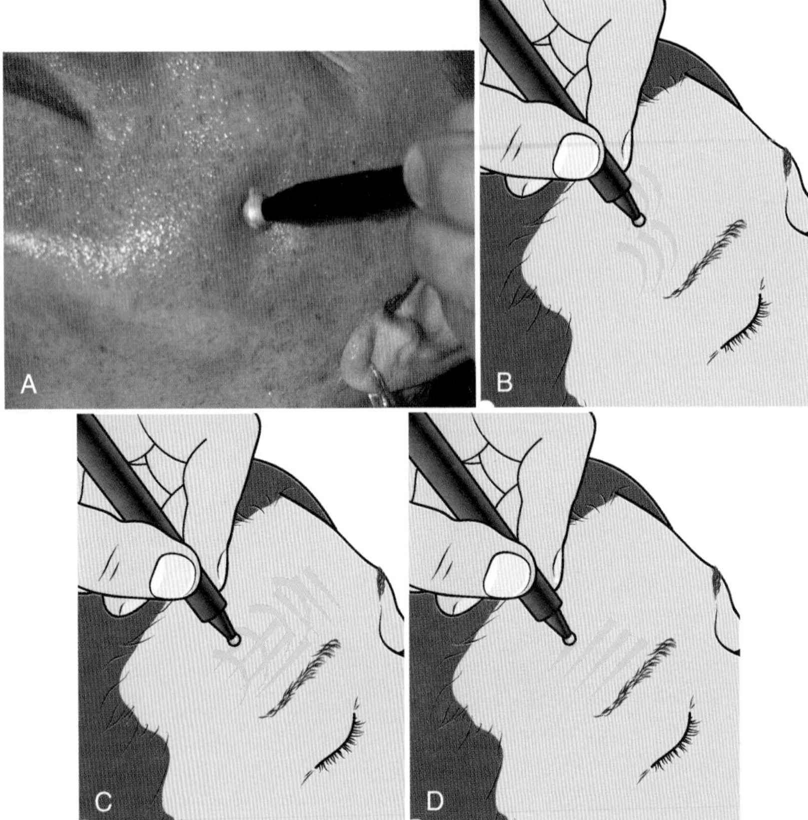

Figure 52-3 The energy is delivered using random geometric patterns such as swirls and horizontal and vertical strokes. The purpose is to deliver a confluent heating to all treated skin and to avoid any nonrandom movement that could theoretically leave a treatment pattern visible in the soft tissues. **A,** The Pelleve probe contacting the skin. **B,** Circular pattern. **C,** Linear and circular patterns (superimposed). **D,** Linear pattern.

epidermal damage. If stretching the skin is desired, hold gauze with a gloved hand on a dry area away from the actual active treatment site to avoid grounding yourself.

With this technique of treating gradually but progressively to the point of apparent maximal skin contraction, every patient should see and feel tightening, smoothing, lifting, or sculpting, depending on the aging characteristics being addressed. The degree of improvement depends on the "skin age" more than chronologic age. The more reversibly bound collagen fibrils remaining, the better, and the more rapid the immediate result. Skin in all areas can be tightened. A photograph of the half-treated face can be taken to document the treatment effects compared with the untreated side.

Figure 52-4 shows a patient before treatment and 2 months after Pelleve. In most patients, *a touch-up treatment* 4 to 8 weeks after the original treatment typically yields an additional 10% to 20% improvement, possibly addressing post-treatment relaxation or incomplete collagen denaturation. These "touch-ups" typically take only two to four passes and always show more rapid heating than the original treatment. The greater the laxity, the greater the response to a second or third procedure. The patient should be advised that treatment results should continue to improve for up to 4 months based on the physiology of thermal tissue injury and that they may repeat the procedure every 1 to 2 years as needed after a desired end point is reached.

Complications

- Very limited
- Discomfort if power is set too high
- Rarely, a burn caused by activating the electrode before making contact or after losing contact
- Possible lack of intended tightening because of inadequate residual collagen
- Inadequate effort

Post-Treatment Care

There should be no downtime with the Pelleve skin tightening procedure when performed properly. Transient reddening of the skin should resolve in 1 to 3 hours, and no change in skin care is required. Makeup can be applied immediately. They are also advised to take 1000 mg of vitamin C daily in oral form for 6 months to ensure an adequate systemic supply for collagen synthesis. Patients are re-evaluated at 6 weeks, 6 months, and 1 year following the procedure. Additional RF treatments are recommended every 6 to 8 weeks for six months, or until the patient is satisfied a maximal result has been achieved (for patients with excessively wrinkled or lax areas). Light peels, filler injections, Botox injections, or surgery can be done any time after the treatment.

Ellman is the sole supplier of the device worldwide. The most significant observed advantages of this device and treatment relative to other RF-based devices and treatments are the tactile control of the treatment; gradual, progressive, continuous heating rather than pulsing; demonstrable results in a single, essentially painless treatment; and the cost of delivery. A bipolar treatment tip is being evaluated at this time and will be available with the same device if additional efficacy is seen.

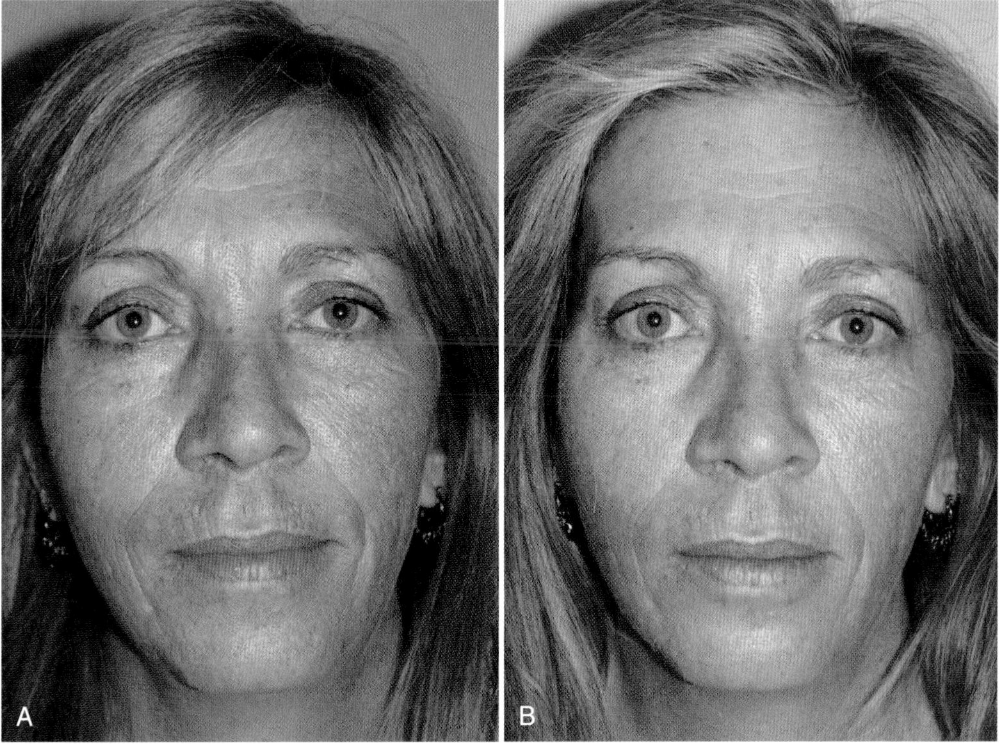

Figure 52-4 Appearance of the skin before (**A**) and after (**B**) Pelleve treatment.

Coding and Billing

This is an aesthetic procedure so there are no CPT/ICD-9 codes.

Patient Education Guides

See patient education and patient consent forms available at www.expertconsult.com.

Suppliers

(Contact information also available online at www.expertconsult.com.)

Ellman International, Inc.
3333 Royal Ave.
Oceanside, NY 11572
800-835-5355/516-594-3333 (phone)
516-569-0054 (fax)
www.ellman.com

Online Resources

www.pelleve.com
www.lookyoungeratanyage.com
www.thebalancingact.com/show_segment.php?id=1266

Bibliography

Arnoczky SP, Aksan A: Thermal modification of connective tissues: Basic science considerations and clinical implications. J Am Acad Orthop Surg 8:305–313, 2000.

Bridenstine JB: Use of ultra-high frequency electrosurgery (radiosurgery) for cosmetic surgical procedures. Dermatol Surg 24:397–400, 1998.

England LJ, Tan M, Shumaker PR, et al: Effects of monopolar radiofrequency treatment over soft tissue fillers in an animal model. Lasers Surg Med 37:356–365, 2005.

Rusciani A, Curinga G, Menichini G, et al: Nonsurgical tightening of skin laxity: A new radiofrequency approach. J Drugs Dermatol 6:381–386, 2007.

Taliaferro C: Submucosal radiosurgical uvulopalatoplasty for the treatment of snoring: Is the monitoring of tissue impedance and temperature necessary? Otolaryngol Head Neck Surg 124:46–50, 2001.

Zelickson BD, Kist D, Bernstein E, et al: Histologic and ultrastructural evaluation of the effects of a radiofrequency-based non-ablative dermal remodeling device: A pilot study. Arch Dermatol 140:204–209, 2004.

CHAPTER 53

Fractional Laser Skin Resurfacing

Gregory A. Buford

History of Laser Resurfacing

Facial aging follows a rather predictable course. As we age, our skin thins and becomes translucent, the collagen fibers in the deep dermis diminish in number and become more randomly organized, and pigmentary changes appear in more superficial layers as a result of years of actinic damage. Some of these changes can be ameliorated or reversed. To do so, the skin must be injured in a predictable manner that stimulates it to reorganize and rejuvenate during the healing process. Chemical peels, microdermabrasion, and laser rejuvenation have been used successfully in the past, but each has its own inherent advantages and disadvantages. In this chapter we focus on laser resurfacing and, most important, *fractional* laser resurfacing.

Lasers were developed in 1960 on the foundation of Einstein's quantum theory of radiation. Over time, the use of different lasing media allowed for the development of specific lasers and ultimately specific applications. Ablative laser resurfacing was first introduced in the 1990s with the advent of the CO_2 laser; soon thereafter, the erbium-doped yttrium aluminum garnet (Er:YAG) laser was released.

Although these two lasers formed the foundation of ablative resurfacing, they provided slightly different outcomes with respect to treatment efficacy, downtime, and risk for adverse events. The shorter wavelength of the erbium laser (2940 nm) versus the CO_2 laser (10,600 nm) allowed for more effective absorption of laser energy by water and thus a significantly higher absorption coefficient (Er = 12,000 vs. CO_2 = 800). As such, residual thermal damage was significantly less with use of the erbium laser than with the CO_2 laser. In addition, faster reepithelialization was noted with the erbium laser. But were these advantages necessarily decisive? Perhaps not: although the erbium laser has been associated with less downtime and erythema and a faster recovery, its overall results have been less dramatic than those attained with use of the CO_2 laser.

In response to the prolonged downtime associated with traditional ablative resurfacing, which is quite aggressive, a number of nonablative technologies were developed with the aim to provide noninvasive facial rejuvenation but to do so with minimal to no downtime. Technologies such as intense pulsed light (IPL), radiofrequency lasers, and infrared lasers were ultimately developed. While the downtime with these devices was definitely less, the overall results also were less impressive.

The next evolution of laser technology involved reintroduction of the erbium laser but in a "fractional pattern," with the first device to pioneer this technology being the Fraxel Laser (Solta Medical, Inc., Hayward, Calif). Fractionated resurfacing uses many small, separate columns of light to create microthermal treatment zones (MTZs) with bridges of untreated tissue in between. In the case of the Lumenis (Santa Clara, Calif) Ultrapulse Encore, spot size varies from 0.12 mm (DeepFX) to 1.3 mm (ActiveFX) and can be applied in a square, rectangular, linear, or other shaped configuration. The treated area appears as many small ablated "dots" as opposed to a single large, homogeneous ablated area. By leaving areas untouched, treated areas heal faster because of ingrowth from the surrounding untreated zones. The result is dramatic improvement with significantly less downtime.

Although fractionated erbium laser technology was a significant step ahead of its predecessors, the disadvantages were also clear. Most patients were seeing improvement, but it came at the cost of at least three to five treatment sessions. So although downtime was minimal, the overall duration of therapy was prolonged. Eventually, fractional technology was extended to a CO_2 platform, which then allowed for more effective rejuvenation in as little as one treatment.

Basics of Laser Therapy

Ablative devices such as the CO_2 and erbium laser use water as a target chromophore. As previously noted, the erbium wavelength is nearly 20 times more highly absorbed than the CO_2 wavelength. This difference effectively differentiates the two lasers. The absorbed laser energy then exerts two effects on the treated tissue: ablation and coagulation. *Ablation* involves actual destruction and removal/vaporization of tissue and can be beneficial in improving the superficial tone, texture, and appearance of the skin. *Coagulation*, on the other hand, is the result of heat transference to the tissue and is thought to encourage collagen remodeling and ultimately tissue tightening.

The amount of ablation and coagulation is controlled by the amount of laser *fluence* (power) and *pulse duration* (or *pulse width*; length of time power is applied). Short pulse durations and high fluence produce greater ablation, whereas longer pulse widths and lower fluencies emphasize coagulation. Settings can therefore be individualized for the desired patient outcome.

The percentage of skin treated is dictated by the *density* setting. Higher density settings affect a greater area within a specific treatment zone (i.e., the columns of light energy are closer together) and can be especially effective for dyschromias. The downside is that there may be a prolonged healing time, depending on the chosen fluence, because there are fewer untreated skin islands surrounding treated areas.

Although there are basic recommendations for treatment parameters for each device, in reality there is considerable variation among practitioners (Table 53-1). In the beginning stages, it is best to incorporate more conservative settings and accept the potential need for additional treatment, versus using more aggressive settings with the greater potential for complications.

Patient Selection

Patient education and selection are essential for achieving optimal results with fractional laser resurfacing. Fitzpatrick skin type

TABLE 53-1 Fractional Technologies Comparison Chart

Supplier Product Name	Device Type	Wavelength	Energy Output	Pulse Length	Price	Accessories
Alma Lasers						
Pixel 2940	Fractional Er:YAG handpiece for Harmony^{XL} system	2940 nm	2500 mJ/p	N/A	Contact mfr.	Pixel 2940 handpiece.
Pixel CO_2	Fractional CO_2 system	10,600 nm	30 W	N/A	$69,900	7 × 7 and 9 × 9 pixel array handpieces, two surgical handpieces.
Pixel Omnifit	Pixelized handpiece for existing CO_2 systems	10,600 nm	N/A	N/A	$34,900	7 × 7 and 9 × 9 pixel array configuration.
Cutera, Inc.						
Pearl Fractional	Fractional 2790 nm YSGG	2790 nm	60–320 mJ per microspot	600 msec	Contact mfr.	Smoke evacuator connector.
Cynosure						
Affirm CO_2	CO_2 with scanner	10,600 nm	30 W	0.2–20 msec ablative, 0.2–2 msec microablative	Contact mfr.	Scanner (microablative and full ablative).
Eclipse, Ltd.						
SmartXide Dot	CO_2 laser and scanner system	10,600 nm	30 W	0.2–80 msec	Contact Eclipse	Scanner offers standard or dot scanning mode.
Ellipse, A/S						
Juvia	Fractional CO_2 laser	10,600 nm	0.1–15 W	N/A	Contact mfr.	Truly flexible fiber delivery. Built-in parameter controls on handpiece. Adjustable scan dwell times: 2 msec, 3 msec, 4 msec, 5 msec, 6 msec, 7 msec. Scan density: 7 × 7; 9 × 9; 11 × 11 MTZ/cm^2. Scan area: 1 cm^2; MTZ (spot) size: 500 μm. No consumables.
Focus Medical						
NaturaLase Er	Er:YAG	2940 nm	Up to 24 J/cm^2	350 msec	$74,900	Fractional handpiece with system. 100–150 μm spots size. Up to 8 Hz.
LASERING USA						
MiXto SX	CO_2 laser	10.6 nm	0.5–30 W	2.5 to 16 msec	$79,000	Patent pending MiXto SX fractional scanner system. 300 μm spot scanner for optimal heat delivery and collagen production. 5% to 40% density adj. Optional 180 μm spot scanner for deep ablation and skin tightening.
Velure S5 MiXto VX	Diode laser	532 nm	0.1–5 W	10–1000 msec	$53,900	MiXto VX fractional scanner. Focusing handpieces with spot sizes of 0.3 mm, 0.5 mm, 1.5 mm.
Lumenis						
UltraPulse ActiveFX	Fractional CO_2 laser	10,600 nm	1–225 mJ	<1 msec	Contact mfr.	Single, minimal downtime treatment for wrinkle/pigment results.
UltraPulse DeepFX	Fractional CO_2 laser	10,600 nm	2.5–50 mJ	<1 msec	Contact mfr.	Fractional CO_2 treatment for wrinkles, scars, and deep collagen treatment.
UltraPulse TotalFX	Fractional CO_2 laser	10,600 nm	1–225 mJ	<1 msec	Contact mfr.	Blended fractional CO_2 treatment for customized patient outcomes.
Lutronic						
eCO2	CO_2 laser	10.6 mm	240 mJ	10.56 msec	Contact mfr.	
Palomar						
StarLux 500 Platform						
Lux2940 Fractional	2940 laser	2940 nm	N/A	N/A	Contact mfr.	
Lux1540 Fractional Laser handpiece	1540 laser	1540 nm	Up to 70 mJ per microbeam	1–500 msec	Contact mfr.	

TABLE 53-1 Fractional Technologies Comparison Chart—cont.

Supplier Product Name	Device Type	Wavelength	Energy Output	Pulse Length	Price	Accessories
LuxDeepIR Fractional Infrared handpiece	Infrared light	850–1350 nm	Up to 175 J	2.5–10 sec	Contact mfr.	
Sandstone Medical Technologies						
Matrix LS-25	CO_2 laser	10,600 nm	25 W	Adjustable to 100 msec	$50,000	Ultrafine-FS Fractional Scanner, 150-mm focusing handpiece.
UltraFine-FS Fractional Scanner	Fractional scanner (adapts to most CO_2 lasers)	10,600 nm	N/A	N/A	$19,995	Fractional scanner.
Sciton						
ProFractional-XC	Tunable laser 2940 μm	2940 μm	Up to 400 J/cm^2	Variable	Contact mfr.	Expandable module.
ProFractional	Tunable laser 2940 μm	2940 μm	Up to 400 J/cm^2	Variable	Contact mfr.	Expandable module/density 1.5% to 60%.
Solta Medical						
Fraxel re:store	Erbium-fiber laser	1550 nm	4–70 mJ/MTZ	N/A	Contact mfr.	Intelligent Optical Tracking System (IOTS). Variable optical spot size using telescope. Maximizes lesion depth for a chosen pulse energy. Ergonomic handpiece and roller tip.
Fraxel re:fine	Single mode fiber laser	1410 nm	5–20 mJ/MTZ	N/A	Contact mfr.	Same as above.
Fraxel re:pair	Fractional CO_2 laser	10,600 nm	5–70 mJ/MTZ	N/A	Contact mfr.	Built-in smokeless evacuation system. Intelligent Optical Tracking System (IOTS). Ergonomic handpiece and roller tip.
Syneron						
eMatrix Matrix RF eMax Matrix RF eLight Matrix RF eLaser Matrix RF	Radiofrequency electrical energy	N/A	Up to 20 J	N/A	Contact mfr.	Spot size 12 × 12 mm, 3-year warranty.

MTZ, microthermal treatment zone.
Data subject to change; please refer to Suppliers section for supplier contact information. Not all devices are FDA cleared for the application(s) indicated.
From The Aesthetic Guides, January–February 2009. www.miinews.com.

classification is a basic way to identify patients at higher risk for pigmentary changes associated with laser resurfacing (see Chapter 46, Introduction to Aesthetic Medicine). Lighter-skinned patients (Fitzpatrick types I to III) are at lowest risk for postprocedure pigmentary changes, whereas darker-skinned patients (Fitzpatrick types IV and V) are at a much higher risk. Although darker-skinned patients can still be treated, more conservative settings must be chosen and they must be carefully counseled about the specific risks they may encounter.

The most important area of patient education, however, is in identification of expectations. Although laser resurfacing can achieve some degree of skin tightening and improve tone and texture, it is no replacement for surgical intervention in the patient who really needs a facelift or necklift. Sagging skin and jowling are surgical problems and cannot effectively be addressed with laser resurfacing alone. Using various combinations of procedures, however, these patients can often achieve synergistic results that go far beyond either intervention (surgical or nonsurgical) alone. In addition, realistic healing and recovery time must be discussed with the patient, as well as the need for patience while waiting for final results, which may take 4 to 6 months. Proper patient selection before treatment is essential for achieving optimal results and can generally allow one to avoid many of the pitfalls associated with unrealistic expectations.

INDICATIONS

- Laser resurfacing can be an effective means for treating the following *age-related conditions*:
  - *Dyschromias (pigment changes)*: Areas of hyperpigmentation can effectively be addressed with fractional resurfacing. Because only light treatment settings are required, the downtime is often as short as 2 to 3 days (Fig. 53-1).
  - *Textural changes*: As aged skin is replaced with new tissue, there is diminishment in the wrinkled, crepey appearance because the collagen matrix is stimulated to regenerate and reorganize (Figs. 53-2 and 53-3).
  - *Fine lines and wrinkles*: Improvement in fine lines and wrinkles has been noted after laser resurfacing, but improvement is known to be enhanced after pretreatment with botulinum toxin type A. With movement stabilized in the treated areas, the newly regenerated skin is allowed to heal in a more stable environment (Fig. 53-4).
  - *Dilated pores*: Many patients notice refinement of pore size, although this effect may take upward of 6 months to fully achieve
- *Scars (surgical vs. traumatic vs. acne vs. burns)*: By effectively planing down the scar and stimulating collagen remodeling, fractional resurfacing can have a beneficial effect on the

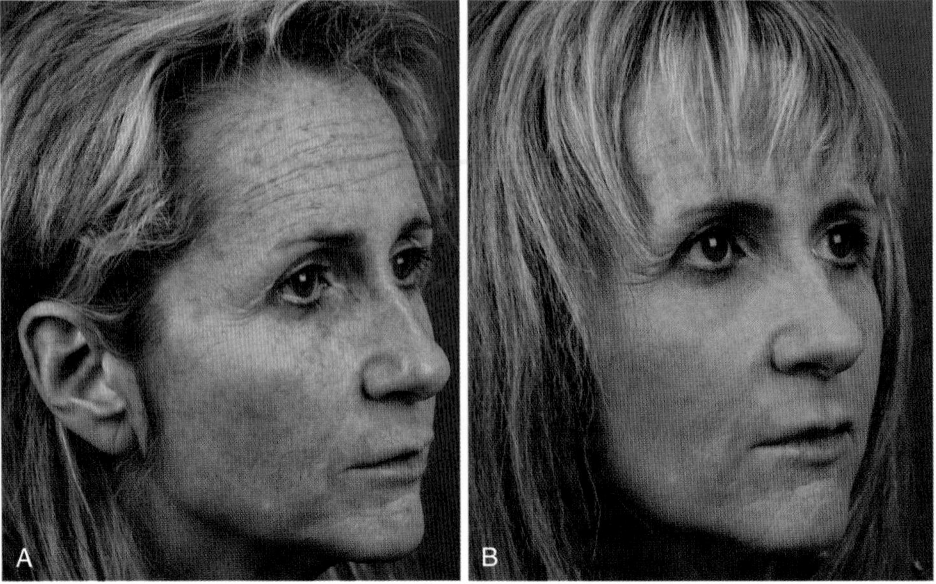

Figure 53-1 Treatment of dyschromias using a Lumenis Ultrapulse Encore Laser. ActiveFX: 100 mJ, 600 Hz, density 100%, single pass; DeepFX: 12.5 mJ, 300 Hz, density 15%, single pass. **A,** Before treatment. **B,** Three months after treatment. (Courtesy of Gregory A. Buford, MD, FACS, Denver, Colo.)

appearance of scars from a variety of sources (Figs. 53-5 through 53-9).

- *Stretch marks (questionable efficacy)*: Although results are variable, some practitioners report improvement in the appearance of stretch marks; however, there are very few well-controlled studies in this area.

CONTRAINDICATIONS

Absolute

- Keloid formers
- Bacterial or viral skin infection
- Use of isotretinoin in the past 12 months
- Scleroderma
- Prior radiation therapy to area
- Localized poor healing
- Melanoma or identified lesions suspect for skin cancer in area to be treated
- Ectropion
- Vitiligo
- History of noncompliance with previous treatments

Relative

- Impaired immune system or known autoimmune disease
- Collagen vascular disorder
- Lower lid laxity

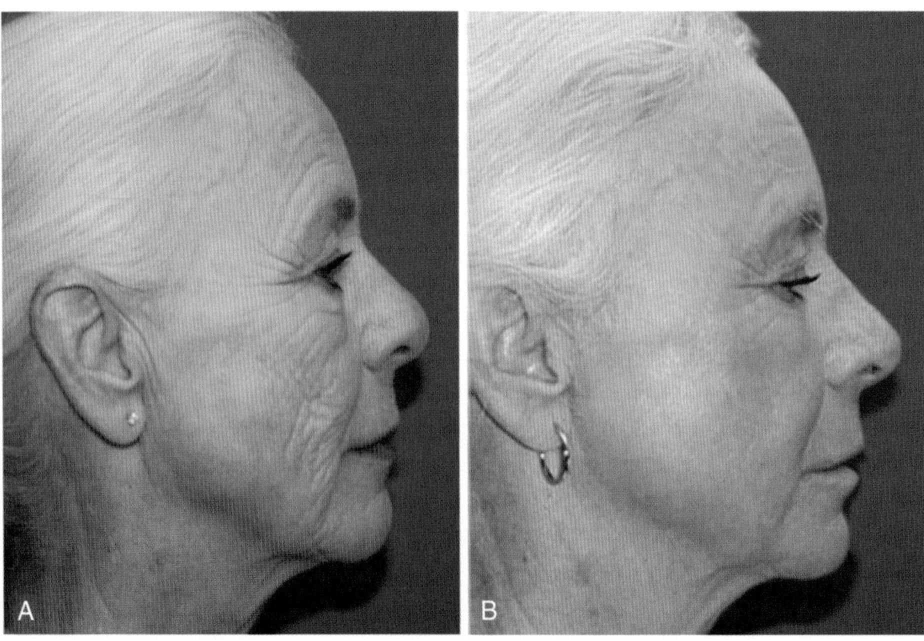

Figure 53-2 Treatment of coarse lines and wrinkles and crepey skin using a Lumenis Ultrapulse Encore Laser. ActiveFX: 125 mJ, 125 Hz, density 82%, double pass. **A,** Before treatment. **B,** After treatment. (Courtesy of Robert Bushman, MD, La Mesa, Calif.)

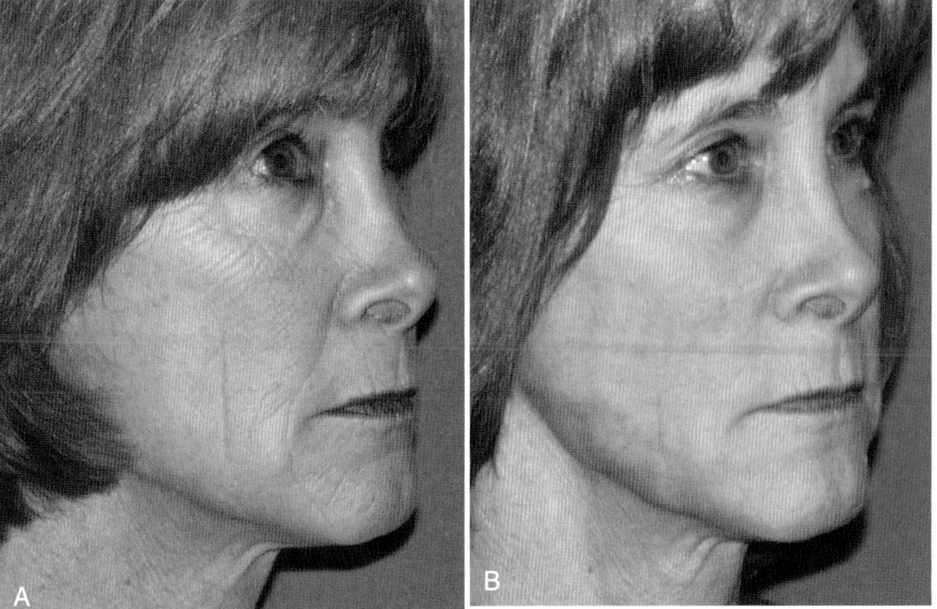

Figure 53-3 Treatment of coarse lines and wrinkles and crepey skin using a Lumenis Ultrapulse Encore Laser. ActiveFX: 125 mJ, 100 Hz, density 82%, single pass. **A,** Before treatment. **B,** One month after treatment. (Courtesy of Gregory A. Buford, MD, FACS, Denver, Colo.)

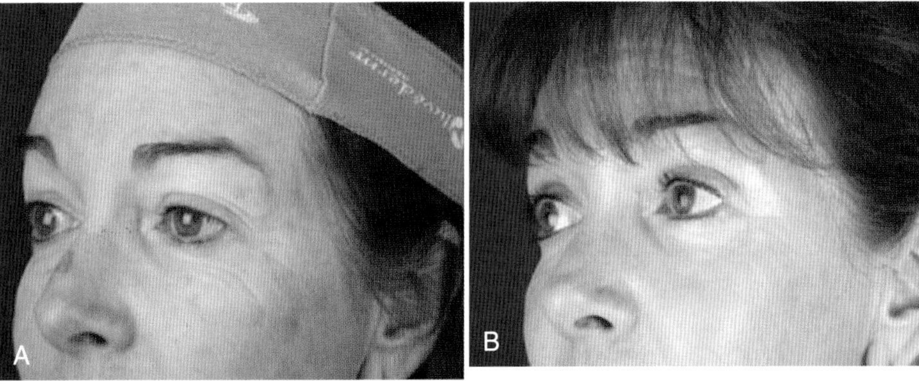

Figure 53-4 Treatment of fine lines and wrinkles (periorbital area) using a Lumenis Ultrapulse Encore Laser. ActiveFX: 90 mJ, 125 Hz, density 68%, single pass; DeepFX: 12.5 mJ, density 5%, single pass. **A,** Before treatment. **B,** Three months after treatment. (Courtesy of Gregory A. Buford, MD, FACS, and Beryl Reker, PMA, Denver, Colo.)

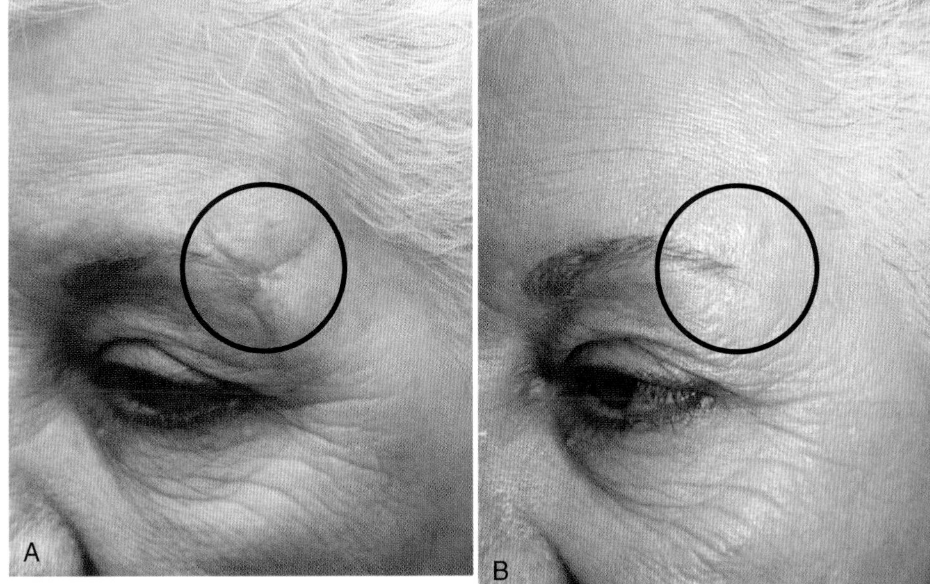

Figure 53-5 Laser scar revision using a Lumenis Ultrapulse Encore Laser. Treatment settings not available. **A,** Before treatment. **B,** After treatment. (Courtesy of Joseph Niamtu III, DMD, Richmond, Va.)

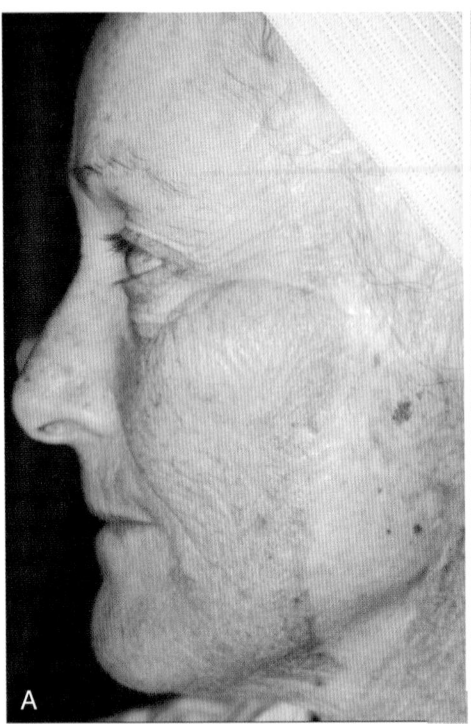

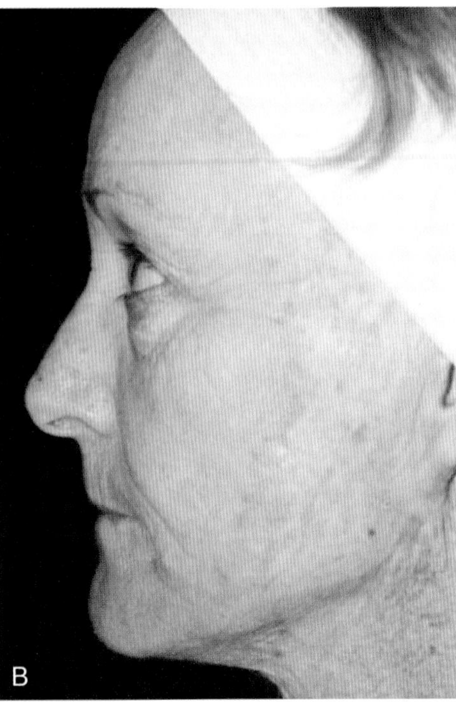

Figure 53-6 Laser scar revision using a Lumenis Ultrapulse Encore Laser. ActiveFX: 80 mJ, 55% coverage, single pass; DeepFX: 12.5 mJ, 15% coverage, single pass. **A,** Before treatment. **B,** After treatment. (Courtesy of Jill Waibel, MD, West Palm Beach, Fla.)

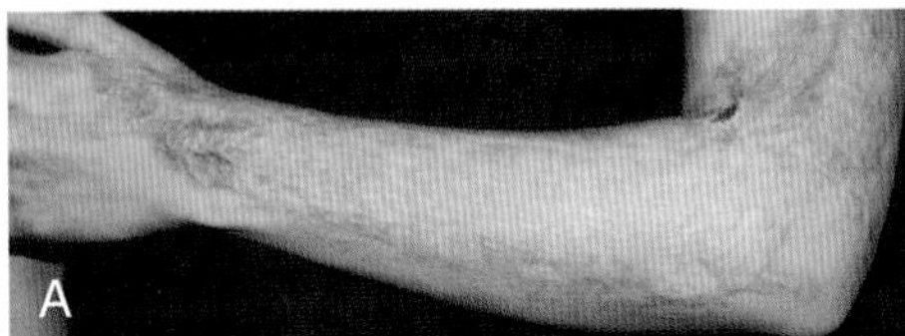

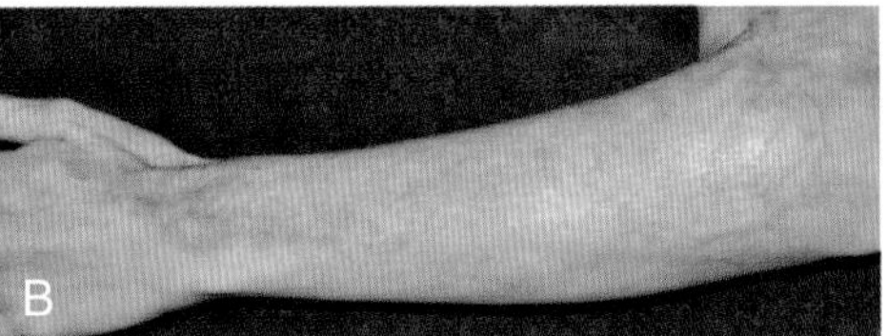

Figure 53-7 Laser scar revision using a Lumenis Ultrapulse Encore Laser. Treatment settings not available. **A,** Patient's arm with 20-year-old burn scar. **B,** After treatment. (Courtesy of Jill Waibel, MD, West Palm Beach, Fla.)

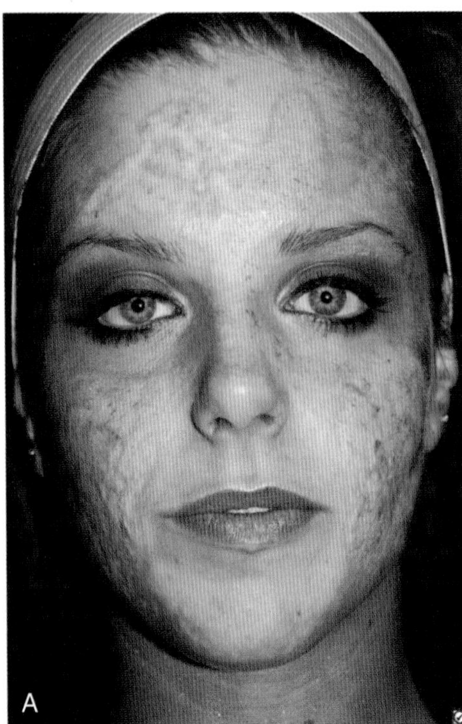

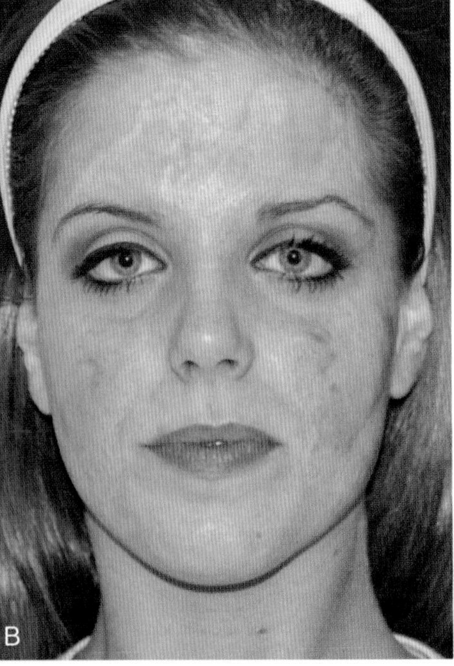

Figure 53-8 Laser scar revision using a Lumenis Ultrapulse Encore Laser. Treatment settings not available. **A,** Before treatment. **B,** Seven months after treatment. (Courtesy of Jill Waibel, MD, West Palm Beach, Fla.)

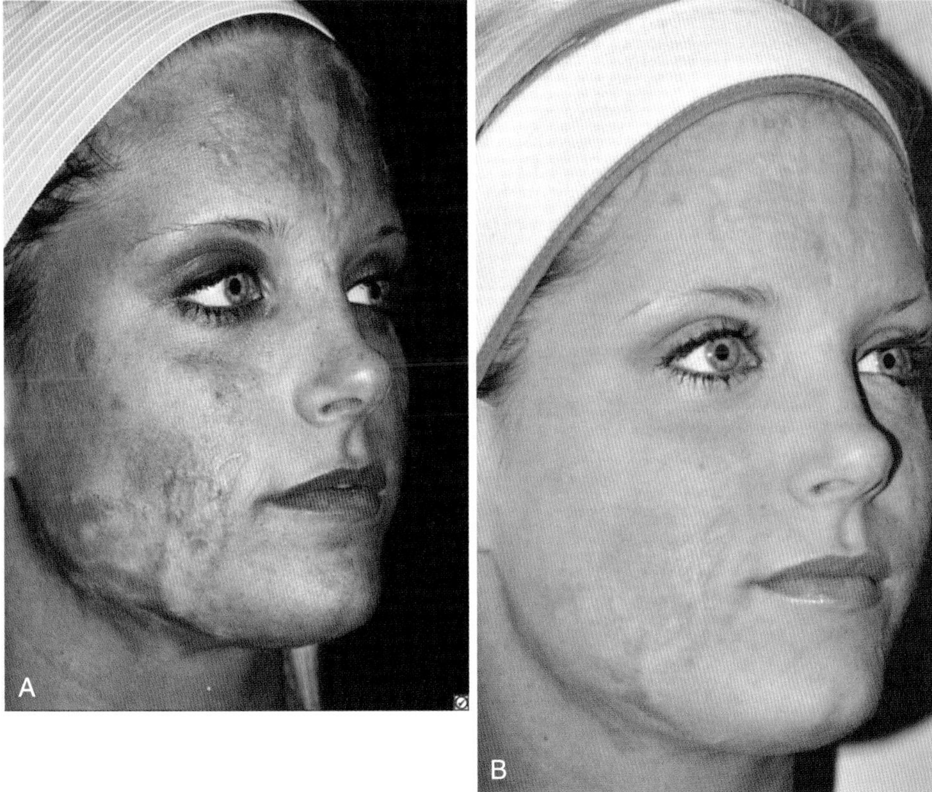

Figure 53-9 Laser scar revision using a Lumenis Ultrapulse Encore Laser. Treatment settings not available. **A,** Before treatment. **B,** Seven months after three total treatments using TotalFX. (Courtesy of Jill Waibel, MD, West Palm Beach, Fla.)

- Photosensitizing medications
- Fitzpatrick skin type IV or V

Pretreatment Patient Evaluation

- *Skin type classification*: Fitzpatrick skin type classification should be determined before treating any patient with fractional or nonfractional laser resurfacing (see Chapter 46, Introduction to Aesthetic Medicine). Darker skin types are at a higher risk for long-term pigmentary changes even with fractional technology, so the degree and number of treatments should be adjusted accordingly.
- *Current medications*: Any medications that will delay or impede wound healing should be discontinued before laser resurfacing.
- *Previous treatment with lasers or deep chemical peels*: Prior treatment with either deep chemical peels or lasers in the same area should be considered before retreatment, given the potential for delayed or impaired healing.
- *Desired end result*: One of the most critical variables in success is patient expectation, so it is important to have an open and honest discussion with each patient before moving forward with any aesthetic procedure. Managing expectations before treatment will better prepare your patient for outcome in both the short and long term. Speak candidly and honestly about the following:
  - Number of treatments
  - Anticipated costs
  - Recovery time
  - Degree of discomfort
- *Pretreatment/post-treatment protocol* (e.g., skin care products, patient instructions): The outcome of any aesthetic procedure is often the result not only of the success of the procedure itself but of the patient's compliance with recommended protocol instructions before and after the treatment. This is especially true with laser resurfacing. Although some experts dispute the importance of an individualized and guided medical skin care regimen before the laser procedure, most agree that it is essential during the healing period.
- *Adjunctive treatment with botulinum toxin type A*: As demonstrated by multiple authors, treatment with botulinum toxin type A allows for more optimal and potentially sustained results when undertaken before laser resurfacing. As one study supports, the practice effectively prevents dynamic facial muscular action in treated areas and potentially minimizes the reestablishment of expressive wrinkles and folds.
- *Discussion of risks/benefits and informed consent*: As with any procedure, informed consent must be obtained after discussion with the patient of associated risks and benefits. Be realistic in describing downtime and discomfort, with the understanding that there is a degree of variation depending on individual patient characteristics, treatment settings, and the specific device used.
- *Pretreatment photographs*: The importance of pretreatment photographs cannot be overemphasized. Aside from the ability to document degree of improvement from the pretreatment to post-treatment stages, taking photographs of your patients also provides you a means with which to educate other patients on the efficacy of these procedures.

Before the Procedure

The laser treatment itself must be performed by a trained laser professional under medical supervision. State laws dictate the actual degree of medical supervision and who can actually perform the procedure.

Pain control should be addressed and individualized, and is really a factor of four variables.

1. Patient pain tolerance
2. Specific device
3. Depth of treatment
4. Area of treatment

With other rejuvenative procedures, some patients require very little analgesia, whereas others have less tolerant pain thresholds. The key is to understand the average patient's needs, begin there, and then fine-tune accordingly. It is always better to make your patients more comfortable than less because their experience will largely be shaped not only by the outcome they eventually receive but by the initial experience they perceive.

A variety of methods can be used to manage pain in an office setting:

- *Topical anesthesia*: For all fractional laser treatments, this is the foundation of pain management and may include a wide variety of topical agents. A frequently used compounded combination is a 23% lidocaine/7% tetracaine cream, which is applied 45 to 60 minutes before treatment. As with any treatment, check for potential allergic reactions before proceeding and watch for signs and symptoms of toxicity. Although with facial resurfacing there is less risk than with extended treatment areas (e.g., laser hair removal), the risk is not zero and so all patients must be observed for evidence of impending toxicity and a resuscitation plan must be in place before any treatment is begun.
- *Nerve blocks* (see Chapter 8, Peripheral Nerve Blocks and Field Blocks, and Chapter 9, Oral and Facial Anesthesia): For more aggressive treatments around the mouth, infraorbital and mental nerve blocks can be used. One milliliter of 2% lidocaine with epinephrine per injection is extremely effective in achieving an acceptable degree of patient comfort. However, warn the patient when transitioning from a blocked to a nonblocked area. Pain control can be so effective using blocks that it can make the transition to an area where only a topical anesthetic was used significantly more sensitive.
- *Oral medications*: Although many practitioners combine some type of either narcotic or non-narcotic (e.g., nonsteroidal anti-inflammatory drugs [NSAIDs]) pain medication with an anxiolytic for their pain management program, it does more to manage acute anxiety than pain. As such, a light anxiolytic (diazepam) may be best so that the patient is still aware of her or his surroundings but, at the same time, lightly relaxed.

Preparing for the Treatment (at Least 1 Week Prior)

- Discuss and obtain informed consent from the patient (see sample consent form online at www.expertconsult.com).
- Review all written postprocedure wound care instructions with the patient and encourage her or him to call the office for any concerns or suspicion of poor healing associated with the treatment.
- Take pretreatment photographs.
- Schedule postprocedure appointments.
- Make sure that the patient has the necessary skin care products for the immediate postprocedure healing period.
- Give the patient Swiss Therapy Eye Masks (if performing periorbital rejuvenation).
- Give the patient prescriptions for all medications related to the treatment and encourage him or her to fill these before the day of the procedure:
  - Antiviral (regardless of prior history of herpes simplex)
  - Ophthalmic antibacterial ointment (if performing periorbital rejuvenation)
  - Anxiolytic or analgesic
- Patients should discontinue the use of aspirin, NSAIDs, vitamin E, St. John's wort, and other dietary supplements, including ginkgo biloba, evening primrose oil, garlic, feverfew, and ginseng, at least 2 weeks before treatment to reduce the risk of bleeding.
- Remind the patient to bring sun-protective clothing (e.g., wide-brimmed hat and sunglasses) on the day of the procedure.
- Arrange for a driver for the day of the procedure (regardless of whether the patient will be medicated for the actual treatment).

Supplies

Before

- Topical anesthetic (to be applied 45 to 60 minutes before the procedure)
- Metal eye shields (intraocular vs. extraocular) plus ophthalmic ointment and anesthetic drops
- Protective laser goggles for all present during the treatment
- Smoke evacuator
- Gloves
- Surgical mask
- 4 × 4 gauze sponges (for wiping away fluid from treated areas and from periorbital area)
- Moistened towels (to be placed below the neck to protect the chest)
- Zimmer Chiller (or other cooling device)
- Laser

After

- 4 × 4 gauze sponges
- Ice water
- Bowl
- Hand towels*
- Aquaphor
- Swiss Therapy Eye Masks

Skin Preparation

Before the actual procedure, the skin must be prepared in the following steps:

1. All makeup removed
2. Skin cleansed with mild cleanser
3. Numbing eye drops placed (when using intraocular eye shields)

Treatment

- The patient should arrive 45 to 60 minutes before the procedure. At that time, all makeup is removed, the skin is cleansed with a mild cleanser, and topical anesthetic is applied to treatment areas. The anesthetic is left in place a minimum of 45 minutes.
- Immediately before the procedure, topical anesthetic cream is removed and the skin is again cleansed with a mild cleanser.
- Position the patient so that both the clinician and patient are comfortable. Whereas some prefer to treat in a flat, supine position, others find it easier to elevate the head of the bed to approximately 30 degrees and treat from the standing position.
- If using eye shields, instill one or two drops of ophthalmic anesthetic solution into each eye. Lubricate the shield side facing the cornea with an appropriate ophthalmic ointment. If the patient is wearing contact lenses, remove them. Gently place the corneal eye shields onto the patient's eyes.
- Make sure that all staff members present have the appropriate laser-protective eyewear.

---

*Before the procedure, the towels are placed in the ice-water slurry to chill. After treatment, the chilled towels are applied to treated areas and left in place for at least 10 minutes. The skin is then gently dried and a thick coating of Aquaphor is applied.

TABLE 53-2 Recommended Treatment Settings for Lumenis Ultrapulse Encore Laser ActiveFX (1.3-mm Spot Size)

Treatment	Energy (mJ)	Scan Size (mm)	Density	Hertz	Repeat Delay (sec)	Cool Scan	No. of Passes
PigmentFX facial	80–125	6–7	2–3	100–150	0.3–1.5	On	1
Moderate photoaging/facial	80–125	6–7	2–3	100–150	0.3–1.5	On	1
Severe photoaging/facial	100–125	6–7	2–3	100–200	0.3–1.5	On	1–2
Skin types V–VI/facial	70	5–6	1–2	75–100	0.3–1.5	On	1
Neck, décolleté	80–100	5–6	1–2	125–150	0.3–1.5	On	1
Hands, forearms	50–60	5–6	1–2	125–150	0.3–1.5	On	1

Courtesy of Lumenis, Inc., Santa Clara, Calif.

- Next, consider the following variables when deciding on specific treatment settings:
  - Specific treatment area
  - Desired depth of treatment
  - Desired effect of treatment
  - Specific skin type
- Choose the *appropriate settings* (i.e., fluence, density, pulse width, shape, repeat time) for the patient and select them for the device. Each particular laser has certain parameters recommended by the company. It will be important to receive training for the unit purchased. Begin with the suggested parameters and adjust them as needed only after gaining experience (Tables 53-2 through 53-4).
- Perform a test spot on a tongue depressor to ensure that the laser is functioning correctly and that you have chosen appropriate treatment settings.
- Begin treatment, observe reactions of the skin to the laser energy, and make any appropriate adjustments. Most practitioners will treat a specific zone as a whole and then move onto the next zone. This provides for a more coordinated approach and allows for differential treatment settings for each individual zone.
- Inform the patient when you are moving onto a different treatment area and be cognizant of her or his pain tolerance. Application of the laser feels like a rubber band snap and can be startling to the patient if the area being treated suddenly shifts from the chin to the upper forehead. Remember, pain tolerance is highly subjective and some patients will need to have their treatment settings adjusted accordingly.
- After standard treatment has been concluded, dial down the settings and "feather" along the jawline and hairline. Feathering blends the treated and untreated areas so there will not be a fine demarcation line between the two when healing is complete. It can be done in several ways: turning the treatment probe at an angle so the penetration is not so deep, or moving the handpiece faster to spread out the density of the columns.
- When treatment is complete, immediately remove the eye shields or protective eyewear and apply cool, damp towels to all treated areas. The towels should remain in place for at least 10 minutes to allow for egress of any residual heat.
- The skin is then dried and an occlusive dressing or ointment applied. This is extremely important, and the patient must understand the importance of keeping the treated tissues moist for the next several days.
- The patient is then discharged and asked to call in the morning for a status report, or earlier if having problems. Encourage plenty of fluids to stay well hydrated because patients tend to lose a significant amount of fluid from their skin during the early healing process. Also suggest avoidance of high-sodium meals because increased salt intake will merely add to the normal and anticipated degree of postprocedure swelling.

Details of an Actual Patient Treatment

The patient is a 65-year-old white woman with advanced facial aging and significant facial laxity. Although she would have benefited from an aggressive ablative CO_2 laser resurfacing, she did not want the associated downtime. The Lumenis Ultrapulse Encore fractionated CO_2 laser treatment was recommended. She underwent this initial treatment in the office with topical anesthetic cream alone and was very comfortable.

Key areas during her treatment session and a few pearls are as follows:

- The patient is a middle-aged white woman with advanced facial aging (a combination of coarse and fine rhytids, facial laxity, and scattered dyschromias; Fig. 53-10A).
- After 45 minutes of topical anesthetic cream use, her skin is degreased, cleansed, and dried. Instill topical anesthetic drops into her eyes and then place lubricated metal eye shields to provide corneal protection during treatment. Once settings have been chosen, test them on a tongue depressor before actual treatment (Fig. 53-10B).
- While the patient is in a semiupright position, treat the forehead first (Fig. 53-10C and D). This area generally requires moderate treatment settings, and this patient was pretreated 2 weeks earlier with botulinum toxin type A to the upper one third of the face to ensure a relaxed post-treatment healing environment.
- Figure 53-10C and D show the application of outward-directed tension to the treated skin to achieve more even penetration of the laser to this area. The pattern is overlapped by around 10% to 20% on the borders. Figure 53-10E shows detail of the fractional pattern, which leaves intact interspersed skin bridges.

TABLE 53-3 Recommended Treatment Settings for Lumenis Ultrapulse Encore Laser DeepFX (0.12-mm Spot Size)

Treatment	Energy (mJ)	Scan Size (mm)	Density	Hertz	Repeat Delay (sec)	No. of pulses	No. of Passes
Deep wrinkles/facial	15–22.5	10	5%–10%	300–400	0.3–1.5	1	2
Periorbital	10–17.5	10	5%–15%	300–400	0.3–1.5	1	1
Perioral	17.5–22.5	10	15%–25%	300–400	0.3–1.5	1	1
Surgical scars	17.5–22.5	10	10%–15%	300–400	0.3–1.5	1–2	1
Hypertrophic scars	15–22.5	10	10%–15%	300–400	0.3–1.5	1–2	1

Courtesy of Lumenis, Inc., Santa Clara, Calif.

TABLE 53-4 Recommended Treatment Settings for Lumenis Ultrapulse Encore Laser TotalFX (ActiveFX + DeepFX)

Treatment	Energy (mJ)	Scan Size (mm)	Density	Hertz	Repeat Delay (sec)	No. of Pulses	No. of Passes
ActiveFX							
Acne scars	100	7	3	100–150	0.3–1.5	N/A	1
Rhinophyma	100–125	6	2	125	0.3–1.5	N/A	1
Burn scars*	80–125	7	1	100	0.3–1.5	N/A	1
DeepFX							
Acne scars	15–22.5	10	10%–20%	300–600	0.3–1.5	1	1
Rhinophyma	20	10	15%–20%	300–600	0.3–1.5	1–2	1
Burn scars	12.5–22.5	10	5%–15%	300–600	0.3–1.5	1–2	1

*Settings depend on thickness of scar tissue and body area treated.
Courtesy of Lumenis, Inc., Santa Clara, Calif.

- Figure 53-10E also shows treatment of the lower perioral subunit and emphasizes the overlap of treatment zones (this provides for more even treatment).
- Figure 53-10F shows application of a second pass. The skin is stretched in this area because the patient has a moderate degree of laxity and, if not stretched, her skin would be unevenly affected. This second pass is reflected as a much darker treatment zone.
- When treating around the eyes, the upper lids are usually done first, followed by the lower lids. This area requires extreme caution. Eyelid skin is the thinnest skin on the body and so great care must be taken to avoid complications. Before treating this area, be sure to assess for lower lid laxity (to minimize the risk for postprocedure ectropion), and always have eye shields in place. Figure 53-10G shows the treatment lines beginning 1 to 2 mm directly above the upper lash line, followed with another row directly above. The skin is stretched to achieve even penetration.
- For the lower lids (Fig. 53-10H), use a tongue depressor to sweep the eyelashes superiorly to reduce the risk of singeing them. Begin about 1 to 2 mm below the lower lash line and then paint a line across the treatment area, followed by blending with the previously treated upper cheek zone. To complete the periorbital area, change to a smaller pattern and effectively fill in the blanks.
- Once all subunits are treated, feather all the edges (see earlier discussion) by dialing down the energy and turning the handpiece at an angle so that the beam appears elongated. Also, move the

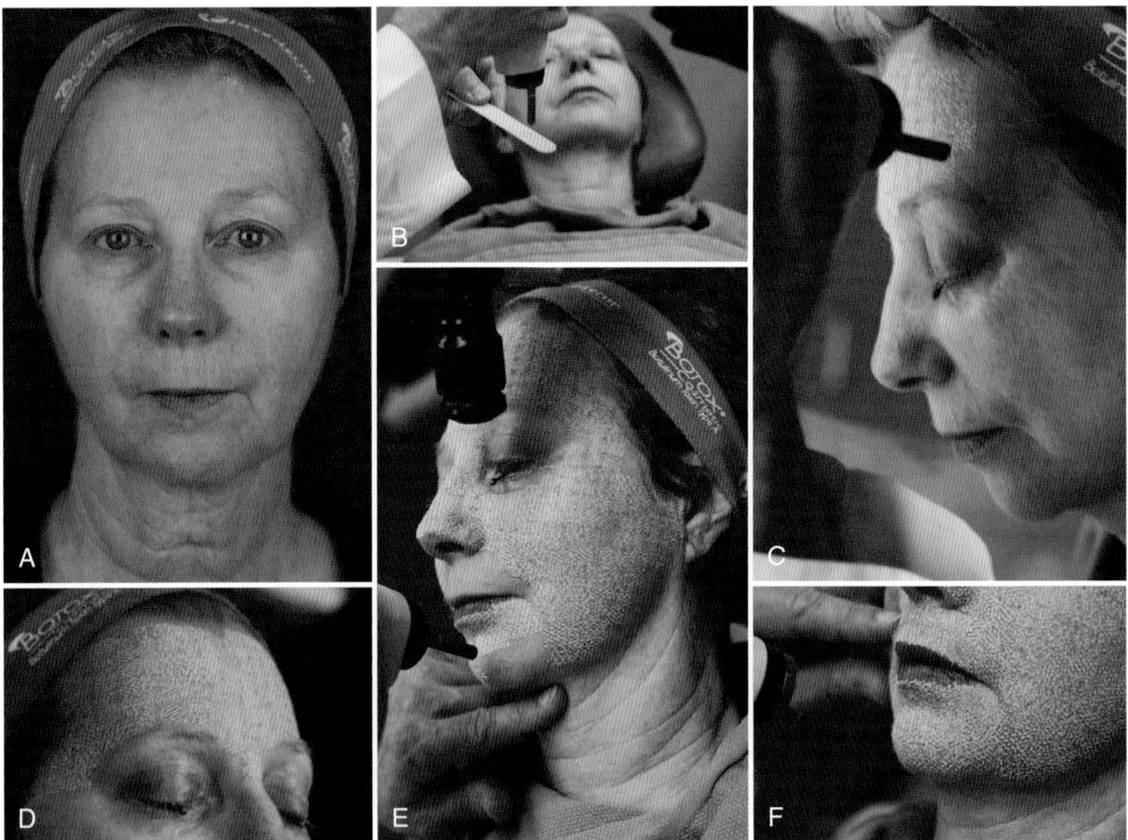

Figure 53-10 Actual client treatment using the Lumenis Ultrapulse Encore fractionated CO_2 laser. **A,** Preprocedure photograph. **B,** Testing settings on a tongue depressor before treatment. **C,** Treatment of the forehead aesthetic subunit. **D,** Completion of treatment of the forehead aesthetic subunit. **E,** Treatment of the perioral subunit with overlapping of pulses with use of the Zimmer cooling unit for intraprocedure pain relief. **F,** Treatment of the perioral subunit with two passes at the same setting to address more advanced localized aging.

wand rather than holding it stationary. Figure 53-10I demonstrates feathering the lower jawline onto the neck.

- Figure 53-10J shows the final appearance after a single ActiveFX pass to the face as well as a second pass to the perioral area. The second pass effect around the mouth creates a slightly denser appearance, but was necessary given the degree of facial aging in this area.
- Remove the patient's eye shields and rinse the eyes with balanced salt solution. Apply cool, moist towels (that have been sitting in an ice-water slurry during the actual treatment) and leave them on for at least 15 minutes to allow heat to dissipate from the patient's skin (Fig. 53-10K).
- Reiterate the essentials of the postprocedure care regimen with both the patient and whoever is accompanying her for discharge. There will be an early striping effect (which is natural) and a mild to moderate degree of swelling (Fig. 53-10L). Emphasize that the swelling will be pronounced for the next 3 days but that it will resolve, how quickly depending on the depth of treatment. During that time, the patient needs to stay upright as much as possible and keep the area cool to facilitate lymphatic drainage and resolution of postprocedure edema.
- Give your office and on-call number and instruct the patient to call for any significant concerns. Complications of laser resurfacing can generally be avoided if the appropriate steps are taken early.

Treatment Caveats

As with any treatment, there are a number of ways to achieve optimal results. There is significant variation among practitioners as to which variables provide the best outcome. Keep in mind that the safest treatment is generally the simplest treatment and that exotic settings, although they may prove successful in highly experienced hands, can be dangerous in the hands of someone in the beginning stages. Use the most basic settings when you start and adapt as you gain experience. Your patients are much more likely to respect an

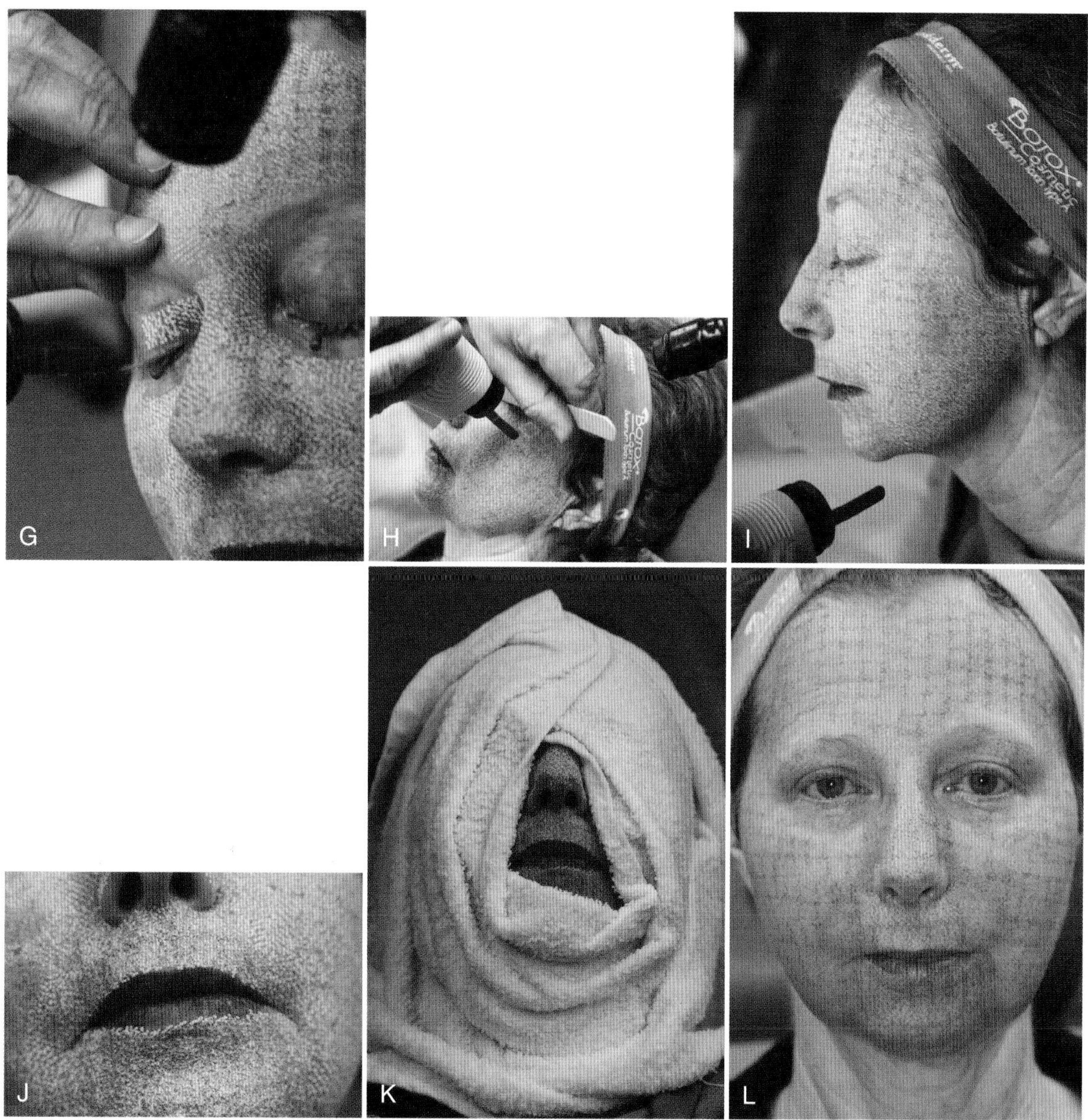

Figure 53-10, cont. **G,** Treatment of the upper and lower lids. **H,** Treatment of the lower lid skin and use of a tongue depressor to decrease eyelash singeing. **I,** Feathering of the junction between treated and nontreated tissue. **J,** Close-up of the perioral treatment area to illustrate appearance of a double pass. **K,** Placement of moist, cool towels to the face immediately after treatment. **L,** Patient appearance after treatment and 15 minutes of cooling. (Courtesy of Gregory A. Buford, MD, FACS, Denver, Colo.)

approach where they may need to come back for a second treatment rather than an overly aggressive approach where they may be at risk for adverse events.

There are a number of controversies in the medical field as to which settings are most important and which should be emphasized when addressing specific needs or end points. With that said, the following are a few suggestions, but they are by no means the only ways to achieve optimal results:

- *Pulse coverage*: Position the coverage area for each pulse so that treatment zones are adjacent with very little (maximum of 10%) to no gapping between them.
- *Density*: Use a density setting right in the middle when treating photoaged skin. *For the patient with dyschromias*, dial down the fluence and dial up the density so that there is a more focused treatment directly over the affected area. For generalized dyschromias, treat the entire area this way; for a localized area of pigmentation, focus simply on the specific area.
- *Fluence*: There is a tremendous amount of controversy as to the optimal fluence. Look at the patient to decide. For a patient with mild photoaging, use a light setting; for an older patient with more advanced photoaging, dial up the setting. However, be very careful in the older patient, whose thinner skin may not tolerate a higher setting, leading to delayed healing.
- *Pulse stacking*: Avoid this until comfort is gained with a specific device. Pulse stacking takes a particular fluence and associated depth of penetration and drives it even deeper. Although there are many advocates of a low fluence doubly stacked, there is still significant controversy as to whether this is more effective than simply increasing the fluence in the first place. There is also the issue of heat dissipation. Keep in mind that double stacking may not allow for adequate heat dissipation, so there may be more of a coagulative effect. That can be good and bad, as discussed earlier. I would strongly discourage you from incorporating this technique until you have considerable experience with your specific laser because the results can often be unpredictable even in the hands of a highly experienced practitioner.
- *Hertz rate*: This is another controversial area. When treating scars, a higher hertz rate may be necessary. However, the science behind this approach is still being actively investigated.
- *Treatment of erythema*: More and more patients want less and less downtime but ultimately the same results. The problem, however, is that the treatment injures the tissue and the tissue needs to fully heal to achieve optimal results. It is best not reduce the erythema for at least 4 to 6 weeks because this enhanced vascularity is part of the overall healing process. Encourage the patient to be patient, and if the erythema is reasonable, wait for at least 4 weeks before intervening with either steroids or intense pulsed light.
- *Combination therapy*: There are a number of excellent reports documenting enhanced long-term results using pretreatment with botulinum toxin type A 1 to 2 weeks before the actual laser treatment. In addition, deep placement of volumizing fillers in conjunction with laser rejuvenation can also provide for a more comprehensive result because laser therapy will do nothing to replace lost volume (Figs. 53-11 through 53-13).
- *Treatment of nonfacial areas*: Extension of laser resurfacing to the neck, chest, and hands allows blending of treated with nontreated areas but it is also carries an increased risk for adverse events. These areas lack the abundant adnexal glands present in the face and so tend to heal less effectively. In addition, tissue of the chest and hands tends to be much thinner with very little underlying subcutaneous tissue. The close proximity of bone to the skin can create a heat sink and actually prevent effective heat dissipation. Aggressive treatment in these areas can lead to delayed healing and worse. Be conservative. Educate your patients about the

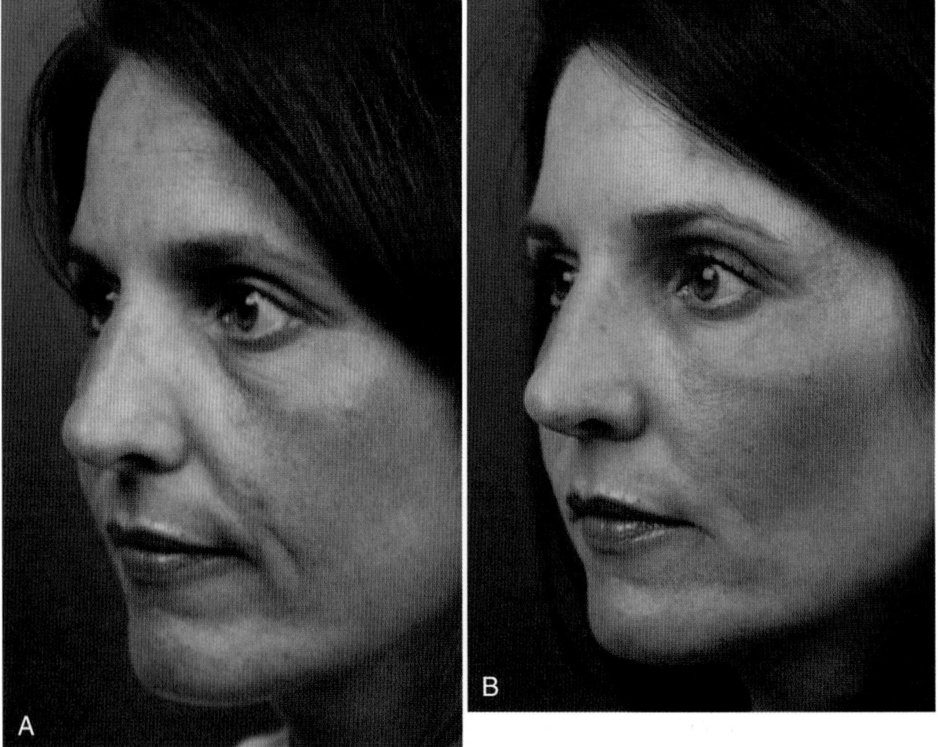

Figure 53-11 Combination therapy using a Lumenis Ultrapulse Encore Laser. *Periorbital area*: ActiveFX: 80 mJ, 125 Hz, density 82%, single pass; DeepFx: 12.5 mJ, 300 Hz, density 15%, single pass. *Remainder of face*: ActiveFX: 125 mJ, 125 Hz, density 82%, single pass; DeepFx: 17.5 mJ, 300 Hz, density 15%, single pass. *Pretreatment with Juvederm Ultra*: medial cheeks and tear trough area. *Pretreatment with botulinum toxin type A*: forehead, glabella, lateral brow, and crow's feet. **A,** Before treatment. **B,** After treatment. (Courtesy of Gregory A. Buford, MD, FACS, Denver, Colo.)

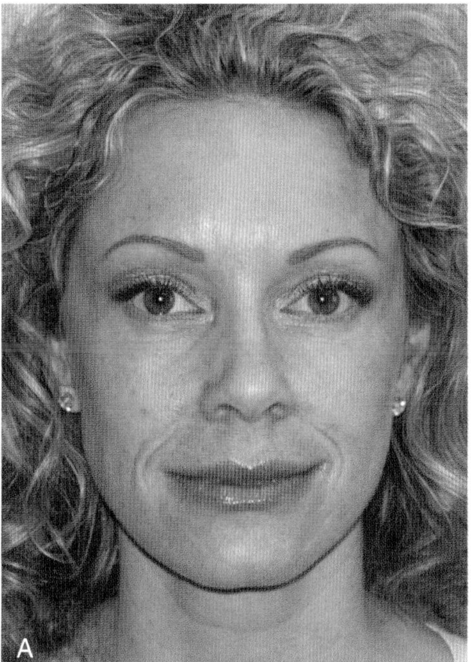

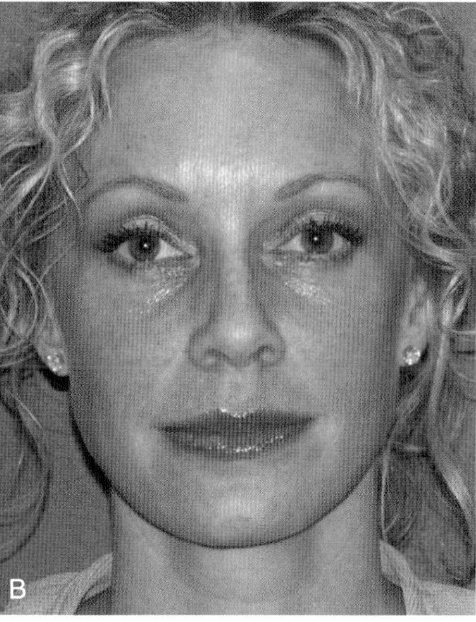

Figure 53-12 Combination therapy using a Lumenis Ultrapulse Encore Laser. *Periorbital area*: ActiveFX: 80 mJ, 125 Hz, density 82%, single pass; DeepFx: 12.5 mJ, 300 Hz, density 15%, single pass. *Remainder of face*: ActiveFX: 125 mJ, 125 Hz, density 82%, single pass; DeepFx: 15 mJ, 300 Hz, density 15%, single pass. *Pretreatment with Juvederm Ultra*: superficial cheek lines. *Pretreatment with botulinum toxin type A*: forehead, glabella, lateral brow, and crow's feet. **A,** Before treatment. **B,** After treatment. (Courtesy of Gregory A. Buford, MD, FACS, Denver, Colo.)

differences in these areas and tell them that it may take several treatments instead of the single treatment that was effective for their face (Fig. 53-14).

Postprocedure Patient Care and Instructions

There are a number of ways to optimize results after laser treatment. The following home care guidelines are one example.

Immediately after Treatment

1. Make a 1-week follow-up appointment.
2. Avoid direct sunlight to the face, even when just driving home from the office.
3. When in the car, turn on the air conditioner or roll down a window to aim cool air at the treated area.
4. Place a piece of gauze between the bridge of the nose and eyeglasses to avoid irritation to the treated skin if that area was treated.

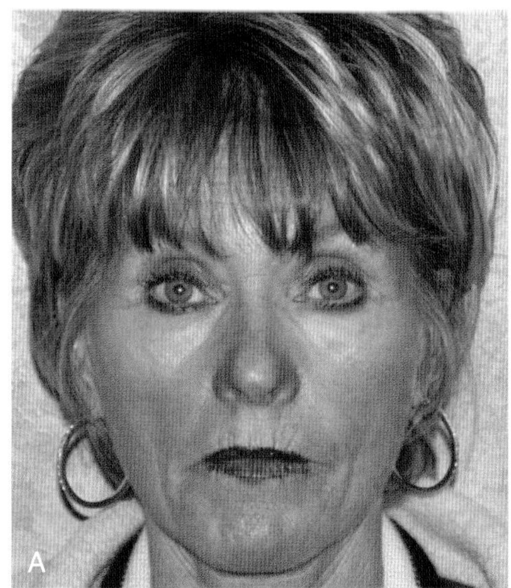

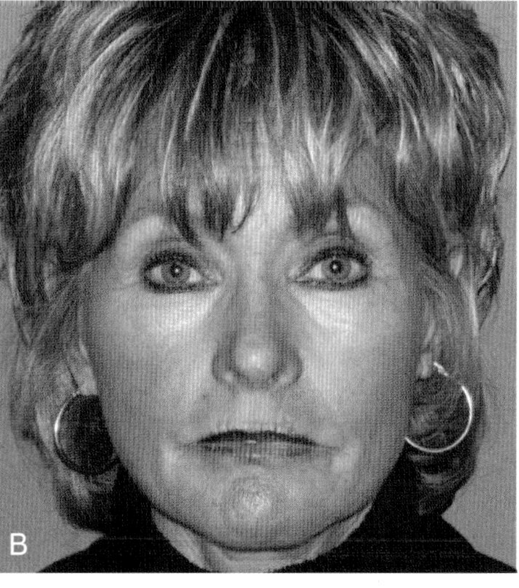

Figure 53-13 Combination therapy using a Lumenis Ultrapulse Encore Laser. *Periorbital area*: ActiveFX: 80 mJ, 125 Hz, density 82%, single pass; DeepFx: 12.5 mJ, 300 Hz, density 15%, single pass. *Perioral area*: ActiveFX: 125 mJ, 125 Hz, density 100%, single pass; DeepFx: 22.5 mJ, 300 Hz, density 20%, single pass. *Remainder of face*: ActiveFX: 125 mJ, 125 Hz, density 82%, single pass; DeepFx: 17.5 mJ, 300 Hz, density 15%, single pass. *Pretreatment with poly-L-lactic acid*: medial and lateral cheeks. *Pretreatment with botulinum toxin type A*: forehead, glabella, lateral brow, and crow's feet. **A,** Before treatment. **B,** After treatment. (Courtesy of Gregory A. Buford, MD, FACS, Denver, Colo.)

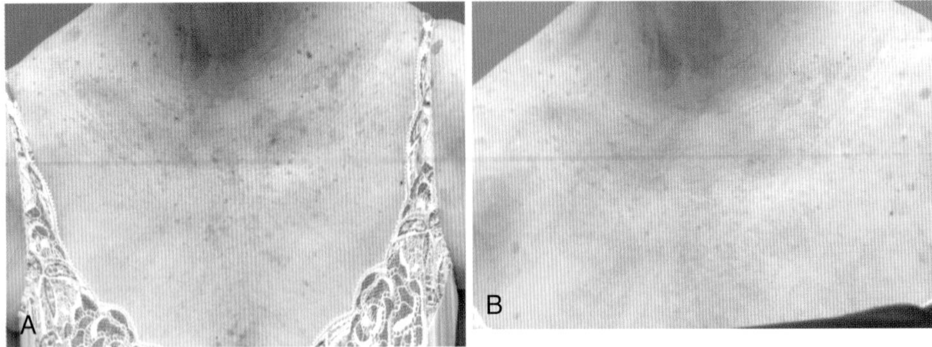

Figure 53-14 Treatment of nonfacial areas using Lumenis Ultrapulse Encore Laser (décolleté). ActiveFX: 100 mJ, 125 Hz, density 68%, single pass. **A,** Pretreatment. **B,** Two months after treatment. (Courtesy of Gordon H. Sasaki, MD, FACS, Pasadena, Calif.)

First 2 to 4 Hours after Treatment

1. Take an analgesic (acetaminophen or ibuprofen) for discomfort.
2. You will be sent home with a container of Thermal Spring Water. Spray this on your skin as often as needed to cool the skin.
3. Avoid direct application of ice to skin. Apply cooling vinegar compresses with cold, wet washcloths using 1 tablespoon of white vinegar in 1 cup of cold water. This will help draw out heat.
4. Blow air from a fan to help with the cooling process.
5. When intense heat subsides, apply Aquaphor Moisturizer, avoiding the area close to the eyes. Keep treated areas covered (thickly) with Aquaphor Moisturizer up to 3 to 4 days, depending on depth of treatment. The skin must not dry out! For the area around the eyes, apply the ophthalmic ointment prescribed and cover with a Swiss Therapy Eye Mask. These will tend to warm and dry out in about 20 to 30 minutes, so always keep an extra one in an ice-water bath and change as necessary.

First Night

1. Sleep on your back and with your head slightly elevated (continue every night until swelling subsides).

   TIP: Place a towel over your pillow to protect it from the Aquaphor Moisturizer.

2. Avoid environmental irritants (e.g., dust, dirt, sun, hairspray) during the healing process.

Day 1 (First Day after Treatment)

1. Stay indoors and avoid direct sunlight.
2. Begin washing treated areas two to three times a day by gently removing Aquaphor Moisturizer with the vinegar/water combination, then cleansing with gentle cleanser and tepid water. Do not rub the skin—gently pat it! Tepid showers and washing the hair is permitted.

   TIP: Stand with your back to the shower.

3. Generously (thickly) reapply occlusive ointment to all treated areas.
4. Hydrate and eat healthy foods. Avoid alcohol because it will tend to dehydrate you. Also avoid exercising until the areas are completely healed.

Day 2

1. Continue to wash the face two to three times a day with gentle cleanser and tepid water.
2. Itching (particularly along the jaw line) begins and is generally an indication that the healing process has started. Mild to moderate itching is normal; if there is severe itching, call the doctor's office.
3. Clinique Medical Recovery Week Complex works well for the itching areas.
4. Continue to apply extra Aquaphor ointment and cool compresses. An oral antihistamine such as diphenhydramine (Benadryl) or loratadine (Claritin) may help.
5. Avoid picking and scratching.

Day 3

1. Continue to wash the face up to two to three times a day with gentle cleanser and tepid water.
2. Itching may persist. Use your Clinique Medical Recovery Week Complex.
3. The central area of the face may begin to exfoliate (peel), leaving behind soft, pink tissue.

Days 4 to 7 (Progress Depends on Depth of Treatment)

1. Itching has usually subsided. If not, continue using an antihistamine, especially at bedtime.
2. Exfoliation begins. Use the NIA 24 Cleansing Scrub if your skin has completely healed.
3. Transition to the Clinique Medical Optimizing Treatment Cream with or without the Recovery Week Complex and spot-treat drier areas with Aquaphor Moisturizer.
4. Start your Clinique Medical sunscreen.
5. Most female patients will be able to apply mineral makeup to treated areas. For male patients, solid sun protection factor is available to help camouflage temporary redness. Be sure to use a fresh applicator and cleanse it with antibacterial soap between applications.

Day 7 and beyond

1. Start your regular skin care program as long as the treated area is healed. Do not use harsh, very active, or strong acids (e.g., Prevage, Retin-A) for 1 month.
2. Continue to apply sunscreen and (female patients) use mineral makeup to protect the treated areas.
3. Avoid exposure to excessive sun for up to 4 weeks. Hat or clothing must be used to protect the treated areas.
4. You may fully return to your normal exercise program.

SIDE EFFECTS

Side effects are common with laser resurfacing, including the following:

- *Erythema*
  - Generally caused by increased blood flow to the area (which is not necessarily a bad thing).
  - Tends to resolve with the overall healing process but may be prolonged in certain patients.
  - Often correlated with depth of treatment and specific type of treatment device.
- *Inflammation*
  - Most people experience moderate swelling after treatment, but individual results vary.
  - The skin may feel tight because of tissue edema in combination with the actual skin-tightening effect of the laser. This effect may wax and wane depending on multiple variables (e.g., treatment depth, individual patient reaction).
- *Allergic reactions*: These usually occur in response to a specific medication or cream.
- *Milia formation*: These are usually the result of use of moisturizers or the injudicious use of irritant cleansers.
- *Acne*
  - Generally associated with the use of heavy emollients during the recovery period
  - Treated by changing topicals or adding oral antibiotics
  - Helpful to use Aquaphor because it is water based
- *Scarring/keloids*: This usually occurs because of some secondary factor (e.g., infection, scratching, poor wound care) that interferes with healing.
- *Xerosis (dry skin)*: This is very common because we are effectively denuding the protective epithelial covering and allowing for greater evaporative water loss from the skin.
- *Desquamation*: Although most patients tend to have some degree of peeling, this is variable and depends on a number of factors, including depth of treatment, skin quality, and so forth.
- *Pruritus*: Although many patients experience some degree of itching that reflects the normal healing process, watch for severe or protracted pruritus because it can herald a more worrisome underlying etiology.

COMPLICATIONS

Complications after laser resurfacing can occur as early as the initial healing phase or as late as several months after the procedure. As such, it is important to educate your patients about signs of an impending complication and ask them to notify the office if they suspect such. The most common complications include the following:

- *Infection*
  - *Bacterial*: Usually seen as adherent yellow crusting papules or increased pain/delayed healing.
  - *Viral (herpes simplex virus)*: Watch for clustered vesicles, although herpes simplex virus infection can have an unusual presentation in the denuded epidermis within a few weeks after treatment.
  - *Yeast*: Symptoms may be subtle and often present simply as increased redness or itching (sometimes confused with contact dermatitis).
- *Pigmentary changes*
  - Although the incidence of pigmentary changes has dramatically decreased with the use of fractional laser resurfacing, pigmentary changes can still occur and steps should be taken before, during, and after treatment to prevent such changes, as well as to identify individuals at higher risk for both hypopigmentation and hyperpigmentation.
  - Contributing factors include the following:
    - Fitzpatrick skin types IV to VI
    - Prior history of pigmentary changes
    - More aggressive treatment settings
  - Treatment options
    - Prevention is the key.
    - Identify increased risk before treating higher Fitzpatrick skin types.
    - Pretreatment (e.g., Tri-Luma) is helpful.
    - Post-treatment protocol generally involves a combination of glycolic acid and hydroquinone.
- *Delayed wound healing*
  - Have high suspicion for potential underlying infection
  - Greater association with more aggressive treatment options
  - Increases potential risk for localized scarring
- Most important ways to *minimize or potentially prevent complications*
  - Patient education
  - Good pretreatment and post-treatment care
  - Early recognition of future problems during the initial consultation
  - Early recognition of issues during the healing period and prompt intervention

SUPPLIERS

(See contact information online at www.expertconsult.com.)

Alma Lasers, Ltd.
Cutera, Inc.
Cynosure, Inc.
Eclipse, Ltd.
Ellipse, A/S
LASERING USA
Lumenis, Inc.
Lutronic, Inc.
Palomar Medical Technologies, Inc.
Sandstone Medical Technologies
Sciton, Inc.
Solta Medical
Syneron, Inc.

ONLINE RESOURCES

American Society for Aesthetic Plastic Surgery: Available at www.surgery.org.

American Society for Aesthetic Plastic Surgery: Fractional Technologies Comparison Chart. Available at http://digital.miinews.com/publication/index.php?i=12807&m=&l=&p=5.

American Society for Laser Medicine and Surgery: Available at www.aslms.org.

American Society of Plastic Surgeons: Available at www.plasticsurgery.org.

eMedicine: Available at www.emedicine.medscape.com.

BIBLIOGRAPHY

The Aesthetic Guide: November/December, 2009, pp 72–73. www.miinews.com.

Alexiades-Armenakas M: Fractional laser resurfacing. J Drugs Dermatol 6:750–751, 2007.

Alster TS, Tanzi EL: Laser skin resurfacing: Ablative and non-ablative. In Robinson JK, Hanke CW, Siegel DM, Sengelmann RD (eds): Surgery of the Skin: Procedural Dermatology. Philadelphia, Mosby, 2005, pp 611–624.

Beer K, Waibel J: Botulinum toxin type A enhances the outcome of traditional fractional resurfacing of the cheek. J Drugs Dermatol 6:1151–1152, 2007.

Carruthers J, Carruthers A: The adjunctive usage of botulinum toxin. Dermatol Surg 24:1244–1247, 1998.

Dierickx C, Khatri K, Alshuler G, et al: Fractionated delivery of Er:YAG laser light to improve efficacy and safety of ablative resurfacing procedure. Lasers Surg Med (Suppl 19):16, 2007.

Goldberg D: Procedures in Cosmetic Dermatology Series: Lasers and Lights, Volume 1: Vascular/Pigmentation/Scars/Medical Applications. Philadelphia, Saunders, 2005.

Goldberg D: Procedures in Cosmetic Dermatology Series: Lasers and Lights: Volume 2: Rejuvenation/Resurfacing/Treatment of Ethnic Skin/Treatment of Cellulite. Philadelphia, Saunders, 2005.

Goldman M: Clinical pearl: Observations on the use of fractionated CO_2 laser resurfacing. J Drugs Dermatol 8:82–86, 2009.

Manstein D, Herron GC, Sink RK, et al: Fractional photothermolysis: A new concept for cutaneous remodeling using microscopic pattern of thermal injury. Lasers Surg Med 34:426–428, 2004.

Perkins SW, Balikian R: Treatment of perioral rhytids. Facial Plast Surg Clin North Am 15:409–414, v, 2007.

Perkins SW, Castellano R: Use of combined modality for maximal resurfacing. Facial Plast Surg Clin North Am 12:323–337, vi, 2004.

Rahman Z, Tanner H, Tournas J, et al: Ablative fractional resurfacing for the treatment of photodamage and laxity. Lasers Surg Med (Suppl 19):15, 2007.

Saluja R, Khoury J, Detweiler S, Goldman M: Histologic and clinical response to varying density settings with a fractionality scanned carbon dioxide laser. J Drugs Dermatol 8:17–20, 2009.

Small R: Anesthesia for cosmetic procedures. In Usatine RP, Pfenninger JL, Stulberg DL, Small R (eds): Dermatologic and Cosmetic Procedures in Office Practice. Philadelphia, Saunders, 2011, Chapter 20 (in press).

Tan KL, Kurniawati C, Gold M: Low risk of postinflammatory hyperpigmentation in skin types 4 and 5 after treatment with fractional CO_2 laser device. J Drugs Dermatol 7:774–777, 2008.

Waibel J, Beer K: Ablative fractional laser resurfacing for the treatment of a third-degree burn. J Drugs Dermatol 8:294–297, 2009.

West TB, Alster TS: Effect of botulinum toxin type A on movement-associated rhytides following CO_2 laser resurfacing. Dermatol Surg 25:259–261, 1999.

Yamauchi PS, Lask G, Lowe NJ: Botulinum toxin type A gives adjunctive benefit to periorbital laser resurfacing. J Cosmet Laser Ther 6:145–148, 2004.

Zimbler MS, Holds JB, Kokoska MS, et al: Effect of botulinum toxin pretreatment on laser resurfacing results: A prospective, randomized, blinded trial. Arch Facial Plast Surg 3:165–169, 2001.

CHAPTER 54

Lasers and Pulsed-Light Devices: Leg Telangiectasia*

Mitchel P. Goldman

Lasers and intense pulsed light (IPL) are used to treat leg telangiectasia for various reasons. *First*, both treatments have a futuristic appeal, not only to the general public but to physicians. By virtue of their advanced technology, they are perceived as state-of-the-art treatment modalities and are sought by the general public because "high tech" is thought of as safer and better than traditional sclerotherapy. Unfortunately, these perceptions have often resulted in unanticipated adverse sequelae (scarring and pain) at an increased cost to the patient (lasers cost considerably more to purchase and maintain than a needle, syringe, and sclerosing solution).

Second, lasers may have theoretical advantages compared with sclerotherapy for treating leg telangiectasia. Sclerotherapy treatment of leg veins has been associated with pigmentation in up to 30% of patients, the development of new blood vessels in up to 10% of patients, and, very rarely, allergenic reactions. These temporary but bothersome adverse effects are perceived not to occur with laser treatment. This chapter discusses the author's experience in treating leg veins with sclerotherapy, lasers, and IPL since 1983.

Mechanism of Action for Lasers and Intense Pulsed Light

Lasers and IPL are *pulsed* so that they act within the thermal relaxation times of blood vessels to produce specific destruction of vessels of various diameters based on the pulse duration (Table 54-1). Lasers of various *wavelengths* and broad-spectrum IPL are used to selectively treat blood vessels by taking advantage of the difference between the light absorption of the components in a blood vessel (oxygenated hemoglobin, deoxygenated hemoglobin, and methemoglobin) and the overlying epidermis and surrounding dermis to selectively thermocoagulate blood vessels. Deoxygenated hemoglobin has distinct optical properties, with two absorption spectrum peaks at approximately 545 and 580 nm, and a broader peak beyond 650 nm (Fig. 54-1). The main feature to note in the curve is the strong absorption at wavelengths below 600 nm, with less absorption at longer wavelengths. This is because the absorption coefficient in blood is higher than that of surrounding tissue for wavelengths between 600 and 1064 nm.

The goal is to deliver sufficient energy to thermocoagulate the target vessel, while the overlying epidermis and perivascular tissue remains unharmed. To accomplish this selective preservation of tissue, some form of epidermal cooling is also required. A number of different laser and IPL systems have been developed toward this end.

*Portions of this chapter are excerpted from Goldman MP, Bergan JB, Guex JJ: Sclerotherapy: Treatment of Varicose and Telangiectatic Leg Veins, 4th ed. London, Mosby, 2006.

An understanding of the appropriate target vessel for each laser or IPL device is important so that treatment is tailored to the appropriate target. As detailed in sclerotherapy textbooks, most telangiectases arise from reticular veins. Therefore, the single most important concept to keep in mind is that feeding reticular veins *must be treated completely before treating telangiectasia*. This minimizes adverse sequelae and enhances therapeutic results. Failure to treat feeding reticular veins and short follow-up periods after the use of lasers may give inflated values to the success rates of laser treatment.

Histology of Leg Telangiectasia

The choice of proper wavelength(s), degree of energy fluence, and pulse duration of light exposure are all related to the type and size of target vessel treated. *Deeper vessels* necessitate a longer wavelength to allow penetration. *Large-diameter vessels* necessitate a longer pulse duration to effectively thermocoagulate the entire vessel wall, allowing sufficient time for thermal energy to diffuse evenly throughout the vessel lumen. The correct choice of treatment parameters is aided by an understanding of the histology of the target telangiectasia.

Venules in the upper and middle dermis typically maintain a horizontal orientation. The diameter of the postcapillary venule ranges from 12 to 35 μm. Collecting venules range from 40 to 60 μm in the upper and middle dermis and enlarge to 100 to 400 μm in diameter in the deeper tissues. Histologic examination of simple telangiectases demonstrates dilated blood channels in a normal dermal stroma with a single endothelial cell lining, limited muscularis, and adventitial layers. Most leg telangiectases measure from 26 to 225 μm in diameter. They are found 175 to 382 μm below the stratum granulosum. The thickened vessel walls are composed of endothelial cells covered with collagen, elastic, and muscle fibers.

Review of Available Lasers

Patients seek treatment for leg veins mostly for cosmetic reasons. Any effective treatment should be relatively free of adverse sequelae.

Krypton Triphosphate and Frequency-Doubled Nd-YAG (532 nm)

Modulated krypton triphosphate lasers have been reported to be effective at removing leg telangiectases using pulse durations between 1 and 50 msec. The 532-nm wavelength is one of the hemoglobin absorption peaks. Although this wavelength does not penetrate deeply into the dermis (about 0.75 mm), relatively specific damage (compared with argon laser) can occur in the vascular target by selection of an optimal pulse duration, enlargement of the spot size, and addition of epidermal cooling (Fig. 54-2).

TABLE 54-1 Thermal Relaxation Times of Blood Vessels

Diameter (mm)	Seconds
0.1	0.01
0.2	0.04
0.4	0.16
0.8	0.6
2.0	4.0

Effective results have been achieved by tracing vessels with a 1-mm projected spot. Typically the laser is moved between adjacent 1-mm spots following the vessels at 5 to 10 mm/sec. Immediately after laser exposure, the epidermis is blanched. Lengthening of the pulse duration to match the diameter of the vessel is attempted to optimize treatment.

We and others have found the *long-pulse 532-nm laser (frequency-doubled Nd:YAG)* to be effective in treating leg veins less than 1 mm in diameter that are not directly connected to a feeding reticular vein. When used with a 4° C chilled tip, a fluence of 12 to 15 J/cm^2 is delivered as a train of pulses in a 3- to 4-mm diameter spot size to trace the vessel until spasm or thrombosis occurs. Some overlying epidermal scabbing is noted, and hypopigmentation is not uncommon in dark-skinned patients. Although individual physicians report considerable variation in results, usually more than one treatment is necessary for maximum vessel improvement, with only rare reports of 100% resolution of the leg vein. Efficacy is technique dependent, with the potential for achieving excellent results. Patients need to be informed of the possibility of prolonged pigmentation at an incidence similar to that with sclerotherapy as well as temporary blistering and hypopigmentation that is predominantly caused by epidermal damage in pigmented skin (type III or above).

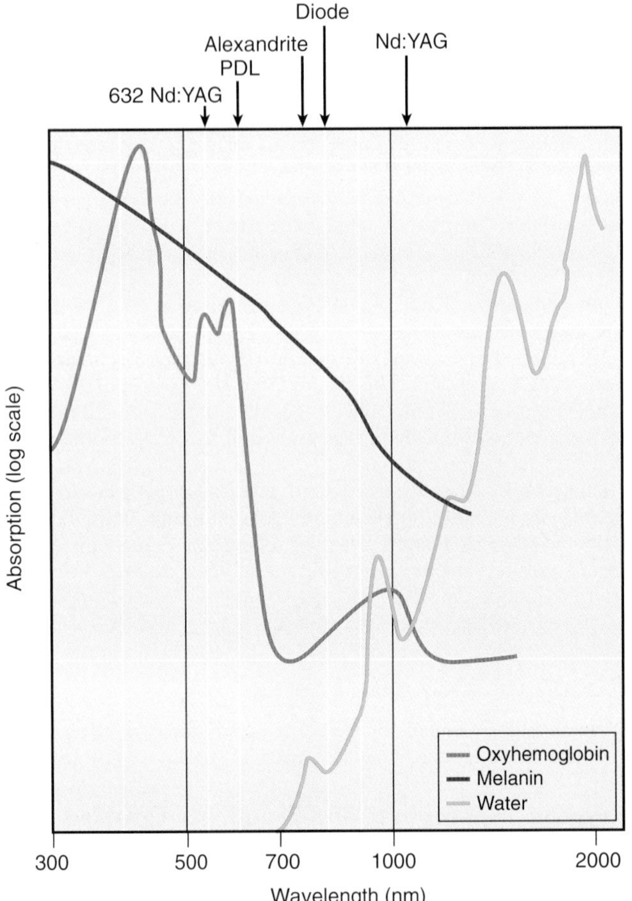

Figure 54-1 **Oxygenated and deoxygenated hemoglobin. Water and melanin absorption curves are given as a function of wavelength.** (Adapted from Boulnois JL: Photophysical processes in recent medical laser developments: A review. Lasers Med Sci 1:47–66, 1986. Reproduced with permission from Goldman MP, Bergan JB, Guex JJ: Treatment of leg telangiectasia with laser and high-intensity pulsed light. In Sclerotherapy: Treatment of Varicose and Telangiectatic Leg Veins, 4th ed. London, Mosby, 2006, p 361, Fig. 13.29.)

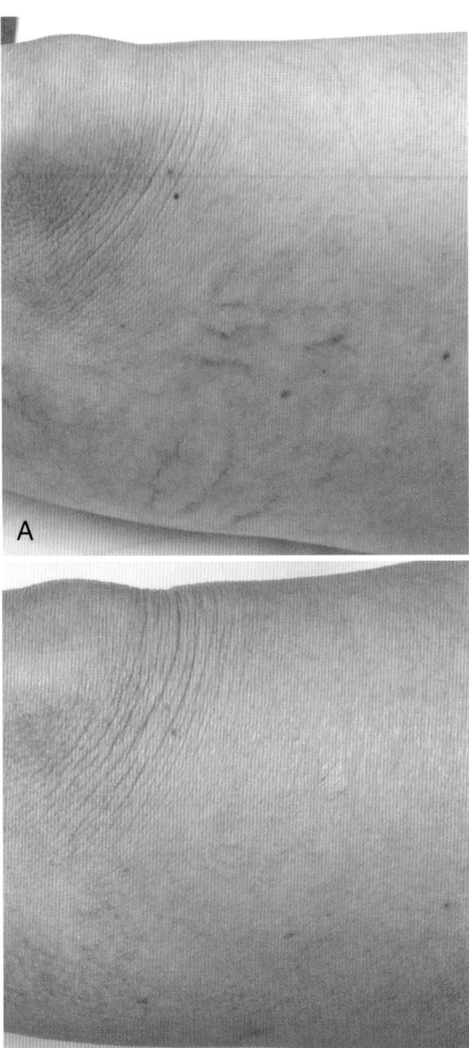

Figure 54-2 Leg telangiectasia. **A,** Before treatment. **B,** After treatment. (Courtesy of David Vasily, MD, Bethlehem, Penn.)

Pulsed-Dye Laser (585 or 595 nm)

The *pulsed-dye laser (PDL)* has been demonstrated to be highly effective in treating cutaneous vascular lesions consisting of very small vessels, including port wine stains (PWSs), hemangiomas, and facial telangiectasia. The depth of vascular damage is estimated to be 1.5 mm at 585 nm and 15 to 20 μm deeper at 595 nm. Consequently, penetration to the typical depth of superficial leg telangiectasia may be achieved. However, telangiectases over the lower extremities have not responded as well, with less lightening and more post-treatment hyperpigmentation. This may be due to the larger diameter of leg telangiectases compared with dermal vessels in PWSs and larger-diameter *feeding* reticular veins, as described previously.

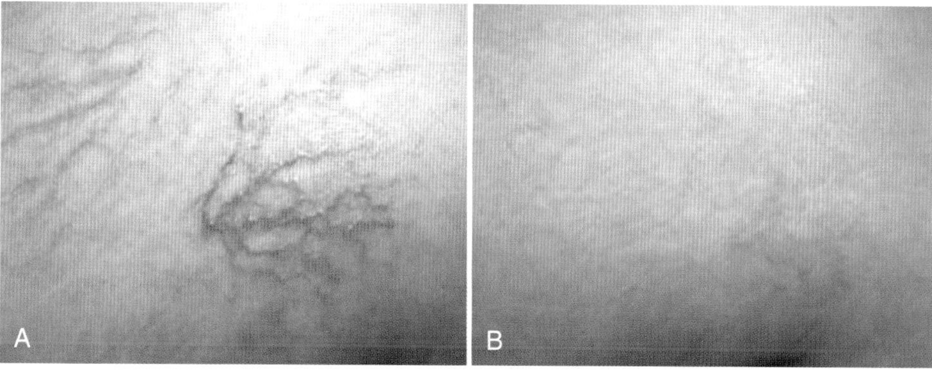

Figure 54-3 Red telangiectasia. **A,** Before treatment. **B,** After treatment. (Courtesy of Khalil A. Khatri, MD, Skin and Laser Surgery Center of New England, Nashua, NH, and Palomar Medical Technologies, Inc., Burlington, Mass.)

Vessels that should respond optimally to PDL treatment are red telangiectases less than 0.2 mm in diameter, particularly those vessels arising as a function of telangiectatic matting after sclerotherapy (Fig. 54-3). This is based on the time of thermocoagulation produced by this relatively short-pulse laser system (see Table 54-1).

In an effort to thermocoagulate larger-diameter blood vessels, pulse duration of PDL has been lengthened to 1.5 to 40 msec and the wavelength increased to 595 nm. This theoretically permits more thorough heating of a larger vessel. These longer pulse durations are created by using two separate laser beams each emitting a 2.4-msec pulse. These lasers operate at 595 nm with an adjustable pulse duration from 0.5 to 40 msec delivered through a 5-, 7-, or 10-mm diameter spot size or a 3 × 10-mm or 5 × 8-mm diameter elliptical spot. Dynamic cooling with cryogen spray is also available, with the cooling spray adjustable from 0 to 100 msec given 10 to 40 msec after the laser pulse or as continuous 4° C air cooling at a variable speed. A fluence of 10 to 25 J/cm^2 can be delivered through a 3 × 10-mm or 5 × 8-mm diameter spot.

We use the PDL at pulse durations matching the thermal relaxation time of the leg veins. The energy fluence used is just enough to produce vessel purpura or spasm. We use stacked pulses to achieve this clinical end point. Because of the necessity for multiple treatments and the significant occurrence of long-lasting hyperpigmentation, we reserve the use of PDL for sclerotherapy-resistant red telangiectases less than 0.2 mm in diameter.

Diode Lasers

Multiple *diode-pumped lasers* are now available, including 532-nm, 810-nm, 915-nm, and 940-nm lasers (Table 54-2). Diode lasers generate coherent monochromatic light through excitation of small diodes. As a result, these devices are lightweight and portable with a relatively small desktop footprint. Diode laser therapy is more painful than sclerotherapy in almost all patients, with equal efficacy noted by the patients who had had both sclerotherapy and laser treatment. A combination diode laser at 915 nm with radiofrequency at levels up to 100 J/cm^2 has been used to treat leg telangiectasia.

Diode lasers are limited by treatment pain and adverse effects. Of note, unless feeding reticular veins are treated, the distal treated telangiectases recur at 6 to 12 months post-treatment. Some authors appear to be able to achieve better results than others using similar parameters. The addition of radiofrequency to the diode appears to offer little advantage.

Intense Pulsed Light

The *high-intensity pulsed light* source was developed as an alternative to lasers to maximize efficacy in treating leg veins (PhotoDerm VL; ESC/Sharplan, now Lumenis, Santa Clara, Calif). This device permits sequential rapid pulsing, longer-duration pulses, and longer penetrating wavelengths than other laser systems. Theoretically, a phototherapy device that produces a noncoherent light as a continuous spectrum longer than 550 nm should have multiple advantages over a single-wavelength laser system. *First*, both oxygenated and deoxygenated hemoglobin absorb light at these wavelengths. *Second*, blood vessels located deeper in the dermis are affected. *Third*, thermal absorption by the exposed blood vessels should occur with less overlying epidermal absorption because the longer wavelengths penetrate deeper and are absorbed less by the epidermis.

With the theoretical considerations just mentioned, IPL emitting in the 515- to 1000-nm range was used at varying energy fluences (5 to 90 J/cm^2) and various pulse durations (2 to 25 msec) to treat venectases 0.4 to 2.0 mm in diameter. Clinical trials using various parameters with the IPL, including multiple pulses of variable duration, demonstrated efficacy ranging from over 90% to total clearance in vessels less than 0.2 mm in diameter, 80% in vessels 0.2 to 0.5 mm, and 80% in vessels 0.5 to 1 mm in diameter. The incidence of adverse sequelae is minimal, with hypopigmentation occurring in 1% to 3% of patients and resolving within 4 to 6 months. Tanned or darkly pigmented Fitzpatrick type III patients are more likely to develop hypopigmentation and hyperpigmentation in addition to blistering and superficial erosions. The choice of a cut-off filter is based on skin color, with light-skinned patients using a 550-nm filter and darker-skinned patients using a 570- or 590-nm filter.

The use of IPL to treat leg veins has produced encouraging results, but these are far from being easily reproduced. This technology requires significant experience and surgical ability to produce good results. Various parameters must be matched to the patient's skin type as well as to the diameter, color, and depth of leg vein. With older machines that do not have integrated cooling through sapphire crystals, a cold gel must be placed between the IPL crystal and skin surface to provide optimal elimination of epidermal heat. There are now dozens of IPL units available from many different manufacturers (see Table 54-2).

Long-Pulse Nd:YAG Laser (1064 nm)

The *1064-nm Nd:YAG laser is probably the most effective laser available to treat leg telangiectasia.* In an effort to deliver laser energy to the depths of leg veins (often 1 to 2 mm beneath the epidermis) with thermocoagulation of vessels 1 to 3 mm in diameter, 1064-nm lasers with pulse durations between 1 and 250 msec have been developed. However, because of the poor absorption of deoxygenated and oxygenated hemoglobin with a 1064-nm wavelength, higher fluences must be used. Depending on the amount of energy delivered, the epidermis must be protected to minimize damage to pigment cells and keratinocytes (Fig. 54-4). Three mechanisms are available to minimize epidermal damage through heat absorption. *First*, the longer the wavelength, the less energy will be absorbed by

TABLE 54-2 Lasers and Light Sources for Leg Veins

Supplier	Product Name	Device Type	Wavelength (nm)	Energy (J)	Pulse Duration (msec)	Spot Diameter (mm)	Cooling
American BioCare	OmniLight FPL	Fluorescent pulsed light	480, 515, 535, 550,580–1200	Up to 90	Up to 500		External continuous
Adept Medical	Ultrawave	Nd:YAG	1064	5–500	5–100	2, 4, 6, 8, 10, 12	None
Alderm	Prolite	IPL	550–900	10–50		10 × 20, 20 × 25	
Asclepion-Meditech	Pro Yellow	Copper bromide	578	55	300	1, 5	None
Candela	Vbeam	Pulsed dye	595	25	0.45–40	5, 7, 10, 12	DCD
	Cbeam	Pulsed dye	585	8–16	0.45	5, 7, 10	DCD
	Gentle YAG	Nd:YAG	1064	Up to 600	0.25–300		DCD
CoolTouch	Varia	Nd:YAG	1064	Up to 500	300–500	3–10	DCD
Cutera	Vantage	Nd:YAG	1064	Up to 300	0.1–300	3, 5, 7, 10	Copper contact
	XEO	Pulsed light	600–850	5–20	?Automatic		None
Cynosure	PhotoGenica V	Pulsed dye	585	20	0.45	3, 5, 7, 10	Cold air
	PhotoGenica V-Star	Pulsed dye	585–595	40	0.5–40	5, 7, 10, 12	Cold air
	SmartEpill II	Nd:YAG	1064	1–200	Up to 100	2, 5, 7, 10	Cold air
	Acclaim 7000	Nd:YAG	1064	300	0.4–300	3, 5, 7, 10, 12	Cold air
	PhotoLight	Pulsed light	400–1200	3–30	5–50	46 × 18; 46 × 10	None
	Cynergie	Pulsed light + Nd:YAG	595 + 1064	20 + 160	0.5–40 + 0.3–300	7	Cold air
DDD	Ellipse	IPL	400–950	Up to 21	0.2–50	10 × 48	
DermaMed USA	Quadra Q4	Pulsed light	510–1200	10–20	60–200	33 × 15	None
Fotana	Dualis	Nd:YAG	1064	Up to 600	5–200	2–10	None
Iridex	Apex-800	Diode	800	5–60	5–100	7, 9, 11	Cooling handpiece
Laserscope	Lyra	Nd:YAG	1064	5–900	20–100	1–5 CA	Cooling handpiece
	Aura	KTP	532	1–240	1–50	1–5 CA	Cooling handpiece
	Gemini	KTP	532	Up to 100	1–100	1–5 CA	Cooling handpiece
		Nd:YAG	1064	Up to 990	10–100	1–5 CA	Cooling handpiece
Lumenis	Quantum	Pulsed light	515–1200				Cooled sapphire crystal
	Vasculite Elite	Pulsed light	515–1200	3–90	1–75	35 × 8	
		Nd:YAG	1064	70–150	2–48	6	Cooled sapphire crystal
	Lumenis One	Pulsed light	515–1200	10–40	3–100	15 × 35, 8 × 15	Cooled sapphire crystal
		Nd:YAG	1064	10–225	2–20	2 × 4, 6, 9	Cooled sapphire crystal
Med-Surge	Quantel Viridis	Diode	532	Up to 110	15–150		
	ProliteII	Pulsed light	550–900	10–50		10 × 20, 20 × 25	None
OpusMed	F1	Diode	800	10–40	15–40	5, 7	None
Orion Lasers	Harmony	Fluorescent pulsed light	540–950	5–20	10, 12, 15	40 × 16	None
		Nd:YAG	1064	35–145	40–60	6	None
		Nd:YAG	1064	35–450	10	2	None
Palomar	MediLux	Pulsed light	470–1400	Up to 45	10–100	12 × 12	None
	EsteLux	Pulsed light	470–1400	Up to 45	10–100	16 × 46	None
	StarLux	Pulsed light/Nd:YAG	550–670/870–1400/1064	Up to 700	0.5–500		
Quantel	Athos	Nd:YAG	1064	Up to 80	3.5	4	None
Sciton	Profile	Nd:YAG	1064	4–400	0.1–200		Contact sapphire crystal
	Profile BBL	Pulsed light	400–1400	Up to 30	Up to 200	30 × 30, 13 × 15	
Syneron	Aurora SR	Pulsed light/RF	580–980	10–30/2–25 RF	Up to 200	12 × 25	
	Polaris	Diode/RF	900	Up to 50/up to 100 RF			
	Galaxy	Diode	580–980	Up to 140/up to 100 RF	Up to 200		
WaveLight	Mydon	Nd:YAG	1064	10–450	5–90	11	Contact or cold air

CA, continous adjustable; DCD, Dynamic Cooling Device; KTP, krypton triphosphate; Nd:YAG, neodymium-doped yttrium aluminum garnet; RF, radiofrequency.
Modified from Goldman MP: Cosmetic and Cutaneous Laser Surgery. Philadelphia, Mosby, 2006.

melanocytes or melanosomes. This will allow darker skin types to be treated with minimum risks to the epidermis because of decreased melanin interaction. *Second*, delivering the energy with a delay in pulses greater than the thermal relaxation time for the epidermis (1 to 2 msec) allows the epidermis to cool conductively between pulses. This cooling effect is enhanced by the application of cold gel on the skin surface that conducts epidermal heat away more efficiently than air. *Finally*, the epidermis can be cooled directly to allow the photons to pass through without generating sufficient heat to cause damaging effects.

Epidermal cooling can be provided in many different ways. The simplest method is continuous contact cooling with chilled water that can be circulated in glass, sapphire, or plastic housings. The laser impulse is given through the transparent housing that should be constructed to ensure that the laser's effective fluence is not diminished. This method is referred to as *continuous contact cooling*.

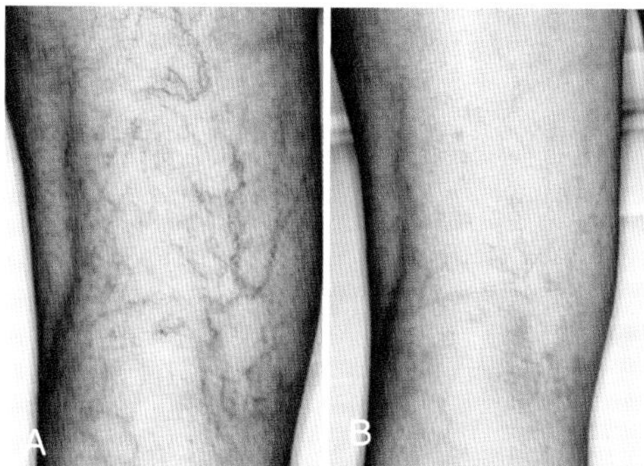

Figure 54-4 Large leg veins. **A,** Before treatment, **B,** After treatment. (Courtesy of Palomar Medical Technologies, Burlington, Mass.)

Its benefit lies in its simplicity. The disadvantage is that the cooling effect continues throughout the time that the cooling device is in contact with the skin. This results in a variable degree and depth of cooling determined by the length of time the cold housing is in contact with the skin. This nonselective and variable depth and temperature of cooling may necessitate additional treatment energy so that the cooled vessel will heat up sufficiently to thermocoagulate.

Another method of cooling is *contact precooling*. In this approach, the cooling device contacts the epidermis adjacent to the laser aperture. The epidermis is precooled and then treated as the handpiece glides along the treatment area. Because the cooling surface is not in the beam path, no optical window is required and better thermal contact can be made between the cooling device and the epidermis. The drawback is the nonreproducibility of cooling levels and degrees, which are based on the speed and pressure with which the practitioner uses the contact cooling device.

Yet another method for cooling the skin is to deliver a *cold spray of refrigerant* to the skin that is timed to precool the skin before laser penetration and also to postcool the skin to minimize thermal backscattering from the laser-generated heat in the target vessel. This method along with continuous air cooling reproducibly protects the epidermis and superficial nerve endings. In addition, it acts to decrease the perception of thermal-laser epidermal pain by providing another sensation (cold) to the sensory nerves. Finally, it allows for efficient use of laser energy because of the relative selectivity of the cooling spray, which can be limited to the epidermis.

Because the target vessel poorly absorbs 1064-nm wavelength, a much higher fluence is necessary to cause thermocoagulation. Whereas a fluence of 10 to 20 J/cm^2 is sufficient to thermocoagulate blood vessels when delivered at 532 or 585 nm, a fluence of 70 to 150 J/cm^2 is required to generate sufficient heat absorption at 1064 nm. Various 1064-nm lasers are available that meet the criteria for selectively thermocoagulating blood vessels (see Table 54-2). All long-pulse 1064 nm Nd:YAG lasers are not the same. Variables include the spot size, laser output (in both fluence and how the long laser pulse is generated), pulse duration, and epidermal cooling.

I have found the 1064-nm, long-pulse Nd:YAG lasers to be beneficial in the treatment of leg telangiectasia not responsive to sclerotherapy or other lasers. The advantage of using a 1064-nm laser is that its longer wavelength can penetrate more deeply, allowing effective thermosclerosis of vessels up to 3 to 4 mm in diameter. In addition, the 1064-nm wavelength permits treatment of patients of skin types I to VI, with or without a tan, because melanin absorption is minimal. The 1064-nm, long-pulse laser systems are not entirely without *side effects*. *Cutaneous burns* with resulting *ulcerations*, *pigmentation*, and telangiectatic *matting* have been observed with each of these systems as parameters are being tested. The dynamically cooled, 1064-nm Nd:YAG laser appears to produce the best clinical resolution with the least pain and adverse effects.

Combination/Sequential 595-nm Pulsed-Dye Laser and 1064-nm Nd:YAG (Cynergy)

The latest laser to enter the market uses a novel sequential 595-nm PDL pulse followed by a 1064-nm Nd:YAG laser pulse. The rationale for enhanced efficacy is that the 595-nm pulse generates methemoglobin, which is more strongly absorbed by 1064-nm wavelengths. Lower energies from both lasers can therefore be used, with the possibility of less pigmentation and adverse sequelae. Preliminary experience is promising in treating bright red vessels less than 0.1 mm in diameter, which are the most difficult vessels to treat with sclerotherapy.

Conclusions

Because sclerotherapy is still considered to be more effective than laser vein therapy and is relatively cost effective compared with laser or IPL treatment, when is it appropriate to use this advanced therapy? Obviously, needle-phobic patients will tolerate the use of this technology even though the pain from lasers and IPL is more intense than that of sclerotherapy with all but hypertonic solutions. Patients who are prone to telangiectatic matting from injected sclerosants are also appropriate candidates. Vessels below the ankle are particularly appropriate to treat with light because sclerotherapy has a relatively high incidence of ulceration in this area owing to the higher distribution of arteriovenous anastomoses. Finally, patients who have vessels that are resistant to sclerotherapy are excellent candidates. A 75% clearance rate with two to three IPL treatments has been documented in sclerotherapy-resistant vessels.

The optimal treatment plan for common leg telangiectasia includes sclerotherapy to treat the feeding venous system and laser or IPL to seal superficial, very tiny vessels to prevent extravasation with resulting pigmentation, recanalization, and telangiectatic matting.

Patent Education Guides

See patient consent form online at www.expertconsult.com.

ONLINE RESOURCE

The American Board of Laser Surgery. Available at www.americanboardoflasersurgery.org.

BIBLIOGRAPHY

Adrian RM: Treatment of leg telangiectasias using a long-pulse frequency-doubled neodymium:YAG laser at 532 nm. Dermatol Surg 24:19–23, 1998.

Alam M, Nguyen TH (eds): Treatment of Leg Veins. Procedures in Cosmetic Dermatology Series, Dover JS, series editor. Philadelphia, Saunders, 2006.

Bernstein EF: Clinical characteristics of 500 consecutive patients presenting for removal of lower extremity spider veins. Dermatol Surg 27:31–33, 2001.

Eremia S, Li CY: Treatment of leg and face veins with a cryogen spray variable pulse width 1064-nm Nd:YAG laser: A prospective study of 47 patients. J Cosmet Laser Ther 3:147–153, 2001.

Garden JM, Tan OT, Kerschmann R, et al: Effect of dye laser pulse duration on selective cutaneous vascular injury. J Invest Dermatol 87:653–657, 1986.

Goldberg D: Procedures in Cosmetic Dermatology Series: Lasers and Lights, Volume 1: Vascular/Pigmentation/Scars/Medical Applications. Philadelphia, Saunders, 2005.

Goldberg D: Procedures in Cosmetic Dermatology Series: Lasers and Lights, Volume 2: Rejuvenation/Resurfacing/Treatment of Ethnic Skin/Treatment of Cellulite. Philadelphia, Saunders, 2005.

Goldman MP: Are lasers or non-coherent light sources the treatment of choice for leg veins? A look into the future. Cosmet Dermatol 14:58–59, 2001.

Goldman MP: Laser and sclerotherapy treatment of leg veins: My perspective on treatment outcomes. Dermatol Surg 28:969, 2002.

Goldman MP, Bergan JB, Guex JJ: Sclerotherapy: Treatment of Varicose and Telangiectatic Leg Veins, 4th ed. London, Elsevier Mosby, 2006.

Kaudewitz P, Kloverkorn W, Rother W: Treatment of leg vein telangiectasias: 1-year results with a new 940 nm diode laser. Dermatol Surg 28: 1031–1034, 2002.

Lupton JR, Alster TS, Romero P: Clinical comparison of sclerotherapy versus long-pulsed Nd:YAG laser treatment for lower extremity telangiectases. Dermatol Surg 28:694–697, 2002.

Sadick NS: Long-term results with a multiple synchronized-pulse 1064 nm Nd:YAG laser for the treatment of leg venulectasias and reticular veins. Dermatol Surg 27:365–369, 2001.

Sadick NS: Laser treatment with a 1064-nm laser for lower extremity class I-III veins employing variable spots and pulse width parameters. Dermatol Surg 29:916–919, 2003.

Sadick NS, Trelles MA: A clinical, histological, and computer-based assessment of the Polaris LV, combination diode, and radiofrequency system, for leg vein treatment. Lasers Surg Med 36:98–104, 2005.

Schroeter CA, Wilder D, Reineke T, et al: Clinical significance of an intense, pulsed light source on leg telangiectasias of up to 1mm diameter. Eur J Dermatol 7:38–42, 1997.

Weiss MA, Weiss RA: Three year results with the long pulsed Nd:YAG 1064 laser for leg telangiectasia. Presented at the Annual Meeting of the American Society for Dermatologic Surgery, Dallas, October 2001.

Weiss RA, Weiss MA: Early clinical results with a multiple synchronized pulse 1064 nm laser for leg telangiectasias and reticular veins. Dermatol Surg 25:399–402, 1999.

CHAPTER 55

Lasers: Tattoo Removal

Kevin Crawford

Decorative tattoos have been a part of human history for thousands of years (Fig. 55-1). The recent discovery of a tattooed, 5000+-year-old, frozen, early European in a glacier in Italy clearly supports this fact. If tattoos have been placed in the skin for over 5000 years, clinicians have likely been trying to remove them for the same amount of time.

It is estimated that 50% or more of all people with tattoos will eventually want them removed completely. Approximately 40% of all tattoo removal patients do *not* want to remove all of the tattoo ink. They in fact desire only to change the existing tattoo and have a new tattoo placed over the old tattoo.

Tattoo Types

Amateur tattoos or home tattoos are usually black tattoos based on "India ink." The carbon-based India ink dyes are, fortunately, the easiest to safely remove. Amateur tattoos are often placed in the dermis by simply dipping the end of a needle into the ink and then dotting the skin to form a design or pattern. The depth of the ink in the dermis is very imprecise. Therefore the density and uniformity of the ink in the design are often very uneven (Fig. 55-2).

Professional tattoos are placed using a repetitively oscillating needle, which in skilled hands will place the ink at a relatively consistent depth in the dermis. Uniform depth can be an advantage for the removal process; therefore, one would think that professional tattoos would have a more consistent removal success rate. However, with professional tattoos, the various colors and the density of the ink complicate the removal process (Fig. 55-3).

Cosmetic tattoos or permanent cosmetics such as lip liners, eyelid liners, and eyebrow color enhancement pose unique challenges when being removed because of location and variety of mixed colors (Fig. 55-4).

Traumatic tattoos are most often the result of an explosion (gunpowder embedded in the skin) or a bicycle or motorcycle accident (asphalt/tar embedded in the skin). Scar tissue often surrounds the embedded particles. The particles are not too deep and can usually be easily removed with a quality-switching (QS) laser (Fig. 55-5).

New Tattoo Pigments

Ink recently developed by Freedom-2, Inc., LLC,* if accepted by the tattoo community, will be much easier to remove. In my area, there are approximately 500 tattoo artists. Many have expressed their reluctance to make tattoos a temporary expression of their art, but may use it for some tattoos (e.g., for names). Freedom-2 ink's micro-encapsulated biocompatible materials address concerns related to adverse skin responses, allergic reactions, infections, inflammation, and adverse systemic reactions. The application of Freedom-2 ink is consistent with today's tattoo technology. However, Freedom-2 ink consists of safe, resorbable pigments microencapsulated in clear, stable polymer beads. Freedom-2 ink can be easily and quickly removed using current laser technology in a much more effective manner than current permanent ink options (see later).

Contraindications

Absolute

- Pregnancy
- Breast-feeding
- Known allergy to pigment
- Uncontrolled systemic disease
- Active untreated bacteria or viral infection
- Use of Accutane in preceding 6 months (this is a matter of debate among many)
- Immunosuppressive disorder

Relative

- Scarring abnormalities
- Bleeding abnormalities
- Hepatitis
- Poorly controlled diabetes mellitus
- Peripheral vascular disease
- Seizure disorder
- Client expectations unreasonable

Former Treatment Methods

Until recently, all tattoo removal modalities resulted in disfiguring scars. In the past, the most popular options included salabrasion (salt-based dermabrasion), mechanical dermabrasion, CO_2 laser ablation, and infrared photocoagulation.

Laser Treatment and Removal

Fortunately, the majority of tattoos are still predominantly composed of *black* ink. However, vibrant colors are becoming more popular and are more difficult to remove. There are three common QS lasers that are frequently used for removing tattoos: the *q-switched ruby laser* (QSRL; 694-nm red), the *q-switched Nd:YAG laser* (QSYL; both 1064-nm infrared and 532-nm [FD-QSYL] green wavelengths), and the *q-switched alexandrite* (QSAL; 755-nm red) laser. *Quality-switching (QS)*, sometimes known as *giant pulse formation*, is a technique by which a laser can be made to produce a pulsed output beam. The technique allows the production of light pulses

*Freedom-2, Inc., 1971 Old Cuthbert Rd., Cherry Hill, NJ 08034, www.freedom2ink.com.

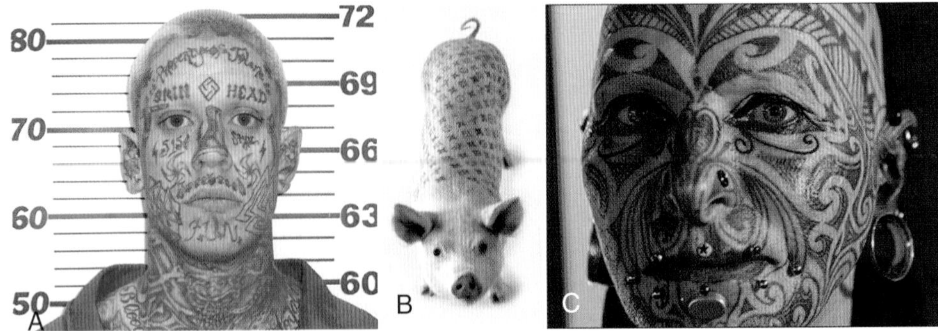

Figure 55-1 **A,** Prison tattoos, Utah State Prison. **B,** Tattooed pig. **C,** Tattoo convention, Berlin, 2007.

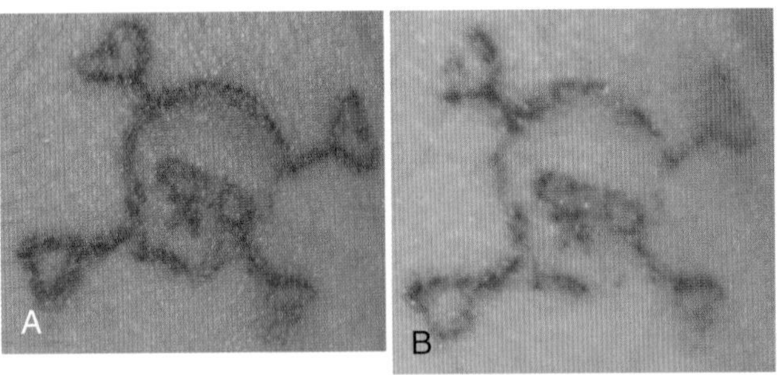

Figure 55-2 Amateur tattoo. Before (**A**) and after (**B**) treatment with HOYA ConBio Revlite, 6.5 J, 6-mm spot size, 1064 nm.

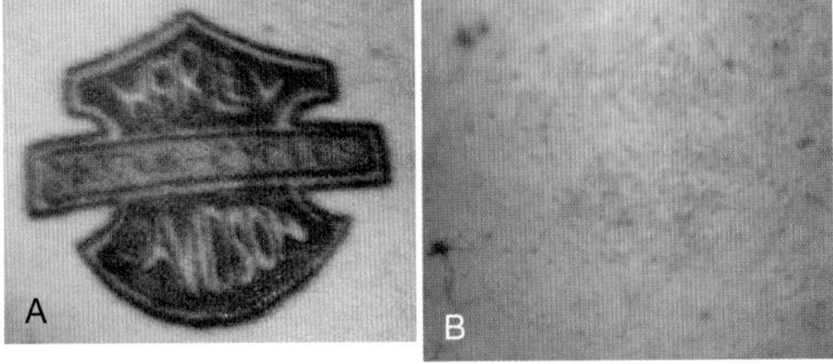

Figure 55-3 Professional tattoo. Before (**A**) and after (**B**) seven treatments over 18 months with VersaPulse-C, 1 to 3 J, 3-mm spot size, 1064 and 532 nm.

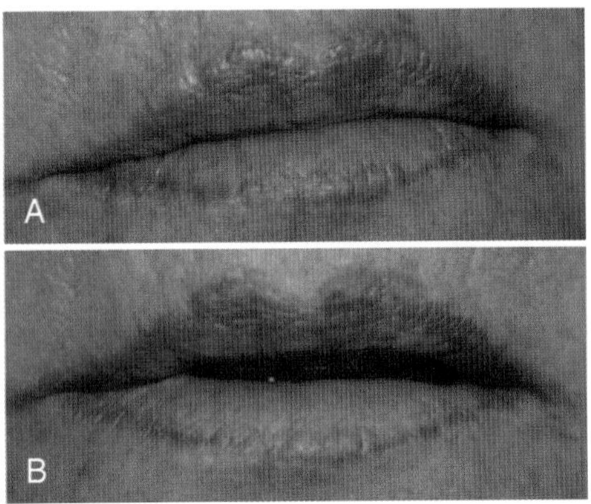

Figure 55-4 Cosmetic tattoo. Before (**A**) and immediately after (**B**) one treatment with HOYA ConBio Revlite, 1.5 J, 4-mm spot size, 1064 nm.

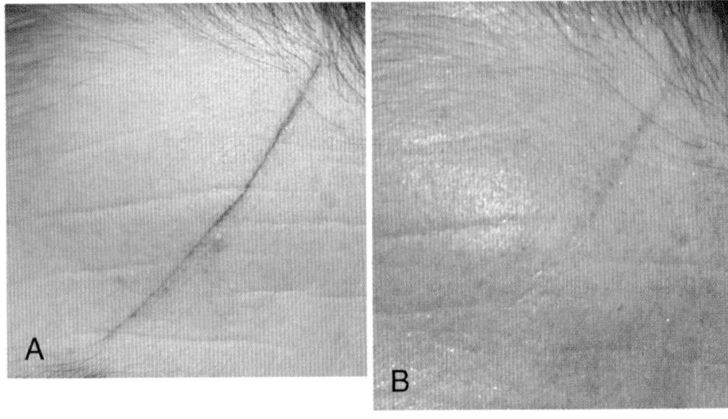

Figure 55-5 Traumatic tattoo. Before (**A**) and after (**B**) 18 treatments over 24 months with VersaPulse-C, 1 to 3 J, 3-mm spot size, 1064 nm. (Courtesy of Richard Burmeier, MD, Perfect Skin Laser Center, Tempe, Ariz.)

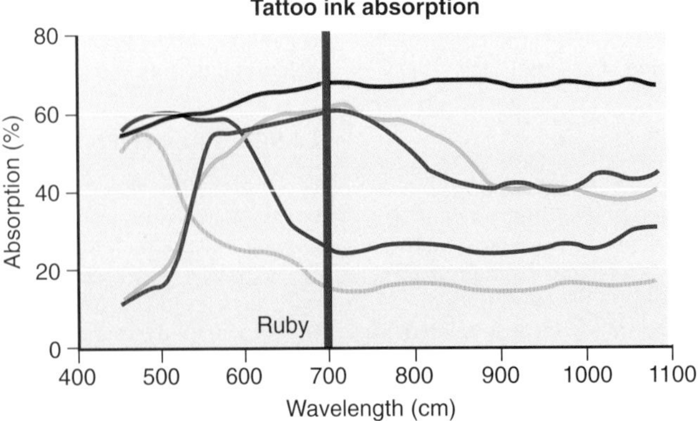

Figure 55-6 Various wavelengths and absorption of different ink colors.

TABLE 55-1 Laser Characteristics for Removal of Different Tattoo Ink Colors

Ink Color	Laser Characteristics*
New black or dark blue	1064 nm, 6 mm, 1.0–2.0 J
Faded black or dark blue	1064 nm, 4–6 mm, 3.0–6.4 J
Red/orange/purple	532 nm, 3 mm, 2.0–3.5 J
Faded red/orange/purple	532 nm, 3–4 mm, 2.0–4.0 J
Green	650 nm, 2 mm (preset)
Sky blue	585 nm, 2–3 mm (preset)

*Wavelength (nm), spot size (mm), energy level (J).

with extremely high (gigawatt) peak power, much higher than would be produced by the same laser if it were operating in a continuous-wave (constant output) mode.

All three of these lasers have strong absorption by *black* ink. The *color* of the ink will determine the wavelength of laser needed (Fig. 55-6). The *amount or density of the ink* and the *depth* of the ink will determine the approximate number of treatments required. The QSYL has been the dominant laser used for removing tattoos. QSYLs, by design, produce shorter, higher peak power pulses than either QSRL, and the QSYL can also produce two very useful output wavelengths. The MultiLite Dye Laser Handpieces, compatible with HOYA ConBio Revlite and C6 lasers, convert the 532-nm wavelength to either 585 nm or 650 nm, effectively offering two additional wavelengths. Candela's AlexTriVantage offers the "Laser-Pumped-Laser" technology with new handpieces that convert the 755-nm wavelength to 532 nm or 1064 nm to improve removal of "all tattoo colors." The choice of an appropriate laser may depend on the prevalence of the type/color of the majority of the tattoos seen in the practice. The QSYL has become popular because of its ability to treat *black, red, orange,* and *blue* inks. The QSYL pulses faster than the ruby- or alexandrite-based laser, so more surface area can be treated in less time.

Treatment Protocol

- For a given color of ink, choose the most appropriate laser based on wavelength and other characteristics (Table 55-1).
- *Cleanse area* of any makeup.
- Laser tattoo removal is painful. Clinicians may decide to apply *a topical anesthetic* with or without occlusion. If this is the case, the topical anesthetic cream must be applied for approximately 45 minutes to 1 hour before commencing treatment (see Chapter 5, Local and Topical Anesthetic Complications). As an alternative to anesthetic creams, a flexible gel ice pack may be used. Apply ice packs for approximately 30 to 45 seconds before laser treatment. Use caution not to freeze the skin.
- *Limit the treatment area* for any given treatment session. Normally the largest area treated at a given time is 24 to 30 square inches. If the tattoo area is larger, the client may come in biweekly to treat additional portions, so that the entire tattoo can be treated every 6 to 10 weeks.
- *Begin* your treatment with the 1064-nm wavelength *to treat the dark ink* in the tattoo. The surface of the skin should turn a mild "hazy white" color each time the laser pulse strikes the skin. Some slight overlap is acceptable from pulse to pulse, but it is not advisable to repeatedly cover the same area because once the skin turns "white" it reflects subsequent laser pulses.
- After the completion of the pass over the black ink in the tattoo, the *red ink* can be treated with the 532-nm wavelength of the QSYL. As with the 1064-nm wavelength, the 532-nm pulses are applied evenly to the red areas of the tattoo until there is "white" color covering the entire treated area (Fig. 55-7).

NOTE: Treating with 532 nm first will cause the skin to reflect the 1064-nm wavelength, minimizing the success in treating the black ink.

- Start off with a lower power setting. There are no "set" parameters to use with tattoo removal as to joules/power, just a range. Setting knowledge comes with time and experience (see Table 55-1).

Common Errors

- *Overtreatment* does not increase the speed of clearance of the tattoo and only increases the risks of negative side effects. It should be noted that it is very common for red ink to blister after treatment.
- In the mid-1990s, *latex-based tattoo ink* was introduced. This ink is vibrant from the first day it is placed in the dermis, and the bright colors remain "glossy." During the initial evaluation the tattoo appears to have the appearance of high-gloss, oil-based paint. *This ink cannot be removed by any laser.* This ink "shrinks" when heated with a laser, causing deep ulcerations that take months to heal and almost certainly resulting in deep, depressed scars.
- *"Cosmetic" tattoos pose other problems.* Generally, cosmetic tattoos are black or dark red and are used to accentuate margins or borders. They include lip liners, eyelid liners, and eyebrow appearance enhancement. When treated with a high-powered QS laser, oxidation occurs and the ink turns black. When the red lip or eye liner changes to a black lip or eye liner, it is very disconcerting for the patient. The *black* ink tattoo can be removed and should be treated as any other black ink tattoo. In general, cosmetic tattoos can be effectively cleared; however, care and a thorough consultation are very important
- *Color changes in dyes: titanium dioxide is a white ink* that, when exposed to a QS pulse of light, can turn black. *Gold atoms* in some inks can change from gold to purple to black depending on the oxidation state change. Again, subsequent treatments usually are successful in removing the changed ink color, but it is very disturbing to the patient to have the tattoo dramatically change color.

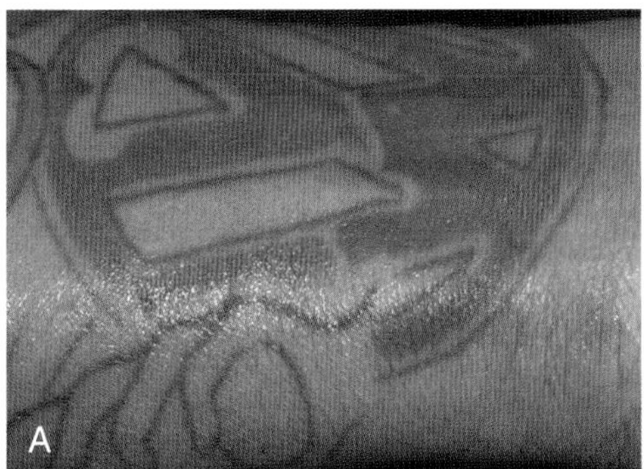

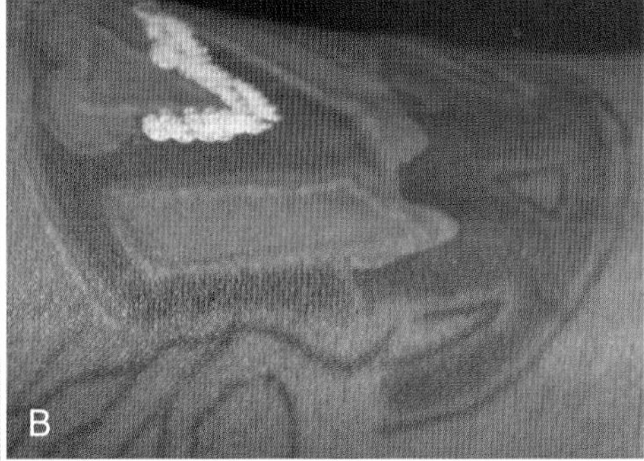

Figure 55-7 Before (**A**) and during (**B**) treatment of red ink tattoo with Palomar Q-YAG 5, 1.5 J, 4-mm spot size, blended 1064/532 nm.

POSTPROCEDURE CARE

- Normally there is erythema and edema immediately after treatment. *Provide an ice pack/ice pillow* after treatment to remove the heat from the treated area and reduce post-treatment discomfort.
- *Ointments* such as Aquaphor are applied to the treated area, which is covered if desired. If epidermal damage does occur, use topical ointments for moist healing to prevent scabbing of the wound (see patient education form for Chapter 30, Radiofrequency Surgery [Modern Electrosurgery], online at www.expertconsult.com).
- In addition to the proper wound care, *sun exposure prevention* of the treated area is very important. Because the treated area has been traumatized by the laser pulses, the skin is more sensitive to hyperpigmentation by exposure to the sun. Encourage SPF 45 use during the entire treatment period. The accepted treatment interval is 6 weeks.
- *Follow-up treatments:* some clinicians feel that *waiting 2 months or even longer between treatment sessions* may be advantageous. Generally, for amateur tattoos, most of the ink can be removed in three to five treatment sessions. Amateur, gang, and prison tattoos are generally easier to remove than professional tattoos. Professional tattoos, depending on the colors of ink, will take from 6 to 10 treatment sessions to remove. In rare instances, some professional tattoos require more than 10 treatments to be successfully removed.

COMPLICATIONS

Although the treatment and removal of tattoos with QS lasers is considered a very safe procedure, potential side effects and risks do exist, including the following:

- Allergic reactions
- Blistering
- Infection
- Pain
- Swelling
- Scabbing
- Bleeding
- Itching
- Hypertrophic scarring
- Atrophic scarring
- Hyperpigmentation
- Hypopigmentation
- Incomplete tattoo removal
- Color changes in dyes

Allergic reactions to tattoo inks are occasionally seen. *Red* inks can produce very severe reactions in patients after QS laser treatments. After treatment of a red tattoo, in particular, patients often complain of itching. This is a sign of an allergic reaction to mercuric oxide in the tattoo ink. These patients should not be treated with a QS laser. Other, nondispersive methods of removal, such as surgical excision or erbium laser resurfacing, may be beneficial.

Although rare, *hypertrophic and atrophic scarring* are the most common complications associated with QS laser tattoo removal. In both cases, the scar formation can be attributed to overly aggressive treatment sessions or poor postoperative wound care by the patient. Keeping the wound clean and covered and preventing the wound from drying out and scabbing are of paramount importance. Conservative post-treatment wound care and strong patient compliance are the keys to preventing hypertrophic scarring.

Because tattoo ink density is always an unknown, the number of treatments necessary to completely remove a tattoo can only be estimated. Patients may become frustrated and impatient during the process. It is not uncommon to find tattoos or parts of tattoos that need greater than 10 treatment sessions, and some patients require 20 or more treatment sessions to remove very stubborn inks. As the number of treatment sessions increases, the degree of *dermal fibrosis* also increases and the texture of the skin changes as well. Patients need to be aware of this.

Postinflammatory hyperpigmentation (PIH) should be considered a transient side effect related to the impact of the high-intensity laser pulse. PIH may fade on its own after the initial treatment, but the need to perform 7 to 10 treatments will, on average, increase the risk of developing PIH. Patients with Fitzgerald skin types IV to VI are more likely to develop PIH and should be advised accordingly. During treatment, portions of the treated area may completely lose pigmentation. This is a more significant problem for darker skin types when treating colored tattoos. When the tattoo removal treatment is completed the treated area will exhibit hypopigmentation or depigmentation in the same shape as the tattoo that was removed, if the melanocytes are permanently disabled. If there are still active, nondamaged melanocytes in the treated area, it should slowly repigment after repeated sun exposure.

One of the most difficult problems to resolve is the *"incomplete" removal* of the tattoo. If the majority of the ink is removed in the first five or six sessions, then extending the intervals between sessions to 12 to 16 weeks will benefit the patient because it will permit more clearance of the ink to take place. At a certain point, further treatments will yield minimal, if any improvement and the decision to discontinue treatment can be made.

PATIENT EDUCATION GUIDES

See patient education and patient consent forms available online at www.expertconsult.com.

SUPPLIERS

(See contact information online at www.expertconsult.com.)

Lasers for tattoo removal
AlexTriVantage
Candela Lasers
Q YAG 5
Palomar Medical
Revlite and C6
HOYA ConBio
VRM 3
Lutronic
Used laser dealers
www.hotlasers.com/
www.medonline.com/
www.medproonline.com

BIBLIOGRAPHY

Alster TS: Q-switched alexandrite laser treatment (755 nm) of professional and amateur tattoos. J Am Acad Dermatol 33:69–73, 1995.

Anderson RR, Parrish JA: Selective photothermolysis: Precise microsurgery by selective absorption of pulsed radiation. Science 220:524–527, 1983.

Goldberg D: Procedures in Cosmetic Dermatology Series: Lasers and Lights, Volume 1: Vascular-Pigmentation-Hair-Scars-Medical Applications. Philadelphia, Elsevier Health Science, 2005.

Goldberg D: Procedures in Cosmetic Dermatology Series: Lasers and Lights, Volume 2: Rejuvenation-Resurfacing-Treatment of Ethnic Skin-Treatment of Cellulite. Philadelphia, Elsevier Health Science, 2005.

Iyengar V, Arndt KA, Rohrer TE: Laser Treatment of Tattoos and Pigmented Lesions. In Robinson JK (ed): Surgery of the Skin. Philadelphia, Mosby, 2005.

Kauvar A, Hruza G: Principles and Practices in Cutaneous Laser Surgery. New York, Taylor and Francis, 2005.

Kilmer SL, Lee MS, Anderson RR: Treatment of multi-colored tattoos with a frequency doubled Q-switched Nd:YAG laser: A dose-response study with comparison to the Q-switched ruby laser. Lasers Surg Med Suppl 5:54, 1993.

Levine V, Geronemus RG: Tattoo removal with the Q-switched ruby laser and the Q-switched ND:YAG laser: A comparative study. Cutis 55: 291–296, 1995.

Removable permanent tattoo ink. Med Lett Drugs Ther 49:75–76, 2007.

Ross V, Naseef G, Lin G, et al: Comparison of responses to picosecond and nanosecond Q-switched ND:YAG lasers. Arch Dermatol 134:167–171, 1998.

CHAPTER 56

Botulinum Toxin

Edward M. Zimmerman

In 1978, a San Francisco ophthalmologist, Alan B. Scott, published the first paper on the use of botulinum toxin in humans. He used it to treat strabismus in 1980. The U.S. Food and Drug Administration (FDA) first approved botulinum A exotoxin (BTX-A or BoNT A) in 1989 for the treatment of strabismus and blepharospasm associated with dystonia, benign essential blepharospasm, and facial nerve (CN VII) disorders in patients 12 years of age or older. It is also used for primary hyperhidrosis of the axillae, palms, and soles, and for treatment of muscular tension headaches and urinary detrusor instability. In 2002, the FDA approved Botox Cosmetic for temporary alleviation of dynamic wrinkles of the glabellar area, and in 2004 Botox was approved for the treatment of primary axillary hyperhidrosis. All other uses are "off-label." This chapter discusses the cosmetic uses of BTX-A, which include the temporary alleviation of dynamic wrinkles of the face and neck; the lifting of nose tips, oral commissures, and brows; the thinning of hypertrophic masseter muscles; and smoothing the pebbly appearance of a "walnut" chin. Botox injections have become the most common cosmetic procedure in the world. Nearly 2.5 million vials of Botox Cosmetic were sold worldwide to perform 4.6 million cosmetic injections in 2008, a continued increase since it was introduced, despite current economic downturns.

BTX-A is available in several forms. Botox, *now called OnabotulinumtoxinA by the FDA*, is a purified neurotoxin complex produced by Allergan, Inc. (Irvine, Calif). It is available in 100-unit vials. Speywood Pharmaceuticals, Ltd., in Maidenhead, England, makes *Dysport* in 500-unit vials. It was FDA approved to be distributed in the United States as Dysport, or AbobotulinumtoxinA, by Medicis Pharmaceuticals (Scottsdale, Ariz). Botox is three to four times as potent per unit as Dysport. Pur-Tox, another BTX-A from Mentor Corporation (Santa Barbara, Calif), is expected to be FDA approved in 2010. Other, non–FDA-approved forms are available outside of the United States, including Xeomin in Germany, Neuronox in Korea, and Chinatox in China.

There are seven serotypes of BTX, designated A through G. Type A is the most potent, and it was the first one commercially available. BTX-A and BTX-E work at the level of the neuromuscular junction of striated muscle, where they irreversibly bind, and after cleaving 9 and 25 amino acids, respectively, from the C-terminus of the SNAP 25 protein, they inhibit the release of acetylcholine. This causes paralysis of that muscle until a new neuromuscular junction is sprouted by the nerve ending, a process that can take weeks to months depending on the density of innervation and on the site, amount, and concentration of the solution injected. The onset of muscle paralysis, reduced sweating, or pain control varies from site to site and patient to patient. Most patients notice a gradual increasing response in 3 to 7 days that plateaus and lasts for 2 to 11 months, with a gradual redevelopment of wrinkles, sweating, or pain. The duration of effect on sweating (6 to 9 months) is significantly longer than on wrinkles (3 to 4 months). Some patients respond more quickly and completely to the injections. A small percentage of patients are minimally responsive, even to large amounts of Botox. Some become resistant to injections. Resistance in patients treated with less than 100 U per session for either blepharospasm or aesthetic purposes is rare. Patients who become resistant to BTX-A because of antibody development after repeated, large doses, and laboratory workers, who are specifically immunized, may respond to BTX-B and BTX-F, which are currently undergoing clinical trials. BTX-B (Myobloc, now called RimabotulinumtoxinB by the FDA) was approved by the FDA in December, 2000, for treatment of patients with cervical dystonia. It is produced by Solstice Neurosciences (South San Francisco, Calif). It has a rapid onset of action (hours to days), loses effect after about 6 to 12 weeks, and is currently used to treat cervical dystonia. BTX-A is about 50 times as potent as BTX-B.

Safety of Botox and Dysport

The LD_{50} of Botox in humans is estimated to be 2500 to 3000 U of toxin for a 70-kg human, or approximately 40 U/kg. For cosmetic purposes, doses of Botox are limited to 100 U; therefore, Botox Cosmetic can be considered a safe and useful chemical. No irreversible clinical effects have been reported.

Similarly, the suggested limit for cosmetic uses of Dysport is 300 U, but up to 1000 U may be used to treat cervical dystonia if needed. No formal drug interaction studies have been conducted with Dysport. However, the package insert lists much the same suggested interactions as could occur with other types of BTX-A.

Indications

FDA-Approved Indications for Botox

- Strabismus
- Blepharospasm with dystonia
- Benign essential blepharospasm
- Cervical dystonia (spasmodic torticollis)
- Primary axillary hyperhidrosis
- Dynamic glabellar rhytids

FDA-Approved Indications for Dysport

- Cervical dystonia
- Dynamic glabellar rhytids

Other Indications for BTX-A

- Cosmetic reduction of dynamic wrinkles in face, lips, and neck
- Hyperhidrosis of the palms, soles, and forehead
- Anal fissures resulting from an increase in rectal sphincter tone (see Chapter 96, Anal Fissure and Lateral Sphincterotomy and Anal Fistula)
- Headaches, both tension and migraine
- Asymmetric face, acquired (e.g., Bell's palsy, hemifacial spasm, or, after facial trauma, the unaffected side causes reduced movement or unopposed muscle tension)

Anecdotally, it is well accepted to perform superficial skin treatments (microdermabrasion, superficial peels, nonablative laser and light treatments) first and then administer BTX-A afterward on the same visit. Injections can also be performed after minor surgeries to different parts of the face (e.g., inject the glabella and brow after blepharoplasty) without causing a deficit in onset or duration of action of BTX-A. More invasive chemical peels, deeper laser resurfacing, and facelifts cause enough inflammation to decrease the duration of action of BTX-A. Injections are usually done 4 to 8 weeks after these procedures.

Contraindications

- Pregnancy.
- Preexisting neuromuscular diseases (this is a relative contraindication; consider obtaining a neurologist's opinion before initiating BTX-A for cosmetic reasons in these patients).
- Sensitivity or allergy to any of the constituents of reconstituted Botox (e.g., BTX-A, human albumin).
- Some medications decrease neuromuscular transmission and may potentiate the effect of large doses of BTX-A (usually not a problem for the small doses used for cosmetic procedures). These include aminoglycosides and similar antibiotics, neuromuscular blocking agents (succinylcholine), penicillamine, quinidine, and calcium channel blockers.
- Sun exposure has been shown to decrease the effect and duration of BTX-A injections.

Equipment

- One vial of Botox (50 U or 100 U) or Dysport (300 U). These are labeled as "single use or single patient use," which some states (e.g., Nevada) are now enforcing—meaning single use on a single patient at a single time. For many years, physicians have reconstituted these drugs and then used separate, sterile syringes of medication on different patients for enhanced economy to the patient with no side effects or problems.
- Sterile normal saline *without preservatives* (single-dose vials). (Although not recommended by the company, saline *with* the preservative benzyl alcohol is commonly used to reconstitute Botox. This solution stores safely in a refrigerator for several weeks and may be less painful to inject because of the numbing effect of the preservative.)
- 20-gauge needle to reconstitute the vial of Botox with saline.
- 1-mL syringes and 30-gauge, ½-inch needles for injection, *or* 0.3-mL insulin syringes with 30- or 31-gauge needles
- Alcohol wipes to cleanse injection sites *(optional)*
- Facial tissues or clean gauze to hold pressure on injection sites
- Nonsterile gloves to wear during injection
- Ice packs or small bags of ice to topically anesthetize the skin and constrict blood vessels at injection sites before injection

Preprocedure Patient Preparation

Botox is delivered by overnight transport in a thick Styrofoam container packed with dry ice to keep the potent toxin stable. Allergan recommends storage of the unmixed toxin at 5° C or lower (frozen). Potency of the toxin is measured in units (U), where 1 U is the amount of toxin that kills 50% (LD_{50}) of a standardized mouse model when injected intraperitoneally. Each vial of Botox contains either 50 U or 100 U of toxin, plus 0.5 mg of human albumin and 0.9 mg of sodium chloride. The toxin is lyophilized and sealed in the vial under negative pressure.

Dysport is supplied in a single-use, sterile vial for reconstitution intended for intramuscular injection. Each vial contains 500 U or 300 U of lyophilized abobotulinumtoxinA, 125 µg human serum albumin, and 2.5 mg lactose. Dysport may contain trace amounts of cow's milk proteins.

The FDA-recommended dose for treatment of dynamic glabellar rhytids with Botox is 20 U, compared with the recommended dose of 50 U for Dysport.

BTX-B (Myobloc) is delivered premixed in several quantities: 2500 U in 0.5 mL, 5000 U in 1 mL, and 10,000 U in 2 mL. (BTX-B may be stored undiluted in the refrigerator at 2° C to 8° C for up to 21 months. If diluted, it should be used promptly because it contains no preservatives.)

An injection site record (Fig. 56-1) should be available before the procedure begins.

Reconstitution and Handling of Botox and Dysport

Alcohol used to cleanse the rubber stoppers and injection sites can inactivate the toxin. Allow it to evaporate completely before proceeding. Allergan recommends that from 1 to 10 mL of sterile saline *without preservatives* (single-dose vials do not contain preservatives—see previous comment) be mixed in the vial of Botox, using the large needle to reconstitute it. A vial that does not demonstrate a vacuum should not be used and will be replaced by the company. The reconstituted Botox should be mixed by gently rolling or swirling the vial. Shaking the vial (i.e., causing foaming) was thought to denature Botox, leading to decreased potency of the solution, but this has proven not to be an issue. Once reconstituted, the toxin should be kept at 2° C to 8° C (refrigerated) and used as quickly as possible. Practitioners may choose to store the solution in the glass vial and use a larger needle to fill the solution into 1-mL syringes as needed or remove the rubber stopper and withdraw the fluid with the small needle on insulin syringes to inject the solution. The package insert recommends using this "single-use vial" of toxin within 4 hours when mixed with sterile saline without preservatives. Group consensus and studies have shown minimal loss of potency in either refrigerated or frozen solution made with saline, with or without preservatives, at 30 days. However, most patients agree that injections reconstituted with saline with preservatives are more comfortable.

Botox dilution varies by use and personal preference. More concentrated dilutions seem to cause effects sooner, but may be more difficult for a clinician to inject accurately and last no longer than injections of more dilute solutions. Most clinicians dilute 100 U of lyophilized Botox with 1 to 6 mL of saline. Dilutions of 100 U/1 mL (10 U/0.1 mL), 100 U/2 mL (5 U/0.1 mL), or 100 U/3 mL (3.3 U/0.1 mL) are commonly used for cosmetic procedures, headache treatments, and hyperhidrosis (Table 56-1). The area of effect associated with each injection point can be up to 2 to 3 cm in diameter.

Dysport can be reconstituted with 1 to 3 mL of saline, depending on the clinician's preference, and used in a similar fashion.

Patient Education

Before injection, the patient should review and sign the informed consent (see the patient consent form online at www.expertconsult.com). The patient should appreciate that the treatment produces temporary results (3 to 4 months) and will take up to 10 days for the full effect. The FDA has recently added a revised form, included with the BTX-A vial, for patient distribution every time BTX-A injections are to be given. It discusses the risk of "potentially life threatening distant spread effects after local injection" because these injections have become so commonplace that some patients may underestimate the associated risk. Conversely, by minimizing the amount of toxin used (to decrease risk of side effects), some wrinkles may not be totally eradicated. However, a "natural" rather than "frozen" face is aesthetically desirable. Efficacy and duration of action vary from patient to patient, but both generally increase with serial injections over time as a result of increasing muscle atrophy. At times, a "touch up" could be of value 2 to 3 weeks after the initial

BOTOX Cosmetic Injection Site Record

Patient Name:________________
Chart#/Ident.:________________

Notes

		Area 1	Area 2	Area 3	Area 4
Location					
Botox Lot Number					
Botox Expiration Date					
Treatment Date					
	Dilution (cc)				
	Units/0.1 cc				
Total Units/Site					
	Site A				
	Site B				
	Site C				
	Site D				
Total Units Used					

Figure 56-1 Sample record of injection sites.

injections, should there be areas where the muscles have not been affected enough or with bilateral symmetry.

Caution the patient against prior use of aspirin, large doses of vitamin E, garlic, ginger, and diet pills, which increase the risk of bruising. Cosmetics covering treatment areas can be removed just before injection and reapplied immediately after, provided the patient *does not rub the treatment areas afterward*. Rubbing the treatment areas can spread the Botox into areas not intended for treatment, increasing the risk of complications such as ptosis. Conversely, the clinician may massage Botox toward or away from areas intentionally.

TABLE 56-1 Dilutions of Botox (100 Units/Bottle as Supplied)

Amount of Saline (mL)	Units/0.1 mL	Units/1 mL
1	10	100
2	5	50
3	3.3	33
4	2.5	25
5	2.0	20

TECHNIQUE

Cosmetic uses for Botox and Dysport include the following:

- *Forehead wrinkles* caused by frontalis muscle contraction
- *Glabellar (frown or "11") lines* and *ridges across the bridge of the nose* caused principally by corrugator and procerus contraction
- *"Bunny lines"* formed across the upper nose (the expression of nose scrunching when someone smells something foul) caused by nasalis muscle contraction

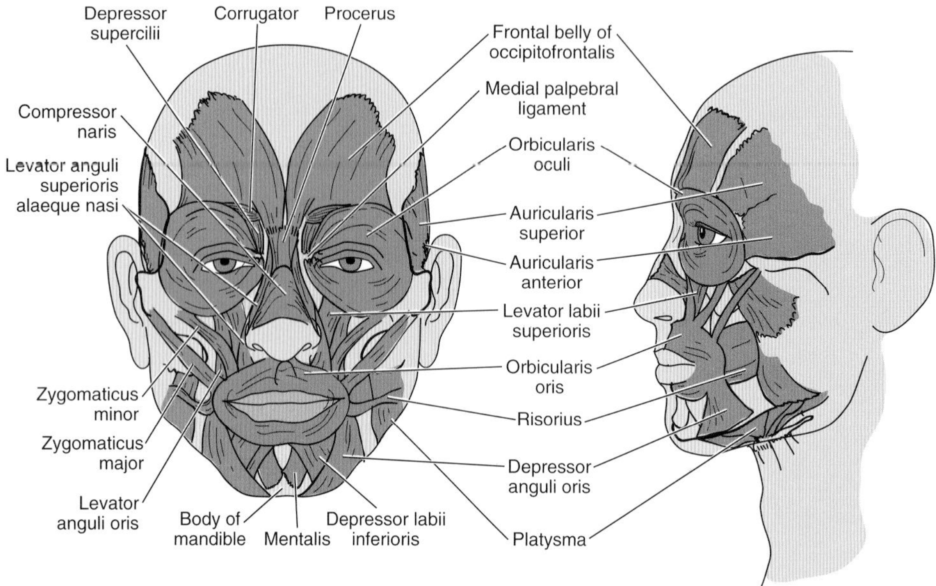

Figure 56-2 Anatomy of the face with masseter muscles noted.

- Lateral *crow's feet, inferior eyelid wrinkles, and ptotic eyebrows* from orbicularis oculi tension
- *Lipstick lines* from orbicularis oris contraction; *chin clefting and elevation* from overactive mentalis muscles
- *Depressed lateral commissures* from overactive depressor anguli
- *Ptotic nose tips and "gummy smiles"* caused by depressor septi nasi and levator labii superioris muscle contraction
- Masseter hypertrophy that causes *lower face broadness* and even *neck bands* from overactive platysma (Fig. 56-2)

Treatment of any site starts with appropriate patient selection, education, and consent. Injections are usually performed in the seated position. It is advisable to take dated, pretreatment photographs of the patient at rest, frowning, smiling, nose scrunching, puckering, and with the brows raised, both front and side views as needed, for later evaluation of treatment efficacy and duration.

1. Cleanse the area to be injected with alcohol and allow it to dry completely.
2. Topically applied anesthesia (e.g., Betacaine, TripleCaine, or equivalent) may be used at injection sites. It should be applied at least 30 minutes in advance to be beneficial.
3. Apply a cold gel pack or glove with ice or water to the proposed injection site to decrease injection discomfort and to cause vasoconstriction.
4. After injection, apply a dry gauze or tissue and ask the patient to hold pressure for a few minutes to reduce bruising and flatten any tissue elevation. Do not let the patient rub the area lest the BTX-A be spread to unwanted areas.
5. Injections are most effective and comfortable when made into the subcutaneous tissue rather than into the muscle or periosteum, or intradermally.

Treatment of Forehead Wrinkles and Frontalis Muscle Contraction Headaches

Horizontal forehead wrinkles and some "stress" or tension headaches are caused by contraction of the frontalis muscle. This muscle usually runs in two bands from the upper margin of the orbits to the scalp. Midforehead creases are usually "sympathy" wrinkles, but this area occasionally requires injection as well. Be aware and careful that inadvertant frontalis contraction may be masking brow ptosis, which would allow excess upper lid skin to collapse down toward or onto the upper lashes. This will be unmasked when Botox or Dysport is administered. Look for this by pushing the forehead down into a fully relaxed/smooth position and see if the patient has or complains of the excess skin on the upper lid.

1. Take pretreatment photographs of the patient.
2. Cleanse the injection sites with alcohol and allow them to dry.
3. Have the patient raise the eyebrows to delineate the muscles.
4. Inject a total of 20 to 30 U of Botox or 50 to 100 U of Dysport *subcutaneously* (Fig. 56-3) into the *ridges* between the wrinkles (furrows) at indicated sites (2.5 to 5 U Botox or 5 to 15 U Dysport per site). Injections can be made relatively perpendicularly to the forehead or threaded under the tissue and injected as the needle is withdrawn. Intramuscular injections tend to bleed more, are less comfortable, and do not provide a better response. Avoid the area between the eyebrows and 1 cm above the superior edge of the orbit lateral to the midpupillary line (or the lowest frontal wrinkle) to decrease the risk of iatrogenic ptosis. Always stay above the lowest line. Eyebrow or upper lid ptosis can last weeks before fading. For treatment of lid ptosis, see the section on Complications.

Treatment of Glabellar Wrinkles (Frown Lines)

Frown lines are caused by the contraction of several muscles; the corrugator runs diagonally from the skin of the medial brow to the bony bridge (root) of the nose. The procerus is a Y-shaped muscle that runs up the bridge of the nose to the forehead. The orbicularis oculi courses around the orbit of the eye. The depressor supercilii muscle is between them. It adds to the depression of the medial brow. Have the patient frown and scrunch his or her nose to identify the dynamic wrinkles, and inject a total of 20 to 40 U of Botox into these areas after each site is cleansed with alcohol, thoroughly dried, and chilled. Toxin is injected into each of the five to seven injection sites proportional to the effect desired. The injection sites are as follows (Fig. 56-4):

- *Site 1:* The bridge of the nose at the level of the lower margin of the upper lid with the eye normally open (5 to 6 U Botox, 10 to 15 U Dysport)
- *Sites 2 and 3:* Directly above *each* medial canthus *at or above* the level of the medial orbital bone (4 to 5 U Botox, 10 to 15 U

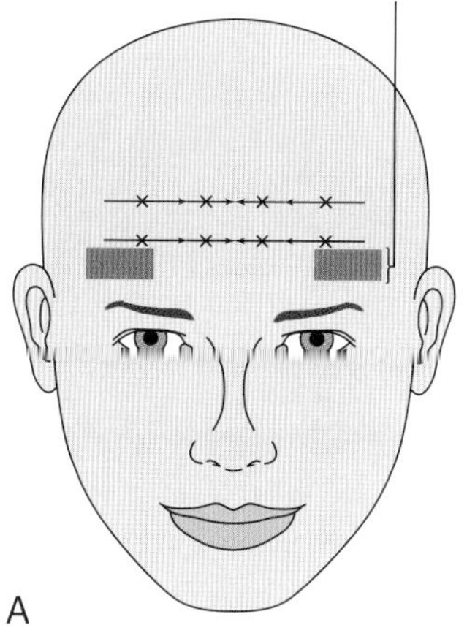
Avoid injections from 1 cm above
down to the superior orbital rim,
and lateral to the midpupillary line,
unless performing a Botox "brow lift"
A
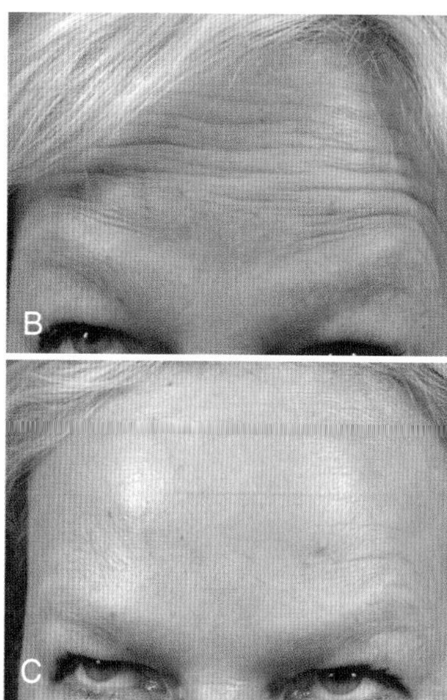
B
C

Figure 56-3 **A,** Treatment of frontalis muscle (forehead wrinkles). See text for details. **B,** Before. **C,** After.

Dysport; injecting below the edge of the orbit may cause lid ptosis)

- *Sites 4 and 5:* About 1 cm above and slightly lateral to sites 2 and 3 following the direction of the corrugator on each side (4 to 5 U Botox, 10 to 15 U Dysport)
- *Sites 6 and 7:* About 1 cm above the brow at each midpupillary line, if necessary (4 to 5 U Botox, 10 to 15 U Dysport; see Fig. 56-4)

Variations in muscular anatomy should be appreciated and treated accordingly in terms of dose and injection location. Do not inject below the superior edge of the orbit, even if the patient has preexisting brow ptosis; this can result in worsening brow ptosis and new upper lid ptosis.

Treatment of Lateral Orbital Wrinkles (Crow's Feet)

Lateral orbital creases are created by contraction of the orbicularis oculi and photoaging. Photoaging and lateral brow ptosis cause static wrinkles, which may not be removed by BTX-A injections alone. Therefore, in older patients who have significant photoaging, the objective of treatment is to minimize rather than abolish the wrinkles entirely. A total of 9 to 15 U of Botox or equivalent dose of Dysport (1 U Botox to 2.5 to 4 U Dysport) is injected in a fanlike pattern into two to five sites on each side, 1 cm lateral to the edge of the orbit (Fig. 56-5). Occasionally, anatomy dictates a second row of injections be placed farther out from the lateral canthus to control a wider orbicularis oculi. Injections made too close to the lower lid margin may cause temporary lower eyelid droop or scleral show, or may worsen infraorbital festoons. Laser treatments and conservative filler injections to the static wrinkles complement the use of Botox in this area. If there are hypertrophic orbicularis oculi muscle folds under the eye with smiling or unapposed, dynamic, inferior orbicularis wrinkles are present, an additional 2 to 4 U of Botox or an equivalent dose of Dysport may be injected subcutaneously at the level of the lower lid crease. Reevaluate results in 2 weeks and retreat as needed.

Insert the needle from a lateral approach to make a smooth entrance into the subcutaneous tissue. Brace or rest your hand(s) on the patient to have the best control over the needle tip and plunger. Start superiorly and inject 2 to 3 U of Botox into each furrow (two to five wrinkles), following the shape of the lateral orbital margin.

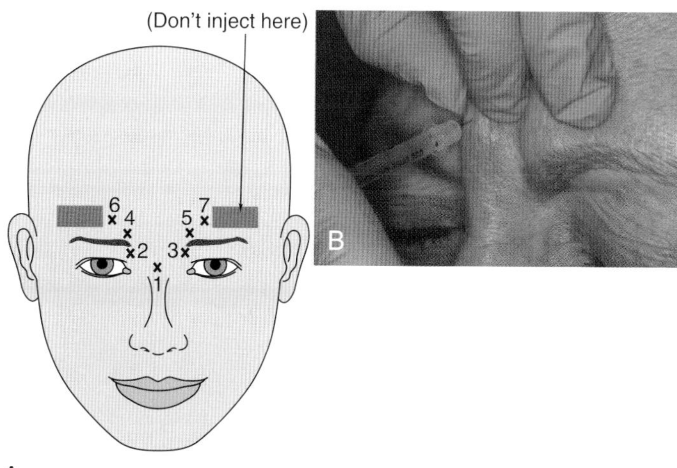
(Don't inject here)
6
4
7
5
2
3
1
A
B

Figure 56-4 **A,** Treatment of frown lines (glabellar muscle). Direct the needle into the bulk of the contracted muscle for corrugator, procerus, and lip injections. All others are directed subcutaneously. See text for details. **B,** Injecting botulinum toxin into the glabellar area for frown lines.

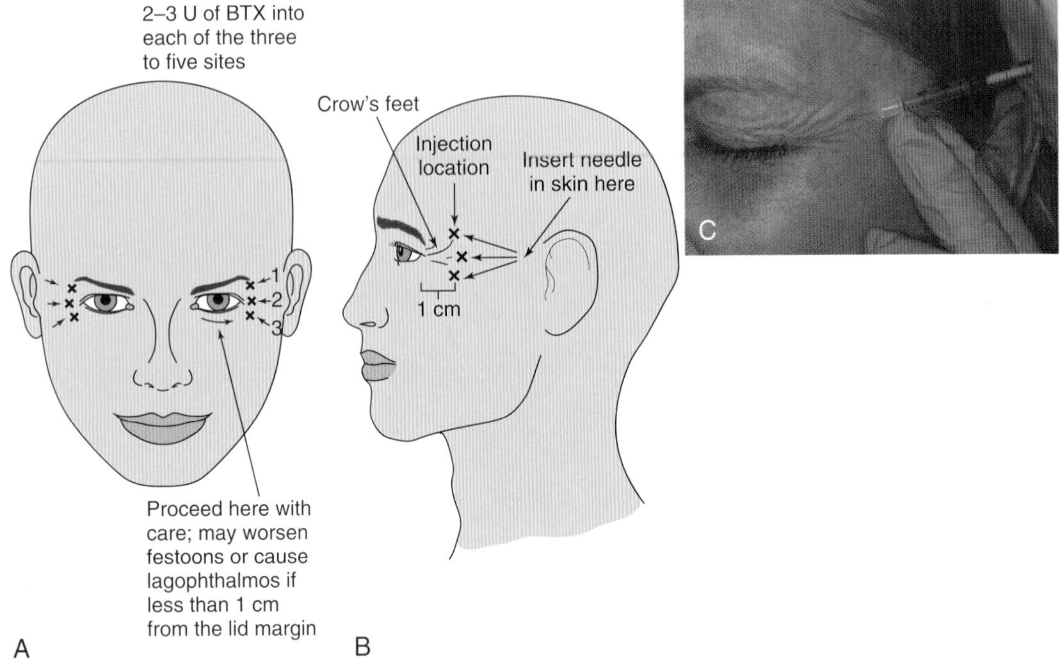

Figure 56-5 Treatment of lateral orbital wrinkles (crow's feet). In this case, three crow's feet wrinkles are treated with three injections. **A,** Frontal view. **B,** Lateral view. **C,** Injecting botulinum toxin for rhytids of the lateral canthal area (crow's feet).

Botox "Brow Lift" and Shaping the Brow

The Botox "brow lift" (Fig. 56-6) relaxes the lateral brow depressors (orbicularis oculi) and medial aspect of the corrugator so that the action of the frontalis muscle is unopposed. To lift the lateral brow, inject 3 to 5 U of Botox at or above the lateral orbit into the brow where you feel the suture line between the frontal and temporal bones on each side. Then inject 3 to 5 U into the corrugator above the medial canthus on each side if the medial brow needs elevation as well. Do not inject the frontalis above these areas, or little lift will be achieved. If there is too much elevation of the medial brow (sad look) or lateral brow ("Spock eyed"), the frontalis muscle may be conservatively injected with a unit or two of Botox at a time until reasonable brow shape and symmetry are restored.

Treatment of Perioral Lines

Contraction of the orbicularis oris can cause vertical lines through and above the vermilion margin, which worsen with smoking and photoaging. Careful injection of 1 to 2 U of Botox into the *valley* of the wrinkle at one or two sites per side into the orbicularis oris muscle helps alleviate contraction (Fig. 56-7). This helps decrease a "gummy smile" in select patients, but they must be warned about the risk of temporary lip droop, which leads to drooling, or lessened or asymmetric smiles. If the "gummy smile" persists, 3 to 5 U of Botox can be injected into the levator labii superioris muscle (see Fig. 56-2 for a depiction of the muscle) in the area of the canine fossa bilaterally. Subtle relaxation of orbicularis allows for an increase in vertical height of the lip (outward pout) by everting the dry vermilion.

After these very precise injections, have the patient avoid rubbing the injection sites to decrease the risk of migration of the toxin to adjacent muscles.

Treatment of Depressed Commissures

Inject 3 to 5 U of Botox along the margin of the jaw directly below each corner of the mouth into the depressor anguli oris muscle (see Fig. 56-2), just anterior to the masseter muscle, which can be

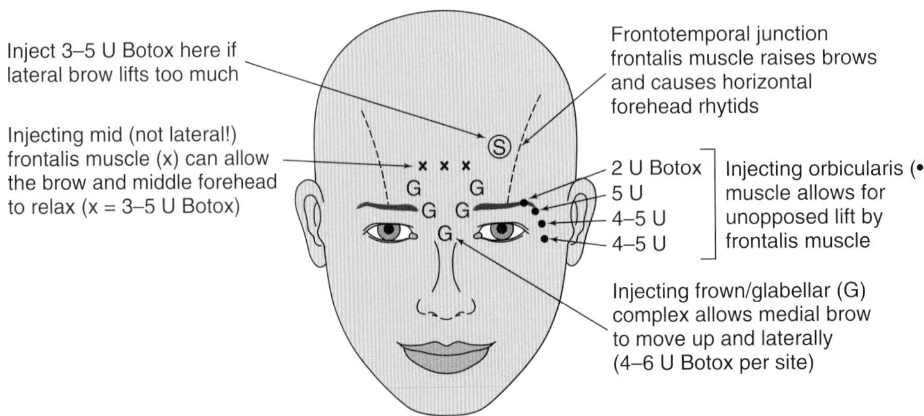

Figure 56-6 Brow lift injection sites.

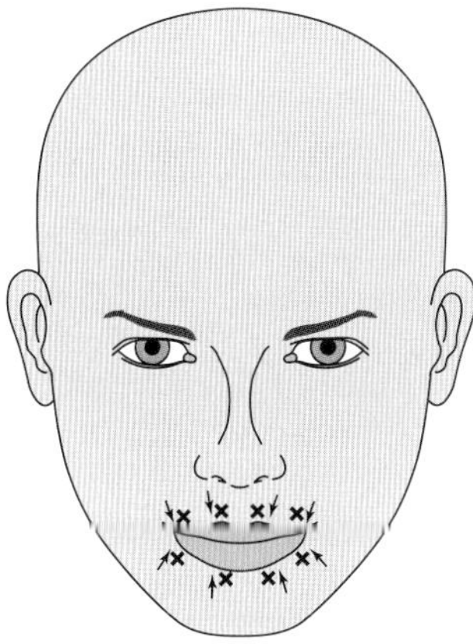

Figure 56-7 Treatment of perioral lines. Inject up to 2 U of botulinum toxin into each valley caused by orbicularis oris contraction.

palpated at the level of the mandible when the patient grits his or her teeth. Check results in 2 weeks. Reinforce with further injections if needed.

Treatment of Wrinkled ("Walnut") or Elevated Chin

Inject 5 to 10 U of Botox centrally into the lower part of the chin (mentalis muscle; see Fig. 56-2) or 5 U/side to a clefted chin. Too high an injection in this area can cause lower lip droop. Check results in 2 weeks. Reinforce with further Botox as needed.

Treatment of Hypertrophic Masseter Muscles

Some (usually female) patients have an angular/squared-off jawline that appears bulky and masculine. Reducing the bulk of the lower half of the masseter muscle helps soften and round that area to obtain a more feminine/oval shape to the face or balance the "pear" shape that patients demonstrate with age. This treatment is more requested by patients of Asian descent. It is also useful for helping to treat patients who chronically grind their teeth or have temporomandibular joint dysfunction.

Draw an imaginary line between the tragus and the corner of the mouth. Inject 20 to 30 U of Botox per side, in three divided doses, below the level of the line, down to the level of the mandible, into the bulk of the masseter muscle (Fig. 56-8). This preserves upper cheek volume while the lower face subjectively thins (masseter muscle atrophies from lack of use) after several months, and can be maintained indefinitely.

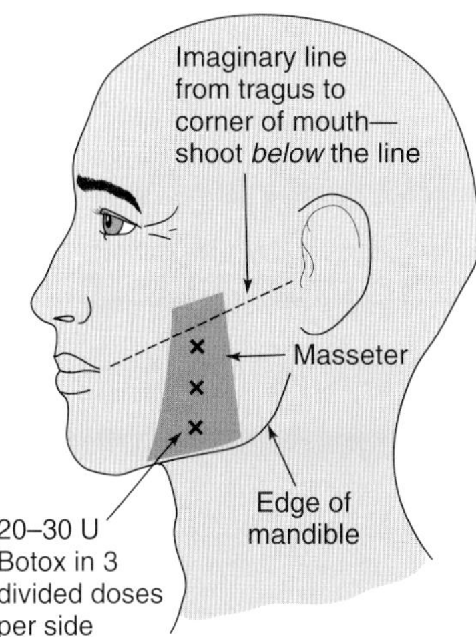

Figure 56-8 Treatment of hypertrophic masseter muscles to narrow lower face.

Treatment of Neck Bands

Botox is more effective on vertical platysmal bands than horizontal bands. Grasp each band where it is most prominent and inject 2 to 5 U of Botox or equivalent dose of Dysport *subcutaneously*, every 1 to 2 cm, and re-evaluate in 2 weeks. Avoid accidently treating the strap muscles or making deep injections that could cause dysphonia, dysphagia, and neck weakness.

Treatment of Primary Hyperhidrosis

Excessive sweat production of the hands and armpits are common conditions that are often treated with topical applications of aluminum salts, iontophoresis, and local and systemic anticholinergic medications. When such treatments fail or give unacceptable side effects, studies have shown that Botox injections may inhibit sweating for 1 to frequently up to 8 months without muscle weakness or other side effects. A 100-U vial of Botox is diluted with 1 to 2 mL of sterile saline, yielding an effective dose of 10 or 5 U per 0.1 mL, respectively. A starch iodine test may be performed to evaluate the major area(s) of hyperhidrosis by thinly applying a liquid iodine solution to the affected areas, allowing it to dry, and then dusting the areas with corn starch. The affected areas will turn blue and can be injected. However, most patients will be able to identify where the area of sweating is most prominent. Roughly 20 small, 2.5-U, subcutaneous blebs are injected, spaced every 1 to 2 cm, into an affected axilla or palm. Topical anesthetics, ice, or continual cold air anesthesia make these injections tolerable. Patients may note some increase in apparent sweat production in surrounding untreated areas and need further treatment.

Sample Operative Report and Progress Note

See Figure 56-1. The following is a sample SOAP (Subjective, Objective, Assessment, Plan) note for Botox treatment of crow's feet:

S—48-year-old woman with no medical problems or contraindications requests Botox chemodenervation of orbicularis oculi muscles to decrease the appearance of dynamic crow's feet.

O—After informed consent and preoperative pictures were obtained, the patient was positioned sitting upright with head supported. Topical anesthetic was applied for 30 minutes and topical ice momentarily applied before 3 injections of 3-plus units of fresh Botox were injected subcutaneously via 30-gauge needle about a centimeter lateral to the lateral orbit on each side. Topical compression was applied to each site. There was no bruising. The injections were tolerated well.

Botox lot no.:_________ Expiration date:_____________ Mix date:__________

A—Botox Chemodenervation of Orbicularis Oculi Muscles; Bilateral; 20 U

P—Patient discharged in stable condition with written instructions. Recheck in 2 weeks or as necessary.

Dysport Use versus Botox Use

Dysport is currently a bit less expensive to effectively treat an area for a similar duration of action as Botox. Dysport is not a household name in the United States, but it has been safely used elsewhere for over 2 decades. The onset of action of Dysport appears to be slightly sooner than that of Botox. The injection techniques are similar once it is understood that 1 U of Botox is equivalent to 2.5 to 4 U of Dysport.

The easiest, least risky place to inject is the glabella. Once you have mastered that area, try the lateral eyes and then the forehead and brow shaping. Lower face injections are mastered once you are comfortable and consistent with upper face treatments and bundling BTX-A treatments with fillers, skin treatments, and skin care programs. Symmetric injection is preferable unless you are trying to correct facial asymmetry. Start with lower doses. Increase the dose to increase the effect and duration. If an area does not respond after 2 weeks, try increasing the dose by 30% to 50%. If it still does not work, you may have one of the few patients who do not respond to these treatments. It is better to inject too high above the brow and leave horizontal forehead rhytids than to drop the brow or upper eyelid. BTX-A is a powerful and forgiving tool for performing minimally invasive, temporary facial shaping. Patients who get the best results are usually working with a physician who integrates various modalities to address loss of facial and neck volume and proportion, skin texture, tone, color, clarity, and elasticity.

Complications

- Brow ptosis
- Ptosis of the upper eyelid
- Double vision
- Temporary discomfort
- Headache, nausea, or flulike symptoms
- Swelling
- Bruising
- Lip droop and drooling
- Temporary facial asymmetry
- Abnormal or lack of facial expression
- Dry mouth (reported after Myobloc injections)
- Incomplete or poor results
- Possible unknown long-term effects (e.g., muscle atrophy, nerve irritability, production of antibodies with unknown effects to general health)

There have been no long-term adverse effects or health hazards related to the use of Botox. Little if any allergy or hypersensitivity has been documented. Repetitive doses of greater than 300 U may lead to production of antibodies, making the patient resistant to further treatment with that particular serotype of BTX. However, it is rare that more than 100 U of Botox is used at any one time for cosmetic uses, or greater than 200 U used at one sitting for the treatment of hyperhidrosis.

Ptosis of the upper eyelid is infrequent (1% to 2%). This temporary side effect of Botox injection can be treated with apraclonidine 0.5% (Iopidine; Alcon Laboratories, Fort Worth, Tex) ophthalmic drops (two drops three times daily to affected eyes). Alternatively, a compounding pharmacy can dilute Neo-Synephrine (phenylephrine) 2.5% ophthalmic drops to 1.25%. Neo-Synephrine drops give relief of lid ptosis in over 80% of patients for 3 to 4 hours, but may cause pupillary dilation with associated photophobia and difficulty with near vision temporarily.

Some patients find injections uncomfortable, which can be minimized by the use of topical anesthetic, ice before injection, small-gauge needles, subcutaneous injections, and topical and verbal distraction during injections. Chilling the tissue to be injected briefly with cold air or direct-contact chilling (e.g., devices available from Zimmer MedizinSystems [www.zimmerusa.com] and ThermoTek [www.thermotekusa.com]) can improve comfort and decrease bruising as well. The risk of bruising and swelling at injection sites is minimized by preinjection chilling and postinjection direct pressure, as described previously. Aspirin and other antiplatelet medications should be avoided for 2 weeks before treatment if possible. Keep injection volumes low. Do not inject below or less than 1 cm above the superior orbital margin lateral to the midpupillary line to prevent brow and upper lid ptosis.

Postprocedure Patient Education

It is important that the patient understands that Botox injections may not entirely alleviate all dynamic wrinkles every time and that the results of the treatment are temporary. Most patients achieve a 60% to 90% improvement 3 to 14 days after their injections. Recheck the patient in about 2 weeks. Review the preinjection photographs, and reinject the areas that have not responded satisfactorily. Remind patients that the objective of treatment is improvement, not perfection, and that some movement is preferred over a frozen face.

It is best if the patient does not lie down or participate in vigorous exercise for at least 4 hours after the injection. Exercising the facial muscles injected by raising the eyebrows, furrowing the brows, and frowning deeply 10 times every 15 minutes for 4 hours will enhance the binding effect of BTX-A.

Conclusion

Botulinum toxin has been used safely in humans since the early 1980s. The FDA approved Botox for cosmetic use in 2002. Botox has been demonstrated to be a safe and effective therapy in a number of studies. It is well accepted in the medical community as a valuable adjunct for the treatment of dynamic wrinkles of the face and neck, control of muscle contraction and vascular headaches, and treatment of hyperhidrosis. The effects of the injections generally last from 3 to 5 months and then fade gradually, with the exception of hyperhidrosis, where they are more likely to be effective for 7 to 9 months.

Patient Education Guides

See the patient education preinjection and postinjection information and patient consent forms online at www.expertconsult.com.

CPT/Billing Codes

Note that for cosmetic purposes, there are no CPT codes nor is there insurance coverage. Insurances vary in their coverage for any Botox injection and it is best to have the patient clarify this with his or her carrier before doing any injections. The fees are often in the thousands of dollars and patients need to be aware of their financial responsibilities.

64612 Chemodenervation of muscle(s); muscles innervated by facial nerve (e.g., blepharospasm, hemifacial spasm). Use for migraines, tension headaches
64613 Neck muscles (e.g., spasmodic torticollis)
64614 Extremity or trunk (e.g., dystonia, cerebral palsy)
64650 Chemodenervation of eccrine glands; both axillae
64653 Chemodenervation of other areas (e.g., scalp, face, neck) per day
64999 For hands or feet (unlisted procedure, nervous system)

ICD-9-CM Diagnostic Codes

The cost of Botox is about $5.25 per unit (100-U vial) in 2009 and under $1.50 per unit for Dysport. Charges for injections range from $8 to $15 per Botox unit, depending on additional overhead, amount used, and prevailing charges in the area.

307.81 Headache: tension
333.81 Blepharospasm
346.9 Headache: migraine
70521 Hyperhidrosis: face, soles, axilla

J Codes

J0585 Botulinum Toxin A per unit (e.g., Botox)
J0587 Botulinum Toxin B per 100 units (e.g., Myobloc)

SUPPLIERS

(See contact information online at www.expertconsult.com.)

Anatomic chart stickers for documenting Botox injections
George Tiemann and Co.
Betacaine LA and Betacaine Plus
Custom Scripts Pharmacy
University Compounding Pharmacy
Botox
Allergan, Inc., sells and distributes the product
Cold Air and Contact Analgesia Units
ThermoTek, Inc.
Zimmer MedizinSystems
Customizable patient education brochures
Contemporary Health Communications
MJD Patient Communications
Dysport
Medicis Aesthetics, Inc.
Topical Anesthetics
See Chapter 5, Local and Topical Anesthetic Complications

ONLINE RESOURCES

Drs. Alistair and Jean Carruthers offer a set of videos at their website, www.carruthers.net (click on Resources, then Educational Resources, and choose from DVDs).

DVDs: Learning to Work with Botox (Botulinum Toxin Type A): A Guide for Clinicians (Paul A. Fox, MD, 2004 [run time: 75 min.]) and Introduction to Botox (Botulinum Toxin Type A) for the Patient are available through www.NPInstitute.com (click on Products, then Physician or Patient DVDs, respectively).

NOTE: There are numerous didactic and clinical training courses for clinicians to attend on cosmetic Botox injection (e.g., National Procedures Institute [www.npinstitute.com] and Creative Health Communications [www.creativehealthcommunications.com]).

BIBLIOGRAPHY

Allergan, Inc.: Botox Cosmetic (botulinum toxin type A) purified neurotoxin complex (Package Insert). Irvine, Calif, Allergan, Inc.

Bartfield JM, May-Wheeling HE, Raccio-Robak N, Lai SY: Benzyl alcohol with epinephrine as an alternative to lidocaine with epinephrine. J Emerg Med 21:375–379, 2001.

Botulinum toxin (Botox Cosmetic) for frown lines. Med Lett Drugs Ther 44:47–48, 2002.

Carruthers A, Carruthers J (eds): Procedures in Cosmetic Dermatology Series: Botulinum Toxin. Philadelphia, Saunders, 2005.

Carruthers A, Carruthers J (eds): Special Issue: Update on Botulinum Toxins. Dermatol Surg 33(Suppl 1):S1–S110, 2007.

Carruthers J, Fagien S, Matarasso SL, Botox Consensus Group: Consensus recommendations on the use of botulinum toxin type A in facial aesthetics. Plast Reconstr Surg 114(Suppl 6):S1–S22, 2004.

Glogau RG: Botulinum A neurotoxin for axillary hyperhidrosis: No sweat Botox. Dermatol Surg 24:817–819, 1998.

Kaminer MS, Hruza GJ: Botulinum A exotoxin injections for photoaging and hyperhidrosis. In Kaminer MS, Dover JS, Arndt KA (eds): Atlas of Cosmetic Surgery. Philadelphia, WB Saunders, 2002, pp 291–311.

Kim JH, Yum KW, Lee SS, et al: Effects of botulinum toxin type A on bilateral masseteric hypertrophy evaluated with computed tomographic measurement. Dermatol Surg 29:484–489, 2003.

Lowe N, Bradbury E, Flynn T, et al: Proceedings of the Facial Aesthetics Conference and Exhibition, Royal College of Physicians, London, 24–25 June 2006. J Cosmet Laser Ther 8:203–222, 2006.

Matarasso SL, Shafer D: Botox(r) cosmetic. In Nahai F, Nahai F, Codner MA (eds): Minimally Invasive Facial Rejuvenation. Techniques in Aesthetic Plastic Surgery Series. Philadelphia, Saunders, 2009, pp 1–20.

Medicis Aesthetics, Inc.: Dysport Package Insert. Scottsdale, Ariz, Medicis Aesthetics, Inc.

Naver H, Aquilonius S-M: The treatment of focal hyperhidrosis with botulinum toxin. Eur J Neurol 4(Suppl 2):S75–S79, 1997.

NOTE: The entire November 1998 issue of *Dermatologic Surgery* is devoted to Botox.

CHAPTER 57

Tissue Filler

Mel Elson

Soft tissue augmentation has been performed since the 15th century, when physicians transplanted fat en bloc to correct defects, usually facial disfigurements related to wartime injuries. The modern era began in 1981, when the U.S. Food and Drug Administration (FDA) approved Zyderm I, a suspension of 3.5% bovine collagen with 0.3% lidocaine. Although not particularly long lasting or effective for a great deal of indications, it was sufficient to treat acne scars and fine lines and wrinkles, such as nasolabial folds, oral commissures, and crow's feet.

Over the past 25 years, products and techniques have evolved so that there are now about 300 different filling materials. Table 57-1 lists the most common filling materials used around the world. Modern techniques and products are used not only for the classic indications for soft tissue augmentation, but also to rebuild and renew faces by replacing lost tissue volume so that they appear much younger.

Indications

The indications for soft tissue augmentation have evolved over the years. Although they remain in the realm of cosmetic treatment, some, such as the soft-tissue injectables for human immunodeficiency virus (HIV) lipoatrophy, are life-changing. The areas of treatment have also expanded from the injection of nasolabial folds (Fig. 57-1), oral commissures, crow's feet, and glabella to neck lines, hands, cheeks (Fig. 57-2), bridge of the nose, chin (Fig. 57-3), and any area of atrophy.

Contraindications

There are both absolute and relative contraindications, as well as those that are generally applicable to all fillers and those that are specific to certain fillers.

- Allergies: Although there is still some limited use of bovine material, it is limited to Zyderm and Zyplast (Inamed, Santa Barbara, Calif) and Artefill (currently off the market). Any *allergy to bovine protein* precludes the use of these materials, and skin testing must take place before use. Animal sources are rarely used for fillers any longer, although there are exceptions. There is one hyaluronic acid product from avian sources (cock's comb); however, this does *not* require skin testing. Most materials are based on hyaluronic acid, which will be discussed in detail and which does not elicit a delayed hypersensitivity response. In addition, only rarely do these materials contain lidocaine, so allergy is not a substantive problem.
- Active infection: Any active infection or skin disease in the area to be injected is a contraindication.
- Location: Injection of robust substances such as Zyplast, Cosmoplast, and biphasic fillers into the glabellar complex must be avoided.
- Patients who are *pregnant or breast-feeding* should not undergo augmentation.

Relative contraindications include the following:

- Unrealistic expectations.
- Body dysmorphic disorder or patients seeking a psychological boost after a life-changing event such as a divorce, death of a family member, or loss of a job. Patients should wait and let things settle down before rushing into a procedure that may or may not be right for them and will not solve the emotional issue.
- Use of anticoagulants. Preparation for the injections *to prevent bruising*, particularly when using biphasic fillers, should consist of discontinuing aspirin and vitamin E for at least 72 hours, and if the patient is on warfarin to consult with the patient's primary care physician regarding the feasibility of discontinuing the drug for a few days. If this cannot be done, the patient should not be injected with biphasic fillers and extreme caution must be taken even with hyaluronic acid fillers. *Topical vitamin K cream* twice a day for a week before and after will significantly decrease the bruising.

Initial Examination and Patient Preparation

A complete *history and physical examination* should be performed before soft tissue augmentation, and particular emphasis should be placed on any prior injections or Botox treatments, what the patient is using for skin care, and any allergic reactions or difficulties with any cosmetic procedures in the past.

Obtaining good-quality *photographs before injection* is strongly encouraged in all patients.

Informed consent should include all the pertinent information regarding possible side effects, cost, and alternative treatments, as well as a statement at the end that the patient has been asked if he or she has any further concerns or questions and stated that he or she does not. It is also prudent, if at all possible, to schedule another session for the patient 2 to 3 weeks after treatment to see if what both the patient and the physician desired has been accomplished. Do not call this a session "for a possible touch-up," but one for injection in case it is needed. When possible, always try to schedule two injection sessions so that if there are any issues they can be easily resolved. The problem with calling a second injection a "touch-up" is that often the patient feels that there was something done incorrectly with the first injection and will be hesitant to pay for a "touch-up."

Equipment for Soft Tissue Augmentation

- Injectable material of choice
- Appropriate-gauge needles for the material of choice
- Anesthetic material
- Ice
- Topical vitamin K
- Alcohol swabs for skin preparation

TABLE 57-1 Most Common Filling Materials Worldwide

Manufacturer	Filling Material	Main Ingredient	Needle Gauge	Indication	Status
Alcon	Silkon 1000	Silicone	30	All except fine work	Off-label use
Allergan	Zyderm I	Bovine collagen	30.32	Fine work	Worldwide
	Zyderm II	Bovine collagen	30	Scars	Worldwide
	Zyplast	Bovine collagen, cross-linked	30	Deeper; lips; base	Worldwide
	CosmoDerm	Human-based collagen	30.32	Same as Zyderm I	Worldwide
	CosmoPlast	Human-based collagen	30	Same as Zyplast	Worldwide
	Juvéderm Ultra	Nonanimal HA	30	All except fine work	Worldwide
	Juvéderm Ultra Plus	Nonanimal HA	27	Deeper; lips; base	Worldwide
Anteis SA	Esthelis	HA	30	Three forms, from fine to deep	Canada, EU, Isreal, Korea
Arters	Artefill	PMMA and bovine carrier	26	All except fine work	Worldwide
Bioform	Radiesse	Acrylic hydrogel + calcium hydroxylapatite	27, 1¾ in.	Contour; not for fine or lips	Increasing
Biopolymer	Matridex	DEAE Sephrades (sephadex)	27 or 30	Medium	CE mark*
	Matridur	HA with cross-linked dextran		Deeper; lips; base	
	Matrigel			Fine work	
ColBar	Evolence	Porcine collagen	30	Like CosmoDerm	EU, Canada, Israel, Korea
Contura	Aquamid	Polyacrylamide gel	27		EU; 30 countries
	Aquamid Recon		27 or 30		
Dermabiol	Rhegecoll	PMMA and bovine carrier	26	Like Artefill	Pending worldwide
Dermatech	Dermalive	HA plus HEMA-EMA	26 or 27	Deep	EU, Canada
	Dermadeep	Larger particles	26	Very deep	EU, Canada
Dermik/Aventis	Sculptra	Polylactic acid	27	All except very fine	EU, US
Fascia Biosystems	Fascian	Human fascia lata	26	Medium depth	Human tissue—not FDA-regulated
FibroGen, Inc.	FG-5017	Human collagen type III	30	Same as CosmoPlast	Not approved yet
FuHua	Amaxingel	Polyacrylamide gel	27	Same as Aquamid	China
FzioMed	Laresse	Carboxymethylcellulose	27 or 30	Medium depth	EU
Isolagen	Isolagen	Autologous fibroblast cells	30	Medium-fine	US
Laboratories ORGéV	MacDermol S	Avian HA, non–cross-linked	30	Moisturizing	CE mark
	MacDermol R	Avian HA, cross-linked	30	Medium depth	CE mark
LCA	Hyaluderm	HA; non–cross-linked	30	Fine lines	CE mark
Medicis; Qmed	Restylane	NASHA	30	Deep; lips	
	Restylane touch	NASHA	32	Contour; not for fine or lips	EU, Canada
	Perlane	NASHA	27	Contour; lips; not for fine lines	CE mark
	Restylane Sub Q	NASHA	27	Medium depth	CE mark
Mentor	Puragen	HA, double cross-linked	27	Medium depth	Some Europe
	Prevelle	HA, cross-linked	30	Finer	Some Europe
Merz	Belotero Soft	Non-animal HA	27	Medium	CE mark
	Belotero Basic	Non-animal HA	30	Lips	CE mark
Polymekon	Bio-Alcamid Face	Polyacrylamide gel	30	Medium	CE mark
	Bio-Alcamid Lips	Polyacrylamide gel	30	Lips	CE mark
	Bio-Alcamid Body	Polyacrylamide gel	30	Same; more material	CE mark
	Bioinblue Lips	Polyvinyl alcohol	30	Lips	CE mark
	Bioinblue DeepBlue	Polyvinyl alcohol	27	Deeper work	CE mark
ProCytech SA	Outline Fine	Polyacrylamide gel	32	Fine work	CE mark
	Outline Original	Polyacrylamide gel	30	Medium depth	CE mark
	Outline Ultra	Polyacrylamide gel	27	Deeper work	CE mark
	Evolution	Polyacrylamide gel + polyvinyl alcohol	30	Medium depth	CE mark
Prollenium	HylaNew	HA, cross-linked	30	Medium	Canada, some Asia
	HyleNew Ultra	Higher concentration	27	Deeper; lips; base	Canada, some Asia
	Hyladex	HA + hypromellose	27	Deeper except lips	Canada, some Asia
Rofil	Reviderm	Dextran (Sephadex)	30	Medium	Worldwide except US
	Rofilan	HA	30	Fine work	Worldwide except US
	Beautical 2	Polyacrylamide gel	30	Fine work	Worldwide except US
	Beautical 5	Polyacrylamide gel	30	Medium depth	Worldwide except US
Teoxane SA	Teosyal 27	HA	27	Medium-deep	CE mark
	Teosyal 30	HA	30	Fine work	CE mark

EMA, ethyl methacrylate; EU, European Union; HA, hyaluronic acid; HEMA, hydroxyethyl methacrylate; NASHA, stabilized nonanimal hyaluronic acid; PMMA, polymethyl methacrylate.

*The CE, or European Conformity, mark indicates the product has met EU consumer safety, health, or environmental requirements. It applies to all countries of the EU, as well as the four countries of the European Free Trade Area (Iceland, Liechtenstein, Norway, and Switzerland) and Turkey.

Material for Injection

This is the point where things become very complicated because there are a myriad of materials available for use. It is not possible to obtain expertise or even experience with all filling materials that are currently available; however, familiarity with a few will provide an armamentarium that will be sufficient for most needs (Table 57-2).

Collagen Products from Human Fibroblasts

CosmoDerm has for the most part replaced Zyderm because it is the same material with the same indications, but with the collagen derived from human foreskin fibroblasts. Therefore it does not require allergy skin testing. *CosmoPlast* is the same as Zyplast except that it is also derived from human tissue.

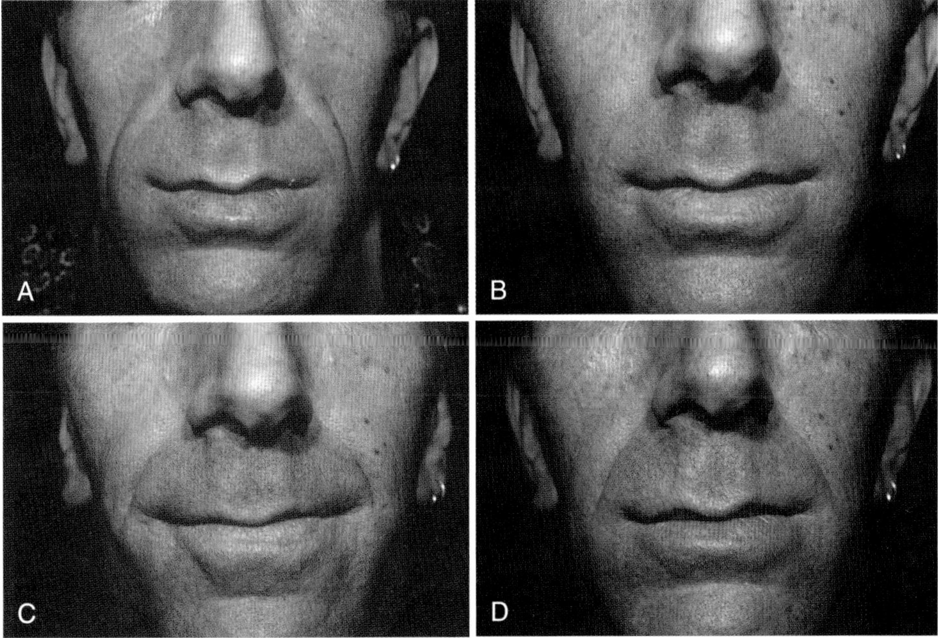

Figure 57-1 Radiesse injection of the nasolabial folds. Before (**A**) and 3 (**B**), 6 (**C**), and 12 (**D**) months after treatment. Volume injected (in milliliters): baseline, 4; 1 month, 0; 6 months, 2; total, 6.

Collagen Products from Bacterial Hyaluronic Acid

Most of the materials available now are based on hyaluronic acid. Hyaluronic acid products have become very popular around the world, and there are indeed many of them, but the most significant in this category are the products from Qmed in Sweden (Restylane, and Perlane Restylane fine lines) and those from Inamed-Allergan (Juvéderm Ultra, Juvéderm Ultra Plus, and Juvéderm Fine Line—also known as Juvéderm 24, Juvéderm 30, and Juvéderm 18). All of these products are manufactured by bacterial fermentation in the laboratory, after which the hyaluronic acid undergoes various degrees of cross-linking and folding to increase the longevity of the implant. Without any manipulation of the molecule to increase cross-linking and molecular weight, the implant would be very short lived because pure hyaluronic acid lasts only hours to a few days when injected into the skin. There is a product in use in Asia called Hyalan that is actually injected into the skin to act as a moisturizer. Hyaluronic acid traps and attracts water to it. This is also the reason that when hyaluronic acid is injected as filler the end result is a smooth surface—because water is absorbed into the area of injection. Although there is great similarity between the two types of hyaluronic acid fillers available, there is much debate as to which is

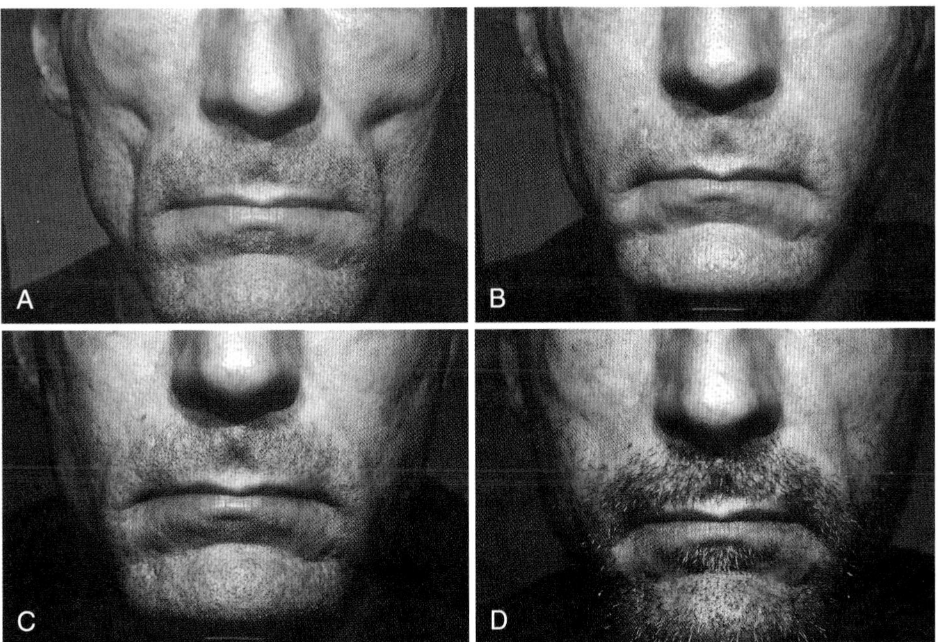

Figure 57-2 Radiesse injection of the cheeks. Before (**A**) and 3 (**B**), 6 (**C**), and 12 (**D**) months after treatments. Volume injected (in milliliters): baseline, 8; 1 month, 5; 6 months, 5.7; total, 18.7.

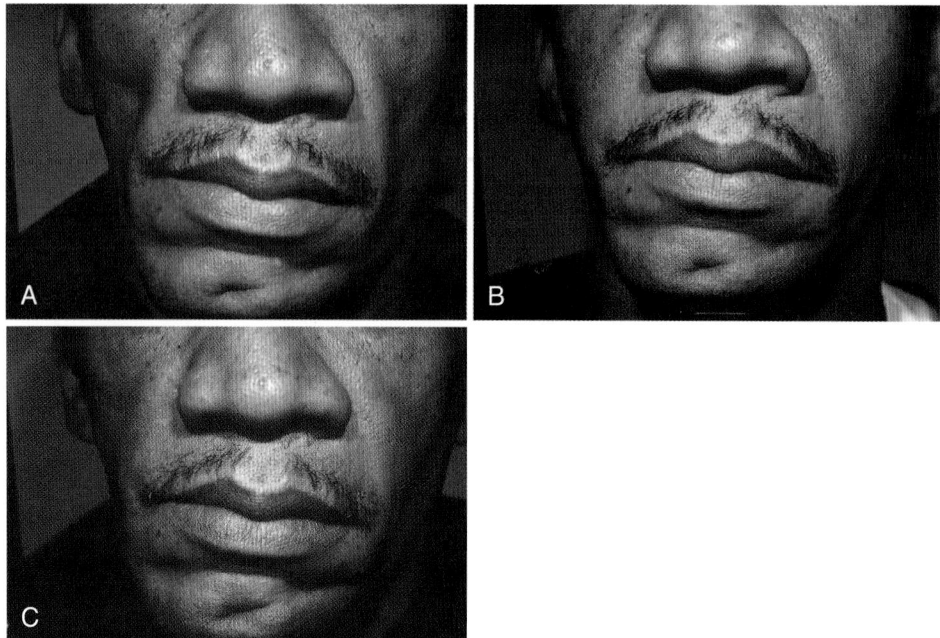

Figure 57-3 Radiesse injection of the chin. Before (**A**) and 3 (**B**) and 12 (**C**) months after treatments (no 6-month postinjection photograph available). Volume injected (in milliliters): baseline, 6; 1 month, 0.8; 6 months, 2; total, 8.8.

the longer lasting, which produces smoother results, and which is more comfortable for the patient. The *higher–molecular-weight products* are used for more aggressive augmentation such as for scars, lip augmentation, and some degree of sculpting. The *lower–molecular-weight products* are used for fine lines such as crow's feet and lip lines. *Midrange products* are used for the majority of augmentation needs such as the treatment of nasolabial folds, oral commissures, and the glabellar area.

The most common fillers used in the United States are Restylane and Perlane (Medicis, Scottsdale, Ariz) and Juvéderm Ultra and Juvéderm Ultra Plus (Allergan, Irvine, Calif), although there are some others available.

Noncollagen, Non–Hyaluronic Acid Products

Some products are not collagen based and do not contain hyaluronic acid—*Sculptra* (called *New-Fill* in Europe) and *Radiesse* are the most widely used at this time. Sculptra (Dermik/Aventis, Bridgewater, NJ) is a polymer of lactic acid that is provided as a powder to be mixed before injection with water or lidocaine. It is very difficult to force into solution, and it is recommended to mix the product the day before use, if possible. It was initially approved in the United States for HIV lipoatrophy and is used in many areas for soft tissue augmentation, including cheek augmentation and postrhinoplasty defects. *It induces new collagen formation* as the implant itself degrades to lactic acid and is absorbed completely by the body. There has been a report of this material inducing correction lasting 40 months, although probably 12 to 24 months is more likely. It is injected into the lowest part of the dermis at the junction with the subcutaneous tissue using a 26-gauge needle, and does require some degree of anesthesia.

Radiesse (Bioform Medical, San Mateo, Calif) is quickly becoming one of the most popular filling materials in the world because it is a biphasic filler that produces long-lasting results (although not permanent because the second phase is biodegradable). A biphasic filler is one that has two phases. Phase one corrects the defect and triggers the second phase, which induces the patient to form collagen from fibroblast infiltration. The key point is that any biphasic material should be both biocompatible and biodegradable so that eventually the only substance that remains is the patient's own collagen producing the correction. Radiesse consists of 70% acrylic hydrogel with 30% calcium hydroxylapatite beads. Calcium hydroxylapatite has been used as a dental material for more than 20 years. Radiesse has been approved by the FDA for vocal fold augmentation, as a radiographic marker, and for maxillofacial augmentation. More recently, the FDA approved the material for the treatment of HIV lipoatrophy and nasolabial fold augmentation. It is injected at the junction of the dermis and subcutaneous tissue using a 27-gauge needle. When augmenting cheeks or correcting nasolabial folds, it is recommended to use a 27-gauge, 1¼-inch needle rather than the more common ½-inch needle, which can be used in shorter areas such as the oral commissures.

The *Radiesse injection technique* is more specific than with other materials. The needle should be inserted through the dermis (where resistance is felt) and then into the subcutaneous space (where there is little resistance). The material is injected in a retrograde fashion *with care taken to discontinue injecting before withdrawal to avoid inadvertent injection into the dermis*. Although this is difficult to master, it is imperative that the injections be done in this manner to avoid

TABLE 57-2 Common Uses of Major Fillers

Filler	NLF	OC	Glabella	Periocular	Lips
Restylane	1.5 mL	1 mL	0.3 mL	0.1 mL	1–2 mL
Juvéderm	1–2 mL	1 mL	0.2 mL	0.1 mL	1–2 mL
Radiesse	0.8 mL	0.4 mL	—	—	—
Teosyal	1 mL	0.5 mL	0.2 mL	0.1 mL	1–2 mL
Revanesse	1 mL	0.5 mL	0.2 mL	0.1 mL	1–2 mL

For this table, it is assumed that the clinician understands the following:

- Every patient is different and the volumes given are averages only.
- There a number of different fillers in each line designated for certain uses that are not interchangeable (e.g., Restylane is for NLF, Perlane is better for lips).
- Teosyal has seven different products in the line, so each product should be used in the appropriate area.
- Never use a biphasic filler in the lips.
- Never use a robust filler around the eyes or in the area of the glabella.
- The volumes refer to each side of treatment.

NLF, nasolabial folds; OC, oral commissures.

foreign body reactions. Rather than a single pass, *multiple passes* are made.

- To correct the *nasolabial fold*, material is injected under the fold in the manner just described, and then closer to the nose, with still a third linear thread just onto the cheek slightly above the fold. *Caution* should also be taken to make the injections in the linear thread smooth without hesitation during the injection so that lumps do not occur. This technique will form a "scaffold" under the nasolabial fold to elevate it.
- To *augment cheeks* the same technique is used, but with an additional triple linear thread at right angles to the first set. This would also apply to correction of *HIV lipoatrophy, rhinoplasty defect, or any other true augmentation.*

Also see later under Plane of Injection, in the Technique section.

The gel and the particles are injected into the desired area of correction. The gel dissipates over a 3- to 4-month period; during this time the particles that have been delivered induce fibroblast collection, stimulating new collagen formation. As the gel disappears, the new collagen remains, producing correction for approximately 18 months or more. The *main advantage to Radiesse* is that the calcium hydroxylapatite particles are biodegradable and disappear over time, avoiding the possible problems of permanent fillers.

This filler also contains no anesthetic, so it is advisable to *provide some form of anesthesia for the patient*. Augmentation of the nasolabial fold, oral commissures, and the like may require only a topical anesthetic such as Ela-Max or Betacaine, but cheek augmentation or treatment of HIV lipoatrophy usually requires a nerve block. Radiesse should not be used for lip augmentation because significant beading may result.

General Guidelines

When using materials for soft tissue augmentation, certain guidelines should be kept in mind.

- The shortest-lasting materials (low molecular weight) are the ones that are injected highest in the dermis with the smallest-gauge needle (30, 32, or 33 gauge), may require overcorrection, can be repeated often, and are forgiving if an error occurs. They usually will last 3 to 4 months.
- Mid–molecular-weight materials should be injected with a 30-gauge needle into the mid-dermis and can be expected to last approximately 6 to 12 months.
- The most robust materials (highest molecular weight) are injected deeper into the tissues, use larger needles (26 or 27 gauge), must *never* be overcorrected, cannot be repeated very often (e.g., no more than twice a year), and may be totally unforgiving in the event of an error on the part of the injector. Inexperienced injectors should begin with more forgiving materials such as CosmoDerm, Restylane, and Juvéderm Ultra and should receive one-on-one instruction from an experienced injector to obtain proper knowledge of soft tissue augmentation.

Preprocedure Patient Preparation

Once a history, physical examination, photographs, and informed consent are obtained, the areas to be injected should be cleansed with alcohol. The patient should not be wearing makeup. Ice can be applied both before and after the procedure for patient comfort. If more anesthesia is desired or required, a field block, nerve block, or mixing the filler material with 0.2 mL of 2% lidocaine with epinephrine will provide more patient comfort.

Technique

The patient should be in the *upright position* for injection. Technique depends on what the goal is for each individual patient. Provide traction by pulling the skin in the direction of the defect and aligning the needle with the defect to be injected. Use the smallest-gauge needle possible (usually provided by the manufacturer with the material). The plane of injection and degree of correction are critical to achieve complete, smooth, and long-lasting correction of the defect.

Basic Technique

Whenever a dermal filler is being injected, regardless of the material being used, the level of injection, or the defect being corrected, the *key technical concept is to inject smoothly*. One should consider the material flowing through the needle, but the syringe–needle unit should be looked on as a continuation of the injector's hand and arm. The action should be smooth, like laying down icing on a cake. Once movement begins, do not stop until the end point is reached.

Plane of Injection

Collagen should be injected into the superficial dermis with some overcorrection. *All hyaluronic acid products* should be injected into the dermis with just slight undercorrection because water will come into the area immediately and continue to do so over time, enhancing the correction. All *biphasic* (e.g., Artefill and Radiesse) and *robust* (e.g., Sculptra) *fillers* must be placed at the dermal–subcutaneous junction with no overcorrection and care taken to avoid placing any material in the dermis.

When injecting biphasic materials, a fanlike scaffold, also known as the *fern technique*, should be formed under the defect to hold up the defect (see the earlier discussion in the section on Noncollagen, Non–Hyaluronic Acid Products). This is performed by entering the subcutaneous space (as soon as resistance gives, one has entered that space) and injecting in the same plane but at varying angles, and not exiting through the dermis before discontinuing the injection so that no material is deposited into the dermis, thus avoiding a possible granulomatous response.

Common Errors in Soft Tissue Augmentation

- Overcorrecting in areas of fine lines (e.g., periorbital and perioral)
- Injecting biphasic fillers into the dermis
- Injecting too robust a filler into the glabellar complex
- Not providing sufficient anesthesia to make the patient comfortable
- Not following up with a second patient visit
- Not taking before and after photographs
- Not obtaining informed consent
- Not taking a complete medical history before injection
- Using a permanent filler of any type
- Not asking patients which type of filler they had injected by a former physician

Complications

- *Bruising:* Some degree of bruising is the most common complication. It can be eliminated or decreased with the application of ice and topical vitamin K before and after the injection session. (See the earlier discussion of relative contraindications.)
- *Erythema:* This is common after injection of any material and is easily addressed with topical vitamin K and ice.
- *Edema:* This is not unusual and is particularly common with hyaluronic acid products; it is temporary and of no consequence.
- *Infection:* Although infection is theoretically possible with dermal fillers, I have never seen this occur in over 25 years of practice.
- *Skin necrosis:* This can occur anywhere on the face from injection of any material; however, the most common area of occurrence

is the glabellar complex owing to the paucity of collateral circulation in this area. The necrosis is not due to injection into a vessel but to the material crimping a vessel in this area, thus occluding the blood supply. If there is sudden blanching and the patient states the injection has become painful, stop immediately and apply nitroglycerin paste or dimethyl sulfoxide (DMSO) to increase the circulation in the area.
- *Uneven results:* The possibility of this occurrence is the primary reason to schedule a second injection session 2 weeks after the first. This is also one of the primary reasons to take pretreatment photographs on every patient; we are not symmetric to begin with, and some patients do not realize that.

Postprocedure Patient Care and Education

- Apply ice immediately after injection.
- Apply topical vitamin K twice daily for at least 5 days.
- No warfarin, aspirin, or vitamin E for 48 hours.
- No significant sun exposure for 48 hours.

Patient should be advised to do the following for overall skin health:

- Apply SPF 30 sunscreen every morning (A and B block).
- Apply retinoids each evening,
- Do not smoke.
- Avoid tanning beds completely.
- Return for another injection session in 2 weeks and then whenever desired in the future, but before all the correction has subsided.

Pearls

- Use the smallest-gauge needle through which the material can flow.
- Use ice before and during the injection session for more patient comfort.
- When injecting the lips, move slightly onto the lip (about 1 mm) to achieve longer-lasting correction.
- To avoid lumpy results, make sure your movements are smooth.
- Try using a 32- or 33-gauge needle for fine lines.
- Change needles before the syringe is empty because the skin dulls needles.
- Always underestimate how long correction will last—in other words, underpromise and overdeliver.
- Do not attempt to learn technique except from an expert (one-on-one, if possible).
- Never talk patients into procedures they are not certain they really want.
- If you are not sure, then don't do it.

Additional Resources

See the treatment record form online at www.expertconsult.com.

Suppliers

(See contact information online at www.expertconsult.com.)

Providers of filler material and videos for injection technique

Allergan
BioForm Medical (Radiesse)
Medicis Aesthetics

VIDEOTAPES AND DVDS

Carruthers J, Carruthers A: Procedures in Cosmetic Dermatology Series: Soft Tissue Augmentation with DVD, 2nd ed. Philadelphia, Saunders, 2007.

Patient Education

Pfenninger JL, Fox PA: Collagen and Newer Tissue Fillers: A Patient's Introduction. 2009. Available at www.creativehealthcommunications.com.

Physician Instruction

Pfenninger JL, Fox PA: Working with Collagen and Newer Tissue Fillers: A Guide for Clinicians. 2009. Available at www.creativehealthcommunications.com.

BIBLIOGRAPHY

Ahn MS: Calcium hydroxylapatite: Radiesse. Facial Plast Surg Clin North Am 15:85–90, 2007.

Busso M, Applebaum D: Hand augmentation with Radiesse (calcium hydroxylapatite). Dermatol Ther 20:385–387, 2007.

Busso M, Voigts R: An investigation of changes in physical properties of injectable calcium hydroxylapatite in a carrier gel when mixed with lidocaine and with lidocaine/epinephrine. Dermatol Surg 34(Suppl 1):S16–S23, 2008.

Duranti F, Salti G, Bovani B, et al: Injectable hyaluronic acid gel for soft tissue augmentation: A clinical and histologic study. Dermatol Surg 24:1317–1325, 1998.

Elson ML: Soft tissue augmentation. In Elson ML (ed): Evaluation and Treatment of the Aging Face. New York, Springer-Verlag, 1986, pp 79–96.

Elson ML: The role of skin testing in the use of collagen injectable materials. J Dermatol Surg Oncol 15:301–303, 1989.

Lowe N, Maxwell CA, Lowe P, et al: Hyaluronic acid skin fillers: Adverse reactions and skin testing. J Am Acad Dermatol 45:930–933, 2001.

Sengelmann RD, Tull S, Pollack SV: Soft-tissue augmentation. In Robinson JK, Hanke CW, Sengelmann RD, Siegel DM (eds): Surgery of the Skin: Procedural Dermatology. Philadelphia, Mosby, 2005, pp 437–462.

Serra M: Facial implants with polymethylmethacrylate for lipodystrophy correction: 30 months follow-up. Antiviral Ther 6(Suppl 4):75, 2001.

Sherman RN: Sculptra: The new three-dimensional filler. Clin Plast Surg 33:539–550, 2006.

Small R: Dermal fillers. In Usatine RP, Pfenninger JL, Stulberg DL, Small R (eds): Dermatologic and Cosmetic Procedures in Office Practice. Philadelphia, Saunders (in press).

Werschler WP: Treating the aging face: A multidisciplinary approach with calcium hydroxylapatite and other fillers. Cosmet Dermatol 20:739–742, 2007.

CHAPTER 58

Microdermabrasion and Dermalinfusion

Basil M. Hantash • Sandy T. Liu

Microdermabrasion: Background

The concept of smoothing the skin by removing or abrading the upper layers can be dated as far back as 1500 BC, when Egyptian physicians used a type of "sandpaper" to treat scars. Modern dermabrasion was developed in Germany in the early 1900s by Kromayer, who used human-powered rotating wheels and rasps as a means of removing the epidermis and superficial portions of the dermis. This new technology was mainly used to treat scars, hyperpigmentation, and keratoses; however, acceptance was not forthcoming. It was not until Kurtin, Burks, and others began using motorized wire brushes in the early to mid-1950s that the power of the technology began to be realized. In spite of the great benefits possible with dermabrasion, there are many potential negatives: need for anesthesia, scarring, prolonged downtime, wound care, infection, and contaminated operative field with aerosolized particles that endanger the practitioner and staff. Many of these problems are also encountered with other techniques, such as laser resurfacing and deep chemical peels. These factors, as well as economic considerations, have pushed for development of a new technology that is less debilitating, safer, and more affordable: microdermabrasion (MDA).

MDA was developed in Italy in 1985 and introduced to the American market during the mid-1990s. MDA has spread at an explosive rate. According to data from the American Society for Aesthetic Plastic Surgery, an estimated 557,131 MDA procedures were performed in the United States in 2008. The aim of this chapter is to help the reader better understand MDA's mechanism of action, clinical indications, contraindications, patient selection and initial evaluation criteria, procedure methods, and complications encountered following treatment.

Mechanism of Action

The most superficial layer of the skin is the *stratum corneum*, which is a lifeless accumulation of protein and lipid material derived from flattened, dead keratinocytes that forms a barrier to protect the skin from a myriad of invasive insults. From the time a keratinocyte is formed in younger skin, it takes approximately 28 days to mature, die, and flake off the skin surface as dander. As humans age, keratinocyte transit times dramatically increase, trapping pigment and debris in the superficial epidermal layers to give the characteristic stained appearance of aging or solar (actinic) damage. Another skin cell of major importance is the dermal fibroblast, which lies within the dermis and synthesizes extracellular matrix (ECM) components, including proteoglycans (e.g., dermatan sulfate), glycosaminoglycans (e.g., hyaluronic acid), collagen, and elastin. This function decreases with aging and actinic damage. The process of MDA addresses both the stained, debris-laden epidermis and the sluggish fibroblast production of ECM, especially collagen.

Epidermal Effects of Microdermabrasion

The micrographs in Figure 58-1 exhibit the immediate sequential thinning and smoothing of epidermal structures as a result of the abrasive effect of the aluminum oxide crystals moving rapidly across the skin surface. The gentle planing of the upper layers of the skin removes pigmentary impurities and debris held within the stratum corneum and yields a smoother, softer skin surface. Each pass of the MDA handpiece is estimated to ablate approximately 15 μm of skin, roughly equal to one pass of the erbium laser. In addition to the immediate smoothing of the skin, the abrasive process seems to stimulate keratinocyte turnover over the long-term. Larson and Shehadi and colleagues have shown increases in epidermal thickness in porcine skin by 9% with MDA.

Dermal Effects of Microdermabrasion

Most MDA machines are quite simple in principle, having a crystal reservoir that supplies abrasive crystals through a flexible tube to a handpiece that is moved across the skin by the operator. The skin is "tented up" by the negative pressure generated in the machine, and abrasive crystals, usually aluminum oxide (corundum), are simultaneously blown and "sucked" across the skin to remove the upper layers of the epidermis. This can be compared with a fine "sandblasting" technique. Other types of particulate materials are occasionally used for the abrasion process, such as sodium chloride crystals, sodium bicarbonate (baking soda), and magnesium oxide crystals. However, aluminum oxide seems ideal because it is widely available, inert, very hard, has multiple sharp edges, does not readily absorb liquid, and is nontoxic even if inadvertently inhaled. Used crystals and cutaneous debris are removed through suction and collected in a separate waste container, thus creating a closed-loop system that avoids the airborne contaminants of open dermabrasion. The handpieces usually can be fitted with reusable metal tips or disposable plastic tips. The metal tips must be sterilized before use with different patients.

Treatments are superficial enough that they do not cause bleeding or "serum ooze." Some patients with very sensitive skin may experience slight discomfort, but treatments are certainly not painful and are generally well tolerated. No topical anesthetics are needed. After each pass, the bulk of crystals should be removed before continuing. The *second pass* should be at right angles, or perpendicular, to the direction of the first pass. An optional *third pass* is performed with a swirling or circular motion, making sure that the skin is taut and the handpiece tip is moving and not stationary over a single skin point. Skilled operators also pay close attention to the direction of lymphatic flow, especially in areas such as the face, in order not to obstruct drainage and prevent unnecessary edema.

Skin changes are cumulative and treatment sessions are recommended at 7- to 14-day intervals. Depending on the type and

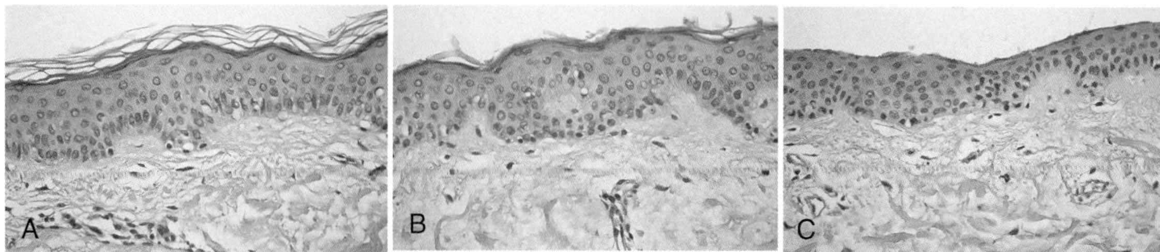

Figure 58-1 **A,** Pretreatment photomicrograph of human skin of the upper back showing fully intact stratum corneum and stratum granulosum. **B,** Upper back skin on same patient after two passes. Note that the stratum corneum has been markedly ablated. **C,** Upper back skin after four passes, same region of the back as (**A**) and (**B**), but separated by 20 minutes, exhibiting total removal of the stratum corneum and most of the stratum granulosum. (Courtesy of Rick Wilson, MD, Dallas, Tex.)

severity of the skin problem(s), usually between 4 and 15 treatments are offered on an as-needed basis between 1 and 4 months. The patient is usually able to return to most normal activities immediately, unless the skin is extremely sensitive. Mild erythema may be observed, and usually resolves within 12 to 24 hours after treatment.

The operator has great flexibility in treating patients and improving outcomes by varying the depth of penetration to match each patient's unique circumstances and requirements. This is accomplished by controlling the following four factors:

1. Density of crystal flow
2. Number of passes completed by the operator
3. Vacuum pressure
4. Handpiece speed over the skin surface

In rare instances (e.g., acne scarring), high vacuum settings (≥20 mm Hg) may be required. The operator should expect variability in vacuum settings and crystal flow with different machines.

Indications

Clinical indications for MDA include the following skin conditions:

- Minor acne scarring
- Postoperative/traumatic scarring
- Fine lines and wrinkles
- Superficial pigmentation such as lentigines and ephelides
- Melasma and other disorders of pigmentation
- Postinflammatory hyperpigmentation (PIH) due to acne or eczema, among other causes
- Blending postlaser hyperpigmentation
- Skin texture irregularities
- Actinic keratoses
- Enlarged pores
- Clogged pores and blackheads
- Whiteheads
- Some mild forms of acne
- Keratosis pilaris
- Rosacea (using dermalinfusion; see later discussion)
- Striae distensae

Patients with stage I, II, or III *acne* have done well when MDA is combined with topical retinoid therapy (Fig. 58-2). In this instance, MDA's action on the stratum corneum allows for better absorption of topical medications. Although MDA does not entirely eliminate stretch marks, it can be an effective treatment option when combined with topical therapies. In a study by Abdel-Latif and Elbendary (2008), better results were seen when treating striae rubra than for striae alba, suggesting that treatment may be limited to more recent-onset stretch marks. Moreover, molecular studies showed that type I collagen expression was upregulated in the skin of patients with striae post-MDA treatment. This provides a biologic mechanism for the clinical benefits of MDA treatment in patients with striae rubra. More recently, cosmeceutical agents such as vitamin C have been proposed as therapies for striae. In addition, work by Lee and colleagues (2003) demonstrated that treatment of ex vivo skin with MDA can significantly increase the uptake of vitamin C. It will be interesting to see whether the combination of MDA and topical vitamin C results in improved clinical outcomes for striae treatment.

Dermalinfusion

Background

Dermalinfusion is an innovative procedure that uses MDA technology to increase delivery of active ingredients to treat specific skin conditions such as hyperpigmentation, telangiectasia, papulopustular acne, eczema, photodamage, dehydration, rosacea, and fine lines. It is unique in that it uses a closed-loop vacuum system with a recessed diamond tip rather than microcrystals to exfoliate the skin while simultaneously infusing the topical dermaceutical into the deeper dermal layers. The size, coarseness of the diamond tip, vacuum, and flow rates can all be adjusted depending on the patient's treatment. A major advantage of dermalinfusion is minimal posttreatment erythema and decreased risk of PIH compared with the harsh and abrasive standard MDA treatments. Furthermore, dermalinfusion is ideal for treatment of the lips, papulopustular acne, as well as rosacea, which are all relatively contraindicated with crystal-based MDA. The optimal treatment regimen involves four to six treatments every 1 to 2 weeks and monthly treatments thereafter.

In an unpublished histologic study conducted by Moy (www.plasticsurgerypractice.com/issues/articles/2007-01_06.asp), patients were pretreated with dermalinfusion in the preauricular area 1 to 3 days before undergoing an elective facelift. During the procedure, the marked dermalinfusion-treated area was removed, fixed with formalin, processed, and then analyzed. The author found that the dermalinfusion treatment created a smooth and uniform abraded

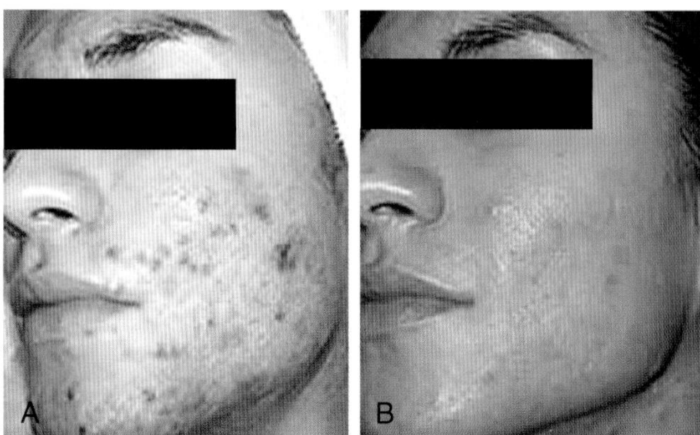

Figure 58-2 **A,** Patient with stage II acne on chronic daily topical retinoids. **B,** Same patient after six SilkPeel treatments combined with dermalinfusion of an antiacne solution.

surface confined to the granular layer approximately 30 to 35 μm deep. The epidermal layer, and the keratinosomes in it that help create the hydrophobic barrier, remained intact after treatment. Moreover, addition of a hydrating serum to the abrasive surface showed vacuolization of keratinocytes, displacement of the nucleus, and edema around collagen fibers near the upper papillary dermis. Furthermore, epidermal thickness was increased by 70% after dermalinfusion, consistent with effective absorption and penetration into the papillary dermis. These findings are consistent with rapid hydration of the underlying dermis and help explain the mechanism for the observed clinical improvement in fine wrinkles after MDA plus dermalinfusion treatment.

Rosacea Treatment

Current treatments of rosacea include avoiding triggers such as sunlight exposure, administration of topical and oral antibiotics, and use of laser and light therapies. Treatment usually lasts 3 to 6 months and is associated with side effects such as skin irritation and dryness, erythema, bruising, and photosensitivity. Moreover, MDA is not recommended for patients with rosacea because it can further aggravate the skin, causing angiogenesis, inflammation, and reactive oxygen species. Dermalinfusion, however, will not exacerbate the deeper epidermal layers and can be considered an alternative monotherapy for patients with rosacea. In a recent study by Desai and colleagues (2006), 30 patients with erythematotelangiectatic or papulopustular rosacea underwent MDA plus dermalinfusion treatment twice a month for a total of 12 weeks. The authors chose to use 2% erythromycin and 2% salicylic acid as their infusion solution to decrease inflammation and induce exfoliation, respectively. Twenty patients completed the entire study: 6 patients with erythematotelangiectatic rosacea and 14 patients with papulopustular rosacea. There was a statistically significant reduction in erythema, papules, and pustules in all patients by the 12th week, with a reduction noted as early as week 4. The authors reported a 42% improvement in erythema in the erythematotelangiectatic group and a 69% decrease in papules and 55% decrease in pustules in the papulopustular group. In addition, photographs taken throughout the study documented an overall improvement in the patients' condition, and there was positive patient feedback regarding tolerability, satisfaction, and overall quality of life. The adverse event most commonly reported by the study participants was transient erythema, which resolved in 3 to 6 hours.

Tattoo Treatment

An interesting case report by Wray and colleagues (2005) documents the first successful treatment of traumatic tattoo with SilkPeel (Envy Medical, Inc., Westlake Village, Calif) MDA treatment during isotretinoin (Accutane) therapy. The adolescent male patient had suffered a traumatic tattoo around the upper and lower eyelids after an explosive accident. The first treatment was performed 48 hours after the accident, with two other treatments on days 3 and 12 postaccident. In addition, comedonal extractors and Vigilon were used as adjunctive therapy for greater efficacy. After the first treatment, more than half of the tattoo marks disappeared, with further improvement reported with each ensuing treatment. The patient was extremely satisfied with the cosmetic outcome, and no complications were reported.

Hyperpigmentation Treatment

More recently, Envy Medical (formerly Emed, Inc.), the manufacturer of the SilkPeel MDA system, has introduced a novel approach for the treatment of hyperpigmentation that involves four MDA treatments spaced 1 week apart, in combination with infusion of a novel skin-lightening solution (Lumixyl) developed by the same company. Although results are preliminary, this new approach represents a potential breakthrough in the treatment of hyperpigmentation because the skin-lightening formulation does not include the more toxic hydroquinone and can thus be used safely in women of child-bearing age, even if pregnant or breast-feeding. In addition, results from the pilot study indicate that no skin irritation or skin thinning would be expected from this treatment because the formulation does not include retinoids or corticosteroids, respectively. Figure 58-3 shows the results for an Asian patient with Fitzpatrick type IV skin before and after four weekly treatments using this approach.

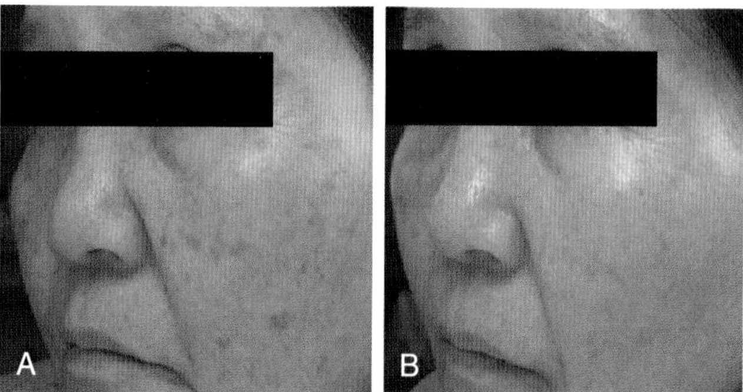

Figure 58-3 **A,** Baseline appearance of patient with Fitzpatrick phototype IV skin and melasma. **B,** Same patient after four SilkPeel treatments combined with dermalinfusion of Lumixyl, a novel skin-lightening formulation that does not contain retinoids or corticosteroids.

Other Dermalinfusion Systems

HydraFacial, manufactured by Edge Systems (Signal Hill, Calif), is another dermalinfusion unit currently used by dermatologists and aestheticians. Similar to SilkPeel, the HydraFacial device simultaneously resurfaces the stratum corneum and delivers active serum into the treated tissue. The exfoliation is achieved with a patented crystal-free tip, patented disposable HydroPeel tip, or a Spa Aggression tip. Various skin-specific solutions such as glucosamine, lactic acid, salicylic acid, and antioxidants (vitamins A and E and white tea extract) are used for infusion. The Tissue Nutrient Solution (TNS) serum developed by SkinMedica (Carlsbad, Calif) is exclusively designed for the HydraFacial system. The serum consists of NouriCel-MD, a patented formulation of human growth factors, cytokines, soluble collagen, antioxidants, and matrix proteins that enables greater skin rejuvenation.

In a study by Freedman (2008), two study groups were randomized to either a series of hydradermabrasion treatments with antioxidant dermalinfusion or treatments with the same antioxidant applied manually. Histologic and clinical assessments showed improvement in skin quality in the hydradermabrasion group. The treated skin showed in a statistically significant increase in antioxidant levels and an increase in epidermal and papillary dermal thickness, collagen hyalinization, and fibroblast density. There was also a decrease in wrinkles, pore size, and hyperpigmentation after hydradermabrasion treatment. The skin with manually applied antioxidant, however, showed no detectable change in structure or antioxidant levels. MDA with antioxidants as an infusion agent may be a reasonable treatment option for those patients who wish to prevent or stop the signs of aging.

In another study by Freedman (2009), 10 patients were treated in split-face fashion with either MDA with infusion of an antioxidant serum or MDA alone. Patients underwent a total of six treatments, each 1 week apart. Histologic assessment of post-treatment biopsy samples revealed that patients treated with MDA plus antioxidants had a marked increase in epidermal and papillary dermal thickness, as well as an increase in fibroblast density and deposition of collagen. Digital photography indicated that skin quality improved more with the combined treatment than MDA alone. Raman spectroscopy was used to measure skin polyphenolic levels. The dermalinfusion-treated skin was found to have a 32% increase in antioxidant levels. Unfortunately, the author did not report the effect of MDA alone on polyphenolic levels, so it remains unclear whether the increase in antioxidant levels is attributable to topical infusion therapy, MDA, or a combination of the two. Further studies are required to clarify this issue.

Although a number of other MDA infusion systems have been commercially developed, only the HydraFacial and SilkPeel systems have appropriate patent protection. Therefore, no other systems are reviewed in this chapter.

Contraindications

SilkPeel has been safely used in patients with inflammatory disorders such as psoriasis or eczema without complication. This is due to its ability to abrade up to specific depths by altering the grit of the diamond used for abrasion. Other MDA systems have not been reported to share this safety advantage. Similarly, many practitioners are using MDA for the treatment of actinic keratoses. However, frank malignancy is a contraindication because of fear of spread of the lesion after treatment. It should be noted that this concern is theoretical and not based on any published reports.

Absolute contraindications to MDA include the following:

- Accutane use within the past 12 months (except SilkPeel)
- Presence of skin malignancy (excluding actinic keratoses; see earlier discussion)
- Presence of herpetic lesion(s)
- Presence of eczema or psoriasis (except SilkPeel)
- Presence of autoimmune disease

Relative contraindications to MDA include the following:

- Accutane use within the past 12 months (for SilkPeel only)
- Patients with thin skin
- Patients with compromised wound healing (e.g., smokers, diabetic patients)
- Patients with compromised immune systems
- Current use of anticoagulation therapy (excludes diamond-based MDA)

Patient Selection

Microdermabrasion is safe and effective; however, proper patient selection is essential. Poor patient selection will cause patient dissatisfaction, staff frustration, and ultimate failure of the MDA program in any given practice.

MDA is an excellent modality for all skin types, even those patients with Fitzpatrick skin types V and VI (see Chapter 46, Introduction to Aesthetic Medicine). These patients are especially vulnerable to hyperpigmentation or hypopigmentation when more aggressive skin resurfacing treatments are administered. MDA is safe in these patients because the depth of penetration is usually limited to the superficial epidermis. Elderly patients with thin skin are not good candidates for MDA unless pretreated with other modalities to improve skin quality. Pregnant women should not undergo MDA because of hormonal changes that cause increased skin sensitivity, delayed wound healing, and increased melanocyte melanin production. Consequently, the risk of PIH and scarring can be significant during pregnancy, and any procedure should be avoided until after delivery. Patients on anticoagulant therapy are also not good candidates for crystal-based MDA and should be treated with caution because it can be difficult for the practitioner to adequately control the abrasion depth, potentially injuring blood vessels in the papillary dermis and causing excessive bleeding.

It is recommended that patients who have had a recent chemical peel or other skin procedure such as collagen injections, waxing, tanning, or sun exposure wait at least 2 weeks before undergoing MDA.

Initial Evaluation

Every patient must be seen and evaluated by the physician before initiation of a treatment protocol. Unfortunately, some offices turn the MDA practice over to an aesthetician and the process runs independent of physician input. This situation is more appropriate for a beauty salon. A physician has the responsibility of seeing and evaluating every patient who is treated in his or her practice. Anything less than this compromises patient care.

After filling out the usual history form, with special attention to current medications, the physician should evaluate the patient with particular attention to the following:

- Fitzpatrick skin typing (see Chapter 48, Lasers and Pulsed-Light Devices: Hair Removal)
- Skin thickness
- Skin tone
- Site-specific rhytids
- Depth and severity of rhytids
- Dryness
- Acne
- Acne scarring
- Other scarring
- Vascular anomalies
- Telangiectases
- Ecchymosis
- Nevi
- Pigmentation problems
- Skin malignancies
- General actinic damage
- Actinic keratoses
- Current tanning status
- Poikiloderma
- Open sores
- Herpetic lesions

Once these and other individual factors are considered, a treatment protocol can be determined for the patient. Instructions should be written or checked off on a patient encounter form and communication with the MDA technician concerning the patient's treatments completed (Fig. 58-4; also see Chapter 46, Introduction to Aesthetic Medicine, Fig. 46-1).

Pretreatment and post-treatment photographs are recommended and are a part of the patient's permanent record. They will also facilitate assessment of clinical outcomes. However, do not expect miracles with every patient. It may be extremely difficult to photographically document improvement in patients whose initial skin quality is good and who just wanted "freshening." Certainly, those patients with major pigment problems, acne scarring, and other extreme conditions yield documentable photographic improvement. More recent advances in digital photographic systems will provide improved sensitivity, allowing detection of less dramatic improvements in patients with reasonable baseline skin quality.

Complications

Complications can result from any type of treatment, regardless of how innocuous the technology may seem. Certainly, MDA is no different. However, the very factor that has contributed to MDA's widespread success is that it has very few, if any, long-term complications. The physician and staff should receive bona fide training before embarking on patient treatments and know the potential complications and treatment options to provide a good outcome.

Erythema is the most common side effect of MDA, and its severity has a nearly linear relationship with the aggressiveness of the treatment. Some patients (e.g., those suffering from dermatographism, rosacea, or certain types of urticaria) have very sensitive skin and will exhibit some erythema no matter how mild the treatment settings. Most erythema resolves spontaneously within a few hours.

Chemical Peel/Microdermabrasion
New Patient Consultation Checklist

Name: ______________________________ Date: __________

Analyze the Skin:
_____ Visually
_____ Patient Profile Form
_____ Consent Form signed (copy to patient)
_____ Fee Schedule Form signed (copy to patient)
_____ Photos taken

Initial Photographs:

Discuss Peel Treatments with Patient:
_____ Expectations
_____ Possible Reactions and Side Effects
_____ Sunblock Use

Home Care Program:
_____ Sample Kit
_____ Instructions
_____ Home Care Regimen
_____ Post Peel Tip Sheet

Peel Appointment:
_____ Preparation for Peel Treatment
_____ Date of First Treatment

Figure 58-4 Sample form: Chemical peel/microdermabrasion new patient consultation checklist. (Courtesy John L. Pfenninger, MD/The Medical Procedures Center, Midland, Mich. Adapted from various sources.)

Inform the patient to avoid sun or tanning bed exposure during the time of his or her treatment sessions because this will surely increase skin irritation. All patients must use daily sunscreen (preferably SPF 30 or greater) to protect their skin.

Most patients experience mild tingling, which is very tolerable. However, a few patients complain of burning and skin discomfort for up to 24 hours after the peel. These patients can be treated effectively with moisturizers.

Purpura, ecchymosis, and petechial hemorrhages are all a function of overly aggressive vacuum settings. They are more common with crystal-based MDA treatments and relatively uncommon with diamond-based ones. Also, poor patient selection, such as treating patients with thin skin or those on anticoagulants (gingko, vitamin E, aspirin, and nonsteroidal anti-inflammatory drugs, among others), can lead to these side effects. Apply ice to the area when first noticed and decrease the vacuum setting to minimize the problem. If one of these complications should occur, do not return to the affected area for peeling at that same treatment session. Skin should return to normal appearance in most patients younger than 50 years of age within 10 to 14 days. It may take longer to resolve these problems in older patients.

Scarring is rare with MDA, but can occur in the following unusual situations:

- Patient circumstance demands aggressive therapy (e.g., treatment of mild to moderate acne scarring on the cheeks, which requires deep planing).
- Aggressive treatments administered to patients currently using Accutane or patients who have been on Accutane within 1 year of initiating MDA.
- Mild skin abrasion in patients who are noncompliant, have compromised immune function and subsequent wound contamination, or have active infection.
- Being too aggressive or allowing the handpiece to stop or dwell on specific skin areas for too long.

Minor skin abrasions can easily occur. Simply having the patient clean these areas and apply petroleum jelly or antibiotic ointment until reepithelialization has occurred should alleviate the situation.

Ocular damage is a potential complication. Protection of the eyes for both the patient and practitioner is absolutely essential. Tsai and associates (1995) discussed development of ocular pain, photophobia, epiphora, and conjunctival congestion with crystal adherence to the cornea and punctate keratopathy resulting from ophthalmologic crystal contamination during MDA. Ocular contamination can be prevented by placing moist, folded 4 × 4 gauze pads over the eyes and holding them in place with suntanning goggles. Alternatively, special eye shields (see next section) can be used alone. After treatment, the technician must meticulously remove crystals from the periorbital region before allowing the patient to get off the treatment table and wash.

Equipment

- MDA unit with tips (sterile, reusable metal; plastic disposable; Fig. 58-5)
- Power examination table and adjustable stool for the technician
- Alcohol wipes
- Crystals (usually aluminum oxide); approximately one-half of a cup (30 to 35 mL) for the face and more for larger areas
- Nonsterile gloves
- Moist 4 × 4 gauzes
- Surgical cap for patient
- Suntanning goggles for patient (alternatively, Derm-Aid Non-Laser Disposable Eye Shields [GPT Glendale, Inc., Lakeland, Fla] work very well)
- Saline eye wash
- Towel or gown to drape around patient's neck
- Protective glasses with shields for operator
- Mask for operator (to reduce inhalation)
- Postoperative moisturizer (e.g., Theraplex, aloe, Kinerase) and sunscreen (with zinc or titanium)
- Flow sheet to record settings and progress
- Digital camera with macro feature for close-up pictures *(ideal but optional)*
- Solutions to be used for dermalinfusion (contact manufacturers)
- Cleaning solutions (contact manufacturers)

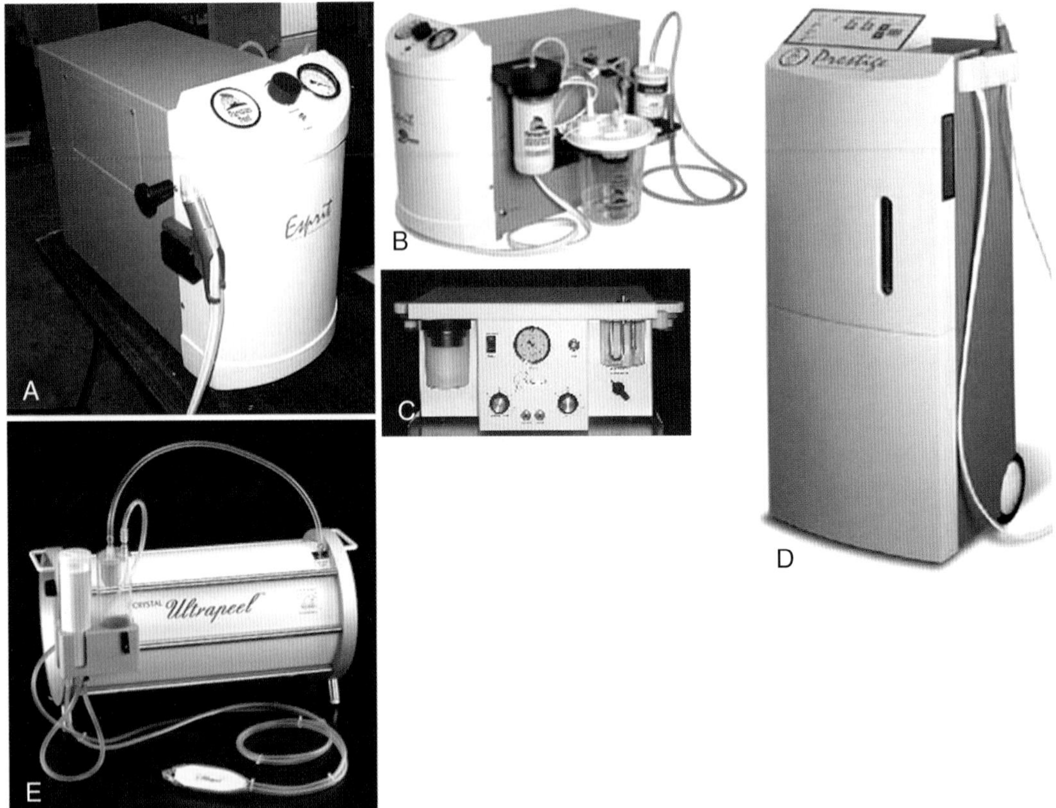

Figure 58-5 **A,** Parisian Peel Esprit. **B,** Inside view of Parisian Peel unit showing the crystal container and collection system. **C,** BellaMed microdermabrasion machine. **D,** Prestige microdermabrasion machine. **E,** Ultrapeel Crystal. (**A, B,** and **D,** Courtesy of Aesthetic Technologies, Broomfield, Colo. **C,** Courtesy of Bella Products, Foothill Ranch, Calif. **E,** Courtesy of Saratoga Diagnostics, Saratoga, Calif.)

Crystals vary widely in quality and cost. Cheaper materials contain variable-sized particles and may not be pure. Fine, powdery substances are not only less effective but aerosolize when the containers are emptied. Not only do these substances cause a sediment in the room, they may be irritating to the patient or clinician. The lower limit of particle size should be 20 μm. Crystals should also be prepared in a "medically clean" way to avoid any type of contamination.

The apertures that the crystals traverse eventually wear larger from the crystal passage. Check to see if the tip needs repair/replacement before each treatment by observing the crystal flow. A wider crystal flow that lacks uniformity indicates the need for tip replacement.

Handpiece tips must be replaced or sterilized (cold or hot) for each patient. Angled handpieces are somewhat more comfortable for the operator to use.

Preprocedure Patient Preparation

- Have the patient wash his or her face to remove all makeup and lotions.
- The patient must wear eye protection and a surgical cap to keep crystals from getting into the eyes and hair. Should crystals get into the eye, they can be very irritating and must be washed out with saline.
- The patient is placed in the supine position on the treatment table. The technician is seated at the head with clear three-sided access to the patient.
- Place a towel or gown around the patient's neck to keep crystals from getting on the patient's clothing.
- Cleanse the patient's face with isopropyl alcohol or acetone to remove any lingering skin oils, makeup, and lotions.
- Examine the skin in the areas to be treated. Open sores should be avoided. Also, be attentive for any type of herpetic outbreak. If the patient does exhibit a herpetic lesion, cancel the treatment for at least 2 weeks and make sure the patient is treated with the appropriate antiviral medication (e.g., Valtrex, Zovirax). Prophylaxis for patients with frequent herpetic outbreaks may be required; however, it should be individualized to each patient's circumstance.

Technique

See specific manufacturers' guidelines for each particular unit.

1. Select the appropriate grit and size of the diamond-tip treatment head. The heads vary in coarseness from smooth (no diamond chips) to fine (120 grit) and coarse (30 grit). The 6-mm head is recommended for the face and the 9-mm head for larger areas such as the arms and legs. The usual power setting for initial treatment starts at 12 to 14 mm Hg and works up to 18 to 20 mm Hg for most patients (those with special problems such as acne scarring may require 20 to 35 mm Hg). *Tip:* The practitioner can make a good estimate of the correct suction level by applying the handpiece to a colored page from a magazine for 3 to 4 seconds. If all color is removed, the power is too high. If most is removed, it is just right. If most color is left, it is too low.
2. With a nonsterile, gloved hand, spread the skin between the thumb and index or middle finger with a moderate amount of tension. Place the MDA treatment head on the skin and move the handpiece parallel to the direction of tension between the two fingers (Fig. 58-6A). Keep the handpiece head moving, and definitely avoid stopping and holding it in contact with one area

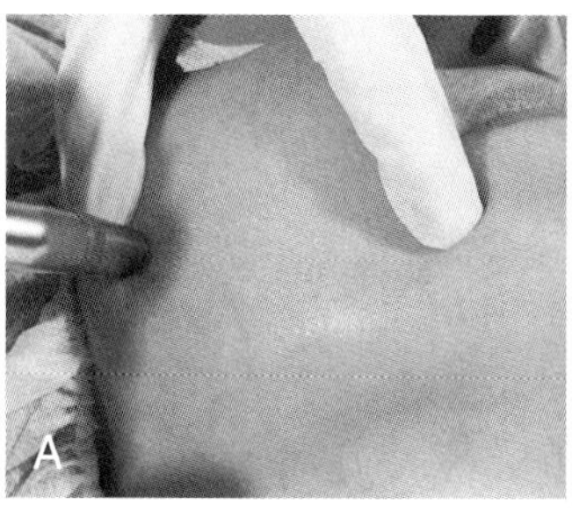
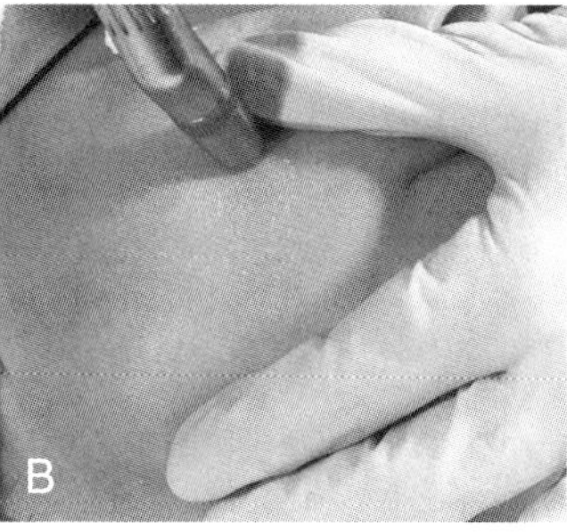

Figure 58-6 **A,** First microdermabrasion pass on the patient's right cheek. The technician's fingers are tensing the skin in a horizontal direction while using parallel movements of the handpiece. **B,** A second pass on the right cheek with the skin tensed in a more vertical orientation, perpendicular to the direction of the first pass in (**A**). Note crystal residue on skin.

of the skin; this could cause deep penetration and seriously damage the skin and cause scarring. Hold the handpiece perpendicular (90 degrees) to the skin.

3. For the first pass, strokes should be from the central face to the periphery. After completing a small area of skin with parallel strokes, move the handpiece for a *second pass* perpendicular to the direction of movement of the first pass (Fig. 58-6B). This crosshatches the area and decreases any streaking or linear erythematous markings. It is recommended to start at the forehead, proceed down the bridge of the nose, and cover the cheeks, chin, and around the mouth.
4. If a third pass is to be made, use a circular or swirling motion. When initiating MDA with a new patient, it may be prudent to see how two passes are tolerated and their effects before making a third.
5. After two or more passes, some patients exhibit a darkened or grayish hue to the skin because of the crystal interaction with skin oils. This is no cause for alarm because it will be removed completely with post-treatment cleansing. (For treatment of the neck, only one pass with vertical strokes is sufficient. For treatment of the chest, use two passes with strokes from the midline to the periphery. For treatment of the hands, have the patient make a fist around a towel and perform two passes with strokes parallel and then perpendicular to the axis of the forearm.)
6. When the treatment is completed, the technician should remove the crystals from the face while the patient is still in the supine position, taking great care to remove all crystal remnants from the periorbital region by suction or gentle removal with a moist cloth.
7. Have the patient cleanse with mild soap and water.
8. A light moisturizer, such as aloe, Theraplex, or Kinerase, will decrease any mild irritation. Also apply sunscreen with SPF 30 or greater (containing zinc or titanium).

After a treatment, it is important to leave the crystal container heater on whenever the machine is not in use to prevent moisturization of the crystals, which would result in poor crystal flow and possible malfunction.

Postprocedure Patient Education

Instruct the patient to avoid applying makeup, if possible, for the next 12 to 18 hours and to avoid significant sun exposure for 3 to 4 days after each treatment. The patient must wear sunblock whenever going outdoors and avoid applying irritant products such as retinoids, astringents, alpha-hydroxy acids, and depilatories for 1 week. See the sample patient education form online at www.expertconsult.com.

Purchasing a Microdermabrasion System

Before purchasing an MDA machine, consider several factors:

- Do you currently have access to a patient base that is appropriate for the use of this technology?
- Can ancillary treatments or therapies be offered to enhance the patient's results and to generate additional income (e.g., skin care products)?
- Do you have the personnel to support these new activities?
- Do you have the office space to dedicate to the MDA unit and a practitioner for the procedure?
- Make sure the local region is not saturated with MDA units. Is there a realistic market potential?
- Evaluate machine functions such as crystal flow, vacuum capacity, and the operator's ability to vary treatment parameters. Machine flexibility is important in treating a variety of skin types, conditions, and problems.
- Evaluate the propensity of the machine to clog, which may occur in a humid, moist environment. Most machines have a crystal heater that maintains dry crystals. The heater is left on continually.
- In today's market, warranty coverage, technical support, and possible shared marketing arrangements have become increasingly important factors in determining purchase decisions.
- Along with designated staff, attend a course that covers the essentials of MDA. These courses are usually sponsored by the equipment manufacturer or physician experts in the field.

Patient Education Guides

See the sample patient education and consent forms online at www.expertconsult.com.

CPT/Billing Codes

15780 Dermabrasion,* total face (e.g., for acne scarring, fine wrinkling, rhytids, general keratosis)
15781 Dermabrasion,* segmental, face
15782 Dermabrasion,* regional, other than face
15783 Dermabrasion,* superficial, any site (e.g., tattoo removal)
15786[†] Abrasion, single lesion (e.g., keratosis, scar)
15787[†] Abrasion, each additional four lesions or less (list separately in addition to code for primary procedure)

ICD-9-CM Diagnostic Codes

695.3 Rosacea
701.8 Wrinkling of skin; rhytides facialis
702.0 Actinic keratosis
706.1 Acne vulgaris
709.0 Dyschromia, unspecified
709.09 Melasma
709.2 Scarring

*No code is available for microdermabrasion as of publication of the 2009 CPT codes. "Dermabrasion" here refers to the traditional, deeper abrasion techniques.
[†]Service includes surgical procedures only.

ACKNOWLEDGMENT

The editors wish to recognize the many contributions by Dexter W. Blome, MD, to this chapter in the previous edition of this text.

SUPPLIERS

(See contact information online at www.expertconsult.com.)

A few examples of MDA machines are shown in Figure 58-5. The following is a list of suppliers:

Aurora/Gemini
Science Innovative Aesthetics
Beauty Skin
Vita Medical Technologies
BellaMed
Bella Products, Inc.
Bio-Brasion
Bio-Therapeutic
ClairDerm
Ageless Aesthetics
Delphia/HydraFacial
Edge Systems
DermaGenesis
Genesis Biosystems
Dermaglide Legacy KS/Microglide
Advanced Laser Centers
Derm-Aid Non-Laser Disposable Eye Shields
GPT Glendale, Inc.
DermaPod
Silhouet-Tone USA
DermaSweep
Cosmetic R & D
DermGlow
Aesthetic Solutions
Esprit Pro-xp
MedSurge Advances, Inc.
Facial H20
Syneron, Inc.
ImageDerm
ImageDerm
MegaPeel
DermaMed, Inc.
MicroGem
Refine USA, LLC
NaturaBrador
Focus Medical, LLC
NewAPeel/DiamondTome
Altair Instruments
Parisian Peel (Prestige, Esprit, Entrée)
Aesthetic Technologies, Inc.
PortaPeel/Setereh
Innovative Med, Inc.
Power Peel
Aesthetic Lasers
Pristine
Viora, Inc.
Salt-A-Peel
Med-Aesthetic Solutions
Sapphire 3 Abrasion
Raja Medical
SilkPeel
Envy Medical, Inc. (formerly Emed, Inc.)
SkinBella
Sybaritic
SmartPeel
SoundSkin Corp.
Synergie Peel
Synergie by Dynatronics
Ultrapeel
Mattioli Engineering
Vibraderm
Vibraderm, Inc.

BIBLIOGRAPHY

Abdel-Latif AM, Elbendary AS: Treatment of striae distensae with microdermabrasion: A clinical and molecular study. J Egypt Womens Dermatol Soc 5:24–30, 2008.

Abu Ubeid A, Wang Y, Zhao L, Hantash BM: Short-sequence oligopeptides with inhibitory activity against mushroom and human tyrosinase. J Invest Dermatol 129:2242–2249, 2009.

American Society for Aesthetic Plastic Surgery: 2008 Statistics on cosmetic surgery. Available at www.surgery.org/sites/default/files/2008stats.pdf.

Ash K, Lord J, Zukowski M, McDaniel DH: Comparison of topical therapy for striae alba (20% glycolic acid/0.05% tretinoin versus 20% glycolic acid/10% L-ascorbic acid). Dermatol Surg 24:849–856, 1998.

Coimbra M, Rohrich RJ, Chao J, Brown SA: A prospective controlled assessment of microdermabrasion for damaged skin and fine rhytides. Plast Reconstr Surg 113:1438–1443, 2004.

Desai TD, Moy LS, Kirby W, et al: Evaluation of the SilkPeel system in treating erythematotelangiectatic and papulopustular rosacea. Cosmet Dermatol 19:51–56, 2006.

Elsaie ML, Baumann LS, Elsaaiee LT: Striae distensae (stretch marks) and different modalities of therapy: An update. Dermatol Surg 35:563–573, 2009.

Fields KA: Skin breakthroughs in the year 2000. Int J Fertil Womens Med 45:175–181, 2000.

Freedman BM: Hydradermabrasion: An innovative modality for nonablative facial rejuvenation. J Cosmet Dermatol 7:275–280, 2008.

Freedman BM: Topical antioxidant application enhances the effects of facial microdermabrasion. J Dermatol Treat 20:82–87, 2009.

Freedman BM, Rueda-Pedraza E, Waddell SP: The epidermal and dermal changes associated with microdermabrasion. Dermatol Surg 27: 1031–1033, 2001.

Hernandez-Perez E, Ibiett EV: Gross and microscopic findings in patients undergoing microdermabrasion for facial rejuvenation. Dermatol Surg 27:637–640, 2001.

Lawrence N, Mandy S, Yarborough J, Alt T: History of dermabrasion. Dermatol Surg 26:95–101, 2000.

Lee WR, Shen SC, Kuo-Hsien W, et al: Lasers and microdermabrasion enhance and control topical delivery of vitamin C. J Invest Dermatol 121:1118–1125, 2003.

Mahuzier F: Microdermabrasion of stretch marks. In Mahuzier F (ed): Microdermabrasion or Parisian Peel in Practice. Marseille, France, Solal, 1999, pp 25–65.

Moy LS, Maley C: Skin management: A practical approach. Plast Surg Pract 2007, January. Available at www.plasticsurgerypractice.com/issues/articles/2007-01_06.asp.

Root LL: A Complete Guide to Microdermabrasion: Treatment, Techniques, and Technology 2001. Scottsdale, Ariz, Esthetic Education Resource, 2001.

Root LL: Microdermabrasion: Technique for the Medical Skin Care Clinic 2001. Scottsdale, Ariz, Esthetic Education Resource, 2001.

Shehadi IE, Larson DL, Archer SM, Zhang LL: Evaluation of histologic changes after micordermabrasion in a porcine model. Aesthet Surg J 24:136–141, 2004.

Shim E, Barnette D, Hughes K, Greenway H: Microdermabrasion: A clinical and histopathologic study. Dermatol Surg 27:524–530, 2001.

Tan MH, Spencer JM, Pires LM, et al: The evaluation of aluminum oxide crystal microdermabrasion for photodamage. Dermatol Surg 27:943–949, 2001.

Tsai RY, Wang CN, Chan HL: Aluminum oxide crystal microdermabrasion: A new technique for treating facial scarring. Dermatol Surg 21:539–542, 1995.

Wray A, Marshall D, Cleaver L: Effective treatment of traumatic tattoo with SilkPeel microdermabrasion during isotretinoin treatment, 2005. Available at www.medisysweb.com/pdfs/TraumaticTattoo.pdf.

CHAPTER 59

SKIN PEELS

Cathy Uecker

With the tremendous increase of older Americans as the "baby boomer" population ages, more and more patients are seeking treatments for photodamage and other conditions commonly seen with aging skin, such as uneven color, tone, and texture. In fact, skin rejuvenation has become one of the most common reasons for patients to consult a plastic surgeon, dermatologist, or clinical skin care provider. Oral isotretinoin (Accutane) prevents much of the deep scarring once seen from acne. However, patients routinely request treatment for minor scarring and postinflammatory hyperpigmentation, usually the result of previous acne lesions. Chemical peels and topical medications continue to be reliable methods used to rejuvenate skin damaged by all of these conditions.

Superficial peels are very common and are deemed so safe that nonclinicians now perform them in health spas and salons. However, many patients would prefer to have even superficial peels performed under the trusted supervision of their primary care clinician if the procedure were made available to them.

Although skin aging is both intrinsic (Table 59-1) and extrinsic (Table 59-2), the majority of damage is from extrinsic causes. *Intrinsically*, chronic use of the muscles of expression and dermal thinning with the loss of collagen fibers due to aging produce wrinkles and skin lines. Most intrinsic aging, such as that associated with hormonal changes, is the result of both chronologic and genetic causes. *Extrinsic aging* is caused by environmental hazards, such as ultraviolet radiation, wind, smoking, and chemical exposure. Years of exposure from the sun and tanning booths can produce wrinkles and pigmentary or surface changes. The stratum corneum thickens and the granulosum and spinosum layers become thinner. Atypical cells develop, the skin becomes less translucent, and pigmentation often becomes markedly irregular. Lentigines (freckles) and actinic precancerous lesions may develop (Fig. 59-1), the papillary dermis thins, and the skin loses elasticity while developing a sallow color. Extrinsic aging causes blood vessels to dilate, telangiectases to proliferate, and collagen to become sparse (clumping in bundles). In turn, the reticular dermis fills with abnormal elastin fibers. Eventually, hair follicles and pores dilate and become filled with desquamated debris.

In America, from the early 1900s until the 1950s, chemical peels were popular for skin rejuvenation. When dermabrasion was developed in the 1950s, it soon became the favored skin resurfacing technique. With newer commercial preparations available and America's "baby boomers" aging, yet able to afford cosmetic treatments, chemical peels became popular again. Recent developments in cryotherapy and laser have also become available for more complex interventions.

TOPICAL TREATMENTS AND ADJUNCTS TO PEELS

Considerable improvements in sun-damaged skin can be achieved with topical therapy alone if the patient is willing to be consistent and compliant with a skin care program. Topical retinoids, such as tretinoin (Retin-A), have been shown to clinically and histologically reverse sun damage. In fact, the more severely damaged the skin, the better the response. Newer tretinoin products have gained popularity owing to advances in their delivery systems geared toward reducing the common side effects of dryness and irritation. For example, *Renova* (Ortho Dermatologics, Skillman, NJ) is delivered in an emollient base. *Retin-A-Micro* (Ortho Dermatologics) has a patented microsphere delivery system, and *Atralin* (Valeant Pharmaceuticals, Aliso Viejo, Calif) is delivered in a water-base, alcohol-free vehicle, with added hydrating and moisturizing ingredients. Compliance and consistency with topical therapy are much greater when dryness and skin irritation are decreased. After the use of topical retinoids, biopsies demonstrate deposition of new dermal collagen, formation of new blood vessels, and normalization of epidermal atypia. Accumulated melanin in the basal layer is transported to the surface and shed, improving pigmentation. Epidermal cell turnover is stimulated, producing a proliferation of new cells and improving skin texture. Improved blood supply to the dermis enhances both skin color and the transportation of nutrients to the skin. However, a minimum of 24 weeks is necessary to manifest visible signs of improvement. Unfortunately, topical treatments must continually be used to maintain improvements. When topical treatments are discontinued, the skin gradually returns to its previous condition.

Fortunately, retinoids are now available generically, so their cost has decreased; however, some dermatologists insist that the generic preparations have a higher risk of skin irritation because of their preservatives. Those likely to benefit the most from retinoids are fair-skinned individuals in their 30s and 40s who have blotchy pigmentation, sunspots, or fine lines around their eyes.

Lustra (Medicis Pharmaceuticals, Phoenix, Ariz) is an antiaging cream that contains 2% glycolic acid, antioxidants, and 4% hydroquinone. *Hydroquinone*, a tyrosinase inhibitor, disrupts the synthesis of melanin, thus lightening the skin or pigmented areas. It is also available in a preparation that contains a complete sunblock (*Lustra AF*). This type of preparation can be used in combination with topical retinoids to treat areas of hyperpigmentation, such as melasma. Use of a combination of topical preparations is likely to be slightly irritating to the skin. To avoid irritation that may cause

TABLE 59-1 Intrinsic (Chronologic and Genetic) Aging of the Skin

Cause	Effect
Decreased vascularity	Yellow skin
Dermal thinning	Atrophy
Decreased dermal cellularity	Irregular texture
Loss of elastic fibers	Fine lines or wrinkles
Decreased mechanical properties with decreased elastic recoil after stretching	Laxity

Adapted from Lewis AB, Gendler EC: Resurfacing with topical agents. Semin Cutan Med Surg 15:139–144, 1996.

TABLE 59-2 Extrinsic (Solar and Environmental) Aging of the Skin

Cause	Effect
Altered cell maturation	Dry, coarse texture, actinic keratoses
Melanocyte alteration (overstimulated or destroyed)	Solar lentigines, mottled pigmentation
Decreased collagen fiber number and strength; elastic fiber curling, branching, and thickening; degeneration into solar elastoses	Fine wrinkling
Loss of collagen support of vessels	Solar (senile) purpura
Alteration of vascular network	Yellow hue, loss of pink color

Adapted from Lewis AB, Gendler EC: Resurfacing with topical agents. Semin Cutan Med Surg 15:139–144, 1996.

patients to discontinue their regimen, it is wise to start with every-other-day application for the first 2 weeks, and then daily.

If skin irritation occurs and becomes problematic, a mild steroid cream or ointment (triamcinolone 0.1%), applied sparingly and concomitantly once a day, may reduce the associated erythema and flaking.

α-Hydroxy acids (AHAs) can be applied at low strength (2% to 20%) by patients as part of their daily skin care regimen to improve collagen and elastin synthesis and promote protein regeneration. AHA is a "blanket" term for a variety of fruit acids. Studies have indicated that both the papillary dermis and the epidermis can be thickened, elastic fibers improved, and melanin dispersed with the use of AHAs. Benefits visible to the patient include the reduction of fine lines and wrinkles along with improved skin color, tone, and texture. At low doses these occur without inflammation. Because AHAs do not cause angiogenesis (as opposed to retinoids), they are the *preferred treatment* for patients with telangiectases from rosacea. In addition, because AHAs work by a different mechanism, they can be used concurrently with retinoids.

The following is a list of some of more commonly used AHAs or ones you may see as ingredients in skin care products:

- *Glycolic acid (GA)*: Derived from sugar cane, by far the most common and widely used. Because it has the smallest molecular size of all the AHAs, it easily penetrates the skin and is often used as a delivery system in skin care products.
- *Lactic acid*: Comes from sour milk and is used as a skin softener and exfoliator.
- *Citric acid*: Vitamin C is most commonly used as an antioxidant.
- *Malic acid*: Derived from unripe and green grapes.

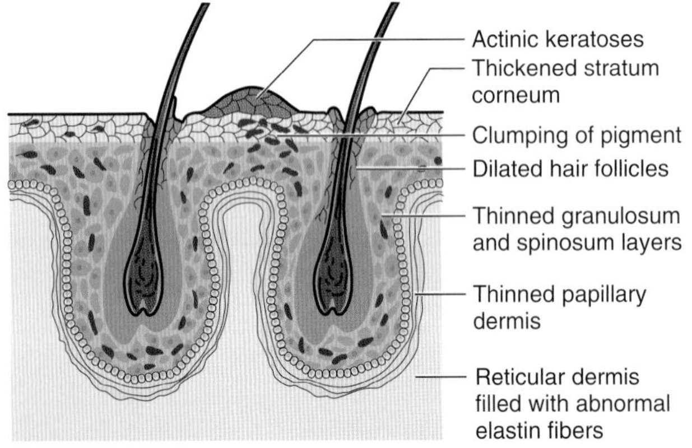

Figure 59-1 Skin damage from years of sun exposure. (Redrawn from Edwards L, Maibach HI, Roenigk HH: What can be done for photoaged skin? Patient Care 30:68, 1996.)

- *Tartaric acid*: A fermentation byproduct from wine making.
- *Mandelic acid*: Derived from almond extract and has antibacterial properties. It is a larger molecule than GA, making it widely tolerated by almost all skin types.

Because of increased sun sensitivity, retinoids are usually applied at night, whereas AHAs are most often applied during the day, along with the recommendation of a sun protection product with an SPF of 15 or greater. Skin texture, and to some degree skin pigmentation, may benefit at any age from retinoids, AHAs, or both. If irregular or abnormal pigmentation is persistent, consider incorporating *hydroquinone*, a tyrosinase inhibitor, or *kojic acid*, a melanin inhibitor, to the patient's treatment program.

There are many AHA preparations available, buffered to various pH levels. It has been theorized that the beneficial or antiaging effects of AHAs are due to activation of transforming growth factor-β, which is increasingly activated at cutaneous pH levels below 5. The prolonged application of "acid" AHAs may reduce the cutaneous pH and thus activate this growth factor. Most unbuffered AHAs have a low pH; however, a low pH also increases the risk of local skin irritation. Buffered preparations with pH levels above 2 are available and may be preferred if skin irritation occurs. In addition, using a low-strength AHA before a chemical peel not only will allow the clinician to judge patient tolerance, but will enhance the penetration of the peel.

Alternative Procedures to Chemical Peels

Alternatives to chemical peels include the following:

- Cryopeels
- Dermaplaning
- Dermabrasion
- Microdermabrasion/dermalinfusion
- Ablative laser resurfacing
- Fractional ablative laser resurfacing
- Nonablative laser (intense pulsed light [IPL])

Of the alternatives to chemical peels, *cryopeels* are the most similar in effect (see Chapter 14, Cryosurgery). Many primary care clinicians already use liquid nitrogen for freezing pigmented spots (lentigines), warts, actinic keratoses, seborrheic keratoses, and angiomas. With considerable experience, and often aided by a special attachment, the clinician can treat the entire face with cryotherapy to produce a cryopeel. It is less expensive for the patient than having a deep chemical peel, and with proper patient selection results may last up to 1 to 2 years. Although a cryopeel may result in more swelling initially, results are often comparable with those of a medium-depth chemical peel.

Originally designed to remove acne scars, *surgical skin planing, or dermaplaning*, was soon found to be useful for scarring from other causes, such as photodamage. After freezing, the skin layers are removed mechanically. Although postoperative healing is slower with dermaplaning and the cost is much higher than for a peel (as much as $4000 for a full-face dermaplane), more severe lesions can be treated, and the results of the skin resurfacing last longer (5 years or more). A more common and less invasive dermaplaning procedure is accomplished by scraping the skin with a no. 12 blade. After cleansing the skin, a light coating of povidone–iodine (Betadine) is applied and allowed to dry. Visualizing the change of color while gently scraping the skin allows the clinician to carefully remove only the most superficial layers of the epidermis. Repeat treatments may be done every 4 to 6 weeks at a cost of $150 to $200 per treatment. Although chemical peels are the procedure of choice for fine wrinkles, dermaplaning has a more prolonged effect and is superior for deep acne scars. *Dermabrasion* is similar to dermaplaning (e.g., preparations, indications) and is most often used to improve the look of facial scars caused by accidents or previous surgery or to smooth out fine facial wrinkles. The patient should be aware that after dermaplaning or dermabrasion, the immedicate postprocedure effects on the face will be quite obvious to friends and colleagues, with an average downtime of at least 10 to 14 days or even longer.

Microdermabrasion (see Chapter 58, Microdermabrasion and Dermalinfusion) is a technique in which the skin is buffed with aluminum oxide crystals. This method has grown in popularity because there is virtually no downtime. It has been coined "the lunchtime peel" and it is much less expensive than dermabrasion (about $50 to $100 per treatment). Three to six treatments are needed at weekly intervals for significant results. Among aesthetic skin care providers, microdermabrasion is the closest equivalent to superficial facial chemical peels. A potential drawback for primary care clinicians is the initial cost of $3500 to $10,000 for equipment.

Carbon dioxide laser resurfacing is another option. Traditionally, lasers were used to obtain a deep resurfacing that often required general or tumescent anesthesia. The cost was as much as $3500 to $5000 per treatment. Although studies have not been published comparing laser surgery with dermabrasion, anecdotal evidence indicates it to be as effective as dermabrasion for removing deep wrinkles around the mouth. There have been no comparative studies showing advantages of laser resurfacing of the whole face over dermabrasion or chemical peeling.

Long-pulse (i.e., 1000 milliseconds) erbium-YAG lasers and CO_2 lasers are now being used to achieve results similar to superficial and medium-depth chemical peels. Using special techniques (fractional ablation techniques), islands of skin are left unaffected within the treated area. This leads to a more rapid recovery time (5 to 7 days) as opposed to previous laser therapy (6 weeks). These lasers can be used anywhere on the body with only topical anesthesia and some oral sedation (see Chapter 51, Lasers and Pulsed-Light Devices: Skin Tightening, and Chapter 53, Fractional Laser Skin Resurfacing). These units require a considerable investment ($70,000 to $140,000).

With the exception of ethnically darker skin types, *IPL therapy* works best for pigment reduction, redness, flushing, or dilated capillaries, and can also be used for overall skin rejuvenation. There is no downtime for patients and minimal discomfort during the four to six required treatments. Unfortunately, the cost of equipment ($40,000 to $80,000) again prevents many primary care clinicians from offering this procedure. Certain IPL technologies can also be successful for hair reduction. However, if using IPL therapy for hair reduction, Fitzpatrick skin types IV through VI will present a challenge in both treatment safety and efficacy (see Chapter 39, Epilation of Isolated Hairs [Including Trichiasis]).

CHEMICAL PEELS

If self-applied over-the-counter AHAs alone are unsatisfactory, they can be used at higher strengths (20% to 70%) or with other agents to cause an inflammatory response or a skin peel. *Chemical peeling relies on penetration of an irritating exfoliant into the dermal level to produce a controlled-depth wound that results in sloughing of the superficial skin layers of the epidermis*. The injury also evokes a nonspecific tissue regeneration that produces a smoother and more youthful-appearing skin. A peel can be used after the skin has been prepared over time with retinoids, AHAs, or both, or it can be used as an alternative to the continuous application of these topicals.

It is not surprising that AHAs improve the skin; fermented food products that contain them have long been used to exfoliate the skin. Ancient Egyptians used the "hemayet" fruit, Greeks used facial masks, and Romans applied various combinations of salts and plants for this purpose.

Four levels of chemical peels are available: (1) *superficial*, (2) *superficial to medium*, (3) *medium*, and (4) *deep* (Table 59-3). The deeper the peel, the higher the risk of complications, patient inconvenience, and discomfort. A downtime of 1 or 2 weeks is to be expected with medium-depth and deeper peels, and it is usually obvious to the patient's friends and colleagues that a cosmetic procedure has been performed. On the other hand, most superficial peels can be performed on a Thursday with the patient able to return to work the following Monday with little noticeable skin damage.

TABLE 59-3 Levels of Chemical Peeling

Type of Peel	Chemical Formula	Indications
Superficial, stratum granulosum/papillary dermis (up to 0.06 mm)	AHA (GA 20%–70%) BHA (SA 20%–30%) 5-Fluorouracil TCA (10%–20%) Jessner solution: 14 g resorcinol 14 g SA 14 g lactic acid 95% ethanol (quantity sufficient to add up to 100 mL) Unna's paste Carbon dioxide (solid)	Fine rhytides (wrinkles) Bad skin texture Acne vulgaris (comedonal/inflammatory, papular-pustular) Acne rosacea (papular-pustular) Pigmentary changes (especially postinflammatory) Superficial actinic keratoses
Superficial to medium (0.06–0.45 mm)	20%–30% TCA Series of AHA (GA 20%–70%) or BHA (SA 20%–30%) peels (see Table 53-4)	Persistent fine rhytides or bad skin texture Persistent acne vulgaris or rosacea Persistent mild pigmentary changes Isolated but deeper actinic keratoses
Medium, upper reticular dermis (0.45–0.6 mm)	50% TCA or 35% TCA plus initial keratolytics Initial keratolytics: Jessner's solution, carbon dioxide (solid), or 70% GA	Moderate rhytides (wrinkles) Chronic photodamage Multiple epidermal/premalignant lesions Pigmentary changes and solar lentigines Multiple actinic keratoses Multiple flat warts
Deep, mid-reticular dermis (0.6–0.8 mm)	Baker-Gordon formula: 3 mL 88% phenol Three drops croton oil Eight drops hexachlorophene 2 mL distilled water	Severe rhytides (wrinkles) Epidermal lesions Superficial neoplasms Deep pigmentary changes

AHA, α-Hydroxy acid; BHA, β-hydroxy acid; GA, glycolic acid; SA, salicylic acid; TCA, trichloroacetic acid.

Because of the potential for postinflammatory hyperpigmentation, scarring, and hypopigmentation, superficial peels are the procedure of choice for individuals with ethnically darker skin.

NOTE: With the ability to achieve many of the effects of deep peels by repeated superficial peels combined with retinoid preparation, the need for deep peels has diminished. For this and other reasons (including a higher risk of permanent skin damage and scarring with deep peels), deep peels should be performed *only* by someone formally trained or significantly experienced in advanced peels. For this chapter, deep peels are discussed only for the sake of completeness and to provide the clinician with an understanding of older, alternative techniques.

Although chemical peels are the least complex of the many cosmetic procedures discussed here, they should not be taken lightly or performed without proper training, experience, and knowledge of managing potential adverse events. With chemical peels, there is less control of the depth of skin penetration and damage than with other skin procedures; therefore, in unskilled hands it is wise to start with superficial peels. Deeper peels should not be performed until the clinician has significant clinical experience with various peeling agents.

Advantages of chemical peels over dermabrasion and laser include the lower cost of equipment and a shorter learning curve, especially for superficial and medium-depth peels.

Various chemicals have been used for skin peels, also known as *chemexfoliation* and *chemabrasion*, in addition to AHAs. These include phenol, trichloroacetic acid (TCA), and β-hydroxy acid (BHA; i.e., salicylic acid [SA]). Combinations are also used. For single agents, lactic, glycolic, and salicylic acids are used most frequently. The difference between BHA and AHA is that AHAs are water soluble, whereas SA (the only BHA) is lipid soluble.

Weaker chemicals such as *resorcinol* have been used and are relatively free of side effects. Resorcinol is rarely used alone; it is most commonly used in Jessner solution (see Table 59-3).

The effects of a single light peel are so subtle that friends, colleagues, and even the patient may not realize that a cosmetic procedure has been performed. For greater patient satisfaction, a series of peels or alternating superficial peels with microdermabrasion treatments is recommended.

Glycolic acid is often the first choice of experts for skin peels. Among the many benefits of using GA is the fact it is stable and water soluble. In addition, GA is colorless, odorless, and nontoxic if ingested. Disadvantages of GA include the fact that the peels are somewhat variable: some patients have a brisk inflammatory response to only 30% GA, whereas others have only a slight response to as high as 70% GA. There is some dispute concerning the degree of buffering to be used with GA. Even though it is water soluble, some controversy also exists on how best to neutralize it after application.

Salicylic acid is "self-limiting" and does not require neutralization after application. Another benefit of SA over GA or any of the AHAs is that the end product is a visible precipitate, or "frost," after application. This allows the clinician to verify that the application is even. If a frost is not clearly visible after the application of one coat, and drying time has been allowed, an additional coat can be applied. SA fluoresces under a Wood's light, which can be used to ensure complete application. These characteristics may be important when clinicians are first learning the procedure. Because it penetrates the epidermal lipids of the skin more deeply than GA, SA usually causes more desquamation (allowing patients to see the peeling and note the changes).

In addition, because SA is lipid (oil) soluble it is naturally comedolytic and is able to penetrate into the pore and exfoliate the buildup of sebum and dead skin cells. Therefore, it is perhaps the best preparation to use with acne rosacea.

With these differences, it would appear that SA is superior to the AHAs; however, in reality most experts do not use these differences to make their choice, but rather their own personal experience.

TCA, AHAs, and SA (at the listed strengths) are not as deeply absorbed through the skin and do not burn the skin nearly as deeply as *phenol*. Therefore, once the clinician is adequately trained on proper patient selection, the application process, and how to manage potential adverse events, using only these preparations avoids most of the long-term sequelae associated with deep phenol peels (e.g., total loss of pigmentation, irregular pigmentation, hypertrophic scars). Because of these risks and a theoretic risk of toxicity if absorbed, phenol peels are used much less frequently than other modalities.

With safe and effective AHA and SA peels available, there is a question as to whether primary care clinicians should even use TCA or phenol, both of which work by coagulating skin proteins. Decreasing the concentration of TCA toward 20% decreases the depth of exfoliation, perhaps making it safer. Before the advent of AHAs and BHA (i.e., SA), TCA was found to be safer than phenol for treating transition zones, such as the area between the face and neck. It was also found to be excellent for treating the thin skin of the hands. In both of these areas, a deeper burn might increase the risk of scar formation.

With AHAs, application of a series of superficial peels, especially if the skin has been prepared by the use of topical retinoids for many weeks, may produce the same effects as one medium peel or even some of the effects of a deep peel. With experience, AHAs allow you to customize the treatment to the area of the body.

INDICATIONS

See Table 59-3.

- Skin rejuvenation—freshen and brighten skin
- Minor to moderate photodamage, especially in 25- to 50-year-old patients
- Dissatisfaction with results from home topical therapy program alone
- Irregular skin texture
- Actinic keratoses
- Acne vulgaris (comedonal and inflammatory, papular and pustular)
- Acne rosacea (papular and pustular)
- Irregular pigmentation (e.g., melasma, freckles, hyperpigmentation, lentigines)
- Superficial acne scars
- Fine wrinkles
- Multiple flat warts

NOTE: If peels are used to treat acne or the complications of acne, the acne should be approximately 75% resolved with whatever primary treatment is being used (e.g., oral antibiotics or topical treatments) before using a peel. In addition, SA is probably the chemical of choice for acne rosacea.

CONTRAINDICATIONS

Absolute

- Concurrent or recent (within 6 months) isotretinoin (Accutane) therapy. It is best to obtain a release from the prescribing physician before performing a chemical peel.
- Concurrent radiation therapy.
- Allergies or hypersensitivities to agents used for chemical peels.
- Presence of melanoma or squamous cell or basal cell carcinoma in the region to be treated (if diagnosis is uncertain, obtain a biopsy first).
- Hemangiomas and nevus flammeus do not respond to chemical peels.
- Alcoholism (heavy alcohol use will impair healing, making it futile to do a peel).

TABLE 59-4 Protocols for Serial Glycolic Acid Peels (Performed 2 to 4 Weeks Apart)

	I		II		III	
Indication	Conc. (%)	Time (min)	Conc. (%)	Time (min)	Conc. (%)	Time (min)
Acne	70	2	35	3	50–70	1–3
Melasma	70	3	35	4	50–70	2–4
Actinic keratoses	70	4	50	3	70	5–7
Fine wrinkles	70	5	50	4	70	4–8
Solar lentigines	70	6	70	3	70	4–8
Back or chest (any indication)	70	7	70	4	70	5–10

Conc., concentration.
Modified from Gendler EC: Topical treatment of the aging face. Dermatol Clin 15:561–567, 1997.

Relative

- Concurrent hormone therapy (increased risk of postinflammatory hyperpigmentation).
- Herpes simplex virus. If there is a history of outbreaks, pretreat with an antiviral medication during the treatment period.
- Inflammatory lesions (e.g., herpes simplex, acute acne papule, cellulitis, severe seborrheic dermatitis) should be avoided during chemical peels. More peeling occurs in areas of inflammation, and hyperpigmentation can result. Dermatitis, areas of broken skin, and infection should be controlled before peels; otherwise the chemicals will penetrate more deeply.
- Smoking results in impaired healing and a greater risk of infection. Changes induced by peels will not counteract the damage to the skin from heavy smoking.
- Medium and deep chemical peels of the neck should be approached with extreme caution. In this area there is difficulty controlling the depth of the peel, thus increasing the risk of hypertrophic scarring.
- Although peels are not absolutely contraindicated, patients with as little as 1/32 Native American heritage may be at increased risk of persistent erythema and subsequent hyperpigmentation after a peel. This may be due in part to a reaction to chemicals.
- Patients with a history of allergy to parabens or perfumes may be at the same risk of excessive reaction and pigmentation.

Every precaution should be taken to prevent an allergic reaction to any agents, preservatives, or perfumes (see the Technique section). Oral and topical steroids for potential allergies should be considered. For patients with the potential for excessive reactions and subsequent hyperpigmentation, consider using a tyrosinase inhibitor (hydroquinone) early in the process (see the Complications section for a formula or the Suppliers section to order Bleacheze from Medical Center Pharmacy).

EQUIPMENT AND SUPPLIES

- Water source in treatment room
- Eye wash or sterile saline
- Headband
- Towels
- Glass beaker for the peel solution
- Gentle facial cleanser
- 4 × 4 gauze pads
- Clock or timer
- Petroleum jelly
- Ultrasound gel
- Cotton-tipped applicators/swabs
- Acetone (for degreasing the skin)
- Hand-held fan for cooling (allows patient to maintain "control" by participating in comfort measure)
- Tepid water or 10% to 15% sodium bicarbonate solution for neutralizing
- Bowls for water
- Nonirritating moisturizer such as Aquaphor (available in drugstores)
- Sunblock to apply immediately after the peel
- Preprocedure photograph
- Postpeel instruction sheet
- Optional topical anesthetic for medium-depth peels (also see Chapter 10, Topical Anesthesia)
  - Lidocaine 2.5% and prilocaine 2.5% (EMLA) mixture
  - Lidocaine 4% (ELA-Max)
  - Lidocaine 7%/tetracaine 7%/benzocaine 20% cream (will need to be compounded)
  - BLT ointment (benzocaine 10%, lidocaine 20%, tetracaine 4%)
  - Quadri-caine (compounded)*
  - Quadri-caine VC (with vasoconstrictor)

Superficial Peels

Kits are available for superficial chemical peels, ranging in price from $4 to $10 per peel. The patient is charged from $65 to $100 per peel. Treatment for photodamage usually obtains optimal benefit after four to six peels, each 1 month apart.

- TCA 10% to 20%
- SA 20% to 30%
- AHAs 20% to 70% (e.g., glycolic, lactic, citric, malic, mandelic, tartaric)

NOTE: Although lower pH (i.e., pH < 2) GA solutions (50% to 70%) create more necrosis, there is no evidence that this leads to a more favorable peel. Additional necrosis produces additional crusting, making it more obvious that the patient has had a procedure performed as well as increasing the risk of complications. Therefore, partially buffered or neutralized GA solutions (i.e., pH > 2) are recommended.

Superficial to Medium-Depth Peels

- TCA 20% to 30%
- A series of AHA or BHA peels (Table 59-4)

Medium-Depth Peels

- TCA 50% or TCA 35% plus initial keratolytics

---

*Quadri-caine enhanced cream is a combination of four anesthetics formulated in a topical cream base containing a penetration enhancer (n-decyl methyl sulfoxide 0.25%). Each gram contains 100 mg of lidocaine USP, 50 mg of tetracaine USP, 50 mg of prilocaine hydrochloride, and 10 mg of bupivacaine hydrochloride.

NOTE: For patient safety and standardization, TCA should be compounded by a weight-to-volume method (i.e., 15% TCA is made by diluting 15 g of TCA crystals in distilled water up to a total volume of 100 mL).

Preprocedure Patient Preparation

Obtain informed consent from the patient before treatment (see sample consent form online at www.expertconsult.com).

In many cases patients will be asked to pretreat the skin with topical retinoids for 3 to 5 weeks before the peel. Benefits of pretreatment include the fact that it accelerates epidermal turnover, which will reduce healing time. If the topical retinoids cause bothersome or severe desquamation, they should be discontinued for several days and then resumed on alternate days.

For superficial and most medium-depth peels, patients can be informed that after the face is cleansed and prepared, applying the chemicals to produce the peel takes very little time, usually less than 1 minute (see Technique section). However, deep peels may require several hours, allowing time to make the patient comfortable, prepare the face, apply the chemical, complete the peel, and permit patient recovery if an antianxiety medication, pain management, or any type of anesthesia was used during the peel.

It is very important to know Fitzpatrick skin types before doing peels (see Chapter 46, Introduction to Aesthetic Medicine). Be aware that anyone of Native American heritage will be much more sensitive. Anyone with allergies to parabens, perfumes, or other skin preparations needs to inform the clinician so that precautions can be used. He or she needs to receive a patient teaching guide and must inform the clinician of any other possible contraindication. (See the sample patient education handouts available online at www.expertconsult.com.)

For superficial peels, patients may experience a stinging or burning sensation during application of the peel. This increases for 2 minutes after application, reaches a peak at 3 minutes, then dissipates over the following few minutes, resulting in a feeling similar to a sunburn. The chemicals themselves cause superficial anesthesia, and patients may find this information psychologically reassuring. In addition, patients usually report a slight tightness and smoothness of the skin immediately after superficial peels.

Within several days, some patients experience slight skin crusting, swelling, and possibly purpura in the lower eyelid areas, which generally resolve over the next 24 to 72 hours depending on the chemical used and the patient's skin type. Erythema almost always resolves in a few weeks.

Whenever the skin is peeled or wounded, there is a risk of scarring and infection. Also, pigmentary augmentation is both a short-term risk (it almost always resolves) and a long-term, permanent risk. The deeper the peel, the higher the risk of all of these side effects and complications.

Superficial peels very rarely cause complications; medium and deep peels are higher risks.

Patients should be aware that their postoperative appearance may be frightening, especially after medium or deep peels. This is rare for superficial peels. Patients should use hypoallergenic, nonscented, complete sunblock (SPF 30 or greater).

For superficial peels, the patient can wear makeup the day of the peel. It will be removed in the clinician's office. Topical retinoids should be stopped 3 days before the procedure. For medium and deep peels, the skin should be washed the evening before the procedure to remove all cosmetics and cleansed again in the office before applying the peeling agent.

NOTE: Disappointment with a chemical peel is most often the result of unrealistically high expectations on either the clinician's or patient's part. Patients should be given a patient teaching guide and made aware that superficial peels yield only modest clinical effects. After multiple peels, patients should be able to better appreciate the benefits. Patients should also be reminded that the effect of a medium-depth peel is not comparable to a face lift. Professional-strength peels increase the effectiveness of GA or other AHA solutions that are used later at home by the patient.

Technique

For a sample documentation form, see Figure 59-2.

Superficial Peels

1. Choose the proper mixture or concentration for the patient. AHA 20% to 70%, BHA (i.e., SA) 20% to 30%, or TCA 10% to 20% causes detachment of keratinocytes at the lower concentrations and epidermolysis at the higher concentrations.
2. Cleanse skin of residual debris, makeup, and body surface oils with alcohol or, preferably, acetone.
3. Using cotton-tipped applicators, apply a thin coat of petroleum jelly at the lash line, taking care to protect the medial and lateral canthi of the eyes, the mouth corners, and the edges of the nose (i.e., nasoalar junction; Fig. 59-3A through C). These are typically dry areas of the face and therefore need protection. Any inflamed lesion, such as an active acne lesion, should be avoided. Ask the patient if there are any other dry areas of the face that need protection from the peel. Patients usually know which areas of their nose and face are the driest.
4. After cleansing and applying protectant jelly, eye patches are placed to prevent accidental eye damage (Fig. 59-3D).
5. Starting on the forehead, apply the acid mixture evenly to the entire face, being careful not to pass your hand directly over the patient's eyes. Gentle stretching of the skin will allow the fluid to coat the depths of wrinkles evenly (Fig. 59-3E and F). In general, facial peels do not need to go beyond, but should generally be feathered just below, the jaw line and the fluid should not be applied closer than a couple of millimeters to the eyelid margin. Feather the solution into the hairline and along the chin to prevent a line of demarcation between the treated and untreated areas. If desired, the solution can also be used to extend the peel to the chest, neck, arms, and hands.
6. Allow the mixture to remain in place for the appropriate time (usually 3 to 5 minutes; Fig. 59-3G). Use a timer or a clock, but even more important, assess the patient and skin; *do not* rely on the timer alone. If there are any areas showing increased penetration, intense redness, or pain ("hot spots"), they can be neutralized with a cotton-tipped applicator dipped in ultrasound gel. The gel does not run like water, so it dilutes the acid effect on the area and decreases discomfort.
7. Neutralize and gently blot the treated areas with either water or sodium bicarbonate solution unless the acid you are using is self-limiting and does not require neutralizing, such as SA or Jessner solution.
8. A hypoallergenic, nonscented moisturizer (e.g., Aquaphor) and complete sunblock should be applied immediately after the peel (Fig. 59-3H).

Superficial to Medium-Depth Peels

1. As for superficial peels, choose the proper mixture technique to obtain a superficial to medium-depth peel. A single agent can be used (TCA 20% to 30%) or superficial peels may be repeated every 2 to 4 weeks for a deeper peel effect or until the desired results are obtained. For AHAs or TCA, three or four treatments may be adequate (see Table 59-4); however, often six to eight SA peels are performed. In most cases, the best results are obtained if the patient waits 1 month between peels.
2. If TCA 20% to 30% is chosen, the skin to be peeled must first be dekeratinized to ensure uniform TCA penetration. AHA or SA superficial peels applied in the office a few days before the TCA procedure can be used for this purpose. Dekeratinization

Chemical Peel Progress Note

Patient Name: ______________________ M/F ____ D.O.B. _________ Date ____________

Allergies: ____

Patient Concern/Goals: ____

Skin Assessment: Fitzpatrick skin type: I II III IV V VI

Check all that apply:

❒ Normal ❒ Sensitive ❒ Telangiectasias ❒ Hyperpigmentation
❒ Oily ❒ Dehydrated ❒ Excoriations ❒ Hypopigmentation
❒ Dry ❒ Rosacea ❒ Scars ❒ Other

Home Program:
Skin care products: ____
Current facial mediations: Retin-A (strength)______ Ranova (strength)______
Taxorac (strength)______ Tazorac (strength)______ Differin (gel or cream)_______
Other: ____

Treatment Plan:
Vitalize Peel Lot #: ____________________ Treatment #: ____________________
Illuminize Peel Lot #: ____________________ Treatment #: ____________________

Treated Area: ❒ Face ❒ Neck ❒ Chest

Step 1: Prepping Solution Lot #: ________ Pressure Applied: ❒ Light ❒ Medium ❒ Strong

Areas of Pressure Applied: ____

Step 2: Prepping Solution Lot #: ________ Pressure Applied: ❒ Light ❒ Medium ❒ Strong

Number of Passes: 1 2 3

Areas of Pressure Applied: ____

Optional Step: Retinoic acid (not supplied with this kit). Number of passes: 1 2

Step 3: Sunscreen

Skin Reaction:
Erythema: ❒ none ❒ mild ❒ moderate ❒ severe Areas affected: ____________________
Burning: ❒ none ❒ mild ❒ moderate ❒ severe Areas affected: ____________________
Frosting: ❒ none ❒ mild ❒ moderate ❒ severe Areas affected: ____________________

Recommendations and Comments: ____

____

Provider's Signature: ____

Figure 59-2 Sample skin peel documentation form. (Courtesy of John L. Pfenninger, MD/The Medical Procedures Center, PC, Midland, Mich.)

can also be performed by the patient before arrival by applying topical retinoids to the skin surface daily for 3 to 5 weeks.

3. Although anesthesia is not necessary, intravenous conscious sedation or topical anesthesia (see earlier discussion) may be used.
4. Protect the necessary areas of the face with petroleum jelly in the same manner as for superficial peels.
5. Using a cotton-tipped applicator with the tip wrung out well to avoid dripping or splashing, apply the TCA to the entire face. It should be applied evenly to produce a smooth, white surface. Greater penetration in certain areas may be achieved by rubbing the applicator vigorously. Gently stretching the skin will allow the fluid to coat the depths of wrinkles evenly. The peel should not be extended below the jaw line. Desired areas of the hands and arms may also be treated.
6. Treatments may be repeated, if necessary, in 1- to 3-month intervals to achieve the desired effect.

Medium-Depth Peels

Pretreatment with 0.1% tretinoin (Retin-A) daily for at least 2 weeks will enhance wound healing from medium-depth peels.

Using a Combination of 70% Glycolic Acid and 35% Trichloroacetic Acid

1. After protecting areas of the face with petroleum jelly in the same manner as for superficial peels, apply a 70% GA mixture to the entire face.
2. Allow the mixture to remain in place for 2 minutes. A fan in the room may ease patient discomfort from the stinging associated with the peel.
3. Wash with water.
4. Optional but effective: Apply a topical anesthetic for 30 minutes without occlusion.

   NOTE: A study comparing two topical anesthetics (EMLA and ELA-Max) with each other and with a placebo found a statistically significant decrease in pain with both topical anesthetics and no difference in efficacy between the two anesthetics. Neither anesthetic affected the depth of penetration of the peel. Other topical anesthetics can be used based on clinician preference.

5. Remove the topical anesthetic and apply 35% TCA to the entire face as previously described.

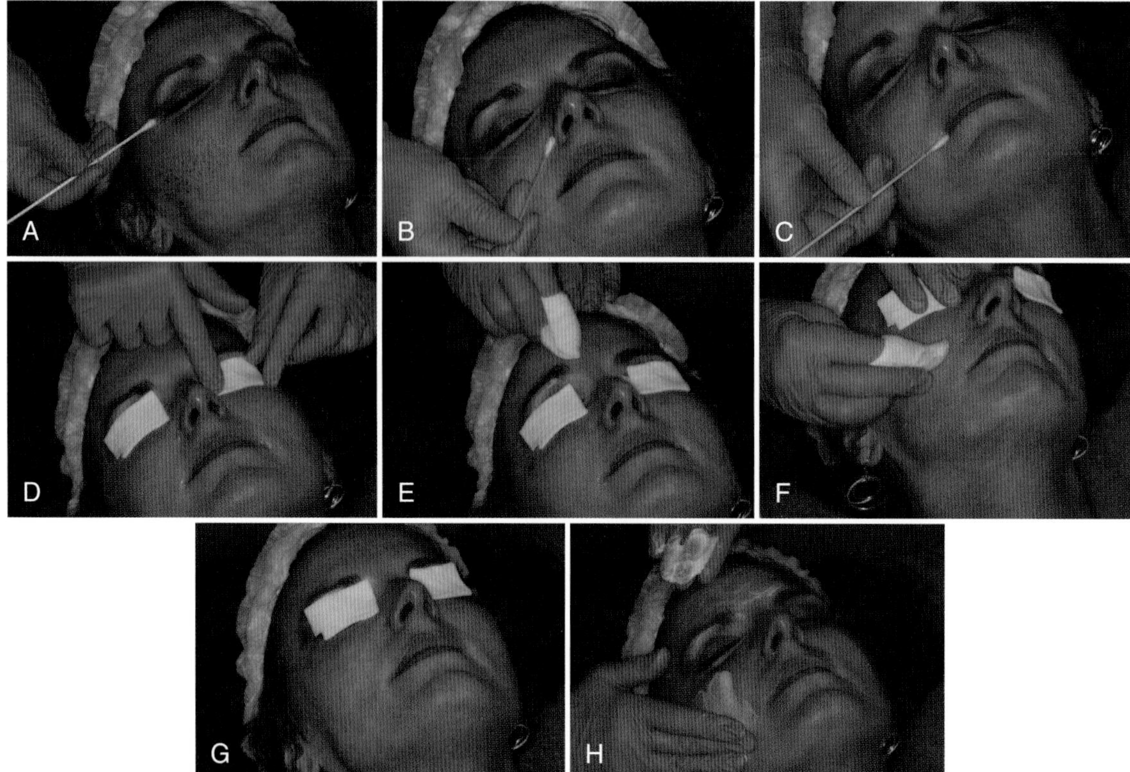

Figure 59-3 Steps in a skin peel procedure (**A–H**). In this case, the Illuminize Peel followed by TNS Ceramide treatment (SkinMedica, Inc., Carlsbad, Calif) were used. See text for a description of each step. (Courtesy of John L. Pfenninger, MD/The Medical Procedures Center, PC, Midland, Mich.)

6. If successful and there are no complications, this technique can be extended to the hands, arms, and chest during the next peel. Depending on the chemical used, be aware of toxicity levels when treating multiple zones and larger surface areas.
7. A cool compress applied to the area after a peel may ease patient discomfort.

Using Trichloroacetic Acid 50%

The technique for a superficial to medium-depth peel with TCA 50% is the same as that noted for the combination 70% GA/35% TCA peel in the previous section.

Complications

Persistent hyperpigmentation is a slight risk, but it is often adequately treated with a tyrosinase inhibitor (hydroquinone, often combined with steroids). One published formula combines 30 g of parabens-free corticosteroid cream, 15 g of 4% hydroquinone, and 20 g of Retin-A 0.1% into a cream to be applied starting 2 weeks after the procedure if hyperpigmentation is developing. Another option is Bleacheze (see the Suppliers section).

The use of oral corticosteroids for 2 weeks after the procedure, followed by a steroid cream, may prevent persistent hyperpigmentation in those at risk or with a history of previous hyperpigmentation.

Postprocedure Patient Education

For superficial peels, the effect is maximal at 48 hours, so the patient should attempt to avoid the sun completely for at least 3 days. If going outside is unavoidable during this time, the patient must use a sunscreen and wear a broad-brimmed hat and large sunglasses. The skin is most vulnerable to damage during this time and sun exposure can cause many problems, including swelling, a deepening of the peel, postinflammatory hyperpigmentation, and potential scarring.

Actual peeling usually begins 2 days after the treatment and can last for up to 7 days. Most patients peel in the central part of the face more heavily than peripherally, and only lightly on the forehead. Some patients peel in fine sheets, but most peel in flakes.

As stated previously, immediately after a superficial peel patients usually report a slight tightness, much like the feeling of a sunburn. A smoothness to the skin is felt and some patients may experience slight skin crusting. Occasionally, swelling occurs, as well as purpura in the lower eyelid areas. These symptoms resolve within a few days. The deeper the peel, the more likely the patient will have these side effects, and the longer they will last.

The effect of a medium-depth peel is maximal at 48 hours. Crusting and some swelling are to be expected and usually subside within the first week. Use of continuous lubrication and sunblock is essential to protect the new skin. If a home care skin regimen is not implemented and maintained, the result of the peel will likely wane by the third month after the procedure.

Aspirin and nonsteroidal anti-inflammatory drugs work very well for postpeel discomfort. A prescription for a mild pain medication may relieve any tingling or throbbing.

In about 7 to 10 days, new skin will be apparent and the patient should be healed sufficiently to return to normal activities. Patients should continue to protect their skin and avoid being in the sun without protection for several months.

After all peels, sunburn may occur at lower doses of sunlight and lead to hyperpigmentation or hypopigmentation. Preservatives, scents, or the chemicals used may also provoke a sensitivity reaction and cause persistent erythema; therefore, a hypoallergenic, non-scented, complete sunblock (SPF 20 or greater) for sensitive skin should be used. Even after healing, the postpeel skin is thinner and more susceptible to sun damage and sunburn. The patient should make a habit of wearing a broad-brimmed hat and large sunglasses, as well as using a complete sunblock every day, and should avoid direct sunlight as much as possible.

Thinner or irritated skin is also more susceptible to desiccation. Thus, a moisturizer should be applied daily.

Patient Education Guides

See the sample patient education handouts online at www.expertconsult.com.

CPT/Billing Codes

15788 Chemical peel, facial; epidermal
15789 Chemical peel, facial; dermal
15792 Chemical peel, nonfacial; epidermal
15793 Chemical peel, nonfacial; dermal

ICD-9-CM Diagnostic Codes

Although most insurers consider chemical peels a cosmetic procedure, occasionally they reimburse for treatment of acne, actinic keratoses, or acne rosacea.

695.3 Acne rosacea
702.0 Actinic keratosis
706.1 Acne
709.00 Dyschromia, unspecified
709.09 Lentigo
709.09 Melasma
709.2 Disfigurement because of scar
709.3 Senile dermatosis

Acknowledgment

The editors wish to recognize the many contributions by Grant C. Fowler, MD, and Stephen F. Ramirez, MD, to this chapter in the previous edition of this text.

Suppliers

(See contact information online at www.expertconsult.com.)

Betacaine and Bleacheze
Custom Scripts Pharmacy

Cosmeceutical skin care, Jessner solution, salicylic acid, and glycolic peels
Allergan, Inc.
Newport Cosmeceuticals, Inc.
SkinMedica, Inc.
Theraplex Company
Visual Changes Skin Care

Glycolic acid
Valeant Pharmaceuticals

Quadri-caine and Quadri-caine VC (vasoconstrictor)
Keystone Pharmacy (compounding pharmacy)
Scripts Pharmacy (compounding pharmacy)

Trichloroacetic acid, glycolic acid, and other supplies
Delasco/Dermatologic Lab and Supply, Inc.

Online Resources

American Society of Plastic Surgeons: Chemical peel. Available at www.plasticsurgery.org/surgery/chempeel.htm.
Plastic Surgery Network: Available at www.plastic-surgery.net.
Plastic Surgery Network: Chemical peels. Available at www.plastic-surgery.net/procedures/chemical_peel.html.
Plastic Surgery Network: Dermabrasion and dermaplaning. Available at www.plastic-surgery.net/dermabrasion.html.

Bibliography

Arndt KA, Kaminer M, Wheeland RG: The promises and limits of cosmetic dermatology. Patient Care 33:97, 1999.

Bernstein EF: Chemical peels. In Kaminer MS, Dover JS, Arndt KA (eds): Atlas of Cosmetic Surgery, 2nd ed. Philadelphia, Saunders, 2009, pp 117–134.

Brody HJ. Chemical Peeling. St. Louis, Mosby-Year Book, 1992.

Brody HJ: Chemical Peeling and Resurfacing, 2nd ed. St Louis, Mosby, 1997.

Brody HJ: Skin resurfacing: Chemical peels. In Freedberg IM, Eisen AZ, Wolff K, et al (eds): Fitzpatrick's Dermatology in General Medicine, 5th ed. New York, McGraw-Hill, 1999, pp 2937–2947.

Coleman WP III, Coleman KM: Techniques for peeling of the face. In Merli GJ (ed): The Clinics Atlas of Office Procedures: Basic Cosmetic Procedures. Philadelphia, WB Saunders, 2000.

Cox SE, Butterwick KJ: Chemical peels. In Robinson JK, Hanke CW, Siegel DM, Sengelmann RD (eds): Surgery of the Skin: Procedural Dermatology. Philadelphia, Mosby, 2005, pp 463–482.

Deprez P: Textbook of Chemical Peels: Superficial, Medium, and Deep Peels in Cosmetic Practice. Abingdon, United Kingdom, Informa Healthcare, 2007.

Edwards L, Maibach HI, Roenigk HH: What can be done for photoaged skin? Patient Care 30:68, 1996.

Farber GA: Prolonged erythema after chemical peel. Dermatol Surg 24: 934–935, 1998.

Fulton JE Jr: Acne: Its causes and treatments. Int J Cosmet Surg Aesthet Dermatol 4:95–105, 2002.

Gendler EC: Topical treatment of the aging face. Clin Dermatol 15: 561–567, 1997.

Kligman D, Kligman AM: Salicylic acid peels for the treatment of photoaging. Dermatol Surg 24:325–328, 1998.

Koppel RA, Coleman KM, Coleman WP: The efficacy of EMLA versus ELA-Max for pain relief in medium-depth chemical peeling: A clinical and histopathologic evaluation. Dermatol Surg 26:61–64, 2000.

Matarasso SL, Hanke CW, Alster TS: Cutaneous resurfacing. Clin Dermatol 15:569–582, 1997.

Moy R, Luftman D, Kakita L: Glycolic Acid Peels. Vol 22: Basic and Clinical Dermatology. Abingdon, United Kingdom, Informa Healthcare, 2002.

Rees TD: Chemabrasion and dermabrasion. In Rees TD, LaTrenta GS (eds): Aesthetic Plastic Surgery, 2nd ed. Philadelphia, WB Saunders, 1994, pp 757–766.

Rubin MG: Procedures in Cosmetic Dermatology Series: Chemical Peels. Philadelphia, Saunders, 2006.

Small R: Chemical peels. In Usatine RP, Pfenninger JL, Stulberg DL, Small R (eds): Dermatologic and Cosmetic Procedures in Office Practice. Philadelphia, Saunders, 2011, Chapter 22 (in press).

Tosti A, Grimes PE, De Padova MP (eds): Color Atlas of Chemical Peels. Berlin, Springer-Verlag, 2005.

Vossen M, Hage JJ, Karim RB: Formulation of trichloroacetic acid peeling solution: A bibliometric analysis. Plast Reconstr Surg 105:1088–1094, 2000.

CHAPTER 60

Photodynamic Therapy

Greta McLaren

The history of photodynamic therapy (PDT) dates back to the early 1900s. Various chemicals, acting as photosensitizers, were found to have cytotoxic effects on specific types of cells after absorption into the cell when followed by activation with light in the presence of oxygen. The principle of PDT is currently used medically to treat various dermatologic conditions, connective tissue disorders, and malignancies. This chapter reviews the various dermatologic conditions, both medical and cosmetic, that can be treated in the office setting using topical PDT. Both U.S. Food and Drug Administration (FDA)–approved applications as well as "off-label" applications are discussed.

PDT using the topical photosensitizer 5-aminolevulinic acid (ALA-PDT) as a procedure to treat various dermatologic conditions has been gaining popularity over the past decade among dermatologists and primary care physicians alike. The procedure received FDA approval in 1999 for the treatment of minimally to moderately thick actinic keratoses of the face and scalp. However, multiple off-label uses have been investigated and found to be safe and effective. Some of the more common off-label treatment protocols that can be performed in the office setting include the treatment of acne, photodamage, sebaceous gland hyperplasia, and hidradenitis suppurativa. Extensive research regarding the "off-label" use of ALA-PDT in the treatment of nonmelanoma skin cancers, including basal cell carcinoma and Bowen's disease, has been published. However, these topics are not covered in this chapter. Please refer to the Bibliography for more information on these subjects (e.g., Gilbert, 2007).

The most common form of ALA used by physicians in the United States is *20% 5-ALA* (Levulan Kerastick; Dusa Pharmaceuticals, Inc., Wilmington, Mass). This photosensitizing chemical has the unique property of being absorbed by the outer layer of the skin and being taken up selectively by cells undergoing rapid turnover. As a result, this procedure allows for the targeting of rapidly reproducing, unhealthy, sun-damaged, precancerous, and cancerous skin cells.

The mechanism by which ALA-PDT works is as follows: once applied to the skin and allowed to incubate and be absorbed, ALA is converted to a potent photosensitizer (PS), protoporphyrin IX (PpIX). When exposed to oxygen and light of various wavelengths, PpIX reacts to produce a cytotoxic effect (singlet oxygen) on the targeted cells. The absorption peaks for PpIX show a maximum peak at 409 nm, with lesser peaks at 509, 544, 584, and 635 nm (Fig. 60-1). Higher fluencies (light energy) are needed for the lesser peaks, although the deeper penetration at the longer wavelengths may have an added benefit.

$$O_2 + PS + \text{light} \rightarrow \text{singlet oxygen (which destroys the target)}$$

ALA-PDT used off label in the treatment of acne vulgaris works in two ways: (1) destruction of *Propionibacterium acnes*, the bacterium associated with the disorder; and (2) shrinkage of the oil glands with less production of oil as a result. The procedure is considered an alternative to isotretinoin (Accutane), with results in some studies lasting for up to 2 years.

In the presence of ALA, *P. acnes* makes a large amount of photosensitive porphyrins, increasing its photosensitivity. The pilosebaceous unit itself selectively accumulates the photosensitizer, PpIX. Light application again produces a chemical reaction that in turn kills the bacteria and also causes involution of the sebaceous gland.

A second PDT photosensitizer, *methyl aminolevulinate* (Metvix, Galderma Laboratories, Paris; and PhotoCure AS, Oslo), has been FDA approved as second-line therapy for the treatment of nonhyperkeratotic actinic keratoses of the face and scalp not amenable to conventional therapy. Despite FDA approval, however, Metvix has not yet been launched in the U.S. market.

Lasers and light sources capable of emitting wavelengths of light that correspond to the absorption peaks for PpIX (see Fig. 60-1) are possible sources for activation of ALA. The activating light source for ALA approved in the FDA protocol for the ALA-PDT procedure is the *BLU-U*, a 417-nm wavelength light manufactured by Dusa Pharmaceuticals. Multiple other light and laser sources noted under the "Equipment" section of this chapter have been found to be effective in activating ALA. Devices such as intense pulsed light (IPL) or pulsed-dye laser (PDL) can be synergistic in that not only are they capable of activating ALA, they are able to target other chromophores such as hemoglobin or melanin. As a result, these devices can simultaneously activate ALA and treat telangiectases and solar lentigines, thereby enhancing the cosmetic result for photodamaged skin. This procedure using a PDL or IPL source is often referred to as *photorejuvenation with ALA*.

Indications

FDA Approved

Actinic keratoses, mild to moderate thickness.

Off-Label Use

- Acne vulgaris
- Acne rosacea
- Cosmetic photorejuvenation
- Sebaceous hyperplasia
- Hidradenitis suppurativa
- Nonmelanoma skin cancers
- Actinic cheilitis
- Warts

Contraindications

Absolute

- Pregnancy
- Breast-feeding (not studied)
- Planned sun exposure within 48 hours
- Isotretinoin (Accutane) use within the previous 6 months

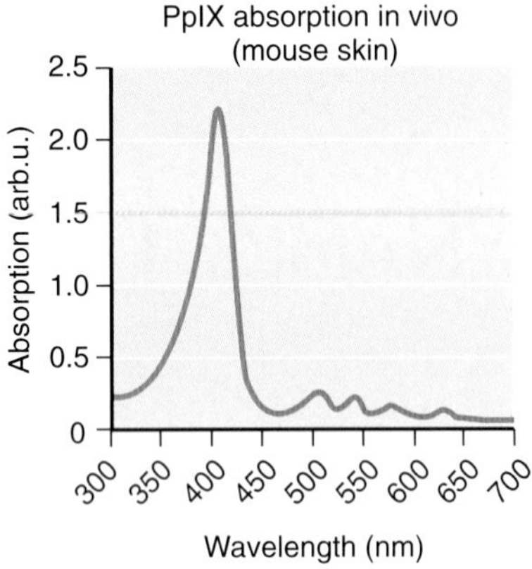

Figure 60-1 The absorption peaks for protoporphyrin IX (PpIX). (Courtesy of Dusa Pharmaceuticals, Inc., Wilmington, Mass.)

Relative

- Seizure disorder
- Diabetes
- Photosensitizing drug use
- Tobacco use

EQUIPMENT

- Acetone and 4 × 4 gauze for skin preparation
- Microdermabrasion machine *(optional)*
- 20% 5-ALA (Levulan Kerastick)
- BLU-U (417 nm), ClearLight (405 to 420 nm; Lumenis, Ltd., Yokneam, Israel), Omnilux Blue Light (415 nm; Photo Therapeutics, Inc., Carlsbad, Calif), PDL (585 or 595 nm), broad-band light source or IPL (410 to 1200 nm)
- Zimmer chiller *(optional)*

PATIENT SELECTION AND PRECAUTIONS

- Photodynamic therapy with ALA can be used on all skin types, Fitzpatrick I through VI, if indicated, using one of the previously noted light devices. Photorejuvenation using an IPL or PDL should be reserved for patients with skin types I through IV only. Patients with *darker skin types* (Fitzpatrick IV and above) are more susceptible to *postinflammatory hyperpigmentation (PIH)* after this procedure. These patients should be well informed of the potential risk of PIH before undergoing the procedure. For the first PDT treatment in skin types IV and above, a shorter incubation time should be considered. The incubation time for subsequent treatments may be gradually increased in 15-minute increments if tolerated (Table 60-1). It is prudent in these patients to take prophylactic measures by prescribing a skin-lightening agent such as hydroquinone 4% gel or cream 2 weeks before and up to 4 weeks after the procedure when treating skin types IV and above.
- The *side effects* and potential downtime with this procedure vary significantly from patient to patient. Some of the more common side effects are *erythema, swelling, peeling, crusting, dryness, and discomfort*. As a general rule, the amount of target tissue present, such as the prevalence of actinic keratoses or severity of acne, along with the length of the incubation period will determine the amount of downtime and side effects.
- *Retinoid use* before the procedure may enhance the results but will also increase the downtime. For better predictability of downtime and side effects, retinoids can be discontinued 1 to 2 weeks before the procedure, unless the enhanced effect, with its potential increased severity of downtime, is desired and discussed with the patient during the consultation.
- ALA-PDT should not be performed on patients who have used *isotretinoin (Accutane) within the previous 6 months.*
- The use of *photosensitizing drugs, including tetracyclines*, must be taken into consideration when performing this procedure. It is acceptable to continue the medication during the treatments; however, the incubation time of ALA is decreased by 15 minutes on the initial treatment to determine if increased side effects due to photosensitivity are likely to occur.
- The discomfort and nerve irritation that may occur with ALA-PDT may stimulate a *herpes simplex virus recurrence* in patients with a history of cold sores. Antivirals should be used prophylactically to prevent this potential side effect in such patients.

PATIENT EDUCATION AND POST-TREATMENT GUIDELINES

Because of the potential severity of side effects and reactions to this procedure, an initial consultation with the patient by a physician with a full explanation of the potential risks, downtime, and side effects is recommended. Once ALA is applied and absorbed in the skin, it may remain reactive to sunlight for the next 24 to 48 hours, regardless of cleansing after the application. It is therefore imperative that patients understand the need to *avoid sunlight*, both direct and indirect, for a minimum of 48 hours after the procedure. An educational handout and informed consent should be reviewed with the patient during the initial consultation.

PROCEDURE

1. Baseline photographs are always helpful.
2. Review consent form and post-treatment guidelines with the patient.
3. Review the history to note any contraindications or use of photosensitizing drugs.
4. Note any cold sore risk and prescribe antivirals if indicated.

TABLE 60-1 Levulan Incubation Time for ALA-PDT Treatment

Area	Treatment Number	Fitzpatrick Skin Type	Disease Severity	Occlusion	Time (in minutes)
Face/scalp	First	I–III	Mild to moderate	No	60
	Second–Fifth	I–III	Same as above	No	60–90*
	First	I–III	Moderate to severe	No	30
	Second–Fifth	I–III	Same as above	No	45–60*
	First–Fifth	IV–VII	All	No	30–45
Chest, back, arms or legs	First–Fifth	I–III	Mild to moderate	Yes	120
	First–Fifth	I–III	Moderate to severe	Yes	90–120
Chest, back	First–Fifth	IV–V	All	Yes	60–90
	First–Fifth	VI	All	Yes	60

*Incubation time may be gradually increased with subsequent treatments if the patient's reaction is well tolerated.

5. Cleanse and prepare the skin with either a vigorous acetone scrub or microdermabrasion.
6. Crush the Levulan Kerastick according to directions and shake the solution for 3 minutes.
7. Protect the patient's eyes and mouth with petrolatum ointment or gauze and apply the Levulan solution to the treatment area (face, neck, chest, back, arms, hands, or legs). Areas with more severe disease may be treated with a second coat of Levulan.
8. Incubate to allow for sufficient absorption of the Levulan depending on area, disease severity, and skin type (see Table 60-1).
9. Areas other than the face and neck, such as chest, back, hands, arms, and legs, require longer incubation times for sufficient absorption of the Levulan. If treating these areas, occluding the area with cellophane (kitchen plastic wrap) and tape will enhance the absorption and decrease the incubation time required (see Table 60-1).
10. When significant acne and or photodamage is present or if the patient has a darker skin type and is at risk for PIH, consider a shorter initial incubation time. Gradually increase incubation times with subsequent treatments, depending on tolerance. Do not exceed a 30-minute incubation time in Fitzpatrick skin type VI because of the increased risk of PIH in these patients (see Table 60-1).
11. Wash the treated area with a gentle cleanser and water after incubation, before starting the light treatment.
12. Activate the Levulan by exposing the treated area to a light source. Narrow-band blue light, IPL, PDL, and light-emitting diode light that falls within the required wavelength absorption spectrum for PpIX (see Fig. 60-1) are all possible sources for activation of Levulan. The operator should use the chosen device in accordance with the individual device's operating protocol. If using the BLU-U light alone, the exposure time is approximately 15 minutes. The recommended energy for the Omnilux 415-nm light, according to the manufacturer, is 48 J/cm^2 for 20 minutes. However, this energy setting can cause significant discomfort, so start with a setting of 24 J/cm^2 for 20 minutes. Energy settings can always be increased. For significant photodamage, actinic keratoses, or deep cystic acne, use IPL at 25 to 45 J/cm^2, depending on the skin type and cooling mechanism, followed by additional exposure using blue light (410 to 417 nm) at 10 to 48 J/cm^2 for 3 to 8 minutes, depending on the energy settings used.
13. Apply a gentle moisturizer or Aquaphor.
14. Inform the patient that the redness and swelling will likely intensify over the next 48 hours. The patient should use a hat or umbrella and sunscreen to guard against any sun exposure for the next 48 hours.
15. Patients appreciate a follow-up by phone or office visit in 24 to 72 hours.
16. To help prevent PIH, prescribe a lightening agent such as hydroquinone 4% cream for darker skin types (IV to VI) once the skin is fully recovered.
17. When IPL with ALA is used for sebaceous gland hyperplasia, at a 7- to 10-day follow-up, hyfrecate the majority of the lesions still present. After two to three treatments with ALA-PDT, there is a significant reduction in the number of newly occurring lesions.

Complications

- *PIH* is a potential complication of this procedure. If this occurs, prescribe a combination cream of hydroquinone 4%, tretinoin 0.05%, and fluocinolone acetonide 0.01% to be used once or twice daily for up to 8 weeks. Microdermabrasion every 2 weeks may also be added.
- Sun exposure in the first 48 hours may result in *blistering, severe discomfort, and peeling*. Cold compresses, pain medication, Aquaphor, and frequent follow-up visits to monitor for infection are recommended.
- *Infection* is rare but can occur. If impetigo occurs, mupirocin (Bactroban) topical ointment or cephalexin 500 mg twice daily may be prescribed for 7 to 10 days. If herpes simplex virus infection occurs, antivirals such as acyclovir should be prescribed.
- Also see some of the common after-effects noted previously.

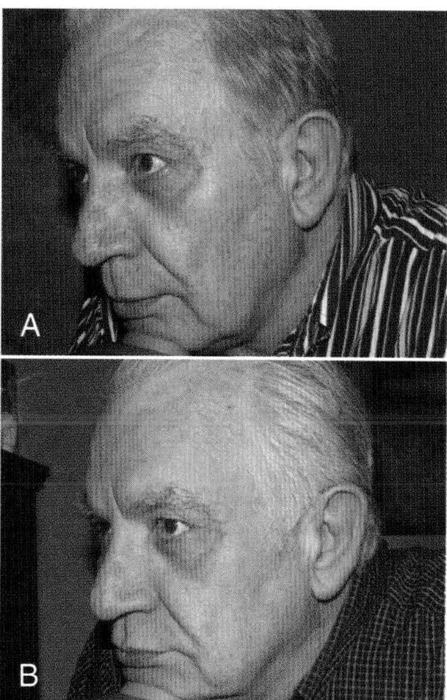

Figure 60-2 **A,** Photodamage before treatment. **B,** Photodamage after three photodynamic therapy treatments with intense pulsed light and BLU-U.

Postprocedure Management

Avoiding sun exposure and keeping the treated area moist are essential. Aquaphor is a preferred healing ointment. To soften any significant crusting, apply wet gauze soaked in a solution of one teaspoon of vinegar to one cup of water. This may be applied for 10 minutes three times daily.

Results

With three to five photorejuvenation treatments with ALA-PDT (60-minute incubation time) in combination with IPL followed by BLU-U for 3 minutes (Fig. 60-2A and B); or with three to five acne treatments with ALA-PDT (60-minute incubation time) and BLU-U exposure alone for 15 minutes (Figs. 60-3 and 60-4), the patient satisfaction rate is very good.

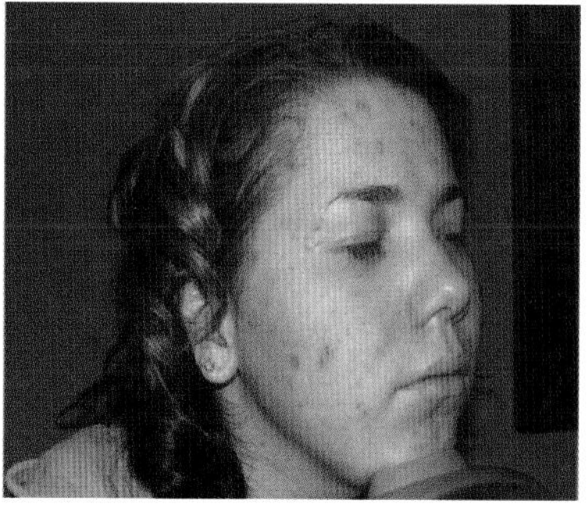

Figure 60-3 Acne before treatment.

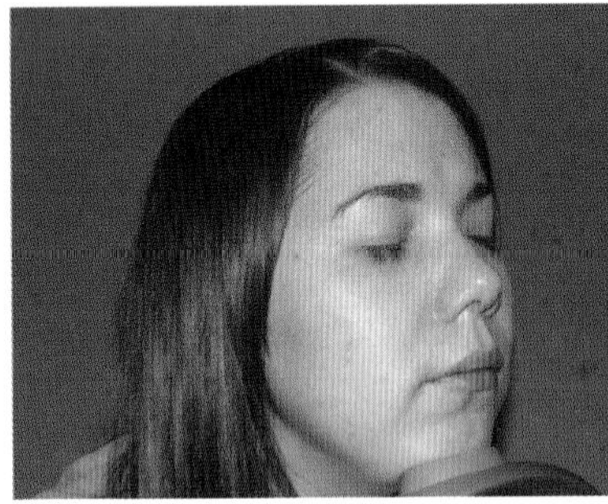

Figure 60-4 Acne after three photodynamic therapy treatments with BLU-U.

Patient Education Guides

See the patient education and patient consent forms available online at www.expertconsult.com.

Billing and Coding

Limited reimbursement for the FDA-approved treatment of actinic keratoses is available through some insurance companies. The majority of the off-label uses of ALA-PDT are considered cosmetic and are unlikely to be covered by insurance.

- For treatment of actinic keratoses, use the CPT code 17004 (destruction premalignant lesions, 15 or more).
- For acne, the ICD-9 code is 706.1 (photodynamic therapy by external application of light to destroy premalignant and/or malignant lesions of the skin and adjacent mucosa, each phototherapy exposure session).
- Use J code 7308 for amino-levulinic acid.

For support in documentation and billing and current CPT codes, Dusa Pharmaceuticals has a reimbursement and coding support center:

Dusa Customer Service and Support: (822) 533-3872 (United States/Canada)
Pinnacle Health Group, Inc. (866) 369-9290 (United States/Canada)
Dusa@thepinnaclehealthgroup.com

Suppliers

(See contact information online at www.expertconsult.com.)

20% 5-ALA (Levulan Kerastick) and light sources for activation of ALA
Dusa Pharmaceuticals, Inc
Broad-band light (BBL)
Sciton
ClearLight and Omnilux Blue
Lumenis
Photo Therapeutics, Inc.
Intense pulsed light
(See Chapters 48 through 55 for other units)
Cutera
Palomar
Pulsed-dye laser
Candela

ONLINE RESOURCE

American Society for Laser Medicine & Surgery. Available at www.aslms.org.

BIBLIOGRAPHY

Alexiades-Armenakas M: Aminolevulinic acid photodynamic therapy for actinic keratoses/actinic cheilitis/acne: Vascular lasers. Dermatol Clin 25:25–37, 2007.
Blume JE, Oseroff AR: Aminolevulinic acid photodynamic therapy for skin cancers. Dermatol Clin 25:5–14, 2007.
Gilbert DJ: Incorporating photodynamic therapy into a medical and cosmetic dermatology practice. Dermatol Clin 25:111–120, 2007.
Gold MH: Introduction to photodynamic therapy: Early experience. Dermatol Clin 25:1–4, 2007.
Gold MH: Photodynamic therapy in dermatology: The next five years. Dermatol Clin 25:119–120, 2007.
Gold MH, Bradshaw VL, Boring NM, et al: The use of novel intense pulsed light and heat source and ALA-PDT in the treatment of moderate to severe inflammatory acne vulgaris. J Drugs Dermatol 3(6 Suppl):S15–S19, 2005.
Goldman MP: Procedures in Cosmetic Dermatology Series: Photodynamic Therapy, 2nd ed. Philadelphia, Saunders, 2007.
Nestor MS: Evolving use of 5-aminolevulinic acid (ALA) topical photodynamic therapy clinically and cosmetically: A clinician's perspective. Cosmetic Dermatol 18:2–5, 2005.
Nestor MS: The use of photodynamic therapy for the treatment of acne vulgaris. Dermatol Clin 25:47–57, 2007.
Nootheti PK, Goldman MP: Aminolevulinic acid-photodynamic therapy for photorejuvenation. Dermatol Clin 25:35–45, 2007.
Richey DF: Aminolevulinic acid photodynamic therapy for sebaceous gland hyperplasia. Dermatol Clin 25:59–65, 2007.
Taub AF: Photodynamic therapy: Other uses. Dermatol Clin 25:101–109, 2007.

CHAPTER 61

Cellulite Treatments

Yves Hébert

Cellulite is a condition that occurs mostly in postpubescent women in which the skin of the lower limbs, abdomen, and pelvic region becomes dimpled. The term was first used in the 1920s in France and began appearing in English-language publications in the late 1960s.

Descriptive names for cellulite include *orange-peel syndrome* and *cottage cheese skin*. Synonyms include *adiposis edematosa*, *dermopanniculosis deformans*, *sclerotic-fibrous-edematous panniculopathy*, and *gynoid lipodystrophy*.

Anatomy of Cellulite

Fat is stored in *fat cells* that lie between the skin and the muscle underneath.

The fat cells are grouped together into large collections that are separated by fibrous strands, or *septa* (Fig. 61-1). These septa run between the muscle and the skin. As the fat cells expand with weight gain, the gap between muscle and skin expands, but unfortunately the septa cannot stretch. This results in the *dimpling* characteristic of cellulite.

The layers of fat are separated into three zones by two planes of connective tissue (Fig. 61-2):

- The *upper zone*, where the fat cell chambers stand vertically separated by radially running septa of connective tissue
- The *middle and lower zones*, where the squat fat chambers and the septa of connective tissue run tangentially to the fascia

Classification

Cellulite is classified using the Nurnberger-Muller scale:

- **Stage 0**: Skin surface is smooth while standing or lying, but *folds or furrows* appear when the skin is pinched.
- **Stage 1**: Skin surface is smooth while standing or lying, but *dimples* appear when the skin is pinched.
- **Stage 2**: Cellulite is present when standing, but disappears when lying.
- **Stage 3**: Cellulite is present regardless of position.

Pathophysiology

The overlying skin begins to bulge as excess fat is stored in the subcutaneous fat cells. With time, the accumulating fatty deposits compress the circulation and create congestion. As congestion increases, fluid and sugars leak out of the vessels to form complex sugar chains that draw even more fluid out of the vasculature through osmolarity. Fat cells begin to organize within fibrous nets to become fatty lobules. Gradually, these fatty lobules invade the skin's dermis and the fibrous nets become more rigid, finally creating skin dimpling ("peau d'orange").

Causes of Cellulite

Currently, the causes of cellulite are poorly understood. It is widely accepted that hormonal factors play a dominant role:

- Estrogens seem to initiate and aggravate cellulite
- Insulin, catecholamines, epinephrine and norepinephrine, thyroid hormones, and prolactin participate in the development of cellulite

Disorders of water metabolism, abnormal hyperpolymerization of the connective tissue, and chronic venous insufficiency are also involved in the pathogenesis of cellulite.

Many predisposing factors are identifiable:

- Sex
- Race
- Phenotype
- Lifestyle
- Smoking status
- Predisposition to circulatory insufficiency
- Abnormal distribution of subcutaneous fat (apple or pear shape)
- Obesity

Treatment of Cellulite

Detoxification Diet

The detoxification diet has been shown to affect the development and amount of cellulite, but it is not a definite cure for cellulite. This diet recommends *less* alcohol, caffeine, refined food (salt), saturated fat, refined carbohydrates, smoking, diet pills, sleeping pills, laxatives, and diuretics, and *more* fresh vegetables and fruits, water, fibers and whole-grain foods, essential nutrients (calcium, potassium, vitamins B and C, glucosamine), and essential fatty acids. All patients wishing to improve the appearance of cellulite should adopt most of the recommendations of this diet but must understand that diet by itself is not a cure for cellulite.

Exercise

Exercise plays an important role in cellulite reduction and is one of the most effective and inexpensive measures for cellulite reduction. Exercise improves the following:

- Muscle tone
- Circulation
- Lymphatic drainage

Aerobic activity, yoga, Pilates, swimming, walking, biking, and stair climbing are excellent forms of exercise for patients with cellulite. Exercise is a fundamental part of the treatment of cellulite and should be strongly encouraged in all patients.

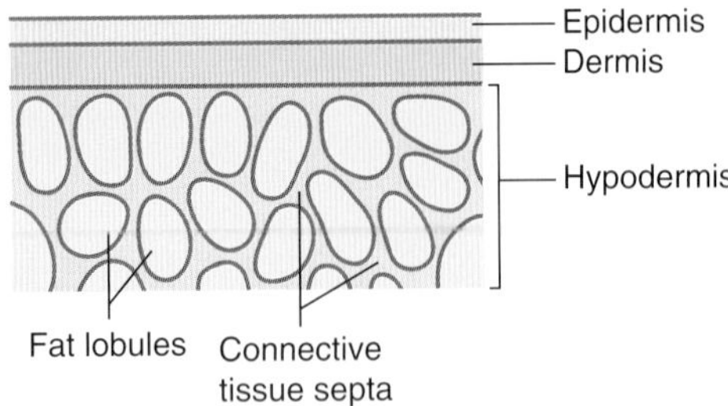

Figure 61-1 Skin and subcutaneous tissue with fat lobules and septa.

Physical and Mechanical Methods

Numerous therapies have been attempted:

- Iontophoresis (transdermal transmission of medication using small electrical charges)
- Ultrasound (high-frequency sound waves)
- Thermotherapy (induced localized hyperthermia)
- Pressotherapy (pneumatic massaging in the direction of the circulation)
- Lymphatic drainage (massage technique to stimulate lymphatic flow)
- Electrolipophoresis (application of a low-frequency electric current)

However, no reports in the scientific literature have shown consistent results. They are possibly helpful in selected patients with lymphatic drainage deficiency.

Pharmacologic Agents

Several drugs that act on fatty tissue have been tried as therapeutic agents. Certain drugs act on the fatty tissue, connective tissue, and the microcirculation. They can be used topically, systemically, or transdermally:

- Methylxanthines (theobromine, theophylline, aminophylline, caffeine), which act through phosphodiesterase inhibition
- Pentoxyphilline, which improves the microcirculation
- β-Adrenergic agonists (isoproterenol and epinephrine)
- α-Adrenergic agonists (yohimbine, piperoxan, phentolamine, dihydroergotamine)
- Methylxanthine enhancers (coenzyme A and the amino acid L-carnitine)
- Drugs with connective tissue activity (silicium and *Centella asiatica*)
- Microcirculation-active drugs (Indian chestnut, gingko biloba, and rutin)

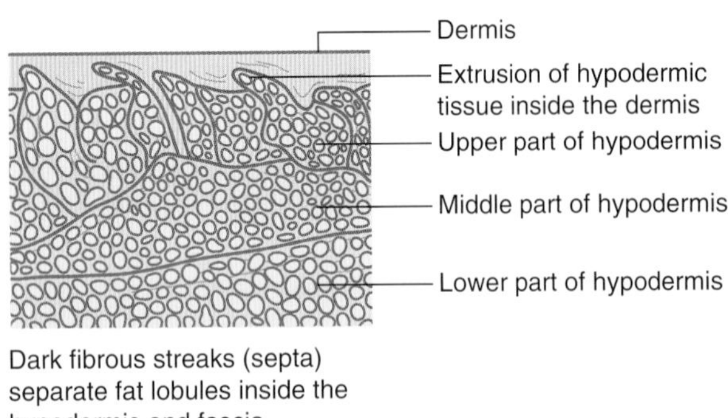

Figure 61-2 Zones of connective tissue in the hypodermis.

None of these medications has been reported in the scientific literature as having a significant effect on cellulite. Some patients could benefit temporarily from an effect on microcirculation.

Anticellulite Creams

Anticellulite creams provide a temporary reduction in cellulite by plumping up the skin and creating a smoother texture. They do not remove the "orange-peel" cellulite appearance. The key ingredients in the creams have antioxidant and anti-inflammatory effects:

- Aminophylline: reduces the bumpy, dimpling effect of cellulite
- Retinol and α-hydroxy acids (AHAs): improve skin texture by exfoliation of dead cells
- Caffeine: reduces fat content in cells by blocking phosphodiesterase, an enzyme that inhibits fat breakdown.

These creams have an indirect effect on cellulite by improving the quality of the skin through skin rejuvenation.

Mesotherapy

Originating in France in the 1950s, mesotherapy is still very controversial in North America. It is practiced extensively in Europe and South America. Small amounts of medications and vitamins are intradermally injected directly into cellulite-affected areas to *increase circulation*, to *decrease fibrosis of the connective tissue*, and to *decrease fat cells*.

Indications

- Spot and cellulite reduction
- Weight loss
- Skin rejuvenation

Side Effects

- Redness and burning that may last for a few days
- Swelling and sensitivity around the treated area for several weeks

Treatment Protocol

Ten to 15 weekly sessions are necessary to achieve visible results.

NOTE: While good reports have come from Europe and South America about the results of this treatment, products are not readily available in North America since the procedure is uncommon.

Lipodissolve

Lipodissolve is a nonsurgical medical procedure that involves the injection of phosphatidylcholine (PPC) into the skin to dissolve fat. The treatment is meant to destroy fat cells, which are eliminated from the body through normal waste removal. The desired end result is precise body contouring in localized areas. PPC is a naturally occurring enzyme and is the main component of soy lecithin. Lecithin has been medically proven to have the ability to break down fat and reduce cholesterol. PPC has been used for fat removal and cellulite reduction by physicians for several years as a safe, noninvasive alternative to surgical procedures such as liposuction.

Treatment Protocol

- Multiple microinjections directly in the subcutaneous tissue
- One to three treatment sessions about 6 weeks apart

The procedure is still very controversial and possibly harmful if done by inexperienced providers because of risk of tissue necrosis. It should be used on selected patients only with localized pockets of fat tissue.

Devices and Technologies

Med Sculpt

See Figure 61-3A. Through a nonmechanical massage and a powerful ultrasound beam, the Med Sculpt system (Sound Surgical Technologies, Louisville, Colo) generates lipoclasis and stimulates the connective layers of the skin for a toned and smoother appearance to the treated areas (mechanical, thermal, and cavitational effects).

PROTOCOL

- Eight sessions twice a week with the vacuum-operated massage
- Four to six sessions at 3-week intervals with the hydrolipoclasia treatment (infiltration of physiologic solution before applying a strong ultrasound beam)
- Ten sessions twice a week of massage only

CLINICAL BENEFITS

- Compact loosening of the fatty tissue matrix
- Stimulation of lymphatic and venous circulation
- Redistribution of subcutaneous fat
- Moderate results on mild cases of cellulite

Endermologie

See Figure 61-3B. Endermologie (LPG Systems, Valence, France) is a temporary cellulite reduction technique. Mechanical rollers and suction provide intense massage to cellulite-affected areas by stimulating circulation to the affected zone. It is said to increase circulation by up to 200%, creating a smoother and toned effect to the cellulite problem areas.

CLASSIC TREATMENT PROTOCOL

- Thirty to 45 minutes per session, one to two times per week until the desired cellulite reduction has been achieved.
- An average of 15 to 18 treatments is required to achieve visible results, and more treatments are required to maintain the results.

LIPOMASSAGE BY ENDERMOLOGIE. This form of Endermologie delivers more intense treatments for faster results with newly designed rollers. Six treatment sessions are recommended.

ENDERMOLOGIE EXPRESS. Sessions are more vigorous and energetic, requiring subject participation. Soliciting the muscles with contraction–relaxation repetitions, the new protocols isolate fat layers and work them more intensively.

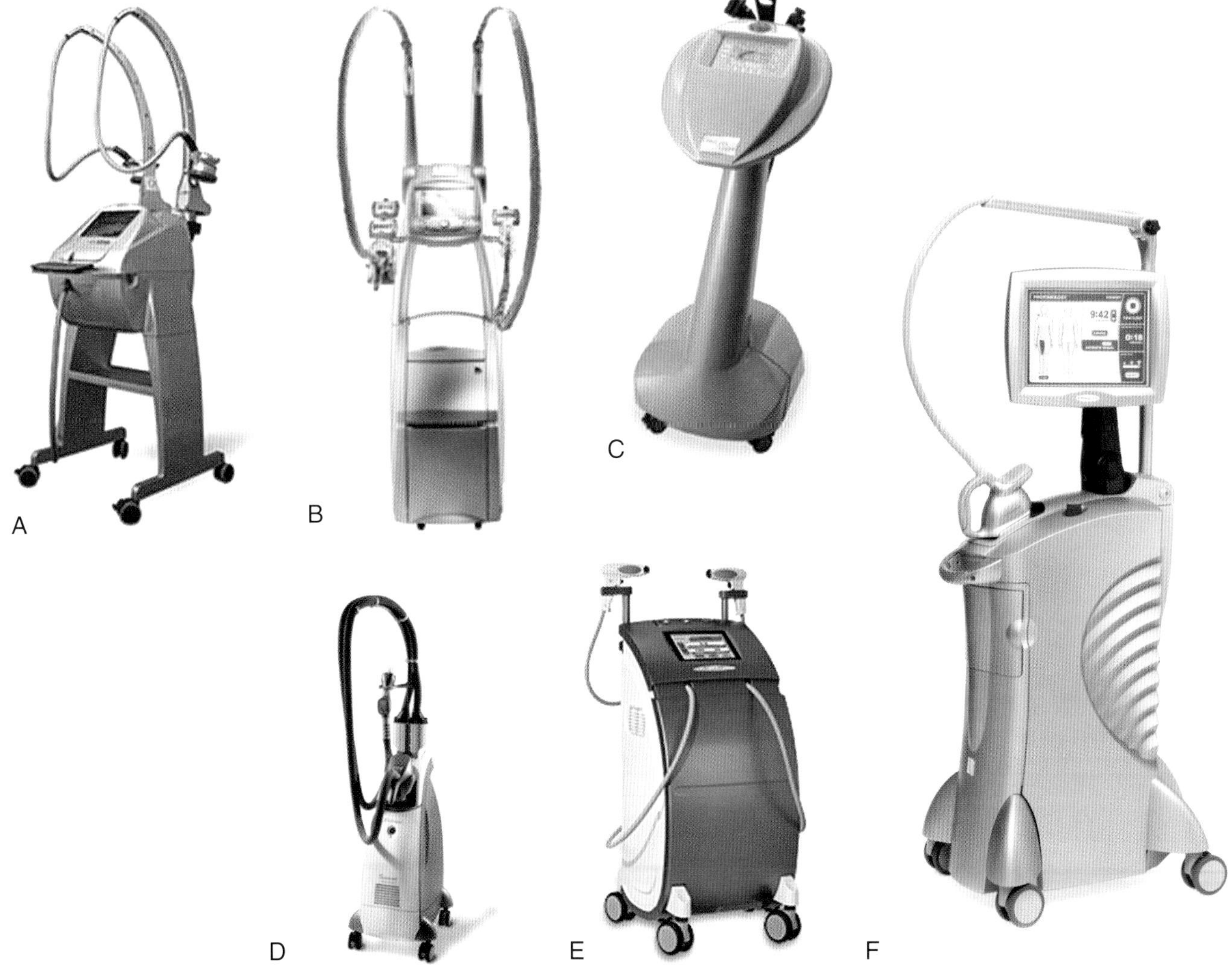

Figure 61-3 **A,** Med Sculpt (Sound Surgical Technologies). **B,** Endermologie (LPG Systems). **C,** TriActive Cellulite Workstation (Cynosure, Inc.). **D,** VelaShape (Syneron, Inc.). **E,** Accent^{XL} (Alma Lasers, Ltd.). **F,** SmoothShapes XV system (Elemé Medical). (**A,** Courtesy of Sound Surgical Technologies, Louisville, Colo.)

NOTE: Enderomologie technology is very operator dependent and patients should inquire about the experience and the training of the technician operating the machine. Results are temporary, as with most of these technologies.

TriActive Cellulite Workstation

See Figure 61-3C. The TriActive Cellulite Workstation (Cynosure, Inc., Westford, Mass) provides a comfortable mechanical massage and rhythmic aspiration to distend the skin in various directions and enhance microcirculation, thereby increasing skin elasticity and improving lymphatic drainage. Six diode lasers penetrate tissues to stimulate fibroblasts for collagen production, yielding smoother, healthier-looking skin. The system can be used in combination with other therapies to enhance the outcomes of surgical and nonsurgical procedures such as liposuction and dermal fillers. This technology provides limited temporary action on superficial cellulite.

VelaShape

See Figure 61-3D. The VelaShape (Syneron, Inc., Irvine, Calif) is a U.S. Food and Drug Administration–cleared system for circumferential reduction through four mechanisms of action:

- The vacuum induces vasodilation and allows deeper penetration of bipolar radiofrequency (RF).
- *Massage* trough roller movements soften tissues and assist in lymphatic drainage.
- *Infrared light* (IR) combined with vacuum provides strong, nonspecific dermal heating, leading to skin toning and firming through collagen stimulation.
- Optimized, controlled RF delivery results in greater depth of penetration and higher peak temperature in the subcutaneous tissue.

TREATMENT PROTOCOL

- Four to eight sessions using both applicators
  - Vsmooth for larger areas
  - Vcontour for smaller areas and localized action

CLINICAL INDICATIONS

- Circumferential reduction
- Cellulite reduction
- Body reshaping through cellulite treatment
- Postliposuction treatment through circumferential reduction
- Postpartum treatment through circumferential reduction

NOTE: The combination of massage, vacuum, and heat (IR and RF) provides interesting results, improving cellulite through skin tightening and circumferential reduction. Patients should be made aware of the short duration of the results and the importance of a maintenance program.

Accent^{XL}

See Figure 61-3E. The Accent^{XL} (Alma Lasers, Ltd., Caesarea, Israel) is an upgradeable, multiapplication, multitechnology, RF-based platform that performs volumetric thermotherapy for the noninvasive treatment of wrinkles and rhytids. A dual-mode RF system tightens and recontours the skin using proprietary unipolar (for deep subcutaneous remodeling) and bipolar (for superficial skin tightening) RF energy, delivered with separate handpieces. Figures 61-4 and 61-5 show the results of treatment with the Accent^{XL}.

TREATMENT PROTOCOL. Four to six sessions 3 to 4 weeks apart.

CLINICAL INDICATIONS

- Skin tightening and rejuvenation
- Cellulite reduction
- Body contouring
- Scar improvement

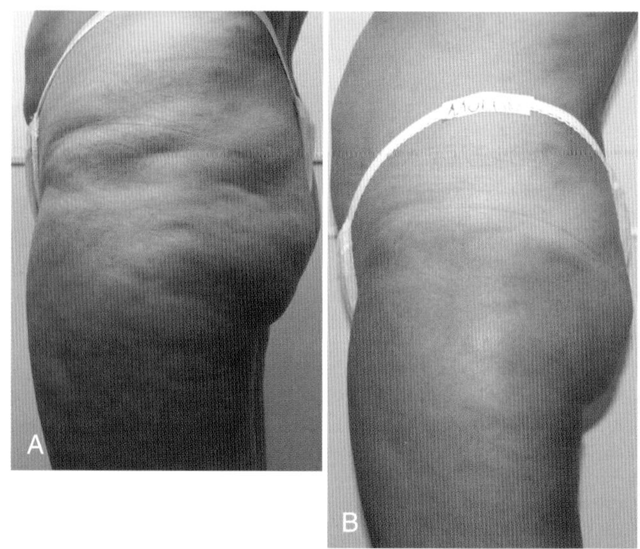

Figure 61-4 Before (**A**) and 2 weeks after (**B**) one Accent^{XL} treatment using the unipolar handpiece. (Courtesy of Emilia del Pino, MD, and Ramon Rosado, MD, Mexico City.)

- Postliposuction touch-ups
- Acne improvement

NOTE: The dual-mode RF system (bipolar and unipolar) improves the appearance of cellulite, but patients should be advised that results are temporary and need maintenance.

SmoothShapes

See Figure 61-3F. The SmoothShapes XV system (Elemé Medical, Merrimarck, NH) effectively treats cellulite by improving the overall condition of enlarged fat cells and inflexible fibrous septae through a proprietary technology called Photomology, which is nondestructive. Photomology restores enlarged cells through a unique mechanism of action that combines dynamic laser and light energy with mechanical manipulation (vacuum and massage) to specifically target problem cellulite resulting in smoother looking skin.

The 915 nm (nanometer) wavelength penetrates well into the tissue and is preferentially absorbed by lipids, causing a thermal effect. The temperature inside the adipocytes is slightly elevated. Contoured rollers move liquefied lipids from the interstitial space to the lymphatic system for dynamic drainage.

TREATMENT PROTOCOL. Eight to 10 sessions on a weekly schedule.

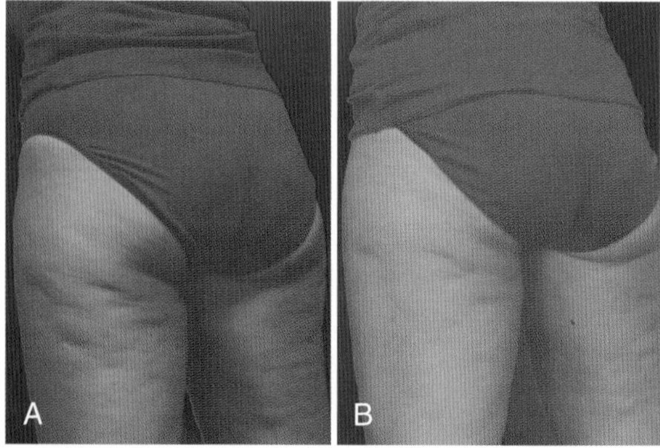

Figure 61-5 Before (**A**) and 4 weeks after (**B**) seven Accent^{XL} treatments using the unipolar handpiece. (Courtesy of David McDaniel, MD, Assistant Professor of Clinical Dermatology and Plastic Surgery, Eastern Virginia Medical School, Norfolk, Va.)

SUPPLIERS

(See contact information online at www.expertconsult.com.)

Alderm
Alma Lasers, Ltd.
Cynosure, Inc.
Elemé Medical
LPG Systems
Syneron, Inc.

BIBLIOGRAPHY

Aesthetic Buyers Guide: www.miinews.com:

Jul/Aug 2007: Mesotherapy controversy: Alma Accent cleared for face and body wrinkles.

Jan/Feb 2008: SmoothShapes targets cellulite.

Sept/Oct 2008: SmoothShapes effectively addresses causes of cellulite.

Jan/Feb 2009: Accent^{XL} adds a new dimension to enhanced body contouring.

May/Jun 2009: SmoothShapes combines dual wavelengths for effective cellulite reduction.

Nov/Dec 2009: MedSculpt provides effective stand-alone or combination therapy.

Alexiades-Armenakas M: Laser and light-based treatment of cellulite. J Drugs Dermatol 6:83–84, 2007.

Draelos Z: Procedures in Cosmetic Dermatology Series: Cosmeceuticals. Philadelphia, Saunders, 2005.

Goldberg D: Procedures in Cosmetic Dermatology Series: Lasers and Lights: Volume 2: Rejuvenation/Resurfacing/Treatment of Ethnic Skin/Treatment of Cellulite. Philadelphia, Saunders, 2005.

Goldman MP, Bacci PA, Leibaschoff G, et al (eds): Cellulite: Pathophysiology and Treatment. New York, Taylor & Francis, 2006.

Madhere S (ed): Aesthetic Mesotherapy and Injection Lipolysis in Clinical Practice. Abingdon, United Kingdom, Informa Healthcare, 2007.

CHAPTER 62

THE THREAD LIFT USING BARBED SUSPENSION SUTURES FOR FACIAL REJUVENATION

Vincent C. Giampapa • Hakan Usal • Oscar Ramirez

Surgeons and patients alike are constantly searching for methods of facial rejuvenation that can be performed with minimal tissue invasion, with the least amount of anesthesia, and with "no" downtime. This is the "holy grail" of aesthetic surgery. One of the latest procedures in this field is the *barbed thread lift*, although suture suspension during lifting has been successfully performed for over two decades. The original type of suture suspension for the midface and neck required an open or a semiopen procedure. Suture suspension worked because of the wide undermining and repositioning of the soft tissues in the elevated position, which was held over the long term by the sutures until scar formation allowed tissue reattachment in the new position. However, when suture suspension was applied in a percutaneous fashion, the general complaint was that the suture tended to act like a "cheese-cutting wire" that would eventually cut through the tissues and diminish the effect over a period of time. The reason this happened was that the sutures were smooth instead of barbed. The advent of the barbed suture represented a new concept in facial lifting because of the ability of barbed sutures to hold and support tissues along their entire length rather than just at the loop made by the smooth sutures. This mechanical advantage provided by the barbed suture permitted its use without the need for tissue undermining.

The barbed suture also makes it easy to insert in one direction and difficult to move in the opposite direction. Once the suture is introduced in the soft tissues, it can be lifted to a position in one direction and the barbs will theoretically prevent the tissues from drooping to their former, original position. Although in principle this made a lot of sense, the early configuration of the barbed sutures was not effective enough. Over time, surgeons modified and improved the configuration of the barbed sutures as well as the surgical principles evolved.

HISTORY OF BARBED SUTURES

In 1964, New Jersey physician J. H. Alcamo patented a roughened suture that offered resistance in one direction only. However, there is no reference to its clinical use. In 1984, Fukuda patented the surgical barbed suture.

The next important landmark was the work done by Russian cosmetic surgeon Marlene Sulamanidze, who, working with Georges Sulamanidze and Tatiana Paikidze from 1986 to 1998, studied a series of subdermal thread insertions using threads from 5 to 18 cm long. This is the first clinical report of the concept and technique of barbed sutures. They described the application of barbed sutures in the subcutaneous plane without undermining. They called their suture design *Aptos (antiptosis) threads*. These sutures were introduced in the United Sates under the name *Featherlift sutures*. However, the Featherlift design did not gain U.S. Food and Drug Administration approval until June 2004.

In the United States in the late 1990s, Gregory Ruff invented what is now called the *Contour Thread*. The difference between the Featherlift and Contour Thread sutures is that the former is a bidirectional, free-floating device that does not require specific anchoring, whereas the latter is a unidirectional barbed suture with needles attached to both ends. The Featherlift requires a hollow cannula for insertion and is not anchored to a fixed structure. It is a self-anchoring device with one barbed segment used to "lift" the lower tissues while the upper barbed segment provides support in a higher position. The first-generation Contour Thread had a unidirectional barb configuration and one needle attached to each end. One long, straight needle is used to thread the suture into the tissues to be lifted (e.g., cheek) and the other end is used to anchor the thread in a fixed structure (e.g., temporal fascia). Subsequently, Leung and Ruff patented other variations and configurations of sutures, such as bidirectional barbed sutures with different types of needles and suture lengths.

BIOMECHANICS OF BARBED SUTURES

Not all barbed sutures are the same. The Aptos barbed sutures are made of 3-0 blue polypropylene with cogs that are relatively longer and thinner than the Contour Thread cogs (Fig. 62-1). The Contour Thread sutures are made of 2-0 clear polypropylene.

The Aptos thread is introduced using a hollow cannula of larger diameter than the suture, whereas the Contour Thread has attached needles of slightly larger diameter than the suture. Because the Aptos suture is inserted through a wider channel, this theoretically may make the cog engagement slightly looser. The Contour Thread needle also widens the channel through which the suture is placed. The flexible needle configuration of the Contour Thread allows the suture to be introduced in a zigzag fashion (Fig. 62-2), which in turn allows better anchoring of the barbs in the tissue. Biomechanical studies have also shown that the shorter the length of the barbs, the stronger their grip on tissues. The Aptos thread has longer barbs than the Contour Thread. Needle attachment at both ends, as well as the bidirectional barb configuration, gives the Contour Thread the additional versatility of permitting a change in direction at the end of the path to apply suture knots if needed or to anchor in a loop of the central, nonbarbed segment. The *newest sutures feature a helicoidal distribution of cogs*, offering an even better grip. A design still in development is an absorbable suture that can be used in semiopen or open methods of tissue lifting.

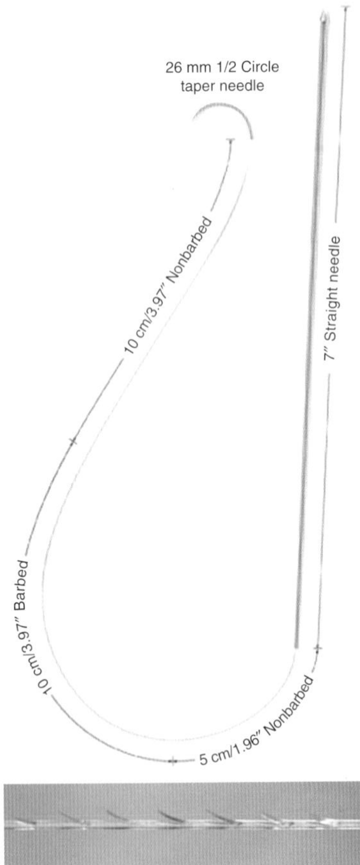

Figure 62-1 The Contour Thread. *Bottom*, Magnified barbed section of thread.

As with all cosmetic surgery procedures, patient selection is the key initial decision in obtaining optimal results. The Contour Thread procedure fulfills the demands of cosmetic patients because it is a minimally invasive yet effective procedure. It offers significant improvement in facial rejuvenation with minimal downtime and potential complications.

Anatomy

There are *four natural aging changes* one needs to consider when seeking to rejuvenate the midface. These were originally described by Hester and colleagues (2000) and include (1) gradual *ptosis of the cheek skin* below the inferior orbital rim with descent of the lax lower eyelid skin (this creates a skeletonized appearance with hollowness around the infraorbital area); (2) *descent of the malar fat pads* with

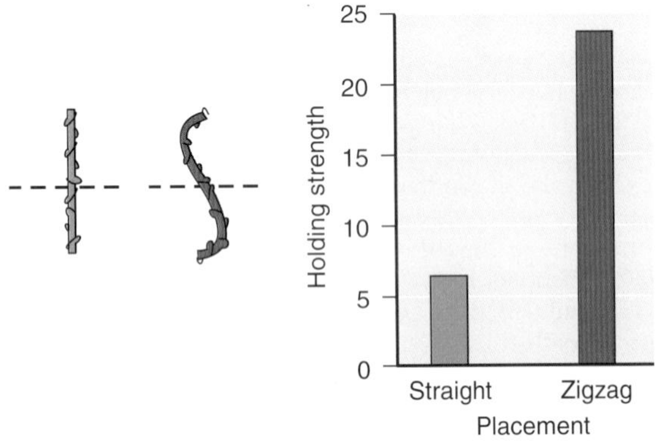

Figure 62-2 Optimized placement patterns.

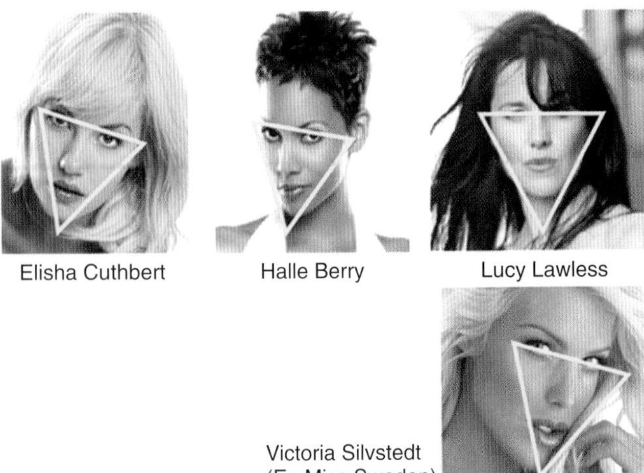

Figure 62-3 The "triangle of youth."

loss of malar prominence in projection; (3) *a prominence and deepening of the tear trough area*; and (4) *a marked enhancement of the nasolabial fold*. These anatomic areas have been called the *triangle of youth* (Fig. 62-3); a youthful facial appearance and contour can be retained by limiting the effects of aging in these areas.

Indications and Uses

- Mild to moderate facial laxity
- Midface laxity
- Neck laxity

The longevity (anywhere from 2 to 4 years) of the rejuvenation obtained depends on the patient's age and quality of facial anatomy. The best result is obtained in a younger individual who displays early signs of facial aging. Patients with strong skeletal support also have better results and greater longevity with the procedure. The poorest candidate is the older individual with severe sagging, redundant skin, and poor skeletal support.

Contraindications

- Older individuals with severely sagging, redundant skin and poor skeletal support
- Uninformed patients with exaggerated expectations
- Patients who are unwilling to comply with a proper postoperative care program

The goal of midface rejuvenation centers around restoring the "triangle of youth," which consists of the malar eminence, nasolabial fold, corners of the mouth, and labiomandibular area (see Fig. 62-3). With the appropriate placement of Contour Threads, specific areas of the midface can be individually targeted for improvement. It is important to inform prospective patients that results using Contour Threads will not equal those obtained with an open facelift, either immediately or in the long term. The ideal patient is one with mild to moderate (class I to III) facial laxity. In particular, patients with laxity in the midface and neck area do very well (Fig. 62-4).

Equipment and Supplies

- 0.5% lidocaine with epinephrine
- Sodium bicarbonate to buffer the lidocaine
- 24-gauge, 4-inch spinal needle
- 27-gauge, 1½ -inch needle
- No. 15 scalpel blade and handle
- 4 × 4 gauze pads

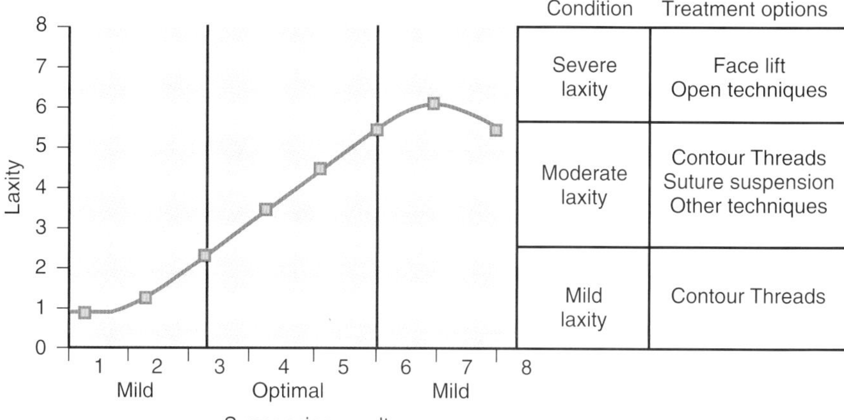

Figure 62-4 Patient selection factors.

- Alcohol wipes
- Lifting thread of choice (e.g., Contour Threads)
- Steri-Strips
- Elastic foam dressing

Preprocedure Patient Preparation

No special preparation is needed before the patient comes to the office for the procedure. Standard consent forms are used.

Technique

Midface Lift

1. The patient is premedicated with oral diazepam (Valium) 5 mg, oxycodone/acetaminophen (Percocet) 5 mg, and Dramamine 10 mg 30 minutes before the procedure.
2. Mark the patient as shown in Figure 62-5.
3. Lidocaine 0.5% with epinephrine 1:200,000 (up to 100 mL) is mixed 10:1 with sodium bicarbonate (buffering lessens the stinging effect). This is injected into the incision sites on the temporal scalp as well as the proposed needle pathways with a 27-gauge needle and a 24-gauge, 4-inch spinal needle.
4. A small, 1- to 2-cm incision is made in a temporal hair-bearing area to introduce the Contour Threads (2-0 polypropylene suture) for the midface lift.
5. The Contour Threads are placed *through the temporal incision and directed downward.* This technique focuses on improving the four key anatomic areas to maximally restore the triangle of youth and provide a more youthful appearance. Each anatomic area is corrected using a specific thread for a specific purpose (see Fig. 62-5).
6. The placement of *thread no. 1* is designed to improve lateral orbital rim and infraorbital rim hollowness, which is a key sign of aging in the triangle of youth. To avoid palpation of the suture, the subcutaneous plane is gently pinched between the thumb and index fingers during suture placement.
7. *Thread no. 2* restores the descent of the malar pad and improves the superior portion of the nasolabial fold. Over the malar eminence and below the zygomatic arch, the suture is placed deeper into the superficial muscular aponeurotic system (SMAS) level and slowly introduced with a weaving action before it exits with a slight curve.

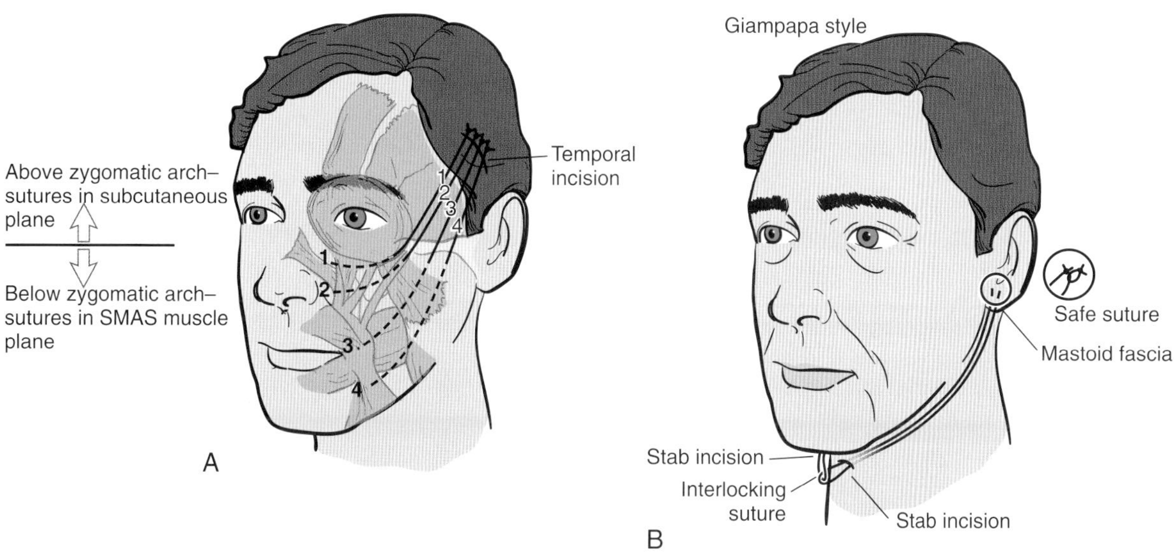

Figure 62-5 **A,** Basic suture placement for midface rejuvenation. (1) Infraorbital hollow and orbital rim depression; (2) malar eminence descent and superior portion of nasolabial fold; (3) ptosis of lateral commissure of mouth and inferior nasolabial fold; (4) labiomandibular fold; SMAS, superficial muscular aponeurotic system. **B,** Neck lift with interlocking suture (Giampapa style).

8. The no. 1 and no. 2 threads are then anchored to the temporal fascia and pulled in a cranial direction. The tension and correction on the tissue will indicate how tight to pull the threads. The barbs are engaged with gentle digital pressure over the entire thread. At the exit points, deeply buried suture knots are tied and kept well below the subcutaneous level to avoid suture palpability.
9. *Thread no. 3* is placed next. This thread corrects descent of the corner of the mouth and improves the lower half of the nasolabial fold and definition of the inframalar area.
10. *Thread no. 4* corrects descent of the labiomandibular area and improves the labiomandibular fold. For the submalar area and corners of the mouth, the same principles are followed and the sutures are placed deep into the SMAS level in the lower third of the face. Sutures are kept lateral to the nasolabial folds.
11. The remaining sutures (nos. 3 and 4) are now secured and tied as described previously.
12. Steri-Strips are then applied to the face with cranial-directed traction.
13. The patient's face and neck are gently dressed with elastic foam dressing for 48 hours to avoid any initial tension in the wrong direction along the barbed section of the sutures.

Postprocedure Patient Care

Patients are advised to avoid excessive facial mimicking/movement and laughter for 96 hours. Patients are seen in the office after 48 hours for dressing removal. Facial cleansing should be performed in a cranial direction to avoid disengagement of the barbed segment of the sutures within the first week. Acetaminophen and other standard pain medications are recommended for pain, as well as the use of an ice compress on the evening after surgery.

Patients are not ready to return to work or engage in social activities until at least 7 to 10 days after the procedure.

Proper early postoperative care is important. The face must be protected from pressure to avoid disengagement of the cogs from the lifted tissues. Patients are instructed to sleep on their backs. Talking and chewing are to be minimal and limited as much as possible. This may restrict the patient's function at work or socially. Facial and scalp cleansing and washing have to be performed in a cranial direction. All of these precautions should be observed for 2 weeks after the procedure, at which time the connective tissue around the cogs may be strong enough for the patient to engage in more liberal activity.

Key Points

All threads are placed in the deep subcutaneous plane *above* the zygomatic arch and then pass into the superficial SMAS plane *below* the zygomatic arch. It is here that the barbed portion of the suture interacts with the SMAS so that it is firmly anchored and supports the underlying tissues in a deeper context, similar to a standard facelift technique. This support of the underlying facial musculature and SMAS level creates the initial improvement as well as the long-lasting results desired.

Common Errors

- Sutures placed too deeply
- Sutures placed too superficially
- Sutures not anchored securely
- Sutures pulled too tight or not tight enough

Complications

- Nerve injury (extremely rare)
- Facial asymmetry
- Ecchymoses
- Skin puckering or dimpling, especially at the suture ends

If any excessive pull or contour deformity is seen after the procedure, the barbs can be released up to 2 weeks after the procedure. This is performed with moderate digital pressure downward over the area that appears to have a "divot" or overtied effect. The bunching effect of skin over the zygoma and postauricular areas and transient tightness and overcorrected look with skin tension improve over the next 1 to 2 weeks, resulting in a very natural appearance.

Furthermore, although it is uncommon, some patients develop significant dimpling at the exit points of the sutures, an uneven contour of facial curvatures with grooving along the cheeks, and waviness and skin folding along the hairline and around the ears. Bruising is rare and resolves within 10 to 14 days. Suture rejection is also rare.

Discussion

The barbed suture technique provides initial marked improvement in the triangle of youth and an extremely high level of patient satisfaction. In our practice we also apply autologous fat injections to the midface as an adjunct procedure to improve midface volume loss. We have noted an initial contraction of the skin in approximately 1 week to 10 days, followed by marked long-term improvement in the patient's overall facial contour. It has been observed that the sutures retain their effect through the formation of a capsule (scarring) around the barbed segments and gradually retract the tissues even more over time. Because the Contour Threads are placed through the SMAS level to ensure final anchoring, it is anticipated that long-term results will be significant, based on the fact that the basic fundamental principles are the same for open facelifting in general.

The "closed form" of the mid-facelift procedure described here can provide approximately 60% to 70% of the results of a standard open facelift procedure. The patient will lose some of the initial lifting results because the immediately apparent postoperative effect relaxes by approximately 30% in the first 6 to 12 weeks (overcorrecting is common because loosening can be performed up to 2 weeks after surgery). The thread lift is certainly not a replacement for the more enduring and proven facelift procedure, nor is it a lunchtime procedure. It is still a surgical procedure that requires local anesthesia and in some select cases intravenous sedation. The degree of facial edema, ecchymosis, discomfort, and tightness can be significant.

If patients have realistic expectations as to the degree of facial rejuvenation attainable with this procedure and understand the need to allow appropriate time for postoperative recovery, then this procedure can yield very good results (Figs. 62-6 and 62-7).

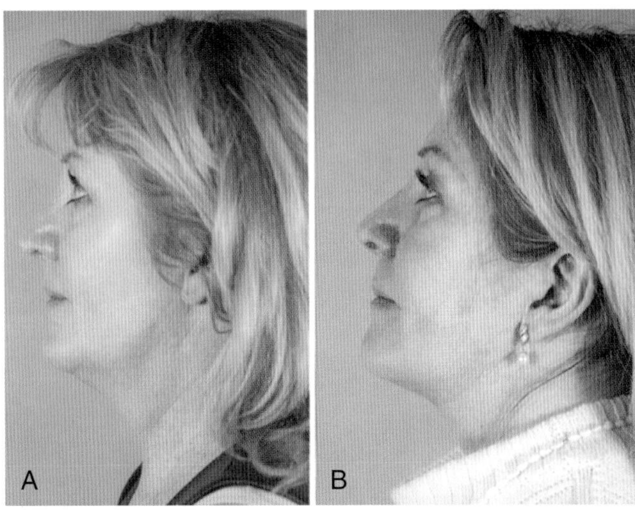

Figure 62-6 Preoperative (**A**) and postoperative (**B**) images of neck lift.

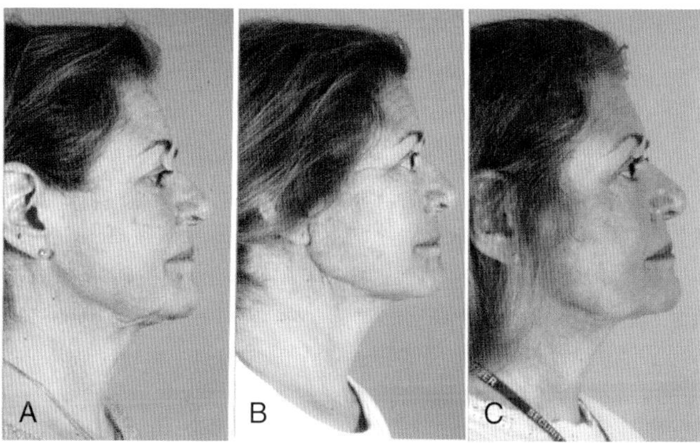

Figure 62-7 Preoperative (**A**), 2-month postoperative (**B**), and 14-month postoperative (**C**) images of combined midface and neck lift.

Barbed suspension sutures for midface rejuvenation are safe and reliable. The technique is relatively easy to perform after a moderate learning curve has been traversed. Nerve injury or facial asymmetry is rare. Like most new procedures, the surgical techniques and technology of barbed sutures have evolved and will likely continue to improve. The final chapter on the barbed suture suspension technique has not yet been written. Despite some controversy, this procedure will certainly find a place in the cosmetic physician's armamentarium and gain popularity in years to come.

SUPPLIER

(See contact information online at www.expertconsult.com.)

Contour threads
Surgical Specialties Corporation

BIBLIOGRAPHY

Badin AZ, Forte MRC, Silva OL: Scarless mid and lower face lift. Aesthetic Surg J 25:340–347, 2005.

Hester TR Jr, Codner MA, McCord CD, et al: Evolution of technique of the direct transblepharoplasty approach for the correction of lower lid and midfacial aging: Maximizing results and minimizing complications in a 5-year experience. Plast Reconstr 105:393–406, 2000.

Sulamanidze MA, Fournier PF, Paikidze TG, Sulamanidze G: Removal of facial soft tissue ptosis with special threads. Dermatol Surg 28:367–371, 2000.

Sulamanidze MA, Shifman MA, Paikidze TG, et al: Facial lifting with APTOS threads. Int J Cosmet Surg Aesthetic Dermatol 4:275–281, 2001.

Wu WTL: Nonsurgical face-lifting with the WOFFLES LIFT. Presented at the American Society of Aesthetic Plastic Surgeons (ASAPS) Annual Meeting, Hot Topics Symposium, Vancouver, Canada, April 16–21, 2004.

Wu WTL: Barbed sutures in facial rejuvenation. Aesthetic Surg J 24: 582–587, 2004.

CHAPTER 63

Radiofrequency-Assisted Upper Blepharoplasty for the Correction of Dermatochalasis

Richard Castillo

Lid droop secondary to redundant skin *(dermatochalasis)* affects nearly all individuals at some point. It is more common on the upper eyelids, but also occurs to a lesser extent on the lower lids. It is typically a bilateral condition, most often manifesting in patients older than 50 years of age. Occasionally, it is observed in younger adults.

Examination of the eyelids reveals redundant, lax skin. An excess fold of skin in the upper lid is characteristic, and the normal upper lid crease may be hidden by the excess tissue. Patients will frequently use the frontalis muscle to augment eyelid opening. This reduces the degree of lid droop, but often results in exaggerated wrinkling or furrowing of the forehead and may lead to muscle tension headaches. Dermatochalasis can present both as a cosmetic problem as well as a functional one by interfering with the superior visual field. In this case, surgical correction is considered *reconstructive* rather than cosmetic.

The introduction of the 4-MHz Dual-Frequency Surgitron (Ellman International, Inc., Oceanside, NY) has made the successful office-based management of dermatochalasis commonplace. The use of the device's unique radiofrequency profile coupled with the proprietary electrode handpieces allow for excellent management of the delicate and highly vascular skin of the eyelid. With proper patient selection, office-based blepharoplasty for the treatment of dermatochalasis is an effective and convenient option (see Chapter 30, Radiofrequency Surgery [Modern Electrosurgery]).

Anatomy

Successful surgery on the eyelids requires a detailed knowledge of the normal anatomic structures and their functional relationships. Good surgical outcomes depend on correcting anomalies while maintaining or reestablishing normal anatomic relationships. The anatomy relevant to the successful correction of dermatochalasis is reviewed here. The bibliography at the end of the chapter contains a few excellent text references practitioners may use to supplement the following review.

In the primary position of gaze (i.e., eyes staring straight ahead), the *palpebral fissure* measures anywhere from 9 to 12 mm vertically. The horizontal dimension is generally 28 to 30 mm. The *upper eyelid margin* lies 1.5 to 2 mm below the superior corneal limbus in the adult. The upper eyelid's marginal contour reaches its highest point slightly nasal to the mid-pupillary line. The lower eyelid margin is normally positioned directly at the inferior corneal limbus.

The *upper eyelid crease* (Fig. 63-1) typically lies 8 to 12 mm above the eyelid margin. It is generally lower in males and higher in females. In *non-Asian eyes*, the crease needs to be reformed as part of the blepharoplasty procedure to reestablish normal cosmetic appearance. In a large percentage of *Asian eyes*, the crease may be lower in position than the aforementioned figures or absent altogether. This factor must be taken into account and discussed with the patient before the procedure so that one does not inadvertently "westernize" an Asian eye against the patient's desires.

The skin of the eyelid is the thinnest skin in the body. The epidermis itself may be only three to four cell layers thick. The combined epidermis and dermis of the eyelid may be only 1 mm thick. The underlying dermis is also scant and poorly defined. It lacks the interdigitations (*rete ridges* and *rete pegs*) with the overlying epidermis that are found in thicker skin. Thus, the epidermis is only loosely adherent to the dermis. We exploit this unique characteristic during blepharoplasty by delivering local anesthetic into this space. The skin of the eyelid also lacks the subcutaneous fat present in skin elsewhere. The skin of the eyelid thus lends itself to healing nicely from properly formed incisions. One tends not to see the depressions found in scars in other areas of the body when the collagen fibers and adipose tissue in the dermis are disrupted.

Below the skin of the eyelid lies the *orbicularis muscle complex* (Fig. 63-2). This is a sheet of striated muscle innervated by branches of the facial nerve that acts to close the eyelid. The muscle is subdivided into an *orbital portion*, which overlies the orbital rim, and a *palpebral portion* overlying the eyelid itself. The palpebral orbicularis is further divided into a superior preseptal portion overlying the orbital septum and a pretarsal portion overlying the tarsus of the lid. The pretarsal portion ends medially and laterally in fibers that form components of the canthal tendons that hold the lid margins against the globe. The medial portion is well developed and forms a structure known as *Horner's muscle*. Care must be taken when excising redundant skin from these areas not to damage these structures or resultant lid malpositions may develop. The orbicularis functions not only in eyelid closure but in the proper functioning of the lacrimal system.

Posterior to the orbicularis is an avascular fascial plane composed of loose areolar tissue. Anatomically it separates the orbicularis from the underlying orbital septum–*levator aponeurosis complex*. This is an important surgical reference plane: it marks the posterior limit of dissection during blepharoplasty for the correction of dermatochalasis.

Note the position of the *supraorbital nerve* in Figure 63-3 as it emerges from the *supraorbital foramen*. Care should be taken to avoid this area during administration of anesthesia as well as while making incisions to avoid trauma to this nerve.

Indications

- Dermatochalasis of the upper eyelids without significant prolapse of orbital fat
- Pseudoptosis of the upper eyelids due to redundant skin folds

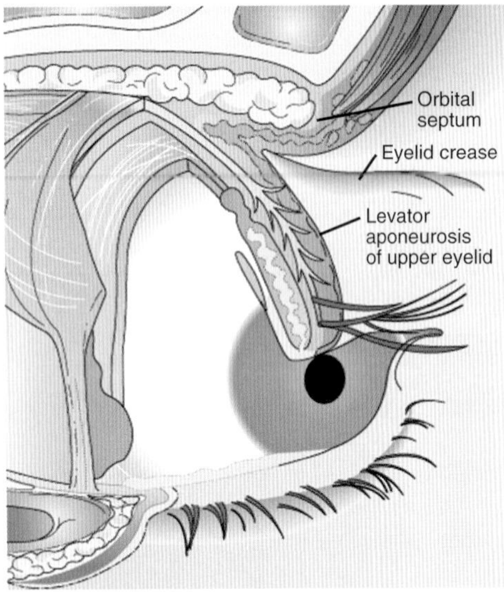

Figure 63-1 Schematic showing the components of the eyelid and the invagination that forms the visible lid crease. (Copyright © 2004, Mosby, Inc. All rights reserved.)

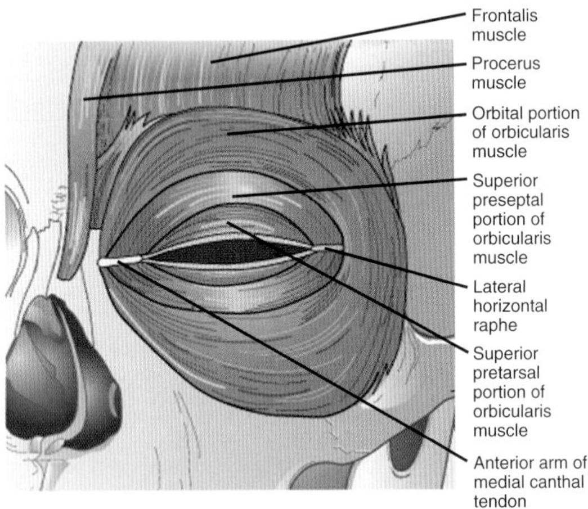

Figure 63-2 Schematic showing the multiple components of the orbicularis muscle. (Copyright © 2004, Mosby, Inc. All rights reserved.)

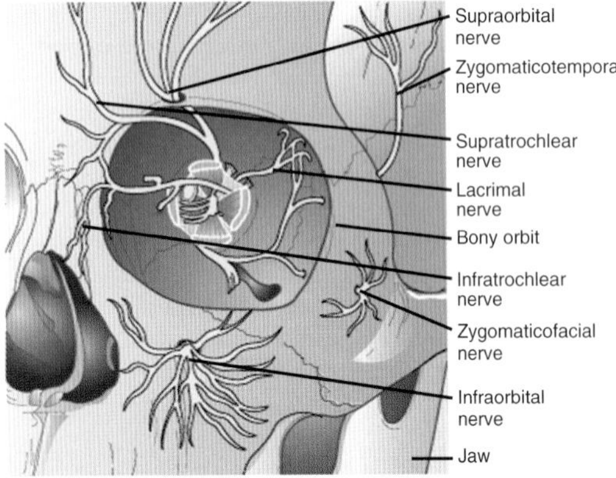

Figure 63-3 Sensory nerves of the periorbital area. Note the position of the supraorbital nerve. (Copyright © 2004, Mosby, Inc. All rights reserved.)

Good surgical outcomes depend as much on accurate diagnosis and proper patient selection as on good surgical technique. In the case of blepharoplasty, mistaking a case of "true" ptosis for pseudoptosis, or lid droop attributed solely to dermatochalasis, will inevitably yield a poor surgical result. The correction of true ptosis involves more than removal of redundant skin. It almost always requires dissection posterior to the orbital septum and into the orbit, manipulation of the levator aponeurosis and the levator palpebrae superioris themselves, and dissection of the preseptal fat pads that are contiguous with the orbital adipose tissue. Depending on the etiology of the ptosis, treatment may require fascial slings or tarsectomy. *A thorough preoperative evaluation is therefore mandatory to establish a proper diagnosis and determine whether one is dealing strictly with dermatochalasis.*

Evaluation of Lid Droop

1. A problem-focused *history* is essential:
   - Rule out systemic conditions possibly associated with ptosis such as myasthenia gravis.
   - History of past ocular disorders (including the lids and surrounding skin)?
   - History of prior ocular surgery?
   - History of wearing contact lenses (giant papillary conjunctivitis secondary to contact lens wear can present as a droopy lid)?
   - Is lid droop congenital or acquired?
   - Gradual or sudden onset?
   - Are there symptoms of visual obstruction, ocular irritation, or *dry eyes*?
   - Are there complaints of diplopia (suggestive of myopathy, neuropathy, or a mass lesion effect)?
2. The *physical examination* should be aimed at determining the etiology of the lid ptosis, as well as detecting conditions that increase the likelihood of surgical complications.
   - *Note the position of the eyebrows.* The brows should be at or above the level of the superior orbital rim; otherwise the patient has brow ptosis, which must be dealt with separately.
   - *Note the amount of dermatochalasis.*
   - *Note the presence of and measure the height of the eyelid crease.*
     An absent crease is a sign of levator dehiscence and cannot be corrected simply by addressing the dermatochalasis component (if present).
     The normal eyelid crease is found anywhere from 8 to 12 mm above the central eyelid margin (in the primary position of gaze).
   - *Note the position of the upper and lower lid margins in both up gaze and down gaze.* The margins should be flush against the globe with lashes directed out. There should be no inversion (entropion) or eversion (ectropion) of the eyelid margins noted.
   - *Measure levator function.* The levator palpebrae superioris is the primary elevator of the eyelid. Measuring levator function is an important component in determining the etiology of the ptosis and can be done as follows: use a millimeter ruler to measure the upper eyelid margin excursion from far down gaze to far up gaze, while blocking frontalis function (manually fix the brow with your hand). Normal for an adult is between 12 to 16 mm of travel. *Less than this usually signifies a problem other than dermatochalasis.*
   - Note any preexisting eyelid scars.
   - Are there any palpable masses?
   - Are the eyes proptotic?
   - Perform a thorough cranial nerve examination.
   - Document any degree of preexisting strabismus or diplopia.
   - Obtain photographs to document findings. Photographs are taken with the eyes in primary position of gaze (Fig. 63-4), as

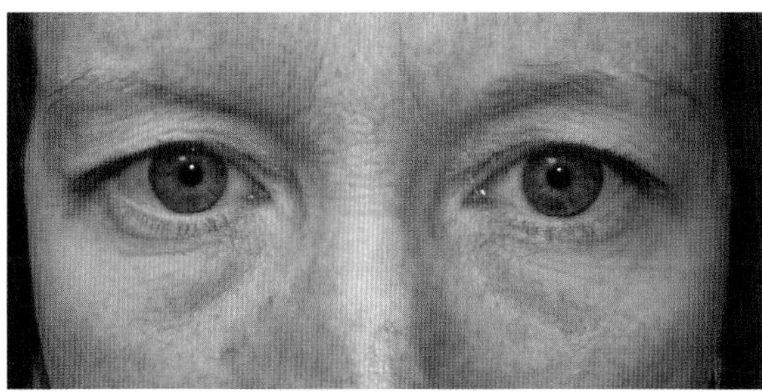

Figure 63-4 Frontal photograph showing redundant skin of the upper lids typical of dermatochalasis (redundant skin). Note the lid margins themselves are in normal position, and pupils free of obstruction. This particular patient would not be expected to show a significant degree of superior visual field restriction.

well as a lateral view (Fig. 63-5). These are essential for reimbursement purposes.

- Perform a screening visual field examination (i.e., tangent screen or automated field) bilaterally with the lids in normal position and then again with the lids held or taped up. To qualify for third-party reimbursement, field testing must show a superior defect within 15 degrees of central vision that improves when the lids are held or taped up. In most cases, an inexpensive tangent screen (Wilson Ophthalmic, Mustang, Okla) testing device can be set up in a small room in the office and the field testing performed by an assistant in less than 5 minutes. One need not perform a full 360-degree field test on each eye. All that is required is one superior isopter mapped out for each eye with the lids in normal position, and then with the lids taped up.
- Note the condition of the external eye.
- Perform ophthalmoscopy.
- Visual acuities (bilateral) are recorded before performing any procedure on or around the eyes.

Once all other potential causes of ptosis have been excluded, a diagnosis of dermatochalasis without other mitigating factors can be established as the cause of the lid droop. Clinically, one should *pay close attention to the position of the eyelid margin*. Sometimes redundant skin folds must be gently lifted up and out of the way to observe the actual eyelid margin. Normally, the lid margin is 1 to 2 mm below the superior limbus. If the lid margin is at or below the superior pupillary border (or within the pupillary zone) with the patient in the primary position of gaze (i.e., staring straight ahead), reconsider the decision to proceed with surgery. In such a case there is likely a secondary cause of the ptosis exclusive of any degree of dermatochalasis.

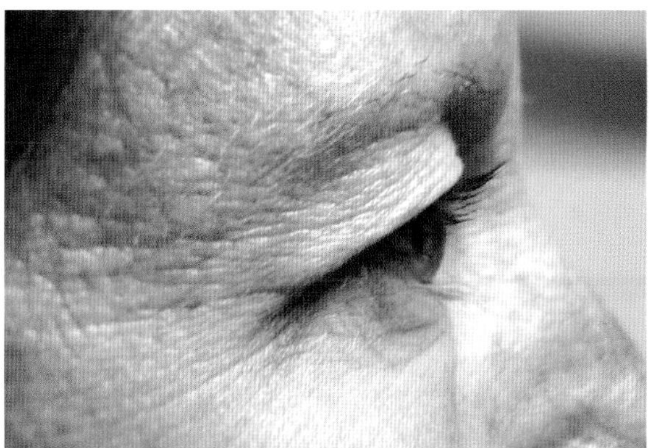

Figure 63-5 Lateral photograph showing skin overhanging the lid margin to rest on the eyelashes.

Contraindications

Dermatochalasis with associated fat prolapse: Correction requires more extensive resection of prolapsed orbital fat posterior to the orbital septum.

Any type of ptosis not due solely to dermatochalasis (redundant skin)

- May require more complicated reconstruction such as advancement of levator aponeurosis, repair of aponeurotic dehiscence, or plication of the aponeurosis tendon.
- May further require frontalis suspension techniques, frontalis sling with tarsectomy, supramaximal levator resection, or other steps that require incising the orbital septum and therefore would not be deemed appropriate to attempt in an office setting.

History of previous eyelid surgery: Previous surgical trauma and distorted anatomy may prevent tissues from responding in the expected manner and therefore make outcomes difficult to predict.

History of thyroid orbitopathy (Graves' disease): Potential for exacerbating lagophthalmos, dry eye syndrome, and exposure keratitis.

History of dry eye syndrome: Potential for exacerbating preexisting condition.

History of corneal disease: Potential for exacerbating preexisting condition.

History of keloid scar formation: May make it difficult to predict outcomes based on poor healing response.

Diabetes: May make it difficult to predict outcomes based on poor healing response. Patients may be more susceptible to postoperative infection.

Hypertension: A heightened risk of intraoperative/postoperative hemorrhage.

Anticoagulants: A heightened risk of intraoperative/postoperative hemorrhage.

Pacemakers: Contraindication for certain radiofrequency devices.

History of myasthenia gravis

- Difficult to predict final lid height/position.
- May inadvertently overcorrect, causing severe lagophthalmos.

Any patient who cannot be properly positioned or would otherwise not be an acceptable risk for office-based surgery.

Equipment and Supplies

- Povidone-iodine (Betadine) 10% skin cleanser
- Proparacaine topical ophthalmic anesthetic
- Corneal shields (Ellman International, Inc.)
- Skin marking pen (fine point)
- Millimeter ruler (disposable)
- Two suture-tying forceps without teeth
- Sterile plastic drapes
- Large cotton-tipped applicators
- Sterile 4 × 4 gauze pads
- Lidocaine 2% with epinephrine 1 : 100,000
- Sterile saline solution
- 0.12-mm toothed forceps
- Westcott scissors (sharp tips)
- Ellman Surgitron Unit (Ellman International, Inc.)
- Empire Micro Needle Electrode for incising the skin (Ellman International, Inc.)
- Coagulation forceps (Ellman International, Inc.)
- 6-0 silk suture
- Needle driver
- Antibiotic ointment

Precautions

- Anticoagulants such as aspirin and warfarin should be discontinued (if possible) at least 7 days before the planned procedure to minimize intraoperative bleeding and postoperative bruising. Vitamin E and fish oil can also increase bleeding tendencies in these lax tissues.

- If signs of blepharitis (lid margin infection) are present (i.e., flaking, crusting, debris between the lashes, erythema of lid margins), surgery should be postponed until lids are treated and clear of infection.
- A corneal shield should always be used while making incisions and carrying out dissection with sharp instruments.
- An etiology of "true" ptosis must be ruled out. This would include congenital, myopathic, neurologic, aponeurotic, and post-traumatic causes of lid droop. Prior evaluation by an ophthalmologist or optometrist is important.

Procedure: Upper Eyelid Blepharoplasty for Dermatochalasis (Without Fat Excision)

1. After a diagnosis of pseudoptosis secondary to dermatochalasis, an informed consent form is reviewed with the patient and signed. The patient is given the opportunity to ask questions. Realistic expectations for the surgery are discussed. Patients are informed that the goal of the procedure is to remove the redundant skin obstructing vision along the superior visual field.
2. The patient is then escorted into the operative suite and placed in supine position. Monitoring devices (electrocardiography, pulse oximetry) and oxygen may be used at the physician's discretion.
3. One drop of a topical ophthalmic anesthetic (e.g., proparacaine) is instilled in each eye.
4. Mark the lower incision line.

   NOTE: Incision lines are marked before administration of subcutaneous anesthetic because administration of an anesthetic bolus will distort normal anatomy and make accurate measurements impossible.

   - The lower incision line is marked with a fine-tipped skin marker and placed within the eyelid crease (if present). Otherwise, a new crease position is planned 9 to 12 mm above the central eyelid margin (slightly higher in women and slightly lower in men).
   - The line is extended and tapered laterally to the lateral canthus (orbital rim) ending approximately 6 mm above the lid margin. It is often helpful to place the lateral incision line in a preexisting rhytid or "crow's feet" wrinkle line.
   - Extend the line medially to the area approximately 5 mm directly above the punctum. Do not extend this line any further medially to avoid trauma to the lacrimal apparatus. The natural contour of the eyelid crease is followed (Fig. 63-6).
5. Mark the upper incision line.
   - With the patient's eyes gently closed (and before administration of subcutaneous anesthetic), determine the upper incision line by grasping the excess skin gently directly above the center of the lid margin with a pair of smooth forceps (Fig. 63-7). Use the forceps to grasp (Fig. 63-8) and bunch up the excess skin until the closed eyelids just begin to open (<1 mm). Mark this point with the skin marker. Repeat this process for an additional three or four points medially and three or four points laterally until the outline of the upper incision line is apparent. Again, the normal contour of the lid should be followed (Fig. 63-9).
   - The "dots" are now connected, creating a smooth continuous line from the medial to the lateral canthus (Fig. 63-10).
   - Care should be taken to ensure that the angle formed by the intersection of the upper and lower incision lines at the lateral and medial canthi does not exceed 60 degrees, or webbing may result if the approach is too steep when the skin margins are sutured together.
6. Recheck the amount of skin to be excised by gently "pinching" the upper and lower incision lines together to confirm that the closed eyelids *do not* open more than 1 mm (Fig. 63-11). If this is the case, the patient may be left with an iatrogenic lagophthalmos that could require subsequent repair.
7. Administer local anesthetic.
   - Inject 1.0 to 1.5 mL of local anesthetic (lidocaine 1% or 2% with epinephrine) subcutaneously beneath the marked area. Care is taken to direct the tip of the needle away from the globe during injection to avoid trauma to the globe itself (Fig. 63-12).
   - Use a 4 × 4 gauze to massage the area to dissipate the bolus of anesthetic.
   - Allow 5 to 10 minutes for the anesthesia to take effect and for the epinephrine to provide some degree of vasoconstriction and hemostasis.
8. Cleanse the skin with Betadine 10% or similar surgical preparation formula. This step can be performed while the anesthesia is taking effect. At a minimum, the forehead, periorbital region, eyelids, nose, and upper cheek should be cleansed bilaterally.
9. Isolate the surgical field with sterile drapes. Disposable plastic sheets with adhesive along one edge work well. A Nevyas drape retractor (Wilson Ophthalmic Corp.) can be used to keep the drape off the patient's nose and mouth.

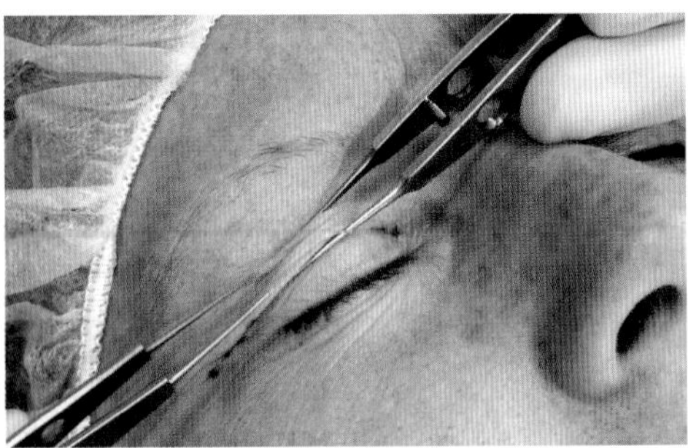

Figure 63-7 The redundant skin is bunched up using smooth forceps to determine the extent of tissue to be excised.

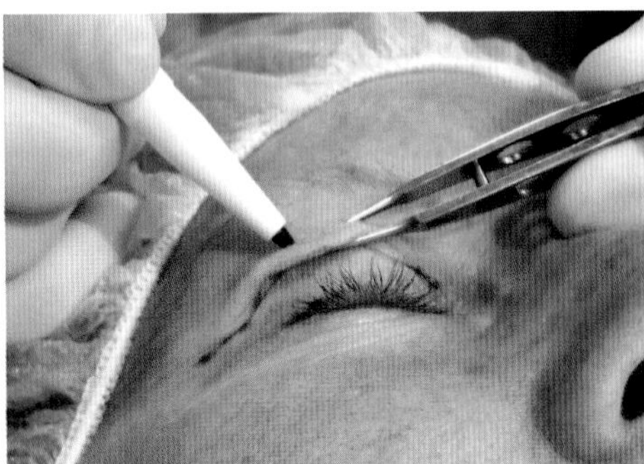

Figure 63-6 Marking the incision lines. The incision is carried and tapered laterally to the orbital rim, and no further medially than the superior punctum.

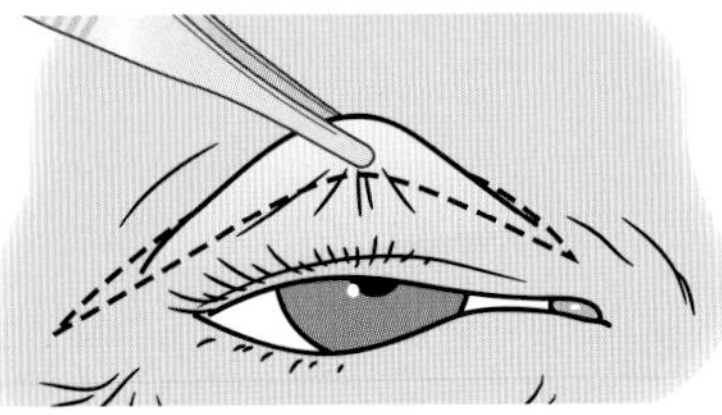

Figure 63-8 Measuring the amount of skin to be excised using the "pinch" method.

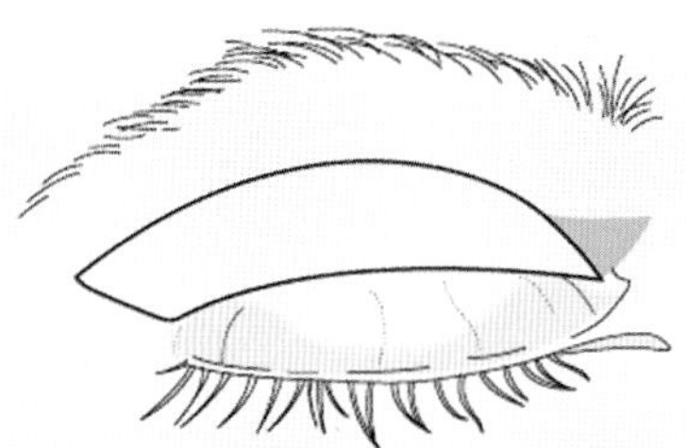

Figure 63-9 Typical skin incision lines for upper blepharoplasty. (Copyright © 2004, Mosby, Inc. All rights reserved.)

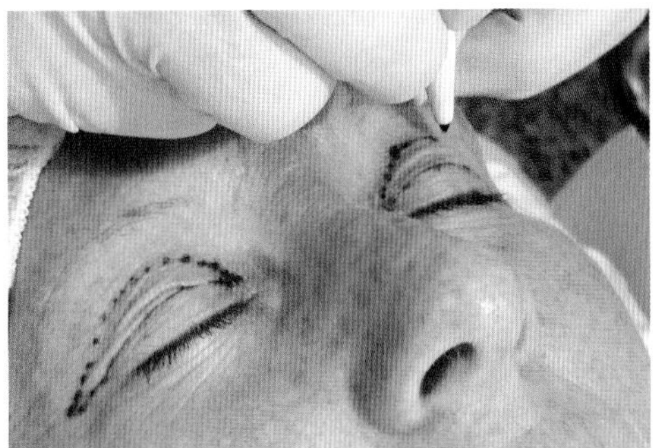

Figure 63-10 Marking the superior incision line.

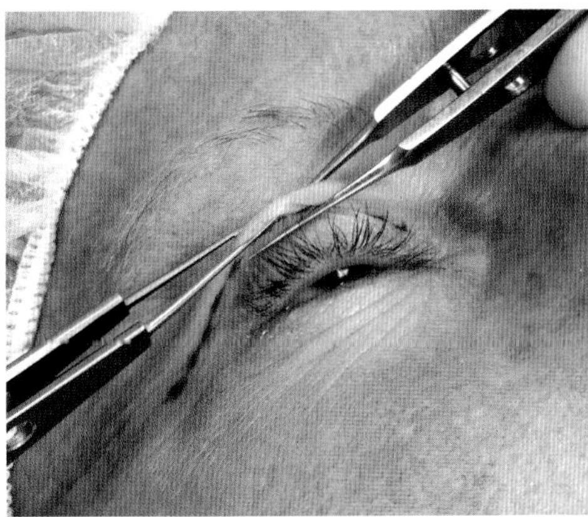

Figure 63-11 Rechecking the amount of skin to be excised using the "pinch" method. Note the eyelid margins should pull apart no more than 1 mm.

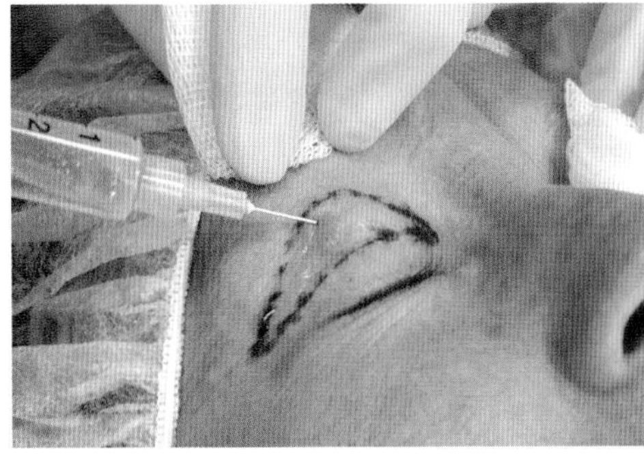

Figure 63-12 Infiltrative subcutaneous anesthesia using lidocaine 1% with epinephrine 1 : 100,000. Drapes omitted for visibility.

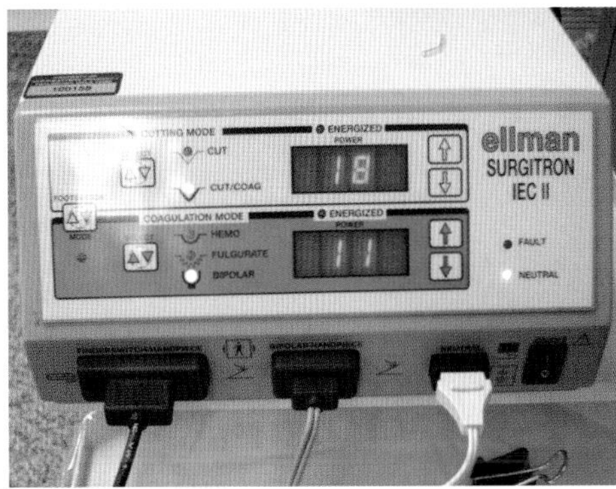

Figure 63-13 The Ellman Dual-Frequency Surgitron II Unit. (Courtesy of Ellman International, Inc., Oceanside, NY.)

10. Check for adequate anesthesia by pinching along the incision lines with toothed forceps. Administer supplementary anesthetic where needed.
11. Place a corneal shield before incising skin.
    A corneal shield (Ellman International, Inc.) is placed directly over the cornea and sclera of the eye being worked on to minimize the risk of trauma while the skin incision/dissection is being performed.
    The shield can be lubricated on the inside with a drop of topical anesthetic and inserted (and removed) with a smooth forceps.
12. The Ellman Surgitron (Fig. 63-13) radiosurgical handpiece with Empire needle electrode tip installed is used to make the skin incisions (Fig. 63-14). The unit is set to the cut/coag blended waveform. Care is taken to keep the power setting to the minimum required to create the skin incision. It is helpful to lightly moisten the skin with a wet 4 × 4 gauze because this facilitates the cutting action of the radiosurgical electrode. Gentle tension along the incision line also facilitates creating the incision. Remember that the total thickness of the epidermis and dermis combined is about 1 mm. The depth of the incision is no greater than that required to visualize the separation of the skin margins as the Empire needle moves along the surface of the incision line. Always cut along the inside of the inked incision line.
13. Dissect and excise an en bloc skin–muscle flap.
    Grasp the lateral corner of the skin flap with toothed forceps and tent up the skin in this area. Using the Empire needle electrode and light horizontal strokes, carefully dissect the skin/orbicularis flap free from the underlying orbital septum along the plane of the suborbicularis fascia (Fig. 63-15). Alternatively, one may remove the skin, leaving the orbicularis intact. Carefully cauterize any bleeders encountered with light cautery using either bipolar coagulation forceps (Fig. 63-16) or the lateral edge of the Empire needle electrode itself.

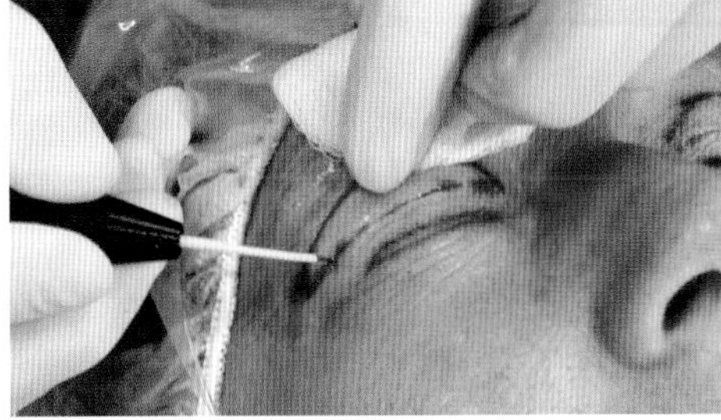

Figure 63-14 The skin incision is created using the Ellman Empire Micro Needle Electrode set to the blended cut/coag waveform.

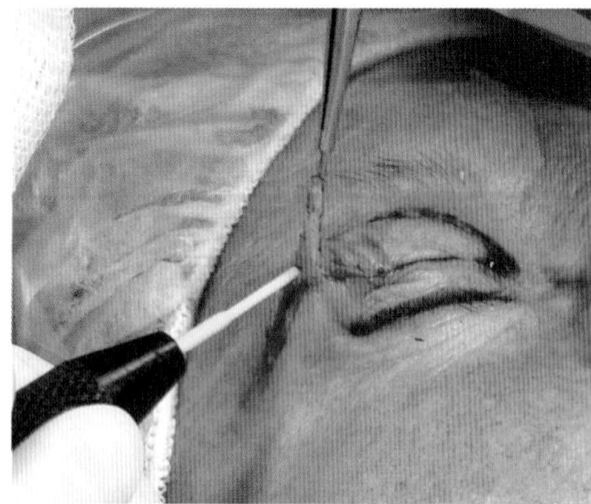

Figure 63-15 The myocutaneous flap is dissected free with the Ellman Empire Micro Needle Electrode.

- Once the myocutaneous flap is dissected free of the underlying tissue bed and significant bleeders controlled with cautery, a 4 × 4 gauze soaked in chilled sterile saline may be placed over the exposed bed to constrict remaining bleeders and achieve hemostasis. This can be done while the skin flap is being excised from the other eye.

14. Close the incision.
    - With the skin flap excised and proper hemostasis achieved, all that remains is to close the incision. The author's preference is 6-0 silk suture placed in simple interrupted fashion (Fig. 63-17). Alternatively, 6-0 Prolene running sutures may be used.
    - The position of the eyelid crease is fixed or reformed by taking a small bite of the underlying fascia as the suture is passed from wound margin to wound margin before it is tied off. Recall that the eyelid crease is usually lower or completely absent in Asian eyes. Both the patient and physician should have a clear understanding of how the eyelid crease will be managed before performing the procedure.
    - Antibiotic ophthalmic ointment is applied to the incision lines, monitoring equipment is removed, the face is gently cleansed, and the patient is escorted to the recovery area.

Sample Operative Report

See the sample operative report online at www.expertconsult.com.

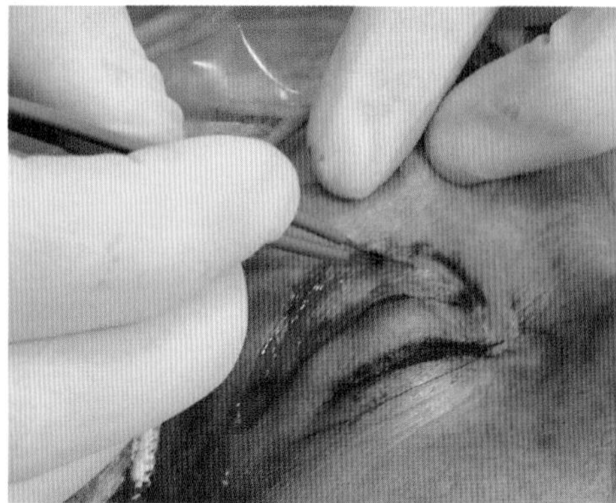

Figure 63-16 Light bipolar cautery being applied to small bleeders. Note the relatively blood-free field that is characteristic of radiofrequency dissection.

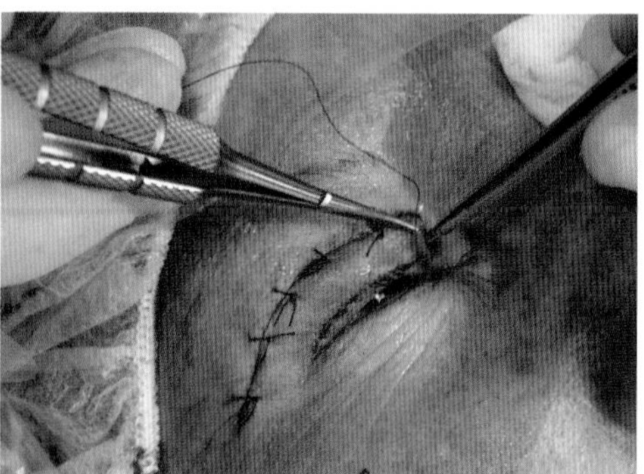

Figure 63-17 Placement of simple interrupted sutures using 6-0 silk. The lid crease is reformed by taking small bites of the underlying fascia as the skin edges are reapproximated.

Complications

Overcorrection (lagophthalmos)

- Usually due to overly aggressive "pinch" estimation while bunching up the excess skin with forceps to establish incision lines.
- A small degree of overcorrection (<2 mm) will usually correct itself with prescribed "force blink exercises" (e.g., blink as hard as you can 10 times then relax. Repeat six to eight times per day for 1 week).
- Overcorrection noticed immediately after surgery may be due to the fact that the orbicularis muscle is still paralyzed from the anesthesia and not functioning fully. This situation is transient and will typically correct itself within a few hours to days.
- If there is any degree of lagophthalmos present, the patient should be given artificial tears to use six to eight times per day to keep the ocular surface (primarily the corneal surface) moist. Antibiotic ointment can be used to protect the ocular surface at night.
- Persistent severe lagophthalmos may require a corrective procedure.

Undercorrection

- Usually due to poor technique or too conservative an estimation of how much skin to remove.
- Postoperative edema can give the false appearance of undercorrection.
  - Cold packs should be started as soon as possible after the procedure and continued for at least 48 hours.
  - In select cases where edema persists, a short course of oral steroids may be helpful.

Dry eye syndrome/tear film dysfunction

- Typically affects older women.
- Lagophthalmos (as mentioned previously) may cause exposure keratitis.
- Transient decreased blink frequency after surgery can cause dry eye symptoms.
- Any degree of dry eye complaint should be treated first with artificial tear supplementation.
- Persistent dry eye complaints or frank lagophthalmos should be referred for evaluation.

Contour deformity

Abnormal/asymmetric lid crease height

Hemorrhage

- Some degree of lid ecchymosis is to be expected.
- Subconjunctival hemorrhage may occur and will resolve spontaneously in 7 to 10 days.
- Retrobulbar hemorrhage is rare but potentially organ threatening. Features of retrobulbar hemorrhage include massive subconjunctival hemorrhage often accompanied by proptosis of

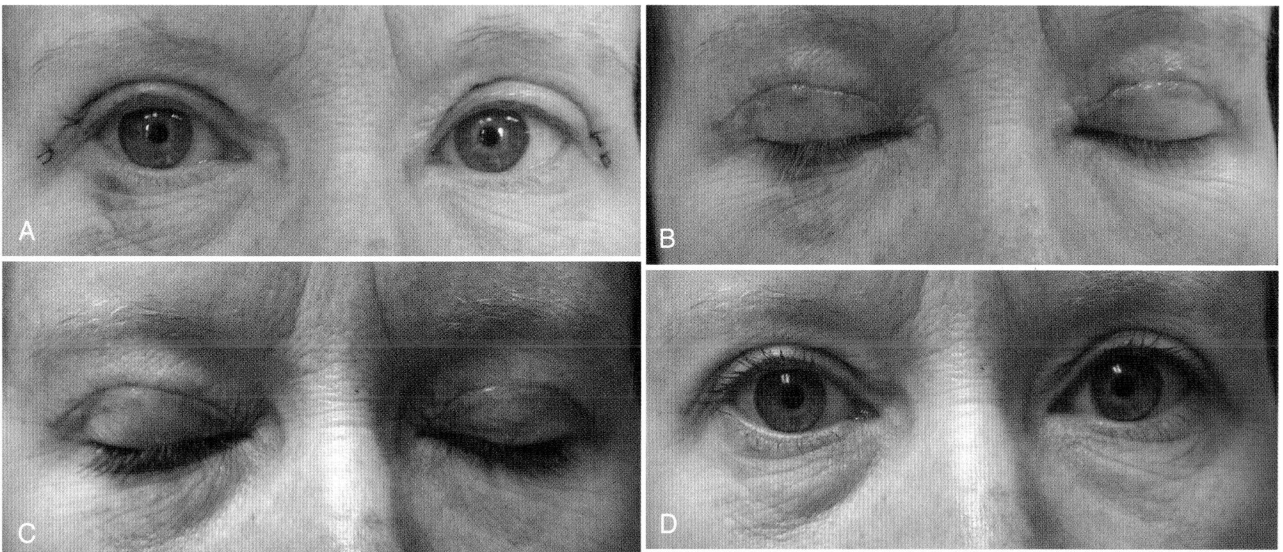

Figure 63-18 **A,** One week after surgery, before suture removal. Mild edema of the lids is evident. This resolves quickly once sutures are removed. **B,** One week after surgery with sutures removed. **C,** Appearance of incisions 2 weeks after surgery. **D,** Front view 2 weeks after surgery.

the globe. Ocular motility may be affected. There may be a ring of erythema/ecchymosis along both upper and lower eyelids. Pain and decreased vision often accompany this complication. Intraocular pressure is elevated. Check the optic nerve head with an ophthalmoscope. If the optic nerve head is swollen, the patient needs to be referred immediately for an emergent lateral canthotomy. Regardless of nerve status, if retrobulbar hemorrhage is suspected, urgent referral is advised.

Infection: Rare; however, the clinician should diligently examine the incisions and the surrounding skin for signs of infection/cellulitis at all follow-up visits and instruct the patient on how to monitor for signs of infection/cellulitis.

Postoperative Management

- Antibiotic ointment is applied sparingly to the incision lines three times per day for 1 week or until the next follow-up visit.
- Cold packs are applied directly to the lids (alternate 15 minutes on with 15 minutes off every hour while awake) for the first 48 hours. If edema persists, this may be extended.
- Area is to be kept clean and dry by gently cleansing with mild soapy solution (e.g., baby shampoo), which is rinsed with clean water and patted dry (do not rub!). Antibiotic ointment is then reapplied during the first week.
- Patient may use his or her usual choice of over-the-counter pain medication (e.g., Tylenol, Motrin) for discomfort if needed. Prescription-strength painkillers are generally not indicated.
- The patient is to return to clinic in 5 to 7 days for suture removal (Fig. 63-18).
- The patient should be advised to try to avoid direct sunlight for prolonged periods. If the patient is going to be outdoors, he or she should wear sunglasses with ultraviolet protection or a hat with a wide brim.
- After discontinuation of the antibiotic ointment at 1 week, the patient should continue to use a good skin moisturizer (preferably with a sunblock) along the incision lines for up to 8 weeks.
- The patient should be advised that the incisions will continue to heal for a period of 3 to 6 months and that the incision lines will gradually fade over the next 6 months to 1 year.

CPT/Billing Codes

15823 Blepharoplasty, upper lid excessive skin weighting down
- For bilateral procedures add -50 modifier.
- Major surgical follow-up global period of 90 days.
- 150% total payment (adjustment) for bilateral procedures applies.

ICD-9-CM Diagnostic Codes

374.33 Mechanical ptosis
374.87 Dermatochalasis

Patient Education Guides

See patient education and sample operative report online at www.expertconsult.com.

Suppliers

(See contact information online at www.expertconsult.com.)

Ellman International, Inc.
Wilson Ophthalmic Corp.

BIBLIOGRAPHY

Chen W: Oculoplastic Surgery: The Essentials. New York, Thieme, 2001.
Collin JRO: A Manual of Systematic Eyelid Surgery, 3rd ed. London, Butterworth-Heinemann, 2006.
Fagien S: Putterman's Cosmetic Oculoplastic Surgery, 4th ed. Philadelphia, WB Saunders, 2007.
Leatherbarrow B: Oculoplastic Surgery. London, Martin Dunitz, The Livery House, 2002.
Moy RL, Fincher EF: Blepharoplasty. In Dover JS (ed): Procedures in Cosmetic Dermatology. Philadelphia, Saunders, 2006.
Tyers AG, Collin JRO: Colour Atlas of Ophthalmic Plastic Surgery, 3rd ed. London, Butterworth-Heinemann, 2007.

CHAPTER 64

GINGIVAL MELANIN HYPERPIGMENTATION

Ali Gürkan • Fatih Arikan

Hyperpigmentation of the gingiva is caused by excessive deposition of melanin. It is more frequently observed in Asian, African, and Mediterranean populations, and has also been called *racial* or *physiologic pigmentation*. Pigmentation may vary not only among subjects of the same ethnic background but within different regions of the mouth. This kind of pigmentation presents as a well-demarcated, bilateral, dark brown, asymptomatic coloration in the keratinized gingiva, mostly in the anterior region. It is due to melanocyte overactivity; both dark- and light-skinned subjects have similar numbers of melanocytes in the gingiva. Because toxic agents in tobacco smoke induce melanocytes to produce melanin, smoking can cause hyperpigmentation in subjects with light skin and may aggravate pigmentation in dark-skinned individuals ("smoker's melanosis"). The severity and extent of melanosis are usually correlated with the duration and quantity of smoking, and the condition improves after the cessation of smoking.

Gingival melanin hyperpigmentation is an aesthetic problem rather than a medical problem. The appearance of the gingiva while smiling is essential to overall personal aesthetics. Because brown-black melanotic lesions mostly involve the anterior vestibular gingiva, they cause an unaesthetic smile. Therefore, depigmentation procedures have attracted much interest, and numerous techniques have been introduced to reverse this change. A novel gingival melanin depigmentation method using radiofrequency (RF) surgery offers advantages over other depigmentation methods, including speed, reliability, lack of postoperative pain, virtually no bleeding, and no discomfort from local anesthetic injection (Table 64-1).

Differential Diagnosis

The patient presenting with pigmented gingiva should be thoroughly evaluated regarding dental and medical history, and have an extraoral and intraoral examination as well as laboratory tests when indicated. Addison's disease (adrenal insufficiency) can also cause gingival hyperpigmentation.

Assess the following:

- Smoking habit (duration and number per day)
- Duration of pigmentation
- Skin pigmentation
- Perioral pigmented lesions (lips, face)
- Systemic diseases (e.g., Addison's)
- Systemic symptoms of malignancy (fatigue, malaise, weight loss)
- Medications
- Lymph nodes
- Characteristics of the pigmented lesions (size, number, distribution, shape, color, surface, and borders)

A biopsy should be performed if a lesion cannot be explained by other factors.

Indication

The removal of gingival melanosis.

Contraindications

- Cardiac pacemakers, cardiac defibrillator implants, cochlear implants (relative contraindication)
- Uncooperative patient

Equipment

- RF device (see Chapter 30, Radiofrequency Surgery [Modern Electrosurgery]).
- Small ball-tip (no. 135; Ellman International, Inc., Oceanside, NY) or, preferably, L-shaped advanced-composition alloy electrode (Ellman no. 136); the L-shaped electrode has a flat end, making it suitable for a "tapping" action.
- 10% lidocaine spray.
- Mouth retractor.

Technique (Dual Frequency)

- Place the retractor and apply anesthetic spray to the region of interest.
- Adjust the device to the cutting mode (10 to 11) for thick gingiva or to the coag mode (7) for thin gingiva.
- Melanocytes are primarily located in the basal and suprabasal cell layers of the epithelium. Therefore, touch the pigmented areas lightly with the electrode tip. Remove the electrode as soon as the tissue around the electrode turns whitish. A "tapping" type approach covering all the pigmented areas works best (Fig. 64-1).
- Repeat the procedure for all pigmented areas.
- During the following week, slight redness is observed around the margins of the RF-treated lesions.
- Epithelialization is completed in 10 days, and at 2 weeks after the first treatment, a second procedure can be performed to treat any residual pigmentation.

Figures 64-2 through 64-5 illustrate the results of RF surgical treatment of gingival hyperpigmentation in a variety of cases.

Postprocedure Care

- Gentle brushing
- Antiseptic rinse
- Analgesic drugs the day of surgery (usually not needed)

TABLE 64-1 Comparison of Gingival Depigmentation Methods

Method	Bleeding	Needle Anesthesia	Post-operative Pain	Periodontal Dressing	Ease of Access to Interdental Papillary Region	Major Disadvantage of Method
Scalpel surgery	+	+	+	+	–	Bleeding
Particle abrasive methods	+	+	+	+	–	Bleeding
Laser	–	+	–	–	+	Expense
Gas cryosurgery	–	–	–	–	–	Safety
Tetrafluoroethane (TFE) cryosurgery (e.g., Envirotech Freezer Spray, Medi-Frig, and Verruca-Freeze)	–	–	–	–	–	Lack of access to interdental papillary region
Radiofrequency surgery	–	–	–	–	+	None

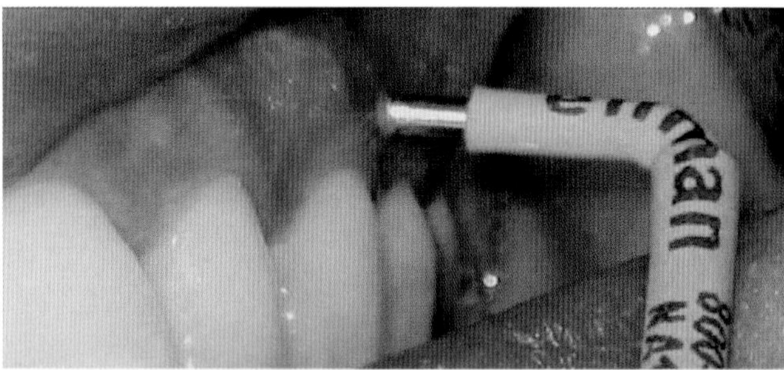

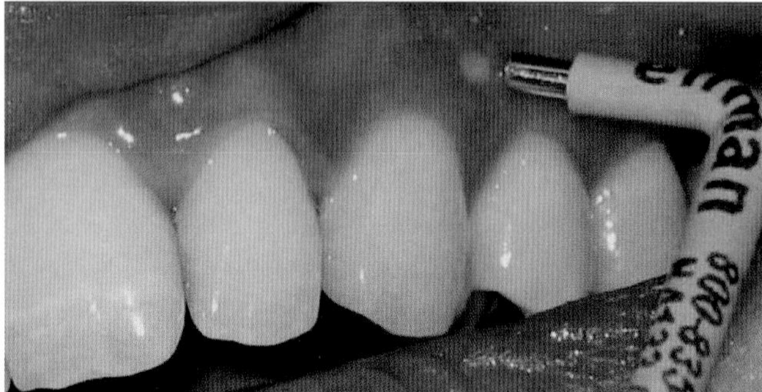

Figure 64-1 Tapping the electrode on the pigmented gingival tissues. A topical anesthetic has been applied.

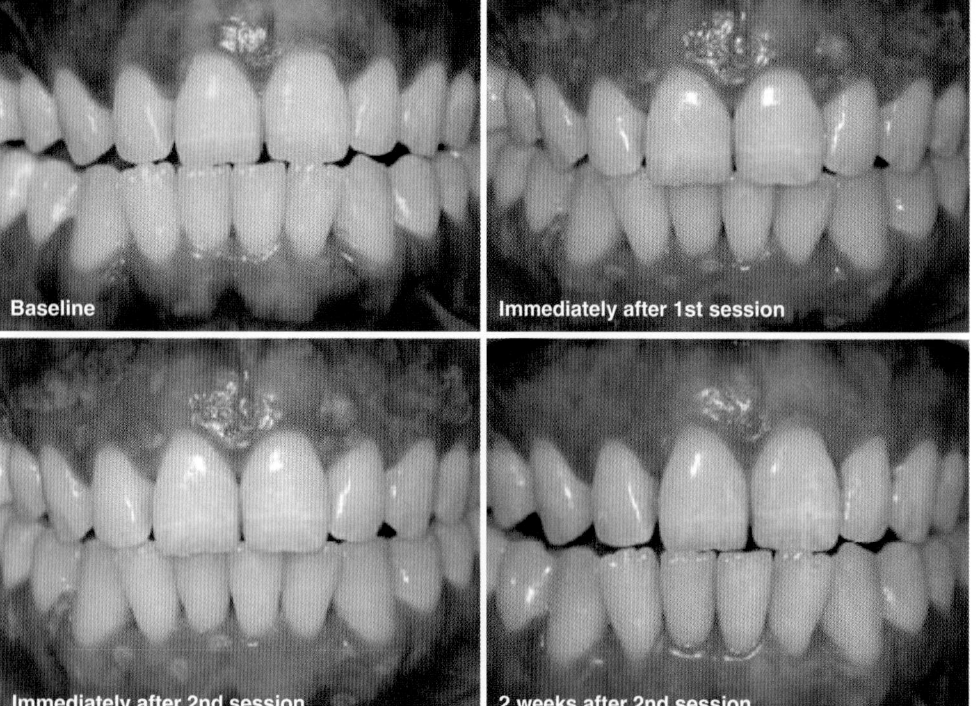

Figure 64-2 Clinical view of a case before and after the procedure.

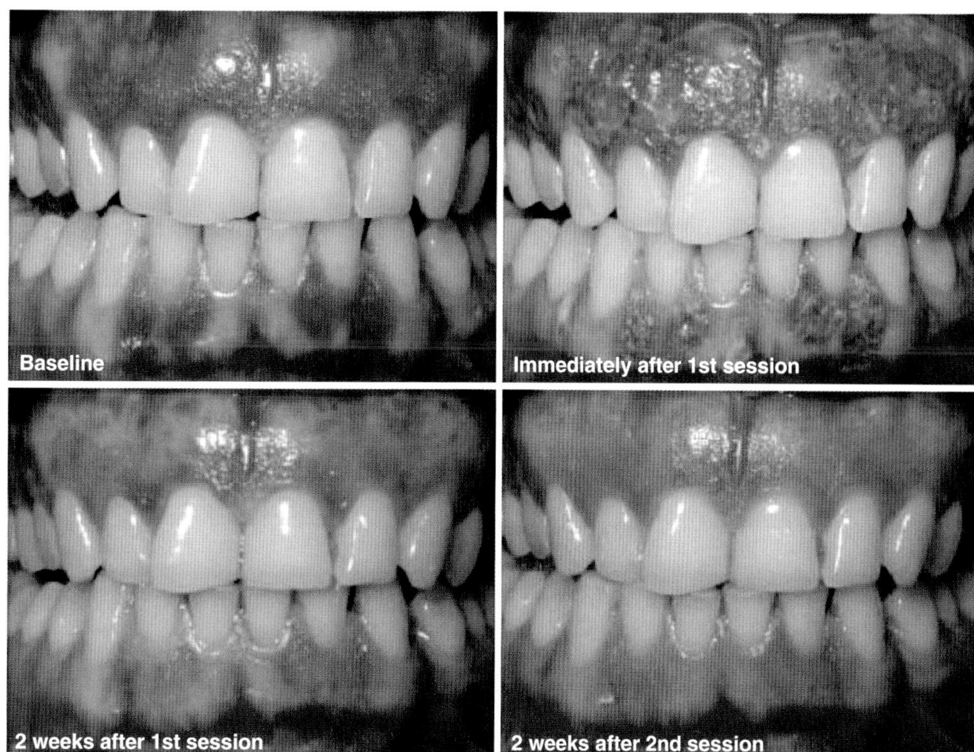

Figure 64-3 Total removal of heavily pigmented lesions with two RF sessions over a 4-week period.

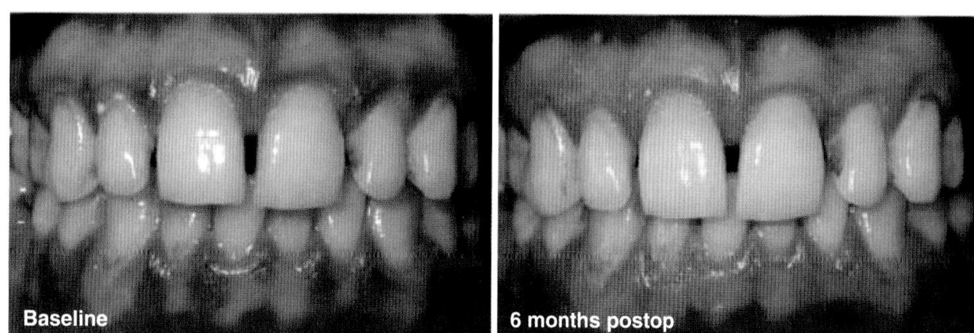

Figure 64-4 Clinical view of a case before and 6 months after RF depigmentation treatment.

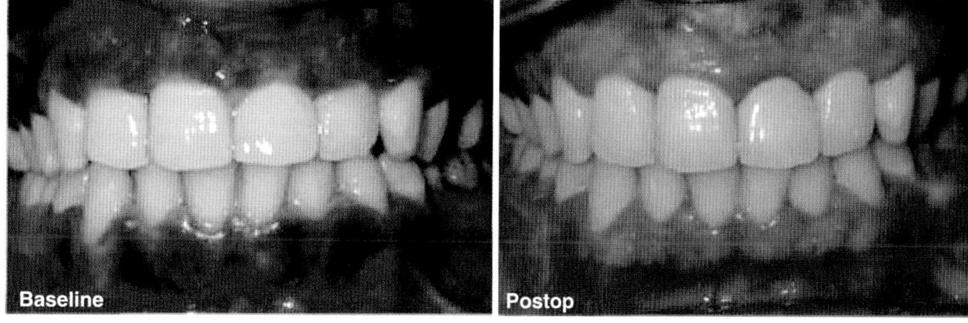

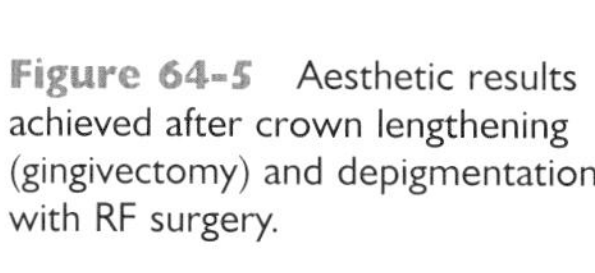
Figure 64-5 Aesthetic results achieved after crown lengthening (gingivectomy) and depigmentation with RF surgery.

COMPLICATIONS

- If the electrode is held in place longer than necessary or if too high a setting is used, excessive tissue necrosis can occur, increasing postoperative pain and compromising healing.
- We have never observed hypopigmentation of the pigmented gingiva after treatment. The brown gingiva becomes pale pink like the neighboring tissues after the healing period at 2 weeks. We have followed these patients for up to 1 year and observed no recurrence, even when they have not changed their smoking habits. In the event of recurrence, the simple procedure can be easily repeated. All of our patients indicated they were willing to repeat the procedure if needed, scoring their satisfaction with the results as "excellent."

BIBLIOGRAPHY

Arikan F, Gürkan A: Cryosurgical treatment of gingival melanin pigmentation with tetrafluoroethane. Oral Surg Oral Med Oral Pathol Oral Radiol Endod 103:452–457, 2007.

Axéll T, Hedin CA: Epidemiologic study of excessive oral melanin pigmentation with special reference to the influence of tobacco habits. Scand J Dent Res 90:434–442, 1982.

Hedin CA: Smokers' melanosis: Occurrence and localization in the attached gingiva. Arch Dermatol 113:1533–1538, 1977.

Kauzman A, Pavone M, Blanas N, Bradley G: Pigmented lesions of the oral cavity: Review, differential diagnosis, and case presentations. J Can Dent Assoc 70:682–683, 2004.

Sherman JA: Oral Radiosurgery: An Illustrated Clinical Guide, 3rd ed. Basingstoke, UK, Taylor & Francis, 2005.

SECTION 4

Eyes, Ears, Nose, and Throat

Section Editor: GRANT C. FOWLER

CHAPTER 65

Chalazion and Hordeolum

James L. Jackson

Patients with a chalazion or hordeolum, focal inflammatory conditions of the eyelids, are frequently encountered in primary care. Invariably they complain of a "stye." Both conditions may be treated by the prudent nonophthalmologist using a minor surgical procedure in the office setting. However, care must be taken not to injure the eye, the eyelid, or sensitive components, particularly the lacrimal drainage system ("tear ducts") or the eyelid margin.

A *chalazion* (Fig. 65-1) is an acute or chronic granulomatous inflammation of a meibomian gland in the eyelid. A *hordeolum* is an acute abscess of a meibomian, Zeis', or Moll's gland (see Fig. 65-10). An *internal hordeolum* points onto the conjunctival surface of the lid, whereas an *external hordeolum* points onto the external surface of the skin or the margin of the lid.

The meibomian glands are basically sebaceous glands located deep within both eyelids (Fig. 65-2). They constantly produce a lipid material that drains through long ducts and emerges from orifices at the eyelid margin. This lipid material then enters the tear film to help keep the surface of the eye lubricated while also slowing evaporation of the tears.

Meibomian secretions are naturally viscous, but under certain conditions they become thick enough to plug the duct of the gland. Because the gland continues to produce secretions, they must go somewhere (similar to a sebaceous cyst); consequently, the secretions eventually leak between the cells of the gland into the surrounding tissue of the eyelid. Here, the secretions incite a chronic granulomatous inflammatory reaction (*chalazion*). As more secretions are produced, the inflammation worsens and it may smolder chronically, sometimes for a year or longer.

Clinically, the inflammation causes localized swelling, edema, or a nodule within the lid, sometimes associated with erythema and mild tenderness. A chalazion may be located at the lid margin or up to a few millimeters away. At times it may be prominent externally, but more commonly a chalazion will be found on the inner (palpebral conjunctiva) surface of the lid. Associated inflammation may cause a soft or even liquid center, and patients may report spontaneous drainage internally, externally, or through the lid margin, which may lead to clinical improvement or resolution. A chalazion may also wax and wane.

Some people experience multiple chalazia over time or even concurrently. Multiple chalazia are more commonly seen in people with acne rosacea or chronic blepharitis. Chronic blepharitis is characterized by eyelid margin inflammation, thickening, and erythema associated with bacterial colonization and crusting at the base of the eyelashes. Chronic blepharitis usually requires a slit-lamp examination to make the diagnosis (see Chapter 67, Slit-Lamp Examination); even with a slit lamp, the findings are often subtle and not easily detected by the nonophthalmologist.

In contrast to a chalazion, a *hordeolum* is an acute bacterial abscess of a meibomian, Zeis', or Moll's gland (see Fig. 65-2). Hordeola are classified as internal or external based on the primary anatomic focus of the inflammation (which is usually obvious). Typically characterized by an acute tender mass within the eyelid, associated with erythema and a collection of pus, hordeola are often accompanied by acute cellulitis of the eyelid. Such cellulitis, in turn, is characterized by erythema, edema, and tenderness of the surrounding skin. ("Eyelid cellulitis" is a different, much more localized entity than the less common "orbital cellulitis," a systemic, vision- and life-threatening condition with which the patient is toxic with a high fever.) A hordeolum usually drains spontaneously at 5 to 7 days, often relieving the symptoms. Hordeola are frequently associated with *Staphylococcus* infections and acute blepharitis, and these both usually respond to antibiotics.

To differentiate a chalazion from a hordeolum can be a clinical challenge. Although a hordeolum is usually more tender and tense with obvious fluctuance, a chalazion may have a liquefied center; however, it is usually not a collection of pus. The presence of significant eyelid cellulitis also usually suggests a hordeolum, but a chalazion may be associated with a degree of surrounding erythema and edema (although it is usually to a lesser degree). The natural history of a hordeolum is usually more acute; yet, a chalazion can present acutely. It may also be important to differentiate a chalazion or hordeolum from other eyelid disorders. If the swelling is located nasal to the medial canthus (the corner where the upper and lower eyelids meet), the patient likely has *dacryocystitis* rather than a chalazion or hordeolum. In this situation, strongly consider prompt referral to an ophthalmologist because dacryocystitis can lead to serious sequelae. Because of the facial anatomy, bacterial dacryocystitis can dissect posteriorly to the cavernous sinus and beyond, with grave consequences.

Chalazion

Medical Management

A chalazion may respond to one or more of the following medical treatments:

- Warm compresses to the eyelid (four times a day if possible).
- Eyelid scrubs of the lid margins at bedtime each night (at base of eyelashes) with commercially available ocular cleansing pads or diluted baby shampoo (diluted to half strength with water, applied with a cotton swab or washcloth).

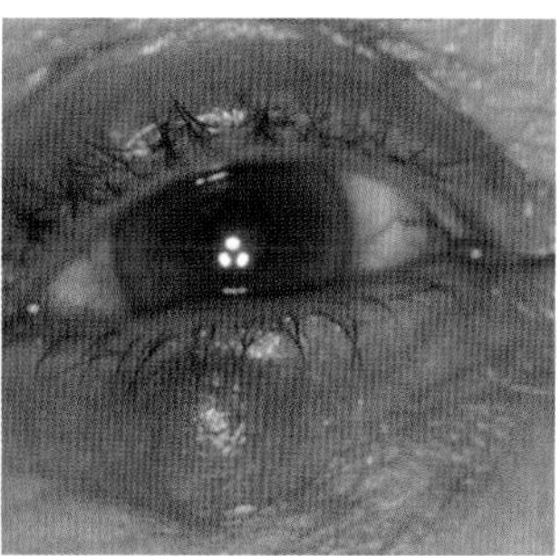

Figure 65-1 Chalazion, lower lid.

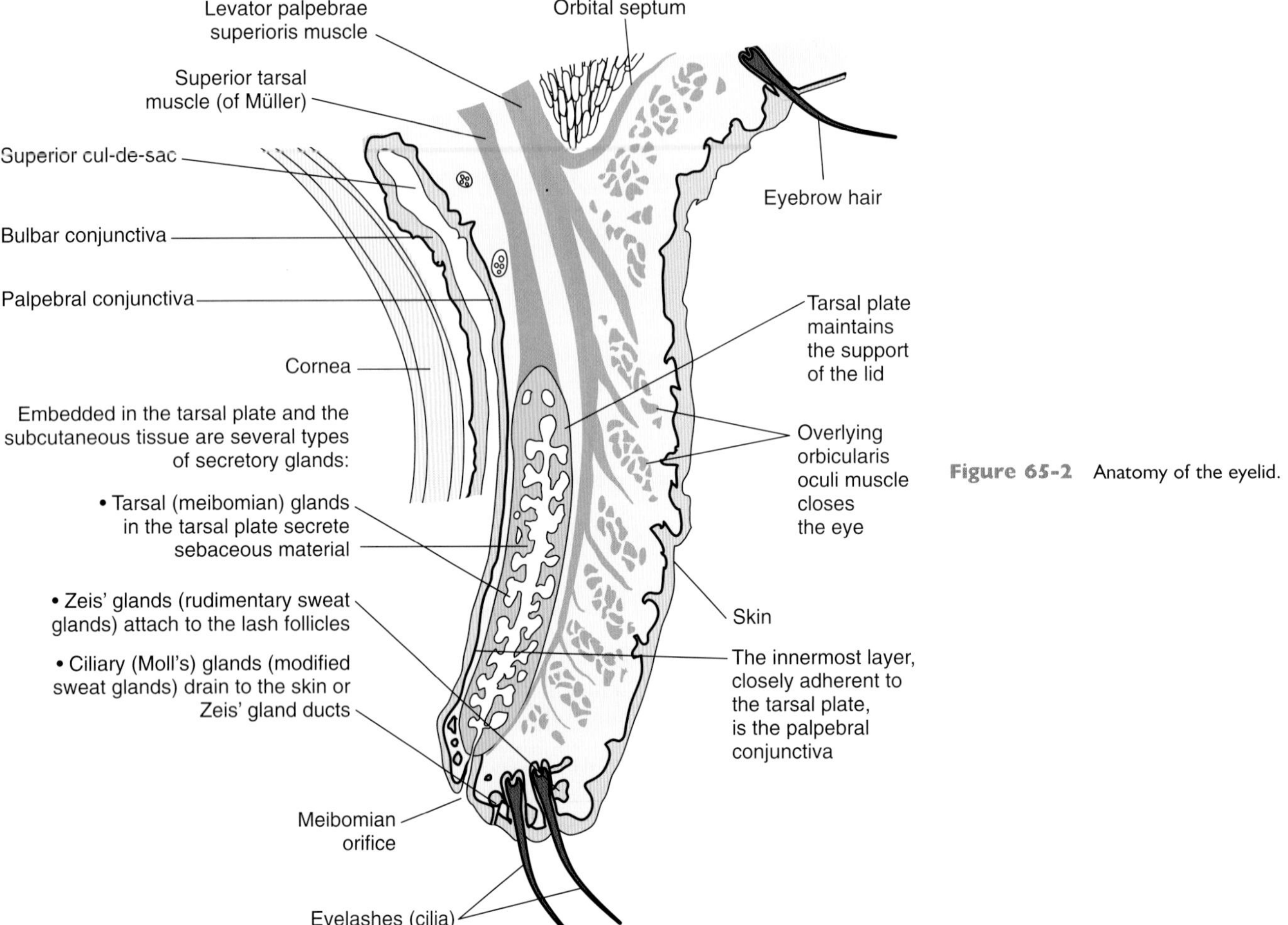
Levator palpebrae superioris muscle
Orbital septum
Superior tarsal muscle (of Müller)
Superior cul-de-sac
Eyebrow hair
Bulbar conjunctiva
Palpebral conjunctiva
Tarsal plate maintains the support of the lid
Cornea
Embedded in the tarsal plate and the subcutaneous tissue are several types of secretory glands:
• Tarsal (meibomian) glands in the tarsal plate secrete sebaceous material
Overlying orbicularis oculi muscle closes the eye
• Zeis' glands (rudimentary sweat glands) attach to the lash follicles
Skin
• Ciliary (Moll's) glands (modified sweat glands) drain to the skin or Zeis' gland ducts
The innermost layer, closely adherent to the tarsal plate, is the palpebral conjunctiva
Meibomian orifice
Eyelashes (cilia)

Figure 65-2 Anatomy of the eyelid.

- Application of antibiotic ointment (usually erythromycin) to eyelid margin after washing.
- Oral doxycycline.
- Intralesional steroid injection (e.g., triamcinolone acetonide) 40 mg/mL, 0.2 to 0.4 mL, 30-gauge needle through the conjunctival (inner) surface of the eyelid, after the use of topical anesthesia (e.g., tetracaine drops). However, steroid injection carries the risk of skin hypopigmentation, especially in dark-skinned individuals.

Indications for Excision

- Chalazion unresponsive to medical management
- Substantial size (large enough to palpate)
- Cosmetic deformity
- Visual problems (e.g., astigmatism, blurry vision)
- Patient desires removal

Contraindications to Excision

- Chalazion that has recently drained through the skin or with very thin overlying skin (relative contraindication, increases risk of a full-thickness "buttonhole" defect of the eyelid, leading to a visible scar and prolonged healing time).
- Skin crusted or markedly inflamed (excision is usually performed from the inner surface of the eyelid and, again, a "buttonhole" defect may result).
- Anticoagulated patient (relative contraindication).
- Chalazion near the lacrimal punctum. The lacrimal punctum is a tiny opening in the nasal aspect of each eyelid margin. Tears drain through the punctum into the canaliculus, which runs just beneath the skin toward the nose. Damage to the punctum or canaliculus may lead to chronic tearing and the need for a complicated surgical repair. If the chalazion is close enough to the punctum that there is a chance it has been damaged, the patient should be referred to an ophthalmologist for excision.

Equipment

See Figure 65-3.

- Mask and goggles to follow universal blood and body fluid precautions
- Sterile tray
- Skin marking pen
- Topical ophthalmic anesthetic drops (e.g., tetracaine)
- Alcohol pads
- Local anesthetic for injection (2% lidocaine with epinephrine), 3-mL syringe, 30-gauge needle
- Povidone–iodine (Betadine) swabs
- Sterile gloves
- Sterile drape, fenestrated
- Chalazion clamps (two or three sizes)
- Scalpel (no. 15 blade)
- Chalazion curettes (two sizes)
- Cotton swabs

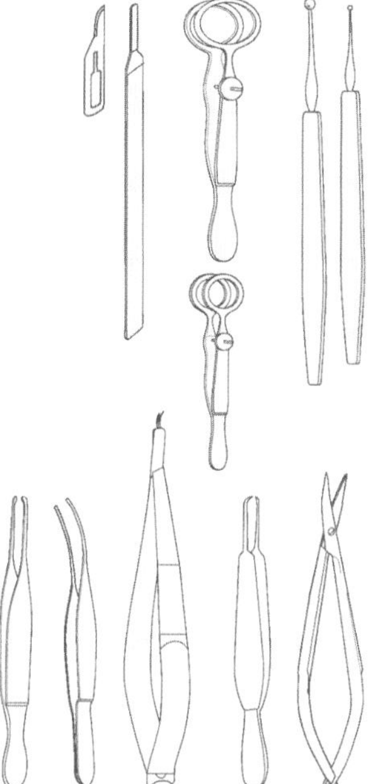

Figure 65-3 Instruments for chalazion excision. *Top row, from left to right:* scalpel (no. 15 or no. 11 blade); chalazion clamps; chalazion curettes. *Bottom row, from left to right:* ocular tissue forceps; needle holder; suturing forceps; Westcott conjunctival scissors.

- Ocular tissue forceps, 0.2 tips
- Westcott conjunctival scissors
- 4 × 4 gauze pads
- Antibiotic–steroid combination ophthalmic ointment (e.g., Maxitrol or TobraDex)
- Eyepatches (two or three) and medical tape
- Suture (6-0 nylon), needle holder, and suture scissors (only in event of full-thickness eyelid defect occurring as a complication)

Preprocedure Patient Preparation

Unless the patient is at high risk of cardiovascular events, he or she should discontinue aspirin or other antiplatelet medications for 1 week and anticoagulants for 4 days before the procedure. The patient should be counseled about the risks for scarring, a possible need for sutures, the risk of recurrence and need for repeat excision, short-term swelling/bruising of eyelid, excessive bleeding, infection, and, rarely, damage to the lacrimal drainage system resulting in chronic tearing. It will be important for the patient to remain motionless during the procedure. The patient may experience some discomfort and tearing with injection of the anesthetic.

Technique

Universal blood and body fluid precautions should be followed. The clinician can achieve good access to the eye by sitting near the top of the head. The patient should lie supine. Good lighting is essential. Injection of the local anesthetic may make palpation of the chalazion difficult, so it is helpful to use a skin marker before injection.

1. Administer several drops of a topical ophthalmic anesthetic. Then inject 2% lidocaine with epinephrine through the skin, infiltrating the area where the chalazion clamp is to be applied (Fig. 65-4A).
2. Place a chalazion clamp over the chalazion, with the open side inside the eyelid (Fig. 65-4B). Avoid damaging the eyelid margin. Tighten the clamp to achieve a firm grip on the eyelid, which will maintain hemostasis during the procedure. Do not overtighten. Evert the eyelid using the clamp as a lever (Fig. 65-5). The chalazion should now be evident and bulging through the opening of the clamp.
3. With a no. 15 blade, make two incisions in the form of a cross, taking care not to go through the eyelid skin but only into the substance of the chalazion (Fig. 65-6; Fig. 65-4C). Some soft material may be released, confirming that the incision is in the correct location.
4. Use the curettes and cotton swabs to remove as much soft, inflamed material as possible (Fig. 65-7; Fig. 65-4D). Remove as much granulation tissue as you can with forceps (Fig. 65-8).
5. Using the Westcott conjunctival scissors and tissue forceps, remove a small amount of the inflamed tarsal plate (the cartilage underneath), if necessary (Fig. 65-4E). Take care not to tent the deeper tissue, which can lead to inadvertent incision of the underlying skin and cause a "buttonhole" defect. Again, avoid damaging the eyelid margin.

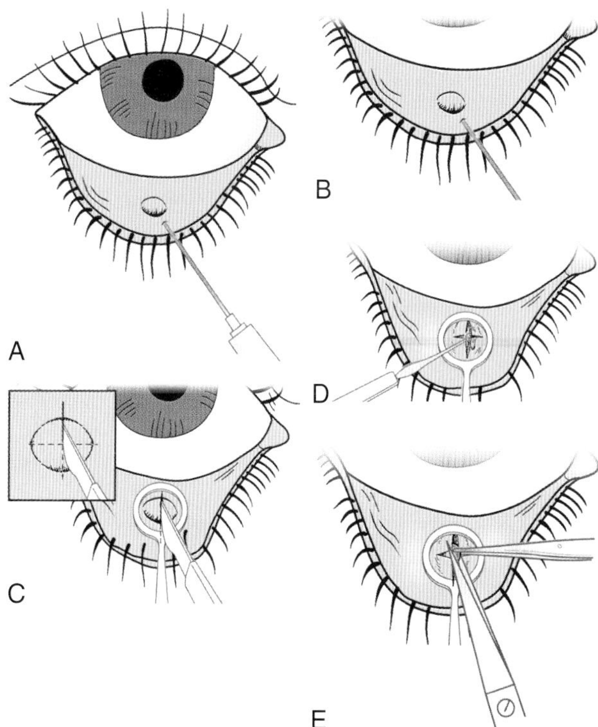

Figure 65-4 Chalazion excision. **A,** Inject anesthetic. **B,** Place chalazion clamp. **C,** Incise with scalpel, making an "X" over the lesion. **D,** Curette interior of chalazion to remove soft, inflamed material. **E,** Remove small amount of inflamed tarsus with Westcott conjunctival scissors and tissue forceps.

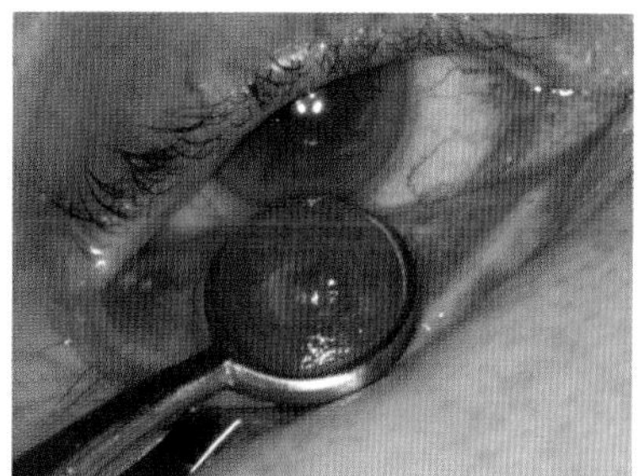

Figure 65-5 After topical anesthetic drops are instilled, a chalazion clamp is used to stabilize and evert lid.

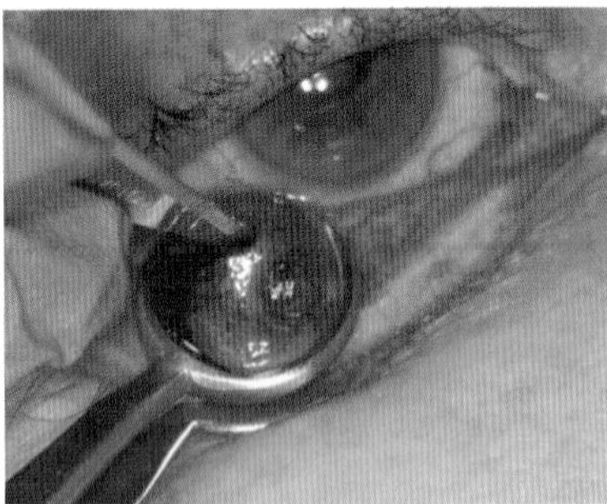

Figure 65-6 Incising the chalazion using a no. 15 blade. Make an "X" over the lesion.

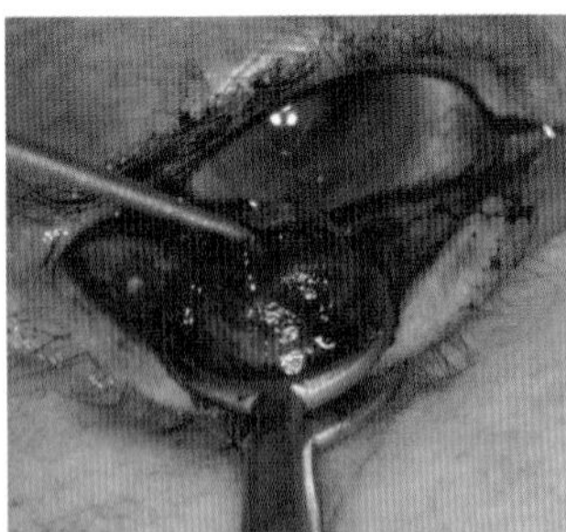

Figure 65-7 Removing contents with a chalazion curette.

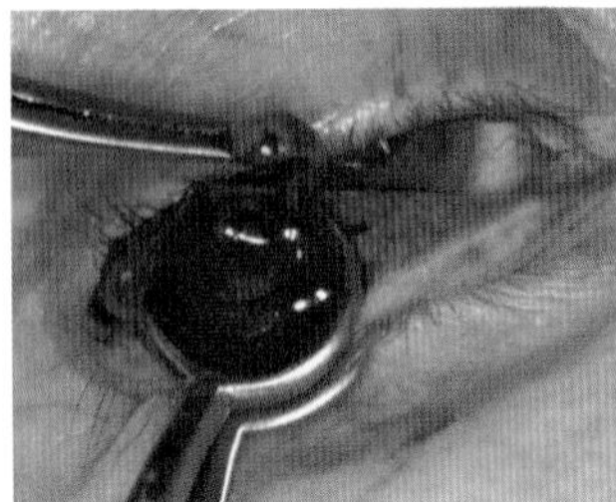

Figure 65-8 Removing granulation tissue with forceps (pickups).

6. Remove the chalazion clamp, which will likely lead to significant bleeding because of the excellent vascularity of the eyelid. Apply direct pressure with cotton swabs or gauze pads to achieve hemostasis. This may take 5 to 10 minutes (Fig. 65-9). Once hemostasis has definitely been achieved, apply an antibiotic–steroid eye ointment and place a pressure patch on the eye (see Chapter 66, Corneal Abrasions and Removal of Corneal or Conjunctival Foreign Bodies, Fig. 66-5, for a technique on pressure patching).
7. If a full-thickness eyelid defect is present, suture the outer skin while taking care that the suture does not include the conjunctival (inner) surface of the eyelid; this would cause a great deal of irritation and possibly a corneal abrasion. If damage to the lacrimal punctum or canaliculus occurs inadvertently, promptly refer the patient to an ophthalmologist.
8. Beware of recurrent or multiple chalazia in older patients, especially with associated ocular inflammation. This could represent sebaceous cell carcinoma, which is very aggressive and not always noted on pathologic examination of an excised chalazion. If a presumed chalazion does not behave as expected after excision, particularly in an elderly patient, sebaceous cell carcinoma should be suspected even if the initial pathology report is negative. In that situation, the patient should be referred to an ophthalmologist.

Postprocedure Patient Education

The patient may remove the patch the evening after the procedure. Tell the patient that he or she can expect a large amount of clotted blood and mattering of the eyelid. The patient should then begin to apply an antibiotic eye ointment (e.g., erythromycin) in the eye twice a day until judged "back to normal." If the eyelid begins to bleed again, the patient should apply pressure until it stops, and should seek medical attention if the bleeding does not stop. If sutures were placed, they should be removed in 5 days.

Hordeolum

Medical Management

If less severe and not yet "pointing," the hordeolum may be treated with frequent warm compresses and an oral antibiotic directed against *Staphylococcus*. In fact, most hordeola respond to this management, with spontaneous drainage and resolution occurring in 5 to 7 days. However, if the patient is being treated medically, he or she should be watched closely in case the need for incision and drainage develops.

Indications for Incision and Drainage

- Hordeolum that fails medical management (Fig. 65-10)
- Hordeolum causing significant pain
- Hordeolum with significant localized accumulation of pus
- Previous or current eyelid cellulitis associated with hordeolum

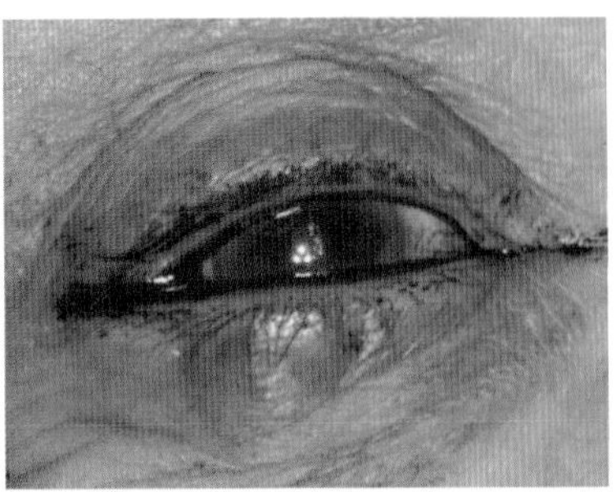

Figure 65-9 Postoperative appearance after chalazion removal.

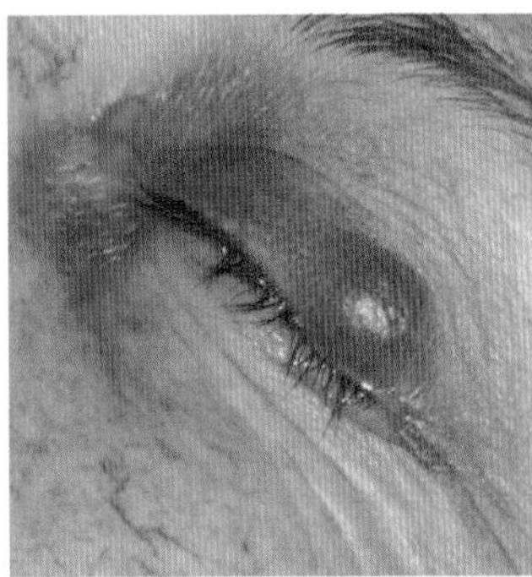

Figure 65-10 Hordeolum of upper lid.

Contraindications to Incision and Drainage

If the hordeolum is located near the lacrimal punctum (i.e., located nasal to the medial canthus), refer the patient to an ophthalmologist because of the risk of damaging the lacrimal drainage system.

Equipment

- Mask and goggles to follow universal blood and body fluid precautions
- Topical ophthalmic anesthetic drops (e.g., tetracaine)
- Alcohol pads
- Local anesthetic for injection, 2% lidocaine with epinephrine, 3-mL syringe, 30-gauge needle
- Nonsterile gloves
- Scalpel (no. 11 blade)
- Cotton swabs
- 4 × 4 gauze pads
- Tongue blade or metal elevator

Preprocedure Patient Preparation

Unless the patient is at high risk of cardiovascular events, he or she should discontinue aspirin or other antiplatelet medications for 1 week and anticoagulants for 4 days before the procedure (although it is usually necessary to perform the procedure without much advanced planning). The patient should be counseled about the risks of scarring, recurrence, and need for repeat incision and drainage, short-term swelling/bruising of eyelid, excessive bleeding, spread of infection, and, rarely, damage to the lacrimal drainage system resulting in chronic tearing. It will be important for the patient to remain motionless during the procedure. The patient may experience some discomfort and tearing with the injection of local anesthetic.

Technique

Universal blood and body fluid precautions should be followed. The hordeolum will point either internally or externally and should be incised from whichever surface allows the best access to the collection of pus (Fig. 65-11A).

1. Administer several drops of topical ophthalmic anesthetic. Then administer 2% lidocaine with epinephrine through the skin, infiltrating the area around the hordeolum. (Remember that anesthesia is more difficult to obtain in the presence of inflammation.) A tongue blade or metal elevator can be inserted behind the lid to protect the eye (Fig. 65-11B). It may be helpful to stabilize the hordeolum and lid with a chalazion clamp (Fig. 65-12).
2. Use a no. 11 scalpel blade to make an incision into the hordeolum until pus is obtained, taking great care to avoid a through-and-through eyelid defect or injury to the eyelid margin or eye. If significant cellulitis is present, it may be prudent to send a sample of the pus for culture and sensitivity testing.
3. After the pus is expressed (Fig. 65-13), apply direct pressure with gauze pads to achieve hemostasis. This may take 5 to 10 minutes. An eyepatch is not necessary.

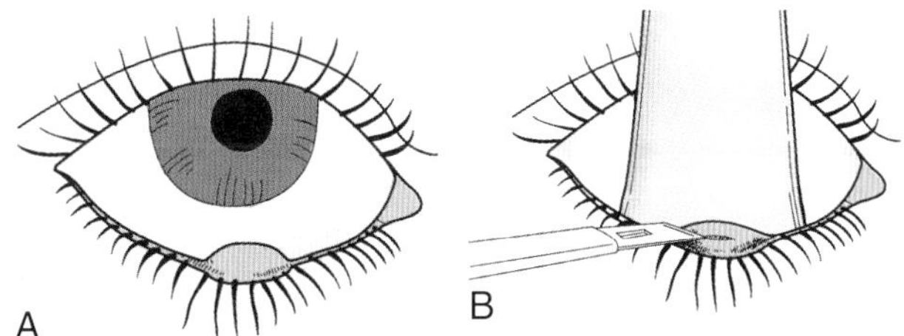

Figure 65-11 Hordeolum excision. **A,** Hordeolum pointing externally. **B,** Incision and drainage of external hordeolum, with a tongue blade or metal elevator protecting the eye.

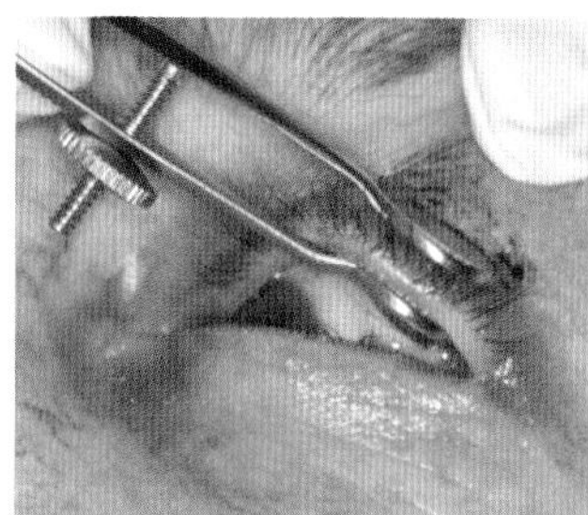

Figure 65-12 Stabilizing the hordeolum with a chalazion clamp.

4. If a full-thickness eyelid defect is present, do not suture the skin because of the presence of acute bacterial infection. Consider appropriate systemic antibiotic therapy for significant cellulitis of the eyelid. If damage to the lacrimal duct occurs inadvertently, promptly refer the patient to an ophthalmologist.

Postprocedure Patient Management

If the eyelid begins to bleed again, the patient should apply pressure until it stops and should seek medical attention if he or she is having difficulty controlling the bleeding. The patient will be given an oral antibiotic (with good coverage for *Staphylococcus*), and should be seen the next day. He or she may need to be seen daily for several days after the procedure until it is evident that the cellulitis is resolving and that pus is not reaccumulating. The patient should make an appointment in 2 to 3 weeks to further assess healing. It may take several weeks for the swelling and tissue distortion to return to normal.

Sample Operative Reports

See sample operative reports online at www.expertconsult.com.

CPT/Billing Codes

For chalazion excision

67800 Excision of chalazion, single
67801 Excision of chalazion, multiple, same lid
67805 Excision of chalazion, multiple, different lids

For incision and drainage of hordeolum

67700 Blepharotomy, drainage of abscess, eyelid

ICD-9-CM Diagnostic Codes

373.2 Chalazion
373.11 Hordeolum, NOS or external
373.12 Hordeolum, internal

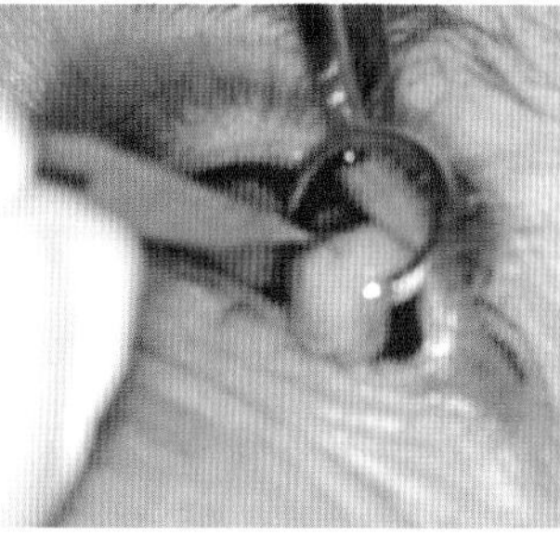

Figure 65-13 Incising the hordeolum: acute infection and drainage are evident.

Patient Education Guides

See the patient education and consent forms online at www.expertconsult.com.

Acknowledgment

The editors wish to recognize the contributions by Lewis E. Mehl, MD, PhD, to this chapter in a previous edition of this text.

Suppliers

(Any medical instrument supplier can provide the necessary equipment. See contact information online at www.expertconsult.com.)

Accutome
Storz (Bausch and Lomb)

Online Resources

For Patients

Medem: Medical Library. Available at http://www.medem.com/medlb/article_detaillb.cfm?article_ID=ZZZBDDQNPGE&sub_cat=37.

RxMed: Illness Information. Available at http://www.rxmed.com/b.main/b1.illness/b1.illness.html.

University of Maryland Health Center: Chalazions and styes. Available at http://www.health.umd.edu/Library/Handouts/Chalazion805.pdf.

For Clinicians

Bessette M: Hordeolum and stye. Available at www.emedicine.com/EMERG/topic755.htm.

Fansler JL, Schraga ED, Santen S: Chalazion. Available at www.emedicine.com/EMERG/topic94.htm.

Bibliography

Jacobs PM, Thaller VT, Wong D: Intralesional corticosteroid therapy of chalazion: A comparison with incision and curettage. Br J Ophthalmol 68:836–837, 1984.

Langston DP: Manual of Ocular Diagnosis and Therapy, 6th ed. Philadelphia, Lippincott Williams & Wilkins, 2008.

Neff AG, Carter KD: Benign eyelid lesions. In Yanoff M, Duker JS (eds): Ophthalmology, 2nd ed. St. Louis, Mosby, 2004, pp 698–710.

Usatine RP: The Color Atlas of Family Medicine. New York, McGraw-Hill, 2009.

CHAPTER 66

Corneal Abrasions and Removal of Corneal or Conjunctival Foreign Bodies

Grant C. Fowler

Patients with "something in the eye," a corneal or conjunctival abrasion or foreign body, are common for primary care clinicians. In most cases, the management is uncomplicated and can be completed in the clinician's office; however, knowledge of certain principles should help avoid impaired vision or blindness.

A detailed history is important, especially knowing what the patient was doing when he or she first noticed a problem. For instance, was the patient wearing eye protection? Was he or she around hammered metal? Did he or she come into contact with a high-velocity foreign body?

NOTE: In the past, corneal abrasions were treated with eye patching and mydriatics; however, there is little evidence to support such therapy, and eye patching may even impede healing. Consequently, most clinicians now use ophthalmic nonsteroidal anti-inflammatory drugs (NSAIDs) and an ophthalmic antibiotic for treatment. Some of the evidence supporting this approach is discussed further in the "Technique" section. Also, if a slit lamp is available, a more thorough evaluation of the eye may be performed for a corneal abrasion or foreign body (see Chapter 67, Slit-Lamp Examination). In the absence of a slit lamp, this chapter indicates when a slit-lamp referral is required.

Fluorescein Examination of the Cornea and Conjunctiva

Indications

- Unilateral foreign body sensation, hypersensitivity to light, excess tearing, or pain—especially on opening or closing the eye
- Red eye
- Eye trauma
- After airbag deployment in automobile accidents
- Unilateral, persistent eye irritation in contact lens wearer
- History of exposure to ultraviolet (UV) light from such sources as a welding torch, sunlight, or a tanning bed (UV light can penetrate the cornea even when the patient's eyes are closed if protective lenses are not worn)
- Mild chemical exposure to eye
- Neonates or infants with persistent crying, unilateral tearing, hypersensitivity to light, or conjunctival inflammation
- Eye discharge in mask-ventilated newborn or heavily sedated or paralyzed adults on a ventilator

NOTE: Hypersensitivity to light, excess tearing, and painful or red eye are also signs and symptoms of glaucoma (see Chapter 68, Tonometry). If there is no foreign body sensation, the patient should be evaluated for acute glaucoma.

Contraindications

Patients with the following symptoms should be referred to an ophthalmologist after they have been provided initial urgent care:

- Suspected high-velocity injury to the eye (e.g., patients exposed to metal hammering or heavy machinery). High-speed metallic or nonmetallic fragments can penetrate the globe while only causing minimal symptoms and damage to the cornea. As a result, significant internal damage must be excluded. If penetration of the globe is apparent, fluorescein staining is usually avoided because it may make further evaluation or surgery more difficult.
- A hyphema, lens opacification, scleral tear, abnormal anterior chamber examination, or irregularity of the pupil. These findings suggest that the globe has been penetrated, and an ophthalmologist needs to be involved. Orbital x-ray films may confirm a metal foreign body. A spiral computed tomography scan or ultrasonography may also confirm a metal foreign body; magnetic resonance imaging is contraindicated if there is a possible ferromagnetic object.
- Long-standing (>24 hours) inflammation as evidenced by iritis, photophobia, or ciliary blush. These findings suggest the presence of an intraocular foreign body or a more serious injury and require slit-lamp examination and evaluation by an ophthalmologist.

  NOTE: A pressure patch is contraindicated in a penetration injury of the globe or a complex lid laceration. For such injuries, a nonpressure protective eye shield should be applied before referral. Metal shields are manufactured for this purpose, or a nonpressure shield can be fashioned from a paper cup (Fig. 66-1). All patches and shields should be taped in the same direction, from the medial forehead across the eye and toward the ear.

- Exposure to caustic or acidic media. Immediate management includes copious irrigation for at least 15 minutes. (It can begin at home with tap water from a shower or hose.)
- Mild chemical exposure. If the clinician is not knowledgeable about or comfortable with managing the case after contacting a Poison Control Center, the patient should be referred.
- Ruptured globe.
- Uncooperative patient. (Infants may have to be sedated; see Chapter 7, Pediatric Sedation and Analgesia.)

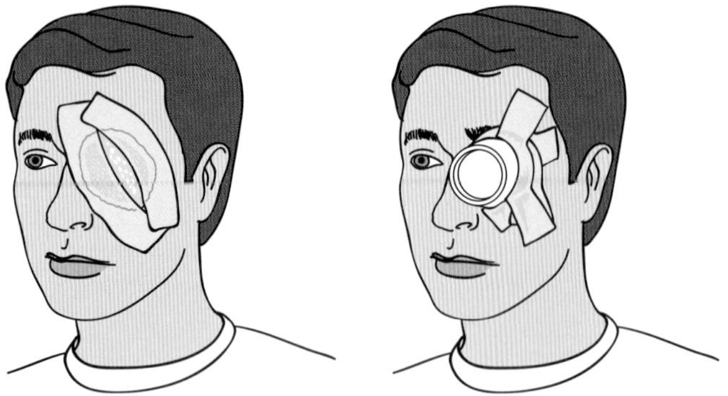

Figure 66-1 Nonpressure patch to protect ruptured globe. A metal shield or a paper cup can be used.

Equipment

- Snellen chart at 6 m (20 ft), or an equivalent visual acuity chart (Fig. 66-2). If a chart is unavailable, ask the patient to read a magazine at arm's length. If the patient cannot do so, measure and record the distance at which the patient can count fingers.
- Topical ophthalmic anesthetic such as 0.5% proparacaine (e.g., Alcaine, Kainair, Ophthaine, Ophthetic, Paracaine, Proparacaine), unless contraindicated (e.g., ruptured globe or allergy to local anesthetics).
- Sterile fluorescein sodium strips. (Because fluorescein is incompatible with preservatives effective against *Pseudomonas* and *Proteus*, multidose dropper bottles of fluorescein solution should not be used. Inoculating abraded corneal epithelium with bacteria could cause infection, permanent scarring, or blindness.)

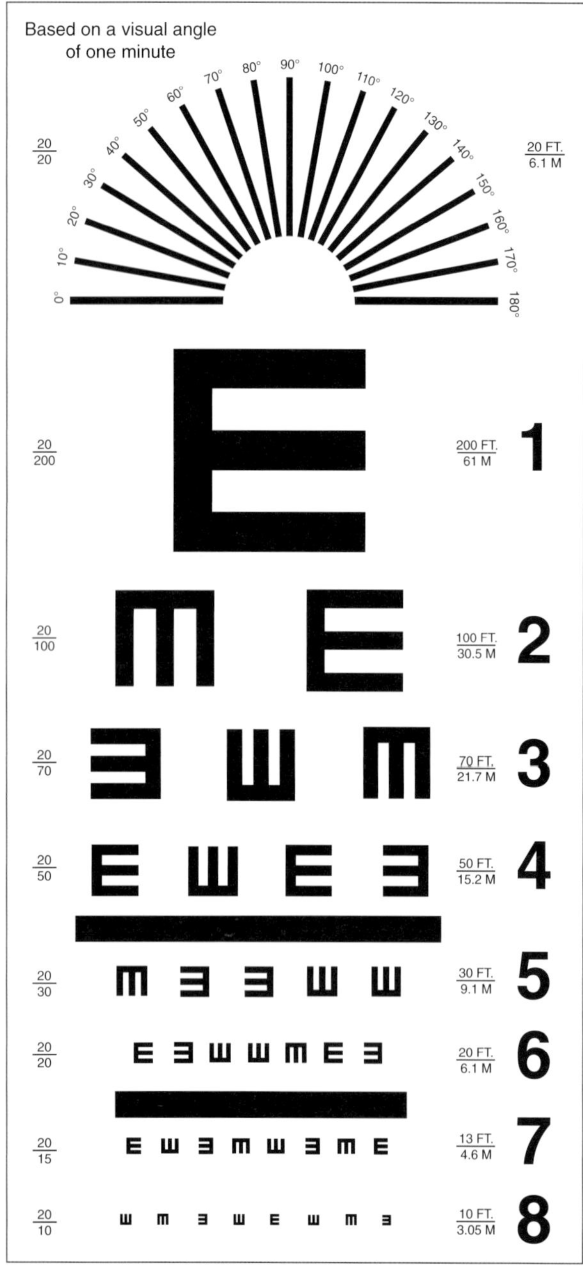

Figure 66-2 **A,** Illiterate E chart. **B,** Near-vision chart.

- Bright white light source (a single-point source such as a penlight is preferable).
- Cobalt-blue light source (Wood's lamp is adequate).
- An 8- to 10-power magnification lens (loupes, a magnifying glass, a colposcope, or an ophthalmoscope on the +20 to +40 diopter setting).
- Sterile cotton-tipped applicators.
- Isotonic ophthalmic irrigant (e.g., Dacriose, Ringer's lactate, normal saline).
- Facial tissues (e.g., Kleenex).

Preprocedure Patient Preparation

The indications for the examination should be explained to the patient as well as any risks or alternatives. The patient needs to know what will occur during the examination, and that he or she may be asked to direct vision to certain locations. Eyedrops and dye will probably be necessary to enhance the examination. Contact lenses should be removed before the eye is stained (fluorescein can stain them permanently). Before instilling fluorescein, the patient should be warned that objects in his or her vision may temporarily appear yellow. Tears may also remain yellow for a short time after the examination and might stain skin or clothing, at least temporarily, so the patient should avoid rubbing his or her eyes or drying tears on something that might stain.

Patients should be instructed to breathe normally and, especially children, may be asked at certain times to remain as still as possible. Children may need assistance with holding still. Patients should know to blink normally unless their eye is being held open by the examiner or they are asked to hold their eye open. They should be aware of the need for the examiner to touch their face and even to pull on their eyelids. Before instilling the topical anesthetic, tell the patient that it may cause a burning sensation until the eye becomes numb. Because patients with a corneal abrasion are usually hypersensitive to light, let them know when you are going to need a bright white light for only a short while, and that the room will otherwise be darkened. The remainder of the examination is done with a blue light, which should be more comfortable. Reassurance that this bright light will not cause permanent visual damage is usually appreciated. In fact, patients should be told that the reason for using this bright light (in most cases) is to *prevent* permanent damage to their vision. After the clinician has located the necessary equipment, the lights in the room can be dimmed during the remainder of the examination.

If an abrasion is diagnosed, emphasize the need for the patient to follow up daily with the clinician until it is completely healed. This will detect early complications such as infection. Instruct the patient to call the office if persistent or recurrent symptoms occur. Patients should also be instructed not to drive if the abrasion impairs their vision or depth perception.

Technique

1. Check and document visual acuity in both eyes *before* instilling topical anesthetic. Documentation of baseline visual acuity *before* the topical anesthetic is applied is important because initial discomfort due to the anesthetic (e.g., burning, stinging) may later be suspected by the patient as having caused impaired vision. If the patient normally wears corrective lenses (e.g., glasses) for refractive error, check visual acuity with refraction. After the acuity check, the patient will probably be most comfortable in the supine position for the remainder of the examination.

   NOTE: If the patient's corrective lenses are not available, a pinhole myopia corrector can be used. These are commercially available, but they are also easy to make. With an 18-gauge needle, punch 8 to 10 holes within a 5-cm (2-inch) circle on an index card. Have the patient select the hole that provides the best vision when viewing the Snellen chart. This effectively corrects the patient's vision.

2. Hand the patient a tissue and instill one to two drops of topical anesthetic into his or her affected eye. (This is not mandatory but does facilitate patient cooperation and comfort.)
3. Inspect the affected eye, briefly but thoroughly, with a bright white light source, and compare it with the opposite eye. The sclera should be intact. The anterior chamber should be free of pus or blood. The iris should be normal in size and shape. The pupil should be normal in size, shape, and reactivity, and it should be symmetric with the other pupil unless there is a history of asymmetry (anisocoria). *If all of these conditions are not met, the patient should be referred to an ophthalmologist.*
4. Eversion of the upper lid is usually necessary to examine the entire conjunctiva (Fig. 66-3). After grasping the lower lid and applying traction, examine the conjunctiva beneath it as well. Inspect the entire bulbar and palpebral conjunctiva for trauma, foreign body, or other sources of symptoms, such as a hordeolum or an ingrown or inverted eyelash. Examine carefully the groove about 2 mm from the lash margin of the everted lid. Tiny objects frequently lodge here and may not be immediately visible. Use the ophthalmoscope for magnification if necessary. For a foreign body, refer to the "Corneal or Conjunctival Foreign Body Removal" section later in this chapter. Older patients often have ingrown hairs (trichiasis) that can cause a foreign body sensation

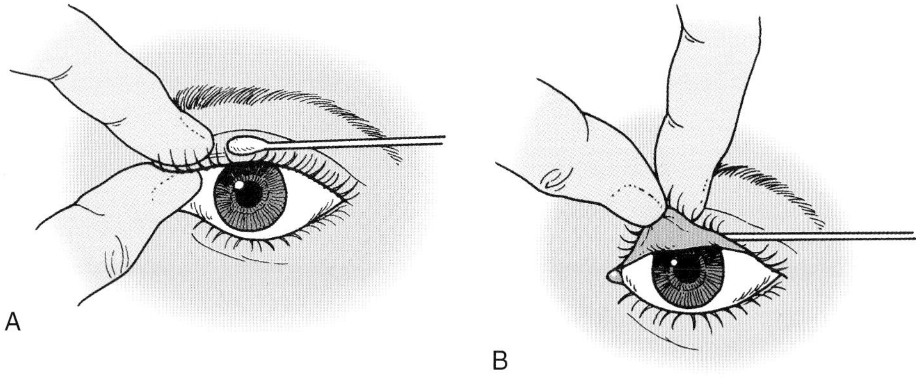

Figure 66-3 **A,** Grasp the upper eyelashes between the thumb and index finger. With the tip of the other index finger or a cotton-tipped applicator, press down gently on the skin of the upper lid. **B,** Pull outward on the lashes and rotate the tarsal plate upward until it forms a right angle with the eyeball. A gentle tug upward should flip the plate into eversion, clearly exposing the conjunctival surface of the upper lid.

(see Chapter 39, Epilation of Isolated Hairs [Including Trichiasis]). Trichiasis most frequently involves the lower lid, and if there are only a few hairs, they can be plucked out with fine forceps. The patient with many hairs should be referred for electrolysis of the roots.

5. Instill fluorescein dye by moistening a sterile fluorescein strip with one or two drops of sterile saline or topical anesthetic, asking the patient to look up, and gently touching the lower conjunctival sac for 3 to 5 seconds. Use a minimal amount of solution when wetting the strip. This usually helps visualize the defect by staining only the defect as opposed to staining the entire eye. Try not to touch the cornea directly with the strip because this may cause iatrogenic staining. After instilling the fluorescein, have the patient blink a few times to remove excess tears, and blot them with the tissue. This is helpful to distinguish true staining from fluorescein saturation of the tear film.
6. Inspect the cornea with magnification under a cobalt-blue light source. If the entire cornea is stained, irrigate the eye again and re-examine. Abraded areas of the cornea should remain highlighted with fluorescein.

   NOTE: Rivulets of fluorescein (Seidel sign) tracking from a puncture site indicate an unsuspected penetration of the globe and require ophthalmologic consultation.

7. Make a drawing of the cornea for later reference, detailing the area(s) of abnormality.
8. If no cause of symptoms is found or if vertical streaking is found on the cornea, suspect an embedded conjunctival foreign body in the eyelid and examine the entire conjunctiva under cobalt-blue light. Keep in mind that fluorescein is taken up by mucus on the conjunctiva; therefore fluorescein staining with a conjunctival injury is less specific than with a corneal injury.
9. At this point, if no cause for the symptoms can be found, the eye should be examined under a slit lamp (see Chapter 67, Slit-Lamp Examination). A slit lamp is helpful when a plain fluorescein examination is nondiagnostic. For deep, dendritic, or central ulcerations or for ulcerations in which infection is suspected (i.e., if there is clouding of the cornea or a purulent discharge), the patient should be referred to an ophthalmologist (Fig. 66-4).

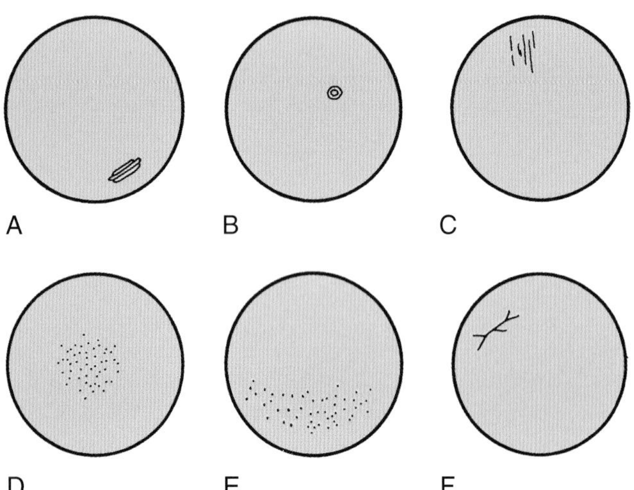

Figure 66-4 Corneal defect staining patterns for specific injuries. **A,** Typical abrasion. **B,** Abrasion around a corneal foreign body. **C,** Abrasion from a conjunctival foreign body under the upper lid. **D,** Abrasion from excessive wearing of a contact lens. **E,** Ultraviolet exposure (resulting from sunlamp exposure, welding, or snow blindness). **F,** Herpetic dendritic keratitis.

Treatment of Uncomplicated Corneal Abrasions

Considerations

Some clinicians working in the emergency department refer all corneal abrasions to ophthalmologists for follow-up. Others rely on their knowledge, skills, and experience to make decisions regarding referral. Knowing that the risk for permanent visual impairment is affected by the magnitude of several factors associated with the abrasion (including depth, size, location, and susceptibility to infection) can be helpful for clinicians when making their decision. Lacking the magnification available with a slit lamp, the depth of the abrasion is often difficult to assess, so referral should be considered. Referral should also be considered for suspected deep or large lesions or for those located centrally in the line of vision. One way to assess a borderline case is to wait until the follow-up examination the next day. The corneal epithelium is one of the fastest-healing areas of the body, and if considerable progress toward healing has not been made by the next day or if there are signs of infection (cloudiness of cornea or pus), the patient should be referred immediately.

Equipment

- Topical ophthalmic anesthetic.
- Isotonic irrigant (Dacriose, Ringer's lactate, sterile saline).
- Ophthalmic antibiotics (ointment is better lubricating and 6 to 10 times less expensive than drops): bacitracin 500 U/g ointment, ciprofloxacin 0.3% solution, erythromycin 0.5% ointment, gentamicin 0.3% ointment or solution, ofloxacin 0.3% solution, sulfacetamide 10% ointment or 10% solution, tobramycin 0.3% solution. Contact lenses wearers need an antipseudomonal antibiotic (e.g., ciprofloxacin, gentamicin, ofloxacin).
- *(Optional)* Cycloplegic, mydriatic drops, such as tropicamide 0.5% or 1% (Tropicacyl, Mydriacyl) or 0.5%, 1%, or 2% cyclopentolate (Cyclogyl, Pentolair), may be useful for pain control. Their duration of action ranges from hours to a day.
- *(Optional)* Sterile eyepatches and 1-inch (preferably nonallergenic) paper tape.

Technique

1. With the patient in the supine position, irrigate the eye copiously with ophthalmic irrigant, with the patient's head turned laterally toward the affected side.
2. Instill one to two additional drops of local anesthetic.
3. Apply an antibiotic ointment or drops. For patients who wear contact lenses, an antipseudomonal antibiotic should be chosen (e.g., ciprofloxacin, gentamicin, ofloxacin). Even under the best of conditions, infection is a possibility because of the avascular nature of the cornea. Prophylaxis with antibiotics is important.

   NOTE: In the past, eye patching was thought to decrease pain from a corneal abrasion by decreasing blinking and reducing eyelid induced trauma. By being a physical barrier, it was also thought to reduce the risk of infection. However, at least one meta-analysis and several subsequent randomized clinical trials have found no benefit to patching regarding either pain or healing. In fact, eye patching was the source of pain in 48% of patients in one study! In various trials, ophthalmic topical NSAIDs provided pain relief that was superior to patching. Furthermore, eye patching decreases oxygen delivery, increases moisture, and may increase the risk of infection.

   As a result of this evidence, many clinicians no longer use eye patching. However, the technique for patching remains in this chapter as an option. Another option that has been studied, for the busy patient who *must* have continuous use of both eyes, is to use a soft contact lens as a protectant barrier. As long as the *cause* of the abrasion was not a contact lens, use of a soft contact lens usually provides comfort and protection and should not impair healing. However, if a soft contact lens is used, the patient should be followed closely and warned for signs of infection.

4. Pain medication should be prescribed in an amount appropriate to the symptoms. However, additional local anesthetic should not be prescribed because it may retard corneal healing and cause corneal scarring. Topical ophthalmic NSAIDs such as ketorolac (Acular) or diclofenac (Voltaren) have been found to reduce pain by about 14% compared with placebo. A systematic review of the literature found that patients using ophthalmic NSAIDs may take fewer oral analgesics, return to work earlier, and take fewer narcotics.
5. In the past, mydriatics were thought to relieve the pain related to ciliary muscle spasm associated with any corneal abrasion. Although there is minimal evidence supporting this practice, it may be reasonable to use a mydriatic when there is obvious spasm, iritis, or irregularity of the pupil (these patients should also be referred to an ophthalmologist). It may also be reasonable to use a mydriatic when the patient presents with photophobia or significant eye discomfort.
6. Re-examine the eye in 24 hours using fluorescein and magnification. If the abrasion has healed, antibiotic ointment or drops should be used for an additional 3 days. If the defect is smaller, instill antibiotic ointment and examine again in 24 hours. If at any time during the follow-up corneal cloudiness or suppuration is seen, refer the patient to an ophthalmologist.
7. The visual acuity test should be repeated and documented just before the patient is discharged from care.
8. Tetanus immunity should be verified or provided.

   NOTE: Abrasions resulting from fingernails or plant matter are notoriously slow to heal. Their progress should be followed patiently, just like any other abrasion, while observing for any signs of early infection.

9. *(Optional)* A double patch (pressure patch) can be used. Before patching, an ophthalmic ointment (as opposed to solution) should be applied. The first patch is then folded and the fold placed immediately under the upper brow (this adds padding and prevents opening of the eye). This patch is covered with the second patch.

   With three to five strips of paper tape, secure the patches by taping from the middle of the forehead, across the eye, and toward the ear (Fig. 66-5).

   If infection is suspected, an eyepatch is contraindicated. Also, abrasions from organic material have fungal potential, so they should not be patched. Abrasions due to contact lenses increase the risk of infection with *Pseudomonas* so they should not be patched. Do not use eyepatches on young children. There is the theoretical risk of permanently affecting the use of one eye or of making amblyopia worse. Very young children typically remove a patch anyway.

Complications

- Infection.
- Scarring (the highest morbidity occurs when the abrasion is near the central line of vision).
- Permanent visual impairment.
- Recurrent corneal erosion (symptoms include foreign body pain, ocular pain, decreased vision, photophobia, increased lacrimation on wakening, blepharospasm). Although the symptoms may be annoying, they do not interfere with activities in most patients.

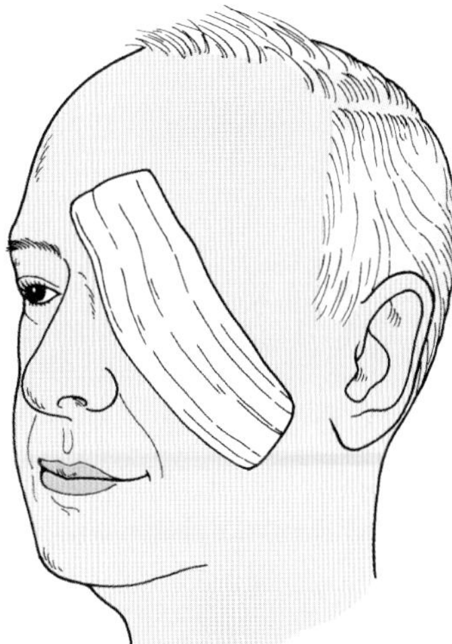

Figure 66-5 Pressure eyepatch.

Postprocedure Patient Education

Instruct the patient not to rub his or her eyes, especially upon wakening in the morning. Rubbing the eye may disrupt new layers of epithelializing cornea. Re-epithelialization can take weeks to complete. Inform the patient that the local anesthetic used during the examination will wear off in a few minutes to hours and that additional pain medication may be necessary. Topical ophthalmic NSAIDs have been found to be safe and somewhat effective. Moist compresses may be applied for some relief if the patient's eye has not been patched. Instruct the patient to return to the office daily until healed or if persistent or recurrent symptoms develop. If a mydriatic was used, inform the patient which one. Also inform the patient to tell any other clinician involved that a mydriatic was used, and which one, if he or she will be seen in another center or referred so that the clinician can know how long to expect the pupil to remain dilated. Instruct the patient not to overuse the affected eye, such as by watching television or reading for prolonged periods. This is especially true for children or anyone with a history of amblyopia. Although there is not a lot of evidence supporting such an intervention, if the abrasion is due to a contact lens, the patient probably should avoid contact lenses until the abrasion is completely healed. It is important to document the degree of healing observed during the discharge examination. Safety goggles or protective glasses should be emphasized if the abrasion was an occupational, exposure, or sports injury. If the eye is patched, the patient should not drive owing to the loss of depth perception. Even if the eye is not patched, the patient should not drive if there is loss of vision or depth perception until the injury heals.

Corneal or Conjunctival Foreign Body Removal

Indications

Noninfected, small, recent corneal or conjunctival foreign body

Contraindications

The contraindications (those that should be referred to ophthalmology) are the same as those for "Fluorescein Examination of the Cornea and Conjunctiva," as well as the following:

- Signs or symptoms that suggest infection, such as edema and clouding of the cornea surrounding the foreign body, ulceration exceeding the size of the foreign body, or purulent discharge

- Large metal foreign body or foreign body with potential to cause a large rust ring (e.g., embedded in the cornea for longer than 24 hours)
- Deeply or centrally embedded foreign body or one that has healed and is covered by epithelium

Equipment

- Topical ophthalmic anesthetic
- Sterile cotton-tipped applicators
- Bright white and cobalt-blue light sources
- Magnification as previously listed (it may be necessary to have an assistant hold the magnifier to allow the operator to use both hands)
- Isotonic ophthalmic irrigant, such as Dacriose, Ringer's lactate, or sterile saline
- Snellen chart or equivalent visual acuity chart
- Sterile 18-gauge needle with small syringe
- Sterile dental burr or cornea drill (optional)

NOTE: Instead of an 18-gauge needle, a tuberculin syringe with a 26-gauge needle, a sterile eye spud, or a small, sterile chalazion curette may be substituted, depending on user experience.

Preprocedure Patient Preparation

Instruct the patient that it will be important to fix his or her gaze on a distant object, maintain that gaze, and hold the head motionless, regardless of what is seen or experienced. The patient will have the urge to blink, but it will be important to keep the eye open. Inform the patient that the eye will be numb from the local anesthetic, but that he or she may feel pressure during the procedure. The patient should know that you will need to touch him or her.

Advise the patient of possible complications and that referral may be necessary regardless of outcome. Some clinicians obtain signed informed consent.

Technique

Controversy exists about the use of a swab or a spud to remove a corneal foreign body and whether this causes more damage. Only experienced users should consider a swab or spud, and they should use them only for a small foreign body. The swab will be more successful with a very recent, superficial foreign body. Irrigation alone is not usually successful unless the foreign object is very recent, consists of carbon, or is water soluble. The patient's tears would normally have already washed away anything that irrigation would remove.

NOTE: Because there may be increased risk of damaging the cornea, it may be prudent to avoid significant corneal procedures in patients who have undergone laser-assisted in situ keratomileusis (LASIK) procedure for nearsightedness. Clinicians should also examine patients who have undergone radial keratotomy very closely under magnification. The corneal incisions in these patients have been known to gape for 6 years postprocedure, and these can entrap a foreign body.

1. Record the patient's visual acuity.
2. With the patient supine, hold the eyelids apart with your thumb and index finger, and position the patient's head so that the foreign object is at the highest point on the eyeball. The patient should fix his or her gaze. For a conjunctival foreign body, the head should be positioned for maximal access.
3. Make an attempt to dislodge the object. Noting the controversy regarding swab or spud use, try to lift the object by lightly touching it with a cotton swab moistened with local anesthetic. This occasionally dislodges the particle. Never use any force to rub the cornea because this will dislodge the epithelium and cause a larger abrasion. The same maneuver can be attempted for a conjunctival foreign body.
4. To use a sterile needle, approach the object from a direction tangential to the eyeball, with the needle bevel upwards and the syringe held with a pencil grip (Fig. 66-6). Rest your hand on the patient's zygoma so that if the patient moves, your hand will move with the patient. Use the needle tip to lift the object gently from its bed. Several attempts may have to be made, but use of a slit lamp (see Chapter 67, Slit-Lamp Examination) or referral should be considered if further corneal damage is anticipated. If several attempts with a needle are unsuccessful, a spud or chalazion curette may be considered (again, noting the controversy discussed). For a conjunctival foreign body, the technique is the same; attempt to lift it from its bed with the same instruments. More vigorous force, if controlled, may be used on the conjunctiva.
5. After removal of the foreign body, if a residual corneal rust ring is found under magnification, it can occasionally be removed with the sterile needle alone. A cornea drill may also be considered. It should have a pressure-sensitive automatic shutoff to minimize corneal damage. Another published technique involves the use of a sterile dental burr held between the thumb and forefinger to approach the rust ring vertically (Fig. 66-7). After the burr has made one gentle rotation, re-examine the eye under magnification to verify complete removal of the ring. Rust is toxic to corneal epithelium and prevents healing; it may also cause night-time visual defects. If attempts to remove the rust ring are unsuccessful or if they will cause further damage to corneal epithelium, referral should be made for management under slit lamp magnification.

NOTE: Some experts suggest that use of a corneal drill or dental burr is contraindicated when the foreign body or rust ring is in the central line of vision. Instead, they recommend referral.

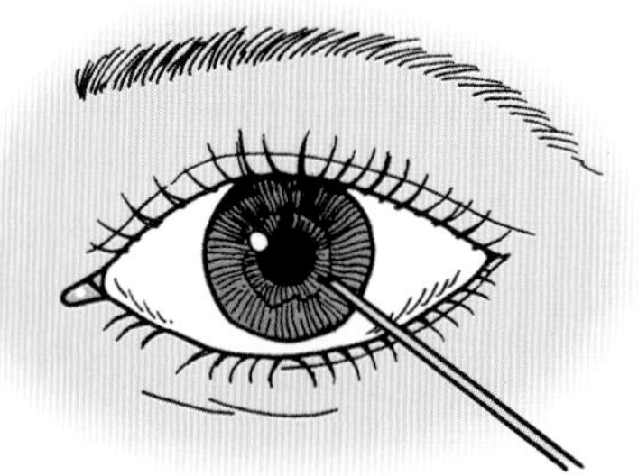

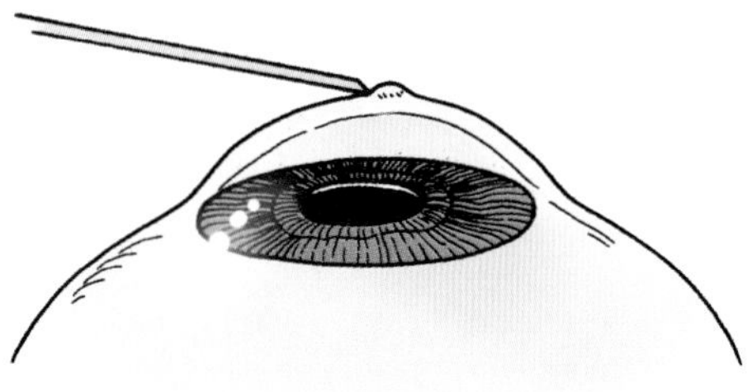

Figure 66-6 Removal of a superficial corneal foreign body. Side view illustrates the thickness of the cornea relative to the beveled needle edge. The needle or eye spud should be held tangential to the cornea, and the object should be gently lifted off of the cornea.

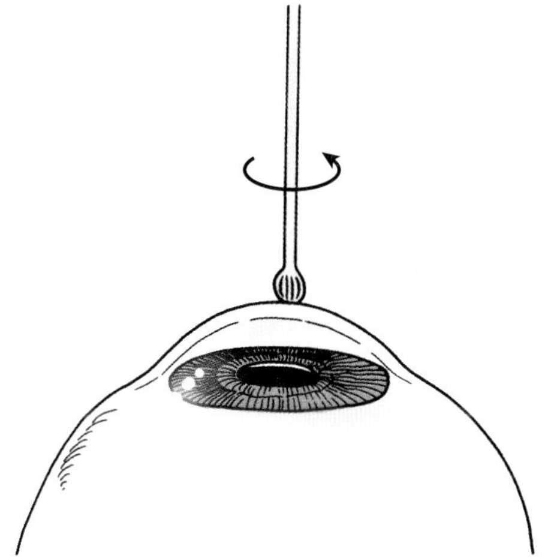

Figure 66-7 Dental burr rotated once to remove corneal rust ring. Note vertical approach.

6. Retest and record the patient's visual acuity. The corneal defect that is present after removal of the foreign body should now be managed the same as a corneal abrasion.

Postprocedure Patient Education

Follow the guidelines for treatment of an uncomplicated corneal abrasion. If the object cannot be removed, the resultant rust ring is too large, or the patient is referred to an ophthalmologist for any other reason, the ophthalmologist should provide further patient education.

Complications

- Same as the complications associated with treatment of a routine corneal abrasion, except the risk of corneal scarring is higher
- Perforation of the cornea or globe
- Incomplete removal of a foreign body
- Failure to heal because of a retained rust ring, infection, or other causes

CPT/Billing Codes

65205 Removal of foreign body, external eye; conjunctival superficial
65210 Removal of foreign body, external eye; conjunctival embedded (includes concretions), subconjunctival, or scleral nonperforating
65220 Removal of foreign body, external eye; corneal without slit lamp
99070 Eye tray: supplies and materials (except spectacles) provided by physician over and above those that are usually included with the office visit or other services rendered (list drugs, trays, supplies, or materials provided)
99173 Screening test of visual acuity, quantitative, bilateral (e.g., Snellen chart)

ICD-9-CM Diagnostic Codes

360.60 Intraocular foreign body, unspecified
361.00 Retinal detachment with retinal defect, unspecified
364.00 Acute iritis
364.70 Adhesions of iris, unspecified
370.20 Superficial corneal keratitis without conjunctivitis
370.24 Photokeratitis
371.82 Corneal injury due to contact lens
918.1 Corneal abrasion
918.2 Superficial injury of conjunctiva
930.0 Corneal foreign body
930.1 Foreign body in conjunctival sac

Suppliers

(See contact information online at www.expertconsult.com.)

Sterile fluorescein sodium strips
Fluor-I-Strip and Fluorets: Bausch and Lomb
Ful Glo: Akorn Pharmaceuticals

BIBLIOGRAPHY

Arbour JD, Brunette I, Boisjoly HM, et al: Should we patch corneal erosions? Arch Ophthalmol 115:313–317, 1997.

Brunette DD: Ophthalmology. In Marx JA, Hockberger RS, Walls RM (eds): Rosen's Emergency Medicine: Concepts and Clinical Practice, 6th ed. St. Louis, Mosby, 2006, pp 1046–1048.

Buttaravoli P: Foreign body, corneal. In Buttaravoli P (ed): Minor Emergencies: Splinters to Fractures, 2nd ed. Philadelphia, Mosby, 2007.

Flynn CA, D'Amico F, Smith G: Should we patch corneal abrasions? A meta-analysis. J Fam Pract 47:264–270, 1998.

Mitchell JD: Ocular emergencies. In Tintinalli JE, Kelen GD, Stapczynski JS (eds): Emergency Medicine: A Comprehensive Study Guide, 6th ed. New York, McGraw-Hill, 2004, pp 1508–1509.

Roberts JR: Myths and misconceptions: An eye patch for simple corneal abrasions. Emerg Med News February:4, 1995.

Thomas SH, Brown DFM: Foreign bodies. In Marx JA, Hockberger RS, Walls RM (eds): Rosen's Emergency Medicine: Concepts and Clinical Practice, 6th ed. St. Louis, Mosby, 2006, pp 859–861.

Usatine RP: The Color Atlas of Family Medicine. New York, McGraw-Hill, 2009.

Wilson SA, Last A: Management of corneal abrasions. Am Fam Physician 70:123–128, 2004.

CHAPTER 67

Slit-Lamp Examination

Christopher J. Bigelow

The slit-lamp biomicroscope is used for a thorough evaluation of the eye as well as for diagnosis of various eye conditions. In short, the eyes remain in a fixed position while the light and microscope are independently moved and adjusted. As with any instrument, repeated use facilitates clinician comfort with the scope as well as his or her ability to obtain the desired or necessary information. With its many levers and knobs (Fig. 67-1), the slit lamp can be somewhat intimidating at first. However, after learning a few simple techniques, even the infrequent user should feel comfortable. Granted, not every primary care clinician's office has a slit lamp. However, if one is available, it can be an invaluable diagnostic opportunity that should not be missed because of lack of experience. Clinicians working in an urgent care center or emergency department would also benefit from knowing how to use a slit lamp. The goal of this chapter is to provide even the novice user with guidance for performing a useful and reproducible slit-lamp examination.

A slit lamp consists of both an illumination and an observation system (see Fig. 67-1). The light source is an incandescent lamp contained in the body of the instrument. Light from the lamp passes through a condenser, the slit mechanism, and an objective lens and is then reflected by an inclined mirror onto the patient's eye. When projected onto the globe, the slit beam of incandescent light creates an optical cross-section of the eye. The height and width of the beam (Fig. 67-2) can be adjusted with controls (often different on each slit lamp). It can be changed from a small pinpoint spot to a slit beam or made even wider for broad illumination. As the beam is narrowed, the scattered light from adjacent tissue is minimized, allowing greater detail to be seen in the cross-section. Beam sizes, their widths, and their usefulness are discussed in the "Technique" section. Light intensity can also be adjusted. In general, brighter illumination settings are better tolerated (e.g., less photophobia) with a short, narrow beam, whereas a long, wide beam is usually better tolerated with a lower-power illumination setting. The observation system is a microscope with a long working distance. Most slit lamps offer a choice of magnification between 5× and 50×. The necessary degree of magnification depends on the tissue being examined.

Use of the slit lamp is indicated in any situation where brighter illumination and increased magnification of the lids, conjunctiva, or anterior segment structures (e.g., cornea, iris, lens) would be helpful. If desired, the clinician could use a slit lamp for most examinations of the eye. With increased magnification, oblique illumination, and a stereoscopic view, a much better evaluation of lesions can be obtained, especially their depth. Attachments are also available to perform applanation (Goldmann) tonometry (see Chapter 68, Tonometry), which is considered the most accurate form of tonometry. In addition, high-powered lenses are available for most slit lamps to allow visualization of the posterior structures (e.g., retina, optic nerve).

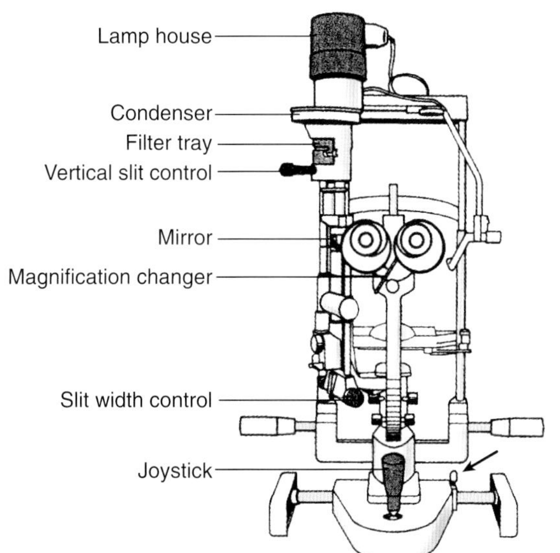

Figure 67-1 A slit lamp and its optics. (From Solley WA, Broocker G: General eye exam. In Palay DA, Krachmer JH: Ophthalmology for the Primary Care Physician. St. Louis, CV Mosby, 1997, pp 1–22.)

Indications

- Need for bright illumination or magnification of lids, conjunctiva, or anterior segment structures (e.g., chronic blepharitis, keratitis, iritis).
- Same indications as for routine fluorescein examination or for foreign body removal (see Chapter 66, Corneal Abrasions and Removal of Corneal or Conjunctival Foreign Bodies). If a slit lamp is available, it will enhance the techniques found in that chapter.

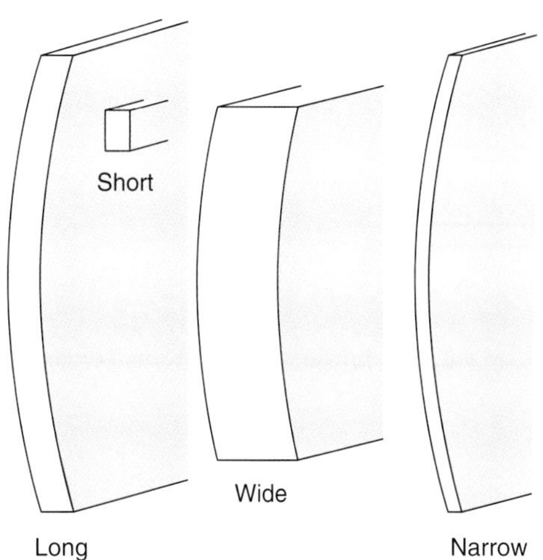

Figure 67-2 Different dimensions of the slit-lamp beam.

- Patient with a foreign body sensation and routine fluorescein examination is negative, or when the routine fluorescein examination is inconclusive or unsuccessful.
- Suspected deep or large abrasions or those centrally located in the line of vision on fluorescein examination. Such lesions increase the risk of vision loss and should be evaluated thoroughly and followed clinically with a slit lamp.
- After several unsuccessful attempts at removing a corneal foreign body in the standard fashion, before additional trauma is inflicted on the cornea, the foreign body and cornea should be evaluated under a slit lamp. It may also be necessary to remove the foreign body with slit-lamp guidance.
- When routine fluorescein examination is relatively contraindicated (e.g., when there is long-standing [>24 hours] inflammation, possible perforation). The presence of iritis, photophobia, or ciliary blush may indicate long-standing inflammation, or it may be the result of an intraocular foreign body or a more serious injury. If the etiology is not evident with a slit-lamp examination, the patient should be referred to an ophthalmologist.
- Recent eye trauma (e.g., to exclude perforation).

Contraindications

After urgent care has been provided, patients with the following symptoms should be referred to an ophthalmologist:

- Suspected high-velocity injury to the eye (e.g., patients exposed to metal hammering or heavy machinery): although a slit lamp may diagnose a perforation, it is possible for high-speed metallic or nonmetallic fragments to penetrate the globe with unnoticeable damage to the cornea. Although there may be minimal symptoms, significant internal damage may have occurred. A hyphema, lens opacification, an abnormal anterior chamber examination, or an irregularity of the pupil may suggest that the globe has been penetrated. Orbital radiographs may confirm a metal foreign body.

  NOTE: A pressure patch is contraindicated in a penetration injury of the globe. Also, for complex lid lacerations, a nonpressure protective eye shield should be applied before referral (see Chapter 66, Corneal Abrasions and Removal of Corneal or Conjunctival Foreign Bodies, Fig. 66-1).

- Exposure to caustic or acidic media: urgent management includes copious irrigation, which should continue for at least 15 minutes. (It can begin at home with tap water from a shower or hose.)
- Other chemical exposure if the clinician is not knowledgeable about its management after contacting a Poison Control Center.
- Ruptured globe.
- An uncooperative patient. (Mild sedation for infants may be helpful; see Chapter 7, Pediatric Sedation and Analgesia.)
- Foreign body removal if there are signs or symptoms that suggest infection (e.g., edema and clouding of the cornea surrounding the foreign body, ulceration exceeding the size of the foreign body, or purulent discharge). If infection is suspected, patching is contraindicated and referral is necessary.
- Large metal foreign bodies or those with potential to cause a large rust ring (i.e., those that have been embedded in the cornea for longer than 24 hours).
- Apparently deeply or centrally embedded foreign bodies.

  NOTE: For these contraindications, although the slit lamp may be helpful for a primary care clinician, management by an ophthalmologist is the usual care.

Equipment

- Topical ophthalmic anesthetic, such as 0.5% proparacaine (Alcaine or Ophthaine) or 0.5% tetracaine (Pontocaine), unless contraindicated (e.g., ruptured globe or allergy to local anesthetics).
- Sterile fluorescein sodium strips. (Because fluorescein is incompatible with preservatives effective against *Pseudomonas* or *Proteus*, multidose dropper bottles of fluorescein solution should not be used. An inoculation of abraded corneal epithelium with either of these bacteria could cause infection, scarring, or permanent blindness.)
- Sterile cotton-tipped applicators.
- Isopropyl alcohol swab.
- Isotonic ophthalmic irrigant (e.g., sterile saline, Dacriose).
- Slit lamp: the two most common slit lamps in use are manufactured by Haag-Streit and Zeiss (see "Suppliers" section).

Preprocedure Patient Preparation

Patients should be informed about the indication(s) for and alternatives to the slit-lamp examination. Once their chins are placed on the scope, patients should be asked to get into a comfortable position that can be maintained for a while. They should be instructed to breathe normally and, especially children, asked to remain as still as possible. Children may need assistance with holding still. Patients should know to blink normally unless their eyes are being held open by the examiner or they are asked to hold their eyes open. They should be aware of the need for the examiner to touch their faces and even to pull on their eyelids. It should be explained that the room is going to be darkened and that a bright light can be expected, especially if the pupil is dilated. Reassurance that this bright light will not cause permanent visual damage is usually appreciated. In fact, patients should be told that the reason for using this bright light (in most cases) is to *prevent* permanent damage to their vision.

The patient needs to know that he or she will be asked to direct his or her vision to certain locations and that eyedrops or dye may be necessary to enhance the examination. Before fluorescein is instilled, the patient should remove contact lenses and be warned that objects in his or her vision may temporarily appear yellow. Tears may also remain yellow for a short time after the examination and might stain skin or clothing, at least temporarily, so they should avoid rubbing their eyes or drying their tears on something that might stain. Before topical anesthetic is instilled, the patient should be warned that it may cause a burning sensation until the eye becomes numb.

Technique

1. Clinicians should be familiar with the anatomy of the external eye before evaluation with a slit lamp (Fig. 67-3). For the novice or infrequent user of a slit lamp, it may also be helpful to get comfortable with the instrument before the patient is in the room. Learn to locate and loosen the locking nut for the mechanical assembly. Practice with the joystick, turn the knobs, and watch the results. The clinician may then benefit from focusing the slit lamp on an object or the skin on his or her hand to gain some sense of perspective. In an urgent care center or emergency department, practicing before the patient is in the room may be important because the slit lamp is often left in complete disarray by others.

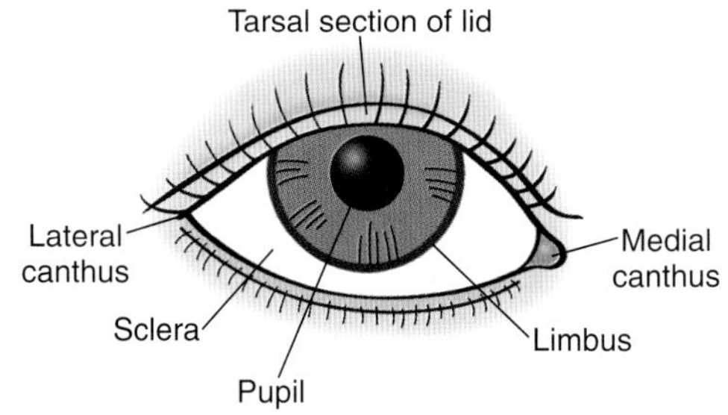

Figure 67-3 External anatomy of the eye.

2. Proper patient positioning is absolutely essential for a satisfactory examination. Both the patient and the examiner should be comfortable. An improperly positioned patient is more likely to move backward and out of focus. He or she is also less likely to maintain positioning for extended periods of time. The patient is seated during the examination. Clean the chin rest with an alcohol swab. The examination chair height should be such that the patient can easily place his or her chin on the adjustable chin rest and forehead against the headrest. Some slit lamps have an eye level marker to assist in gauging head positioning. If the patient is unable to place his or her forehead against the headrest, either elevate the chair or lower the chin rest. If the patient is not positioned against the headrest, it will be difficult to focus on deeper ocular structures. This common mistake often causes a great deal of frustration for the novice slit-lamp user. After the patient is positioned, loss of focus may indicate that he or she has moved his or her head backward. It should be repositioned. Small children should sit in the chair on their knees, stand up on the footrest, or sit in their parent's lap.
3. Examiner positioning is also important. The clinician should be able to reach the patient's eye comfortably and easily rest an elbow on the slit-lamp table. Such a position is important if the eyelids need to be manipulated or for holding instruments used in foreign body removal. The examiner should also be seated comfortably in the chair so that his or her eyes easily reach the eyepiece without leaning forward. This description may seem overly simplistic, but many a novice slit-lamp examiner looks like a baseball catcher coming up from a crouch. This is not a position that can be maintained for very long.
4. Turn on the power to the lamp (the switch is usually located on the left lower side, just under the table base), and select anywhere from a low power (preserves bulb life the longest) to the next-to-highest power illumination setting. The illumination power setting rheostat is usually part of the power switch or located nearby. The eyepieces can then be adjusted to correct the clinician's refractive error, although it is often simpler for the clinician to set the eyepieces at zero (1×) and wear his or her spectacles or contact lenses. Once the eyepieces are adjusted, the interpupillary distance is set. After this adjustment, no further manipulation of the eyepieces should be necessary. Magnification can be changed with a knob found anterior to the eyepieces on some slit lamps, or by shifting a lever found below the eyepieces on other models.
5. After positioning and eyepiece adjustment, darken the examination room as much as possible. The eyepieces (and thus the examiner) should remain perpendicular to the chin rest throughout the examination. The light source, not the oculars, should be moved to facilitate viewing. Move the light source vertically by using the control lever located at the base of the slit lamp. Horizontal movement is accomplished by moving the swing arm with the examiner's other hand. Position the slit beam at an oblique angle, starting at the temporal side of each eye and moving the light nasally. Beware when moving the light source from the temporal side of the eye: from this position, if the examiner is not careful, the patient's nose is often struck by the mirror or light source. To view the nasal portion of an eye, have the patient gaze temporally on that side, which should bring the desired area into focus.
6. The depth of focus is adjusted by moving the slit lamp backward and forward. Focusing is typically accomplished at the same time as vertical positioning with the joystick. Remember to examine both eyes, even if the symptoms are monocular. The "normal" eye can be used for comparison with any pathology in the other eye.
7. At the start of the examination, the patient should be instructed to look toward the examiner's ear opposite to the eye being examined (i.e., the patient looks at the examiner's left ear while the right eye is being examined). Some slit lamps have a fixation light to direct the patient's gaze, but it is often simpler to instruct the patient to focus on a larger, nonmoving object such as the examiner's ear.
8. Evaluation of the ocular structures has already begun with a focused history, the measurement of visual acuity in both eyes, and a gross handlight examination of the eyelid skin and surrounding structures. The slit-lamp examination should then proceed in a systematic manner from external (lids and lashes) to internal (vitreous). Failing to be systematic can cause the examiner to get caught up in the fine detail that the slit lamp provides. As a result, the examiner may "miss the forest for the trees."
9. Choose the white light beam filter lens. A long, wide beam is useful for scanning tissues such as the lids and lashes. For these structures, a low-power magnification (e.g., 10× to 16×) should be adequate.

   NOTE: Avoid focusing the light into the pupil for an extended period. This can be very uncomfortable for the patient and may result in injury.

   - Observe the general appearance of the lid margin; the lid's color, position, and vascularity; and any meibomian gland openings. Thickening, crusting, and erythema of the eyelid margins are consistent with blepharitis. Examine the lashes and eyebrows for the presence of inflammation, scaling, or elevated or ulcerated lesions. Also examine the lashes for evidence of lid debris and for missing or additional lashes. Scan for the misdirection of lashes (trichiasis), which can cause a severe foreign body sensation in an otherwise normally positioned lid. If there are only a few misdirected eyelashes, pluck them with fine forceps. If there are many, the patient should be referred for electrolysis (see Chapter 39, Epilation of Isolated Hairs [Including Trichiasis]) of the roots. Also evaluate lid position for being turned in (entropion) or out (ectropion). Note discrete changes in lid pigmentation.
   - Examination of the lower lid is aided by having the patient look up while pulling the lower lid down with your index finger. This exposure provides a good view of the posterior lid margin and the lower palpebral conjunctiva. Eversion of the upper lid is necessary to properly examine the upper palpebral conjunctiva (e.g., to exclude foreign bodies). Lid eversion can be performed by having the patient close his or her eyes and look down (see Chapter 66, Corneal Abrasions and Removal of Corneal or Conjunctival Foreign Bodies, Fig. 66-3). Grasp the upper lid margin gently between thumb and index finger. A cotton-tipped swab is then placed about 15 mm from the lid margin. The lid is then moved out, up, and over the cotton-tipped swab. A drop of local anesthetic often enhances patient comfort with this procedure. Carefully examine the few millimeters proximal to the lid margin. This is a common location for small foreign bodies missed on the routine examination.
10. A long, wide beam is also used to examine the conjunctiva. Low-power magnification (e.g., 10× to 16×) should be adequate. The examiner gently separates the eyelids with the opposite hand while the patient is asked to look in all directions of gaze. The conjunctiva is normally a transparent tissue with the white sclera visible beneath. Occasionally, there are slightly elevated, yellow lesions at the 3- and 9-o'clock positions at the limbus (edge of cornea) called *pinguecula.* These benign lesions are more common with advancing age. Areas of pigmentation of the conjunctiva can also be seen. These are commonly benign nevi, most often translucent and flat. For irregularly shaped or pigmented lesions suspect for melanoma, the patient should be referred to an ophthalmologist.
11. A long, narrow beam, which produces an optical cross-section, is usually best for examining the cornea. Higher-power

magnification (e.g., >20×) may be useful when examining the cornea in minute detail. Within this cross-section, the epithelium or tear film is seen as the most anterior band. The stroma can be seen as the large middle layer, and the posterior band represents the endothelium (Fig. 67-4). The examiner brings the slit-lamp beam across the cornea from the temporal to the nasal limbus while paying attention to the regularity of the corneal surface. Any disruption in the corneal surface such as an abrasion should be easily noted as an irregular, distorted, or dulled light reflex. When the light is shone from a lateral position, it produces greater shadows, which in turn enhances the ability to determine the depth and texture of corneal lesions.

- One way of screening for a corneal lesion or foreign object is to use limbal scatter. To do this, light is directed from the laterally placed scope to the closest portion of the limbus. The cornea then simulates a fiberoptic element, and light is transmitted through the cornea medially to the limbus on the other side. A lesion or foreign body in the cornea should cause light to backscatter; consequently, the lesion should be seen clearly against the dark pupillary background.
- Deeper focus allows examination of the corneal stroma, which makes up 90% of the corneal tissue. A narrow slit beam allows for accurate determination of the depth of either a foreign body or a penetrating injury involving this area. Opacities or haze may be noted, both of which are indicative of previous trauma, infection, or inflammation. Old lesions tend to be more circumscribed, whereas an active keratitis usually produces a diffuse pattern of corneal haze.
- The endothelium is visible as the posterior line in the optical section. Abnormalities may present either as folds in the endothelium or as changes that resemble the surface of a golf ball called *corneal guttae*. Both of these changes may be indicative of endothelial cell loss.

12. The anterior chamber is the space between the corneal endothelium and the iris. Continuing to use a narrow beam, gauge the anterior chamber depth by estimating the distance between the corneal endothelium and the front surface of the iris. This distance is normally 3 mm or more. When shining from the temporal to the nasal side, a normal anterior chamber will allow this narrow light beam to project evenly from side to side. A narrowed anterior chamber will have a lighted temporal side and a narrowed nasal side.
13. The aqueous humor is normally clear, with light passing through it without change. To examine the aqueous humor for the presence of cells or flare, a short (3 or 4 mm), narrow beam with bright illumination and high magnification (e.g., >20× to 30×) should be used. Cells in the aqueous humor may indicate inflammation (iritis) or hemorrhage (hyphema). While keeping the beam centered on the pupil, any white (i.e., white blood cells, indicating iritis) or red (i.e., red blood cells, indicating a hyphema) specks will be highlighted against the dark pupillary background. Protein in the aqueous humor (i.e., intraocular inflammation) causes a visible flare (Tyndall effect). This effect is similar to that seen when shining a flashlight through smoke (Fig. 67-5). Take care to examine the lower aspect of the anterior chamber because cells and inflammatory products tend to settle in this part of the eye and may form a meniscus when the patient is seated upright.
14. The iris has numerous crypts that should be plainly visible with the slit lamp. Nevi, surgical openings, neovascularization, atrophy, tears, or abnormally pigmented lesions may be seen with magnification. If the iris is scarred to the lens (posterior synechiae) or cornea (anterior synechiae), it should be noted. Of interest in those patients who have undergone cataract extraction, a tremulousness of the iris called *iridodonesis* is often seen. It is caused by removal of the support usually provided by the lens.
15. Next, use a long, narrow slit beam to examine the layers of the lens. Dilating the pupil allows for the most thorough evaluation of the lens. Any opacity in the crystalline lens is called a *cataract*. The slit beam passes through multiple layers from anterior to posterior: anterior capsule, anterior cortex, nucleus, posterior cortex, and posterior capsule (Fig. 67-6). Cortical cataracts resemble spokes radiating from the lens equator. Nuclear cataracts are central and are often seen as a yellow or amber hue discoloring the normally clear lens. Posterior subcapsular cataracts often appear as clustered punctate vacuoles. These can be seen either directly or with retroillumination.

    Retroillumination uses the red reflex and will often provide a striking view of a lens opacity, especially through a dilated pupil. The slit beam is directed parallel to the visual axis to either the nasal or temporal side of the lens. The examiner then views the red reflex, which is the light reflected off the retina and back through the lens. Against this red background, lens opacities such as capsular cataracts are prominently displayed.

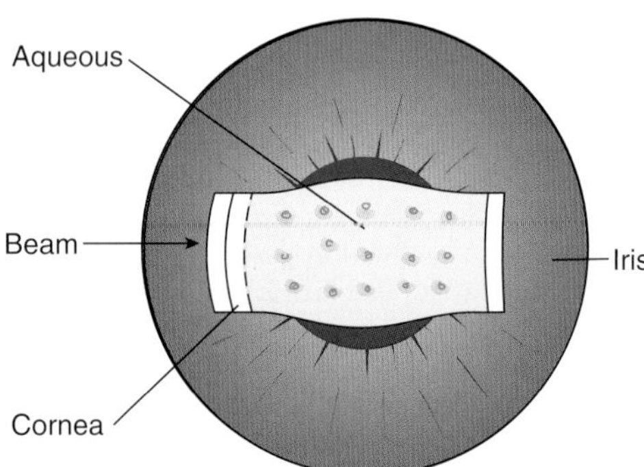

Figure 67-5 Optical cross-section of the anterior chamber showing cell and flare.

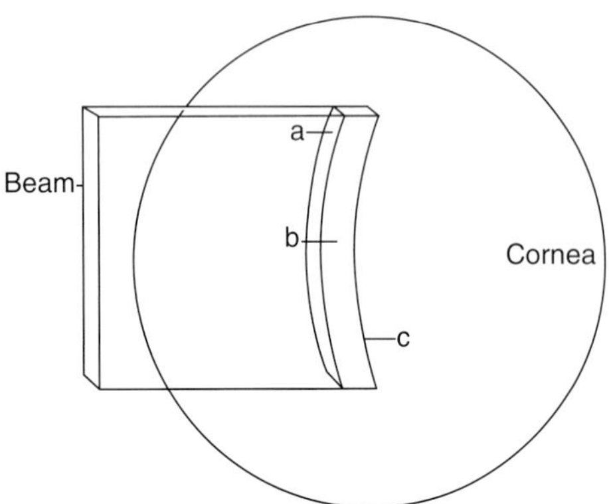

Figure 67-4 Optical cross-section of the cornea: Corneal epithelium (a); corneal stroma (b); corneal endothelium (c).

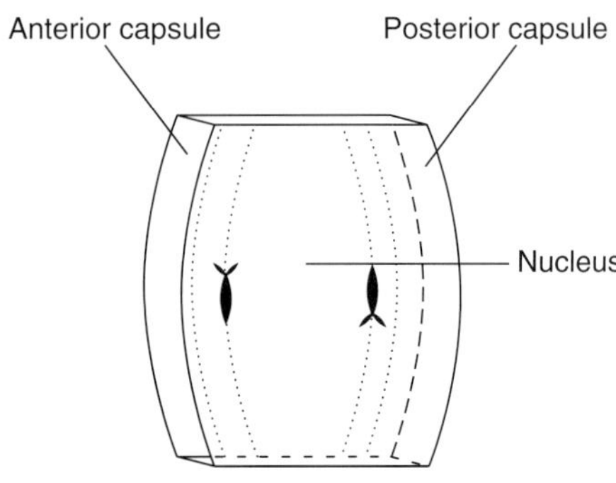

Figure 67-6 Optical cross-section of the lens.

16. After examining the posterior lens capsule, examine the anterior vitreous humor. Normally, the vitreous humor is a relatively clear fluid with minimal cellular material. If cellular material is noted, refer the patient to an ophthalmologist. Gross vitreous opacities, such as floaters, can also be seen with the slit beam.
17. At this point, if a corneal abrasion is suspected but not yet seen, a fluorescein strip should be used. It will stain areas of absent epithelium bright green when viewed with a cobalt-blue light filter. A wider slit beam is better tolerated by patients (i.e., causes less photophobia) if it is blue. (For instilling fluorescein, see Chapter 66, Corneal Abrasions and Removal of Corneal or Conjunctival Foreign Bodies.) Be careful to use minimal amounts of fluorescein to avoid flooding the eye and obscuring the abnormal epithelium. (Also, avoid staining the patient's skin and clothing with fluorescein!) Avoid touching the cornea directly with a fluorescein strip because this may result in an iatrogenically stained cornea. If either of these occurs, have the patient blink, blot the excess fluorescein away, and then reexamine. If the eye is still flooded, flush it with ophthalmic saline and again have the patient blot away the excess. The fluorescein examination is usually performed after the remainder of the eye has been examined with the slit lamp to avoid any "light scatter" that could be caused by fluorescein adsorbed to a corneal abrasion.
18. Using special lenses, often through a dilated pupil, the vitreous body, retina, and optic nerve can also be viewed with a slit lamp. For example, a Hruby lens can be attached by inserting the lens spindle into the groove of the lens guide plate on the slit lamp. A handheld lens positioned in front of the patient's eye can also be used in the same manner. When using a lens, the slit beam is positioned parallel to the visual axis. (Distracting light reflections off the lenses can often be resolved by tilting the lens slightly.) The posterior structures of the eye can then be examined. This part of the examination should probably not be performed if the patient has an iritis or a corneal abrasion because of the associated severe photophobia.

Postprocedure Patient Education

The findings should be discussed with the patient, as well as any needed postprocedure care. Any necessary referrals should be made. For corneal foreign bodies or abrasions, see Chapter 66, Corneal Abrasions and Removal of Corneal or Conjunctival Foreign Bodies, for management and postprocedure patient information.

CPT/Billing Codes

65222 Removal of foreign body, external eye; corneal with slit lamp
92002 Ophthalmologic services: medical examination and evaluation with initiation of diagnostic and treatment program; intermediate, new patient
92012 Intermediate, established patient

NOTE: Intermediate examination includes biomicroscopy.

99070 Eye tray: supplies and materials (except spectacles) provided by physician over and above those that are usually included with the office visit or other services rendered (list drugs, trays, supplies, or materials provided)

ICD-9-CM Diagnostic Codes

364.00 Acute or subacute iritis
364.01 Acute, primary iritis
364.02 Acute, primary recurrent
364.03 Iritis, secondary, infectious
364.04 Iritis, secondary
364.10 Iritis, chronic
364.70 Adhesions of iris, unspecified
918.1 Corneal abrasion
370.20 Superficial or unspecified keratitis
370.24 Welder's or photokeratitis
370.40 Superficial corneal keratitis with conjunctivitis
371.82 Corneal injury due to contact lens
918.2 Superficial injury of conjunctiva
930.0 Corneal foreign body
930.1 Foreign body in conjunctival sac
361.00 Retinal detachment with retinal defect, unspecified
360.60 Intraocular foreign body

Suppliers

(See contact information online at www.expertconsult.com.)

Sterile fluorescein sodium strips
Haag-Streit
Zeiss

BIBLIOGRAPHY

Coles WH: Ophthalmology: A Diagnostic Text. Baltimore, Williams & Wilkins, 1989.

James D: Use of the slit lamp: In James DM (ed): Field Guide to Urgent and Ambulatory Care Procedures. Philadelphia, Lippincott Williams & Wilkins, 2001, pp 1–3.

Knoop KJ, Dennis WR, Hedges JR: Ophthalmologic procedures. In Roberts JR, Hedges JR (eds): Clinical Procedures in Emergency Medicine, 4th ed. Philadelphia, Saunders, 2004, pp 1241–1279.

Miller D, Greiner JV: Corneal measures and tests. In Albert DA, Jakobiec FA (eds): Principles and Practice of Ophthalmology, 2nd ed. Philadelphia, WB Saunders, 2000.

Schabowski S: Eye examination. In Reichman EF, Simon RR (eds): Emergency Medicine Procedures. New York, McGraw-Hill, 2004, pp 1191–1210.

CHAPTER 68

TONOMETRY

Deepa A. Vasudevan • Grant C. Fowler

Tonometry is used to detect increased intraocular pressure, which is common in patients at risk for glaucoma. Glaucoma is actually caused by a group of conditions, all of which can lead to optic nerve damage and a loss of visual function. More than 2 million persons in the United States are estimated to have some degree of blindness caused by glaucoma. It is the third most common cause of blindness, and its incidence increases with age. Despite the fact that most blindness caused by glaucoma is preventable, or at least able to be delayed, there are estimates that less than half of patients with glaucoma have been diagnosed. Tonometry remains one of the easiest methods of screening for glaucoma; however, patients with glaucoma can have normal intraocular pressures and, vice versa, not all patients with increased intraocular pressures have glaucoma. Researchers are currently pursuing other risk factors associated with glaucomatous changes in the eye to develop additional practical screening techniques. When this succeeds, glaucoma will be more readily diagnosed, even in those with normal intraocular pressure. Until then, tonometry, in combination with funduscopic examination and visual field testing, is the most sensitive and specific method for detection of glaucomatous changes in the eye. Patients at high risk for glaucoma should be screened with all three.

There are three basic types of tonometry. *Impression tonometry* measures the depth of the impression produced on the ocular wall by a given force, and the Schiøtz tonometer uses this method. *Noncontact/air-puff tonometry*, originally considered the least accurate and therefore designed for screening (especially for children), has turned out to be fairly accurate even when compared with applanation tonometry, the "gold" standard. *Applanation (Goldmann) tonometry* measures the force necessary to flatten an area of the cornea. Because applanation tonometry is more accurate than Schiøtz tonometry, most optometrists and ophthalmologists use this technique; however, it requires the ability to use a slit lamp (see Chapter 67, Slit-Lamp Examination). Consequently, the Schiøtz tonometer is still the standard for measuring intraocular pressure in the offices of primary care clinicians, in urgent care centers, and in emergency departments. The Schiøtz tonometer is also less expensive (about $300). Many urgent care centers and emergency departments also now have available a hand-held portable device (e.g., Tono-Pen; Reichert, Inc., Depew, NY) that uses applanation technology, although it is somewhat more expensive (about $3000) than the Schiøtz tonometer. Regardless of the method of tonometry, the clinician may recommend other tests or a referral if the initial test result is abnormal. This chapter discusses the techniques used in impression (Schiøtz and Tono-Pen), and applanation (Goldmann) tonometry.

INDICATIONS

Screening Those with Risk Factors

- Age older than 45 years (>35 years in African Americans).
- Family history of glaucoma (fourfold to ninefold increased risk).
- African Americans (fourfold to sixfold higher risk than whites).
- Hispanics age older than 60 years.
- Asian Americans (increased risk of angle-closure glaucoma, but this causes <10% of glaucoma).
- Diabetes mellitus.
- Hypertension.
- Decreased visual acuity (myopia or hyperopia).
- Central corneal thickness less than 0.5 mm.
- Prior injury: blunt or penetrating trauma, eye surgery, eye inflammation (e.g., uveitis) can cause glaucoma acutely or years later.
- Prior or current medications: use of corticosteroids (including high-dose inhaled corticosteroids), mydriatics, phenothiazines, and sympathomimetics can precipitate glaucoma.

Diagnosis

- Ocular pain (especially if associated with signs or symptoms of angle-closure glaucoma such as acute-onset red eye, cloudy or smoky cornea, fixed mid-position pupil, blurry vision, halos around lights, nausea and vomiting, frontal headache)

  NOTE: Patients with angle-closure glaucoma may complain more about nausea and vomiting than eye symptoms.

- Red eye (especially if associated with signs or symptoms of angle-closure glaucoma)
- History of visual field loss

Determining Baseline Intraocular Pressure

- Uveitis: patients with iritis or uveitis can develop both open- and closed-angle glaucoma. Corticosteroid treatment of uveitis can also cause glaucoma.
- After blunt ocular trauma: patients with hyphema often have an acute rise in intraocular pressure.
- Orbital fracture: an intraocular pressure greater than 22 mm Hg or a difference greater than 3 mm Hg between eyes is a reasonable marker for ocular injury in the patient with an orbital fracture.

CONTRAINDICATIONS

- Eye infection (Although Tono-Pen can be used because it uses disposable tip covers, noncontact tonometry may be preferred.)
- Corneal abrasion (Although Tono-Pen can be used in another area of the cornea, tonometry is commonly deferred until a subsequent visit.)
- Recent eye trauma (Tono-Pen/Schiøtz tonometry should not be performed in patients with suspected penetrating ocular injury; pressure on the globe can result in extrusion of intraocular contents. Slit-lamp examination should be performed to exclude perforation.)
- Patients who cannot keep their eyes still or open (Schiøtz and applanation tonometry cannot be used in patients with severe eyelid swelling or those unable to open their eyes; however, the Tono-Pen can sometimes be used.)

EQUIPMENT

- Topical ophthalmic anesthetic drops, such as proparacaine hydrochloride 0.5% or tetracaine 7%
- Gloves, mask, goggles (whatever is needed to follow universal blood and body fluid precautions)
- For Schiøtz: Schiøtz tonometer kit (each kit contains the tonometer, three plunger weights, a concave test block, conversion tables, pipe cleaners, and instructions for care)
- For Tono-Pen: Tono-Pen unit, condom-style disposable tip covers, optical-grade canned air for cleaning
- For applanation: Slit lamp with Goldmann applanation device attached, sterile fluorescein strips

PREPROCEDURE PATIENT PREPARATION

Explain the reason for measuring the intraocular pressure with the tonometer (e.g., presence of risk factors, symptoms, or positive physical findings). Briefly explain the procedure as well as the fact that this test only detects increased intraocular pressure. The patient should know that anesthetic ophthalmic drops may sting a little as they are instilled. The patient should also know that having normal intraocular pressures does not completely exclude glaucoma. If glaucoma is suspected, even with normal intraocular pressures, tonometry should be combined with the other tests mentioned previously.

TECHNIQUE

Schiøtz or Tono-Pen

1. Check and record the patient's visual acuity. Examine the eyes. Immediately after the funduscopic examination, place two drops of topical ophthalmic anesthetic in each eye. (The anesthetic will have time to take effect while you prepare the tonometer.) The clinician should follow universal blood and body fluid precautions.
2. Assemble the Schiøtz tonometer with the 5.5-g weight in place, and test for accuracy on the convex metal test block (Fig. 68-1). The Schiøtz tonometer is precalibrated by the manufacturer and must be returned for repair if it does not read "0" when resting on the test block. The Tono-Pen (Fig. 68-2) should also be calibrated before each use. Turn the transducer tip straight down and push the operation button twice within 1.5 seconds. It will beep and the liquid crystal display (LCD) will read "CAL." Although it may take up to 15 seconds, the Tono-Pen will then beep and display "UP." Immediately invert the tip straight upward, and if it is functioning properly, it should beep again and display "Good" in the LCD, which means it is calibrated. It is now ready for use, so the tip should be covered with a disposable cover.

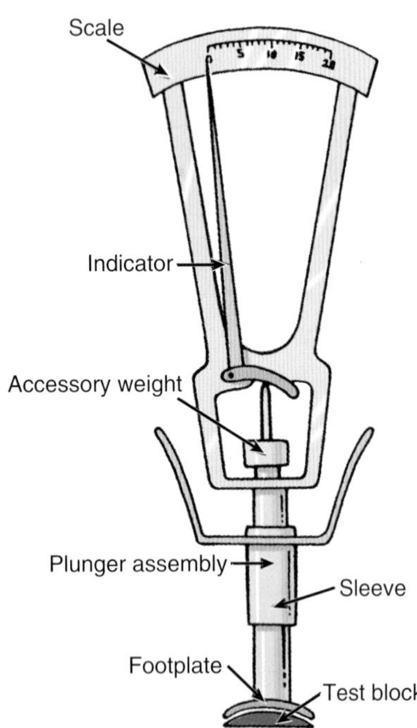

Figure 68-1 Schiøtz tonometer.

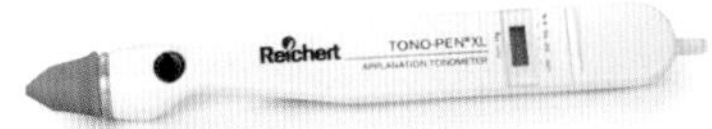

Figure 68-2 Hand-held tonometer (Tono-Pen XL). (Courtesy of Reichert, Inc., Depew, NY.)

NOTE: Beware of latex allergy in patients if latex Tono-Pen tip covers are being used.

Press the operation button again, and the instrument will display "[8.8.8.8]" followed by a single row of dashes and then a double row of dashes followed by a beep. Proceed with obtaining intraocular pressure readings within 15 seconds.

NOTE: Any time the operation button is depressed twice within 1.5 seconds, the instrument will attempt to calibrate and will display "CAL." While attempting to calibrate, if "Bad" is displayed in the LCD, repeat the process. If further attempts are unsuccessful, press the RESET button and repeat the process. If still unsuccessful, use optical-grade canned air to clean the probe tip for about 2 seconds, wait 3 minutes for the instrument to stabilize thermally, and then repeat the calibration process. If still not working, the batteries should be replaced and the process repeated. ("Lob" on the display also indicates low batteries.) Further unsuccessful attempts to calibrate warrant a call to technical support (1-800-866-6736 [TONO-PEN], www.tonopen.com, or see the supplier information in Appendix D).

3. For Schiøtz tonometry, have the patient lie on a table in the supine position and keep both eyes wide open. Ask the patient to relax and fix his or her gaze on a spot on the ceiling, with the line of vision perpendicular to the table. Retract the lids of the eye against the bony margin of the orbit with one hand, being careful to touch only the orbital margin because pressure directed into the orbit will cause the tonometer reading to be falsely elevated. Hold the tonometer by its handles with the thumb and middle finger of the other hand. After the patient has relaxed from the involuntary muscle contraction that occurs when the tonometer is first placed in his or her line of sight, center the foot plate of the tonometer over the cornea and gently lower the tonometer until it is resting on the cornea (Fig. 68-3). The indicator will come to rest at a position to the right of 0. The tonometer should be perpendicular to the cornea in a vertical position. Record the scale reading. If it is less than 4, repeat the reading because this indicates an elevated intraocular pressure. Perform another reading after adding the 7.5- or 10-g weight, as necessary, to obtain a scale reading between 4 and 8. Convert the scale reading to millimeters of mercury using the calibration scale included with the kit (Table 68-1). Record the intraocular pressure in the patient's chart. If the intraocular pressure in the other eye is going to be measured, immediately clean the foot plate with an alcohol swab and allow it to air dry for 1 to 2 minutes.
4. If the Tono-Pen is used, the patient can be in any position. However, the head should be supported so that the patient cannot pull away when the Tono-Pen is placed in his or her line of vision. Have the patient fix his or her line of vision by looking straight ahead.

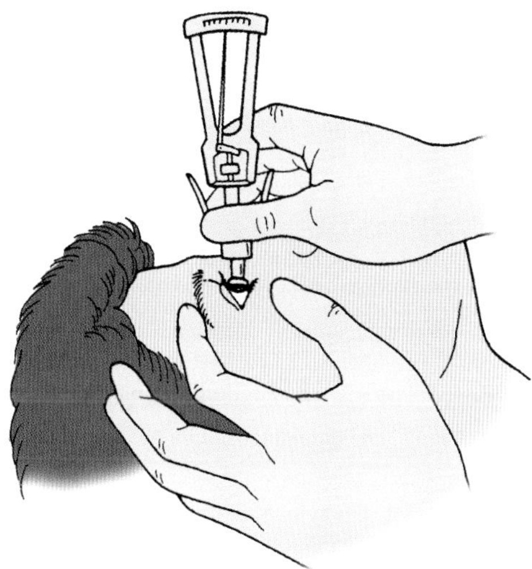

Figure 68-3 Examination with the Schiøtz tonometer.

TABLE 68-1 Sample Calibration Scale for Schiøtz Tonometer

Scale Reading	Intraocular Pressure (mm Hg) by Plunger Load 5.5 g	7.5 g	10.0 g	15.0 g
0	41	59	82	127
0.5	38	54	75	118
1.0	35	50	70	109
1.5	32	46	64	101
2.0	29	42	59	94
2.5	27	39	55	88
3.0	24	36	51	82
3.5	22	33	47	76
4.0	21	30	43	71
4.5	19	28	40	66
5.0	17	26	37	62
5.5	16	24	34	58
6.0	15	22	32	54
6.5	13	20	29	50
7.0	12	19	27	46
7.5	11	17	25	43
8.0	10	16	23	40
8.5	9	14	21	38
9.0	9	13	20	35
9.5	8	12	18	32
10.0	7	11	16	30
10.5	6	10	15	27
11.0	6	9	14	25
11.5	5	8	13	23
12.0		8	11	21
12.5		7	10	20
13.0		6	10	18
13.5		6	9	17
14.0		5	8	15
14.5			7	14
15.0			6	13
15.5			6	11
16.0			5	10
16.5				9
17.0				8
17.5				8
18.0				7

From Schiøtz Tonometer Kit literature, courtesy of Gulden Ophthalmics, Elkins Park, Pennsylvania.

NOTE: Regardless of technique used, to assist patients in fixing their gaze, ask them to extend an arm straight upward or out and to stare at their thumbnail placed over a spot on the wall or ceiling.

5. The clinician should consider bracing the heel of his or her hand on the patient's cheek for stability and then touching the tip of the Tono-Pen lightly to the central cornea directly over the pupil (the cornea does not need to be indented; indentation may lead to inaccurate readings). If the cornea is abraded over the pupil, touch the Tono-Pen to the cornea elsewhere. While holding the Tono-Pen perpendicular to the corneal surface, tap the cornea lightly several times. The Tono-Pen will chirp after each valid intraocular pressure reading is obtained. After four valid readings, the Tono-Pen will sound a final beep and display a mean intraocular pressure (mm Hg) with a horizontal line under it on the LCD. The statistical reliability of the measurement is also displayed, and if the reliability measure (standard deviation) is 20% or higher, a repeat measurement is recommended. Likewise, a single row of dashes in the LCD indicates an insufficient number of valid readings were collected, so after pressing the operation button, additional measurements should be made. When a valid intraocular pressure is displayed, record it in the patient's chart.

   NOTE: The tip of the Tono-Pen is a very sensitive probe that can be easily damaged, so it should never be touched by anything except a tip cover and then the cornea or the airflow from the optical-grade canned air when it needs to be cleaned.

6. Carefully clean the Schiøtz tonometer after each use to prevent transmission of disease. It can then be soaked in a special stand that soaks the tip only. A sterilizing solution that can eliminate human immunodeficiency virus should be used. Rinse carefully and allow to dry before using again. Alternatively, set the tonometer in an ultraviolet sterilizer stand. The tonometer should be disassembled at the end of each day and a pipe cleaner soaked with sterilizing solution run through the barrel to remove any debris. Accumulated debris could interfere with the motion of the plunger. Next, a dry pipe cleaner should be used to dry the barrel. The tonometer should not be oiled. If a Tono-Pen is used, it should not be immersed in fluids because the electronics will be damaged. Instead, the tip of the Tono-Pen should be cleaned of accumulated dust with optical-grade canned air; this step should be completed after it has been used for about 30 to 40 patients, or at least once a month. The tip cover should be changed after each use. A fresh tip cover should also be in place when the Tono-Pen is stored in the provided storage case. If the Tono-Pen is not going to be used for an extended period of time, the batteries should be removed.

Applanation

1. Check and record the patient's visual acuity. Examine the eyes. Immediately after the funduscopic examination, place two drops of anesthetic in each eye. (The anesthetic will have time to take effect while you prepare the slit lamp and attached Goldmann tonometer tip.) The clinician should follow universal blood and body fluid precautions.
2. Stabilize the patient's head by putting his or her chin on the chin rest and placing the forehead firmly against the headrest of the slit lamp (see Chapter 67, Slit-Lamp Examination). Each eye should be stained with fluorescein and the patient then asked to gaze straight ahead. His or her vision can be further fixated by asking him or her to focus on the clinician's ear on the side opposite the eye being examined.
3. The slit lamp should be on low-power magnification, the light filter switched to cobalt blue, and the slit diaphragm opened completely. Angle the light arm at about 45 to 60 degrees to the

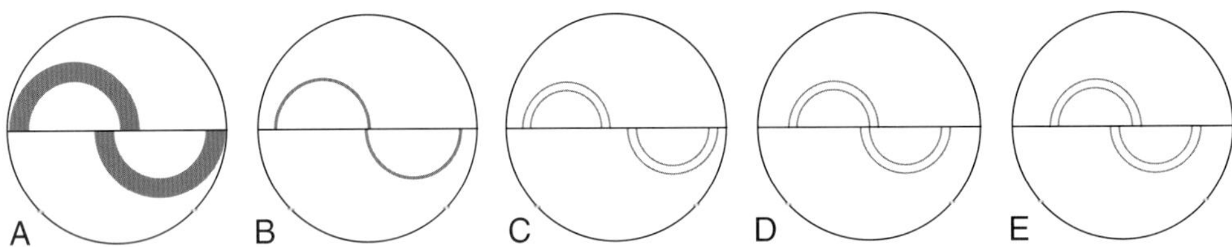

Figure 68-4 **A,** Semicircles too wide: excessive moisture. **B,** Semicircles too thin: excessive dryness. **C,** Intraocular pressure greater than knob setting (semicircles are correct width). **D,** Intraocular pressure equals knob setting (applied pressure). **E,** Intraocular pressure less than knob setting.

clinician's line of observation while shining the light on the plastic tonometer tip.

4. Set the pressure knob on the tonometer to 1 g (10 mm Hg). The patient should hold his or her eyes wide open and try to avoid blinking. The clinician may have to help the patient hold the lids open by applying pressure on the lids (only on the orbital rim).
5. Watching from the side (not through the slit lamp), the joystick should be used to move the tonometer tip up to the center of the patient's cornea, and then gentle contact is made. When contact is made, an immediate bluish glow should be noted all the way to the margin of the cornea. Avoid touching the lid margins with the tonometer tip because it will provoke blinking.
6. Through the slit lamp, the clinician should see two blue semicircles, each bordered by an arc of green light. These semicircles should be of equal extent above and below a horizontal dividing line. If the dividing line is not horizontal, the tonometer tip should be withdrawn and rotated on the holder until it is horizontal and reapplied to the cornea. If the semicircles extend beyond the illuminated field, there is too much pressure on the tonometer tip, so it should be backed away slightly from the eye.
7. The width of the arcs can be used to judge whether enough or excessive moisture is present. The width should be approximately 1/10 the diameter of the flattened surface contained within the arc. If the width is greater than 1/10 the diameter of the flattened area (Fig. 68-4A), too much moisture is present, either because of the tonometer tip being wet before application or because of excessive tears. The tip should be withdrawn from the patient's eye, dried, and reapplied. If the width of the arc is too narrow (Fig. 68-4B), the tear film has dried excessively. The tip should be withdrawn from the patient's eye and he or she should be asked to blink several times.
8. The blue semicircles and the surrounding green light will pulsate synchronously with the cardiac rate. If the intraocular pressure is greater than 10 mm Hg, the semicircles will not touch (Fig 68-4C). The clinician should turn the pressure knob up until the semicircles are touching (Fig. 68-4D). If the knob is turned up too far, the semicircles will overlap (Fig. 68-4E). Because the semicircles will move with cardiac pulsations, readings should be taken when the semicircles touch about midway between systole and diastole. In other words, when the knob pressure matches intraocular pressure, the semicircles should glide back and forth past each other through excursions of equal distance. If the width of the semicircles suddenly shrinks, either the patient has withdrawn from the scope or the instrument has been inadvertently backed away from the eye.
9. Record the intraocular pressure reading in the chart. Clean the tip of the tonometer with an alcohol swab immediately after use, and let it air dry for 1 to 2 minutes. Repeat the procedure on the contralateral eye if needed for comparison.

Postprocedure Patient Education

Routine prophylactic topical antibiotics are no longer prescribed after the procedure. The patient should be instructed to avoid rubbing, touching, or traumatizing the eyes for 1 or 2 hours after the test to avoid injuring the cornea. A contact lens should not be worn until the eye regains sensation. Patients should be warned that an anesthetized eye is easily traumatized and they should call the clinician's office immediately if symptoms of a corneal abrasion occur. If the result is abnormal (increased intraocular pressure), follow-up care should be discussed. Most clinicians recommend consultation with an ophthalmologist if the pressure in either eye is greater than 20 mm Hg. Intraocular pressure less than 9 mm Hg with recent eye surgery or trauma should also be discussed with an ophthalmologist. Emergent consultation with an ophthalmologist or treatment should be considered if the pressure is greater than 26 mm Hg. Patients need to know the importance of follow-up; however, they should be aware that increased intraocular pressure does not always mean that they have glaucoma and, vice versa, that normal intraocular pressure does not always exclude glaucoma.

Complications

- Trauma to the cornea during tonometry is uncommon; however, a corneal abrasion can occur after the procedure while the cornea is still anesthetized.
- Infection can usually be avoided by properly cleaning the tonometer and using fresh Tono-Pen tip covers or applanation tips.
- Low-pressure glaucoma may be missed; therefore, patients with suspiciously cupped disks on ophthalmic examination should be referred.

Limitations

Falsely elevated intraocular pressure readings can be a normal variant, or they can be the result of an inflamed cornea, a scarred cornea, or pressure placed on the globe during the procedure. They can also occur with a thick or steeply curved cornea (Tono-Pen minimally affected). Falsely low measurements can be a normal variant, or they can result from high-grade myopia or rapidly repeated measurements.

CPT/Billing Codes

Ophthalmological services constitute integrated services. Itemization of tonometry is not applicable.

92002 Ophthalmological services: medical examination and evaluation with initiation of diagnostic and treatment program; intermediate, new patient

92012 Ophthalmological services: medical examination and evaluation with initiation or continuation of diagnostic and treatment program; intermediate, established patient

92100 Serial tonometry (separate procedure) with multiple measurements of intraocular pressure over an extended time period with interpretation and report, same day (e.g., diurnal curve or medical treatment of acute elevation of intraocular pressure)

99173 Screening test of visual acuity, quantitative, bilateral (e.g., Snellen chart) (This cannot be used with 92002 or 92012)

Patient Education Guides

See patient education and patient consent forms available online at www.expertconsult.com.

Suppliers

(See contact information online at www.expertconsult.com.)

Schiøtz tonometer kit
Gulden Ophthalmics

Tono-Pen and applanation (Goldmann) tonometry equipment
Reichert, Inc.

Online Resources

Eye Care America: Foundation of the American Academy of Ophthalmology. Available at www.eyecareamerica.org (offers glaucoma risk assessment, educational materials, and access to care).

Glaucoma Research Foundation. Available at www.glaucoma.com (has patient information in Spanish).

National Eye Institute. Available at www.nei.nih.gov/ (has patient information in Spanish).

The Glaucoma Foundation. Available at www.glaucomafoundation.org/.

Bibliography

James DM: Tonometry. In James DM (ed): Field Guide to Urgent and Ambulatory Care Procedures. Philadelphia, Lippincott Williams & Wilkins, 2001, pp 4–8.

Knoop KJ, Dennis WR, Hedges JR: Ophthalmologic procedures. In Roberts JR, Hedges JR (eds): Clinical Procedures in Emergency Medicine, 5th ed. Philadelphia, Saunders, 2009, pp 1164–1169.

Morse RM, Heffron WA: Preventive health care in family practice. In Rakel RE (ed): Textbook of Family Practice, 6th ed. Philadelphia, Saunders, 2002.

Verplanck MW, Rolain M: Intraocular pressure measurement (tonometry). In Reichman EF, Simon RR (eds): Emergency Medicine Procedures. New York, McGraw-Hill, 2004, pp 1226–1233.

Wightman JM, Hamilton GC: Red and painful eye. In Marx J, Hockberger R, Walls R, et al (eds): Rosen's Emergency Medicine e-dition, 6th ed. Philadelphia, Mosby, 2006, pp 286–287.

CHAPTER 69

AUDIOMETRY

Gerald A. Amundsen

Hearing is measured according to its two main components: frequency/pitch and intensity/loudness. Audiometry is a procedure used to measure and graph an individual's hearing over a range of frequencies (measured in cycles per second [Hz, for Hertz]) at various intensity levels (measured in decibels [dB]). Although it is used frequently to test young children and the elderly (the groups at highest risk for hearing loss), audiometry is also an important component of any successful occupational hearing loss prevention program. In many instances, formal audiometry is performed by an audiologist; however, because screening audiometry is not a complex procedure and only a minimal amount of equipment is required, it is often performed by primary care clinicians. Even if not performing audiometry, primary care clinicians should have a basic understanding of not only the procedure but also the possible results.

An audiometer consists of a variable frequency oscillator that produces electrical impulses across the audible/perceptible frequencies, a transducer to convert the electrical impulses into sound or vibrations, and an attenuator to create variations in intensity. The device may be a stationary part of a designated testing facility or a portable unit with the flexibility to be used in a variety of settings. When sound is transmitted through headphones or an earpiece worn by the patient, and the patient responses are then recorded, an *air conduction audiogram* is produced. Air conduction audiometry evaluates both sensorineural and conductive hearing.

Sensorineural hearing refers to that produced by the cochlea of the inner ear, the auditory nerve, and the cochlear nuclei of the brain. There are both acquired and congenital causes of sensorineural hearing loss (Box 69-1). To test sensorineural hearing alone, a *bone conduction audiogram* is performed. With this procedure, similar to using a tuning fork when performing a physical examination, a bone conduction oscillator or vibrator is held against the mastoid process or forehead. Usually secured by a headband, the vibrator sets the skull into oscillation, producing a disturbance of the fluid in the cochlea. This disturbance is sensed by the cochlea and transmitted down the auditory nerve to the cochlear nuclei, *all without use of the middle ear system*. Results are graphed as the bone conduction audiogram. With pure sensorineural hearing loss, both air and bone conduction are impaired, and the impairments are about the same.

With air conduction hearing loss (usually due to middle or outer ear problems), air conduction is impaired but bone conduction is preserved. In the normal ear, the differences between the air and bone conduction thresholds, or the air–bone gap, should not exceed 10 dB. A gap larger than this indicates an air conduction problem (again, usually due to a middle or outer ear problem) as the source of hearing loss. Patients with air conduction hearing loss frequently respond to surgery; new surgical treatments for sensorineural hearing loss are also on the horizon. In many patients, hearing impairment is due to a combination, or a *mixed hearing loss*, and these also usually respond somewhat to surgery.

The symbols used on an audiogram (Fig. 69-1) have been standardized by the American Speech-Language Hearing Association (ASHA; www.ahsa.org). Traditionally, symbols representing the right ear were recorded in red, whereas results from the left ear were recorded in blue. Because color is potentially lost in photocopying, different symbols specific to each ear are now used on most audiograms.

Frequency is represented on the horizontal axis of the graph from low to high, from left to right. Although the normal human ear is capable of hearing a range from 20 to 20,000 Hz, an audiogram usually tests the range most necessary for hearing and the understanding of speech (usually 250 to 8000 Hz). Intensity, the measurement of "loudness," is represented on the vertical or left axis of the graph, and usually ranges from 0 to 120 dB. Data points plotted on the graph represent the lowest decibel intensity that can be heard by the individual 50% of the time at each frequency, and this is the *auditory threshold* for that particular frequency.

Results are interpreted relative to 0 dB, or *audiometric zero*. *Audiometric zero* is defined as "normal" by the American National Standards Institute (ANSI) and is derived from sampling a large

Box 69-1. Causes of Sensorineural Hearing Loss

Newborn

- Anoxia, asphyxia, hypoxia
- Bacterial infections
- Birth trauma
- Congenital syphilis
- Genetic causes, expressed at birth
- Hyperbilirubinemia requiring exchange transfusion
- Prematurity
- TORCH syndrome (toxoplasmosis, other agents, maternal rubella, cytomegalovirus, herpes simplex)

Acquired

- Autoimmune inner ear disorders
- Bacterial meningitis
- Congenital or acquired syphilis
- Cranial radiation therapy
- Excessive occupational noise or exposure to loud music
- Genetic
- Glomus tumors
- Head trauma (temporal bone fractures or labyrinthine concussion)
- Herpes zoster
- Human immunodeficiency virus infection/acquired immunodeficiency syndrome
- Labyrinthitis
- Lyme disease
- Measles
- Meniere's disease
- Mumps
- Ototoxic medications
- Vascular disorders

Modality	Response*		
	Ear		
	Left	Unspecified	Right
Air conduction: earphones			
Unmasked	X		O
Masked	□		△
Bone conduction: mastoid			
Unmasked	>	^	<
Masked	]		[
Bone conduction: forehead			
Unmasked	└	v	┘
Masked	┌		┐
Air conduction: sound field	X	S	∅

Figure 69-1 Standardized symbols for recording audiogram results. *For "no response," use a downward 45-degree arrow pointing to the left for the right ear symbols, and to the right for left ear symbols (e.g., ⌕ for no response in the right ear unmasked).

population of ear-disease–free young adults. In other words, if a person's threshold at a given frequency is 20 dB, it means that the individual can hear sound at that frequency only when it is 20 dB louder than that needed by an average disease-free young adult.

NOTE: From 1 to 6 of 1000 newborns have severe hearing loss, usually sensorineural in origin. The Joint Committee on Infant Hearing and the National Institutes of Health Consensus Statement recommend screening all infants for hearing loss at no later than 1 month of age. If the screening test result in the very young is abnormal, they should have comprehensive audiologic evaluation at no later than 3 months of age (e.g., behavioral observation audiometry, auditory brain stem response, otoacoustic emissions testing, visual reinforcement audiometry, conditioned play audiometry). Such an evaluation is beyond the scope of this text.

Indications

- General screening in children at the earliest age possible
- Exposure to one (or more) of the causes for sensorineural hearing loss (see Box 69-1)
- Speech delay in children
- Persistent behavioral problems or changes in children or the elderly
- Screening of the elderly, especially when performing geriatric assessment (see Chapter 232, Special Considerations in Geriatric Patients)
- Patient complaints of hearing loss
- Persistent serous otitis media, especially bilateral in children
- Anyone undergoing tympanometry with suspected sensorineural hearing loss (an abnormal tympanogram usually implies conductive hearing loss; however, sensorineural hearing loss may also be present)
- Formal audiometric evaluation of a failed screening test

NOTE: Up to 5% of school-age children will have fluctuating hearing loss during the school year because of middle ear effusions. Retesting is imperative.

- Patient complaints of tinnitus, dizziness, or vertigo
- After severe head trauma
- After use of ototoxic drugs
- After meningitis, encephalitis, or other serious viral or bacterial infections that could affect hearing
- Occupational screening and follow-up for individuals with noisy work environments

Contraindications

- Inexperienced technician
- Acute otitis media
- Local pinna infection that would cause pain from the earphone or earpiece application
- Uncooperative patient
- Uncontrollable background noise in the room when testing
- Occlusion of the canal by cerumen (see Chapter 72, Cerumen Impaction Removal) or a foreign body (see Chapter 76, Removal of Foreign Bodies from the Ear and Nose)

Equipment

- Audiometer: These range from simple hand-held screening instruments that test one ear at a time with a limited range of frequencies and intensities to more comprehensive devices. Audiometers may test air conduction alone or may be equipped to test both bone and air conduction. The most comprehensive units test frequencies from 125 to 8000 Hz at 0 to 100 dB. Audiometers are either stationary or portable, and many modern units interface directly with a laptop computer to record, store, and interpret patient evaluations.
- An individual trained in proper techniques for obtaining reliable, reproducible, and valid test results. (For occupational/industrial screening, the individual should be certified by the Council for Accreditation of Occupational Hearing Conservationists [www.caohc.org].)
- Quiet or sound-treated room, preferably tested (by an outside company) for acceptable background/ambient noise levels. If ambient noise levels are too high, thresholds may be artificially elevated, particularly in the lower frequencies.

Preprocedure Patient Preparation

The indications for the procedure should be explained to patients, and they should be reassured that the process is painless. Patients should know that they will be hearing tones of varying degrees of loudness and pitch, and that they should signal both when they first hear a tone and when the tone disappears. They should know how they are expected to demonstrate or signal when they hear the tone (e.g., raising their hand, pushing a button). Patients should sit in a relaxed and comfortable position and look straight ahead. If they can hear noise from outside the earphones or earpiece, they should inform the clinician. If bone conduction testing will be performed, the source and nature of the vibrations should be explained to the patient.

Technique

1. The examination must be administered using a properly calibrated instrument in a room with an acceptable level of background noise. The ear canal should have been checked for patency by the clinician.
2. The patient should be comfortably seated facing neither the monitor nor the examiner. (Usually patients are seated in a position that provides a side profile view to the examiner.)
3. Anything that may interfere with earphone application (or earplug insertion) should be removed (earrings, glasses, hats), and the headphones must be appropriately seated on the patient's head (or the earplugs properly inserted), sealing the ears from environmental noise.
4. Instruct the patient to respond to the faintest detectable sound at each frequency. Responses can consist of raising a hand or finger or pressing a test button when sound is first heard. The patient should continue to signal for the duration of audible sound. Having the patient indicate the entire duration of audible sound allows the examiner to determine if the responses

are reproducible. If reproducible, the threshold should be the same at the beginning and at the end for a particular frequency, at least 50% of the time; this can then be recorded. Patients should be tested from low to high decibels and then back to low. This step helps the examiner exclude false-positive responses.

5. Threshold testing is initiated in the better ear (or the right ear if hearing is equal in both) with the following recommended sequence of frequencies: 1000, 2000, 4000, 8000, 1000 (repeated), 500, and 250 Hz. Start with 0 dB hearing levels and produce the tones for 1 to 2 seconds unless the patient responds.
6. Increase the tone by 5 dB, and, if the patient responds, reduce it by 10-dB increments until it is inaudible.
7. Continue repeated ascents in 5-dB increments and descents in 10-dB increments until a 50% reproducible response is obtained. Generally this requires three to four repetitions, with the patient attaining the same response at least half of the time. This result is then entered with the appropriate symbol on the audiogram.
8. Test through the frequencies sequentially as previously noted, starting 15 to 20 dB below the threshold of the previously tested frequency. Continue testing until all frequencies have been tested.
9. If bone conduction testing is planned, this same sequence can be applied and the results recorded with the appropriate symbols.
10. It may be necessary to mask or obscure one sound with another when the difference in hearing loss between the ears is great (e.g., a 40-dB difference for air conduction testing, a 5-dB difference for bone conduction hearing) or there is a 10-dB air–bone gap in the ear being tested. In these situations, crossover of sound to the better ear may occur and artificially lower the threshold of the impaired ear, so masking is applied to the nontest ear. Audiometers are calibrated so that a 10-dB masking noise will block a 10-dB pure signal.

INTERPRETATION

Air conduction testing alone can approximate the degree of hearing loss. However, to differentiate between conductive, sensorineural, and mixed hearing loss, it is often best to test both air and bone conduction hearing.

A threshold of up to 20 dB is considered normal. Above that, hearing loss can be divided into degrees of severity (Table 69-1). Certain patterns of hearing loss, especially unilateral, can indicate specific diseases. Hearing asymmetry of more than 20 dB, especially if it is suspected to be sensorineural in origin, may indicate a retrocochlear lesion or mass (Fig. 69-2). Such patients should be evaluated further with imaging or referred. The tympanometer may be used as an additional tool to assess mobility of the tympanic membrane when conductive hearing loss is diagnosed by audiometry. Conversely, audiometry is often used as an adjunct to tympanometry when a persistently abnormal tympanogram is present (see Chapter 75, Tympanometry, for more details).

Figures 69-2 through 69-11 illustrate classic patterns of hearing loss. In the examples, hearing thresholds have been converted to hearing loss (HL). In addition, because each ear was recorded separately, the standardized symbols were not necessary to distinguish left from right.

TABLE 69-1 Classification of Severity of Hearing Loss

Degree of Hearing Loss (dB)	Level of Severity
0–20	Normal
21–40	Mild
41–55	Moderate
56–70	Moderately severe
71–90	Severe
>90	Profound

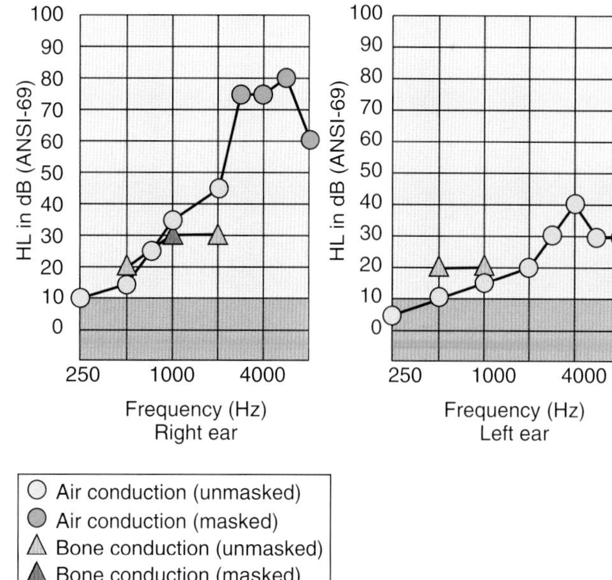

Figure 69-2 Sixty-year-old man with suspected right acoustic neuroma. Note the unilateral hearing loss. (The corresponding tympanograms would be type A or normal.) (Redrawn from Jacobsen JT, Northern JL [eds]: Diagnostic Audiology. Austin, Tex, Pro-Ed, 1991.)

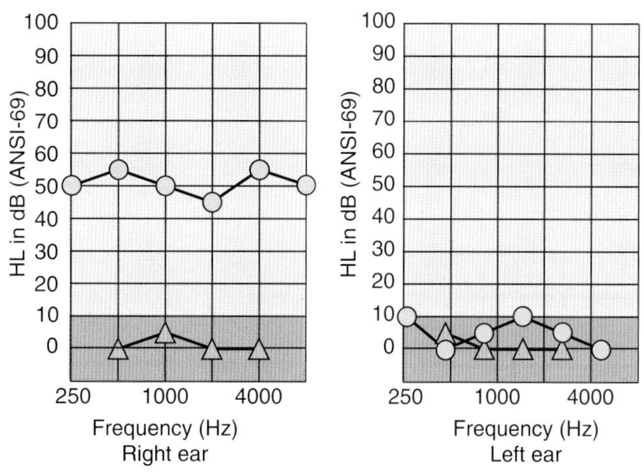

Figure 69-3 Nine-year-old boy with right acute otitis media with effusion. Using masking, the curves would probably appear the same; however, there would be slightly more assurance of the accuracy of the study. (The corresponding tympanogram would be type B.) (Redrawn from Jacobsen JT, Northern JL [eds]: Diagnostic Audiology. Austin, Tex, Pro-Ed, 1991.)

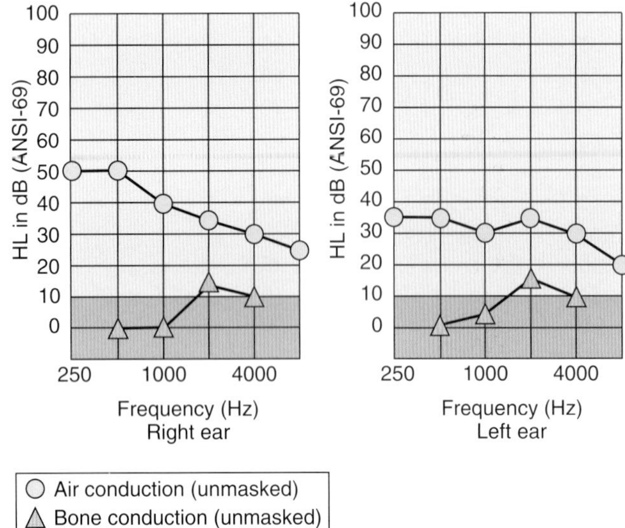

Figure 69-4 Forty-year-old woman with bilateral otosclerosis. (The corresponding tympanograms would be type A or A_S.) This disorder is autosomal dominantly inherited with about 40% penetrance. (Redrawn from Jacobsen JT, Northern JL [eds]: Diagnostic Audiology. Austin, Tex, Pro-Ed, 1991.)

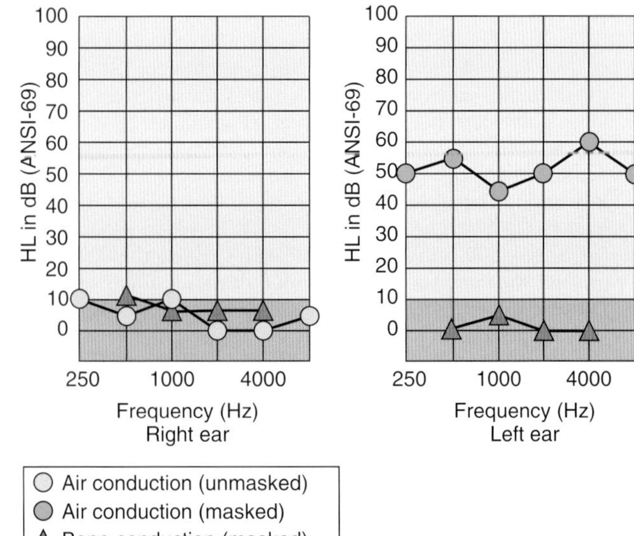

Figure 69-5 Twenty-year-old man with ossicular disruption on the left after mild head trauma. (The corresponding left ear tympanogram would be type A_D.) (Redrawn from Jacobsen JT, Northern JL [eds]: Diagnostic Audiology. Austin, Tex, Pro-Ed, 1991.)

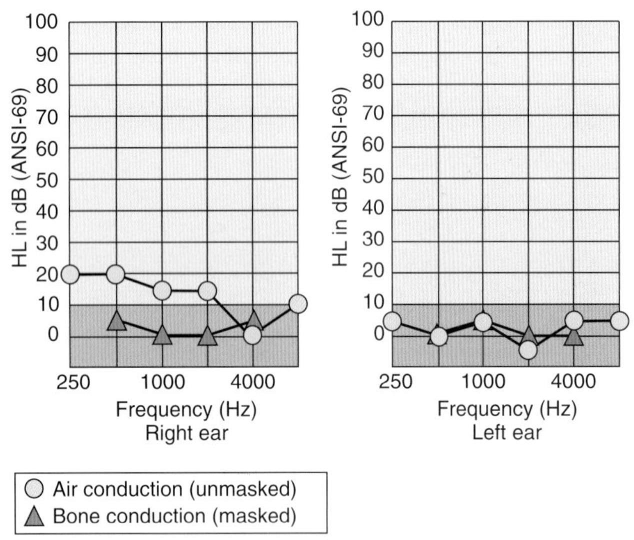

Figure 69-6 Fifteen-year-old girl with right tympanic membrane perforation. (The corresponding right ear tympanogram would be type B.) (Redrawn from Jacobsen JT, Northern JL [eds]: Diagnostic Audiology. Austin, Tex, Pro-Ed, 1991.)

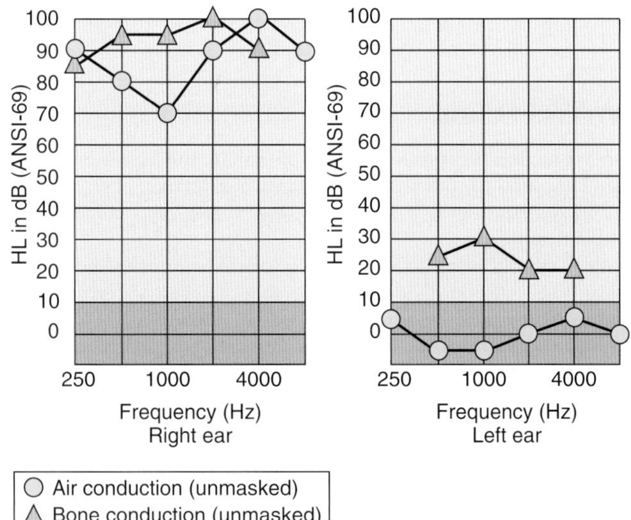

Figure 69-7 Forty-year-old man with suspected functional (factitious) hearing loss after industrial accident with a single exposure to high-intensity noise (e.g., an explosion). Bone conduction should be intact after a single exposure. (The corresponding tympanograms would be type A or normal.) (Redrawn from Jacobsen JT, Northern JL [eds]: Diagnostic Audiology. Austin, Tex, Pro-Ed, 1991.)

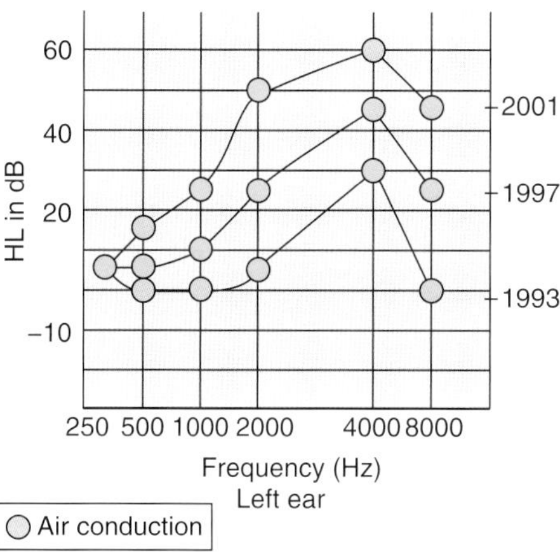

Figure 69-8 Fifty-five-year-old man with gradually progressive left neurosensory hearing loss over several years. Such a hearing loss can be seen in a person who hunts and shoots left-handed. In most such cases, the audiogram differs from that of presbycusis because it spares the upper frequencies (8000 Hz). (The corresponding tympanogram would be type A or normal.) (Redrawn from Jacobsen JT, Northern JL [eds]: Diagnostic Audiology. Austin, Tex, Pro-Ed, 1991.)

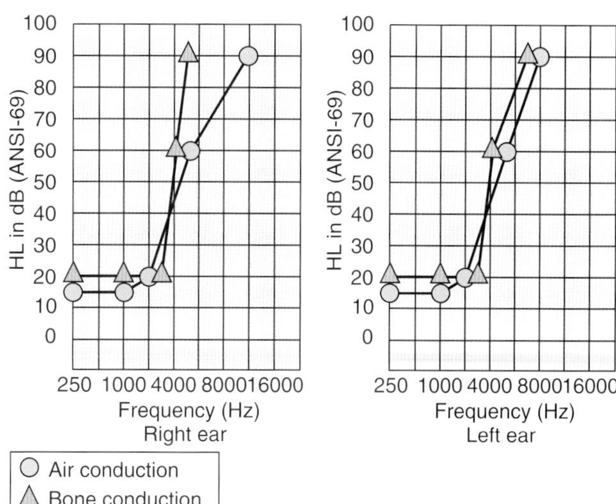

Figure 69-9 Eighty-year-old man with presbycusis, or hearing loss caused by advancing age. It is usually bilateral, and in men it often affects the higher frequencies more severely. In women, in addition to symmetric high-frequency loss, there may be hearing loss in the lower frequencies. (The corresponding tympanograms would be type A or normal.) (Redrawn from Jacobsen JT, Northern JL [eds]: Diagnostic Audiology. Austin, Tex, Pro-Ed, 1991.)

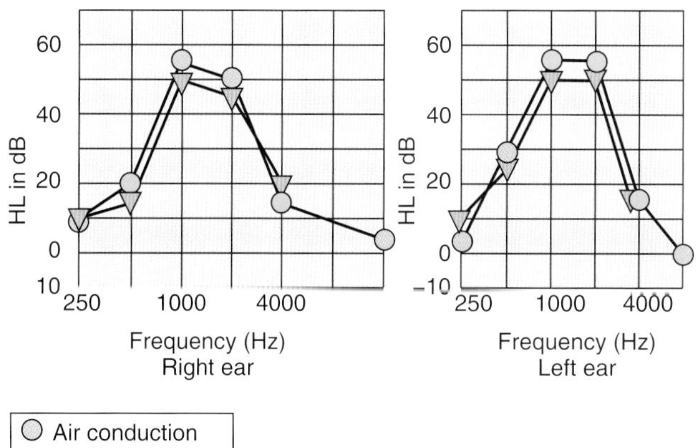

Figure 69-10 Fifty-year-old woman with long-term exposure to loud occupational noise, which could include loud music. Note the speech frequencies are more affected than the higher frequencies. (The corresponding tympanogram would be type A or normal.) (Redrawn from Jacobsen JT, Northern JL [eds]: Diagnostic Audiology. Austin, Tex, Pro-Ed, 1991.)

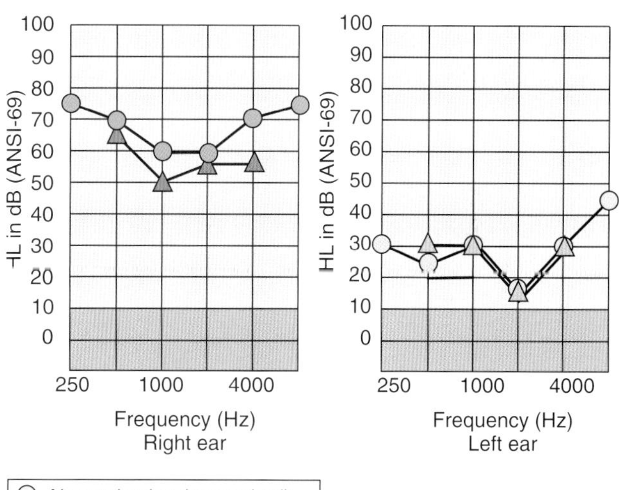

Figure 69-11 Fifty-two-year-old man with Meniere's disease, predominantly affecting right ear. This hearing loss is often associated with episodes of tinnitus and vertigo, frequently at the same time. Remission can occur, as well as exacerbation. Over time, the hearing loss typically progresses to moderate or moderately severe and persistent. (The corresponding tympanograms would be type A or normal.) (Redrawn from Jacobsen JT, Northern JL [eds]: Diagnostic Audiology. Austin, Tex, Pro-Ed, 1991.)

CPT/Billing Codes

92551 Screening test, pure-tone, air only (e.g., single-decibel-level device with selected frequencies)
92552 Pure-tone audiometry, threshold; air only
92553 Pure-tone audiometry, threshold; air and bone
92555 Speech audiometry, threshold
92556 Speech audiometry, threshold; with speech recognition
92557 Comprehensive audiometry, threshold evaluation and speech recognition (92553 and 92556 combined)

ICD-9-CM Diagnostic Codes

388.2 Hearing loss, sudden, unspecified
389.00 Hearing loss, conductive, unspecified
389.02 Hearing loss, tympanic membrane, conductive
389.03 Hearing loss, middle ear, conductive
389.04 Hearing loss, inner ear, conductive
389.05 Hearing loss, conductive, unilateral
389.06 Hearing loss, conductive, bilateral
389.2 Hearing loss, mixed conductive and sensorineural
389.8 Hearing loss, high or low frequency
389.9 Deafness
389.10 Hearing loss, sensorineural, unspecified
389.14 Hearing loss, central
389.15 Hearing loss, sensorineural, unilateral
389.18 Hearing loss, sensorineural, bilateral
951.5 Traumatic deafness
V19.2 Family history of hearing loss
V72.11 Hearing exam following failed hearing screening
V72.19 Hearing exam

Acknowledgment

The editors wish to recognize the many contributions by Gregory J. Forzley, MD, to this chapter in the previous two editions of this text.

Suppliers

(See contact information online at www.expertconsult.com.)

Benson Medical Instruments
Castle Group
Gordon Stowe
Grason-Stadler, Inc.
Maico Diagnostics
Micro Audiometrics
Otometrics
Welch Allyn, Inc.

BIBLIOGRAPHY

American Academy of Family Physicians; American Academy of Otolaryngology-Head and Neck Surgery; American Academy of Pediatrics Subcommittee on Otitis Media with Effusion: Otitis media with effusion [clinical practice guideline]. Pediatrics 113:1412–1429, 2004.

American Academy of Pediatrics, Joint Committee on Infant Hearing: Year 2007 position statement: Principles and guidelines for early hearing detection and intervention programs. Pediatrics 120:898–921, 2007.

American Speech-Language-Hearing Association: Guidelines for audiometric symbols. ASHA 32(Suppl. 2):25, 1990.

American Speech-Language-Hearing Association: Guidelines for the Audiologic Assessment of Children from Birth to 5 Years of Age. 2004. Available at www.asha.org/policy. Accessed November 2007.

Cunningham M, Cox EO; Committee on Practice and Ambulatory Medicine and Section on Otolaryngology and Bronchoesophagology: Hearing assessment in infants and children: Recommendations beyond neonatal screening. Pediatrics 111:436–440, 2003.

Hall JW III, Antonelli PJ: Assessment of peripheral and central auditory function. In Newlands SD, Calhoun KH, Curtin HD, et al (eds): Head and Neck Surgery—Otolaryngology, 4th ed. Philadelphia, Lippincott Williams & Wilkins, 2006, pp 1927–1942.

Isaacson JE, Vora NM: Differential diagnosis and treatment of hearing loss. Am Fam Physician 68:1125–1132, 2003.

CHAPTER 70

Auricular Hematoma Evacuation

George D. Harris

The external ear is subject to a wide variety of injuries. Traumatic injury to the ear is commonly seen in athletes, particularly wrestlers, boxers, and rugby players. Such trauma can also be the result of motor vehicle accidents, assaults, fights, and falls. Although a cushion of subcutaneous fat on the medial surface of the auricle can dissipate a direct force, allowing the skin to slide over the underlying cartilage, the lateral surface lacks this layer of fat. Consequently, blunt trauma over the lateral surface causes shearing forces between the perichondrium and the underlying cartilage, resulting in torn blood vessels in the perichondrium and the formation of a hematoma. The location of the hematoma has classically been described as between the perichondrium and cartilage; however, the hematoma can arise within the cartilage itself.

Untreated lesions affecting the external ear (pinna) can lead to overt disfigurement (cauliflower or wrestler's ear), especially if there is a delay in diagnosis and management.

With trauma, swelling can occur immediately or up to several hours later. Auricular hematomas can also occur spontaneously in older patients and in patients with a blood dyscrasia. A hematoma between the auricular cartilage and the perichondrium deprives the cartilage of its nutrient supply. If left untreated, a hematoma is at risk for secondary infection, perichondritis, cartilage necrosis, contracture, and neocartilage formation. The goals of treatment are to evacuate the hematoma, provide compression in the area, prevent the reaccumulation of fluid, and maintain the cartilage contour. Early treatment helps prevent aseptic necrosis and the loss of cartilage, and, it is hoped, avoids the permanent cosmetic ear deformity (cauliflower ear) from clot organization with fibrin deposition.

This chapter gives primary care clinicians, especially those involved in sports medicine, the information necessary to become familiar with the clinical presentation, appropriate treatment, and complications encountered when faced with an auricular hematoma.

NOTE: Patients presenting 7 to 10 days after the time of injury need extensive management. By this time, there is newly formed cartilage and perichondrium; treatment of these patients is beyond the scope of this chapter.

Indications

Auricular hematoma: red, reddish-purple, or bluish fluctuant swelling, usually involving the entire lateral auricle. It is also usually quite tender.

Contraindications

- Hematoma accompanied by auricular laceration
- Injury beyond the abilities of the clinician

Equipment

- Topical antiseptic, such as povidone–iodine (Betadine)
- For aspiration, 18- or 20-gauge needle and syringe
- Adhesive plastic ear drape or fenestrated drape
- Sterile gloves
- No. 15 scalpel blade and holder
- Curved hemostat
- Forceps
- For anesthesia, 30-gauge needle and syringe
- Local anesthetic such as lidocaine 1% (optional, mixed with 1 : 100,000 epinephrine)
- Small suction catheter or curette
- Penrose drain or sterile rubber band and scissors
- Gauze dressing
- Petrolatum gauze, or cotton balls soaked with petroleum jelly or mineral oil
- For alternative compression techniques: (1) cotton dental roll or tightly folded gauze, and monofilament nylon suture (3-0 or 4-0) with needle and a needle holder; or (2) otolaryngologist's (ear, nose and throat [ENT]) silicone putty or dental impression material (Exaflex type O putty [GC America, Inc., Alsip, Ill])
- Topical antibiotic ointment (bacitracin/polymyxin or mupirocin)
- Eye protection

Preprocedure Patient Preparation

Explain the indications for, alternatives to, and possible complications of the procedure as well as the possible complications from not performing the procedure to the patient. Obtain informed consent, if possible. Also explain the discomfort of injected local anesthetic, and the necessity for the patient to remain very still during the procedure. The patient should be prepared for some mild discomfort during hematoma removal, even with use of the local anesthetic.

Technique

Treatment requires the complete drainage of the hematoma to prevent deformity. This can be done in multiple ways, but the predominant methods are needle aspiration and incision and evacuation. Both should be followed by some type of compression dressing to prevent reaccumulation. There is controversy about which method of drainage is superior. In addition, there are no randomized trials, case-controlled trials, or cohort studies to support one treatment over another regarding the best cosmetic result with the least permanent deformity. Because of the difficulty in removing the entire hematoma, the difficulty in eliminating the dead space, the consequent high risk of recurrence, and the frequent need for a second procedure after needle aspiration, many experts prefer the incision and evacuation technique.

1. Position the patient comfortably in the supine position with the injured ear accessible. Universal blood and body fluid precautions should be followed.
2. Cleanse the helix with antiseptic solution. Examine for associated lacerations. Anesthesia is achieved by performing a regional block (see Chapter 8, Peripheral Nerve Blocks and Field Blocks)

or by placing a skin wheal of local anesthetic over the hematoma. Many clinicians prefer a regional block because it is very difficult to inject local anesthetic at the site (there is no subcutaneous layer of fat below the skin; consequently, the skin is tightly adherent to perichondrium). The hematoma should not be injected because the anesthetic will only cause the hematoma to expand and increase the damage.

3. Attempt aspiration of the most fluctuant area of the hematoma using an 18- or 20-gauge needle (Fig. 70-1). To ensure complete evacuation of the hematoma, it may be helpful to express the hematoma between the thumb and index finger of the opposite hand while aspirating. This technique may be all that is necessary to evacuate the hematoma, especially if the injury is quite recent and the hematoma is small. If so, proceed to step 9 and then to the "Alternative Compression Techniques" section.

   NOTE: Using a simple aspiration technique is not adequate for preventing recurrence; consequently one must also use a compression technique. If the hematoma has been present for 6 to 8 hours, it is likely an organized clot. This will be difficult to aspirate, and incision and drainage will probably be required. However, if the patient presents 1 week postinjury, the clot usually has broken down and aspiration once again can be attempted. Larger hematomas may require an open approach or the placement of a drain.

4. If aspiration does not completely evacuate the hematoma, incision and evacuation will need to be performed. While maintaining a sterile field, a regional block should be performed. (A regional block is necessary for reasons previously mentioned, including the lack of a subcutaneous layer of fat.)
5. While waiting 10 to 15 minutes for the anesthetic to take effect, drape the patient in a manner that keeps his or her hair away from the involved area.
6. Note the anatomy of the external ear (Fig. 70-2). With the no. 15 scalpel, make a curvilinear incision over the hematoma, usually 4 to 5 mm in length (and no longer than 1 cm). For the best cosmetic result, the incision should follow the natural recessions of the ear between the helix and antihelix, or the antihelix and the concha (Fig. 70-3). Multiple incisions may be needed. The hematoma may then be expressed or removed using the forceps, gentle suctioning, or curettage.
7. Probe the cavity with the hemostat to ensure complete evacuation. Additional manipulation can be performed, if necessary, with digital pressure applied to assist with complete evacuation. Apply pressure until hemostasis is obtained.
8. Insert a piece of the Penrose drain or rubber band into the incision. (This should be removed within 48 hours to minimize the risk of infection.)
9. Apply antibiotic ointment to the area of the aspiration or incision.

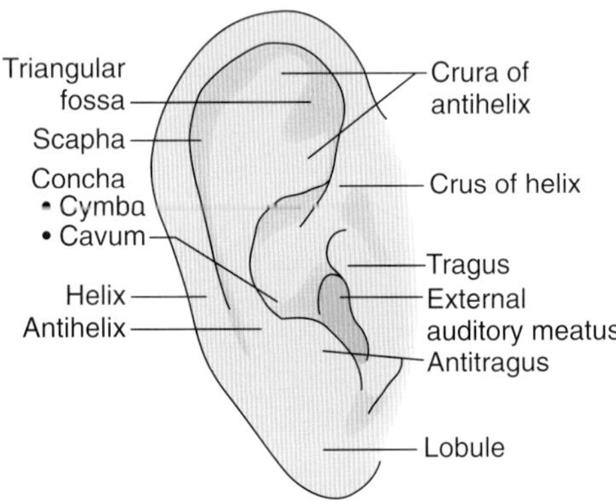

Figure 70-2 Anatomy of the external ear. (From Bisaccia E, Lugo A, Johnson B, Scarborough D: The surgical correction of protuberant ears. Skin Therapy Lett 10:7–9, 2005.)

10. Place a piece of sterile dry cotton in the external auditory canal. Then, fit petroleum jelly–treated gauze or petroleum jelly– or mineral oil–soaked cotton balls externally onto the contours of the ear. They should be placed in layers until level with the lateral helical rim. Trimmed gauze squares should then be placed between the ear and the head. Finally, over these layers of gauze or cotton, apply an elastic gauze compression dressing to the ear (Fig. 70-4).
11. Prescribe prophylactic oral antibiotics and appropriate analgesia. Antibiotics are important if the hematoma has been present for more than 24 hours, if the hematoma recurs and requires repeated incision and drainage, or if there are signs of cellulitis. They should cover *Staphylococcus aureus*, *Pseudomonas aeruginosa*, and a variety of other gram-negative bacteria.
12. Instruct the patient to remove the elastic gauze bandage daily to evaluate the auricle. He or she should return in 48 hours for complete dressing removal and reevaluation. Redrain the ear or reapply the dressing as needed to maintain ear compression for 1 week.

Alternative Compression Techniques

Cotton Dental Rolls

The alternative compression technique uses cotton dental rolls for compression *after* evacuation. First, follow steps 1 through 7, as described previously.

8. Next, cut a dental roll to fit over most of the hematoma. The smaller remnant of the cut roll will be stitched medially. (Two

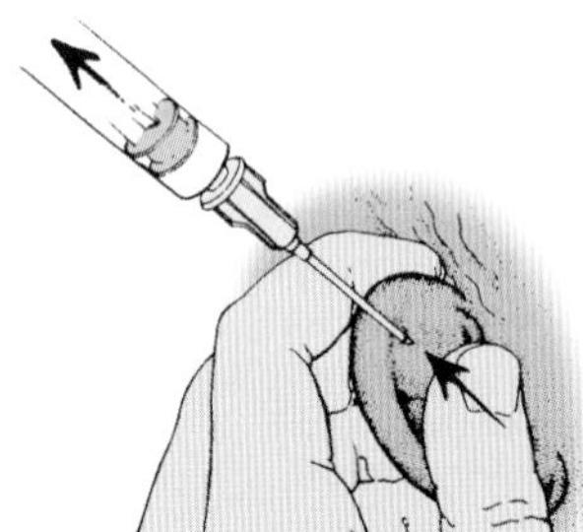

Figure 70-1 While stabilizing the pinna with the thumb and fingers, puncture the most fluctuant part of the hematoma. Use the thumb and index finger to "milk" the hematoma into the syringe.

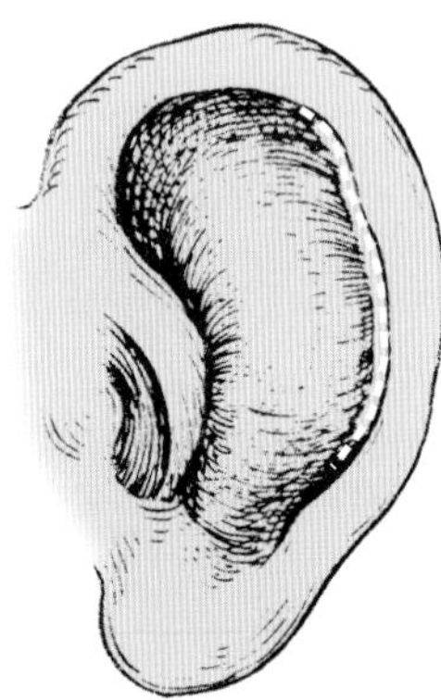

Figure 70-3 A curvilinear incision is made.

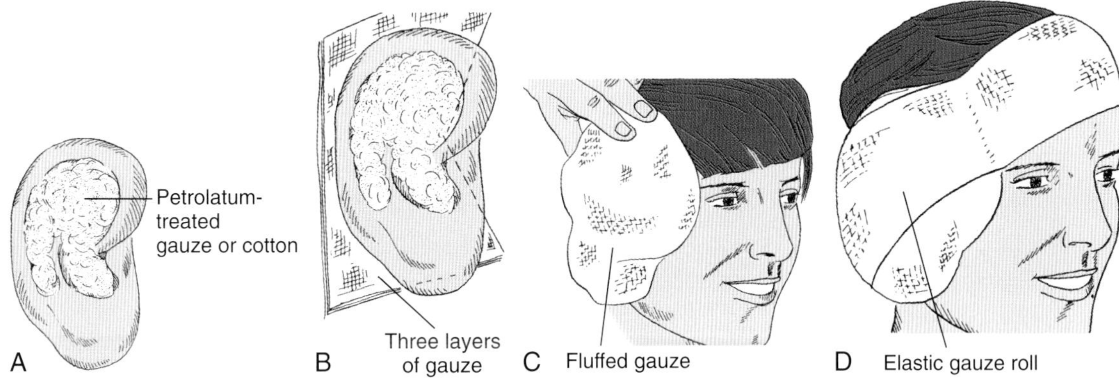

Figure 70-4 External gauze compression dressing. **A,** Dry cotton is first placed into the ear canal. A conforming material is then carefully molded into all the convolutions of the auricle. **B,** When the convolutions are fully packed, a medial gauze pack is placed behind the ear. A V-shaped section has been cut from the gauze to allow it to easily fit behind the ear. **C,** Multiple layers of fluffed gauze are placed over the packed ear. **D,** The entire dressing is held in place with Kling or an elastic gauze roll. The ear is thus compressed between two layers of gauze, and the packing ensures even distribution of pressure to all parts of the auricle.

tightly packed pieces of gauze can be stitched in a similar manner, with similar effects.)

9. After slightly straightening the suture needle, pass it through one end of the cut dental roll.
10. Pass the needle through the most cephalic end of the hematoma from lateral to medial. To use the smaller remaining piece of dental roll as medial compression, pass the needle back and forth through the smaller roll (Fig. 70-5).
11. Next, pass the needle through the inferior portion of the hematoma from medial to lateral and then through the other end of the lateral dental roll. If necessary, multiple rolls can be used (Fig. 70-6).
12. Tie the suture securely. This creates both lateral and medial compression of the hematoma.
13. Apply antibacterial ointment liberally over the dental rolls and the ear. Next, apply an elastic gauze dressing. Oral antibiotics are given as in preceding step 11.
14. Ask the patient to return in 24 hours, at which time the elastic gauze dressing is removed. Instruct the patient to continue applying antibacterial ointment until the dental roll dressing is removed in 2 weeks.

NOTE: This technique requires an aseptic procedure, anesthesia, and frequent daily dressings. Patients frequently complain of auricular pain for several days after a stitched compressed dressing is applied. The stitched compressed dressing can sometimes lead to pressure necrosis of the auricle.

ENT Silicone Putty or Dental Impression Material

The technique using ENT silicone putty or dental impression material first follows steps 1 through 7, described previously.

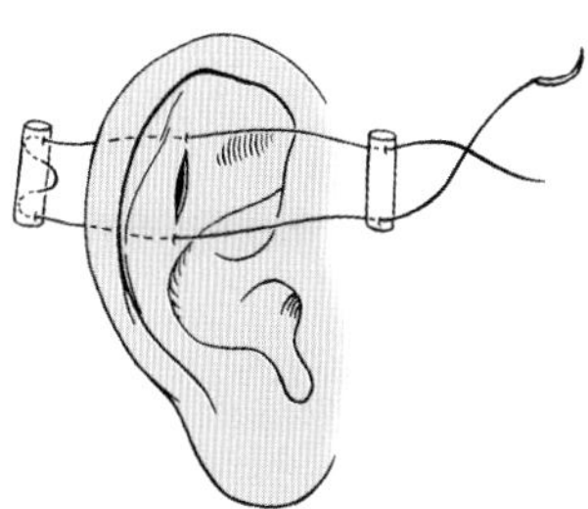

Figure 70-5 Alternative technique using cotton dental roll for compression.

8. Next, mold ENT silicone putty to fit the lateral ear just lateral to the external auditory meatus. Wrap the putty medially to match the pinna (Fig. 70-7). The putty contains a hardener, causing it to solidify in a few minutes. Dental impression material can be mixed and used in the same manner (Fig. 70-8).
9. An elastic gauze head bandage is then applied for 2 days. It can then be removed. The ENT putty or hardened dental impression material mold should be left in place for a week. Use oral antibiotics as described previously. Instruct the patient to return in 48 hours for reevaluation.

Postprocedure Patient Education

The patient should be aware of the importance of maintaining compression for at least a week. He or she should understand the risk of complications, regardless of management, and should see a clinician if there are signs of infection (e.g., increasing redness, drainage, tenderness, warmth, pain at site). If an external elastic gauze is used to cover the site (see Fig. 70-4), it should be removed daily to check for signs of infection or complications and then reapplied. Oral antibiotics are indicated with any puncture, incision, or laceration of the auricle, so patients should know how to take them

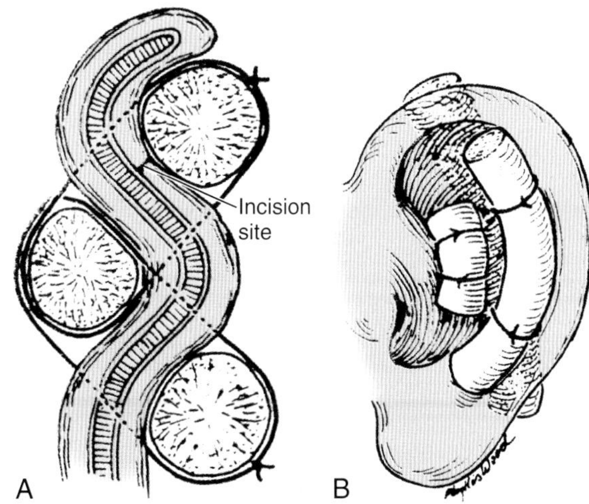

Figure 70-6 Multiple dental rolls used for compression after evacuation of a large hematoma. **A,** Medial auricular. **B,** Lateral auricular. (From Cummings CW [ed]: Otolaryngology: Head and Neck Surgery, 2nd ed. St. Louis, Mosby, 1993.)

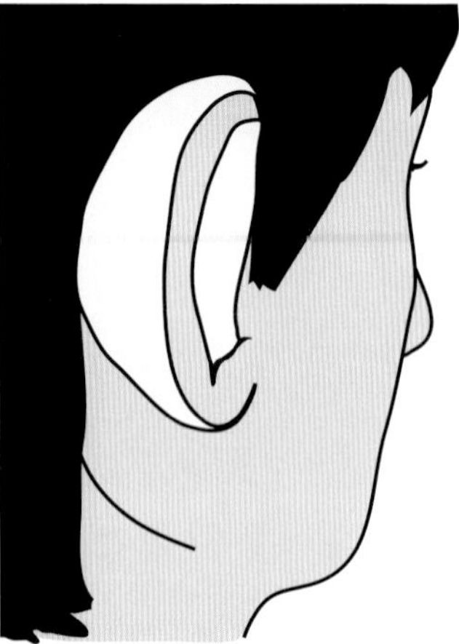

Figure 70-7 ENT putty used for compression. The putty is molded to fit the ear, and an external compression dressing is used for 2 days. By then the putty is hardened and can be left open to air.

and the importance of taking them. He or she should know when to return to the clinician's office and what possible complications to report.

COMPLICATIONS

- Bleeding or recurrence of hematoma
- Scar at the site of the incision
- Infection including perichondritis (risk minimized by prophylactic oral antibiotics)
- Auricular deformity, either in spite of appropriate treatment, or because the treatment is inadequate

CPT/BILLING CODES

69000 Drainage external ear, abscess or hematoma; simple
69005 Complicated

ICD-9-CM DIAGNOSTIC CODE

380.31 Auricular hematoma

ACKNOWLEDGMENT

The editors wish to recognize the many contributions by Gregory J. Forzley, MD, to this chapter in the previous two editions of this text.

BIBLIOGRAPHY

Ghanem T, Rasamny JK, Park SS: Rethinking auricular trauma. Laryngoscope 115:1251–1255, 2005.

James DM: Management of auricular hematoma. In James DM (ed): Field Guide to Urgent and Ambulatory Care Procedures. Philadelphia, Lippincott Williams & Wilkins, 2001, pp 33–35.

Jones SE, Mahendran S: Interventions for acute auricular hematoma. Cochrane Database Syst Rev 2:CD004166, 2004.

Lee D, Sperling N: Initial management of auricular trauma. Am Fam Physician 53:2339–2344, 1996.

Reichman EF: Auricular hematoma evacuation. In Reichman EF, Simon RR (eds): Emergency Medicine Procedures. New York, McGraw-Hill, 2004, pp 1276–1285.

Riviello RJ, Brown NA: Otolaryngologic procedures. In Roberts JR, Hedges JR (eds): Clinical Procedures in Emergency Medicine, 5th ed. Philadelphia, Saunders, 2009, pp 1195–1198.

Schuller DE, Dankle SD, Strauss RH: A technique to treat wrestlers' auricular hematoma without interrupting training or competition. Arch Otolaryngol Head Neck Surg 115:202–206, 1989.

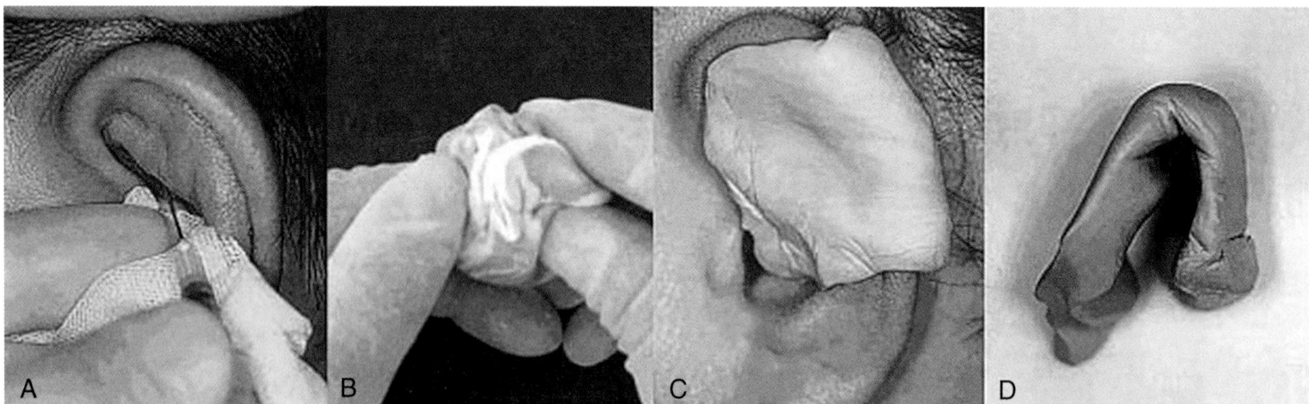

Figure 70-8 Technique for treatment of auricular hematoma using dental impression material. **A,** Follow steps 1 through 7 of the procedure. **B,** The impression material is prepared using equal parts (one scoop) of base and catalyst of Exaflex type O putty (GC America, Inc., Alsip, Ill), which is composed of vinyl polysiloxane and spontaneously cures after base and catalyst are mixed. The materials are kneaded in the hands for 1 minute or until uniform in color. **C,** The mixed impression material is placed on both the lateral and medial surfaces of the auricle. Make sure the lateral surface of the auricle is adequately covered, including the cavum concha area, to maintain the normal contour of the auricle. It takes about 3 to 5 minutes for the Exaflex mixture to cure spontaneously. **D,** The dental impression material is contoured into the shape of an inverted "U," which acts to stabilize the frame. The cured dental frame is fixed and stabilized with paper tape and then dressed simply with gauze. The patient is checked again 3 days after the procedure, and then on day 7. At that time, the impression material is removed. (From Choung YH, Park K, Choung PH, Oh JH: Simple compressive method for treatment of auricular haematoma using dental silicone material. J Laryngol Otol 119:27–31, 2005.)

CHAPTER 71

Earlobe Repair

Dennis LaRavia

Constant or repetitive traction by jewelry worn in a pierced earlobe may eventually cause a large, elongated hole (Figs. 71-1A and 71-2). Over time, the defect may even extend through the tip of the lobe, creating a bifid lobe that is completely reepithelialized (Fig. 71-1B). More acutely, an earring can be pulled or ripped through the lobe, resulting in a laceration. This area is also a common site for cysts. Regardless of the cause, the results are often unacceptable cosmetically to the patient; it may also become impossible to wear a pierced earring at that site. Although some patients will opt for clip-ons or piercing at an adjacent site and wear large earrings to cover the defect, others will choose to repair the lobe.

Primary care clinicians can repair the earlobe in the office, often bringing great satisfaction to a patient by improving both cosmetic appearance and convenience with jewelry. The usual charge from a plastic surgeon for such a repair is $450 to $650; consequently, primary care clinicians can usually work something out that is beneficial to both the patient and the clinician.

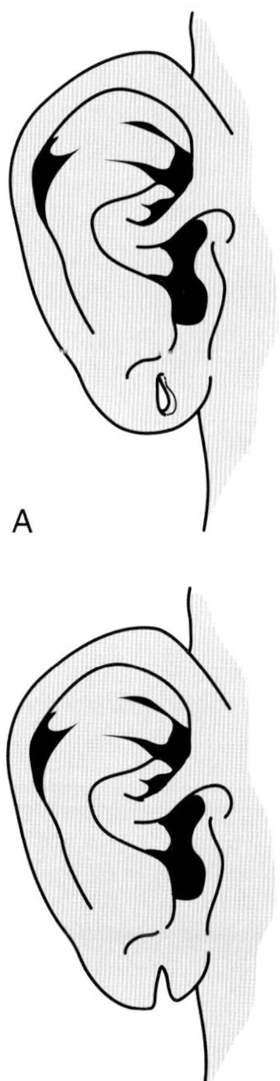

Figure 71-1 The torn earlobe defect. **A,** Incomplete tear with resulting large hole defect. **B,** Complete tear.

Equipment

- Sterile preparation and setup (alcohol or chlorhexidine, sterile drapes and gloves).
- Lidocaine 1% or 2%, *without epinephrine*.
- Laceration repair kit including skin hooks and 6-0 nylon suture.
- Scalpel with a no. 15 or 15c blade, and possibly a no. 11 blade.
- Antibacterial ointment or petroleum jelly.
- Sterile dressing.
- If available, an electrosurgical or radiofrequency unit (e.g., Ellman Surgitron) with a fine cutting needle or wire works well to excise the tissue (see Chapter 30, Radiofrequency Surgery [Modern Electrosurgery]).

Preprocedure Patient Preparation

In spite of the fact that the patient desires this procedure, it is often considered a cosmetic procedure by insurance companies and may not be a covered expense. Explain this possibility, as well as the possible complications of the procedure, which may include discomfort, bleeding, infection, and a cosmetic defect. The patient should be aware that there will be a scar after repairing an earlobe, and that his or her earlobe will not be identical to the contralateral one. However, every attempt will be made to minimize any additional cosmetic defect. If the patient tends to develop keloids or hypertrophic scars, these may result from the procedure. Obtain informed consent. Also explain the discomfort of injected local anesthetic and the necessity for the patient to remain very still during the procedure.

Technique

1. After a sterile preparation is performed, sterile technique is used, and the clinician should observe universal blood and body fluid precautions.
2. A wheal of lidocaine *without epinephrine* placed circumferentially around the entire base of the ear will provide good anesthesia (ear block; see Chapter 8, Peripheral Nerve Blocks and Field Blocks). The concha and ear canal retain sensation. Use of the circumferential block as opposed to injection directly into the lobe avoids distortion of the local anatomy.
3. Excise the defect with a no. 15 or 15c blade, a no. 11 pointed blade, or with the electrosurgical or radiofrequency unit (e.g., Ellman Surgitron; level 2, pure cut, Varitip or fine needle; Figs. 71-3 through 71-5). If the defect is a large hole, it is often easier just to excise all the way through the lobe to create a "V" (see Fig. 71-3). Various sterilized objects with a flat surface have been used to support the lobe during the excision because it is so flaccid, but with gentle traction by the nondominant hand, the lobe should remain stable. The radiofrequency unit makes this step easier, especially if the defect is a hole and you are trying to

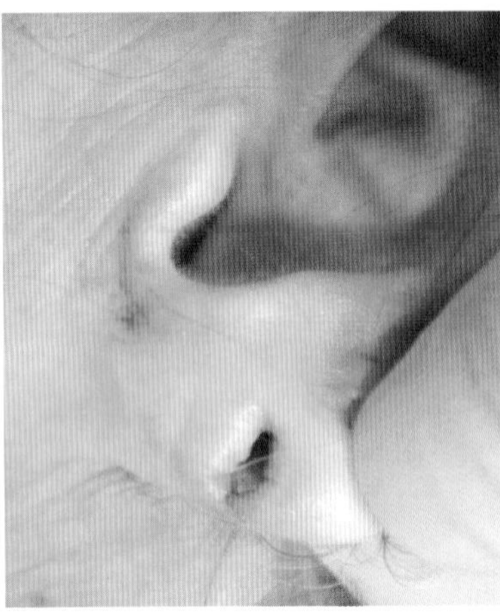

Figure 71-2 Chronic earlobe laceration.

preserve the lower intact rim of tissue (see Figs. 71-4 and 71-5). Care should be taken to excise a smooth line and to treat the exposed subcutaneous tissue and wound edges extremely gently. If needed, skin hooks should be used. Absolutely avoid grasping the skin edges with forceps; this delivers a crushing-type force, induces unnecessary trauma, and increases scarring. Earlobe cysts are removed and repaired in the same manner (Fig. 71-6).

4. Control bleeding with pressure.
5. Close the skin edges anteriorly to posteriorly with interrupted 6-0 nylon. It is wise to begin suturing anteriorly first so that any malalignment is confined to the posterior aspect. Also, sutures may be placed intermittently at first, and then the gaps filled in to conclude the repair. Proper approximation at the tip of the lobe is important (Fig. 71-7; see also Figs. 71-3 and 71-4). The wound edges may try to invert, and a vertical mattress stitch may help prevent this.
6. Apply antibacterial ointment or petroleum jelly.
7. Place a pack behind the earlobe and against the mastoid to secure the lobe and ensure that it will not suffer trauma or excessive motion. Cover the wound with a sterile pressure dressing. Overall, patients generally appreciate the final result (Fig. 71-8).

Postprocedure Patient Education

1. For the first few hours, the patient should lie on the side that was repaired to compress the area and reduce bleeding.
2. The patient should remove the dressing in 12 to 24 hours, and thereafter wash the area gently twice a day with alcohol or hydrogen peroxide on cotton-tipped applicators. All blood and crusts should be removed to minimize the risk of scarring and infection. A small amount of antibacterial ointment (avoid neomycin, which can inhibit reepithelialization) or petroleum jelly should then be applied with a new cotton-tipped applicator.
3. The patient should return for suture removal in 5 days. Some clinicians use Steri-Strips to give additional support for several days.
4. Repiercing of the ear may be performed after 6 to 8 weeks in a location off of the wound line.
5. The patient should be instructed to avoid heavy, dangling, or large loop earrings in the future to avoid repeated, undue traction on the lobe.

CPT/Billing Codes

12011 Repair, simple, of superficial wounds of ear (2.5 cm or less)
12051 Repair, intermediate, layer closure of ear (2.5 cm or less)

ICD-9-CM Diagnostic Codes

872.01 Laceration, external ear (pins), without mention of complication
872.11 Laceration, external ear (pins), complicated
873.40 Wound or laceration, face
906.0 Late effect of open wound or laceration, head, neck, trunk

Patient Education Guides

See the sample patient education form available online at www.expertconsult.com.

Acknowledgment

The editors wish to recognize the many contributions by Stephen K. Toadvine, MD, to this chapter in a previous edition of this text.

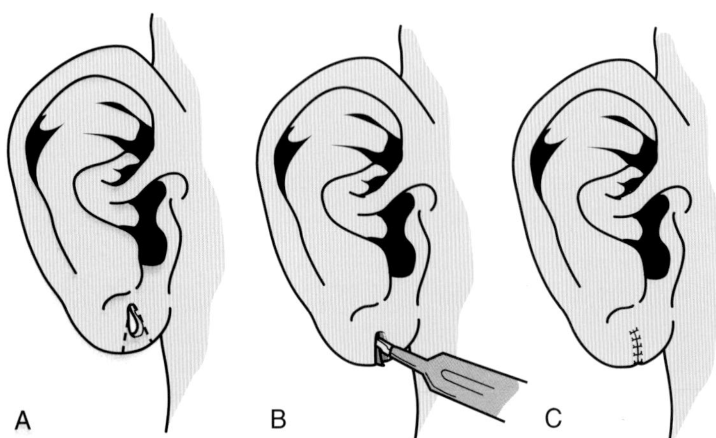

Figure 71-3 Excising reepithelialized skin within the defect using a no. 11 blade. **A,** Area to be excised. In this case, a large opening is being converted into a "V." Alternatively, for a smaller hole, a small elliptical excision could be made around it to preserve the lower margin of the lobe. **B,** Making the excision. **C,** Appearance after closure.

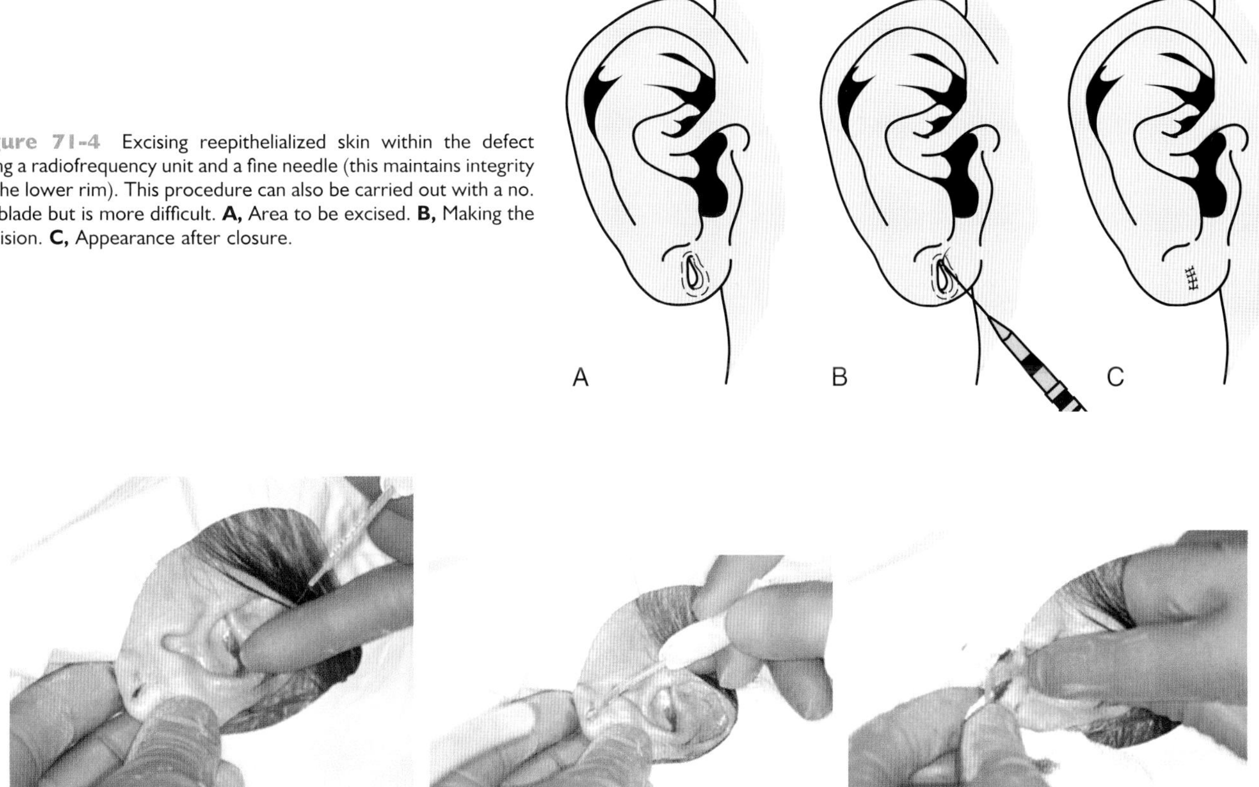

Figure 71-4 Excising reepithelialized skin within the defect using a radiofrequency unit and a fine needle (this maintains integrity of the lower rim). This procedure can also be carried out with a no. 11 blade but is more difficult. **A,** Area to be excised. **B,** Making the excision. **C,** Appearance after closure.

Figure 71-5 Excising reepithelialized skin with a radiofrequency unit. **A**, Chronic earlobe laceration from earring. Anesthetic ear block has been obtained. **B**, Using the radiofrequency unit, the healed margins of the wound are excised. **C**, Wound margins can now be approximated using fine nylon suture.

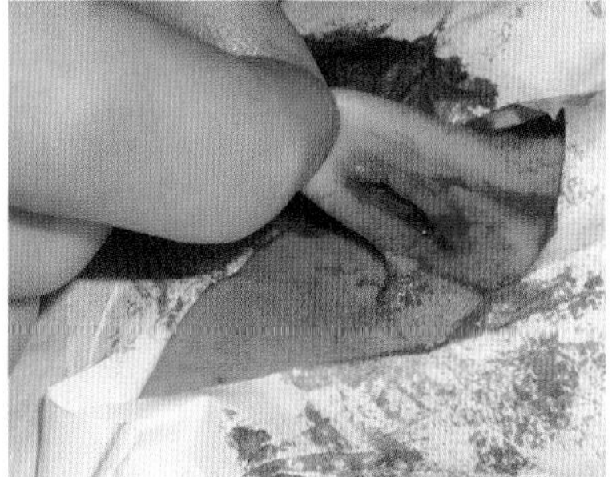

Figure 71-6 Earlobe cysts are removed and repaired in the same manner.

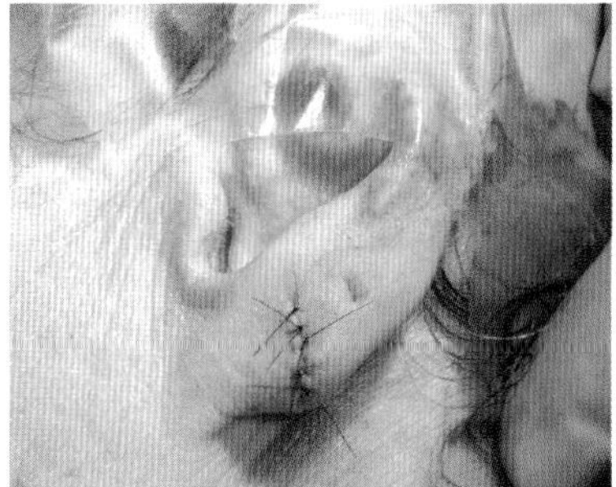

Figure 71-7 Appearance after suture closure.

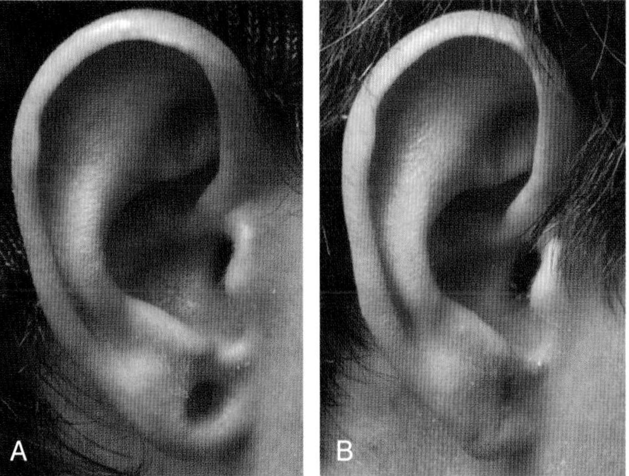

Figure 71-8 Before (**A**) and after (**B**) earlobe repair using radiofrequency unit. (Courtesy of Greg Lawrence.)

BIBLIOGRAPHY

Agarwal R: Repair of cleft earlobe using double opposing Z-plasty. Plast Reconstr Surg 102:1759–1760, 1998.

Harter DA, Miller S: Management of specific soft tissue injuries. In Reichman EF, Simon RR (eds): Emergency Medicine Procedures. New York, McGraw-Hill, 2004, pp 748–761.

Nikko A, Hsu S, Quan LT, Greenbaum SS: Surgical pearl: Repair of partially torn earlobes: Punch technique versus conversion to complete tear. J Am Acad Dermatol 43:99–101, 2000.

Silapunt S, Goldberg LH: Repair of the split earlobe, ear piercing and earlobe reduction. In Robinson JK, Hanke DW, Sengelmann RD, Siegel DM (eds): Surgery of the Skin: Procedural Dermatology. Philadelphia, Mosby, 2005, pp 291–310.

Smith C, Glaser DA: Surgical pearl: Repair of split or deformed ear lobe with tongue blade for stabilization during surgery. J Am Acad Dermatol 38:990–991, 1998.

CHAPTER 72

CERUMEN IMPACTION REMOVAL

Michael McHenry

Cerumen impaction is one of the most common otologic problems encountered by primary care clinicians (approximately 150,000 ears are irrigated per week in the United States to remove cerumen). Cerumen is a naturally occurring lubricant and protectant of the external auditory canal. The predominant form is a wet, sticky, honey-colored wax that can darken, but a dry, scaly form occurs in some patients. Normally cerumen is carried from inside the canal to the outside by tiny cilia. Accumulation of cerumen can cause decreased hearing, tinnitus, vertigo, infection, or a sensation of increased pressure. The hearing loss is usually quite sudden when the cerumen seals off the canal and is often described by the patient as a "blocked ear." Accumulation is common in elderly patients and in patients working in dusty environments. Patients often do a poor job of removing cerumen with cotton-tipped sticks or over-the-counter preparations, leaving the clinician to complete the procedure. In fact, overzealous use of these applicators frequently disrupts the natural ciliary cleaning process. For removal by the clinician, topical anesthesia may be desired; foreign bodies may also need to be removed (see Chapter 76, Removal of Foreign Bodies from the Ear and Nose, which also describes a technique for injecting anesthetic for external canal field block). The overall goal of this procedure is to remove cerumen under direct visualization or by irrigation without causing injury. The risk of injury is not to be taken lightly because ear irrigation is one of the more common causes of iatrogenic injuries cared for by otolaryngologists. Asymptomatic cerumen buildup does not require removal; rather, the patient should be taught how to perform his or her own ear irrigation to clean the ears.

INDICATIONS

- Tympanic membrane or ear canal obscured by cerumen with otologic complaint
- Patient complaint of decreased hearing, otalgia, tinnitus, vertigo, or unsteady gait associated with cerumen
- External otitis associated with cerumen (the ear should be dried meticulously after the procedure)
- Clinician needs to examine an ear canal or tympanic membrane obscured by cerumen
- Patient needs hearing tested and ear canal(s) obscured by cerumen

CONTRAINDICATIONS

- Uncooperative patient or infant who cannot be adequately restrained.
- Clinician unfamiliar with or unable to define anatomy of the external auditory canal.
- Patient with distorted anatomy (e.g., prior or current injury obscuring normal anatomy), although this is a relative contraindication.
- Previous ear surgery with resultant scarring and increased risk of perforation (relative contraindication).
- Known or suspected cholesteatoma.
- The affected ear is the only hearing ear (relative contraindication, but referral should be considered).
- For irrigation, acute otitis media or known/suspected perforation of the tympanic membrane is a contraindication. In these situations, the curette or suction catheter should be used under direct visualization.

EQUIPMENT

- Equipment necessary for clinician to observe universal blood and body fluid precautions (gloves, mask, goggles)
- Ear curette
  - Metal: *rigid*, Buck, Shapleigh, or Yankauer; *flexible*, Billeau flexible earloop
  - Plastic: Flex-loop ear curette, disposable ear curette, or infant ear scoop
- Otoscope with moveable posterior lens or shield, or ear speculum and light source
- Ear forceps
- Ball-tipped ear hook
- Local anesthetic solution or suspension (e.g., lidocaine solution)
- For suction: Various ear suction catheters with suction source (Fig. 72-1)

NOTE: Hollow ear candles have been found ineffective.

- For irrigation
  - Ear syringe (large stainless steel syringe with irrigant deflector), *or* a commercially available jet irrigator (on "ENT table units," or an oral Waterpik [Water Pik, Inc., Fort Collins, Colo]), *or* a 22-gauge butterfly intravenous catheter tubing (with needle and butterfly removed) and a 20- to 50-mL syringe. An 18-gauge Angiocath type IV catheter can also be used with a syringe.
  - Lukewarm tap water ("lukewarm" is confirmed when a drop placed on the inner forearm of the examiner is comfortable, similar to testing baby formula).
  - Towels, Chux, or plastic drape.
  - Cotton gauze strip.
  - Emesis or ear basin to collect irrigant.
  - Aqueous-based ceruminolytics, in contrast to the traditional organic or oil-based preparations, have been found to be most effective in in vitro studies. Distilled water can be used, but 3% hydrogen peroxide or 5% to 10% sodium bicarbonate was superior in studies. Olive oil was not useful. Sialic acid took twice as long as distilled water to dissolve cerumen. The sodium bicarbonate solution can be made at home by dissolving ¼ teaspoon sodium bicarbonate (baking soda) in 10 mL of water.

PREPROCEDURE PATIENT PREPARATION

- For curette and suction removal, discuss the chance of perforation and minor trauma to the ear canal associated with pain.
- For irrigation removal, discuss the risk of perforation and potential dizziness during the irrigation. Local discomfort may also be experienced, especially when the ear syringe is used.

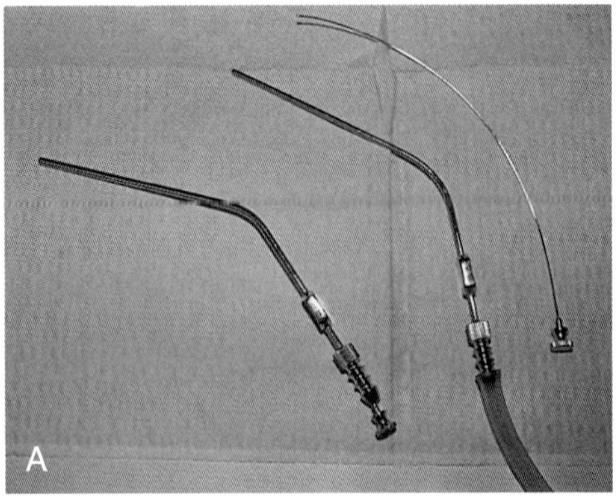

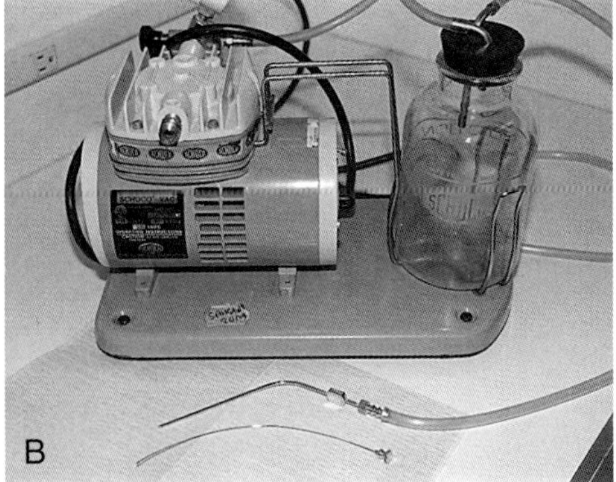

Figure 72-1 Suction catheters (including Frazier) (**A**) and basic suction pump (**B**) can assist in managing ear canal obstruction.

- Stress the importance of remaining still during the procedure.
- The patient should expect to hear occasional loud noises while the clinician is working in the ear, especially if suction is used.
- Patients should be aware that firmly adherent cerumen frequently tears the skin lining the ear canal when removed, regardless of the technique used. As a result, there may be some bleeding. Slight bleeding does not indicate perforation. There is also a slightly increased risk of external otitis after cerumen removal. For both reasons, antibiotic ear drops are frequently prescribed.

TECHNIQUE

The clinician should follow universal blood and body fluid precautions when performing these procedures.

Curette or Suction Technique

A curette is usually the fastest way to remove cerumen and may be preferred for small amounts of easily visible and reachable wax. It is also usually the easiest method for children, who may find it difficult to remain still for suction or irrigation. In adults, suction can be used for deeper or slightly more adherent impactions. Suction works best for multiple tiny fragments or for soft cerumen; it often fails when there is a single, hard, irregular, and impacted cerumen plug. Young children are often frightened by the noise suction makes. For children and adults, irrigation will be necessary for dense, adherent, or circumferential impactions.

1. Seat the patient on the examination table. If available, a neck rest, such as those on a dental or otolaryngology (ears, nose, throat [ENT]) chair, may help adults remain immobile. Children often tolerate the procedure better if held securely or swaddled with a sheet in a parent's lap or, if supine, with the parent or assistant stabilizing the head.
2. Using the otoscope, first visualize the opposite canal to become familiar with the patient's anatomy. Next, visualize the cerumen in the affected canal by applying traction on the helix as necessary. In adults, traction is usually applied posteriorly and upward on the pinna while simultaneously pulling it slightly out from the head. In the small child, the pinna is pulled down, back, and slightly out from the head. Five to 10 mL of local anesthetic instilled in the ear will usually result in increased patient comfort for the duration of the procedure; however, it may obscure the canal briefly, so sometimes it is better just to remove the cerumen.
3. Using the selected curette, ear hook, or suction catheter, reach through the partially open magnifying posterior lens of the otoscope and gently remove the impacted cerumen. Take care to avoid traumatizing the bony ear canal. Work either through the scope (Fig. 72-2A) or, after identifying the location of the cerumen, by direct visualization (Fig. 72-2B).

   NOTE: The clinician's hand should be stabilized by remaining firmly in contact with the patient's head at all times to minimize the risk of scraping the wall of the external canal or perforating the tympanic membrane. Even the most cooperative patient may move involuntarily because of a stimulated vagal nerve cough reflex.
4. If hard wax is encountered, installation of 8 to 10 drops of 3% hydrogen peroxide or 5% to 10% sodium bicarbonate for 5 to 10 minutes should facilitate removal. For wax adherent to the tympanic membrane, irrigation or suction may be necessary. Suction catheters (see Fig. 72-1) are quite loud when used in the external canal, so if suction is used, the patient should be warned and instructed not to pull away from the noise.
5. Firmly adherent cerumen frequently tears epithelium as it is removed. Consider prescribing topical otic antibiotics if epithelium is disrupted.

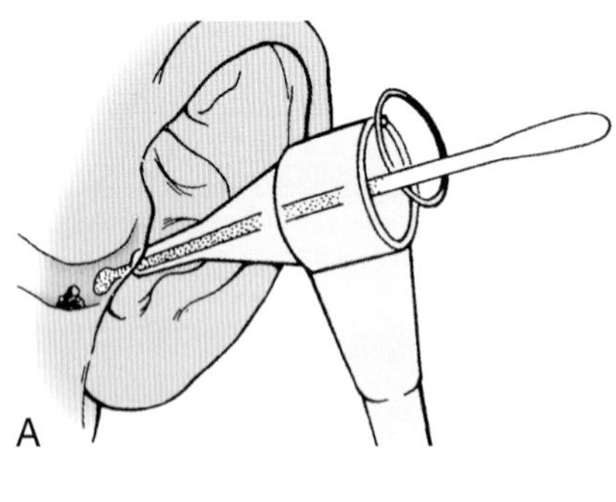

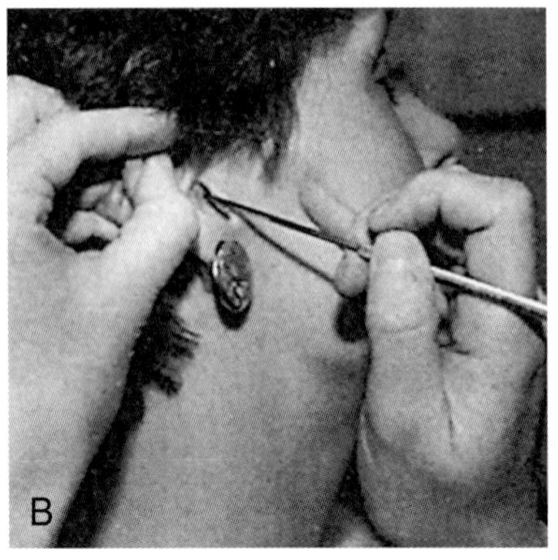

Figure 72-2 **A,** Removal through the otoscope. **B,** Often, foreign bodies or cerumen in the ear canal can be removed with direct visualization after careful, magnified, otoscopic examination is completed. Notice how the patient's head is supported and the clinician's hand rests on the patient's face.

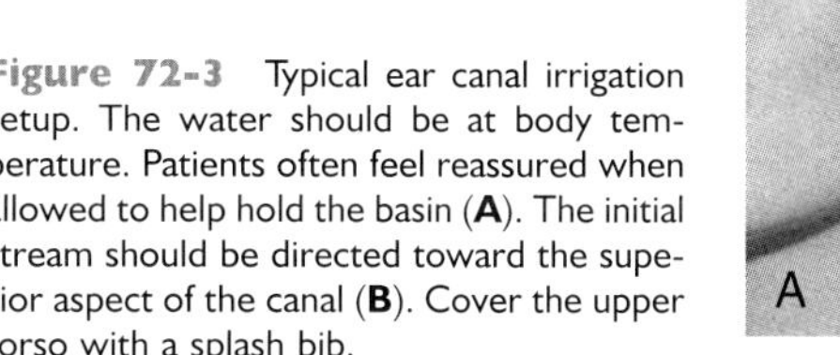

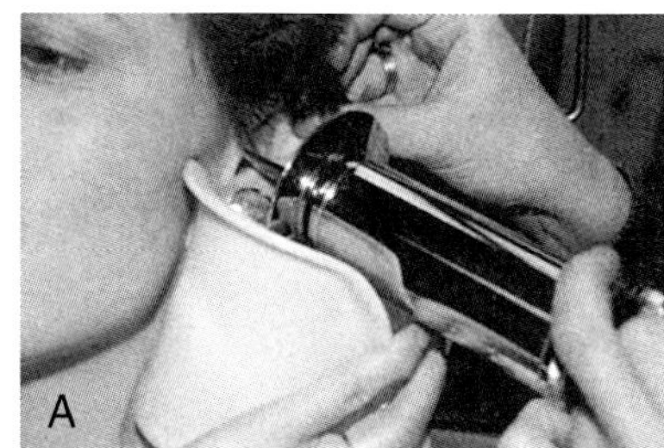

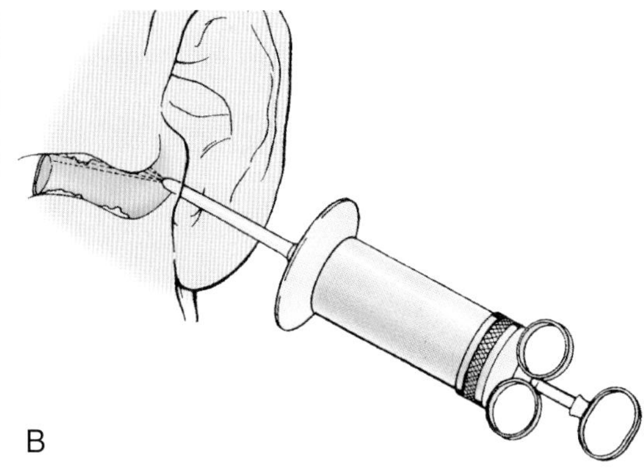

Figure 72-3 Typical ear canal irrigation setup. The water should be at body temperature. Patients often feel reassured when allowed to help hold the basin (**A**). The initial stream should be directed toward the superior aspect of the canal (**B**). Cover the upper torso with a splash bib.

Irrigation Technique

The irrigation technique (Figs. 72-3 through 72-5) takes longer than the curette or suction technique. However, irrigation rarely fails; it is the safest technique; it is the technique used most often by non-otolaryngologists; and it is often used when other techniques have failed or caused pain.

1. Fill the irrigator (syringe) with *body-temperature* tap water. Using water at this temperature reduces the chance for stimulation of the vestibular reflex, causing nystagmus and nausea. Test the water temperature by placing a drop on the inner forearm of the examiner. It should feel neither warm nor cold to touch.

   NOTE: If the jet irrigator (e.g., Waterpik) is used, adjust the pressure to the *lowest* setting to reduce the risk of perforation or acoustic trauma. Even at low pressures, jet irrigators have been known to rupture the tympanic membrane; therefore, some experts no longer recommend use of jet irrigators for cerumen removal. If a jet irrigator is used, the clinician may want to use a "safe" irrigation tip (see Suppliers section).

2. Protect the patient with a towel, Chux, or plastic sheet to collect excess water.
3. Have the patient tilt his or her head to the side being irrigated, and hold the ear basin (Fig. 72-6) below the patient's earlobe. Patients often feel reassured when allowed to help and hold the basin. Advise the patient not to pull his or her head away from the irrigating tip.
4. Using the selected device, direct the water jet superiorly toward the occiput, allowing space for the return of the water and cerumen. Directed in this manner, water circulates first above and behind the cerumen, and then it pushes the cerumen out of the ear. The irrigation should *not* be directed onto the tympanic membrane. No irrigation device should be inserted more than 1 cm into the canal.
   - If the ear syringe is used, fairly vigorous force may be needed. The use of large (25- to 50-mL) syringes prevents excessive pressure. Be sure that air bubbles are removed from the syringe before use.
   - If the jet irrigator or catheter–syringe unit is used, after directing the flow superiorly, rotate the tip back and forth to change the direction of spray.
5. Often the cerumen washes out in one or two large pieces in a few seconds, at which point the canal is reexamined. If the canal is clear, stop the irrigation and dry the canal by inserting and removing a small length of cotton gauze. If the patient has otitis externa, the ear canal should be dried meticulously.
6. Occasionally the impacted cerumen will need to be prodded with an ear curette. If irrigation is still unsuccessful after a few moments, terminate the procedure and send the patient home to use a liquid ear wax softener. Have the patient return in a few days for a repeat irrigation.
7. Consider prescribing topical otic antibiotics if the epithelium was disrupted to provide prophylaxis against external otitis.

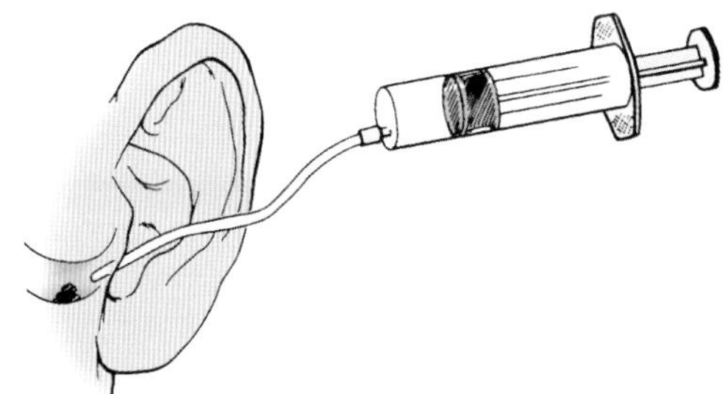

Figure 72-4 Alternative irrigation setup. Use an 18-gauge plastic intravenous catheter or butterfly tubing with needle and butterfly removed.

COMPLICATIONS

- Tympanic membrane perforation and damage to ossicles with possible hearing loss
- Otitis externa
- Vertigo or nausea and vomiting
- Minor canal wall abrasions—as mentioned earlier, some bleeding may occur if hard wax is adherent to the epithelium and causes desquamation with removal (if noted, antibiotic otic drops should be used for a few days)
- Tinnitus

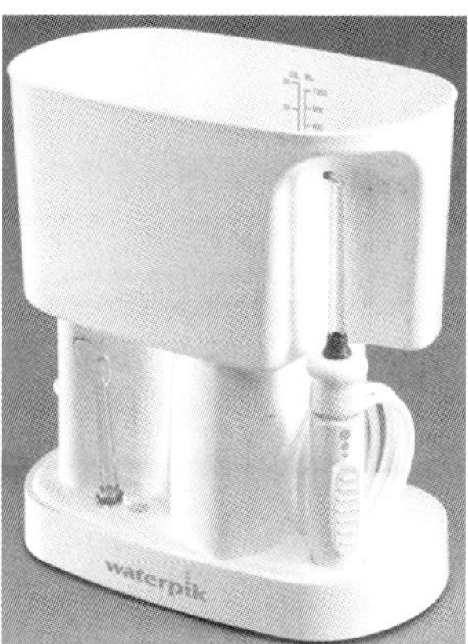

Figure 72-5 Waterpik oral cleaning system (not marketed by the company for cerumen impaction removal). (Courtesy of Water Pik, Inc., Fort Collins, Colo.)

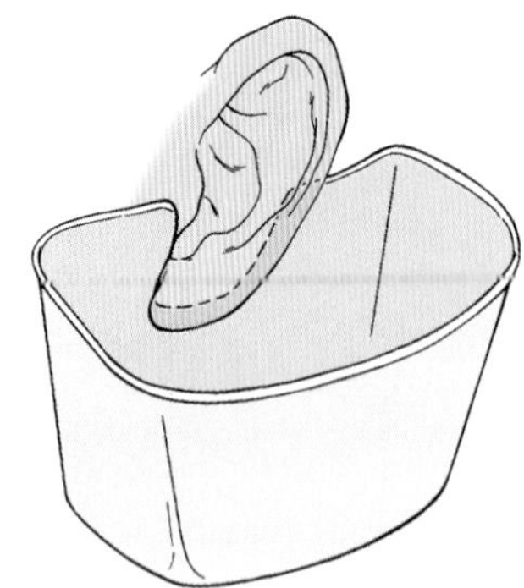

Figure 72-6 Basin cup that fits under ear.

Postprocedure Patient Education

Instruct the patient to contact the clinician's office for fever or vertigo or for decreased hearing, purulent drainage, or pain in the affected ear. Slight bleeding from the affected ear may be expected if the skin was disrupted. Diabetic and other immunocompromised patients should be especially observant for signs of infection because they are prone to development of malignant otitis externa (often due to *Pseudomonas*), with its resultant high morbidity and mortality rates.

Inform patients with recurring cerumen impactions, unless contraindicated, to perform monthly or bimonthly ear cleansing using hydrogen peroxide, 5% to 10% sodium bicarbonate (mixed as previously described in Equipment section), or distilled water as an irrigant from a squeeze bulb ear syringe (similar to nasal bulb syringe used in newborns; both are available at local pharmacies). Advise the patient to avoid self-instrumentation of the ear canal with cotton-tipped applicators or any other instrument. It may be helpful to explain that cotton-tipped applicators or other instruments often disrupt the cilia and other natural ear cleansing mechanisms, even *causing* an accumulation of cerumen. Cotton-tipped applicators should be used only on the external ear and never inserted into the canal. Another option is the instillation of two to three drops of mineral oil, pure vegetable oil, or liquid docusate sodium every couple of weeks in the ear canal to soften the wax (these are contraindicated with suspected perforation). There is no consistent evidence that one ceruminolytic is better than another. Patients who use hair spray should cover the ears when spraying to avoid hardening the cerumen.

CPT/Billing Code

69210 Removal impacted cerumen (separate procedure), one or both ears

ICD-9-CM Diagnostic Codes

380.4 Cerumen impaction
380.10 Otitis externa (secondary diagnosis)

Acknowledgment

The editors wish to recognize the many contributions by Gregory J. Forzley, MD, and Gary R. Newkirk, MD, to this chapter in the previous two editions of this text.

Suppliers

(See contact information online at www.expertconsult.com.)

Metal and plastic disposable curettes
- Cardinal Health
- Miltex, Inc.
- Spectrum Surgical Instruments

Plastic curettes and safe irrigation tips
- Bionix Corporation

Bibliography

Dinces EA: Cerumen. Available at www.uptodate.com.

Dinsdale RC, Roland PS, Manning SC, Meyerhoff WL: Catastrophic otologic injury from oral jet irrigation of the external auditory canal. Laryngoscopy 101:75–78, 1991.

Kamien M: Practice tip: Which cerumenolytic? Aust Fam Physician 28:817, 828, 1999.

Murtagh J: Ear wax and syringing. In Murtagh J: Practice Tips, 4th ed. Sydney, Australia, McGraw-Hill, 2004.

Roberts RR: Cerumen impaction removal. In Reichman EF, Simon RR (eds): Emergency Medicine Procedures. New York, McGraw-Hill, 2004, pp 1267–1272.

Robinson AC, Hawke M: The efficacy of ceruminolytics: Everything old is new again. J Otolaryngol 18:263–267, 1989.

CHAPTER 73

Tympanocentesis and Myringotomy

Mark S. Grubb

Tympanocentesis is a puncture of the tympanic membrane performed with a hollow needle to aspirate fluid for diagnostic or therapeutic purposes. A myringotomy is an incision in the tympanic membrane made with a myringotomy knife. Ventilation of the middle ear space by either method instantly relieves pain and pressure associated with acute otitis media. Culture of middle ear aspirate establishes disease etiology and enables precisely targeted antibiotic therapy. Tympanocentesis or myringotomy can also relieve hearing loss and discomfort associated with chronic middle ear effusions.

At this time, myringotomy is performed almost exclusively during tympanostomy tube insertion, for which the patient is under general anesthesia. Tympanocentesis is the more suitable procedure for primary care settings. Needle puncture of the tympanic membrane is easy to accomplish, requires only local anesthesia, poses less risk than a myringotomy incision, and permits drainage for up to 5 days.

The ear that would benefit from tympanocentesis will have fluid behind the tympanic membrane, and the membrane will have either a bulging or retracted appearance resulting from positive or negative pressure in the middle ear space. Despite this distorted appearance, the location of the umbo and the orientation of the manubrium usually remain discernible. Tympanocentesis is performed on the inferior half of the membrane at the location of maximal bulge, usually in the anterior quadrant. The puncture or incision should be performed nearer to the tip of the manubrium than to the fibrous annulus. Do not perform the procedure on the fibrous annulus, over the incus or stapes, or directly over the round window (Fig. 73-1).

Indications

Tympanocentesis

- For immediate relief of pain and pressure associated with acute otitis media
- For aspiration of middle ear fluid for culture to select precisely targeted antibiotic therapy
- As an adjunct to watchful waiting for acute otitis media; tympanocentesis relieves symptoms and promotes therapeutic drainage during the observation period, and enables accurate drug selection for patients who remain symptomatic after 48 hours
- For identifying pathogens in persistent acute otitis media or in episodes that have failed to respond to antibiotic therapy
- For otitis media diagnosed in immunocompromised patients or those with multiple antibiotic allergies
- For complicated otitis media such as that associated with unusually severe pain, signs of toxicity, facial nerve palsy, mastoiditis, meningitis, encephalitis, brain abscess, or dural sinus thrombosis
- For alleviation of conductive hearing loss or discomfort associated with chronic serous otitis media
- As an alternative therapy for patients who wish to avoid antibiotics

Myringotomy

- For immediate relief of pain and pressure associated with acute otitis media
- For placement of tympanostomy tubes

Contraindications

- Known anomalous positioning of the jugular bulb
- Cochlear implant
- Acute otitis externa (relative contraindication)
- Uncooperative patient (relative contraindication)
- Obscure landmarks (consider referral to otolaryngologist)

Equipment

- Local anesthesia: 0.5 mL of 8% tetracaine otic solution, eyedropper, cotton balls, 3% hydrogen peroxide, tissue wicks
- Tympanocentesis
  - CDT (channel directed tympanocentesis) speculum method: A CDT (Walls Precision Instruments, Baker City, Ore) 3- or 5-mm Speculum and Aspirator bulb, and a Welch-Allyn otoscope with pneumatic, diagnostic, or operating head. The CDT instrument has a protected needle and other safety features enabling safe completion of the procedure without restraints for most patients (Fig. 73-2).
  - Tympanocentesis collector method: A 3-inch 20- or 21-gauge spinal needle, a Medtronic Xomed Tympanocentesis Collector (Medtronic ENT, Jacksonville, Fla), an otoscope with operating head, a papoose board or other patient restraint (as needed), and a vacuum pump or wall suction (Fig. 73-3).
  - Syringe method: A 3-inch 20- or 21-gauge spinal needle bent at the hub to about 60 degrees, a 3-mL syringe, an otoscope with operating head, and a papoose board or other patient restraint (as needed; Fig. 73-4).
- Myringotomy
  - Myringotomy knife, an otoscope with operating head, and a papoose board or other patient restraint (as needed; Fig. 73-5).
  - Aspiration after myringotomy will require a vacuum pump, and either a Juhn Tym-Tap aspirator (Medtronic) or a Baron suction tube combined with an inline suction trap.

NOTE: In all instances where an operating otoscope head is used, the clinician may elect to move the lens of the otoscope out of the

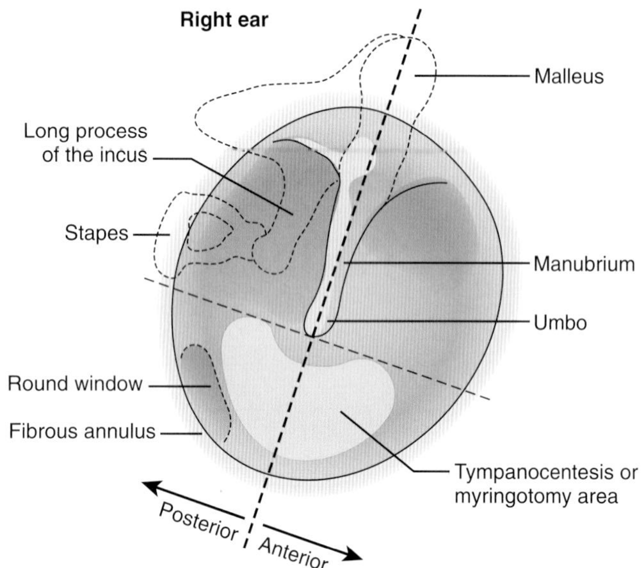

Figure 73-1 Tympanic membrane of the right ear. (Courtesy of David Spaugh.)

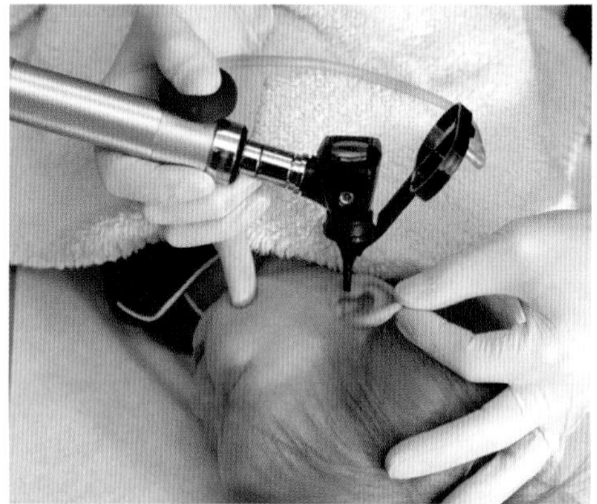

Figure 73-2 Tympanocentesis with CDT Speculum and CDT Aspirator bulb.

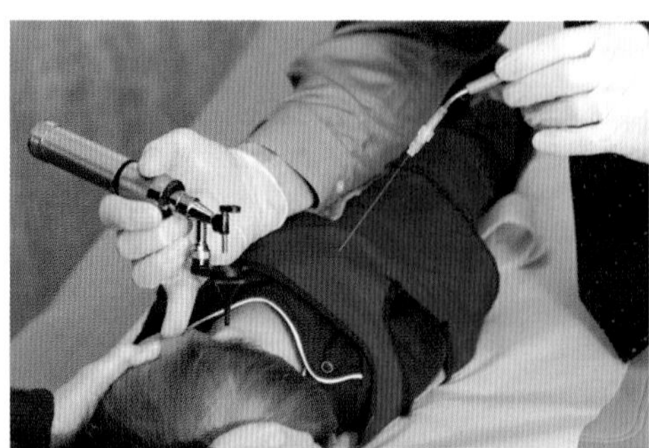

Figure 73-3 Tympanocentesis with Xomed Tympanocentesis Collector attached to vacuum pump.

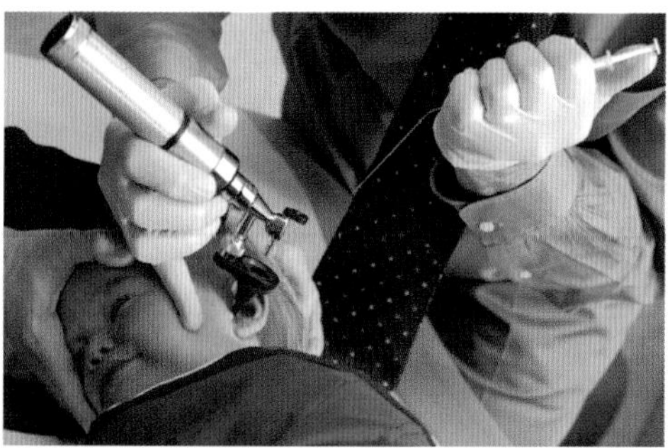

Figure 73-4 Tympanocentesis with spinal needle attached to 3-mL syringe.

field of view and use a head-mounted portable binocular microscope instead.

Preprocedure Patient Education and Forms

Explain the indications, the procedure, risks of the procedure, options for procedural anesthesia, and available alternative therapies. The patient should be warned that working near the tympanic membrane can be noisy. Unless conscious sedation is used, they should also be aware that they will experience some discomfort. Obtain signed informed consent and document it in the patient's chart. A sample patient education form is available online at www.expertconsult.com.

Technique

Tympanocentesis

1. Remove any cerumen from the canal (see Chapter 72, Cerumen Impaction Removal).
2. Initiate the desired preprocedure anesthesia or analgesia. The methods most frequently used are the following:
   - 8% tetracaine otic solution applied topically to the membrane, held in place for 15 minutes with a cotton dam or wick
   - Acetaminophen with codeine, given orally 30 minutes before the procedure
   - Midazolam (requires training in conscious sedation; see Chapter 2, Procedural Sedation and Analgesia) or pediatric sedation (see Chapter 7, Pediatric Sedation and Analgesia)

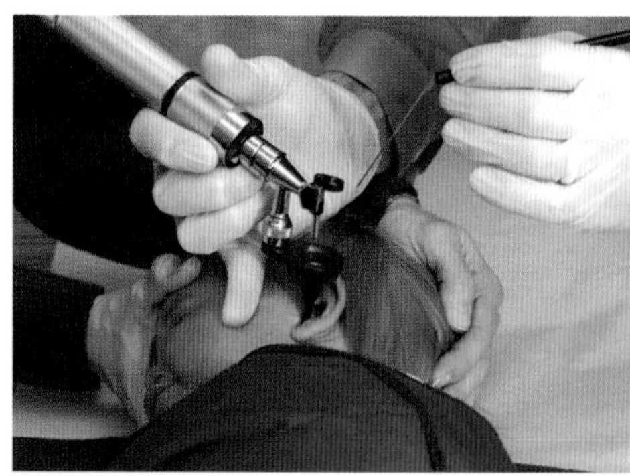

Figure 73-5 Myringotomy with Xomed disposable myringotomy knife.

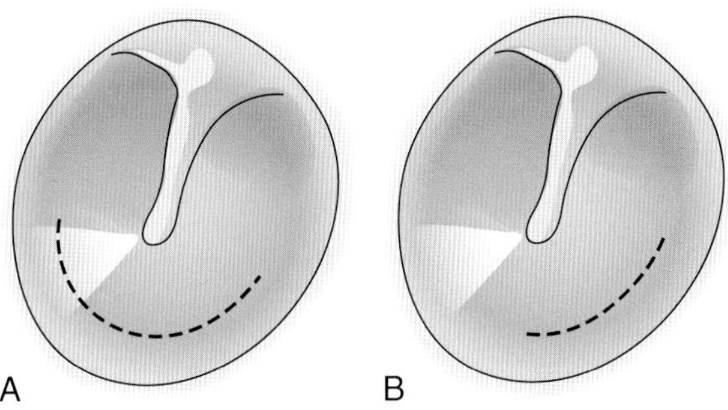

Figure 73-6 Locations for myringotomy. A tympanocentesis could precede either of these myringotomy incisions in the same location. **A,** Wide myringotomy incision through the tympanic membrane might be used in patient with refractory purulent otitis media or for prolonged drainage of pus if necessary. **B,** More limited myringotomy incision.

NOTE: Topical anesthetic solutions are typically bacteriostatic. If the clinician intends to culture aspirated fluid, excess anesthetic solution must be removed from the external auditory canal before the procedure.

3. Lay the patient in the supine position with head turned to one side. A papoose restraint is usually necessary when the procedure is performed with an unprotected sharp. Use a tissue wick to remove excess anesthetic solution from the canal and membrane.
4. Insert the speculum into the ear canal, and visually determine the point of the intended perforation.
5. Extend the needle 2 mm through the tympanic membrane at the point of maximal bulge in the inferior portion.
6. Aspirate fluid while the tip of the needle is in the middle ear space, as follows:
   - CDT method: Release thumb pressure on the aspirator bulb (see Fig. 73-2).
   - Collector method: Occlude the trap opening with a finger (see Fig. 73-3). An assistant can be helpful with this step.
   - Syringe method: Retract the syringe plunger with the thumb (see Fig. 73-4).
7. Retract the needle and then the speculum from the patient's ear.
8. Irrigate the canal with 3% hydrogen peroxide solution and remove excess fluid with a tissue wick.

Myringotomy

1. The steps for office myringotomy are essentially the same as for tympanocentesis, except a myringotomy knife is used to make a curved incision in the tympanic membrane (see Fig. 73-5). A myringotomy may be preceded by tympanocentesis in the same location (Fig. 73-6).
2. If aspiration is to accompany myringotomy, it is accomplished by reentering the myringotomy incision with aspiration equipment before removing the speculum from the patient's ear. (If fluid is sent for culture, this would be the method to obtain it. Postprocedure aspiration of exudate directly from the canal is not recommended for culture because the aspirate may be contaminated by canal flora.)
3. Do not irrigate the ear canal or use peroxide-saturated wicks after myringotomy.
4. Other than applying topical antibiotic solutions, the ear canal should be kept dry for 5 days after myringotomy.

COMPLICATIONS

Potential complications include chronic perforation, puncture of abnormally positioned bulb of jugular vein, a scar on the tympanic membrane, and hearing loss (if using a method with unrestricted needle traverse). Authors of the current medical literature and those who use tympanocentesis in clinical settings describe a zero incidence for these complications. Otitis externa is also a potential, less threatening complication.

POSTPROCEDURE MANAGEMENT

Tympanocentesis

Purulent drainage may continue for up to 5 days. Twice-daily cleaning of the external canal with peroxide and tissue wicks will remove residual drainage and prevent external otitis.

Myringotomy

Purulent drainage may continue for up to 5 days. Peroxide rinse of the external canal is not recommended after myringotomy. Patients should be instructed to keep the ear dry for 5 days after myringotomy, with particular attention to care when bathing or washing hair. A cotton ear plug coated with a thin film of petroleum jelly works well during these times.

A sample postprocedure patient education form is available online at www.expertconsult.com.

CPT/BILLING CODES

NOTE: Presently, there is no differentiating CPT code for tympanocentesis. The procedure is coded and billed using the myringotomy code set.

69420 Myringotomy including aspiration and/or eustachian tube inflation (also used for tympanocentesis)
 69420.LT or 69420.RT (Use LT or RT modifiers for the left or right ear)
 69420.50 (Use the .50 modifier for bilateral procedures)
69421 Myringotomy including aspiration and/or eustachian tube inflation requiring general anesthesia

ICD-9-CM DIAGNOSTIC CODES

381.00 Otitis media, NOS, with effusion
381.01 Otitis media, acute serous
381.4 Otis media, nonsuppurative (allergic, exudative, transudative, secretory, mucoid)
381.4 Otis media, nonsuppurative with effusion
381.10 Otitis media, chronic serous, simple
382.00 Acute suppurative otitis media without spontaneous rupture of eardrum
382.01 Acute suppurative otitis media with spontaneous rupture of eardrum
382.3 Otitis media, chronic suppurative
388.70 Otalgia
993.0 Otitis media due to barotrauma
909.4 Otitis media due to barotrauma, late effect

PATIENT EDUCATION GUIDES

See patient education and patient consent forms available online at www.expertconsult.com.

ACKNOWLEDGMENT

The editors wish to recognize the contributions by Gregory J. Forzley, MD, to this chapter in the previous two editions of this text.

SUPPLIERS

(See contact information online at www.expertconsult.com.)

CDT (channel directed tympanocentesis) Speculum kits
Walls Precision Instruments

Tympanocentesis Collector, Tym-Tap, and Baron suction catheters
Medtronic ENT
Xomed (Medtronic)

ONLINE RESOURCES

CDT Speculum. Available at www.tympanocentesis.com.

Outcomes Management Educational Workshops, Inc.: Featured Articles. Brook I: Tympanocentesis in the diagnosis and treatment of otitis media. Available at www.omew.com/research/tympanocentesis.htm.

Tympanocentesis Collector, Tym-Tap, and Baron suction catheters. Available at www.xomed.com.

University of Pittsburgh School of Medicine: Pediatrics education—enhancing proficiency in otitis media. http://pedsed.pitt.edu/06_browse.asp.

University of Texas Medical Branch: Improving accuracy in diagnosis of acute otitis media. www.utmb.edu/pedi_ed/AOM-Otitis/default.htm.

BIBLIOGRAPHY

Block SL, Harrison CJ: Diagnosis and Management of Acute Otitis Media. New York, Professional Communications, 2005.

Brook I: Tympanocentesis in the diagnosis and treatment of otitis media. Infect Med 18:363–366, 2001.

Dudley JP: Making tympanocentesis easier. J Emerg Med 8:765–767, 1990.

Hoberman A, Paradise JL, Wald ER: Tympanocentesis technique revisited. Pediatr Infect Dis J 16(2 Suppl):S25–S26, 1997.

Jones PJ: Tympanocentesis. In Reichman EF, Simon RR (eds): Emergency Medicine Procedures. New York, McGraw-Hill, 2004, pp 1273–1275.

Pichichero ME, Wright T: The use of tympanocentesis in the diagnosis and management of acute otitis media. Curr Infect Dis Rep 8:189–195, 2006.

CHAPTER 74

REDUCTION OF DISLOCATED TEMPOROMANDIBULAR JOINT (WITH TMJ SYNDROME EXERCISES)

Robert S. Tan • Grant C. Fowler

Although anyone may dislocate his or her temporomandibular joint (TMJ), such a dislocation occurs more commonly in older patients. Although the cause is often uncertain, TMJ dislocation can be associated with rheumatoid arthritis or osteoarthritis. Excessive laughter or yawning may also cause a luxation of the TMJ. Trauma can cause a TMJ dislocation; the history often reveals a blow to the chin while the mouth is slightly open. Dystonic reactions to medications can also cause dislocation. Patients who have had one dislocation are prone to further dislocations. Anterior dislocation occurs when the muscles and ligaments supporting the mandible are relaxed enough to allow the condyle to jump anteriorly over the articular eminence of the fossa. (Although posterior dislocation can occur, it is rare and usually the result of a direct blow to the chin that does not break the condylar neck.) Once the dislocation occurs, trismus and muscle spasms prevent the joint from returning to its natural position. Consequently, the patient presents to the clinician with an open mouth that cannot be closed and difficulty swallowing and talking. For anterior dislocation, pain is localized anterior to the tragus, and there will be a visible and palpable preauricular depression from the displacement of the mandibular condyle. Although unilateral dislocation causes a deviation away from the affected side, the more common bilateral dislocation prevents the mouth from being closed.

For clicking or tender TMJs, splinting by a dentist or oral surgeon is a common treatment. In the "Postprocedure Patient Education" section, three published alternatives to splint therapy are described, and a TMJ "rest" program is elucidated. For an acutely painful TMJ, as described in the "Passive Reduction" section, the joint can also be injected with a lidocaine/corticosteroid mixture.

INDICATIONS

Unilateral or bilateral TMJ dislocation(s) without fractures (the dislocation should be confirmed with a radiograph, which also rules out a fracture)

CONTRAINDICATIONS

Fractured condyle(s) (patient should be referred to a maxillofacial surgeon)

EQUIPMENT

- Gloves, mask, goggles
- Gauze to protect the clinician's thumbs
- Parenteral muscle relaxant may be helpful (e.g., diazepam, lorazepam, midazolam)
- Examination chair with firm neck rest
- *(Optional)* 5 mL of 2% lidocaine (Xylocaine) in a 10-mL syringe with a 25-gauge needle, 4 × 4 inch gauze sponges, povidone–iodine (Betadine) solution
- *(Optional)* Injectable corticosteroid

PREPROCEDURE PATIENT PREPARATION

Inform the patient which technique(s) will be attempted, whether passive or active, and the indications for, risks of, and alternatives to these techniques. If the passive technique is to be attempted, explain how muscle spasm is inhibiting reduction of the dislocated TMJ, and that an intravenous muscle relaxant may be all that is necessary.

NOTE: If an intravenous muscle relaxant is used, the patient should be accompanied by someone and not be allowed to drive that day. The patient should also be aware that his or her urine would test positive for benzodiazepines should drug testing be done.

Alternatively, an injection of local anesthetic into the TMJ may allow patients to reduce the dislocation themselves. If the active technique is necessary, patients should know that while the joint is being reduced, they may experience considerable pressure on the molars. They may also experience some referred pain to the neck, face, or ear, as well as mild, aching TMJ arthralgia after the reduction. Stress the importance of trying to remain relaxed and immobile while the joint is being reduced.

TECHNIQUE

Passive Reduction

One theory suggests that muscle spasm is all that is inhibiting reduction; therefore, an intravenous muscle relaxant should suffice. However, another theory suggests that painful stimuli arising from the capsule cause the muscle spasm to maintain the dislocation. Consequently, injection of lidocaine into the joint would be needed to overcome these painful stimuli and allow for passive reduction. The choice of technique may be determined by patient desire or by what is available in the clinic setting. Universal blood and body fluid precautions should be followed when performing this procedure.

1. If *intravenous muscle relaxation* is chosen, administer titrating doses of a muscle relaxant (e.g., diazepam, lorazepam, midazolam).

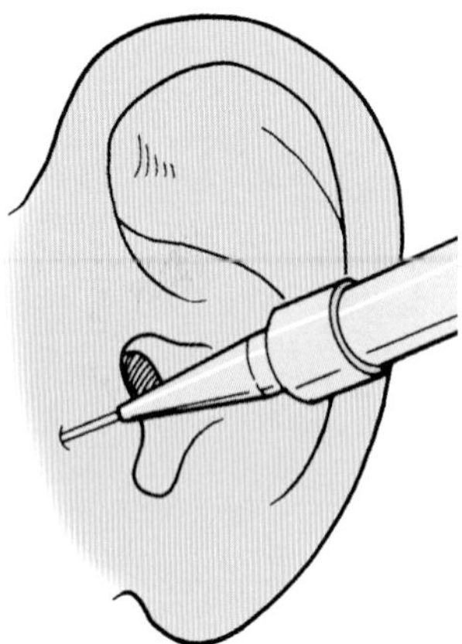

Figure 74-1 Injection of lidocaine into the joint.

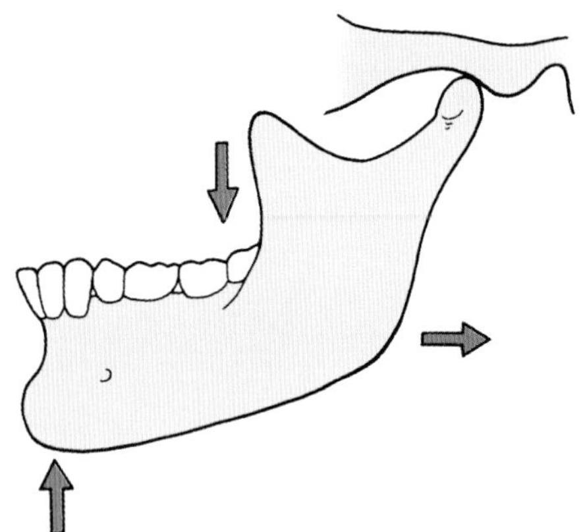

Figure 74-2 Direction of combined forces necessary for reduction.

Often, as the medication is titrated, the joint reduction occurs spontaneously.

NOTE: When benzodiazepines are administered intravenously, appropriate airway and hemodynamic monitoring is required. Moderate (conscious) procedural sedation privileges may also be required (see Chapter 2, Procedural Sedation and Analgesia).

2. If *TMJ injection* is chosen, have the patient open his or her mouth at least 4 cm. Palpate the joint line anterior to the tragus of the ear and the condyle of the mandible located immediately beneath the zygomatic arch. These landmarks are further confirmed by having the patient open and close the jaw while the clinician is palpating the joint line. After preparing the site with povidone–iodine, 3 to 5 mL of lidocaine should be injected into the joint. The needle should be inserted just below the zygomatic arch, one fingerbreadth anterior to the tragus, and directed inward and slightly upward. It will move freely when the tip is in the joint cavity.

   NOTE: For an acutely painful TMJ, injection with a combination of 0.5 mL corticosteroid and 0.5 mL local anesthetic may be helpful. Joint rest, as described in the "Postprocedure Patient Education" section, may also be helpful.
3. The injection of lidocaine alone may allow for spontaneous reduction (Fig. 74-1). Otherwise, a few minutes after the injection, even with bilateral dislocation, the patient might be able to close his or her mouth and retract the mandible into its normal position.
4. If passive reduction by muscle relaxation or TMJ injection is unsuccessful, active reduction may be necessary.

Active Reduction

This technique can be used for unilateral or bilateral dislocation.

1. The patient's head should be placed against a wall or high headrest to prevent backward movement. Take care to protect your thumbs because the mandible usually snaps sharply back into place with tremendous pressure, and this is an involuntary reflex. At a minimum, gauze should be wrapped over the gloved thumbs to protect them.
2. While standing in front of the patient, have the patient open his or her mouth slightly and place your thumbs on the occlusal surfaces of his or her posterior lower teeth.
3. Firmly grasp the mandible on the outside with your fingertips. Exert downward force on the molars (Fig. 74-2) in a slow and firm manner.
4. For anterior dislocation, after 30 to 60 seconds of downward pressure, apply very light pressure in a posterior direction and elevate the chin. (Pressure should be exerted in the opposite direction for a posterior dislocation.) This light posterior pressure and chin elevation can be accomplished by rotating the posterior or inferior mandible with your fingertips. At this point, the condyles should clear the articular eminence and allow the mandible to slide into its normally closed position (Fig. 74-3). If unsuccessful, this step may be repeated once or twice. With posterior dislocation, because the condyle may have prolapsed into the external auditory canal, baseline hearing should be documented (see Chapter 69, Audiometry).
5. Should these procedures fail, attempt to reduce the TMJ under more aggressive procedural sedation (see Chapter 2, Procedural Sedation and Analgesia). Should this also fail, consultation should be considered because reduction may need to be done under general anesthesia.
6. If the patient can swing his or her jaw from side to side, the reduction has been successful. Postprocedure radiographs are not required unless the procedure was difficult or traumatic, or there is significant postreduction pain. If the jaw immediately dislocates after successful reduction, a Kerlix-type gauze or a Barton bandage (elastic fabricated bandage) should be wrapped around the jaw and over the top of the head, producing a pressure-type dressing to keep the jaw closed. In this situation, the patient should also be referred to a dentist or an oral or maxillofacial surgeon.

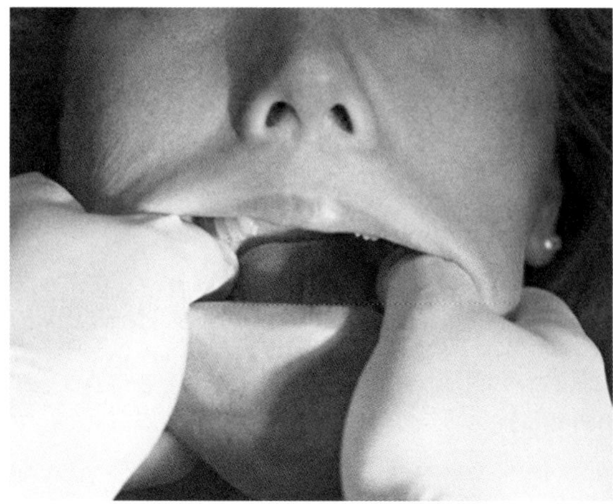

Figure 74-3 Reduction of a dislocated mandible from a position in front of the patient.

NOTE: For recurrent dislocations, search for possible causes (e.g., occlusal disharmony causing muscle spasm, medication-induced trismus, or rheumatoid arthritis).

COMPLICATIONS

All of the following complications occur only rarely.

- Posterior dislocation of the TMJ from reduction of anterior dislocation, and vice versa.
- Iatrogenic fracture or avulsion of the articular cartilage.
- Anesthesia complications (e.g., allergic reaction to lidocaine).
- Nerve damage.
- Permanent TMJ arthritis related to an improperly managed or undiagnosed condylar fracture; this is particularly a risk if the fracture extends into the articular surface. Prolonged disarticulation (several days) or recurrent disarticulation is also associated with TMJ arthritis.

POSTPROCEDURE PATIENT EDUCATION

Patients should be instructed to avoid opening their mouth more than 2 cm (the width of their thumb) for 2 weeks, and they should not yawn widely, take large bites of food, or laugh excessively for 4 to 6 weeks. They should also be placed on a soft diet for 2 weeks, and acetaminophen or nonsteroidal analgesics may be helpful for any discomfort after reduction. Patients should be taught to support the mandible with a hand when they yawn. In some instances, immobilization of the jaw is needed after reduction. For immobilization, refer the patient to a dentist. Some dentists immobilize the jaw for up to 2 weeks to give the stretched muscles and ligaments an opportunity to heal. This also allows the edema to subside. Inadequate immobilization may lead to recurrence of dislocation. If the dislocation was not traumatic, inform the patient that repeating the action that caused it will again cause dislocation. This is particularly true in the 4 to 6 weeks after reduction when the ligaments are not fully healed. Also warn the patient that recurrent dislocations may lead to permanent TMJ arthritis. In recurrent TMJ dislocation, the patient should be referred and the jaw immobilized for 4 to 6 weeks.

Three Alternatives to Splint Therapy for a Tender or Clicking Temporomandibular Joint

Patients with a tender or clicking TMJ are frequently referred to a dentist or oral surgeon for internal splinting or "splint therapy." A custom splint is made to be inserted between the upper and lower molars and provide constant tension on the TMJ by separating the molars. Such constant tension and immobilization of the TMJ hopefully allows it to heal. Some primary care clinicians use a "boil and bite" mouthpiece (which can be bought in most sporting goods stores to protect teeth during contact sports) in the same manner. The following exercises have been published as alternatives to splinting. If they fail, rest therapy (as noted in the section to follow) may be an option.

Method A

1. Have the patient obtain a soft wooden or plastic rod, approximately 15 cm long and 1.5 cm in diameter (e.g., a wooden dowel).
2. At least three times a day, the patient should thrust the mandible forward and grasp the rod with his or her back molars.
3. For 2 to 3 minutes, the patient then rhythmically bites on the rod with a grinding movement (Fig. 74-4).

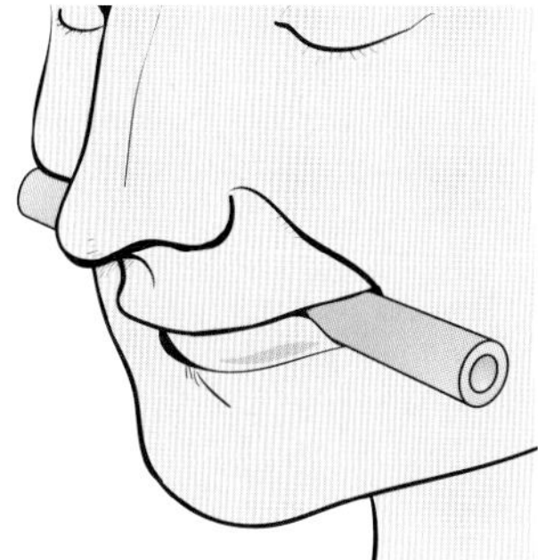

Figure 74-4 Wooden rod chewing exercise.

Method B

1. Although it may be initially uncomfortable, this exercise should eventually lead to some relief in uncomplicated TMJ syndrome.
2. At least four to five times a day, for 15 repetitions, the patient should rhythmically thrust the lower jaw forward and backward, in an anterior-posterior direction. The mouth should be slightly open, and when the exercise is performed correctly, the patient will look like a cheeky schoolchild exposing the bottom lip (Fig. 74-5).

Method C

This method consists of six exercises to be repeated six times per day (6 × 6).

NOTE: These exercises were recommended by an oral surgeon and should not cause pain while being performed. If performance causes discomfort, the intensity, rather than the number and frequency of the repetitions, should be reduced.

1. Have the patient hold the front third of his or her tongue to the roof of the mouth and take six deep breaths.
2. Next, have the patient hold his or her tongue to the roof of the mouth and open the mouth six times. The jaw should not click.
3. Have the patient hold the chin with both hands, keeping the chin still. *Without actually letting it move*, the patient should *attempt* to move his or her chin up, down, and to each side.
4. Next, with the chin between the heels of both hands, and the fingertips behind the neck, have the patient pull his or her chin toward the neck. Hold for 6 seconds.
5. Next, have the patient push his or her upper lip back *as if* to push the head straight back while using the neck muscles to *prevent* the head from being pushed back. Hold for 6 seconds.
6. To finish the exercises, have the patient pull the shoulders back, as if to touch the shoulder blades together, and hold for 6 seconds.

Temperomandibular Joint "Rest" Program

The following instructions may be given to patients:

1. Avoid biting any food with your front teeth—use small, bite-size pieces.

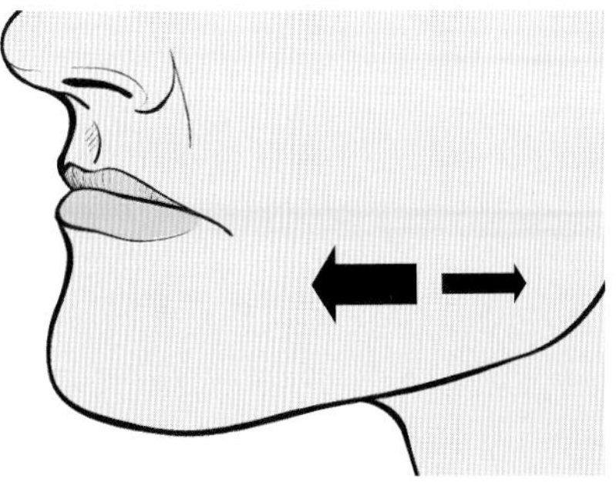

Figure 74-5 Lower jaw thrust exercise.

2. Food should be in small enough pieces to avoid opening your mouth wider than the thickness of your thumb.
3. Avoid eating food that requires prolonged chewing (e.g., raw vegetables, tough meat, hard crusts of bread).
4. Avoid protruding your jaw (e.g., talking, applying lipstick) or your tongue.
5. Try to breathe through your nose at all times.
6. Do not sleep on your jaw; attempt to always sleep on your back.
7. Avoid clenching your teeth—keep your lips together and your teeth apart.
8. Avoid chewing gum.
9. Always try to open your mouth in a hinge or arc motion.
10. Practice a relaxed lifestyle so that your jaws and face muscles feel relaxed.

CPT/Billing Codes

21480 Closed uncomplicated treatment of temporomandibular dislocation, initial or subsequent

21485 Closed complicated treatment of temporomandibular dislocation (e.g., recurrent requiring intermaxillary fixation or splinting), initial or subsequent

ICD-9-CM Diagnostic Codes

524.60 Temporomandibular joint-pain-dysfunction syndrome

524.62 Temporomandibular joint arthralgia

524.64 Temporomandibular joint sounds on opening/closing the jaw

524.69 Dislocation of temporomandibular joint, recurrent

830.0 Dislocation of temporomandibular joint, closed

BIBLIOGRAPHY

Amsterdam JT: Oral medicine. In Marx JA, Hockberger RS, Walls RM (eds): Rosen's Emergency Medicine, 6th ed. St. Louis, Mosby, 2006, pp 1041–1042.

Haddon R, Peacock WF IV: Face and jaw emergencies. In Tintinalli JE, Kelen GD, Stapczynski JS (eds): Emergency Medicine: A Comprehensive Study Guide, 6th ed. New York, McGraw-Hill, 2004, pp 1475–1476.

James DM: Reduction of a dislocated mandible. In James DM (ed): Field Guide to Urgent and Ambulatory Care Procedures. Philadelphia, Lippincott Williams & Wilkins, 2001, pp 44–47.

Murtagh J: Musculoskeletal medicine. In Murtagh J: Practice Tips, 4th ed. Sydney, Australia, McGraw-Hill, 2004, pp 128–130.

CHAPTER 75

Tympanometry

Gerald A. Amundsen

The tympanometer is a tool that has been used since the 1970s to assist in evaluation of middle ear and eardrum (tympanic membrane) function. Despite the current availability of multiple other tools and measuring instruments, tympanometry, with or without pneumatic otoscopy, continues to be a useful tool in the primary care clinic. The tympanogram, a graphic display of the information obtained from the tympanometer, provides the clinician an ability to objectively evaluate *otitis media with effusion*, *acute otitis media*, suspected or known *perforation of the tympanic membrane*, *patency of pressure equalization tubes* (PE tubes), *ossicular chain function*, and suspected *eustachian tube dysfunction*. When added to the history, clinical signs, and otoscopic findings, a tympanogram usually improves the clinician's diagnostic accuracy as well as his or her ability to monitor treatment.

The tympanometer consists of the probe, which is inserted into the external ear canal, and the associated hardware that produces stimuli (air and sound) to be directed toward the tympanic membrane, measures the response, and records the results. The probe has three ports, each of which has an independent function. The speaker port transmits the tone toward the tympanic membrane, and the air port transfers air to vary the pressure in the canal between the probe tip and the tympanic membrane. The third port has a microphone to gather sound waves reflected from the tympanic membrane. The remaining components of a tympanometer include the air pump, the oscillator (produces the tone transmitted through the speaker port), a manometer, a recorder, and an impedance bridge to translate information received through the microphone.

Ultimately, the tympanometer evaluates *immittance*, a measurement of the performance of the tympanic membrane and the middle ear. *Immittance* is the term used to describe the flow of energy into the middle ear (*admittance*) or the opposition to this flow of energy (*impedance*). The word *immittance* was coined by combining the words *impedance* and *admittance*.

Indications

- Any patient with complaints of ear pain, vertigo, or hearing loss
- If patency of PE tubes is in question
- Abnormalities (e.g., fluid, tympanic membrane retraction, perforation) visualized on otoscopic examination
- Possible tympanic membrane perforation (or to follow-up previously diagnosed perforation)
- Eustachian tube dysfunction when the tympanic membrane appears normal on examination
- Persistent middle ear effusion or otitis media with effusion

Contraindications

- Fulminant otitis externa
- Occlusion of the canal by cerumen (see Chapter 72, Cerumen Impaction Removal) or a foreign body (see Chapter 76, Removal of Foreign Bodies from the Ear and Nose)
- Age younger than 7 months (relative contraindication)

NOTE: Age younger than 7 months is a relative contraindication because although a positive result (type B curve) likely indicates an effusion, a negative result may be falsely negative. Even in the presence of a significant effusion, the soft, highly compliant ear canals in infants may result in a normal tympanogram.

Equipment

- Probe covers of various sizes to create a good seal in ear canals of different sizes (universal to all models).
- A tympanometer with air pressure range of −400 to +100 mm H_2O is preferable. Air pressure is also measured in decapascals (daPa, 1.0 daPa = 1.02 mm H_2O).
- Oscillator in tympanometer that produces a tone of 226 cycles per second (hertz [Hz]; 220 Hz is actually optimal).
- Most units, even the hand-held units, have some version of a printer for documentation.
- *(Optional)* Memory (may store data from one to eight patients, with one or two tests per patient).
- Units range from hand-held models to more expensive models equipped with a graphic acoustic reflex display or the instrumentation to perform audiometry. Although the basic tympanometer is a generally affordable tool for the office, these other features can increase the cost of equipment.

Preprocedure Patient Preparation

After educating the patient about the indication(s) for the procedure, reassure him or her that the process is painless. Describe the tone that may be heard and the slight bursts of air that will be felt in the canal. Emphasize the importance of remaining still during the test to ensure accuracy and ease of data collection.

Technique

1. Check the ear canal for patency and visualize the tympanic membrane with the otoscope. At this point, the use of pneumatic otoscopy may improve diagnostic accuracy.

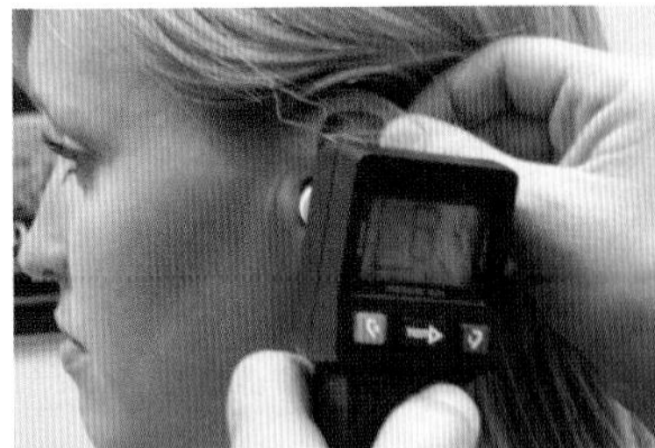

Figure 75-1 With the patient seated upright, apply traction to the helix and insert the probe.

2. Select the probe tip; choose the size that occludes the canal and creates a seal without entering too deeply.
3. Place the patient upright in the seated position, or in the lap of a parent in the case of a young child.
4. Apply posterior-superior traction to the helix to straighten the ear canal (posterior-inferior traction in the young child), and place the probe into the outer canal (Fig. 75-1).
5. Once a seal has been obtained, the tympanometer will automatically deliver the sound, vary the air pressures, and record the various parameters.

Common Errors

- Failure to remove cerumen impaction or a foreign body leads to false-positive results (type B curves) or inability to complete the test owing to "occlusion."
- Inappropriate probe tip size leads to "occlusion" or "air leak."

NOTE: Typical devices display results on a graphic screen when a test is successfully completed. Error messages such as "occlusion" or "leak" indicate the need for repositioning the probe or selection of a more appropriate tip size. The test will usually not run to completion unless occlusions in the canal have been removed and an appropriate seal has been achieved and maintained.

TABLE 75-1 Interpretation of the Tympanogram

Tympanogram Result	Characteristics	Possible Diagnoses
Type A	The "normal' curve Peak compliance is at 0 mm H_2O or daPa	Normal or negative tympanogram
Type A_D	Tall peak at 0 mm H_2O or daPa indicating high compliance	Monomeric (one layer) tympanic membrane due to healing perforation, disruption of the ossicular chain
Type A_S	Short peak at 0 mm H_2O or daPa indicating low compliance	Thickened tympanic membrane, ossicular fixation, presence of middle ear fluid
Type B	Flat or minimal peak indicating minimal compliance	*With low canal volume:* Cerumen impaction, foreign body, wrong probe *With high canal volume:* Pressure equalization tubes, perforation *With normal canal volume:* middle ear fluid
Type C	Peak compliance at negative pressure (<−100 mm H_2O or daPa)	Retracted membrane, eustachian tube dysfunction with or without effusion

daPa, decapascals.

Interpretation

The tympanogram is a graph of middle ear compliance on the vertical axis and pressure on the horizontal axis. From this graph, four useful pieces of information can be obtained for interpretation (Fig. 75-2 and Table 75-1):

- **Canal volume** is a measurement of the approximate volume between the probe tip and the tympanic membrane. It is usually 0.2 to 2.0 mL, but varies with age and bony structure. Abnormally high volume is indicative of a patent PE tube or a perforation. Abnormally low volume may indicate obstruction or a bulging tympanic membrane due to effusion.
- **Compliance** of the tympanic membrane when receiving sound at various pressures. The peak of the curve (maximal compliance) typically occurs when the air pressure is equal on both sides of the tympanic membrane (0 mm H_2O or daPa).
- **Pressure** (mm H_2O or daPa) at which the compliance peaks: usually 0 mm H_2O, but may be negative with eustachian tube dysfunction or a retracted tympanic membrane, or greater than 0 mm H_2O or daPa when the membrane is bulging.
- **Width of the curve** is calculated by the device. This may be too wide with early or resolving effusion or tympanosclerosis. This is the least useful portion of the data because the result is quite variable and the diagnostic reliability for middle ear pathology is uncertain.

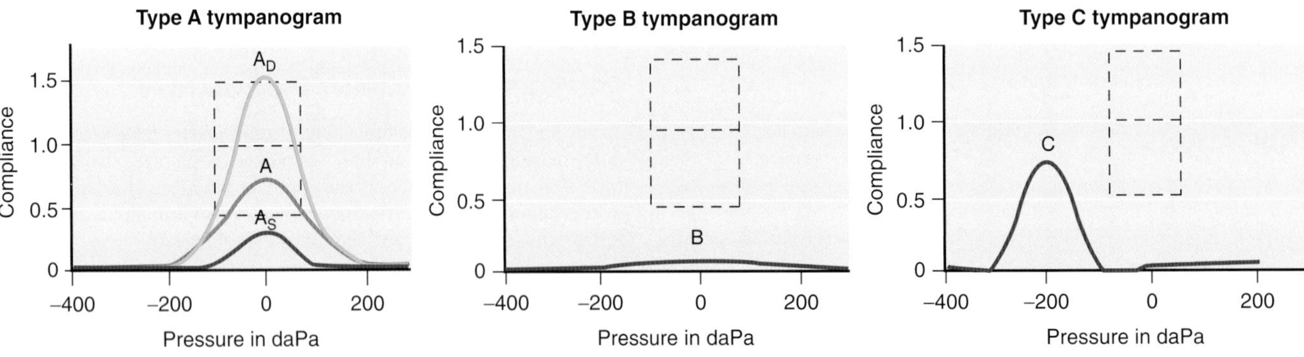

Figure 75-2 Tympanograms. Compliance and pressure are normal for adults if the curve crosses into the rectangles at any point and normal for children younger than 10 years of age if the curve crosses into the lower rectangle. See Table 75-1 for interpretation.

It should be noted that a localized abnormality (e.g., perforation of the tympanic membrane) may obscure the ability to evaluate the rest of the middle ear system. However, compared with pneumatic otoscopy, the tympanogram is usually more accurate: pneumatic otoscopy may elicit movement of a tympanic membrane despite a pinpoint perforation, whereas a tympanogram will likely make the correct diagnosis. In contrast, middle ear mucosal edema may be sufficient to mask even a large perforation on tympanometric evaluation.

Postprocedure Patient Education

The tympanogram is used to help direct treatment and monitor progress. The patient should be informed of the result and treatment plan. Appropriate consultation should be requested when indicated.

CPT/Billing Code

92567 Tympanometry (impedance testing)

ICD-9-CM Diagnostic Codes

380.4 Cerumen impaction
381.00 Acute otitis media with effusion
381.01 Acute serous otitis
381.30 Chronic serous otitis with effusion
382.90 Acute otitis media
382.90 Chronic serous otitis
384.20 Perforation tympanic membrane
384.81 Healed tympanic membrane perforation
388.7 Ear pain
872.61 Perforation: traumatic

Acknowledgment

The editors wish to recognize the many contributions by Gregory J. Forzley, MD, to this chapter in the previous two editions of this text.

Suppliers

(See contact information online at www.expertconsult.com.)

Tympanometers
Gordon Stowe
Grason-Stadler, Inc.
Maico Diagnostics
Micro Audiometrics
Welch Allyn, Inc.
Madsen

BIBLIOGRAPHY

American Academy of Family Physicians; American Academy of Otolaryngology-Head and Neck Surgery; American Academy of Pediatrics Subcommittee on Otitis Media with Effusion: Otitis media with effusion [clinical practice guideline]. Pediatrics 113:1412–1429, 2004.

Green LA, Culpepper L, de Melker RA, et al: Tympanometry interpretation by primary care physicians: A report from the International Primary Care Network (IPCN) and the Ambulatory Sentinel Practice Network (ASPN). J Fam Pract 49:932–936, 2000.

Hall JW, Antonelli PJ: Assessment of peripheral and central auditory function. In Bailey BJ, Johnson JT, Newlands SD (eds): Head and Neck Surgery-Otolaryngology, 4th ed. Philadelphia, Lippincott William & Wilkins, 2006, pp 1927–1942.

Onusko E: Tympanometry. Am Fam Physician 70:1713–1720, 2004.

Ramakrishnan K, Sparks RA, Berryhill WE: Diagnosis and treatment of otitis media. Am Fam Physician 76:1650–1658, 2007.

CHAPTER 76

Removal of Foreign Bodies from the Ear and Nose

John Harlan Haynes III • Michael Zeringue

The nasal orifice and external auditory canal occasionally collect small objects such as beads, insects, peanuts, pebbles, or beans. Foreign bodies in this area are especially common in pediatric and mentally impaired individuals. Knowledge of the type of foreign body and how long it has been lodged in the orifice is very helpful. If an expandable material is suspected (e.g., organic materials, beans, seeds), irrigation with water or saline may be contraindicated because it may cause additional expansion of the object. Timeliness may be a priority because the object may become more firmly lodged in place as the mucosa swells. Reactive debris may accumulate as a local response to the irritation. Manual removal or suction may be required to remove these objects and the accompanying debris.

Various techniques are available for removing foreign bodies with instruments; however, simple attempts at removal should generally be pursued before instrumentation. In children with a nasal foreign body, a nebulized decongestant can be used to assist expulsion with simple nose blowing. A positive-pressure technique (as in mouth-to-mouth resuscitation) using a pediatric bag valve mask (Ambu bag) may be used in infants and young children. Block the unaffected nostril and, while not exceeding recommended maximal pressure with the bag valve mask (by cardiopulmonary resuscitation guidelines), force air briskly through the oropharynx and out the obstructed nostril to dislodge the object. In older children and adults, vasoconstrictive nasal solutions (e.g., phenylephrine, epinephrine, oxymetazoline) may be used to reduce mucosal edema. Wait 10 minutes after application, then have the patient obstruct one nostril and then blow our forcefully through the other nostril to dislodge the object. Even if the object does not come out, the relaxed and decongested mucosa will give the clinician more room to work.

In the external ear canal, pulsing saline irrigation through an 18-gauge plastic catheter and directing it posteriorly may dislodge the impacted object. If tympanic membrane perforation is suspected, however, irrigation is contraindicated.

The use of strong acrylic glue (cyanoacrylate) has been advocated for removing beads from the nose or external canal but the patient must be able to remain very still. The ultimate goal when removing a foreign body with this technique, as well as with all techniques, is to remove the object with as little trauma as possible and to avoid pushing it further back toward the posterior nasal passage or tympanic membrane. If this technique is to be used, make sure acetone is available to remove any misplaced cyanoacrylate (see section on "Alternate Technique: Glue").

Having acetone available may also be helpful if the foreign body turns out to be chewing gum or polystyrene (e.g., Styrofoam) foam or beads. In addition to dissolving cyanoacrylate glue, acetone has been reported in the literature to dissolve or soften polystyrene; it also reduces the adherence of particles consisting of these substances or gum. Ethyl chloride has been used in the same manner. It should be noted that there have been no studies regarding any possible toxicity from acetone, dissolved polystyrene, or ethyl chloride in contact with a mucous membrane. Therefore, only a few drops of the acetone or ethyl chloride should be dripped directly onto the foreign body under guidance with an otoscope. After being left in place for 5 minutes or less, the resulting combination should be removed with forceps, suction, or irrigation. Ultimately, the ear should be irrigated to remove any residual chemicals after the object is removed. If there is a possibility or a history of a perforated tympanic membrane, this process is contraindicated.

Both reassurance and immobilization are important in manual removal of nasal or external canal foreign bodies. Availability of the proper tools and an adequate light source are also critical. To minimize the risk of lacerations or abrasions, all attempts to remove foreign bodies should be made under direct visualization with magnification if at all possible. The clinician should set realistic limits on the amount of time to be spent and number of attempts to be made. Referral to an ear, nose, and throat (ENT) specialist may be prudent (1) if the examiner is dealing with an expandable material (unless there is a high probability of successful removal); (2) when the nasal passage or external ear canal is completely occluded and surrounded by marked edema and inflammation; (3) if the object is adherent or adjacent to the tympanic membrane; or (4) if attempts to remove the object have been unsuccessful or will worsen the scenario. For such difficult removals, local anesthesia, conscious sedation, or even general anesthesia may be necessary. If an ENT specialist agrees, and if the patient is in considerable pain, instillation of topical anesthetic drops before transportation may be appreciated.

NOTE: Miniature button or disk batteries are commonly used in watches, calculators, cameras, hearing aids, travel clocks, and even greeting cards that play music. Consequently, they are frequently found as foreign objects in noses and ears. Removal is a high priority because permanent damage can result (usually localized electrical burns, but bone and cartilage can be destroyed) if they are allowed to remain for more than a short time. Although miniature batteries contain toxic heavy metals such as mercury and other poisonous substances, their greater danger lies in the fact that they can produce electrochemical current. They should be removed promptly, and irrigation, nose drops, or eardrops are strictly contraindicated.

NOTE: If a recent foreign body turns out to be a moth, take the patient into a dark room and shine a flashlight into the ear or nose. The moth will likely fly out toward the light!

Indication

A known foreign body is the indication for treatment.

NOTE: A general rule for foreign bodies in the ear is that if the object is in the outer two thirds of the canal and is easily accessible, it can usually be removed. If it is closer to the eardrum and cannot be removed by irrigation, referral should be considered.

Contraindications

Consider referral if any of the following contraindications apply.

- Lack of knowledge of normal anatomy of nasal passage or external ear canal.
- Nasal passage or external ear canal is obscured because of trauma. With a foreign body that has perforated the tympanic membrane, removal may cause further damage to the tympanic membrane, possible damage to middle ear ossicles, as well as loss of hearing.
- The airway is in danger from a nasal foreign body.
- A large foreign body is impaled into the external ear canal.
- The patient is uncooperative and cannot be sedated (see Chapter 7, Pediatric Sedation and Analgesia) or anesthetized (see the section on "Anesthesia for Auditory Canal" and Chapter 4, Local Anesthesia, Chapter 9, Oral and Facial Anesthesia, and Chapter 10, Topical Anesthesia).
- For a miniature battery, do not use nose or ear drops.
- For organic or expandable materials, unless the clinician is fairly certain of a successful removal, flushing with saline or water is contraindicated. Flushing can hasten or enhance the swelling.
- Irrigation is contraindicated with an acute or chronic ruptured tympanic membrane.
- For other contraindications to removal from ear, see Chapter 72, Cerumen Impaction Removal.

Equipment

- Traditional foreign body extraction tools such as a Frazier suction tip; ear curette (Fig. 76-1) or wire loop curette; nasal bayonet (see Fig. 76-1), alligator (Fig. 76-2; see Fig. 76-1), or Hartmann forceps; fine tissue or Adson forceps; right-angle hook (can be made from 21-gauge needle; Fig. 76-3) or ball-tipped right-angle hook.
- Cotton-tipped swabs.
- Nasal or ear speculum (select the largest that will fit the orifice or canal; visibility and room for instrumentation is better with a speculum than with an otoscope).
- Magnification, in the form of either an otoscope with an operating head or a loupe.
- Bright light that can be directed or focused. If a headlamp is available, both hands will be free to perform the procedure.
- Topical anesthetic such as 2% to 5% lidocaine (see the section on "Anesthesia for Auditory Canal" and see Chapter 10, Topical Anesthesia). Benzocaine spray (14%, Cetacaine) can be used for nasal anesthesia; 20% benzocaine solution can be used for the external ear canal.
- For a local field ear block, use a 27-gauge, 1½-inch needle. An anesthetic such as 1% lidocaine with epinephrine can be used on the external canal. For subcutaneous injections deeper inside the canal, plain 2% lidocaine may be useful (see also Chapter 4, Local Anesthesia, and Chapter 9, Oral and Facial Anesthesia). Adding a 1:10 mixture of 8.4% sodium bicarbonate to lidocaine helps reduce the pain of injection.
- Nasal decongestant such as phenylephrine (0.25% to 2%; Neo-Synephrine, Vicks), epinephrine (1:50,000; Adrenalin), or oxymetazoline hydrochloride (0.05%; Afrin, Neo-Synephrine 12 hour) spray. An atomizer is helpful if available.
- Irrigant such as saline.
- Wall or portable suction unit.
- Equipment necessary for clinician to follow universal blood and body fluid precautions, especially when working near mucous membranes of a patient.
- Strong magnet and magnetizable nail for retrieving metal foreign bodies.
- Irrigation equipment (e.g., surgical Chux, kidney basin) as noted in Chapter 72, Cerumen Impaction Removal.
- *Optional:* 2- to 6-Fr diameter Fogarty (biliary or cardiovascular), Foley, Swan-Ganz or Schuknecht FB catheter, or Katz oto-rhino foreign body remover (single-use balloon-tipped catheter attached

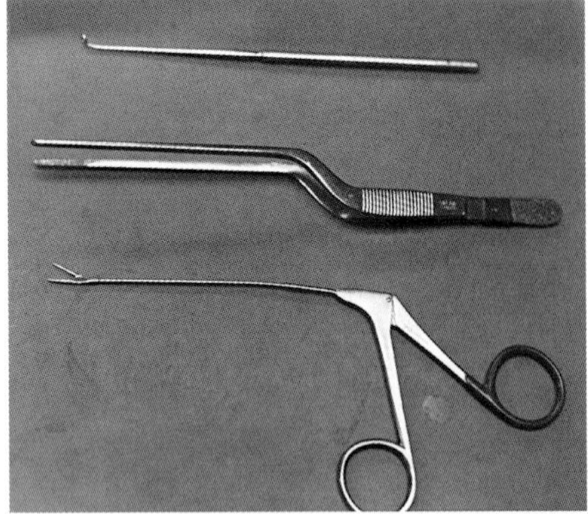

Figure 76-1 Traditional instruments used for foreign-body extraction: Ear curette (*top*), nasal (bayonet) forceps (*middle*), and alligator forceps (*bottom*).

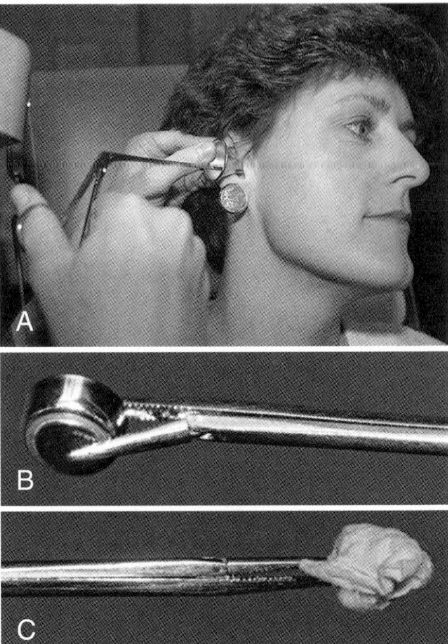

Figure 76-2 Alligator forceps (**A**) for retrieving small batteries (**B**) and paper balls (**C**) from auditory canal.

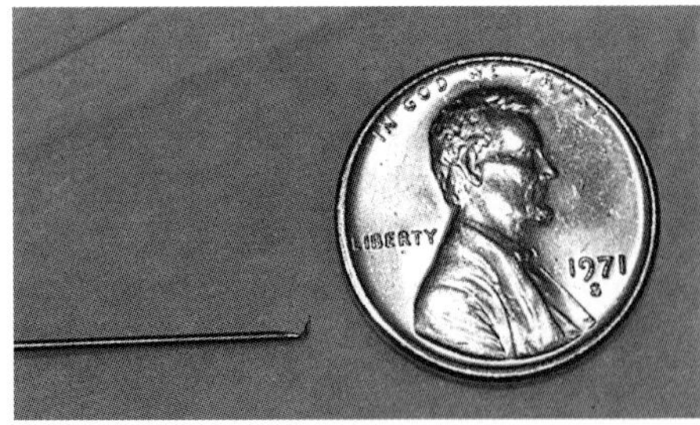

Figure 76-3 Precise right-angle hook made from bending a 1½-inch, 21-gauge needle tip at a right angle is an excellent tool for removing smooth objects such as beans and corn kernels.

to syringe). The balloons on the Fogarty, Foley, or Swan-Ganz catheters will need to be inflated with a 2-mL syringe.

- *Optional:* Commercially available, single-use, disposable, Hognose (4-, 5-, or 6-mm) or Gatornose (small or large) otoscope tip.
- *Alternate technique, suction:* 30-inch plastic intravenous extension tubing or 10-Fr suction catheter, heat source (e.g., burner, alcohol lamp, lighter), blunt end of metal ear curette handle or atomizer tip, and hemostat.
- *Alternate technique, glue:* Dacron-tipped applicator, thin paintbrush, plastic ear curette, straightened paperclip, toothpick, or the wooden end of cotton-tipped swab and strong acrylic glue (cyanoacrylate; Dermabond or Superglue), with acetone to remove the glue if necessary.

Preprocedure Patient Preparation

- Stress the importance of remaining immobile during the procedure.
- For nasal or otic foreign body removal, discuss the chance of minor trauma. This may be associated with discomfort during the procedure or some bleeding after the procedure.
- For nasal foreign bodies, the risk of aspiration should be discussed.
- For ear irrigation or instrument removal, discuss the risk of perforation and dizziness.
- Alternatives, risks, and benefits should be explained and informed consent obtained.
- If instrumentation is to be performed, after the topical anesthetic is applied, touch the mucosa with the instrument slightly inside the orifice so that the patient knows what to expect and to avoid being startled.

Technique: Nasal Foreign Body

1. Topical anesthesia and vasoconstriction can be applied as a spray or with drops (e.g., a mixture of 2% to 5% lidocaine and 0.25% to 2% phenylephrine hydrochloride or 0.5% oxymetazoline hydrochloride). After waiting a few minutes for the mixture to work, carefully examine the nostril and determine the best instrument or technique. Alternatively, the decongestant can be sprayed first; after waiting a few minutes for the decongestant to work, if the topical anesthetic is then sprayed, it may last longer. The disadvantage of spraying the decongestant and topical anesthetic separately is that the clinician then has to wait a few more minutes for the topical anesthetic to work.
2. The patient may be sitting or lying. Extend the patient's head. Apply pressure on the tip of the nose in a superior and posterior direction to help visualize the nasal canal. Irrigation should not be used in the nasal cavity because it may push the object into the oropharynx or larynx, causing aspiration.
3. Smooth, round objects can be removed using suction or right-angle hooks. For the right-angle hook, slide it past the object with the tip parallel to the nasal sidewall. Once it has passed the object, rotate it 90 degrees so that the tip is behind the object, and then gently pull the object out.
4. An alligator or bayonet forceps may be used to grasp an object that has a small leading edge.
5. A lubricated, small Fogarty, Foley, Swan-Ganz, or Schuknecht FB catheter, or a Katz oto-rhino foreign body catheter can be passed beyond the foreign body. After inflating the balloon or opening the umbrella, gentle traction will either facilitate removal or stabilize the foreign body to prevent oropharyngeal aspiration. This technique may slightly increase the risk of trauma and epistaxis; it is rare to visualize much of the catheter tip during insertion.
6. In all cases, instruments introduced into the nasal passage require a steady hand resting on the patient's head in case of sudden movements, which can be involuntary if pain is elicited.
7. After removal, examine the orifice closely to make sure that another foreign body was not behind the first and that all debris has been removed. Any particles left behind can lead to irritation, inflammation, drainage, or chronic granulation. Also check the unaffected nasal and ear orifices for any other surprises.

Technique: Otic Foreign Body

1. Many clinicians perform hearing testing (see Chapter 69, Audiometry) to determine the baseline before inserting instruments. Some also perform tonometry (see Chapter 68, Tonometry) to attempt to determine if the tympanic membrane has been perforated.
2. Small children may need to be sedated (see Chapter 7, Pediatric Sedation and Analgesia). If an attempt is to be made without sedation, they may want to sit on the lap of a parent or attendant with the ear facing the clinician. Adults usually want to remain seated with the affected ear facing the clinician. The patient may also be comfortable lying down with the affected ear facing upward.
3. With the ear turned upward, instill a topical anesthetic. After several minutes, use suction to remove pus, topical anesthetics, or blood as necessary to visualize the object. The patient should be warned that suction can be very loud.
4. With adults, visualization of the external ear canal is aided by pulling the auricle upward and backward to straighten the canal. In small children, the auricle is pulled downward. If an instrument is to be used, it should be used only under direct visualization. Insert it slightly inside the auricle, at first, to help the patient accommodate to the noise and sensation of instrumentation. Compared with the internal canal, the external third of the canal has a thicker layer of skin and subcutaneous tissue that covers cartilage; the internal two thirds has a thinner, more fragile layer of skin covering only bone.
5. The depth and surface qualities of the object usually suggest which tool(s) to use. Grasp fibrous objects (e.g., cotton, plant matter) with the alligator forceps (see Fig. 76-2). Smooth objects (e.g., beans, seeds, popcorn kernels) that are blocking no more than half the diameter of the canal might be dragged out by passing an ear curette or wire loop beyond the object and gently withdrawing it. Larger, smooth, and hard items such as small batteries and BBs may be teased out with a fine, 1-mm, right-angle hook (see Fig. 76-3) or ball-tipped right-angle hook. Slide the right-angle hook past the object with the tip parallel to the canal sidewall. Once it has passed the object, rotate it 90 degrees so that the tip is now behind the object, and gently pull the object out. Objects with sharp projections, such as earrings and screws, may need to be grasped with forceps to avoid laceration of sensitive membranes.
6. Irrigation may move a foreign body far enough away from the eardrum to increase the chance of extraction.
7. Occasionally, iron-containing items such as a BB can be removed with a small magnet probe. A probe can be fashioned from a nail that has been blunted and magnetized by drawing it across any strong permanent magnet. Permanent magnets are available in hardware stores or can be found in the rear of stereo speaker cones.
8. Irrigation may be useful in certain instances after object removal, such as when small fragments of debris remain.
9. Insects in the auditory canal should be drowned or smothered by instilling lidocaine or a benzocaine solution. The liquid kills the insects, which halts their disturbing and painful movements. An alligator forceps can then be used to grasp and remove the insect. Suction can also be used to remove both the insect and the liquid. Some clinicians suggest that mineral oil immobilizes insects faster; however, mineral oil does not provide anesthesia for the patient, and other clinicians say mineral oil is more likely to cause the insects to break into fragments during attempts to remove them.

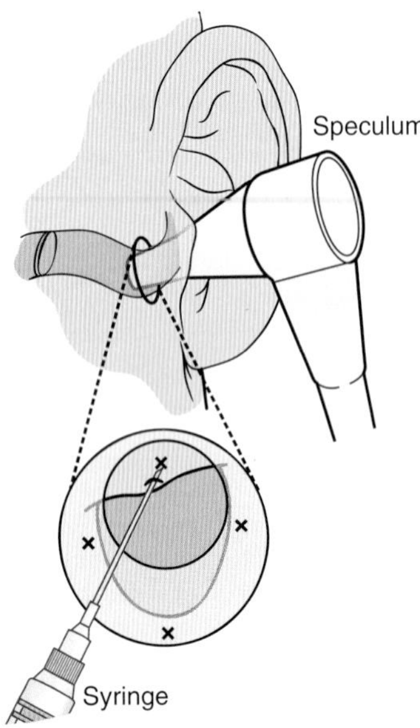

Figure 76-4 Four-quadrant field block anesthesia of the external auditory canal. Local anesthetic is injected subcutaneously in the four quadrants of the lateral portion of the ear canal. The largest speculum that will fit is used to guide the injections. The speculum is withdrawn slightly, tilted toward each of the four quadrants, and the needle is inserted subcutaneously (x). A very small amount of anesthetic (0.25 to 0.5 mL) is injected to produce a slight bulge in the soft tissue. A total of 1.5 to 2 mL of anesthetic is usually sufficient to anesthetize the ear canal and permit painless removal of a foreign body. (Riviello RJ: Otolaryngologic procedures. In Roberts JR, Hedges JR [eds]: Clinical Procedures in Emergency Medicine, 4th ed. Philadelphia, Saunders, 2004, pp 1280–1316.)

10. In all situations, instruments introduced into the auditory canal require a steady hand resting on the patient's head in case of sudden movements, which can be involuntary if pain is elicited.
11. Light, moderate (e.g., intramuscular or intravenous), or general anesthesia may be needed to remove foreign bodies in individuals who cannot tolerate instrumentation with or without local agents. Field block anesthesia of the external auditory canal may be helpful, if tolerated (Fig. 76-4).
12. After removal, make sure that another foreign body is not behind the first and that all debris has been removed. Any particles left behind can lead to irritation, inflammation, drainage, or chronic granulation. Some clinicians repeat hearing tests after removing a foreign body to compare with baseline. Also check the unaffected nasal and ear orifices for any other surprises.

Alternate Technique: Suction

Suction is especially useful for removing round foreign bodies from the ear or nasal cavity.

1. Cut off the tip of the tubing or suction catheter (Fig. 76-5A). Heat the end of the curette handle or metal atomizer tip (Fig. 76-5B). Flange the cut tube end with the preheated handle or tip so that it molds to the blunt, rounded metal (Fig. 76-5C and D). An alternative to this self-made catheter is the commercially available Hognose otoscope tip.
2. Clamp the tubing with a hemostat and attach the opposite end to the suction unit (Fig. 76-5E). Alternatively, apply low to medium suction to the Hognose suction line.
3. Gently insert the flanged end into the orifice containing the foreign body under direct visualization and advance it to the object.
4. When the flange is in contact with the object, quickly unclamp the suction catheter tubing (Fig. 76-5F) and apply full suction immediately through the suction cup onto the foreign object. Alternatively, using the Hognose otoscope tip, apply suction when the soft tip is in contact with the object.
5. While suctioning, gently extract the tubing and the suction-attached foreign body (Fig. 76-5G).

Alternate Technique: Glue

This technique is especially useful for removing smooth, round objects that are difficult to grasp (e.g., plastic beads) from the nasal cavity or ear. It may be more useful in adults because cooperation is required.

1. Place a small drop of acrylic glue (cyanoacrylate such as Dermabond or Superglue) on the blunt end of an applicator (e.g., Dacron-tipped applicator, thin paintbrush, curette, straightened paper clip, toothpick, or the wooden end of cotton-tipped swab). Allow the glue to become tacky.
2. Quickly, but carefully, touch the glue on the end of the applicator to the foreign body. Establish and maintain contact. Avoid contacting the mucosa en route or pushing the object any farther inward. Hold the applicator still and maintain contact for 30 seconds until the glue hardens.
3. Gently pull the applicator out of the orifice with the foreign body stuck to it.

Anesthesia for Auditory Canal

For local anesthesia, instill five drops of 2% to 5% lidocaine or 20% benzocaine solution into the canal and allow it to remain for 5 to 10 minutes. Suction to remove fluid and canal debris before injection of a local anesthetic (if needed) under direct visualization. If tympanic membrane rupture is suspected, eardrops and irrigation are contraindicated.

For local field anesthesia of the external half of the auditory canal, inject small amounts (usually <2 mL total) of 1% lidocaine with epinephrine at three or four sites equally spaced along the exterior verge of the canal (see Fig. 76-4). For deeper canal anesthesia (much more sensitive area), subcutaneous injections (0.5 to 1 mL) of plain 2% lidocaine may be considered but is not recommended because the need for multiple injections is usually much more traumatic than the actual foreign body removal. This is especially true for the pediatric population, where in many instances it is more appropriate to use sedation. If subcutaneous injections are used, they are placed in the canal just external to the junction of the cartilaginous and bony canal (approximately one third of the way into the canal). Beginning at the posterior and superior aspect of the canal, use a 27-gauge, 1½-inch needle to slowly infiltrate lidocaine. Repeat this at two or three spots equally spaced around the canal. Allow the lidocaine to dissect down, "blanching" the ear canal and drum, if visible. Topical lidocaine or benzocaine applied to the auditory canal before an injection is often useful. Wait 5 to 10 minutes before instrumentation.

Complications

- Trauma to mucous membranes (e.g., excoriation, laceration) with the possibility of trauma-related infection or bleeding.
- Injury to a nasal passage, external canal, tympanic membrane, or middle ear.
- Deeper progression of the object leading to the inability to extract in the office.
- Aspiration (nasal passage foreign bodies).
- With delayed or incomplete removal of nasal foreign bodies, the patient may be at risk of obstructive sinusitis and even meningitis from local extension of the sinusitis.

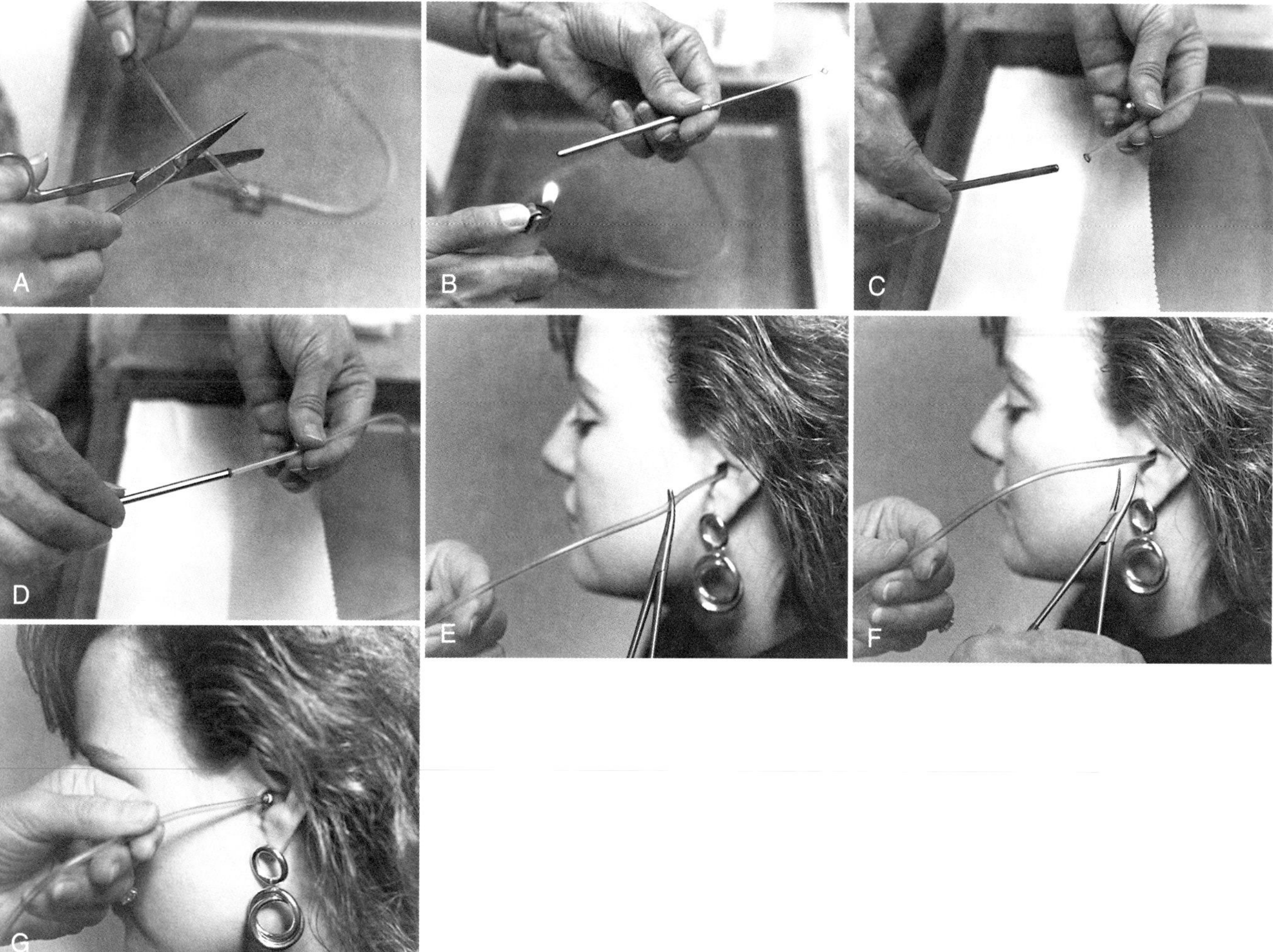

Figure 76-5 **A–G,** Technique for removing spherical foreign bodies from the ear. See text for details.

- With foreign bodies of the ear, acute otitis externa is common and may result from injury caused by the foreign body itself or by its removal. Also, when instruments are placed in the ear, the patient may experience bradycardia, or nausea or vomiting (or both).
- Complications of using cyanoacrylate glue include abrading or excoriating the mucosa with the applicator, dripping or spilling the glue on the mucosa, or gluing the applicator to the mucosa. Acetone can be used to remove the glue.

Postprocedure Patient Education

Inform the patient to watch for signs of infection (see Chapter 72, Cerumen Impaction Removal). The patient should follow up with the clinician in 1 to 2 days. He or she should report a headache, fever, or drainage after removal of a foreign body. These symptoms could indicate sinusitis or meningitis or other serious infection. After removal of nasal foreign bodies, the patient should use saline irrigation, two to three times a day for 2 or 3 days. Many clinicians prescribe several days of antibiotic otic drops to prevent external otitis after the mucosa has been possibly abraded, excoriated, or lacerated with irrigation or removal of a foreign body.

Patient Education Guides

See the sample patient education and consent forms online at www.expertconsult.com.

CPT/Billing Codes

30300 Removal foreign body, intranasal; office type procedure
30310 Removal foreign body, intranasal; requiring general anesthesia
69200 Removal foreign body from external auditory canal; without general anesthesia
69205 Removal foreign body from external auditory canal; with general anesthesia

ICD-9-CM Diagnostic Codes

931 Foreign body in ear, auditory canal or auricle
932 Foreign body in nose, nasal sinus or nostril

Acknowledgment

The editors wish to recognize the many contributions by Gary Newkirk, MD, to this chapter in a previous edition of this text.

Suppliers

(See contact information online at www.expertconsult.com.)

Hognose and Gatornose otoscope attachments/specula
IQDr., Inc.
Katz oto-rhino foreign body remover
Inhealth Industries

BIBLIOGRAPHY

Backlin SA: Positive-pressure technique for nasal foreign body removal in children. Ann Emerg Med 25:554–555, 1995.

Douglas AR: Use of nebulized adrenaline to aid expulsion of intra-nasal foreign bodies in children. J Laryngol Otol 110:559–560, 1996.

Finkelstein JA: Oral Ambu-bag insufflation to remove unilateral nasal foreign bodies. Am J Emerg Med 14:57–58, 1996.

Friedman EM, Munter DW, Richards JR, et al: When and how to retrieve foreign bodies. Patient Care 13:186–200, 1997.

Hanson RM, Stephens M: Cyanoacrylate-assisted foreign body removal from the ear and nose in children. J Paediatr Child Health 30:77–78, 1994.

Jensen JH: Technique for removing a spherical foreign body from the nose or ear. Ear Nose Throat J 55:270–271, 1976.

Kadish H: Ear and nose foreign bodies: "It is all about the tools." Clin Pediatr (Phila) 44:665–670, 2005.

Kadish HA, Corneli HM: Removal of nasal foreign bodies in the pediatric population. Am J Emerg Med 15:54–56, 1997.

Provenza M: Nasal foreign body removal. In Reichman E, Simon R (eds): Emergency Medicine Procedures. New York, McGraw-Hill, 2004, pp 1286–1290.

Riviello RJ: Otolaryngologic procedures. In Roberts JR, Hedges JR (eds): Clinical Procedures in Emergency Medicine, 4th ed. Philadelphia, Saunders, 2004, pp 1280–1316.

Roberts JR, Hedges JR (eds): Clinical Procedures in Emergency Medicine, 4th ed. Philadelphia, Saunders, 2004.

Roberts R: External auditory canal foreign body removal. In Reichman E, Simon R (eds): Emergency Medicine Procedures. New York, McGraw-Hill, 2004, pp 1259–1266.

Usatine RP: The Color Atlas of Family Medicine. New York, McGraw-Hill, 2009.

CHAPTER 77

NASOLARYNGOSCOPY

Grant C. Fowler • Rolf O. Montalvo

Fortunately, the incidence and mortality rates for cancers of the oral cavity, pharynx, and larynx have declined slightly over the last 20 years. That said, cancers of the pharynx and larynx remain two of most common cancers in the upper aerodigestive tract, with 12,400 and 12,250 new cases diagnosed, respectively, each year in the United States. Both types of cancer can be diagnosed with nasolaryngoscopy, and the earlier the diagnosis, the better the cure rate. At the same time, the number of nasopharyngeal complaints in the offices of primary care clinicians has increased. For example, sinusitis is now one of the most common chronic diseases in the United States. These facts—combined with the fact that many primary care clinicians have difficulty visualizing the nasal passages, oropharynx, and larynx—have led many practitioners to seek alternatives to nasolaryngoscopy. Nasolaryngoscopy has now been used for over 30 years. The ease of learning the technique (especially for clinicians already performing endoscopic procedures), its low risk (no need for sedation), the rapidity of the procedure (most procedures can be completed in 10 to 20 minutes), and the relatively low cost of equipment ($3500 to $7000) have resulted in increasing numbers of primary care clinicians using this valuable diagnostic tool. In addition, patients appreciate the immediately available diagnostic results, especially when nasolaryngoscopy is performed in the familiar and comfortable environment of their primary care clinician's office. Recent developments include biopsy ports, smaller-diameter scopes, and distal-chip optical systems (improve visualization and may be less prone to fogging). Narrow-band imaging, an image enhancement system, is now available in some models and increases the contrast in the background when visualizing capillaries and veins. This may allow clinicians to diagnose smaller lesions at an earlier stage. In addition, biopsies, dilations, botulinum toxin (Botox) injections, and in-office laser procedures can now be performed through these small-diameter scopes. Although these scopes may in turn be replaced by those capable of performing transnasal esophagoscopy, at present nasolaryngoscopy remains a popular procedure.

The indications for nasolaryngoscopy by primary care clinicians are chronic upper respiratory complaints, especially in smokers or those with unilateral conditions. Nasolaryngoscopy is also helpful in patients with certain acute disorders (e.g., one study found nasolaryngoscopy more effective than sinus films for diagnosing acute maxillary sinusitis). Nasolaryngoscopy is helpful when there is difficulty examining the larynx with an indirect mirror (see Chapter 79, Indirect Mirror Laryngoscopy), such as when there is unusual anatomy or persistent gagging. A large (n = 20,000) ongoing trial in France (Trial of Head and Neck Cancer Screening, THANCS) will attempt to answer whether nasolaryngoscopy combined with esopharyngeal brush biopsy will be effective for screening patients with a history of heavy alcohol consumption and smoking, perhaps decreasing the mortality rate from head and neck cancer.

INDICATIONS

Chronic Conditions

- Chronic hoarseness (>3 weeks)
- Chronic sinusitis or sinus discomfort, especially unilateral
- Chronic serous otitis media or eustachian tube dysfunction in an adult, especially unilateral
- Recurrent otalgia
- Suspected neoplasm
- Chronic cough
- Chronic nasal obstruction or postnasal drip
- Chronic rhinorrhea
- Chronic pharyngeal pain
- Halitosis
- Previous head and neck cancer
- Previous conservative treatment of laryngeal polyps
- Head or neck mass or adenopathy
- Recurrent epistaxis
- Dysphagia
- Globus hystericus
- Foreign body sensation in pharynx
- Evaluation of snoring
- Vocal cord paralysis
- Further reassurance against serious disease in any chronic upper respiratory condition, especially in smokers
- Chronic acid (reflux) laryngitis

NOTE: More than 60% of patients with reflux laryngitis do not have the classic gastroesophageal symptoms of heartburn and reflux. Instead, they may present with chronic intermittent hoarseness, vocal fatigue, chronic cough, dysphagia, sore throat, stridor, croup, postnasal drip, frequent throat clearing, globus sensation, or a choking sensation. They may also have associated asthma, pulmonary fibrosis, chronic bronchitis, or pneumonia.

Acute Conditions

- Hemoptysis
- Acute sinusitis
- Acute epistaxis (without profuse hemorrhage)
- Suspected nasal foreign body
- Suspected laryngeal foreign body
- Acute onset of hoarseness after straining voice

CONTRAINDICATIONS

- Acute epiglottitis (may precipitate complete airway obstruction)
- Acute epistaxis (bleeding source may be difficult to visualize with profuse hemorrhage)

- Uncooperative patient
- Facial fractures, especially midface, or basilar skull fractures with possible cribriform plate injuries (relative contraindication, orolaryngoscopy may be a better option, but see text regarding a bite block)
- Recent nasal or oropharyngeal surgery (may be relative contraindication, depending on nature and location of the surgery)

EQUIPMENT

- Flexible nasolaryngoscope with light source. Like recently manufactured gastroscopes and colonoscopes, newer nasolaryngoscopes are available with distal-chip digital optical systems (i.e., camera at the tip) where the cameras have basically replaced the fiberoptic technology. However, fiberoptic nasolaryngoscopes are still manufactured and tend to be less expensive. Recently manufactured scopes (both fiberoptic and distal-chip) are also completely immersible, which simplifies cleaning and disinfection. Frequently, light sources used for other endoscopes in the office may be adaptable to a nasolaryngoscope. This might be an important consideration when purchasing a flexible sigmoidoscope, gastroscope, or colonoscope.

  NOTE: Although distal-chip technology improves visualization enough in colonoscopy to sometimes overcome an inadequate preparation, thereby allowing the clinician to complete a procedure that might be impossible with a fiberoptic scope (the lens in fiberoptic scopes is more easily occluded by stool when the prep is poor), there is no preparation necessary with nasolaryngoscopy. Therefore, there is less need to increase the cost by upgrading to distal-chip from fiberoptic technology for nasolaryngoscopy.
- Nasal speculum
- Sterilizing solution, such as glutaraldehyde (Cidex)
- Decongestant*: phenylephrine (0.25% to 2%) spray (Neo-Synephrine, Vicks) or epinephrine 1:50,000 (Adrenalin) or oxymetazoline hydrochloride 0.05% spray (Afrin, Neo-Synephrine 12 hour)
- Anesthetic: lidocaine (2% to 5%) solution in an atomizer spray bottle or benzocaine spray (14%) (Cetacaine)†
- Goggles, mask, and gloves (equipment necessary to follow universal blood and body fluid precautions)
- Optional supplies include cotton balls or pledgets soaked in either a decongestant or anesthetic. Three ear, nose, and throat spuds with soaked cotton applicators are another option. Cocaine solution (4% to 10%) can be used for both decongestion and anesthesia. At this strength, it does not produce a euphoric effect; however, many clinicians choose not to stock cocaine because of the mandatory record keeping and the risk of burglary. If cocaine is considered for the anesthetic, patients should be informed of the risk of finding its metabolites in their urine in case they have on-the-job drug screening.

PREPROCEDURE PATIENT EDUCATION

After explaining the procedure, inform the patient that he or she may experience an intense tickling sensation on insertion of the scope. Warning the patient beforehand can minimize his or her response. Use of a topical decongestant or an anesthetic may decrease this sensation. Although nasolaryngoscopy can be performed without these, visualization and patient tolerance are usually improved with their use. This may be especially helpful with inexperienced operators or anxious patients. The patient should be informed if a decongestant or anesthetic will be used. Next, the objectives of the procedure should be described carefully. Explain to the patient that he or she may speak during the procedure, and that you should be told if the patient is having any significant discomfort other than pressure. The patient will be asked to say certain words or sounds and may be asked to swallow or to avoid swallowing at different stages. The patient should keep his or her eyes open and focused straight ahead to minimize the gag reflex. Breath holding can also trigger the gag reflex, so the patient should be encouraged to breathe through the mouth.

TECHNIQUE

1. Before performing the procedure, a thorough head and neck history and examination, as well as the remainder of a complete history and physical examination, should be performed. The procedure is brief enough to be performed on the initial visit. If nasolaryngoscopy is not performed on the initial visit, when the patient returns obtain the interval history and again examine the head and neck. Explain the procedure again.
2. Before applying decongestant or anesthetic, the patient should be asked to gently blow his or her nose to clear the nasal passage. Give the patient some tissues to hold in one hand and a plastic emesis basin in the other. The patient should have an absorbent sheet draped over the shoulders that is then tucked inside the collar. The clinician should follow universal blood and body fluid precautions.
3. With the patient sitting up, apply decongestant generously by spraying the atomized solution into both nostrils. If the same spray nozzle is to be used with another patient, it should not touch him or her. One spray should be directed superiorly and a second posteriorly. After spraying, have the patient tilt his or her head back to allow the liquid to drain as far back as possible. The patient should then swallow any residual. Unless both nares need to be intubated, determine by visual inspection which nostril is the least obstructed. After decongestion, this is the nostril that should be anesthetized for scope insertion.
4. After waiting 5 to 10 minutes for the decongestant to take effect, anesthetize the nostril(s) chosen for scope insertion. Spray liberal amounts of lidocaine or benzocaine aerosol spray; direct the spray superiorly for 1 second and then posteriorly for about 1 second with the patient tilting his or her head back and again swallowing any residual. The patient should be warned that lidocaine has a sour taste. Swallowing the anesthetic assists with suppression of the gag reflex. For patients with a hyperactive gag reflex, gargles with lidocaine solution or a generous spraying of the pharynx with benzocaine may be helpful. The patient is ready for the procedure when he or she reports a lack of sensation at the back of the throat.

   As an alternative to spraying, soaked cotton balls or pledgets can be inserted with offset or bayonet forceps through the nasal speculum. One cotton ball (or pledget) should be inserted superiorly, another inserted in the middle meatus, and a third posteriorly. They should remain in place for 5 to 10 minutes and then removed before insertion of the scope. Three ENT spuds with cotton applicators can be used in the same manner. If cotton balls, pledgets, or spuds are used, the back of the pharynx should also be sprayed with anesthetic to suppress the gag reflex.
5. Before insertion of the scope and while waiting for the anesthesia to take effect, the clinician may want to become reacquainted with the scope (for those who do not regularly perform endoscopic procedures). Deflect the tip both ways to observe which direction and how far it moves for a given movement of the deflector. The focal length on most scopes is about 5 mm or greater, and viewing an object through the scope (e.g., a penny, a piece of gauze) before insertion may give the clinician a better sense of distance and magnification. In general, as it is advanced, the tip of the scope moves toward whatever structure is directly

*Should be used with caution in those who are severely hypertensive or have a history of sensitivity to the agent.

†Should be used with caution in those who have a history of an allergy or sensitivity to the agent.

in the center of the field of view. Note that for these very small scopes, a slight deflection of the tip can cause a marked change in direction of the scope. It should also be noted that the most difficult aspect of nasolaryngoscopy may not be manipulating the scope, but rather maintaining familiarity with the complex anatomy of the nose and throat. Clinicians who do not frequently perform the procedure may benefit from a brief review of the anatomy before each procedure. Atlases and CD-ROMs/DVDs are available for such reviews (see the "Bibliography" section).

6. Place the patient in either an erect (sitting) or supine position. Both examiner and patient should be in a position that they can maintain comfortably for 20 minutes. The patient is reasonably protected from injury caused by his or her own sudden movements or by jumping away from the scope if in the supine position. Patients who are sitting can be protected by placing their head all the way back against a high, firm headrest. A small child may want to sit in a parent's lap; the parent should then hold the child firmly, especially the head, to help protect from any injury that might be caused by sudden involuntary movements.
7. Rest the hand you will be using to guide the endoscope on the patient's cheek. Your middle, ring, and little fingers should form a tripod to support the index finger and thumb while handling and guiding the tip of the scope. As you gain more experience, you may wish to rest this tripod on the patient's forehead to sense for tensing of the frontalis muscle, which is often the first sign that the patient is experiencing significant discomfort. Turn on the light source. Tell the patient to close his or her eyes and to expect a bright light and possibly a tickling sensation. Insert the tip through the least-obstructed nostril and past the nasal hairs at the vestibule. If the scope is prone to becoming fogged, rest it against the nasal septum to warm it. Warming the scope usually defogs it.
8. The floor of the nasal cavity, which is in the inferior meatus, usually offers the most open channel and the best passage for intubations (Fig. 77-1). (The meatus is the space below each turbinate.) Advance the scope only toward visualized objects; avoid advancing the scope blindly or against significant resistance. As with other endoscopic procedures, if only white is visible (a "whiteout"), the scope is probably resting against mucosa and should be withdrawn until the actual structure that the mucosa is covering is visualized. A deviated septum or large maxillary ridge may impede advancement of the endoscope along the floor. In this situation, make an attempt to pass the scope through the middle meatus, keeping in mind that the patient usually experiences discomfort whenever the scope is directed or advanced superiorly. If this is unsuccessful, withdraw the scope and intubate the other nostril.

NOTE: If unable to intubate either nostril, after spraying the back of the pharynx with benzocaine to suppress the gag reflex, the scope can be passed through the oropharynx. In this situation, the patient might damage the scope by biting it. To minimize this risk, the barrel of a 10-mL syringe (minus the plunger) can be cut in half (cut crosswise or across the diameter), and the remaining barrel placed between the patient's upper and lower front incisors. If the scope is then inserted through the barrel, it should serve as a bite-block.

9. As the scope is advanced along the floor, the feet of the medial crura (of the lower lateral septal cartilages) can frequently be seen protruding from the medial aspect of the nasal passage. The inferior turbinate is visualized about 1 cm into the passage. Note the texture and size of the inferior turbinate, as well as any polypoid degeneration or any swelling of the covering mucosal membranes. Flexion of the scope slightly upward often illuminates the middle turbinate in the distance and its meatus. The nasolacrimal duct drains into the inferior meatus and is usually not seen; however, purulent fluid draining from it is evidence of a nasolacrimal gland infection. If the patient has had surgical antral windows placed into the maxillary sinus, the openings are frequently located in the inferior meatus. These openings can often be entered with a scope (Fig. 77-2). Note the condition of the mucosa if the antral windows are entered.
10. Next, pass the scope posteriorly about 4 to 5 cm until the choana comes into view. The choana is the junction between the nasal fossa and the nasopharynx, and it looks just like a posterior "nostril." It should form a halo in front of adenoid tissue. If desired, move the scope laterally and superiorly to allow entry into the middle meatus. However, because superior reflection of the scope may result in discomfort to the patient, it may be prudent to examine the middle meatus on the way out after visualizing the larynx. Again, if the nasal floor is obstructed, there may be no choice but to attempt passage of the scope through the middle meatus.
11. On entering the choana, the adenoid pad appears on the posterior wall of the pharynx. Star-shaped scarring may be all that is seen if the patient has had an adenoidectomy. Advance the endoscope into the nasopharynx, and when the posterior margin of the septum is passed (when it is no longer seen), slightly flex the tip of the endoscope and rotate 90 degrees laterally to observe the torus tubarius. The torus is the valve at the opening of the eustachian tube (Fig. 77-3). Ask the patient to say "key, key, key" while you observe valve function. The eustachian tube should open and close slightly. Adenoid or lymphoid hyperplasia may be noted in this area or elsewhere throughout the procedure. It may actually block the torus tubarius. By advancing the scope slightly and rotating 180 degrees

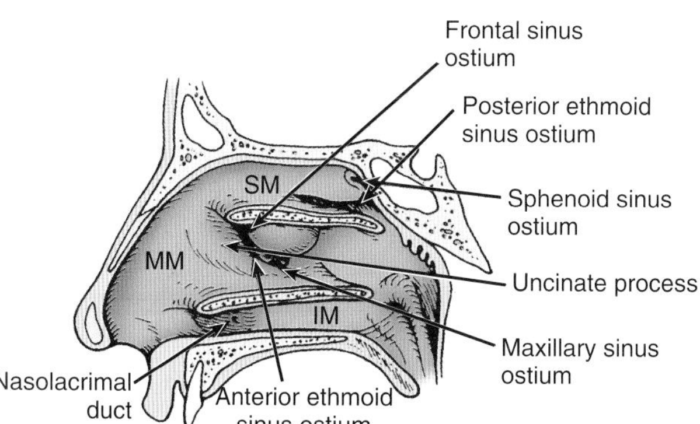

Figure 77-1 Sagittal section of the head with the turbinates removed to demonstrate ostia of the paranasal sinuses and the nasolacrimal duct. IM, inferior meatus; MM, middle meatus; SM, superior meatus.

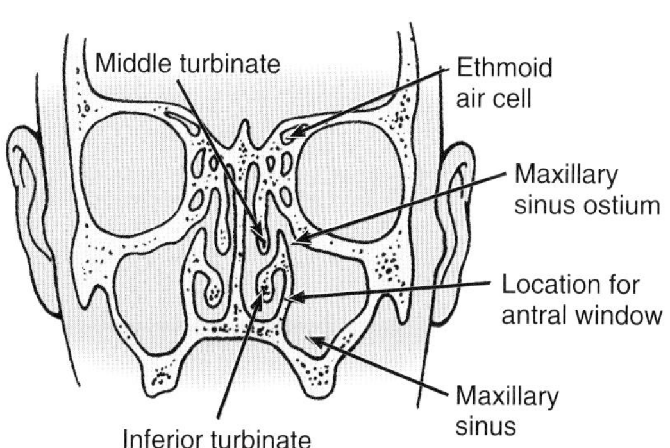

Figure 77-2 Frontal section of the head. In this section, eight ethmoid air cells (four on each side) are shown in their locations medial to the orbit. A rather large maxillary sinus ostium is demonstrated, as well as the location in the inferior meatus for surgical placement of antral windows.

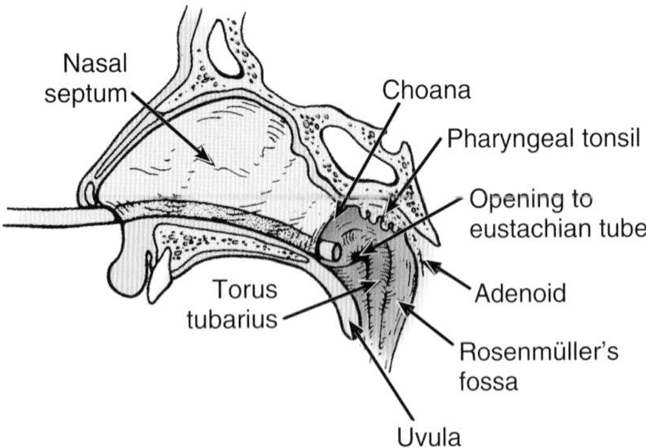

Figure 77-3 Anatomy of nasopharynx and oropharynx.

while avoiding the septum (make sure to avoid contacting the septum!), the opposite torus is illuminated. Its function should also be observed. Purulent fluid may be seen draining from a eustachian tube and should be noted. Posterior to both tori and anterior to the adenoid pad lie the clefts of Rosenmüller, each of which should be carefully inspected. Most nasopharyngeal malignancies are found in this area.

12. Next, advance the scope inferiorly and toward the posterior wall of the oropharynx (Fig. 77-4).

NOTE: If possible, avoid touching the posterior pharynx or the base of the tongue, which may elicit the gag reflex.

Instruct the patient to breathe through his or her nose to keep the soft palate from obstructing the view. As the patient swallows or talks, the normal movement of the soft palate can be seen. Downward flexion and slight rotation of the scope as it nears the posterior wall will allow for inspection of the uvula, the soft palate, and the lateral and posterior walls of the pharynx. The epiglottis should be seen in the distance. Note the presence of any masses, scarring, inflammation, exudate, mucosal irregularities, or pulsations. In some cases, dysphagia may be explained by lymphoid hyperplasia in this area, especially if the hyperplasia is associated with enlarged palatine tonsils and an exudate.

13. When the scope has passed the soft palate, it enters the oropharynx. Again, for the remainder of the procedure, attempt to avoid touching the posterior pharynx while keeping the scope as close as possible to it. If the scope becomes fogged, tell the patient to swallow; this often clears the scope. With slight flexion and rotation, examine the posterior tongue, lingual tonsils, palatine tonsils, epiglottis, and medial and lateral glossoepiglottic folds. Avoid touching the base of the tongue, which can trigger the gag reflex. Examine the valleculae from above (Figs. 77-5 and 77-6). Ask the patient to stick out his or her tongue to improve visualization of the valleculae.

14. When the scope has passed the epiglottis, it enters the hypopharynx (see Fig. 77-4). Ask the patient to refrain from swallowing; at this level, swallowing can induce an unusual foreign body sensation or provoke coughing. Assure the patient that if it is unavoidable, it is all right to swallow; however, he or she may experience the sensation of swallowing the scope. If this sensation becomes too strong, the scope may be withdrawn until the sensation passes. The arytenoid cartilages, the corniculate and cuneiform cartilages, and the aryepiglottic folds can be visualized at this level. The piriform sinuses posterior to the cords should be at least partially inspected. Closely examine the

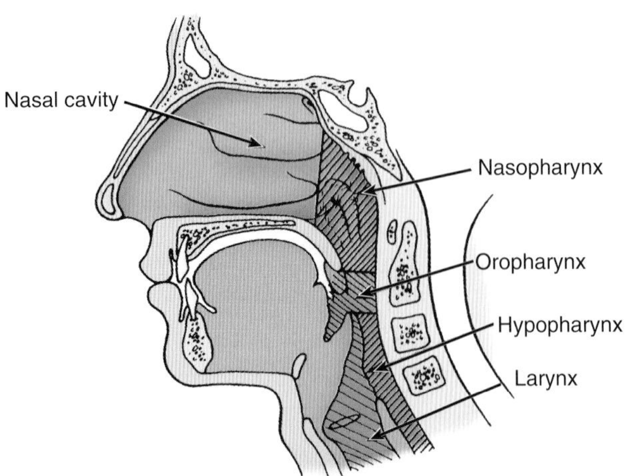

Figure 77-4 Anatomic divisions of the upper airway. All five divisions may be inspected with a fiberoptic nasolaryngoscope.

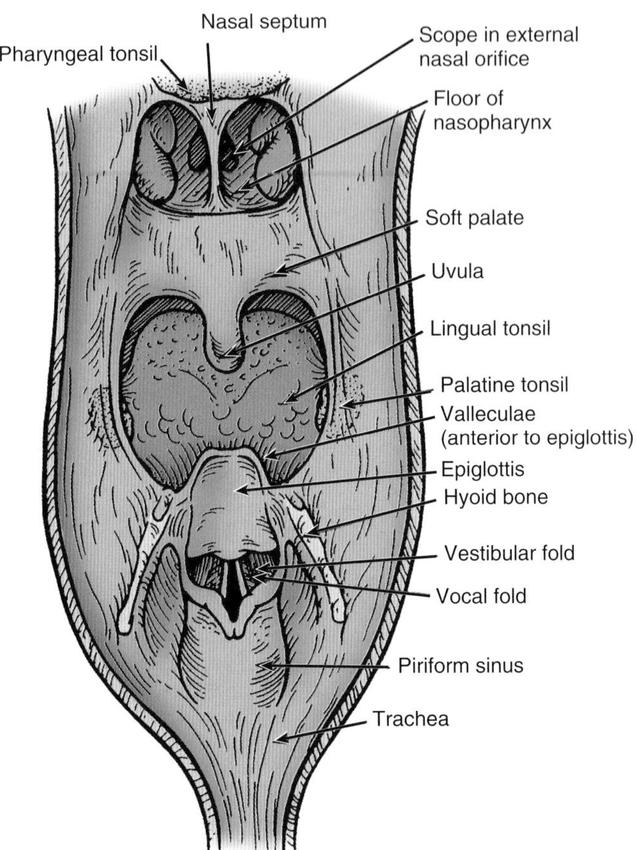

Figure 77-5 Oropharyngeal and laryngeal areas, viewed from posterior.

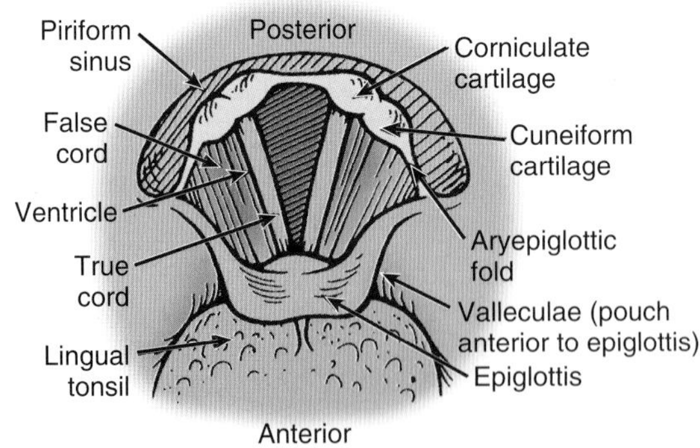

Figure 77-6 Larynx viewed from above and oriented as it would be seen with a fiberoptic nasolaryngoscope.

false and true vocal cords and the ventricles during quiet respiration (see Fig. 77-6). Tell the patient to hold a prolonged high "eee" sound while you watch for symmetry of cord mobility as well as edema, hemorrhages, erythema, nodules, or masses of the cords or surrounding structures. Record any mucosal or structural abnormalities.

Vocal cord nodules, cysts, and polyps usually occur at the junction of the anterior and middle third of the cord. Nodules are generally caused by vocal abuse and are usually bilateral, small, white, sessile, and firm. Vocal cord cysts are usually unilateral and filled with caseous material, and can be due to vocal abuse (i.e., epidermoid). Mucous retention cysts are also usually unilateral due to an obstructed duct and filled with mucoid material. Polyps are also caused by vocal abuse, are usually unilateral, and can be sessile or pedunculated with a prominent feeding vessel on the superior aspect of the vocal cord. There may be evidence of preceding hemorrhage. Reinke's edema, also known as *polypoid degeneration of the vocal cords*, appears as sausage-shaped edematous vocal cords. It is usually due to tobacco abuse, but can also be at least partly due to vocal abuse and gastroesophageal reflux disease. Other findings associated with reflux laryngitis can be diffuse or limited to the vocal cords. The ventricles can be obliterated, the arytenoids thickened, and there may be erythema, edema, or "cobblestoning" of the posterior aspect of the larynx or trachea.

NOTE: The scope should *never* touch or pass below the cords. When nearing the cords, if the patient accidentally swallows, the operator should be prepared to quickly withdraw the scope enough to avoid touching them. If the cords are touched, severe laryngospasm can occur with resultant patient asphyxia.

15. Next, withdraw the scope to a position just anterior to the choana and direct it very superiorly, almost inverted on itself (Fig. 77-7). With the tip in this position, carefully withdraw the scope slightly again, and the sphenoid bone should appear. (The sphenoid bone will appear in what was previously an inferior position in scope orientation, before inversion.) The superior turbinate may be seen, as might an anatomic variant, the supreme turbinate. The ostia of the sphenoid sinus—medial to the superior turbinate—should be visible. The sphenoid sinus, which can be thought of as a large posterior ethmoid air cell (Fig. 77-8), is usually the only sinus in the posterior ethmoid group with a visible ostium (see Fig. 77-1). Again, care is necessary when directing the scope superiorly. This is an area where anesthesia is frequently incomplete, and this maneuver may cause the patient some discomfort.

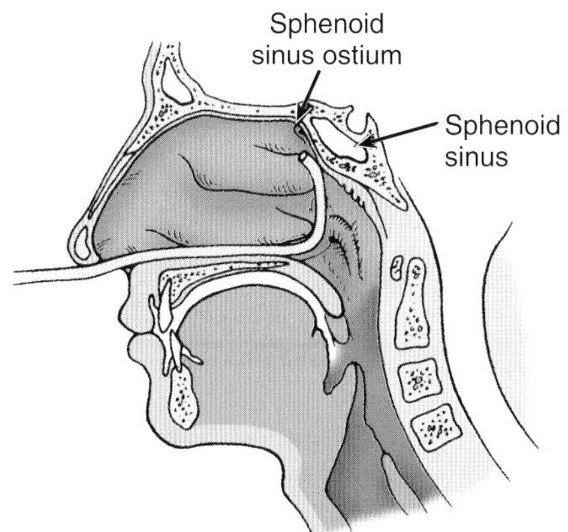

Figure 77-7 Nasolaryngoscope is withdrawn to a position just anterior to the choana and retroflexed.

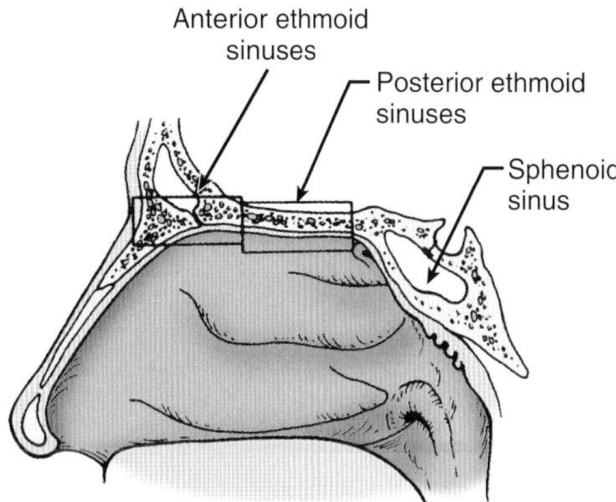

Figure 77-8 Parasagittal section of the head showing the relationship of the anterior and posterior ethmoid sinuses. The bone in this area is eggshell thin.

16. Straighten the scope and withdraw to the level where the complete choana comes into view. Move the scope in a superior and lateral direction to allow examination of the middle meatus. In most cases it is easier to examine the middle meatus from posterior to anterior. The frontal sinus, anterior ethmoid cells, and maxillary sinus ostia are located in the middle meatus, with the maxillary sinus ostia the most likely to be visualized. Observe for any drainage from ostia.

    NOTE: Drainage of pus from an ostium is diagnostic of acute sinusitis, with accuracy possibly greater than radiographs.

    Inflammation should be recorded, and attempts should be made to identify the source of any purulent fluid or polyps protruding from or occluding the ostia. The majority of polyps are seen in the middle meatus, originating from the anterior ethmoid cells. Typical polyps are slightly yellow, translucent, and relatively avascular. They can originate from nasal mucosa (most common) or they can result from polypoid degeneration of a turbinate. Polyps can be filled with mucus or fluid. Frequently they have a stalk, or extension of mucosa, that can be traced back to their sinus of origin. Through air drying and subsequent keratinization, polyps can develop benign squamous metaplastic changes, becoming more opacified and whiter or grayer in appearance.
17. On completion of the examination, withdraw the scope and explore the opposite nasal cavity, if indicated.

    NOTE: As with any endoscopic procedure, the natural tendency during nasolaryngoscopy is for the examiner to move toward whatever is being visualized. This action may form a tight loop in the scope outside the patient's nose. Such a tight loop may actually break the scope or the fibers in the scope (if a fiberoptic scope). To prevent this tendency, remember to relax and maintain the same distance from the patient throughout the procedure. If you straighten the scope at the end of the procedure before removing it from the patient's nose, the patient is usually grateful.

CARE AND CLEANING OF EQUIPMENT

Although nasolaryngoscopes are fairly indestructible, they are composed of fibers/lenses or cameras that can be broken; hence, avoid bending the scope into tight angles (especially a fiberoptic scope) or traumatizing the tip. Wash the scope with soap and water between procedures, and then soak it for 10 minutes in glutaraldehyde. Make sure the glutaraldehyde is thoroughly rinsed from the scope, before air drying, to prevent chemically irritating the next patient's mucosa. Clean the lens with lens cleaner and paper.

Complications

- An adverse reaction to anesthetic or decongestant (most common)
- Sneezing and gagging severe enough to prevent completion of the procedure
- Laryngospasm with possible asphyxia; prevented by remaining above the level of the vocal cords
- Blood pressure elevation (very rare and usually related to an adverse drug reaction)
- Vasovagal reaction (rare)
- Epistaxis (it is possible to dislodge eschar or to traumatize a tumor)
- Vomiting with possible aspiration

CPT/Billing Codes

92511 Nasopharyngoscopy with endoscope
99070 Supplies and materials (except spectacles) provided by the clinician over and above those usually included with the office visit or other services rendered (list drugs, trays, supplies or materials provided)

ICD-9-CM Diagnostic Codes

V10.21 Laryngeal cancer, history
161.9 Laryngeal cancer, NEC
300.11 Globus hystericus
306.1 Psychogenic dysphonia or cough
382.3 Otitis media, chronic suppurative, unspecified
382.4 Otitis media, suppurative, unspecified
382.9 Otitis media, unspecified, chronic or acute
388.70 Earache, unspecified
471.0 Nasal polyp
471.8 Sinus polyp
472.0 Rhinitis, chronic
472.1 Pharyngitis, chronic
473.0 Sinusitis, chronic, maxillary
473.1 Sinusitis, chronic, frontal
473.2 Sinusitis, chronic, ethmoidal
478.4 Laryngeal or vocal cord polyp
478.30 Vocal cord paralysis, unspecified
491.0 Cough, smoker's
784.2 Neck mass
784.7 Epistaxis
784.41 Aphonia (loss of voice)
784.49 Hoarseness
784.99 Halitosis or choking sensation
786.05 Dyspnea, chronic
786.09 Snoring
786.1 Stridor
786.2 Cough, chronic
786.3 Hemoptysis
787.2 Dysphagia
933.0 Foreign body in hypopharynx, nasopharynx, or pharynx
933.1 Foreign body, larynx

Suppliers

(See contact information online at www.expertconsult.com.)

Flexible nasolaryngoscopes with light source
Fujinon Medical
Olympus America Inc.
Pentax Precision Instruments Corporation
Vision-Sciences, Inc. (manufactures a scope as well as disposable sheath covers for various brands of scopes)
Welch Allyn Corporation

Bibliography

American Academy of Family Physicians: Nasolaryngoscopy for the family physician (CD-ROM or DVD). Leawood, Kan, American Academy of Family Physicians, 1998.

Corey GA, Hocutt JE, Rodney WM: Preliminary study of rhinolaryngoscopy by family physicians. Fam Med 20:262–265, 1988.

Deutsch ES, Yang JY, Reilly JS: Introduction to peroral endoscopy and laryngoscopy. In Snow JB, Ballenger JJ (eds): Ballenger's Otorhinolaryngology Head and Neck Surgery, 16th ed. Hamilton, Ontario, BC Decker, 2003, pp 1513–1514.

Hayes JT, Houston R: Flexible nasolaryngoscopy: A low-risk, high-yield procedure. Postgrad Med 106:107–110, 114, 1999.

Hocutt JE, Corey GA, Rodney WM: Nasolaryngoscopy for family physicians. Am Fam Physician 42:1257–1268, 1990.

Holsinger FC, Kies MS, Weinstock YE, et al: Videos in clinical medicine. Examination of the larynx and pharynx. N Engl J Med 358(3):e2, 2008. Available at http://content.nejm.org/cgi/content/short/358/3/e2.

Olympus Corporation: Fiberoptic examination of the pharynx and larynx (videotape). Melville, NY, Olympus Corporation, 1994.

Olympus Corporation: Nasolaryngoscopy: The inside view (videotape). Greenville, NC, East Carolina University School of Medicine, Center for Medical Communications, 1988.

Patton D, DeWitt DE: Flexible nasolaryngoscopy: A procedure for primary care. Prim Care Cancer 12:13–21, 1992.

Pentax Corporation: Current concepts in examination of the nasopharynx and larynx (videotape). New York, Pentax Corporation, 1995.

Postma GN, Belafsky PC, Amin MR, et al: Endoscopic evaluation of the upper aerodigestive tract. In Bailey BJ, Johnson JT, Newlands SD (eds): Head and Neck Surgery–Otolaryngology, 4th ed. Philadelphia, Lippincott William & Wilkins, 2006, pp 745–754.

Riviello RJ: Otolaryngologic procedures. In Roberts JR, Hedges JR (eds): Clinical Procedures in Emergency Medicine, 4th ed. Philadelphia, Saunders, 2004, pp 1280–1316.

Usatine RP: The Color Atlas of Family Medicine. New York, McGraw-Hill, 2009.

CHAPTER 78

MANAGEMENT OF EPISTAXIS

Scott Savage

Nosebleed is a common complaint with an incidence of approximately 1 per 1000 patients annually in the United States. Ninety percent of nosebleeds resolve, either spontaneously, with the aid of pinching the outer soft tissue of the nose (Fig. 78-1), or by applying an ice pack to the bridge (Fig. 78-2). Managing the other 10% is the topic of this chapter.

The most common cause of minor nosebleed is dry nasal mucosa (i.e., low-humidity environment such as in the desert or in a cold climate where heating is used). Moderate nosebleed is usually caused by nasal trauma; severe nosebleed is often a complication of a medical condition such as a coagulopathy caused by medications, cancer, or cirrhosis. Although hypertension is often seen in patients with nosebleeds, studies have been unable to confirm this condition as a cause. Rather, it appears that nosebleeds are associated with anxiety, and anxiety leads to hypertension. Localized causes of nosebleeds also include inflammation from colds and allergies, foreign bodies, nasal septum deformities, and sinonasal neoplasms. Systemic causes include coagulopathies, Osler-Weber-Rendu disease (hereditary hemorrhagic telangiectasia), and use of nonsteroidal anti-inflammatory drugs or anticoagulants. Osler-Weber-Rendu disease is an autosomal dominant condition in which the vascular walls lack contractile elements; consequently, prolonged and heavy bleeding can occur despite a normal coagulation profile. The diagnosis can be suspected when there is a family history compatible with the disease.

Nosebleeds can be divided into three groups: anterior, posterior, and mixed. Anterior bleeds account for approximately 90% of epistaxis. Posterior and mixed bleeds can be clinically suspected in patients who have brisk, bilateral, nontraumatic bleeding that does not abate with anterior packing. Posterior bleeding can be life-threatening and is more common in patients older than 40 years of age. Usually the patient can tell you which side of the nose started bleeding. With posterior bleeding, blood also usually runs down the back of the throat.

Understanding the anatomy of the nasal cavity is useful for obtaining efficient and effective control of bleeding. The blood supply for the nasal septum arises from both the internal and external carotid arteries. A primary source for the posteroinferior septum is the sphenopalatine artery, a branch of the internal maxillary artery, which in turn is a branch of the external carotid system. The uppermost part of the nasal septum is supplied by the anterior and posterior ethmoid arteries, which arise indirectly from the internal carotid system. The blood supply for the anterior nasal septum is the superior labial artery, which is also indirectly a branch of the internal carotid system. All of these arteries anastomose in the anterior central portion of the nasal septum, an area known as *Kiesselbach's plexus* (Fig. 78-3). It is estimated that 95% of anterior nasal bleeds occur there. An occasional source of anterior bleeding is an exposed edge from a perforated nasal septum. Anterior bleeding from the lateral nasal cavity is rare, although telangiectases from Osler-Weber-Rendu disease can be seen here. Trauma can also result in lateral bleeding.

The clinician treating epistaxis must understand the normal anatomy of the nose and be familiar with the nasal septum and its appropriate midline position. He or she should be able to identify the inferior and middle turbinates. With an understanding of normal anatomy, when a patient has a nosebleed, the examiner should quickly notice if there are any anatomic abnormalities (e.g., deviated nasal septum, a nasal polyp, a mass). Bleeding is not unusual on either side of a deviated nasal septum.

INDICATIONS

- Nosebleed lasting longer than 10 minutes despite pinching outer nasal tissue or application of ice
- Recurrent nosebleeds despite treatment
- Traumatic nosebleed with suspected nasal fracture
- Nosebleed associated with a septal perforation or other nasal abnormality
- Nosebleed in patient with high-risk medical condition
- Nosebleed in frail patient

CONTRAINDICATIONS (RELATIVE)

- Patients with advanced chronic obstructive pulmonary disease (COPD) or other advanced cardiac or pulmonary conditions (nasal packing can induce the nasopulmonary reflex, causing the arterial oxygen pressure to drop by as much as 15 mm Hg).
- Untreated coagulopathy, a displaced fracture, or Osler-Weber-Rendu disease (nasal packing can disrupt friable tissue, especially posterior packing, and should be done with caution in these patients; attempts should be made to normalize clotting factors, if possible, before instrumentation).
- Other critical conditions, such as a threatened airway or other problem that should be managed first, may mandate a delay in managing a nosebleed.

EQUIPMENT

Preparing a "nosebleed tray" in advance is useful.

- Headlight
- Tongue depressor
- Yankauer suction catheter
- Frazier suction catheters, no. 5 and no. 7
- Nasal speculums, short and medium length
- Bayonet or offset forceps (see Chapter 76, Removal of Foreign Bodies from the Ear and Nose, Fig. 76-1)
- Fine Adson forceps
- Emesis (kidney) basin
- Cotton balls
- Cotton-tipped swabs (wooden handle preferred if applying Gelfoam or Surgicel)

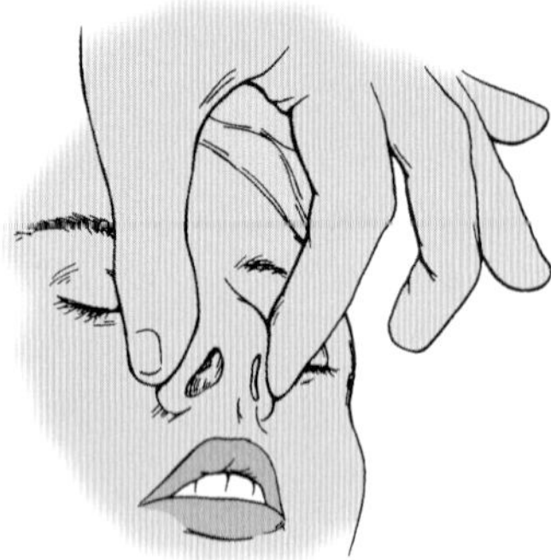

Figure 78-1 Apply pressure by pinching the nose to stop the bleeding.

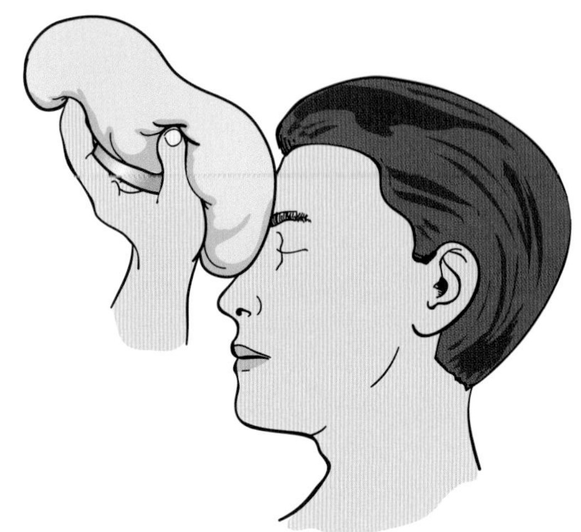

Figure 78-2 An ice pack can be applied to the bridge of the nose.

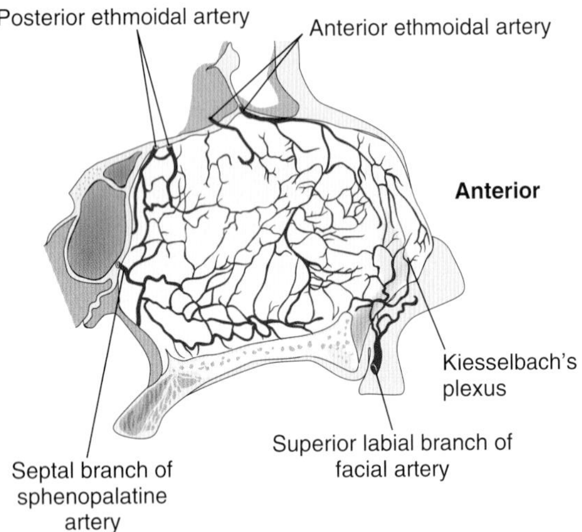

Figure 78-3 Anatomy of the septal blood supply.

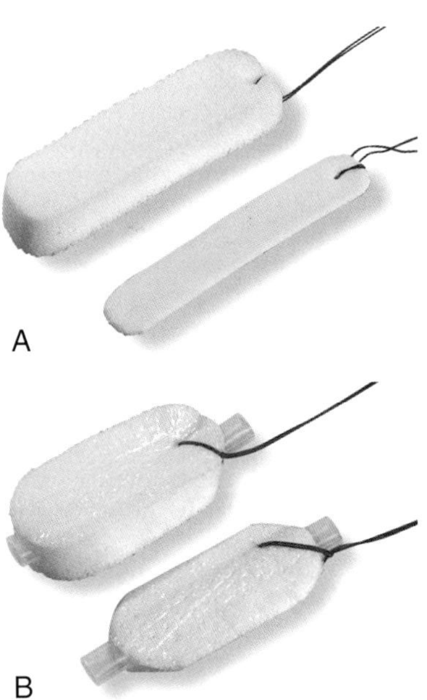

Figure 78-4 Nasal sponges. **A,** Pope pack. **B,** Nasal sponge with airway (Merocel 2000 4.5 cm). (**A** and **B,** Courtesy of Medtronic Xomed ENT, Inc., Jacksonville, Fla.)

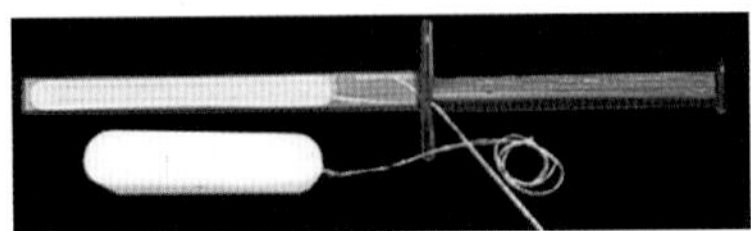

Figure 78-5 Rhino Rocket nasal sponge system. (Courtesy of Shippert Medical Technologies, Centennial, Colo.)

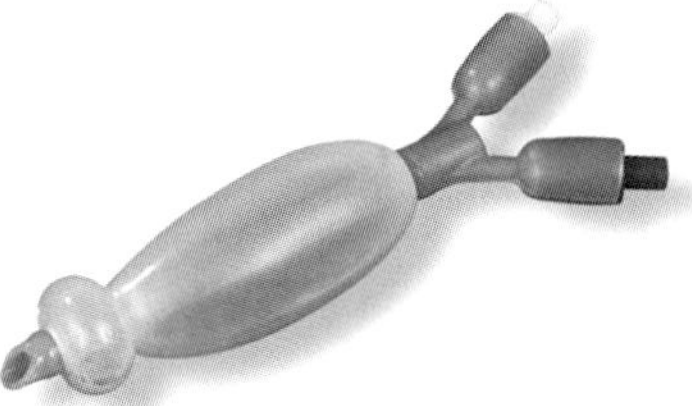

Figure 78-6 Nasal balloon device. The *Medtronic Xomed EpiStat I* (pictured) is a double (anterior and posterior) balloon catheter. The *EpiStat II* is a posterior balloon catheter with anterior soft packing attached. It also contains an airway and can be used for bleeding from an indeterminate site, whether posterior, anterior, or both. If posterior bleeding stops, the balloon catheter and airway can be removed, leaving the anterior packing in place. (Courtesy of Medtronic Xomed ENT, Inc., Jacksonville, Fla.)

- Gelfoam or Surgicel (Surgicel may be better for coagulation but may delay healing, so it is often reserved for when Gelfoam is not effective or available)
- 4 × 4 gauze sponges
- Silver nitrate sticks
- Petroleum impregnated gauze, ½-inch wide, up to 72 inches long
- Nasal sponges/tampons (Fig. 78-4) or Rhino Rocket (Fig. 78-5)
- Nasal balloon devices (Fig. 78-6)
- 12- to 14-Fr Foley catheter with 30-mL balloon, umbilical clamp and padding
- Red rubber (in and out or Robinson) soft catheter(s)
- Bite block
- 3-inch dental gauze roll
- Umbilical tape or heavy silk (nonabsorbable) sutures, two pieces at least 18 inches long each
- Petroleum jelly (Vaseline) or other lubricant
- Phenylephrine 2% or oxymetazoline 0.05%
- Epinephrine 1 : 1000
- Local anesthetic such as lidocaine 2% to 5%, benzocaine 14% spray or 20% solution, or tetracaine 2%
- Gowns, gloves, and face shield as necessary for clinician to follow universal blood and body fluid precautions
- Chux or towels

Preprocedure Patient Education

The patient or guardian should know about the risks (as listed in the Complications section), benefits, and any options for the procedure as well as the procedure itself. Obtain written informed consent if the patient's condition allows (see consent form online at www.expertconsult.com). Warn the patient that the procedure may be painful, especially initially, but that everything possible will be done to minimize the discomfort. If the patient is stable, a mild narcotic or sedative may be helpful, especially for posterior packing.

Technique

Patient and Clinician Preparation

1. Obtain vital signs and address any significant vital sign abnormalities. Apply pulse oximetry (vasoactive drugs will be used; packing can provoke the nasopulmonary reflex with subsequent decreases in oxygen saturation).
2. Have the patient sit back on a procedural chair or gurney with the head elevated approximately 45 degrees. Gown and drape the patient appropriately; the patient can also be given an emesis basin. While getting the patient positioned, ask which side started bleeding first and which side is currently bleeding the most. Have the patient continue to apply ice or pressure while the equipment is being assembled.
3. Connect the suction tubing and catheters to wall suction. Don the headlamp. *Good lighting is critical to the procedure.*
4. Inspect the oropharynx for trauma, or any other abnormality. Plan to inspect the nasal cavity that is not actively bleeding first. If both are bleeding, and the patient cannot state which side started bleeding first, inspect the side of the patient's dominant hand. Many nosebleeds are caused by nose-picking, and people are less clumsy with their dominant hands. This side will generally be easier to examine.
5. Have the patient blow his or her nose gently to remove any loose clots that may obstruct the examination. Insert the short nasal speculum and open it vertically. Suction any blood or clots and inspect the nasal cavity, specifically looking at the floor, vestibule, turbinates, and septum. Forceps may be helpful for manual removal of large clots.

NOTE: If you are able to get behind the source of the bleeding with the suction tip, the condition can be managed in the office.

6. Vasoconstrict and anesthetize the nasal mucosa using appropriate agents. If using separate agents for these purposes, apply the anesthetic first unless bleeding is so rapid that the anesthetic is likely to be washed out before being effective. Having the patient sniff an aerosolized solution is the easiest way. If time allows, best results are obtained if the anesthetic has been in place at least 15 minutes.
7. Alternatively, pledgets soaked with an agent can be applied. Monitor the patient's vital signs when using vasoconstrictive agents.

NOTE: The offset forceps can be used to make a pledget. First, flatten and grasp with the forceps most of the length of an appropriate amount of cotton pulled from a cotton ball. Next, grasp the opposite end of the cotton with the other hand, and while holding this end, twirl the forceps to twist the cotton in and around the long blades. Finally, relax the forceps and slip the pledget off the end. It is now ready to be soaked and inserted.

Absorbable Dressings

Although several types of absorbable dressings are now available, the two most commonly used are still Gelfoam and Surgicel. These dressings form a scaffold for the formation of a blood clot. Although Surgicel may be better for stimulating coagulation, it is more expensive and may delay healing; therefore, Gelfoam is usually preferred. Surgicel is often reserved for when Gelfoam is not effective or available. These dressings may be used as a primary technique for discrete bleeding, as a bandage over a previously cauterized site, or as a mucosal sheet over an area of diffuse bleeding (e.g., coagulopathy) before packing is applied. If these are in place before packing is removed, it may prevent the clot from being dislodged.

1. When applying these dressings it is helpful to use forceps and a cotton-tipped swab stick with a wooden handle to manipulate the dressing, to press it onto the bleeding site, and especially to hold it down when releasing the forceps so the dressing does not dislodge.
2. Before using the swab stick, remove about half of the cotton to make it small enough to be useful, and moisten the tip with saline or tap water to prevent the dressing from sticking to it.

Cauterization

Cauterization is suitable for discrete areas of bleeding in the anterior nares. The preferred method is to use silver nitrate sticks, which are especially useful in children. Do not perform cautery at the same location on both sides of the septum because it may interrupt the entire blood supply to the septum, resulting in damage or necrosis. Electrocautery should be done only by an experienced operator because damage to the septal cartilage may occur.

1. First, suction the nares and keep a small Frazier suction catheter ready to suction excessive blood. Attempt to dry the surrounding mucosa with a dry cotton swab; this will not only make the silver nitrate more effective, it will also minimize spread beyond the area.
2. Apply the silver nitrate stick with gentle pressure for 3 to 10 seconds. Do not use the stick for more than 10 seconds in any area or septal cartilage may be damaged. Do not cauterize an area greater than 1 cm in diameter, which is equivalent to about four dabs of the stick if only the bulb portion is used. As mentioned previously, do not cauterize both sides of the septum at the same location. Silver nitrate causes a burning sensation, so the patient will appreciate having the anesthetic in place for at least 15 minutes. Some authors apply the silver nitrate peripherally (approximately 0.5 cm from site) and in a circular motion around the offending area or vessel. They then gradually move toward

the center of the site until the bleeding stops. Electrocautery should be applied in the same manner. Some clinicians apply electrocautery directly down the Frazier suction tip by touching it with the cautery unit.

3. After hemostasis is obtained, use Gelfoam, Surgicel, or an equivalent specialized dressing to protect the cauterization site. If these are not available, use a small amount of petroleum jelly and gently place it on the cautery site.
4. Antibiotic therapy is considered optional in these cases. If cauterization fails, consider the use of packing or a balloon device.

Expandable Nasal Sponge and Tampon Packing

This technique is generally easy and effective in mild to moderate anterior bleeding. The sponges/tampons come in a variety of sizes and shapes, and the 4- to 6-cm sizes are usually ideal (see Fig. 78-4). They are initially rigid, but soften when saline or tap water is applied or blood is absorbed.

1. Prepare the sponge/tampon by opening the package and removing the string (the string is not necessary and is usually irritating to the patient). If necessary, trim the sponge to a size and shape that appears consistent with the patient's nasal opening, usually about 4 to 6 cm in length. An exact fit is not required, but using a wide, 10-cm-long sponge in a small patient is uncomfortable, unnecessary, and more difficult to remove. Likewise, if only a small sponge is available, and the patient has a large nasal opening, then consider using two sponges side by side. When cutting the sponge, make sure to avoid leaving any corners or other sharp edges.
2. Coat all but the distal tip of the sponge in petroleum jelly to avoid premature softening of the sponge. Use of an antibiotic ointment is more expensive, not necessary, and not beneficial to the patient; the antibacterial activity lasts only 2 to 4 hours. If using the Rhino Rocket (see Fig. 78-5), remove the sponge from the syringe-like device before inserting it. The syringe can generate enough force to damage the nasal mucosa, septum, or other structures.
3. Insert the sponge in a smooth motion, entering in a near vertical direction, and then rotating it to a horizontal direction. Continue passing the sponge along the inferior nasal floor until it is completely inside the nasal passage. When in place, the trailing tip of the sponge should be visible inside the nostril but not protruding from it.
4. Slowly drip about 2 mL of saline or tap water onto the tip to help the sponge expand more quickly.
5. Closely monitor the patient for 3 to 5 minutes for complications and to see if the technique was adequate to abate the bleeding. Keep the patient in observation status for approximately 30 minutes after completing the packing.
6. If successful, packing should be left in place for 48 hours and the patient should be placed on oral antibiotics. Persistent bleeding may be due to a bowed septum; inserting the same size sponge on the contralateral side may halt bleeding. If bleeding persists, choices include removing the sponge to insert a larger sponge or two smaller sponges or proceeding to anterior packing or insertion of a nasal balloon (see Fig. 78-6).

Anterior Packing

Packing is a time-consuming process, but is a viable alternative where there is diffuse bleeding but a nasal sponge/tampon is either unavailable or insufficient.

1. Because of the amount of discomfort caused by this technique, it is generally advisable to give the patient a narcotic or sedative medication, or both, unless a contraindication exists. If using a combination analgesic, take caution to use one that does not increase bleeding.

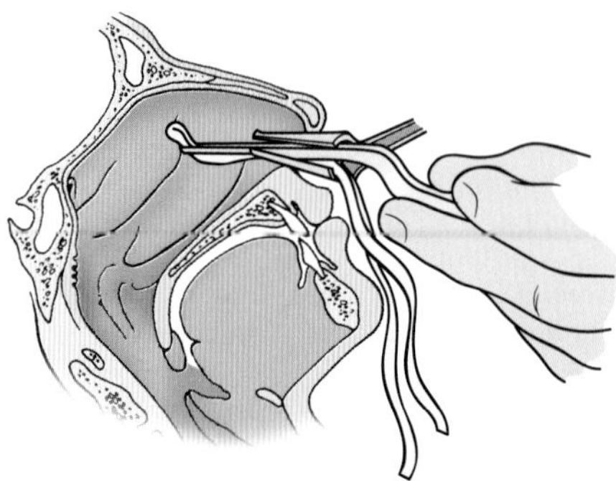

Figure 78-7 Insert anterior pack with folded end inserted first.

2. Fold a ½- by 72-inch piece of petrolatum gauze in half. Using bayonet forceps, place the center-folded end (not the free end) into the nostril (Fig. 78-7). Make sure the gauze is placed back all the way to the posterior soft tissue.
3. Pat down the gauze, and continue to layer it in an accordion fashion, patting down each layer. Gauze should be layered from nasal floor to turbinates (Fig. 78-8). Approximately 4 to 5 feet of gauze will be required.
4. Leave at least an inch of gauze protruding from the nostril. This should be taped to the patient's cheek to avoid inadvertent removal.
5. If successful, leave the packing in place for 48 hours. Also place the patient on antibiotics. If this incompletely stops the bleeding, then packing the contralateral nostril in a similar fashion may buttress the original dressing by preventing bowing of the septum. If bleeding persists, choices include removing the packing to insert an anterior nasal balloon, a posterior balloon, or posterior packing.

Balloon Tamponade

These devices are fast and easy to place. They come in several sizes, shapes, and configurations (e.g., single-balloon, dual-balloon). The most versatile device is the dual-balloon (see Fig. 78-6); it can be used for both anterior and posterior bleeding. Although nasal balloon devices are more expensive than sponges or gauze, they often save the clinician time.

1. Place the balloon in a basin of water, inflate it with air according to manufacturer specifications, and observe for air leaks. Then deflate the balloon and coat the tip of the device with petroleum jelly or other lubricant.
2. Insert the catheter with the longer portion of the bevel toward the nasal septum to prevent damage to the turbinates or mucosa.
3. Inflate the anterior balloon with air according to manufacturer specifications. Do not use saline or tap water. (If the balloon

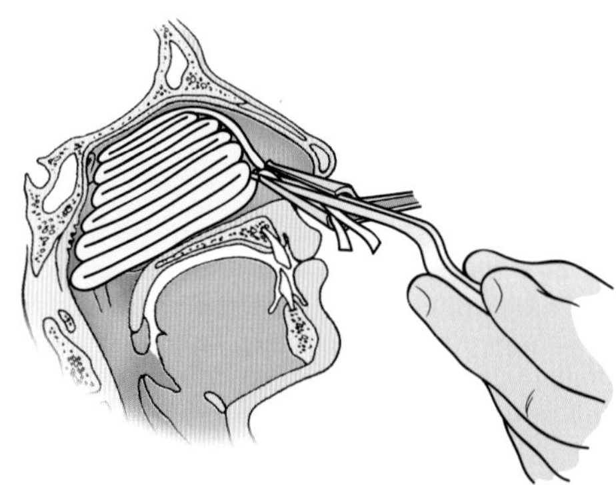

Figure 78-8 Pack folded gauze in layers, from nasal floor to turbinates.

were fluid-filled and it leaked, the patient might aspirate the contents.) If the patient complains of pain at a pressure lower than manufacturer specifications, the balloon may be larger than the nasal cavity. Deflate the balloon until the pain subsides. Do not inflate the posterior balloon at this time unless the patient has such significant bleeding that there is risk of aspiration or exsanguination.

4. Observe the patient for further bleeding. If bleeding has stopped, appropriate antibiotic therapy is indicated. These devices are uncomfortable, so analgesics and even sedative medications are generally indicated. If bleeding persists, it is likely due to an area high in the nasal cavity, where the balloon does not reach. One solution is to deflate the balloon, leave it in place, and use anterior petroleum gauze packing on top of it. The balloon can then be reinflated to seal the packing in the upper portion of the anterior nasal cavity. Persistent bleeding may also be due to a bowed septum; packing the contralateral side may halt bleeding by correcting the bowing. If these maneuvers fail to relieve the bleeding, then it is likely the patient has a posterior bleed. At this time, inflate the posterior balloon.
5. It is important to document the procedure, notify the follow-up clinician if there is additional packing, and tell the patient that this second packing is present so that it is not left behind when the balloon is removed.

Foley Catheter

If posterior bleeding is suspected, this technique may be used. It may also be used to provide a posterior buttress for anterior packing. Use a catheter with a 30-mL balloon.

1. Prepare the catheter by cutting off the portion of the catheter that is distal to the balloon. Test the balloon by inflating with air and checking for leaks. Deflate the balloon and lubricate the distal catheter with petroleum jelly or equivalent.
2. If present, remove the anterior packing.
3. Have the patient open his or her mouth widely. Pass the catheter along the floor of the nasal cavity until a small portion of the balloon is visible in the mouth. Inflate the balloon with 7 to 10 mL of air.
4. Retract the balloon until it gently lodges against the soft tissue of the choanal arch. If it withdraws into the nasal cavity, advance it back into the nasopharynx and add an additional 3 to 5 mL of air. Keep adding air in 3- to 5-mL aliquots until the balloon lodges upon withdrawal. The balloon is overinflated if the soft palate bulges or the patient complains of pain.
5. While an assistant maintains gentle traction on the catheter, place or replace anterior packing with a sponge or gauze as clinically indicated. Place an umbilical clamp on the catheter just outside the nares to secure the device (Fig. 78-9). Pad the umbilical clamp to prevent pressure necrosis.
6. Secure the proximal portion of the catheter by taping it to the side of the face. Do not tape it to the neck; if the patient were to turn his or her head, the device might be dislodged. Avoid cutting the proximal catheter—this may cause the balloon to deflate.
7. This procedure can be repeated on the opposite side if necessary. Use antibiotics and analgesics as indicated.

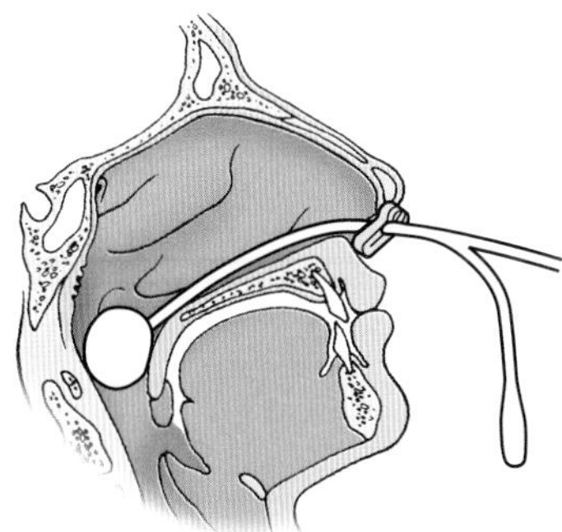

Figure 78-9 Foley catheter as posterior pack.

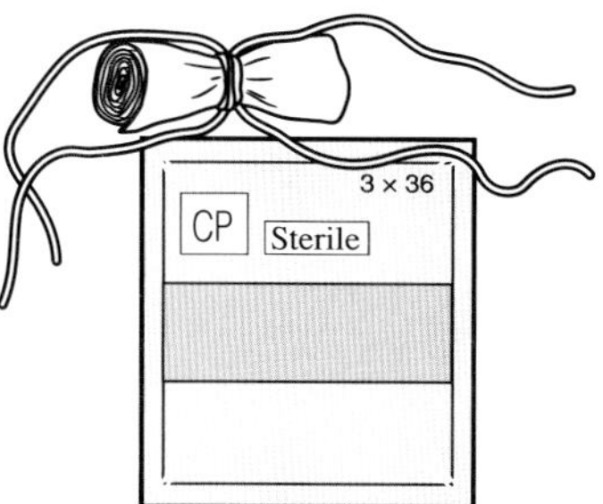

Figure 78-10 Prepare posterior pack.

Posterior Packing

Although posterior packing is described in many textbooks, in practice it is a technically difficult procedure and very time consuming. The author believes it is best left to the otolaryngologist. A simpler technique is to use either a commercially available dual-balloon tamponade device or, failing that, the Foley catheter technique previously described. Balloon tamponade devices are available with channels for the patient to breathe through, making them a more acceptable alternative. A long, expandable sponge may also be attempted, but these are of limited success. Posterior packing is included in this chapter for the sake of completeness or for when the otolaryngologist is not available.

1. A posterior pack can be made from a 3 × 36-inch piece of petrolatum gauze rolled into a tight, cylindrical, 3-inch long pack. Two 18-inch pieces of umbilical tape (or heavy nonabsorbable suture) should be tied around the middle of the pack (Fig. 78-10).
2. Before inserting the pack, spray the posterior pharynx with anesthetic (e.g., benzocaine spray).
3. Next, insert a soft red rubber catheter through the bleeding nostril. Visualize the catheter tip through the patient's open mouth as it passes behind the palate. Pull the tip from the pharynx and out the patient's mouth with forceps. Tie both ends of umbilical tape around the catheter (Fig. 78-11). Pull the catheter back through the nose and snug the roll of gauze against the posterior aspect of the choanal arch (Fig. 78-12). While using something to protect yourself from being bitten (e.g., bite block), guide the pack into this location after pushing it around the soft

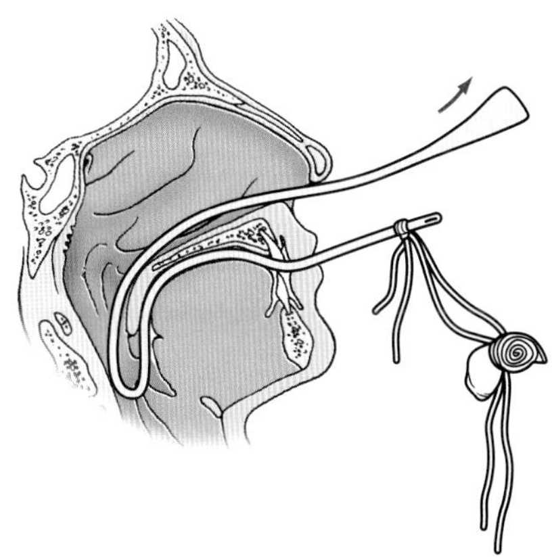

Figure 78-11 Tie or suture posterior pack to catheter.

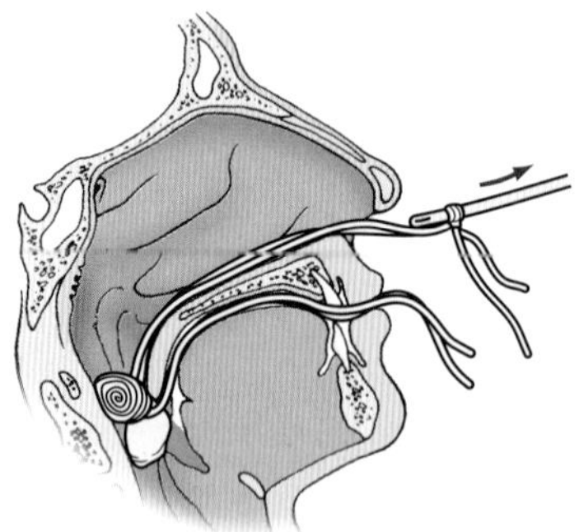

Figure 78-12 Pull pack into position.

palate with your finger. Leave the second piece of umbilical tape hanging from the mouth for pack removal in the future.

NOTE: Some clinicians use two soft red rubber catheters to perform posterior packing, inserting one through each nostril and then tying the umbilical tape from each side of the posterior pack to the respective red rubber catheter.

4. Secure the posterior pack by tying the piece of umbilical tape that is in the patient's nose around rolled 4 × 4 gauze pads. These rolls should be fitted flush, but not too firmly, against the nares (Fig. 78-13).
5. If bleeding slows but does not subside, it will be necessary to place an anterior nasal sponge/tampon or gauze packing.

NOTE: Nasal packing fails to stop epistaxis in up to 25% of cases. If bleeding does not subside with these techniques, otolaryngology consult is indicated. Sinus endoscopes can be used to locate the site of bleeding and cauterize it. Septoplasty or ligation of the anterior or posterior ethmoid, internal maxillary, sphenopalatine, or external carotid artery may be necessary. Arterial embolization is another option.

Removing Packing

Posterior packing should be removed by a specialist. Anterior packing may be removed in the medical office if the patient is medically stable and healthy, does not take anticoagulant medications, and has not had significant complications of therapy. Have an epistaxis tray in the room in case the nosebleed recurs. *Having good lighting is critical to the procedure.*

1. Soften and rehydrate the dressing with saline, taking care not to use so much as to cause the patient to aspirate. Usually, 3 to 5 mL of saline is sufficient. Give the fluid a few minutes to diffuse through the material.
2. Follow universal precautions and protect the patient, furniture, and flooring from potential blood spills. Have the patient sit up and lean forward, bracing him- or herself with arms grasping a supporting surface—the mattress of the examination table, or the arm of the chair. Instruct the patient to mouth breathe, remain still, and not blow his or her nose or snort.
3. With a basin in one hand, and bayonet forceps in the other, gently and smoothly remove the packing.
4. Inspect the nasal mucosa for residual bleeding and retained packing. If present, treat appropriately. Often there will be some mild drainage that is nasal mucus mixed with old blood. This drainage rapidly subsides and does not require further treatment.

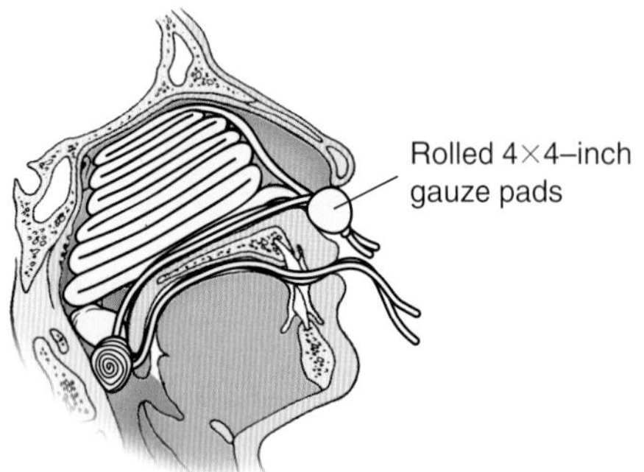

Figure 78-13 Securing posterior pack after placing anterior pack.

Complications

- Hypoxia, causing cardiac or respiratory distress
- Cardiac dysrhythmias
- Pressure necrosis of soft tissue
- Sinusitis
- Nasal septal perforation
- Otitis media
- Toxic shock syndrome
- Aspiration
- Bacteremia
- Allergic reaction to materials or anesthetics

Postprocedure Care

Acetaminophen or narcotics can be used for pain; use of aspirin and other nonsteroidal anti-inflammatories should be minimized because they may encourage bleeding. Patients should be cautioned against nose picking, straining, and bending over. Children's nails should be trimmed short to avoid trauma (parents may want them to wear mittens or socks over their hands at night to protect the nose during sleep). If patients feel that sneezing is imminent, instruct them to keep their mouth open. Patients treated with cautery alone should keep the nasal mucosa moist with petroleum jelly or A&D ointment three times daily for a week. Patients with packing require antibiotics that cover common nasal pathogens such as *Staphylococcus aureus*, *Streptococcus pneumoniae*, *Moraxella catarrhalis*, and *Haemophilus influenzae*. All patients should be instructed to notify health care providers if increasing pain, rebleeding not controlled with 15 minutes of nose pinching/ice application, or fever occurs. Patients should also receive instructions on how to keep the packing moist with a humidifier at home and frequent applications of nasal saline drops. Patients with anterior packing should have the packing removed by an experienced health care provider in 48 to 72 hours. If the patient is medically frail or had significant bleeding, hospital admission may be indicated. Patients needing posterior packing or insertion of a Foley or posterior balloon device generally require admission to an intensive care unit and specialist consultation. Nearly 40% of these patients will eventually require intubation.

Patient Education Guides

See the sample patient education and consent forms online at www.expertconsult.com.

CPT/Billing Codes

30901	Control nasal hemorrhage, anterior, simple (limited cautery and/or packing), any method
30901-50	(use modifier "-50" for bilateral)
30903	Control nasal hemorrhage, anterior, complex (limited cautery and/or packing), any method
30903-50	(bilateral)
30905	Control nasal hemorrhage, posterior, with posterior nasal packs and/or cautery, any method, initial
30906	(subsequent)

ICD-9-CM Diagnostic Codes

478.19 Other diseases of nasal cavity and sinuses (necrosis of nose [septum], ulcer of nose [septum], nasal septal perforation [nontraumatic])

784.7 Epistaxis (acute)

Acknowledgment

The editors wish to recognize the many contributions by Nancy Schantz, MD, Robert Beck, MD, and Jerry Hizon, MD, to this chapter in previous editions of this text.

Suppliers

(See contact information online at www.expertconsult.com.)

Boston Medical Products
Nasostat Gottschalk

Rhino Rocket
Shippert Medical Technologies

Xomed EpiStat I & II
Medtronic Xomed Surgical Products, Inc.

BIBLIOGRAPHY

Buttaravoli P: Minor Emergencies, 2nd ed. St. Louis, Mosby, 2007.

Kelanic SM, Caldarelli DD: Epistaxis management. In Reichman EF, Simon RR (eds): Emergency Medicine Procedures. New York, McGraw-Hill, 2004, pp 1307–1319.

Marx JA, Hockberger RS, Walls RM (eds): Rosen's Emergency Medicine: Concepts and Clinical Practice, 5th ed. New York, Mosby, 2004.

Riviello RJ: Otolaryngologic procedures. In Roberts JR, Hedges JR (eds): Clinical Procedures in Emergency Medicine, 4th ed. Philadelphia, Saunders, 2004, pp 1280–1316.

Tintinalli JE, Kelen GD, Stapczynski JS (eds): Emergency Medicine: A Comprehensive Study Guide, 6th ed. New York, McGraw-Hill, 2004.

Wurman LH, Sack JG, Flannery JV Jr, Lipsman RA: The management of epistaxis. Am J Otolaryngol 13:193–209, 1992.

CHAPTER 79

Indirect Mirror Laryngoscopy

Grant C. Fowler • Carlos A. Dumas

Although flexible nasolaryngoscopy is often available for visualization of the upper respiratory tract, indirect mirror laryngoscopy remains the simplest, fastest, least expensive, and often most helpful method of examining the upper tracheal rings, vocal cords, epiglottis, larynx, and hypopharynx. In certain cases, mirror laryngoscopy combined with an adequate history will be all that is needed to make the diagnosis. Experienced clinicians appreciate the glare-free lighting of the laryngeal structures provided by mirror laryngoscopy, which allows for observation of subtle color variations. Mirror laryngoscopy requires very little preparation, very little time to perform, and very little effort to care for only a few inexpensive instruments. The upper respiratory tract in most adults and children older than 6 or 7 years of age will be easily visualized by experienced clinicians. Examples of when mirror laryngoscopy may be useful include when nasolaryngoscopy is not available, in patients at low risk of malignancy, and during follow-up for a known lesion after complete nasolaryngoscopy has excluded other lesions. It may also be useful as a preliminary examination before nasolaryngoscopy. To keep oriented, clinicians should recall that when using a mirror, everything is seen in reverse. Before performing the procedure, it may be helpful for clinicians to refamiliarize themselves with the anatomy of the oropharynx, hypopharynx, and larynx (see Figs. 77-4 through 77-6 in Chapter 77, Nasolaryngoscopy).

NOTE: When not done on a regular basis, the necessary coordination of patient and instruments to perform mirror laryngoscopy may make it difficult, and occasionally impossible, to examine the patient's larynx—even for expert laryngologists. This fact was highlighted when a survey in the 1980s found that less than 30% of primary care clinicians practicing in Ohio were able to visualize a larynx, and that less than 4% included inspection of the larynx as part of their complete physical examination. Primary care clinicians in Ohio are probably representative of those elsewhere, and a few commented anonymously that they had never visualized a larynx!

Indications

- Chronic hoarseness (>3 weeks)
- Suspected or previous neoplasm
- Chronic cough
- Chronic dyspnea
- Halitosis
- Head or neck mass or adenopathy suggestive of malignancy
- Dysphagia
- Phonation disturbance such as vocal weakness in the elderly or psychogenic dysphonia
- Chronic foreign body sensation in pharynx
- Hemoptysis
- Suspected laryngeal foreign body
- Acute onset of hoarseness after straining voice
- Stridor, particularly inspiratory stridor
- Post-traumatic evaluation
- Any chronic unilateral upper respiratory complaint in a smoker
- Any clinical situation in which visualization of the oropharynx, hypopharynx, and larynx will aid in diagnosis or therapy

Contraindications

- Acute epiglottitis. (Patient usually has a toxic appearance, will be leaning forward, drooling secretions, and may not be able to talk.) Laryngoscopy may precipitate complete airway obstruction.
- Infants and young children who are unable to cooperate.
- Acute inflammation or infection of the throat *(relative contraindication)*.
- Patient who cannot open his or her mouth adequately *(relative contraindication)*.

Equipment

- Bright headlight or head mirror with external light source
- No. 4 and no. 5 laryngeal mirrors; smaller sizes for children
- 4 × 4 inch gauze sponges
- Local anesthetic: lidocaine* spray (2% to 4%) or benzocaine* spray (14%)
- Goggles, gloves, and mask (to follow universal blood and body fluid precautions)
- Alcohol lamp or bowl of hot water to warm mirrors *(optional)*

Preprocedure Patient Preparation and Evaluation

After obtaining and performing a thorough head and neck history and examination, as well as the remainder of a complete history and physical examination, explain the indications and alternatives for the procedure as well as what will happen during the procedure. Every effort should be made to relax the patient. The clinician should maintain a gentle, unhurried manner, and perhaps show the patient the instruments by touching the patient with the instruments in a nonthreatening area such as the hand or arm. Gently inform the patient that it will be important to try to relax and that the mirror will be placed in the top of the back of his or her mouth, avoiding the throat and the gag reflex. The patient should know that if the procedure is performed properly and an anesthetic is used, the risk of gagging should be minimized, especially if the patient keeps his or her eyes open and looks straight ahead (which diminishes the gag reflex). Possible complications should be explained, and the patient should remove any dentures.

Technique

1. The patient should sit upright and straight, preferably in a high-backed chair with a headrest. Tell the patient to lean slightly forward. The head and jaw should be jutted forward in a "sniffing" position (Fig. 79-1). The chin should be up.

*Should be used with caution in those who have a history of an allergy or sensitivity to the agents (see Chapter 4, Local Anesthesia).

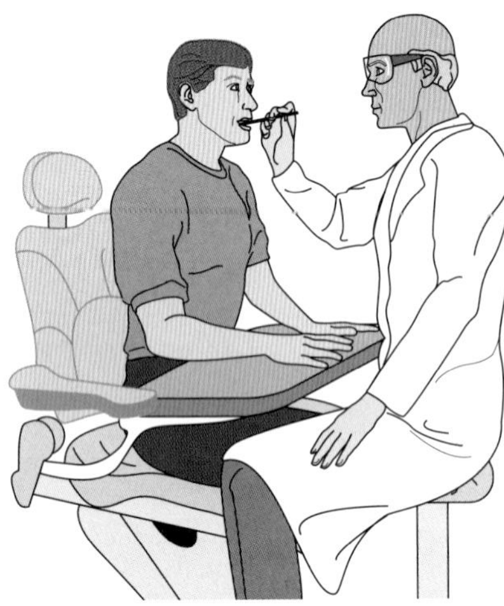

Figure 79-1 Proper positioning of the patient is essential for successful visualization of the larynx.

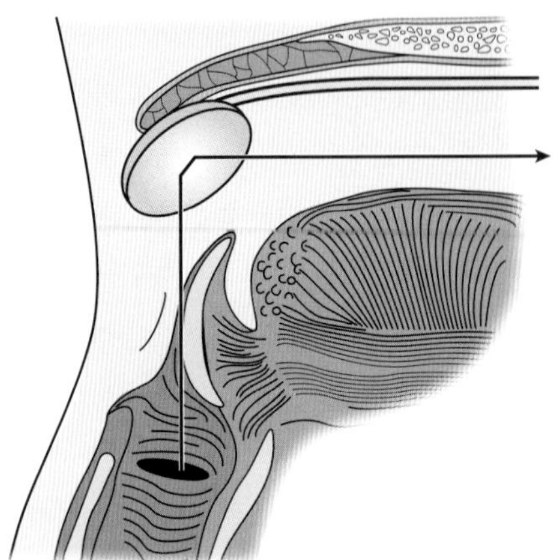

Figure 79-2 Laryngeal mirror is inserted into the pharynx, lifting the uvula but avoiding contact with the posterior pharyngeal wall.

2. Sit slightly to the side of the patient. Sitting slightly higher than the patient will also facilitate visualization of the laryngeal structures. Position the light source so that the light is directed parallel to your visual axis and focused on the patient's posterior pharynx. The examiner should be comfortable and understand that the use of a hurried approach can make this procedure more difficult. The clinician should follow universal blood and body fluid precautions.
3. Spray the patient's pharynx with the anesthetic and have him or her gargle and spit it out.
4. Select the largest mirror that will fit comfortably into the back of the throat, and warm it over the alcohol lamp, in the warm water, or inside the patient's cheek. Warming the mirror should prevent fogging. If the mirror is externally warmed, check its temperature on the back of your hand to make sure that it is not too hot before inserting. In addition, you can touch the warmed mirror to the hand or arm of the patient, not only to reassure the patient that the temperature is acceptable, but to demonstrate that the mirror is nonthreatening.
5. Have the patient protrude his or her tongue. Cover it with gauze and grasp it firmly between the thumb and middle finger of your nondominant hand. In effect, the ventral surface of the tip of the tongue is rolled over your middle finger. Do not pull so hard as to cause discomfort. Use your index finger to retract the patient's upper lip.
6. Ask the patient to breathe in and out through the mouth or to "pant like a puppy." This opens the space between the soft palate and the tongue. Remind the patient to keep his or her eyes open, and to perhaps focus on your forehead or headband to serve as a distraction.
7. With the warm mirror in your dominant hand and the glass surface pointing downward, slowly introduce the mirror and visualize the epiglottis. Next, slowly and gently apply the posterior aspect of the mirror to the uvula and a portion of the soft palate. With a smooth, gentle movement, slowly lift them upward and backward out of the way. Avoid touching either the posterior pharyngeal wall or the base of the tongue. Touching these might stimulate the gag reflex (Fig. 79-2).

   NOTE: In certain patients, adequate anesthesia is not attainable for this portion of the procedure. In those cases, flexible nasolaryngoscopy should be performed.

8. With the mirror gently lifting the uvula and soft palate out of the way, tilt it in various directions to visualize the larynx, the hypopharynx, and the anterior oropharynx, including the base of the tongue. Move your head toward and away from the mirror to focus the light source maximally on visualized objects (Fig. 79-3). Continue to encourage the patient to breathe gently in and out through the mouth. If the structures are not adequately visualized after lifting the soft palate and uvula out of the way, check the positioning of the patient's chin and neck. Reposition if necessary.
9. With the larynx visualized (see Fig. 77-6 in Chapter 77, Nasolaryngoscopy), observe vocal cord activity during quiet respiration. Next, observe cord activity while the patient holds a prolonged high "eee" sound. This lengthens the vocal cords and moves the larynx upward vertically, which should allow visualization of the anterior commissure. Observe for symmetry of cord mobility and for edema, hemorrhage, erythema, nodules, or a mass on the cords or in the surrounding structures. Note any other mucosal or structural abnormalities.

   NOTE: All structures viewed will be seen in mirror image (upside-down and backward).

10. If the mirror fogs during the procedure, it needs to be reheated. If externally heated, it needs to be tested again on your hand or arm before use. For those patients whose pharynx is not suitably visualized by this technique, or for those in whom a closer evaluation of an abnormality is indicated, nasolaryngoscopy should be performed or referral to an otolaryngologist considered.

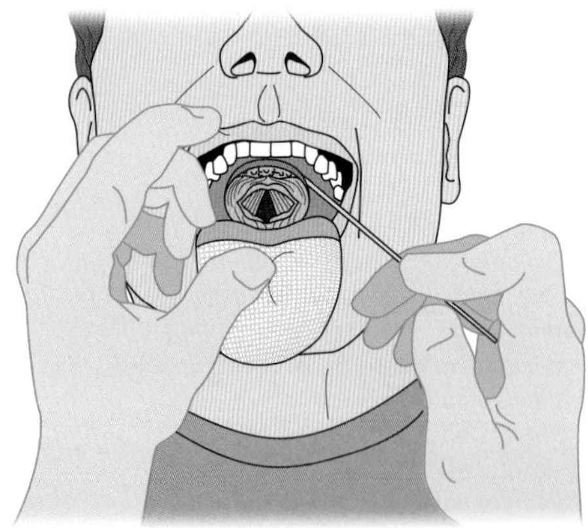

Figure 79-3 The tongue is pulled forward with gauze, and the mirror is tilted in various directions to visualize the larynx, hypopharynx, and anterior oropharynx.

Findings

- Epiglottis: Usually has a slightly curved and regular upper edge but is sometimes acutely curved and conical ("infantile type"). It may hang backward and obscure the view of the cords in the relaxed state or hang forward to hide the valleculae. If the epiglottis is floppy, small lesions on the laryngeal surface of the epiglottis may be difficult to see. The apices of the pyriform sinuses are also not usually visualized. The epiglottis rises upward and forward during phonation.
- Aryepiglottic folds: May have swelling or ulceration.
- Interarytenoid area: May be thickened or covered with papilla.
- False cords: May show swelling or ulceration.
- Vocal cords must be examined for the following:
  - *Color*: Normal color is pearly white.
  - *Movement*: May be restricted by paresis or by infiltration of tumor. Arthritis of cricoarytenoid joint may also cause limited movement.
  - *Surface*: May be intact or ulcerated.
  - *Edge*: May be irregular.
  - *Anterior commissure*: Not always seen because of anatomic variations.
- Subglottic space: Difficult to examine, but swellings may be seen below the level of the vocal cords.

Complications

- Possible laceration of the undersurface of the tongue from stretching the tongue over the teeth
- Possible adverse reaction to anesthetic
- Vomiting, with possible aspiration
- Failure to diagnose an abnormality because of inadequate visualization

CPT/Billing Code

No separate code is available for this procedure. Consider using a more comprehensive E/M code.

ICD-9-CM Diagnostic Codes

161.9	Laryngeal cancer, NEC
305.1	Nicotine addiction, or addiction in remission
306.1	Psychogenic dysphonia
784.2	Neck mass
784.41	Aphonia
784.49	Hoarseness
784.99	Halitosis
786.05	Dyspnea, chronic
786.1	Stridor
786.2	Cough, chronic
786.3	Hemoptysis
787.2	Dysphagia
933.0	Foreign body in hypopharynx, nasopharynx, oropharynx, or pharynx
933.1	Foreign body, larynx

Bibliography

Deutsch ES, Yang JY, Reilly JS: Introduction to peroral endoscopy. In Snow JB, Ballenger JJ (eds): Ballenger's Otorhinolaryngology Head and Neck Surgery, 16th ed. Hamilton, Ontario, BC Decker, 2003, pp 1513–1514.

Wilson KM, Padhya TA: Clinical tests. In Seiden AM, Tami TA, Pensak ML, et al (eds): Otolaryngology: The Essentials. New York, Thieme, 2002, p 242.

CHAPTER 80

Peritonsillar Abscess Drainage

Roger K. Waage

Peritonsillar abscess, an infection in the space between the palatine tonsil and the pharyngeal constrictors, is the most common deep infection or abscess of the head and neck. Approximately 45,000 cases of peritonsillar abscess occur annually in the United States, usually in patients in the second or third decade of life; it rarely occurs in immunocompetent children younger than 6 years of age. Symptoms include fever, malaise, severe sore throat, trismus, odynophagia, and dysphagia with drooling. The patient may be dehydrated from a lack of oral intake. Pain is often referred to the ear, and the patient may have a voice with muffled resonance known as a "hot potato" voice. Signs of peritonsillar abscess include nonexudative pharyngitis in the majority of cases, marked edema of the soft palate, and a fluctuant fullness of the tonsil, which is covered superiorly by a shiny membrane. The classic sign is deflection of the swollen uvula to the opposite side (Fig. 80-1). There is often inferior and medial displacement of the affected tonsil. Tender cervical adenopathy is usually present.

The local anatomy must be understood before attempting to aspirate or drain a peritonsillar abscess. The palatine tonsils lie between the palatoglossal and palatopharyngeal arches. These two pillars form the anterior and posterior borders of the tonsil. The surface of each tonsil has a covering of mucosa with an irregular number of indentations known as *tonsillar crypts*. Beneath the mucosa, each tonsil is surrounded by a fibrous capsule. A peritonsillar abscess is a collection of pus between the fibrous capsule of the tonsil and the superior constrictor muscle of the pharynx, which forms the lateral wall of the tonsil. Progression of pus formation and lateral extension of cellulitis irritate the surrounding musculature, particularly the internal pterygoids, resulting in spasm and trismus. It is also important to note for this procedure that the internal carotid artery lies approximately 2.5 cm posterolateral to the tonsil and that the facial artery lies lateral to the tonsil.

Historically, it was thought that a peritonsillar abscess developed as a progression of an acute exudative tonsillitis. Currently, a peritonsillar abscess is thought to originate in Weber's salivary glands, which are found in a space just above the tonsil known as the *supratonsillar fossa*. Weber's salivary glands are a group of about 20 mucous salivary glands that assist with digestion of food particles trapped in the tonsillar crypts. They are connected to the palatine tonsil by a duct that extends to the surface of the tonsil. Supporting the theory that Weber's glands are involved in the pathogenesis of peritonsillar abscess are the facts that a peritonsillar abscess can occur after tonsillectomy, even while the patient is on appropriate antibiotics, and the majority of abscesses are found in the superior pole of the palatine tonsil. Only 20% of abscesses are found in the mid-tonsil, and only 10% occupy the lower pole.

A peritonsillar abscess is usually polymicrobial. The most common aerobic organisms are *Streptococcus pyogenes* (group A beta-hemolytic *Streptococcus*) and *Staphylococcus aureus*. The most common anaerobes are *Bacteroides* and *Fusobacterium*. Throat cultures are of no benefit, and cultures from the aspirate have rarely been found to be helpful for selection of antibiotics.

The differential diagnosis of peritonsillar abscess includes unilateral tonsillitis, peritonsillar cellulitis, neoplasm, retropharyngeal abscess, leukemia, herpes simplex tonsillitis, infectious mononucleosis, foreign body aspiration, aneurysm of the internal carotid artery, and retromolar abscess. The most common entity that is confused with peritonsillar abscess is peritonsillar cellulitis. Peritonsillar cellulitis has the same symptoms, and perhaps similar physical findings, but because there is no pus between the tonsil and the lateral muscles, there is no fluctuance in the peritonsillar area. Ultrasonography may help distinguish between cellulitis and abscess, noninvasively. However, intraoral ultrasonography requires a skilled and experienced sonographer and the examination may be limited by trismus. Intraoral ultrasonography is probably most useful for locating the abscess when aspiration or incision and drainage is unsuccessful. Transcutaneous ultrasonography can also be performed by placing the transducer over the submandibular gland and scanning the tonsillar area, but there is a loss in the resolution of the image because of the distance from the transducer, so this is rarely used. Computed tomography (CT) is occasionally helpful. The CT should be done with contrast and may be helpful for ruling out an extension of the abscess.

The initial treatment of all patients with peritonsillar abscess should include adequate pain relief, hydration, and antibiotics. There is no consensus on choice of antibiotics. Penicillin, clindamycin, or cephalosporins are all reasonable as a first choice. Use of oral penicillin in doses of 500 mg four times daily has resulted in reasonable cure rates. Some clinicians add metronidazole if the clinical response in 24 hours is less than expected. Other clinicians advocate combining steroids with antibiotics. A recent study of rural field hospitals in the Indian Health Service suggested that high-dose steroids combined with cephalosporins, intravenous hydration, and analgesia were effective in reducing the number of patients needing to be air-evacuated from remote locations (see Lamkin and Portt, 2006).

Historically, the surgical treatment of peritonsillar abscess has been either abscess tonsillectomy or incision and drainage. If untreated, the abscess can rupture, possibly resulting in laryngeal aspiration, pneumonia, sepsis, or death. An untreated abscess can also spread locally or hematogenously, causing extensive local infection or even meningitis. Patients with a peritonsillar abscess and a history of three episodes of tonsillitis in the past year should probably be sent for an abscess tonsillectomy. However, for those patients without recurrent tonsillitis, there is growing evidence that needle aspiration is the treatment of choice. Needle aspiration has been shown to have an 85% to 100% success rate. Of those patients who respond initially, only 10% will have a recurrence. A second needle aspiration should also have a high success rate. Patients who fail a second or third needle aspiration should probably have an abscess tonsillectomy. (Even those patients who respond to a third aspiration should probably have a tonsillectomy, especially if this is the third infection in a year; see Chapter 83, Tonsillectomy and Adenoidectomy). The small percentage of patients whose abscess fails to resolve with a needle aspiration should probably have an

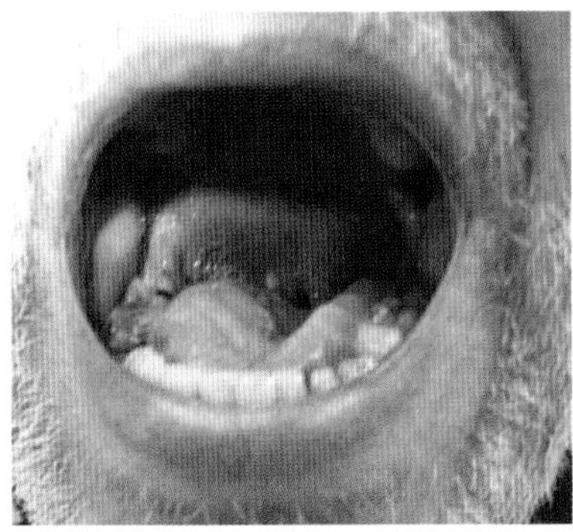

Figure 80-1 Peritonsillar abscess on patient's right side. Note fluctuance, lack of exudate on tonsil, soft palate edema, and deviation of uvula to the opposite side.

incision and drainage procedure or be referred to an otolaryngologist to rule out a possible pterygomaxillary space abscess. An algorithm for the management of peritonsillar abscess is shown in Figure 80-2. Considering that the incision and drainage technique is now typically reserved for more difficult cases, it is not surprising that the recurrence rate is slightly higher than in the past, ranging from 6% to 24%.

Needle aspiration does have some drawbacks. It is painful, invasive, and performed somewhat blindly. A series of 12 patients evaluated by Haeggstrom and associates demonstrated that abscesses were located within 4 to 25 mm from the carotid artery. In addition, needle aspiration samples only one area in the tonsillar fossa and may require repeated attempts. From 12% to 24% of abscesses are missed on the first aspiration attempt. However, it is relatively simple to perform, even by those with little experience and who are not ear, nose, and throat specialists, and it does not require expensive or specialized equipment. A study performed in 1980 (Herzon and Aldridge) on the efficacy of needle aspiration showed that 80% of aspirations were performed by interns and 20% by emergency medicine specialists. Successful aspiration or incision and drainage may also help the patient avoid a hospitalization.

Indications

Peritonsillar abscess in a patient who is not indicated for abscess tonsillectomy

Contraindications (Absolute and Relative)

- Septic shock or impending respiratory compromise (patient should first be stabilized)
- Uncooperative patient
- Operator unfamiliar with anatomy
- Anticoagulated patient or patient with coagulopathy (either the anticoagulation/coagulopathy should be reversed or otolaryngology consulted)
- Inadequate equipment

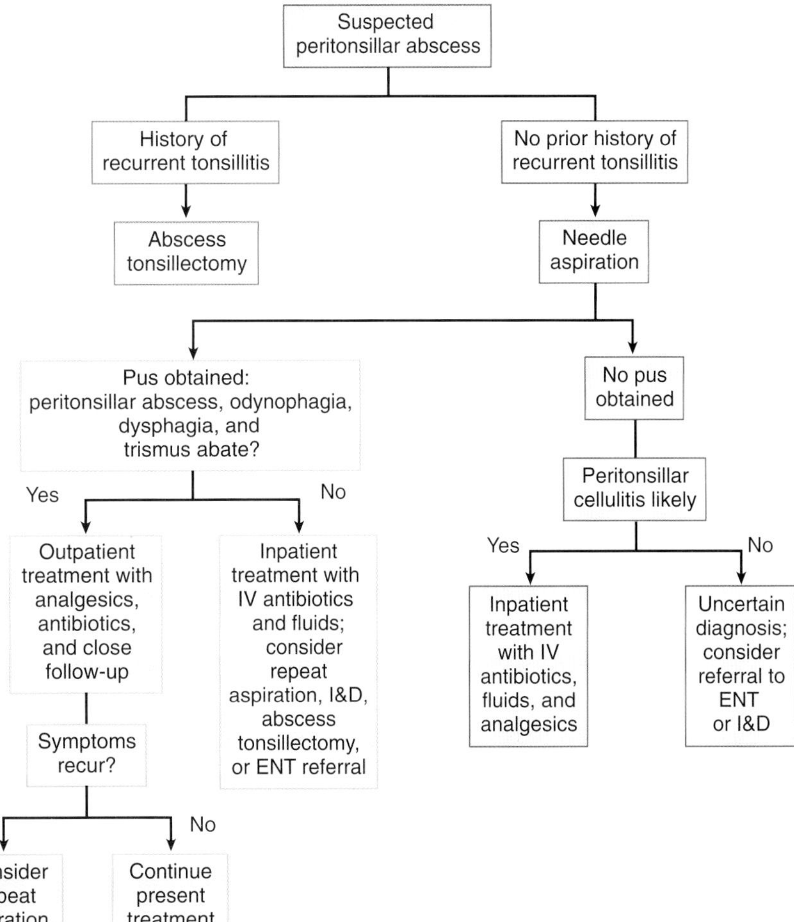

Figure 80-2 Algorithm for management of peritonsillar abscess. ENT, ear, nose, and throat; I&D, incision and drainage.

EQUIPMENT

Needle Aspiration

- Topical anesthetic—lidocaine, tetracaine, or benzocaine (Cetacaine) spray or 4% cocaine
- 2% lidocaine with epinephrine 1 : 100,000 in a 3- to 5-mL syringe with a 25- or 27-gauge, 1.5-inch needle or tonsil needle
- 18-gauge 1.5-inch or longer needle or spinal needle
- 10-mL syringe

NOTE: As a guide to keep from going too deep, place a piece of tape or Steri-Strip 8 mm proximal to the needle tip or cut 8 mm off the end of the needle cover and put it back on the needle, leaving 8 mm of needle exposed.

- Suction: tonsillar or no. 8 Frazier
- Good lighting: headlight or head mirror with gooseneck lamp
- Kidney basin
- Tongue depressor
- Bite block or heaped gauze (as thick as the clinician's finger) folded over the patient's incisor teeth to help the clinician avoid being bitten when palpating the area
- Surgical assistant to help with the equipment and procedure
- Gloves and mask for the clinician to observe universal blood and body fluid precautions

Incision and Drainage

All of the aforementioned, plus a curved Kelly or tonsillar clamp and a no. 15 scalpel blade marked with tape or Steri-Strip 8 mm from the tip

PREPROCEDURE PATIENT EDUCATION

The procedure of choice for most patients is needle aspiration, so this procedure should be explained, as well as the risks and any alternatives. Advise the patient that he or she may experience some discomfort while attempting to hold the mouth (or as it is held) open and when the local anesthetic is injected (even though the pharynx will be sprayed first with a topical anesthetic). The patient may also experience some discomfort when the abscess is aspirated or incised and drained. If aspiration fails, the procedure may shift to incision and drainage, and the patient should know the difference. He or she may gag or experience fluid running down the throat. Fortunately, the pus can usually be aspirated or incised and drained successfully, and, if so, the symptoms will improve dramatically. If this is successful, the patient can be treated with oral antibiotics and analgesics, and hospitalization can be avoided. If the abscess is not successfully drained or if the symptoms do not resolve, further treatment and hospitalization may be required. The patient should also be told that there is a 10% chance of recurrence after aspiration and a 6% to 24% chance of recurrence after incision and drainage. If the abscess recurs after successful aspiration, there is a high success rate for merely repeating the aspiration. However, even if aspiration is successful three times, the patient would probably benefit from tonsillectomy, especially if three infections have occurred in the same year. Fortunately, there are new methods available for tonsillectomy and adenoidectomy (see Chapter 83, Tonsillectomy and Adenoidectomy) that can usually be performed in the outpatient setting and that minimize postoperative pain and recovery time. Obtain a signed informed consent from the patient or his or her representative for all of these procedures.

TECHNIQUE

Precautions

One disaster to avoid is aspiration or incision of the carotid or facial arteries or an undiagnosed carotid artery aneurysm. (Fortunately, there are no recent reports in the literature of this occurring, so it is extremely rare.) Another disaster to avoid is patient aspiration of purulent material into his or her lungs. The risk of the first can be minimized by directing the needle or scalpel only posteriorly when performing the procedure (the major vessels are located laterally) and never inserting it more than 8 mm. The risk of the latter can be minimized by ensuring adequate wall operative suction at the time of incision and drainage.

Procedure

1. Seat the patient leaning slightly forward, in the sniffing position, at eye level with the operator. His or her neck should be supported posteriorly to prevent the patient from moving abruptly. A kidney basin should be available for the patient to expectorate. Suction must be readily available with either a tonsillar or no. 8 Frazier tip. Good lighting is necessary, provided by either a headlight or a head mirror with a bright light source behind the patient.
2. Have the patient open his or her mouth as wide as possible. If trismus restricts jaw motion, the patient may need some encouragement to open more widely. Mild pressure on the lower jaw may also be necessary to help open the mouth. The cheek may be retracted laterally to improve visualization. Your assistant can help provide exposure by placing mild pressure on the jaw and lateral traction on the cheek. For moderate to severe trismus, sedation may be beneficial (see Chapter 2, Procedural Sedation and Analgesia). Palpate the soft palate and tonsil to localize the fluctuant area, and administer topical anesthetic to the affected side. A bite block or some heaped gauze folded over the patient's incisor teeth may help the clinician avoid being bitten. Be prepared to avoid a bite when palpating the area because the patient may not be able to hold his or her mouth open for very long. The patient may also gag when the area is palpated. When the topical anesthetic has taken effect, inject 2% lidocaine with epinephrine (using a 25- to 27-gauge, 1.5-inch needle, or tonsil needle) into the mucosa, just above and lateral to the tonsil. Avoid injecting into the abscess.
3. After a few minutes, attempt aspiration. Hold the tongue depressor in your nondominant hand and the aspirating syringe in your dominant hand. You may need to ask your assistant to create suction with the syringe. Insert the 18-gauge long or spinal needle on a 10-mL syringe, and direct it straight posteriorly. When inserted, attempt aspiration (Fig. 80-3). The needle should not be inserted more than 8 mm. If you aspirate pus, continue until no more pus returns. Scientific evidence suggests there is no reason to culture the aspirated fluid, which is usually between 2 and 14 mL of pus.
4. If you do not aspirate any pus, withdraw the needle slightly and redirect inferiorly. When performing this procedure, be aware that the carotid artery lies approximately 2.5 cm posterior and lateral to the tonsillar pillars. In addition, the more the needle is directed toward the lower pole of the tonsil, the more likely it is to enter the carotid artery. Therefore, make sure it is only directed posteriorly. Never aspirate lateral to the molar. If blood returns on aspiration, the procedure should be stopped, the needle should be removed, and direct pressure should be applied to the puncture site. An otolaryngologist should be consulted immediately.
5. If the aspiration is unsuccessful and the diagnosis of peritonsillar abscess is certain, immediate incision and drainage can be performed. With a no. 15 scalpel blade directed posteriorly, make an incision just through the mucosa in the upper pole of the tonsil at the point of maximum fluctuance (prominence; Fig. 80-4). Maximum fluctuance (prominence) is usually demonstrated as a shiny membrane over the abscess. Avoid inserting the scalpel blade more than 8 mm. After an incision is made through this membrane, there is often prompt expression of pus. Immediate and aggressive suction is required. Having the surgical assistant ready

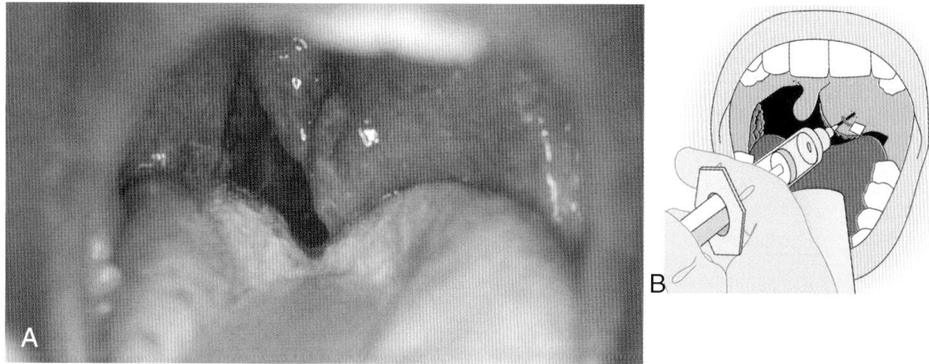

Figure 80-3 Aspiration of peritonsillar abscess. **A,** Abscess. **B,** The abscess should be anesthetized topically, injected with 2% lidocaine with epinephrine, and then aspirated with an 18-gauge long needle or spinal needle at the point of maximal fluctuance (prominence).

with the suction placed at the incision site, before the incision is made, often reassures the patient and keeps him or her comfortable. It may also help the patient avoid any gagging or drowning sensation that can occur when pus is released into the pharynx.

NOTE: When surveyed, the initial procedure performed by most otolaryngologists for a peritonsillar abscess is incision and drainage, whereas the initial procedure by most nonotolaryngologists is aspiration.

6. Sometimes the incision needs to be widened with a curved Kelly or tonsillar clamp. Any loculations that are apparent should be opened. Loculations are especially common inferiorly. Any remaining pus or blood should be suctioned before the procedure is finished. The patient can then rinse his or her mouth with tap water, normal saline, or peroxide. The patient should be observed directly for a few minutes after incision and drainage for any persistent drainage. If drainage persists, the patient should be admitted for intravenous antibiotics. The patient should also be observed for at least an hour before discharge to ensure stable vital signs and absence of bleeding.
7. All patients successfully treated by needle aspiration or incision and drainage may be sent home with penicillin (or erythromycin if they are allergic to penicillin). Liquid elixirs are much easier for the patient to swallow. Anaerobic coverage with metronidazole or clindamycin is probably not necessary.

Complications

- Hemorrhage
- Tracheal aspiration of purulent material
- Respiratory distress
- Pneumonia
- Failed aspiration or incision and drainage, persistent cellulitis
- Recurrence

Sample Operative Reports

See sample operative reports online at www.expertconsult.com.

Postprocedure Patient Education

All patients who have been treated for a peritonsillar abscess need adequate antibiotics and analgesia, preferably in the liquid form. Warm gargles may help keep the area clean and provide mild analgesia. The patient will want to maintain a liquid or soft diet until the discomfort has resolved. Patients should be instructed to return if they experience a recurrence of symptoms, fever greater than 101° F, severe pain, significant bleeding, or trouble breathing or swallowing. A follow-up appointment within 48 hours should be scheduled.

CPT/Billing Codes

42700 Incision and drainage of peritonsillar abscess
88170 Needle aspiration (location needs to be recorded for insurance billing)

ICD-9-CM Diagnostic Code

475 Peritonsillar abscess, quinsy, peritonsillar cellulitis

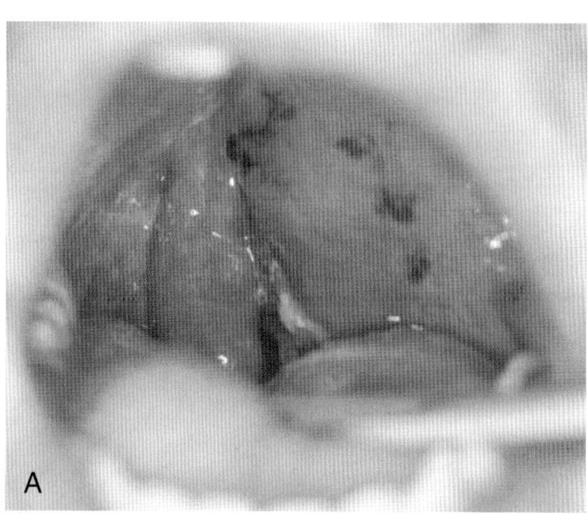

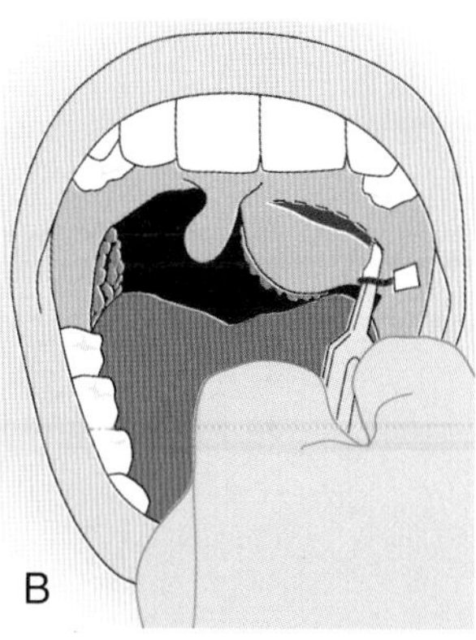

Figure 80-4 Incision and drainage of peritonsillar abscess. **A,** Abscess. **B,** After topical and local anesthesia, the incision should be made in the upper pole of the tonsil at the point of maximal fluctuance (prominence). The incision may need to be probed or widened with a curved Kelly or tonsillar clamp.

ONLINE RESOURCES

eMedicineHealth: Peritonsillar abscess. Available at www.emedicinehealth.com/peritonsillar_abscess/page7_em.htm.

Medline Plus: Peritonsillar abscess. Available at www.nlm.nih.gov/medlineplus/ency/article/000986.htm.

BIBLIOGRAPHY

Epperly T, Wood T: New trends in the management of peritonsillar abscess. Am Fam Physician 42:102–112, 1990.

Galioto NJ: Peritonsillar abscess. Am Fam Physician 77:199–202, 2008.

Haeggstrom A, Gustafsson O, Engquist S, et al: Intraoral ultrasonography in the diagnosis of peritonsillar abscess. Otolaryngol Head Neck Surg 108:243–247, 1993.

Herzon F, Aldridge J: Peritonsillar abscess: Needle aspiration. Otolaryngol Head Neck Surg 89:910–911, 1980.

Lamkin RH, Portt J: An outpatient medical treatment protocol for peritonsillar abscess. Ear Nose Throat J 85:658, 660, 2006.

Riviello RJ: Otolaryngologic procedures. In Roberts JR, Hedges JR (eds): Clinical Procedures in Emergency Medicine, 4th ed. Philadelphia, Saunders, 2004, pp 1280–1316.

Silva JC: Peritonsillar abscess incision and drainage. In Reichman EF, Simon RR (eds): Emergency Medicine Procedures. New York, McGraw-Hill, 2004, pp 1335–1341.

Steyer T: Peritonsillar abscess: Diagnosis and treatment. Am Fam Physician 65:93–96, 2002.

CHAPTER 81

Management of Dental Injuries and Reimplantation of an Avulsed Tooth

Grant C. Fowler

Dental trauma, ranging from a slight chip of the enamel to avulsion of a tooth, causes some of the most common injuries to the face. An occlusive misadventure (e.g., biting a hard object or a seizure) or a blow to the face can cause dental trauma. Up to 10% of emergency department visits are due to dental trauma. Injuries to the maxillary central incisors account for 70% of dental injuries, subluxations account for about 50% of injuries to the teeth, and up to 5 million avulsions occur annually in the United States. It is estimated that 50% of children will experience dental trauma. Management depends on the age of the patient and the nature of the injury. Often, the primary care clinician is the first to evaluate such an injury. Occasionally, the clinician will receive a phone call from a patient requesting guidance after a fracture, subluxation, luxation, or avulsion has occurred. Proper management of dental trauma may minimize pain and disfigurement. For example, knowledge of proper storage and treatment of an avulsed tooth is crucial to optimize the chances of successful reimplantation.

NOTE: If a tooth or portion of a tooth is missing and it cannot be unequivocally located by history or physical examination, attempts should be made to locate it with radiographs. Facial films may find it in a maxillary sinus (which may necessitate surgery), a chest radiograph may document that it has been aspirated (requiring bronchoscopic retrieval), or abdominal films may document that it has been swallowed. Also, with a luxation or avulsion, care should be taken to determine whether a tooth is primary (i.e., deciduous, milk, temporary) or permanent in children because it may change the management (Fig. 81-1). This determination may be tricky in children between the ages of 6 and 12 years who may have "mixed" dentition. In addition, patients (parents) should be aware that it may not always be possible to detect the presence or extent of a dental fracture with the initial examination and radiographs. Root fractures (although rare), which may require extensive dental care, are notorious for avoiding detection by radiography; they may be diagnosed only later by radiography, as they are healing.

Management of a dental fracture is based on the extent of the fracture (Fig. 81-2) and the age of the patient. Ellis I fractures involve only the enamel of the tooth. They may be a mere "chip" off of the tooth. Management is necessary only if a resultant sharp edge is disturbing the adjacent soft tissues. In that case, a nail file (emery board) can be used to file down the edge. Referral can be made to a general dentist for cosmetic restoration. Patients or parents may appreciate being reassured that the tooth can usually be restored to its natural appearance with the use of enamel-bonding plastic materials.

Ellis II fractures, which account for 70% of tooth fractures, not only involve the enamel but also expose the dentin layer, which has a creamy- or ivory-yellow color compared with the white enamel. Beneath the dentin lies the pulp, which continually lays down dentin for the life of the tooth, and the goal of emergency management is to maintain the vitality of this pulp. Patients usually complain of sensitivity to hot, cold, or even air passing over the exposed surface when breathing. They should be warned that any trauma to a tooth may lead to pulpal necrosis or tooth resorption, regardless of management, and that dental referral is required within 24 hours. Patients younger than 12 years of age have less dentin, so there is usually less discomfort. However, because dentin is a microtubular structure that can allow bacteria to penetrate the pulp, tooth fractures in children and adolescents involving the dentin are more serious because the pulp is more likely to be contaminated. Fortunately, this age group also has much greater pulpal regenerative ability. Early treatment may prevent contamination of the pulp and

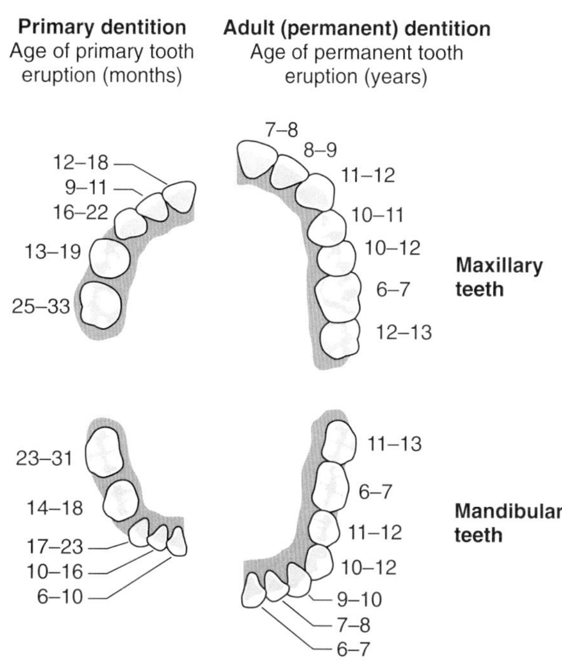

Figure 81-1 The normal eruptive patterns of primary and permanent teeth. Extra or fewer teeth are common in both types of teeth. (Redrawn from Upadhye S, Ross DJ: Fractures tooth management. In Reichman EF, Simon RR [eds]: Emergency Medicine Procedures. New York, McGraw-Hill, 2004, pp 1397–1402.)

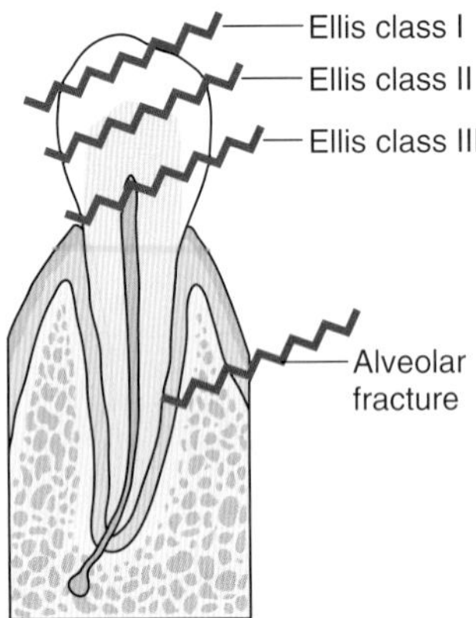

Figure 81-2 Ellis classification for fractures of anterior teeth. (From James DM: Immediate management of tooth fracture and avulsion. In James DM [ed]: Field Guide to Urgent and Ambulatory Care Procedures. Philadelphia, Lippincott Williams & Wilkins, 2001, pp 36–39.)

the need for subsequent root canal, so a pediatric or general dentist should be notified right away. For patients older than 12 years of age, because they have more dentin and less pulp, referral can be made for the next working day. Regardless of age, warming the sterile saline before flushing may decrease temperature sensitivity. A thin layer of a protective dressing that is also a sedative to the pulp (e.g., calcium hydroxide paste or zinc oxide with eugenol; see Suppliers section), or even toothpaste, should be applied with a small applicator. The exposed dentin should be covered and then the paste covered with a dry gauze. To maintain a dry field while working, cotton gauze or rolls can be placed on either side of the tooth. Patients older than 12 years of age should then be advised to avoid extremes of intraoral temperatures. A piece of dental foil or aluminum foil placed over the paste-covering gauze may provide additional protection from discomfort associated with temperature extremes until the dentist can see the patient. If available, instead of gauze, three to four coats of dental varnish (see Suppliers section) or clear nail polish can be painted over the paste. Allow time to dry between coats; this may help protect against temperature extremes.

Ellis III fractures expose the pulp of the tooth. Again, because there is more pulp relative to dentin in children, fractures involving the pulp are more common in children. Pulp can easily be distinguished from dentin because exposed pulp produces a red blush or a drop of blood when brushed with sterile gauze. These fractures are a dental emergency, and the usual treatment is removal of the pulp (pulpotomy). Significant delay in care can lead to long-term pain

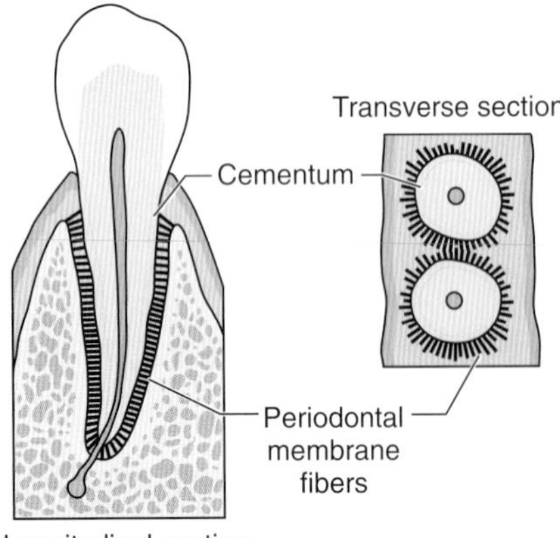

Figure 81-3 Arrangement of periodontal fibers. The cementum is a thin cell layer lining the root between the root and the periodontal fibers. Together, the cementum, periodontal fibers, and alveolar bone form the *attachment apparatus*.

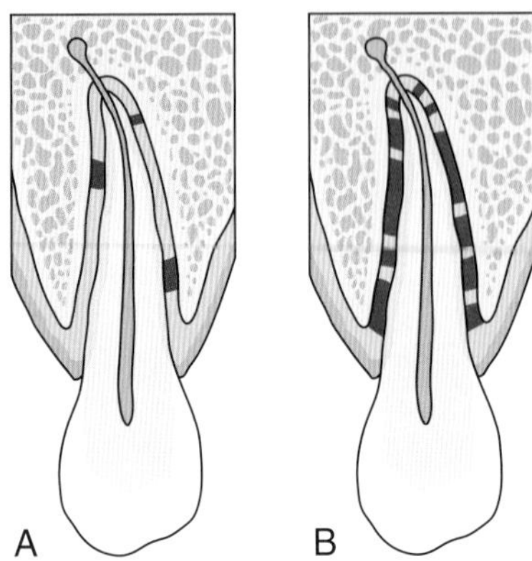

Figure 81-4 Slightly (**A**) and moderately (**B**) concussed tooth.

and abscess formation. The clinician should not attempt to probe the pulp or remove any material; instead, the affected area should be covered with aluminum foil, adequate analgesia should be provided, and oral antibiotics effective for mouth flora should be prescribed. Such a fracture can cause considerable pain, so a dental anesthetic nerve block may be appreciated. The patient should then consult a dentist immediately because definitive treatment for all but the smallest pulpal exposures is endodontic or root canal therapy. If a dentist will not be available, bleeding can be stopped by dripping dilute epinephrine (or lidocaine with epinephrine) over the site. Injection of lidocaine with epinephrine around the tooth also often provides hemostasis. If unsuccessful, pressure can be applied with a saline-moistened, sterile cotton-tipped applicator. It may take 3 to 5 minutes for hemostasis. A thick coat of calcium hydroxide or zinc oxide with eugenol paste can then be applied to the tooth and an adjacent tooth (for stability), making sure that it is not so thick as to interfere with occlusion. If a dentist is not available, a minimal Ellis III fracture (<1 to 2 mm pulp exposure) can be treated as an Ellis II fracture and followed up by a dentist in 24 hours, although this alternative is less than ideal.

Teeth are held in place by surrounding periodontal membrane fibers and ligaments, a fragile cell layer lining the root known as the *cementum*, and alveolar bone (Fig. 81-3). These structures combined are known as the *attachment apparatus*. The crown is the hard enamel portion of the tooth located above the gum line. With trauma, periodontal fibers and the attachment apparatus may be concussed (Fig. 81-4), a tooth may be subluxed (ligaments damaged) or luxated (dislocated) extrusively, intrusively, or laterally, or an entire tooth may be avulsed (Fig. 81-5). Concussion is defined as injury to the tooth, and although the tooth will be tender to palpation, there will be no increased mobility. The radiograph will be negative. If examination of the surrounding gingiva reveals blood, there has also usually been ligamentous damage, which is confirmed if the tooth can be wiggled. Ligamentous damage can be caused by subluxation or luxation, with subluxation resulting in a loose tooth that may or may not be sensitive to touch. Extrusive luxation results in a misaligned, loose tooth that is often elevated above those bordering it.

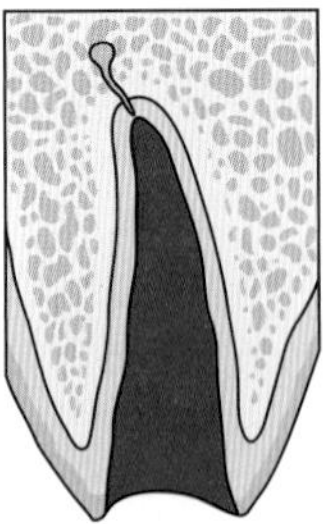

Figure 81-5 Avulsed tooth.

The patient frequently complains of malocclusion because this tooth contacts the opposing teeth early when chewing. Intrusive luxation is a more severe form of luxation in which the tooth is driven into the alveolar bone. With primary teeth, this process can cause damage to the permanent tooth bud. Depending on the force involved, the tooth can even be driven into the maxillary sinus and appear avulsed. If intrusive luxation is suspected and the tooth is not visible, a radiograph may be needed to locate the tooth. Although an extrusive luxation is the result of a partial avulsion or dislodgment of the tooth, there is no fracture, so the radiograph will be negative. Lateral luxation is the result of an alveolar bone fracture with lateral displacement of the tooth in the mesial, distal, buccal, or lingual direction. A radiograph should confirm the fracture.

Treatment of a concussed tooth is directed by the severity of the discomfort. Nonsteroidal anti-inflammatory drugs (NSAIDs) and a soft diet may be all that is necessary to manage the pain. For subluxation, a minimally mobile tooth will usually "firm up" over a week or two, and splinting usually is not required. Severely subluxed primary teeth should be extracted; otherwise, concussed and subluxed primary teeth are treated in the same manner as permanent teeth. For subluxed teeth, the patient should maintain a soft diet and avoid undue pressure on the affected tooth during that time, and may benefit from NSAIDs for pain control. For either concussion or subluxation, referral to a dentist may be prudent, not only to confirm the diagnosis, but also to exclude more serious injury.

An extrusively luxated primary tooth should be removed; conversely, and extrusively luxated permanent tooth needs to be repositioned. Firm, gentle pressure will usually realign the tooth to its original position, and this maneuver may be better tolerated if a local anesthetic is injected. Avoid excessive pressure when attempting this maneuver; a hematoma may be blocking repositioning and require more definitive care by a dentist. If repositioning is successful, splinting should be provided to stabilize the tooth for 1 to 2 weeks during healing, either by a dentist with flexible wire splinting or by a primary care clinician using a cold-curing periodontal pack (see Suppliers section) or dressing until a dentist, oral surgeon, or maxillofacial surgeon can provide definitive care (ideally within 24 hours). To use a cold-curing periodontal pack, thoroughly mix equal portions of the epoxy and catalyst on an uncontaminated surface until it has the consistency of putty. It should be allowed to dry slightly for a few minutes and then applied by molding it to the exterior, buccal surface of the tooth and adjacent teeth on either side. Avoid covering any of the occlusal surface. The patient should remain in the clinic until the splinting material has completely hardened; reexamination ensures the absence of impingement of an occlusal surface or soft tissue sufficient to cause local irritation. Dental utility wax or beeswax may be used in the same fashion if a cold-curing periodontal pack is not available.

Intrusive luxation is a more serious injury, resulting in alveolar fracture. Management consists of defining the extent of injury (e.g., is a sinus involved?), locating the tooth, providing analgesics, and referral. Laterally luxated primary teeth should be extracted. With permanent teeth, because lateral luxation causes a fracture, repositioning the tooth may be more difficult. However, by grasping the tooth firmly between thumb and forefinger, the clinician will usually be able to realign the tooth. After referral, stabilizing with a splint is necessary for a minimum of 2 weeks.

In the event of avulsion, the neurovascular supply is disrupted. Although primary teeth are usually not reimplanted (to avoid damaging the developing permanent teeth), the more rapidly a permanent tooth is reimplanted, the more likely the tooth will remain viable. If the tooth can be replanted within 5 minutes, there is a greater than 80% chance that the tooth will remain vital. Given this urgency, bystanders or clinicians should not be overly concerned about cleaning or flushing the socket or tooth before reimplanting. When preparing for reimplantation, only the crown should be touched; touching the root can devitalize it. Significant debris and large clots can merely be brushed off; small clots or dirt can be removed by the patient by placing the tooth under his or her tongue for a few seconds. If it is going to be reimplanted immediately, the tooth can be flushed with saline or tap water. Reimplantation should then be performed with follow-up by a dentist.

For the tooth that is not immediately reimplanted, proper storage is crucial. Prognosis for later reimplantation deteriorates rapidly—within minutes—if the tooth dries out, causing pulpal and periodontal damage. Storage media available to prevent drying, in order from most to least successful, are Hanks' balanced salt solution (a pH-balanced cell culture medium), Viaspan (used for preservation of transplant donor tissue), milk, physiologic (normal) saline, and saliva. An egg white may also be used. These fluids have an osmotic pressure similar to those of the pulp and periodontal tissues and therefore help preserve these structures. Tap water is not an appropriate storage medium because of its hypotonicity.

Although Hanks' solution, Viaspan, and milk are superior to saliva as storage media, the prevention of desiccation is much more important than waiting until Hanks' solution, Viaspan, or milk is available. If none of these is *immediately* available, the tooth can be stored in saliva. Perhaps the most readily available preservative other than saliva is fresh whole milk on ice (between 4° C and 20° C); however, parents, schools, teams, and facilities that sponsor sporting events now often have Hanks' solution in a kit. Hanks' solution has been shown to keep periodontal ligaments alive for 4 to 6 hours. Successful results have been reported with teeth suspended in Hanks' solution for up to 96 hours. It has also been found to restore cell viability in a tooth that has been avulsed for longer than 60 minutes. These kits contain a basket and net or a similar system to suspend, clean, and store the tooth in Hanks' solution while it is being transported for reimplantation (see Suppliers section). A basket allows the clinician to remove the tooth from the solution without touching it with fingers or forceps.

INDICATIONS

- Avulsed permanent tooth with minimal pulpal and periodontal damage, especially a tooth from the front of the mouth
- Tooth out of its socket for only a brief period of time
- Tooth stored in the proper physiologic medium

NOTE: One readily available source of saliva is the patient's mouth, and the tooth can be stored under the tongue. Another option is the mouth of a relative if the patient is unconscious or uncooperative. If stored in the patient's mouth, he or she needs to concentrate on not swallowing the tooth! Universal blood and body fluid precautions should be remembered if considering storing the tooth in someone else's mouth.

CONTRAINDICATIONS

- Primary (i.e., deciduous, milk, temporary) teeth should not be reimplanted. (Reimplanting these teeth may result in their fusion to the supporting bone and possible facial deformity. It may also damage or interfere with the development of the permanent teeth.)
- Avulsed teeth with gross caries or fractures should not be reimplanted.
- Patients with significant loss of periodontal support (periodontitis) should not have teeth reimplanted.

EQUIPMENT

- Adequate light
- Equipment necessary to follow universal blood and body fluid precautions (gloves, eye protection, mask)
- Sterile normal saline
- Irrigation syringe
- Local anesthetic (lidocaine with epinephrine), syringe (dental aspirating type or 3 mL), and 2-inch, 25- to 27-gauge needle

- Sterile 2 × 2 inch cotton gauze squares or cotton rolls
- Nail file or emery board for tooth fracture, dental drill if available
- Tooth forceps
- Fraser suction catheter, suction source, and tubing
- Calcium hydroxide or zinc oxide and eugenol paste (protective and sedative for pulp; see Suppliers section) or toothpaste
- Dental dry foil or aluminum foil
- Small brush and cavity varnish (see Suppliers section) or clear nail polish
- Cold-curing periodontal pack (i.e., elastic quick setting dressing), dental utility wax, or beeswax (see Suppliers section)
- Applicator sticks (e.g., tongue depressor, wooden end of cotton swabs)
- Dental radiography equipment and supplies
- Penicillin VK 500-mg tablets (18 to 26 tablets) or clindamycin (parenteral antibiotics for those at risk; see Chapter 221, Antibiotic Prophylaxis)
- Hanks' balanced solution, a pH-balanced cell culture medium (*optional* is Viaspan, used to preserve transplant tissue)
- Tooth-saving system (*optional*, contains Hanks' balanced solution; see Suppliers section)
- Citric acid, 2% stannous fluoride, doxycycline syrup or suspension (*optional*, especially useful if a dentist is not available and tooth has dried more than an hour)
- Cyanoacrylate glue (*optional*, especially useful if a dentist is not available)
- Paper clip (*optional*, especially useful if a dentist is not available)

Preprocedure Patient Preparation

Explain to the patient the procedure, possible complications, benefits, and the need for follow-up. The patient will need to remain still during the procedure, but discomfort should be minimal. Informed consent should be obtained.

NOTE: Immediate reimplantation (within 5 minutes) is one of the most critical factors related to periodontal healing. Unless stored in proper media, if the interval is more than 30 minutes before reimplantation, the success rate falls to less than 20% and the tooth inevitably requires endodontic therapy. If the patient or family member calls and is more than 5 minutes away from clinical care, an immediate attempt to reimplant the tooth provides the best outcome. Have the patient rinse the tooth under cold water or place it under his or her tongue for a few seconds, and then reimplant it at once. Instructions or words of encouragement may be needed. However, accident-associated factors such as the person's emotional state, a lack of knowledge of proper first aid, a lack of confidence by bystanders, or informed consent issues are often obstacles at the accident site. If these obstacles cannot be overcome, the only choice may be to store the tooth in the best medium available and to transport it and the patient to the clinic.

Technique

1. If the tooth is stored in Hanks' solution, Viaspan, or milk on arrival, leave it in the medium. If it is stored in saliva or no media, place the avulsed tooth in Hanks' solution, Viaspan, or normal saline as soon as possible. If the tooth has been dry for from 20 to 60 minutes, it should be soaked in Hanks' solution for 30 minutes. If it has been dry for more than an hour, the periodontal cells are dead and the goal is to reduce root resorption. In that situation, dentists often recommend soaking the tooth for 5 minutes in each of three different solutions before reimplantation: citric acid, followed by 2% stannous fluoride, and finally doxycycline syrup or suspension. The tooth should not be merely discarded; attempts should be made to contact a dental professional for guidance.
2. If the patient is at risk for bacteremia, administer parenteral antibiotics.
3. Conduct a rapid medical history and systematic evaluation of the traumatized individual:
   - Where, how, and when did the trauma occur? Are there fractures?
   - Is there any neurologic damage? Unconsciousness? Amnesia? Headache? Nausea?
   - Are there any underlying medical conditions? Immunocompromise? Diabetes? Prostheses? Severe mitral valve prolapse? Heart murmurs? If any of these are life- or limb-threatening, they should be managed first. If not, make mental notes of other problems while rapidly preparing to reimplant the tooth.
4. When the patient is stable, administer local anesthetic to the socket area if necessary. The clinician should follow universal blood and body fluid precautions.
5. Perform a brief clinical examination:
   - Are there any other intraoral lacerations or disturbances?
   - Is the bite disturbed by other displaced teeth?
   - Make mental notes of these findings while rapidly preparing to reimplant the tooth.
6. Examine the tooth socket and flush with normal saline. Remove all clot material.

   NOTE: Although flushing the socket is commonly suggested in practice guidelines, there is little scientific evidence to support this activity, so the socket should be manipulated as little as possible. (That is why reimplanting the tooth at the scene of the accident, if it can be accomplished within 5 to 10 minutes, is much more important than waiting to flush the socket or tooth.)
7. Remove the tooth from its soaking medium and, while holding the crown with gauze or tooth forceps, reimplant it as close as possible to its normal position, using finger pressure. *Do not touch the root.* The patient can assist the reimplantation by gently biting on gauze; this maneuver can also be used to help stabilize the tooth after reimplantation until more permanent stabilization can be arranged. Make sure the alignment is anatomic (remember that the curved side faces the tongue!). Observe the patient for malocclusion. If the tooth contacts another tooth with occlusion, it may be better to transport the tooth in preservation medium to a dental professional for definitive reimplantation.
8. Take a radiograph of the area, if possible.
9. Refer to a dentist for semirigid splinting and follow-up. If a dentist is unavailable, a cold-curing periodontal pack, aluminum foil wrapped over the tooth and the neighboring teeth, or dental wax or beeswax can act as a splint. For a more rigid splint, a small paper clip bent to conform to the buccal side of the neighboring teeth can be glued to the reimplanted tooth as well as two or three neighboring teeth with cyanoacrylate glue. The dentist can later remove the glue with a dental pick.
10. Immediately administer penicillin VK 1 g orally (for those not already given parenteral dose), then 500 mg orally four times a day for 4 to 6 days (clindamycin for those allergic to penicillin).
11. Administer tetanus toxoid if the patient has not had a booster within 5 years.

Postprocedure Patient Education

Nonsteroidal anti-inflammatory drugs and an occasional narcotic analgesic may be all that is necessary to manage the pain. The patient should avoid chewing in the area of the tooth; he or she should follow a soft diet and avoid extremes of temperature. Patients should be warned that any trauma to the tooth may cause pulpal necrosis or tooth resorption, regardless of management. For an avulsed tooth, inform the patient that the prognosis depends on the

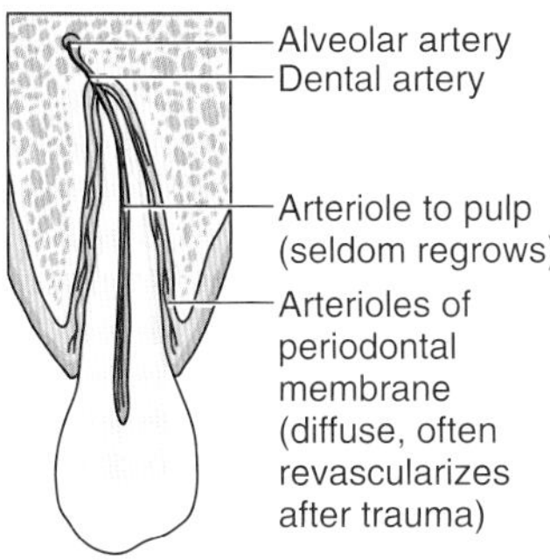

Figure 81-6 Blood supply to tooth.

length of time the tooth was out of the socket and the medium in which it was stored. Fortunately, a tooth has two sources of blood supply (Fig. 81-6). However, pulpal revascularization through the pulpal arterioles is almost nonexistent in teeth after complete root development (adult teeth). It is unusual even with immature root development. Periodontal ligament preservation is also infrequent, depending on the length of drying time to which the tooth was exposed. Fortunately, the periodontal ligament has a more diffuse blood supply and revascularizes more readily than the pulp. However, the importance of consulting a dentist for the appropriate follow-up care should be stressed, especially if further splinting is necessary.

Complications

- Necrosis of the pulp or periodontal ligament or complete loss of the tooth can occur. (Necrotic pulp tissue necessitates subsequent endodontic work.)
- An inadequately splinted tooth can remain loose, cause further damage to the attachment apparatus, and decrease the chance of tooth viability. If the tooth becomes dislodged it could result in aspiration.
- With a nonvital periodontal ligament, ankylosis or osteoclastic root resorption can occur, which requires a root canal.
- Localized infection or bacteremia can occur, but it is very rare.
- If avulsed teeth are unaccounted for, the possibility of aspiration or entrapment in soft tissues should be considered.

CPT/Billing Code

D7270 Tooth reimplantation and/or stabilization of accidentally avulsed or displaced tooth (HCPCS Code)

ICD-9-CM Diagnostic Codes

521.81 Cracked tooth
525.11 Loss of teeth due to trauma
873.63 Tooth broken or fractured due to trauma

Suppliers

(See contact information online at www.expertconsult.com.)

Calcium hydroxide paste
Dycal by Dentsply International
Ultracal by Ultradent Products, Inc.
Cavity varnish
Copalite by Cooley and Cooley
Cold-curing periodontal packs
Coe Pak Automix and Coe Pak Perio by GC America, Inc.
Periocare Periodontal Dressing by Pulpdent Corporation
Tooth-saving systems
EMT Tooth Saver by Smart Practice
Save-A-Tooth System
Viaspan by Barr Pharmaceuticals

Bibliography

Amsterdam JT: Oral medicine. In Marx JA, Hockberger RS, Walls RM (eds): Rosen's Emergency Medicine, 6th ed. St. Louis, Mosby, 2006, pp 1036–1040.

Beaudreau RW: Oral and dental emergencies. In Tintinalli JE, Kelen GD, Stapczynski JS (eds): Emergency Medicine: A Comprehensive Study Guide, 6th ed. New York, McGraw-Hill, 2004, pp 1489–1492.

James DM: Immediate management of tooth fracture and avulsion. In James DM (ed): Field Guide to Urgent and Ambulatory Care Procedures. Philadelphia, Lippincott Williams & Wilkins, 2001, pp 36–39.

Upadhye S, Ross DJ: Fractured tooth management. In Reichman EF, Simon RR (eds): Emergency Medicine Procedures. New York, McGraw-Hill, 2004, pp 1397–1402.

Upadhye S, Ross DJ: Subluxed and avulsed tooth management. In Reichman EF, Simon RR (eds): Emergency Medicine Procedures. New York, McGraw-Hill, 2004, pp 1388–1396.

CHAPTER 82

TONGUE-TIE SNIPPING (FRENOTOMY) FOR ANKYLOGLOSSIA

Gary R. Newkirk • Mary Jane Newkirk

"Tongue-tie," or ankyloglossia, results from underdevelopment of the lingual frenum (frenulum) and occurs in nearly 5% of infants. Infants differ substantially in the degree to which their frenum attaches to the tongue. Most cases of tongue-tie are thought to resolve spontaneously by adulthood with little likelihood of feeding or speech development problems. However, the condition is often not noticed until later in life and has been associated with such symptoms as a speech defect (e.g., a lisp), dental problems with the lower teeth, and accumulation of food in the floor of the mouth. If noticed in an infant or child, parents are usually the ones to bring this to the clinician's attention (Fig. 82-1). The condition can easily be overlooked during the newborn examination because infants typically retract and roll the tongue downward when their mouth is open, which effectively hides the frenum from view. Furthermore, newborns rarely stick their tongues out for more than brief periods, so no one notices if the tongue cannot be protruded because of ankyloglossia.

Because tongue-tie is a fairly common and often unnoticed condition that lacks a precise definition, there are few formal outcome studies comparing infants having undergone frenotomy versus not. On one side of the debate, problems with sucking, breast-feeding, chewing, swallowing, dentofacial growth and development, gingival hygiene, and speech have been attributed to tongue-tie. On the other side, some researchers feel that the parents, not the child, have the problem. That is countered, again, by the fact that partial frenotomy, also referred to as *tongue-tie snipping*, remains a quick, easy, and safe procedure with benefits even if performed for cosmetic reasons or parental "dis-ease." Clinicians are more likely to perform partial frenotomy if they believe that ankyloglossia contributes to poor infant sucking and other breast-feeding problems, such as insufficient infant weight gain or sore nipples or recurrent mastitis in the mother. Simple frenotomy for infants and small children who have partial ankyloglossia can be performed safely in the outpatient setting.

The best method and timing for frenotomy remain debatable. When ankyloglossia *severely* interferes with lingual function (e.g., "frozen tongue"), few would argue the need for reduction, but in this case formal Z-plasty is necessary. The patient should be referred to an experienced surgeon because this procedure requires general anesthesia and sometimes a complicated reconstruction.

Anatomically, the frenum of the tongue is a triangular fold of mucous membrane extending back from the lower midline gingival tissue along the floor of the mouth and then arching to the midline of the undersurface of the tongue. The extent to which the tongue portion of the frenum extends along the undersurface to the tip of the tongue is variable. Tongue-tie occurs when the frenum (or an abnormal portion of the frenum) continues distally toward the tip of the tongue so that the height/length of the frenum is so short that it prevents normal elevation or protrusion of the tongue.

INDICATIONS

Clinical evidence of short lingual frenum in an infant with resultant perceived speech problems or inhibited tongue protrusion, feeding, or swallowing.

RELATIVE AND ABSOLUTE CONTRAINDICATIONS

- Lack of clinical evidence or suspicion that ankyloglossia is a problem for the infant or child.
- Unstable medical conditions, such as a bleeding disorder (in many cases, this can be reversed).
- Evidence of dental or oral infection. (The procedure should be postponed until the infection is adequately treated or resolves.)
- Severe ankyloglossia, which requires frenectomy under general anesthesia. (Usually this procedure involves Z-plasty or a similar plastic surgery procedure.)
- Orofacial abnormalities. It is recommended that infants or children with ankyloglossia combined with other orofacial abnormalities be referred.

EQUIPMENT

- Straight or curved mosquito hemostat
- Surgical scissors (some clinicians prefer iris or other straight scissors, others use curved Metzenbaum scissors)
- Tongue retractor (e.g., small spoon, wooden tongue blade)
- Ice, ice chips, popsicle, or teething ring (*optional*)
- Topical anesthetic (e.g., viscous lidocaine, benzocaine [Cetacaine spray or Hurricaine syrup]) (*optional*)
- Infant restraint (e.g., swaddling sheets, circumcision or papoose board) (*optional*)
- Lidocaine with epinephrine, to control bleeding afterward (*optional*)

PREPROCEDURE PATIENT EDUCATION

Describe the risks to the parents, including discomfort; possible medication reaction (if used); recurrence of ankyloglossia during or after healing; injury to tongue or sublingual mucosa or tissue; infection; or bleeding. Parents may help by holding their small child in their lap and, while doing so, holding the child's head still and the

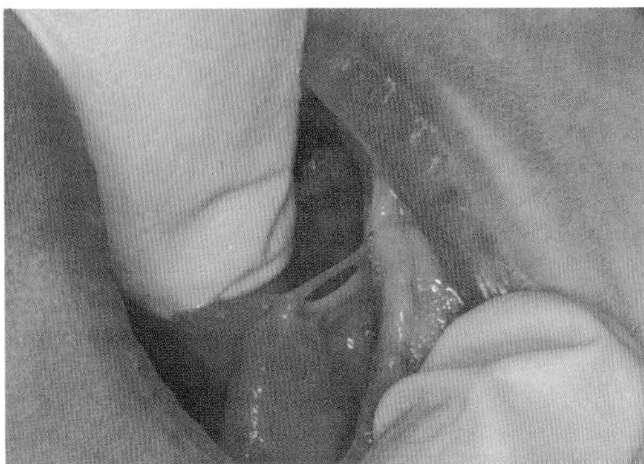

Figure 82-1 Ankyloglossia in a 2-week-old infant experiencing feeding difficulties.

child's mouth open. However, for newborns and infants—for the same reasons as for a circumcision—parents may want to leave the room. After examining the child, if more than one technique is possible, the clinician should explain the various techniques to the parents. Attempt to obtain their input on the desired technique. Parents should be aware that while performance of partial frenotomy may improve tongue function, it does not prevent all tongue, feeding, or speech problems.

Technique

1. With assistance as necessary, position or hold small infants or children in such a way that they will remain still. Wrapping an infant with sheets or a blanket is a very effective method of immobilization. Parents can still hold an infant that is "swaddled" in this manner in their lap. A "circumcision board" is effective if an assistant also stabilizes the head.

   NOTE: Crying often improves exposure of the frenum.

2. Identify the frenum, the abnormal portion of the frenum (causing ankyloglossia), and the necessary degree of surgical lysis. A limited "snipping" of the lucent, membranous portion of the distal frenum is usually all that is required.
3. Many clinicians snip a lucent membranous or very thin fibrinous distal frenum without topical agents or the use of a hemostat, especially for infants younger than 4 months of age. While this technique may increase local bleeding, for a thin membrane there should be no more bleeding than when a child falls and bites his or her lip or tongue. This technique may also cause less overall trauma than with the use of a hemostat. If the child is old enough not to aspirate, have him or her suck on ice, ice chips, or a popsicle before and after the procedure for a certain degree of anesthesia and to minimize bleeding. Younger children may appreciate a frozen teething ring.
4. For a thicker or coarser frenum, topical anesthesia may be beneficial. For example, a cotton-tipped swab can be moistened in benzocaine syrup or sprayed with benzocaine (Fig. 82-2) and focally applied to the lower mouth and bottom of the tongue for excellent local anesthesia (Fig. 82-3). Viscous lidocaine or benzocaine spray can be applied directly to the area in the same manner. Mild sedation may also be beneficial (see Chapter 7, Pediatric Sedation and Analgesia).

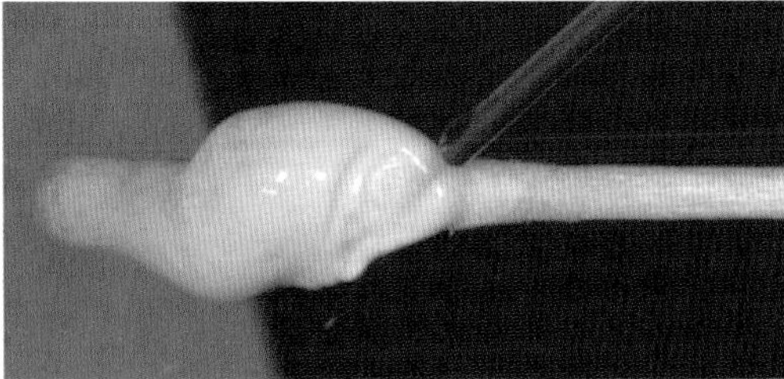

Figure 82-2 Spraying topical anesthetic on a cotton-tipped applicator.

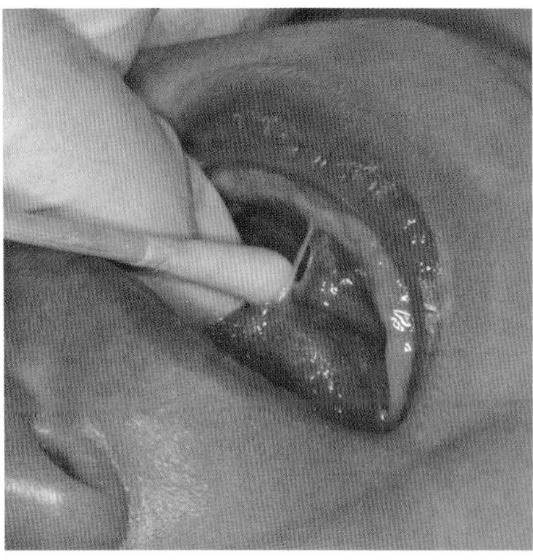

Figure 82-3 Applying topical anesthetic to the frenum and surrounding area.

5. If necessary, retract and gently elevate the tongue. A small spoon or wooden tongue blade with a slit fashioned in the end may be helpful.
6. As an option, with the tip of the mosquito clamp, grab and crush the frenum to the depth and at the position where the scissor snip will be made (Fig. 82-4A). After the discomfort from crushing the tissue has resolved, a certain degree of anesthesia is experienced in the crushed area.
7. Snip the crushed portion of the frenum (Fig. 82-4B). *Warning:* If tissue is snipped outside or beyond the crushed area of the frenum, it will result in more bleeding and pain.

   NOTE: Although crushed tissue is somewhat anesthetized, a patient experiences some discomfort at the time of the crush. A child's immediate memory of pain as the result of an instrument being placed in the mouth may make it difficult to open the mouth again to snip the crushed frenum. This is why some clinicians perform the procedure by simply snipping (Fig. 82-5) without using a hemostat (especially when the frenum is very thin). However, for a thicker and coarser frenum, crushing the tissue with a hemostat will be necessary. For older children, there may be value in telling them that the painful part of the procedure is over after the hemostat has been applied and removed.

8. Use a dry cotton-tipped swab, or one moistened with 1% lidocaine with epinephrine, to control any bleeding or oozing. Ice, a popsicle, or a teething ring may also help control oozing. Figure 82-6 shows the appearance of the completed procedure.

Sample Operative Report

See a sample operative report online at www.expertconsult.com.

Postprocedure Patient Education

- No special care of the surgical site is necessary.
- Ask the patient (or parent) to report significant bleeding or signs of infection.
- Instruct the parent to allow infants and children to resume normal feeding habits immediately.
- Ice chips, an ice cube, or a popsicle for children old enough to not aspirate, or a frozen teething ring for infants, may help stop any later bleeding or oozing.

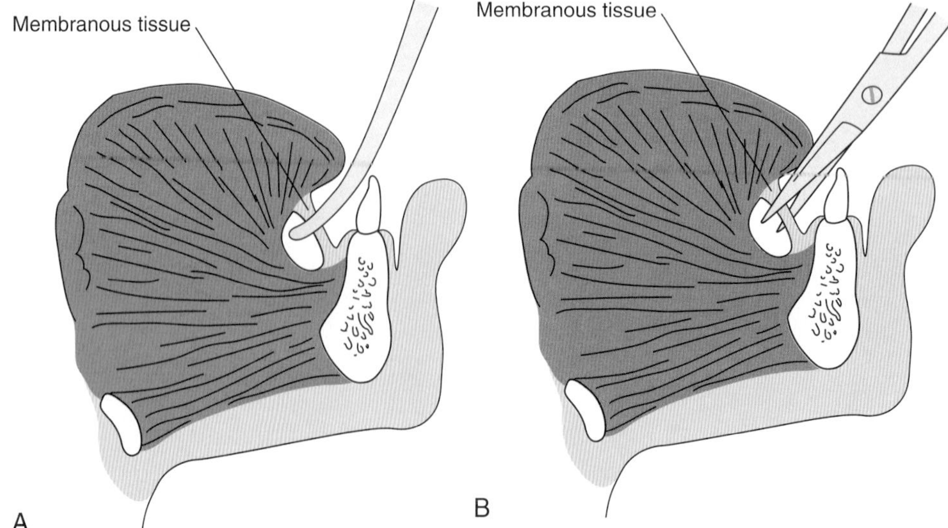

Figure 82-4 Tongue-tie snipping technique. **A,** Crush the abnormal portion of the frenum where the snip is to be made. **B,** Cut through the crushed area.

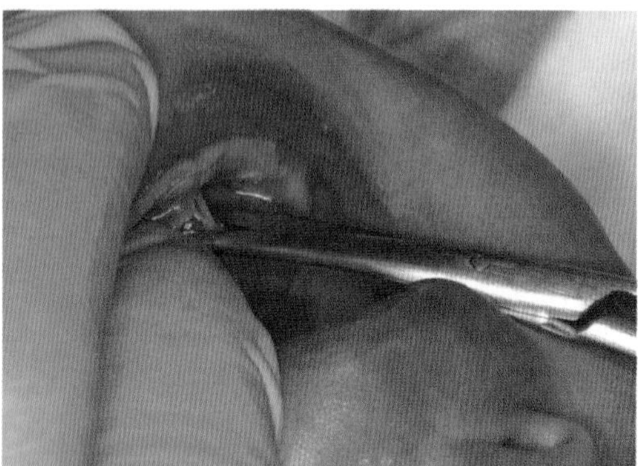

Figure 82-5 Incising the abnormal portion of frenum (causing ankyloglossia) using curved Metzenbaum scissors.

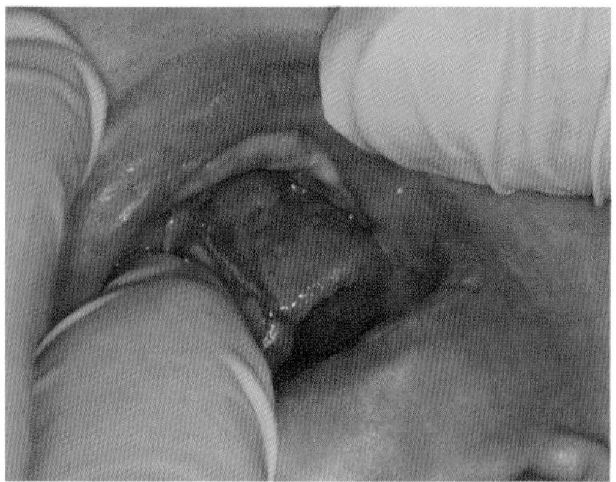

Figure 82-6 Appearance of the normal remaining frenum after partial frenotomy is completed.

- Ask the patient (or parent) to report any feeding difficulties or significant swelling.
- Inform the patient (or parent) to return for follow-up in 2 weeks, or sooner if complications arise.

CPT/Billing Code

41010 Incision of lingual frenum (frenotomy)

ICD-9-CM Diagnostic Code

750.0 Ankyloglossia

Supplier

(See contact information online at www.expertconsult.com.)

Hurricaine Syrup
Beutlich LP Pharmaceuticals

ONLINE RESOURCES

MedlinePlus: Tongue tie. Available at www.nlm.nih.gov/medlineplus/ency/article/001640.htm.

Tongue Tie: From Confusion to Clarity. Available at www.tonguetie.net.

BIBLIOGRAPHY

Hogan M, Westcott C, Griffiths M: Randomized, controlled trial of division of tongue-tie in infants with feeding problems. J Paediatr Child Health 41:246–250, 2005.

Messner AH, Lalakea ML, Aby J, et al: Ankyloglossia: Incidence and associated feeding difficulties. Arch Otolaryngol Head Neck Surg 126:36–39, 2000.

Murtagh J: Release of tongue tie (frenulotomy). In Murtagh J: Practice Tips, 4th ed. Sydney, McGraw-Hill, 2004, p 205.

Ricke LA, Baker NJ, Madlon-Kay DJ, et al: Newborn tongue-tie: Prevalence and effect on breast feeding. J Am Board of Fam Pract 18:1–7, 2005.

Wright JE: Tongue-tie. J Paediatr Child Health 31:276–278, 1995.

CHAPTER 83

TONSILLECTOMY AND ADENOIDECTOMY

Thomas N. Todd

Tonsillectomy is one of the oldest surgeries known. It was first described in 50 A.D. by Celsus, who used a hook to grasp the tonsil and his finger to excise the bulk of the tonsillar tissue. By the 6th century, hygienic concerns had led to the use of knives and other instruments to complete the surgery. These early surgeons were quick to recognize the importance of following the correct tissue planes to be successful, a fact that holds true today. The pain of doing surgery without anesthesia led to the development of instruments that would remove the tonsils quickly. These methods often failed to remove all the tonsillar tissue and obstruction would recur. Throughout the first half of the 20th century, tonsillectomy was performed under local anesthesia and later general anesthesia without airway protection. The procedure was often performed with very few indications in healthy individuals. Adenotonsillectomy reached its peak when 1.4 million procedures were performed in the United States in 1959.

Over the last 50 years the frequency of tonsillectomy and adenoidectomy has declined among American clinicians; however, it still remains the most common surgery performed on children younger than 15 years of age. There are many techniques and innovations that have been tried through the years, from snares to lasers. Many fell out of favor because of concerns over excessive blood loss, tissue damage, excessive postoperative pain, or extended intraoperative time.

This chapter focuses on three of the most popular techniques used today. These are *cold knife and snare* with or without electrocautery, *harmonic ultrasonic scalpel (Ethicon Endosurgery)*, and *bipolar radiofrequency ablation* or *Coblation (Arthrocare)*.

Most studies agree that the less heat introduced into the pharyngeal tissue, the less postoperative pain experienced by the patient. Cold knife and snare removal puts no heat into the system, but cold steel does nothing to stop the bleeding. Bleeding is the most feared complication of tonsillectomy, and electrocautery or sutures must be used as a supplemental measure to control the brisk bleeding. Electrocautery produces considerable heat at the operative site (400° C; Fig. 83-1A). Electrocautery and figure-of-eight sutures also cause collateral tissue damage for several millimeters around the bleeding site. This heat and tissue damage nullifies any benefits the cold knife procedure may have had with respect to lower pain levels or prompter healing rates. Both the harmonic ultrasonic scalpel and the radiofrequency Coblation wand cut and coagulate at the same time, resulting in very little blood loss. Hemostasis is achieved by the production of a protein plug in the end of the cut vessel from the ultrasonic or plasma energy of the devices. The harmonic scalpel generates operative site temperatures of 70° C to 80° C, and the radiofrequency Coblation wand produces a slightly lower temperature of 60° C (Fig. 83-1B). Less heat translates into slightly lower postoperative pain scores for the Coblator compared with the harmonic ultrasonic scalpel. However, recovery time is nearly identical, so the temperatures should not be a significant factor when deciding between these two techniques. All studies agree that lower pain scores and decreased recovery time also come from gentle and careful removal of all of the tonsillar tissue. Therefore, the best method for tonsillectomy is the technique with which the operating clinician is most comfortable, or has the most experience.

ANATOMY OF THE TONSIL BED

See Figure 83-2 for an overview of tonsil bed anatomy.

- **Superior:** soft palate
- **Inferior:** lingual tonsil
- **Deep:** superior constrictor muscle
- **Anterior:** palatoglossus muscle
- **Posterior:** palatopharyngeus muscle
- Vascular supply to the tonsil (Fig. 83-3)
  - Superior pole
    - Ascending pharyngeal artery
    - Lesser palatine artery
  - Inferior pole
    - Tonsillar branches of facial artery
    - Dorsal lingual artery
    - Ascending palatine artery

NOTE: The key to controlling brisk tonsillar bed bleeding is to direct efforts toward the superior or inferior poles first before trying to control every bleeder in the tonsillar bed because the poles are the vascular points of entry.

INDICATIONS FOR TONSILLECTOMY

Absolute Indications

- Hypertrophy resulting in obstructive sleep symptoms in adults or children that lead to adverse pulmonary or cardiovascular conditions
- Hypertrophy and airway obstruction leading to malformation of the facial bones or malocclusion of the teeth requiring dental attention
- Hypertrophy resulting in dysphagia and poor weight gain
- Recurrent peritonsillar abscesses requiring drainage that fail to heal with appropriately dosed medications (see Chapter 80, Peritonsillar Abscess Drainage)
- Tonsillitis that spawns febrile convulsions
- Tonsils that exhibit suspect growth or anatomic characteristics that may require biopsy for the exclusion of malignancy

Relative Indications

- Three or more documented episodes of acute tonsillitis within a year that result in lost time from work or school and require

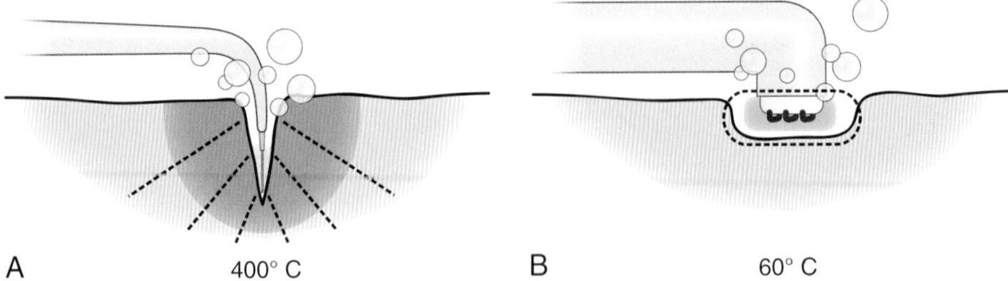

Figure 83-1 **A,** Electrocoagulation produces excessive heat at the operative site and results in a wide area of thermal damage (400° C). **B,** The bipolar radiofrequency ablation (Coblation) wand and the ultrasonic cutting and coagulating instrument (harmonic scalpel) produce low heat (60° C) at the tissue interface while achieving good hemostasis. (Courtesy of ArthroCare ENT, Sunnyvale, Calif.)

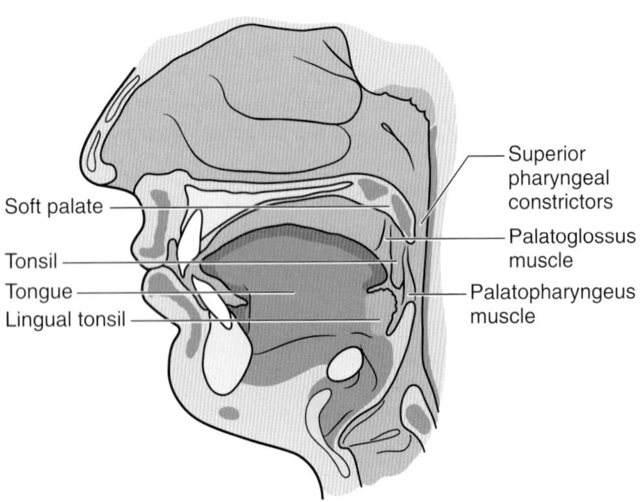

Figure 83-2 Anatomy of the tonsil bed.

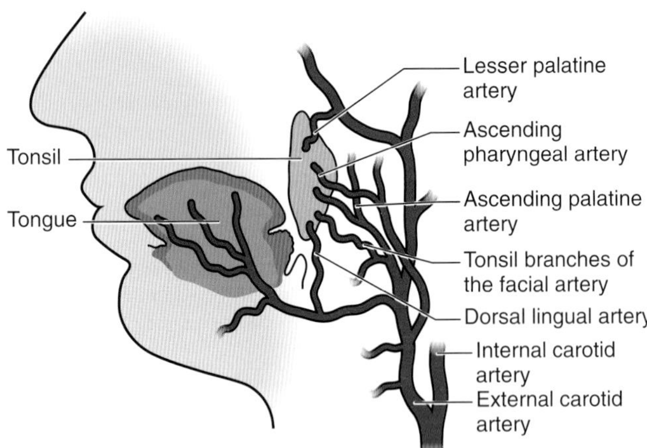

Figure 83-3 The tonsil is sustained by a rich supply of vessels that enter through the inferior pole. Only two branches enter the superior pole. Directing maximum hemostatic effort to the inferior pole controls most of the potential intraoperative bleeding.

treatment by a clinician. (Some clinicians recommend tonsillectomy in children who miss 2 or more weeks of school annually because of tonsillar infections.)
- Persistent episodes of a foul taste in the mouth or malodorous breath that do not clear with appropriate medical therapy.
- Chronic bouts of tonsillitis in a streptococcal carrier that do not respond to beta lactamase–resistant antibiotics.
- Nocturnal enuresis where upper airway obstructive sleep disorder also is present from large tonsils and adenoids.
- Attention deficit hyperactivity disorder resistant to treatment with coexistent upper airway obstructive sleep disorder.

Contraindications to Tonsillectomy and Adenoidectomy

- Poor anesthetic risk
- Uncontrolled medical illness
- Anemia
- Acute bilateral infections
- Anticoagulated patient or patient with coagulopathy (either the anticoagulation/coagulopathy should be reversed or otolaryngology consulted)

Complications of Tonsillectomy and Adenoidectomy

- Hemorrhage during surgery, immediately in the postoperative period, or 5 to 7 days after surgery when the scabs slough off the adenotonsillar bed. Intraoperative bleeding around the endotracheal tube may form a clot and lead to airway obstruction after extubation. Swallowed blood can lead to postoperative nausea and vomiting.
- Dehydration.
- Temporary weight loss during the postoperative period.
- Perforation of the anterior or posterior tonsillar pillars, a benign complication.
- Airway obstruction.
- Death.
- *Specific to adenoidectomy:* nasopharyngeal stenosis and velopharyngeal insufficiency (nasal regurgitation of food and hypernasal speech).

NOTE: Patients with significant airway obstruction due to adenotonsillar hypertrophy may be at risk for postobstructive pulmonary edema syndrome once the obstruction is removed.

Preprocedure Patient Evaluation and Considerations

- Complete blood count, prothrombin time/international normalized ratio (INR), and bleeding time if there is a suspicion or a history of a bleeding disorder.
- Caution in children younger than 3 years of age, or with history of prematurity, seizures, neuromuscular conditions, or asthma, and in anyone with a significant history of obstructive sleep apnea or other severe medical conditions or extenuating circumstances.

NOTE: These patients may have to be monitored more closely in the postoperative period, and some may have to remain overnight to exclude delayed complications.

- Children with cardiovascular defects or heart murmurs must receive appropriate preoperative and postoperative antibiotic treatment.
- Evaluate and possibly remove extremely loose deciduous teeth that could be dislodged during the course of the surgery and threaten the airway.
- Patients should not eat solid foods for 8 hours before surgery.
- Intraoperative intravenous (IV) antibiotics such as ampicillin followed by a 1-week course of oral antibiotics have been shown to significantly reduce postoperative morbidity.
- Injection of local anesthetics into the tonsillar or adenoid beds at the start of surgery may decrease hemorrhage and improve postoperative recovery.
- Universal blood and body fluid precautions should be followed, whichever technique is performed.

TYPES OF TONSILLECTOMY

Figure 83-4 illustrates the two types of tonsillectomy.

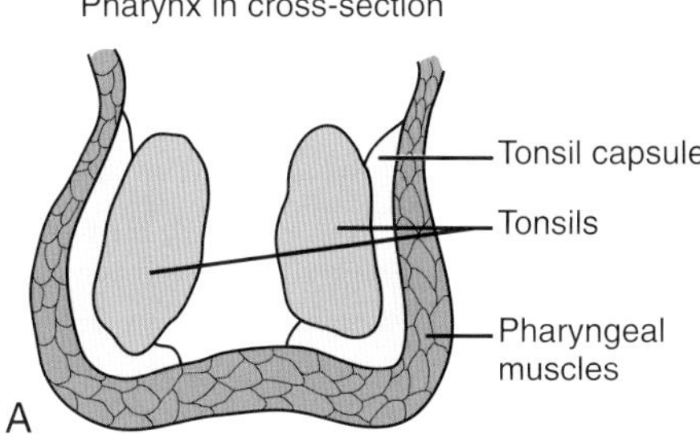

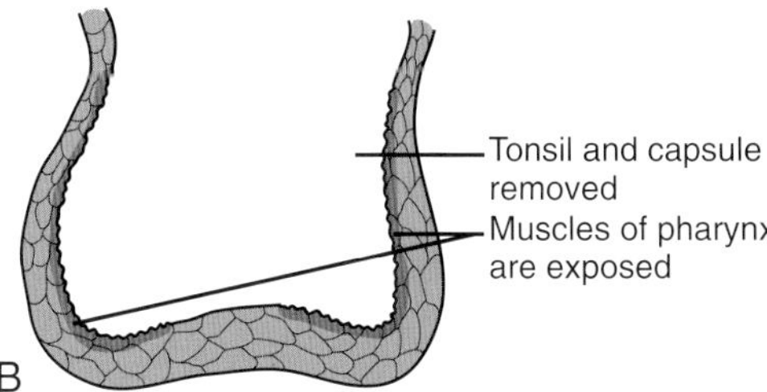

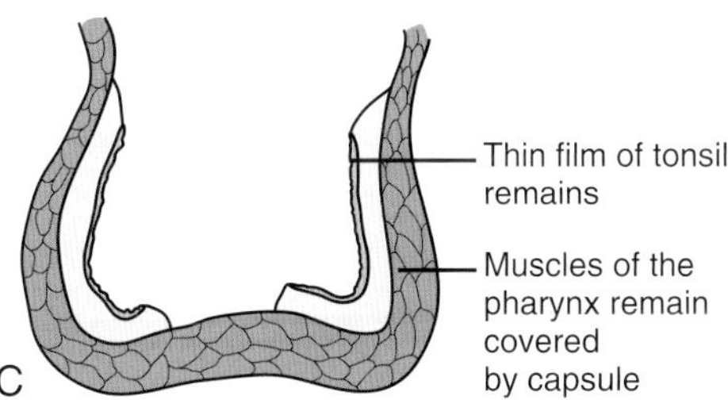

Figure 83-4 **A,** The tonsil is separated from the pharyngeal muscle by a fibrous capsule. **B,** Extracapsular (subcapsular) tonsillectomy removes the tonsil and capsule, leaving the pharyngeal muscle to epithelialize in several weeks. **C,** Intracapsular tonsillectomy leaves the capsule and some tonsil attached. Tonsil regeneration is greater with this procedure.

Intracapsular (Tonsillotomy)

This method removes only the body of the tonsil down to the level of the capsular membrane, which remains in contact with the pharyngeal musculature. The tonsillar tissue is removed in small pieces using suction along with some type of tissue ablation, such as electrocautery, Coblation, or a harmonic scalpel. The incremental removal is useful when extremely friable tonsillar tissue will not allow grasping or traction with a tonsillar forceps to perform a subcapsular procedure. This procedure also theoretically decreases postoperative pain and recovery time. *All the tonsillar tissue must be removed to reduce the risk of bleeding and recurrence.*

Subcapsular

This technique is the favored method in use today. It involves the gentle traction and careful dissection of the tonsil and the capsule from the musculature surrounding the tonsillar bed. Using blunt cold dissection, dissection with the aid of a harmonic ultrasonic scalpel, or radiofrequency ablation, the entire tonsil with accompanying capsule is removed from the tonsillar bed. No redundant capsule or tonsillar tissue is left behind, reducing the risk of delayed complications.

COLD KNIFE AND SNARE METHOD

This is the oldest and most widely recognized method of tonsil removal. Bleeding must be controlled by other means such as electrocautery, vasoactive topical agents, packing, or placement of absorbable sutures.

Equipment

See corresponding numbers in Figure 83-5.

- Self-retaining mouth gag and tongue retractor (1)
- Three sizes of tongue blades
- Operative suction and cautery (2)
- Curved tonsillar tenaculum (3)
- Posterior throat pack with attached retrieval string and small hemostat (4)
- Tonsil dissector and pillar retractor (5)
- Curved tonsil knife (6)
- Tonsillar bed hemostat (7)
- Needle holder (8)
- 0 or 2-0 plain gut suture on tonsil needle (9)
- Laryngeal mirror (10)
- Tonsil snare and wire (11)

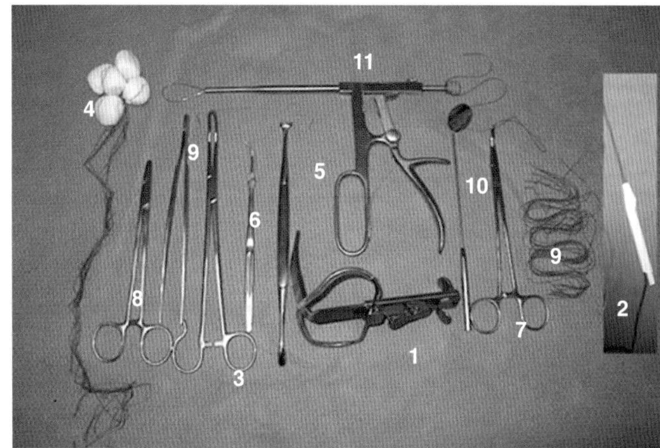

Figure 83-5 Equipment for tonsil removal. See the "Equipment" section under "Cold Knife and Snare Method" for corresponding numbered parts.

Technique

1. The patient is placed supine on the operating table, and the head is hyperextended using a dropped headrest or a shoulder roll. The head must be secured on a donut-style headrest or on head pads.
2. The airway is protected by endotracheal intubation. A self-retaining mouth gag and tongue retractor is placed in the mouth to expose the tonsils. Exposure can be increased by suspending the handle of the tongue retractor from the Mayo stand. Some clinicians prefer to retract the soft palate with a small red rubber catheter placed through the nose and out of the mouth. It can then be secured over the mouth gag with a clamp; however, such a catheter is not always necessary for adequate exposure.

   NOTE: The mouth gag and tongue retractor places pressure on the base of the tongue, so it should be released intermittently to restore circulation to the tongue and, it is hoped, reduce postoperative pain.

3. A throat pack is placed in the posterior pharynx. There should be a string or umbilical tape firmly applied to the pack for later retrieval. A hemostat is placed on the tape and left in place to ensure the pack is removed at the end of the procedure.
4. The tonsil is then grasped at its midpoint using a tonsillar tenaculum. Care should be taken not to grasp the anterior (palatoglossus muscle) or posterior pillars (palatopharyngeus muscle) when grasping the body of the tonsil. The tenaculum is used to apply medial traction on the tonsil, thereby tenting the tonsil into the tonsillar fossae and oral cavity.
5. Begin the dissection superiorly. Using a curved tonsil knife, an incision is made down to the palatoglossus muscle along the posterolateral aspect of the muscle in the plane of the muscle fibers.
6. Using a tonsillar dissector, the tonsil is bluntly and gently dissected away from the bed and removed. The dissection should start from the superior portion of the tonsillar bed and work downward toward the lower one third or inferior portion of the tonsillar bed.
7. Leaving the inferior portion of the tonsil attached to the tonsillar bed, the snare is then applied. (The snare can then be applied over the tonsillar tenaculum's special handle [Fig. 83-6] or the tenaculum removed and then replaced through the loop of the snare.)

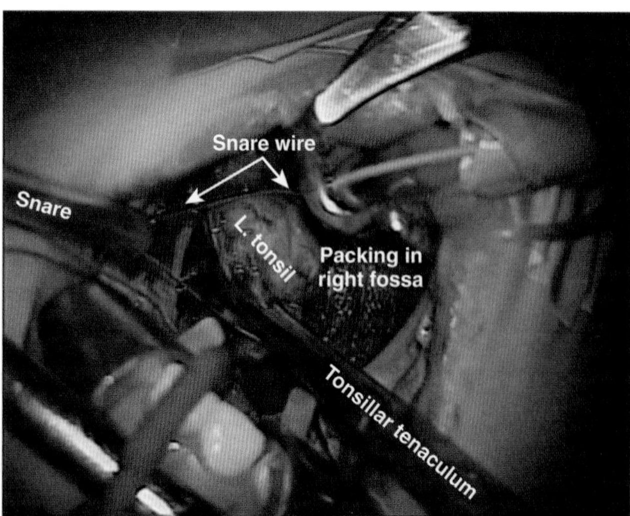

Figure 83-6 The right tonsil has been removed and is packed. The left tonsil has been bluntly dissected from superior to medial, and the tonsil snare is being applied to clip off the inferior pole. Note the generous amount of bleeding in the throat and mouth. (Courtesy of Kevin T. Kavanaugh, MD.)

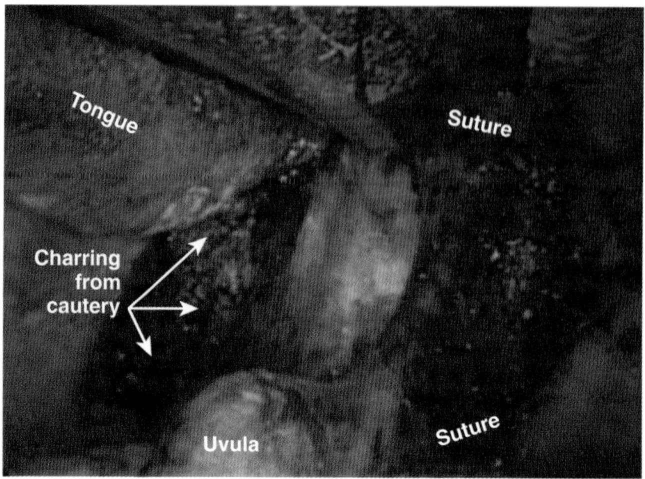

Figure 83-7 If simple packing fails to control postoperative bleeding, then suture ligatures and suction cautery need to be used. The photograph shows the charring of conventional cautery on the left and the area on the right for most effective suture placement to control hemorrhage. (Photograph by Thomas N. Told, DO.)

8. The snare is now tightened slightly so that it nearly approximates the size of the body of the tonsil, but it is not yet tightened around the tonsil.
9. The tip of the snare is then moved to the back of the pharynx, to a point posterior to the body of the tonsil. The wire loop will be bent slightly inferiorly and medially relative to the body of the tonsil.
10. This snare is then closed briskly and firmly, which bluntly dissects the inferior portion of the tonsil away from the tonsillar bed. Bleeding will be brisk from the superior and inferior aspects of the tonsillar fossae. This can be controlled by placing packs into the bleeding tonsillar bed and waiting for the bleeding to stop. Applying figure-of-eight sutures to the superior and inferior aspects of the tonsillar fossae using 0 or 2-0 plain gut sutures on a tonsil needle may help with hemostasis. (Avoid placing the sutures too deeply, which could damage nearby structures, including blood vessels such as the carotid artery.) Unipolar or bipolar cautery, with or without suction, can also be used to ablate the bleeding areas (Fig. 83-7).
11. The procedure is repeated on the opposite side.

Harmonic Scalpel Method

This procedure requires the use of an ultrasonic generator that passes energy to a special titanium rod that vibrates at 55,000 times per second (Hz). This generates enough energy to vaporize tissue at the point of contact with the tip, and this can be limited to the width of a knife blade. The ultrasonic energy also generates enough heat (70° C to 80° C) to form protein plugs in the severed ends of blood vessels (Fig. 83-8).

There are two energy settings on the generator, a low setting (level 3) and a high setting (level 6). Unlike conventional electrocautery, where higher settings result in greater cautery power, the ultrasonic harmonic scalpel creates more hemostasis on the lower settings. The best setting for tonsillectomy is level 3.

The vapor that is generated from cell destruction helps undermine the tissue layers as well.

The tip is disposable and contains a blunt, curved back portion, a sharply hooked front, and large flat sides (Fig. 83-9). Most of the surgery is performed with the blunt, curved back part of the tip because it produces better bleeding control than the sharp, hooked front of the tip (see Fig 83-9). The large, flat side surfaces can also

Figure 83-8 **A,** The ultrasonic generator forms a high-frequency sound wave that is transmitted to the handpiece, where it causes a titanium rod to vibrate at 55,500 Hz. **B,** A special torque wrench ensures proper fit between handle and titanium rod to prevent loss of energy. (Courtesy of Ethicon Endo-Surgery, Inc., Cincinnati, OH.)

be used for hemostasis in areas like the superior and inferior tonsillar poles where the major blood vessels enter. The sharp, hooked portion of the front of the blade can be used to divide the nonvascular membranes or the thick, tough tissue that has been cauterized by the curved back part of the tip. Although the harmonic scalpel can control the usual bleeding that occurs during the course of a normal procedure, other measures such as unipolar cautery or sutures may be required to control larger, more brisk bleeders that cannot be occluded by the harmonic scalpel tip.

Equipment

See the corresponding numbers in Figure 83-10.

- Harmonic scalpel generator and disposable hooked dissection tip (1)
- Self-retaining mouth gag and tongue retractor (2)
- Three sizes of tongue blades (3)
- Curved tonsillar tenaculum (4)
- Posterior throat pack with attached retrieval string and small hemostat (5)
- Operative suction and cautery (6)
- Laryngeal mirror
- Sucralfate liquid
- 0 or 2-0 plain gut tonsil suture, and curved, long-handled needle holder on standby

Technique

1. The patient is placed supine on the operating table with the neck hyperextended and the head secured.
2. The airway is protected by endotracheal intubation. A self-retaining mouth gag and tongue retractor is placed in the mouth, exposing the tonsils. Exposure can be increased by suspending the handle of the tongue retractor from the Mayo stand. Some clinicians prefer to retract the soft palate with a small red rubber catheter placed through the nose and out of the mouth. It can then be secured over the mouth gag with a clamp; however, such a catheter is not always necessary for adequate exposure.
3. The body of the tonsil is grasped with the tonsillar tenaculum and retracted medially into the tonsillar fossae/oral cavity. This will tent the palatoglossus muscle and accentuate the boundaries of the tonsillar body.
4. The dissection begins near the boundary of the palatoglossus muscle with the anterior aspect of the body of the tonsil.
5. Using the blunt, curved back portion of the tip as a scalpel (see Fig. 83-9), and extremely light downward pressure, the tip is

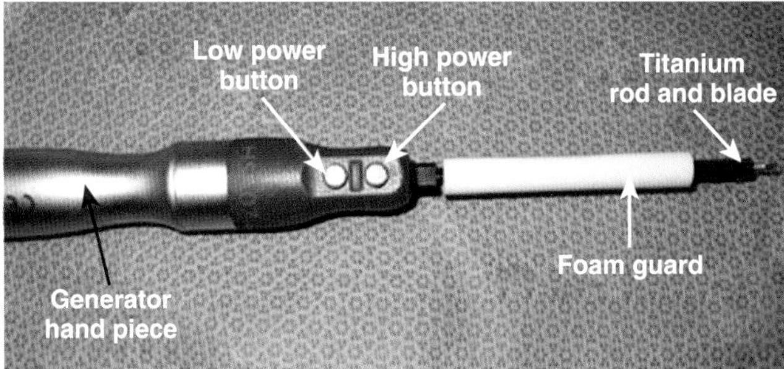

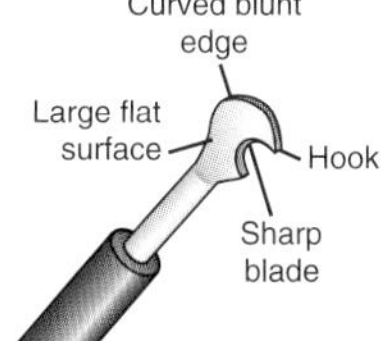

Figure 83-9 Heat can be generated along the rod, so a foam guard covers the rod where it could touch lip and other mouth parts. High power cuts quickly but gives less hemostasis. Low power controls bleeding the best. *Bottom,* Magnified view of the hooked blade shows the operative surfaces. (Courtesy of Ethicon Endo-Surgery, Inc., Cincinnati, OH.)

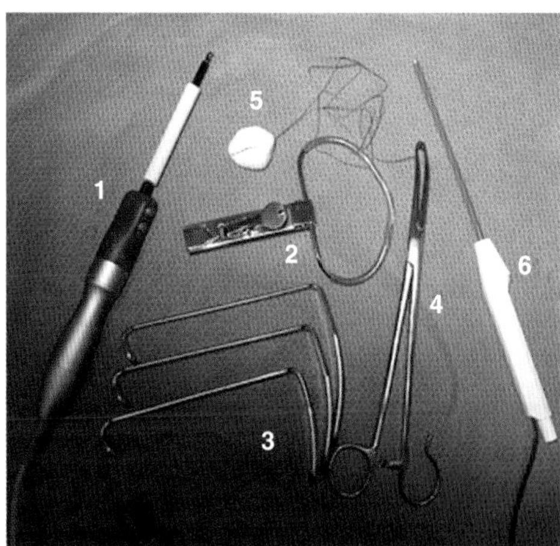

Figure 83-10 Harmonic scalpel method equipment. See the "Equipment" section under "Harmonic Scalpel Method" for corresponding part numbers. (Courtesy of Ethicon Endo-Surgery, Inc., Cincinnati, OH.)

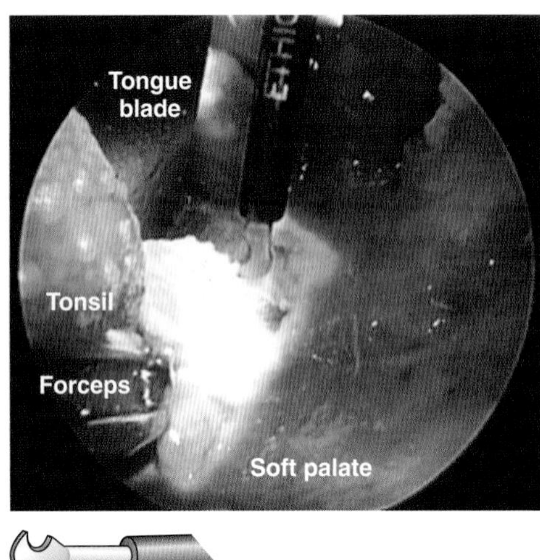

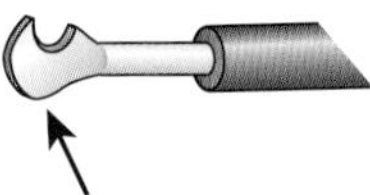

Figure 83-11 Dissection of the middle and superior portion is done with the blunt, curved side of the hooked blade. The traction on the tonsil clamp is in the direction opposite to the plane being operated. Note the white hemostatic capsular plane under the scalpel. *Bottom,* The curved edge *(arrow)* is the best dissector and is used to do most of the procedure. (Photograph by Thomas N. Told, DO.)

energized and moved back and forth a few millimeters each way. Proceed slowly and carefully to deliver the tonsil (Fig. 83-11).

6. There will be some vapor and foam released by the tip. This vapor tends to separate the tissue planes and make the dissection easier. The capsular tissue under the tip will turn white to slightly brown; it is important to stay in this plane. The tonsillar capsule will remain a white and glistening membrane, whereas the delivered tonsil will have an egglike appearance. Continue this maneuver in a lateral and inferior or superior direction until the entire anterior portion of the tonsil is released.
7. If the tip of the harmonic scalpel penetrates the body of the tonsil, the tonsillar tissue will bubble up with the appearance of fresh-cooked oatmeal. If this happens, change the direction and pressure of the tip slightly until you again enter the correct plane.
8. The dissection can then proceed inferiorly or superiorly, depending on which direction the tonsil releases easiest from the bed.
9. The tonsillar tenaculum can be manipulated and twisted to more easily expose the different surfaces of the tonsil (Fig. 83-12).
10. The largest vessels enter the tonsil from the inferior aspect of the tonsillar bed near the lingual tonsil. When dissecting this area, most clinicians use the larger, flat side of the harmonic scalpel tip to create a greater area of hemostasis and less bleeding (Fig. 83-13).
11. When the body of the tonsil is completely released from the superior or inferior tonsillar bed, the tenaculum can then be reapplied to facilitate removal of the tonsil from the palatopharyngeus muscle of the posterior pillar.

    NOTE: When removing the tonsil body from the muscle where tissue planes have been destroyed by infection, it is important to confine the dissection to the tonsillar side rather than the muscular side.

12. When the tonsil is completely removed, residual bleeding can be controlled by placing the flat portion of the dissection tip against the bleeding site and gently tamponading the bleeding. The tip can be placed on low power for 10 seconds to coagulate the bleeding. Small amounts of capillary bleeding can also be controlled by lightly moving the activated tip over the bleeding site until the bleeding stops or a light char appears.

    NOTE: When controlling bleeders, it is important that the clinician be very careful not to apply excessive downward pressure to the tip because it will quickly bury the tip into deeper layers and cause serious bleeding.

13. The procedure is repeated on the opposite tonsil.
14. The tonsillar beds are painted with sucralfate liquid, and the self-retaining retractor released to check for any residual bleeding. The posterior throat pack is removed and the posterior pharynx is then thoroughly suctioned, if necessary.

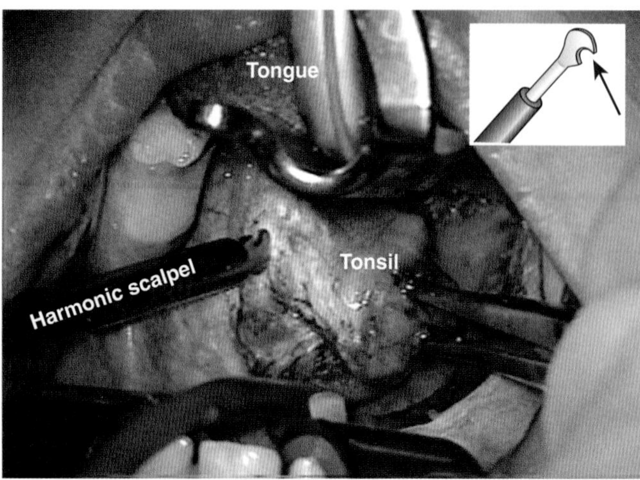

Figure 83-12 The sharp, hooked portion of the harmonic scalpel is not frequently used because it cuts too rapidly to provide effective hemostasis. It is best used on thin tissue in the superior portion of the tonsil, or to cut tough, thick capsule. *Inset:* The sharp, hooked blade *(arrow)* can be used to do fine dissection or transect large avascular tissue.

COBLATION METHOD

This technique is the favorite for many surgeons because it is relatively fast and produces less heat and pain, all leading to shorter recovery times. The wand in this unit contains both suction and

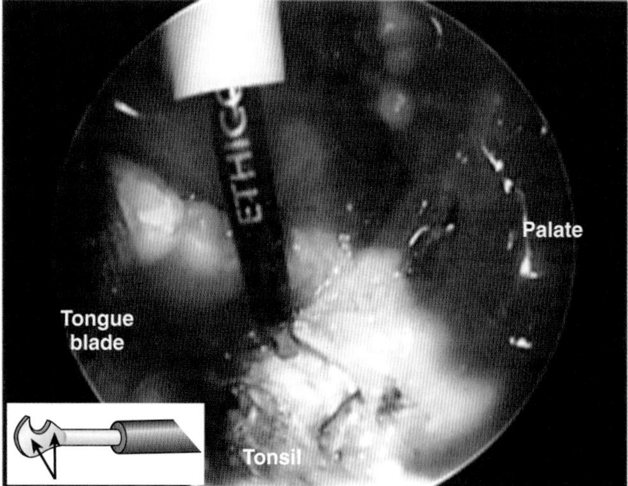

Figure 83-13 The flat portion of the hooked blade is used on the inferior aspect of the tonsil near the tongue blade, where the major blood vessels enter. This achieves maximum hemostasis. Extremely large vessels are gently compressed with the large, flat surface of the blade and power applied for 5 to 10 seconds. *Inset:* The flat surface of the blade *(arrows)* provides the best hemostasis. (Photograph by Thomas N. Told, DO.)

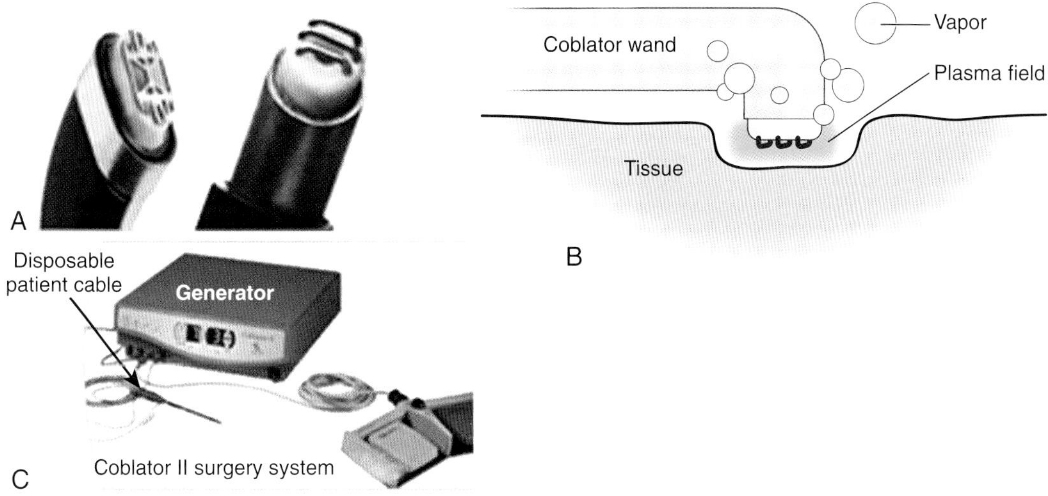

Figure 83-14 The Coblation wand contains both suction and bipolar cautery (**A**). It produces tissue vaporization by passing a bipolar radiofrequency current through normal saline (**B**). The Coblator is the only device that can do both tonsillectomy and adenoidectomy (**C**). (Courtesy of ArthroCare ENT, Sunnyvale, Calif.)

bipolar cautery. It produces tissue vaporization by passing a bipolar radiofrequency current through normal saline (Fig. 83-14A). This results in the production of a plasma field of sodium ions (Fig. 83-14B). This plasma field is able to vaporize tissue at low temperatures (60° C) and coagulate blood in any severed vessels. As previously mentioned, the instrument possesses a built-in suction feature that removes excess water and blood. Larger vessels that are not controlled with the plasma field can be cauterized with the built-in electrocautery. Set the electrocautery feature on the lowest settings that will work to avoid collateral tissue damage. The Coblator is the only device that can do both tonsillectomy and adenoidectomy (Fig. 83-14C). The power of the Coblator's plasma field also can be varied so that the operator can perform either dissection or ablation.

The Coblation wand is more than twice the diameter of the harmonic scalpel, but its curved tip makes it easy to use. Like the harmonic scalpel, the Coblation wand must be used slowly and carefully during dissection for the best results. This device can also perform either an intracapsular or a subcapsular tonsillectomy without requiring extra equipment.

Equipment

See Figure 83-10 for pieces 2 through 5.

- Bipolar radiofrequency Coblator unit and wand (see Fig. 83-14C)
- Self-retaining mouth gag and tongue retractor (2)
- Three sizes of tongue blades (3)
- Curved tonsillar tenaculum (4)
- Posterior throat pack with attached retrieval string and small hemostat (5)
- Laryngeal mirror
- Sucralfate liquid

Technique

1. The patient is placed supine on the operating table with the neck hyperextended and the head secured.
2. The airway is protected by endotracheal intubation. A self-retaining mouth gag and tongue retractor is put in place and, if necessary, suspended from the Mayo stand to increase exposure.
3. The tonsil is grasped with a tonsillar tenaculum and retracted medially.
4. The tip of the wand is used to carefully dissect the anterior portion of the tonsil away from the surrounding muscle. The tip of the wand is always pointed toward the tonsillar tissue to prevent injury to underlying tissue (Fig. 83-15). The tonsil is manipulated to expose the lateral and inferior surfaces to the tip of the wand.
5. Larger vessels are point cauterized with the electrocautery feature. Care must be taken to use the lowest setting to avoid excess tissue damage.
6. The procedure is repeated on the opposite tonsil.
7. The tonsillar fossae are painted with sucralfate solution.
8. The mouth gag is released and the beds are inspected for bleeding.
9. The posterior throat pack is removed and the posterior pharynx is suctioned, if necessary.
10. Both fossae are inspected for the presence of any tonsil tissue (Fig. 83-16).

Indications for Adenoidectomy

- Large adenoids causing upper airway obstruction and resulting in obstructive sleep apnea.
- Children with large adenoids, with or without large tonsils, resulting in snoring and mouth breathing.

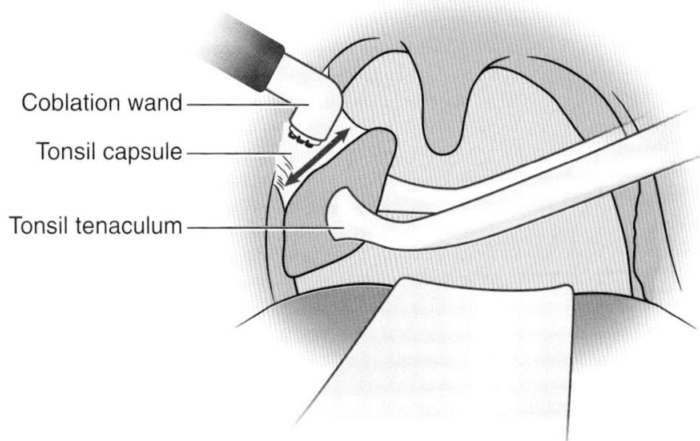

Figure 83-15 The Coblation wand uses a sodium ion cloud at the tissue interface to cut tissue and coagulate blood vessels. Bipolar cautery is also provided to coagulate large bleeding vessels. The wand also contains a suction tip that removes vapor and blood obscuring the operative field. Traction is maintained in an opposing direction to the wand, which aids in separating the tissue planes. (Courtesy of ArthroCare ENT, Sunnyvale, Calif.)

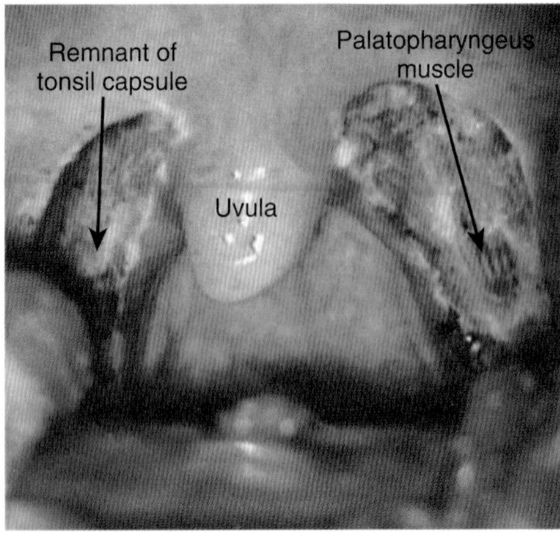

Figure 83-16 Photograph showing the pharynx with both tonsils ultrasonically removed, exposing the posterior tonsil pillars with a thin film of capsule and exposed palatopharyngeus muscle. Note the absence of the charring usually present with conventional electrocautery. (Courtesy of ArthroCare ENT, Sunnyvale, Calif.)

NOTE: There is no evidence that adenoidectomy improves chronic otitis media; therefore, its use is *discouraged* for this condition.

Contraindications to Adenoidectomy

Only conservative adenoidectomy should be performed in the presence of occult submucous cleft palate; therefore, both the hard and soft palates should be examined visually and manually for a cleft palate.

Equipment

See the corresponding numbers in Figure 83-17.

- Self-retaining mouth gags and tongue retractor (1)
- Palate retractor (2)
- Adenoid curettes (3)

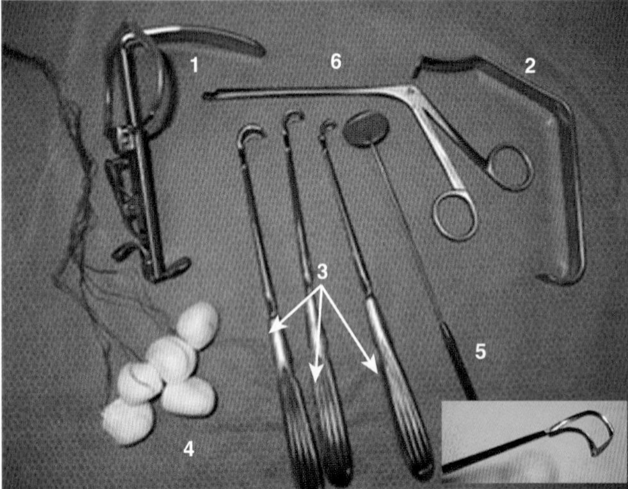

Figure 83-17 Adenoid curettes come in three widths, and care must be taken to choose one that is not too wide. A curette that is too wide may injure the opening to the eustachian tube adjacent to the adenoid tissue. Adenoid tissue around the eustachian tube can be removed with the punch adenotome. See the "Equipment" section under "Adenoidectomy" for corresponding part numbers. *Inset:* Curette blade. (Photograph by Thomas N. Told, DO.)

- Punch adenotome (6)
- Posterior throat pack with attached retrieval string and small hemostats (4)
- Laryngeal mirror (5)
- Suction cautery (optional)
- Nasal suction catheter of appropriate caliber
- Coblation equipment and wand (for coblation method)

Technique

Curette Method

1. A self-retaining mouth gag is placed in the mouth and suspended from the Mayo stand.
2. The hard and soft palates are inspected visually and manually for occult submucous cleft palate. If there is no cleft palate, the soft palate is then retracted with a red rubber catheter that is placed through the nose and out the mouth and clamped over the retractor to expose the adenoid bed.
3. The adenoid bed is inspected with the laryngeal mirror for the presence of adenoid tissue. Adenoid tissue decreases with age and is often gone by the teenage years.
4. An adenoid curette is placed on the adenoid tissue extending superior to the soft palate. It is placed high in the nasopharynx, basically abutting the posterior aspect of the nasal septum.
5. Downward pressure is applied to the curette while the curette is moved along the plane of the posterior pharyngeal muscle (Fig. 83-18). Take care not to penetrate deeply into the prevertebral tissue.
6. The bulk of the adenoid tissue is removed with the first pass.
7. Occasionally a second pass may be needed with grossly enlarged adenoids. Take care not to venture too far laterally to avoid injuring the torus tubarius or eustachian tube opening.

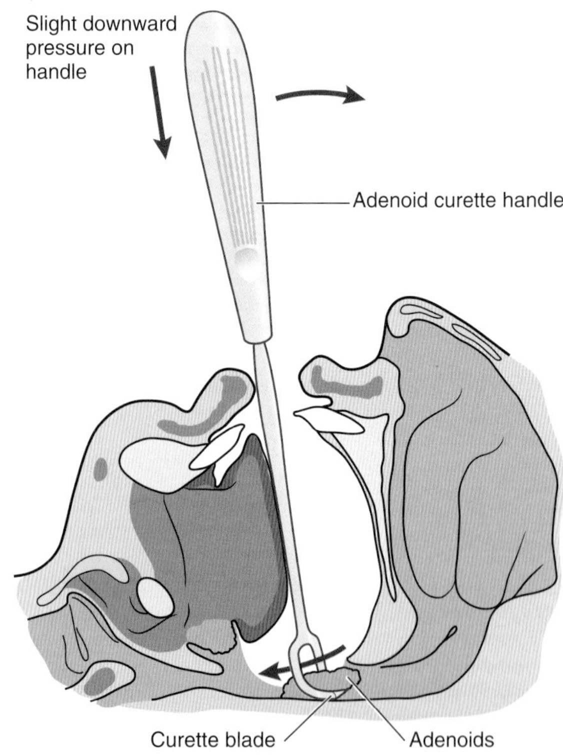

Figure 83-18 The handle of the adenoid curette moves back slightly as the blade moves forward, curetting the tissue. Slight downward pressure is applied to keep the blade in contact with the posterior pharyngeal wall.

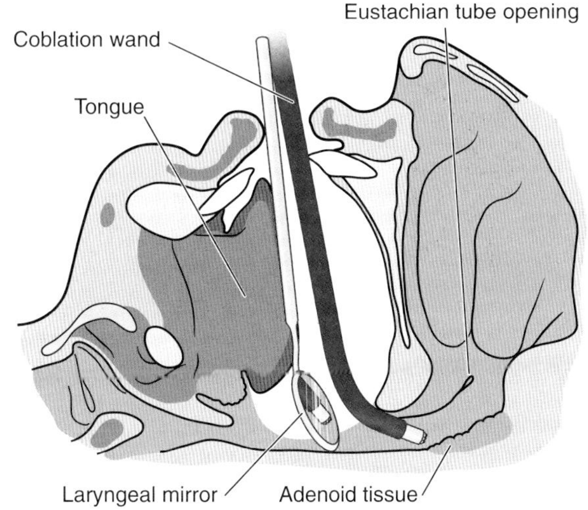

Figure 83-19 Coblation adenoidectomy. (Courtesy of ArthroCare ENT, Sunnyvale, Calif.)

8. Redundant tissue around the opening of the eustachian tube can be carefully removed with a punch adenotome.
9. A nasal suction catheter is inserted and continuous suction is applied for 2 to 3 more minutes, until bleeding stops. Nasopharyngeal packing may also help.
10. Rarely does this technique produce enough bleeding for cautery to be required. Persistent postoperative oozing may be controlled somewhat by nasal decongestant drops.

Coblation Method

1. Patient preparation and exposure are the same as with the curette method.
2. The soft palate is retracted with a red rubber catheter placed through the nose and out the mouth and then clamped over the retractor to expose the adenoid bed.
3. Using a laryngeal mirror, the area to be ablated is inspected.
4. The Coblator is set on level 6 or 7 and the tip of the wand is energized. The tissue is removed to the level of the pharyngeal muscle (Fig. 83-19). Take care not to venture too far laterally, which increases the risk of injury to the openings of the eustachian tubes on both sides of the pharynx.
5. Bleeding can be controlled with the built-in electrocautery feature.

Postprocedure Evaluation and Orders after Tonsillectomy and Adenoidectomy

- Most procedures can be done in same-day surgery.
- Continue IV maintenance fluids until the patient tolerates oral fluids.
- Oral fluids can be started after surgery when the patient is awake enough to protect the airway.
- Some children benefit from postoperative ice collars and cool mist vaporizers.
- Nausea can be controlled with promethazine 12.5 to 25 mg IV every 4 to 6 hours in adults or 0.25 to 1 mg/kg IV every 4 to 6 hours in children. Ondansetron (Zofran) 6 to 8 mg IV every 6 hours in adults and 0.15 mg/kg IV every 4 to 6 hours in children also works well.
- Give IV analgesics such as meperidine 25 to 50 mg IV every 3 hours in adults, and 0.25 to 0.5 mg/kg IV every 3 hours in children for severe pain.
- Morphine sulfate 2.5 to 10 mg every 2 to 4 hours in adults, 0.05 to 0.2 mg/kg every 4 hours in children, also can be given for severe pain.
- If the patient can tolerate oral fluids, give acetaminophen/hydrocodone 500/7.5/15 mL 2.5 to 5 mL orally every 4 hours to children, and 10 to 15 mL orally every 4 hours to adults.
- The role of sucralfate to reduce pain in the postoperative period is still debated, but 1 teaspoon orally four times a day can be of benefit in both children and adults.
- Dexamethasone elixir 0.03 to 0.3 mg/kg/day in children, 0.75 to 9 mg/day in adults, divided into two doses can be used in the postoperative period to reduce swelling and nausea. Given in the immediate postoperative period, dexamethasone is probably of greatest benefit to those patients at risk of laryngeal edema or airway obstruction. In other patients, it may be of benefit to wait until the third postoperative day, when most patients seem to suffer the greatest discomfort. Instituting oral dexamethasone for 3 or 4 days during this time can reduce pain and increase oral intake, and is relatively free of side effects.
- Amoxicillin given orally for 1 week after surgery has been shown to decrease morbidity.
- Children who cannot tolerate oral opioids usually do very well on regular doses of acetaminophen, but they should avoid all aspirin or nonsteroidal anti-inflammatory drug (NSAID)–containing products.
- Adults who can tolerate oral tablets can be sent home on oral analgesics that contain no aspirin or NSAIDs.

CPT/Billing Codes

42825 Tonsillectomy, primary or secondary, younger than age 12
42826 Tonsillectomy, primary or secondary, age 12 or over
42830 Adenoidectomy, primary, younger than age 12
42831 Adenoidectomy, primary, age 12 or over

ICD-9-CM Diagnostic Codes

474.00 Tonsillar hypertrophy with chronic tonsillitis
474.01 Tonsillar enlargement with chronic adenoiditis
474.02 Tonsillar hypertrophy (hyperplasia) with chronic adenoiditis and tonsillitis
474.8 Tonsillar remnant or tag
474.9 Tonsillar disease, chronic
474.10 Tonsillar hyperplasia with adenoid hyperplasia
474.11 Tonsillar enlargement or hyperplasia

Patient Education Guides

See patient education form available online at www.expertconsult.com.

Suppliers

(See contact information online at www.expertconsult.com.)

Coblator
ArthroCare ENT
Harmonic scalpel
Ethicon Endo-Surgery, Inc. (Johnson & Johnson)

Online Resources

ENT USA: Tonsillectomy: Tonsil and adenoid surgery (video presentation of tonsillectomy and adenoidectomy using various methods). Available at www.entusa.com/tonsils_adenoid_surgery.htm.

BIBLIOGRAPHY

Tonsillectomy and adnoidectomy. In Cummings CW, Haughey BH, Thomas JR (eds): Cummings Otolaryngology: Head and Neck Surgery, 4th ed. St. Louis, Mosby, 2005.

Wein RO, Chandra RK, Weber RS: Disorders of the head and neck. In Brunicardi FC, Andersen DK, Billiar TR, et al (eds): Schwartz's Principles of Surgery, 8th ed. New York, McGraw-Hill, 2005, pp 369–395.

SECTION 5

Cardiovascular and Respiratory System Procedures

Section Editor: JOE ESHERICK

CHAPTER 84

Ambulatory Blood Pressure Monitoring

Russell D. White • Thomas H. Mitchell

Ambulatory blood pressure monitoring (ABPM) is an automated, noninvasive technique for obtaining blood pressure measurements at predetermined intervals over an extended period of time (usually 24 hours or more) while the patient goes about his or her daily activities. The process involves attaching a measuring and recording device to the patient. These devices are lightweight and use either the auscultatory (i.e., microphone and Korotkoff's sounds) or the oscillometric method (i.e., senses arterial waves) to determine blood pressure. Although the auscultatory method needs low ambient noise levels to obtain its most accurate results, it tolerates patient movement better than the oscillometric method. In contrast, although the oscillometric method tolerates high levels of environmental noise, it is most accurate when the patient is less physically active. The recordings can be downloaded for analysis.

Hypertension has traditionally been defined as an office systolic blood pressure of 140 mm Hg or higher and diastolic blood pressure of 90 mm Hg or higher; however, it is now defined at lower levels for patients with diabetes or target organ damage (e.g., left ventricular hypertrophy, heart failure, angina or prior myocardial infarction, prior coronary revascularization, stroke or transient ischemic attack, dementia, chronic kidney disease [glomerular filtration rate <60 mL/min], peripheral arterial disease, retinopathy), and elevated systolic blood pressure is frequently isolated (i.e., elevated in the absence of elevated diastolic blood pressure). Over 50 million Americans are hypertensive, a major risk factor for such common diseases as cardiovascular disease, stroke, aortic aneurysm rupture, renal failure, and retinopathy. Because some patients are hypertensive only during specific hours of the day, documentation of adequate blood pressure control over 24 hours is imperative to prevent sequelae. Studies have shown that hypertension diagnosed with ABPM more often correlates with target organ damage than hypertension noted on sporadic blood pressure measurements in the office setting (especially in patients with albuminuria or echocardiographically determined left ventricular hypertrophy). Patients whose average pressures by 24-hour ABPM are greater than 135/85 mm Hg have twice the risk for a cardiovascular event compared with those with 24-hour mean blood pressures less than 135/85 mm Hg, regardless of the blood pressures measured in the office. In most people, blood pressure decreases by 10% to 20% at night; those without such a reduction (i.e., nondippers) are at increased risk of cardiovascular events. Conversely, overtreatment of hypertension can lead to complications such as transient hypotension, dizziness, and myocardial ischemia. In addition, as many as 21% of patients with mild blood pressure elevation in the office are *incorrectly* diagnosed with and treated for hypertension. Likewise, although having the patient monitor his or her blood pressure at home (i.e., self-monitored blood pressure) can improve blood pressure control, it has been difficult to correlate such a practice with fewer cardiovascular events. Therefore, ABPM offers an alternative to both office and home blood pressure measurements, facilitating both the diagnosis and the management of hypertension.

Indications

Routine sporadic blood pressure measurements in the office setting remain the recommended method to screen for and monitor hypertension. ABPM should not be used indiscriminately as a screening device. However, because blood pressure measurements in the office can lead to both false-positive and false-negative results, ABPM can be useful for finalizing the diagnosis. Figure 84-1 provides a helpful algorithm. Indications may include the following:

- Normal or borderline office hypertension with target organ damage (defined by the American Heart Association [AHA] and the National Institutes of Health [NIH] Joint National Committee's [JNC] Seventh Report as left ventricular hypertrophy, heart failure, angina or prior myocardial infarction, prior coronary revascularization, stroke or transient ischemic attack, dementia, chronic kidney disease [glomerular filtration rate <60 mL/min], peripheral arterial disease, retinopathy)
- Persistent office hypertension without target organ damage
- Discrepancy between office and home blood pressure measurements (especially in diabetic and elderly patients)
- Considerable blood pressure variability found during same office visit or over different visits
- Episodic hypertension (e.g., smoking raises blood pressure acutely, and the level returns to baseline about 15 minutes after stopping)
- Episodic angina or pulmonary congestion *unrelated* to exercise
- Determination of the duration or efficacy of antihypertensive medications during the 24-hour treatment cycle
- Dosage adjustment of antihypertensive medications
- Documented hypertension unresponsive to treatment ("drug resistance")
- Suspected pressor ("white coat") hypertension and no target organ damage
- Office blood pressure elevated during pregnancy and preeclampsia suspected
- Autonomic dysfunction
- Hypotensive symptoms while on antihypertensive medication
- Evaluation of syncope or pacemaker syndromes

Contraindications and Limitations

- Cost: some insurance companies may not reimburse for ABPM
- Irregular, rapid heart rate: limits ability to obtain blood pressure measurements and limits the accuracy of ABPM
- Severe obesity: limits ability to obtain blood pressure measurements and limits the accuracy of ABPM
- Severe patient anxiety regarding instrument

Ambulatory blood pressure monitoring

Persistent office hypertension

CCD/TOD?

Yes → Start treatment

No

Home blood pressure

Persistently low/normal → White coat hypertension 24-hr mean ABPM <135/85 mm Hg → Continue to monitor

Persistently elevated → Start treatment

Difficult to interpret/unavailable → 24-hour ABPM

Ambulatory hypertension 24-hr mean ABPM >135/85 mm Hg

Nondipping SBP reduction from day to night <10% → Start treatment

Dipping SBP reduction from day to night >10%

<1 risk factor*; no diabetes, or CCD/TOD, and blood pressure load[†] >30% → Continue to monitor

>1 risk factor; diabetes, CCD/TOD, or blood pressure load >30% → Start treatment

Figure 84-1 Algorithm for appropriate use of ambulatory blood pressure monitoring (ABPM). CCD, clinical cardiovascular disease; SBP, systolic blood pressure; TOD, target organ damage. *Major cardiovascular risk factors in patients with hypertension (Joint National Congress VI) include smoking, dyslipidemia, diabetes, age older than 60, gender (men and postmenopausal women), and family history of early cardiovascular disease. [†]The proportion of blood pressures during the monitoring period that are increased relative to preset thresholds (140/90 mm Hg awake, 120/80 mm Hg asleep). (Updated from Ernst ME, Bergus GR: Ambulatory blood pressure monitoring: Technology with a purpose [editorial]. Am Fam Physician 67:2262–2263, 2003; with permission.)

Preprocedure Patient Preparation

The procedure should be explained to the patient as well as its risks, benefits, and any alternatives. Obtain either verbal or written consent. Patients should be instructed to record any symptoms or events that occur during the monitoring period and any medications they are taking (and when they take them). In most cases, they should be instructed not to speak or move during cuff deflation (recording phase). Patients should also usually avoid strenuous activity (e.g., running or racquet sports) during the study. They should know how long they will be monitored, where to go to have the equipment removed, and when they might expect the results. If not contraindicated, the clinician may choose to offer the patient a sleep medication to minimize the equipment's interference with sleep.

Equipment

- Monitor (with instructions) for ABPM
- Automatic blood pressure cuff and sphygmomanometer
- Connectors and tubing
- 24-hour diary for events, activities, and medications

Technique

1. The clinician should follow the manufacturer's instructions for attaching the equipment and performing the procedure. However, this usually means placing the microphone/sensor over the brachial artery proximal to the elbow of the *nondominant* arm (Fig. 84-2). *Proper positioning of the microphone/sensor is critical.*
2. Select the appropriate cuff size. The bladder inside the cuff should encircle 80% of the upper arm circumference without overlap.
3. Attach and secure the automatic cuff to the upper arm. To prevent shifting of the cuff on the arm, an adhesive-backed strap is usually placed on the arm. The cuff is then placed around the arm and secured to the adhesive-backed strap, often by snapping it in place.
4. Connect the cuff–microphone/sensing unit to the monitor.
5. The connecting tubing is passed under upper body clothing to the monitor worn on the waist in a carrying pouch.
6. Calibrate the monitor for each patient in the lying, sitting, and standing positions. Measure blood pressure simultaneously with a manual cuff and sphygmomanometer or sphygmomanometer attached to the monitor through a T-tube device. (Three consecutive measurements should be within 3 to 5 mm Hg of one another.)
7. Secure the hose and microphone/sensor cable in a manner that will minimize patient discomfort.
8. Set the frequency of recordings. (Typical is three to four times per hour during waking hours and one to two times per hour during sleeping hours.)
9. Instruct the patient to record any symptoms or events, his or her activities, and which medications were taken and when they were taken during the monitoring period.
10. Instruct the patient to not speak or move during cuff deflation (i.e., recording phase).

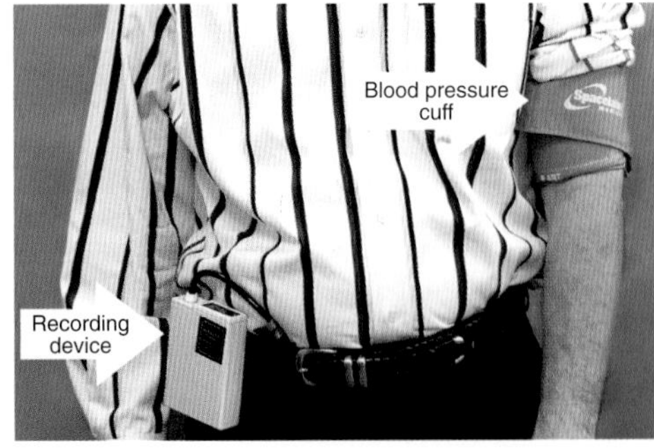

Figure 84-2 Placement of ambulatory blood pressure monitoring unit.

11. Instruct the patient to avoid strenuous activity (e.g., running or racquet sports) during the study.
12. Remove the monitoring and recording device at the end of the study period and retrieve the recorded data.

Complications

- Inaccurate or incomplete results
- Interference with normal sleep patterns
- Inconvenience related to device
- Petechiae at measurement site
- Arm edema distal to cuff
- Transient arm discomfort
- Dermatitis
- Ulnar nerve palsy (rare)

Interpretation of Results

Information acquired from ABPM normally includes (1) *average* blood pressures (usually average systolic, diastolic, and mean blood pressures); (2) *diurnal fluctuations* in blood pressure; and (3) *short-term variability* of blood pressure.

Most normotensive individuals exhibit a circadian pattern of blood pressure, reaching a peak during the daytime hours and a nadir after midnight (however, shift workers may reverse this pattern). Hypertensive patients also usually follow this diurnal pattern, with (as mentioned previously) an average blood pressure greater than 135/85 mm Hg when awake and greater than 120/75 mm Hg during sleep. Blood pressure usually increases after awakening and with increased activity in the early morning. Staessen and colleagues (1991) reviewed several studies and summarized average diurnal blood pressures (Table 84-1). Combining these data with the criteria of the JNC 7 report (Chobanian et al., 2003), the 2007 European Society for Hypertension–European Society for Cardiology guidelines (Table 84-2), and other data, the following diagnostic criteria are suggested:

- *Hypertension* is diagnosed if more than 30% of the 24-hour systolic readings are greater than 140 mm Hg, or greater than 90 mm Hg for diastolic readings (Fig. 84-3). This is an abnormal *blood pressure load* (percentage of elevated systolic and diastolic pressures during a 24-hour period). In patients with diabetes or target organ damage, hypertension should be diagnosed if more than 30% of the 24-hour systolic readings are greater than 130 mm Hg, or greater than 80 mm Hg for diastolic readings.
- Average systolic arterial pressure greater than 130 mm Hg or average diastolic pressure greater than 80 mm Hg is considered *hypertension*. Also, daytime average systolic pressure greater than 135 mm Hg or daytime average diastolic pressure greater than 85 mm Hg, or night-time average systolic pressure greater than 120 mm Hg or night-time average diastolic pressure greater than 70 mm Hg is considered *hypertension* (2007 European Society for Hypertension–European Society for Cardiology guidelines).
- A *nondipper* is diagnosed if the patient's blood pressure does not decrease by at least 10% at night. If the patient is being treated for hypertension, medications may need to be given at bedtime or a medication with a longer half-life chosen.
- Finally, patients whose blood pressure recordings *vary widely* during 24-hour ABPM may require medication changes to provide control during the entire 24 hours.

TABLE 84-1 Average Normal Ambulatory Blood Pressure Monitoring Values

	Day	Night	24-Hour
Average blood pressure (mm Hg)	123/76	106/64	118/72
Systolic range (mm Hg)	101–146	86–127	97–139
Diastolic range (mm Hg)	61–91	48–79	57–87

From Staessen JA, Fagard RH, Lijnen PJ, et al: Mean and range of the ambulatory pressure in normotensive subjects from a meta-analysis of 23 studies. Am J Cardiol 67:723–727, 1991.

TABLE 84-2 Blood Pressure Thresholds (mm Hg) for Definition of Hypertension with Different Types of Measurement

Measurement	Systolic Blood Pressure	Diastolic Blood Pressure
Office or clinic	140	90
24-hour	125–130	80
Day	130–135	85
Night	120	70
Home	130–135	85

From Mancia G, De Backer G, Dominiczak A, et al: 2007 Guidelines for the management of arterial hypertension: The Task Force for the Management of Arterial Hypertension of the European Society of Hypertension (ESH) and of the European Society of Cardiology (ESC). Eur Heart J 28:1462–1536, 2007.

CPT/Billing Codes

93784 Ambulatory blood pressure monitoring, utilizing a system such as magnetic tape and/or computer disk, for 24 hours or longer, including recording, scanning analysis, interpretation and report
93786 Recording only
93788 Scanning analysis with report
93790 Physician review with interpretation and report

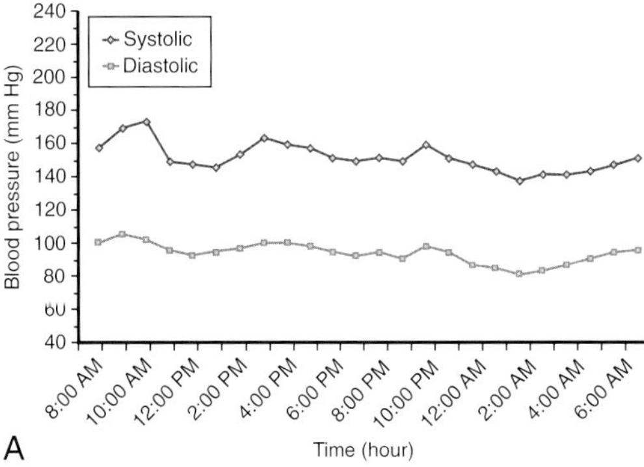

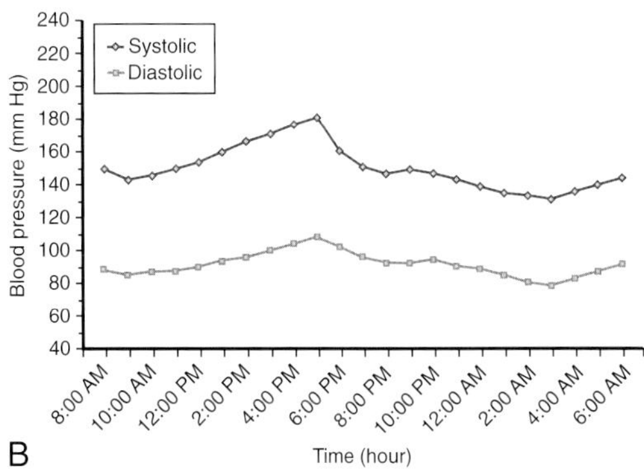

Figure 84-3 Two examples of 24-hour ambulatory blood pressure monitoring (ABPM) recordings in hypertensive patients. **A,** The first patient is newly diagnosed and needs to be treated. **B,** This report is for a different patient on a low-dose antihypertensive medication and the dose needs to be increased. If the patient is having symptoms, it is unlikely to be due to the medication.

ICD-9-CM Diagnostic Codes

Hypertension

X means additional digit required.

401 Hypertension, essential
- 401.0 Malignant
- 401.1 Benign
- 401.9 Unspecified

402 Hypertensive heart disease (e.g., cardiomegaly, cardiomyopathy, cardiovascular disease)
- 402.00 Malignant, without heart failure
- 402.01 Malignant, with heart failure
- 402.9 Unspecified
- 402.10 Benign, without heart failure
- 402.11 Benign, with heart failure

403 Hypertensive chronic kidney disease
- 403.00 Malignant, stage 1 through IV
- 403.01 Malignant, stage V or end stage
- 403.1X Benign
- 403.9X Unspecified

404 Hypertensive heart and chronic kidney disease
- 404.02 Malignant, stage I through IV
- 404.03 Malignant, stage V or end stage
- 404.1X Benign
- 404.9X Unspecified

405 Secondary hypertension
- 405.01 Malignant, renovascular
- 405.9 Unspecified
- 405.11 Benign, renovascular
- 405.19 Benign, other

796.2 Elevated blood pressure reading without diagnosis (incidental without diagnosis)

Hypotension

458.0 Orthostatic or postural
458.1 Chronic hypotension, permanent, idiopathic
458.2 Iatrogenic, abnormally low blood pressure due to medical treatment
458.8 Other specified hypotension
458.9 Hypotension, unspecified

Syncope

780.2 Syncope, cardiac, vasovagal, fainting, pre- or near-syncope
337.0 Carotid sinus or idiopathic peripheral autonomic neuropathy
337.9 Disorder of autonomic nervous system, unspecified

Cardiomyopathy

425.1 Hypertrophic obstructive cardiomyopathy
425.3 Endocardial fibroelastosis
425.4 Other primary cardiomyopathies (congestive, constrictive, familial, hypertrophic, idiopathic, nonobstructive, obstructive, restrictive, cardiovascular collagenosis)
425.5 Alcohol cardiomyopathy
425.7 Nutritional/metabolic cardiomyopathy
425.8 Cardiomyopathy in other diseases classified elsewhere (e.g., progressive muscular dystrophy, sarcoidosis)
425.9 Secondary cardiomyopathy, unspecified

Patient Education Guides

See patient education form available online at www.expertconsult.com.

Acknowledgment

The editors wish to recognize the contributions by Peter Hanson, MD, and Diane Lillis, RN, to this chapter in a previous edition of this text.

Suppliers

(See contact information online at www.expertconsult.com.)

Advanced BioSensor, Inc.
Colin Medical (Omron)
Lifesource Medical (A & D Medical)
SpaceLabs Healthcare
SunTech Medical
Welch Allyn

BIBLIOGRAPHY

Appel LJ, Robinson KA, Guallar E, et al: Utility of blood pressure monitoring outside of the clinic setting. Evidence Report/Technology Assessment Number 63. AHRQ publication no. 03-E003. Rockville, Md, Agency for Healthcare Research and Quality, 2002.

Chobanian AV, Bakris GL, Black HR, et al, Committee on Prevention, Detection, Evaluation, and Treatment of High Blood Pressure. National Heart, Lung, and Blood Institute; National High Blood Pressure Education Program Coordinating Committee: Seventh Report of the Joint National Committee on Prevention, Detection, Evaluation, and Treatment of High Blood Pressure: JNC 7. Hypertension 42:1206–1252, 2003.

Clement DL, De Buyzere ML, De Bacquer DA, et al: Prognostic value of ambulatory blood-pressure recordings in patients with treated hypertension. N Engl J Med 348:2407–2415, 2003.

Ernst ME, Bergus GR: Ambulatory blood pressure monitoring: Technology with a purpose [editorial]. Am Fam Physician 67:2262–2263, 2003.

Gardner SF, Schneider EF: 24-Hour ambulatory blood pressure monitoring in primary care. J Am Board Fam Pract 14:166–177, 2001.

Mancia G, De Backer G, Dominiczak A, et al: 2007 Guidelines for the management of arterial hypertension: The Task Force for the Management of Arterial Hypertension of the European Society of Hypertension (ESH) and of the European Society of Cardiology (ESC). Eur Heart J 28:1462–1536, 2007.

Mancia G, Facchetti R, Bombelli G, et al: Long-term risk of mortality associated with selective and combined elevation in office, home, and ambulatory blood pressure. Hypertension 47:846–853, 2006.

Marchiando RJ, Elston MP: Automated ambulatory blood pressure monitoring: Clinical utility in the family practice setting. Am Fam Physician 67:2262–2270, 2003.

Ohkubo T, Kikuya M, Metoki H, et al. Prognosis of “masked” hypertension and “white-coat” hypertension detected by 24-h ambulatory blood pressure monitoring: 10-year follow-up from the Ohasama study. J Am Coll Cardiol 46:508–515, 2005.

Sheps SG, Clement DL, Pickering TG, et al: Ambulatory blood pressure monitoring: Hypertensive Diseases Committee, American College of Cardiology. J Am Coll Cardiol 23:1511–1513, 1994.

Staessen JA, Fagard RH, Lijnen PJ, et al: Mean and range of the ambulatory pressure in normotensive subjects from a meta-analysis of 23 studies. Am J Cardiol 67:723–727, 1991.

Verdecchia P: Prognostic value of ambulatory blood pressure: Current evidence and clinical implications. Hypertension 35:844–851, 2000.

White WB, Berson AS, Robbins C, et al: National standard for measurement of resting and ambulatory blood pressures with automated sphygmomanometers. Hypertension 21:504–509, 1993.

CHAPTER 85

AMBULATORY PHLEBECTOMY

Karl S. Hubach

The treatment of venous disease has undergone considerable change in the past two decades. Ambulatory phlebectomy (AP) remains popular as a surgical means of removing large varicose veins. This chapter introduces the basic techniques and ideas behind AP, which is an in-office surgical technique used to remove varicose veins through multiple small incisions. It is performed using only a local anesthetic and yet provides excellent cosmetic and functional results. When the compression bandage is in place, ambulation is allowed immediately after the procedure. Because the highest (most proximal) point of reflux in the venous system must be corrected for AP to remain successful, AP is frequently done in conjunction with another procedure such as junctional ligation, ultrasonography-guided sclerotherapy, an ablation procedure with laser or radiofrequency, or venous stripping (see Chapter 86, Endovenous Vein Ablation, and Chapter 92, Sclerotherapy).

Benefits of AP include the following:

- It is performed in an outpatient setting.
- It is a convenient, safe, and cost-effective treatment for varicose veins.
- The patient is able to walk out of the office following the procedure with little to no change in his or her level of activity.
- The rate of complications is extremely low.
- The procedure can be performed without hospitalization or general anesthesia and it allows for a return to normal activity; thus the expense to the patient and the health care system is markedly reduced.

Therefore, AP provides an excellent addition to the total care and treatment of varicose veins and venous disease.

INDICATIONS

- To remove veins of most sizes for symptomatic or cosmetic reasons
- Primarily used for the removal of symptomatic, visible varicose veins of the lower extremities

CONTRAINDICATIONS

Absolute

- Known metastatic carcinoma
- Allergy to the local anesthetic
- Hypercoagulable or hypocoagulable state
- Severe arterial occlusive diseases (see Chapter 88, Noninvasive Venous and Arterial Studies of the Lower Extremities)
- Hemodynamically important secondary varicosities
- Poor general health
- Incapacitated elderly patient
- CREST syndrome (calcinosis, Raynaud's phenomenon, esophageal involvement, sclerodactyly, and telangiectasia) involving the lower extremities

Relative

- Superficial thrombophlebitis
- Bacteremia and certain other blood-borne infectious diseases
- Pregnancy
- Coagulopathies
- Propensity to keloid formation
- Significant fibrosis of the vein
- Acute deep venous thrombosis
- Overlying infection or significant skin compromise
- Deep venous insufficiency

EQUIPMENT AND SUPPLIES

- Camera
- Surgical marking pen
- Vein transilluminator (e.g., Veinlite)
- 10-mL syringe with a 25-gauge, 1½-inch needle
- 0.5% lidocaine with epinephrine
- Povidone–iodine (Betadine) or chlorhexidine (Hibiclens) prep
- Sterile draping
- Sterile gloves and Occupational Safety and Health Administration (OSHA)–approved attire for the clinician to observe universal blood and body fluid precautions
- Set of phlebectomy hooks
- Curved iris scissors
- Minimum of six curved micro mosquito forceps
- Four towel clamps
- Needle holder (to hold the blade at proper location to produce desired depth and length of incision [see Fig. 85-5])
- No. 11 scalpel blade (alternative, 18-gauge needle)
- 3-0 absorbable suture (e.g., Vicryl)
- 4 × 4 gauze
- Steri-Strips (plain or saturated with povidone–iodine)
- Benzoin spray
- 4-inch web roll (as an absorbent wrap over the 4 × 4 dressing)
- Nonstretch compression dressing (e.g., Comprilan, Coban)
- Class II thigh-high compression stockings
- Shower bag to cover dressing, when needed
- Written postoperative instructions
- Consent form

ANATOMY AND PATHOLOGY OF VENOUS DISEASE

Before proper treatment options can be determined, the clinician must have a clear understanding of the patient's underlying anatomy and disease process. The clinician should also have undertaken some advanced study of the overall anatomy and diseases of the lower extremity venous system; some specialized training should have been obtained before performing AP. This section serves only as a brief overview and is far from comprehensive. (The reader is again referred to Chapter 86, Endovenous Vein Ablation, Chapter 88,

Noninvasive Venous and Arterial Studies of the Lower Extremities, and Chapter 92, Sclerotherapy.)

There are primarily three venous systems in the leg: the superficial venous system lies above the deep fascia, the deep venous system lies under the deep fascia, and the perforator vein system connects the superficial with the deep systems (Fig. 85-1). The muscular pump of the leg produces a distal-to-proximal compression to facilitate blood flow back to the cardiopulmonary system. If the valvular system is intact, normal veins allow only unidirectional flow.

The superficial venous system consists of a network of veins that feed two primary vessels, the great saphenous vein and the short saphenous vein. The great saphenous vein terminates at the saphenofemoral junction after it has coursed proximally from the dorsal arch vein of the foot and medially along the medial leg and thigh. The short saphenous vein also begins with the dorsal arch vein but travels behind the lateral malleolus and along the lateral leg. After reaching the popliteal fossa, the short saphenous vein empties into the popliteal vein of the deep venous system at the saphenopopliteal junction. It should be noted that the location of this junction is variable (see Chapter 92, Sclerotherapy, Figs. 92-2 and 92-3).

Perforator veins allow blood to flow from the superficial to the deep system. By doing so, more than 90% of blood flows through the deep venous system on its way back to the heart. The importance of competent venous valves for enforcing unidirectional flow in such a low-pressure system is often unappreciated. Once venous reflux occurs through incompetent valves, normal blood flow is altered, intraluminal pressure increases, and the disease process worsens. The increased flow and pressure to the superficial system leads to dilated vessels and the development of varicosities. As chronic venous insufficiency develops, approximately one third of patients also develop problems with superficial thrombophlebitis, dermatitis, lipodermatosclerosis, or ulceration.

It is also important for the phlebologist to have a clear understanding of the sensory nerves and lymphatic vessels of the leg. Both of these systems lie close to the superficial veins. Consequently, complications can develop from damage to these structures. The most frequent nerve damage occurs to the saphenous or the sural nerve or their branches. The saphenous nerve is most vulnerable at the location where it lies along the distal portion of the great saphenous vein near the dorsal foot veins. The sural nerve is vulnerable along its entire course as it runs beside the short saphenous vein

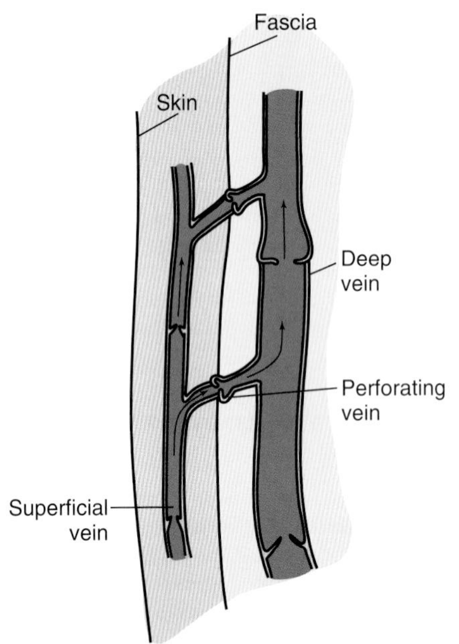

Figure 85-1 Venous compartments of the leg consist of the superficial venous system, the deep venous system, and the perforator vein system.

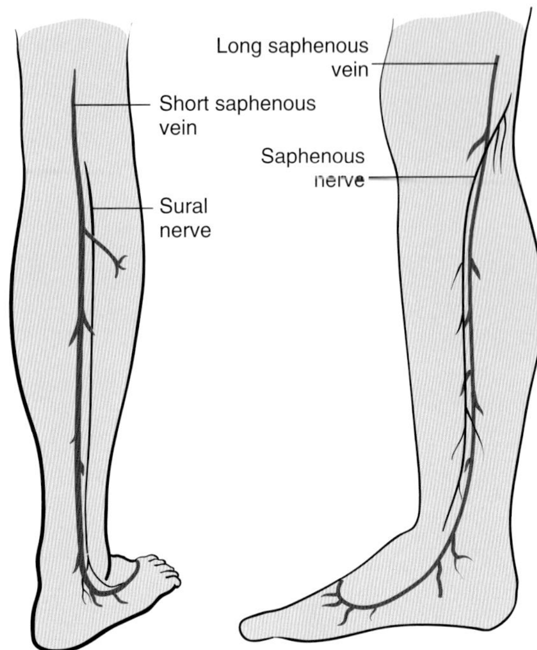

Figure 85-2 Important sensory nerves and their location relative to vessels of the leg.

(Fig. 85-2). Damage to the lymphatic vessels most commonly occurs below the medial knee in the anterior tibial region near Boyd's perforators.

Preprocedure Patient Preparation

An accurate patient history and physical examination will allow the clinician to formulate a better diagnosis and treatment plan, one that is best suited for the patient's needs. The examination must also exclude any potential contraindications. Additional studies, such as an electrocardiogram, complete blood count, bleeding studies, and serum electrolytes, glucose, urea nitrogen, and creatinine levels, may be required. Figure 85-3 shows a general history form with a focus on venous-related symptoms or diseases.

The venous examination should result in an accurate map of the veins of the lower extremities. The clinician should also note if chronic venous changes are present. Dermatitis, edema, corona phlebectatica, and lipodermatosclerosis or ulcerative disease may raise a suspicion for deep venous disease or long-standing chronic venous insufficiency.

The handheld Doppler is often referred to as the "phlebologist's stethoscope." It is an invaluable instrument for examining the patient for venous reflux. The Doppler examination is performed with the patient in the standing position, bearing his or her weight on the opposite leg. The Doppler probe is placed at a 45-degree angle over the vein to be examined. Compression of the calf muscle distal to the probe induces blood flow in a proximal direction. In a diseased vein, reflux is heard as a loud rumbling sound after the sudden release of compression of the calf muscle. A normal vein has only a monophasic (unidirectional) signal. By performing this simple maneuver, the examiner can locate the highest, most proximal source of reflux. (See also Chapter 88, Noninvasive Venous and Arterial Studies of the Lower Extremities.)

Duplex ultrasonographic examination provides information useful for producing an even better venous map. The examination is typically performed with a 7.5- to 13-MHz linear probe and the patient in a standing position. Areas of venous dilation or large perforators can reveal sources of proximal venous reflux. The deep venous system can also be visualized to assess for thrombus or incompetence. Areas of reflux in the superficial system, which may be difficult to visualize or palpate, can be studied easily. Duplex scanning also provides a hard copy (image and often a blood velocity graph) for documentation of the venous disease before and after treatment.

Many phlebologists evaluate the leg function with an additional test, photoplethysmography. This is most helpful to document normal or correctable deep venous function in those patients with evidence of stasis changes (see Chapter 92, Sclerotherapy).

Once a thorough understanding of the underlying disease process is obtained, an accurate treatment plan can be formulated. It needs to be emphasized that the highest, most proximal point of reflux must be corrected. This often requires a procedure in addition to AP. Ablation of the saphenous vein, ultrasonography-guided sclerotherapy (often referred to as "chemical ablation"), or a partial stripping or ligation of the great or short saphenous vein may be needed in conjunction with AP. If the venous incompetence cannot be treated with these techniques or the clinician does not have the training or skills to perform them, the clinician may choose to consult another surgeon. This consultation helps to ensure a lower recurrence rate and better relief of the symptoms from venous insufficiency.

See the sample patient education form available online at www.expertconsult.com.

Technique

1. On the night before surgery the patient should shave his or her legs carefully, minimizing any nicking. Instead of shaving, patients (especially men) may prefer to use "Magic Hair Removal" or a depilatory.
2. Preoperative pictures are highly recommended.
3. Just before surgery, have the patient stand for venous marking with a surgical marking pen. Proper lighting in a warm room, and having the patient stand for a period of time, will maximize venous dilation and visibility. In turn, this will improve the clinician's ability to mark the veins. Some clinicians mark the most superficial and easily palpable portion of the vein with a crosshatch. A vein transilluminator (Veinlite) is helpful for ensuring accurate marking.
4. Once the visible veins have been marked, use a focused Duplex examination to locate and mark the perforator veins (and any large branches along the vein) that are to be excised (Fig. 85-4).
5. Place the patient in 10 to 15 degrees of Trendelenburg to empty the veins during surgery. The foot can be propped on a pillow or cushion.
6. Prepare the area with a 5-minute povidone–iodine (Betadine) or chlorhexidine (Hibiclens) scrub and then apply sterile drapes to the area.
7. Inject 0.5% lidocaine with epinephrine on each side of the marked veins using a 25-gauge, 1½-inch needle.

   NOTE: Many clinicians use a tumescent technique, originally developed for use in liposuction surgery. Larger amounts of dilute local anesthetic (0.2% lidocaine with a 1:500,000 concentration of epinephrine) are instilled perivascularly with a 22-gauge spinal needle. These clinicians believe that instilling larger volumes into the perivascular space provides additional local compression and further minimizes risk of bleeding after the procedure.

8. Starting proximally, make a small 2- to 3-mm vertical incision over or adjacent to the marked vein. A no. 11 scalpel blade or an 18-gauge needle may be used for the incision. A no. 11 blade can be held in a needle holder at the proper location to produce the desired depth and length of the incision (Fig. 85-5).
9. Gently insert a phlebectomy hook through the incision (Fig. 85-6). It may be necessary to break up adhesions and fibrous attachments to the vein, before extraction, by undermining the vein and surrounding skin and subcutaneous tissue with the stem of the phlebectomy hook. However, be careful not to damage any nearby structures such as nerves or lymphatics.
10. Hook the vein with a gentle rotation and retraction technique. When the vein is pulled through the incision, it will be identified by its distinguishing pearly white appearance (Fig. 85-7).
11. The vein is grasped with a set of fine curved mosquito hemostats. As the vein is exteriorized, the tension on the vein will produce a palpable cord under the skin. The next incision is made at the distal point of the palpable cord, or the next crosshatch.
12. The most proximal end of the vein being excised is tied off with absorbable suture (e.g., 3-0 Vicryl). The author also chooses to tie off as many perforators as possible, and these were easily located and marked with Duplex before surgery. Many phlebologists choose to simply tear the vein loose from the perforator and have an assistant apply constant pressure to the area for 5 to 10 minutes.
13. The vein is sequentially pulled through successive distal incisions until it is totally excised. When removed in pieces, these can be laid out along the course to ensure total removal of the vein (Fig. 85-8).
14. With extensive varicosities, the surgeon may choose to perform the AP in stages, separated by 7 to 14 days between each surgery. The procedure, when performed in stages, typically begins on the distal part of the limb. With experience it will take the surgeon less time to remove the same length of vein. Several hours should be allowed for each surgery, and only one leg should be done at a time.
15. Clean the limb with sterile water and pat dry. Benzoin spray is used to increase the adhesion of the Steri-Strips applied over the incisions.
16. Apply gauze or an absorbent padding along the course of the excised vein.
17. Wrap the leg in a distal-to-proximal direction with a nonstretch compression bandage (e.g., Comprilan, Coban).
18. Place a thigh-high, class II compression stocking over the dressing.

Common Errors

- Not making sure the highest, most proximal point of reflux is corrected
- Administration of the anesthetic too deep into the tissue
- Making incisions too large, resulting in excessive scaring
- Overzealous hook movement and pulling, resulting in superficial nerve damage or skin damage
- Poor approximation of incisions
- Not providing sufficient padding at pressure points or leaving creases under the compression dressing
- Not ensuring and stressing the importance of walking regularly after the procedure

Complications

Box 85-1 shows a list of complications seen in a review of the literature done by Ramelet (1997). The rate of transient, patient-perceived complications might be as high as 5% to 10%, including such things as skin blisters, hyperpigmentation, and contact dermatitis (Table 85-1). True complications that require professional attention or that have long-term sequelae are quite rare.

Complications can be divided into cutaneous, vascular, and neurologic. Most *cutaneous complications* can be avoided with the proper use and application of the postoperative dressing. The size and type of vessels operated on, the anatomic location of the surgery, and the individual patient's history of previous sclerotherapy, phlebitis,

Name:__________ Date:________ Age:______ Ht:_____ Wt:_____

When did you first notice your enlarged or discolored veins?__________

Which leg bothers you the most? Right______ Left______ Both______

What symptoms are you having?

1. Sharp pain	Yes ____	No ____	8. Burning	Yes ____	No ____
2. Dull pain	Yes ____	No ____	9. Heaviness	Yes ____	No ____
3. Aching legs	Yes ____	No ____	10. Cramps	Yes ____	No ____
4. Swelling	Yes ____	No ____	11. Throbbing	Yes ____	No ____
5. Itching	Yes ____	No ____	12. Restless legs	Yes ____	No ____
6. Leg ulcers	Yes ____	No ____	13. Appearance	Yes ____	No ____
7. Tiredness	Yes ____	No ____			

Have you ever had any of the following:

1. Phlebitis (clots in legs)	Yes____	No______	When ________
2. Deep vein thrombosis	Yes____	No______	When ________
3. Pulmonary embolus (blood clot in lung)	Yes____	No______	When ________
4. Leg or ankle ulcers	Yes____	No______	When ________
5. Painful varicose veins	Yes____	No______	When ________
6. Venogram (vein x-rays)	Yes____	No______	When ________

Have you ever been pregnant? Yes______ No______

How many times? __________

How many deliveries? __________

Are you currently pregnant? Yes______ No______

List all medicines you are currently taking (including aspirin, if applicable):

__________ __________ __________

__________ __________ __________

List any hormones you are taking:

__________ __________ __________

Birth control pills: Yes______ No______

List all allergies:

__________ __________ __________

__________ __________ __________

Have you ever had any adverse reactions with scars? Yes______ No______

Have you ever had any of the following:

AIDS or HIV positive	Yes ____	No ____
Diabetes	Yes ____	No ____
Migraine headaches	Yes ____	No ____
High blood pressure	Yes ____	No ____
Heart disease	Yes ____	No ____
Jaundice or hepatitis	Yes ____	No ____
Cancer	Yes ____	No ____
Recent weight change	Yes ____	No ____
Major injury or surgery in your legs	Yes ____	No ____
Leg pain at night	Yes ____	No ____
Leg pain caused by walking	Yes ____	No ____
Leg pain caused by standing	Yes ____	No ____
Clotting or blood problems	Yes ____	No ____

Figure 85-3 Sample general patient history form with a focus on venous-related history.

Have you ever used prescription compression hose for your legs? Yes______ No______ When______

Have you ever had sclerotherapy before? Yes______ No______ When______

Have you ever smoked? Yes______ No______ Packs/day______ Number of years______

Are you currently smoking? Yes______ No______ Packs/day x years______

List any and all family members with vein problems:

______ ______ ______

______ ______ ______

Whom can we thank for referring you to our office?______

FOR DOCTOR USE ONLY

Movie seen: Yes______ No______

Telangiectasias: Right______ Left______ Severity______

Reticulars: Right______ Left______ Severity______

Varicose veins: Right______ Left______ Severity______

V. V.: Size:______mm

SFJ reflux: Right______ Left______

SPJ reflux: Right______ Left______

PPG: Yes______ No______ Right______ Left______ Ven______ Art______ Both______

U.S.: Yes______ No______ Right______ Left______

Appt. for sclero: Yes______ No______

R L   L R   R L   R L

Figure 85-3, cont.

or lipodermatosclerosis will all affect the likelihood of a vascular complication. Many of the *vascular complications* are avoidable by applying adequate compression and stressing the importance of postoperative ambulation. *Neurologic complications* can occur from the local anesthetic, directly from the phlebectomy, or from the postoperative dressing. The most problematic nerve injury is damage to the sural nerve; this must be avoided by dealing carefully with the short saphenous vein. Damage to sensory nerves can often be avoided because the patient will usually complain of pain if the surgeon is too close to the nerve; this awareness allows the surgeon to avoid damaging or destroying the nerve. Excessive compression to the dorsal foot can induce a painful tarsal syndrome.

The primary care clinician does not require special training to handle the complications that occur with AP. Emphasis must be placed, however, on adequate training to perform AP and on the proper understanding of the underlying pathophysiologic process.

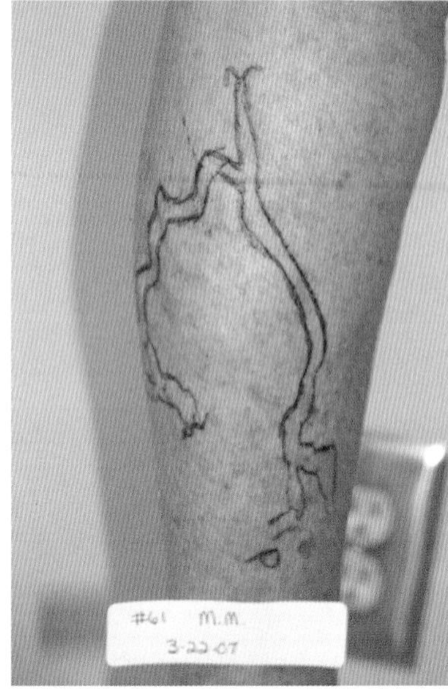

Figure 85-4 Venous marking with surgical marking pen.

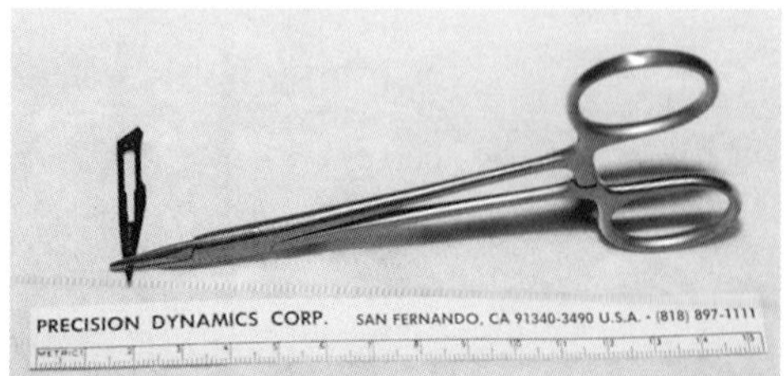

Figure 85-5 No. 11 blade placed in needle holder in preparation for incision.

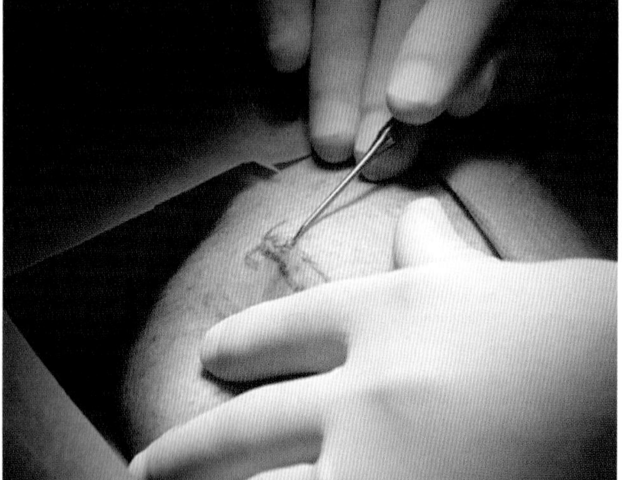

Figure 85-6 Phlebectomy hook gently inserted through incision.

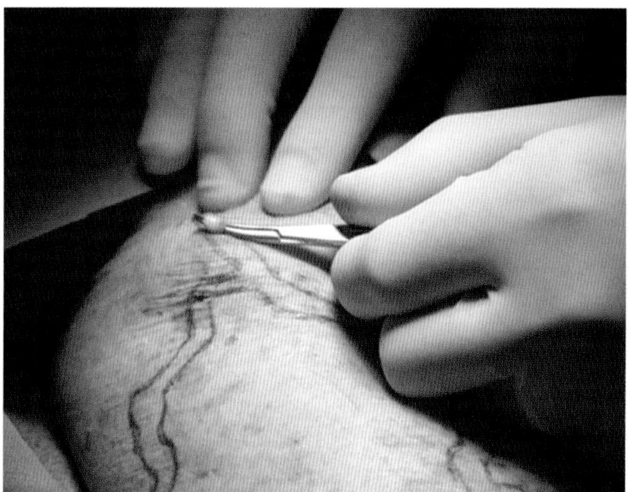

Figure 85-7 Vein pulled through incision.

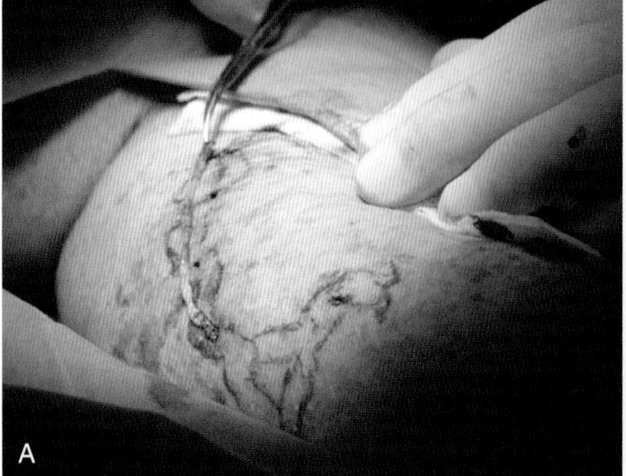

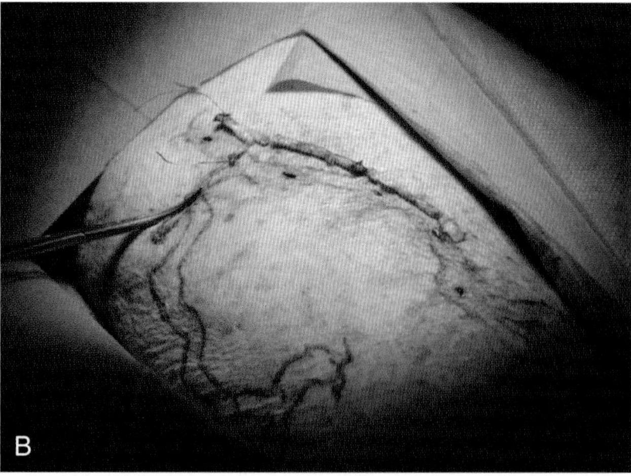

Figure 85-8 **A–C,** Vein is sequentially pulled through successive distal incisions.

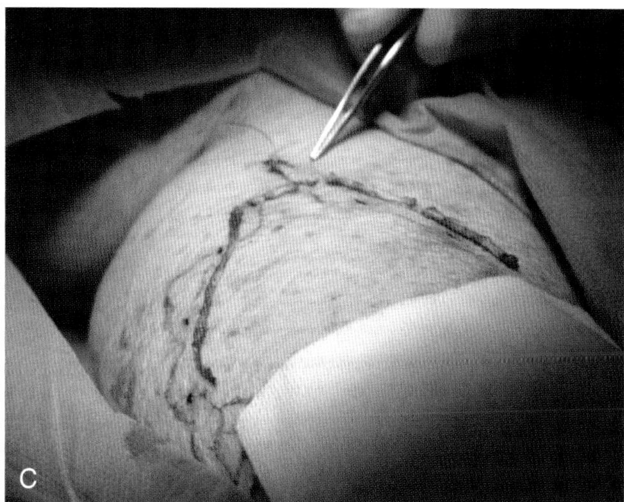

Figure 85-8, cont.

Postprocedure Management and Patient Education

Written and oral postoperative instructions should be provided to the patient (see the sample patient education form available online at www.expertconsult.com). All patients should be encouraged to walk approximately one half mile immediately after surgery, then 1 to 3 miles per day for the next 2 weeks. They should start taking one aspirin daily for 2 weeks, starting 12 to 16 hours after surgery. Strenuous workouts, heavy lifting, and standing for long periods of time should be avoided for 2 weeks. Over-the-counter ibuprofen should be sufficient for any discomfort that may occur after surgery. The dressing should remain in place and be kept dry until the follow-up appointment 1 week later. At that time, the dressing will be removed and the incisions inspected. The compression stocking alone is worn during the day for an additional week. The Steri-Strips are removed 2 weeks after surgery, and then any further surgeries or required therapy can be scheduled.

Box 85-1. Complications of Ambulatory Phlebectomy

Cutaneous Complications

Skin blisters from dressing
Transient hyperpigmentation
Visible scars
Contact dermatitis
Infection
Keloid and hypertrophic scars
Tattooing with pen
Koebner's phenomenon
Skin necrosis

Neurologic Complications

Postoperative pain
Paresthesia

Vascular Complications

Hematomas
Postoperative hemorrhage
Superficial phlebitis
Matting
Lymphatic pseudocyst
Lymphorrhea
Persistent edema
Deep venous thrombosis with potential pulmonary embolus

Data from Ramelet A: Complications of ambulatory phlebectomy. Dermatol Surg 23:947–954, 1997.

TABLE 85-1 Frequency of Complications of Ambulatory Phlebectomy

Rank	Type	No. of Events/ Phlebectomy	Percentage/ Phlebectomy
1	Blister formation	214	5.4%
2	Pigmentation (transitory)	183	4.6%
3	Telangiectasia matting	145	3.6%
4	Localized superficial phlebitis	110	2.8%
5	Temporary dysesthesia	15	0.4%
6	Lymphocele	6	0.2%
7	Extensive superficial phlebitis	5	0.1%
8	Delayed bleeding	4	0.1%
9	Hematoma	4	0.1%
10	Dimpling	3	0.07%
11	Skin necrosis	3	0.07%
12	Tattooing	3	0.07%
13	Wound infection	3	0.07%
14	Allergic reaction to wrappings	3	0.07%
15	Keloid	3	0.07%
16	Local anesthetic overload	2	0.05%
17	Deep venous thrombosis	1	0.02%
	Totals	**707**	**17.79%**

Data from Olivencia JA: Complications of ambulatory phlebectomy: A review of 4000 consecutive cases. Am J Cosmet Surg 17:161–165, 2000.

Patient Education Guides

See the sample patient education and consent forms online at www.expertconsult.com.

Other Resources

Phlebology Societies

American College of Phlebology
101 Callan Avenue, Suite 210
San Leandro, CA 94577
Phone: 510-346-6800
Website: www.phlebology.org

Training Courses

The National Procedures Institute
12012 Technology Blvd, Suite 200
Austin, TX 78727
Phone: 1-800-462-2492
Website: www.npinstitute.com

CPT/Billing Codes

37700 Ligation and division of great saphenous vein at saphenofemoral junction, or distal interruptions
37765 Stab phlebectomy of varicose veins, one extremity, 10 to 20 stab incisions
37766 Stab phlebectomy, more than 20 stab incisions
37799 Stab phlebectomy, less than 10 stab incisions. Also, use for any unlisted procedure, vascular surgery
37780 Ligation and division of the short saphenous vein at saphenopopliteal junction
37785 Ligation, division, and/or excision of varicose vein cluster(s), one leg

ICD-9-CM Diagnostic Codes

454.1 Varicose veins of lower extremities with inflammation
454.8 Varicose veins of the lower extremities with complications (edema, pain, swelling)
459.81 Venous (peripheral) insufficiency, chronic or unspecified

Acknowledgment

The editors wish to recognize the many contributions by Roger Murray, MD, to this chapter in a previous edition of this text.

Suppliers

(See contact information online at www.expertconsult.com.)

An excellent general resource for all sclerotherapy and phlebotomy instruments and equipment
Wagner Medical
Clinician and patient education DVDs or VHSs
Phlebology and Aesthetic Concepts
Compression stockings
Beiersdorf-Jobst, Inc. (also manufactures Comprilan dressing)
Juzo (Julius Zorn), Inc.
Medi USA
Sigvaris
Venosan
Compression wrap
3M (Coban)
3M Center
STD Pharmaceutical
Phlebectomy hooks
Aesculap
Venosan
Shower bag cover
Gill Podiatry Supply and Equipment

Bibliography

Brown JS: Stab-avulsion varicose veins. In Brown JS (ed): Minor Surgery: A Text and Atlas, 4th ed. New York, Oxford University Press, 2000, pp 372–377.

Flynn JC: Procedures in Phlebotomy, 2nd ed. Philadelphia, WB Saunders, 1999.

Goldman M, Bergan J: Ambulatory Treatment of Venous Disease: An Illustrative Guide. St. Louis, CV Mosby, 1995.

Goldman MP, Weiss RA: Endovenous ablation techniques with ambulatory phlebectomy for varicose veins. In Robinson JK, Hanke CW, Siegel DM, Sengelmann RD (eds): Surgery of the Skin. Philadelphia, Mosby, 2005, pp 645–656.

Olivencia JA: Maneuver to facilitate ambulatory phlebectomy. Dermatol Surg 22:654–655, 1996.

Ouriel K: Lower Extremity Vascular Disease. Philadelphia, WB Saunders, 1995.

Ramelet A: Complications of ambulatory phlebectomy. Dermatol Surg 23:947–954, 1997.

Ricci S, Georgiev M, Goldman M: A Practical Guide for Treating Varicose Veins. St. Louis, CV Mosby, 1995.

Sadick NS: Manual of Sclerotherapy. Philadelphia, Lippincott Williams & Wilkins, 2000.

Tibbs D, Sabiston D, Davies M, et al: Varicose Veins, Venous Disorders, and Lymphatic Problems in the Lower Limbs. Oxford, Oxford University Press, 1997.

Weiss R, Weiss M: Ambulatory phlebectomy compared to sclerotherapy for varicose and telangiectatic veins: Indications and complications. Adv Dermatol 11:3–16, 1996.

Weiss RA, Dover JS: Leg vein management: Sclerotherapy, ambulatory phlebectomy, and laser surgery. In Kaminer MS, Dover JS, Arndt KA (eds): Atlas of Cosmetic Surgery. Philadelphia, Saunders, 2002.

CHAPTER 86

ENDOVENOUS VEIN ABLATION

Jerry Ninia

Primary venous insufficiency is characterized by the development of varicose veins of the lower extremities. The great saphenous vein (GSV) is the largest and longest vein of the superficial venous system, and reflux in the GSV is often associated with the development of large superficial varices. In addition to cosmetic issues and symptoms of leg pain and fatigue, varicose veins can give rise to ambulatory venous hypertension with its associated skin changes and ulceration. In fact, up to 80% of leg ulcers are due to venous disease. If incompetence of the saphenofemoral junction (SFJ) or a perforator vein is detected, treatment is medically indicated. In addition, reflux in other veins such as the small saphenous vein (SSV), anterior accessory saphenous vein, and vein of Giacomini may contribute to the development of varicose veins. This chapter describes ultrasonography-guided percutaneous techniques for treating patients with varicose veins who are ambulatory and whose sonographic findings include the documentation of reflux.

Knowledge of lower extremity duplex ultrasonography is an absolute necessity for the performance of these procedures. The venous anatomy is described in Chapter 92, Sclerotherapy. Patients need to be evaluated before surgery with ultrasonographic mapping and marking, during surgery with guiding and checking, and after surgery for response to treatment. *Mapping* refers to diagramming the findings on the patient's chart. *Marking* pertains to outlining vein findings on the patient's skin. Intraoperative *guiding and checking* refers to proper performance of the procedure and proper instrumentation and application of tumescent anesthesia. Response to treatment is assessed at 1 week, 1 month, and longer intervals as needed to determine the effectiveness of the procedure.

ENDOVENOUS CHEMICAL ABLATION

Also see Chapter 92, Sclerotherapy, which discusses many of the concepts and the anatomy involved in treating venous diseases.

Commonly referred to as "ultrasonography-guided sclerotherapy," *endovenous chemical ablation (ECA)* involves injecting a sclerosing solution under ultrasonographic guidance directly into the lumen of the vein being treated. Even if the vein has significant tortuosity the sclerosant (liquid or foam) will distribute itself within the vein lumen. An example is the use of ECA in the treatment of patients with *groin neovascularization*—a phenomenon seen in patients who have previously undergone surgical vein stripping. As such, ECA is especially helpful in treating these patients with postsurgical recurrences and an anatomically variable SSV with its associated tortuous tributaries. Equipment needed is very similar to that used for basic injection–compression sclerotherapy, with the addition of a 7.5- to 15-MHz linear-array ultrasound transducer. Ultrasonography provides real-time feedback to confirm intraluminal placement of the needle tip or catheter, intraluminal injection without extravasation, and attainment of the treatment end point (i.e., vasospasm; Fig. 86-1). Vasospasm is an indicator of the immediate efficacy of the foam injection; however, the final therapeutic effects of foam sclerotherapy should be evaluated clinically according to symptoms and follow-up duplex ultrasonography. Tumescent anesthesia is not required. Graduated class II (30 to 40 mm Hg) compression stockings need to be worn *continuously* for 24 to 36 hours, then during the daytime for 6 days postinjection.

The *direct needle injection* technique involves ultrasonographic visualization of the vein in a longitudinal plane (Fig. 86-2). A 21- to 25-gauge, 1- to 1½-inch needle is inserted obliquely into the lumen of the vessel with the bevel directed up. Slow aspiration is performed to verify correct needle placement. A small amount (1 to 2 mL) of sclerosant foam or liquid (1% to 3% sodium tetradecyl sulfate [STS]) is injected slowly; a "snowstorm" sonographic pattern is appreciated on injection (Fig. 86-3).

Foam Sclerotherapy

Although liquid sclerosants can be used, for larger veins the effect of sclerotherapy is enhanced by creating a sclerosant *foam*. Foam is created using the *Tessari technique* (Fig. 86-4). The Tessari technique involves using one syringe with liquid *detergent* sclerosant (e.g., STS 0.1% to 3%, polidocanol 1% to 2%, and others) and another syringe with air. The ratio of air to sclerosant is 4:1. The syringes are connected by a two- or three-way stopcock. By forcing the air and fluid back and forth numerous times, foam is created. The sclerosant is supposedly concentrated on the bubbles and thus has greater potency, leading to more efficacious treatment. The foam reconstitutes into liquid very quickly, within a matter of minutes, so it needs to be injected rather quickly. Although not mandatory, using rubber-free and Silicone-free syringes (e.g., B. Braun Injekt) prolongs the foam state. This technique is simple and economical and produces good-quality foam. Ultrasonography will demonstrate more of a "snowstorm" pattern when foam is injected. Amounts and concentrations depend on the size and number of veins injected. Although foam can be used for telangiectases, complications may be more frequent and hence the technique is more commonly reserved for larger veins.

Whether foam or liquid is used, injections are administered with the patient supine, starting in the distal leg and progressing proximally to the point of reflux in order to minimize the volume of sclerosant and number of injections. Alternatively, injections can be administered starting 8 to 10 cm distal to the point of reflux, then proceeding from proximal to distal as previously injected segments undergo vasospasm. If 3% liquid STS is used, the maximum amount of solution during a treatment session is 10 mL. *If foam is used, the volume limit is 10 mL of foam sclerosant as well, regardless of the concentration of the liquid detergent sclerosant used to create the foam* (Breu and colleagues, 2008).

Needle versus Catheter Infusion

The *syringe-and-needle technique* is technically less difficult than the *catheter infusion technique*; however, it has a narrower margin of safety. This is due to the need for multiple injections and the potential for vein laceration and subsequent sclerosant extravasation.

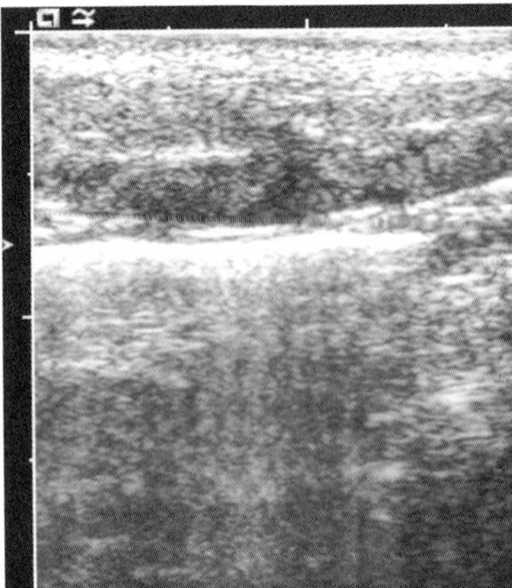

Figure 86-1 Vasospasm end point. (Courtesy of Nick Morrison, Scottsdale, Ariz.)

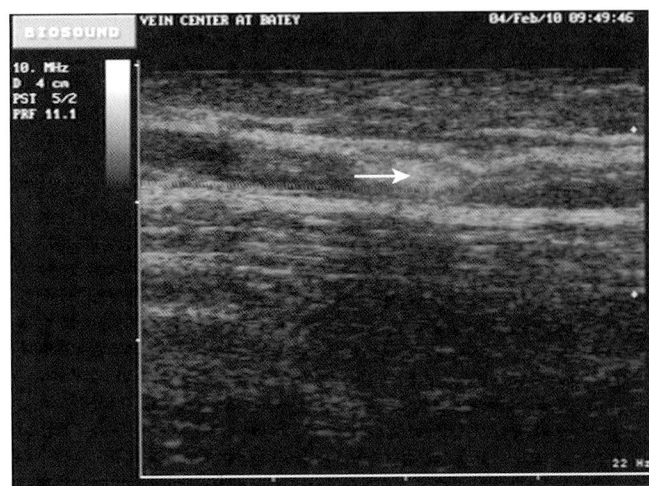

Figure 86-3 "Snowstorm" pattern *(arrow)* after injection. (Courtesy of John Mauriello, MD, Bradenton, Fla.)

The *catheter infusion technique* involves the introduction of a peripherally inserted central catheter line or a 2.5-inch, 18-gauge intravenous catheter fully inserted directly into the lumen of the vein. The catheter tip is initially located 8 to 10 cm distal to the point of reflux (Fig. 86-5). The sclerosant is injected slowly as the catheter is withdrawn. Subsequent percutaneous catheter placements are made distally and injections are directed cephalad as previously injected segments undergo vasospasm. Often, incompetent perforator veins do not require direct injection because they respond to treatment of the overlying superficial vein.

NOTE: When using the catheter infusion method, venipuncture sites are placed sequentially moving distally, with injections of the foam directed proximally (cephalad). When using the syringe-and-needle technique, injections are made from proximal to distal, with injections also directed cephalad.

Complications of ECA include those that may occur with standard injection–compression sclerotherapy. *Deep venous thrombosis* (extremely rare—incidence is between 0% to 5.7%) may occur if sclerosant finds its way into the deep venous system, especially in cases of inadequate post-ECA compression and lack of ambulation. Other side effects reported after ECA include *transient visual disturbances*, with no long-term visual or neurologic sequelae reported to date. *Intra-arterial injection*—the most feared complication of sclerotherapy—has been reported more frequently in association with ECA. This can cause severe skin necrosis; limb amputations have been reported as well. Therefore, performance of ECA must not be undertaken lightly. Detailed knowledge of the vascular sonographic anatomy is essential to perform ECA properly, safely, and effectively.

Endovenous Radiofrequency and Laser Ablation

Over the past several years, in addition to ECA, there has been the introduction of newer procedures in the treatment of chronic venous insufficiency. *Endovenous radiofrequency ablation* (RFA) and *endovenous laser ablation* (ELA) have emerged as less invasive and more effective alternatives to vein stripping. Performed in an office setting using *tumescent anesthesia*, these procedures can often be completed in under 1 hour. Procedure times depend on how long it takes to access the vein percutaneously, the length of the vein, and whether it is necessary to perform any ancillary procedures such as sclerotherapy or ambulatory phlebectomy. Graduated compression stockings are required post-treatment, as they are for ECA.

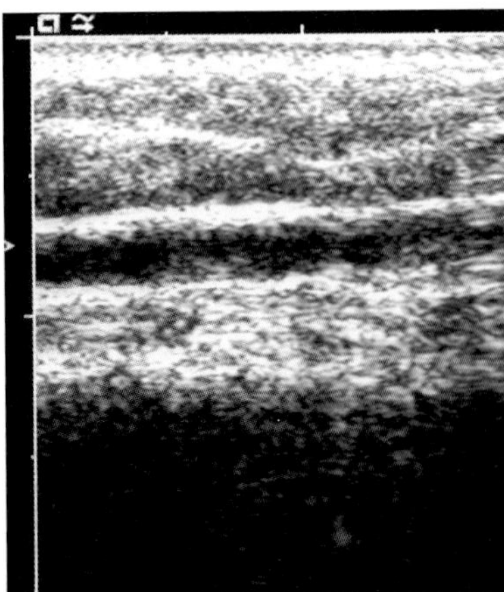

Figure 86-2 Vein imaged longitudinally. (Courtesy of Nick Morrison, Scottsdale, Ariz.)

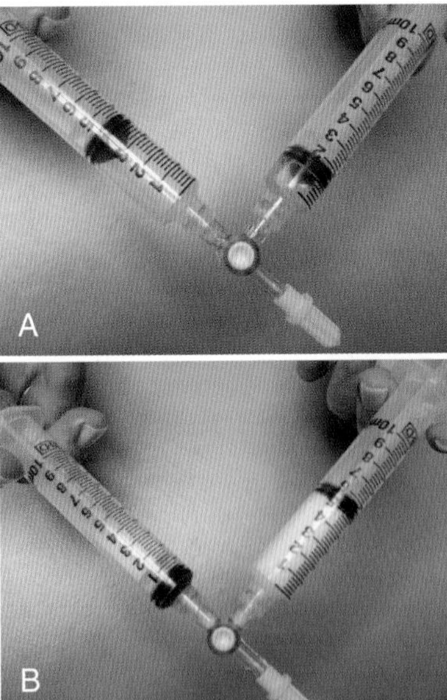

Figure 86-4 The Tessari technique. **A**, A 4 : 1 ratio of air to liquid sclerosant. **B**, The product after foam is created.

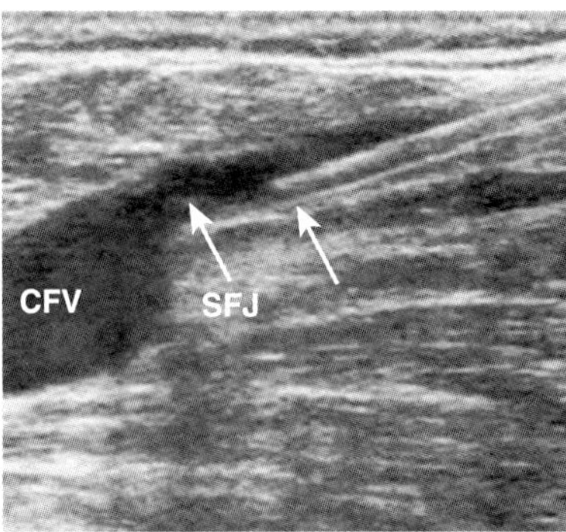

Figure 86-5 Catheter tip *(arrow)* 1 cm below the saphenofemoral junction (SFJ).

With RFA, radiofrequency energy is delivered to the vein lumen to heat, shrink, and occlude refluxing saphenous veins. Occlusion results from the contraction of collagen in the vein wall. *VNUS ClosureFAST* (VNUS Medical Technologies, San Jose, Calif) uses a specially designed catheter to treat 7-cm segments of the vein while maintaining intraluminal temperature at 85° C to 90° C (Fig. 86-6). A 35-cm-long vein can be treated in 2 minutes. With ELA, laser energy of varying wavelengths is delivered to the vein lumen. Examples of wavelengths used for ELA include 810 nm (AngioDynamics, Latham, NY), 980 nm (Biolitec, East Long Meadow, Mass, and AngioDynamics, Latham, NY), and 1320 nm (CoolTouch, Roseville, Calif). Laser treatment generates steam by heating blood inside the vein, producing fibrosis and subsequent occlusion of the vein. Deoxygenated hemoglobin is the main chromophore of the 810- and 980-nm lasers, whereas the energy of the 1320-nm laser is directed toward water in the vein wall. If treatment failure (recanalization) occurs (10%), it usually develops within the first year. If the vein is closed at 1-year follow-up, it is unlikely to recanalize.

Indications

The following are indications for RFA and ELA:

- Fully ambulatory patient without any contraindications
- Bulging varicose veins with or without symptoms (e.g., leg heaviness, throbbing, aching)

  NOTE: In some female patients, symptoms may occur only premenstrually (see Ninia, 2008).

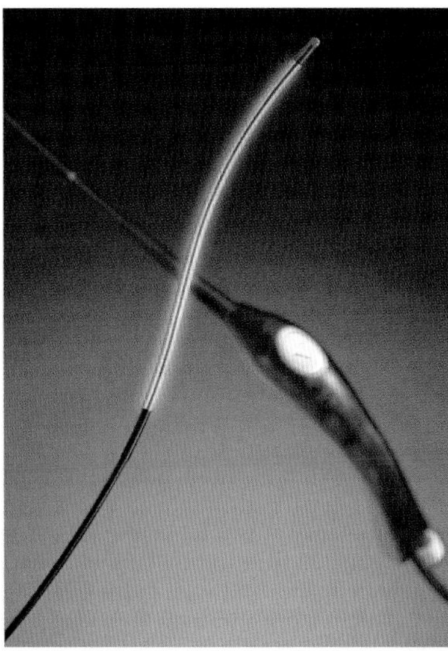

Figure 86-6 Catheter. (Courtesy of Covidien, Mansfield, Mass.)

- Bulging varicose veins with or without dermatologic signs of chronic venous insufficiency (e.g., edema, hyperpigmentation, lipodermatosclerosis, ulceration)
- Duplex ultrasonographic findings consistent with incompetence of the GSV or SSV
- Minimal tortuosity of the GSV or SSV to permit catheter placement

Contraindications

- RFA cannot be used in patients with *pacemakers*.
- Contraindications to treatment with all methods include *inability to ambulate, active superficial or deep venous thrombosis, hypoplastic deep veins, poor health, and pregnancy*.

Equipment and Supplies

- Basic equipment for ELA and RFA (Total Vein Solutions, Houston, Tex; Vascular Solutions, Minneapolis, Minn)
- *Duplex ultrasonography* equipment, available as portable or stationary units (Fig. 86-7)
- *Povidone–iodine and sterile drapes*
- Sterile gloves
- Drapes
- Ultrasound probe cover
- *1% lidocaine without epinephrine*, 5-mL syringe, and 30-gauge needle for local anesthesia before inserting the angiocatheter
- No. 11 blade
- 18-gauge angiocatheter
- Luer-Lok syringes
- Class II graduated compression stockings
- J-wire (guidewire)
- Sheath and vein dilator
- Micropuncture kits, available for veins less than 3 mm in diameter

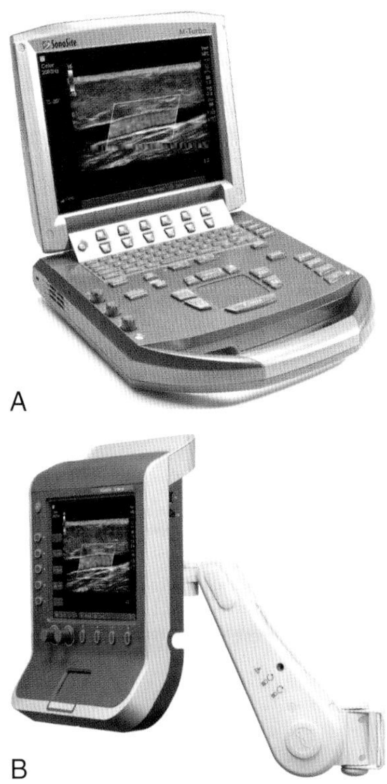

Figure 86-7 Duplex ultrasonography equipment is available as portable (**A**) or stationary (**B**) units. (Courtesy of Sonosite, Bothell, Mass.)

- Protective *eyewear* for use during laser procedures
- Skin *marking pen*
- Fluid for *tumescent anesthesia*. Various preparations of tumescent solutions have been used, with studies showing the maximum safe dose of lidocaine to be 35 mg/kg. In general, a dilute solution of lidocaine can be prepared by taking a 250-mL bag of 0.9% normal saline, removing 15 mL, and replacing it with an equal amount (15 mL) of 1% lidocaine. A small amount (5 mL) of sodium bicarbonate can be added as a buffer to decrease the stinging sensation.

NOTE: Supplies are available commercially from various sources (e.g., Vein Solutions, Total Vascular Solutions, Cook Medical [Bloomington, Ind]). The endolaser and radiofrequency companies preassemble kits that contain necessary supplies.

Preoperative Patient Education

See patient education forms online at www.expertconsult.com.

Procedure

A *preoperative evaluation* is carried out, usually on a date before that of the procedure, and begins with a directed history and physical examination with an emphasis on the lower extremities of patients with varicose veins. Type and duration of symptoms along with any improvement with support stockings should be documented. Skin changes related to ambulatory venous hypertension, such as edema, hyperpigmentation, corona phlebectasia, lipodermatosclerosis, atrophie blanche, and ulceration, are best documented with photography.

1. Patients are premedicated orally with 0.5 mg of the anxiolytic alprazolam 30 minutes before the procedure.
2. The *ultrasonographic examination* is performed with the patient standing and the weight shifted onto the opposite leg (see Chapter 88, Noninvasive Venous and Arterial Studies of the Lower Extremities). For the GSV, start at the groin and work caudad along the medial thigh. The GSV is identified in its characteristic location at the SFJ and then within the fascial sheath (Fig. 86-8). Its course is marked on the skin. Vein diameter should be measured along with documentation of reflux by Doppler analysis (Fig. 86-9). Reflux is demonstrated by an audible retrograde flow of greater than 0.5 to 1 second while manually compressing and releasing the calf muscles. Significant reflux of 2 seconds or more is often associated with skin changes characteristic of venous insufficiency. Documentation of this finding is necessary to secure reimbursement as a medically necessary procedure.
3. After venous duplex mapping and marking, a *percutaneous entry point is chosen*.

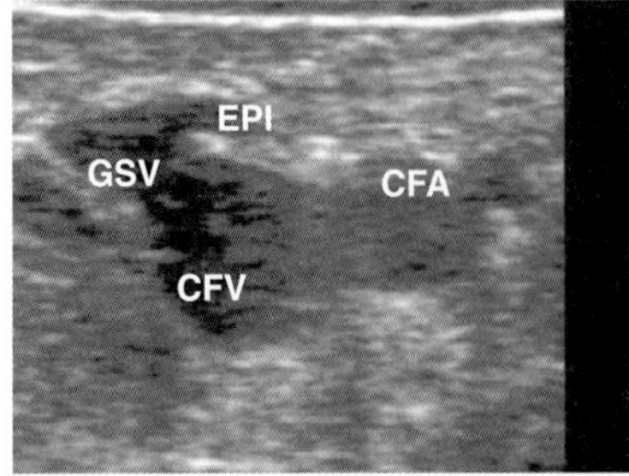

Figure 86-8 Sonographic appearance of great saphenous vein (GSV) joining common femoral vein (CFV) at the saphenofemoral junction. EPI, superficial epigastric artery; CFA, common femoral artery.

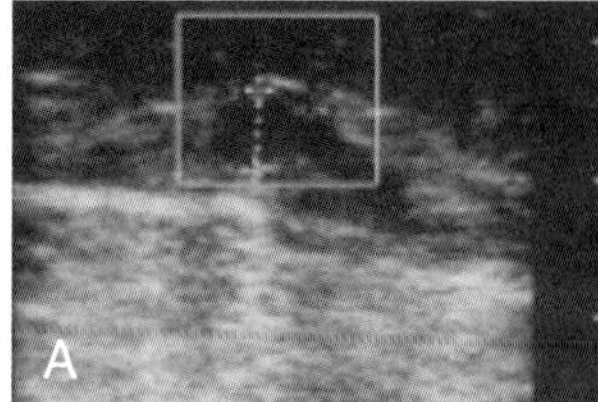

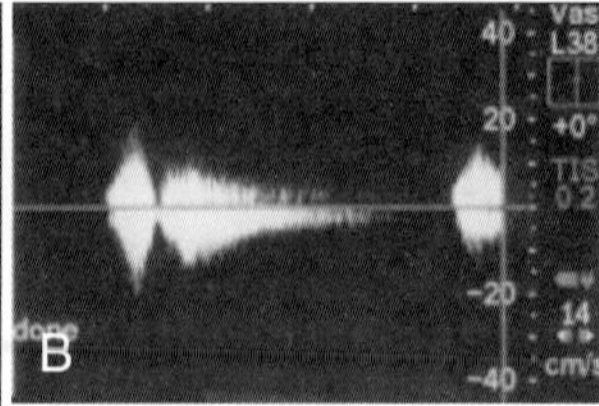

Figure 86-9 **A,** Great saphenous vein (GSV) within the fascial sheath. This vessel was measured at midthigh and noted to be approximately 0.57 cm in diameter. **B**, Quantification of reflux of the GSV in (**A**). After manual compression of the calf muscles, reflux lasts approximately 2 seconds.

4. The *leg is prepared and draped* in sterile fashion using povidone–iodine, and the access site is visualized longitudinally with ultrasonography.
5. A *1% lidocaine wheal* is raised at the access site.
6. An 18-gauge, 2-inch *angiocatheter is inserted* into the vein (Terumo, Somerset, NJ). A 0.035-inch-diameter J-wire (guidewire) is placed through the angiocatheter and directed toward the SFJ. The angiocatheter is removed. The percutaneous entry site is slightly widened and a 5-Fr sheath with a dilator is placed over the guidewire. The sheath is positioned 1 cm below the SFJ. This serves to preserve the superficial epigastric vein. A competent superficial epigastric vein preserves venous drainage of the anterior abdominal wall and prevents the phenomenon of neovascularization—the condition associated with vein recurrences after surgical ligation and stripping. The J-wire and dilator are then removed. Venous return is confirmed by aspirating the syringe attached to the sheath.
7. At this point, either an RFA or an ELA *catheter is introduced* into the sheath. *In the case of laser*, the aiming beam of the 600-μm laser fiber tip is transilluminated through the skin. If the aiming beam is not seen, it suggests that the laser fiber tip is incorrectly placed in the deep venous system. In this circumstance, the laser fiber and sheath need to be withdrawn until the aiming beam is visualized.
8. *Tumescent anesthesia* is administered after the laser fiber or the RFA catheter has been inserted. It is injected manually or with the use of a mechanical pump (Klein pump, HK Surgical, San Clemente, Calif) perivascularly into the saphenous sheath with ultrasonographic guidance, and the GSV is then "floated" in the anesthetic fluid (Fig. 86-10). In addition to providing anesthesia, this compresses the diameter of the GSV and causes the vein to spasm. The fluid surrounding the vein also provides for a "heat sink" to prevent injury to adjacent tissue.

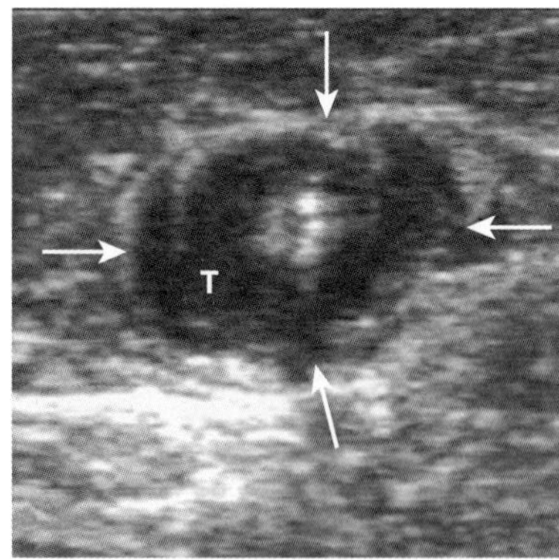

Figure 86-10 Saphenous vein "floated" in its sheath *(arrows)* after perivascular administration of tumescent anesthetic. The "T" represents the tumescent liquid surrounding the vein. Note how, in transverse view, the vein spasms around the echogenic laser fiber after the tumescent fluid is administered. This liquid now serves as a heat sink to absorb heat energy from the laser.

9. *Delivery of RF or laser energy is now administered*. For RF, using a "segmental heating" approach, the ClosureFAST catheter is positioned as described.. The exposed 7-cm heating element portion is activated with RF energy for a 20-second heating cycle. When the cycle is complete, energy delivery is automatically terminated by the generator. The catheter is then repositioned to the next treatment zone as indicated by the markings on the catheter. Spaced at increments of 6.5 cm, the catheter shaft allows for a 0.5-cm overlap between each treated segment to ensure complete treatment along the length of the vein. In addition to speed, an advantage of RFA over ELA is that the energy delivered is controlled by the temperature sensor on the catheter. This minimizes the risk of vein perforation and associated postoperative pain and bruising.

   In general, for all laser units, a minimum of 70 J/cm is needed to successfully occlude the vein. This can be accomplished by delivering 14 W of power and using a fiber withdrawal rate of 2 mm/sec, the latter of which is accomplished simply and accurately by using the 10-cm markings along the sheath in conjunction with the time display in seconds on the individual laser unit.
10. A class II (30 to 40 mm Hg) thigh-high, open-toe graduated compression stocking is immediately applied to the treated leg.

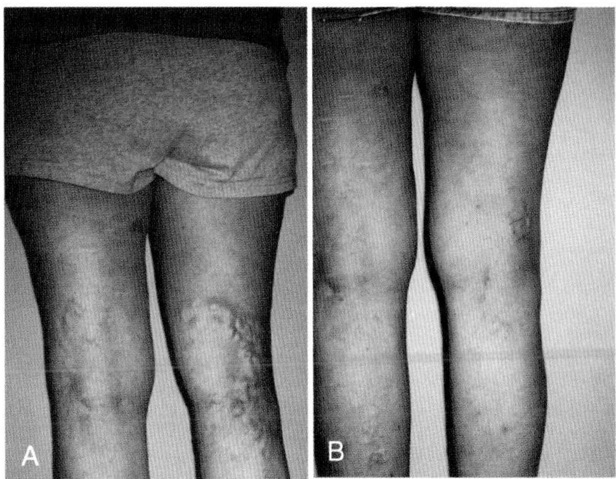

Figure 86-11 Appearance before (**A**) and after (**B**) endovenous laser ablation.

Common Errors

- If the vein spasms, application of a small amount of 2% nitroprusside may help correct the vasospasm. Alternatively, the patient may ambulate for 10 minutes and venepuncture may be reattempted.
- The room temperature is too cold.
- The patient is in the wrong position (reverse Trendelenburg is correct).
- Not attending to the needs of a nervous patient. Anxiolytics (lorazepam 0.5 to 1 mg) work well. "Vocal anesthesia" and speaking to the patient during the procedure may also help allay anxiety.

Postprocedure Patient Care and Education

See the patient education forms online at www.expertconsult.com. Patients are encouraged to ambulate and resume their normal activities.

- The compression hose is worn overnight and then for 6 more days while the patient is up and ambulating. The stocking may be removed at bedtime and for showering.
- Ibuprofen 600 mg three times daily is prescribed for 3 days and is to be taken, then used every 6 hours as needed afterward for pain.
- Physical examination and ultrasonographic follow-up are performed 3 to 7 days post-treatment (Fig. 86-11).

The treated vein wall will be thickened and fibrotic. Adequate flow in the deep venous system should be noted (Fig. 86-12). Although a resolution of symptoms and an improved cosmetic appearance are often noted within 1 month of treatment, most patients will need additional therapy in the form of sclerotherapy or ambulatory phlebectomy of residual varices to attain maximum results. Telangiectases will need to be treated separately as well. Some operators perform these procedures at the time of the endovenous ablation procedure. Others prefer to wait 1 month postprocedure to see what, if any, additional procedures need to be performed.

Complications

Significant complications of RFA and ELA are rare.

- Bruising and discomfort tend to be more common with ELA.
- Local paresthesias can occur with both modalities (<5% with ELA and <15% with RFA) but typically resolve within 2 to 3 months. Application of adequate tumescent anesthesia by floating the vein at least 10 mm below the skin will reduce this risk.
- The incidence of deep venous thrombosis is reported to be less than 1% with both modalities. This is very rare, especially when immediate ambulation and compression are used.
- Failure rates for either RFA or laser are less than 2% at 5-year follow-up.

Conclusions

Results of endovenous therapies have been very encouraging. Compared with vein stripping, these office-based procedures offer the advantages of lower procedural risks and cost. Patients are awake during the procedures and remain fully ambulatory, with no downtime afterward. Over the past several years there has been an increased understanding and interest in the management of venous disease. Over the next several years, these promising minimally invasive endovenous ablative procedures will essentially replace vein stripping.

Patient Education Guides

See sample patient education and consent forms online at www.expertconsult.com.

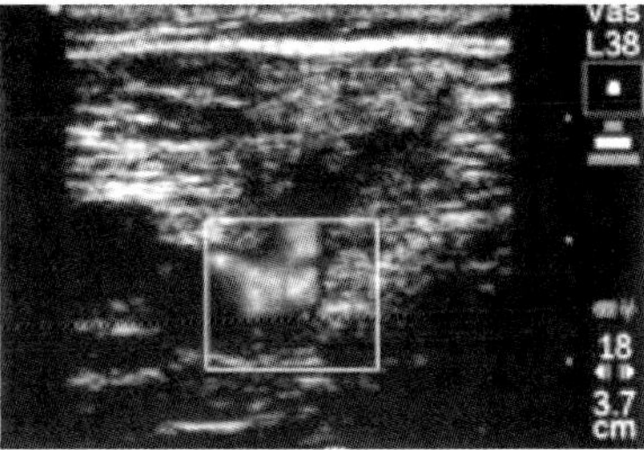

Figure 86-12 Postprocedure blood flow in a common femoral vein (CFV). Because this is a deep vein, one would want to see blood flow in its lumen both before and after the procedure. Compromised blood flow in the CFV postprocedure raises concern over an iatrogenic deep venous thrombosis.

CPT/Billing Codes

36475 Endovenous ablation therapy of the incompetent vein, extremity, inclusive of all imaging guidance and monitoring, percutaneous, radiofrequency; first vein treated
36476 Second and subsequent veins treated in a single extremity, each through separate access sites
36478 Endovenous laser ablation therapy of incompetent vein, extremity, inclusive of all imaging guidance and monitoring, percutaneous, laser; first vein treated
36479 Second and subsequent veins treated in a single extremity, each through separate access sites

ICD-9-CM Diagnostic Codes

459.3 Chronic venous hypertension
454.8 Varicose veins with complications
454.9 Varicose veins with skin changes/ulceration
454.9 Varicose veins lower extremity
459.81 Venous (peripheral) insufficiency

Suppliers

(See contact information online at www.expertconsult.com.)

Laser ablation
- Angiodynamics
- Biolitec
- CoolTouch

Radiofrequency ablation
- VNUS Medical

Support hose
- BSN-Jobst Institute, Inc.
- Carolon Health Care Products
- MediUSA
- Sigvaris

Ultrasonography
- Biosound Esaote
- Sonosite
- TeraRecon
- Terason
- Terumo Medical Corporation
- United Medical

Online Resource

American College of Phlebology: Available at www.phlebology.org. A good reference for frequently asked questions.

Bibliography

Alam M, Dover JS, Nguyen TH (eds): Procedures in Cosmetic Dermatology Series: Treatment of Leg Veins. Philadelphia, Saunders, 2006.

Breu FX, Guggenbichler S, Wollman JC: 2nd European Consensus Meeting on Foam Sclerotherapy 2006, Tegernsee, Germany. Vasa 37(Suppl 71): 1–30, 2008.

Darte SG, Baker SJ: Ultrasound-guided foam sclerotherapy for the treatment of varicose veins. Br J Surg 93:969–974, 2006.

Geroulakos G: Foam sclerotherapy for the management of varicose veins: A critical reappraisal. Phlebolymphology 13:202–206, 2006.

Goldman MP, Weiss RA: Endovenous ablation techniques with ambulatory phlebectomy for varicose veins. In Robinson JK, Hanke CW, Siegel DM, Sengelmann RD (eds): Surgery of the Skin: Procedural Dermatology. Philadelphia, Mosby, 2005, pp 645–656.

Luebke T, Brunkwall J: Systematic review and meta-analysis of endovenous radiofrequency obliteration, endovenous laser therapy, and foam sclerotherapy for primary varicosis. J Cardiovasc Surg 49:213–233, 2008.

Merchant RF, Pichot O: Long-term outcomes of endovenous radiofrequency obliteration of saphenous reflux as a treatment for superficial venous insufficiency. J Vasc Surg 42:502–509, 2005.

Navaro L, Min RJ, Boné C: Endovenous laser: A new minimally invasive method of treatment for varicose veins—preliminary observations using an 810 nm diode laser. Dermatol Surg 27:117–122, 2001.

Ninia JG: Premenstrual symptoms in lower limbs and duplex scan investigations. Phlebolymphology 15:125, 2008.

Winterborn RJ, Taiwo F, Slim F, et al: The incidence of deep vein thrombosis following ultrasound-guided foam sclerotherapy. Br J Surg 96(Suppl 1):A10, 2009.

CHAPTER 87

Ambulatory Electrocardiography: Holter and Event Monitoring

David Flinders • Scott Akin

Norman Holter developed ambulatory electrocardiography in the form of Holter monitoring in the early 1960s. The first device weighed about 85 pounds, and was worn as a backpack. As the technology, availability, and convenience of equipment have improved, use of ambulatory electrocardiography (AECG) has increased. Although in the past Holter recordings were primarily requested, provided, and interpreted by cardiologists, this procedure, as well as other forms of AECG, have become increasingly popular among primary care clinicians. As our population ages, the prevalence of arrhythmias will increase, along with the prevalence of cardiovascular disease. Routine use of AECG generally involves evaluation of patients who report symptoms possibly related to cardiac arrhythmias, such as unexplained palpitations, unexplained syncope, presyncope, or episodic dizziness. More advanced (and in some cases more controversial) uses of AECG include arrhythmia detection in asymptomatic patients with cardiac risk factors, ST segment monitoring for silent myocardial ischemia in the patient with coronary artery disease (CAD), assessment of antiarrhythmic drug therapy, and assessment of pacemaker/implantable cardioverter-defibrillators (ICD) function.

As primary care clinicians have increased their competence in use of AECG devices, they have become more comfortable providing access to them in their offices. Benefits include more readily, and perhaps more rapidly, available data for their patients. These data allow for more complete and definitive care for many patients. AECG is attractive because it requires little of the clinician's time to interpret the results and is therefore a time-efficient, income-generating test. With more widespread use, the cost of equipment has also decreased. However, acquisition of an office monitoring system is not a decision to be taken lightly. Although it is relatively easy to interpret the results, it is considerably more difficult to apply them clinically. The clinician must have a clear interest in cardiac arrhythmias and be willing to invest the time needed to learn the system. The clinician must also make the commitment to promptly interpret the results of all tests performed. Realistically, with training and a modicum of practice, clinicians can interpret and dictate the results of most Holter reports within 5 to 15 minutes. Interpretation of event monitoring usually takes even less time. However, despite being more readily available, ambulatory monitoring should not be considered a routine procedure. From the patient's and insurer's perspective, it is expensive and time consuming. It should be reserved for specific indications. This chapter outlines the different types of AECG, their indications, and the techniques necessary for use, and provides a foundation for basic AECG interpretation.

Overview and Comparison of Available Methods of Evaluation and Arrhythmia Monitoring

12-Lead ECG and Rhythm Strip

- Only monitors cardiac rhythm for a short period. Therefore, unless the patient is symptomatic at time of ECG, it is difficult to correlate clinically.
- Can diagnose certain conditions associated with worrisome arrhythmias (hypertrophic cardiomyopathy, Brugada syndrome, long QT syndrome, etc.).
- Inexpensive and readily available.

24-Hour Holter Monitor (Often Extended to 48 Hours)

- Standard monitoring modality for arrhythmias that occur frequently (i.e., several times daily).
- Patient wears two to three electrodes on the chest with leads attached that communicate continuously with a data-collecting device worn on the patient's belt.
- Patient completes a diary that enables a correlation of symptoms with the timing of arrhythmias.
- Because the recording period is short (24 to 48 hours), it only detects arrhythmias that are responsible for symptoms approximately 10% of the time. It may miss infrequent but potentially dangerous arrhythmias.
- Can identify subjects with worrisome arrhythmias (as well as quantify the frequency, duration, etc.) and silent ischemia. However, the interpreter must be aware of the tremendous spontaneous variability in frequency not only of ectopy, but also of ST segment changes that may or may not indicate ischemia (see later discussion).
- Moderately expensive ($250 to $500 per test in most institutions).

Postevent Recorders

- The device is kept by the patient at all times for up to several weeks. While experiencing symptoms, the patient places the device on the chest and activates the device (the device does not record the ECG until the patient activates it). The patient can then transmit the recording over the telephone.
- The patient keeps the device until several recordings have been made, or for an agreed-upon time frame (usually between 2 to 6 weeks).

- The patient must be aware of arrhythmias when they occur and must maintain consciousness long enough to activate the device.
- Short-lived arrhythmias, and those preceding activation of the device, may be missed.
- Some newer devices are credit card size—small enough to carry in a wallet or to be worn as a necklace or wristwatch.
- Use is not recommended in the setting of arrhythmias that may cause serious symptoms such as syncope.
- Compliance can be problematic because of waning patient motivation without recurrent symptoms or patient error in correctly activating the device.
- Cost is more expensive than Holter monitoring.

External Pre-Event Recorders ("Loop Recorders")

- The patient wears a recording device and electrodes (that are changed by the patient every several days and removed for bathing), usually over the period of a month.
- The standard device continuously records 5 to 10 minutes of ECG data. When the device is activated, the preceding data are captured or "frozen" and additional data are saved for a few minutes following activation at the time of an event. The data can then be transmitted over the telephone to a center for analysis. If the button is not pushed, the ECG loop continuously replaces the old data. Technicians may be on call 24 hours a day to interpret the data when transmitted. If necessary, they can coordinate a trip to the emergency department.
- The device can be programmed to detect asymptomatic arrhythmias and alert the patient to transmit data for evaluation.
- It is the recommended initial monitoring modality for patients with syncope because the activation button can be pressed once consciousness has been regained.
- It is the recommended initial monitoring modality in the workup of most patients with palpitations for which AECG monitoring is deemed appropriate.
- Compliance can be problematic (similar to postevent recorders), and in addition some patients report problems with electrode attachment and skin irritation.
- Cost is more expensive than Holter monitoring.

Implantable Loop Recorders

- For extremely infrequent arrhythmias, a device the size of a pack of gum is implanted subcutaneously in the chest under local anesthesia and is left in place for up to 24 months.
- Like other loop recorders it stores ECG data, which can be telephonically transmitted. The device can be programmed to store 1 minute of data prior to and 1 minute of data after automatic activation for a total of approximately 20 events. The device can also be activated externally and programmed to record up to 8 minutes of preactivation data and 2 minutes of postactivation data.
- It can be programmed to detect bradyarrythmias or tachyarrhythmias on a prespecified basis.
- This device is generally used in the patient who has undergone previous noninvasive testing that was nondiagnostic but who continues to have infrequent symptoms.
- This method is not a good choice for high-risk patients (those with prior myocardial infarction [MI] or conduction abnormalities on ECG) in whom other testing, such as tilt-table or electrophysiologic testing, may make a diagnosis earlier and thus allow for earlier treatment.
- Cost is more expensive than pre-event external loop recorders.

Electrophysiology Studies

- Electrophysiology (EP) studies are helpful when Holter or event monitoring results are equivocal, particularly in patients with a low ejection fraction, documented ischemic heart disease, and a history of syncope or near syncope.
- Used in post-MI patients at high risk of a life-threatening arrhythmia.
- Can determine whether an arrhythmia is inducible.
- Very expensive and higher risk (can provoke refractory or life-threatening arrhythmias).

Signal Averaged ECG

- Signal averaged ECG (SAECG) enables detection of the substrate for potentially dangerous arrhythmias, such as ventricular tachycardia (VT), by using computed filtering and averaging of ECG complexes, which facilitates the detection of very low amplitude cardiac potentials not detectable by routine ECG.
- Generally 200 to 400 QRS complexes with the same morphology are averaged over approximately 3 to 7 minutes to record an adequate SAECG.
- Can be used to stratify risk for ventricular arrhythmias and sudden cardiac death, but only in specific settings such as post-MI, cardiomyopathies, Brugada syndrome, arrhythmogenic right ventricular dysplasia, mitral valve prolapse, ventricular aneurysms, and idiopathic VT.
- Used more widely in the past, it is now known that the positive predictive value of SAECG is poor. As a result, utility is more for its negative predictive accuracy.
- It does not quantitate the frequency of premature ventricular complexes (PVCs).
- The procedure has limited availability and is moderately expensive.

Exercise ECG (Stress) Testing

See also Chapter 93, Exercise Electrocardiography [Stress] Testing.

- Commonly used as a screening or diagnostic test for underlying cardiac ischemia or significant CAD.
- May confirm ischemia as the etiology of an arrhythmia or document its association with an arrhythmia.
- Demonstrates the effect of activity on ventricular arrhythmias.
- May detect some forms of complex ventricular ectopy not detected by Holter monitoring.
- ST segment depression in the absence of chest pain may alert the clinician to silent ischemia (but may be falsely positive).
- Not nearly as sensitive as Holter monitoring for the detection of PVCs.
- Systems are now available to check for T wave alternans, a risk factor for ventricular arrhythmias, particularly in patients with a dilated cardiomyopathy or post-MI with a decreased ejection fraction.

Mobile Cardiac Outpatient Telemetry

- Continuous ECG monitoring from three leads that communicate with a palm-sized monitor. On detection of arrhythmia, real-time data are automatically transmitted via cell phone to a remote monitoring center. The device generally can store data for transmission if the patient is temporarily in an area where cell phone transmission is unavailable.
- Allows up to 2 weeks of continuous monitoring.
- Does not require the patient to activate the device, unlike post-event and loop recorders. Technicians are on call 24 hours a day to interpret the data when transmitted. If necessary, they can coordinate a trip to the emergency department.
- May have a higher yield of arrhythmia detection or exclusion than loop recorders, though validation is still in progress.
- Expensive.

Benefits and Drawbacks of Available Monitoring Methods

Physical examination and cardiac auscultation are unreliable for differentiating supraventricular from ventricular premature beats. The least expensive yet reliable method to document these arrhythmias is a standard 12-lead ECG with a short rhythm strip. Unfortunately, with an ECG the cardiac rhythm is monitored only for a short period. Considering that the commonly accepted definition of "frequent" ventricular ectopy is more than 10 to 30 PVCs an hour, it becomes easy to see how even "frequent" PVCs can be overlooked by this method. On the other hand, if any PVCs are noted on a short rhythm strip, it is likely that the patient has both frequent and complex ventricular ectopy. Both would probably be detected during a longer period of monitoring, such as a Holter monitor study.

In the past, Holter recordings of only a few hours' duration were used for arrhythmia detection. Although practical and economical, such brief recordings do not accurately reflect the severity of cardiac arrhythmias in many individuals. This point is best illustrated by reviewing what is known about the frequency of ventricular arrhythmias over the course of a 24-hour period. Simply stated, even with the same patient, a tremendous amount of spontaneous variability in PVC frequency exists between one Holter recording and another. Similarly, marked variability in PVC frequency also occurs in patients with chronic ventricular arrhythmias. PVC frequency varies greatly from one day to the next, between successive 8-hour monitoring periods, and even from hour to hour within a single day. Certain individuals exhibit PVCs primarily during the day; others manifest them principally at night. As might be expected, PVC frequency often varies with physical activity and emotional state. However, in many individuals, marked spontaneous variability in PVC frequency persists even when monitoring conditions are kept absolutely constant.

Because of such fluctuations in PVC frequency, a monitoring period of at least 24 hours has become the standard for adequate characterization of an arrhythmia, and thus Holter monitors are generally worn for 24 hours, though occasionally the time period is extended to 48 hours. For most individuals, 24-hour monitoring not only permits recognition of diurnal variations in arrhythmias, but it also allows detection of the maximal grade of ectopy.

The key caveat of 24-hour Holter monitoring is that no conclusions can be reached about whether a symptomatic arrhythmia exists unless symptoms occur during the 24 hours of monitoring. As noted previously, a patient may even have a malignant symptomatic ventricular arrhythmia that occurs only intermittently, sometimes as infrequently as once every few weeks. Event monitors, either in the form of a "postevent" device that necessitates patient activation or more commonly a continuously recording pre-event ("loop") device, circumvent the short time limitation of the Holter monitor, as patients use these devices for several weeks at a time.

Although many variations of event monitoring exist, patients are generally issued a device that transmits the patient's rhythm over the telephone. Usually the equipment remains with the patient for a few days or weeks. For cases of extremely infrequent arrhythmias, subcutaneously implanted units may be used for months. The principal weakness of the postevent monitor is that patients must be aware of arrhythmias when they occur, and they must maintain consciousness long enough to capture or transmit the rhythm. In the case of pre-event ("loop") recorder, the patient can activate the device after regaining consciousness, and the preceding data will be saved. Some loop recorders can be programmed to detect asymptomatic arrhythmias and alert the patient to transmit data for evaluation. These automatic detection devices typically have greater data storage capability because they may not reliably discriminate arrhythmias from artifact, potentially creating a lot of false-positive events.

In the past, most clinicians began with full 24-hour Holter monitoring and then proceeded to event monitoring only for those cases when symptoms persisted despite negative Holter findings. However, because asymptomatic Holter results are often complicated and confusing and there is a low yield of positive findings on Holter monitoring when arrhythmias are infrequent, event monitoring is now more commonly ordered than Holter monitoring. Overall, event monitoring is at least as effective as Holter monitoring for detection of symptomatic arrhythmias; event monitoring also has the advantage of less frequently recording asymptomatic background arrhythmias (for which treatment is unnecessary). In the case of syncope and the evaluation of unexplained palpitations, the diagnostic yield of pre-event loop recorders over Holter monitors has been validated, and is the preferred initial AECG modality (Kinlay and colleagues, 1996).

When Holter or event monitoring results are equivocal, EP studies may be helpful. Although EP is an invasive study, the information obtained may be critical. Patients in whom a clinically relevant arrhythmia can be induced during EP testing usually have a worse prognosis, even if asymptomatic, than patients in whom an arrhythmia cannot be induced. However, EP testing does have a small but significant false-negative rate; results in patients with nonischemic cardiomyopathy are also difficult to interpret.

SAECG is a noninvasive test that has been advocated for risk stratification in potentially lethal ventricular arrhythmias. Although its main initial use was following MI, SAECG use has expanded to include patients with cardiomyopathies, Brugada syndrome, arrhythmogenic right ventricular dysplasia, mitral valve prolapse, ventricular aneurysms, and idiopathic VT. By computer-averaging signals for several hundred recorded beats, background "noise" can be filtered out to allow detection of low-amplitude, high-frequency late potentials after the QRS. These late potentials are suggestive of areas of slower conduction that may facilitate development of ventricular reentry. Unfortunately, the positive predictive accuracy of late potentials on SAECG following MI is less than optimal, around 15% to 20% for prediction of VT or ventricular fibrillation (VF). Therefore, negative findings on this test are more useful. SAECG is of established value in the evaluation of the syncope patient, but only in the setting of ischemic heart disease, and again its value is in its negative predictive accuracy.

Exercise ECG testing (EET; see Chapter 93, Exercise Electrocardiography [Stress] Testing) is a common method for evaluating PVCs (especially in older patients or those with coronary risk factors) and other arrhythmias (especially exercise-induced arrhythmias). It serves as a convenient, noninvasive test to screen for or to diagnose underlying CAD. EET may be indicated if ischemia is diagnosed with AECG. If CAD is diagnosed, EET can also evaluate its severity and assist with its management. EET also demonstrates what effect exercise has on arrhythmias. In general, PVCs that diminish with progressively increasing activity are less worrisome and tend to be associated with a better prognosis than those brought on by low levels of exercise. Recent evidence suggests that PVCs occurring during recovery from EET are associated with increased mortality, whereas PVCs during the EET are not (Dewey and colleagues, 2008). Although not nearly as accurate as Holter monitoring for quantitative or qualitative assessment of PVCs, complex ventricular arrhythmias (including VT) and symptoms are sometimes elicited only by vigorous exercise. Chronotropic incompetence (unable to obtain heart rate >120 beats per minute) on EET may suggest sick sinus syndrome, which is best diagnosed with a Holter monitor. Holter monitoring and EET may thus be complementary procedures that provide different information, and both tests should sometimes be considered for the complete evaluation of patients with ventricular arrhythmias.

It should be emphasized that detection of PVCs per se on EET is not indicative of an ischemic response. However, PVCs are cause for more concern when they occur in association with evidence of ischemia, such as ST segment depression or substernal chest pain in patients who are likely to have CAD. Thus, it is inadvisable to allow a middle-aged individual who has coronary risk factors to exercise in an unsupervised manner if EET produces frequent PVCs and ST segment depression or symptoms. Instead, further evaluation for CAD or ischemic or structural heart disease may be warranted.

On the other hand, many clinicians are much more comfortable allowing healthy young adults who have frequent PVCs to exercise vigorously if EET does not produce ST segment depression or if PVCs resolve with exercise. When these younger, asymptomatic, and otherwise healthy adults go out and exercise, their PVCs and symptoms will probably resolve with activity. Moreover, such individuals are much less likely to have underlying ischemic heart disease. Rare, life-threatening complex arrhythmias, seen only at peak exercise, will also be excluded with EET.

Mobile cardiac outpatient telemetry (MCOT) is an emerging technology that allows up to 2 weeks of continuous "real-time" ECG monitoring. Data collected are automatically transmitted via cell phone to a monitoring center. Benefits include less patient error because the device does not require patient activation, unlike post-event and loop recorders. A small industry-sponsored study suggested that MCOT devices may have a higher yield of arrhythmia detection or exclusion than loop recorders, although full validation is still in progress (Rothman and colleagues, 2007).

An all-too-often-ignored adjunct for monitoring is the patient's history (perception) of symptoms compatible with an arrhythmia. Although many individuals are totally unaware of their arrhythmias, others are able to sense each and every ectopic beat. For individuals with non-life-threatening arrhythmias who have this awareness—and in whom AECG has confirmed a temporal relation between symptoms and the occurrence of their arrhythmias—the *patient's account of symptoms* may serve as a fairly reliable and cost-effective adjunct for long-term monitoring (i.e., it may greatly reduce the need for [and expense of] repeated Holter recordings for judging the effect of treatment).

Consider the case of a young patient who is markedly symptomatic from extremely frequent ventricular ectopy. Baseline Holter monitoring reveals several thousand PVCs during the day of monitoring but no runs of VT and no evidence of ischemia. The echocardiogram is normal; there is no evidence of pericarditis, cardiomyopathy, or a metabolic cause for the PVCs, and the patient's diary confirms a definite temporal relationship between symptoms and periods of greatest ectopy. If treatment with a beta-blocker (or a reduction in stimulants such as caffeine) leads to complete resolution of symptoms, does the Holter recording need to be repeated? The answer to this key question is often found by asking two additional questions: Would repeating the Holter recording alter treatment? Will the patient's account of symptoms (i.e., the "poor person's Holter") be adequate for guiding management? In many instances, such as in this particular case, experts would consider monitoring the patient's symptoms alone to be adequate.

INDICATIONS

Evaluation of Patients with Symptoms Possibly Related to Rhythm Disturbances

Symptoms of patients with VT or VF include palpitations (i.e., a sensation in the chest of a rapid or irregular cardiac rhythm), dizziness, and unexplained syncope. These symptoms may suggest a hemodynamically compromising arrhythmia.

However, not all patients with symptoms such as palpitations, dizziness, and syncope need Holter monitoring. An occasional episode of skipped, dropped, or racing beats is not suggestive of VT or VF. Symptom duration and severity, the likelihood of underlying cardiac disease based on a history of risk factors or echocardiogram result, the existence and effect of potentially reversible extracardiac factors (e.g., caffeine, alcohol, sleep deprivation, viral illness, electrolyte abnormalities, hyperthyroidism, nonessential medications, normal sedimentation rate), the patient's or clinician's "need to know," and cost concerns should all be considered. Therefore, on a patient's first visit, do *not* routinely order Holter monitoring for patients who lack underlying heart disease or risk factors, especially if symptoms are of recent onset and are not particularly bothersome to the patient. On the other hand, you probably should consider some form of AECG monitoring for a patient with activity-limiting symptoms, especially when the symptoms are persistent, and especially when the patient has possible underlying structural heart disease or multiple risk factors for CAD.

Ambulatory electrocardiography can be of use in evaluating the patient with unexplained syncope, presyncope, or episodic dizziness. The most recent American College of Cardiology/American Heart Association (ACC/AHA) guidelines give a class I recommendation for an AECG in such patients "in whom the cause is not obvious" (Crawford and colleagues, 1999). Although syncope is a prevalent disorder, it is only infrequently secondary to a cardiac cause. However, mortality rate is quite high in patients with a cardiac cause of syncope, and it is an independent predictor of sudden death. (One pearl: The older the patient is with the first episode of syncope, the more likely the syncope is due to a cardiac cause and the worse the prognosis.) Unfortunately, the yield of AECG monitoring in the patient with syncope is low because most patients do not have symptoms during the time they are being monitored. In fact, it is estimated that AECG establishes a diagnosis in only 2% to 3% of syncope patients. Because syncope can be a symptom of a potentially serious underlying problem, an AECG is prudent to pursue in the high-risk patient. In the evaluation of syncope, the most appropriate type of AECG monitoring is usually the loop recorder, which can be activated by the patient once he or she regains consciousness. The higher yield of loop recorders over Holter monitors was demonstrated in a prospective randomized trial (Sivakumaran and colleagues, 2003). Sometimes results of the AECG can determine whether the patient with syncope would benefit from being evaluated in the electrophysiology laboratory. For example, the syncope patient with structural heart disease noted to have nonsustained VT on AECG has a high likelihood of having a serious underlying ventricular tachyarrhythmia induced in the electrophysiology laboratory.

Evaluation of unexplained recurrent palpitations, a widely accepted indication for AECG monitoring, was also given a class I recommendation by the ACC/AHA. Unexplained palpitations may be secondary to a potentially dangerous underlying arrhythmia, and it is prudent to identify high-risk patients. Although the diagnostic yield of identifying the cause of frequent palpitations from a 24-hour Holter monitor is approximately 35%, the percentage is doubled if one uses a loop recorder. Therefore, it is considered more cost-effective to start the AECG evaluation of palpitations with a loop recorder rather than a Holter monitor. Often (perhaps in one third of patients) a symptom is reported in the patient's symptom diary that does not correlate with any abnormality on the ECG, a scenario that is helpful to exclude a cardiac cause, reassure the patient, and consider pursuing other noncardiac causes of the patient's symptoms.

Evaluation of palpitations with AECG is a special case, with insight provided in a study (Weber and Kapoor, 1996) showing that one third of patients coming to an emergency facility with palpitations as their chief complaint had a psychological cause for this symptom (either generalized anxiety or panic disorders). Four factors were found in this study to be independently predictive of a cardiac (arrhythmia) cause: male gender, a history of heart disease, subjective sensation of an irregular heartbeat, and symptom duration (palpitations) of more than 5 minutes. Awareness of these findings may help in the decision of when to order an objective form of arrhythmia detection.

Evaluation of Antiarrhythmic Drug Therapy

Although in the past AECG was commonly used to evaluate the efficacy of an antiarrhythmic drug, it is now used less frequently for this indication because interpretation is limited by a high spontaneous variability in the frequency and type of arrhythmia within each individual, and lack of correlation between suppressing an arrhythmia and patient outcome. This limitation was particularly evident in the Cardiac Arrhythmia Suppression Trial (CAST; Echt and colleagues, 1991), in which attempted arrhythmia suppression with flecainide, encainide, and moricizine resulted in an increased mortality rate. This study outcome led to class I antiarrhythmics no longer being recommended as long-term therapy for arrhythmia suppression, resulting in less AECG monitoring. Furthermore, approximately 25% of patients with ventricular arrhythmias have spontaneous resolution within 12 to 17 months, making it difficult to establish benefit (or causality) after antiarrhythmics are started. When AECG is chosen for monitoring drug response it is done so under three specific circumstances: (1) to document drug response in a patient with known baseline of arrhythmias that are reproducible; (2) to detect proarrhythmic response to an antiarrhythmic drug; or most commonly, (3) to assess rate control in chronic atrial fibrillation.

A review of the statistics behind spontaneous variability in PVC frequency is essential if the practitioner is to use Holter recordings to evaluate the effectiveness of antiarrhythmic therapy, especially now that nonrepetitive ventricular ectopy is treated much less often than it was in the past. To *statistically* exclude a spontaneous variation in response following antiarrythmic therapy, a reduction in PVC frequency of at least 70% to 90% between Holter recordings is required.

Evaluation for Silent Myocardial Ischemia

Silent myocardial ischemia, defined as objective evidence of ischemia without chest discomfort or any anginal equivalent, is the most common manifestation of CAD. It is estimated that over 75% of ischemic episodes occur without symptoms while patients go about their activities of daily living, and because episodes of silent myocardial ischemia are not alarming to the patient, they frequently go undetected and untreated. AECG monitoring to detect ST segment changes was first investigated in the mid-1970s, but there was much skepticism, particularly regarding a high number of false-positive results. In monitoring for silent ischemia, the Holter monitor continuously records ST segments, which can be assessed for flat or downsloping ST depression of 1 to 2 mm or more (see discussion of Equipment Settings). However, because of large day-to-day variability of ST segment changes, ST segment depression as detected by Holter monitors may not be indicative of ischemia. In recent years, technologic improvements have resulted in increased specificity for ischemia particularly in certain population subgroups. We now know that ischemia detected by Holter monitoring is associated with increased coronary events and increased mortality risk, but this applies only to patients with known CAD, particularly those who have had an MI. At this point, there is no role for monitoring for silent myocardial ischemia in patients without CAD. For this reason, the ACC/AHA do not strongly support the routine use of AECG to assess for silent myocardial ischemia (with one exception being the patient with suspected variant [Prinzmetal's] angina). Furthermore, Holter monitoring should not be used as an alternative to EET to diagnose ischemia. It has been suggested that Holter monitoring may allow for further risk stratification in patients who have had a positive EET, by assessing for ischemia while patients perform their routine activities. Such detection of ischemia by Holter monitoring may help to identify groups of patients who would benefit most from more aggressive antiplatelet and anti-ischemic therapy.

Risk Assessment in High-Risk Asymptomatic Patients

There are approximately 450,000 sudden cardiac deaths per year in the United States; most are due to ventricular tachyarrhythmias such as VF or VT. One key role of AECG is, in certain high-risk patient populations, to detect arrhythmias that are precursors to sudden death so that there is time to consider an intervention that may reduce the patient's chance of sudden death. Patients who survive VF or sustained VT are likely to have recurrences (particularly if they have CAD or structural heart disease), and unfortunately many such recurrences are fatal. Much attention has been given to the prevention of sudden cardiac death, particularly with the development of ICDs, which have shown a mortality risk benefit in select patient populations. Antiarrythmic drugs, although less effective in certain subgroups for primary and secondary prevention of sudden cardiac death, are often used in conjunction with ICDs to reduce the frequency of shocks.

Conditions associated with ventricular arrhythmias and sudden cardiac death include CAD, dilated or hypertrophic cardiomyopathy, right ventricular dysplasia, long QT syndrome, electrolyte abnormalities, use of antiarrhythmic drugs, and valvular heart disease. As noted earlier, AECG can be used to identify high-risk patients who may be at risk for sudden cardiac death. Currently there are only three conditions for which the ACC/AHA support (albeit weakly with class IIb recommendations) risk assessment in the absence of symptoms: post-MI patients with left ventricular ejection fraction (LV EF) less than 40%, patients with congestive heart failure, and patients with hypertrophic cardiomyopathy.

In general, patients with ischemic heart disease, especially those with a history of MI, have a very high risk for a serious or fatal arrhythmic event. Frequent and complex PVCs are an independent risk factor associated with a two- to fivefold increased risk of death after an MI. AECG (particularly Holter monitoring) is sometimes performed in post-MI patients with a low EF (<40%) as a risk assessment tool.

It is well established that patients with congestive heart failure and underlying cardiomyopathy have an increased risk of sudden death. Much attention has been paid to the possible role of AECG as a way to further identify which of these patients may or may not benefit from ICDs. However, the data are conflicting and the role for using AECG in this population is not well established.

Patients with hypertrophic cardiomyopathy have an increased risk of sudden death. AECG monitoring for nonsustained VT (NSVT) has been proposed in this patient population, with the idea that NSVT may be a marker for sudden death. However, this has not been clearly established, and arrhythmia treatment has not been shown to improve mortality risk. Therefore, AECG for risk assessment in this population remains unclear.

Evaluation of Pacemaker or Implantable Cardioverter-Defibrillator Function

In the past, Holter monitors were commonly used to assess the function of a pacemaker or an ICD, and the data were used to guide programming, for example, by changing pacing thresholds. This practice is becoming less frequent because newer generation devices generally have the ability to store ECG data that can be retrieved and analyzed. However, AECG is still recommended in several situations, such as to evaluate for device failure or malfunction (e.g., pacemaker-induced tachycardia in the setting of frequent palpitations, syncope, or near syncope) or to assess the response to adjunctive pharmacologic therapy in patients receiving frequent ICD discharges.

Contraindications

As with other office-based procedures, AECG monitoring can be overutilized. More information is not necessarily better, particularly when the information could be misleading, such as may be the case with a false-positive result in a low pretest probability setting (e.g., a low-risk patient with a constellation of vague symptoms). AECG should not be used as a screening tool in the low-risk asymptomatic patient, or for the evaluation of chest pain in low-risk patients who can exercise. Similarly, the ACC/AHA discourages AECG for patients with syncope or palpitations in whom another etiology has been identified, or in the assessment of a patient who has had a cerebrovascular accident but with no evidence of arrhythmia.

Preprocedure Patient Education and Preparation

- Explain to the patient why Holter or event monitoring is necessary.
- Explain to the patient the need for a symptom diary.

An essential part of the Holter recording is the patient's symptom diary. Consider how often supraventricular and ventricular ectopy are found in the general population as well as how frequently patients come to a clinician with symptoms suggestive of cardiac arrhythmias; the importance of establishing a cause-and-effect relationship between the two should be evident. For example, if symptoms are noted at 10 AM, 2 PM, 5 PM, and 11 PM, but no cardiac arrhythmias are seen at these times, it is unlikely that the symptoms are cardiac related. Therefore, much useful information may be obtained from Holter recordings even in the absence of arrhythmias—provided the diary is completed carefully.

In symptomatic individuals who actually demonstrate cardiac arrhythmias on Holter monitoring, one can determine whether the arrhythmias are likely to be the cause of their symptoms by the temporal relationship in the diary. For example, if long runs of ventricular bigeminy occur while the patient is relaxed and totally unaware of the arrhythmia—and palpitations or chest discomfort are noted only during periods of sinus rhythm—ventricular bigeminy is probably not related to the patient's symptoms.

Unfortunately, in clinical practice, completion of the diary is all too often neglected. As a result, consider the following:

- Emphasize the importance of filling out the diary to your patient.
- Be sure that the patient can read and write before providing the diary. If the patient is illiterate, see if someone can help the patient fill out the diary.
- For hospitalized patients, consider actively involving the nursing staff to ensure accurate completion of the patient diary.

NOTE: Use of event monitoring is much more conducive to correlating symptoms with arrhythmias than Holter monitoring because the occurrence of symptoms is what prompts the patient to initiate the event monitor recording.

Equipment

- Holter, event, or other AECG monitor with desired capabilities (check for cracked or broken wires and for damage to the carrying case)
- Fresh, alkaline batteries
- Printer paper, ink, extra cassettes (for the Holter report to be printed out for interpretation)
- Razor
- Rubbing alcohol
- Electrodes
- Lead attachment kit

Most of the time, hospitals and commercial Holter or event laboratories employ trained technicians to scan Holter recordings for the interpreting clinician. This is a tremendous time-saving feature because the technician can highlight the principal findings, thus sparing the clinician the need to meticulously scan each of the full-disclosure printouts.

On the other hand, the luxury of having a trained technician to scan tracings is not available to many clinicians who have purchased their own Holter monitoring system. In this case options include the following:

- Having the hard copy of the Holter recording processed and scanned by a commercial laboratory—an expensive and rarely used option.
- Hiring or training a technician to scan, which may be the most cost-effective solution for the busy practitioner who has a nurse or technician with interest and expertise in arrhythmia interpretation.
- Not printing 24-hour full disclosure. (Full disclosure means that the Holter device prints out a miniaturized strip of each hour of the 24-hour tracing.) Depending on the area's third-party payment regulations, the practitioner may not receive full reimbursement unless 24-hour full disclosure is printed out.
- Printing but ignoring the 24-hour full disclosure, or looking only at those portions of the printout that seem relevant to the clinical problem (i.e., looking at full disclosure only at times when symptoms are noted in the diary, or at times of densest ectopy as suggested on the hourly summary). This saves time, but if something is missed, it will be documented.
- Printing 24-hour full disclosure and scanning the printout yourself. Although this takes a greater amount of time to accomplish, it may be time well spent.
- Purchasing a Holter system that does not provide full disclosure. If reimbursement for this modality in your area is comparable to that for full-disclosure systems, this alternative may be both cost and time effective, especially if the practitioner does not have great interest or expertise in arrhythmia interpretation. However, such systems are more likely to yield equivocal findings, and they may overlook potentially important arrhythmias. Personal interpretation of Holter data recorded on such systems is only as good as the system's computer software.

NOTE: The authors feel that full 24-hour disclosure is indispensable for optimal Holter interpretation. Many experts suggest that it is essential for the interpreter to scan the entire recording, even when trend analyses, hourly summaries, and selected rhythm strips are normal.

Systems that offer data compression do not provide full disclosure. Using signal averaging to evaluate "compressed" data, and then re-expanding it, does not allow every QRS complex to be reproduced.

Technique

1. The patient's report form (see Fig. 87-14) should be completed with relevant patient information such as date of birth and indications for procedure. Recorded data such as cardiac risk factors, medications, activity level, and other medical problems that may affect the management following interpretation would also be helpful.
2. Monitoring parameters on the equipment should be set.
3. Attach the ECG electrodes in the locations indicated for the particular model of Holter or event monitor (see the operating instructions or illustrations provided by the monitor manufacturer). In general, limb leads are placed more centrally than with an office ECG.

Equipment Settings

Most Holter systems provide the operator some flexibility in selecting the parameters used to scan for abnormalities. Some routine settings are shown in Table 87-1. In this example, the computer will record a full-size rhythm strip for those tachycardias that are faster than 120 beats per minute (automatic high rate); for bradycardias slower than 40 beats per minute (automatic low rate); and for pauses longer than 2 seconds (automatic pause). Since automatic abnormal is set at three events, the machine should record the first three

TABLE 87-1 Equipment Settings

Automatic high rate	120 bpm
Automatic low rate	40 bpm
Automatic pause	2.00 sec
Automatic supraventricular ectopic	25%
Automatic ST level	2 mm
Automatic abnormal	3/hr
Periodic storage	2 hr
Strips per hour	5

incidents of tachycardia that occur during any given hour, to a maximum of five strips per hour for any reason—which may potentially yield a total of 120 rhythm strips to review (up to 5 strips per hour × 24 hours = 120 strips).

Because periodic storage is set at 2 hours, the computer should record at least 1 rhythm strip every 2 hours, even if no abnormalities occur. This guarantees that the interpreter will have at least 12 rhythm strips to view, even if the Holter result is completely normal.

NOTE: The authors are generally uncomfortable accepting the computer's reading of "normal" unless a minimal number of normal full-size rhythm strips are displayed.

One reason for favoring 120 beats per minute as the upper rate limit is that lower numbers (e.g., 100 or 110 beats per minute) are more likely to produce an excessive number of benign sinus tachycardia strips, whereas higher numbers (e.g., 130 or 140 beats per minute) might prevent the detection of significant tachycardias with relatively slow rates, such as VT at 125 beats per minute.

NOTE: Selection of equipment settings always involves a compromise, and the setting of 120 beats per minute may occasionally yield a monotonous deluge of sinus tachycardia strips at 120 to 125 beats per minute.

For similar reasons, a lower rate limit of 40 beats per minute is favored. For example, selecting a lower rate limit of 50 beats per minute might result in a deluge of benign sinus bradycardia strips if the Holter examination was performed on an otherwise healthy individual who happened to have a slow resting heart rate.

Pauses of up to 2 seconds are common, especially in the elderly, and are usually benign. Longer pauses, especially those accompanied by frequent episodes of bradycardia with rates of fewer than 40 beats per minute, suggest the possibility of sick sinus syndrome, particularly in the setting of structural heart disease.

The automatic supraventricular ectopic (SVE) setting of 25% should record rhythm strips demonstrating a greater than 25% variation in R-R interval. This record is how atrial fibrillation or premature atrial contractions (PACs) are detected. Setting the SVE lower (e.g., at 10%) would detect many more PACs but would also pick up sinus arrhythmia. Higher settings might miss too many PACs. Even with a setting of 25%, imagine the number of strips that would result when the underlying rhythm is atrial fibrillation!

The most controversial parameter is the automatic ST segment level, which is usually set at 2 mm, unless the reason for performing the Holter monitoring is to "seek and search for" silent ischemia (which is only recommended in the known CAD patient). Resolution of ST segment images may be less than ideal, and because of marked day-to-day variability of ST segment changes, in an otherwise unselected population the majority of episodes of ST segment depression between 1 and 2 mm will be false-positive results; that is, they will not represent true silent ischemia. Setting the ST segment parameter at 2 mm greatly increases the specificity for true silent ischemia. The tradeoff is that some patients with CAD may have frequent episodes of silent ischemia with lesser degrees of ST segment depression. Although the ST segment trend analysis (see Fig. 87-4) should reflect this, it is important to document the phenomenon by recording at least a few full-size strips that demonstrate definite ST segment depression. This is one benefit of lowering the ST segment parameter to 1 mm when the principal reason for performing the Holter test is to evaluate the patient with known CAD for silent ischemia.

NOTE: The technique and equipment settings for event monitors are usually similar to those for Holter monitors.

Interpretation of Results

Appreciation of the wide range of normal is essential for meaningful interpretation of ambulatory ECG recordings. Premature supraventricular and ventricular contractions, as well as certain other cardiac arrhythmias, are common in otherwise healthy, asymptomatic individuals without underlying structural heart disease or CAD. Additional evaluation of such individuals is potentially expensive and may be harmful.

Although a detailed description of all of the variants of "normal" is beyond the scope of this chapter, a brief discussion of the prevalence of ventricular arrhythmias and then an overview of the clinical perspective of the process may be helpful.

Prevalence of Premature Ventricular Contractions in the General Population

Premature ventricular contractions are common. They are found in up to 50% of otherwise healthy, asymptomatic young adults. Their frequency increases with age; thus most adults over 60 have some ventricular ectopy during a 24-hour period of monitoring. Less well appreciated is the fact that in the absence of underlying heart disease, complex forms of ventricular ectopy (e.g., ventricular couplets, salvos, or longer runs of VT) are uncommon and when present in this population are generally associated with low risk of sustained VT or sudden death. The excellent prognosis for such patients has been documented in patients with primary electrical disease (Kennedy and colleagues, 1985) and competitive athletes. In contrast, both frequent and complex ventricular ectopy are common when underlying heart disease is present.

The term *frequent* when used to quantify ventricular ectopy is subject to interpretation. In a population of middle-aged individuals with underlying heart disease, frequent ventricular ectopy is most often defined as an average of more than 10 to 30 PVCs per hour over 24 hours of monitoring (i.e., at least 240 PVCs per day). In contrast, among otherwise healthy, asymptomatic young adults, a much lower number to define *frequent* should probably be used. As noted earlier, although up to half of these individuals have some PVCs during 24 hours of monitoring, it is unusual for them to have as many as 100 PVCs per day.

Clinical Significance of Premature Ventricular Contractions

The significance of ventricular ectopy depends on the clinical setting in which it occurs. Patients with PVCs who do not have underlying heart disease tend to have a benign prognosis. Even among individuals with primary electrical disease and frequent, complex PVCs (as noted previously), treatment may not be indicated in the absence of both symptoms and underlying heart disease, as demonstrated by the Cardiac Arrythmia Suppression Trials (CAST I and II), which found that antiarrhythmic treatment was associated with an increased mortality rate.

In a study of 355 athletes ages 14 to 35 years of age who underwent a 24-hour Holter study because of palpitations or frequent PVCs noted on routine ECG (Biffi and colleagues, 2002), there were no deaths during a mean 8-year follow-up in the group (284 athletes) noted to have fewer than 2000 PVCs in 24 hours. The 71 athletes who had 2000 or more PVCs per day were excluded from competitive athletics. There was only one sudden death in this excluded group in an individual with arrhythmogenic right ventricular cardiomyopathy; it occurred while playing field hockey against medical advice.

In contrast, in the setting of acute ischemia, especially if associated with angina, any ventricular ectopy at all must be viewed as significant and as a potential trigger of VF. Data suggest that this is particularly true of PVCs that occur in recovery following exercise, for example, during exercise ECG (stress) testing (Dewey and colleagues, 2008).

Although left ventricular function is the most important predictor of death during the year following acute MI, PVCs are also an independent risk factor. Death in this year is related to the frequency of ventricular ectopy, as detected by Holter monitoring before discharge from the hospital. Patients with less than one PVC per hour tend to have a low (<10%) mortality rate. This figure rises sharply as a function of PVC frequency. About half of the total PVC-associated deaths happen at PVC frequencies as low as three per hour. A mortality rate plateau (20% to 30% for the ensuing year) is reached above PVC frequencies of 10 per hour. Thus, a predischarge Holter monitor recording obtained for a post-MI patient needs to be interpreted in a different light than that of one obtained on a patient with chronic ventricular ectopy. The definition of "frequent" ventricular ectopy should probably be adjusted downward in post-MI patients.

The frequency of ventricular arrhythmias detected in the postinfarction period is time dependent. PVCs are infrequent for 3 to 5 days following infarction. They tend to increase in frequency over the next 6 to 12 weeks, and then the frequency levels off. Despite the tendency of PVC frequency to increase after discharge from the hospital, it may be more practical to obtain a baseline Holter monitor in selected patients *before* they go home.

Repetitive forms of ventricular ectopy (e.g., ventricular couplets, and especially salvos and longer runs of VT) are additional cause for concern. Their presence more than doubles the first-year mortality risk after MI over that of patients who do not demonstrate repetitive forms. In contrast to previous thinking, multiform PVCs and R-on-T complexes are considered much less worrisome than repetitive forms.

Much less can be said about the clinical benefit of drug treatment for PVCs in postinfarction patients. Beta-blockers are generally favored as first-line therapy because they are well tolerated, have a low proarrhythmia effect, and reduce both postinfarction mortality *and* ventricular ectopy rates. As mentioned, the CAST studies demonstrated a two- to threefold *increase* in mortality rate when postinfarction patients with ventricular arrhythmias were routinely treated with flecainide or encainide. Treatment of such patients with a class Ia, Ib, or Ic antiarrhythmic agent when beta-blockers cannot be used is not recommended. Because these antiarrhythmic drugs may produce significant side effects, increase mortality risk, or be proarrhythmic or ineffective, the decision to use them should never be taken lightly.

Fortunately, there are alternatives to pharmacologic therapy. ICDs are often lifesaving, but expensive, and may be associated with morbidity from repetitive shocks. That said, ICDs are often recommended in patients with prior MI who have an EF less than 30%, and in survivors of sudden cardiac arrest. Most patients with VT and normal LV function may not require or be candidates for ICDs. Catheter ablation of the ectopic focus or reentry circuit is another potential alternative in some of these patients.

SAMPLE HOLTER MONITOR

Many types of Holter monitor systems are on the market. Each has its own advantages and disadvantages. The field continues to evolve at an amazingly rapid pace, so that current drawbacks of a particular system may be corrected by the next version of that system. It behooves the interested clinician to become familiar, at least in general terms, with the pros and cons of several types of Holter systems. This familiarity will assist the clinician in selecting those operative features that are likely to be most applicable for a particular practice setting.

In the following section, the information provided by one particular full-disclosure Holter system is illustrated. Although resolution quality of P wave and ST segment morphology is admittedly less than optimal with this system, it should still be adequate for office monitoring. The general principles illustrated by this Holter system are applicable to other systems, as well as to many of the principles involved in event monitoring. The main difference with event monitoring is that 24-hour full disclosure is not included.

CASE STUDY

A 60-year-old man has dyspnea on exertion, which has been increasing for 1 month. He had an MI in the distant past, but he has been active for years and is otherwise doing well and is not on cardiac medications. He has not complained of chest pain or palpitations but recently described frequent episodes of intense dyspnea, weakness, and dizziness, most often associated with activity. Physical examination is unremarkable, and a resting ECG reveals normal sinus rhythm without any acute changes. Because of the frequent occurrence of symptoms with activities of daily living, the practitioner has decided to obtain a Holter monitor before exercise testing.

Patient Diary

It is important for patients to keep a diary to aid in interpreting the results of Holter monitoring. As mentioned earlier, symptoms of potential cardiac etiology and arrhythmias are common in the general population. The only way to prove that symptoms are cardiac related is to document a temporal correlation between their occurrence and the occurrence of arrhythmias on a Holter monitor.

As emphasized earlier, completion of a diary can provide the clinician with much useful information, even if the Holter result is entirely normal. Thus, if multiple symptoms are noted on the day of monitoring and no arrhythmias are detected on the Holter, the patient can be reassured that symptoms are unlikely to be cardiac in origin. The diary (Fig. 87-1) is especially helpful in this case because it indicates eight symptomatic episodes of weakness, dizziness, or shortness of breath.

12-Lead Electrocardiogram

Many clinicians obtain a preprocedure 12-lead ECG on all patients scheduled for Holter monitoring to screen for baseline artifact. If there is significant artifact on the 12-lead ECG, such artifact will likely be seen on the Holter recording and might preclude accurate assessment of the rhythm strip. However, this additional step may

Time	Activity	Symptoms
1PM	Lunch, relax	
2PM	Rake leaves	Weak, dizziness
4PM	Sitting, resting	Weak, dizziness
6PM	Resting	Weak
7PM	Watching TV	Dizziness
9PM	Went to bed	Dizziness
7AM	Breakfast	Short of breath
8AM	Resting	Short of breath, dizzy
9AM	Drove to doctor's office	Weak, dizziness

Figure 87-1 Patient diary for Holter monitoring.

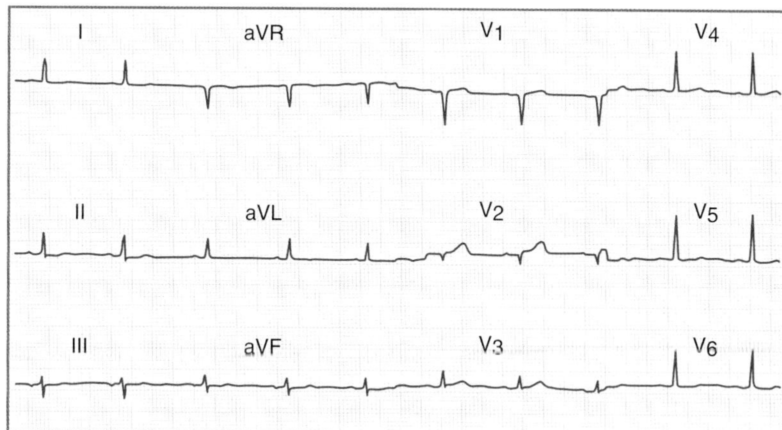

Figure 87-2 Baseline 12-lead electrocardiogram.

be considered unnecessary and time consuming by technicians because the patient has usually undergone a 12-lead ECG at a recent clinical visit. In most cases, proper attention to lead placement precludes baseline artifact.

If there has been a frequent problem with the quality of Holter results, certain systems offer the ability to test the three or five leads of a Holter recording through a 12-lead ECG at the time of lead attachment. Others require the use of a "block," a conversion device available from the manufacturer, to connect the Holter monitor to a 12-lead ECG for testing.

In this case example, despite the fact that the P wave amplitude is small on the patient's 12-lead ECG (Fig. 87-2), the underlying rhythm fortunately turns out to be clearly identified as sinus on the eventual Holter (since the P wave is upright in lead II). Although this overall Holter study is interpretable, on many of the selected rhythm strips, as predicted by the 12-lead, a sinus rhythm is harder to identify with certainty.

Other benefits of obtaining a baseline 12-lead ECG include accurate determination of intervals (PR, QRS, and QT), and a much better appreciation of the baseline ST segment (many patients have baseline ST depression, which is not indicative of ischemia). As a result, determination of ST segment shifts (i.e., possible silent ischemia) is greatly facilitated. In this Holter study example, all intervals are normal. There is some nonspecific ST-T wave flattening in the inferolateral leads, but no significant ST segment depression and no acute changes.

Narrative Summary

Some Holter monitors produce a narrative summary (Box 87-1) that consolidates the principal findings detected by the computer. Practically speaking, the main task of the interpreter is to verify that this computed summary of pertinent findings is accurate.

In this case example, the narrative summary indicates a number of abnormal findings. The interpreter will certainly want to see representative samples of the following:

- Episodes of tachycardia (with a heart rate of up to 160 beats per minute)
- Episodes of bradycardia (with a heart rate between 36 to 39 beats per minute)
- Pauses (between 2.14 and 3.29 seconds in duration)
- Rhythm strips at the time the patient activated the event button (which occurred on two occasions)
- "Abnormal beats" (1151 were detected), including the two episodes of "successive abnormal episodes"

The clinician–interpreter does not need to find each of the 1144 abnormal beats. Nevertheless, he or she should verify that the beats are truly abnormal (not artifactual), whether the "abnormal" beats are truly PVCs, and whether these PVCs seem to be occurring frequently enough to explain the computer count. Practically speaking, it matters little if there are 1144 abnormal beats or 1100 abnormal beats—or 800 or 500, for that matter—since the difference between 1151 and 800, or 500, is still well within the range for spontaneous variability. Clinically, it is unlikely that treatment would differ for a patient who has 1151 PVCs or 500 PVCs. In both situations, it is probably sufficient to say that there are "frequent" PVCs.

REMEMBER: Evaluate any intervention; a reduction of at least 70% to 90% of the PVCs from one Holter to the next must be demonstrated to rule out the possibility of spontaneous variation. Therefore, in this particular case, the number of PVCs would have to be reduced from 1144 to *less than* 350 to eliminate this possibility.

Finally, this particular Holter system does not indicate whether the PVCs are uniform or multiform; it simply gives the sum of all

Box 87-1. Narrative Summary of Holter Recording*

- During this period the average heart rate was 75 bpm with a maximum heart rate of 160 bpm at 16:45 and a minimum heart rate of 36 bpm at 03:38.
- There were 29 tachycardic episodes detected during the monitoring period.
- These episodes ranged in rate from 120 bpm to 160 bpm.
- There were 7 bradycardic episodes detected during the monitoring period.
- These episodes ranged in rate from 36 bpm to 39 bpm.
- There were 57 pause episodes detected during the monitoring period.
- These episodes ranged in duration from 2.14 sec to 3.29 sec.
- There were 25 SVE episodes detected during the monitoring period.
- The patient pressed the event button two times during the monitoring period.
- There were no ST segment episodes detected during the monitoring period.
- During the monitoring period there were 1144 abnormal beats detected.
- There were two successive abnormal episodes detected during the monitoring period.

SVE, supraventricular ectopy.
*The patient was monitored for a period of 23:36 (hours and minutes).

"abnormal" beats. Once again, practically speaking, this really does not matter in view of the following facts:

- The prognostic implications of multiformity are not nearly as ominous as previously thought. Much more important than multiform PVCs are *repetitive* PVCs (e.g., couplets, salvos, and longer runs of VT).
- Almost all individuals with frequent ventricular ectopy over a 24-hour period demonstrate at least some degree of multiformity.

Trend Analysis of Abnormal Beats

The trend analysis of abnormal beats allows the interpreter, at a glance, to see what time of day PVC frequency peaks. In this case, minimal ventricular ectopy occurs at night and maximal ectopy occurs during the daytime and evening hours (e.g., between noon and midnight) when the patient is active (Fig. 87-3).

Identifiable periods of peak ventricular ectopic activity may suggest a specific approach to treatment. For example, patients who manifest diurnal variation or increased ectopic activity during the hours of maximal daily activity often have an increase in sympathetic tone as part of their etiology. Therefore, these patients are optimal candidates for beta-blocker therapy. Patients on antiarrhythmic therapy who demonstrate a peak in ectopic activity 6 to 10 hours after the last dose of their medication may benefit from an increased dosing frequency or by use of a sustained-release product.

Trend Analysis of Heart Rate and ST Segment Level

The heart rate trend analysis demonstrates, at a glance, heart rate variations throughout the day. In this case, it is easy to see that a tachycardia of approximately 150 beats per minute was sustained for most of the period between 16:00 and 17:00 (Fig. 87-4). The ST segment level trend analysis shows that 1 mm of ST segment depression was sustained throughout much of this same period (*arrow*), suggesting that the ST segment depression is likely to be at least partially rate related.

The ST segment level trend analysis may facilitate quantitative assessment of the type and duration of ST segment depression in patients with silent ischemia.

Hourly Summary

Most Holter systems produce an hourly summary in some type of tabular format. Although it usually takes some time and practice to become familiar with this type of format, doing so tremendously facilitates interpretation. The hourly summary shows exactly where to look on the full-disclosure tracings to verify abnormal findings.

The hourly summary in this case (Fig. 87-5) indicates the following:

- The lowest heart rate (36 beats per minute) was recorded between 03:00 and 04:00. The fastest heart rate (160 beats per minute) was recorded between 16:00 and 17:00. The greatest hourly frequency of PVCs, or "isolated abnormalities," (235) occurred between 16:00 and 17:00.
- The event button was activated twice (once between 15:00 and 16:00, and once between 09:00 and 10:00).
- All 57 pause episodes (38 + 19) occurred between 19:00 and 21:00.

Selected (Full-Size) Rhythm Strips

Inspection of selected representative full-size rhythm strips is essential for verifying pertinent computer findings and is generally performed next. These strips have usually been selected by the reviewing technician as discussed previously. The rhythm strips should include portions of the tracings that were patient activated (i.e., the patient was symptomatic at the time the device recorded the strip) as well as abnormalities noted by the technician. Thus, in this case, the patient had a 10-beat run of paroxysmal atrial fibrillation at 13:03:20 (Fig. 87-6). He was in a regular, presumably sinus rhythm of 80 beats per minute at 15:03:20 (Fig. 87-7). An ever-so-slightly irregular supraventricular tachycardia (rapid atrial fibrillation) is evident at 15:51:09 (Fig. 87-8).

Another rhythm strip was automatically recorded at 15:55:53 (Fig. 87-9), presumably because of the rapid, irregular rhythm and associated ectopic activity. Finally, a rhythm strip is shown at 21:56:13 (Fig. 87-10) when the computer probably interpreted the tracing, mistakenly, as representing ventricular ectopic beats. Close inspection suggests that the baseline irregularity is in fact due to artifact.

Full-Disclosure Strips

Many insurance carriers now require full disclosure as a prerequisite for maximal financial compensation. The obvious benefit of full disclosure is that it enables the interpreter to review any or all events of the day. The interpreter can also print out a full-size rhythm strip of any abnormality not initially recognized by the computer or technician. Interpretation of full-disclosure tracings probably seems like an overwhelming task to the uninitiated; however, this need not be the case.

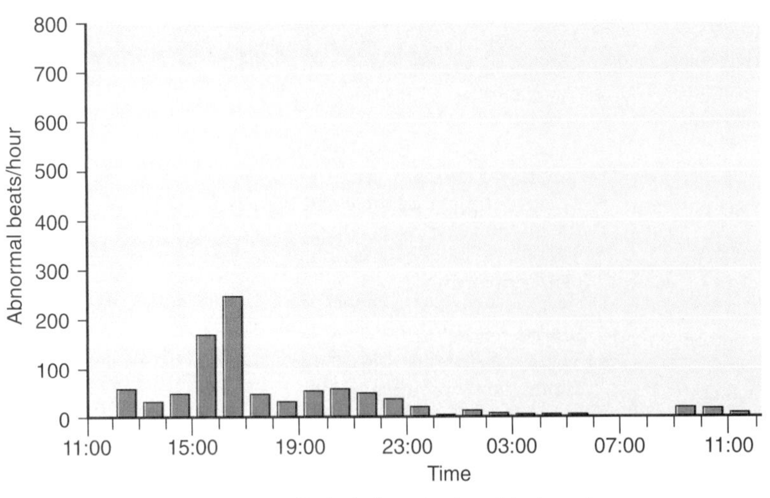

Figure 87-3 Trend analysis of abnormal heartbeats during 24-hour Holter monitoring.

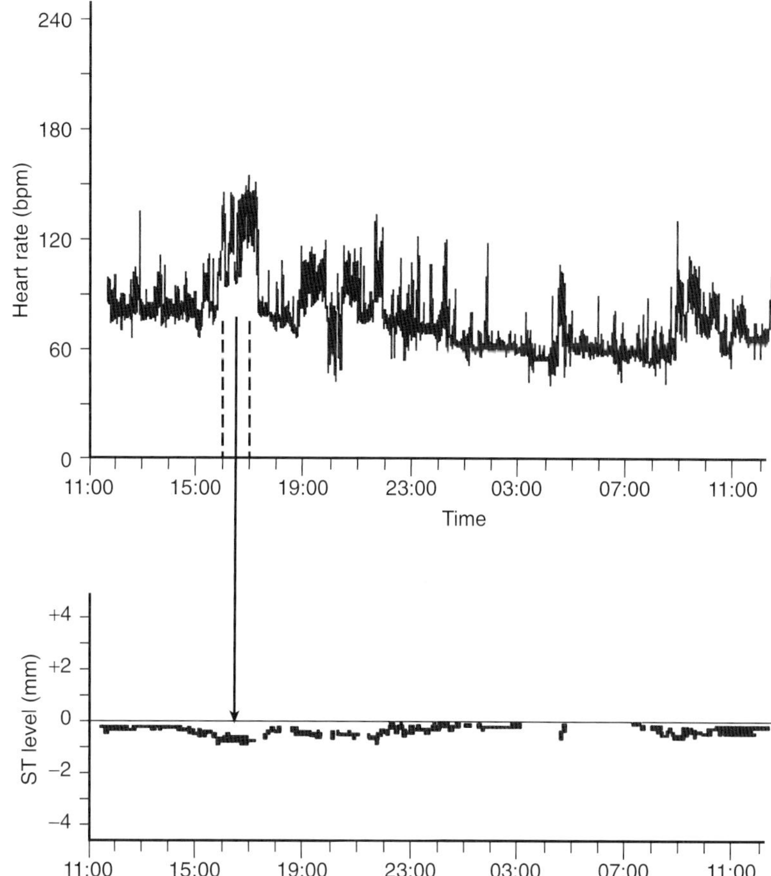

Figure 87-4 Heart rate and ST segment trend analysis during Holter monitoring.

Time	Heart Rate Avg	Heart Rate Max	Heart Rate Min	S/T LEV	S/T SLP	Tachy EPS	Brady EPS	Pause EPS	SVE	Iso. abn.	Coup.	Succ. abn.	Pat. event
11:00	87	105	70	−0.4	−02	0	0	0	0	5	0	0	0
12:00	82	105	62	−0.4	−02	0	0	0	0	64	0	0	0
13:00	80	139	63	−0.4	−01	0	0	0	1	40	0	0	0
14:00	81	114	68	−0.4	−02	0	0	0	0	67	0	0	0
15:00	94	153	63	−0.8	−09	3	0	0	2	176	0	0	1
16:00	129	160	89	−1.0	−17	8	0	0	10	235	0	0	0
17:00	83	159	67	−0.4	−04	4	0	0	3	71	0	0	0
18:00	82	136	63	−0.2	−01	2	0	0	0	57	0	0	0
19:00	85	141	37	−0.4	−01	4	3	38	1	79	0	0	0
20:00	87	129	44	−0.4	−02	4	0	19	0	86	0	0	0
21:00	84	144	50	−0.4	−06	4	0	0	1	62	0	0	0
22:00	73	126	51	−0.2	−03	0	0	0	1	51	0	0	0
23:00	73	124	56	−0.2	−03	0	0	0	0	32	0	0	0
00:00	62	94	43	0.0	−04	0	0	0	0	9	0	0	0
01:00	61	122	53	0.0	−05	0	0	0	0	16	0	0	0
02:00	58	81	39	0.0	−04	0	1	0	2	9	0	0	0
03:00	58	110	36	0.0	−05	0	1	0	0	6	0	1	0
04:00	63	105	42	0.0	−03	0	0	0	0	7	0	1	0
05:00	58	91	50	0.0	−03	0	0	0	1	4	0	0	0
06:00	56	91	39	0.0	−03	0	1	0	0	3	0	0	0
07:00	56	99	38	0.0	−03	0	1	0	1	4	0	0	0
08:00	87	137	53	−0.4	−01	0	0	0	1	23	0	0	0
09:00	72	101	55	−0.2	−01	0	0	0	0	20	0	0	1
10:00	70	93	48	−0.2	−01	0	0	0	1	13	0	0	0
11:00	70	105	55	−0.2	−03	0	0	0	0	5	0	0	0
Avg	75			−0.2	−04	1	0	2	1	48	0	0	0
TOTAL						29	7	57	25	1144	0	2	2

Figure 87-5 Hourly summary for 24-hour Holter study. Abn., abnormality (i.e., primarily premature ventricular contractions); Avg, average; Brady, bradycardia; Coup., couplets; EPS, events per section; Iso., isolated; LEV, level above (+) or below (−) baseline in mV; max, maximum; min, minimum; pat., patient; S/T, ST segment; SLP, slope; Succ., successive; SVE, supraventricular ectopy; Tachy, tachycardia.

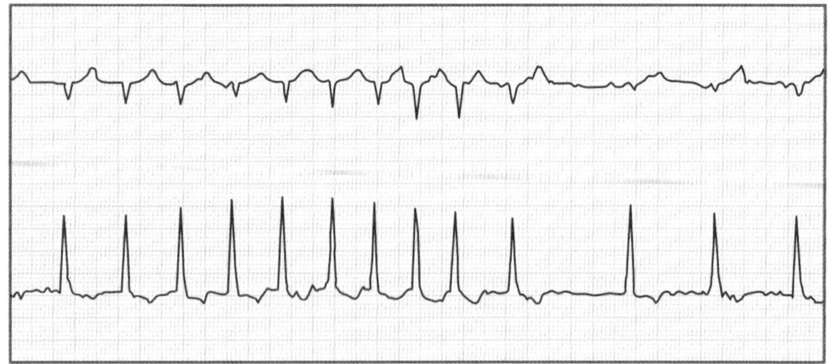

Figure 87-6 Selected rhythm strip at 13:03:20.

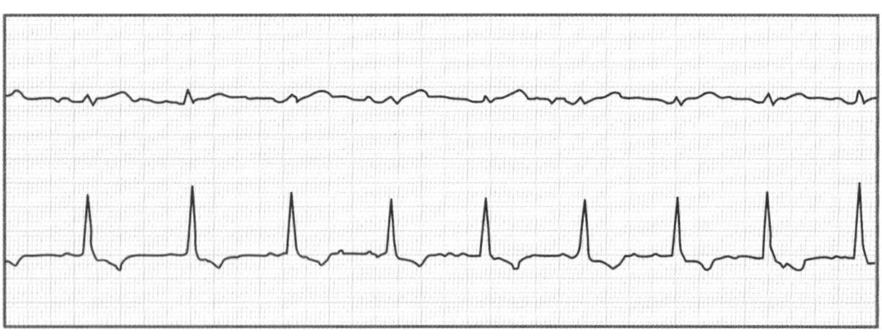

Figure 87-7 Selected rhythm strip at 15:03:20.

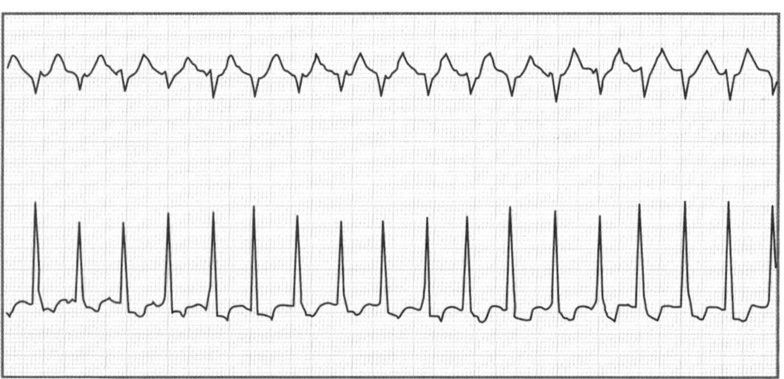

Figure 87-8 Selected rhythm strip at 15:51:09.

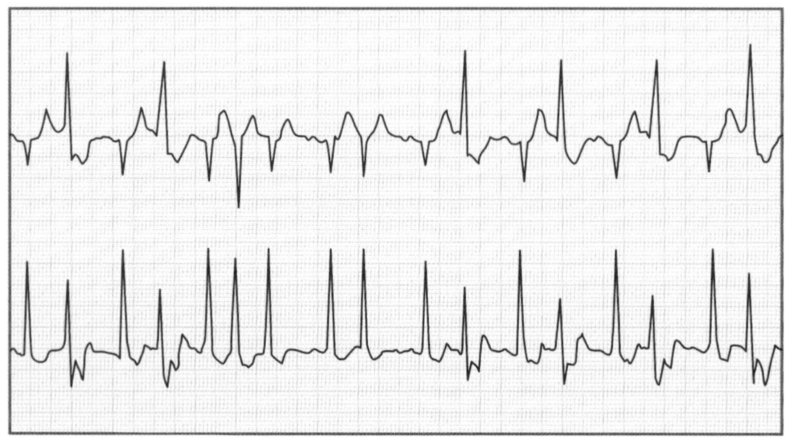

Figure 87-9 Selected rhythm strip at 15:55:53.

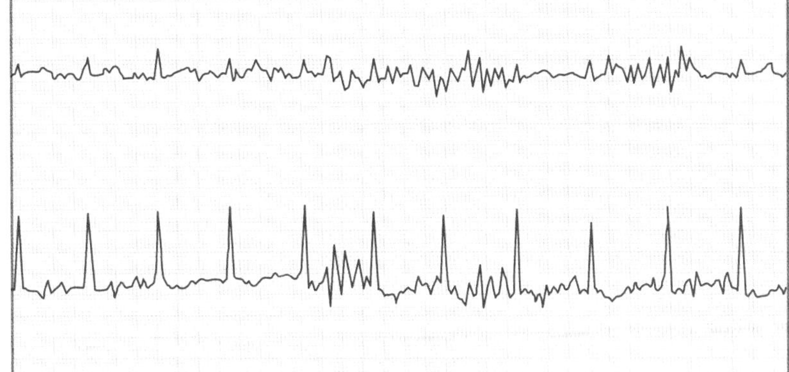

Figure 87-10 Selected rhythm strip at 21:56:13.

For orientation to full-disclosure tracings, portions of three pages from the case example Holter study are displayed. Normally, each page contains a miniaturized account of a full hour of Holter recording from a single monitoring lead. One minute of recording is represented by each of the 60 lines on the page. Because of space constraints for this chapter, only half of a page (30 minutes) is used for each demonstration. Thus, the period from 13:00 to 13:29 is shown in Figure 87-11; from 15:30 to 15:59 in Figure 87-12; and from 16:00 to 16:29 in Figure 87-13.

A scan of the first few lines of Figure 87-11 shows how relatively easy it is to identify the short run of supraventricular tachycardia that occurs between 13:03:10 and 13:03:20. (See Fig. 87-6 for the full-size recording of this short burst of tachycardia.) Also note how easy it is both to spot the "different looking" (i.e., abnormal) beats, which are PVCs, and to see that the baseline undulation on the 13:06 and 13:12 lines is likely due to artifact.

With practice, self-discipline, and diligent concentration, the interpreter should be able to scan each page (i.e., each hour of recording) rapidly (in <10 seconds) and still be able to identify most major abnormalities on the page.

Now look at Figure 87-12. The selected full-size rhythm strips previously reviewed demonstrated rapid atrial fibrillation at 15:51:09 (see Fig. 87-8) and rapid atrial fibrillation with frequent ventricular ectopy at 15:55:53 (see Fig. 87-9). Find these arrhythmias on the full-disclosure tracing.

Once a particular abnormality has been seen on the miniaturized full-disclosure tracing, it becomes relatively easy to spot other episodes of that abnormality. Thus, other short runs of frequent ventricular ectopy on lines 15:52, 15:53, 15:54, and 15:56 are easily noticed. Finally, look at Figure 87-13. Note how the patient has a sustained tachycardia for a substantial portion of this monitoring period. Actual-size rhythm strips reveal persistence of rapid atrial fibrillation during much of the hour.

Interpretation of Case Study

This case study is an excellent example of how to use a Holter system to determine the cause of a patient's symptoms. In this case, the patient's symptoms were not well defined; they included increasing dyspnea, weakness, and dizziness over the previous month. There were no palpitations, and apart from some nonspecific ST-T wave changes, the patient's baseline ECG was unremarkable. With this history, although most clinicians would include a cardiac arrhythmia in the differential diagnosis, other possibilities would merit

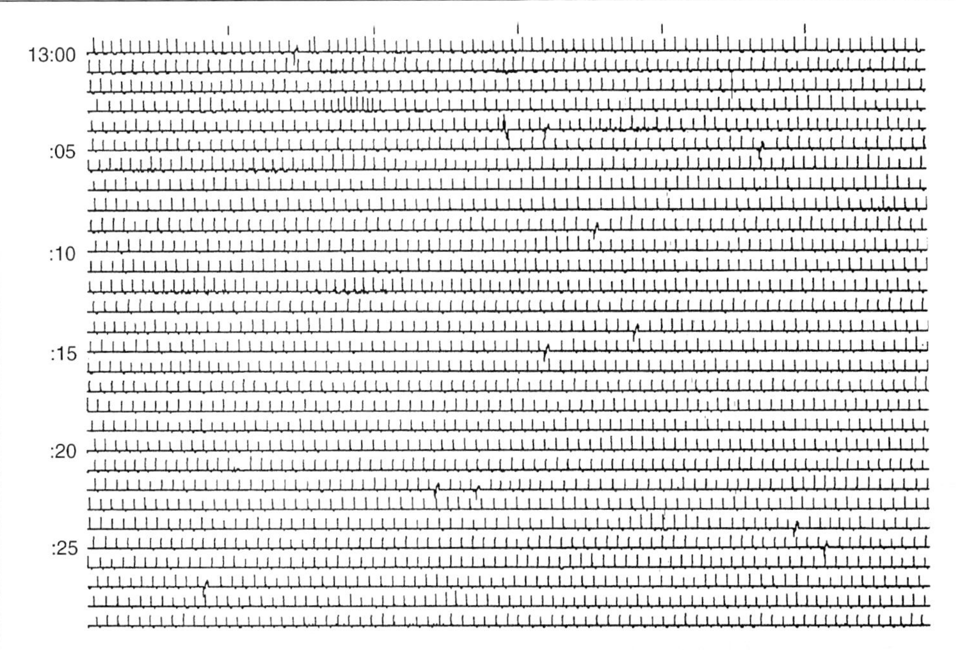

Figure 87-11 Full-disclosure strip between 13:00 and 13:29.

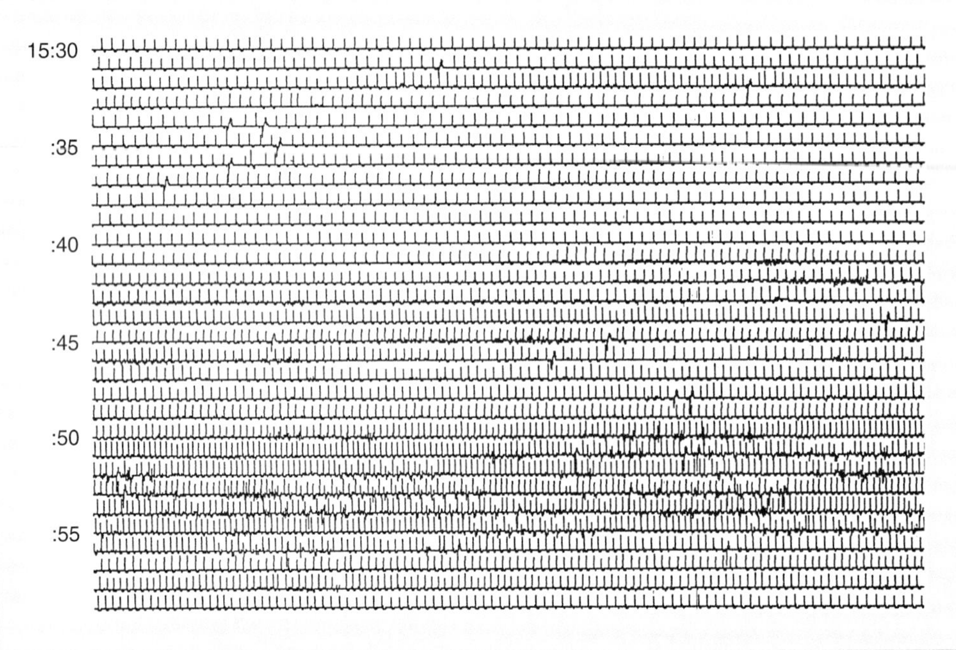

Figure 87-12 Full-disclosure strip between 15:30 and 15:59.

equal attention. However, after combining the results of this Holter data with the diary, there is little doubt as to the final diagnosis.

Final Interpretation

- Sinus rhythm with periods of sinus bradycardia down to 36 to 40 beats per minute.
- Several episodes of rapid, paroxysmal atrial fibrillation lasting minutes, with heart rate up to 160 beats per minute.
- Normal intervals.
- No significant ST segment shifts.
- Frequent PVCs (1144 recorded), especially during the waking hours—but virtually no repetitive forms.
- Diary indicates eight symptomatic episodes of weakness, dizziness, and dyspnea that correlate precisely with episodes of rapid, paroxysmal atrial fibrillation. These findings strongly suggest that the patient's symptoms are cardiac related (and should be treated).

Despite notation on the narrative summary of 57 pause episodes of up to 3.29 seconds, close inspection of full-disclosure tracings did not reveal any sustained pauses, suggesting that this count may reflect computer error.

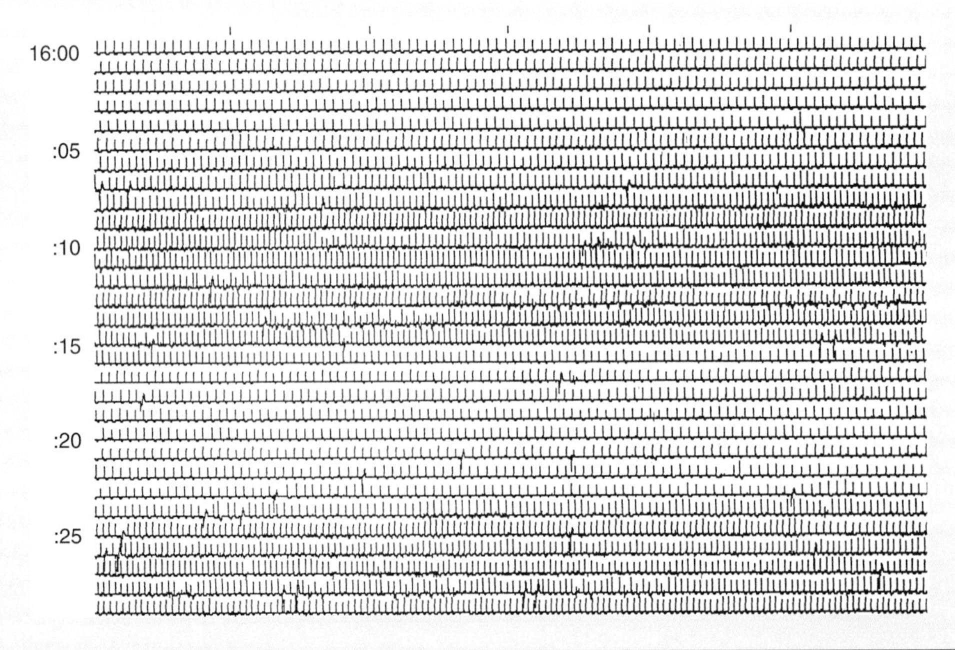

Figure 87-13 Full-disclosure strip between 16:00 and 16:29.

Standard Interpretation Form

Use of a standardized form greatly facilitates the task of Holter interpretation. The two-sided form (Fig. 87-14) organizes the key components of an ambulatory ECG study. In so doing, it not only saves time, but also ensures consistency in interpretation, provides clear documentation of findings, and facilitates the reporting of information in an easily understood, clinically relevant manner.

Several components of this form deserve special mention. Because artifact is often misread by the computer as ventricular ectopy, a boxed commentary (under "Arrhythmias") is included on the form to reflect the interpreter's assessment of the computer's PVC count. The interpreter should indicate whether the count is likely to be accurate or a distortion produced by artifact. Rather than focusing exclusively on the number of ectopic beats, a greater emphasis is placed on whether the occurrence of premature atrial, junctional, and ventricular contractions (including couplets and runs of VT) is "common," "occasional," or "rare/absent."

Finally, it is occasionally difficult to convey the clinical relevance of a patient's diary, especially when attempting to correlate it with the ambulatory ECG recording. The relative scales on the back of the interpretation form help resolve this problem. They attempt to clarify the interpreter's assessment of the validity of the patient's diary and the correlation (if any) between patient symptoms and the arrhythmias that are noted.

ICD-9-CM Diagnostic Codes

412 Old MI (healed; past MI diagnosed on ECG, but currently no symptoms)
414.01 Coronary atherosclerosis, of native coronary artery
414.02 Coronary atherosclerosis, of autologous vein bypass graft
414.04 Coronary atherosclerosis, of artery bypass graft
414.8 Chronic coronary insufficiency
426.3 Left bundle branch block, complete
426.4 Right bundle branch block
426.7 Anomalous atrioventricular excitation (Wolff-Parkinson-White syndrome)
426.9 Conduction disorder, unspecified
426.11 Atrioventricular block, first degree
426.12 Atrioventricular block, Mobitz type II
426.13 Atrioventricular block, Mobitz type I (Wenckebach's)
426.82 Long QT syndrome
427.0 Paroxysmal supraventricular tachycardia
427.1 Paroxysmal ventricular tachycardia
427.5 Cardiac arrest
427.31 Atrial fibrillation
427.32 Atrial flutter
427.41 Ventricular fibrillation
427.60 Premature beats, unspecified
427.61 Supraventricular premature beats
427.69 Ventricular premature beats, contractions, or systoles
427.81 Sinoatrial node dysfunction, sick sinus syndrome, sinus bradycardia
427.89 Other rhythm disorder, including bradycardia
428.1 Dyspnea, cardiac, also includes left-sided heart failure
780.2 Syncope, presyncope and collapse, including vasovagal and cardiac syncope
780.4 Dizziness
785.1 Palpitations

CPT/Billing Codes

Holter Monitor Studies

93224 Wearable electrocardiographic rhythm derived monitoring for 24 hours by continuous original ECG waveform recording and storage, *with visual superimposition scanning*; includes recording, scanning analysis with report, physician review, and interpretation
93225 Recording (which includes hook-up, recording, and disconnection)
93226 Scanning analysis with report
93227 Physician review and interpretation
93230 Wearable electrocardiographic rhythm derived monitoring for 24 hours by continuous original ECG waveform recording and storage, *without superimposition scanning* using a device capable of producing a full miniaturized printout; includes recording, microprocessor-based analysis with report, physician review, and interpretation
99231 Recording (which includes hook-up, recording, and disconnection)
99232 Microprocessor-based analysis with report
99233 Physician review and interpretation
93235 Wearable electrocardiographic rhythm derived monitoring for 24 hours by continuous computerized monitoring and noncontinuous recording, and *real-time data analysis using a device capable of producing intermittent full-size waveform tracings*, possibly patient activated; includes monitoring and real-time data analysis with report, physician review, and interpretation
93236 Monitoring and real-time data analysis with report
93237 Physician review and interpretation
93268 Wearable patient activated electrocardiographic rhythm derived event recording with presymptom memory loop, 24-hour attended monitoring, *per 30-day period of time*; includes transmission, physician review and interpretation
93270 Recording (includes hook-up, recording and disconnection)
93271 Monitoring, receipt of transmission, and analysis
93272 Physician review and interpretation

Cardiac Pre-Event ("Loop Recorder") Studies

93268 Patient demand single or multiple event recording with presymptom memory loop, per 30-day period; includes transmission, physician review, and interpretation

Acknowledgment

The editors wish to recognize the many contributions by David Feller, MD, and Ken Grauer, MD, to this chapter in a previous edition of this text.

Suppliers

Holter systems

Cardiac Science Corporation
3303 Monte Villa Parkway
Bothell, WA
866-469-3800
www.cardiacscience.com/cardiology-products/

GE Healthcare
3000 N. Grandview
Waukesha, WI
www2.gehealthcare.com/portal/site/usen/menuitem.d9d1e5260a507013d6354a1074c84130/?vgnextoid=15466f6bba930210VgnVCM10000024dd1403RCRD&plCode=205&pcChannelObj=Diagnostic+ECG&pcChannelId=e9fda52fcea2d110VgnVCM100000258c1403

Philips Medical Systems N.A.
3000 Minuteman Rd.
Andover, MA 01810-1099
1-800-345-6443
www.healthcare.philips.com/main/products/cardiography/products/holter/holter.wpd

Holter Interpretation Form

Name of patient __________ Name of clinician __________ Date ______

Indications for testing __________

Baseline ECG interpretation __________

PR interval ______ QRS duration ______ QTc: Normal ❒ Borderline ❒ Long ❒

Trend analysis:

The heart rate varies from ____ to ____, with an average rate of ____/min.

ST segment shifts? ❒ Yes ❒ ***No significant ST segment shifts***

ST elevation? ❒ ST depression? ❒ with Sx? ❒ without Sx? ❒

Estimated duration of ST segment depression over 24 hours ______.

Rhythm:

Selected strips show the rhythm to be ______.

Arrhythmias:

Number of **PVCs** *counted* by computer ______.

Probable ***accuracy*** of computer **PVCs count**

Poor (PVCs are rare; much artifact present) — Moderate — Excellent (Computer count is probably accurate)

True **PVCs appear to be:** Common ❒ Occ ❒ Rare/absent ❒ Multiform? ❒

Number of ventricular couplets ______. Couplets are: Common ❒ Occ ❒ Rare/absent ❒

Number of runs of VT (≥ 3 PVCs) ______. VT runs are: Common ❒ Occ ❒ Rare/absent ❒

Number of **PACs/PJCs** counted by computer ______.

PACs/PJCs are: Common ❒ Occ ❒ Rare/absent ❒

Longest tachyarrhythmia (type) ______. ***No significant tachyarrhythmias*** ❒

Duration of run ______. Time ______ with Sx? ❒ without Sx? ❒

Longest bradyarrhythmia (type) ______. ***No significant bradyarrhythmias*** ❒

Duration of run ______. Time ______ with Sx? ❒ without Sx? ❒

Longest pause (type) ______. ***No significant pauses*** ❒

Number of pauses >2.0 sec ______at ______. with Sx? ❒ without Sx? ❒

Figure 87-14 Standardized interpretation form. PAC, premature atrial contraction; PJC, premature junctional contraction; PVC, premature ventricular complex. (Modified from Grauer K, Leytem B: A systematic approach to Holter monitor interpretation. Am Fam Physician 45:1641, 1992.)

Pre-event recorders ("loop recorders")

Instromedix
O'Hare International Center II
10255 W. Higgins Rd.
Suite 100
Rosemont, IL 60018
800-633-3361
http://www.instromedix.com/pdf/products/cardiac/KOH_Express.pdf

NOTE: The authors recommend a system from a company with a proven track record. Many companies have come and gone over the years. Often, the companies with a proven track record also produce equipment for other procedures, such as exercise ECG (stress) testing. Choosing such a company may simplify service contracts.

BIBLIOGRAPHY

Abbott AV: Diagnostic approach to palpitations. Am Fam Physician 71:743, 2005.

Adan V: Diagnosis and treatment of sick sinus syndrome. Am Fam Physician 67:1725, 2003.

Biffi A, Pelliccia A, Verdile L, et al: Long-term clinical significance of frequent and complex ventricular tachyarrhythmias in trained athletes. J Am Coll Cardiol 40:446, 2002.

Cain ME, Anderson JL, Arnsdorf MF, et al: Signal averaged electrocardiography: ACC expert consensus document. J Am Coll Cardiol 27:238, 1996.

Crawford MH, Bernstein SJ, Deedwania PC, et al: ACC/AHA guidelines for ambulatory electrocardiography: Executive summary and recommendations. A report of the American College of Cardiology/American Heart Association task force on practice guidelines (Committee to revise the guidelines for ambulatory electrocardiography) developed in collaboration with the North American Society for Pacing and Electrophysiology. Circulation 100:886, 1999.

Dewey FE, Kapoor JR, Williams RS, et al: Ventricular arrhythmias during clinical treadmill testing and prognosis. Arch Intern Med 168:225, 2008.

Echt DS, Liebson PR, Mitchell LB, et al: Mortality and morbidity in patients receiving encainide, flecainide, or placebo. The Cardiac Arrythmia Suppression Trial. N Engl J Med 323:781, 1991.

Enseleit R, Duru R: Long-term continuous external electrocardiographic recording: A review. Europace 8:225, 2006.

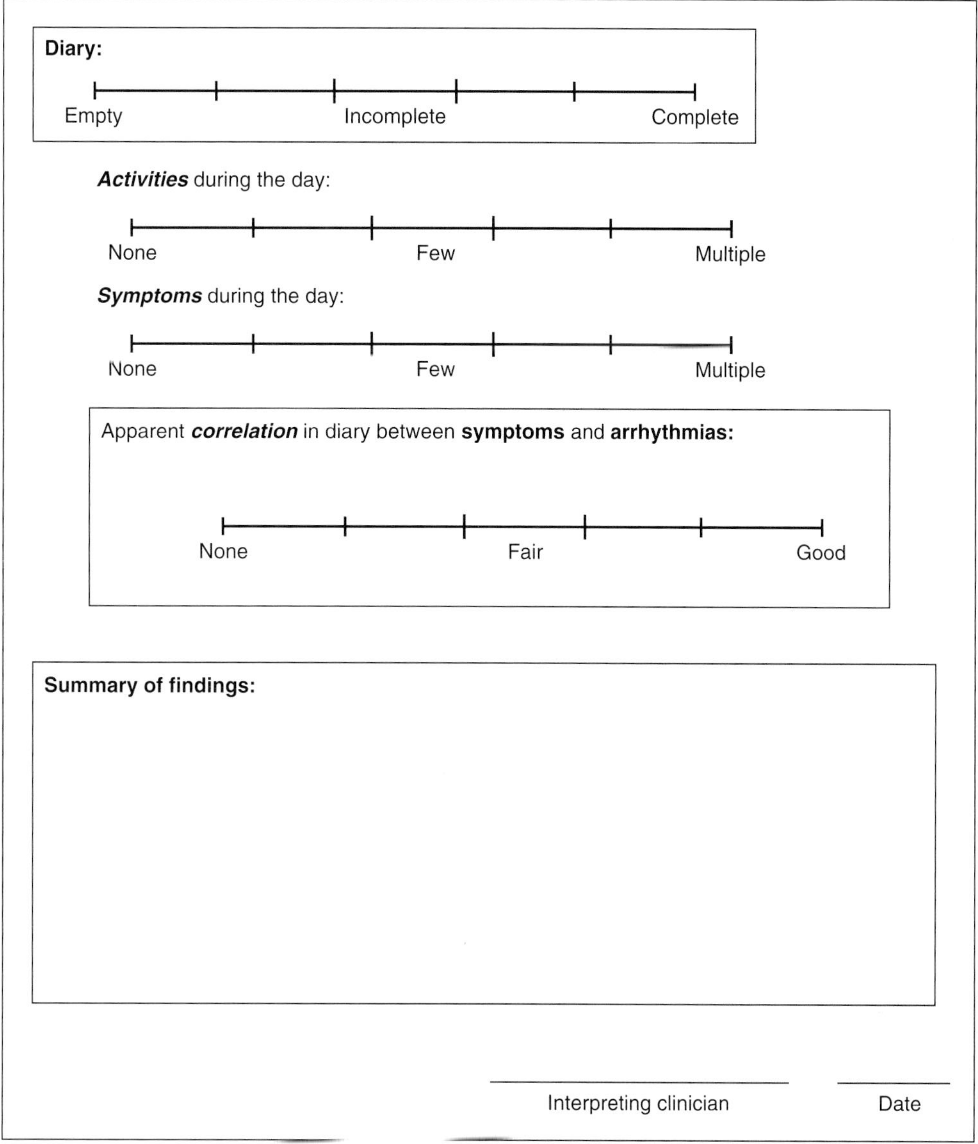

Figure 87-14, cont.

Gibson CM, Ciaglo LN, Southard MC, et al: Diagnostic and prognostic value of ambulatory ECG (Holter) monitoring in patients with coronary heart disease. J Thromb Thrombolysis 23:135, 2007.

Hatch R, Grauer K, Gums J: Cardiac arrhythmias. In Taylor RB (ed): Family Medicine: Principles and Practice, 4th ed. New York, Springer-Verlag, 1993, pp 601–616.

Kennedy HL, Whitlock JA, Sprague MK, et al: Long-term follow-up of asymptomatic healthy subjects with frequent and complex ventricular ectopy. N Engl J Med 312:193, 1985.

Kinlay S, Leitch JW, Neil A, et al: Cardiac event recorders yield more diagnoses and are more cost-effective than 48-hour Holter monitoring in patients with palpitations: A controlled clinical trial. Ann Intern Med 124:16, 1996.

Miller TH, Kruse JE: Evaluation of syncope. Am Fam Physician 72:1492, 2005.

Rothman SA, Laughlin JC, Seltzer J, et al: The diagnosis of cardiac arrythmias: A prospective multi-center randomized study comparing mobile cardiac outpatient telemetry versus standard loop event monitoring. J Cardiovasc Electrophysiol 18:241, 2007.

Sivakumaran S, Krahn AD, Klein GJ, et al: A prospective randomized comparison of loop recorders versus Holter monitors in patients with syncope or presyncope. Am J Med 115:1, 2003.

Solomon H, DeBusk RF: Contemporary management of silent ischemia: The role of ambulatory monitoring. Int J Cardiol 96:311, 2004.

Weber B, Kapoor W: Evaluation and outcomes of patients with palpitations. Am J Med 100:138, 1996.

SUGGESTED READING ON ECG INTERPRETATION AND CARDIAC ARRYTHMIAS

Dubin D: Rapid Interpretation of EKGs. Tampa, FL, Cover Publishing, 2000.

Grauer K: A Practical Guide to ECG Interpretation. St Louis, Mosby, 1998.

Huff J: ECG Workout: Exercises in Arrhythmia Interpretation. Philadelphia, Lippincott Williams & Wilkins, 2005.

Thaler M: The Only EKG Book You'll Ever Need. Philadelphia, Lippincott Williams & Wilkins, 2006.

CHAPTER 88

Noninvasive Venous and Arterial Studies of the Lower Extremities

Grant C. Fowler • Bal Reddy

The accuracy of noninvasive vascular studies depends not only on the skills of the operator and the interpreter, but also on the quality of the equipment or assay. That said, with state-of-the-art equipment or laboratory tests, many clinicians will manage anticoagulation therapy on the basis of noninvasive venous studies, alone, and some vascular surgeons will perform arterial surgery without preoperative arteriography.

The literature has clearly demonstrated the accuracy and benefit of compression ultrasonographic scanning, or duplex ultrasonographic scanning if it is available, in the emergency department. This is often performed by emergency medicine clinicians to exclude deep venous thrombosis (DVT). As a result, ultrasonography has basically become the standard of care for excluding DVT in the emergency department (see Chapter 225, Emergency Department, Hospitalist, and Office Ultrasonography [Clinical Ultrasonography]). As more primary care clinicians become comfortable performing duplex scanning, there is little doubt that they will extend its use into arterial and other studies.

In the remainder of the hospital and in vascular laboratories, duplex or color Doppler ultrasonography has basically become the standard for evaluation of lower extremity veins; computed tomography (CT) or magnetic resonance (MR) angiography has become the standard for evaluation of arteries. Not only have older noninvasive techniques been replaced, but venography has also essentially been replaced by duplex ultrasonographic studies; consequently, the risk of complications from invasive techniques and contrast dye has decreased. However, it should be noted that many vascular laboratories continue to use older noninvasive techniques for veins because duplex or color Doppler ultrasonography is not always available. Most centers can afford only one or two duplex units, and they are often kept very busy. In some settings, the cost of equipment for even one duplex or color Doppler ultrasonography unit is prohibitive. In the meantime, very sensitive D-dimer assays have become available with algorithms that can be used to effectively rule out DVT. These algorithms can be used in conjunction with older noninvasive diagnostic techniques; consequently, these techniques remain in this chapter. Older noninvasive techniques may yet see a resurgence in popularity because not only is there evidence supporting their use, but they are very cost effective and less operator dependent. In fact, they may find permanent use as a preliminary screening test to determine who should undergo compression ultrasonographic, duplex, or color Doppler scanning.

Noninvasive Venous Studies

Each year in the United States, approximately 200,000 patients die from a pulmonary embolus. DVT can be found in about 80% of patients with a pulmonary embolus. See Figure 88-1 for the most common sites for DVT; the incidence increases with age, and DVT is more common in women. One third to one half of patients older than 40 years of age who experience an acute myocardial infarction, a hip fracture, major surgery (especially orthopedic, pelvic, or urologic), or a stroke develop venous thrombi. Box 88-1 lists traditional risk factors in hospitalized patients. Lower limb DVT affects 1% to 2% of hospitalized patients. In addition, as a result of previous DVT, the prevalence of postphlebitic sequelae in the adult population is estimated to be 5%.

Early diagnosis of DVT is important because approximately 50% of untreated proximal DVT cases will result in a pulmonary embolism. Diagnosis of DVT is also important to minimize long-term complications such as venous stasis or ulceration from chronic venous insufficiency. Accurate diagnosis is crucial to limit anticoagulation therapy to those who really need it. Venous thrombi usually arise at bifurcations and in valve cusps. An aging thrombus

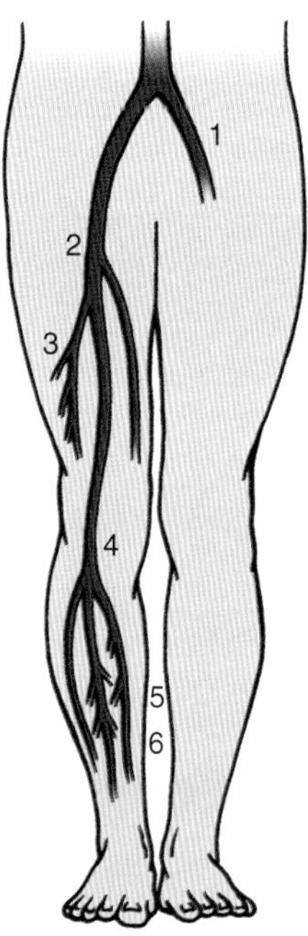

Figure 88-1 Six most common sites of deep venous thrombosis (DVT) in the lower body. 1, Left iliac vein; 2, common femoral vein; 3, termination of deep femoral vein (profunda femoris); 4, popliteal vein at adductor canal; 5, posterior tibial vein; 6, intramuscular veins of calf.

Box 88-1. Traditional Risk Factors for Deep Venous Thrombosis (Especially in Hospitalized Patients)

Acute myocardial infarction
Acute respiratory failure
Acute stroke with paresis
Blood type (persons with type A may be at higher risk than those with type O)
Fractures, especially spine, pelvis, long bone fractures, or multiple fractures
Heart disease, especially congestive heart failure
Hypercoagulable states
Local injury to veins
Malignancy
Mechanical ventilation
Myeloproliferative disorders
Nephrotic syndrome
Oral contraceptive use
Paroxysmal nocturnal hemoglobinuria
Persons older than 40 years of age
Persons with paralysis or otherwise immobilized
Postoperative state from major surgery
Pregnancy or postpartum, especially postcesarean section
Previous DVT or pulmonary embolism
Trauma
Ulcerative colitis or Behçet's syndrome
Venous stasis

can adhere to the vein wall and damage or destroy nearby valves. The two most important valves for controlling venous hydrostatic pressure are those of the proximal superficial femoral vein and the distal popliteal vein. Destruction of these valves is more likely to lead to sequelae. The goal is to diagnose DVT before a thrombus either embolizes or becomes extensive enough to permanently damage these or any other valves.

Clinical diagnosis of acute DVT, without the benefit of radiographic or noninvasive techniques, has been reported to be notoriously inaccurate for years, with only about a 50% accuracy rate. However, this accuracy was probably underestimated because it was based on older studies performed on seriously ill, hospitalized patients. Since then, various scoring systems have been developed in an attempt to predict pretest likelihood of DVT in ambulatory patients. The best known and studied is the Wells scoring system, which was first proposed in 1995 and updated in 2003. Although patients in this study were ambulatory, they were seen in either the emergency department or hospital, so these data may not be as applicable to patients in a primary care clinic. However, the Wells system has since been studied in 1082 ambulatory patients presenting to 5 major academic medical centers. Of these, 495 patients were thought likely to have DVT, whereas 587 were categorized as unlikely. Diagnostic evaluation followed by 3 months of observation confirmed DVT or pulmonary embolism in 28% of those thought likely to have DVT and in only 5.5% of those deemed unlikely to have DVT (Table 88-1). Combining the Wells system with further diagnostic studies can be used to virtually exclude DVT. For instance, a negative D-dimer test result in those thought unlikely to have DVT effectively excluded DVT (<1%) during the 3-month follow-up.

TABLE 88-1 Wells Scoring System for Predicting Deep Venous Thrombosis

Clinical Variable	Score*
Active cancer (ongoing treatment or active within the last 6 mo or palliative care for cancer)	1
Paralysis, paresis, or recent plaster immobilization of the lower extremities	1
Recently bedridden for 3 or more days, or major surgery within the last 12 wk requiring regional or general anesthesia	1
Localized tenderness along the distribution of the deep venous system	1
Entire leg swelling	1
Calf swelling at least 3 cm larger in circumference than that of the asymptomatic leg, measured 10 cm below the tibial tuberosity	1
Pitting edema confined to the affected leg	1
Distended collateral superficial veins (not varicosities)	1
Previously documented DVT	1
Alternative diagnosis at least as likely as DVT	−2

DVT, deep venous thrombosis.
*Scoring method: if 1 or less, DVT unlikely; if 2 or greater, DVT likely.
From Wells PS, Owen C, Doucette S, et al: Does this patient have deep vein thrombosis? JAMA 295:199–207, 2006.

Alternatives for Diagnosis of Deep Venous Thrombosis, Their Limitations, and Evidence Supporting Their Use

1. *Contrast venography* is regarded as the gold standard for diagnosis of DVT; however, it is not without its own risks—including allergic reactions, congestive heart failure, acute renal insufficiency, and postvenography syndrome. (After venography, postvenography syndrome affects 10% to 20% of patients. Although it usually causes only transient discomfort in the calf for 24 to 48 hours, and in most cases it resolves without treatment, it may actually progress to DVT.) In addition, venography is not easily repeated, and it is usually performed only in one limb. Venography may be impossible to perform in patients with poor venous access, especially obese patients and those with severe edema or cellulitis. It may also be difficult to perform in urgent situations without proper support staff. Furthermore, contrast venography cannot be performed in 20% to 25% of patients because of previous DVT. Although a study of postmortem contrast venograms reported a sensitivity rate of 95% and a specificity rate of 97% for diagnosis of DVT, a more recent multicenter study evaluating the degree of interobserver variation questions these high sensitivities and specificities. For these reasons, as well as the fact that compression and duplex ultrasonography have become more readily available, they have basically replaced contrast venography for making the diagnosis of DVT.
2. *Compression ultrasonographic imaging (high-frequency, B-mode, real-time)* has limitations in obese and asymptomatic postoperative patients. Ultrasonography's ability to visualize the venous system above the inguinal ligament (i.e., pelvic, iliac veins) or distal to the popliteal vein is also limited. That said, for symptomatic proximal DVT, sensitivities ranging from 93% to 100% and specificities ranging from 97% to 100% have been reported since the 1980s (Appelman and colleagues, 1987; Vogel and colleagues, 1987; Cronan and colleagues, 1987; Lensing and colleagues, 1989). Compression ultrasonography is less operator dependent than duplex scanning, and this may explain why it is the most common technique used in large urgent-emergent care centers and after hours in hospitals. Because it is a less expensive technique, many centers have developed algorithms for its use; they either use compression ultrasonography alone in low-risk patients or use compression ultrasonography as a screen to determine whether a duplex scan is needed. Although approximately 10% of isolated calf DVTs will be missed with compression ultrasonography, calf DVT by itself is not life-threatening and may only need to be followed to exclude proximal progression. Benefits of compression ultrasonography include the ability actually to visualize the veins, valves, and thrombus. Compression ultrasonography may be necessary in special cases in which (other than

obese or asymptomatic postoperative patients) impedence plethysmography (IPG) has unclear results or limitations. Compression ultrasonography is also usually performed during duplex scanning.

3. *Duplex ultrasonographic scanning* combines velocity measurements using Doppler technology with ultrasonographic imaging. Duplex scanning may be used to confirm findings from compression ultrasonography. Duplex scanning is accurate and reproducible, and compared with venography, its sensitivity and specificity for DVT are more than 90%. Both the positive and negative predictive values for DVT are in the 90% to 95% range. Studies have shown that color enhancement of the Doppler velocities also improves accuracy in areas where compression may be difficult, such as at the inguinal ligament, the adductor canal, or in the calf veins. It may also be used to determine the patency of the pelvic and iliac veins and the inferior vena cava.
4. *Electrical impedance plethysmography* was previously the most extensively studied and commonly used noninvasive technique. It remains the least expensive and least operator-dependent alternative to venography. IPG provides a functional evaluation of the venous system for outflow obstruction. Compared with contrast venography, a sensitivity of 92% and a specificity of 95% were reported for IPG from studies in the 1990s. However, the range for sensitivity dropped to 66% in one study. High false-positive rates are found in the presence of certain conditions (e.g., obesity, congestive heart failure, external venous compression from gravid uterus in pregnancy) and chronic DVT. IPG is inaccurate in the diagnosis of thrombi in calf veins, profunda femoris, or internal iliac veins. It is also limited for diagnosing nonoccluding DVT, asymptomatic or moderately symptomatic DVT, and, therefore, postoperative DVT. IPG is limited for diagnosing clots in paired veins or determining the progression of disease. For these situations, duplex or color Doppler imaging has mostly replaced IPG. That said, a number of prospective studies (Hull and colleagues, 1985; Huisman and colleagues, 1986; Heijboer and colleagues, 1993) have demonstrated that serial negative IPGs are sufficiently sensitive to justify withholding anticoagulation, even in symptomatic patients.
5. *Hand-held (pocket) Doppler* (with or without recorded velocities) can be used to assess venous function. Pooled data from several studies found an overall sensitivity of 84% and specificity of 88% for detection of lower extremity DVT in symptomatic outpatients. However, individual studies report sensitivities ranging from 31% to 100% and specificities ranging from 59% to 100%, thereby indicating the shortcoming of this technique and the fact that it is very operator dependent (Turnbull and Dymowski, 1989). Consequently, hand-held Doppler is probably most useful when combined with another study such as compression ultrasonography or IPG, and was therefore included in the protocols of many of the original noninvasive venous studies. When combined with compression ultrasonography or IPG, hand-held Doppler can add information about the calf veins.
6. *D-dimer*, a degradation product of cross-linked fibrin, is usually elevated in patients with DVT. After determining pretest likelihood, the results of a high-sensitivity D-dimer assay can be used in place of IPG, ultrasonography, or duplex scanning in patients unlikely to have DVT and is especially useful in symptomatic patients with a suspected first episode of DVT. It can also be checked in addition to IPG, ultrasonography, or duplex scanning. A D-dimer test is most effective in excluding DVT in outpatients because hospitalized patients frequently have other conditions that cause an elevated result (i.e., false positives). Increasing age also increases the likelihood of false-positive results. Although there are at least seven commercial assays available, the enzyme-linked immunosorbent (ELISA) technique is considered a high-sensitivity test. From a recent meta-analysis (Wells and colleagues, 2006), a negative high-sensitivity D-dimer test combined with a low-probability score (pretest likelihood) resulted in a 0.1% likelihood of DVT during 3-month follow-up *without using ultrasonography*. Although semiquantitative slide agglutination assays are probably not accurate enough to use for exclusion of DVT (low sensitivity), newer quantitative agglutination methods (moderate sensitivity) have increased the accuracy to acceptable levels (<0.5% during 3-month follow-up) in patients unlikely to have DVT by the Wells scoring system. Likewise, bedside assays that use whole blood are also now available and are considered to be of moderate sensitivity and useful when combined with the Wells scoring system (Fig. 88-2).

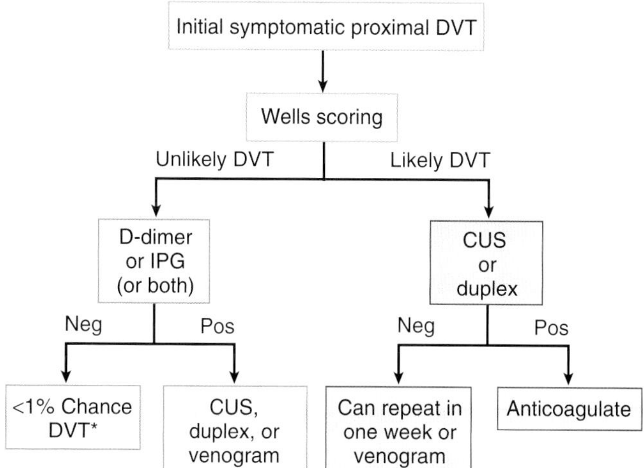

Figure 88-2 Algorithm for incorporating Wells scoring system into testing for deep venous thrombosis (DVT). (1) If DVT is unlikely (see Table 88-1) and the moderate or high-sensitivity D-dimer test (or impedence plethysmography [IPG], or both) result is negative, no further testing is required. (2) Symptomatic patients with an abnormal compression ultrasonography (CUS) or duplex study result can be treated without any further testing, or (3) if the patient has a negative CUS or duplex study result, yet DVT is likely, options include venography or serial CUS or duplex studies (i.e., repeat in 1 week). This algorithm provides a safe and cost-effective manner of excluding DVT. *Because this algorithm has not been studied prospectively and there is some subjectivity in using the Wells scoring system, some clinicians will always perform another noninvasive test before excluding DVT.

7. *Radionuclide scintigraphy or magnetic resonance venography (MRV)* may be useful in selected patients. Scintigraphy uses radiolabeled albumin or tagged red blood cells as the contrast for venography. However, it may be unreliable in the calf and not helpful in those with previous DVT. Radiolabeled autologous platelets or peptides can also be used to detect active thrombus formation. These techniques may be helpful in symptomatic patients with a previous history of DVT. MRV is particularly useful in the diagnosis of portal, inferior vena caval, pelvic vein, or calf vein DVT. However, MRV is highly operator dependent, expensive, and not always available in urgent situations. It should probably be reserved for cases in which scintigraphy is contraindicated. Both radionuclide scintigraphy and MRV are beyond the scope of this textbook.

Indications

Nongravid

- Verification of clinically suspected acute DVT. (This may require serial studies if calf thrombosis is suspected, and especially if IPG or compression ultrasonography is the diagnostic study used. Neither of these techniques is highly sensitive for calf thrombosis and serial studies are recommended to monitor for more proximal progression of a thrombus, which will occur in approximately 25% of patients. Asymptomatic calf vein thrombosis seems to progress proximally as frequently as that in symptomatic patients.)
- Diagnosis of recurrent DVT.
- Evaluation before discontinuation of anticoagulation for DVT. (E.g., IPG has been used to verify collateral flow or lysis of the thrombus by repeating every 4 to 6 weeks until the results return

to normal. However, it should be noted that insurers often reimburse only for symptomatic patients.)
- Venous evaluation of patient with pulmonary embolism.
- Preoperative study before saphenous vein stripping.
- Preoperative study before venous sclerotherapy.
- Venous insufficiency.

Gravid

- Gravid patients with superficial venous thrombosis should be evaluated thoroughly because up to 17% will also have DVT. DVT in a gravid patient places her at very high risk of pulmonary embolism. (One review of maternal deaths revealed that pulmonary embolism was the second leading cause of death.)

Considerations

- Unilateral or unexplained edema of the lower extremity, especially if associated wtih pain in area
- Screening of certain high-risk patients (e.g., postoperative, especially with multiple risk factors; see Table 88-1)
- Suspected pulmonary embolus (in combination with either a multidetector CT pulmonary angiogram or a V/Q scan)

Compression Ultrasonographic Scanning

Real-time, B-mode ultrasonography in the higher frequency ranges (5 to 10 MHz) allows direct "visualization" (imaging) of the venous system, and it allows the technician or clinician to search for a thrombus. Sound waves are best transmitted in fluid; therefore, large veins and arteries are easily visualized with the proper probe and adequate acoustic gel interface. Arteries are differentiated from veins by their thicker walls and pulsatile nature. They are also not as easily compressed when pressure is applied on the leg with the probe. In addition, arteries do not engorge with a Valsalva maneuver or vary with respiration.

Compression ultrasonography is currently the most widely used noninvasive test for diagnosis of DVT. In some situations, such as after 5:00 PM in some emergency departments, compression ultrasonography is the only diagnostic modality available. Studies of such situations have indicated that accuracy of diagnosis of DVT by compression ultrasonography approaches that of venography.

Personnel and Equipment

- A clinician or technician familiar with venous anatomy (Fig. 88-3) as well as ultrasonographic technology
- 5- to 10-MHz probe (transducer) and scanner (2- to 3.5-MHz probe in obese patients)
- Acoustic gel

Technique

1. Place the patient in the supine position with the lower extremities lowered about 20 or 30 degrees (reverse Trendelenburg), slightly separated and externally rotated. This position increases the fluid volume in the veins and facilitates scanning. The patient should be relaxed, comfortable, and bearing most of the weight on the contralateral side to avoid venous compression by tense muscles.
2. Apply ample acoustic gel. With the probe perpendicular to the vessel and beginning at the groin, scan the common femoral vein, the saphenofemoral junction (the most common location for a thrombus to extend from superficial to deep veins), and then the superficial femoral vein. Scan distally in the longitudinal and transverse dimensions. Longitudinal scanning is usually used to locate and follow the vein, whereas transverse scanning is used to check for compressibility. Have the patient perform a Valsalva maneuver, which should expand the veins, enhancing visualization as far distal as the popliteal veins. *Echogenic* matter (which appears white) within the vessels should be studied carefully to exclude a possible thrombus. Presence or absence of thrombus should be recorded. Partially obstructing thrombi may be confused with scarred, thickened venous walls; therefore, it is important to record and comment about wall thickness. If a thrombus is found in the femoral veins, attempt to scan the iliac veins and inferior vena cava for the presence of additional thrombi.
3. If no thrombus is visualized, turn the probe transversely and apply gentle pressure to compress the vessel walls. Compressions should be made every 3 to 5 cm, progressing distally. If the vein is not compressible, continue to apply increasing pressure until the diameter of the adjacent artery is reduced slightly. At this pressure, if the vein is not compressible, an early thrombus is preventing compression; it may not have become organized or

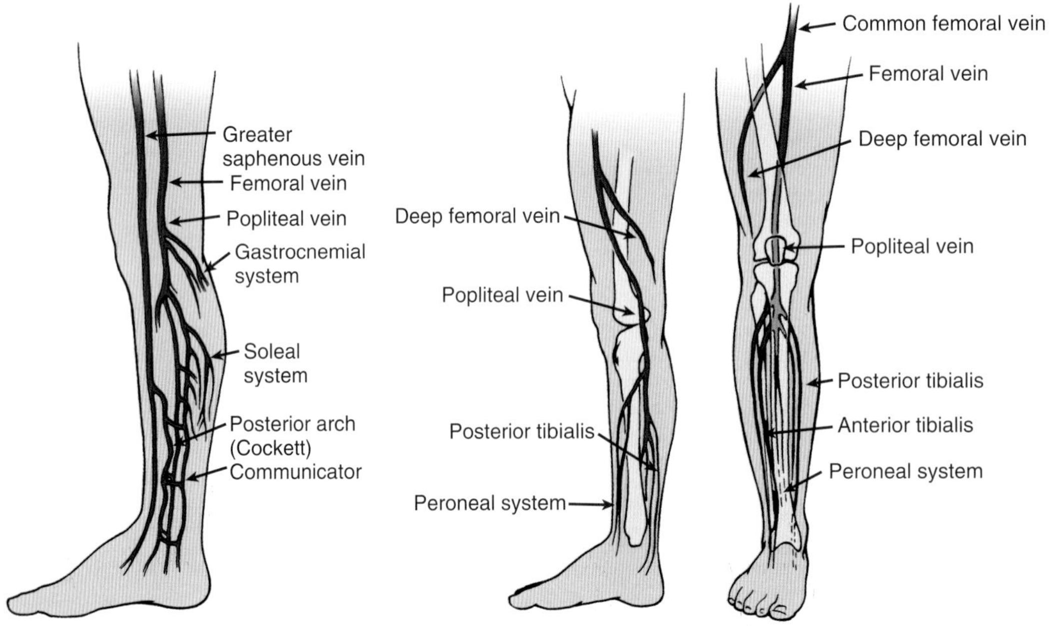

Figure 88-3 Venous system of the lower extremity.

dense enough to be visualized or cause echoes. Compressibility of the vein walls (or lack thereof) should be recorded.

4. Proceed distally and continue scanning vessels in the longitudinal and transverse dimensions to the mid-medial and then the distal thigh. In the distal thigh, fascial planes at the adductor hiatus (Hunter's canal) may obscure the superficial femoral vein.
5. Next, scan the popliteal vein either with the patient in this position or by rotating the patient to a prone position with the knees flexed 20 or 30 degrees. A pillow placed under the feet may facilitate this position and enhance patient comfort.
6. In about 30% of patients, infrapopliteal vessels can be scanned, with the anterior and posterior tibial veins visualized more easily than the peroneal veins. Sitting the patient up and allowing his or her legs to dangle over the edge of the bed may enhance imaging of the calf veins.
7. Valve thickness and motion should be recorded when observed.
8. Vein response to a Valsalva maneuver and deep inspiration should be recorded at the level of the common femoral, superficial femoral, and popliteal veins.

Interpretation

- Visualization of an intraluminal thrombus is diagnostic. A thrombus is further confirmed when a Valsalva maneuver produces minimal changes in vein diameter and the vessel wall is incompressible. Early studies indicate that these diagnostic criteria are superior to all other techniques, except venography, for diagnosing DVT. In a symptomatic patient, treatment (anticoagulation) can be initiated with the visualization of a thrombus alone.
- A *probable positive* study is one in which the veins are incompressible or do not distend with a Valsalva maneuver. Consider duplex scanning for confirmation if a thrombus is not visualized during compression ultrasonography. The accuracy and outcomes of duplex scanning have been studied extensively, and it produces diagnostic results similar to venography in cases in which a thrombus is not visualized.
- Occasionally, an acute thrombus can be differentiated from a chronic thrombus. Acute thrombi can have low-level echoes and tend to have a homogeneous texture, can be free-floating, and are somewhat compressible. The vein is often dilated. A chronic thrombus increases in echogenicity and decreases in size. With a chronic thrombus, although the vein is usually back to its normal diameter (i.e., the same diameter as the corresponding vein on the contralateral side), it will still contain an echogenic clot partially obstructing the lumen. Lateral veins will often form alongside. Chronic thrombi usually are not compressible, have heterogeneous echogenicity, and are firmly attached to the walls.
- Increased wall thickness, especially compared with veins of the contralateral extremity, can be due to previous or chronic DVT or to a partially obstructing thrombus. All of these possibilities should be strongly considered in a symptomatic patient because all of these scenarios also place the patient at risk for DVT.
- At least one published study indicates safety in withholding treatment with a negative compression ultrasonographic study result. This result should be weighed against the pretest likelihood of DVT and availability of duplex scanning. However, even in patients likely to have DVT by the Wells scoring system, two negative compression ultrasonographic studies, performed a week apart, reduces the risk of DVT to less than 1% (see Fig. 88-2).
- Although superficial thrombophlebitis is not life-threatening, patients with saphenous vein phlebitis should be scanned very thoroughly; one prospective study found 33% of patients with a thrombus in the above-knee segment of the greater saphenous vein had a documented episode of pulmonary embolism. Likewise, although isolated calf vein thrombosis is not life-threatening, it propagates proximally into the popliteal vein and thigh in approximately 25% of patients, so there is value in repeating the scan in 1 week. If the result is negative, it reduces the risk of proximal DVT to less than 2%. The risk of proximal propagation is apparently as high in asymptomatic calf vein thrombosis as in symptomatic.
- Because of the lack of a validated clinical model, making the diagnosis of recurrent DVT can be challenging. The diagnosis is easier if it occurs in a new location or in the contralateral extremity. However, if it recurs in the same venous segment of prior DVT, it requires comparison with a prior study. Clearly, a newly noncompressible segment confirms recurrent DVT. Certain experts consider an increase of greater than 2 mm in the compressed diameter (or 4 mm in the uncompressed diameter) of the previously thrombosed venous segment to be diagnostic for recurrent DVT. An extension of the length of the thrombus by 9 mm is also considered recurrent DVT by most sonographers. Conversely, fully compressible deep veins or no significant increase in diameter excludes recurrent DVT.

DUPLEX SCANNING

Duplex scanning adds another parameter—venous blood velocity—to the data obtained from a compression ultrasonographic study. With duplex scanning, Doppler technology is incorporated into the probe of an ultrasonographic scanner. The drawbacks to duplex scanning include its cost to the patient (averaging $300 to $600 per study), the cost and nonportability of equipment, the time required for a complete examination, and the experience required for the technician or clinician to perform and interpret the study. In many centers, it is not available at all hours or in urgent situations. As with compression ultrasonography, the ability to study the venous system above the inguinal ligament, and occasionally the superficial femoral and tibial veins at the adductor hiatus, is poor compared with IPG.

Duplex scanning has advantages over compression ultrasonography in areas where the vein cannot be compressed because of physical restrictions, such as with smaller vessels (e.g., infrapopliteal). With duplex scanning, other measurable or demonstrable parameters of venous function can be evaluated if a suspected thrombus is not clearly visualized with compression ultrasonography.

Technique

The technique of duplex scanning is the same as for compression ultrasonography, except that most of the velocity data are gathered with the probe turned longitudinally along the vein. Duplex scanning allows the evaluation of venous physiologic parameters, and there are three additional criteria for a positive result: (1) the absence of phasicity (i.e., variation) during quiet respiration, (2) the absence of spontaneous blood flow, and (3) the absence of augmentation of flow when the limb is compressed distal to the site of probe placement. The effect of a Valsalva maneuver should also be observed (e.g., should reduce venous flow to the heart). Even with a thrombus that is clearly visualized, confirmation by an alteration of these four factors can be comforting before anticoagulation therapy is initiated. In addition, valve function can be assessed; functional valves should not allow augmentation of reverse flow with proximal compression. The extent of valve function at the level of the common femoral, femoral, and popliteal veins should be routinely recorded. They should also be evaluated and recorded as far distally as possible.

Interpretation

Treatment decisions in most large centers are based on duplex scans alone. Occasionally, venography and duplex results differ. If clearly abnormal findings on a duplex scan are contradicted by normal findings on venography, the disparity may be due to the presence of a duplicate vein (up to 20% of patients), which may

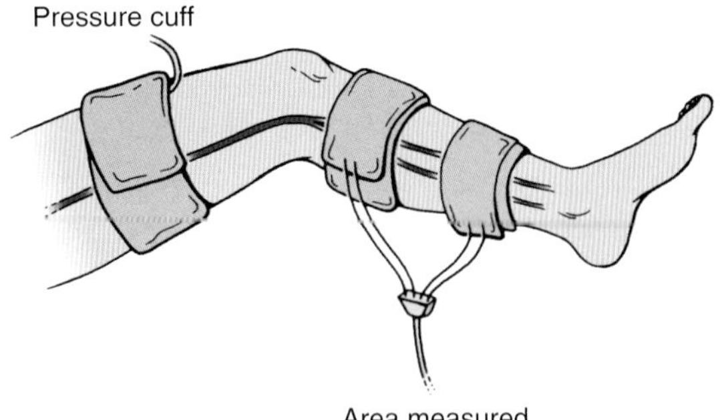

Figure 88-4 For impedance plethysmography testing, elevate the leg 25 to 30 degrees. Apply electrodes around the calf and place a pressure cuff around the thigh.

appear normal on venography despite the presence of a thrombus in the other vein. Also, thrombosis of a superficial femoral or popliteal vein can be missed by a venogram. Therefore, for a patient with a normal venogram despite significant symptoms, and a clearly abnormal duplex scan, treatment is not out of the question.

ELECTRICAL IMPEDANCE PLETHYSMOGRAPHY

Various plethysmography techniques are available to study a change in physical function as a result of a change in volume (e.g., strain gauge, air, IPG). Electrical IPG records the impedance (the inverse of conductivity) of the lower extremity as the blood volume varies. When venous return is restricted in the lower extremity by a cuff, venous volume in the lower extremity increases. Because blood is a good conductor of electricity, conductivity in the lower extremity also increases (i.e., resistance or impedance decreases). This is evaluated by administering a weak electrical current that is imperceptible to the patient, and then measuring the current's strength after it passes through the area. When the cuff is released, conductivity should rapidly decrease if the deep venous system is patent. In patients with a thrombus, the rate of change of electrical conductivity is reduced, especially if the thrombus is in the popliteal or more proximal vein. IPG has been proven to be safe, painless, reliable, and cost effective (cost to the patient is about the same as for an electrocardiogram, usually $50 to $100).

Relative Contraindications

- Patients with risk of false-positive result (e.g., patient with significant pain [involuntary muscle restriction], full bladder [especially elderly patients] or the inability to relax [involuntary muscle restriction], congestive heart failure [elevated central venous pressure], external vein occlusion [pregnancy, popliteal cyst or mass], obesity, or chronic DVT). In these patients, the risk of a false-positive result is increased and initiation of anticoagulation should be weighed against the risks of waiting for the availability of another, more accurate venous study.
- Patients who are unable to remain supine, such as those with severe orthopnea.

Personnel and Equipment

- A clinician or technician trained to perform and record IPG
- A clinician trained to interpret IPG
- IPG recorder
- Appropriate 8-inch cuff and electrodes

Technique

1. Place the patient in the supine position, with the leg to be examined elevated 25 to 30 degrees (Fig. 88-4). This can be accomplished by placing a pillow under the calf and heel. All tight garments should be removed, and the leg to be studied should be well exposed. To relax the patient, the leg is allowed to rotate externally at the hip. The knee is slightly flexed—10 to 20 degrees—to prevent compression of the popliteal vein.
2. Place an 8-inch-wide pneumatic cuff around the thigh and place electrodes circumferentially around the calf.
3. After the instrument has been electrically balanced and a stable baseline has been obtained, inflate the cuff to the manufacturer's specification, which is usually 50 mm Hg. This blocks the venous outflow but does not impair arterial inflow.
4. After the cuff has been inflated for 2 minutes and the pressure tracing has reached a stable plateau, suddenly release the pressure in the compression cuff.
5. The total rise of the IPG tracing during cuff occlusion and the fall during the first 3 seconds of deflation are now plotted on a two-way graph (Fig. 88-5 shows normal and abnormal IPG tracings, and Fig. 88-6 shows plotting).

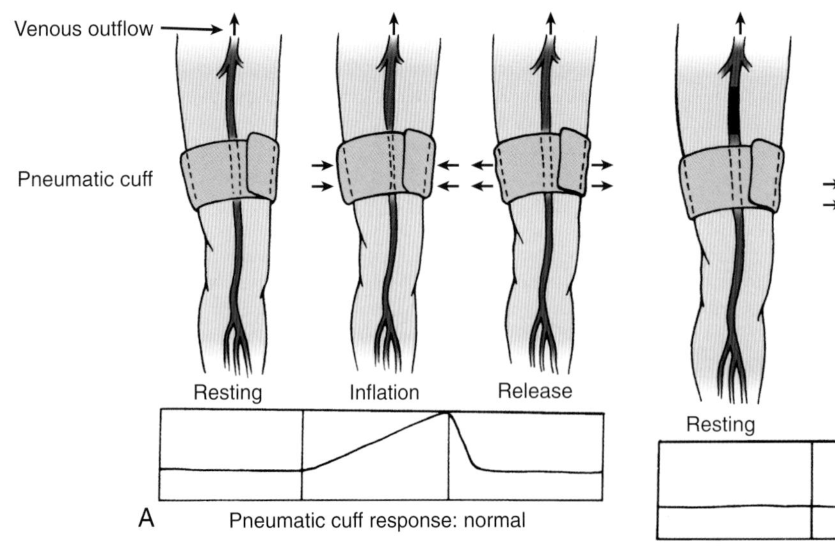

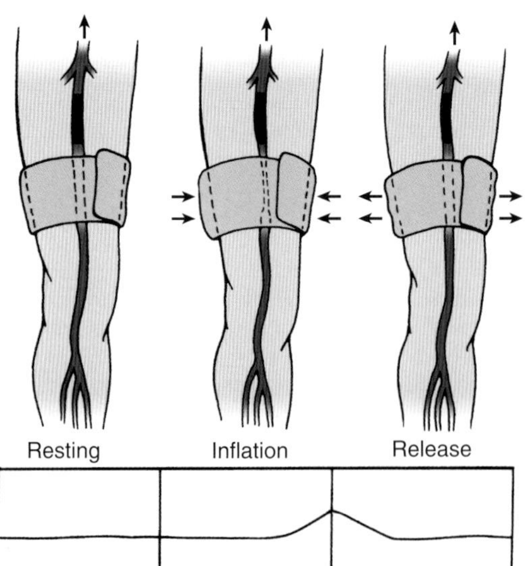

Figure 88-5 Normal (**A**) and abnormal (**B**) impedance plethysmography tracings.

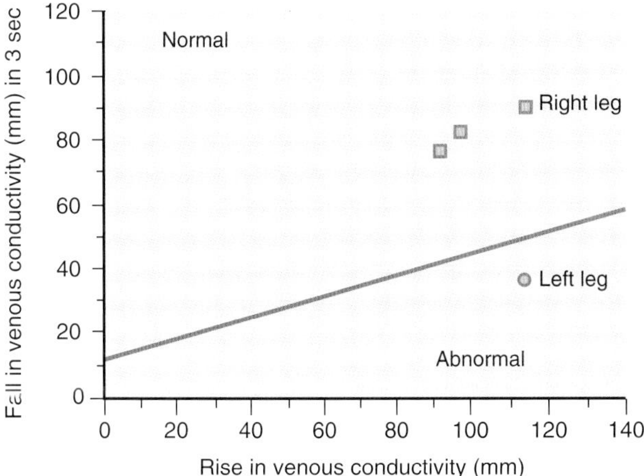

Figure 88-6 Typical result of impedance plethysmography. This reading suggests deep venous obstruction in the left leg, with normal venous function in the right leg.

Interpretation and Sources of Error

Overall, the major shortcoming of IPG is a false-positive rate of approximately 5%. Sensitivity increases in the symptomatic patient and is reduced during evaluation for silent proximal thrombosis, such as with postoperative screening. The error rate can be minimized by a clinician with experience who takes into consideration the following factors:

- Positive predictive accuracy is improved for those with a high pretest likelihood of DVT (see Table 88-1).
- If the first result falls below the discriminant line, it is not necessarily abnormal. With repeated testing, the values may fall above the discriminant line, where they are considered normal. In the presence of true outflow obstruction, the result remains fixed. To improve the accuracy of IPG, a five-test sequence can be used with occlusion times of 45, 45, 120, 45, and 120 seconds.
- The closer the result falls to the discriminant line on either side, the more likely that it is abnormal. Such test results (close to the line) should be confirmed with either venography or duplex scanning.
- Some experts suggest that if abnormal results are found with both lower extremities, they are likely false-positive results; therefore, the patient should be evaluated further with another technique.
- Excessive tightness of the cuff, particularly in obese patients, may cause tension on the skin during cuff occlusion and thus a false-positive result.
- Any systemic disease limiting arterial inflow or venous outflow will interfere with results.

Hand-Held Venous Doppler

Hand-held Doppler studies (without imaging) can be used to qualitatively assess the venous system. The hand-held Doppler probe translates the velocity of venous blood into an audible signal or onto a chart recorder. Velocities are evaluated while the patient undergoes various maneuvers. This technology has not been studied as extensively as IPG or duplex scanning. Advantages to hand-held Doppler studies include inexpensive and, in most cases, more portable equipment. However, the safety of withholding anticoagulant treatment in patients with normal hand-held Doppler results has never been evaluated formally. For anyone performing noninvasive venous studies, a working knowledge of this technique is important to understand basic venous physiology.

Indications

Practical indications are slightly different than those previously discussed; for example, hand-held Dopplers may be used alone when other diagnostic methods are unavailable to confirm proximal DVT in a symptomatic patient, or they may be used to diagnose postphlebitic syndrome. This technique can also be used to screen patients for determining whether duplex scanning or IPG is indicated, especially if those studies are not readily available. If the screening test is positive, the additional cost or effort of obtaining a duplex or IPG study may be warranted. A hand-held Doppler is more reliable than IPG for the diagnosis of DVT in patients with severe arterial insufficiency or with a leg in traction. Used alone, a hand-held Doppler provides mainly qualitative evidence of venous function.

Relative Contraindications

Obese patients and patients with massive leg swelling may be difficult to study.

Personnel and Equipment

- A clinician or technician familiar with venous anatomy and Doppler ultrasonographic technology. (Because the vein cannot be visualized with this technique, a better knowledge of anatomy is required than with ultrasonography [see Fig. 88-3]. Experience significantly increases the accuracy of this examination.)
- 5- to 10-MHz hand-held Doppler with audio. It can often be used for listening to fetal heart tones as well.
- Acoustic gel.

Technique

1. Prepare the room and patient. The room temperature should be warmer than 70° F to prevent vasoconstriction. Place the patient in the supine position with the head slightly elevated. All tight garments should be removed and the leg well exposed (tight-fitting garments may interfere with venous return). The leg should be slightly abducted, externally rotated, and slightly flexed at the knee. It should also be relaxed to prevent compression of the deep veins. Support the knee with a pillow for better muscle relaxation.
2. Locate the common femoral vein by first finding the artery and then moving the probe medially until the characteristic venous flow or tone is found. The best tone is usually obtained with the probe angled toward the heart (in the direction of venous flow). Use minimal probe pressure to keep from compressing the vein. Arterial flow is characterized by a high-pitched, usually abrupt, tone. Venous flow is usually lower pitched and more continuous.
3. Evaluate the patient with the Doppler from the level of the common femoral vein distally to the superficial femoral, popliteal, and posterior tibial veins (Fig. 88-7). When the level of the popliteal vein is reached, the patient may be turned to a prone position with knees slightly flexed. Rest the patient's feet on two pillows.
4. Compare the sound or tracing from one leg with that of the other leg at each level of the examination and record the results.

Interpretation

Four characteristics describe *normal venous flow* (*physiology*):

- It is *patent* if flow is heard at the anatomic level of the vein.
- It is *spontaneous* if it can be heard at all levels of the vein.
- It varies with respiration, or is *phasic*.
- It is *augmented* by distal compression of the limb or by release of proximal compression.

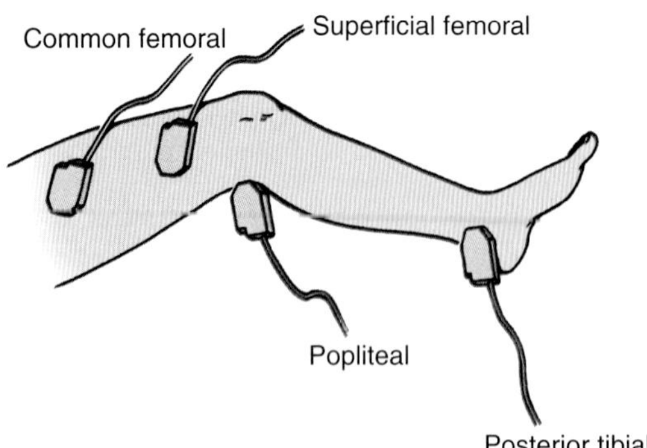

Figure 88-7 Doppler sonographic examination. The patient is supine with the head slightly elevated. Examine the common femoral, superficial femoral, popliteal, and posterior tibial veins sequentially.

Patent

Rarely does the flow completely disappear with DVT because some flow is usually preserved around a thrombus or through collateral vessels. Differences between one side and the other may be more important, and DVT is frequently associated with a continuous, high-pitched signal. A pulsatile tone that varies with the cardiac cycle is not normal and indicates increased venous pressure.

Spontaneous

Deep venous thrombosis causes loss of spontaneous flow. Other causes of loss of spontaneity include anything leading to vasoconstriction. As previously stated, low ambient room temperature or patient anxiety can cause vasoconstriction. The posterior tibial vein may not have a spontaneous signal in normal individuals. Spontaneity is usually found when venous flow is phasic.

Phasic

This characteristic variation of flow with respiration may be lost with DVT. With normal veins, a Valsalva maneuver should decrease the signal, whereas a deep breath should augment the signal.

Augmented

Firm, gentle compression of the limb for a few seconds distal to the vein should cause augmentation of the flow. Release of proximal compression should also result in augmentation. DVT causes a more abrupt and shorter augmentation—if augmentation remains present at all—compared with that of a normal leg. Presence of augmentation provides support that the vein is patent. Reverse augmentation produced by proximal compression or after releasing distal compression indicates valvular incompetence.

False-negative results may occur in patients with incomplete venous obstruction by thrombi and false-positive results may be caused by extrinsic venous compression. When treatment decisions are made, the fact that no outcome studies are available using hand-held Doppler alone must be weighed against the availability of compression ultrasonography, duplex, IPG, or contrast studies. Abnormal Doppler results are frequently confirmed with another technique. It should be noted that portable hand-held Doppler equipment, similar to various types of plethysmography equipment (other than electrical IPG), is relatively inexpensive. Either can be used alone, but in combination they may complement each other and provide additional types of quantitative data. These supplementary studies may be helpful to the clinician when determining which patients need further evaluation.

Noninvasive Arterial Studies

Peripheral artery disease (PAD) affects 29% of patients in a primary care clinician's office who are older than 70 years of age (or older than 50 years of age with a history of diabetes or smoking). Although only a small proportion of individuals with PAD and intermittent claudication develop skin breakdown or limb loss, the associated pain and disability from PAD often restrict ambulation. The restriction of ambulation not only interferes with the quality of life, it may interfere with the ability to prevent coronary artery disease (CAD) with exercise. PAD can progress to pain at rest, ulceration, and gangrene. Men are affected more frequently than women. Diabetic patients and smokers develop this disease more frequently and at an earlier age, and the prognosis is grave in diabetic patients because PAD almost always progresses. Diabetic patients also have a greater incidence of vessel involvement between the knee and ankle. Diabetic PAD is responsible for about half of all amputations.

A history of intermittent claudication and absent or diminished peripheral pulses are unreliable signs or symptoms of PAD. PAD most frequently involves the superficial femoral and popliteal arteries, followed by the distal aorta and iliac arteries, in order of decreasing frequency. The absence of a posterior tibial pulse is a more useful finding on examination than the absence of a dorsalis pedis pulse because 10% to 15% of persons have congenitally absent dorsalis pedis pulses. However, neither finding is very accurate.

Multiple noninvasive techniques are available for the diagnosis of lower extremity PAD. A comprehensive history and physical examination and a combination of at least two noninvasive tests should be performed to both confirm the diagnosis and determine the location of the lesion. If the location of a hemodynamically significant lesion is known, the risks associated with tests involving contrast dye can be minimized; this knowledge can also guide the radiologist's, cardiologist's, or surgeon's approach for optimal contrast visualization. Different and sometimes more useful information can be gained from noninvasive studies than with contrast studies; as a result, some radiologists/cardiologists/surgeons operate without subjecting the patient to preoperative contrast studies. Although it can be very operator dependent for a small artery (e.g., popliteal artery), the accuracy of MR or CT angiography is similar to that of a contrast study. Contrast studies may also be avoided if noninvasive studies fail to demonstrate a hemodynamically significant lesion consistent with the patient's symptoms.

NOTE: The clinician must always consider the possibility of cardiac and cerebrovascular disease in patients with PAD. Intermittent claudication is often the first sign or symptom of generalized atherosclerosis, and these patients most frequently succumb to myocardial infarction or stroke. National guidelines consider PAD a cardiovascular risk equivalent, meaning the patient with PAD has at least as high a risk of a myocardial infarction over the next decade (i.e., 20%, if not higher) as a patient who has previously experienced a myocardial infarction. Using routine coronary angiography in patients with claudication, CAD was identified in 90% of patients and severe CAD in 28% of patients. The Framingham Study demonstrated a 10% risk of fatal stroke in patients with claudication. Therefore, treatment should be targeted to prevent myocardial infarction and stroke as much as to prevent complications of PAD.

Regarding screening, although noninvasive studies are more accurate than physical examination, the literature does not demonstrate a benefit to early detection of PAD. Even though noninvasive diagnosis of PAD may be one of the easiest methods to diagnose generalized atherosclerosis, additional data are needed before noninvasive testing should be considered for routine screening.

Risk Factors

- Older age
- Male
- Diabetes
- Cigarette smoking
- Hypertension (greater risk factor for women)
- Hyperlipidemia (not a consistent independent risk factor for claudication)
- Family history of PAD (although a risk factor for CAD, this may not be a risk factor for claudication)

- Homocystinemia, hyperfibrinogenemia, hypercoagulable states (probable risk factors)

Indications (Especially in Diabetic Patients)

- Intermittent claudication
- Nonhealing foot ulcer
- Exertional leg pain of unknown etiology
- Possible trauma to an artery

Considerations

- To screen before lower extremity surgery in a diabetic patient
- To screen patients with neuropathy who may have ischemia without symptoms (numbness from neuropathy)
- To follow a patient after reconstructive arterial surgery or percutaneous intervention (angioplasty or stent) or for whom nonoperative therapy is selected

It has been said that an experienced clinician can diagnose PAD in most patients by using the history and physical examination alone. However, many clinicians who evaluate patients with extremity pain are neither experienced nor current in the management of vascular disease. Noninvasive studies provide an objective, definitive diagnosis so that clinicians can either rule in PAD or search for another cause for the symptoms.

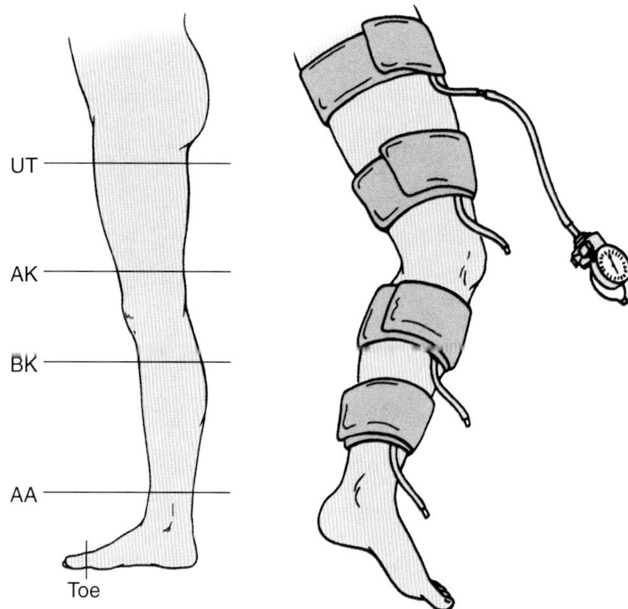

Figure 88-8 Segmental arterial pressure measurement. Cuff positions: AA, above ankle; AK, above knee; BK, below knee; UT, upper thigh.

Segmental Pressure Measurement

The segmental pressure study is the most generally accepted and widely applied noninvasive arterial test. Segmental pressures are often evaluated as the initial test for a possible arterial abnormality.

Personnel and Equipment

- A clinician or technician familiar with arterial anatomy of the foot and Doppler ultrasonographic technology
- 5- to 10-MHz hand-held Doppler probe (transducer) with audio
- Acoustic gel
- Aneroid (gauge) manometer
- Four cuffs for each leg (they can be of the same diameter; if eight are available, study time is considerably reduced)

With arterial stenosis, and especially with collateral flow, arterial resistance is significantly increased. This increased resistance leads to a large or asymmetric drop in arterial blood pressure over the particular arterial segment with obstruction. The brachial pressure can also be used as a standardized reference for the pressures of the lower extremity. At a minimum, brachial pressure should always be recorded along with its ratio to the pressure at the ankle (i.e., ankle–brachial index [ABI]).

When using a pressure gauge (aneroid as opposed to mercury manometer), artifact is not a concern if the same gauge is used throughout the study (ratios and gradients are the values obtained rather than absolute blood pressure measurements). Likewise, the same cuff widths can be used throughout the lower extremities without concern for cuff artifact. (Interpretation has taken cuff artifact into account.) In most cases this technique produces a high-thigh systolic pressure greater than the brachial artery pressure, which is acceptable for calculating ratios.

Technique

1. With the patient in the supine position, measure systolic pressures in both arms and record them.
2. On one lower limb apply four segmental cuffs (Fig. 88-8). The systolic values recorded refer to the cuff level rather than the artery studied.
3. Using the hand-held Doppler, evaluate the three major arteries of the foot (dorsalis pedis, posterior tibial, and peroneal) for the strongest signal. Use this artery for the remainder of the study. When determining pressures, hold the Doppler probe consistently over the artery at the angle and in the direction that produces the strongest signal.
4. Using the same pressure gauge throughout, attach it to a cuff and inflate the cuff until the Doppler signal in the foot disappears.
5. Deflate the cuff slowly until the first signal is audible in the foot and record this systolic pressure for that cuff level.
6. Sequentially inflate and deflate and record the systolic pressures for each cuff level. Repeat at the same four levels on the other lower extremity.
7. Calculate the ABI, which is the highest ankle systolic pressure divided by the highest brachial systolic pressure.

Sources of Error

Most errors arise when the examiner moves the probe off the artery while inflating the cuff. One limitation of this technique is that, even though it is fairly sensitive for diagnosing PAD, it is not as helpful for localizing lesions.

Vessel calcification, such as that found in patients with diabetes and chronic renal failure, may lead to an arterial segment that is compressible only at very high pressures (e.g., >300 mm Hg) and may produce unusual results. In fact, segmental pressures may appear to follow a reverse gradient. Suspect vessel calcification when the ABI is higher than 1.4.

With an ABI less than 1.0, always consider the possibility of an obstructed aorta or bilaterally obstructed iliac arteries. Because of cuff artifact, high-thigh pressures may be greater than brachial pressures and mask aortic or iliac obstruction.

With an abnormal study result, consider comparing the systolic pressures in all the arteries of the foot. This prevents the artifact that might be produced if there is localized obstruction of just one pedal artery.

Interpretation

The single best method of quantitative screening for PAD is an ABI determined by Doppler ultrasonography. Normally, the ankle pressure is equal to or slightly greater than the arm pressure. An ABI less than 0.95 is abnormal. Typically, patients with rest claudication or gangrene have ABIs less than 0.5, which often indicates multisegmental disease. Patients with intermittent claudication usually have ABIs between 0.5 and 0.9, generally associated with single-segment disease.

During a follow-up evaluation, a change in the ABI of more than 0.15 is considered clinically significant. A decrease in this amount usually indicates disease progression or a problem with a reconstructive procedure. An increase suggests improvement in circulation resulting from the development of collaterals. There is no current consensus on how often studies should be repeated.

A high-thigh pressure less than the arm pressure, any pressure drop of 30 mm Hg or more from one segment to the next, or a difference of 30 mm Hg or more between extremities at the same segmental level signifies a probable obstruction in that segment. Some asymmetry of results in the lower extremities is normal. Remember that pressure drops may represent the sum of more than one lesion.

NOTE: Many clinicians use the ABI alone to screen for PAD, and studies have verified its value for use in this manner (Hirsch and colleagues, 2001); however, it requires staff time to perform, document, and interpret the findings. This must be weighed against the fact that although Medicare and other insurers now reimburse for this procedure (CPT-93922), many insurers reimburse only for symptomatic patients. Beckman and colleagues (2006) recently demonstrated that an automatic blood pressure cuff (using the oscillatory technique) can be used to check ABI (and save time), with a sensitivity of 88%, specificity of 85%, and a negative predictive value of 96%. If normal, a screening ABI performed in this manner probably does not need to be repeated more than once every 5 years.

Waveform Analysis

Velocity or pulse volume waveform analysis is indicated whenever there is an abnormal ABI or segmental pressure study. These studies can confirm each other and assist in localization of the obstruction.

Velocity Waveform Analysis

Personnel and Equipment

- A clinician or technician familiar with arterial anatomy of the lower extremity and Doppler ultrasonographic technology
- 5- to 10-MHz probe (transducer) with audio and chart recorder
- Acoustic gel

NOTE: The same equipment can often be used for venous Doppler studies.

Technique

1. Prepare the room and patient. The room temperature should be greater than 70° F to prevent vasoconstriction. The patient should rest in the supine position for at least 10 minutes. The leg should be well exposed, slightly abducted, externally rotated, and slightly flexed at the knee. Supporting the knee with a pillow may increase patient comfort.
2. Beginning at the common femoral artery, apply acoustic gel and auscultate with the probe for maximal tone and amplitude on the recorder. The best tone is usually obtained with the probe pointed away from the heart in the direction of arterial flow. Arterial flow is characterized by a high-pitched, usually abrupt tone. This should be differentiated from the sound of venous flow, which is usually lower pitched and more continuous.
3. Obtain tracings from common femoral, popliteal, and posterior tibial arteries. For the popliteal arteries, the patient may be turned to a prone position with knees slightly flexed and feet resting on two pillows if this position is more comfortable.
4. Compare the sound and tracing from one leg with the other leg at each level of the examination and record.

Sources of Error

- Dense objects or tissue (e.g., local excess fat, hematoma, scar tissue, or plaque on the anterior wall of the vessel) may significantly interfere with ultrasound transmission, making it more difficult to obtain a tracing.
- Prosthetic vessels are almost impossible to study.
- In severe disease, tracings may be unattainable in spite of being able to hear a tone, especially in distal extremities.
- With an incorrect probe angle, the multiphasic components of a tracing can be missed or lost.

Interpretation

The normal arterial velocity signal is multiphasic, characterized by one systolic and one or more diastolic components. With a directional Doppler study, the diastolic component should at first be briefly negative followed by a positively directed systolic flow component (Fig. 88-9). The diastolic component may be decreased in a vasodilated individual and increased in a vasoconstricted individual.

The arterial velocity signal produced *just proximal* to an occlusion is usually of low amplitude and short duration (Fig. 88-10A). The arterial velocity signal produced *over* a stenotic segment is characteristically high pitched with less prominent diastolic components (Fig. 88-10B). The arterial velocity signal produced *distal* to a stenotic segment usually lacks a diastolic component and has a dampened systolic signal. It is not as high pitched as the stenotic signal (Fig. 88-10C). The arterial signal *far distal* to a stenotic segment is like the poststenotic segment but is likely to have an even lower amplitude. *Collateral* signals are high pitched and nearly continuous.

To differentiate the contour of normal arterial signals from the contour of obstructed arterial signals, clinicians often describe them as "teepees" and "igloos." "Teepee" refers to the shape of the velocity tracing of a normal artery with its rapid upstroke and resultant high amplitude. The sluggish upstroke tracing with minimal amplitude, as seen with the typical postobstructed artery, might well be described as an "igloo."

A rule of thumb: the presence of a *multiphasic* Doppler signal in a distal vessel, such as that of the foot, strongly suggests that the proximal artery is normal.

Pulse Volume Waveform Analysis

Pulse volume recordings (PVRs) are less operator dependent, are not limited by calcification of the vessel walls, and are readily and rapidly obtained using the same cuffs already in place for segmental

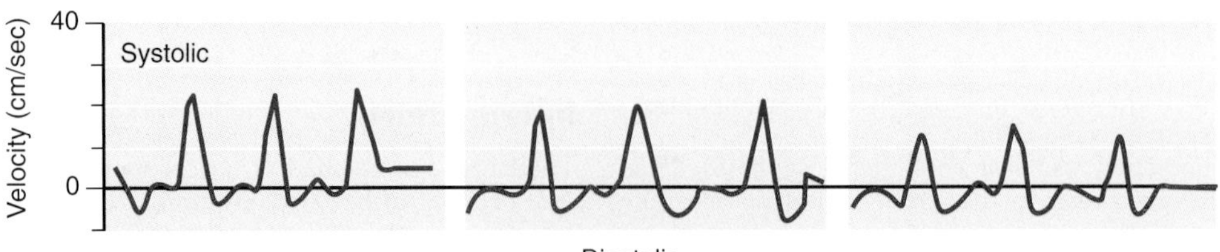

Figure 88-9 Normal arterial Doppler velocity tracings.

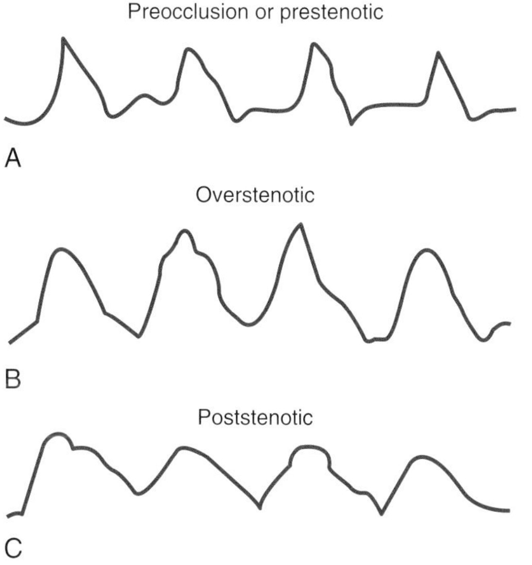

Figure 88-10 Examples of prestenotic (**A**), overstenotic (**B**), and poststenotic (**C**) tracings.

pressure measurements. This is a quantitative measurement that allows reasonably accurate localization of a lesion or lesions.

Personnel and Equipment

- A clinician or technician familiar with PVR technology
- Pulse volume recorder
- Four cuffs for each leg (they can be of the same diameter; if eight are available, the study time is reduced)

Technique

1. Place the patient in the supine position. Cuffs are placed in the same locations as for segmental pressure determinations and are inflated to 65 mm Hg.
2. Record the PVR at each level.

Source of Error

With severe proximal disease it may be difficult to assess the degree of distal disease because the PVRs are often flat throughout the extremity.

Interpretation

Changes in waveforms with progression of PAD are shown in Figure 88-11. First noted is the loss of the reflected diastolic wave. Next, with more progressive disease, a decrease is seen in the rate of fall of the catacrotic limb, or the downsloping portion. Finally, a further delay in the rise of the anacrotic limb, or the upsloping initial portion of the wave, is noted. With moderate to severe disease, an "igloo" is the predominant feature.

OTHER STUDIES

For the patient with a history of claudication or intermittent claudication, and yet normal vascular studies, additional testing is available.

1. Vascular treadmill stress testing is probably the most commonly used next study. Because of the cost of equipment, a referral to a vascular laboratory may be necessary. For those with a treadmill, after recording ankle systolic pressures, have the patient walk at a speed of 2 miles per hour with a 12% grade until pain begins or 5 minutes elapses. Patients older than 50 years of age should have continuous electrocardiographic monitoring. The time it takes to induce pain is noted as the maximal walking time. Once the pain begins, or 5 minutes has elapsed, the patient is placed in a supine position and the ankle systolic pressure is again recorded. It should be recorded every minute until it returns to baseline. In healthy individuals, strenuous exercise causes a transient fall in ankle systolic pressure, which quickly returns to baseline at rest. In contrast, when a patient with PAD exercises, pain usually commences before 5 minutes and the ankle pressure falls precipitously, often to unrecordable levels. It usually does not recover for several minutes. A fall in systolic pressure of more than 20 mm Hg from baseline and a recovery time of more than 3 minutes are considered abnormal. (Note that when using the resting brachial pressure to calculate a postexercise ABI, some

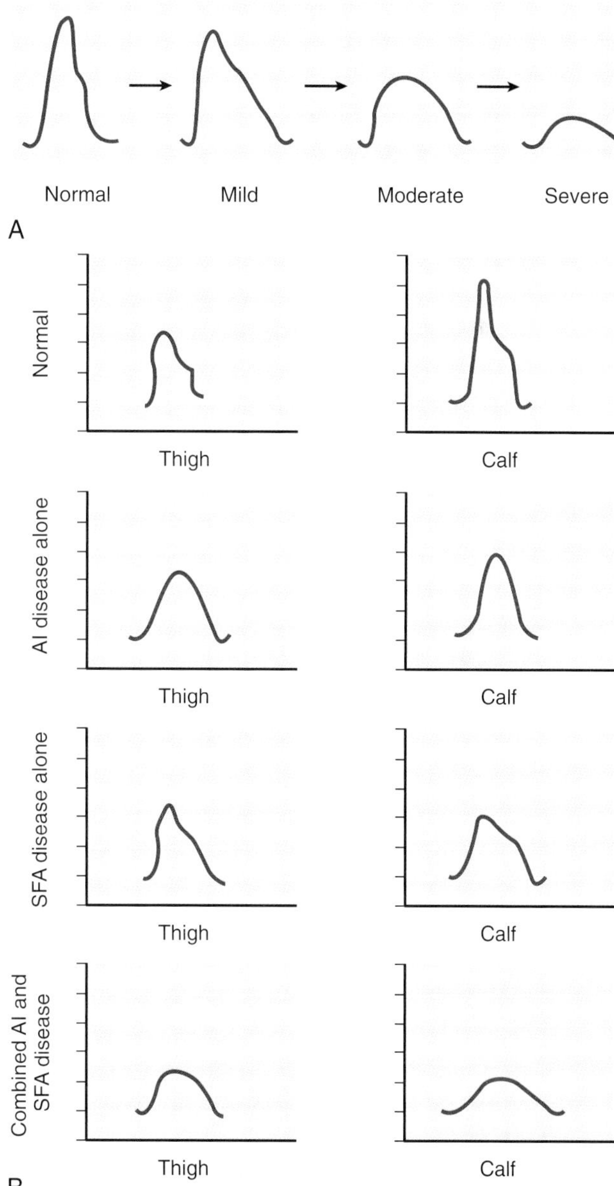

Figure 88-11 **A,** Alterations seen in pulse volume waveform as arterial occlusive disease progresses from mild to moderate to severe. **B,** Various thigh and calf waveform patterns characteristic of aortoiliac and superficial femoral arterial occlusive disease. In the normal example, notice the contour of both the thigh and calf waveforms as well as the characteristic increase in amplitude of the calf pulse volume recordings. AI, aortoiliac; SFA, superficial femoral artery.

sources consider a postexercise ABI abnormal if it falls more than 20% from baseline and remains low for more than 3 minutes.) If a postexercise ABI returns to normal in 5 minutes, it suggests a single PAD lesion; delays of more than 10 minutes suggest multilevel PAD.
2. Toe raises, up to 50 repetitions, have been substituted in many vascular laboratories for treadmill walking with good results, and this can be performed in the office setting.
3. MRA—although sometimes a long, complex, and expensive procedure, some clinicians have replaced contrast angiography with MRA and perform contrast angiography only while they are performing a percutaneous intervention (angioplasty or stent).
4. Multislice CT angiography—although it requires considerable radiation and as much contrast dye as a regular angiogram, multislice CT angiography may replace percutaneous angiography.

CPT/Billing Codes

93922 Noninvasive physiologic studies of upper or lower extremity arteries, single level, bilateral (e.g., ankle/brachial indices, Doppler waveform analysis, volume plethysmography, transcutaneous oxygen tension measurement)
93923 Noninvasive physiologic studies of upper or lower extremity arteries, multiple levels or with provocative functional maneuvers, complete bilateral study (e.g., segmental blood pressure measurements, segmental Doppler waveform analysis, segmental volume plethysmography, segmental transcutaneous oxygen tension measurement, measurements with postural provocation tests, measurements with reactive hyperemia)
93924 Noninvasive physiologic studies of lower extremity arteries, at rest and following treadmill stress testing, complete bilateral study
93925 Duplex scan of lower extremity arteries or arterial bypass grafts, complete bilateral study
93926 Duplex scan of lower extremity arteries or bypass grafts, unilateral or limited study
93965 Noninvasive physiologic studies of extremity veins, complete bilateral study (e.g., Doppler waveform analysis with responses to compression and other maneuvers, phleborheography, impedance plethysmography)
93970 Duplex scan of extremity veins including responses to compression and other maneuvers; complete bilateral study
93971 Duplex scan of extremity veins including responses to compression and other maneuvers; unilateral or limited study

ICD-9-CM Diagnostic Codes

415.11 Pulmonary embolism, iatrogenic
415.19 Pulmonary embolism, other
440.20 Atherosclerosis of native arteries of the extremities, unspecified
- 440.21 with intermittent claudication
- 440.22 with rest pain
- 440.23 with ulceration
- 440.30 of unspecified graft
- 440.31 of autologous vein bypass graft

451.0 Phlebitis and thrombophlebitis, superficial vessels, lower extremity
- 451.11 femoral vein (deep or superficial)
- 451.19 other
- 451.81 iliac vein

459.1 Postphlebitic syndrome
459.2 Edema, leg, resulting from venous obstruction
459.81 Venous (peripheral) insufficiency, unspecified
707.1 Chronic ulcer of skin, lower extremity
729.5 Pain, leg
782.3 Edema, legs

Suppliers

(See contact information online at www.expertconsult.com.)

For compression ultrasonography suppliers and equipment, see Chapter 225, Emergency Department, Hospitalist, and Office Ultrasonography (Clinical Ultrasonography).

Hand-held (pocket) Dopplers
MedaSonics (Cooper Surgical)
Vascular equipment, including duplex
BioMedix
Vascular equipment, including duplex and hand-held Dopplers
Cardinal Health (Viasys Healthcare/Nicolet Vascular/IMEX)
Parks Medical Electronics

BIBLIOGRAPHY

Anderson DR, Kovacs MJ, Kovacs G, et al: Combined use of clinical assessment and D-dimer to improve the management of patients presenting to the emergency department with suspected deep vein thrombosis (the EDITED Study). J Thromb Haemost 1:645–651, 2003.
Appelman PT, De Jong TE, Lampmann LE: Deep venous thrombosis of the leg: US findings. Radiology 163:743–746, 1987.
Beckman JA, Higgins CO, Gerhard-Herman M: Automated oscillometric determination of the ankle-brachial index provides accuracy necessary for office practice. Hypertension 47:35–38, 2006.
Brodsky CM, Martin R: Ultrasound and Doppler examination of veins and arteries. Atlas Off Proced 3:421, 2000.
Creager MA, Dzau VJ: Vascular diseases of the extremities. In Wiener CM, Kasper DL, Braunwald E, Hauser S (eds): Harrison's Principles of Internal Medicine, 16th ed. New York, McGraw-Hill, 2005, pp 1486–1494.
Cronan JJ, Dorfman GS, Scola FH, et al: Deep venous thrombosis: US assessment using vein compression. Radiology 162:191–194, 1987.
Heijboer H, Büller HR, Lensing AW, et al: A comparison of real-time compression ultrasonography with impedance plethysmography for the diagnosis of deep-vein thrombosis in symptomatic outpatients. N Engl J Med 329:1365–1369, 1993.
Heit JA, O'Fallon WM, Petterson TM, et al: Relative impact of risk factors for deep vein thrombosis and pulmonary embolism: A population-based study. Arch Intern Med 162:1245–1248, 2002.
Hirsch AT, Criqui MH, Treat-Jacobson D, et al: Peripheral arterial disease detection, awareness, and treatment in primary care. JAMA 286: 1317–1324, 2001.
Huisman MV, Büller HR, ten Cate JW, Vreeken J: Serial impedance plethysmography for suspected deep venous thrombosis in outpatients: The Amsterdam General Practitioner Study. N Engl J Med 314:823–828, 1986.
Hull RD, Carter CJ, Jay RM, et al: Diagnostic efficacy of impedance plethysmography for clinically suspected deep-vein thrombosis: A randomized trial. Ann Intern Med 102:21–28, 1985.
Hunt D: Determining the clinical probability of deep venous thrombosis and pulmonary embolism. South Med J 100:1015–1021, 2007.
Kearon C, Julian JA, Newman TE, Ginsberg JS: Noninvasive diagnosis of deep venous thrombosis: McMaster Diagnostic Imaging Practice Guidelines Initiative. Ann Intern Med 128:663–677, 1998.
Labropoulos N, Tassiopoulos A: Vascular diagnosis of venous thrombosis. In Mansour MA, Labropoulos N (eds): Vascular Diagnosis. Philadelphia, Saunders, 2005, pp 429–438.
Lensing AW, Prandoni P, Brandjes D, et al: Detection of deep-vein thrombosis by real-time B-mode ultrasonography. N Engl J Med 320:342–345, 1989.
Nordness PJ, Money SR: Evaluation of claudication in vascular diagnosis. In Mansour MA, Labropoulos N (eds): Vascular Diagnosis. Philadelphia, Saunders, 2005, pp 429–438.
Turnbull TJ, Dymowski JJ: Emergency department use of hand-held Doppler ultrasonography [review]. Am J Emerg Med 7:209–215, 1989.
Vogel P, Laing FC, Jeffrey RB Jr, Wing VW: Deep venous thrombosis of the lower extremity: US evaluation. Radiology 163:747–751, 1987.
Wells PS, Anderson DR, Rodger M, et al: Evaluation of D-dimer in the diagnosis of suspected deep-vein thrombosis. N Engl J Med 349:1227–1235, 2003.
Wells PS, Owen C, Doucette S, et al: Does this patient have deep vein thrombosis? JAMA 295:199–207, 2006.

CHAPTER 89

Office Electrocardiograms

Russell D. White • George D. Harris

The electrocardiogram (ECG) is a graphic description of the electrical activity of the heart, recorded from skin surface electrodes positioned to demonstrate this activity from a variety of spatial perspectives. The waves of electrical activity are represented as a sequence of deflections on the ECG (P wave, QRS complex, and T wave). The resting ECG is the most widely used cardiovascular diagnostic test in the United States. Current estimates are that half are performed or interpreted by clinicians without fellowship training in cardiology. The clinician supervising, performing, or interpreting ECGs must be familiar with the proper use of the machine and electrode placement. In addition, guidelines and clinical competency statements are available (see the Bibliography).

The validity of using the resting 12-lead ECG as a screening test for cardiovascular disease in asymptomatic individuals has never been demonstrated convincingly. One reason is the relatively low prevalence of ECG abnormalities in the general population (ranges from 1% to 10%) . Such a low prevalence limits the ECG's sensitivity for screening, its predictive accuracy, and its usefulness (Fig. 89-1). Likewise, the ECG can appear completely normal in patients experiencing an acute coronary event. Therefore, it is important for the clinician to consider each ECG in the context of the clinical situation. Pertinent to each ECG are the patient's age, risk factors, medications, symptoms, physical findings, and laboratory results as well as findings from any previous ECGs (for comparison).

Indications

In the office, the following situations are the most common to warrant an ECG:

- Chest pain, especially if suspected to be of cardiac origin
- Palpitations
- Acute-onset dyspnea
- Syncope
- Presence of a new cardiac finding on examination (e.g., murmur, gallop, rub)
- Dysrhythmia recognition and management
- Baseline or longitudinal data for patients with hypertension, diabetes, chronic kidney disease (defined as glomerular filtration rate <60 mL/min), or other chronic diseases that might cause ECG changes or increase cardiac risk
- Preoperative screen for patients with known coronary artery disease (CAD) or who are at high risk for adverse cardiac events
- Electrolyte abnormalities that may cause ECG alterations (e.g., potassium, calcium)
- Before administration of pharmacologic agents that are known to have a high incidence of cardiovascular effects (e.g., medications causing a QT prolongation, cancer chemotherapy) and after starting therapy
- Before exercise testing (to note any contraindications)
- Individuals in special occupations that require high cardiovascular performance or who would immediately endanger others if they experienced a cardiovascular event
- Possibly for a baseline during a physical examination of those older than 40 years of age, especially patients with risk factors for CAD

Patients can be classified into three major groups when undergoing an ECG: (1) patients with known cardiovascular disease or dysfunction, (2) patients who are suspected of having or who are at increased risk of developing cardiovascular disease or dysfunction, and (3) patients with no apparent or suspected heart disease or dysfunction. For patients in the first two groups, an ECG is indicated if there has been a change in symptoms or if the therapy may change the ECG. The ECG may show changes during symptoms and in response to treatment, which would confirm a cardiac basis for symptoms. It also may demonstrate preexisting structural or ischemic heart disease (e.g., left ventricular hypertrophy, Q waves).

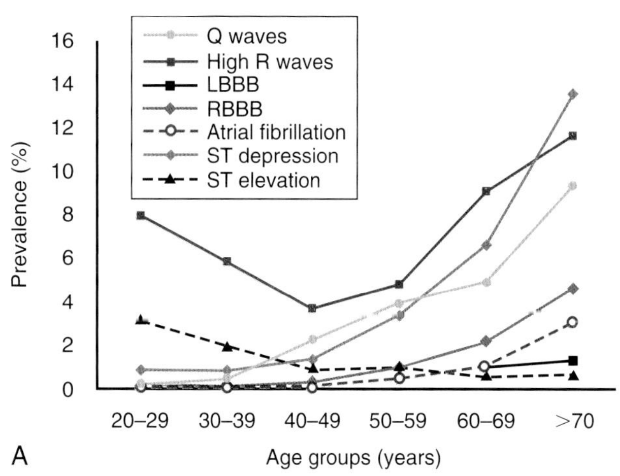

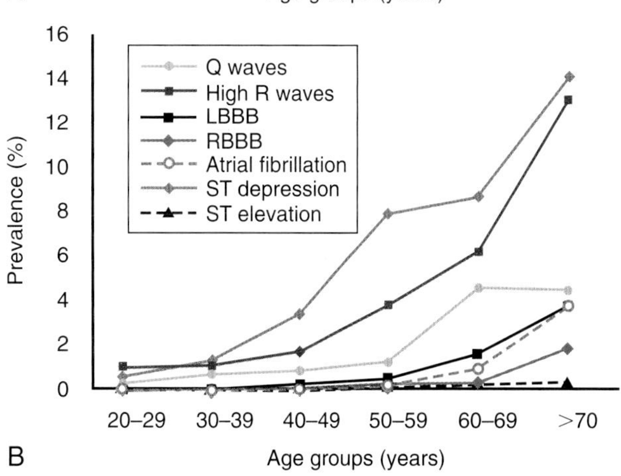

Figure 89-1 Prevalence of ECG abnormalities in men (**A**) and women (**B**). LBBB, left bundle branch block; RBBB, right bundle branch block.

However, a normal ECG or one that remains unchanged from the baseline does not exclude the possibility that chest pain is ischemic in origin. The last group (group 3) represents a large proportion of the patients treated in the usual office practice.

NOTE: The routine use of a resting ECG to screen for CAD in asymptomatic adults is not recommended by the American College of Physicians or the Canadian Task Force on Preventive Health Care. The American Academy of Family Physicians and the U.S. Preventive Services Task Force recommend *against* routine screening for CAD with resting ECG in asymptomatic adults at low risk for events from CAD. They also find insufficient evidence to recommend for or against routine screening with resting ECG in patients at increased risk for events from CAD.

Although the American Heart Association likewise does not recommend routine or repeated ECGs for risk assessment, various ECG abnormalities have been reported to have predictive power. For example, the most common abnormal ECG findings (Q waves, ST segment depression, nonspecific T-wave abnormalities, left ventricular hypertrophy [LVH], and bundle branch blocks) on the resting ECG have been found to have independent predictive power for both coronary mortality and total cardiovascular mortality. In some studies, patients with one or more of these abnormalities were associated with two to four times increased cardiovascular risk (i.e., multivariate-adjusted relative risks between 2.0 and 4.0). These study results indicate that ECG abnormalities might suggest an increased clinical risk in certain patients and therefore warrant further investigation or risk reduction. Persistent abnormalities on the resting ECG on serial tracings are associated with a higher clinical risk than transient findings alone.

Contraindications

- Emergent need for airway maintenance or management of breathing or circulation (these needs should be addressed before an ECG procedure is performed)
- Patient phobia, refusal, or inability to remain still or in one position (relative contraindication in life-threatening situation)
- Skin conditions (e.g., burns, infections) that would interfere with electrode placement (relative contraindication in life-threatening situation)

Equipment

- Electrodes.
- ECG machine with appropriate patient cables and paper.
- If computerized storage is expected, a floppy disk (or other digital media) should be inserted or a connection made to the Internet, Intranet, or telephone line.

Preprocedure Patient Preparation

Explain the procedure to the patient and discuss why the patient needs to remain as immobile as possible, maintain normal respirations, and not talk during the procedure. Occasionally, there is a need to reassure the patient that the procedure is safe and will not cause an electrical shock (e.g., "It takes electricity out of you and does not put it in"). The patient should be aware that further cardiac work-up may be necessary regardless of the outcome of the ECG. The patient should also be aware that a normal ECG result does not eliminate the possibility of CAD or significant heart disease. Moreover, abnormal ECGs do not always indicate significant cardiac disease.

Technique

Most modern ECG machines are so simple that an operator's manual is not needed. Standardization is accurate with digital machines, which often automatically adjust for excessive voltage. Perform the ECG procedure in a room away from powerful electrical equipment (e.g., electric motors, x-ray equipment), if possible. Electrode placement remains the biggest challenge.

1. Place the patient in the supine position on the table. Generally, the patient has a pillow under his or her head. Arms should rest at the sides of the torso. Legs should be flat, apart, and not touching each other. If the patient is in a position other than supine (e.g., head elevated to relieve orthopnea), the heart's electrical axis is altered, possibly an issue when comparing serial tracings. In such cases, a note should be made on the ECG strip of degree or angle of patient elevation so that future ECGs can be obtained with the patient at the same angle for comparison. Although the patient's chest and distal extremities are exposed, keep the rest of the body covered. This protects patient dignity and should prevent shivering, which can cause a tremor artifact on the ECG tracing.
2. Bring the ECG machine near the table and turn it on. The usual paper speed is 25 mm/sec and the amplitude 1 mV/10 mm.

   NOTE: Older equipment, especially analog equipment, occasionally needs to be standardized. If available, review the operator's manual regarding standardization. Standardize the machine when it is tracing at 25 mm/sec by briefly depressing the standardization button. One millivolt should deflect exactly 10 mm, and full standardization should be used if possible. If standardization is not performed or is allowed to vary, evaluation of serial tracings is less accurate.

3. Wipe the areas for electrode placement with an alcohol swab. It may be necessary to shave some areas so that the electrodes stick. We recommend shaving *after* using the alcohol swab to avoid applying alcohol to any abrasions resulting from shaving. Gentle abrasion with a fine-grit sandpaper or equivalent may also reduce noise and artifact and improve the quality of the ECG. We also recommend using adhesive electrodes with a tab for fastening the clips from the cable lead.
4. Place the limb electrodes. The red electrode is for the left leg and is labeled "left leg." The electrode for the right leg is universally green and is labeled "right leg." The electrode for the right arm is often banded in white and labeled "RA." The electrode for the left arm is banded in black and labeled "LA." Traditionally, limb electrodes were placed on the wrists and ankles. However, with the development of high-quality disposable electrodes, many clinicians have started applying the limb electrodes below the hips and on the upper arms. Applying the electrodes more proximally may reduce motion artifact.
5. Place the chest electrodes in the following order (Fig. 89-2):
   - V_1 (red): fourth intercostal space at right sternal border
   - V_2 (yellow): fourth intercostal space at left sternal border

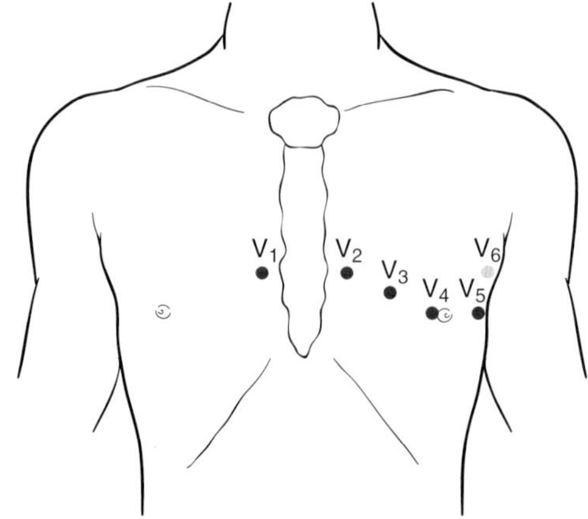

Figure 89-2 Placement of electrodes. Note that V_6 is in the same horizontal plane as V_4 and V_5, but more lateral, in the mid-axillary line.

- V_4 (blue): fifth intercostal space at the mid-clavicular line
- V_3 (green): halfway between V_2 and V_4
- V_5 (tan): anterior axillary line at the same level as V_4 (directly lateral and in the same transverse plane)
- V_6 (violet): mid-axillary line at the same level as V_4 and V_5 (again, directly lateral to V_5)

For a landmark in men, the nipples are usually in the mid-clavicular line and overlie the fourth intercostal space. For consistent placement, use only bony landmarks for precordial electrodes. The sternal angle, between the manubrium and body of the sternum, is immediately above the second intercostal space. The V_4 through V_6 electrodes are placed in the same horizontal plane (not necessarily in the same intercostal space).

6. Perform the ECG procedure with the electrodes in their proper locations. For dysrhythmias, an extended rhythm strip or another attempt at a 12-lead ECG may be indicated for improved technical quality. Multichannel machines are superior to single-channel machines for rhythm strips. When a second channel is available, it is best to display lead II for rhythm and V_5 for ischemia. If three channels are available, it is best to display leads aVF, V_2, and V_5.

   NOTE: For continuous monitoring (telemetry), any lead can be used; however, most coronary care units use a modified bipolar chest lead. The negative electrode is near the left shoulder and the positive is the traditional V_1. A third is placed at a more remote area of the chest and serves as a ground. However, of all leads, V_5 is the most sensitive for the diagnosis of ischemia. Ventricular arrhythmias are more ominous when ischemia is present (see Chapter 87, Ambulatory Electrocardiography: Holter and Event Monitoring). If a single channel is all that is available and ischemia is a concern, V_5 should be used.

7. Remove the electrodes from the patient, dispose of them, and clean the areas on the patient where the electrodes were attached. Modern adhesive electrodes are dry and leave very little residue.

INTERPRETATION

Although computer interpretive programs provide the noncardiologist with a quick and convenient second opinion, they do not provide advice on what to do with an abnormality. The following discussion is aimed at supplementing the available interpretive programs with a suggested course of management, including troubleshooting for errors.

Limb Lead Reversal

Limb lead reversal is the most common noticeable error involving the frontal leads. It usually occurs between the right and left arm electrodes, probably because these leads are usually grouped, bundled, or connected together. Lead reversal has become more common as inexperienced personnel replace ECG technicians. Fortunately, the right and left leg electrodes can be switched without affecting the recorded ECG. The clinician should consider arm lead reversal as a possibility whenever the computer interpretation is *marked right axis deviation*, especially if it is new compared with a previous tracing, or when precordial leads do not exhibit the normal R-wave progression. Also, the precordial leads and aVF will be normal, whereas limb lead I will be inverted. Normally, limb lead I somewhat matches V_6 in terms of morphology of the P-wave and QRS direction; this will not be the case with arm lead reversal. When every tracing from an ECG machine exhibits this pattern, the actual ECG leads may be mislabeled.

The second most common placement error is reversal of V_1 and V_3 (again, frequently in the same group or bundle of leads). This should be considered a possibility when R-wave amplitude does not increase from V_1 to V_3 and there is T-wave inversion in V_3.

Management includes repeating the ECG procedure after checking previous ECGs from the patient, checking the ECG machine, and verifying lead placement. If limb lead reversal is excluded and the finding is still not explained, check the precordial leads for normal R-wave progression. If the R waves do not progress normally, move the precordial leads to the patient's right side and record for the possibility of dextrocardia. If dextrocardia is confirmed, correlation with a chest radiograph is the next step.

Wolff-Parkinson-White

Wolff-Parkinson-White (WPW) is an ECG pattern characterized by a short PR interval followed by a delta wave and a prolonged QRS duration. The QRS duration may be longer than 120 milliseconds (msec), but it may also be shorter, depending on the degree of fusion of conduction. These characteristics are due to aberrant conduction of activation through an accessory pathway. WPW occurs in 1 of 10,000 individuals and can be entirely asymptomatic, or it can be associated with tachycardia and palpitations. When WPW is present, the ST segments cannot be used to identify ischemia. Q waves are actually negative delta waves and are not due to infarction. Individuals who are incidentally found to have this ECG finding are usually otherwise normal. However, they should be questioned about symptoms of palpitations or syncope. Also, a family history of syncope or sudden death could have significance. If either of these symptoms has occurred or the family history is positive, referral to an electrophysiology cardiologist is appropriate.

Right Atrial Abnormality (Not Present on Prior ECGs)

If the right atrial abnormality or P-pulmonale is new compared with previous ECGs, consider the clinical possibilities of a pulmonary embolus (e.g., tachycardia, pleuritic chest pain, cough, fever, hypoxia, presence of cancer, or immobilization) versus an exacerbation of lung disease.

Right Atrial Abnormality (Present on Prior ECGs)

If the right atrial abnormality is a consistent finding, examine the patient for chronic lung disease (e.g., prolonged expiration, hyperresonance, rhonchi and distant breath sounds, lowered diaphragms) and consider the overall history, including possible exposure to asbestos, coal dust, or cigarette smoke. Pulmonary function testing may be indicated.

Left Atrial Abnormality (Not Present on Prior ECGs)

If the left atrial abnormality or P-mitrale is new compared with previous tracings, consider the clinical possibilities of new congestive heart failure (CHF) or mitral valvular insufficiency. Mitral valvular insufficiency is confirmed by a holosystolic murmur radiating into the axilla and, if necessary, by echocardiography.

Left Atrial Abnormality (Present on Prior ECGs)

If the left atrial abnormality or P-mitrale is consistent compared with previous tracings, evaluate the ECG for additional LVH criteria. LVH plus left atrial abnormality can be an ominous marker for future events such as CHF, stroke, or death. Physical examination and an echocardiogram can confirm the findings.

Right Axis Deviation (Not Present on Prior ECGs)

When right axis deviation is a new finding, it can be due to an exacerbation of lung disease, a pulmonary embolus, or simply a tachycardia. If right axis deviation is a change from previous ECGs, question the patient for symptoms consistent with an exacerbation of lung disease or a pulmonary embolus. If the patient has findings consistent with embolus, a nuclear ventilation/perfusion ($\dot{V}/\dot{Q}$) scan or computed tomographic (CT) angiogram is usually indicated. If a $\dot{V}/\dot{Q}$ mismatch or thrombus is noted, anticoagulation is appropriate.

Right Axis Deviation (Present on Prior ECGs)

Chronic right axis deviation is normal in those younger than 21 years of age and in athletes. It can also be a chronic finding in patients with lung disease, right ventricular hypertrophy, an old lateral wall myocardial infarction, or a left posterior hemiblock.

Left Axis Deviation

Left axis deviation (LAD) is the most common "abnormality" in adults, occurring in over 8% of patients. It can be part of the criteria for LVH, but in isolation it has little significance. Marked LAD (45% or more) is called *left anterior hemiblock* or *left anterior fascicular block*. If LAD is present and the patient is not known to be hypertensive, it may be worth efforts to exclude the diagnosis of hypertension with frequent blood pressure checks or ambulatory blood pressure monitoring (see Chapter 84, Ambulatory Blood Pressure Monitoring). LAD can also be seen after an old inferior wall myocardial infarction.

Right Bundle Branch Block

Right bundle branch block (RBBB) can be normal (occurring without underlying disease) or due to trauma, increased right ventricular pressure, ischemia, or infarction. An incomplete RBBB has a QRS duration of less than 120 msec and an RSR′ pattern in V_1 and V_2 without an R wave greater than the amplitude of the S wave. It sometimes is simply called an *RSR′ pattern* and usually is a normal finding. Very rarely, it can be associated with an atrial septal defect. Incomplete RBBB or right ventricular conduction delay (RVCD) is not necessarily a precursor of RBBB or any conduction abnormality. Such atypical right ventricular conduction patterns are seen more frequently in people younger than 21 years of age and in athletes, and they can also be normal variants. Although wide splitting of the second heart sound is a very common finding among normal patients, fixed splitting of the second heart sound can also be associated with an atrial septal defect. Remember that the abnormalities of the second heart sound must be heard in the sitting position because splitting is often wide in normal individuals when supine. If present, an echocardiographic air contrast ("bubble") study is indicated. Any pulmonary disease process can be associated with RVCD, and RVCD can occur acutely with exacerbation of lung disease or a pulmonary embolus. Clinical correlation is necessary; either treatment of the lung disease or a $\dot{V}/\dot{Q}$ scan/CT angiogram might be indicated.

Left Bundle Branch Block

Left bundle branch block (LBBB) can result from severe trauma (car accident), ischemia, or infarction. It is often associated with LVH or left ventricular dilation. LBBB can also result from fibrosis of the conduction system. LBBB has a weak predictive power in a young, asymptomatic population (consistent with Bayes' rule), but is quite ominous in an older population as a marker for an increased risk of death, stroke, and CHF. Incomplete LBBB and the hemiblocks are usually not associated with cardiac disease. Clinical correlates, including the cardiac examination, should direct any further studies in response to a new LBBB. If the patient has an enlarged heart with signs or symptoms of CHF, an echocardiogram is usually indicated. If a patient with LBBB has prolonged ischemic-type chest pain, the patient is experiencing an ST-elevation myocardial infarction until proven otherwise. Percutaneous coronary intervention, or thrombolysis if percutaneous coronary intervention is not available, is indicated. If the patient is asymptomatic and clearly not having an acute myocardial infarction, unfortunately neither the resting nor the exercise ECG can be used as a diagnostic tool. Instead, a stress echocardiogram or a nuclear perfusion test is required.

Right Ventricular Hypertrophy

Right ventricular hypertrophy can be a normal finding in people younger than 21 years of age and in athletes. It can be associated with chronic obstructive pulmonary disease, primary and secondary pulmonary hypertension, some types of congenital heart disease, pulmonary embolus, and CHF. Clinical correlation is indicated. If the right ventricular hypertrophy is new compared with previous tracings, consider the clinical presentation for pulmonary embolus or exacerbation of lung disease. The patient may require hospitalization and treatment with heparin for pulmonary embolism, or bronchodilators, antibiotics, and steroids for chronic obstructive pulmonary disease. If the pulmonary disease ECG criterion is not a new finding, examine the patient for chronic lung disease (e.g., prolonged expiration, hyperresonance, rhonchi and distant breath sounds, lowered diaphragms) and consider the overall medical history, including possible exposure to asbestos, coal dust, or cigarette smoke. Pulmonary function testing as well as an echocardiogram may be indicated.

Left Ventricular Hypertrophy

Left ventricular hypertrophy requires clinical correlation, beginning with blood pressure measurement and physical examination for cardiac size and murmurs and morbid obesity. A complete medical history should be obtained with emphasis on symptoms of aortic valve disease (e.g., angina, syncope) and CHF. If CHF or aortic stenosis is suspected after the history or examination or there is an abnormal cardiac examination, an echocardiogram may be indicated. LVH is one of the most ominous ECG indicators of risk for future cardiovascular events in patients older than 30 years of age.

ST Segment Depression

Acute ST segment depression can be associated with ischemia, unstable angina/non–ST segment elevation myocardial infarction (acute coronary syndrome), electrolyte abnormalities, osmolality changes, hyperventilation, standing up, and certain drugs. An ECG should be obtained in any patient with chest pain of uncertain etiology because an acute ST shift can confirm that it is due to ischemia. ST segment depression may also be associated with subendocardial damage, as opposed to Q waves, which are usually associated with transmural damage from infarction. Although *chronic ST segment depression* is nonspecific as a marker for cardiac disease, it is associated with a poor outcome. It can be due to electrolyte abnormalities and drugs, particularly digoxin. The patient should be questioned about a past or present history of cardiac ischemic pain. Blood chemistries, including electrolytes, glucose, calcium, magnesium, blood urea nitrogen (BUN), and creatinine, should be obtained. All medications should be recorded carefully and any nonprescription drugs that the patient may be taking should be noted. Many nonprescription drugs, especially from other countries, contain diuretics and even digoxin.

Prolonged QT Interval

Diagnosis of prolonged QT interval is complicated by the inherent difficulty in identifying T-wave end and the inaccuracy of Bazett's formula when correcting for heart rate. It may be preferable to judge the QT interval prolonged when it changes in length or when it exceeds 50% of the R-R interval. QT prolongation can be due to multiple causes, but its importance is its association with premature ventricular contractions, ventricular tachycardia, and ventricular fibrillation; in other words, it is associated with vulnerability to a lethal arrhythmia. The following is a list of some of the conditions that can cause QT prolongation: hereditary syndromes (rare), electrolyte–metabolic abnormalities (hypokalemia, hypomagnesemia, or hypocalcemia), medications (e.g., type Ia antiarrhythmics such as quinidine; tricyclic antidepressants, antihistamines, anticholinergic drugs, antibiotics [e.g., macrolides], and antifungals), central nervous system disorders, systemic illnesses, and myocardial infarction. Obtain blood chemistries, including electrolytes, glucose, calcium, magnesium, BUN, and creatinine. Take a careful medication history, including noncardiac drugs such as decongestants, anti-GERD (gastroesophageal reflux disease) medications, and antibiotics. Ask specifically about any family history of syncope or sudden death.

Troubleshooting

- Arm lead reversal can result in false-negative or false-positive signs of ischemia.
- Older ECG machines use thermal-head printers that automatically adjust for tracing intensity. Some newer machines use laser printers that actually write the grid. They use regular paper rather than the more expensive, heat-sensitive grid papers. Extra paper, styluses, or printer cartridges should always be available.
- For a wandering baseline, there is either poor electrode contact or a bad cable, or the patient is slowly moving or breathing deeply. For older equipment, especially analog equipment, the machine may not be warmed up adequately.
- A jagged baseline is from wall current (AC) interference, a broken wire, improper grounding, or other electrical interference.
- For older equipment with heat-sensitive paper, if the baseline is too light or thin, the stylus is not hot enough. If the baseline is too thick, the stylus is too hot (refer to the operating manual). Improper stylus pressure is detected by using the standardization pulse. With proper pressure, the standardization pulse should produce a tracing with sharp corners. Rounded or exaggerated angles indicate improper pressure.
- Technicians and other medical personnel responsible for obtaining ECGs should have training and periodic retraining in skin preparation, lead placement, and patient positioning.

Complications

- Local skin irritation or allergic reaction to electrode placement or adhesive
- Patient distress over abnormal ECG
- Incorrect interpretation because of improper lead placement, ECG performance, or computer or clinician error
- Unnecessary diagnostic work-up or treatment (and the adverse events associated with these additional interventions) because of false-positive results, no prior ECG tracing with which to compare, an inadequate clinical correlation, or a normal ECG variant

Postprocedure Patient Education

For persistent symptoms, the patient should schedule a follow-up visit with his or her clinician, regardless of the ECG result. The patient should be given the results of the ECG, as well as instructions for medications, follow-up, or further work-up, as necessary. The clinician may wish to give the patient a copy of the ECG or ECG interpretation for his or her personal records.

Patient Education Guides

See patient education form available online at www.expertconsult.com.

CPT/Billing Codes

93000 Electrocardiogram, routine, with at least 12 leads; with interpretation and report
93005 Tracing only, without interpretation and report
93010 Interpretation and report only

NOTE: An ECG is usually needed to rule out a contraindication to exercise testing; however, Medicare will not reimburse for an ECG on the same day as an exercise test. For this and other reasons, it is usually better to bring the patient back on another day for an exercise test. Before every exercise test, another comparison ECG is performed; it is just not reimbursable by Medicare.

ICD-9-CM Diagnostic Codes

401.0 Hypertension, malignant
401.1 Hypertension, benign
405.01 Hypertension, renovascular, malignant
405.11 Hypertension, renovascular, benign
410.00 MI, acute, anterolateral
410.10 MI, acute, anterior, NOS
410.20 MI, acute, inferolateral
410.30 MI, acute, inferoposterior
410.40 MI, acute, other inferior wall, NOS
410.50 MI, acute, other lateral wall
410.60 MI, acute, true posterior
410.70 MI, acute, subendocardial
410.90 MI, acute, unspec.
412 MI, old
414.01 Coronary atherosclerosis, native coronary artery
414.8 Ischemic heart disease, chronic, other
414.9 Ischemic heart disease, chronic, unspec.
426.0 Atrioventricular block, third degree
426.3 Bundle branch block, left
426.4 Bundle branch block, right
426.11 Atrioventricular block, first degree
426.12 Atrioventricular block, Mobitz II
426.13 Atrioventricular block, Wenckebach's
426.82 Long QT syndrome
427.0 Tachycardia, paroxysmal SVT
427.31 Atrial fibrillation
427.32 Atrial flutter
427.41 Ventricular fibrillation
427.89 Sinus bradycardia, NOS
428.0 Heart failure, congestive, unspec.
428.20 Heart failure, systolic, unspec.
428.21 Heart failure, systolic, acute
428.22 Heart failure, systolic, chronic
428.30 Heart failure, diastolic, unspec.
428.32 Heart failure, diastolic, chronic
428.40 Heart failure, combined, unspec.
429.3 Cardiomegaly
440.9 Atherosclerosis, NOS (not heart/brain)
785.0 Tachycardia, NOS
785.1 Palpitations
786.50 Chest pain, unspec.

ACKNOWLEDGMENT

The editors wish to recognize the contributions by Mark Clasen, MD, PhD, Jerry Hizon, MD, and Victor Froelicher, MD, to this chapter in the previous two editions of this text.

SUPPLIERS

See Chapter 93, Exercise Electrocardiography (Stress) Testing, for a list of suppliers.

ONLINE RESOURCES

American Academy of Family Physicians: ICD-9 Coding Tools from FPM. Available at www.aafp.org/fpm/icd9.html.

American Heart Association. Available at www.americanheart.org.

Canadian Task Force on Preventive Health Care. Available at www.ctfphc.org.

Cardiology.org (Clinical Exercise Physiology Consortium). (Examples of ECG abnormalities and what to do about them.) Available at www.cardiology.org.

KG-EKG Press: (ECG interpretive aids.) Available at www.kg-ekgpress.com.

www.atforum.com/SiteRoot/pages/addiction_resources/QTDrugs%209-03-02.pdf.

BIBLIOGRAPHY

Ashley EA, Raxwal VK, Froelicher VF: The prevalence and prognostic significance of electrocardiographic abnormalities. Curr Probl Cardiol 25:1–72, 2000.

Fowler-Brown A, Pignone M, Pletcher M, et al: Exercise tolerance testing to screen for coronary artery disease: A systematic review for the technical support for the U.S. Preventive Services Task Force. Ann Intern Med 140:W9–W24, 2004. Also available online at www.ncbi.nlm.nih.gov/books/bv.fcgi?rid=hstat3.chapter.32532. Accessed July 15, 2008.

Friedland S, Sedehi D, Soetikno R: Colonoscopic polypectomy in anticoagulated patients. World J Gastroenterol 15:1973–1976, 2009.

Froelicher V, Quaglietti S: Handbook of Ambulatory Cardiology. Philadelphia, Lippincott-Raven, 1997.

Grauer K: 12-Lead ECGs: A "Pocket Brain" for Easy Interpretation, 2nd ed. Gainesville, Fla, KG EKG Press, 2007.

Grauer K: A Practical Guide to ECG Interpretation, 2nd ed. St Louis, Mosby, 1998.

Grundy SM, Bazzarre T, Cleeman J, et al: Prevention Conference V: Beyond secondary prevention: Identifying the high-risk patient for primary prevention: medical office assessment: Writing Group I. Circulation 101: E3–E11, 2000.

Kadish AH, Buxton AE, Kennedy HL, et al, American College of Cardiology/American Heart Association/American College of Physicians-American Society of Internal Medicine Task Force; International Society for Holter and Noninvasive Electrocardiology: ACC/AHA clinical competence statement on electrocardiography and ambulatory electrocardiography: A report of the ACC/AHA/ACP-ASIM task force on clinical competence (ACC/AHA Committee to develop a clinical competence statement on electrocardiography and ambulatory electrocardiography) endorsed by the International Society for Holter and noninvasive electrocardiology. J Am Coll Cardiol 38:2091–2100, 2001.

Kligfield P, Gettes LS, Bailey JJ, et al, American Heart Association Electrocardiography and Arrhythmias Committee, Council on Clinical Cardiology; American College of Cardiology Foundation; Heart Rhythm Society: Recommendations for the standardization and interpretation of the electrocardiogram: Part I: The electrocardiogram and its technology. A scientific statement from the American Heart Association Electrocardiography and Arrhythmias Committee, Council on Clinical Cardiology; the American College of Cardiology Foundation; and the Heart Rhythm Society endorsed by the International Society for Computerized Electrocardiology. J Am Coll Cardiol 49:1109–1127, 2007.

Mason JW, Hancock EW, Gettes LS, et al, American Heart Association Electrocardiography and Arrhythmias Committee, Council on Clinical Cardiology; American College of Cardiology Foundation; Heart Rhythm Society: Recommendations for the standardization and interpretation of the electrocardiogram: Part II: Electrocardiography diagnostic statement list. A scientific statement from the American Heart Association Electrocardiography and Arrhythmias Committee, Council on Clinical Cardiology; the American College of Cardiology Foundation; and the Heart Rhythm Society Endorsed by the International Society for Computerized Electrocardiology. J Am Coll Cardiol 49:1128–1135, 2007.

Schlant RC, Adolph RJ, DiMarco JP, et al: Guidelines for electrocardiography: A report of the American College of Cardiology/American Heart Association Task Force on Assessment of Diagnostic and Therapeutic Cardiovascular Procedures (Committee on Electrocardiography). J Am Coll Cardiol 19:473–481, 1992.

U.S. Preventive Services Task Force: Screening for coronary heart disease. Guide to Clinical Preventive Services. February 2004. Online. Available at www.ahrq.gov/clinic/uspstf/uspsacad.htm.

CHAPTER 90

ECHOCARDIOGRAPHY

Grant C. Fowler • Terry Reynolds

The prevalence of heart disease will continue to increase in the United States as the population ages. The amount of heart disease managed by primary care clinicians will also continue to increase. In many cases, both the management and the prognosis of heart disease are based on the amount of remaining viable myocardium. This is especially true for patients with congestive heart failure (CHF), cardiomyopathy, arrhythmias, and ischemic heart disease. One method of quantifying the remaining viable myocardium is to assess the ejection fraction. In fact, the most common reason echocardiography is currently performed in the United States is to determine the ejection fraction.

Many common symptoms, signs, or diagnoses of heart disease (e.g., palpitations, cardiomegaly on electrocardiogram [ECG] or chest x-ray, atrial fibrillation, CHF) are evaluated or managed based on data from echocardiography (Table 90-1). In certain situations, the more readily available the echocardiogram, the better the management. For example, acute chest pain is managed differently when echocardiography is immediately available. Even extracardiac causes for acute chest pain, some of which can be life threatening (e.g., pulmonary embolus, aortic dissection), can be diagnosed with echocardiography. If an acute myocardial infarction (MI) is diagnosed, risk stratification can be performed immediately. Complications from an acute MI can also often be diagnosed early.

Other common diagnoses that can be made or evaluated in the primary care clinician's office with echocardiography include mitral valve prolapse, dilated left atrium (important for patients with atrial fibrillation), left ventricular hypertrophy, transient ischemic attack, and ischemic heart disease. Whether in the clinician's office, the hospital, or the emergency department, a rapid diagnosis of pericardial tamponade or a pericardial effusion may be life-saving. Furthermore, if pericardiocentesis is needed, the risk of complications is significantly reduced if it is performed under ultrasonic guidance (see Chapter 214, Pericardiocentesis).

Improvements in image quality, portability, and affordability for real-time sonography have allowed it to become a valuable adjunct for the clinician in the office, in the hospital, or in the emergency department. Albeit not by much, the cost of echocardiography equipment has also decreased as the technology has expanded and improved. Consequently, echocardiography has seen some of the most rapid growth among procedures performed by primary care clinicians (see Chapter 94, Stress Echocardiography). For those clinicians with a large number of adult patients, two-dimensional (2D) and M-mode echocardiography may be a welcome addition to their practice. If the primary care clinician is uncomfortable performing echocardiography, contractors are available to provide sonographers. Over-reading services are also available (see the "Suppliers" section). This chapter predominately describes the performance of a 2D/M-mode echocardiogram with a brief summary of common findings. Since color and Doppler flow imaging are helpful for almost all echocardiograms, especially for those assessing the hemodynamic severity of an abnormality, they will also be discussed briefly. For a discussion of ultrasound principles and concepts, and for information regarding limited echocardiography, see Chapter 225, Emergency Department, Hospitalist, and Office Ultrasonography (Clinical Ultrasonography). Electromechanic dissociation, pericardial effusion, pericardial tamponade, and assessing intravascular volume status, right ventricular strain/dysfunction, and acute pulmonary hypertension (e.g., pulmonary embolism) are briefly discussed in that chapter. (Assessing for possible pulmonary hypertension is also discussed in the Interpretation section of this chapter.)

Two-dimensional echocardiography provides the clinician with cross-sectional, real-time images of various cardiac structures. Using 2D, cardiac chambers, walls, valves, and other structures can be observed as they move through the cardiac cycle. Freeze-framing and the use of calipers allow the clinician to measure certain structures, if needed, at various points during the cardiac cycle.

M-mode echocardiography produces graphic images in which time makes up the horizontal axis and the structures in motion being scanned compose the vertical axis. In other words, wherever the cursor is placed on the image, a linear beam of ultrasound is directed through the corresponding tissue and movement of the structures is graphically imaged over time. The resultant M-mode tracing can then be used to look at excursion and contraction patterns as well as to precisely measure distances from the various horizontal structures over time. Chamber dimensions, wall thicknesses, and valve excursions can be measured precisely throughout the cardiac cycle. From chamber dimensions, an ejection fraction can be estimated.

Doppler flow imaging is used to measure the velocity of blood flowing over certain structures. Using the Bernoulli equation, pressure gradients (e.g., across a valve) can also be determined. As with M-mode, time and the cardiac cycle are graphed along the horizontal axis while the vertical axis consists of blood velocity in meters per second. By convention, flow *toward* the transducer is depicted above the baseline and flow *away* from the transducer is depicted below the baseline. Pulsed wave (PW) technology and measurements utilize tiny, three-dimensional sample volumes to detect the exact location of any abnormalities. However, PW Doppler is limited when there is high-velocity flow. Continuous wave (CW) technology utilizes two crystals (one continuously emitting sound waves, the other continuously listening for echoes) and can measure high velocities (e.g., stenotic valves). However, it is of limited use for localizing abnormalities. As a result of these limitations, both PW and CW should be utilized with every valve. Color flow Doppler is a special adaptation of PW technology. It uses thousands of sampling volumes to produce a color image of velocities. By convention, flow *away* from the transducer is *blue* and flow *toward* the transducer is *red*. The intensity of the color increases with the velocity.

INDICATIONS

- Determine ejection fraction (most common indication)
- Acute chest pain
- Acute or old myocardial infarction
- Atrial fibrillation
- Cardioversion preparation

TABLE 90-1 Common Symptoms and Differential Diagnosis for Echocardiography

Reason for Echocardiography	Differential Diagnosis
Chest pain	Aortic dissection Coronary artery disease: acute myocardial infarction or angina Hypertrophic cardiomyopathy Pericarditis Pulmonary embolism Valvular stenosis
Heart failure	Dyspnea Hypotension Left ventricular diastolic dysfunction Left ventricular systolic dysfunction (global or segmental) Pericardial disease Right ventricular dysfunction Valvular heart disease
Palpitations	Congenital heart disease (e.g., atrial septal defect, Ebstein's anomaly) Left ventricular systolic dysfunction Mitral valve disease Pericarditis Structural cardiac disease
Murmur: systolic	Aortic stenosis, subaortic obstruction, hypertrophic obstructive cardiomyopathy Flow murmur (valve abnormality) Mitral regurgitation Pulmonic stenosis Tricuspid regurgitation Ventricular septal defect
Murmur: diastolic	Aortic regurgitation Mitral stenosis Pulmonic regurgitation Tricuspid stenosis
Cardiomegaly on chest x-ray	Dilated cardiomyopathy Pericardial effusion Specific chamber enlargement (e.g., left ventricle in chronic aortic regurgitation)
Systemic embolic event	Aortic valve disease Left atrial thrombus (only diagnostic if seen, otherwise transesophageal echo needed) Left ventricular systolic function and segmental wall motion abnormalities (aneurysms) Left ventricular thrombus Mitral valve disease Patent foramen ovale

Adapted from Otto CM: Textbook of Clinical Echocardiography, 2nd ed. Philadelphia, WB Saunders, 2000.

- Cardiomegaly on chest radiograph
- Congestive heart failure
- Dyspnea (possibly due to cardiac origin)
- Embolus (systemic or pulmonary)
- Hypotension (possibly due to cardiac origin)
- Hypertensive heart disease
- Ischemic heart disease
- Mitral valve prolapse
- Murmur
- Palpitations
- Pericardial effusion, electromechanical dissociation, or suspected pericardial tamponade
- Suspected cardiomyopathy
- Suspected infectious endocarditis
- Suspected left ventricular hypertrophy (e.g., LVH on ECG)
- Transient ischemic attack
- Valvular defect, stenosis, regurgitation, or insufficiency
- Ventricular arrhythmias (with suspected cardiac structural abnormality)

CONTRAINDICATIONS

- Patient too unstable or too uncooperative to be scanned
- Patient needs Doppler flow imaging or a color Doppler scan, and the equipment does not have this capability

PREPROCEDURE PATIENT PREPARATION

Indications for the study and possible findings should be explained to the patient. The patient should be prepared to change positions, if possible, while being scanned. The patient should be prepared for adequate gel and pressure from the transducer to be applied to the parasternal, apical, suprasternal, and, possibly, subxiphoid areas of the chest and abdominal walls. The patient should be gowned and in the supine or left lateral decubitus position.

EQUIPMENT

- For best images, an ultrasound machine with several probes of different frequency should be available. Among these probes, a low-frequency (e.g., 2.5 MHz) probe with 2D, M-mode, and cardiac Doppler capabilities is necessary. An ultrasound machine with harmonic imaging ensures high-quality images. A method of recording and storing the data (e.g., server, DVD, VCR) is also needed for documentation. For limited scans in emergency situations, a machine without Doppler capability can be used.
- Ultrasonic jelly (and towels to clean up after scanning).
- Patient gown.

TECHNIQUE

Two-Dimensional Echocardiography

Viewing the front of the chest, if the 12 o'clock position is considered cephalad and the 6 o'clock direction caudal, the axis of the heart is usually located in a line drawn between the 10 o'clock and the 4 o'clock positions. Placing the marker dot of the transducer at about the 10 o'clock position usually produces the long-axis view of the heart, especially if the probe is located parasternally. A line drawn between the patient's right shoulder and left hip also approximates the long axis of the heart. The long-axis view is essentially the longitudinal view of the heart, if described in the conventional terminology of ultrasound for the remainder of the body. Rotating the marker dot almost 90 degrees or perpendicular to the long axis, to the 2 o'clock position, produces the short-axis view of the heart. This is essentially a transverse view of the heart (Fig. 90-1). A line drawn between the left shoulder and the right hip also approximates this axis.

Because the patient is usually lying in the left lateral decubitus position while being scanned and the transducer is placed on the anterior chest wall (or abdominal wall for the subxiphoid view), the

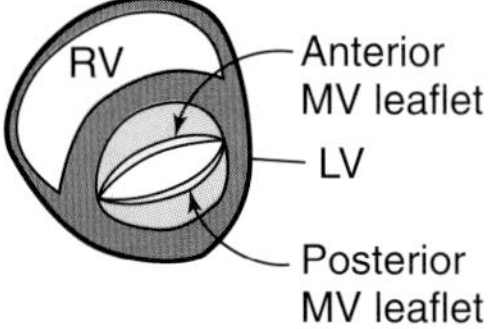

Figure 90-1 Parasternal short-axis view at the level of the mitral valve (MV). LV, left ventricle; RV, right ventricle. (From Reynolds T: The Echocardiographer's Pocket Reference, 2nd ed. Phoenix, School of Cardiac Ultrasound at Arizona Heart Institute, 2000.)

transducer edge will be noted at the top of the image. Posterior cardiac structures will be located at the bottom (inferior aspect) of the image. With the usual orientation, if the directional marker is noted on the right side of the image, objects to the right of the screen will correspond to objects near the marker dot on the transducer.

1. With the patient in the left lateral decubitus position, attempt to scan by first placing the transducer in the parasternal location (third to fourth intercostal space, next to the sternum) or the apical location (inferolateral to the left nipple at the point of palpated maximal cardiac impulse [PMI]). These same two traditional auscultatory points are used for a stethoscope. If the best window is found at the apical location, skip to step 12.
2. When scanning parasternally, the probe will be rotated so that the marker dot is either in the 10 o'clock (long-axis) or the 2 o'clock (short-axis) position. The short-axis view at the level of the mitral valve is often a good view for assessing the adequacy of the window, since the mitral valve is usually prominent and easily located (see Fig. 90-1).

   NOTE: Some ultrasound equipment places the marker dot 180 degrees away from this standard orientation (that is, the 4 o'clock position is what would typically be the 10 o'clock position). To determine the orientation of the probe, the directional marker on the image should be found. It corresponds with the marker dot on the probe and should be displayed on the right side of the display for cardiac imaging.
3. Small changes in patient position (e.g., rolling the patient further onto his or her left side) or working with the patient's breathing may improve the quality of the image. These adjustments cause the lingula of the lung to fall away from the heart, often providing a better window.
4. For unresponsive patients, those who cannot be moved, patients with chronic obstructive pulmonary disease, or other technical difficulties impairing the use of ultrasound in the parasternal position, the subxiphoid position will often provide a good window. Place the transducer directly below the xiphoid and angle it toward the patient's left shoulder with the marker dot toward the patient's left side. If this is the only location where an adequate window can be obtained, skip to step 16.
5. If a good window can be found at the parasternal short-axis view, rotate the transducer 90 degrees to the parasternal long-axis view (Fig. 90-2). With this view, observe the anterior and posterior leaflets of the mitral valve as it is scanned lengthwise. With prolapse, the leaflets will close beyond 90 degrees or cross the plane of the mitral annulus. True prolapse is often associated with thickened valves. Also with this view, the right ventricle is seen at the superior portion of the image, and the interventricular septum is noted as the inferior border of the right ventricle. Beneath the interventricular septum to the left of the image is the left ventricular chamber bordered by its posterior wall. Note that the ventricular walls thicken during systole, reducing the size of the ventricular cavity. Very little of the apex can be visualized with this view, because it is beyond the left side of the image. The left atrium is to the right side of the image, immediately inferior to the aortic root. The left atrial diameter should be about the same as the aortic root diameter. If either is markedly larger than the other or more than 4 cm in their anteroposterior diameter, they are considered dilated. The descending thoracic aorta is noted behind the left atrium. Rotate the transducer slightly clockwise if a better longitudinal view of the aorta is desired.

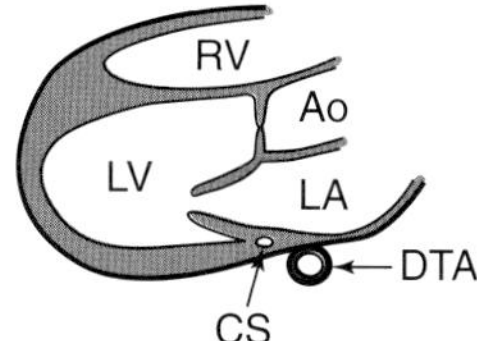

Figure 90-2 Parasternal long-axis view. Ao, aortic root; CS, coronary sinus; DTA, descending thoracic aorta; LA, left atrium; LV, left ventricle; RV, right ventricle. (From Reynolds T: The Echocardiographer's Pocket Reference, 2nd ed. Phoenix, School of Cardiac Ultrasound at Arizona Heart Institute, 2000.)

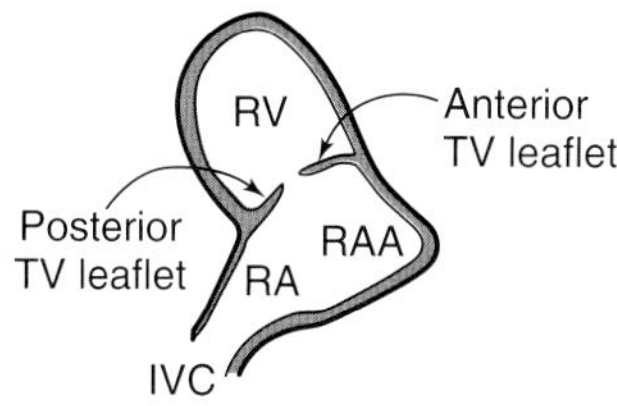

Figure 90-3 Parasternal long-axis view of the right ventricular inflow tract (RVIT view). IVC, inferior vena cava; RA, right atrium; RAA, right atrial appendage; RV, right ventricle, TV, tricuspid valve. (From Reynolds T: The Echocardiographer's Pocket Reference, 2nd ed. Phoenix, School of Cardiac Ultrasound at Arizona Heart Institute, 2000.)

6. To obtain the long-axis view of the right ventricular inflow tract (RVIT) view, from the parasternal long-axis view, tilt the transducer inferomedially or toward the right hip. This is a good view in which to study the tricuspid valve, right atrium, and the right ventricle (Fig. 90-3). The posterior and anterior tricuspid leaflets separate the right atrium from the right ventricle. In fact, this is about the only view where the posterior leaflet of the tricuspid valve can be seen. Liver tissue is usually noted adjacent to the diaphragmatic wall of the right ventricle.
7. After angling the probe back again to the parasternal long-axis view, rotate the transducer 90 degrees so that the marker dot is at the 2 o'clock position. This will produce the parasternal short-axis view again (see Fig. 90-1). Note the appearance in real time of the opening and closing mitral valve. Some have likened this image to that of a "fish mouth" opening and closing, especially if there is any stenosis. Without stenosis, the lateral and medial commissures of the valve are easy to distinguish. At this level, the ventricular wall can be divided into six segments, and the contractility of all of the segments should be observed (see step 10). In the normal heart, the segments should be contracting uniformly and symmetrically. The tricuspid valve may be seen above and to the left of the mitral valve.
8. Next, without actually moving or rotating the transducer, merely angle it more cephalad toward the base of the heart to observe the aortic valve (Fig. 90-4). In this transverse view of the aortic valve, it produces a characteristic "Y sign" when the leaflets are closed. If the valve itself is viewed as the face of a clock, the commissures are noted in the 2, 6, and 10 o'clock positions at the edges of the Y. When the valve is open in systole, it should produce a triangular shape. If it produces an oval shape with opening, the aortic valve is bicuspid. This is one of the most common abnormal findings on adult echocardiography, occurring in 1% to 2% of the population. If it is

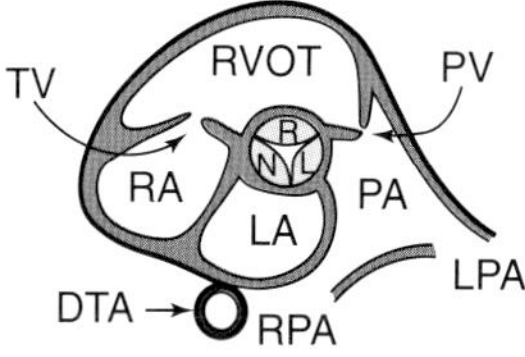

Figure 90-4 Parasternal short-axis view at the level of the aortic valve. DTA, descending thoracic aorta; L, left coronary cusp; LA, left atrium; LPA, left pulmonary artery; N, noncoronary cusp; PA, pulmonary artery; PV, pulmonary valve; R, right coronary cusp; RA, right atrium; RPA, right pulmonary artery; RVOT, right ventricular outflow tract; TV, tricuspid valve. (From Reynolds T: The Echocardiographer's Pocket Reference, 2nd ed. Phoenix, School of Cardiac Ultrasound at Arizona Heart Institute, 2000.)

found the patient should also be scanned for coarctation of the aorta, because 50% to 80% of those with aortic coarctation will have a bicuspid aortic valve (see the suprasternal notch view, step 21). At this level of the parasternal short-axis view, the right ventricular outflow tract (RVOT) can be seen curving above and around the aortic valve. The tricuspid valve is noted to the left of the aortic valve and the pulmonary valve is located superiorly and to the right. The right ventricle is located between the two. The right atrium is located in the inferior portion of the image to the left of the aortic valve. The left atrial appendage can often be seen to the far right of the aortic valve, and the left atrium is noted inferior or posterior to the aortic valve. Part of the atrial septum can be noted between the atria. The three cusps of the aortic valve are labeled the right, left, and noncoronary cusps. The right cusp is located next to the right ventricular outflow tract, the noncoronary cusp closest to the right atrium, and the left coronary cusp next to the left atrium. In a normal heart, the corresponding right and left coronary arteries originate from the same-labeled cusps.

9. Tilting the transducer yet more superiorly, beyond the aortic valve, the aortic root can be visualized in its short axis (transversely). At this level, on the right side of the image of the aortic root, the pulmonary artery can often be noted to bifurcate into the right and left pulmonary arteries.
10. Next, angle the probe back through the mitral valve, down to the level of the papillary muscles (Fig. 90-5). This level provides an excellent view for assessing left ventricular wall motion and the severity of left ventricular hypertrophy if it is present. At this level, the left ventricular wall can again be divided into six segments—the anterior, anteroseptal, anterolateral, inferolateral (posterolateral), inferoseptal (posteroseptal), and inferior (posterior) segments—which are all visualized. This same segmentation system can be used on the parasternal short-axis view at the level of the mitral valve. Each of the segments should contract in a uniform manner. With coronary artery disease, determining which wall becomes hypokinetic with ischemia may predict which coronary artery is obstructed (see "Findings and Interpretation" section). Usually two papillary muscles are visualized at this level, one located anterolaterally and the other posteromedially. At this level, only part of the right ventricle can usually be visualized, and it will be to the left of the image.
11. Next, slide the transducer slightly toward the apex and obtain a short-axis view of the ventricles at the apex (Fig. 90-6). By convention, the left ventricular wall is divided into only four segments (anterior, lateral, septal, and inferior [posterior]) at this level. In the normal heart, all four segments will contract uniformly.
12. By moving the transducer to the apex, which can be located by palpating the PMI inferolateral to the left nipple, the apical four-chamber view can be obtained (Fig. 90-7). At this position, the majority of scanning is usually performed with the marker dot at the 3 o'clock position. Angle the transducer back up toward the base of the heart to obtain the best possible four-chamber image. To confirm the orientation while scanning, note that the septal leaflet of the tricuspid valve is closer to the apex than the anterior leaflet of the mitral valve. By convention, the tricuspid valve and the right ventricle should be on the left side of the image. The right ventricle can usually be distinguished from the left ventricle because the right ventricle has the echogenic moderator band extending from the apex to the septal wall. Again, the right ventricular wall is more trabeculated than the left ventricular wall. With this view, again observe the ventricular wall motion for uniformity of contraction. From this transducer position, observe the valves again for abnormalities.
13. Tilt the transducer slightly anteriorly, toward the anterior chest wall (tail of transducer is tilted downward slightly), from the apical four-chamber view to obtain the apical five-chamber view (Fig. 90-8). This view provides an excellent image of the left ventricular outflow tract as well as an excellent view to exclude hypertrophic obstructive cardiomyopathy.
14. Return to the apical four-chamber view and rotate the transducer 90 degrees counterclockwise and tip it slightly laterally to obtain the apical two-chamber view (Fig. 90-9). The left ventricle and atrium will be visualized, separated by the mitral valve. With this image, the full length of the inferior wall of the left ventricle can be visualized. Observe this wall, along with the anterior wall of the left ventricle, for uniform contractility.

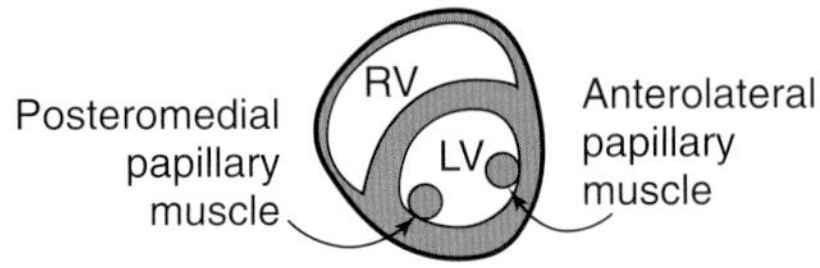

Figure 90-5 Parasternal short-axis view of the left ventricle at the level of the papillary muscles. LV, left ventricle; RV, right ventricle. (From Reynolds T: The Echocardiographer's Pocket Reference, 3rd ed. Phoenix, School of Cardiac Ultrasound at Arizona Heart Institute, 2007.)

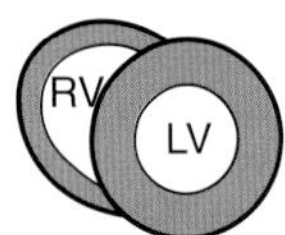

Figure 90-6 Parasternal short-axis view at the level of the apex. LV, left ventricle; RV, right ventricle. (From Reynolds T: The Echocardiographer's Pocket Reference, 2nd ed. Phoenix, School of Cardiac Ultrasound at Arizona Heart Institute, 2000.)

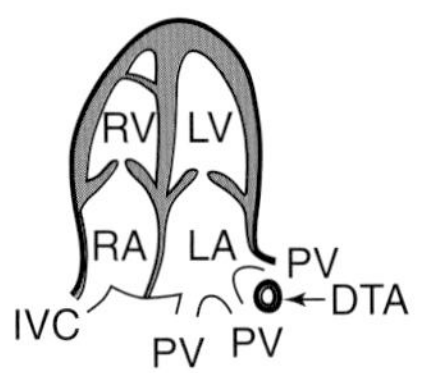

Figure 90-7 Apical four-chamber view. DTA, descending thoracic aorta; IVC, inferior vena cava; LA, left atrium; LV, left ventricle; PV, pulmonary vein; RA, right atrium; RV, right ventricle. (From Reynolds T: The Echocardiographer's Pocket Reference, 2nd ed. Phoenix, School of Cardiac Ultrasound at Arizona Heart Institute, 2000.)

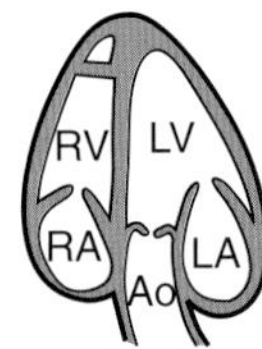

Figure 90-8 Apical five-chamber view. Ao, aortic root; LA, left atrium; LV, left ventricle; RA, right atrium; RV, right ventricle. (From Reynolds T: The Echocardiographer's Pocket Reference, 2nd ed. Phoenix, School of Cardiac Ultrasound at Arizona Heart Institute, 2000.)

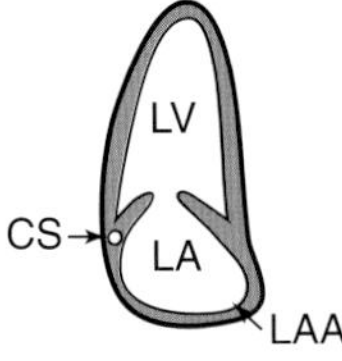

Figure 90-9 Apical two-chamber view. CS, coronary sinus; LA, left atrium; LAA, left atrial appendage; LV, left ventricle. (From Reynolds T: The Echocardiographer's Pocket Reference, 2nd ed. Phoenix, School of Cardiac Ultrasound at Arizona Heart Institute, 2000.)

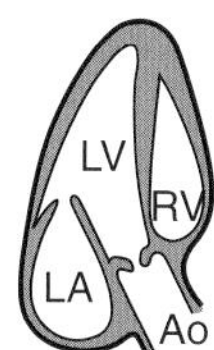

Figure 90-10 Apical long-axis view. Ao, aortic root; LA, left atrium; LV, left ventricle; RV, right ventricle. (From Reynolds T: The Echocardiographer's Pocket Reference, 2nd ed. Phoenix, School of Cardiac Ultrasound at Arizona Heart Institute, 2000.)

15. Rotate the transducer counterclockwise so that the sector plane passes through the long axis of the heart to obtain the apical long-axis view (Fig. 90-10). The aortic root can be evaluated, while the aortic valve is noted to be contiguous with the base of the anterior mitral leaflet. This view is very similar to the parasternal long-axis view, but the apex is visualized from this position. With this image, the anterior interventricular septum and the inferolateral ventricular wall can be inspected for uniform contractility.
16. Moving the transducer to below the xiphoid, the subxiphoid (subcostal) four-chamber view (Fig. 90-11) can be obtained with the marker dot to the patient's left side. Usually a portion of the liver is used as a window. The ventricles will be to the right side of the image and the atria to the left side. The left ventricle and atrium will be located behind (below) the right ventricle and atrium. Inspect both the mitral valve and the tricuspid valve, and observe wall motion for uniformity of contraction.
17. From the subxiphoid four-chamber view, by tilting the transducer anteriorly, visualize the aortic valve lengthwise. This will again provide an image similar to that seen with the parasternal long-axis view. This technique of imaging may be very valuable if the standard parasternal long-axis image cannot be obtained because of technical difficulties.
18. From the subxiphoid four-chamber view, it is also possible to angle the transducer to visualize the entire atrial septum. This position is the most reliable for evaluating patients for atrial septal defects and patent foramen ovale.
19. From the subxiphoid view, the inferior vena cava (IVC) can be imaged (Fig. 90-12) and its diameters measured. The diameter of the IVC can be used to estimate right atrial pressure (RAP). With the marker dot toward the patient's feet and the transducer located in the midline, the long-axis view of the IVC can be obtained by angling slightly to the patient's right side. Normally the IVC is less than 2 cm in diameter and collapses more than 50% with inspiration. It will also normally collapse with pressure from the transducer. If it does not collapse, the formula in the "Findings and Interpretation" section can be used to estimate RAP. The IVC is thin-walled compared with the aorta, and it may appear to pulsate as a result of pulsations transmitted through solid tissue from the aorta. When it collapses with inspiration, these pulsations will be minimized.
20. In addition to what has been described, almost all of the parasternal short-axis views can be obtained scanning from the subxiphoid position. However, because of the depth of tissue necessary to scan from this position, there is usually some loss of resolution. This is especially true when compared with scanning from the parasternal position.

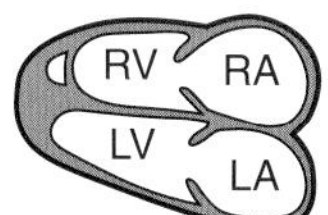

Figure 90-11 Subxiphoid four-chamber view. LA, left atrium; LV, left ventricle; RA, right atrium; RV, right ventricle. (From Reynolds T: The Echocardiographer's Pocket Reference, 2nd ed. Phoenix, School of Cardiac Ultrasound at Arizona Heart Institute, 2000.)

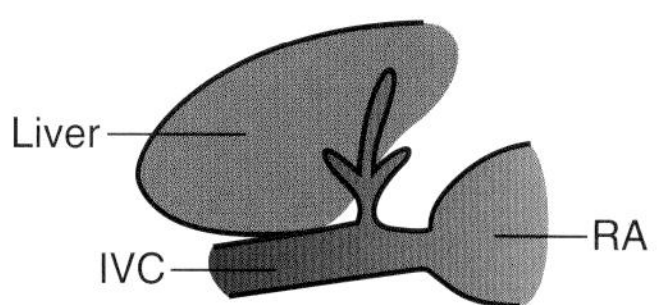

Figure 90-12 Subxiphoid long axis view of inferior vena cava. IVC, inferior vena cava; RA, right atrium. (From Reynolds T: The Echocardiographer's Pocket Reference, 2nd ed. Phoenix, School of Cardiac Ultrasound at Arizona Heart Institute, 2000.)

21. Placing the transducer in the suprasternal notch with the marker dot to the patient's left side, scan the aortic arch in its long axis (Fig. 90-13) to provide what some call the "candy cane" view. With this image, the ascending aorta, its horizontal arch, and the proximal descending thoracic aorta can often be visualized. The origins of the left subclavian and left carotid arteries off of the aorta can usually be visualized, and occasionally the origin of the brachiocephalic artery can be seen. The right pulmonary artery is usually noted in short-axis view beneath the arch. This is the best view for excluding coarctation of the aorta.
22. From the suprasternal view, by angling the transducer anteriorly and to the patient's right, the aortic root can often be visualized.
23. Further clockwise rotation can be used to obtain short-axis views from the suprasternal notch (Fig. 90-14). The right pulmonary artery can often be visualized in this manner. The right pulmonary artery is located between the aorta and the left atrium. It may be possible to visualize where the pulmonary veins drain into the left atrium.

NOTE: With the incidence of abdominal aortic aneurysm (AAA) increasing (5% to 7% of individuals over the age of 60), there is a strong correlation between individuals having an AAA and having an echocardiogram for other indications. With the patient already gowned and covered with jelly, it may be an excellent opportunity to screen for an AAA, even if no one is charged for the service.

M-Mode Echocardiography

From the parasternal position, with either the long-axis or the short-axis view, M-mode images are usually obtained at three different levels: the level of the aortic valve, the level of the mitral valve, and the level of the papillary muscles in the left ventricle (Fig. 90-15). The subxiphoid transducer position can also be used for M-mode scanning when there is difficulty obtaining the standard parasternal images.

1. At the mitral valve level, the anterior mitral leaflet makes an M-shaped pattern. The posterior leaflet moves as its mirror image to make a W-shaped pattern. The point of maximal early opening excursion is labeled E (Fig. 90-16). Next, the rapid filling phase

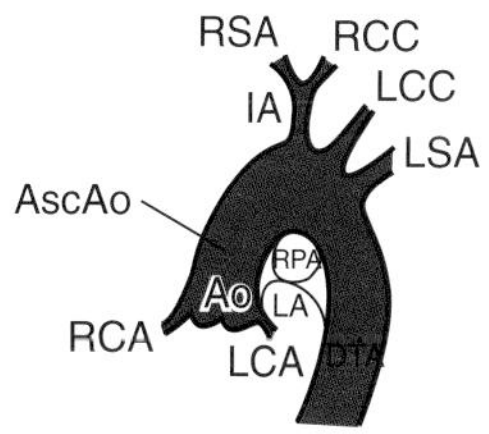

Figure 90-13 Suprasternal notch long-axis view of aortic arch. Ao, aortic root; AscAo, ascending aorta; DTA, descending thoracic aorta; IA, innominate artery; LA, left atrium; LCA, left coronary artery; LCC, left common carotid; LSA, left subclavian artery; RCA, right coronary artery; RCC, right common carotid; RPA, right pulmonary artery; RSA, right subclavian artery. (From Reynolds T: The Echocardiographer's Pocket Reference, 2nd ed. Phoenix, School of Cardiac Ultrasound at Arizona Heart Institute, 2000.)

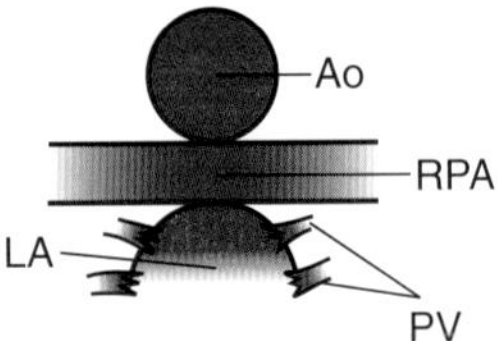

Figure 90-14 Suprasternal notch short-axis view of aortic arch. Ao, aortic root; LA, left atrium; PV, pulmonary veins; RPA, right pulmonary artery. (From Reynolds T: The Echocardiographer's Pocket Reference, 2nd ed. Phoenix, School of Cardiac Ultrasound at Arizona Heart Institute, 2000.)

of early diastole occurs, and then the valve closes partially. While it is closing partially, the valve moves along the E to F slope. Note that this slope will be flatter if there is any condition impairing left ventricular filling. The E to F slope is followed by the remainder of diastole. During this phase, the A point indicates atrial systole. After atrial systole, the valve moves to the fully closed position labeled C. The closed leaflets then move together in ventricular systole until they separate at the D point. The B point is labeled but does not exist for normal patients. It only occurs if the A to C line is interrupted due to elevated left end-diastolic pressure or diastolic dysfunction (see Fig. 90-16).

To determine the E to F slope, first draw diagonal Line 4 through Line 1 (i.e., basically a continuation of Line 1). Draw a horizontal line (Line 5) near the bottom of the tracing where Line 4 intersects one of the time lines on the tracing. Draw Line 5 horizontal to the left for a distance corresponding to exactly 1 second on the tracing. Next, draw a vertical line (Line 6) from Line 5 to where it intersects Line 4. Line 6 should be perpendicular to Line 5. The length of Line 6 in millimeters is the E to F slope of the anterior leaflet in mm/sec (normal range 70 to 150 mm/sec). The E-point septal separation (EPSS) is the vertical distance between the E-point and the septal wall. It is enlarged for dilated cardiomyopathy and suggests a reduced ejection fraction.

2. With M-mode imaging at the aortic valve level (Fig. 90-17), typically only two aortic cusps are identified. At the onset of systole, they separate abruptly; at the end of systole they close abruptly, producing a "square box" on the image. Because normal aortic valves are very thin and often difficult to follow throughout the M-mode tracing, if the cusps are easily visualized, they may in fact be thickened. Following closure of the valve, the cusps normally remain opposed (closed) throughout diastole.

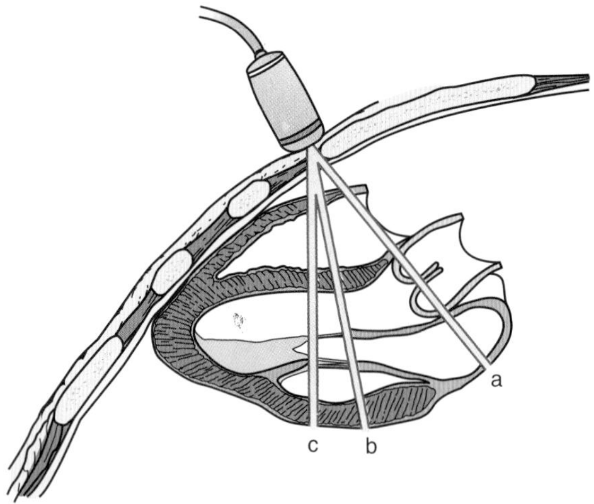

Figure 90-15 Levels to obtain M-mode images: Level of aortic valve (a); level of mitral valve (b); level of papillary muscle (c). (From Reynolds T: The Echocardiographer's Pocket Reference, 2nd ed. Phoenix, School of Cardiac Ultrasound at Arizona Heart Institute, 2000.)

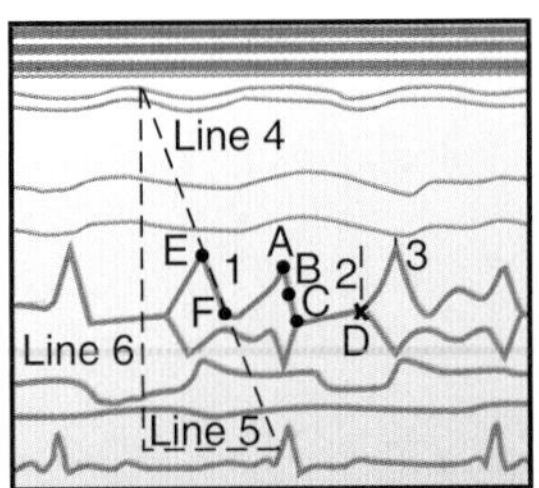

Figure 90-16 M-mode at the level of the mitral valve. E, E-point (point of anterior leaflet maximal early opening); line 1, MV E–F (mitral valve, E to F slope); line 2, MV EXC, vertical distance, mitral valve excursion (normal range 18 to 28 mm); line 3, EPSS (E-point septal separation [normal range 2 to 7 mm]); A, atrial systole; B, see text for explanation; C, valve fully closed; D, leaflets separate (valve opens). See text for explanation of lines 4, 5, and 6 and how to calculate E to F slope. (From Reynolds T: The Echocardiographer's Pocket Reference, 2nd ed. Phoenix, School of Cardiac Ultrasound at Arizona Heart Institute, 2000.)

The image at the level of the aortic valve is the most difficult to obtain with M-mode. Measurements of the left atrium, the aorta, and the valve cusp separation (opening diameter) are also taken at this level.

3. To obtain measurements of systolic time intervals, calipers can be used. The ejection time (LVET) is the time from the opening of the aortic valve until it closes. The pre-ejection period (PEP) is the time from the onset of the QRS to the onset of aortic valve opening (see Fig. 90-17).
4. Left ventricular measurements (e.g., systolic and diastolic dimensions) are best made slightly above the level of the papillary muscles, at the level of the chordae tendineae (Fig. 90-18). This is also an excellent view and level for obtaining right ventricular internal dimensions. Precise measurements of the thickness of all walls can also be made, in both diastole and systole.
5. For tricuspid valves, usually only one leaflet is traced with the M-mode for normal individuals. The RVIT view is an excellent view for tracing this single tricuspid leaflet. The pattern of motion for a single leaflet is similar to that of a mitral leaflet.
6. For pulmonary valve M-mode tracings, the parasternal short-axis view at the level of the aortic valve can be used. Once again, usually only one leaflet is traced for normal individuals. Because normal tricuspid cusps are very thin, it is often difficult to follow the leaflet motion throughout the cycle.

Color and Doppler Flow Echocardiography

Multiple views can be used for this application, but inevitably the apical four-chamber view provides the best view for evaluating three of the valves. The parasternal short-axis view is often utilized to complete the evaluation of the valves. As each valve is being studied, the transducer should be placed so that it is as close as

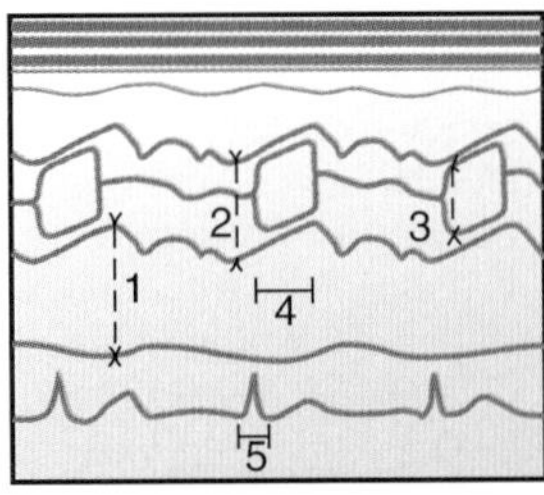

Figure 90-17 M-mode at the level of the aortic valve. 1, LA (left atrium end-systolic dimension; normal range 1.9 to 4 cm); 2, AoR (aortic root end-diastolic diameter; normal range 2 to 3.7 cm); 3, ACS (aortic cusps separation in systole; normal range 1.5 to 2.6 cm); 4, LVET (left ventricular ejection time); 5, PEP (pre-ejection period). (From Reynolds T: The Echocardiographer's Pocket Reference, 2nd ed. Phoenix, School of Cardiac Ultrasound at Arizona Heart Institute, 2000.)

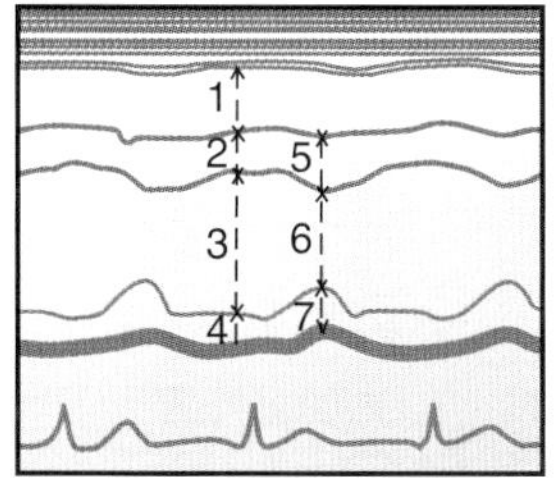

Figure 90-18 M-mode at the level of the mitral valve chordae tendineae. 1, RVIDd (right ventricular internal diameter in diastole); 2, IVSd (interventricular septal thickness in diastole); 3, LVIDd (left ventricular internal diameter, diastole); 4, LVPWd (left ventricular posterior wall thickness in diastole); 5, IVSs (interventricular septal thickness in systole); 6, LVIDs (left ventricular internal diameter, systole); 7, LVPWs (left ventricular posterior wall thickness in systole). (From Reynolds T: The Echocardiographer's Pocket Reference, 2nd ed. Phoenix, School of Cardiac Ultrasound at Arizona Heart Institute, 2000.)

possible to being in line with the maximal flow across the valve. Transducer positioning can be guided by the resultant 2D image, by obtaining the maximal velocity on graphic image, by maximizing the sound, or by all three. Each operator develops his or her own technique for performing a complete examination and he or she should follow this technique with every evaluation (Fig. 90-19). A sample technique is provided here.

1. From the apical position, evaluate the left ventricular inflow tract with PW. Next, evaluate the left ventricular outflow tract.
2. The right ventricular or tricuspid inflow tract should then be evaluated. Next, either continuing to use the apical four-chamber view or shifting to the parasternal short-axis view at the level above the aortic valve, the right ventricular/pulmonary outflow tract should be evaluated.
3. Repeat the evaluation with CW.
4. If available, repeat the evaluation with color Doppler.

Findings and Interpretation

Two-Dimensional and M-Mode Echocardiography

Overview of Study

The quality of every study should be described in the report (e.g., good, fair, poor). This determination often depends on the quality of the window, the equipment used, and the body habitus of the patient. Every report should also have at least a *qualitative* comment about the ejection fraction and segmental wall motion (e.g., normal, mildly impaired, moderately impaired, severely impaired). These parameters can also be measured *quantitatively*.

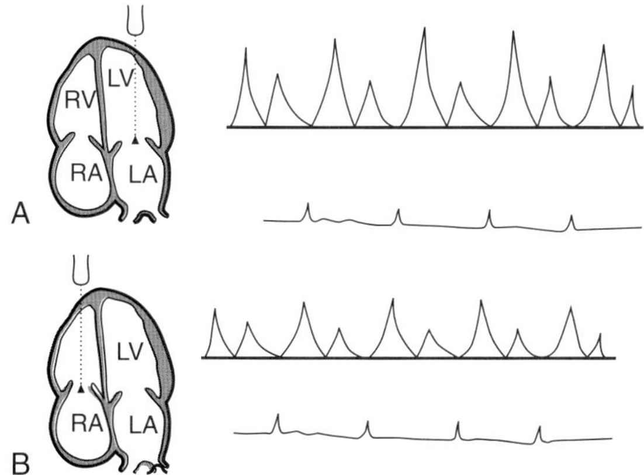

Figure 90-19 Normal Doppler tracings. **A,** Left ventricular inflow tract (mitral valve). **B,** Right ventricular inflow tract (tricuspid valve). LA, left atrium; LV, left ventricle; RA, right atrium; RV, right ventricle. (From Reynolds T: The Echocardiographer's Pocket Reference, 2nd ed. Phoenix, School of Cardiac Ultrasound at Arizona Heart Institute, 2000.)

EJECTION FRACTION. With 2D, the ejection fraction can be calculated by summing a series of discs, if the equipment software is capable of tracing the ventricular cavity. It can also be calculated using M-mode measurements applied to Table 90-2.

$$\text{Ejection fraction} = [(\text{EDV} - \text{ESV})/\text{EDV}] \times 100$$

End-diastolic volume (EDV) and end-systolic volume (ESV) are both obtained from Table 90-2 using the left ventricular internal diameter in diastole (LVIDd) and then the left ventricular internal diameter in systole (LVIDs) as the dimension in the table. LVIDs is measured at the lowest vertical point of the septum. (See Table 90-3 for normal ranges.)

NOTE: At the Arizona Heart Institute, M-mode echocardiography is no longer used for determining the ejection fraction. Instead, at the end of every 2D study, the ejection fraction is either quantitatively measured using calipers or cavity tracings or estimated as normal (60%), moderately impaired (40%), or severely impaired (20%). As it turns out, various studies have compared qualitative

TABLE 90-2 Ventricular Volumes for Calculating Ejection Fraction

Ventricular volumes (EDV and ESV) calculated from ventricular dimensions (LVIDd and LVIDs, respectively), using the formula of Teichholz:

$$\text{Volume} = \frac{7}{2.4 + D} \times D^3$$

Dim.	Vol.	Dim.	Vol.	Dim.	Vol.
2.0	13	4.0	70	7.0	254
2.1	14	4.1	74	7.1	265
2.2	16	4.2	79	7.2	272
2.3	18	4.3	83	7.3	280
2.4	20	4.4	88	7.4	288
2.5	22	4.5	92	7.5	300
2.6	25	4.6	97	7.6	307
2.7	27	4.7	103	7.7	315
2.8	30	4.8	107	7.8	327
2.9	31	4.9	113	7.9	336
3.0	35	5.0	118	8.0	343
3.1	38	5.1	123	8.1	356
3.2	41	5.2	129	8.2	364
3.3	44	5.3	135	8.3	372
3.4	47	5.4	142	8.4	385
3.5	51	5.5	148	8.5	393
3.6	55	5.6	155	8.6	407
3.7	59	5.7	159	8.7	415
3.8	62	5.8	166	8.8	429
3.9	66	5.9	174	8.9	439
		6.0	180		
		6.1	187		
		6.2	194		
		6.3	202		
		6.4	209		
		6.5	216		
		6.6	224		
		6.7	232		
		6.8	240		
		6.9	246		

EDV, end-diastolic volume; ESV, end-systolic volume; LVIDd, left ventricular internal diameter in diastole; LVIDs, left ventricular internal diameter in systole. From Teichholz LE, Cohen MV, Sonnenblick EH, Gorlin R: Study of left ventricular geometry and function by B-scan ultrasonography in patients with and without asynergy. N Engl J Med 291:1220, 1974.

TABLE 90-3 Normal M-Mode Measurements

	Mean	Range
Mitral Valve		
E–F slope	80 mm/sec	70–150 mm/sec
D–E excursion	20 mm	18–28 mm
EPSS	5 mm	2–7 mm
Aortic Root and Valve		
Root diameter	2.7 cm	2–3.7 cm
Root index	1.5 cm/m^2	1.2–2.2 cm/m^2
Valve systolic separation	1.9 cm	1.5–2.6 cm
Left Atrium		
LA diameter	2.9 cm	1.9–4 cm
LA index	1.6 cm/m^2	1.2–2.2 cm/m^2
LA/Ao ratio	1	0.87–1.11
Left Ventricle		
LVIDd	4.7 cm	3.7–5.6 cm
LVIDd index	2.6 cm/m^2	1.9–3.2 cm/m^2
LVIDs	3.1 cm	2–3.8 cm
LVIDs index	1.6 cm/m^2	1.3–1.9 cm/m^2
Interventricular Septum and Left Ventricular Posterior Wall		
IVS diastolic thickness	0.9 cm	0.6–1.1 cm
IVS excursion	0.7 cm	0.44–1.2 cm
LVPW diastolic thickness	0.9 cm	0.6–1.1 cm
LVPW excursion	1.2 cm	0.9–1.4 cm
Maximum velocity of LVPW excursion	61 mm/sec	40–78 mm/sec
IVS/LVPW ratio	$<1.3:1$	$<1.5:1$ hypertensive patient
Right Ventricle		
RVIDd (left lateral)	1.7 cm	0.9–2.6 cm
RVIDd index	0.9 cm/m^3	0.4–2.5 cm/m^2
RVIDs	1.8 cm	1.5–2.2 cm
RVIDs index	0.9 cm/m^2	0.7–1.1 cm/m^2
RV free wall excursion	0.9 cm	0.7–1 cm
RV free wall systolic thickening	50	30–38
RV velocity of systolic free wall excursion	41 mm/sec	36–55 mm/sec
RV wall thickness		0.5–0.8 cm
Pulmonary Valve		
"A" dip		2–7 mm
E–F slope		6–115 mm/sec
Left Ventricular Systolic Function		
IVS % thickening[a]	46%	27%–70%
LVPW % thickening[b]	45%	25%–80%
Fractional shortening[c]	33%	28%–41%
Ejection fraction[d]	62%	45%–90%
Mean circumferential fiber shortening[e]	1.2 circ/sec	1–1.9 circ/sec
Relative wall thickness[f]	37	30–45
Left Ventricular Mass		
American Society of Echocardiography 1.04 [(LVIDd + IVSd + LVPWd)^3 – (LVIDd^3)] 0.8 + 0.6 g		
Penn Convention 1.04 [(LVIDd + IVSd + LVPWd)^3 – (LVIDd^3)] – 13.6 g		

Ao, aortic root; EDV, end-diastolic volume; EPSS, E-point septal separation; ESV, end-systolic volume; IVS, interventricular septum; LA, left atrium; LVIDd, left ventricular internal diameter in diastole; LVIDs, left ventricular internal diameter in systole; LVPW, left ventricular posterior wall; RV, right ventricle; RVIDd, right ventricular internal diameter in diastole; RVIDs, right ventricular internal diameter in systole.

[a]IVS % thickening = [(IVSs – IVSd)/IVSd] × 100

[b]LVPW % thickening = [(LVPWs – LVPWd)/LVPWd] × 100

[c]Fractional shortening = [(LVIDd – LVIDs)/LVIDd] × 100

[d]Ejection fraction = [(EDV – ESV)/EDV] × 100

[e]Mean Vcf = (LVIDd – LVIDs)/(LVIDd × LVET)

[f]Relative wall thickness = 2 LVPWd/LVIDd or IVSd + LVPWd/LVIDd

From Reynolds T: The Echocardiographer's Pocket Reference, 2nd ed., Phoenix, School of Cardiac Ultrasound at Arizona Heart Institute, 2000.

estimates of ejection fraction with calculated ejection fractions, especially for those patients with suboptimal imaging. Qualitative estimates have been found to be fairly accurate.

SEGMENTAL WALL MOTION. The American Society of Echocardiography has established the convention of dividing the heart into 17 segments (Fig. 90-20). These segments are distributed across three levels. Anything above the level of the head of the papillary muscle, where it joins the mitral leaflet, is defined as the basal level of the heart. The mid-level of the heart is defined by the entire length of the papillary muscle. Anything below the level of the base of the papillary muscle, where it attaches to the ventricular wall, is designated the apical level.

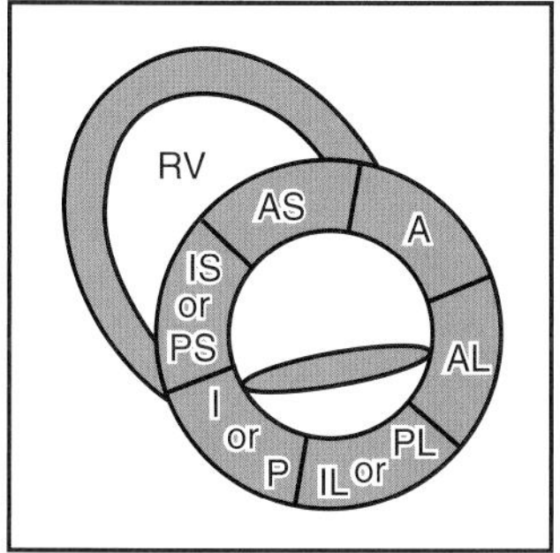

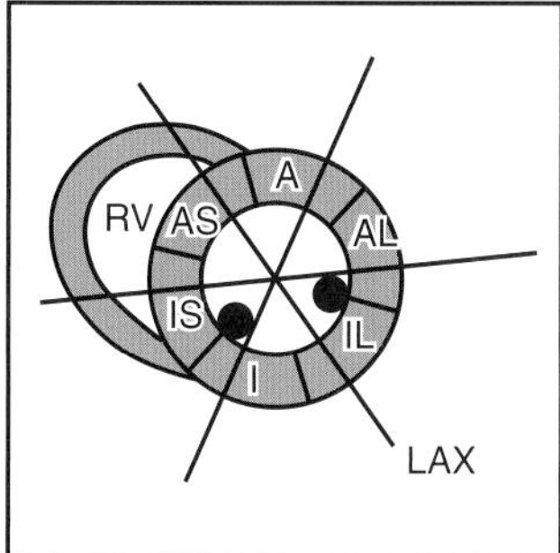

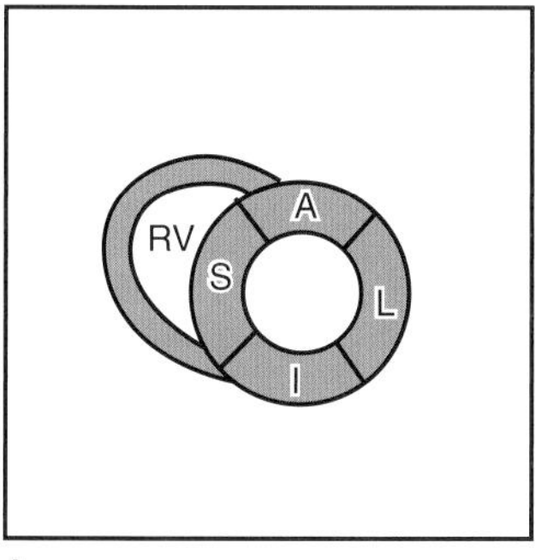

Figure 90-20 American Society of Echocardiography's 17-segment model of heart. A, anterior; AL, anterolateral; AS, anteroseptal; I, inferior; IL, inferolateral; IS, inferoseptal; L, lateral; LAX, long axis; P, posterior; PL, posterolateral; PS, posteroseptal; RV, right ventricle; S, septal. (From Reynolds T: The Echocardiographer's Pocket Reference, 2nd ed. Phoenix, School of Cardiac Ultrasound at Arizona Heart Institute, 2000.)

Each wall segment has a corresponding coronary artery that perfuses it. In general, the anterior and anteroseptal walls and the entire apex are supplied by the left anterior descending coronary artery (LAD). Therefore, even though the apex is divided into four segments—anterior, lateral, septal, and inferior (posterior) segments—all of these segments are usually perfused by the LAD. Both the mid-level of the heart and the basal level are divided into six segments. The inferior (posterior) wall and the inferoseptal (posteroseptal) walls at the basal and mid-levels are supplied by septal perforators (posterior descending artery [PDA]) from the dominant coronary artery on the inferior (posterior) surface of the heart. The lateral walls of the ventricle (anterolateral and inferolateral [posterolateral]) above the apex are supplied by the left circumflex artery.

Wall motion in each segment is scored based on the recommendations of the American Society of Echocardiography:

Normally contracting segment (or hyperkinetic segment) = 1
Hypokinesia = 2
Akinesis = 3
Dyskinesis = 4
Aneurysmal segment (i.e., deformed during diastole) = 5

The wall motion score index is derived from the sum of all scores divided by the number of segments visualized. A normally contracting left ventricle has a wall motion score index (WMSI) of 1 (i.e., each of the 17 segments receives a wall motion score of 1; thus, the total score is 17 and the WMSI is 17/17 = 1). Patients at increased risk for future cardiac events after an acute MI can be identified in part by a high WMSI (≥1.7).

Multiple views should be obtained with 2D echocardiography to compare the wall motion between various segments and to obtain the wall motion scores. Hypokinesis is defined as a less than 30% increase in wall thickening during systole and akinesis is defined as a less than 10% increase in thickening. Dyskinesis is present when the wall moves paradoxically outward when systolic thickening should be occurring. Comments should be made about wall motion, but more important, the walls should be scanned carefully for systolic thickening, which can be blunted by ischemia or infarction. Although wall motion scores may slightly overdiagnose the severity of an acute MI (e.g., severe ischemia can mimic an infarction), echocardiography is still much more accurate than an ECG. Of note, M-mode echocardiography has limited value when scanning for ischemia.

Acute Myocardial Infarction

In the setting of acute MI, 2D is very helpful because it provides immediate information, is noninvasive, and can be performed at the bedside. It can usually determine not only the location of the infarct, but also the extent of the infarct. Because 2D is noninvasive, serial scans can be performed to track progression. An abnormal wall motion score or evidence of a complication on 2D is valuable prognostic data. These patients should be triaged for aggressive therapy, as opposed to those patients who can be safely discharged early. In comparison, when using an ECG to determine risk (either high or low), the severity or the location of the lesion cannot be predicted by ECG changes. Although an ECG may be helpful for diagnosing the acuity of an infarct, 2D is usually much more helpful overall because it can be used to actually stratify the patient's risk.

Mechanical complications of an acute MI that can be diagnosed early with 2D include pericarditis, pericardial effusion, pericardial tamponade, electromechanical dissociation, ventricular aneurysm, acute ischemic cardiomyopathy, mural thrombus, rupture of a papillary muscle (posteromedial much more commonly than anterolateral), and rupture of the ventricular free wall or septum.

Atrial Fibrillation

A left atrial dimension of greater than 4.5 cm indicates an increased risk of developing atrial fibrillation as well as a high probability of unsuccessful cardioversion. For more than 20 years, left atrial dilation in conjunction with mitral stenosis and atrial fibrillation has been associated with an increased risk of peripheral embolism and stroke. Such a finding should be managed aggressively with anticoagulation (if not contraindicated).

NOTE: Atrial appendage thrombi are best excluded by transesophageal echo.

Cardiac Tumors

Cardiac tumors are seen as echogenic masses, and the majority (75% to 80%) of primary cardiac tumors are benign and curable. Thirty percent of benign tumors are myxomas, and they are usually attached by a stalk to the interatrial septum. They often partially or completely prolapse into the left ventricle during diastole.

Cardiac Tamponade and Pericardial Effusion

Cardiac tamponade and pericardial effusion (as well as electromechanical dissociation [EMD]) are discussed in Chapter 225, Emergency Department, Hospitalist, and Office Ultrasonography (Clinical Ultrasononography).

Cardiomyopathy

DILATED CARDIOMYOPATHY. Cardiomyopathy is defined as a primary disease of the myocardium and, by definition, is not due to ischemia or valvular disease. Dilated cardiomyopathy is by far the most common type of cardiomyopathy. It is characterized by dilation of all four chambers and reduced systolic function in both ventricles. Left ventricular dimensions (end-diastolic and end-systolic) and volumes are increased, whereas wall thicknesses are usually normal or slightly decreased. There will be a spherical configuration to the left ventricle with decreased left ventricular posterior wall and interventricular septal wall systolic thickening. As a result, there will be a decreased left ventricular ejection fraction. On M-mode, the left ventricular ejection time will be shortened with a resultant prolonged PEP/LVET ratio (>0.40). The distance of the anterior mitral leaflet from the septal wall (EPSS) is increased. The presence of a B-bump on the mitral valve tracing indicates increased left ventricular end-diastolic pressure (>15 mm Hg). There may be pulmonary hypertension, and for an ejection fraction less than 35%, an echogenic mural thrombus (in either ventricle) must be excluded. Mitral regurgitation is present to some degree in most patients with dilated cardiomyopathy.

HYPERTROPHIC CARDIOMYOPATHY. This form is much less common than dilated cardiomyopathy, and is an autosomal dominantly inherited disease with variable penetrance. The hypertrophy is usually asymmetrical and the interventricular septum is often involved (asymmetrical septal hypertrophy [ASH]). Less commonly, the left ventricular free wall or the apex can be asymmetrically involved. ASH can also be associated with obstruction of the left ventricular outflow tract, frequently as a result of the proximity of the anterior mitral leaflet to the septal wall (hypertrophic obstructive cardiomyopathy [HOCM]). Anterior motion of this leaflet during systole (systolic anterior motion [SAM]) can be noted on real-time or M-mode echocardiography to obstruct the outflow tract. Ventricular chambers are usually small. Most patients have mitral regurgitation as a result of SAM. On M-mode, midsystolic closure of the aortic valve can also be noted.

RESTRICTIVE (NONDILATED/NONHYPERTROPHIC) CARDIOMYOPATHY. This type is rare and is characterized by normal ventricular wall thicknesses and cavity size at initial presentation. The systolic function is normal and the heart failure is due to a stiff, hypertrophied ventricle with resultant impaired diastolic function. Biatrial enlargement is usually noted. The etiology is usually a fibrotic or infiltrative process such as hemochromatosis, sarcoidosis, or hypereosinophilic syndrome. As the disease progresses, the patient can develop a dilated cardiomyopathy. Although amyloid heart has a separate definition than fibrotic or restrictive, it can appear very similar on echocardiography. It is common to find an associated pericardial effusion with amyloid heart.

Ischemic Heart Disease

Ischemic heart disease is assessed by looking at (1) global ventricular function (quantified with an ejection fraction) and (2) segmental wall function. Both should be assessed because both ischemia and infarction can cause significant segmental wall dysfunction without markedly impacting the ejection fraction.

Left Ventricular Hypertrophy

A common cause of LVH is hypertensive heart disease, initially with concentric hypertrophy, increased left ventricular mass, impaired diastolic function, and normal systolic function. As LVH progresses toward end-stage heart disease, systolic dysfunction develops and the left ventricle dilates. The left atrium will eventually dilate because of decreased left ventricular compliance and possibly mitral regurgitation. (A left atrial dimension greater than 4.5 cm indicates an increased risk of developing atrial fibrillation.) Frequently, the aortic root will dilate and there will be associated aortic valve sclerosis. There may also be mitral annular calcification.

Concentric Hypertrophy

With concentric hypertrophy there is an equally distributed (uniform or globular) increase in ventricular wall thicknesses with normal ventricular dimensions (e.g., patients with valvular aortic stenosis or systemic hypertension). Left ventricular mass can be calculated to follow progression of LVH (see Table 90-3).

Eccentric Hypertrophy

Eccentric hypertrophy is commonly seen with aortic or mitral regurgitation. There is a spherical configuration to the left ventricle with normal wall thicknesses.

Mitral Valve Prolapse

In past years, MVP was overdiagnosed with echocardiography. As a result, a more formal definition was developed. Because the mitral valve, when closed, bulges normally or is "saddle-shaped" in the plane of the mitral annulus, true prolapse should be diagnosed only if a portion of the anterior leaflet prolapses beyond this plane. By new criteria, it must prolapse more than 2 mm beyond the mitral annular plane on the parasternal long-axis view or more than 1 cm on the apical four-chamber view. Posterior leaflet prolapse is diagnosed if any of the leaflet prolapses beyond the mitral annular plane in the parasternal long-axis view, the apical four-chamber view, or by more than 2 mm on the apical two-chamber view. The mitral annular plane is defined by drawing an imaginary line from the base of the anterior leaflet to the base of the posterior leaflet.

Myxomatous degeneration is the result of an increase in the middle layer of the valve, the spongiosa. With proliferation, the spongiosa replaces part of the fibrosa layer and the valve is weakened. Eventually, the valve becomes thickened, redundant, and elongated. In fact, it can develop the physical appearance of a hemorrhoid in its short-axis view. Myxomatous degeneration is usually diagnosed with 2D echocardiography; however, the thickness of the valve can be measured with either 2D or M-mode. The leaflets are considered redundant if they are 5 mm or more thick on the parasternal long-axis view during diastole, or more than 1.4 times the wall thickness of the posterior wall of the aorta during diastole. On M-mode, the thickness is considered abnormal if 5 mm or greater.

Preliminary 2D and M-Mode Scanning before Using Color and Doppler Flow

Diastolic function is best determined with color and Doppler flow imaging. As mentioned previously, color and Doppler flow imaging also assist with determining the hemodynamic severity of lesions and are therefore helpful for assessing valvular abnormalities. Color-flow Doppler also produces jets that are characteristic for certain abnormalities. Eccentric jets are very helpful for aligning CW Doppler when attempting to optimize the spectrum. Such spectrum analysis is helpful for further quantifying regurgitant lesions.

NOTE: When assessing tricuspid valve regurgitation (TR) with color and Doppler flow imaging, note that TR is very common (90% of population). As a result, the regurgitation itself does not always need to be assessed. More importantly, the severity of the tricuspid regurgitation can be used to determine right-sided ventricular pressures. Pulmonary valve regurgitation is less common than TR, and mitral regurgitation is much less common. Aortic valve regurgitation is somewhat rare and its presence is always considered pathologic.

Despite the fact that the following disorders are best scanned with color and Doppler flow imaging, some information is usually obtained during preliminary 2D/M-mode scanning before using Doppler. This preliminary scanning is usually being performed while 2D/M-mode measurements are being taken (see Table 90-4 for normal values).

TABLE 90-4 Normal Echo Measurements by TTE

Structure	Measurement by TTE
Normal values of the right heart chambers	
RV anteroposterior, diastole (cm)	2.5–3.8
RV anteroposterior, systole (cm)	2–3.4
RV mediolateral, diastole (cm)	2.1–4.2
RV mediolateral, systole (cm)	1.9–3.1
RV area, diastole (cm^2)	11–36
RV area, systole (cm^2)	5–20
RV ejection fraction (%)	>40
RV free-wall thickness (mm)	2–5
RV outflow tract, systole (cm)	1.8–3.4
RA anteroposterior, systole (cm)	—
RA mediolateral, systole (cm)	2.9–4.6
RA volume (mL)	15–58 in men, 14–44 in women
RA area (cm^2)	8.3–19.5
Normal measurements of the left heart valves and great vessels	
Mitral valve area (cm^2)	4–6
Mitral annulus, diastole (cm)	2–3.4
Mitral leaflets thickness (mm)	4
Mitral regurgitation (overall %)	38–45
Pulmonary veins (mm)	8–15
Aortic valve area (cm^2)	3–5
Aortic annulus, systole (cm)	1.4–2.6
Aortic regurgitation (overall %)	0–2
Aortic root sinuses, diastole (cm)	2.1–3.5
Aortic root tubule, diastole (cm)	1.7–3.4
Aortic arch (cm)	2–3.6
Descending aorta (cm)	
Normal measurements of the right heart valves and great vessels	
Tricuspid valve area (cm^2)	4–6
Tricuspid annulus, diastole (cm)	2–4
Tricuspid leaflet thickness (cm)	4
Tricuspid regurgitation (overall %)	15–78
Superior vena cava (cm)	—
Proximal inferior vena cava (cm)	1.2–2.3
Hepatic vein (cm)	0.5–1.1
Coronary sinus (cm)	—
Pulmonic valve area (cm^2)	3–5
Pulmonic valve annulus (cm)	1–2.2
Pulmonic regurgitation (overall %)	28–88
Right ventricular outflow tract, systole	1.8–3.4
Main pulmonary artery	1–2.9
Right or left pulmonary artery	0.7–1.7
Normal values of the left heart chambers	
LV anteroposterior, diastole (cm)	3.5–5.7
LV anteroposterior, systole (cm)	2.5–4.3
LV mediolateral, diastole (cm)	3.7–5.6
LV mediolateral, systole (cm)	2.5–4.8
LV volume, diastole (mL)	59–157
LV volume, systole (mL)	16–68
LV area, diastole (cm^2)	18–47
LV area, systole (cm^2)	8–32
LV fractional shortening (%)	30–35
LV ejection fraction (%)	55
LV interventricular septal thickness, diastole (cm)	0.6–1.1
LV posterior wall thickness, diastole (cm)	0.6–1
LV mass (g)	<294 in men, <198 in women
LV outflow tract, systole (cm)	1.8–3.4
LA anteroposterior, systole (cm)	2.2–4.1
LA mediolateral, systole (cm)	2.5–4.5
LA volume (mL)	20–77 in men, 15–59 in women
LA area (cm^2)	9–23
LA appendage length (cm)	—
LA appendage diameter (cm)	—

LA, left atrial; LV, left ventricular; RA, right atrial; RV, right ventricular; TTE, transthoracic echocardiography.

From Reynolds T: The Echocardiographer's Pocket Reference, 2nd ed. Phoenix, School of Cardiac Ultrasound at Arizona Heart Institute, 2000.

Aortic Stenosis

Aortic stenosis (AS) is usually the result of a degenerative process, rheumatic heart disease, or a bicuspid valve. With *degenerative/rheumatic aortic stenosis*, the aortic cusps are usually thickened and there is associated concentric left ventricular hypertrophy, a dilated aortic root, a dilated left atrium, mitral annular calcification (50%), and a decreased mitral valve E–F slope.

As discussed earlier, the most common abnormality in adult echocardiography is a bicuspid aortic valve. With AS resulting from a *bicuspid valve*, thickened leaflets are often noted as well as the characteristic oval shape to the valve opening. All of the findings of rheumatic/degenerative AS are also seen, except for the mitral annular calcification.

Aortic Regurgitation

With aortic regurgitation, all of the findings of bicuspid aortic stenosis can be seen, except that the aortic root may not be dilated. Additional findings include premature closure of the mitral valve and premature opening of the aortic valve. Ventricular hypertrophy may be noted, either the eccentric or the globular type. There may also be an anatomic reason for the regurgitation (e.g., ascending aortic aneurysm, bicuspid aortic valve, valvular vegetation).

Mitral Stenosis

Mitral stenosis causes a decreased E–F slope and a decreased A wave on the M-mode tracing. The mitral leaflets may be thickened or they may be noted to have decreased mobility. In addition, the mitral valve opening orifice may be decreased, giving it the appearance of a "fish mouth" on 2D. The clinician should attempt to determine the degree of commissural and subvalvular involvement with the stenosis and scan for calcification of either the valve or the annulus. Possible associated findings include atrial dilation, a steep A–C slope, pulmonary hypertension, and an atrial septal defect. If the atrium is dilated, the clinician should scan for the presence of an echogenic thrombus. There may be right ventricular hypertrophy or dilation and evidence of right-sided volume overload. Clinicians should also scan for involvement of other valves. Doppler is needed to determine the orifice opening diameter when the leaflets are densely calcified, when there is an inadequate parasternal short-axis image, when there has been a surgical commissurotomy, or when there is extensive subvalvular involvement (e.g., a secondary orifice located below the valve).

Mitral Regurgitation

With mitral regurgitation, there is usually echocardiographic evidence of left atrial and left ventricular volume overload patterns, as well as an associated right-sided overload pattern. Pulmonary hypertension may be noted. LVH may be present, and serial scans may be needed to monitor the progression of LVH. In addition, the mitral annulus may be dilated (normal 2.3 ± 0.5 cm) on the apical four-chamber view. There may be an anatomic basis for the regurgitation: myxomatous degeneration of the valve with subsequent prolapse is the leading cause for regurgitation in the United States, but flail leaflets, annular calcification, or LV dysfunction (e.g., from ischemia) can be noted. The clinician should scan carefully to exclude flail leaflets.

Pulmonary Hypertension

With pulmonary hypertension, RAP will be elevated. The dimensions of the IVC can be used to estimate RAP (Table 90-5).

With pulmonary hypertension, there will also usually be evidence of right ventricular hypertrophy (>5 mm thickness), especially if it is chronic. This hypertrophy may cause impingement on the left ventricle, resulting in a D-shaped left ventricle. The right atria and pulmonary artery may also be dilated. The interatrial septum may be deviated toward the left atrium.

TABLE 90-5 Estimating Right Atrial Pressure

	RAP (mm Hg)
With pulmonary hypertension, RAP will be elevated. The dimensions of the IVC can be used to estimate RAP.	
IVC <2 cm diameter and collapses >50% with inspiration	5
IVC <2 cm diameter and collapses <50% with inspiration	10
IVC >2 cm diameter and collapses <50% with inspiration	15
IVC >2 cm diameter and does not collapse with inspiration	20

IVC, inferior vena cava; RAP, right atrial pressure.

On M-mode, mitral valve disease may be diagnosed. Paradoxic septal motion as well as an increased septal wall thickness may be noted. There will also be abnormalities of the pulmonary valve cusp motion.

Tricuspid Regurgitation

With TR, there is usually evidence of a right ventricular volume overload pattern, including right atrial dilation. A "B-bump" of the anterior tricuspid leaflet is often noted on M-mode. The tricuspid valve annulus may be dilated (3.4 cm diameter in systole, ≥3.2 cm in diastole). There may be signs of pulmonary hypertension. For regurgitation, there may be an anatomic etiology (e.g., valvular vegetation, ruptured chordae tendineae).

Tricuspid Stenosis

With tricuspid stenosis, thickened valve leaflets may be noted. The right atrium is usually dilated as well as the IVC (normal 1.2 to 2.3 cm) on M-mode. There will be decreased tricuspid valve excursion (D–E) and a decreased or absent A wave of the anterior leaflet.

Color and Doppler Flow Imaging

A complete listing of all of the possible findings and interpretation with color and Doppler flow imaging is beyond the scope of this book. However, there are some rules of thumb:

- Any velocity greater than 2 m/sec in the heart must be explained. Something as simple as a hyperdynamic heart from anemia can cause it; however, pathologic causes should be excluded.
- The Bernoulli equation can be used to determine pressure drops across values:

$$\Delta P\ (\text{mm Hg}) = 4 \times [\text{velocity}\ (\text{m/sec})]^2$$

- An approximation for right ventricular systolic pressure (RVSP) is

$$\text{RVSP}\ (\text{mm Hg}) = 4\ \Delta\ \text{P}\ [\text{tricuspid valve}\ (\text{mm Hg})] + 10\ \text{mm Hg}$$

  The actual method of calculating RSVP is

$$\text{RSVP}\ (\text{mm Hg}) = 4 \times (\text{TR peak velocity})^2 + \text{RAP}$$

  See the "Pulmonary Hypertension" section for estimation of RAP; for most patients, RAP can be approximated at 10 mm Hg.

- Normal aortic and pulmonary valves produce a "bullet-shaped" pattern on spectral analysis. Normal mitral and tricuspid valves produce an "M-shaped" pattern on spectral analysis.
- Laminar flow produces linear spectral analyses, but turbulent flow fills in the area under the curve. Regurgitant flow is always turbulent.
- With color Doppler, a green hue indicates turbulent flow. Highly turbulent flow is mosaic in appearance.

Complications

- Failure to provide an adequate scan
- Failure to diagnose
- Clinical deterioration while scanning in the acute setting

CPT/Billing Codes

93307 Echocardiography, transthoracic, real-time with image documentation (2D), includes M-mode recording, complete, without spectral or color Doppler echocardiography
93308 Follow-up or limited study
93320 Doppler echocardiography, pulsed wave and/or continuous wave with spectral display (list separately in addition to codes for echocardiographic imaging); complete
93321 Follow-up or limited study

ICD-9-CM Diagnostic Codes

214.2 Myxolipoma, intrathoracic organs
394.0 Mitral stenosis, rheumatic
394.2 Mitral stenosis with insufficiency, rheumatic
402.10 Hypertensive heart disease or hypertensive LVH, benign, without CHF
402.11 Hypertensive heart disease, benign, with CHF
410.00 Acute myocardial infarction, of anterolateral wall, episode of care unspecified
410.20 Acute myocardial infarction, of inferolateral wall, episode of care unspecified
410.90 Myocardial infarction, acute, unspecified site and episode
412 Old myocardial infarction
414.00 Coronary atherosclerosis, of unspecified type of vessel, native or graft
414.01 Coronary atherosclerosis, of native coronary artery
414.9 Ischemic heart disease, chronic
414.10 Aneurysm of heart wall
415.11 Iatrogenic pulmonary embolism and infarction
416.0 Pulmonary hypertension, primary, chronic
416.8 Pulmonary hypertension, secondary, chronic
420 Pericardial effusion, acute
420.91 Pericarditis, acute, idiopathic
420.99 Pericarditis, acute, purulent
422.90 Myocarditis, acute
423.0 Hemopericardium
423.3 Cardiac tamponade
423.9 Pericardial effusion, unspecified disease of pericardium
424.0 Mitral valve disorders, nonrheumatic (incompetence, insufficiency, regurgitation, prolapse)
424.1 Aortic valve disorders (incompetence, insufficiency, regurgitation, stenosis)
425.4 Cardiomyopathy, congestive, constrictive, familial, hypertrophic, idiopathic, restrictive, obstructive, nonobstructive, NOS)
425.5 Cardiomyopathy, alcoholic
426.3 Left bundle branch block, complete or NOS
426.4 Right bundle branch block
427.5 Cardiac arrest
427.31 Atrial fibrillation
428.0 Congestive heart failure
428.1 Congestive heart failure, left, acute
428.4 Combined systolic and diastolic heart failure
428.21 Systolic heart failure, acute
428.22 Systolic heart failure, chronic
428.31 Diastolic heart failure, acute
429.1 Cardiomyopathy, arteriosclerotic
429.3 Cardiomegaly
429.79 Mural thrombus (atrial, ventricular) acquired following myocardial infarction
434.1 Cerebral embolism
435.8 Cerebral ischemia, transient
435.9 Transient ischemic attack
441.01 Aortic dissection, thoracic
785.1 Palpitations
786.50 Chest pain, unspecified

SUPPLIERS

There are several manufacturers with products ranging from the basic to the very sophisticated. Small hand-held machines are now available. Acuson Siemens, Biosound Esaote, General Electric Healthcare, Medison, Phillips, and Toshiba all offer a range of devices from hand-held to research oriented (see the "Suppliers" section in Chapter 172, Obstetric Ultrasounography, for the Internet and mailing addresses as well as the phone numbers for many manufacturers). An excellent way to review the equipment is to visit the company websites. Used equipment is also available, but the cost and inconvenience of service and repairs are often a disadvantage. Over-reading services are also available.

ONLINE RESOURCES

Arizona Heart Institute, School of Cardiac Ultrasound (CME and DVDs on echocardiography): www.azheart.com/scripts/forceframe.pl? and www.azheart.com/proed/ultrasound/index.asp. Accessed April 1, 2010.

Mayo Clinic (CME and DVDs on echocardiography): cmestore.mayo.edu/index.php. Accessed April 1, 2010.

BIBLIOGRAPHY

ACC/AHA: Clinical competence statement on echocardiography. Circulation 107:1068–1089, 2003. Also available online at http://circ.ahajournals.org/cgi/reprint/107/7/1068. Accessed March 28, 2010.

ACC/AHA/ASE: Guideline update for the clinical application of echocardiography: Summary article: A report of the American College of Cardiology/American Heart Association Task Force on Practice Guidelines (ACC/AHA/ASE Committee to Update the 1997 Guidelines for the Clinical Application of Echocardiography). Circulation 108:1146–1162, 2003.

ACCF/ASE/ACEP/ASNC/SCAI/SCCT/SCMR: Appropriateness criteria for transthoracic and transesophageal echocardiography. J Am Coll Cardiol 50:187–204, 2007. Also available online at http://content.onlinejacc.org/cgi/content/full/j.jacc.2007.05.003v1. Accessed August 4, 2010.

Armstrong WF, Ryan T: Feigenbaum's Echocardiography, 7th ed. Philadephia, Lippincott, Williams & Wilkins, 2009.

Otto CM: Textbook of Clinical Echocardiography, 4th ed. Philadephia, Saunders, 2009.

Reynolds T: The Echocardiographer's Pocket Reference, 3rd ed. Phoenix, School of Cardiac Ultrasound at Arizona Heart Institute, 2007.

CHAPTER 91

Pulmonary Function Testing

Michael A. Altman

Pulmonary function testing (PFT) is an important tool used by clinicians to evaluate individuals for lung disease. The parameters commonly measured include lung volume, airflow (timed volume), and airway reactivity. As it turns out, clinicians cannot reliably identify obstructive or restrictive patterns from history taking and physical examination alone. In one study, when clinicians were asked to predict the results of PFTs, they correctly predicted an obstructive pattern 83% of the time. However, when predicting a normal or restrictive pattern, they were correct only about half of the time. Besides identifying abnormalities, PFTs allow the severity of an abnormality to be quantified and the amount of reversibility to be determined. This ability to quantify abnormalities also allows a clinician to follow treatment in an objective manner.

A spirogram is a recording of exhaled and inhaled volume (liters) over time (seconds). Spirometric examination is the most widely used tool to assess pulmonary function in office practice. It can be used to evaluate patients suspected of having disease on the basis of clinical findings or to monitor changes in a patient over time. Although formal PFTs are more comprehensive and, if necessary, can provide an objective measure of impairment, spirometry is sufficient most of the time.

In fact, spirometry is underused. Such examinations should be readily available in most medical offices. The National Asthma Education Program (NAEP) recommends an objective measurement of lung function (either spirometry or PFTs) whenever diagnosing or managing asthma. There is evidence that both patients and clinicians have inaccurate perceptions of the severity of asthma in the absence of PFTs, thereby increasing the risk of mortality. The American Thoracic Society (ATS), the European Respiratory Society (ERS), and the Global Initiative for Chronic Obstructive Lung Disease (GOLD) have published guidelines urging the use of spirometry to correctly diagnose chronic obstructive pulmonary disease (COPD). Even the National Committee for Quality Assurance (NCQA), which grades quality of care, lists spirometry use in patients with newly diagnosed COPD as one indicator of clinician performance for the Health Plan Employer Data and Informed Set (HEDIS). Some experts suggest that the use of spirometry should be as common as the use of a blood pressure cuff in a primary care clinician's office, especially for patients with asthma or COPD.

NOTE: Although useful information can be obtained from spirometry and PFTs, these physiologic tools alone do not establish a diagnosis. The test results must be carefully correlated with clinical and chest radiographic findings.

Definitions and Pathology

Common lung volumes measured by spirometry are illustrated in Figure 91-1. The simplest test of lung function is based on a forced expiration. It is one of the most informative tests and requires minimal equipment and calculations. The *vital capacity* is the total volume of gas that can be exhaled after a full inspiration. The vital capacity measured with a forced expiration may be less than that measured with a slower exhalation, so the term *forced vital capacity (FVC)* is generally used.

Any reduction in FVC affects the ventilatory capacity. The FVC can be affected by conditions affecting the thoracic cage (kyphoscoliosis), diseases affecting the nerve supply to the thoracic muscles, intrinsic diseases of the muscles, abnormalities of the pleural cavity, space-occupying lesions, lung tissue pathology, or stagnation of blood flow in the lungs (as seen in congestive heart failure). In addition, chronic, severe diseases of the airways such as asthma and chronic bronchitis cause peripheral small airways to close prematurely during expiration. This limits the volume that can be exhaled rapidly.

Forced expiratory volume (FEV_1) is the volume of gas (liters) exhaled in 1 second by a forced expiration from full inspiration. The FEV_1 is affected by the airway resistance of the medium to large airways. *Forced expiratory flow ($FEF_{25\%-75\%}$)* is the flow over the middle half of the FVC, the average flow from the point at which 25% of the FVC has been exhaled to the point at which 75% has been exhaled. It is measured in volume (liters) divided by time (seconds). It is the most sensitive office measurement of small airway obstruction or disease. Any increase in airway resistance reduces the ventilatory capacity. Of note, older patients, especially those with obstructive disease, may take a long time to exhale completely for an FVC, as long as 12 to 15 seconds. This is a long time to maintain maximal expiratory effort and may cause discomfort or even lightheadedness. Consequently, certain experts now suggest measuring FEV_6 (forced expiratory volume at 6 seconds) as a substitute for FVC in adults. Subsequently, FEV_6 has been shown to be equivalent to FVC for identifying obstructive and restrictive patterns in adults,

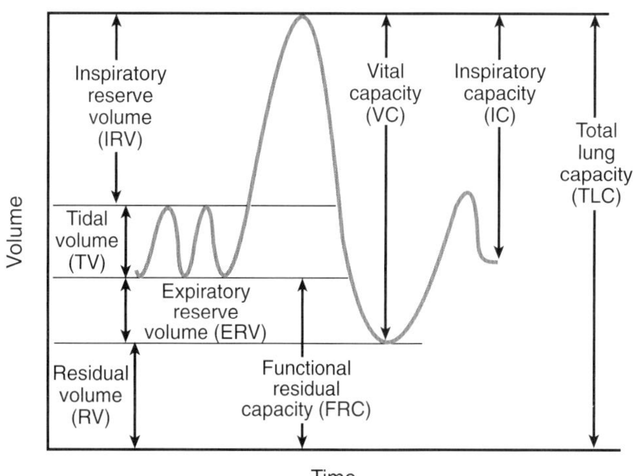

Figure 91-1 Spirogram showing tidal breathing and the divisions of total lung capacity. The residual volume is measured by indirect techniques. (From Mueller GA, Elgen H: Pulmonary function testing in pediatric practice. Pediatr Rec 15:403–411, 1994.)

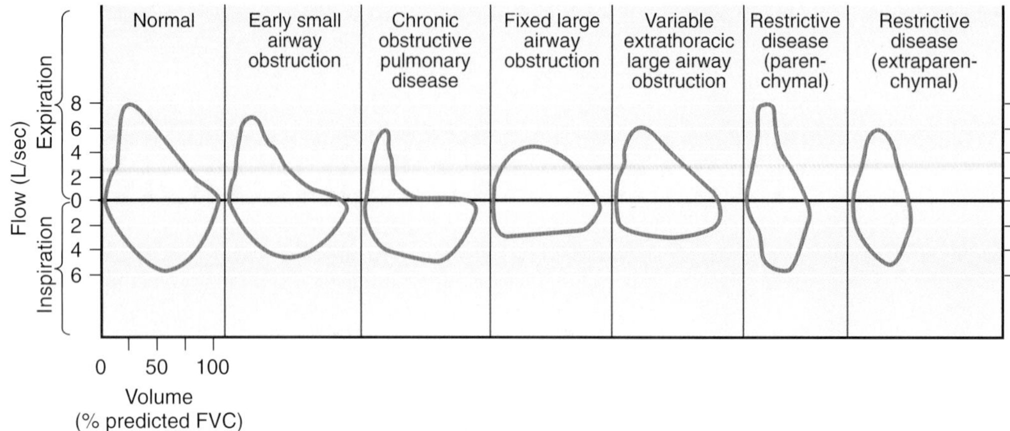

Figure 91-2 Characteristic flow–volume curves of restrictive disease and various types of obstructive diseases compared with normal. The top part of the curve represents maximal forced expiration, whereas the bottom represents maximal inspiration. FVC, forced vital capacity.

and to be more reproducible and less demanding. The flow–volume loop (Fig. 91-2) has two components: the expiratory flow–volume (top half of curve) and the inspiratory flow–volume (bottom half of curve). The top half is where 95% of the information is obtained (expiratory flow).

The inspiratory flow–volume curve is not affected by anything causing dynamic compression of the airways because the pressures during inspiration always expand the bronchi. However, a large (fixed or variable) airway obstruction will cause flattening of the curve because maximal flow is limited. The expiratory flow–volume curve will also be flattened by a fixed large airway obstruction. With restrictive airway disease, the flow–volume curve will be smaller or narrower. One important place to review the inspiratory flow–volume curve is when factitious asthma is suspected. With factitious asthma, there is inappropriate vocal cord closure, also known as *vocal cord dysfunction*, and although the subsequent wheezing may mimic asthma (or exercise-induced asthma), the inspiratory curve is notched or attenuated, which does not occur in true asthma. With true asthma, only the expiratory curve is usually affected.

The expiratory flow–volume curve may take on different morphologies. Notice how the downward loop becomes more scalloped as airway obstruction increases. However, a large (fixed or variable) airway obstruction will cause flattening of the curve because maximal flow is limited. In restrictive lung disease, the flow–volume curve will be *narrow* (almost up-and-down), with little to no "terminal tail" like that seen with COPD.

Two "pearls" should be borne in mind: (1) examination of the shape of the curve is just as important as the actual numerical data generated by spirometry testing; and (2) restrictive lung disease can be ruled out in 95% to 99% of cases with a normal-appearing flow–volume loop. However, if suspected on clinical grounds, formal PFTs measuring the total lung volumes are indicated. (Spirometry falsely identifies restrictive lung disease in 58% of flow–volume loops that suggest a restrictive defect.)

INDICATIONS

Diagnostic Indications

- To evaluate symptoms, signs, or abnormal results of other diagnostic tests in individuals older than 5 years of age.
  - Symptoms: cough, dyspnea, wheezing, orthopnea, or chest pain
  - Signs: overinflation, expiratory slowing, cyanosis, chest deformity, wheezing, or unexplained crackles
  - Abnormal results of diagnostic tests: hypoxemia, hypercapnia, polycythemia, or abnormal chest radiographs
- To measure the effect of disease on pulmonary function.
- To screen persons at risk for pulmonary disease (e.g., persons with occupational exposure to injurious substances or who have active or passive smoke exposure). The evidence does *not* support the widespread use of spirometry to improve smoking cessation rates.
- To assess preoperative risk in patients with COPD or asthma. However, there are few published data comparing spirometric data with clinical data for predicting postoperative pulmonary complications in patients undergoing nonthoracic surgery. Hence, even a poor FEV_1 result is *not* sufficient grounds to withhold surgery in *non*-thoracic cases.
- To screen patients undergoing lung resection surgery.
- To assess prognosis of lung disease.

Monitoring Indications

- To assess effectiveness of a therapeutic intervention (e.g., bronchodilator therapy, steroid treatment for asthma or interstitial lung disease). For asthma, according to NAEP guidelines, PFTs are indicated after therapy is initiated and symptoms and peak flow have stabilized, during periods of progressive or prolonged loss of control, and at least every 1 to 2 years.
- To track the course of a disease affecting lung function in patients who identify activity-limiting symptoms, especially when FEV_1 is less than 50% (e.g., obstructive airway disease, interstitial lung disease, or neuromuscular disease, such as Guillain-Barré syndrome).
- To assess current status of persons with occupational exposure to injurious substances.
- To detect adverse reactions to drugs with known pulmonary toxicity.

Evaluation of Disability or Impairment

- To assess patients as part of a rehabilitation program (e.g., medical, industrial, vocational).
- To assess risks for an insurance evaluation (no evidence of benefit).
- To assess the condition of persons for legal reasons (e.g., Social Security or other program involving government compensation, personal injury lawsuits).

Public Health

- Epidemiologic surveys
- Derivation of normal values for PFTs

CONTRAINDICATIONS

- Severe debilitation and excessive tiring (patients who cannot expend the required effort for testing)
- Severe or moderately severe respiratory distress
- Patients not motivated or desiring to take the test
- Children too young to conduct testing (PFTs are usually helpful if the patient is older than 5 years of age; however, some children cannot conduct testing adequately until after age 7 years)

EQUIPMENT

- Pulmonary function testing machine/spirometer
- Comfortable chair and private area of office for testing (avoids patient embarrassment)
- Nose clips (soft clips are preferred and recommended to prevent air leaks)
- Various inhalants for testing response to bronchodilators (e.g., albuterol inhaler with 90 μg/puff), if indicated

The office spirometer should conform to minimal requirements or specifications established by the American Thoracic Society (Table 91-1). Not all commercially available spirometers meet these standards. Ideally, the computerized spirometer should have software that allows formulas and algorithms to be modified. Routine preventive maintenance, cleaning, and quality control measures are necessary to ensure accurate results in spirometric testing. Frequent (if not daily) calibration according to the manufacturer's instructions is highly recommended. The spirometer should also be evaluated frequently for leaks. Instructions for maintenance, as well as how to perform tests for quality control, should be provided by the manufacturer. The clinician is responsible for ensuring that the office personnel are trained to carry out the recommended maintenance.

NOTE: Peak flow meters are advantageous for patients to use at home, but they do not provide the documentation needed in the office.

PREPROCEDURE PATIENT PREPARATION

Before performing a PFT, review the patient's respiratory history, including any medications the patient may be taking for respiratory problems. A clear explanation of the test and what is to be expected is essential to the patient's performance. The PFT has both an effort-dependent and an effort-independent portion. The best overall result is obtained when the patient gives a maximal effort. Patients with no prior experience with PFTs should make two to three practice attempts until a maximal effort is obtained. A demonstration of the test may be helpful.

Usually the patient is seated to perform the test. The thorax should be erect and the head should be in a neutral position. Explain that this test measures lung function and that the best results are obtained when the patient takes a deep breath and then blows out as hard, as fast, and as long as possible (with the exception of older patients, for whom at least 6 seconds may be necessary to obtain a result [FEV_6]). Smokers should try to abstain from smoking for at least 1 hour before testing.

TECHNIQUE

1. Prepare the equipment to test for FVC. Machine calibration and parameter setups vary between spirometers. See the individual instructions pertaining to the particular instrument for this portion of the procedure.
2. Document the patient's position (usually seated). If for some reason the patient is standing, it will increase FVC.
3. Have the patient breathe in and out several times with the nose clips in place, to become comfortable.
4. Ask the patient to take in as deep a breath as possible, to completely fill the lungs.
5. Then have the patient quickly insert the mouthpiece. It should be between the teeth with a tight seal being held around it using the lips.
6. Next, have the patient blow out as hard, as fast, and as long as possible (try for at least 6 seconds; Fig. 91-3). Enthusiastically coach the patient to breathe out until the forced vital curve flattens out (usually 5 to 6 seconds).
7. When the lungs are completely emptied, have the patient breathe in as deeply as possible, to obtain the inspiratory parameter and complete the evaluation. To follow the diagram (see Fig. 91-1), the patient first takes several normal (tidal) breaths, after which he or she will perform a maximal inspiration to total

TABLE 91-1 Minimal Recommendations (Specifications) for Diagnostic Spirometry*

Test	Range/Accuracy (BTPS)†	Flow Range (L/sec)	Time (sec)	Resistance and Back Pressure	Test Signal
VC	0.5 to 8 L ± 3% of reading or ± 0.05 L, whichever is greater	0–14	30		3-L Cal syringe
FVC	0.5 to 8 L ± 3% of reading or ± 0.05 L, whichever is greater	0–14	15	<1.5 cm H_2O/L/sec	24 standard waveforms 3-L Cal syringe
FEV_1	0.5 to 8 L ± 3% of reading or ± 0.05 L, whichever is greater	0–14	1	<1.5 cm H_2O/L/sec	24 standard waveforms
Time zero	The time point from which all FEV_1 measurements are taken			Back extrapolation	
PEF	Accuracy: ± 10% of reading or ± 0.4 L/sec, whichever is greater				
	Precision: ± 5% of reading or ± 0.2 L/sec, whichever is greater	0–14		Same as FEV_1	26 standard waveforms
$FEF_{25\%-75\%}$	7.0 L/sec ± 5% of reading or ± 0.2 L/sec, whichever is greater	±14	15	Same as FEV_1	24 standard waveforms
V	± 14 L/sec ± 5% of reading or ± 0.2 L/sec, whichever is greater	0–14	15	Same as FEV_1	Proof from manufacturer
MVV	250 L/min at TV of 2 L within ± 10% of reading or ± 15 L/min, whichever is greater	±14 ± 3%	12–15	Pressure < ±10 cm H_2O at 2-L TV at 2.0 Hz	Sine wave pump

FEF, forced expiratory flow; FEV_1, forced expiratory volume; FVC, forced vital capacity; L/sec, liters per second; MVV, maximal voluntary ventilation; PEF, peak expiratory flow; TV, tidal volume; V, volume; VC, vital capacity.

*Unless specifically stated, precision requirements are the same as the accuracy requirements.

†BTPS, body temperature pressure saturated (37° C and ambient pressure).

From American Thoracic Society: Standardization of spirometry: 1994 update. Am J Resp Crit Care Med 152:1107–1136, 1995.

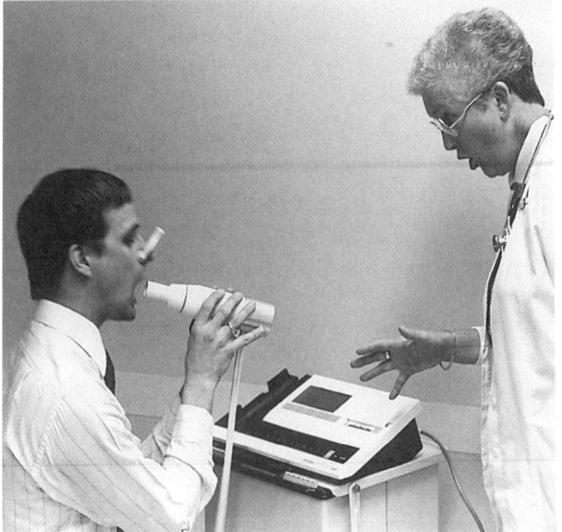

Figure 91-3 Patient takes a deep breath, inserts the mouthpiece, and blows out as fast and as hard as possible.

lung capacity (TLC). The patient then exhales fast and hard, as much as he or she can (FVC or FEV_6).

8. Repeat the test three times. A minimum of three and a maximum of eight maneuvers are performed until three acceptable curves are obtained. Two or three maneuvers that have values within a 5% difference of each other indicate reproducibility. The best effort is then saved and reported. Acceptability and reproducibility criteria are summarized in Box 91-1.
9. If prebronchodilator and postbronchodilator comparison PFTs are needed, administer a short-acting β-adrenergic agonist (e.g., albuterol two to four puffs of 90 μg/puff) or other bronchodilator through a hand-held inhaler.
10. Wait about 20 minutes for bronchodilation to occur. Then repeat the FVC (FEV_6 for older patients with obstructive disease) for the postbronchodilation measurements, as in steps 1 through 8.

Box 91-1. Acceptability and Reproducibility Criteria: Summary

Acceptability Criteria

Individual spirograms are "acceptable" if

1. They are free from artifacts, such as
   - Cough or glottis closure during the first second of exhalation
   - Early termination or cut-off
   - Variable effort
   - Leak
   - Obstructed mouthpiece
2. They have good starts
   - Extrapolated volume <5% of FVC or 0.15 L, whichever is greater; *or*
   - Time to peak expiratory flow <120 msec (optional until further information is available)
3. They have a satisfactory exhalation
   - Six seconds of exhalation or a plateau in the volume–time curve; *or*
   - Reasonable duration or a plateau in the volume–time curve; *or*
   - If the subject cannot or should not continue to exhale

Reproducibility Criteria

After three acceptable spirograms have been obtained, apply the following tests:

- Are the two largest FVCs within 0.2 L of each other?
- Are the two largest FEV_1 values within 0.2 L of each other?
- If both of these criteria are met, the test session may be concluded.
- If both of these criteria are not met, continue testing until
  - Both of the criteria are met with analysis of additional acceptable spirograms *or*
  - A total of eight tests have been performed *or*
  - The patient/subject cannot or should not continue

  Save, at a minimum, the three best maneuvers.

From American Thoracic Society: Standardization of spirometry: 1994 update. Am J Respir Crit Care Med 152:1107–1136, 1995.

INTERPRETATION

Some of the factors that influence the normal values of PFTs include the formula used to predict the normal values, test quality, height, age, weight, sex, ethnicity, posture, effort, smoking, and even circadian rhythm. The results and interpretation depend on the clinician paying careful attention to the characteristics of the equipment used, the patient's performance and clinical condition, and the reference values chosen. A patient's own baseline values will provide the best reference data for assessing a patient with chronic pulmonary disease over time.

Interpretation of PFTs can be categorized into three basic patterns: normal function, obstructive, and restrictive (Fig. 91-4). A diagnosis is then made by correlating the test results with the clinical findings from the history, physical examination, and radiographs.

An obstructive process, such as asthma or COPD, is characterized by flow that is low relative to lung volume. Characteristically, timed volume (FEV_1) and flow ($FEF_{25\%-75\%}$) are decreased. A decrease in $FEF_{25\%-75\%}$ may detect obstruction in the smaller airways early in the course of the disease, before a change in FEV_1 is evident. This is especially common in smokers, and may be their best early warning before permanent lung damage. A reduction in $FEF_{25\%-75\%}$ from small airway obstruction gives the flow–volume curve a characteristic concave shape. Other causes of small airway obstructive patterns in children include cystic fibrosis, bronchiolitis, bronchiectasis, and heart disease. Causes of large airway obstructive patterns in children include a foreign body, vocal cord dysfunction, vascular rings or laryngeal webs, laryngotracheomalacia, tracheal or bronchial stenosis, enlarged lymph nodes, or tumor. In adults, causes of obstructive patterns include asthma, COPD, congestive heart failure, pulmonary embolism, mechanical obstruction of the airway (benign and malignant tumors), pulmonary infiltration with eosinophilia, vocal cord dysfunction, and cough due to medications (e.g., angiotensin-converting enzyme inhibitors).

Distinguishing between asthma and COPD can be challenging because there can be overlap between the two. However, the following points can be helpful.

For asthma

1. The history. Diagnosis is typically picked up in childhood (although it can be missed) with cough, wheezing, dyspnea, chest tightness; occurring or worse at night; identifiable triggers (e.g., infections, stress, allergies, changes in weather, strong emotional expression [laughing or crying hard], menstrual periods); a clearly reversible component when a bronchodilator is added (e.g., increase FEV_1 >200 mL, >12% from baseline, or >10% over predicted FEV_1).
2. FEV_1—the gold standard—<80% if moderate; also, FEV_1/FVC ratio <80%. In fact, FEV_1/FVC ratio (i.e., FEV_1%) is a better measure of asthma severity than FEV_1.

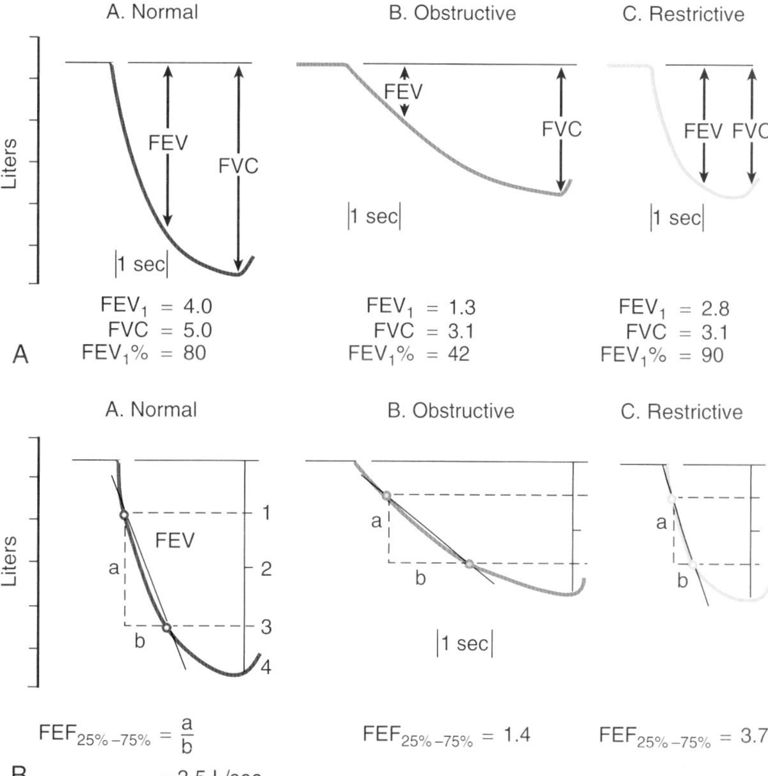

Figure 91-4 **A,** Normal, obstructive, and restrictive patterns of a forced expiration. **B,** Calculation of forced expiratory flow between 25% and 75% of the FVC ($FEF_{25\%-75\%}$). FEV_1, forced expiratory volume at 1 second; FVC, forced vital capacity. $FEV_1\% = (FEV_1/FVC) \times 100$. (From West JB: Pulmonary pathophysiology. In Respiratory Physiology: The Essentials, 6th ed. Philadelphia, Lippincott Williams & Wilkins, 2003.)

For COPD

1. The history. Almost always there will be an explanation or cause: tobacco abuse (most common, especially if at least a 20–pack-year history; note, however, that only about 20% of cigarette smokers develop clinically significant COPD), α_1-antitrypsin deficiency (accounts for 1% of COPD cases; consider if smoking history absent or very early COPD [age <55 years] in smokers), exposure to airway toxins (e.g., industrial chemicals, mineral dust, silica, dust, coal dust, and inhaled endotoxins [e.g., farm worker]).
2. COPD-related airflow obstruction is less reversible to inhaled bronchodilator challenges and less variable than asthma.
3. FEV_1/FVC ratio <70% of normal, and FEV_1 <80% of normal.

Postbronchodilator FEV_1 is also recommended for the diagnosis and assessment of severity of COPD.

Low volumes and normal flows characterize a restrictive lung process. The primary criterion for this diagnosis is a reduction in TLC; however, the presence of restriction is commonly inferred from a decreased FVC. It should be kept in mind that a decreased FVC only *infers* a restrictive process because FVC can also be reduced in the presence of airflow obstruction. Significant decreases in FEV_1 and the FEV_1/FVC ratio are key findings that will help differentiate an obstructive from a restrictive pattern when FVC is reduced (see Fig. 91-4A). In addition, when there is both airflow obstruction and reduced FVC, the possibility of restriction can usually be eliminated with evidence of overinflation on the physical examination or a chest radiograph.

Spirometry falsely identifies restrictive patterns in 59% of cases in which FVC was low, consistent with restrictive defect. Unless dictated on clinical grounds, restrictive defects should be confirmed by total lung volume measurements. Measuring TLC requires referral to a pulmonary function laboratory. Measurement of lung volume by helium dilution, nitrogen washout, or body plethysmography can definitively confirm a diagnosis of a restrictive lung condition. Although a reduced TLC defines restriction, measuring FVC has frequently been demonstrated to be more useful for following the course of the disease process. Restrictive disease is uncommon and can be divided into parenchymal and extraparenchymal etiologies. Parenchymal causes include silicosis, pneumoconiosis, idiopathic pulmonary fibrosis, sarcoidosis, and drug- or radiation-induced interstitial lung disease. Extraparenchymal disease can be due to loss of lung volume (e.g., pleural effusion, pneumothorax), chest wall deformity, extrathoracic compression (e.g., ankylosing spondylitis, ascites, kyphoscoliosis, obesity), or neuromuscular problems (e.g., Guillain-Barré syndrome, myasthenia gravis, muscular dystrophy, cervical spine injury, or diaphragmatic weakness or paralysis). Suspicion of restrictive disease warrants referral. Table 91-2 summarizes the characteristic patterns of obstructive and restrictive lung diseases as measured by spirometry.

Many systems are available to quantify the severity of pulmonary impairment; however, there is currently no universal standard based

TABLE 91-2 Characteristic Patterns of Obstructive and Restrictive Lung Disease as Measured by Spirometry*

	Obstruction	Restriction
FVC	Normal or ↓	↓
FEV_1	↓	Normal or ↓
FEV_1/FVC	Normal (early) or ↓	↑
$FEF_{25\%-75\%}$	↓	Normal, ↑ or ↓

FEF, forced expiratory flow; FEV_1, forced expiratory volume; FVC, forced vital capacity.

*Low flows with normal volumes characterize obstructive disease, whereas normal flows with low volumes characterize restrictive disease. In severe obstruction, gas trapping reduces FVC because of an increased residual volume.

on differences between ethnic populations.* In practice, severity is usually described as a percentage of either predicted FEV_1 for obstructive conditions or predicted TLC for restrictive conditions. ("Normal" predicted test values are obtained by testing a large group of people who have been determined to be free of lung disease.) The test results for a given patient are then expressed as a percentage of the predicted value for age, height, sex, and race. In reality, no one set of equations will be entirely accurate for every person in a given population. For the final report, the ATS recommends that clinicians define the lower limits of normal by using calculations of the lower 95th percentiles (from the specific set of prediction equations that have been selected as standard reference values); these should be recorded, rather than just the percentages of predicted function (e.g., 80% for FEV_1/FVC%). The patient should be comparable in age, race, and sex to the reference population. In computerized equipment, it is essential for population standards to be defined in the software.

Although using percentage of predicted function to evaluate results may not be recommended, some guidelines the clinician can use to get a general clinical picture of pulmonary function follow:

Vital Capacity

FVC	
80% to 120% of predicted value	Normal
70% to 79% of predicted value	Mild reduction
50% to 69% of predicted value	Moderate reduction
<50% of predicted value	Severe reduction

Again, *restrictive* lung disease is characterized by reduced vital capacity and relatively normal airflow rates. If obstruction is present (see "Flow Rates" section), the reduction in vital capacity may only be reported as "probably secondary to obstruction" if the severity of the reduced vital capacity and that of the obstructive findings are approximately equal. In comparing vital capacities obtained at different times (including those obtained before and after bronchodilator administration), the expiratory time must be considered and compared. The raw curves should also be compared.

Flow Rates

FEV_1 can be plotted as the percentage of vital capacity [(FEV_1/FVC) × 100], or FEV_1%.

FEV_1%	
>75%	Normal
60% to 75%	Mild obstruction
50% to 59%	Moderate obstruction
<50%	Severe obstruction

NOTE: For patients less than 25 years old, add 5% to these figures; for those more than 60 years old, subtract 5%.

$FEF_{25\%-75\%}$	
>79% of predicted value	Normal
60% to 79% of predicted value	Mild obstruction
40% to 59% of predicted value	Moderate obstruction
<40% of predicted value	Severe obstruction

In most cases of *obstructive* lung disease, the percentage of the predicted value of the $FEF_{25\%-75\%}$ will be "worse" than the percentage of the predicted value of the FEV_1. However, the modifier used to describe the type of *obstruction* (i.e., mild, moderate, or severe) should be that associated with the value of the FEV_1, not the $FEF_{25\%-75\%}$. The $FEF_{25\%-75\%}$ may be separately referred to with such statements as "... particularly affecting small airways, as reflected in the $FEF_{25\%-75\%}$." Should the $FEF_{25\%-75\%}$ *alone* be abnormal, the diagnosis of obstructive lung disease should not be assumed; rather, the reduction should be interpreted as compatible with "early small airways disease." Again, for comparison over time, the raw curves should be examined to determine adequacy of effort.

Therefore, an FEV_1% less than 75% indicates some loss of elastic recoil (e.g., emphysema) or obstructive disease (e.g., asthma), whereas reduced FVC and FEV_1 (but FEV_1% >75%) indicates restrictive disease. Again, suspicion of restrictive disease warrants referral.

For the final interpretation, the flow–volume loops can be useful in conjunction with the volume–time spirogram. A flow–volume loop can help determine whether an obstruction is in the larger or the smaller airways. It can also help determine whether a restrictive pattern is due to a parenchymal or an extraparenchymal cause. The most useful information obtained from flow–volume loops is usually in the expiratory portion of the flow loop (see Fig. 91-2). However, flow–volume loops may be derived only if the spirometer is accurate in displacement and time.

*There are referenced "normal" data sets now on the Internet for different parts of the world.

Application of Spirometry in Asthma and Chronic Obstructive Pulmonary Disease Management

The following flow rates (FEV_1; from NAEP Guidelines, 2007) can be used to assess asthma:

≥80%	Mild asthma (if associated with symptoms)
60% to 79%	Moderate asthma
≤60%	Severe asthma

Low FEV_1 is associated with increased risk of severe asthma exacerbations. However, in children, exacerbations can happen even with normal FEV_1. Consequently, recent emphasis has shifted to FEV_1% (FEV_1/FVC × 100, with levels of impairment listed in the "Flow Rates" section) because it may be a more sensitive indicator of asthma severity. Ultimately, in children and adults, treatment decisions should be based on symptoms and frequency and severity of past exacerbations, combined with PFTs as an additional guide.

Spirometry can also be very helpful in staging COPD severity. More important, it provides a basis for medical decisions based on objective data. Revised guidelines (2006) by GOLD through the National Heart Lung and Blood Institute (NHLBI) and the World Health Organization (WHO) are briefly summarized in Table 91-3.

The FEV_1 and FEV_1/FVC data generated in the clinician's office using a spirometer define when to "step up" treatment and which drugs should be used.

Errors and Rules of Thumb in Pulmonary Function Testing

Some technical errors and their effects in pulmonary function testing include the following:

- An air leak due to a poorly fitting nose clip or mouthpiece can result in a wandering baseline, which can lead to underestimation of many spirometric measurements.
- An incomplete expiration may give a falsely low reading of FVC and a spurious increase in $FEF_{25\%-75\%}$.
- Poor initial expiratory effort may give a falsely low reading of the FEV_1 and $FEF_{25\%-75\%}$.

PFTs have a false-positive rate of approximately 5%. Borderline values should be interpreted cautiously. In addition to the ranges listed in Table 91-3, the changes in spirometric results over time for an individual can affect the interpretation of the results. The coefficient of variation relates the standard deviation to the main value and is a measure of test-to-test variability in a given individual. The

TABLE 91-3 Change in Spirometric Indexes over Time

	Percent Changes Required to Be Significant		
	FVC	FEV_1	$FEF_{25\%-75\%}$
Within a Day			
Normal subjects	≥5%	≥5%	≥13%
Patients with COPD	≥11%	≥13%	≥23%
Week to Week			
Normal subjects	≥11%	≥12%	≥21%
Patients with COPD	≥20%	≥20%	≥30%
Year to Year			
Normal subjects	≥15%	≥15%	
Patients with COPD	≥15%	≥15%	

COPD, chronic obstructive pulmonary disease; FEF, forced expiratory flow; FEV_1, forced expiratory volume; FVC, forced vital capacity.
Adapted from American Thoracic Society: Lung function testing: Selection of reference value and interpretive strategies. Am Rev Respir Dis 144:1202–1218, 1991.

interval between tests, the intrinsic variability of the test, and the presence of disease are among the factors that determine the coefficient of variation.

Lung function declines with age. It is estimated that vital capacity decreases 60 mL/year after peaking during young adulthood. Differentiating "real" decline in lung function from expected test variability across time can be difficult. Recommended requirements for significant spirometric changes (normal variability) have been calculated and are listed in Table 91-3.

Adolescents should not be compared with adult standards until growth and puberty are complete. This recommendation is necessary because leg length, thorax height, and total body height proportions change throughout puberty.

Other sources of error include inadequate preventive maintenance of the equipment, inadequate training of the staff, inadequate patient motivation, not correlating the results with the entire clinical picture (e.g., history, physical examination, radiographic findings), and not ordering more definitive tests when the results are unclear (e.g., obtaining a formal TLC measurement when both FVC and flow are reduced).

In the past, when managing patients with COPD, if the FEV_1 went below 1.0 L, the prognosis was thought to worsen dramatically (similar to a cardiac ejection fraction <20%). We now know that patients occasionally can survive for years with an FEV_1 less than 1.0 L if they stop smoking and have a good exercise capacity (e.g., can walk several blocks).

For final values that are confusing or do not make sense (e.g., hyperinflation on chest radiograph and abnormal PFTs, yet no history of smoking and no other risk factors for COPD), cardiopulmonary exercise testing (expired gas exercise testing) may be helpful. In addition, one of the most common causes of emphysema (or premature emphysema in nonsmokers) is α_1-antitrypsin deficiency. This tends to run in families and can be excluded by a simple blood test that many laboratories perform.

CPT/Billing Codes

94010 Spirometry, including graphic record, total and timed vital capacity, expiratory flow rate measurement(s), with or without maximal voluntary ventilation
94060 Bronchodilation responsiveness: spirometry as in 94010, before and after bronchodilator administration
94375 Respiratory flow volume loop

ICM-9-CM Diagnostic Codes

491.0 Chronic bronchitis, simple
491.2 Chronic bronchitis, obstructive
491.9 Chronic bronchitis, unspecified
492 Emphysema
493.00 Asthma, extrinsic, without mention status asthmaticus
493.90 Asthma, unspecified, without mention status asthmaticus
514 Pulmonary edema

Acknowledgment

The editors wish to recognize the contributions by Edward A. Jackson, MD, and Jose Bayona, MD, to this chapter in the previous two editions of this text.

Suppliers

(See contact information online at www.expertconsult.com.)

Nova Medical Systems Corporation
Puritan Bennett (Tyco Healthcare)
SDI Diagnostics, Inc.
Vitalograph
Welch Allyn

BIBLIOGRAPHY

Aaron SD, Dales RE, Cardinal P: How accurate is spirometry at predicting restrictive pulmonary impairment? Chest 115:869–873, 1999.
American Thoracic Society: Lung function testing: Selection of reference value and interpretative strategies. Am Rev Respir Dis 144:1202–1218, 1991.
American Thoracic Society: Standardization of spirometry: 1994 update. Am J Respir Crit Care Med 152:1107–1136, 1995.
Ferguson GT, Enright PL, Buist AS, Higgins MW: Office spirometry for lung health assessment in adults: A consensus statement from the National Lung Health Education Program. Chest 117:1146–1161, 2000.
Holten KB: Revisiting spirometry for the diagnosis of COPD. J Fam Pract 55:51, 2006. Online. Available at www.jfponline.com.
Lee TA, Bartle B, Weiss KB: Spirometry use in clinical practice following diagnosis of COPD. Chest 129:1509–1515, 2006.
Margolis M: PFT principles and bronchodilator testing in clinical practice: A guide for primary care physicians. Compr Ther 24:441–445, 1998.
Marseglia GL, Cirillo I, Vizzaccaro A, et al: Role of forced expiratory flow at 25–75% as an early marker of small airways impairment in subjects with allergic rhinitis. Allergy Asthma Proc 28:74–78, 2007.
McIvor RA, Taskin DP: Underdiagnosis of chronic obstructive pulmonary disease: A rationale for spirometry as a screening tool. Can Respir J 8:153–158, 2001.
National Asthma Education Program, National Heart, Blood, and Lung Institute: Expert Panel Report 3: Guidelines for the Diagnosis and Management of Asthma. Bethesda, Md, Department of Health and Human Services, National Institutes of Health, 2007.
Petty TL: Simple office spirometry. Clin Chest Med 22:845–859, 2001.
Qaseem A, Snow V, Fitterman F, et al, Clinical Efficacy Assessment Subcommittee of the American College of Physicians: Risk assessment for and strategies to reduce perioperative pulmonary complications for patients undergoing noncardiothoracic surgery: A guideline from the American College of Physicians. Ann Intern Med 144:575–580, 2006.
Rabe KF, Hurd S, Anzueto A, et al, Global Initiative for Chronic Obstructive Lung Disease: Global strategy for the diagnosis, management, and prevention of chronic obstructive pulmonary disease: GOLD executive summary. Am J Respir Crit Care Med 176:532–555, 2007.
Sly M: Decreases in asthma mortality in the United States. Ann Allergy Asthma Immunol 85:121–127, 2000.
Smetana FW: Preoperative pulmonary evaluation. N Engl J Med 340: 937–944, 1999.
Spahn JD, Chipps BE: Office-based objective measures in childhood asthma. J Pediatr 148:11–15, 2006.
West JB: Pulmonary pathophysiology. In Respiratory Physiology: The Essentials, 6th ed. Philadelphia, Lippincott Williams & Wilkins, 2003, pp 3–15.

CHAPTER 92

SCLEROTHERAPY

Jerry Ninia

Sclerotherapy is a technique used to eliminate unwanted veins (both varicosities and spider veins). This is accomplished by injecting a noxious agent into the lumen of the vein, which causes destruction of the endothelium with an inflammatory response. When used with compression, it results in obliteration of the vessel. The goal of treatment is to eradicate abnormal veins while preserving healthy veins.

BACKGROUND

Ancient physicians, scholars, and poets, including Hippocrates and Homer, recognized varicose veins. Improvements in syringes and needles and the development of more effective and safe sclerosing solutions allowed sclerotherapy to become a modern and effective method of treatment. Clinicians now use sclerosants developed in the 20th century (e.g., hypertonic glucose, hypertonic saline, sodium morrhuate, chromated glycerin, ethanolamine oleate, and stabilized polyiodide iodine). However, the most popular agents used in sclerotherapy are sodium tetradecyl sulfate (Sotradecol), polidocanol (Aethoxysklerol), and hypertonic saline (Table 92-1).

Organizations worldwide—including the American College of Phlebology and the American Venous Forum in the United States—have been formed to further research and education in venous disease. Recently, the American Medical Association has recognized phlebology as a separate and distinct medical specialty.

ANATOMY

The venous system is divided into three levels: *deep*, *perforating*, and *superficial* veins. The veins treated with sclerotherapy are the perforating and the superficial veins.

Deep veins are encased in fascia and muscle. In ascending order, they are the anterior and posterior tibial veins, the peroneal vein, the tibioperoneal trunk, the popliteal vein, the superficial femoral vein, the deep femoral vein, the common femoral vein, and the iliac vein. These veins convey blood from the lower limb back to the heart (Fig. 92-1).

The superficial venous system is confined to the veins above the fascia in the subcutaneous tissue and involves the great and small saphenous veins and their tributaries, in addition to the lateral subdermal veins (of Albanese) around the knee (Figs. 92-2 and 92-3).

Approximately 150 perforating veins connect the superficial and deep systems. Many of these veins are eponymous with the anatomists who demonstrated them (Fig. 92-4). In the middle area of the thigh are the Hunterian perforators, and in the distal thigh are the Dodd perforators. These veins connect the thigh portion of the great saphenous vein to the femoral vein. Below the knee is Boyd's perforator, connecting the great saphenous vein to the popliteal vein. The infrapopliteal perforating veins along the medial aspect of the leg connect a major branch of the saphenous vein, the posterior tibial arch vein, to the posterior tibial vein.

There are also important perforating veins along the posterior aspect of the calf, which connect the small saphenous system to the tibial venous system, and perforators along the lateral aspect of the knee that connect the lateral subdermal plexus of Albanese to the deep venous system.

There are several important connections from the superficial venous system to the deep femoral vein. The posterior thigh perforator connects the superficial veins of the posterior thigh to the deep femoral vein. In addition, the inferior gluteal vein and the veins of the medial thigh connect through the internal pudendal system to the deep pelvic veins. It is the latter system that results in the vulvar varicosities seen frequently in pregnancy. Although it is not necessary to remember all of the proper names of these perforators, it is important for the clinician to have knowledge of their location so that sclerotherapy can be carried out in a logical and effective manner.

In general, unwanted veins are referred to as *telangiectases*, *reticular varicosities*, or *varicose veins* (Table 92-2).

PHYSIOLOGY

Primary Varicose Veins

The veins of the lower limb carry blood against the force of gravity back to the heart. This is accomplished by two principal means. When the muscles of the calf contract, they compress the soleal sinuses and the deep veins encased in fascia and muscle, achieving a pressure of up to 300 cm H_2O. Because the veins of the lower limb have valves that allow blood to flow only in a proximal direction, the column of blood is forced into the valveless veins of the abdomen.

If a person is standing still, the pressure of the veins on the dorsum of the foot will equal the distance from the foot to the right heart. This results in an average pressure of approximately of 70 to 80 cm H_2O. As evidenced by the pressure relationship mentioned previously, the pressure exerted by the contraction of the calf muscles is sufficient to overcome the effects of gravity and propel blood in a proximal direction. The flow of venous blood from the calf back to the heart may be considered the systolic phase. During this phase, blood is prevented from going into the superficial venous system by the valves of the perforating veins. During the relaxation phase, when the pressure in the calf compartment is diminished, blood can flow from the superficial veins through the perforators into the deep veins. Therefore, the superficial venous system may be likened to an atrium of the heart, and the deep veins of the calf may be likened to a ventricle.

This physiologic system breaks down when the walls of the veins dilate, causing the valves to become incompetent. The manner in which veins become incompetent is somewhat controversial. The belief has been that the problem is initiated by a malfunctioning valve. The incompetent valve allows blood to flow in a reverse direction as gravity pulls it down toward the foot. The resulting increase in venous pressure causes the veins to dilate and

TABLE 92-1 Most Common Sclerosing Agents in the United States

Agent	Food and Drug Administration Approval	Supply	Maximum Dose Per Visit	Indications	Companies	Comments
Sodium tetradecyl sulfate (Sotradecol, STS)	Yes	2-mL ampules (1%, 3%)	10 mL 3% solution	0.1%–0.25% up to 2 mm; 0.25%–0.5% reticular; 0.5%–1% <4 mm; 1%–3% >4 mm	Elkin-Sinn, Inc. (Cherry Hill, NJ); Wyeth-Ayerst (Philadelphia, PA)	Painless; can cause extravascular necrosis
Hypertonic saline	Yes, as abortifacient	30-mL ampules (23.4%); dilute as needed with lidocaine 1% (may be stored dilute for up to 12 wk)	10 mL; more can cause leg cramps, significant salt load	11.7% <2 mm (especially for matting); 23.4% >2 mm (many use the 18.7% solution for all vessels; see text)		Major advantages: no anaphylaxis and inexpensive; some discomfort on injection
Polidocanol (Aethoxysklerol)	No	2-mL and 30-mL ampules (0.5%, 1%, 2%, 3%)	2 mg/kg	0.25%–1% telangiectases and reticulars <4 mm	Kreussler & Co. (Wiesboden-Bielsrich, Germany)	Painless; less extravascular necrosis; need to have compounded or obtain out of United States

sequentially creates incompetence in the more distal valves. Although this incompetence still may occur, especially in patients who have had phlebitis, which can destroy the valve structure, it now seems likely that in patients who develop primary varicose veins the initiating event is dilation of the vein itself.

The most proximal valve of the superficial system is at the saphenofemoral junction. This valve normally allows blood to flow from the great saphenous vein into the common femoral vein. When this valve becomes incompetent, blood will flow from the common femoral vein into the great saphenous vein, causing progressive dilation of the saphenous vein. This dilation can affect more distal valves, causing them to become incompetent; thus a cycle is begun that eventually causes dilation of the entire saphenous system.

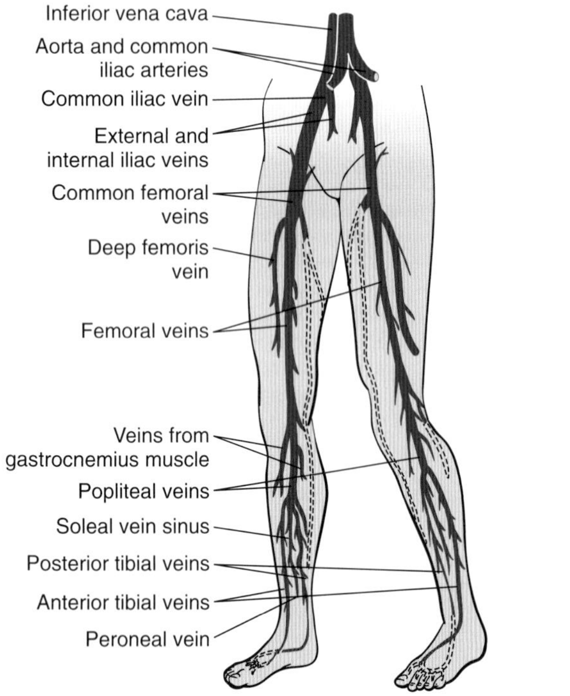

Figure 92-1 Main venous conduits formed by the deep veins of the lower limbs; numerous branch veins join these.

Another mechanism for the development of varicose veins is incompetence of the perforating vein valves. When the calf muscles contract, blood is prevented from flowing through the perforating veins into the superficial system by closure of their valves. If a valve is not working properly, blood will flow from the deep veins into the superficial venous system. The flow of blood from the deep system into the superficial system diminishes the blood flow back to the heart, and it greatly increases the venous pressure in the leg. This increase of the venous pressure, termed *venous hypertension*, is the

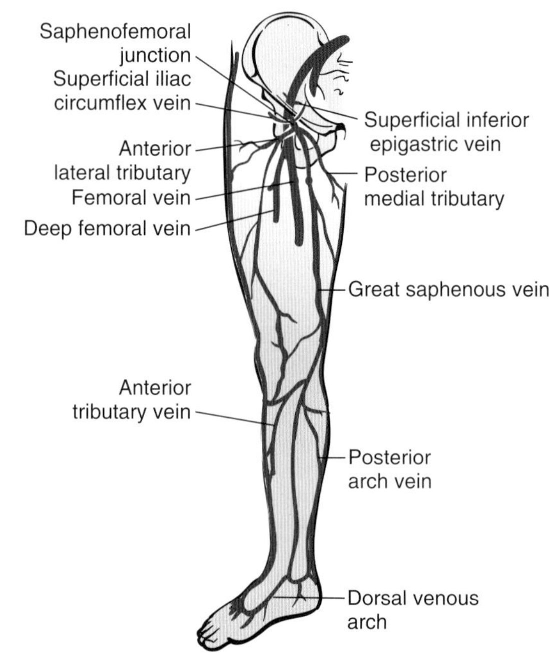

Figure 92-2 Normal anteromedial superficial venous anatomy is depicted. The great saphenous vein ascends from the dorsal venous arch and dominates the anteromedial superficial drainage system. It receives the posterior arch vein (vein of Michelangelo). It also receives variable anterior and posterior tributary veins in the anteromedial calf just below the knee. As the saphenous vein reaches its termination, it receives important tributaries medially and laterally. These tributaries are commonly visualized in duplex ultrasonographic examinations, which may identify reflux in one or both of these vessels.

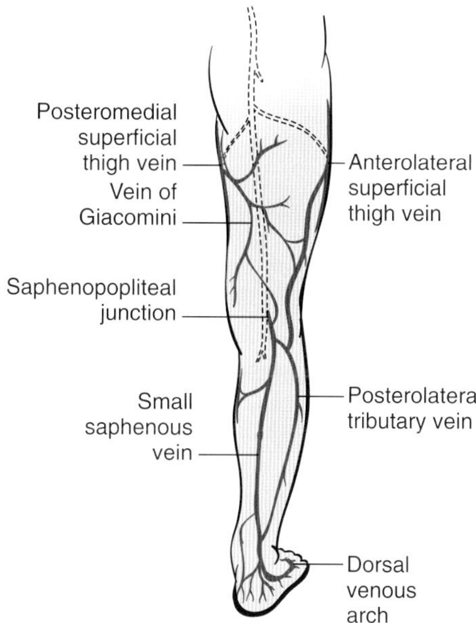

Figure 92-3 The small saphenous vein dominates the posterolateral superficial venous drainage. It originates in the dorsal venous arch; at the posterolateral ankle, it is intimately associated with the sural nerve. Note the important posterolateral tributary vein and the posterior thigh vein, which ascends and connects the small saphenous venous system with the great saphenous venous system. The anterolateral superficial thigh vein and the posterolateral tributary vein can be very important in congenital venous anomalies, such as Klippel-Trénaunay syndrome.

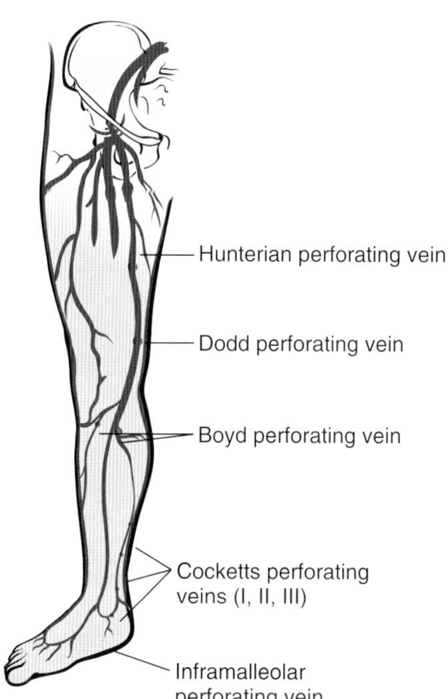

Figure 92-4 Locations of the most important perforating veins associated with the great saphenous system are shown. Note that the Cocketts and inframalleolar perforating veins are actually separate from the great saphenous system. The Boyd perforating vein is constantly present, but it may drain the saphenous vein or its tributaries. Perforating veins in the distal third of the thigh are referred to as *Dodd perforators*, whereas those in the middle third of the thigh are referred to as *Hunterian perforators*.

TABLE 92-2 Vessel Classification

Type	Vessel Classification	Characteristics	Color
I	Telangiectases ("spider veins")	0.1–1 mm	Red
Ia	Telangiectatic matting	<0.2 mm, very fine; can occur after injection or surgery	Red
II	Venulectasia	1–2 mm	Violaceous
III	Reticular veins	2–4 mm	Blue
IV	Nonsaphenous varicosities (second-degree incompetent perforators)	3–8 mm	Blue
V	Saphenous varicosities	7–8 mm	Blue

Adapted from Sadick NS: Manual of Sclerotherapy, Philadelphia, Lippincott Williams & Wilkins, 2000.

cause of many of the sequelae seen in chronic venous insufficiency, such as edema, stasis dermatitis, pigmentation from hemosiderin, and ultimately the development of lipodermatosclerosis and venous ulceration.

Secondary Varicose Veins

Secondary varicose veins can occur as a result of a superficial or deep venous thrombosis (DVT) or from an arteriovenous fistula with resulting high venous pressure. All of these conditions may cause venous dilation and lead to valve incompetence.

INDICATIONS

- Small, bulging varicose veins up to 0.6 cm in diameter (some phlebologists treat larger veins)
- Venulectasia
- Telangiectasia (commonly called *spider veins)*
- Pain, itching, burning, tiredness, and heaviness in the lower limb (previously mentioned indications, regardless of size, may cause these symptoms)
- Cosmesis in the absence of other symptoms
- Venous stasis ulcer
- Venous stasis pigmentation
- Recurrent bleeding of a vessel of any size

Injection of facial telangiectases has been done and reported. It is efficacious. However, venous sinus thrombosis (in the brain) has occurred. Radiofrequency ablation or various laser/light methodologies are often as helpful without the associated risks.

CONTRAINDICATIONS

- Saphenofemoral junction or saphenopopliteal junction reflux.
- Reflux from deep system into superficial creates high venous pressure, making it difficult to obliterate vein.
- Veins larger than 0.6 cm in diameter.
- If the vein has a large diameter, it is difficult to obtain coaptation of intimal surfaces for permanent obliteration; it is more likely that a thrombus will develop within the lumen of the vein and recanalize over time.
- Some practitioners do inject these large vessels, but recurrence and complications are more common and phlebectomy might be a wiser choice of treatment.
- Arterial insufficiency.
- Ankle-to-brachial index less than 0.7 or other signs of inadequate arterial flow.
- Diabetic neuropathy.
- Acute superficial or deep thrombophlebitis.

- Massive obesity.
- Anticoagulation.
- Obstruction of the deep venous system.
- Severe systemic disease (especially collagen vascular disease, malignancy, or severe cardiac problems).
- Pregnancy.
- Lack of mobility, such as seen in stroke, arthritis, or other musculoskeletal disorders.
- Unwillingness to comply with a program of compression.
- Acute febrile illness.

NOTE: The clinician should use caution in patients with asthma or numerous allergies (unless hypertonic saline is used) to avoid potential hypersensitivity. Age is not a contraindication if the patient is active and has reasonably good skin turgor.

EQUIPMENT

- Camera for pictures *(optional)*.
- Examination table. (A power table is helpful but not mandatory.)
- Patient stand. (The examination can be performed more optimally if the patient's feet are 24 inches off the floor. Usually this requires a made-to-order stand that includes a strong railing. The stand can be used for both examination and treatment.)
- Good lighting. (A gooseneck lamp is sufficient; however, some therapists use a more intense light source, such as a headlamp.)
- Magnification loupes (3×).
- Syringes (3.0 and 1.0 mL); 1/2-inch, 30-gauge needle.
- Handheld Doppler probe.
- Sclerosing solution:
  - *Sodium tetradecyl sulfate* (preferred by the author) in dilutions of 0.2%, 0.5%, 1.0%, and (rarely) 3.0%.
  - *Hypertonic saline* in a dilution of 18.7% is also commonly used (and preferred by the editor). It can be prepared by injecting 2 mL of 2% lidocaine into a 30-mL, multiple-dose vial of 23.4% saline (0.5 mL of this solution is injected per site). It is sterile and can be left diluted for up to 12 weeks.
  - *Polidocanol* is another common sclerosant but is not approved by the U.S. Food and Drug Administration (FDA).

NOTE: The assistant should have 5 to 10 1-mL syringes drawn up for use, depending on the sclerosant and the quantity of veins to be injected. Each agent has benefits and risks. Hypertonic saline is effective and there are no allergic reactions; however, it is painful and the risk of extravasation necrosis of the skin is significant (Box 92-1). Polidocanol (0.05% to 3%) is a weak sclerosant, but it works well on small veins. Allergic reactions are possible but rare, and it is not FDA approved (in phase III trials). However, it is frequently used in the United States even now (Box 92-2 and Table 92-3). Sodium tetradecyl sulfate is medium in potency and relatively painless, but it must be injected carefully to avoid skin necrosis. Allergy and anaphylaxis can occur, although this is rare (see Table 92-1).

Box 92-1. Hypertonic Saline Description

True allergic reactions are nonexistent, but side effects are more common.
The degree of endothelial damage is directly proportional to the concentration used.
Dilution with heparin or anesthetics can decrease effectiveness, depending on amounts.
It destroys *all* cells: endothelium and red blood cells (RBCs).
Significant extravasation can produce cutaneous necrosis.
Hemolysis of RBCs can cause cutaneous hemosiderin staining.

Box 92-2. Polidocanol Description

Polidocanol was originally developed as a topical anesthetic under the trade name Sch 600.
There are three groups of local anesthetics:
1. Esters: procaine, benzocaine, tetracaine
2. Amides: lidocaine, prilocaine, mepivacaine, procainamide, dibucaine
3. Urethane: polidocanol

It is generally classified as a weak detergent solution.
It should be diluted with distilled sterile water.
Patients should be warned about an Antabuse–alcohol reaction.
Elimination half-life is 4 hours, with 90% elimination within 12 hours; it does not cross the blood–brain barrier.
Injection is painless and cutaneous necrosis difficult to produce.

- Cotton balls with isopropyl alcohol or benzalkonium chloride (Zephiran).
- Tape (1 inch wide). (Some patients require paper tape.)
- Compression stockings. Some clinicians stock them in the office. Patients can also be given a prescription to purchase them at a medical supply store (with proper measurements noted on the prescription) or they may be fitted at certain retailers. Pantyhose, full-length stockings, thigh-high stockings, or calf-high stockings are selected based on the areas being injected. Rubber gloves are helpful to apply the stocking(s).
- Elastic wraps (4 to 6 inches wide; e.g., Ace bandages).
- Nonsterile gloves.

NOTE: Additional instruments that may be helpful, but not necessary, include a photoplethysmograph, light reflection rheograph, and a duplex scanner. Duplex ultrasound has become very important in phlebology, especially in the proper evaluation and treatment of patients with advanced venous disease.

PREPROCEDURE PATIENT PREPARATION

It is best if the patient receives patient education materials before the office visit (see the patient education handouts online at www.expertconsult.com). An initial visit is scheduled for 30 minutes. The patient is evaluated, venous testing is done, the legs are measured for hose, and counseling is completed. Future visits of 15 to 30 minutes are scheduled for the injections at 2- to 4-week intervals. It is best not to reinject the same area any sooner than 3 to 4 weeks. Average patients will require three 30-minute injection visits.

A careful history and physical examination must be performed (Fig. 92-5), and those problems that might affect treatment with sclerotherapy (e.g., anticoagulation, history of phlebitis, vein surgery, arterial disease, bleeding problems, diabetes, history of severe allergic reactions) should be sought.

Physical examination must include a careful evaluation of the pedal pulses. If they are not readily felt, it is necessary to obtain an ankle-to-brachial index. The only equipment needed for this is a blood pressure cuff, stethoscope, and handheld Doppler probe.

TABLE 92-3 Maximum Daily Doses of Polidocanol

	Dose (mL) According to Body Weight of Patient				
Concentration	50 kg	60 kg	70 kg	80 kg	90 kg
0.5%	20	24	28	32	36
1.0%	10	12	14	16	18
2.0%	5	6	7	8	9
3.0%	3.3	4	4.6	5.3	6

It is essential to look for the presence of saphenofemoral or saphenopopliteal reflux, also known as *axial vein reflux*. Its presence is a contraindication to sclerotherapy, and many insurance companies will not cover sclerotherapy if it is present. This determination can be accomplished with a careful hand-held Doppler examination. The patient must be standing. The tip of the Doppler probe is held at the saphenofemoral or saphenopopliteal junction while the calf muscle is firmly and sharply compressed. This creates a sound when the blood is propelled forward. As the muscle is released, there should be no retrograde flow (only silence). If flow is heard, it means there is reflux at these junctions. Newer techniques are indicated, including saphenous vein ablation with a radiofrequency or laser catheter (see Chapter 54, Lasers and Pulsed Light Devices: Leg Telangiectasia).

Patients are often screened with *photoplethysmography* (PPG) and *light reflection rheography*. These are means of measuring the venous refilling time of the lower limb using a transducer to shine a certain wavelength of light into the skin about 10 cm proximal to the medial malleolus. Hemoglobin specifically absorbs this wavelength. With the patient seated, he or she dorsiflexes the foot 8 to 10 times. This compresses and empties the normal dermal venous plexus. The light that is not absorbed by hemoglobin is reflected back to the transducer and is measured. This reflection back is greater when the veins are empty (less hemoglobin to absorb the light) and decreases when the veins are full because the vessels filled with blood (hemoglobin) absorb more light. The instrument then records how long it takes for the blood of the dermal plexus to return to baseline. A refilling time of less than 25 to 30 seconds indicates that the venous plexus is filling partially in a retrograde fashion and demonstrates incompetence of the venous system. If the test result is abnormal, a tourniquet should be applied just above and then below the knee. The test is repeated; if values normalize, it suggests that the problem is within the superficial venous system (Figs. 92-6 through 92-8) and that sclerotherapy can proceed. If the filling time does not normalize with above- and below-knee tourniquets, it suggests deep venous insufficiency and further evaluation (i.e., duplex ultrasonography) may be indicated.

PPG findings have been found to correlate well with venograms for the determination of DVT. In this instance, outflow of blood is blocked, and thereby the tracing is flat.

A duplex scan performed when the patient is standing allows an estimate of the location of venous reflux and its magnitude. The clinician can also look for DVT, venous obstruction, and incompetent perforators. Duplex ultrasound has emerged as the most reliable, cost effective, reproducible way to evaluate the lower extremity venous system. In recent years, units have become less expensive and training in ultrasonography is available.

Photographs of the lower limbs may be necessary. Some insurance companies require them. More important, photographs provide baseline information to which the patient's limbs can be compared as treatment progresses. Many phlebologists first draw the veins in on diagrams.

The technique of sclerotherapy must be carefully explained to the patient, including possible complications and what will happen over the course of treatment. The patient must be cautioned not to expect perfection. A well-educated patient is more cooperative and satisfied.

Technique

Before injecting the patient, obtain a signed consent (see the sample patient consent form online at www.expertconsult.com).

Wipe the area to be injected with Zephiran or alcohol. This not only cleanses the area but improves visualization of the vessels. Use a small syringe (1 or 3 mL). Stretch the skin surrounding the vessel with the nondominant hand. It is helpful to bend up the tip of the 30-gauge needle about 20 to 30 degrees to cannulate these tiny veins (Fig. 92-9).

Direct cannulation of the vein is absolutely essential. Extraluminal injections may lead to skin necrosis. For the treatment of veins 2 mm in diameter or less, 0.2% sodium tetradecyl sulfate is used. Although some therapists suggest a concentration of 0.1%, it is not necessary to decrease the concentration (Table 92-4, p. 615). Aspiration of blood from the small vessels cannot be accomplished. If a small wheal forms at the time of injection, the needle is not in the lumen and injection must be stopped. If the needle is properly inserted, the vessel should blanch. Once the blanching stops, withdraw the needle and go to the next vessel. More is *not* better unless new vessels continue to blanch. The injection is carried out with extremely gentle pressure, and only 0.1 to 0.3 mL is used. Too much pressure can rupture the vein and lead to unnecessary inflammation.

For injection of veins 3 to 5 mm, 0.5% sodium tetradecyl sulfate is used in a quantity of 0.5 mL to a maximum of 1.0 mL. Because a stronger solution is being used, it is more likely that subcutaneous injection may lead to tissue necrosis. Therefore, aspiration of blood into the hub of the needle is recommended before the injection of sclerosant.

For veins 5 to 6 mm in diameter, 1.0% sodium tetradecyl sulfate is used with a volume of 0.5 mL to a maximum of 1.0 mL (see Table 92-4). Aspiration before injection is essential.

All of the previously mentioned procedures can be performed with the patient supine. Spider veins will remain visible, but at times it may be difficult to cannulate large veins in a supine patient because the veins are not dilated and collapse when the patient lies down. In this case the patient should be asked to stand and the vein cannulated with a no. 27 butterfly that is taped in place. The patient can then be placed in a supine position and the vein injected as previously described. Alternatively, the veins are marked with a skin-marking pen in the standing position and can be injected when the patient lies down.

A compression dressing consisting of a folded piece of gauze is placed over each site and covered with a piece of Dermicel or similar tape. Paper tape is necessary for some patients to avoid allergic responses. A cotton ball and tape are used by many phlebologists and work well. The limb is then compressed either by elastic wraps or compression stockings, as discussed in the section on Compression.

NOTE: It is often quicker and easier to just wrap Coban or Co-Flex around the entire leg, followed by the compression hose. This keeps the blood off the hose and makes it easier to get the hose on the leg. These rolls are 4 inches wide and 9 yards long.

A complete note should be dictated (or a form used) for at least the first injection visit (Fig. 92-10, p. 616). After this, we recommend flow sheets to save time (Fig. 92-11, p. 617).

Pearls

Injection sclerotherapy using hypertonic saline solution or sodium tetradecyl sulfate is a safe, relatively painless method of ablating small varicose veins, reticular venules, and spider telangiectases, with a minimum of complications. The attending physician will have better results and happier patients if several important concepts are remembered:

- Although spider veins may be symptomatic, most patients seek treatment because they are unhappy with the appearance of their legs. The clinician should be cautious and conservative to avoid creating a blemish worse than what the patient already has.
- Sclerotherapy should be viewed as a semicosmetic procedure, and the patient's expectations must be carefully considered.
- Careful preinjection discussion of risks must occur with patients so that they are fully aware of the protracted and tedious nature of sclerotherapy, as well as the potential complications.
- The effect of gravity and incompetent venous valves must always be remembered. Varicose veins and spider veins tend to

Patient Questionnaire/Evaluation: Vein Injection (Sclerotherapy)

Date ________ Name ____ Birthdate ______________ Age __________
Sex ________ Height ________ Weight ________
Referred by: ______________________________

1. How many years have you noticed this problem? ___
2. Have you ever been previously treated for this problem?
   Yes ____ No ____
   By whom and when? ____________________________
   ____

   With what method?
   - Injection __________
   - Electrocautery __________
   - Laser __________
   - Surgery __________
3. When did the problem with your veins occur?
   - Age __________
   - Before pregnancy __________
   - After pregnancy __________
   - After trauma or Premarin therapy __________
   - Other __________
4. Is there a family history of varicose or spider veins?
   - Mother __________
   - Father __________
   - Sister __________
   - Brother __________
   - Children __________
   - Aunts __________
   - Uncles __________
5. Do you have a history of
   - Smoking __________
   - Blood clots __________
   - Lupus __________
   - Bleeding disorders __________
   - Easy bruisability __________
   - Dark spots after skin injury or surgery __________
   - Easy scarring __________
6. Are you developing new veins? ______
7. Are your present veins getting bigger? ______
8. After prolonged standing or sitting do your legs ache? ______
9. Do your legs or veins ache before menses? ______
10. Does walking or exercise relieve or aggravate the pain? (circle)
11. Describe any symptoms you have from your veins: ____________
    ____
12. Are you required to be on your feet for long periods? ______
13. Do you jog, run, jump rope, or do aerobics? (circle)
    How often per week? ______
14. Are you pregnant or planning a pregnancy soon? ______
15. Did you read and understand the patient education materials given to you? ______
16. Do you understand the risks and benefits as well as possible complications to vein injection? ______
17. Are you prepared to wear hose on a regular basis as described? ______
18. Is your problem cosmetic or medical? ______

PMH: MI: ____
ALL: ____
MEDS: ____
FH: ____

Figure 92-5 Patient questionnaire for sclerotherapy. (Modified from Mitchel P. Goldman, MD, Dermatology Associates of San Diego County, Inc., La Jolla, Calif.)

recur. The wearing of compression stockings in the immediate postinjection period is mandatory. Compression stockings worn on a long-term basis will significantly reduce recurrence.

- Meticulous technique is essential in sclerotherapy.
  - The clinician must be sure the needle is in the vein.
  - The solution should be injected slowly.
  - A maximum of 0.5 mL of solution should be used per injection, and large bolus injections should be avoided.
  - The clinician should watch the needle tip and stop injecting if there is any extravasation.
- The larger vessels should be injected first.
- The clinician should begin injections proximally and work down the leg. If injections are started distally, the proximal vessels often go into spasm and it is very difficult to inject them.
- Telangiectases will be visible when the patient lies down, but varicosities may disappear. It helps to mark them with a marking pen while the patient is standing.
- The clinician should not attempt to withdraw blood before injecting telangiectases; however, it is essential to withdraw blood before injecting larger vessels to be sure the needle is in the lumen.
- If a wheal is seen, the clinician should stop injecting immediately. The magnification loupes help identify this early in the procedure. If recognized early and the injection is stopped, the small blebs that occur generally do not lead to any tissue necrosis. Older texts recommended diluting the area with saline for extravasation, but it is not needed with these small amounts.

NOTE: With careful and precise technique, the majority of small telangiectatic (i.e., spider) veins can be eliminated. Patient satisfaction with the procedure is high.

Compression

The amount and duration of compression used with sclerotherapy remain somewhat controversial. Initially, Irish sclerotherapists who were treating large, bulging varicose veins used 6 weeks of continuous compression, a regimen quite difficult for the patient. Later studies suggested that 3 weeks of compression for large veins is adequate. Whether this should be used for 24 hours a day or only while the patient is standing is still an unsettled issue.

When injecting spider veins, elastic compression bandages (4 inches wide) can be used for the first 24 hours. The patient then removes the elastic bandage and the underlying dressings and wears lightweight, measured compression pantyhose (15 mm Hg–gradient hose). Many therapists use 20 to 30 mm Hg–gradient hose or even 30 to 40 mm Hg–gradient hose. The patient is asked to wear the hose during the course of treatment whenever he or she is out of

Patient Questionnaire/Evaluation: Vein Injection (Sclerotherapy)

Varicosities

	R	L
Vulvar		
Groin		
Thigh		
Below knee		

Pulses

	R	L
Femoral		
Popliteal		
Dorsalis pedis		
Posterior tibial		

Presence of

	R	L
Edema		
Stasis pig		
Cellulitis		
Active ulcer		
Healed ulcer		
Venules		
Tenderness		

	R	L
PPG		
PRG		
Doppler		

Impression: ______________________________

Plan: Discussed

- Method
- Cost
- Complications
  - hyperpigmentation
  - blistering
  - recurrence
  - pain
  - phlebitis
  - matting
- Stockings
- Number of anticipated visits

Measurements

Ankle ____________
Calf ____________
Thigh ____________
Length ____________
Shoe size ____________
Type:
Panty
Thigh high
Knee high
20/30 or 30/40

cc: ____________ ____________ Physician signature ____________ Date

Figure 92-5, cont.

bed. If the patient has sclerotherapy appointments every 2 to 3 weeks, for example, and requires three visits, the patient will wear the stockings for 9 or 10 weeks. After the last treatment, the clinician can suggest that the patient wear the stockings while out of bed for at least 10 more days (preferably for 3 weeks). A recent review confirmed that wearing support hose continuously for 3 days, then while ambulatory for 3 more weeks, markedly reduced complications and recurrence.

When larger veins are injected, 30- to 40-mm Hg–gradient compression hose are recommended. The type of stocking depends on the areas being injected. If the thighs and both lower limbs are involved, panty hose are best. Otherwise, a full-length stocking, thigh-high stocking, or calf-high stocking can be used if it compresses the areas that were injected. The physician can prescribe the stocking at the time of the patient's initial visit and the patient can then bring it to the first therapeutic session. Many of the stocking

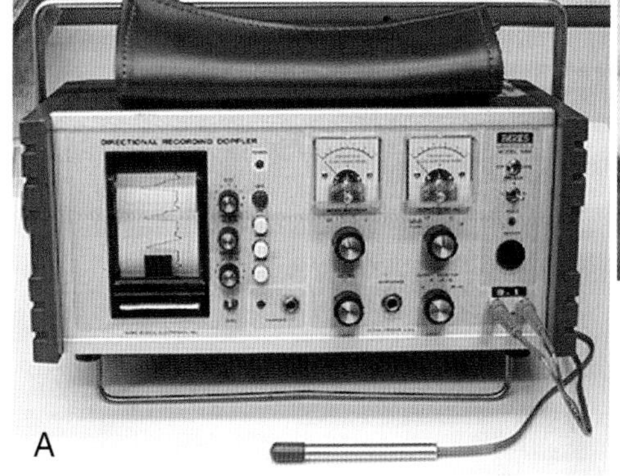

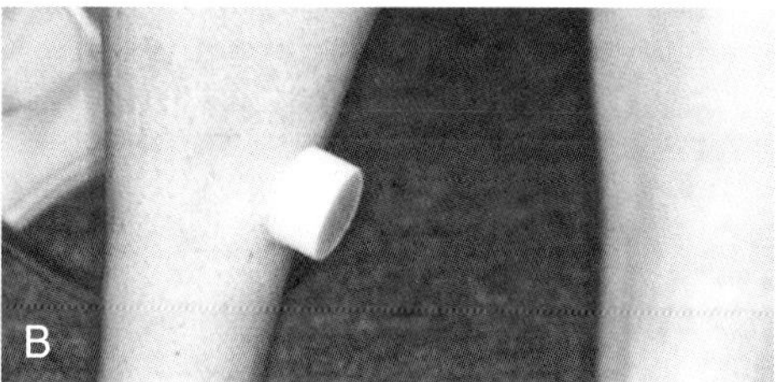

Figure 92-6 **A,** Photoplethysmography (PPG) machine. **B,** PPG machine attached to a patient. (*Author's note:* PPG has been important in the vascular laboratory, but in a clinical setting PPG has been largely replaced by duplex ultrasonography.)

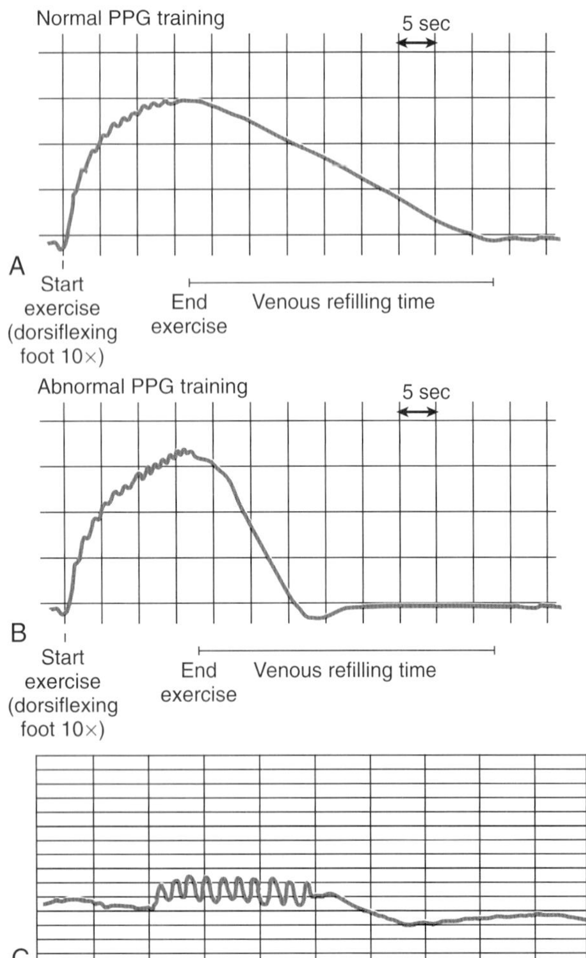

Figure 92-7 Tracings of photoplethysmography (PPG) readings. **A,** Normal. After dorsiflexing the foot 10 times, the blood has been "squeezed out" of the ankle, so less light is absorbed and more is reflected back. This gives a higher reading. As the veins refill with blood, more light is absorbed so less is reflected back. Thus, a lower amplitude is recorded. A refill time over 25 seconds is normal. **B,** Abnormal. Rapid refill indicating venous insufficiency. Refill time is only 15 to 17 seconds. (Without tourniquets, this could be deep or superficial; if tourniquets are in place, this is most likely indicative of deep venous insufficiency.) **C,** Abnormal. No indication of emptying, suggesting deep venous obstruction or marked insufficiency ("picket fence" pattern).

companies are quite good in supplying physician's offices with stockings and providing prompt, next-day delivery service. Ancillary personnel can learn to measure the patient for ready-made or custom stockings. The patient may then receive the stockings from the physician's office.

It is recommended that patients wear lightweight compression pantyhose as much as possible on an indefinite basis to diminish the recurrence of varicose veins or the development of new ones; however, many patients are resistant to such a regimen. Compression stockings are also used in the management of patients with post-thrombotic syndrome, healed venous ulcers, lymphedema, and other problems. Although patients can purchase cheaper over-the-counter hose, these generally provide only uniform compression and not a gradient of more to less pressure as the hose goes up the leg.

COMPLICATIONS

- *Bruising.* Patients must understand that they will look worse before they look better. It may take 4 to 8 weeks before the postsclerotherapy changes have resolved.

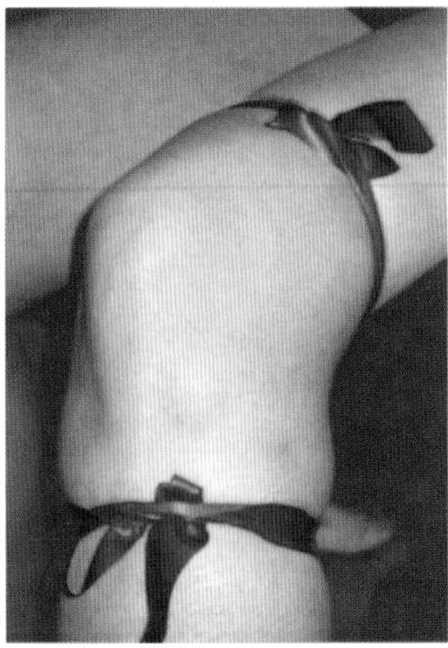

Figure 92-8 Placement of tourniquets above and below the knee when the photoplethysmogram is abnormal. If the tracing normalizes, it indicates superficial venous incompetence. If it remains abnormal with rapid refilling, deep venous insufficiency is suggested.

- *Hemosiderin staining (hyperpigmentation).* This occurs transiently in almost every case. It is considered a complication when it lasts for more than several weeks. In about 5% to 10% of patients, it can take up to 1 year to diminish. The discoloration follows the outline of the previously injected vein and can also be seen after stripping or phlebectomy. The larger the vein, the more likely it is to occur—especially if compression hose are not worn long enough. Unfortunately, in spite of trying many bleaching creams, little can be done to hasten resolution. If clots are evident, their removal lessens the duration of pigmentation. Prevention (with the use of compression hose) is the key.
- *Matting (neoangiogenesis).* This is the development of tiny vessels at or near the site of previous injection and occurs in 3% to 10% of patients. It may result from an injection under too high a pressure (causing rupture of the vessel) or because either the volume of the sclerosing solution was too large or the solution was too strong. Matting probably develops as part of the inflammatory response that occurs as the result of these errors in technique.

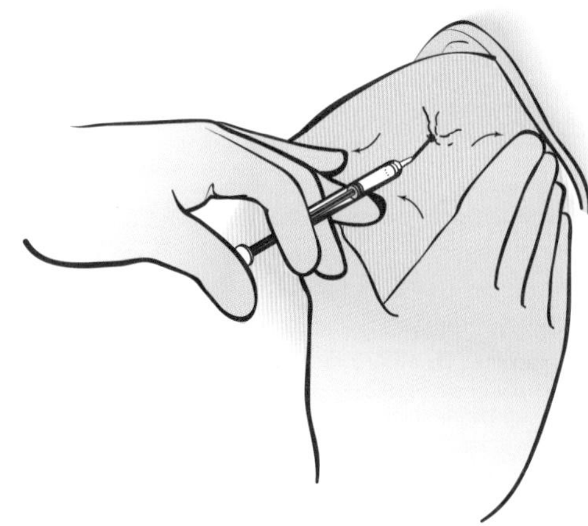

Figure 92-9 Proper injection technique. The nondominant hand stretches the skin around the vessels. The needle bevel is up and the needle itself is bent 30 degrees upward. (Redrawn from Sadick NS: Manual of Sclerotherapy. Philadelphia, Lippincott Williams & Wilkins, 2000.)

TABLE 92-4 Rapid Guide for Selection of Sclerosing Solution by Vessel Type*

Vessel	Solution/Concentration	Volume (per Injection Site)
Telangiectatic matting (after previous treatment)	**Hypertonic saline, 11.7%** **Sodium tetradecyl sulfate, 0.1%** Polidocanol, 0.25% (Go slow with low injection pressures)	0.1–0.2 mL
Telangiectasia (up to 1 mm)	**Hypertonic saline, 11.7%†** **Sodium tetradecyl sulfate, 0.1%–0.2%** Polidocanol, 0.25%	**0.1–0.3 mL**
Venulectasia (1–2 mm)	**Hypertonic saline, 11.7%–23.4%†** **Sodium tetradecyl sulfate, 0.1%–0.25%** Polidocanol, 0.5%–0.75%	**0.2–0.5 mL**
Reticular veins (2–4 mm, subcutaneous blue veins)	**Hypertonic saline, 18.7%–23.4%†** **Sodium tetradecyl sulfate, 0.33%–0.5%** Polidocanol, 0.75%–1.5%	0.5 mL (may increase to 1 mL if filling of reticular vein is observed)
Nonsaphenous varicose veins (3–8 mm)	**Hypertonic saline, 18.7%–23.4%** **Sodium tetradecyl sulfate, 0.5%–1.0%** Polidocanol, 1.0%–3.0%	0.5 mL (may increase to 1 mL per injection site in large-capacity vein)
Saphenous varicose trunks (usually >5 mm)	**Hypertonic saline, 18.7%–23.4%** **Sodium tetradecyl sulfate, 1.0%–3.0%** Polidocanol, 3.0%–5.0%	0.5 mL (low-volume injection critical at high concentrations)

*Solutions in **bold** approved by the U.S. Food and Drug Administration.
†Many use standard 18.7% for all these indications.

However, even with excellent technique, matting may occur. It may disappear in a few months. If it does not, the clinician should make a very careful search for a reticular vein leading into the area and try to obliterate it. Sometimes the matting itself can be injected or treated with light therapy, such as PhotoDerm or laser. If reinjection is done, the clinician should use low concentrations of sclerosants and inject slowly.

- *Skin slough with ulceration*. Usually this is related to extravasation of the solution. It may occur because of improper placement of the needle, rupture of the vein, having only part of the needle in the lumen, or injection of an arteriole. A tiny arteriole may also connect to a vein. In these cases, closure of the arteriole can cause a skin infarct. Ulcerations can even occur with a perfectly performed injection when the solution erodes through the wall of the vein into unhealthy skin. The ulceration often takes 4 to 8 weeks to resolve.
- *Arterial injection*. This is a dreaded complication. It will result in a large slough and even limb loss if a large artery it is injected. It is more likely to occur around the ankle, especially in the area of the posterior tibial artery.
- *Syncope*. This is more common if injections are done with the patient standing. At times standing is necessary when inserting butterfly needles; then have the patient assume a recumbent position for the injection of large veins.
- *Allergic reaction*. This will not occur with hypertonic saline, and it occurs extremely rarely with sodium tetradecyl sulfate (approximately 0.3%). When it does occur, it is usually a mild response, although anaphylaxis has been reported. Necessary equipment to treat this problem, such as an Ambu-bag, artificial airways, epinephrine for injection, steroid for injection, and an injectable anticonvulsant should be on hand (see Chapter 220, Anaphylaxis). Pretreatment of allergic patients with 50 mg of diphenhydramine (Benadryl) will obviate this problem.
- *Superficial thrombophlebitis*. Injection of sclerosant creates a chemical thrombophlebitis that is controlled and affects only the treated area. However, at times the solution can travel proximally or distally and create an area of thrombus within the veins. The area overlying this often becomes red and tender. In most cases careful technique using only a small amount of solution (0.5 to 1 mL) will prevent this outcome. It is more likely to occur when injecting larger veins. When it does occur, the patient must be reassured that nothing serious has happened. Treatment consists of compression and an anti-inflammatory drug (e.g., ibuprofen).
- *Thrombus formation*. Clots can form in small veins or especially in the larger ones. They can be aspirated with a needle or incised and drained. Usually for the larger ones, a small amount of lidocaine is injected, then a no. 11 blade used to open the skin over the area. Pressure will expel the clot. No suture is needed. Thrombi are more common when larger veins are injected and if compression is not optimal postinjection. If a clot has been present for more than 4 weeks, it often organizes and then is difficult to remove.
- *Postinjection itching and pain*. Patients often complain of a transient itching after injection; some phlebologists apply steroid cream immediately after injection, but this is not necessary. The site of injections may become painful. Over-the-counter pain medication, including nonsteroidal anti-inflammatory drugs (NSAIDs), is adequate to control this and does not interfere with the effectiveness of treatment. Pain during the injection is minimal and well tolerated.
- *DVT and pulmonary emboli*. Fortunately, this is a rare complication. It is most likely to occur if too much solution is used and it gets into the deep system. Patients who have had a prior venous thromboembolic event or who have an underlying thrombophilia are more likely to have this problem. Birth control pills and estrogen may slightly increase the tendency toward this complication, but it is rare and their use does not contraindicate sclerotherapy. DVT may be reduced or eliminated by having the patient walk for 20 to 30 minutes after injection of large veins to avoid pooling in the deep venous system.

Postprocedure Patient Education

Patients are asked to walk immediately after a session of sclerotherapy. Some therapists recommend 30 minutes, but even 5 or 10 minutes seems to be enough. Walking diffuses the solution that may have gone into the deep system and, more important, increases circulating fibrinolysins. (See the sample patient education form online at www.expertconsult.com.)

The same area should not be injected again for 3 to 4 weeks (Fig. 92-12). The patient can return at weekly intervals for treatment of alternate sites until treatment is complete. Patients should be able to resume normal activities, including high-impact aerobics

Sclerotherapy Treatment Note

Name: ______________________ Birthdate: ______________
Referring physician: ______________________ Date: ______________
Chief Complaint: Sclerotherapy injection

S: The patient has thought over what we have discussed on the last visit and has read over multiple patient education materials supplied. He/she has elected to go ahead and have the sclerotherapy performed today. We explained again the nature of the complications: hyperpigmentation, matting, recurrence, slight ulceration, phlebitis, and blebs. He/she understands these and has elected to go ahead and have the injections done. There were no further questions and subsequently we proceeded.

O: Venous sclerotherapy

Areas: ______________________
Sclerosant: ______________
Amount: ______________ mL
Number of complexes injected: ______________
Complications: None or ______________________

Procedure Note: The patient was once again examined in the supine position. The complexes of veins that were to be injected were noted. These areas were all wiped with Zephiran. Individual 1-mL syringes were used with 30-gauge needles. Each syringe was used no more than 3 to 4 times and no more than 0.5 mL of the solution was injected per vein site. In the majority of cases the vein was cannulated but in a few areas there was minimal extravasation of the sclerosant. After injection, a rolled 4 × 4 was immediately placed over the area and secured with paper tape. Upon completion of injection of the various veins, the Sigvaris/MediUSA/Jobst pantyhose/thigh high/above the knee support stockings, which were measured for the patient, were used to hold the pressure dressings in place. They were of the 20/30 gradient type. The patient tolerated this well and was discharged home.

Changes to routine: ______________________

Impression:
1. ______________________
2. ______________________

P: The patient will wear the stockings for at least __ days and __ nights without removing them. Cool baths can then soak off the tape making it easier to remove the pressure dressings. He/she is to wear the support hose for at least 4 weeks during the day but may remove them at night. After injection, he/she is to walk at least 30 minutes. Hot baths are to be avoided for at least 2 weeks. It is best to wear some type of support hose for the rest of his/her life since venous disease is an ongoing problem and the source of the problem is not resolved by the injections. It may be necessary to come back every 1–2 years to have "touch-ups" on new or recurrent veins. There may be some pigmentation from the veins. The patient should call should there be any significant problems. Follow-up in ____ weeks for a recheck and for any possible further injections.

Other: ______________________
cc: ______________ ______________ ______________
Physician signature Date

Figure 92-10 Sample form of a sclerotherapy treatment note. (Courtesy of The National Procedures Institute, Midland, Mich.)

and jogging, 24 hours after injections for spider veins; however, some therapists would further restrict patients for 1 week. No good prospective studies indicate the effect of robust activity on sclerotherapy.

Conclusion

Sclerotherapy, when practiced properly, is a highly effective means of treating small to medium-sized varicose veins and telangiectases. Many therapists treat even large varicosities in this manner. Laser and other forms of light therapy are not as efficient and effective in most instances. At best they are useful for treating veins 3 mm in diameter or smaller. Equipment and methods may improve the results of light therapy, but sclerotherapy remains the gold standard for treating such veins. Careful work-up and management of patients with special attention to proper technique should provide good to excellent results in more than 90% of patients.

CPT/Billing Codes

Injections for telangiectasia, even if symptomatic, are rarely covered by insurance. Coverage for varicosities is quite variable. It is often necessary to document that conservative therapy (e.g., use of compression stockings) has failed. Frequently, preapproval and photographs will be required.

Most sclerotherapists do not deal with insurance companies and ask the patient to pay at the time of service. Some will charge by the number of injections and others by the amount of solution used; still others will inject for a certain time period (15 to 30 minutes). There are no routine standards.

10140 I&D, hematoma
10160 Aspiration, hematoma
36468 Injection; multiple telangiectases, leg
36469 Injection; multiple telangiectases, face (see caution in the "Indications" section)

Follow-up Sclerotherapy

Patient :____________________ DOB: __________ Date: ____________________

Initial evaluation: __________________ Referring physician: ____________________

PPG: ____________________ Sclerosant:

Working diagnosis: Support hose/Ace wrap/other:

Date	Subjective/Examination	Treatment	Impression	Plan

Figure 92-11 Sample flow sheet for follow-up sclerotherapy appointments. (Courtesy of The National Procedures Institute, Midland, Mich.)

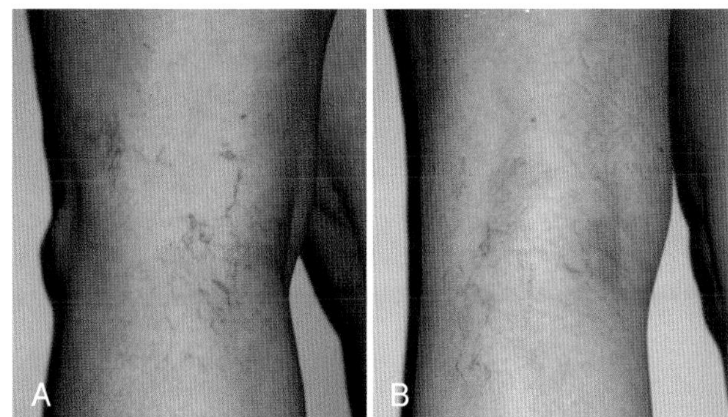

Figure 92-12 Telangiectasia treatment with hypertonic saline. **A**, Treatment was administered at time of initial photograph. **B,** Photograph obtained 2 months later.

36470 Injection of single varicose vein
36471 Injection of multiple varicose veins, same leg
-50 Modifier for bilateral procedure
93965 Impedance plethysmography
93970 Duplex scan

ICD-9-CM Diagnostic Codes

448.1 Spider vein/telangiectasia
448.9 Capillary vein
454.1 Varicosity with inflammation
454.1 Stasis dermatitis
454.2 Varicosity with ulceration
454.9 Varicose vein, leg
457.1 Lymphedema
459.1 Postphlebitic syndrome
459.81 Chronic venous insufficiency

709.0 Dyschromia of skin (hyperpigmentation)
729.5 Pain in leg
729.81 Swelling in leg
782.0 Burning, hyperesthesia
782.3 Edema
924.5 Hematoma, lower extremity

Patient Education Guides

See patient education and consent forms available online at www.expertconsult.com.

Acknowledgment

The editors wish to recognize the many contributions by Stanley A. Hirsch, MD, and John L. Pfenninger, MD, to this chapter in the previous edition of this text.

Suppliers

(See contact information online at www.expertconsult.com.)

Headlamp and ocular loupes
Luxtec
Welch Allyn
Hypertonic saline/Sotradecol
Delasco
Patient education materials
American Academy of Dermatology Association
Contemporary Health Communications
MJD Patient Communications
Website: www.mjdpc.com
Polidocanol
Pharmacy Specialists (Sam Pratt, RPh)
Support hose
BSN-Jobst Institute, Inc.
MediUSA
Sigvaris
Syringes and needles
Air-Tite Products Company
Venous noninvasive diagnostic equipment (e.g., PPG, Doppler) and assistance with all sclerotherapy supplies
Sam Wagner
PO Box 431
202 Dodd St.
Middlebourne, WV 26149
304-758-2370

NOTE: This is a superb resource.

Bibliography

Alam M, Nguyen TH (eds): Treatment of Leg Veins. Procedures in Cosmetic Dermatology Series, Dover JS, series editor. Philadelphia, Saunders, 2006.
Bergan JJ, Kistner RL (eds): Atlas of Venous Surgery. Philadelphia, WB Saunders, 1992.
Conrad P, Malouf GM, Stacey MC: The Australian polidocanol (Aethoxysklerol) study: Results at 2 years. Dermatol Surg 21:334–336, 1995.
Goldman MP, Beaudoing D, Marley W, et al: Compression in the treatment of leg telangiectasia: A preliminary report. J Dermatol Surg Oncol 16:322–325, 1990.
Goldman MP, Bergan JJ (eds): Ambulatory Treatment of Venous Disease. St. Louis, Mosby, 1996.
Goldman MP, Bergan JB, Guex JJ: Sclerotherapy: Treatment of Varicose and Telangiectatic Leg Veins, 4th ed. London, Elsevier Mosby, 2006.
NOTE: This is the "bible" and a must for anyone performing sclerotherapy.
Goldman MP, Sadick NS, Weiss RA: Cutaneous necrosis, telangiectatic matting, and hyperpigmentation following sclerotherapy: Etiology, prevention, and treatment. Dermatol Surg 21:19–29, 1995.
Goldman MP, Weiss RA: Endovenous ablation techniques with ambulatory phlebectomy for varicose veins. In Robinson JK, Hanke DW, Sengelmann RD, Siegel DM (eds): Surgery of the Skin: Procedural Dermatology. Philadelphia, Mosby, 2005, pp 645–656.
Goldman MP, Weiss RA, Bergan JJ (eds): Varicose Veins and Telangiectasias. St. Louis, Quality Medical, 1999.
Goldman MP, Weiss RA, Brody HJ, et al: Treatment of facial telangiectasia with sclerotherapy, laser surgery, and/or electrodesiccation: A review. J Dermatol Surg Oncol 19:899–906, 1993.
Green D: Sclerotherapy for varicose and telangiectatic veins. Am Fam Physician 46:827–837, 1992.
Isaacs MN: Symptomatology of vein disease. Dermatol Surg 21:321–323, 1995.
Kanter AH: The effect of sclerotherapy on restless legs syndrome. Dermatol Surg 21:328–332, 1995.
Olivencia JA: Varicose veins: Not just a cosmetic problem. Patient Care 15:140–158, 1996.
Pfeifer JR, Hawtof GD: Injection sclerotherapy and CO_2 laser sclerotherapy in the ablation of cutaneous spider veins of the lower extremity. Phlebology 4:231, 1989.
Sadick NS: Manual of Sclerotherapy. Philadelphia, Lippincott Williams & Wilkins, 2000.
NOTE: This source is superb, concise, thorough, and practical.
Tibbs DJ, Sabiston DC, Davies MG, et al. (eds): Varicose Veins: Venous Disorders and Lymphatic Problems in the Lower Limb. New York, Oxford University Press, 1997.
Tretbar LL: Injection sclerotherapy for spider telangiectasias: A 20-year experience with sodium tetradecyl sulfate. J Dermatol Surg Oncol 15: 223–225, 1989.
Weiss RA, Dover JS: Leg vein management: Sclerotherapy, ambulatory phlebectomy, and laser surgery. In Kaminer MS, Dover JS, Arndt KA (eds): Atlas of Cosmetic Surgery. Philadelphia, WB Saunders, 2002, pp 407–432.
Weiss RA, Sadick NS, Goldman MP, Weiss MA: Post-sclerotherapy compression: Controlled comparative study of duration of compression and its effect on clinical outcome. Dermatol Surg 25:105–108, 1999.

CHAPTER 93

EXERCISE ELECTROCARDIOGRAPHY (STRESS) TESTING

Grant C. Fowler • Michael A. Altman

Seventeen million Americans have known coronary artery disease (CAD); however, in more than half of everyone else in whom CAD will be diagnosed, the diagnosis will *follow a bad outcome*—namely, a myocardial infarction (MI) or sudden cardiac death. Approximately one third of all deaths (more than half a million per year) in the United States are caused by CAD, the leading cause of death in both sexes. Exercise electrocardiography (ECG) testing (EET) is not only a safe (<1 event per 10,000 properly selected patients) and cost-effective method for diagnosing CAD, it is probably the most cost-effective method to screen for and manage CAD. EET can also be used to reassure patients about the safety of exercise and to customize their exercise prescription.

For the diagnosis of CAD, although much money, time, and effort have been spent designing and applying other tests with greater sensitivity, the sensitivity of EET exceeds 90% (perhaps 95%) for *significant* CAD—meaning left main CAD or multivessel disease with resultant left main equivalent CAD (i.e., left ventricular [LV] dysfunction resulting from ischemia). Supporting this, several studies have examined the incremental value of exercise myocardial perfusion imaging compared with EET for diagnosis and risk stratification of CAD. In an analysis of these studies, the modest incremental benefit of imaging did not appear to justify its cost (which has been estimated at $20,550 per additional patient correctly classified). Consequently, the American College of Cardiology (ACC) and the American Heart Association (AHA) recommend a stepwise strategy for diagnosing CAD in patients with an intermediate pretest likelihood, using an EET as the initial test, and not an imaging procedure, if the patient is able to exercise, has a normal resting ECG, and is not taking digoxin* (ACC/AHA/ASNC Guidelines). (See chapter 94, Stress Echocardiography, for testing patients with an abnormal resting ECG or who are taking digoxin, and for a dobutamine echo protocol for patients unable to exercise.)

With medical management of CAD more successful than ever, primary care clinicians' skills in managing CAD have become more important. Performing EET is one method of maximizing these skills. In fact, using the Duke Treadmill Score (DTS) or nomogram for positive tests, primary care clinicians can now risk-stratify and prognose CAD as well as their cardiologist colleagues. It should be noted that in the latest guidelines (2002, 2007) from AHA/ACC for management of stable CAD, an EET is a reasonable test for risk stratification in patients with a normal resting ECG and who are able to exercise. In part, these guidelines are based on "the simplicity, lower cost, and widespread familiarity with the performance and interpretation of the standard EET." Also, when patients divided into risk groups using EET have been studied with imaging (Gibbons and colleagues, 1999), few patients (<5%) who have a low-risk DTS (≤1% annual cardiac mortality rate) will be identified as high risk after imaging, and thus the cost of identifying these patients again argues against routine imaging. Those patients identified as high risk (≥3% per year annual cardiac mortality) should probably be referred directly for cardiac catheterization and a possible intervention (again, see Chapter 94, Stress Echocardiography). Only those patients with an intermediate DTS (>1% and <3%) seem to benefit from an imaging study to further differentiate low-risk patients from those who might benefit from an intervention.

Performing a maximal EET provides additional information valuable for predicting prognosis, such as exercise capacity and heart rate in recovery (HRR, explained later), even if the ECG cannot be used for interpretation or predicting prognosis. From a study of 7163 patients (Diaz and colleagues, 2001) with known or suspected CAD undergoing myocardial perfusion imaging at the Cleveland Clinic and for whom a DTS could not be calculated (e.g., patient taking digoxin, resting ECG abnormalities), the independent prognostic values of exercise capacity and HRR were determined. Patients were followed for an average of 6.7 years, and, when compared with results of myocardial perfusion imaging, not only did exercise capacity and HRR provide additional prognostic information, but if exercise capacity and HRR were both abnormal, it portended a higher risk of mortality than the result from the myocardial perfusion test in nonrevascularized patients.

Primary care clinicians can also use EET to screen certain asymptomatic individuals. Such screening may be especially helpful for diabetic patients, firefighters, anyone about to undergo noncardiac surgery, high-risk patients after revascularization, patients about to undergo cardiac rehabilitation, and older individuals about to embark on a vigorous exercise program. Although the ACC/AHA are not currently recommending EET to screen all asymptomatic individuals, there is emerging evidence that this will be a future growth area for the procedure. A negative EET demonstrating good exercise capacity combined with a negative multidetector (>32-slice) computed tomography (CT) angiogram, which has a false negative rate of less than 2% for CAD, will likely be our ultimate screening test for CAD. In the meantime, with estimates that 12% of deaths in the United States are due to a lack of exercise, any method to motivate patients to exercise should be beneficial. EET can be used not only to reassure individuals of the safety of exercise, but to customize their exercise prescription. After almost every EET, patients should receive some type of customized exercise prescription based on their true maximal heart rate (MHR), their exercise (aerobic) capacity, and the test results. We now know that almost every patient benefits from an exercise program, even cardiac transplant recipients. In fact, of all the options available, exercise may be the single best method for improving endothelial function.

Benefits of performing EET in the primary care clinician's office include having test results immediately available, improving communication and referral patterns to cardiologists, and improving primary care clinicians' ECG reading skills. Clinicians performing EET also naturally improve their understanding of CAD pathophysiology as well as exercise physiology. With results immediately

*EET has a higher specificity in the absence of 1 mm ST segment depression due to resting ST segment changes, LV hypertrophy, and digoxin use.

available, patient satisfaction is usually improved and liability from failure to diagnose should be decreased. Using the DTS when there is a positive study, the patient can immediately be counseled from an outcomes or prognosis perspective. Such data allow a patient to make a truly informed decision before undergoing a major procedure, such as coronary artery bypass graft (CABG) surgery. With personalized data, the patient can weigh his or her known risks of forgoing surgery against available known risks of an intervention, with interventions reserved for those who choose to accept the risks.

For primary care clinicians covering emergency departments or urgent care centers, or those working as hospitalists, knowledge of a patient's recent EET results may be helpful for perioperative evaluation. Management of patients with an acute chest pain syndrome is also greatly facilitated when EET is available. For many patients, after myocardial damage has been excluded by serial blood tests, resolution of the symptoms, and stabilized ECG findings, an EET may be useful for triage or early discharge. National guidelines with algorithms are available, and they have been demonstrated to be both safe and useful.

Physiology of Exercise ECG Testing

Performing exercise increases *total* oxygen demand and consumption, with the amount of increase depending on the size of the muscles used. In other words, the larger the muscles, the more oxygen is consumed. Oxygen demand and consumption also increase as the intensity of exercise increases. In response to increased exercise and oxygen demand, the body increases ventilation, oxygenation, cardiac output, and oxygen extraction by tissues. Unless there is moderate to severe lung disease (e.g., chronic obstructive pulmonary disease) or a process severely limiting oxygen transport or extraction (e.g., severe anemia), cardiac output is usually the factor limiting an individual's maximal exercise capacity. In turn, the limiting factor for cardiac output in those with obstructive CAD is usually coronary blood flow. Maximal exercise capacity can therefore be limited by coronary blood flow. In fact, maximal exercise capacity is usually quantified by measuring or estimating an individual's maximal oxygen uptake ($\dot{V}O_2$ max). In other words, maximal exercise with large muscles can be used both to estimate $\dot{V}O_2$ max and to evaluate limitations in coronary blood flow.

Cardiac output is calculated by multiplying the stroke volume by the heart rate; therefore, increases in either the stroke volume or the heart rate will increase the cardiac output. Increasing the stroke volume is generally a more efficient method of increasing cardiac output (i.e., requires less oxygen). However, unless the patient is taking a beta blocker, the initial physiologic response to increased demand for cardiac output is usually an increase in heart rate. (In part, this is why beta blockers work for treating angina; they block the increase in heart rate when there is a need for increased cardiac output, thereby forcing an increase in stroke volume and keeping the increased myocardial oxygen demand to a minimum.) Therefore, as intensity of exercise increases, heart rate increases up to a maximum (MHR), usually when the patient has reached maximal voluntary effort or exertion.

In normal patients there is a linear relationship between *myocardial* oxygen demand and heart rate. In other words, the faster the heart rate, the more oxygen the heart requires. Because the heart rate continues to increase as exercise intensity increases, so does the myocardial oxygen demand. MHR can be crudely *estimated* based on age (i.e., 220 − age in years ≅ MHR) or by using graphs; however, *true* MHR is best determined with a maximal EET. MHR is the heart rate noted when the patient is at maximal voluntary effort (voluntarily fatigued), and this number should be recorded and given to the patient at the completion of each EET when the clinician is customizing an exercise prescription.

There is also a linear relationship between myocardial oxygen demand and systolic blood pressure (SBP). In other words, the higher the SBP, the harder the heart is working (and consequently the higher the myocardial oxygen demand). Therefore, one method of quantifying the overall *myocardial* oxygen demand is to multiply the SBP by the heart rate; the product obtained is the *double product*, also known as the *rate–pressure product (RPP)*. At any given moment the RPP is therefore an estimate of total myocardial oxygen demand; as long as the demand has not exceeded the supply, it is also a measure of total myocardial oxygen uptake or consumption. In other words, the higher the RPP, the more oxygen the heart is demanding; if supply is matching demand, the higher the capacity the heart has to deliver its own oxygen.

When the myocardium demands more oxygen, there are two options for supplying it: either the coronary arterial *flow* increases or the *extraction* of oxygen from the flow increases. As it turns out, increased myocardial oxygen demand during exercise is met primarily through an increase in coronary arterial flow rather than through increased oxygen extraction. This is because myocardial tissue is very efficient at extracting almost all of the available oxygen from the coronary arterial flow, even in the resting state. Therefore, coronary arterial *flow* is usually the limiting factor for cardiac oxygenation. This is especially true in patients with obstructive CAD.

With gradually increasing levels of exertion in the patient with obstructive CAD, a threshold is eventually reached where the heart's supply of oxygen cannot meet the demand. At this threshold, the heart becomes ischemic, initially at the subendocardial layer. With subendocardial ischemia, the patient usually demonstrates ECG changes in the form of ST segment depression. Usually, and eventually, this is followed by chest discomfort (i.e., angina). Because in most cases the ischemia is due to a fixed lesion, patients develop these ECG changes at about the same threshold or RPP every time. If symptoms occur, they also occur at the same RPP and follow the same pattern every time. In other words, angina caused by a fixed lesion does not radiate only into the left arm one day and into the right arm another day. If ST segment depression occurs (due to ischemia) and angina is not experienced, the diagnosis is silent ischemia.

Large muscles, such as leg muscles, rapidly increase the oxygen demand with increased exertion (e.g., using a treadmill or bicycle). $\dot{V}O_2$ max is the greatest amount (i.e., volume) of oxygen that a person can extract from inspired air while performing dynamic exercise. It is usually reached when the patient is in the anaerobic range. Measuring $\dot{V}O_2$ max is a method of quantifying maximal exercise capacity, and $\dot{V}O_2$ max varies with body weight, heredity, sex, and exercise habits. It often decreases progressively with age, but this decrease may be purely due to inadequate exercise habits. Performing aerobic exercise on a regular basis may maintain a constant $\dot{V}O_2$ max for life. There is a nearly linear relationship between $\dot{V}O_2$ max and the maximum cardiac output; therefore the $\dot{V}O_2$ max is a measure of the functional capacity of the cardiovascular system. It can be measured directly with inspired/expired gas analysis or more easily estimated from a maximal EET. As mentioned previously, in those with CAD, $\dot{V}O_2$ max may be limited by coronary blood flow. With prognosis data discussed later in this chapter, estimating $\dot{V}O_2$ max is very important for predicting outcomes from a cardiovascular perspective.

Basal oxygen consumption, or 1 metabolic equivalent (1 MET), defines the amount of oxygen an average individual consumes sitting at rest, which is approximately 3.5 mL/kg/min (i.e., 1 MET = 3.5 mL/kg/min O_2). $\dot{V}O_2$ max is often quantified as a multiple of the basal oxygen consumption in METs. For instance, walking 2 miles per hour (mph) on level ground requires approximately 2 METs. Walking 4 mph on level ground requires approximately 4 METs. Moderately active young men usually have a $\dot{V}O_2$ max of at least 42 mL/kg/min, or 12 METs. This means they are able to consume 12 times the amount of oxygen that they consume at rest. Obviously METs can also be used as a conversion factor between types of exercise. Charts are available (Fig. 93-1) to estimate a patient's exercise capacity or maximal METs by cross-referencing MET levels with different daily activities. This estimate may then be used to predict performance before placing a patient on a treadmill. Performing a maximal EET remains one of the more accurate methods

VETERANS' ADMINISTRATION SPECIFIC ACTIVITY QUESTIONNAIRE

Instructions to patient: Draw a line below the activities done routinely with minimal or no symptoms, such as shortness of breath, chest discomfort, and fatigue.

1 MET:	Eating, getting dressed, working at desk
2 METs:	Taking a shower
3 METs:	Walking slowly on a flat surface for one or two blocks Doing a moderate amount of work around the house, such as vacuuming, sweeping the floors, or carrying groceries
4 METs:	Doing light yard work (e.g., raking leaves, weeding, light carpentry, or painting)
5 METs:	Walking briskly (5 mph), dancing
6 METs:	Playing nine holes of golf carrying own clubs, performing heavy carpentry or mowing lawn with a push mower
7 METs:	Playing tennis (singles), carrying 60 lbs
8 METs:	Moving heavy furniture Jogging slowly, climbing stairs quickly, carrying 20 lbs upstairs
9 METs:	Bicycling at a moderate pace, sawing wood, jumping rope (slowly)
10 METs:	Swimming briskly, bicycling up a hill, walking briskly uphill, jogging 6 mph
11 METs	Skiing cross-country Playing basketball (full court)
12 METs:	Running briskly and continuously (level ground, 8-minute miles)
13 METs:	Rowing, backpacking, any competitive activity, including those that involve intermittent sprinting, running competitively

Figure 93-1 Veterans' Administration specific activity questionnaire.

of estimating maximal METs. An individual's maximal METs, whether determined on a bicycle or a treadmill, has significant management and prognosis implications if the person has CAD. Even if the test is positive for CAD, achieving certain MET thresholds can be very reassuring for prognosis.

During a maximal EET, a perceived exertion scale (PES) may be helpful for monitoring the patient. The PES is similar to a pain scale; however, the patient quantifies "effort" or "exertion" instead of "pain" during testing. Originally studied and published with a scale from 5 to 20 (with 20 being the subjective maximum that an individual could work and 5 being minimal or no work at all), it has now been modified. Most clinicians in the United States use a range from 1 to 10 (Box 93-1) for the PES. Although it is a subjective measurement, in most patients the PES level is very reproducible; in other words, if they were asked to repeat the EET in 2 weeks, they would report the same PES level at the same workload and

Box 93-1. Perceived Exertion Scale

0	Nothing at all
0.5	Very, very weak
1	Very weak
2	Weak
3	Moderate
4	Somewhat strong
5	Strong
6	
7	Very strong
8	
9	
10	Very, very strong

duration for both EETs. Interestingly, their heart rate is also usually very similar at a given PES. As a result, a PES target can be given to most patients to use as part of their exercise prescription. This replaces the patient's need to check the heart rate during exercise, and anything that simplifies an exercise prescription will, it is hoped, increase the chance of adherence/compliance.

A positive test result occurs when subendocardial ischemia causes *ST segment depression* on the ECG tracing. Because this is a "global" phenomenon, meaning much of the subendocardial layer is affected, it is almost always seen in more than one lead; if suspected it should be confirmed in an area of the ECG tracing where the baseline is relatively flat. True ischemia will cause ST segment depression for at least three beats in a row, and the ischemia (ST changes) usually persists or worsens during the recovery period. ST segment depression occurs because ischemia impairs the sodium/potassium adenosine triphosphatase (Na^+/K^+ ATPase) pump at the cellular level. Such an ST segment change can also be noted in patients taking digitalis, whose site of action is the Na^+/K^+ ATPase pump. When the pump is affected, there is a resultant change in the Na^+/K^+ intracellular gradient and a subsequent small shift in polarity. This shift in polarity is what is noted on the ECG tracing as ST segment depression.

With exercise-induced ischemia, ST segment depression becomes a global phenomenon, meaning it involves the entire subendocardium. When one area of the subendocardium becomes ischemic, there is a "fail-safe" mechanism that responds, meaning this subendocardial segment reduces its workload or shuts down before becoming permanently damaged. As a result, the remaining and surrounding subendocardium must work harder to compensate. This surrounding area subsequently becomes ischemic, and a domino effect occurs, cascading around the entire subendocardium. Consequently, ST segment depression is usually seen in multiple leads. In fact, this is such a global phenomenon that the coronary vessels involved cannot be predicted by which of the leads are demonstrating ST segment depression. (If knowledge of the coronary vessels involved or the total burden of ischemia is needed, an imaging test [myocardial perfusion or echocardiogram, see Chapter 94, Stress Echocardiography] should be added to the stress test.)

If the entire wall of the myocardium (full thickness) becomes ischemic, such as from severe CAD, *ST segment elevation* may be noted. It may appear very similar to that seen with a transmural/ST-elevation infarct or a ventricular aneurysm. In this situation, unless the clinician is certain that the finding is due to a ventricular aneurysm (e.g., associated with Q waves, or the clinician previously diagnosed/managed the infarct), the EET should be stopped. If either transmural ischemia or a new infarction is occurring, the potential for an arrhythmia is very high. However, transmural ischemia is rare in a community setting. In almost all positive EETs, *ST segment depression* is what is noted, the same as with what used to be called a *subendocardial infarct*. The subendocardial layer is usually the first to become ischemic because it is the "watershed" area of the heart, or the farthest from the arteries that are located in the epicardium (Figs. 93-2 and 93-3).

Certain other conditions may also make it difficult to perfuse the subendocardial layer, even in the absence of CAD. Normally the subendocardial layer is perfused during diastole and relies on perfusing "downhill" from 80 to 90 mm Hg of diastolic blood pressure (DBP) to an area where there is only 5 to 10 mm Hg pressure (i.e., end-diastolic pressure [EDP]). Thus, the pressure gradient, or the difference between "uphill" DBP and "downhill" EDP, is 80 or 90 minus 5 or 10, which is a 75 to 85 mm Hg difference (DBP – EDP = 75 to 85). If hypertension is poorly controlled, EDP may be elevated, reaching as high as 30 to 40 mm Hg, with the resultant drop in this pressure gradient (DBP – EDP = 40 to 60). In other words, there is much less "pressure" for blood to flow "downhill." Anything causing diastolic dysfunction, such as profound hypothyroidism or severe valvular disease, can also result in an elevated EDP, a decreased pressure gradient, and a false-positive EET result. A thickened myocardial wall, as seen in left ventricular hypertrophy, can

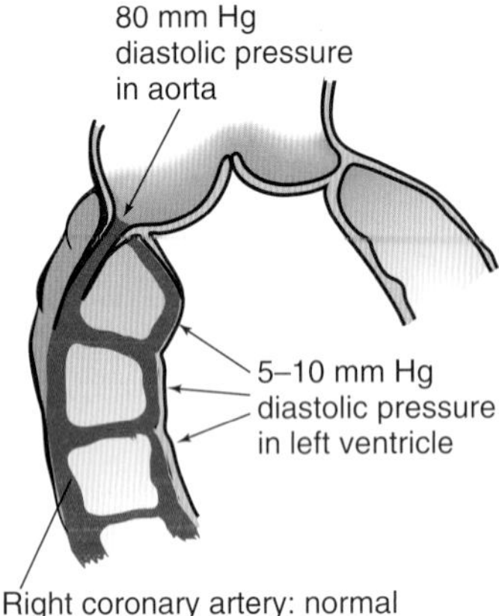

Figure 93-2 Normal myocardial perfusion. Note perfusion gradient is from 80 mm Hg to 5 to 10 mm Hg. (Redrawn from Ellestad MH: Stress Testing: Principles and Practice, 4th ed. Philadelphia, FA Davis, 1996.)

make it physically difficult to perfuse through the wall, thereby causing subendocardial ischemia and ST segment depression, even without CAD. In addition to physical causes, other situations that can cause false-positive results include hypokalemia and other electrolyte imbalances. Inadequate potassium prevents the Na^+/K^+ ATPase pump from functioning correctly, resulting in ST segment changes. As mentioned previously, digitalis may also result in ST segment depression, even at physiologic doses.

Normal Clinical Responses to Exercise ECG Testing

1. A gradual increase in heart rate to MHR where MHR is estimated by the formula 220 − age (i.e., 220 − age ≅ MHR). If a heart rate of 120 beats per minute (bpm) cannot be achieved, the diagnosis of *chronotropic incompetence* is possible (see "Interpretation" section).
2. Return of the heart rate to resting values within the first few minutes after exercise. The rate of return of the heart rate to its resting value depends partly on the exercise conditioning effect on vagal tone (i.e., frequent exercise or "being fit" increases vagal tone). An *abnormal* HRR is declared when the heart rate does not decrease by at least 12 bpm in the first minute of recovery (see "Interpretation" section).
3. A gradual rise in SBP. SBP is usually the highest at maximal workload. A drop in SBP during the exercise phase of EET, especially if it drops below resting standing SBP, may indicate severe CAD. An SBP greater than 214 mm Hg is designated a *systolic hypertensive response to exercise* (see "Interpretation" section).
4. A return of SBP and DPB to resting values by approximately 3 minutes after exercise. Failure of return of either blood pressure to normal by 3 minutes of recovery is also a *hypertensive response to exercise* (see "Interpretation" section).
5. Minimal change or a decrease in DBP during exercise. During exercise, the legs produce lactic acid, one of the most potent vasodilators known. As a result, a significant amount of blood volume flows into the legs. Because of this vasodilation, and the effects of exercise on Korotkoff sounds, diastolic pressure by auscultation can decrease all the way to zero in normal individuals. An increase in DBP of more than 10 mm Hg is also designated a *diastolic hypertensive response to exercise* (see "Interpretation" section).
6. Most patients perceive an increase by 1 to 3 points on the PES per stage of exercise. Few ever admit to reaching a full 10 points on the scale. For many patients, PES level increases rapidly from 7 to 9 when they are near maximal effort.

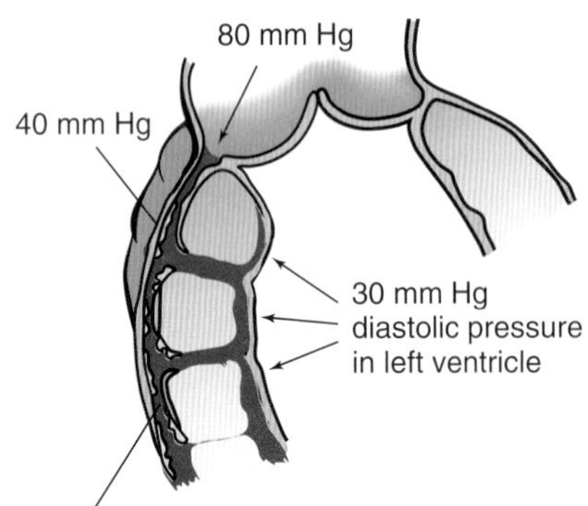

Figure 93-3 Myocardial perfusion in coronary artery disease (CAD). Note perfusion gradient is only from 40 mm Hg to 30 mm Hg. (Redrawn from Ellestad MH: Stress Testing: Principles and Practice, 4th ed. Philadelphia, FA Davis, 1996.)

Indications

Comprehensive, national guidelines are available regarding the appropriate use of EET, including special cases and situations (e.g., diabetic patients, patients in the emergency department, firefighters, before noncardiac surgery, before and after revascularization). There are three general indications for EET: *diagnosing CAD* (especially helpful when evaluating atypical chest pain and screening asymptomatic patients at significant risk), *managing CAD*, and *providing data for an exercise prescription* while determining exercise capacity and safety. In certain cases, several of these indications are evaluated during the same procedure. An example would be a patient who has an intermediate pretest likelihood and is found to have CAD when performing the EET. Because the diagnosis has now been made, if it is considered safe to continue the procedure, prognosis may also be determined. Exercise capacity (i.e., aerobic capacity) could be determined if the patient were allowed to complete a maximal EET; this is helpful for determining prognosis. Based on the results, an exercise prescription along with cardiac rehabilitation might be initiated. In this manner, the diagnosis, management (e.g., prognosis, cardiac rehabilitation), and exercise prescription could all be determined during the same test.

General Indications

1. Diagnosing CAD
   - Patients with an intermediate (20% to 70%) pretest probability of CAD based on sex, age, and symptoms (see "Determination of Pretest Likelihood," later; Fig. 93-4 and Table 93-1).
   - Asymptomatic patients with multiple risk factors, possible myocardial ischemia on ambulatory ECG monitoring, or an abnormal coronary calcium score from electron-beam computed tomography (EBCT) scan. It should be noted that asymptomatic patients are included in the graphs and tables (see Fig. 93-4 and Table 93-1) used to determine pretest probability.

   NOTE: For diagnosing CAD, determining pretest likelihood is important. This is explained for patients with symptoms by examples in the section "Determination of Pretest Likelihood."
2. Managing CAD*
   - Patients with known or highly probable CAD, for initial assessment or for a change in symptoms
   - After MI or revascularization (especially those at high risk), for prognostic assessment, activity prescription, evaluation of medical therapy, or cardiac rehabilitation
   - Demonstrating proof of ischemia before revascularization
   - Consider for perioperative evaluation of patients with CAD *only* if results would change management

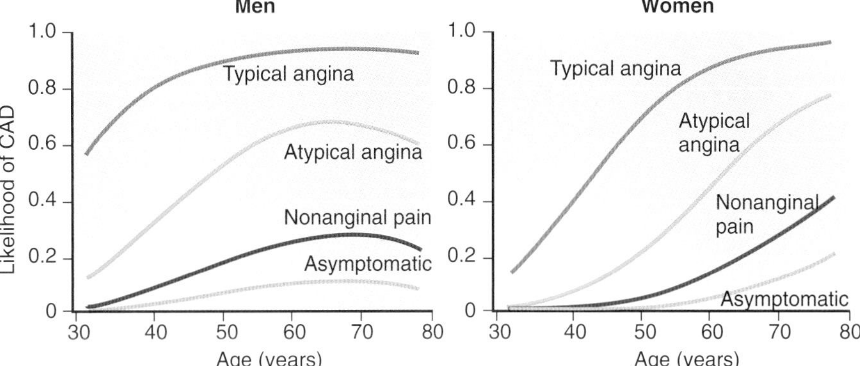

Figure 93-4 Pretest likelihood of coronary artery disease (CAD). (Redrawn from Diamond GA, Forrester JS: Analysis of probability as an aid in the clinical diagnosis of coronary-artery disease. N Engl J Med 300:1350–1358, 1979.)

TABLE 93-1 Pretest Likelihood of Coronary Artery Disease Based on Symptoms

Age (yr)	Asymptomatic	Nonanginal Chest Pain	Atypical Angina	Typical Angina
Women				
35	0.3	1	4	26
45	1	3	13	55
55	3	8	32	79
65	8	19	54	91
Men				
35	2	5	22	70
45	6	14	46	87
55	10	22	59	92
65	12	28	67	94

Adapted from Diamond GA, Forrester JS: Analysis of probability as an aid in the clinical diagnosis of coronary artery disease. N Engl J Med 300:1350–1358, 1979. In Fowler GC, Evans CH, Altman MA: Office procedures: Exercise testing. Prim Care 24:375–406, 1997.

3. Determining exercise prescription data, exercise capacity, and safety
   - Evaluation of exercise-related symptoms, including possible exercise-induced arrhythmias* (also see Chapter 87, Ambulatory Electrocardiography: Holter and Event Monitoring).
   - Graded treadmill EET is one of the best methods for determining an individual's MHR. The exception is the elite athlete, for whom a sport-specific EET should be used.
   - True MHR must be known to calculate a training heart rate range, which can be used as a guideline for aerobic training.
   - An EET can also be used to estimate an individual's $\dot{V}O_2$ max, which is helpful in determining the current level of fitness or conditioning.

Specific ACC/AHA Indications

For the sake of completeness of this chapter, most of the indications for EET in adults from the ACC/AHA guidelines will be listed. Guidelines for special cases (e.g., children, EET with expired ventilatory gas analysis) may be found in the ACC/AHA reference or on the AHA website (www.americanheart.org), under "Science and Professional, Scientific Publications, Scientific Statements." The ACC/AHA guidelines use the following classification system for indications:

Class I: Conditions for which there is evidence and/or general agreement that a given procedure or treatment is useful and effective.
Class II: Conditions for which there is conflicting evidence and/or a divergence of opinion about the usefulness/efficacy of a procedure or treatment.
Class IIa: Weight of evidence/opinion is in favor of usefulness/efficacy.
Class IIb: Usefulness/efficacy is less well established by evidence/opinion.
Class III: Conditions for which there is evidence and/or general agreement that the procedure or treatment is not useful/effective and in some cases may be harmful.

Exercise ECG Testing in Diagnosis of Obstructive CAD

Class I: Adult patients (including those with complete right bundle branch block [RBBB] or less than 1 mm of resting ST segment depression) with an intermediate pretest probability of CAD based on sex, age, and symptoms (see "Determination of Pretest Likelihood," Fig. 93-4, and Table 93-1).
Class IIa: Patients with vasospastic angina.
Class IIb: Patients with a high or low pretest probability of CAD by age, symptoms, and sex; patients with less than 1 mm of baseline ST segment depression and taking digoxin; patients with ECG criteria for LV hypertrophy (LVH) and less than 1 mm of baseline ST segment depression.
Class III: Patients with the following baseline ECG abnormalities: preexcitation syndrome (i.e., Wolff-Parkinson-White [WPW] syndrome), electronically paced ventricular rhythm, greater than 1 mm of resting ST segment depression, complete left bundle branch block (LBBB); patients with a documented MI or prior coronary angiography demonstrating significant disease and who have an established diagnosis of CAD. (Note that for diagnostic purposes, EET may not be useful. However, overall risk for individuals can be determined from obtaining $\dot{V}O_2$ max if it is deemed safe to test [see following sections "Risk Assessment and Prognosis in Patients with Symptoms or a History of CAD," "Exercise ECG Testing after Myocardial Infarction," and "Exercise ECG Testing before and after Revascularization"].)

Risk Assessment and Prognosis in Patients with Symptoms or a History of CAD

Class I: Patients undergoing initial evaluation with suspected or known CAD. Patients with suspected or known CAD previously evaluated but now with a significant change in clinical status (specific exceptions noted in Class IIb). Low-risk patients with unstable angina (moderate or high likelihood of CAD with new-onset or progressive angina with walking) 8 to 12 hours after presentation or intermediate-risk unstable angina (prolonged [>20 minutes] or at rest angina; patients with prior MI, CABG,

*Patients with LV dysfunction, history of recent (within 7 to 10 days) acute coronary syndrome, severe valvular (aortic) stenosis, or complex or life-threatening arrhythmias are considered a higher-risk group. Exercise testing for them should be performed in the hospital by a clinician with significant experience treating patients with CAD or with consultation by a cardiologist.

atherosclerotic cerebrovascular disease [ASCVD], or peripheral artery disease; aspirin use; age older than 70 years; or troponins negative or slightly elevated [<0.1 mg/mL]) 2 to 3 days after presentation; both groups of patients with unstable angina should have been free of active ischemic or heart failure symptoms.

Class IIa: Intermediate-risk patients with unstable angina who have initial cardiac markers that are normal, a repeat ECG without significant change, cardiac markers 6 to 12 hours after the onset of symptoms that are normal, and no evidence of ischemia during observation.

Class IIb: Patients with the following resting ECG abnormalities: preexcitation (i.e., WPW syndrome), electronically paced ventricular rhythm, greater than 1 mm of resting ST segment depression, complete LBBB. Patients with a stable clinical course who undergo periodic monitoring to guide treatment.

Class III: Patients with severe comorbidity likely to limit life expectancy or candidacy for revascularization. Patients with high-risk unstable angina (prolonged, ongoing >20 minutes pain at rest; pulmonary edema; new or worsening mitral regurgitant murmur; new/worsening rales; hypotension; bradycardia; tachycardia; age older than 75 years; transient ST segment changes; or elevated troponin [>0.1 mg/mL]).

Exercise ECG Testing after Myocardial Infarction

Class I: Before discharge for prognostic assessment, activity prescription, or evaluation of medical therapy (submaximal at about 4 to 7 days). Early after discharge for prognostic assessment, activity prescription, evaluation of medical therapy, and cardiac rehabilitation if the predischarge EET was not done (do a symptom-limited EET at about 14 to 21 days). Late after discharge for prognostic assessment, activity prescription, evaluation of medical therapy, and cardiac rehabilitation if the early EET was submaximal (do a symptom-limited EET at about 3 to 6 weeks).

Class IIa: After discharge for activity counseling or exercise training as part of cardiac rehabilitation in patients who have undergone coronary revascularization.

Class IIb: Patients with preexcitation syndrome (i.e., WPW syndrome), electronically paced ventricular rhythm, greater than 1 mm of resting ST segment depression, complete LBBB, digoxin therapy, LVH. Periodic monitoring in patients who continue to participate in exercise training or cardiac rehabilitation.

Class III: Patients with severe comorbidity likely to limit life expectancy or candidacy for revascularization. At any time after MI if there is uncompensated congestive heart failure (CHF), cardiac arrhythmia, or noncardiac conditions that limit the patient's ability to exercise.

Exercise ECG Testing in Asymptomatic Patients without Known CAD

Class I: None.

Class IIa: Evaluation of asymptomatic persons with diabetes mellitus who plan to start vigorous exercise.

Class IIb: Evaluation of patients with multiple risk factors as a guide to risk reduction therapy. Evaluation of asymptomatic men older than 45 years of age and women older than 55 years of age planning to start vigorous exercise (especially if physically inactive), or involved in occupations in which impairment might affect public safety, or at high risk for CAD because of other diseases (e.g., peripheral vascular disease, chronic renal failure).

Class III: Routine screening of asymptomatic men or women.

NOTE: The class IIb indication evokes controversy because of the increased risk of false-positive results. However, with good clinical judgment or consultation of a table (e.g., Fig. 93-4, Table 93-1), the clinician may determine that the patient has a pretest likelihood as high as 15% to 20%, making the patient a reasonable candidate for EET.

Exercise ECG Testing for Valvular Heart Disease

Class I: In chronic aortic regurgitation, assessment of functional capacity and symptomatic responses in patients with a history of equivocal symptoms.

Class IIa: In chronic aortic regurgitation, evaluation of symptoms and functional capacity before participation in athletic activities. For prognostic assessment before aortic valve replacement in asymptomatic or minimally symptomatic patients with LV dysfunction.

Class IIb: Evaluation of exercise capacity in patients with valvular heart disease.

Class III: Diagnosis of CAD in patients with moderate to severe valvular disease or with baseline ECG abnormalities (preexcitation, electronically paced ventricular rhythm, >1 mm ST segment depression, complete LBBB).

Exercise ECG Testing before and after Revascularization

Class I: Demonstration of proof of ischemia before revascularization. Evaluation of patients with recurrent symptoms suggesting ischemia after revascularization.

Class IIa: After discharge for activity counseling or exercise training as part of cardiac rehabilitation in patients who have undergone coronary revascularization.

Class IIb: Detection of restenosis in selected, high-risk (multivessel CAD, proximal left anterior descending CAD, family history of sudden cardiac death, diabetes, hazardous occupations, suboptimal results from the revascularization, saphenous vein graft,* CHF*) asymptomatic patients within the first 12 months after percutaneous coronary intervention (PCI). Periodic monitoring of selected, high-risk asymptomatic patients for restenosis, graft occlusion, or disease progression.

Class III: Localization of ischemia for determining site of intervention. Routine, periodic monitoring of asymptomatic patients after PCI or coronary artery bypass grafting without specific indications.

Exercise ECG Testing for Investigation of Heart Rhythm Disorders

Class I: Identification of appropriate settings in patients with rate-adaptive pacemakers.

Class IIa: Evaluation of patients with known or suspected exercise-induced arrhythmias. Evaluation of medical, surgical, or ablative therapy in patients with exercise-induced arrhythmias (including atrial fibrillation).

Class IIb: Investigation of isolated ventricular ectopic beats in middle-aged patients without other evidence of CAD. Investigation of prolonged first-degree atrioventricular block or type I second-degree Wenckebach, LBBB, RBBB, or isolated ectopic beats in young patients considering participation in competitive sports.

Class III: Investigation of isolated ectopic beats in young patients.

Noninvasive Stress Testing before Noncardiac Surgery

Class IIa: Noninvasive stress testing of patients with three or more clinical risk factors (e..g, CAD, CHF, ASCVD, diabetes mellitus, renal insufficiency) and poor functional capacity (<4 METs or cannot walk up a flight of stairs) who require high-risk (often >5% risk of serious complications) surgery (e.g., vascular, defined as aortic or other major vascular, peripheral vascular surgery) is reasonable if it will change management.

Class IIb: Noninvasive stress testing may be considered for patients with at least one to two clinical risk factors and poor functional capacity (<4 METs) who require intermediate-risk (1% to 5% risk of serious complications) noncardiac surgery (e.g.,

---

*Although not listed as high risk in ACC/AHA guidelines, patients with these conditions have worse long-term outcomes postrevascularization.

intraperitoneal; intrathoracic; carotid or aortic stent; carotid endarterectomy; head and neck, orthopedic, or prostate surgery) if it will change management. Noninvasive stress testing may be considered for patients with at least one to two clinical risk factors and good functional capacity (≥4 METs) who are undergoing high-risk/vascular surgery.

Class III: Noninvasive testing is not useful for patients with no clinical risk factors undergoing intermediate-risk or low-risk (<1% risk of serious complications) noncardiac surgery (e.g., endoscopic, superficial, cataract, breast, ambulatory).

Indications for Diabetic Patients

Because of a disproportionate burden of CAD in diabetic patients, the American Diabetes Association (ADA) has developed indications for cardiac testing in diabetic patients. They include the following:

1. Patients with typical or atypical cardiac symptoms
2. Patients with an abnormal resting ECG, especially if suggestive of ischemia or infarction

The ADA has recognized additional risk factors for obstructive CAD in diabetic patients, including renal disease (40% risk of coronary event in 5 years), evidence of other atherosclerotic disease (90% of their deaths are due to CAD), cardiovascular autonomic neuropathy (e.g., tachycardia, bradycardia, orthostatic hypotension, inadequate heart rate acceleration with exertion), older age, and female sex.

Indications in the Emergency Department

Patient has or had chest pain and fulfills the following requirements:

1. Two sets of negative cardiac markers from each of two different types of assays (troponin, myoglobin, or creatinine kinase MB) at 4-hour intervals.
2. Pre-exercise 12-lead ECG shows no significant changes compared with original ECG at the time of presentation to the emergency department.
3. Absence of baseline (resting) ECG abnormalities that would preclude accurate assessment of the EET.
4. From admission to the time that results are available from the second set of cardiac markers, the patient has become asymptomatic, has had lessening of chest pain symptoms, or has had persistent atypical symptoms.
5. Absence of ischemic chest pain at the time of EET.

Indications for Firefighters

The following guidelines were recommended by the National Fire Protection Association (NFPA) in 2000:

1. At age 40 years, periodic treadmill testing should be performed. The frequency should increase with age, but at a minimum the test should be done every 2 years.
2. At age 35 years, periodic treadmill testing should be performed for individuals with one or more coronary risk factors (premature family history [younger than age 55 years], hypertension, diabetes mellitus, cigarette smoking, and hypercholesterolemia [total cholesterol >240 or high-density lipoprotein <35]).

Indications before Noncardiac Surgery

Half of serious complications related to noncardiac surgery are cardiovascular. Although older patients have the highest risk of a cardiovascular complication with surgery, they also make up the largest group of patients undergoing surgery. Consequently, as the population ages, the cardiovascular risk of surgery will increase. Guidelines are available for screening patients before noncardiac surgery, and the ACC/AHA guidelines have been studied from an outcomes perspective. Box 93-2 provides some shortcuts for determining need for noninvasive testing. Patients about to undergo low-risk surgery (<1% risk; e.g., endoscopic, superficial, cataract, breast, ambulatory surgery) or with at least a fair functional/exercise capacity do not need further testing. If the patient has undergone revascularization (PCI or CABG) within the past 5 years or a thorough evaluation of the coronary arteries (e.g., EET, stress imaging) within the past 2 years, and there has not been a change in symptoms suggestive of ischemia, then according to ACC/AHA guidelines no further testing is necessary. Conversely, if high-risk (often >5% risk of serious complications) vascular surgery is planned and the patient has three or more clinical risk factors (i.e., CAD, CHF, ASCVD, diabetes, or renal insufficiency [creatinine ≥2 mg/dL]), noninvasive testing is reasonable if the results will change the management. It should be kept in mind that the goal of perioperative cardiac assessment is to detect the patient who would benefit from revascularization anyway, not just to get him or her through surgery. (See also Chapter 230, Preoperative Evaluation.)

Noninvasive testing is also probably indicated if the patient has poor functional/exercise capacity and one or more clinical risk factors. For intermediate-risk (1% to 5% risk of serious complications) surgery (e.g., intraperitoneal; intrathoracic; carotid or aortic stent; carotid endarterectomy; head and neck, orthopedic, or prostate surgery) or high-risk surgery with only one or two clinical predictors, there is insufficient evidence to determine the best

Box 93-2. Shortcuts to Determine Indicators for Noninvasive Testing before Noncardiac Surgery

No testing necessary if "Yes" to any of these four questions:

1. Is this low-risk surgery (e.g., endoscopic, superficial, cataract, breast, ambulatory surgery)?
2. Does the patient have fair functional/exercise capacity (≥4 METs) and no symptoms?
3. Has the patient undergone revascularization (CABG or PCI) within past 5 years without a change in symptoms indicating ischemia?
4. Has the patient had a thorough cardiac evaluation within past 2 years without a change in symptoms indicating ischemia?

Conversely, if vascular surgery is planned and the patient has three or more clinical risk factors, noninvasive testing is reasonable if the results will change the management.

Also, if "Yes" to both the following questions, noninvasive testing is reasonable*:

1. Poor functional/exercise capacity by questionnaire or specific questioning (<4 METs, or inability to climb one flight of stairs)?
2. Clinical risk factor present (CAD, CHF, ASCVD, diabetes, or renal insufficiency)?

*For intermediate- or high-risk surgery with only one or two clinical predictors present, there is insufficient evidence to determine the best management, beta blockade therapy versus noninvasive testing.

From Fleisher LA, Beckman JA, Brown KA, et al: ACC/AHA 2007 guidelines on perioperative cardiovascular evaluation and care for noncardiac surgery: Executive summary. A report of the American College of Cardiology/American Heart Association Task Force on Practice Guidelines (Writing Committee to Revise the 2002 Guidelines on Perioperative Cardiovascular Evaluation for Noncardiac Surgery). Circulation 116:1971–1996, 2007.

management, beta blockade therapy versus noninvasive testing. Also, high-risk surgery (e.g., aortic/major vascular surgery, peripheral vascular surgery) may be managed like intermediate-risk surgery if only one or two clinical risk factors are present.

Indications before and after Revascularization (PCI or CABG)

In recent years, at least nine studies (BARI, CABRI, RITA-1, EAST, GABI, Toulouse, MASS, Lausanne, ERACI) have been published comparing PCI with CABG in patients with symptomatic CAD. Most were smaller studies, but BARI (the Bypass Angioplasty Revascularization Investigation) included 1829 patients, CABRI (Coronary Angioplasty vs. Bypass Revascularization Investigation) 1054 patients, and RITA-1 (first Randomized Intervention Treatment of Angina trial) 1011 patients. Although these trials differ slightly in their design and in the sort of patients who were included, the findings have all been remarkably consistent. At almost any point after initial treatment, whether the patient was treated with PCI or CABG, the rates of death or nonfatal MI are essentially the same. However, at the time of these trials, patients undergoing PCI usually received percutaneous transluminal coronary angioplasty (PTCA). Consequently, the reintervention rate was much higher among patients initially treated with PCI than for those undergoing CABG. There have been several additional trials (ERACI II, ARTS, SOS) using stents for PCI and comparing outcomes with CABG. Although the reintervention rate remains higher with PCI than CABG, it has been significantly reduced with the use of stents. Mortality and nonfatal MI rates have again remained basically the same whether the patient is treated with PCI or CABG. The BARI trial 10-year follow-up data are now published; overall, the annual mortality rate was 2.8%. Consequently, there are going to be many patients having undergone revascularization living a long time.

From the BARI trial, we also learned about EET postrevascularization. Per protocol, at years 1, 3, and 5, 1388, 1208, and 1097 patients, respectively, underwent EET (Krone and colleagues, 2001). Only 9% experienced angina when taking the EET, consistent with the "protocol- not symptom-driven" indication for EET. Overall, patients taking EET during the first 3 years of the study not only had a very low risk of mortality or MI, but very rarely did EET results affect management. The authors concluded that their study supported ACC/AHA guidelines, which do not recommend routine testing for 3 to 5 years after successful revascularization. The authors also speculated that exercise imaging would not have been helpful because such a low-risk population would have likely produced a large percentage of false-positive results. Consequently, only a fraction of those with a significant perfusion or echocardiographic defect would have had a subsequent event.

From the BARI trial, we also learned about risk stratification postrevascularization, including the risk of not undergoing EET according to protocol. In the asymptomatic population that did not follow the protocol, *not taking the EET* was a stronger predictor of mortality than results of the EET in those who followed the protocol. Overall, nonexercisers had a 3- to 10-fold increased risk of mortality compared with exercisers. Diabetic nonexercisers who had undergone CABG had a 30% 5-year mortality rate. Even more striking, diabetic nonexercisers who *had undergone PTCA had a 52.4% 5-year mortality rate!*

We have long known that patients with CAD and poor functional or exercise capacity (<4 METs) are at high risk for cardiovascular events, and that is one of the criteria for considering EET or other noninvasive testing when evaluating patients before surgery. Such a low exercise capacity may correlate with what the BARI investigators found to be nonexercisers. Regardless, clinicians should be aware that patients unable to exercise are at high risk postrevascularization.

How then should we monitor patients postrevascularization? Interestingly, of the nine studies comparing PCI with CABG, most used EET at various points to monitor patients for safety. Although the ACC/AHA guidelines suggest that an exercise imaging test is the preferred method of evaluating patients postrevascularization, the experts designing these trials considered EET to be adequate. Regardless, ACC/AHA guidelines also list certain situations where EET may or may not be helpful in the revascularized patient.

A reasonable use for EET in the revascularized patient is after discharge for activity counseling or exercise training as part of a cardiac rehabilitation program (indication: class IIa). Although the evidence is less well established, EET may be considered for the detection of restenosis in the first months after PTCA in selected, high-risk (Box 93-3), asymptomatic patients (indication: class IIb). And although the evidence is likewise less well established, EET may be considered for periodic testing for restenosis, graft occlusion, or disease progression in selected, high-risk (see Box 93-3), asymptomatic individuals postrevascularization (indication: class IIb).

What about the patient who has remained asymptomatic, is more than 5 years postrevascularization, and needs to be evaluated before surgery? Figure 93-5 incorporates the ACC/AHA guidelines for these patients as well as most asymptomatic patients postrevascularization.

Box 93-3. Criteria for High-Risk Patients Postrevascularization

Multivessel CAD
Proximal left anterior descending CAD
Family history of sudden cardiac death
Diabetes
Hazardous occupations
Suboptimal results from the revascularization
Saphenous vein graft*
Congestive heart failure*

*Although not listed as high risk in ACC/AHA guidelines, patients with these conditions have worse long-term outcomes postrevascularization compared with other patients.

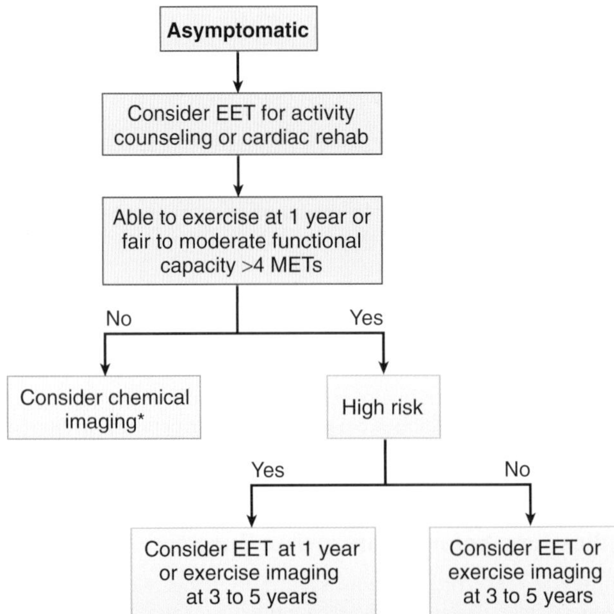

Figure 93-5 Algorithm for exercise ECG testing (EET) in the asymptomatic patient postrevascularization. *Especially those with prior MI and/or renal insufficiency.

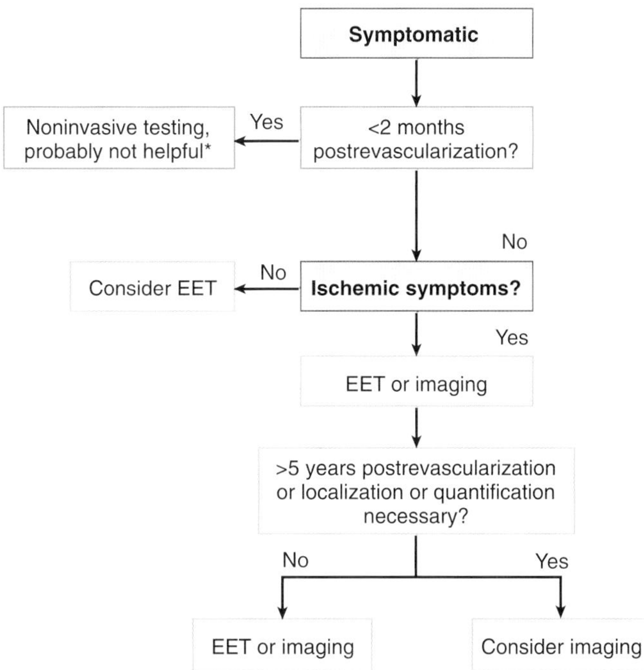

Figure 93-6 Algorithm for exercise ECG testing (EET) in the symptomatic patient postrevascularization. *However, CT angiography may be helpful (≥16-slice post-CABG; ≥32-slice post-PCI).

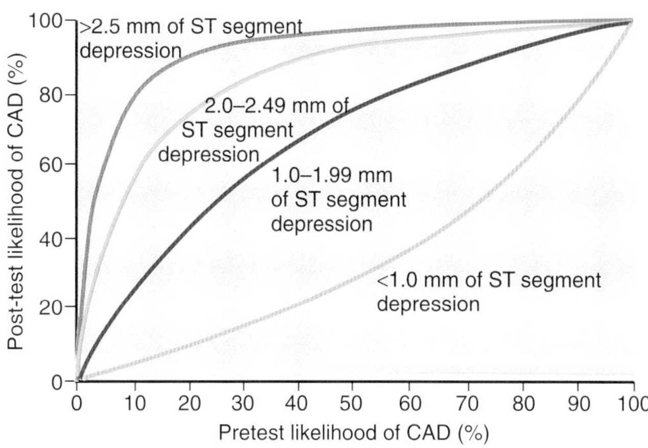

Figure 93-7 Post-test likelihood of coronary artery disease (CAD) with positive (>1 mm ST segment depression) and negative (<1 mm ST segment depression) test results. (Redrawn from Epstein SE: Implications of probability analysis on the strategy used for noninvasive detection of coronary artery disease: Role of single or combined use of exercise electrocardiographic testing, radionuclide cineangiography and myocardial perfusion imaging. Am J Cardiol 46:491–499, 1980.)

What tests should be used if the patient becomes symptomatic postrevascularization? Figure 93-6 provides an algorithm for these patients. As multislice CT angiography becomes more readily available, combining it with an EET may be the screening and diagnostic procedure of choice for revascularized patients.

Determination of Pretest Likelihood

If the goal of the EET is to exclude CAD, determining pretest likelihood will help decide whether EET is the indicated and proper procedure. For diagnostic purposes, EET is most valuable for patients with an intermediate (20% to 70%) pretest likelihood. Simple graphs and tables are available that require only three variables to estimate pretest likelihood in symptomatic individuals (see Fig. 93-4 and Table 93-1). With a pretest likelihood in the 20% to 70% range, an abnormal or positive EET result provides strong justification for additional studies, including invasive studies. A negative EET may provide justification for merely close observation with frequent follow-up visits.

The value of using this range (20% to 70%) is further demonstrated with a graph of post-test likelihood of CAD (Fig. 93-7). From this graph, the clinician should be able to see that the most information is obtained from patients with an intermediate pretest likelihood. In other words, for Figure 93-7 the vertical gap is largest between what would be a positive EET and a negative EET for patients in the intermediate pretest range. In this group, positive studies are most clearly delineated from negative studies; therefore, the most information is obtained. For example, a patient with a pretest likelihood of 40% with 2 mm or more of ST segment depression now has more than an 85% post-test likelihood of CAD. Such a post-test likelihood would justify an invasive procedure. However, in the same patient, less than 1 mm of ST segment depression (a negative EET) lowers the risk of CAD to less than 20%. Close follow-up of this patient may be adequate.

For patients with a low (<20%) pretest likelihood, although there may be other benefits of performing EET (e.g., customized exercise prescription), positive studies are more likely to be bothersome false-positive results that lead to unnecessary patient anxiety and further expensive diagnostic testing. On the other hand, a negative test in the high pretest likelihood group (>70%) may not be sufficient to exclude CAD. For the young or very active individual with a high pretest likelihood, coronary angiography is diagnostic and might be a more appropriate study. Again, to use an example, a patient with a pretest likelihood of 90% who has a positive study (>2 mm ST segment depression) has approximately a 96% post-test likelihood (using Fig. 93-7). This is only a 6% gain in probability, which is very little information. If the EET is negative, the patient still has a 75% likelihood of CAD. For diagnostic purposes, this probability certainly does not rule out CAD, so EET has apparently been of little value. (Again, even in patients for whom little diagnostic information is gained with EET, performing it may be helpful for other reasons, such as for managing CAD.)

Pretest likelihood can be estimated by a description of the chest pain and the patient's sex and age. *Typical angina* is described (Diamond and Forrester, 1979) as substernal, exertional, and relieved by rest or nitroglycerin. Chest discomfort with two of these three characteristics is *atypical angina*; with only one it is *nonanginal chest pain*. Using these three descriptions, pretest likelihood tables and their corresponding graphs (see Fig. 93-4 and Table 93-1) can be readily applied to determine pretest likelihood.

Although Figure 93-4 and Table 93-1 also include asymptomatic patients, in general asymptomatic patients never reach an intermediate (20%) pretest likelihood. This is why mass screening of the asymptomatic population with EET is not recommended. It should be kept in mind that the data for Figure 93-4 and Table 93-1 were compiled from *a community* with an average number of risk factors (at the time, not many *individuals* had multiple risk factors). Therefore, for an individual patient with *severe* abnormalities in each of the risk categories, such as severe hypertension, heavy smoking, and severe hypercholesterolemia, or possessing *multiple* risk factors, pretest likelihood should be increased even if he or she is asymptomatic. Tables similar to Table 93-1 have been developed that attempt to adjust for severity of risk factors, but few experts use them because they have mostly been developed from patients seen in referral centers as opposed to the community. In the asymptomatic group, the Framingham calculator (available online at http://hp2010.nhlbihin.net/atpiii/calculator.asp) or tables (including international tables similar to those developed for the

Framingham Study) can also be used to help quantify risk. Although the Framingham calculator is designed to estimate absolute risk of a coronary event over the next 10 years, combining this result with clinical gestalt, clinicians can estimate which asymptomatic patients with risk factors would possibly reach the 20% pretest likelihood and benefit from EET. It should also be kept in mind that approximately one third of individuals who developed CAD in the Framingham Study had none of the usual risk factors, so generous estimates should be made when assessing pretest likelihood. As newer risk factors (e.g., chronic kidney disease; elevated homocysteine, ferritin, high-sensitivity C-reactive protein, fibrinogen, apolipoprotein [B], LDL particle number, or lipoprotein [A] levels) are studied, the clinician may again have to use clinical judgment or gestalt to correctly estimate pretest likelihood for an individual with these risk factors.

CONTRAINDICATIONS

Absolute

- Very recent acute MI (within 2 days) or other acute cardiac event
- High-risk unstable angina
- Severe symptomatic LV dysfunction or uncontrolled symptomatic CHF
- Potentially life-threatening or uncontrolled cardiac arrhythmias causing symptoms or hemodynamic compromise
- Acute pericarditis, myocarditis, or endocarditis
- Symptomatic severe aortic stenosis
- Acute aortic dissection
- Acute pulmonary edema, embolus, or infarction

Relative

- Left main coronary stenosis
- Moderate stenotic valvular heart disease
- Third-degree atrioventricular block or second-degree Mobitz type II block without pacemaker
- Tachyarrhythmias or bradyarrhythmias
- Severe arterial hypertension (resting >200 mm Hg systolic or >110 mm Hg diastolic)
- Hypertrophic cardiomyopathy or other form of outflow obstruction
- Acute thrombophlebitis, deep venous thrombosis, or intracardiac thrombi
- Electrolyte abnormality
- Acute or serious general illness or infection
- Neuromuscular, musculoskeletal, or arthritic condition that precludes exercise
- Uncontrolled metabolic disease, such as diabetes, thyrotoxicosis, or myxedema
- Medication intoxication from drugs such as digoxin, sedatives, or psychotropic agents
- Patient inability or lack of desire or motivation to perform the test, including severe emotional distress
- Unavailability of advanced cardiac life support (ACLS) equipment or of an individual certified to perform ACLS

NOTE: In selected cases, a skilled cardiologist may perform testing for patients with one of these diagnoses (generally in a referral center). All are contraindications to EET in the office.

Contraindications in the Emergency Department

- New or evolving abnormalities on the resting ECG
- Abnormal cardiac markers
- Inability to perform exercise
- Worsening or persistent ischemic chest pain symptoms from admission to the time of EET
- Clinical risk profiling indicating coronary angiography is likely
- Any routine contraindications from the previous section

Additional Relative Contraindications

There are certain conditions that produce a study that is difficult to interpret or that will have results that add very little clinical information. Such relative contraindications include:

- Ventricular aneurysm
- Chronic infectious disease (e.g., mononucleosis, hepatitis, advanced human immunodeficiency virus infection)
- Fixed-rate pacemaker (rarely used)
- Advanced or complicated pregnancy
- Frequent or complex ventricular ectopy

EQUIPMENT

- A treadmill with adjustable speed and grade and adequate weight capacity: This is by far the most common equipment used for EET in the United States. Advantages include the ability to test most patients under the actual physiologic conditions of exercise. The most common types of exercise performed in the United States are walking and running. In addition, patient motivation wavers less during the treadmill test than with the bicycle EET. Disadvantages include the fact that the treadmill may be difficult to use for patients with lower extremity or low-back problems or for patients who are very obese. The equipment is also more expensive, causes more motion artifact, and is noisier than a bicycle ergometer.

  NOTE: If a treadmill is chosen, it should have a warm-up speed of about 0.5 to 1.5 mph, with testing speeds ranging from 2.0 mph up to 12 mph. For elite athletes, the speed may need to reach 15 mph. The slope or grades possible should range from 0% (flat) to 20%. If testing elite athletes, the grade may need to reach 25%. It should also be able to accommodate the patient's weight; capacity for some models is now 500 pounds.

- Bicycle ergometers: Bicycle ergometers use adjustable resistance and pedal frequency to exert the patient (Fig. 93-8). Advantages with the bicycle ergometer include easier-to-obtain blood pressure (BP) measurements and the ability to terminate the test instantly. Many patients feel more secure sitting on the bicycle. Unfortunately, in the United States leg fatigue is common because most patients do not bike. In fact, as a result of leg fatigue the procedure often fails to determine $\dot{V}O_2$ max. Bicycle ergometry also depends on motivation throughout its duration. As a result, if the patient can tolerate the treadmill, most U.S. clinicians prefer it.
- Arm ergometer: The arm ergometer (Fig. 93-9) enables patients with severe orthopedic problems to be tested. However, muscle fatigue often occurs before the maximum heart rate is achieved.
- Continuous ECG monitor: A three- to six-lead model with a screen-freeze or capture/replay option is desirable (Fig. 93-10). Although previous models provided only 3 or 4 beats in each lead

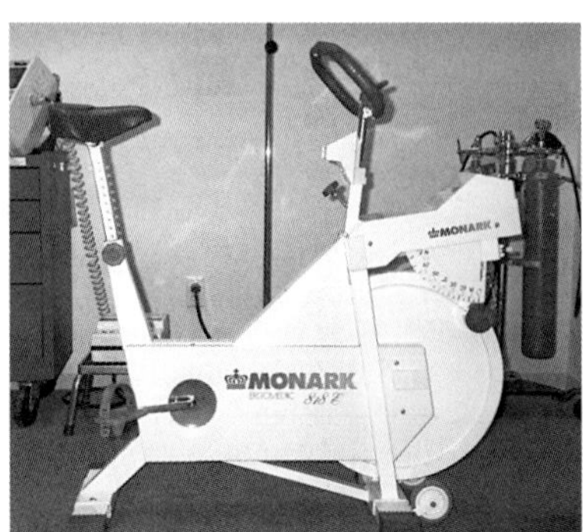

Figure 93-8 Bicycle ergometer.

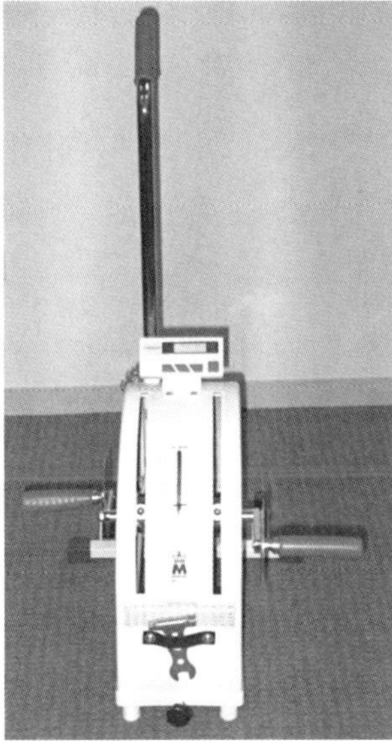

Figure 93-9 Arm ergometer.

if 6 or more leads were monitored, newer equipment often allows clear simultaneous monitoring of all 12 leads.

- 12-Lead ECG recorder: With modern equipment, the recorder also runs the treadmill. Recent developments for primary care offices (e.g., wider wheelbase) allow the recorder to be wheeled from room to room for routine ECGs. Interpretive packages for 12-lead ECGs are also convenient. Most equipment is now digital, allowing data to be filtered to provide a smooth baseline. However, it is important to avoid overfiltering the data and, in so doing, filtering out ST segment depression. Newer models are personal computer–based and can use either thermal paper or a laser printer. Many are compatible with electronic medical records.
- Sphygmomanometer, including various cuff sizes: A gauge manometer is adequate because the most important readings are those relative to resting pressures (not the absolute pressures).
- Stethoscope.
- Razor, rubbing alcohol, skin abrasive.
- Electrodes: Disposable electrodes designed for EET (regular ECG electrodes are not adequate and will cause artifact).
- Cables and belt: A disposable or washable belt is preferred because patients usually sweat.
- Emergency equipment (see Fig. 220-4 in Chapter 220, Anaphylaxis): Defibrillator; oxygen; airway, intubation, and suction equipment; and an emergency drug kit containing intravenous fluids, tubing, and medications to support ACLS protocols.

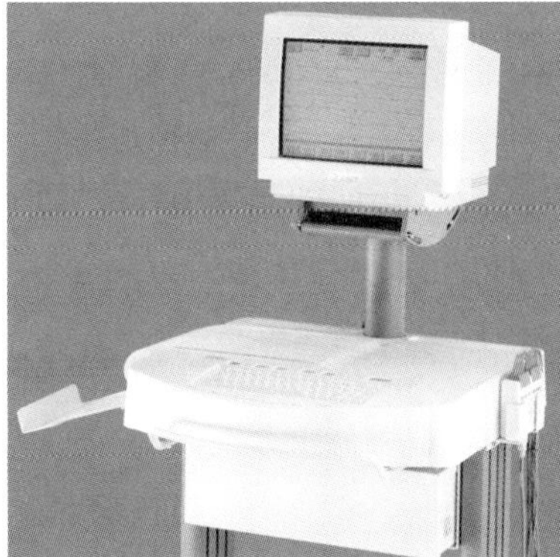

Figure 93-10 ECG monitor. (Courtesy of Cardiac Science/Burdick, Inc., Deerfield, Wisc.)

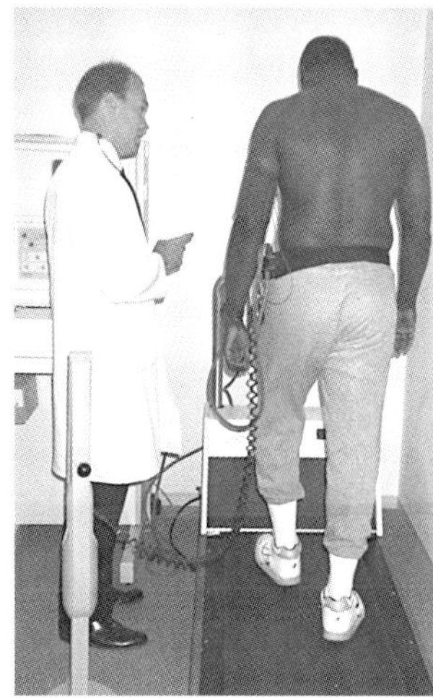

Figure 93-11 Trained technician monitoring patient.

NOTE: It is also helpful to have a trained technician (Fig. 93-11) to assist during the procedure. Technician certification for EET is available through the American College of Sports Medicine. In many centers the technician prepares the patient; monitors the ECG, the patient's response to exercise, the heart rate, and the BP; and prepares the results for interpretation. For low-risk patients, the technician may actually perform the entire study without a physician being present. Otherwise, the clinician should examine the patient before, during, and after the procedure, confirm which protocol to use, and terminate the study. The clinician should monitor the ECG tracing when the technician is taking BP readings, and the clinician should interpret the final results.

Written Procedure Protocols

- Informed consent (see the sample consent form "Cardiac EET" in Appendix B)
- Medical history, physical examination, handwritten report form (Fig. 93-12)
- Criteria for stopping EET (see the section on "Test Termination Criteria," later)
- Emergency response plan (should be designed for every office and kept on file in event of a complication from EET)
- Quality assurance plan, including calibration and testing of equipment

NOTE: All emergency equipment should be checked daily and medications should be checked weekly to monthly, depending on their use. The EET equipment should be inspected and calibrated periodically, based on manufacturer recommendations. ACLS certification cards should be kept on file along with the information and protocols listed previously.

Preprocedure Patient Preparation

Deconditioned patients or those anticipated to have a poor exercise capacity (see the Veterans' Administration [VA] Specific Activity Questionnaire, Fig. 93-1):

- In the geriatric or physically inactive population, it is safe to exercise to a heart rate of 100 bpm, regardless of age, without prior testing. In those anticipated to have very poor exercise capacity, if they are not in urgent need of a cardiovascular intervention, it may be reasonable to help them increase their exercise capacity before undergoing an EET. This may be achieved with a walking program for several weeks or even months, four or five times a week, with a target heart rate of 100 bpm. In this manner

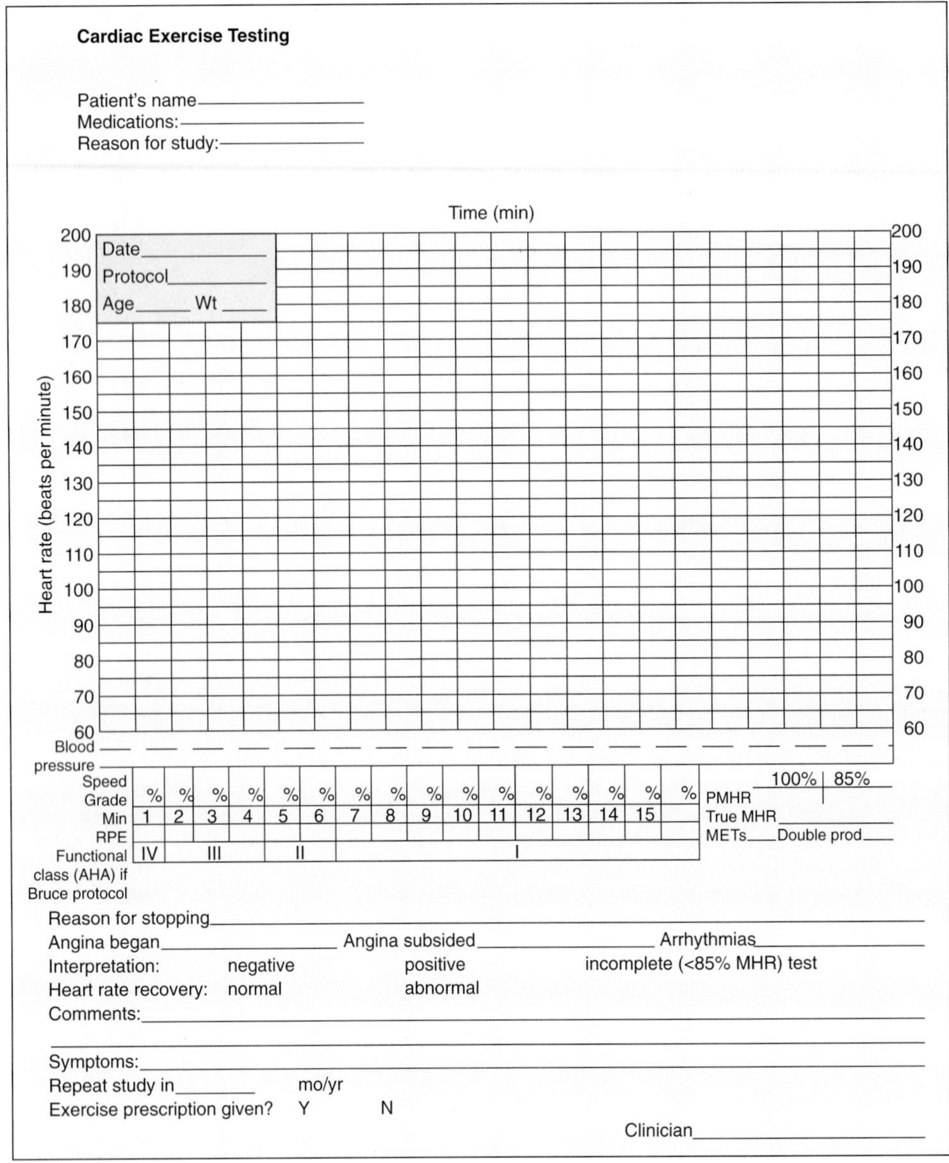

Cardiac Exercise Testing

Patient's name________________

Medications:________________

Reason for study:________________

Time (min)

Date________

Protocol________

Age______ Wt______

Heart rate (beats per minute): 200, 190, 180, 170, 160, 150, 140, 130, 120, 110, 100, 90, 80, 70, 60

Blood pressure

Speed															
Grade	%	%	%	%	%	%	%	%	%	%	%	%	%	%	%
Min	1	2	3	4	5	6	7	8	9	10	11	12	13	14	15
RPE															
Functional class (AHA) if Bruce protocol	IV		III		II				I						

PMHR 100% | 85%

True MHR________

METs____Double prod____

Reason for stopping________________

Angina began________ Angina subsided________ Arrhythmias________

Interpretation: negative positive incomplete (<85% MHR) test

Heart rate recovery: normal abnormal

Comments:________________

Symptoms:________________

Repeat study in________ mo/yr

Exercise prescription given? Y N

Clinician________________

Figure 93-12 Exercise test results form. METs, metabolic equivalents; PMHR, predicted maximum heart rate (220 − age). (Modified from Evans CH, Karunaratne HB: Exercise stress testing for the family physician: Part I. Performing the test. Am Fam Physician 45:121–132, 1992.)

it may be possible to avoid some uninterpretable or incomplete tests.

Before arrival

- The patient should be instructed to minimize consumption of alcohol, over-the-counter medications, and caffeine, both the day before and the day of the procedure. The patient should be encouraged to get a good night's sleep the night before the procedure. Patients should not eat for 2 hours before the test. It might be advisable for the most recent meal to be a small and predominately liquid meal. To minimize the risk of patient fatigue, many clinicians prefer performing EET in the morning. They then instruct the patient to avoid breakfast or to have only a liquid breakfast that day.
- The procedure should be rescheduled, if possible, if the patient has a cold or other viral illness or is not feeling well in general.
- If the indication for the test is to diagnose CAD (as opposed to managing CAD) or to screen for CAD, the clinician should instruct the patient to avoid taking beta blockers (or rate-limiting calcium channel blockers) the day of the test.

NOTE: Digoxin can cause artifact even at therapeutic doses. If possible, digoxin should not be taken for 2 weeks before a test, the amount of time necessary for its elimination. However, a negative EET in a patient taking digitalis is a good study. Estrogen and tricyclic antidepressants can have similar effects and can be managed the same way. Beta blockers can suppress the heart rate and prevent determination of the MHR. Patients who discontinue beta blockers should watch closely for "rebound" symptoms and, if they develop, should restart their beta blockers. Because angiotensin-converting enzyme inhibitors or angiotensin receptor blockers have little or no effect on performance of an EET, frequently they may be used as a substitute antihypertensive. If necessary, they can be taken on the day of the test and usually work within an hour. Clonidine may be used in the same manner.

- If the indication for the test is to determine pharmacologic efficacy in patients with CAD, obviously beta blockers should be taken the day of the study.
- The clinician should instruct the patient to bring shoes and clothing that are comfortable for walking and possibly for

jogging. Bras with underwiring are contraindicated; sports bras work well.

- To minimize patient worry and stress (which often cause an elevated resting SBP), the clinician should explain that the risk of death for patients being tested using a treadmill is very small, and even less in an office setting (<1 per 10,000 patients).

After arrival

- The clinician should again explain the reasons for the test and answer any questions.
- The procedure should be explained again to the patient (e.g., how frequently the workload will be increased, how BP measurements will be taken, how the PES works).
- The patient should be assured that close monitoring will take place and reassured that although the procedure exerts the heart, it is a relatively safe procedure (<1 : 10,000 mortality rate).
- The patient should know what symptoms to report during the test.
- The clinician should explain to the patient how to terminate the procedure should he or she have severe symptoms or an emergency.
- Signed, written informed consent should be obtained (see sample online at www.expertconsult.com).

Determining Protocol

There are many excellent protocols available; the choice usually depends on the patient's predicted exercise capacity and clinician preference. The VA Specific Activity Questionnaire (see Fig. 93-1) may be very helpful for predicting exercise capacity and deciding between a regular protocol and a modified (less aggressive) protocol. If a patient can walk up a flight of stairs carrying a bag of groceries, he or she should be able to tolerate a regular Bruce or Balke protocol. Choose a protocol that starts at a low level of exertion (2 to 3 METs) and then gradually increases.

1. A protocol with stage durations of at least 3 minutes (2 minutes for bicycle ergometer) allows more physiologic adaptation to the workload of each stage.
2. Workload increases that are no greater than 1 to 3 METs per stage also allow more physiologic adaptation.
3. Choose a protocol (Fig. 93-13) with a target of completing the EET in less than 15 minutes (even more preferable is 10 minutes or less). EETs that last more than 15 minutes may produce fatigue and overheating, which can independently affect results.

The Bruce protocol (Table 93-2) is the most frequently used protocol and has been the most extensively studied and validated. It is especially useful in active patients and takes less time than other protocols because it rapidly increases workload. Conveniently, the number of METs the patient will achieve is about the same as the number of minutes it takes to complete an EET using the Bruce protocol. A formula is available for estimating maximal exercise capacity in METs for the Bruce protocol. In men, this is METs = (2.94 × [min Bruce] + 7.65)/3.5. For women, the formula is METs = (2.95 × [min Bruce] +3.74)/3.5.

The Bruce protocol also has its disadvantages; by the fourth or fifth stage, the patient will need to run, which increases artifact. In addition, the patient often experiences difficulty accommodating increases in both slope and speed at the same time. Elderly patients usually have decreased proprioception in their toes and some degree of impairment in both vision and balance, making it especially difficult for them to adjust to changes in slope and speed at the same time.

In general, most "modified" protocols, such as the modified Bruce or modified Balke protocols, have a reduced progression of workload and are better tolerated by debilitated patients. Modified protocols usually maintain the same speed and vary only the elevation.

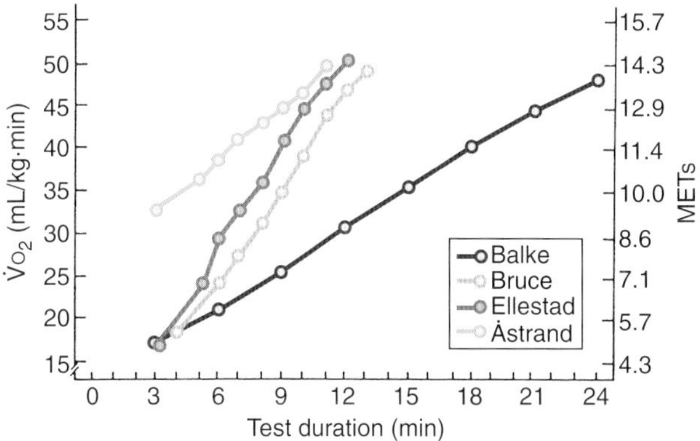

Figure 93-13 Oxygen uptake measured according to time of exercise on four different protocols. (From Pollock MI, Bohannon RL, Cooper KH, et al: A comparative analysis of four protocols for maximal treadmill stress testing. Am Heart J 92:39–46, 1976.)

Gradual but continuously increasing workload protocols (e.g., ramp) are also available. Table 93-3 indicates various protocols and Figure 93-13 graphically compares METs per minute and $\dot{V}O_2$ max as measured for four protocols. If the clinician chooses the ramp protocol, the VA questionnaire is helpful for estimating $\dot{V}O_2$ max in METs; most clinicians program the equipment to reach maximal METs in about 10 minutes.

With additional equipment that measures expired gases (e.g., oxygen, carbon dioxide) and total ventilation, the clinician can do four things: (1) actually measure the maximal aerobic capacity; (2) determine the anaerobic threshold (i.e., the point during exercise when marked lactic acid production begins); (3) give a more accurate exercise prescription; and (4) decide if impaired exercise capacity is due to a pulmonary condition or a cardiac cause (more common). Such equipment is becoming smaller and more affordable, which broadens the indications for EET in the office and (some experts say) increases the potential for greater reimbursement (see the "Suppliers" section). To avoid large capital equipment costs, there are service companies that will bring portable equipment to your office for this procedure and split the fees.

Technique

1. Review the patient's interval medical history and examine the patient. Based on the history and reexamination, make sure no contraindication has developed since the last time the patient was seen.
2. Select the mode of EET (e.g., treadmill, bicycle ergometer, arm ergometer), based on the individual's ability to exercise.
3. Select the protocol.
4. Obtain the resting BP.

TABLE 93-2 Standard Bruce Protocol

Stage*	Speed (mph)	Grade (%)	Metabolic Equivalents	Oxygen Consumption (mL/kg/min)
I	1.7	10	4	13
II	2.5	12	6.6	25
III	3.4	14	10	34
IV	4.2	16	14.2	46
V	5.0	18	17.2	58
VI	5.5	20	20.5	70

*Each stage lasts 3 minutes.

From Fowler GC, Evans CH, Altman MA: Office procedures: Exercise testing, Prim Care 24:375–406, 1997.

TABLE 93-3 Various Exercise Protocols

AHA Functional Class	Clinical Status	O_2 Cost (mL/kg/min)	METs	Bicycle Ergometer	Bruce (Treadmill)		Balke-Ware	USAFSAM		"Slow" USAFSAM		McHenry		Stanford		ACIP		CHF		METs
				1 W •• 6.1 kpm/min For 70 kg body weight kpm/min	3-min stages mph	percent grade	Percent grade at 3.3 mph 1-min stages	mph	percent grade	mph	percent grade	mph	percent grade	Percent grade at 3 mph	Percent grade at 2 mph	mph	percent grade	mph	percent grade	
					5.5	20														
Normal and I	Healthy, Dependent on Age, Activity	56.0	16		5.0	18	26, 25													16
		52.5	15				24	3.3	25							3.4	24.0			15
		49.0	14	1500			23, 22					3.3	21							14
		45.5	13		4.2	16	21	3.3	20					22.5		3.1	24.0			13
		42.0	12	1350			20, 19					3.3	18	20		3.0	21.0			12
	Sedentary Healthy	38.5	11	1200	3.4	14	18, 17							17.5		3.0	17.5	3.4	14.0	11
		35.0	10	1050			16	3.3	15	2	25	3.3	15	15				3.0	15.0	10
		31.5	9	900			15, 14					3.3	12	12.5		3.0	14.0	3.0	12.5	9
	Limited	28.0	8	750			13, 12	3.3	10	2	20	3.3	9	10	17.5	3.0	10.5	3.0	10.0	8
		24.5	7		2.5	12	11							7.5	14.0	3.0	7.0	3.0	7.5	7
II	Symptomatic	21.0	6	600			10, 9	3.3	5	2	15	3.3	6	5	10.5			2.0	10.5	6
III		17.5	5	450	1.7	10	8, 7			2	10			2.5	7.0	3.0	3.0	2.0	7.0	5
		14.0	4	300	1.7	5	6	3.3	0	2	5	2.0	3	0	3.5	2.5	2.0	2.0	3.5	4
		10.5	3				5, 4	2.0	0	2	0					2.0	0.0	1.5	0.0	3
		7.0	2	150	1.7	0	3, 2											1.0	0.0	2
IV		3.5	1				1													1

MET, metabolic equivalents.

From Froelicher VF: Exercise and the Heart: Clinical Concepts, 3rd ed. St Louis, Mosby, 1993.

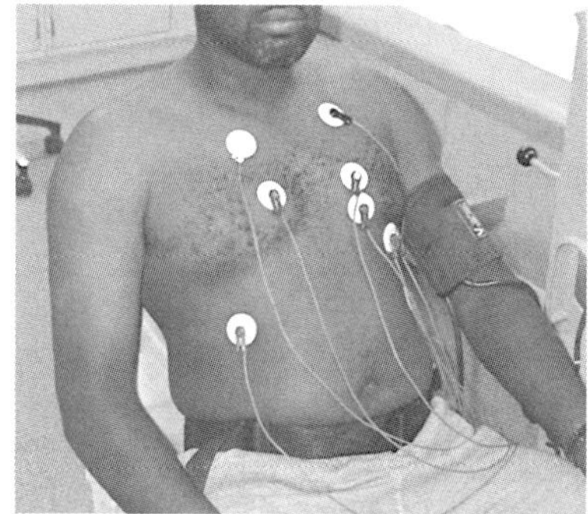

Figure 93-14 Patient with electrodes attached.

5. Prepare the patient for the ECG leads and apply them.
   - Locate sites on the chest for electrode placement, which are the same as for the office ECG (see Chapter 89, Office Electrocardiograms), except that the arm electrodes are placed in the infraclavicular fossae (mid-clavicle) and the leg electrodes are placed on the lower abdomen above the beltline (Fig. 93-14).
   - Cleanse the skin at these sites with an alcohol prep and let the sites dry thoroughly.
   - Shave any hair from the electrode sites. The cornified outer layer of skin should then be removed with gentle dermabrasion. Fine sandpaper or other abrasives are usually provided in the preparation kit for this purpose.
   - Apply electrodes to these sites.
   - Attach lead wires from the *octopus* to the appropriate electrodes. (An ECG octopus is the set of leads usually provided by the equipment manufacturer.)
   - Stabilize the EET octopus with a belt around the patient's waist. The octopus can be bundled and affixed to the patient with extra expansion loops to allow variation in distance from the ECG machine and to minimize motion artifact. Fortunately, most equipment is now digital and can use filters to minimize motion artifact.
   - If desired, for female patients, a gown or loose-fitting shirt can be worn over the lead wires. Jog bras work well; bras with underwire should be avoided.
6. Obtain the supine, resting ECG. Because a recent MI is a contraindication to EET, if there is even the remote chance of a recent MI or an interval MI since the last clinician visit, a routine ECG must be repeated. For maximal diagnostic sensitivity, this supine routine ECG should be obtained with the leads in the standard limb positions to allow for comparison with any prior standard ECGs. If this ECG reveals no changes, the limb leads can then be moved back to the exercise positions to obtain the baseline supine preexercise ECG.

NOTE: In an occasional patient, hyperventilation alone will produce ST segment depression. Because patients naturally hyperventilate during exercise, if there is ST segment depression during the procedure, it may be difficult to determine whether hyperventilation caused it or if there is true ischemia. However, hyperventilation artifact is rare enough that most authorities now recommend hyperventilating only those patients with a positive EET, after recovering them, to determine if hyperventilation caused the ST segment deviation. This technique of hyperventilating only those patients with a positive result saves not only time but expense, including the expense of ECG paper. This method is especially effective in the office setting, where fewer positive results typically occur.

Treadmill EET

7. Have the patient stand and obtain an ECG. This is the resting standing ECG, which becomes the baseline ECG. If the equipment is digital, it will often take 15 to 20 seconds to acquire the resting standing ECG. During this time, the equipment is acquiring an average of 15 to 20 seconds of ECG tracings to provide the "signal average" that it measures against for later comparison.

   NOTE: Occasionally, ST segment depression is provoked by having the patient stand. Therefore, the isoelectric standard to measure against for ST segment depression during exercise is the resting standing baseline ECG before the EET.

8. Begin the EET using the selected protocol. Try to discourage the patient from gripping the handrail during the study because this will falsely elevate the maximal exercise capacity; it may also increase ECG artifact and falsely elevate BP. Time may be saved if staff demonstrates the procedure and allows the patient to practice before the clinician arrives. Staff should show the patient how to rest two fingers or the wrists on the handrail while walking near the front of the treadmill and looking straight ahead. (If the patient looks down, dizziness often results.)

Bicycle Ergometer EET

7. After completing steps 1 through 6 for treadmill EET, have the patient sit on the bicycle and obtain a sitting ECG.
8. Begin the EET using the preselected protocol. The usual protocol starts at 25 W of resistance and increases by 25 W every 2 minutes.

For Both Treadmill and Bicycle Ergometer EET

9. Monitor and record the patient's symptoms, overall condition, heart rate, and ECG at all times. *Instruct the patient to try to give adequate warning before he or she needs to stop the test.* With the exception of submaximal testing, encourage the patient to go as far and as long as possible.
10. Record a 12-lead ECG at the end of each stage, at any time an abnormality is noted on the monitor, immediately on stopping, and every minute postexercise during recovery.

    NOTE: Real data are obtained only from a hard copy of the 12-lead ECG. The monitor merely provides ongoing information, estimates of ST segment changes, and allows the clinician to monitor for arrhythmias. If there is any question regarding ST segment changes, print a hard copy for measurement and interpretation.

11. During each stage, at the start of the final minute, ask the patient if there is any chest discomfort, at what point he or she has reached on the PES, and whether he or she wants to continue into the next stage. Also record the BP and heart rate near the end of each stage or at the time of any problems.

    NOTE: For most patients, their perceived exertion (see Box 93-1) is reproducible at a given level of exercise and tracks fairly linearly with their heart rate. Ask patients to indicate on a scale of 0 to 10 how hard they feel they are working with each stage. On the average, most patients feel they increase by 2 to 3 on the PES with each stage in the early part of the study. PES then usually increases more rapidly, from 7 to 9, near the end of the study. Rarely will anyone declare a 10. Individuals with good perception may not have to measure their pulse as frequently while following their exercise prescription. They can simply be instructed to exercise to the level of perceived exertion that matched their appropriate heart rate for the aerobic range (60% to 80% MHR). On the other hand, patients who highly underestimate their effort must be taught to measure their pulse before receiving an exercise prescription.

12. After completion of the EET, if it has been done for diagnostic purposes and the study has been negative, immediately ask the

patient to lie down. Although this may not be comfortable for certain patients, especially if they are overweight or having slight difficulty breathing, it minimizes false-positive results during the recovery. Make sure to record the heart rate at 1 minute (HRR).

13. If the EET is positive or being performed for CAD management purposes, keep the patient exercising for 3 to 4 minutes during recovery at a very low workload to prevent venous pooling and to minimize the risk of an arrhythmia. The patient may then either sit or lie down for the remainder of recovery.

    NOTE: For positive studies—even for those profoundly positive—very rarely is it necessary to administer medications. Simply stopping the exertion and having the patient sit up to improve oxygenation should be adequate. If there is strong suspicion that a plaque has been destabilized (MI has occurred), aspirin, if not contraindicated, is the best choice for a medication. In the absence of contraindications, oxygen may also be considered. Sublingual nitroglycerin is risky in a vasodilated patient because it may drop the BP. Sublingual calcium channel blockers are contraindicated.

14. Monitor the BP, heart rate, any symptoms, and the ECG tracing during recovery.
15. The patient should be monitored for at least 8 minutes in recovery or until symptoms or ECG abnormalities have resolved (some clinicians monitor only for 4 minutes postexercise for negative EETs in low-risk patients, such as those being tested as part of a wellness program).

Test Termination Criteria

A good rule of thumb for stopping an EET is *after* the necessary information is obtained and *before* there is a complication. In the young or fit individual, when he or she reaches the predicted MHR (220 − age), it may be prudent to explain that all the necessary information has been obtained; however, the patient may continue to exercise for as long as he or she desires. (Allowing the patient to make this choice is also indirectly obtaining informed consent.)

NOTE: In the past, authorities denoted two possible definitions of a maximal EET: (1) achieving a target heart rate of greater than 85% of the predicted MHR for that patient's age (i.e., roughly 85% of 220 − age); or (2) exercise to the point of symptoms or maximal voluntary fatigue. *Most authorities now encourage patients to exercise to the point of symptoms or maximal voluntary fatigue.*

Predicted MHR (220 − age) is not patient specific and is frequently a poor prediction. The only contraindications to going to the point of symptoms are for debilitated or elderly patients or if a submaximal test is indicated. Maximal voluntary fatigue/maximal effort is usually indicated by maximal perceived exertion and the inability to continue at that workload.

Benefits to using the point of symptoms as the end point include the ability to measure true exercise capacity and to determine the patient's true MHR. It also gives the clinician knowledge about a patient's cardiac response at a level of exercise beyond what the patient is likely to reproduce on his or her own. This is certainly reassuring to the clinician when giving an exercise prescription (i.e., it should be safe for the patient to exercise at a lower level of exertion). Disadvantages include discomfort for the patient, especially if he or she is significantly deconditioned.

How does the clinician know if the patient gave a maximal effort? Following the PES is often helpful. Also, an RPP greater than 25,000 generally indicates that the patient has given a good effort. Many other physiologic parameters have been studied in an attempt to predict maximal effort (e.g., heart rate, respiratory rate, BP response), and none has been found to be predictive. However, if patients are aware that it is important to give maximal effort to exclude heart disease, they are usually motivated.

Absolute Indications to Terminate a Study

- As exertion increases during EET, if SBP drops below resting standing value, especially after the first minute or two of the EET (most dangerous if it reflects LV dysfunction; in that situation there is a high risk of life-threatening arrhythmias).
- Worsening anginal chest pain (severe enough that the patient desires to stop); it is not prudent for patients to exercise beyond the point where they obtain their "usual" amount of chest discomfort. In other words, there is no reason for the patient to demonstrate his or her worst chest pain while performing the study.
- Central nervous system symptoms (e.g., dizziness, disorientation).
- Signs of poor perfusion (e.g., cyanosis, pallor) or severe ventricular dysfunction (e.g., dyspnea).
- Serious arrhythmias (e.g., three or more premature ventricular contractions [PVCs] in a row [e.g., a salvo, ventricular tachycardia] is an indication to terminate the test), increasingly frequent PVCs associated with ischemia (chest pain or ST segment changes), or atrial arrhythmia with cardiovascular compromise.
- Technical problems with equipment, ECG monitor, or SBP monitoring.
- Marked ECG changes (>3 mm of horizontal or downsloping ST segment depression, or 1 mm of ST segment elevation).
- When maximal voluntary exertion/maximal effort has been attained.
- Patient wants to stop the test (especially elderly patients, where there may be little warning of a complication about to happen).

Relative Indications to Terminate a Study

- Worrisome ST or QRS segment changes (e.g., excessive junctional depression, marked axis shift)
- Significant fatigue, shortness of breath, wheezing, leg cramps, or intermittent claudication
- Worrisome appearance (especially important in the elderly, where stability can deteriorate very rapidly; poor perfusion may be indicated solely by a loss of color in an elderly patient)
- Elevated BP (SBP >250 mm Hg, DBP >120 mm Hg)
- Less serious dysrhythmia, including supraventricular tachycardia
- Development of a bundle branch block pattern that cannot be distinguished from ventricular tachycardia or an ST segment elevation MI

INTERPRETATION

Incomplete Exercise ECG Tests

Failure to attain at least 85% of the age-predicted MHR is an incomplete EET.

Medications (e.g., beta blockers, rate-limiting calcium channel blockers) are a common cause of this; therefore, another reason to withhold such medications is if the EET is being performed for diagnostic purposes. If the EET is being performed to manage CAD, use of beta blockers may increase the patient's exercise capacity, which is also a goal of cardiac rehabilitation. One hopes that increased exercise capacity is a surrogate marker for improved prognosis. If the EET is being performed for diagnostic purposes and the incomplete EET is not deemed due to a medication, options at this point include an exercise imaging test, a chemical (e.g., regadenoson, adenosine, dipyridamole, dobutamine, arbutamine; see Chapter 94, Stress Echocardiography, for a dobutamine echo protocol) imaging test, cardiology consultation, or getting the patient on an exercise program and repeating the EET in 3 to 6 months. Given the choice, many patients will choose to start an exercise program.

Normal ECG Responses to Exercise

- P-wave amplitude increases.
- T-wave amplitude often increases.

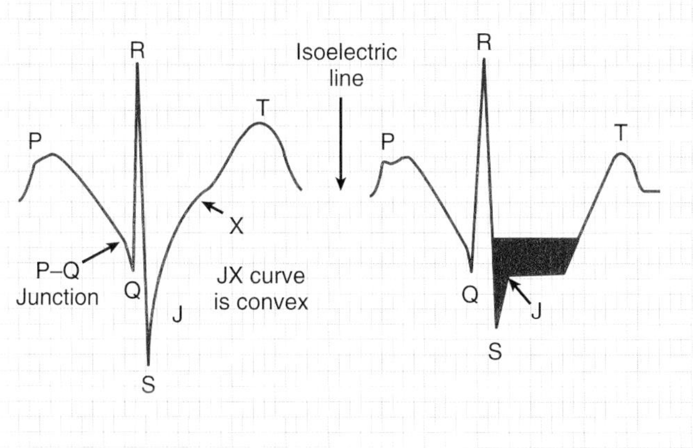

Figure 93-15 *Left,* Normal exercise ECG complex. Note that the P-Q junction is deflected below the resting isoelectric line. This point is considered to be the baseline for determining ST segment deviations. *Right,* A horizontal ST segment depression of 2.0 mm as measured from the P-Q junction. (From Ellestad MH: Stress Testing: Principles and Practice, 4th ed. Philadelphia, FA Davis, 1996.)

- RR and PR intervals decrease in length.
- Below a heart rate of 150 bpm, the R-wave amplitude is unchanged or increased; above 150 bpm or near maximal exercise, the R wave in a healthy heart usually decreases in amplitude, and the overall QRS amplitude also usually decreases, especially in the lateral leads (the so-called Brody effect).
- J-point (i.e., the junction between the S wave and ST segment) is depressed in the lateral (possibly all) leads, especially at maximum exercise, and gradually returns to normal during recovery. The P–Q junction is also usually depressed (Fig. 93-15).
- ST segment slope is usually upsloping; however, from the J-point, the tracing rapidly returns to baseline. In other words, at 0.04 to 0.06 second after the J-point, the final position of the ST segment is at the baseline level.

ST Segment Analysis

- A positive EET is determined by ECG criteria. However, the EET results should not be labeled simply as normal, positive, or abnormal, but rather the specific responses to exercise should be identified and documented.
- Age and risk factors for CAD should be taken into account when interpreting results.
- Many conditions and circumstances can cause a false-positive or a false-negative EET (Box 93-4).
- The lateral leads (e.g., V_4, V_5, V_6) are the most important leads to monitor for ischemia. Their electrodes are located directly over the left ventricle and are the most likely to show ischemic ST segment changes. Although it is always recommended to use at least three leads, studies have found that lead V_5 is the most sensitive lead if a single lead were to be used.

NOTE: The actual data are the hard copy printouts of the 12-lead recordings. It is recommended that these be interpreted separately, in a quiet room, scanning the entire printout, before giving the patient the results and recording them.

1. An EET is considered positive when 1 mm of ST segment depression occurs in at least three beats in a row, in more than one lead, and in an area of the tracing where the baseline is relatively flat. If it is truly positive, ST segment depression usually occurs in almost all of the leads; in most cases it will continue more than 1 minute into recovery. In fact, the ST segment depression may worsen in recovery, especially if the patient is asked to lie down immediately after exercise is discontinued (recommended if EET is being performed for diagnostic purposes).
2. ST segment deviation (depression or elevation) should be measured down or up from the level of the PQ junction. A line drawn horizontally from the PQ junction denotes the isoelectric line (see Fig. 93-15).
3. ST segment deviation (depression or elevation) should be measured at the J-point (i.e., ST zero, also known as the beginning of the ST segment or end of the QRS complex).
4. Most experts now consider the study positive only if the slope for 80 msec after the J-point is horizontal or downsloping. The ACC/AHA guidelines suggest this is the best definition of a positive EET. Other experts also consider a slow upsloping ST

Box 93-4. Causes of False-Positive and False-Negative Test Results

Causes of False-Positive Test Results

Preexisting abnormal resting ECG (e.g., ST segment abnormalities and bundle branch block, especially left bundle branch block)
Cardiac hypertrophy (LVH)
Female sex (see section on "ST Segment Analysis in Women," under "Interpretation")
Wolff-Parkinson-White syndrome and other preexcitation variants
Short PR interval
Anemia, hypothyroidism
Hypertension (poorly controlled)
Hyperventilation
Medications (e.g., digitalis, estrogen, tricyclic antidepressants)
Nonfasting state
Cardiomyopathy
Hypokalemia and other electrolyte abnormalities
Hypoxemia
Vasoregulatory abnormalities
Excessive rate–pressure product (>45,000)
Sudden intense exercise
Mitral valve prolapse syndrome and valvular heart disease
Congenital heart disease
Pericardial disorders
Ventricular pacemaker
Pectus excavatum
Inadequate recording equipment, incorrect criteria, improper interpretation, or improper lead system or placement
Technical or observer error
Atrial repolarization (usually seen in inferior leads only, and short PR interval occurs on resting ECG)

Causes of False-Negative Test Results

Right bundle branch block
Failure to reach an adequate exercise workload
Insufficient number of leads to detect ECG changes
Failure to use other information (e.g., systolic blood pressure drop, symptoms, arrhythmia, heart rate response) in test interpretation
Single-vessel disease
Excessive digital filtration on tracing
Technical or observer error
Medications (tricyclic antidepressants; also medications like long-acting nitrates, beta blockers, and calcium channel blockers have antianginal effects; they may "prolong the positive" or prolong the time of the study before the test becomes positive)

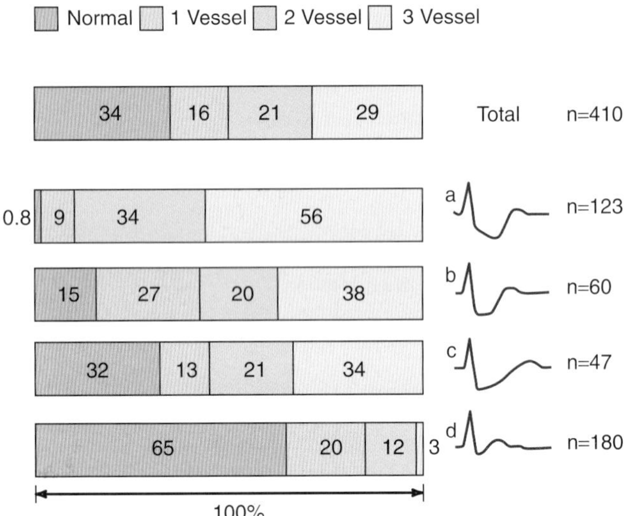

Figure 93-16 Three patterns of ST segment depression. Although the downsloping pattern, *a*, usually represented three-vessel disease (56%) and the flat pattern, *b*, occasionally represented three-vessel disease (38%), the slow-uploading pattern, *c*, had three-vessel disease in 34% and at least one-vessel disease in 68% (these usually convert to flat or downsloping in recovery). The rapid-upsloping pattern, *d*, has been accepted as the normal physiologic pattern. (Redrawn from Goldschlager N, Selzer A, Cohn K: Treadmill stress tests as indicators of presence and severity of coronary artery disease. Ann Intern Med 85:277–286, 1976.)

segment pattern as positive, although this was based on much older data from the 1970s (Fig. 93-16). They will consider a slow upsloping pattern positive if the tracing fails to reach within 1.5 mm of the baseline level of the PQ junction at 80 msec after the J-point. It should be understood that although a slow upsloping pattern may be positive, it is much more likely to be a false-positive result or represent insignificant CAD; however, accepting this pattern as a possible positive result slightly increases the sensitivity of the test for CAD. Therefore, increased sensitivity must thus be weighed against the increased likelihood of a false-positive result. A slow upsloping pattern is more likely to be a true-positive result if it persists beyond 1 minute into recovery and is seen not only in the inferior leads (i.e., II, III, aVF), but in other leads. If the proper technique of immediately laying the patient down during recovery is followed, slow upsloping ST segments that truly represent ischemia usually convert to flat or downsloping ST segments with depression.

5. Although occasionally ST segment elevation (i.e., transmural ischemia) can indicate the vessel involved, ST segment depression does not localize ischemia. In other words, it cannot detect which blood vessel is involved. Subendocardial ischemia is a "global" phenomenon (i.e., for significant CAD, ST segment changes will be seen in most leads).
6. If ST segment elevation occurs over or adjacent to diagnostic Q waves, it may be caused by a ventricular aneurysm or a wall motion abnormality. If it occurs in a patient with a normal resting ECG or without a history of previous infarction, it probably indicates transmural ischemia and the test should be stopped. Transmural ischemia is extremely arrhythmogenic.
7. If downsloping or flat-pattern ST segment depression occurs, and it is less than 1 mm or only in recovery, it may be indicative of early CAD. This is an "equivocal" result. Management options are discussed in a following section.

EET Indicators of Significant or Extensive CAD (Three-Vessel CAD with LV Dysfunction or Left Main CAD)

- Markedly positive ST segment response in multiple leads (>2.5 mm downsloping or horizontal ST segment depression)
- Early positive ST segment response (stage 1 or 2 of Bruce protocol or at ≤4 to 5 METs)
- Unable to complete stage 2 of Bruce protocol (especially if unable to complete stage 1)
- Typical angina chest pain, especially if associated with ST segment depression
- Worrisome ventricular arrhythmias (especially if associated with ST segment depression or at a heart rate <130 bpm)
- Fall in exercise SBP (>10 mm Hg below resting standing baseline), especially when associated with angina or significant ST segment changes
- Prolonged positive ST segment response (>6 minutes of recovery)

ST Segment Analysis in Special Situations

Baseline Abnormalities

When the ST segments are abnormal on the resting ECG, certain criteria can be used to declare a test positive (Table 93-4).

ST Segment Analysis in Women

False-positive results are less common in women older than 50 years of age. The following data are from a study by Pratt and colleagues (1989).

1. True-positive results are associated with four factors:
   - Absence of mitral valve prolapse
   - An exercise duration of less than 5 minutes
   - The ability to reach the target heart rate
   - The ST segment takes 6 minutes or more to normalize
2. False-positive results are associated with two factors:
   - The ability to exercise to stage 3 of the Bruce protocol
   - Rapid (<4 minutes) normalization of the ST segment shift after cessation of exercise

NOTE: In general, if slow upsloping ST segments are used to define a positive EET, they are associated with a high false-positive rate in women. If the proper technique of laying the patient down during recovery is followed, slow upsloping ST segments that truly represent ischemia usually convert to flat or downsloping ST segments with depression.

Scenarios with Decreased Sensitivity and False-Positive and False-Negative Results

- If LBBB or WPW syndrome is present, ST segment depression does not necessarily indicate ischemia.

TABLE 93-4 Recommended Criteria to Declare an EET Positive When There Are Baseline ECG Abnormalities

Abnormal Resting ST Segment T-Wave Configuration	Exercise or Postexercise ST Segment Configuration	ST Segment Depression and Point of Measurement
Flat or sagging ST segment and T wave	Horizontal	1.0 mm more depressed than at rest
	Upsloping	1.5 mm more depressed than at rest at 80 msec from J-point
	Downsloping	1.0 mm more depressed than at rest
Inverted T wave	Horizontal	1.5 mm at 60 msec from J-point
	Upsloping	1.5 mm at 80 msec from J-point
	Downsloping	1.5 mm at 20 msec from J-point

Note that these current criteria are slightly different depending on the configuration of the resting ST segment and T wave.
From Ellestad MH: Horizontal and downsloping ST segments. In Stress Testing: Principles and Practice, 4th ed, Philadelphia, FA Davis, 1996.

- If RBBB is present, the ST segments can be analyzed only in V_4, V_5, or V_6, and the sensitivity of the test may be decreased.

  NOTE: Recent data indicate that the presence of complete RBBB on the resting ECG is associated with a 50% greater risk of death over the next 20 years, a rate similar to that of LBBB. The mechanism underlying the relationship is unclear.

- If ST segment depression occurs only in inferior leads II, III, or aVF and not in the lateral leads, it is usually a false-positive result caused by atrial repolarization. When reviewing, these patients frequently have a short PR interval on the resting ECG (the atrial repolarization wave, which is negative, "pulls down" the ST segment when superimposed). Frequently, the ST segment depression returns to normal in less than 1 minute of recovery in the false-positive cases.
- If coronary artery bypass surgery has been performed, sensitivity of the test may be decreased.
- If anterior or lateral Q waves or both are present (after MI), the sensitivity of the test may be decreased.
- See Box 93-4 for a complete listing of causes of false-positive and false-negative test results.

Arrhythmias

- Prognosis in supraventricular and ventricular arrhythmias appears to be more related to underlying or coexisting conditions, especially ischemia. Patients who are symptomatic should be treated or referred.
- If the arrhythmia is associated with signs or symptoms of ischemia, in most cases management should be directed at treating the ischemia to minimize the arrhythmia.
- PVCs are common. They are ominous only in patients with LV dysfunction, severe ischemia, valvular heart disease, a cardiomyopathy, or a family history of sudden cardiac death.
- Three unifocal PVCs in a row is defined as a "salvo" and an indication to terminate the test. Interestingly, asymptomatic, nonsustained ventricular tachycardia in an individual with a normal ejection fraction is not associated with increased cardiovascular mortality. However, a Holter monitor, echocardiogram, or both may be indicated.
- Young (i.e., <40 years of age) but otherwise healthy individuals with no CAD risk factors may have frequent PVCs at rest that resolve with exercise. If the EET is negative, further evaluation is often not necessary. PVCs that go away with exercise in this population are almost always benign.

Exercise Capacity and Heart Rate Recovery

- The ability to achieve 15 METs indicates an excellent prognosis, even in those with known three-vessel CAD. The ability to achieve 10 METs indicates that medical management is reasonable, even in patients with a positive EET. An inability to achieve 5 METs indicates a poor prognosis, especially if the EET is positive.
- $\dot{V}O_2$ max can be estimated from various exercise protocols using standard formulas, tables, or graphs. Using estimated $\dot{V}O_2$ max, an individual's approximate level of aerobic conditioning can be determined using age- and sex-matched tables. Figure 93-17 also estimates the exercise capacity based on the number of METs a patient can achieve.
- Failure of the heart rate to decrease 12 bpm in the first minute of recovery is an abnormal HRR. This indicates a fourfold increased risk of mortality over the next 5 years.
- As mentioned previously, in patients where ECG changes during EET could not be used to predict prognosis (e.g., baseline ECG abnormalities, digoxin use)—in other words, the DTS could not be used—Diaz and colleagues (2001) at the Mayo Clinic found exercise capacity and HRR to be better predictors of risk over 6.7 years than radionuclide imaging in nonrevascularized patients.

Other Parameters Followed

- *Heart rate:* Failure to obtain a heart rate of 120 bpm is chronotropic incompetence with a resultant poor prognosis

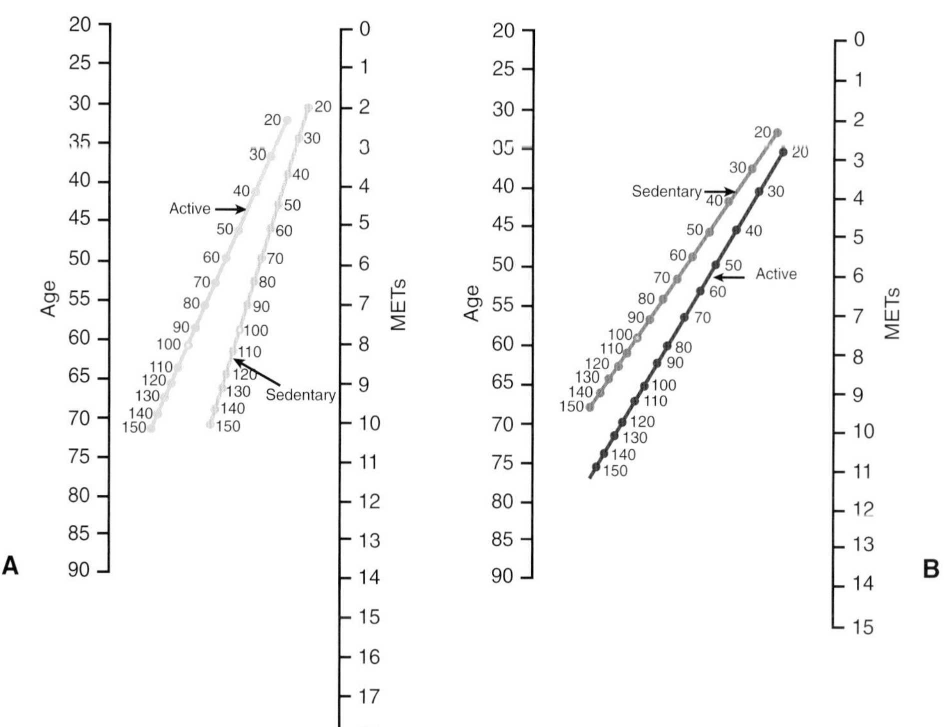

Figure 93-17 Nomograms of percentage normal exercise capacity. **A,** Percentage of normal in healthy men. **B,** Percentage of normal in referred men. (Redrawn from Kenney WL [ed]: ACSM's Guidelines for Exercise Testing and Prescription, 5th ed. Baltimore, Williams & Wilkins, 1995.)

(approximately 15% per year will experience a coronary event); it may also indicate early sick sinus syndrome.

- *BP:* As exertion increases during EET, if the SBP drops below resting standing baseline, it predicts either a poor prognosis or severe CAD. In one study, men with a maximal exercise SBP of less than 140 mm Hg also had a 15-fold increase in the annual rate of sudden death compared with those whose pressures exceeded 200 mm Hg.

  A DBP increase of more than 10 mm Hg, an SBP greater than 214 mm Hg, or failure of DBP and SBP to return to normal 3 minutes into recovery is a *hypertensive response to exercise.* In otherwise healthy individuals, a hypertensive response to exercise increases the likelihood that they will develop hypertension over the next few years. However, EET should not be used to screen for hypertension because ambulatory BP monitoring is much more effective. In individuals with known hypertension, a hypertensive response to exercise may indicate poorly treated hypertension. Poorly treated hypertension may have a negative impact on exercise tolerance.
- *BP and heart rate in diabetic patients:* Diabetes can cause an elevated resting heart rate; BP and heart rate responses are frequently blunted in diabetic patients.
- *Symptoms:* Substernal chest pain in men being tested on a treadmill, even without ECG changes, is 90% predictive of CAD in studies from a few decades ago.
- *Lack of symptoms:* Painless ST segment depression (i.e., silent ischemia) is common in diabetic patients and those older than 70 years of age.

Determining Prognosis

Normal ECG Responses and Negative EET (Prognosis Is Excellent)

- Absence of any change in the ST segment at maximal or near MHR.
- Junctional or J-point depression with rapidly rising ST segment slope.
- Development of isolated T-wave inversion without ST segment displacement.
- Ventricular ectopic beats occur infrequently, especially those occurring at heart rates exceeding 130 bpm and not associated with any evidence of ischemia.
- Although rare, even a poorly controlled atrial arrhythmia without cardiovascular compromise has a good prognosis.
- Although rare, development of RBBB with exercise has a good prognosis.

Patients can be reassured that if they achieve a heart rate of 160 bpm (regardless of age) and achieve 13 METs (basically equivalent to completing 12 minutes on the Bruce protocol), even with ECG evidence of ischemia, they have a very good 4- to 5-year prognosis. They basically have less than a 1% per year risk of a cardiac event for that time span. The same is true if they achieve an RPP greater than 35,000; they are extremely unlikely to have significant CAD. Even for positive studies, periodic evaluation with a retest in 6 to 12 months may be the most aggressive management needed.

If patients are unable to achieve these end points, it may indicate either inadequate effort by the patient or the presence of CAD. For a strong clinical suspicion of disease, additional testing such as imaging or angiography should be considered.

Positive and Abnormal EETs

To obtain prognosis data for abnormalities of heart rate or blood pressure, see "Other Parameters Followed" in the previous section. Otherwise, prognosis is poor for patients unable to achieve 5 METs or for patients demonstrating a positive EET at less than 5 METs. For those patients in whom an intervention is appropriate or if the clinician is unsure of the diagnosis, prognosis, or management, a cardiologist should be consulted.

For those patients with a positive EET and able to achieve 5 METs, a heart rate of 120 bpm, and an RPP of more than 25,000, a nomogram is available for determining prognosis, counseling, and follow-up. As opposed to other similar nomograms available, women (although not as many) were included in the studies resulting in the nomogram in Figure 93-18. Therefore, this nomogram can be used when counseling women.

Most large coronary artery bypass surgery centers have known or published complication rates. The AHA's website (www.americanheart.org) also has excellent data for predicting complications from coronary artery bypass surgery. Using the nomogram (see Fig. 93-18), patients can evaluate their annual risk of a cardiovascular event with medical management versus a surgical intervention. These are very powerful tools for what is usually a very important decision for patients to make.

Based on several studies, for patients with CAD and able to achieve 10 METs, which is basically the level of exertion necessary to complete approximately 9 minutes of a Bruce protocol, medical management is prudent or reasonable. It is also very unlikely that these patients have significant disease if they achieve a RPP of 25,000 or greater. With an outstanding exercise capacity, even patients with multivessel CAD do well. One study revealed that in patients with known three-vessel CAD and able to complete 15 minutes of a Bruce protocol, the 5-year survival rate was 100%.

Complications

- Hypotension
- Congestive heart failure exacerbation
- Severe cardiac arrhythmia
- Cardiac arrest
- Acute MI
- Acute central nervous system event, such as syncope or stroke
- Death

NOTE: The overall safety of EET has been confirmed with multiple studies. For patients being tested on a treadmill, the mortality rate is approximately 1 in 10,000. The hospital admission rate related to arrhythmia, prolonged chest pain, or MI is approximately 4 in 10,000. However, it should be noted that these numbers include patients with known CAD, perhaps even taking antiarrhythmics. A much smaller risk can be maintained if patients are selected carefully, which is what must be done for office testing.

Postprocedure Patient Education

Patients should be informed that EET, just like any other noninvasive study for diagnosing CAD, is not 100% accurate. Individuals with a change in symptoms or symptoms of chest discomfort, palpitations, or any other symptoms that could be caused by CAD should be evaluated by their clinician regardless of the result of the EET.

In patients with CAD or a high probability of CAD, counseling should be directed at modifying risk factors. Exercise prescriptions should be given and discussed.

Giving an Aerobic Exercise Prescription

- Exercise capacity or endurance is increased by performing regular (i.e., three episodes per week) aerobic exercise. For primary prevention, although a fourth episode further increases exercise capacity, after the fourth per week the incremental benefit is less. The greatest benefit of additional episodes of exercise per week

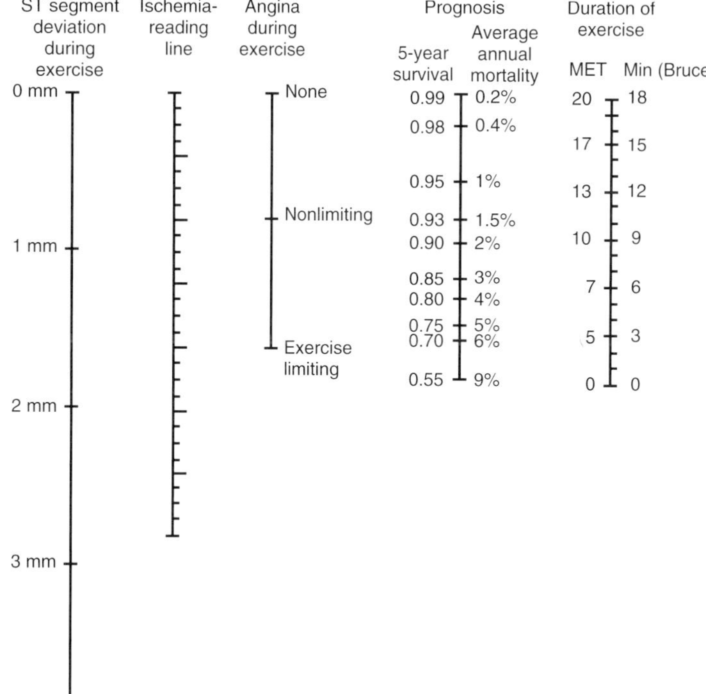

Figure 93-18 Nomogram for Duke University Prognostic Score. (Redrawn from Mark DB, Shaw L, Harrell FE, et al: Prognostic value of a treadmill exercise score in outpatients with suspected coronary artery disease. N Engl J Med 325:849–853, 1991.)

is to assist with weight loss. For secondary prevention, there continues to be improvement in exercise capacity with additional episodes per week. Consequently, most cardiac rehabilitation programs recommend exercising most days of the week for an hour a day.

- For primary prevention, aerobic exercise can be performed 3 days in a row to maintain fitness; however, the risk of an injury increases without adequate rest between episodes. It is therefore recommended that individuals exercise, at an aerobic level, every other day. Participating in a less intense walking program on intervening days may also assist with weight loss.
- Aerobic exercise involves raising the heart rate to a specified point (60% to 80% of MHR) and maintaining that level of exercise for 30 to 45 minutes per session. Three 10-minute episodes in the same day accomplish the same effect as one 30-minute episode.
- After EET, a safe aerobic training range is at a heart rate of 60% to 80% of MHR. This range is called the *target heart rate*. A PES of 5 to 7 can also be used in most patients; however, some patients have a poor perception of level of exertion, and therefore PES cannot be used.
- Patients should avoid dehydration and weather extremes. Unlike what was done if the EET was performed for diagnostic purposes, they should warm up and cool down after each episode, especially older patients.
- A repeat EET can evaluate the improvement after implementation of an aerobic exercise program. After introduction of an exercise program, it takes approximately 12 weeks of regular exercise to achieve a new level of exercise capacity.
- To avoid boredom, it is recommended that an exercise prescription include more than one kind of aerobic exercise (e.g., swimming, biking, race walking, jogging, aerobic dance).
- An exercise prescription should include a target heart range or level of PES, duration of exercise sessions, frequency of sessions, and types of exercises that can be used to achieve the goals of cardiovascular conditioning (aerobic). For new exercise prescriptions, the rate of progression needs to be explained.
- Competitive athletes want to use their training program to raise their anaerobic threshold (i.e., level of exercise at which they can no longer oxygenate all tissues). Anaerobic thresholds are now best measured with ventilator-expired gas analysis EET.

Patient Education Guides

See the sample patient consent form available online at www.expertconsult.com.

CPT/Billing Codes

93000 Electrocardiogram, routine ECG with at least 12 leads; with interpretation and report
93015 Cardiovascular stress test using maximal or submaximal treadmill or bicycle exercise, continuous ECG monitoring, and/or pharmacologic stress; with physician supervision, with interpretation and report
93016 Physician supervision only, without interpretation and report
93017 Tracing only, without interpretation and report
93018 Interpretation and report only

ICD-9-CM Diagnostic Codes

412 Old MI (healed; past MI diagnosed on ECG, but currently no symptoms)
413.9 Other and unspecified angina pectoris
414.01 Coronary atherosclerosis, of native coronary artery
414.02 Coronary atherosclerosis, of autologous vein bypass graft
414.04 Coronary atherosclerosis, of artery bypass graft
414.05 Coronary atherosclerosis, of unspecified type of bypass graft
414.8 Chronic coronary insufficiency
427.69 Ventricular premature beats, contractions, or systoles
785.1 Palpitations
786.51 Precordial chest pain

SUPPLIERS

(See contact information online at www.expertconsult.com.)

NOTE: Most manufacturers in the following list also sell defibrillators. Purchasing these as part of a package is often cost effective.

Cardiac Science (from merger of Burdick and Quinton Instrument Co).
General Electric Healthcare
Mortara
Welch Allyn Schiller

Emergency/ACLS medication kits
Banyan International Corp.

Expired gas analysis or cardiopulmonary exercise testing
Medical Graphics

BIBLIOGRAPHY

BARI Investigators: The final 10-year follow-up results from the BARI randomized trial. J Am Coll Cardiol 49:1600–1606, 2007.

Diamond GA, Forrester JS: Analysis of probability as an aid in the clinical diagnosis of coronary-artery disease. N Engl J Med 300:1350–1358, 1979.

Diaz LA, Brunken RC, Blackstone EH, et al: Independent contribution of myocardial perfusion defects to exercise capacity and heart rate recovery for prediction of all-cause mortality in patients with known or suspected coronary heart disease. J Am Coll Cardiol 37:1558–1564, 2001.

Douglas PS, Khandheria B, Stainback RF, et al: ACCF/ASE/ACEP/AHA/ASNC/SCAI/SCCT/SCMR 2008 appropriateness criteria for stress echocardiography: A report of the American College of Cardiology Foundation Appropriateness Criteria Task Force, American Society of Echocardiography, American College of Emergency Physicians, American Heart Association, American Society of Nuclear Cardiology, Society for Cardiovascular Angiography and Interventions, Society of Cardiovascular Computed Tomography, and Society for Cardiovascular Magnetic Resonance: Endorsed by the Heart Rhythm Society and the Society of Critical Care Medicine. Circulation 117:1478–1497, 2008. Available at circ.ahajournals.org/cgi/reprint/CIRCULATIONAHA.107.189097. Accessed March 22, 2009.

Ellestad MH: Stress Testing: Principles and Practice, 5th ed. New York, Oxford University Press, 2003.

Evans CH: Exercise testing. Prim Care Clin Off Pract 28, 2001.

Evans CH, Karunaratne HB: Exercise stress testing for the family physician. Part I: Performing the test. Am Fam Physician 45:121–132, 1992.

Evans CH, Karunaratne HB: Exercise stress testing for the family physician. Part II: Interpretation of the results. Am Fam Physician 45:679–688, 1992.

Fleisher LA, Beckman JA, Brown KA, et al: ACC/AHA 2007 guidelines on perioperative cardiovascular evaluation and care for noncardiac surgery: Executive summary. A report of the American College of Cardiology/American Heart Association Task Force on Practice Guidelines (Writing Committee to Revise the 2002 Guidelines on Perioperative Cardiovascular Evaluation for Noncardiac Surgery). Circulation 116:1971–1996, 2007. Available at circ.ahajournals.org/cgi/content/full/116/17/1971. Accessed March 11, 2009.

Fletcher GF, Balady GJ, Amsterdam EA, et al: American Heart Association Scientific Statement: Exercise standards for testing and training: a statement for healthcare professionals from the American Heart Association. Circulation 104:1694–1740, 2001.

Fletcher GF, Mills WC, Taylor WC: Update on exercise stress testing. Am Fam Physician 74:1749–1754, 2006.

Fowler G, Altman M: Exercise testing after bypass or percutaneous coronary intervention. In Evans CH, White RD (eds): Exercise Stress Testing for Primary Care and Sports Medicine Physicians. New York, Springer-Verlag, 2009, pp 231–254.

Fowler GC, Evans CH, Altman MA: Exercise testing. Prim Care 24:375–406, 1997.

Fraker TD Jr, Fihn SD; 2002 Chronic Stable Angina Writing Committee; American College of Cardiology; American Heart Association, Gibbons RJ, et al: 2007 Chronic angina focused update of the 2002 guidelines for the management of patients with chronic stable angina: A report of the American College of Cardiology/American Heart Association Task Force on Practice Guidelines Writing Group to develop the focused update of the 2002 guidelines for the management of patients with chronic stable angina. J Am Coll Cardiol 50:2264–2274, 2007. Available at circ.ahajournals.org/cgi/reprint/CIRCULATIONAHA.107.187930. Accessed March 11, 2009.

Froelicher VF, Myers J: Exercise and the Heart, 5th ed. Philadelphia, Saunders, 2006.

Froelicher VF, Quaglietti S: Handbook of Exercise Testing. Boston, Little, Brown, 1996.

Gibbons RJ, Abrams J, Chatterjee K, et al: ACC/AHA 2002 guideline update for the management of patients with chronic stable angina—summary article: A report of the American College of Cardiology/American Heart Association Task Force on Practice Guidelines (Committee on the Management of Patients With Chronic Stable Angina). Circulation 107:149–158, 2003. Available at circ.ahajournals.org/cgi/content/full/107/1/149. Accessed March 11, 2009.

Gibbons RJ, Balady GJ, Bricker JT, et al: ACC/AHA 2002 guideline update for exercise testing: summary article: a report of the American College of Cardiology/American Heart Association Task Force on Practice Guidelines (Committee to Update the 1997 Exercise Testing Guidelines). Circulation 106:1883–1892, 2002. Available at circ.ahajournals.org/cgi/content/full/106/14/1883. Full text also available online at www.americanheart.org/downloadable/heart/1204037436515exercise_clean.pdf. Accessed March 11, 2009.

Gibbons RJ, Hodge DO, Berman DS, et al: Long-term outcome of patients with intermediate-risk exercise electrocardiograms who do not have myocardial perfusion defects on radionuclide imaging. Circulation 100:2140–2145, 1999.

Klocke FJ, Baird MG, Lorell BH, et al: ACC/AHA/ASNC guidelines for the clinical use of cardiac radionuclide imaging: Executive summary. A report of the American College of Cardiology/American Heart Association Task Force on Practice Guidelines (ACC/AHA/ASNC Committee to Revise the 1995 Guidelines for the Clinical Use of Cardiac Radionuclide Imaging). Circulation 108:1404–1418, 2003. Available at circ.ahajournals.org/cgi/content/full/108/11/1404. Accessed March 11, 2009.

Knox MA: Optimize your use of stress tests: A Q&A guide. J Fam Pract 59:262–268, 2010.

Krone RJ, Hardison RM, Chaitman BR, et al: Risk stratification after successful coronary revascularization: The lack of a role for routine exercise testing. J Am Coll Cardiol 38:136–142, 2001.

Mark DB, Shaw L, Harrell FE Jr, et al: Prognostic value of a treadmill exercise score in outpatients with suspected coronary artery disease. N Engl J Med 325:849–853, 1991.

Mattera JA, Arain SA, Sinusas AJ, et al: Exercise testing with myocardial perfusion imaging in patients with normal baseline electrocardiograms: Cost savings with a stepwise diagnostic strategy. J Nucl Cardiol 5:498–506, 1998.

Nishime EO, Cole CR, Blackstone EH, et al: Heart rate recovery and treadmill exercise score as predictors of mortality in patients referred for exercise ECG. JAMA 284:1392–1398, 2000.

Pratt CM, Francis MJ, Divine GW, Young JB: Exercise testing in women with chest pain: Are there additional exercise characteristics that predict true positive test results? Chest 95:139–144, 1989.

Rodgers GP, Ayanian JZ, Balady G, et al: American College of Cardiology/American Heart Association Clinical Competence Statement on Stress Testing: A report of the American College of Cardiology/American Heart Association/American College of Physicians-American Society of Internal Medicine Task Force on Clinical Competence. Circulation 102:1726–1738, 2000. Available at circ.ahajournals.org/cgi/reprint/102/14/1726. Accessed March 11, 2009.

Stein RA, Chaitman BR, Balady GJ, et al: Safety and utility of exercise testing in emergency room chest pain centers: An advisory from the Committee on Exercise, Rehabilitation and Prevention, Council on Clinical Cardiology, American Heart Association. Circulation 102:1463–1467, 2000.

Usatine RP: The Color Atlas of Family Medicine. New York, McGraw-Hill, 2009.

CHAPTER 94

Stress Echocardiography

Grant C. Fowler • Al Smith

Although one of every three deaths (more than half a million deaths a year) in the United States is caused by coronary artery disease (CAD), which is the leading cause of death in both genders, we are doing a better job at keeping these patients alive. Consequently, primary care clinicians will continue to manage an increasing number of patients with known CAD. Not only is stress echocardiography ("stress echo") a safe, cost-effective, and noninvasive method for diagnosing CAD, but it is also helpful for managing CAD, including determining the prognosis. Some clinicians also use stress echo to screen high-risk asymptomatic individuals or to stratify risk in preoperative evaluations. With medical management of CAD more successful than ever, primary care clinicians' skills in diagnosing and managing CAD have become more important. Performing stress echo is one method of maximizing these skills.

With improved ultrasound technology and image quality, adequate imaging can now be produced from 85% to 90% of patients undergoing stress echo. Improved digital imaging recording capabilities are also more likely to provide adequate pre- and postexercise stress echo images for comparison, side by side. The cost of echo equipment has also decreased significantly as the technology has expanded and improved. Consequently, echo has seen some of the most rapid growth among procedures performed by primary care clinicians.

Adding a cardiac imaging test to an exercise electrocardiography (ECG) test (EET) or a pharmacologic stress test is indicated when there is need to define the location, overall extent, or functional significance of CAD. Differing from an EET, which cannot predict which obstructed coronary artery is causing a positive test, stress echo is able to determine which coronary artery is obstructed by noting which ventricular wall becomes ischemic (Table 94-1). Although coronary angiography may not be the best method for determining the functional significance of CAD, it can be used as the gold standard when comparing the accuracy of nuclear myocardial perfusion imaging with stress echo. In the revascularized patient, several meta-analyses compared the accuracy of these two tests for detection of restenosis. Based on results showing very similar sensitivities, specificities, and accuracies for diagnosis of CAD, the choice of imaging for CAD after revascularization will likely depend upon clinician experience and other local factors, such as availability and expertise. Regarding prognosis for patients with CAD, several other meta-analyses compared stress echo with myocardial perfusion imaging and demonstrated comparable results. If echo images are excellent, stress echo may be more accurate than myocardial perfusion imaging.

Further, when evaluating patients for cardiac problems, stress echo can diagnose other possible causes such as hypertrophic cardiomyopathy, aortic dissection, valvular heart disease, diastolic dysfunction, and pericardial effusion, which sets it apart from myocardial perfusion imaging. Stress echo is also faster to complete, is less expensive, and does not require irradiation.

In addition to greater convenience to the patient, benefits for primary care clinicians performing stress echo (especially in the office setting) include having test results immediately available, improving communication and referral patterns to cardiologists, and improving their echo reading skills. Clinicians performing stress echo also naturally improve their understanding of CAD pathophysiology as well as exercise physiology. With immediately available results, patient satisfaction is usually improved and liability for the clinician from failure to diagnose should be decreased.

Physiology of Stress Echocardiography

Normally, as the heart rate increases with exercise, the walls of the left ventricle increase contractility, increase endocardial excursion (>5 mm), become hyperdynamic, and thicken in systole. Depending upon the exercise protocol utilized, the ejection fraction will also normally increase. Consequently, the end-systolic volume, which is the actual size of the left ventricle at end-systole, decreases. In the patient with obstructive CAD, with increasing exercise, a threshold is eventually reached at which the heart's demand for oxygen exceeds the supply. At this threshold, the heart becomes ischemic, first regionally or in segments, and then often globally. Although it is best to obtain echo images within the first minute of discontinuing exercise, this blunting of wall motion will typically persist for 3 to 5 minutes depending on the severity and duration of the preceding ischemia. Interpretation of a stress echo test consists of quantifying these transient regional wall motion abnormalities (Fig. 94-1) as well as the global function (i.e., ejection fraction/end-systolic volume). Transient ischemia is assessed and quantified by comparing pre- and postexercise echo images. (Depending on the protocol, images are also sometimes obtained at maximal exertion.)

From an ECG perspective, with subendocardial ischemia, the patient usually demonstrates ST segment depression (i.e., a positive exercise EET; see Chapter 93, Exercise Electrocardiography [Stress] Testing) in several leads. Usually this depression is followed by chest discomfort (i.e., angina) as the "ischemic cascade" progresses. The term "ischemic cascade" describes the predictable sequence of events that occur after the onset of ischemia. With stress echo, earlier aspects of this ischemic cascade can be noted. Soon after the metabolic abnormalities are produced from ischemia, diastolic abnormalities appear, and these can be seen with stress echo. The appearance of these abnormalities is rapidly followed by myocardial perfusion defects and, in turn, by wall motion abnormalities again seen on stress echo. In other words, ischemic changes can be seen on perfusion imaging and stress echo prior to the development of ECG changes on EET. Eventually chest pain may develop, the exception being patients who experience so-called "silent angina" (typically patients >70 years of age, possibly earlier in diabetics). In patients with silent angina, dyspnea or dyspnea with exertion is a common presentation of an anginal equivalent.

Because exercise capacity is an important, separate predictor of outcome from a cardiovascular perspective, for those patients able to exercise, exercise echo is recommended over pharmacologic stress echo. For those able to walk on a treadmill, it is probably the preferred mode of exercise testing because the workload achieved as well as the maximal heart rate is usually higher than with a bicycle.

TABLE 94-1 Left Ventricular Wall Segments and Corresponding Coronary Artery Supply

Echocardiographic Segment	Coronary Artery
Basal, mid-, and apical anterior	LAD
Basal, mid-, and apical anterior septum	LAD
Apical lateral	LAD
Basal and mid-anterolateral	LAD/LCA
Basal and mid-inferior	RCA
Basal and mid-inferior septum	RCA
Apical inferior	RCA/LAD
Basal and mid-inferolateral	LCA

LAD, left anterior descending artery; LCA, left circumflex artery; RCA, right coronary artery.

The most common forms of exercise in the United States are walking and jogging, so patients are often more comfortable with a treadmill and it is possibly less effort- or motivation-dependent. However, the maximal blood pressure achieved is usually higher on a bicycle than with a treadmill, and images can be obtained during exercise and at peak workload with use of a supine bicycle. A bicycle is also often the preferred form of exercise for patients with orthopedic problems.

INDICATIONS

AUTHOR'S NOTE: The American College of Cardiology (ACC)/ American Heart Association (AHA) suggest that for the patient capable of exercise with no baseline ECG abnormalities affecting the ability to monitor or interpret an EET (e.g, left bundle branch block [LBBB], digitalis effect, Wolff-Parkinson-White [WPW] syndrome, left ventricular hypertrophy [LVH], >1 mm ST segment depression), EET is the preferred method of evaluation to exclude CAD. *Not every patient* needs to be evaluated with imaging. Even in the patient with an intermediate pretest probability of disease, the ACC/AHA recommend a stepwise strategy for diagnosing CAD; in these patients, an EET is the preferred initial test. That said, there are plenty of indications for stress echo:

- Detection of CAD.
- Dyspnea possibly due to CAD.

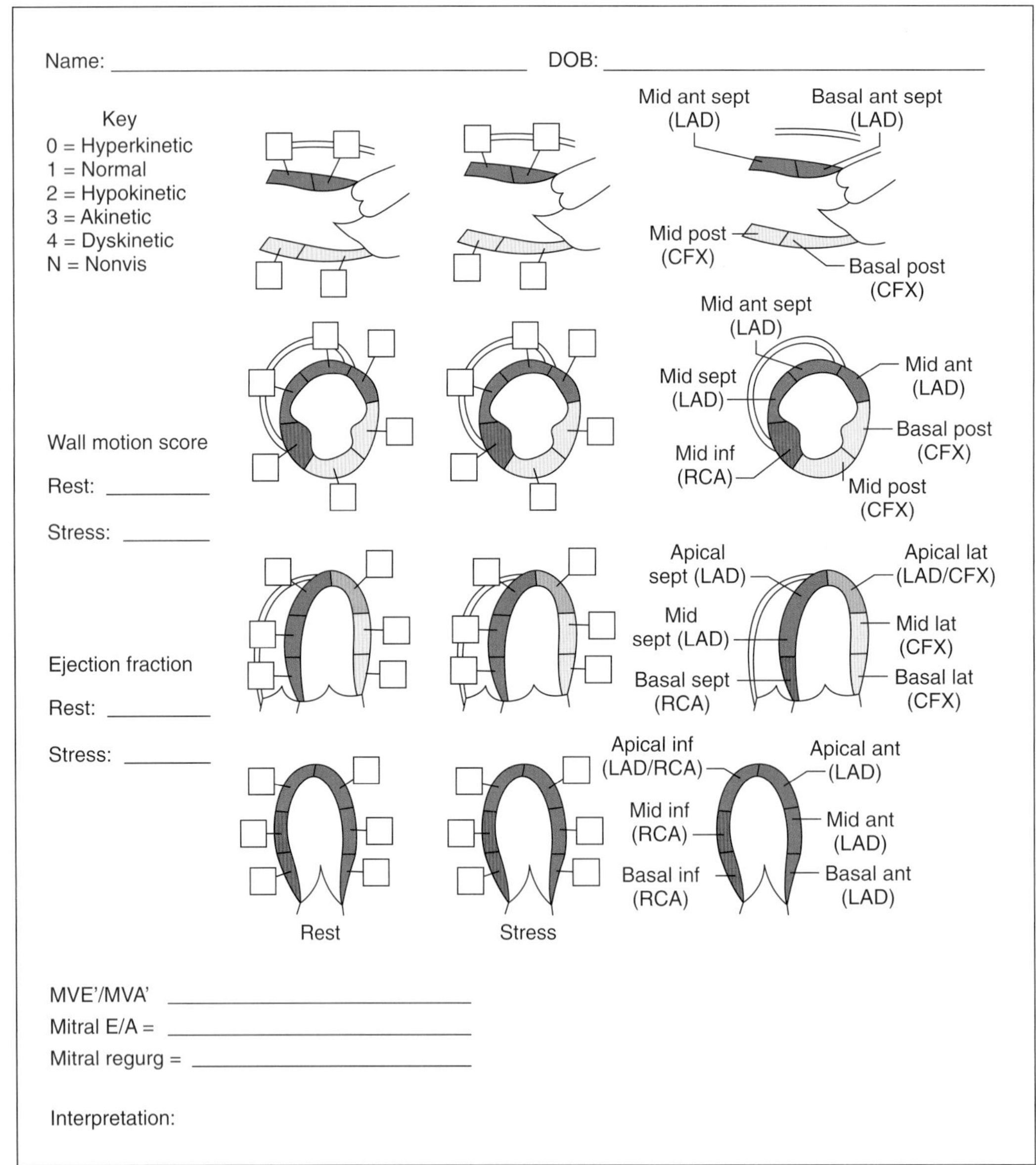

Figure 94-1 Stress echocardiography test score form. CFX, circumflex coronary artery; DOB, date of birth; LAD, left anterior descending coronary artery; MVA', mitral valve annulus velocity; MVE', mitral inflow velocity; RCA, right coronary artery.

- Equivocal, uninterpretable, or suspected false-positive EET.
- High probability of false-positive EET (e.g., women, mitral valve prolapse).
- Baseline ECG abnormalities that would affect the ability to monitor or interpret an EET (e.g., LBBB, digitalis effect, WPW syndrome, LVH, >1 mm ST segment depression).
- New-onset atrial fibrillation or heart failure, especially if there is an intermediate pretest probability of CAD.
- Need to define extent, location, or functional significance of CAD.
- Risk stratification/prognostic assessment in patient with known CAD (preoperative, post–myocardial infarction).

AUTHOR'S NOTE: Dobutamine echo is probably the preferred method of evaluating a patient preoperatively for high-risk or vascular surgery. See Box 94-1 for shortcuts to determine indications for noninvasive testing prior to noncardiac surgery. (See also Chapter 230, Preoperative Evaluation.)

- Risk stratification after coronary revascularization (percutaneous coronary intervention or coronary artery bypass graft) procedures.
- Viability assessment in candidate for revascularization.
- Radionuclide perfusion imaging not available.
- High probability of false-positive radionuclide perfusion imaging (e.g., correction software package not available for perfusion imaging when likely to have attenuation artifact due to nearby adipose tissue such as in women or large-chested men).

Box 94-1. Shortcuts to Determine Indicators for Noninvasive Testing before Noncardiac Surgery

No testing necessary if the answer is *Yes* to any of these four questions:

1. Is this low-risk surgery (e.g., endoscopic, superficial, cataract, breast, ambulatory surgery)?
2. Does the patient have fair functional/exercise capacity (≥4 METs) and no symptoms?
3. Has the patient undergone revascularization (CABG or PCI) within last 5 years without a change in symptoms indicating ischemia?
4. Has the patient had a thorough cardiac evaluation within last 2 years without a change in symptoms indicating ischemia?

Conversely, if vascular surgery is planned and patient has three or more clinical risk factors (CAD, CHF, ASCVD, diabetes, or renal insufficiency), noninvasive testing is reasonable if the results will change the management.

Also, if the answer is *Yes* to both of the following two questions, noninvasive testing is reasonable*:

1. Poor functional/exercise capacity by questionnaire or specific questioning? (<4 METs or inability to climb one flight of stairs)
2. Clinical risk factor present? (CAD, CHF, ASCVD, diabetes, or renal insufficiency)

*For intermediate- or high-risk surgery with only one or two clinical predictors present, there is insufficient evidence to determine the best management—β-blockade therapy versus noninvasive testing.
ASCVD, atherosclerotic cardiovascular disease; CABG, coronary artery bypass graft; CAD, coronary artery disease; CHF, congestive heart failure; METs, metabolic equivalents; PCI, percutaneous coronary intervention.
From ACC/AHA: 2007 Guidelines on perioperative cardiovascular evaluation and care for noncardiac surgery. Circulation 116: 1971–1996, 2007.

- Asymptomatic patients with multiple risk factors for CAD, or high-risk coronary calcium score from electron beam computed tomography scan (EBCT) or on ambulatory ECG (Holter or event) monitoring (see Chapter 87, Ambulatory Electrocardiography: Holter and Event Monitoring).
- Incomplete EET (failure to achieve 85% of predicted maximal heart rate; pharmacologic testing may be indicated).
- A pharmacologic agent may be indicated with stress echo (dobutamine, arbutamine preferred for stress echo over vasodilator infusion; vasodilator infusion usually preferred for myocardial perfusion imaging) in patients unable to exercise (e.g., peripheral artery disease, orthopedic problems, low exercise tolerance, contraindications to exercise [acute coronary syndrome with negative serial cardiac markers, equivocal aortic stenosis with low cardiac output]). Vasodilator (e.g., adenosine, dipyridamole, regadenoson) infusion produces only mild to moderate increases in heart rate and a mild decrease in blood pressure.
- Contrast study may be indicated with stress echo if two or more segments are not seen on noncontrast images.
- Permanent or transesophageal pacing may be indicated with stress echo (the pacing rate can be increased until the desired heart rate is achieved; however, these techniques are beyond the scope of this chapter).
- Mitral and aortic valve stenosis and regurgitation can be assessed, usually involving color Doppler (these techniques are beyond the scope of this chapter).
- Careful assessment of aortic stenosis by noting rapid change in pre– and post–aortic valve peak pressures.

Results of a comprehensive, expert survey are available regarding the appropriate use of stress echo. The most common and appropriate indications for primary care clinicians include diagnosing CAD (especially when EET is uninterpretable or equivocal or there is a high risk of a false-positive EET or myocardial perfusion imaging test) and managing CAD (especially when it is necessary to define the extent, location, or functional significance of CAD such as in the revascularized patient). These guidelines also cover special situations in which stress echo is useful (e.g., dyspnea, pulmonary hypertension, valvular stenosis, new-onset atrial fibrillation, or heart failure), especially if combined with intermediate probability of CAD. The use of stress echo often helps sort out whether the symptom or problem is coming from CAD or another source. As previously discussed, clinicians should recall that by the age of 70 (possibly earlier for diabetics), the most common symptom for presentation of an acute myocardial infarction (MI) is dyspnea as opposed to chest pain. This is the so-called "silent angina" or anginal equivalent that patients often develop resulting in dyspnea with exertion.

Indications for Diabetics

Because of a disproportionate burden of CAD in diabetic patients, the American Diabetes Association has suggested indications for cardiac testing in diabetic patients. Although these indications have varied over the years, two indications have persisted:

1. Typical or atypical cardiac symptoms
2. Abnormal resting ECG (especially if suggestive of ischemia or myocardial infarction)

Many diabetic patients are unable to undergo an EET due to peripheral artery disease or neuropathy. Such patients are generally at higher risk for cardiovascular events than those able to undergo an EET. Dobutamine stress echo has been shown to provide independent prognostic information in this group.

Determination of Pretest Probability

Determining pretest probability may help the clinician decide whether stress echo is the indicated and proper diagnostic procedure. Stress echo is probably not indicated in patients with a low pretest probability of CAD (<10%) if they are able to exercise and have an interpretable electrocardiograph (i.e., absence of baseline ECG abnormalities such as LBBB, digitalis effect, WPW syndrome, LVH, >1 mm ST segment depression).

Pretest probability can be estimated by a description of the chest pain and the patient's gender and age. *Typical angina* is described as substernal, exertional, and relieved by rest or nitroglycerine. Chest discomfort with two of these three characteristics is *atypical angina*. Chest discomfort with only one of these characteristics is considered *nonanginal chest pain*. Using these three descriptions, pretest probability tables and their corresponding graphs (see Table 93-1 and Fig. 93-4 in Chapter 93, Exercise Electrocardiography [Stress] Testing) can be readily applied to determine pretest probability. Determining pretest probability may also be helpful when assessing prognosis.

Contraindications

- Unable to obtain adequate resting echo images
- Very recent acute MI (within 2 days) or other acute cardiac event (submaximal testing may be indicated unless patient has undergone angioplasty or stent placement)
- High-risk unstable angina
- Severe symptomatic left ventricular dysfunction or uncontrolled symptomatic heart failure
- Potentially life-threatening or uncontrolled ventricular arrhythmias causing symptoms or hemodynamic compromise
- Third-degree atrioventricular block or second-degree Mobitz type II block without pacemaker
- Acute pericarditis, myocarditis, or endocarditis
- Severe aortic stenosis, hypertrophic cardiomyopathy, or other form of outflow obstruction (can be excluded by performing echo prior to test)
- Suspected dissecting aneurysm
- Severe arterial hypertension (resting >200 mm Hg systolic or >115 mm Hg diastolic)
- Electrolyte abnormality
- Acute pulmonary edema, embolus, or infarction
- Acute thrombophlebitis, deep vein thrombosis, or intracardiac thrombi
- Acute or serious general illness or infection
- Neuromuscular, musculoskeletal, or arthritic condition that precludes exercise (pharmacologic testing may be an option)
- Uncontrolled metabolic disease, such as diabetes, thyrotoxicosis, or myxedema
- Medication intoxication from drugs such as digoxin, sedatives, or psychotropic agents
- Advanced or complicated pregnancy
- Patient inability or lack of desire or motivation to perform the test, including severe emotional distress
- Nonavailability of advanced cardiac life support (ACLS) equipment or of an individual certified to perform ACLS

NOTE: Some of these contraindications are relative. In selected cases, a skilled cardiologist may perform testing for patients with these diagnoses (generally in a referral center). All are contraindications to testing in the office.

Equipment

- For best images, an ultrasound machine with several probes of varying frequency should be available. Among these probes, a low frequency (e.g., 2.5 MHz) probe with two-dimensional (2D), M-mode, and cardiac Doppler capabilities is necessary. An ultrasound machine with harmonic imaging ensures high-quality images. A method of recording the examination (e.g., server, DVD, VCR) is also needed for documentation.
- Ultrasonic jelly and towels to clean up after scanning.
- Patient gown.
- A treadmill with adjustable speed and grade (see Fig. 93-11 in Chapter 93, Exercise Electrocardiography [Stress] Testing)—this is the most common equipment used for stress echo. Advantages include the ability to test most patients under the actual physiologic conditions of exercise. Disadvantages include the fact that the treadmill may be difficult to use for patients with lower-extremity or lower-back problems or for patients who are very obese. The equipment is also more expensive, causes more motion artifact, and is noisier than a bicycle ergometer.
- Bicycle ergometers (see Fig. 93-8 in Chapter 93, Exercise Electrocardiography [Stress] Testing) use adjustable resistance and pedal frequency to exert the patient. Advantages with the bicycle ergometer include the capability to terminate the test instantly. If a bicycle ergometer is utilized, images can be obtained at peak workload, especially if a supine bicycle ergometer is utilized. These images are especially useful for evaluating diastolic and valvular dysfunction, especially with use of color Doppler. Many patients feel more secure sitting on the bicycle. This method is also associated with less artifact, and blood pressure (BP) measurements are easier to obtain. Unfortunately, in the United States leg fatigue is common because most patients do not bike. In fact, as a result of leg fatigue the procedure often fails to determine $VO_{2\ max}$. Bicycle ergometry is also dependent on motivation throughout its duration. As a result, in the United States if the patient can tolerate the treadmill, most clinicians prefer to use it.
- Arm ergometer (see Fig. 93-9 in Chapter 93, Exercise Electrocardiography [Stress] Testing) enables patients with severe orthopedic problems to be tested. However, muscle fatigue often occurs before the maximum heart rate is achieved.
- ECG machine (see Fig. 93-10 in Chapter 93, Exercise Electrocardiography [Stress] Testing)—A continuous monitor is needed (a three-channel model with continuous tracing and a screen-freeze option is desirable) as well as a 12-lead ECG recorder. With modern equipment, the recorder also runs the treadmill. Most equipment is now digital, allowing data to be filtered to provide a smooth baseline.
- Electrodes, cables, and belt—A disposable or washable belt is preferred because patients usually sweat.
- Sphygmomanometer, including various cuff sizes—A gauge manometer is adequate because the most important readings are those relative to resting pressures (not the absolute pressures).
- Stethoscope.
- Razor, rubbing alcohol.
- Intravenous (IV) setup and medications for pharmacologic testing, if planned, including atropine.
- Emergency equipment (see Fig. 220-4 in Chapter 220, Anaphylaxis) includes a monitor/defibrillator; oxygen; airways, intubation, and suction equipment; and an emergency drug kit containing IV fluids and tubing (available drugs should be able to support ACLS protocols).

All emergency equipment should be checked daily, and medications should be checked weekly to monthly, depending on their use. The exercise testing equipment should be inspected and calibrated periodically, based on manufacturer recommendations. ACLS certification cards should be kept on file along with any other information or written protocols.

NOTE: It is also helpful to have a trained technician assisting (see Fig. 93-11 in Chapter 93, Exercise Electrocardiography [Stress] Testing). Technician certification for exercise testing is available through the American College of Sports Medicine. In many centers the technician prepares the patient; monitors the electrocardiograph and the patient's response to exercise, his or her heart rate, and BP; obtains the pre- and postexercise echo images; and prepares the results for interpretation. For low-risk patients, the technician may actually perform the entire study without a physician being present. Otherwise, the clinician should examine the patient before, during, and after the procedure; confirm which protocol to use; and terminate the study. The clinician should also monitor the ECG tracing when the technician is taking BP readings, and the clinician should interpret the final results.

Preprocedure Patient Preparation

Before arrival

- The clinician should instruct the patient to minimize alcohol, over-the-counter medications, and caffeine consumption the day before and the day of the procedure. The patient should be encouraged to get a good night's sleep the night before the procedure and should not eat for 2 hours before the test. It might be advisable for the most recent meal to be a small and predominately liquid meal. To minimize the risk of patient fatigue, many clinicians prefer performing exercise testing in the morning. They then instruct the patient to avoid breakfast or to have only a liquid breakfast that day.
- The procedure should be rescheduled, if possible, if the patient has a cold or other viral illness or is not feeling well in general.
- If the indication for the test is to screen for disease or to make the diagnosis of CAD, the clinician should instruct the patient to avoid taking β-blockers the day of the test.

  NOTE: β-Blockers can suppress the heart rate, diminish segmental wall contractility, and prevent determination of the maximal heart rate (MHR). Patients who discontinue β-blockers should watch closely for "rebound" symptoms and, if they develop, should restart their β-blockers. Because angiotensin-converting enzyme (ACE) inhibitors have little or no effect on performance of a stress test, frequently they may be used as a substitute for other antihypertensive agents. If necessary, they can be taken on the day of the test and usually work within an hour. Clonidine may be used in the same manner.

- If the indication for the test is to determine pharmacologic efficacy in patients with CAD, obviously β-blockers should be taken the day of the study.
- Depending upon the exercise protocol or mode of stress anticipated, the clinician may want to instruct the patient to bring shoes and clothing that are comfortable for walking, possibly for jogging, or for riding a bicycle.
- To minimize patient worry and anxiety (which often cause an elevated resting systolic BP), the clinician should explain that the risk of death for patients being tested using a treadmill is very small (1:10,000 patients). Because exercise testing in an office setting is an elective procedure, patients should never be exposed to excess risk (i.e., patients should be chosen very carefully to ensure that the actual risk of death is much less than even 1:10,000). With dobutamine infusion, the risk of myocardial infarction or ventricular fibrillation is slightly higher, about 1:2,000; however, it has been shown to be safe to use even in patients with left ventricular dysfunction, aortic and cerebral aneurysms, and implantable cardioverter defibrillators.
- With dobutamine infusion, the patient may experience palpitations, nausea, headache, chills, urinary urgency, and anxiety. Symptoms related to high or low blood pressure or chest pain may also be experienced. Patients should know it is very rare for the symptoms to be severe enough to stop the test.

After arrival

- The clinician should again explain the reasons for the test and answer any questions.
- The procedure should be explained again to the patient (e.g., how frequently the workload will be increased or what to expect with pharmacologic infusion, how BP measurements will be taken, when the echo images will be obtrained, how the perceived exertion scale [PES] works; see Box 93-1 in Chapter 93, Exercise Electrocardiography [Stress] Testing).
- The patient should be assured of close monitoring and reassured that although the procedure stresses the heart, it is a relatively safe procedure (<1:10,000 mortality rate for exercise, 1:2000 event rate for dobutamine infusion).
- The patient should know what symptoms to report during the test.
- The clinician should explain how the patient can terminate the procedure should he or she have severe symptoms or an emergency.
- A signed, written consent form should be obtained (see a sample consent form [Chapter 93] online at www.expertconsult.com).
- Confirm the mode of exercise (e.g., treadmill, bicycle ergometer, arm ergometer) or method of evoking stress (e.g., pharmacologic), based on the individual's ability to exercise or any contraindications to exercise.
- If using exercise, select the protocol. There are many excellent protocols in use; therefore the choice is often dependent on the patient's predicted exercise capacity and on clinician preference. The Veterans' Administration (VA) Specific Activity Questionnaire (see Fig. 93-1 in Chapter 93, Exercise Electrocardiography [Stress] Testing) may be very helpful for predicting exercise capacity and helping decide between a standard protocol and a less aggressive, modified protocol. One MET is the amount of oxygen consumed while sitting quietly at rest, or basal oxygen consumption, and it can be used as a conversion unit for exercise capacity (e.g., 2 METs is an exercise capacity that consumes twice the amount of oxygen as basal consumption). If the patient can walk up a flight of stairs, he or she has an exercise capacity of approximately 4 METs. If the patient can walk up a flight of stairs carrying a sack of groceries, he or she can probably tolerate a regular protocol. Otherwise, a modified protocol will probably be necessary. Choose a protocol that starts at a low level of exertion (2 to 3 METs).
  - A protocol with stage durations of at least 3 minutes (2 minutes for bicycle ergometer) allows more physiologic adaptation to the workload of each stage.
  - Workload increases that are no greater than 1 to 3 METs per stage also allow more physiologic adaptation.

The Bruce protocol (see Table 93-2 in Chapter 93, Exercise Electrocardiography [Stress] Testing) is the most frequently used protocol with stress echo; overall, it has been the most extensively studied and validated. The number of METs the patient will achieve is about the same as the number of minutes an individual can complete on the Bruce protocol. It is especially useful in active patients and takes less time than other protocols because it rapidly increases workload. It does have its disadvantages: By the fourth or fifth stage, the patient usually must run, which increases artifact on the EET. In addition, the patient often experiences difficulty in accommodating increases to both slope and speed at the same time. This difficulty is especially seen in elderly patients because they usually have decreased proprioception in their toes and some degree of impairment of vision. In general, most "modified" protocols, such as the modified Bruce or modified Balke protocol, have a reduced progression of workload and are better tolerated by elderly or debilitated patients. Modified protocols usually maintain the same speed and only vary the elevation. Table 93-3 in Chapter 93, Exercise Electrocardiography (Stress) Testing, indicates various protocols, and Figure 93-15 graphically compares METs per minute and VO_{2max} as measured for four protocols.

- Prepare the patient for the ECG machine to be used in the test. Locate sites on the chest for electrodes, which are the same locations as for the office ECG (see Chapter 89, Office Electrocardiograms), except that the arm electrodes are placed in the infraclavicular fossae (midclavicle) and the leg electrodes are placed on the lower abdomen just above the beltline (see Fig.

93-14). The location of the lateral leads may need to be adjusted to allow application of the transducer to sites for the parasternal and apical windows.

- Prepare the patient for the echo after exercise or dobutamine infusion. The patient should know that it is very important to obtain the recovery images within the first minute, so it will be very important to move in a safely and timely manner to the echo examination table. The patient will then need to lie fairly still in the supine position position until the images are obtained.

TECHNIQUE

Getting Started and Resting Echo

1. Review the patient's interval medical history and examine the patient. Based on the history and re-examination, make sure that no contraindication has developed since the last time the patient was seen. Again, determine that in this particular clinicial scenario stress echo is the preferred technique for testing.
2. With the patient lying down, obtain and record the resting heart rate, BP, and electrocardiograph.
3. Using the left parasternal and apical windows, obtain the supine, resting 2D echo images. A screening assessment should be made of ventricular function, chamber sizes, wall motion thicknesses, aortic root, and valves, unless this assessment has already been performed.
4. Perform the exercise or pharmacologic stress test (see Chapter 93, Exercise Electrocardiography [Stress] Testing, about performing and monitoring the standard EET).

Exercise Treadmill Echocardiography

5. With the patient standing beside the treadmill, an electrocardiograph should be obtained. At this point, most equipment records data to provide the signal-averaged ECG for future monitoring.
6. Begin the exercise treadmill test using the preselected protocol.
7. Monitor the patient's symptoms, overall condition, pulse rate, and ECG at all times. *Instruct the patient to give adequate warning if the test needs to be stopped.* With the exception of submaximal testing, encourage the patient to go as far and as long as possible.
8. Record a 12-lead electrocardiograph at the end of each stage, at any time when an abnormality is noted on the monitor, immediately on stopping, and every minute for 8 minutes after exercise during recovery.
9. During each stage, at the start of the final minute, ask the patient if there is any chest discomfort, what point he or she has reached on the PES, and whether he or she wants to continue into the next stage. Also record the BP and heart rate near the end of each stage or at the time of any problems.

NOTE: For most patients, their perceived exertion (see Box 93-1 in Chapter 93, Exercise Electrocardiography [Stress] Testing) is reproducible at a given level of exercise and correlates fairly well with their heart rates. Ask patients to indicate on a scale of 0 to 10 how hard they feel they are working with each stage. On the average, most patients feel they increase by 2 to 3 on the exertion scale with each stage in the early part of the study. PES usually increases more rapidly, from 7 to 9, near the end of the study. Rarely will anyone declare a 10. Use of the PES will not only help the clinician plan for gathering data during the stress echo, but it may also help with giving an exercise prescription (see Chapter 93, Exercise Electrocardiography [Stress] Testing, for additional information about giving a customized exercise prescription).

10. After completion of the exercise treadmill test, immediately ask the patient to lie down. Be aware that this step may be uncomfortable for certain patients, especially if they are overweight or having slight difficulty breathing; reassure them that they will not be required to lie down for long. Obtain the needed images within 1 minute and then record the BP and heart rate. If an assistant is available, it is best to be obtaining the vital signs at the same time as the images.

Exercise Bicycle Ergometer Echocardiography

5. With the patient sitting on the bicycle, an electrocardiograph should be obtained. At this point, most equipment records data to provide the signal-averaged ECG for future monitoring. There may be value in again explaining to the patient the importance of moving safely and rapidly to the echo examination table immediately after the exercise has stopped in order to obtain the images.
6. Begin the exercise test using the preselected protocol. The usual bicycle protocol starts at 25 W of resistance and increases by 25 W every 2 minutes. (A higher initial workload may be appropriate for younger patients or those with a higher estimated exercise capacity.) If images are to be obtained during exercise, many clinicians obtain them at a workload of 25 W and again at peak exercise.
7. Monitor the patient's symptoms, overall condition, pulse rate, and ECG at all times. *Instruct the patient to give adequate warning if the test needs to be stopped.* With the exception of submaximal testing, encourage the patient to go as far and as long as possible.
8. Record a 12-lead ECG at the end of each stage, at any time an abnormality is noted on the monitor, immediately on stopping, and every minute for 8 minutes after exercise during recovery.
9. During each stage, at the start of the final minute, ask the patient if there is any chest discomfort, what point he or she has reached on the PES, and whether he or she wants to continue into the next stage. Also record the BP and heart rate near the end of each stage or at the time of any problems.
10. After completion of the upright-bicycle exercise test, immediately ask the patient to lie down. Be aware that this step may be uncomfortable for certain patients, especially if they are overweight or having slight difficulty breathing; reassure them that they will not be required to lie down for long. Obtain the needed images within 1 minute and then record the BP and heart rate. If an assistant is available, it is best to be obtaining the vital signs at the same time as the images.

Dobutamine Stress Echocardiography

AUTHOR'S NOTE: Vasodilator infusion (e.g., adenosine, dipyridamole, regadenoson) can be used in a similar manner for perfusion imaging using contrast stress echo.

5. The patient can remain in the supine position for dobutamine infusion. Begin the dobutamine infusion following the standard or low-dose protocols. Dobutamine can be initiated at the standard rate of 5 μg/kg/min and increased in 3-minute intervals to 10, 20, 30, and 40 μg/kg/min. (For those with moderate to severely depressed left ventricular function, multivessel disease, or at high risk for an arrhythmia, a low-dose protocol can be used with the infusion initiated at 2.5 μg/ kg/min and increased more gradually to 5, 7.5, 10, and 20 μg/kg/min.) At the Mayo Clinic, echo images are also attained at lower doses (5 to 10 μg/kg/min), prepeak, and at peak dose (or after administration of atropine).
6. Vigilant monitoring is indicated with the use of dobutamine, especially in patients with moderately to severely depressed left ventricular function or multivessel disease because of the high risk for an arrhythmia. Monitor the patient's symptoms, overall condition, pulse rate, and ECG at all times. Record a 12-lead electrocardiograph at any time an abnormality is noted on the monitor.
7. The test is terminated if the target heart rate is achieved (85% of predicted MHR; predicted MHR = 220 − age) or with the

appearance of new or worsening wall-motion abnormalities of moderate degree, significant arrhythmias, hypotension, severe hypertension, or intolerable symptoms. If the test is being done for assessment of viability (low-dose protocol), it should be terminated if there is no functional improvement in segments that are akinetic at baseline. Likewise, worsening of function in hypokinetic segments should trigger termination of the test. Conversely, if there is improvement in function using the low-dose protocol and no untoward side effects, the dose can be escalated to match the high-dose protocol (up to 40 μg/kg/min).

8. If the target heart rate is not readily achieved, atropine can be given IV in divided doses of 0.25 to 0.5 mg to a total of 2 mg. The minimum dose of atropine needed to obtain the target heart rate should be used to minimize the risk of the rare complication of central nervous system toxicity. Use of atropine increases the sensitivity of the test in patients taking β-blockers or those with single-vessel CAD.

   AUTHOR'S NOTE: Patients given atropine at the 30 μg/kg/min dobutamine infusion stage reach target heart rate more quickly and with fewer side effects.

9. Obtain the needed images and then record the BP and heart rate. If an assistant is available, it is best to be obtaining the vital signs at the same time as the images. For persistent symptoms, tachycardia, or severe tachycardia, short-acting IV β-blockers (e.g., metoprolol, esmolol) are effective at reversing the dobutamine effects.

After Exercise or Pharmacologic Stress Testing

1. Immediately after exercise or pharmacologic testing, the patient can be placed in the left lateral recumbent position. Obtain the apical four-chamber images, then the two-chamber images, and finally the parasternal long-axis followed by short-axis images (some laboratories obtain the parasternal images first). Observe recovery of ischemic wall motion abnormalities (usually 3 to 5 minutes after exercise).
2. Monitor the BP, heart rate, any symptoms, and the ECG tracing during recovery. Observe the patient in recovery until symptoms, echo, or ECG changes have resolved completely (or for at least 8 minutes if symptoms, echo, or ECG changes resolve earlier).

Test Termination Criteria

A good rule of thumb for stopping the study is *after* the necessary information is obtained and *before* there is a complication. In young or fit individuals, when they reach their predicted maximal heart rate (again, predicted MHR = 220 – age), it may be prudent to explain that all the necessary information has been obtained; however, they may continue to exercise for as long as they desire. (Allowing the patient to make this choice is also indirectly obtaining informed consent.) In older, less fit, or more debilitated patients, those with multivessel disease, and those with a positive test, obtaining at least 85% of predicted MHR is usually adequate for a stress echo. The benefit of going beyond predicted MHR is the ability to give patients a customized exercise prescription based upon their true MHR.

NOTE: In the past, authorities denoted two possible definitions of a maximal stress exercise test: (1) achieving a target heart rate greater than 85% of the predicted MHR for that patient's age (i.e., roughly 85% of [220 – age]) or (2) exercise to the point of symptoms. Most authorities now encourage patients to exercise to the point of symptoms (usually generalized or voluntary fatigue or the usual amount of chest pain).

Predicted MHR is not patient specific and is frequently inaccurate. Proceeding to the point of symptoms is contraindicated only for debilitated or elderly patients or if a submaximal test is indicated. Maximal effort is usually indicated by maximal perceived exertion and the inability to continue at that workload. Also, for stress echo, a rate pressure product (RPP = systolic blood pressure × heart rate) greater than 20,000 indicates to the clinician that the patient has given a good effort.

Indications to terminate a study include the following:

- Significant elevated BP (systolic blood pressure >250 mm Hg, diastolic blood pressure >115 mm Hg) occurs.
- Significant heart rate abnormalities (inability to obtain 120 beats per minute [bpm] or excessive high heart rate for level of exertion) appear.
- Systolic blood pressure drops more than 20 mm Hg below resting value, especially after the first minute or two of the study (most dangerous if it reflects LV dysfunction; in that situation there is a high risk of life-threatening arrhythmias).
- Anginal chest pain worsens (severe enough that the patient desires to stop); it is not prudent for patients to exercise beyond the point at which they obtain their "usual" amount of chest discomfort. In other words, there is no reason for the patient to demonstrate his or her worst chest pain while performing the study.
- Central nervous system symptoms (e.g., dizziness, disorientation) appear.
- Signs of poor perfusion (e.g., cyanosis, pallor) or severe ventricular dysfunction (e.g., dyspnea) occur. Remember that in the elderly, stability can deteriorate very rapidly; poor perfusion may be indicated solely by a loss of color in an elderly patient.
- Serious arrhythmias develop.
- Target heart rate has been attained.
- Patient wants to stop the test (especially elderly patients, in whom there may be little warning of a complication about to happen).
- Technical problems with equipment (e.g., ECG monitor, systolic blood pressure monitoring) occur.

INTERPRETATION

Chapter 93, Exercise Electrocardiography (Stress) Testing, discusses interpretation of the EET. ECG criteria are used to determine whether the EET is positive or negative. The test result can also be abnormal because of other responses (e.g., BP, symptoms). Rather than just labeling the result as normal, positive, or abnormal, the specific responses to exercise should be identified and documented. It should be noted that occasionally the EET is falsely positive or falsely negative; if the echo images are good, the results of the stress echo take precedence over the EET results.

Normal Echocardiographic Responses to Exercise

- Myocardial segments visualized have normal contraction at rest and become hyperdynamic with exercise or infusion of dobutamine.
- A normal stress echo is defined as normal left ventricular wall motion at rest and with stress.
- Ejection fraction normally increases with exercise.
- Left ventricular end-systolic volume normally decreases with exercise.

Abnormal Echocardiographic Responses to Exercise

- Cardiac segment changes from normal to hypokinetic, from hypokinetic to akinetic, and from akinetic to dyskinetic are considered wall motion abnormalities.
- Resting wall motion abnormalities, unchanged with stress, are classified as "fixed" and most often represent regions of prior

TABLE 94-2 Typical Rest and Stress Wall Motion Responses

Rest	Stress	Interpretation
Normal	Hyperkinetic	Normal
Normal	Hypokinetic/akinetic	Ischemic
Akinetic	Akinetic	Prior infarction
Hypokinetic	Akinetic/dyskinetic	Ischemic or prior infarction
Hypokinetic/akinetic	Normal	Viable

infarction. Fixed wall motion abnormalities that develop new or worsening wall motion abnormalities are indicative of ischemia.

- Typical patterns are seen with normal, ischemic, and prior infarction responses to stress echo (Table 94-2).
- Function in each segment is graded at rest and with stress as normal or hyperdynamic, hypokinetic, akinetic, dyskinetic, or aneurismal. Table 94-3 provides a scoring system).
- Images from low or intermediate stages of supine bicycle or dobutamine infusion should be compared with peak stress images to maximize the sensitivity for detection of CAD.
- Stress-induced changes in left ventricular shape, increase in cavity size, and lack of increase in global contractility indicate ischemia.
- Ischemia also delays the onset of contraction and relaxation and decreases the maximum amplitude of contraction.

Segmental Wall Motion Analysis

- One expert (Ellestad) feels the standard four-chamber view provides the most information.
- The American Society of Echocardiography (ASE) suggests that either a 16- or 17-segment model of the left ventricle (see Fig. 90-20 in Chapter 90, Echocardiography) be used for segmental wall motion analysis. The extra segment in the 17-segment model is the "apical cap," which is the portion of the left ventricle located below where the ventricular cavity is seen.
- Although there is some variability among data reported when segmental wall analysis is used to evaluate stress echo results (i.e., thresholds from calculated sum ratios of wall motion abnormalities used to define patients at high risk have been variable), the authors still use Figure 94-1 to quantify the results. Each segment is evaluated and scored at rest and during stress (bicycle or pharmacologic) or after stress (treadmill). The sum of all the segments from the stress echo is divided by the sum of the resting segments. Patients considered high risk have a score greater than 1.4.

Ejection Fraction and End-Systolic Volume Analysis

The ejection fraction should increase on the postexercise echo images and the end-systolic volumes decrease (with the exception of recumbent bicycle protocol). On these images, no change in the ejection fraction or end-systolic volume, a decrease in the ejection fraction, and an increase in the end-systolic volume are all indicative of CAD and increased patient risk of a cardiovascular event.

TABLE 94-3 Wall Motion Scoring

Description	Score
Hyperkinetic (hyperdynamic)	0
Normal	1
Mildly hypokinetic*	1.5
Hypokinetic	2
Severely hypokinetic*	2.5
Akinetic	3
Dyskinetic	4
Aneurysm	5

*Optional scores used by some clinicians.

Other Parameters Followed

- *Heart rate*. Failure to obtain a heart rate of 120 bpm is chronotropic incompetence with a resultant poor prognosis (approximately 15% per year will experience a coronary event); it may also indicate early sick sinus syndrome or multivessel CAD (often small-vessel CAD).
- *Heart rate recovery*. Failure of the heart rate to decrease 12 bpm in the first minute of recovery is an abnormal heart rate recovery. This indicates a two- to fourfold increased risk of death over the next 5 years.
- *Blood pressure*. If the systolic BP drops below resting, it predicts either a poor prognosis or severe CAD. In one study, men with a maximal exercise systolic blood pressure below 140 mm Hg had a 15-fold increase in the annual rate of sudden death when compared to those whose BPs exceeded 200 mm Hg.

False-Positive Results

Box 94-2 lists causes of false-positive results on stress echocardiography. Advanced age, marked hypertension, a cardiomyopathy, or taking a β-blocker can blunt the normal hypercontractile response to exercise.

False-Negative Results

Box 94-2 also lists causes of false-negative results on stress echocardiography. Suboptimal stress is a primary cause of false-negative tests. An adequate level of stress is frequently defined as achievement of 85% or more of the patient's age-predicted maximal heart rate for exercise or dobutamine stress or a rate pressure product of 20,000 or more for exercise testing.

DETERMINING PROGNOSIS

Normal Stress Echocardiogram

A negative stress echo is very reassuring because prognosis is excellent. Patients have less than 1% annual risk of MI or cardiac events, which is equivalent to that of an age- and sex-matched population (Box 94-3). These patients do not require further diagnostic evaluation unless there is a change in signs or symptoms. Patients with a negative pharmacologic stress echo have a slightly higher risk of cardiovascular events, perhaps due to their inability to exercise, other comorbidities, or typically older age at the time of testing. However, a negative pharmacologic stress echo still implies less than 2% annual risk of MI or cardiac death (see Box 94-3).

Uninterpretable or Incomplete Exercise Test Results

This result is caused by failure to attain at least 85% of the age-predicted MHR, with absence of ischemic changes in a well-motivated patient (β-blockers are a common cause of this).

Positive and Abnormal Studies

In addition to segmental wall analysis and evaluation of the ejection fraction/end-systolic volumes, other factors are known to affect risk (Box 94-4). While the degree that each of these factors affects risk is variable, we know that the more factors a patient possesses, the higher the risk. Certain investigators also attempt to combine the results of the EET to estimate risk using the Duke Treadmill Nomogram (see Fig. 93-18 in Chapter 93, Exercise

Box 94-2. Causes of False-Positive and False-Negative Results on Stress Echocardiography

Causes of False-Positive Results

Hypoxemia or anemia—can cause ischemia unrelated to CAD
Apical hypokinesis due to LVH—can cause wall motion abnormalities
Hypertension (poorly controlled)—can cause ischemia or wall motion abnormalities
Cardiomyopathy—idiopathic cardiomyopathy can cause ischemia; other cardiomyopathies can cause wall motion abnormalities
Long-standing hypertension—can cause wall motion abnormalities, even without resting left ventricular function and in absence of LVH
Mitral valve prolapse syndrome and valvular heart disease
Coronary spasm (Prinzmetal's or variant angina)
Mitral valve replacement or annulus calcification can lead to decreased motion of the basal inferior and basal inferoseptal segments due to tethering
Left bundle branch block, right ventricular pacing, and previous open heart surgery can lead to decreased septal wall motion (abnormal septal motion usually present at rest)
Inadequate recording equipment, incorrect criteria, improper interpretation, or improper transducer placement
Technical or observer error
Advanced age
β-blocker therapy

Causes of False-Negative Results

Failure to achieve an adequate workload (heart rate >85% of age-predicted MHR for exercise or pharmacologic stress, or rate pressure product of at least 20,000 for exercise echo)
Single vessel, especially left circumflex, CAD (supine bicycle testing has higher sensitivity)
Concentric remodeling or LVH (especially for dobutamine stress, because affected patients have increased relative wall thickness and smaller left ventricular cavity volume)
Significant aortic or mitral valve regurgitation (due to resulting hyperdynamic state)
Failure to use other information (e.g., EET results, systolic blood pressure drop, symptoms, dysrhythmia, heart rate response) in test interpretation
Inadequate recording equipment, incorrect criteria, improper interpretation, or improper transducer placement
Technical or observer error

CAD, coronary artery disease; EET, exercise electrocardiography testing; LVH, left ventricular hypertrophy; MHR, maximal heart rate.

Electrocardiography [Stress] Testing). This nomogram is most accurate for those patients with a positive study and able to achieve 5 METs, a heart rate of 120 bpm, and an RPP of more than 25,000. Box 94-3 is utilized for further quantifying those patients considered high risk (greater than fourfold increased risk over the low-risk group previously defined).

Viability Studies

The highest sensitivity of the dobutamine test for viability is noted when there is improvement in wall motion with the low-dose

Box 94-3. Stress Echocardiography Predictors of Risk

Low Risk

<1% per year risk of MI or cardiac events: Normal exercise echo and good exercise capacity (≥7 METs in men, 5 METs in women)
<2% per year risk of MI or cardiac death: Normal pharmacologic stress echo (defined as HR > 85% of age-predicted MHR for dobutamine stress echo and low to intermediate pretest probability*)

High Risk[†]

Extensive resting wall motion abnormalities (four to five segments)
Baseline ejection fraction <40%
Extensive ischemia (four to five segments)
Multivessel ischemia
Resting wall motion abnormalities and remote ischemia
Low ischemic threshold
Ischemia with 20 μg/kg/min dobutamine
Ischemic wall motion abnormalities, no change or decrease in ejection fraction

HR, heart rate; MHR, maximum heart rate; MI myocardial infarction.
*See Determination of Pretest Probability in Indications section in this chapter.
[†]Greater than fourfold increase over low risk.
From American Society of Echocardiography Recommendations for Performance, Interpretation and Application of Stress Echocardiography. J Am Soc Echocardiogr 20:1021–1041, 2007.

Box 94-4. Factors Increasing Risk in Patients with Normal Stress Echocardiography Results*

Increasing age
Male sex
Diabetes
High pretest probability[†]
History of dyspnea or CHF
History of MI
Limited exercise capacity
Inability to exercise
EET demonstrates ischemia
Resting wall motion abnormalities
LVH
Ischemia on stress echo
Baseline reduced ejection fraction
No change or increase in end-systolic volume with exercise
No change or decrease in ejection fraction with exercise
Increasing wall motion score with stress

CHF, congestive heart failure; EET, exercise electrocardiography testing; LVH, left ventricular hypertrophy; MI, myocardial infarction.
*The degree to which each factor increases risk is variable.
[†]See Determination of Pretest Probability in Indications section of this chapter (>90% by calculations in that section).
From American Society of Echocardiography Recommendations for Performance, Interpretation and Application of Stress Echocardiography. J Am Soc Echocardiogr 20:1021–1041, 2007.

protocol. Viability is defined by improvement by at least one grade in two or more wall segments (see Table 94-3). Patients with a large area of viable myocardium (>25% of left ventricle) have a greater chance of improving ejection fraction and a better outcome (decreased remodeling, persistent improvement in heart failure, lower incident of cardiac events) when revascularized.

Complications

- Hypotension
- Congestive heart failure exacerbation
- Severe cardiac arrhythmia
- Cardiac arrest
- Acute MI
- Acute central nervous system (CNS) event, such as syncope or stroke
- Death

Postprocedure Patient Education

Patients should be counseled appropriately regarding their risk and whether consultation with a cardiologist is indicated. Patients should be informed that stress echocardiography, just like any other noninvasive study for diagnosing CAD, is not 100% accurate. However, it usually diagnoses those coronary arteries with greater than 70% obstruction. Medical management is probably best for those vessels with less than 70% obstructions and the patient should probably be reassured that this is already ongoing (i.e., management of diabetes, hypertension, lipids). Regardless, individuals with a future change in symptoms or symptoms suggestive of coronary ischemia such as chest discomfort, palpitations, or shortness of breath with exertion should be evaluated by their clinician regardless of the result of the stress echocardiogram.

In patients with CAD or a high probability of CAD, counseling should be directed at modifying risk factors and medical management. Exercise prescriptions should be given and discussed. See Chapter 93, Exercise Electrocardiography (Stress) Testing, for how to give an aerobic exercise prescription if not contraindicated. A cardiac rehabilitation program should be considered.

CPT/Billing Codes

93016 Cardiovascular stress testing using maximal or submaximal treadmill or bicycle exercise, continuous ECG monitoring, and pharmacologic stress; physician supervision only, without interpretation and report
93017 Tracing only, without interpretation and report
93018 Interpretation and report only
93350 Echocardiography, transthoracic, real-time with image documentation (2D), with or without M-mode recording, during rest and cardiovascular stress test using treadmill, bicycle exercise, and pharmacologically induced stress, with interpretation and report (Stress testing codes 93016 to 93018 should be reported, when appropriate, in conjunction with 93350 to capture the cardiovascular stress portion of the study. Do not report 93015 in conjunction with 93350.)
93351 Including performance of continuous electrocardiographic monitoring, with physician supervision (Do not report 93351 in conjunction with 93015 to 93018, 93350.)

ICD-9-CM Diagnostic Codes

394.0 Mitral stenosis, rheumatic
394.2 Mitral stenosis with insufficiency, rheumatic
402.10 Hypertensive heart disease or hypertensive LVH, benign, without congestive heart failure (CHF)
402.11 Hypertensive heart disease, benign, with CHF
410.00 Acute MI, of the anterolateral wall, episode of care unspecified
410.20 Acute MI, of the inferolateral wall, episode of care unspecified
410.90 MI, acute, unspecified site and episode
412 Old MI (healed or no symptoms)
413.9 Other and unspecified angina pectoris
414.00 Coronary atherosclerosis, of unspecified type of vessel, native or graft
414.01 Coronary atherosclerosis, of native coronary artery
414.02 Coronary atherosclerosis, of autologous vein bypass graft
414.04 Coronary atherosclerosis, of artery bypass graft
414.05 Coronary atherosclerosis, of unspecified type of bypass graft
414.8 Chronic coronary insufficiency or ischemic heart disease
414.9 Chronic ischemic heart disease, unspecified
414.10 Aneurysm of heart wall
416.0 Pulmonary hypertension, primary, chronic
416.8 Pulmonary hypertension, secondary, chronic
420.90 Pericardial effusion, acute
420.91 Pericarditis, acute, idiopathic
422.90 Myocarditis, acute
423.9 Pericardial effusion, unspecified disease of pericardium
424.0 Mitral valve disorders, nonrheumatic (incompetence, insufficiency, regurgitation, prolapse)
424.1 Aortic valve disorders (incompetence, insufficiency, regurgitation, stenosis)
425.4 Cardiomyopathy, congestive, constrictive, familial, hypertrophic, idiopathic, restrictive, obstructive, nonobstructive, NOS)
425.5 Cardiomyopathy, alcoholic
426.3 Left bundle branch block, complete or NOS
426.4 Right bundle branch block
427.5 Cardiac arrest
427.31 Atrial fibrillation
427.69 Ventricular premature beats, contractions, or systoles
428.0 Congestive heart failure
428.1 Congestive heart failure, left, acute
428.4 Combined systolic and diastolic heart failure
428.21 Systolic heart failure, acute
428.22 Systolic heart failure, chronic
428.31 Diastolic heart failure, acute
429.1 Cardiomyopathy, arteriosclerotic
429.3 Cardiomegaly or cardiac dilation or hypertrophy
429.79 Mural thrombus (atrial, ventricular) acquired following myocardial infarction
441.01 Aortic dissection, thoracic
785.1 Palpitations
786.50 Chest pain, unspecified
786.51 Precordial pain

Suppliers

(For full contact information go to www.expertconsult.com.)

For stress testing equipment, see the Suppliers section in Chapter 93, Exercise Electrocardiography [Stress] Testing. Most manufacturers on that list also sell defibrillators. Purchasing these as part of a package is often cost effective. For echo equipment, there are several manufacturers with products ranging from the very basic to the very sophisticated. Small hand-held machines are now available. Acuson Siemens, Biosound Esaote, General Electric Healthcare, Medison, Phillips, and Toshiba all offer a range of devices from hand-held to research oriented (see the Suppliers section in Chapter 172, Obstetric Ultrasonography, and the Suppliers listings in Appendix D for the Internet and mailing addresses and the phone numbers for many manufacturers). An excellent way to review the equipment is to visit the company websites. Used equipment is also available, but the cost and inconvenience of service and repairs are often a disadvantage. To avoid large capital equipment costs, service companies will bring portable echocardiography equipment to the physician's office for this procedure and split the fees. Over-reading services are also available. The following are two companies with which the authors are familiar:

Echocardiography equipment
General Electric Healthcare
Toshiba America Medical Systems
Emergency/ACLS medication kits
Banyan International Corp.

ONLINE RESOURCE

See the sample patient consent form (Chapter 93) online at www.expertconsult.com.

BIBLIOGRAPHY

ACC/AHA: Clinical competence statement on stress testing: A report of the American College of Cardiology/American Heart Association/American College of Physicians–American Society of Internal Medicine Task Force on Clinical Competence. Circulation 102:1726, 2000. Also available online at http://circ.ahajournals.org/cgi/reprint/102/14/1726. Accessed March 28, 2010.

ACC/AHA: Clinical competence statement on echocardiography. Circulation 107:1068–1089, 2003. Also available online at http://circ.ahajournals.org/cgi/reprint/107/7/1068. Accessed March 28, 2010.

ACC/AHA: Guidelines on perioperative cardiovascular evaluation and care for noncardiac surgery. Circulation 116:1971–1996, 2007.

ACC/AHA/ASE: Guideline update for the clinical application of echocardiography: Summary article: A report of the American College of Cardiology/American Heart Association Task Force on Practice Guidelines (ACC/AHA/ASE Committee to Update the 1997 Guidelines for the Clinical Application of Echocardiography). Circulation 108:1146–1162, 2003.

ACC/AHA/ASNC: Guidelines for the clinical use of cardiac radionuclide imaging—Executive summary. Circulation 108:1404, 2003. Also available online at http://circ.ahajournals.org/cgi/content/full/108/11/1404. Accessed March 28, 2010.

ACCF/ASE/ACEP/AHA/ASNC/SCAI/SCCT/SCMR: Appropriateness criteria for stress echocardiography. Circulation 117;1478–1497, 2008. Also available online at http://circ.ahajournals.org/cgi/reprint/117/11/1478 or http://content.onlinejacc.org/cgi/reprint/j.jacc.2007.12.005v1.pdf. Accessed March 28, 2010.

AHA Scientific Statement: Exercise standards for testing and training: A statement for healthcare professionals from the American Heart Association. Circulation 104:1694, 2001.

American Diabetes Association: Consensus development conference on the diagnosis of coronary heart disease in people with diabetes. Diabetes Care 21:1551–1559, 1998.

Armstrong WF, Ryan T: Feigenbaum's Echocardiography, 7th ed. Philadephia, Lippincott, Williams & Wilkins, 2009.

Chin AS, Goldman LE, Eisenberg MJ: Functional testing after coronary artery bypass graft surgery: A meta-analysis. Can J Cardiol 19:802–808, 2003.

Dori G, Denekamp Y, Fishman S, Bitterman H: Exercise stress testing, myocardial perfusion imaging and stress echocardiography for detecting restenosis after successful percutaneous transluminal coronary angioplasty: A review of performance. J Intern Med 253:253–262, 2003.

Ellestad MH: Stress Testing, Principles and Practice, 5th ed. New York, Oxford University Press, 2003.

Fowler G, Altman M: Exercise testing after bypass or percutaneous coronary intervention. In Evans CH, White RD (eds): Exercise Stress Testing for Primary Care and Sports Medicine Physicians. New York, Springer Verlag, 2009, pp 231–254.

Froelicher VF, Myers J: Exercise and the Heart, 5th ed. St Louis, Mosby, 2006.

Garzon PP, Eisenberg MJ: Functional testing for the detection of restenosis after percutaneous transluminal coronary angioplasty: A meta-analysis. Can J Cardiol 17:41–48, 2001.

Mattera JA, Arain SA, Sinusas AJ, et al: Exercise testing with myocardial perfusion imaging in patients with normal baseline electrocardiograms: Cost savings with a stepwise diagnostic strategy. J Nucl Cardiol 5:498, 1998.

Nguyen P: Stress echo. In Evans CH, White RD (eds): Exercise Stress Testing for Primary Care and Sports Medicine Physicians. New York, Springer Verlag, 2009, pp 143–165.

Oh JK, Seward JB, Tajik AJ: The Echo Manual, 3rd ed. Philadelphia, Lippincott, Williams & Williams, 2006.

Otto CM: Textbook of Clinical Echocardiography, 4th ed. Philadephia, Saunders, 2009.

Pellikka PA, Nagueh SF, Elhendy AA, et al: American Society of Echocardiography recommendations for performance, interpretation and application of stress echocardiography. J Am Soc Echocardiogr 20:1021–1041, 2007. Also available online at http://www.asefiles.org/stress2007.pdf. Accessed March 28, 2010.

Reynolds T: The Echocardiographer's Pocket Reference, 3rd ed. Phoenix, School of Cardiac Ultrasound at Arizona Heart Institute, 2007.

Roldan CA, Abrams J: Evaluation of the Patient with Heart Disease. Integrating the Physical Exam and Echocardiography. Philadelphia, Lippincott, Williams & Wilkins, 2002.

CHAPTER 95

THORACENTESIS

Terry S. Ruhl • Jennifer L. Good

Pleural effusions are common in primary care. Sampling the fluid may yield information important for treatment decisions or may help the patient feel better. Similar techniques can also be used to treat certain pneumothoraces.

ANATOMY

The pleural "space" is a potential space between the visceral pleura, which is adherent to the lung, and the parietal pleura, which is adherent to the chest wall. Normally, it contains only a thin film of lubricating fluid. When this space becomes filled with air or extra fluid, it may become painful or increase the work of breathing.

INDICATIONS

- Any significant (>10 mm on lateral decubitus radiograph) pleural effusion of unknown etiology (effusions with an easily explained cause, such as congestive heart failure, may be observed for response to therapy)
- Large symptomatic effusion
- Spontaneous pneumothorax (a minimally symptomatic, spontaneous pneumothorax of less than 20% may be merely observed if the patient has no significant underlying lung disease)

CONTRAINDICATIONS

Absolute

- Patient refuses the procedure
- When chest tube placement is planned and would be more appropriate
  - Known or suspected hemothorax
  - Empyema or complicated parapneumonic effusion
  - Large spontaneous pneumothorax
  - Spontaneous pneumothorax in a patient with underlying lung disease

Relative

- Coagulopathy or patient undergoing anticoagulant therapy (international normalized ratio >1.5, consider reversing the coagulopathy or anticoagulant before performing thoracentesis).
- Thrombocytopenia (platelet count <50,000).
- Inability to cooperate or sign informed consent.
- Very small pleural effusions (<10 mm thick on lateral decubitus chest radiograph), unless aided by real-time ultrasonography.
- Local skin compromise (e.g., cellulitis, burn, pyoderma, herpes zoster infection).
- Unstable medical condition.
- Positive-pressure ventilation (though one study has found thoracentesis to be as safe in ventilator-dependent patients as in patients not being mechanically ventilated).
- Radiographic evidence of loculated pleural effusions making localization of fluid uncertain unless aided by real-time ultrasonography.
- Patients with chronic obstructive pulmonary disease are at increased risk for complications.

EQUIPMENT AND SUPPLIES

Commercial thoracentesis trays are available. If a commercial tray is used, the manufacturer's instructions *must* be reviewed because equipment varies. Alternatively, the equipment described in the following sections can be assembled.

Preparation and Anesthesia

- Povidone–iodine solution or chlorhexidine and applicators
- Fenestrated drape or sterile towels
- 10-mL Luer-Lok syringe
- 25-gauge or smaller needle
- 1½- to 2-inch, 22-gauge needle
- Lidocaine 1% to 2% with epinephrine

Insertion

- Sterile gloves
- 50-mL Luer-Lok syringe, three-way stopcock
- 2½-inch, 18-gauge needle (for air), 2½-inch, 15-gauge needle (for fluid), or 16-gauge catheter over needle (can decrease risk of pneumothorax, but kinks can increase the "dry tap" rate).

  NOTE: Obese people may require longer needles.

- Specimen tubes: one red top, one lavender top, culture tubes (aerobic and anaerobic), 10- to 50-mL red top for cytology, possibly 1 green top, ice for pH

Optional

- Sterile plastic tubing
- Curved clamp for marking insertion depth on needle
- 500- or 1000-mL vacuum bottles
- Telemetry, oximetry, blood pressure monitoring, and supplemental oxygen

Dressing

Use sterile gauze pads and adhesive tape or adhesive bandage with antibiotic ointment.

PRECAUTIONS

The use of real-time ultrasonographic guidance is helpful in situations where there is a small effusion (<10 mm free-flowing pleural fluid on lateral decubitus radiograph), there is presence of a loculated pleural effusion, the patient is receiving positive-pressure mechanical ventilation, or in other high-risk situations. "Marking" the location for later drainage is unhelpful because fluid shifts, but marking at the time of aspiration may be helpful. Use of ultrasonography may also help determine needle depth and the angle at which the needle should be directed. Removal of large amounts of fluid may increase the incidence of postprocedure complications, although many advocate "draining it dry."

TECHNIQUE

Patient Positioning and Insertion Site

1. Seat the patient comfortably (Fig. 95-1) with arms supported on a table. The lower back should be kept as vertical as possible so that the most dependent portion of the hemithorax is posterior, thereby keeping free-flowing fluid in a posterior location.

   NOTE: Debilitated patients can be placed in the lateral decubitus position, lying on the side of the effusion with their back near the edge of the bed. The procedure would then be performed in the mid-scapular line or the posterior axillary line.

2. Confirm the location and extent of fluid or air by percussion, auscultation, and study of posteroanterior, lateral, and lateral decubitus (fluid-affected side down) chest radiographs.

   NOTE: If available, ultrasonography may be very helpful for completing this step (see Chapter 225, Emergency Department, Hospitalist, and Office Ultrasonography [Clinical Ultrasonography]).

3. Select the needle insertion site. Use an area one or two interspaces below the fluid level and 5 to 10 cm lateral to the spine. Do not insert below the eighth intercostal space.
4. Mark insertion site with marker or by applying pressure from the hub of a needle or pen.
5. Verify the patient's identity, ensure the insertion site is correctly marked, and take a "time out" to verify this with everyone present.

Preparation and Anesthesia

1. Prepare the skin with povidone–iodine or chlorhexidine. Use sterile technique and universal blood and body fluid precautions. Drape with sterile towels or fenestrated drape. Some experts monitor all patients with telemetry, oximetry, and automatic blood pressure equipment and have supplemental oxygen available during this procedure, especially if the patient has underlying pulmonary disease.

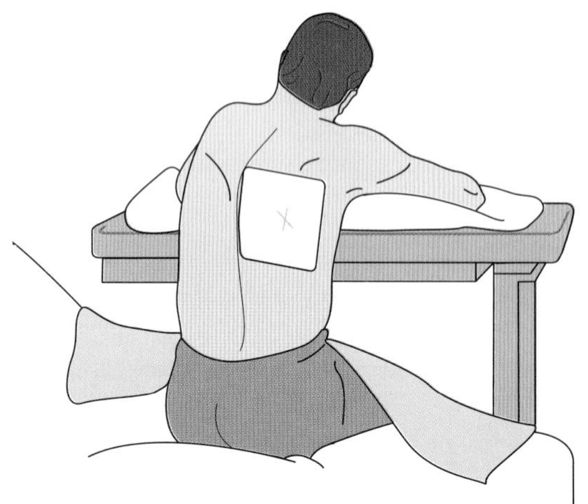

Figure 95-1 Position for fluid removal.

2. Raise a skin wheal using lidocaine with epinephrine and a 25-gauge or smaller needle attached to a 10-mL syringe.
3. Angle a ½-inch 22-gauge needle slightly downward, and insert it through the skin wheal so that the needle tip touches the superior border of a rib, aspirating and injecting as you advance. "Walk" the needle over the superior margin of the rib and deeper into the interspace, anesthetizing the intercostal muscle layers (Fig. 95-2A).
4. To confirm the presence of fluid or air with the small anesthesia needle, continue advancing the needle while aspirating and injecting until the parietal pleura has been penetrated. (A "pop" may be felt, or fluid/air aspirated.) Warn the patient that there may be a twinge of pain as you go through the pleura. Inject more lidocaine. Note the depth. Consider placing a clamp on the needle at the skin level to mark the depth (Fig. 95-2B). Withdraw the needle. If no fluid is obtained, ultrasonographic guidance is recommended. If air is unexpectedly obtained, try a lower intercostal space.

Aspiration Option 1 (If No Kit Available): Needle-Only Insertion Technique

1. Prepare the equipment. Attach a 15-gauge needle to a 50-mL syringe with a three-way stopcock. Mark the previously measured depth on this needle with a clamp. Test the equipment to be sure you are well acquainted with the use of the stopcock. Open the stopcock to the syringe.
2. Insert the thoracentesis needle in the same track as the anesthesia needle, and advance it to the level of the clamp. ("Walk" over the rib, not under it, to avoid damaging vessels and nerves). Aspirate to confirm placement. Keep the clamp attached to prevent penetrating too deeply.

Aspiration Option 2: Catheter-over-Needle Insertion Technique

(Use a commercially prepared thoracentesis tray. Read the manufacturer's instructions carefully.)

1. Prepare the equipment. Familiarize yourself with the stopcock. Visualize the measured insertion depth on the needle.
2. Insert the thoracentesis needle in the same track as the anesthesia needle, aspirating with the syringe until fluid is obtained.
3. Making sure the stopcock is turned off to the environment, completely withdraw the needle, leaving the catheter in the pleural space. As the needle is removed, quickly turn the stopcock to close the catheter to the environment. Alternatively, a gloved finger can be used to quickly cover the catheter hub after the needle is removed to prevent air from entering the pleural cavity.

Completing the Procedure

1. *For stopcock and evacuated container:* Attach one end of the tube to the stopcock and the other end to a second 15-gauge needle. Insert the needle through the seal of an evacuated container, and open the stopcock to the evacuated container (Fig. 95-2C).

   For stopcock and open container: Pull the fluid into the syringe. Turn the stopcock off to the needle, being careful not to open the needle to the environment. Push the fluid out of the syringe into the container. Alternate aspiration into the syringe and emptying into the container.
2. After withdrawal of the necessary amount of fluid, remove the needle while the patient is exhaling.
3. Dress the site with an occlusive, sterile dressing.
4. Send the fluid for analysis (see "Interpretation of Results" for details). In most cases, a volume of 50 to 60 mL is sufficient for diagnostic tests.

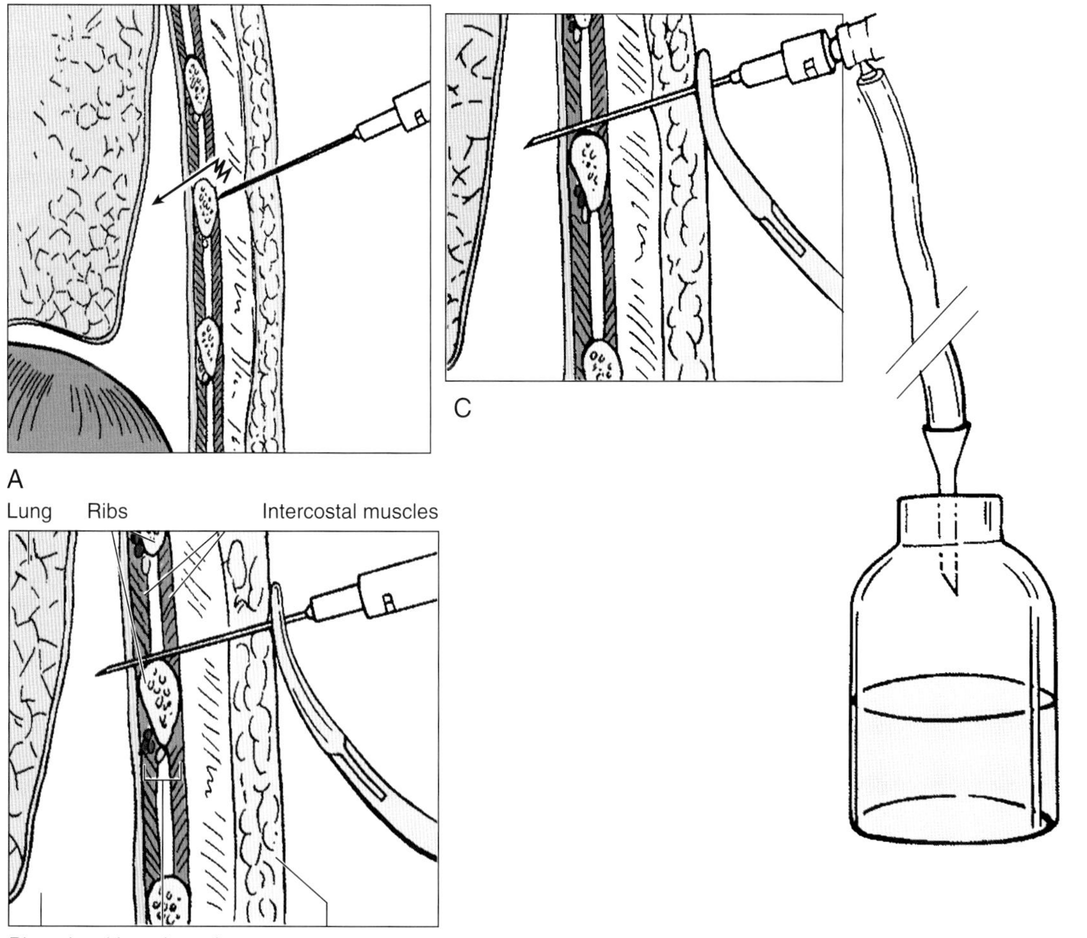

Figure 95-2 **A,** Anesthetizing the intercostal muscle layers. Needle is "walked" over the rib. **B,** Clamp is placed to mark the depth to the effusion. **C,** Needle in pleural space with fluid draining into evacuated bottle.

5. Consider an end-expiratory chest radiograph to check for a pneumothorax. Some experts repeat this radiograph in 4 to 6 hours to look for delayed pneumothorax.

Thoracentesis for Aspiration of a Simple Spontaneous Pneumothorax

1. Position the patient supine with the head of the bed elevated at a 30- to 45-degree angle and infiltrate local anesthetic into the second or third intercostal space in the mid-clavicular line (Fig. 95-3). (Alternatively, the patient can be placed in the lateral decubitus position and the fourth or fifth intercostal space in the mid-clavicular line can be used.)
2. Using a catheter over a needle (at least 16 Fr and 2 inches long), enter the pleural space and withdraw the needle. As described earlier, "walk" the needle over the cephalic surface of the rib.
3. When the pleural space is entered, remove the needle from the catheter during exhalation and attach a three-way stopcock and 60-mL Luer-Lok syringe to the catheter. Be sure to occlude the hub of the catheter during this maneuver to prevent air entry into the pleural space.
4. Using the three-way stopcock, manually aspirate air into the 60-mL syringe. Stop when resistance to aspiration is felt, the patient coughs excessively or experiences chest pain or dyspnea, or more than 2 L of air is removed (this suggests the need for a chest tube). Remove the catheter.
5. Obtain a chest radiograph. If the pneumothorax is very small or has resolved, the procedure has been successful. Monitor for another 4 to 6 hours and discharge if a subsequent chest radiograph shows no recurrence of the pneumothorax.

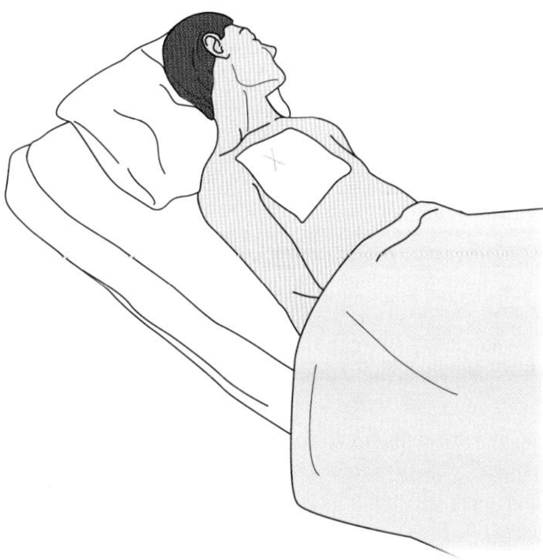

Figure 95-3 Position for air removal.

Sample Operative Report

See a sample operative report online at www.expertconsult.com.

Common Errors

- Stopcock confusion—mistakenly opening the needle or catheter to the environment
- Missing the effusion—by shifting patient position or not using ultrasonography for small effusions
- Wrong side procedure—may occur if radiographs are malpositioned, mislabeled, or not confirmed by physical examination
- Kit changes—being given an unfamiliar kit without reviewing the instructions

Complications

- Pneumothorax may result if air is introduced through the needle or catheter, or if the visceral pleura is punctured. Between 3% and 20% of procedures produce a pneumothorax, which requires treatment with a chest tube about 20% of the time. Pneumothorax incidence may be reduced with ultrasonography-guided thoracentesis. Insert the needle only as far as needed to obtain fluid. Get comfortable with the equipment, especially the stopcock, before insertion. Use of smaller needles and short bevels, and removal of less fluid, may also decrease the risk of pneumothorax.
- Hemothorax may result from laceration of intercostal vessels or internal mammary vessels, but is rare. To reduce the risk of hemothorax, insert the needle just above the rib, avoiding the neurovascular bundle that runs below each rib. Never puncture medial to the mid-clavicular line.
- The spleen, liver, or diaphragm may be lacerated. To avoid lacerations to these organs, do not insert the needle lower than the eighth intercostal space posteriorly.
- Risk of hypovolemia and reexpansion pulmonary edema can be minimized by removing less than 1.5 L of fluid at a time (although many experts advocate draining the effusion dry). Remove fluid slowly and stop if the patient develops a cough, dyspnea, or chest pain.
- A catheter fragment may be left in the pleural space. To avoid this possibility, *never* withdraw a catheter over the needle.
- Failure to obtain fluid can occur. For improved success rates, pay close attention to landmarks obtained by auscultation, percussion, and radiographic examination. Consider ultrasonographic guidance.
- Infection can occur. To minimize this possibility, use sterile technique and avoid inserting through infected skin.
- Pain is associated with thoracentesis. Use adequate local anesthesia, especially at the pleura.
- Hypoproteinemia is a possibility. To reduce the risk of this problem, avoid repeated thoracenteses.

Postprocedure Management

Because the risk of complications is low, a post-thoracentesis chest radiograph is necessary only if air was obtained during the thoracentesis, or if the patient is mechanically ventilated or develops cough, chest pain, hypoxia, or dyspnea during or after the procedure. If a thoracentesis is performed for the management of a small, primary spontaneous pneumothorax, a chest radiograph should be obtained and the patient should be observed for recurrent pneumothorax for at least 6 hours.

Hypoxemia is very common after thoracentesis and occurs because of ventilation–perfusion mismatching in the newly expanded lung. Oxygenation should be checked periodically by pulse oximetry after thoracentesis and supplemental oxygen provided if necessary.

Postprocedure Patient Education

The dressing should stay on for 24 hours. The patient should inform someone if shortness of breath increases, there is fever, or there is redness at the puncture site.

Interpretation of Results

The first important distinction is whether the fluid is a transudate (unbalanced hydrostatic forces) or an exudate ("leaks in the system"). If the lactate dehydrogenase (LDH) levels in the fluid and the pleural fluid/serum ratios for LDH and protein are all normal, the fluid is a transudate and further studies are unlikely to give useful information. Most transudates are from congestive heart failure, with the rest associated with hypoalbuminemia, hepatic hydrothorax, hydronephrosis, pulmonary embolism, peritoneal dialysis, or trapped lung. Occasionally, pleural effusions that appear to be due to congestive heart failure may be classified as an exudate using traditional measures of LDH and total protein, particularly if the patient has been treated with diuretics. In this case, the use of a serum–pleural effusion albumin gradient (SEAG) can be useful. A SEAG of greater than 1.2 g/dL will classify the pleural effusion as transudative, and less than 1.2 g/dL as exudative (Roth and colleagues 1990). One diagnostic approach is to send some of the fluid for protein, pH, LDH measurement, and possibly aerobic and anaerobic culture and sensitivities while storing the remaining fluid for the other tests if the fluid proves to be an exudate (Fig. 95-4). Causes of exudates include cancer, pneumonia, trauma, tuberculosis, pulmonary embolism, pancreatitis, rheumatoid arthritis, and systemic lupus erythematosus. Up to 50% of patients with a pulmonary malignancy will have neoplastic cells in the pleural fluid, so sending exudates for cytology is important. Low pH (<7.2) can indicate a complicated parapneumonic effusion, which may require chest tube drainage. See Table 95-1 for potentially useful tests and their significance.

CPT/Billing Codes

32000 Thoracentesis, puncture of pleural cavity for aspiration, initial or subsequent
99070 Surgical tray (when performed in a clinician's office)

ICD-9-CM Diagnostic Codes

012.00 Pleural effusion, tuberculous, unspecified
197.2 Pleural effusion, malignant
511.1 Pleural effusion, bacterial
511.9 Pleural effusion, unspecified
512.0 Pneumothorax, tension
512.1 Pneumothorax, iatrogenic or postoperative
512.8 Pneumothorax, spontaneous, acute or chronic
860.0 Pneumothorax, tension, traumatic

Additional Resources

See patient education and patient consent forms available online at www.expertconsult.com.

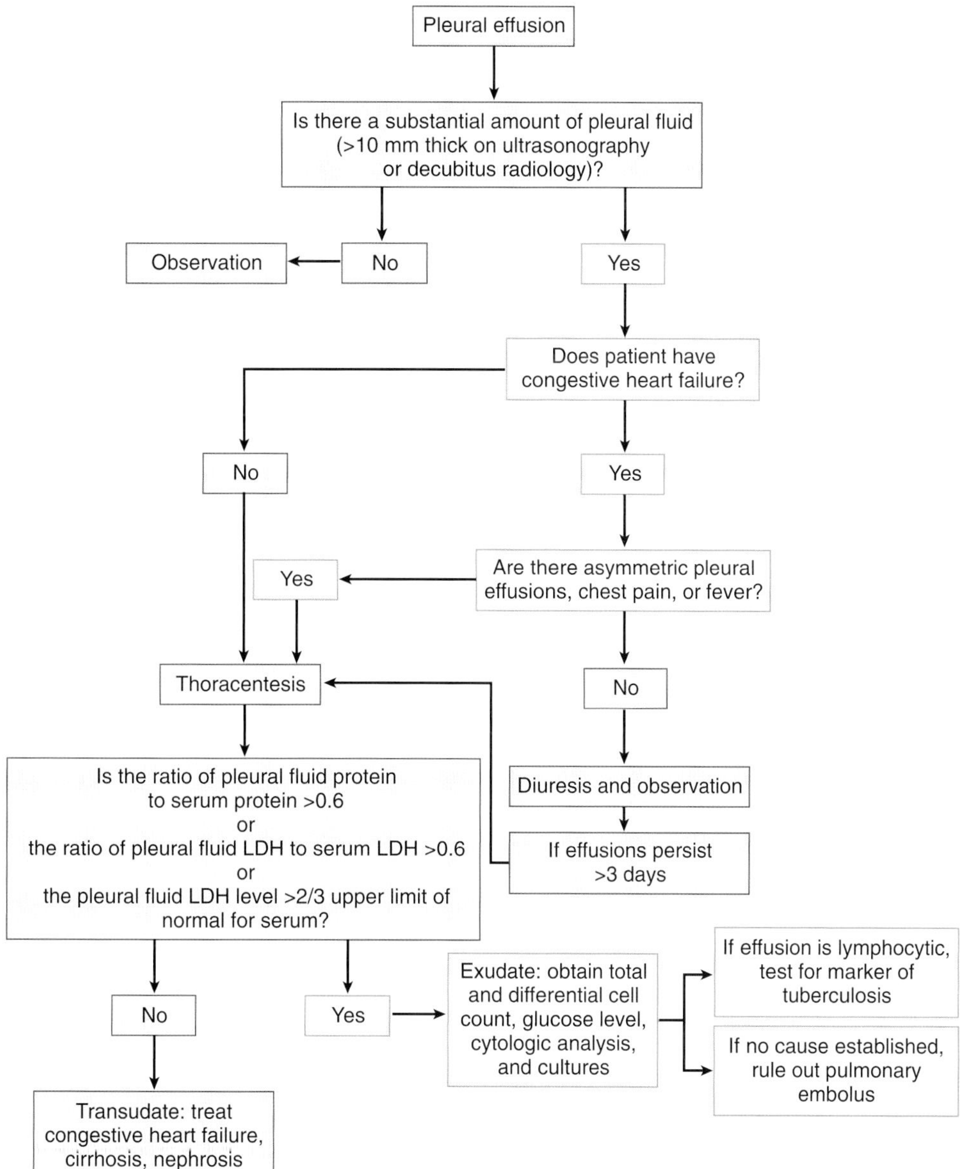

Figure 95-4 Diagnostic scheme for pleural effusion. LDH, lactate dehydrogenase. (From Light RW: Pleural effusion. N Engl J Med 346:1971–1977, 2002.)

TABLE 95-1 Potentially Useful Tests in the Evaluation of Pleural Effusions

Pleural Fluid Test	Abnormal Values	Frequently Associated Condition
Protein (PF/S)	>0.5	Exudate
LDH (PF/S)	>0.6	Exudate
LDH (IU)	>2/3 upper limit of normal for serum	Exudate
Red blood cells (per mm^3)	>100,000	Malignancy, trauma, pulmonary embolism, tuberculosis
White blood cells (per mm^3)	>10,000	Pyogenic infection
Neutrophils (%)	>50	Acute pleuritis
Lymphocytes (%)	>90	Tuberculosis, malignancy, sarcoidosis, fungal infection
Eosinophilia (%)	>10	Asbestos effusion, pneumothorax, resolving infection
Mesothelial cells	Absent	Tuberculosis
Glucose (mg/dL)	<60	Empyema, tuberculosis, malignancy, RA, SLE
pH	<7.20	Complicated parapneumonic process (needs chest tube), empyema, esophageal rupture, tuberculosis, malignancy, RA, urinothorax, SLE
Amylase (PF/S)	>1	Pancreatitis
Bacteria	Positive	Infection
Cytology	Positive	Malignancy

IU, concentration in international units; LDH, lactate dehydrogenase; PF/S, pleural fluid/serum ratio; RA, rheumatoid arthritis; SLE, systemic lupus erythematosus.
Adapted from Kinasewitz GT: Pleural fluid dynamics and effusions. In Fishman AP (ed): Fishman's Pulmonary Diseases and Disorders, 3rd ed, vol 1. New York, McGraw-Hill, 1998, pp 1389–1410.

SUPPLIERS

(See contact information online at www.expertconsult.com.)

Thoracentesis trays

Arrow International
CardinalHealth
Kendall Healthcare Products

ONLINE RESOURCES

Kaufmann DA: Thoracentesis. Medline Plus Medical Encyclopedia. Available at http://www.nlm.nih.gov/medlineplus/ency/article/003420.htm. Patient education handout linked to other information.

Porcel JM, Light RW: Diagnostic approach to pleural effusion in adults. Am Fam Physician 73:1211–1220, 2006. Available at http://www.aafp.org/afp/20060401/1211.html.

Sonosite. Teaching videos for ultrasonically directed thoracentesis. Available at www.sonosite.com.

Thomsen TW, DeLaPena J, Setnik GS: Thoracentesis. N Engl J Med Videos in Clinical Medicine. Available at http://www.youtube.com/watch?v=6-9W-Y2dbpc. Accessed November 16, 2009.

Tuggy M, Garcia J: Procedures Consult. Available at www.proceduresconsult.com.

BIBLIOGRAPHY

Decker MC: Thoracentesis. In Reichman EF, Simon RR (eds): Emergency Medicine Procedures. New York, McGraw-Hill, 2004, pp 237–249.

Ferrer JS, Muñoz XG, Orriols RM, et al: Evolution of idiopathic pleural effusion: A prospective, long-term follow-up study. Chest 109:1508–1513, 1996.

Fishman AP (ed): Fishman's Pulmonary Diseases and Disorders, 3rd ed, vol 1. New York, McGraw-Hill, 1998.

Light RW: Pleural effusion. N Engl J Med 346:1971–1977, 2002.

McCartney JP, Adams JW, Hazard PB: Safety of thoracentesis in mechanically ventilated patients. Chest 103:1920–1921, 1993.

Miller AC, Harvey JE: Guidelines for the management of spontaneous pneumothorax. BMJ 307:114–116, 1993.

Peterson WG, Zimmerman R: Limited utility of chest radiograph after thoracentesis. Chest 117:1038–1042, 2000.

Roth BJ, O'Meara TF, Cragun WH: The serum-effusion albumin gradient in the evaluation of pleural effusions. Chest 98:546–549, 1990.

SECTION 6

Gastrointestinal System Procedures

Section Editor: JOHN L. PFENNINGER

CHAPTER 96

Anal Fissure and Lateral Sphincterotomy and Anal Fistula

James A. Surrell

Anal Fissure

Anal fissure is defined as a painful linear ulcer (tear) of the distal anal canal, located just inside the anal opening and extending cephalad toward the dentate line (Fig. 96-1). The most common cause of an anal fissure is from passing a large, firm, forced bowel movement. The history of a patient with anal fissure is so characteristic that the diagnosis can usually be made accurately based on the history alone. Patients complain of moderate to severe pain during and after bowel movements and have a variable amount of bleeding. The painful symptoms nearly always resolve within 15 to 30 minutes. Rarely, the patient with an anal fissure complains of severe and constant pain, but this is usually seen only with a severe, deep anal fissure with associated significant anal spasm. A small amount of bleeding with bowel movements is common ("just on the toilet paper"), with frank bleeding rare.

The severe pain, "like glass is cutting me," is thought to be secondary to tearing the fissure open and associated *internal anal sphincter spasm*. Subsequently, avoiding constipation and keeping the bowel movements soft along with relieving the anal muscle spasm is the goal of all therapies.

The *internal* anal sphincter is a totally involuntary muscle and responds to pain by contracting, which leads to more pain and a smaller opening through which the stool must pass, thus creating a vicious cycle. The *external* sphincter generally acts in an involuntary fashion but is under voluntary control. Both sphincters form a ring of muscle around the anus (Fig. 96-2).

The history must include whether the fissure is acute or chronic. *Chronic fissure* can arbitrarily be defined as one that has been present with signs and symptoms of pain or bleeding for more than 3 months. Unless the symptoms are extremely disabling, all fissures should be given a trial of conservative management, as discussed later. If conservative management fails, lateral internal sphincterotomy is the procedure of choice for treatment of an anal fissure.

Once the history suggests an anal fissure, the diagnosis can usually be made easily on visual examination of the external anus and with gentle digital examination. The left lateral decubitus position is recommended for patients undergoing anorectal examination. With gentle eversion of the anoderm, one can usually directly visualize the fissure. Touching the fissure with a cotton-tipped applicator confirms the diagnosis if this reproduces the painful symptoms experienced with bowel movements. If necessary, a digital examination with good lubrication will confirm not only pain but marked increased sphincter tone due to spasm. Finally, if the diagnosis is in doubt, the anoscopic examination can provide more direct visualization. In classic cases, the insertion of the anoscope may be so painful that it should be deferred. It should be performed at a later time to identify other possible diseases.

Anal fissures occur most commonly in the posterior midline. Approximately 90% of fissures are in this location, and 10% are located in the anterior midline. If the clinician sees an anal fissure in any location other than the anterior or posterior midline, a thorough gastrointestinal work-up is necessary to rule out the presence of inflammatory bowel disease (IBD) or other very rare causes such as tuberculosis, syphilis, occult abscess, leukemic infiltrates, carcinomas, herpes, or acquired immunodeficiency syndrome.

If it is present, IBD with an atypical fissure is most commonly Crohn's disease. Another physical examination feature that should raise the suspicion of perianal Crohn's disease is the presence of fleshy, edematous skin tags (see Chapter 108, Removal of Perianal Skin Tags [External Hemorrhoidal Skin Tags]). If the examiner suspects IBD, upper gastrointestinal with small bowel x-ray films are necessary, as well as colonoscopy or barium enema radiography combined with flexible sigmoidoscopy. Magnetic resonance imaging enterography also may be used to evaluate for Crohn's disease and other bowel lesions.

Treatment

If the patient has symptoms of moderate to severe pain or bleeding during and after bowel movements, he or she probably has an anal fissure. As noted, the initial goal of therapy is to keep the bowel movements soft and easy to pass while providing pain relief. If these symptoms are severe, disabling, and constant, surgical intervention should be considered sooner rather than later.

However, for most fissures, a 1- to 3-month trial of *conservative management* is indicated. This management includes a *high-fiber diet* of at least 30 g of dietary fiber, six to eight glasses of water, and 3 to 6 g of commercially available fiber supplements per day. If the fissure pain is severe, consider prescribing 5% *lidocaine ointment* to be applied to the fissure on arising and at bedtime, as needed throughout the day, and again after bowel movements. Commercially available nonprescription ointments and creams are minimally effective in the treatment of anal fissures. They may, however, be used to lubricate the anal canal for bowel movements. Steroid preparations may or may not be helpful, but they are not intended for long-term use.

Specifically advise patients not to use any ointment or cream with a rectal tube-tipped applicator or any suppositories because these products and devices tend to worsen the symptoms of an anal fissure. Advise patients to apply a small amount of any recommended ointment or cream directly to the fissure with a finger

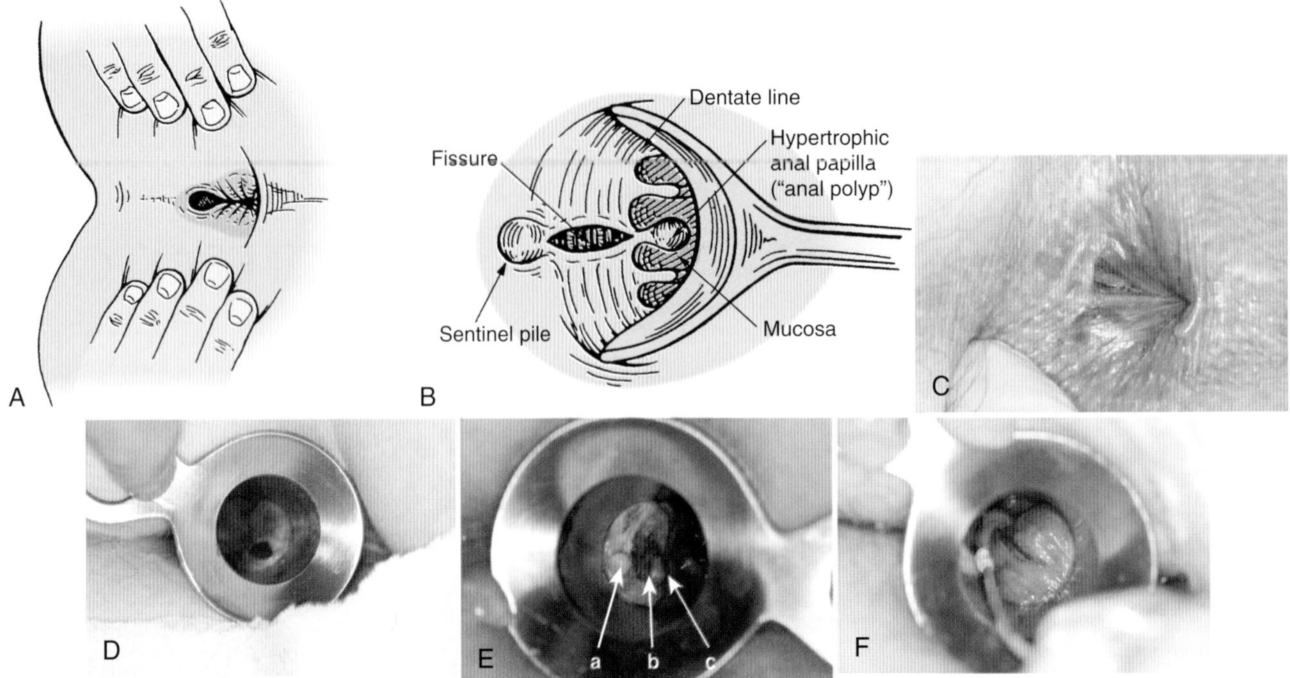

Figure 96-1 Anal fissures. Patient is in the left lateral decubitus position. **A,** External examination. Gentle eversion of the buttocks reveals a posterior midline anal fissure. **B,** Anoscopic examination. Chronic posterior anal fissure with a distal "sentinel pile/tag" and a proximal hypertrophic anal papilla at the level of the dentate line. **C,** Superficial anal fissure visualized easily with manual retraction of perianal tissues. **D,** Acute anal fissure diagnosed with use of an Ives slotted anoscope. **E,** Chronic anal fissure. *Arrows* point to sentinel tag (a), fissure (b), and anal polyp (c). **F,** Large acute anal fissure obscured by hemorrhoids until fold retracted with cotton-tipped applicator. (**C–F,** Courtesy of John L. Pfenninger, MD, The Medical Procedures Center, PC, Midland, Mich.)

because an anal fissure is always located just inside the anal verge. The application of silver nitrate to or the use of electrocautery on the fissure site is *not* recommended and may even exacerbate the symptoms. Anal dilators should *not* be used because of the unpredictable disruption of the anal sphincters and the potential for causing incontinence.

For persistent fissures, a trial of *0.2% to 0.5% nitroglycerin ointment or jelly* may be tried. It is recommended that a small amount of this ointment (about the size of a pencil eraser) be applied directly to the fissure three to four times a day, and that it be gently rubbed onto the fissure and not just applied superficially. Patients must be cautioned that if they experience a headache, they are using too much nitroglycerin ointment. Usually, using a lesser amount will eliminate the headaches. The 0.2% to 0.5% nitroglycerin ointment formulation is not yet commercially available (it comes as 2%), but it can be made up by any reputable local pharmacist from a physician's prescription. The prescription usually reads as follows: "Rx: 0.2% nitroglycerin ointment, DISP: 60 g, SIG: apply small amount to anal fissure, as directed, three to four times a day for 6 to 8 weeks for anal fissure pain." (Be sure to clarify 0.2%, not 2.0%.) Most studies use soft white paraffin to dilute it, or lidocaine or Anusol ointment. If headache does occur, the patient should take an aspirin 1 hour beforehand and lessen the volume applied to the fissure.

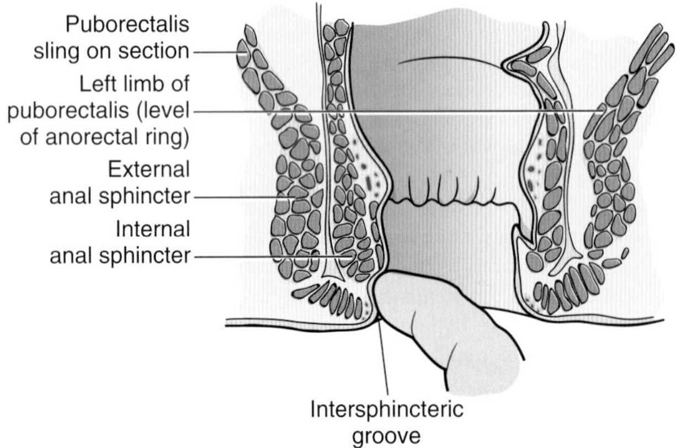

Figure 96-2 Sagittal section of the anal canal to illustrate the palpation of the intersphincteric groove by the surgeon's examining finger. (Also see Chapter 97, Clinical Anorectal Anatomy and Digital Examination.)

Some practitioners now question the efficacy of nitroglycerin and have switched to using *nifedipine gel 0.2%*. The mixture is rubbed in two to three times a day. (Nifedipine gel 0.2%. Mix #10, 20-mg capsules of nifedipine in 100 mL surgical lubricant. Apply to rectal area qid [100 mL].) Some add bethanechol to make 0.1%. K-Y Jelly or 2% lidocaine jelly can be used instead of surgical lubricant.

Both medications pharmacologically relax the anal sphincter to reduce spasm and pain and to assist with the healing process (a "chemical sphincterotomy").

Botulinum toxin (Botox) injected into the anal sphincter is also an option for medical management of anal fissures. The mechanism of action appears to be inhibition of anal sphincter spasm. Initial response is favorable, but long-term follow-up in some studies shows a high recurrence rate. Botox is contraindicated in pregnant and nursing patients and those with neuromuscular disease.

Botulinum Toxin Type A Injection Technique

Botulinum toxin type A (Botox) is generally available in 100-U aliquots. (See storage and mixing instructions, Chapter 56, Botulinum Toxin.) The dosage most commonly used for anal fissures is a *total* of 40 U, with half injected on the right and the remainder injected into the left lateral side of the anal verge. (Remember, most "routine" anal fissures are located anteriorly and posteriorly.) Although various techniques are used, the best results are apparent when the Botox is injected away from the fissure. Usual and customary sterile technique is used, and the perianal area is prepared with povidone–iodine (Betadine). A local anesthetic injection is not recommended because this will likely cause a similar amount of discomfort as the Botox injection itself. This procedure may be done with or without an anoscope. If the patient is not in too much pain from the anal fissure, a small and well-lubricated anoscope is gently placed into the anal canal in the usual fashion. It is recommended that an open-sided anoscope (Ives slotted anoscope) be used to facilitate palpation of the intersphincteric groove on the right and left sides (see Fig. 96-2). This will obviously require withdrawal and replacement of the anoscope to identify the intersphincteric groove on the contralateral side and may cause significant pain. Each side needs to be injected. The specific technique is to inject a total of 20 U of Botox into the intersphincteric groove using a 30-gauge needle at a depth of approximately 1 cm. (Some choose to inject directly into the internal sphincter.) The two sites of injection are in the middle of both the right and left perianal tissues, directly into the intersphincteric groove. The intersphincteric groove is palpable and usually easily identified on digital examination by slowly withdrawing the gloved examining finger from just within the anal canal out onto the perianal area. In this manner, one should be able to identify this palpable groove without difficulty. It is important to accurately identify the intersphincteric groove site for the subsequent Botox injection into the intersphincteric space.

The effect of botulinum toxin (relaxing the internal sphincter) is not permanent and lasts only 2 to 4 months. If the patient also follows a high-fiber diet, however, this is usually enough time for the fissure to heal. If there is relief but the fissure persists, a second injection can be tried. If there is little relief, a second injection can be made with a smaller dosage of toxin 4 to 6 weeks after the first.

Mild, transient incontinence of gas or feces is not uncommon with this treatment.

Lateral Internal Sphincterotomy

Indications

Lateral internal sphincterotomy is indicated if conservative management has been recommended, the patient has complied for approximately 1 month, and the symptoms of pain or bleeding are still present during and after bowel movements, without improvement.

Contraindications

- An atypical location of the fissure (other than anterior or posterior) until a work-up for secondary causes is completed (see previous discussion)
- Preexisting anal incontinence, although the coexistence of an anal fissure and incontinence is uncommon

Equipment

The only special equipment required for lateral internal sphincterotomy is an assortment of various-sized anoscopes and a surgical electrocautery unit. The Hill-Ferguson anal retractor is available in small, medium, and large sizes. Any modern electrosurgery device with a cutting and coagulation setting should suffice.

Preprocedure Patient Preparation

Although some will perform lateral sphincterotomies in the office, most procedures are performed in day surgery. They take approximately 15 minutes and can be performed in either the left lateral decubitus knee–chest position or in the dorsal lithotomy (pelvic) position.

Inform the patient that lateral internal sphincterotomy is a procedure to divide only the fibers of the *involuntary* internal sphincter to allow the anal canal to relax during bowel movements. The *external* sphincter remains intact and allows for anal control. There is an approximate 5% recurrence rate and a 3% to 5% infection rate. Patients should expect mild to moderate postprocedure pain, which usually is well controlled with oral analgesics. Generally no more than 1 or 2 days is required for recovery, and postoperative pain is minimal compared with the preoperative discomfort from the fissure. There will be minimal bleeding and spotting for up to 6 weeks after the procedure. With proper technique combined with a thorough understanding of anal sphincter anatomy, alteration of anal continence is uncommon.

As always, before any surgical procedure patients should be made aware of nonoperative treatment options, as discussed previously. If the fissure is not resolved with either conservative or surgical treatment, the patient generally experiences intermittent, persistent symptoms. Fibrosis of the internal anal sphincter can lead to anal stenosis. A subcutaneous fistula originating through the base of a long-standing anal fissure may develop, but is not common.

Technique

This is an outpatient procedure, usually performed in the operating room, under monitored anesthesia care using intravenous sedation and local anesthesia. Complete familiarity with the anorectal anatomy is essential.

1. Place the patient on the operating table in the left lateral decubitus position, with the buttocks just off the edge of the table and the knees flexed. Identify the intersphincteric groove between the internal and external sphincters so that only the fibers of the internal sphincter are divided (see Fig. 96-2); this is done to preserve anal continence for both flatus and feces.
2. Use the electrocautery unit to make a superficial 1-cm radial incision just distal and parallel to the palpable intersphincteric groove in the left lateral quadrant of the anal area (Fig. 96-3).
3. Grasp the skin edge and clearly identify the intersphincteric groove using the dissecting scissors. The darker-red external sphincter should not be divided or damaged in any way. The lighter-colored internal sphincter is bluntly elevated with forceps. It normally extends 1 to 1.5 cm into the canal.
4. Divide the full thickness of the internal sphincter from its distal margin up to the level of the dentate line, which is visible in the anal canal. The internal sphincter is immediately subjacent to the internal hemorrhoidal vessels, and significant bleeding may occur if these vessels are divided. If proper hemostasis cannot be obtained by using pressure or electrocautery, figure-of-eight suture ligation of these vessels may be necessary for persistent bleeding (rare).
5. It is very important to leave the primary incision site open and allow it to close secondarily because this technique will almost completely eliminate the chance of a postoperative infection developing at the operative site. If there is a prominent sentinel skin tag ("pile") *distal* to the fissure site or a prominent hypertrophic anal papilla *proximal* to the fissure site, you may excise the tag or the papilla with the electrocautery unit at the time of the sphincterotomy procedure. Generally, no specific operative treatment is performed at the fissure site itself. The average operative time is 15 minutes or less.

Postprocedure Patient Education

After lateral internal sphincterotomy, provide a prescription for nonconstipating pain medication (e.g., ibuprofen). The patient should continue to follow a high-fiber diet of at least 30 g of dietary fiber per day and to use psyllium-based powder fiber supplements once or twice a day. He or she should expect some discomfort, slight bleeding, and discharge from the operative site because the wound is generally left open. Bed rest is not recommended, inasmuch as the pain from the sphincterotomy is often minimal and may even be less than that of a severe fissure.

Complications

- Approximately 5% of patients have *nonhealing fissures* after sphincterotomy and may need repeat sphincterotomy.
- Various studies have shown a postoperative *infection* rate of approximately 3% to 5%, and a very small percentage of these patients will go on to develop an associated *anal fistula*.

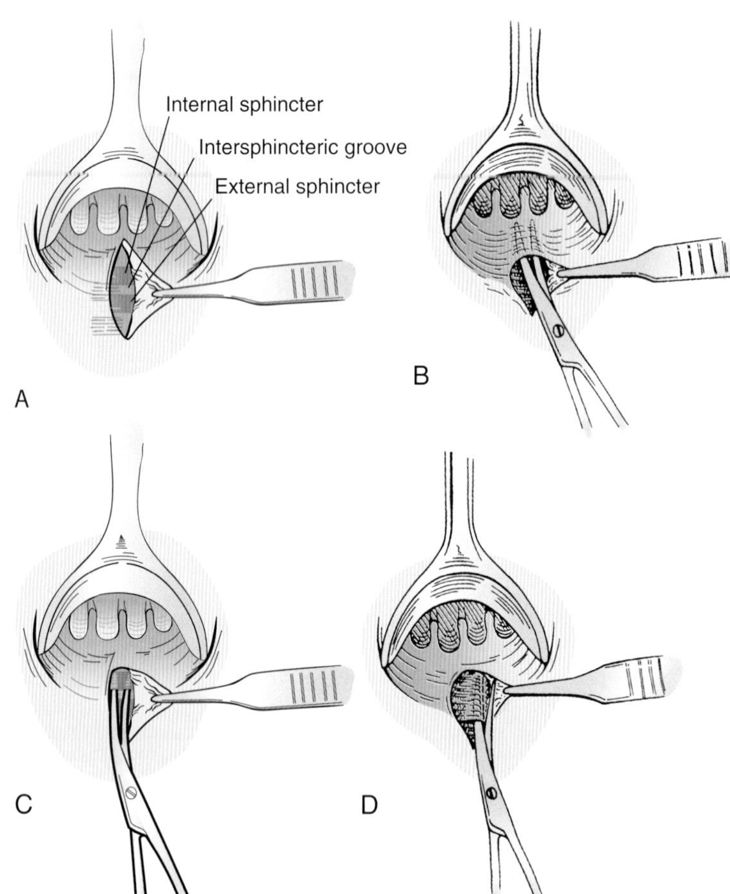

Figure 96-3 Lateral internal anal sphincterotomy using the open technique. The patient is placed in the lateral or the prone (jackknife) position. **A,** A radial incision is made across the intersphincteric groove. A narrow Hill-Ferguson retractor is in place. **B** and **C,** The internal sphincter is separated from the anoderm by blunt dissection. **D,** The internal sphincter is divided. The wound may be closed or left open.

- The most morbid long-term complication is the development of *anal incontinence*, either of flatus or feces. Postoperative anal incontinence can result from technical operative error during the procedure, whereby muscle fibers other than those of the internal sphincter muscle are divided. Another factor that can contribute to postoperative anal incontinence is unrecognized preexisting anal incontinence.

Patient Education Guides

See the sample patient education handout available online at www.expertconsult.com.

CPT/Billing Code

46080 Anal sphincterotomy

ICD-9-CM Diagnostic Code

565.0 Anal fissure

Suppliers

(See contact information online at www.expertconsult.com.)

Anal retractors
Allegiance Healthcare Corp.
CareFusion

NOTE: Anoscope product codes are SU180, SU181, and SU182.

Davol Surgical Electrocautery Unit
Davol, Inc.

Also refer to Chapter 30, Radiofrequency Surgery (Modern Electrosurgery).

Anal Fistula

Fistula is the Latin word for "pipe." The medical definition of fistula is an abnormal "pipelike" communication between any two anatomic body parts that do not normally communicate. Anal fistulas are caused by (1) infection, (2) an inflammatory process, or (3) malignancy. The most common cause of a fistula is infection, usually as a secondary complication from a perianal abscess (see also Chapter 107, Perianal Abscess Incision and Drainage). Fortunately, not all patients who present with a perianal abscess develop a subsequent anal fistula. The diagnosis of an anal fistula, like most medical conditions, is made based on a focused history, followed by a careful anorectal examination. Because of the pain involved, if a perianal abscess is present the assessment for an anal fistula should be deferred, unless one is conducting an examination under anesthesia. Treat the abscess first; if symptoms persist, further evaluation is needed.

Anatomy

A perianal abscess is adjacent to the anal canal and slowly enlarges to cause increased tissue damage. The abscess likely started as a superficial infection at the dentate line in one of the crypts ("cryptitis"), but rather than spontaneously draining into the anal canal without consequence, the infection spread laterally into the perianal tissues. This now becomes a potential tract, or "pipe," that may develop into a fistula. Development of both a perianal abscess and an anal fistula is increased in the immune-compromised patient (e.g., on steroids) and in patients with IBD (specifically, Crohn's disease), diabetes, status postperianal radiation, and other

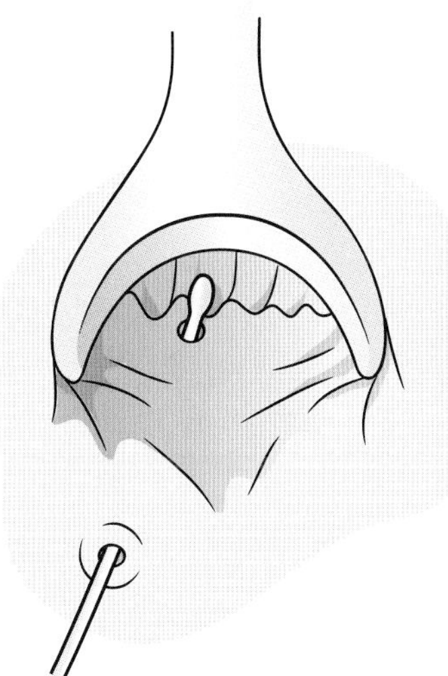

Figure 96-4 Simple fistula tract with blunt fistula probe in place.

conditions. However, fewer than 20% of patients who develop a *single* perianal abscess will ever develop an anal fistula. If, however, a patient presents with a *recurrent* perianal abscess, one must strongly consider the presence of an anal fistula because the odds of a fistula being present are at least 50%, and even higher if the perianal abscess is in the same anatomic location.

An anal fistula may be *simple* or *complex*. A *simple* anal fistula is generally defined as a single tract, as noted in Figure 96-4. A *complex* fistula has multiple tracts and may involve more than two anatomic locations. The discussion here focuses on the more common simple anal fistula.

An anal fistula always has an internal opening and an external opening. By definition, the *external opening* of a simple anal fistula is located on the perianal skin, usually within 3 cm of the anal opening (anal verge), and can be readily visualized on gross examination (see Fig. 96-4). The *internal opening* is within the anal canal and is most commonly located at the level of the dentate line, which is located within 2 cm proximal to the anal verge (Fig. 96-5). The external opening of the fistula may appear to be inflamed, and often there is a varying degree of discharge. In fact, this discharge may be the symptom that brings the patient in for evaluation, and represents a chronically draining infection. As long as the external opening remains open, a perianal abscess does not develop. The chance of an established anal fistula spontaneously closing without surgical intervention is essentially zero.

Three anal muscles provide anal continence: the internal anal sphincter, the external anal sphincter, and the puborectalis muscle (anorectal ring). Further, the external anal sphincter has three components: subcutaneous, superficial, and deep. In general, involuntary anal continence is provided by the internal sphincter and voluntary anal continence is provided by the external sphincter and the puborectalis muscle, the latter of which essentially comprises the anorectal ring. It is very important to thoroughly understand this anatomy and to clearly identify these three muscles, and the extent of their involvement in any fistula tract, before performing anal fistulotomy.

History and Physical Examination

A focused patient *history* is very important. The patient likely will have a history of a perianal abscess, with a nonhealing, chronically draining site, usually at the location of the previous perianal abscess. The external opening may not always be active and may swell and drain only infrequently. Typically, however, a patient with an anal fistula presents with a small, palpable, firm nodule within 3 cm of the anal verge, and this site will periodically swell, cause minor discomfort, and drain. The frequency of these symptoms is highly variable.

On *physical examination*, the examiner should carefully and gently palpate all around the anal verge and perianal area. Ask the patient where he or she can feel any swelling, discomfort, or site of drainage. The external opening will not necessarily appear as a true opening, or "hole," and may appear only as a small, erythematous papule (see Fig. 96-5). Usually the external opening will feel indurated, and this firmness may extend for several centimeters from the external opening. Palpate for a subcutaneous tract leading from the external opening toward the anal canal. If present, this suggests a superficial fistula tract and will feel like a small, firm "pipe" just under the skin.

A *digital anorectal examination* should be completed, with careful palpation all around the level of the dentate line to feel for any

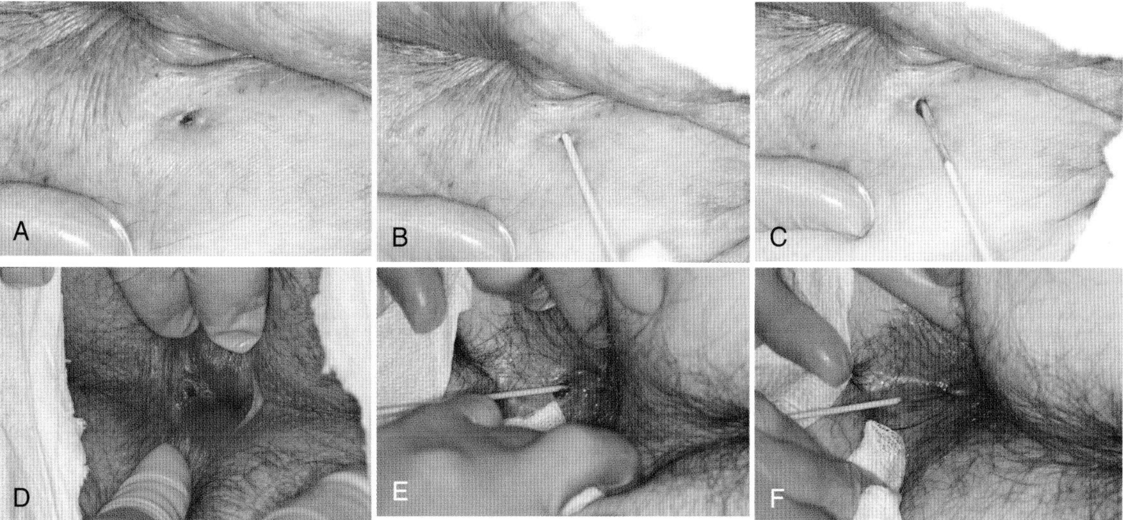

Figure 96-5 The clinical appearance and confirmation of a suspected fistula using a blunt probe. **A,** Papular, small, pustular-appearing lesion in left buttock. **B,** Blunt wooden end of cotton-tipped applicator is easily and gently inserted into fistula. The probe is inserted only a short distance to confirm diagnosis. **C,** The blood on the wooden probe shows the fistula is at least 2 cm deep. **D,** Another clinical presentation under an anal tag. **E,** Probe inserted. **F,** Probe removed. Blood staining shows depth probe was inserted to confirm diagnosis. (Courtesy of John L. Pfenninger, MD, The Medical Procedures Center, PC, Midland, Mich.)

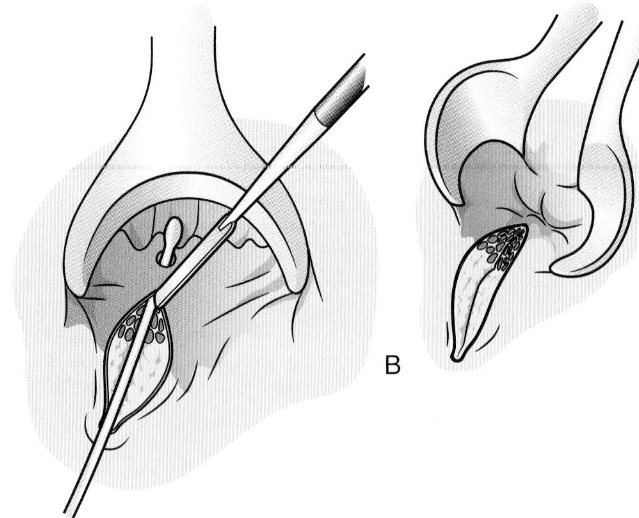

Figure 96-6 Performing a fistulotomy. **A,** Use of electrocautery to perform simple fistulotomy. **B,** Completed fistulotomy with wound left open to heal by secondary intention.

induration or scar tissue, which may suggest the location of the internal opening. Carefully evaluate the anal canal and anoderm with the specific goal of locating any internal opening. Finding the internal opening is ultimately necessary for treatment but is not entirely necessary to establish the diagnosis.

Very gently attempt to pass a blunt fistula probe into the external opening to assess for an established tract. This is usually a small, malleable, 1- to 2-mm-diameter "silver probe" with a tiny bulbous end. The wooden end of a cotton-tipped applicator can also be used, but may be more painful. However, and this cannot be emphasized strongly enough, *do not pass the fistula probe against any resistance at all.* Creating a false tract will worsen the situation and make treatment much more difficult. If a fistula probe is used, it is most commonly done with the anoscope in the anal canal to offer concurrent visualization of the anoderm and dentate line. The fistula probe is touched to the area of the suspected external opening, and *minimal* pressure is applied. If this is a true fistula, the probe will literally "drop" into the opening. If it passes easily toward the anal canal, there is really no need to probe further at this time. The suspected anal fistula diagnosis has now been confirmed (see Fig. 96-5).

See Chapter 97, Clinical Anorectal Anatomy and Digital Examination, and the previous discussion of anal fissure and lateral sphincterotomy.

Treatment with Seton or Anal Fistulotomy

The treatment for anal fistula is anal fistulotomy. It is absolutely essential to precisely establish the locations of both the internal and external openings of a simple fistula before fistulotomy can be performed. Once these are established, the examiner must carefully assess how much anal sphincter muscle will be divided as a result of simple fistulotomy. If the internal opening is at or distal to (below) the dentate line, a simple fistulotomy may be performed with little to no likelihood of altering anal continence. During fistulotomy, one can generally divide the fibers of the subcutaneous and *superficial* portions of the external and the internal sphincters, usually with little impact on subsequent anal continence.

Anal fistulotomy is usually performed under sedation with monitored anesthesia care. In the left lateral decubitus knee–chest position, with the patient's buttocks just off the edge of the operating room table and with the anoscope in place, local anesthetic with epinephrine is injected along the sides of the fistula tract. This is used primarily for hemostasis and early postoperative comfort. Once the fistula tract anatomy is accurately identified, the blunt fistula probe is placed into the tract with an anoscope in place so both the internal and external openings are clearly visualized, as noted in Figures 96-4 and 96-5. Fistulotomy may now be performed with electrocautery to divide the tissue overlying the indwelling fistula probe within the fistula tract. Essentially, you are converting an infected "pipe" to an open "ditch." Bleeding points are cauterized. This chronically infected wound is always left open to heal by secondary intention. Dry sterile dressings are applied.

A nearly completed simple fistulotomy, performed with electrocautery, is shown in Figure 96-6. The resulting wound after simple fistulotomy is left open to heal by secondary intention, as noted in Figure 96-7.

Although a *seton* (a suture placed into the fistula and tied in place) can also be used for simple fistulas, it is usually reserved for the treatment of complex ones. If the course of the fistula tract is lateral to the external sphincter or the internal opening extends above the dentate line, this is *not* a simple anal fistula, and complete fistulotomy should *not* be performed. This is now a *complex fistula*, and surgical treatment should be performed only by an experienced surgeon thoroughly trained in anorectal surgery because of the potential for altering anal continence.

If the internal opening to the fistula tract extends above the dentate line near the anorectal ring, then the fistulotomy becomes a staged operation and will almost certainly involve the use of a seton. The *seton* is usually a nonabsorbable, doubled, heavy silk suture (see Fig. 96-7A) placed into the fistula tract and tied around to itself to permit a slow cutting through of the fistula tract. The seton is placed into the fistula tract using a blunt fistula probe with an "eye" on the leading end. The long silk seton is threaded through this eye and the probe is replaced into the fistula tract, permitting placement of the doubled suture into the fistula tract. After the probe exits the internal opening, the suture is grasped with a hemostat, and the fistula probe is removed, with the doubled silk suture remaining in the fistula tract. The two ends of the seton are now *snugly tied together*, as noted in Figure 96-7B, to permit continued slow cutting through the overlying muscle. This produces an inflammatory response and scarring. The few remaining fibers of muscle that overlie the fistula are fully divided, usually with cautery, no sooner than 6 weeks later. The sphincter muscle will not retract and separate now because of the scarring, thereby preserving anal continence.

Contraindications

- Immunocompromised patient
- History of radiation to fistula location
- Uncontrolled diabetes
- Recent steroid use

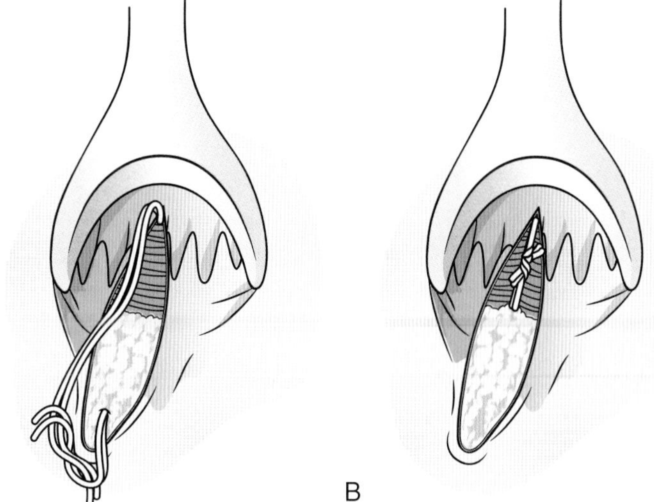

Figure 96-7 Placement of a seton for complex fistula. **A,** The doubled heavy silk suture is threaded through the fistula and tightly tied to put some tension on the skin, **B,** Six weeks later, the overlying remaining tissue is separated using electrocautery and the suture is removed.

- Significant medical comorbidities such as severe cardiac or respiratory disease

Common Errors and Potential Complications

- Dividing excess muscle length overlying the fistula tract, leading to varying degrees of anal incontinence
- Not recognizing as-yet-undiagnosed perianal Crohn's disease
- Not diagnosing and draining an associated occult perianal abscess
- Not recognizing a complex fistula with multiple tracts
- Creating a false fistula tract with overly aggressive use of the fistula probe

Postoperative Management

After fistulotomy, the patient has an open wound extending into the anal canal. Patients are often fearful of this wound becoming infected because of exposure to fecal material, but an open wound cannot become infected. The patient should shower or tub bathe to irrigate the wound twice a day for the first week, then once a day for 3 to 4 weeks, and apply dry dressings to absorb the expected discharge. The wound will attempt to close prematurely, and the usual wound care measures should be taken to be certain the wound closes from "the inside out." The skin edges must be the last portion of the wound to close; this will dramatically minimize the chance of recurrence. If the skin edges close before the fistula tract is totally closed down by the healing and scarring process, another fistula, often more superficial, has been created. The patient must be instructed that efforts must be made to keep the wound open as long as possible, with complete healing usually occurring within 4 to 6 weeks. The patient should be seen on a weekly basis to ensure this proper healing process.

CPT/Billing Codes

46020 Placement of seton
46030 Removal of seton
46270 Surgical treatment of anal fistula (fistulectomy/fistulotomy); subcutaneous
  46275 Submuscular
  46280 Complex or multiple, with or without seton

ICD-9-CM Diagnostic Code

565.1 Anal fistula

BIBLIOGRAPHY

Altomare DF, Rinaldi M, Milito G, et al: Glyceryl trinitrate for chronic anal fissure—healing or headache? Results of a multicenter, randomized, placebo-controlled, double-blind trial. Dis Colon Rectum 43:174–179, 2000.

American Gastroenterological Association medical position statement: Diagnosis and care of patients with anal fissure. Gastroenterology 124: 233–234, 2003.

Antropoli C, Perrotti P, Rubino M, et al: Nifedipine for local use in conservative treatment of anal fissures: Preliminary results of a multicenter study. Dis Colon Rectum 42:1011–1015, 1999.

Arroyo A, Perez F, Serrano P, et al: Long-term results of botulinum toxin for the treatment of chronic anal fissure: Prospective clinical and manometric study. Int J Colorectal Dis 20:267–271, 2005.

Baraza W, Boereboom C, Shorthouse A, Brown S: The long-term efficacy of fissurectomy and botulinum toxin injection for chronic anal fissure in females. Dis Colon Rectum 51:239–243, 2008.

Boushey RP, Roberts PL (eds): Recent advances in the management of benign and malignant colorectal diseases. Surg Clin North Am 86(4), 2006.

Brisinda G, Cadeddu F, Brandara F, et al: Randomized clinical trial comparing botulinum toxin injection with 0.2 per cent nitroglycerin ointment for chronic anal fissure. Br J Surg 94:162–167, 2007.

Brisinda G, Maria G, Bentivoglio AR, et al: A comparison of injections of botulinum toxin and topical nitroglycerin ointment for the treatment of chronic anal fissure. N Engl J Med 341:65–69, 1999.

Carapeti EA, Kamm MA, Evans BK, Phillips RK: Topical diltiazem and bethanechol decrease anal sphincter pressure without side effects. Gut 45:719–722, 1999.

Corman ML: Colon and Rectal Surgery, 6th ed. Philadelphia, Lippincott Williams & Wilkins, 2005.

Fruehauf H, Fried M, Wegmueller B, et al: Efficacy and safety of botulinum toxin injection compared with topical nitroglycerin ointment for the treatment of chronic anal fissure: A prospective randomized study. Am J Gastroenterol 101:2107–2112, 2006.

Gordon P, Nivatvongs S (eds): Principles and Practice of Surgery for the Colon, Rectum, and Anus, 3rd ed. Abingdon, United Kingdom, Informa Healthcare, 2007.

Gorfine SR: Topical nitroglycerin therapy for anal fissures and ulcers. N Engl J Med 333:1156–1157, 1995.

Jost WH, Schimrigk K: Therapy of anal fissure using botulinum toxin. Dis Colon Rectum 37:1321–1324, 1994.

Loder PB, Kamm MA, Nicholls RJ, Phillips RK: "Reversible chemical sphincterotomy" by local application of glyceryl trinitrate. Br J Surg 81:1386–1389, 1994.

Lund JN, Scholefield JH: A randomised, prospective, double-blind, placebo-controlled trial of glyceryl trinitrate ointment in treatment of anal fissure. Lancet 349:11–14, 1997.

Madoff RD, Fleshman JW: AGA technical review on the diagnosis and care of patients with anal fissure. Gastroenterology 124:235–245, 2003.

Mazier W, Levien D, Luchtefeld M, Senagore A (eds): Surgery of the Colon, Rectum, and Anus. Philadelphia, WB Saunders, 1995.

Minguez M, Herreros B, Espi A, et al: Long-term follow-up (42 months) of chronic anal fissure after healing with botulinum toxin. Gastroenterology 123:112–117, 2002.

Pernikoff BJ, Eisenstat TE, Rubin RJ, et al: Reappraisal of partial lateral internal sphincterotomy. Dis Colon Rectum 37:1291–1295, 1994.

Practice parameters for the treatment of fistula-in-ano. The Standards Practice Task Force, The American Society of Colon and Rectal Surgeons. Dis Colon Rectum 39:1361–1362, 1996.

Richard CS, Gregoire R, Plewes EA, et al: Internal sphincterotomy is superior to topical nitroglycerin in the treatment of chronic anal fissure: Results of a randomized, controlled trial by the Canadian Colorectal Surgical Trials Group. Dis Colon Rectum 43:1048–1057, 2000.

Rosen L: Anorectal abscess-fistulae. Surg Clin North Am 74:1293–1308, 1994.

Schouten WR, Briel SW, Auwerda JJA, de Graaf EJR: Ischemic nature of anal fissures. Br J Surg 83:63–65, 1996.

Sharp RF: Patient selection and treatment modalities for chronic anal fissure. Am J Surg 171:512–515, 1996.

Tranqui P, Trottier DC, Victor CJ, Freeman JB: Nonsurgical treatment of chronic anal fissure: Nitroglycerin and dilatation versus nifedipine and botulinum toxin. Can J Surg 49:41–45, 2006.

Whiteford MH, Kilkenny J 3rd, Hyman N, et al: Practice parameters for the treatment of perianal abscess and fistula-in-ano (revised). The Standards Practice Task Force, The American Society of Colon and Rectal Surgeons. Dis Colon Rectum 48:1337–1342, 2005.

Witte ME, Klaase JM: Botulinum toxin A injection in ISDN ointment-resistant chronic anal fissures. Dig Surg 24:197–201, 2007.

CHAPTER 97

Clinical Anorectal Anatomy and Digital Examination

James A. Surrell

A practical knowledge of anorectal anatomy is necessary for the proper evaluation and treatment of patients with anorectal complaints, hemorrhoids, and anal fissures. A basic anorectal examination includes *visual inspection* of the perianal tissues and *digital palpation* of the anorectal area. Depending on patient complaints, anoscopy and sigmoidoscopy or colonoscopy may also be necessary. This chapter describes the practical and the clinically important features of anorectal anatomy. See Chapter 98, Anoscopy, for the anoscopic examination.

Basic Anatomy

Figure 97-1 is a diagram of the anatomy of the anal canal and lower rectum.

- *Rectum:* The distal 10 to 12 cm of the colon.
- *Anus:* The outlet of the gastrointestinal tract, consisting of the lower 6 to 8 cm of the bowel.
- *Anal verge:* Most distal extent of the anal canal, just at the opening.
- *Dentate or pectinate line:* The squamocolumnar junction located 2 to 3 cm proximal to the anal verge where there is an abrupt change from squamous, sensory anoderm to columnar or mucosal epithelium. There are no sensory nerve fibers above the dentate line, only visceral-type fibers that sense pressure.
- *Transitional zone:* Composed of mixed columnar and squamous epithelium; where the anal canal merges with the rectum.
- *Internal sphincter:* The innermost circular muscle.
- *External sphincter:* Located outside (lateral to) the internal sphincter. Note that the external sphincter is external to the internal sphincter not only from a medial to lateral aspect, but from a cephalic to caudal aspect at the anal verge.
- *Puborectalis muscle (anorectal ring):* Located about 1 to 2 cm above the dentate line. The distal rectum and anal canal are surrounded by two sleeves of circular muscles. This palpable anorectal ring represents the puborectalis muscle, which encircles the very distal rectum from its anterior point of attachment at the pubis.
- *"Valves of Houston":* These are not really "valves" but just folds of mucosa. There are generally three located at approximately 8, 11, and 13 cm (inferior, middle, and superior, respectively).
- *Anal papillae:* The mucosal tips of the anal glands at the dentate line. (They can become hypertrophied and elongated and be confused with a polyp.)
- *Anal crypt:* A small pocket along the dentate line. Usually the site of cryptitis, which can lead to a fistula.
- *Anal glands:* Located at dentate line. They secrete mucus to lubricate the canal and can become infected or plugged (cryptitis).
- *Columns of Morgagni:* Folds of tissue above the anal crypts/dentate line.
- *Internal hemorrhoids:* Located at and just proximal to the dentate line.
- *External hemorrhoids:* Located distal to the dentate line at the anal verge.
- *Arteriovenous vessels:* Located above, below, or at the dentate line, or both above and below the dentate line.

Patient Position

A complete anorectal examination can be accomplished with the patient on the examining table in the left lateral decubitus position (Fig. 97-2). The patient's knees are flexed and drawn toward the chest and the buttocks are drawn toward the examiner to a point just slightly off the table. The patient's head and shoulders should remain well toward the middle of the examination table so that the patient is confident that he or she will not fall. This position also directs the axis of the anal canal and rectum directly toward the examiner. Alternatively, the rectum may be examined with the patient in the pelvic position after a genital examination or in a flexed position while bending 90 degrees over an examination table.

External Anal Examination

After appropriately advising the patient, visually inspect the external anus. Look for any sign of perianal inflammation that may suggest pruritus ani or other dermatologic conditions. Gently separate the buttocks; this will generally evert the anoderm to a sufficient degree so that a posterior or anterior anal fissure may be directly visualized.

If there is a *sentinel skin tag* present in either the posterior or anterior midline, be diligent in evaluation for a fissure, especially if the history is consistent with anal fissure (see Chapter 96, Anal Fissure and Lateral Sphincterotomy and Anal Fistula). If present, anal skin tags, perianal abscess, or thrombosed external hemorrhoids should be readily visible at this time. Internal and external hemorrhoids are classically located in the right anterior, right posterior, and left lateral quadrants.

Internal hemorrhoids are located at and just proximal to the dentate line. Because they are above the dentate line, any condition involving them is usually painless. *External hemorrhoids* are located distal to the dentate line at the anal verge, and pathology or treatment in this area is generally quite painful. Hemorrhoids are collections of arteries and veins that, if not enlarged, represent normal anatomy and are not considered varicosities (see Chapter 106, Office Treatment of Hemorrhoids).

It is recommended that clinical anorectal findings be described in terms of the anatomy (i.e., right anterior, right posterior, left anterior, left posterior, right lateral, and left lateral) to provide consistency, regardless of the position of the patient.

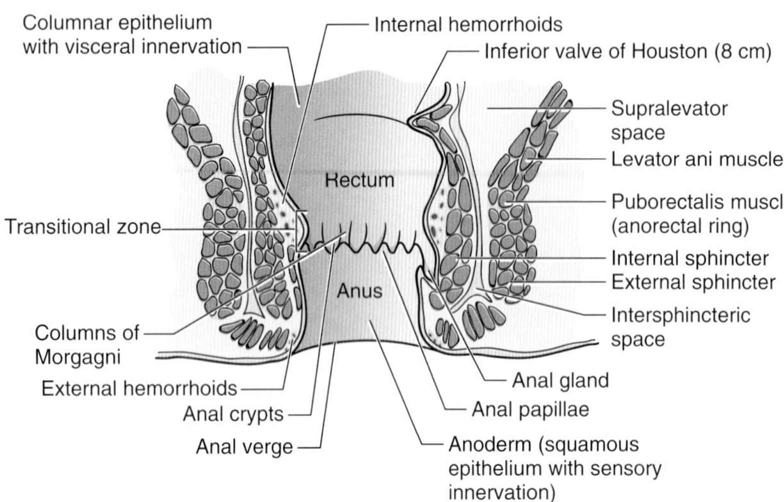

Figure 97-1 Anal and rectal anatomy.

Digital Anorectal Examination

Inform the patient that the anus will be touched with a well-lubricated, gloved examining finger. Apply gentle pressure to the anal verge to allow the examining finger to enter the anal canal. If an anal fissure is present, you may feel palpable induration, most commonly in the posterior midline and less commonly in the anterior midline. Increased tone will also be noted. If the patient complains of severe pain, *do not persist*, because you will lose the patient's confidence. You may wish to reattempt the digital examination after applying 5% lidocaine ointment to the anus and waiting 10 to 15 minutes. The most common causes of severe anal pain on examination are a deep symptomatic anal fissure or a perianal abscess. Fissures are found most commonly anteriorly and posteriorly. Rarely, you may need to consider offering the patient an examination under sedation or refer for examination under anesthesia. Consciously palpate all around the anorectal area (360 degrees).

In men, assess the prostate gland with your gloved examining finger in the anal canal.

To assess continence and anal sphincter function, flex your index finger slightly posteriorly and ask the patient to "squeeze down" as if to try to stop a bowel movement. If the patient has normal anatomic sphincter function, you will feel the tightening of the distal extent of the external sphincter at the base of your examining finger.

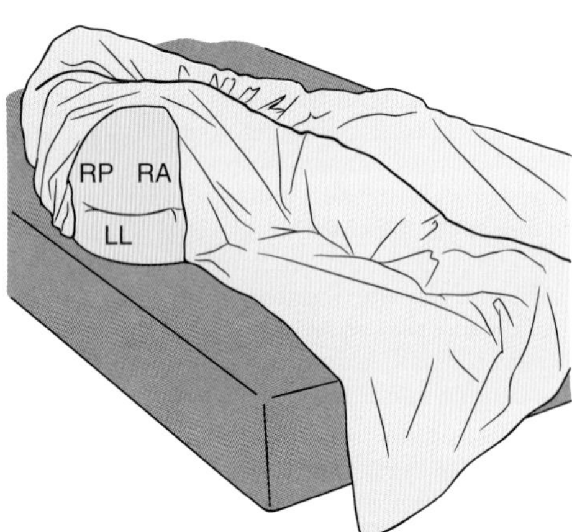

Figure 97-2 Placing the patient in the left lateral decubitus position (Sims' position). Digital examination, flexible sigmoidoscopy, and most anorectal procedures can be performed in this position. LL, Left lateral hemorrhoidal quadrant; RA, right anterior; RP, right posterior.

The puborectalis muscle of the anorectal ring will also contract, pulling the tip of the examining finger from posterior to anterior. You should then be able to sweep the examining finger around the circumference of the distal rectum at the level of the anorectal ring and note the point of fixation of the puborectalis muscle at the symphysis pubis. Advise the patient to relax as the examination continues.

In general, internal hemorrhoids and the dentate line are not palpable to the gloved examining finger. However, a large hypertrophic anal papilla present at the level of the dentate line may be palpable. If necessary, obtain a small sample of stool on the tip of the gloved examining finger for occult blood testing.

The procedure for anoscopic examination can be found in Chapter 98, Anoscopy. Anal fissures are discussed in Chapter 96, Anal Fissure and Lateral Sphincterotomy and Anal Fistula.

Anal Continence

The external sphincter and puborectalis muscle of the anorectal ring are the two muscles generally thought to afford *voluntary* anal continence. The external sphincter extends from the anal verge to the anorectal ring. The anorectal ring consists primarily of the puborectalis muscle, which encircles the very distal rectum. From a practical standpoint, it is generally accepted that either an intact functional external sphincter or an anorectal ring can provide near-perfect anal continence. The internal sphincter plays little role in maintaining voluntary anal continence. This is important when counseling patients during consideration of surgical treatment of anal fissures (see Chapter 96, Anal Fissure and Lateral Sphincterotomy and Anal Fistula).

Summary

A practical understanding of the anatomy of the anal canal is essential to conducting an adequate anorectal examination. Lesions commonly seen may include pruritus ani or perianal dermatitis, anal fissures, fistulas, thrombosed external hemorrhoids, prolapsing bleeding internal hemorrhoids, hypertrophic anal papillae, perianal abscess, pilonidal disease, condylomata, polyps, cancer, and others. When anal continence is an issue, the physician must be able to evaluate the function of the external sphincter and of the puborectalis muscle of the anorectal ring on digital anorectal examination. With appropriate patient preparation and technique, the anorectal examination should not be an uncomfortable or painful experience. See Chapter 98, Anoscopy, for a description of the anoscopic examination.

BIBLIOGRAPHY

Corman ML: Colon and Rectal Surgery, 6th ed. Philadelphia, Lippincott Williams & Wilkins, 2005.

Gordon P, Nivatvongs S: Principles and Practice of Surgery for the Colon, Rectum, and Anus, 3rd ed. Portland, Me, Informa Health, 2007.

Marvin CL: Colon and Rectal Surgery. Philadelphia, Lippincott Williams & Wilkins, 2004.

Mazier W, Levien D, Luchtefeld M, Senagore A: Surgery of the Colon, Rectum, and Anus. Philadelphia, WB Saunders, 1995.

Pfenninger JL, Zainea G: Common anorectal conditions: Part I. Symptoms and complaints. Am Fam Physician 63:2391–2398, 2001.

Pfenninger JL, Zainea G: Common anorectal conditions: Part II. Lesions. Am Fam Physician 64:77–88, 2001.

CHAPTER 98

ANOSCOPY

Peter L. Reynolds • Thad Wilkins

Anoscopy is a common procedure in both ambulatory and emergency medical care. It is used primarily to evaluate the patient with perianal and anal complaints. It may also be performed just before or after withdrawing the colonoscope or flexible sigmoidoscope. Chapter 97, Clinical Anorectal Anatomy and Digital Examination, includes a review of clinical anatomy. High-resolution anoscopy (HRA) refers to an evolving technique to evaluate patients at high risk for anal human papillomavirus (HPV) infection. This includes men who have sex with men and human immunodeficiency virus–infected women with cervical dysplasia. With HRA, the anus is stained with acetic acid and then evaluated using magnification—usually a colposcope (see Chapter 99, High-Resolution Anoscopy).

INDICATIONS

- Initial evaluation of rectal bleeding
- Anal or perianal pain
- Perianal itching (pruritus ani)
- Anal discharge
- Prolapse of the rectum
- External or internal hemorrhoids
- Fissures in ano
- Fistulas in ano
- Painful digital rectal examination
- Perianal condylomata
- Palpable masses on digital examination
- In association with sigmoidoscopy and colonoscopy (screening or diagnostic)
- Evaluation of intra-anal trauma
- Follow-up of inflammatory bowel
- Retrieval of foreign body
- Evaluation of sexual abuse
- Fecal impaction
- Anal polyps, cancer
- Screening for anal HPV in high-risk individuals

CONTRAINDICATIONS

- Unwilling patient
- Severe debilitation
- Acute myocardial infarction or similar cardiovascular condition
- Acute abdomen (relative contraindication)
- Marked anal canal stenosis
- Severe pain

EQUIPMENT

- Anoscope
- Light source
- Gloves
- Lubricant
- Large-tipped cotton swabs
- Biopsy forceps, if needed (the cervical biopsy forceps or the flexible wire biopsy forceps used during sigmoidoscopy or colonoscopy work well)
- Monsel's solution (ferric subsulfate solution)
- 3% acetic acid solution *(HRA only)*
- Colposcope with 10× to 40× magnification *(HRA only)*

The anoscope consists of two parts: a hollow, gently tapering cylinder and a solid obturator that fits inside. The components are made of disposable plastic or reusable metal (Fig. 98-1). Clear plastic anoscopes may provide better visualization of the rectal and anal mucosa than opaque devices, but they do tend to compress the tissues and may obscure some findings. The size varies from 7 to 10 cm in length. They may or may not have handles. The distal diameter is approximately 2.5 cm.

Some anoscopes are readily attachable to battery light sources. Others require an external light source (e.g., a gooseneck lamp or headlight).

The *Ives slotted anoscope* is made of metal but has an open slot on one half of the upper side of the device (see Fig. 98-1D and E). The slot provides an unobstructed view of the walls of the anal canal. This instrument is extremely useful not only for evaluation but when treating various conditions. The advantage of the slotted instrument is that the mucosa is not compressed; thus, small lesions and hemorrhoids may be more readily visible and treated. The diameter is also larger than most other anoscopes, and instruments are more easily manipulated within the lumen. Rather than looking through the end of the tube, the operator can visualize the mucosal wall in a more direct fashion (Fig. 98-2).

PREPROCEDURE PATIENT PREPARATION

Patients dread inspection of the anal canal. They perceive this examination as unpleasant and uncomfortable, if not painful. There are always concerns of embarrassment. This mandates that the patient be prepared mentally for what is involved. However, these concerns should not dissuade the clinician from doing the examination when it is indicated. Far too often the "assumed" diagnosis by the patient or the physician is made without a visual examination completed. This is not only unacceptable, it can place the patient at great risk for missed diagnoses such as cancer, inflammatory bowel disease, and other significant problems. The patient must be cooperative and relaxed. Frank admission that the procedure will be unpleasant and uncomfortable, but not painful, is helpful. Explain the reasons necessitating the examination and the implications of not performing it. Reassure the patient that there are no significant complications resulting from anoscopy alone. However, if a biopsy sample is obtained or a lesion is removed, there may be some bleeding. If the biopsy is from below the dentate line, it will also be painful and local anesthetic will be needed.

If the reason for the examination is to evaluate anal pain (e.g., possible fissure), patients can be extremely tender and apprehensive. In addition, the anal sphincter contracts, making the examination

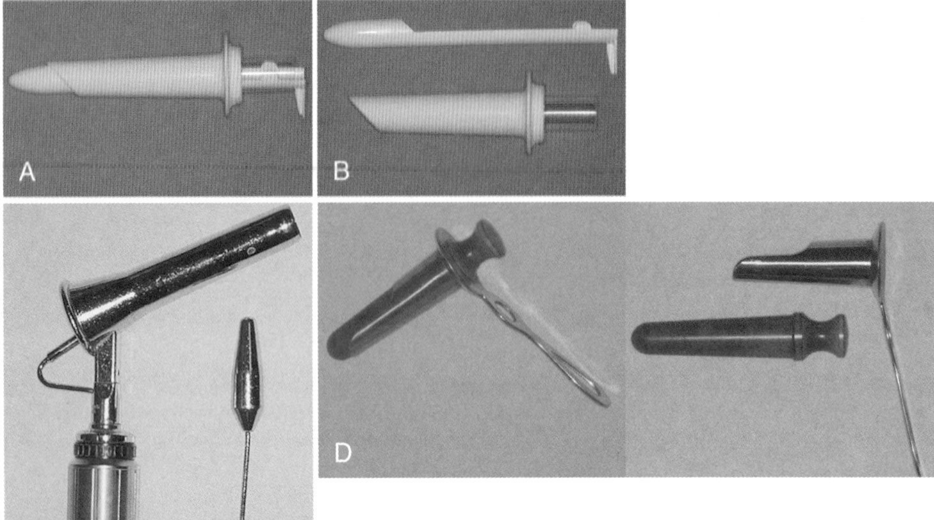

Figure 98-1 Disposable plastic opaque anoscope requiring external light source with obturator in place (**A**) and obturator removed (**B**). Reusable type for use with battery-powered light source; inserting trocar has been removed (**C**). **D,** Ives slotted anoscope with obturator in place (*left*) and obturator removed (*right*). The Ives slotted anoscope provides the best visualization and the most operative space for any interventional procedures.

difficult. Application of a topical anesthetic, such as 5% lidocaine, 30 minutes before the examination can markedly reduce discomfort (see Chapter 10, Topical Anesthesia). If pain is so severe that the examination needs to be deferred, the presumptive diagnosis is an anal fissure, but the examination, perhaps at a later date after treatment, is necessary to confirm that there is no other pathologic process.

Technique

An assistant is helpful and gender-appropriate chaperones recommended. Both physician and assistant must wear gloves on both hands. An enema is usually not needed but may be helpful. Consider eye protection.

1. Place the patient in the left lateral position and drape. This position is most comfortable for the patient and is adequate in at least 95% of situations. At times, placing the patient in stirrups or in the head-down position may be indicated.
2. Have the assistant separate the glutei laterally, allowing full visibility of the perianal area. Alternatively, have the patient pull up on the right gluteus. Check for any obvious lesions and possible fistulous tracks.
3. Inspect the tissue closely. Ask the patient to bear down, and observe for hemorrhoid or polyp prolapse.
4. Perform a careful circumferential digital examination with an index finger that has been lubricated with K-Y Jelly or 2% lidocaine jelly. Note the sphincter tone. (See Chapter 97, Clinical Anorectal Anatomy and Digital Examination.)
5. In male patients, palpate the prostate for size and masses.
6. Lubricate the anoscope well with K-Y Jelly with the obturator in place (see Fig. 98-1).
7. Gently insert the anoscope into the anal aperture, gradually overcoming the resistance of the sphincters. Advance the instrument in the direction of the umbilicus until the full length of the anoscope is inserted (subject to patient acceptance and tolerance). The procedure is better tolerated and accomplished by asking the patient to gently take a few deep breaths at the beginning of the procedure and to bear down just slightly. If the patient complains of pain with insertion, the quality and location should be noted and correlated with clinical symptoms.
8. After inserting the full length of the instrument, remove the obturator so that the mucosa of the anal canal can be visualized. Fecal material is often encountered and can be removed with a large swab. Note the gross appearance of the mucous membrane, the pectinate (dentate) line, and the vasculature, as well as the presence of blood, mucus, pus, hemorrhoidal tissue, and so forth.
9. Gradually withdraw the instrument with the obturator still removed. Observe the anal canal as the anoscope is extracted. Figure 98-3 shows a small, bleeding internal hemorrhoid as seen through the opening of the anoscope. For reference, the same area is shown in Figure 98-4 as visualized through a retroflexed colonoscope. With opaque devices, rotate the long-cylinder anoscopes to the right and left to ensure that the entire canal has been visualized. The Ives slotted instrument must be

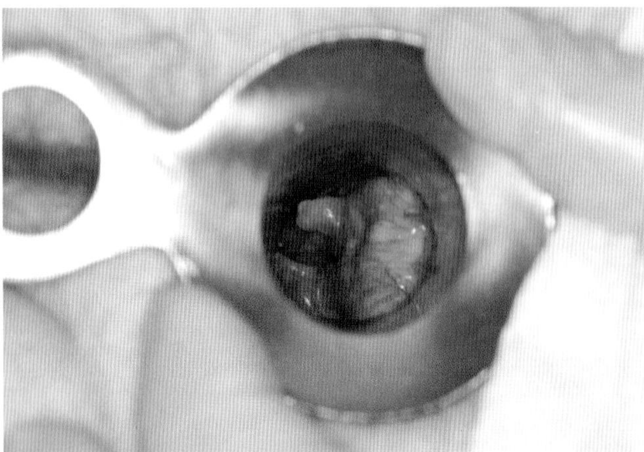

Figure 98-2 Hypertrophic papilla found on anoscopic examination (Ives slotted anoscope). This is often palpable as a firm mass.

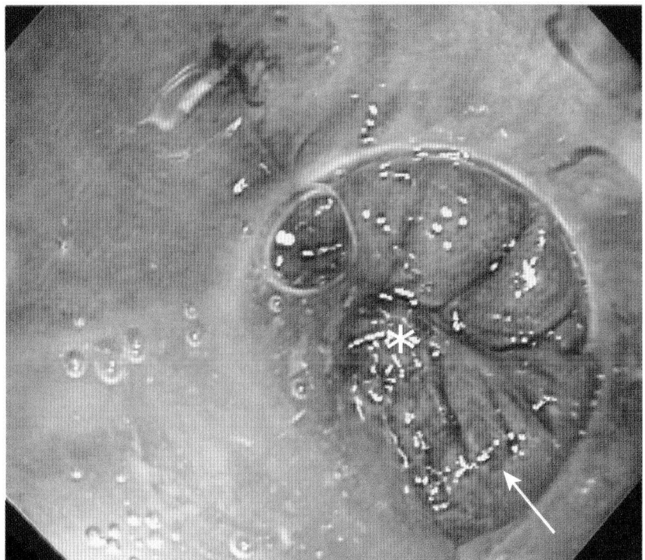

Figure 98-3 Pectinate (dentate) line *(arrow)* and small bleeding internal hemorrhoid *(asterisk)* seen as anoscope is slowly withdrawn.

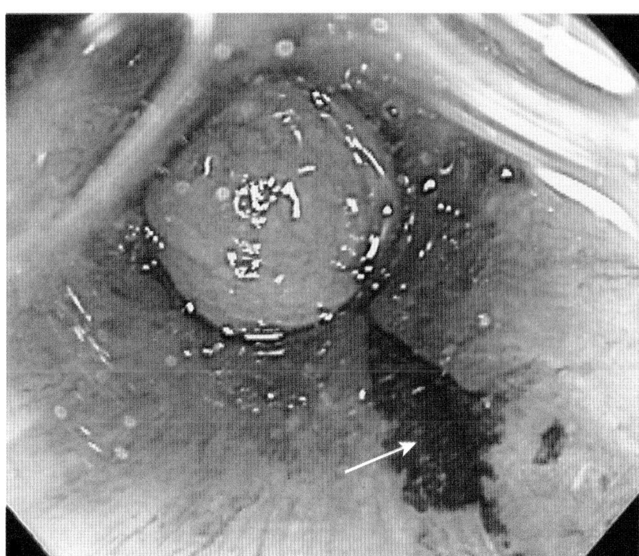

Figure 98-5 Anal fissure seen through the wall of a clear plastic anoscope *(arrow)*.

inserted four times so that each quadrant can be examined. Keeping it in place for a minute or two allows any hemorrhoids that are present to engorge with blood and be more readily visible. Do not rotate this instrument because it causes discomfort. The clear plastic anoscope allows the examiner to visualize the mucosa both through the anoscope as well as at the opening of the device. Figure 98-5 shows an anal fissure as seen through the wall of the anoscope.

10. If a biopsy specimen is to be obtained, a variety of long-handled biopsy instruments can be used. The instruments used for cervical biopsy work well (obtain the smallest "bite" possible). The clinician can also use the biopsy forceps normally used for flexible sigmoidoscopy. In this case it is applied with direct visualization of the areas. Expect some bleeding, but it is usually readily controlled with Monsel's solution or silver nitrate and natural pressure when the anoscope is removed. Stay superficial; only 3 or 4 mm of tissue is necessary.

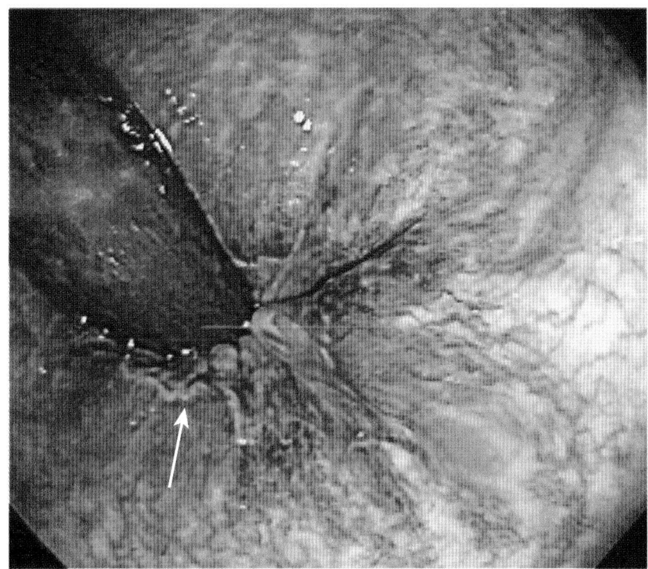

Figure 98-4 View of same patient as in Figure 98-3 using a retroflexed colonoscope. Pectinate line is indicated by the *arrow*. (Note that internal hemorrhoids are flattened by insufflated air.)

11. *HRA:* After an anoscope is inserted in the rectum, gauze soaked in 3% acetic acid solution is applied to the rectal mucosa. After 1 minute, the gauze is removed and the anoscope is repositioned as needed. Visualization is performed using a colposcope at 10–40x magnification. Abnormal lesions can be sampled and hemostasis obtained with Monsel's solution. An anal Pap smear should be done in conjunction with HRA. Additional references on this subject are included in this chapter and in Chapter 99, High-Resolution Anoscopy.
12. Complete the procedure form (Fig. 98-6).

Complications

Anoscopy, when performed gently, has few if any complications. Likely or possible complications include discomfort, tearing of the perianal skin or mucosa, and abrasion or tearing of hemorrhoidal tissue. There may be bleeding after biopsy, but infection almost never occurs.

Postprocedure Patient Education

Thoroughly explain the findings to the patient, and use pictures and drawings in the explanation. Discuss the etiology, treatment, and course of resolution of each finding as thoroughly as possible.

CPT/Billing Codes

(See also CPT billing codes for Chapter 106, Office Treatment of Hemorrhoids.)

46600 Anoscopy, diagnostic
46604 Anoscopy with dilation
46606 Anoscopy with biopsy, single or multiple
46608 Anoscopy with removal of foreign body
46610 Anoscopy with polypectomy, hot or bipolar forceps
46611 Anoscopy with polypectomy, snare technique
46614 Anoscopy with control of bleeding
46615 Anoscopy with ablation of tumor(s), polyp(s), or other lesion(s)
46900 Destruction, lesions (e.g., condyloma), chemical
46910 Destruction, lesions, electrodessication
46916 Destruction, lesions, cryocautery
46917 Destruction, lesions, laser
46922 Destruction, lesions, excision

ANOSCOPY

Patient name ______________________ B.D. ________ Sex ______
Patient ID # ______________________
Procedure ______________________ Date ________
Chief complaint: ______________________
Subjective: ______________________
Past medical history: ______________________

Medications: ______________________

Family history: ______________________

FINDINGS	**Normal**	**Abnormal**
Perianal skin		
Prostate		
Sphincter tone		
Anal canal		
Dentate line visualized?		
Mucosa		
Tears/fissure		
Vasculature		
Tumor/polyps		
Bleeding		
Hemorrhoids		

Imp ______________________

Follow-up date ______________________
Physician ______________________ Date ______________________

Figure 98-6 Procedure form for anoscopy.

ICD-9-CM Diagnostic Codes

154.1 Cancer, rectum
154.2 Cancer, anus
211.4 Benign neoplasm, colon
455.0 Internal hemorrhoids
455.1 Internal hemorrhoid, thrombosed
455.2 Internal hemorrhoid, bleeding
455.3 External hemorrhoid
455.9 Hemorrhoidal skin tags
555.1 Crohn's disease: colon
556.9 Ulcerative colitis
558.1 Radiation colitis
558.9 Colitis, nonspecific
564.0 Constipation
564.1 Irritable colon
565.0 Anal fissure
565.1 Fistula
566.0 Perirectal abscess
566.0 Perianal abscess
566.0 Ischiorectal abscess
566.0 Intersphincteric abscess
569.0 Anal polyp
569.3 Anal hemorrhage
569.42 Anal pain
698.0 Pruritus ani
787.6 Stool incontinence
787.99 Tenesmus
937.0 Foreign body, anus

	Malignant					
	Primary	Secondary	Carcinoma in situ	Benign	Uncertain behavior	Unspecified
Anus	173.5	198.2	232.5	216.5	238.2	239.2
Gluteal region	173.5	198.2	232.5	216.5	238.2	239.2
Perianal	173.5	198.2	232.5	216.5	238.2	239.2

BIBLIOGRAPHY

Fox PA, Seet JE, Stebbing J, et al: The value of anal cytology and human papillomavirus typing in the detection of anal intraepithelial neoplasia: A review of cases from an anoscopy clinic. Sex Transm Infect 81:142–146, 2005.

Goldstone SE, Winkler B, Ufford LJ, et al: High prevalence of anal squamous intraepithelial lesions and squamous-cell carcinoma in men who have sex with men as seen in a surgical practice. Dis Colon Rectum 44:690–698, 2001.

Mathews WC, Sitapati A, Caperna JC, et al: Measurement characteristics of anal cytology, histopathology, and high-resolution anoscopic visual impression in an anal dysplasia screening program. J Acquir Immune Defic Syndr 37:1610–1615, 2004.

Stier EA, Krown SE, Chi DS, et al: Anal dysplasia in HIV-infected women with cervical and vulvar dysplasia. J Low Genit Tract Dis 8:272–275, 2004.

Tuggy M, Garcia J: Procedures Consult. Available at www.proceduresconsult.com.

CHAPTER 99

High-Resolution Anoscopy

J. Michael Berry • Naomi Jay

High-resolution anoscopy (HRA) is the examination of the anus and perianal region using a colposcope for magnification. It is a technique pioneered at the University of California, San Francisco (UCSF) in the Anal Neoplasia Study to determine the natural history of human papillomavirus (HPV)–related anal neoplasia. Similar to examination of the cervix, 3% acetic acid is applied to the anus and a colposcope is used to carefully examine the anal mucosa and perianal skin. Lesions can be identified using standard colposcopic criteria and sampled for histologic confirmation.

High-risk HPV types are found in up to 93% of anal cancers. High-grade anal intraepithelial neoplasia (HGAIN), including AIN grade 2 or 3 (moderate or severe dysplasia) or carcinoma in situ, are considered potentially precancerous lesions. It is believed that identification and eradication of HGAIN may prevent anal cancer, but studies demonstrating this principle have yet to be performed. The anus and cervix are similar biologically: both have a squamocolumnar junction, both are susceptible to the same types of HPV, and both demonstrate a similar spectrum of lesions. Because of these similarities, techniques for cervical cancer screening have been adapted for the anus.

In the United States in 2009 it was estimated that there were 5290 new cases of anal cancer, 2100 in men and 3190 in women. The incidence in the general population is 1.5/100,000. In human immunodeficiency virus (HIV)–negative men-who-have-sex-with-men (MSM), before the HIV epidemic, the incidence was estimated to be 35/100,000. Since the introduction of highly-active antiretroviral therapy, studies demonstrate an incidence twice that in several cohorts of HIV-positive patients, ranging from 78.2 to 92/100,000. The relative risk for anal cancer is increased to 4.68 (95% confidence interval 3.87–5.62) in women with a history of grade 3 cervical intraepithelial neoplasia (CIN) compared with women with no history.

Anal HPV infection can be found in more than 90% of HIV-positive MSM and approximately 60% of HIV-negative MSM. HRA with biopsy of suspect lesions found HGAIN in 52% of HIV-positive MSM, and in 16% of HIV-negative MSM at baseline in a cohort of men enrolled in the UCSF Anal Neoplasia Study between 1998 and 2000. A more recent population-based sample found rates of anal HPV infection of 57% in HIV-negative versus 88% in HIV-positive MSM. HGAIN was detected during HRA-guided biopsy in 25% and 43%, respectively.

In a study of 470 HIV-positive and 185 HIV-negative women, anal HPV was found in 80% of HIV-seropositive women compared with 50% of HIV-seronegative women. HGAIN was found in 9% of HIV-positive women and in 1% of HIV-negative women. In HIV-negative women with a history of CIN, 58% had anal HPV (slightly more than 30% had cervical HPV) and 15% had abnormal anal cytology. In women without a history of CIN who presented for sexually transmitted infection testing, 53% had anal HPV and 11% had anal squamous intraepithelial lesions. A group of 40 women with vulvar cancer were compared to 80 age-matched control women who were all examined with HRA. Coexistent HGAIN in 15 patients and 1 invasive anal cancer were found in the patients with vulvar cancer, compared with no cases of HGAIN in the control subjects.

Markov modeling demonstrated that *anal cytology* for *anal cancer screening is cost effective every 2 to 3 years in HIV-negative* MSM *and every 1 to 2 years in HIV-positive* MSM. In spite of these data, except for the state of New York, there are no official public health recommendations for screening programs. There are several reasons why routine screening programs have not been recommended in spite of convincing epidemiologic data. Data are just emerging demonstrating that HGAIN can progress to cancer. Currently, no controlled clinical trials have been initiated or completed demonstrating that screening and treatment of HGAIN prevent anal cancer. Another main limiting factor for screening is the lack of providers trained and experienced in performing HRA.

Ideally, HRA should be used to identify and target lesions for treatment because these lesions are largely invisible without the application of acetic acid and magnification. Data from several papers demonstrate that HGAIN can be effectively eradicated in many patients using an office-based procedure known as *infrared coagulation*. Patients with more *extensive lesions* are effectively managed with a combination of targeted surgical therapy of HGAIN guided by HRA coupled with office-based infrared coagulation to manage the inevitable recurrences. There was no evidence of HGAIN in 192 of 246 (78%) patients treated with this combined approach at their last follow-up visit.

Screening HIV-positive MSM with anal cytology and referring those with any level of cytologic abnormality can be recommended based on demonstrated cost effectiveness and increased prevalence of HGAIN and anal cancer. Some providers believe that if resources are available, HIV-positive MSM could be examined with HRA to maximize detection of HGAIN. For similar reasons, all MSM could be offered anal cytology screening. Because of the known association between high-risk HPV, high-grade CIN and vulvar intraepithelial neoplasia, and cervical and vulvar cancer, anal cytology screening may also be useful in women with these findings, followed by referral for HRA for any cytologic abnormalities.

Solid organ transplant recipients are at increased risk of anogenital cancer and may benefit from screening as well. Patients with *perianal condylomata* regardless of sex or sexual orientation may also benefit from screening.

Anal cytology screening in patients at increased risk for anal cancer requires that providers experienced in performing HRA be available to follow up on any abnormal results. HRA is a necessary requisite for a successful program in managing anal neoplasia because in the absence of palpable or visible lesions such as condylomata or anal masses, *most HGAIN lesions are not visible or palpable*.

Formal programs for certification, training, and standards in performing HRA have been created only recently. The first course in HRA was conducted in San Francisco in conjunction with the American Society for Colposcopy and Cervical Pathology (ASCCP) and coupled with this group's Comprehensive Colposcopy course in August 2005. It is now offered annually.

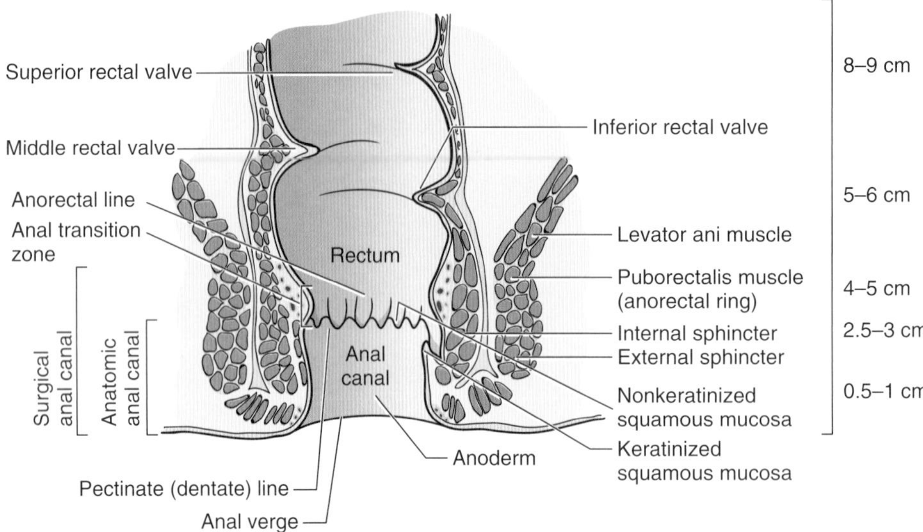

Figure 99-1 Anal anatomy.

Before learning HRA, providers should attend a formal colposcopy course and a formal didactic course in HRA, if possible. After basic colposcopy skills have been gained, attending an existing anal neoplasia clinic and spending several days observing HRA and the performance of anal biopsies in multiple patients is helpful. Further experience can be gained only by performing the procedure. Novices are advised to keep a logbook of all of their patients and to record their clinical and colposcopic impression. This can then be correlated with the cytologic and histologic results when they become available. This allows not only for patient follow-up, triage, and disposition, but for the clinician to develop and hone his or her clinical skills.

Anatomy

Like the cervix, the anus has a *transformation zone (AnTZ)* and a *squamocolumnar junction (SCJ)* where the anal squamous mucosa is adjacent to the colon columnar epithelium (Fig. 99-1). The SCJ is above the *dentate* or *pectinate line*. A similar process of squamous metaplasia occurs in the AnTZ, and dysplastic changes can occur during this dynamic time of transformation. When performing anal cytology, it is important to sample all areas of the AnTZ, just like in the cervix, so that cells are sampled from all areas. An adequate cytologic sample will have columnar or squamous metaplasia, which indicates that the AnTZ was sampled.

Indications

Other than for a formal screening program for those at risk (MSM, anal-receptive intercourse, women with high-grade cervical and vulvar dysplasias/cancers, and organ transplant recipients), reasons patients may be referred for HRA include the following:

- Abnormal anal cytology of any degree
- Incidentally detected condylomata or HGAIN during colonoscopy
- Before hemorrhoidectomy or surgery for other benign anorectal conditions to rule out concurrent disease and allow treatment at the same time
- Perianal lesions, including condylomata, hyperpigmented lesions typical of Bowen's disease, erythematous lesions, ulcerations, or masses
- Evaluation of anal symptoms such as irritation, itching, pain with bowel movements, bleeding or discomfort with receptive intercourse
- Self-detected lump or bump
- Prior history of anal condylomata, HGAIN, or anal cancer
- CIN, vulvar dysplasia

Contraindications

Severe neutropenia (<1000) is the one absolute contraindication to performing HRA. Current or past neutropenia or thrombocytopenia may indicate the need to defer biopsies or have current blood work available to determine the safety of performing biopsies.

Equipment and Supplies

Most of the equipment is the same as that used for a cervical examination (see Chapter 137, Colposcopic Examination). A procedure tray for HRA is shown in Figure 99-2. The tray includes the following:

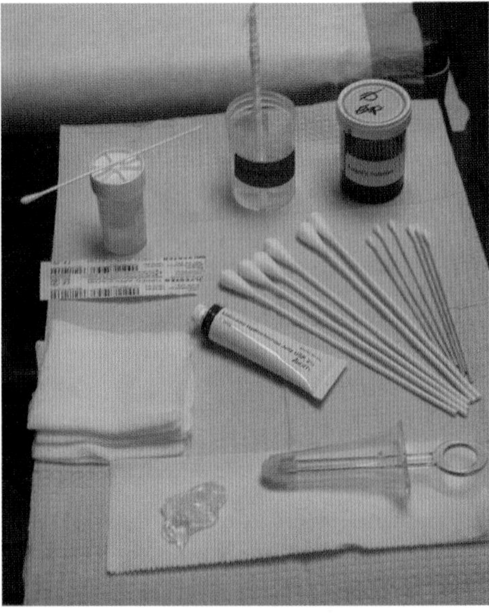

Figure 99-2 A typical equipment tray for high-resolution anoscopy.

- Cytology liquid medium (or conventional slide with fixative solution)
- Dacron swab ("Q tip")
- Anoscope (disposable plastic or sterilized metal)
- 3% acetic acid
- Nonsterile cotton swabs
- Nonsterile scopettes
- Nonsterile 4 × 4 gauze pads
- Lugol's solution
- K-Y jelly mixed with 1% to 5% lidocaine gel
- A 4 × 4 gauze wrapped around a cotton swab

Additional Equipment for Biopsies

- Formalin bottles
- Baby Tischler or mini-Townsend cervical punch biopsy or endoscopy forceps
- Monsel's solution

Additional Equipment for Perianal Biopsies

- 1% lidocaine with epinephrine and sodium bicarbonate (2 mL per 10 mL of lidocaine)
- 22-gauge needle (to fill syringe)
- 30-gauge needle (for injection)
- 1-mL syringe
- Small pickup Adson forceps, generally without teeth, punch biopsy
- Silver nitrate used for hemostasis

Colposcope

The following specifications are helpful for performing HRA with a colposcope:

- Double objective lens with magnification up to 25×
- Angled eyepieces (the straight-on view is ergonomically difficult for HRA unless the height of the table is adjustable)
- Side-swing arm

Preprocedure Patient Education

Patients should be told to refrain from inserting anything per anus for 24 hours before the procedure. This includes anal sex and insertion of any toy, medication, or enemas.

When discussing the procedure with patients, explain that a normal examination with biopsies will take 10 to 20 minutes. There are no pain nerve endings in the anal canal above the dentate line, only below it. The majority of lesions are above the dentate line and so biopsies are rarely felt beyond a sensation of minor pressure. The examination itself is not painful, but often there is mild discomfort associated with the pressure of the anoscope on the sphincter. Incontinence is rare, but patients should be told that the pressure will make them feel as if they need to have a bowel movement.

Medical history should include prior anal diseases, including abnormal cytology results, diagnoses of condylomata, low-grade anal intraepithelial neoplasia (LGAIN), HGAIN, or cancer, and any treatments used. In women, prior or current genital HPV-associated disease is important. A history of rectal abscesses, fistula tracts, fissures, or hemorrhoids can help determine potential sources of pain, bleeding, and scar tissue. Evaluate for history of immunosuppression or immune-suppressing drug therapy for organ transplantation, lupus, Crohn's disease, or any disease requiring ongoing steroid therapy.

Complications such as severe bleeding and infection are rare. Scant bleeding after a biopsy may occur over a 1- to 2-day period and is not cause for alarm. Vasovagal reactions occur rarely.

Procedure

Anal Cytology

Anal cytology results are categorized according to the Bethesda classification system using terminology similar to that for cervical cytology. Anal cytology sensitivity for detection of anal neoplasia is comparable to that of cervical cytology, with a 25% or higher miss rate. The goal of anal cytology screening is to identify patients with HGAIN, who can then be treated. Cytology should be repeated every 2 to 3 years in low-risk patients and more frequently in high-risk patients (Fig. 99-3).

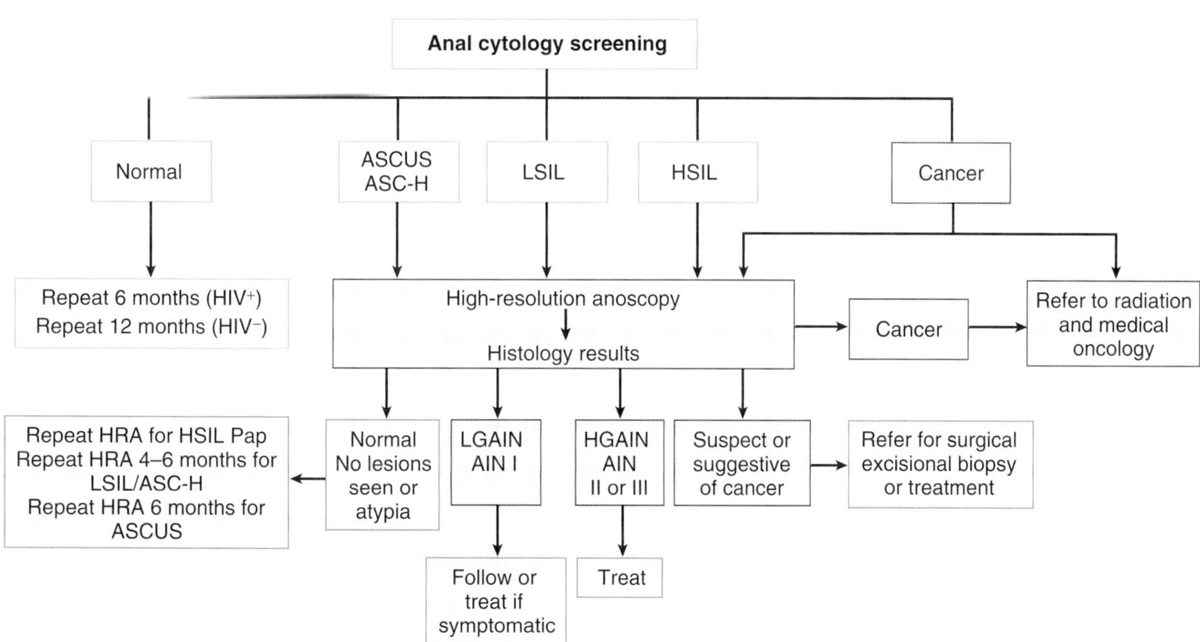

Figure 99-3 Anal cytology screening triage algorithm. AIN, anal intraepithelial neoplasia; ASC-H, atypical squamous cells, cannot exclude high-grade lesion; ASCUS, atypical squamous cells of undetermined significance; HGAIN, high-grade anal intraepithelial neoplasia; HIV, human immunodeficiency virus; HRA, high-resolution anoscopy; HSIL, high-grade squamous intraepithelial lesion; LGAIN, low-grade anal intraepithelial neoplasia; LSIL, low-grade squamous intraepithelial lesion.

Anal cytology is used to identify those populations and individuals most likely to have HPV-associated disease. *An anal cytology result of ASCUS (a typical squamous cells of undetermined significance) or higher grade is considered abnormal*, and HRA is advised based on research showing that the sensitivity for cytology screening improved when ASCUS was used as the threshold for abnormal. *The cytology result is considered a screening test and is not diagnostic*. The diagnosis will be provided through HRA-identified and sampled lesions. Figure 99-3 provides a screening and HRA algorithm.

Performing Anal Cytology

The anal cytology specimen should be obtained before HRA and any digital examination in order to obtain the highest yield of cells without interference from lubricants.

1. The left lateral position provides adequate comfort for the patient and good visualization for the clinician. However, the lithotomy position can be used, and if a proctology table is available patients can lean forward and lie prone.
2. Gently separate the buttocks. Patients can hold their buttock to facilitate the view.
3. Insert a moistened Dacron swab approximately 4 to 5 cm into the anus. For most patients this will ensure adequate sampling of the AnTZ. (However, the depth for location of the AnTZ and SCJ varies in individuals. In some it is a significant distance in [5 to 6 cm], whereas in others it is just inside the anal verge.) The swab should be inserted just past the internal sphincter until it abuts the rectal wall. If initial resistance is encountered, change the angle of the swab and reinsert. It should be possible to insert the swab with very little discomfort. Use a nonscored Dacron swab because the scored swabs can break when pressure is applied (Fig. 99-4).
4. While slowly withdrawing the swab, apply pressure against the anal sidewalls and sample the entire circumference of the canal, going in a circular motion. This facilitates sampling cells from all aspects of the canal. A slight bending in the "stick" while removing the swab indicates that adequate pressure is being used. Count slowly to 10 as you remove it to maximize the yield of exfoliating cells.
5. Preserve the sample quickly on slides for a conventional smear, or in liquid medium. Fewer cells exfoliate from the anal canal than the cervix, and air-dried artifacts can be more problematic. If using conventional slides it is better to quickly immerse the slides in cytology fluid rather than spraying them.
6. *Digital rectal examination* may be the most sensitive way of detecting an actual cancer and therefore should be performed in all patients after a cytologic sample has been obtained.

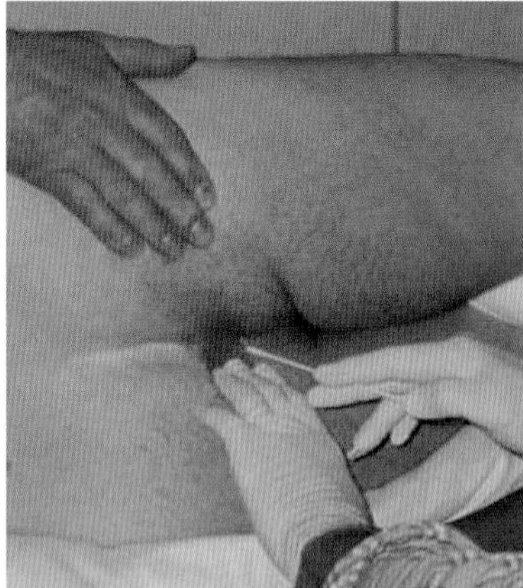

Figure 99-4 Insertion of Dacron swab for anal cytology. Retracting the buttocks facilitates more comfortable insertion of the swab.

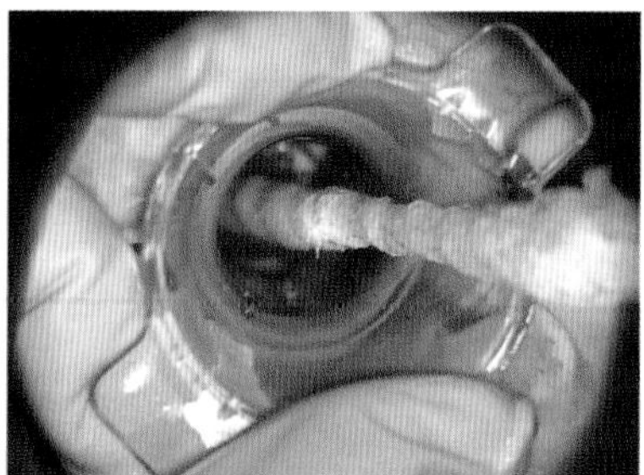

Figure 99-5 Insertion of the acetic acid–soaked gauze through the anoscope. The anoscope is then withdrawn, leaving the gauze in place.

Performing High-Resolution Anoscopy

After an abnormal cytology result, or for a routine baseline examination in an at-risk individual, HRA is used to inspect the AnTZ, SCJ, anal canal, anal verge, and perianal areas. The clinician identifies lesions based on clinical impression and obtains biopsies to determine the level and extent of disease for treatment.

Although basic colposcopy skills form a foundation for HRA, there are several unique differences in the skill sets required to accurately recognize lesions and to manage anal neoplasia. Mucosal folds and hemorrhoidal bulges make visualization of the entire SCJ difficult because it is common for lesions to be hidden within the folds. Additional acetic acid must be applied during the examination to the entire SCJ and canal. Lesions may be more subtle in their presentation, with variations of acetowhitening and epithelial changes. Similar to colposcopy, having a low threshold for taking biopsies is necessary, particularly in the early stages of learning HRA.

1. The same position can be used for HRA as for the cytologic collection. If a cervical examination is also being performed, the lithotomy position can be used, but most women prefer to switch to the left lateral position for HRA. A prone position can be used if an overhead colposcope is available. If in the lithotomy position, patients should lie as close to the bottom edge of the table as possible to ensure adequate focusing of the colposcope. In the left lateral decubitus position, they should lie as close to the edge of the table as possible with the anus directed at the examiner. A power table facilitates the use of a colposcope.
2. After a cytologic sample has been obtained (if indicated), perform a digital rectal examination. Lubricate the anal canal with K-Y jelly mixed with 2% to 5% lidocaine gel. Palpate for warts, masses, ulcerations, fissures, and focal areas of discomfort or pain. The presence of hard, fixed, or painful lesions should increase your index of suspicion for cancer because warts and

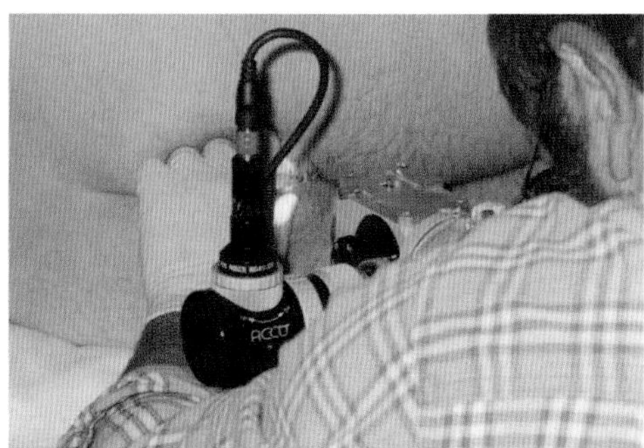

Figure 99-6 The colposcope is focused with one hand while the other hand holds the anoscope in place.

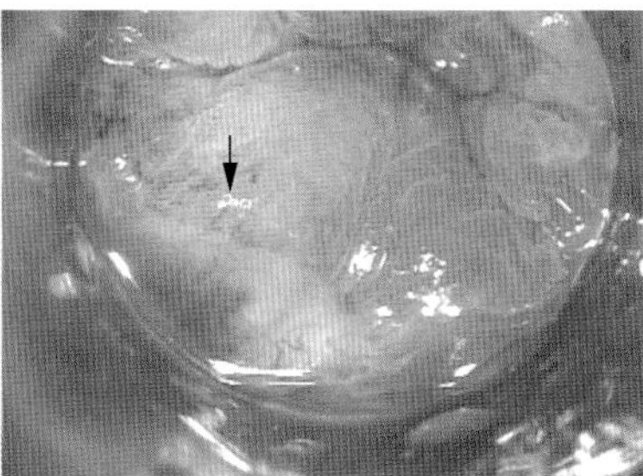

Figure 99-7 The anal transformation zone (AnTZ) is seen as a thin white line adjacent to the columnar epithelium. The anal mucosa is lighter than the colon, which is darker red.

hemorrhoids do not usually present in these ways. Make note of scar tissue, which will feel less elastic and may have thickening, ridges, and firm areas. Prior abscess, fistula repair, and surgery for warts are possible causes for scarring.

3. Insert a well-lubricated anoscope and remove the obturator (see Chapter 98, Anoscopy). Wrap a 4 × 4 gauze that has been soaked in acetic acid around a cotton swab and insert it through the anoscope. Remove the anoscope, leaving the cotton swab–wrapped gauze inside (Fig. 99-5).
4. Allow the acetic acid to soak for 1 to 2 minutes; 3% acetic acid is better tolerated in the anus but 5% can be used.
5. Remove the gauze and reinsert the anoscope with the obturator. Remove the obturator. Control the anoscope with one hand, while focusing the colposcope with the other hand (Fig. 99-6).
6. Observe through the anoscope as you slowly withdraw it. Focusing the colposcope requires manipulating the anoscope and colposcope simultaneously so that the anus is always in focus.
7. Withdraw the anoscope until the AnTZ comes into focus. The AnTZ is rarely viewed in its entirety in one field of view. Adjusting and re-angling the anoscope as well as using cotton swabs to manipulate the folds, hemorrhoids, or prolapsing mucosa will allow all aspects of the AnTZ to be viewed (Fig. 99-7).
8. A thorough examination requires reapplication of acetic acid to the entire SCJ multiple times. Not only does the staining of the abnormalities fade, it is essential that all areas, including those between the folds, be stained.
9. Lugol's solution may be applied judiciously to help better define lesions or their margins. Normal glycogenated squamous epithelium stains dark mahogany. *Abnormal lesions lack glycogen and may stain partially or not at all.* Columnar epithelium and scar tissue also will not stain with Lugol's. We also do not use Lugol's solution on the fully keratinized perianal area because the staining patterns are not sensitive enough. It is important to observe directly through the colposcope while the Lugol's solution is applied to differentiate areas not expected to pick up the Lugol's stain from true nonstaining areas that are lesions. Most HGAIN lesions will be Lugol's negative. As much as half of LGAIN lesions also are Lugol's negative. However, lesions that are partially or positively stained with Lugol's solution are rarely HGAIN. As such, choosing a Lugol's-negative lesion to sample may help increase the yield for HGAIN (Figs. 99-8 and 99-9).
10. Once the entire AnTZ has been observed, continue the examination of the anal canal as the anoscope is slowly withdrawn. Continue to apply more acetic acid using a scopette or cotton-tipped swabs. Lesions seen at the SCJ may radiate distally into the canal and even to the verge. A complete evaluation includes assessment of the extent of all lesions so that a treatment recommendation can be made.
11. Examine the verge and perianal skin applying additional acetic acid. By consensus, the perianal area is considered to radiate 5 cm beyond the verge. Perianal lesions are more difficult to evaluate and may require applying a gauze soaked in 5% acetic acid for 3 to 5 minutes (Fig. 99-10).

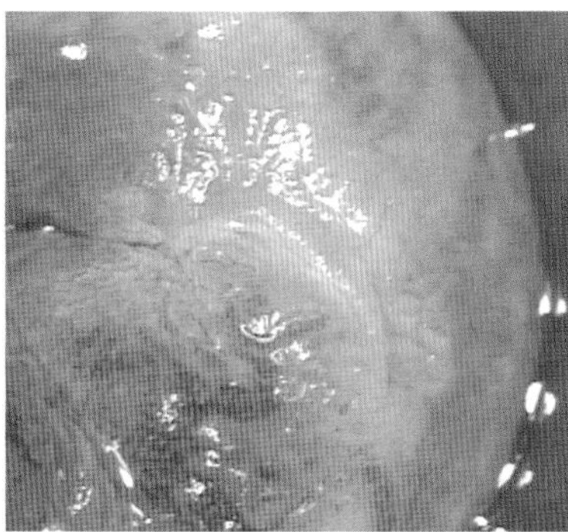

Figure 99-8 This high-grade anal intraepithelial neoplasia is faintly acetowhite with a mosaic pattern noted in the bottom edge of the lesion.

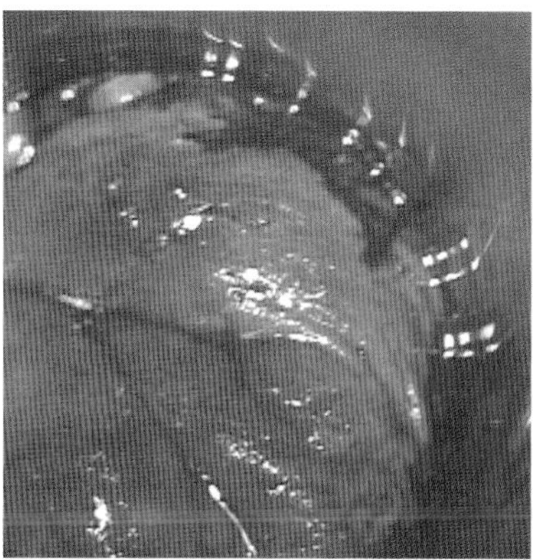

Figure 99-9 High-grade anal intraepithelial neoplasia is more clearly delineated with application of Lugol's staining.

Performing Anal Biopsy

1. Biopsies are directed at areas thought to represent the highest grade of abnormality (see Chapter 137, Colposcopic Examination, which reviews colposcopic findings) to determine (1) the severity of the disease present and (2) the extent of involvement in order to determine treatment options. If there are many different lesions, sampling multiple areas will help define the extent of HGAIN or LGAIN to clarify therapeutic options.
2. Anal biopsies are smaller than cervical biopsies. Forceps no larger than 2 to 3 mm should be used, such as the baby Tischler or mini-Townsend.
3. Insert the forceps through the anoscope while it is closed. Directly visualize the area for biopsy to determine that the correct area is

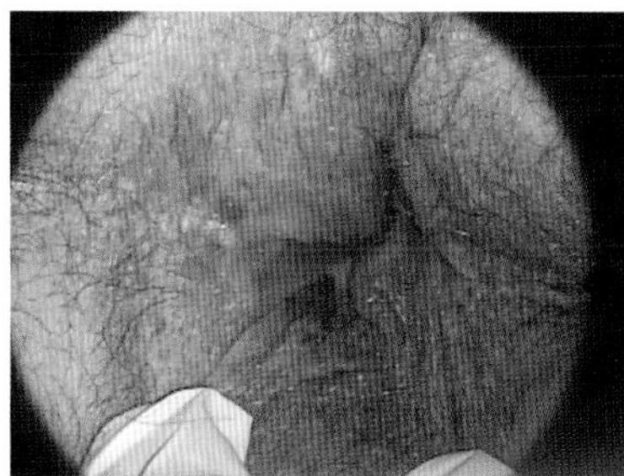

Figure 99-10 Perianal high-grade anal intraepithelial neoplasia with acetowhite changes, shallow ulcerations, and hyperpigmentation.

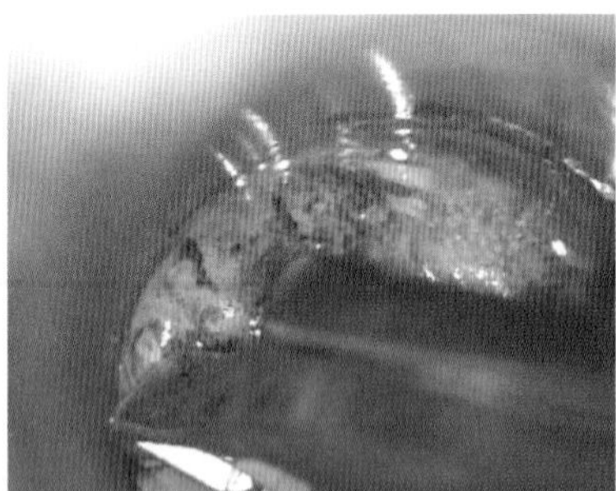

Figure 99-11 Opening the forceps partially is wide enough for an anal specimen and will help minimize bleeding.

being sampled. A *common mistake of novice providers* is to look around instead of through the colposcope to visualize the lesion during biopsy.

4. Sample lower lesions first so bleeding does not obscure other lesions (which can happen if superior lesions are sampled first).
5. When the lesion is visualized, adjust the forceps so it is partially open and adjacent to the lesion. A partially opened forceps will provide an adequate specimen and only minimal bleeding. Open it in the direction that allows the forceps to grasp the tissue most easily. For some lesions the forceps must be positioned sideways or upside down (Fig. 99-11).
6. The normal pressure of the anus after removing the anoscope is often sufficient to stop bleeding, but a small amount of Monsel's solution can be applied to promote hemostasis. Do not use Monsel's solution until all biopsies are complete because it can interfere with the pathology reading.
7. HRA-directed biopsy is a "one-handed" procedure because one hand will always be holding the anoscope. It takes practice to adeptly manipulate the specimens into the formalin containers with one hand while holding the anoscope in place for the remainder of the procedure. If available, an assistant can place biopsy specimens in containers.
8. Anal biopsies do not require anesthesia. Perianal biopsies, however, are similar to vulvar biopsies and require a small amount of injectable 1% lidocaine with epinephrine. Buffering the lidocaine with sodium bicarbonate (2 mL $NaHCO_3$:10 mL lidocaine) improves the comfort of the procedure.

High-Resolution Anoscopy Observations

1. Squamous epithelium usually appears lighter and pinker compared with columnar or rectal epithelium, which is darker and redder. In most people, the anoscope is longer than the anal canal and, if inserted fully, the colonic mucosa will be noted first as the obturator is removed.
2. The anal canal of most women is shorter compared with men. The AnTZ is much closer to the verge in some women and it may seem as if the anoscope is nearly outside before the AnTZ is viewed. In people with anal prolapse, the AnTZ may also be noted at the verge or at times seen externally. Those who have had surgery may also present with the SCJ closer to the verge. Acetic acid is still helpful in delineating the AnTZ and SCJ.
3. If the AnTZ does not appear readily, generously apply acetic acid while manipulating the anoscope. Eventually a thin white line should begin to appear. Once an area of the AnTZ has been located, the remainder should be visible with manipulation of the anoscope and continued application of acetic acid.
4. *Clinical/colposcopic terminology for describing anal lesions* is similar to that for cervical lesions. Lesions are described by *color (acetowhite), contour (raised or flat), surface vascularity (punctation, mosaic patterns, atypical vessels), margins (distinct and indistinct), and Lugol's staining (negative, partial, positive)*. Lesion margins are not very well defined in anal mucosa. Frequently one or more parts of the lesion margins are not observed, especially adjacent to the columnar epithelium.
5. Lesions appear as demarcated acetowhite areas with characteristics similar to those seen on the cervix. Refer to the Chapter 137, Colposcopic Examination, for a more thorough discussion of lesion characteristics.
6. A typical raised LGAIN lesion is acetowhite and raised, has warty, looped capillary vessels and papillae, and is often partially stained with Lugol's solution. A typical HGAIN lesion is acetowhite and flat, has punctation and mosaic patterns, and is Lugol's negative (Table 99-1 and Figs. 99-12 and 99-13).
7. Be consistent when describing the location of the lesions. The anal "clock" is different from the cervical "clock." By convention, the 12:00 position is posterior in the anus if the patient is standing and bent over a table, but anterior if in the lithotomy position. Because referrals are frequently made to colorectal surgeons it is helpful to provide the locations anatomically (posterior, anterior, left or right lateral; Fig. 99-14).

Common Errors

- Applying lubricant or doing a digital examination before obtaining cytology
- Not sampling the entire AnTZ when obtaining cytology
- Not being persistent and examining the entire AnTZ with the colposcope
- Looking around (not through) the colposcope when obtaining biopsies
- Obtaining too large a sample for biopsy, causing excessive bleeding

Interpretation of Results

Cytology is considered a screening test and is not diagnostic. Diagnosis is based on the histologic result. HGAIN is considered the cancer precursor lesion, and LGAIN is considered a benign abnormal lesion. Results that are described as "atypia suggestive of LGAIN" are considered atypical but not abnormal. "Atypia cannot rule out HGAIN" is also an atypical finding and an indicator for HRA. A higher grade on cytology than the biopsy histologic grade

TABLE 99-1 Typical Features of Anal Intraepithelial Neoplasia and Cancer on High-Resolution Anoscopy

	DRE	Surface Characteristics	Epithelial Characteristics	Vascular Characteristics	Lugol's Staining
LGAIN	Granular, soft warty nodularity	Raised or flat	Papillae, micropapillae	Fine or coarse punctation, warty vessels	Negative, partial or complete
HGAIN	Nonpalpable or subtle thickening	Flat or slightly raised	Smooth	Coarse punctation, mosaic patterns, increased vascularity	Negative
Cancer	Firm mass, indurated or distinct thickening	Raised, ulcerated, occasionally flat	Peeling or denuded, heaping edges	Atypical, large, nonbranching vessels, grossly dilated, friable	Negative

DRE, digital rectal examination; HGAIN, high-grade anal intraepithelial neoplasia; LGAIN, low-grade anal intraepithelial neoplasia.

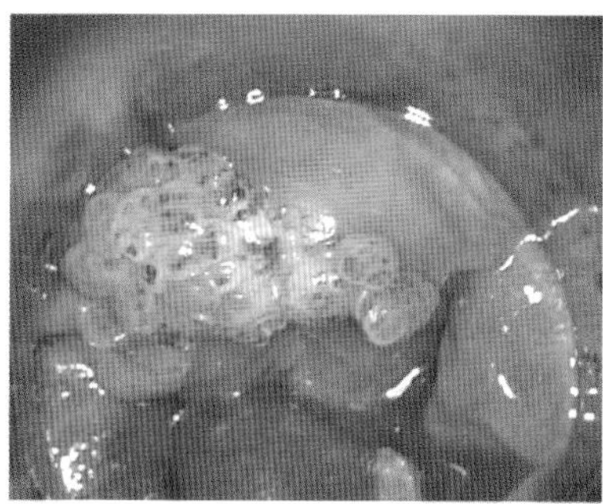

Figure 99-12 Typical low-grade anal intraepithelial neoplasia.

suggests that the lesion was not seen on HRA and the examination may have to be repeated. Repeat HRA examination is indicated if HGAIN was found on cytology but not on biopsy.

Reasons for discordant results include inadequate examinations due to obscuring hemorrhoids or warts (diffuse circumferential warts may obscure smaller areas of HGAIN) or that the highest-grade lesions were missed on HRA because of lack of adequate staining. The learning curve for HRA is steeper than for cervical colposcopy because of differences between anal and cervical anatomy. Discordant results are not unusual for novices and occur even for experienced providers.

A thorough discussion of *treatment* is beyond the purview of this chapter. The threshold for treatment depends on the situation (see Fig. 99-2). LGAIN can be treated when it is symptomatic, when the patient requests it to be removed, and when it is diffuse and obscures the ability to perform an adequate examination. HGAIN should be treated unless the patient is medically fragile or treatment is otherwise contraindicated. These patients should be followed carefully by cytology and digital rectal examination every 3 to 4 months. Most HGAIN can be treated as an office procedure using the infrared coagulator. Diffuse circumferential disease or patients who cannot tolerate long procedures may require referral to a colorectal surgeon for surgical removal or ablation.

Ablation is the mainstay of therapy. Office ablation techniques include cryotherapy (only for external lesions), trichloroacetic acid or bichloroacetic acid for small-volume disease, and electrocautery or infrared coagulation for larger-volume disease. Small lesions can sometimes be excised with the forceps or snipped off using sharp tissue scissors such as Metzenbaums. Laser has been used for both office and surgical ablation but requires a smoke evacuator. In surgery, most patients receive fulguration or electrocautery.

CPT/Billing Codes

There is no CPT code for HRA. 46999 is an "unlisted anoscopy code." It can be used to describe intraoperative HRA to guide treatment of anal high-grade squamous intraepithelial lesions, but must include a letter explaining why it is medically justified. Not dictating a report or sending a letter may delay reimbursement.

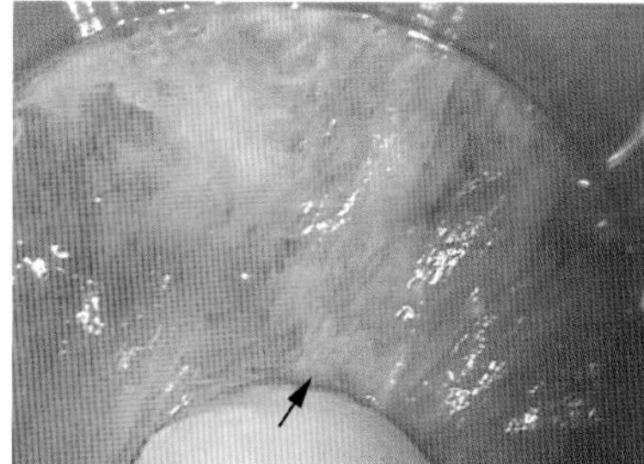

Figure 99-13 Typical high-grade anal intraepithelial neoplasia.

Anal clock in the left lateral HRA position

Posterior = 12:00 Anterior = 6:00

R lateral
Post. Ant.
L lateral
Internal

R lateral
Post. Ant.
L lateral
External

Figure 99-14 The "anal clock" from the perspective of the left lateral high-resolution anoscopy (HRA) position. Note that posterior = 12:00 and that this is the opposite of the "cervical clock."

46600	Anoscopy
46606	Anoscopy with biopsy
46610	Anoscopy with polypectomy
46614	Anoscopy with destruction
46900	Destruction, chemical, simple
46910	Destruction, electro, simple
46916	Destruction, cryosurgical, simple
46922	Destruction, surgical excision
46924	Destruction, extensive lesions
46937	Cryosurgical destruction, benign rectal tumor

For initial visits, or if the patient is referred to you and you send a letter to the referring provider, you can bill for a consultation (99243 or 99244) and also for the anoscopy procedure with or without biopsy (46600 or 46606). This is the only time you can bill for both. Medicare has eliminated consultation codes as of 2010, and other insurances may do the same.

If the patient presents with an additional problem and has anoscopy, you may be able to bill for an established office visit (99213 or 99214 with a –25 modifier and 46600 or 46606), but you must specify using the appropriate ICD-9 code for the additional problem.

Some providers also use the code for transanal excision of rectal tumor when treating lesions that are proximal to the dentate line, but this is somewhat controversial and may be subject to scrutiny.

ICD-9-CM Diagnostic Codes

042	HIV infection
078.11	Condyloma
154.2	Anal cancer
211.4	Benign neoplasm of anus (low-grade squamous intraepithelial lesion or AIN 2)
230.5	Carcinoma in situ of anal canal (AIN 3)

Online Resources

American Society for Colposcopy and Cervical Pathology: Sponsors course in colposcopy and HRA. Available at www.asccp.org.

University of California at San Francisco (UCSF) Anal Neoplasia Research and Treatment Group: Describing approach to patients at UCSF and listing providers. Available at www.analcancerinfo.ucsf.edu.

BIBLIOGRAPHY

Apgar BS, Brotzman GL, Spitzer M (eds): Colposcopy: Principles and Practice. An Integrated Textbook and Atlas, 2nd ed. Philadelphia, Saunders, 2008.

Bower M, Powles T, Newsom-Davis T, et al: HIV-associated anal cancer: Has highly active antiretroviral therapy reduced the incidence or improved the outcome? J Acquir Immune Defic Syndr 37:1563–1565, 2004.

Caseli M, Darragh TM, Jay N, et al: Prevalence and risk factors for anal human papillomavirus (HPV) infection and anal squamous intraepithelial lesions (ASIL) in low-risk human immunodeficiency virus (HIV)-negative women. Presented at the 22nd International Papillomavirus Conference, Vancouver, Canada, April 30–May 6, 2005.

Chin-Hong PV, Berry JM, Cheng SC, et al: Comparison of patient- and clinician-collected anal cytology samples to screen for human papillomavirus-associated anal intraepithelial neoplasia in men who have sex with men. Ann Intern Med 149:300–306, 2008.

Cranston RD, Hirschowitz SL, Cortina G, Moe AA: A retrospective clinical study of the treatment of high-grade anal dysplasia by infrared coagulation in a population of HIV-positive men who have sex with men. Int J STD AIDS 19:118–120, 2008.

Daling JR, Weiss NS, Klopfenstein LL, et al: Correlates of homosexual behavior and the incidence of anal cancer. JAMA 247:1988–1990, 1982.

D'Souza G, Wiley DJ, Li X, et al: Incidence and epidemiology of anal cancer in the multicenter AIDS cohort study. J Acquir Immune Defic Syndr 48:491–499, 2008.

Edgren G, Sparen P: Risk of anogenital cancer after diagnosis of cervical intraepithelial neoplasia: A prospective population-based study. Lancet Oncol 8:311–316, 2007.

Goldie SJ, Kuntz KM, Weinstein MC, et al: The clinical effectiveness and cost-effectiveness of screening for anal squamous intraepithelial lesions in homosexual and bisexual HIV-positive men. JAMA 281:1822–1829, 1999.

Goldie SJ, Kuntz KM, Weinstein MC, et al: Cost-effectiveness of screening for anal squamous intraepithelial lesions and anal cancer in human immunodeficiency virus-negative homosexual and bisexual men. Am J Med 108:634–641, 2000.

Goldstone SE, Hundert JS, Huyett JW: Infrared coagulator ablation of high-grade anal squamous intraepithelial lesions in HIV-negative males who have sex with males. Dis Colon Rectum 50:565–575, 2007.

Goldstone SE, Kawalek AZ, Huyett JW: Infrared coagulator: A useful tool for treating anal squamous intraepithelial lesions. Dis Colon Rectum 48:1042–1054, 2005.

Hessol NA, Holly EA, Efird JT, et al: Anal intraepithelial neoplasia in a multisite study of HIV-infected and high-risk HIV-uninfected women. AIDS 23:59–70, 2009.

Jay N, Berry JM, Hogeboom CJ, et al: Colposcopic appearance of anal squamous intraepithelial lesions: Relationship to histopathology. Dis Colon Rectum 40:919–928, 1997.

Joseph DA, Miller JW, Wu X, et al: Understanding the burden of human papillomavirus-associated anal cancers in the US. Cancer 113(10 Suppl): 2892–2900, 2008.

Ogunbiyi OA, Scholefield JH, Robertson G, et al: Anal human papillomavirus infection and squamous neoplasia in patients with invasive vulvar cancer. Obstet Gynecol 83:212–216, 1994.

Palefsky JM, Holly EA, Efirdc JT, et al: Anal intraepithelial neoplasia in the highly active antiretroviral therapy era among HIV-positive men who have sex with men. AIDS 19:1407–1414, 2005.

Palefsky JM, Shiboski S, Moss A: Risk factors for anal human papillomavirus infection and anal cytologic abnormalities in HIV-positive and HIV-negative homosexual men. J Acquir Immune Defic Syndr 14:415–422, 1994.

Patel P, Hanson DL, Sullivan PS, et al: Incidence of types of cancer among HIV-infected persons compared with the general population in the United States, 1992–2003. Ann Intern Med 148:728–736, 2008.

Pineda CE, Berry JM, Jay N, et al: High-resolution anoscopy targeted surgical destruction of anal high-grade squamous intraepithelial lesions: A ten-year experience. Dis Colon Rectum 51:829–835, 2008; discussion 35–37.

Pineda CE, Berry JM, Welton ML: High resolution anoscopy and targeted treatment of high-grade squamous intraepithelial lesions. Dis Colon Rectum 49:126, 2006.

Scholefield JH, Castle MT, Watson NF: Malignant transformation of high-grade anal intraepithelial neoplasia. Br J Surg 92:1133–1136, 2005.

Spitzer M, Brotzman GL, Apgar BS: Practical therapeutic options for treatment of cervical intraepithelial neoplasia. In Apgar BS, Brotzman GL, Spitzer M (eds): Colposcopy: Principles and Practice. An Integrated Textbook and Atlas, 2nd ed. Philadelphia, Saunders, 2008, pp 505–520.

Stier EA, Goldstone SE, Berry JM, et al: Infrared coagulator treatment of high-grade anal dysplasia in HIV-infected individuals: An AIDS Malignancy Consortium pilot study. J Acquir Immune Defic Syndr 47:56–61, 2008.

Watson AJ, Smith BB, Whitehead MR, et al: Malignant progression of anal intra-epithelial neoplasia. ANZ J Surg 76:715–717, 2006.

CHAPTER 100

Colonoscopy*

John Bartels Pope

Colonoscopy is a procedure that allows for visual inspection of the entire large bowel from the distal rectum to the cecum. The procedure is generally well accepted by patients and, in the proper hands, is a safe and effective means of examining the large bowel. A well-trained endoscopist can usually perform a total colonoscopy in 30 to 45 minutes, achieving cecal intubation in greater than 90% of attempted procedures under optimal conditions (excellent bowel preparation, high-quality equipment, technical support, appropriate sedation, and low-risk patient population).

Colonoscopy has a greater sensitivity and specificity for the detection of colonic polyps and colorectal cancers (CRCs) than fecal occult blood testing, air-contrast barium enema, or computed tomographic (CT) colonography (virtual colonoscopy), and greater sensitivity than flexible sigmoidoscopy because more of the colon is visualized. Colonoscopy is the procedure of choice in the work-up of most cases of lower gastrointestinal bleeding. A significant advantage of colonoscopy over radiologic evaluation of the large intestine is the ability to perform additional diagnostic and therapeutic measures, such as biopsy, polypectomy, and control of bleeding. Although traditionally performed in the hospital, colonoscopy can also be performed in free-standing offices or in ambulatory endoscopy centers.

It is widely accepted that the vast majority of colon cancers arise from adenomatous (neoplastic) polyps. It has been shown that the removal of adenomatous polyps by colonoscopic polypectomy can reduce the incidence of colorectal cancer by 76% to 90%. Colonoscopy then provides an opportunity to greatly influence the incidence of colorectal cancer by allowing the removal of polyps throughout the entire colon.

Anatomy

The colon is approximately 150 cm in length from anal verge to cecum.

Anus
- The outlet to the gastrointestinal tract

Rectum
- Dentate (pectinate) line demarcating junction between pain-sensitive squamous epithelium of anus and pain-insensitive columnar epithelium of rectum
- Approximately 15 cm in length with capacious lumen
- Prominent folds (valves of Houston) that may create potential blind spots
- Mucosal transparency with prominent hemorrhoidal venous plexus visible

Sigmoid colon
- Variably mobile (key to successful colonoscopy)
- Loops anteriorly, then posteriorly to be retroperitoneal
- 35 to 45 cm in length

Descending colon
- Fixed, straight course up left paracolic gutter
- Narrowest portion of colon
- Retroperitoneal
- Approximately 20 to 30 cm in length

Transverse colon
- Longer than the distance it traverses and may sag into umbilical region
- Lumen generally has a triangular appearance
- Approximately 45 to 55 cm in length

Ascending colon
- Capacious lumen with straight course
- Retroperitoneal into right paracolic gutter
- Terminates at ileocecal valve, which demarcates beginning of cecum
- Approximately 10 to 20 cm in length

Cecum
- Variable mobility and capacious lumen
- Landmarks include ileocecal valve, appendiceal orifice, and terminal portion of taeniae coli ("crow's foot")
- Transillumination is frequently seen
- Approximately 5 to 8 cm in length

Indications

Diagnostic Indications

- Total colon evaluation after the finding of adenomatous polyps, especially high-risk polyps (i.e., those >1 cm, small polyps with advanced histopathology, or multiple small adenomatous polyps), during flexible sigmoidoscopy.
- Evaluation of abnormal or equivocal barium enema.
- Evaluation of overt or occult colonic or rectal bleeding.
- Evaluation of abnormal findings on CT colonography.
- Evaluation of iron-deficiency anemia of undetermined cause.
- Surveillance of neoplastic disease after removal of polyps or cancer.
- Screening for neoplastic disease in patients with family history of colorectal cancer or adenomatous (neoplastic) polyps before age 60 years; screening should begin at 40 years of age or 10 years before the age of discovery in relative.
- Screening and surveillance for neoplastic disease in hereditary cancer syndromes
  - Familial adenomatous polyposis syndrome (FAP). Gene carriers or at-risk family members who have not had genetic testing or are from families in whom the gene test is uninformative should be offered a flexible sigmoidoscopy or colonoscopy every 12 months starting at around 10 to 12 years of age and continuing until 35 to 40 years of age if negative. Colonoscopy is necessary in attenuated FAP, where the usual presentation of thousands of polyps is reduced to less than 100 polyps, which may be more proximally located.

*EDITOR'S NOTE: Much of the information in Chapter 103, Flexible Sigmoidoscopy, is very pertinent to colonoscopy. Material will not be repeated here. The reader is encouraged to review that chapter also.

- Hereditary nonpolyposis colon cancer syndrome (HNPCC). HNPCC is defined as CRC in three or more family members, two of whom are first-degree relatives of the third, with at least two generations involved and at least one person diagnosed with CRC before 50 years of age. Use of the term *nonpolyposis* is a misnomer. Polyps do indeed occur in HNPCC, just not to the extent seen with FAP. Individuals at risk for HNPCC should undergo colonoscopy every 1 to 2 years starting at 20 to 25 years of age or 10 years younger than the age of the earliest diagnosis of cancer in the family, whichever is earlier.
- Evaluation and surveillance of inflammatory bowel disease (after 8 years in pancolitis and after 12 years in left-sided colitis).
- Evaluation of chronic diarrhea of undetermined cause.
- Intraoperative evaluation of polypectomy site, bleeding lesions, or anastomotic leaks.
- Endosonography for local staging (primary tumor, regional nodes, and metastasis [TNM]) of colorectal cancer.
- Screening in average-risk population (>50 years of age) and in the increased-risk groups (Table 100-1).
- Evaluation of significant weight loss.
- Evaluation of abdominal pain.

NOTE: Colonoscopy is often of little benefit in determining the causes of chronic lower abdominal pain or changes in bowel habits in the absence of rectal bleeding, weight loss, or anorexia.

Therapeutic Indications

- Biopsy of suspect lesion
- Polypectomy
- Therapy of bleeding lesions
- Removal of foreign body
- Reduction of sigmoid volvulus
- Decompression of pseudo-obstruction of colon
- Dilation of colonic strictures and placement of colonic stents
- Laser therapy of lesions

CONTRAINDICATIONS

Absolute

- Acute abdomen
- Suspected peritonitis
- Acute diverticulitis with systemic symptoms
- Acute exacerbation of inflammatory bowel disease
- Documented or suspected bowel perforation
- Patient refusal
- Risk to patient outweighs benefits of procedure

Relative

- Unstable cardiopulmonary status
- Recent myocardial infarction or pulmonary embolism
- Significant pelvic or abdominal adhesions
- Blood coagulation abnormalities
- Recent (within 1 week) bowel surgery
- Hyperplastic polyps on flexible sigmoidoscopy with no other indication
- Poorly prepared patient
- Uncooperative patient
- Metastatic adenocarcinoma of unknown primary site in the absence of colonic symptoms when it will not influence management
- Severe neutropenia
- Pregnancy (second or third trimester)
- Large abdominal aortic aneurysm
- Splenomegaly

EQUIPMENT

Basic equipment necessary to perform colonoscopy includes the following:

- Fiberoptic colonoscope
- Light source (i.e., halogen or xenon)
- Suction apparatus
- Biopsy forceps
- Polypectomy snares
- Electrosurgical unit
- Conscious sedation setup (see Chapter 2, Procedural Sedation and Analgesia)

Additional instruments that may also be useful include injection needle catheter, heater probe or multipolar cautery probe, polyp retrieval baskets, endoscopic clips, and three-prong grasping forceps. Lubricating jelly, gauze pads, saline, sterile water, protective gowns, and protective eyewear are also recommended.

The *colonoscope* is similar in design to the sigmoidoscope, only longer. The outside diameter of the insertion tube varies from 11 to 13 mm, and the length of the shaft varies from 105 to 185 cm. The narrower scopes are typically used in pediatric settings and are generally lighter with a more flexible shaft. The scopes have an eyepiece with focusing controls; control wheels to deflect the tip through a range of positions, including deflection over 180 degrees; a biopsy port; suction and air and water control knobs; and locking levers to fix control wheels in a particular position (see Chapter 103, Flexible Sigmoidoscopy).

Most colonoscopies are now performed with video endoscopes. Videoscopes are fiberoptic devices; however, they use a charge-coupled device to convert light energy into electronic signals that can be converted by a computer processor into images. Videoscopes provide recording capability of entire procedures, and they also allow transmission of images to remote sites. Videoscopes also provide for a more comfortable posture for the endoscopist during the procedure. The newest video colonoscopes offer optional features such as variable stiffness capability, forward water jet,

TABLE 100-1 Guidelines for Screening and Surveillance for the Early Detection of Colorectal Adenomas and Cancer in Individuals at Increased Risk or at High Risk

Risk Category	Age to Begin	Recommendation	Comment
Increased Risk—Patients with History of Polyps at Prior Colonoscopy			
Patients with small rectal hyperplastic polyps	—	Colonoscopy or other screening options at intervals recommended for average-risk individuals	An exception is patients with a hyperplastic polyposis syndrome. They are at increased risk for adenomas and colorectal cancer and need to be identified for more intensive follow-up.
Patients with 1 or 2 small tubular adenomas with low-grade dysplasia	5 to 10 years after the initial polypectomy	Colonoscopy	The precise timing within this interval should be based on other clinical factors (such as prior colonoscopy findings, family history, and the preferences of the patient and judgment of the physician).

TABLE 100-1 Guidelines for Screening and Surveillance for the Early Detection of Colorectal Adenomas and Cancer in Individuals at Increased Risk or at High Risk—Cont.

Risk Category	Age to Begin	Recommendation	Comment
Patients with 3 to 10 adenomas or 1 adenoma >1 cm or any adenoma with villous features or high-grade dysplasia	3 years after the initial polypectomy	Colonoscopy	Adenomas must have been completely removed. If the follow-up colonoscopy is normal or shows only 1 or 2 small, tubular adenomas with low-grade dysplasia, then the interval for the subsequent examination should be 5 years.
Patients with >10 adenomas on a single examination	<3 years after the initial polypectomy	Colonoscopy	Consider the possibility of an underlying familial syndrome.
Patients with sessile adenomas that are removed piecemeal	2 to 6 months to verify complete removal	Colonoscopy	Once complete removal has been established, subsequent surveillance needs to be individualized based on the endoscopist's judgment. Completeness of removal should be based on both endoscopic and pathologic assessments.
Increased Risk—Patients with Colorectal Cancer			
Patients with colon and rectal cancer should undergo high-quality perioperative clearing	3 to 6 months after cancer resection, if no unresectable metastases are found during surgery; alternatively, colonoscopy can be performed intraoperatively	Colonoscopy	In the case of nonobstructing tumors, this can be done by preoperative colonoscopy. In the case of obstructing colon cancers, CTC with intravenous contrast or DCBE can be used to detect neoplasms in the proximal colon.
Patients undergoing curative resection for colon or rectal cancer	1 year after the resection (or 1 year following the performance of the colonoscopy that was performed to clear the colon of synchronous disease)	Colonoscopy	This colonoscopy at 1 year is in addition to the perioperative colonoscopy for synchronous tumors. If the examination performed at 1 year is normal, then the interval before the next subsequent examination should be 3 years. If that colonoscopy is normal, then the interval before the next subsequent examination should be 5 years. Following the examination at 1 year, the intervals before subsequent examinations may be shortened if there is evidence of HNPCC or if adenoma findings warrant earlier colonoscopy. Periodic examination of the rectum for the purpose of identifying local recurrence, usually performed at 3- to 6-month intervals for the first 2 or 3 years, may be considered after low-anterior resection of rectal cancer.
Increased Risk—Patients with a Family History			
Either colorectal cancer or adenomatous polyps in a first-degree relative before age 60 years or in 2 or more first-degree relatives at any age	Age 40 years or 10 years before the youngest case in the immediate family	Colonoscopy	Every 5 years
Either colorectal cancer or adenomatous polyps in a first-degree relative ≥age 60 years or in 2 second-degree relatives with colorectal cancer	Age 40 years	Screening options at intervals recommended for average-risk individuals	Screening should begin at an earlier age, but individuals may choose to be screened with any recommended form of testing.
High Risk			
Genetic diagnosis of FAP or suspected FAP without genetic testing evidence	Age 10 to 12 years	Annual FSIG to determine if the individual is expressing the genetic abnormality and counseling to consider genetic testing	If the genetic test is positive, colectomy should be considered.
Genetic or clinical diagnosis of HNPCC or individuals at increased risk of HNPCC	Age 20 to 25 years or 10 years before the youngest case in the immediate family	Colonoscopy every 1 to 2 years and counseling to consider genetic testing	Genetic testing for HNPCC should be offered to first-degree relatives of persons with a known inherited MMR gene mutation. It should also be offered when the family mutation is not already known, but 1 of the first 3 of the modified Bethesda Criteria is present.
Inflammatory bowel disease, chronic ulcerative colitis, and Crohn's colitis	Cancer risk begins to be significant 8 years after the onset of pancolitis or 12 to 15 years after the onset of left-sided colitis	Colonoscopy with biopsies for dysplasia	Every 1 to 2 years; these patients are best referred to a center with experience in the surveillance and management of inflammatory bowel disease

CTC, Computed tomographic colonography; DCBE, double-contrast barium enema; FAP, family adenomatous polyposis; FSIG, flexible sigmoidoscopy; HNPCC, hereditary nonpolyposis colon cancer; MMR, mismatch repair.

From Levin B, Lieberman DA, McFarland B, et al: Screening and surveillance for the early detection of colorectal cancer and adenomatous polyps, 2008: A joint guideline for the American Cancer Society, the US Multi-Society Task Force on Colorectal Cancer, and the American College of Radiology. CA Cancer J Clin 58:130–160, 2008.

high-resolution HDTV imaging, narrow-band imaging, close focusing, and 170-degree field of view. Video endoscopy setups are significantly more expensive than conventional setups.

Cleaning and disinfecting the instrument and equipment are very important to prevent iatrogenic infections. Strict adherence to appropriate cleaning protocols virtually eliminates these risks. The American Society for Gastrointestinal Endoscopy (ASGE) provides practice guidelines for infection control during gastrointestinal endoscopy. Company representatives also provide excellent guidelines and videotapes demonstrating the process.

Preprocedure Patient Preparation

Informed consent is a necessary component of colonoscopy. Consent should be obtained by the physician and should include discussion of the nature of the procedure (how it is performed), expected benefits of the procedure, risks of the procedure (including those from sedation, procedure complications [perforation and bleeding], and the possibility of missed lesions), and alternatives to the procedure. The consent process may be facilitated with the use of *patient education videotapes* or written materials available from various organizations (e.g., ASGE, Society of American Gastrointestinal Endoscopic Surgeons, and The National Procedures Institute). Sample consent forms and patient education handouts are also available online at http://drpearlman.btrtest.com/patient_education.htm and http://springfieldasc.com/patient-information/patient-forms.

A *focused history* should be obtained before the procedure to ensure that an appropriate indication exists for the procedure and to identify factors that may influence safe and effective performance of the procedure and subsequent management of the patient. Pertinent history should include present illness, past medical and surgical history (hysterectomy or abdominal surgeries may increase intubation difficulty), current medications, allergies, and tobacco and alcohol use. The patient should also be asked about any previous complications from anesthesia, as well as any history of coagulation abnormalities or chronic use of narcotics or tranquilizers, which may influence the ability to properly sedate (Fig. 100-1).

Physical examination should include (as a minimum) assessment of vital signs and sensorium and heart, lung, and abdominal examination.

Laboratory testing is not routinely performed before colonoscopy; however, in specific circumstances testing may be warranted (e.g., severe anemia with anticipation of polypectomy, known fluid and electrolyte abnormality, anticoagulation).

A clean bowel is essential for colonoscopy. Two of the most common and effective *preparations for cleansing the bowel* include the following:

1. Polyethylene glycol (PEG) solution (4 L) taken orally (Colyte, GoLYTELY) over a 1- to 3-hour period
2. Magnesium citrate solution (10 oz) taken with four bisacodyl tablets (5 mg) the afternoon before the procedure, and repeat the magnesium citrate the morning of the procedure

Although commonly used in the past as a bowel preparation agent, aqueous phosphosoda (NaP) colon preparations (e.g., Fleet) are no longer approved for that purpose by the U.S. Food and Drug Administration because of the risk of renal toxicity and renal failure. The over-the-counter Fleet preparation is no longer manufactured. Tablet formulations of NaP (Visicol, Osmoprep) are available by prescription but now carry a black-box warning. *Caution should be used when administering any phosphosoda-type preparation to patients with renal insufficiency, ascites, or congestive heart failure.* Acute renal failure has been reported with these preparations. The use of NaP preparations is declining, and future use should probably be avoided in light of the current restrictions and risk.

Polyethylene glycol bowel preparations should be administered starting at 4 PM the day before colonoscopy. After beginning the preparation the patient can have only clear liquids until midnight, then NPO. One or two tap water enemas administered 1 or 2 hours before the procedure may also be helpful if particulate matter or dark-colored bowel contents are still present. In general, enemas should be avoided because they are unpleasant for the patient and may cause punctate erosions/inflammation in the colonic mucosa, falsely suggesting colon pathology. This phenomenon can also be seen when NaP preparations are used.

It is important for the clinician to individualize the preparation for each patient and to take time to explain the reasons for the bowel cleansing preparation. *If patients are chronically dependent on laxatives or have had a previous inadequate bowel preparation*, it may be advisable to add an additional day of clear liquids before beginning the preparation. Optimal examination may be better accomplished if the patient has received a PEG solution (i.e., GoLYTELY, NuLYTELY, Colyte); however, many physicians claim "less is best." PEG solutions may be more palatable when taken chilled or mixed with a sugar-free drink mix (red-colored mixes should be avoided). Smaller-volume PEG-type preparations (e.g., Half-Lytely) are now available that reduce the volume necessary for the patient to consume and add a mild laxative agent to the process. A less expensive, better-tasting alternative preparation combines 238 g of over-the-counter PEG laxative (MiraLax powder) with 0.5 gallon of Gatorade or similar drink that is consumed over 1 to 2 hours. Four bisacodyl tablets are taken about 2 hours before drinking the preparation the afternoon before the procedure.

It is important to *maintain adequate hydration* of the patient before, during, and after the administration of any colon preparation to minimize possible adverse events. This is especially important in older individuals and in those with known renal disease or who are on medications that may predispose to fluid and electrolyte disturbances.

Diabetic patients will be NPO for an extended time during the colon preparation and should generally refrain from taking their diabetes medications beginning the day of the preparation. It also is advisable to *withhold iron therapy* beginning 4 to 5 days before the preparation because iron tends to darken and thicken the stool, thereby decreasing preparation effectiveness.

Bowel cleansing is essential, not only to provide an unobstructed view but to minimize the rare, but possible, risk of combustion from methane gas should cautery be used during polypectomy or to stop bleeding. Good bowel preparation may also help improve surgical outcomes in the case of perforation and subsequent repair.

Antibiotic Prophylaxis

The American Heart Association, American College of Cardiology, and the Standards of Training and Practice Committee of the ASGE have recently updated their recommendations regarding antibiotic prophylaxis for prevention of bacterial endocarditis. Both groups no longer recommend periprocedural antibiotic prophylaxis for the prevention of infective endocarditis for any gastrointestinal endoscopic procedure, regardless of the patient's cardiac risk status. When used, antibiotic prophylaxis regimens usually include ampicillin and gentamicin, or vancomycin in penicillin-allergic patients.

Anticoagulation

The Standards of Practice Committee of the ASGE has developed practice guidelines for the use of colonoscopy in conjunction with anticoagulated patients. *Management is determined by establishing risk of bleeding versus risk of thromboembolic events.* Colonoscopy with polypectomy is considered a high-risk procedure for bleeding. *Conditions considered high risk for thromboembolic events are* chronic atrial fibrillation with associated valvular heart disease, mechanical valve in the mitral position, and mechanical valve and prior thromboembolic event. *High-risk procedures (i.e., colonoscopy with polypectomy) performed in high-risk conditions* should be managed by discontinuing warfarin 3 to 5 days before the procedure. Consider heparin while

Colonoscopy, Biopsy, and Polypectomy

Name: ________________________ DOB __________ Age ________
Telephone (H) ______________ (W) ______________
Your referring doctor: ________________________________
Primary care doctor: ______________________ Want a copy sent to him/her? Y N
Blood pressure: __________________ Received, read, and understood handouts? Y N

SYMPTOMS/HISTORY:
Reason for consult: ______________________
787.99 Change in stools
285.9 Anemia, NOS
578.9 Blood
783.2 Weight loss
455.6 Hemorrhoids, NOS
780.9 Chills
Frequency ______ daily _______ weekly
Pain: 780.9 Abdomen Where? __________
569.42 Rectum
w/BM

564.0 Constipation
780.6 Fevers
578.1 Black stools
562.11 Diverticulitis/diverticulosis
787.91 Diarrhea
211.3 Polyps
V10.05 Personal Hx colon Ca
V16.0 Family Hx Colon Ca
Who? ______________
Age ______________

Hemoccults: Date ____________ Neg Pos Not done
Previous sigmoid: Date ____________ Who? ______________ OR findings: __________
Findings: ____
____
Previous barium enema: Date ____________ Findings ______________________
Previous abdominal surgery: ____________________________________
Hysterectomy (for women) Y N

PMH:
Bleeding problems
Artificial joints
Artificial heart valve
Asthma

Coronary artery disease
Heart murmur needing prophylaxis
COPD
Smoker _______ PPD 3 ______ years

Other medical problems: 1. ________________ 2. ________________
3. ________________ 4. ________________
Medications ____
Allergies ____

OBJECTIVE:
General:
Neck:
Lungs:
Cor:
Abd:

IMPRESSION: ________________________________
____
____

COUNSELING:
Indications
Sedation
Bowel prep Mag Citrate-Dulcolax-Fleet or GoLYTELY
Alternatives Not performing examination/flex sig and ACBE
Risks Bleeding
Perforation
Infection
Need for hospitalization
Sedation related
Expected results
Monitoring: BP Pulse Oxygen concentration

RECOMMENDATIONS:
1. Mag Citrate-Dulcolax-Fleet bowel prep or GoLYTELY bowel prep
2. Driver when receiving sedation
3. Sedation type IV ____________________ oral ____________________
4. ____
5. ____

________________________ __________
Physician Date

Figure 100-1 Sample patient counseling form for colonoscopy, biopsy, and polypectomy.

the international normalized ratio (INR) is below the therapeutic level. *Low-risk conditions* require only discontinuation of warfarin 3 to 5 days before the procedure without use of heparin. The ASGE no longer considers *recent aspirin or nonsteroidal anti-inflammatory drug use* a contraindication to colonoscopy with polypectomy in the absence of a preexisting bleeding disorder.

An alternative is to use "bridge anticoagulation" with low-molecular-weight heparin. Although low-molecular-weight heparin bridging is being used more frequently, prospective, controlled data supporting this method are currently lacking.

SEDATION

Most colonoscopic examinations are performed while the patient is under conscious sedation (see Chapter 2, Procedural Sedation and Analgesia), although *unsedated colonoscopy is possible* in some circumstances with motivated patients. Sedation may allow for a more thorough examination of the colon because of increased patient comfort and decreased anxiety. Appropriate equipment must be available to monitor blood pressure, pulse, and respiration. A pulse oximeter is now commonly used to monitor oxygen saturation as well. During colonoscopy, it is mandatory to have an assistant available to monitor the patient. Intravenous (IV) access should be established and maintained during the entire procedure in patients receiving IV sedation.

Benzodiazepines are the drugs most commonly used for sedation and include *midazolam (Versed)* 2 to 5 mg or *diazepam (Valium)* 5 to 10 mg. *Meperidine (Demerol)* 25 to 100 mg or *fentanyl (Sublimaze)* 25 to 100 μg is often used in conjunction with benzodiazepines to achieve optimal sedation. These medications should be administered slowly through the IV route. Dangerous side effects can be reversed with *flumazenil (Romazicon)* or *naloxone (Narcan)*, although properly titrating these medications will minimize the need for these drugs. *Propofol (Diprivan)* given as repeated boluses (10 to 20 mg) IV is becoming more commonly used as a sedation agent in colonoscopy because of its rapid, profound sedative effect and subsequent clearance, with faster patient recovery time. Endoscopists should be thoroughly familiar with the pharmacology of all these drugs. Further discussion is found in Chapter 101, Esophagogastroduodenoscopy, and Chapter 2, Procedural Sedation and Analgesia.

A "crash cart" should be immediately available in case of cardiopulmonary arrest. See Chapter 220, Anaphylaxis, and the discussion regarding Banyan kits for the office.

TECHNIQUE

Colonoscopy

The procedure for colonoscopy is as follows (also see Chapter 103, Flexible Sigmoidoscopy, because the technique is virtually identical for the first 70 cm):

1. Place the patient on the examining table in the *left lateral decubitus position.*
2. *Check all of the equipment* for proper functioning.
3. After appropriately sedating the patient, perform a *digital anorectal examination* with a well-lubricated, gloved examining finger.
4. *Lubricate the shaft of the colonoscope and gently insert its tip into the anal canal.* The lumen of the bowel should be directly visualized at all times during the colonoscopy procedure.
5. *Insufflate air* into the *rectum* until the lumen becomes readily apparent. The three "valves" of Houston (i.e., prominent mucosal folds) are often seen as consistent landmarks. The plexus of blood vessels is usually very apparent in the rectal mucosa (Fig. 100-2). The scope can usually be advanced without difficulty as far as the rectosigmoid junction at 15 to 18 cm.
6. Enter the *sigmoid* colon by passing the scope through the rectosigmoid angle. The sigmoid colon is the most common site of difficulty in passage of the instrument. There may be fixation of the bowel from diverticular disease or adhesions from prior surgery, including a hysterectomy. The *sigmoid colon is the most common site of perforation* during colonoscopy. Successful passage through the sigmoid colon may require a series of maneuvers including torquing to the right and withdrawing the scope to reduce loops, applying abdominal pressure, repositioning the patient (even into a supine position), or deflating the lumen of excess air. *An essential but difficult lesson to learn is that when passage of the scope is impeded, torque the shaft to the right and* withdraw *the scope to straighten out the bowel.* Although intubation should optimally occur while the lumen is being visualized, occasionally a "slide-by" technique is used to negotiate abrupt angulations in the bowel. In these acute turns the lumen cannot be well visualized without extreme deflection of the scope tip. Exaggerated deflections of the scope tip may provide complete views of the lumen, but they often impair forward intubation. In the "slide-by" technique, the lumen view is partially sacrificed to allow the scope to be gently advanced while the mucosa is seen to slide past the scope tip. The endoscopic view of the mucosa appears reddish from the underlying vasculature. A blanching of the mucosa could indicate excessive pressure against the bowel wall, and further insertion should be discontinued as the bowel is straightened using other techniques described previously. Although most endoscopists use the slide-by technique occasionally, it should not characterize the intubation technique.
7. The *descending colon* can be recognized by a relatively straight passage through the circular-shaped bowel (Fig. 100-3) to the *splenic flexure*. Traversing the angle of the splenic flexure may resemble passage through the rectosigmoid junction because this angle may be abrupt and may require a small degree of slide-by for passage. The *transverse colon* can be recognized by its characteristic triangular appearance (Fig. 100-4), and it generally has a fairly straight configuration. The *hepatic flexure* is often recognizable by the "liver shadow" (Fig. 100-5), which appears as a bluish-brown area where the liver is in direct

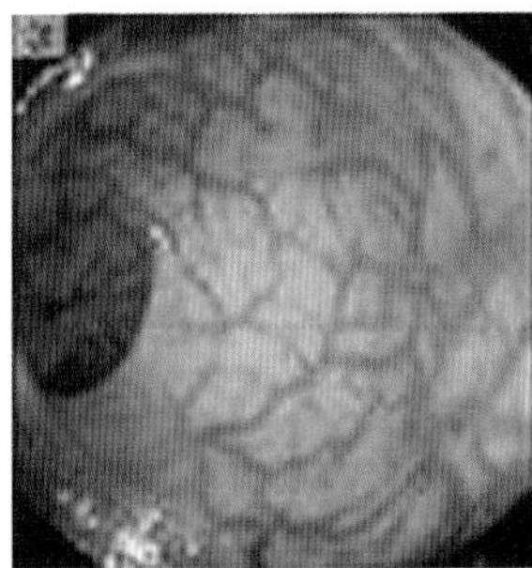

Figure 100-2 Endoscopic view of hemorrhoidal plexus of blood vessels in normal rectum mucosa.

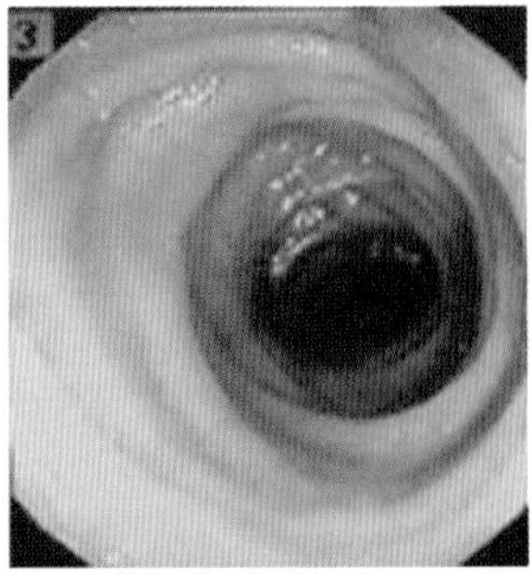

Figure 100-3 Endoscopic view of descending colon.

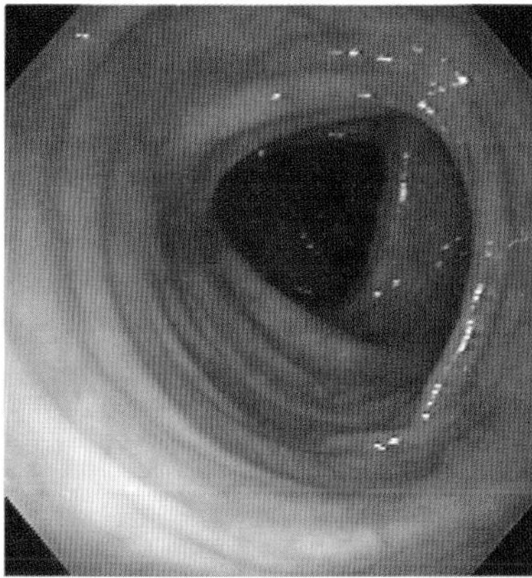

Figure 100-4 Endoscopic view of transverse colon.

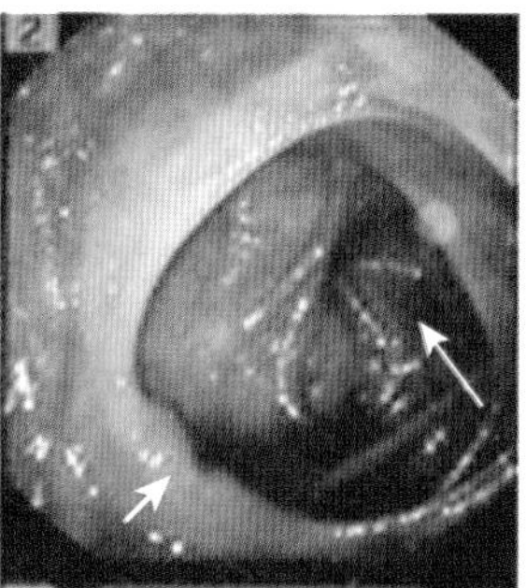

Figure 100-6 Endoscopic view of ileocecal valve *(small white arrow)* and "crow's foot" *(large white arrow)* in cecum.

contact with the bowel wall. The hepatic flexure is seen as another angle to traverse with the scope. The *ascending colon* may also appear triangular.

8. Advance the scope into the *cecum* by pulling back, keeping the tip of the scope in the center of the lumen, and applying full suction to pull the cecum toward the scope tip. The cecal landmarks, which may or may not be prominent, include the *ileocecal valve* (Fig. 100-6) and the *appendiceal orifice* (Fig. 100-7). Convergence of the terminal portion of the taenia coli in the cecum forms a characteristic appearance known as the *"crow's foot"* or *cecal strap* (see Fig. 100-6). *Other methods to ascertain if the cecum has been reached* are to check for ballottement externally above the right inguinal canal or for transillumination in the right lower quadrant (less consistent findings).
9. *Intubate the terminal ileum* by advancing the tip just beyond the ileocecal valve and then deflecting the tip toward the valve as the scope is carefully withdrawn. As the tip of the scope meets the valve opening, torque the scope gently clockwise to allow the tip to advance briefly into the terminal ileum.
10. *Carefully inspect the colon wall as the scope is withdrawn.* Use a circular motion of the tip to inspect behind every mucosal fold. Lavage with water any areas of the bowel with inadequate preparation and carefully reinspect. Obtain any necessary *biopsy* specimens and *remove polyps* during this portion of the procedure.

Endoscopists use various combinations of the techniques described in the foregoing discussion in a time-efficient manner to safely intubate the colon to the cecum in a high percentage of cases. It is important to recognize that not every colonoscopy can safely be completed to the cecum. Most colonoscopies take an average of 30 to 45 minutes, although this is variable. Time spent examining the colon during withdrawal may be a more important indicator of quality than overall procedure time. It has been suggested that withdrawal time should be at least 6 minutes because data have shown a lower polyp detection rate when withdrawal time is shorter than this.

11. *Inspect the distal rectum and anorectal junction* before completely withdrawing the scope. As the tip of the scope passes the dentate line, reinsert the scope approximately 5 to 10 cm while simultaneously rotating both control wheels counterclockwise to completely deflect the tip back upon itself (*retroflexion or turnaround maneuver*). Torque the shaft to inspect all around the anorectal junction. *Alternatively, use an anoscope* (Ives' slotted anoscope is recommended) to complete the examination of this area.

General principles for safe and efficient intubation of the colon to the cecum include the following:

- Minimize air insufflation.
- Keep the instrument straight.
- Avoid loop formation (pull back frequently).
- Avoid advancing the scope blindly (i.e., slide-by technique) when at all possible.
- Do not sedate the patient more than is necessary to maintain comfort.

Polypectomy

Polyps may be *sessile* (i.e., broad-based polyps) or *pedunculated* (i.e., with a stalk; Figs. 100-8 and 100-9). Almost all pedunculated polyps and many sessile polyps can be easily removed with the electrocautery snare with a low risk of perforation and bleeding. Risk may be higher in larger polyps and in those located in the right colon. Sessile polyps may also be removed with hot or cold forceps (Fig. 100-10). The patient experiences no pain with polypectomy.

There has been recent attention in the literature to the concept of *"flat" or "depressed" polyps*. These polyps are not exophytic and may actually lie below the regular surface of the mucosa, often making their detection difficult during colonoscopy. There is concern that these lesions may have a higher likelihood of

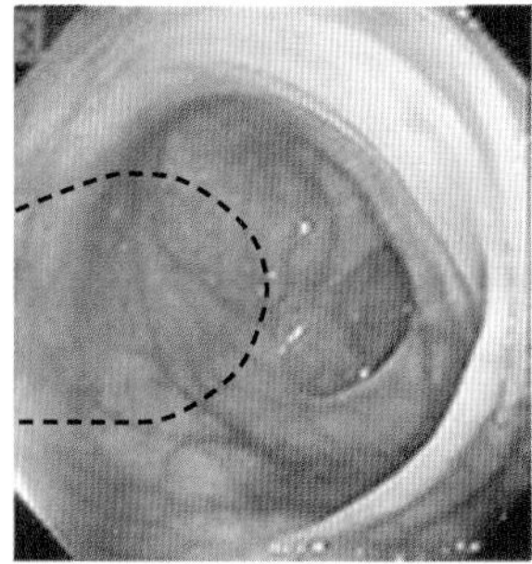

Figure 100-5 Endoscopic view of hepatic flexure. The characteristic liver shadow is outlined by the *dashed line*.

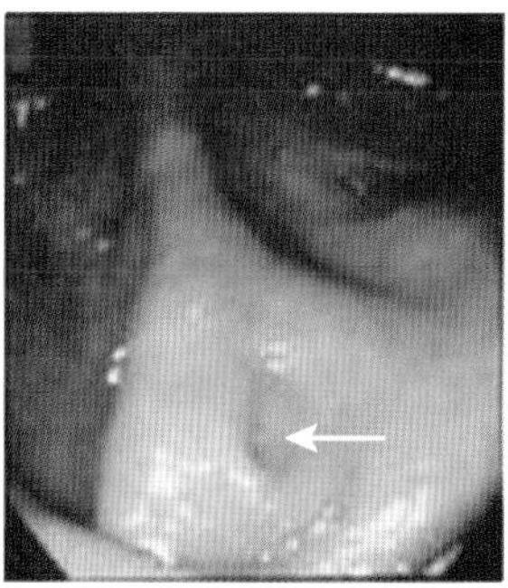

Figure 100-7 Endoscopic view of appendiceal orifice *(arrow)*.

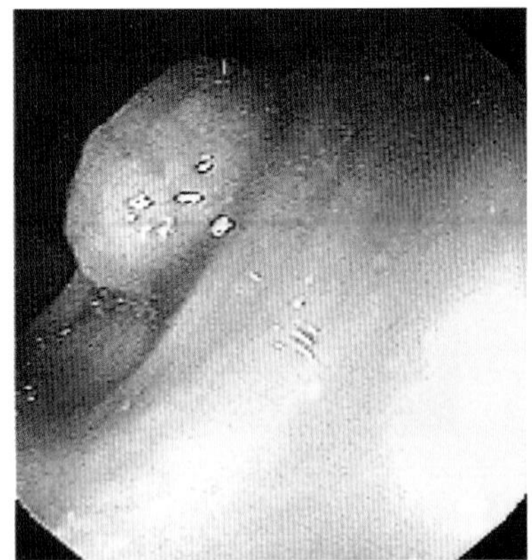

Figure 100-8 Endoscopic view of sessile polyp.

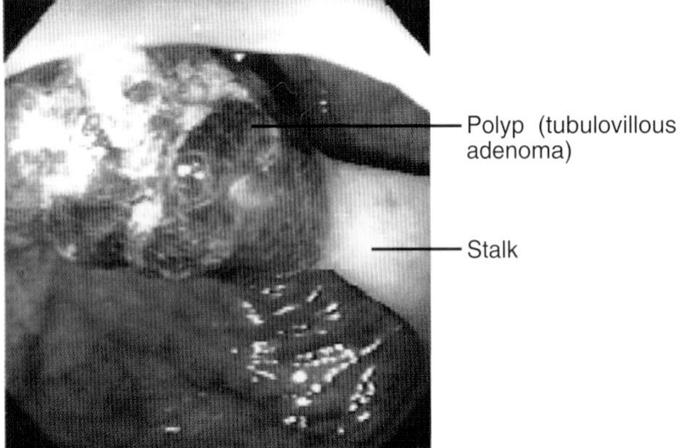

Figure 100-9 Endoscopic view of pedunculated polyp.

malignant degeneration, and yet may go undetected. Careful inspection of the mucosa is imperative as well as insistence on a high-quality bowel preparation to improve early detection of these lesions. Novel techniques are in development that may assist in detection of these lesions, including use of high-magnification colonoscopes with mucosal stains (chromoscopy) and narrow-band imaging.

Biopsies of mucosal lesions are commonly obtained during colonoscopy as well as from normal-appearing mucosa when indicated. Generally, 4 to 6 biopsy specimens should be obtained of mucosal abnormalities and 8 to 10 biopsy specimens should be obtained from larger mass lesions. Pathologic interpretation is generally more sensitive if specimens are obtained from the junction of normal and abnormal mucosa. Avoid sampling areas of apparent necrosis or deep ulceration because these areas tend to provide poorer tissue specimens.

The procedure for polypectomy is as follows:

1. Position the scope so that the polyp can be visualized approximately 2 to 3 cm beyond the tip of the colonoscope. Positioning the polyp at the 5 o'clock position where the port for the electrocautery snare exits can be helpful for biopsy and polypectomy.
2. Under direct vision at all times, pass the electrocautery snare catheter through the colonoscope port. Position the tip of the sheath of the snare near the polyp, advance the wire loop, and open it, always under direct vision. Manipulate the snare and maneuver the tip of the colonoscope to place the snare around the polyp. Slowly secure the wire loop around the pedicle or polyp base as the snare catheter is advanced toward the stalk to avoid excessive pull on the stalk or a tangential cut. Maneuver the colonoscope to draw the polyp and snare away from the bowel wall to avoid excess burn injury and possible perforation.
3. Apply the electrocautery current (coagulation only) until a white eschar forms around the polyp stalk. Use the least amount of current necessary to achieve the eschar in 2 to 3 seconds (amount varies with the diameter of the stalk and with each electrocautery unit, but generally set at 10 to 15 W). Tighten the snare as coagulation continues until the stalk is transected.
4. Retrieve the excised polyp using suction or forceps, or simply regrasp the polyp with the snare. At times this may require removal and reinsertion of the entire colonoscope. Unretrieved polyps may occasionally need to be retrieved later by straining stools after further bowel preparation solutions and cathartics are given, although recovery of polyps using this method is often unsuccessful. Large polyps may require multiple snare-resection excisions. *Tissue desiccation without prior biopsy should be avoided because it is very important to have pathologic diagnosis of all colonic lesions*.
5. Cancerous polyps do not need further resections if the tumor is well differentiated, if there is no lymphatic or vascular invasion, and if there is at least 2 mm between the tumor and the line of resection. With an obvious advanced colon cancer that is friable or ulcerated, biopsies will usually provide sufficient tissue for diagnosis. However, because only tiny samples can be obtained, the cancer may occasionally be missed and the specimens reveal only benign adenomatous tissue. If a strong clinical suspicion of cancer exists, the lesion should be reexamined and resampled. Surgical consultation may be warranted.

Operative Report

A well-documented procedure note is essential. Notes can be dictated (Fig. 100-11) or hand-written on standardized endoscopy forms (Fig. 100-12). Endoscopy report templates are available for

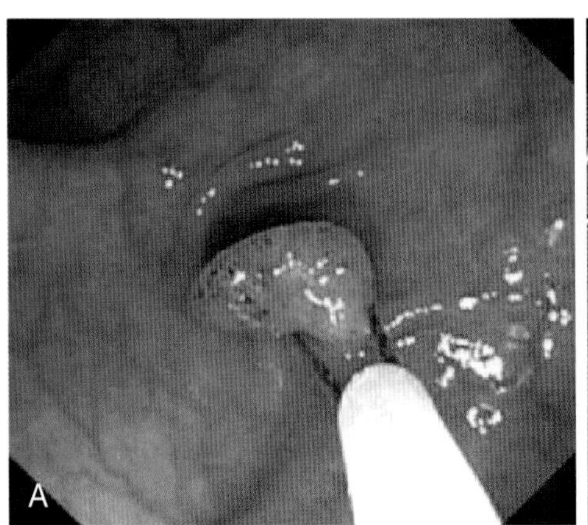

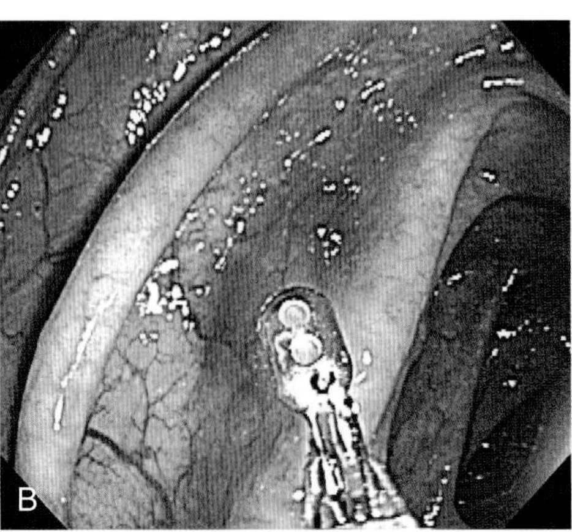

Figure 100-10 **A,** Polyp being snared. **B,** Polyp being removed with cold forceps.

Procedure: Colonoscopy
Equipment: Olympus Colonoscope
Pre-op diagnosis: History of previous colon polyps
Post-op diagnosis: Diminutive polyp
Endoscopist:
Assistant:

HPI:
Patient is a 71-year-old African-American male who was seen by Dr. Smith on 6-26-2001 and scheduled for screening colonoscopy. The patient was asymptomatic at the time. The patient had a history of colonic polyps dating back to 1996. The patient was found on that colonoscopy to have a colonic polyp reported as an adenoma by pathology report. Patient was recommended at that time to have a repeat colonoscopy in one year. The patient denied any history of colon cancer. Patient had no iron-deficiency anemia. Patient received one gallon of GoLYTELY yesterday, and the patient was NPO for the procedure today.

Informed consent was obtained from the patient after a full discussion of the risks, benefits and alternatives to the procedure. Patient was also advised of the risk of missed lesions with this procedure. He expressed an understanding of these issues and desired to continue with the colonoscopy. All questions were answered.

Medications: Conscious sedation was obtained with 50 mg of Demerol IV push with Versed 1 mg IV push. Conscious sedation was maintained throughout the procedure.

Procedure: After conscious sedation was obtained, the patient was placed in the left lateral position. Digital rectal examination was performed, which showed normal sphincter tone, no masses, no external hemorrhoids. Prostate gland was not enlarged. After rectal examination was performed, the regular colonoscope was introduced via the anus and advanced inside the colon into the cecum. The procedure was difficult as a result of redundancies of the colon. External compressions of the abdomen and multiple changes in the position of the patient were required throughout the procedure in order to advance into the cecum. The bowel preparation was adequate. The extent of the exam was to the cecum. The cecum was identified by the ileal-cecal valve, and the appendiceal orifice was clearly visualized. After reaching the cecum, the scope was slowly withdrawn with careful inspection of all aspects of the colon in a circular fashion. Retroflexion was performed inside the rectum before completely straightening the scope, and the scope was subsequently removed from the patient. Patient was transported to recovery area and monitored for 30 minutes until return to baseline state was observed.

Complications: None

Findings: There was a diminutive polyp approximately 3 mm in size in the ascending colon that was removed with cold-force biopsy forceps. The colonic mucosa was otherwise normal. Neither diverticula nor internal hemorrhoids were seen.

Impression: Diminutive polyp

Recommendation: Given the small size of this polyp and patient's previous history, I would recommend that the patient repeat colonoscopy in 5-10 years. Other methods of colon cancer screening would not be necessary over this 10 year period (i.e., no need for checking fecal occult blood test). Patient will return to the primary care doctor for follow-up, and I have ordered Metamucil, 1 Tbsp mixed with a glass of water once a day for constipation. This can be increased to twice a day if needed.

Figure 100-11 Sample procedure note for colonoscopy.

use with electronic medical records. Procedure notes should include clear recommendations for future management and surveillance of the patient, and this information should be imparted to the referring clinician and the patient.

Common Errors

- Failure to properly insufflate the colon with air
- Failure to identify landmarks
- Failure to monitor the patient during and after the procedure
- Failure to terminate the procedure when appropriate (lack of progression despite optimal technique, patient instability or intolerance, or risk outweighs benefit)
- Failure to adequately inspect the colonic mucosa
- Failure to straighten the sigmoid loop during insertion
- Failure to ensure an adequate preparation

Complications

Complications occur infrequently with diagnostic colonoscopy and only slightly more frequently with therapeutic colonoscopy. Major complications include the following:

- Cardiopulmonary—over 60% related to sedation and medications used
  - Vasovagal reactions (i.e., hypotension, bradycardia)
  - Arrhythmias (including ventricular tachycardia and fibrillation)
  - Myocardial infarction

Procedure Note
Date:
Patient Name:
Identification Number:
Procedure:
Equipment:

Pre-op diagnosis:

Post-op diagnosis:

Endoscopist:

Assistant:

HPI:

Informed consent:

Medications:

Procedure:

Complications:

Findings:

Impression:

Recommendations:

Signature

Figure 100-12 Sample procedure form for colonoscopy.

- Colon perforation
- Postpolypectomy bleeding
- Postpolypectomy syndrome
- Missed lesions
- Painful experience for patient

Other rare complications include the following:

- Preparation complications
  - Aspiration
  - Dehydration
  - Hyperphosphatemia, hyponatremia
  - Toxic megacolon
  - Renal failure
- Infections without perforation
  - Bacteremia
  - Scope transmission of infectious agent
- Sigmoid or cecal volvulus
- Splenic rupture
- Pancreatitis
- Diverticulitis
- Incarcerated snare or colonoscope

Perforation of the colon occurs at a rate of 0.1% to 0.8% (approximately) for diagnostic colonoscopy and 0.3% to 3% for therapeutic colonoscopy. Perforations can occur for a number of reasons but are most commonly caused by excessive force of insertion of the endoscope tip or with the side of the scope during slide-by, loop formation, loop reduction, or advancement despite presence of fixating lesions. Other causes of perforation include rupture of diverticulum, rupture of stricture site, transmural injury with electrocautery current with subsequent perforation, or polypectomy- and biopsy-induced perforations. Perforations may also rarely occur from pneumatic rupture of the proximal colon.

Perforations are more common with patients who are oversedated or who are under general anesthesia. It is uncommon for the scope tip to actually penetrate the bowel, but this type of perforation is usually noticed immediately. More frequently the perforation is small and occurs away from the scope tip. It may go unrecognized until the patient later experiences *abdominal pain, fever, and distention*. A radiographic film of the abdomen or chest will show *pneumoperitoneum*. In the majority of perforations, immediate surgery is indicated. With fecal soiling a diverting colostomy is needed; however, in the absence of obvious contamination, primary closure may be sufficient. Perforation can occur even in experienced hands and does not per se imply negligence on the part of the endoscopist.

Bleeding postcolonoscopy and postpolypectomy occurs in approximately 1 in 1000 procedures. Bleeding may occur immediately or up to 4 weeks postprocedure. Most cases of bleeding resolve spontaneously, but some may require repeat colonoscopy with attempts to coagulate the area (i.e., epinephrine injection followed by multipolar cautery or heater probe) or laparotomy. Avoiding aspirin prophylaxis for 10 days postpolypectomy may decrease late bleeding risk.

Postpolypectomy syndrome is caused by a transmural thermal injury (i.e., burn) resulting in full-thickness bowel necrosis, which may lead to serosal inflammation. Postpolypectomy syndrome may be accompanied by fever, leukocytosis, and localized and rebound tenderness over the polypectomy site without evidence of intraperitoneal air. A conservative approach generally leads to a good outcome.

Missed neoplastic lesions have been shown to occur even with "expert" endoscopists. In one study, colonoscopy detected 95% of all lesions present. Of the 5% missed, half were not appreciated because of inability to pass the scope far enough; however, in the other half, lesions were passed without being seen. Other studies report a miss rate for advanced lesions (>1 cm) of 12% to 17% for skilled colonoscopists using CT colonography as a reference standard (Pickhardt and colleagues, 2004; Van Gelder and colleagues, 2004).

Postprocedure Management

After colonoscopy, monitor the patient (i.e., clinical assessment, blood pressure, pulse, oxygen saturation) for at least 30 minutes and until a return to baseline cognitive function has occurred. Explain the results of the procedure to the patient, including the treatment plan and follow-up appointments. Patients may resume a normal diet on discharge even when polypectomy has been performed. Clearly explain precautions concerning possible delayed bleeding or unrecognized perforation when clinically indicated. Patents should be cautioned not to drive, operate heavy machinery, or sign legal documents for 24 hours after conscious sedation.

Interpretation and Follow-up of Results

Table 100-2 explains the current recommendations for follow-up of polyps. Pathology results should be communicated to the patient and the referring clinician, and appropriate follow-up or surveillance should be arranged based on the findings.

Learning Colonoscopy

For a basic overview of colonoscopy principles and technique, the reader is directed to Raskin and Nord's *Colonoscopy: Principles and Techniques*, which contains excellent diagrams, photographs, tips, and techniques. Additional information on endoscopic technique is found in Williams' chapter on insertion technique in Waye's *Colonoscopy: Principles and Practice*. Silverstein and Tytgat's *Atlas of Gastrointestinal Endoscopy*, Forbes' *Atlas of Clinical Gastroenterology*, and Wilcox's *Atlas of Clinical Gastrointestinal Endoscopy* contain excellent photographs of colorectal pathology as well as information on gastrointestinal diseases. Anatomy is thoroughly illustrated in *Netter's Gastrointestinal Anatomy and Motility*. For an in-depth review of colonoscopic polypectomy, see Chapter 12 in Tytgat and colleagues' *Practice of Therapeutic Endoscopy* and Chapter 38 of Ginsberg's *Clinical Gastrointestinal Endoscopy*.

Before attempting to perform colonoscopy, it is useful to become proficient and skilled in flexible fiberoptic sigmoidoscopy. The instrument controls and techniques used for flexible sigmoidoscopy are identical to those used to perform colonoscopy. *Formal (CME) courses* are available to teach colonoscopy concepts, skills, and techniques through the American Academy of Family Physicians (AAFP; phone: 1-800-274-2237), The National Procedures Institute (phone: 1-866-674-2631), and the American Association for Primary Care Endoscopy (phone: 913-906-6000, ext. 6706).

One method often used for obtaining colonoscopy skills in the postresidency environment is to form a teaching relationship with a proficient endoscopist willing to act as a preceptor until adequate proficiency is obtained. Colonoscopy can be mastered without fellowship training. Studies show that high-quality care and complication rates essentially identical to those for fellowship-trained gastroenterologists can be attained (Hopper and colleagues, 1996; Wilkins and colleagues, 2009), and that physician assistants and nurses may also become qualified to perform colonoscopy (Lieberman and Ghormley, 1992; Lomas, 2009). The AAFP has published a position paper on family physicians performing colonoscopy. It can be found on the organization's website (www.AAFP.org/policy/issues/c-colonoscopyposition.html) and includes guidelines for establishing and maintaining proficiency and suggestions for obtaining privileges in colonoscopy. ASGE videotapes on endoscopy technique can be ordered through ASGE at www.asge.org/TrainingEducationIndex.aspx?id=410. Free endoscopy technique and pathology videos may be viewed at The DAVE Project—Gastroenterology (see Atlases, under Online Resources).

Endoscopy simulators can be a useful adjunct in basic colonoscopy training, particularly when used before actual experience with colonoscopy in patients. Simulators have improved in haptic (touch) feedback technology and also offer various polypectomy

TABLE 100-2 Surveillance Protocols for History of Colonic Neoplasia

Finding	Colonoscopy Interval
Small hyperplastic polyps	10 yr
1–2 tubular adenomas (<1 cm) and only low-grade dysplasia	5 yr
>3 adenomas, villous elements, or high-grade dysplasia, or >1 cm	3 yr
> 10 adenomas	Within 3 yr
Large sessile adenomas (especially if removed piecemeal)	2–6 mo
Negative follow-up examination	No earlier than 5 yr
Previous colon cancer	High-quality clearance at or around time of resection followed by colonoscopy at 1 yr, then 3 yr and 5 yr if normal
Previous rectal cancer	Clearance of remainder of colon at time of resection, then colonoscopy at 1 yr and 4 yr after resection, then 5-yr intervals

From Rex DK, Petrini JL, Baron TH, et al: Quality indicators for colonoscopy. Gastrointest Endosc 63(4 Suppl):S16–S28, 2006.

Box 100-1. Overview of Colonoscopy Privileges

From the American Academy of Family Physicians Position Paper

- "It is the position of the American Academy of Family Physicians (AAFP) that clinical privileges should be based on the individual physician's documented training and/or experience, demonstrated abilities and current competence, and not on the physician's specialty."
- More than 1440 family physicians across the United States perform colonoscopy in the hospital setting.
- In the 1998 AAFP Practice Profile Survey, 1163 family physicians reported performing colonoscopy in their offices.
- Twenty-six percent of family practice residencies provide training in colonoscopy.
- "Skills for performing colonoscopy are most often acquired during three years of family practice residency training. Another possible route to acquire colonoscopy skills is through preceptorship with a physician who already has such training and privileges. Established experience in flexible sigmoidoscopy examination is helpful in developing colonoscopy skills."
- "The American Society for Gastrointestinal Endoscopy (ASGE) recommends that physicians perform a minimum of 100 diagnostic colonoscopies and 20 snare polypectomies as a threshold for determining clinical competence. However, this recommendation was based on expert opinion, not scientific data."
- "...the AAFP strongly believes that all medical staff members should realize that there is overlap between specialties, and that no one department has exclusive rights to privileges."
- "A legal opinion on privileges for endoscopy submitted to the AAFP in 1993 stated the following:
  A. Hospitals and peer review participants risk liability under state law if they base credentialing decisions solely on whether or not a physician has obtained specialty certification.
  B. The Council on Ethical and Judicial Affairs of the AMA has issued the opinion that competitive factors must be disregarded in making decisions about credentials and privileges.
  C. There is no evidence that only board-certified gastroenterologists are qualified to perform endoscopic procedures.
  D. Hospitals violate the Medicare Conditions for Participation if they base credentialing decisions solely on specialty board certification.
  E. Hospitals and peer review participants risk loss of federal and state immunity from liability by basing credentialing decisions solely on whether or not a physician has obtained specialty certification."

From the American Medical Association Clinical Privileges

Regarding clinical privileges, the 1993 AMA Policy Compendium states, "The accordance and delineation of privileges should be determined on an individual basis, commensurate with an applicant's education, training and experience, and demonstrated current competence." It also states that "in implementing these criteria, each facility should formulate and apply reasonable nondiscriminatory standards for the evaluation of an applicant's credentials, free of anticompetitive intent or purpose."

From the American Society for Gastrointestinal Endoscopy

- "Competency is the minimum level of skill, knowledge, and/or expertise, attained through training and experience, required to perform a procedure safely and proficiently."
- "Departments often develop criteria for recommending privileges and, not surprisingly, these suggested criteria may vary significantly depending on the particular departmental discipline and whether the department represents mainly generalists or specialists."
- "Highly motivated family physicians or internists can acquire a level of training adequate to perform endoscopic examinations of high quality."

Adapted from Worthington DV: AAFP position paper. Colonoscopy: Procedure skills. Am Fam Physician 62:1177–1182, 2000; American Medical Association: Clinical privileges. In AMA Policy Compendium. Chicago, American Medical Association, 1993; and American Society of Gastrointestinal Endoscopy (ASGE): President's message, October, 1999.

simulations. Simulators are manufactured by the Immersion Corporation (www.immersion.com).

Obtaining Hospital Privileges

Most hospitals have credentialing standards regarding colonoscopy privileges. Hospitals vary widely in those standards but generally require a minimum number of procedures and possible proctoring of applicants until competency is established. In general, credentialing becomes more restrictive where a high number of specialists perform colonoscopy in the hospital. It is advisable to carefully document all endoscopy experience and related experience and provide a plan for continued medical education and quality assurance when applying for colonoscopy privileges.

See the AAFP Colonoscopy Position Paper for further information (Box 100-1). For articles that may assist in obtaining colonoscopy privileges, see the bibliography (AMA, 1993; ASGE, 1999; Worthington, 2000). A position paper on endoscopy privileging was recently released by the American Association of Primary Care Endoscopists (AAPCE) and can be accessed at www.AAPCE.org. The AAPCE recommends that 50 colonoscopies be used as a target number for hospitals requiring a certain number before privileging, which is in accord with surgical society recommendations as well.

CPT/Billing Codes

45378* Colonoscopy beyond splenic flexure
45379* Colonoscopy with foreign body removal
45380* Colonoscopy with biopsy (single or multiple)
45382* Colonoscopy with control of bleeding (any method)
45383* Colonoscopy with ablation of tumor
45384* Colonoscopy with removal of lesion by hot forceps or bipolar cautery
45385* Colonoscopy with removal of lesion by snare technique
G0105 Screening colonoscopy in patients at high risk for CRC, if 23 months since last screening colonoscopy or barium enema (Medicare)

*The Health Care Financing Administration (HCFA) allows additional payment for a tray for this procedure when performed in a physician's office. Charge appropriately using code "99070—surgical tray."

G0121 Screening colonoscopy in patients at least 50 years of age at average risk for CRC, if 119 months since last screening colonoscopy or barium enema (Medicare)

If colonoscopy is abnormal, the applicable CPT and ICD-9-CM codes (not G-codes) should be used. Conscious sedation is considered part of the colonoscopy and is not billed separately unless performed by a different provider.

ICD-9-CM Diagnostic Codes

153.0 Ca, colon-hepatic flexure
153.1 Ca, colon-transverse
153.2 Ca, colon-descending
153.3 Ca, colon-sigmoid
153.4 Ca, colon-cecum
153.6 Ca, colon-ascending
154.1 Ca, rectum
211.3 Benign neoplasm, colon, or familial adenomatous polyposis (FAP)
211.4 Benign neoplasm, rectum-anus
455.0 Internal hemorrhoids
455.3 External hemorrhoids
555.1 Crohn's disease, colon
556.9 Ulcerative colitis
558.9 Colitis, nonspecific
562.1 Diverticulosis
562.12 Diverticulosis with hemorrhage
564.0 Unspecified constipation
564.5 Chronic diarrhea
569.84 Angiodysplasia
578.9 GI hemorrhage
787.6 Stool incontinence
789.0 Abdominal pain
793.4 Radiographic abnormality, GI tract
V76.51 Screening, cancer, colon (to be used with G-codes; see previous discussion)

Patient Education Guides and Additional Resources

See patient education and patient consent forms available online at www.expertconsult.com.

Sample consent forms and patient education handouts are also available online at http://drpearlman.btrtest.com/patient_education.htm and http://springfieldasc.com/patient-information/patient-forms.

Suppliers

(See contact information online at www.expertconsult.com.)

Extensive marketing and technical information about colonoscopy equipment is readily available. When selecting a supplier, the clinician should consider local availability for education, equipment service, and technical support. It may be desirable to ask for local references from suppliers.

New equipment

- Fujinon Corp.
- Olympus Corp.
- Pentax Corp.

Used or refurbished equipment

- B-Met Endoscopic, Inc.
- Cardinal Health
- Corthel, Inc.
- Endoscopy Support Services, Inc.
- Instrument Specialists, Inc.
- Integrated Medical Systems, Inc.
- Karl Storz Endoscopy–America
- Matlock Endoscopic
- Medical Optics
- Medical Replacement Parts LLC
- Mobile Instrument Service
- Nuell, Inc.
- SOS Medical
- Spectrum Surgical Instruments
- SterilMed
- Surgical Optics LLC
- Surgical Repair Technologies
- United Endoscopy
- Universal Endoscopic Services
- Used Medical Equipment and Devices Medline

Online Resources

American Association for Primary Care Endoscopy: www.aapce.org.
American College of Gastroenterology: www.acg.gi.org.
American Gastroenterological Association: www.gastro.org.
American Society for Gastrointestinal Endoscopy: www.asge.org.
Colorectal-cancer.net: www.colorectal-cancer.net/colorectal.htm
GastroSource: www.gastrosource.com.

Atlases

The Atlas of Gastrointestinal Endoscopy: www.endoatlas.com.
The DAVE Project—Gastroenterology (good video library): http://dave1.mgh.harvard.edu/.
Colonoscopy Atlas: http://lib-sh.lsuhsc.edu/fammed/atlases/colon/Colon_Atlas_TOC_11.html.
El Salvador Atlas of Gastrointestinal Video Endoscopy: www.gastrointestinalatlas.com/index.html.
Feldman's GastroAtlas Online: www.gastroatlas.com.
Gastrolab: www.gastrolab.net/.
Jackson/Siegelbaum Gastroenterology: Images of the colon: www.gicare.com/Endoscopy-Center/Images-Colon.aspx.
http://www.gastrosource.com/content/landingpage/endoscopy-atlas-jaramillo?utm_internal_banner=Jaramillo+endoscopy+atlas&utm_internal_campaign=text.
www.endoskopischer-atlas.de/indexe.htm.

Bibliography*

Accreditation Council for Graduate Medical Education (ACGME): Memorandum: Changes in minimum requirements for laparoscopy and endoscopy. February 1, 2006. Available at www.acgme.org/acWebsite/RRC_440/440_minReqLaparoscopy.asp

Ackermann RJ: Performance of gastrointestinal tract endoscopy by primary care physicians: Lessons from the US Medicare database. Arch Fam Med 6:52–58, 1997.

American Medical Association: Clinical privileges. In AMA Policy Compendium. Chicago, American Medical Association, 1993.

American Society for Gastrointestinal Endoscopy (ASGE): Standards of Practice Committee: Guideline on the management of anticoagulation and antiplatelet therapy for endoscopic procedures. Gastrointest Endosc 55:775–779, 2002.

American Society for Gastrointestinal Endoscopy (ASGE): Standards of Practice Committee: The management of low-molecular weight heparin and nonaspirin antiplatelet agents for endoscopic procedures. Gastrointest Endosc 61:189–194, 2005.

American Society for Gastrointestinal Endoscopy (ASGE): Standards of Practice Committee: Antibiotic prophylaxis in endoscopy. Gastrointest Endosc 67:791–798, 2008.

American Society for Gastrointestinal Endoscopy, the Society of American Gastrointestinal Surgeons, and the American Society of Colorectal Surgeons: Principles of privileging and credentialing for endoscopy and colonoscopy. Gastrointest Endosc 55:145–148, 2002.

Atkin WS, Whynes DK: Improving the cost-effectiveness of colorectal cancer screening. J Natl Cancer Inst 92:513–514, 2000.

Bauer JJ: Colorectal Surgery Illustrated: A Focused Approach. St. Louis, Mosby, 1993.

*For additional pertinent references, also see Chapter 2, Procedural Sedation and Analgesia, and Chapter 103, Flexible Sigmoidoscopy.

Bittner JG 4th, Marks JM, Dunkin BJ, et al: Resident training in flexible gastrointestinal endoscopy: A review of current issues and options. J Surg Educ 64:399–409, 2007.

Brooks DD, Winawer SJ, Rex DK, et al: Colonoscopy surveillance after polypectomy and colorectal cancer resection. Consensus guidelines from the U.S. Multi-Specialty Task Force on Colorectal Cancer and The American Cancer Society. Am Fam Physician 77:995–1002, 1003–1004, 2008.

Brunelli SM, Feldman HI, Latif SM, et al: A comparison of sodium phosphosoda purgative to polyethylene glycol bowel preparations prior to colonoscopy. Fam Med 41:39–45, 2009.

Cotton PB, Connor P, McGee D, et al: Colonoscopy: Practice variation among 69 hospital-based endoscopists. Gastrointest Endosc 57:352–357, 2003.

Forbes A: Atlas of Clinical Gastroenterology, 3rd ed. Philadelphia, Mosby, 2005.

Frazier AL, Colditz GA, Fuchs CS, Kuntz KM: Cost-effectiveness of screening for colorectal cancer in the general population. JAMA 284:1954–1961, 2000.

Friedland S, Sedehi D, Soetikno R: Colonoscopic polypectomy in anticoagulated patients. World J Gastroenterol 15:1973–1976, 2009.

Ginsberg GG: Clinical Gastrointestinal Endoscopy. Philadelphia, Saunders, 2005.

Harper MB, Pope JB, Mayeaux EJ: Colonoscopy experience at a family practice residency: A comparison to gastroenterology and general surgery services. Fam Med 29:575–579, 1997.

Herman FN: Avoidance of sedation during total colonoscopy. Dis Colon Rectum 33:70–72, 1990.

Hopper W, Kyker K, Rodney WM: Colonoscopy by a family physician: A 9-year experience of 1048 procedures. J Fam Pract 43:561–566, 1996.

Imperiale TF, Glowinski EA, Lin-Cooper C, et al: Five-year risk of colorectal neoplasia after negative screening colonoscopy. N Engl J Med 359: 1285–1287, 2008.

Kim DH, Pickhardt PJ, Taylor AJ, et al: CT colonography versus colonoscopy for the detection of advanced neoplasia. N Engl J Med 357: 1403–1412, 2007.

Knox L, Hahn RG, Lane C: A comparison of unsedated colonoscopy and flexible sigmoidoscopy in the family medicine setting: An LA net study. J Am Board Fam Med 20:444–450, 2007.

Kolber M: Outcomes of 1949 endoscopic procedures performed by a Canadian rural family physician. Can Fam Physician 55:170–175, 2009.

Leard LE, Savides TJ, Ganiats TG: Patient preferences for colorectal cancer screening. J Fam Pract 45:211–218, 1997.

Leung FW: Unsedated colonoscopy—Question: Is it worth staying awake for: Answer: Yes, for those who know what it is. Presented at the Digestive Disease Week, Washington, DC, 2007.

Leung FW: Promoting informed choice of unsedated colonoscopy: Patient-centered care for a subgroup of U.S. veterans. Dig Dis Sci 53:2955–2959, 2008.

Leung FW, Aharonian S, Guth PH, et al: Unsedated colonoscopy: Time to revisit this option? J Fam Pract 57:E1–E14, 2008.

Levin B, Lieberman DA, McFarland B, et al: Screening and surveillance for the early detection of colorectal cancer and adenomatous polyps, 2008: A joint guideline for the American Cancer Society, the US Multi-Society Task Force on Colorectal Cancer, and the American College of Radiology. CA Cancer J Clin 134:1570–1595, 2008.

Lieberman D, et al: Standardized colonoscopy reporting and data system: Report of the Quality Assurance Task Group of the National Colorectal Cancer Roundtable. Gastrointest Endosc 65:757–766, 2007.

Lieberman DA, Ghormley JM: Physician assistants in gastroenterology: Should they perform endoscopy? Am J Gastroenterol 87:940–943, 1992.

Lieberman DA, Holub JL, Moravec MD, et al: Prevalence of colon polyps detected by colonoscopy screening in asymptomatic black and white patients. JAMA 300:1459–1461, 2008.

Lieberman DA, Weiss DG: One-time screening for colorectal cancer with combined fecal occult-blood testing and examination of the distal colon. N Engl J Med 345:555–560, 2001.

Lin OS, Kozarek RA, Schembre DB, et al: Screening colonoscopy in very elderly patients: Prevalence of neoplasia and estimated impact of life expectancy. JAMA 295:2357–2365, 2006.

Lomas C: Endoscopy nurses "equal" doctors. Nurs Times 11(Feb 16):56, 2009. http://www.nursingtimes.net/whats-new-in-nursing/endoscopy-nurses-equal-doctors/1991298.article. Accessed April 23, 2010.

Netter F: Netter's Gastrointestinal Anatomy and Motility. Teterboro, NJ, Icon Custom Communications, 2001.

Newman RJ, Nichols DB, Cummings DM: Outpatient colonoscopy by rural family physicians. Ann Fam Med 3:122–125, 2005.

Pickhardt PJ, Nugent PA, Mysliwiec PA, et al: Location of adenomas missed by optical colonoscopy. Ann Intern Med 141:352–359, 2004.

Pierzchajlo RP, Ackermann RJ, Vogel RL: Colonoscopy performed by a family physician: A case series of 751 procedures. J Fam Pract 44:473–480, 1997.

Raskin JB, Nord HJ: Colonoscopy: Principles and Techniques. New York, Igaku-Shoin, 1995.

Reed DN, Collins JD, Wyatt WJ, et al: Can general surgeons perform colonoscopy safely? Am J Surg 163:257–259, 1992.

Rex DK, Johnson DA, Anderson JC, et al: American College of Gastroenterology Guidelines for Colorectal Cancer Screening 2008. Am J Gastroenterol 104:739–750, 2009.

Rex DK, Petrini JL, Baron TH, et al: Quality indicators for colonoscopy. Gastrointest Endosc 63(4 Suppl):S16–S28, 2006.

Roetzheim RG, Pal N, Gonzalez EC, et al: The effects of physician supply on the early detection of colorectal cancer. J Fam Pract 48:850, 1999.

Schoenfeld P, Cash B, Flood A, et al: Colonoscopic screening of average-risk women for colorectal neoplasia. N Engl J Med 352:2061–2068, 2005.

Sedlack RE, Baron TH, Downing SM, Schwartz AJ: Validation of a colonoscopy simulation model for skills assessment. Am J Gastroenterol 102: 64–74, 2007.

Silverstein FE, Tytgat G: Atlas of Gastrointestinal Endoscopy, 3rd ed. London, Mosby, 1997.

Singh H, Turner D, Xue L, et al: Risk of developing colorectal cancer following a negative colonoscopy examination: Evidence for a 10-year interval between colonoscopies. JAMA 295:2366–2373, 2007.

Smith RA, Cokkinides V, Eyre HJ: American Cancer Society guidelines for the early detection of cancer, 2006. CA Cancer J Clin 56:11–25, 2006.

Soetikno RM, Kaltenbach T, Rouse RV, et al: Prevalence of nonpolypoid (flat and depressed) colorectal neoplasms in asymptomatic and symptomatic adults. JAMA 299:1027–1035, 2008.

Tytgat GNJ, Classen M, Waye JD, Nakazawa S (eds): Practice of Therapeutic Endoscopy, 2nd ed. Philadelphia, WB Saunders, 2002.

U.S. Preventive Services Task Force (USPSTF): Screening for colorectal cancer: Recommendation statement. October 2008. Available at www.ahrq.gov/clinic/uspstf08/colocancer/colors.htm.

Van Gelder RE, Nio CY, Florie J, et al: Computed tomographic colonography compared with colonoscopy in patients at increased risk for colorectal cancer. Gastroenterology 127:41–48, 2004.

Volkers N: How can physicians define and improve procedural competency? Ann Intern Med 125:I39, 1996.

Wilcox CM: Atlas of Clinical Gastrointestinal Endoscopy, 2nd ed. Philadelphia, Saunders, 2007.

Wilkins T, LeClair B, Smolkin M, et al: Screening colonoscopies by primary care physicians: A meta-analysis. Ann Fam Med 7:56–62, 2009.

Wilkins T, Reynolds PL: Colorectal cancer: A summary of the evidence for screening and prevention. Am Fam Physician 78:1385–1392, 1393–1394, 2008.

Wilkins T, Wagner P, Thomas A, et al: Attitudes toward performance of endoscopic colon cancer screening by family physicians. Fam Med 39:578–584, 2007.

Williams C: Insertion technique. In Waye JD, Rex DK, Williams CB (eds): Colonoscopy: Principles and Practice. Oxford, Blackwell, 2003, pp 318–338.

Wilson W, Taubert KA, Gewitz M, et al., for the American Heart Association Rheumatic Fever, Endocarditis and Kawasaki Disease Committee; Council on Cardiovascular Disease in the Young; Council on Clinical Cardiology; the Council on Cardiovascular Surgery and Anesthesia; and the Quality of Care and Outcomes Research Interdisciplinary Working Group. Prevention of infective endocarditis [published correction appears in Circulation]. Circulation 116:1736–1754, 2007.

Winawer SJ, Zauber AG, Fletcher RH, et al: Guidelines for colonoscopy surveillance after polypectomy: A consensus update by the US Multi-Society Task Force on Colorectal Cancer and the American Cancer Society. CA Cancer J Clin 56:143–159, 2006.

Worthington DV: AAFP position paper. Colonoscopy: Procedural skills. Am Fam Physician 62:1177–1182, 2000.

Xirasagar S, Hurley TG, Sros L, Hebert JR: Quality and safety of screening colonoscopies performed by primary care physicians with standby specialist support. Med Care 48:703–709, 2010.

CHAPTER 101

Esophagogastroduodenoscopy

Edward G. Zurad

During the past four decades, performing flexible fiberoptic esophagogastroduodenoscopy (EGD), or gastroscopy, has revealed a myriad of diseases and conditions of the upper gastrointestinal tract to primary care physicians, surgeons, and gastroenterologists. Refinements in equipment and technology have dramatically improved endoscopic diagnosis. Advancements have also permitted any interested physician, in a variety of settings, to evaluate and treat patients with both simple and complex problems of the esophagus, stomach, and the duodenum. Rapid diagnosis of upper gastrointestinal (GI) pathology with appropriate pharmaceutical and surgical management assures a high level of cost-effective care that any primary care physician can provide.

EGD is relatively quick and can be completed within 5 to 20 minutes. The procedure can be performed in various clinical environments, including the office, outpatient endoscopic suite, the hospital, or surgical center. The procedure can even be completed in the intensive care unit (ICU) or emergency room (ER) setting with a portable endoscopy cart. One study (Rodney and colleagues, 1990) indicated that when primary physicians performed EGD, it was associated with enhanced management and improved diagnostic accuracy in 89% of cases. Primary care physicians now perform flexible sigmoidoscopy, EGD, and colonoscopy on an increasingly frequent basis in their offices.

In EGD, a small flexible endoscope is introduced through the mouth (or with newer thinner diameter scopes, through the nose) and advanced through the pharynx, esophagus, stomach, and usually into the second portion of the duodenum. Both the fiberoptic and video gastroscopes are similar in construction to the flexible sigmoidoscope, the device with which many primary care physicians began to develop skills over the past three decades. Most modern endoscopes use a video chip (charge coupled device) for improved and more definitive imaging, as opposed to the older endoscopes, in which fiberoptics are used for image transmission. The tip of the scope can be moved in multiple directions. The endoscope has *channels for air insufflation, air aspiration, biopsy, and water instillation.*

The procedure is usually performed while the patient is under conscious sedation, although it can be completed with only topical anesthesia (a common practice in Asia). General anesthesia is reserved for a select group of patients who are difficult to sedate because of chronic narcotic drug usage or who may have allergies to the very effective agents now available for conscious sedation.

The EGD technique is also utilized when performing endoscopic ultrasound (EUS) and endoscopic interventions that are outside the realm of this chapter, including endoscopic retrograde cholangiopancreatography (ERCP) and transthoracic echocardiography.

Indications

Symptoms

In many instances, it is one of the following symptoms that prompt the physician's decision to consider an EGD:

- Dyspepsia (abdominal pain)
- Dysphagia (difficulty swallowing)
- Odynophagia (painful swallowing)
- Early satiety
- Recurrent regurgitation or gastroesophageal reflux disease (GERD)
- Epigastric pain
- When swallowing, sensation of food sticking or a foreign body
- Meal-related heartburn
- Severe indigestion
- Chronic nausea and vomiting
- Substernal or paraxiphoid pain
- Severe weight loss
- Persistent anorexia
- Noncardiac chest pain

Because over-the counter (OTC) proton pump inhibitors (PPIs) and histamine-2 (H_2) antagonist therapy are available, many patients independently initiate therapy for their upper gastrointestinal symptoms. They present to their primary care physician only after failing a self-directed trial of PPIs or H_2 antagonists. In addition, many patients have tried antacids or other agents for their upper gastrointestinal symptoms that have failed, which results in their concern for detection of the etiology of recalcitrant symptoms. EGD provides a precise evaluation to obtain a direct endoscopic assessment of the esophagus, stomach, and duodenum. Furthermore, EGD permits the physician to retrieve tissue specimens for pathologic analysis during this brief invasive procedure, which is of increasing importance.

Signs

- Unexplained anemia
- Gross or occult gastrointestinal bleeding
- Radiographic abnormality of the upper GI tract
- Weight loss
- Abdominal mass
- Hematemesis

Preexisting Conditions

Conditions that require further evaluation or surveillance with direct EGD include the following:

- Cancer surveillance in high-risk patients (e.g., those with Barrett's esophagitis, gastric polyposis, pernicious anemia)
- Esophageal stricture
- Acute or chronic duodenitis
- Acute or chronic esophagitis
- Acute or chronic gastritis
- Symptomatic hiatal hernia
- Gastric ulcer monitoring
- Gastric retention
- Duodenal ulcer disease

- Pyloroduodenal stenosis
- Esophageal or gastric varices
- Angiodysplasia in other area of the GI tract

CONTRAINDICATIONS

There are relatively few contraindications to the performance of EGD. The diameter of the currently available fiberoptic endoscopes is similar to the diameter of the nasogastric (NG) tubes that are inserted on a daily basis in most hospitals. The safety of the procedure is readily acknowledged. Most primary care physicians inserted NG tubes during their early medical school education and residency training. Recalling the simplicity of these early experiences should help clinicians feel more confident about the insertion of an EGD scope.

Contraindications to EGD include the following.

Absolute

- History of a bleeding disorder (e.g., platelet dysfunction, hemophilia)
- History of profusely bleeding esophageal varices
- Cardiopulmonary instability from any cause
- Recent myocardial infarction
- Suspected perforated viscus
- Uncooperative patient
- Absence of informed consent

Relative

Anticoagulants

Diagnostic EGD is considered a low-risk procedure for bleeding in patients taking anticoagulants and, therefore, can be performed without adjustment of anticoagulants prior to the procedure by physicians *extremely* familiar with EGD technique. Difficult or traumatic intubation of the scope could result in cricopharyngeal hematoma, which could theoretically cause carotid artery occlusion. A risk of retropharyngeal hematoma also may be present in patients with severe coagulation abnormalities.

If biopsy or polypectomy is contemplated, then the patient's coagulation profile should be normalized. Certain therapeutic procedures (i.e., dilations, percutaneous gastrostomy, polypectomy, endoscopic sphincterotomy, EUS-guided fine-needle aspiration, laser ablation, coagulation) are considered high-risk procedures for bleeding, and adjustment of anticoagulation is required. The use of low-molecular-weight heparin bridge therapy may be necessary for individuals with chronic atrial fibrillation or valvular heart prostheses in order to prevent the risk of embolic events.

EQUIPMENT

Endoscopes are produced by several different manufacturers (e.g., Olympus, Pentax, Fujinon, Visions Sciences).

The typical esophagogastroscope consists of an "*umbilical cord*" (containing transmitted light and imaging capabilities), *control head* (with hand-operated wheels for up/down and left/right, air/water control buttons, and a suction button), and the *long insertion* tube, which is approximately 100 cm long and 7.8 to 11 mm wide. The bending section at the tip of the scope allows up to 180 degrees of deflection for retroflexion of the tip of the endoscope.

The endoscope contains a *lumen* for insufflation of *air* and *water*, a *working channel* of 2 to 3 mm diameter (larger channel diameter for therapeutic endoscopes) used for suctioning and passage of instruments, *control wires* for moving the tip of the endoscope, and the *imaging system* that is either fiberoptic (rare) or video (widely available). The endoscope light source and imaging source (either video monitor or direct-view through the eyepiece) are critical aspects of the scope. Images and video can be recorded and printed depending on the equipment used.

Flexible ultrathin fiberoptic and video endoscopes can be used without sedation for office-based EGD. Commonly used without conscious sedation, these endoscopes are inserted transnasally or perorally and have a working length of 925 to 1100 mm, an external diameter of 5.3 to 6 mm, and a working channel diameter of 2 mm. With *interventional scopes*, multiple instruments have been developed that can be introduced through the working channel of the endoscope. These instruments include biopsy *forceps*, *snares*, *sclerotherapy needles*, *heater probes*, *electrocautery probes*, *balloon-dilation devices*, *nets*, *and baskets*. Guidewires can be placed, and, when the endoscope is withdrawn, wire-guided bougie *dilators* can be utilized. Devices can also be placed onto the end of the endoscope for *banding* of esophageal varices and endoscopic mucosal resection.

Some of the newer endoscopes provide *high resolution and magnification*. Such scopes are used for the evaluation of certain upper gastrointestinal diseases. The upper endoscope is also used to guide endoscopic treatment of GERD, such as with the Bard EndoCinch endoscopic suturing device and the NDO full-thickness plicator. One of the more recent advances in video endoscopy is *narrow band imaging* (NBI). NBI uses optical filters and high relative intensity of blue light for imaging and assessment of mucosal morphology and topography, such as mucosal and superficial vascular patterns. NBI has been studied in patients with Barrett's esophagus, early gastric tumors, and colorectal lesions and has had promising results. Its full clinical utility has yet to be realized. In addition to the endoscope, other important equipment should be in operational order prior to starting an EGD:

- Light source (halogen light source versus xenon)
- Camera source
- Color video printer
- Video monitor
- Video recorder
- Biopsy forceps/brush
- Endoscopy table/cart
- Intravenous (IV) stand and IV sets
- Mouth guard
- Stool with wheels for the endoscopist (if he or she sits during the performance of the procedure)
- Sphygmomanometer versus continuous blood pressure monitor
- Stethoscope
- Electrocardiogram (ECG) machine or continuous cardiac monitor
- Oxygen saturation monitor (pulse oximeter) (consider Welch Allyn system that performs all necessary monitoring functions)
- Dextrose 5% and 0.45% sodium chloride solution (1 L) or lactated Ringer's solution
- Suction equipment and tubing
- Specimen jars with formalin solution
- Syringes and needles
- K-Y Jelly (water-soluble) scope lubricant
- Protective gloves (remember latex sensitivity in sensitive patients)
- Rapid urease test (CLO test) materials
- Anesthetic, sedative, and narcotic medications (see Chapter 2, Procedural Sedation and Analgesia)
- Oxygen and delivery mask or nasal cannula
- "Crash cart" supplies (consider the Banyan kit—"a crash cart in suitcase"—if procedure is being performed in the office)
- Toothpicks to remove tissue from biopsy forceps
- Dictation capabilities or computer for immediate completion of the procedural record
- Sink/supplies for cleaning the scope

Cleaning Supplies

- Plastic containers for the endoscope tube
- Surgical scrub solution and water (follow the manufacturer's recommendations)
- Enzyme solution

- 70% isopropyl alcohol
- Glutaraldehyde soaking solution (follow the manufacturer's recommendations)
- Brushes and various channel insertion devices provided by manufacturer for internal channel cleaning

Preprocedure Patient Preparation

As with any procedure, EGD needs to be explained to the patient in detail prior to the procedure. The possible risks, benefits, and complications must be reviewed. It is wise to include a *patient education handout* and instructions for the patient to follow before the procedure (see the patient education handout online at www.expertconsult.com). The patient should also be given a copy of these to take home to share with a spouse or other family members.

Informed consent must be obtained before performance of EGD (see the patient consent form online at www.expertconsult.com). A preprocedure video or DVD that the patient and spouse or family member can view will reduce anxiety regarding the upcoming EGD. This video, which can be obtained from various pharmaceutical companies free of charge, will also introduce the subject of conscious sedation and review contraindications to the procedure. Figures 101-1 to 101-6 show other helpful forms for office use.

Antibiotic Prophylaxis

According to the latest American Heart Association guidelines, antibiotic prophylaxis for endoscopy with or without gastrointestinal biopsy is not recommended (see Chapter 221, Antibiotic Prophylaxis). No published data demonstrate a conclusive link between procedures of the GI tract and the development of bacterial endocarditis. No studies exist that demonstrate that the administration of antimicrobial prophylaxis prevents endocarditis in association with procedures performed on the upper GI tract.

Sedation

See Chapter 2, Procedural Sedation and Analgesia, and Chapter 7, Pediatric Sedation and Analgesia.

EGD has traditionally been performed in a hospital procedure room specializing in gastrointestinal disorders (a "GI suite"). It has also commonly been performed in an emergency room setting, an outpatient surgery facility, or a hospital operating room specially equipped for endoscopic procedures. Facility fee costs and sedation fees exceed physician reimbursement severalfold. Many physicians have completed the procedure in their offices simply using a topical anesthetic spray (Table 101-1).

Most physicians who perform EGD in their offices use a combination of a benzodiazepine and a narcotic to achieve appropriate sedation and pain control for EGD. An angiocath is usually placed when IV medications are to be used during the performance of EGD. The angiocath is connected to an IV line with IV fluids that are usually composed of D_5 (5% dextrose and one half normal saline) and normal saline. It is essential that resuscitation equipment and reversal drugs are readily available throughout the course of the procedure.

Many endoscopists now routinely use oxygen delivered through nasal cannula at 2 L/min to prevent any likelihood of hypoxemia that can occur during EGD, resulting from the mechanical nature of the tube in the upper airway region. This allows for a continuous source of oxygen delivery. The patient can be stimulated to inhale by simply advising him or her to take a deep breath. If oxygen is not used in a continuous fashion during the performance of the

Staff Gastroscopy Instructions Guidelines

1. Be sure the patient has a copy of the patient teaching guides and that he or she understands and has read the instructions.
2. Advise the patient that the purpose of the study is to insert a tube through the mouth into the stomach and into the beginning of the small intestine in order to inspect the upper GI tract. We will be looking for inflammation, ulcers, growths, bleeding points, a hiatal hernia, and abnormal growths.
3. The following medications will probably be used: a "Caine" topical anesthetic, Demerol, and Valium or Versed. Be sure to inquire about sensitivity or allergy to any of the medications just mentioned. These medications act to depress the central nervous system. The patient's current medications, particularly tranquilizers, sedatives, sleeping pills, and muscle relaxants, must be reviewed, and their effects when taken with preprocedure medication must be considered.
4. Possible serious side effects are extremely unlikely, but they include bleeding, perforation of the GI tract, tearing of the vocal cords (voice box), aspiration of stomach contents into the lungs, tearing of the mucosa, or even death from a severe reaction (e.g., to medications).
5. All patients will have gagging, but very few (if any) will experience any discomfort with gagging if they take the full prep. Patients who take the full prep will be groggy, sleepy, or lethargic for a variable period after the procedure. They must not drive or do anything "delicate" for at least 4 hours following the procedure if they received a prep. If grogginess persists, they should wait until they are fully alert. We recommend waiting 8 hours, if possible. If patients have a medical condition that affects medication metabolism, the wait will most likely be longer.
6. The procedure can be performed in a highly motivated patient without any preparation, but the gagging is uncomfortable and tends to persist throughout the procedure. It does, however, decrease after the scope is partially inserted. A topical anesthetic spray will greatly decrease gagging in the patient who chooses to not have IV sedation.

EGD Checklist

Be sure to be aware of the following:

Recent use of:	ASA	Persantine	Motrin	Advil	NSAIDs	Coumadin	Plavix
Preexisting disease:	Asthma	Heart disease	COPD	Phlebitis	Prosthetic valves or joints		

If plans to deal with any of the above medications or preexisting diseases are not recorded in the chart, please discuss with the physician how to handle the situation.

Notes:________________________________

Figure 101-1 Sample form of instruction guidelines for gastroscopy staff. (From The Medical Procedures Center, Midland, Mich.)

Counseling for Office EGD (Upper Endoscopy)

Name: ______________________ DOB______________ Age________

Telephone (H)____________________ (W)________________

Your referring doctor:____

Primary care doctor:____________________________ Want a copy sent to him/her?________

Blood pressure______________________ Received, read, and understood handouts?____________

SYMPTOMS/HISTORY: Reason for consult: ________________________________

Nausea
Vomiting
Heartburn
Need for antacids/H2 blockers
Early satiety
Positive *H. pylori* test
Family Hx of stomach Ca

Previous gastric ulcer
Duodenal ulcer
Esophagitis
Bloating
Pain with swallowing
Difficulty swallowing
Who?____________________

Food getting stuck
Black, tarry stools
Anemia
Belching
Atypical chest pain

PAST MEDICAL HISTORY:

Ulcer treatment
Ex-smoker–quit
Aspirin use
NSAID use
Bleeding problems
Pulmonary disease
Heart disease

Other medical problems
(1)____________________
(2)____________________
(3)____________________
(4)____________________
(5)____________________

Current Medications
(1)____________________
(2)____________________
(3)____________________
(4)____________________
(5)____________________

Allergies ____

OBJECTIVE:
General
Mouth Dentures or partials Teeth: chips
Neck: ability to hyperextend
Lungs
Heart
Abdomen

IMPRESSION:
(1) Good candidate for EGD
(2)
(3)
(4)

COUNSELING:
Bleeding
Aspiration
Perforation

Sore throat
Infection
Medication reaction

Sedation options:
Halcion/Stadol vs. IV sedation (Demerol/Versed) or topical only. Other____________________
Driver if sedated

PLAN:
(1) Halcion 0.25 mg 2 tablets PO 1 hr PRN with sip of water or IV sedation or topical
(2) NPO after midnight
(3) Driver if sedation
(4) Scheduled for EGD
(5)
(6)

____ Date______________
Physician's signature

Figure 101-2 Sample form for esophagogastroduodenoscopy (EGD) counseling. (From The Medical Procedures Center, Midland, Mich.)

Guidelines for Monitoring the Patient Receiving Sedation and Anelgesia for Gastrointestinal Endoscopy: A Summation

1. Patient monitoring is one aspect of the overall quality assurance program for the endoscopy unit.
2. A well-trained gastrointestinal assistant, working closely with the endoscopist, is the most important part of the monitoring process.
3. The use of equipment to monitor patients may be a useful adjunct to patient surveillance, but it is never a substitute for conscientious clinical assessment.
4. Although changes in blood pressure, pulse, cardiac rhythm, and oxygen saturation do occur during endoscopy, no controlled studies address the question of whether noninvasive monitoring with equipment decreases complications.
5. The amount of monitoring should be proportional to the perceived risk of the patient undergoing the procedure. It may vary from one procedure to the next.
6. The minimal clinical monitoring advised for all sedated patients should include the determination of heart rate, blood pressure, and respiratory rate before sedation, during the procedure, immediately after the procedure, and when the patient is released from the endoscopy area.
7. The proper role for pulse oximetry and continuous electrocardiographic monitoring during endoscopic procedures is controversial and unsettled.
8. Given the cost of the equipment and the manpower to use it, the best decision as to whether such monitoring should be used would be based on data showing an effect on clinical outcome. Such data do not exist; however, in those situations in which the individualized need of the patient indicates that measurement of cardiac rhythm or oxygen saturation will complement the clinical assessment, the use of cardiac monitoring or pulse oximetry may be beneficial.

Figure 101-3 Sample form of monitoring instructions for gastroscopy staff. (From Fleischer D: Monitoring the patient receiving conscious sedation for gastrointestinal endoscopy: Issues and guidelines. Gastrointest Endosc 35:262, 1989.)

EGD Nursing Checklist

Patient______________________________ Date__________ Age__________

Notify the physician if an unexpected, unusual, or negative answer is obtained.
Have the patient change into a gown.
Orient the patient to the room and the equipment.
Confirm the patient read the handouts and took oral medication at home.
Consent signed.
NPO since____________________
Someone is present to drive the patient home.
Current meds______________________________
Drug allergies______________________________
Recent use of anticoagulants
Preexisting and/or existing disease: None Heart Lung Other
Biopsy forceps, specimen cups, and slides ready.
Gloves, lubricant, and 4x4s available.
Resuscitation equipment available and ready, including oxygen.
Scope leakage tested.
Suction and water bottles prepared and connected.
If needed: IV 500 mL D5W /D51⁄2 NS /NS started in LUE/RUE with #__________ Intracath/butterfly
by______________ at__________ AM/PM.
Assist with obtaining and processing biopsies.
Secure the safety of the patient after the procedure.
Print record of vital signs and disconnect monitoring equipment.
Vital signs record attached.
Clean the equipment.
Disconnect IV fluids if used.
Prepare the patient for the physician conference.
Escort patient out with instruction sheets.

	Time
Patient in room	
Sedation started	
Procedure started (scope inserted)	
Procedure ended	
Patient discharged	

Medications	Dosage	Time

Figure 101-4 Sample form of esophagogastroduodenoscopy (EGD) nursing checklist. (From The Medical Procedures Center, Midland, Mich.)

EGD Procedure

Name:____ BD:____________ Date:____________

The patient gave informed consent for the procedure. Intravenous access was obtained in the R/L upper extremity. Topical anesthesia was used in the pharynx. The patient was placed in the left lateral position, and the neck flexed to the chest. The bite block was placed gently, and the scope lubricated and passed through the bite block over the tongue. The hypopharynx was visualized, the vocal cords visualized, and the scope passed through the cricopharyngeus. The scope was passed into the distal esophagus with the GE junction seen and diaphragmatic indentation noted by the sniff test. The scope was advanced into the stomach and the gastric lake suctioned. The scope was passed through the pylorus and maneuvered into the descending duodenum. The duodenum and duodenal bulb were visualized and the scope brought back into the stomach. A biopsy for CLO testing was obtained. The scope was retroflexed to view the cardia. The scope was pulled into the esophagus and the esophagus closely examined. The scope was withdrawn, and the patient tolerated the procedure well. Monitoring showed normal cardiac/oxygen status. The patient was informed of the procedure results. Pulse oximetry monitoring was used throughout the procedure to evaluate the patient for hypoxemia. A printed report is attached.
Changes to above procedure: None or ____

Anesthesia:	Versed________ mg IV Demerol________ mg IV Topical Cetacaine spray Xylocaine 2% liquid	Monitoring:	Oximetry Cardiac monitoring Blood pressure

Complications: ____
Areas not well visualized:____
Abnormalities noted:

Bleeding	Erythema	Friability	Erosion	Polyp	Tumor
Ulcer, gastric	Ulcer, duo	Barrett's	Diverticula	Gastric bile	Varices
Dilation	Hiatal hernia	Carcinoma	Stenosis	Scarring	Angiodysplasia

Biopsies performed:____

Diagnoses:

535.00	Gastritis, acute	531.00	Gastric ulcer, acute with hemorrhage
530.81	Esophageal reflux	535.60	Duodenitis
532.00	Duodenal ulcer	553.3	Hiatal hernia, acute with hemorrhage
530.1	Esophagitis, reflux	Other	

Plan: ________________________	Stop smoking Avoid NSAIDs Avoid chocolate/mints Avoid offending foods	Low fat diet Elevate head of bed 4–6 inches Do not eat 2 hours before bedtime

cc:________________________ Physician________________________________

Figure 101-5 Sample form for the esophagogastroduodenoscopy (EGD) procedure. (From The Medical Procedures Center, Midland, Mich.)

procedure, oxygen must be available in the event that hypoxemia occurs.

Midazolam (Versed) is a sedative/hypnotic commonly used for sedation. The peak effect of midazolam is seen within 3 to 5 minutes. It has a duration of action of 1 to 3 hours. Some of the major adverse effects include respiratory depression, hypotension, and rarely seen paradoxic agitation. The typical starting dose is 0.5 to 1 mg IV, which can be titrated to achieve a desirable level of sedation (usually in 1-mg increments every 2–3 minutes). Lower doses of midazolam should be administered to elderly patients with cardiopulmonary problems to avoid serious respiratory depression.

Diazepam (Valium) may be used instead of midazolam for sedation during EGD, but many centers prefer midazolam (over diazepam) because of its well-received amnestic effect and reduced tendency to cause local vein phlebitis. Diazepam is initiated at 1 to 2 mg IV and titrated at 2-mg doses given every 1 to 2 minutes. This agent can also cause respiratory depression and should be used carefully in elderly patients. Paradoxic excitation can be seen with this sedative.

Benzodiazepines can rarely cause paradoxic excitement. If it occurs, however, pure narcotics can usually be used to complete the procedure. In extreme cases cancel the procedure and reschedule it when assistance with sedation is available.

Meperidine (Demerol) is a narcotic analgesic that has mild sedative properties, slow onset of action, long duration, and long recovery time. When coadministered with benzodiazepines, potential complications include respiratory depression and sedation. The peak effect of meperidine is approximately 10 minutes, with a duration of action of 2 to 3 hours. Adverse effects include respiratory depression, hypotension, nausea, and vomiting. The typical starting dose is 12.5 to 50 mg IV, with subsequent doses not to exceed 25 mg/dose.

Fentanyl (Sublimaze) is a mildly sedative narcotic analgesic that has a rapid onset of action and short recovery time. In many endoscopy centers, fentanyl is the preferred agent for outpatient EGD. The peak effect is 5 to 8 minutes, and the duration of action is 1 to 3 hours. One of the major adverse effects is respiratory depression. The typical starting dose is 0.03 to 0.1 mg IV, with subsequent doses of 0.02 to 0.05 mg/dose.

When IV sedation is used, the end point to be titrated is slurred speech with the patient still able to be aroused.

Several agents are used as *reversal agents* for conscious sedation. Physicians employing conscious sedation should be very familiar with these agents. Naloxone (Narcan) reverses opioid-induced analgesia, central nervous system (CNS) effects, and respiratory depression. Naloxone has a peak effect of 1 to 2 minutes and a potential duration of action of 1 to 3 hours. Adverse effects include pain, agitation, nausea, vomiting, arrhythmias, sudden death, pulmonary edema, and withdrawal syndrome in patients with chronic opioid abuse. The typical dose is 0.04 mg IV for reversal of

Role of the Assistant

The well-trained and motivated assistant makes the EGD examination a pleasant task for the physician. It is not necessary for the attendant to attend a special course, but it is necessary to spend time learning each step of the procedure. Representatives from the endoscope manufacturer will assist in training assistants in the cleaning and care of the scopes. It is important to have assistants trained in CPR.

Before the patient arrives for the procedure, the assistant must do the following:
1. Prepare the room.
2. Have the IV set up, medications, endoscope, and the resuscitation equipment ready (but not opened).
3. Prepare the paperwork.

When the patient arrives, the assistant must do the following:
1. Bring the patient to the procedure room.
2. Orient the patient to the room and the equipment.
3. Make sure consent forms are signed, and that the patient has read and understands the instructions.
4. Verify that the patient is properly prepared (NPO, has a qualified adult to accompany the patient home). Check patient allergies.

Review and record current patient medications.
5. Review the EGD procedure with the patient.
6. Record baseline vital signs.
7. Place EKG monitor pads and initiate oximetry and cardiac monitoring if indicated.
8. Initiate IV fluids at KVO if IV sedation used.
9. Give the patient topical anesthesia within 3 to 5 minutes of starting the procedure.

During the procedure, the assistant must do the following:
1. Record vital signs every 15 minutes during the procedure.
2. Assist the endoscopist with the scope, if needed.
3. Watch the monitoring equipment, and notify the physician of changes in patient status.
4. Assist with obtaining multiple biopsies and brushings.
5. Receive and process biopsy specimens and paperwork.

After the procedure, the assistant must do the following:
1. Monitor the patient's vital signs for 15 minutes.
2. Secure the safety of the patient, raise the gurney rails, etc.
3. Complete the paperwork associated with the procedure.
4. Remove monitoring equipment from the patient.
5. Clean the equipment.
6. Discontinue the IV fluids, if used.
7. Clean the room for the next procedure.
8. Prepare the patient for the physician conference.
9. Give the patient the instruction sheets.
10. Inform the person accompanying the patient of signs to observe.

Figure 101-6 Sample form detailing the role of the assistant. (From The Medical Procedures Center, Midland, Mich.)

analgesia/sedation and 0.4 mg for narcotic overdose and respiratory arrest.

Flumazenil (Romazicon) is typically used for reversal of benzodiazepine-induced sedation and respiratory depression. Flumazenil has a peak effect of 3 to 5 minutes and a duration of action of 1 to 2 hours. Potential adverse effects include resedation and seizures. The typical dose is 0.2 to 0.5 mg IV for reversal of sedation (up to 1 mg total) and 1 to 3 mg IV for benzodiazepine overdose. This agent must be used with care in patients who are chronic anxiolytic users because it could cause the onset of seizures.

The use of monitored anesthesia care (MAC) and propofol (Diprivan) has developed widespread patient acceptance because of the short recovery time required for the patient. Such an approach is typically utilized in outpatient surgical centers, hospitals, or GI endoscopic suites. Many institutions have special guidelines regarding the use of propofol due to its possible potent adverse effects, which include apnea and hypopnea.

Sufficient anesthesia or sedation can often be accomplished without IV drug administration, using new approaches that are called *non-IV conscious sedation*. With this technique, a patient can be given diazepam 10 mg orally 1 hour before the procedure, or lorazepam 1 to 2 mg sublingually 30 to 60 minutes before the procedure. Halcion, 0.5 mg orally, can also be used. An optional intramuscular dose of ketorolac (Toradol) 60 mg may be given 30 to 60 minutes before the procedure.

Butorphanol tartrate (Stadol), 1 to 2 sprays (intranasally), can be added if needed to the preceding regimen, or used alone. It generally provides both sedation and analgesia sufficient to carry out EGD. In many countries, EGD is performed with topical anesthesia only. Topical anesthesia with a benzocaine and tetracaine mixture (Cetacaine) or lidocaine has the advantages of requiring less time for the overall procedure, eliminating the risks of conscious sedation, and decreasing the cost of the procedure by reducing or eliminating recovery time and nursing staff and anesthesia personnel. The spray is directed toward the posterior osopharynx while advising the patient to avoid breathing during the application. Inhaling the spray can cause significant coughing and gagging.

The disadvantages of using only topical anesthesia are patient discomfort and problems in performing the procedure on an uncooperative patient. An *alternative choice* for *topical anesthesia* is the *"popsicle stick" method*. In this scenario, lidocaine ointment (2%) is squeezed on a tongue blade that is covered with the patient's favorite food flavoring, and this is placed into the back of the patient's throat. The patient sucks on the tongue blade while vital signs are completed and the patient is prepared for the procedure. A tongue blade can be pressed into the posterior oral pharynx to ascertain that appropriate topical anesthesia has been obtained before insertion of the endoscope. Lack of a gag reflex ensures the desired effect. With the cost-saving trends in medicine, and with the newer, smaller scopes, EGD without sedation will likely become more

TABLE 101-1 Drugs Used for Esophagogastroduodenoscopy

Medication	Dose
Narcotics	
Meperidine (Demerol) IV	10–75 mg (0.5–1 mg/kg)
Fentanyl (Sublimaze) IV	1–2 mg
Butorphanol tartrate (Stadol Nasal Spray)	1–2 mg (1–2 sprays in nostril)
Propofol	Variable*
Benzodiazepines	
Diazepam (Valium) IV	1–10 mg
Midazolam (Versed) IV	2–5 mg (0.035–0.1 mg/kg)
Lorazepam (Ativan) SL (onset in 10 min)	1–2 mg
Triazolam (Halcion) PO	0.5 mg
Anticholinergic	
Glycopyrrolate (Robinul)	0.002 mg (0.01 mL/kg) IM 1 hour before procedure or 0.1 mg (0.5 mL) repeated every 2–3 minutes as needed
Miscellaneous	
Simethicone (Mylicon) drops	0.6 mL (30–40 mg) in 30 mL of water PO (can also be flushed through the gastroscope with 5 mL of water)
Ketorolac (Toradol)	60 mg IM; 15 mg IV
Topical Local Anesthetics	
Lidocaine 2% viscous solution gargle	
Benzocaine 20% (Hurricaine) spray	
Benzocaine 14% and tetracaine 2% (Cetacaine)	
Antagonists	
Naloxone (Narcan) IV	0.2–0.8 mg
Flumazenil (Romazicon) IV	0.2–1 mg (start with 0.2 mg; repeat every 60 sec. to a maximum of 1 mg or until reversal of benzodiazepine effect has been achieved)
Nalmefene hydrogen chloride (Revex)	1–2 mL IV

IM, intramuscular; IV, intravenous; PO, orally; SL, sublingually.
*Sedation may be initiated by infusing propofol at 100 to 150 mcg/kg/min (6 to 9 mg/kg/h) for a period of 3 to 5 minutes and titrating to the desired clinical effect while closely monitoring respiratory function.

commonplace in the future. With the introduction of the previously described smaller caliber endoscopes that can be passed through the nose, EGD without sedation may be more acceptable to patients.

Currently available small-diameter scopes allow for a comfortable examination with little manipulation or trauma to the cricopharyngeal region. As stated previously, the diameter of the scope is similar to that of an NG tube inserted daily by hospital nursing staffs.

It is important to select patients wisely for office-based EGD. This is a critical step. In individuals who are in the high-risk group (Box 101-1), the clinician should consider performing EGD in a facility where complications can be handled and more aggressive monitoring procedures can be carried out. The utilization of MAC is suggested in such cases.

Monitoring

The current move to office endoscopy was initiated because of its many benefits, including safety and cost effectiveness. The American Academy of Family Physicians and the Joint Commission for Accreditation of Hospitals and Organizations do not recommend continuous ECG monitoring or continuous pulse oximetry for low-

Box 101-1. High-Risk Groups for Esophagogastroduodenoscopy

Agitated, uncooperative patient
Barium administration within a few hours of the procedure
Cardiopulmonary instability of any type
Current active bleeding
Older than 70 years old
Prosthetic cardiac valves
Recent cerebrovascular accident
Significant bleeding disorder or coagulopathy
Significant chronic obstructive pulmonary disease
Significant valvular heart disease
Uncontrolled coronary artery disease
Younger than 12 years old

risk patients. More extensive monitoring becomes necessary under the following conditions:

- Procedures that last longer than 30 minutes
- Large-bore scopes
- Individuals with significant cardiopulmonary disease
- Elderly patients (over 70)
- High-risk patients (see Box 101-1)
- Situations in which more than "light" sedation is used

In these scenarios more extensive clinical monitoring, including continuous ECG monitoring and pulse oximetry, is wise. All patients should have clinical monitoring of skin color, degree of sedation, loss of reflexes, blood pressure, pulse, and respiratory rate in a well-lighted room.

Technique

It is essential to ensure that aspirin, clopidogrel (Plavix), and platelet-inhibiting nonsteroidal anti-inflammatory drugs (NSAIDs) have been discontinued at least 7 days before the procedure. The patient must take nothing by mouth after midnight on the day of the examination (or at least 8 hours must have elapsed since eating).

The assistant should initiate the IV angiocath and connect it to the IV line. If pulse oximetry and continuous ECG monitoring are to be utilized, connect them at this time. Blood pressure, pulse, and respiration monitoring can also be started at this time and recorded.

1. Examine the oral cavity while the patient is in a sitting position. *Any dentures or foreign objects should be removed.*
2. If using a fiberoptic scope, ask the patient to swallow 40 mg of *simethicone* in 30 mL of tap water before the initiation of the procedure. This tends to minimize the reflective bubbles in the stomach (Fig. 101-7) that present considerable impediment to visibility during the procedure. Alternatively, simethicone can be used only if needed during the procedure (0.6 mL of simethicone liquid can be injected down the gastroscope followed by 5 mL of water).

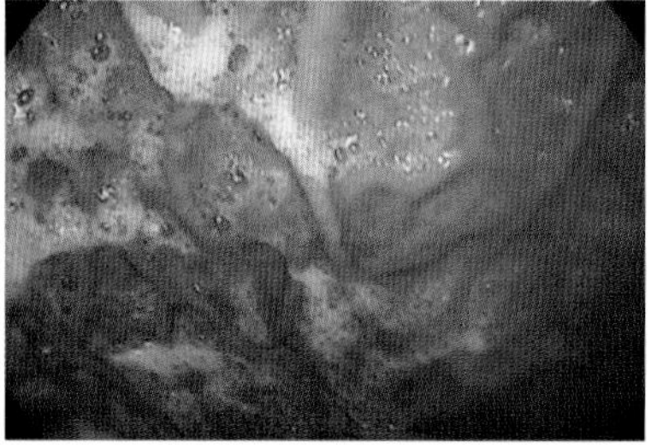

Figure 101-7 Bubbles in the stomach.

3. The topical anesthesia should be completed at this point, as noted previously.
4. After good *topical anesthesia* is ensured, the patient should be placed in the left lateral decubitus position, especially if sedated. Unsedated ECDs are often performed in the sitting position with the patient bent 45 degrees forward at the waist.
5. *Lubricate the distal 10 cm of the scope* with a minimal amount of water-soluble gel (an excessive amount may induce coughing or sneezing).
6. *Insert the mouth guard* into the patient's mouth; the teeth should grip this guard. The guard not only protects the patient's teeth, tongue, and oral mucosa but it also prevents the patient from damaging the scope. Introduce the scope through the mouth guard and direct it across the superior aspect of the tongue into the posterior oral pharynx.

   In the edentulous patient, the mouth guard can be placed over the scope and the scope can then be introduced through a channel created by placing the left second and third fingers of the examiner's hand over the back of the tongue.

   Guide the scope across the back of the tongue into the cricopharyngeal region. This is usually the first point of resistance encountered (approximately 17 cm from the incisor teeth and at the level of the vocal cords) (Fig. 101-8).

   Under direct vision, or blindly, ask the patient to swallow repeatedly while applying gentle pressure. The scope will easily pass through the *cricopharyngeus region* without difficulty and can then be advanced down through the esophagus (Fig. 101-9A and B).
7. *Never* use force as the scope passes the cricopharyngeus region. The patient's normal swallowing mechanism will assist in advancing the endoscope.
8. Once the tip of the endoscope has entered the esophagus, insufflate a small puff of air to open the esophagus to easily visualize the mucosa throughout the cylindric esophagus. Additional air will need to be insufflated after the scope reaches the stomach and duodenum.

   NOTE: Identify the channel in front of the scope before attempting to pass the scope to prevent injury to the patient. The lumen should always be seen during EGD.

   The endoscope should be advanced quickly but gently through the esophagus. The first landmark seen is the *bronchioaortic constriction* (Fig. 101-10).
9. As the scope is advanced, the *gastroesophageal (GE) junction (Z line)* is typically found at approximately 40 cm from the incisor teeth. It is essential to evaluate the esophagus and GE junction during this "first pass," because the mucosa may become irritated by the passage of the scope. This irritation can distort the appearance of the GE junction (Fig. 101-11A and B). There is a typical mucosal color demarcation that occurs at the GE junction, with the esophageal lining being pale pink and the gastric mucosa represented by a darker pink or orange hue.
10. At this time, *ask the patient to sniff* through his or her nose (i.e., the "sniff test") if the patient is partially conscious. As the patient sniffs, the crura of the diaphragm extrinsically compress the GE junction at the esophageal hiatus. If the Z line is visualized above the level of the extrinsic compression seen from the

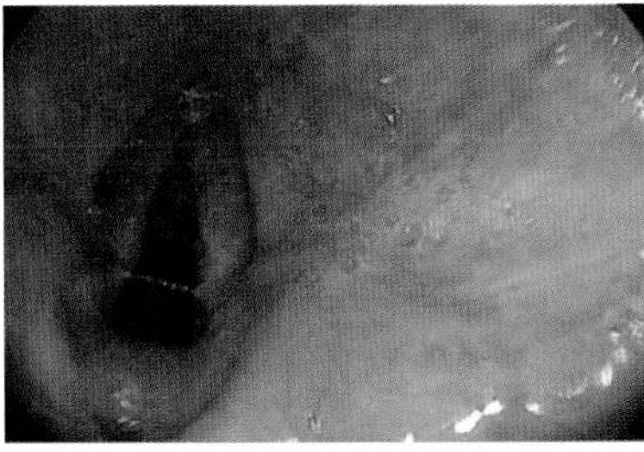

Figure 101-8 Open vocal cord.

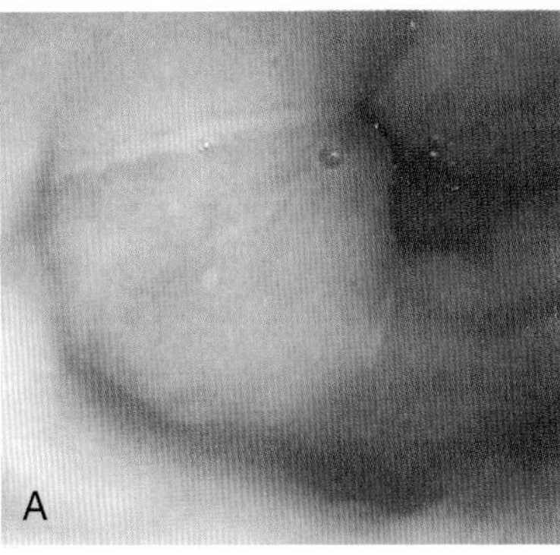

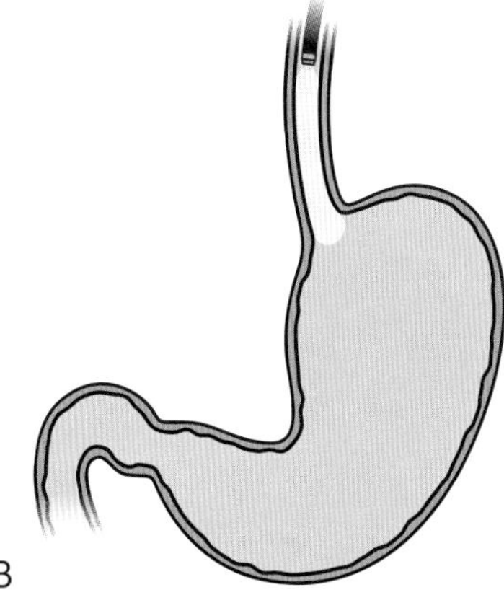

Figure 101-9 **A,** Proximal esophagus. **B,** Unshaded area is seen by lighted scope.

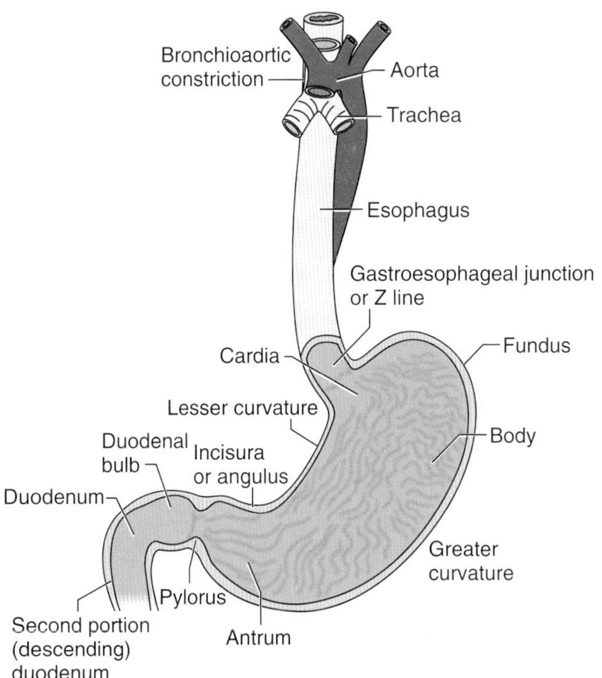

Figure 101-10 Relevant anatomy for gastroscopy. The *cardia* is that portion of the stomach immediately surrounding the esophageal opening. The *gastroesophageal junction* is also known as the GE junction, the Z line, ora serrata, or gastric rosette. The upper end or dome of the stomach is the *fundus*. The upturn of the J of the stomach is separated from its vertical portion by the *angular* notch (also known as the angulus, angularis, or incisura). The *antrum* lies to the right of the angulus and ends at the *pylorus*, or greatly thickened muscular wall. The *duodenum* lies beyond the pylorus. The *lesser curvature* is the upper right border of the stomach, whereas the *greater curvature* is the left inferior margin.

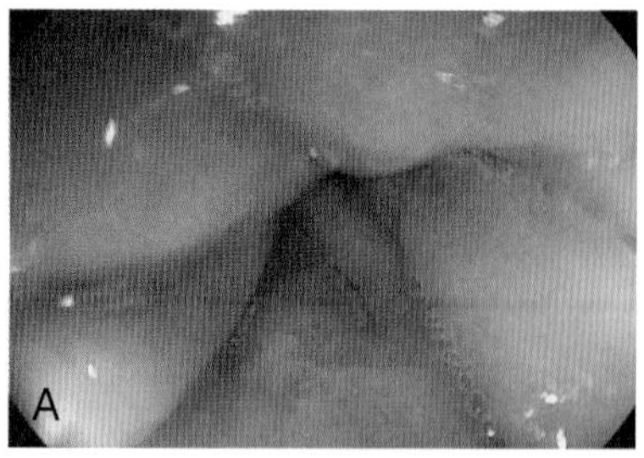

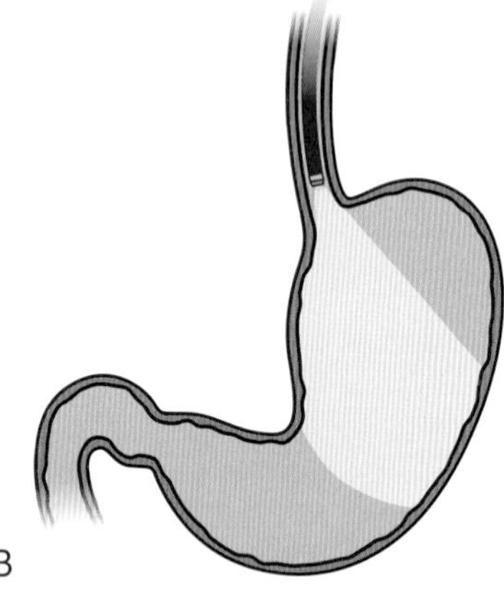

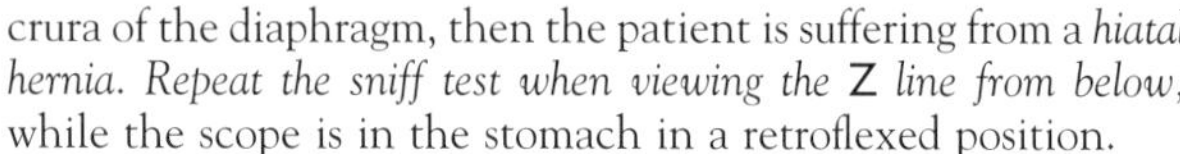

Figure 101-11 **A,** Distal esophagus Z line. **B,** Unshaded area is seen by lighted scope.

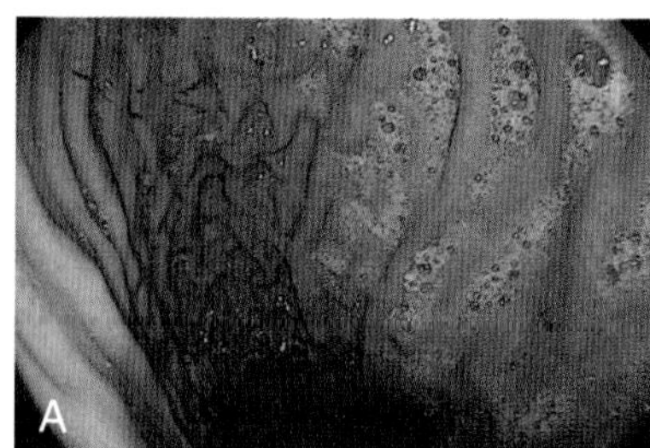

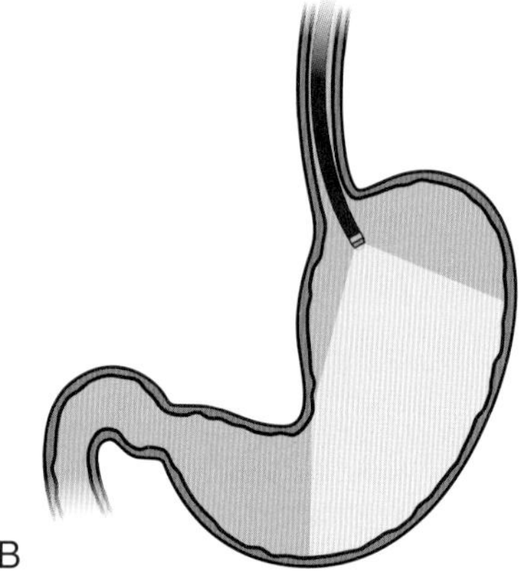

Figure 101-12 **A,** Gastric lake with reflective bubbles/fluid seen from 1 to 3 o'clock. **B,** Unshaded area is seen by lighted scope.

crura of the diaphragm, then the patient is suffering from a *hiatal hernia. Repeat the sniff test when viewing the Z line from below,* while the scope is in the stomach in a retroflexed position.

NOTE: Use air, water, suction, and "miniwithdrawals" as needed to pass the scope and to fully evaluate all surfaces of the mucosa.

11. After passing through the GE junction, the endoscope is inserted into the *stomach.* After the scope reaches the stomach, the gastric lake, which is a collection of fluids in the dependent portion of the stomach, will typically impair visibility (Fig. 101-12A and B). Air should be insufflated sufficiently to spread the mucosal walls apart so that this fluid can be aspirated. Some clinicians aspirate the gastric fluid and test the pH of the fluid to record the acidity of the gastric lake. After the fluid is removed and the lumen again is clearly visualized, the scope can rapidly be advanced following the rugae along the lesser curvature to the *angular notch.* The scope is subsequently passed below the angularis, then into the antrum and up to the pylorus (Figs. 101-13A to E, and see Fig. 101-10).

    NOTE: The scope should be adjusted so that the small black arrow is at the top of the field and so it corresponds with the incisura. This adjustment provides proper orientation with the patient in the left lateral position.

12. Guide the endoscope through the relaxed pyloric sphincter into the duodenal bulb (Fig. 101-14A and B). Do not attempt to pass the scope through a tightly closed pylorus. The repetitive trauma of attempting to do this will simply cause greater pylorospasm and prevent good evaluation of the duodenum. When the scope is passed through the pylorus into the duodenal bulb, it is common to encounter a *white-out* or a *red-out.* This is because the scope typically tends to rapidly advance to the junction of the first and second portions of the duodenum and press against the mucosal. At this point it is wise to withdraw the scope very slowly to reestablish the lumen and complete the duodenal examination. Biopsies are rarely needed in this area.
13. The second portion of the duodenum becomes retroperitoneal. Thus, it is wise to turn the scope to the right and pass the scope downward so that it can enter the second portion of the duodenum (see Fig. 101-13). The *second portion of the duodenum* is recognizable because of the vertical, cylindric nature of the viscera in this region. In addition, the *Kerckring's folds* (Fig. 101-15A) will readily appear. The *ampulla of Vater* (Fig. 101-15B) can be seen along the medial aspect of the second portion of the duodenum 20% to 30% of the time. It is not essential to evaluate this area for the completion of an EGD.
14. The scope can be advanced occasionally into the *third portion of the duodenum* or the horizontal portion of the duodenum.

    NOTE: At this point of the procedure, the insertion portion is complete, and it is time to withdraw the scope.

15. *Withdraw the endoscope* slowly with the attempt to evaluate the entire 360-degree circumferential portion of the mucosal surface. The second and sometimes the third portions of the duodenum can be evaluated readily.
16. The *duodenal bulb* is difficult to assess because, as it is being withdrawn, the scope typically tends to rapidly retract through the pyloric junction, back into the stomach. It is therefore necessary to reinsert it through the pylorus so that the duodenal bulb mucosa can be closely examined to rule out disease.
17. Once back into the stomach, it is helpful to deflect the scope tip up and down as the control head is rotated right and left to ensure that the entire gastric mucosal surface has been evaluated. If not previously performed, retroflex the scope so that it is viewing itself and observe the GE junction. Examine the cardia and fundus (Fig. 101-16A to D).
18. *Straighten the scope tip deflections before removing the scope through the GE junction.* One way to do this is to align the letters on the large inner wheel (up/down control) and the small outer wheel (left/right control) before withdrawing the instrument. If the scope is withdrawn with the tip retroflexed, it could result in mucosal damage of the GE junction or an esophageal tear.

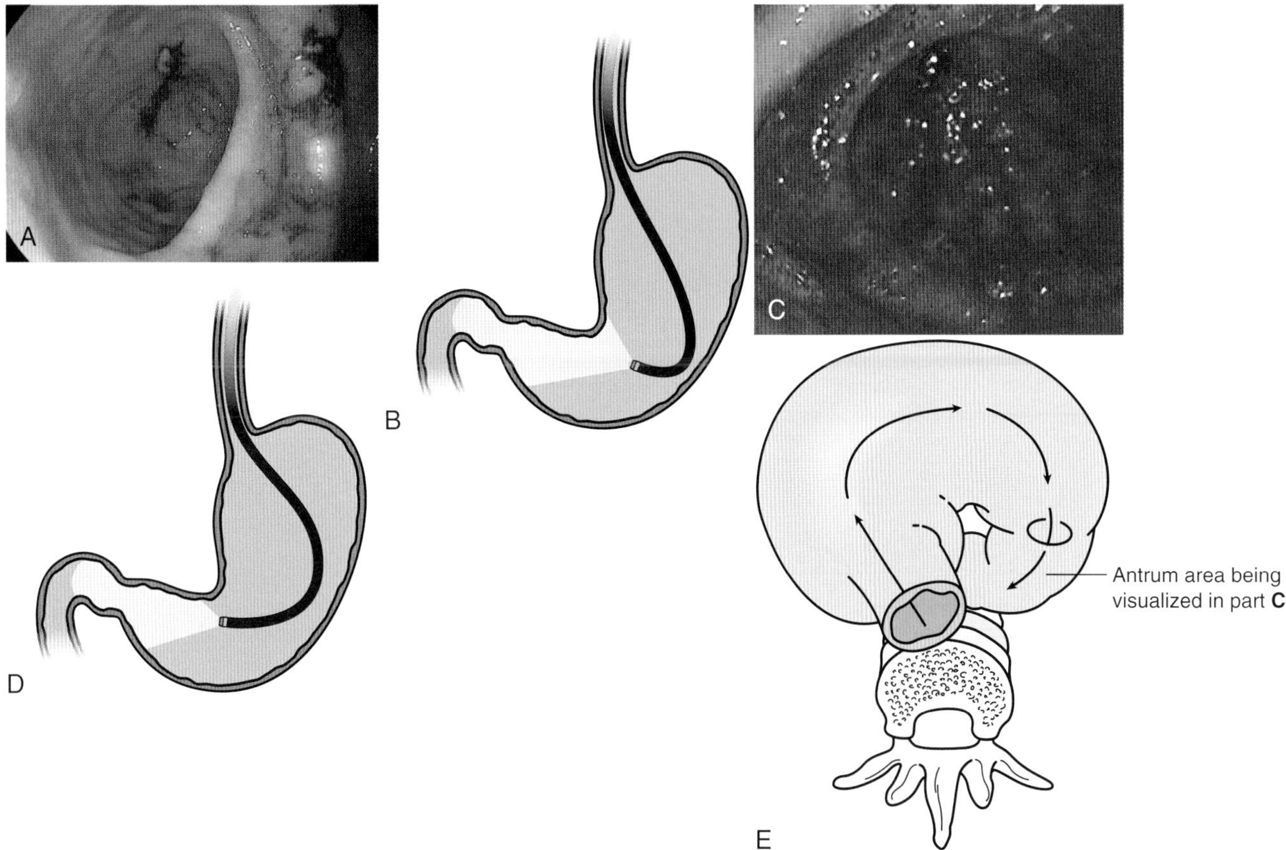

Figure 101-13 **A,** Angularis is along the right side of visual field. Pyloris is in the distance but cannot be seen due to angularis obstructing the view. Prepyloric ulcer is seen at 11 o'clock. **B,** Unshaded area is seen by lighted scope. **C,** Antrum at the 6 o'clock position. Pyloric opening and angularis at the 12 o'clock position. **D,** Unshaded area is seen by lighted scope. **E,** To reach the pylorus, the clinician should make a clockwise spiral around the vertebral column.

19. The scope is withdrawn through the GE junction slowly. Again, close evaluation of the GE junction is completed. *Complete a sniff test at this region one final time.*
20. As the procedure is being carried out, photographs can be taken on a continuing basis, both during the initial insertion and during withdrawal.
21. *Biopsies* during EGD are completed as the scope is withdrawn to prevent significant downstream bleeding that can impair visibility of the mucosal surface (see the "Biopsy" section).
22. It is important to *record the appearance of the vocal cords* before the scope is withdrawn. The documentation of an attempt to view the vocal cords is an important component of EGD before the removal of the scope, even if they cannot be seen because of coughing or gagging.
23. The assistant should complete the monitoring process of the patient after the scope is withdrawn. The mouth guard should also be removed, and the physician may want to reexamine the patient before discharge from the facility. A 30-minute observation period after the procedure is typical if minimal sedation is used (Box 101-2).
24. Discuss the findings with the patient (and the person who has accompanied the patient to the office) before discharge. If the patient has received significant administration of benzodiazepines, such as midazolam (Versed), he or she may be amnestic

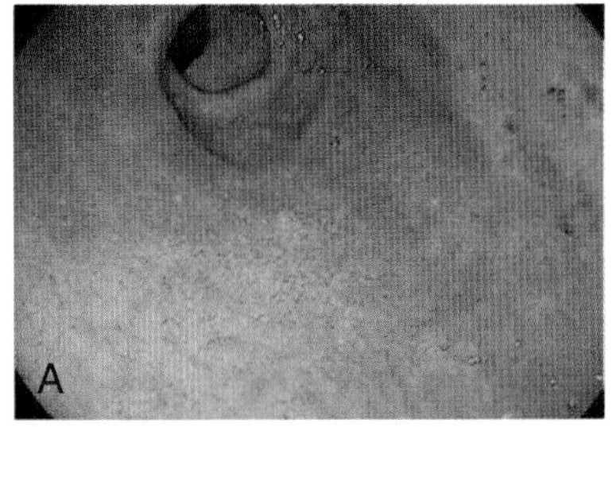

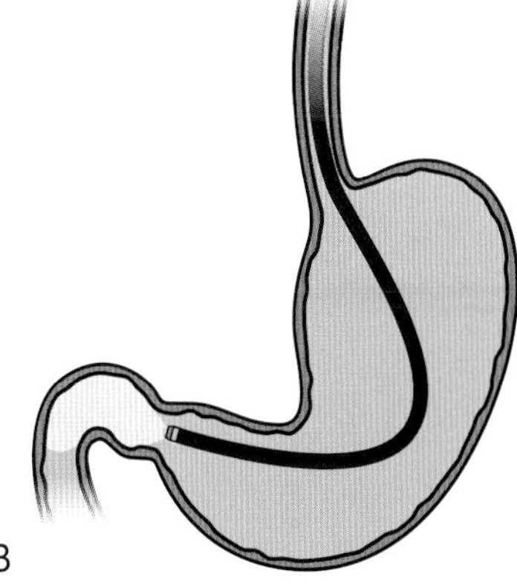

Figure 101-14 **A,** Duodenal bulb. **B,** Unshaded area is seen by lighted scope.

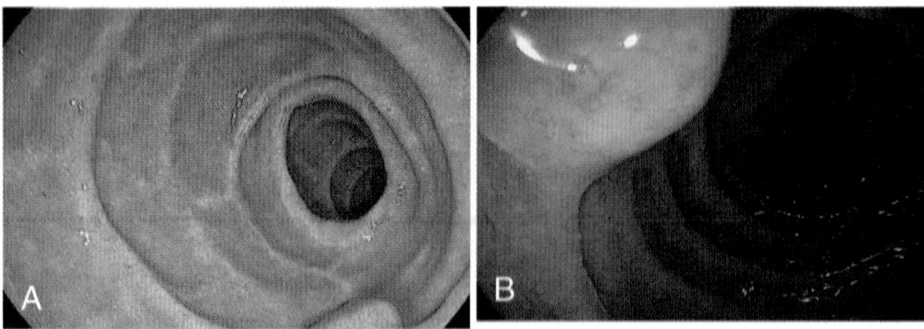

Figure 101-15 **A,** Folds of Kerckring. **B,** Ampulla of Vater.

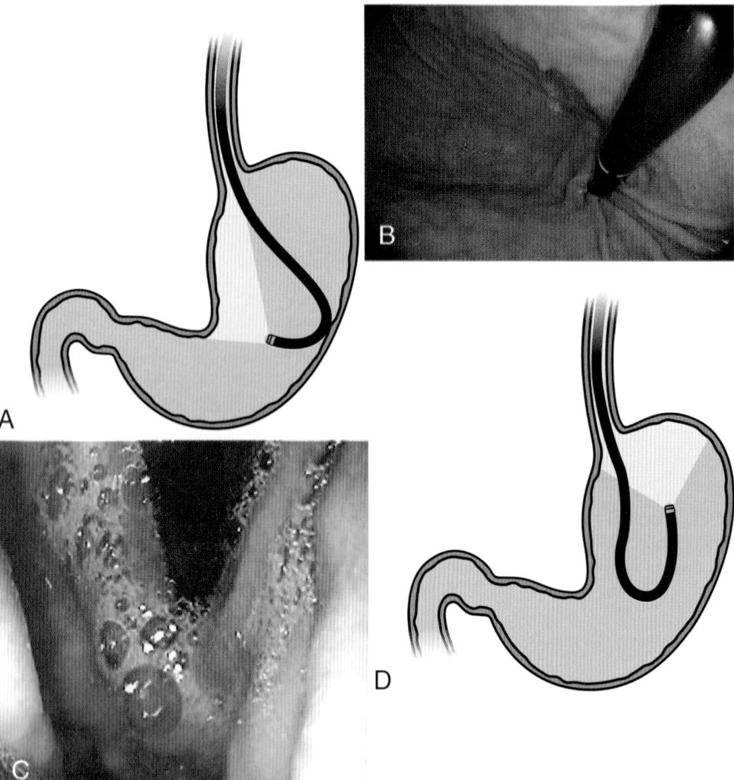

Figure 101-16 **A,** A 180-degree angulation retroflexes the tip to see the lesser curve. **B,** Retroflexion view. **C** and **D,** Reflexion view of the cardia.

Box 101-2. Intravenous Sedative Administration Recovery Nursing Documentation Parameters

- Note and record level of consciousness on arrival.
- Note and record response and anxiety level.
- Note and record patency of airway, spontaneous respiratory effort.
- Note and record status of intravenous (IV) access site (redness or edema).
- Note and record respiratory effort and degree of chest movement.
- Note and record vital signs every 5 min.
- Place the cardiac monitor.
- Place the pulse oximeter.
- Note and record body temperature.
- Administer oxygen at 2 L through a nasal cannula.
- Raise head of the bed 30 to 45 degrees.
- Note and record skin turgor.
- Note and record quality of speech (clarity and ease of speech).
- Note and record presence or absence of nausea, gagging, spasmodic coughing, and ability to swallow.
- Note and record presence or absence of abdominal distention or tenderness.
- Note and record quality of bowel sounds.
- Note and record expulsion of gas.
- Note and record abdominal cramping.
- On admission, perform an assessment of the patient's medical conditions.
- Note and record any untoward symptoms as they occur.
- Note and record the patient's condition after 15 min.
- Note and record discharge status.
- Record vital signs every 5 min and post monitor strips, with a simple explanation, every 15 min or when there is an unusual occurrence.
- Report any unusual responses immediately to the physician.

and forget any information provided by the physician. Photographic records of the findings, along with graphic demonstration or written comments, are extremely helpful in reviewing the results of the procedure with the patient and his or her family. Complete and review all monitoring forms.

25. The gastrointestinal assistant should document the condition in which the patient was discharged.
26. It is helpful to call the patient at home at the end of the day (before the office closes) to document that the patient is not experiencing any untoward effects after the completion of EGD.

Unsedated Transnasal Esophagogastroduodenoscopy

With the advent of newly developed ultrathin diameter endoscopes (5.1- to 6-mm insertion tube), unsedated transnasal EGD (T-EGD) has become possible. Unsedated EGD obviously eliminates the danger of medication-related complications from sedative drugs. More than half of the morbidity and mortality attributed to EGD is due to cardiopulmonary complications from sedation effects.

Significant cost reduction is associated with the absence of fees for sedation and monitoring equipment. This alone has become a significant motivational factor to encourage office-based T-EGD.

Previously, either the patient or the physician may have opted for an empiric therapeutic trial of medications for a myriad of upper gastrointestinal complaints rather than having an EGD. Such choices may have been based on patient anxiety or physician concerns about the procedure. Such a delay in diagnosis is no longer necessary because T-EGD can be completed easily and rapidly in the office, eliminating the need for nursing time and anesthesia personnel. Also preoperative, concurrent, and postoperative monitoring with a pulse oximeter are no longer issues.

Other hidden costs can also be eliminated. Such costs include the drain on the economy's workforce associated with the current need for family members or friends taking time off to assist and transport patients for EGD. Patient convenience is enhanced, because endoscopies can be performed during office hours. No lengthy recovery period or check-in or discharge time is required. Patients can return to work almost immediately following T-EGD. Physicians can perform more endoscopies in less time after they are trained and familiar with the unsedated technique.

A remaining hurdle is the fact that most patients experiencing EGD have come to expect that they will sleep through their procedure and awaken with little or no awareness of what was done. Patient apprehension can be a major obstacle. This concern can be overcome with good patient education (such as videos of actual procedures), which will increase acceptability and tolerance. Patients can actually watch their anatomy on the screen and actively communicate (talk during the procedure), providing feedback to the physician. Immediate demonstration and explanation of the pathology are possible with a conscious patient who is viewing the procedure as it occurs. Biopsies can now be performed with newer generation transnasal endoscopes to allow for tissue retrieval.

Biopsy

Biopsy samples are taken when visible changes are seen in the stomach or esophagus. Routine, blind biopsy specimens of the esophagus, stomach, or duodenum are *not* indicated. The clinician should perform a biopsy on any gastroesophageal abnormality, unless it is vascular in appearance (i.e., pulsating or bluish in color). Any intended areas of biopsy should be approached with a closed biopsy forceps to assess the vascularity and induration of the subject area. The clinician should ensure that the intended biopsy site can be successfully reached with the scope in its current position. Biopsy of duodenal ulcers is rarely necessary because the risk of cancer is extremely small in this region.

During biopsy, the forceps are advanced through the end of the scope by the examiner, and the assistant is in charge of the operating controls. The closed forceps are directed at the area to be biopsied (Fig. 101-17A).

After reaching the desired site with the closed forceps, the forceps are withdrawn a few centimeters, the assistant is advised to open the forceps, and the forceps are passed directly into the biopsy area. The examiner asks the assistant to close the forceps. A gentle tug is given, and the biopsy forceps are pulled through the opening of the scope by the examiner. Tenting of the mucosa can be seen with the removal of the tissue (Fig. 101-17B).

The assistant then retrieves the tissue by opening the biopsy forceps over a container with formalin. A toothpick is placed into the teeth of the open biopsy forceps, dislodging the tissue material into the formalin container.

For gastric ulcers, the clinician should *biopsy all four quadrants at the edges*. Removal of tissue from the center of the ulcer will not result in adequate tissue examination. If diffuse *intestinal gastritis* is present, multiple biopsies are indicated. Because the biopsies are small, there is generally minimal bleeding. In most cases bleeding from esophageal biopsies stops within 4 to 5 minutes.

It is unnecessary to continuously monitor a biopsy site during the performance of the procedure. Commonly, the examiner can complete the examination by looking at other areas of the upper GI tract and then return to reevaluate a biopsy site before the completion of the procedure. If bleeding does occur and is profuse, it must be controlled before withdrawing the scope and noted on the operative report. In most cases, the acidic milieu of the stomach coagulates bleeding sites. Occasionally the distal esophagus will bleed more persistently after the completion of a biopsy; therefore, many examiners perform brush "biopsies" in this region rather than the surgical biopsy.

Gastric biopsies are also commonly done to obtain tissue samples for CLO tests or for histologic analysis for *Helicobacter pylori*. *H. pylori*–associated gastritis often cannot be diagnosed by endoscopic appearance alone. *When assessing a patient with chronic dyspepsia, the*

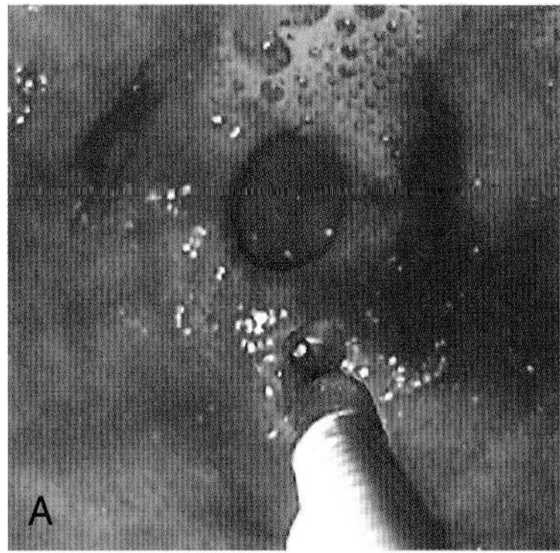

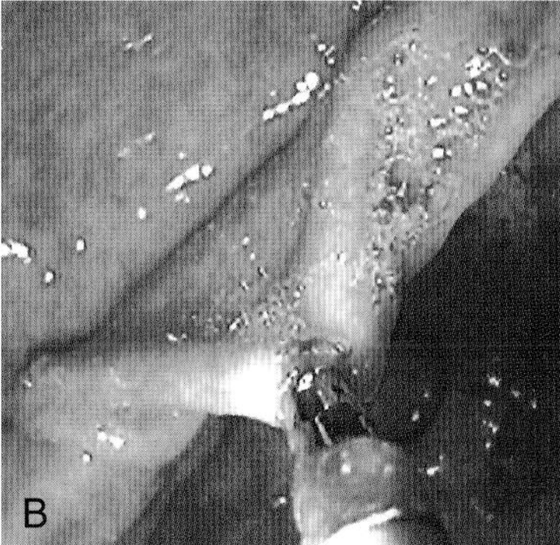

Figure 101-17 **A,** Closed biopsy forceps. **B,** Tenting of the mucosa during biopsy.

clinician should remember that normal-appearing gastric mucosa may exhibit marked histologic gastritis.

When performing the CLO test, the examiner should warm the slide to room temperature before the endoscopy. The absence of bismuth preparations and a 4-week abstinence from antibiotics should be documented before the performance of the procedure.

When performing *H. pylori* biopsies, the clinician should obtain tissue samples from the *normal-appearing* portions of the gastric antrum. The normal-appearing area of the mucosa is chosen because *H. pylori* may be scarce in areas where the epithelium is eroded or where the mucous layer is denuded.

Many physicians read and interpret the results of a CLO test (a simple color change) themselves. However, the tissue can be sent to a pathologist. Some physicians collect two specimens: one for a CLO test and one for histologic analysis (the histologic analysis specimen is sent only if the CLO test is negative but there is a strong suspicion of *H. pylori*). A single biopsy has a sensitivity of approximately 95%, whereas two biopsies approach 100% sensitivity. *H. pylori* have a patchy distribution.

Complications

The complication rate of endoscopy performed by primary care physicians from eight clinical sites was 0.0014 (1 in 717). All cases were collected sequentially from the beginning of each physician's experience (Rodney and colleagues, 1990). The complication rate in large subspecialty populations is 0.0013 (1.3 in 1000). Therefore, complications from EGD are extremely rare. Sixty percent of the adverse effects associated with EGD are due to cardiopulmonary complications that arise directly from the conscious sedation used in the procedure. True complications might include the following:

- Perforation
- Bleeding secondary to trauma or biopsy
- Infection
- Cardiopulmonary complications from conscious sedation
- Inadequate interpretation

The risk of perforation is increased when therapeutic procedures (not discussed in the text) are performed at the time of endoscopy. Risk increases as follows:

- Esophageal dilation, 0.5%
- Esophageal dilation for achalasia, 1.7%
- Endoscopic thermal therapy, 1% to 2%
- Endoscopic variceal sclerotherapy, 1% to 6%
- Endoscopic laser therapy, 5%
- Photodynamic therapy, 4.6%
- Esophageal stent placement, 5% to 25%

Completion of the EGD Report

The final EGD report can be completed on a preconstructed template (Fig. 101-18) or a computer template macro, or it can be dictated into a transcription system. The report should include the diagnosis and the symptoms or signs that led to the performance of the EGD. Inclusion of the sedative agents and doses is important to incorporate especially if future endoscopy is contemplated. All of the findings should be detailed. A listing of the final diagnoses and treatment plan is essential to include. The physician should also note the number of biopsies and the location from which they were obtained.

Training

Most physicians who are performing primary care endoscopy have received training either in a residency situation or in short courses such as those through The National Procedures Institute. Both of these training situations provide excellent introduction to the technique of EGD, the use of conscious sedation, and the interpretation of common pathologic conditions seen with the endoscope.

It is essential for the clinician to obtain preceptor training from a skilled endoscopist who can assist with the proper insertion technique and the proper interpretation of anatomic findings during the performance of EGD.

There is no common agreement concerning how many procedures a clinician who is already competent at other endoscopic procedures (e.g., flexible sigmoidoscopy, colonoscopy) should perform before performing EGD without supervision. Many skilled primary care endoscopists believe that approximately 5 to 15 examinations under supervision are adequate. This number is significantly less than a specialist who will be doing more advanced therapeutic/interventional care rather than diagnostic evaluation.

Obtaining Hospital Privileges

Hospital privileges remain a strongly contested area; the debate over who should receive these privileges is primarily motivated by subspecialty concerns. There are absolutely no study-supported data in the literature denoting a minimal number of procedures that should be supervised before obtaining hospital privileges. Although many numbers are reported by subspecialty organizations as a proposed minimum, these numbers are subject to debate and are not in any way a demonstration of individual competency. Thus, it is essential to have a skilled endoscopist act as preceptor to an individual to ascertain adequate eye-hand coordination and good visual-spatial skills. For more information, the clinician should review the American Academy of Family Physicians' position paper on endoscopy at www.expertconsult.com.

Patient Education Guides

See the sample patient education and consent forms online at www.expertconsult.com.

CPT/Billing Codes

36000	Introduction of needle or intracatheter, vein
43200*	Esophagoscopy with or without brush
43202*	Esophagoscopy with biopsy, single or multiple
43215*	Esophagoscopy foreign body removal
43234*	Simple upper endoscopy
43235*	EGD with or without brushings
43239*	EGD with biopsies
43247*	EGD with foreign body removal
90780	IV therapy 1 hour
90781	IV therapy each additional hour
90784	IV injection
94761	Oximetry
99070	Surgical tray/IV tubing/supplies

ICD-9-CM Diagnostic Codes

150.3	Carcinoma (Ca), esophagus, upper third
150.4	Ca, esophagus, middle third
150.5	Ca, esophagus, lower third
151.1	Ca, stomach, pylorus
151.2	Ca, stomach, antrum
151.3	Ca, stomach, fundus
151.4	Ca, stomach, body
152.0	Ca, duodenum

*Health Care Financing Administration (HCFA) allows additional payment for a tray for this procedure when performed in a physician's office. Charge appropriately using code "99070—surgical tray."

Upper Endoscopy Report—EGD

Date:____________ Referring Physician: ____________________

Endoscopist:____________________________

Indications/preprocedure diagnosis: ____

Physical Exam:

Neurologic Status: ❒ Alert Airway: ❒ patent Dentures Y/N

Heart: ❒ RRR ❒ No murmur

Lungs: ❒ Normal breath sounds

Abdomen: ❒ Nondistended ❒ Nontender ❒ No masses

Medications: Versed _______mg Demerol ________mg Fentanyl_______ mcg

Propofol_________mg

Findings: endoscope passed to ______________ part of duodenum ___________

Vocal Cords:

Esophagus:

Sniff Test:

Stomach:

Cardia

Fundus

Body

Antrum

Pylorus

Duodenum:

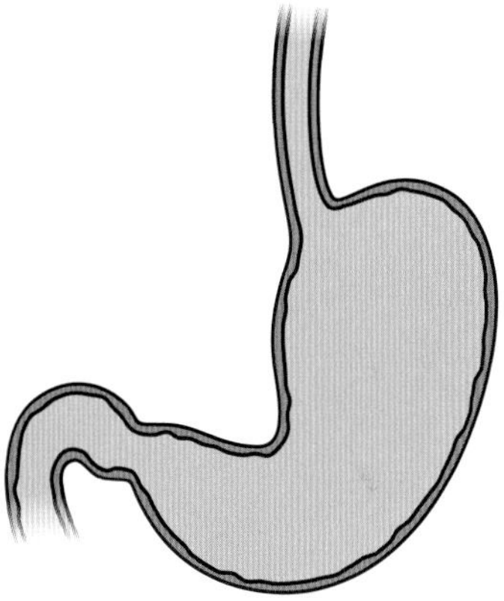

Bx for H. pylori ___x4

Pyloritek results ____

Complications:____

Impression:

Recommendations:

Signature of Endoscopist (____dictated)

cc ____

Physician

Figure 101-18 Upper endoscopy report.

211.0 Benign lesion, esophagus
211.1 Benign lesion, stomach
211.2 Benign lesion, duodenum
464.0 Acute laryngitis/tracheitis
476.1 Chronic laryngitis
530.2 Esophageal ulcer
530.3 Esophageal stricture
530.6 Esophageal diverticulum
530.7 Mallory-Weiss tear
530.10 Esophagitis, unspecified
530.11 Esophagitis, reflux
530.12 Acute esophagitis
530.81 Esophageal reflux
530.82 Esophageal hemorrhage
530.83 Esophageal leukoplakia
531.0 Gastric ulcer, acute with hemorrhage (hem)
531.40 Gastric ulcer, chronic with hem
531.70 Gastric ulcer, chronic
532.0 Duodenal ulcer, acute with hem
532.40 Duodenal ulcer, chronic with hem
532.70 Duodenal ulcer, chronic
532.91 Gastric ulcer, chronic with obstruction
532.91 Duodenal ulcer, chronic with obstruction
535.00 Acute gastritis
535.01 Acute gastritis with hem
535.10 Atrophic gastritis
535.60 Duodenitis
536.2 Persistent vomiting
536.8 Dyspepsia
537.1 Gastric diverticulum
553.3 Hiatal hernia
578.0 Hematemesis
784.49 Hoarseness
786.09 Wheezing
786.50 Chest pain
787.01 Nausea and vomiting
787.1 Heartburn (i.e., pyrosis)
787.2 Dysphagia
787.3 Belching
789.0 Abdominal pain
793.4 X-ray abnormality, GI tract
V16.0 Family history, GI tract Ca (not primary diagnosis)
V18.5 Family history, GI disorders (not primary diagnosis)

SUPPLIERS

Full contact information is available online at www.expertconsult.com.

CME Courses for learning
The National Procedures Institute
Gastroscopes
Fujinon Medical
Olympus America
Pentax Medical Company
Other organizations of interest
Association for Primary Care Endoscopy
Patient education materials
American Society for Gastrointestinal Endoscopy
Transnasal esophagoscope (with sterile disposable sheath)
Vision Sciences
Videotapes
The National Procedures Institute
Welch Allyn vital signs monitor
Welch Allyn

BIBLIOGRAPHY

Ables AZ, Simon I, Melton ER: Update on *Helicobacter pylori* treatment. Am Fam Physician 2007;75:351–358.

American Academy of Family Physicians: Colonoscopy (position paper). Available at http://www.aafp.org/online/en/home/policy/policies/c/colonoscopypositionpaper.html. Accessed Feb. 20, 2009.

American Society for Gastrointestinal Endoscopy (ASGE): Methods of granting hospital privileges to perform gastrointestinal endoscopy. Gastrointest Endosc 55:780–783, 2002.

Behrman SW: Management of complicated peptic ulcer disease. Arch Surg 140:201–208, 2005.

Bittner JG, Marks JM, Dunkin BJ, et al: Resident training in flexible gastrointestinal endoscopy: A review of current issues and options. J Surg Educ 64:399–409, 2007.

Cappell MS, Friedel D: The role of esophagogastroduodenoscopy in the diagnosis and management of upper gastrointestinal disorders. Med Clin North Am 86:1165–1216, 2002.

Ebell MH: Prognosis in patients with upper GI bleeding. Am Fam Physician 70:2348–2350, 2004.

Eisen GM, Dominitz JA, Faigel DO, et al: An annotated algorithmic approach to acute lower gastrointestinal bleeding. Gastrointest Endosc 53:859–863, 2001.

Hernandez-Diaz S, Rodriguez LA: Incidence of serious upper gastrointestinal bleeding/perforation in the general population: Review of epidemiologic studies. J Clin Epidemiol 55:157–163, 2002.

Huang JQ, Sridhar S, Hunt RH: Role of *Helicobacter pylori* infection and non-steroidal anti-inflammatory drugs in peptic ulcer disease: A meta-analysis. Lancet 359:14–22, 2002.

Kalyanakrishnan R, Salinas R: Peptic ulcer disease. Am Fam Physician 76:1005–1012, 1013, 2007.

Kovacs TO, Jensen DM: Recent advances in the endoscopic diagnosis and therapy of upper gastrointestinal, small intestinal, and colonic bleeding. Med Clin North Am 86:1319–1356, 2002.

Layke JC, Lopez, PP: Gastric cancer: Diagnosis and treatment options. Am Fam Physician 69:1133–1140, 1145–1146, 2004.

Lewis JD, Brown A, Localio AR, Schwartz JS: Initial evaluation of rectal bleeding in young persons: A cost-effectiveness analysis. Ann Intern Med 136:99–110, 2002.

Reed W, Kilkenny J, Dias D, Wexner S, SAGES EGD Outcomes Study Group: A prospective analysis of 3525 esophagogastroduodenoscopies performed by surgeons. Surg Endosc 18:11–21, 2004.

Rodney WM, Hocutt JE Jr, Coleman WH, et al: Esophagogastroduodenoscopy by family physicians: A national multisite study of 717 procedures. J Am Board Fam Pract 3:73–79, 1990.

Sharma VK, Coppola AG, Raufman JP: A survey of credentialing practices of gastrointestinal endoscopy centers in the United States. J Clin Gastroenterol 39:501–507, 2005.

Society of American Gastrointestinal Endoscopic Surgeons: Granting of Privileges for Gastrointestinal Endoscopy. SAGES Publication No. 0011, printed 09/01.

Talley NJ, Vakil NB, Moayyedi P: American Gastroenterological Association technical review on the evaluation of dyspepsia. Gastroenterology 129:1756–1780, 2005.

CHAPTER 102

Management of Fecal Impaction

George G. Zainea

Fecal impaction is a common condition that typically occurs in the bedridden or nursing home patient. Individuals who suffered a cerebrovascular accident are at particular risk. Fecal impaction is the most common gastrointestinal disorder occurring in patients with a spinal cord injury. Medications such as narcotics predispose to this problem. It is also a common complication of anorectal procedures as a result of reflex spasm of the anal sphincter. Painful anal fissures may cause the same problem.

Diagnosis

Fecal impaction should be suspected when a patient has unexplained constipation or diarrhea. Diarrhea occurs as liquid stool passes around the hard fecal bolus. Rectal distention from the fecaloma causes reflex relaxation of the internal anal sphincter. The patient may have acute or chronic large bowel obstruction, both clinically and by radiographic examination. The chronic obstruction will increase mucosal water and electrolyte secretion, leading to frequent, loose, watery stools that pass around the bolus. The patient with spinal cord injury may demonstrate autonomic hyperreflexia with pain, fever, tachycardia, and abdominal distention.

Digital rectal examination reveals impacted feces palpated in the rectum. It is important to assess for size and consistency of the bolus as well as for the presence of blood. In the normal situation, the rectal ampulla remains empty. A fecal bolus does not pass beyond the rectosigmoid junction until the act of defecation commences.

Complications of fecal impaction can include acute or chronic bowel obstruction, mucosal ulceration, and hemorrhage.

After disimpaction, particularly in the recurrent setting, it is important to rule out an anatomic cause of obstruction. This may require proctosigmoidoscopy or a water-soluble contrast examination. Impaction may be associated with an anal or rectal stricture. The practitioner must assess for the presence of a tumor. Last, a deep mucosal ulcer may cause bleeding or infection as a result of fecal impaction. This is known as a *stercoral ulceration*.

Technique

An attempt at *medical therapy* in an otherwise ambulatory patient is a reasonable first step. Careful administration of one or two Fleet enemas into the bolus to soften and hydrate the stool should be followed in 1 hour by the administration of a mineral oil enema to assist in passage of the softened stool. Soapsuds, hot water, or hydrogen peroxide enemas are discouraged because they may irritate the mucosa and result in bleeding. An alternative is an attempt at antegrade cleansing with either mineral oil or polyethylene glycol (PEG) solution lavage. The dose of mineral oil is 30 mL/10 kg orally in two divided doses for 2 consecutive days. The dose of PEG solution is 20 mL/kg daily for 2 consecutive days.

Manual disimpaction is required in most patients. This is best performed after a *circumanal block* of the anal musculature with local anesthetic. A four-quadrant field block allows for complete muscle relaxation and a painless disimpaction. Use 0.5% lidocaine drawn up in a 10-mL syringe. A 22-gauge, 1½-inch needle is used. Insert the needle all the way to the hub in each of the right, left, anterior, and posterior positions 1 cm away from the anal verge (Fig. 102-1). "Fan it out" in three directions at each of the injection sites, depositing a total of 2 to 3 mL of local anesthetic in each of the four sites as the needle is slowly withdrawn. The left decubitus position with hips and knees flexed to the chest is the most comfortable for the patient.

Gentle *digital dilation* of the sphincter is then performed as the fecal bolus is fragmented and extracted. A large, rigid proctoscope may be necessary to soften and break up stool residing higher in the rectum. After passing the rigid scope up to the fecal bolus, phosphate enema solution is passed through the scope to soften the stool. A long rigid aspirator is then passed through the scope to break up the softened stool and allow for evacuation. This process is repeated as many times as necessary to empty the bowel of stool.

Disimpaction may be facilitated by intravenous or intramuscular administration of a narcotic or anxiolytic. Early posthemorrhoidectomy impaction may be managed best in the operating room under general or regional anesthesia.

After disimpaction, it is prudent to institute a bowel habit program that includes laxatives, stool softeners, or enemas along with a regular time for evacuation to prevent reimpaction. PEG

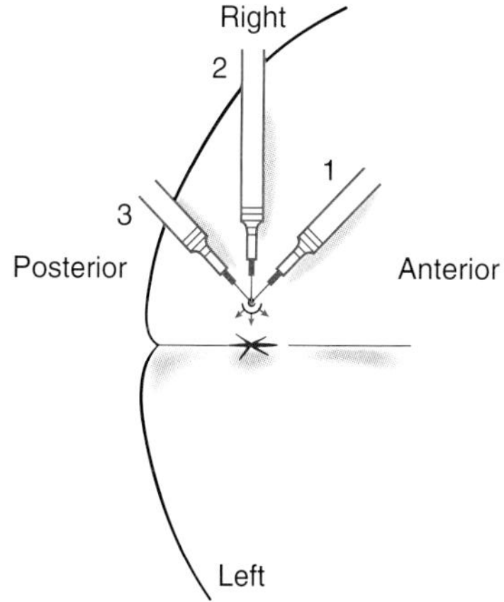

Figure 102-1 Technique of circumanal block with local anesthetic. Patient is in the left lateral decubitus position. Repeat the injection as shown, 1 cm from the anal verge, in all four quadrants (right, left, posterior, and anterior).

solution can be useful to treat patients with chronic constipation prone to develop recurrent impaction.

CPT/Billing Codes

45300 Rigid proctosigmoidoscopy
45915 Removal of fecal impaction or foreign body under anesthesia
45999 Procedure rectum (unspecified)

ICD-9-CM Diagnostic Code

560.39 Fecal impaction

BIBLIOGRAPHY

Araghizadeh F: Fecal impaction. In: Clinics in Colon and Rectal Surgery, vol 18. New York, Thieme, 2005, pp 116–119.

Wexner SD, Bartolo DC: Constipation: Etiology, Evaluation, and Management. Oxford, Butterworth-Heinemann, 1995.

CHAPTER 103

Flexible Sigmoidoscopy

Michael B. Harper

The flexible sigmoidoscope has become a standard instrument in the primary care physician's office to detect and prevent colorectal cancer (CRC). Approximately 150,000 cases of CRC occur each year in the United States, with 55,000 deaths. It is the second-highest cause of cancer deaths in this country. The sigmoidoscope may be used to decrease morbidity and mortality of CRC either through early detection or by preventing it by removing precursor polyps. Well-designed, case-controlled studies have demonstrated the effectiveness of using sigmoidoscopy to screen for CRC, and sigmoidoscopy combined with annual fecal occult blood testing (FOBT) can be expected to yield an 80% reduction in mortality from CRC. In addition to screening for CRC, the sigmoidoscope is a valuable tool in evaluating symptomatic patients.

All major sources of guidelines for preventive medicine recommend screening for CRC, and physicians who fail to perform or recommend screening face medical-legal issues. Debate continues, however, regarding the best method of screening for this cancer. FOBT and sigmoidoscopy continue to be the most commonly used methods of screening for CRC in average-risk patients. Screening colonoscopy is becoming more popular, especially in high-risk patients, but direct evidence of mortality reduction is lacking. An extensive review of the literature (Frazier and colleagues, 2000) concluded that the best and most cost-effective method for CRC screening in average-risk patients was flexible sigmoidoscopy every 5 years, along with FBOT every year. In another screening model, colonoscopy once every 10 years was more cost effective than sigmoidoscopy every 5 years, but this model did not combine sigmoidoscopy and FOBT screening (Sonnenberg and colleagues, 2000). A recent study demonstrated that screening flexible sigmoidoscopy performed only once on people between ages 55 and 64 years, conferred a substantial (31% reduction in mortality) and long lasting protection from colorectal cancer (Atkin and colleagues, 2010).

Studies have concluded that patients will undergo whatever test their physician recommends. Unfortunately, in 2004 only 57% of adults in the United States had been screened by currently recommended methods. *It is imperative for physicians to implement and encourage proper screening.*

Indications

- Screening: The American Society of Gastroenterology (ASGE), the American Cancer Society (ACS), the American College of Physicians (ACP), the National Cancer Institute (NCI), the American College of Obstetricians and Gynecologists (ACOG), the American Academy of Family Physicians (AAFP), and the United States Preventive Services Task Force (USPSTF) all recommend routine screening of not-at-risk patients 50 years of age and older for colon polyps and colon cancer. Note that no one is considered at "low risk" for screening purposes. The 2008 clinical summary of the USPSTF recommendations for screening for CRC are included in Table 103-1. (Also see "Colon Cancer Screening Options Vary" online at www.expertconsult.com.)
- Surveillance after previous polypectomy.
- Surveillance for effectiveness of treatment for ulcerative colitis/Crohn's disease.
- Abdominal pain.
- Rectal bleeding (bright red or occult).
- Constipation or diarrhea.
- Persistent change in usual bowel habits.
- Unexplained weight loss, fever, or anemia.
- Suspected inflammatory bowel disease or antibiotic-associated colitis.
- Anorectal symptoms. (Note, however, that hemorrhoids alone are not an absolute indication for flexible sigmoidoscopy or air-contrast barium enema [ACBE] and must be put into the context of the entire patient history and examination. Medicare does not reimburse for an endoscopy procedure with the sole diagnosis of "hemorrhoids.")
- Evaluation of radiographic abnormality or to confirm a radiologic finding with a biopsy.

Although flexible sigmoidoscopy may be used for the initial evaluation of some complaints, it is limited by the amount of colon it can evaluate. Certainly with selected symptoms, if the sigmoidoscopy is negative, a more extensive work-up is still indicated. Thus, for many patients, obtaining a colonoscopy as the primary procedure may be more cost effective. On the other hand, availability and cost concerns may lead to sigmoidoscopy as the initial procedure of choice.

Because of redundant loops of sigmoid colon and because the insertion tube that is used for barium enema can obscure a lesion, flexible sigmoidoscopy (or, at the minimum, anoscopy) is generally needed along with ACBE if the entire bowel must be visualized. Individual circumstances dictate whether a flexible sigmoidoscopy alone or in conjunction with an ACBE is needed.

Contraindications

Absolute

- Acute abdomen
  - Suspected perforation abscess
  - Peritonitis or intraabdominal sepsis
  - Diverticulitis
  - Bowel infarct
  - Fulminant colitis
- Severe cardiopulmonary disease
- Inadequate bowel preparation
- Uncooperative patient
- Marked bleeding disorder

Relative

The following conditions require additional caution before performing flexible sigmoidoscopy:

TABLE 103-1 Screening for Colorectal Cancer: Clinical Summary of U.S. Preventive Services Task Force Recommendation*

Population	Adults Age 50 to 75 Years†	Adults Age 76 to 85 Years†	Adults Older than 85 Years†
Recommendation	**Screen with high-sensitivity FOBT, sigmoidoscopy, or colonoscopy** **Grade: A**	**Do not screen routinely** **Grade: C**	**Do not screen** **Grade: D**
	For all populations, evidence is insufficient to assess the benefits and harms of screening with computed tomographic colonography and fecal DNA testing. **Grade: I (insufficient evidence)**		
Screening Tests	High-sensitivity FOBT, sigmoidoscopy with FOBT, and colonoscopy are effective in decreasing colorectal cancer mortality. The risks and benefits of these screening methods vary. Colonoscopy and flexible sigmoidoscopy (to a lesser degree) entail possible serious complications.		
Screening Test Intervals	Intervals for recommended screening strategies: Annual screening with high-sensitivity FOBT Sigmoidoscopy every 5 years, with high-sensitivity FOBT every 3 years Screening colonoscopy every 10 years		
Balance of Harms and Benefits	The benefits of screening outweigh the potential harms for 50- to 75-year-olds.	The likelihood that detection and early intervention will yield a mortality benefit declines after age 75 years because of the long average time between adenoma development and cancer diagnosis.	
Implementation	Focus on strategies that maximize the number of individuals who get screened. Practice shared decision making; discussions with patients should incorporate information on test quality and availability. Individuals with a personal history of cancer or adenomatous polyps are followed by a surveillance regimen, and screening guidelines are not applicable.		
Relevant USPSTF Recommendations	The USPSTF recommends against the use of aspirin or nonsteroidal anti-inflammatory drugs for the primary prevention of colorectal cancer. This recommendation is available at http://www.preventiveservices.ahrq.gov.		

FOBT, fecal occult blood testing.

*This document is a summary of the 2008 recommendation of the U.S. Preventive Services Task Force (USPSTF) on screening for colorectal cancer. For a summary of the evidence systematically reviewed in making these recommendations, the full recommendation statement, and supporting documents please go to http://www.preventiveservices.ahrq.gov.

†These recommendations do not apply to individuals with specific inherited syndromes (Lynch syndrome or familial adenomatous polyposis) or those with inflammatory bowel disease.

From U.S. Preventive Services Task Force: Screening for Colorectal Cancer: Clinical Summary of U.S. Preventive Services Task Force Recommendation. AHRQ Publication No. 08-05124-EF-4. Rockville, Md, Agency for Healthcare Research and Quality, October 2008. Available at http://www.ahrq.gov/clinic/uspstf08/colocancer/colosum.htm.

- Pregnancy
- Recent abdominal surgery
- Distorted pelvic anatomy
- History of pelvic irradiation
- Recent barium enema (if still passing barium because it can occlude the scope's port)
- When colonoscopy is indicated (such as in high-risk patients with inflammatory bowel disease who should receive a colonoscopy 8 years after the diagnosis was first made and every 5 years thereafter, for follow-up of polyps and colon cancer, and for patients with familial polyposis syndromes)

EQUIPMENT

The flexible sigmoidoscope is available as either a fiberoptic endoscope or video endoscope. Although the fiberoptic scope has been the most commonly used version, the video sigmoidoscope is state of the art, using computer chip and video technology. The image from the tip of the scope is transmitted to a video monitor. This equipment facilitates videotape recording, sound narration, and other patient information storage.

The following basic equipment is necessary to carry out routine flexible sigmoidoscopy:

- 60- to 70-cm-long submersible scope consisting of the body with controls (Fig. 103-1) and the shaft of the scope with tip and apertures (Figs. 103-2 and 103-3)
- Light source (most have air supply and wash bottle attached; Fig. 103-4)
- Suction apparatus (Fig. 103-5)
- Biopsy forceps (Fig. 103-6)
- Water-based lubricant (e.g., K-Y Jelly)
- 4 × 4 gauze pads
- Nonsterile gloves
- Shielded glasses
- Anoscope (Ives slotted anoscope preferred; see Chapter 98, Anoscopy)
- Basin of soapy water (immediately on completion of the procedure, suction water through the scope, then place the scope in the basin)
- Formalin jars
- Disinfecting cleanser
- Nursing assistant (to assist with equipment and procedure)
- Video unit and monitor (for video endoscopes only)

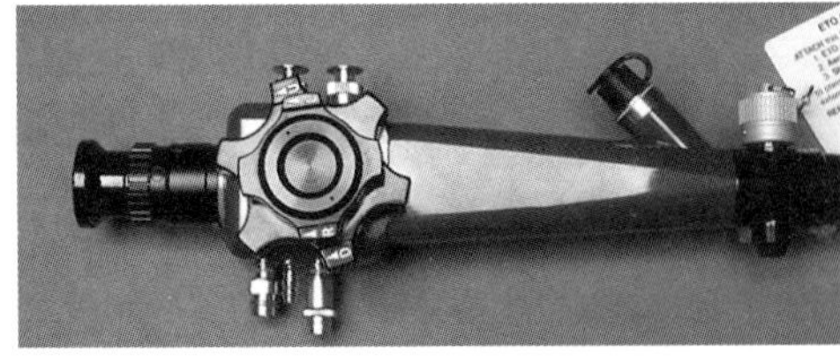

Figure 103-1 Control head and body of the fiberoptic sigmoidoscope.

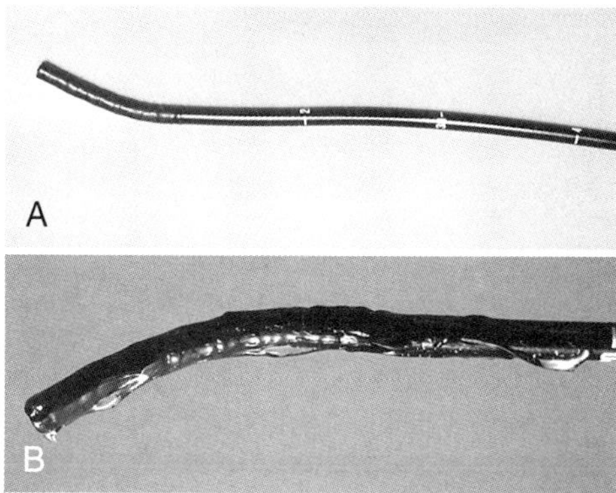

Figure 103-2 **A,** Tip of the sigmoidoscope. **B,** Tip lubricated with K-Y Jelly.

PREPROCEDURE PATIENT PREPARATION

A good history (present and past) is essential before performing any procedure. Not only should the patient's overall medical risk status be determined, but the risk for CRC and any associated symptoms must be assessed to ensure that flexible sigmoidoscopy is indeed the proper procedure and that there are no contraindications to performing it.

Flexible sigmoidoscopy in most patients is easily performed in less than 15 minutes. However, for some patients the very thought of a tube in the rectum provokes anxiety, apprehension, and reluctance. This makes it necessary for the clinician to reassure the patient and allay apprehension and anxiety with a thorough explanation. Use simple words with the aid of charts and figures. Explain the procedure to be performed, why and how it will be done, and the possible complications. The components of this patient education process include the following:

1. Bowel cleansing instructions (usually two enemas; see the sample patient education handout online at www.expertconsult.com)
2. Equipment used
3. Anatomy of the colon
4. Explanation of procedure
5. Discomfort experienced during the procedure ("crampy distention," especially at the second curve around 40 cm and with insufflation of air)

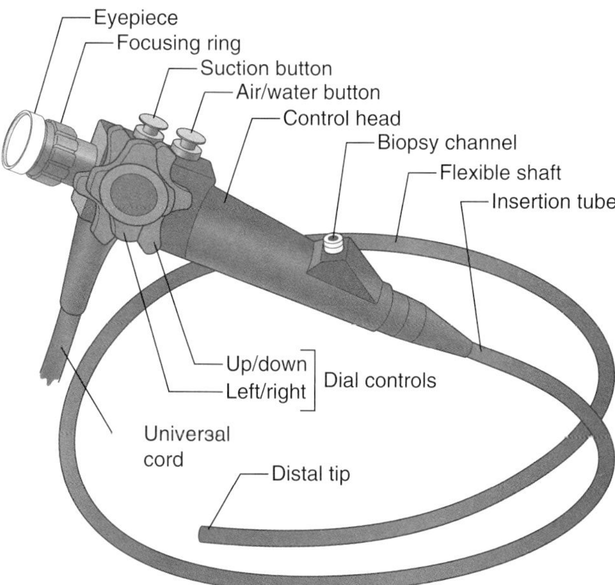

Figure 103-3 Schematic diagram of a fiberoptic sigmoidoscope.

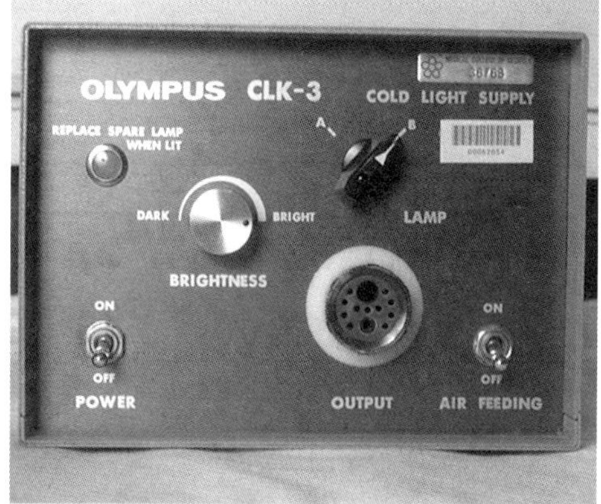

Figure 103-4 Light source with air supply.

6. Complications that are remotely likely (e.g., perforation, bleeding)
7. Possible diseases likely to be detected
8. Biopsy technique, if needed
9. Whether photography or videotape will be used
10. Management of any findings
11. The need to continue all prescribed medications

It is highly advisable to have the patient sign the informed consent form for this procedure after reading the patient information materials. (See the sample patient education handout and consent form online at www.expertconsult.com.)

Flexible sigmoidoscopy is well tolerated by the vast majority of patients. Mild analgesia or sedation, whether given orally or intramuscularly, is rarely needed. Oral diazepam or ibuprofen can be used as needed in the individual situation. Atropine 0.5 mL intramuscularly can be given for those who have a tendency to faint or experience vasovagal symptoms.

Patient Bowel Preparation

Simple enemas (tap water, Phospho-Soda) administered until clear fluid is passed is the only requirement. This usually entails two enemas (occasionally three) 30 to 60 minutes before the procedure. Patients are allowed to take their medications and eat normally. If the patient tends to be constipated, a laxative should be given the day before the procedure. Keeping the regimen simple is more likely to ensure compliance.

In one study (Sharma and Chockalingham, 1997), two Fleet enemas given on arrival to the endoscopy suite were compared with one bottle of magnesium citrate and two Dulcolax tablets the evening before the procedure. Both patients and endoscopists preferred the oral method. Another study (Manoucheri and colleagues,

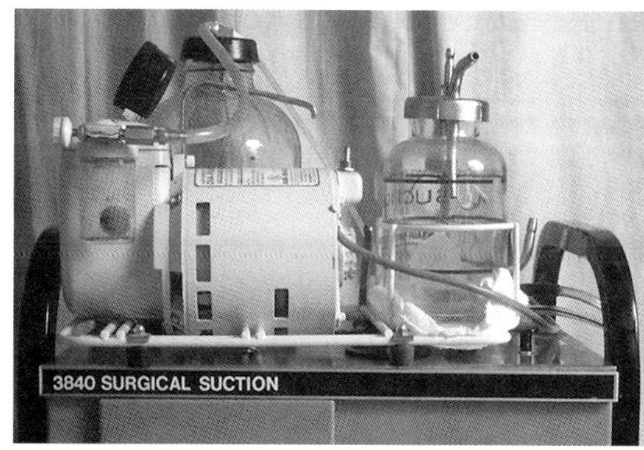

Figure 103-5 Suction apparatus.

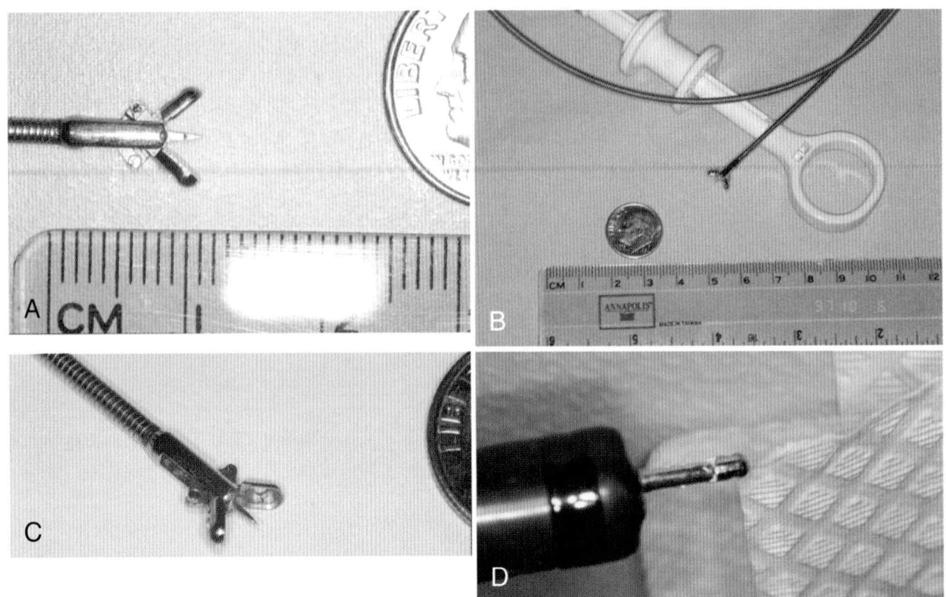

Figure 103-6 Biopsy forceps. **A,** Relative size of forceps. **B,** Control handle. **C,** Stabilizing needle. **D,** Biopsy forceps protruding from end of scope, closed on a piece of paper. (Courtesy of John L. Pfenninger, MD, The Medical Procedures Center, PC, Midland, Mich.)

1999) showed no difference in results comparing four bowel preparation regimens.

Antibiotic Prophylaxis

Antibiotics for subacute bacterial endocarditis prophylaxis are no longer recommended for lower endoscopy procedures with or without the performance of biopsies, even in high-risk patients (see Chapter 221, Antibiotic Prophylaxis).

TECHNIQUE

A specific terminology has developed around the procedure of flexible sigmoidoscopy. Box 103-1 summarizes this "language" that must be understood before learning the procedure.

1. Before beginning the procedure, *all functions of the endoscope must be checked.* The light source should be turned on and clarity of view confirmed. White balance must be performed for videoscopes. The "button" to insufflate air and the water button are the same (see Fig. 103-2). Just covering the air/water button introduces air, whereas pushing it down all the way ejects a small amount of water to clean the lens. This button is the one closest to the patient. The second button, closer to the eyepiece, is for suction. *Remember: the button closest to the patient puts things in and is usually colored blue, the button closest to the endoscopist "sucks" things out and is usually colored red.* Air function is confirmed by inserting the scope tip in water and seeing bubbles when the air port is occluded. Suction is confirmed by suctioning a small amount of water through the endoscope. Tip deflection is checked by rotating both control wheels fully in both directions while observing and feeling for free movement. After checking all functions, the fiberoptic unit may be turned off temporarily. Many video endoscopes have to be white balanced each time they are turned off, so leaving them on is preferable.
2. *If sedation is to be used,* record the patient's temperature, pulse, respiration, blood pressure, and results of heart/lungs auscultation and abdominal examination.
3. Position the patient in the *left lateral Sims' position* (see Chapter 97, Clinical Anorectal Anatomy and Digital Examination, Fig. 97-2).
4. The endoscopist and assistant should wear *nonsterile gloves* on both hands. Double glove the right hand. (Remove the extra glove after the tip has been lubricated, the rectal examination performed, and the scope initially inserted.) Place the body and shaft of the scope on the cart. *Lubricate the distal 3 to 4 cm of the shaft tip with K-Y Jelly* (avoid the lens). Notice where the dials are positioned when the shaft is completely straight.
5. Separate the gluteal folds laterally with the hands to expose the anal area and the anal aperture for inspection. *Perform a digital rectal examination* with K-Y Jelly or lidocaine ointment to ensure there is no obstruction or stool in the anal canal. In male patients, examine the prostate carefully. A painful examination should alert the endoscopist to a fissure, proctitis, or colitis. The examination is uncomfortable but should not be painful if it is done gently. The digital examination helps to relax the sphincter and lubricates the anal canal. (See Chapter 97, Clinical Anorectal Anatomy and Digital Examination.)
6. Now hold the body of the scope in your left hand (Fig. 103-7). *Hold the end of the scope shaft in the right hand, and, with the index finger alongside and stabilizing the very end, gently insert it.* Hold the tip at an oblique angle pointing posteriorly, and stretch the sphincter as the tip is slipped into the anal canal. The shaft tip can be blindly inserted 10 to 20 cm. Stop when resistance is felt. Remove the second glove on the right hand.
7. With the distal 10 cm or more of the scope in the anal canal, *switch on the light source, air, and suction,* if these had been turned off. Check the view in the eyepiece or on the video screen.
8. Keep holding the body of the scope in your left hand so that your thumb controls the large dial and your index finger controls the suction, irrigation, and air valves. *Hold the shaft and advance it* with your right hand, which is also available to control the small dial. *Alternatively, an assistant may advance the scope,* and you may use your right hand to manipulate the dials. The assistant must be cautioned never to advance the scope against resistance and to advance the scope only when told to do so. This latter method is easier and faster for some physicians, but solo operation may allow better coordination of movements of the shaft and deflecting tip. Use the technique that accomplishes the procedure in the fastest manner with minimal patient discomfort.
9. Insufflation advance technique
   - *Air is needed* to maintain patency of the lumen and to obtain a clear view adjacent to the tip and a few centimeters beyond. Remember, the air button and water button are the same.

Box 103-1. Flexible Fiberoptic Sigmoidoscopy Terminology

Tip: Distal end of the shaft of the sigmoidoscope (see Fig. 103-2).

Dials: Tip control knobs. Large inner dial moves the tip up and down. Small outer dial moves the tip left and right (see Fig. 103-3). The clinician should note the neutral position for future reference when in the bowel.

Biopsy channel: The slot through which the biopsy forceps and also the brush wire are passed through the body and shaft of the scope (see Figs. 103-1, 103-3, and 103-6D).

Suction control button (nearest the operator): When pressed all the way down, this button allows the suction to operate continuously.

Air insufflation/lens cleaner (water) button (farthest from the operator): This button has a small opening that can be occluded to allow air to pass into the colon continuously (see Fig. 103-3). Pressing the button completely down will squirt water across the lens at the tip and will clear away debris.

Suction, air, and water connection ports: The location of tubes connecting on the bottom of the handpiece that go to suction, air, and water sources.

Slide-by: A technique of passing the flexible sigmoidoscope where the advancing tip of the scope is advanced proximally into the colon without complete visualization of the lumen. As the scope advances, the practitioner sees the vascular mucosa "slide by." This maneuver is often unavoidable but should be used very sparingly, and the scope should be advanced only 5 to 10 cm. If the lumen is not fully visualized or if pressure, resistance, or pain is encountered, the clinician should pull back and look again for the lumen.

Pullback: Withdrawing the shaft of the scope to diminish or eliminate whiteout, redout, stretching, or looping.

One-on-one: As the scope is advanced into the rectum, there is an equal advance of the scope into the segment of colon (versus just stretching the colon without true advancement).

Redout: The tip of the scope lies flat against the mucosal surface, resulting in a red appearance through the lens.

Whiteout: The mucosal surface is stretched by the tip of the scope pressing against the mucosal surface. The vessels are thus blanched, giving a white appearance.

Tip deflection: The tip can be directed in four directions by rotating the dials: up ("north"), down ("south"), left ("west"), and right ("east"). The deflection should always be moderate and gentle. Alternatively, the head of the scope itself can be rotated right and left to turn the tip to the right or left after being flexed up or down.

Dithering: A to-and-fro advance-and-withdrawal process performed with an amplitude of 5 to 6 cm and repeated every 2 to 4 seconds, coupled with a clockwise torque on the shaft on the pullback motion and a counterclockwise torque on the inward motion. This maneuver helps straighten the sigmoid colon, allowing it to compress like an accordion over the scope (see Fig. 103-9).

Jiggling: A to-and-fro, 5- to 6-cm inward-and-outward motion of the shaft performed every 2 to 4 seconds. It helps in the visualization of a segment of colon and can often aid scope advancement (see Fig. 103-10).

Alpha maneuver: Used only after much practice by the experienced endoscopist to assist in shortening or pleating the segments of the colon (see Fig. 103-11 and text for explanation).

Torquing: Twisting the distal shaft of the scope by rotating the head either clockwise or counterclockwise.

Retroflexion: Maximally flexing the tip of the scope, enabling it to look back on itself. This is often used to evaluate the rectum.

Just covering the button introduces air, whereas pushing it down all the way diverts air into the water bottle and ejects a stream of water across the lens to clean it. A sufficient amount of air must be used to expand the bowel, but too much air may cause cramping or, in extreme cases, even

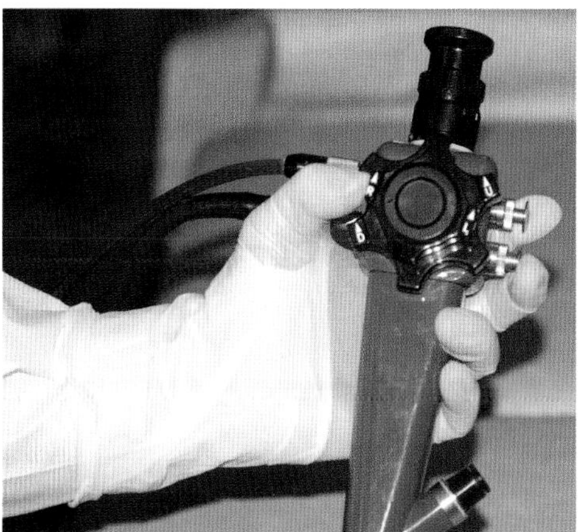

Figure 103-7 Control head of the sigmoidoscope should be held in the left hand so that the thumb rests on the up/down control dial and the index finger can regulate the suction and air/water buttons. (Courtesy of Michael B. Harper, MD.)

perforation. Excess air also lengthens the bowel and may cause sharper bends. Use patient comfort as a guide. With a clear view ahead, gently advance the shaft forward. The scope is usually advanced up to 15 to 18 cm without difficulty. There are three "valves" that are encountered in the rectum: the valves of Houston. These are semilunar in shape, are not really "valves," and are located 6, 9, and 12 cm from the anal verge. Negotiating advancement into the rectosigmoid can be hampered by these folds, and the tip needs to be deflected away from the fold and toward the lumen to avoid redout or whiteout. The clinician can get "lost" in the vast arena of the rectal vault and have difficulty in locating the rectosigmoid orifice. This is more likely if too much air is insufflated, which causes the ampulla to expand upward.

There is always a question of how much air to use. The answer: enough! Generally, as long as the patient is not sedated, he or she will tell if too much pressure is being generated. Some clinicians are too timid and will never see the lumen if "enough" air is not used.

At this stage, you do not need to attempt to visualize the entire circumference of the bowel. Rather, the primary goal is to insert the scope as far as possible. Deflect the tip only enough to clearly see the direction of the lumen. By minimizing tip deflection the force of insertion will be directed more toward the tip and the tendency to form a loop is decreased. It is critical that the complete circumference of the bowel be closely inspected, lest a lesion be missed, but this is usually performed during withdrawal of the scope.

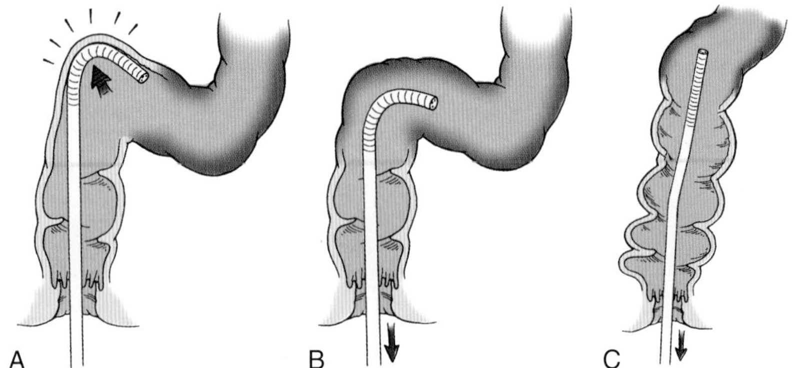

Figure 103-8 Method of advancement at the rectosigmoid junction. Various maneuvers are needed. **A,** The scope is entering into the anus, but the view from the end of the sigmoidoscope is not changing. There is no "one-on-one" advancement; rather, the segment of colon is merely being stretched, often causing pain. **B,** Try the simple hook-and-pullback technique initially. **C,** Pulling back on the scope causes an accordion effect and straightens the curve.

- It is ideal if the scope is passed only when the lumen is seen, but, practically speaking, *the slide-by method is used commonly* and is safe as long as the scope passes easily and the patient (unsedated) is not feeling excessive pain (see Box 103-1). To perform this maneuver, first determine the direction of the lumen. If you do not see the lumen it is easily located by moving the controls toward neutral, then releasing the controls and slowly withdrawing the scope (*this is a basic maneuver to find the lumen with any gastrointestinal endoscopy*). The lumen will usually come into view after withdrawing only a few centimeters. Once the lumen direction is determined, deflect the tip toward the lumen and gently advance the scope while watching for movement of mucosa. Continue to advance as long as the patient is comfortable and you see mucosal movement. The lumen should come back into view after advancing a few centimeters. Stop the slide-by if you have a redout or whiteout, or cause excessive patient discomfort.

10. *Advancing the scope into the sigmoid and descending colon may require using different maneuvers* in the presence of redundancy, adhesions, angulation, and loops. At times, especially in young persons, the scope can be advanced all the way up to the transverse colon without any difficulty. In older patients, especially those who have had abdominal or pelvic surgery, the presence of adhesions may make further advancement difficult. The rectosigmoid junction is at 15 to 18 cm. Advancement may be hampered here by the angulation of the bowel toward the left into the left iliac fossa. The length of the sigmoid itself varies from 20 to 45 cm. Certain maneuvers—individually or in combination—can then be attempted to advance the scope through the descending colon and into the distal portion of the transverse colon.
    - *Advancement by hook, rotation, and pullback*. When the scope will not advance, deflect the tip of the shaft 30 to 90 degrees behind a mucosal fold (Fig. 103-8) and withdraw the shaft 5 to 10 cm, pulling the segment of the colon downward, twisting the head of the scope to the right, and creating a pleating and straightening-out effect. Repeat this maneuver several times as needed to achieve the desired goal of compressing the bowel over the shaft of the scope, much like an accordion. It should be done very gently with minimal (if any) resistance. *When you cannot go forward, flex the tip down, torque to the right, and withdraw. It is a difficult concept to master, but to go forward you must pull back, as noted.*
    - *Dithering-torque maneuver* (Fig. 103-9). The dithering-torque maneuver is a to-and-fro advance-and-withdrawal process performed with an amplitude of 5 to 6 cm every 2 to 4 seconds. It is coupled with a clockwise torque of the shaft of about 45 to 60 degrees on the pullback motion and a counterclockwise torque on the inward motion. This process "accordionizes" the colon onto the shaft of the scope, thereby shortening the colon and enabling a larger length of the colon to be traversed and examined. Gentle tip deflection of 30 degrees with the torque motion is recommended. The *clockwise* torque tends to loop the sigmoid, whereas the *counterclockwise* torque tends to straighten it. This is an effective maneuver in shortening the sigmoid, and it is of greatest use in a redundant sigmoid colon. Excessive tip deflection can become a hindrance to further advancement; therefore it should be kept to the minimum to maintain visualization of the lumen. If the tip needs greater deflection at the moment, it should be straightened soon after the lumen is located.
    - *Jiggling* is merely an in-and-out motion deflecting the tip slightly, trying to get the scope to advance. In performing flexible sigmoidoscopy, it is best to keep the scope moving in some manner to maximize the opportunity of seeing the lumen (Fig. 103-10).
    - *Alpha maneuver* (for experienced endoscopists). Advance the scope into the sigmoid. At about 25 to 30 cm, deflect the tip to visualize the lumen anteriorly, and then torque the shaft counterclockwise about 145 to 180 degrees (Fig. 103-11A). This swings the proximal part of the sigmoid over the distal part, so that the sigmoid colon forms a loop over itself (Fig. 103-11B and C). Here, minimally deflect the tip to locate the lumen and then straighten it as much as possible. Further advancement of the scope will lead it into the descending colon. If resistance is encountered, rotate the shaft clockwise and withdraw to "accordionize," or shorten, the sigmoid (Fig. 103-11D). The shaft can then be advanced into the descending colon, to the splenic flexure (see Fig. 103-12D). The alpha maneuver is rarely needed but may be necessary in the redundant bowel. It should be used only by the experienced endoscopist.
11. Opinions vary as to whether *changing patient position* will improve visualization or aid in advancement of the scope. Many

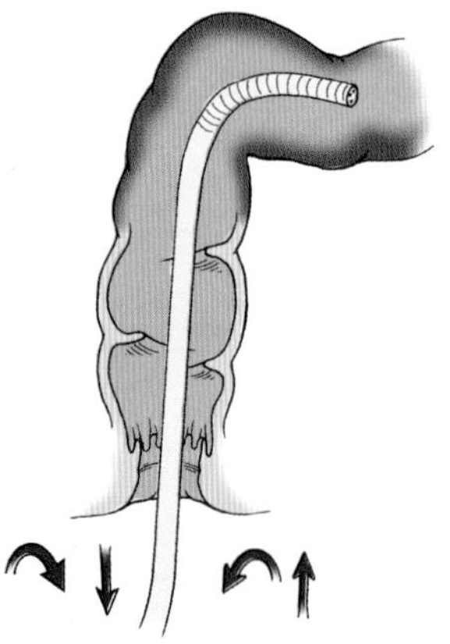

Figure 103-9 Dithering maneuver. Rotate counterclockwise when withdrawing and clockwise when inserting. See text for details.

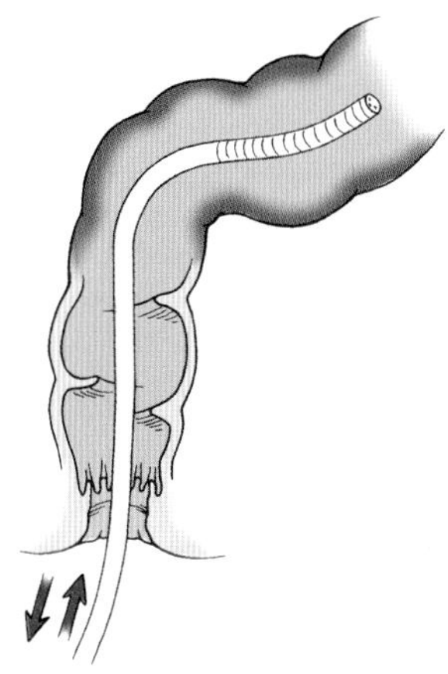

Figure 103-10 Jiggle maneuver. See text for details.

will roll patients onto their backs. Try it if other maneuvers do not work.

12. Once past the "second curve," the scope is generally advanced with minimal manipulation into the descending colon by jiggling, hooking, and pulling back; simply maintaining mild inward pressure on the shaft usually suffices.

    The area of the splenic flexure can often be recognized by the bluish hue superiorly, which represents the transmitted vascularity of the spleen sitting on the colon exteriorly. The colon takes a turn anteriorly and to the patient's right at this point, and the triangular folds of the transverse colon can be identified easily (see Fig. 103-12E).
13. *Inspection: Withdrawal of the scope is easy but probably the most important part of the procedure*. Using a combination of tip deflection and torquing in both directions, gradually withdraw the shaft, visually inspecting the entire circumference of the intubated colon. Pay careful attention to all areas of the mucosal surface, particularly behind mucosal folds. Make note of diverticula and any masses. (See the Biopsy section, later.) If any segment is not seen completely, advance and withdraw again. Continue withdrawing until the rectum is reached.

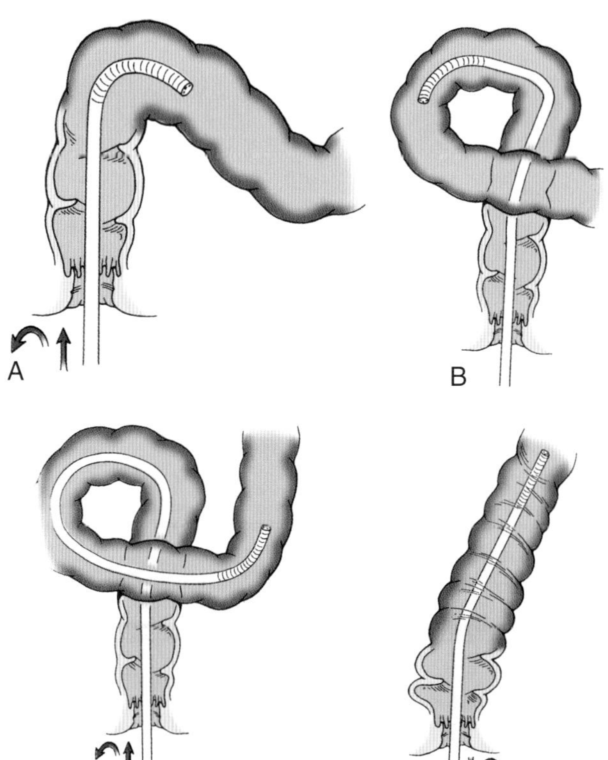

Figure 103-11 **A–D,** Alpha maneuver. See text for details.

14. *Retroflexion: The anal canal and distal rectum must be inspected* thoroughly in one of two ways: by using an anoscope or by completely deflecting the sigmoidoscope tip to look back on itself (i.e., retroflexion; see Fig. 103-12N through Q). Either procedure is performed after completing the examination of as much proximal bowel as possible with the sigmoidoscope. The sigmoidoscope can simply be withdrawn completely and the anal canal examined with the anoscope. Or, to accomplish the retroflexion maneuver, withdraw the endoscope to the anal verge, then gently advance the scope about 10 to 12 cm while simultaneously turning both controls counterclockwise to full deflection. You will be looking back onto the shaft of the scope and will see it passing through the anal canal. By torquing the shaft you can perform a 360-degree visual inspection of the distal rectal vault and the inner aspect of the anal canal and papillae to detect masses and hemorrhoids (although these are much better appreciated with an Ives slotted anoscope). After completing the examination, straighten the tip and withdraw it very slowly. Grasp the tip of the scope as it slips out of the anus so that it does not drop on the table, damaging its delicate construction.
15. *Remove all the air: You may do this before completely removing the scope or reinsert the scope 5 to 6 cm. Apply intermittent suction* and use a to-and-fro motion with rotation to prevent the mucosa from being drawn into the suction port, thus occluding it (see following Step 16). After the patient indicates that the air is gone, remove the scope and immediately draw soapy water through the suction port. Also, occlude the air port to "blow out" any accumulated debris. The latter two steps will enhance cleaning and preserve proper functioning of the scope.
16. *Removing colonic fluid and air.* Do not attempt to suction any solid material through the scope. The channels are extremely small and are easily plugged. When suctioning (button closest to the endoscopist), intermittently push the button all the way down while instilling air and moving the scope back and forth a few centimeters. Constant suctioning at one position will suck mucosa into the scope, causing what appears to be a polyp ("suction polyp" or "pseudopolyp"). This artifact should disappear or flatten if the bowel lumen is expanded with air but may temporarily leave a circular mark on the mucosa. Keeping the scope in motion and compressing the suction button intermittently will help avoid unnecessary biopsy procedures and confusing findings.
17. The scope should be cleaned and disinfected as soon as possible after the procedure is completed (see later discussion).

Biopsy

There are many opinions about when and if biopsies should be obtained during flexible sigmoidoscopy. Some points of view with countering arguments include the following:

- *Primary care physicians should not perform a biopsy on any lesion.* (*Counter:* The biopsy technique is simple and virtually without complication when only the cold [without electrocautery] biopsy forceps are used. It samples only 2 to 3 mm of the mucosa, and unless the tissue is pulsating, ulcerated, or inside a diverticulum, perforation is almost impossible.)
- *It is useless to obtain a biopsy sample because the colonoscopist will need to remove the polyp anyway.* (*Counter:* If the biopsy result shows only a hyperplastic polyp [see Fig. 103-12H], there is no need for colonoscopy. Documentation of an abnormality aids in categorizing the patient's risk status and reinforces the physician's rationale for the patient to have the often-resisted colonoscopy performed. It also confirms the diagnosis for the colonoscopist and mandates that the lesion be found.)

- *Do not perform a biopsy on small polyps (<5 mm)*. (*Counter:* It is precisely these lesions that are difficult to diagnose accurately with an endoscope, so they require biopsy to determine if they are adenomatous and thus require full colonoscopy. Even very small, "diminutive" polyps, that appear to be benign, can be advanced adenomas [villous histology or high-grade dysplasia], and cause the patient to be in the same high-risk group as patients with larger adenomatous polyps [Schoen and colleagues, 2006].)
- *Performing a biopsy may increase malpractice insurance*. (*Counter:* Not doing it may miss a crucial diagnosis. In general, premiums are not increased for this very–low-risk diagnostic procedure. If the lesion is not sampled and the colonoscopist cannot find it on a later examination, it may prolong the procedure, and the patient's actual status remains unknown.)
- Performing a biopsy provides pathology feedback to the endoscopist, which increases the learning curve for clinical diagnoses in the future.

EDITOR'S NOTE: It is our practice to perform a biopsy on essentially all nonvascular lesions. No complications have been encountered. If it does not look like the mucosa on the inside of your mouth, if it is not pulsating, if you are not inside a diverticulum, and if you do not know what it is, perform a biopsy!

Precautions

The following are some caveats regarding biopsy:

- A vascular lesion (especially if pulsating!) may best be left for later biopsy under more controlled situations.
- Do not perform electrosurgical removal of a polyp except in a fully prepared bowel (bowel gases in the colon can explode).
- After the procedure, ensure and document that all bleeding has stopped.
- Document the location from which each polyp was removed and, except for small polyps in close proximity to each other, place each polyp in a separate specimen container.

Biopsy Technique

Position the scope tip is so the selected biopsy site is 2 to 4 cm away and at 6 o'clock on video endoscopes or opposite the black triangle on fiberoptic scopes. Pass the closed forceps down the biopsy channel while keeping the lumen in view to avoid risk of damaging the bowel wall. The assistant should maintain gentle pressure on the forceps controls to keep the jaws closed. Excessive closing pressure causes the forceps to become stiff and can make passage through a deflected tip difficult or damage the endoscope. Once the forceps tip has emerged from the distal tip of the scope, ask the assistant to open the jaws of the forceps. Advance the open forceps against the desired site and ask the assistant to close the jaws. Gently pull out on the forceps to "tent" the mucosa and confirm the desired site is in the jaws, and then sharply withdraw the forceps to remove the tissue by applying a quick jerk to the line. The biopsy sample is placed in formalin and the site observed for bleeding. Occasionally, a second or even a third biopsy sample of the lesion may be indicated (see Fig. 103-5). If the forceps have a central needle, a second biopsy can often be obtained on a single passage.

FINDINGS

See Figure 103-12.

- Polyps (iatrogenic "suction polyps," hyperplastic, and adenomatous [tubular, tubulovillous, and villous adenomas])
- Cancer
- Inflammation (inflammatory bowel [Crohn's and ulcerative colitis], antibiotic-associated colitis)
- Diverticula
- Melanosis coli
- Arteriovenous malformations
- Foreign bodies
- Condylomata
- Hemorrhoids (internal)

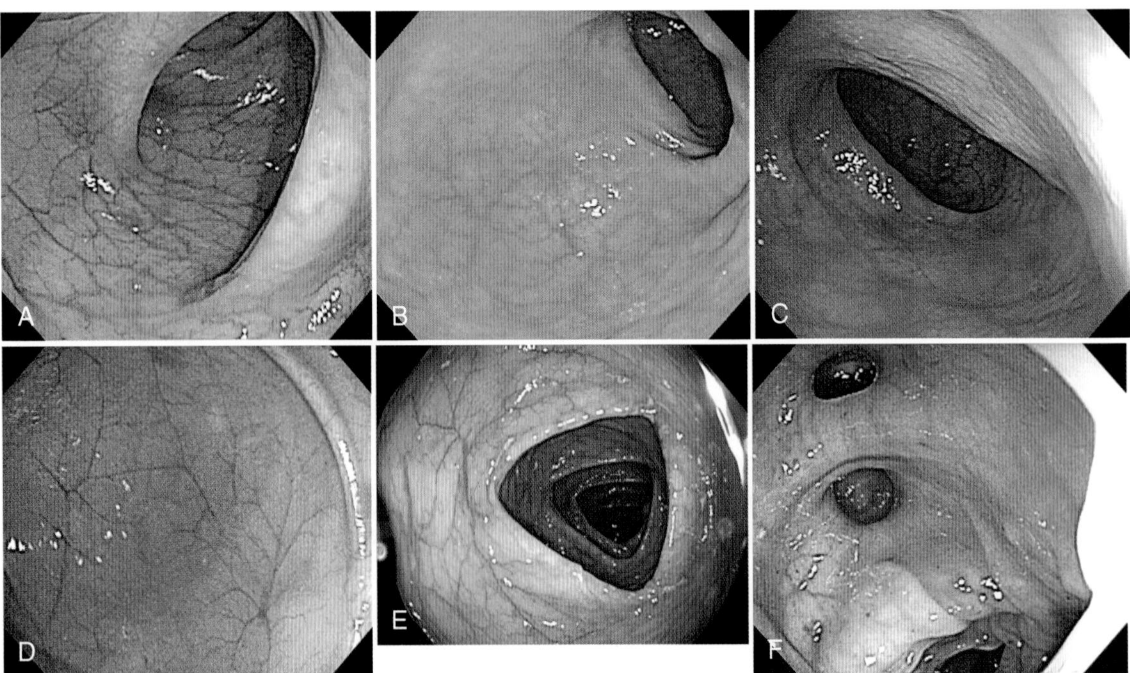

Figure 103-12 Normal and abnormal findings during sigmoidoscopy. **A,** Semilunar valves of Houston. **B,** Rectosigmoid area. **C,** Sigmoid colon. **D,** The splenic flexure. The spleen projects a cyanotic hue through the colon wall. **E,** The transverse colon with characteristic triangular appearance of the folds. **F,** Diverticulosis.

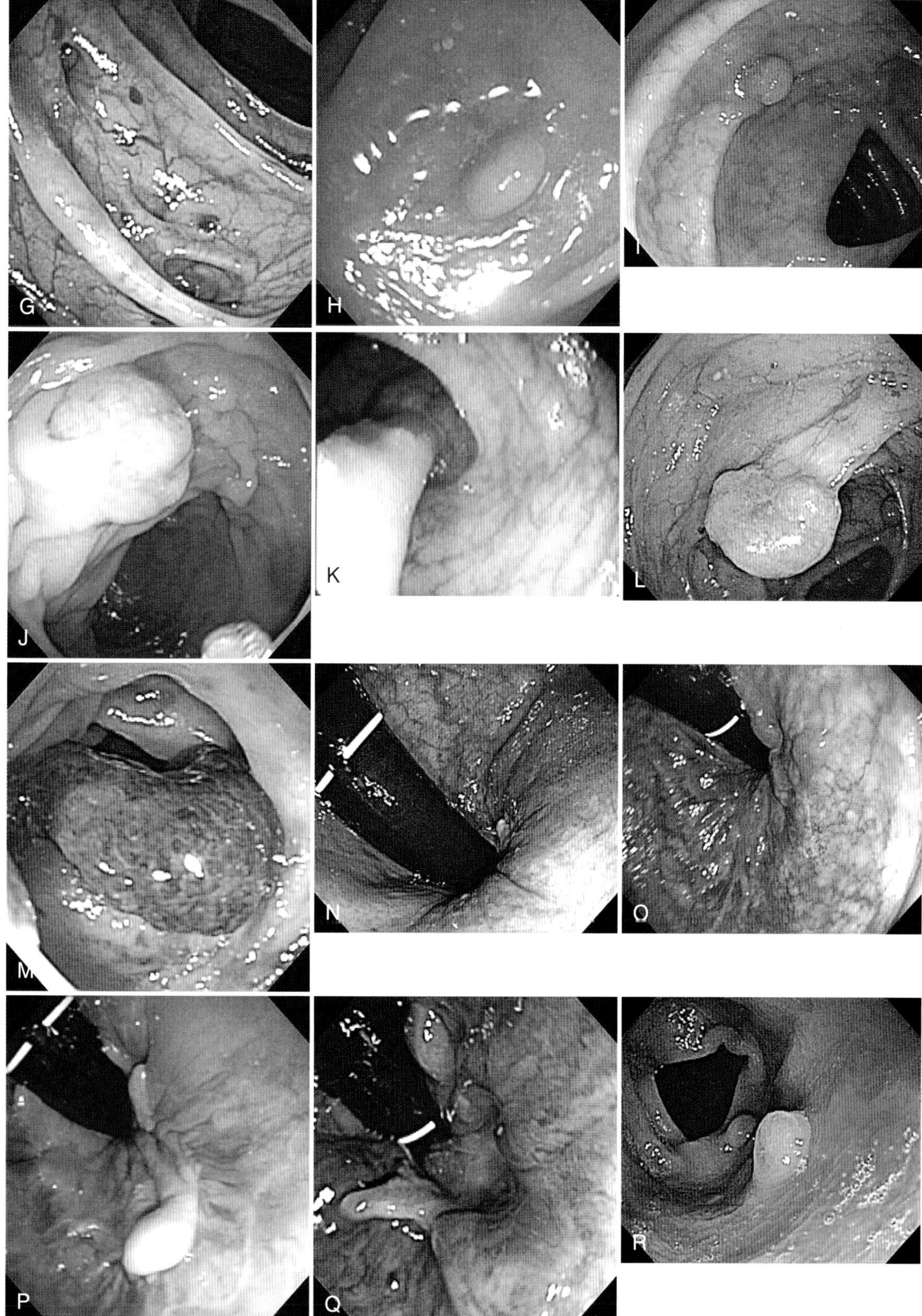

Figure 103-12, cont. **G,** Multiple diverticula. **H,** Small polyp that was hyperplastic on biopsy. **I,** Small adenomatous polyp at the splenic flexure. The scope is looking across the transverse colon, which can be identified by its triangular shape. **J,** Pedunculated polyp. **K,** Another pedunculated polyp. **L,** Large sessile polyp in the sigmoid colon. **M,** Large colon mass that was a cancer on biopsy. **N,** The retroflexion maneuver in a normal rectum performed just before the scope is totally removed. Note that the scope is turned upon itself in a "big U" and the view is of the scope coming through the anus. Note the normal vascular pattern of the bowel. **O,** Internal hemorrhoids seen on retroflexion. **P,** Hypertrophied anal papilla. **Q,** Hypertrophied papilla along the dentate line. Internal hemorrhoids also present. **R,** Everted diverticulum, confirm by probing with closed forceps, do not snare these. (**K,** Courtesy of John L. Pfenninger, MD, The Medical Procedures Center, PC, Midland, Mich.)

Documentation

It is important that all findings be noted and documented. A comment should be made on each of the following: scope used, distance inserted by anatomic location and centimeters, quality of preparation, patient tolerance, vascular and mucosal patterns, size of any polyps identified and location where they were found, ease of biopsy and control of any bleeding, final impression, and follow-up recommendations (Fig. 103-13).

Significance of Various Polyps

It is beyond the scope of this chapter to provide an extensive discussion of the significance of various polyps. More information is included in Chapter 100, Colonoscopy. In brief, all adenomatous (neoplastic) polyps (tubular, tubulovillous, and villous lesions) have a malignant potential. Recent articles document the reduction of CRC if all neoplastic polyps are removed. Most experts agree that hyperplastic polyps have little prognostic significance. Colonoscopy

Flexible Sigmoidoscopy

Name: ____________ Birth date: ____________ Phone: (H) ____________
Age: ____________ (W) ____________

Your usual doctor: ____________ Send a copy of report to him/her? Y N
Blood pressure: ____________ Received and understood handouts? Y N

SYMPTOMS/HISTORY

Frequency ____________ Pain: Abdomen Rectum w/BM
Consistency: Loose Formed Hard Anemia ____________
Change in stools ____________ Weight loss ____________
Diarrhea ____________ Fever ____________
Constipation ____________ Polyps ____________
Blood ____________ Hemorrhoids ____________
Black stools ____________ F.H. ____________

TESTS

Hemoccult: Date ____________
positive/negative not done
Previous sigmoidoscopy/colonoscopy: Date ____________
Findings ____________
Previous barium enema: Date ____________
Findings ____________

PMH

Bleeding problems? Yes No
Artificial joints? Yes No
Artificial heart valve? Yes No
Heart murmur needing prophylaxis? Yes No

Allergies ____________
Other medical problems? ____________
Medications? ____________
Health maintenance? ____________

PROCEDURE **Scope: OSF-3**

Abdominal exam: Megaly Y N Mass Y N Tenderness Y N
Preparation: Adequate/Inadequate Fleet given in office Y N
Rectal: ____________
Depth: ____________
Reason for stopping: Limits of scope or ____________
Tolerance: ____________
Complications: none or ____________
Findings: ____________
Biopsy: ______ cm ______ cm ______ cm Bleeding controlled Y N
Proctoscopy: ____________

IMPRESSION: ____________
RECOMMENDATIONS: ____________
Daily aspirins, vitamins, diet, estrogen
Repeat exam ____________
cc: ____________ ____________ ____________
Physician's signature Date

Figure 103-13 Sample procedure form for flexible sigmoidoscopy. (Courtesy of John L. Pfenninger, MD, The Medical Procedures Center, PC, Midland, Mich.)

is not recommended for hyperplastic polyps, whereas it is essential with neoplastic polyps.

Complications

- Bowel perforation (very rare, <1 : 20,000)
- Bleeding (more likely if a biopsy sample was obtained, but still very uncommon)
- Abdominal distention and pain, often due to the insufflated air (be sure it is all removed)
- Infection (although very rare, inadequate cleaning of scopes can transmit disease)
- Vasovagal symptoms
- Missed disease

Complications from flexible sigmoidoscopy are very rare. Their incidence is higher in patients with previous bowel or pelvic surgery, or irradiation. These patients have more adhesions, which tether the bowel to a fixed position, predisposing it to perforation. If the scope is advanced blindly, without seeing the lumen, the risk of perforation also increases. However, at times this is necessary and safe as long as no resistance is felt and the patient is not overly uncomfortable.

Care must be taken in the presence of diverticulosis. The mouth of the diverticulum can be interpreted as the bowel lumen, and if the scope is inserted, perforation can occur.

Missed disease can occur if the endoscopist is unable to adequately insert the endoscope. This problem occurs more commonly in women and elderly patients (Walter and colleagues, 2004). Disease in the rectum can also be missed if retroflection or anoscopic examination is not performed.

Cleaning and Disinfection of Scopes

The various instrument representatives will detail the exact cleaning mechanism for each brand of scope. Tremain and colleagues (1991) present an excellent review, and reading of this article is strongly encouraged. Jackson and Ball (1997) also summarize the essential steps in disinfecting scopes. It is *essential that the clinician's staff pay meticulous attention to cleaning directions for the scope*. The orifices are very small and a small amount of debris can prevent optimal functioning.

Postprocedure Patient Education

After completion of the procedure, explain the following to the patient:

- Findings.
- Where the biopsy samples have been taken from and the necessity for pathologic evaluation.
- Further management or referral, and future surveillance plans.
- Implications of the presence of cancer or polyps for the patient's siblings and children.
- Necessity of reporting any excessive bleeding or abdominal pain.
- Reinforce that proximal lesions are certainly possible and that if any symptoms develop (or persist if present), then further evaluation is necessary.
- Primary prevention methods include the possible use of a nonsteroidal anti-inflammatory drug (NSAID), not smoking, and a high-bulk, low-fat diet with at least five helpings of fruits and vegetables a day. A multivitamin a day (folic acid and vitamin D), estrogen use, and statins may also reduce the incidence of CRC. The USPSTF recommends against the routine use of aspirin and NSAIDs to prevent CRC in individuals at average risk for CRC since side effects may outweigh the benefits.

CPT/Billing Codes

45330 Sigmoidoscopy, flexible fiberoptic; diagnostic with or without collection of specimen by brushing or washing
45331 Sigmoidoscopy with biopsy, single or multiple
45332 Sigmoidoscopy with removal of foreign body
45333 Sigmoidoscopy with removal of polypoid lesion(s) by hot biopsy forceps or bipolar cautery
45334 Sigmoidoscopy with control of hemorrhage (e.g., electrocoagulation)
45338 Sigmoidoscopy with removal of polypoid lesion(s) by snare technique
45339 Sigmoidoscopy with ablation of tumor or mucosal lesion not amenable to removal by hot biopsy, or snare technique
46600 Anoscopy; diagnostic (separate procedure)

Medicare will pay for *screening* flexible sigmoidoscopy after 47 months have passed since the flexible sigmoidoscopy or barium enema. The code GO104 should be used. If a biopsy is taken, the code 45331, not the "G" code, should be used.

ICD-9-CM Diagnostic Codes

078.11 Condyloma
153.2 Cancer, colon—descending, left
153.3 Cancer, colon—sigmoid
154.1 Cancer, rectum
154.2 Cancer, anus
153.9 Cancer, colon, unspecified
211.3 Benign neoplasm, colon
211.4 Benign neoplasm, rectum/anus
455.0 Internal hemorrhoids
455.2 Internal hemorrhoids, bleeding
555.1 Crohn's disease—colon
556.9 Ulcerative colitis
558.1 Radiation colitis
558.9 Colitis, nonspecific
562.10 Diverticulosis without hemorrhage
562.12 Diverticulosis with hemorrhage
562.13 Diverticulitis with hemorrhage
564.00 Unspecified constipation
564.1 Irritable colon
565.0 Anal fissure
566 Perirectal abscess
569.0 Anal polyp
569.3 Anal hemorrhage
569.42 Anal pain
569.82 Ulcer, colon
569.84 Angiodysplasia, colon
578.1 Melena
578.9 Gastrointestinal hemorrhage, hematochezia
783.21 Weight loss
787.4 Hyperperistalsis
787.6 Stool incontinence
787.99 Tenesmus
789.00 Abdominal pain
793.4 X-ray abnormality, gastrointestinal tract
V10.05 Personal history colon cancer (not primary diagnosis)
V16.0 Family history colon or other GI cancer (not primary diagnosis)
V18.51 Family history colon polyps
V18.59 Family history other gastrointestinal disorders (not primary diagnosis)

Medicare-covered codes include history adenomatous polyps (V6700, V12.72), malignant and benign gastrointestinal tract neoplasm (150.0–154.8, 159.0, 159.8, 211.0–211.4), and ca-in-situ

(230.1–230.7, 235.2, 235.5, 239.0); infectious gastrointestinal diseases and colitis (555.0–556.9, 558.2–558.9), ischemic lesions (557.0–557.1), other diseases (560.0–566, 568.0–569.9, 619.1, 759.6, V12.70); hematochezia, melena, change in bowel habits, abdominal pain, abdominal or pelvic mass, occult blood, anemia, abnormal x-ray examination, personal history of gastrointestinal cancer.

ACKNOWLEDGMENT

The editors wish to recognize the many contributions by John L. Pfenninger, MD, to this chapter in the previous edition of this text.

SUPPLIERS

(See contact information online at www.expertconsult.com.)

Sigmoidoscopes

Fujinon, Inc.
Olympus America, Inc.
Pentax Medical

(Also see the "Used or refurbished equipment" list in the Suppliers section of Chapter 100, Colonoscopy.)

ONLINE RESOURCES

American Association for Primary Care Endoscopy: Available at www.aapce.org.

American Gastroenterological Association (AGA): Available at www.gastro.org.

American Society of Colon and Rectal Surgeons: Available at www.fascrs.org.

CA: *A Cancer Journal for Clinicians* (American Cancer Association): Available at www.ca-journal.org.

The DAVE Project—Gastroenterology: Available at http://daveproject.org/index.cfm.

BIBLIOGRAPHY

Anderson ML, Pasha TM, Leighton JA: Endoscopic perforation of the colon: Lessons from a 10-year study. Am J Gastroenterol 95:3418–3422, 2000.

Atkin WS, Edwards R, Kralj-Hans I, et al: Once-only flexible sigmoidoscopy screening in prevention of colorectal cancer: A multicentre randomised controlled trial. Lancet 375:1624–1633, 2010.

Brill JR, Baumgardner DJ: Establishing proficiency in flexible sigmoidoscopy in a family practice residency program. Fam Med 29:580–583, 1997.

Brooks DD, Winawer SJ, Rex DK, et al: Colonoscopy surveillance after polypectomy and colorectal cancer resection. Am Fam Physician 77: 995–1002, 2008.

Centers for Disease Control and Prevention: Increased use of colorectal cancer tests—United States, 2002 and 2004. MMWR Morb Mortal Wkly Rep 55:308–311, 2006.

Esber EJ, Yang P: Retroflexion of the sigmoidoscope for the detection of rectal cancer. Am Fam Physician 51:1709–1711, 1995.

Frazier AL, Colditz CA, Fuchs CS, et al: Cost-effectiveness of screening for endorectal cancer in the general population. JAMA 284:1954–1961, 2000.

Gatto NM, Frucht H, Sundararajan V, et al: Risk of perforation after colonoscopy and sigmoidoscopy: A population-based study. J Natl Cancer Inst 95:230–236, 2003.

Holman JR, Marshall RC, Jordan B, Vogelman L: Technical competency in flexible sigmoidoscopy. J Am Board Fam Pract 14:424–429, 2001.

Jackson FW, Ball MD: Correction of deficiencies in flexible fiberoptic sigmoidoscope cleaning and disinfection technique in family practice and internal medicine offices. Arch Fam Med 6:578–582, 1997.

Jemal A, Siegel R, Ward E, et al: Cancer statistics, 2008. CA Cancer J Clin 58:71–96, 2008.

Levin B, Lieberman DA, McFarland B, et al: Screening and surveillance for the early detection of colorectal cancer and adenomatous polyps, 2008. A joint guideline from the American Cancer Society, the US Multi-Society Task Force on Colorectal Cancer, and the American College of Radiology. CA Cancer J Clin 58:130–160, 2008.

Levin TR, Conell C, Shapiro JA, et al: Complications of screening flexible sigmoidoscopy. Gastroenterology 123:1786–1792, 2002.

Levin TR, Palitz A, Grossman S, et al: Predicting advanced proximal colonic neoplasia with screening sigmoidoscopy. JAMA 281:1611–1617, 1999.

Lin OS, Schembre DB, McCormick SE, et al: Risk of proximal colorectal neoplasia among asymptomatic patients with distal hyperplastic polyps. Am J Med 118:1113–1119, 2005.

Loeve F, Brown ML, Boer R, et al: Endoscopic colorectal cancer screening: A cost-saving analysis. J Natl Cancer Inst 92:557–563, 2000.

Manoucheri M, Nakamura DY, Lukman RL: Bowel preparation for flexible sigmoidoscopy: Which method yields the best results? J Fam Pract 48:272–274, 1999.

Pfenninger JL, Zainea GG: Common anorectal conditions: Part I. Symptoms and complaints. Am Fam Physician 63:2391–2398, 2001.

Pfenninger JL, Zainea GG: Common anorectal conditions: Part II. Lesions. Am Fam Physician 64:77–88, 2001.

Provenzale D, Garrett JW, Condon SE, Sandler RS: Risk for colon adenomas in patients with rectosigmoid hyperplastic polyps. Ann Intern Med 113:760–763, 1990.

Read TE, Kodner IJ: Colorectal cancer: Risk factors and recommendations for early detection. Am Fam Physician 59:3083–3092, 1999.

Roetzheim RG, Pal N, Gonzalez EC, et al: The effects of physician supply on the early detection of colorectal cancer. J Fam Pract 48:850–858, 1999.

Schoen RE, Weissfeld JL, Pinsky PF, Riley T: Yield of advanced adenoma and cancer based on polyp size detected at screening flexible sigmoidoscopy. Gastroenterology 131:1683–1689, 2006.

Sharma V, Chockalingham S: Randomized, controlled comparison of two forms of preparation for screening flexible sigmoidoscopy. Am J Gastroenterol 92:809–811, 1997.

Sonnenberg A, Delco F, Inadomi JM: Cost-effectiveness of colonoscopy in screening for colorectal cancer. Ann Intern Med 133:573–584, 2000.

Tremain SC, Orientale E, Rodney WM: Cleaning, disinfection, and sterilization of gastrointestinal endoscopes: Approaches in the office. J Fam Pract 32:300–305, 1991.

UK Flexible Sigmoidoscopy Screening Trial Investigators: Single flexible sigmoidoscopy screening to prevent colorectal cancer: Baseline findings of a UK multicentre randomised trial. Lancet 359:1291–1300, 2002.

U.S. Preventive Services Task Force: Screening for Colorectal Cancer: U.S. Preventive Services Task Force Recommendation Statement. Ann Intern Med 149:627–637, 2008.

Walter LC, de Garmo P, Covinsky KE: Association of older age and female sex with inadequate reach of screening flexible sigmoidoscopy. Am J Med 116:174–178, 2004.

Wilson W, Taubert KA, Gewitz M, et al: Prevention of infective endocarditis: Guidelines from the American Heart Association. A guideline from the American Heart Association Rheumatic Fever, Endocarditis, and Kawasaki Disease Committee, Council on Cardiovascular Disease in the Young, and the Council on Clinical Cardiology, Council on Cardiovascular Surgery and Anesthesia, and the Quality of Care and Outcomes Research Interdisciplinary Working Group. Circulation 116:1736–1754, 2007.

CHAPTER 104

VIDEO CAPSULE ENDOSCOPY*

Matti Waterman • Edward G. Zurad • Ian M. Gralnek

Video capsule endoscopy (VCE) of the small bowel is one of the major advances in small bowel imaging in the last several years. Compared with other existing imaging modalities, VCE has been demonstrated to have the highest yield in the diagnosis of gastrointestinal (GI) hemorrhage of obscure origin, iron-deficiency anemia (IDA), small bowel tumors, suspected or early Crohn's disease (CD), and several other medical conditions involving the small intestine. This relatively easy-to-use, minimally invasive procedure, requiring limited or no patient preparation and no sedation, has acquired enormous worldwide popularity since its clearance by the U.S. Food and Drug Administration (FDA) in 2001. The original wireless capsule endoscope was the M2A small bowel capsule (now called Pillcam SB; Given Imaging, Ltd., Yoqneam, Israel). In September 2007, the FDA cleared the Olympus Corporation's EndoCapsule. Other companies have also started to produce small bowel capsule endoscopes, including the MiroCam from South Korea and the OMOM capsule from the People's Republic of China. Neither of those products has FDA clearance for use in the United States. In 2008 it was estimated that over 600,000 capsules have been ingested worldwide and over 600 scientific articles regarding VCE have been published. Its growing popularity and simplicity make VCE a viable option in the office work-up of patients with suspected small bowel disease by primary care physicians. In this chapter, we discuss indications for the procedure, the procedure itself, the image reviewing process and interpretation of common findings, patient instructions, and procedure-related complications and how to minimize them. Capsule endoscopy for the esophagus and the colon is still not widely accepted and practiced, and therefore these procedures are not discussed.

INDICATIONS

Indications for VCE of the small bowel are listed in Box 104-1.

Obscure Gastrointestinal Bleeding

The source of GI bleeding remains unidentified in approximately 5% of patients and is thus referred to as *obscure*. Obscure GI bleeding may be overt, as evidenced by clinical signs (melena or hematochezia), or occult and manifested as positive fecal occult blood testing or IDA. By definition, obscure GI bleeding occurs when esophagogastroduodenoscopy (EGD) and colonoscopy are negative. In such cases, further work-up is required. The role of VCE in obscure GI bleeding has been validated in two meta-analyses and is outlined in Figure 104-1. In patients presenting with IDA, VCE has a less validated role (Fig. 104-2). As has been validated in the aforementioned meta-analyses, VCE is the most sensitive diagnostic modality and is considered the first line in the diagnostic work-up for obscure GI bleeding. Figure 104-3 shows an example of bleeding in the small bowel as captured by the Pillcam.

*Conflict of interest statement: Drs. Waterman, Zurad, and Gralnek are consultants of Given Imaging, Yoqneam, Israel, the maker of Pillcam SB.

Crohn's Disease

Crohn's disease is an idiopathic inflammatory disease involving the small bowel in approximately 75% of cases. Because no diagnostic gold standard exists, the diagnosis of CD in the small bowel is based on clinical, endoscopic, radiologic, and histologic findings. However, available diagnostic modalities are neither sensitive nor specific. As a result, appropriate drug therapy may be delayed. Furthermore, available endoscopic procedures (e.g., push enteroscopy) fail to visualize the entire small bowel distal to the ligament of Treitz; thus, significant small bowel involvement may be missed. VCE has a role both in diagnosing suspected CD (Fig. 104-4) and in determining the extent of small bowel involvement in CD. VCE also has been shown to be more sensitive than other imaging modalities in detecting small bowel mucosal breaks and thus is very helpful in diagnosing early CD (Fig. 104-5) and in assessing mucosal healing after drug treatment and disease recurrence after surgery.

Small Bowel Tumors

The advent of VCE has resulted in a major shift in the diagnosis of small bowel tumors (Fig. 104-6). In the past, small bowel tumors were usually diagnosed only during the work-up of persistent abdominal pain or when obstructive symptoms appeared. Today, approximately 80% of small bowel tumors that are detected by VCE are from referrals to VCE due to obscure GI bleeding evaluation. The estimated prevalence of small bowel tumors in VCE for obscure bleeding is 6.3% to 12.3%. There is preliminary evidence that VCE

Box 104-1. Indications for Small Bowel Video Capsule Endoscopy

- Celiac disease
- Crohn's disease
  - Assessment of small bowel mucosal healing
  - Identification of postoperative disease recurrence
  - Indeterminate colitis
  - Suspected Crohn's disease
- Evaluation of abnormal small bowel imaging
- Evaluation of drug-induced small bowel injury
- Obscure gastrointestinal bleeding
  - Iron-deficiency anemia
  - Occult (positive fecal occult blood test)
  - Overt (hematemesis, coffee-ground vomiting, melena, hematochezia)
- Suspected small bowel tumor
- Surveillance of inherited polyposis syndromes

Adapted from Eliakim AR: Video capsule endoscopy of the small bowel (PillCam SB). Curr Opin Gastroenterol 22:124–127, 2006.

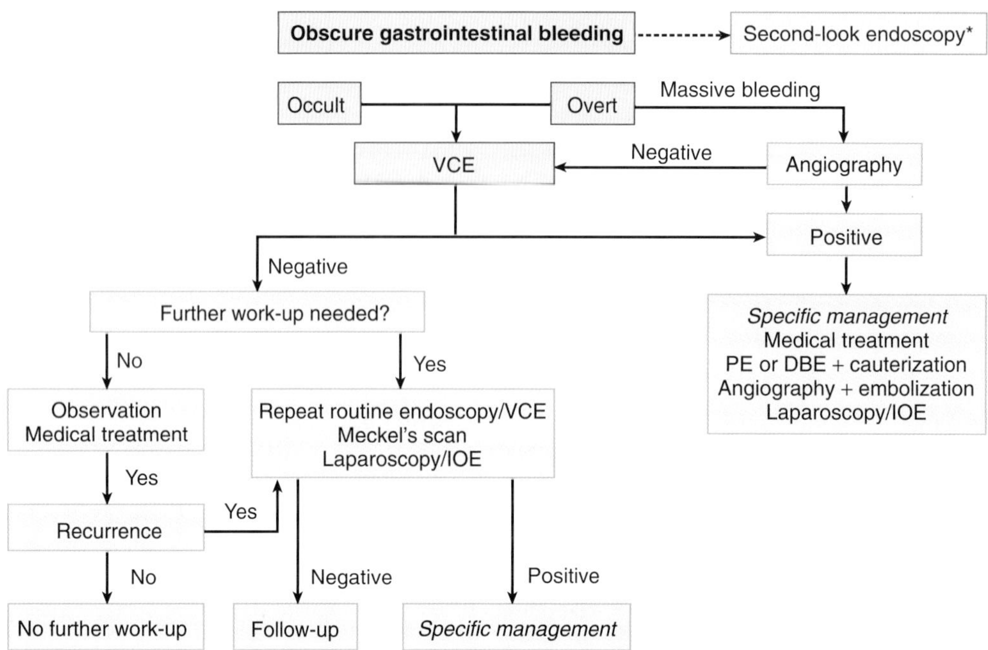

Figure 104-1 The diagnostic algorithm of obscure gastrointestinal hemorrhage. DBE, double-balloon enteroscopy; IOE, intraoperative enteroscopy; PE, push enteroscopy; VCE, video capsule endoscopy. *Some experts suggest a second-look endoscopy prior to capsule endoscopy to ensure that no pathology was missed.

favorably changes the clinical outcome in such cases. Note that when small bowel obstructive symptoms are present the initial work-up should be push enteroscopy or double-balloon enteroscopy rather than VCE.

Inherited Polyposis Syndromes

The lifetime risk of duodenal and small bowel tumors in familial adenomatous polyposis may be as high as 5% to 12%. Other polyposis syndromes, including Peutz-Jeghers syndrome and juvenile polyposis, also portend increased risk for small bowel and duodenal cancers, with a relative risk of 13% for small bowel tumors in Peutz-Jeghers syndrome. This risk has led to a recommended screening schedule including EGD or small bowel barium series every 1 to 3 years. VCE has been shown be a sensitive surveillance tool for detecting small bowel polyps in this high-risk population, with a reported sensitivity of over 90%.

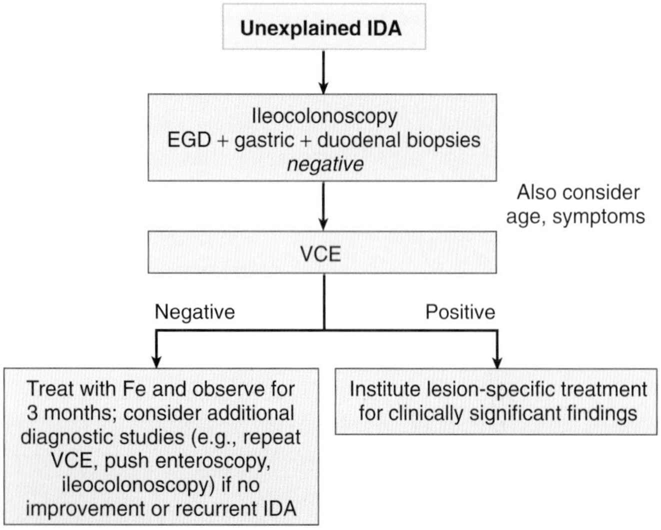

Celiac Disease

Celiac disease has a prevalence of approximately 1% in the general population and is diagnosed by clinical suspicion, serologic and histologic findings obtained by small bowel biopsy ranging from partial to total villous atrophy, and patient response to a gluten-free diet. VCE, which provides a high-resolution magnified view of the small bowel mucosa, can detect mucosal changes such as scalloping, mosaic pattern, loss of normal villous architecture, loss of small bowel folds, and nodularity (Fig. 104-7). These findings by capsule endoscopy have been correlated with the typical histologic findings of celiac disease. Moreover, VCE has been shown to have good sensitivity and excellent specificity in the diagnosis of celiac disease

Unexplained IDA

Ileocolonoscopy
EGD + gastric + duodenal biopsies
negative

Also consider
age, symptoms

VCE

Negative

Positive

Treat with Fe and observe for 3 months; consider additional diagnostic studies (e.g., repeat VCE, push enteroscopy, ileocolonoscopy) if no improvement or recurrent IDA

Institute lesion-specific treatment for clinically significant findings

Figure 104-2 The diagnostic algorithm of iron-deficiency anemia (IDA). EGD, esophagogastroduodenoscopy; VCE, video capsule endoscopy.

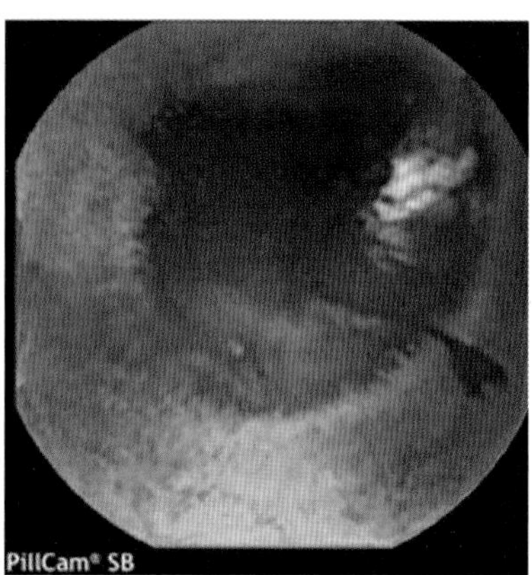

Figure 104-3 Active small bowel bleeding.

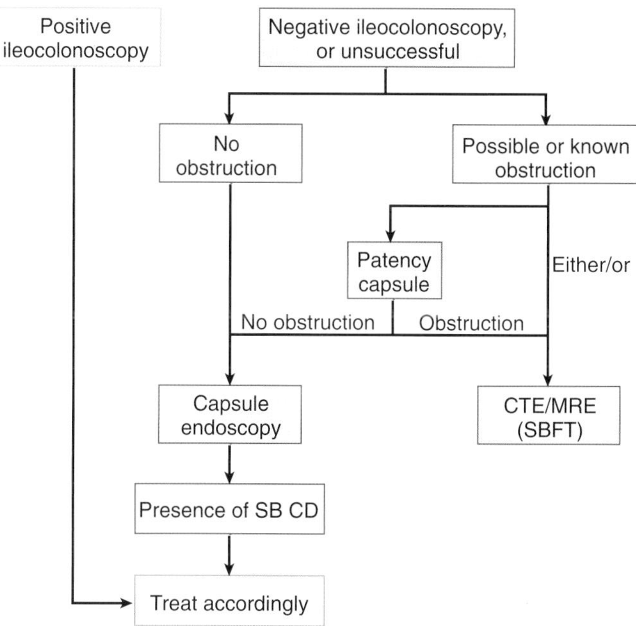

Figure 104-4 The role of capsule endoscopy in the diagnosis of Crohn's disease. CTE, computed tomographic enterography; MRE, magnetic resonance enterography; SB CD, small bowel Crohn's disease; SBFT, small bowel follow-through.

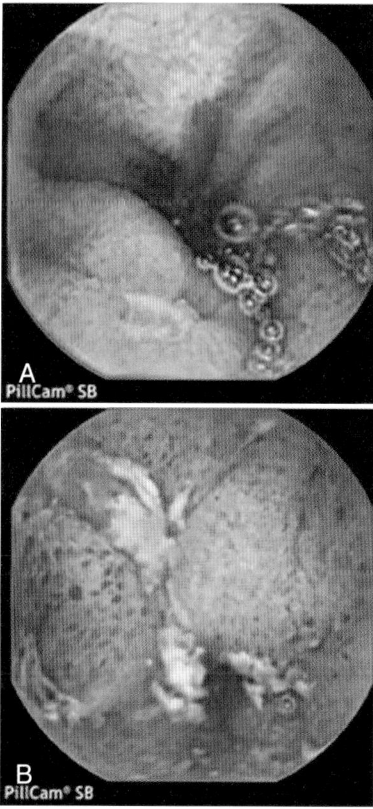

Figure 104-5 Small bowel Crohn's disease. **A,** Aphthous ulcer. **B,** Inflammatory stricture.

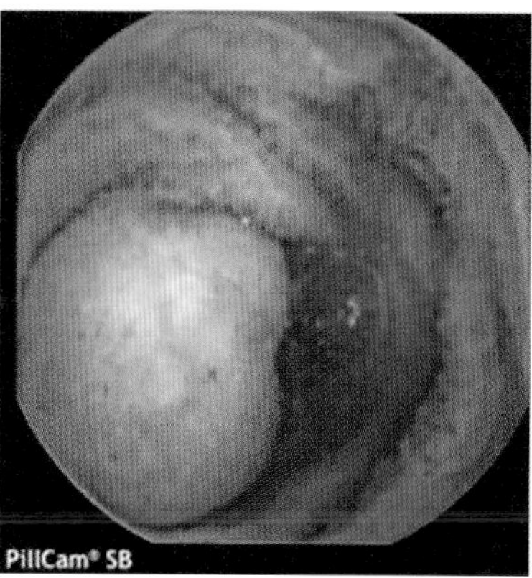

Figure 104-6 Small bowel tumor.

even in a "real life" setting and in the detection of more subtle histologic changes. It appears that VCE has a role in the diagnosis of celiac disease when there is a strong clinical suspicion (typical symptoms or positive serology) and EGD with small bowel biopsy is either negative or inconclusive, or the patient does not tolerate or is unwilling to undergo EGD. Furthermore, when patients with diagnosed celiac disease on a strict gluten-free diet develop worrisome symptoms such as weight loss, anemia, fever, bleeding, abdominal pain, or recurrence of malabsorption, or when results of abdominal imaging are abnormal (except for stricture), VCE is indicated to evaluate for small bowel malignancy or enteropathy-associated lymphoma. However, the diagnosis of the typical injury pattern seen with VCE in celiac disease requires considerable expertise, and such patients probably should be referred to specialized centers.

Monitoring Small Bowel Drug Effects or Side Effects

Several studies have shown that VCE is a sensitive tool to demonstrate small bowel injury caused by nonsteroidal anti-inflammatory drugs (NSAIDs). In fact, VCE can readily detect erythema, erosions, ulcerations, and weblike strictures caused by NSAIDs, even in asymptomatic subjects. There have also been recent reports on VCE being used to monitor response to immunosuppressive therapy to manage intestinal graft-versus-host disease.

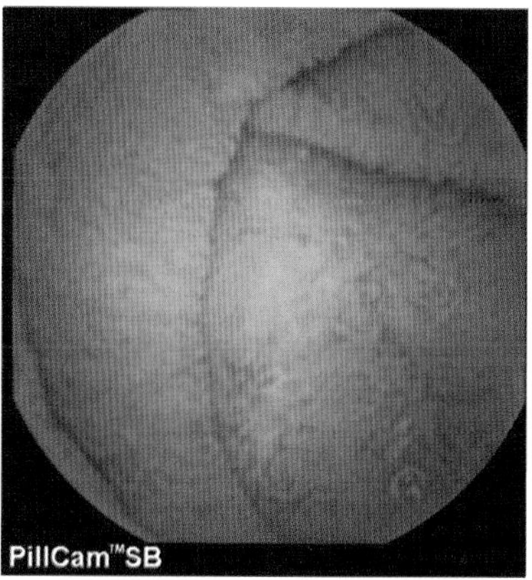

Figure 104-7 Celiac disease: mucosal scalloping.

Contraindications

Video capsule endoscopy is contraindicated for use under the following conditions (Box 104-2):

- Patients with known or suspected GI obstruction, strictures, or fistulas based on the clinical picture or preprocedure testing
- Patients with cardiac pacemakers, cardiac defibrillators, or other implanted electromedical devices
- Patients with swallowing disorders

Also, see the pertinent history in the Preprocedure Patient Preparation section.

Equipment and Overview of Video Capsule Endoscopy System

The capsule (Pillcam SB2; Given Imaging, Ltd.) is a disposable device (11 × 26 mm) composed of a light source, lens, metal oxide semiconductor imager, battery, and transmitter (Fig. 104-8). The capsule has a slippery coating that allows easy ingestion and transit with normal intestinal peristalsis. The capsule coating also prevents adhesion of luminal contents and obstruction of the visual field. The battery life is approximately 7 to 8 hours, during which two images per second are acquired and transmitted to a recording device worn by the patient (Fig. 104-9). The images are acquired through the optical dome, creating a visual field of 140 to 176 degrees and a magnification of 8:1. In total, 50,000 to 60,000 images are acquired and transmitted by a sensor array (8 sensors) located on the chest and abdominal wall of the patient to the recording device worn on the patient's belt (see Fig. 104-9). After 7 to 8 hours, the recorder and sensors are removed from the patient and the images are downloaded into a reporting and processing of images and data (RAPID) computer workstation (Fig. 104-10). A continuous video movie is created. Additional features that are currently used include an approximate localization system for each image, a blood detector, an image magnifier, and simultaneous viewing of two to four images.

In summary, the required equipment to perform small bowel VCE includes the following:

- Capsule endoscope
- Computer workstation including a data recorder, battery-charging cradle for the data recorder (Fig. 104-11), a sensor array set with disposable adhesive sleeves for sensor placement on the abdominal wall, and color printer
- A diagram that describes how to locate the sensors on the abdominal wall according to anatomic landmarks
- Drinking water and (disposable) cups for capsule ingestion
- Dark/dimmed light viewing room with a comfortable chair

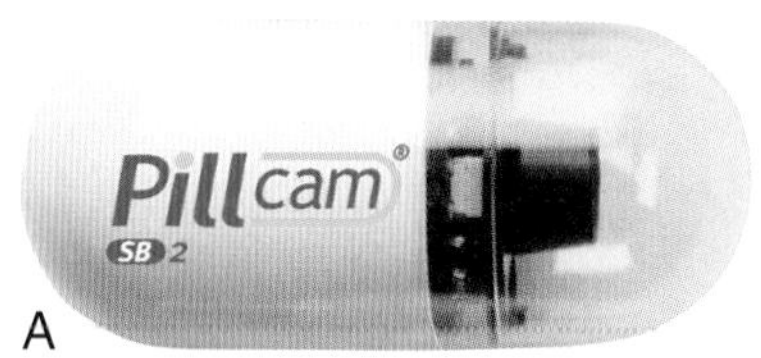

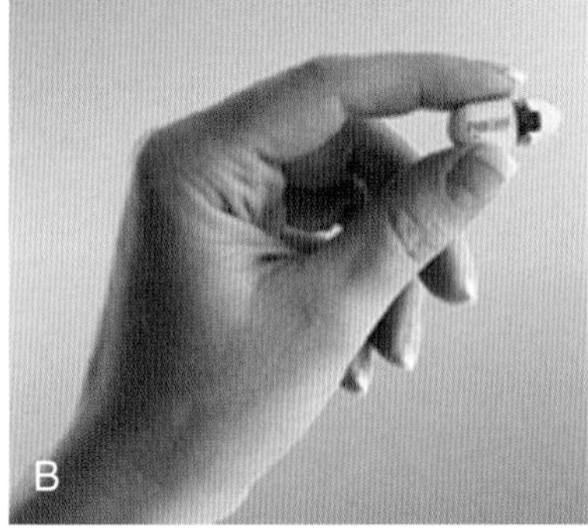

Figure 104-8 **A,** PillCam SB2. **B,** A patient holding a capsule. (**A,** Courtesy of Given Imaging, Yoqneam, Israel.)

Box 104-2. Relative and Absolute Contraindications to Video Capsule Endoscopy

Absolute

Clinical or radiographic evidence of bowel obstruction
Extensive and active Crohn's disease of the small bowel, with or without strictures
Intestinal pseudo-obstruction
Young children (<10 years)

Relative

Cardiac pacemakers or other implanted electromedical devices
Dysphagia
Extensive intestinal diverticulosis
Pregnancy
Previous abdominal or pelvic surgery

Adapted from Ho KK, Joyce AM: Complications of capsule endoscopy. Gastrointest Endosc Clin N Am 17:169–178, 2007.

Preprocedure Patient Preparation

Although VCE is a minimally invasive procedure, there are potential procedure-associated risks that need to be explained in detail to the patient before performing the procedure. Emphasis should be put on the *risk of capsule retention* (see later) and the capsule ingestion procedure (mainly to reduce patient anxiety at swallowing a large capsule). For further information, the patient may be referred to several Internet sites (e.g., www.givenimaging.com). The patient should also be provided with a detailed information sheet explaining the VCE procedure (available online at www.expertconsult.com). Immediately before the procedure, explain the alternatives and risks and have the patient sign an informed consent document (available online at www.expertconsult.com).

Any *history of dysphagia or neuromuscular disease* that may interfere with swallowing the capsule should be carefully sought before

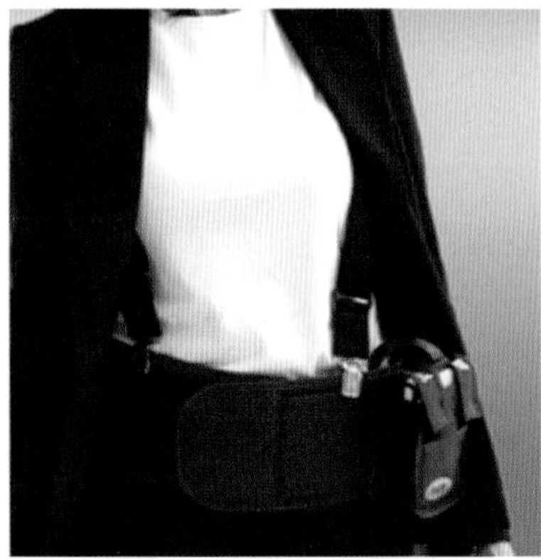

Figure 104-9 Recorder and belt.

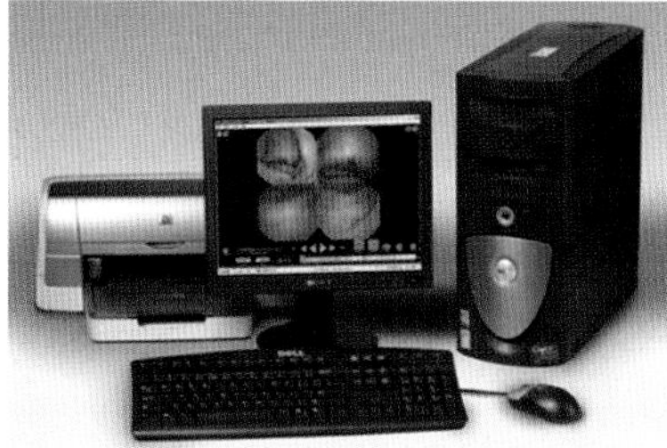

Figure 104-10 RAPID computer workstation.

capsule ingestion. *History of bowel obstruction* or symptoms suggesting partial obstruction such as postprandial cramps, bloating, nausea, or vomiting should be reviewed with the patient. If any positive history exists, a small bowel barium series should be obtained looking for possible strictures or fistulas. Similarly, any *history of prior small bowel or other intra-abdominal surgery* and any abnormal findings on small bowel imaging suggesting *obstruction, stricture, or fistula* should be carefully sought and addressed before capsule ingestion.

Before capsule ingestion the patient should adhere to the following regimen:

- Refrain from aspirin or NSAID therapy for a minimum of 14 days before capsule examination. (Even the sporadic use of NSAIDs has been shown to cause erosions and bleeding. Indeed, erosions, aphthous ulcers, and strictures mimicking CD have been reported at VCE in patients who have used NSAIDs. NSAID therapy may not be reported (or even considered) by the patient because many of these medications are sold over the counter or not believed to be significant by patients. Thus, the physician should specifically ask about regular or sporadic NSAID use in the weeks before VCE and recommend that it be discontinued if not mandatory.)
- Refrain from ingesting oral iron therapy, including iron-containing multivitamins, in the 7 days before the VCE procedure.
- Refrain from eating seeds, nuts, or grains the day before VCE. It is also advisable to refrain from dairy products and any other dark-colored or high-fiber foods. Ample intake of clear fluids the day before the procedure is also recommended.
- Fast for 10 hours.
- Consult his or her physician regarding regular medication (e.g., insulin and other diabetes-related medications, antihypertensives) use before VCE examination.

Use of Prokinetics, Laxative, and Osmotic Bowel Preparations

It has been reported that in as many as 20% of VCE examinations, incomplete small bowel imaging (defined as the capsule not reaching the ileocecal valve/cecum) may occur because of decreased gastric emptying or prolonged small bowel transit time. Furthermore, turbid or dark intraluminal contents of the small bowel may interfere with the quality of the examination, particularly in the distal ileum. *Prokinetics* are medications given with the aim of accelerating gastric emptying or small bowel transit time, thereby improving the proportion of cases in which the cecum is reached. Bowel preparations are medications given with the primary aim of cleansing the small bowel.

Although current evidence is limited, the International Conference on Capsule Endoscopy in 2006 (ICCE 2006) concluded that small bowel preparation (e.g., polyethylene glycol [PEG], Phospho-Soda, clear liquids) before VCE may not significantly improve small bowel cleanliness and that there is no definitive evidence that such preparations increase the diagnostic yield of small bowel VCE. Therefore, at present, *there is no convincing evidence for recommending the routine use of bowel preparations in clinical practice*. However, if the use of a bowel preparation is desired by the practitioner, there are several regimens that may be used (Table 104-1). Prokinetic agents (e.g., metoclopramide and erythromycin) may shorten gastric emptying and small bowel transit times, but because they have been less well studied than bowel preparations, no recommendation for their use can be made. Simethicone, an oral antifoaming agent/defrothicant, may be given in its liquid suspension form to improve visualization of the bowel mucosa. Although older age, diabetes mellitus, and inpatient status may be predictive factors for prolonged gastric emptying or small bowel transit time, no firm evidence supports the use of prokinetics or bowel preparation even in these patient subgroups.

Technique

It is mandatory to verify that the patient has completed the following steps:

- Fasted for the 10 hours immediately preceding the capsule study
- Maintained a clear liquid diet since lunch the day before the procedure
- Stopped oral iron therapy seven days before the procedure and refrained from aspirin/NSAID use for fourteen days before the procedure
- Signed the informed consent form

The physician should verify, preferably by a checklist or a structured preprocedure visit form, that the indication for VCE is clear and that no contraindications to the procedure exist.

Preparing the Equipment

Because the procedure takes approximately 7 to 8 hours to complete, it is convenient to schedule the patient for VCE examination first thing in the morning. Therefore, disconnecting the sensor array and downloading the data recorder will take place in the middle to late

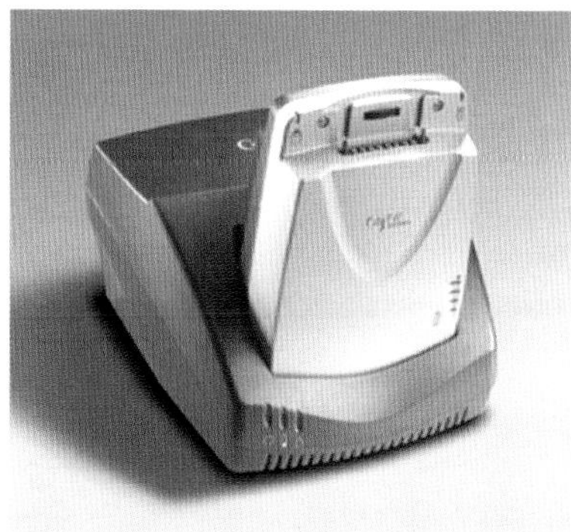

Figure 104-11 Data recorder and charging cradle.

TABLE 104-1 Bowel Preparation Regimens

Medication	Dosing
Sodium phosphate*	90 mL the night before procedure
PEG	2 L ingested 16 hr before procedure
PEG	4 L: 3 L ingested the evening before + 1 L ingested 3 hr immediately before the procedure

PEG, polyethylene glycol.

*Sodium phosphate preparations should not be used in patients with renal or cardiac insufficiency/failure and are to be avoided in older patients because of the increased risk of hyperphosphatemia.

Adapted from Villa F, Signorelli C, Rondonotti E, de Franchis R: Preparations and prokinetics. Gastrointest Endosc Clin North Am 16:211–220, 2006.

afternoon. The following items should be readily available at the time of patient presentation:

- A fully charged data recorder (as indicated by the battery indicator light), after patient check-in procedure has been launched using the RAPID workstation
- PillCam SB in its original sealed package
- One disposable cup of water, a sensor array with adhesive sleeves, a sensor location diagram for correct sensor placement on abdomen, and a belt for the data recorder

Getting Started

The patient should lie supine and the sensor array should be placed on the abdomen at the locations indicated by the sensor location diagram. Care should be taken to be sure that the sensors are firmly attached in the correct location. The patient should then stand, wearing his or her clothes, and make sure that no discomfort is caused by the sensors. The belt, with the data recorder in place, is worn over the patient's clothing (see Fig. 104-9). The capsule should then be removed from its packaging. Once the capsule is detached from its cell (and magnet) it is important to verify that the eight light-emitting diodes (LEDs) start to work (lights on the capsule will begin to flash immediately on detachment) and that the capsule transmission indicator on the data recorder starts flashing blue. This indicates that the data recorder is acquiring the signal from the capsule. The patient then takes the capsule (see Fig. 104-8), taking great care not to drop it, and places it in his or her mouth (the orientation of the capsule in the mouth is not important). The patient is then instructed to swallow the capsule while drinking a full glass of water. In cases when swallowing is unsuccessful, a repeat attempt should be made. If further attempts are unsuccessful, the capsule should be put back into its cell and magnet so that battery life is preserved.

Endoscopic placement of the capsule into the stomach or duodenum is possible using a video endoscope and a dedicated capsule-holding suction cup, snare, or endoscopic net. However, this procedure should be performed only by an experienced endoscopist, and as soon as possible, because the battery may not completely stop and capsule battery life span may be shortened.

After capsule ingestion the patient should be instructed as follows:

- Remain in the clinic area for approximately 15 to 30 minutes to make sure that no technical problems occur.
- Pay attention that the flashing blue LED on the data recorder is on.
- Treat the data recorder with the utmost care.
- Refrain from being near areas of magnetic fields such as magnetic resonance imaging (MRI) machines, security gates, and the like. Certain industrial magnetic fields may interfere with transmission of the images.
- Refrain from liquid intake for 2 hours and food intake for 4 hours after capsule ingestion.
- Contact the medical staff in case of severe abdominal pain, nausea, or vomiting.
- Note capsule excretion. In case of any doubt, any symptoms of bowel obstruction, or before MRI, an abdominal radiograph should be performed to verify capsule excretion. For patients who do not visualize/observe capsule excretion and in whom the colon is not visualized on the video imaging, an abdominal radiograph should be performed on day 14 to identify those with capsule retention.

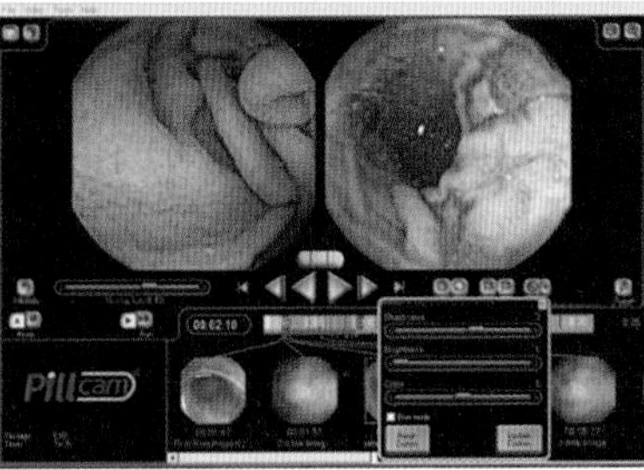

Figure 104-12 RAPID viewing screen.

Video Reviewing

General Information

- The average reviewing time for small bowel VCE is usually 30 to 60 minutes.
- Video reviewing should take place in a semidarkened room and, because video reviewing requires considerable concentration, no visual distractions should be allowed. However, listening to music is possible.
- Before attempting to review VCE videos it is imperative to be familiar with the software and to have experience in interpretation of VCE findings. We strongly encourage attending Capsule Endoscopy courses such as those provided by the American Society for Gastrointestinal Endoscopy (www.asge.org). Furthermore, the authors strongly recommend reviewing your initial 10 to 20 capsule videos with proctoring from a colleague experienced in VCE.

Video Reviewing Procedure

- We recommend using the simultaneous two-picture viewing mode (Fig. 104-12), setting the video speed to 18 to 22 in the manual mode (M-mode, preferable) or lower speed using the automated mode (A-mode).
- It is of utmost importance to determine and mark the following anatomic landmarks:
  - First image of the gastric folds
  - First duodenal image (identified by the first image where villi on the mucosa are seen [Fig. 104-13]; usually passage of the capsule through the pylorus is seen immediately before this point of transit)

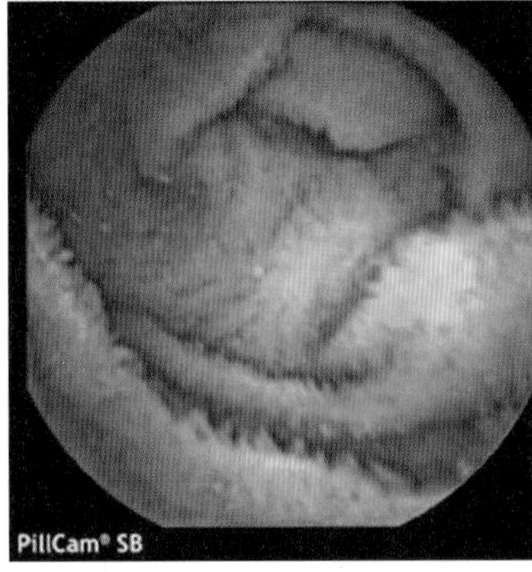

Figure 104-13 Small bowel: normal villi.

- First cecal image (the first image where villi are absent, fecal matter is dominant, and typically where there is a lack of the characteristic peristalsis of the small bowel)
- *Capsule findings* should be reported by creating a thumbnail from the image. Preferably, each pathologic finding should be defined and noted in the thumbnail's comment. In cases where the nature of the finding is unclear, refer to the image atlas in the product software or an endoscopic atlas or VCE atlas (e.g., Keuchel and colleagues, 2006).
- *Capsule transit time* through the stomach and small bowel is another aspect of video interpretation. Transit delays may suggest stricture or obstruction, and should be noted. If the capsule fails to reach the ileocecal valve or did not traverse the ileocecal valve into the cecum during the time of recorded video, this should be noted in the report. Careful follow-up of these patients is warranted to verify capsule excretion in the following days and that no symptoms or signs of small bowel obstruction appear. A capsule present for more than 14 days after the capsule examination is considered to be retained.
- Use of the *suspected blood identification system*: The RAPID software provides an accessory tool for detecting blood in the small bowel. This software tool has limited sensitivity and specificity. The blood detector does not replace careful reviewing of the entire video for bleeding and bleeding sources.
- *Localization of findings*: Each clinically significant finding detected during video reviewing should be considered for further management (e.g., referral for surgery, enteroscopy, or ileocolonoscopy). This is usually done by referring to the anatomic landmarks. Although the software system provides an estimated location for each image by using the localization system, exact localization of findings in the small bowel is difficult. It is useful to use terms such as *duodenum*, *proximal jejunum*, *distal jejunum/proximal ileum*, *distal ileum*, and *terminal ileum* when describing the location of a finding. This description is completed using noted anatomic landmarks, transit times, and the timing of each thumbnail, but because of the variable speed of the capsule's peristaltic movement through the intestine, this method is not very accurate.
- *Creating the report*
  - Verify that the patient demographic details and reason(s) for capsule endoscopy referral are reported and inserted into the appropriate report fields during patient check-in. If not, you may do this when creating the VCE report.
  - A brief summary of the VCE findings (e.g., gastric and small bowel) should be typed in the box specified for procedure information and findings.
  - The final diagnosis and recommendations for further work-up or treatment should be stated and typed in the appropriate field.

COMPLICATIONS

Clinical Complications

Clinical complications include complications of capsule ingestion, capsule retention, and incomplete examination. Capsule retention (defined as presence of capsule 14 days after capsule ingestion) is by far the most serious of these. An incomplete examination may be considered a technical problem rather than a clinical complication, and therefore is not discussed here. The safety of VCE has not been examined systematically in pregnant women and in children younger than 10 years of age. Therefore, we do not recommend the use of VCE in the primary care setting in these patients.

Capsule Retention

At the 2005 ICCE, capsule retention was defined as an endoscopic capsule remaining in the digestive tract for more than 14 days. Capsule retention has been further defined as failure of the capsule to be excreted unless surgical, endoscopic, or medical interventions are performed. The prediction of this serious complication is difficult in that no single modality, including small bowel follow-through, may accurately predict it. However, experts believe that obtaining a careful history is perhaps the best single method to identify high-risk patients. Important clues to possible small bowel stricture/stenosis include the following:

- Chronic NSAID use
- Suspected or known CD
- History of intestinal surgery
- Suspected small bowel tumor
- History of abdominal radiation therapy
- Suspected mesenteric ischemia

Symptoms such as pain, nausea or vomiting, and abdominal distention may also indicate increased potential for capsule retention. The overall incidence of capsule retention is 1% to 2%, with two thirds of capsule retentions occurring in CD-related strictures. The relative incidence rates of capsule retention are shown in Table 104-2.

PREVENTION OF CAPSULE RETENTION

- Careful history taking and risk stratification according to the aforementioned groups.
- Small bowel follow-through: This is currently the best way to establish the presence of small bowel strictures. Possible disadvantages include false-negative results and radiation exposure.
- Patency capsule (Agile Patency System; Given Imaging, Ltd.): Made of lactulose, this capsule is specifically designed to dissolve spontaneously after 40 hours in the bowel. The capsule has a radiopaque tag, a timer, and a radiofrequency identification tag. It is readily detected by plain abdominal radiographs and by the detection device of the Agile System, thus enabling localization of the stricture causing the obstruction. The patency capsule disintegrates completely after 80 to 100 hours. Current experience with the patency capsule is that it is no more sensitive than small bowel follow-through or computed tomographic enteroclysis in detecting small bowel strictures. Moreover, 2 of 22 (11%) patients who swallowed the patency capsule developed small bowel obstruction that required surgery. Thus, given the comparable sensitivity and the risk for capsule-associated bowel obstruction, we do not recommend the use of the patency capsule in the work-up of a suspected small bowel stricture.

TABLE 104-2 Capsule Retention Rates According to Video Capsule Endoscopy Indication

Indication	Retention Rate
Healthy volunteers	0%
All comers	0.75%
Suspected Crohn's disease	1.4%
Obscure gastrointestinal bleeding	Up to 5%
Known Crohn's disease	Up to 8%
Suspected bowel obstruction	21%

Modified from Eliakim AR: Video capsule endoscopy of the small bowel (PillCam SB). Curr Opin Gastroenterol 22:124–127, 2006.

MANAGEMENT OF CAPSULE RETENTION

- Immediate referral to plain abdominal radiographs and possible surgery in cases of clinical symptoms and signs of small bowel obstruction.
- Extraction of the retained capsule by means of push enteroscopy, double-balloon enteroscopy, or surgery. Because most patients with capsule retention are asymptomatic, the extraction is not urgent. Thus, referral for further evaluation by a gastroenterologist or a surgeon is warranted promptly but not urgently.
- A prokinetic agent such as metoclopramide or erythromycin may also be prescribed to accelerate the small bowel transit time and induce capsule passage.

Swallowing Disorders

Inability to swallow the capsule or (rarely) aspiration of the device has been reported in up to 1.5% of VCE procedures. Difficulty in swallowing may be overcome by introduction of the capsule by means of an oroesophageal overtube or EGD with a snare with a basket or foreign object retrieval device. Thus, patients who are unsuccessful in swallowing the capsule may be referred to a center dedicated to VCE. Aspiration of the capsule can usually be overcome simply by coughing. In cases of suspected aspiration, referral for a chest radiograph or bronchoscopy is indicated.

Technical Complications

In the largest series to date, Rondonotti and colleagues (2005) reported an overall 9% technical failure rate in 733 patients. These technical failures included gaps in image recording; shortened battery operation; malfunction of the battery package; and failure of capsule activation, image downloading, and the localization system. In 33% of cases with technical problems, the diagnosis was hampered. Overall, a total of 3% of all hampered diagnoses were attributed to technical problems. Interference with communication between the capsule and recorder is also a technical problem. This interference may be caused by nearby electromagnetic devices such as cardiac pacemakers, electronic article surveillance systems, and cellular telephones. Because radiofrequency electrosurgery and cellular telephones have been reported to interfere with cardiac pacemaker functioning, the presence of an implantable cardiac device is considered a relative contraindication to VCE. However, a small series of patients with pacemakers who underwent VCE have been reported to have no arrhythmias or pacemaker malfunction on Holter electrocardiographic monitoring during VCE. Similarly, the pacemakers did not interfere with VCE in these patients. Leighton and colleagues (2005) have reported similar results in a small series of five patients with an implantable cardiac defibrillator.

Current and Future Developments in Video Capsule Endoscopy

Since the FDA approval of the first M2A capsule in 2001, many new developments have been put into clinical use. New capsules, such as PillCam ESO with double-sided cameras and acquisition of 14 frames per second for the detection of esophageal diseases, including Barrett's esophagus and esophageal varices, and PillCam SB2 with better illumination technology and a wider visual field of 156 degrees for improved accuracy in the diagnosis of small bowel diseases, have recently been approved by the FDA for clinical use. Moreover, a new capsule, PillCam Colon, for the diagnosis of colonic mucosal disease is currently under investigation and has been approved (given a CE mark) for use in the European Union. Improvements in the diagnostic software allow for simplified viewing modes and shorter video review time, making this procedure even easier to use and more widely accepted. It is therefore imperative for any physician involved in VCE to be familiar with current and future developments in this rapidly evolving technology.

BIBLIOGRAPHY

Bailey AA, Debinski H, Appleyard M, et al: Diagnosis and outcome of small bowel tumors found by capsule endoscopy: A three-center Australian experience. Am J Gastroenterol 101:2237–2243, 2006.

Burt RW: Colon cancer screening. Gastroenterology 119:837–853, 2000.

Cave D, Legnani P, de Franchis R, et al: ICCE consensus for capsule retention. Endoscopy 37:1065–1067, 2005.

Cellier C, Green PH, Collin P, et al: ICCE consensus for celiac disease. Endoscopy 37:1055–1059, 2005.

Delvaux M, Soussan EB, Laurent V, et al: Clinical evaluation of the use of the M2A patency capsule system before a capsule endoscopy procedure, in patients with known or suspected intestinal stenosis. Endoscopy 37:801–807, 2005.

Denkler K: A comprehensive review of epinephrine in the finger: To do or not to do. Plast Reconstruct Surg 108:114–124, 2000.

Eisen GM, Eliakim R, Zaman A, et al: The accuracy of PillCam ESO capsule endoscopy versus conventional upper endoscopy for the diagnosis of esophageal varices: A prospective three-center pilot study. Endoscopy 38:31–35, 2006.

Eliakim R, Fireman Z, Gralnek IM, et al: Evaluation of the PillCam Colon capsule in the detection of colonic pathology: Results of the first multicenter, prospective, comparative study. Endoscopy 38:963–970, 2006.

Eliakim R, Sharma VK, Yassin K, et al: A prospective study of the diagnostic accuracy of PillCam ESO esophageal capsule endoscopy versus conventional upper endoscopy in patients with chronic gastroesophageal reflux disease. J Clin Gastroenterol 39:572–578, 2005.

Fischer D, Schreiber R, Levi D, Eliakim R: Capsule endoscopy: The localization system. Gastrointest Endosc Clin N Am 14:25–31, 2004.

Gay G, Selby W: Tumors, ICCE Consensus 2006.

Goldstein JL, Eisen GM, Lewis B, et al: The use of capsule endoscopy to prospectively assess the incidence of small bowel lesions with celecoxib, naproxen plus omeprazole, and placebo. Clin Gastroenterol Hepatol 3:133–141, 2005.

Graham DY, Opekun AR, Willingham FF, Qureshi WA: Visible small intestinal mucosal injury in chronic NSAID users. Clin Gastroenterol Hepatol 3:55–59, 2005.

Gralnek IM: Obscure-overt gastrointestinal bleeding. Gastroenterology 128:1424–1430, 2005.

Ho KK, Joyce AM: Complications of capsule endoscopy. Gastrointest Endosc Clin N Am 17:169–178, 2007.

Holden JP, Dureja P, Pfau PR, et al: Endoscopic placement of the small-bowel video capsule by using a capsule endoscope delivery device. Gastrointest Endosc 65:842–847, 2007.

Hopper AD, Sidhu R, Hurlstone DP, et al: Capsule endoscopy: An alternative to duodenal biopsy for the recognition of villous atrophy in coeliac disease? Dig Liver Dis 39:140–145, 2007.

Itzkowitz SH, Rochester J: Colonic polyps and polyposis syndromes. In Feldman M, Friedman LS, Brandt LJ (eds): Sleisenger and Fordtran's Gastrointestinal and Liver Disease: Pathophysiology, Diagnosis, Management, 8th ed. Philadelphia, Saunders, 2006, pp 2741–2743.

Keuchel M, Hagenmueller F, Fleicher DE (eds): Atlas of Video Capsule Endoscopy. Heidelberg, Springer-Verlag, 2006.

Krunic AL, Wang LC, Soltani K, et al: Digital anesthesia with epinephrine: An old myth revisited. J Am Acad Dermatol 51:755–759, 2004.

Leighton J, Sharma V, Srivathsan K, et al: Safety of capsule endoscopy in patients with pacemakers. Gastrointest Endosc 59:567–569, 2004.

Leighton J, Srivathsan K, Carey E, et al: Safety of wireless capsule endoscopy in patients with implantable cardiac defibrillators. Am J Gastroenterol 100:1728–1731, 2005.

Lewis B: How to prevent endoscopic capsule retention. Endoscopy 37: 852–853, 2005.

Maiden L, Thjodleifsson B, Theodors A, et al: A quantitative analysis of NSAID-induced small bowel pathology by capsule enteroscopy. Gastroenterology 128:1172–1178, 2005.

Marmo R, Rotondano G, Rondonotti E, et al: Capsule enteroscopy vs. other diagnostic procedures in diagnosing obscure gastrointestinal bleeding: A cost-effectiveness study. Eur J Gastroenterol Hepatol 19:535–542, 2007.

Mergener K, Ponchon T, Gralnek I, et al: Literature review and recommendations for clinical application of small-bowel capsule endoscopy, based on a panel discussion by international experts. Consensus statements for small-bowel capsule endoscopy, 2006/2007. Endoscopy 39:895–909, 2007.

Mishkin DS, Chuttani R, Croffie J, et al: ASGE technology status evaluation report: Wireless capsule endoscopy. Gastrointest Endosc 63:539–545, 2006.

Neumann S, Schoppmeyer K, Lange T, et al: Wireless capsule endoscopy for diagnosis of acute intestinal graft-versus-host disease. Gastrointest Endosc 65:403–409, 2007.

Payeras G, Piqueras J, Moreno J, et al: Effects of capsule endoscopy on cardiac pacemakers. Endoscopy 37:1181–1185, 2005.

Radovic P, Smith RG, Shumway D: Revisiting epinephrine in foot surgery. J Am Podiatr Med Assoc 93:157–160, 2003.

Rockey DC: Gastrointestinal bleeding. In Feldman M, Friedman LS, Brandt LJ (eds): Sleisenger and Fordtran's Gastrointestinal and Liver Disease: Pathophysiology, Diagnosis, Management, 8th ed. Philadelphia, Saunders, 2006, pp 289–290.

Rondonotti E, Herrrerias J, Pennazio M, et al: Complications, limitations, and failures of capsule endoscopy: A review of 733 cases. Gastrointest Endosc 62:712–716, 2005.

Rondonotti E, Spada C, Cave D, et al: Video capsule enteroscopy in the diagnosis of celiac disease: A multicenter study. Am J Gastroenterol 102:1624–1631, 2007.

Sachdev MS, Leighton JA, Fleischer DE, et al: A prospective study of the utility of abdominal radiographs after capsule endoscopy for the diagnosis of capsule retention. Gastrointest Endosc 66:894–900, 2007.

Sands BE: Crohn's disease. In Feldman M, Friedman LS, Brandt LJ (eds): Sleisenger and Fordtran's Gastrointestinal and Liver Disease: Pathophysiology, Diagnosis, Management, 8th ed. Philadelphia, Saunders, 2006, pp 2459–2498.

Schoofs N, Deviere J, Van Gossum A: PillCam colon capsule endoscopy compared with colonoscopy for colorectal tumor diagnosis: A prospective pilot study. Endoscopy 78:971–977, 2006.

Schulmann K, Hollerbach S, Kraus K, et al: Feasibility and diagnostic utility of video capsule endoscopy for the detection of small bowel polyps in patients with hereditary polyposis syndromes. Am J Gastroenterol 100: 27–37, 2005.

Schwartz GD, Barkin JS: Small bowel tumors detected by wireless capsule endoscopy. Dig Dis Sci 52:1026–1030, 2007.

Selby W: Complete small-bowel transit in patients undergoing capsule endoscopy: Determining factors and improvement with metoclopramide. Gastrointest Endosc 61:80–85, 2005.

Sharma P, Wani S, Rastogi A, et al: The diagnostic accuracy of esophageal capsule endoscopy in patients with gastroesophageal reflux disease and Barrett's esophagus: A blinded, prospective study. Am J Gastroenterol 103:525–532, 2008.

Signorelli C, Villa F, Rondonotti E, et al: Sensitivity and specificity of the suspected blood identification system in video capsule enteroscopy. Endoscopy 37:1170–1173, 2005.

Thomson CJ, Lalonde DH, Denkler K, Feicht AJ: A critical look at the evidence for and against elective epinephrine use in the finger. Plast Reconstruct Surg 119:260–266, 2007.

Triester SL, Leighton JA, Leontiadis GI, et al: Meta-analysis of the yield of capsule endoscopy compared to other diagnostic modalities in patients with obscure gastrointestinal bleeding. Am J Gastroenterol 100:2407–2418, 2005.

Triester SL, Leighton JA, Leontiadis GI, et al: A meta-analysis of the yield of capsule endoscopy compared to other diagnostic modalities in patients with non-stricturing small bowel Crohn's disease. Am J Gastroenterol 101:954–964, 2006.

Yakoub-Agha I, Maunoury V, Wacrenier A, et al: Impact of small bowel exploration using video-capsule endoscopy in the management of acute graft versus host disease. Transplantation 15:1697–1701, 2004.

CHAPTER 105

INGUINAL HERNIA REDUCTION

George G. Zainea

The *indirect inguinal hernia* is the most common type of groin hernia. It occurs lateral to the inferior epigastric vessels. The hernia sac passes through the internal inguinal ring. It is associated with patency of the processus vaginalis. This hernia is typically seen in children and young adults (Figs. 105-1 and 105-2).

The *direct inguinal hernia* occurs medial to the inferior epigastric vessels. It protrudes through the posterior inguinal floor. It is more commonly seen in adults (see Figs. 105-1 and 105-2). The risk of incarceration is less than that of indirect inguinal hernia.

Femoral hernias, usually found in adult women, are seen far less commonly. The protrusion occurs beneath the inguinal ligament just medial to the femoral vessels in the upper thigh. The risk of incarceration and strangulation is high with this type of hernia (see Figs. 105-1 and 105-2).

DIAGNOSIS

Diagnosis involves palpation with the patient both supine and standing. An incarcerated groin hernia manifests as a nonreducible, painful groin bulge. Associated intestinal obstruction may also be present.

A Valsalva maneuver (grunting or coughing) allows the appreciation of a palpable impulse in a true hernia. Auscultation may reveal bowel sounds. Transillumination can be performed to assist with diagnosis.

DIFFERENTIAL DIAGNOSIS

The history and physical examination usually allow the physician to exclude other disorders that may mimic an incarcerated groin hernia, such as an *inflamed lymph node*, which is usually evident by history and on palpation; a *dilated varicose vein*, which may appear as a bulge in the inguinal region; a large lipoma; and a *hydrocele* of the spermatic cord, which typically is not tender, does transilluminate, and rarely is associated with an acute presentation. Other disorders to consider include *testicular torsion*, which manifests as extreme scrotal pain and swelling. With torsion, pain may be intensified with scrotal elevation, and swelling is usually confined to beneath the pubic tubercle. Finally, an *undescended testicle* may appear as an isolated groin bulge. This should be suspected if the gonad is not present in the scrotal sac.

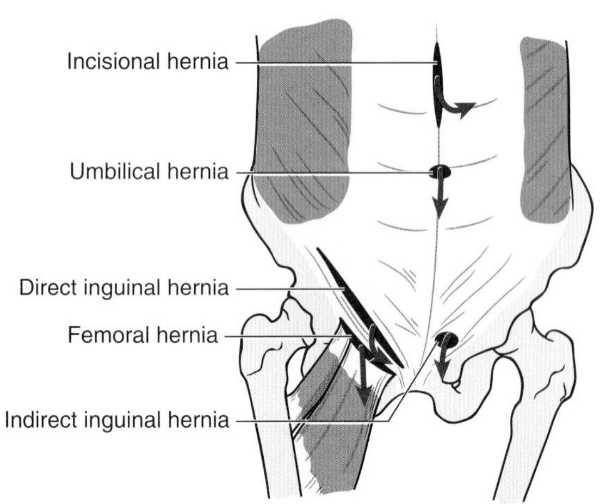

Figure 105-1 Hernia locations in the abdominal wall. (Modified from Abel ME, Glassman SL, Harris RJ, Gibson TJ: The Hernia Surgery Book: How Hernias Develop and How They're Repaired. San Bruno, Calif, StayWell, 1999.)

TECHNIQUE

By definition, a hernia that is nonreducible is *incarcerated*. Incarceration usually involves either the bowel or the omentum. The practitioner may see intestinal obstruction with bowel incarceration; however, the most feared complication of incarceration is strangulation. With strangulation, the blood supply to the intestine is compromised, and ischemic necrosis and gangrene may result.

The decision to reduce incarcerated hernias requires clinical judgment. If strangulation is suspected, the situation is best dealt with immediately in the operating room. Patients with strangulation typically appear ill, and may be febrile. The bulge is extremely tender, and overlying skin erythema may be present.

If strangulation is not suspected, the clinician may attempt closed reduction as follows:

1. Place the patient in the supine Trendelenburg position. This allows gravity to assist with hernia reduction.
2. Administer a narcotic for analgesia and intravenous diazepam for muscle relaxation. After sedation, allow for passive reduction of the hernia over a 30- to 40-minute period.
3. If the attempt at passive reduction is unsuccessful, proceed with an attempt at active reduction. Place one hand over the neck of

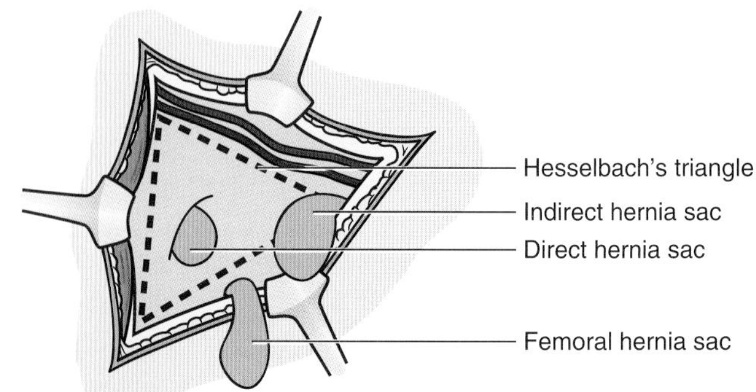

Figure 105-2 Operative view of inguinal and femoral hernias.

the hernia sac to guide its contents into the peritoneal cavity. Use the other hand to provide gentle and steady distal-to-proximal compression over the hernia (Fig. 105-3).

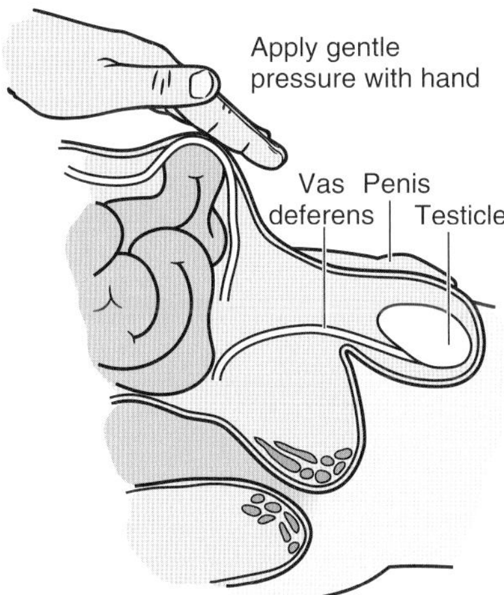

Figure 105-3 Application of gentle pressure to reduce inguinal hernia. (Modified from Abel ME, Glassman SL, Harris RJ, Gibson TJ: The Hernia Surgery Book: How Hernias Develop and How They're Repaired. San Bruno, Calif, StayWell, 1999.)

Using these techniques, the clinician should be able to reduce one third to one half of incarcerated groin hernias. Patients with irreducible groin hernias or incarcerated femoral hernias (which are seldom reducible) should be referred to a surgeon immediately.

Infants and children who successfully undergo closed reduction of inguinal hernias should be admitted to the hospital for surgical repair. An adult patient with suspected compromised bowel in the reduced hernia should be admitted to the hospital for observation. Adults who undergo successful closed reduction and return home should soon thereafter undergo elective hernia repair. A truss should be used only temporarily to prevent recurrent protrusion before surgery can be performed.

BIBLIOGRAPHY

Kauffman HM, O'Brien DP: Selective reduction of incarcerated inguinal hernia. Am J Surg 119:660–673, 1970.

Leape LL, Holder TM: Pediatric surgery. In Sabiston DC (ed): Davis-Christopher Textbook of Surgery, 12th ed. Philadelphia, WB Saunders, 1981, pp 1351–1400.

Shandling B: Hernias. In Behrman RE, Vaughn VC (eds): Nelson Textbook of Pediatrics, 13th ed. Philadelphia, WB Saunders, 1987.

Ziegler MM: Lumps and bumps. In Schwartz MW, Charney EB, Curry TA, Ludwig S (eds): Principles and Practice of Clinical Pediatrics. St. Louis, Mosby, 1990.

CHAPTER 106

Office Treatment of Hemorrhoids

George G. Zainea • John L. Pfenninger

Hemorrhoidal disease occurs in approximately 50% to 80% of the U.S. population. Although this disease is rarely fatal, it accounts for a great deal of human pain and suffering. Internal hemorrhoids are the most common cause of lower gastrointestinal (GI) bleeding. Nonetheless, it is imperative that the clinician confirm that bleeding is indeed originating from hemorrhoidal disease and not from a more proximal lesion. Occasionally, bleeding can be severe and is associated with anemia.

Most hemorrhoidal symptoms can be managed with medical therapies that include suppositories, topical agents, and fiber supplementation. Patients who fail medical therapies are appropriate candidates for in-office treatments of hemorrhoids. Only a minority of individuals requires definitive treatment for severe symptomatic hemorrhoids with a surgical hemorrhoidectomy or hemorrhoidopexy. A hemorrhoidectomy requires general or regional anesthesia and is associated with significant discomfort and loss of time from work and usual activities after surgery.

Rubber-band ligation is a time-tested and proven method for treating *internal hemorrhoids*. However, other approaches have been developed, with infrared photocoagulation (IRC) being used most frequently and, rarely, sclerotherapy. Direct-current (Ultroid) and radiofrequency (Bicap) techniques were described in the first edition of this text. Bicap is no longer available, and although Ultroid has recently been reintroduced to the market, the time required and the cost of the probes make it less likely to be used. Cryotherapy was also used in the past but not currently because of the availability of more cost-effective modalities. These therapies can be used selectively or in combination depending on the extent and severity of internal disease. Lasers have also been used for the treatment of internal disease. The treatment for *external hemorrhoid disease* has been unchanged for decades.

Two meta-analyses have been reported on the treatment of internal hemorrhoids. One concludes that band ligation is best, whereas the other supports IRC. In both instances, hemorrhoid symptoms resolved in 80% to 90% of properly selected cases.

The physician must know the anorectal anatomy (see Chapter 97, Clinical Anorectal Anatomy and Digital Examination) and must be able to perform a thorough anoscopic examination (see Chapter 98, Anoscopy) to appropriately assess and treat hemorrhoids.

After completion of any of these procedures, a medical program to regulate bowel habits should be implemented to prevent recurrence, which is as important as the surgical intervention itself.

Classifications and Symptoms

Hemorrhoids are enlarged arteriovenous vessels within fibrous tissue and are classified according to their origin either above or below the dentate (pectinate) line. Those developing from *above the dentate line are internal hemorrhoids*; those from *below are external hemorrhoids*. It should be clear that classification depends on *origin*, not on the location of the most distal portion of the hemorrhoid (Fig. 106-1).

Hemorrhoids above the dentate line—*internal hemorrhoids*—are covered by mucosa and do not have somatic sensory innervation. Thus, internal hemorrhoids are well suited for treatment in the office setting without anesthesia because they lack pain fibers. Those below the dentate line—*external hemorrhoids*—are covered by skin (anoderm) and are extremely sensitive. Treatment of external hemorrhoids requires some form of anesthesia. *Mixed hemorrhoids* refers to those vessels that originate right at the dentate line or to the presence of both internal and external hemorrhoidal tissue in continuity.

The anal canal can be divided into eight segments. With the patient lying in the left lateral decubitus position, they are as noted in Figure 106-2A. Internal hemorrhoids usually occur in three major positions based on the vascular architecture of the anal canal: the right anterior, right posterior, and left lateral positions (Fig. 106-2B). However, they can occur anywhere and even be circumferential. They also seem to "shift" with insertion of the anoscope, so absolute position is not that critical.

Internal hemorrhoids are also characterized by their size and degree of prolapse from grades I to IV, as noted in Table 106-1 and Figure 106-3. Symptoms of internal hemorrhoids include *painless* bleeding, prolapse, aching after defecation, and discharge. The key step in diagnosis and classification of internal hemorrhoids is anoscopic examination (see Chapter 98, Anoscopy). External hemorrhoids can form clots that are *painful*. Patients then present with a "painful lump."

Hemorrhoidal skin tags are residual fibrotic masses of stretched skin. Their size can vary significantly. They are generally asymptomatic except for occasional pruritus. Most commonly, when larger, they can cause problems with hygiene.

Approximately 25% of internal hemorrhoid symptoms do not respond adequately to medical treatment and require further therapy. Most thrombosed external hemorrhoids require evacuation or excision to provide symptomatic relief.

Internal Hemorrhoids

Indications

Bleeding or other symptomatology, such as prolapse, from internal hemorrhoids that has failed medical management (i.e., bulk agents, suppositories, topical preparations, and sitz baths) is an indication for treatment.

NOTE: The mere presence of hemorrhoids alone, without symptoms, is not necessarily an indication for treatment.

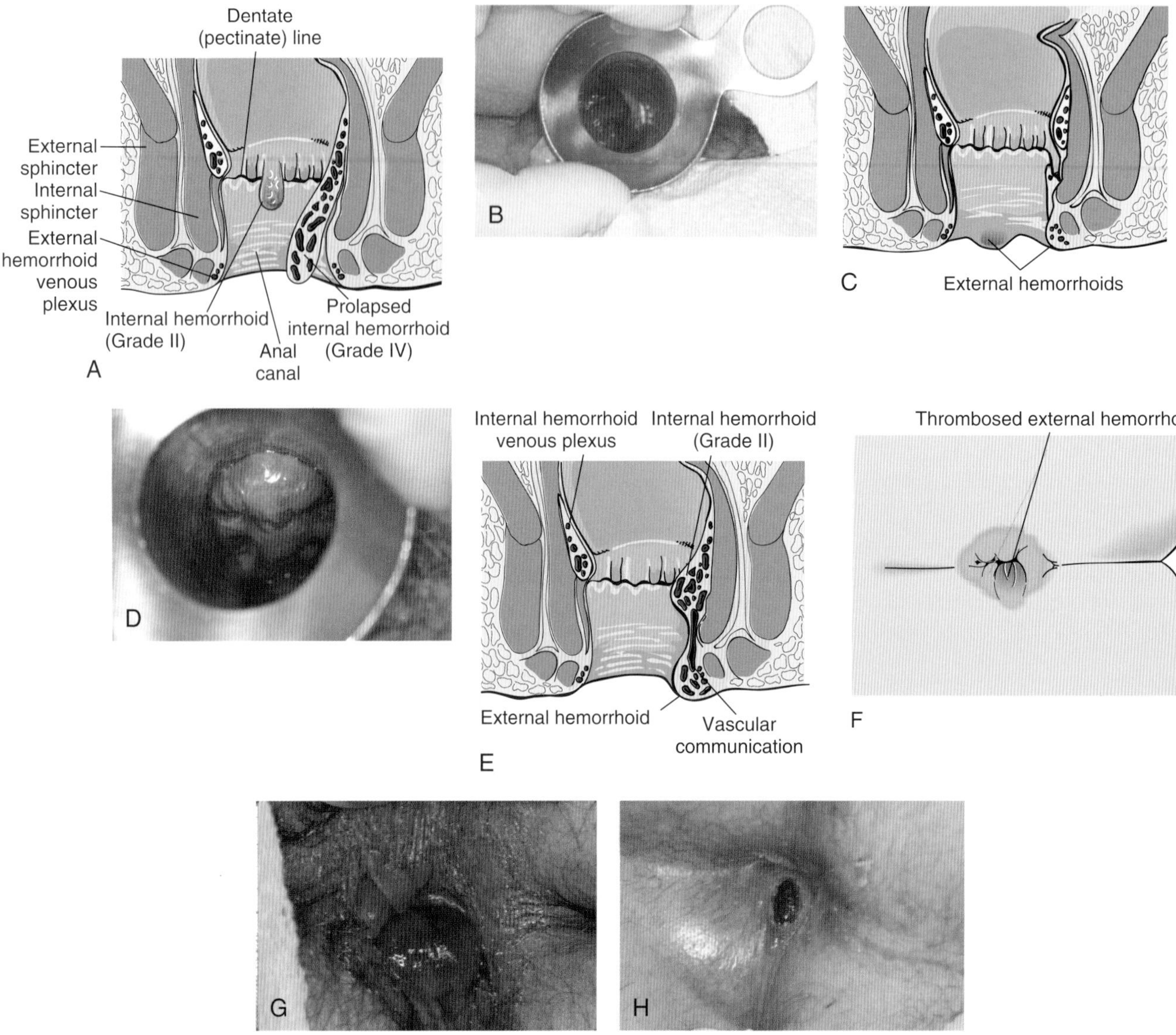

Figure 106-1 Various types of hemorrhoids. **A,** Internal hemorrhoid. Note that although an internal hemorrhoid may be visible "externally" (grade IV), it is classified by its origin, which, as shown here, is above the dentate line. **B,** Internal hemorrhoid as seen through the Ives slotted anoscope. **C,** External hemorrhoids. **D,** External hemorrhoid as seen through the Ives anoscope. **E,** Mixed hemorrhoid disease (both internal and external hemorrhoids with a vascular communication). **F,** Thrombosed external hemorrhoid. **G,** Large acute thrombosed hemorrhoid. **H,** Normal progression of a thrombosed external hemorrhoid 4 to 5 days after occurrence. The skin over the top becomes necrotic and appears to be a thin membrane. (**A, C, E,** and **F,** Redrawn from Pfenninger JL, Surrell J: Nonsurgical treatment options for internal hemorrhoids. Am Fam Physician 52:821–837, 1995. Original art copyrighted by Steve Oh. **B, D, G,** and **H,** Courtesy of John L. Pfenninger, MD, The Medical Procedures Center, PC, Midland, Mich.)

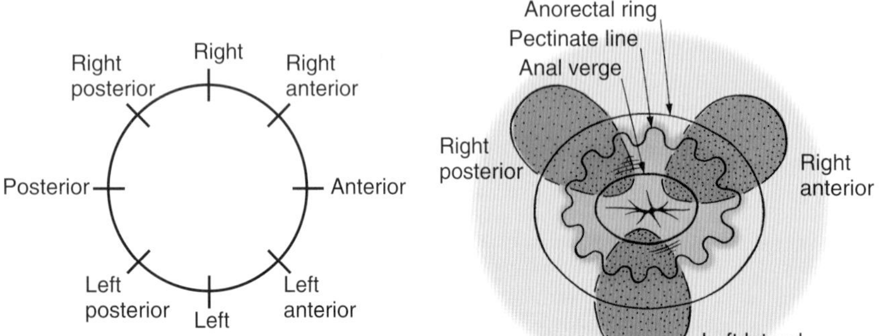

Figure 106-2 **A,** Representation of eight segments in the rectum as seen through a slotted (Ives) anoscope, with the patient in the left lateral decubitus position. **B,** Usual three primary hemorrhoidal groups.

TABLE 106-1 Classification of Internal Hemorrhoids

Grade	Description
I	Small, do not prolapse
II	Medium, prolapse and return spontaneously
III	Large, prolapse but reduce manually
IV	Largest, prolapse, not reducible

Contraindications

- Bleeding diathesis (relative). If on warfarin, the international normalized ratio (INR) should be in the therapeutic range. There is always an increased risk of bleeding if the patient is on aspirin or clopidogrel, but generally this is not a contraindication to treatment.
- Pregnancy or immediately postpartum (<8 weeks).
- Inflammatory bowel disease.
- Anorectal fissures.
- Active anorectal infections.
- Acquired immunodeficiency syndrome or other immunodeficiency states.
- Portal hypertension (relative).
- Rectal wall mucosal prolapse.
- Anorectal tumors.

Recommendations for antibiotic subacute bacterial endocarditis prophylaxis have been updated (see Chapter 221, Antibiotic Prophylaxis). Basically, antibiotics are *not* indicated for hemorrhoidal procedures. For those in the very–high-risk categories, they would be optional.

Preprocedure Patient Preparation

1. Give the patient one or two enemas before the procedure. Although not absolutely necessary, it is aesthetically helpful and improves visualization of the anatomy.
2. Ask the patient to avoid aspirin or clopidogrel for 1 week before treatment in low-risk situations.
3. Provide a patient education handout to ensure informed consent (see the sample patient education handouts online at www.expertconsult.com).
4. A complete history of the complaints as well as the pertinent past medical history and physical examination are essential. Record these on the sample encounter forms (go to www.expertconsult.com) that summarize the information.
5. The patient may be examined and treated in the left lateral decubitus position, which is usually more comfortable, the prone jackknife position, or even in the customary stirrups. The latter two positions can be used when exposure is difficult. No sedation is necessary for a patient having only anoscopy and internal hemorrhoid treatment. The patient may take four ibuprofen 200-mg tablets 1 to 2 hours before the office visit. Before performing anoscopy, perform an external visual and a digital anorectal examination. Ask the patient to perform a Valsalva maneuver (bearing down) to rule out full-thickness rectal prolapse. (Occasionally, examination with the patient sitting on the commode is necessary to assess for this.)

NOTE: Only internal hemorrhoids are treated by IRC, banding, or sclerotherapy. Treatment of external hemorrhoids requires excision and is associated with pain, so at least local anesthetics are needed.

Treatment

Rubber-band ligation (Barron or McGivney ligation), IRC, and sclerotherapy for internal hemorrhoids are discussed in the following sections. A summary of techniques and their indications is found in Table 106-2. The treatment of external hemorrhoids is covered later in this chapter and the treatment of perianal skin tags is dealt with separately in Chapter 108, Removal of Perianal Skin Tags (External Hemorrhoidal Skin Tags). Because of the associated discharge and poor patient acceptance, cryotherapy is not covered in this discussion.

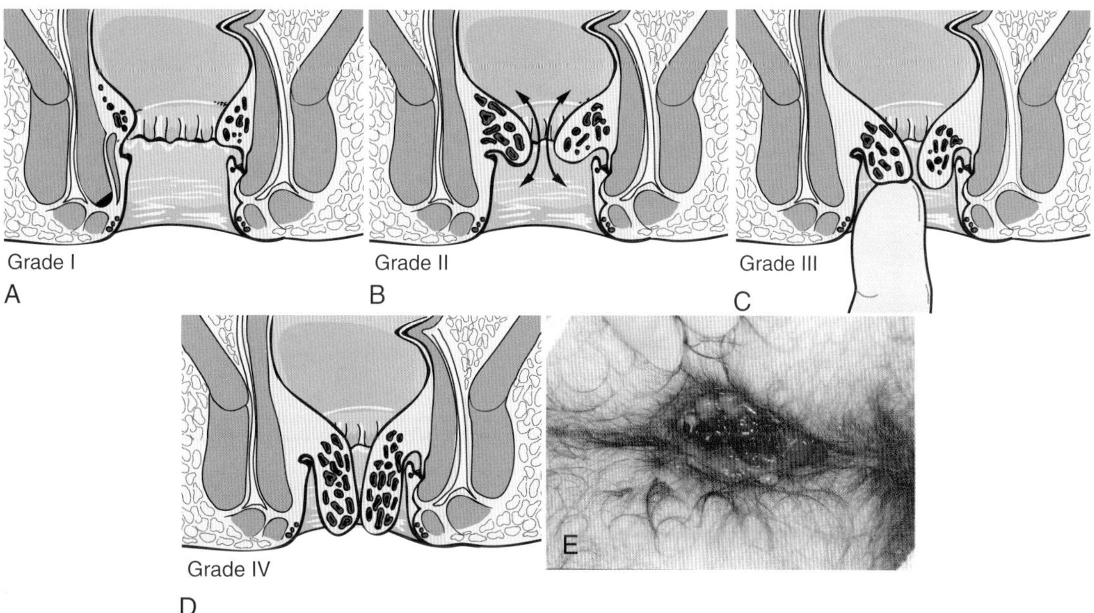

Figure 106-3 Grading of *internal* hemorrhoids. **A,** Grade I hemorrhoids are present and identifiable. **B,** Grade II hemorrhoids prolapse with a bowel movement but return spontaneously. **C,** Grade III hemorrhoids prolapse and can be replaced manually. **D,** Grade IV hemorrhoids remain prolapsed in spite of all efforts at reduction and are often associated with varying amounts of mucosal prolapse. **E,** Grade IV prolapsed internal hemorrhoid. (**A–D,** From Pfenninger JL, Surrell J: Nonsurgical treatment options for internal hemorrhoids. Am Fam Physician 52:821–837, 1995. Original art copyrighted by Steve Oh.)

TABLE 106-2 Comparison of Therapeutic Modalities for Treatment of Internal Hemorrhoids

Method	Grade of Internal Hemorrhoid I	II	III	IV	Ease of Performance	Complications	Location
Infrared coagulator	+++	+++	±	–	+++	Rare	Office
Rubber band	±	+++	+++	–	++	Some	Office
Sclerotherapy	++	+++	±	–	+	Common	Office
Stapled hemorrhoidopexy	–	–	+++	+++	+	See text	OR
Surgical excision	–	–	++	+++	+	Common	OR

OR, operating room.
Scale: –, not recommended (does not work); +++, easiest (best suited).

Rubber-Band Ligation

Rubber-band ligation involves placing a rubber band around the base of an internal hemorrhoid. The ensnared tissue undergoes necrosis and sloughs. Rubber-band ligation is used for treatment of second- or third-degree bleeding or prolapsing internal hemorrhoids.

EQUIPMENT

- Slotted Ives anoscope (see Chapter 98, Anoscopy, Fig. 98-1)
- McGivney ligator with bands (or an acceptable alternative device; Fig. 106-4) is the traditional applicator. Alternatively, a disposable hemorrhoid ligator is available, the O'Regan Hemorrhoid Banding System (Fig. 106-5).
- Alligator forceps (similar to long-handled Allis clamp)
- External light source
- Large obstetric/gynecologic cotton swabs

TECHNIQUE. See Figure 106-6.

1. Load the ligating drum with two bands. Insert the cone into the drum and slide the bands over it. A small amount of liquid soap on the cone will facilitate this. Hold the handle with the other hand to prevent the inadvertent sliding of the outer drum over the inner drum of the ligator while loading.
2. Insert the anoscope and visualize the hemorrhoid to be ligated. Treat the largest hemorrhoid group, or the obviously bleeding source, first. Have an assistant stabilize the anoscope.
3. With one hand, draw the hemorrhoidal tissue into the ligating drum with an alligator forceps. If the patient experiences pain, grasp the hemorrhoidal tissue more proximally. Pull only hemorrhoidal tissue into the ligator; avoid excessive mucosa.
4. With the other hand, grasp the handle of the ligator and push forward slightly. Squeeze the handle. The outer drum slides over the inner drum, displacing the rubber bands around the hemorrhoid.
5. Reposition or withdraw the anoscope. Patient tolerance is highest if only one hemorrhoid group is treated per visit. However, some physicians treat more than one segment per visit. Avoid circumferential ligation because it may increase pain, and the tension on the mucosa may lead to nonhealing fissures.

COMPLICATIONS

- Spotting can be expected for 8 to 10 days. Profuse bleeding, although rare, occurs 1 to 2 weeks after the procedure, when the hemorrhoidal tissue sloughs. Bleeding can be significant and occasionally requires active intervention.
- Patients may experience a dull ache for 2 days after the procedure. If severe pain is experienced during the procedure, the band will need to be removed with scissors. It was applied too far distally.
- Thrombosis of external hemorrhoids occurs rarely and is treated symptomatically or with excision.
- Sepsis with pelvic cellulitis (perineal sepsis) is a serious complication, but it rarely occurs. Patients complain of fever, increasing perineal pain, swelling, inability to urinate, or dysuria. Treatment requires hospitalization, broad-spectrum antibiotic administration, and débridement.
- Slow healing or nonhealing of the treatment site can lead to formation of an anal fissure.

ADVANTAGES

- The instrument itself is inexpensive, and there are no disposable tips to replace.
- Higher grades of hemorrhoids can be treated.
- The procedure is quick.
- The procedure is easy to learn.

DISADVANTAGES

- The procedure is somewhat more uncomfortable than other techniques, and significant complications have been reported (e.g., perineal sepsis).

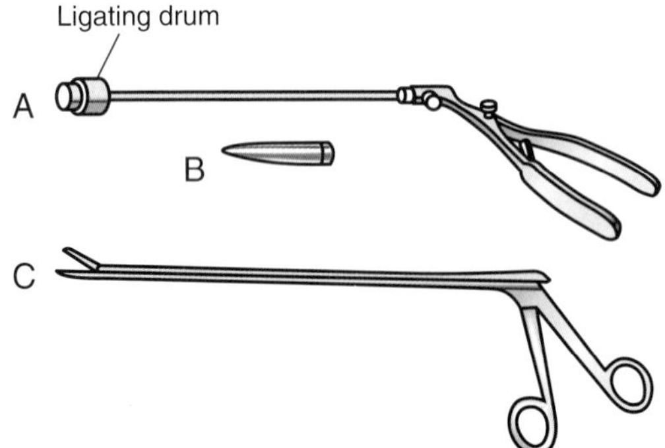

Figure 106-4 McGivney ligator. **A,** Ligator. **B,** Cone to load bands. **C,** Forceps to grasp hemorrhoid.

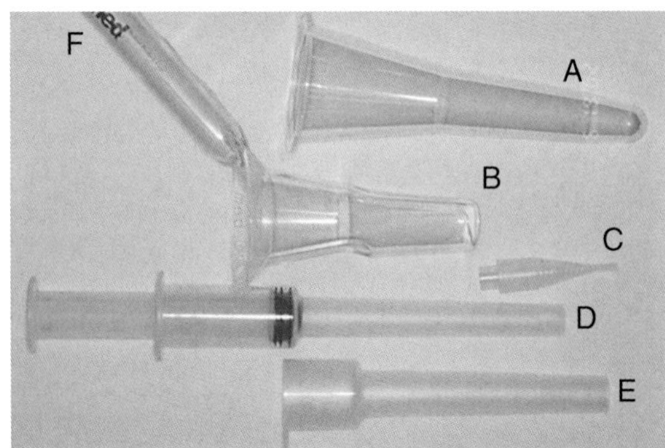

Figure 106-5 O'Regan disposable banding unit. **A,** Trocar for insertion of anoscope. **B,** Anoscope. **C,** Loading cone for bands. **D,** Syringe for suction to pull up hemorrhoid. **E,** Sleeve that fits over syringe apparatus that pushes bands off onto hemorrhoids. **F,** Penlight inserted into anoscope handle for light.

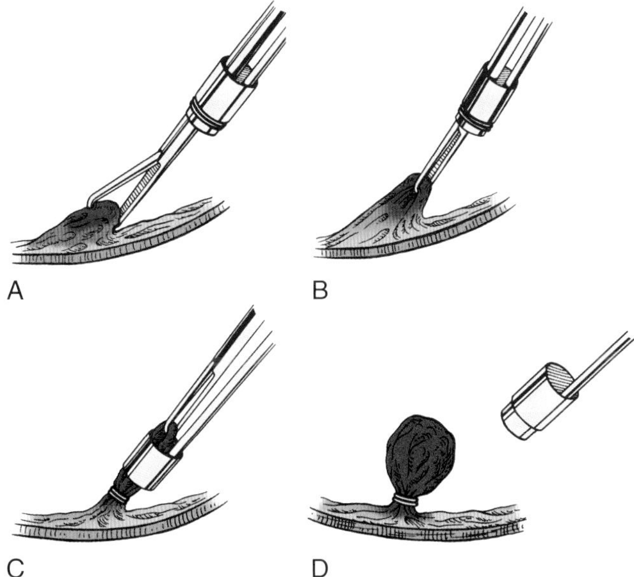

Figure 106-6 Rubber-band ligation. The hemorrhoid is gently grasped (**A**) and brought into the drum of the ligator (**B**). Two rubber bands are released (**C**). Appearance of the ligated hemorrhoid after equipment is removed (**D**). If the patient tolerates the grasping of the hemorrhoid with forceps, ligation can be performed with minimal or no discomfort.

- Two people are needed to perform the procedure (the operator and the assistant, who holds the anoscope).

POSTPROCEDURE PATIENT EDUCATION. See the patient education handouts online at www.expertconsult.com.

- Inform the patient that mild aching discomfort may be experienced over the next 2 days.
- Ask the patient to report any excessive bleeding, fever, dysuria, inability to urinate (a sign of perineal sepsis), or increasing pain.
- Ask the patient to follow up in 4 to 6 weeks for reexamination and further banding, as needed.

Infrared Coagulation

EQUIPMENT

- Infrared coagulator (Redfield Corporation, Rochelle Park, NJ; Fig. 106-7)
- Slotted Ives anoscope (Redfield Corporation; see Chapter 98, Anoscopy, Fig. 98-1)
- External light source
- Large obstetric/gynecologic cotton swabs

NOTE: IRC units are not submersible for cleaning. Instead, they use a disposable sheath that is changed for each visit (see Fig. 106-7B). It is imperative not to immerse the newer units (in contrast to the older units) in sterilizing solutions.

TECHNIQUE. Infrared light is applied to the *base* of the internal hemorrhoid, forming a white coagulum that ulcerates and then forms a scar. The diameter of burn correlates with the size of the probe tip, which is usually 6 mm. The depth of penetration correlates with the time of the pulse, which is generally 1.5 to 2 seconds. Infrared coagulation is used for first- and second-degree and smaller third-degree internal hemorrhoids. It can be used for larger hemorrhoids (use a 2- to 2.5-second setting), but treatment may need to be repeated in 4 to 6 weeks. It is a painless procedure, and although more than one hemorrhoid group is sometimes treated, most clinicians begin by treating only one complex to determine patient tolerance. Treatment of more than one complex of hemorrhoids at a time may increase post-treatment discomfort and the other complications, especially bleeding. A teaching video describing this technique is available from Redfield Corporation.

1. With the patient in the left lateral decubitus position, insert the Ives slotted anoscope and identify the hemorrhoid to be treated. Insert the 6-mm IRC probe.
2. Press the probe tip onto the hemorrhoid itself, or preferably on the most proximal portion of the hemorrhoid. Only light pressure is needed.
3. Pull the trigger and keep it compressed. The unit has an incorporated time switch that limits exposure and will turn off automatically. The typical setting is 1.5 seconds. Generally, four to six separate applications are made for each hemorrhoid group.

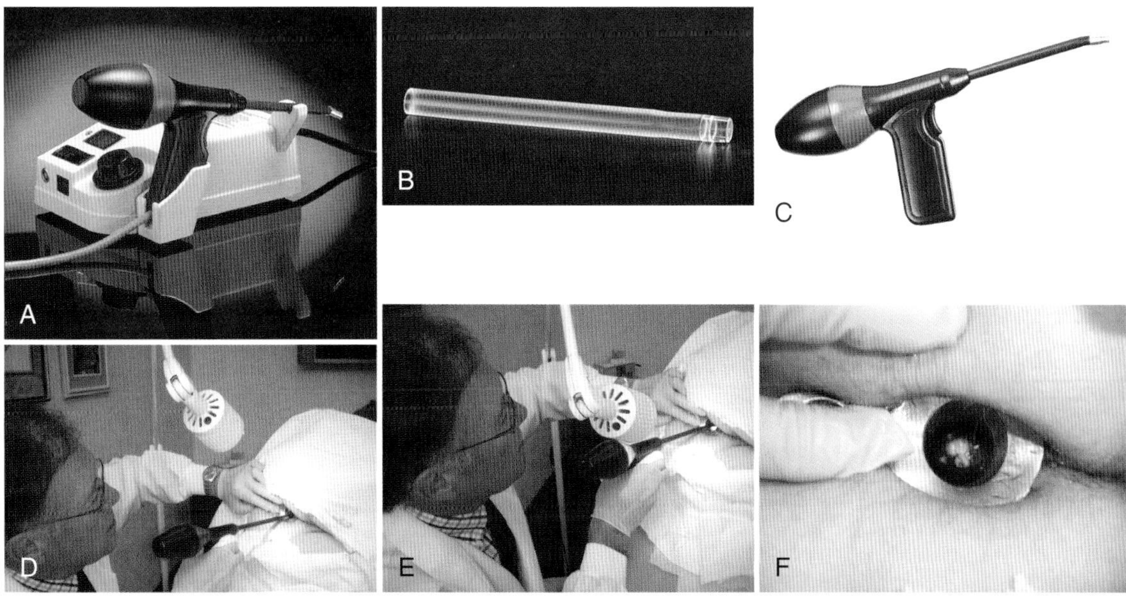

Figure 106-7 Infrared coagulator (IRC) unit (**A**), sheath (**B**), and handpiece (**C**). The tip of the IRC is inserted through the Ives slotted anoscope and placed on the base of the hemorrhoid (**D**). When the unit is activated (**E**), a light is visible (noted here in the bulb of the handpiece) that automatically shuts off after the programmed time, usually 1.5 to 2 seconds. The internal hemorrhoid appears white over the treated area (**F**). (**A–C,** Courtesy of Redfield Corporation, Rochelle Park, NJ; **D–F,** Courtesy of John L. Pfenninger, MD, The Medical Procedures Center, PC, Midland, Mich.)

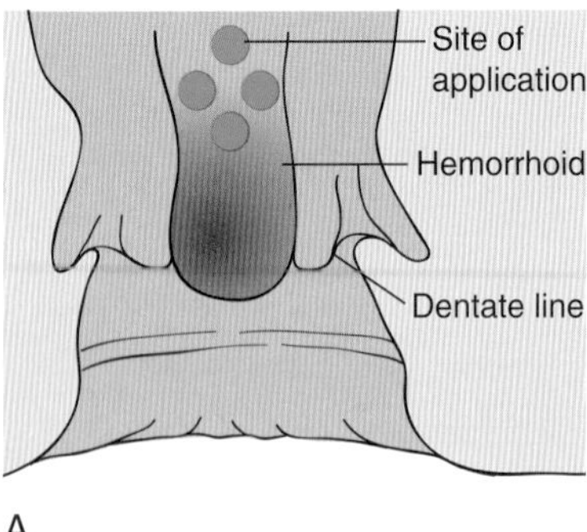

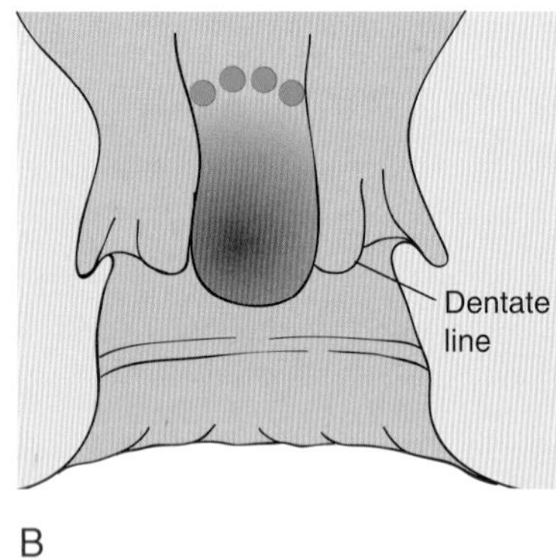

Figure 106-8 Treatment of base (proximal portion) of the internal hemorrhoids using infrared coagulation. **A,** Diamond shape. **B,** Linear method. Each circle indicates a single application for 1.5 to 2 seconds. Up to six applications per visit may be needed per hemorrhoid segment.

One group is treated per visit at 4- to 6-week intervals. For the first treatment, select the hemorrhoid that is bleeding or that is the largest. Larger hemorrhoids and grade III hemorrhoids may require more than one treatment session or a longer exposure (2 seconds).

CAUTION: Do not overlap treatment sites. Overlapping increases the depth of burn. Place the probe adjacent to a previous site in a linear fashion or in a diamond shape, but do not overlap if possible (Fig. 106-8). If overlapping does occur, it rarely causes a significant problem, but purposely avoid it *if possible.*

4. *Wipe off the tip with saline-soaked gauze between applications.* This allows the tip to cool and cleans the end. If a loud "pop" is heard, there is debris or mucus between the tip and the mucosa. No damage is done, but the sudden noise can be frightening to the patient (and the clinician). It will sound much like a small firecracker.
5. Realign the anoscope and apply treatment to another hemorrhoidal group if more than one group is to be treated.
6. Remove the anoscope. No special aftercare is needed.

COMPLICATIONS

- Patients may experience a mild, dull, aching pain lasting up to 2 days after treatment.
- Minor bleeding may be encountered for up to 2 weeks after the procedure. More bleeding can be expected at 10 to 14 days when the eschar sloughs. This can usually be managed conservatively but very rarely will require topical astringents or maybe even a suture.
- Rarely, patients experience a thrombosed external hemorrhoid in the area after treatment.
- Rarely, slow-healing ulcers can be encountered.
- Slow healing or nonhealing of the treatment site can lead to formation of an anal fissure.

ADVANTAGES

- It is an essentially painless procedure.
- There have been no reported cases of perineal sepsis.
- The procedure is quick, simple to learn, and cost effective.
- The procedure is well tolerated by patients.
- There are no costs for disposable probes, but disposable vinyl sheaths are used.
- It can be used in patients with pacemakers.
- The unit can also be used to remove tattoos, reduce nasal turbinates, stop bleeding from biopsy and hair donor sites, and treat verrucae and condylomata.
- The unit is well made and requires little maintenance.

DISADVANTAGES

- The procedure is not very effective for advanced third-degree hemorrhoidal disease and works poorly for fourth-degree hemorrhoidal disease.
- The unit costs more than the materials for band ligation.

POSTPROCEDURE PATIENT EDUCATION. See the patient education handouts online at www.expertconsult.com.

- Ask the patient to follow up in 4 to 6 weeks to treat residual disease or another group of hemorrhoids. In the elderly or compromised patient (e.g., diabetes), it is best to wait longer.
- Ask the patient to report any severe symptoms of pain, fever, or inability to urinate.

Sclerotherapy

Sclerotherapy is used for treatment of first- or second-degree internal bleeding hemorrhoids. Injection of 1 to 2 mL of sclerosant into the internal hemorrhoid causes sclerosis and fixation of the submucosa to the underlying muscularis. This technique is relatively quick. All three major hemorrhoidal groups can be treated at one sitting. It is a useful technique for a patient on warfarin. Unfortunately, it has not been as effective as other modalities and has been associated with impotence, the reason for which is unknown.

EQUIPMENT

- Ives slotted anoscope
- 5-mL syringe
- 21-gauge spinal needle
- Sclerosant (sodium morrhuate, sodium tetradecyl sulfate, hypertonic saline, or phenol in almond oil)

TECHNIQUE. See Figure 106-9.

1. Insert the anoscope and visualize the hemorrhoid group to be injected.
2. Insert the spinal needle into or immediately above the hemorrhoid group in the submucosal space. Withdraw the plunger of the syringe and aspirate for blood to ensure that the sclerosant will *not* be injected directly into a vein.
3. Inject 1 to 2 mL of sclerosant. *A wheal should be noted during injection.* Take care to inject well *above* the level of the dentate line.
4. Document the location of the injection and the amount of sclerosant used.
5. Reposition the anoscope to visualize the next hemorrhoid group to be treated.

COMPLICATIONS

- The procedure is painful if the sclerosant is injected below the level of the dentate line.
- Thrombosis of internal or external hemorrhoids may occur, causing pain. Thrombosis is managed with topical creams, analgesics, and sitz baths.
- Bleeding is usually the result of injection into the mucosa rather than the submucosa. Necrosis and ulceration with bleeding

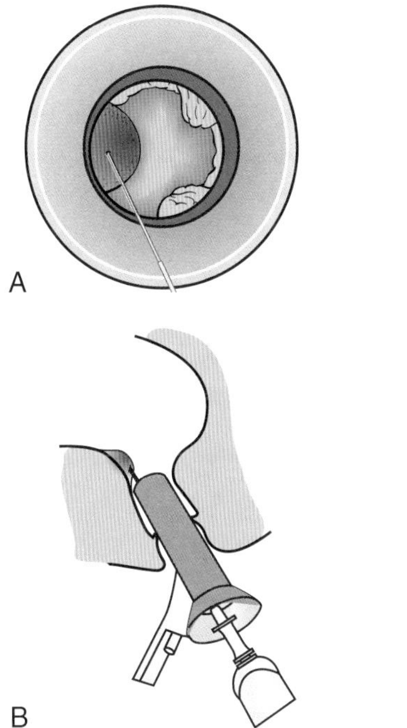

Figure 106-9 **A,** Sclerotherapy as viewed through the anoscope. If a wheal is not produced, the injection is too deep and the needle should be withdrawn. An injection that is too superficial will produce necrosis of the anal canal lining. **B,** Injection technique.

occur 2 to 3 weeks after injection. Healing usually occurs in 3 to 6 weeks.
- Abscess occurs very rarely.
- Anaphylaxis from the sclerosant is rare.
- Impotence has been reported, but the etiology is uncertain.

ADVANTAGES

- The procedure is effective.
- It can be used in a patient on warfarin.
- The equipment cost is minimal.
- It can be used concomitantly with banding or other therapies.

DISADVANTAGES

- The procedure is associated with more significant complications than other methods.
- The technique is harder to master.

POSTPROCEDURE PATIENT EDUCATION. See the sample patient education handouts online at www.expertconsult.com.

- Inform the patient that mild rectal discomfort may occur after treatment, and tell the patient to report any severe symptoms.
- Instruct the patient to return to the office in 4 weeks for repeat examination and further treatments if necessary.

Stapled Hemorrhoidopexy

Recently, stapled hemorrhoidopexy (SH or PPH, "procedure for prolapse and hemorrhoids") has been introduced as a novel method of correcting third- and fourth-degree hemorrhoids. During this procedure, a specialized stapling device reduces hemorrhoidal prolapse by excising a circumferential band of prolapsed mucosa and submucosa between the distal rectum and proximal anal canal (Fig. 106-10). This procedure interrupts the terminal branches of the hemorrhoidal arteries and resuspends the anal canal mucosa to a more physiologic location. The stapling device is know as the PPH 03 and is manufactured Ethicon Endo-Surgery, Inc. (Cincinnati, Ohio).

INDICATIONS. This procedure can be used with minimally symptomatic external disease. Other clinicians will perform PPH and add single- and multiquadrant excision or external hemorrhoids or tags.

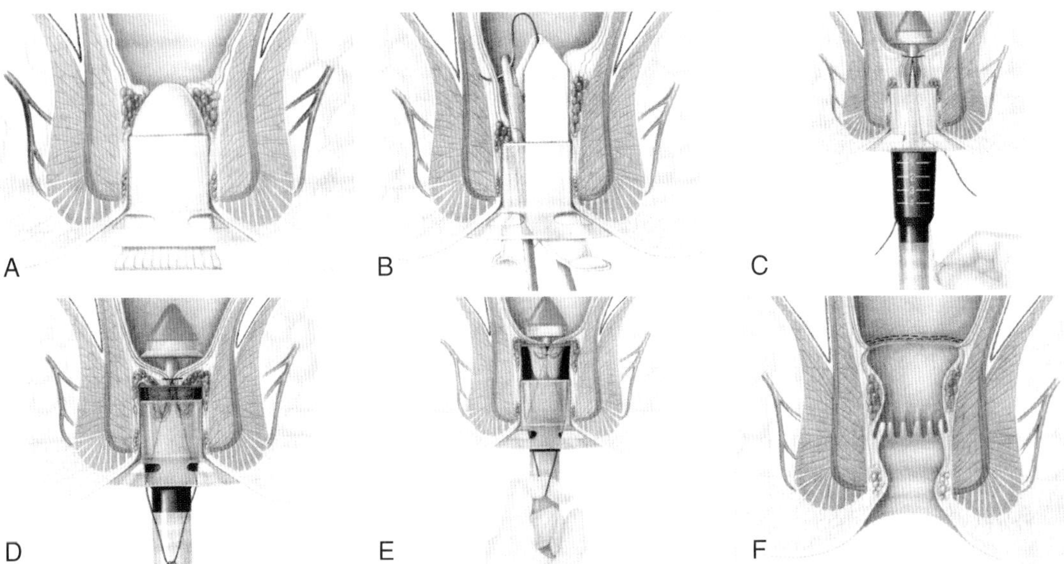

Figure 106-10 Procedure for prolapse and hemorrhoids, or stapled hemorrhoidopexy. **A,** A circular anal dilator/obturator is inserted into the anal canal to push the prolapse back and lift the hemorrhoidal tissue into place. **B,** The internal hemorrhoids are held back while a pursestring suture is prepared in the rectal mucosa/submucosa approximately 4 to 6 cm from the dentate line. **C,** A fully opened hemorrhoidal circular stapler is inserted beyond the pursestring suture. The pursestring is tied around the anvil to secure the excess mucosal tissue. With the suture threader, each limb of the suture is brought through the channel of the instrument. **D,** After the ends of the retraction suture are knotted, the stapler is tightened and gently pushed into the anal canal. Moderate traction on the pursestring must be maintained so that the prolapse is drawn into the stapler casing. **E,** The stapler is then closed completely, fired in one fluid motion, and withdrawn gently. The anal canal wall is reconnected and restored, and the hemorrhoidal artery's terminal branches, which feed internal hemorrhoids, are interrupted. **F,** Successful completion of the procedure for prolapse and hemorrhoids corrects the prolapse, restores internal hemorrhoids to their normal anatomic position, and alleviates the patient's symptoms. (From Senagore AJ, Abcarian H, Chiu YSY, Ellis CN: Current treatment options for patients with grades III and IV hemorrhoids. Contemp Surg Supplement:S5–S11, 2006.)

CONTRAINDICATIONS

- Anal stenosis
- Large external hemorrhoids or tags
- Gangrenous or strangulated hemorrhoids
- Perianal sepsis
- Full-thickness rectal prolapse
- Anal-receptive intercourse

ADVANTAGES

- Less postoperative pain and more rapid return to normal activities than with a surgical hemorrhoidectomy
- No external wounds to care for
- Less incontinence and constipation reported than with conventional hemorrhoidectomy

COMPLICATIONS

- Anal stenosis.
- Secondary bleeding.
- Urinary retention.
- Pelvic sepsis.
- Incontinence.
- Prolonged, intractable pain has been reported.

POSTPROCEDURE PATIENT EDUCATION

- There are usually no external wounds to care for. This is case dependent.
- Prescribe an oral analgesic.
- Discomfort lasts for 1 to 2 weeks.
- Warm tub soaks may relieve discomfort.
- The patient should take a bulk laxative to maintain soft stool.

THROMBOSED EXTERNAL HEMORRHOIDS

External hemorrhoids occur below the dentate (pectinate) line. Patients with thrombosed external hemorrhoids have a painful, tender, swollen, bluish lump at the anal orifice. If the patient is seen within 48 hours of the onset of symptoms, the thrombosed hemorrhoid should be incised or excised. After 48 to 72 hours, symptoms have usually improved and symptomatic care is recommended if the pain is minimal, especially for smaller lesions. However, *if the patient is still experiencing significant pain*, the hemorrhoid can be surgically relieved at any time.

There are three basic surgical approaches: (1) excise an ellipse over the clotted hemorrhoid and evacuate the clot, (2) excise the hemorrhoid completely, and (3) make a simple incision over the clot and express the contents.

Equipment

- No. 11 blade and tissue scissors
- Mosquito hemostats
- Fine tissue forceps
- Lidocaine (2%) with epinephrine; 27-gauge, 1½-inch needle, and 3-mL syringe
- Antiseptic solution
- 4-0 or 5-0 absorbable suture (if closure is desired, but best if left open)

Technique

See Figures 106-11 and 106-12.

1. Cleanse the perianal area with antiseptic solution.
2. Infiltrate the skin over the thrombosed external hemorrhoid with lidocaine with epinephrine (1 to 2 mL).
3. Excise the entire hemorrhoid as an ellipse, or *perform an elliptical excision* over the *top* of the hemorrhoid and remove the skin. Be sure to evacuate all clots.
4. Control any bleeding with electrocautery or silver nitrate sticks if pressure alone is not adequate.
5. The wound is best left open to heal by secondary intention, which it usually does without adverse sequelae. The skin edges may also be approximated with interrupted, fine absorbable suture (unless silver nitrate was used), but this is generally discouraged.
6. Alternatively, after anesthesia, the base of the clotted hemorrhoid can be clamped (under the clot) with a hemostat. The tissue over the hemostat is excised with a blade. With the hemostat still in place, a suture is placed proximal to the tip. If interrupted sutures are used, leave the ends of the first stitch long and use them for traction to pull down the upper portion of the incision. If a running stitch is used, the long end can be used in the same manner. Then remove the hemostat and complete the closure. This ensures that the entire excisional site has been sutured closed.
7. Some physicians *simply incise* over the thrombus and evacuate the clot. If this is done, it is imperative that *all* clots be removed. After the incision is made, express the clot, and then explore the cavity with hemostats to break down any septa. Another incision inside the cavity may be necessary. Frequently more than one clot will be evacuated. Reexpress the area to be sure all clots have been removed. This technique is quicker, but warn the patient that there is a higher likelihood of reaccumulation with this approach. Consider this method when the clot has been present for several days and the acute clotting process has resolved.

Complications

- Bleeding
- Pain
- Recurrence
- Chronic fissure
- Infection

Postprocedure Patient Education

See the sample patient education handouts online at www.expertconsult.com.

- Recommend that the patient take sitz baths two to three times per day for 1 week.
- Oral analgesics, topical anesthetic cream/ointment (e.g., lidocaine 5%), and stool softeners are helpful.
- A follow-up examination should be scheduled for 4 weeks.
- Emphasize that the patient avoid prolonged sitting on the toilet to prevent recurrent thrombosis. Also, avoid any activity (e.g., weight lifting) that induces a Valsalva maneuver.
- Explain to the patient that a high-bulk, high-fluid diet is essential.

EXTERNAL HEMORRHOIDAL TAGS

See Figures 106-13 and 106-14 (also see Chapter 108, Removal of Perianal Skin Tags [External Hemorrhoidal Skin Tags]).

External hemorrhoidal tags are usually the result of previous external hemorrhoidal disease. Occasionally, a patient has experienced a thrombosis that resolved spontaneously but the skin remains stretched out. These lesions no longer have dilated vessels and are often quite fibrotic. The major symptoms include pruritus and problems with cleanliness. Generally, when removed in the office, only one area is removed at a visit unless the attachments are quite small.

Equipment

- Alcohol wipe
- 3% to 5% lidocaine with epinephrine

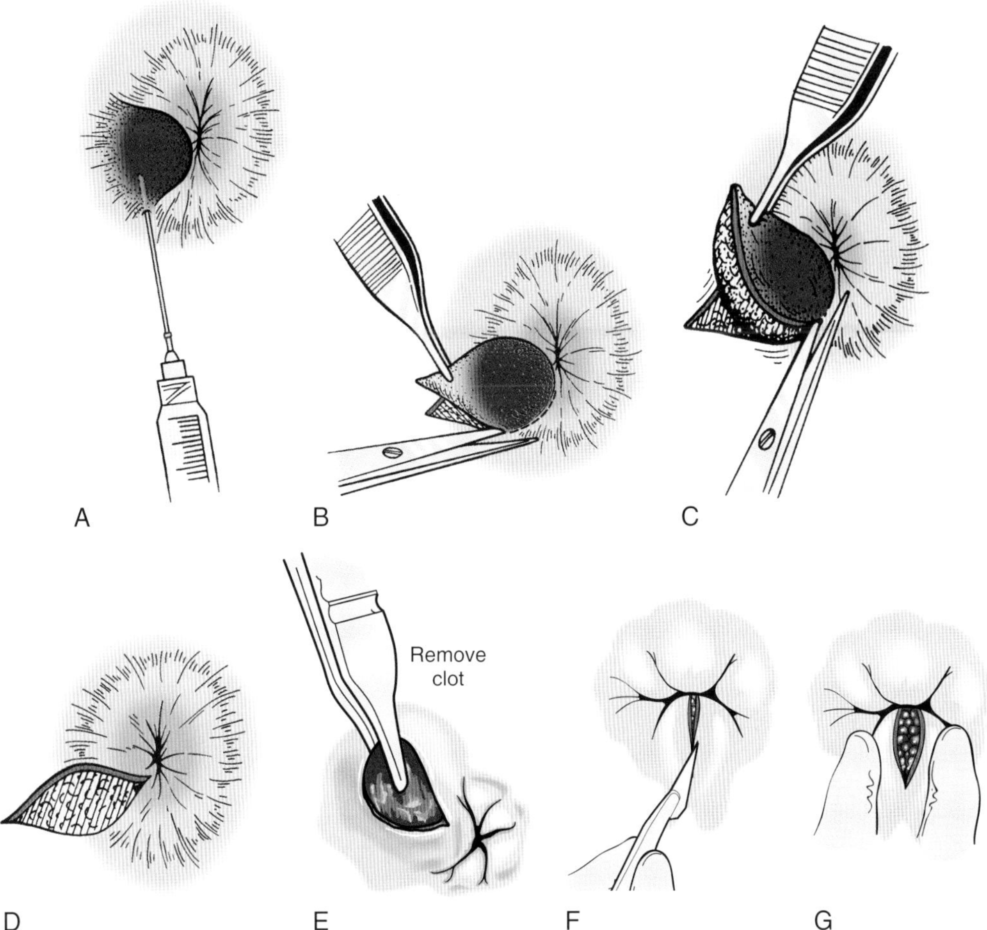

Figure 106-11 Excision of a thrombosed hemorrhoid. **A,** The area is infiltrated with 2% lidocaine with epinephrine. **B** and **C,** The thrombosed hemorrhoid is excised along with a small wedge of skin. **D,** Skin edges are sufficiently separated to permit adequate drainage, thereby preventing clot reaccumulation. They can also be closed with fine absorbable suture. **E,** Instead of removing the entire hemorrhoid, a small elliptical incision is made over the hemorrhoid and the clot is expressed. No suture closure is needed. **F,** A simple incision and drainage with expression of all clots can also be performed. Multiple clots are often present and should be removed. **G,** After the initial clot is removed, spread the incision to expose the base of the hemorrhoid to remove other thrombi. The disadvantage of this approach is that the incision can seal over, allowing the clot to reaccumulate.

- No. 15 scalpel blade
- Monsel's solution to control bleeding
- Cautery (ball electrode or bipolar forceps)
- 5% lidocaine ointment
- Ives slotted anoscope
- Lubricant
- Nonsterile gloves
- Formalin pathology jar

Indications

Symptomatic as noted previously.

Contraindications

The treatment is contraindicated if the patient is unwilling to tolerate pain for several days.

Technique

1. Place the patient in left lateral decubitus position. Perform digital and anoscopic examinations.
2. Identify the lesion to be removed and wipe with alcohol or other antiseptic.
3. Inject the lidocaine in a field block pattern. Be careful not to tent up the area too much under the tag, which may lead to excision of too much tissue.
4. If using a radiofrequency unit, set at cut and coag (level 3, or 30 W) and use either a Vari-Tip wire or a loop and remove the lesion. Control the bleeding with Monsel's solution or cautery.
5. Alternatives are to use a blade or scissors to remove the lesion. There may be more bleeding with this method. If the base of the tag is quite large, a hemostat can be applied and left in place for several minutes, and then the tissue excised. This ensures approximation of the skin margins. No sutures are placed because they increase the chances of infection. Control bleeding as indicated previously.
6. Apply antibiotic ointment mixed with 5% lidocaine ointment.

Complications

- Pain
- Bleeding
- Infection
- Chronic fissure

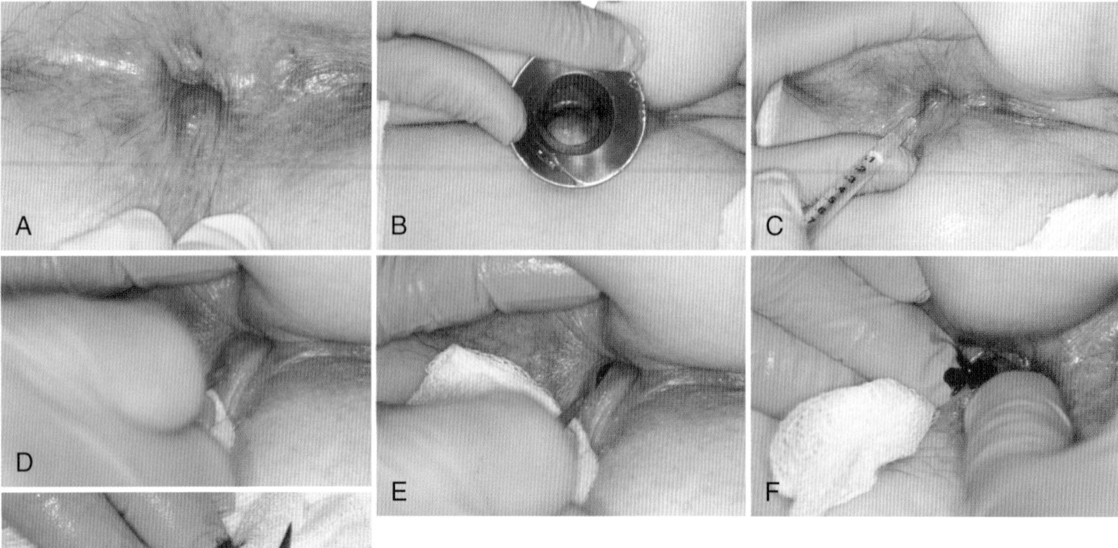

Figure 106-12 Incision and drainage of thrombosed external hemorrhoid using small ellipse technique. **A,** Thrombosed external hemorrhoid. **B,** View through Ives slotted anoscope. **C,** Injection of 1 mL 2% lidocaine with epinephrine. **D,** Initial incision with no. 11 pointed blade. **E,** Forming the ellipse. **F,** Expressing the clot. **G,** Clot and no. 11 blade. (Courtesy of John L. Pfenninger, MD, The Medical Procedures Center, PC, Midland, Mich.)

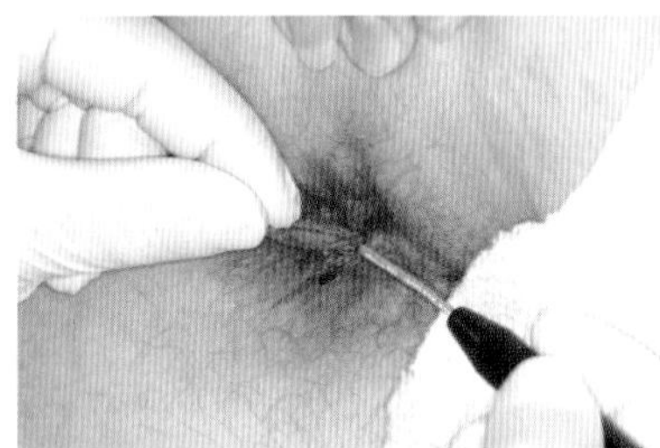

Figure 106-13 Removal of small hemorrhoidal tag using radiofrequency loop after anesthetic injection. (Courtesy of John L. Pfenninger, MD, The Medical Procedures Center, PC, Midland, Mich.)

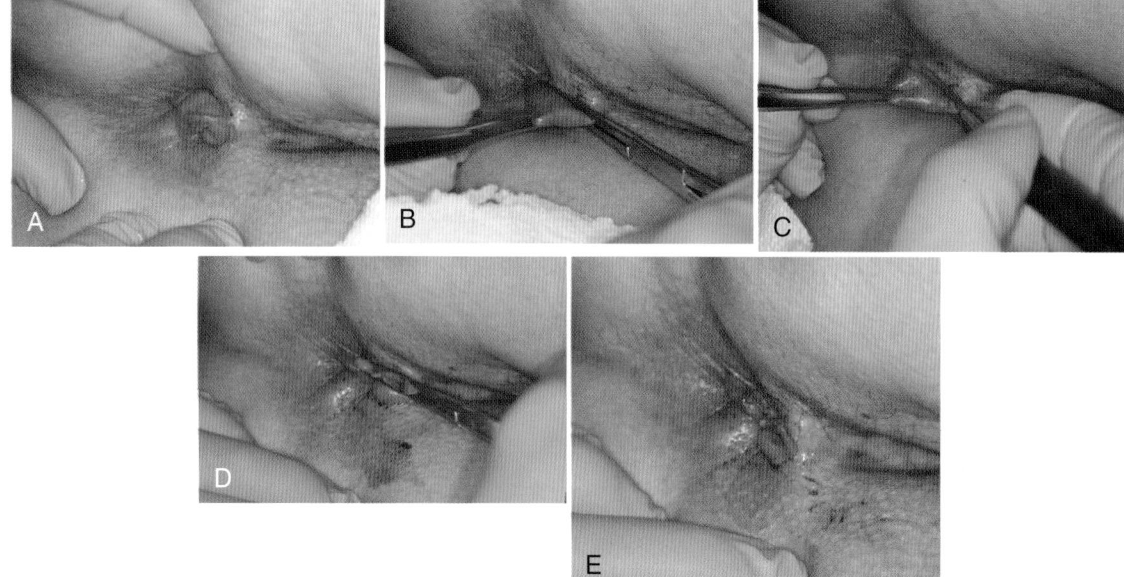

Figure 106-14 Removal of hemorrhoidal tag with large base. **A**, Tag. **B**, Applying large clamp or hemostats. **C**, Electrosurgical cutting/removal of tag. **D**, Appearance after removal of tag with clamp in place. **E**, No sutures are used to close the wound. (Courtesy of John L. Pfenninger, MD, The Medical Procedures Center, PC, Midland, Mich.)

Postoperative Patient Care

Nonsteroidal anti-inflammatory drugs are the mainstay for pain control. Narcotics can cause constipation. Lidocaine 5% ointment is helpful to control and reduce abrasive rubbing of clothes or other skin. Sitz baths are very helpful and the area should be cleansed three to four times a day. It may be best to stay off work for 2 to 3 days, depending on the size of the lesion.

CPT/Billing Codes

46083 Incision and drainage of thrombosed external hemorrhoid
46220 Excision, single anal tag
46221 Hemorrhoidectomy, by simple ligature (e.g., rubber band)
46230 Excision of external hemorrhoid tags and/or multiple papillae
46320 Enucleation or excision of external thrombosed hemorrhoid
46500 Injection of sclerosing solution, hemorrhoids
46600 Anoscopy
46934 Destruction of hemorrhoids, any method; internal (e.g., IRC)
46935 Destruction of hemorrhoids, any method; external
46936 Destruction of hemorrhoids, any method; internal and external
46947 Hemorrhoidopexy (e.g., prolapsing internal hemorrhoids) by stapling

NOTE: The last code is inappropriate when only IRC, band ligation, or sclerotherapy techniques are used for treatment of internal hemorrhoids.

ICD-9-CM Diagnostic Codes

455.0 Internal hemorrhoids
455.1 Internal hemorrhoids, thrombosed
455.2 Internal hemorrhoids, bleeding
455.3 External hemorrhoids
455.4 External hemorrhoids, thrombosed
455.9 Hemorrhoid tag

Suppliers

(See contact information online at www.expertconsult.com.)

Band ligator
Redfield Corporation
Infrared coagulator (IRC)
Redfield Corporation
Ives slotted anoscope
Redfield Corporation
O'Regan Hemorrhoid Banding System
Medsurge Medical, Inc.
Sclerosing agents
See Table 92-1.

BIBLIOGRAPHY

Bleday R, Pena JP, Rothenberger DA, et al: Symptomatic hemorrhoids: Current incidence and complications of operative therapy. Dis Colon Rectum 35:477–481, 1992.

Bullock N: Impotence after sclerotherapy of haemorrhoids: Case report. BMJ 314:419–420, 1997.

Corman ML (ed): Colon and Rectal Surgery, 5th ed. Philadelphia, Lippincott Williams & Wilkins, 2004.

Dennison AR, Whiston RJ, Rooney S, Morris DL: The management of hemorrhoids. Am J Gastroenterol 84:475–481, 1989.

Devine R, Ory S: Treatment of hemorrhoids in pregnancy. J Fam Pract 17:65, 1992.

Gordon P, Nivatvongs S (eds): Principles and Practice of Surgery for the Colon, Rectum, and Anus, 3rd ed. New York, Informa Healthcare, 2007.

Johanson JF, Rimm A: Optimal nonsurgical treatment of hemorrhoids: A comparative analysis of infrared coagulation, rubber band ligation, and injection sclerotherapy. Am J Gastroenterol 87:1600–1606, 1992.

MacRae HM, McLeod RS: Comparison of hemorrhoidal treatment modalities: A meta-analysis. Dis Colon Rectum 38:687–694, 1995.

Pfenninger JL: Modern treatments for internal haemorrhoids. BMJ 314:1211–1212, 1997.

Pfenninger JL, Surrell J: Nonsurgical treatment options for internal hemorrhoids. Am Fam Physician 52:821–837, 1995.

Pfenninger JL, Zainea GG: Common anorectal conditions: Part I. Symptoms and complaints. Am Fam Physician 63:2391–2398, 2001.

Pfenninger JL, Zainea GG: Common anorectal conditions: Part II. Lesions. Am Fam Physician 64:77–88, 2001.

Russell TR, Donahue JH: Hemorrhoidal banding: A warning. Dis Colon Rectum 28:291–293, 1985.

Simon T: Minor office procedures. Clin Colon Rectal Surg 18:225–260, 2005.

Smith LE: Hemorrhoidectomy with lasers and other contemporary modalities. Surg Clin North Am 3:665–679, 1992.

Standards Task Force of the American Society of Colon and Rectal Surgeons: Practice parameters for the treatment of hemorrhoids. Dis Colon Rectum 36:1118–1120, 1993.

Templeton JL, Spence RA, Kennedy TL, et al: Comparison of infrared coagulation and rubber band ligation for first and second degree haemorrhoids: A randomised prospective clinical trial. BMJ 286:1387–1389, 1983.

Tuggy M, Garcia J: Procedures Consult. Available at www.proceduresconsult.com, and as an application at www.apple.com/iTunes.

Usatine RP: The Color Atlas of Family Medicine. New York, McGraw-Hill, 2009.

Walker AJ, Leicester RJ, Nicholls RJ, Mann CV: A prospective study of infrared coagulation, injection and rubber band ligation in the treatment of haemorrhoids. Int J Colorectal Dis 5:113–116, 1990.

Zinberg SS, Stern DH, Furman DS, Wittles JM: A personal experience in comparing three non-operative techniques for treating internal hemorrhoids. Am J Gastroenterol 84:488–492, 1989.

CHAPTER 107

Perianal Abscess Incision and Drainage

James A. Surrell

A perianal abscess is one of the most painful anal conditions seen in the outpatient setting. The pain of a perianal abscess is severe, disabling, and progressive, and the only relief these patients obtain is with spontaneous rupture of the abscess or when they seek medical attention for incision and drainage (I&D). The most common etiology of perianal abscess is thought to be an infection originating at the dentate line in the anal crypts (see Chapter 97, Clinical Anorectal Anatomy and Digital Examination). The infection then usually migrates through the path of least resistance to the perianal tissues, where there is a closed-space environment ideal for proliferation of this mixed bacterial infection.

The four locations where abscesses can occur and their relative incidence are shown in Figure 107-1. The most common site of an abscess in the anal area is in the *perianal* tissues immediately adjacent to the anal verge (60%). If the abscess is located 2 to 3 cm away from the anal verge, then it is most likely in the *ischiorectal* location (25%), just outside the anal sphincters. An *intersphincteric* abscess occurs in the intersphincteric plane, between the internal and external sphincters. An abscess in this location may not be externally visible or palpable in the perianal tissues. The pain of an abscess is present but the diagnosis will be confirmed only on digital anorectal examination, where the fluctuant mass is easily palpable. The least common abscess in this area is in the *supralevator* location, and is more correctly identified as a peri*rectal* abscess as opposed to a peri*anal* abscess. Most clinicians would agree that if a supralevator abscess is diagnosed, they must look for an intra-abdominal or pelvic source. A supralevator abscess may be associated with appendicitis, diverticulitis, pelvic inflammatory disease, or other pelvic or abdominal disease.

Patients with a perianal abscess may develop an associated fever and often have a marked leukocytosis, depending on the severity of the infection. Once the diagnosis of perianal abscess is made, it is essential to proceed with adequate I&D treatment without delay. This is especially important in any patient who may be immunocompromised, is on steroids, or who has diabetes or any other debilitating comorbidity. The treatment of choice for a perianal abscess is clearly I&D—*not* antibiotic therapy. If adequate I&D of a perianal abscess is not performed, patients can rapidly develop severe infectious problems such as *necrotizing fasciitis*, which can become life-threatening, or *perineal sepsis*, which is a medical emergency identified with the classic triad of pain, fever, and inability to void.

Indications

Nearly every perianal abscess should be incised and drained. The only reason not to perform this procedure would be if spontaneous drainage of the abscess has occurred and if, in the judgment of the examining clinician, adequate drainage has resulted. These abscess cavities can have multiple loculations, and if spontaneous drainage has occurred, the abscess cavity must still be explored with a digital examination or hemostats to break down any loculated areas within the abscess.

Contraindications

Patients with underlying hematologic diseases may have perianal abscesses. The associated hematologic disease may include leukemia, granulocytopenia, and lymphoma. The infecting organisms seen with this type of perianal abscess may be quite different from those seen with an otherwise uncomplicated perianal abscess. In those patients with an associated hematologic disorder and a perianal abscess—for example, with leukemia under poor control—conservative treatment with antibiotics combined with local radiation therapy may be advised. Other clinicians recommend aggressive surgical management of perianal abscess in patients with hematologic disorders, but clearly this is never to be attempted in the outpatient setting.

Equipment

A minor surgical instrument setup includes the following:

- Local anesthesia (2% lidocaine with epinephrine)
- 25- to 30-gauge, 1½-inch needle with 5-mL syringe
- Hemostats
- No. 11 blade
- 4 × 4 gauzes
- Penrose drain or iodoform gauze
- Suction may be needed if the abscess is large
- Surgical electrocautery unit is often helpful to achieve hemostasis at the I&D site of the infected and hyperemic tissue
- Ives slotted anoscope or various-sized Hill-Ferguson rectal retractors to facilitate visualization (available from most medical supply companies)

Preprocedure Patient Preparation

Advise the patient that, in all likelihood, rather dramatic pain relief will follow the procedure. Further advise the patient that, unless adequate I&D is accomplished, further tissue damage may result. Clearly, the most effective way to afford adequate pain relief is to drain the abscess. Recurrence, bleeding, and pain are all possible. Further work-up may also be necessary to rule out other disease processes, such as inflammatory bowel, once the infection is controlled.

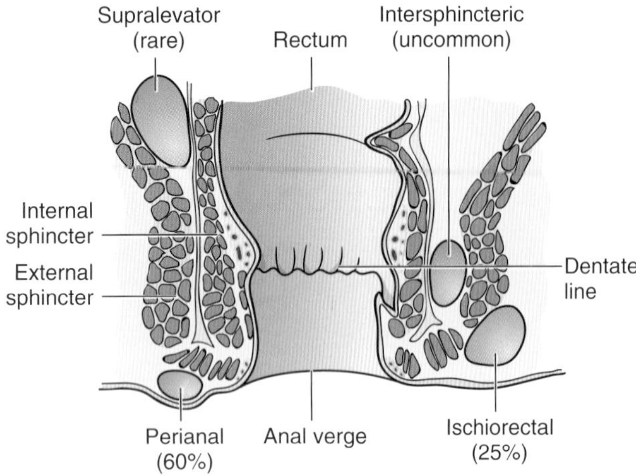

Figure 107-1 Anatomic locations of anorectal abscesses.

Technique

Patients with a perianal abscess have a clear need for prompt pain relief. Local anesthesia may be used in an attempt to anesthetize the skin at the intended I&D site, but this is often only marginally effective. The infected perianal tissues usually do not respond well to local anesthetic agents because of the highly acid environment. Either spinal or general anesthesia for this outpatient procedure may be required, depending primarily on the size of the abscess and on the specific patient circumstances. Before the actual I&D of the abscess cavity, it is appropriate, if not essential, to perform anoscopy to look for an internal opening of a fistula tract feeding the abscess cavity. The advantage of doing the anoscopy before I&D of the abscess is that, with gentle pressure on the abscess cavity, the physician may see pus expressed from an internal opening at the level of the dentate line. This then clearly establishes the diagnosis of an associated anal fistula. Textbooks of colon and rectal surgery vary widely on the incidence of associated fistula with perianal abscess, but most experts would agree that it is at least in the range of 50%.

1. Anesthetize the area using 2% lidocaine with epinephrine and a 27- or 30-gauge needle.
2. Make an incision over the fluctuant area near the anal canal in a plane radial to the circumference of the anal canal. The advantage of this type of incision is that it can be extended easily to perform anal fistulotomy if a fistula is present and if fistulotomy is indicated. Another option is to remove an ellipse of tissue such that you can easily place a gloved examining finger into the abscess cavity (if it is that large) to break down any loculations and to place drains. At this time, express all of the purulence. Cultures may be obtained at this time in the more complicated cases, if desired.
3. Irrigate the abscess cavity and, if deemed necessary, place a Penrose drain loosely into the abscess cavity and suture it at the skin edge level. A Penrose drain will not adhere to surrounding tissue, which makes its subsequent removal generally painless. (Alternatively, pack small wounds with ¼- or ½-inch iodoform gauze.)
4. Remove the Penrose drain within 24 to 48 hours. With a small perianal abscess, in the office setting, the iodoform gauze is removed in 10 to 14 days. Earlier removal may lead to recurrence of the abscess.
5. In selected patients with a well-defined, fluctuant perianal abscess, drainage can be accomplished without anesthesia by placing a large-bore, 16-gauge needle (attached to suction or a large syringe) into the abscess (Fig. 107-2). This can be an effective *temporizing* measure to afford dramatic and prompt pain relief if definitive surgical treatment is not readily available. The disadvantage of this needle suction technique is that evaluation for an associated anal fistula becomes more difficult.
6. Postoperative antibiotics are generally not required. Consider them in immunocompromised patients or if there is extensive cellulitis or sepsis.

Complications

Recurrence is the most common complication after I&D of a perianal abscess. The most common cause of recurrence is an unrecognized, and therefore untreated, associated fistula. The patient with a recurrent perianal abscess must be thoroughly evaluated for the presence of an associated anal fistula. Another possible cause of recurrent perianal abscess is inflammatory bowel disease, most commonly Crohn's disease. Postprocedure bleeding and excess pain are rare complications.

Postprocedure Patient Education

After an adequate drainage procedure of a perianal abscess, advise the patient to take sitz baths for 10 to 15 minutes two to four times a day. Spend some time with the patient and his or her family to reinforce the fact that the infected wound must heal from the inside out. Most patients understand that they must keep the wound from closing with either sitz baths or showering along with the gauze packing. Explain that daily wound irrigations may be needed (if gauze is not used) to prevent the skin edges from closing prematurely before the abscess cavity has resolved. This will help to avoid a secondary infection and a recurrent abscess. These instructions usually serve as adequate motivation to follow the recommended postprocedure care.

CPT/Billing Codes

10060 Incision and drainage of one abscess, skin, and subcutaneous structures
10061 Incision and drainage of multiple abscesses, or complex (e.g., placement of drain, packing)
10180 Incision and drainage, complex, postoperative wound infection
45005 Incision and drainage, submucosal rectal abscess
45020 Incision and drainage of deep supralevator, pelvirectal, or retrorectal abscess
46040 Incision and drainage of ischiorectal and/or perirectal abscess

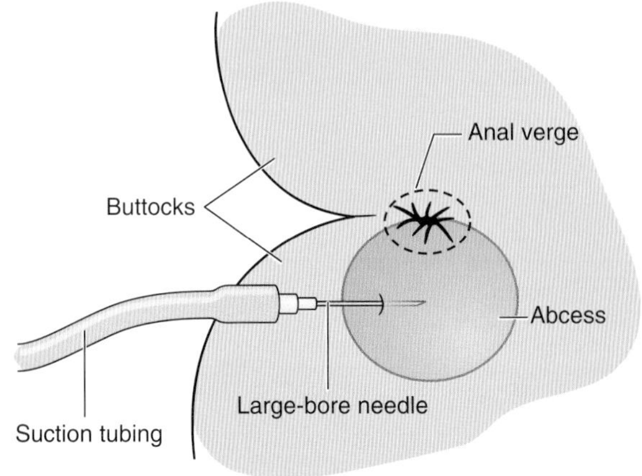

Figure 107-2 Needle (16 gauge or larger) and suction aspiration of a perianal abscess.

46045 Incision and drainage of intramural, intramuscular, or submucosal abscess, transanal under anesthesia
46050 Incision and drainage of superficial perianal abscess

ICD-9-CM Diagnostic Codes

566 Perirectal abscess
566 Perianal abscess
566 Ischiorectal abscess
566 Intersphincteric abscess

BIBLIOGRAPHY

Corman ML: Colon and Rectal Surgery, 5th ed. Philadelphia, Lippincott Williams & Wilkins, 2004.
Gordon P, Nivatvongs S: Principles and Practice of Surgery for the Colon, Rectum, and Anus, 3rd ed. St. Louis, Informa Health, 2006.
Mazier W, Levien D, Luchtefeld M, Senagore A (eds): Surgery of the Colon, Rectum, and Anus. Philadelphia, WB Saunders, 1995.
Pfenninger JL, Zainea G: Common anorectal conditions: Part I. Symptoms and complaints. Am Fam Physician 63:2391–2398, 2001.
Pfenninger JL, Zainea G: Common anorectal conditions: Part II. Lesions. Am Fam Physician 64:77–88, 2001.

CHAPTER 108

Removal of Perianal Skin Tags (External Hemorrhoidal Skin Tags)

James A. Surrell

Perianal skin tags represent a stretching and enlargement of the normal perianal skin (Fig. 108-1). As such, they are not true external hemorrhoids. Perianal skin tags are believed to occur as a result of large external hemorrhoids that have receded. A previously thrombosed external hemorrhoid may also leave redundant skin after resolving. Patients most often seek treatment for them when they begin to interfere with anal hygiene. It is important to note that perianal skin tags do not cause pain, bleeding, or itching. If these symptoms are present, then another source must be sought as the cause of these symptoms.

Indications

- Large perianal skin tags limiting anal hygiene
- Perianal skin tags that annoy the patient or are symptomatic (e.g., pruritus)

NOTE: The only time anal skin tags cause itching is when the patient is doing excessive perianal cleansing, thereby irritating the skin tag and the surrounding perianal tissues.

Generally, a conservative approach to the management of perianal skin tags is recommended because the vast majority of these benign lesions are asymptomatic. If the patient is bothered by pruritus, try local measures first. (See patient education form available online at www.expertconsult.com.)

Contraindications

- If the patient with perianal skin tags complains of pain, bleeding, or itching, then another source for these symptoms must be sought. Skin tag excision will *not* relieve these symptoms. Even when the patient complains of pruritus "from the tag," be sure he or she is following proper hygiene practices noted in the aforementioned patient education handout because the tag itself may not be the cause of symptoms.
- If the perianal skin tags have a fleshy, edematous appearance, a diagnosis of anal Crohn's disease must be strongly considered. Nearly all patients with anal Crohn's disease will develop fleshy, edematous skin tags and have associated signs and symptoms of pain, discharge, bleeding, and atypical anal fissures (see Chapter 96, Anal Fissure and Lateral Sphincterotomy and Anal Fistula). Excision of perianal skin tags in Crohn's disease may lead to significant morbidity because of the creation of an indolent, nonhealing wound.

Equipment

- 2% lidocaine with epinephrine, 3 to 5 mL
- 25-gauge, 1½-inch to 30-gauge, ½-inch needle
- 4 × 4 gauze pads
- Hemostat, straight not curved
- Pickups
- No. 10 or no. 15 blade or sharp tissue scissors (alternatively, a radiofrequency/electrocautery unit)
- Monsel's solution (ferric subsulfate)
- Cautery unit should there be bleeding
- Absorbable suture in case of uncontrolled bleeding
- Lidocaine 5% ointment
- Feminine Peri-Pad

Because the perianal skin tags are external to the anal canal, no anal retractor is needed. Any standard surgical forceps are adequate to grasp the skin tag, which is usually removed with electrocautery. The electrocautery unit should have both coagulation and cutting capability. (See Chapter 30, Radiofrequency Surgery [Modern Electrosurgery], and Chapter 149, Loop Electrosurgical Excision Procedure for Treating Cervical Intraepithelial Neoplasia, for listings of suppliers of various modern electrosurgery units.) Alternatively, the lesion can be excised with sharp tissue scissors or a knife blade, but this will increase the likelihood of bleeding.

Preprocedure Patient Preparation

Most patients should be discouraged from having their perianal skin tags excised. Because perianal skin tags per se usually cause no significant symptoms, question the patient in depth about his or her reasons for wanting the skin tags excised. Advise the patient that there will be some mild to moderate "burning" postoperative pain at the site of the excision for up to 2 weeks, possibly more. Postoperative bleeding is usually negligible but can be a problem, and infection is rare because the cauterized operative site is usually left open. The chances for infection increase if the site is sutured (Vicryl, chromic).

Technique

1. Place the patient in the left lateral decubitus position on the procedure table.
2. Infiltrate the base of the skin tag with approximately 1 mL of local anesthetic (e.g., 2% lidocaine with epinephrine). To minimize discomfort, inject the anesthetic solution (at room

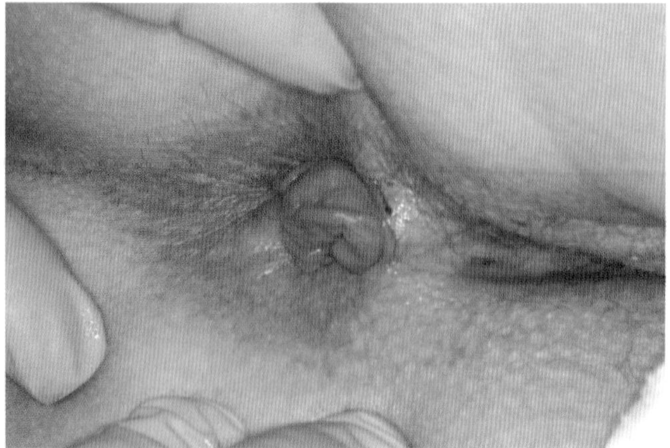

Figure 108-1 Large perianal tag.

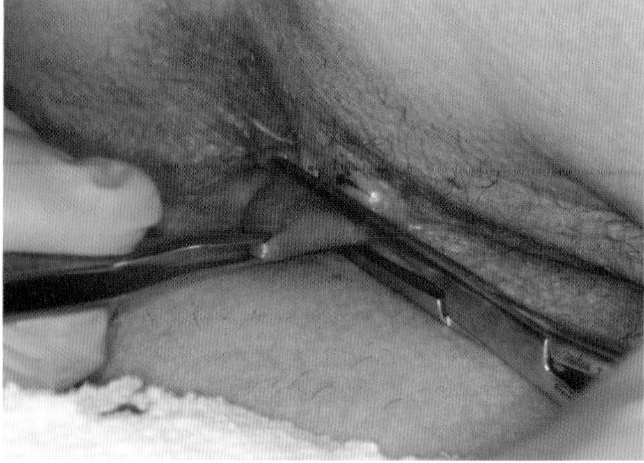

Figure 108-3 Clamping the base of tag for hemostasis.

temperature) very slowly at the base of the skin tag with a 25- or 30-gauge, ½-inch hypodermic needle. When performed properly, this injection technique affords minimal discomfort to the patient. Do not use too much volume because this will distort the area to be excised and may leave an excessively large wound. Alternatively, do a field block around the lesion to maintain undisturbed anatomy near the tag.

3. After approximately 1 minute, grasp the skin tag with a 4 × 4 gauze pad between the thumb and index finger and compress it to reduce the edema caused by infiltration of the local anesthetic. This also restores the skin tag to its "normal" anatomy so the site of excision can be identified properly.
4. Grasp the skin tag with forceps (which will confirm that appropriate anesthesia has been induced) and hold it perpendicular to its base on the perianal skin. *Care must be taken not to put any undue tension on the skin tag* because this will also serve to "tent up" and broaden the base of the skin tag and create an excision site that is much larger than needed.
5. Excise the skin tag, using the electrocautery unit in the cutting or blend mode. The site of excision should be approximately 3 mm above the normal perianal tissues because there will be electrocautery tissue destruction below the site of excision. If the skin tag is held taut or excised right at the level of the perianal skin, the resulting wound defect and patient discomfort will be greater than needed (Fig. 108-2).
6. Cauterize any residual small bleeding sites. No more than three perianal skin tags are recommended to be excised during any one procedure.

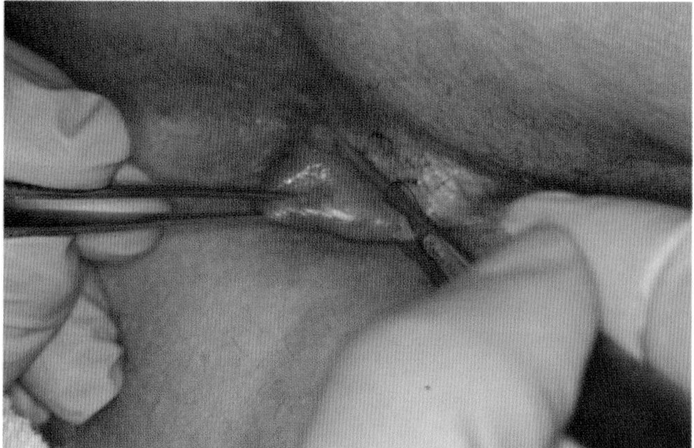

Figure 108-4 Scalpel excision of tag.

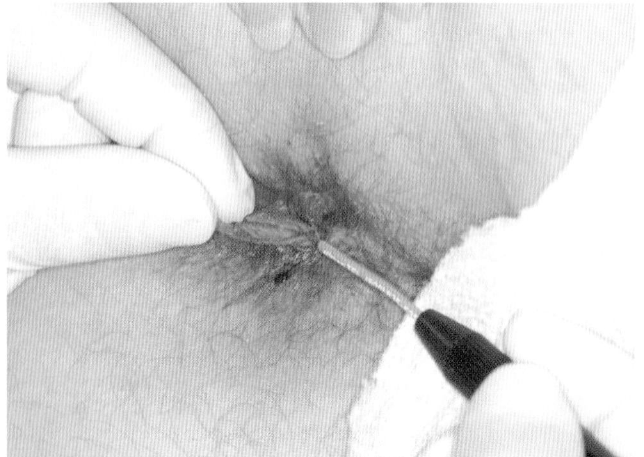

Figure 108-2 Removing perianal tag using cutting electrosurgery.

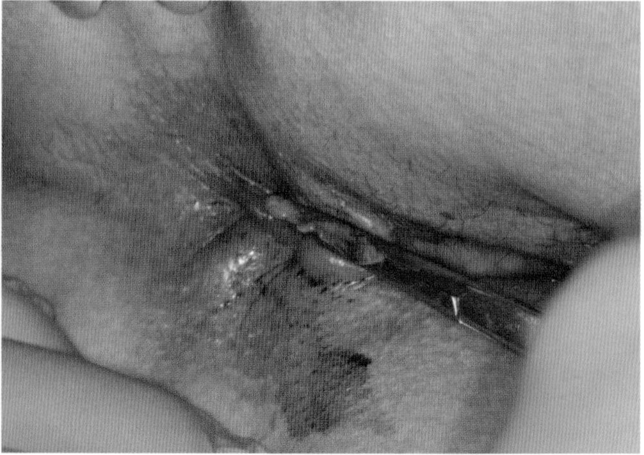

Figure 108-5 Appearance immediately after removing tag.

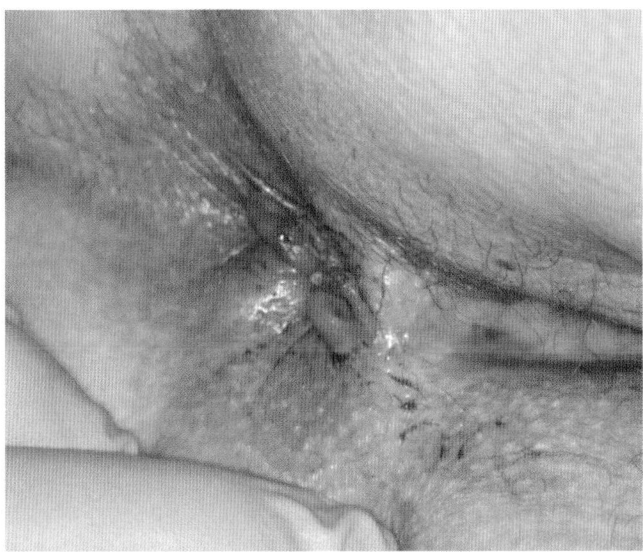

Figure 108-6 Final result. No sutures are used for closure.

7. Leave the site of excision open because suture closure contributes to an increase in postoperative pain and a greater likelihood of perianal abscess.
8. For larger tags, apply a straight hemostat at the base of the lesion, being careful not to grasp too much tissue. Leave it in place several minutes to control potential bleeding. Shave off the excess tissue using desired method. Remove clamp (Figs. 108-3 to 108-6).
9. Control bleeding.
10. Apply antibiotic ointment to soothe the area and prevent it from drying/sticking to clothing.
11. Give the patient a Peri-Pad to prevent blood from reaching clothing.
12. It is probably best to excise only one tag at a time if the procedure is being done in the office. This limits pain and the potential for bleeding, and decreases tension on the healing wound. This is especially true with larger-based lesions.

COMPLICATIONS

- A perianal abscess can develop at the site of excision of a skin tag, although this is uncommon and occurs less than 1% of the time. If an abscess does occur, appropriate incision and drainage will be necessary.
- If the skin tag excision site is very close to the anal verge, a chronic fissure may develop, although this is also very uncommon. Should a fissure develop and persist, lateral internal sphincterotomy would be recommended.
- Perianal cellulitis can rarely occur. Should this be diagnosed, appropriate antibiotic therapy should be instituted. Topical antibiotics can be used with the lidocaine ointment to alleviate this potential.
- Bleeding or hematoma may occur within the first 24 hours after the procedure. Usually, applying ice or having the patient sit on a rolled-up washcloth provides enough pressure to tamponade a bleeder. Occasionally, a suture(s) may be required.

Excision of skin tags should not alter anal continence because of the lack of involvement of this procedure with the anal sphincters.

POSTPROCEDURE PATIENT EDUCATION

Wash the area gently three to four times a day and after defecation with mild soap and water. Lidocaine ointment 5% or an antibiotic ointment may be used to decrease discomfort. Prescribe a nonconstipating pain medication (e.g., ibuprofen). Further advise the patient to follow a high-fiber diet with commercial fiber supplements and four to six glasses of water per day. Time off from work is usually minimal and would range from 0 to 3 days, depending on the extent of excision. Total healing time may take up to 6 weeks for complete new skin coverage. Perianal discomfort is usually present for 1 week or less.

PATIENT EDUCATION GUIDES

See patient education form online at www.expertconsult.com.

CPT/BILLING CODE

46230 Excision of perianal skin tag

ICD-9-CM DIAGNOSTIC CODE

4559 Hemorrhoidal tag

BIBLIOGRAPHY

Corman ML: Colon and Rectal Surgery, 5th ed. Philadelphia, Lippincott Williams & Wilkins, 2004.

Gordon P, Nivatvongs S: Principles and Practice of Surgery for the Colon, Rectum, and Anus. St. Louis, Quality Medical, 1992.

Mazier W, Levien D, Luchtefeld M, Senagore A: Surgery of the Colon, Rectum, and Anus. Philadelphia, WB Saunders, 1995.

Pfenninger JL, Zainea GC: Common anorectal conditions: Part I. Symptoms and complaints. Am Fam Physician 63:2391–2398, 2001.

Pfenninger JL, Zainea GC: Common anorectal conditions: Part II. Lesions. Am Fam Physician 64:77–78, 2001.

Tuggy M, Garcia J: Procedures Consult. Available at www.proceduresconsult.com.

CHAPTER 109

Pilonidal Cyst and Abscess: Current Management

James A. Surrell

A *pilonidal cyst* or *abscess* is located in the gluteal crease, usually within 5 to 10 cm of the anal verge. This lesion was originally described in the mid-1800s, and there has been considerable debate in the literature over whether it is an acquired or a congenital lesion. Most experts now believe that this is an acquired lesion resulting from penetration of the skin at this level from shafts of hair. A pilonidal sinus frequently contains multiple hairs that are microscopically noted to be tapered at both ends like shed hairs. The existence of hair follicles in the wall of the pilonidal sinus tract has never been demonstrated conclusively. Pilonidal sinus and abscess is a disease of the younger population, and 75% of cases are seen in males. Most patients develop symptoms of pilonidal disease between the ages of 20 and 25 years. A typical patient develops an abscess or experiences recurrent infection and drainage at the base of the spine. The disease is characterized by the development of multiple sinus tracts in this location.

Examination of the patient with suspected pilonidal disease generally reveals an area of inflammation in the midline of the gluteal crease, with one or more sinus openings (Fig. 109-1). The openings may be slightly off the midline. Careful inspection of this site often reveals loose hairs projecting from the sinus openings. Note that these hairs are *not* growing in the pilonidal sinus cavity, but rather are shed loose hairs that have migrated to this dependent site in the gluteal crease. If the pilonidal sinus has an associated abscess, the patient will complain of pain and the examiner may note swelling and erythema at this site. Spontaneous and ongoing drainage is the common indicator, however, and if an abscess is present it is usually small. As a general guideline, if the patient gives a history of recurrent infection at the base of the spine, this in itself is almost diagnostic of a pilonidal sinus disease. Some difficulty in diagnosis may occur if the pilonidal sinus is located in the more caudal position closer to the anal canal. This position raises the possibility of an anal fistula as the cause of the infection. If, however, hairs are found in the lesion, this offers convincing confirmatory evidence that the physician is dealing with a pilonidal sinus or abscess.

Indications

Surgical treatment should be performed for the following:

- Acute abscess formation in the superior gluteal crease area (simple incision and drainage [I&D] may be adequate but recurrences are common).
- Patients with a history of recurrent infections and drainage at the base of the spine are better treated with complete excision of the area. (Antibiotic therapy should be considered only as temporizing and palliative because recurrence will be the rule until adequate I&D or excision is accomplished.)

Contraindications

- Patient with a paucity of symptoms, such as only minimal drainage with little or no discomfort or inflammation occurring perhaps only once or twice per year
- History of bleeding disorder

Equipment

- Local anesthesia.
- No special equipment is necessary to perform a simple I&D; a no. 11 blade is adequate.
- Only a minor surgical setup is required for excision plus a dermal curette.

Preprocedure Patient Preparation

The procedure of choice is I&D; for recurrent abscesses or persistent draining, excision of the involved area is needed. The wound is left open to heal by secondary intention. With this technique the patient needs to be informed of a prolonged healing time. The wounds are not at all disabling and they can be expected to close, but it takes 8 to 12 weeks. Other options for treatment of pilonidal disease must be reviewed to include excision with primary closure, as well as using a skin flap or other plastic procedures for more extensive and complex involvement.

Technique

A simple I&D may be all that is needed for a small abscess or first-time presentation. For recurrent disease, perform an elliptical incision at the site of the pilonidal disease to include the obvious sinus tract(s) (Fig. 109-2). The lateral and deep margins should extend to noninfected tissue that appears healthy. This procedure can be performed under local anesthesia (with or without intravenous sedation) or under general anesthesia in the operating room. Because of the proximity of the infected site, spinal anesthesia is *not* recommended. Thoroughly inspect the wound during the procedure, and curette all chronically infected granulation tissue so that the remaining wound defect is lined with healthy-appearing tissue with no obvious remaining sinus tracts. If the resultant wound defect is not too deep, depending on the extent of the disease and the body habitus of the patient, consider marsupialization of the wound by tacking the skin edges to the base of the wound with an absorbable running simple suture (Fig. 109-3) to help prevent premature secondary wound closure. Total procedure time is generally 30 minutes or less.

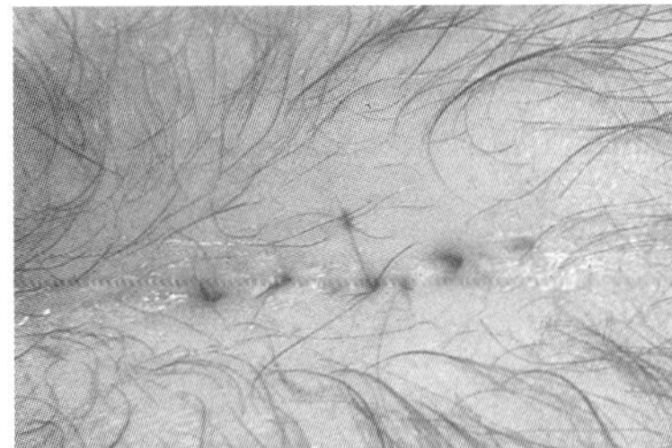

Figure 109-1 Multiple (six) pilonidal sinus openings in the natal cleft. (From Thomson J: Disorders of the anus and anal canal. In Misiewicz JJ, Bartram CI, Cotton PB, et al [eds]: Slide Atlas of Gastroenterology. London, Gower Medical, 1986.)

Complications

Clearly, the most common complication of surgery for pilonidal disease is *recurrence*. The results are variable, but most physicians report that the open technique has less of a recurrence rate than the closed technique. The obvious disadvantage to the open technique is the prolonged healing time, but these wounds generally do not afford significant morbidity to the patient during this longer healing process. With the open technique, *bleeding, excessive pain*, and *infection* are rare. Two randomized trials have compared a surgical "flap" procedure with primary closure. Both studies found the flap procedure to be superior in terms of pain, healing, complications, and return to work, but these surgical procedures are more extensive and should be performed only by an experienced surgeon. The flap procedure may be the best option for persistently recurrent pilonidal disease.

Postprocedure Patient Education

If the procedure is performed with the pilonidal disease excised and the wound left open, instruct the patient on proper wound management. An open wound should be cleansed several times daily with soap and water, either by showering or other irrigation.

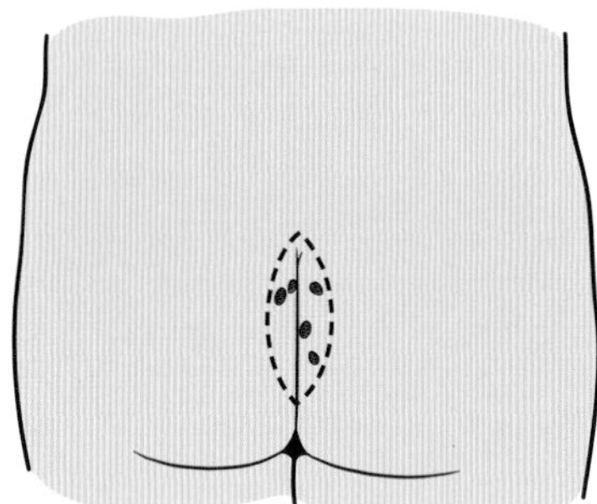

Figure 109-2 Area of elliptical excision for pilonidal sinus.

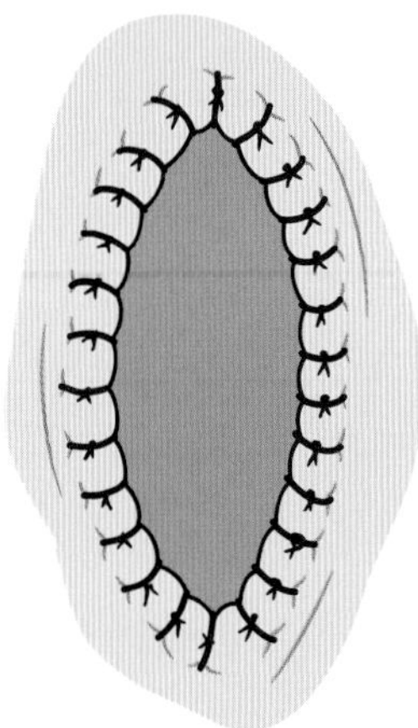

Figure 109-3 Marsupialization after excision of pilonidal sinus, closed with interrupted absorbable sutures.

During the early stages of wound healing, the wound is packed with moistened gauze sponges changed twice daily. During the early phases of postprocedure recovery, examine the patient on a weekly basis to assess adequate progress. At this time, if hair regrowth is occurring, wound edges may be shaved. Every effort to prevent loose hairs from entering the healing wound should be made. Instruct the patient on the concept of the wound's healing from the inside out so that premature skin bridging does not occur before the entire cavity is obliterated. Typical time off from work is approximately 1 week.

CPT/Billing Codes

10080 Incision and drainage of pilonidal cyst, simple
10081 Incision and drainage of pilonidal cyst, complicated
11770 Excision of pilonidal cyst or sinus, simple
11771 Excision of pilonidal cyst or sinus, extensive
11772 Excision of pilonidal cyst or sinus, complicated

ICD-9-CM Diagnostic Codes

685.0 Pilonidal cyst with abscess
685.1 Pilonidal cyst, without mention of abscess

Bibliography

Corman ML: Colon and Rectal Surgery. Philadelphia, Lippincott Williams & Wilkins, 2004.

Gordon P, Nivatvongs S: Principles and Practice of Surgery for the Colon, Rectum, and Anus, 3rd ed. St. Louis, Informa Health, 2006.

Mazier W, Levien D, Luchtefeld M, Senagore A: Surgery of the Colon, Rectum, and Anus. Philadelphia, WB Saunders, 1995.

SECTION 7

Urinary System Procedures

Section Editor: JAMIE BROOMFIELD

CHAPTER 110

Bladder Catheterization (and Urethral Dilation)

Robert E. James • Grant C. Fowler

Bladder catheterization may be performed for diagnostic or therapeutic indications (or both). This procedure is the most common retrograde manipulation performed in the urinary tract. Familiarity with the anatomy of the urethra and the available catheters will increase the ease and success of this procedure. Like all procedures in urology, this should be performed in a gentle fashion; instruments need not be forced. This is considered by patients to be among the five most painful emergency procedures, so, when possible, anesthetic jelly should be used. Indications and contraindications for infants and children are basically the same as for adults.

In the adult male patient, there are two points where obstruction is commonly encountered when passing a catheter. The first is at the point of acute upward angulation located between the bulbous and the membranous urethra. The second is at the bladder neck, where a bladder neck stenosis or an enlarged median lobe of the prostate gland may be present (Fig. 110-1). In younger male patients, urethral folds or valves may resist the insertion of a catheter.

In the female patient, the urethra is much shorter, averaging only 2 inches in an adult. The angle between the urethra and the bladder neck increases with age. Consequently, in the older patient, the urethra is normally directed toward the sacrum, whereas in the younger patient it is angled toward the umbilicus. Keeping these urethral angles in mind will improve the clinician's technique, thereby increasing patient comfort and facilitating passage of the catheter. Catheter size is measured in French units. As the number increases, the size increases (i.e., a 16-Fr catheter is larger than a 12-Fr catheter). One "French unit" is approximately 0.33 mm.

Indications

Short-Term Catheterization

- Acute urinary retention
- Collection of uncontaminated urine specimen for analysis, culture, and sensitivity (especially for female patients)
- Diagnostic studies of the lower urinary tract (e.g., cystogram, voiding cystourethrogram, urodynamics)
- Monitoring of urinary output
- Measurement of postvoid residual urine volume
- Irrigation of the bladder or instillation of medication
- Surgery on the urinary tract or adjacent structures
- Bladder drainage during and after surgical procedures requiring anesthetics
- Intermittent (in and out) catheterization for neurogenic bladder

Long-Term Catheterization

- Chronic urinary retention
- Neurogenic bladder in patient with inability to intermittently self-catheterize
- Incontinence with complicating skin breakdown
- As a comfort measure for terminally ill or severely disabled patient with incontinence

NOTE: A Cochrane review found that patients requiring catheterization for up to 14 days had less discomfort, bacteriuria, and need for recatheterization when suprapubic catheters were used compared with urethral catheters. Similarly, in a recent meta-analysis of patients having abdominal surgery, suprapubic catheters were found to cause less bacteriuria and discomfort and were preferred by patients (see Chapter 113, Suprapubic Catheter Insertion and/or Change).

Contraindications

- Known or suspected urethral disruption resulting from pelvic trauma (be suspicious if there is blood at the urethral meatus, a perineal hematoma, or a high-riding prostate)
- Recent reconstructive surgery of the urethra or bladder neck *(relative contraindication, but should consult urology)*
- Known urinary tract obstruction, such as a urethral stricture *(relative contraindication, may be able to dilate)*
- A combative or uncooperative patient *(relative contraindication;* see Chapter 2, Procedural Sedation and Analgesia)
- An acute infection of the prostate and/or urethra *(relative contraindication)*

Equipment

- Urethral catheters
  - *Robinson catheter:* A straight, rounded-tip catheter used for short-term catheterization; one version is the red rubber catheter. Low-friction, hydrophilic-coated catheters have been found to increase patient satisfaction and decrease urinary tract infection and hematuria in patients who practice clean, intermittent self-catheterization.
  - *Foley catheter:* A straight, self-retaining catheter that may have two or three lumina. While urine flows through the main, large lumen, and the secondary, smaller lumen is connected to a port used to inflate the retaining balloon (Fig. 110-2A), a Foley with a third lumen may be selected if irrigation will be necessary, such as for ongoing hematuria. A 16- to 18-Fr Foley catheter may be used for adults or adolescents (smaller sizes are used for infants and children) who require either a temporary or a chronic indwelling catheter. Foley catheters have short- or long-nose tips. Silicone or silicone-coated versions tend to be preferred over rubber catheters for long-term use because they produce less tissue reaction, have less encrustation, and have a larger lumen. By design, the retaining balloons can be overinflated, if necessary, to twice their stated capacity.

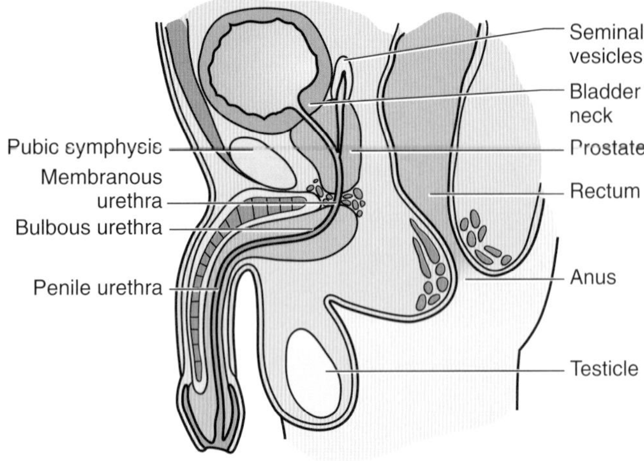

Figure 110-1 Male urethral anatomy.

- *Coudé catheter:* This catheter is similar to a Foley catheter with some slight variations: the terminal 2 inches are curved upward (*coudé* is the French word for "elbow"; Fig. 110-2B) and there is a small ball on the tip. This catheter is used in adult men for whom a Robinson or Foley catheter cannot be inserted because of an enlarged median lobe of the prostate or an elevated bladder neck. Some clinicians advocate using a coudé catheter in all men older than 50 years of age. Coudé catheters are available with or without a self-retaining balloon. A 16- to 18-Fr catheter is normally used.
- *Filiforms and followers:* Filiforms are very thin, very pliable solid catheters that range in size from 1 to 6 Fr and are used to dilate a male urethral stricture. They may be straight or pig-tailed, or have a coudé tip, but they all have a female screw tip on the opposite end for attachment of followers. Followers are larger in diameter (12 to 30 Fr), have a male screw tip to attach to the filiforms, and are usually hollow with an open end. (Avoid the solid or closed-end followers; it may be impossible to tell when the forward tip has reached the bladder, so significant damage can occur. With the hollow, open-ended followers, you can tell when you are in the bladder because urine starts to flow.) Both filiforms and followers have a smooth-coated surface and are made of plastic or have a woven fiber core.

NOTE: Silastic catheters are available for latex-sensitive patients. Although a Cochrane review found that silver alloy–impregnated catheters compared with standard catheters were associated with decreased rates of urinary tract infections, this is considered controversial and they are expensive.

- Lubricant: either a water-soluble lubricant (K-Y Jelly) or a lubricant with a local anesthetic (2% lidocaine jelly) may be used. When available, the latter is preferred; 10 mL is sufficient for adult and adolescent female patients and 10 to 20 mL for adult and adolescent male patients, with smaller amounts for infants and children.
- Sterile towels and gloves
- Sterile cotton-tipped applicators
- Antiseptic solution
- Closed urinary drainage system (bedside overnight drainage bag, leg bag, or abdominal drainage system [belly bag])

Preprocedure Patient Preparation

The specific indications for catheterization, as well as the risks, benefits, alternatives, and technique, should be reviewed with the patient, parent, or caregiver. Long-term catheter care should be discussed if the catheter is to remain in place. (See the sample patient education form available online at www.expertconsult.com.) Informed consent is not always necessary for catheterization; however, at least verbal consent should be obtained and documented in the chart. Self-catheterization should be taught to the patient (or parent or caregiver) with the neurogenic bladder. Adequate lubrication and sufficient frequency are more important than sterile conditions if the patient is going to intermittently self-catheterize. If dilation is necessary, the patient should also understand the risks, benefits, alternatives, and technique. Informed consent should be obtained. It may be comforting to reassure the patient that everything possible will be done to maintain his or her modesty.

Technique

Bladder Catheterization

1. The *female patient* is placed in the dorsal lithotomy or the supine position with the legs abducted (i.e., frog-legged position). The *male patient* is placed in the supine position; the legs may be either abducted slightly or straight. The clinician should observe universal blood and body fluid precautions.
2. Identify the urethral meatus. For men, the penis should be grasped by the clinician's nondominant hand and positioned pointing toward the umbilicus. Although the meatus should be easily identified in the circumcised man, gentle retraction of the foreskin (prepuce) may be necessary to identify the meatus in the

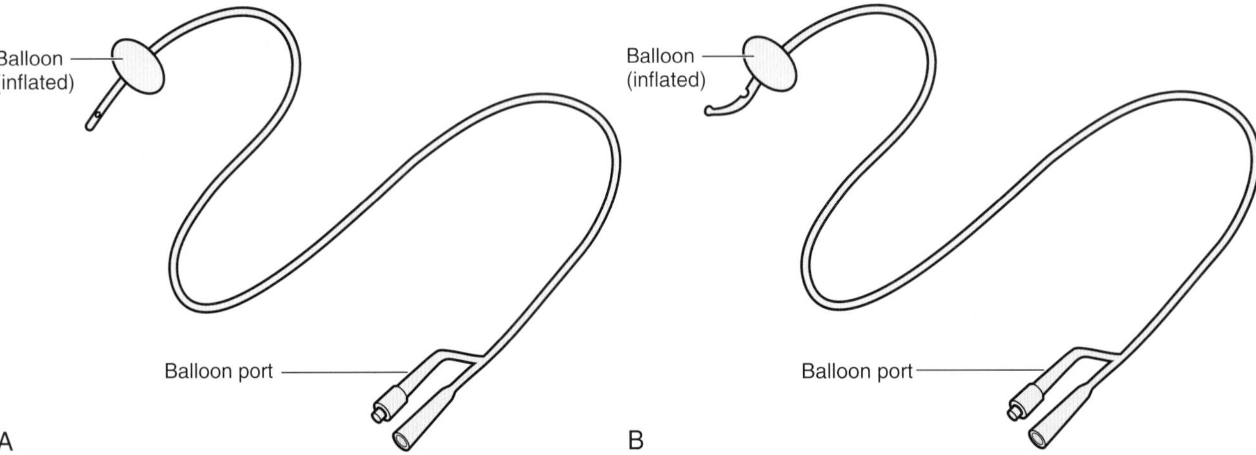

Figure 110-2 **A,** Foley catheter with balloon inflated. **B,** Coudé catheter with balloon inflated.

uncircumcised man. Lateral and outward traction on the labia by the clinician's nondominant hand may help identify the meatus in women. Applying downward pressure with the posterior bill of a vaginal speculum may also be helpful in women. In female infants or girls, hymenal folds may obscure the meatus, but again, lateral traction by the nondominant hand will usually help identify the meatus. If not, downward pressure with a cotton-tipped applicator placed over the introitus will usually improve visualization. Women who will be self-catheterizing can be taught to identify the meatus with a mirror. For repeat catheterizations in women, a finger inserted into the vagina can help guide the catheter.

3. Cleanse the urethral meatus and surrounding area with antiseptic solution, and isolate the genitalia with sterile drapes or towels. Maintain sterile technique throughout the remainder of the procedure.

NOTE: Bladder catheterization is considered by patients to be among the top five most painful emergency procedures. If possible, anesthetic jelly should be used.

4. Insert the lubricant into the urethra with a syringe. If anesthetic jelly is used, leave it in place for approximately 5 to 10 minutes (longer is better to maximize effect). Some manufacturers place the lubricant in a syringe with a smooth conical end that can be inserted into the urethra. Otherwise, draw it into a 10-mL syringe. Place the end of the syringe (*without a needle*) gently inside the urethral meatus and inject the jelly into the urethra. Less lubricant is needed for infants, children, and women because the urethra is shorter. An alternative to injecting anesthetic jelly into the female urethra is to place it on a sterile cotton-tipped applicator and insert it gently into the urethra. This method allows the clinician to also determine the angle of the urethra to follow for later insertion of the catheter. After injecting the jelly, the *male patient* should be asked to compress the mid-urethra between his index finger and thumb to prevent the jelly from leaving the urethra.

5. Insertion technique for male and female patients:
   - For *adult or adolescent female patients*, select a 16- or 18-Fr Foley or Robinson catheter (use appropriately sized pediatric feeding tubes in female newborns and infants; smaller Foley or Robinson catheters can be used in larger girls). Following the anticipated course of the urethra, pass the catheter into the bladder. Catheter placement is confirmed when urine is obtained, and this is usually after advancing about 3 inches in adults (less for infants and children). For a Foley catheter, the balloon may be inflated with 5 mL of normal saline or water. The catheter is then gently pulled outward until the balloon rests against the bladder neck.
   - For *adult or adolescent male patients younger than 50 years of age*, a 16- or 18-Fr Foley or Robinson catheter may be used (use appropriately sized pediatric feeding tubes in male newborns and infants, smaller Foley or Robinson catheters in larger boys). With the nondominant hand, hold the penis taut while directing it toward the umbilicus in order to straighten the urethra. With the dominant hand, pass the catheter into the bladder the full length, up to the junction of the Foley catheter and the inflation port for the balloon (Fig. 110-3), or until it reaches the hub of a Robinson catheter.

CAUTION: In male patients, if the Foley is not passed all the way to the port, the balloon may be inflated within the urethra, causing significant damage. The balloon is normally inflated with 5 mL of normal saline or water. If the balloon does not inflate easily, or if the patient experiences discomfort in the perineum or penis as the balloon is being inflated, you should suspect that the balloon is located within the urethra. In such a case, the balloon should then be deflated and the catheter reinserted.

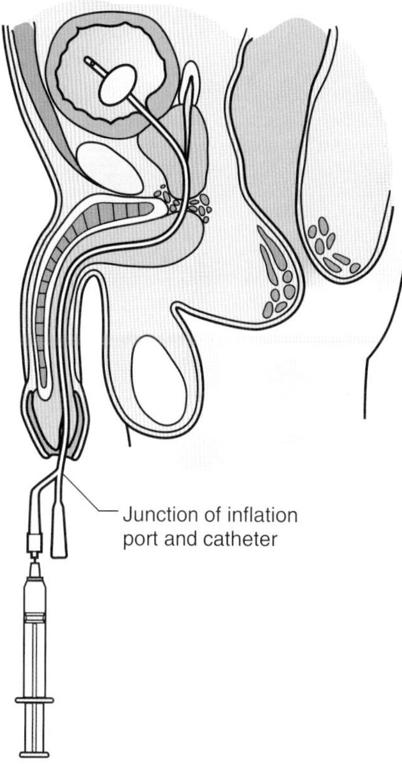

Figure 110-3 In the male patient, the Foley catheter is passed into the bladder until the junction of the catheter and inflation port for the balloon is met.

Once the balloon has been inflated, the catheter is then gently pulled outward until the balloon rests against the bladder neck.

   - For *male patients older than 50 years of age*, consider a coudé catheter. The curve at the tip of the catheter should be directed at the 12 o'clock (anterior) position. This will permit the catheter to glide over an enlarged median lobe of the prostate gland or an elevated bladder neck. If the catheter does not pass easily, it should be removed and the procedure repeated. Occasionally, the tip of the catheter will rotate as it is being inserted. If this occurs, the catheter will not pass through the prostatic urethra into the bladder. If you cannot pass a 16-Fr Foley or coudé catheter into the male urethra, there is usually a urethral stricture, bladder neck stenosis, or very large median lobe of the prostate gland. *Or, if the prostatic urethra has been previously resected*, the tip of the catheter may hang up at the widened outlet of the prostatic urethra. In any of these cases, you may consider using a 12-Fr Foley or coudé catheter. The catheter tip may be caught in a posterior urethral fold, right before it can enter the prostatic urethra. Upward pressure with three fingers from the nondominant hand on the perineum, between the scrotum and the rectum, may direct the catheter tip upward enough to enter the urogenital diaphragm on its way into the prostatic urethra. Alternatively, if the patient has an enlarged prostate, directing the catheter tip into the prostatic urethra with the dominant hand while a gloved finger from the other hand is in the rectum may also be helpful. If the smaller catheter does not pass after these maneuvers, either dilation with filiform and followers is necessary or a urology consultation should be sought.

6. Once in place, the catheter needs to be secured to the leg with tape or other means to prevent trauma to the urethra. If urine does not flow freely, the tip of the catheter may be obstructed by

lubricating jelly. Suprapubic pressure on a full bladder will usually flush the lubricant from the lumen. If the bladder is not full, gentle flushing from below with a 60-mL syringe full of sterile saline may open the lumen. It may take more than one syringe full in a dehydrated patient, but there should be return of fluid with gentle aspiration after injecting sterile saline. If not, remove the catheter from the urethra and repeat the procedure.

Difficult Catheterizations

WOMEN. Postmenopausal women with a narrow introitus, obese women, or women with a recessed or high-riding urethra may be very difficult to catheterize because the urethral meatus is difficult to visualize. In these cases, the following technique is usually successful. After preparing the patient as previously described, identify the urethral meatus with the tip of one of your index fingers. Then, slide a 16-Fr catheter along the index finger and into the urethra. If this cannot be accomplished, the patient may have a stenotic meatus. Applying the same technique, use a 12-Fr Foley or coudé catheter. If this attempt is unsuccessful, a urology consult is advised.

MEN. In uncircumcised male patients, to avoid the complication of a paraphimosis, always reduce the foreskin after catheter placement. In men with a severe phimosis, the foreskin cannot be retracted enough to see the urethral meatus. If the os of the foreskin is large enough to pass a catheter, you may be successful using the following technique. Fix the glans penis in its normal position with the meatus at the 6 o'clock position. Using a coudé catheter, rotate the catheter tip to the 6 o'clock (posterior) position. The tip of the catheter will be directed through the os of the foreskin in this position. Once the catheter has entered the urethra, it may be rotated until the tip is pointed up, to the 12 o'clock position. The catheter may then be advanced into the bladder. If the os of the foreskin will not permit the passage of a catheter, a dorsal slit of the foreskin may be performed (see Chapter 119, Dorsal Slit for Phimosis) and the catheter inserted. Otherwise, a suprapubic catheter may need to be inserted. To minimize the risk of stricture formation in male patients with a long-term indwelling catheter, the catheter should be secured to the anterior abdominal wall (i.e., abdominal drainage system or belly bag).

The optimal amount of time to leave a catheter in place for men with benign prostatic hyperplasia (BPH) is unknown. For men catheterized to relieve acute urinary retention due to BPH, up to 70% will have recurrent urinary retention within a week if the bladder is simply drained. However, the use of α-adrenergic blockers (e.g., alfuzosin, tamsulosin) for 3 days starting at the time of catheter insertion has been shown to increase the likelihood of a successful voiding trial without a catheter at 2 to 3 days after catheter removal. American Urological Association (AUA) guidelines recommend at least one attempted trial of voiding after catheter removal before considering surgical intervention. Prevention of acute urinary retention in BPH may be achieved by long-term treatment (4 to 6 years) with dutasteride, finasteride, or a combination of finasteride and doxazosin. The AUA guidelines recommend using only the 5-α-reductase inhibitors finasteride and dutasteride in men with demonstrable prostate enlargement by digital rectal examination.

Filiforms and Followers

After unsuccessful Foley and coudé catheterization attempts in male patients these methods are tried.

1. Reinstill anesthetic jelly into the urethra of the patient who has already been prepared and draped for prior catheterization attempts.
2. With the nondominant hand, hold the penis taut while directing it toward the umbilicus in order to straighten the urethra. With the dominant hand, grasp a filiform, dip it into anesthetic jelly, and gently insert it into the urethra. Advance the filiform into the urethra until resistance is met. The filiform should be rotated slightly while it is being advanced. Grasp a second filiform, dip it into anesthetic jelly, and advance it likewise into the urethra, while rotating it, until resistance is again met. Attempt to advance the first filiform further. If the first filiform will not advance, insert a third filiform after dipping it in anesthetic jelly, and advance it with slight rotation until it meets resistance. Attempt to advance the first and second filiforms, again. At this point, the filiform tips are either in a false lumen or the resistance is due to a fold or stricture. Inserting additional filiforms will either dilate the stricture or pass the fold or false lumen. Continue to insert filiforms, while each time attempting to advance the previously inserted filiforms, until one advances. Advance this filiform until only approximately 1 inch remains outside the penis. Remove all other filiforms except this one.
3. Lubricate a follower catheter and attach it to the inserted filiform. Use only a hollow, open-ended follower catheter so that you can tell when the bladder has been reached or entered. When the bladder has been reached by the follower, urine should flow through it spontaneously. Gently advance the follower into the bladder until only 1 or 2 inches remains outside the penis. (The tip of the filiform will curl up inside the bladder for the follower to advance.) If resistance is met, withdraw the tip connected to the filiform until it is an inch or more outside the penis. Select, lubricate, and attach a follower that is 1 or 2 Fr smaller than the previous one, and attempt to insert this gently into the bladder. Continue this process until a follower is able to be inserted into the bladder (i.e., up to the point where only 1 or 2 inches remains outside the penis). The urethra may then need to be dilated using the process described in the next step.
4. If the follower catheter is 16 or 18 Fr in diameter, remove it and insert a Foley catheter. If it is less than 16 Fr, the urethra must be dilated. Withdraw the tip connected to the filiform until it is 1 or 2 inches outside the penis. Select, lubricate, and attach a follower that is 1 or 2 Fr larger than the previous one, and attempt to gently insert this into the bladder. Continue this process until a 16- or 18-Fr follower can be inserted and then converted to a Foley.

Catheter Management

With indwelling catheters, many patients experience discomfort at the junction of the urethral meatus with the catheter. This may be mitigated by applying petroleum jelly or vitamin E ointment to the meatus daily. (Otherwise, daily meatal care should be avoided because it has been associated with increased risk of infection.) Chronic indwelling catheters are usually replaced every 6 weeks, or sooner if not draining properly. Robinson and non–self-retaining coudé catheters need to be secured to the penis. Clinicians should note that tape should never be applied circumferentially around the penis because it may cause ischemia. Instead, three thin strips of tape applied along the penis and attached to the catheter will usually prevent inadvertent removal.

Antibiotic Therapy

If a urinary tract infection is suspected or the patient has a history of mitral valve prolapse, valvular heart disease or replacement, a penile prosthesis, an artificial urinary sphincter, or a recent prosthesis such as a total knee or joint, a urine culture and sensitivity should be obtained and the patient placed on a broad-spectrum antibiotic for at least 3 days. If the patient is not allergic to fluoroquinolones, ciprofloxacin or levofloxacin is an appropriate choice. Alternatively, an intravenous dose of a cephalosporin, quinolone, or other antibiotic that covers skin and perineal flora may be given just before inserting the catheter.

Box 110-1. Centers for Disease Control and Prevention Guidelines for Prevention of Catheter-Associated Urinary Tract Infection

Category I: Strongly Recommended

Catheterize only when necessary.
Educate personnel in correct techniques of catheter insertion and care.
Emphasize handwashing.
Insert catheter using aseptic technique and sterile equipment.
Secure catheter properly.
Maintain closed sterile drainage.
Obtain urine specimens aseptically.
Maintain unobstructed urine flow.

Category II: Moderately Recommended

Periodically reeducate personnel in catheter care.
Use smallest suitable catheter bore.
Avoid irrigation unless needed to prevent or relieve obstruction.
Refrain from daily meatal care.
Do not change catheter at arbitrary intervals.

From Cravens DD, Zweig S: Urinary catheter management. Am Fam Physician 61:369–376, 2000. Information from Wong ES: Guideline for prevention of catheter-associated urinary tract infections. February 1, 1981. Available at http://aepo-xdv-www.epo.cdc.gov/wonder/prevguid/p0000416/p0000416.asp. Accessed June 20, 2008.

Complications

- Urinary tract infection (see Box 110-1 for prevention guidelines)
- Transient hematuria
- Creation of a false passage or perforation resulting from the use of a small catheter or excessive force, or the presence of a urethral stricture
- Conversion of a partial urethral tear into a complete tear in a trauma patient with urethral injury
- Urethral stricture
- Obstruction of flow
- Epididymitis, pyelonephritis, and urosepsis are often seen with prolonged catheterization. Increased mortality was found in nursing home patients with an indwelling catheter at 1 year, but that statistic is probably confounded by other factors such as protein-calorie malnutrition.

CPT/Billing Codes

51700 Bladder irrigation, simple, lavage and/or instillation
51701 Insertion of non-indwelling bladder catheter (e.g., straight catheterization for residual urine)
51702 Insertion of temporary indwelling bladder catheter; simple (e.g., Foley)
51703 Insertion of temporary indwelling bladder catheter; complicated (e.g., altered anatomy, fractured catheter/balloon)
53620 Dilation of urethral stricture by passage of filiform and follower, male; initial

ICD-9-CM Diagnostic Codes

344.61 Neurogenic bladder, with cauda equina syndrome
596.0 Bladder neck obstruction, acquired
596.54 Neurogenic bladder, NOS
598.1 Urethral stricture, caused by trauma
598.9 Urethral stricture, unspecified
599.60 Urinary obstruction, unspecified
600.0 Prostatism, hypertrophy (benign) of prostate
600.91 Hyperplasia of prostate, unspecified, with urinary obstruction
602.8 Prostatic stricture
605 Phimosis
625.6 Stress urinary incontinence, female
753.6 Bladder neck obstruction, congenital
788.20 Urinary retention or stasis, unspecified
788.30 Urinary incontinence, unspecified
788.32 Stress urinary incontinence, male

Patient Education Guides

See the sample patient education form available online at www.expertcosult.com.

Suppliers

(See contact information online at www.expertconsult.com.)

General
Bard Medical
Cook Medical
Catheters and closed drainage systems
Rusch, Inc. (Teleflex Medical)

Online Resource

Urinary Catheters. University of Maryland Medical Center. Available at www.umm.edu/ency/article/003981.htm.

Bibliography

Brosnahan J, Jull A, Tracy C: Types of urethral catheters for management of short-term voiding problems in hospitalised adults. Cochrane Database Syst Rev 1:CD004013, 2004.

Cravens DD, Zweig S: Urinary catheter management. Am Fam Physician 61:369–376, 2000.

McPhail MJ, Abu-Hilal M, Johnson CD: A meta-analysis comparing suprapubic and transurethral catheterization for bladder drainage after abdominal surgery. Br J Surg 93:1038–1044, 2006.

Moore KN, Kelm M, Sinclair O, Cadrain G: Bacteriuria in intermittent catheterization users: The effect of sterile versus clean reused catheters. Rehabil Nurs 18:306–309, 1993.

Niel-Weise BS, van den Broek PJ: Urinary catheter policies for short-term bladder drainage in adults. Cochrane Database Syst Rev 3:CD004203, 2005.

Selius BA, Subedi R: Urinary retention in adults: Diagnosis and initial management. Am Fam Physician 77:643–650, 2008.

Stokes S III, Ray PS, Meer J: Urethral catheterization. In Reichman EF, Simon RR (eds): Emergency Medicine Procedures. New York, McGraw-Hill, 2004, pp 1117–1127.

Tuggy M, Garcia J: Procedures Consult. Available at www.proceduresconsult.com.

Wong ES: Guideline for prevention of catheter-associated urinary tract infections. February 1, 1981. Available at http://aepo-xdv-www.epo.cdc.gov/wonder/prevguid/p0000416/p0000416.asp. Accessed June 20, 2008.

CHAPTER 111

DIAGNOSTIC CYSTOURETHROSCOPY

Grant C. Fowler

The construction of the cystoscope has progressed from the original tube-and-candle, first described in the early 1800s, to the flexible fiberoptic cystoscope available today. The standard rigid cystourethroscope is composed of three components: the telescope, the sheath, and the bridge. (Rigid urethroscopes are also available, designed exclusively for evaluation of the urethra, and are a modification of the cystoscope.) Once the sheath is in place, the telescope can be removed and changed as needed for different lenses to view different aspects of the bladder. Various instruments useful for procedures (e.g., biopsy, cautery, injection), both rigid and flexible, can also be inserted.

Unlike the rigid cystoscope, the flexible cystoscope combines the optical systems and irrigation/working channel into a single unit. The flexible cystoscope also has a smaller diameter and a tip that can be deflected as much as 290 degrees in a single plane; it can be used without a working sheath, and is generally more comfortable for the patient. The patient can be in the recumbent position as opposed to the dorsal lithotomy position. This makes it ideal for use in the office or outpatient setting. However, the image from a flexible cystoscope is not as clear as that obtained with a rigid cystoscope, and because the diameter of the flexible cystoscope is smaller, operative and diagnostic procedures are limited by the decreased capacities of the irrigating and working channels. Because there is no sheath, the flexible cystoscope has to be removed completely to change the lens, and reinserted to assess residual urine and to reevacuate the irrigant. Therefore, the flexible cystoscope is used more commonly in the office setting for routine diagnostic viewing of the bladder and urethra (hematuria or tumor surveillance, double-J stent retrieval) as opposed to operative procedures. That said, either type of cystoscope, rigid or flexible, can be useful in the diagnosis of various conditions ranging from urinary incontinence to pain syndromes.

EDITOR'S NOTE: It might be helpful to review Chapter 110, Bladder Catheterization (and Urethral Dilation), along with this chapter.

INDICATIONS

- Urethral stricture or diverticulum on radiograph (for diagnostic or therapeutic purposes; e.g., using the rigid cystourethroscope or urethroscope, a cold knife incision of a limited stricture can be performed or a catheter placed into a diverticulum for localization during open surgical repair)
- Suspected urethral calculi (rare), foreign body, or condylomata (for diagnosis or removal)
- Urinary incontinence
  - Intrinsic sphincter deficiency (cystourethroscopy confirms the diagnosis and allows treatment with periurethral bulking agents)
  - Obstructive or irritative voiding symptoms (e.g., urgency, frequency, urge incontinence) unresponsive to conservative measures
- Suspected or known bladder diverticulum or fistula, or ectopic ureter (e.g., seen on radiograph)
- Gross or microscopic hematuria
- Known or suspected urogynecologic malignancy
  - Staging or surveillance for bladder, cervical, or endometrial cancer
- Recurrent urinary tract infections
- Pelvic pain symptoms
  - Dyspareunia
  - Suspected interstitial cystitis, urethritis, or trigonitis (see also Chapter 12, Office Testing and Treatment Options for Interstitial Cystitis [Painful Bladder Syndrome])
  - Endometriosis of the bladder
- Traumatic injury to the lower genital tract
- Intraoperative assessment of the bladder or urethra
  - Exclusion of inadvertent intraluminal suture placement or bladder trauma after incontinence or prolapse correction procedures
  - Assessment of coaptation of the urethra after suburethral sling procedures
  - Evaluation of ureteral patency with intravenous indigo carmine dye

CONTRAINDICATIONS

- Acute cystitis, prostatitis, or pyelonephritis should be treated before cystourethroscopy is performed because sepsis has been reported after cystoscopy in an infected patient.
- Anticoagulated patient or patient with coagulopathy (either the anticoagulation/coagulopathy should be reversed or urology consulted).

EQUIPMENT

- Rigid cystoscope and sheath (Fig. 111-1).
  - Sterile rigid telescopes with 0-, 30-, 70-, and 120-degree lenses.
  - The 0-degree lens (forward looking) is useful for intraurethral work, the 30-degree lens (forward oblique) is useful for evaluation of the urethra and bladder, the 70-degree lens (lateral) is useful for inspecting the interior of the bladder, and the 120-degree lens (retrograde) is useful for retrograde viewing of the bladder neck.
  - Sterile sheath of 17- to 26-Fr diameter with inflow and outflow ports.
  - Sterile scope-to-sheath bridge. This bridge may have one or two operative ports that admit the passage of biopsy instruments or urethral catheters.
  - A light cable and light source compatible with the telescope.
  - Urethral dilators, including a range from 14 to 32 Fr.
- Flexible cystoscope and light source.
- Irrigation tubing.
- Distension medium in 500-mL to 3-L bags. Saline or Ringer's lactate may be used if electrocautery is not anticipated. If electrocautery is anticipated, then a nonconductive medium such as sterile water, mannitol, sorbitol, or glycine should be used, with

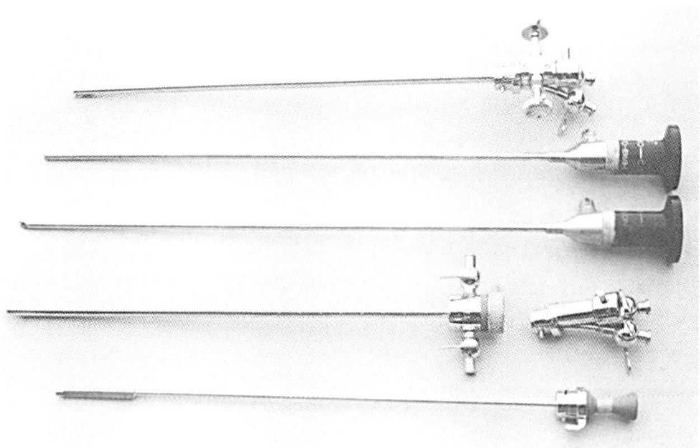

Figure 111-1 Cystoscope components, including *(from top to bottom)* operative sheath, telescopes (two), sheath and bridge, and obturator.

water having the advantages of increased visibility and, because it is hypotonic, lysing tumor cells.

- Cotton balls moistened with an antiseptic solution (e.g., povidone–iodine).
- Sterile gloves.
- Sterile cotton-tipped applicators.
- 1% or 2% lidocaine (Xylocaine) gel.
- Blue towel for tray top.
- Basin to capture irrigation runoff.

Although optional and expensive, video equipment, such as a camera, high-resolution monitor, video recorder, and printer, has its advantages. Video equipment provides a magnified, binocular view, allows the clinician the ability to maintain a more comfortable position when performing the procedure, is helpful for teaching or when an assistant is available, and provides the clinician greater eye protection from body fluids.

Preprocedure Patient Preparation

Indications for, alternatives to, and risks of cystourethroscopy should be explained to the patient, and informed consent obtained before the procedure. The patient should be informed of the possibility of discomfort during and after the procedure, as well as the potential for postprocedure urinary tract infection.

If a urinary tract infection is suspected or the patient has a history of mitral valve prolapse, valvular heart disease or replacement, or a recent prosthesis such as a total knee or joint, a urine culture and sensitivity should be obtained and the patient placed on a broad-spectrum antibiotic for at least 3 days. If the patient is not allergic to fluoroquinolones, ciprofloxacin or levofloxacin is an appropriate choice (see Chapter 221, Antibiotic Prophylaxis).

Technique

Before routinely performing cystoscopy, clinicians should familiarize themselves with the equipment and feel comfortable recognizing abnormalities or pathology on visualization of the urethra or bladder. Universal blood and body fluid precautions should be followed throughout the procedure.

Preparation

1. After the patient has emptied the bladder, *cleanse the urethral meatus* with an antiseptic solution.
2. Generously *lubricate the cotton-tipped applicator* with 1% or 2% lidocaine gel and insert it into the urethral meatus to the level of the bladder neck. Observe the angle of the urethra as an aid to inserting the cystoscope.

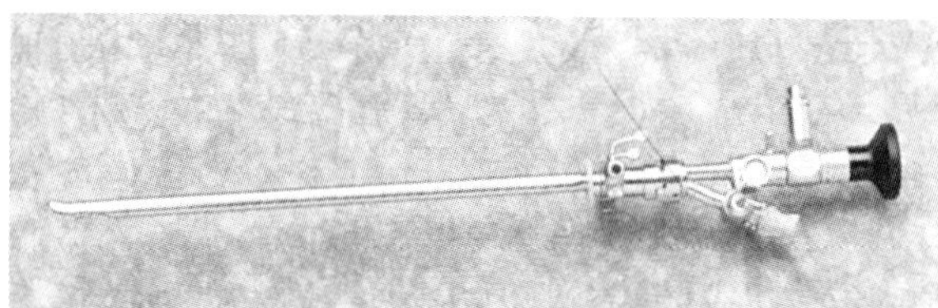

Figure 111-2 Assembled cystoscope with telescope, bridge, and sheath.

NOTE: Use sterile technique and wear sterile gloves from this point onward throughout the procedure.

Rigid Cystourethroscopy

3. Prepare the cystourethroscope as follows:
   - *Assemble the cystourethroscope* by attaching the 0-degree telescope to the bridge and sheath (Fig. 111-2).
   - *Attach the light cable* to the cystourethroscope and the light source. Turn on the light source before insertion to ensure proper illumination.
   - *Attach the infusion tubing* to the infusion port on the sheath, and attach this in turn to the appropriate instillation medium hung on a nearby intravenous pole. The tubing is then flushed.
4. *Lubricate the distal portion of the cystoscope* sheath with 1% or 2% lidocaine gel. Remove the applicator. After ensuring that all ports are in the closed position, *start the flow of the infusion medium* by opening the stopcock of the inflow port. The operator should have sole control of the fluid infusion through this port.

Urethroscopy

5. *Insert the lighted and assembled cystoscope* into the urethral meatus, following the line of the urethra. Initial insertion may be achieved using fluid as the obturator. Fluid is infused during inspection to a maximum of 350 to 500 mL or until the patient is uncomfortable. If resistance is encountered, the scope should not be forced; rather, the angle of insertion of the cystoscope should be reassessed. Continued difficulty in inserting the cystourethroscope may be an indication for urethral dilation before proceeding. Dilation can be performed serially using urethral dilators beginning with 14 Fr and dilating up to 32 Fr. Alternatively, a smaller-sized sheath can be used.
6. *Advance the cystoscope* under direct visualization into the bladder lumen. Then withdraw it slowly until the internal urethral meatus is visualized. While slowly withdrawing the cystourethroscope, examine the entire length of the urethral mucosa for pathology (Fig. 111-3). Gentle palpation of the anterior vaginal

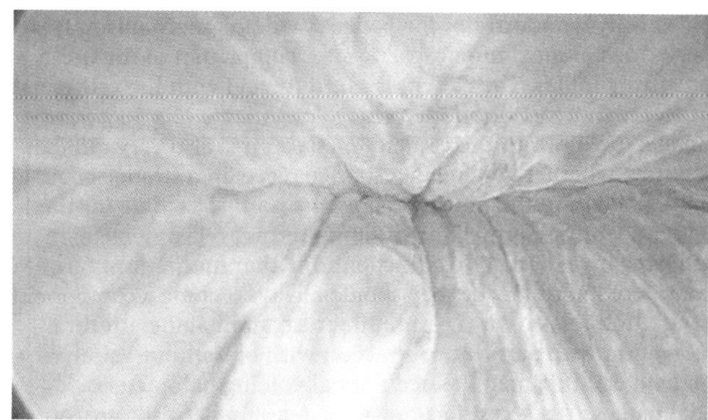

Figure 111-3 View of normal urethral mucosa.

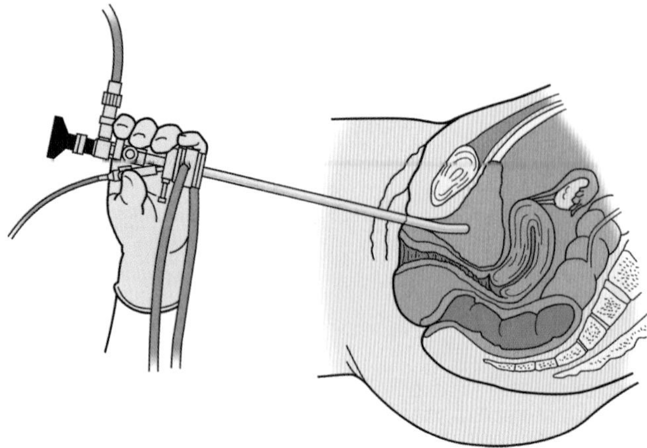

Figure 111-4 Technique of cystoscopy using angled telescopic lens.

wall during withdrawal may help to identify a urethral diverticulum, which tend to occur on the posterior aspect of the urethra.

Cystoscopy

7. *Remove the cystoscope* and discontinue the infusion flow. *Replace the 0-degree telescope with an angled-lens (30- or 70-degree) telescope and reinsert* the reassembled cystoscope as described previously. For adequate cystoscopy the bladder should be filled to approximately 250 mL or greater. If the patient notes discomfort from overdistention of the bladder, open the outflow port on the sheath and drain an appropriate amount of fluid from the bladder.
8. *Perform a systematic examination of the bladder lumen*, apply suprapubic pressure to facilitate visualization, and identify a small air bubble, which is usually present at the bladder dome. With this as a landmark, examine the anterior and lateral sidewalls in a stepwise fashion. To visualize the entire bladder dome, rotate the angled lens about the long axis of the telescope while keeping the camera in a fixed orientation (Fig. 111-4). Lateral torque, with the urethral meatus as the fulcrum, can cause pain and should be avoided. Intraluminal pathology, including the presence of tumor, endometriosis, trabeculations, stones, chronic cystitis, or hemorrhage, should be noted (Fig. 111-5). The bladder should be examined at various levels of filling; glomerulations and ecchymoses are frequently seen only with full distention. Intraluminal sutures inadvertently placed at the time of a previous urethropexy are generally identified on the lateral sidewalls at the 2 and 10 o'clock positions.
9. *Visualize the trigone*, located posteriorly just proximal to the internal urethral meatus at the 6 o'clock position. Any abnormalities should be noted. Rotating the scope 20 to 30 degrees to each side will allow visualization of the *ureteral orifices*. If one orifice is visualized, identification of the *interureteric ridge* will lead to the contralateral orifice. (In patients with large cystoceles, reduction of the prolapse may be necessary to see the orifices.) If possible, *identify ureteral peristalsis with efflux of urine*.
10. Concurrent vaginal examination in women may be helpful for evaluating a cystocele. A concurrent rectal examination in men may be useful for assessing prostate size and length of the prostatic urethra.
11. For patients with pelvic pain or interstitial cystitis, bladder distention with at least 600 to 1000 mL may be therapeutic but usually requires general anesthesia because of poor tolerance in the office as a result of severe pain.
12. After completing the procedure, *turn off the infusion of distention medium and drain the patient's bladder* with the ancillary port on the cystoscope sheath. Samples of this drainage can be sent for cytologic analysis if desired (e.g., patient with prior history of malignancy). Remove the cystoscope and turn off the light source to prevent accidental injury from the hot light.
13. Disassemble the cystoscopic telescopes, bridge, and sheaths and clean them by immersion in glutaraldehyde solution (Cidex) for 20 minutes before reuse.

Flexible Cystoscopy

14. Lubricate the distal portion of the cystoscope with 1% or 2% lidocaine gel.
15. Advance the cystoscope under direct visualization into the bladder lumen. (The flexible cystoscope is passed in a manner similar to a Foley catheter, except the lumen is visualized as it is passed.) Flex and torque the instrument to obtain a view of the same structures as visualized with rigid cystourethroscopy. The same maneuvers may be used as with rigid instruments to enhance visualization of various structures and pathology.
16. Withdraw the cystoscope slowly until the internal urethral meatus is visualized. While slowly withdrawing the cystoscope, examine the entire length of the urethral mucosa for pathology. The prostatic urethra will not be seen as clearly as with rigid instruments, but a general impression of prostatic size can be obtained.
17. Clean the flexible cystoscope and flush all channels and ports with soap and water. This should be followed by immersion in glutaraldehyde solution (Cidex) for 20 minutes before reuse.

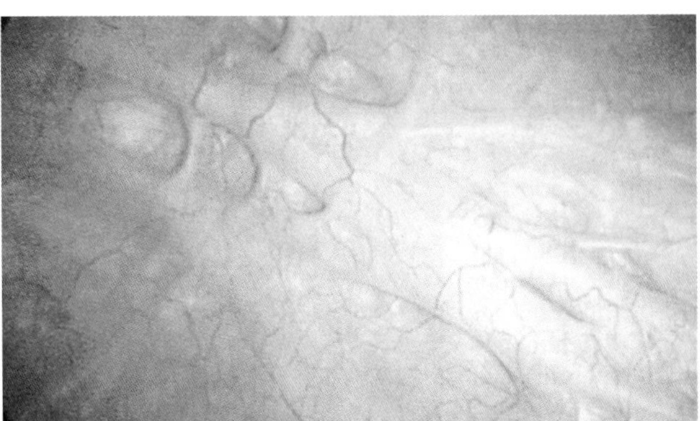

Figure 111-5 Cystoscopic evaluation of bladder lumen demonstrating coarse trabeculations (ridges).

Biopsy

Bladder or urethral mucosa biopsy is useful for evaluation and histologic confirmation of suspect lesions, including possible interstitial cystitis or malignancy. Although it can be performed in the office, bladder biopsy usually requires a larger sheath to accommodate the biopsy forceps, is associated with patient discomfort, and occasionally requires electrocautery to control bleeding. Given these considerations, it is recommended that cystoscopic biopsies be performed in the ambulatory surgical suite. Flexible biopsy forceps are available for the rigid scopes and may be helpful for reaching areas of the bladder that are difficult to reach with rigid forceps such as the dome and anterior wall; however, rigid biopsy forceps can remove tissue samples up to 5 mm in diameter, whereas the size of fragments obtained with flexible biopsy forceps is usually less than 2 mm.

Complications

- Bacteriuria
- Sepsis
- Urethral or bladder neck trauma
- Bleeding
- Pain

Complications after cystourethroscopy are rare. The reported rate of bacteriuria after this procedure is 2% to 7%. Rare cases of systemic sepsis associated with performance of cystoscopy in the presence of untreated infection have been reported. Rarely, trauma to the urethra and bladder neck can result from instrumentation.

Interpretation of Results

A complete review of abnormal findings at the time of cystoscopy is beyond the scope of this chapter. However, the clinician who routinely performs cystoscopy should be familiar with the normal appearance of the bladder and urethra. Abnormal anatomic findings should correlate with the patient's symptoms. In patients with overactive bladder symptoms (urgency, frequency, nocturia, enuresis, or urge incontinence), the urethra should be inspected for a stricture or diverticulum and the bladder inspected for trabeculations, infectious changes, and foreign bodies.

For the evaluation of incontinence, cystoscopy is useful in the evaluation of intrinsic sphincter deficiency (the internal urethral meatus is open at rest) and vesicovaginal and urethrovaginal fistulas. In patients with genitourinary pain syndromes, the urethra may appear atrophic and the bladder may reveal petechial hemorrhages, ecchymoses, glomerulations, or Hunner's ulcers consistent with interstitial cystitis (see also Chapter 112, Office Testing and Treatment Options for Interstitial Cystitis [Painful Bladder Syndrome]). Bladder distention, which is often therapeutic, can be accomplished at the time of cystoscopy with instillation of 600 to 1000 mL of solution.

Cystoscopy is useful for evaluation of lower urinary tract injury. Cystoscopy may reveal a bladder laceration or penetration of the bladder by sutures placed during surgery. To assess ureteral integrity and patency, patients can be given 5-mL intravenous indigo carmine at the time of cystoscopy. Both ureteral orifices should be noted to eject dye 5 to 10 minutes after intravenous injection. In some cases dye spillage may be delayed up to 15 minutes.

Postprocedure Patient Education

Each patient should be provided with instructions concerning expected postprocedure symptoms. A preprinted informational handout may be useful for this purpose. Specific information should include the following:

1. Patients should take antibiotic prophylaxis, if prescribed. They should be instructed to follow up immediately if dysuria, pyuria, or fever greater than 100.4° F develops within 72 hours of the procedure.
2. A small amount of transient hematuria within the first few hours after cystoscopy is normal. If it persists or is excessive, the patient should be instructed to follow up immediately.
3. The patient may have some discomfort after the procedure. A short course of the bladder analgesic, phenazopyridine, may be used to alleviate this. If the discomfort persists, the patient should be instructed to follow up for evaluation.

CPT/Billing Codes

52000 Cystourethroscopy (separate procedure)
52005 Cystourethroscopy, with ureteral catheterization
52204 Cystourethroscopy, with biopsy
52260 Cystourethroscopy, with dilation of bladder for interstitial cystitis; general or conduction (spinal) anesthesia
52281 Cystourethroscopy, with calibration and/or dilation of urethral stricture or stenosis
52285 Cystourethroscopy for treatment of the female urethral syndrome with any or all of the following: urethral meatotomy, urethral dilation, internal urethrotomy, lysis of urethrovaginal septal fibrosis, lateral incisions of the bladder neck, and fulguration of polyp(s) of urethra, bladder neck, and/or trigone

ICD-9-CM Diagnostic Codes

592.1 Calculus: ureteral
594.2 Calculus: urethral
595.1 Cystitis: interstitial
595.2 Cystitis: other chronic
596.2 Fistula: bladder, not elsewhere classified
597.80 Urethritis, unspecified
597.81 Urethral syndrome, NOS
598.0 Urethral stricture due to infection
599.1 Fistula: urethral
599.2 Diverticulum: urethral
599.7 Hematuria
625.6 Incontinence: stress
753.6 Bladder neck obstruction
788.1 Dysuria
788.20 Urinary retention, unspecified
788.21 Incomplete bladder emptying
788.30 Incontinence: unspecified
788.31 Incontinence: urge
788.33 Incontinence: mixed
788.37 Incontinence: continuous leakage
788.41 Urinary frequency
867.0 Injury: bladder/urethra, without mention of open wound

Acknowledgment

The editors wish to recognize the many contributions by Andrew C. Steele, MD, and Neeraj Kohli, MD, to this chapter in a previous edition of this text.

Suppliers

(See contact information online at www.expertconsult.com.)

Gyrus ACMI Corporation (Olympus)
Karl Storz Endoscopy-America, Inc.
Stryker

Online Resources

Agency for Health Care Research and Quality: Urinary Incontinence in Adults: Clinical Practice Guideline Update. (Patient information on incontinence from the AHCRQ.) Available at www.ahrq.gov/clinic/uiovervw.htm.

Gyrus ACMI. (Official website for a leading supplier of endoscopic equipment; this site also has a number of instructional videos available on performing cystoscopy.) Available at www.circoncorp.com.

HealthWorld Online: Urinary Incontinence in Adults: Acute and Chronic Management. (Patient information.) Available at www.healthy.net/scr/article.asp?ID=409.

Karl Storz. (Another major supplier of endoscopy equipment.) Available at www.karlstorz.com.

National Institute of Diabetes and Digestive and Kidney Diseases. (Information on a wide range of topics on urologic conditions from the National Kidney and Urologic Diseases Information Clearinghouse and National Institutes of Health.) Available at www.niddk.nih.gov.

BIBLIOGRAPHY

American College of Obstetricians and Gynecologists: Practice bulletin no. 63. Urinary incontinence in women. Obstet Gynecol 105:1533–1545, 2005.

American College of Obstetricians and Gynecologist: Practice bulletin no. 104. Antibiotic prophylaxis for gynecologic procedures. Obstet Gynecol 113:1180–1189, 2009.

Grossfeld GD, Litwin MS, Wolf JS Jr, et al: Evaluation of asymptomatic microscopic hematuria in adults: The American Urological Association best practice policy—part II. Patient evaluation, cytology, voided markers, imaging, cystoscopy, nephrology evaluation, and follow-up. Urology 57:604–610, 2001.

McDonald MM, Swagerty D: Assessment of microscopic hematuria in adults. Am Fam Physician 73:1748–1754, 2006.

Metts JF: Interstitial cystitis, urgency and frequency syndrome. Am Fam Physician 64:1199–1206, 2001.

Stoller ML: Retrograde instrumentation of the urinary tract. In Tanagho EA, MacAninch JW (eds): Smith's General Urology, 17th ed. New York, McGraw-Hill, 2008, pp 163–174.

Wen CC, Babayan RK: Instrumentation of the lower urinary tract. In Siroky MB, Oates RD, Babayan RK (eds): Handbook of Urology: Diagnosis and Therapy, 3rd ed. Philadelphia, Lippincott Williams & Wilkins, 2004, pp 63–78.

CHAPTER 112

Office Testing and Treatment Options for Interstitial Cystitis (Painful Bladder Syndrome)

Stephen A. Grochmal

Interstitial cystitis (IC), also known as *painful bladder syndrome* (PBS, which is actually a slightly broader category of disorders), is characterized by bladder pain of varying intensity, lasting over a prolonged period. IC is more prevalent in women but can also affect men, and the overall prevalence appears greater than was previously estimated. Identification, diagnosis, and treatment of IC are controversial, similar to other medical conditions of unknown etiology that are difficult to treat.

Anatomy

The urinary and reproductive systems are related embryologically, and both systems develop from the intermediate mesoderm of the embryo. The endoderm that ultimately gives rise to the epithelium of the bladder trigone and urethra is the same as that which develops into the lower third of the vagina and vestibule. Therefore, conditions that affect the bladder throughout life may also produce a variety of vaginal or vulvar symptoms, and vice versa.

The superior surface of the bladder is covered with peritoneum that separates it from the coils of the ileum and the sigmoid colon. As the bladder fills (maximum capacity is about 500 mL), this superior surface bulges upward into the abdominal cavity and the covering peritoneum separates from the lower part of the anterior abdominal wall so that the bladder comes into direct contact with the anterior abdominal wall.

The glycosaminoglycan layer normally coats the urothelial bladder surface and renders it impermeable to any solutes. Defects in this layer may permit urinary irritants to penetrate the urothelium and activate the underlying nerve and muscle tissues. This process can lead to additional tissue damage, hypersensitivity, and pain. This ongoing bladder damage may also be propagated by mast cells in the bladder.

The pelvic floor and bladder are both innervated from sacral nerve roots S2, S3, and S4. These nerve roots include motor/efferent and sensory/afferent pathways of both the visceral and somatic systems.

Because of the proximity of the bladder to other surrounding structures, including the bowel, pelvic floor musculature, and reproductive organs, it is not surprising that if one of the pelvic organs becomes diseased, the other pelvic organ systems may exhibit similar symptoms. This should be kept in mind when evaluating pelvic pain of bladder origin.

Clinical Presentation

Interstitial cystitis is defined by suprapubic pain related to bladder filling and is frequently accompanied by urinary frequency and urgency and nocturia in the absence of proven infection or other obvious pathologic process. Furthermore, the term *interstitial cystitis* is reserved for those patients with PBS symptoms who also have characteristic (but not pathognomonic) cystoscopic findings or histologic evidence during bladder hydrodistention.

Patients may also describe chronic pelvic pain (CPP) not due to their bladder pain, but associated with other ongoing symptoms or disorders such as dysmenorrhea, endometriosis, adenomyosis, vulvodynia, irritable bowel syndrome, and fibromyalgia.

Although the etiology of IC is clearly multifactorial, recent evidence suggests a strong correlation between IC and (1) dysfunctional, abnormal bladder epithelial permeability and (2) increased mast cell activity. The abnormal bladder epithelial permeability appears to be due to changes found in the bladder mucous layer. This layer contains defective glycosaminoglycans that increase the permeability of the urothelium to irritants, especially potassium. It is still unclear whether mast cells play a causative or secondary role in the disease.

IC is expressed as a continuum from mild to severe disease, and can persist for decades. The mild to moderate stages are often associated with symptom flares and remissions. Flares may occur in association with sexual intimacy or before menses, complicating the process of distinguishing IC from other gynecologic disorders. Subsequently, women often consult multiple clinicians (an average of five over a period of 4 or more years) before the correct and precise diagnosis is made; unfortunately, the causes of IC or any associated CPP cannot always be determined with a simple gynecologic examination.

Additional factors known to cause IC exacerbations include allergies, emotional or physical stress, exercise, sexual intercourse, remaining seated for prolonged periods (e.g., air travel), and ingestion of foods and drinks with a high potassium content (e.g., oranges, strawberries, coffee). Most patients in the early stages of IC complain of urgency and frequency; however, dysuria and dyspareunia can also be seen. The symptoms may vary from day to day but are usually gradual in onset and worsen over a period of months. Pain of increasing severity often becomes the predominant complaint.

IC or PBS symptoms can be associated with chronic pain and fatigue, a disturbance of the patient's home and work life, and a decreased overall quality of life. From a review of multiple surveys, up to 70% of patients claim sleep disturbance, more than 50% are unable to work full time, and almost 80% complain of dyspareunia leading to decreased sexual intimacy. More than 90% of patients surveyed claim that the symptoms of IC or PBS affect their daily activities.

Patient Investigation and Diagnosis

The work-up for IC should include a careful pelvic examination; during this examination, care should be taken to evaluate for tenderness of the anterior vaginal wall/bladder base. A urinalysis and urine culture should be obtained to rule out hematuria and infection. Conditions for which IC may be mistaken include recurrent urinary tract infection, overactive bladder, vulvar and vaginal conditions, and abdominopelvic adhesions. It is important to be aware of signs, symptoms, and risk factors for bladder cancer. Microscopic hematuria is the main sign, and, if present, cancer should be ruled out with a thorough urologic work-up, including cystoscopy (see Chapter 111, Diagnostic Cystourethroscopy). Risk factors for bladder cancer include age greater than 40 years, long-standing symptoms, and smoking.

Although additional procedures such as cystoscopy/cystourethroscopy (with or without bladder hydrodistention) can be performed at the clinician's discretion, these procedures are not required for the diagnosis and treatment of IC or PBS. Bladder biopsy is not required except to rule out other disorders. Additional diagnostic tools such as biomarkers (e.g., antiproliferative factor) may play a future role in the diagnosis of IC or PBS, but further studies are needed. Urodynamic testing does not currently have a role in identification or diagnosis of IC or PBS.

Tools for Diagnosing Interstitial Cystitis

The majority of patients with IC or PBS, even early disease, can be identified with the Pelvic Pain and Urgency and/or Frequency (PUF) questionnaire or the optional potassium sensitivity test (PST).

Pelvic Pain and Urgency and/or Frequency Questionnaire

When the clinical presentation and physical examination suggest IC, the PUF questionnaire (Fig. 112-1) is a rapid (<5 minutes), self-administered tool available to screen for IC. The PUF has been

PELVIC PAIN and URGENCY/FREQUENCY
PATIENT SYMPTOM SCALE

Please circle the answer that best describes how you feel for each question.

	0	1	2	3	4	SYMPTOM SCORE	BOTHER SCORE
1 How many times do you go to the bathroom during the day?	3–6	7–10	11–14	15–19	20+		
2 a. How many times do you go to the bathroom at night?	0	1	2	3	4+		
b. If you get up at night to go to the bathroom does it bother you?	Never	Mildly	Moderate	Severe			
3 Are you currently sexually active? YES ____ NO ____							
4 a. IF YOU ARE SEXUALLY ACTIVE, do you now have or have you ever had pain or symptoms during or after sexual intercourse?	Never	Occasionally	Usually	Always			
b. If you have pain, does it make you avoid sexual intercourse?	Never	Occasionally	Usually	Always			
5 Do you have pain associated with your bladder or in your pelvis (vagina, lower abdomen, urethra, perineum, testes, or scrotum)?	Never	Occasionally	Usually	Always			
6 Do you have urgency after going to the bathroom?	Never	Occasionally	Usually	Always			
7 a. If you have pain, is it usually		Mild	Moderate	Severe			
b. Does your pain bother you?	Never	Occasionally	Usually	Always			
8 a. If you have urgency, is it usually		Mild	Moderate	Severe			
b. Does your urgency bother you?	Never	Occasionally	Usually	Always			
SYMPTOM SCORE = (1, 2a, 4a, 5, 6, 7a, 8a)							
BOTHER SCORE = (2b, 4b, 7b, 8b)							
TOTAL SCORE = (Symptom Score + Bother Score)							

Figure 112-1 A score of 15 or greater is highly suggestive of interstitial cystitis. In some patients, especially adolescents, even a score in the range of 6 to 10 may warrant further investigation and treatment.

validated against the intravesical PST in both urologic patients suspected of having IC and gynecologic patients with pelvic pain. This questionnaire has proven to be of tremendous value for identifying patients with IC. Unlike other IC questionnaires, the PUF gives balanced attention to pelvic pain, urgency/frequency, and dyspareunia. (The cut-off score for a definitive IC/PBS diagnosis based on the PUF is 15 or higher; however, some patients have IC with a PUF score of 12 or higher. It is also the author's experience that in some patients with IC, particularly adolescent women not yet sexually active, the PUF score may be much lower than 12 because these patients fall out of the questionnaire's parameters.)

Potassium Sensitivity Test

The PST is an optional test that involves instilling potassium chloride solution into the bladder (Fig. 112-2). If the patient experiences urgency or pain, the presence of abnormal epithelial permeability is strongly suggested. During the PST, 40 mL of sterile water is instilled into the bladder and notation made of any associated pain. The bladder is then drained and filled with a 40-mL solution of 0.4 M potassium chloride (40 mEq KCl/100 mL water); a finding of increased pain during this second filling is considered indicative of bladder hypersensitivity and suggestive of IC or PBS. The PST can be an uncomfortable procedure; therefore, an intravesical "rescue" solution should be available to alleviate symptoms provoked by the test.

Some studies claim that the PST should not be used routinely because its results are nonspecific for IC or PBS. Although most patients with IC have a positive PST result, a small percentage will have a negative result, and the reason for this is unknown. More important, to minimize the use of the PST, one study found an 84% correlation with positive PST findings among individuals with PUF scores of 15 or higher. This has resulted in the PUF questionnaire gaining acceptance as a sensitive and easy-to-use surrogate for the PST.

Recently, investigators have reported that intravesical instillation of 2% lignocaine solution is useful for excluding patients with pelvic pain originating from organs other than the bladder (Taneja, 2010). Further studies are needed to substantiate this claim.

Indications

Potassium Sensitivity Test

- Validation of patient symptom scale (PUF questionnaire)/confirmation of bladder epithelial dysfunction
- Assessment or monitoring of current disease state/treatment
- Patient seeking second opinion concerning treatment of IC previously investigated by an unremarkable cystoscopy or hydrodistention
- Confirmation for "new to treat" clinicians of their clinical impression
- Validation for suffering patients that their disease is real

Intravesical Instillation Therapy

- Provide rapid relief as needed in patients suffering with bladder pain, symptoms, or flares
- "Jump start" therapy to complement initiation of oral treatment in newly diagnosed patients
- Adjunctive second-line therapy to multimodal oral treatment regimens
- In patients unable to tolerate oral treatment or when oral therapy is ineffective
- "At home" elective intravesical instillation treatments by patients

Contraindications

- *Absolute:* Known allergy or sensitivity to any of the components used in the test or instillation treatment solutions (e.g., lidocaine, heparin)
- *Relative:* Acute urinary tract infection

Equipment and Supplies

Potassium Sensitivity Test

- Examination table with or without pelvic tilt/stirrups
- Impermeable drapes
- Surgical prep solution (e.g., povidone–iodine, chlorhexidine)
- Gloves

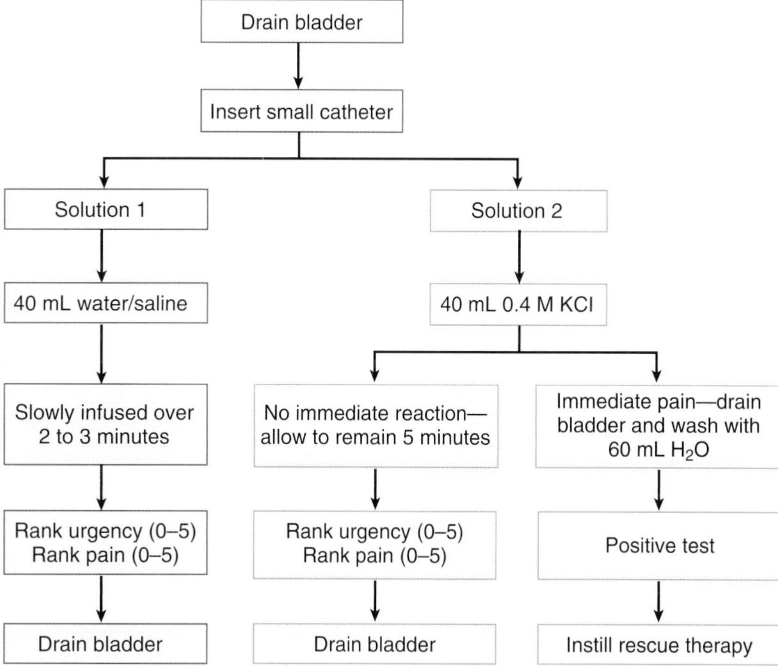

Figure 112-2 Flow diagram of the potassium sensitivity test. The rescue solution or cocktail should be prepared in advance in the event of an uncomfortable or positive reaction to the test. The rescue solution is composed of 10,000 U heparin, 10 mL of 1% lidocaine, and 3 mL of 8.4% sodium bicarbonate.

- LoFric catheter (Astra Tech, Inc., Urology Division, Torrance, Calif; 8 to 10 Fr, 8 inches for female patients, 12 Fr for male patients)
- Solution no. 1: 40 mL of sterile water or saline
- Solution no. 2: 40 mL of 0.4 M KCl (40 mEq of KCl/100 mL sterile water)
- One bottle of 100 mL sterile water for diluent
- Two 60-mL syringes
- 20-mL syringe
- 18-gauge needle
- Permeability Study Record Sheet (available online at www.expertconsult.com)

*Rescue Solution**

- 20-mL syringe
- Heparin sulfate, 10,000 U
- 10 mL lidocaine 1%
- 3 mL 8.4% NaOH (sodium bicarbonate)
- 100 mL sterile water for dilution

NOTE: 100 to 200 mg of oral pentosan polysulfate sodium (PPS) emptied from its capsule, dissolved in 10 mL of buffered normal saline per 100-mg capsule, may be substituted for heparin.†

Intravesical Instillation ("Jump Start" Therapy)

- LoFric catheter (8 to 10 Fr, 8 inches for female patients, 12 Fr for male patients)
- 20- or 30-mL syringe(s)
- 100 to 200 mg of oral PPS emptied from its capsule, dissolved in 10 mL of buffered normal saline per 100-mg capsule†
- 10 mL lidocaine 1% or 16 mL lidocaine 2%
- 3 mL 8.4% NaOH (sodium bicarbonate)
- Dimethyl sulfoxide (DMSO, is FDA approved for intravesical therapy)
- 100 mL sterile water for dilution

Technique

Potassium Sensitivity Test

1. The patient is awake and without anesthesia for this procedure.
2. Have the patient void completely.
3. Position patient in the dorsal position, preferably in stirrups.
4. Place an impermeable, waterproof drape under the patient's buttock.
5. Cleanse/prepare the vulvar/urethral area as if you were inserting a Foley catheter. This is a clean, not sterile procedure.
6. Insert the straight catheter, drain any residual urine, and attach the syringe filled with solution no. 1 (see Fig. 112-2).
7. Instill solution no. 1, wait, and record observations on Permeability Study Record Sheet (available online at www.expertconsult.com).
8. Drain the bladder.
9. Attach the second syringe, instill solution no. 2 into subject's bladder, and wait 5 minutes.
10. Record patient's degree of provoked urgency and pain. Patients are rated on a scale of 0 to 5 (with 0 = no provocation and 5 = severe provocation). A score of 2 or more in the pain or urgency scale is considered a positive test. If the patient's bladder is abnormally permeable, the PST will provoke urinary urgency or pain well above the patient's baseline levels.
11. If necessary (e.g., if patient has an immediate reaction to solution no. 1 on instillation or after test is concluded and patient voids), instill rescue solution immediately and have patient lie semiupright for approximately 10 to 20 minutes or until bladder discomfort dissipates.
12. Make a notation in the patient's records regarding the outcome of the test, any reaction, and administration of rescue solution, if used, and maintain a copy of Permeability Study Record Sheet.

*Prepare this solution in advance of performing the PST. Use sterile water to bring volume up to at least 20 mL.

†Intravesical administration of PPS is an off-label use of the drug.

Treatment Options for Interstitial Cystitis or Painful Bladder Syndrome

Because of the multiple possible etiologies for IC or PBS, therapy should generally use a multimodal approach. The foundation of oral therapy for IC is PPS, 100 mg three times a day. Additional medications are added as needed. Currently, PPS is the only oral medication approved by the U.S. Food and Drug Administration (FDA) for the treatment of IC; it has been evaluated in five placebo-controlled trials. PPS is a compound that mimics the glycosaminoglycan layer on the surface of the bladder and is believed to help correct the dysfunctional bladder epithelium. Hydroxyzine (25 mg/day in the evening, 50 to 100 mg/day during allergy season) is prescribed to control histamine discharge associated with allergic flares, which can in turn provoke exacerbations of IC or PBS. Amitriptyline (25 mg/day at bedtime) can be added to block both peripheral and central neural activity. Occasionally, an anticholinergic is also used to control severe urinary urgency complaints. In many patients with IC or PBS, PPS must be administered for at least 3 to 6 months before its full effectiveness can be realized (Fig. 112-3).

If a more rapid treatment response is needed, intravesical "jump start" therapy can be initiated at the time of diagnosis. This consists of various therapeutic "cocktails" made from heparin, PPS, 8.4% sodium bicarbonate, lidocaine, or DMSO (Fig. 112-4). These cocktails are instilled directly into the bladder through a catheter to facilitate immediate relief, as opposed to the several weeks to months it may take for PPS alone to take effect. It should be noted that DMSO is the only FDA-approved medication for intravesical instillation. The current use of all other combinations of medications for intravesical therapy is considered off-label.

Evaluation of ongoing treatment can be accomplished with a repeat PUF questionnaire, looking for a change (decrease) in score as treatment progresses. Another form that may be useful is the Patient Overall Rating of Improvement of Symptoms (PORIS). The PORIS helps in assessing patient progress with long-term treatment regimens. This form should be maintained as part of the patient record (available online at www.expertconsult.com).

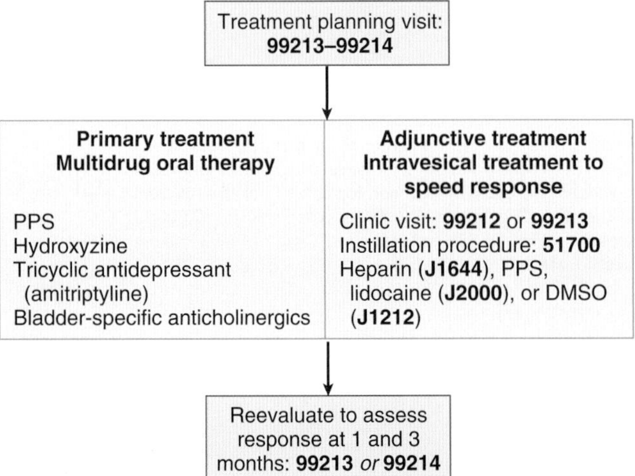

Figure 112-3 Synopsis of treatment options with appropriate codes. DMSO, dimethyl sulfoxide; PPS, pentosan polysulfate sodium.

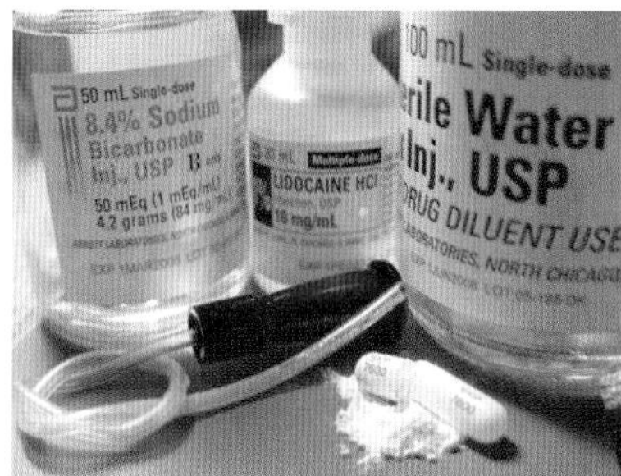

Figure 112-4 Example of components used for intravesical instillation, including 8-Fr catheter and open capsule of pentosan polysulfate sodium.

Surgical intervention is rarely indicated or beneficial. In addition to pharmacologic therapy, various supportive or behavioral measures may be helpful. Effective self-care options for patients with IC or PBS include stress reduction and comfort activities such as pet therapy, meditation, and even prayer. Improvement in IC symptoms has been reported using self-hypnosis and posthypnotic suggestion in patients refractory to conventional medical treatments.

Technique for Intravesical Instillation Therapy

1. Prepare the therapeutic cocktail solution in a single syringe.
2. Follow steps 1 through 5 as described in PST Technique section.
3. Place catheter into bladder (10 Fr, 8 inches for female patients, 12 Fr for male patients).
4. Drain the bladder.
5. Attach the syringe and instill the therapeutic solution.
6. Have the patient retain the instilled solution for 10 to 20 minutes.
7. Remove the catheter.
8. Direct the patient to void the solution.
9. Make a notation in the patient's record of the solution used, amount, and the patient's tolerance for the procedure.

Assuming that the bladder is the source of pain in the patient with IC, direct treatment of the bladder surface with a therapeutic solution may result in immediate and profound relief and improvement of symptoms. This symptom improvement resulting from the instillation therapy may aid in differentiating bladder-based pain from other forms of pelvic discomfort. Some clinicians use a purely anesthetic cocktail, such as lignocaine or bupivacaine with 2% lidocaine jelly, for this purpose.

Common Errors

- Mix-up between solutions nos. 1 and 2 during the PST (label each syringe after preparation and before use).
- Incorrect quantities of components for cocktail solutions (record components as you prepare the solution).
- Failure to record the patient reactions during the PST (keep record sheet handy during the PST).
- Failure to have the rescue solution available at the start of the PST (should be prepared along with testing solutions).
- Failure to observe the patient at least 15 minutes post-PST voiding for any delayed response of pain or discomfort requiring you to administer the rescue solution.

Complications

- Rarely, an expected adverse effect may include a worsening of symptoms when the effects of the rescue solution or therapeutic solution have ceased. Reassure the patient that this exacerbation will dissipate within a few hours.

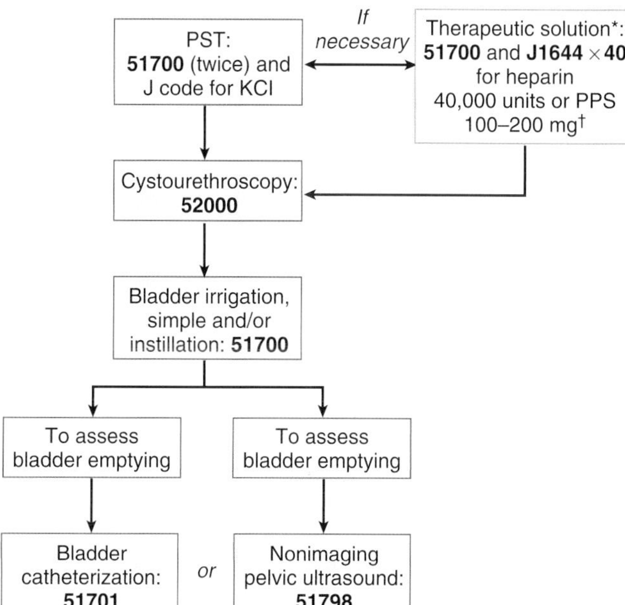

Figure 112-5 Listed CPT and J codes for the PST, catheterization, and cystourethroscopy procedures performed in-office. KCl, potassium chloride; PPS, pentosan polysulfate sodium; PST, potassium sensitivity test. *Solution also includes 10 mL of 1% lidocaine or 16 mL of 2% lidocaine and 3 mL of 8.4% sodium bicarbonate (not billable). †PPS 100 to 200 mg (not billable) may be substituted for heparin. Intravesical instillation of PPS is an off-label use of this product.

- Rarely, urinary retention. Treat as needed with catheterization to relieve discomfort.

CPT/Billing Codes

For all newly diagnosed patients with IC there are specific codes for these procedures listed on the flow chart in Figure 112-5.

Laboratory Testing

81000	Urinalysis
87086, 87088, 87181, 87184, P9612	Urine culture
51700 (twice) and J code for KCl	Potassium sensitivity test

Therapeutic Solution

51700	Bladder irrigation, simple and/or instillation
J1644 (x40)	Heparin

NOTE: 8.4% NaOH is not billable.

J2000 Lidocaine (for rescue cocktail)

Ancillary Procedures

51701	Bladder catheterization
52000	Cystourethroscopy
A4123	Syringes
A4351	Catheter supplies, home use
J1212	DMSO

ICD-9-CM Diagnostic Codes

595.1	Chronic interstitial cystitis
788.9	Bladder pain

SUPPLIERS

(See contact information online at www.expertconsult.com.)

LoFric catheter (8 to 10 Fr for female patients, 12 Fr for male patients)
Astra Tech, Inc., Urology Division

Pentosan polysulfate sodium 100-mg capsules
Ortho-McNeil-Janssen Pharmaceuticals

Lidocaine (1% or 2%), 8.4% sodium bicarbonate, heparin 10,000-U vials, sterile water diluent, DMSO, 60-mL syringes
Moore Medical

ONLINE RESOURCES

Grochmal SA: How to Perform the PST [video for physicians]. Contact: Endoreprogyne@aol.com.
Interstitial Cystitis Association (ICA): Available at www.ichelp.org.
Interstitial Cystitis Network (ICN): Available at www.ic-network.com.
Ortho-McNeil-Janssen Pharmaceuticals: Elmiron web page. Available at www.myortho360.com/myortho360/elmiron/welcome.html.

BIBLIOGRAPHY

Abrams L, Cardozo M, Fall M, et al: The standardisation of terminology of lower urinary tract function: Report from the Standardisation Sub-committee of the International Continence Society. Am J Obstet Gynecol 187:116–126, 2002.

Chung MK, Chung RR, Gordon D, Jennings C: The evil twins of chronic pelvic pain syndrome: Endometriosis and interstitial cystitis. JSLS 6: 311–314, 2002.

Dasgupta J, Tincello DG: Interstitial cystitis/painful bladder syndrome: An update. Maturitas 64:212–217, 2009.

Dell JR, Grochmal SA, Chandakas S, et al: Intravesical "jump start" therapy using a therapeutic cocktail for the treatment of interstitial cystitis. JSLS 10:S1–S77, 2006.

Driscoll A, Teichman JMH: How do patients with interstitial cystitis present? J Urol 166:2118–2120, 2001.

Forrest JB, Mishell DR Jr: Breaking the cycle of pain in interstitial cystitis/painful bladder syndrome: Toward standardization of early diagnosis and treatment. Consensus Panel Recommendations. J Reprod Med 54:3–14, 2009.

Grochmal SA, Shulman L, Dell JR, et al: Continued chronic pelvic pain in adolescent women with failed treatment for endometriosis: Identification and treatment outcome in patients with bladder origin of CPP (interstitial cystitis). J Minim Invasive Gynecol 13(5 Suppl):S151, 2006.

Hanno P: Is the potassium sensitivity test a valid and useful test in the diagnosis of interstitial cystitis? Against. Int Urogynecol J Pelvic Floor Dysfunct 16:428–429, 2005.

Henry R, Patterson L, Avery N, et al: Absorption of alkalized intravesical lidocaine in normal and inflamed bladders: A simple method for improving bladder anesthesia. J Urol 165:1900–1903, 2001.

Langenberg PW, Wallach EE, Clauw DJ, et al: Pelvic pain and surgeries in women before interstitial cystitis/ painful bladder syndrome. Am J Obstet Gynecol 202:286.e1–286.e6, 2010.

Lynch DF Jr: Empowering the patients: Hypnosis in the management of cancer, surgical disease and chronic pain. Am J Clin Hypnosis 2:122–130, 1999.

Marszalek M, Wehrberger C, Temml C, et al: Chronic pelvic pain and lower urinary tract symptoms in both sexes: Analysis of 2749 participants of an urban screening project. Eur Urol 55:499–508, 2009.

Mishell DR Jr, Dell J, Sand PK: Evolving trends in the successful management of interstitial cystitis/painful bladder syndrome. J Reprod Med 53:651–657, 2008.

Moore J, Kennedy S: Causes of chronic pelvic pain. Best Pract Res Clin Obstet Gynecol 14:389–342, 2000.

Mulholland SG, Hanno P, Parsons CL, et al: Pentosan polysulfate sodium for therapy of interstitial cystitis: A double-blind placebo-controlled clinical study. Urology 35:552–558, 1990.

Neis KJ, Neis F: Chronic pelvic pain: Cause, diagnosis and therapy from a gynaecologist's and an endoscopist's point of view. Gynecol Endocrinol 25:757–761, 2009.

Nickel JC, Barkin J, Forrest J, et al, the Elmiron Study Group: Randomized double-blind, dose-ranging study of pentosan polysulfate sodium for interstitial cystitis. Urology 65:654–658, 2005.

Papandreau C, Skapinakis P, Giannakis D, et al: Antidepressant drugs for chronic urological pelvic pain: An evidence-based review. J Urol 174:1–9, 2009.

Parsons CL: Interstitial cystitis: Epidemiology and clinical presentation. Clin Obstet Gynecol 45:242–249, 2002.

Parsons CL: Evidence-based strategies for recognizing and managing IC. Contemp Urol 15:22–35, 2003.

Parsons CL: Argument for the use of the potassium sensitivity test in the diagnosis of interstitial cystitis. Int Urogynecol J Pelvic Floor Dysfunct 16:430–431, 2005.

Parsons CL: The role of the urinary epithelium in the pathogenesis of interstitial cystitis/prostatitis/urethritis. Urology 69(4 Suppl):S9–S16, 2007.

Parsons CL, Bullen M, Kahn BS, et al: Gynecologic presentation of interstitial cystitis as detected by intravesical potassium sensitivity. Obstet Gynecol 98:127–132, 2001.

Parsons CL, Dell JR, Stanford JL: Increased prevalence of interstitial cystitis: Previously unrecognized urologic and gynecologic cases identified using a new symptom questionnaire and intravesical potassium sensitivity. Urology 60:573–578, 2002.

Parsons CL, Housley T, Schmidt JD, et al: Treatment of interstitial cystitis with intravesical heparin. Br J Urol 73:504–507, 1994.

Parsons CL, Mulholland SG: Successful therapy of interstitial cystitis with pentosan-polysulfate. J Urol 138:513–516, 1987.

Pontari MA, Hanno PM: Oral therapies for interstitial cystitis. In Sant GR (ed): Interstitial Cystitis. Philadelphia, Lippincott-Raven, 1997, pp 173–176.

Sant G, Theoharides TC: The role of the mast cell in interstitial cystitis. Urol Clin North Am 21:41–53, 1994.

Sidman J, Lechtman MD, Lyster EG: A unique hypnotherapeutic approach to interstitial cystitis: A case report. J Reprod Med 54:523–524, 2009.

Taneja R: Intravesical lignocaine in the diagnosis of bladder pain syndrome. Int Urogynecol J 21:321–324, 2010.

van Ophoven A, Hertle L: Long-term results of amitriptyline treatment for interstitial cystitis. J Urol 174:1837–1840, 2005.

Webster DC, Brennan T: Self-care effectiveness and outcomes in women with interstitial cystitis: Implications for mental health clinicians. Issues Ment Health Nurs 19:495–519, 1998.

CHAPTER 113

Suprapubic Catheter Insertion and/or Change

Robert E. James • James R. Palleschi

Suprapubic catheters are normally used to provide short-term urinary drainage. If the patient's age or comorbid conditions preclude corrective surgery, the temporary catheter may be left in place or, with the aid of an exchange wire and appropriate dilators, may be replaced with a permanent suprapubic catheter.

Indications

- An impassable urethral stricture, bladder neck contracture, or obstruction
- Inability to pass a urethral catheter over an elevated bladder neck or an enlarged median lobe of the prostate gland
- Urethral trauma
- Recent urethral or bladder neck reconstructive surgery
- Inability to tolerate a urethral catheter and unwilling or unable to perform intermittent self-catheterization
- Bladder drainage required in the presence of a significant urethral or prostate infection
- Severe phimosis precluding the insertion of a urethral catheter (see Chapter 119, Dorsal Slit for Phimosis)

Contraindications

- Uncooperative patient
- Anticoagulated patient or patient with coagulopathy (either the anticoagulation/coagulopathy should be reversed or urology consulted)
- Cellulitis over the insertion site
- Surgical scar in suprapubic area, or bladder or pelvic anatomic abnormality from previous surgery, cancer, or trauma (small bowel may be interposed in the retropubic space; however, ultrasonographic guidance may be helpful for avoiding small bowel; see Chapter 225, Emergency Department, Hospitalist, and Office Ultrasonography [Clinical Ultrasonography])

Equipment

- Local anesthetic: 10-mL lidocaine 1% to 2%
- 10-mL syringe; $1\frac{1}{2}$-inch, 22-gauge spinal needle
- Antiseptic skin preparation (e.g., povidone–iodine)
- Sterile towels
- Sterile saline, to possibly fill the bladder, irrigate the catheter, or inflate a Foley bulb
- Mask and sterile gloves
- Mounted scalpel blade (no. 11 or no. 15)
- Suture scissors, needle holder, and 2-0 nylon suture
- Closed urinary drainage system
- Suprapubic catheter set

NOTE: There are many manufacturers of suprapubic catheters and insertion kits, including the Bonnano catheter (Becton-Dickinson Corp.), Stamey percutaneous suprapubic catheter set (Cook Medical/Urological), and the Simplastic suprapubic catheter/SupraFoley suprapubic catheter introducer (Rusch, Inc./Teleflex Medical).

The principal components of each set, except for the SupraFoley suprapubic catheter introducer, are a metal obturator and the suprapubic catheter. The metal obturator is placed down through the suprapubic catheter and is subsequently removed when the catheter is appropriately positioned within the bladder. The end of the catheter may consist of a *coudé tip (with balloon)*, *Malecot tip*, or *Foley*. Unlike the red rubber catheter (also known as the *Robinson*), which is not self-retaining, all of these catheters are equally effective in retaining themselves within the bladder (Fig. 113-1).

Preprocedure Patient Preparation

Explain the indications for, alternatives to, and risks of the procedure to the patient. Informed consent should be obtained. The patient should know what to expect during the procedure, including the need for injection of local anesthetic before the procedure. Also explain to the patient that mild to moderate suprapubic discomfort may be experienced for a few hours to days after this procedure.

Technique

1. Place the patient in the supine position. If the bladder is not palpable, either the procedure should be delayed until the bladder can be easily identified or else the insertion should be completed with ultrasonographic guidance (see Chapter 225, Emergency Department, Hospitalist, and Office Ultrasonography [Clinical Ultrasonography]).

   NOTE: If the patient has a bladder or pelvic anatomic abnormality from previous surgery, cancer, or trauma, the procedure should be performed only with the aid of ultrasonographic guidance.

2. Maintain sterile technique and observe universal blood and body fluid precautions. Prepare the suprapubic skin with an antiseptic solution and drape with sterile towels. Inject the local anesthetic into the skin overlying the abdominal wall, into the subcutaneous layer, into the fascia, and down to the dome of the bladder. After penetrating the subcutaneous layer, aspirate before injection to avoid intravascular injection.
3. With the scalpel, make a 1-cm horizontal skin incision (some clinicians also incise the anterior rectus fascia) 5 cm above the symphysis pubis in the midline (in both adult and pediatric patients). At this point, some clinicians prefer to pass a 22-gauge

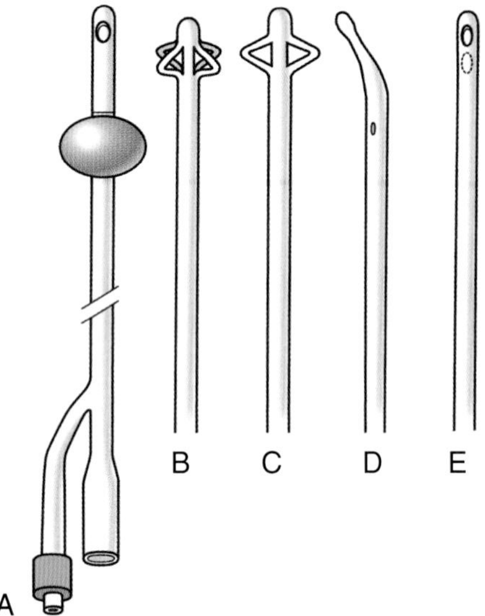

Figure 113-1 Commonly used catheters. **A,** Foley-type balloon catheter. **B,** Malecot self-containing, four-wing urethral catheter. **C,** Malecot self-retaining, two-wing catheter. **D,** Coudé hollow, olive-tip catheter. **E,** Robinson urethral catheter. (From Walsh PC, Retik AB, Vaughan ED Jr, Wein AJ [eds]: Campbell's Urology, 7th ed. Philadelphia, WB Saunders, 1998.)

spinal needle down and into the bladder. This will verify the bladder location before the suprapubic catheter is inserted. If the bladder is distended, this procedure is not necessary. If the bladder is not distended sufficiently to guide the obturator, the long needle can also be used to fill the bladder with sterile saline solution. Alternatively, ultrasonography can be used to determine if the bladder is full and for guidance.

4. Once the incision has been made, place the metal obturator into the lumen of the suprapubic catheter, with the sharp oblique end of the obturator extending beyond the tip of the catheter (Fig. 113-2). Advance the obturator and catheter together through the incision at a 60-degree caudal angle toward the bladder neck (approximately the mid-perineal area; Fig. 113-3). With momentary pressure, advance the catheter through the rectus sheath and muscle and into the dome of the bladder. This requires inserting it a total of approximately 5 cm below the skin in adults.
5. Advance the catheter and obturator an additional 5 cm in adults to ensure appropriate positioning. Remove the obturator; urine will be seen passing from the suprapubic catheter. After the obturator is removed, the wings of the Malecot type of catheter (Stamey suprapubic catheter) will expand, or the pigtail tip of the Bonnano catheter will coil inside the bladder to prevent it from falling out. If the catheter has a balloon tip, once it has been appropriately positioned within the bladder, inflate the balloon with sterile saline.

   Alternatively, the SupraFoley suprapubic catheter introducer consists of a plastic sheath, through which a sharp, plastic obturator is inserted. Advance the obturator through the incision and the rectus sheath, into the bladder. Then remove the obturator and advance a Foley catheter down through the plastic sheath into the bladder. The balloon is filled with 5 to 10 mL of water or saline. A tab is located on the top edge of the plastic sheath; pull down and remove it. This removes a strip of the sheath,

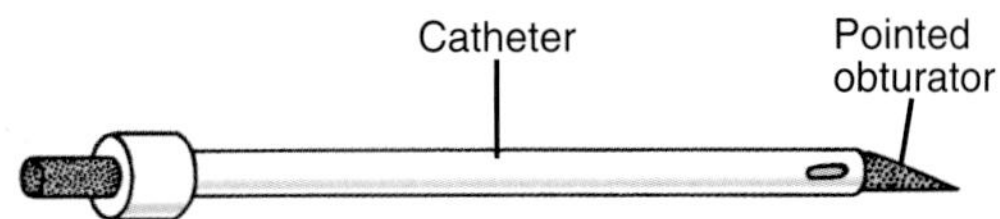

Figure 113-2 Suprapubic catheter with obturator in place.

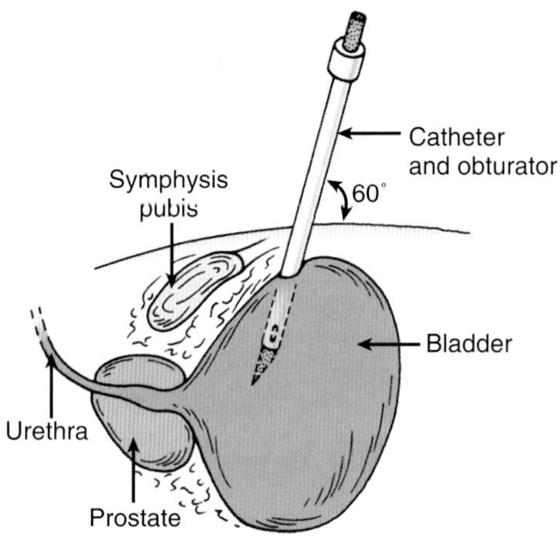

Figure 113-3 Insertion and advancement of the catheter and obturator.

   allowing the removal of the sheath and leaving the catheter in place in the bladder.
6. Pull back the catheter until the wings, coil, or balloon is resting against the dome of the bladder.
7. Secure the catheter in place with a nylon suture.
8. Using sterile saline, irrigate the catheter to ensure appropriate drainage and position.
9. Connect a drainage bag to the catheter, using an overnight or bedside drainage bag, leg bag, or abdominal drainage system (belly bag).

Complications

- Perivesicular bleeding
- Gross hematuria
- Failure to drain
- Infection
- Intestinal perforation (more likely when the bladder is not distended, when the normal anatomy is distorted by previous surgery, cancer, irradiation, or trauma, or when the obturator and catheter are not introduced at the correct angle; normally, a small perforation will seal spontaneously without consequence)

Suprapubic Catheter Replacement

Usually, a suprapubic catheter is replaced every 6 weeks, or whenever it is not draining properly. If the catheter has been in place for several weeks and a mature tract is established, the existing catheter may be removed and replaced with a similar catheter. First, place an obturator in the new catheter. Next, fill the bladder with sterile saline or water, and remove the catheter. The sterile water or saline will begin to pass through the suprapubic catheter site, and, consequently, the catheter needs to be replaced promptly. Advance the new catheter with obturator down the tract until the sterile water or saline begins to exit through or around the catheter. Usually a local anesthetic is not required.

If the catheter needs to be replaced before the tract is mature, the bladder should be filled with sterile saline or water before removing the catheter. If the catheter is obstructed, it should be removed and another catheter inserted once a distended bladder can be palpated. At that time, a new catheter may be inserted in the same tract, using the technique described previously. Ultrasonographic guidance should be used if the bladder cannot be positively identified or palpated.

With a Malecot or winged-tip catheter, frequently the wings are soft enough that they will retract as the catheter is removed. If there is difficulty removing the catheter, insert the obturator in the catheter to straighten the wings before removing the catheter. The tension in the pigtail is maintained by a silk suture that runs through the catheter and exits near its end. There it is tied around a small post. When the suture is cut or released, the pigtail will uncurl and can be removed.

If an open suprapubic cystotomy has been performed, a mature tract between the skin and the bladder usually is formed within 4 to 6 weeks. If the catheter must be replaced, select a similar-sized catheter. Normally, a catheter guide or obturator is not required. The new catheter should be introduced into the bladder immediately after removing the original one. After inflating the balloon with 5 to 10 mL of sterile saline, irrigate the bladder to ensure that the catheter is draining properly.

After catheter replacement, connect an overnight or bedside drainage bag, leg bag, or abdominal drainage system (belly bag).

Use of Antibiotics

For suprapubic catheter placement, if a urinary tract infection is suspected or the patient has a history of mitral valve prolapse, valvular heart disease or replacement, or a recent prosthesis such as a total knee or joint, a urine culture and sensitivity should be obtained and the patient placed on a broad-spectrum antibiotic for at least 3 days. If the patient is not allergic to fluoroquinolones, ciprofloxacin or levofloxacin is an appropriate choice.

Prophylactic antibiotic therapy is not required when changing a suprapubic catheter. If a clinically significant urinary tract infection is suspected, a specimen of urine should be obtained for a culture and sensitivity and an oral antibiotic ordered until the culture results are available. Appropriate choices, depending on the patient's allergy history, include nitrofurantoin or a fluoroquinolone.

Postprocedure Patient Education

Explain again to the patient that mild to moderate suprapubic discomfort may be experienced for a few hours to days after this procedure. As long as the catheter is in place, intermittent hematuria and irritating voiding symptoms may be present. The patient should know to take good care of the catheter system, to keep it clean and dry, and to not let the bag drag on the floor. Review additional catheter care, including the use of an overnight or bedside drainage bag, leg bag, or abdominal drainage system (belly bag). Once a day, the patient should wash his or her hands with soap and water and then use a clean, soapy washcloth to clean the catheter and the skin around it. Hydrogen peroxide should be useful for removing any crustiness that does not come off with soap and water. After washing with soap or peroxide, the catheter should be rinsed with clean water and patted dry. The patient should take care not to pull too much on the catheter. If the patient wants it, a slit gauze can be placed over the catheter. Tell the patient to contact the clinician if increasing pain, excessive bleeding, temperature greater than 101° F, or a nonfunctioning catheter is noticed.

After the catheter is removed, patients should be aware that they will have lost some of the ability to sense a full bladder; therefore, they should urinate every 2 hours for 1 to 2 weeks, even after going to bed. They should drink plenty of fluids, but not force them, and they should refrain from fluids for 2 hours before going to bed. Patients should expect the site to drain small amounts of urine for a few days, so they should keep it covered with gauze. They should clean the site with soap and water at least once a day.

CPT/Billing Codes

51010 Insertion of a percutaneous suprapubic catheter
51705 Changing a cystostomy tube (suprapubic catheter), simple

ICD-9-CM Diagnostic Codes

596.0 Bladder neck contracture/obstruction
596.54 Neurogenic bladder, NOS
597.80 Urethritis, unspecified
598.9 Urethral stricture, unspecified
599.60 Urinary obstruction, unspecified
600.91 Hyperplasia of prostate, unspecified, with urinary obstruction
601.0 Acute prostatitis
602.8 Prostatic stricture
605 Phimosis
867.0 Urethral and bladder injury, with no open wound
867.1 Urethral and bladder injury, with open wound into cavity

Suppliers

(See contact information online at www.expertconsult.com.)

BD Bonnano suprapubic trays and kits
Becton-Dickinson Corp.

Stamey percutaneous suprapubic catheter kit and many other suprapubic catheter sets
Cook Medical/Urological

Simplastic, SupraFoley suprapubic catheters and introducers
Rusch Inc. (Teleflex Medical)

Online Resources

Cincinnati Children's Hospital: Kidney, Bladder and Genitals Home Care. (Patient education.) Available at www.cincinnatichildrens.org/health/info/urinary/home/suprapubic.htm.

Medline Plus: Urinary catheters. (Patient education.) Available at www.nlm.nih.gov/medlineplus/ency/article/003981.htm.

University of Maryland Center: Urinary catheters—overview. (Patient education.) Available at www.umm.edu/ency/article/003981.htm.

Bibliography

Carter BH: Instrumentation and endoscopy. In Walsh PC, Retik AB, Vaughan ED Jr, Wein AJ (eds): Campbell's Urology, 7th ed. Philadelphia, WB Saunders, 1998, pp 159–169.

McPhail MJ, Abu-Hilal M, Johnson CD: A meta-analysis comparing suprapubic and transurethral catheterization for bladder drainage after abdominal surgery. Br J Surg 93:1038–1044, 2006.

Niel-Weise BS, van den Broek PJ: Urinary catheter policies for short-term bladder drainage in adults. Cochrane Database Syst Rev 3:CD004203, 2005.

Wen CC, Babayan RK: Instrumentation of the lower urinary tract. In Siroky MB, Oates RD, Babayan RK (eds): Handbook of Urology: Diagnosis and Therapy, 3rd ed. Philadelphia, Lippincott Williams & Wilkins, 2004, pp 63–78.

CHAPTER 114

SUPRAPUBIC TAP OR ASPIRATION

Robert E. James • James R. Palleschi

Suprapubic aspiration is a valuable diagnostic procedure, and, occasionally, it may even be a valuable therapeutic tool. In most cases, suprapubic aspiration can be performed safely at the bedside or in the clinician's office. (For insertion of suprapubic catheters, see Chapter 113, Suprapubic Catheter Insertion and/or Change.)

To review the anatomy, clinicians should be aware that the dome of the bladder has peritoneal attachments and that needle penetration into this area can cause injury to bowel or an intraperitoneal bladder perforation. The colon lies posterior and inferior to the bladder, so the clinician should avoid advancing the needle through both walls of the bladder. Alongside the bladder, in the pelvis, lie significant vascular structures, including the common iliac and hypogastric vessels. Aspiration in this area may lead to inadvertent and significant hemorrhage.

A properly directed needle will penetrate only the skin and subcutaneous tissue of the lower anterior abdominal wall, the rectus sheath, the peritoneum, and the anterior bladder wall.

INDICATIONS

- Collection of a urine specimen for analysis, culture, and sensitivity using sterile technique
- Temporary relief of acute urinary retention in patient not able to be catheterized

CONTRAINDICATIONS

- Anticoagulated patient or patient with coagulopathy (either the anticoagulation/coagulopathy should be reversed or urology consulted)
- An uncooperative patient (see Chapter 2, Procedural Sedation and Analgesia)
- Infection or cellulitis of the suprapubic area
- Full bladder not palpable*
- Patient not able to lay supine or have his or her bladder palpated*
- Surgical scar in suprapubic area, or bladder or pelvic anatomic abnormality from previous surgery, cancer, or trauma (small bowel may be interposed in the retropubic space)*
- Abnormalities of genitourinary anatomy, enlargement of pelvic organs (e.g., ovarian cysts, uterine fibroids), distention or enlargement of abdominal viscera (including intestinal obstruction)*

EQUIPMENT

- Local anesthetic: 10 mL lidocaine 1%
- Needles:
  - *For anesthetic:* 1½-inch, 25- to 30-gauge needle
  - *Localization needle:* 4-inch, 22-gauge spinal needle
  - *Aspiration needle:* In most cases, the localization needle will be sufficiently large to obtain an adequate urine specimen. If not, an 18- or 20-gauge intravenous needle may be used.
- 10-mL syringe
- Microscope slide for direct examination, methylene blue, and Gram's stain
- Sterile urine culture collection container

*Ultrasonographic guidance may allow suprapubic aspiration to be performed in these situations and may be helpful for avoiding complications (see Chapter 225, Emergency Department, Hospitalist, and Office Ultrasonography [Clinical Ultrasonography]).

PREPROCEDURE PATIENT PREPARATION

Review the purpose of the procedure, risks, alternatives, and the technique with the patient and family. The patient may experience some pain in the suprapubic area with injection of the local anesthetic and during the procedure. He or she may also experience some hematuria for 24 to 48 hours after this procedure. Obtain informed consent.

TECHNIQUE

1. Place the patient in the supine position on the examination table. Examine the suprapubic area by palpation and percussion to identify the distended bladder. If the distended bladder cannot be identified positively, the procedure should be delayed until the bladder can be identified, or the procedure may be performed with ultrasonographic guidance.
2. Cleanse the suprapubic area with an antiseptic solution and drape in a sterile fashion. Maintain the sterile technique and observe universal blood and body fluid precautions.
3. In the midline, anesthetize the skin approximately 2 inches above the symphysis pubis (in both the adult and the pediatric patient). Next, inject sequentially down to the fascia and bladder, aspirating each time before injection. In the adult, usually 10 mL is required to anesthetize the skin, abdominal wall, and abdominal bladder. In a child, the same can be accomplished with 3 to 5 mL of anesthetic.
4. Direct the 22-gauge spinal needle caudad toward the bladder neck, with the obturator in place (Fig. 114-1), through the anesthetized skin at a 60-degree angle to the skin. If the bladder is distended, the needle will enter the abdominal bladder after it has been advanced approximately 2 inches in the adult.
5. Remove the obturator and connect a sterile syringe (Fig. 114-2) to aspirate urine from the bladder. If urine is not obtained, slowly advance the needle, applying continuous suction on the syringe. If the specimen cannot be obtained after advancing the needle an additional 2 inches, terminate the procedure and start again, as described previously, but direct the needle at a 50-degree angle to the skin. If you are unsuccessful a second time, the procedure should be delayed until the bladder is further distended, or the procedure should be performed with ultrasonographic guidance. If continued difficulties are encountered, a urology consultation should be obtained.

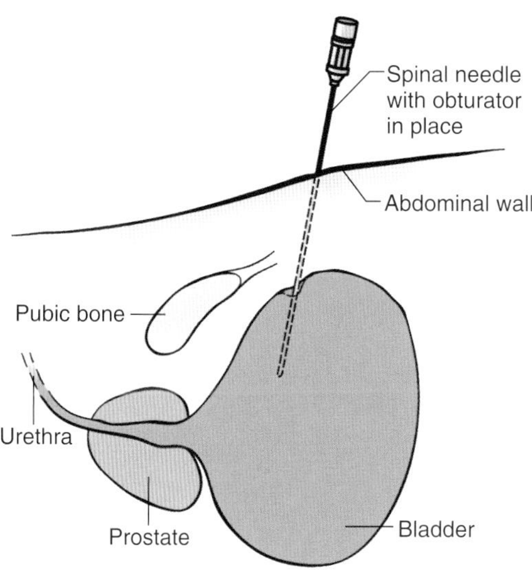

Figure 114-1 Insertion of the spinal needle with the obturator in place.

Complications

- Transient hematuria
- Perivesicular hematoma
- Intestinal perforation (if this occurs with a 22-gauge needle, it should seal spontaneously and not be a problem)

Postprocedure Patient Education

The patient may have some discomfort or soreness in the area for a day or so, which should be relieved by acetaminophen or a nonsteroidal anti-inflammatory drug. The patient should notify the clinician in case of persistent (lasting longer than 2 days) or increasing blood in the urine, increasing abdominal pain, difficulty urinating, or a temperature above 101° F.

CPT/Billing Code

51000 Suprapubic bladder aspiration by needle

ICD-9-CM Diagnostic Codes

599.0 Urinary tract infection, site not specified
780.6 Fever

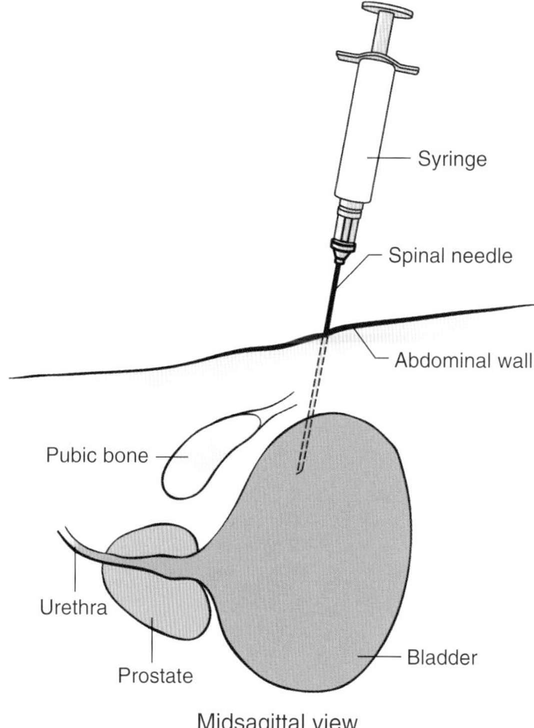

Figure 114-2 Connection of the syringe to aspirate urine from the bladder.

788.20 Urinary retention or stasis, unspecified
995.91 Sepsis
995.92 Severe sepsis (acute organ dysfunction)

BIBLIOGRAPHY

Hagen IK: Instrumental examination of the urinary tract. In Smith DR (ed): General Urology. East Norwalk, Conn, Lange Medical Publications, 1984.

Nguyen HT: Bacterial infections of the genitourinary tract. In Tanagho EA, MacAninch JW (eds): Smith's General Urology, 17th ed. New York, McGraw-Hill, 2008, pp 203–227.

Roth DR: Suprapubic aspiration. Emedicine, February 10, 2006; updated April 5, 2009. Available at http://emedicine.medscape.com/article/82964-overview.

Stokes S III, Kulkarni A: Suprapubic bladder aspiration. In Reichman EF, Simon RR (eds): Emergency Medicine Procedures. New York, McGraw-Hill, 2004, pp 1128–1133.

CHAPTER 115

Bedside Urodynamic Studies

Jeffrey R. Dell

The diagnosis and management of urinary incontinence and voiding dysfunction (e.g., frequency, dysuria, retention) are often challenging. Urinary incontinence has many etiologies, but it is most often the result of urethral incompetence *(genuine stress incontinence)*, detrusor instability *(urge incontinence)*, a combination of both *(mixed incontinence)*, or poor bladder emptying *(overflow incontinence)*. Urodynamic testing, specifically the cystometrogram, is used to demonstrate and differentiate among these conditions. Establishing the correct diagnosis is critical for developing an effective management plan. Although the patient history and physical examination may provide preliminary data regarding the underlying cause of incontinence or other urinary tract dysfunction, urodynamic testing provides an objective assessment while increasing the sensitivity and specificity of the diagnostic work-up.

Urodynamics is the study of the hydrodynamics and muscle activity of the lower urinary tract, with cystometry and uroflowmetry being the mainstays. Cystometry assesses the filling–storage phase by measuring the pressure–volume relationship of the bladder as it distends and contracts. It helps diagnose abnormalities of detrusor activity, sensation, capacity, and compliance. In contrast, uroflowmetry evaluates the voiding phase by measuring the urine volume voided over time. The combination of cystometry and uroflowmetry allows detection of both anatomic (obstructive) and physiologic (functional) voiding abnormalities.

Studies have shown that bedside (simple) urodynamic testing has a sensitivity of *up to 75%* for the correct diagnosis in the evaluation of urinary incontinence. It is easy to perform and cost effective in the office setting, and is frequently performed by the office personnel. A correlation of these test results with the patient history and physical examination usually determines the cause of urinary incontinence or other voiding dysfunction. Most conservative management protocols can be initiated on the basis of these results alone, without the need for formal multichannel urodynamic studies (see Chapter 116, Urodynamic Testing [Multichannel]).

However, in certain patients, greater sensitivity or specificity or more precise measurements may be needed. Examples include patients with diabetes; individuals with neurologic disorders; and patients needing surgery for incontinence, especially if they are at high surgical risk. Male patients also frequently require multichannel urodynamic testing. Additional examples include following pelvic radiation or surgery or for patients with incontinence and a confusing diagnosis or mixed etiology. Incontinence after failed surgery for incontinence or failing routine treatment or where the treatment progress needs to be monitored quantitatively may require more precise measurements. For all of these situations, formal uroflowmetry or formal cystometry is indicated, each being a part of formal multichannel urodynamic testing.

Indications

- Urinary incontinence
- Overactive bladder symptoms (urgency, frequency, nocturia, enuresis)
- Urinary retention or incomplete bladder emptying (ultrasonography can also be used to determine postvoid residuals; see Chapter 225, Emergency Department, Hospitalist, and Office Ultrasonography [Clinical Ultrasonography])
- Pelvic pain
- Painful voiding syndromes

Contraindications

- Active cystitis
- Recurrent cystitis or gross hematuria (after cystoscopy and imaging have ruled out malignancy and stones, bedside urodynamics may be helpful)
- Intolerance of urethral catheterization
- Uncooperative patient
- Formal, multichannel urodynamic testing indicated (see Chapter 116, Urodynamic Testing [Multichannel])

Patients with active cystitis, recurrent cystitis, or gross hematuria should be evaluated and treated before urodynamic testing. Patients unable to tolerate urethral catheterization in the office or who are uncooperative are not candidates for bedside urodynamic testing.

Equipment

See Figure 115-1.

- Nonsterile gloves
- Stopwatch
- Graduated voiding container
- Iodine swabs
- Water-based lubricating gel (nonanesthetic)
- 14-Fr red rubber urinary catheter
- Sterile urine specimen container
- Urinalysis Chemstrips
- 50-mL catheter-tip syringe with bulb or plunger removed
- 500 mL of room-temperature sterile saline or sterile water
- Sterile cotton-tipped swab with anesthetic gel

Preprocedure Patient Preparation

All patients should be counseled regarding the indications, techniques, alternatives, and complications associated with urethral catheterization and bedside urodynamics. Clear communication and instructions should improve patient comfort during testing and thereby improve the results obtained. Patients should be instructed to come to the office with a full bladder to maximize information obtained from initial uroflowmetry. Each step of the procedure should be explained to the patient before proceeding.

Technique

Clinicians should follow universal blood and body fluid precautions when performing this procedure.

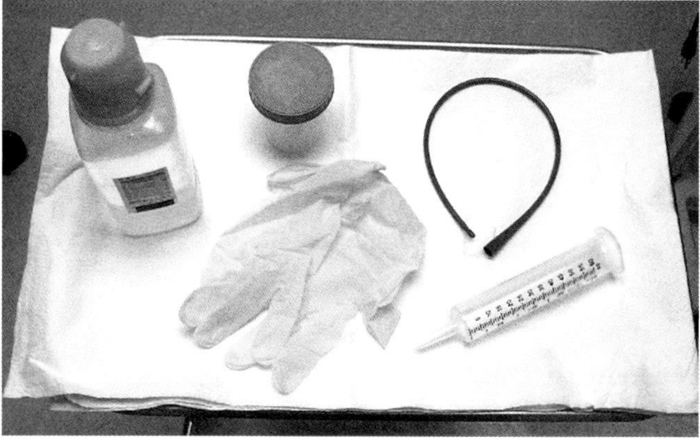

Figure 115-1 Equipment used for urodynamic testing.

Simple Uroflowmetry

1. The patient's bladder should be very full. If not, provide fluids and time for the patient to fill the bladder. Because urine flow parameters depend on the volume voided, the patient needs to be able to void at least 200 mL for this test to be reliable.
2. In a relaxed, private setting, tell the patient to void into a graduated container in hand or placed over the commode. The total time to void is recorded with the stopwatch, the total volume voided measured, and both are documented.

Simple Cystometry

3. After the patient has voided, clean the external urethral meatus with iodine swabs and insert the lubricated tip of the urinary catheter into the bladder lumen. Drain the residual urine into the sterile specimen container and record the postvoid residual volume. After completion of the cystometry and cough stress test, perform a urinalysis on this specimen to rule out urinary tract infection. In patients with a positive urinalysis, send the specimen for urine culture.
4. With the urinary catheter in place, attach the 50-mL syringe (with bulb or plunger removed) to the proximal end of the urinary catheter and hold it approximately 15 cm above the pubic symphysis. Fill the bladder by slowly pouring the sterile saline or sterile water through the open-top syringe in increments of 50 mL (Fig. 115-2). Take care to keep the tip of the catheter within the bladder lumen (i.e., avoid withdrawing it into the urethra).
5. During filling, ask the patient to report when he or she feels the first sensation of fullness and then the first urge to void, as well as when he or she has reached maximum bladder capacity. Record the total volume infused for each of these sensations.
6. Observe the water level in the syringe during filling; it should fall steadily. A sudden rise in the water level with or without associated urgency or incontinence may indicate an uninhibited detrusor contraction or detrusor instability (Fig. 115-3). Other causes of a "water hiccup" may be artifact (e.g., Valsalva maneuver, cough by the patient) or the catheter tip slipping into the proximal urethra.

Cough and Valsalva Stress Tests

7. After the bladder is filled to maximum capacity, remove the catheter and examine the patient in the supine dorsolithotomy position. The patient is asked to cough or perform a Valsalva maneuver, and the external urethral meatus is observed for signs of urine leakage. Abrupt urine leakage with a cough suggests *stress urinary incontinence*, whereas prolonged leakage after cessation of the cough indicates cough-induced *detrusor instability*. In women, if urinary leakage is observed in the vagina from the anterior vaginal wall, a *vesicovaginal fistula* should be considered.
8. Repeat the test with the patient standing.

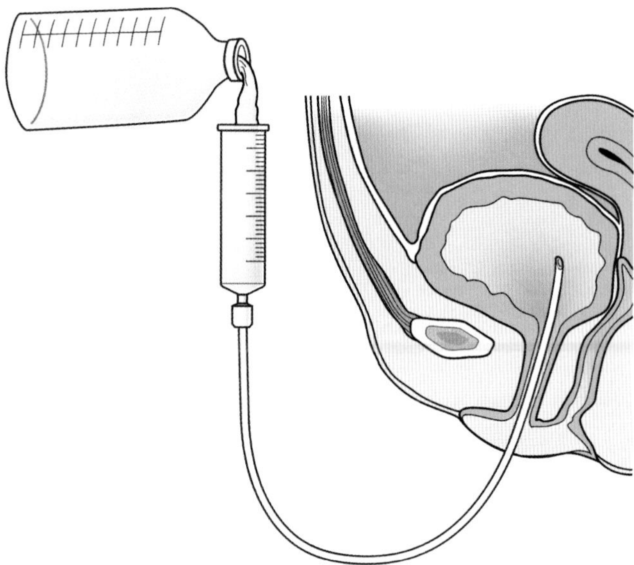

Figure 115-2 Cystometry.

Cotton Swab Test (Q-Tip Test) for Women

9. After the supine and standing cough stress test, place the patient in the supine dorsolithotomy position and reexamine her. Insert a cotton-tipped swab with anesthetic gel into the urethra until resistance is overcome; this indicates its position at the bladder neck. Record the swab resting angle relative to the horizontal plane. Ask the patient to cough or perform a Valsalva maneuver again, and measure the maximum angle of

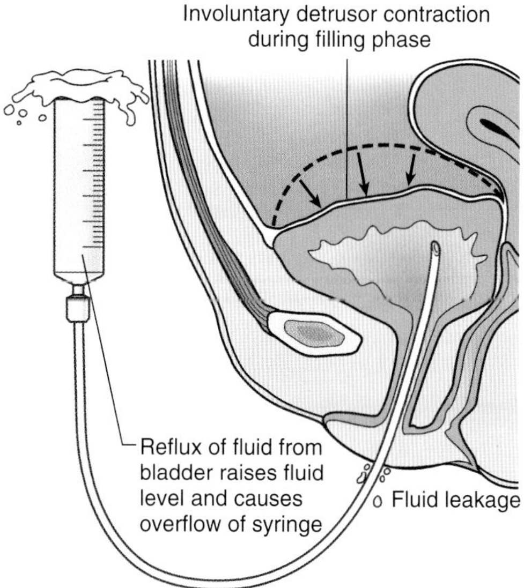

Figure 115-3 Involuntary detrusor contraction.

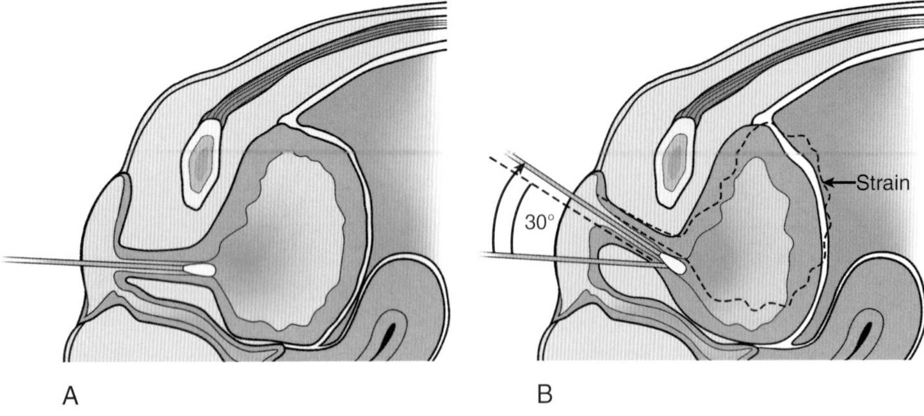

Figure 115-4 Cotton swab test for ureterovesical junction mobility. **A,** Cotton swab at rest. **B,** Cotton swab with strain (Valsalva).

deflection. The difference between this value and the resting angle is the *angle of change*. An angle of change of greater than 30 degrees indicates *urethral hypermobility* (Fig. 115-4).

Measurement of Postvoid Residual

10. Next, instruct the patient to void into the graduated container. Measure and record the amount voided (total void).
11. Determine a second postvoid residual by subtracting the measured total void from the maximum bladder capacity noted on filling cystometry.

Complications

- Urinary tract infection (rare)
- Transient gross hematuria
- Urethral discomfort, transient
- Pelvic pain, transient

Bedside urodynamics are associated with few complications. In rare cases, patients may develop a urinary tract infection after the procedure. These patients should be treated accordingly. Routine prophylactic antibiotics after the procedure are not usually indicated.

Transient gross hematuria may be noted after the procedure, especially after a difficult catheterization in a postmenopausal woman with urethral atrophy. This usually resolves spontaneously within 48 hours. Some patients may complain of urethral discomfort or pelvic pain after testing. These symptoms are usually self-limited, but these patients may benefit from a short course of phenazopyridine (Pyridium). Cystoscopy-urethroscopy should be considered in patients with hematuria or lower urinary tract pain that persists beyond 48 to 72 hours (see Chapter 111, Diagnostic Cystourethroscopy).

Interpretations of Results

Uroflowmetry with measurement of a postvoid residual assesses bladder emptying and evaluates for overflow incontinence. Most experts consider uroflowmetry to be normal if the patient *voids at least 200 mL in the course of 15 to 20 seconds*. More specific normal flow rates have been determined by age and sex (Abrams and Torrens, 1979). For men younger than 40 years, between 40 and 60 years, and older than 60 years of age, normal rates are 22 mL/sec, 18 mL/sec, and 13 mL/sec, respectively. In women younger than 50 years of age, the flow rate be should be greater than 25 mL/sec; for women older than 50 years of age, it should be greater than 18 mL/sec. The normal flow pattern (volume over time) is bell-shaped and continuous. Prolonged voiding times may indicate an obstructed voiding pattern resulting from increased outlet resistance (*e.g., urethral obstruction, external sphincter dyssynergia)* or poor propulsive force *(detrusor dysfunction)*. An interrupted pattern suggests straining to void or lack of coordination between detrusor muscle contraction and sphincter relaxation.

Cystometry evaluates bladder function, including sensation, compliance, and detrusor activity during filling. Most patients experience a *first sensation of filling at 100 to 150 mL, first urge to void at 200 to 350 mL*, and *maximum bladder capacity at 400 to 550 mL*. *Urge incontinence* should be considered in patients with reduced bladder capacity, with or without a spontaneous detrusor contraction and coexisting overactive bladder symptoms. Patients with increased bladder capacity should be evaluated for a *neurogenic bladder*. *Urge incontinence from detrusor instability* is documented when an involuntary contraction results in an overflow of the filling syringe (see Fig. 115-3). A cystometrogram is the best method for differentiating between bladder outlet obstruction and poor detrusor muscle contractility.

Normal values for a postvoid residual are not universally established, but various experts have defined *a normal postvoid residual measurement as less than 200 mL and less than 20% of the total void*. Patients with urinary frequency or incontinence and a normal postvoid residual have a bladder storage problem, and this can result from disorders of bladder compliance, involuntary bladder contractions, bladder hypersensitivity, or bladder outlet abnormalities. Bladder outlet abnormalities can be due to lack of support, fibrosis, or neurologic insult.

A positive cough stress test indicates *genuine stress incontinence* (GSI). In patients with GSI and a positive Q-Tip test, *urethral hypermobility* is suspected. In patients with GSI and a fixed urethra on Q-Tip test, *intrinsic sphincter deficiency* is the presumed diagnosis. These patients require complex multichannel urodynamics for further evaluation (see Chapter 116, Urodynamic Testing [Multichannel]).

Postprocedure Patient Education

The results of the testing and various management options should be discussed in detail with the patient. Patients should be instructed to call the clinician's office for pain or hematuria lasting longer than 48 hours and for symptoms of a urinary tract infection. Patients with persistent incontinence despite conservative therapy are candidates for complex urodynamics.

CPT/Billing Codes

51725 Simple cystometrogram (e.g., spinal manometer)
51736 Simple (nonelectronic) uroflowmetry (e.g., stopwatch flow rate, mechanical uroflowmeter)
81000 Urinalysis, by dip stick or tablet reagent

ICD-9-CM Diagnostic Codes

595.0 Cystitis, acute
619.0 Vesicovaginal fistula
625.6 Incontinence, stress, female
625.9 Unspecified symptom associated with female genital organs (i.e., pelvic pain)
788.1 Dysuria
788.21 Incomplete bladder emptying
788.30 Urinary incontinence, unspecified
788.31 Incontinence, urge
788.32 Incontinence, stress, male
788.33 Incontinence, mixed (male or female)
788.36 Nocturnal enuresis
788.41 Urinary frequency

Acknowledgment

The editors wish to recognize the many contributions by Neeraj Kohli, MD, and Judy Wynn Neff, RN, BSN, to this chapter in a previous edition of this text.

ONLINE RESOURCES

Agency for Health Care Research and Quality: Urinary Incontinence in Adults: Clinical Practice Guideline Update. (Patient information on incontinence from the AHCRQ.) Available at www.ahrq.gov/clinic/uiovervw.htm.

National Institute of Diabetes and Digestive and Kidney Diseases. (Information on a wide range of topics on urologic conditions from the National Kidney and Urologic Diseases Information Clearinghouse and National Institutes of Health.) Available at www.niddk.nih.gov.

BIBLIOGRAPHY

Abrams PH, Torrens MJ: Urine flow studies. Urol Clin North Am 6:71–79, 1979.

Berni KC, Cummings JM: Urodynamic evaluation of the older adult: Bench to bedside. Clin Geriatr Med 20:477–487, 2004.

Fantl A, Newman DK, Colling J, et al. Urinary incontinence in adults: Acute and chronic management. Clinical Practice Guideline No. 2, 1996 update. AHCPR publication no. 96-0682. Rockville, Md, Agency for Health Care Policy and Research, U.S. Department of Health and Human Services, 1996.

Holroyd-Leduc JM, Tannenbaum C, Thorpe KE, Straus SE: What type of urinary incontinence does this woman have? JAMA 299:1446–1456, 2008.

Kohli N, Karram MM: Urodynamic evaluation for female urinary incontinence. Clin Obstet Gynecol 41:672–690, 1998.

CHAPTER 116

Urodynamic Testing (Multichannel)

Jeffrey R. Dell • Grant C. Fowler

Incontinence, dysuria, urinary retention and frequency, and other urinary symptoms are common problems among a growing population, the elderly. Given the broad range of etiologic factors that can cause incontinence (Box 116-1) and other urinary symptoms, accurate diagnosis is the cornerstone for formulating an effective treatment plan. In addition to a careful history and physical examination, urodynamic testing—the study of hydrodynamics and muscle activity to define the functional status of the lower urinary tract—can quantify abnormalities in order to make an accurate diagnosis. Urodynamic testing is also useful for objective assessment of patient improvement after a prescribed treatment protocol.

Although simple urodynamics (see Chapter 115, Bedside Urodynamic Studies), which can be performed in the office setting and provide objective qualitative data, are useful for conservative treatment in the uncomplicated patient, some patients require more precise quantitative analysis of lower urinary tract function. Formal, multichannel urodynamics (MCUD) provides specific quantitative information about detrusor and urethral function during filling, storage, and emptying of urine.

MCUD involves the simultaneous measurement of pressure from multiple sites during bladder filling and emptying and allows precise measurement of intravesical, intraurethral, and intra-abdominal pressure (Fig. 116-1). *Complex uroflowmetry* measures and graphs urine volume voided over time, allowing detection of anatomic (obstructive) and physiologic (functional) voiding abnormalities. *Complex cystometry*, a filling test of the bladder, measures and graphs the pressure–volume relationship of the bladder as it distends and contracts, determining abnormalities of detrusor activity, sensation, capacity, and compliance consistent with urge incontinence or detrusor instability. *Urethral pressure profilometry* evaluates the urethral continence mechanism as a possible cause of stress urinary incontinence (SUI). *Pressure–flow studies* allow determination and quantification of a patient's voiding mechanism, helping establish the etiology of voiding dysfunction. *Electromyography (EMG)* evaluates contractile activity and innervation of the perineal muscles involved with voiding. *Bethanechol testing* can be used to diagnose a neurogenic bladder. If a contrast medium is used for the infusion, a *voiding cystourethrogram* can be performed.

When performing MCUD, bladder (P_{ves}) and urethral (P_{ura}) pressures are measured directly with a single intravesical catheter that contains two microtransducers, one located in the bladder and the other in the urethra. A separate, single microtransducer catheter is placed in either the rectum or the vagina and indirectly measures simultaneous intra-abdominal pressure (P_{abd}). Detrusor pressure (P_{det}) and urethral closure pressure (P_{ucp}) are derived from electronic subtraction of one measured pressure from a second measured pressure. Detrusor pressure is derived by subtracting intra-abdominal pressure from intravesical pressure ($P_{det} = P_{ves} - P_{abd}$), whereas urethral closure pressure is the difference between urethral pressure and intravesical pressure ($P_{ucp} = P_{ura} - P_{ves}$; Fig. 116-2).

Box 116-1. Differential Diagnosis of Urinary Incontinence

Genitourinary
- Genuine stress incontinence
- Detrusor instability (idiopathic)
- Detrusor hyperreflexia (neurologic)
- Mixed incontinence
- Overflow incontinence
- Fistula (vesical, ureteral, urethral)
- Congenital abnormalities (ectopic ureter)

Nongenitourinary
- Functional
- Neurologic
- Cognitive
- Environmental
- Pharmacologic
- Metabolic

Definitions

Valsalva leak point pressure (VLPP): The pressure required to open the urethra.

Urethral pressure profile (UPP): The pressure along the functional length of the urethra. The maximal urethral closure pressure (MUCP) is recorded as maximal pressure minus the baseline urethral pressure (P_{ura}). It reflects the highest pressure the sphincter has at rest in order to keep it closed.

Intravesical pressure (P_{ves}): The pressure within the bladder.

Intra-abdominal pressure (P_{abd}): The pressure surrounding the bladder. It is approximated by the pressure within the rectum or the vagina.

Detrusor pressure (P_{det}): The component of the intravesical pressure that is created from the force in the bladder wall alone. It is estimated by subtracting intra-abdominal pressure from intravesical pressure. The simultaneous measurement of both intra-abdominal and intravesical pressure is required to obtain this measurement.

Urethral pressure (P_{ura}): The pressure within the urethra, which reflects both the urethral closure pressure and the vesical pressure.

Functional bladder capacity: The amount of urine the bladder can hold under natural conditions.

Cystometric capacity: A subjective measure of the total volume of fluid the patient can tolerate comfortably during bladder filling.

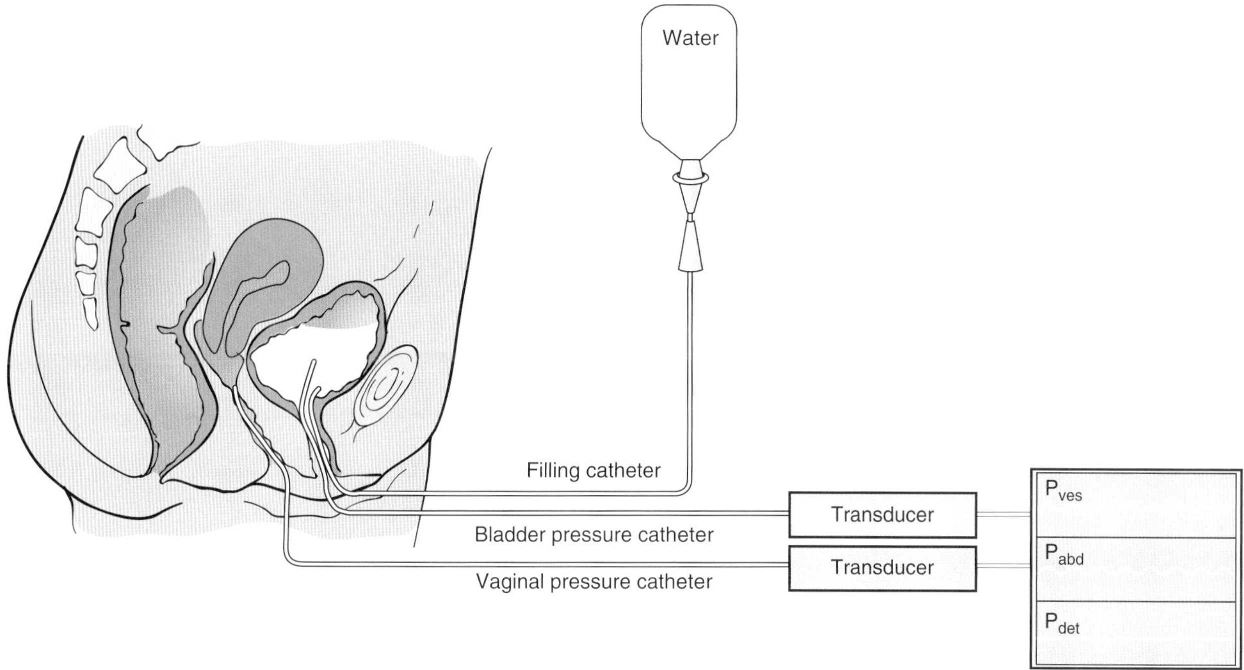

Figure 116-1 Multichannel urodynamics (MCUD) with measurement of vesical and abdominal pressure using separate catheters. P_{abd}, intra-abdominal pressure; P_{det}, detrusor pressure; P_{ves}, bladder pressure.

Indications

History

- Mixed incontinence
- Unclear etiology of incontinence
- Continuous leakage
- Coexisting neurologic disorder or diabetes
- Male patients (frequently require MCUD)

After Bedside Urodynamic Studies

- Simple cystometry or flowmetry that is ambiguous or inconclusive
- Mixed incontinence results
- Failure of treatment based on bedside urodynamics results

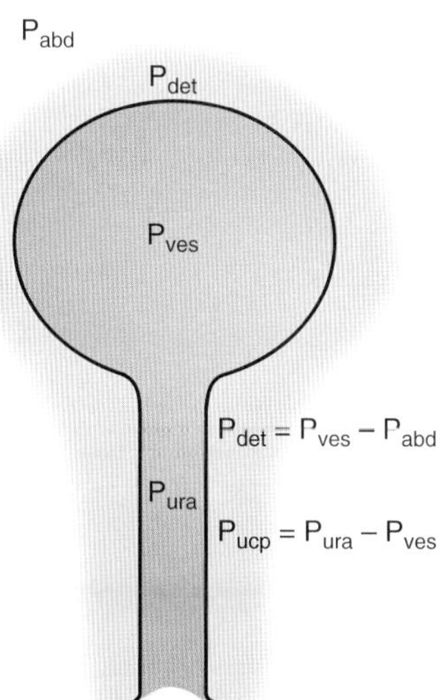

Figure 116-2 Mathematical formulas deriving detrusor pressure and urethral closure pressure from multichannel urodynamics measurements. P_{abd}, intra-abdominal pressure; P_{det}, detrusor pressure; P_{ucp}, urethral closure pressure; P_{ura}, urethral pressure; P_{ves}, bladder pressure.

Stress Incontinence

- Before surgical correction (especially if patient is high surgical risk)
- Potential SUI with significant pelvic prolapse
- Recurrent incontinence after previous surgery for SUI

Therapeutic Failures

- Urge incontinence
- Frequency, urgency, and pain syndrome
- Nocturnal enuresis

Miscellaneous

- Lower urinary tract dysfunction after pelvic radiation
- Lower urinary tract dysfunction after radical pelvic surgery
- To monitor treatment precisely

Contraindications

- Untreated cystitis
- Unevaluated and untreated gross hematuria
- Uncooperative patient
- Inability to tolerate urinary catheterization

There are few contraindications to MCUD. Patients with active cystitis or gross hematuria should be evaluated and treated before urodynamic testing. Patients who are unable to tolerate urethral catheterization or are uncooperative in the office setting should not be considered candidates for MCUD testing.

Equipment

- Nonsterile gloves
- Commode with attached uroflowmetry instrument
- Adjustable urodynamics chair (recommended)
- Urodynamics unit (includes cystometer and uroflowmeter) with printer
- Microtip or dual-lumen measuring catheters

- Intravenous pole with 1-L bag of room-temperature infusion solution (sterile water, saline, lactated Ringer's solution, or radiographic contrast media)
- Iodine swabs
- Water-based lubricating gel (nonanesthetic)
- Red rubber urinary catheter or 14-Fr straight catheter
- Sterile urine specimen container
- Urinalysis Chemstrips
- Roll of tape (to secure the measuring catheters in place)
- Large cotton-tipped applicators or vaginal speculum (to reduce uterine prolapse)

Preprocedure Patient Preparation

All patients should be counseled regarding the indications, techniques, and complications associated with urethral catheterization (see the sample patient education form available online at www.expertconsult.com). Clear communication and instructions improve patient comfort during testing, thereby improving the results obtained. Patients should be instructed to come to the office with a full bladder to maximize information obtained from initial uroflowmetry. Each step of the procedure should be carefully explained to the patient before proceeding. Drug allergies should be noted before prescribing prophylactic antibiotics or phenazopyridine. Patients will be asked about symptoms and their usual voiding pattern during the testing.

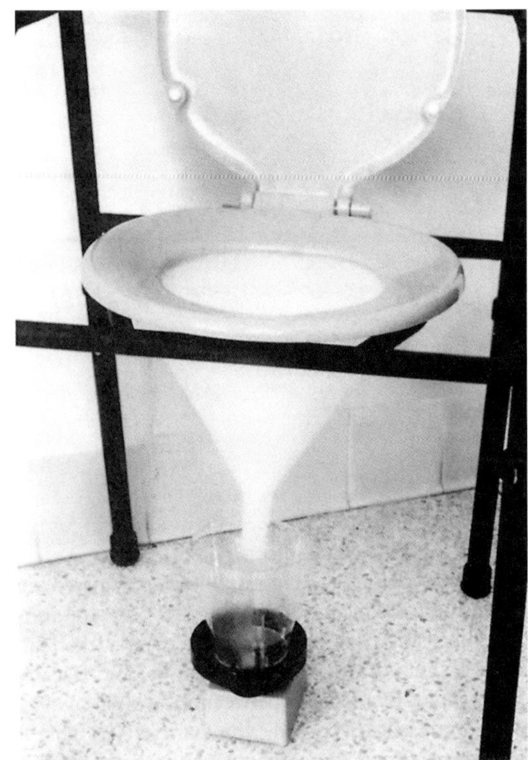

Figure 116-3 Typical complex uroflowmetry setup with commode and uroflow instrument.

Technique

Clinicians should follow universal blood and body fluid precautions when performing this procedure. Because the primary goal of MCUD is to reproduce and quantify the patient's symptoms, patients should be asked if their usual voiding pattern and their symptoms are reproduced during testing.

Complex Uroflowmetry

1. The patient is asked to come to the office with a full bladder because urine flow parameters depend on the volume voided (the patient should void at least 150 mL, and preferably 200 mL, for the test to provide reliable data).
2. In a relaxed, private setting, the patient is instructed to void into a commode with a uroflow instrument attached (Fig. 116-3). Uroflowmetry measurements, including time and flow rate, are recorded with the urodynamic unit set to "uroflowmetry."

Complex Cystometry

3. After the patient has voided, place him or her in the sitting position and cleanse the external urethral meatus with iodine swabs. Insert the lubricated tip of the red rubber catheter into the bladder lumen. The residual urine is drained into the sterile specimen container and the postvoid residual volume is recorded. The red rubber catheter is then removed and dipstick urinalysis is routinely performed. In patients with a positive test for leukocytes, MCUD should be postponed until after treatment of the urinary tract infection. The catheterized specimen may be sent for urine culture.
4. Turn on the urodynamic unit and printer and attach the pressure catheters to the appropriate channels. Connect the bladder catheter infusion port to the intravenous tubing of the infusion solution, which is attached to a water pump to regulate flow (Fig. 116-4).
5. Calibrate the urodynamic unit by flushing all bubbles from the catheters with infusion solution and setting all channels to zero. Introduce the bladder catheter into the bladder through the external urethral meatus with the microtransducer at the 3

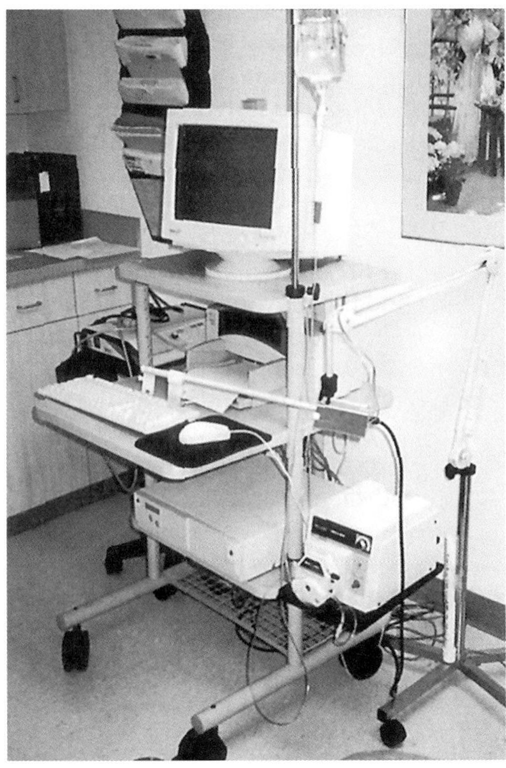

Figure 116-4 Complex cystometry setup with fluid, water pump, multichannel transducers, computer, and recording device.

TABLE 116-1 Correlation of Interval Bladder Sensations to Normal Experiences

	Sensation	Normal Volume (mL)	Life Circumstance
First	Awareness of bladder filling	100–200	While watching TV, aware that urine is in the bladder
Second	Normal desire to void	200–300	Sensation that the patient would usually and normally empty his or her bladder
Third	Strong desire to void	300–400	Patient would attempt to hold urine during good TV program
Fourth	Urgent desire to void		Patient would go straight to the bathroom at a department store during a sale
Fifth	Maximum capacity	400–600	Patient would consider pulling the car off the road to urinate in the woods

o'clock position. Take care to place the proximal transducer near the midurethra. Then place the abdominal catheter into the rectum or the vagina. If a woman has pelvic prolapse beyond the hymenal ring, the probe should be placed into the rectum. The catheters are secured to the patient's inner thigh with tape. In women with significant prolapse, to reduce artifact, even if the probe is placed in the rectum, we recommend performing the cystometry with the prolapse reduced using a large cotton-tipped applicator.

6. Activate the cystometrogram recording device and ask the patient to cough to confirm correct placement. A cough should produce a pressure spike on both the intra-abdominal and the intravesical tracings. The bladder is then filled with infusion solution at a medium fill rate, which is usually 50 mL/min (but can be 10 to 100 mL/min).
7. Record bladder volumes corresponding to first sensation, normal desire to urinate, strong desire, urgency, and maximum bladder capacity. This is most easily accomplished by correlating bladder sensations with normal experiences (Table 116-1). Instruct the patient to periodically cough (cough stress test), and inspect the external urethral meatus for sudden urine loss. Determine the minimum volume at which leakage occurs (when leakage is first noted). If leakage is continuous, it can usually be minimized with gentle traction on the catheter or by manual occlusion of the male penile urethra to obtain maximum bladder capacity.
8. The infusion should be stopped when a contraction occurs or any leakage is noted, after which the infusion should be restarted. Continue bladder filling until bladder pressure shows a progressive rise above baseline (reduced compliance) or maximum bladder capacity. At maximum bladder capacity, the patient usually has a contraction and he or she should be asked to try to inhibit the contraction, a test for detrusor instability of hyperreflexia. If no images or pressure flow studies are needed, the catheter is then opened and the infusion solution drained.

Urethral Pressure Profile and Functional Urethral Length

9. After completion of the cystometry, a urethral pressure profile and functional urethral length (UPP/FUL) is recorded by graphing the pressure while pulling the transducer from the internal to the external urethral meatus at a constant speed (usually 0.5 cm/sec). It can be pulled by hand or with a mechanical pulling device. This test commonly uses a transducer-containing, side-hole catheter that is perfused at 2 mL/min. Multiple measurements can be performed by reinserting and withdrawing the pressure catheter. The MUCP is calculated by subtracting the baseline urethral pressure from the maximum (Fig. 116-5).

Pressure–Flow Studies

10. If a pressure–flow study is required to evaluate voiding dysfunction, the catheters are left in place and the patient is instructed to void into the commode. Intravesical, intra-abdominal, and intraurethral pressures are measured and, using subtraction analysis, the mechanism of voiding is evaluated.

Electromyography

11. Contractile activity and innervation can be checked using EMG. Surface electrodes (including anal-vaginal plugs) are usually adequate for checking contractile activity, especially in children. Needle electrodes are usually necessary for checking innervation.

Bethanechol Testing

12. For an acontractile bladder, subcutaneous bethanechol (5 mg in patients weighing >75 kg, or 0.3 mg/kg) can be used to determine if a neurogenic bladder is the cause. Cannon's law of denervation supersensitivity suggests that a denervated organ produces an exaggerated response to its natural neurotransmitter. To perform the test, baseline cystometric pressures should be measured with the bladder filled to 100 mL, and then the bladder drained. About 15 minutes after administering subcutaneous bethanechol (in those for whom it is not contraindicated), there will be evidence of its systemic effect with increased salivation and flushing. At that time, an increase in pressure of 20 cm H_2O over baseline when the bladder is again filled to 100 mL suggests supersensitivity due to denervation. Atropine 0.4 mg (given intramuscularly) should be available to reverse bethanechol if necessary.

COMPLICATIONS

- Bladder infection
- Gross hematuria

Like bedside urodynamics, MCUD is associated with few complications. In rare cases, patients may develop a urinary tract infection after the procedure. Routine prophylactic antibiotics as well as phenazopyridine, a bladder analgesic, are recommended after the procedure. Transient gross hematuria may also be noted after the procedure, especially after difficult catheterization in a postmenopausal woman with urethral atrophy. This usually resolves spontaneously within 48 hours. Cystoscopy-urethroscopy should be considered in patients with persistent hematuria or lower urinary tract pain beyond 48 to 72 hours.

INTERPRETATION OF RESULTS

Given the complexity of the lower urinary tract, results of MCUD should always be correlated with the physical examination and clinical history.

Uroflowmetry, with measurement of a postvoid residual, assesses bladder emptying and evaluates for overflow incontinence. Urine flow rate depends on initial bladder volume. Specific normal flow rates for greater than 150 mL voided have been determined by age and sex (Abrams and Torrens, 1979), and for men younger than 40 years, between 40 and 60 years, and older than 60 years of age, normal rates are 22 mL/sec, 18 mL/sec, and 13 mL/sec, respectively. In women younger than 50 years of age, the flow rate should be greater than 25 mL/sec; in women older than 50 years of age, it should be greater than 18 mL/sec. The normal flow pattern (volume

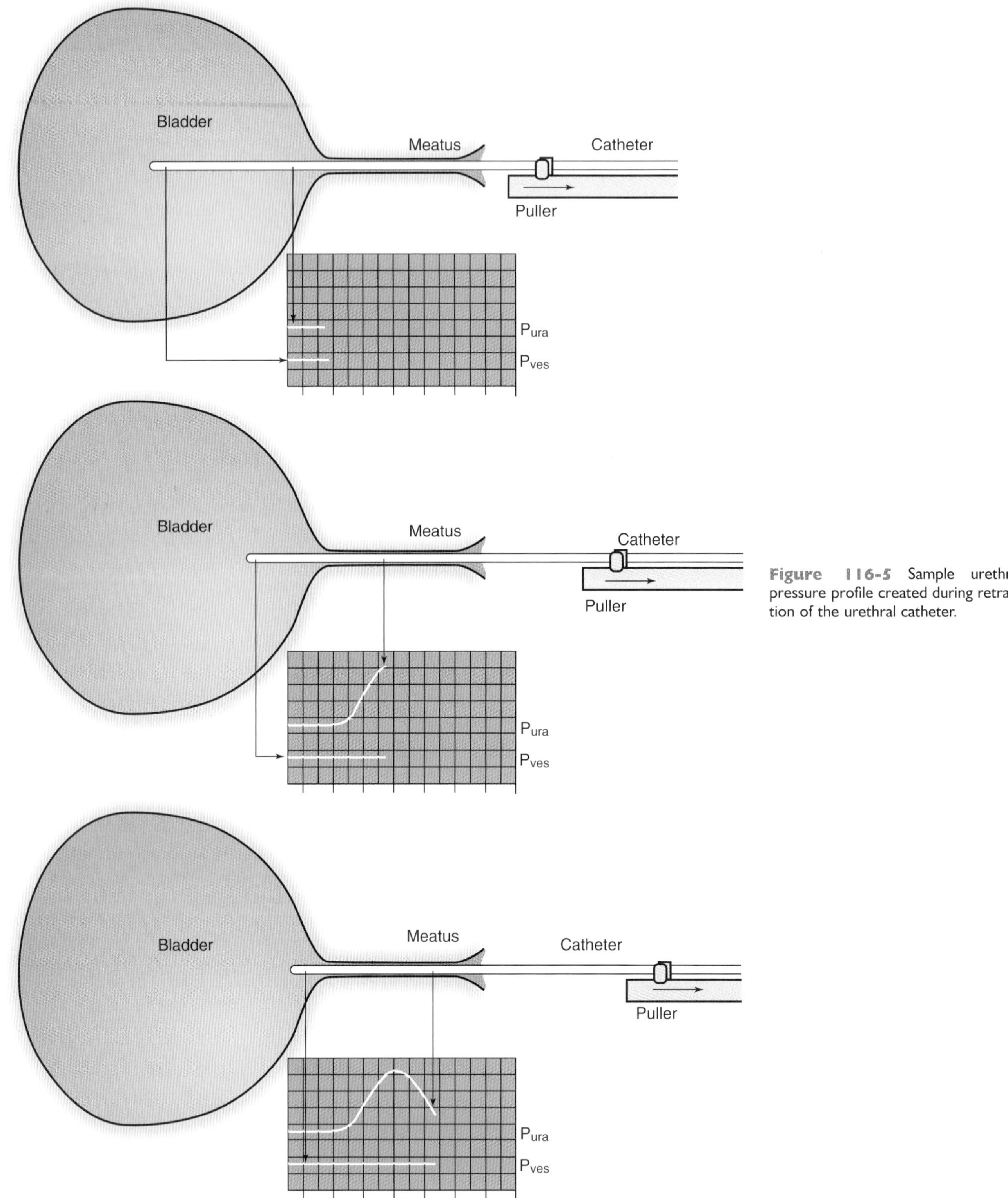

Figure 116-5 Sample urethral pressure profile created during retraction of the urethral catheter.

over time) is bell-shaped (Fig. 116-6) and continuous. An interrupted pattern suggests straining to void or lack of coordination between detrusor muscle contraction and sphincter relaxation. Prolonged voiding times may indicate an obstructed voiding pattern resulting from increased outlet resistance (e.g., urethral obstruction, external sphincter dyssynergia) or poor propulsive force (detrusor dysfunction).

Normal values for a postvoid residual are not universally established, but previous investigators have advocated a normal postvoid residual measurement to be less than 200 mL and less than 20% of

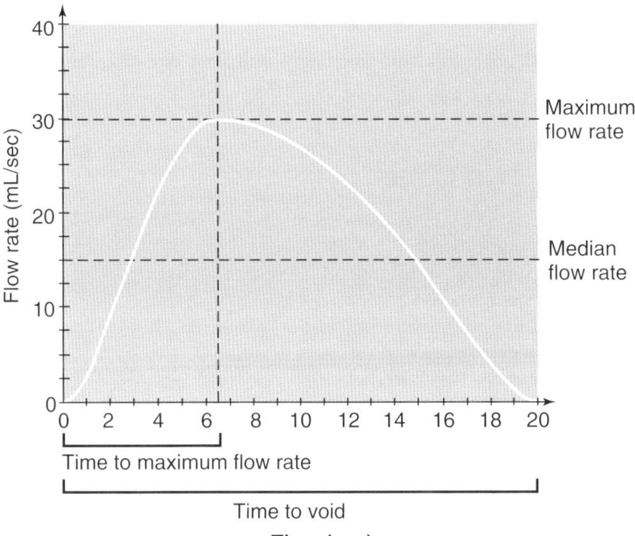

Figure 116-6 Normal uroflow tracing in woman without obstruction.

the total void. Patients with urinary frequency or incontinence and a normal postvoid residual have a bladder storage problem, and this can result from disorders of bladder compliance, involuntary bladder contractions, bladder hypersensitivity, or bladder outlet abnormalities. Bladder outlet abnormalities can be due to lack of support, fibrosis, or neurologic insult.

Cystometry will document abnormalities of bladder sensation and compliance (Box 116-2). With a normal bladder capacity and compliance, the detrusor pressure should remain stable (<15 cm H_2O change) throughout filling. A rise and decline of the detrusor pressure indicates detrusor instability, which may or may not be associated with observable urge incontinence episodes. A large-capacity bladder due to chronic urinary retention may demonstrate increased compliance with little or no increase in pressure despite a large volume of infusion. A gradual persistent rise in detrusor pressure indicates decreased compliance, with possible causes being chronic inflammation, radiation cystitis, interstitial cystitis, and bladder carcinoma. A gradual persistent rise could also be due to a low-grade contraction. Discontinuing the filling can help differentiate between decreased compliance and a low-grade contraction; the pressure stops rising or falls slightly with decreased compliance. Sudden urine loss associated with periodic coughing or Valsalva maneuver during filling cystometry is diagnostic of SUI (Fig. 116-7).

Most patients can suppress a detrusor contraction completely, if asked to do so, even when the bladder is very full. Detrusor overactivity usually declares itself with a contraction when less than 200 mL has been infused. If there is a known neurologic lesion preventing this inhibition, it is known as *detrusor hyperreflexia*. The term *detrusor instability* is usually reserved for non-neurogenic or idiopathic causes. *Acontractile detrusor* is defined by an inability to contract the detrusor when it is full. However, in 10% of men and 50% of women, acontractile detrusor is due to psychological inhibition, one of the most common causes for overinterpretation of MCUD. Bethanechol testing should be used if a neurogenic bladder is suspected as the cause of acontractile detrusor.

Box 116-2. Bladder Capacity Abnormalities: Diagnoses and Predisposing Conditions

Reduced Bladder Capacity

Diagnoses

Detrusor instability (idiopathic)
Detrusor hyperreflexia (neurogenic)
Genuine stress incontinence
Hypersensitive bladder (sensory urgency)

Predisposing Conditions

Urinary tract infection
Interstitial cystitis
Bladder tumor
Radiation cystitis or fibrosis
Emotional factors

Elevated Bladder Capacity

Diagnoses

Neuropathy
Tabes dorsalis
Lumbar spinal disk disease
Multiple sclerosis
Diabetes mellitus
Hypothyroidism
Pernicious anemia

Predisposing Conditions

Chronic outlet obstruction
Urethral stricture
Uterovaginal prolapse
Urethral tumor
Previous radical pelvic surgery
Habitual infrequent voiding

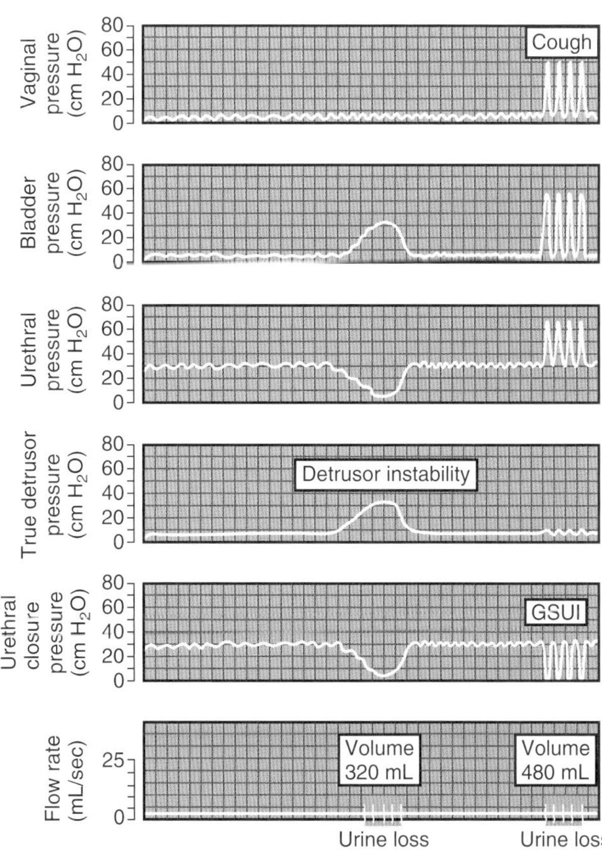

Figure 116-7 Typical complex cystogram tracing in woman with mixed incontinence, detrusor instability (at 320 mL), and genuine stress urinary incontinence (GSUI) (at 480 mL).

TABLE 116-2 Normal Values for MUCP and FUL

	Age (yr)	MUCP (cm H_2O)	FUL (cm)
Male	≤50	65–105	3.5–4.5
	>50	65–105	4.0–4.5
Female	≤50	60–90	2.0–3.5
	>50	50–80	2.0–3.5

FUL, functional urethral length; MUCP, maximal urethral closure pressure.

Urethral pressure profiles and urethral length provide static evaluation of the urethral sphincter mechanism. MUCP values less than 20 cm H_2O are consistent with intrinsic sphincter deficiency, and values between 20 cm H_2O and normal are considered borderline. Normal values for both MUCP and FUL are listed in Table 116-2, and Figure 116-8 shows a normal urethral pressure profile curve as well as demonstrating FUL. In men, the FUL normally increases with age, whereas the MUCP decreases with age in women.

Postprocedure Patient Education

After MCUD testing, results should be reviewed in detail with the patient. The diagnosis should be confirmed on the basis of careful review of the urodynamic tracing, and management options should be discussed. Patients with voiding dysfunction may benefit from urethral dilation, smooth muscle relaxants, or intermittent self-catheterization. For patients who demonstrate detrusor instability or reduced bladder capacity with coexisting overactive bladder symptoms, nonsurgical treatment modalities, including anticholinergic medications, bladder retraining, dietary modification, and neuromodulation, should be considered. Patients with SUI should be offered both surgical and nonsurgical treatment modalities (see Chapter 153, Pessaries), depending on the severity of their incontinence, the anticipated outcomes, and surgical risk factors.

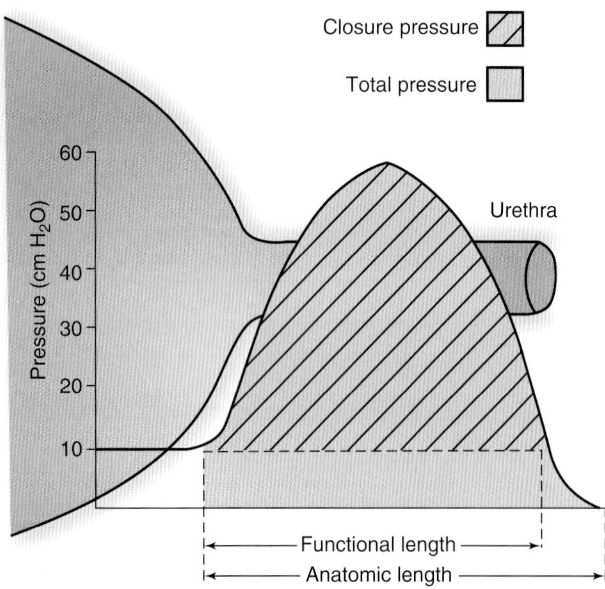

Figure 116-8 Normal urethral pressure profile curve. Functional urethral length is also demonstrated.

Patient Education Guides

See patient education form available online at www.expertconsult.com.

CPT/Billing Codes

51726 Complex cystometrogram (e.g., calibrated electronic equipment)
51741 Complex uroflowmetry (e.g., calibrated electronic equipment)
51772 Urethral pressure profile (UPP) studies, any technique
51784 Electromyography studies of anal or urethral sphincter, other than needle, any technique
51795 Voiding pressure studies, bladder voiding pressure, any technique
51797 Voiding pressure studies, intraabdominal voiding pressure (rectal, gastric, intraperitoneal)

When multiple procedures are performed in the same session, either modifier -51 or code 09951 is used. All the preceding procedure codes imply that procedures were performed by or under the direct supervision of a physician, and include supplies.

ICD-9-CM Diagnostic Codes

595.0 Cystitis, acute
596.5 Bladder dysfunction, other
596.51 Hypertonicity of bladder
596.52 Low bladder compliance
596.54 Neurogenic bladder
596.55 Detrusor sphincter dyssynergia
596.59 Other functional disorder of bladder (e.g., detrusor instability)
599.82 Intrinsic (urethral) sphincter deficiency (ISD)
625.6 Incontinence, stress, female
625.9 Unspecified symptom associated with female genital (e.g., pelvic pain)
788.1 Dysuria
788.20 Urinary retention, unspecified
788.21 Incomplete bladder emptying
788.30 Urinary incontinence, unspecified
788.31 Incontinence, urge
788.32 Incontinence, stress, male
788.33 Incontinence, mixed (male or female)
788.36 Nocturnal enuresis
788.37 Incontinence, continuous leakage
788.41 Urinary frequency
788.35 Incontinence with postvoid dribbling
788.43 Nocturia

Acknowledgment

The editors wish to recognize the many contributions by Neeraj Kohli, MD, and Briana Walton, MD, to this chapter in a previous edition of this text.

Suppliers

(See contact information online at www.expertconsult.com.)

Cooper Surgical (Lumax)
Laborie Medical Technologies
Life-Tech, Inc.
Medtronic Functional Diagnostics

ONLINE RESOURCES

Agency for Health Care Research and Quality: Urinary Incontinence in Adults: Clinical Practice Guideline Update. (Patient information on incontinence from the AHCRQ.) Available at www.ahrq.gov/clinic/uiovervw.htm.

HealthWorld Online: Urinary Incontinence in Adults: Acute and Chronic Management. (Patient information.) Available at www.healthy.net/scr/article.asp?ID=409.

Laborie Medical Technologies. (Leading manufacturer of urodynamic equipment; training materials available.) Available at www.laborie.com.

National Institute of Diabetes and Digestive and Kidney Diseases. (Information on a wide range of topics on urologic conditions from the National Kidney and Urologic Diseases Information Clearinghouse and National Institutes of Health.) Available at www.niddk.nih.gov.

Small D: A Urodynamics Home Page. (Comprehensive review of various urodynamic tests.) Available at www.sghurol.demon.co.uk/urod/index.htm.

BIBLIOGRAPHY

Abrams PH, Torrens MJ: Urine flow studies. Urol Clin North Am 6:71–79, 1979.

Berni KC, Cummings JM: Urodynamic evaluation of the older adult: Bench to bedside. Clin Geriatr Med 20:477–487, 2004.

Fantl A, Newman DK, Colling J, et al. Urinary incontinence in adults: Acute and chronic management. Clinical Practice Guideline No. 2, 1996 update. AHCPR publication no. 96-0682. Rockville, Md, Agency for Health Care Policy and Research, U.S. Department of Health and Human Services, 1996.

Holroyd-Leduc JM, Tannenbaum C, Thorpe KE, Straus SE: What type of urinary incontinence does this woman have? JAMA 299:1446–1456, 2008.

Kohli N, Karram MM: Urodynamic evaluation for female urinary incontinence. Clin Obstet Gynecol 41:672–690, 1998.

Wen CC, Siroky MB: Urodynamic studies. In Siroky MB, Oates RD, Babayan RK (eds): Handbook of Urology: Diagnosis and Therapy, 3rd ed. Philadelphia, Lippincott Williams & Wilkins, 2004, pp 87–97.

SECTION 8

Male Reproductive System

Section Editors: JOHN L. PFENNINGER AND JAMIE BROOMFIELD

CHAPTER 117

Adult Circumcision

John R. Holman

Adult circumcision is a procedure about which little is written, even in urologic literature. It is often performed for reasons that are not purely medical, yet it also has clearly defined medical indications. Some patients have their own nonmedical reasons.

General anesthesia may be necessary, but usually local anesthesia is sufficient in the outpatient setting, including the properly equipped office. Informed consent should be obtained after a thorough discussion with the patient (and partner, if appropriate), during which the indications, procedure, postprocedure care, and potential complications are explained. (See the sample patient education and consent forms online at www.expertconsult.com.) This consent is required for all patients, and it must always be documented to serve as a record of the authenticity of the patient's presenting symptoms. Thorough documentation is important because individual physicians may vary in their judgments of surgical necessity. The physician must make sure that the patient's reasons for requesting circumcision are medically sound and that the patient's expectations of the results are realistic. There is evidence circumcision does not change sexual experience or satisfaction.

Anatomy

Identify normal male anatomy before proceeding. Patients with an occult hypospadias or epispadias should be referred to a urologist.

Indications

- Phimosis (tightness of the foreskin so that it cannot be drawn back from over the glans); possibly related to complaints of pain with erections and intercourse
- Paraphimosis (retraction of a narrow, inflamed foreskin that cannot be replaced)
- Penile hygiene; recurrent balanitis (inflammation of the glans penis)
- Posthitis (inflammation of the prepuce) not relieved by medical treatment
- Preputial neoplasms (e.g., erythroplasia of Queyrat, which is severe squamous dysplasia)
- Excessive foreskin redundancy
- Frenular tears
- Patient or partner preference after informed discussion

Patients may also have social, religious, or personal reasons for requesting a circumcision. Exploration of these reasons ensures a thorough understanding of the risks and benefits as well as alternatives to the procedure. Circumcision can reduce the rate of human immunodeficiency virus infection by 50% to 60% and decreases penile human papillomavirus infection. However, it does not appear to prevent other sexually transmitted infections.

Contraindications

Relative

- Psychiatric disorder or history (relative contraindication; these patients must be screened carefully)
- Bleeding dyscrasias (evaluate appropriately)
- History of penile surgery, significant trauma, or unusual-appearing or ambiguous genitalia (consider a referral to a specialist)

Absolute

- Active inflammation in the genital area
- Infection in the genital area

Equipment and Supplies

- 10-mL syringe with a 1- to 1½-inch, 27-gauge needle and a ½-inch, 30-gauge needle
- Prep bowl with a dozen 4 × 4 gauze sponges
- Iodine solution or other antiseptic for scrub
- Ring forceps
- Pack of sterile 4 × 4 gauze bandages
- One fenestrated drape
- 6-inch segment of half-inch Penrose drain
- Six straight mosquito forceps
- One large straight forceps
- One curved Mayo scissors
- One medium-size straight Metzenbaum scissors
- One suture scissors
- 5-inch needle holder
- One Brown-Adson thumb forceps
- 4-0 or 5-0 absorbable suture (e.g., Vicryl, Dexon)
- Petrolatum gauze
- 1-inch Kling bandage
- One malleable 4- to 6-inch silver probe *(optional)*
- Needle-tip electrocautery unit
- Sterile marking pen

Preprocedure Patient Education and Forms

The patient should be properly counseled and evaluated before the surgery. A patient education handout is provided, and a consent form is signed. (See the sample patient education and consent forms online at www.expertconsult.com.) If the patient is anxious, a preprocedural dose of an oral, sublingual, intramuscular, or intravenous anxiolytic (e.g., diazepam 10 mg) may be administered. If such a dose is used, someone must drive the patient home after the procedure. (See the sample patient education handout online at www.expertconsult.com.)

PROCEDURE

The patient should be supine and comfortable. Shaving and clipping of hair should be avoided to minimize the infectious complications. Surgically prepare the entire genitalia, scrotum, and pubic area with an appropriate antiseptic solution. Use a fenestrated drape.

Anesthesia

Ring Block

1. Using a 10-mL syringe filled with 1% lidocaine *without* epinephrine and a 1-inch, 27-gauge needle, inject 0.5 to 1 mL subcutaneously over the superficial dorsal vein so that the wheal is raised at the junction of the penis and the pubis (Fig. 117-1).
2. Without withdrawing the needle, angle it toward both sides of the dorsal vein and inject additional lidocaine.
3. Extend the needle subcutaneously downward to the deep fascia of the penis—an area of firm resistance—and continue injecting circumferentially, staying close to the deep fascia of the penis. The penile skin is loose; therefore, complete circumferential deployment of the anesthetic agent can be accomplished, and the ventral surface can be reached from both sides. This is called a *ring block*. Inject approximately 4 mL in this manner on each side. Do not penetrate the fascia.
4. Wait a few minutes, and then inject 1 mL of the local anesthetic subcutaneously into the frenulum using a ½-inch, 30-gauge needle (Fig. 117-2).
5. Wait several more minutes and then test the depth of local anesthesia by cautiously grasping the edge of the foreskin with a mosquito hemostat. Should more anesthesia be required, use a Penrose drain as a tourniquet around the midportion of the penis. Tie the tourniquet tightly or hold the Penrose drain with a clamp to obstruct venous return. Inject an additional 2 mL of lidocaine into both corpora cavernosa just distal to the tourniquet (Fig. 117-3).
6. After approximately 5 minutes, retest for anesthesia; if anesthesia is adequate, remove the tourniquet.

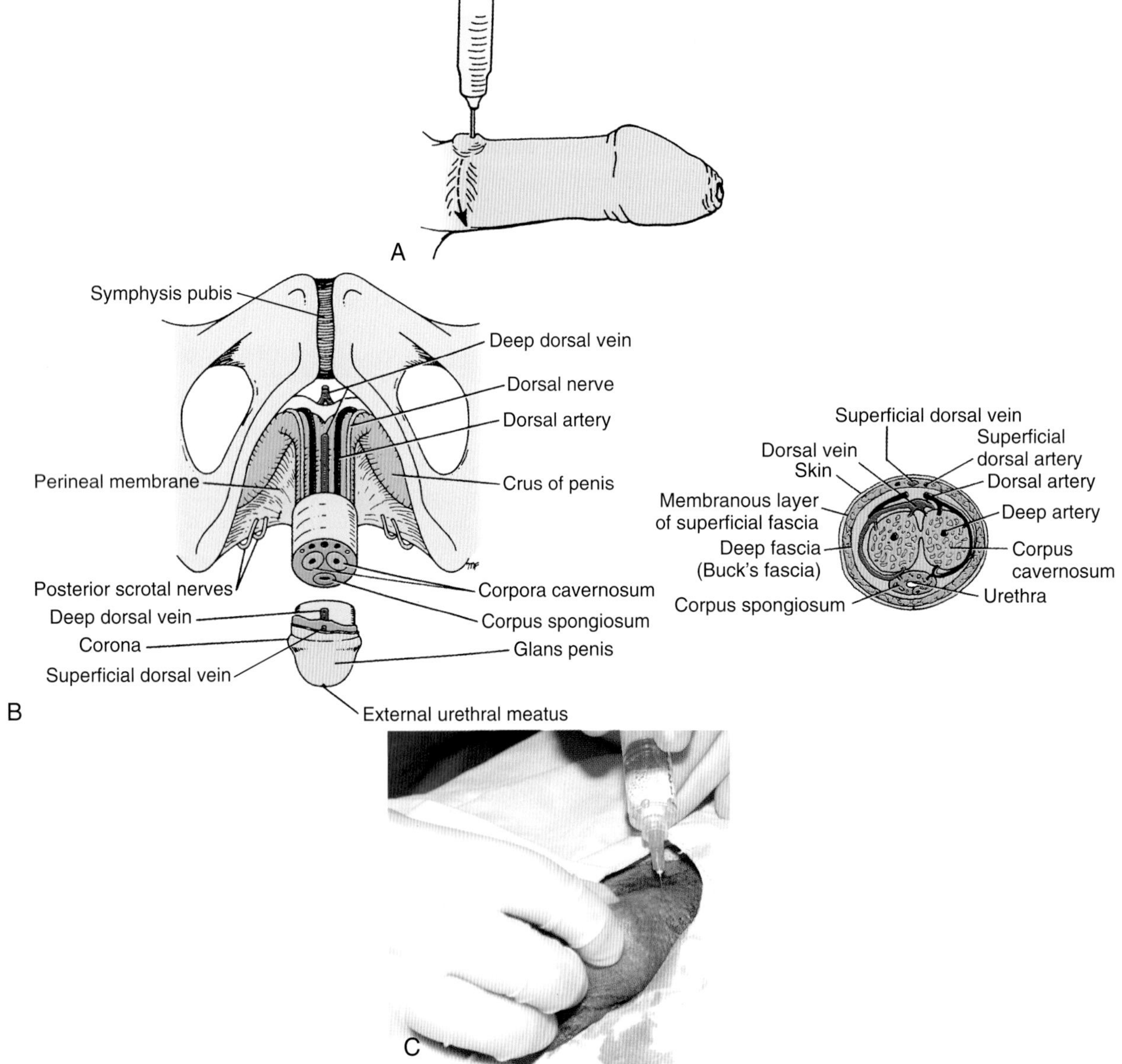

Figure 117-1 Ring block of the penis. **A,** Site of initial injection over dorsal vein. **B,** Cross-sectional view of the penis. **C,** Operative view. (**B,** From Snell RS, Smith MS: Clinical Anatomy for Emergency Medicine. St. Louis, Mosby, 1993.)

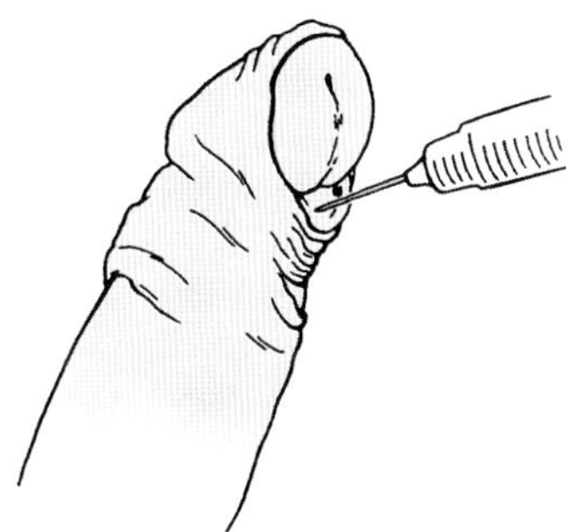

Figure 117-2 Additional anesthetic injected into the frenulum.

Dorsal Penile Nerve Block

As an alternative to or in addition to the ring block, the surgeon may perform a *dorsal penile nerve block.* The dorsal penile nerve is blocked by injecting local anesthetic solution deep to Buck's fascia, where the nerves emerge from under the pubic bone (see Fig. 117-1B).

1. The patient is placed in the supine position.
2. After preparation of the skin, two injection sites are identified over the inferior edge of the pubic bone at approximately the 10 and 2 o'clock positions relative to the base of the penis.
3. A 27-gauge (1½-inch) needle is inserted directed ventrally until the pubic bone is contacted.
4. The needle is "walked" caudad off the pubis and through Buck's fascia.
5. After aspiration, 5 mL of local anesthetic is injected at each site. A mixture of equal volumes of 0.5% bupivacaine (Marcaine) and 1% or 2% lidocaine without epinephrine provides rapid onset of anesthesia and suitable duration for circumcision.

Dorsal Slit Technique

The dorsal slit technique is preferred if the patient has phimosis or paraphimosis. An assistant is of considerable help in carrying out this procedure.

1. Using small straight hemostats, grasp the distal foreskin at the 11, 1, 5, and 7 o'clock positions, and gently pull the foreskin over the glans.
2. Use a malleable silver probe or the hemostats on the undersurface of the dorsal foreskin to determine a point 1 cm distal to the corona.
3. Place a large straight hemostat at the 12 o'clock position, close it firmly, and compress and crush the foreskin to the point that you previously determined with the silver probe (Fig. 117-4). Repeat this procedure of clamping at the 6-o'clock position, going up to the base of the frenulum.
4. After the dorsal and ventral areas are clamped, mark a line where the circumferential excision of the foreskin is to occur. Use a marking pen to connect the dorsal point with the inferior point on each side.

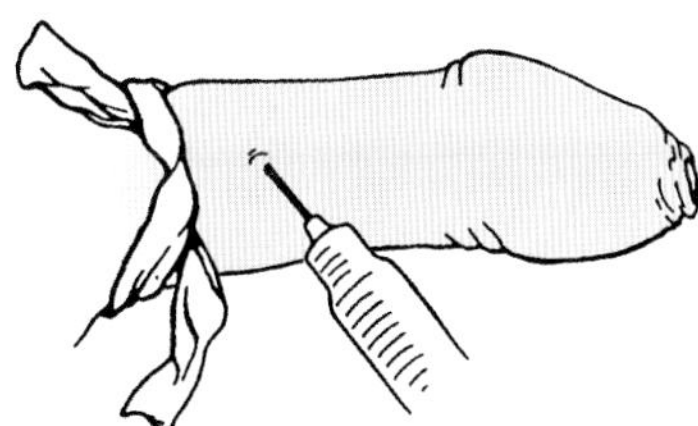

Figure 117-3 Injection of anesthetic into corpora cavernosa with tourniquet applied.

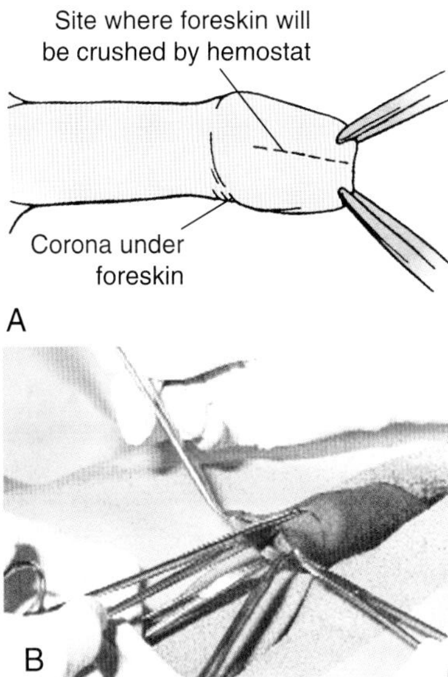

Figure 117-4 Straight hemostats (four) applied at the dorsal and ventral aspects of the tip of foreskin at the 11, 1, 5, and 7 o'clock positions. **A,** Schematic. **B,** Operative view.

5. After 5 or more minutes (time it by the clock), remove the forceps and use a straight Metzenbaum scissors to incise through the *center* of the crushed areas (Fig. 117-5). Crushing the tissue reduces the bleeding from this incision.
6. Using a curved Mayo scissors, carefully excise these two lateral tissue flaps, *maintaining a 1-cm margin from the corona,* except at the frenulum, where the foreskin is tapered only 2 to 3 mm (Fig. 117-6). Fulgurate all bleeders or tie with a 5-0 plain catgut.
7. If the large dorsal vein is cut, ligate with absorbable sutures.
8. After complete hemostasis, sew the outer layer of skin just proximal to the glans to the underlying mucosal layer (1-cm skin remnant of prepuce) with multiple 4-0 or 5-0 absorbable sutures (Fig. 117-7). If performing the procedure alone, leave some sutures long dorsally. These can be used (and cut off later) for retraction to stabilize the penis when suturing ventrally. Use hemostats to fix the long suture to the drape.
9. Place two layers of petrolatum gauze dressing, which is nonadherent, over the suture line around the entire circumference and overlay with a light layer of Kerlix or Kling (Fig. 117-8).

Sleeve Technique

The sleeve technique uses two circumferential incisions. One is made on the internal aspect of the foreskin distally, near the coronal sulcus. The other is made on the external part of the foreskin proximally and defines an amount of prepuce removed. A "sleeve" of tissue between the two incisions will be excised.

1. The external preputial incision is outlined with a marking pen at the level of the corona (Fig. 117-9A and B).
2. After retracting the foreskin, the internal preputial incision is marked with the pen approximately 1 cm proximal to the coronal sulcus. It is important to apply gentle downward pressure on

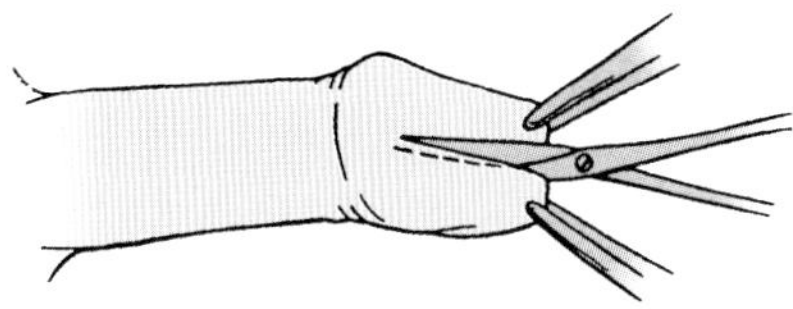

Figure 117-5 Cutting through crushed tissue.

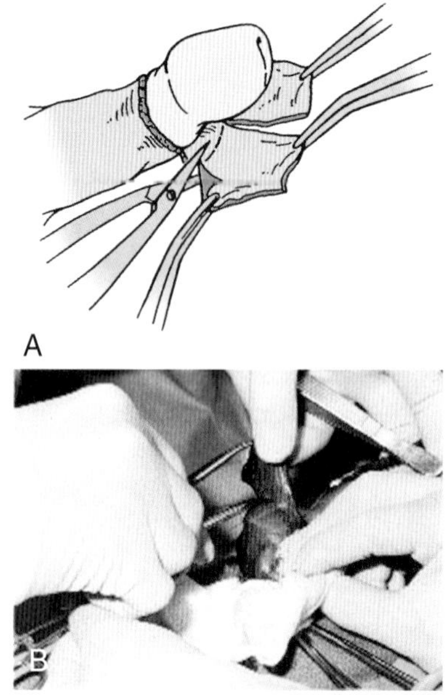

Figure 117-6 Excision of foreskin. **A,** Schematic. **B,** Operative view.

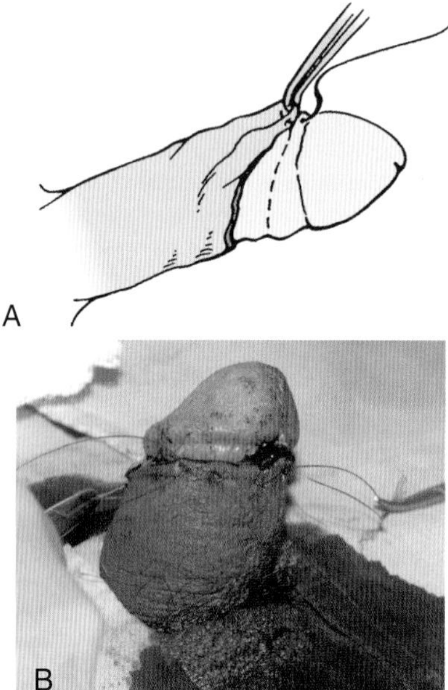

Figure 117-7 Suturing of the skin to the shaft mucosa just proximal to the corona. **A,** Schematic. **B,** Operative view.

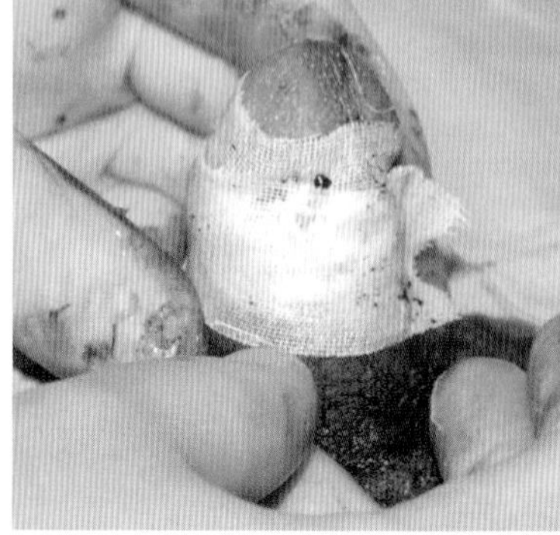

Figure 117-8 Suture covered with gauze dressing.

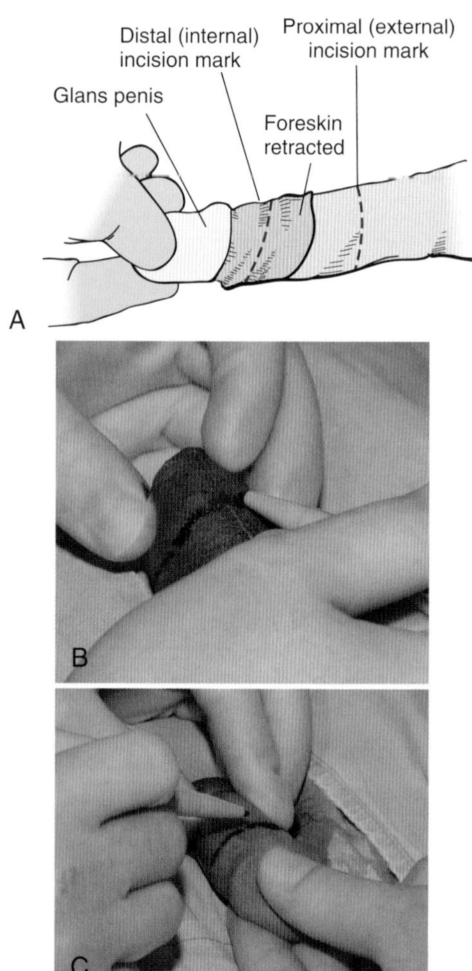

Figure 117-9 External and internal preputial skin incision sites are marked. **A,** Schematic. **B,** Operative view, internal incision mark. **C,** Operative view, external incision mark. (**A**, Redrawn from images in Holman JR, Stuessi KA: Adult circumcision. Am Fam Physician 59:1514–1518, 1999.)

the *prepubic* fat pad at the base of the penis while making the initial outlines to remove the correct amount of skin (Fig. 117-9A and C).

3. The external proximal *circumferential* preputial incision is made with the scalpel and carried to Buck's fascia.
4. After retracting the foreskin, a second circumferential incision is made in the inner prepuce at the previous mark. The internal incision is carried straight across the frenulum ventrally.
5. A sleeve of tissue now exists between the two incisions. This sleeve is the foreskin. Hemostats are placed dorsally for traction (Fig. 117-10).
6. After making a superficial linear incision on the sleeve with the electrocautery tool, subcutaneous attachments are separated between Buck's fascia and the prepuce. The sleeve is excised with electrocautery (Fig. 117-11).
7. The frenulum is reapproximated initially with the "U" stitch.
8. Four quadrant sutures are placed on the dorsum and both sides, and the remaining interrupted sutures are placed at 4- to 7-mm intervals (see Fig. 117-7).
9. A sterile dressing of petroleum gauze can be applied (see Fig. 117-8).

Sample Operative Report

See the sample operative report online at www.expertconsult.com.

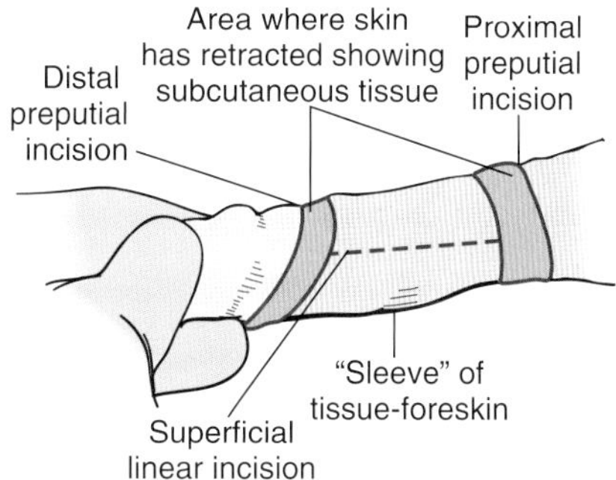

Figure 117-10 After incisions are made, a "sleeve" of preputial skin remains. The shaded *(pink)* areas show where the skin has retracted, showing subcutaneous tissue. (Redrawn from images in Holman JR, Stuessi KA: Adult circumcision. Am Fam Physician 59:1514–1518, 1999.)

Common Error

Removal of too much or too little foreskin is a common error. Correct planning of the incision is crucial to avoid this mistake.

Complications

- *Bleeding*—direct pressure, cautery, or suture ligature can be used.
- *Hematoma*—avoid with management of bleeding before skin closure. Apply pressure.
- *Infection*—sterile technique during surgery is important.
- *Pain with erection*—prevented by leaving an adequate "cup" (1-cm margin) of coronal skin (see step 6 under the "Dorsal Slit Technique" section).
- *Stricture and scarring* (rare).
- *Dehiscence* resulting from nocturnal erections (see next section).

Postprocedure Management

- Prescribe 5 days' worth of adequate analgesics appropriate for the patient's pain tolerance. A combination product containing codeine (such as Tylenol no. 3), a nonsteroidal anti-inflammatory drug, or a similar product is sufficient. Topical 5% lidocaine ointment can also be helpful.
- Instruct the patient to soak in a tub of warm water 24 to 36 hours later and to remove all of the dressing at that time. Replace the dressing daily after soaking off.
- One ampule of amyl nitrate (crush and inhale one to six times as needed; may be repeated once after 5 minutes) can be used as abortive therapy for erections during the 1-week recovery period.

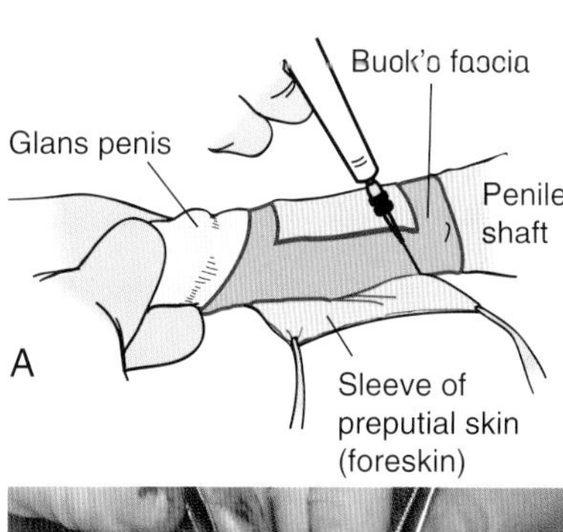

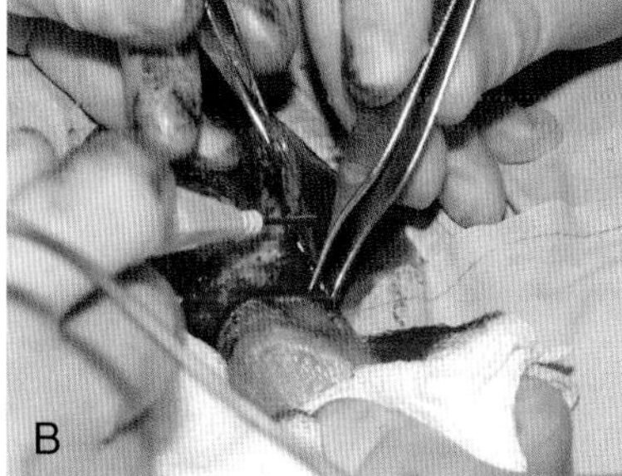

Figure 117-11 Sleeve excised with electrocautery, tissue scissors, or scalpel. **A,** Schematic. **B,** Operative view. (**A,** Redrawn from images in Holman JR, Stuessi KA: Adult circumcision. Am Fam Physician 59:1514–1518, 1999.)

Postprocedure Patient Education

- Instruct the patient on how to replace the petroleum gauze and Kling gauze, which should be done every day until the patient returns to the office for the follow-up visit in 1 week.
- Tell the patient to call if there is any undue pain, active bleeding, or signs of infection (e.g., streaks of redness, fever, purulent drainage).
- Instruct the patient to avoid sexual arousal and sexual intercourse for about 4 weeks.

Patient Education Guides

See the sample patient education, operative report, and consent forms online at www.expertconsult.com.

CPT/Billing Code

54161 Circumcision, surgical excision other than clamp device, or dorsal slit, other than newborn

ICD-9-CM Diagnostic Codes

605 Phimosis and paraphimosis
607.1 Balanitis
607.9 Penile pain
302.70 Psychosexual dysfunction

Acknowledgment

The original chapter on adult circumcision was written by Donald E. DeWitt, MD. John M. Holman, MD, has revised and updated this chapter for the previous two editions. The opinions contained herein are those of the author and should not be construed as official or as reflecting the views of the Departments of the Navy or Defense.

Bibliography

Fakjian N, Hunter S, Cole GW, Miller J: An argument for circumcision: Prevention of balanitis in the adult. Arch Dermatol 126:1046–1047, 1990.

Holman JR, Stuessi KA: Adult circumcision. Am Fam Physician 50: 1514–1518, 1999.

MacLean R: Odds of penile HPV are reduced for circumcised men and condom users. Int Fam Plan Perspect 31:42, 2005.

Mehta SD, Moses S, Agot K, et al: Adult male circumcision does not reduce the risk of incident *Neisseria gonorrhoeae*, *Chlamydia trachomatis*, or *Trichomonas vaginalis* infection: Results from a randomized, controlled trial in Kenya. J Infect Dis 200:370–378, 2009.

Pienkos EJ: Circumcision at the 121st Evacuation Hospital: Report of a questionnaire with cross-cultural observations. Mil Med 154:169–171, 1989.

Pories WJ, Thomas FT: Office Surgery for Family Physicians. Stoneham, Mass, Butterworth, 1985.

Senkul T, Iseri C, Sen B, et al: Circumcision in adults: Effect on sexual function. Urology 63:155–158, 2004.

Szmuk P, Ezri T, Ben Hur H, et al: Regional anaesthesia for circumcision in adults: A comparative study. Can J Anaesth 41:1181–1184, 1994.

Wakefield SE, Elewa AA: Adult circumcision under local anaesthetic. Br J Urol 75:96, 1995.

White RG, Glynn JR, Orroth KK, et al: Male circumcision for HIV prevention in sub-Saharan Africa: Who, what and when? AIDS 22:1841–1850, 2008.

CHAPTER 118

Androscopy

John L. Pfenninger

Androscopy is an office procedure mainly used to identify condylomata. It examines the male genitalia under magnification after acetic acid has been applied. It can be used to evaluate any dermatologic disorder/lesion in the genital areas and also to ensure complete removal of lesions. Another term for this procedure is *penoscopy*.

Recent literature documents that the human papillomavirus (HPV) is the cause of cervical dysplasia and cervical cancer. Whether the virus *alone* leads to cancer is unknown. Yet, HPV is the necessary, if not the single sufficient cause for cervical cancer. HPV is very contagious and it is most readily spread through sexual contact. Intromission is not necessary because skin-to-skin contact is enough. It may also be transmitted in yet-unknown ways in a minority of cases. Fomites do not transmit the disease. Condoms provide only partial protection from HPV but do help prevent spread.

The clinical significance of condylomata and HPV in men is less serious than it is in women, but men act as carriers and may transmit the disease to sexual partners. Although rare, HPV can cause penile carcinoma. Anal-receptive homosexual men have 50 times the rate of anal carcinoma compared to the incidence in the average population. An increased rate of anal carcinoma in anal-receptive women can also be anticipated, but there is no literature to document this.

There are over 100 types of HPV. Eight to 10 of these characteristically infect the genital areas. Condylomata acuminata, the visible lesions that we commonly see, are caused by noncarcinogenic strains, such as types 6 and 11. The subclinical types, identified only by examination under magnification after acetic acid staining, are more likely to cause neoplastic changes; frequently these are types 16 and 18. (See Chapter 137, Colposcopic Examination, Chapter 142, Human Papillomavirus DNA Typing, and Chapter 155, Treatment of Noncervical Condylomata Acuminata.)

There is no evidence that treatment of male partners of women who have dysplasia lessens the likelihood of persistence or recurrence in the woman. It is uncertain why condom use is beneficial because the infection is a regional disease. In men, it is present on the penis, scrotum, perineum, and perianal areas. What is visible is only a focal manifestation of a diffuse involvement. In women, it is present on the cervix, vagina, vulva, and the perineal and perianal areas. Winer and colleagues (2006), however, in a well-designed study showed significant protection in women with consistent condom use by their male partners.

Some clinicians question the value of carrying out an androscopic examination. Identification and treatment of condylomata is not the only reason to perform androscopy. Patient education is perhaps the most valuable aspect of this procedure. The man must be informed of the significance of his disease and the necessity of maintaining a single-partner committed relationship. It is no longer a matter of moral or religious persuasion, but rather a good health practice to be monogamous (as are exercising, not smoking, eating low-fat foods, and so forth). Men spread the disease even when visible lesions are not apparent. Only through education can they change their habits.

Men who have HPV can affect their partners in several ways. Not only do they spread the virus by skin-to-skin contact, but HPV has been shown to be present in the semen and in the sperm cell itself. Men who smoke have nicotine and its byproducts in their ejaculate as well as on their hands (important during manual stimulation), which may be a cofactor in HPV persistence. Those who are subject to passive smoking have lower folate levels—a known risk factor for cervical cancer.

The common factors for penile carcinoma include lack of hygiene, sex outside of marriage, smoking, and HPV infection. Clinically differentiating mild, moderate, and severe dysplasia of the penis (penile intraepithelial neoplasia [PIN]) is nearly impossible without obtaining biopsy samples. Anorectal cancer frequently contains the HPV, and some now recommend obtaining a Papanicolaou (Pap) smear of the pectinate (dentate) line on a regular basis to detect anal dysplasias in high-risk individuals. High-resolution anoscopy (HRA), which uses magnification (usually a colposcope) and acetic acid staining, can identify precursor lesions for treatment (see Chapter 99, High-Resolution Anoscopy).

Indications

- *Visible condylomata on the penis, scrotum, or anus.* Staining and examination with magnification will identify smaller lesions that are easier to treat and often not visible to the naked eye. This is likely to decrease recurrences. Androscopy also confirms that the entire lesion has been removed when surgical or ablative therapies are used. Early and complete treatment may reduce the recurrence of the disease. Figure 118-1 shows an example of large condylomata. Examination under magnification will aid in completing removal once the bulk of the lesion has been removed and also identify any smaller lesions that are not immediately obvious. Completing the removal under magnification helps in limiting the depth of excision because penile skin is so thin.
- *Partner with recurrent or persistent condylomata acuminata or cervical dysplasia.* There is some evidence that if the male partner presents with a high viral load, the immune system response of his partner may be overwhelmed by the virus. High viral load may exist if the man has extensive visible acuminate lesions or a diffuse acetowhite staining of the penis (Fig. 118-2).
- *Psychological reassurance.*
- *Chronic perineal or perianal irritation.*
- *Recurrent condylomata.* This could be from incomplete previous removal or failure to identify smaller lesions.
- *Medical–legal examinations in child abuse cases.*
- *History of other sexually transmitted infections.* Although rarely performed for this reason, androscopy with a negative result helps reassure patients that currently there are no HPV lesions.
- *Necessity for patient education.* Performing a procedure is better received by the patient than just "coming in to talk." A biopsy-proven diagnosis speaks a thousand words of reinforcement.
- *Penile lesions of uncertain significance.*

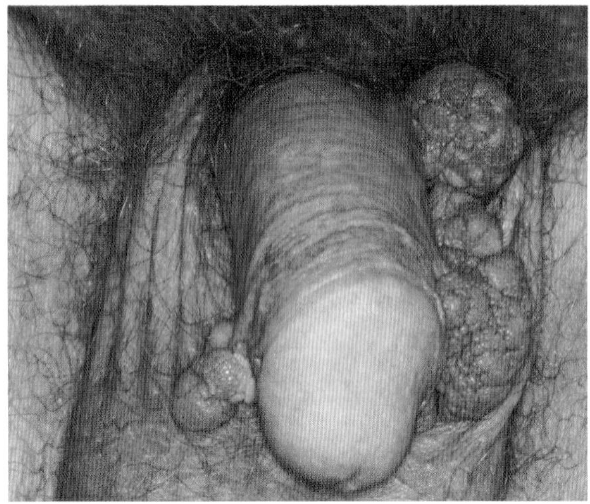

Figure 118-1 Large condylomata. (Courtesy of John L. Pfenninger, MD, The Medical Procedures Center, PC, Midland, Mich.)

EQUIPMENT

- Spray bottle with 5% acetic acid (white vinegar).
- Colposcope (or a high-quality hand-held magnifying lens).
- High-quality fine tissue scissors (e.g., 5-inch curved Metzenbaum scissors) or sharp dermal curettes to obtain a biopsy/remove lesions.
- Pickups.
- Formalin jars.
- Aluminum chloride (Drysol) for hemostasis. Monsel's solution may cause an extended period of hyperpigmentation but is also acceptable.
- 1 to 5 mL lidocaine 1% or 2% without epinephrine.
- 30-gauge needle.
- 1- to 5-mL syringe (depending on size and number of lesions).
- Radiofrequency unit with smoke evacuator, 85% trichloroacetic acid (TCA), or an infrared coagulator if condylomata are to be treated. (See Chapter 155, Treatment of Noncervical Condylomata Acuminata.)

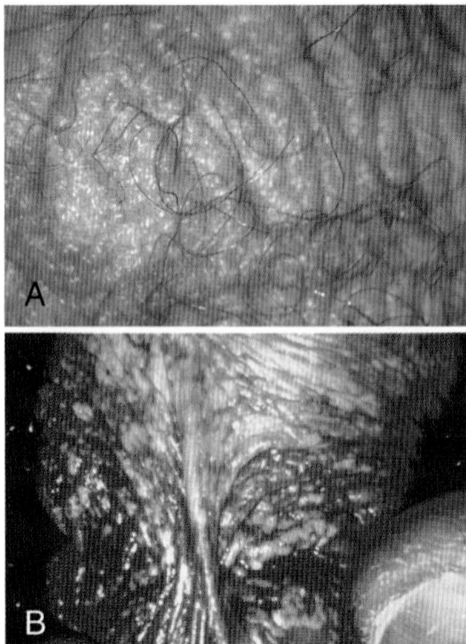

Figure 118-2 **A,** White epithelium seen on the scrotum after application of 5% acetic acid. **B,** Condylomata seen on the penis after application of 5% acetic acid. Lesions were not visible before staining. (Courtesy of John L. Pfenninger, MD, The Medical Procedures Center, PC, Midland, Mich.)

PREPROCEDURE PATIENT PREPARATION

It is always best if the patient is well informed about the nature of the disease before the procedure. Provide the patient with educational material. Prior to the visit, encourage the patient to watch a 21-minute videotape (available from Creative Health Communications/The National Procedures Institute, Midland, Mich) that discusses the implications of HPV infection in men and women. Viewing the videotape will help the patient focus on questions that he or his partner may have, and it will allow the practitioner to avoid repetitious explanations of the same counseling information. Written handouts are also available from many organizations. No preoperative medication is needed for the procedure, and the patient can be reassured that there will usually be minimal discomfort, even if biopsies are obtained. More discomfort may be experienced should treatment be undertaken, however.

TECHNIQUE

Although the examination may take only 10 minutes, patients frequently have numerous questions and concerns. Unless the patient is well known to the practitioner, at least 20 minutes should be allotted for this examination—longer if treatment is undertaken.

1. After the patient is placed in the examination room, the nurse instructs him to spray the entire genital and anal area with 5% acetic acid (white vinegar) and allow it to soak for 5 minutes.
2. Obtain a detailed sexual history (Fig. 118-3, Androscopy Encounter Form).
3. Place the patient on an examination table with stirrups, and position as a woman is positioned for a Pap smear. Conduct a visual inspection first and note any lesions.
4. Spray the entire genital and perineal area again. Allow the solution to run freely over the perineum and anus.
5. Inspect the entire anogenital area under magnification, including the meatus of the penis. Generally a colposcope is used on low power (3× to 5×). Move the penis and scrotum forward and back to bring them into focus (unlike colposcopy, where the cervix is stationary and the scope is adjusted into focus). There is no study comparing good hand-held magnification to colposcopy.
6. Grossly apparent warts that were previously seen will generally turn white with the acetic acid. Previously unseen, small, "flat," or subclinical lesions will also now be identifiable on the penis, scrotum, perineum, or rectum. They will show up as white areas, referred to as *acetowhite changes* (see Fig. 118-2).
7. Sample any atypical lesions with an unusual vascular pattern (mosaicism or punctation; see Chapter 137, Colposcopic Examination) or pigmentation. The pigmentation in lesions that predicts dysplasia will look different from that of a freckle or nevus; it will be a nondiscrete, brownish discoloration (Fig. 118-4). If no atypical lesions are seen, sample one or two of the acuminate lesions or the acetowhite areas to document the presence of HPV and that there is no dysplasia (Fig. 118-5). It is very convincing to have the pathology report confirm your clinical diagnosis, which reinforces the findings to the patient. It also is not always possible to tell clinically what the lesions are.
8. A penile biopsy specimen is easily obtained by using sharp tissue scissors. (A punch biopsy is not needed—you are not sampling the cavernosa!) If only one or two small lesions are to be sampled, simply tent up the skin by pinching it at its base (Fig. 118-6). Looking through the colposcope, obtain a 3- to 4-mm sample with the sharp tissue scissors or remove the entire lesion. No anesthetic is required if only one to two small lesions will be sampled, and this method is often less painful than the injection with anesthesia. Only a very superficial sampling is needed. If the lesions are larger, or more than two samples are to be obtained, it is best to anesthetize with 1% to 2% lidocaine

Androscopy Patient Encounter Form

Patient to fill out:

Name____________________ Date__________

Birth date____________ Age: _____ Referring physician __________

Phone____________________ Reason for exam__________

History				
Smoker	Y N		History of sexual abuse	Y N
Packs per day_____	Since _____		History of genital warts	Y N
Age at first intercourse _____			Treated previously How? _____	
No. of sexual partners (Total in lifetime)_____			Visible warts now	Y N
Family history of cancer	Y N		Partners with warts	Y N
			Previous partners w/abnormal Pap	Y N

Other history of venereal disease (circle): Gonorrhea Syphilis AIDS Herpes Hepatitis

Do you desire testing for any of the above diseases: Y N Advised:__________

Other __________

Physician Section

Illnesses: __________

Medications: __________

Allergies: __________

Health maintenance: __________

Family history: __________

Procedure:

Gross inspection:
5% acetic acid and
examination with colposcope: penis
urethra
scrotum
groin
perineum
rectum

Biopsy:__________

Impression:__________

Treatment:__________

Plan: Discourage smoking
Counseling regarding safer sex, cause for cancer, reporting penis lesions, partner evaluation, vaccines
Instruction sheets on androscopy/HPV? Y N Videotapes viewed? Y N
Consider other VD testing? Y N
Follow-up in _____ weeks

Physician signature: __________ Date __________

cc: __________

Figure 118-3 Patient encounter form. (Courtesy of John L. Pfenninger, MD, The Medical Procedures Center, PC, Midland, Mich.)

without epinephrine. Using a 30-gauge needle minimizes any discomfort.

Alternatively, a 3- to 4-mm, disposable, sharp dermal curette can be used for the biopsy or removal. This is a particularly effective method for small lesions, but the curette *must be sharp*. Use disposable units because the reusables are never sharp enough.

9. If the condylomata are numerous (see Fig. 118-5), diffuse, or large, they may need to be treated with radiofrequency fine loop surgical removal, ball electrocautery, 85% TCA (Fig. 118-7), cryosurgery, 5-fluorouracil (Efudex; Valeant Pharmaceuticals, Aliso Viejo, Calif), imiquimod (Aldara; Graceway Pharmaceuticals, Bristol, Tenn), podofilox (Condylox; Oclassen Pharmaceuticals, San Rafael, Calif), the infrared coagulator, laser, or excisional (shave) therapy. Excision with suture closure is virtually contraindicated. A dorsal penile nerve block may facilitate this removal. (See Chapter 155, Treatment of Noncervical Condylomata Acuminata.)
10. Aluminum chloride (Drysol; Person & Covey, Inc., Glendale, Calif), ferric subsulfate (Monsel's solution), or light

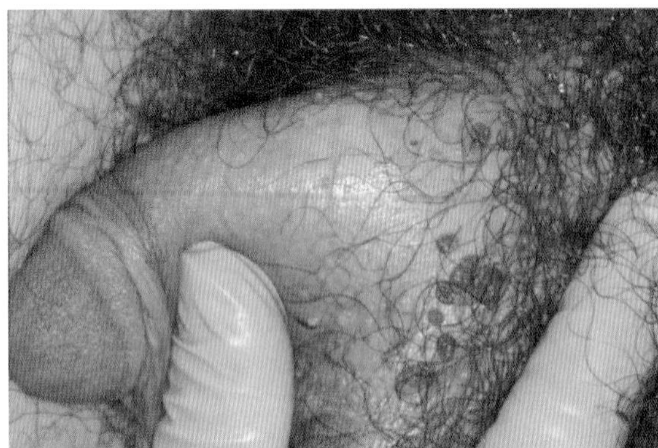

Figure 118-4 Pigmented condylomata. These lesions are more likely to be dysplastic. (Courtesy of John L. Pfenninger, MD, The Medical Procedures Center, PC, Midland, Mich.)

electrocautery/desiccation may be needed as an astringent to limit postoperative bleeding.

11. If only flat, asymptomatic acetowhite changes appear on the penis, anus, or scrotum, treatment is unnecessary, although the biopsies will confirm HPV.
12. Unless the patient has had an extensive area of warts treated, he can return to full activity with no modification of his daily routine.
13. Sample any lesion of uncertain significance. The differential of penile and anal lesions and the approach to evaluation are noted in Box 118-1 and Figure 118-8.
14. Cystoscopy and anoscopy are not routinely recommended for men with condylomata. If lesions are present around the anus and if the man is not anal receptive (which occurs very frequently), treat all perianal lesions first. Anoscopy is indicated but only after resolving the external lesions. Frequently more lesions will be found proximally around the dentate line; these can be removed as biopsies, treated with 85% TCA, frozen, or ablated with ball electrocautery (see Chapter 99, High-Resolution Anoscopy).

PRECAUTION

Not everything that turns acetowhite (white epithelium) is HPV. Chronic irritation, tinea, and other similar conditions can also appear white after the application of acetic acid.

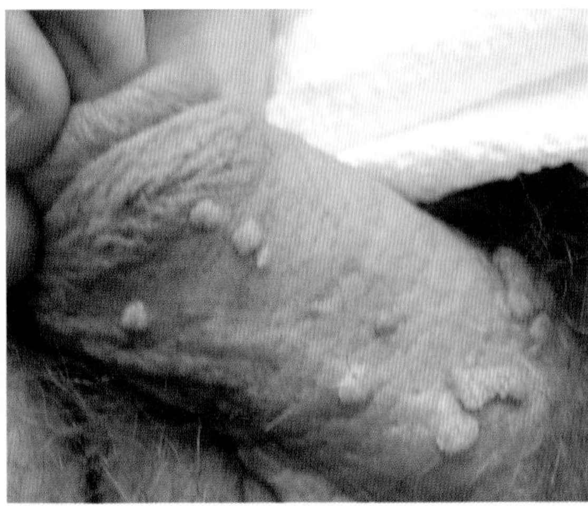

Figure 118-5 Extensive condylomata. (Courtesy of John L. Pfenninger, MD, The Medical Procedures Center, PC, Midland, Mich.)

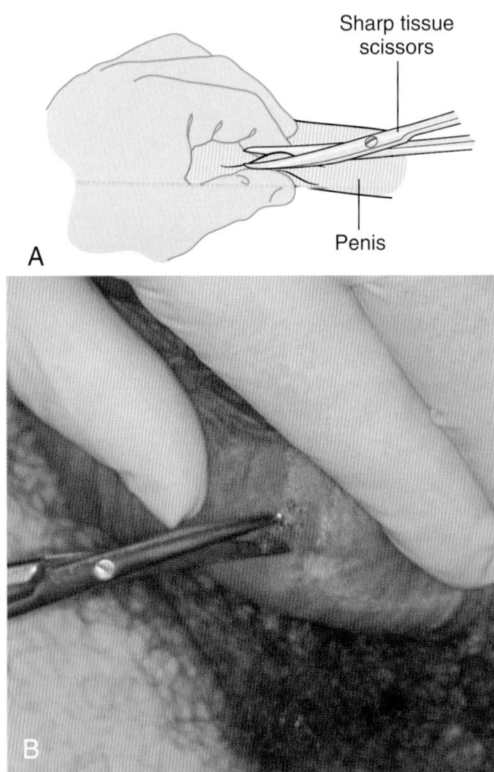

Figure 118-6 **A,** Tenting up the penile skin to obtain a biopsy. **B,** Penile biopsy using curved Metzenbaum scissors.

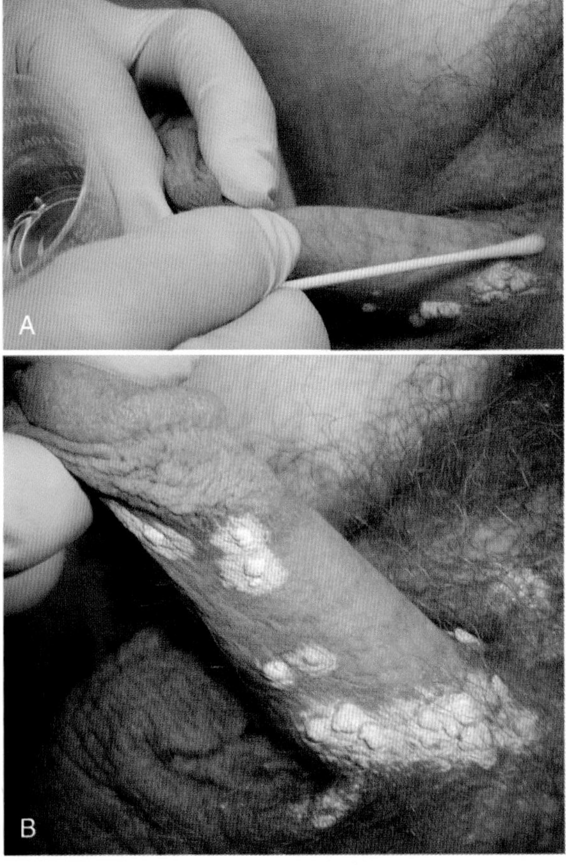

Figure 118-7 **A,** Application of 85% trichloroacetic acid (TCA) with a cotton-tipped applicator. **B,** Appearance of condylomata immediately after application of 85% TCA. (Courtesy of John L. Pfenninger, MD, The Medical Procedures Center, PC, Midland, Mich.)

Box 118-1. Differential Diagnosis of Anogenital Lesions in Men

Infectious Lesions

Chancre
Condylomata acuminata
Condylomata lata
Herpes simplex virus
Molluscum contagiosum
Syphilis
Tinea pubis

Noninfectious Benign Lesions and Conditions (Including Normal Variants)

Anal polyp
Contact dermatitis
Cyst
Nevus
Normal-variant, papular lesions of the corona (pearly penile papules)
Normal-variant, papular lesions of the frenulum
Seborrheic keratosis
Sentinel "polyp" on a chronic fissure
Skin tags

Preneoplastic and Neoplastic Lesions

Bowen's disease (severe dysplasia)
Bowenoid papulosis
Cancer (squamous cell carcinoma of the penis and anus, prolapsing adenocarcinoma of the rectum)
Erythroplasia of Queyrat (squamous cell cancer in situ)
Penile intraepithelial neoplasia (PIN I, PIN II, PIN III)

From Pfenninger JL: Androscopy: Examination of the male partner. In Apgar B, Brotzman G, Spitzer M (eds): Colposcopy: Principles and Practice. An Integrated Textbook and Atlas, 2nd ed. Philadelphia, Saunders, 2008, pp 483–496.

Common Errors

- Not allowing enough time during the visit to counsel the patient and partner adequately.
- Not performing a complete examination, including retracting the foreskin (Fig. 118-9).
- Sampling or treating a normal variant of the corona, pearly penile papules (Fig. 118-10).
- Failing to perform a biopsy and continuing to treat lesions when they do not respond (Fig. 118-11).
- Using expensive prescription topicals when a simple surgical procedure or application of TCA will quickly and more cost-effectively treat the lesion.
- Not using magnification when removing lesions, which increases the likelihood of incomplete removal or missing smaller lesions, thereby increasing the likelihood of recurrence/persistence. Without magnification, it is also more common to perform any removal too deeply, leading to scarring.
- Treating all acetowhite lesions. Even when biopsies confirm the presence of HPV, if the lesions are totally asymptomatic and not visible to the naked eye, treatment is probably unnecessary. Remember that treatment does not eliminate the virus, but only the external manifestations of the disease. It is likely that the virus persists at a subclinical level. There is no evidence that treatment of the male partner in such cases reduces recurrences in female partners.

Postprocedure Patient Care

Topical 5% lidocaine ointment not only soothes the area but prevents treated sites from adhering to the undergarments. A nonsteroidal anti-inflammatory drug (NSAID) is recommended to reduce pain and swelling if more than just a biopsy was done.

No definite recommendations can be made regarding treatment of dysplastic lesions on the penis because studies with long-term follow-up have not been conducted. Between 1% and 5% of the sampled lesions will be reported as mild or moderate bowenoid dysplastic change. Rarely, a severe dysplasia will be found. (Unlike dysplastic cervical lesions in women, it is difficult to predict the degree of dysplastic change observed during the clinical examination, even with magnification, in the man.) In such situations, the patient should return for reexamination in 6 weeks to confirm that the entire dysplastic lesion(s) was removed. The patient should report any unusual growths or ulcerations at once, and he should discuss his HPV history with his physician during future examinations. Sexual partners should be examined and should obtain regular Pap smears. Smoking is strongly discouraged. Supplemental vitamins with folic acid may reduce recurrences. See Chapter 155, Treatment of Noncervical Condylomata Acuminata, for post-treatment patient instructions.

Complications

Complications are minimal. There may be some depigmentation, scarring, pain, or bleeding, regardless of the technique used. The penile skin is very thin and the biopsy/removal should be kept very superficial. Condylomata acuminata can be confused with other lesions, such as condylomata lata, molluscum contagiosum (commonly seen), keratoses, bowenoid dysplasia, nevi, hemorrhoidal tags, and other nondescript papular lesions. Care must be taken that men do not experience undue psychological difficulty because of HPV infection, but at the same time know that each new sexual partner is at risk of contracting the wart virus and should receive annual Pap smears for several years before going to more lengthy intervals.

Conclusion

Androscopy is a simple procedure to perform that enhances the evaluation and treatment of genital lesions in the male patient. The colposcope is expensive, but if it is available in the office for colposcopic examinations, it can aid male patients also. Studies have not been completed using simple magnification devices, but they may also be an aid. HPV vaccines (Gardasil) for men have just been approved, and appear promising.

Patient Education Guides

See patient education and consent forms available online at www.expertconsult.com.

CPT/Billing Codes

There currently is no CPT code for androscopy. Use 55899, unlisted procedure, male genital system (documentation suggested). Insurance companies still rarely pay. Consider charging for a more extended visit with a higher category E&M code (if a new patient or a consult) and for treatment of warts or penile biopsy rather than for "androscopy."

54100 Biopsy, penis, cutaneous
54050 Simple destruction of penile lesions: chemical
54055 Simple destruction of penile lesions: electrosurgical
54056 Simple destruction of penile lesions: cryocautery
54057 Simple destruction of penile lesions: laser
54060 Simple destruction of penile lesions: excision
54065 Destruction of penile lesions, extensive, any method
54105 Biopsy of penis, deep (generally not applicable with HPV)

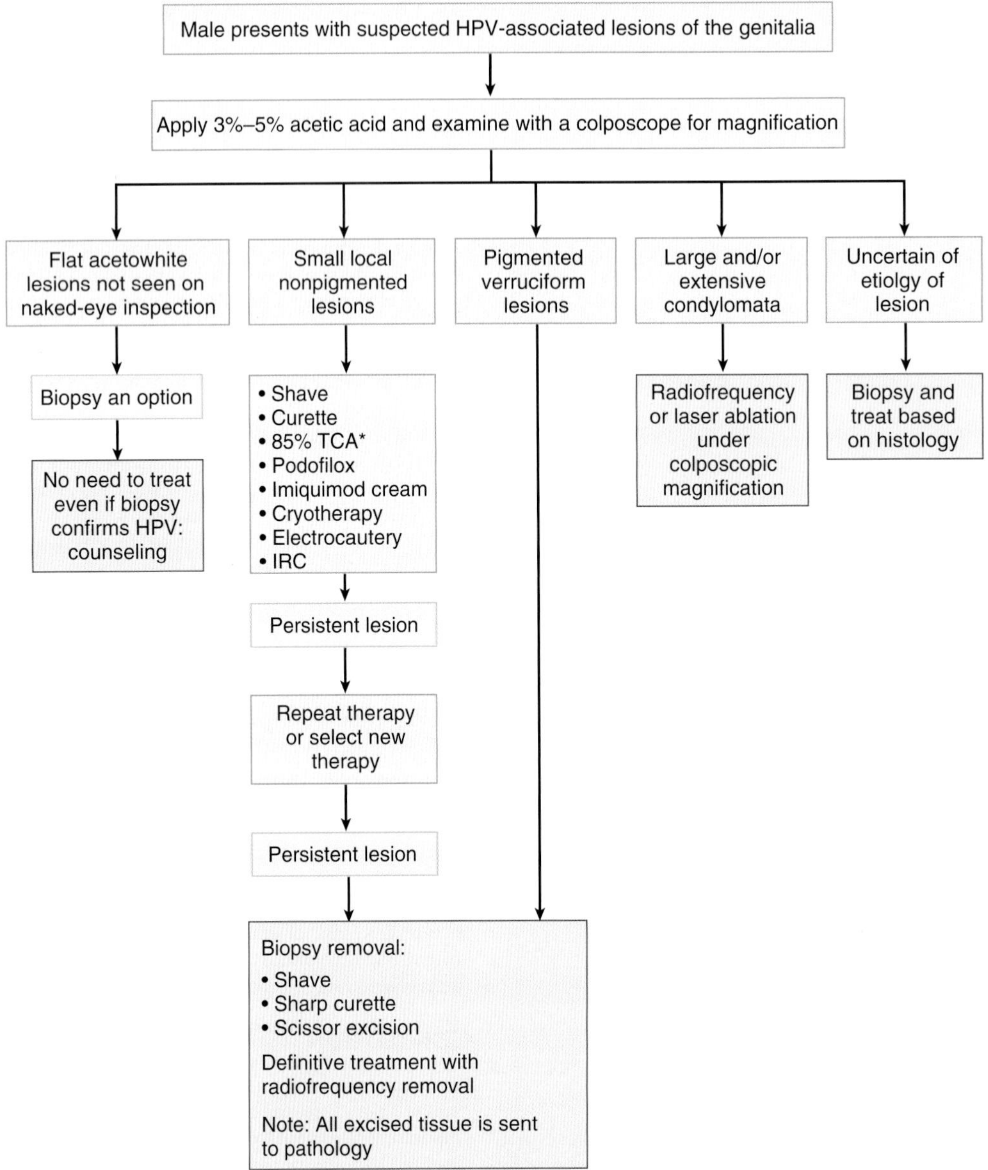

Figure 118-8 Summary of evaluation and treatment options for lesions of the male genitalia. HPV, human papillomavirus; IRC, infrared coagulation. *Eighty-five percent trichloroacetic acid (TCA) is often a first choice for therapy. It is effective 70% of the time, is quick acting, and can treat extensive lesions during the office visit if they are not too large. It is inexpensive compared with other treatments; however, it does burn for 5 minutes after application. (Adapted from Pfenninger JL: Androscopy: Examination of the male patient. In Apgar BS, Brotzman GL, Spitzer M [eds]: Colposcopy: Principles and Practice. An Integrated Text and Atlas, 2nd ed. Philadelphia, Saunders, 2008, pp 483–496.)

ICD-9-CM Diagnostic Codes

07811 Condyloma
607.9 Penile pain

Skin Lesions

173.5 Anus, primary malignancy
187.4 Penis, primary malignancy
187.7 Scrotum, primary malignancy
198.82 Penis, scrotum, metastatic
198.2 Anus, metastatic
216.5 Anus, benign
232.5 Anus, cancer-in-situ
233.5 Penis, cancer-in-situ
233.6 Scrotum, cancer-in-situ
222.1 Penis, benign
222.4 Scrotum, benign
236.6 Penis, uncertain
238.2 Anus, uncertain
239.2 Anus, unspecified
239.5 Penis, scrotum, unspecified

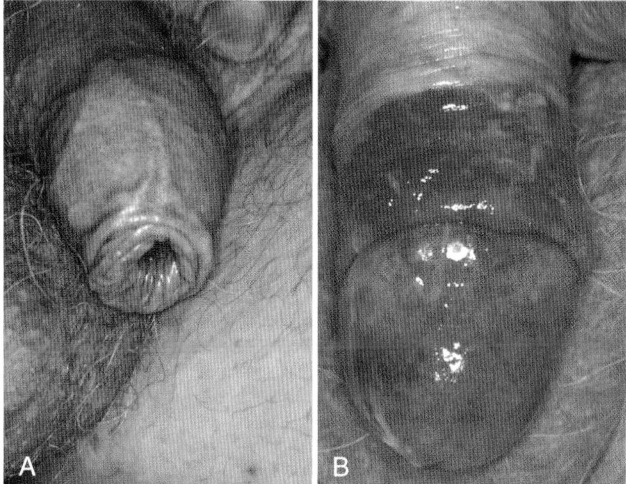

Figure 118-9 **A,** Appearance of uncircumcised penis on presentation. **B,** Erythroplasia of Queyrat (bowenoid carcinoma in situ) after retraction of foreskin. A biopsy can easily be obtained with the technique noted previously using sharp tissue scissors after local anesthesia. (Courtesy of John L. Pfenninger, MD, The Medical Procedures Center, PC, Midland, Mich.)

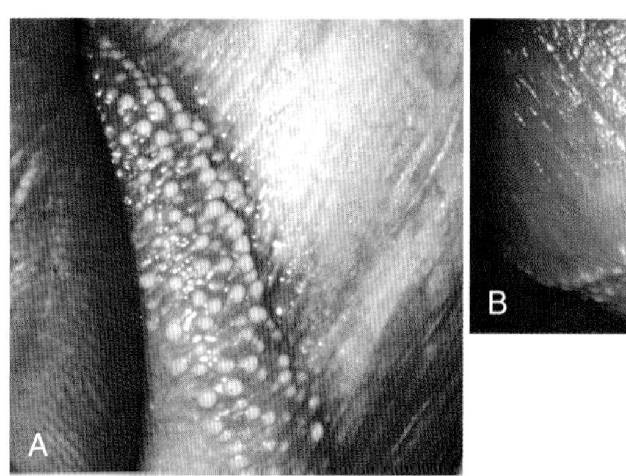

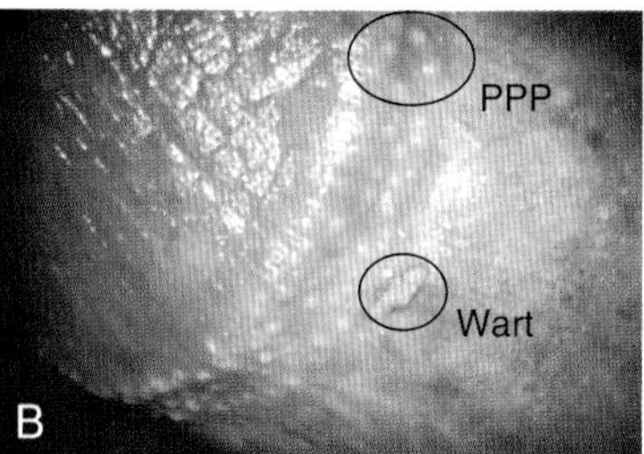

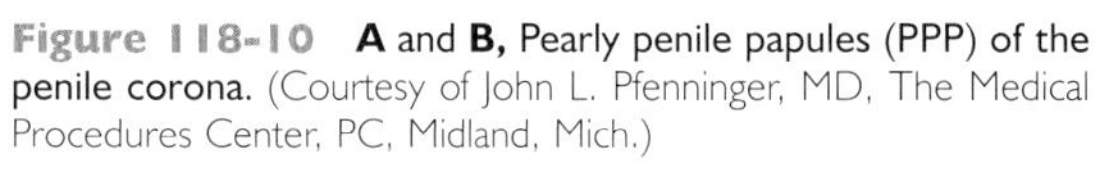

Figure 118-10 **A** and **B,** Pearly penile papules (PPP) of the penile corona. (Courtesy of John L. Pfenninger, MD, The Medical Procedures Center, PC, Midland, Mich.)

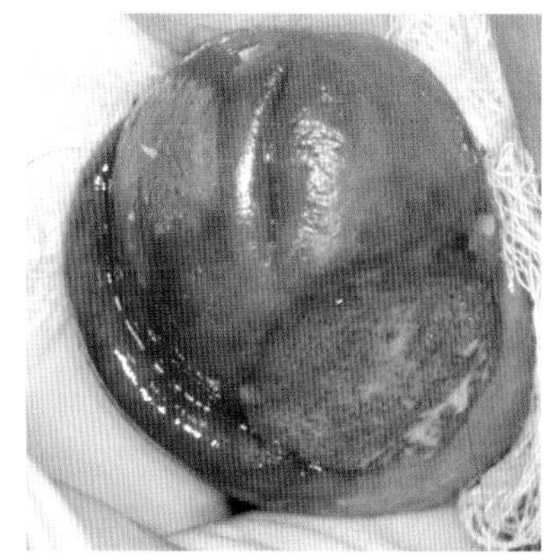

Figure 118-11 Penile squamous cell carcinoma appearing as a "simple condyloma" clinically. Patient was referred to us for definitive treatment after he had been treated four times with 85% TCA and cryotherapy. (Courtesy of John L. Pfenninger, MD, The Medical Procedures Center, PC, Midland, Mich.)

BIBLIOGRAPHY

Barrasso R, DeBrux J, Croissant O: High prevalence of papillomavirus-associated penile intraepithelial neoplasia in sexual partners of women with cervical intraepithelial neoplasia. N Engl J Med 317:916–923, 1987.

Block SL: Comparison of the immunogenicity and reactogenicity of a prophylactic quadrivalent human papillomavirus (types 6, 11, 16, 18) L1 virus-like particle vaccine in male and female adolescents and young adult women. Pediatrics 18:2135–2144, 2006.

Bosch FX, Castellsague X, Muñoz N, et al: Male sexual behavior and human papilloma DNA: Key risk factors for cervical cancer in Spain. J Natl Cancer Inst 88:1060-1067, 1996.

Brinton LA, Li JY, Rong SD, et al: Risk factors of penile cancer: Results from a case-control study in China. Int J Cancer 47:504–509, 1991.

Burmer GC, True LD, Krieger JN: Squamous cell carcinoma of the scrotum associated with human papillomavirus. J Urol 149:374–377, 1993.

Christopher A: Hearing addresses condoms for HPV prevention. J Natl Cancer Inst 96:985, 2004.

Daling JR, Weiss NS: Are barrier methods protective against cervical cancer? Epidemiology 1:261–262, 1990.

Darragh TM, Berry TM, Jay M, Palefsky J: Anal disease. In Apgar B, Brotzman G, Spitzer M (eds): Colposcopy: Principles and Practice. An Integrated Textbook and Atlas, 2nd ed. Philadelphia, Saunders, 2008, pp 451–482.

EDITOR'S NOTE: This chapter is an excellent review of HPV and anal disease, including anal cytology smears and high-resolution anoscopy (HRA).

Demeter LM, Stoler MH, Bonnez W, et al: Penile intraepithelial neoplasia: Clinical presentation and an analysis of the physical state of human papilloma DNA. J Infect Dis 168:38–46, 1993.

Epperson WJ: Androscopy for anogenital HPV. J Fam Pract 33:143–146, 1991.

Frisch M, Fenger C, van den Brule AJ, et al: Variants of squamous cell carcinoma: Cancer of the anal canal and perianal skin and their relation to human papillomavirus. Cancer Res 59:753–757, 1999.

Goldie SJ, Kuntz KM, Weinstein MC: The clinical effectiveness and cost-effectiveness of screening for anal squamous intraepithelial lesions in homosexual and bisexual HIV-positive men. JAMA 281:1822–1829, 1999.

Holmes KK, Levine R, Weaver M: Effectiveness of condoms in preventing sexually transmitted infections. Bull World Health Org 82:454–461, 2004.

Koutsky L: Epidemiology of genital human papillomavirus infections. Am J Med 102(5 Suppl 1):3–8, 1997.

Krebs HB: Management of human papilloma virus-associated genital lesions in men. Obstet Gynecol 73:312–316, 1989.

Krebs HB, Helmkamp F: Does the treatment of genital condylomata in men decrease the treatment failure rate of cervical dysplasia in the female sexual partner? Obstet Gynecol 76:660–663, 1990.

Krogh G: Clinical relevance and evaluation of genito-anal papillomavirus infections in the male. Semin Dermatol 11:229–240, 1992.

Lai YM, Yang FP, Pao CC: Human papillomavirus deoxyribonucleic acid and ribonucleic acid in seminal plasma and sperm cells. Fertil Steril 65:1026–1030, 1996.

Malek RS, Goellner JR, Smith T, et al: Human papillomavirus infection and intraepithelial, in-situ, and invasive carcinoma of the penis. Urology 42:159–170, 1993.

Noel JC, Vandenbossche M, Peny MO, et al: Verrucous carcinoma of the penis: Importance of human papillomavirus typing for diagnosis and therapeutic decisions. Eur Urol 22:83–85, 1992.

Palefsky JM: Anal cancer and its precursors: An HIV-related disease. Hosp Physician 29:35, 1993.

Palefsky JM, Holly EA, Gonzales J, et al: Detection of human papillomavirus DNA in anal intraepithelial neoplasia and anal cancer. Cancer Res 51:1014–1019, 1991.

Patton D, Rodney WM: Androscopy of unproven benefit. J Fam Pract 332:135–136, 1991.

Pfenninger JL: Androscopy: Technique for examining men for condyloma. J Fam Pract 29:286–288, 1989.

Pfenninger JL: Letter to the editor. J Fam Pract 33:566, 1991.

Pfenninger JL: Androscopy: Examination of the male partner. In Apgar B, Brotzman G, Spitzer M (eds): Colposcopy: Principles and Practice. An Integrated Textbook and Atlas, 2nd ed. Philadelphia, Saunders, 2008, pp 483–496.

Pineda CP, Berry JM, Welton ML: High resolution anoscopy and targeted treatment of high-grade squamous intraepithelial lesions. Dis Colon Rectum 49:126, 2006.

Poblet E, Alfaro L, Fernander-Segoviano P, et al: Human papillomavirus-associated penile squamous cell carcinoma in HIV-positive patients. Am J Surg Pathol 23:1119–1123, 1999.

Rando RF: Human papilloma virus: Implications for clinical medicine. Ann Intern Med 108:628–630, 1988.

Richart R: Men and HPV. Prim Care Cancer 8:5, 1995.

Rosemberg SK: Sexually transmitted papillomaviral infections: IV. The white scrotum. Urology 33:462–464, 1989.

Teichman JMH, Sea J, Thompson IM, Elston DM: Noninfectious penile lesions. Am Fam Physician 81:167–174, 2010.

Tokudome S: Semen of smokers and cervical cancer risk [letter]. J Natl Cancer Inst 89:96, 1997.

von Krogh G: Clinical relevance and evaluation of genitoanal papilloma virus infection in the male. Semin Dermatol 11:229–240, 1992.

Weiner JS, Liu ET, Walther PJ: Oncogenic human papillomavirus type 16 in association with squamous cell cancer of the male urethra. Cancer Res 52:5018–5023, 1992.

Whidden P: Cigarette smoking and cervical cancer [letter]. Int J Epidemiol 23:1099, 1994.

Wikström A, Hedblad MA, Johansson B, et al: The acetic acid test in evaluation of subclinical genital infection: A competence study on penoscopy, histopathology, virology and scanning electron microscopy findings. Genitourin Med 68:90–99, 1992.

Winer RL, Hughes JP, Feng Q, et al: Condom use and the risk of genital human papillomavirus infection in young women. N Engl J Med 354:2645–2654, 2006.

Winer RL, Lee SK, Hughes TP, et al: Genital human papilloma virus infection: Rates and risk factors in a cohort of female university students. Am J Epidemiol 157:218–226, 2003.

Xi LF, Critchlow CW, Wheeler CM, et al: Risk of anal carcinoma-in-situ in relation to human papillomavirus type 16 variants. Cancer Res 58:3839–3844, 1998.

Zabbo A, Stein BS: Penile intraepithelial neoplasia in patients examined for exposure to human papillomavirus. Urology 41:24–26, 1993.

CHAPTER 119

Dorsal Slit for Phimosis

Morteza Khodaee • Gary Yen

Although the exact definition of phimosis is still controversial, this condition has been recognized since ancient times. Phimosis can be physiologic, congenital, or acquired as a result of inflammation or infection. About 90% of boys have a fully retractable foreskin by the age of 3 years. American literature describes phimosis as *scar formation of the foreskin secondary to any injury or inflammatory condition, with the inability to retract the foreskin over the glans penis* (Wein and colleagues, 2007). Poor hygiene, diabetes, and zipper injuries are conditions that may increase the risk of phimosis. *Acute phimosis* may occur with infection or as a complication of various treatments for conditions such as verrucae, which can cause inflammation (e.g., 85% trichloroacetic acid, electrocoagulation).

Phimosis may lead to urinary retention or infection as well as *paraphimosis* (nonreducible retracted foreskin), which may require urgent or emergent intervention (Fig. 119-1). A debate exists over medical versus surgical management of phimosis. In countries in which circumcision is not widely practiced, nonsurgical and conservative surgical methods are often used. Recent worldwide studies demonstrated the efficacy of topical steroids (0.05% betamethasone cream once or twice a day for 4 to 6 weeks).

Surgical options for phimosis include dorsal slit, ventral slit, preputioplasty, and circumcision. Various preputioplasty techniques (including sutureless prepuceplasty, triple incision plasty, La Vega slit) have been developed to accomplish better cosmetic results. These techniques usually involve a longitudinal incision in an attempt to release the tight prepuce ring. Dorsal slit is a simple procedure involving a single cut along the dorsal foreskin that allows rapid access to the urethral meatus and glans penis.

Indications

- To gain emergency access to the urethral meatus for bladder catheterization in the presence of phimosis
- To prevent recurrent balanitis with abscess formation
- As an adjunct treatment before circumcision or after phimotic ring incision for paraphimosis

Contraindications

- Active infection of the genitalia
- Anatomic abnormalities of the external genitalia (refer to urologist)

Equipment

- 10-mL syringe with 1-inch, 27-gauge needle
- 1% to 2% lidocaine without epinephrine
- Three small, straight hemostats
- Straight iris or small Metzenbaum scissors
- Suture scissors
- Absorbable suture (4-0) on small reversed cutting needle
- Needle driver
- Fenestrated drape
- Iodine solution or other antiseptic scrub
- Preparation bowl with 4 × 4 gauze sponges
- Adson forceps

Preprocedure Patient Preparation

Provide appropriate information to the patient about the procedure while obtaining informed consent (see the patient consent form online at www.expertconsult.com). Risks include pain, bleeding, infection, damage to the glans, poor cosmetic result, and hematoma formation. Benefits include resolution of phimosis, prevention of paraphimosis, increased ease of hygiene, decreased risk of urinary retention, and decreased pain with intercourse.

Place the patient in a comfortable supine position on an examination table in a well-lit room. Using sterile technique, surgically prepare the genital area with an antiseptic solution. Place the penis through a fenestrated drape and onto the surgical field.

Technique

Anesthesia

1. *Dorsal penile nerve block* or modified "ring block" is used to obtain anesthesia after preparing and draping the penis (see Chapter 179, Subcutaneous Ring and Dorsal Penile Block for Newborn Circumcision). A dorsal penile nerve block anesthetizes the right and left dorsal nerves where they branch from the pudendal nerve from under the pubic bone. The lateral and ventral portions of the penile shaft are innervated by branches arcading from the dorsal midline, radiating toward the ventral surface. The axons innervating the glans are in a constant dorsal, midline location along most of the penile shaft.
2. A 27-gauge, 1-inch needle is inserted at the base of the penis just under the pubic bone and into Buck's fascia at the 2 o'clock and 10 o'clock positions (Fig. 119-2A and B).
3. After aspirating, inject 3 to 5 mL of lidocaine into the base of the penis at the 2 o'clock and 10 o'clock positions deep to Buck's fascia at the inferior edge of the pubic bone.
4. Wait 5 minutes and test for the adequacy of anesthesia by grasping the dorsal foreskin with a hemostat.
5. A *modified ring block* can be used if anesthesia is incomplete. This is performed by interconnecting the two positions across the dorsal midline at the base of the penis in a subcutaneous fashion (Fig. 119-2C).

Procedure

1. After achieving local anesthesia, the operator grasps the distal dorsal foreskin in the 2 o'clock and 10 o'clock positions with two of the small, straight hemostats (Fig. 119-2D). Use the instruments to apply countertraction when performing the procedure.
2. Identify the corona of the glans with the foreskin in a relaxed position or with just gentle straightening. The corona determines the proximal extent of the dorsal slit.

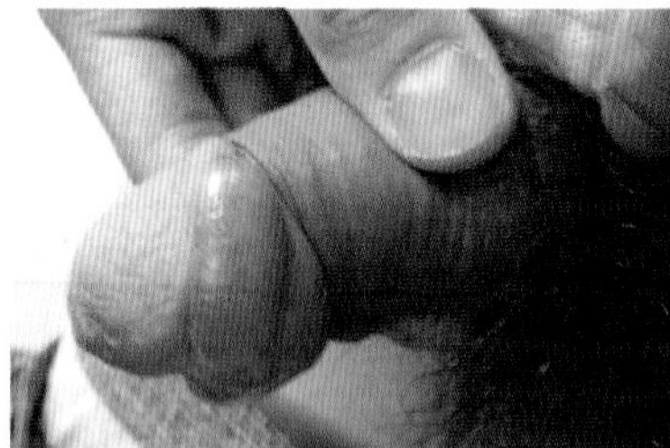

Figure 119-1 Paraphimosis.

3. Gently retract the foreskin and attempt to identify the urethral meatus.
4. A closed small, straight hemostat is horizontally introduced into the opening of the foreskin between the inner layer of the foreskin and the glans penis. Advance it proximally to the coronal sulcus. Avoid entering the urethral meatus.
5. Tent up the foreskin and spread open the hemostat. Withdraw the instrument and twist to the right and left to break up adhesions around the circumference of the glans (Fig. 119-2E).
6. When lysis of adhesions is complete, the hemostat is withdrawn. Reinsert it open with one jaw of the hemostat in the plane between the glans and the inner layer of the foreskin while the other is placed on the outer skin. This should be at the 12 o'clock position with the instrument in a longitudinal position. Advance the instrument to the level of the coronal sulcus and clamp tightly. This crushes the interposed anesthetized foreskin. Leave in place for 3 to 5 minutes (Figs. 119-2F and 119-2G).
7. Remove the hemostat and cut the foreskin longitudinally with iris or Metzenbaum scissors along the entire distance of the serrated, crushed foreskin, being careful to leave 1 or 2 mm of crushed tissue at the apex lest uncrushed skin be incised, which can lead to significant bleeding.
8. If crush hemostasis is inadequate or if the incision does extend too far and there is bleeding after cutting the dorsal slit, absorbable sutures should be used to obtain adequate hemostasis. This

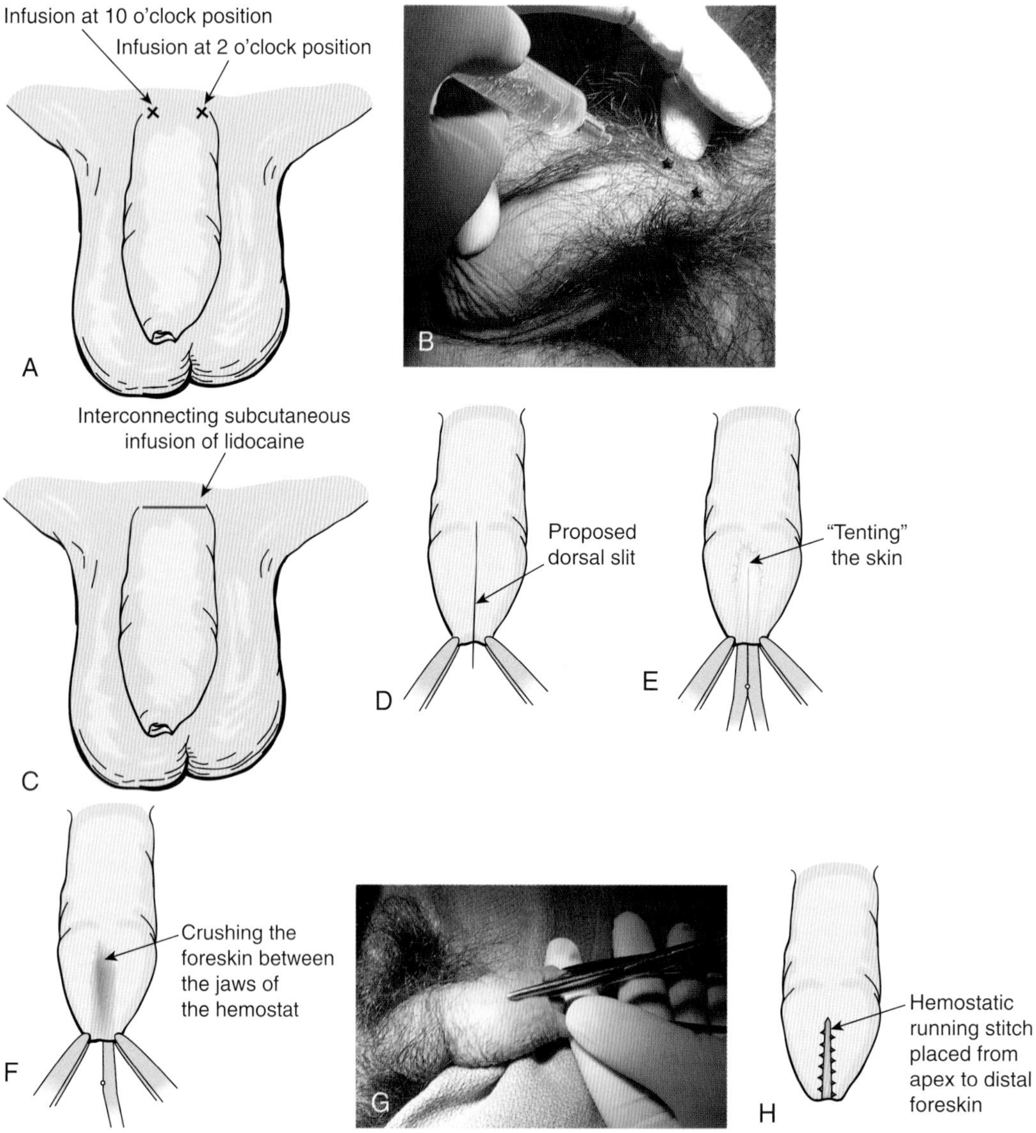

Figure 119-2 Dorsal penile nerve block. **A** and **B,** Inject at 10 and 2 o'clock positions. **C,** Partial ring block. **D,** Grasp foreskin at the 10 and 2 o'clock positions. Attempt to identify urethral meatus. **E,** Lysing adhesions. Separate the foreskin from the glans by spreading while withdrawing the hemostat. **F** and **G,** Place clamp longitudinally in the 12 o'clock position for 3 to 5 minutes. **H,** Placement of sutures to control bleeding if needed.

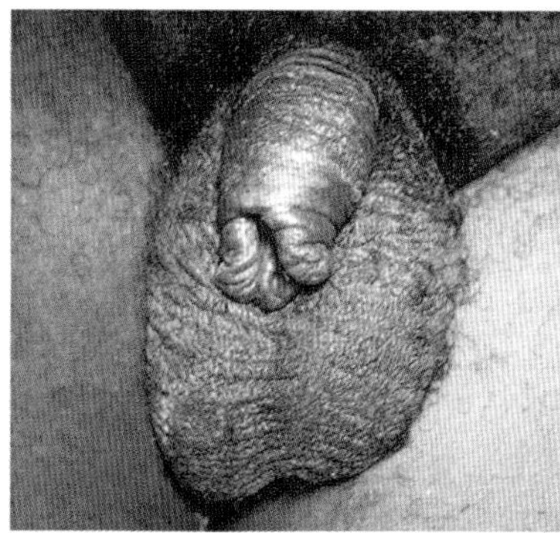

Figure 119-3 "Dog-ear" appearance that results from the dorsal slit procedure. A formal, complete circumcision can be performed if desired and the inflammation has resolved. (From Roberts JR, Hedges JR [eds]: Clinical Procedures in Emergency Medicine, 5th ed. Philadelphia, Saunders, 2009.)

is performed by placing two running 4-0 Vicryl or Dexon sutures beginning at the apex of the dorsal slit and running distally to reapproximate the two layers of each side of the incision of the foreskin (Fig. 119-2H).

9. Application of sterile petroleum jelly or antibiotic ointment on the wound edges prevents the dressing from adhering to the wound.

Complications

- *Bleeding*: Late bleeding can be controlled with direct pressure, Monsel's solution, Gelfoam, or the placement of hemostatic ligatures.
- *Injury to the urethral meatus or glans*: Avoid blind introduction of hemostat and scissors when performing the procedure to prevent injury to the urethral meatus or glans.
- *Infection*: Antibiotics can be used to control infection commonly due to skin pathogens such as *Streptococcus* or *Staphylococcus*.
- *Pain*: Hyperesthesia with intercourse may occur.
- *Anesthesia complications*: There may be hematoma formation at the site of injection.
- *Poor cosmetic result*: Elective circumcision may be recommended if the patient is not satisfied with the "dog-ear" appearance of the foreskin (Fig. 119-3).

Postprocedure Patient Education

- After successful dorsal slit for phimosis, the prepuce is easily retracted to access the urethral meatus and cleanse the glans penis.
- After completion of catheterization or cleansing, the foreskin should be reduced to avoid iatrogenic paraphimosis.
- Between 3 and 5 days of analgesics should be prescribed for postprocedure pain.
- The patient should wear loose briefs and gently cleanse the wound for 5 to 7 days with soap and water three to four times a day.
- The patient should avoid intercourse or masturbation for 4 to 6 weeks to prevent disruption of the wound.
- The patient should be instructed to return for postprocedure wound check in 1 to 2 weeks and to return immediately if excessive bleeding occurs.
- Instruct the patient on signs of infection that should not be confused with fibrinous exudate (a straw-colored exudate), which is part of normal healing.

Conclusion

Dorsal slit is an effective procedure that permits easy retraction of the foreskin, without the need for circumcision. It can be performed in the office setting or emergency department for complications related to phimosis.

Patient Education Guides

See the sample patient education and consent forms online at www.expertconsult.com.

CPT/Billing Code

54160 Dorsal slit for phimosis

ICD-9-CM Diagnostic Codes

605 Phimosis
605 Paraphimosis

Acknowledgment

The editors wish to recognize the many contributions by Scott A. Cota, MD, to this chapter in the previous edition of this text.

BIBLIOGRAPHY

Christianakis E: Sutureless prepuceplasty with wound healing by second intention: An alternative surgical approach in children's phimosis treatment. BMC Urol Mar 4 8:6, 2008.

Cuckow PM, Rix G, Mouriquand PD: Preputial plasty: A good alternative to circumcision. J Pediatr Surg 29:561–563, 1994.

Esposito C, Centonze A, Alicchio F, et al: Topical steroid application versus circumcision in pediatric patients with phimosis: A prospective randomized placebo controlled clinical trial. World J Urol 26:187–190, 2008.

Holman JR, Stuessi KA: Adult circumcision. Am Fam Physician 59:1514–1518, 1999.

Munro NP, Khan H, Shaikh NA, et al: Y-V preputioplasty for adult phimosis: A review of 89 cases. Urology 72:918–920, 2008.

Roberts JR, Hedges JR (eds): Clinical Procedures in Emergency Medicine, 4th ed. Philadelphia, Saunders, 2004.

Santucci RA, Kim H, Terlecki RP: Phimosis, adult circumcision and buried penis. eMedicine 2006, updated April 15, 2009. Available at www.emedicine.com/med/topic2873.htm.

Steadman B, Ellsworth P: To circ or not to circ: Indications, risks, and alternatives to circumcision in the pediatric population with phimosis. Urol Nurs 26:181–194, 2006.

Sugita Y, Ueoka K, Tagkagi S, et al: A new technique of concealed penis repair. J Urol 182(4 Suppl):1751–1754, 2009.

Szmuk P, Ezri T, Ben Hur H, et al: Regional anaesthesia for circumcision in adults: A comparative study. Can J Anaesth 41:1181–1184, 1994.

Van Howe RS: Cost-effective treatment of phimosis. Pediatrics 102:E43, 1998.

Wein AJ, Kavoussi LR, Novick AC, et al. (eds): Campbell-Walsh Urology, 9th ed. Philadelphia, Saunders, 2007.

Yang CC, Bradley WE: Neuroanatomy of the penile portion of the human dorsal nerve of the penis. Br J Urol 82:109–113, 1998.

CHAPTER 120

PROSTATE MASSAGE

Robert E. James • James R. Palleschi

Prostate massage has been used therapeutically and diagnostically in the management of recurrent or chronic prostatitis and prostatodynia. At this time, its primary benefit are to aid in the diagnosis of chronic prostatitis and for collecting a specimen of urine for a *PCA3* (prostate cancer gene 3) test.

The urinary *PCA3* test has been found by some investigators to be helpful in screening for prostate cancer. After performing a prostate massage, the patient is asked to provide a urine specimen, which is sent to the lab to complete the *PCA3* analysis. The *PCA3* gene is overexpressed in patients with prostate cancer, but not in men with prostatitis or an enlarged prostate gland.

INDICATIONS

- Diagnosis of chronic or subacute prostatitis
- Management of prostatitis and prostatodynia (infrequent)

CONTRAINDICATIONS

- Acute prostatitis
- Prostatic abscess
- Significant difficulty voiding

EQUIPMENT

- Examination glove and water-soluble lubricant
- Microscope
- Sterile culture container

PREPROCEDURE PATIENT PREPARATION

Tell the patient that he may have an urge to urinate and may feel rectal pressure for 15 to 60 minutes after prostatic massage. Tell the patient to contact the physician or the nearest emergency department if he experiences chills, myalgia, rigors, or temperature above 101° F.

TECHNIQUE

1. Place the patient in a comfortable position for the prostate examination. A variety of positions may be used: the knee–chest position, left lateral decubitus position, or bent over the examination table. (With this position, the patient should place his elbows on the examination table and spread his heels apart. The patient is thus immobilized, which facilitates the prostate examination and the subsequent massage.) In addition, the patient may assist you in collecting the expressed prostatic fluid by holding the microscope slide below the urethral meatus of the glans penis.
2. Apply a generous amount of lubricant to the anus and to your gloved index finger. The examination will be more comfortable for the patient if he performs a mild Valsalva maneuver as the finger passes through and into the anal opening. In patients with a high-riding prostate, a Valsalva maneuver may bring the gland down to the examining finger.
3. For the prostate massage, press the pad of your index finger into the substance of the prostate. Start on the superior and lateral aspect of the prostate and move your index finger toward the midline or median sulcus. Gradually work from the base or superior aspect of the prostate gland down to the inferior portion or apex (Fig. 120-1). This motion is carried out several times bilaterally. Last, massage the median furrow, or mid-aspect, of the prostate gland, from the base to the apex. The prostatic secretions are massaged toward the prostatic urethra. These secretions then pass through the distal urethra and can be collected for microscopic examination and culture and sensitivity if desired. Normally, you need to repeat the prostatic massage for a period of 30 to 90 seconds before any secretions are obtained. The quantity collected may vary from a few drops to 2 to 3 mL. Some patients will not discharge any secretions (despite correct performance of the prostate massage as described) or may have discomfort sufficient to abort the procedure. Clinically, more than 15 white blood cells per high-power field suggest an infectious process.

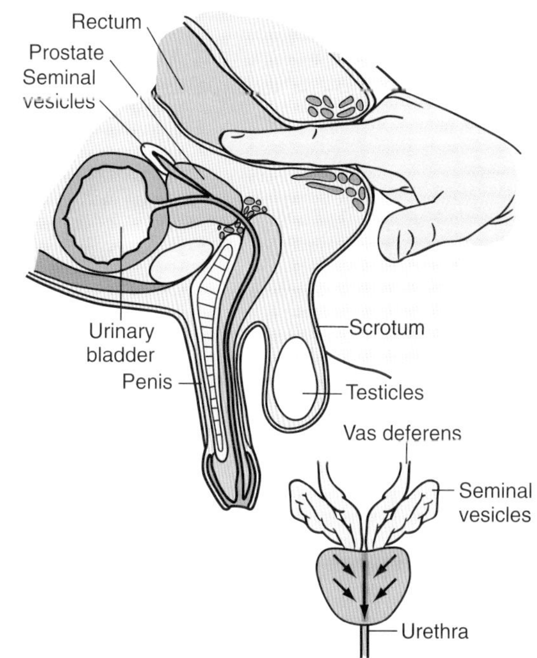

Figure 120-1 Technique of prostatic massage. The glandular substance is compressed from its lateral edges to the urethra, which lies in the center. The *arrows* in the inset drawing show the direction of pressure. The seminal vesicles are then stripped from above downward.

Complications

- Rarely, bacteremia or urosepsis may occur after a prostate massage. These problems can be avoided by not performing prostate massage on a patient suspected of having acute prostatitis or a prostate abscess.
- Occasionally, a patient with significant prostatism resulting from prostatic hypertrophy may develop prostatic edema after a massage, leading to temporary difficulty urinating or urinary retention.
- Hematuria and hematospermia occur infrequently after a prostate massage.

NOTE: Any manipulation or trauma to the prostate gland may elevate a patient's serum prostate-specific antigen (PSA) for several weeks. Therefore, after performing a digital rectal examination, I would wait one week before performing a PSA and after a prostate massage, I would wait two weeks. An acute prostatitis or prostate infarct may cause an elevated PSA for up to six weeks.

CPT/Billing Code

87205 Prostatic smear

There is no CPT code for prostate massage.

ICD-9-CM Diagnostic Codes

600.0 Prostatitis, hypertrophic
600.9 Prostatitis
601.0 Prostatitis, acute
601.1 Prostatitis, subacute or chronic
601.3 Prostatocystitis
601.2 Abscess of prostate (note: avoid prostate massage)
601.9 Prostatitis (congestive)
602.1 Congestion or hemorrhage of prostate
602.9 Unspecified disorder of prostate, prostatodynia

Bibliography

Campbell-Walsh Urology, 9th ed. Philadelphia, Saunders, 2007.
Tanagho EA: Physical examination of genitourinary tract. In Tanagho EA, McAninch JW (eds): Smith's General Urology, 12th ed. Norwalk, Conn, Appleton & Lange, 1988, pp 38–45.

CHAPTER 121

PROSTATE AND SEMINAL VESICLE ULTRASONOGRAPHY AND BIOPSY

Philip J. Aliotta • Grant C. Fowler

Transrectal ultrasonography of the prostate (TRUSP) and seminal vesicles (SVs) is an essential tool in the assessment of these organs. Useful for defining anatomy, evaluating blood flow, and diagnosing and treating benign and malignant diseases of these glands, it is now the standard in most urologists' practices.

Although TRUSP-SV has proved helpful in the investigation of the infertile couple, more importantly, the introduction of TRUSP-SV has improved the accuracy of prostate tissue sampling. Even though a digital rectal examination (DRE)–guided fine-needle or core (e.g., Tru-Cut, Biopty) biopsy may confirm cancer, it is not as useful for excluding cancer; DRE is more helpful for guiding biopsy of a palpable nodule. TRUSP-SV improves the ability of the clinician to exclude cancer in more regions of the gland and has somewhat become the standard for evaluation of possible prostate cancer.

One important recent development for TRUSP-SV, especially for underserved areas, is that technicians or sonographers are now making services available on-site for primary care clinicians, even to guide biopsy. Overreading services for TRUSP-SV by a radiologist are also now available over the Internet (see the "Suppliers" section). This may revolutionize the management of suspected prostate cancer. However, an understanding of anatomy is necessary before scanning or biopsy. The prostate can be described by its general, vascular, zonal, tissue, or ultrasonographic anatomy.

Although recent large studies in the United States and Europe have failed to clarify whether men benefit from screening for prostate cancer, most organizations are now recommending at least a discussion of this topic with their clinician, especially in men younger than 75 years of age and with at least a 10-year life expectancy. A prostate biopsy may be indicated if the examination or laboratory result is suspect for cancer (Fig. 121-1). Although certain ethnic groups (e.g., African Americans) were thought to be at increased risk of prostate cancer in the past, more contemporary analyses suggest that this discrepancy is disappearing. Much of any remaining variation may be more strongly related to education, insurance status, and access to health care.

GENERAL ANATOMY

Figure 121-2 shows the general anatomy of the prostate and seminal vesicles.

Prostate

The prostate is a chestnut-shaped gland surrounded by a pseudocapsule of dense fibrous tissue and smooth muscle that connects with the muscular layers of the prostatic urethra. The pseudocapsule cannot be separated from the gland itself. It has an anterior, posterior, and lateral surface. The prostate base is contiguous with the bladder superiorly. The apex of the prostate is contiguous with the striated urethral sphincter. Lateral to the prostate is the pubococcygeal portion of the levator ani and endopelvic fascia. Denonvilliers' fascia, which separates the prostate from the rectum, is posterior to the prostate.

Vas Deferens and Seminal Vesicles

Arising from the tail of the epididymis, the vas deferens consists of a tortuous proximal portion and a dilated terminal portion called the *ampulla*. The ampulla is capable of storing sperm and lies posterior to the bladder. Bordering the base of the bladder, posteriorly, are the seminal vesicles. They also lie adjacent to the ampullae of the vasa deferentia and the distal ureters.

VASCULAR ANATOMY

The prostatic artery is a branch of the internal iliac artery. It divides into capsular and urethral arteries. The capsular arteries supply two thirds of the gland; the urethral arteries supply the remaining third. Branches of the inferior vesical artery supply the seminal vesicles, and occasionally the base of the prostate gland. The neurovascular bundles located posterolaterally (at the confluence of the seminal vesicle and prostate bilaterally) provide the main neurovascular supply and drainage system of the prostate.

ZONAL ANATOMY

Traditionally, the prostate was divided into five major lobes (anterior, middle, posterior, and two lateral lobes) and two minor lobes (trigonal and subcervical lobes). McNeal derived a three-dimensional model of the prostate, as illustrated in Figure 121-3.

TISSUE ANATOMY

The normal prostate consists of a combination of *glandular tissue* and *fibromuscular structures*.

Glandular Tissue

Glandular tissue accounts for about 66% of the prostate. There are four identified glandular zones, each with a distinct ductal system draining into a specific part of the urethra. The first three zones share similar histologic and embryologic origin. The fourth zone is the central zone (CZ) and differs histologically from the rest of the gland. It is derived from the Wolffian duct.

1. *Peripheral zone (PZ; as much as 75% of the glandular tissue)*. The largest area of glandular tissue is in the PZ, which comprises the lateral and most of the posterior aspect of the prostate (except at the base). The PZ ducts drain into the distal urethral segment. The majority (>65%) of prostate cancers occur in the PZ.

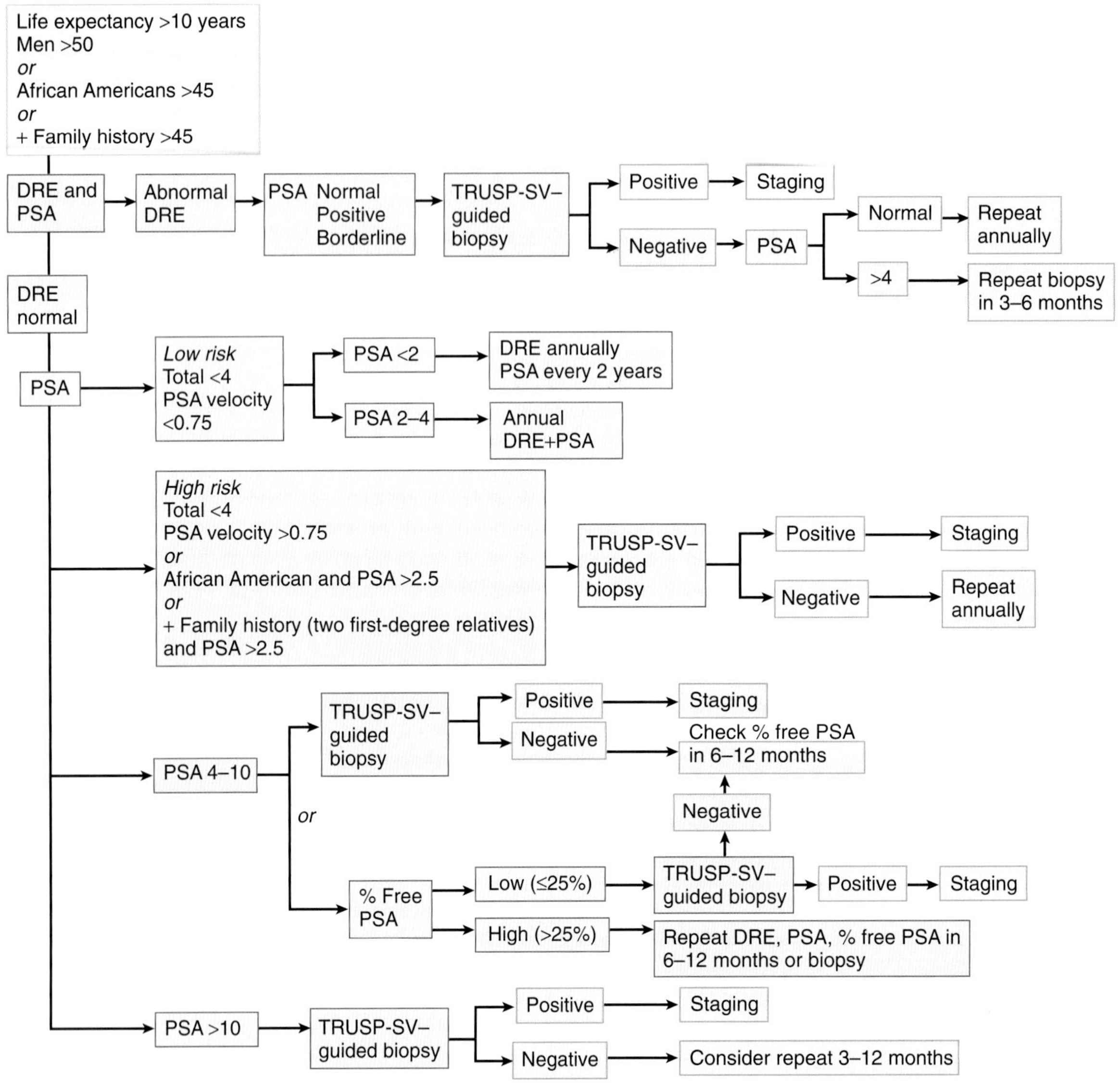

Life expectancy >10 years
Men >50
or
African Americans >45
or
+ Family history >45

- DRE and PSA → Abnormal DRE → PSA Normal / Positive / Borderline → TRUSP-SV–guided biopsy
  - → Positive → Staging
  - → Negative → PSA
    - → Normal → Repeat annually
    - → >4 → Repeat biopsy in 3–6 months
- DRE normal → PSA
  - → *Low risk* Total <4, PSA velocity <0.75
    - → PSA <2 → DRE annually, PSA every 2 years
    - → PSA 2–4 → Annual DRE+PSA
  - → *High risk* Total <4, PSA velocity >0.75 *or* African American and PSA >2.5 *or* + Family history (two first-degree relatives) and PSA >2.5 → TRUSP-SV–guided biopsy
    - → Positive → Staging
    - → Negative → Repeat annually
  - → PSA 4–10
    - → TRUSP-SV–guided biopsy
      - → Positive → Staging
      - → Negative → Check % free PSA in 6–12 months
    - *or* → % Free PSA
      - → Low (≤25%) → TRUSP-SV–guided biopsy → Positive → Staging; → Negative → Check % free PSA in 6–12 months
      - → High (>25%) → Repeat DRE, PSA, % free PSA in 6–12 months or biopsy
  - → PSA >10 → TRUSP-SV–guided biopsy
    - → Positive → Staging
    - → Negative → Consider repeat 3–12 months

Figure 121-1 Sample algorithm for men who desire early cancer detection after discussion of pros and cons with their clinician. DRE, digital rectal examination; PSA, prostate-specific antigen; TRUSP-SV, transrectal ultrasonography of the prostate and seminal vesicles. Contemporary analyses of African American men suggest that ethnic discrepancies are disappearing. Much of any ethnic variation still noted may be more strongly related to education, insurance status, and access to health care rather than ethnicity. (Redrawn from Braunwald E, Fauci AS, Kasper DL, et al. [eds]: Harrison's Principles of Internal Medicine, 15th ed. New York, McGraw-Hill, 2001.)

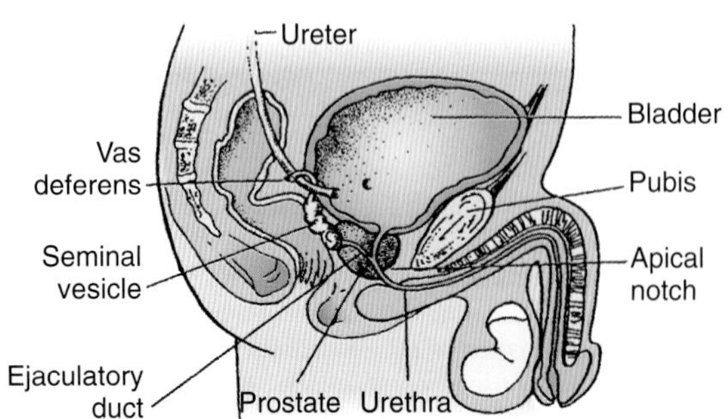

Figure 121-2 General anatomy of prostate and seminal vesicles. (From Brooks JD: Anatomy of the lower urinary tract and male genitalia. In Walsh PC, Retik AB, Vaughan ED Jr, Wein AJ [eds]: Campbell's Urology, 7th ed. Philadelphia, WB Saunders, 1998, pp 112–117.)

2. *Transition zone (TZ; 5% or more of the glandular tissue)*. Between 5% and 10% of the glandular tissue is in the TZ. The TZ comprises two small lobules on either side of the proximal urethral segment just lateral to the periprostatic sphincter. The TZ is the origin of most symptomatic benign prostatic hyperplasia (BPH) and approximately 20% of carcinomas.
3. *Periurethral glands (PUGs; 1% or more of the glandular tissue)*. These glands are embedded in the smooth muscle wall of the urethra, entirely within the preprostatic sphincter. Involved in the BPH process, these glands can give rise to an enlarged middle lobe.
4. *Central zone (CZ; as much as 25% of the glandular tissue)*. The CZ is cone shaped and surrounds the ejaculatory ducts. The major distinction between the CZ and the PZ is that the CZ is relatively resistant to the development of cancer. Only 10% of cancers occur in the CZ. Interestingly, BPH does not seem to occur in the CZ.

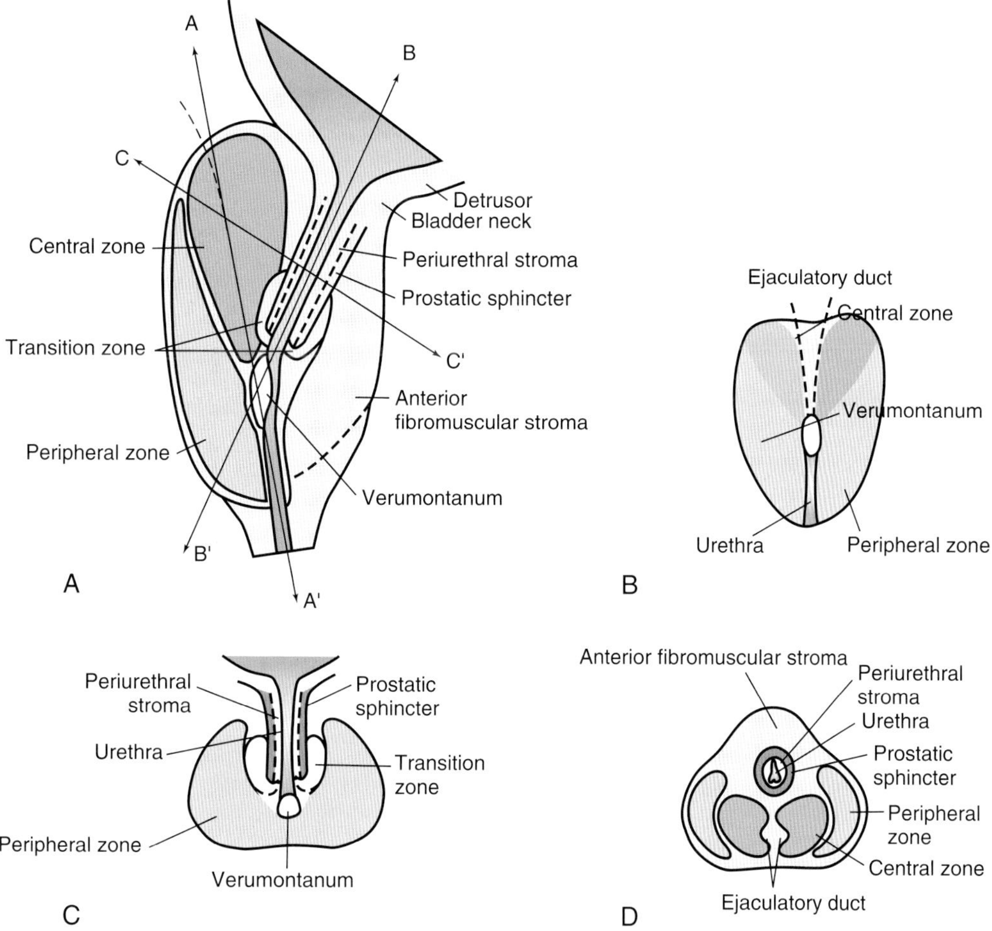

Figure 121-3 Anatomy of the prostate. **A,** Midsagittal plane. **B,** Coronal section (through the plane A-A′ in **A**). **C,** Oblique coronal section (through the plane B-B′ in **A**). **D,** Transverse section (through the plane C-C′ in **A**). (**A,** Redrawn from McNeal JE: Normal and pathologic anatomy of prostate. Urology 17[Suppl 3]:11–16, 1981. **B–D,** Redrawn from Muldoon LD, Resnick MI: Normal anatomy of the prostate. In Resnick MI [ed]: Prostatic Ultrasonography. Philadelphia, BC Decker, 1990.)

Fibromuscular Structures

Fibromuscular structures make up 33% of the prostate. There are four fibromuscular structures:

1. Anterior fibromuscular stroma (AFS)
   - A continuation of the detrusor muscle
   - Covers the anterior and anterolateral aspects of the glandular tissue from base to apex
2. Preprostatic sphincter (PPS)
   - Smooth muscle fibers of the lower ureters and superficial trigone
   - Intimately related to the TZ
   - Prevents pooling of urine in the proximal segment of the urethra
   - Prevents retrograde ejaculation
3. Postprostatic sphincter (POPS)
   - The proximal extension of the striated external urethral sphincter muscle covering the anterior and lateral aspects of the distal urethra
   - Contributes to continence
4. Longitudinal smooth muscle (LSM)
   - Part of the urethra

The key to understanding prostate tissue anatomy is to understand the anatomy of the prostatic urethra, which is approximately 3 cm long. It should be used as a primary reference point. After traveling through the proximal prostate, the urethra takes a 35-degree turn, angling anteriorly. The point of angulation divides the urethra into its proximal and distal urethral segments. The proximal urethral segment is related to two tiny glandular regions, the TZ and PUG, and to the preprostatic sphincter. The verumontanum lies entirely in the distal segment. In addition, the distal urethral segment is related to the function of ejaculation. The ejaculatory ducts and the excretory ducts (PZ and CZ) empty into the distal urethral segment.

Ultrasonographic Anatomy

(For definitions of *hyperechoic*, *isoechoic*, and *hypoechoic*, see the "Interpretation" section.)

With ultrasonography, the anatomy is divided into two general areas that are immediately obvious to the examiner:

1. The outer area, or *outer gland*, is close to the rectum and generally described as isoechoic.
2. The inner area, or *inner gland*, is more hypoechoic in appearance.

Composition of the Inner and Outer Glands

Inner Gland

- Anterior fibromuscular stroma
- Preprostatic sphincter
- Periurethral glands
- Longitudinal smooth muscle
- Postprostatic sphincter

Outer Gland

- Transition zone
- Central zone
- Peripheral zone

Basic Ultrasound Physics

Ultrasound imaging is based on the "pulse echo" principle, whereby a short burst of ultrasound is emitted from a transducer and directed into the tissue. Echoes are produced as a result of the interaction of sound with tissue, and some of these echoes travel back to the transducer. By timing the period elapsed between the emission of the pulse and the reception of the echo, the distance between the transducer and the echo-producing structure can be calculated and an image produced (see Chapter 225, Emergency Department, Hospitalist, and Office Ultrasonography [Clinical Ultrasonography]).

Sound consists of longitudinal vibrations that propagate through a medium such as water or soft tissue. It consists of the repetitive (or periodic) production of such compressions, which travel in regular succession. The number of compressions produced each second is the *frequency* (measured in hertz [Hz]), and the distance between successive compressions, which depends on the speed at which the sound travels in the medium, is the *wavelength* (measured in millimeters). Tissues that are very elastic, dense, or compressible tend to transmit sound waves through them. Inelastic, less dense, or noncompressible tissues tend to reflect the sound waves.

Gain adjustment refers to the amount of amplification applied to a returning echo signal. *Contrast and brightness* adjustments can also be made to provide a homogeneous midrange echo pattern of the normal peripheral zone.

Sound Frequency

The characteristics of sound transmission are as follows:

- The lower the frequency, the longer the wavelength.
- The higher the frequency, the shorter the wavelength.
- The lower the frequency of sound, the greater the ability to penetrate tissue, but the poorer the quality (resolution) of the ultrasonographic picture obtained.
- The higher the sound frequency, the poorer the tissue penetration by sound, but the better the quality (resolution) of the picture.

The ideal frequency for imaging the prostate is about 7 MHz. Although a 10-MHz probe provides better resolution of smaller objects, it has a more limited field of view; it shows only the part of the prostate closest to the rectum. A 3-MHz probe, with its lower frequency, delivers higher penetration, but the image quality and resolution usually suffer (Fig. 121-4).

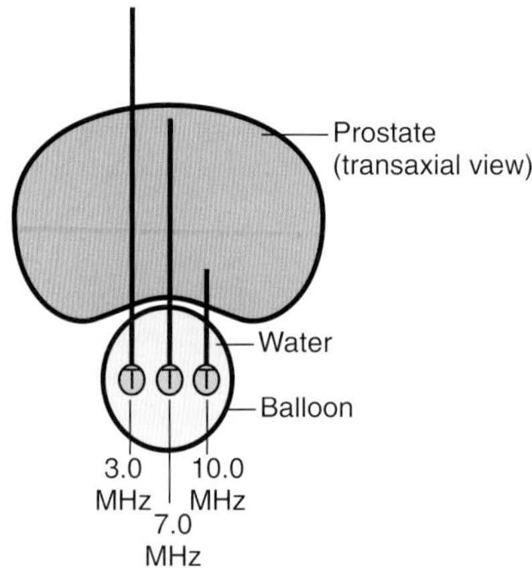

Figure 121-4 Ideal frequency for imaging the prostate is about 7 MHz. (From Cooner WH: Physical principles of prostate ultrasonography. Monogr Urol 11:18, 1990.)

Indications

TRUSP-SV

- Suspicion of prostatic abscess
- Azoospermia
- Brachytherapy
- Prostatitis
  - Acute
  - Chronic
  - Chronic pelvic pain syndrome
  - Prostatitis with an elevated prostate-specific antigen (PSA)
- Prostate volume study
- Detection of post-treatment prostate cancer recurrence
- Prostatic intraepithelial neoplasia on prior biopsy
- Prostate cancer staging
- Adenosis on prior biopsy

NOTE: In the patient with cancer, when attempting to determine the extent of local disease, TRUSP-SV is generally restricted to determining whether the tumor has invaded the seminal vesicles.

TRUSP-SV and Prostate Biopsy

- Evaluation of a palpable prostatic nodule or induration
- Abnormal PSA (Fig. 121-1 shows an algorithm combining PSA, free PSA, PSA velocity, and TRUSP-SV.)
  - Elevated PSA
  - Low free PSA (<25%) in individual with PSA in the range of 4 to 10 ng/mL
  - Elevated PSA velocity (doubling in <6 months or >0.75 ng/mL rise in PSA per year; optimally these have been done by same laboratory)
  - Elevated PSA density (>0.1 to 0.15 ng/mL)
- Detection of post-treatment prostate cancer recurrence
- Prostatic intraepithelial neoplasia on prior biopsy

Contraindications

TRUSP-SV and Prostate Biopsy

- Bleeding disorders
- Anticoagulant therapy
- Significant rectal disease
  - Obstructing lesions
  - Fissures
  - Thrombosed hemorrhoids
  - Proctitis
- Untreated bacterial urinary tract infection
  - Cystitis
  - Prostatitis
- Operator not familiar with the procedure, the anatomy, or the interpretation of TRUSP-SV
- Patient life expectancy less than 10 years, or age 75 years or greater *(relative contraindications)*

NOTE: If a hypoechoic area is seen on transrectal ultrasonography (TRUSP-SV), it probably should be sampled for biopsy, regardless of PSA. Therefore, some experts warn against performing TRUSP unless a biopsy is indicated; it should probably not be used for screening. The primary role of ultrasonography is to ensure accurate sampling of any lesions and of the entire gland during biopsy.

Preprocedure Patient Preparation

1. Serum PSA on record
2. Documented DRE
3. Informed consent signed and copy on chart
4. Fleet enema 1 to 2 hours before the procedure
5. Fluoroquinolone therapy
   - The authors prefer a 3-day regimen using a quinolone the day before, the day of, and, if a biopsy is performed, the day after.
   - For patients undergoing repeat TRUSP-SV and biopsy (for persistent abnormalities in PSA despite negative biopsies and normal DRE), use a 5-day protocol of quinolone therapy, extending the quinolone for 3 days after the biopsy. Also, add metronidazole 500 mg twice a day by mouth for 3 days after the biopsy.
6. Patient vital signs before procedure
7. Patient positioning options
   - Knee–chest
   - Lithotomy
   - Left lateral decubitus with knees flexed 90 degrees (Fig. 121-5)

Indications, alternatives, risks, potential benefits, and expected results should be discussed with the patient and signed informed consent obtained. The patient should expect some discomfort with either TRUSP-SV or biopsy. He should also expect some discomfort with injection of the local anesthetic and the prostate biopsy. Let the patient know he will be warned before a biopsy. It will also be important for him to remain very still during certain portions of the procedure.

Equipment

An available assistant to help with the equipment is useful, especially if a biopsy is to be performed.

TRUSP-SV

- Transducer sheath or condom (should be sterile if biopsy is to be performed)
- Nonsterile gloves (also sterile gloves if biopsy is to be performed)
- Ultrasonic gel
- Eye protection and gown (sterile gown if biopsy is to be performed)

Types of Prostate Ultrasonography

- Transabdominal
- Transperineal
- Endourethral
- Transrectal (with and without color flow Doppler enhancement)

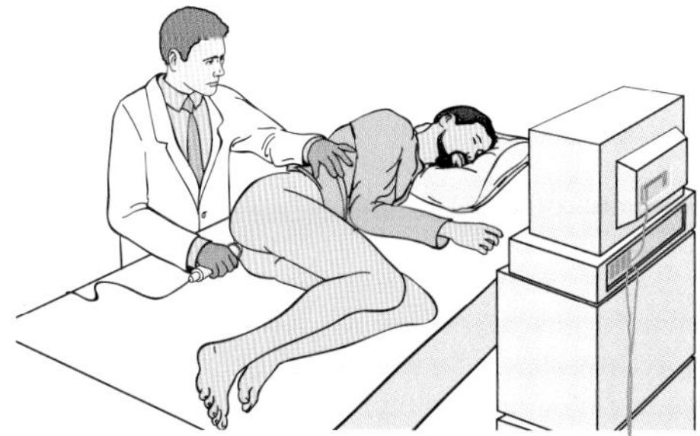

Figure 121-5 Positioning of patient.

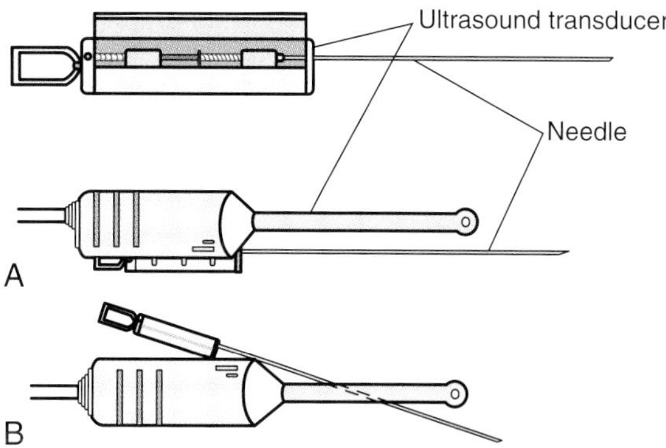

Figure 121-6 Biopsy instrument can be introduced through an internal (**A**) or an external (**B**) needle guide or puncture guide. (Redrawn from Brackman J, Denis LJ: Prostate ultrasound and needle biopsy. In Graham SD Jr [ed]: Glenn's Urologic Surgery, 5th ed. Philadelphia, Lippincott-Raven, 1998.)

Types of Transducer Design

- Radial array (with cephalocaudad or right-to-left oscillation)
- Linear array (piezoelectric crystals are placed in a line, and each crystal fires and receives echoes in sequential order)

Recent advancements in ultrasound technology have resulted in the following:

- The development of biplanar probe transducers
- The development of a single probe to image the gland in both the transverse and sagittal planes
- A single probe that can have one of the following:
  - Two perpendicularly positioned transducers
  - A single transducer that can rotate
  - An end-fire transducer that can provide either a transverse or sagittal view by merely rotating the probe 90 degrees.

Prostate Biopsy

- Biopsy instrument, usually spring-loaded, and needle guide (Fig. 121-6)
- Sterile tray and sterile drapes for patient
- Bottles containing specimen preservative (formaldehyde)
- Lidocaine 1%, 22-gauge, 15- to 20-cm spinal needle and 10-mL syringe (*optional*)

Technique

TRUSP-SV

General Principles

The performance of prostate ultrasonography requires the examiner to know which aspects of the procedure are operator dependent so that the best possible study can be obtained. No mandatory technical standards exist for performance of prostatic ultrasonography. The examination sequence remains a matter of personal preference. Practitioners should develop a technique that is thorough and reproducible and with which they are comfortable.

Prostate ultrasonography and examination should be carried out in at least two planes:

1. Transaxial–transverse (across the long axis). Images from this orientation offer several advantages in the assessment of the prostate:

- Increased information about the lateral margins
- Assessment of capsular integrity
- Accurate volume assessment

2. Longitudinal–sagittal (parallel to the body axis or long axis). Images from this orientation provide more information about the apex and base of the prostate and facilitate biopsy.

Procedure

1. Perform a DRE before insertion of the probe. This procedure serves many purposes:
   - Dilates the anal sphincter, reducing discomfort from probe insertion.
   - Assesses the gland for size, shape, and areas of irregularity or suspicion. This enables the sonographer to associate palpable lesions with what is being viewed during the study.
   - Rules out a rectal obstructive process of either benign or malignant etiology.
2. Position the patient. Various positions will work, but the left lateral decubitus position is often more comfortable for the patient and may reduce bowel gas interference (see Fig. 121-5).
3. Prepare the probe. A small amount of ultrasonic gel is placed either in the tip of the probe sheath or on the tip of the probe. The cover is then inserted over the probe. Any air bubbles over the tip of the probe should be smoothed away.
4. Have the patient perform a slight Valsalva maneuver during probe insertion to relax the sphincter and further facilitate probe insertion.
5. After insertion, while scanning in the transaxial mode, advance the probe to the level of the seminal vesicles. Making parallel images (cuts), scan from superior to inferior (Fig. 121-7). Examination of the seminal vesicles should focus on the following:
   - Symmetry
   - Size
   - Echo pattern
   - Any masses
   - Cystic changes

   Because the seminal vesicles do not always lie symmetrically in the body, it is occasionally difficult to comment on their symmetry on a cut-by-cut basis. Often they must be studied and their images interpreted as they appear in their entirety. If prostate cancer is present, it is important to determine whether there has been local invasion to the seminal vesicles (see "Interpretation" section).
6. From the seminal vesicles, the probe is withdrawn to the level of the base of the prostate and all areas from the base to the apex should be scanned. Evaluate the prostate for symmetry, its lateral margins, and the integrity of the capsule. Assess the inner and outer gland for irregularities. The periprostatic "environment" is also assessed at this time. Normal peripheral zone echogenicity represents the *baseline* or is *isoechoic*. Any lesion that is less echogenic is labeled *hypoechoic*; anything giving rise to more echoes is *hyperechoic*.
7. The probe should then be rotated (or a perpendicular plane in the probe activated) to scan the prostate longitudinally. The clinician should be thorough and evaluate the entire prostate and surrounding tissue in each longitudinal plane. Particular emphasis should be placed on scanning and evaluating the apex and base of the prostate.
8. Volume determination should be performed. Various software applications or technical features of individual ultrasound machines enable the examiner to estimate prostate volume. An option is a formula for calculating estimated prostate volume: prostate volume (mL) = $(\pi/6) \times$ (anterior-posterior diameter [cm]) $\times$ (transverse diameter [cm]) $\times$ (sagittal diameter [cm]). Regardless of technique used, the error in measuring prostate volume may approach 25%.

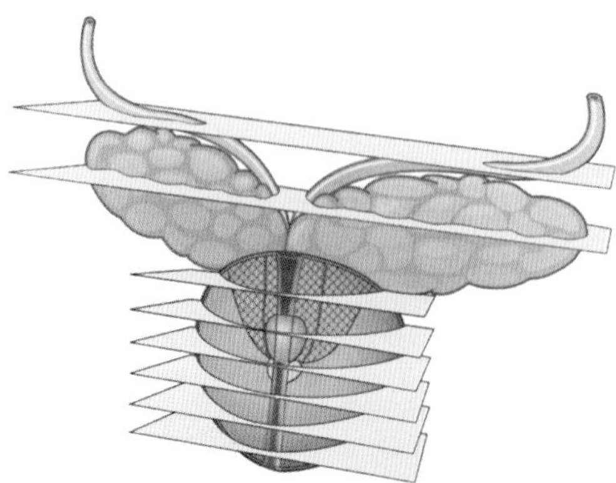

Figure 121-7 **Ultrasonographic transaxial examination of the seminal vesicles and prostate using parallel images from superior to inferior.** (From Rifkin MD: Ultrasound of the Prostate: Imaging in the Diagnosis and Therapy of Prostatic Disease, 2nd ed. Philadelphia, Lippincott-Raven, 1997.)

SPECIAL CASE: Ultrasonography and/or biopsy of a man without a rectum: this requires transperineal ultrasonography in conjunction with magnetic resonance imaging (MRI). The MRI defines the areas of suspicion as a region of low signal intensity on T2-weighted sequences. Although transperineal ultrasonography may help localize the abnormal area of the prostate, it seldom demonstrates the specific lesion. The transperineal approach to biopsy is more painful but carries a lower risk of infection than the transrectal approach.

Prostate Biopsy

1. With eye protection in place, the clinician is gowned in a sterile manner and the patient draped likewise. A small amount of ultrasonic gel should be placed either on the tip of the probe sheath or on the tip of the probe. The needle guide and transducer are then covered with the sterile sheath. The sterile sheath often has an extension that can be unrolled over the transducer cord. Any air bubbles located over the probe tip should be smoothed away.
2. After having the patient perform a slight Valsalva maneuver, the probe is inserted in the same manner as for TRUSP-SV.
3. *Prostate anesthetic block:* It is the authors' opinion that providing a local anesthetic block with 1% lidocaine before prostate biopsy is beneficial. It may not only reduce anxiety and discomfort, but it may enhance patient compliance (especially if a repeat biopsy is ever necessary). After the probe is in the rectum, a 22-gauge, 15- to 20-cm spinal needle is introduced through the needle guide on the probe. The needle is then advanced into Denonvilliers' fascia and the area adjacent to the apex in the longitudinal plane. Lidocaine is injected between the gland and the rectum. The authors usually inject 4 mL of local anesthetic in the apical region and then switch to the horizontal plane to inject the remaining 3 mL into the right and left neurovascular bundles. After waiting 5 to 10 minutes for the anesthetic to take effect, one can proceed with the biopsy. At this point, some clinicians also use moderate (conscious) sedation (see Chapter 2, Procedural Sedation and Analgesia).
4. The biopsy instrument, usually a spring-loaded biopsy gun, is then inserted until the tip of the instrument can be seen at the edge of the prostate. For an *outer gland lesion*, the tip of the instrument is placed just in front of the lesion, at the edge of the mass and before the prostatic capsule is penetrated. For an *inner gland lesion*, the tip of the instrument must first penetrate the capsule and outer gland before it is placed just in front of the lesion, at the edge of the mass.

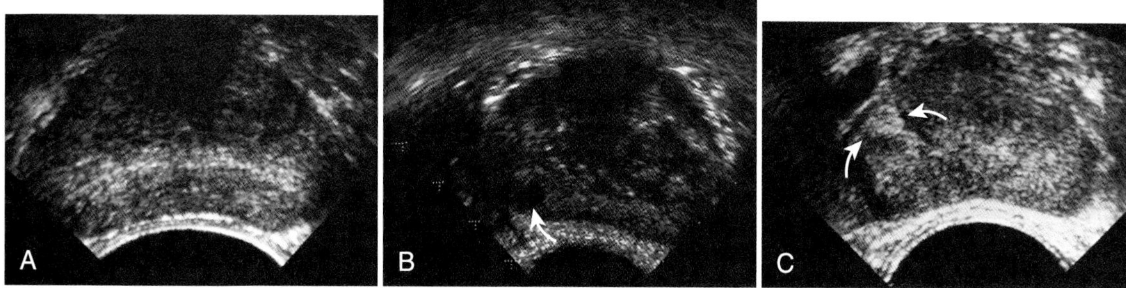

Figure 121-8 Echogenic patterns of the prostate. **A,** Isoechoic patterns. The images are typically produced by the glandular areas of the prostate and appear as low-level gray. The images are in a midrange and a medium percentage of sound waves are reflected back to the transducer. **B,** Hypoechoic patterns *(arrow)* are seen typically in the fibrous and muscular structures of the prostate and with cancers of the prostate. With hypoechoic patterns, fewer echoes are reflected back and more actually pass through the tissues, making them appear darker. **C,** Hyperechoic patterns *(arrows)* result when more sound waves are reflected back to the transducer, producing images that are light gray to white. The periprostatic fat is hyperechoic, as are some cancers. (From Rifkin MD: Ultrasound of the Prostate: Imaging in the Diagnosis and Therapy of Prostatic Disease, 2nd ed. Philadelphia, Lippincott-Raven, 1997.)

5. If the patient is awake, to avoid any surprises, he should be warned just before the instrument is fired. The instrument is then fired. Any additional suspect areas on TRUSP-SV should likewise be sampled.
6. Additional random passes are then made, obtaining biopsies in the superior, central, and inferior portions of the prostate. Emphasis should be placed on obtaining tissue from the peripheral zone. The specific number of biopsies varies by clinician, but the current literature recommends 12 to 18 passes (6 to 9 on each side). Various systems are used to label the biopsies, with "1" or "A" commonly used to label the right superior gland, "2" or "B" for right middle, "3" or "C" for right inferior (apex), "4" or "D" for left superior, "5" or "E" for left middle, and "6" or "F" for left inferior. When in doubt about which system to use, the clinician can merely be descriptive with the labeling (e.g., "right superior").

Interpretation and Evaluation of the Prostate

Interpretation

From the prostate, three types of echogenic pattern are described: isoechoic (Fig. 121-8A), hypoechoic (Fig. 121-8B), and hyperechoic (Fig. 121-8C). Unfortunately, no single finding on ultrasonography permits universal distinction between malignant and benign conditions. However, most cancers are hypoechoic. Cancers less than 5 to 7 mm, those that are well differentiated, and those located in the TZ are difficult to distinguish from normal prostate.

Evaluation

- General appearance
- Inner gland status
- Outer gland status
- Anterior prostate status
- Any focal intraprostatic abnormalities
- Status of the internal architecture
  - Normal
  - Disrupted
- Integrity of capsule
- Urethral position
- Focal lesion(s)
  - Number
  - Location
  - Echogenic pattern: hypoechoic, isoechoic, hyperechoic, mixed, anechoic
  - Margin of the focus: well defined, poorly defined
  - Calculi
  - Cysts
- Ejaculatory duct status
  - Normal
  - Dilated
  - Infiltrated
- Neurovascular bundles present?
- Lymph nodes visible?
- Seminal vesicles
  - Overall, symmetric or asymmetric
  - Size
  - Shape
  - Echo pattern
  - Cystic changes
  - Solid mass effect
- Rectal wall integrity

Normal Ultrasonographic Appearance of the Prostate Gland*

- The peripheral zone is isoechoic and the transitional zone hypoechoic.
- The appearances change with enlargement—the peripheral zone becomes thinner.
- The gland shape depends on the type of TRUSP-SV probe used.
- The central zone is not identifiable as a separate area.
- The prostatic capsule, although seen, is not a true capsule.
- Flow on color Doppler is symmetric.

Abnormal Ultrasonographic Appearance of the Prostate Gland

Most prostate cancers appear as a hypoechoic lesion in the peripheral zone.

Hints for Staging

- Findings consistent with extracapsular extension of prostate cancer include bulging of the prostate contour and an angulated appearance of the lateral margin.
- Findings consistent with seminal vesicle invasion include a posterior bulge of the prostate contour at the base of the seminal vesicle and asymmetry of echogenicity in the seminal vesicles associated with hypoechoic areas at the base of the prostate.

*Patel and Rickards, 2002.

COMPLICATIONS

TRUSP-SV and Prostate Biopsy

- Rectal bleeding from the following:
  - Hemorrhoidal vessels
  - Rectal wall laceration
  - Arteriovenous malformation
- Hematuria
- Hematospermia
- Urinary retention
- Urosepsis
- Bacteremia
- Vasovagal response with or without seizure

Prostate Biopsy (Rare)

- Perirectal or pelvic hematoma or hemorrhage
- Needle tract seeding of cancer

POSTPROCEDURE PATIENT EDUCATION

Postprocedure vital signs should be performed and fluids offered or provided (e.g., sport drink, fruit juice). The TRUSP-SV findings and any instructions should be reviewed with the patient. A follow-up appointment should be made. If biopsies were performed, the results will be discussed with the patient at the follow-up appointment. Patients should be aware that even with a negative biopsy, they may have microscopic cancer in a small area of the prostate. If the biopsy was for an abnormal PSA and it remains abnormal, a repeat biopsy may be necessary at a later date. After TRUSP-SV or biopsy, the patient should call the facility for difficulty urinating, rectal bleeding, high fever, or further questions.

PATIENT EDUCATION GUIDES

See the sample patient education and consent forms available online at www.expertconsult.com.

CPT/BILLING CODES

55700 Prostate biopsy; needle or punch, single or multiple, any approach
76872 Ultrasound, transrectal
76942 Ultrasonic guidance for needle placement (e.g., biopsy, aspiration, injection, localization device), imaging supervision and interpretation

ICD-9-CM DIAGNOSTIC CODES

185 Malignant neoplasm of prostate
187.8 Malignant neoplasm of seminal vesicles
600.00 Hypertrophy (benign) of prostate without urinary obstruction
600.01 Hypertrophy (benign) of prostate with urinary obstruction
600.10 Nodular prostate without urinary obstruction
600.11 Nodular prostate with urinary obstruction
600.20 Benign localized hyperplasia of prostate without urinary obstruction
600.21 Benign localized hyperplasia of prostate with urinary obstruction
601.0 Prostatitis, acute
601.1 Prostatitis, chronic
602.0 Calculus of prostate
602.3 Dysplasia of prostate
608.82 Hematospermia

ACKNOWLEDGMENT

The editors wish to recognize the contributions by Robert S. Tan, MD, to this chapter in a previous edition of this text.

SUPPLIERS

(See contact information online at www.expertconsult.com.)

Transrectal ultrasonography units with needle guides
Available from most ultrasonography equipment manufacturers (see Chapter 172, Obstetric Ultrasonography, and Chapter 185, Musculoskeletal Ultrasonography, for lists of manufacturers).
Bard biopsy cut instruments and needle
Bard Peripheral Technologies
Overreading services
APEX Radiology, Inc.
Nighthawk Radiology Services

NOTE: These services require T1 internet access; DSL is not compliant with the Health Information Privacy Act (HIPA).

Probes and scans
See Figures 121-9 to 121-14.

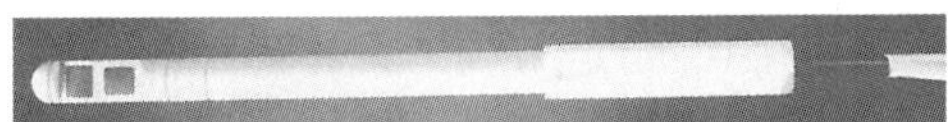

Figure 121-9 **Biplane probe.** (From Rifkin MD: Ultrasound of the Prostate: Imaging in the Diagnosis and Therapy of Prostatic Disease, 2nd ed. Philadelphia, Lippincott-Raven, 1997.)

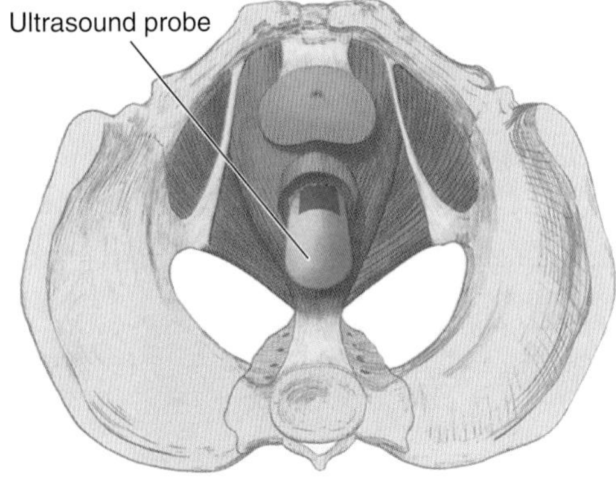

Figure 121-10 **Endorectal scan. Note probe is located very near and posterior to prostate.** (From Rifkin MD: Ultrasound of the Prostate: Imaging in the Diagnosis and Therapy of Prostatic Disease, 2nd ed. Philadelphia, Lippincott-Raven, 1997.)

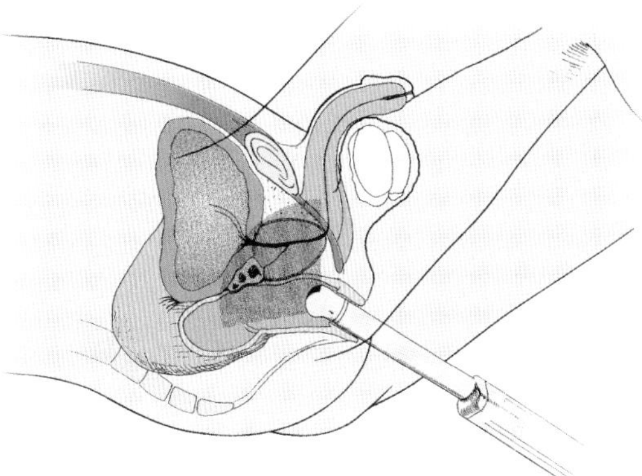

Figure 121-11 End-fire endorectal probe scanning longitudinally. (Modified from Rifkin MD: Ultrasound of the Prostate: Imaging in the Diagnosis and Therapy of Prostatic Disease, 2nd ed. Philadelphia, Lippincott-Raven, 1997.)

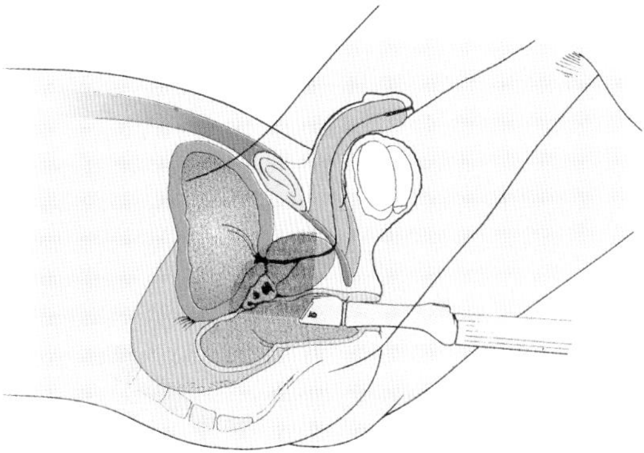

Figure 121-12 Oblique end-fire probe scanning longitudinally. (From Rifkin MD: Ultrasound of the Prostate: Imaging in the Diagnosis and Therapy of Prostatic Disease, 2nd ed. Philadelphia, Lippincott-Raven, 1997.)

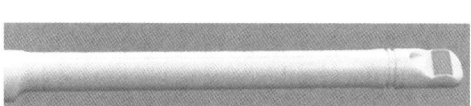

Figure 121-13 Side-fire probe. (From Rifkin MD: Ultrasound of the Prostate: Imaging in the Diagnosis and Therapy of Prostatic Disease, 2nd ed. Philadelphia, Lippincott-Raven, 1997.)

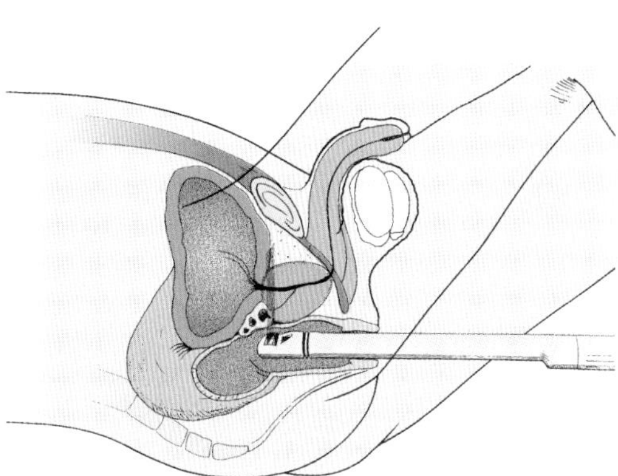

Figure 121-14 Side-fire probe scanning transaxially. (From Rifkin MD: Ultrasound of the Prostate: Imaging in the Diagnosis and Therapy of Prostatic Disease, 2nd ed. Philadelphia, Lippincott-Raven, 1997.)

BIBLIOGRAPHY

Bieker T: Prostate: Prostate carcinoma, benign prostatic hypertrophy. In Sanders RC, Winter TC (eds): Clinical Sonography: A Practical Guide, 4th ed. Philadelphia, Lippincott Williams & Wilkins, 2007, pp 251–260.

Brawer MK: Techniques of examination in prostatic ultrasonography. In Resnick MI (ed): Prostatic Ultrasonography. Philadelphia, BC Decker, 1990.

Brawer MK, Chetner MP: Ultrasonography of the prostate and biopsy. In Walsh PC, Retik AB, Vaughan ED Jr, Wein AJ (eds): Campbell's Urology, 7th ed. Philadelphia, WB Saunders, 1998, pp 2506–2517.

Brooks JD: Anatomy of the lower urinary tract and male genitalia. In Walsh PC, Retik AB, Vaughan ED Jr, Wein AJ (eds): Campbell's Urology, 7th ed. Philadelphia, WB Saunders, 1998, pp 112–117.

Cooner WH: Physical principles of prostate ultrasonography. Monogr Urol 11:18, 1990.

Kaye KW: Ultrasound of the normal prostate. Contemp Urol 3:64–75, 1991.

McNeal JE: The prostate gland: Morphology and pathology. Monogr Urol 9:36, 1988.

Muldoon LD, Resnick MI: Normal anatomy of the prostate. In Resnick MI (ed): Prostatic Ultrasonography. Philadelphia, BC Decker, 1990.

Patel U, Rickards D: Transrectal Ultrasound & Biopsy of the Prostate. London, Martin Duntz, 2002.

Presti KC Jr, Kane CJ, Shinohara K, Carroll PR: Neoplasms of the prostate gland. In Tanagho EA, McAninch JW (eds). Smith's General Urology, 17th ed. New York, McGraw-Hill, 2008, pp 367–385.

Rifkin MD: Ultrasound of the Prostate. Imaging in the Diagnosis and Therapy of Prostatic Disease, 2nd ed. Philadelphia, Lippincott-Raven, 1997.
This book is a must-read for the individual who is serious about prostate ultrasonography.

CHAPTER 122

Self-Injection Therapy for the Treatment of Erectile Dysfunction

Robert E. James • James R. Palleschi

Significant advances have been made in the diagnosis and treatment of erectile dysfunction. Although the introduction of oral drugs has decreased the need for and the use of injection therapy, it is still indicated in some patients. The self-injection of vasoactive agents into the corpora cavernosa now enables many patients to resume satisfactory sexual activities without surgery.

Oral medications (sildenafil, tadalafil, and vardenafil) are most effective in patients with mild to moderate impotence. This category would include men who are able to obtain a good erection but cannot maintain it and those men who have an erection that is at least a 5 out of 10 in rigidity, where "10" is defined as the best erection they can remember.

The *transurethral form of alprostadil (MUSE)* is most effective in men who have difficulty maintaining an erection and in those who have a partial erection, or 5 out of 10 in rigidity.

Despite the advances in the treatment of erectile dysfunction, *vacuum erection devices* remain an option or adjunct. These devices are attractive to patients who have failed oral therapy and decline or fail intraurethral or intracavernosal alprostadil. Patients using intracavernosal therapy who want to have intercourse more than three times a week usually meet their goal by using vacuum erection devices (see Chapter 125, Vacuum Devices for Erectile Dysfunction).

In the treatment of moderate to severe erectile dysfunction, intracavernosal therapy with vasoactive agents still has a very important role.

In July of 1995, the U.S. Food and Drug Administration (FDA) approved *injectable alprostadil (prostaglandin E_1 [PGE_1])* for the treatment of organic erectile dysfunction. The American Urological Association's guidelines for the treatment of erectile dysfunction recommend alprostadil as the drug of choice, and it is the only intracavernosal vasoactive agent approved by the FDA.

There is also *papaverine hydrochloride*, a nonspecific smooth muscle relaxant. In addition to alprostadil, which is a vasodilator and a smooth muscle relaxant, papaverine hydrochloride may be used with *phentolamine mesylate*, a smooth muscle relaxant that enhances the effect of papaverine. For several years these agents have been used extensively for impotence, although this remains an unlabeled indication.

These vasoactive agents induce an erection by increasing arterial blood flow, relaxing the sinusoidal spaces within the cavernosal tissue, and increasing venous resistance. An excellent erection that lasts for 30 to 90 minutes usually occurs in patients with mild to moderate arterial insufficiency, mild to moderate venous incompetence, psychogenic impotence, neurogenic impotence, and medication-induced impotence.

Indications

- Impotence resulting from arterial insufficiency.
- Impotence resulting from mild to moderate venous incompetence.
- Psychogenic impotence. (Patients with performance anxiety may be treated with counseling, oral agents, short-term intracavernosal agents, or a combination of these methods.)
- Neurogenic impotence.
- Medication-induced impotence, when drug therapy cannot be altered or terminated.
- Diagnostic erection.
- Intolerance to or ineffective oral drugs.

Contraindications

- Blood dyscrasia, coagulation disorder, or anticoagulation drug therapy
- Unstable cardiovascular disease
- Impaired manual dexterity or vision
- Presence of a prosthetic penile device
- Valvular heart disease
- Intolerance to the test dose of the vasoactive agent
- Patients taking monoamine oxidase (MAO) inhibitors
- Patients with a propensity toward secondary forms of priapism, such as individuals with sickle cell disease or trait, leukemia, and multiple myeloma

NOTE: If a physician elects to use intracavernosal pharmacotherapy to treat erectile dysfunction in men with Peyronie's disease, a special informed consent is advised.

Equipment

- 1- to 3-mL syringes with ½-inch, 27- and 30-gauge needles
- Alcohol swabs
- Vasoactive agents
  - *Papaverine HCl* 30 mg/mL is available in 10-mL multidose vials.
  - *Papaverine and phentolamine* solution: Inject 5 mg (or 10 mg) of phentolamine (Regitine; Novartis, East Hanover, NJ) into a 100-mL vial of papaverine 30 mg/mL. The (approximate) concentrations will be papaverine 30 mg/mL and phentolamine 0.5 or 1.0 mg/mL.
  - *PGE_1 (alprostadil):* There are two proprietary forms of injectable alprostadil for the treatment of erectile dysfunction available in the United States: Caverject and Edex (Schwarz Pharma, Mequon, Wis). The clinical dose range varies from 2

to 40 μg per injection. Each manufacturer has provided alprostadil in a ready-to-use, easily assembled syringe that does not require refrigeration. The syringes are meant for single use only.

- PGE_1 *(alprostadil)* is also available in 1-mL ampules from Upjohn (Kalamazoo, Mich) as Prostin VR Pediatric 500 mg/mL. For the desired concentration, inject 0.2 mL of this preparation into each of five 10-mL vials of bacteriostatic normal saline for injection. Each vial will contain PGE_1 10 mg/mL.

Bennett and coworkers in 1991 developed *a trimix combination therapy* for the treatment of erectile dysfunction. This three-drug mixture contains 2.5 mL of papaverine (30 mg/mL), 0.5 mL of phentolamine (5 mg/mL), and 0.05 mL of alprostadil (500 μg/mL) for intracavernous injection. Most patients require less than 0.25 mL per injection.

Open vials or compounded solutions should be refrigerated to maintain sterility and effectiveness. A 30-day expiration date is recommended; however, sufficient effectiveness has been reported for up to 3 months.

α-Adrenergic agents will cause vasoconstriction and thus will usually result in prompt detumescence should priapism occur. Some of the available agents include *ephedrine sulfate, epinephrine*, and *phenylephrine hydrochloride* (Neo-Synephrine). (See the "Treatment of the Persistent Erection [Priapism]" section for dilutions and use.)

Preprocedure Patient Preparation

Discuss the self-injection program, alternatives, and potential complications with the patient and, when possible, his partner. Patients using this program may experience *bruising* at the injection site and local or systemic infection (<0.05% incidence). *Chronic fibrosis* at the injection site may occur with repeated injections, and this may result in *pain or penile curvature*. Papaverine may elevate the results of *liver function tests*. Consequently, patients should obtain pretreatment liver function tests and should be retested every 3 months while using papaverine. If the liver function test values begin to rise, the medication should be discontinued. If the initial liver function test results are elevated, use PGE_1 instead of papaverine. Approximately 20% of patients using PGE_1 may experience an *ache in the penis* that may last for several hours and that may recur with each injection. *Priapism*, an erection lasting longer than 4 hours, may occur in up to 10% of patients receiving any of the vasoactive agents, but it reportedly occurs less frequently with PGE_1. Systemic side effects, such as dizziness and orthostatic hypotension, occur in 2% of patients receiving these vasoactive agents and are believed to be secondary to penile venous incompetence.

Instruct the patient to contact the physician if he experiences a significant erection that persists for more than 4 hours. This condition will need to be treated promptly to prevent intracorporeal fibrosis and failure to respond to future therapy.

Technique

1. Complete the patient's history and physical examination to provide a preliminary diagnosis.
2. Select the agent and the dose. If psychogenic or neurogenic impotence is suspected, use a smaller dose of the vasoactive agent. In patients with psychogenic impotence, one fourth of the maximum dose should be used; in patients with neurogenic impotence, no more than one sixth of the maximum dose should be used initially. The maximum dose of *papaverine* is 60 mg, and that of PGE_1 is 20 μg. To reduce the risk of priapism and to prevent other untoward reactions, even when vascular disease is suspected as the cause of impotence, the initial dose should not exceed 30 mg of papaverine or 10 μg of PGE_1. If a satisfactory erection does not occur, the dose may be appropriately increased at the time of the next office appointment. Although the usual dose of *alprostadil* is between 10 and 20 μg, urologists have used up to 40 μg in some cases. In patients with psychogenic or neurogenic impotence, you should begin with 2 to 5 μg and gradually increase the dose as needed. Otherwise, the usual starting dose is 10 μg.
3. Once the desired dose of the vasoactive agent has been selected, extend the patient's penis and prepare the lateral surface with an alcohol swab. Locate the neurovascular bundle at the 12 o'clock position and the urethra at the 6 o'clock position (Figs. 122-1 and 122-2). Select as the injection site an area between these two structures (1 to 5 o'clock on the patient's left, 7 to 11 o'clock on the patient's right) in which there are no superficial veins. The injection site may be anywhere between the base of the penis and just proximal to the glans penis. It is strongly recommended that only Caverject or Edex be used. With the patient standing, gently direct the penis to the left or the right to expose its lateral surface. Introduce a 27- or 30-gauge needle perpendicular to the skin and tunica albuginea and into the corpus cavernosum. Normally, the needle is advanced 0.5 inch. Inject the vasoactive agent rapidly as a bolus into the corpus cavernosum. The medication will enter the opposite corpus cavernosum through cross-circulation. If resistance is met as the medication is injected, withdraw the needle slowly as you continue to inject. The resistance normally occurs because the needle is against the opposite wall of the corpus cavernosum. To prevent injection of the medication into the subcutaneous space, *advance the needle the entire 0.5 inch and then withdraw slowly*.
4. Once the injection is completed, have the patient apply pressure to the injection site for 2 minutes.
5. Evaluate the condition of the patient periodically during the first 15 minutes after the injection. The patient's comfort, presence of side effects, and the quality of the erection should be evaluated at 15-minute intervals for 30 to 60 minutes. To evaluate the quality of the erection the patient will experience with sexual stimulation, you may ask the patient to apply manual stimulation. The patient may be discharged from the office within 30 to 60 minutes after the injection, provided he is comfortable and not experiencing any side effects. Instruct the patient to contact you if priapism occurs. Once the appropriate dose has been determined and the patient is skilled and comfortable with self-injection therapy, he may perform it independently, but *no more than three times per week*. Priapism rarely occurs after the appropriate dose has been determined, unless the patient independently increases the dose.

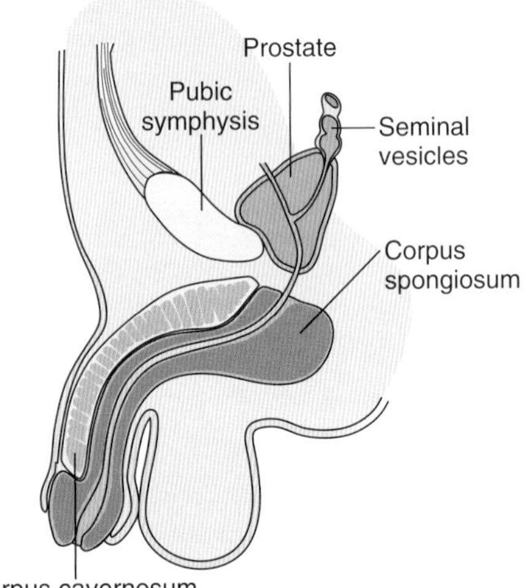

Figure 122-1 Side view of penis and scrotum.

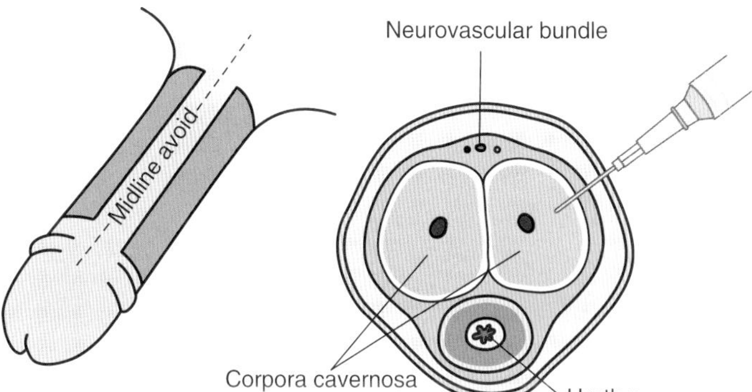

Figure 122-2 Intracavernous injection site. The clinician grasps the glans and pulls firmly outward to tense penis without rotating.

Treatment of the Persistent Erection (Priapism)

If the patient does not have significant hypertension or unstable cardiac or cerebrovascular disease, an intracavernosal α-adrenergic agonist is safe and very effective in the treatment of priapism. Priapism is defined as an erection that lasts over 4 hours. Before injecting the antidote, you should attempt to treat the priapism by first irrigating blood from the corpus cavernosum with saline. Inject the skin over the aspiration site (shaft of the penis) with 0.5 to 1 mL of local anesthetic (1% to 2% lidocaine). If ineffective, the patient may benefit from a penile block with 1% to 2% lidocaine and intravenous morphine sulfate. Then irrigate using aseptic technique with a 30-mL syringe and a 16- to 18-gauge needle. Insert the needle 0.5 inch into the midlateral corporal body and irrigate with saline. If the priapism does not resolve with irrigating with 250 to 500 mL of saline, proceed with injection of ephedrine, epinephrine, or phenylephrine, as discussed in the following section.

The following agents may be considered for the treatment of priapism if aspiration and irrigation of blood are unsuccessful:

- *Ephedrine sulfate:* A vial contains 50 mg (25 mg/mL). Initially inject 10 to 25 mg into the corpus cavernosum. If detumescence does not begin within 15 to 30 minutes, the dose may be repeated. A maximum of 50 mg may be given. Ephedrine is the drug of choice because of its efficacy, simplicity, and safety. If ineffective, a urology consult is advised.
- *Epinephrine:* Inject 1 mL of diluted epinephrine (10 to 20 μg/mL) slowly into the corpus cavernosum every 5 to 10 minutes. This may be repeated twice, and if satisfactory detumescence does not occur, a urology consultation should be obtained. (To prepare the proper dilution, use epinephrine 1:10,000 solution. For 10 μg/mL, dilute 0.1 mL of epinephrine with 0.9 mL of normal saline. For 20 μg/mL, dilute 0.2 mL of epinephrine with 0.8 mL of normal saline.)
- *Phenylephrine hydrochloride (Neo-Synephrine) 1%:* Inject 1 mL slowly into the corpus cavernosum every 5 to 10 minutes. If satisfactory detumescence does not occur after the second dose, a urology consultation should be obtained. (To prepare the proper dilution, use phenylephrine hydrochloride 0.1 mL diluted with 0.9 mL of normal saline for 100 μg/mL. Use phenylephrine hydrochloride 0.2 mL diluted with 0.8 mL of normal saline for 200 μg/mL.)

These medications should be given individually and never in combination. Monitor the blood pressure and pulse closely in all patients. Cardiac arrhythmias and significant hypertension may occur. If these measures are ineffective, obtain a urology consultation. Surgical intervention may be required at this time.

Complications

- Priapism (an erection that lasts over 4 hours)
- Infection
- Subcutaneous ecchymosis or hematoma
- Fibrosis to the corpus cavernosum with repeated injections
- Curvature of the penis occurring after repeated injections
- Painful erections
- Dizziness or postural hypotension
- Myocardial infarction, stroke, or both, in patients with unstable cardiac or cerebrovascular disease
- Elevated liver function test results (papaverine)

Postprocedure Patient Education

As many as 50% of men using self-injection therapy will discontinue this treatment within 1 year. There may be many reasons for this cessation, including lack of a suitable partner; fear of needles; inadequate response to therapy; fear of complications; lack of sexual spontaneity; and the desire for alternative therapy, including a permanent solution, such as a penile prosthesis. Consequently, the patient should be seen periodically and should be asked about his sexual activity and satisfaction with self-injection therapy.

Patient Education Guides

See the sample patient education form available online at www.expertconsult.com.

CPT/Billing Codes

54235 Injection of corpus cavernosum
54250 Nocturnal tumescence and/or rigidity test

J-Codes

J0170 Epinephrine, adrenalin up to 1 mL
J0270 Alprostadil injection 1.25 μg
J0275 Alprostadil urethral suppository
J2370 Phenylephrine HCl up to 1 mL
J2440 Papaverine HCl up to 60 mg

ICD-9-CM Diagnostic Codes

302.72 Impotence (sexual, psychogenic)
607.84 Impotence, organic origin NEC

ONLINE RESOURCES

Pfizer, Inc.: Caverject Impulse. Available at www.caverject.com.
Pfizer, Inc.: Viagra. Available at www.viagra.com.
Sexual Medicine Society of North America, Inc. Available at www.smsna.org.

BIBLIOGRAPHY

Armstrong DK, Convery A, Dinsmore WW: Intracavernosal papaverine and phentolamine for the medical management of erectile dysfunction in a genitourinary clinic. Int J STD AIDS 4:214–216, 1993.

Barada JH, McKimmy RM: Vasoactive pharmacotherapy. In Bennett AH (ed): Impotence. Philadelphia, WB Saunders, 1994, pp 229–250.

Bennett AH, Carpenter AJ, Barada JH: An improved vasoactive drug combination for a pharmacological erection program. J Urol 146:1564–1565, 1991.

Bernard F, Lue TF: The roles of urologist and patient autoinjection therapy for erectile dysfunction. Contemp Urol 4:21–26, 1990.

Brant WO, Bella AJ, Gracia MM, Lue TF: Priaprism. In Hohenfellner M, Santucci RA (eds): Emergencies in Urology. Berlin, Springer-Verlag, 2007, pp 301–312.

Bucher A, Mrstik C, Stogermayer F: Therapeutic effect of PGE_1 in the treatment of erectile dysfunction. Aktuel Urol 21:17–18, 1990.

Floth A, Schramek P: Intracavernous injection of prostaglandin E_1 in combination with papaverine: Enhanced effectiveness in comparison with papaverine plus phentolamine and prostaglandin E_1 alone. J Urol 145: 56–59, 1991.

Fritsche HMA, Usta MF, Hellstrom WJG: Intracavernous, transurethral, and topical therapies for erectile dysfunction in the era of oral pharmacotherapy. In Broderick GA (ed): Oral Pharmacotherapy for Male Sexual Dysfunction: A Guide to Clinical Management (Current Clinical Urology). Totowa, NJ, Humana Press, 2005, pp 253–277.

Gerber GS, Levine LA: Pharmacological erection program using prostaglandin E_1. J Urol 146:786–789, 1991.

Kerfoot WW, Carson CC: Pharmacologically induced erections among geriatric men. J Urol 146:1022–1024, 1991.

Kulmala RV, Tamella TL: Effects of priapism lasting 24 hours or longer caused by intracavernosal injection of vasoactive drugs. Int J Impot Res 7:131–136, 1995.

Lee M, Cannon B, Sharifi R: Chart for preparation of dilutions of alpha-adrenergic agonists for intracavernous use in treatment of priapism. J Urol 153:1182–1183, 1995.

Lewis R: Review of intraurethral suppositories and iontophoresis therapy for erectile dysfunction. Int J Impot Res 12(Suppl 4):S86–S90, 2000.

Lue TF: Priapism after transurethral alprostadil. J Urol 161:725–726, 1999.

Lui S M-C, Lin J S-N: Treatment of impotence: Comparison between the efficacy and safety of intracavernous injection of papaverine plus phentolamine (Regitine) and prostaglandin E_1. Int J Impot Res 2(Suppl): 147–151, 1990.

Padma-Nathan H: Corporal pharmacotherapy for erectile dysfunction and priapism. Monogr Urol 17:51–64, 1996.

Padma-Nathan H: Erectile dysfunction. Patient Care 17(Suppl 4):2, 1998.

Peterson A, Wessells H: Improving prospects for patients with priapism. Contemp Urol 14:30–32, 35, 39–40, 42, 2002.

Porst H, Adaikan G: Self-injection, trans-urethral, and topical therapy in erectile dysfunction. In Porst H, Buvat J (eds): Standard Practice in Sexual Medicine. Malden, Mass, Blackwell, 2006, pp 94–108.

Seftel AD (ed): Muse and intracavernous therapies. In Male and Female Sexual Dysfunction. St. Louis, Mosby, 2004, pp 121–128.

Sundaram CP, Thomas E, Pryor LB, et al: Long-term follow-up of patients receiving injection therapy for erectile dysfunction. Urology 49:932–935, 1997.

Sur RL, Kane CJ: Sildenafil citrate-associated priapism. Urology 55:950, 2000.

Virag R, Shoukry K, Floresco J, et al: Intracavernous self-injection of vasoactive drugs in the treatment of impotence: 8-year experience with 615 cases. J Urol 145:287–292, 1991.

CHAPTER 123

Sperm Banking

Dan B. French • Edmund S. Sabanegh, Jr.

Men undergoing some types of medical therapy such as chemotherapy, radiation therapy, or surgery face the real possibility of temporary or permanent infertility. An option to preserve fertility potential is to freeze (cryopreserve) sperm before undergoing these other medical treatments. Cryopreservation of sperm, or sperm banking, involves the freezing of sperm in liquid nitrogen followed by long-term storage for future use. Unfortunately, patients who may benefit from cryopreservation of sperm are not always aware of their options or may not even be considering their future fertility, considering the stress of their present situation. Therefore, a well-informed health care provider who is able to appropriately discuss cryopreservation with the patient is an invaluable resource.

Cryopreserved sperm was first used to achieve successful pregnancy in 1953. Because of moral controversy surrounding assisted reproductive techniques at the time, it would be another 10 years before use of cryopreserved sperm for artificial insemination would gain popularity. A technique using liquid nitrogen for freezing of sperm was developed in 1963. Over the years, other technical developments, such as the addition of cryoprotectants and the advancement of assisted reproductive techniques, have been introduced. With the advent of in vitro fertilization (IVF) and intracytoplasmic sperm injection (ICSI), even men with very few, poor-quality sperm can achieve fertility, with pregnancy rates approaching 50% per cycle.

Indications

One of the most important patient populations that may need this service is reproductive-age men who will undergo gonadotoxic chemotherapy for malignancy. Testicular cancer, leukemia, and lymphoma are the most common malignancies that may have reproductive consequences, either from the treatment or the disease itself. Cytotoxic chemotherapeutic regimens often result in acute azoospermia as defined by the absence of sperm in the ejaculate. Depending on the regimen used, only half of these men will recover spermatogenesis, and there is no precise way to predict who will do so. Even before receiving any cytotoxic therapy, these patients often have suboptimal semen quality as a result of their systemic disease, and therefore every effort should be made to cryopreserve any sperm they might have before initiating chemotherapy.

Radiation therapy, often used for certain testicular tumors and Hodgkin's disease, is also gonadotoxic, and appropriate individuals should be offered sperm cryopreservation before treatment. Even if the radiation is administered to distant sites and the testes are shielded, fertility can be impaired owing to scatter radiation.

Nonmalignant conditions may also require gonadotoxic treatment. Conditions such as autoimmune disorders, inflammatory bowel disease, or organ transplants may require immunosuppressive or cytotoxic therapies that impair fertility. These patients should be offered sperm banking if it is known that their treatment may lead to infertility.

Because up to 5% of men receiving a vasectomy will eventually request a restoration of their fertility, it is reasonable to offer sperm banking before vasectomy. Men who are undergoing vasectomy reversal may choose to have sperm extracted at the time of reconstructive surgery in the event that the reconstruction fails in the future.

Men with a history of spinal cord injury may require electroejaculation or surgical extraction for sperm retrieval. They may also choose to have sperm banked as a matter of convenience instead of undergoing repeated procedures.

Contraindications

The main contraindication to sperm cryopreservation is the *presence of a disease communicable through the sperm*. For this reason, donors are screened for human immunodeficiency virus, hepatitis B and C, chlamydia, gonorrhea, syphilis, cytomegalovirus, and human T-lymphotropic virus. Specimens are incubated for 6 months to confirm absence of any of these conditions before use.

Although not a contraindication, it should be noted that sperm with damaged DNA do not thaw as well as healthy sperm. With the development of IVF/ICSI, even semen samples with elevated levels of sperm DNA damage or severe oligospermia can be used effectively. Among the thousands of conceptions that have occurred from frozen sperm, the incidence of birth defects has been no different than that among children conceived through intercourse.

Procedure

The patient will complete various forms, including a *consent form*, agreement of fee schedules, and, most important, a legal document clearly outlining the fate of the sperm should the patient die or otherwise become incapacitated. Blood samples are drawn for screening for various sexually transmitted infections. Before freezing, a semen analysis is performed to assess the concentration, total number, and quality of sperm. The sample is then mixed with cryoprotectants such as egg yolk or glycerol.

Sperm can be collected for banking from various sources, depending on the clinical circumstances. These include ejaculated semen specimens, sperm recovered from the bladder in patients with retrograde ejaculation, and surgically retrieved specimens from either the epididymis or testicular tissue. If the specimen is an ejaculate, it should be produced by masturbation at the collection site or at least brought to the collection site immediately after collection. The donor should not have had any ejaculations within the preceding 48 to 72 hours if at all possible. Depending on semen quality, several collections separated by 48 to 72 hours of abstinence may be required. Once collected, the sample is allowed to liquefy at room temperature.

The specimen is labeled with the pertinent data, including but not limited to patient name, identification number, and date of collection. This information is verified by the donor. Sometimes photographs of the donor are used as an additional security feature. The sample is divided into a certain number of straws or vials for freezing based on the concentration of sperm. One of these aliquots is thawed the next day to assess for viability following thaw. This test is used as a predictor of future viability for the entire batch. Samples, once preserved, can be stored for many years without fear of deterioration.

The cost of sperm cryopreservation varies between institutions. Cost for an initial analysis and freezing ranges from $150 to $600. This price is even higher when specimens must be shipped, usually when using a commercial cryobank. Most cryobanks assess annual storage fees ranging from $50 to $365.

Conclusion

The incidence of cancer in reproductive-age men has been increasing worldwide over the past 25 years. Although cancer cure and the management of acute toxicities remain the paramount issues for both the medical professional and the patient, future fertility is a major concern for young patients. With advances in both cryopreservation technology and assisted reproductive techniques, cryopreservation of sperm has become a valuable tool in the treatment of male infertility. Men of reproductive age embarking on gonadotoxic treatments for cancer as well as other selected groups of patients need to be aware that cryopreservation of sperm is an option, and it is incumbent on the provider to educate them about this option. The procedure is relatively simple and affordable and, unfortunately, remains underutilized.

CPT/Billing Codes

89259 Sperm cryopreservation
89343 Storage per year
89353 Thawing of cryopreserved sperm/each aliquot

ICD-9-CM Diagnostic Codes

V26.52 Status vasectomy
V66.2 Status post chemotherapy
186.9 Testicular tumor
201.9 Hodgkin's disease
202.80 Lymphoma
208.90 Leukemia
606.0 Azoospermia
606.1 Oligospermia

Online Resources

American Society for Reproductive Medicine. Available at www.asrm.org.

CryoChoice: For information on sperm cryopreservation using the mail system. Available at www.cryochoice.com.

RESOLVE: The National Infertility Association. Available at www.resolve.org.

Society for the Study of Male Reproduction. Available at www.ssmr.org.

Sperm Bank Directory: For a listing of local sperm banks. Available at www.spermbankdirectory.com.

Bibliography

Agarwal A, Sidhu RK, Shekarriz M, Thomas AJ Jr: Optimum abstinence time for cryopreservation of semen in cancer patients. J Urol 154:86–88, 1995.

Anger JT, Gilber BR, Goldstein M: Cryopreservation of sperm: Indications, methods and results. J Urol 170:1079–1084, 2003.

Kliesch S, Kamischke A, Nieschlag E: Cryopreservation of human semen. In Nieschlag E, Behre HM (eds): Andrology: Male Reproductive Health and Dysfunction, 2nd ed. Berlin, Springer, 2000, pp 349–356.

Nalesnik JG, Sabanegh ES Jr, Eng TY, Buchholz TA: Fertility in men after treatment for stage 1 and 2a seminoma. Am J Clin Oncol 27:584–588, 2004.

Peterson PM, Giwercman A, Skakkebaek NE, Rorth M: Gonadal function in men with testicular cancer. Semin Oncol 25:224–234, 1998.

Witt MA: Sperm banking. In Lipshultz LI, Howards SS (eds): Infertility in the Male, 3rd ed. St. Louis, Mosby, 1997, p 501.

CHAPTER 124

Implantable Hormone Pellets for Testosterone Deficiency in Adult Men

John Harlan Haynes III • Terrance S. Hines

Testosterone is responsible for normal growth and development of male sex organs and maintenance of secondary sex characteristics. As the primary androgenic hormone, its production and secretion are the end products of hormonal and biochemical interactions. Gonadotropin-releasing hormone (GnRH) is secreted by the hypothalamus and controls the pituitary secretion of luteinizing hormone (LH) and follicle-stimulating hormone (FSH). LH regulates production of testosterone by the testes, and FSH stimulates spermatogenesis. Testosterone can be converted in the body either to dihydrotestosterone by 5-α reductase or to estradiol by aromatase. Dihydrotestosterone preferentially binds to androgen receptors and becomes the more active form involved in hair growth and sebum production. Estradiol may be important in maintaining libido and bone mass, but may contribute to truncal obesity and feminine characteristics.

Testosterone deficiency is common, occurring in 1 in 200 men. The prevalence increases with age as testosterone levels decrease and sex hormone–binding globulin levels increase (causing a further decrease in free or bioavailable testosterone). More than 50% of men older than 55 years of age may have low testosterone, increasingly referred to as *andropause*. Treatment should be considered in all men with testosterone deficiency as long as contraindications do not exist.

Abnormally low testosterone levels are associated not only with sexual dysfunction, but with other comorbid conditions such as lipid disorders, cardiovascular disease, insulin insensitivity, osteoporosis, and cognitive and mood changes. Testosterone deficiency may be a cause of sarcopenia, a condition of aging senescence characterized by muscular weakness and atrophy.

In general, there are two basic types of testosterone deficiency:

1. *Primary*, or hypergonadotropic, hypogonadism results from primary testicular failure. In this situation, testosterone levels will be low and levels of pituitary gonadotropins (LH or FSH) will likely be high-normal or elevated.
2. *Secondary*, or hypogonadotropic, hypogonadism is the result of inadequate secretion of pituitary gonadotropins. In addition to a low testosterone level, LH or FSH levels will be low or low-normal.

Satisfactory replacement of testosterone is possible regardless of the type of deficiency.

Hypogonadism is defined as a free testosterone level that is below the lower limit of normal for young adult control subjects. Age-related decreases in free testosterone were once accepted as "normal." Currently, they are not considered normal. No agreement exists on the exact normal level of testosterone as men age or the serum testosterone level at which a man loses his sexual function.

The definition of *relative hypogonadism* is also uncertain. Many men have perfectly normal sexual function even if their testosterone levels decline into the age-adjusted lower normal range. Patients with low-normal to subnormal testosterone levels may warrant a clinical trial of testosterone. The threshold of response to and dosage of testosterone vary with age. If LH is increased and the testosterone level is low, the patient will have decompensated primary testicular failure. Testosterone replacement therapy can be essential to maintain physiologically normal levels. Testosterone replacement improves sexual function and mood, increases lean muscle mass and strength, and decreases fat mass in hypogonadal men.

An effect of testosterone on endothelial function in men is supported by a recent study that reported on the effects of intravascular administration of physiologic doses of testosterone on coronary blood flow in men with coronary artery disease. The results showed an increase in coronary vasodilation and blood flow in the testosterone test subjects.

Health Implications of Testosterone Deficiency

Testosterone deficiency can result in the following:

- Anemia
- Decreases in or loss of libido and erectile function
- Absence or regression of secondary sexual characteristics
- Oligospermia or azoospermia
- Decrease in energy, increased fatigue
- Depressed mood
- Increase in fat mass
- Progressive decrease in lean body mass and in muscle strength
- Decrease in bone density and increased risk of osteopenia/osteoporosis

Men with testicular failure may suffer from sexual dysfunction, as well as osteoporosis, muscle weakness, depression, and lassitude, which is the clinical spectrum of hypogonadism. The sexual dysfunction, especially decreased libido and decreased erectile capacity, often reverses with testosterone replacement therapy. Ideally, testosterone therapy should provide physiologic-range testosterone levels (400 to 800 ng/dL). The variability of response in some patients may be related to comorbid medical illnesses, vascular dysfunction causing erectile dysfunction at the penile level, or psychological factors (Box 124-1).

Box 124-1. Testosterone Deficiency Screening Questions

The "low-testosterone syndrome" often seen in healthy older men is thought to play a role in a number of clinical problems seen in the growing elderly male population. A checklist has been developed to help raise awareness of the presence of testosterone deficiency in the older man. Physicians may find the following questions helpful in screening their older patients:

1. Do you have a decrease in libido (sex drive)?
2. Do you have a lack of energy?
3. Do you have a decrease in strength or endurance?
4. Have you lost height?
5. Have you noticed a decreased "enjoyment of life"?
6. Are you sad or grumpy?
7. Are your erections less strong?
8. Have you noted a recent deterioration in your ability to play sports?
9. Are you falling asleep after dinner?
10. Has there been a recent deterioration in your work performance?

Men at Increased Risk for Testosterone Deficiency

- Decreased secondary sexual characteristics
- Erectile dysfunction or reduced libido
- An unexplained decrease in energy, or muscle weakness
- Unexplained osteopenia or osteoporosis
- Testicular atrophy
- Human immunodeficiency virus infection/acquired immunodeficiency syndrome with weight loss
- Long-term systemic glucocorticoids
- Chronic alcoholism or substance abuse
- Chronic systemic diseases (e.g., chronic renal failure, chronic inflammatory diseases)
- Recent-onset gynecomastia
- Morbid obesity
- Family history of endocrine failure
- Hypothyroidism

Diagnosis of Testosterone Deficiency

In symptomatic men, these suggested guidelines may be followed:

- Measure total testosterone (total T) by blood measurement taken between 7 and 10 AM.
- A total T above 400 ng/mL is considered normal.
- If total T is between 300 and 400 ng/mL, use the free or bioavailable testosterone level and clinical judgment to guide therapy.
- If total T is less than 300 ng/dL
    - Rule out treatable endocrine causes and transient hypogonadism due to reversible illness, drugs, or nutritional deficiency.
    - Repeat the test and measure free or bioavailable testosterone, LH, and FSH levels.
- If repeat total T or free T is confirmed as low, consider initiating testosterone replacement therapy.
- LH, FSH, or both, are measured to distinguish between primary (testicular) and secondary (pituitary hypothalamic) hypogonadism.
- If FSH and LH are low or normal, this is secondary hypogonadism, and in the presence of very low total T (<150 ng/dL), a prolactin level and other pituitary hormones should be obtained. If the prolactin level is elevated or other signs of a tumor mass exist, obtain magnetic resonance imaging of the sellar and pituitary region to rule out a pituitary tumor. Referral to an endocrinologist is indicated for further evaluation.
- With a low total T and a high FSH and LH, Klinefelter's syndrome must be considered, which is a common identifiable cause of primary testicular failure and may be diagnosed by obtaining a karyotype.
- A dual-energy x-ray absorptiometry (DEXA) scan may considered to evaluate bone mineral density in men with severe androgen deficiency and fracture risk.

Contraindications

- Known or suspected prostate cancer or breast cancer
- Palpable prostate nodule or prostate-specific antigen (PSA) greater than 3 ng/mL without further urologic evaluation
- Severe benign prostatic hypertrophy (BPH) related bladder outlet obstruction or other urinary tract symptoms
- Erythrocytosis (hematocrit >50%)
- Hyperviscosity of blood (hyperviscosity syndrome)
- Treatment for improved athletic performance, body building, or short stature
- Untreated sleep apnea
- Untreated or severe congestive heart failure

Patients in Whom Treatment Requires Careful Monitoring

- Prostate problems and uncorrected obstructive symptoms caused by BPH
- Edema, fluid retention
- Gynecomastia
- Polycythemia or exacerbated erythropoiesis
- Hypogonadal adolescent boys because treatment may increase physical aggression
- Anyone whose epiphyses have not yet closed, because premature closure and permanent short stature can result from treatment

NOTE: It is important to closely monitor those patients with a family history (i.e., presence in a first-degree relative) of prostate cancer, although the relationship between the cancer and testosterone replacement therapy is controversial. A double-blind, randomized, placebo-controlled trial of 237 men 60 to 80 years of age, conducted in the Netherlands from 2004 to 2005 and published in the *Journal of the American Medical Association* in 2008 (Emmelot-Vonk and colleagues), showed an increase in lean body mass, a decrease in fat mass, increased insulin sensitivity, and no short-term negative effects on the prostate or on cognition. In a review of the literature by Rhoden and Morgentaler in the *New England Journal of Medicine* in 2004, prospective studies demonstrated a low frequency of prostate cancer in association with testosterone replacement therapy. The conclusion was that there is no compelling evidence at present to suggest that men with higher testosterone levels are at greater risk of prostate cancer or that treating men who have hypogonadism with exogenous androgens increases this risk. It should be recognized that prostate cancer becomes more prevalent exactly at the time of a man's life when testosterone levels decline.

Treatment

Testosterone should be administered only to men who are testosterone deficient, as evidenced by distinctly subnormal serum testosterone levels (<400 ng/dL, or subnormal based on specific assay used). The Endocrine Society's 2006 Clinical Practice Guidelines recommend testosterone therapy for symptomatic men with androgen deficiency who have low testosterone levels, to induce and maintain secondary sex characteristics and to improve their sexual function, sense of well-being, muscle mass and strength, and bone mineral density.

The principal goals of testosterone therapy are to alleviate symptoms and to reduce health risks by restoring the serum testosterone concentration to the normal range.

The currently acceptable modes of testosterone delivery are transdermal, intramuscular (IM), implantable, and buccal.

NOTE: *Oral androgens* (methyltestosterone, fluoxymesterone) are not as effective and are associated with a significant risk of hepatotoxicity (e.g., cholestatic jaundice, peliosis hepatis, and hepatoma) and are therefore not recommended.

Transdermal testosterone (Testoderm, Androderm): Unlike the original patches applied to scrotal skin, Androderm is worn on the arm or torso and delivers approximately 5 mg in 24 hours. Transdermal therapeutic systems are replaced every 24 hours. Transdermal preparations provide a relatively stable concentration of testosterone compared with other routes. Serum levels of testosterone peak 2 to 8 hours after application of a patch. Anecdotally, as much as one third of men do not tolerate this route because of severe skin rash. This rash may be prevented by pretreating with a topical corticosteroid.

Testosterone gel (AndroGel 1%, Testim 1%) 5-mg packs or tubes: Applied daily to skin, "T gel" is a translucent hydroalcoholic gel that may cause less skin irritation and lower discontinuation rates compared with the transdermal patch. These positive results occur within 30 days. Because of the amount of skin to which the gel is applied, the serum concentrations are more even and higher over 24 hours than with the patch. Testim is dosed at 50 to 100 mg and has a musky aroma. All T gel formulations have a warning about secondary exposure because virilization has been reported in children who were secondarily exposed to testosterone gel. The black box warning states that children should avoid contact with unwashed or unclothed application sites in men using testosterone gel and that health care providers should advise patients to strictly adhere to recommended instructions for use.

Injectable testosterone esters: The principal esters available in North America are testosterone enanthate and testosterone cypionate. Injections of testosterone enanthate or testosterone cypionate may be given at intervals ranging from 7 to 14 days. Dosing typically is 100 mg IM per week to 300 mg IM per 3 weeks. A weekly injection of 100 mg causes less variation outside of the normal range. Although biologically effective, disadvantages of this route include the need for frequent deep IM administration and pronounced fluctuations in energy, mood, and libido (particularly as the dosing interval is increased). Testosterone undecanoate (Nebido) is available in several countries and is dosed at 100 mg every 3 months.

Implantable hormone pellets (Testopel): The implantable pellets are perhaps the most convenient, dependable, and best-tolerated method of testosterone delivery. Subcutaneous pellets are viewed as a more cost-effective and convenient therapy with potentially much greater compliance and tolerance than other methods. Placed subcutaneously in the buttocks through a special trocar device, 8 to 10 pellets (600–750 mg) usually provide sustained adequate physiologic blood levels (e.g., 400 to 800 ng/dL) for 4 to 6 months (Box 124-2).

Buccal tablet: The U.S. Food and Drug Administration approved Striant (30 mg, twice a day) in June 2003. It is adhered to a depression in the gum above the upper incisors.

Finally, although not an androgen, human chorionic gonadotropin (hCG) stimulates production of testosterone and sperm by the testes.

Box 124-2. Insurance Criteria for Reimbursement for Testosterone Pellets

Aetna, U.S. Healthcare, BlueCross/Blue Shield, and Medicare cover U.S. Food and Drug Administration–approved implantable testosterone pellets (Testopel pellets) subject to the following patient selection criteria only:

- As *second-line testosterone replacement therapy* in men with congenital or acquired endogenous androgen absence or deficiency associated with primary or secondary hypogonadism when neither transdermal nor intramuscular testosterone replacement therapy is effective or appropriate.
- Primary hypogonadism includes conditions such as testicular failure as a result of cryptorchidism, bilateral torsion, orchitis, vanishing testis syndrome, inborn errors in testosterone biosynthesis, or bilateral orchiectomy.
- Secondary hypogonadism (hypogonadotropic hypogonadism) includes conditions such as gonadotropin-releasing hormone deficiency and pituitary–hypothalamic injury as a result of surgery, tumors, trauma, or radiation, and is the most common form of hypogonadism seen in older adults.

Monitoring Patients on Testosterone Replacement

- Clinical symptoms and signs of testosterone deficiency
- Frequency and duration of erections
- Acne and oiliness of skin, breast size and tenderness
- Possible skin irritation with transdermal therapy
- Serum testosterone levels
- Lipid profiles
- Sleep apnea

Transdermal testosterone delivery systems: Serum testosterone should be drawn 8 to 12 hours after application or per patch label instructions. Because concentrations fluctuate in an unpredictable way when using the gel preparation, at least two measurements should be obtained. Skin irritation at the site of the patch is common.

Injectable or implantable testosterone: Monitor nadir testosterone levels at 3 months (implants) or before the next injection/implantation. Levels that exceed 800 ng/dL or are less than 200 ng/dL require adjustment of the dose or frequency.

Digital rectal examination (DRE) and PSA: DRE should be performed and a PSA level checked in all men before initiating treatment, again at 3 months, and then annually in men older than 40 years of age. An abnormal DRE, a confirmed increase in PSA of more than 1.4 ng/mL in any 1-year period, a total PSA of more than 4.0 ng/mL, or a PSA velocity of greater than 0.4 ng/mL per year (beginning 6 months after therapy initiation) requires evaluation by a urologist. Exacerbations of obstructive uropathy related to BPH are a concern, and, if warranted, urine flow rate and postvoid residuals should be measured.

Hematocrit: Testosterone replacement therapy has been associated with increased hematocrit and hemoglobin. The hematocrit should be checked at baseline, then at 3 months and yearly. A hematocrit of more than 52% warrants evaluation for hypoxia and sleep apnea or a reduction in the dose of testosterone therapy. Testosterone is known to stimulate erythropoiesis.

Sleep apnea: Screening for sleep apnea includes interrogation of symptoms (e.g., excessive daytime sleepiness, snoring, or witnessed apnea) and polysomnography when indicated.

Liver function, cholesterol, and high-density lipoprotein (HDL) cholesterol: Levels should be checked periodically. Testosterone lowers total cholesterol, low-density lipoprotein, and HDL.

Breast examination: Regular breast examinations are recommended.

Bone mineral density: Measurement of bone mineral density of the lumbar spine or the femoral necks at 1-year intervals may be considered in hypogonadal men with osteopenia, especially those younger than 80 years of age.

Equipment

- Trocar implanter kit (includes the trocar and stylet plunger)
- Disposable 5-cm trocar pellet implanter (3.2-mm bore diameter)
- Forceps
- Stainless steel tray
- Sterile gloves
- 1% lidocaine with epinephrine 2 to 3 mL
- 3-mL syringe; 27-gauge, 1½-inch needle
- No. 11 scalpel blade
- 75-mg testosterone pellets (Testopel; Slate Pharmaceuticals), 3 × 8 mm (most common total dose for 4 to 6 months is 10 pellets), in individual sterile glass tubes
- Lidoderm 5% patch or topical anesthetic placed 15 minutes before the procedure at site of insertion *(optional)*
- 2.0 chromic suture or Steri-Strips and tincture of benzoin

NOTE: The disposable trocar *should be sterile and individually packaged.* If an older stainless steel trocar is used, it should be sterilized by steam in an autoclave at 121° C for a minimum of 15 minutes. The standard procedures for sterilizing surgical instruments should be followed.

Preprocedure Patient Preparation

All potential risks, benefits, and alternatives to testosterone replacement therapy should be discussed, specifically the potential complications regarding trocar insertion subcutaneously (including infection and bleeding). The patient should understand that once the pellets are inserted, they are not typically removed unless the risks outweigh the benefits. The pellets slowly dissolve and the effects will last for 4 to 6 months.

Technique

The office procedure usually takes approximately 15 minutes. The testosterone pellets should be implanted into the subdermal fat of the buttocks using a special trocar implanter under sterile conditions and using a local anesthetic. The 75-mg pellets are fat soluble and so are implanted subcutaneously. In most men, an area on either lateral buttock between the gluteus maximus and the tensor fasciae latae muscle is preferred so that implantation is made below the skin and above the muscle and fascia, just inferior to the iliac spine, directed inferiorly along the line of the femur. The skin is marked 3 cm below the halfway mark between the iliac crest and the sacroiliac joint and the line is extended about 10 cm inferiorly parallel to the femur. Anecdotally, pellets implanted more superiorly near the belt line or in the buttock on the side under the wallet pocket have been subject to inadvertent extrusion (Fig. 124-1A).

Preparation

1. Place patient comfortably in the lateral jackknife or fetal position.
2. Cleanse the skin over the insertion site with Hibiclens, alcohol, and povidone–iodine (Fig. 124-1B).
3. Sterile technique is used.
4. Create a skin wheal using lidocaine 1% with epinephrine (1:100,000; Fig. 124-1C).
5. Inject 2 to 3 mL of 1% lidocaine with epinephrine along the intended tract of the trocar insertion to a depth of 2 cm.

Implantation

1. Place pellets as indicated in the sterile container (the most common dose is ten 75-mg pellets).
2. After adequate local anesthesia, make a small (4-mm) puncture incision with a no. 11 scalpel blade (Fig. 124-1D).
3. Insert the trocar with stylet (solid rod in metal sheath with pointed end), direct it subcutaneously pointed at a 30-degree angle to the skin surface, and advance it inferiorly to a depth of 2 cm.
4. The trocar and stylet are then angled horizontal to the skin surface and advanced beneath the skin through the

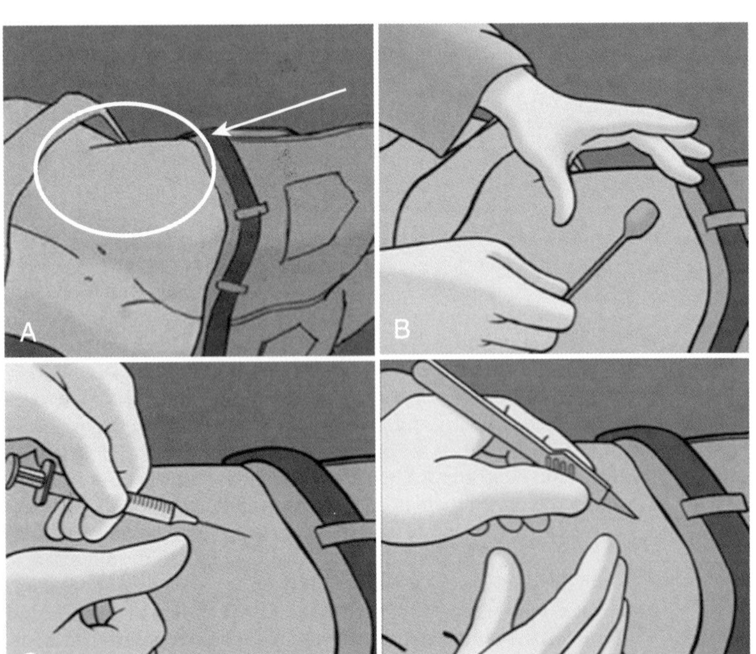

Figure 124-1 Preparation for implantation of testosterone pellets. **A** and **B,** Cleanse skin with Hibiclens, alcohol, and povidone–iodine. **C,** Create skin wheal using lidocaine 1% with epinephrine. **D,** Make small incision with no. 11 blade. (Courtesy of Slate Pharmaceuticals, Inc., Durham, NC.)

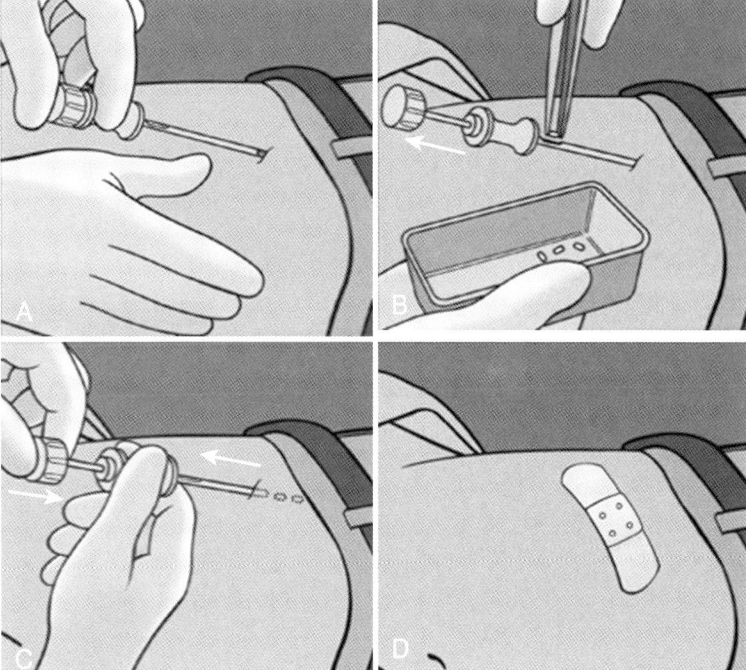

Figure 124-2 Implantation of testosterone pellets. **A,** Insert the trocar implanter with the stylet in place and direct it subcutaneously to the depth of the bolt (about 5 cm). **B,** Remove the stylet and place all the pellets in the lumen of the implanter with sterilized tissue forceps. **C,** Insert the stylet and, while stabilizing and slowly pulling back the implanter, push the pellets through the bore and into the fatty tissues. **D,** Close the puncture site. (Courtesy of Slate Pharmaceuticals, Inc, Durham, NC.)

subcutaneous tissue above the muscle and parallel to the trajectory of the femur to full depth (about 5 cm) until reaching the pellet slot (Fig. 124-2A).

5. The pointed stylet is then removed, and, using sterile tissue forceps, pellet implants are carefully placed in the slot of the hollow tube of the implanter. Usually, three to five pellets per tract are placed (Fig. 124-2B). (A sterile tray or cup may be held beneath the implanter as a "safety net" to catch pellets that may be inadvertently misplaced.)
6. The stylet is then inserted into the trocar to be used as a plunger. The implanter is stabilized with one hand as the pellets are pushed through the bore and advanced within the hollow trocar sheath. The stylet is advanced inside the trocar as the trocar is slowly withdrawn, and the pellets are pushed out and deposited into the fatty tissue (Fig. 124-2C).
7. This insertion process may be repeated through the same incision in a fanlike fashion until the total dose (usually 10 pellets) is deeply inserted. Extrusions may be minimized by placing pellets in tracts arranged in a fanlike pattern (e.g., three, four, and three at 45, 90, and 135 degrees, respectively).
8. After all the pellets have been inserted, the stylet is advanced within the trocar and the trocar is withdrawn using a clockwise–counterclockwise twisting motion.
9. Give the patient a dry pressure dressing to apply pressure for a few minutes.
10. Clean and then close the puncture site using Steri-Strips or a chromic suture, and cover with an adhesive bandage (Fig. 124-2D). Cold compression using body weight on an ice pack is advised for 10 minutes.

The pellets are slowly absorbed and are not removed. The procedure may be repeated on the opposite buttock in 4 to 6 months, depending on the adequacy of serum testosterone. Have the patient return in 3 months to check for efficacy and tolerability.

Complications and Risks

The chief adverse reactions with testosterone pellets include the following:

- Pellet extrusion
- Minor bleeding (typically insignificant and controlled by applying pressure to the surgical wound)
- Infection (infrequent and may also result in pellet extrusion)

The use of povidone–iodine skin disinfectant before the procedure appears to lower pellet extrusion rates. The likelihood of pellet extrusion may decline with increasing operator experience. Preoperative and postoperative oral antibiotics (e.g., cephalexin 1000 mg) may reduce the incidence of infection. Some patients develop fibrosis (scarring, nodules) around implantation sites, but this typically does not prevent further implantations.

Other, rare, complications include the following:

- Pain at insertion site
- Increased fluid retention
- Gynecomastia
- Worsening sleep apnea
- Increased hematocrit
- Worsening prostate symptoms
- Testicular atrophy
- Mood swings
- Oligospermia or azoospermia

Postprocedure Patient Education

Most patients return to work the day of, or the day after, implantation but are advised to avoid bending or vigorous physical activity. For the first 24 hours, the patient should keep a dry pressure bandage on the insertion site and limit strenuous activity. He should watch for any complications as noted previously.

Regulations

Testopel pellets are classified as a Schedule III controlled substance under the Anabolic Steroids Act of 1990. Physicians should restrict usage to avoid long-term on-site storage. As with other Schedule III substances, it is necessary to strictly follow state pharmacy and federal Drug Enforcement Agency regulations, and always document and copy. A prescription may be written and the patient may obtain the pellets and bring them to the clinic for insertion, or the pellets and trocar may be ordered directly from Slate Pharmaceuticals (Durham, NC). Slate has an updated website for additional reference (www.Testopel.com).

CPT/Billing Codes

S0189 Testosterone pellet (75 mg)
11980 Subcutaneous implantation of testosterone pellets

ICD-9-CM Diagnostic Codes

253.4 Pituitary hypogonadism
257.2 Male hypogonadism, testicular, primary or secondary
257.8 Other testicular dysfunction
353.4 Hypogonadotropic hypogonadism

Supplier

(See contact information online at www.expertconsult.com.)

Slate Pharmaceuticals

BIBLIOGRAPHY

Bhasin S, Cunningham GR, Hayes FJ, et al: Testosterone therapy in adult men with androgen deficiency syndromes: An Endocrine Society clinical practice guideline. J Clin Endocrinol Metab 91:1995–2010, 2006.

Cavender RK: Subcutaneous pellet implantation procedure for treatment of testosterone deficiency syndrome. J Sex Med 6:21–24, 2009.

Cavender RK, Fairall M: Subcutaneous testosterone pellet implant (Testopel) therapy for men with testosterone deficiency syndrome: A single-site retrospective safety analysis. J Sex Med 6:3177–3192, 2009.

Cunningham GR, Snyder PJ, Swerdloff RS, Tenover JS: Testosterone replacement therapy in men: Emerging clinical issues. Newsletter from the Endocrine Society's 82nd Annual Meeting, June 24, 2000, Toronto, Ontario, Canada.

Emmelot-Vonk MH, Verhaar HJ, Nakhai Pour HR: Effect of testosterone supplementation on functional mobility, cognition, and other parameters in older men: A randomized controlled trial. JAMA 299:39–52, 2008.

Guay AT, Nankin HR: AACE clinical practice guidelines for the evaluation and treatment of male sexual dysfunction (developed by the American Association of Clinical Endocrinologists and the American College of Endocrinology), 1980. Available at http://www.aace.com/pub/pdf/guidelines/sexdysguid.pdf.

Handelsman DJ, Mackey MA, Howe C, et al: An analysis of testosterone implants for androgen replacement therapy. Clin Endocrinol (Oxf) 47:311–316, 1997.

Jockenhovel F, Vogel E, Kreutzer M, et al: Pharmacokinetics and pharmacodynamics of subcutaneous testosterone implants in hypogonadal men. Clin Endocrinol (Oxf) 45:61–71, 1996.

Leichtnam M, Rolland H, Wüthrich P, Guy RH: Testosterone hormone replacement therapy: State-of-the-art and emerging technologies. Pharm Res 23:1117–1132, 2006.

Mäkinen J, Järvisalo M, Pöllänen P, et al: Increased Carotid Atherosclerosis in Andropausal Middle Aged Men. J Am Coll Cardiol 45:1603–1608, 2005.

Nieschlag E, Behre H, Bouchard P, et al: Testosterone replacement therapy: Current trends and future directions. Hum Reprod Update 10:409–419, 2004.

Petak SM, Nankin HR, Spark RF, et al: AACE clinical practice guidelines for the evaluation and treatment of hypogonadism in adult male patients: 2002 update (developed by the American Association of Clinical Endocrinologists and the American College of Endocrinology), 2002. Available at http://www.aace.com/pub/pdf/guidelines/hypogonadism.pdf.

Rhoden EL, Morgentaler A: Risks of testosterone-replacement therapy and recommendations for monitoring. N Engl J Med 350:482–492, 2004.

Rosano GM, De Ziegler D, Pagnotta P, et al: Plasma testosterone levels in males with coronary disease. Eur Heart J 19(Suppl):141, 1998 [abstract].

Snyder PJ, Peachey H, Berlin JA, et al: Effects of testosterone replacement in hypogonadal men. J Clin Endocrinol Metab 85:2670–2677, 2000.

Tenover JL: Male hormone replacement therapy including "andropause." Endocrinol Metab Clin North Am 27:969–987, 1998.

Wang C, Swerdloff RS, Iranmanesh A, et al: Transdermal testosterone gel improves sexual function, mood, muscle strength, and body composition parameters in hypogonadal men. J Clin Endocrinol Metab 85:2839–2853, 2000.

Webb CM, McNeill JG, Hayward CS, et al: Effects of testosterone on coronary vasomotor regulation in men with coronary heart disease. Circulation 100:1690–1696, 1999.

CHAPTER 125

Vacuum Devices for Erectile Dysfunction

John R. Holman

Erectile dysfunction is a common medical problem occurring in nearly 30 million American men. Vacuum devices to promote erection are safe and have overall clinical success rates of approximately 90% but are considered second-line therapy given the efficacy, favorable side effect profile, and ease of use of phosphodiesterase inhibitors. They are useful in nearly all men with erectile dysfunction except those with severe cavernous fibrosis. Therapy depends on the ability to transfer blood into the corpus cavernosa, which is limited if fibrosis is present.

A number of devices are available for use. The majority have *three common components*: a vacuum chamber or cylinder, a vacuum pump that creates a negative pressure within the chamber, and an elastic constriction band.

The devices create a nonphysiologic erection by trapping blood in both the intracorporeal and extracorporeal compartments of the penile shaft by means of the negative-pressure vacuum. The constrictor band is then placed before the chamber, over the proximal shaft, constricting blood flow into and out of the penis and maintaining an erection for sexual intercourse. Erection is maintained distal to the constricting band. Most manufacturers recommend that the vacuum-induced erection be maintained for less than 30 minutes because penile distention, edema, and cyanosis may ensue with prolonged use. The American Urologic Association, in its erectile dysfunction clinical practice guideline, reviewed and validated in 2009 and based on panel consensus, recommends only vacuum constriction devices containing a vacuum limiter–relief valve should be used, whether purchased over-the-counter or procured with a prescription.

Indications

Erectile dysfunction resulting from

- Vascular disorders
- Neurologic disorders
- Psychogenic disorders
- Hormonal disorders
- Medications, when the medication cannot be altered or terminated

Contraindications

- Blood dyscrasias, coagulation disorders, or anticoagulation drug therapy
- Impaired manual dexterity to operate the device

Equipment

- Vacuum erection device, including chamber, vacuum pump, and constriction bands (Fig. 125-1A). Battery-operated suction devices may be preferable in patients with impaired manual dexterity or after debilitating neurologic events such as stroke or quadriplegia. Constriction bands come in a variety of sizes to fit the penile shaft.
- Lubricant as needed.

Preprocedure Patient Preparation

Discuss use of the suction device, alternatives, relative benefits, and potential complications with the patient and, when possible, his partner. The patient should be aware that a vacuum-induced erection, unlike a physiologic erection, causes rigidity distal to the constrictor band and may allow the penis to pivot at its base, requiring positioning for vaginal penetration. Although it is generally well tolerated, patients using this device may experience *painful ejaculation*, *penile pain*, *ecchymoses*, *hematomas*, *petechiae*, and *decreased penile temperature or numbness* distal to the constriction band. Most men have normal ejaculations with vacuum devices. Delayed or painful ejaculations have been reported in 10% to 15% of men, along with a feeling of trapped semen during ejaculation. The use of constriction rings with a "cut out" on the ventral aspect of the ring can help prevent this (Fig. 125-1B). Otherwise, the semen drains out the penile meatus once the constriction band is removed. *Hematomas* have been reported in 9.8% and local *skin injury* in 2.2% of long-term users. These complications can be reduced or eliminated by increased experience with the device and by emphasizing the need to remove the constriction band after 30 minutes. Most manufacturers provide instructional materials, videos, and customer service availability by phone to assist with appropriate use of their equipment.

Technique

1. Complete the patient's history and physical examination to establish a diagnosis of erectile dysfunction.
2. Select a desired device for use.
3. Apply the open end of the vacuum chamber over the penis. A seal should be made with the skin at the base of the penis, usually with the help of lubricant jelly.
4. Activate the vacuum pump to create negative pressure within the chamber, thereby drawing blood into the penis and producing an erection-like state. Most devices have release valves in the chamber that prevent formation of excessive pressure (Fig. 125-1C).
5. Once adequate tumescence is achieved, slide the constrictor band at the base of the chamber onto the penile shaft. This effectively traps blood in the penis to maintain the erection. The chamber and pump may now be removed. Constrictor bands are available in a variety of sizes.

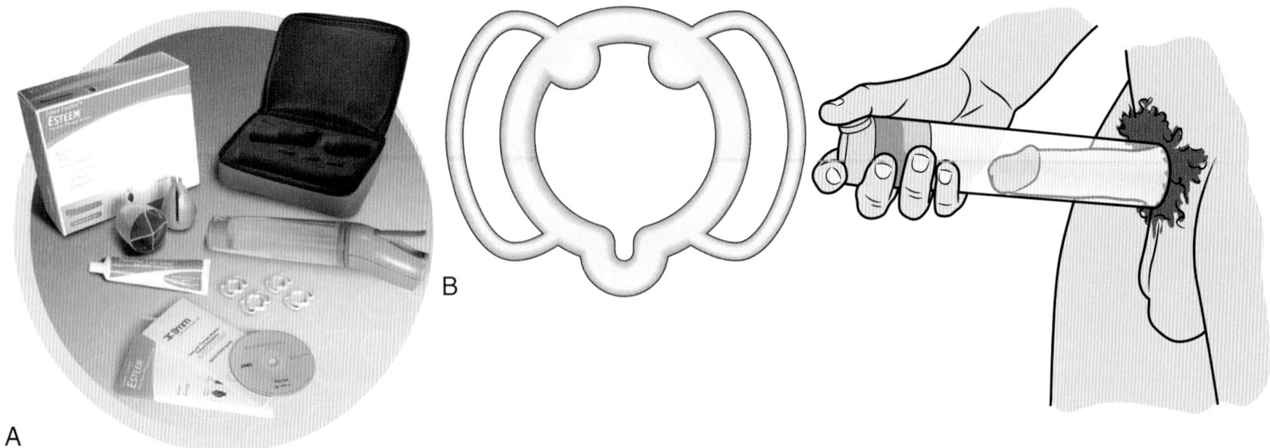

Figure 125-1 **A,** Typical vacuum device for erectile dysfunction. **B,** Constricting rings on device, cross-sectional view. **C,** How to activate the pump. (**A,** Courtesy of TIMM Medical Technologies, Eden Prairie, Minn. **B,** Redrawn from TIMM Medical Technologies.)

6. After intercourse, remove the band from the penile shaft. The vacuum-induced erection will subside.
7. Inspect the penis for evidence of injury.
8. After use, submerge all parts of the suction devices, except the vacuum pump, in soapy water for cleaning.

Complications

- Decrease in penile temperature or numbness distal to the constriction band.
- Local skin injury.
- Painful ejaculation.
- No ejaculation.
- Penile pain.
- Subcutaneous ecchymoses, petechiae, or hematoma.
- With prolonged use (>30 minutes), progressive penile distention, edema, and cyanosis may occur.

Patient Education Guides

See the sample patient education and consent forms online at www.expertconsult.com.

CPT/Billing Code

55899 Unlisted procedure, male genital system (documentation suggested)

ICD-9-CM Diagnostic Codes

302.72 Psychosexual dysfunction
607.84 Impotence of organic origin

Acknowledgment

The author would like to thank Chad J. Smith, DO, for his contributions to this chapter in the previous edition.

Suppliers

(See contact information online at www.expertconsult.com.)

ErecAid
TIMM Medical Technologies
SOMAerectSTF
Augusta Medical Systems

Bibliography

Derouet H, Caspari D, Rohde V, et al: Treatment of erectile dysfunction with external vacuum devices. Andrologia 31(Suppl 1):89–94, 1999.

Lewis RW, Witherington R: External vacuum therapy for erectile dysfunction: Use and results. World J Urol 15:78–82, 1997.

Montague DK, Jarow JP, Broderick GA, et al, for the American Urological Association Erectile Dysfunction Update Panel: The management of erectile dysfunction: An update. 2007. Available at www.auanet.org/content/guidelines-and-quality-care/clinical-guidelines/main-reports/edmgmt/content.pdf. Accessed December 1, 2009.

NIH Consensus Development Panel on Impotence: NIH Consensus Conference: Impotence. JAMA 270:83–90, 1993.

Raina R, Agarwal A, Alamaneni SS, et al: Sildenafil citrate and vacuum constriction device combination enhances sexual satisfaction in erectile dysfunction after radical prostatectomy. Urology 65:360–364, 2005.

Wylie KR, Jones RH, Walter S: The potential benefit of vacuum devices augmenting psychosexual therapy for erectile dysfunction: A randomised controlled trial. J Sex Marital Ther 29:227–236, 2003.

CHAPTER 126

VASECTOMY

Charles L. Wilson

Vasectomy is a safe, inexpensive, permanent form of contraception. Ten per 1000 men 25 to 49 years of age have a vasectomy annually in the United States, totaling between 500,000 and 600,000 per year. In comparison, there are somewhere between 600,000 and 700,000 tubal ligations per year, with about half being performed postpartum. Unlike tubal ligation, vasectomy is usually performed in an office setting, is less expensive, and is associated with fewer and less severe complications. No mortality from vasectomy has been reported, whereas approximately 10 women die annually from complications of tubal ligation in the United States. Although both procedures have low failure rates, a failure of tubal ligation is discovered only when pregnancy occurs, whereas failure of vasectomy can be detected by routine postvasectomy semen testing. Thus, vasectomy offers high efficacy with lower morbidity and lower cost, yet it continues to be underused.

The decision process that leads up to the choice of vasectomy often starts with a general discussion of birth control options and family planning, which may involve the primary care physician or the partner's gynecologic care provider. It is essential that these providers be knowledgeable and prepared to provide accurate information about vasectomy to the man and his partner.

Patient education handouts for this chapter are available online at www.expertconsult.com. Explicit patient instructions are imperative, especially in this procedure. The patient education handouts are highly recommended for this purpose.

As discussed later in the section on Technique Variations, vasectomy can be performed in many ways. In the mid-1980s, EngenderHealth (formerly AVSC International) helped popularize the *no-scalpel vasectomy* (NSV), a method devised in China by Dr. Li Shunqiang. China was at that time struggling against a 2:1 bias favoring tubal ligation over vasectomy. Dr. Li designed a vas fixation clamp and sharp dissecting forceps (SDF), which allowed him to perform vasectomy in a "refined" and less invasive manner. NSV became widely accepted by Chinese men. Whether NSV is, in practice, less invasive than the traditional methods depends entirely on the training, skill, and experience of the surgeon. Certainly it has been demonstrated in some hands to be a quick, virtually bloodless, and often painless procedure. It lends itself to a significant psychological advantage with the apprehensive patient.

Similarly, the "no-needle no-scalpel vasectomy," or more simply, *no-needle vasectomy* (NNV) technique, devised by the author in 1999, replaces the previous skin wheal and vasal block anesthetic with a jet injection, and helps relieve patients' fear of needle administration of anesthetic in this sensitive area (Wilson, 2001).

In any case, the no-needle and no-scalpel approaches simply define *methods of anesthesia and of entry and access to the vas deferens*. How the vas deferens is then occluded is variable and a matter of preference.

The term *laser vasectomy* has been used to refer to the minimally invasive techniques, but in reality there is no practical use or value for a laser in the vasectomy procedure.

The long-sought goal of a completely reversible vas occlusion method has spawned experimental models of occlusion without dividing the vas deferens. Such methods include simply clamping the vas with metal vascular clips or with the plastic VasClip (VMBC, LLC, Roseville, Minn), injecting glues or scarifying agents into the lumen, implanting silicone plugs, or simply cauterizing a length of the lumen transcutaneously. None of these methods has proven sufficiently successful or reversible.

ANATOMY

The *scrotal epidermis* is very thin and the *dermis* is supported by the thick and elastic dartos muscle. These layers are well endowed with blood vessels, which makes them susceptible to bleeding and ecchymosis; however, they are also particularly resistant to infection and capable of rapid healing after surgical incision. The *scrotum* can vary widely among patients in its size, shape, and texture (from that of a full, round, tense cyst that resists palpation; to a thin, smooth, droopy sac with nearly visible contents; or a flat, rugous thickening along the dependent fold of an abdominal panniculus). Individual anatomy plays the largest role in determining whether a vasectomy will be easy or difficult to perform. A *septum* separates the left and right sides of the scrotum, and loose connective tissue cushions the scrotal contents. In single-incision vasectomy, the septum does not present a practical barrier, and bleeding risk is less than with two separate incisions.

The *epididymis* is a soft, comma-shaped attachment on the testis that originates at the superior pole and wraps around the back down to the inferior pole, clinging to the smooth, firm surface of the testis, but separated by a sulcus. (See patient education worksheet online at www.expertconsult.com.)

The *vas deferens* originates as a *convoluted*, tenuous duct from the tail of the epididymis at the inferior pole of the testis. As it courses cephalad along the posteromedial aspect of the spermatic cord, it becomes *straight* and sturdy, with thick walls of smooth muscle tissue, which give it a dense, almost gritty texture to palpation. In a cross-section of the scrotum above the level of the testicles, the vas is a prominent tubular structure surrounded by tiny vasal nerves and supplied by its own small deferential artery (Fig. 126-1). It is deep within the scrotum, separated from the skin surface by nine tissue layers, the deepest of which is the *internal spermatic fascia*, which also contains the testicular artery, lymphatics, and nerves, and the pampiniform plexus. At that level it is usually distinctly palpable and firm, about 3 mm in thickness, like a hard-cooked spaghetti noodle or a ball-point pen refill. But anatomic variation accounts for vasa that may be as thin as 1.5 mm or as thick as 4.5 mm. Occasionally, the convoluted portion extends all the way to the inguinal canal. Some patients have congenital absence of the vas on one side, although they are rarely aware of it.

Sensation in the anterior scrotum is mediated by the ilioinguinal nerves and the perineal nerves arising from the pudendal nerves. Complete anesthesia for vasectomy depends on blocking not only these somatic sensory paths, but the autonomic afferents that supply the vas deferens with its visceral sensation.

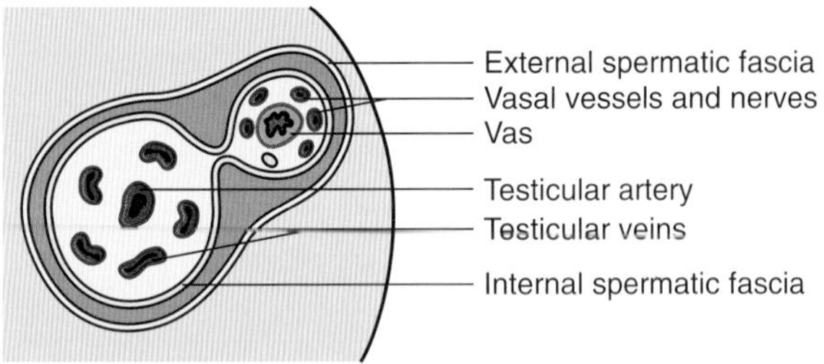

Figure 126-1 Schematic coronal view of spermatic cord and internal structures. Note location of vas deferens with its associated vessels and nerves, as well as the testicular artery and veins, all located within the internal spermatic fascia.

Indications

- Vasectomy is appropriate for a man when he (and usually his partner) have decided they do not wish to have children, or to have any more children.
- For some couples there is a medical contraindication to pregnancy in the female partner or a commitment to adopt children in lieu of having their own.
- Occasionally a man seeks vasectomy as extra assurance even though his partner has had a tubal ligation or a history of infertility.
- A man diagnosed with a genetic contraindication to fathering a child may desire vasectomy.

Contraindications

Absolute

- Bacterial skin infection
- Uncontrolled coagulation disorders
- Inability to palpate and elevate both vasa
- Hypersensitivity to palpation, precluding isolation of the vas
- Lack of adequate informed consent
- Depression, psychosexual impairment, or impaired decision making

Relative

- Anticoagulant or antiplatelet therapy. Aspirin and clopidogrel (Plavix) should ideally be stopped for 5 days before the surgery and for 2 to 3 days afterward. Each case should be evaluated individually and if the medications cannot be stopped, meticulous hemostasis must be ensured at the time of surgery.
- Impending infertility, such as menopause or hysterectomy in partner.
- Unresolved conflict or stress, for example recent childbirth, marital discord, divorce or financial setback.
- Inappropriate expectations of vasectomy (e.g., improving a troubled marriage, curing sexual problems).
- Excessive, unreassured concerns regarding sexual functioning after the vasectomy.

Preprocedure Patient Preparation

Patient education materials and handouts are widely used and are of great value in preparing the patient for vasectomy. The vasectomy questionnaire, patient education handouts, and patient consent forms help achieve fully informed consent. (See all of these forms online at www.expertconsult.com.)

Schedule a preoperative consultation and evaluation at least several days before the scheduled procedure. This allows time for the patient and his partner to think about the decision and the information provided before the procedure. This appointment will generally take 15 minutes if prior patient education material has been reviewed by the patient or if he has reviewed a counseling video. Without these materials, it may take 30 minutes to properly inform the patient and answer all questions.

Many now recognize the educational value of patient education videotapes/DVDs. The patient can review the material several times privately at home. A vasectomy counseling videotape is available from Creative Health Communications through The National Procedures Institute (see the Suppliers section). With portable DVD players, the patient can easily view the material in the office before seeing the physician.

The patient should sign the formal consent form. The consent form may be titled "Request for Vasectomy" to emphasize the patient's role in decision making. The physician still retains responsibility to help the patient make a decision that will be in his best long-term interest. It is wise to include the wife or partner, if any, in the consent process; however, a man has the right to choose vasectomy even in the absence of spousal consent. Similarly, a patient who is young, unmarried, or without children should not be denied vasectomy on these grounds alone.

The *preprocedure counseling visit can be documented* using the encounter form, which reviews the patient's pertinent history, physical examination, and counseling points, and documents the follow-up semen specimen checks. The form can be found online at www.expertconsult.com.

At the conclusion of the session, perform a careful *genital examination*, noting any anomalies of the area and especially the size, texture, and position of the vasa deferentia as they course through the upper scrotum. Be alert to the possible absence of a vas or presence of a third or fourth vas, although such cases are extremely rare. Make a mental note of the ease or difficulty of mobilizing each vas to the anterior midline, and make a final decision whether to proceed with this vasectomy or stop and refer. Check for testicular masses, varicoceles, inguinal hernias, and possible granulomas. Note any tenderness to palpation. Groin rashes should be resolved before surgery.

Also helpful is the Patient Education Worksheet, which also is available online at www.expertconsult.com. This is a checklist of the counseling material to be reviewed with the patient. The original sheet is for the patient and a copy is made for the chart. Not only is it a good summary of all points covered, but it serves as a reminder for the patient of what to do just before and after the surgery. (For a more detailed description of the preprocedural counseling visit, see Pfenninger [1984b].)

The clinician should note the questions, "*How well do you tolerate pain?*" and "*Do you have a tendency to faint?*" on the encounter form. If the patient tolerates pain poorly or has a tendency to faint, *atropine 0.5 mg* may be given intramuscularly on arrival to the office before surgery to reduce vasovagal effects of nausea, bradycardia, and syncope. This optimizes the "vasectomy experience" for both the patient and physician. *Oral sedation* with either diazepam 10 mg or alprazolam 1 mg 1 hour before surgery may be used in addition to the atropine or alone to help relax the nervous patient. Sedation, however, requires that he avoid driving and other activities requiring alertness for the rest of the day. One may plan to prescribe a narcotic *analgesic* for patients who indicate above-average sensitivity to pain based on their prior experiences. However, a nonsteroidal anti-inflammatory drug (NSAID) such as ibuprofen 800 mg is usually adequate and safe. Some now use tramadol (Ultram) 100 mg.

To minimize risk of bleeding complications, patients on antiplatelet therapy should have their platelet function restored by the time of surgery. This requires abstaining from aspirin-containing products and clopidogrel for 5 days. NSAIDs (except cyclooxygenase-2 inhibitors) in very rare instances are associated with bleeding. If a patient does have a questionable history, NSAIDs should be withheld for 48 hours before and after surgery. If there is no history of bleeding disorder or prior complications of surgery, normal platelet function can usually be assumed.

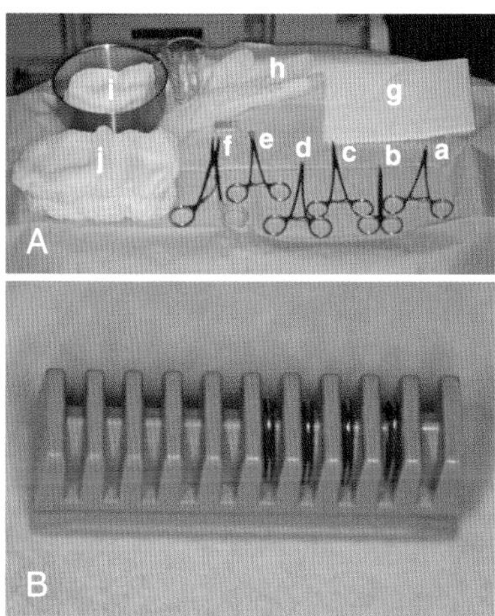

Figure 126-2 **A,** The surgical tray: sharp dissecting forceps (a); scissors (b); straight mosquito hemostats (c); curved mosquito hemostats (d); Wilson vasectomy forceps (e); hemoclip applicator with clips (f); pack of 4 × 4 gauze (g); battery cautery in sterile glove (h); basin of wet gauze pads (i); large number of "fluffed-up" gauze pads to place inside scrotal supporter (j). **B,** Close-up of hemoclip pack with four clips remaining.

Federal agencies require that a specific consent form be executed for the physician to be compensated. These are usually available from local health departments or the state Medicaid agency. Forms must be completed fully and accurately to avoid denial of payment. Note that consents are valid only for surgery performed more than 30 days and less than 180 days after the counseling session at which the form is signed.

Equipment and Supplies

The preparation for vasectomy includes gathering the necessary equipment and supplies and arranging the sterile items on a surgical tray (Fig. 126-2). Each setup depends on the surgical setting and the surgeon's preferred technique and choice of available supplies. A checklist for the staff to use in preparing for the procedure is a good way to avoid omissions and oversights.

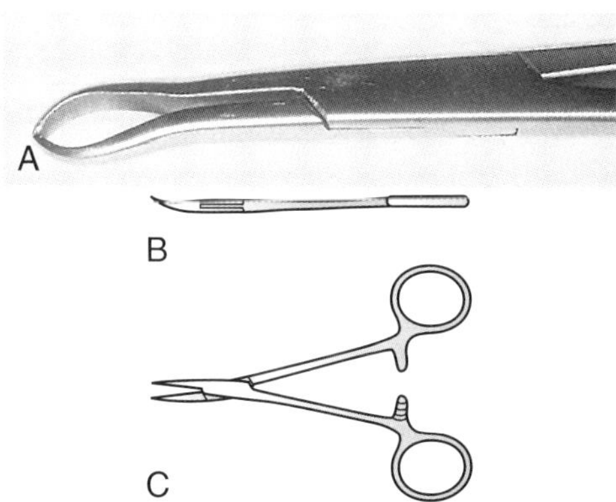

Figure 126-3 No-scalpel instruments. **A,** Wilson vasectomy forceps. **B** and **C,** Sharp dissecting forceps. (**B** and **C,** From Li SQ, Goldstein M, Zhu J, Huber D: The no-scalpel vasectomy. J Urol 145:341–344, 1991.)

Figure 126-4 Battery-operated cautery unit with disposable tip. (Courtesy of Advanced Meditech International, Flushing, NY).

- *Vas-fixing forceps (VFF;* one or two pairs) are locking clamps used to secure the vas during puncture and dissection (Fig. 126-3A). Historically, sharp or blunted towel clips have been popular. The *Wilson* vasectomy forceps (Advanced Meditech International [AMI], Flushing, NY; Marina Medical, Sunrise, Fla) provide a secure yet atraumatic grasp of the vas for incisional vasectomy, and work equally as well as VFF in the no-scalpel technique. The *Li* vasectomy forceps (AMI) were introduced in China as VFF for NSV. They feature a cantilever design to limit closing force.
- *Sharp dissecting forceps* (*SDF*; AMI, Marina Medical) are the key to atraumatic dissection of the vas and are used to puncture the skin instead of a scalpel incision and to hook and deliver the vas. They are essentially sharp-pointed hemostats (Fig. 126-3B and C).
- If a *scalpel* will be used for incision or sharp dissection, include a disposable scalpel or scalpel handle with a no. 15 blade.
- *Cautery unit*, either an electrocautery unit and handpiece, with a fine-needle electrode (unit should be set at the lowest level that quickly cauterizes small "bleeders"), or a battery unit. Battery-powered thermal cautery units with disposable sterile sheaths and disposable specialized vasectomy tips are available from AMI (Fig. 126-4). Based on Schmidt's (1992) findings, a battery-powered cautery unit may be the instrument of choice for optimal sealing of the vas ends compared with an electrosurgical unit.
- *Three mosquito hemostats.*
- *Adson tissue forceps* (1 × 2 teeth) with suture platform for holding the vas or fascia.
- *Tissue scissors* for dividing or hemitransecting the vas.
- Method to seal vas sheath: Either a needle holder with a *4-0 absorbable plain, chromic, or polyglycolic acid suture* on an atraumatic needle *or a medium hemoclip applicator with clips.*
- A method to anesthetize the area: Traditionally, a *10-mL syringe* (1½-inch, 27-gauge needle) with lidocaine (2%) without epinephrine (10 mL) was used. In the NNV anesthesia technique (see later discussion), an instrument called the *MadaJet* is used to administer the lidocaine. Only 0.1 mL of lidocaine is used per side with this instrument, but it requires at least 1 mL in the chamber to prime and function correctly.
- *Sterile sodium bicarbonate solution* to mitigate pain during anesthetic infiltration if needle injection is used *(optional)*. Just before injection of the anesthetic, the clinician should draw up 1 mL of sodium bicarbonate with 9 mL of the lidocaine. This reduces the "sting and burning" associated when lidocaine is injected. Sodium bicarbonate is not needed if the MadaJet is used.
- Large pack of 4 × 4 gauze.
- A povidone–iodine (Betadine) or chlorhexidine (Hibiclens) preparation.
- Fenestrated sterile drape and nonfenestrated drape.
- Sterile gloves and mask.
- Single sterile glove (into which the cautery device is placed if the sterile cautery sheaths are not used). This is not needed if a sterile cautery handset is used.
- Pair of nonsterile gloves for preparation.
- Specimen jar with formalin.

No-Needle Vasectomy Anesthesia Technique

In the NNV technique, the traditional vasal block method is replaced by the no-needle technique. This is accomplished using a piston-like instrument (MadaJet 401UR; Mada Medical, Inc., Carlstadt, NJ; Fig. 126-5A), which uses the force of fluid under pressure to "push" the anesthetic into the tissues. The jet injection is a fine stream (about 0.006 inch in diameter) that instantly

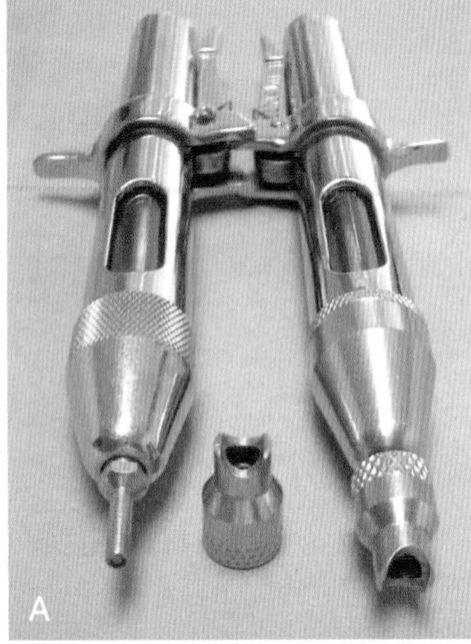

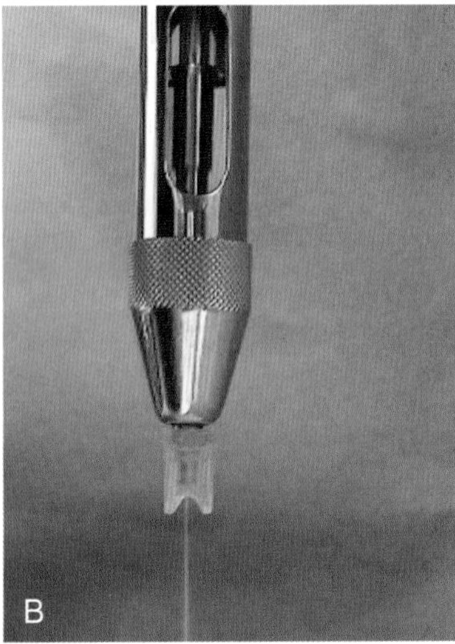

Figure 126-5 **A,** MadaJet model 401UR with metal sheath that fits over the nozzle tip to align the stream with the vas. **B,** Stream of lidocaine emitted from the MadaJet orifice.

penetrates about 4 mm through the skin and vas deferens, producing an almost immediate and complete anesthetic effect (Fig. 126-5B).

The vas should be isolated as described later in step 3 of the No-Scalpel Vasectomy Procedure section. However, now both the index and middle fingers are placed behind the scrotum with the thumb in front. The straight segment of vas spans a small "safe" space between the index and middle fingers. The MadaJet is cocked and the tip is then placed firmly over the vas next to the thumb, directed into the "safe" space, and actuated by pushing the button. Each injection will be 0.1 mL of lidocaine. When beginning, it may help to mark the intended site of the scrotum with a marking pen and then isolate the vas to this spot for anesthesia. The marked spot will make it easier to bring the other vas to the same location. It also identifies where the opening should be made. A second application can be made over each vas to ensure a good block if desired. The total amount of anesthetic will then be 0.2 to 0.4 mL.

CAUTION: Be careful *not* to have fingers positioned behind the vas in line with the jet injection stream. Lidocaine can penetrate through the patient's tissues and into the surgeon's fingers. This is the reason for the special finger positions for NNV.

The MadaJet 401UR is supplied with the proper settings for NNV and comes with a stainless-steel spacer, which is notched to conform to the vas. The MadaJet design incorporates air space between the tip of the injector and the skin, so it does not require disposable parts like other injectors do. It does, however, demand careful attention to cleaning, sterilization, and maintenance procedures between uses according to the manufacturer's instructions.

After each patient use, careful sterilization of the MadaJet is essential. The entire MadaJet may be routinely autoclaved, but that is not necessary between patient uses. After use, the device is fired once to clean the exit port, then the tip, spacer, and body are cleaned, and the entire tip end of the device is cold sterilized by immersion in Madacide-FD solution for at least 10 minutes. The reservoir tube holds 4 mL of lidocaine, enough for about 40 actuations. At the end of each day, the MadaJet is disassembled, cleaned, and autoclaved. Periodic maintenance, at least annually, is required and is performed by the manufacturer.

There are several *advantages to NNV*. First, no needle penetrates the skin, reducing the risk of bleeding complications related to needle damage. Second, needlestick risk for surgical personnel is avoided, and medical waste is reduced. Third, it relieves patients of fears they may have about needles—this benefit cannot be overestimated. (The hypospray is very efficient. In over 11,000 NNVs by the author, 97% required only one injection for each vas. That is only 0.2 mL of lidocaine per patient, or about 1/30 the usual amount required for the complete vasectomy. It is so effective that even "slow responders" to local anesthetics experience rapid numbness.)

The major limitation of NNV is the small area of numbness, about the size of a dime. With advanced skills and precision in NSV technique, a physician can incorporate the no-needle anesthetic technique successfully. Otherwise, more injections to include adjacent tissues will be required to keep the patient comfortable.

Physicians will find a myriad of other applications for the MadaJet among the procedures they perform in the office. "No-needle anesthesia" will be embraced by many patients in addition to men undergoing vasectomy. A single "snap" suffices for a punch biopsy, injecting scars with steroids, skin tag excision, or skin anesthesia before needling for joint aspiration or injection or fine-needle aspiration of the breast, to name a few examples. A special dermatologic tip is needed for these applications.

Technique Variations

Traditional Vasectomy versus No-Scalpel Vasectomy Technique

In both techniques, the anesthetized vas is manipulated to lie under the skin of the scrotum where the opening will be made. Traditional technique may involve two separate anterolateral incisions (one for each vas) in the scrotum, although increasingly a single midline entry is used. The NSV technique specifies a single opening located in the anterior midline of the scrotum, between the upper one third and the lower two thirds of the scrotum.

The *essential difference is in the method of entry through the skin* and in the delivery of the vas. *In the traditional technique*, a typical surgical incision 1 to 2 cm long is made in the skin with a scalpel, then carried through the dartos and fascial layers sequentially until the vas is exposed and bluntly dissected free of the fascia. Bleeding is controlled at each layer, as needed, usually with cautery.

In the NSV technique, the method of entry is reduced to three smooth, precise movements, eliminating most of the operating time, tissue trauma, bleeding, and hemostatic maneuvers of traditional vasectomy. The key is the SDF. It is held and used in a precise manner to puncture the skin, all layers of fascia, and the anterior wall of the vas deferens in one smooth motion. It is then used to dilate the resulting 2-mm tract by stretching, not cutting, all layers at once. Finally, the tip of the SDF is precisely placed in the vas and rotated to hook the vas and deliver it cleanly from the fascial sheath, minimizing dissection.

Once the vas is delivered, there is no distinction between traditional and NSV in how one proceeds with occlusion of the vas, and alternatives are discussed in the following section. After occlusion of the vasa, traditional scalpel incisions are usually closed with one or two sutures, whereas the small stretched opening of NSV contracts and rarely requires closure.

Occlusion Methods

A number of occlusion techniques have been used, with varying degrees of success, but existing evidence is insufficient to recommend one specific technique (Sokal and Labrecque, 2009).

Traditional division of the vas and suture ligation of both ends has a 1% to 3% failure rate and is discouraged at this time.

Intraluminal cautery alone is superior to ligation of the vas in any way, regardless of whether cautery is also used. In other words, ligation or placing a hemoclip over the *vas itself* is discouraged.

Interposing fascia between the cut and cauterized ends results in very low failure rates of 0.1% to 0.5%. The fascia can be closed with absorbable suture or with hemoclips. The latter are quicker and avoid the bleeding seen occasionally when placing a suture. (For an excellent discussion of various techniques, see Lipshultz and Benson [1980]. Although it is a dated article, the material remains an excellent review.)

Excision of a vas segment greater than 4 cm is 100% successful, but causes excess morbidity and leaves little possibility of reversal. Labrecque and colleagues (2002) found that excising a longer (15 mm) segment of vas did not improve recanalization rates over shorter excisions. In some settings, specimens for pathologic examination may be required by policy; however, there is little or no benefit, and substantial added cost, in having histologic confirmation. The optimal length of excised segment is thought to be 1 to 2 cm. Experienced surgeons may not remove any tissue once they are able to identify the vas in vivo with certainty, and are certain of their *cautery and fascial interposition* techniques. The American Urology Association has stated that sending vas segments for histologic confirmation is not necessary. Instead of sending the segments for histologic examination, some clinicians give the 1-cm vas segments in formalin to the patient and instruct him to keep the segments in a medicine cabinet, away from children, until he has had two negative semen checks. The patient can then dispose of the segments once sterility is confirmed. Considering that 500,000 vasectomies are performed each year in the United States, that each pathology specimen costs between $150 and $200 to process, and that some physicians put each side in separate bottles, clinicians can save the health care system $75 million to $150 million per year by not sending the vas segments to the laboratory! If the patient keeps the specimens, and if the vasectomy should fail (which is rare), the patient can then submit the tissue to the laboratory for evaluation, if desired.

Open-Ended versus Closed-Ended

The "*open-ended*" technique uses cautery only on the *prostatic* end of the cut vas, along with closing the fascia over that end. It differs from other techniques in that the testicular end of the vas remains unoccluded, or "open." The open-ended technique was first recommended and used more than 50 years ago. Errey and Edwards (1986) reported an improvement in postoperative complaints. The technique is assumed to minimize back-pressure on the testicle, which could be associated with long-term pain in the occasional patient (i.e., postvasectomy pain syndrome). The trade-off is that symptomatic sperm granulomas and vasectomy failure could be increased because of the open pathway from the testicle. Careful attention to proper technique of cautery and fascial interposition helps prevent failure; however, most surgeons still routinely cauterize both the prostatic *and* testicular ends in the belief that this "*closed-ended*" method is the best assurance against failure. Some surgeons use the open-ended technique only for men younger than 30 years of age on the basis that they may be more likely to request reversal, which would then be theoretically easier, while routinely using the closed-ended technique in those older than 30 years.

No-Scalpel Vasectomy Procedure

1. *Examination and positioning of patient*: Have the patient lie down undressed but draped from the waist down. As described earlier in the section on Preprocedure Patient Preparation, it is recommended that a genital examination be performed at the conclusion of the counseling process. Review those findings and, if necessary, reexamine the patient to be confident about the position and mobility of each vas. Clip any remaining excess scrotal hair.
2. *Skin anesthesia* (this step is *not required* with NNV): After cleaning the site with an alcohol wipe, the anesthetic may be administered before the sterile preparation and draping. Use 0.5 to 1 mL of lidocaine to raise a wheal in the median raphe. The small volume helps prevent distortion at the site of entry. Lidocaine may be mixed with sodium bicarbonate to reduce the brief burning sensation during injection. Epinephrine is generally not used in the deep injection to avoid arterial constriction. However, some physicians prefer to use lidocaine with epinephrine in the skin wheal because the area of anesthesia is later identified by the resulting blanching.
3. *Isolating the vas with the three-finger technique*: The right-handed surgeon stands at the patient's right side. The left-handed surgeon will use reverse handedness throughout. Identify the left vas in the upper third of the scrotum by palpating from the midline laterally. The vas is firm to compression and about the diameter of a cooked spaghetti noodle or a ball-point pen refill. Use the *three-finger fixation method* to secure the vas, as follows. Reaching across the patient, place the middle finger of the left hand (if right-handed) under the scrotum and press up from behind the scrotum, elevating the vas to the anterior surface. Press down from the front of the scrotum with both the thumb and index finger, securing the vas in place (Fig. 126-6A). The space between the thumb and index finger is where you will access the vas.

   Although the vas can be occluded close to the epididymis (even in the convoluted portion), it is desirable to choose a site more distal (i.e., closer to the groin), where the straight segment of vas is more easily mobilized, less likely to spontaneously recanalize, and more amenable to surgical reanastomosis. Secure the vas then in the midline between the upper third and the lower two thirds of the scrotum.
4. *Anesthetizing the vas*: Use NNV (see earlier discussion) or the following traditional vasal block technique (Fig. 126-7): With needle and syringe, enter the skin from the anesthetized midline spot, advance the needle tip several centimeters cephalad along the vas, and inject 3 to 5 mL around the vas high on the left. If the needle tip lies very close to the vas, the anesthetic will flow around the vas, within the internal spermatic fascia, and it will effectively block the perivasal nerves without having to repeatedly insert the needle. The anesthetic effect will extend along the vas toward the epididymis without distorting the tissues where you will be dissecting the vas. Let the vas fall back, then grasp the right vas (Fig. 126-6B). Here the three-finger fixation method does not require reaching across the patient, but directly placing the left middle finger behind the right side of the scrotum to elevate the right vas, and applying counterpressure with the thumb and index finger anteriorly. Reinsert the needle through the midline, advance the tip along the right vas, and inject another 3 to 5 mL.
5. *Surgical preparation and draping*: The anesthetic will have time to take effect while the preparation is taking place. Nonsterile gloves are used with *warm* disinfectant solution. Warm solutions will help relax the scrotum, which allows easier palpation of the

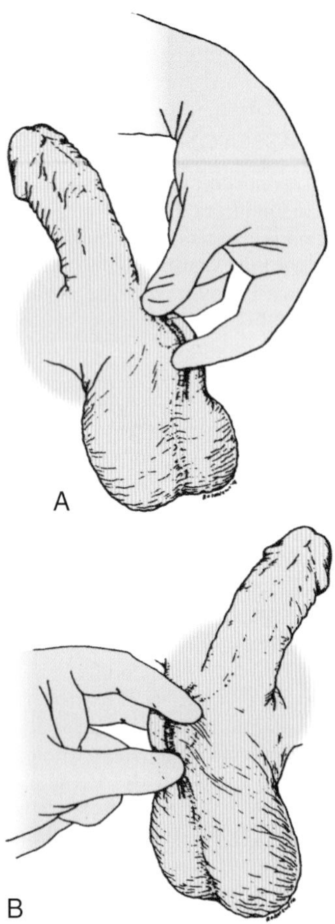

Figure 126-6 **A,** Three-finger fixation of the left vas beneath the skin in the midline. **B,** Three-finger fixation of the right vas. (From Li SQ, Goldstein M, Zhu J, Huber D: The no-scalpel vasectomy. J Urol 145:341–344, 1991.)

vas. A 50% solution of chlorhexidine (Hibiclens) smoothes the skin during palpation of the vas, unlike the stickier povidone–iodine solutions. Prepare well down onto the perineum because the hands will often be in this area when manipulating the vas. Cover the area with sterile surgical drapes. A fenestrated drape usually goes over the scrotum, whereas a nonfenestrated drape may be placed over the thighs.

6. *Fixing the vas in the clamp*: Isolate the *left* vas using the three-finger technique described step 3. Next, use the VFF to pinch the skin to demonstrate for both you and the patient the effect of the anesthetic. (If necessary, reposition your grasp or inject more lidocaine.) Now spread the tips of the VFF approximately 4 mm and place them against the skin, straddling the vas, which is in the space between your thumb and index finger. Gradually increase downward pressure against your middle finger. Warn the patient that he will feel pressure for the next few seconds. When you feel the pressure of the two tips of the forceps distinctly on the pad of your middle finger, begin *slowly* closing the VFF. Just before locking the forceps closed, slightly relax the downward pressure, so as not to pinch the posterior scrotum, but while completely encircling the vas in the grasp of the VFF (Fig. 126-8A).
7. *Repositioning your grasp*: At this point, release the three-finger grasp and reposition your left hand to hold only the VFF in the manner shown (Fig. 126-8B). Note that there are no fingers behind the scrotum at this point. The tips of the VFF are elevating the vas and the handles are lowered.
8. *Penetrating the skin*: While holding the vas firmly fixed in position in the VFF, use the SDF with the tips spread apart to pierce the skin where it is tensed over the vas, penetrating down into the lumen of the vas with one of the tapered tips (Fig. 126-8C). This tract will be dilated to deliver the vas to the surface. So, carefully slip the single tip out of the tract, close the forceps, and reinsert the two tips while closed together to the depth of the tract.
9. *Exposing the vas*: While keeping the tips deep in the tract, spread the handles of the SDF widely to spread the tips 4 to 8 mm, dilating all layers of skin and fascia down to the vas in one step. This mode of dissection is remarkably free of bleeding compared with a layer-by-layer approach or sharp dissection using a scalpel. The vas is distinguishable as grayish-white, slightly translucent tissue with a low-sheen surface. A very shiny surface indicates the vas is still covered by a layer of fascia. In that case, pierce again and spread just the thin fascia to reveal the bare vas. It is not necessary to expose more than a few millimeters of vas to proceed with delivery (Fig. 126-8D).
10. *Delivering the vas*: Now open the sharp dissecting forceps with *the curve facing down* and the handles held below the level of the tips. Insert one jaw, the far tip of the SDF, into the vas just 1 to 2 mm. Using care to keep the tip buried in the vas, rotate clockwise about the long axis of the instrument. As the curve of the SDF *points upward*, the vas will rise through the skin (Fig. 126-8E). With the vas poised in this position, use your left hand to unlock and remove the VFF (Fig. 126-8F).

Provided that the fascia has been adequately dissected and there are no fascial adhesions from previous infections, trauma, or surgery, a bare loop of vas will slide out of the fascia. Now *regrasp* the vas by pinching it at the top of the loop with the VFF. Avoid encircling the vas at this point; rather, grasp into the vas tissue itself (Fig. 126-8G).

If a loop of vas does not slide out easily, replace the VFF around (vs. through) the vas once again and try removing any adherent fascia by inserting the closed SDF under the vas fascia and spreading the tips against the vas surface. Alternatively, try

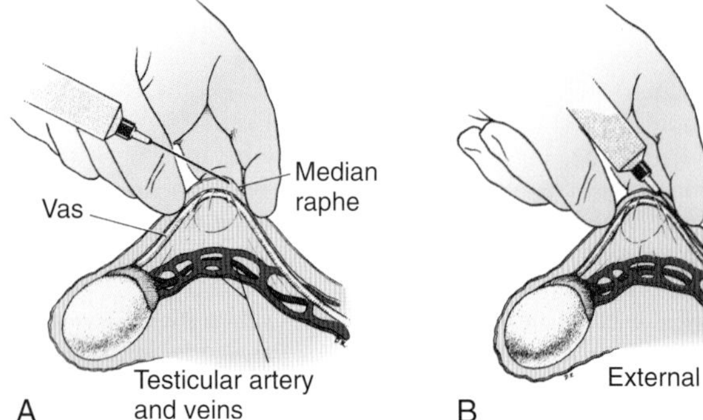

Figure 126-7 Technique of vasal block anesthesia, using the traditional syringe and needle method. **A,** To anesthetize the skin, a wheal of anesthetic is placed intradermally in the median raphe. **B,** To anesthetize the vas, the 1½-inch needle is inserted through the midline wheal and advanced along the vas toward the inguinal area. The anesthetic diffuses around the vas. This is then repeated with the other vas. (From Li SQ, Goldstein M, Zhu J, Huber D: The no-scalpel vasectomy. J Urol 145:341–344, 1991.)

passing the closed SDF or hemostat under the vas to elevate about a 1-cm section.

11. *Baring a loop of vas*: With the vas held securely, create a "window" in the "web" of fascia under the loop. Start near the top of the loop by passing one tip of the SDF through the loop, close enough to the vas that the deferential artery and all fascial vessels are cleanly separated from the vas. The artery often may not be visible, but meticulous dissection at this step will be rewarded with a bloodless field. Dilate the opening by spreading the two tips of the SDF within the loop to "strip" the tissue off about 1 cm of vas (Fig. 126-8H).
12. *Securing the loop*: A measure of safety may be added by applying hemostats to the fascia at one or both ends of the isolated vas segment (Fig. 126-8I).
13. *Accessing the vas lumen*: If a segment of vas is going to be removed, *hemitransect* the vas but do not cut completely through, making two *partial* incisions 1 to 1.5 cm apart (Fig. 126-8J). *If a portion of the vas is not going to be removed*, the lumen of the vas may be accessed through the initial puncture of the vas if it is visible, or through an incision (Fig. 126-8K). Alternatively, the wall of the vas may be penetrated using a sharp electrocautery needle or a hot thermal cautery tip.
14. *Cauterizing the vas:* Cauterize the lumen of the prostatic end only (open-ended technique) or of both ends of the vas (closed-ended technique) by inserting the cautery tip 10 mm into the lumen, activating the cautery unit, and then withdrawing the tip (Fig. 126-8L). Whether using electrocautery or thermal cautery, the objective is to create a graduated injury to the duct lining, minimal at the upper portion and maximal at the cut tip so that fibroblasts are stimulated to form scar tissue that will occlude the vas somewhere in between. If a section of vas is excessively desiccated to the point that the muscular wall is devitalized, the entire tip may slough.
15. *Completing transection/removing segment of vas*: With the hemostats still in place, complete the transection through the entire vas. If a segment of vas is to be removed, it is placed in formalin (Fig. 126-8M).
16. *Creating fascial interposition*: *With 4-0 chromic*, create a purse-string closure and draw the fascia over the *prostatic* end of the vas, being careful that the open *testicular* end does not fall back into the sheath (Fig. 126-8N). *Alternatively, a medium hemoclip* is applied (only on the fascia). This is quicker and may cause less bleeding (Fig. 126-8O). In a similar alternative, the edges of fascia may be approximated with a hemostat and then ligated with a free tie, avoiding the use of a suture needle. Release the hemostat only from the prostatic end at this point. (There is no research evidence to conclude which side should have the fascial interposition to optimize results, or if it really makes a difference.)

    NOTE: The suture is placed only through the fascia, not on the vas itself. Ligating the vas itself is not recommended because if it is not tight enough, the suture serves no purpose, allowing sperm to pass through. If it is too tight, the end necroses, often leaving an open tip.

17. *Releasing the vas*: Lower the vas into the scrotum while still grasping the fascia with one hemostat. This can reveal a bleeder that was not previously evident owing to constriction by the tight skin edges. After hemostasis is ensured, drop the vas back into the scrotum. If a bleeding point is identified at any time during the procedure, use the least amount of cautery necessary to control it. For bleeding from the vasal artery, clamp and ligate with suture or a hemoclip. Often the bleeding will be from the skin opening and not the deeper tissues, so check this area closely. In general, skin edge bleeding can be ignored until the end of the procedure, and then managed with 5 minutes of gently pinching the wound closed.
18. *Repeat entire procedure on right side*: Now identify the right vas. (If a second incision is made, provide additional anesthesia on the skin.) Isolate the right vas in the VFF. *Confirm that it is the right vas* by tugging gently to move the right testicle. The procedure that was carried out on the left side is now carried out on the right.
19. *Care for the scrotal opening*: The scrotal incision may occasionally require a suture if it gapes or continues to bleed from the skin edge after cautery or 10 minutes of firm pinching between gauze. A single 4-0 absorbable suture should suffice. Tell the patient to expect the suture knot to fall off after the period of absorption.
20. *Dressing*: Antibiotic ointment on the wound is optional. Several 4 × 4 gauze pads provide a loose dressing, held in place with the patient's tight briefs or an athletic supporter.
21. *Postoperative instructions*: Give the patient appropriate instructions for care. Provide two containers for semen samples, and caution the patient to use alternative birth control until the semen checks are clear.
22. *Discharge the patient* once he is ambulatory with no lightheadedness.
23. *Document the procedure* with the appropriate operative report (Box 126-1).

Clinical photographs of the procedure are shown in Figures 126-9 through 126-11.

Cautery Instrument Sterility

Sterile, disposable, single-use, battery-powered thermal cautery units are available and inexpensive for use in vasectomy. More environmentally friendly reusable units are provided with replaceable tip elements and sterile sheaths to envelop the handle.

For *electrocautery* users, sterile single-use, or reusable autoclavable handle and cord sets are available, but a clean, nonsterile cord set and handle can be safely reused, if the cord is maintained out of contact with the sterile field and the surgeon's sterile gloves. After the physician is gloved, have an assistant lower the cautery handle into a spare sterile glove by holding the cord (Fig. 126-12). Place a sterile electrode tip into the handpiece right through the glove. The handpiece can now be safely placed on the sterile tray. Reusable battery-powered units can be used in a similar fashion.

Postprocedure Patient Care

All of this information should be discussed with the patient during the preoperative counseling session. It is important to reinforce it on the day of surgery.

No routine postprocedure office visit is necessary. For the physician who is just beginning to perform vasectomy procedures, it may be advisable to see the patients in 1 to 2 weeks to gain an appreciation for the normal postprocedure changes.

An uneventful recovery thus depends on the patient following good self-care principles and the specific written instructions he received in the office. Sample postoperative handouts can be found online at www.expertconsult.com. These sample instructions describe expected conditions and those that should prompt a call to the physician. It is always best to thoroughly review the instructions with the patient, as well as providing them in written format for later reference.

Patients usually report minimal to mild discomfort after NSV. Severe pain is rare enough that it should prompt a call to the physician. NSAIDs such as naproxen sodium (Aleve) or ibuprofen will keep most patients comfortable and may be routinely taken the day of surgery and the first day after surgery. They can be continued if the patient is feeling an ache or fullness. Some patients will simply rest easier knowing they have a prescription analgesic medication on hand, should they need it. Narcotics (rarely needed) can

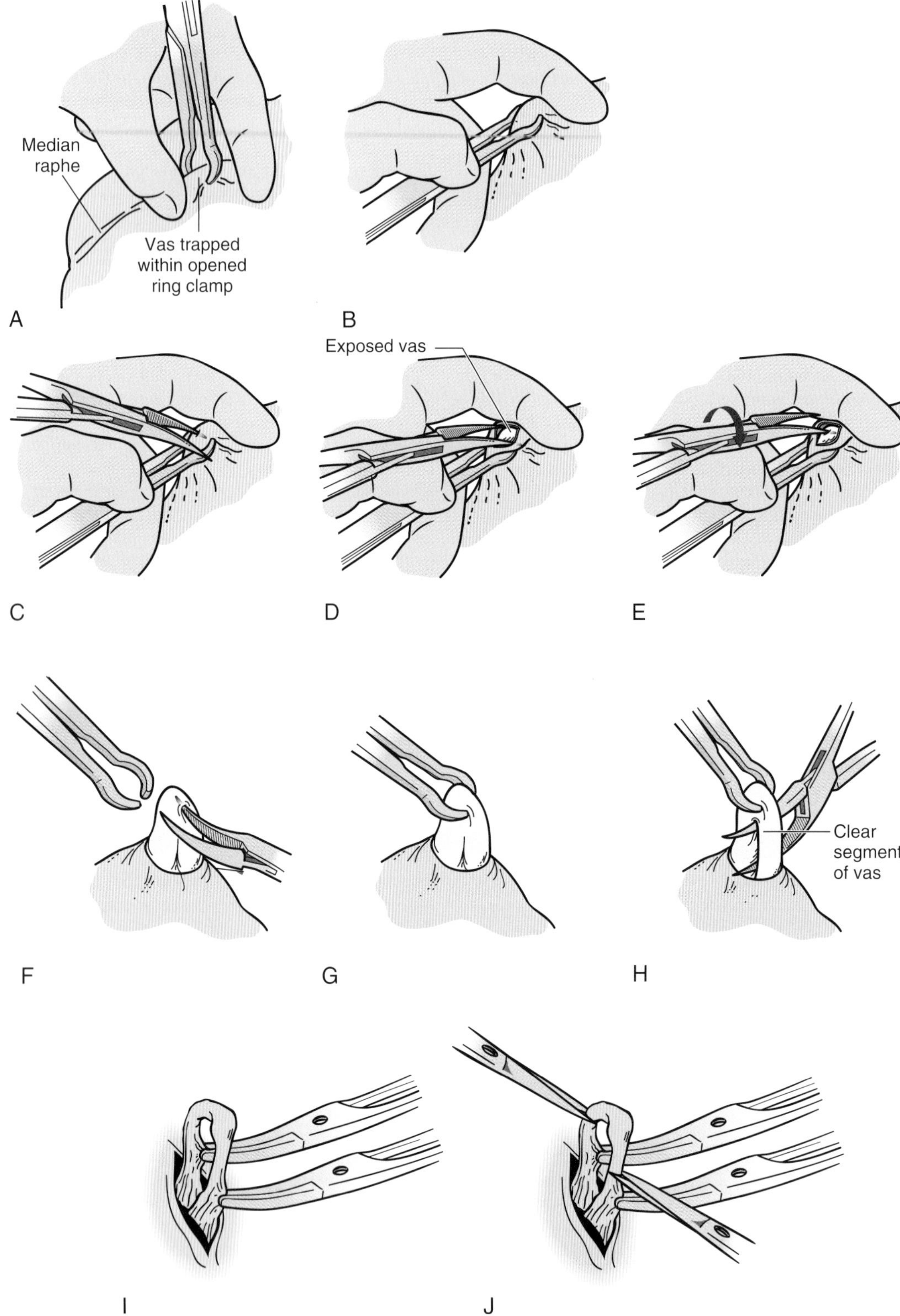

Figure 126-8 **A–H,** Sequence of the no-scalpel vasectomy procedure. See text for details. **A,** Percutaneous clamping with Li forceps. **B,** Tenting up vas. **C,** Incising with single jaw of dissecting forceps. **D,** Spreading perivasal tissue down to vas. **E,** Inserting single jaw into vas. **F,** Holding vas. **G,** Grasping through vas with clamp. **H,** Further stripping of perivasal tissue. **I–O,** Several alternatives for occlusion. See text for details. **I,** Grasping perivasal tissue just below intended resection sites. **J,** Hemisection of vas at intended sites of resection.

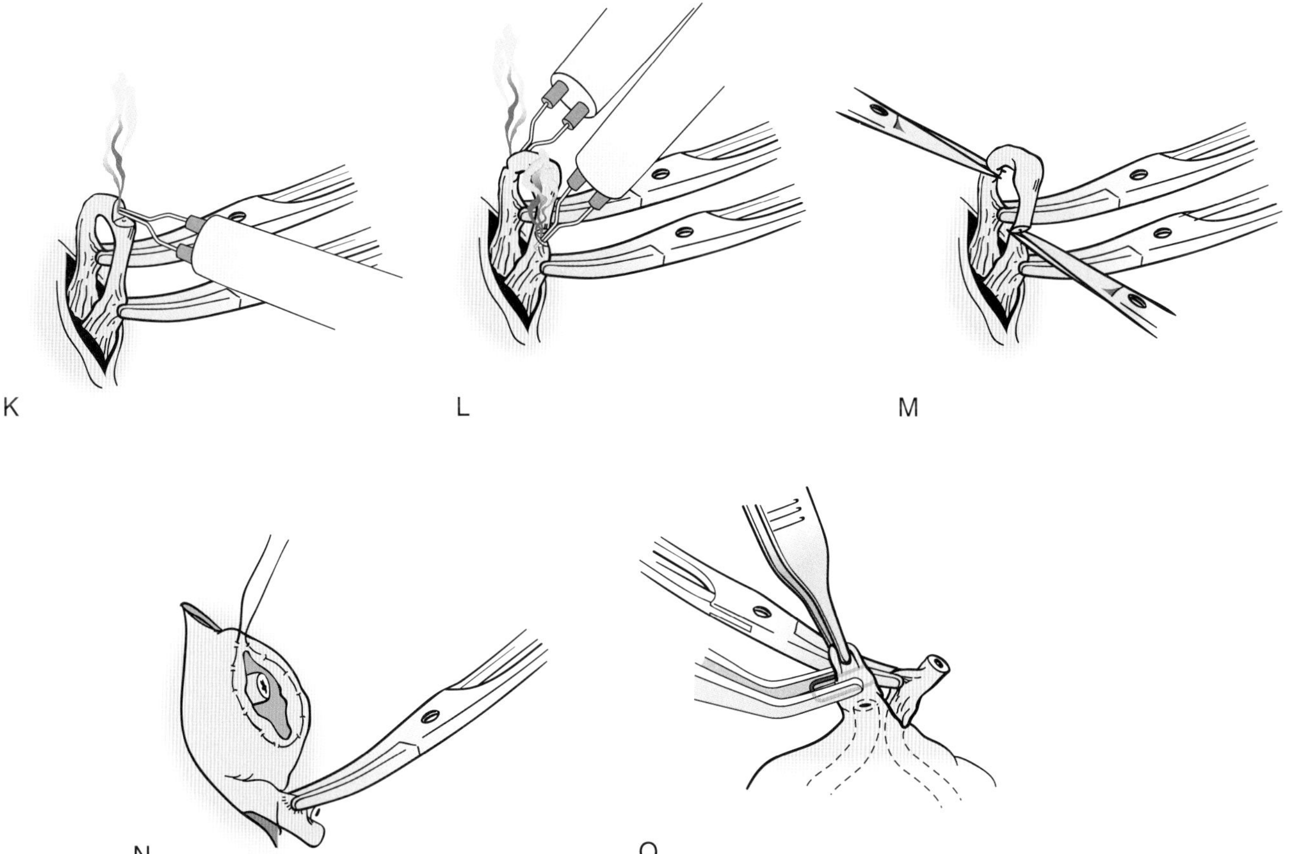

Figure 126-8, cont. **K,** Open-ended technique (cauterize only the prostate end, no piece removed). **L,** Cauterizing both ends (piece to be removed). **M,** Removing a 1.5-cm segment of vas. **N,** Using the pursestring suture to close the perivasal tissue. **O,** Alternatively, a medium hemoclip occludes the fascia over the vas end.

Box 126-1. No-Scalpel Vasectomy Operative Report

Patient ______________________________
DOB:____________Date ______________
The patient comes in today for a vasectomy. He understands the risks, benefits, and possible complications. He has read over the handouts and viewed the instructional tapes. All questions were answered before the start of the procedure. He does understand that alternative contraceptive choices are available and that vasectomy must be considered a permanent procedure. He has no further questions, and subsequently we proceeded.

Procedure note:
Procedure: Bilateral no-scalpel, no-needle vasectomy.
Surgeon: John L. Pfenninger, MD
Assistant: ______________________________
Present in the room: wife, partner, friend, family member
Driver: ______________________
Anesthesia:

________cc of a 50/50 mixture of 2% lidocaine with epinephrine and 1% lidocaine without epinephrine
or
________cc of 2% lidocaine with epinephrine using the MadaJet.

Premedication: 800 mg ibuprofen Valium 10 mg atropine 0.5 mg Dt
Tolerance (*circle one*): Excellent Good Poor
Estimated blood loss: ______________ cc
Complications: None or ________________________
____

The patient was laid supine and the anterior scrotum was prepped with alcohol. The left vas was grasped and 0.1 cc of 2% lidocaine with epinephrine was deposited around the vas in the upper scrotum using the MadaJet technique, in the midline. Similarly a vasal block was carried out on the right. The entire scrotum, penis, and suprapubic and inguinal areas were then prepped with Betadine. Sterile draping was carried out.

Betadine was wiped clear of the scrotum. The left vas was identified, brought to the midline, and isolated with the ring forceps. The skin over the vas was then punctured using the sharp dissecting vas forceps. A small opening was made and the perivasal tissue was stripped clear. The sharp dissecting forceps were then inserted under the vas and the ring clamp removed and replaced through the vas itself for stabilization. Dissection of the perivasal fascia was completed providing 1 to 1.5 cm of vas deferens. The vas was then hemitransected on both sides of the elevated loop. The proximal and distal ends of the vas were cauterized using the battery cautery unit. The proximal vas (testicular end) was then fully transected and allowed to retract below the fascial tissues. The fascia over the proximal vas was then occluded using a medium metal hemoclip. The clip was placed up to, but not on, the distal vas. This completed a good fascial interposition between the two ends. The distal vas end protruded above the hemoclip. The distal end was then fully transected and the tissues returned to the scrotum. The 1 cm of transected vas was placed in

Continued on following page.

Box 126-1. No-Scalpel Vasectomy Operative Report—cont.

formalin. Good hemostasis was noted. Attention was then turned to the right side where the vas was isolated and brought through the same midline opening. The same technique carried out. The right vas was confirmed by gently tugging the vas and noting testicular movement on the right.

After completion of the procedure, the scrotum was washed with sterile saline. Good hemostasis was noted at the skin site. Antibiotic ointment was placed over the entry wound and gauze applied. An athletic supporter was placed.

The patient was given postoperative instructions and will watch for signs of infection and report any excessive pain or bleeding. Guidelines for complete rest today with gradual increase in activity were reviewed. Acetaminophen and ibuprofen are to be used for discomfort. Ice is to be applied to the scrotum until the evening. Gauze packing should be used inside the scrotum until the morning. The athletic supporter should be used for at least 48 hours. The patient should refrain from heavy lifting, straining, running, jogging, and sexual activity for one week. He is aware that live sperm may be present in the ejaculate for up to 15 ejaculations. It was emphasized to use contraception until two sperm evaluations at 6 and 12 weeks show no sperm. Containers were given to the patient and methods of collection were explained. The patient shall keep the two pieces of transected vas in the medicine cabinet, in the formalin jar, until the two negative semen checks. At that time, he can dispose of them. The patient should call if there are any other problems. Postoperative instruction sheets were also given. Once again, the patient had no further questions.

Changes to procedure: None or ________________________

____

Impression: Uncomplicated no-scalpel, no-needle vasectomy

Other instructions: ________________________________

____

Cc: ________________________

Physician:______________________________

Date:____________

supplement, but should not replace anti-inflammatory medication, except when the latter is contraindicated.

Most men will do better if they use a scrotal supporter ("jock strap") for a few days. These are often reinforced with gauze or a washcloth to provide more support/pressure.

Activity should be limited. The day of surgery, it is best to relax with the feet up such as in a recliner. It is permissible to go to the bathroom and to the table to eat, but otherwise the feet should be up. On the first postoperative day the patient may walk around inside the house. A cool shower is acceptable. On the second postoperative day limited activities outside the house, such as going to church, to a movie, or to a restaurant, are permitted. On the third day, most activities can be resumed, except for strenuous ones like jogging, riding a bike, weight lifting, and having sex. These should be delayed for a week. Most men can return to work and gradually ease back into their usual activities.

Be sure to reinforce that the patient must use another form of contraceptive until he has two negative semen checks at 6 weeks (after 15 ejaculations) and again at 12 weeks. Samples can be obtained by self-stimulation, collecting secretions from a condom, or withdrawing after intercourse and collecting the ejaculate. It is best to examine the specimen within 2 hours of collection.

A routine telephone call to the patient on the first or second day after the vasectomy can provide valuable reassurance, promote compliance with activity restrictions, and address any questions or concerns that might have arisen on the part of the patient or his partner.

COMPLICATIONS

Minor

Minor complications, causing discomfort and inconvenience but no serious threat to health, occur in 5% to 10% of vasectomy patients.

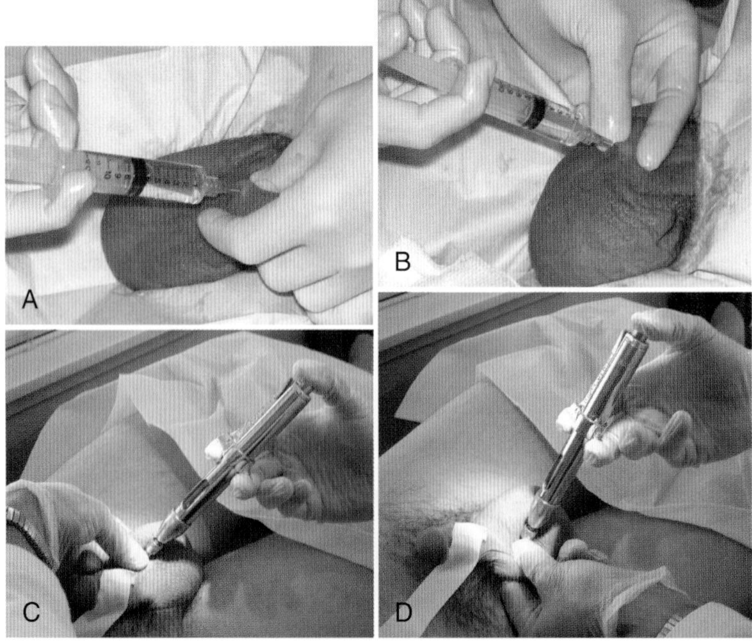

Figure 126-9 Vasectomy anesthesia: vasal block of left vas (**A**) and right vas (**B**). No-needle anesthetic using MadaJet to left vas (**C**) and right vas (**D**).

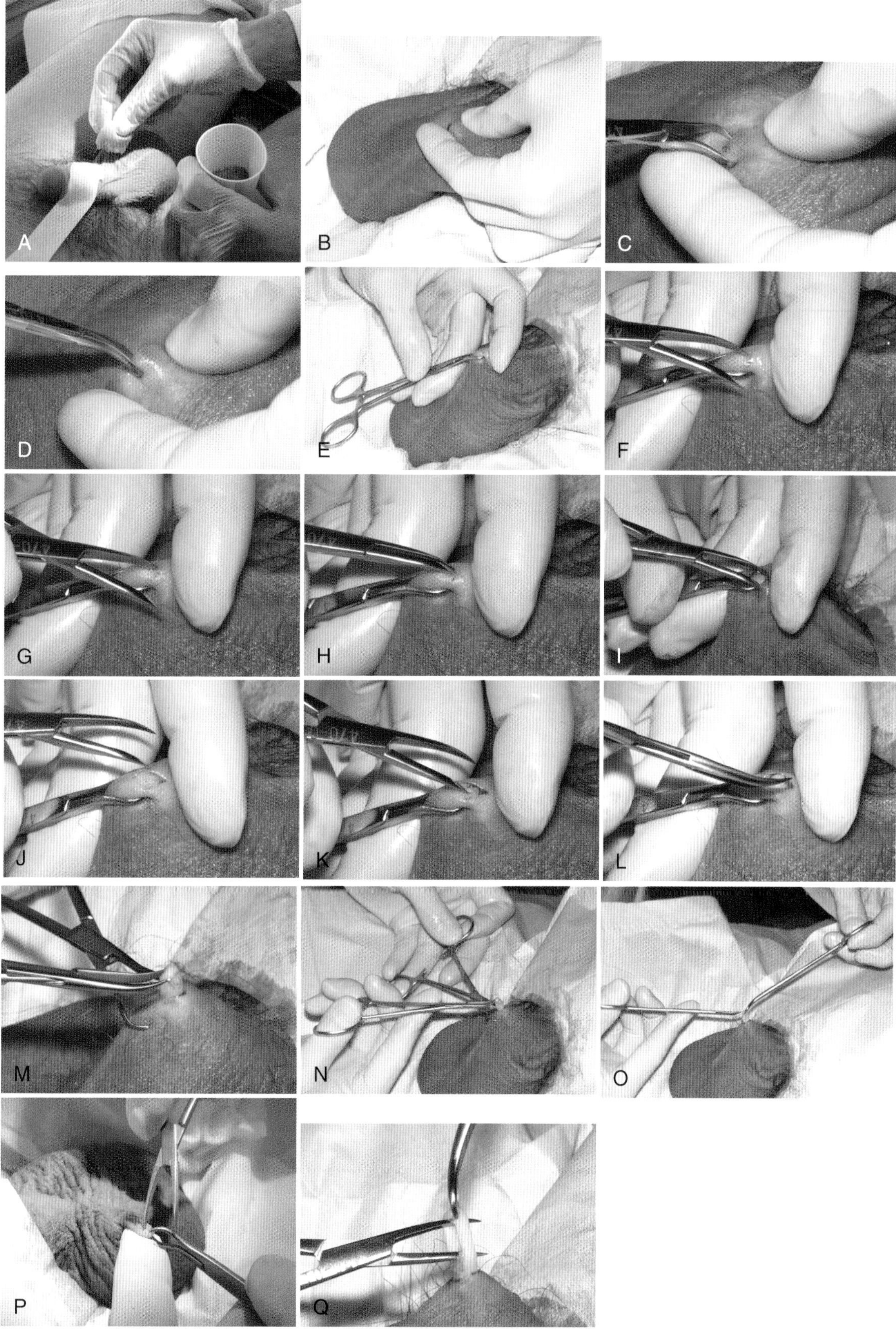

Figure 126-10 The no-scalpel vasectomy procedure. **A,** Warmed chlorhexidine (Hibiclens) preparation. **B,** Three-finger grasp of left vas. **C,** Straddling left vas with vas-fixing forceps (VFF). **D,** Vas is securely fixed in place with the VFF. **E,** Regrasping the VFF, the handles are lowered and skin is tensed over the prominent segment of the vas. **F,** Sharp dissecting forceps (SDF) poised over vas. **G,** SDF tip in the lumen of vas. **H,** Both tips now in lumen. **I,** Spreading all layers, skin to vas, in one motion. **J** and **K,** The SDF tip is placed into the lumen. **L** and **M,** The hand is rotated palm up, so the SDF tip hooks and delivers the vas. **N,** The VFF is unlocked and released. **O,** The vas loop is then regrasped. **P,** The fascia is sharply dissected from loop. **Q,** Fascia is stripped from a bare loop of vas, allowing occlusion to proceed with no bleeding from the plethora of fascial vessels.

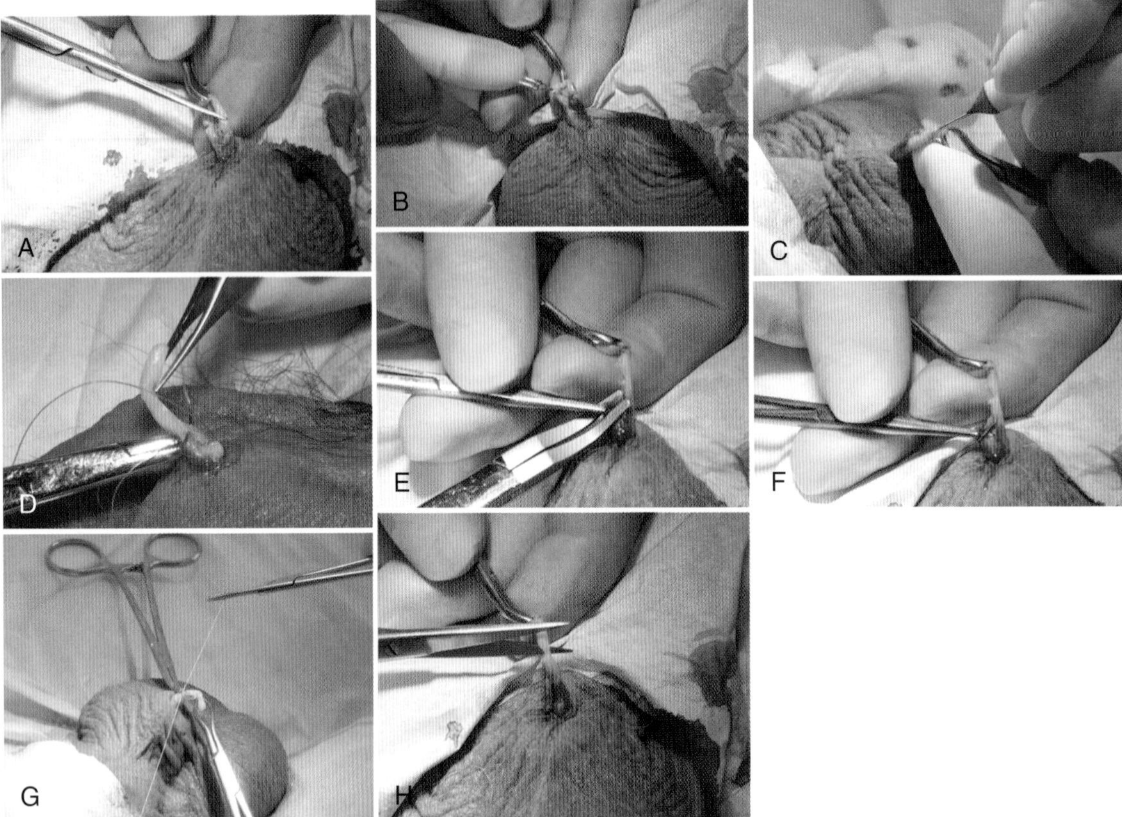

Figure 126-11 Various occlusion steps. **A,** Hemitransecting the vas in two areas approximately 1.5 cm apart. **B,** Cauterizing the two ends of the hemitransected vas. (In the open-ended technique, only the prostatic end would be occluded.) Here, a battery cautery unit within a sterile glove is being used. **C,** Intraluminal electrocautery. The sharp tip has penetrated the vas wall and 1 cm of the needle electrode lies within the lumen before the current is applied and the electrode is gradually withdrawn. **D,** Fascial interposition may be accomplished using a pursestring suture to close the edges of the fascial opening. **E,** Here the fascia is approximated with a hemostat, covering over the vas end. A hemoclip is then applied to secure fascial closure. **F,** Note the hemoclip does not include the vas. **G,** Alternatively, the fascial closure is secured with a free tie. **H,** Excising the segment of vas by completing the other hemitransection. (**A, B, E, F,** and **H,** Courtesy of Jan Drlik, MD, The Medical Procedures Center, PC, Midland, Mich.)

- *Swelling and discomfort* are prevented routinely by using an ice pack, mild analgesic (acetaminophen or ibuprofen), a tight athletic supporter packed with gauze or a wash cloth, and bed rest. The ice is usually placed over the supporter but may need to be applied directly to the skin if bleeding is suspected.
- *Bleeding from the skin incision* is normally nil or less than a 3-cm spot on the gauze overnight. Persistent bleeding is controlled with pressure by pinching the skin incision between gauze for 10 minutes.
- *Ecchymosis*, a purple discoloration, makes the scrotum look bad but is harmless. Careful cautery of any bleeding, especially on the skin margins of the incision, usually prevents it. Ecchymosis may become extensive, involving the entire scrotum, and can extend to the penis and even to the groin and thighs. It may present in the first day or several days later. It will be alarming to the patient, but in the absence of a hematoma (see later discussion), ecchymosis is harmless and usually painless and results from minor amounts of blood extravasated into the skin or subcutaneous layers. The color may evolve through red, yellow, and green as the blood is resorbed. Prevention is by meticulous hemostasis. Icing the area intermittently during the first day may be effective.
- *Superficial wound infection* is rare because of the excellent blood supply to the scrotum. A minimal infection responds to local treatment and oral antibiotics. The key to prevention may lie in dissuading the curious patient from touching the wound.
- *Skin reaction* to the surgical antiseptic solution may present with rash and itching.
- *Neuroma* is a tender nerve ending buried in scar tissue, where a small sensory nerve was severed or damaged. It is rarely reported after vasectomy and is more often a curiosity than a hindrance to normal activities. A single injection of procaine combined with an equal dose of reassurance can provide a definitive cure.
- *Suture rejection* can present weeks after vasectomy. Absorbable plain gut suture may prove the least reactive for fascial closure.
- *Hemospermia* occurs very rarely in the first few months after vasectomy. It clears up spontaneously and has no clinical significance.
- *Sperm granuloma* is a reaction to sperm leakage into the tissue at the site of the vas division or a rupture in the epididymis. Although such leakage is common, only about 1.5% of patients report finding a tender nodule there. Treatment is an NSAID and reassurance. Rarely, the nodule will require excision or injection with steroids. Abstaining from sexual stimulation in the first week is thought by some to reduce the incidence of sperm leaking from an unhealed vas, but data are lacking on the question. Patients with open-ended vasectomy do not present more frequently with this complaint, suggesting that leakage and scarring are not factors.
- *Congestive epididymitis* usually presents with a new, unilateral, or occasionally bilateral, tenderness and achy pain localized to the epididymis and radiating to the ipsilateral groin, aggravated by movement. It can occur weeks or years after the procedure. The epididymis feels enlarged and boggy to palpation and may be somewhat tender. It is self-limited, but may linger for 1 to 3 weeks

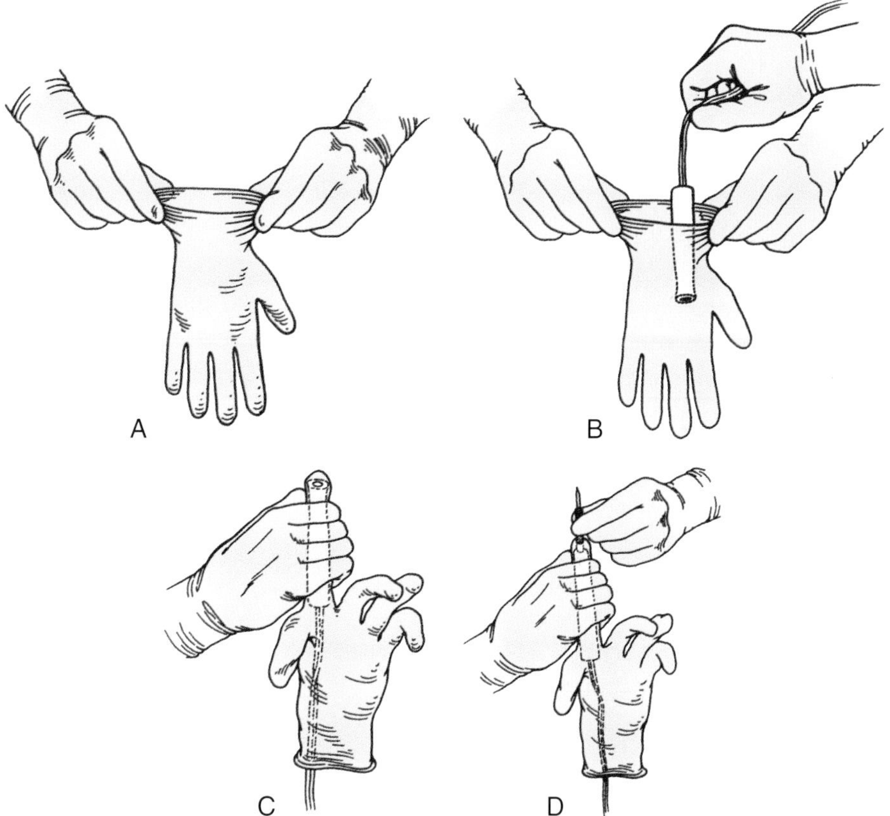

Figure 126-12 Maintaining a sterile cautery instrument. **A,** Gloved physician holds the sterile glove. **B,** Assistant holds the cautery handpiece without the tip by the cord and carefully drops it into a finger of glove. **C,** Gloved physician grasps the cautery handle inside the glove finger. **D,** Sterile tip is punctured through rubber glove. The unit can now be handled in a sterile fashion; the clinician is careful not to contaminate the surgical field with the cord. (If it is a battery unit without wire, the unit can be activated so that the tip will burn through the glove to be exposed for use.)

if untreated. It responds within 48 hours to a full regimen of NSAIDs, such as naproxen sodium 1100 mg per day or ibuprofen 800 mg three times a day, and sexual abstinence for 10 to 14 days.

- *Postvasectomy pain syndrome* is a term applied to various types of chronic pelvic and scrotal pain in men who have previously had a vasectomy. The incidence is low and, in most cases, the symptoms eventually abate spontaneously. Its causation and relationship to vasectomy and to chronic pain that occurs in men without vasectomy are unknown. Management may be enhanced by a supportive, multidisciplinary approach including urologic evaluation, psychological support, and pain clinic management of medications and therapies (an extremely rare occurrence). Surgery has provided little if any benefit to patients with postvasectomy pain syndrome.
- *Persistent sperm in the ejaculate*. Depending on the study and technique used, *vasectomy failure* rates vary from 1/100 to 1/1200. The latter efficacy is obtained by using resection of 1 cm of vas, cautery of the ends, and fascial interposition. Most often failure is due to the process of spontaneous recanalization, by which a channel forms between the cut ends of a vas and conducts fresh sperm from the testicle. If recanalization occurs, it generally takes place in the first few weeks after surgery and is detectable by routine semen testing (see later discussion). In half of those cases the channel will close permanently and sperm will disappear from the semen as the scar around the vas matures. If motile sperm persist over time, however, a repeat vasectomy is performed on each vas.
- If a *true surgical failure* is suspected based on semen analysis, it may be advisable to have the patient produce a specimen in the office before proceeding with repeat vasectomy. However, genetically proven paternity has occurred with men whose semen tests were clear of visualized sperm both before and after impregnation. Couples dealing with unexplained postvasectomy pregnancy should be made aware of such rare possibilities.
- One of the most common causes of persistent sperm in the ejaculate is *not having had at least 15 ejaculations before the check*. Sperm that may have refluxed into the prostate and seminal vesicles can persist for 8 to 10 weeks or more.
- *Misidentification of one or both of the vasa deferentia* (very rare) could be detected by submitting excised specimens for histologic examination by a pathologist. This is advisable when any doubt exists at the time of surgery. However, when gross tissue identification is certain, histologic examination is not cost effective and does not provide assurance against failure.
- Despite hearsay evidence of vasectomies failing because of a *third vas deferens*, documented cases of supernumerary vasa are extremely rare.
- *Prematurely abandoning other contraceptive methods* before achieving a clear test can result in pregnancy with a successful vasectomy as well as with a failed vasectomy. If two clear semen checks are obtained (no sperm seen), the incidence of late (secondary) failure is very rare, and pregnancy risk is even lower.

Major

Major complications, which cause temporary disability and require medical or surgical intervention, occur in less than 1% of patients and include scrotal hematoma and infection.

- *Hematoma* is a mass of blood accumulated in the scrotum from a leaking blood vessel. It is a major concern because the loose connective tissue of the scrotum may allow a hematoma to expand

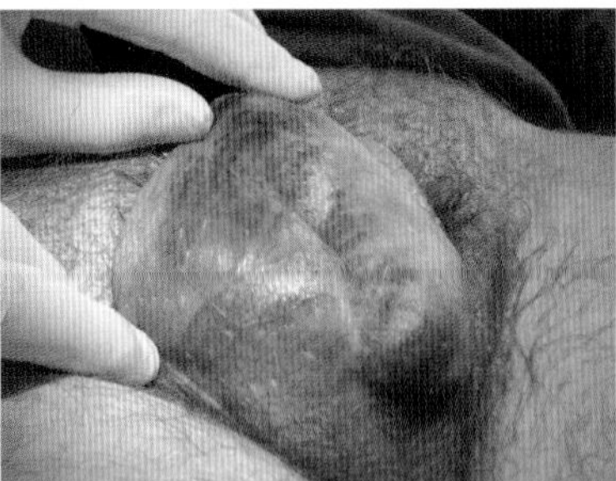

Figure 126-13 Left hemiscrotal hematoma postvasectomy.

from a few centimeters to the size of a grapefruit (Fig. 126-13) Thus, early *(nonsurgical)* intervention is critical. It is generally not possible to apply direct pressure on the site of internal bleeding, but the supporter can be packed tight with gauze or a washcloth. Strict bed rest, elevating the scrotum on a folded towel, and applying ice packs intermittently (30 minutes on and 15 to 20 minutes off to prevent injury) will usually stop progression. Attempts at *surgical evacuation* may be unwise because clots are not easily extracted and surgical trauma to neurovascular structures may contribute to excess morbidity. Close monitoring for signs of infection is combined with progressive mobilization with scrotal support. Complete resolution may take from several weeks to many months. Prevention is by meticulous surgical hemostasis during the surgery and by limiting patient activity after surgery. With the current NNV methods, patients feel so good after surgery that they tend to overdo it. *Proper postoperative rest and care cannot be stressed enough.*

- *Scrotal infection* after vasectomy is a rare but potentially serious complication. Fever, chills, redness, warmth, swelling, and induration are signs of infection. Prompt evaluation and early consultation are important. Very localized signs around the incision with an otherwise negative scrotal examination and no systemic symptoms might safely be treated on an outpatient basis with oral antibiotics and warm packs if careful observation for progressive symptoms and follow-up within 48 hours is ensured. Signs of cellulitis or the presence of systemic symptoms would usually warrant parenteral antibiotics. If fluctuance is detected, surgical drainage of an abscess should not be delayed. Preexisting skin infections, diabetes mellitus, and immunodeficiency contribute to risk of infection. Careful attention to sterile technique is essential to prevention. Also important is reducing tissue trauma in surgery by handling tissues gently, minimizing cautery and suture ligation, and using atraumatic forceps. Early recognition and careful evaluation of symptoms are keys to correct diagnosis. A low threshold for hospitalization and for parenteral antibiotic use to arrest an infection may prove critical to management of resistant infections.

Regardless of one's surgical skills, some complications cannot be avoided. The most important thing is to be prepared to handle them properly so as to minimize the adverse effect on your patient.

Be sure patients know to call you if symptoms arise, and ensure that you or someone equally knowledgeable is available to take their calls.

Stay in touch, providing open communication that is compassionate, informative, and honest. Even when a consultant is making treatment decisions, be sure to stay involved and obtain information on your patient. Contribute to his care through active listening and ensuring his needs are met. He should know that you care about his recovery. Even a patient who has a good outcome may become resentful and litigious if he feels neglected or uncared for. On the other hand, a patient who has suffered a major complication may advocate for his physician if he feels genuinely well cared for throughout the experience. Remember, too, the common wisdom that one patient's unhappiness can have widespread repercussions with other men considering vasectomy in the community.

In large, long-term studies of vasectomy, *no increase* in mortality or incidence of *chronic disease*, including, among other entities, hypertension, diabetes, autoimmune diseases, cardiovascular diseases, and prostate cancer, has been found. There is no decreased libido or sexual experience. Basically, what is present before the procedure will persist after the procedure.

Studies show patients are 98% to 99% satisfied with the vasectomy decision. However, some *regret* having the procedure, either because of the complications discussed previously or later desire for children.

Postoperative Semen Testing

A postoperative semen check is a waived CLIA (Clinical Laboratory Improvement Amendments) test. It is customary to require two postprocedure semen tests. Because sperm can persist in the ejaculate for many weeks, the first specimen is tested after 6 weeks or 15 ejaculations (whichever is later) and the second after 3 months.

Allow the freshly collected semen specimen to stand at room temperature for 30 minutes (or 10 minutes at body temperature) until the viscous mucus component is autolyzed by enzymes in the semen. The clinician places a drop of unspun fresh ejaculate onto a slide (no staining is necessary). The sample is covered with a coverslip and examined under high power (40× magnification) for the presence of live or dead sperm (higher power with oil immersion is not necessary). Figure 126-14 shows the appearance of many sperm in one high-power field in a *failed* vasectomy (no sperm should be seen).

Some define a positive specimen as having any visualized sperm under high power (unspun specimen). Sequential semen testing in a study of 364 patients showed that a single sample with "severe oligospermia" (<100,000 sperm/mL) at 12 weeks predicted success of vasectomy with 99.7% accuracy. That would correspond to seeing approximately one sperm per high-power field using the aforementioned technique. Observing live sperm after 6 weeks suggests, however, that a second specimen should be examined.

NOTE: The author's approach is to require that a single specimen pass an examination of 100 high-power fields with no more than 2 sperm seen (approximately 10,000/mL) and no motile sperm. Specimens are accepted up to 24 hours after collection to improve patient compliance. The editor prefers two samples at 6 and 12 weeks. A few dead sperm are acceptable at 6 weeks but usually are not seen. If any sperm persist at 12 weeks, another sample is requested. Any live sperm after 12 weeks should be regarded as a possible failure. Unprotected intercourse is allowed after the two negative checks.

An early pregnancy does not mean a failed surgical technique. Pregnancy can occur either because contraception was not used until the sperm were cleared or because of spontaneous recanalization in spite of proper technique.

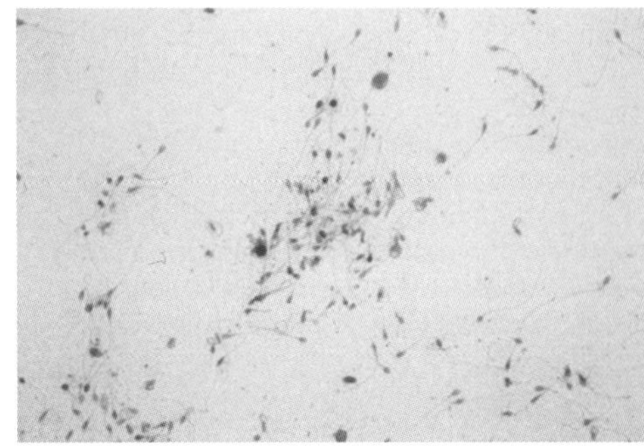

Figure 126-14 Postoperative semen check: the appearance of sperm in the ejaculate of a failed vasectomy. (Courtesy of Nicholas Hruby, MD, Saginaw, Mich.)

Semen tests are included as part of the vasectomy procedure code (55250) if performed in the physician's office. (They are separately billable if performed by an independent laboratory.)

REVERSAL

With fully informed consent, patient and partner satisfaction with vasectomy is extremely high. (Rosenfeld and colleagues [1993] showed it is the only contraceptive method with which 100% of women are satisfied. For tubal ligation, the method with next-highest acceptance rate, only 78% of women are satisfied.) Occasionally, however, patients request vasectomy reversal, usually because a new partner wishes to have children. Reversal can be accomplished using either a macroscopic or microscopic approach, and results in pregnancy approximately 50% to 80% of the time. The sooner it is reversed, and the longer the testicular remnant of the vas, the better the chances of reversal. Observation of live sperm from the testicular vas end at the time of surgery is another good prognosticator. Although patency is often achieved, the presence of sperm antibodies that persist after reversal can inactivate sperm efficacy to impregnate the egg. Intracytoplasmic sperm injection can be used, but is much more costly. The use of previously frozen sperm is the least expensive option, if available (see Chapter 123, Sperm Banking).

PATIENT EDUCATION GUIDES

See the following forms online at www.expertconsult.com:

- Patient Consent
- Patient Education
  - Preoperative
  - Postoperative
  - Postsedative
  - Worksheet
- Vasectomy Questionnaire

CPT/BILLING CODES

55250 Vasectomy, unilateral or bilateral (separate procedure), including postoperative semen examination(s)
89321 Semen analysis, presence and/or mobility of sperm (if vasectomy performed elsewhere)
99203 Counseling visit(s), new patient
99214 Counseling visit(s), established patient

Other routine office visit codes can also be used for the counseling sessions.

ICD-9-CM DIAGNOSTIC CODES

V25.0 Contraceptive management
V25.09 Family planning advice
V25.2 Sterilization advice
V25.8 Other specified contraceptive management, postvasectomy sperm count
V25.40 Contraceptive surveillance, unspecified
V26.52 Sterilization status (vasectomy)

ACKNOWLEDGMENT

The editors wish to recognize the many contributions by George C. Denniston, MD, to this chapter in the previous edition of this text.

SUPPLIERS

(See contact information online at www.expertconsult.com.)

Battery-operated cautery
Advanced Meditech International (AMI)
Ellman

NOTE: Most medical suppliers also carry battery-operated cautery equipment.

Forceps
Miltex, Inc.

Hemoclips and clip applicators
Advanced Meditech International (AMI)
Ethicon, Inc.
Weck Closure Systems

No-needle instruments
Mada Medical, Inc.

No-scalpel instrument suppliers
Advanced Meditech International (AMI)
Marina Medical (Wilson clamp and dissecting forceps)

Other patient information
Advanced Meditech International (AMI)
EngenderHealth

Teaching models
Advanced Meditech International (AMI)
Dr. Charles Wilson
The National Procedures Institute (NPI)

Technique videotapes for physicians
Advanced Meditech International (AMI)
American Academy of Family Physicians
Creative Health Communications
Dr. Charles Wilson
EngenderHealth
Health Sciences Center for Educational Resources, University of Washington
The National Procedures Institute (NPI)

Videotapes for patient education
Creative Health Communications
EngenderHealth
The National Procedures Institute (NPI)

Written patient education handouts
Advanced Meditech International (AMI)
American Urological Association
EngenderHealth
Krames Communications
Procter & Gamble Pharmaceuticals

ONLINE RESOURCES

Vasectomy.com: This website provides balanced, well-written information for patients on vasectomy, no-needle vasectomy, and vasectomy reversal. One can locate doctors nearby who provide services. Available at www.vasectomy.com.

VasectomyMedical.com: An excellent Internet resource on vasectomy and vasectomy reversal that includes physician directories for providers. This popular site walks the prospective patient through the decision-making process, explaining in simple, understandable language all that should be considered. Available at www.vasectomymedical.com.

BIBLIOGRAPHY

Alderman PM: Complications in a series of 1224 vasectomies. J Fam Pract 33:579–584, 1991.

Alderman PM: Standard incision in non-scalpel vasectomy. J Fam Pract 48:719–721, 1999.

Barone MA, Hutchinson PL, Johnson CH, et al: Vasectomy in the United States, 2002. J Urol 176:232–236, 2006.

Barone MA, Irsula B, Chen-Mok M, Sokal DC, the Investigator Study Group: Effectiveness of vasectomy using cautery. BMC Urol 4:10, 2004.

Benger JR: Persistent spermatozoa after vasectomy: A survey of British urologists. Br J Urol 76:376–379, 1995.

Cox B, Sneyd MJ, Paul C, et al: Vasectomy and risk of prostate cancer. JAMA 287:3110–3115, 2002.

Davis JE: Male sterilization. Curr Opin Obstet Gynecol 4:522–526, 1992.

Denniston GC: The effect of vasectomy on childless men. J Reprod Med 21:151–152, 1978.

Denniston GC: Vasectomy by electrocautery: Outcomes in a series of 2,500 patients. J Fam Pract 21:35–40, 1985.

Denniston GC, Kuehl L: Open-ended vasectomy: Approaching the ideal technique. J Am Board Fam Pract 7:285–287, 1994.

DerSimonian R, Clemens J, Spirtas R, Perlman J: Vasectomy and prostate cancer risk: Methodological review of the evidence. J Clin Epidemiol 46:163–172, 1993.

Edwards IS: Early testing after vasectomy, based on the absence of motile sperm. Fertil Steril 59:431–436, 1993.

Errey BB, Edwards IS: Open-ended vasectomy: An assessment. Fertil Steril 45:843–846, 1986.

Giovannucci E, Ascherio A, Rimm EB, et al: A prospective cohort study of vasectomy and prostate cancer in US men. JAMA 269:873–877, 1993.

Giovannucci E, Tosteson TD, Speizer FE, et al: A long-term study of mortality in men who have undergone vasectomy. N Engl J Med 326:1392–1398, 1992.

Greenberg MJ: Vasectomy technique. Am Fam Physician 39:131–138, 1989.

Guess HA: Is vasectomy a risk factor for prostate cancer? Eur J Cancer 29A:1055–1060, 1993.

Hartanto VH, Chenven ES, DiPiazza DJ, et al: Fournier gangrene following vasectomy. Infect Urol 14:80–82, 2001.

Haws JM, Feigin J: Vasectomy counseling. Am Fam Physician 52: 1395–1399, 1995.

Haws JM, Morgan GT, Pollack AF, et al: Clinical aspects of vasectomies performed in the US in 1995. J Urol 52:685–691, 1998.

Healy B: From the National Institutes of Health: Does vasectomy cause prostate cancer? JAMA 269:2620, 1993.

Hendry WF: Vasectomy and vasectomy reversal. Br J Urol 73:337–344, 1994.

Howards SS, Peterson HB: Vasectomy and prostate cancer: Chance, bias, or a causal relationship? JAMA 269:913–914, 1993.

John EM, Whittemore AS, Wu AH, et al: Vasectomy and prostate cancer: Results from a multicentric case-control study. J Natl Cancer Inst 87: 662–669, 1995.

Kendrick JS, Gonzales B, Huber DH, et al: Complications of vasectomy in the United States. J Fam Pract 25:245–248, 1987.

Labrecque M, Hoang D, Turcot L: Association between the length of the vas deferens excised during vasectomy and the risk of postvasectomy recanalization. Fertil Steril 79:1003–1007, 2003.

Labrecque M, Nazerali H, Mondor M, et al: Effectiveness and complications associated with 2 vasectomy occlusion techniques. J Urol 168:2495–2498, 2002.

Labrecque M, St-Hilare K, Turcot L: Delayed vasectomy success in men with a first postvasectomy semen analysis showing motile sperm. Fertil Steril 83:1435–1441, 2005.

Leslie TA, Illing RO, Cranston DW, Guillebaud J: The incidence of chronic scrotal pain after vasectomy: A prospective audit. BJU Int 100:1330–1333, 2007.

Li PS, Li SQ, Schlegel PN, Goldstein M: External spermatic sheath injection for vasal nerve block. Urology 39:173–176, 1992.

Li SQ, Goldstein M, Zhu J, Huber D: The no-scalpel vasectomy. J Urol 145:341–344, 1991.

Lipshultz LI, Benson GS: Vasectomy—1980. Urol Clin North Am 7:89–105, 1980.

Magnani RJ, Haws JM, Morgan GT, et al: Vasectomy in the United States, 1991 and 1995. Am J Public Health 89:92–94, 1999.

McDonald S: Is vasectomy harmful to health? Br J Gen Pract 47:381–386, 1997.

McKay W, Morris R, Mushlin P: Sodium bicarbonate attenuates pain on skin infiltration with lidocaine, with or without epinephrine. Anesth Analg 66:572–574, 1987.

O'Brien TS, Cranston D, Ashwin P, et al: Temporary reappearance of sperm 12 months after vasectomy clearance. Br J Urol 76:371–372, 1995.

Pfenninger JL: Complications of vasectomy. Am Fam Physician 30:111–115, 1984a.

Pfenninger JL: Preparation for vasectomy. Am Fam Physician 30:177–184, 1984b.

Raspa RF: Complications of vasectomy. Am Fam Physician 48:1264–1268, 1993.

Reynolds RD: Vas deferens occlusion during no-scalpel vasectomy. J Fam Pract 39:577–582, 1994.

Reynolds RD: Evaluating vasal occlusion methods for vasectomy. Am Fam Physician 78:697, 2008.

Rosenfeld JA, Zahorik PM, Saint W, Murphy G: Women's satisfaction with birth control. J Fam Pract 36:169–173, 1993.

Schmidt SS: Prevention of failure in vasectomy. J Urol 109:296–297, 1973.

Schmidt SS: Vasectomy: Principles and comments. J Fam Pract 33:571–573, 1991.

Schmidt SS: The vas after vasectomy: Comparison of cauterization methods. J Urol 40:468–470, 1992.

Sokal D, Irsula B, Hays M, et al: Vasectomy by ligation and excision, with or without fascial interposition: A randomized controlled trial. BMC Med 2:6, 2004.

Sokal D, Labrecque M: Effectiveness of vasectomy techniques. Urol Clin North Am 36:317–329, 2009.

Stockton MD, Davis LE, Bolton KM: No-scalpel vasectomy: A technique for family physicians. Am Fam Physician 46:1153–1167, 1992.

Tuggy M, Garcia J: Procedures Consult. Available at www.proceduresconsult.com.

Wilson CL: No-needle anesthesia for no-scalpel vasectomy [letter]. Am Fam Physician 63:1295, 2001.

Wilson CL: No-scalpel vasectomy: A self-study program for the family physician. Videotape/DVD. Leawood, Kan, American Academy of Family Physicians, 2002.

Wilson CL: Re: No-needle jet anesthetic technique for no-scalpel vasectomy [letter]. J Urol 174:1504–1505, 2005.

Vasectomy: Procedures for your practice. Patient Care 24:116, 1991.

SECTION 9

Gynecology and Female Reproductive System Procedures

Section Editor: DALE A. PATTERSON

CHAPTER 127

PREGNANCY TERMINATION: FIRST-TRIMESTER SUCTION ASPIRATION

Lawrence Leeman • Emily Godfrey

First-trimester surgical termination of pregnancy (suction aspiration) is one of the safest surgical procedures performed in the United States, with 1.2 million procedures performed each year. By the time a woman reaches 45 years of age, approximately one in three will have had an abortion. About half of these are performed at 8 weeks or less in gestational age, and 88% are completed in the first trimester of pregnancy. Although abortion has been legal in all 50 states since the 1973 *Roe v. Wade* Supreme Court decision, many states have imposed laws such as parental consent for minors, mandatory waiting periods, and compulsory state-directed counseling that may limit availability of the procedure or discourage a woman from having an abortion. *Therefore, clinicians performing abortion must be aware of any state and local restrictions that govern it.*

Virtually all first-trimester surgical abortions are accomplished with vacuum aspiration. This chapter contains specific information about uterine aspiration using manual vacuum aspiration (MVA) and electric suction abortion in the first trimester. The most commonly used MVA device is a 60-mL syringe with locking valves and a plunger that provides identical suction pressure (26 inches of mercury) as an electric pump until the cylinder reaches approximately 80% capacity. The aspirator can be quickly emptied and reused if more capacity is needed. It is small, portable, and quiet and thus very practical for a variety of settings, including offices, emergency departments, and hospital-based locations. Although there is still some suction sound, there is no mechanical noise. When MVA and electric suction have been compared in studies, some patients prefer MVA because the sound of electrical suction can be disquieting. Clinicians may prefer MVA for aspiration at early gestational ages because it causes less disruption of the gestational sac, the presence of which confirms a successful aspiration procedure. Electrical suction may be preferred for later first-trimester gestational ages because of the larger amounts of products of conception (POC) and the need for repeat passes if MVA is used.

The suction technique described in this chapter for first-trimester abortion *can also be used for surgical completion of spontaneous abortion*, including missed and incomplete abortion. Many institutions use operating room settings for completion of spontaneous abortion. In most circumstances, however, spontaneous abortion treatment can be integrated into outpatient settings. Expectant management to await spontaneous passage of the POC and medical management with misoprostol are also safe options. The highest patient satisfaction is achieved when patients can make their own choice of a management plan. The relative and absolute contraindications to first-trimester abortion would also apply to treatment of spontaneous abortion.

ANATOMY

Anatomic variations can increase the likelihood of complications occurring during uterine aspiration. A *vaginal septum* may interfere with visualizing and accessing the cervix. *Cervical stenosis* may occur and can be caused by prior surgical procedures including loop electrical excision, cryotherapy, and cold knife cone biopsy. Dilation may be more difficult in *nulliparous* teenagers because of a tight cervical os, particularly at early gestational ages. *Mullerian anomalies* including uterus didelphys, bicornuate uterus (Fig. 127-1), and an intrauterine septum may interfere with successful uterine aspiration. Intraoperative ultrasonography can facilitate the procedure. *Adnexal masses or uterine fibroids* may result in inaccurate gestational age dating; fibroids can interfere with cervical dilation.

INDICATIONS

- Elective abortion up to 12 weeks' estimated gestational age
- Treatment of early pregnancy failure or spontaneous abortion for uterine sizes up to 12 weeks
- Postabortal hematometra
- Backup for medical abortion (mifepristone/misoprostol or methotrexate/misoprostol; see Chapter 128, Pregnancy Termination: Medication Abortion)

CONTRAINDICATIONS

Medical contraindications are rare. It is important for clinicians to be aware that some clinical scenarios require stabilization before abortion or that the procedure be performed in a hospital setting.

Absolute

Absolute contraindications to first-trimester abortion in an outpatient setting include the following:

- Hemodynamic instability
- Active pelvic infection

Relative

Relative contraindications include the following:

- Uncontrolled hypertension
- Uncontrolled diabetes
- Molar pregnancy (based on gestational age)
- Coagulopathy

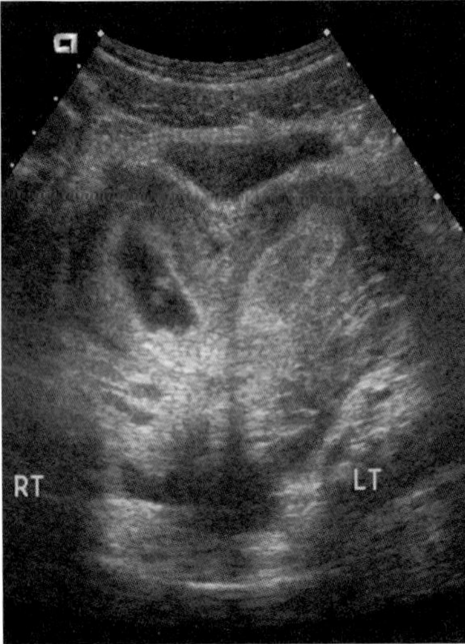

Figure 127-1 Ultrasonographic scan of bicornuate uterus with gestational sac in the right horn.

Equipment and Supplies

- Medium Graves speculum (size and type varies based on patient habitus).
- Single-tooth or atraumatic tenaculum.
- Syringe with 22- to 27-gauge, 3-inch spinal needle, or 22- to 27-gauge needle on 3-inch needle extender.
- Anesthetic agent for cervical block (e.g., 0.5% or 1% lidocaine with epinephrine or vasopressin).
- Rigid cervical dilators for mechanical dilation: Pratt, Hegar, or Denniston (see Chapter 136, Cervical Stenosis and Cervical Dilation).
- Osmotic dilators: Sterilized seaweed stem (*Laminaria japonicum*) available in a variety of sizes (2 to 10 mm); when used, they should be inserted into the cervical os 6 to 18 hours before the procedure (see Chapter 136, Cervical Stenosis and Cervical Dilation).
- Cervical softening agents: misoprostol (prostaglandin E_1 analog), available in 200-μg dose.
- Povidone–iodine or other antiseptic solution or sterile water.
- Ring forceps.
- 4 × 4 gauze pads.
- Manual vacuum syringe (Ipas MVA Plus; Fig. 127-2).
- Disposable suction cannulas, which come in a variety of sizes or flexibility, including flexible, semiflexible, or rigid (curved and straight; see Fig. 127-2). It is essential that the clinician identify which cannula produces adequate seal and suction with the type of MVA device that is being used.
- Suction machine with tubing as an alternative to MVA syringe (Fig. 127-3).

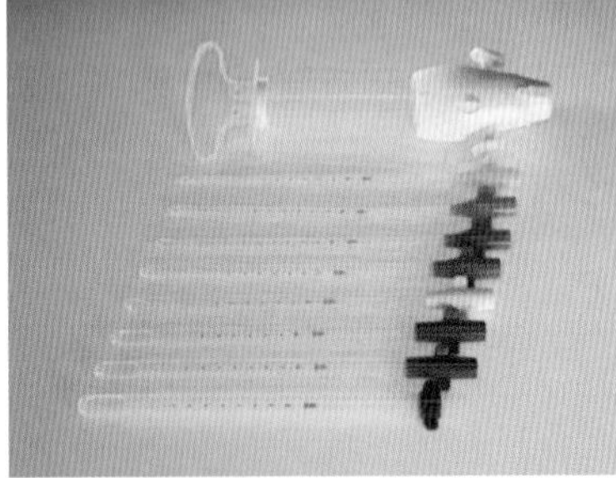

Figure 127-2 Ipas Plus syringe with flexible plastic cannulas for manual vacuum aspiration. (From ARHP [Association of Reproductive Health Professionals]: www.arhp.org.)

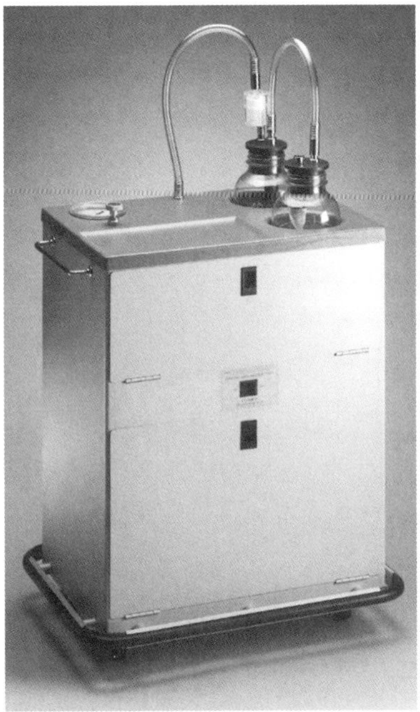

Figure 127-3 Berkeley Synevac vacuum curettage machine.

- Metal bowl for POC (if using MVA)
- Medium-sharp uterine curette
- Formalin jar (POC may be sent to pathology; however, many physicians performing aspiration abortion examine their own POC)
- Intravenous solutions, tubing, and oxytocics (for treatment of excessive bleeding)

Precautions

With the availability of portable office ultrasonography, pregnancies can be detected at very early gestational ages. In the past, women were frequently asked to defer pregnancy termination until they were at least 7 weeks' gestation, when a change of uterine size can be detected on physical examination and cervical softening occurs naturally. Now that these pregnancies can be verified earlier with ultrasonography and cervical softening agents are available, women can routinely be offered uterine aspiration or medical abortion as soon as a gestational sac is identified on transvaginal ultrasonography. Women who present for a first-trimester abortion with a positive urine pregnancy test in whom ultrasonography cannot confirm an intrauterine pregnancy can pose a management dilemma. In these cases, an algorithm has been suggested by Creinin and Edwards (Fig. 127-4). Outpatient uterine aspiration under local analgesia with a cervical block works well for most women. Some women, including those with a history of anxiety disorder, substance abuse, or poor tolerance to gynecologic examinations may be best cared for in clinical sites where conscious sedation or general anesthesia is provided. These patients should be identified during options counseling and offered referral to a clinic that can offer a greater range of anesthetic options.

Preprocedure Patient Education

It would be impossible provide a full discussion of counseling here, but several techniques and general principles can be outlined.

1. *Explore the patient's feelings*. This may be done by asking nonjudgmental and open-ended questions as well as through active listening. The clinician should empathize and help the patient

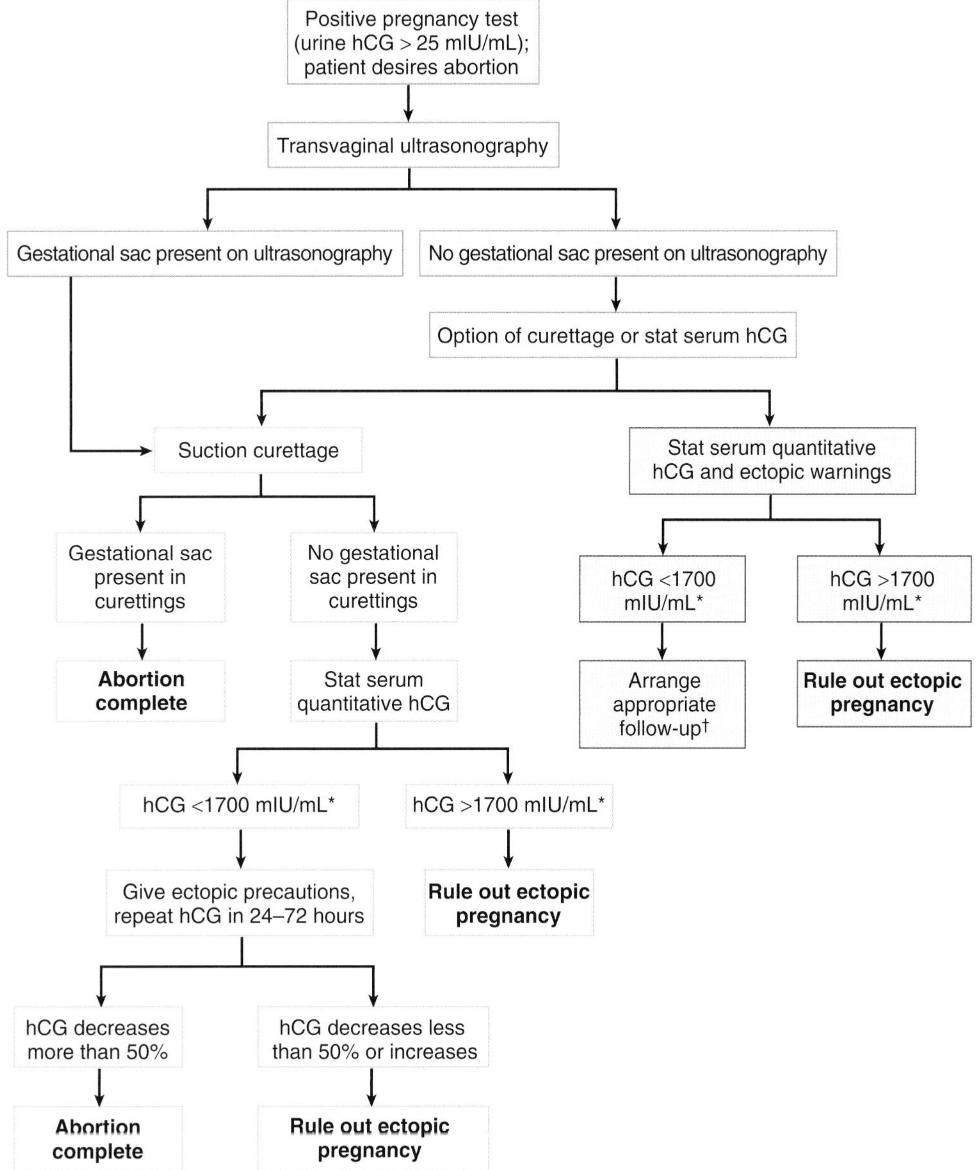

Figure 127-4 Algorithm for early surgical abortion. hCG, human chorionic gonadotropin. *Discriminatory zone. †The timing of follow-up serum quantitative hCG test or ultrasonography (or both) may vary according to patient's risk factors for ectopic pregnancy. (Adapted from Creinin MD, Edwards J: Early abortion: Surgical and medical options. Curr Probl Obstet Gynecol Fertil 20:1–32, 1997.)

reflect on her own feelings. Ambivalence should be acknowledged and discussed.

2. *Explore options*. The patient's options regarding her pregnancy include terminating or continuing the pregnancy. If she chooses to continue the pregnancy, she has the additional option of parenting or making an adoption plan. The risks, advantages, and disadvantages of each option should be explored in the context of the woman's particular life situation. If she chooses pregnancy termination, appropriate options based on gestational age should be discussed.
3. *Making decisions*. Strategies for decision making and the need for any additional counseling may be explored. The patient should be encouraged to seek advice from others she trusts: partner, parents, siblings, friends, teachers, or spiritual counselors. It is imperative that a timetable for decision making be established based on the gestational age.
4. *Screening for special problems*. Extreme anxiety, ambivalence, drug or alcohol use, medical problems, or psychological problems may require special and individualized measures.
5. *Informed consent*. The risks of the procedure must be reviewed and any questions answered. The patient's ability to give informed consent must be reviewed with regard to her age, mental status, and any possibility of coercion. A support person may be present during any procedure.
6. *Postprocedure issues*. These include the need for any additional counseling, contraception, follow-up visits, and reporting any complications. Emerging evidence indicates that increasing use of contraceptive implants and intrauterine devices (IUDs) could reduce repeat pregnancy among adolescent mothers and repeat abortions among women seeking induced abortion. IUDs can be inserted immediately after a first-trimester surgical abortion.

Procedure

Before starting the procedure, the following steps must be completed:

1. *Pregnancy must be confirmed*. A home pregnancy test may not have been performed correctly, and therefore it is best to

confirm a pregnancy with an in-office urine pregnancy test or ultrasonography demonstrating an intrauterine pregnancy.

2. *Gestational age must be determined.* This can be accomplished by correlating weeks from the last normal menstrual period with a pelvic examination to size the uterus. Abnormal bleeding in pregnancy, contraception use, menstrual irregularities, and poor recall of dates, denial, and even the possibility of falsification may hinder a clinician in calculating an accurate gestational age from historical data. A pelvic examination to size the uterus requires practice and may be complicated when a patient is obese or uncooperative, has uterine fibroids or adnexal masses, or has a retroverted uterus. As a rough guideline, up to the sixth week of pregnancy, the uterus is the size of a plum in nulliparous women and the size of a pear in parous women. By 8 to 9 weeks the uterus is the size of a small orange but is softer and often asymmetrically enlarged. By 10 weeks the uterus is the size of a medium orange. By 12 weeks the uterus is as large as a grapefruit and becomes palpable suprapubically in thin or normal-weight women. A retroverted uterus will pop forward out of the pelvis between 12 and 13 weeks. By 15 or 16 weeks the uterus is the size of a cantaloupe. Ultrasonographic examination is highly accurate in dating a pregnancy, regardless of historical data or results of the physical examination. Ultrasonography also sheds light on several important complications of pregnancy such as first-trimester fetal demise, ectopic pregnancy, and gestational trophoblastic disease or molar pregnancy. Many clinicians routinely perform a dating ultrasonographic examination before planning abortion by uterine aspiration. Ultrasonography can also be useful during or after the procedure to confirm completion of the procedure. Intraoperative ultrasonographic guidance is recommended for women with uterine anomalies or fibroids. It can also be used if the clinician has difficulty with dilation or uterine aspiration.
3. Perform a *hematocrit or hemoglobin* if there is a history or clinical suspicion of anemia.
4. *Optional testing*, depending on patient risk factors, the nature of the practice, and financial considerations, includes wet prep, Papanicolaou smear, gonorrhea and chlamydia screening, and blood tests for syphilis and human immunodeficiency virus.
5. *Determine Rh factor status (mandatory)*. Rh-negative women who have been pregnant less than 13 weeks should receive a 50-μg dose of D immunoglobulin (MICRhoGAM 50 μg) within 48 hours of the procedure. It is ideally given during the procedure or immediately after. Some give the MICRhoGAM injection intracervically at the anterior lip where the cervical block was placed.
6. *Premedication* is recommended 30 to 60 minutes before the procedure with a nonsteroidal anti-inflammatory medication such as ibuprofen 600 to 800 mg orally. Diazepam (5 or 10 mg) or an oral narcotic may be given an hour before the procedure in selected cases.
7. Establishment of an *intravenous (IV) line generally is unnecessary* in an outpatient setting. Oxytocin, methylergonovine (Methergine), and other injectable drugs must be readily available should an unexpected hemorrhage occur. They can be administered intramuscularly when an IV line is not in place.
8. *Conscious sedation may be offered*. It is important that clinicians be aware of the rules and regulations regarding conscious sedation at their institutions before instituting this level of care. A simple and effective regimen is midazolam (Versed) given IV at the rate of 1 mg/min up to 5 mg, accompanied by fentanyl 50 to 100 μg IV. The patient should be monitored for respiratory depression with a pulse oximeter and frequent vital signs, and a crash cart should be available (see Chapter 2, Procedural Sedation and Analgesia).
9. *Atropine* 0.4 mg may be given IV or subcutaneously in patients with a history of a vagal reaction to prior cervical manipulations (e.g., bradycardia, fainting/loss of consciousness, diaphoresis, nausea).
10. *Prophylactic antibiotics* are a standard of care. A common regimen is doxycycline 100 mg twice daily for 3 days. Metronidazole (500 mg orally, twice daily for 2 days) is an option if the patient is allergic to doxycycline. Special consideration must be given to women with active infections, cardiac defects, prostheses, and other high-risk conditions (see Chapter 221, Antibiotic Prophylaxis).

Initial Steps

1. Position the patient in the dorsal lithotomy position using stirrups. The patient should have her buttocks at or slightly beyond the edge of the table.
2. If not already done, assess the shape, size, and position of the uterus by performing a bimanual examination.
3. Remove osmotic dilators, if placed previously.
4. After inserting the speculum, cleanse the cervix with sterile water or other antiseptic solution such as povidone–iodine.

Paracervical Block

1. Paracervical block (see Chapter 173, Paracervical Block, for additional information) is a simple, safe, and effective means of providing local anesthesia for abortion in the office setting (Fig. 127-5). The technique can vary, including the site of injection, type of anesthetic, and quantity of solution injected. Most clinicians limit the total amount of 1% lidocaine injected to 20 mL (or 0.5% lidocaine to 40 mL) to avoid lidocaine toxicity.

Cervical Preparation

The cervix may be dilated mechanically with plastic or metal dilators, or with the assistance of preprocedural *prostaglandins such as misoprostol*. Prostaglandins cause softening and dilation of the cervix as well as some uterine cramping. Misoprostol is the prostaglandin of choice because it is inexpensive, stable at room temperature, and effective in a variety of dosing routes, and has been shown to be

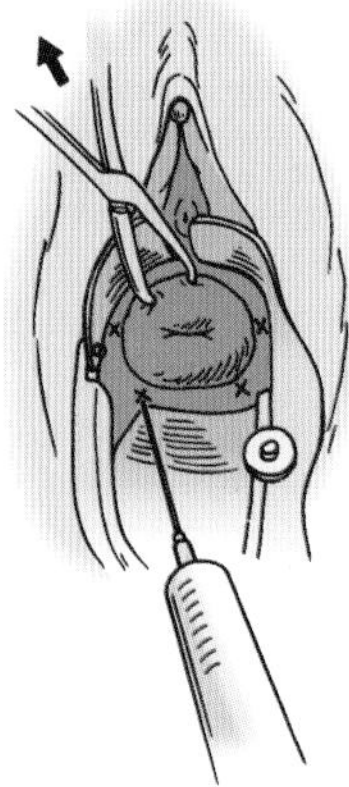

Figure 127-5 Paracervical block technique. "X" marks the locations where submucosal injections can be made. Ten milliliters of local anesthetic (1% lidocaine or 2% chloroprocaine) are injected with a 22-gauge needle into four sites at the 3, 5, 7, and 9 o'clock positions. (Some clinicians prefer to inject in the 4 and 8 o'clock positions only.) Ideally, the injection should be given submucosally, near the junction of the cervix and vagina. The injection should be superficial enough to raise a bleb or wheal under the mucosa. Because the area is vascular, care must be taken not to inject the anesthetic directly into a vessel. The tenaculum may be used to elevate the cervix and hold it to either side for better exposure of the injection sites.

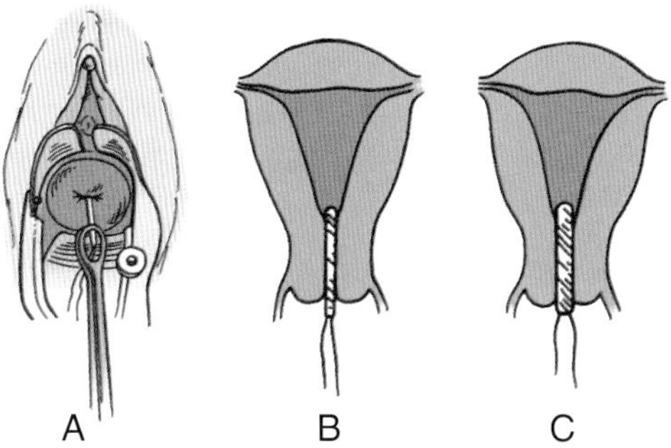

Figure 127-6 **A,** Insertion of the laminaria. **B,** Immediately after insertion. **C,** Twelve to 24 hours after insertion.

effective in first-trimester abortion. Several studies show that misoprostol, given vaginally, is more effective than given orally; buccal and sublingual dosing have also been documented as effective, but they both have more unwanted side effects than the vaginal route. Studies examining various doses found that 400 μg (vaginal or sublingual) is most effective and that higher doses were not necessary. Although not well studied, 400 μg by the buccal route is a commonly used alternative. Optimal dosing occurs when misoprostol is given 2 to 4 hours before the procedure; however, administration as late as 1 hour before the procedure can be helpful with cervical softening. Patients commonly experience some cramping and bleeding before the actual surgical procedure with this drug.

Laminaria is an option for dilation but it is less popular because it requires two visits to the office (Fig. 127-6). Some clinicians routinely use misoprostol for all women undergoing uterine aspiration in the outpatient setting regardless of gestational age. Other providers prefer laminaria for primiparous women over 10 to 12 weeks and multiparous women with an estimated gestational age of 12 weeks or greater. The Society of Family Planning guidelines for first-trimester abortion state that cervical ripening be *considered* for all adolescents and is recommended for any women at 12 to 14 weeks or if an initial attempt at dilation has been unsuccessful.

"No-Touch" Technique

Bacteria invariably contaminate the vagina and perineum during outpatient uterine aspiration procedures despite attempts at cleansing with povidone–iodine or other preparations. The operator's fingers are likely to become contaminated from the vagina and perineum during the introduction of the speculum despite the use of sterile gloves. The "no-touch" technique is based on the operator not touching the parts of the instruments that will enter the cervix. The dilators are grasped only in their midportion (Fig. 127-7), the cannula tip is not touched, and care is taken to prevent instruments that have been used from contaminating unused instruments.

Mechanical Dilation with Surgical Dilators

1. Apply a single-tooth tenaculum to the anterior or posterior cervical lip.
2. Gradually open the cervix by introducing progressively larger dilators (Fig. 127-8). Hold the dilator with a delicate pencil grip, in the middle of the dilator, using the no-touch technique.

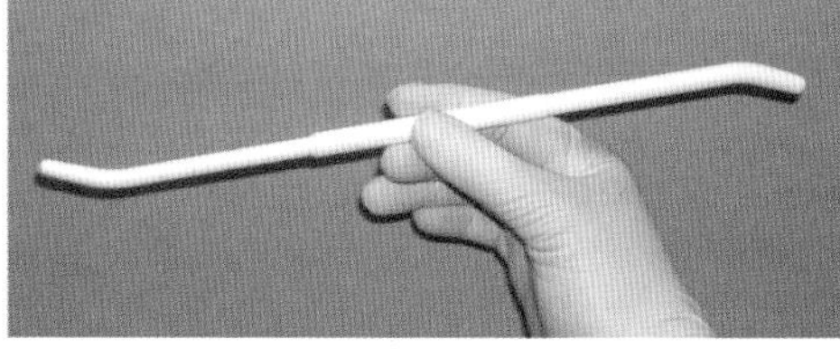

Figure 127-7 A Denniston dilator held using the "no-touch" technique.

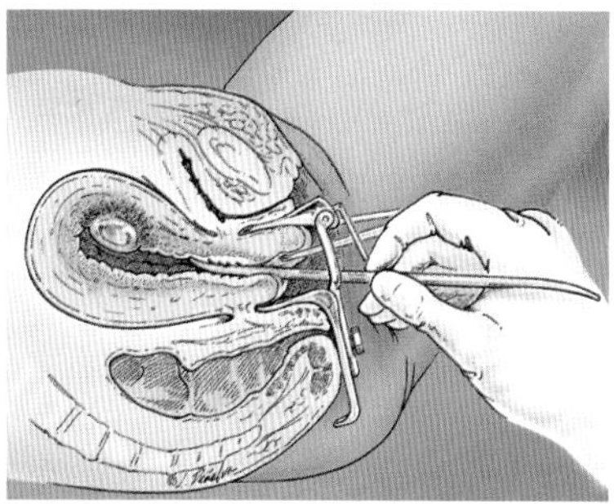

Figure 127-8 Dilation is needed when the cervical canal will not permit passage of a cannula of the appropriate size. (From ARHP [Association of Reproductive Health Professionals]: www.arhp.org.)

3. Pull gently on the cervix using the tenaculum to straighten out the endocervical canal while moving instruments into the uterus.
4. Apply enough pressure to move the dilator forward through the os and feel for a slight "pop" or giving sensation as the dilator passes through the internal os (see Fig. 127-8). Sometimes this sensation is not present if the patient has already undergone cervical ripening with misoprostol or laminaria.
5. Each dilator should be left in place for a few seconds before going to the next larger one.
6. Dilation is complete when the size of dilator matches the intended size of curette. Many clinicians prefer a cannula size with the millimeter diameter equal to or one size smaller than the gestational age of the patient. For example, if the patient is 9 weeks gestational age, an 8- or 9-mm cannula is used. Most patients experience some cramping during dilation.

Manual Vacuum Aspiration

A key component of MVA is the preparation and use of the syringe (Fig. 127-9).

1. Place the cannula into the cervical os of the uterus (Fig. 127-10). Take care to maintain the no-touch technique by touching only the end of the cannula that attaches to the aspirator, being careful not to touch the tip of the cannula with hands, the perineum, or the vagina.
2. With the Ipas-type MVA, suction is created by first pushing the buttons on the unit down and forward (see Fig. 127-9[1]).

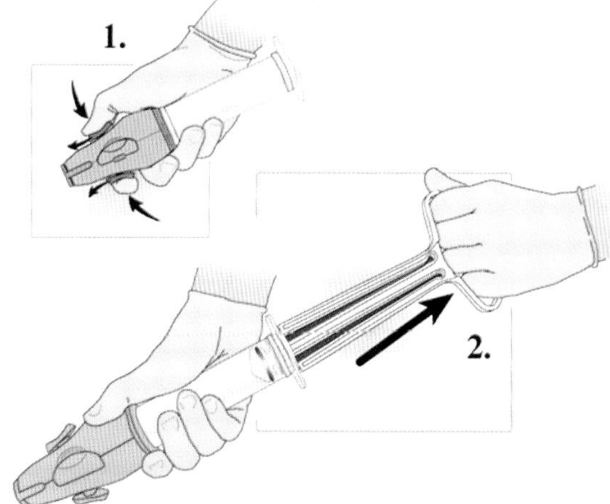

Figure 127-9 **1,** Begin with the valve buttons open and the plunger pushed all the way into the barrel. Close the valve by pushing the buttons down and forward until they lock into place. **2,** Pull the plunger back until its arms snap outward over the end of the syringe barrel. Make sure the plunger arms are positioned over the wide edges of the barrel. (Adapted from images of Ipas [www.ipas.org].)

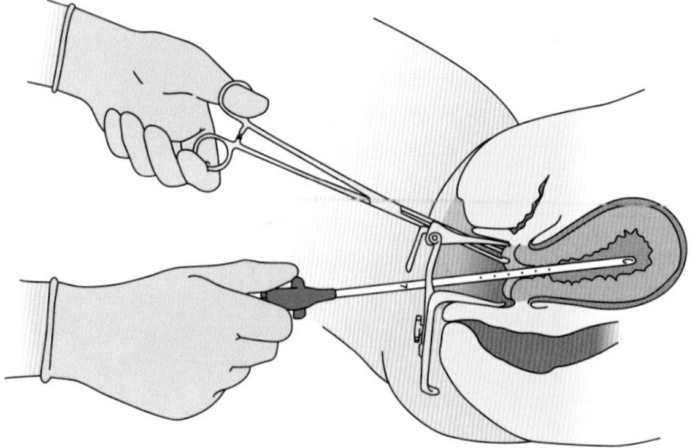

Figure 127-10 The cannula is inserted through the cervix with traction on the tenaculum to straighten the endocervical canal. (Adapted from images of Ipas [www.ipas.org].)

3. Draw back the plunger using a moderate amount of force to create the vacuum, until the wings of the plunger spring outward over the end of the syringe barrel (see Fig. 127-9[2]). This preserves the vacuum until the valve is opened.
4. Attach the aspirator to the cannula that has been placed into the uterus (Fig. 127-11).
5. Releasing the buttons in a backward direction activates the vacuum (Fig. 127-12).
6. Uterine aspiration is performed by holding the cylinder of the MVA device and using a combination of quick rotation and gentle back-and-forth movements (Fig. 127-13).
7. Watch the tissue that appears in the cannula and MVA cylinder to confirm correct cannula placement. Frequently, clear fluid is noted initially, followed by light tan, "fluffy" material, which is the remnants of the placenta and decidua mixed with blood. The appearance of abnormal tissue (such as omental fat or bowel) in the cannula is a sign of *perforation*. Absence of tissue is also important to note.
8. Withdraw the cannula and break suction to clear tubing. Empty the contents of the MVA cylinder into a metal bowl or emesis basin. The MVA device is emptied by pushing the plunger down through the cylinder.
9. The cannula can be reinserted into the cervical os, should an additional pass be desired. The MVA device can be recharged and attached to the cannula for additional passes into the uterus for aspiration.
10. Aspiration should be repeated until there is no tissue noted in the cannula or syringe.
11. As the uterus is evacuated, it tends to clamp down, creating a gritty sensation with the cannula. Patients will experience more discomfort at this point.
12. If the abortion is not complete based on clinical or ultrasonographic diagnosis, then a medium-sharp uterine curette can be used to curette and feel all quadrants of the uterine cavity. A clean uterus will have a firm, slightly gritty or rough feel. Additional tissue adherent to the uterine walls feels spongy or slippery. Alternatively, a small ring forceps or stone polyp forceps may be used to grasp within the uterine cavity for any additional tissue. Particular caution should be used to avoid perforation when placing metal instruments into the uterus.
13. If sharp curettage is used, a final pass with the cannula and MVA device should be done to remove any debris or blood.
14. Follow-up transvaginal ultrasonography may be performed immediately after the procedure to demonstrate that the gestational sac and POC have been removed from the uterus.
15. The procedure is now completed. Remove the tenaculum and clean the vagina with gauze and check for signs of bleeding or cervical tears.
16. Once the vaginal check is complete, the speculum should be removed and the perineum should be wiped down to clear any blood or other fluids that may have collected from the procedure.
17. Observe the patient for 10 to 15 minutes for bleeding or any unusual reaction. If sedation or general anesthesia was used, follow the appropriate guidelines for postprocedure monitoring.
18. The patient is then free to leave, with appropriate follow-up information (see the sample patient education handout, "Instructions after Termination of Pregnancy," online at www.expertconsult.com).
19. Examine all tissue using the "float test" to identify POC immediately after the procedure. This step is particularly important in very early abortions, procedures in which scant tissue is obtained, and in patients who are at risk for ectopic pregnancy. The tissue obtained should be washed free of blood with saline or tap water in a strainer. Fragments of tissue can then be suspended in any clear fluid—saline, tap water, and formalin all work—and carefully inspected. Placental tissue has a characteristic "fronding" or finely arborized appearance because of the villi. Backlighting and low-power magnification such with as a colposcope or a magnifying glass is helpful. With a little

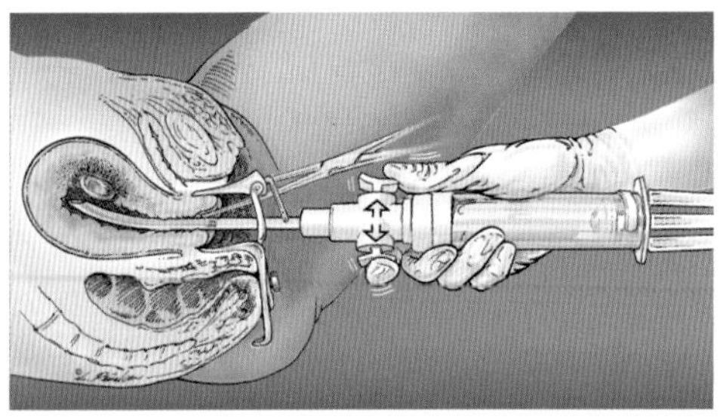

Figure 127-12 Releasing the pinch valve transfers the vacuum through the cannula to the uterus. (From ARHP [Association of Reproductive Health Professionals]: www.arhp.org.)

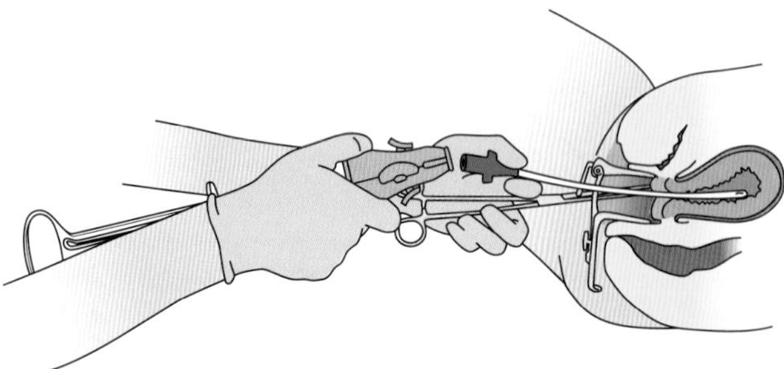

Figure 127-11 Aspirator is attached to the cannula. Alternatively, the cannula may be attached to the aspirator at the time of initial insertion of the cannula. (Adapted from images of Ipas [www.ipas.org].)

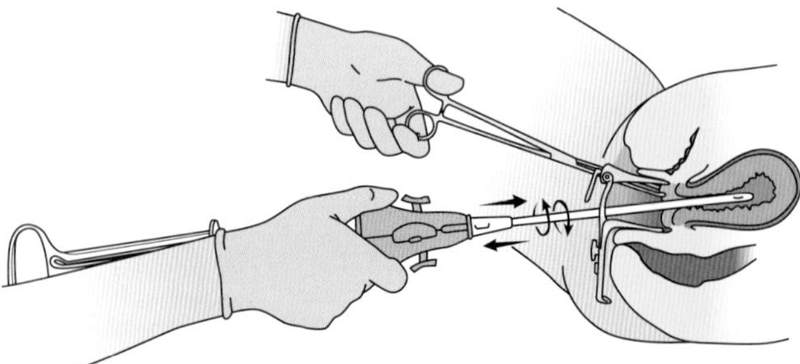

Figure 127-13 Rotating the syringe moves the cannula gently back and forth. Do not withdraw cannula aperture(s) beyond cervical os. Do not grasp syringe by the plunger arms. Blood, tissue, and bubbles will flow through the cannula into the syringe. (Adapted from images of Ipas [www.ipas.org].)

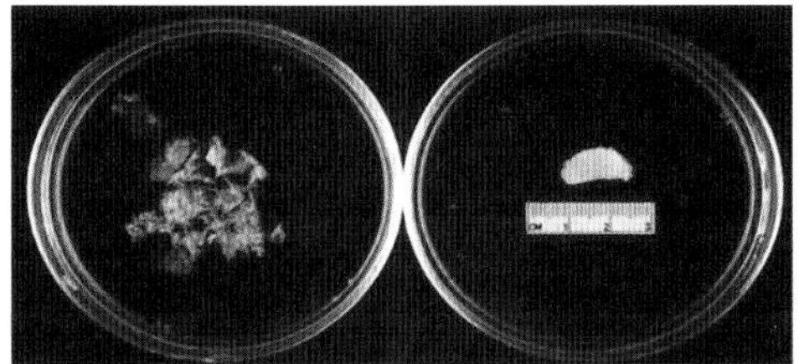

Figure 127-14 Five-week gestational sac aspirated by manual *(right)* or electric *(left)* vacuum aspiration. Note that the sac appears intact after manual vacuum aspiration. (From ARHP [Association of Reproductive Health Professionals]: www.arhp.org.)

practice, the gestational sac and placental tissue can be distinguished easily from decidua and clot (Fig. 127-14).

20. In some states, the uterine contents must be sent for confirmation of tissue by a pathologist. It is important that clinicians be aware of the laws in their states.

Suction Abortion (Electrical Pump)

An electrical vacuum pump is the predominant mode of aspiration in many U.S. clinics. Electric power allows for constant flow of suction, which many providers find convenient—particularly for later first-trimester gestations. Rigid disposable plastic cannulas are usually used with machine suction. The *disadvantages* of machine suction are the cost of the machine itself, which may not be affordable in offices that perform uterine aspiration only periodically, as well as the noise, which may not be acceptable in some clinical settings. Performing uterine aspiration with machine suction is similar to using MVA, except that the machine creates suction with an electrical pump.

1. Attach the suction machine to the cannula by means of the tubing. Do not activate the suction yet. *The suction is controlled with the slide control on the handle*. It is *not* necessary to turn the machine on and off. Insert the cannula into the uterus.
2. Close the valve on the handle to create intrauterine suction. A suction pressure of 55 to 75 mm Hg or greater is required to accomplish the procedure. If suction is inadequate, there is probably a leak in the system that should be identified and corrected.
3. Rotate the handle on the tubing as you would with the MVA, and watch the tissue that appears in the curette and tubing.
4. After several rotations in each direction, remove the curette while the suction is still on. Reinsert it into the uterus with the suction off. Turn the suction back on, rotate, and remove it again, repeating this until no further tissue is seen in the curette. Even with disposable rigid cannulas, the uterus should feel smaller at the end of the procedure and the operator should feel some sense of "grittiness," although not as great as felt when using MVA.
5. Inspect the uterine contents as described in step no. 19 under Manual Vacuum Aspiration.

Sample Procedure Note

The patient presents to clinic today requesting an elective abortion. She is a G**P** with an LMP of (date) and estimated gestational age (weeks). She is Rh+. The patient was counseled on all of her options and she is sure of her decision. The patient was informed of the risks and benefits of the manual vacuum aspiration procedure and all questions were answered. The patient was informed about the possibility of perforation, infection, bleeding, pain, and missing some tissue. Diazepam (Valium) 10 mg PO and ibuprofen 800 mg PO were given preoperatively. Patient was taken to the procedure room and placed in the dorsal lithotomy position. Bimanual exam revealed an anteverted uterus measuring about 8 weeks' gestation. Speculum placed without difficulty. Cervix cleansed with Betadine. Approximately 2 mL of 1% lidocaine with epinephrine was placed at the anterior lip. A sharp-tooth tenaculum was placed on the anterior lip. Another 8 mL of lidocaine was placed at the cervicovaginal junction at 4 o'clock and 8 mL placed at 8 o'clock. Cervix was dilated with Dennison dilators to 8 mm. An 8-mm cannula was inserted without difficulty and uterine contents were aspirated without incident. The uterine cavity was explored with forceps and no residual tissue was found. Tenaculum removed. Minimal bleeding at tenaculum site. Patient tolerated procedure well. No complications. Estimated blood loss (EBL) = 30 mL.

Gross inspection of the POC revealed villi and gestational sac consistent with 8-week gestation. POC were then placed in sterile urine cup with formalin and sent to pathology.

Patient recovered in procedure room for 20 minutes after procedure. Vital signs were reassessed and were stable, and patient reported minimal cramping. Patient was released to home at (time) and given printed instruction sheets as well as emergency numbers of the clinic. She was also given an oral contraceptive pill prescription to start this evening. (Alternatively, the Copper T 380A IUD was inserted without difficulty.) Patient agreed with plan and verbalized understanding of instructions. Patient is to follow up for a postoperative visit in 1 to 2 weeks or if experiencing any problems whatsoever.

Common Errors

1. *Poor speculum placement* is a common error that can make the procedure more cumbersome than necessary. A speculum placed too anterior to the cervix elongates and narrows the working space needed to perform the procedure. In addition, it can lead to expulsion of the speculum, which can be problematic, particularly if instruments are already on or in the cervix.
2. *Inadequate traction on the tenaculum* placed on the cervix. Tenaculum traction is essential so that the endocervical canal can straighten and decrease the angle between the cervix and the uterine cavity during dilation. This is important to decrease the risk of creating a false passageway or uterine perforation. Some clinicians fear traction will cause the patient to feel pain or cause the tenaculum to rip away from the cervix. It is important that the tenaculum is placed with a large enough "bite" so that there is adequate tissue to hold the tenaculum. A vertical placement of the tenaculum through the cervical os often provides a firm purchase on the cervix when it is short.

Complications

Less than 0.5% of women experience a complication during a first-trimester surgical abortion, and the risk of death is about one-tenth that during childbirth. However, complications can and do occur, including those resulting in major disability or even death. Careful attention to technique and constant vigilance for complications are mandatory. Complications may occur before the uterine aspiration procedure (*misdiagnosis, problems with laminaria, or problems with a paracervical block*), during the process of dilation and aspiration (*hemorrhage, uterine perforation, inability to evacuate the uterus*), or after the patient has returned home (*infection, retained POC, hematometra*).

Preprocedure Complications

- *Misdiagnosis* may occur when a woman presenting for a first-trimester abortion procedure has an ectopic pregnancy, a miscarriage, or advanced gestational age. *Ectopic pregnancy* may be suspected when preprocedure ultrasonography does not show a gestational sac with a yolk sac or fetal pole and the float test of the tissue obtained from such a procedure shows only decidua and not the actual POC. In these cases, additional studies, such as

ultrasonography and serial quantitative β-human chorionic gonadotropin (hCG) determinations, are indicated.
- *Miscarriage* or early pregnancy failure occurs in about 15% of clinically diagnosed pregnancies. Symptoms include bleeding, cramping, and passage of tissue. Modern means of diagnosing miscarriage in the first trimester include transvaginal ultrasonography and serial quantitative hCG determinations. Patients who are already bleeding may request an abortion and may want to have uterine aspiration even if a nonviable pregnancy is diagnosed or suspected. Alternatively, a woman may elect to initiate expectant management for miscarriage and defer uterine aspiration.
- *Advanced gestational age can become a complication* if the practitioner initiates a procedure that is beyond his or her training or clinical setting because of inaccurate gestational age dating based on misinterpretation of ultrasonographic or bimanual examination findings. Adnexal masses or uterine fibroids may render bimanual examination less accurate. Fortunately, this will usually result in an overestimation of gestational age rather than underestimation.
- If *laminaria* have been placed they *may fall out, migrate up into the uterus, or fragment*. If the laminaria falls out before dilation is effected, mechanical dilation or replacement of the laminaria will be required. Occasionally, the internal os will be stenotic and the laminaria may assume an hourglass configuration, which makes it difficult to remove because the part of the laminaria that is in the intrauterine space is larger than the narrowed, stenotic os. If migration or fragmentation (a piece breaks off and remains intrauterine) is suspected, a careful search of the uterine cavity must be carried out to remove it. Occasionally, a patient will change her mind after the laminaria has been placed. The laminaria can be removed at any time, and in most cases the pregnancy will continue unaffected. However, the patient must be warned of the risk of miscarriage.
- Some patients may experience a *vasovagal reaction* during laminaria placement or at other times during or after the procedure. Vasovagal reactions involve bradycardia, diaphoresis, nausea, and (rarely) convulsions. Atropine may be administered for treatment and prevention (0.4 mg IV or subcutaneously); the patient's legs should be elevated and her head lowered. If the patient admits to having a low pain threshold or tendency to faint easily, atropine may be given prophylactically 15 to 30 minutes before laminaria placement or the aspiration procedure. Alternatively, atropine may be added to the paracervical block.

Procedural Complications

- The *paracervical block injection can cause some bleeding* at the sites of injection. Intravascular injection is common despite efforts to prevent it. Patients may experience dysphoria, tinnitus, an unusual taste in the mouth, and visual disturbances. These sensations are transient. Severe reactions, such as convulsions or allergic reactions, are rare.
- The clinician may be *unable to successfully dilate the cervix* and enter the uterine cavity. A decision can be made to defer the procedure until after the placement of laminaria or use of misoprostol for cervical ripening.
- *Uterine fibroids* may prevent or limit access to the uterine cavity. Performing the procedure under ultrasonographic guidance may be the only recourse. *Duplication anomalies of the female genital tract* result from the failure of the uterus to fuse completely during embryonic development; these anomalies range from arcuate uterus to total duplication of the cervix and uterus in uterus didelphys. The critical point in abortion in a woman with a duplicated system is determining the location of the pregnancy and gaining access to it. Rarely, a pregnancy in a hemiuterine horn is inaccessible to surgical evacuation. Mifepristone medical abortion might be the preferred method in women at less than 63 days' estimated gestational age with complex uterine anomalies or fibroids preventing easy access to the uterine cavity.
- *Uterine perforation* is an uncommon but feared complication that occurs in less than 1 per 1000 procedures. It is generally asymptomatic if caused during the dilation phase. If it occurs with suctioning, then the *perforation may be* identified by increased pain, hemorrhage, or signs of an acute abdomen. Fat or bowel tissue observed in the suction apparatus is diagnostic, as is passing a blunt instrument up through the perforation. Visualization of the cul de sac by transvaginal or abdominal ultrasonography may point to the possibility of internal bleeding. A culdocentesis is another option to help confirm bleeding (see Chapter 136, Cervical Stenosis and Cervical Dilation). Treatment must be individualized and depends on whether the abortion is complete and whether there is the likelihood of intra-abdominal injury. Minimum treatment includes close observation for 2 to 4 hours or overnight in an inpatient setting. Outpatient observation is reasonable if the perforation did not result in fat or bowel tissue aspiration and there is no abdominal pain or rebound tenderness or evidence of intra-abdominal bleeding. If the risk of hemorrhage or visceral injury is great, laparoscopy or laparotomy may be necessary. If perforation occurs before the uterus is emptied, the procedure may be completed under laparoscopic guidance.
- *Hemorrhage* occurring during the procedure *suggests laceration or perforation or, more commonly, uterine atony* with incomplete evacuation of the uterus. Coagulopathy is an uncommon cause of hemorrhage. *Lacerations* of the cervix can sometimes occur on the ectocervix because of a tenaculum tearing off during the process of cervical dilation. These are usually quite superficial, and bleeding will usually stop with tamponade. Suturing is rarely needed. Puncture sites on the cervix can also bleed briskly and respond to tamponade with the clamping of the ring forceps for a few minutes. Monsel's solution or silver nitrate may be applied to achieve hemostasis if bleeding does not resolve with pressure or packing.
- *Atony* occurs infrequently but the risk increases when the pregnancy is greater than 10 weeks' gestation. Methylergonovine (Methergine) 0.2 mg intramuscularly or orally may be helpful, and some clinicians use methylergonovine routinely when terminating pregnancies of 8–10 weeks and beyond. Misoprostol may be given in an 800-μg dose by rectal or buccal route for atony. Carboprost tromethamine injection (Hemabate; Pharmacia-Upjohn Pharmaceuticals [Pfizer], NY) given intramuscularly or directly into the cervix is indicated if atony is severe. Retained POC because of incomplete evacuation may be present along with atony. The procedure must be repeated if retained POC are suspected. If bleeding is severe, repeating the procedure may require deeper anesthesia to ensure complete evacuation of all tissue.

Postprocedure Complications

- *Excessive bleeding* in the days or weeks after the abortion suggests incomplete abortion, which may be accompanied by infection. Alternatively, a hematometra may have developed in which blood clots gradually fill the uterine cavity and are unable to easily pass through the cervix. Repeating the procedure is the best course for retained POC or hematometra.
- *Postabortal infection*, or endometritis, is relatively common but not usually severe. Symptoms of endometritis include uterine tenderness, lower abdominal pain, fever, and elevated white blood cell count. Oral antibiotics may be prescribed; however, repeat suction curettage may be required. Rarely, a patient will have severe sepsis or septic shock and require aggressive treatment, including hospital admission, broad-spectrum IV antibiotics (e.g., gentamicin and clindamycin), fluids, and even hysterectomy.
- *Late sequelae*, such as *infertility, premature labor, and incompetent cervix*, have been studied extensively and are not thought to be associated with first-trimester aspiration procedures using modern

methods. Asherman's syndrome is the formation of intrauterine or cervical adhesions after curettage. Because uterine aspiration has replaced curettage as the primary technique of first-trimester abortion Asherman's syndrome is a very uncommon complication and usually involves cervical rather than intrauterine adhesions. The cervical adhesions can be treated by using small dilators to reopen the endocervical canal.

Postprocedure Management

Doxycycline 100 mg orally twice a day for 3 days is recommended as routine surgical prophylaxis, with the first dose given before or soon after the procedure. *Methylergonovine* 0.2 mg administered orally every 6 hours for six doses is occasionally given to assist in contracting the uterus and preventing bleeding in women having aspiration abortion after 10–12 weeks gestational age or experiencing postprocedure bleeding because of uterine atony. If the provider is concerned that the patient may have more bleeding than usual, *misoprostol* can be given, although the U.S. Food and Drug Administration has not approved its use in this manner. *Effective contraception* should be offered to the patient and prescribed or provided the same day the abortion is performed. Intrauterine devices may be placed immediately after the conclusion of a first-trimester uterine aspiration abortion. Hormonal contraceptives may be started the same day of an abortion procedure.

Postprocedure Patient Education

No sexual activity is advisable for 1 week. Also see the sample patient education form available online at www.expertconsult.com.

Interpretation of Results

The POC must be examined after the procedure either by the float test or by sending them to a laboratory for pathology. In states that do not require pathologic examination, many operators will defer sending POC for pathologic analysis. If scant tissue is noted or a molar pregnancy is suspected based on ultrasonographic findings or gross review of the POC, evaluation by a pathologist should be considered. If the pathology is read as consistent with a molar or partial molar pregnancy, then appropriate follow-up with a clinician skilled in the management of gestational trophoblastic disease is essential. In addition, a pathology report that notes trophoblastic tissue inconsistent with preprocedural gestational age assessment requires follow-up. The patient should be contacted and reassessed with a repeat bimanual examination, ultrasonography, or serial quantitative hCG determinations, as indicated.

Patient Education Guides

See the sample patient education and consent forms available online at www.expertconsult.com.

CPT/Billing Codes

59200 Insertion of cervical dilator (e.g., laminaria, prostaglandin)
59812 Treatment of incomplete abortion, any semester, completed surgically
59820 Treatment of missed abortion, completed surgically, first trimester
59821 Treatment of missed abortion, completed surgically, second trimester
59830 Treatment of septic abortion, completed surgically
59840 Induced abortion, by dilation and curettage
59841 Induced abortion, by dilation and curettage and evacuation
59855 Induced abortion, by one or more vaginal suppositories (e.g., prostaglandin) with or without cervical dilation (e.g., laminaria), including hospital admission and visits

ICD-9-CM Diagnostic Codes

622.4 Cervical stenosis
632 Abortion, missed
634.91 Abortion, spontaneous, incomplete
634.92 Abortion, spontaneous, complete
635.90 Abortion, elective
637.90 Abortion, inevitable
637.91 Abortion, incomplete
637.92 Abortion, complete
640.00 Abortion, threatened, unspecified
646.30 Abortion, habitual or recurrent

Acknowledgment

The editors wish to recognize the contributions by Steven H. Eisinger, MD, to this chapter in the previous edition of this text, titled First-Trimester Abortion and Emergency Oral Contraceptives.

Suppliers

(See contact information online at www.expertconsult.com.)

All special equipment, including suction machines,* hosing, curettes, dilators, laminaria, and ancillary instruments
Berkeley Medevices, Inc.
Manual vacuum aspiration syringes
HPSRx Enterprises, Inc.
Ipas
Most instruments are available from general medical suppliers or the following sources:
Cheshire Medical Specialties, Inc.
Gynex
MedGyn
Wallach Surgical Devices, Inc.
Portable ultrasonography
SonoSite Inc.

ONLINE RESOURCES

Additional Resources for Clinicians

Advancing New Standards in Reproductive Health (ANSIRH), Early Abortion Project: A group that has developed training resources for primary care clinicians learning to provide abortion care. Online and downloadable versions of the Early Abortion Training Workbook available at www.ansirh.org/training/workbook.php.

Association of Reproductive Health Professionals (ARHP): Offers up-to-date slide presentations and Internet presentations on the use of MVA for the treatment of miscarriage or induced abortion. Available at www.arhp.org.

Ipas: Provides additional information regarding MVA and electrical aspiration. Available at www.ipas.org.

National Abortion Federation (NAF): The NAF provides many resources for physicians providing abortion services. Available at www.prochoice.org. Information on surgical abortion services and the NAF Clinical Practice Guidelines is available at www.prochoice.org/education/resources/surgical.html.

Reproductive Health Access Project: Website includes guidelines, office forms, consents, and other resources for primary care clinicians offering abortion services. Available at www.reproductiveaccess.org/.

RHEDI: RHEDI, the Center for Reproductive Health EDucation In Family Medicine, is dedicated to the goal of integrating high-quality comprehensive abortion and family planning training into U.S. family medicine residency programs. Available at www.rhedi.org.

Society of Family Planning provides evidence-based insight to improve clinical care in the areas of contraception and abortion. Evidence-based clinical guidelines are available on their website: www.societyfp.org.

---

*A Gomco suction unit, which many offices have for other purposes, can also be used. The pressure is set between 50 and 60 mm Hg.

Counseling Resource for Patients

Exhale: A talk line for women who would like to discuss their experience with abortion (available in other languages, including Spanish, Vietnamese, Chinese). Available at www.4exhale.org.

BIBLIOGRAPHY

Allen R, O'Brien BM: Use of misoprostol in obstetrics and gynecology. Rev Obstet Gynecol 2:159–168, 2009.

Allen RH, Goldberg AB, Board of Society of Family Planning: Cervical dilation before first trimester surgical abortion (<14 weeks' gestation). SFP Guideline 2007. Contraception 76:139–156, 2007.

American College of Obstetricians and Gynecologists: Medical management of abortion. ACOG Practice Bulletin No. 67. Washington, DC, ACOG, October 2005.

American College of Obstetricians and Gynecologists: Antibiotic prophylaxis for gynecologic procedures. ACOG Practice Bulletin No. 104. Washington DC, ACOG, May 2009.

American College of Obstetricians and Gynecologists: Misoprostol for postabortion care. ACOG Committee Opinion No. 427. Obstet Gynecol 113:465–468, 2009.

American College of Obstetricians and Gynecologists Committee on Gynecologic Practice, Long-Acting Reversible Contraception Working Group: Increasing use of contraceptive implants and intrauterine devices to reduce unintended pregnancy. ACOG Committee Opinion No. 450. Obstet Gynecol 114:1434–1438, 2009.

Blumenthal PD, Remsburg RE: A time and cost analysis of the management of incomplete abortion with manual vacuum aspiration. Int J Gynaecol Obstet 45:261–267, 1994.

Christin-Maitre S, Bouchard P, Spitz I: Medical termination of pregnancy. N Engl J Med 342:946–956, 2000.

Creinin MD, Edwards J: Early abortion: Surgical and medical options. Curr Probl Obstet Gynecol Fertil 20:1–32, 1997.

Fiala C, Gemzell-Danielsson K, Tang OS, von Hertzen H: Cervical priming with misoprostol prior to transcervical procedures. Int J Gynaecol Obstet 99(Suppl 2):S168–S171, 2007.

Glick E: Surgical Abortion. Reno, Nev, West End Women's Medical Group, 1998.

Goldberg AB, Dean G, Kang MS, et al: Manual versus electric vacuum aspiration for early first-trimester abortion: A controlled study of complication rates. Obstet Gynecol 103:101–107, 2004.

Keder LM: Best practices in surgical abortion. Am J Obstet Gynecol 189:418–422, 2003.

Lichtenberg ES, Shott S: A randomized clinical trial of prophylaxis for vacuum abortion: 3 versus 7 days of doxycycline. Obstet Gynecol 101:726–731, 2003.

Lyus RJ, Gianutsos P, Gold M: First trimester procedural abortion in family medicine. J Am Board Fam Med 22:169–174, 2009.

Macisaac L, Grossman D, Balistreri E, Darney P: A randomized controlled trial of laminaria, oral misoprostol, and vaginal misoprostol before abortion. Obstet Gynecol 93:766–770, 1999.

National Abortion Federation: Clinical Policy Guidelines. Washington, DC, National Abortion Federation, 2005.

National Abortion Federation: Medical Education Series—Early Options: A Provider's Guide to Medical Abortion [training and resource binder]. Washington, DC, National Abortion Federation, 2001.

Panchal HB, Godfrey EM, Patel A: Buccal misoprostol for cervical ripening prior to first trimester abortion. Contraception 81:161–164, 2010.

Paul M, Lichtenberg S, Borgatta L, et al (eds): Management of Unintended and Abnormal Pregnancy: Comprehensive Abortion Care. San Francisco, Wiley-Blackwell, 2009.

Paul M, Stewart FH, Goodman S, Wolfe M, for the TEACH Trainers Collaborative Working Group: Early Abortion Training Workbook, 2nd ed. San Francisco, UCSF Center for Reproductive Health Research & Policy, 2004.

Policar MJ, Pollack AE: Clinical Training Curriculum in Abortion Practice. Washington, DC, National Abortion Federation, 1995.

Sawaya GF, Grady D, Kerlikowske K, et al: Antibiotics at time of induced abortion: The case for universal prophylaxis based on a meta-analysis. Obstet Gynecol 87:884–890, 1996.

Stubblefield PG, Carr-Ellis S, Borgatta L: Methods for induced abortion. Obstet Gynecol 104:174–185, 2004.

Swingle HM, Colaizy TT, Zimmerman MB, Morriss FH Jr: Abortion and the risk of subsequent preterm birth: A systematic review with meta-analysis. J Reprod Med 54:95–108, 2009.

CHAPTER 128

Pregnancy Termination: Medication Abortion

Ruth Lesnewski • Linda Prine

Medication abortion is the elective termination of a pregnancy using pharmaceuticals. Since 2000, when mifepristone became available in the United States, mifepristone/misoprostol has been the most commonly used medication abortion regimen in this country. Alternate regimens use methotrexate/misoprostol or misoprostol only. Medications can be used to end an unintended pregnancy of up to 7 to 9 weeks' gestational age, depending on the regimen available. Medication abortion has proven to be remarkably safe and effective, and it provides women with an alternative to surgical abortion.

Selecting Medication or Surgical Abortion

Women with unintended pregnancy often present to their primary care provider for pregnancy diagnosis and counseling, treatment, or referral. Physicians who do not offer abortion in their office can counsel women about the factors influencing selection of medication or aspiration abortion methods. Table 128-1 provides an overview of both methods. Although aspiration abortion is quicker and slightly more effective, medication abortion offers women more privacy, less instrumentation, and a feeling of control over the experience (see Chapter 127, Pregnancy Termination: First-Trimester Suction Aspiration). Because medication regimens involve cramping and bleeding at home, women who choose medication abortion should have a safe, supportive environment available to them. Women who select medication abortion must agree to return for a follow-up visit and to have an aspiration procedure if the medications fail.

Indication

Elective termination of pregnancy (up to 63 days' gestation with some regimens) is the indication for medication abortion.

Contraindications

Absolute

- Ectopic pregnancy (mifepristone/misoprostol protocols)
- Uncertain gestational age (must establish gestational age before procedure)

Relative

- Adrenal failure
- Severe asthma
- Long-term systemic glucocorticoid therapy
- Intrauterine contraceptive device in place (must be removed before procedure)
- Anticoagulation
- Severe anemia

Equipment and Supplies

Physicians must order mifepristone directly from its manufacturer and have a prescriber's agreement in place with the manufacturer (available at www.earlyoptionpill.com). This medication cannot be obtained from pharmacies. If possible, physicians should order misoprostol as well and dispense it directly to patients; otherwise, patients may have difficulty obtaining misoprostol as quickly as needed. Routine ultrasonography is not required. However, clinicians need access to ultrasonography (either in-office or by referral) for women with an uncertain last menstrual period, size/dates discrepancy, or increased risk of ectopic pregnancy.

Preprocedure Patient Education

Patients who undergo mifepristone/misoprostol abortion must read the Medication Guide (see Guide online at www.earlyoptionpill.com/userfiles/file/Med%20Guide%204-22-09%20Final.pdf) produced by Danco Laboratories (New York), mifepristone's sole

TABLE 128-1 Comparison of Medication and Aspiration Abortion

Medication Abortion	Aspiration Abortion
Suitable for early pregnancy only	Suitable for early and later pregnancy
Medications only	Surgical procedure
Higher level of patient involvement	Lower level of patient involvement
Abortion may take place in the clinician's office (FDA protocol) or at home (updated protocol)	Occurs in office, clinic, or hospital
Takes two to three visits over several days; sometimes longer	Takes one to two visits; the actual procedure is brief
High success rate (>96%), but some chance of failure	Very high success rate (>98%)
Requires careful patient follow-up	Requires follow-up
Oral pain medication over several hours	Local or intravenous sedation or general anesthesia
Treats missed abortion	Treats missed abortion
Does not treat ectopic pregnancy (mifepristone/misoprostol)	Does not treat ectopic pregnancy
Resembles miscarriage	Surgical procedure
May be more private	Requires office or clinic visits during surgical hours; may be less private

FDA, U.S. Food and Drug Administration

U.S. manufacturer (see Online Resources). Patients must then sign Danco's Patient Agreement (Fig. 128-1). Clinicians must also provide patients with an office-specific consent form (Fig. 128-2; see also at www.expertconsult.com), which describes the risks, benefits, and possible complications as well as the correct dosing and administration of both medications. After obtaining informed consent, clinicians should have women sign the consent form. Clinicians should also review the misoprostol aftercare instructions (Figs. 128-3 and 128-4) with their patients carefully to ensure that they understand guidelines for administering misoprostol at home, and to ensure that the practitioner's contact information is clear.

Procedure

Mifepristone and Misoprostol

Mifepristone is a progestin blocker that causes decidual necrosis. *Misoprostol* is a prostaglandin analog that causes uterine contraction and expulsion of pregnancy. Mifepristone/misoprostol abortion involves several steps and at least two office visits. The physician determines, by history, ultrasonography, or bimanual sizing with a quantitative human chorionic gonadotropin (hCG) level, that the pregnancy is less than 7 to 9 weeks (depending on regimen). After pregnancy dating confirmation, options counseling, selection of method, and completion of necessary paperwork, the patient takes mifepristone orally in the physician's office. Six to 72 hours later (depending on the protocol in use), she takes misoprostol at home. Misoprostol can be used orally, vaginally, or buccally. The dosing and timing of administration vary according to route; see Table 128-2 for details. Soon after she takes misoprostol, the patient experiences cramping and bleeding. At first, cramps can be quite intense, often requiring a combination of nonsteroidal anti-inflammatory drug and a mild narcotic. The bleeding that follows may be heavy, with large clots. The patient should call her clinician if she bleeds enough to soak through more than two pads per hour for 2 consecutive hours. Cramps and bleeding decrease in intensity after the first few hours but can persist in a milder form for 3 weeks or more. Bleeding sometimes lasts long enough to blend into the woman's next menses.

Rh-negative women should receive Rh immune globulin. A 50-μg dose (MICRhoGAM) should be given before using misoprostol or within 72 hours of bleeding. Patients should be informed that this medication is a human blood derivative. Patients who refuse the injection should sign a statement documenting their decision.

Four to 14 days after the initial visit, the patient returns for follow-up. At this visit, the physician confirms the procedure's success by history and by either repeating the ultrasonographic examination or repeating the quantitative hCG (depending on which was done at the initial visit). The physician also revisits the woman's choice of an ongoing contraceptive method. If the quantitative hCG is repeated, it will drop by 75% from the previous week, indicating the success of the medication abortion.

The U.S. Food and Drug Administration (FDA) approved mifepristone in 2000, using evidence from studies completed in 1996 and earlier. After 1996, further research on medication abortion led to simpler, more convenient protocols with higher efficacy and lower cost. Table 128-2 compares the FDA protocol with two updated protocols. Most clinicians in the United States use an updated protocol for mifepristone/misoprostol abortion.

Methotrexate and Misoprostol and Misoprostol-Only Regimens

Of the three most commonly used medication abortion regimens, mifepristone/misoprostol has the highest efficacy and best side effect profile. Methotrexate/misoprostol, used in the United States before mifepristone's release, works over weeks rather than days, requires multiple office visits, and can be used in pregnancies of less than 8 weeks' gestation. Methotrexate has the advantage of treating early ectopic pregnancy, whereas mifepristone and misoprostol regimens do *not* end ectopic pregnancies. Misoprostol-only regimens require several doses, each with significant side effects. This regimen has widespread lay use in countries where abortion remains legally restricted or is too expensive.

Sample Procedure Notes

See Initial Visit Note and Follow-up Visit Note (Figs. 128-5 and 128-6) for examples of documentation for the mifepristone/misoprostol regimen.

Complications

Mifepristone causes far fewer side effects than does misoprostol. *Misoprostol's side effects include nausea, vomiting, fever, chills, and uterine cramping.* Vaginal or buccal administration causes fewer side effects than oral administration. Misoprostol is believed to be a teratogen when administered in early pregnancy if abortion should fail to occur.

Although all are uncommon, the major complications of mifepristone/misoprostol abortion are continuation of the pregnancy, retained products of conception, heavy bleeding, and infection. Continuation of pregnancy may occur slightly more often with later gestational age. Overall, the rate of continuing pregnancy is under 1%. Incomplete abortion—that is, failure to expel all pregnancy tissue with medications alone—occurs in 0.6% to 3% of women. The rate depends in part on clinicians' and patients' threshold for resorting to an aspiration procedure. Cramping and bleeding are expected with medication abortion, but bleeding heavy enough to require emergency care (or heavy enough to require transfusion) occurs in fewer than 0.1% of patients. The treatment for continuing pregnancy, retained products of conception, and heavy bleeding is the same: a uterine aspiration procedure.

Endometritis after medication abortion is extremely rare. The rate varies from 0.09% to 0.5%, and treatment requires broad-spectrum antibiotics. Over the past few years, five North American women have died because of toxic shock after mifepristone/misoprostol abortion. Four of these deaths were associated with a specific pathogen, *Clostridium sordellii.* Although the death rate associated with medication abortion remains exceedingly low—under 1 in 100,000—and very little is known about the risk factors for *C. sordelli* infection, many clinicians began to advise buccal rather than vaginal administration of misoprostol after these deaths.

Postprocedure Management and Education

The mifepristone aftercare instruction sheets explain misoprostol administration, use of pain medications, and initiation of contraception (see Figs. 128-3 and 128-4).

Patient Education Guides

See the Medication Guide for Mifeprex at www.earlyoptionpill.com/userfiles/file/Med%20Guide%204-22-09%20Final.pdf.

See the consent form online at www.expertconsult.com. See Figures 128-1 through 128-4 for patient information.

PATIENT AGREEMENT
Mifeprex (mifepristone) Tablets

1. I have read the attached MEDICATION GUIDE for using Mifeprex* and misoprostol to end my pregnancy.
2. I discussed the information with my health care provider.
3. My provider answered all my questions and told me about the risks and benefits of using Mifeprex and misoprostol to end my pregnancy.
4. I believe I am no more than 49 days (7 weeks) pregnant.
5. I understand that I will take Mifeprex in my provider's office (Day 1).
6. I understand that I will take misoprostol in my provider's office two days after I take Mifeprex (Day 3).
7. My provider gave me advice on what to do if I develop heavy bleeding or need emergency care due to the treatment.
8. Bleeding and cramping do not mean that my pregnancy has ended. Therefore, I must return to my provider's office in about 2 weeks (about Day 14) after I take Mifeprex to be sure that my pregnancy has ended and that I am well.
9. I know that, in some cases, the treatment will not work. This happens in about 5 to 8 women out of 100 who use this treatment.
10. I understand that if my pregnancy continues after any part of the treatment, there is a chance that there may be birth defects. If my pregnancy continues after treatment with Mifeprex and misoprostol, I will talk with my provider about my choices, which may include a surgical procedure to end my pregnancy.
11. I understand that if the medicines I take do not end my pregnancy and I decide to have a surgical procedure to end my pregnancy, or if I need a surgical procedure to stop bleeding, my provider will do the procedure or refer me to another provider who will. I have that provider's name, address and phone number.
12. I have my provider's name, address and phone number and know that I can call if I have any questions or concerns.
13. I have decided to take Mifeprex and misoprostol to end my pregnancy and will follow my provider's advice about when to take each drug and what to do in an emergency.
14. I will do the following:
    - Contact my provider right away if in the days after treatment I have a fever of 100.4°F or higher that lasts for more than 4 hours or severe abdominal pain.
    - Contact my provider right away if I have heavy bleeding (soaking through two thick full-size sanitary pads per hour for two consecutive hours).
    - Contact my provider right away if I have abdominal pain or discomfort, or I am "feeling sick," including weakness, nausea, vomiting or diarrhea, more than 24 hours after taking misoprostol.
    - Take the MEDICATION GUIDE with me when I visit an emergency room or a provider who did not give me Mifeprex, so that they will understand that I am having a medical abortion with Mifeprex.
    - Return to my provider's office in 2 days (Day 3) to check if my pregnancy has ended. My provider will give me misoprostol if I am still pregnant.
    - Return to my provider's office about 14 days after beginning treatment to be sure that my pregnancy has ended and that I am well.

Patient Signature: ______________________
Patient Name (print): ______________________
Date: ______________________

The patient signed the PATIENT AGREEMENT in my presence after I counseled her and answered all her questions.
I have given her the MEDICATION GUIDE for mifepristone.

Provider's Signature: ______________________
Name of Provider (print): ______________________
Date: ______________________

After the patient and the provider sign this PATIENT AGREEMENT, give 1 copy to the patient before she leaves the office and put 1 copy in her medical record. Give a copy of the MEDICATION GUIDE to the patient.
Rev 2: 7/19/05

*Mifeprex is a registered trademark of Danco Laboratories, LLC.

Figure 128-1 Patient agreement form. (Courtesy of Danco Laboratories, New York.)

Consent for Mifepristone/Misoprostol Abortion

Write your initials before each statement to show that you understand and agree with it.

___ I understand that this consent form differs from the Mifeprex patient agreement.

___ I understand that my three choices for this pregnancy are parenthood, adoption and abortion.

___ "Medication abortion" means an abortion using drugs. A suction abortion uses instruments to empty the uterus or womb. I know that I should not begin a medication abortion unless I am sure that I want to end my pregnancy. I am willing to have a suction abortion if the medication abortion fails.

___ I understand that medication abortion must be done within the first 9 weeks of pregnancy. A physical exam, a blood test and/or an ultrasound exam will be done to confirm the size of my pregnancy.

___ I will take 2 medications. The first is mifepristone, which blocks a hormone needed to continue a pregnancy. I will take a 200 mg dose because research shows this dose is effective. The second drug is misoprostol. It causes the cramps which expel the pregnancy.

___ Before I take these medications, I may have blood tests to check for anemia and to check my Rh type. If I am Rh negative, I will get a shot of MICRhoGAM.

___ I will swallow the mifepristone tablet before I leave the health center. I know that this can cause some nausea and diarrhea, and later cramps.

___ I know that I will take 4 misoprostol tablets home with me.

___ BUCCAL MISOPROSTOL: I will put 2 misoprostol tablets in each cheek no sooner than 24 hours after I swallow the mifepristone, but before 48 hours have passed.

or

___ VAGINAL MISOPROSTOL: I will put 4 misoprostol tablets in my vagina no sooner than 6 hours after I swallow the mifepristone, but before 72 hours have passed.

___ I will receive prescriptions for pain medications.

___ I understand that 1 to 6 hours after I insert the misoprostol, I will have cramping and bleeding. The cramping can be very strong for a few hours, but usually not for more than 24 hours. The bleeding can be quite heavy with clots for a few hours. I may see some pregnancy tissue (usually white or gray in color).
If the heavy bleeding lasts for more than 12 hours, or if I soak more than two maxi pads each hour for two hours in a row, I should call my provider. I know that I should also call if I do NOT bleed within 24 hours of inserting the misoprostol.

___ If I start to feel very ill, I will call the health center. Very rarely, women have had "toxic shock" type illness after a medication abortion.

___ I know that I should return for my one-week check-up to be sure that the abortion is complete. At this visit, an ultrasound or a blood test may be done. If the abortion is not complete, I may need a vacuum aspiration (a suction procedure to empty the uterus) to end the pregnancy.

___ The abortion must be complete because misoprostol can cause serious birth defects if a pregnancy continues.

___ I have read this form and have had time to think about it. I have had all of my questions answered.

___ If a complication occurs, I request and allow the physician to do whatever is necessary to protect my health and welfare.

___ I hereby consent that ______________________________ give me the medications mifepristone and misoprostol for an early medication abortion.

Signature of patient: ____

Date: ____________________

Witness: ____

Date: ____________________

Figure 128-2 Patient consent form.

Medication Abortion (Vaginal Misoprostol) Patient Aftercare Sheet

Today, _________________, you took mifepristone to end your pregnancy. You took 200 milligrams of mifepristone at ____am/pm. You may have some vaginal bleeding after taking this pill.

Any time from 6 to 72 hours from now, _____am/pm, you must take another medicine, misoprostol (also called Cytotec). **Choose a time when you have had a good meal and plenty of rest.** Swallow one ibuprofen pill one hour before you take the misoprostol—this will help decrease your cramps. You must take the misoprostol even if you have started to bleed.

Each misoprostol pill is 200 micrograms. **Place 4 misoprostol pills in your vagina.** Lie down for 30 minutes. It's OK if the pills fall out after 30 minutes.

What to expect
Misoprostol causes cramping and bleeding, often with clots. The cramps and bleeding may be much more than you get with a period. The cramps usually start 2 to 4 hours after you insert the pills, and may last for 3 to 5 hours. This heavy bleeding means that the treatment is working. The bleeding often lasts 1 to 2 weeks, and it may stop and start a few times.

You may have a lot of pain or cramps—if so, take pain medicine. You can take ibuprofen (Motrin or Advil) up to 800 milligrams every 8 hours and/or hydrocodone up to 2 pills every 4–6 hours. You can also use a heating pad to relieve the pain. Some women get nausea, diarrhea or chills. This should get better in a few hours.

You **should** call me if
- Your bleeding soaks through more than 2 maxi pads per hour for 2 hours.
- You do **not** bleed within 24 hours after inserting the misoprostol.
- You start to feel very ill after the heavy cramping and bleeding are over.

To reach me
Call my 24-hour number: _________________________. If you have any questions or think something is going wrong, call this number and I will call you back. It may take me 10 to 15 minutes to return your call. No question is too small. **Please feel free to call me.**

Follow-up
You have an appointment to come back to my office on __________at _________ am/pm. At this visit I will make sure that the abortion is complete.

Birth control
If you want to use birth control pills, patch, or ring, I have given you a prescription. You should start these on ___________, even if you are still bleeding.

Figure 128-3 Aftercare information for vaginal misoprostol.

Medication Abortion (Buccal Misoprostol) Patient Aftercare Sheet

Today, ________________, you took mifepristone to end your pregnancy. You took 200 milligrams of mifepristone at ____am/pm. You may have some vaginal bleeding after taking this pill.

Any time from 12 to 48 hours from now, _____am/pm, you must take another medicine, misoprostol (also called Cytotec). **Choose a time when you have had a good meal and plenty of rest.** Swallow one ibuprofen pill one hour before you take the misoprostol—this will help decrease your cramps. You must take the misoprostol even if you have started to bleed.

Each misoprostol pill is 200 micrograms. **Place 2 misoprostol pills in each cheek.** Leave them in your cheeks for 30 minutes. After 30 minutes, swallow the pills with water.

What to expect
Misoprostol causes cramping and bleeding, often with clots. The cramps and bleeding may be much more than you get with a period. The cramps usually start 2 to 4 hours after you insert the pills, and may last for 3 to 5 hours. This heavy bleeding means that the treatment is working. The bleeding often lasts 1 to 2 weeks, and it may stop and start a few times.

You may have a lot of pain or cramps—if so, take pain medicine. You can take ibuprofen (Motrin or Advil) up to 800 milligrams every 8 hours and/or hydrocodone up to 2 pills every 4–6 hours. You can also use a heating pad to relieve the pain. Some women get nausea, diarrhea or chills. This should get better in a few hours.

You **should** call me if

- Your bleeding soaks through more than 2 maxi pads per hour for 2 hours.
- You do **not** bleed within 24 hours after taking the misoprostol.
- You start to feel very ill after the heavy cramping and bleeding are over.

To reach me
Call my 24-hour number: ______________________. If you have any questions or think something is going wrong, call this number and I will call you back. It may take me 10 to 15 minutes to return your call. No question is too small. **Please feel free to call me.**

Follow-up
You have an appointment to come back to my office on _________at _________ am/pm. At this visit I will make sure that the abortion is complete.

Birth control
If you want to use birth control pills, patch, or ring, I have given you a prescription. You should start these on __________, even if you are still bleeding.

Figure 128-4 Aftercare information for buccal misoprostol.

TABLE 128-2 Medication Abortion Protocol Comparison

		Updated Regimen	
Protocol	**FDA Regimen**	**Vaginal Misoprostol**	**Buccal Misoprostol**
Maximum gestational age	49 days from LMP	63 days from LMP	63 days from LMP
Mifepristone dose	600 mg orally in office	200 mg orally in office	200 mg orally in office
Misoprostol dose	400 μg orally (two tablets)	800 μg vaginally (four tablets)	800 μg buccally (four tablets)
Misoprostol timing	48 hr after mifepristone	6–72 hr after mifepristone	24–36 hours after mifepristone
Misoprostol location	Clinician's office	Home	Home
Follow-up visit	14 days after mifepristone	4–14 days after mifepristone	4–14 days after mifepristone
Minimum number of office visits	Three	Two	Two
Cost	Higher	Lower	Lower

FDA, U.S. Food and Drug Administration; LMP, last menstrual period.

Medication Abortion Initial Visit Note

Subjective:

_______________ is here with an unintended pregnancy. We fully discussed all of her options. The patient has indicated that this is not a good time for her to become a parent and would like to end the pregnancy. The options, including medication abortion, suction abortion with local anesthesia, and referral for suction abortion under general anesthesia, were discussed. She has chosen a medication abortion with mifepristone and misoprostol.

Past Medical History:

Past Surgical History:

G___P___

Her obstetric and gynecologic history is __________. Her prior methods of contraception: _______________.

She ❐ IS ❐ IS NOT in a safe situation at home and ❐ DOES ❐ DOES NOT describe a situation that might be high risk for abuse.

The patient ❐ DOES ❐ DOES NOT meet the following criteria: There is no IUD in place, she is not allergic to prostaglandins/mifepristone, there is no chronic adrenal failure, no long-term systemic corticosteroid use, no concurrent anticoagulant therapy, and no hemorrhagic disorders.

Rh status: ___

Physical examination
Vital signs:

General appearance: _________

Uterus: ___ weeks size

ULTRASOUND (limited study for the purpose of determining gestational age):
Performed: ❐ YES ❐ NO ❐ Not applicable
Gestational sac: ❐ YES ❐ NO ❐ Not applicable
Yolk sac: ❐ YES ❐ NO ❐ Not applicable
Crown–rump: ❐ YES ❐ NO ❐ Not applicable, ___mm
Gestational age: _____ days by ultrasound

Assessment
_____________ is a good candidate for medical abortion with a pregnancy at less than 63 days gestational age. She has no medical contraindications. She understands the protocol and possible side effects, the need for a follow-up visit, and the need for a suction procedure if the medical abortion fails. She knows how to contact me in case of an emergency.

Plan
Mifeprex medication guide given: ❐ YES ❐ NO
Mifeprex provider / patient agreement signed: ❐ YES ❐ NO
Updated consent form signed: ❐ YES ❐ NO
Pain medication prescribed as per orders.
Mifeprex lot number recorded: by nursing, see nursing note.
Dispensed 4 tablets of misoprostol (200 mcg each) for home use.
Patient information sheet given; this sheet details the self-insertion of the misoprostol and the expected bleeding patterns.
RhoGAM given: ❐ YES ❐ NO ❐ Not applicable
The certificate of induced termination was sent to the health department ❐ YES ❐ NO ❐ Not applicable
The sonogram (if done) is to be scanned into the record along with the Mifeprex and alternative consent form.
She has chosen ____________ as her ongoing contraceptive method and has been instructed on when to begin this method. (OCP users to start one or two days after the insertion of the misoprostol)

Quantitative hCG level ordered: ❐ YES ❐ NO
Follow-up visit scheduled in approximately 1–2 weeks

Figure 128-5 Procedure note for initial visit.

Medication Abortion Follow-up Visit Note

_______________________ presents for follow-up after medical abortion.
Within 24 hours after taking misoprostol, she had cramping and bleeding.
Bleeding now reported as: _________
She has no symptoms of pregnancy.

Objective
Vital signs:
General appearance:
Ultrasound (if done) shows absence of gestational sac and thickening of the endometrial lining:
❒ YES ❒ NO ❒ Not applicable

Assessment
Abortion completion assessed by:
History: ❒ YES ❒ NO
Sonogram: ❒ YES ❒ NO ❒ Not applicable

Plan
Contraception plan reviewed: ❒ YES ❒ NO
Repeat hCG level ordered: ❒ YES ❒ NO ❒ Not applicable
Discussed duration of bleeding and potential complications.
No restrictions on activity.

Figure 128-6 Procedure note for subsequent visit.

Billing and Coding

The following codes can be used to bill for medication abortion.

Visit 1

The first visit includes verification of pregnancy and pregnancy date, counseling, and administration of mifepristone:

CPT 99204 or 99214	Level 4 new or established patient E/M visit
ICD-9 635.92	Legally induced abortion, without mention of complication, complete
J8499	Prescription drug, oral, nonchemo, not otherwise specified
	or
J3490	Unclassified drug

If J codes are not accepted by insurance carrier, use 99070 (a cost-of-materials CPT code) or S0190 for mifepristone. *Each insurance carrier may reimburse for mifepristone using a different code.* The name of the drug (mifepristone), the dosage (200 mg), and the 11-digit national drug code (NDC) from the drug package must accompany this claim. In addition, submit a copy of the drug invoice to show the cost of the drug.

76815	Limited ultrasound, pregnant uterus
	or
76817	Transvaginal ultrasound, pregnant uterus

In addition, submit codes for appropriate laboratory tests or MICRhoGAM (90385) if done in office.

Visit 2

The second visit is to verify that the pregnancy has ended.

CPT 99213 or 99214	Level 3 or 4 E/M visit for established patient
CPT 76817 or 76815	Ultrasound
ICD-9 635.92	Legally induced abortion, without mention of complication, complete

Online Resources

Association of Reproductive Health Professionals: Available at www.arhp.org. A resource for clinical education in reproductive health topics.

Center for Reproductive Health Education in Family Medicine: Available at www.rhedi.org. A resource for family medicine residency programs expanding their reproductive health education and services.

Gynuity Health Projects: Available at www.gynuity.org. A research and technical assistance organization.

Mifepristone information (Danco Laboratories, mifepristone's U.S. manufacturer): Available at www.earlyoptionpill.com.

Mifepristone medication guide: Available at www.earlyoptionpill.com/userfiles/file/Med%20Guide%204-22-09%20Final.pdf.

National Abortion Federation: Available at www.prochoice.org. Medication abortion information.

Reproductive Health Access Project: Available at www.reproductiveaccess.org. A resource for community family physicians offering medication abortion.

Bibliography

American College of Obstetricians and Gynecologists: Medical management of abortion: ACOG practice bulletin no. 67. Obstet Gynecol 106:871–882, 2005.

American College of Obstetricians and Gynecologists: ACOG Committee Opinion no. 450: Increasing use of contraceptive implants and intrauterine devices to reduce unintended pregnancy. Obstet Gynecol 114:1434–1438, 2009.

Blanchard K, Shochet T, Coyaji K, et al: Misoprostol alone for early abortion: An evaluation of seven potential regimens. Contraception 72:91–97, 2005.

Borgatta L, Burnhill MS, Tyson J, et al: Early medical abortion with methotrexate and misoprostol. Obstet Gynecol 97:11–16, 2001.

Creinin MD: Medical abortion regimens: Historical context and overview. Am J Obstet Gynecol 183(2 Suppl):S3–S9, 2000.

Kulier R, Gülmezoglu AM, Hofmeyr GJ, et al: Medical methods for first trimester abortion. Cochrane Database Syst Rev 2:CD002855, 2004.

Swingle HM, Colaizy TT, Zimmerman MB, Morriss FH Jr: Abortion and the risk of subsequent preterm birth: A systematic review with meta-analysis. J Reprod Med 54:95–108, 2009.

Tuggy M, Garcia J: Procedures Consult. Available at www.proceduresconsult.com.

CHAPTER 129

EMERGENCY CONTRACEPTION

Steven H. Eisinger • Eric A. Smith

Emergency contraception (EC) is treatment intended for women who have had unprotected intercourse and wish to avoid pregnancy. Ingestion of high doses of sex steroids administered within 120 hours of exposure is known to prevent pregnancy. The mechanism remains unclear but appears to involve either inhibition or delay of ovulation or interference with implantation of a fertilized ovum. Some regard this as a form of abortion, but others believe that abortion occurs only after implantation. If taken by an already pregnant patient, current commercially available medical EC does not interrupt the pregnancy and there is no proven harm to the developing fetus. Studies in China have shown that mifepristone used as a form of EC is equally or more efficacious, but this use is not approved and could potentially harm an established pregnancy. Other selective progesterone receptor modulator drugs, such as ulipristal, are under active investigation.

Lack of knowledge and access to EC appear to be the major barriers to the provision of EC. Both doctors and patients are often unaware of EC. Critical delays in treatment may occur when doctors require an office visit before prescribing or the patient has to search for a pharmacy that carries the prescription. For these reasons, the American College of Obstetricians and Gynecologists has advocated the practice of discussing EC with all patients who are sexually active and at risk for a contraceptive failure. In the primary care setting, this should include both female and male patients of reproductive age. Telephone prescribing appears to be safe.

The cost of EC varies from $21 to $50 retail. Availability has been sporadic in the past. Indeed, the safety profile of the progestin-only method resulted in the U.S. Food and Drug Administration (FDA) approving Plan B (Duramed Pharmaceuticals, Cincinnati, Ohio) for nonprescription sale to adults in August of 2006. In April of 2009, the FDA decreased the minimum age of over-the-counter (OTC) purchase of EC to 17 years old. However, the medication remains behind the pharmacy counter and requires a prescription for patients younger than 17 years of age. Access may still be limited by pharmacists' unwillingness to dispense the medication and the lack of privacy when requesting EC from a pharmacist.

INDICATIONS

Women who have had intercourse within 5 days and who have used no contraception during intercourse, whose method of contraception failed (e.g., a broken condom), or who have been victims of sexual assault are candidates for EC if they are at risk for pregnancy. Women at midmenstrual cycle who may be near ovulation are at greatest risk, but risk exists at any time in the cycle and EC need not be "timed" to coincide with an individual's menstrual cycle. See Figure 129-1 for an approach to EC use.

CONTRAINDICATIONS

The progestin-only method (Plan B One Step, Next Choice, or their equivalent) has *no known medical contraindications*. The World Health Organization has stated that the only contraindication to EC is an ongoing pregnancy. No teratogenic effects have been identified, however. Medical contraindications to oral contraceptives, such as severe hypertension and history of thromboembolism, should be considered but have not been shown to be significant with the short dosage schedule.

PRECAUTIONS

An accurate timeline of exposure is critical to the use of EC. A pregnancy test can be considered before administration. Testing for and treatment of sexually transmitted infections should be offered and encouraged. An adequate plan for contraception after EC use should be recommended.

PREPROCEDURE PATIENT EDUCATION

Because the product is available OTC, preprocedure counseling may not be possible. If the patient contacts her physician before taking EC, she should be informed of the risks and benefits of the medication as outlined in this chapter and the patient education handout. Educating patients about the availability of EC at health maintenance visits may be appropriate.

PROCEDURE

Medical

Plan B One Step (Duramed Pharmaceuticals, Cincinnati, OH) and Next Choice (Watson Pharma, Morristown, NJ) are commercial oral EC regimens available by prescription (for those <17 years of age) and OTC (for those >17 years of age). Plan B One Step consists of a single tablet containing 1.5 mg of levonorgestrel. Plan B (being phased out) and Next Choice consist of two tablets, each containing 0.75 mg of levonorgestrel. Following the FDA-approved regimens, the first or single pill is taken as soon as possible within 72 hours after exposure and, if part of the prescription, the second pill is taken 12 hours later. An alternate and equally effective regimen to the two-pill prescription is to take both tablets (1.5 mg levonorgestrel) as a single dose. Further research has also demonstrated effectiveness of the method up to 120 hours (5 days) after exposure, with declining success as delay increases.

A dual-hormone brand of EC known as Preven is no longer available by prescription, but hormones found in certain common oral contraceptives, including a number of generic preparations, can be used to replicate it. It may be advantageous to know how to provide the *dual-hormone ("Yuzpe") method* because it may be more readily available and less expensive than commercially available EC if the patient has access to oral contraceptive pills. Two widely used forms of progestin can be used: levonorgestrel (like Plan B, Plan B One Step, and Next Choice) and norgestrel. Twice as much norgestrel is required for the same therapeutic effect (0.75 mg levonorgestrel or 1.50 mg norgestrel per dose). Determining the

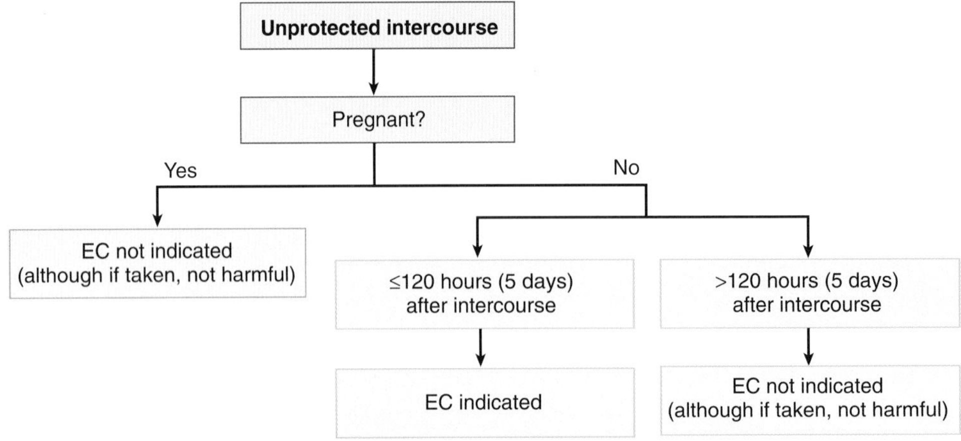

Figure 129-1 Emergency contraception (EC) decision pathway.

correct number and color of active pills available to the patient may require help from the local pharmacy (Table 129-1).

The prescribing regimen is similar for all the options: *the first dose is taken immediately, and, when indicated, the second dose is taken 12 hours later*. Only Plan B has been proven to be equally effective if both of the tablets are taken as a single dose, and thus received FDA approval for Plan B One Step. Evidence shows that early administration enhances efficacy. The greatest efficacy occurs when the regimen starts within 24 hours of exposure, but the treatment may be initiated up to 120 hours after exposure.

In a head-to-head randomized, blinded study the progestin-only method had an efficacy up to 85%, whereas the dual-hormone method had an efficacy up to 57%. Thus, progestin-only EC is the better option when available.

Female patients may be given a prescription to be held in reserve in case of an exposure. A *national telephone hotline* (not associated with the manufacturers) has been established to provide the names and numbers of local clinics that provide emergency contraceptive services: 888-NOT-2-LATE (888-668-2528).

Intrauterine Contraceptive Device

Another approach to EC is the placement of a copper intrauterine device (IUD), ParaGard. The IUD is effective up to 1 week after exposure and is significantly more effective than oral methods, with a reduced risk of pregnancy of 99% if inserted within 5 days of unprotected intercourse. IUD insertion has its own risks and disadvantages, but placement for EC has the advantage of immediate and continuous contraception. See Chapter 145, Intrauterine Device Insertion, for a full discussion of IUD insertion.

Complications

With the *dual-hormone* method, *nausea and vomiting* are common problems. Therefore, a prophylactic antiemetic is recommended before the hormones are administered. *Breast tenderness* may also occur. Side effects are less frequent with the progestin-only methods. *Menses may be early, on time, or delayed* after treatment. If the menstrual delay is 21 days or more from the date of treatment, a pregnancy test should be performed. If the medication is vomited within the first hour of ingestion, repeat administration with an antiemetic is indicated. If vomited more than 1 hour post-ingestion, repeat administration is still advised.

Postprocedure Management

Discuss a post-EC plan for contraception and ensure that the patient understands that EC is not an effective method of continuous

TABLE 129-1 Commercially Available Emergency Oral Contraceptives and Their Equivalents from Regular Oral Contraceptive Brands*

Name	Formulation	Dosage
Dedicated Progestin-Only Product		
Next Choice	0.75 mg levonorgestrel	1 pill immediately and in 12 hr *or* 2 pills immediately
Plan B One Step	1.5 mg levonorgestrel	1 pill immediately
Plan B	0.75 mg levonorgestrel	1 pill immediately and in 12 hr *or* 2 pills immediately
Equivalent Progestin-Only from Oral Contraceptive Brand		
Ovrette	0.075 mg norgestrel	20 pills immediately and in 12 hr *or* 40 pills immediately
Common Combined-Hormone Oral Contraceptive Brands*		
Alesse	0.1 mg levonorgestrel, 20 μg EE	5 pills immediately and in 12 hr
Alesse-28	Same as above (pink tablets)	Same as above
Levlen	0.15 mg levonorgestrel, 30 μg EE	4 pills immediately and in 12 hr
Tri-Levlen	0.125 mg levonorgestrel, 30 μg EE (yellow tablets)	Same as above
Levlite	0.1 mg levonorgestrel, 20 μg EE (pink tablets)	5 pills immediately and in 12 hr
Levora	0.15 mg levonorgestrel, 30 μg EE	4 pills immediately and in 12 hr
Nordette	0.15 mg levonorgestrel, 30 μg EE (light orange tablets)	Same as above
Ogestrel	0.5 mg norgestrel, 30 μg EE	2 pills immediately and in 12 hr
Low-Ogestrel	0.3 mg levonorgestrel, 30 μg EE	4 pills immediately and in 12 hr
Ovral	0.5 mg norgestrel, 50 μg EE	2 pills immediately and in 12 hr
Ovral-28	Same as above (white tablets)	Same as above
Lo/Ovral	0.3 mg norgestrel, 30 μg EE	4 pills immediately and in 12 hr
Lo/Ovral-28	Same as above (white tablets)	Same as above
Triphasil	0.125 mg levonorgestrel, 30 μg EE (yellow tablets)	4 pills immediately and in 12 hr
Trivora	0.125 mg levonorgestrel, 30 μg EE (pink tablets)	4 pills immediately and in 12 hr

EE, ethinyl estradiol.
*All regimens must begin within 72 hr of the unprotected intercourse.

contraception. If the patient has no menses within 21 days, test for pregnancy. Screen for sexually transmitted infections when indicated.

Patient Education Guides

See the patient education form online at www.expertconsult.com.

CPT/Billing Codes

There is no specific CPT code for EC. The appropriate office visit or telephone consultation should be documented and billed.

ICD-9-CM Diagnostic Codes

V25.03 Emergency contraception
V25.1 IUD insertion
V25.4 Contraceptive surveillance
V69.2 High-risk sexual behavior

Online Resources

Association of Reproductive Health Professionals: Emergency Contraception. Available at www.arhp.org/ec.

The Emergency Contraception Website. Available at http://ec.princeton.edu; and www.not-2-late.com.

Bibliography

American College of Obstetricians and Gynecologists: Emergency oral contraception. ACOG practice bulletin no. 69. Obstet Gynecol 106:1443–1452, 2005.

Cheng L, Gülmezoglu AM, Piaggio GGP, et al: Interventions for emergency contraception. Cochrane Database Syst Rev 2:CD001324, 2008.

Grimes D, Raymond E, Jones B: Emergency contraception over-the-counter: The medical and legal imperatives. Obstet Gynecol 98:151–155, 2001.

Ngai SW, Fan S, Li S, et al: A randomized trial to compare 24 h versus 12 h double dose regimen of levonorgestrel for emergency contraception. Hum Reprod 20:307–311, 2005.

Trussell J, Raymond EG: Emergency contraception: A cost-effective approach to preventing unintended pregnancy. Updated December 2009. Available at http://ec.princeton.edu/questions/ec-review.pdf.

CHAPTER 130

Barrier Contraceptives: Cervical Caps, Condoms, and Diaphragms

Beth A. Choby

Cervical barriers are relatively safe and inexpensive options for contraception. They are immediately effective and reversible and have few side effects. Barrier methods are options for women who have contraindications to hormonal contraceptives, cannot tolerate intrauterine devices, or are not ready for sterilization. Additional benefits include ease of transportability, safety during lactation, and the convenience of flexible timing of insertion. Current barrier methods are 80% effective in preventing pregnancy when used correctly and consistently. Table 130-1 lists various barrier options, contraceptive failure rates, and costs.

Although more options for barrier contraception are available today than ever before, the percentage of women choosing barrier methods is small. Only 0.3% of women used a diaphragm for contraception in 2002; in the 1980s, 8.1% of women selected this method. A possible protective effect against sexually transmitted infection (STI) has focused renewed attention on barrier contraception. Protection is thought to occur through mechanical blocking of exposure to semen and bodily fluids. Most barrier devices are used in combination with nonoxynol-9, but spermicide itself does not enhance protection against STIs. The Centers for Disease Control and Prevention recommends that women at high risk for human immunodeficiency virus (HIV) infection avoid nonoxynol-9 spermicides because they offer no protection against STIs and may increase the risk of HIV infection.

Cervical Caps

Cervical caps are small, firm silicone cups that adhere to the cervix by suction. Four types of cervical cap are available internationally. The *Prentif* cap was approved by the U.S. Food and Drug Administration (FDA) in May 1988, but was voluntarily removed from the U.S. market by the manufacturer in March 2005. The only cervical cap currently available in the United States is the FemCap (Fig. 130-1). The FemCap is silicone based and shaped like a sailor's hat. Initial efficacy studies of the FemCap were based on the first-generation product, which is no longer available. A Cochrane Database Review comparing the first-generation FemCap with the diaphragm found that the FemCap was less effective in preventing pregnancy. Fourteen percent of nulliparous women using the FemCap became pregnant during the first year with typical use; parous women had a 29% failure rate. The first-generation FemCap is now considered obsolete and has been replaced with a second-generation design. Although research on the effectiveness of the second-generation FemCap is limited, the typical failure rate is estimated to be 7.6%. Failure rates with perfect use are 2% to 4%. Dislodgement of the first-generation device occurred in one third of users; the second-generation FemCap dislodgement rate is estimated at 2%. Future studies should better clarify long-term efficacy. The cap has a high level of patient acceptability, and FemCap users may have decreased risk of urinary tract infections compared with women using a diaphragm. The Prentif cap was associated with cervical dysplasia when the device was used for longer than 3 months. Although small trials do not link cytologic abnormalities with FemCap use, baseline Papanicolaou screening (Pap smear) and annual surveillance are reasonable in women choosing this method.

Anatomy

The FemCap has a dome that fits over the cervix. An asymmetric brim flares outward to fit against the vaginal fornices (see Fig. 130-1).

Indications

- Prevention of pregnancy
- Possible protection against STIs

Contraindications

Absolute

- Allergy to silicone
- Less than 10 weeks postpartum
- History of toxic shock syndrome
- History of recent cervical surgery or abortion
- Cancer of the vulva, vagina, cervix, or uterus
- Anatomic abnormalities of the vagina, uterus, or cervix

Relative

- Uterine prolapse
- Patient unable to be properly fitted
- Patient unable to understand instructions for use or proper insertion/removal of the device
- Current genital tract infection
- Poor vaginal muscle tone
- Vaginal or cervical tissue breakdown

Equipment and Supplies

The FemCap is a clear silicone device that covers both the cervix and vaginal fornices. A strap over the dome augments removal.

TABLE 130-1 Comparison of Female Barrier Contraceptives

Method	Over-the-Counter	Multiuse/ Reusable	1 Year Failure Rate with Typical Use (%)	Timing of Insertion (Maximum Hours Prior to Intercourse)	Time to Be Left in after Intercourse (Hours)	Maximum Duration of Use (Hours)	Cost (US$)
Diaphragm	No	Yes	16	6	6	24	50*
FemCap	No	Yes	7.6†	40	6	48	65: includes video/DVD, device and instructions*
FC2 female condom	Yes	No	21	8	Remove after intercourse	One time use	2.50
Lea's shield	No	Yes	15	Prior to intercourse	8	48	65; direct order from internet*
Sponge	Yes	No	13–17	24	6	30	7.50–9 for pack of 3
Male condom	Yes	No	85	Prior to intercourse	Remove after ejaculation		0.50

*Does not include costs for spermicide.
†Based on limited-duration trials of second-generation FemCap.

Spermicide is applied in the groove between the brim and the dome. The cap is available in three sizes. Determining the correct size depends in general on the user's childbearing history:

- 22 mm (Small): use in nulliparous women
- 26 mm (Medium): use in women with a previous abortion or cesarean delivery
- 30 mm (Large): use in women with history of vaginal delivery

The FemCap kit contains the device, physician instructions for fitting, and a patient education DVD/video detailing product use. Cost of the kit averages $65.

Precautions

- Perform a pelvic examination before a cervical cap fitting. A Pap smear is recommended at baseline and then annually. Cervical cultures should be obtained in women at risk for STIs.
- Cervical cap fitting is contraindicated during pregnancy or the postpartum period (10 weeks).

Patient Education: Cervical Cap Use for Contraception

- Before use, one third of the inner side of the dome should be filled with spermicidal jelly.
- The jelly should not be applied to the inner surface of the rim.
- The cap may be inserted at any time from immediately before intercourse up to 40 hours before intercourse. It is most easily inserted in a squatting or semireclining position.
- The cap should be left in place for at least 6 hours following intercourse.

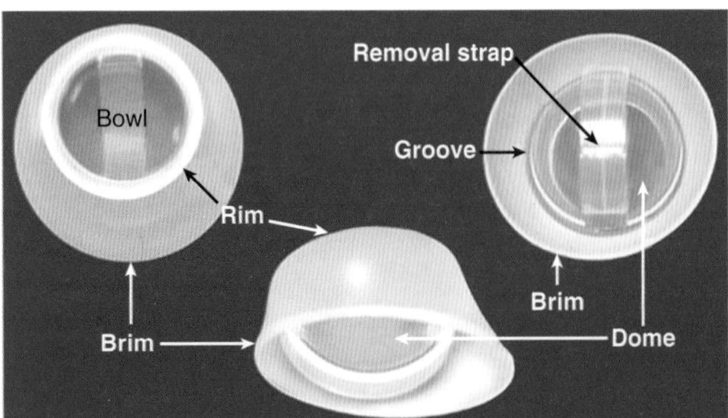

Figure 130-1 The FemCap cervical cap. (Courtesy of FemCap, Inc., Del Mar, Calif; with permission.)

- The cap may be left in place for up to 48 hours.
- If intercourse occurs more than once while the cap is in place, no additional spermicide is needed. However, the wearer should check for correct positioning of the cap before each episode.
- An additional contraceptive method should be used the first three times the cap is worn during intercourse (to ensure protection should the cap become dislodged). If dislodgement occurs, cap use should be discontinued and the cap should be refitted.
- The cap should not be used during menses.
- Refitting is necessary after abortion or childbirth.
- The cap should not be used in the presence of vaginal infection, discharge, pain, or odor. If these occur, medical evaluation is necessary.
- If lubrication is needed for intercourse, only water-based lubricants should be used. (Spermicide works well for this purpose.)
- The cap should be washed carefully after use with soap and water. If an odor develops, it can be soaked in vinegar or a cup of water with a teaspoon of lemon juice. Alternatively, the cap can be cleaned with a 25% bleach solution for 20 minutes, after which it should be rinsed thoroughly.
- A Pap smear should be taken 3 months after beginning use of the cap. If this is negative, then a Pap smear should be obtained every year thereafter.
- The cap should be replaced yearly (sooner if thin spots or tears occur). The patient should make an appointment with her physician to check if it still fits adequately.
- If the cervical cap is used properly, 6% of women will become pregnant after using the device for a year.
- If the device is left in too long, infections can occur, so the patient must follow the previously listed guidelines.

Procedure

1. Review the instructions from the FemCap kit.
2. Put on gloves and select the appropriate size of FemCap (described in the equipment section).
3. Lubricate the edges of the device, compress it, and insert vaginally. The FemCap should be inserted with the long brim first and pushed into the vagina until the dome fits snugly over the cervix (Fig. 130-2).
4. The cap should cover the entire cervix and adhere to it by self-generated suction.
5. The rim of the cap should fit evenly around the circumference of the vaginal fornices.
6. No gaps should be felt between the rim of the cap and the cervix.
7. Tug gently on the removal strap to guarantee that the cap will not dislodge.

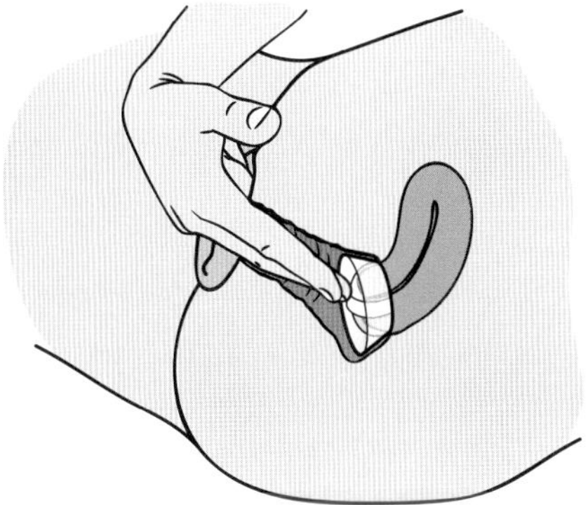

Figure 130-2 Proper placement and positioning of the FemCap. (Courtesy of FemCap, Inc., Del Mar, Calif; with permission.)

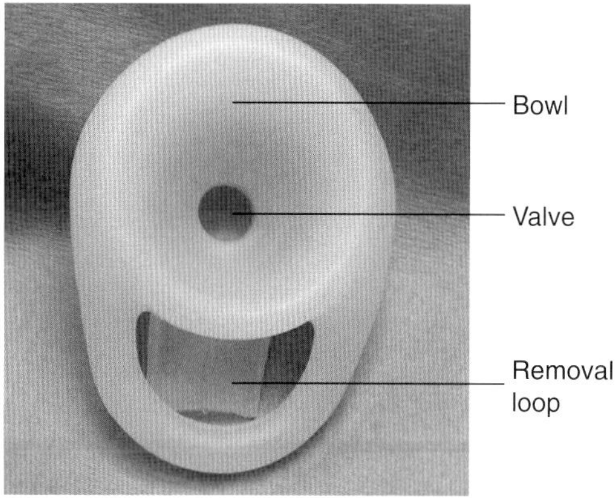

Figure 130-3 Lea's shield. (Courtesy of Yama, Inc., Union, NJ; with permission.)

8. If the cap does not fit satisfactorily, try one of the other two sizes.
9. *Remove the cap* by gripping the strap and rotating the FemCap. Push on the dome to break the suction and pull the cap out using the strap.
10. Have the patient repeat the insertion and removal process to demonstrate understanding.

Complications

- Pregnancy is possible if the cap dislodges during intercourse. This was one of the major reasons women discontinued the first-generation cervical cap, although dislodgement is much less common with the second-generation FemCap. Counseling patients about emergency contraception and providing a prescription for emergency use may be a desired option for certain women (see Chapter 129, Emergency Contraception).
- Vaginal odor or discharge occurs in 5% to 27% of users.
- Vaginal or cervical lacerations and abrasions are possible if the cap is left in place too long.
- Vaginal discomfort occurs in less than 3% of users.
- Toxic shock syndrome is uncommon.

Postprocedure Management

The patient should sit and also ambulate to ensure that the cap does not dislodge. No discomfort should be noted when the cap is correctly applied.

Postprocedure Patient Education

- The FemCap should be used with a one-quarter teaspoon of spermicide. Spermicide should be applied in the dome and spread over the brim.
- The FemCap must be placed before intercourse.
- The cap must be left in place for 6 hours after intercourse.
- It may be safely worn for up to 48 continuous hours.
- After removal, the FemCap should be washed with mild soap and water and allowed to air dry.
- FemCaps generally last approximately 1 year.

SHIELD

Lea's shield is a one-size silicone barrier (Fig. 130-3). It has a valve that allows for passage of cervical secretions while the shield is in place. The device was FDA approved in 2002; data on efficacy of Lea's shield are limited to one 6-month clinical trial. The 6-month pregnancy rate in this study was 5.6 per 100 when spermicide was used and 9.3 per 100 without spermicide. Women who are parous have slightly higher failure rates with this method. Shield dislodgement occurs in less than 3% of users.

Although the shield does not require fitting by a medical provider, health care providers should be comfortable discussing use of the shield. Most women can learn how to insert and remove the shield by reading the user's manual.

Anatomy

Lea's shield has an elliptical bowl that fits over the cervix and acts as a reservoir for spermicide. It is held in place by its volume and the vaginal musculature.

Indication

Lea's shield is use to prevent pregnancy.

Contraindications

Absolute

- Allergy to silicone
- Vaginal delivery within the past 6 weeks
- History of toxic shock syndrome
- Others similar to cervical cap contraindications

Relative

- Breaks in the cervical or vaginal tissue
- Frequent urinary tract infections
- Genital tract infection
- Others similar to cervical cap contraindications

Equipment and Supplies

- Lea's shield
- Spermicide

Preprocedure Patient Education and Forms

Please refer to the patient education form available online at www.expertconsult.com.

Procedure

1. Review the instructions for placement of Lea's shield. The shield is one size and does not require fitting by a medical provider. Most women can master insertion and removal of the shield after reading the Lea's shield user's manual.

2. The user should wash her hands with soap and water.
3. Coat the inside of the area around the bowl, the front rim, and the outer valve with spermicide.
4. Separate the labia with one hand and pinch the shield's rim.
5. With the thickest end first, insert the shield into the vagina. The valve should be facing out (down).
6. Push the shield up into the vagina as far as is comfortable.
7. The valve vents air and allows the shield to create a correct fit. The valve can be pressed to make sure all air is removed.
8. The removal loop should not protrude from the vagina.

Common Errors and Complications

- Three percent of users experience shield dislodgement; shield inversion occurs in 4% to 5% of users. A discussion of emergency contraception and a provisional prescription are helpful in cases of contraceptive failure.
- Failure to use spermicide may increase the rate of contraceptive failure.
- Increased frequency of urinary tract infections occurs in some shield users. Women should be encouraged to urinate before shield insertion and after intercourse.
- Shield removal before 8 hours after intercourse increases the failure rate. The shield should be left in place for a minimum of 8 hours.

Postprocedure Management

The patient should not feel discomfort with the shield in place. Have the patient ambulate and squat to ensure correct fit and placement of the shield. A 2-week follow-up after prescribing is recommended by the manufacturer.

Postprocedure Patient Education

- Shield position should be checked before each episode of intercourse to rule out dislodgement.
- The shield should not be used for more than 48 consecutive hours.
- When removing the shield, grasp the loop with a finger, rotate to break suction, and pull the device out of the vagina.
- Thoroughly wash the shield with a mild soap for 2 minutes, air dry, and store in the provided pouch.
- Replace the shield annually.

DIAPHRAGM

Diaphragms were first produced in the United States in 1925, and current diaphragm design is not significantly different. Of the three models currently available, two are made of latex whereas the third is silicone. Contraceptive efficacy studies of newer barrier methods are usually judged against the diaphragm. Although diaphragms are traditionally used with spermicidal jelly, a recent Cochrane Review was unable to distinguish a difference in effectiveness when diaphragm use with spermicide was compared with diaphragm use alone.

Barrier contraceptive efficacy is highly dependent on proper and consistent use. Sixteen of 100 women using the diaphragm become pregnant annually with typical use. Perfect use of the diaphragm has a 6 per 100 failure rate.

Indications

- Pregnancy prevention
- Contraception for women with contraindications to other methods and who do not desire to be sterilized
- Desire for additional STI protection in combination with other contraceptive methods that do not confer protection

Contraindications

Absolute

- Latex or spermicidal jelly allergy/hypersensitivity
- Postpartum (<6 weeks)

Relative

- Vaginal stenosis or significant pelvic abnormalities
- Recurrent urinary tract infections
- Aversion to manipulation of the genitals
- Uterine prolapse
- Significant cystocele or rectocele

Equipment

- Diaphragms (sizes 65 to 90) are of three types:
  1. *Arching spring:* Molded one-piece spring and firm-rimmed dome that form an arc when the rim is compressed in the center. It requires no introducer and is recommended for women with decreased pelvic support, cystocele or rectocele, or retroverted uterus, or for those who find a firmer rim easier to insert. This is the most popular type in the United States.
  2. *Coil spring:* Molded one-piece spring and dome with a softer, more flexible rim. It may be used with an introducer and is recommended for women with good vaginal support and no cystocele, rectocele, or pelvic floor relaxation; the cervix should be midplane or anterior.
  3. *Flat spring:* Molded one-piece spring and dome with a softer and more flexible rim than the arching spring or coil spring. It has flat-plane flexibility, may be used with an introducer, and is recommended for smaller women with a narrow or shallow pelvic shelf. It is excellent for nulliparous women or athletic women with strong pelvic musculature.
- Fitting ring kit. Kits can be obtained from most diaphragm manufacturers at minimal to no cost. The rings are graduated sizes that differ by increments of 5 mm. Fitting with domed rings provides a more realistic sensation for the patient as to how a diaphragm will feel (Fig. 130-4).
- Diaphragm introducer *(optional)*.
- Spermicidal jelly (usually nonoxynol-9).

Precautions

- Poor vaginal tone, a shallow vaginal shelf, or a cystocele or rectocele may prevent effective use of the diaphragm.
- Refitting is often necessary after pregnancy, pelvic surgery, or weight gain of more than 15 pounds.
- Women with a latex allergy are candidates for the wide seal rim diaphragm (latex free).

Preprocedure Patient Education and Forms

Diaphragm fitting by a health care provider is required. The fitting process should be discussed with the patient. Efficacy rates and the

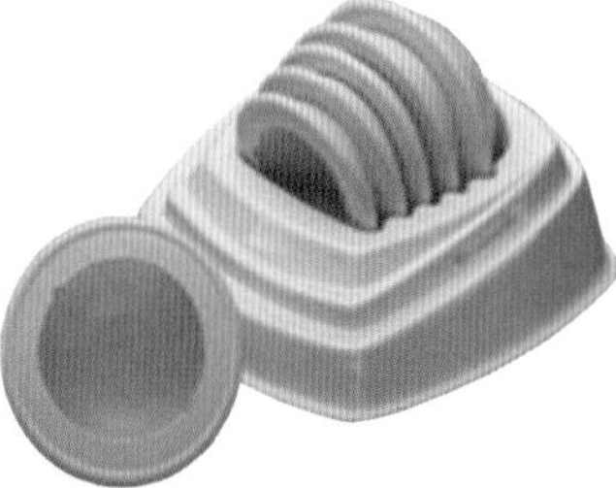

Figure 130-4 Diaphragm fitting kit. (Courtesy of CooperSurgical, Inc., Trumbull, Conn.)

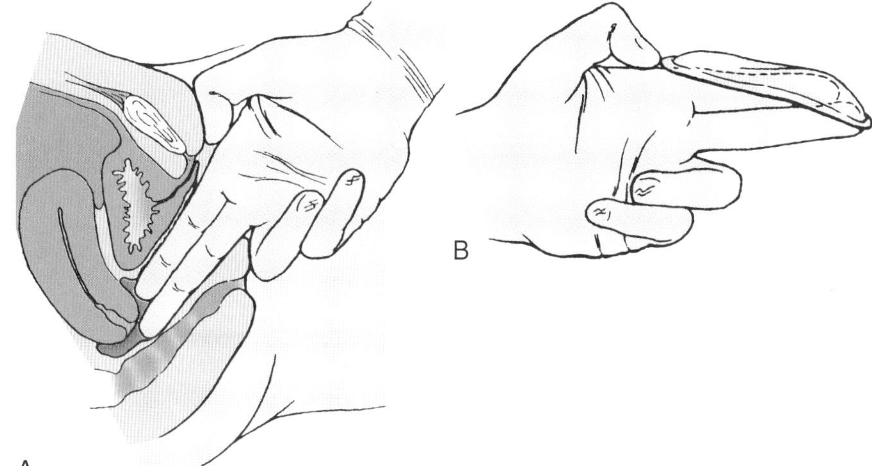

Figure 130-5 Clinical examination to determine proper diaphragm size. **A,** Insert the gloved index and middle fingers into the vagina, aiming for the posterior fornix with the middle finger. Mark the spot on the glove where the index finger touches the inferior pubic symphysis. **B,** Place the fitting ring or diaphragm over the end of the middle finger, and place the opposite side of the ring over the line marked on the gloved index finger.

proper and consistent use of the diaphragm should be stressed. Please refer to the patient education form available online at www.expertconsult.com.

Procedure

1. Place the patient in dorsal lithotomy (pelvic) position.
2. Don examination gloves and apply surgical lubricant to the index and middle fingers.
3. To estimate the size of the diaphragm, insert the gloved index and middle fingers into the vagina. Aim for the posterior fornix with the middle finger (Fig. 130-5A).
4. Note the spot where the index finger touches the inferior pubic symphysis.
5. Mark this spot on the glove using either a marker or instrument, or your thumb.
6. Remove the fingers from the vagina.
7. Place the fitting ring or diaphragm over the end of the middle finger.
8. Place the opposite side of the ring over the line marked on the gloved index finger (75 mm is a common size; Fig. 130-5B).
9. Apply surgical lubricant to the outer surface of the fitting *ring* (only) that most closely approximates the determined diameter.
10. Fold this fitting ring in half by pressing the sides together with the thumb and fingers (Fig. 130-6A).
11. Insert the folded diaphragm vaginally while the other hand holds open the vulva. Direct the diaphragm toward the posterior fornix (Fig. 130-6B).
12. Check for correct positioning by feeling for the cervix through the dome of the fitting diaphragm or in the center of the fitting ring (Fig. 130-6C).
13. Gently manipulate the anterior rim until it rests directly behind the pubic symphysis.
14. Have the patient perform a Valsalva maneuver and squat to confirm the fit.
15. *Remove the diaphragm* by hooking the index finger up and around the anterior rim and pulling the diaphragm down and out through the introitus (Fig. 130-7).
16. The patient should demonstrate proper technique for both insertion and removal of the diaphragm. Check that the patient can feel the cervix through the diaphragm dome and confirm placement of the anterior rim behind the pubic symphysis.
17. Describe the proper application of spermicide to the diaphragm. One tablespoon of spermicidal jelly containing nonoxynol-9 is applied to the concave side of the dome (for use) in addition to around the rim.

Common Errors

- Improper fitting. A diaphragm that is *too small* does not lodge behind the pubic symphysis and falls out. An inappropriately large diaphragm protrudes out in front of the pubic symphysis.
- Failure to leave the diaphragm in place for a minimum of 6 hours *after* intercourse. Patients should be counseled not to douche or remove the diaphragm immediately after coitus.

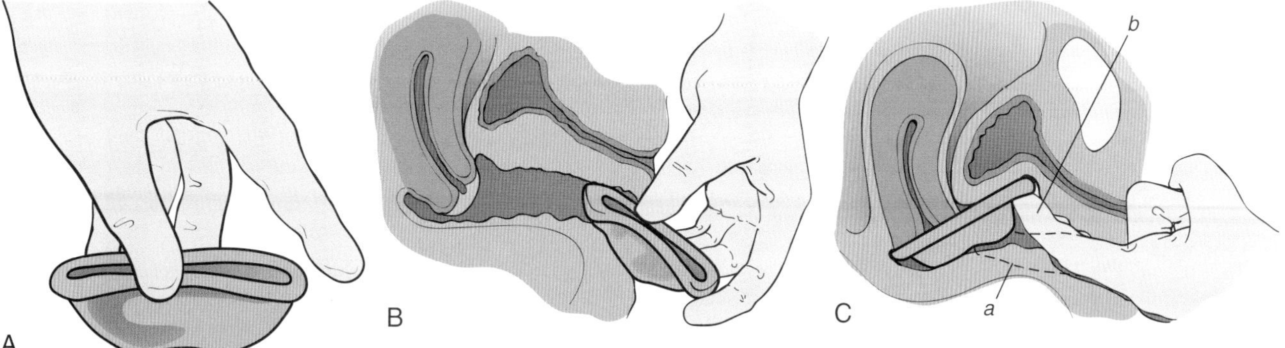

Figure 130-6 **A,** Diaphragm is folded for insertion. **B,** Insertion of the folded diaphragm. **C,** Proper diaphragm position: The cervix is palpable behind the diaphragm (*a*); the rim fits snugly behind the symphysis pubis (*b*).

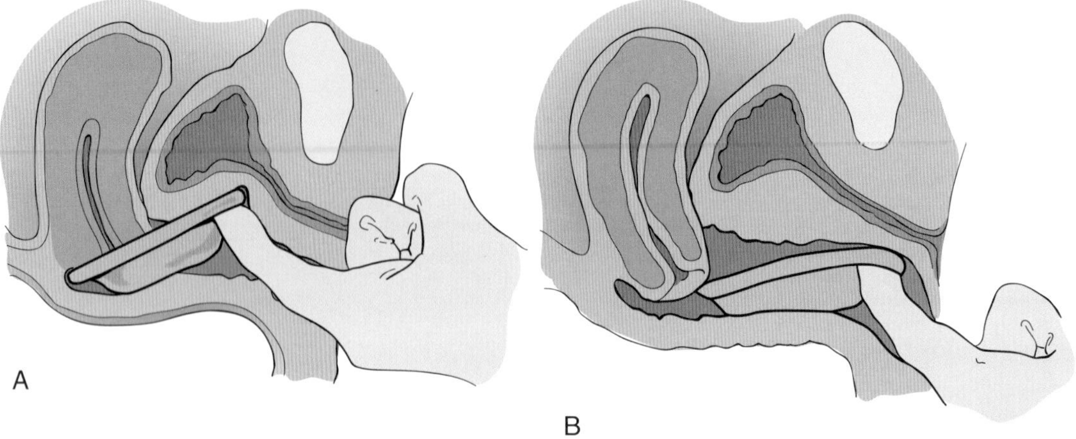

Figure 130-7 Removal of the diaphragm. **A,** Finger is hooked under the rim. **B,** Diaphragm is pulled through the introitus.

Complications

- Continuous diaphragm use for longer than 24 hours increases the risk of toxic shock syndrome (incidence of 2.4 per 100,000 women).
- Ulceration can result from excessive pressure of the diaphragm against the vaginal sidewalls with a poorly fitting device.
- Urinary tract infections are the most frequent side effect of diaphragm use.

Postprocedure Patient Education

- Patients should be shown and should practice diaphragm insertion and removal techniques, including how to apply spermicidal jelly to the rim and the dome. One tablespoon should be applied to the concave surface of the dome and the rim of the diaphragm so that the uterus is sealed off mechanically and chemically.
- Make sure that the diaphragm rim is firmly in place behind the pubic bone and below and behind the cervix. The patient should feel for the cervix through the dome of her diaphragm to ensure correct placement.
- Warn the patient not to douche or remove the diaphragm for 6 hours after intercourse. Leave the diaphragm in place and apply more spermicide if additional coitus occurs during this time.
- The patient should walk around the examination room with the diaphragm in place to ensure a comfortable fit.
- The diaphragm prescription should include the manufacturer's name, the type, and the size. A refill can be prescribed in case a new diaphragm is needed and the provider is unavailable.

Please refer to the sample patient education form available online at www.expertconsult.com.

SPONGES

The sponge is a nonprescription, single-use barrier contraceptive made of polyurethane foam impregnated with nonoxynol-9 spermicide. The concave side fits against the cervix, whereas the loop on the opposite side augments sponge removal. Although the Protectaid sponge is available in Canada, the Today Sponge is the only contraceptive sponge currently available in the United States (Fig. 130-8).

Sponges are sold in packs of three ($7.50 to $9). Effectiveness rate is 89% to 91% for perfect use and 84% to 87% with typical use. Parous women may have higher rates of failure than women who have not been pregnant. The sponge does *not* reduce the risk of STIs or HIV/acquired immunodeficiency syndrome (AIDS).

Anatomy

The sponge is inserted transvaginally and placed with the concave side covering the cervix.

Indications

- Prevention of pregnancy
- Contraception for women who are breast-feeding
- Birth control for women with contraindications to other methods or who need backup for the pill

Contraindications

Absolute

- Allergies to polyurethane, nonoxynol-9, or medications containing sulfa
- History of toxic shock syndrome
- History of recent delivery, miscarriage, or abortion (<8 weeks)
- Vaginal obstruction/anatomic abnormalities

Relative

- Current menstruation
- Active genital tract infection

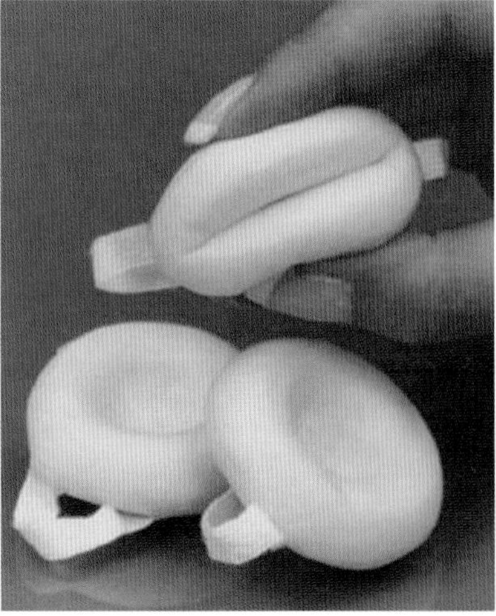

Figure 130-8 The Today Sponge. (Courtesy of Allendale Pharmaceuticals, Allendale, NJ; with permission.)

- Patient difficulty in understanding instructions for use
- Patient difficulty correctly inserting or removing the sponge
- Patient discomfort touching genitals

Precautions

The sponge offers no protection against STIs or HIV/AIDS.

Procedure

1. The patient should read the package insert before use.
2. Wash hands with soap and water.
3. Wet the sponge with a minimum of two tablespoons of clean water.
4. Squeeze the sponge to help activate the spermicide.
5. Fold the sponge in half with the loop toward the outside.
6. Slide the folded sponge into the vagina and push it inside until the cervix is covered. The sponge will unfold.
7. Check sponge placement by sliding a finger around the edge to guarantee that it covers the cervix. The loop should be palpable.
8. Insert up to 24 hours before intercourse; the sponge must be left in place for 6 hours after intercourse.
9. Remove the sponge after 30 hours of continuous use.
10. *To remove*, insert a finger intravaginally and pull the sponge out using the loop.

Common Errors

- Failure to hydrate the sponge before use. The spermicide is most effective if the sponge is dampened with at least two tablespoons of water and then squeezed.
- Failure to place the correct side of the sponge directly against the cervix. After placement, check that the sponge edges are well applied against the fornices and that the loop is on the side that faces the vagina.

Postprocedure Patient Education

The sponge should be left in for a minimum of 6 hours after intercourse. It should not be left in place for longer than 30 continuous hours. Sponges are for one-time use only. Used sponges should be disposed of in a trash receptacle and not in a toilet.

Male and Female Condoms

The *male condom* is a barrier contraceptive device that covers the penis and isolates sperm. It is unrolled onto the erect penis while leaving a space at the end to contain the ejaculate. Although most modern male condoms are made of latex, animal-product and polyurethane-based prophylactics are inexpensive and all are available without a prescription. The clinician should discuss appropriate use with patients because male condoms are frequently used incorrectly and patients are often reticent about asking questions. When combined with spermicide, pregnancy rates range from 2 to 10 pregnancies per 100 users per year. Male condoms serve as a barrier and can decrease the transmission of STIs.

The *FC Female Condom* is an over-the-counter, FDA-approved condom for women (Fig. 130-9). It is one size and does not require fitting. Made of soft, flexible polyurethane, it is a lubricated sheath with flexible rings on each end. The sealed ring is inserted into the vagina like a diaphragm, whereas the open ring rests against the vulva. Female condoms made of nitrile (FC2 condoms) are one-third the cost of the polyurethane condom, but are not available in the United States. Of 100 women who use female condoms, 21 become pregnant within 1 year with typical use; perfect use has a 5 in 100 failure rate.

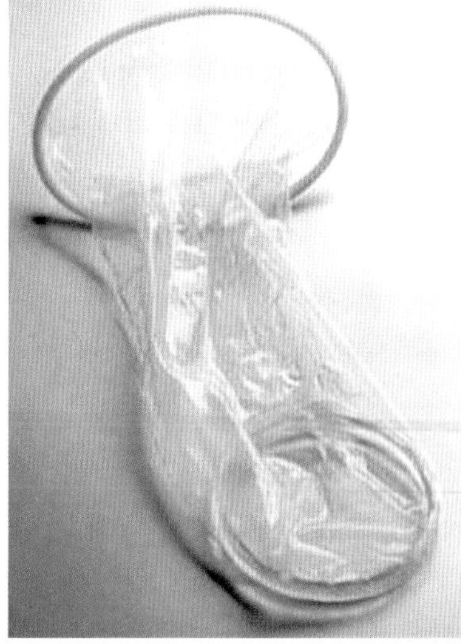

Figure 130-9 The FC female condom. (Courtesy of The Female Health Company, Chicago, Ill; with permission.)

Indications

- Pregnancy prevention
- Prevention of STIs
- Adjunct to other contraception for STI prevention

Absolute Contraindications

- Allergy or hypersensitivity to latex (latex condoms)
- Allergy or hypersensitivity to spermicide (condoms containing spermicide)
- Allergy to polyurethane (female condom)

Precautions

The availability of emergency contraception should be discussed.

Preprocedure Patient Education and Forms

The female condom can be inserted up to 8 hours before intercourse but usually is inserted immediately before use. The FC2 condom is available over the counter and is for one-time use only. The cost is around $2.50 per condom.

Please see the patient education form available online at www.expertconsult.com.

Procedure (Female Condom)

1. Detailed instructions for use are available in the product packaging.
2. Squeeze the sides of the inner ring (closed end of condom) and insert it into the vaginal vault.
3. Push the inner ring until it encircles the cervix
4. Let the outer ring overlap an inch over the perineum.
5. For condom removal, squeeze and twist the outer ring to keep semen from leaking out. Pull the condom from the vagina and dispose of it in the trash.

Common Errors

- Condom efficacy is decreased with use of certain lubricants or oil-based compounds (Box 130-1).
- Use of old/dated condoms may result in contraceptive failure. Keep condoms properly stored and use by the expiration date printed on the wrapper.

Box 130-1. Common Oil-Based Preparations that Adversely Affect Condom Efficacy

Baby oil
Butoconazole (Femstat)
Butter
Cocoa butter
Cold cream
Conjugated estrogens (Premarin)
Estradiol (Estrace)
Hand lotion
Lubricants
Medications
Miconazole (Monistat)
Mineral oil
Petroleum jelly Hand lotion
Shortening
Suntan oil
Tioconazole (Vagistat-1)
Vegetable oil

Complications

- Vaginal irritation with female condom use.
- Condom rupture can result in pregnancy. Emergency contraception may be considered if the risk of pregnancy is high (see Chapter 129, Emergency Contraception).
- Hypersensitivity or allergy to latex or polyurethane. Male and female condoms made from plastic or nitrile are an option.

CPT/Billing Code

57170 Diaphragm or cervical cap fitting with instructions

ICD-9 Diagnostic Codes

V25 Encounter for contraceptive management
V25.0 General contraceptive counseling and advice
V25.02 Initiation of other contraceptive measures: fitting of diaphragm, prescribing of other agents
V25.09 Other family planning advice
V25.40 Surveillance of a previously prescribed unspecified contraceptive
V25.9 Unspecified contraceptive management

Suppliers

(See contact information online at www.expertconsult.com.)

Cervical cap
FemCap
Diaphragm
Milex Wide-Seal silicone diaphragm
Milex Products, Inc.
Ortho All-Flex Arcing Spring and Ortho Coil Spring diaphragms
Ortho-McNeil Janssen Scientific Affairs, LLC
Female condoms
FC Female Condom
Female Health Company
Lea's shield
Yama, Inc.
Sponge
Today Sponge contraceptive
SYNOVA Healthcare Inc.

Online Resources

Cervical Barrier Advancement Society (CBAS). Available at www.cervicalbarriers.org/information/methods.cfm.
Female Health Company: The product. Available at www.femalehealth.com/theproduct.html.
FemCap: News. Available at www.femcap.com/news.htm.
Lea's Shield. Available at www.leasshield.com/.
Planned Parenthood: Birth control. Available at www.plannedparenthood.org/birth-control-pregnancy/birth-control/prescription.htm.

Bibliography

Allen R: Diaphragm fitting. Am Fam Physician 69:97–100, 103, 105–106, 2004.
Cook L, Nanda K, Grimes D: Diaphragm versus diaphragm with spermicides for contraception. Cochrane Database Syst Rev 1:CD002031, 2003.
Gallo M, Grimes D, Schulz K: Cervical cap versus diaphragm for contraception. Cochrane Database Syst Rev 4:CD003551, 2002.
Kuyoh M, Toroitich-Ruto C, Grimes D, et al: Sponge versus diaphragm for contraception. Cochrane Database Syst Rev 3:CD003172, 2002.
Minnis A, Padian N: Effectiveness of female controlled barrier methods in preventing sexually transmitted infections and HIV: Current evidence and future research directions. Sex Transm Infect 81:193–200, 2005.
Narrigan D: Women's barrier contraceptive methods: Poised for change. J Midwifery Womens Health 51:478–485, 2006.
Usatine RP: The Color Atlas of Family Medicine. New York, McGraw-Hill, 2009.

CHAPTER 131

Bartholin's Cyst and Abscess: Word Catheter Insertion, Marsupialization

Michael L. Tuggy

Bartholin's glands are located at the vaginal opening between the hymenal ring and labia minora (at approximately the 5 and 7 o'clock positions). Simple incision and drainage (I&D) of a Bartholin's duct cyst or gland abscess may give immediate results with significant pain relief, but recurrence after such a procedure is common. Bartholin's cysts and abscesses are best treated using a *Word catheter* to induce the formation of an epithelialized tract from the *vulvar vestibule* to the cyst. This allows continued functioning of the Bartholin's gland, proper drainage, and minimal recurrence. The recurrence rate using this technique is between 2% and 15%. The Word catheter has a short latex stem with an inflatable bulb at the distal end (Fig. 131-1) and can be used for both conditions.

For patients with noninflamed and recurrent Bartholin's cysts, *marsupialization* is a permanent cure. The procedure can be performed in the office but often is done as a same-day surgical procedure. It is very well tolerated by patients, with a rapid healing time and minimal postprocedure discomfort. Complications are rare and the technique is easily learned, especially by those physicians familiar with perineal repairs.

Indications

- Treatment of symptomatic Bartholin's duct cyst (painful, growing)
- Treatment of Bartholin's gland abscess

Contraindications

Any condition that would preclude normal I&D of a vulvar cyst or abscess would preclude use of the Word catheter. Small, asymptomatic glands do not need to be drained.

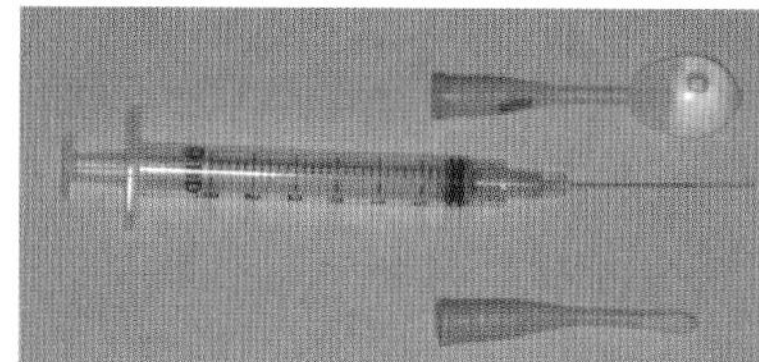

Figure 131-1 Word catheter (*bottom*). 3-mL syringe filled with water and 25-gauge needle (*middle*). Word catheter inflated with water (*top*).

Equipment

- Word catheter (Rusch and Milex; most medical suppliers will have on hand)
- 3-mL syringe (for catheter inflation)
- 22-gauge, 1-inch needle (for catheter inflation)
- 2% lidocaine for anesthesia, usually with epinephrine
- 30-gauge, $1\frac{1}{2}$-inch needle (for anesthesia)
- 3-mL syringe (for anesthesia)
- No. 11 blade
- Pickups with teeth
- Small hemostats (two)
- 4 × 4 gauze pads
- Normal saline for irrigation
- Antiseptic solution (povidone–iodine if not allergic)
- 4-0 Vicryl suture (if marsupialization is done)

Preprocedure Patient Education

The clinician should explain the procedure to the patient and obtain informed consent. A non-narcotic oral analgesic may be administered before the procedure, if desired.

Procedure

Word Catheter Placement

1. Place the patient in the dorsal lithotomy position.
2. Prepare the labia and vagina with the antiseptic solution. It is preferable to enter the cyst (Fig. 131-2A) or abscess from the vaginal side of the introitus unless this would require a much deeper incision (Fig. 131-2B). Inject lidocaine over the intended site of entry. If the incision is to be made external to the introitus where the abscess is "pointing," plan to insert the catheter approximately in the area of the original duct orifice, immediately adjacent the hymenal ring (Fig. 131-2C).
3. Lance or incise the cyst or abscess with a no. 11 scalpel blade (see Fig. 131-2C). It is essential that the stab wound penetrate the cyst or abscess wall, which will be evidenced by the free flow of pus or mucus. *Culture* contents if indicated. Although the majority of simple cysts are sterile, abscesses are typically

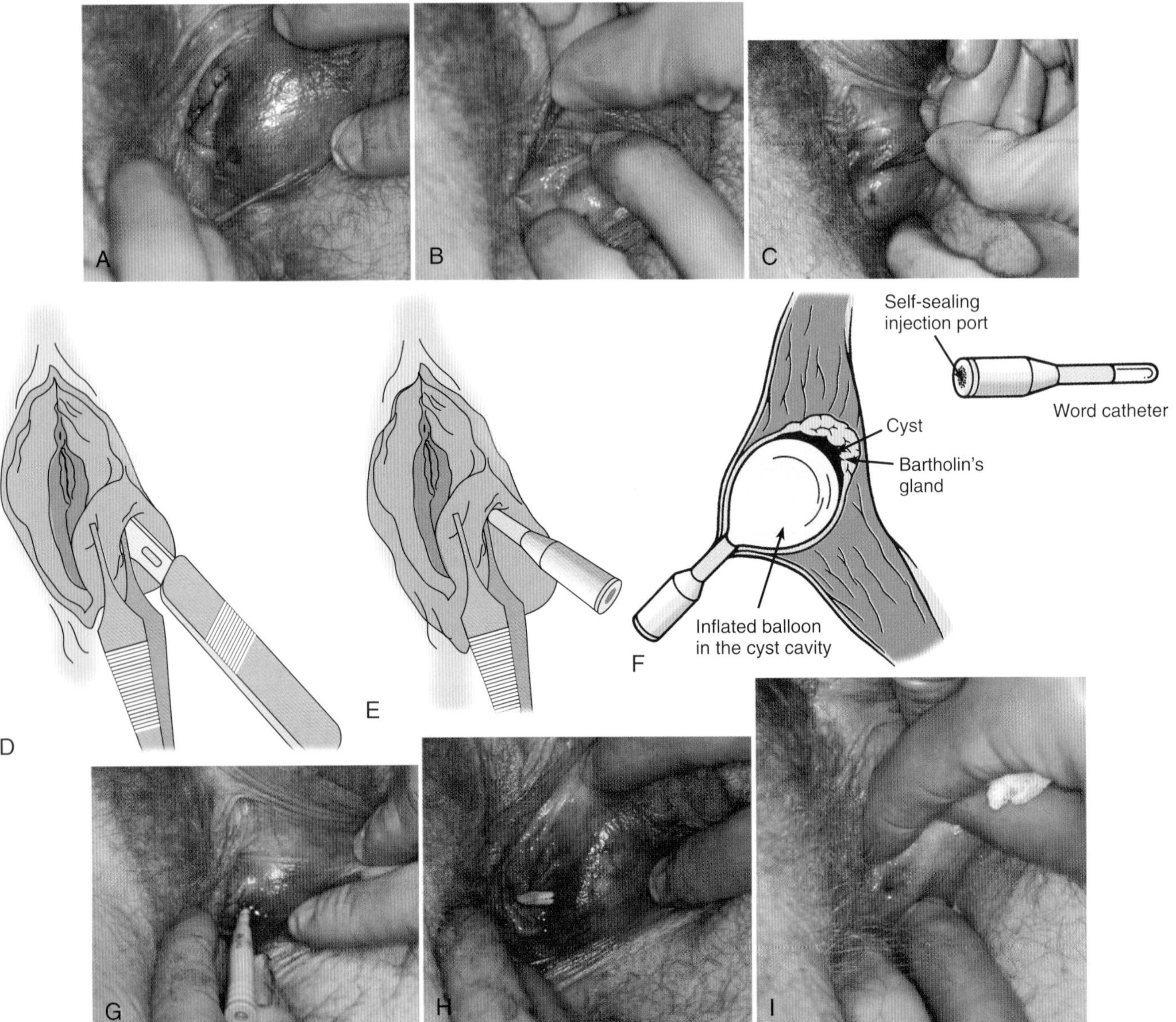

Figure 131-2 Insertion of Word catheter. **A,** Bartholin cyst after local anesthetic has been injected superficially. **B,** No. 11 blade points to ideal location inside the hymenal ring for the incision. However, the cyst is more prominent externally, so incision will be made there. **C,** Incising the cyst. Make the opening just large enough for the uninflated Word catheter tip to enter. **D,** Slide Adson forceps with teeth along the blade (which is in the cyst/abscess) and gently grasp the tissue. This will define the tract into the cyst. If this is not done, especially in smaller cysts, a false cavity may be created when inserting the catheter. **E,** The blade is removed but the forceps are kept in place. Insert the catheter along the forceps. **F,** Remove the forceps. Inflate the balloon with saline. Gently tug the catheter after inflation to ensure it does not fall out of the opening. **G,** Balloon is inflated within the cavity of the cyst so that it will not fall out through the stab wound. **H,** Tuck the exposed portion of the catheter into the vagina. **I,** Appearance of the area immediately after removal of the catheter.

polymicrobial, and many others contain *Neisseria gonorrhoeae*. Culture usually will not change initial management. The stab wound must be *just large enough* for the catheter to be inserted, usually 3 to 4 mm.

It may be difficult to insert the catheter into the cyst cavity if the incision is made, the contents are extruded, and the cyst/abscess has collapsed. Attempting to insert the catheter blindly may create a false tract and the catheter may not be in the cyst/abscess itself, which is necessary. *To avoid creating a false tract and to ensure proper placement of the catheter*, incise carefully through the skin until the cyst/abscess fluid drains. Before removing the blade, but after the incision is made, insert pickups (with teeth) down the side of the blade into the lumen and grasp gently (Fig. 131-2D). This stabilizes the tissue and identifies the cavity. Remove the blade. Insert the Word catheter (Fig. 131-2E).

4. Once inserted, inflate the catheter bulb by injecting 3 mL of saline through the sealed-stopper end (Fig. 131-2F). Use just that quantity of saline necessary to ensure that the catheter will not fall out with normal activity (usually 2.5 to 3 mL). Do *not* use air to inflate the catheter. Remove the pickups (Fig. 131-2G).
5. If the incision was made inside the hymen, tuck the catheter stem into the vagina, where it will rest perpendicular to the perineum (Fig. 131-2H). With the catheter in the vagina, the patient has freedom of movement and activity without the added awareness of protrusion of the catheter stem, which can occur if an external incision site is used. Most patients tolerate the catheter without discomfort if excessive amounts of saline are not introduced into the catheter bulb.
6. The catheter can be removed after withdrawing the saline in 4 to 6 weeks, leaving a small ostium for the gland (Fig. 131-2I).

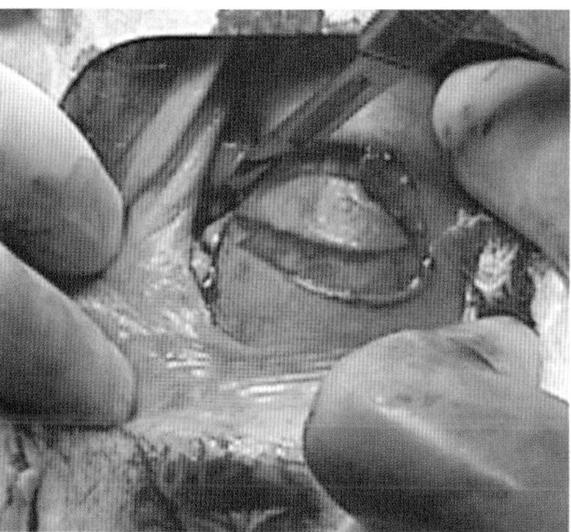

Figure 131-3 Incision for marsupialization on vaginal sidewall (retracted).

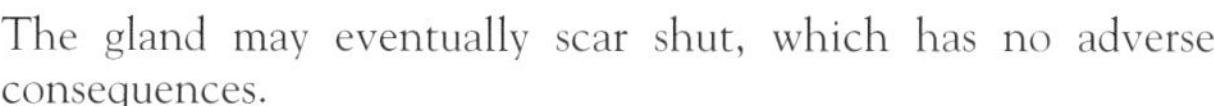

The gland may eventually scar shut, which has no adverse consequences.

Bartholin's Cyst Marsupialization

1. Place the patient in the dorsal lithotomy position. Block the incision site with local anesthetic with 2% lidocaine with epinephrine or use a pudendal block with 2% lidocaine without epinephrine. Some patients may prefer spinal or general anesthesia, but this requires the procedure be done in a same-day surgery center.
2. Clean the perineum with povidone–iodine solution (if not allergic).
3. Inspect the external genitalia to determine the extent of the duct cyst. Retract the labium laterally to identify the incision site *internal* to the hymeneal ring. Make the incision longitudinal with respect to the vagina (Fig. 131-3). Incisions can also be done following the circumferential folds of the vaginal mucosa, but lack the natural tension of the mucosa and could lead to premature closure and incomplete marsupialization. Generally, a fusiform incision 1 or 2 cm in width at the center is needed to allow for removal of a substantial portion of the Bartholin's cyst wall. Avoid excising any portion of the external skin (vs. mucosa).
4. Usually during this excision of the ellipse, the cyst contents and the cyst wall will collapse. Therefore, the mucosa over the cyst should be excised first and the cyst wall grasped with two small hemostats before the segment is removed. Explore the cyst with small hemostats and remove any loculated portions of the cyst. Patients older than 40 years of age are at higher risk for cancer in Bartholin's gland, so look for signs of neoplastic-appearing epithelium in the cyst (Fig. 131-4).
5. Thoroughly irrigate the cyst cavity with normal saline.

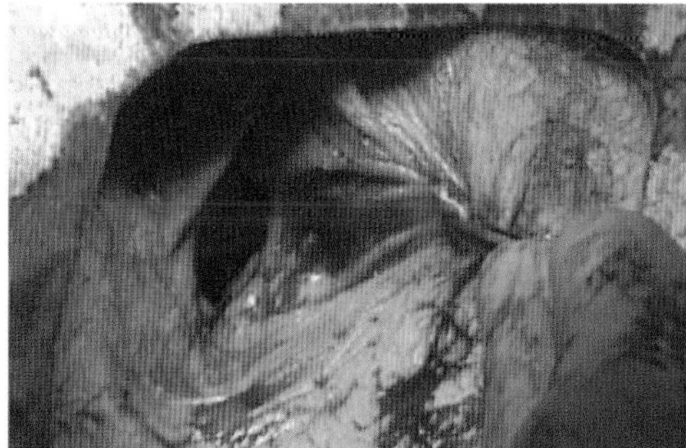

Figure 131-4 Bartholin's cyst opened with roof removed.

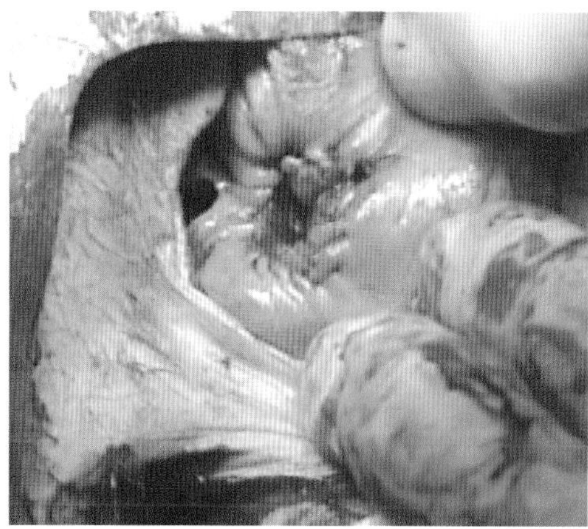

Figure 131-5 Marsupialized Bartholin's cyst with sutures in place.

6. When suturing the Bartholin's cyst wall, approximate the cut edge of the cyst wall to the adjacent edge of the vaginal mucosa. This allows for more rapid transformation of the Bartholin's cyst wall into a normal mucosal lining that will blend into the vaginal mucosa. Use 4-0 Vicryl and place interrupted sutures around the excisional margins.
7. Place an anchoring stitch with long tags proximally to grasp and stabilize the tissue. Pass the stitches from the inside through just the Bartholin's cyst wall. Bring the needle to the surface between the cyst wall and submucosal layer. Now insert the needle under the vaginal epithelium and pull it to the surface of the vaginal wall. This effectively imbricates the two layers (cyst wall and vaginal mucosa) over the submucosal tissue, which allows them to heal together (Fig. 131-5). The intent is to suture the cyst cavity open.
8. After the entire site has been sutured open, irrigate the wound and inspect it for bleeding. There should be a gap of at least 1 cm across the open marsupialization. Normally no dressing is needed. A pad is placed to allow for collection of blood or drainage from the wound.
9. Instruct the patient to perform sitz baths daily for 3 or 4 days and to return for follow-up in about a week (see the postoperative patient handout available online at www.expertconsult.com). At that time, the cavity will be probed for patency. Use of prophylactic antibiotics is unnecessary in most cases and the need should be assessed individually. Excessive induration in the local tissue or risk factors for infection, such as pregnancy or diabetes, may prompt the need for antibiotic therapy. Sutures will absorb without further intervention.

Common Errors

- Creating a false tract for the catheter placement (see earlier).
- Catheter falls out before it is time to be removed. This may lead to recurrence of the cyst/abscess. The error occurs after the balloon is inserted into the cyst/abscess and after the fluid is injected into the balloon (but the syringe is still in the port), when the clinician releases the pressure on the syringe plunger to check the tightness of the balloon in the cavity by tugging on it. Although it may seem secure then, the increased pressure in the balloon will push some saline back up into the syringe (unless pressure is maintained on the plunger). The balloon then in effect deflates to a smaller size and the catheter may inadvertently fall out prematurely. To prevent this from occurring, *maintain pressure on the syringe plunger while checking the bulb placement and snugness in the cavity*. The catheter could also fall out because of too large of a stab wound.

- Continuous pain after insertion of the Word catheter may occur. The bulb may be too large for the cyst cavity, which may be corrected by withdrawing some of the fluid, thus reducing the size of the bulb. Also, if the bulb is not in the true cavity but in the space between the fascia and the cyst wall, the patient will complain of significant pain. In this case, catheter removal and reinsertion will need to be repeated under local anesthesia.
- With an abscessed Bartholin's gland, there may be cellulitis around the vulvar opening of the duct. Insertion of the catheter may not correct the cellulitis and antibiotics may need to be administered for 48 to 72 hours after insertion of the catheter. If *N. gonorrhoeae* is cultured, appropriate actions need to be taken.
- If the needle used to introduce the saline into the catheter punctures the stem, the catheter will gradually deflate and fall out before epithelialization is complete.
- If the stab wound is too large, the catheter will fall out. It may be necessary to suture the stab wound around the catheter to keep it in place. If the catheter falls out in less than 4 weeks, the likelihood of recurrence is high. Because of only partial formation of a new tract, placement of another Word catheter is indicated, but it may not be possible because of constriction of the opening.

Complications

- Excessive bleeding (rare)
- Discomfort (usually only a few days)
- Recurrence
- Scarring (usually minimal)
- Infection
- Premature expulsion of the catheter

Postprocedure Patient Education

Word Catheter

- Tell the patient to expect a discharge because the catheter will allow for drainage of the cyst or abscess.
- The Word catheter is left in place for 4 to 6 weeks until epithelialization of the new tract is complete.
- Advise the patient that sexual activity may be resumed after 2 weeks, but it may increase the risk of expulsion of the catheter. If this happens, another catheter may need to be inserted. It is best to defer sexual activity until the catheter is removed.
- Encourage daily showers or tub baths.
- Schedule a return visit in 4 to 6 weeks. At that time, the catheter is removed by inserting a needle into the catheter sealed-stopper end and drawing out the saline. The catheter is then withdrawn from the incision.

Marsupialization

- Daily sitz baths are encouraged for 3 to 5 days.
- Avoid sexual activity until after the first postoperative check at 1 week, although waiting for an additional week would be most prudent to allow for more complete healing.

CPT/Billing Codes

56405 I&D of vulvar or perineal abscess
56420 I&D of Bartholin's gland cyst/abscess
56440 Marsupialization of Bartholin's gland cyst
56740 Excision of Bartholin's gland or cyst

ICD-9-CM Diagnostic Codes

616.2 Bartholin's cyst
616.3 Bartholin's abscess
616.4 Other vulvar abscess

Acknowledgment

The editors wish to recognize the contributions by Barbara S. Apgar, MD, to this chapter in the previous two editions of this text.

Suppliers

(See contact information online at www.expertconsult.com.)

Word Bartholin's gland catheter
Milex Products, Inc.
Rusch, Inc.

BIBLIOGRAPHY

Goldberg JE: Simplified treatment for disease of Bartholin's gland. Obstet Gynecol 35:109–110, 1970.

Heah J: Methods of treatment for cysts and abscesses of Bartholin's gland. Br J Obstet Gynaecol 95:321–322, 1988.

Lashgari M, Curry S: Preferred methods of treating Bartholin's duct cyst. Contemp Obstet Gynecol 40:38–41, 1995.

Omole F, Simmons BJ, Hacker Y: Management of Bartholin's duct cyst and gland abscess. Am Fam Physician 68:135–140, 2003.

Tuggy M, Garcia J: Procedures Consult. Available at www.proceduresconsult.com.

Wechter MD, Wu JM, Marzano D, Haefner H: Management of Bartholin duct cyst and abscesses: A systematic review. Obstet Gynecol Surv 64:395–404, 2009.

Word B: New instrument for office treatment of cyst and abscess of Bartholin's gland. JAMA 190:777–778, 1964.

CHAPTER 132

BREAST BIOPSY

Helen A. Pass

An excisional breast biopsy is a technically straightforward outpatient procedure readily performed under local anesthesia. With appropriate training and experience, primary care physicians can become qualified to perform most simple breast biopsies. The challenge is to correctly identify which lesions are amenable to biopsy and which require referral to a breast (general) surgeon. The goals in the management of a patient with a breast mass should be to obtain the diagnosis in the most expedient manner, to achieve good cosmesis, and to preserve all therapeutic options if the mass is unexpectedly found to be malignant at biopsy.

The only definitive method for ensuring that a mass is benign is to remove tissue for pathologic examination. The missed or delayed diagnosis of a breast mass that ultimately proved to be cancerous is currently the most litigious aspect of medical practice. Failure to be impressed with physical examination findings was cited as the most common reason for the delay in the diagnosis of breast cancer. Benign masses are usually smooth, well circumscribed (round), and freely mobile; however, many cancers (e.g., colloid, medullary, and expansive intraductal) may mimic this presentation. Similarly, even though the incidence of breast cancer rises dramatically after age 65 years, 63% to 80% of lawsuits resulted from the missed diagnosis of cancer in women younger than 50 years of age. In addition, whereas the presence of a significant positive family history increases the suspicion that a palpable abnormality may prove to be malignant, two thirds of all women with the diagnosis of breast cancer have no identifiable risk factor. Nevertheless, it is important to remind our patients and ourselves that not all breast masses are cancerous.

The role of mammography in women with a breast mass is twofold. First, it can offer clues as to the degree of suspicion that the mass may be malignant. Worrisome mammographic features include the findings of a spiculated lesion, a mass associated with pleomorphic microcalcifications, or dermal edema and retraction. Second, it allows assessment of the remainder of the breast parenchyma in both the involved and contralateral breasts. Before proceeding with excisional biopsy, a baseline mammogram must be obtained to rule out the presence of an occult synchronous lesion that may alter the surgical approach. Moreover, if the mass is highly suspect, *referral to a surgeon* may be indicated to facilitate management of a presumed breast cancer. *It is crucial to realize that failure of mammography or ultrasonography to visualize a discrete, palpable abnormality should not be construed as evidence of the benignity of the lesion.* Up to 10% of breast cancers are radiographically occult. Thus, a lesion should be removed if it meets the criteria for biopsy based on the clinical breast examination, regardless of the breast imaging characteristics. Likewise, if a woman identifies an area of change in her breasts, the complaint should be taken seriously.

In addition to highly suspect lesions, *referral to a breast (general) surgeon* should be considered for an additional small subset of patients. *Masses in prepubertal or pubescent girls* (prepubertal gynecomastia) could represent the forming breast buds and must not be sampled for biopsy unless highly suspect because lifelong cosmetic deformity may result. *Masses greater than 4 cm* are best approached by core biopsy provided that if the lesion proves to be malignant, consideration should be given to neoadjuvant chemotherapy. In addition, if the lesion is benign, special surgical techniques will be necessary to minimize the cosmetic deformity associated with subsequent removal. Finally, biopsy of *lesions requiring preoperative mammographic localization with wire placement* should be performed by physicians who have received specific training in this technique.

Consideration should be given to performing fine-needle aspiration (FNA) before core or excisional biopsy (see Chapter 226, Fine-Needle Aspiration Cytology and Biopsy). FNA is both diagnostic and therapeutic for simple cysts, thereby avoiding unnecessary anxiety and surgery. If the mass is solid, a specimen for cytologic examination can be obtained, and breast cancer can be diagnosed before excisional biopsy. The false-negative rate of FNA is 0.4% to 35% and the false-positive rate is less than 1%. Thus, concordance among the clinical breast examination, the breast imaging, and the FNA (the triple test) must be established, especially if the decision is made not to proceed to biopsy.

ANATOMY

Anatomically, the breast extends superiorly to the level of the clavicle, inferiorly to the sixth or seventh rib, medially to the lateral border of the sternum, and laterally to the border of the latissimus dorsi muscle. The glandular structure sits atop the pectoralis major muscle, and deep breast biopsies may extend to the level of the fascia. The *blood supply* originates from the internal mammary, axillary, and intercostal arteries. The venous outflow parallels this arterial supply. The only *innervation* to the breast is cutaneous, extending from the plexus of nerves in the neck for the superior half of the breast and the intercostal nerves for the lower half of the breast. There is no direct innervation to the glandular structure. The *lymphatic vessels* in the breast drain to the axilla and the internal mammary lymph nodes.

In the center of the breast is the *nipple and areolar complex*. Surrounding the edge of the areolar complex are Montgomery tubercles, which provide lubrication important for breast-feeding.

The breast mound itself is composed of fat and glandular milk-producing tissue. About 15 to 20 ducts converge to exit the nipple. *Cooper's ligaments* run from the deep fascia to the dermis, traversing the breast gland and serving as suspensory ligaments of the breast. The lack of named structures within the breast glandular tissue simplifies breast biopsy because hemostasis usually is readily achieved with electrocautery. Except with circumareolar incision placement, numbness is rare in the peri-incisional area.

INDICATIONS

- The presence of a palpable, dominant abnormality in a male or female patient
- A cystic lesion if
  - The FNA contained bloody fluid
  - A palpable abnormality remains after FNA
  - The cyst recurred after two FNAs

- After an FNA that was equivocal, nondiagnostic, or not concordant with the clinical breast examination or breast imaging
- Unresolved patient anxiety and a desire for removal of the mass
- Physician uncertainty about the true nature of the lesion

Contraindications

Relative

- Mass that is highly suspect for breast cancer (refer to breast or general surgeon)
- Mass greater than 4 cm (consider diagnosis by core biopsy or referral to surgeon)
- Mass in a prepubertal or pubescent female (consider referral)
- Lesion requiring preoperative mammographic localization (i.e., it is nonpalpable; consider referral)

Absolute

Uncorrected bleeding disorder or other unstable medical condition is an absolute contraindication.

Equipment and Supplies

- Surgical marking pen
- Povidone–iodine or other antiseptic skin preparation solution
- Fenestrated drape
- Local anesthetic (the addition of 1 mL of 8.5% sodium bicarbonate solution to each 10 mL of 1% lidocaine without epinephrine creates a buffered solution with a more neutral pH, allowing less discomfort during infiltration and a more rapid onset of action)
- Sterile 4 × 4 gauze
- Scalpel with no. 15 blades
- Two curved hemostats
- Needle driver
- Adson pickups
- DeBakey pickups *(optional)*
- Metzenbaum tissue scissors
- Allis clamp
- Small self-retaining retractor (e.g., mastoid retractor or small Weitlaner retractor) *(optional)*
- Army-Navy or Senn retractor
- Electrocautery unit
- 3-0 or 4-0 Vicryl suture
- 4-0 or 5-0 Monocryl or polydioxanone suture
- Steri-Strips or Dermabond
- Jobst postoperative brassiere *(optional)*

Precautions

Immediately before any planned procedure, the woman must be examined. The surgeon must verify with the patient that the palpable abnormality still persists, concur on its location, and mark it with indelible ink. As with any surgical procedure, standard presurgical clearances and permits should be obtained.

Preprocedure Patient Preparation

All women older than 30 years of age should have a preprocedure mammogram. Provide calm reassurance to the patient because the discovery of a breast mass and the knowledge that biopsy is necessary is a highly stressful event for the patient. Provide detailed explanations of the procedure supplemented by written educational material.

Procedure

The abnormality should be identified and marked before the procedure with the patient's assistance. Determining the optimal placement of the incision for an excisional breast biopsy is a balance between achieving the most desirable cosmetic result and preserving further surgical options should the lesion prove to be cancerous. Use of preoperative FNA or core biopsy can minimize the number of breast masses unexpectedly found to be malignant. Generally, incisions placed along Langer's lines—the natural lines of skin tension and creasing—produce the best cosmetic result (Fig. 132-1A). However, a radial incision may be preferable in the most medial part of the breast (much easier to reexcise if a mastectomy is subsequently required) or in the lower half of the breast if the mass is larger, or subsequent removal of skin will be required (e.g., with reexcision lumpectomy; Fig. 132-1B). A better cosmetic result is achieved in the lower half of the breast by narrowing the breast when removing breast volume through a radial incision than by shortening the distance between the areolar complex and inframammary fold with a curvilinear incision. In a young woman in whom the mass is likely benign, consideration may be given to placing the incision in a circumareolar location.

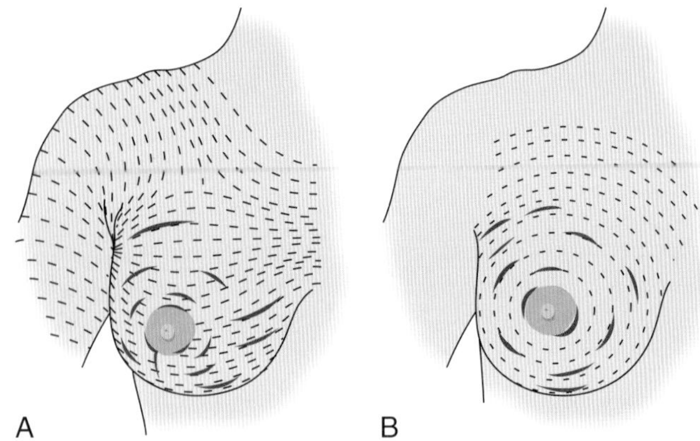

Figure 132-1 Proper planning of incisions limits postoperative scarring. See text for details.

Benign lesions may either be enucleated or removed with a small rim of normal tissue. Care should be taken to ensure that the mass is not morcellated. The specimen should be oriented for pathologic examination in case it is found to be malignant and reexcision is necessary.

After removing the breast mass, most surgeons no longer reapproximate the remaining deep breast parenchyma ("dead space"). This eliminates the breast distortion with poorer cosmesis and greater mammographic distortion that occurs when the "dead space" is reapproximated. Meticulous hemostasis must be achieved to avoid hematoma formation. Drains should *not* be used. Closure of the superficial fascia provides good restoration of the breast contours. The skin is then closed in a subcuticular fashion.

1. Obtain written informed consent.
2. Using sterile technique, cleanse and drape the breast.
3. Using a surgical marking pen, outline the incision and the borders of the mass (Fig. 132-2).
4. Give local anesthesia (1% lidocaine without epinephrine mixed 10:1 with 8.5% sodium bicarbonate). Infiltrate the incision with the local anesthetic to create a dermal wheal. Use the anesthetized wheal for all subsequent needle inserts, and infiltrate circumferentially around the lesion to be removed. Excess local anesthetic directly overlying the mass may obscure palpation of the nodule, hindering identification. (Alternatively, do a field block by injecting circumferentially around the lesion but not over the lesion itself. This allows easier palpation of the mass in the center of the field without the distortion created by the volume of anesthetic [Fig. 132-3].)
5. Incise the skin with a no. 15 blade, making sure to hold the blade at right angles to the skin edges to avoid beveling

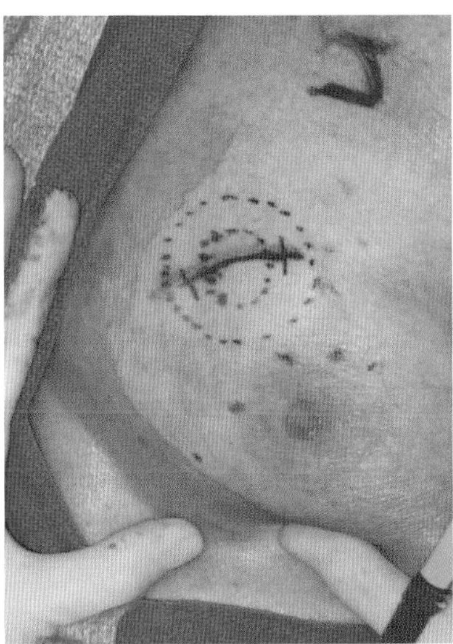

Figure 132-2 Palpable lesion marked for biopsy.

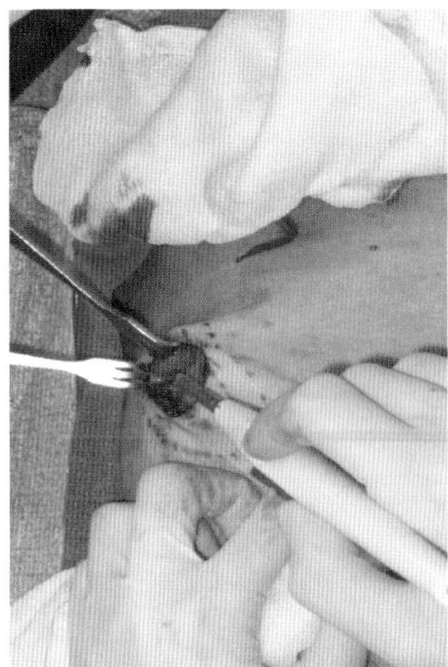

Figure 132-4 Dissection with electrocautery.

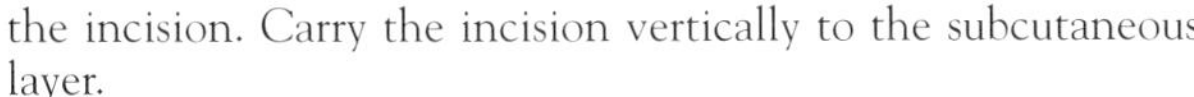

the incision. Carry the incision vertically to the subcutaneous layer.

6. Use tissue scissors or cautery to dissect down to the level of the mass (Fig. 132-4).
7. Cauterize bleeders with the electrocautery.
8. Circumferentially excise the specimen using the tissue scissors, a no. 15 blade, or the electrocautery unit (Fig. 132-5). Exercise care to avoid harming the skin edges. An Allis clamp may be used on the mass to provide countertraction, facilitating removal of the mass. Provide more local anesthesia in the deeper layers as needed).
9. Orient the specimen for pathologic evaluation using marking sutures (this can facilitate localization of inadequate margins should the lesion be found to be an incompletely excised malignancy).
10. Submit all specimens for pathologic evaluation. Use of frozen-section analysis is optional because hormone receptor analysis is now routinely performed on paraffin-embedded tissue in case of malignancy.
11. Obtain meticulous hemostasis with electrocautery.

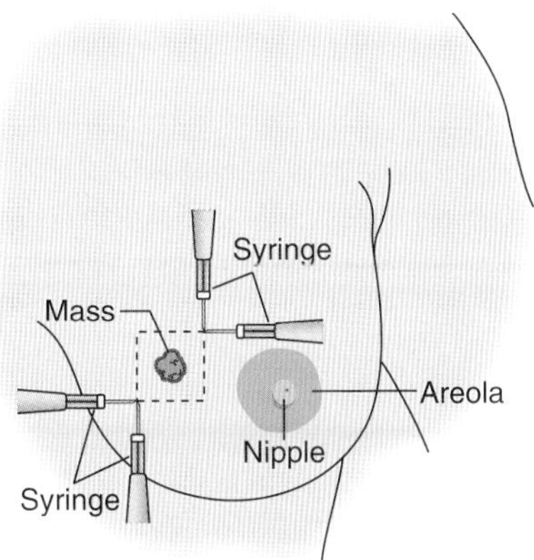

Figure 132-3 Field block local anesthesia technique to preserve the ability to palpate the lesion in the center of the field. Infiltration of excessive amounts of local anesthetic directly over the mass makes palpation of the abnormality difficult.

12. Reapproximate the subdermal tissue with buried interrupted Vicryl sutures. To prevent deformity, do not reapproximate the deep tissues, and do not incorporate excessively large amounts of tissue because this may lead to dimpling (Fig. 132-6).
13. Close the skin with a running subcuticular suture of 4-0 or 5-0 Monocryl or polydioxanone (Fig. 132-7).

Sample Operative Report

See the sample operative report online at www.expertconsult.com.

Common Errors

- Failure to sample a palpable, dominant mass because the lesion is radiographically occult
  Resolution: Because up to 10% of cancers can be radiographically occult, biopsy must be performed if clinical examination confirms the presence of a dominant mass.
- Failure to obtain a mammogram before biopsy
  Resolution: All women older than 30 years of age should have a recent mammogram before biopsy to rule out the presence of occult synchronous lesions that may modify the surgical approach.
- Poor orientation of the surgical incisions
  Resolution: Proper planning can ensure a better cosmetic outcome and allow for subsequent surgery if malignancy is identified (see Fig. 132-1).

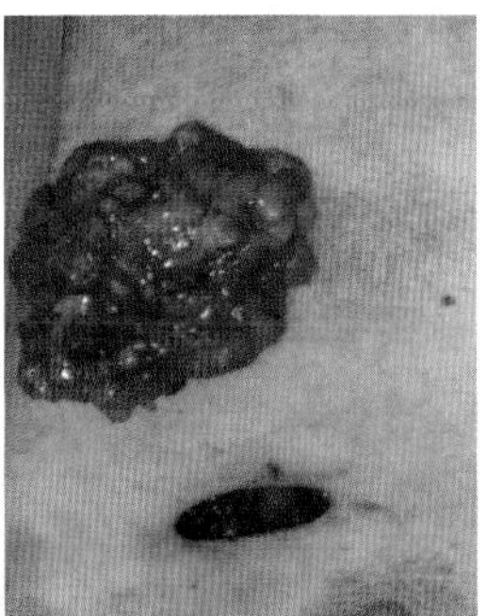

Figure 132-5 Lesion excised.

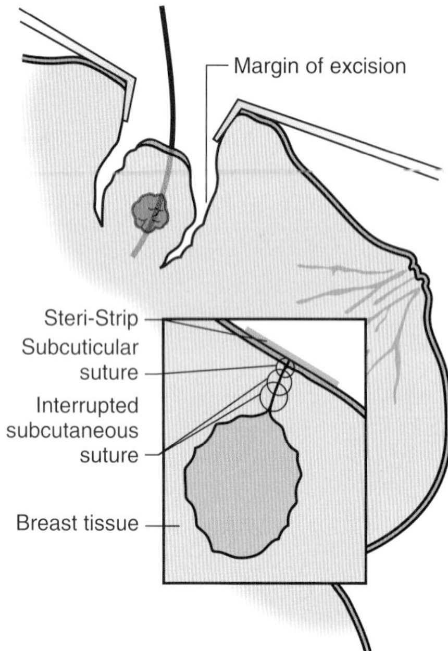

Figure 132-6 Schema for closure technique.

Complications

- Hematoma (may mimic recurrence of the mass)
  Resolution: (1) Confirm patient does not have an unsuspected bleeding diathesis. (2) If the hematoma is symptomatic, reoperate with evacuation of the hematoma. Search for and cauterize or ligate of any site of bleeding. Use a compressive dressing. (3) If asymptomatic, reassurance, use of a supportive brassiere, and passage of time will allow spontaneous resolution.
- Infection (cellulitis or abscess formation)
  Resolution: Seroma aspiration can differentiate between cellulitis and cellulitis with abscess formation (send fluid for Gram stain, culture, and sensitivity even if the fluid is clear). Cellulitis without abscess formation usually responds to oral antibiotic therapy. Resolution is usual with the use of a first-generation cephalosporin. If no response is obtained in 7 to 10 days, culture and sensitivity data may be helpful. For cellulitis with abscess formation, drainage of the abscess is necessary. Complete aspiration under ultrasonographic guidance and initiation of oral antibiotic therapy may be tried initially. If abscess recurs, drain placement with or without surgical evacuation and irrigation may be necessary. Again, culture and sensitivity data can help with antibiotic selection.

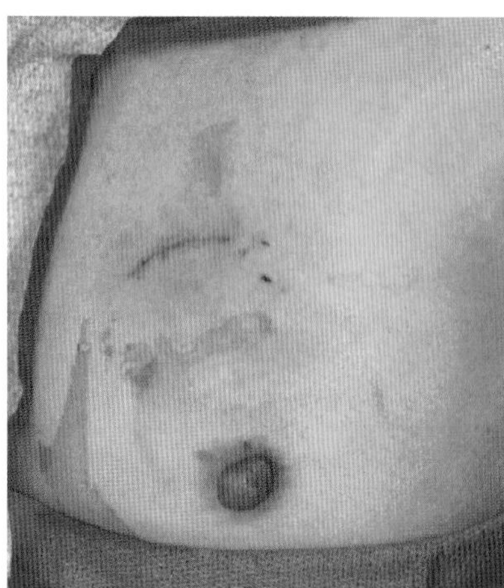

Figure 132-7 Cosmetic closure: appearance on completion of the surgery.

- Scarring or skin distortion
  Resolution: Be sure the patient understands that a fine scar should be expected. If the patient tends to form hypertrophic or keloid scars, a small amount of triamcinolone (10 mg/mL) can be used with the local anesthesia in the incision tract. Avoid scarring with appropriate preoperative planning. After surgery, silicone sheeting, Mederma cream application, or cross-scar massage may improve appearance of scarring.
- Pain (usually minimal)
  Resolution: The use of oral analgesics, use of supportive brassiere, and topical application of ice or heat should provide adequate relief.
- Fluid collection (seroma)
  Resolution: May require aspiration but only if symptomatic. The presence of an asymptomatic seroma is *not* an indication for drainage.
- Failure to identify the correct mass or incomplete removal of the lesion
  Resolution: Can be avoided by proper preoperative localization, marking, and patient confirmation. Before closure, palpate the biopsy bed to confirm the absence of residual palpable abnormality. If it is recognized after surgery, prompt reoperation is indicated.
- Need for subsequent surgery
  Resolution: If the mass is malignant or incompletely excised, promptly refer to a breast (general) surgeon.

Postprocedure Management

Wash off any remaining skin preparation solution, and then apply Steri-Strips and a sterile bandage or use a cyanoacrylate surgical glue (e.g., Dermabond [Ethicon, Somerville, NJ]). If adequate hemostasis has been ensured, there is no need for bulky, pressure dressings. A surgical brassiere may be used to enhance postoperative comfort.

The patient must be provided with prescriptions for adequate analgesia by mouth, emergency phone numbers, and written postoperative instructions.

The patient may remove the dressing in 24 to 48 hours and resume showering. If Dermabond or Opsite (Smith & Nephew, London) is used over gauze-covered Steri-Strips, the patient may shower immediately. Submersion of the incision (e.g., swimming) and vigorous exercise should be avoided for 1 week. The sutures will dissolve and should not require removal.

Postprocedure Patient Education

Give the patient written instructions regarding removal of the dressing, resumption of showering, and follow-up appointment. The patient should report excessive pain, drainage from the wound, redness, fever, or abnormal swelling. A follow-up appointment will ensure the lesion has been removed, although induration may be palpable for several weeks. See the patient education form online at www.expertconsult.com.

Special Considerations

- The appearance of the incision is all the patient sees; your surgical skill will be judged by the scar left on the breast. Plan the incision carefully and use plastic surgical technique for skin closure.
- It is imperative to communicate the pathology results in a timely manner and to refer to specialists if necessary.
- Avoid biopsy of large or complicated lesions; refer instead.

- Management of breast complaints is very litigious. Adequately document the work-up. Obtain informed consent. Diligently follow up all biopsy results, and recognize when referral is appropriate.

Conclusion

Accurate interpretation of the clinical breast examination can be difficult. Any persistent palpable abnormality or asymmetric finding must be evaluated with physical examination, breast radiologic imaging (mammography or ultrasonography), and tissue diagnosis. All findings must be concordant; if they are not, work-up must proceed even if the mammogram is negative. With sufficient training and experience, most primary care practitioners can perform excisional breast biopsies in the office setting expeditiously and with a good cosmetic outcome. Complex or highly suspect masses may prompt referral to a breast specialist.

Patient Education Guides

See patient education and patient consent forms available online at www.expertconsult.com.

CPT/Billing Codes

10021	Fine-needle aspirate (FNA)
10022	Fine-needle aspiration with imaging guidance
19000	Needle aspiration, cyst—one
19001	Needle aspiration, each additional cyst
19100	Biopsy of breast, core needle
19101	Biopsy of breast, incisional
19102	Biopsy of breast, core needle using imaging guidance
19103	Biopsy of breast, incisional using imaging guidance
19120	Excision of cysts or breast lesions
19125	Excision of breast lesion identified by preoperative placement of radiological marker
19126	Excision radiographically guided, each additional lesion

ICD-9-CM Diagnostic Codes

174.9	Malignant neoplasm of breast (female), unspecified
217	Benign neoplasm of the breast
611.72	Lump or mass in the breast
793.80	Abnormal mammogram, unspecified
793.81	Mammographic microcalcification
793.89	Other abnormal findings on radiological examination of the breast

Supplier

(See contact information online at www.expertconsult.com.)

Jobst postoperative brassiere
Fredericks–Jobst Institute, Inc.

Online Resource

National Comprehensive Cancer Network has online breast cancer screening and diagnosis guidelines, which are updated annually. www.nccn.org.

The Susan G. Komen for the Cure website contains medically reviewed material on screening, diagnosis, and treatment of breast diseases authored by the largest breast cancer patient advocacy group. www.komen.org.

Bibliography

Cady B, Steele GD, Morrow M, et al: Evaluation of common breast problems: Guidance for primary care providers. CA Cancer J Clin 48:49–63, 1998.

Conry C: Evaluation of a breast complaint: Is it cancer? Am Fam Physician 49:445–450, 453–454, 1994.

Donegan WL: Evaluation of a palpable breast mass. N Engl J Med 327: 937–942, 1992.

Gamble WG: Breast surgery. In Benjamin RB (ed): Atlas of Outpatient and Office Surgery, 2nd ed. Philadelphia, Lea & Febiger, 1994.

Layfield LJ, Glasgow BJ, Cramer H: Fine-needle aspiration in the management of breast masses. Pathol Annu 24:23–62, 1989.

Physician Insurers Association of America: Breast Cancer Study. Lawrenceville, NJ, Physician Insurers Association of America, 1990.

CHAPTER 133

Cervical Cerclage

Madeline R. Lewis • Mark Lewis

Cerclage is a procedure designed to manage cervical insufficiency, which is defined as a painless dilation of the cervix with expulsion of the products of conception in the second or early third trimester. Most often cerclage is used to prevent preterm deliveries in women with a history of previous second-trimester pregnancy losses or known shortened cervices.

The incidence of cervical insufficiency is uncertain because of the lack of clear diagnostic criteria and inadequate reporting methods. The success rate of cerclage is also difficult to assess owing to a paucity of adequate data. Available studies suggest a 75% to 90% success rate with cerclage when used in a subsequent pregnancy after recurrent pregnancy loss.

There are several different cerclage techniques; the most common and simplest is the McDonald procedure. Other techniques include the Shirodkar cerclage and transabdominal approaches. The McDonald cerclage involves inserting a pursestring stitch at the cervicovaginal junction using monofilament suture. This procedure is best done as an elective procedure but may also by used in an urgent or emergent setting.

American College of Obstetricians and Gynecologists (ACOG) guidelines recommend performing an elective cerclage at 14 to 16 weeks' gestation after verifying fetal life by ultrasonography. The cerclage is removed after the 37th week of pregnancy or the onset of premature labor.

Anatomy

The relevant anatomy is shown in Figure 133-1. The area of importance is the proximal cervix, near the area where the cervix meets the vaginal wall. The orientation of the cervix is important, and this chapter uses the clock method of describing locations on the cervix. This method assumes that the patient is in the dorsal lithotomy position and that the anterior cervix is defined as 12 o'clock.

Indications

Cervical insufficiency may be due to many factors. Cerclage may be considered for all. Indications include the following:

- Most frequently, a history of cervical insufficiency that resulted in three or more unexplained second-trimester pregnancy losses or preterm labor. When possible, medical records from these pregnancies should be carefully reviewed to verify cervical insufficiency.
- Surgical trauma from cone biopsy, loop electrosurgical excision procedure, obstetric laceration, or overdilation during pregnancy termination.
- Congenital anomalies of the patient.
- Cervical length abnormalities (e.g., foreshortened cervix).
- Deficiencies in cervical collagen and elastin.
- In utero diethylstilbestrol exposure.
- Funneling of amniotic membranes into the cervical canal on ultrasonography.
- Placenta previa if associated with cervical dilation. Some advocate the use of cerclage with placenta previa alone, but this has not been shown to prolong pregnancy in these patients. Cerclage is not contraindicated in patients with placenta previa who otherwise should have the procedure performed.

Contraindications

Absolute

- Nonviable pregnancy
- Undiagnosed vaginal bleeding
- Ruptured membranes
- Active preterm labor
- Acute cervical or intrauterine infection

Relative

- Known or suspected abnormal pregnancy
- Prolapse of fetal membranes through the external cervical os (higher risk of iatrogenic rupture of membranes)

Equipment and Supplies

Cerclage is considered an outpatient procedure and is performed in the operating room. Sterile preparation and proper drapes and equipment are necessary. Specific instruments include the following:

- Bladder catheter
- Weighted vaginal speculum
- Retractor (Deaver or right-angle)
- Ring forceps
- Nonabsorbable suture material (no. 5 Mersilene band, Ethibond; not to be confused with a 5-0 suture, which is much smaller) and curved needle
- Pickups
- Metzenbaum scissors
- Needle driver

Precautions

Be aware that an urgent or emergent cerclage will have an increased incidence of complications. A cerclage is best performed in a scheduled setting with clear indications. Be certain to confirm a viable pregnancy before starting the procedure.

Preprocedure Patient Education

- Inform patient that there are few data to prove the exact benefits and risks of the procedure.
- Review the risks of the procedure with the patient:
  - Rupture of membranes (may be up to 65% within 2 weeks)
  - Chorioamnionitis (may occur in up to 30% of cases)
  - Suture displacement

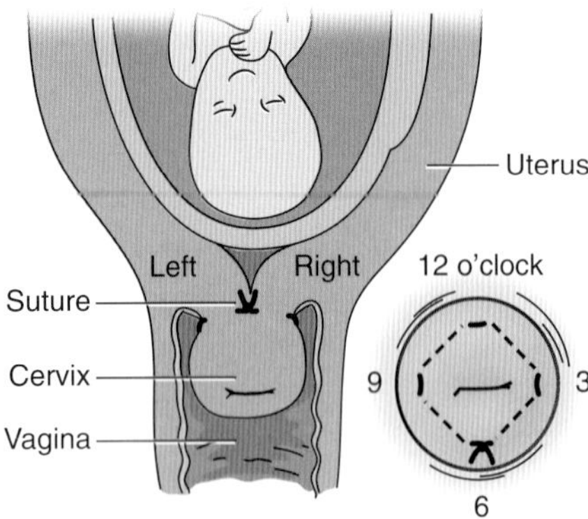

Figure 133-1 Cervical cerclage and relevant anatomy. Note that the initial suture is placed at 6 o'clock to allow the knot to reside in the posterior vagina.

- Uterine rupture
- Maternal septicemia
- Preterm labor and delivery
- Fetal loss
- Preoperative testing may be indicated to rule out cervical infection (gonorrhea/chlamydial infection).
- Ultrasonography is done before the procedure to confirm a normal intrauterine pregnancy.
- The procedure is done in an operating room and requires anesthesia (general or regional); the patient will need to have someone with her to drive her home after procedure.
- The procedure is usually done as an outpatient, same-day procedure.
- The patient will be placed on a fetal monitor before and after the procedure to document fetal viability
- After the procedure, acetaminophen (Tylenol) usually provides adequate pain control, if necessary.
- The patient may experience significant vaginal discharge for weeks after the procedure.
- The patient will need to be seen more frequently throughout the remainder of the pregnancy.
- Pelvic rest is often recommended; instruct the patient to limit physical activity for at least 1 week and to abstain from vaginal intercourse for at least 1 week and up to the entire pregnancy.

PROCEDURE

1. Obtain informed consent (see sample patient consent form online at www.expertconsult.com).
2. Document intrauterine viability.
3. The patient is brought to the operating room and either a general or regional anesthetic is given. Local anesthesia or paracervical anesthesia is avoided because of concern for alteration in uterine blood flow.
4. Place the patient in the dorsal lithotomy position; prepare and drape in sterile fashion.
5. Drain the bladder (a Foley catheter is not necessary).
6. Place a weighted speculum in the posterior vagina.
7. Place a Deaver or right-angle retractor in the vagina to provide adequate exposure; have an assistant hold it carefully to avoid bladder trauma.
8. Using a ring forceps, grasp the anterior lip of the cervix and displace it superiorly.
9. Place a stitch at the 6 o'clock position in the mid-portion of the cervix equidistant from the ectocervix and the vaginal reflection (near the cervicovaginal junction). Place the suture through the mid-portion of the cervical stroma, being careful not to enter the cervical canal. Sutures that are too shallow may tear out when drawn tight. Be aware of the cervical vascularity. By starting at the 6 o'clock position instead of the 12 o'clock position, the patient may have decreased bladder irritation from the suture because the knot will rest in the posterior vagina. Direct the needle toward the 3 o'clock position *within* the cervical tissue.
10. Proceeding in a counterclockwise manner (clockwise if left-handed), pass the suture to the 3 o'clock position. Remove it from the cervix and then immediately loop it back into the cervix. Pass the stitch to the 12 o'clock position, again, within the tissue itself. Withdraw it and then reinsert in same area. Again pass the stitch to the 9 o'clock position, withdraw, and reinsert. Finally, pass the stitch to the starting position (6 o'clock) and withdraw the suture (see Fig. 133-1).
11. Cinch down the suture like a pursestring without drawing too tightly and tie it, leaving ends long enough to grasp with ring forceps for removal.
12. Some surgeons prefer to place a second cerclage lower than the first, but no improvement in outcome has been documented and complications like membrane rupture or bladder perforation may be more frequent.
13. The patient then recovers while being placed on a fetal monitor to ensure fetal viability.
14. The patient is usually discharged after a period of adequate observation. Antibiotics are not recommended and tocolytic agents have no proven benefit.
15. Complete a postoperative note indicating the type of cerclage placed (McDonald), the suture type, the anesthesia, the location of the suture placement, and the number of knots placed. A diagram is helpful. Place a copy of the operative report in the pregnancy record.

REMOVAL

The cerclage is left in place until the 37th week of the pregnancy, at which time it can usually be removed easily in the office. The patient is placed in the usual examination position with the speculum placed. The knot is then grasped with the pickups (e.g., a Russian), the knot is elevated, and the Metzenbaum scissors are used to cut the cerclage stitch, which is then easily removed. If, however, difficulty arises when attempting to remove the stitch, the clinician should not hesitate to proceed to the operating room. If preterm labor is encountered later in the pregnancy and tocolysis is not successful, the cerclage should be removed at that time to avoid damage to the cervix.

SAMPLE OPERATIVE REPORT

Procedure:	McDonald cervical cerclage
Preop diagnosis:	Cervical insufficiency at ________ wks gestation
Postop diagnosis:	Same
Surgeon:	
Anesthesiologist:	
Estimated blood loss:	________ cc
Specimen:	None
Drains:	None
Complications:	None
Disposition:	To Labor and Delivery for observation

History and Indications

Ms. ____________________________ is a ________ year old G________ P________ at ________ weeks' gestation with a viable fetus. She had ________ prior 2nd trimester pregnancy losses with a history suggestive of cervical insufficiency. The plan was to place a cervical cerclage at 14 weeks. The patient was informed of the risks and benefits of the procedure and signed the appropriate consent form.

Procedure

Fetal heart tones were documented and the patient was seen by me and the anesthesiologist. The patient was then taken to the operating room, room no. ________, where she received a spinal anesthetic by Dr. __________________________. She was then placed in the dorsal lithotomy position. After verifying the adequacy of the spinal anesthetic, the patient was prepped and draped in the usual manner and her bladder was drained of ________ cc of urine.

A weighted speculum was placed in the vagina and the anterior lip of the cervix was gently grasped. No membranes protruded through the external cervical os.

A no. 5 Mersilene tape suture was placed at the 6 o'clock position at the level of the internal os with the suture exiting at the 3 o'clock position, reinserted in this same area, exiting at the 12 o'clock position. The suture was reinserted at the 12 o'clock position and removed at the 9 o'clock position, reinserted in this same area, exiting at the 6 o'clock position. The suture was tied with three knots at the 6 o'clock position. No significant bleeding was noted.

The weighted speculum and ring forceps were removed and the patient transferred from the operating table to a bed and then transported to Labor and Delivery in the care of the anesthesiologist, Dr. __________________________, in stable condition.

Signature, date, and time: ______________________________

Common Error

Placing a suture too shallowly so that it pulls out when tightened is a common error.

Complications

- Rupture of membranes (incidence may be up to 65% within 2 weeks)
- Chorioamnionitis (may occur in up to 30% of cases)
- Uterine rupture
- Maternal septicemia
- Pregnancy loss
- Scarring of the cervix, which may cause cervical and potential uterine injury during labor
- Suture may migrate; may need to replace cerclage if still early in pregnancy (<24 weeks)
- Significant vaginal discharge from the foreign body reaction of the cervical suture
- Increased frequency of contractions

Postprocedure Patient Care

- Monitor the patient until adequately recovered from anesthesia and patient is able to ambulate and void.
- Fetal viability must be documented before discharge.
- Acetaminophen should provide any necessary pain relief.
- Patient discharge instructions should include the following:
  - Vaginal discharge after the procedure is normal and may continue for weeks.
  - Call office with any leakage of fluid from the vagina, fever, severe cramping or pain.
  - Pelvic rest and limited physical activity for at least 1 week if procedure was elective; if procedure was emergent, pelvic rest and limited activity throughout remainder of pregnancy.
- See patient frequently (weekly or biweekly) for cervical checks.

Postprocedure Patient Education

- The patient should avoid vaginal intercourse and limit physical activity for the first week after the procedure. Consider no intercourse and no heavy physical activity until after delivery.
- Vaginal discharge may be normal for weeks after this procedure. The patient should contact her physician if she experiences severe cramping, fever, or any vaginal bleeding.
- Acetaminophen is helpful for any pain or discomfort after this procedure.
- Monitor the patient closely with checks every 1 to 2 weeks.
- Advise that a second stitch may be needed if the first stitch does not remain tightly secured.
- The stitch will be removed at around 37 weeks' gestation, and this is usually done in the office.

Be aware that there is little evidence to support these recommendations, and they may be modified to fit the individual situation. Any emergently placed cerclage is monitored more closely.

CPT/Billing Codes

59320 Cerclage
59871 Removal of cerclage suture under anesthesia (other than local)

No CPT code exists for removal of a cerclage without anesthesia.

ICD-9-CM Diagnostic Codes

622.5 Incompetent cervix
654.53 Incompetent cervix in pregnancy
761.0 Incompetent cervix in pregnancy affecting fetus or newborn

Acknowledgment

The editors wish to recognize the many contributions by Charles E. Werner, Jr., MD, to this chapter in the previous two editions of this text.

Bibliography

Althuisius SM, Dekker GA, Hummel P, et al: Final results of the Cervical Incompetence Prevention Randomized Cerclage Trial (CIPRACT): Therapeutic cerclage with bed rest versus bed rest alone. Am J Obstet Gynecol 185:1106–1112, 2001.

American College of Obstetricians and Gynecologists: ACOG practice bulletin no. 48: Cervical insufficiency. Obstet Gynecol 102:1091–1099, 2003.

Cunningham FG, Leveno KL, Bloom S, et al (eds): Williams Obstetrics, 22nd ed. New York, McGraw-Hill, 2005, pp 863–865, 918.

Drakeley AJ, Roberts D, Alfirevic Z: Cervical stitch (cerclage) for preventing pregnancy loss in women. Cochrane Database Syst Rev 1:CD003253, 2003.

Gabbe SG, Niebyl JR, Simpson JL (eds): Obstetrics: Normal and Problem Pregnancies, 5th ed. New York, Churchill Livingstone, 2007, pp 655–664.

Hassan SS, Romero R, Maymon E, et al: Does cervical cerclage prevent preterm delivery in patients with a short cervix? Am J Obstet Gynecol 184:1325–1329, 2001.

McDonald IA: Suture of the cervix for inevitable miscarriage. J Obstet Gynaecol Br Emp 64:346–350, 1957.

Neilson JP: Interventions for suspected placenta praevia. Cochrane Database Syst Rev 2:CD001998, 2003.

Novy MJ, Gupta A, Wothe DD, et al: Cervical cerclage in the second trimester of pregnancy: A historical cohort study. Am J Obstet Gynecol 184:1447–1454, 2001.

Rust OA, Atlas RO, Reed J, et al: Revisiting the short cervix detected by transvaginal ultrasound in the second trimester: Why cerclage therapy may not help. Am J Obstet Gynecol 185:1098–1105, 2001.

Te Linde RW, Rock JA, Thompson JD (eds): Te Linde's Operative Gynecology, 10th ed. Philadelphia, Lippincott Williams & Wilkins, 2003, pp 760–782.

CHAPTER 134

Cervical Conization

Lydia A. Watson

In most cases, proper evaluation of abnormal Pap smears and cervical lesions includes colposcopy, multiple-punch biopsy sampling, and endocervical curettage. However, conization of the cervix plays an important role in both the diagnosis and the management of abnormalities of the cervix. Cold-knife conization (CKC) is considered the gold standard by which all other outpatient techniques are critiqued. "Cold knife" refers to a surgical blade versus the old "hot-wire" cone, or the loop procedure.

Conization of the cervix consists of the removal of a cone-shaped wedge of tissue from the cervix uteri. To be considered an adequate specimen, the tissue removed must include the entire transformation zone with the squamocolumnar junction and the entire lesion surrounded by uninvolved margins. The large loop electrical excision procedure is described in Chapter 149, Loop Electrosurgical Excision Procedure for Treating Cervical Intraepithelial Neoplasia. A review of Chapter 137, Colposcopic Examination, and Chapter 138, Cryotherapy of the Cervix, is also recommended.

Indications

A conization may be indicated for diagnosis or treatment, or both. Usually any conization method can be used interchangeably, although using a knife blade causes less tissue artifact (pathologic distortion) than other methods and may allow a better histologic examination.

For Diagnosis

- Inadequate colposcopic evaluation of the cervix
  - The lesion is not seen on colposcopic examination, but Pap smear is significantly abnormal
  - Incomplete visualization of a lesion that extends into the endocervical canal (ECC) on colposcopic examination
  - Inadequate visualization of entire transformation zone, including the squamocolumnar junction (e.g., goes into the os, where it cannot be evaluated)
- Positive endocervical curettings (i.e., dysplasia or cancer)
- Inconsistencies between cytologic findings, histologic diagnoses, and colposcopic impression (e.g., a Pap smear that is at least two stages worse than colposcopic biopsy)
- Inability of colposcopic examination to exclude invasive cancer

For Therapy

- Cytology or biopsy specimen suggests microinvasive carcinoma of the cervix (clinician must rule out frank invasion to define the proper treatment; in this case, procedure may also be therapeutic)
- High-grade dysplasia (i.e., moderate or severe dysplasia by biopsy) greater than 2 cm or in more than two quadrants
- Cervical cryotherapy is contraindicated (see Chapter 138, Cryotherapy of the Cervix)
  - Lesion too large for cryotip
  - Markedly irregular surface of cervix with crevices that cryotherapy will not reach
  - Glandular involvement on biopsy (relative)
  - Lesion extends more than 5 mm into the os
- Noncompliance (e.g., patient unlikely to be compliant with follow-up after cryotherapy and during attempts to monitor lesser cervical intraepithelial neoplasia without treatment)
- Correction of cervical stenosis (although the os is more likely to be opened using a shallow LEEP than a CKC)

Contraindications

Absolute

- Known frank invasive carcinoma of the cervix or endocervix ("Carcinoma in situ" is not a cancer, but rather a severe dysplasia. With microinvasive cancer, a conization procedure must be performed to rule out frank invasion.)
- Patient with contraindications to general or regional anesthesia
- Unstable medical conditions (rarely is conization an emergency)

Relative

- Unstable bleeding disorders
- Inflammatory cervicitis (causes increased bleeding)
- Heavy menses at time of surgery (makes the procedure more difficult)
- Pregnancy

NOTE: Although pregnancy is not an absolute contraindication to conization, only a well-trained physician capable of managing complications should perform the procedure on a pregnant patient (see the "Complications" section).

Preprocedure Patient Education

- The procedure and potential complications should be explained to the patient, and written informed consent should be obtained. (See the patient education handout titled "Cold-Knife Conization of the Cervix [Cone Biopsy]" available online at www.expertconsult.com.)
- The need for general, local, or regional anesthesia should be explained.
- All options for treatment and evaluation should be explained.

Equipment

- Povidone–iodine
- Colposcope with green filter
- Acetic acid and full-strength Lugol's solution
- Vasopressin 20 U in 20 mL of normal saline for infiltration of the cervix
- Long scalpel handle with no. 11 blade

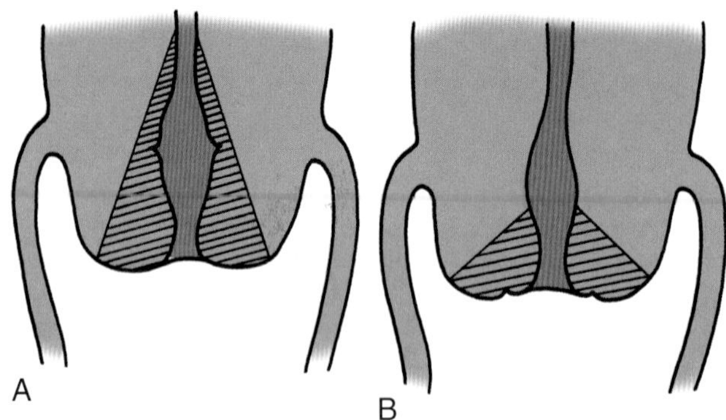

Figure 134-1 Variation in size and shape of cervical tissue removed during conization. **A,** For large ectocervical lesion. **B,** For canal lesions.

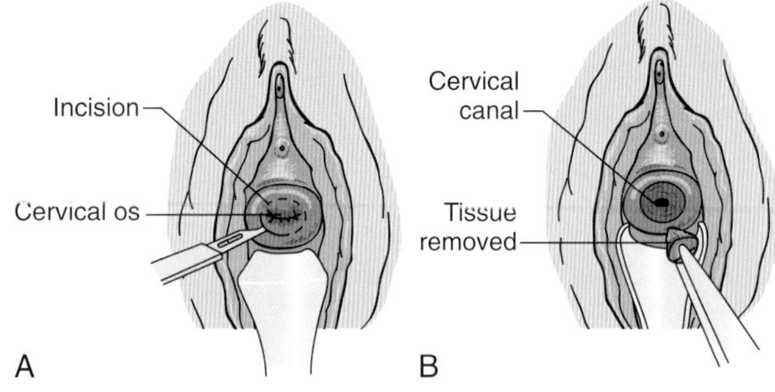

Figure 134-3 Conization technique (see text for details). **A,** Incision. **B,** Removal of tissue.

- Long, fine-tooth forceps
- Kevorkian endocervical curette
- Electrocautery unit
- 0-chromic or 0-Vicryl suture (or Surgicel, Gelfoam, or Avitene) for hemostasis; long needle holders
- Large Graves speculum
- Uterine sound

Procedure

1. *Special considerations:* Most lesions are found on the ectocervix in premenopausal women, so the cone should have a broad base and the top should have a wide angle (Fig. 134-1A). In postmenopausal women, the specimen will be long and narrow, with an acute angle at the cone top. The squamocolumnar junction in these patients has generally moved inside the ECC, and lesions are more likely to be endocervical. The transformation zone in older women is usually quite small (Fig. 134-1B).
2. Administer general, local (intrastromal), or regional anesthesia to the patient, and obtain adequate exposure of the cervix. The bladder should be drained.
3. Apply full-strength Lugol's solution to the cervix to aid in determining the width of the cone base. All areas that do not stain will be removed. Alternatively, perform colposcopy using acetic acid and the green filter to demarcate the lesion and the transformation zone.
4. Obtain hemostasis by circumferentially infiltrating the cervical stroma with a solution of 20 U of vasopressin diluted in 20 mL of normal saline (Fig. 134-2).

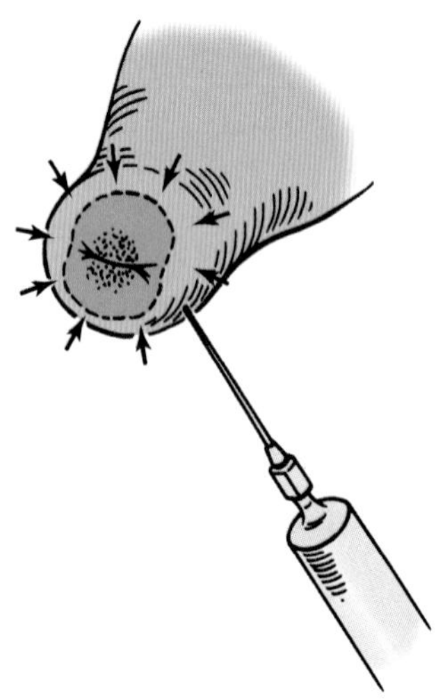

Figure 134-2 Intracervical injection.

NOTE: Hemostatic retention sutures are no longer routinely used.

5. Gently sound the uterine canal to determine position and size of the uterus.
6. Incise the cervix in a circular fashion, making the incision outside of the Lugol's-negative or acetowhite area. Begin at the 6 o'clock position. This will prevent the blood that runs down from obscuring the incision line (Fig. 134-3A). Angle the blade centrally to the width and depth desired.
7. Use a fine-tooth forceps to elevate the cone away from the underlying bed. Avoid damaging the cervical epithelium (Fig. 134-3B).
8. Mark the 12 o'clock position of the specimen for the pathologist with a single suture placed into the cervical stroma. Consider measuring the specimen because it may shrink before it is measured by the pathologist.
9. Curette the remainder of the ECC with a small curette to rule out disease above the upper margins of the cone.
10. Perform a dilation and curettage, *if indicated,* at this time.
11. Obtain hemostasis with superficial electrocoagulation by using a ball electrode or individual suture ligatures to control bleeding. The cone site may also be packed with an absorbable gelatin sponge (e.g., Gelfoam) or similar hemostatic material. Most apply Monsel's solution to the base of the excision after coagulation.
12. Place the cone specimen in fixative to send for pathologic interpretation.

Complications

Complications for the nonpregnant patient include the following (overall complication rate 10%):

- Pain and cramping (generally minimal).
- Immediate or delayed hemorrhage. (Eschar sloughs in 7 to 10 days. Delayed hemorrhage can occur at this time; some spotting is to be expected for 10 to 14 days.) If bleeding is excessive at the time of surgery, inject 1 mL of 2% lidocaine with epinephrine into each bleeding spot. This will usually slow bleeding enough to allow electrocoagulation. Alternatively, and rarely, a "figure-of-8" stitch may need to be placed over the bleeding vessel.
- Cervical stenosis (<3 mm) that prevents menses or obtaining a good endocervical Pap smear.
- Uterine perforation.
- Pelvic cellulitis (very rare) or cervicitis.
- Damage to the bladder or rectum. (This is usually seen in cases of significant vaginal atrophy with shallow vaginal fornices.)
- Cervical incompetence.
- Infertility caused by loss of mucus-producing endocervical glands.
- Anesthetic complications.

- Positive margins or positive ECC. (If ectocervical margins show only dysplasia, the patient should be followed closely but a repeat cone is not indicated. Usually the lesion will resolve during the inflammatory healing process. A repeat cone may be indicated in older patients who are at a high risk and do not desire pregnancy, those who have had pelvic irradiation, or in whom both the margins and ECC are positive. If the ECC above the excisional site is positive with a high-grade lesion, repeat conization should be considered.)
- Missing the lesion (rare).

In addition to the complications mentioned for the nonpregnant patient, complications for the pregnant patient include the following:

- Fetal loss rate of 10% (secondary to rupture of the membranes, premature labor, and excessive hemorrhaging).
- Postoperative hemorrhage rate of 30%.

Postprocedure Management

- A follow-up appointment should be scheduled for 4 to 6 weeks.
- The patient should be instructed to avoid intercourse, douching, and tampon use until follow-up examination confirms healing.
- The patient should be asked to notify the clinician of elevated temperature, excessive vaginal bleeding, or purulent discharge.
- The first follow-up Pap smear should be scheduled in 3 to 4 months if all margins are clear.

CPT/Billing Codes

57520 Conization, with or without fulguration, with or without dilation and curettage (D&C), with or without repair, cold knife or laser
57522 Conization, loop electrode
57505 Endocervical curettage (not done as part of D&C)
99070 Surgical tray

ICD-9-CM Diagnostic Codes

078.11 Condyloma
079.4 Human papillomavirus infection
180.9 Cervical neoplasm, malignant (excludes carcinoma in situ)
219.0 Benign neoplasm, cervix
233.1 Carcinoma in situ, cervix (includes CIN III, severe dysplasia of cervix)
622.0 Cervical erosion or ulcer
622.1x Dysplasia of cervix (5th digit required, 0 unspecified, 1 mild [CIN I], 2 moderate [CIN II])
622.2 Cervical leukoplakia
622.4 Cervical stenosis
622.7 Cervical polyp

Patient Education Guides

- See the sample patient education handout, "Cold-Knife Conization of the Cervix (Cone Biopsy)," available online at www.expertconsult.com.
- See the sample patient consent form, "Cervical Conization," available online at www.expertconsult.com.

BIBLIOGRAPHY

American College of Obstetricians and Gynecologists: Cervical cytology: Evaluation and management of abnormalities. ACOG technical bulletin number 183, August 1993. Int J Gynaecol Obstet 43:212–219, 1993.

Disaia P, Creasman W (eds): Clinical Gynecologic Oncology, 5th ed. St. Louis, Mosby, 1997.

Narducci F, Occelli B, Boman F, et al: Positive margins after conization and risk of persistent lesion. Gynecol Oncol 76:311–314, 2000.

Parsons L, Ulfelder H: An Atlas of Pelvic Operations. Philadelphia, WB Saunders, 1968.

Pfenninger JL: Good things still come in old packages: Cryosurgery vs LEEP. Loop electrosurgical excision procedure. J Am Board Fam Pract 12:416–418, 1999.

Ryan KJ, Berkowitz R, Barbieri RL (eds): Kistner's Gynecology: Principles and Practice. Chicago, Year Book, 1990.

Schaefer G, Graber A (eds): Complications in Obstetrics and Gynecologic Surgery. New York, Harper & Row, 1981.

Thompson D, Rock JA (eds): Te Linde's Operative Gynecology, 7th ed. Philadelphia, JB Lippincott, 1992.

Turner RJ, Cohen RA, Voet RL, et al: Analysis of tissue margins of cone biopsy specimens obtained with "cold knife," CO_2 and Nd:YAG lasers and a radiofrequency surgical unit. J Reprod Med 37:607–610, 1992.

Wheeless CR (ed): Atlas of Pelvic Surgery, 2nd ed. Philadelphia, Lea & Febiger, 1988.

White CD, Cooper WL, Williams RR: Cervical intraepithelial neoplasia extending to the margins of resection in conization of the cervix. J Reprod Med 36:635–638, 1991.

CHAPTER 135

Cervical Polyps

Beth A. Choby

Cervical polyps affect 4% of women. Although their etiology is poorly understood, polyps are associated with obstructed cervical blood vessels, pregnancy, chronic inflammation, and an abnormal response to increased estrogen. Women with diabetes or recurrent vaginitis may be at increased risk. Most cervical polyps are benign, although 1% of lesions undergo malignant transformation. Because of this risk, polyps are generally removed and histologically examined to rule out precancerous change.

The incidence of cervical polyps increases with age. Cervical polyps are rarely seen in girls who have not reached menarche. Polyps are fairly common in parous women in their 20s. Diagnosis is often made during a routine speculum examination. Multiparous women 30 to 50 years of age and perimenopausal women are most often affected. The influence of hormone therapy on the progression of cervical polyps is not well defined. Postmenopausal cervical polyps are often associated with endometrial polyps. Women taking tamoxifen who have a cervical polyp are significantly more likely to have concomitant endometrial polyps. Evaluation with hysteroscopy is indicated in this situation.

Most cervical polyps are asymptomatic and found by chance during routine gynecologic examination. When present, symptoms are usually vague and include vaginal spotting or bleeding after exercise, douching, or intercourse. Vascular congestion and edema cause ulceration of the polyp tip and postcoital bleeding. Larger polyps are associated with intermenstrual spotting. Defecation or straining can cause bleeding. Abnormal menses or nonpurulent vaginal discharge is sometimes noted. When cervical polyps cause postmenopausal vaginal bleeding, further work-up to exclude malignancy is mandatory.

Cervical polyps range in size from a few millimeters to several centimeters. Polyps on longer pedicles (stalks) sometimes protrude from the vaginal orifice. Large endocervical polyps cause cervical dilation and pain.

The differential diagnosis for cervical polyps is given in Box 135-1. Because cervical polyps often coexist with endometrial polyps, hysteroscopy has been suggested as the first-line therapy in the management of cervical polyps. Older recommendations include performing a suction dilation and curettage with all cervical polypectomies. Current literature fails to support either intervention as substantially improving outcomes compared with routine simple polyp removal. In low-risk, asymptomatic women, most physicians still proceed with in-office cervical polypectomy.

Anatomy

Cervical polyps are pedunculated tumors arising from endocervical or ectocervical tissue. *Endocervical* polyps originate within the endocervical canal, are most common in premenopausal women, and can prolapse through the cervix (Fig. 135-1). *Ectocervical* polyps more often affect postmenopausal women (Fig. 135-2). Polyps are bright red to pink and appear spongy. Polyps are most often solitary, although multiple polyps are sometimes encountered.

Endometrial polyps are sometimes confused as being of cervical origin. Endometrial polyps can protrude through the endocervical canal. Management of endometrial polyps is more complicated because the polyp's blood supply is usually more extensive and the attachment is much higher up (Fig. 135-3).

Some lesions can mimic cervical polyps and be benign (Fig. 135-4), whereas malignant conditions such as adenocarcinoma can also masquerade as a polyp. Histologic study is often the only way to be certain of the true nature.

Indications for Removal

- Asymptomatic cervical polyps found on routine gynecologic examination
- Cervical polyps associated with pain, bleeding, or other symptoms

Contraindications

Absolute

- Patient unwilling/unable to consent to procedure
- Patient unwilling/unable to cooperate with vaginal examination

Relative

- Endometrial polyps or cervical polyps with a dense, thick pedicle/blood supply
- Polyps larger than several centimeters (may be better removed in a surgical suite)
- Pregnancy
- Blood dyscrasias
- High likelihood of multiple polyps (consider hysteroscopy)

Box 135-1. Differential Diagnosis of Cervical Lesions

Cervical malignancy
Cervical polyp
Condyloma
Endometrial polyp
Nabothian cyst
Prolapsed myoma
Retained products of conception
Sarcoma
Squamous papilloma

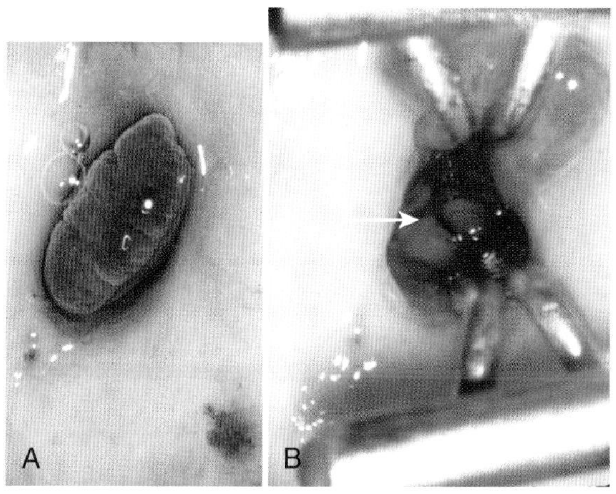

Figure 135-1 **A,** Endocervical polyp. **B,** Identification of polyp base *(arrow)* using an endocervical speculum. (Courtesy of Duane Townsend, MD.)

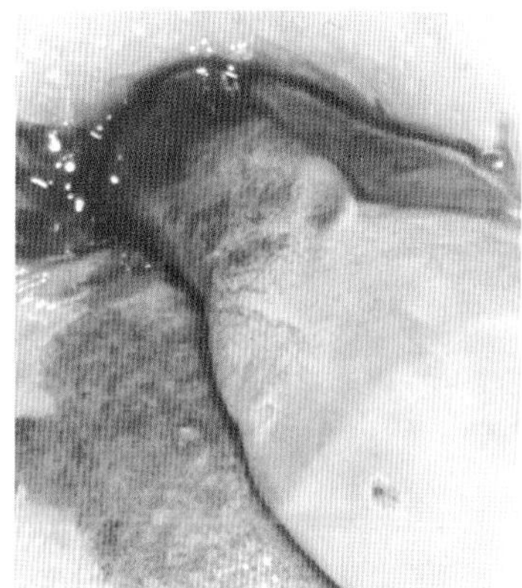

Figure 135-3 Dysplastic endometrial polyp. Stalk originates in endometrial cavity. (Courtesy of Duane Townsend, MD.)

Equipment and Supplies

- Nonsterile gloves
- Vaginal speculum
- Colposcope *(optional)*
- Ring forceps
- Cervical biopsy forceps (may not be needed)
- Endocervical curette (Kevorkian)
- Pathology specimen containers
- Silver nitrate sticks
- Topical anesthetic (lidocaine jelly or benzocaine solution), though this is usually not needed
- Kogan's endocervical speculum

Precautions

- Identify the base of the polyp stalk to exclude an endometrial polyp. Endometrial polyps are often larger with more vascular stalks. Suspect an endometrial polyp if the stalk extends into the cervix or remains visible after polypectomy. Endometrial polypectomy is most often done by hysteroscopy.
- Cervical polyps have increased vascularity during pregnancy. Asymptomatic polyps that do not change in size or appearance may be observed and removed after delivery. If bleeding necessitates removal during pregnancy, electrocautery or loop electrosurgical excision procedure is sometimes required.
- Remove large cervical polyps in an outpatient surgical suite. Hysteroscopy is useful for confirming the size and origin of polyps found deeper inside the endocervical canal.

Preprocedure Patient Education and Forms

Naproxen (500 mg) or a similar nonsteroidal anti-inflammatory drug is given orally 1 hour before the procedure. The procedure should not be scheduled during menses. Discuss risks and benefits of the procedure with the patient and obtain informed consent. Please see the consent form available online at ww.expertconsult.com.

Procedure

1. Don nonsterile gloves and insert a vaginal speculum. If a recent Pap examination has not been performed, it can be completed before the procedure.
2. Visualize the polyp. The use of a colposcope may improve visualization.
3. Gently manipulate the cervical os using ring forceps to identify the polyp base. Use a Kogan's endocervical speculum if the stalk extends into the endocervical canal.
4. Determine whether the polyp is cervical or endometrial in origin.
5. Remove the polyp using one of the following methods:
   - Cut through the tissue at the base of the polyp using cervical biopsy forceps.

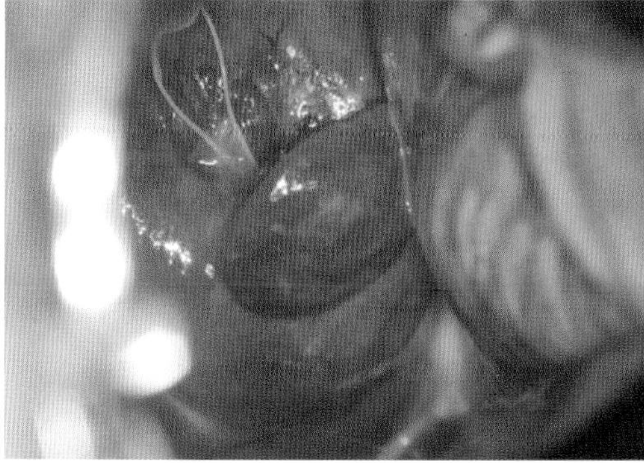

Figure 135-2 Ectocervical polyp. Stalk is attached to the ectocervix. Note the intrauterine device strings. (Courtesy of The Medical Procedures Center PC, Midland, Mich.)

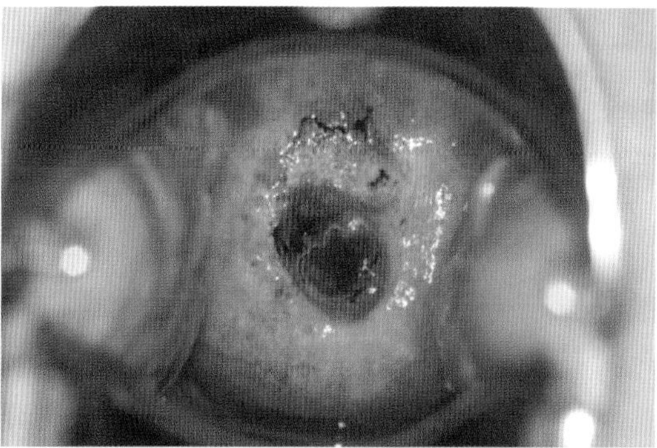

Figure 135-4 Suspected cervical polyp, which is actually a large nabothian cyst. (Courtesy of The Medical Procedures Center PC, Midland, Mich.)

- Grasp the polyp with the ring forceps and twist the forceps around the stalk until it comes off. Patients may complain of mild discomfort.
- If the polyp is small, scrape it off in its entirety using a sharp curette.

6. Place the cervical polyp and stalk into a specimen container with formalin.
7. Perform an endocervical curettage using a Kevorkian curette (see Chapter 137, Colposcopic Examination). Although this step is optional, it ensures that all of the abnormal tissue has been removed. Place the tissue in a separate specimen container from the cervical polyp.
8. Control bleeding using silver nitrate, Monsel's solution, or cautery. Bleeding is usually minimal. Silver nitrate also destroys residual polyp tissue and minimizes the chance of recurrence.

Sample Operative Report

See the sample operative report online at www.expertconsult.com.

Common Errors

- Failure to remove the polyp, stalk, and base entirely. The use of a colposcope to identify the origin of the polyp before excision may facilitate complete removal.

  When multiple polyps are present, it is best to thoroughly curette the endocervical canal. If the patient is postmenopausal, has irregular bleeding, or takes tamoxifen, a dilation and curettage or hysteroscopy may be a better option.
- Misidentification of a prolapsed endometrial polyp as a cervical polyp.

Complications

- Postprocedure bleeding or spotting
- Postprocedure pain
- Recurrence

Postprocedure Management

- Monitor the patient for vasovagal reactions.
- Provide the patient with a sanitary pad.
- Advise the patient to take a nonsteroidal anti-inflammatory drug for 24 hours as needed for abdominal cramping.

Postprocedure Patient Education

Patients should avoid tampon use, douching, or sexual intercourse for 1 week after cervical polypectomy. Active vaginal bleeding warrants timely reevaluation. Patients are followed up at 6 to 8 weeks. Because polyps are generally benign and no further treatment usually needed, routine gynecologic surveillance is appropriate.

Patient Education Guides

See patient education and consent forms and sample operative report available online at www.expertconsult.com.

CPT/Billing Codes

There is no separate CPT code for cervical polyp removal.

57500 Biopsy of the cervix, single or multiple, or local excision of lesion, with or without fulguration
57505 Endocervical curettage (not performed as part of dilation and curettage)

ICD-9-CM Diagnostic Codes

078.11 Condyloma acuminatum
219.0 Benign neoplasm of the cervix (adenomatous polyp of the cervix)
236.0 Neoplasm of uncertain behavior: uterus
621.0 Polyp endometrium/uterus NOS
622.7 Polyp of cervix NOS
625.9 Unspecified symptoms associated with female genital organs
626.6 Metrorrhagia. Bleeding unrelated to menstrual cycle; irregular intermenstrual bleeding
627.1 Postmenopausal bleeding

Online Resources

Martin E: Cervical polyp. Discovery Health: Diseases and Conditions. Available at http://health.discovery.com/encyclopedias/illnesses.html?article=1991.

MedlinePlus Encyclopedia: Cervical polyps. Available at www.nlm.nih.gov/medlineplus/ency/article/001494.htm.

Bibliography

Bajo J, Moreno-Calvo F, Uguet-de-Resayre C, et al: Contribution of transvaginal sonography to the evaluation of benign cervical conditions. J Clin Ultrasound 27:61–64, 1999.

Golan A, Ber A, Wolman I, David MP: Cervical polyp: Evaluation of current treatment. Gynecol Obstet Invest 37:56–58, 1994.

Hassa H, Tekin B, Senses T, et al: Are the site, diameter, and number of endometrial polyps related with symptomatology? Am J Obstet Gynecol 194:718–721, 2006.

Neri A, Kaplan B, Rabinerson D, et al: Cervical polyp in the menopause and the need for fractional dilatation and curettage. Eur J Obstet Gynecol Reprod Biol 62:53–55, 1995.

Speiwankiewicz B, Stelmachow J, Sawicki W, et al: Hysteroscopy in cases of cervical polyps. Eur J Gynaecol Oncol 24:67–69, 2003.

Tuggy M, Garcia J: Procedures Consult. Available at www.proceduresconsult.com.

CHAPTER 136

CERVICAL STENOSIS AND CERVICAL DILATION

Linda Prine

Cervical stenosis is a stricture or narrowing of the cervix. It is diagnosed by the inability to pass a 2-mm dilator into the uterus. Cervical stenosis can be either *congenital* or *acquired*. *Acquired* stenosis can result from postoperative scarring (from conization, whether it be cold knife, large loop electrosurgery, or laser; cautery; or cryotherapy of the cervix), cancer (endometrial or endocervical), radiation complications, infections, or atrophy from lack of estrogen (most common). In acquired cases the external os is most frequently affected (Fig. 136-1). In *congenital cases*, seen most often in nulliparous cervices, the stenosis is usually at the internal os.

Narrowing of the cervical canal can impede menstrual flow, causing intrauterine pressure during menses. Premenopausal women with cervical stenosis may have pelvic pain, dysmenorrhea, amenorrhea, infertility, or abnormal bleeding. In some cases retrograde menstrual flow may occur, causing endometriosis. Women may have a soft, slightly tender midpelvic mass as a result of hematometra. Postmenopausal women may have pyometra, which is highly suspect for endometrial carcinoma.

Ultrasonography can assess canal anatomy while evaluating the patient for hematometra and a pyometra. Most often, cervical stenosis is discovered when the physician is attempting to enter the uterus for a Pap smear, hysteroscopy, intrauterine device (IUD) insertion, endometrial biopsy, uterine aspiration for elective or spontaneous abortion, or placement of Essure devices.

CERVICAL DILATION

Treatment of cervical stenosis consists of dilation by using (1) progressive metal or plastic dilators, (2) osmotic tents, or (3) prostaglandin analogs. *Laminaria tents* are made from the stems of seaweed, usually *Laminaria japonica*, that is dried and made into sticks. Self-expanding cervical dilators (Dilateria, Lamicel) that resemble laminaria tents can also be used. Once the tents are placed into the endocervical canal, they rehydrate and expand, thereby causing dilation of the cervical canal (Figs. 136-2 and 136-3). Laminaria tents should not be used if pyometra is present or infection is suspected. The os and canal must be patent enough to admit the tents, which are available in several diameters. Some mechanical dilation may be necessary to allow their placement. Another option for the treatment of external os stenosis is the use of the carbon dioxide laser or a small radiofrequency loop excision. The latter two methods can remove a stricture that is readily visible externally.

Recently, clinicians have come to depend on the administration of *misoprostol* for softening and dilating the cervix. Misoprostol is most effective on the pregnant uterus, and very small doses are used to soften the cervix for labor. Documentation of efficacy is best in the pregnant uterus. In nonpregnant uteri, efficacy has been shown clearly in women of reproductive age. Studies of misoprostol use on postmenopausal women are conflicting regarding its effectiveness. In nonpregnant uteri or in the first trimester, two to four 200-μg tablets administered vaginally, buccally, or sublingually 1 to 2 hours before the procedure is usually effective.

The majority of dilations can be performed in the office. For extremely anxious patients or if pain cannot be controlled easily, the procedure may need to be performed in the operating room.

INDICATIONS

- Symptomatic stenosis (e.g., dysmenorrhea)
- Inability to obtain adequate Pap smears
- IUD insertion
- To perform an indicated endocervical curettage or dilation and curettage
- To perform an aspiration abortion
- If needed for hysterosalpingogram
- Before hysteroscopy
- Before endometrial ablation techniques
- To perform an endometrial biopsy
- To insert Essure devices for mechanical tubal occlusion

CONTRAINDICATIONS

Absolute

The procedure is absolutely contraindicated in a patient who is trying to become pregnant.

Relative

- Laminaria tents are not to be used in cases of pyometra
- Pelvic inflammatory disease; vaginal or cervical infections (treat before dilation)

EQUIPMENT

- Table that allows the patient to be placed in the lithotomy position
- Needle extender or long spinal needle to provide local anesthesia, if needed (see Chapter 149, Loop Electrosurgical Excision Procedure for Treating Cervical Intraepithelial Neoplasia)
- 5 mL 1% lidocaine
- Adequate light source
- Appropriately sized vaginal speculum
- Nonsterile gloves; use sterile gloves if a procedure entering the uterus is to be performed
- Ring forceps
- Uterine sound—plastic, malleable preferred
- Denniston plastic dilators (1 to 8 mm; Fig. 136-4) or metal dilators (1 to 6 mm) and/or osmotic tent (various sizes; see Fig. 136-2)
- OS Finder or os locator or small silver probe (like a tear duct probe)
- Cervical single-tooth tenaculum
- Paracervical block kit with 10 mL 1% lidocaine in a 10-mL syringe with a 6-inch, 20-gauge needle; may be helpful if dilation

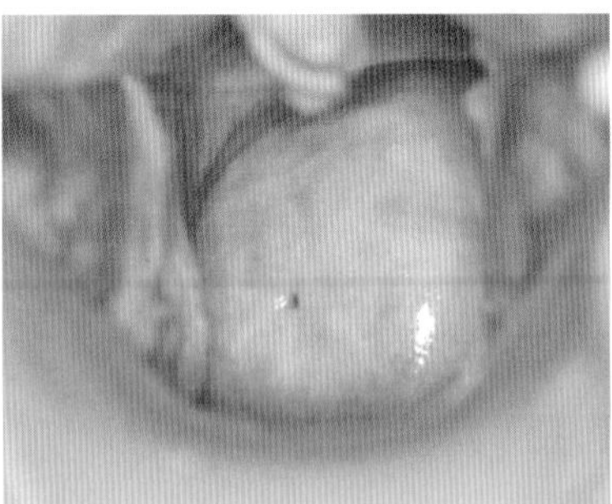

Figure 136-1 External os stenosis after loop electrosurgical excision procedure.

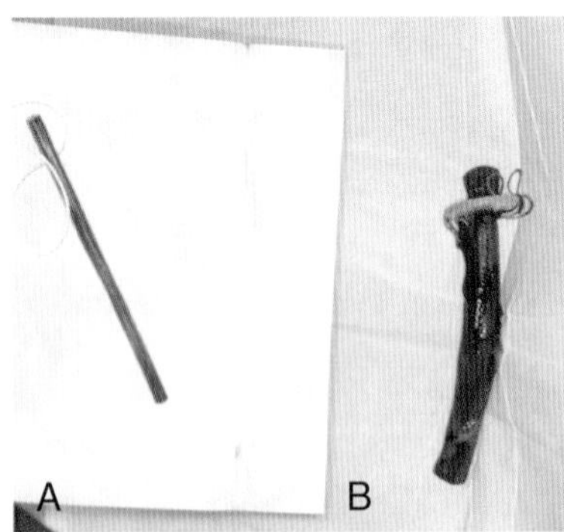

Figure 136-2 **A,** Laminaria before insertion. **B,** Swollen laminaria after removal.

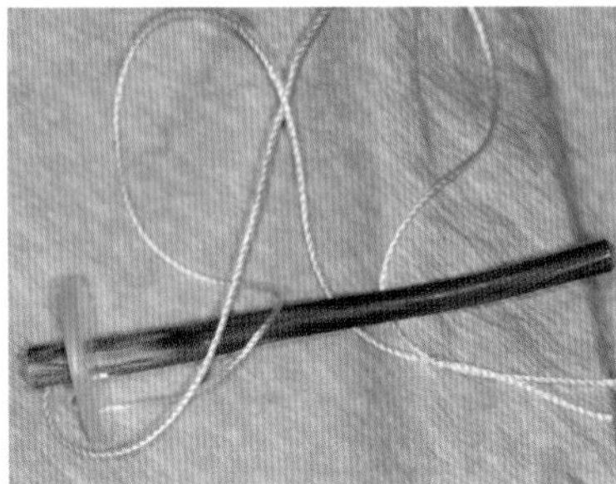

Figure 136-3 Close-up of laminaria in Figure 136-2A.

Figure 136-4 Denniston plastic dilators, 5 mm to 14 mm sizes.

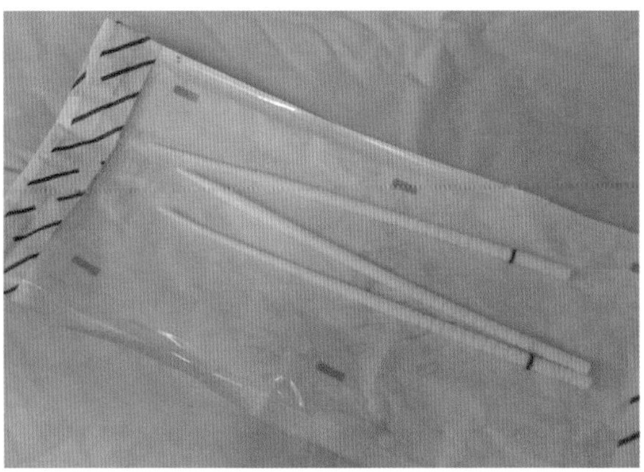

Figure 136-5 OS Finder.

of more than 4 to 6 mm is done (see Chapter 173, Paracervical Block)

- 4 × 4 gauze; povidone–iodine (Betadine) solution
- Ultrasonography machine with abdominal probe if needed for guidance *(optional)*

Preprocedure Patient Education

- Obtain informed consent from the patient. (See the patient consent form available online at ww.expertconsult.com.)
- The patient can insert 400 to 800 μg of misoprostol at home before the procedure, or the clinician can insert it at the time of the procedure when the stenosis is discovered.
- Generally 800 mg of ibuprofen 1 hour before the procedure helps with pain management. Consider diazepam 10 mg by mouth for the anxious patient.
- If further sedation is needed, see Chapter 2, Procedural Sedation and Analgesia.

Procedure

1. Place the patient in the lithotomy position.
2. Perform a pelvic examination to evaluate the uterine size and position.
3. Prepare the cervix and vagina with povidone–iodine (or diluted chlorhexidine if the patient is allergic to povidone–iodine).
4. Try to cannulate the cervical canal with a small silver probe, the 2-mm dilator, or the OS Finder or os locator (Fig. 136-5). If the patient becomes uncomfortable, administer 5 mL of a local anesthetic *submucosally* at the 12, 3, 6, and 9 o'clock positions on the cervix (see Chapter 149, Loop Electrosurgical Excision Procedure for Treating Cervical Intraepithelial Neoplasia), or use a paracervical block with 5 mL lidocaine at the 4 and 8 o'clock positions (see Chapter 173, Paracervical Block). Aspirate for blood before injecting to ensure that the needle is

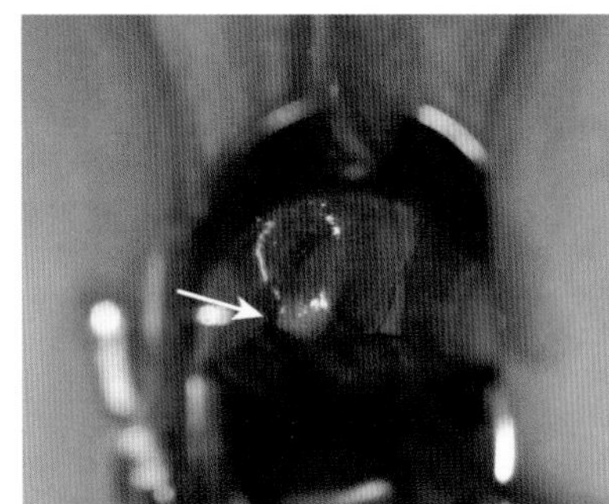

Figure 136-6 Single-tooth tenaculum placed posteriorly *(arrow)* on the cervix.

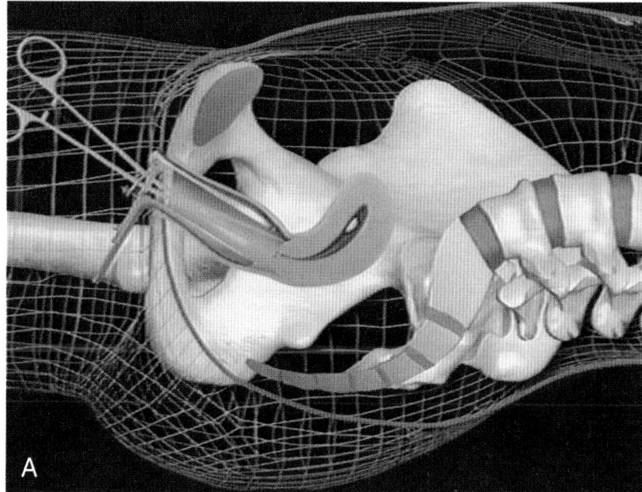

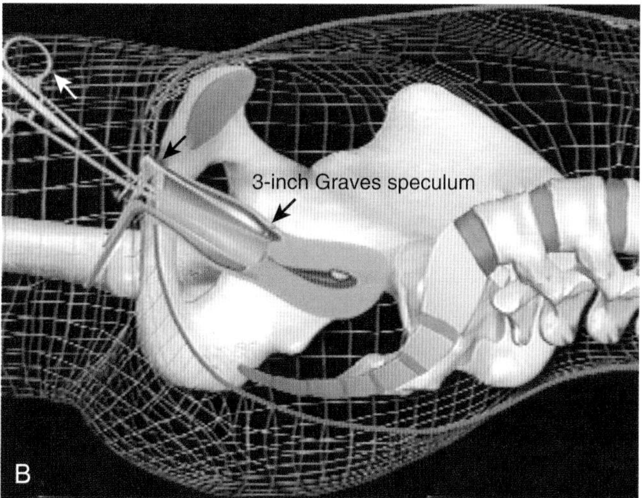

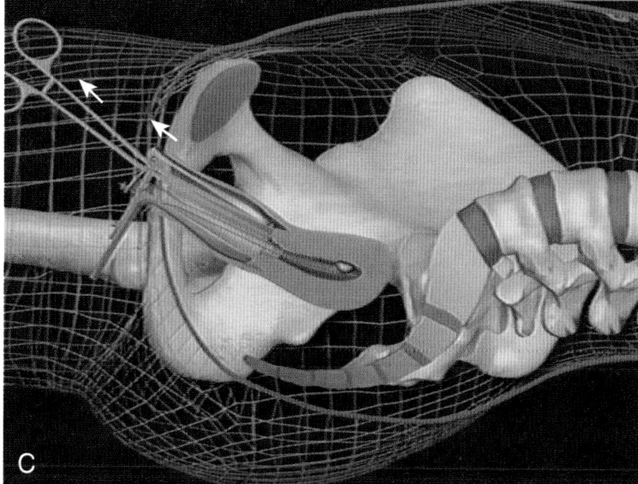

Figure 136-7 Applying traction to the cervix is often the solution to the problem of uteri with extremes of anatomic flexion. **A,** A tenaculum has been applied to the cervix of an anteroflexed uterus. **B,** By applying outward traction (*arrows*) on the tenaculum, the uterus is straightened. **C,** Dilators can now be inserted. Additional pressure on the speculum against the perineum is sometimes needed for the acutely ante-flexed uterus in order to create a straightened passageway.

not in a blood vessel. The use of a local injection into the cervix may obviate the need for the more complicated and uncomfortable paracervical block.

5. If the cervix is too mobile, place a tenaculum at the 12 o'clock or 6 o'clock position and use it to apply traction on the cervix while dilating it (Fig. 136-6). The straightening action of placing traction on the cervix (Fig. 136-7) is often the solution to the problem of uteri with extremes of anatomic flexion. Use progressively larger dilators and proceed slowly.
6. Once the external os is entered, the most difficult part of the procedure is passing through the internal os. If the sound/dilator does not pass readily, apply the tenaculum if not already done. The OS Finder or os locator usually enters the lumen without creating a false passage. It often takes firm, steady pressure on dilators to penetrate the internal os. To avoid perforation, the plastic Denniston dilators are strongly recommended. (This step causes significant anxiety in the clinician!) The clinician should be able to feel the smooth contour of the cervical canal. A rough surface as the dilator advances is a strong indicator that a false passage is being created. (If the roughness is felt, this would be a good time to confirm orientation with ultrasonography, if not already in use.) As the tenaculum is pulled outward, the dilator is pushed forward until a "give" is felt. Insert the dilator finder just through the internal os.
7. Gradually insert larger dilators until the degree of dilation needed for the particular procedure is attained.
8. A plastic, malleable or metal uterine sound can be inserted to determine the size of the uterine cavity, if needed. If a metal sound is used, bend it to conform to the position of the uterus as determined on the pelvis (anteverted or retroverted). The sound should pass easily before resistance is felt. For the normal-size uterus, this should be no more than 10 cm (possibly 12 cm). If the sound goes beyond this, suspect perforation unless the clinical examination or ultrasonography suggested a large uterus. If a perforation occurs, stop further efforts. (See later discussion.)
9. Dilation to 4 to 6 mm is sufficient for most non–pregnancy-related procedures and is usually readily accomplished in the office. When inserting the dilator, rest your fourth and fifth fingers on the perineum and buttocks to prevent uncontrolled movements of the dilator (Fig. 136-8).
10. Perform the procedure indicated.

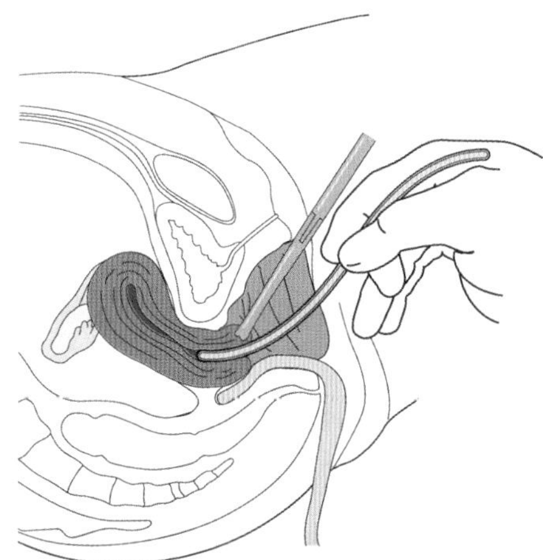

Figure 136-8 Cervical dilation using a Hegar dilator. During the procedure, the fourth and fifth fingers rest against the perineal area in order to prevent uncontrolled movements of the dilator, which can lead to uterine perforation. A weighted speculum is in the posterior vagina. The tenaculum is applied to the anterior lip of the cervix. (Adapted from Cunningham FG, MacDonald PC, Gant NF, et al. [eds]: Williams Obstetrics, 20th ed. Stamford, Conn, Appleton & Lange, 1997.)

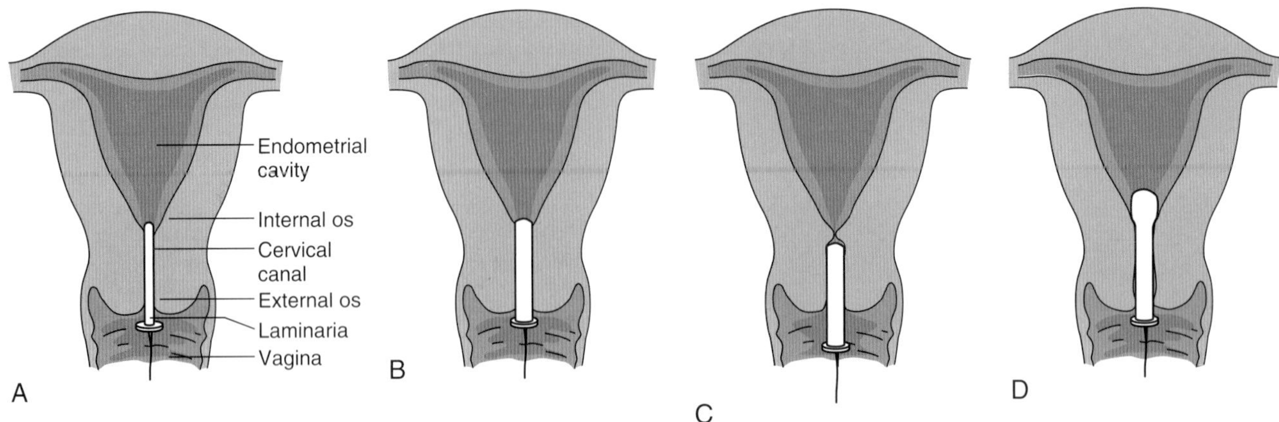

Figure 136-9 Insertion of a laminaria tent. **A,** The laminaria tent immediately after placement. Note that the upper end is just through the internal os. It is difficult to determine this "optimal" position, and it is not possible to obtain it with internal os stenosis. **B,** The laminaria tent 24 hours later. **C,** The laminaria tent not placed far enough to dilate the internal os. **D,** The laminaria tent inserted too far, making it difficult to remove. (Adapted from Cunningham FG, MacDonald PC, Gant NF, et al. [eds]: Williams Obstetrics, 20th ed. Stamford, Conn, Appleton & Lange, 1997.)

Laminaria Tent Placement

1. For laminaria tents to be used, the external os must be patent. Subsequently, they are used either for internal os stenosis or for a gradual dilation of the canal for larger procedures. They come in various sizes, and more than one may be inserted for greater dilation if needed.
2. Prepare the patient and cervix as described previously.
3. Sound the endocervix if possible.
4. Grasp the cervix with the tenaculum, if necessary, and use it to apply traction on the cervix (see Fig. 136-6).
5. Hold the *string end* of the laminaria with ring forceps and insert it into the os, ensuring that the laminaria tent does not extend into the uterine cavity. Use the largest laminaria tent that will fit into the os. Sometimes, this may be quite small. If unable to insert the laminaria tent, you may have to dilate the os further before its insertion (Figs. 136-9 and 136-10).
6. Laminaria are quite long and usually protrude out of the cervix for several millimeters.
7. Cover the cervix and the inserted laminaria with a sterile 4 × 4 gauze that has been dipped into *dilute* povidone–iodine solution, and tuck the edges in the fornices. Then place several dry 4 × 4 gauzes over the first one to hold the laminaria tent in place (Fig. 136-11).
8. Remove the speculum while holding the gauze in place with the ring forceps.
9. To prevent infection, the laminaria tent should be removed within 24 hours by grasping it with a ring forceps, rotating it 360 degrees, and pulling it out. Lesser procedures may only require 8 to 12 hours. Often the laminaria is inserted at the end of the day and removed the next morning. Alternatively, the patient can be the first one seen during the morning, with the laminaria removed when she is seen again as the last patient of the day. It may be necessary to replace the initial smaller laminaria with a larger one if the dilation is not adequate on removal.
10. Dilation can cause significant cramping, and ibuprofen 600 mg every 6 hours is advised.

Common Errors

- The most common error is *failure to straighten the uterus*. This occurs by not placing sufficient traction on the tenaculum or by using a speculum with long blades, trapping a flexed uterus in its flexed position. Failure to make this adjustment can result in uterine perforation, the most common complication of a difficult dilation.
- The laminaria may fail to dilate the canal because it has not been inserted far enough. Sounding the canal and marking the laminaria will aid in knowing when it has been inserted far enough (see Fig. 136-9C).
- The laminaria can be inserted too far, making it difficult to remove because of a bulbous swelling inside the uterine cavity (see Fig. 136-9D).

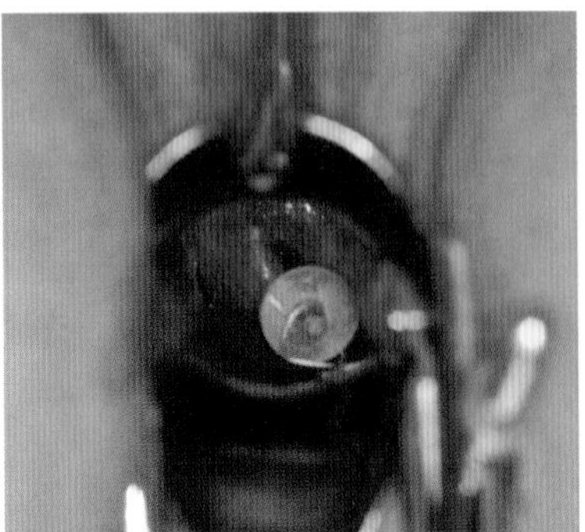

Figure 136-10 Laminaria tent has been inserted. It is difficult to appreciate that the tent actually protrudes 2 mm outside the cervix.

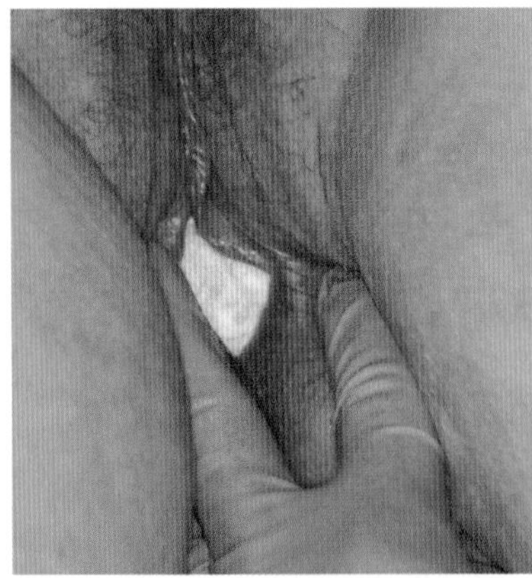

Figure 136-11 Laminaria held in place with 4 × 4 gauze inserted in the vagina. Patients tolerate this surprisingly well.

Complications

- Pain
- Hemorrhage
- Infection (especially if the laminaria tent is left in over 24 hours)
- Anaphylaxis or allergic reaction to the laminaria tent or misoprostol (rare)
- Inability to dilate the os
- Laminaria tents can break or separate on removal, making retrieval of the pieces difficult
- Inability to remove the laminaria because of an excessively deep placement

Many physicians are fearful of a *perforation*, but it is generally uneventful unless it is not recognized. The perforation can be complicated if further procedures are attempted and the instruments are introduced beyond the uterine cavity. If perforation is suspected, no further instrumentation should be done. Explain to the patient what is suspected. After 30 minutes of observation she can go home if vital signs are stable and there is no pain. She should report any fever, pain, or excessive bleeding. A follow-up visit or phone call within 24 hours is advisable. Repeat cannulation or dilation can be attempted after 6 to 8 weeks.

Postprocedure Patient Education

See also Chapter 141, Dilation and Curettage.

- If a laminaria tent is placed, the patient should be instructed to return within 24 hours for removal of the laminaria tent. Eight to 12 hours is often adequate.
- The patient should not engage in sexual intercourse while the laminaria is in place.
- If dilation was performed for cervical stenosis causing hematometra or pyometra, or after an excisional procedure, the patient should be instructed to return in 4 to 6 weeks for repeat examination and possible repeat dilation.
- The patient should return or call for fever, abdominal or pelvic pain, purulent vaginal discharge, or bleeding.
- In postmenopausal women not on estrogen replacement, or those with low estrogen states (e.g., Depo-Provera or Implanon users), estrogen cream helps maintain patency of the os. This is especially important if dilation was done for postsurgical (conization) scarring complications.

Conclusion

Cervical stenosis may require cervical dilation several times on a monthly basis to keep the os patent. Pregnancy and vaginal delivery may actually lead to a more lasting cure. As long as the patient is menstruating and is asymptomatic, and a Pap smear can be obtained, then physician intervention is not needed.

Patient Education Guides

See patient education and consent forms available online at www.expertconsult.com.

CPT/Billing Codes

57505 Endocervical curettage
57800 Dilatation of cervical canal, instrumental
58120 Dilation and curettage, diagnostic and/or therapeutic (nonobstetrical)
59200 Cervical dilation, laminaria

ICD-9-CM Diagnostic Code

622.4 Cervical stenosis

Acknowledgment

The editors wish to recognize the many contributions by Kathleen T. Dor, MD, to this chapter in the previous edition of this text.

Suppliers

(See contact information online at www.expertconsult.com.)

Denniston dilators
Ipas
Laminaria
Norscam
Laminaria and Lamicel, all mechanical dilators, os locator, canal finder
MedGyn
Mechanical dilators and os locators
CooperSurgical

Online Resource

The following site provides a good review of the topic: http://www.ihs.gov/medicalprograms/MCH/m/documents/MisoIUD4306.doc.

Bibliography

Cunningham FG, Keveno KJ, Bloom SL, et al. (eds): Williams Obstetrics, 22nd ed. New York, McGraw-Hill, 2005.

Hammoud AO, Deppe G, Elkhechen SS, Johnson S: Ultrasonography-guided transvaginal endometrial biopsy: A useful technique in patients with cervical stenosis. Obstet Gynecol 107:518–520, 2006.

Li YT, Kuo TC, Kuan LC, Chu YC: Cervical softening with vaginal misoprostol before intrauterine device insertion. Int J Gynaecol Obstet 89: 67–68, 2005.

Ngai SW, Chan YM, Liu KL, Ho PC: Oral misoprostol for cervical priming in non-pregnant women. Hum Reprod 12:2373–2375, 1997.

CHAPTER 137

COLPOSCOPIC EXAMINATION

Gary R. Newkirk

Colposcopy is the examination of the cervix, vagina, and genital organs with light and magnification to identify abnormal areas for biopsy, so that the patient can be triaged to appropriate care. Topical application of saline, acetic acid, and iodine solutions helps identify biopsy sites.

Addressing the widespread human papillomavirus (HPV) and genital epithelial dysplasia epidemic requires mastery of the skills to perform colposcopy, cervical biopsy, and endocervical curettage (ECC). The most frequent indications for these procedures include evaluation of an abnormal Papanicolaou (Pap) smear (see Chapter 151, Pap Smear and Related Techniques for Cervical Cancer Screening), visible cervical abnormalities, evidence of clinical HPV infection, and follow-up of prior cervical treatment. Most cases of cervical dysplasia can be managed entirely in the outpatient setting. Successful colposcopy requires *strict compliance with established protocol* and often the support of the pathologist, urologist, and gynecologist. Mechanisms for excellent documentation and rigorous follow-up are mandatory. Physicians who assimilate colposcopy skills into their practices will respond to a major public health problem and enhance their patients' access to care.

The *colposcope* is essentially a stereoscopic, portable operating microscope (3× to 40×) with a focal distance appropriate to examine the genitalia and cervix. The colposcopic examination serves to (1) identify normal landmarks, (2) identify abnormal areas in relation to these landmarks, (3) facilitate directed biopsy of abnormal areas for histologic diagnosis, and (4) rule out invasive cancer. Based on the findings, patients are triaged for observation, for procedures (e.g., cryotherapy, loop electrosurgical excision procedure [LEEP], cervical cold conization), and for definitive staged therapy for invasive carcinoma.

Colposcopic-directed *biopsy* provides histologic clarification of abnormal Pap smears; this is mandatory before definitive therapy. Premalignant and malignant cervical conditions produce colposcopically identifiable epithelial changes that are often characteristic and generally occur within the transformation zone (TZ), which can be examined carefully during the colposcopic examination. Ultimately, the pathologist is the one who provides the histologic diagnoses for abnormalities identified during the colposcopic examination. Therefore, the major challenge for the colposcopist is to *distinguish the normal from the abnormal and to sample the most abnormal-appearing changes for histologic confirmation*. When there is any question about the colposcopic impression, biopsy should be undertaken. The ECC, or other cervical assessment methods such as endocervical brushing techniques, is performed as part of the routine colposcopic examination (contraindicated in pregnancy) to confirm the absence of occult disease in the endocervical canal. Nearly all agree that traditional ECC *should be performed* (1) if there is any question of invasive disease within the canal; (2) before ablative therapy such as cryotherapy or laser ablation; (3) as part of the work-up for atypical glandular cell abnormalities; (4) when either the initial or follow-up cytology indicates a high-grade squamous intraepithelial lesion and colposcopy of the cervix does not yield a clear source; and (5) when the entire TZ/squamocolumnar junction (SCJ) cannot be evaluated (known as an "unsatisfactory colposcopy"). Other common reasons for performing a traditional ECC include follow-up of the treatment of severe dysplasia, especially when a cone resection (including LEEP) was performed and histology indicates positive margins with significant dysplasia, or if the ECC immediately after a cone resection was positive.

Colposcopy itself, without the benefit of histologic confirmation, is not considered a diagnostic tool. Even though colposcopically defined visual abnormalities correlate with cervical dysplasia or frank carcinoma, the ultimate diagnosis rests on the traditional histologic interpretation of submitted samples and not with the visual pattern recognition. Accordingly, diagnostic accuracy requires that the colposcopist perform *liberal* biopsy of the abnormal cervix.

In the past decade, major changes in our understanding of the epidemiology and science of cervical carcinoma have yielded efforts to develop a unified terminology to be used throughout the international scientific community. The International Federation for Cervical Pathology and Colposcopy (IFCPC) approved a basic colposcopic terminology at its 7th World Congress in Rome in May 1990 and further refined the terminology at its 11th World Congress in Barcelona, June 9, 2002 (Fig. 137-1). These terms should be used to describe findings during the colposcopic examination. Those terms marked with an asterisk are correlated with a higher likelihood of the histology demonstrating more severe dysplasia or cancer.

COLPOSCOPIC ANATOMY AND FINDINGS

The prudent colposcopist must be completely familiar with the normal findings and the visual abnormalities that correlate with dysplasia and malignancy on the cervix. Basic Pap smear terminology and cervical anatomy are reviewed in Chapter 151, Pap Smear and Related Techniques for Cervical Cancer Screening. Colposcopy terminology is summarized in Figure 137-1. It is also important to consider the appearance of the cervix in different age groups because the anatomy varies developmentally in response to hormonal stimulation (Figs. 137-2 to 137-4).

Normal Colposcopic Findings

See Figures 137-2 and 137-3.

Original Squamous Epithelium

This is a featureless, smooth, pink epithelium on the outer aspects of the ectocervix going back to the cervicovaginal reflection. There are no features suggesting columnar epithelium, such as gland

Colposcopic Terminology*

I. Normal colposcopic findings
  A. Original squamous epithelium
  B. Columnar epithelium
  C. Normal transformation zone
  D. Squamous metaplasia
II. Abnormal colposcopic findings
  A. Within the transformation zone
    1. Acetowhite epithelium (areas of white after application of acetic acid-vinegar)†
      (a) Flat
      (b) Micropapillary or microconvoluted
    2. Punctation (red dots)
    3. Mosaicism (linear, tilelike patterns)
    4. Leukoplakia (white change *before* application of vinegar)
    5. Iodine-negative epithelium (tissue that is *not* deeply stained by iodine [full-strength Lugol's solution])†
    6. Atypical vessels
  B. Outside the transformation zone (ectocervix, vagina)
    1. Acetowhite epithelium
      (a) Flat
      (b) Micropapillary or microconvoluted
    2. Punctation
    3. Mosaicism
    4. Leukoplakia
    5. Iodine-negative epithelium
    6. Atypical vessels
III. Colposcopically suspect invasive carcinoma
IV. Unsatisfactory colposcopy
  A. Squamocolumnar junction not visible
  B. Severe inflammation or severe atrophy
  C. Cervix not visible
  D. Entire lesion not seen (i.e., goes into canal)
  E. Most advanced lesion not sampled (i.e., in canal)
V. Miscellaneous findings
  A. Nonacetowhite micropapillary surface (micropapillomatosis vaginalis)
  B. Exophytic condyloma
  C. Inflammation
  D. Atrophy
  E. Ulcer
  F. Other (polyp, hemorrhage, cysts, etc.)

Figure 137-1 Colposcopic terminology. ***See text for definitions. †For the effects of acetic acid and iodine to be appreciated, the cervical and vaginal tissues must have estrogen stimulation.** (Adapted from Stafl A, Wilbanks GD: An international terminology of colposcopy: Report of the Nomenclature Committee of the International Federation of Cervical Pathology and Colposcopy. Obstet Gynecol 77:313–314, 1991.)

openings or nabothian cysts. The epithelium was "always" squamous and was not transformed from columnar to squamous after birth.

Columnar Epithelium

This is a single layer of mucus-producing, tall epithelium that extends between the endometrium and the cervical squamous epithelium. Columnar epithelium appears irregular, with stromal papillae and clefts. With acetic acid application and magnification, columnar epithelium has a grapelike or "sea anemone" appearance. It turns mildly acetowhite. Columnar epithelium is found in the endocervix, surrounding the cervical os, and is generally visible on the ectocervix in the reproductive age group.

Transformation Zone

As a woman ages, and under the influence of various hormones, the columnar epithelium that is originally found on the ectocervix is covered and transformed into squamous epithelium. The *transformation zone* is the geographic area between where the *original* squamous epithelium ended medially and where the outer lateral edge of the columnar epithelium currently exists. It is occupied by metaplastic epithelium in varying degrees of maturity because the columnar epithelium is being "transformed" into squamous epithelium. There is no way to discern where the *original* squamous epithelium was and what has been transformed. What can be identified is the *active TZ*, which contains gland openings, nabothian cysts, and, typically, islands of columnar epithelium surrounded by metaplastic squamous epithelium. The recognizable TZ is the area of most active metaplasia and transformation. The *active TZ* then extends from the SCJ (see later) laterally to the outermost visible gland. For all practical purposes, when the term "transformation zone" is used, it is generally referring to the active TZ because that is where disease processes occur. The progression, then, from central to lateral, is columnar epithelium, SCJ, active TZ, squamous epithelium that has been transformed, and original squamous epithelium.

Squamous Metaplasia

Columnar epithelium on the ectocervix is transformed over time into mature squamous epithelium by undergoing squamous metaplasia. Squamous metaplasia typically occupies the TZ to varying degrees. Metaplasia appears as a "ghost white" film when acetic acid is applied and it looks like a denser line of this white where the columnar epithelium and squamous epithelium meet.

Squamocolumnar Junction

Generally, this is a clinically visible line seen on the ectocervix or within the distal canal (e.g., postcryotherapy or in the

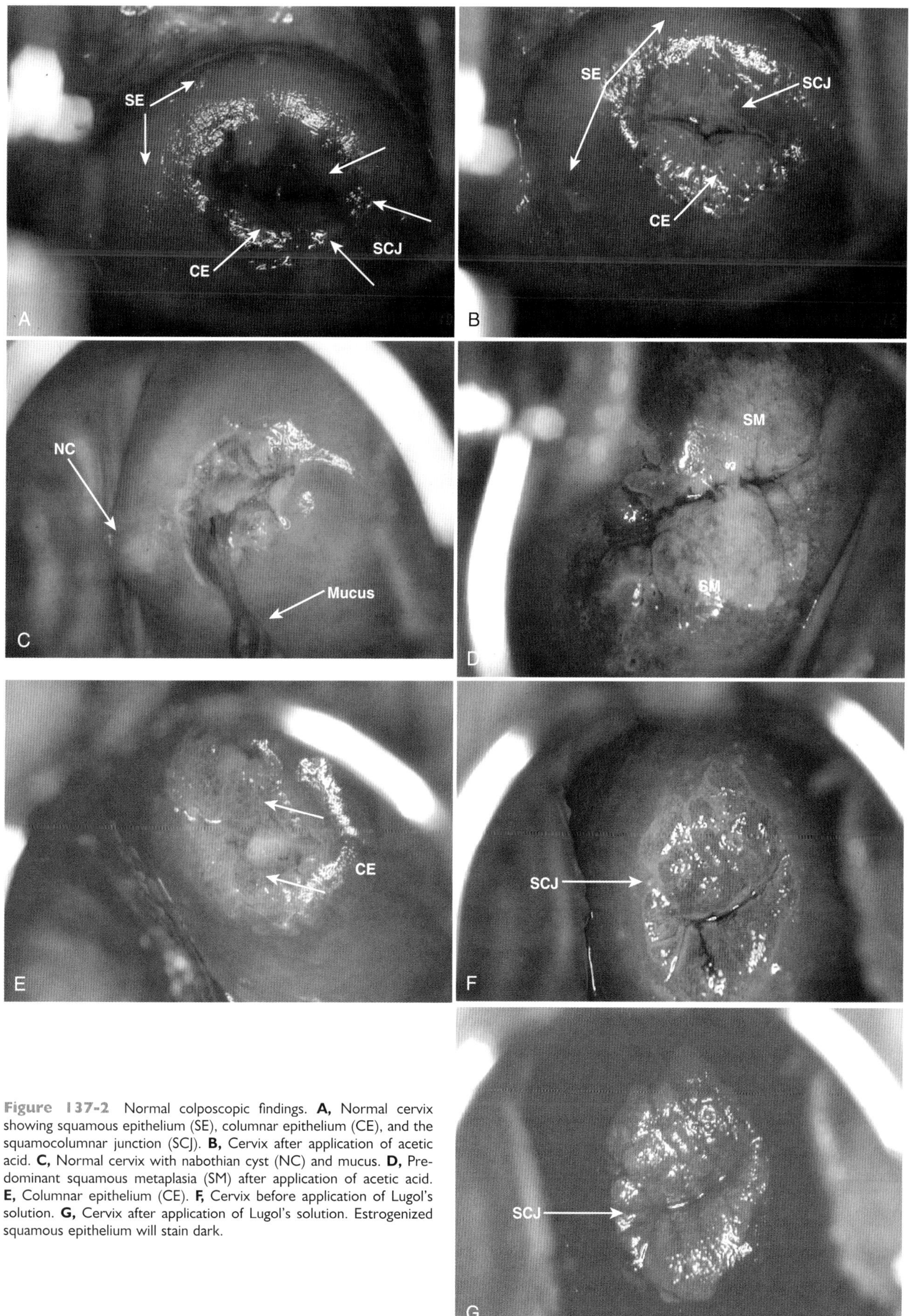

Figure 137-2 Normal colposcopic findings. **A,** Normal cervix showing squamous epithelium (SE), columnar epithelium (CE), and the squamocolumnar junction (SCJ). **B,** Cervix after application of acetic acid. **C,** Normal cervix with nabothian cyst (NC) and mucus. **D,** Predominant squamous metaplasia (SM) after application of acetic acid. **E,** Columnar epithelium (CE). **F,** Cervix before application of Lugol's solution. **G,** Cervix after application of Lugol's solution. Estrogenized squamous epithelium will stain dark.

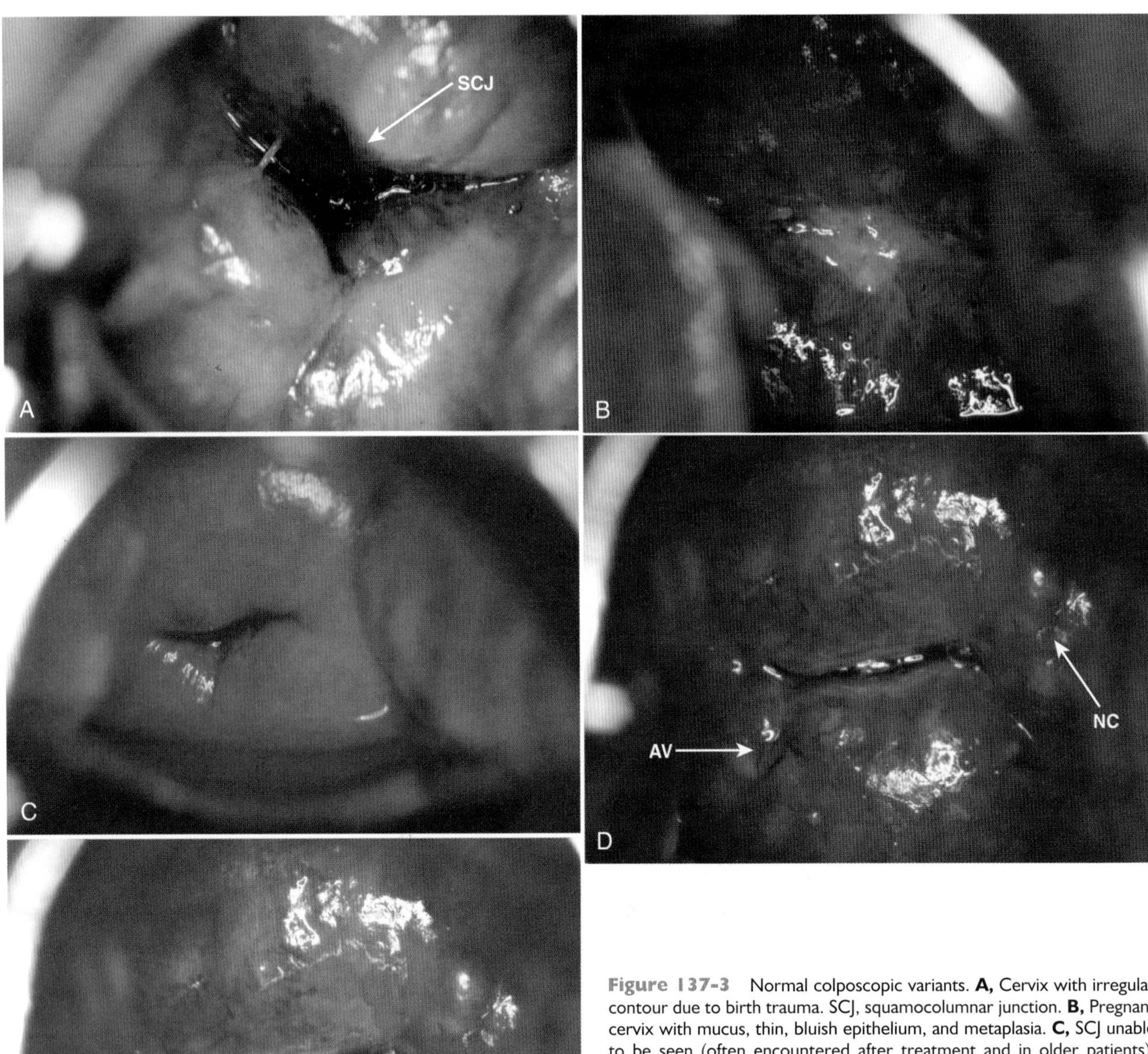

Figure 137-3 Normal colposcopic variants. **A,** Cervix with irregular contour due to birth trauma. SCJ, squamocolumnar junction. **B,** Pregnant cervix with mucus, thin, bluish epithelium, and metaplasia. **C,** SCJ unable to be seen (often encountered after treatment and in older patients). **D,** Prominent vessels can overlie nabothian cysts (NC), some of which may appear atypical. Biopsy is recommended if there is any doubt. AV, atypical vessel. **E,** Blue/green filter can enhance visualization of vessels, allowing the red vessels to appear black against a greenish background.

postmenopausal age group) that demarcates endocervical tissue from squamous tissue. Conceptually, the SCJ is comparable with the vermilion border around the mouth and the dentate or pectinate line in the rectum, where the mucosa meets squamous epithelium. The SCJ is the inner (medial) border of the TZ.

Abnormal Colposcopic Findings

See Figure 137-4.

Atypical Transformation Zone

A TZ with findings suggesting cervical dysplasia or neoplasia is considered abnormal. Usually, acetic acid (3% to 5% vinegar) is applied and the cervix is viewed under magnification with the colposcope.

1. *Acetowhite epithelium (AWE):* Epithelium that transiently whitens after the application of acetic acid. Areas of acetowhite correlate with higher nuclear density. The white staining fades within minutes. The more abnormal the changes, the more quickly they will turn white, the more dense they will be, and the longer they will last. All AWE is not necessarily abnormal because metaplasia also has a higher nuclear ratio owing to a more rapid growth rate and turns white with acetic acid.
2. *Punctation:* A stippled appearance of capillaries viewed end-on; often found within acetowhite areas, where they appear as fine to coarse red dots.

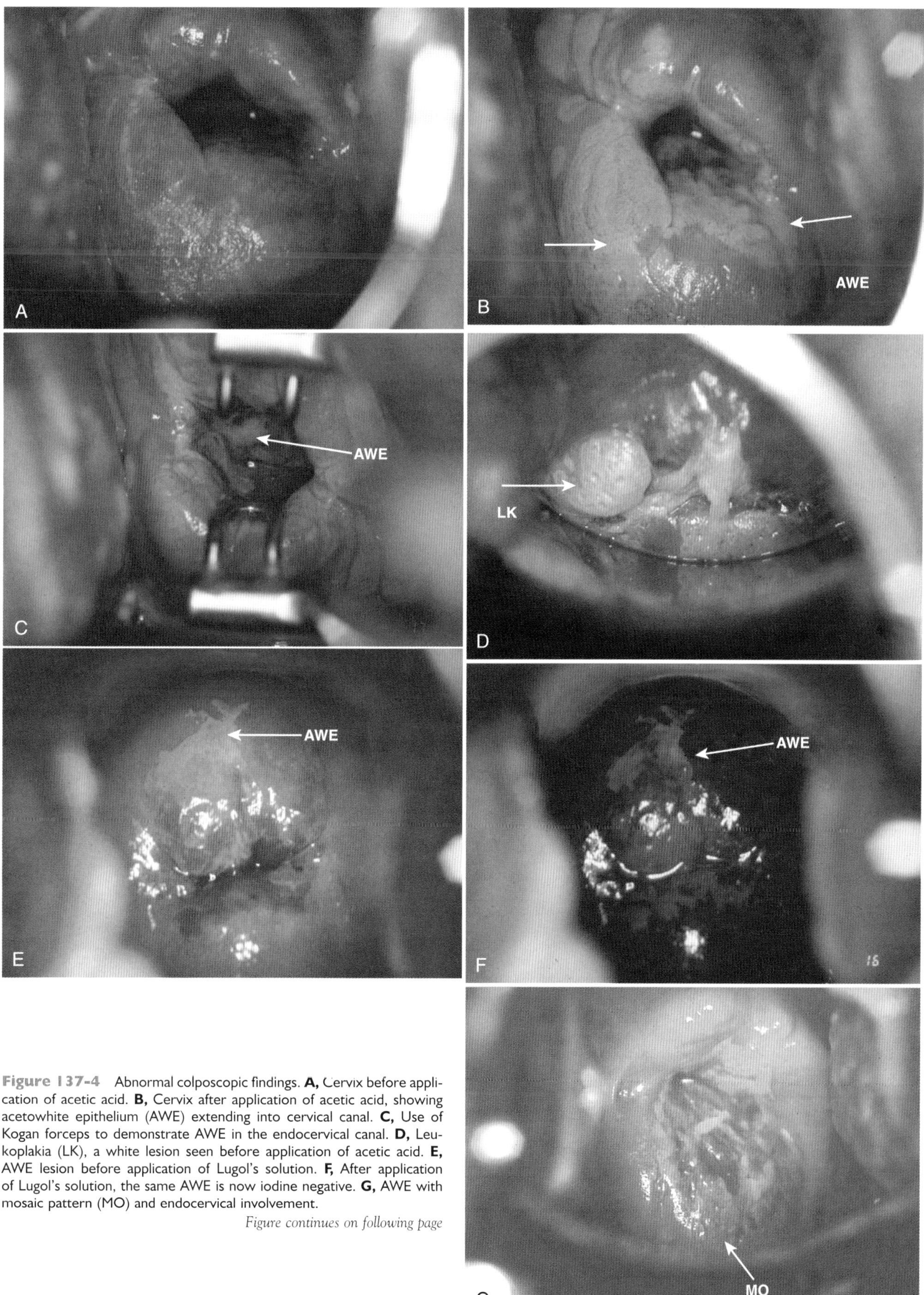

Figure 137-4 Abnormal colposcopic findings. **A,** Cervix before application of acetic acid. **B,** Cervix after application of acetic acid, showing acetowhite epithelium (AWE) extending into cervical canal. **C,** Use of Kogan forceps to demonstrate AWE in the endocervical canal. **D,** Leukoplakia (LK), a white lesion seen before application of acetic acid. **E,** AWE lesion before application of Lugol's solution. **F,** After application of Lugol's solution, the same AWE is now iodine negative. **G,** AWE with mosaic pattern (MO) and endocervical involvement.

Figure continues on following page

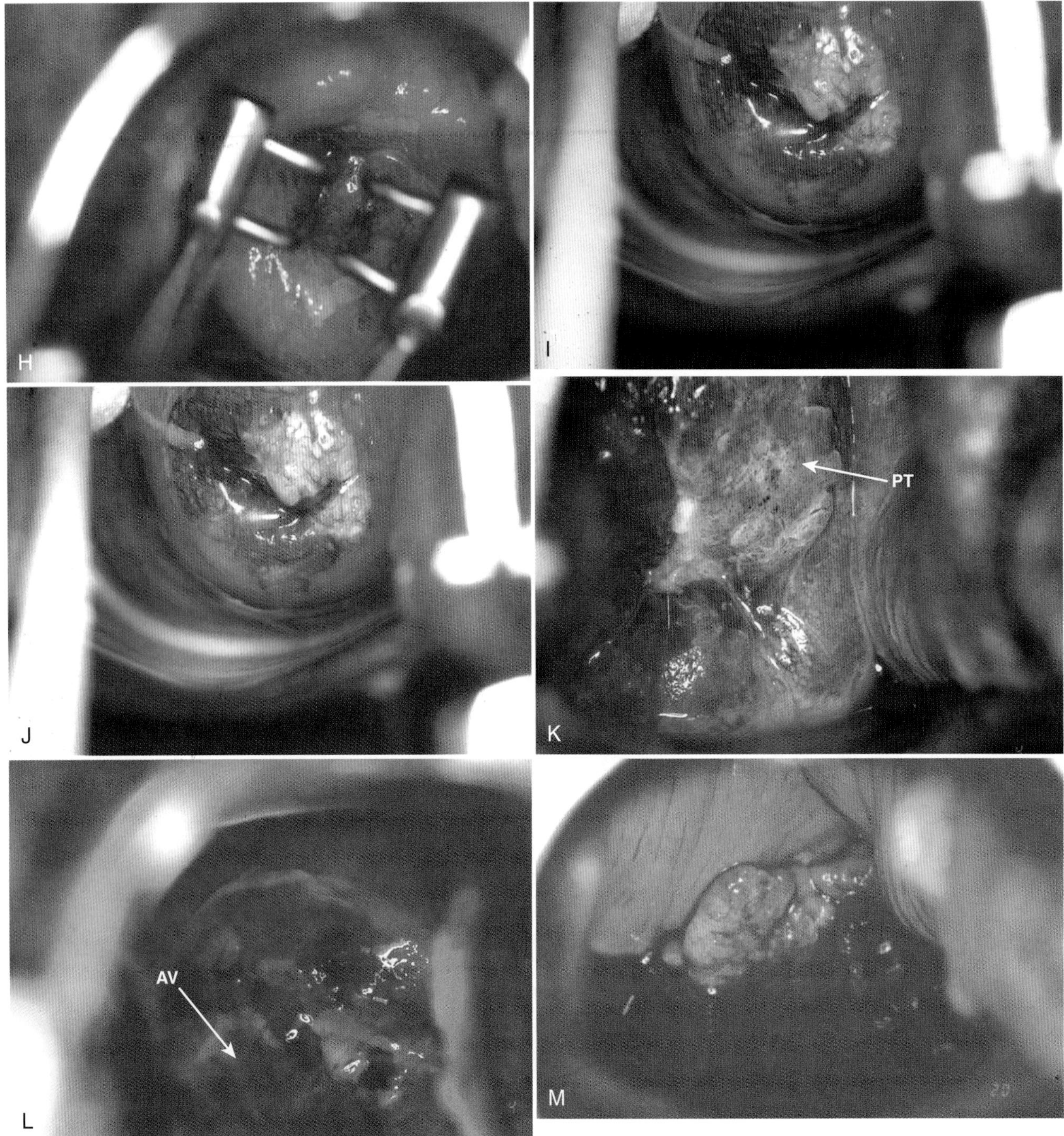

Figure 137-4, cont. **H,** AWE with endocervical involvement seen with Kogan endocervical dilators. **I,** AWE showing a coarse mosaic pattern before green light application. **J,** AWE showing a coarse mosaic pattern after green light application. **K,** Large, protruding lesion with coarse punctation (PT). **L,** Friable, peeling cervical epithelium and atypical vessels (AV) suspect for invasive carcinoma are seen in this example of invasive cervical carcinoma. **M,** Grossly deformed mass replacing the cervix consistent with invasive carcinoma.

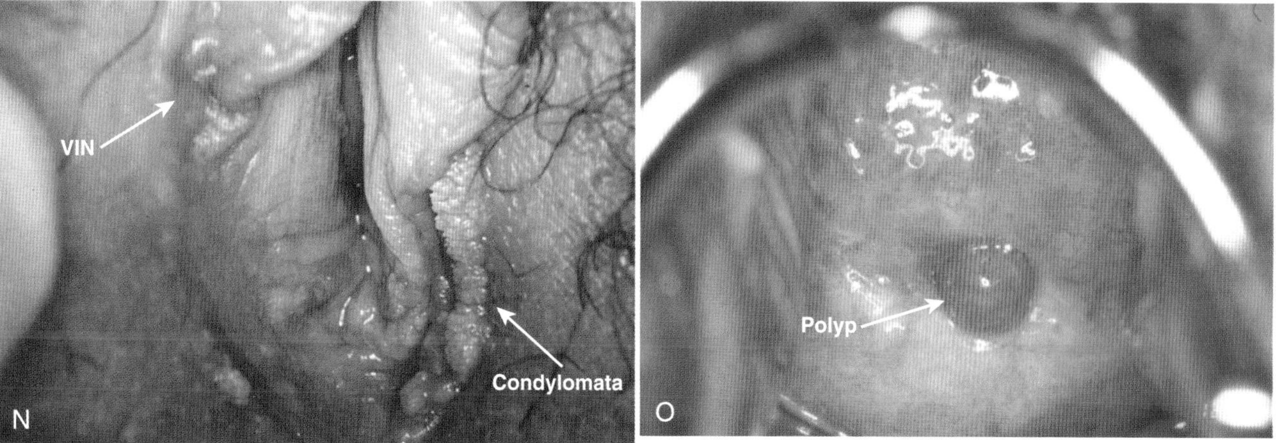

Figure 137-4, cont. **N,** Colposcopic view of the vulva with both condylomata and vulvar intraepithelial neoplasia (VIN). Remember, colposcopy includes inspection of the vulva. **O,** Central cervical polyp.

3. *Mosaicism:* An abnormal change made up of small red blood vessels appearing in linear form, suggesting a confluence of tile or chicken-wire patterns. This is best viewed after staining with acetic acid under magnification.
4. *Leukoplakia (hyperkeratosis):* Typically an elevated white plaque seen *before* the application of acetic acid. There is generally no change, or the area becomes more densely white, after application of acetic acid.
5. *Abnormal blood vessels:* Atypical, irregular, true vessels with abrupt courses and patterns; often appear as commas, corkscrews, or spaghetti-like shapes. No definite pattern is recognized, as there is with punctation or mosaicism. Abnormal blood vessels are seen in cancer and occasionally in advanced dysplasias.
6. *Iodine-negative epithelium:* Estrogenized epithelium will stain with Lugol's solution to a deep brown color. Abnormal tissue and nonestrogenized tissue do not stain.

Suspect Invasive Cancer

A complex pattern consisting of roughened, irregular cervical epithelium, typically with abundant abnormal vessel patterns and dense acetowhite change, often with a dense eggshell-white or slightly yellowish hue. It may also appear as ulcerated, friable, necrotic tissue. There may be a bulk effect or tumor-like appearance.

Unsatisfactory Colposcopy

In an unsatisfactory colposcopy, the entire SCJ or the limits of all lesions cannot be completely visualized. Proper examination can also be hampered if an active inflammatory process is present, if the patient is not estrogen primed (e.g., postmenopausal without replacement therapy, on progesterone-only types of contraception, lactation), or if heavy menses is present.

Other Colposcopic Findings

- Vaginocervicitis
- Traumatic erosion
- Atrophic epithelium
- Endocervical polyps
- Changes from diethylstilbestrol (DES)
- Abnormal pigmentation
- Nabothian cysts
- Post-traumatic clefts, deformities from birth or treatment
- Vaginal, vulvar, perineal, perianal lesions

Guidelines regarding visual colposcopic findings help ensure sampling of the most advanced sites of cervical dysplasia. The classic hallmark of cervical dysplasia includes the change that dysplastic epithelium undergoes after the application of 3% to 5% acetic acid (vinegar) or Lugol's (concentrated iodine) solution.

After the application of acetic acid to estrogenized tissue, *dysplastic epithelium* typically turns whiter than the surrounding normal epithelium (*AWE*). More advanced dysplasia typically appears more densely white, thicker, and smoother with raised borders. The surface of advanced dysplasia often becomes rougher or thicker as the severity of dysplasia advances and satellite lesions (multiple small abnormal areas) are less common. There may begin to be a "yellowish" hue. Changes in the vasculature pattern also correlate with cervical dysplasia. These abnormal patterns, which often occur in an acetowhite or leukoplakia patch, include *punctation, mosaicism,* and frankly *abnormal vessel variations.* The more coarse the punctation or mosaicism, the more severe the dysplasia is. Frankly abnormal vessel patterns imply severe dysplasia or potential invasive carcinoma.

After the *application of Lugol's solution* to estrogenized tissue, there is an immediate blackening (staining) of normal epithelium (iodine uptake is high in normal cells that are rich in cytologic glycogen). Abnormal dysplastic tissue, which has cells that contain much less intracellular glycogen, are not stained by iodine *(Lugol's-negative epithelium)* and remain white or faint yellow. The same pattern is seen if there is little or no estrogen stimulation.

Squamous metaplasia, a normal finding, may appear slightly acetowhite and may take up Lugol's solution incompletely; therefore, this tissue can cause some degree of confusion for the colposcopist. Squamous metaplasia is the physiologically normal tissue present where the columnar epithelium is being transformed into mature squamous epithelium. This occurs in the TZ—the same site where dysplasia generally occurs. Squamous metaplasia is especially prominent with certain conditions, such as active cervicitis, and where healing and reparative activities occur, such as after treatment. *Questionable areas always warrant biopsy.* If squamous metaplasia without dysplasia is reported on biopsy, but the Pap smear was abnormal, the prudent colposcopist must look elsewhere to explain the finding of dysplasia on the Pap smear (see Appendix K). A report of squamous metaplasia among other biopsies revealing dysplasia reflects the difficulty encountered by the colposcopist in evaluating this normal variant of acetowhite change. (Indeed, neither are all appendices removed for an acute abdomen the source of the pain!) The only other common areas that normally turn slightly white with acetic acid are the *endocervical (columnar) cells,* which are typically located in the cervical canal and extend a variable distance onto the exocervix. Endocervical tissue can usually be differentiated from abnormal areas by colposcopic examination because of its grapelike appearance on high-power magnification. Biopsy is still warranted if there is any confusion.

This chapter focuses on the evaluation of the abnormal Pap smear as it typically relates to cervical disease. *The complete examination also includes the colposcopic examination of the remainder of the genital system in women*. The colposcope can also be used for other purposes, such as to examine male genitalia or the anus, and to evaluate sexual abuse victims (see Chapter 99, High-Resolution Anoscopy, Chapter 118, Androscopy, and Chapter 157, Treatment of the Adult Victim of Sexual Assault). Ultimately, the patient's cytologic, colposcopic, and histologic data are used in concert to direct appropriate management. A well-managed colposcopy program provides effective evaluation and treatment for all patients with identified abnormalities of the cervix and genital tract.

Many colposcopists keep their scopes immediately available to augment the routine Pap and pelvic examination, especially if abnormalities are seen and both time and patient preference are favorable. Although complete formal colposcopic examination and biopsy can be performed when visual abnormalities are identified, many clinicians prefer to reschedule patients for full colposcopic examination at a later date. This allows more time for patient education and thorough evaluation.

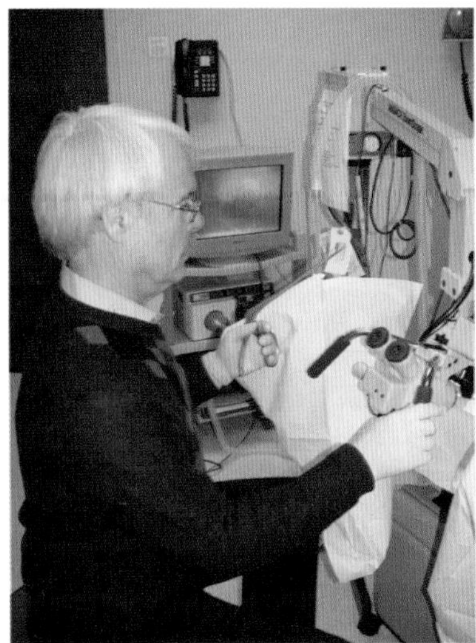

Figure 137-5 A contemporary colposcopy suite with motorized table with leg stirrups, boom-mounted video colposcope, and available loop electrosurgical excision procedure unit.

Indications

Refer to Appendix K for the 2006 American Society for Colposcopy and Cervical Pathology (ASCCP) Consensus Guidelines on the management of cytologic and histologic cervical abnormalities, and the indications and clinical scenarios in which colposcopy is indicated. The most common indications include the following:

- Pap smear consistent with dysplasia or cancer (see Chapter 151, Pap Smear and Related Techniques for Cervical Cancer Screening, for detailed recommendations regarding abnormal Pap smears)
- *Pap smear with atypical glandular cells* (*always* perform colposcopy)
- Worrisome history despite normal Pap smear findings (e.g., postcoital bleeding)
- An atypical Pap smear in which the patient tests positive for high-risk HPV
- Suspect visible lesion or palpable lesion of the cervix
- Abnormal vaginal bleeding, especially if postcoital, regardless of Pap smear status
- History of intrauterine DES exposure
- Evaluation or follow-up of previously treated or high-risk patients

The colposcope can be used for other reasons, such as removal of a cervical polyp, to find a lost intrauterine contraceptive device string, or to evaluate a rape victim, but in these instances a full colposcopic examination protocol is generally not indicated.

Contraindications

There are no absolute contraindications to colposcopy. Most contraindications relate to temporary or treatable conditions that alter the timing of the colposcopic examination rather than absolutely prevent it from occurring. The satisfactory colposcopic examination requires excellent visualization with a compliant and cooperative patient.

Relative

- Active inflammatory cervicitis
- Uncooperative patient
- Heavy menses (may prevent adequate examination)

NOTE: Pregnancy is not a contraindication to colposcopy, including biopsy, although a slightly different protocol is used and more bleeding can be expected from the biopsies.

Equipment and Supplies

The equipment and supplies used during routine colposcopy should be within easy reach in the colposcopy examination room (Figs. 137-5 through 137-7).

- Colposcope: variable fixed-power or zoom lens (3× to 7× low power to 15× to 40× high power).
- Biopsy forceps* (e.g., Tischler, baby Tischler, mini-Townsend, Kevorkian).
- Endocervical curette* (Kevorkian, no basket).
- Endocervical speculum† (Kogan, both narrow and wide types).
- Ring forceps.*
- Tenaculum† (rarely used).
- Cervical hook† (rarely used).
- Pap smear materials.†
- Vaginal speculums (e.g., metal Graves or disposable plastic speculum) in various sizes and lengths (use largest tolerated), or a clear, lighted, plastic speculum setup (e.g., Welch Allyn) for selected cases.
- Acetic acid solution 3% to 5% (white vinegar; 4 to 6 oz, or 120 to 180 mL).‡
- Full-strength Lugol's iodine solution (30 mL) (not always necessary after experience is gained but must be readily available).†,§
- Monsel's solution (ferric subsulfate), 1 mL.§ Monsel's is a topical astringent and is used to control bleeding after biopsy. It should be thoroughly shaken in its original bottle and then allowed to evaporate in a separate container until it is the consistency of a thick, yellowish-brown paste; this renders it a potent astringent to control biopsy-induced bleeding. Monsel's solution should be prepared several days in advance in order to achieve proper consistency. If the solution becomes too thick, it can be diluted with liquid solution from the original bottle.

*Included in the "colpo pack." These must be sterilized before procedures. "No-touch" technique is used on the ends of instruments touching the patient. Reusable instruments are sterilized, but colposcopy is not a "sterile" procedure per se.
†Available in colposcopy room but not used at every procedure.
‡Grocery store or mix to make 3% to 5% acetic acid.
§Hospital pharmacy.

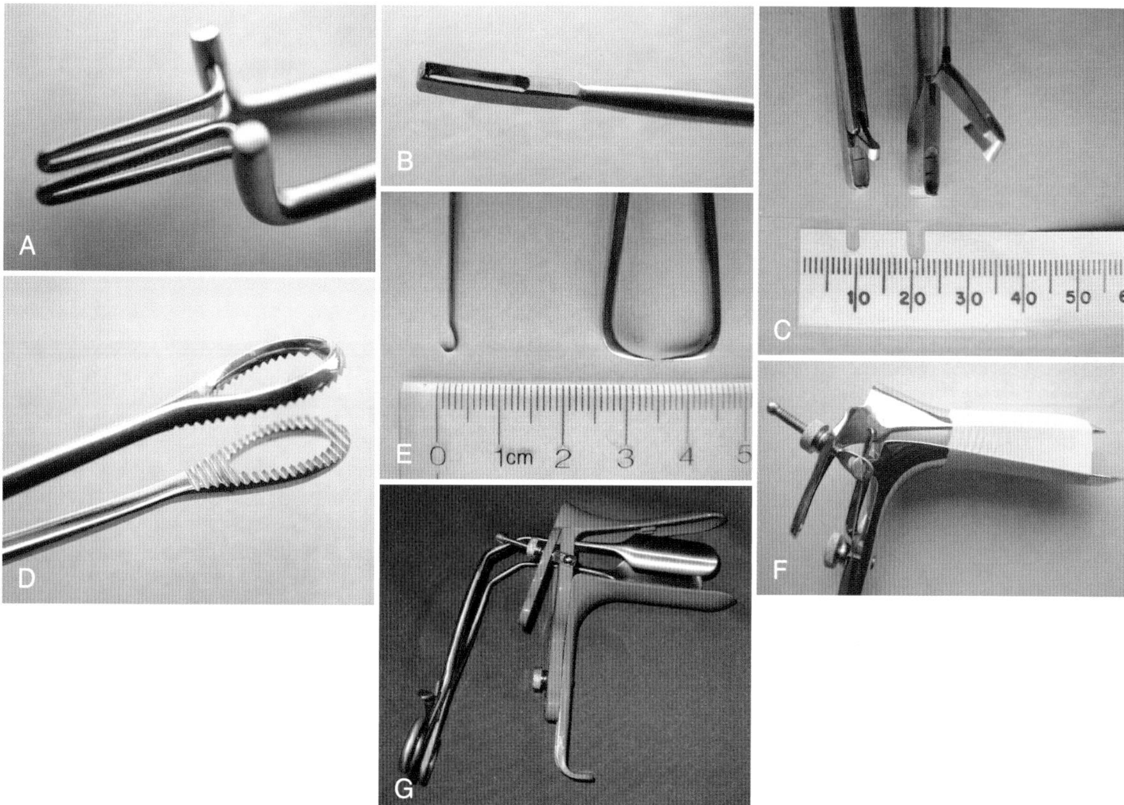

Figure 137-6 **A,** Narrow Kogan endocervical speculum. **B,** Kevorkian endocervical curette without basket. **C,** Tischler "wide jaw opening" biopsy forceps in both the large and small ("baby") options. **D,** A 1-cm ring forceps used to apply vinegar with folded gauze or cotton balls, or assist in visualizing the vaginal fornices and manipulating the cervix. **E,** A small cervical hook and tenaculum to help move the cervix (rarely needed). **F,** Vaginal speculum with glove finger applied and used as vaginal wall retractor. **G,** Vaginal speculum with vaginal wall retractor inserted.

- Cotton- or rayon-tipped swabs (8 to 10)
- Junior scopettes/OB-GYN applicators (6 to 10)
- 4 × 4–inch gauze
- Urine or sputum cups for vinegar
- Vaginal sidewall retractor
- Underpads ("chuck pads") (17 × 24 inch)
- Cotton balls (15 to 20)
- Power-assisted patient examination table that can be raised or lowered (Minimum height should be no more than 24 inches from floor, or older and disabled patients will have a difficult time getting on to it.)

Optional items include a preprocedural dose of an oral nonsteroidal anti-inflammatory agent, aromatic ammonium capsules ("smelling salts") for vasovagal responses, and a camera-video attachment.

Some clinicians now use a Pap smear sampling or similar brush to obtain the endocervical assessment instead of performing a formal ECC. Disposable ECC devices are also available and may be substituted for the reusable Kevorkian device.

Colposcopes come in a variety of "shapes and sizes" (Figs. 137-8 through 137-11), but all are basically the same. The stand may be

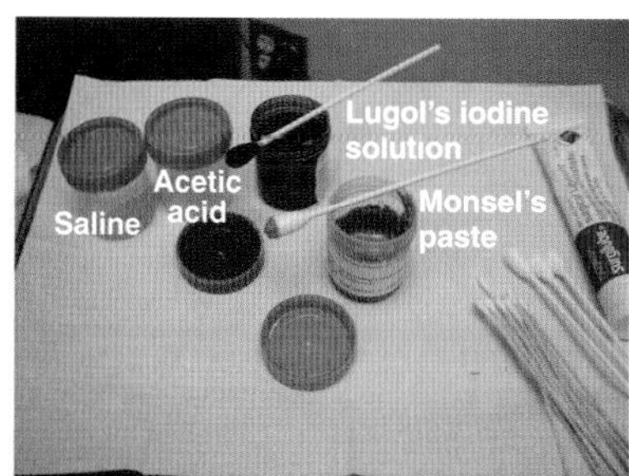

Figure 137-7 Common items on the colposcopy tray in addition to the equipment in Figure 137-6: cups of normal saline, acetic acid, Lugol's solution, Monsel's solution that has dehydrated to a paste, small and large swabs, lubricant. Formalin bottles and Pap smear supplies are not included here.

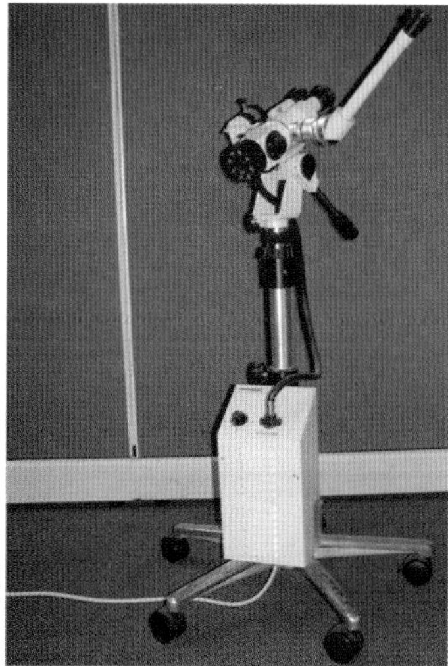

Figure 137-8 A pedestal-mounted colposcope with teaching head attached and fiberoptic light source.

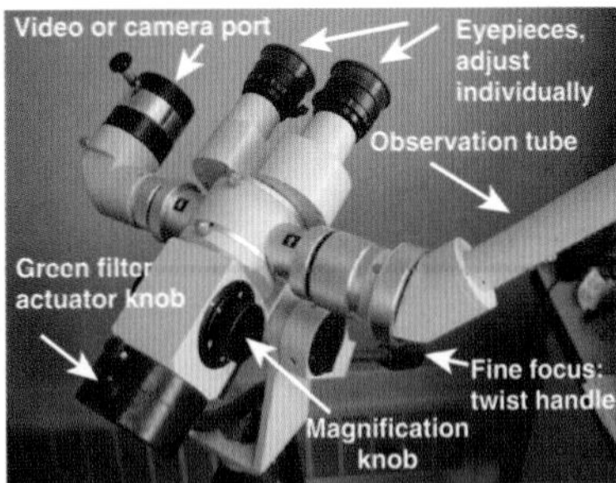

Figure 137-9 Features of the colposcopic head: fixed magnification knob, green filter knob, twisting handle for fine focus. Magnification changes are available between 4× and 25× in five steps. The camera/video port and observation (teaching) tube are optional features.

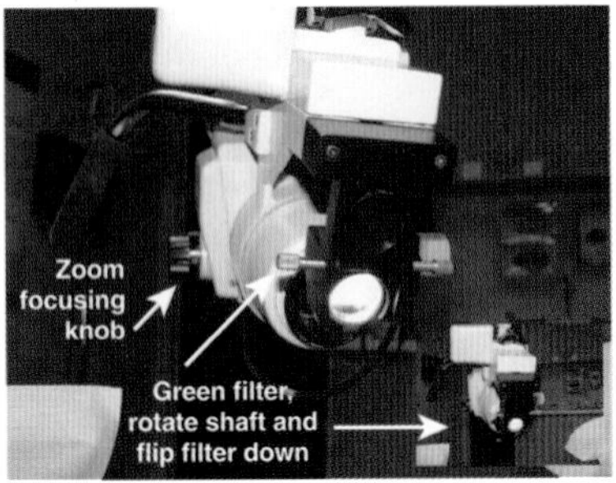

Figure 137-10 A zoom power colposcope head with green filter and zoom focus knob. Magnification smoothly zooms from 3× to 20×.

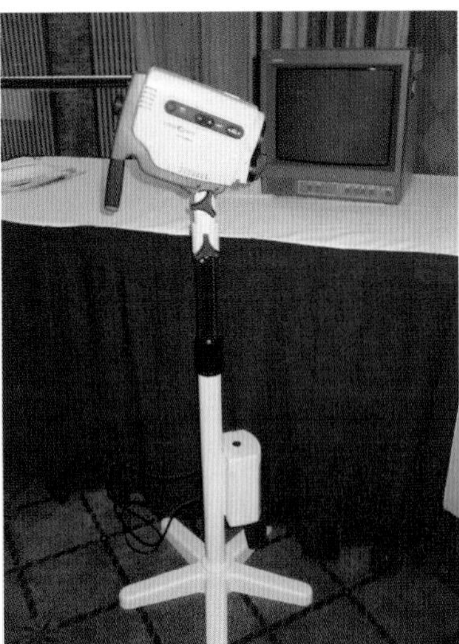

Figure 137-11 A dedicated video colposcope with traditional binocular optical viewing replaced with a monitor for viewing. (Courtesy of Welch Allyn, Skaneateles Falls, NY.)

a pedestal, may be on rollers, or may project out on an arm. There is a knob for changing magnification and another for fine focusing. The eyepieces also focus independently. A simple mechanism is usually available for inserting a *green filter* into the visual field, which makes identifying vascular abnormalities easier. The unit is turned on to the highest light intensity and then used essentially as a three-dimensional, short-range set of binoculars, but with an intense light source and variable magnification.

Some scopes have *video options* that project the image on a screen instead of using the binocular option (i.e., Welch Allyn; see Fig. 137-11). Most other scopes can be adapted for video use. In teaching situations, some type of video mode or teaching head adapter is mandatory. It is not necessary to take pictures or video for routine colposcopic examinations.

Preprocedure Patient Education and Forms

Providing educational materials to the patient and the patient's partner before the procedure can help alleviate the fear and uncertainty surrounding not only the procedure, but all of the issues surrounding HPV infection. Brochures are available from the American College of Obstetricians and Gynecologists (ACOG), ASCCP, and several other organizations (see the sample patient education handout online at www.expertconsult.com). An excellent patient education videotape is available from The National Procedures Institute (Midland, Mich). By providing materials beforehand, the clinician can focus on questions rather than try to take the time to explain a very complex topic with every patient.

- *Discuss the indications for colposcopy* with the patient. The patient should acknowledge the importance of long-term follow-up. The patient should advise the physician's clinic of change of address or telephone number.
- *Instruct the patient to continue contraceptive practices* before and after the colposcopic examination until treatment or management decisions have been made. There is no evidence that any type of contraception or estrogen replacement therapy causes progression of cervical dysplasia.
- Explain to the patient that a *pregnancy test* may be performed on the day of the procedure if pregnancy is a possibility, but colposcopy with or without biopsies carries very low risk in the pregnant woman. ECC is contraindicated in pregnancy.
- Instruct the patient to consume a *regular diet on the day of the procedure and not to skip a meal* before the procedure. This lessens the possibility of a vasovagal episode.
- *Advise against taking aspirin*, or medications containing aspirin, for 7 days before the procedure. Aspirin consumption within the past week does not ordinarily contraindicate colposcopy with biopsy, but you should be aware of the potential for more bleeding. Normally, nonsteroidal anti-inflammatory drugs, such as ibuprofen, do not significantly prolong bleeding; therefore they may be taken before the procedure for pain control.
- *Review the medical history* with particular attention to in utero exposure to DES; drug allergies; asthma; diabetes mellitus; history of vagal sensitivity (frequent fainting); bleeding disorder; recent symptoms of cervicitis or pelvic inflammatory disease; symptoms or history suggesting pregnancy; symptomatology suggestive of an endometrial disorder that may require endometrial sampling; and history of prior cervical treatment, including conization, laser therapy, or cryotherapy. Latex or iodine allergy history would contraindicate the use of latex gloves or iodine-containing solutions (Lugol's or povidone–iodine).
- *Explain that the procedure will take about 20 to 30 minutes*. Most clinics ask patients to arrive at least 15 minutes early to allow for appropriate education, a pregnancy test, and questions.
- If *pictures* will be taken, inform the patient and establish consent before the actual procedure.

- *Review the risks* before the procedure: pain, infection, bleeding, discharge, and missed disease. Menstrual-type cramping and limited discharge are common, but persistent pain, bleeding, or infection is rare.
- *Explain* that colposcopy with biopsy ordinarily renders a *diagnosis and is not a therapeutic procedure* per se. Definitive therapy will be determined by correlation of historical, colposcopic, cytologic, and histologic data.
- *Discuss treatment options*. Ordinarily, cervical cryotherapy, if indicated, is performed after the cervix has had time to heal from the biopsy and pathology reports are available. This typically can be performed as early as 2 weeks after colposcopy or after the next menstrual cycle.
- If applicable, inform the patient that she will probably receive a separate bill for the interpretation of the pathology samples obtained during the biopsy procedure.
- *Subacute bacterial endocarditis prophylaxis is not necessary*.

PROCEDURE

Figure 137-12 includes forms for documenting the colposcopic examination for both initial and follow-up visits. Clinicians are also advised to either dictate or record their findings in the medical record to supplement the colposcopic examination form, if necessary.

In addition to the necessary technical skills, the successful colposcopy program requires close attention to data interpretation and careful patient follow-up. The patient who has an abnormal Pap smear and who ultimately has biopsy-confirmed cervical dysplasia remains at an increased lifetime risk for recurrence of genital malignancy.

1. *Prepare the colposcopy room*. Make sure the room is warm. Some patients benefit from quiet background music. Have all necessary solutions and equipment ready at hand. Make sure the appropriate culture media, potassium hydroxide (KOH), and wet preparation materials are in the room. Keep all sizes of specula in your colposcopy room; prewarming is appreciated.
2. *Prepare the patient*. Mail information before the procedure. Answer her questions. (See section on Preprocedure Patient Education.) Ibuprofen 800 mg may be offered 30 minutes before the procedure. Check for medication, latex, and iodine allergies.
3. *Obtain informed consent*. Before the office visit, allow the patient to review a written description of the procedure, its risks, and complications (see the sample patient education handout online at www.expertconsult.com). Address questions and concerns. Obtain informed consent, which should include a signed consent.
4. *Obtain a pregnancy test as necessary. ECC is contraindicated in pregnancy*. Unexpected early pregnancy at the time of colposcopy is common. Even if ECC is performed, it rarely, if ever, has any adverse consequence.
5. *Perform a bimanual examination if one has not been done recently*. If a Pap smear is to be collected/repeated, complete that *before* the bimanual examination. The bimanual examination can also be performed after the colposcopy, but it may be more difficult if biopsies are taken. Care should be taken not to traumatize the cervix. Is the uterus enlarged or tender? What position is the cervix? Can the cervix be moved? How long is the vagina? Are there palpated abnormalities of the introitus, vagina, fornices, or cervix? Examine the vulva for obvious condylomata.
6. *Warm and insert the speculum*. Colposcopy requires the widest speculum the patient can comfortably tolerate. The examination requires greater cervical and vaginal exposure than a screening Pap smear. Because of the relative duration of the colposcopic examination, the vaginal walls may migrate inward, which makes visualization more difficult. A carefully inserted, wide, large Graves speculum is far more comfortable in the long run than constant prodding and manipulating of the vagina to move the vagina out of the field of view if an inappropriately narrow speculum is used. If necessary, use a vaginal sidewall retractor. Alternatively, a surgical glove finger or condom can be stretched over the speculum blades and the end cut before insertion of the speculum to facilitate visualization. A thin layer of water-soluble vaginal lubricant can be applied on the speculum. This thin coating significantly facilitates the insertion and removal of the speculum and does not interfere with biopsy or Pap smear interpretation. Use both thumbscrew dimensions of the speculum to gain maximum exposure. Ideally, the colposcopic examination is facilitated by having the cervix facing anteriorly and virtually "suspended" between the blades of the speculum.
7. *Grossly (using the naked eye) examine the cervix and vaginal fornices*. Does the cervix appear inflamed or infected? An active cervicitis confuses colposcopic detail. Characterize the vaginal and cervical discharge. Are there areas of obvious vessel atypia? Scan the cervix for gross leukoplakia before applying acetic acid. Although acetic acid greatly enhances the elucidation of diseased areas, its mild vasoconstricting properties can render significant vessel detail less obvious. Use magnification to quickly scan the unstained cervix to identify landmarks, such as the TZ with its SCJ, and identify any possible abnormalities.
8. *Obtain specimens for cultures, KOH and wet preparations, HPV DNA probe, and Pap smear, as necessary* (see Chapter 142, Human Papillomavirus DNA Typing, Chapter 151, Pap Smear and Related Techniques for Cervical Cancer Screening, and Chapter 160, Wet Smear and KOH Preparation). Even a correctly performed Pap smear irritates the cervix, may cause bleeding, and may change fine colposcopic detail. The Pap smear may need to be repeated because the original Pap smear was performed at a different laboratory; because more than 3 months have elapsed since the last Pap smear; because the patient is pregnant (Pap smears are less reliable during pregnancy and because colposcopy is more difficult, it is important to maximize clinical assessment); and because of the need to allay any concern or confusion regarding the adequacy or interpretation of the original Pap smear results. Once the Pap smear, KOH, or wet preparation is obtained as deemed necessary, it is permissible to gently blot (not rub) excess secretions to view the cervix more clearly.
9. *Apply 3% to 5% acetic acid*. One method is to use 4 × 4 gauze rolled up tightly and held longitudinally in a ring forceps. This saturates the cervix with vinegar quickly and without trauma. Cotton balls or large swabs also work well. Use large swabs to repeat the application. Refer to acetic acid as "vinegar" or simply as "douche solution" when discussing it with the patient. Warn her of brief stinging and coldness. Repeat application as necessary, usually every few minutes because the changes fade rapidly.
10. *Perform the colposcopic examination*. Start with low power (typically 5×). Scan the entire cervix with bright white light. Use a vinegar-soaked, cotton-tipped swab to help manipulate the cervix and TZ into view. It is almost never necessary to use the tenaculum to move the cervix. The cervical hook can be used; however, it is rarely needed. The Kogan endocervical speculum aids in the examination of the distal endocervical canal. It should be used when either the entire SCJ or the entire lesion cannot be seen because it (or they) is inside the endocervical canal. Use this instrument gingerly to prevent bleeding and pain. (Proper application of the Kogan endocervical speculum, although generally not needed, requires skill and practice. Using it routinely, especially for those new to colposcopy, will assist in learning the technique for when it is needed.) Now use higher magnification to carefully document abnormal findings.

COLPOSCOPY

PATIENT INSTRUCTIONS: Please complete questions down to "Procedure."

Date________________________________ Age_____________ Birthdate______________________________
Name________________________________ Referring physician______________________________________
Phone (home)_______________(work)________________ Reason for colposcopy______________________

HISTORY

Previous abnormal Paps?	Y	N	Age of first Pap_________ How often__________		
History of previous cryocautery (freezing)?	Y	N	Number of pregnancies______ Children_______		
History of previous cervical surgery?	Y	N	Date of last menstrual period________________		
Personal history of cancer?	Y	N	Type of contraception_______________________		
Family history of cancer?	Y	N	Number of sexual partners (lifetime)__________		
History of venereal diseases (circle)			Age at first sexual intercourse________________		
• gonorrhea • AIDS • herpes • syphilis			Do you smoke?	Y	N
Do you desire testing for any of these diseases?	Y	N	Partner(s) with warts?	Y	N
History of genital warts?	Y	N	History of sexual abuse?	Y	N
Visible warts now?	Y	N	Other PMH:		
Previously treated?	Y	N	Meds:______________________________		
If so, how?____________________			Allergies:___________________________		
			Other: ______________________________		

PROCEDURE (Doctor will fill out)

Observation without staining: ____

Pap repeated?	Y	N
SCJ seen?	Y	N
Endo spec needed?	Y	N
EGG done?	Y	N
Entire lesion seen?	Y	N

LK = Leukoplakia
WE = While epithelium
PN = Punctation
MO = Mosaicism
ATZ = Abnormal transformation zone
AV = Abnormal vessel
BE = Bulk effect
AG = Atypical glands
X = Biopsy sites

Vaginal vault:

Urethra:

Labia:

Perineum:

Rectum:

IMPRESSION: Adequate colposcopy? Y N

____

____

RECOMMENDATIONS:

Cryocautery	Y	N	Tip: __________
Referral to specialist	Y	N	
LEEP	Y	N	
Other:			

PLAN:
Discourage smoking
Partner needs information
Need at least annual Paps for rest of life no matter what others say
Handout on cryocautery/LEEP/Andro/HPV/vitamins/smoking

cc:____________________________________

____
Physician's Signature

Figure 137-12 Examples of initial colposcopy procedure and follow-up documentation forms. (Courtesy of John L. Pfenninger, MD, The Medical Procedures Center, PC, Midland, Mich.)

Follow-up Colposcopy Visits

Name_______________________________________ Referred by________________________________
Initial colposcopy date:________________________ Findings: Cervix __________________________
ECC __________________________
Other __________________________

Laser

Cryo

Treatment date: _______________ TCA

Efudex

LETZ: Ecto _______ Endo ______ ECC _______

Problem: ____
Partner evaluated? Y N Viewed tapes: Self? Y N
Partner? Y N
Smoker? Y N
Diet: _____________________________________
Vitamins? Y N

Date	History Findings/Treatments	Pap/Bx's: Done	Pap/Bx's: Results	Plan	Copy Sent

____
Physician

Figure 137-12, cont.

The entire TZ, including the SCJ, must be seen and evaluated. Abnormalities will usually turn white (AWE).

11. *Use the green filter to enhance vascular detail.* The green filter helps highlight vascular detail by rendering the red vascular patterns as black against a greenish background, similar to its use with the ophthalmoscope during the funduscopic examination. All abnormal areas require biopsy.
12. *Consider the use of Lugol's solution.* Lugol's solution aids with the identification of abnormal (dysplastic) areas, but its use is not mandatory (it is unnecessary and messy). Both dysplastic and reparative (metaplastic) tissue will incompletely stain with concentrated iodine because of low levels of cellular glycogen (compared with the staining of healthy, mature squamous epithelium). The sharply outlined borders afforded by Lugol's staining can be dramatic, and this can help clarify biopsy sites. Iodine staining does not interfere with histologic investigation. However, Lugol's will obscure the underlying vascular pattern. Lugol's solution should be used when further clarification of potential

biopsy sites is necessary or when no lesion is seen with acetic acid. Applying Lugol's solution will also help delineate the SCJ for the beginning colposcopist (endocervical cells do not stain with Lugol's), and Lugol's solution is used for performing cervical loop electrosurgical procedures (LEEP, large loop excision of the TZ) because its effects last longer than those of acetic acid. Lugol's solution is also helpful in the examination of the vagina because acetowhite changes there can be more subtle.

13. *Mentally map the cervix. The main goal of colposcopy is to identify areas for biopsy.* The colposcopist must be able to differentiate normal tissues from abnormal. *Tips on the findings include the following:*
    - Acetowhite areas that are unifocal; have sharp, flat, straight borders; stain white quickly; and appear thick or raised are likely to be more abnormal histologically.
    - The presence of *coarse* punctation or mosaic patterns, or of frankly abnormal vessels, is associated with a more severe degree of dysplasia. Ultimately, however, the histopathologist is the one who makes the diagnosis from biopsy samples.

    Be prepared to draw a careful record of what is observed and where biopsy samples were taken. The colposcopic impression of severity of disease *must be recorded* to compare and correlate later findings. Coppleson and associates (1986) proposed scoring indexes to help discern colposcopically identifiable lesions. Many physicians find these helpful when beginning colposcopy (Reid, 1993), but their utility and ability to predict the degree of disease present have been called into question.

14. *Is the colposcopic examination satisfactory?* The entire TZ, including all the SCJ, must be visualized. The borders of all lesions must be seen in their entirety (lesions should not disappear into the canal, for example). Patients who are uncooperative or who have a severely flexed uterus with inadequate visualization are potential "real-world" causes of unsatisfactory colposcopy. An unsatisfactory colposcopic examination coupled with cytologic evidence of significant dysplasia may necessitate a cervical conization for evaluation. It is a very important principle that all criteria be met to have an adequate examination. In summary, then, *the satisfactory colposcopic examination requires the following:*
    - Visualizing the entire TZ, including the SCJ
    - Identifying the area of abnormality producing the abnormal Pap smear
    - Confirming that the limits of all abnormal areas are clearly seen
    - Obtaining a biopsy sample of all abnormal areas
    - Verifying no colposcopic evidence of malignancy

15. *Perform the ECC.* Some colposcopists elect to omit ECC in instances where a clear source of cervical dysplasia is identified on the ectocervix, the SCJ is clearly seen, and the canal appears colposcopically clear of dysplasia. This is especially true if a low-grade squamous intraepithelial lesion (LGSIL) is the indication for colposcopy, the colposcopic examination supports cervical intraepithelial neoplasia (CIN) 1 or less, and visual inspection of the canal is negative. Others consider replacing ECC with careful endocervical brush sampling of the canal at the time of the colposcopic examination. Nonetheless, most colposcopists still perform ECC as a necessary component of the colposcopic examination, especially for a high-grade squamous intraepithelial lesion (HSIL) on a Pap smear, a marginally satisfactory colposcopy, a canal that is impossible or difficult to evaluate, suspicion of any degree of atypical adenomatous or glandular dysplasia, and always when ablative therapy such as cervical cryotherapy may be performed later (see Chapter 138, Cryotherapy of the Cervix, and Appendix K). Usually, neither local nor topical anesthesia is necessary.

    Use a Kevorkian curette *without* a basket (or other appropriate curette). Insert gently until the internal cervical os is reached, about 1.5 to 2 cm within the canal. This can be manifested by a slight puckering of the cervix with further advancement. In multiparous women the internal os is not well defined; the curette should not be advanced farther than 2 cm. Scrape the entire lining of the canal (360 degrees) *twice*. The procedure may be done with or without colposcopic observation. Use caution that the curette does not sample any tissue on the ectocervix and thus provide a false impression that there is disease within the canal. The curetted sample appears as a coagulum of mucus, blood, and small gray or tan tissue fragments. Sometimes a Cytobrush is used to retrieve the remnants of the ECC sample, which may persistently remain stuck in the canal. Submit the ECC sample in a separate bottle on a piece of paper towel, lens paper, or Telfa. Ordinarily, it is not necessary to place a sample pad in the posterior vaginal fornix, as it is with formal dilation and curettage.

    Do *not* perform an ECC on pregnant patients or patients with evidence of active cervicitis or pelvic inflammatory disease. All other patients must have a documented negative ECC before ablative therapy.

    Some physicians prefer to perform ECC after the cervical biopsy samples are obtained because (1) bleeding caused by the ECC can obscure lesions on the lower lip (but a cervical biopsy can bleed and "wash away" or dilute the curettage sample); and (2) the ECC, which takes only 30 seconds, is still the most uncomfortable part of the procedure. If performed first, however, the patient can be reassured early on that "the worst is over." Also, the chance of including dislodged tissue from a previous biopsy in the ECC specimen is minimized. This could again cause a false-positive ECC result, leading to more invasive treatment.

16. *Obtain cervical biopsy samples.* Sample the *posterior (lower) areas first* to prevent blood from dripping over future biopsy sites. Select the areas that appear most abnormal. "Blind random biopsies" are generally discouraged. The average number of biopsies taken is often in the range of two to five, but may be as few as one or as many as six or seven. It all depends on experience and the size, appearance, and number of lesions. The cervix can be manipulated with a cotton-tipped swab (preferred) or a hook (rarely) to provide an adequate angle for obtaining the biopsy sample. A 3-mm–deep sample is all that is necessary. It is *not* necessary to include normal-appearing tissue with biopsy samples (i.e., to include the margins of lesions in the sample). Beginning colposcopists can enhance their skills by placing samples from different biopsy sites in separate bottles and subsequently correlating them with colposcopic impression. After sufficient experience colposcopists can place all biopsy samples together. The cervix will be treated based on the most severe lesion as well as the size of the lesion. *Putting different biopsies in separate containers only increases cost, but it does not change therapy.* For anyone, to enhance the learning experience, an unusual or atypical-appearing lesion may be placed in a separate container to provide better feedback.

    If bleeding is profuse from a particular site and more samples are needed, hold a cotton-tipped swab to the area and proceed with obtaining the next sample. (To control persistent bleeding, see the Complications section.) Do not apply Monsel's solution until all samples are obtained. Monsel's solution in a biopsy specimen can affect histologic interpretation. As noted previously, some physicians prefer to obtain the cervical biopsy samples before the ECC.

17. *Apply Monsel's solution to bleeding areas after all biopsies have been obtained.* To be most effective, the Monsel's solution should be as thick as toothpaste. This consistency can be achieved by allowing the solution to evaporate down to a pasty consistency. Once bleeding is controlled, swab out the excess Monsel's and bloody debris in the posterior vaginal vault, which appears as a black mass of coagulum that may alarm the patient when it appears as a black discharge and irritates the vulva. Observe the cervix until all evident bleeding ceases.

18. *Examine the vagina while removing the speculum*. Reapply acetic acid to the vaginal sidewalls. Gently retract the speculum with a back-and-forth twisting motion to the right and left and observe through the colposcope as the vaginal wall collapses around the receding blades. Are abnormal vaginal areas apparent? If there is any question, Lugol's solution may help clarify the situation because condylomata and dysplasia (vaginal intraepithelial neoplasia [VAIN]) do not stain. Be sure to colposcopically examine any vaginal areas that felt abnormal during the bimanual examination. Biopsies of the vagina can be obtained with the same biopsy forceps but are placed in separate containers. It is not necessary to take deep bites.
19. *Examine the vulva and anus*. Acetic acid application will produce an acetowhite effect in most sites with condylomata or dysplasia (vulvar intraepithelial neoplasia [VIN]). It is mandatory to do a careful vulvar colposcopic examination with acetic acid in these women who are at high risk for vulvar dysplasia, especially those with unexplained vulvar itching or other symptoms, smokers older than 40 years of age, those with abnormal-appearing areas of vulvar tissue, and those with human immunodeficiency virus infection.

    The easiest way *to examine the vulva* is to begin superiorly. Use two hands to separate the vulva and slowly raise the power table with the foot pedal. Examine carefully from clitoris to anus. *The finding of perianal condylomata warrants anoscopy, especially if they have been persistent*. The Ives slotted anoscope is ideal (see Chapter 98, Anoscopy). If condylomata are grossly visible, it may be best to resolve the external lesions first before inserting the anoscope and risking spread internally. Acetic acid can be used in the anal canal but is rarely necessary. Small anal canal condylomata can usually be palpated. For the technique for sampling the vulva, see Chapter 159, Vulvar Biopsy. For high-resolution anoscopy, which is a colposcopic examination of the anal area, see Chapter 99, High-Resolution Anoscopy.
20. *Allow the patient to recover*. Have the patient rest supine for at least several minutes, then sit up slowly and rest again. Offer juice or cookies, especially if the patient has a history of syncope or missed the meal before her colposcopy.
21. *Document your findings*. Carefully draw a picture of lesions and biopsy sites. Photographs of the cervix do not replace accurately drawn diagrams of the colposcopic cervical findings. These should be included regardless of whether the colposcopic examination is considered adequate.

    Chart whether the colposcopic impression supports outpatient cervical cryotherapy or if excisional treatment will be needed, and which cryotip or loop electrode should be used (size and shape). This is not a decision based solely on colposcopic appearance. It requires correlation of cytologic, colposcopic, and histologic data to define the appropriate therapeutic intervention. Factors such as lesion location, grade of dysplasia, and number and size of lesions also dictate treatment options. For instance, large lesions (>25 mm in diameter, >15 mm from the os, or involving more than two cervical quadrants), even if they are only mildly dysplastic, are treated more appropriately with loop excision or laser therapy, as opposed to a small focal severe dysplasia, which may respond to ambulatory cryotherapy very well. (See Chapter 138, Cryotherapy of the Cervix, and Chapter 149, Loop Electrosurgical Excision Procedure for Treating Cervical Intraepithelial Neoplasia.) In general, the patient is a candidate for ablative therapy if the colposcopy is adequate (see earlier) and the following criteria are met:
    - No lesion extends more than 5 mm into the canal
    - The ECC is negative
    - There is no colposcopic evidence of malignancy
    - Any high-grade lesion is only focal in size (<1 cm)
    - There is correlation between the Pap smear findings, the colposcopic impression, and histology
22. *Discuss the findings and give postprocedure instructions*. After the patient has recovered and is dressed, review your impressions but withhold the specific diagnosis until the histology report has returned and all the clinical data have been examined. Provide careful postprocedure instructions (see the sample patient education handout online at www.expertconsult.com). Advise abstaining from intercourse for 24 hours and using tampons for 5 days. Instruct the patient to return if she experiences unusual vaginal odor, discharge, pelvic pain, or fever. Make a specific agreement as to how the results of the biopsy are to be reported. Unless a problem arises, the patient does not need a follow-up pelvic examination. Discussing the results of the biopsy sampling and subsequent treatment options on the telephone may be an appropriate follow-up mechanism for some patients; however, most will appreciate a visit to the physician for this important interaction.

Sample Operative Note

A prepared colposcopy procedure form, including patient identification materials, history, and a written diagram of findings, is an excellent way to document and archive findings (see Fig. 137-12).

Common Errors

1. *Losing track of patients* who have a significantly abnormal Pap smear or biopsy-proven dysplasia, and for whom treatment is necessary. This can place the patients at risk for delayed management and treatment. "No-shows" are a significant problem. Develop a follow-up tracking system.
2. *Finding an abnormal-appearing cervix on visual inspection when obtaining a Pap smear but then relying on the Pap result to determine if colposcopy is needed*. Visual abnormalities take precedence over the Pap report as an indication for colposcopy. If the cervix appears to be abnormal, colposcopy with biopsy is indicated.
3. *Omitting the ECC* in patients for whom cervical ablative treatment may be an option, especially for high-grade dysplasia (see Chapter 138, Cryotherapy of the Cervix).
4. *Failing to inspect the vulva, cervical fornices, and vagina during colposcopy*. Significant dysplasia can be a comorbid condition to cervical disease.
5. *Performing too few biopsies*, especially for large, high-grade appearing lesions where there is risk of missing invasive cancer. Studies continue to emphasize the importance of obtaining enough biopsies.
6. *Canceling colposcopy in women who are having routine menses*. Colposcopy can be performed in most patients regardless of bleeding.
7. *Trying to perform colposcopy with an active cervicitis*. Culture and reschedule soon.
8. *Failing to take the time to address all the emotional issues* surrounding HPV and other sexually transmitted infections, and condylomata/abnormal Pap smear concerns.
9. *Putting biopsies in separate formalin containers*. This usually is not necessary.

Complications

- *Bleeding*. Most *biopsy* or *ECC bleeding is minimal* and handled readily with Monsel's solution. Rarely, the patient experiences a fresh, bloody discharge. Often, a simple reapplication of Monsel's solution is all that is necessary. Silver nitrate sticks may also be used to cauterize small areas of bleeding (see Chapter 40, Topical Hemostatic Agents). Some clinicians will saturate the end of a vaginal tampon with Monsel's solution and insert this to provide pressure and astringent action for persistent cervical oozing. The tampon can then be removed several hours later by the patient. Very rarely, a simple *stitch of 4-0 absorbable suture* across a particularly deep biopsy site may be required. At times, it may be necessary to *cauterize* the biopsy site. An effective way to control fairly brisk bleeding is to *inject 1 to 2 mL of 2% lidocaine with epinephrine* into the bleeding site. This will either stop or reduce the bleeding enough to effectively apply Monsel's solution or cauterize the site. Use a needle extender (see Chapter 149, Loop Electrosurgical Excision Procedure for Treating Cervical Intraepithelial Neoplasia) or a spinal needle to reach the cervix. If possible, try to avoid obtaining a cervical biopsy sample immediately before the menses; subsequent bleeding may be confused with menstrual flow. This may not be very practical in the busy daily routines.

- A *foul cervical discharge*, *fever*, or *pelvic pain* may indicate postprocedure infection. Infection is almost unheard of, but typically occurs on the third or fourth day after the biopsy sample has been taken. A cervical biopsy should be avoided if there is clinical evidence of significant, extensive cervicitis identified by erythematous changes and marked friability. Not only will pathology be more difficult to interpret, but bleeding can be quite brisk.
- Despite correct technique, there is the potential risk that the most advanced *cervical disease may be missed* by the colposcopist at the time of the biopsy sampling or potentially by the histologist at the time of tissue analysis. Careful, timely transport of all samples to a reputable laboratory is important. The ECC sample should remain separate from cervical biopsies. The colposcopist is well advised to be liberal in obtaining biopsies of all abnormal-appearing areas of the cervix for histologic interpretation; costs can be controlled by placing all biopsies in one container. Widespread, four-quadrant cervical disease challenges the colposcopist to identify areas most likely to contain cervical carcinoma. Lack of correlation between the Pap cytologic results and subsequent histologic findings can suggest a situation in which potentially the worst area has not been sampled. The main goal of colposcopy is to rule out invasive cervical cancer and to select patients who are candidates for outpatient treatment. When the colposcopist cannot safely accomplish this goal, cervical conization—rarely, but importantly—is the only way of accomplishing this task. "Blind biopsies" in which random samples are obtained are, again, generally discouraged.
- Some women will experience *vaginal discharge* that often looks like coffee grounds after a cervical biopsy sample is obtained. This will typically last 1 or 2 days and should diminish with time. It is often due to the Monsel's solution used to control bleeding.
- Cervical biopsy sampling typically causes *brief pain and discomfort*. Ordinarily, this pain is well tolerated by most women. Careful explanation of the procedure, a warm room, and a caring, careful manner all minimize the discomfort. Studies have shown preoperative oral nonsteroidal anti-inflammatory drugs decrease discomfort associated with the procedure. Topical anesthetics generally are not left on long enough to make any difference.
- Rarely, *vasovagal reactions* occur with the procedure but are much more likely to occur with cervical cryotherapy.

Postprocedure Patient Education

See the sample patient education handout online at www.expertconsult.com.

- Agree on a time to discuss and interpret biopsy findings by phone or follow-up visit.
- Explain that mild vaginal discharge may occur after a cervical biopsy procedure, especially if Monsel's solution was used to control bleeding. This discharge is often grainy and black, like coffee grounds, which is the result of Monsel's solution mixing with mucus and blood. This discharge may last approximately 24 hours.
- Advise the patient that she may have spotting for at least 48 hours. Although there may be some spotting, it is safe to resume intercourse after 24 to 48 hours.
- Instruct the patient to report passage of clots, onset of fresh, profuse bleeding, foul vaginal odor, fever, or pelvic pain. Women with these complaints after a cervical biopsy procedure require evaluation.
- Encourage the patient to continue contraception.
- Patients rarely require vaginal creams after a cervical biopsy has been obtained. Nonetheless, some women may have vaginitis caused by organisms such as yeast, bacteria, or *Trichomonas*, and therapy aimed at these pathogens may be helpful and is not contraindicated after biopsy.
- *Emphasize the importance of returning for definitive therapy*. Reemphasize the relationship of cervical dysplasia with sexually transmissible disease, poor diet, smoking, and nonmonogamous sexual practices. Be sure the patient understands the lifelong risks of HPV infection.

Interpretation of Results

If at all possible, the same pathologist (or at least the same group of pathologists) should interpret both the cytologic and histologic results for a given patient. The clinician should be concerned *if a significant discrepancy is found between the Pap smear cytology, the colposcopic appearance of the cervix, and the biopsy histology*. In general, a report that a *more advanced lesion* was found on the biopsy compared with the Pap smear (e.g., Pap = CIN 2; biopsy = CIN 3) is common and acceptable. The clinician should be concerned, however, if biopsy-generated histology results are significantly *less advanced* than the Pap cytology. In general, most will accept a biopsy diagnosis one degree less, but if it is two degrees, the discrepancy must be explained. For instance, a cytology smear indicating carcinoma in situ, with biopsy samples of only mild dysplasia, might indicate that the worst area was missed on evaluation and that the patient may have in situ or invasive carcinoma in another site. The clinician is advised not to freeze or ablate any cervix until the discrepancy between histology and cytology has been explained adequately and sufficiently. Repeating colposcopy with biopsy to reconcile the difference is indicated. Freezing invasive cancer is never acceptable.

A *negative* ECC sample will show strips or fragments of orderly, benign columnar epithelium with mucus and blood. Lack of identifiable endocervical tissue constitutes an *inadequate* ECC sample. An inadequate ECC sample is not uncommon, and in the overwhelming majority of patients it simply means that the ECC must be repeated before definitive ablative therapy. If the ECC sample indicates dysplasia, it is a *positive* ECC and an indication for an excisional procedure (see Chapter 134, Cervical Conization, and Chapter 149, Loop Electrosurgical Excision Procedure for Treating Cervical Intraepithelial Neoplasia). Current protocol does not support freezing the canal with a long, narrow probe to treat endocervical dysplasia. Some "positive" ECCs result from contamination with dysplastic lesions at the verge of the os. *Nonetheless, do not assume this!* The beginning colposcopist must remain comfortable referring patients with equivocal or problematic colposcopic, cytologic, and histologic correlation. Know your limitations and seek help.

Patient and Physician Educational Resources

(See full contact information online at www.expertconsult.com under "Suppliers.")

American College of Obstetricians and Gynecologists
American Social Health Association
American Society for Colposcopy and Cervical Pathology: National society for promotion of quality education and patient care for cervical/vaginal disease
Krames Communications
The National Procedures Institute (videotapes)

CPT/Billing Codes

56605 Biopsy of vulva, single
56606 Biopsy of vulva, each additional
56820 Colposcopy of the vulva
56821 Colposcopy of the vulva; with biopsy(s)
57100 Biopsy of vaginal mucosa, simple
57105 Biopsy of vaginal mucosa, extensive
57420 Colposcopy of the entire vagina, with cervix if present
57421 Colposcopy of the entire vagina, with cervix if present; with biopsy(s) of vagina
57452 Colposcopy of the cervix including upper/adjacent vagina
57454 Colposcopy of the cervix including upper/adjacent vagina with biopsy(s) of the cervix and endocervical curettage
57455 Colposcopy of the cervix including upper/adjacent vagina with biopsy(s) of the cervix
57456 Colposcopy of the cervix including upper/adjacent vagina; with endocervical curettage
57460 Colposcopy of the cervix including upper/adjacent vagina with loop electrode biopsy(s) of the cervix
57461 Colposcopy of the cervix including upper/adjacent vagina; with loop electrode conization of the cervix (do not report 57456 in addition to 57461)
57500 Biopsy of cervix only, single or multiple (also use this code for removal of a cervical polyp since there is no other specific code)
57505 Endocervical curettage (not done as part of a D&C)
57510 Electrocautery of cervix
57511 Cryosurgery of cervix
57513 Laser ablation of cervix
57520 Conization of cervix, laser or cold knife
57522 Conization, LEEP technique

ICD-9-CM Diagnostic Codes

078.11 Condyloma acuminatum
180.9 Cervical neoplasm, malignant (excludes carcinoma in situ)
219.0 Benign neoplasm, cervix
233.1 Carcinoma in situ, cervix
233.1 CIN III
233.31 Vagina dysplasia, severe
233.32 Vulvar dysplasia VIN III
616.0 Cervicitis
616.10 Vaginitis
622.0 Cervical ectropion
622.0 Cervical erosion/ulcer
622.1 Cervical atypia
622.2 Cervical leukoplakia
622.4 Cervical stenosis
622.7 Cervical polyp
622.8 Cervical atrophy
622.8 Nabothian cyst
622.10 Cervical dysplasia (unspecified)
622.11 CIN I
622.12 CIN II
623.0 Vagina, dysplasia
623.1 Vaginal leukoplakia
623.5 Vaginal leukorrhea
623.7 Vaginal polyp
623.8 Vaginal cyst
624.01 Vulvar dysplasia, leukoplakia VIN I
624.02 Vulvar dysplasia VIN II
624.1 Vulvar atrophy
624.6 Vulvar or labial polyp
795.XX Abnormal Pap (requires five digits for specificity, see Chapter 151, Pap Smear and Related Techniques for Cervical Cancer Screening for details)

Suppliers

(See contact information online at www.expertconsult.com.)

Colposcope and instrument manufacturers
Carl Zeiss Surgical, Inc.
Claflin Medical Equipment
CooperSurgical, Inc. (acquired Leisegang)
Gyne-Tech Instrument Corp.
Gyrus ASMI Distributor (Olympus)
MedGyn
Seiler Colposcope
Wallach Surgical
Welch Allyn, Inc.

Other colposcopy equipment and supplies
CooperSurgical (Medscand [Cytobrush])
Delasco
Milex
Wallach Surgical (Papette, Pap smear samplers)
Welch Allyn, Inc.

Also see Chapter 138, Cryotherapy of the Cervix, and Chapter 149, Loop Electrosurgical Excision Procedure for Treating Cervical Intraepithelial Neoplasia.

Online Resource

American Society for Colposcopy and Cervical Pathology (ASCCP): Available at www.asccp.org.

Bibliography

Apgar BS, Brotzman GL, Spitzer M (eds): Colposcopy: Principles and Practice, 2nd ed. Philadelphia, Saunders, 2008.
Baggish MS: Colposcopy of the Cervix, Vagina, and Vulva. Philadelphia, Mosby, 2003.
Coppleson M, Pixley E, Reid B: The tissue basis of colposcopic appearances. In Colposcopy: A Scientific and Practical Approach to the Cervix, Vagina, and Vulva in Health and Disease, 3rd ed. Springfield, Ill, Charles C Thomas, 1986.
Ferris DG, Cox JT, O'Connor DM, et al: Modern Colposcopy: Textbook and Atlas, 2nd ed. American Society for Colposcopy and Cervical Pathology. Dubuque, Iowa, Kendall/Hunt, 2004.
Newkirk GR (ed): Colposcopy for the Family Physician, 2nd ed [includes video instruction on colposcopy, cryotherapy, and LEEP]. Kansas City, Mo, American Academy of Family Physicians, 2005.
Reid R: Biology and colposcopic features of human papillomavirus–associated cervical disease. Obstet Gynecol Clin North Am 20:123–151, 1993.
Spitzer M, Jones HW 3rd, Runowicz CD, Waggoner SE: Advanced Colposcopy [CD ROM]. Washington, DC, American College of Obstetricians and Gynecologists, 2002; joint publication of the American Society for Colposcopy and Cervical Pathology.
Tuggy M, Garcia J: Procedures Consult. Available at www.proceduresconsult.com.
Usatine RP, Smith MA, Mayeaux EJ Jr, et al: The Color Atlas of Family Medicine. New York, McGraw-Hill, 2008.

CHAPTER 138

Cryotherapy of the Cervix

Madeline R. Lewis • John L. Pfenninger

Cryotherapy is the treatment of choice for select small cervical intraepithelial lesions (cervical intraepithelial neoplasia [CIN] 1, 2, and 3, or mild, moderate, and severe dysplasia). This procedure is easy to learn, is well tolerated by the patient, and has a success rate similar to other therapies, including LEEP (the large loop electrical excision procedure) and laser. It requires a refrigerant gas under pressure, such as nitrous oxide, and an applicator probe. The cryoprobe allows rapid freezing of cervical tissue, causing a controlled destruction of the transformation zone and the epithelial lesion. Cellular destruction is greatest when a rapid freeze, slow thaw, and refreeze method is used. This efficacious procedure has few complications, can be performed quickly, is low in cost, and preserves cervical tissue.

The *only negative aspect* is that there is no tissue specimen available to confirm removal of all abnormalities. However, considering that up to 18% of patients experience pregnancy complications after LEEP, cryotherapy should be strongly considered for women who meet the criteria for treatment.

Cryotherapy treats cervical dysplasia by destroying the lesion and the transformation zone. Cell death occurs as a result of ice crystal penetration into the intracellular space. The depth of destruction is directly proportional to the lateral spread of the freeze, which is measured by the *size of the ice ball* that forms around the tip of the cryoprobe. An ice ball of 5 to 7 mm will result in adequate cellular destruction, because severe dysplasia (CIN 3) can extend to a depth of 3 to 5 mm into the glands in the transformation zone. The frequency and depth of gland involvement seem to be directly proportional to the grade of the squamous intraepithelial lesion. However, the overall success of cryotherapy is related more to the size of the lesion than the grade of the lesion. Small high-grade lesions (<1 cm) may be adequately treated with cryotherapy. Low-grade lesions should be less than 3 cm in diameter (some recommend <2 cm). For all lesions, they should involve no more than two quadrants of the cervix and extend no more than 5 mm into the endocervical canal. Large high-grade lesions (>1 cm), microinvasive lesions, and invasive lesions need more aggressive treatment such as LEEP, conization, or even hysterectomy.

Treatment failures may occur with cryotherapy as with any other treatment modality. "Cure rates" have been in the 95% range for CIN 1 and CIN 2, which is consistent with other modalities. For CIN 3 the cure rate drops to 89% overall, but this has been correlated more to lesion size and depth, not to severity of disease. High-grade lesions are often larger and extend deeper into the glands, making them more difficult to treat.

Anatomy

Cervical anatomy is discussed in detail in Chapter 137, Colposcopic Examination.

Indications

Also see the current American Society for Colposcopy and Cervical Pathology recommendations in Appendix K.

Cryotherapy may be used for *treatment of squamous dysplasia* that was confirmed with a biopsy after a complete and adequate colposcopic examination and if all criteria noted later have been met. It is *essential* that the Pap smear results, the appearance of the cervix on colposcopic examination, and the histologic report from the biopsy do not vary by more than one degree of severity. That is, colposcopic impression and histologic findings can only be one degree less severe than the Pap smear findings. If there is *lack of correlation*, this must be resolved or a LEEP or conization of the cervix is indicated because it is presumed the most advanced lesion has not been identified. It is common for histology to be worse than the Pap smear because the Pap smear is a screening test only. However, the Pap smear is essentially never two grades worse than tissue pathology or biopsy. If the correlation principle is met, the patient would then be treated *based on biopsy findings*. Cryotherapy may be used to treat low-grade squamous intraepithelial lesions (LSILs) and small, focal high-grade intraepithelial lesions (HSILs). Large high-grade lesions usually have deeper gland involvement, and these patients will need to have an excisional treatment, such as LEEP or conization. *Cryotherapy is not appropriate for any invasive lesion.* The practitioner must be sure to differentiate between "carcinoma in situ" and "microinvasive cancer." Although select patients with carcinoma in situ who meet the criteria may be treated with cryotherapy, *microinvasive lesions should never be treated this way*. Patients with microinvasive disease need a conization procedure to determine the true extent of the disease.

Criteria for cryotherapy of the cervix include the following:

- Complete colposcopic examination with good correlation between Pap smear results, visual examination, and histologic biopsy report.
- Entire squamocolumnar junction and the entire lesion must be visible ("adequate colposcopy").
- Lesions should be less than 2 to 3 cm in diameter and involve no more than two quadrants of the cervix.
- The probe tip must be able to cover the entire lesion and the entire transformation zone.
- The lesion does not extend more than 5 mm into the endocervical canal.
- The endocervical canal sampling is negative for dysplasia.
- The cervix should be relatively flat without large crevices.
- There should be no significant glandular involvement on biopsy.
- The patient must be reliable for follow-up.

Cryotherapy may also be useful *to treat patients with chronic cervicitis* that is culture negative and unresponsive to antibiotic therapy, and has negative colposcopy and biopsy findings. External genital human papillomavirus lesions may be treated with cryotherapy, although a different freezing technique is used (see Chapter 14, Cryosurgery, and Chapter 155, Treatment of Noncervical Condylomata Acuminata).

Contraindications

Absolute

- Patients with colposcopic or histologic findings more than one degree less severe than the Pap smear findings. These patients need to have a complete reevaluation before any treatment (see previous discussion).
- Positive endocervical curettage or other canal sampling that is positive (dysplasia or cancer).
- Large lesion that the cryoprobe will not cover completely.
- Lesion extends into the endocervical canal more than 5 mm.
- Large high-grade lesions or carcinoma in situ (>1 cm). LEEP is the treatment of choice for most of these lesions and will result in a better cure rate than cryotherapy.
- Invasive lesions (including microinvasion); these will need more aggressive treatment.
- Pregnancy.
- Cryoglobulinemia.
- Significant glandular involvement on endocervical curettage or biopsy.

Relative

- Patient is within 1 week of menses or is having heavy menstrual flow. The resulting canal edema from cryotherapy could obstruct the normal menstrual outflow.
- Acute cervicitis. In these patients it is best to treat the acute infection before cryotherapy.
- Immunosuppressed patients.
- Women exposed to diethylstilbestrol (DES) in utero, because they are at greater risk for cervical stenosis.
- Markedly irregular cervix where the indentations are deep and the cryoprobe will not reach these areas.
- Noncompliant patient (consider doing definitive excisional procedure).

Many would suggest that all CIN III lesions (i.e., carcinoma in situ) be treated with conization procedures. However, the data strongly support the efficacy of properly performed cryotherapy for small lesions that meet the aforementioned criteria. Cryotherapy is much more cost effective, with potentially fewer and less significant complications.

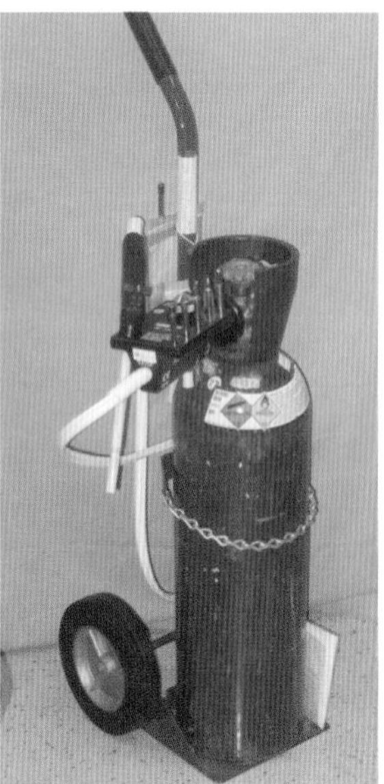

Figure 138-1 Nitrous oxide tank with the yoke adapter for the cryogun. Several cryotips are attached.

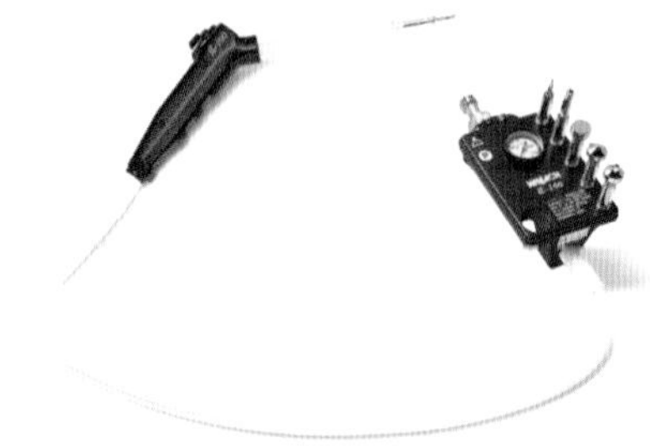

Figure 138-2 Close-up views of yoke adapter with pressure gauge, cryogun, and cryotips. (Courtesy of Wallach Surgical Devices, Milford, Conn.)

Equipment and Supplies

- Nitrous oxide 20-lb tank with a pressure gauge and gas cut-off valve (Figs. 138-1 and 138-2).
- Flexible tubing from tank to probe.
- Probe handle.
- Probe tips: 19- and 25-mm-diameter tips, slightly coned or flat; do not use any tips with nipples that are more than 5 mm in length (Fig. 138-3).
- Water-soluble lubricant, such as K-Y Jelly.
- Vaginal speculum.
- A minute timer.
- Vaginal sidewall retractors or glove to place over the speculum (to prevent injury to vaginal sidewalls in patients with redundant vaginal walls; see the "Technique" section of Chapter 151, Pap Smear and Related Techniques for Cervical Cancer Screening, for instructions on how to retract sidewalls with a "homemade" device).
- O-ring supply for some older cryo units. These are round rubber washers that attach at the base of the probe tip. They may crack over time, which could result in leakage of the refrigerant at the joint between the probe and the rod tip. They are easily and quickly replaced by simply removing the old one and sliding on the new one.

Precautions

- Verify the patient is not pregnant before the procedure. A good history is usually adequate, but if in doubt obtain a pregnancy test. Although it is unlikely that there would be any harm, it is best to avoid cryotherapy in the pregnant patient.
- Be certain that vaginal walls are away from the cryotip to avoid freezing these tissues.
- Check the pressure in the tank to ensure it is adequate. The gauge dials are generally self-explanatory.

Preprocedure Patient Education

- Provide the patient with a patient education handout (see the patient education handout available online at www.expertconsult.com).

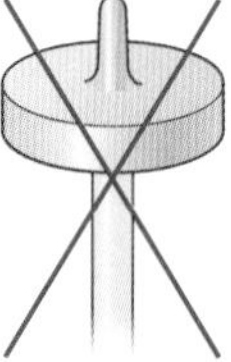

Figure 138-3 Older cryotherapy tips with endocervical nipples longer than 5 mm should be avoided.

- Discuss the risks, the benefits, and the possible complications of cryotherapy.
- Before the procedure, review the indications with the patient.
- Obtain written informed consent.
- Confirm that this patient is willing to return for follow-up.
- Update the menstrual history and do a pelvic examination if one has not been done within the previous few months.
- Verify the patient is not pregnant; perform a pregnancy test if there is any doubt.
- Confirm the biopsy report and note any area where disease is concentrated to ensure that the cryoprobe readily covers the area.
- Premedicate the patient on her arrival to the office (if appropriate) with ibuprofen 800 mg or another nonsteroidal anti-inflammatory drug (NSAID) to reduce cramping that may occur with the procedure (if not already taken). For maximum effectiveness, the NSAID should be taken approximately 30 to 60 minutes before the procedure.

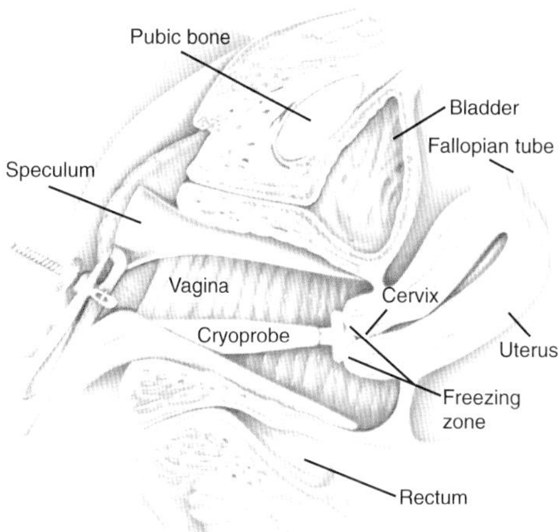

Figure 138-4 Proper application of the cryotip to the cervix.

PROCEDURE

Prepare Equipment

1. Ensure that the tank has adequate pressure; for most tanks the needle on the pressure gauge will be in the "green zone."
2. Ensure that the O-ring (the small rubber washer) at the base of the probe tip is intact, if applicable (mainly on older units).
3. Select the proper size and shape of probe tip. If the 19-mm tip covers the entire lesion and the entire transformation zone, it can be used. If all areas are not covered, use the larger, 25-mm tip. If the lesion is near the os or extends slightly (<5 mm) into the os, use the conical tip. If the lesion and squamocolumnar junction are well out on the ectocervix, a flat probe tip may be more appropriate to use. Avoid tips with long extensions because these may cause cervical stenosis (see Fig. 138-3).
4. Select the proper size vaginal speculum; the entire cervix and transformation zone must be well visualized, so consider using the largest speculum the patient can tolerate.

Prepare the Patient

1. Place the patient in a comfortable dorsal lithotomy position in stirrups.
2. In select cases, consider using a submucosal cervical injection with lidocaine (see Chapter 149, Loop Electrosurgical Excision Procedure for Treating Cervical Intraepithelial Neoplasia). Some clinicians use topical anesthetics, but unless they are in place for 20 to 30 minutes they have little effect.
3. Insert the speculum. If necessary, use a speculum cover or vaginal sidewall retractor to prevent vaginal injury in those with redundant mucosa.

Perform Cryotherapy

1. Apply water-soluble lubricant (e.g., K-Y Jelly) to the cryoprobe tip.
2. Turn on the gas valve (pressure gauge in the "green zone").
3. Apply the probe firmly to the cervix and begin freezing by pulling the trigger or pushing the freeze button. The tip will adhere in about 3 to 5 seconds (Fig. 138-4). After the tip adheres, pull back slightly. *Avoid the tendency to push in on the probe*, which stretches the uterosacral ligaments and causes discomfort. Pulling back slightly will cause the vagina to "billow out," reducing the likelihood of the probe sticking to the sidewalls.
4. Watch the probe tip carefully to monitor the rim of ice. A 5- to 7-mm ice ball around the perimeter of the tip is required for cellular destruction (Fig. 138-5). This formation usually takes at least 3 minutes. *A timed freeze alone is not recommended* because the size of the tip used, the amount of cervical vascularity and fibrous tissue, and the pressure in the nitrous tank all alter the amount of time required to form the 5- to 7-mm ice ball. In the majority of cases, *at least* a 3-minute freeze is used, after which the cervix is inspected to judge the size of the ice ball around the tip. If there is any question, continue the freeze. "Overfreezing" generally does not cause a significant problem.
5. When the ice ball around the probe tip reaches 5 to 7 mm, defrost by pushing the defrost button (on most machines) or releasing the freeze button. The probe tip will detach in about 15 seconds. Do not try to pull the probe off until it has thawed because that may result in laceration of cervical tissue. (The "active" defrost requires that the gas be left on—do not turn off the gas valve on the tank itself. A "passive" defrost takes at least 5 minutes just for the probe to release from the tissues.) If the probe does not easily release, check to be sure no one has turned off the gas. Switch back and forth between freeze and defrost. Sometimes the valve can stick.
6. Allow for a complete thaw of the cervix, which is seen when the cervix resumes a normal pink color. This may take 8 to 10 minutes. The patient often feels "flushed" during this period. Now, refreeze; the second freeze may take less time. Again, a 5- to 7-mm ice ball is required. *A rapid freeze, slow defrost, and rapid refreeze technique* has been shown to be the most efficacious method of treatment.
7. Thaw as described previously.
8. Remove the speculum and turn off the tank.
9. Have the patient sit up slowly to avoid any vasovagal symptoms, such as lightheadedness or flushing. These may occur up to 10 minutes after completing the procedure.

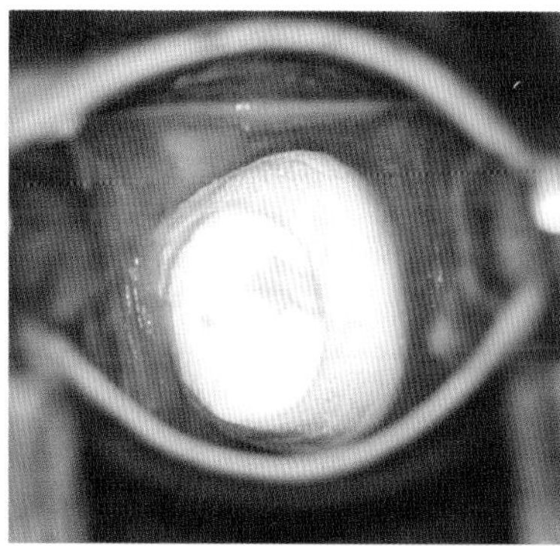

Figure 138-5 Appearance of the cervix immediately after cryotherapy. (Courtesy of John L. Pfenninger, The Medical Procedures Center, PC, Midland, Mich.)

10. Give the patient follow-up information. She will have a profuse, watery or blood-tinged discharge for 2 to 4 weeks. The next Pap smear should be scheduled for 6 months after this procedure (see the sample patient education handout online at www.expertconsult.com).
11. Consider prescribing a vaginal cream that aids in healing the cervix and potentially decreasing the discharge. Such a cream was previously available as Amino-Cerv Vaginal Crème, but it is no longer offered. It now must be compounded with the following ingredients:

Urea	8.34% (6.672 g)
Sodium propionate	0.50% (0.4 g)
Methionine	0.83% (0.664 g)
Cysteine	0.35% (0.28 g)
Inositol hexanicotinate	0.83% (2.988 g)

Ingredients are buffered to pH of 5.5 in a water-miscible emollient cream base to make 80 g. Prescribe one vaginal application at bedtime for 2 weeks.

Common Errors

- The patient may experience vasovagal symptoms after the procedure; avoid this by having the patient sit up slowly and rest a while before standing. Caution her to sit down immediately if she feels lightheaded.
- The anticipated postprocedure copious vaginal discharge can be mistaken for cervicitis.
- Turning off the gas at the tank before the probe has been released from the cervix.
- "Timing" the application as the sole criterion for the length of freeze. The size of the ice ball is the most important factor.
- Not emphasizing adequately to the patient that there will be a copious discharge but that this temporary inconvenience is worth it to avoid other, more severe complications associated with other methods of treatment.

Complications

- *Vaginal mucosal injury* is possible; avoid this by being certain that the cryoprobe does not touch the vaginal sidewalls. Use a speculum cover or vaginal wall retractors if necessary. If small areas are frozen, there are usually no significant adverse outcomes. If it appears that large areas of mucosa are being frozen, stop the procedure, take measures to protect the sidewalls, and start over.
- *Pain and cramping* may occur during cryotherapy; medicate patients with an NSAID about 30 to 40 minutes before the procedure. On rare occasions an anxiolytic may be helpful. In an especially anxious patient, consider a mucosal block. Avoid aggressive pulling on the cryoprobe during freezing because this may cause more intense cramping.
- The *profuse watery discharge* that follows cryotherapy is the most unpleasant consequence. It usually begins within the first day or two and lasts at least 2 weeks. The compounded cream noted earlier may help and may be used for a total of 4 weeks. Do not confuse this discharge, which always happens, with an infection.
- A *cervicitis* is possible after therapy. If the discharge is not improving after 2 weeks, consider oral metronidazole.
- A *pelvic inflammatory infection* is extremely rare. Consider it if there is extreme pelvic tenderness and fever.
- Should the patient surprisingly start her period within 4 to 5 days of cryotherapy, she may *retain menses*, causing severe discomfort. The cervix can be probed with a cotton-tipped applicator, which will usually release the blood.
- A very rare complication is *cervical stenosis*; using the proper probe tip should prevent this. Avoid any cryotip with projections greater than 5 mm.
- *Asymmetric freeze of the cervix.* If the cervix is very irregular in shape, consider freezing in segments, starting with the small, slightly nippled tip, then use the flat tip to cover the remaining areas.
- *Treatment failure.* Close follow-up is essential.

It is important to reassure the patient that there have been no documented long-term follow-up complications with future pregnancies after cryotherapy treatment.

Postprocedure Management

See the patient education handout available online at www.expertconsult.com.

1. Give the patient written follow-up information. She will have a profuse, watery or blood-tinged discharge for 2 to 4 weeks.
2. Consider a compounded cream to decrease the discharge (see earlier discussion). A peri-pad is needed for a few weeks.
3. Regular bathing is acceptable. Showers are preferable over baths.
4. Tampons should be avoided because they can irritate the friable cervix and cause bleeding.
5. Intercourse should be avoided for 2 to 3 weeks to allow adequate cervical healing and to prevent infection.
6. A follow-up Pap smear should be performed 6 months after cryotherapy, which allows adequate repair time of the cervical tissues. If that Pap smear is normal, it should be repeated in another 6 months. Colposcopy or human papillomavirus DNA testing may be performed along with either of these Pap tests, and may be especially useful if the patient had an initial high-grade lesion (see the American Society for Colposcopy and Cervical Pathology Guidelines in Appendix K). If follow-up laboratory results are normal, routine Pap examinations are resumed. Most recurrences occur within the first year after cryotherapy. If any of the postcryotherapy test results are abnormal, a complete reevaluation should be performed, including colposcopy, biopsy, and especially endocervical sampling. The cervix will have an altered appearance after cryotherapy, taking up to 4 months to return to a totally normal appearance (Figs. 138-6 to 138-10).

NOTE: Although some authors previously recommended bringing a patient back to the office after 2 to 7 days to "débride the cervix" to reduce the discharge, this procedure has been found to be of little or no value.

Patient Education Guides

See the patient education and patient consent forms available online at www.expertconsult.com.

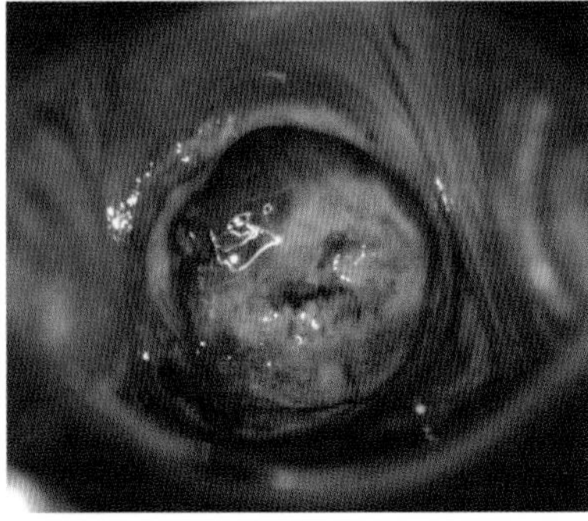

Figure 138-6 Appearance of the cervix with large eschar 10 days after cryotherapy. (Courtesy of John L. Pfenninger, The Medical Procedures Center, PC, Midland, Mich.)

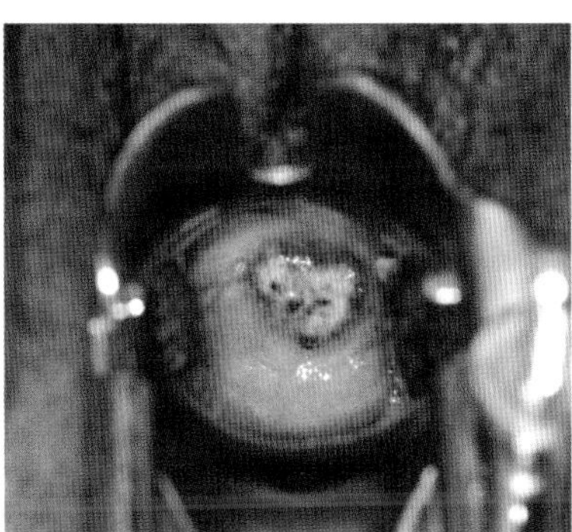

Figure 138-7 Appearance of the cervix 6 weeks after cryotherapy. (Courtesy of Duane Townsend, MD, Midway, Utah.)

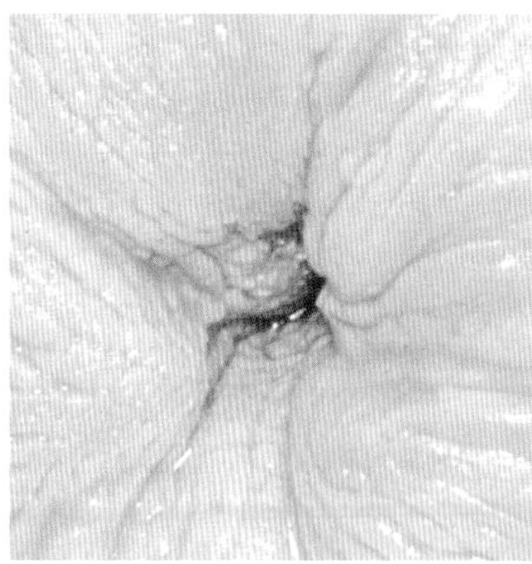

Figure 138-8 Appearance of the cervix 8 to 10 weeks after cryotherapy. Note radial striations. (Courtesy of Duane Townsend, MD, Park City, Utah.)

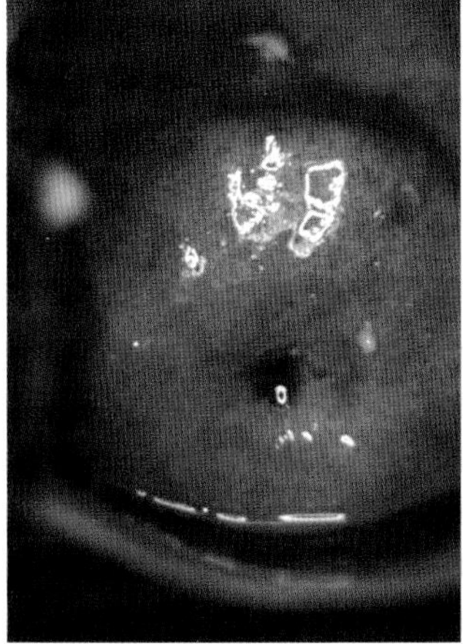

Figure 138-9 Appearance of the cervix 8 months after cryotherapy. Note the smooth ectocervix and lack of ectocervical transformation zone. The squamocolumnar junction is located right at the os. (Courtesy of Duane Townsend, MD, Park City, Utah.)

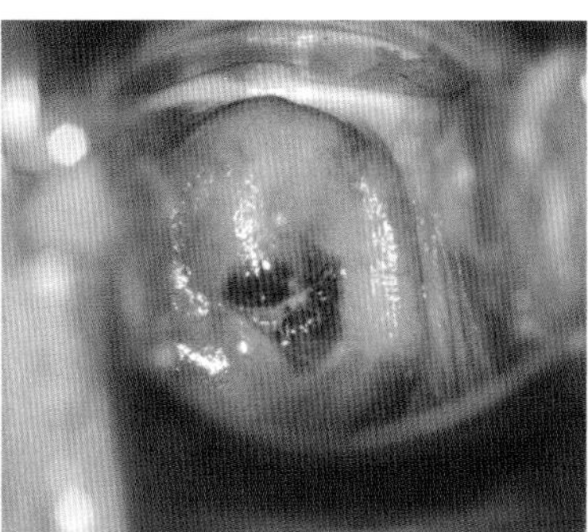

Figure 138-10 Inadequate cryotherapy because the transformation zone has not been eliminated. Retreatment is not necessary unless significant abnormalities recur.

CPT/Billing Code

57511 Cryocautery of cervix, initial or repeat

ICD-9-CM Diagnostic Codes

078.11 Condyloma acuminatum
622.11 Mild dysplasia of cervix (CIN 1)
622.12 Moderate dysplasia of cervix (CIN 2)
233.1 CIN 3/carcinoma in situ of cervix
616.0 Chronic cervicitis

Suppliers

(See contact information online at www.expertconsult.com.)

CooperSurgical, Inc.
Wallach Surgical Devices, Inc.

ONLINE RESOURCE

American Society for Colposcopy and Cervical Pathology: 2006 Consensus guidelines for the management of women with cervical intraepithelial neoplasia. Available at www.asccp.org/consensus/histological.shtml.

BIBLIOGRAPHY

Castro W, Gage J, Gaffikin L, et al: Effectiveness, safety, and acceptability of cryotherapy: A systematic literature review. Seattle, Wash, Program for Appropriate Technology in Health, 2003. Available at www.path.org/publications/details.php?i=687.

Cuzick J, Clavel C, Petry KU, et al: Overview of the European and North American studies on HPV testing in primary cervical cancer screening. Int J Cancer 119:1095–1101, 2006.

Denny L, Kuhn L, De Souza M, et al: Screen-and-treat approaches for cervical cancer prevention in low-resource settings: A randomized controlled trial. JAMA 294:2173–2181, 2005.

Luciani S, Gonzales M, Munoz S, et al: Effectiveness of cryotherapy treatment for cervical intraepithelial neoplasia. Int J Gynaecol Obstet 101:172–177, 2008.

Sherris J, Wittet S, Kleine A, et al: Evidence-based, alternative cervical cancer screening approaches in low-resource settings. Int Perspect Sex Reprod Health 35:147–154, 2009.

Spitzer M, Brotzman GL, Apgar BS: Practical therapeutic options for treatment of cervical intraepithelial neoplasia. In Apgar BS, Brotzman GL, Spitzer M (eds): Colposcopy: Principles and Practice, 2nd ed. Philadelphia, Saunders, 2008, pp 505–520.

World Health Organization: Comprehensive Cervical Cancer Control: A Guide to Essential Practice. Geneva, World Health Organization, 2006.

Wright TC Jr, Massad LS, Dunton CJ, et al: 2006 consensus guidelines for the management of women with cervical intraepithelial neoplasia or adenocarcinoma in situ. Am J Obstet Gynecol 197:340–345, 2007.

CHAPTER 139

CULDOCENTESIS (COLPOCENTESIS)

Steven H. Eisinger

Culdocentesis is a procedure for female patients designed to detect and sample free fluid in the peritoneal cavity. The classic application of this test is for the diagnosis of *hemoperitoneum* due to ruptured ectopic pregnancy, but it can also be used to detect acute *pelvic inflammatory disease* and to sample *ascites*. Modern imaging modalities, such as ultrasonography, have greatly reduced the need to perform culdocentesis, but occasionally in an emergency or where imaging resources are unavailable, culdocentesis can be extremely useful—even life-saving.

ANATOMY

The cul de sac is the lowest point in the abdominal cavity of a woman (when upright). The tissue septum between the posterior fornix of the vagina and the posterior cul de sac consists of vaginal mucosa, peritoneum, and little else. It is about 1 cm in thickness and contains no major blood vessels or organs. Thus, a needle introduced from the vagina into the cul de sac can easily access free fluid in the peritoneal cavity (Fig. 139-1).

INDICATIONS

Ectopic Pregnancy

Ruptured ectopic pregnancy is the classic indication. Signs and symptoms of ruptured ectopic pregnancy include amenorrhea, abdominal pain with rebound tenderness, vaginal bleeding, shoulder pain, and a positive pregnancy test. Hemodynamic instability and acute anemia may be present. On speculum examination the posterior fornix of the vagina may bulge into the vagina from the weight of the blood behind it. This 3-minute test can offer definitive proof of hemoperitoneum requiring immediate surgery.

Acute Salpingitis

Acute salpingitis can also be diagnosed by culdocentesis. This is the only means, short of abdominal surgery, to obtain pus from within the abdominal cavity for diagnosis and culture.

Other

Ascitic fluid may be sampled for analysis such as for cytology for ovarian cancer, or even for therapeutic withdrawal.

CONTRAINDICATIONS

Absolute

A mass (e.g., a neoplasm, an abscess, an endometrioma, or an unruptured ectopic pregnancy, whose rupture could be harmful) in the cul de sac is an absolute contraindication.

Relative

Severe, fixed retroversion of the uterus is a relative contraindication since culdocentesis may be unsuccessful because the cul de sac is obliterated and the needle will strike the corpus of the uterus.

EQUIPMENT AND SUPPLIES

The equipment for culdocentesis is simple and should be available in any emergency department or medical office with gynecologic capabilities (Fig. 139-2). The following are required:

- Speculum
- Single-tooth tenaculum
- 10- or 20-mL syringe (a three-finger control syringe will allow aspiration with one hand)
- 20-gauge spinal needle or a 3-inch needle extender with a 20-gauge needle attached
- Sterile swabs or sponges
- Ring forceps
- Antiseptic solution
- Local anesthetic (optional)

The instruments should be sterile and gloves should be used to perform the procedure. Face mask and drapes are unnecessary.

PRECAUTIONS

Universal blood precautions should be observed.

PREPROCEDURE PATIENT EDUCATION

Verbal discussion is recommended. A procedure consent form should be completed. The listed risks should include bleeding, bowel perforation, rupture of a cyst, infection, and failure to detect blood (or fluid).

PROCEDURE

1. *Perform a standard pelvic examination* before the procedure. During the speculum examination, vaginal cultures may be obtained or other tests performed. A bulging of the cul de sac into the posterior fornix of the vagina is a finding suggestive of the presence of intraperitoneal fluid. It is important to detect fixed masses in the cul de sac, or fixed retroversion of the uterus, both of which contraindicate culdocentesis.
2. *Position the patient.* After first obtaining orthostatic vital signs allow the patient to stand or sit up for a minute before the procedure to permit blood to collect in the cul de sac. The procedure may be performed on any regular examination table with stirrups. The head and shoulders should be slightly raised.
3. *Place the speculum.* A medium Graves speculum is suitable for most patients. Open it widely with the blades deeply placed in

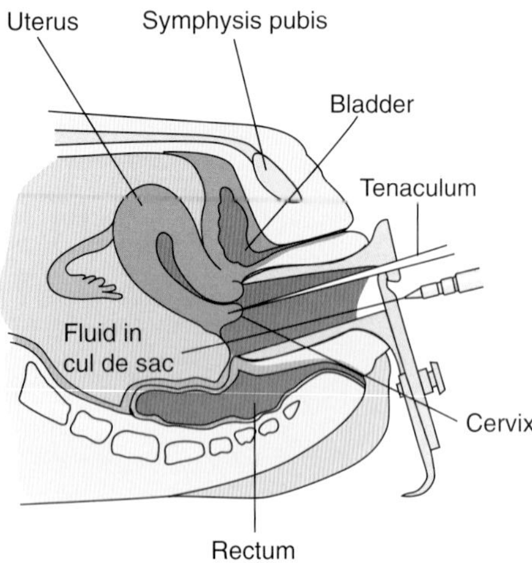

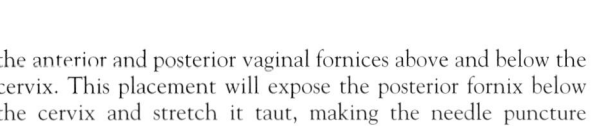

Figure 139-1 Midline sagittal view of pelvis during culdocentesis showing anatomic relationships and position of instruments. (Redrawn from Eisinger SH: Procedures in family practice: Culdocentesis. J Fam Pract 13:95–101, 1981.)

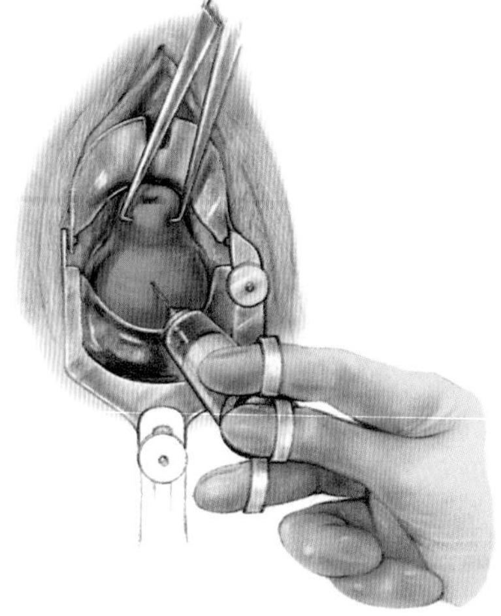

Figure 139-3 Operator's view of culdocentesis. (From Eisinger SH: Procedures in family practice: Culdocentesis. J Fam Pract 13:95–101, 1981.)

the anterior and posterior vaginal fornices above and below the cervix. This placement will expose the posterior fornix below the cervix and stretch it taut, making the needle puncture easier.

4. *Cleanse the vagina* with a suitable antiseptic solution.
5. *Grasp the cervix with a tenaculum* (Fig. 139-3). The tenaculum may be placed vertically or horizontally on the anterior or posterior lip, as the clinician desires. One milliliter of local anesthetic injected into the tenaculum site before placement is optional.
6. *Choose the puncture site*. Manipulate the cervix gently with the tenaculum by pulling either in and out or up and down. This maneuver will identify the line of reflection where the mucosa sweeps off the cervix and crosses or covers the cul de sac. The needle puncture site should be about 1 cm below this reflection, in the midline.
7. *Administer anesthesia*. This step is optional. Culdocentesis is usually perceived as quite painful. Some clinicians recommend injecting a small amount of local anesthetic into the mucosa at the puncture site. Alternatively, intravenous medication such as midazolam or hydromorphone may be given. The patient should be reassured that although the pain may be sharp, it will last only for a few seconds.
8. *Make the puncture*. Elevate the cervix in the vagina with the tenaculum to expose and stretch the mucosa of the posterior fornix. A small amount of air (1 to 2 mL) may be placed into the syringe before the puncture. The needle should be held approximately horizontal. Make the puncture itself with a bold, smooth movement, inserting the needle 3 to 4 cm through the mucosa, in the midline.
9. *Inject the air in the syringe*. Usually the air passes freely, and sometimes it can be heard bubbling through fluid. If the air does not pass freely, the needle tip is in a solid organ such as the uterus, and should be repositioned. Some practitioners may choose not to inject air.
10. *Aspirate by pulling back on the syringe plunger*. If blood or fluid fills the syringe, stop when it is full. If no fluid is obtained, then a second or even third attempt may be made at a slightly different angle or location.
11. *Terminate the procedure when fluid is obtained*, or when three attempts fail to yield any fluid.
12. *Examine the fluid from the cul de sac*. Observe free-flowing blood for several minutes for clotting because this may indicate a traumatic tap. Blood-tinged or frankly bloody fluid should be spun for a hematocrit. Clear or turbid fluid should be examined microscopically, and cultures, both aerobic and anaerobic, should be obtained. Fluid can also be sent for cytology if indicated.
13. *A brief handwritten note* or dictated paragraph in an operative note will suffice for documentation.

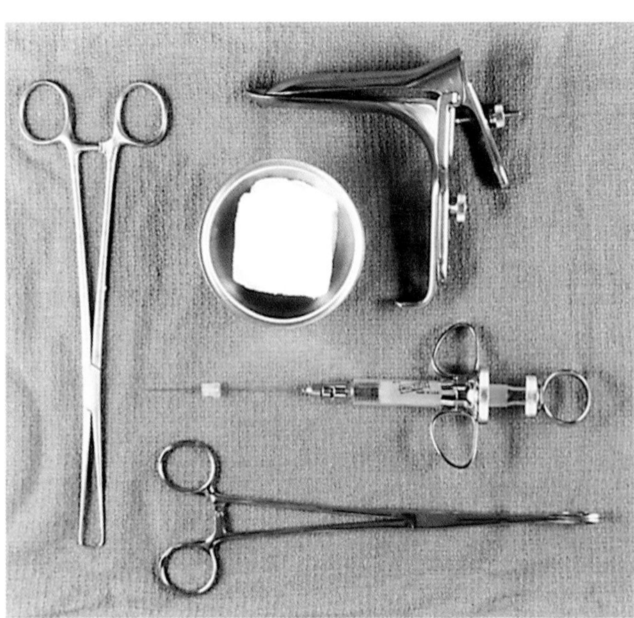

Figure 139-2 Equipment required to perform culdocentesis.

SAMPLE OPERATIVE REPORT

Indication: Suspected ruptured ectopic pregnancy.

Procedure: Informed consent was obtained. Speculum placed allowing good visualization of the cervix and vagina. Area cleansed with iodine swabs. 2 mL of 1% lidocaine injected at aspiration site. Culdocentesis performed with 20-gauge spinal needle with insertion in the posterior fornix. First stick obtained 10 mL of free-flowing, nonclotting, bloody fluid with hematocrit of 20%. Patient tolerated procedure well with no signs of hemodynamic instability.

Common Errors

The most common error is incorrect angle or depth of needle puncture. This results in a failure to obtain fluid. This is corrected by repositioning the needle.

Complications

Complications of culdocentesis are rare. *Bowel may be punctured* on occasion. This usually resolves without sequelae. *Puncturing a neoplasm or abscess* is an unlikely possibility. *Intra-abdominal bleeding* is unlikely as long as the needle is kept in the midline, away from the great vessels of the pelvis. The *most serious complication is a confusing result* that prevents necessary treatment or leads to unnecessary intervention.

Postprocedure Management

Vaginal bleeding is usually minimal and stops quickly. Patients should be provided with appropriate postprocedure instructions related to the diagnosis made as a result of the procedure (e.g., pelvic infection, ectopic pregnancy).

Interpretation of Results

Blood obtained from the cul de sac should be tested for clotting and hematocrit. Pooled blood taken from within the peritoneal cavity is usually defibrinated and will not clot. However, in exceptional cases bleeding from a ruptured ectopic pregnancy is so brisk that the blood has not had time to become defibrinated and will therefore clot in the syringe. Peritoneal fluid may appear bloody even with a very low hematocrit. As a rough rule, a hematocrit below 15% suggests slight bleeding or a bloody tap, whereas a hematocrit over 15% indicates hemoperitoneum and confirms a surgical emergency.

Pus or turbid fluid should be Gram stained and cultured. White blood cells and bacteria may be noted. Appendicitis and pelvic inflammatory disease can cause a turbid exudate.

Clear fluid may result from a ruptured cyst, ascites, or normal peritoneal fluid.

Somewhat less than half the time no fluid can be obtained despite multiple taps. This phenomenon should be referred to as a *dry tap*, not a negative tap. No diagnostic assumptions should be made on the basis of a dry tap.

CPT/Billing Code

57020 Colpocentesis (culdocentesis)

ICD-9-CM Diagnostic Codes

098.17 Salpingitis (acute)
625.9 Unspecified symptom associated with female genital organs (pelvic pain)
633.90 Ectopic pregnancy, ruptured

BIBLIOGRAPHY

Eisinger SH: Procedures in family practice: Culdocentesis. J Fam Pract 13:95–101, 1981.

Hager WD, Eschenbach DA, Spence MR, Sweet RL: Criteria for diagnosis and grading of salpingitis. Obstet Gynecol 61:113–114, 1983.

Mishell DR Jr: Ectopic pregnancy: Etiology, pathology, diagnosis, management, fertility prognosis. In Stenchever MA, Droegemueller W, Herbst AL, Mishell DR Jr (eds): Comprehensive Gynecology, 4th ed. St. Louis, Mosby, 2001, p 457.

Romero R, Copel JA, Kadar N, et al: Value of culdocentesis in the diagnosis of ectopic pregnancy. Obstet Gynecol 65:519–522, 1985.

Vermesh M, Graczykowski JW, Sauer MV: Reevaluation of the role of culdocentesis in the management of ectopic pregnancy. Am J Obstet Gynecol 162:411–413, 1990.

CHAPTER 140

HYSTEROSCOPY

Stephen A. Grochmal • Lydia A. Watson • Dale A. Patterson

Hysteroscopy is one of the oldest endoscopic procedures described in the medical literature and was first performed in 1807 by Bozzini. Unfortunately, few gynecologists and even fewer primary care physicians actually perform office hysteroscopy today. The hysteroscope is an extremely valuable tool for viewing the endocervical canal and uterine cavity, and hysteroscopy is now recognized as the method of choice for diagnosing, sampling, and treating intrauterine disease. Hysteroscopy provides an immediate direct visualization of the topography and contents of the uterine cavity, resulting in a more accurate diagnosis than that obtained from a dilatation and curettage (D&C) or blind endometrial biopsy. More important, a hysteroscopic inspection increases the accuracy of diagnosis when there is an abnormally shaped endometrial cavity or other pathologic condition present. Visually directed biopsies (via hysteroscopy) are preferable to D&C, especially for focal rather than global disease. Direct visualization provided by the hysteroscope confirms that the suspicious pathology has been sampled appropriately. Hysteroscopy can be performed in the office or in an operating room and typically is *most easily accomplished when performed during the proliferative phase of the menstrual cycle*, when the endometrium is the thinnest.

ANATOMY

The uterus is a muscular organ that is partially covered by peritoneum. The cavity of the uterus is lined by the endometrium. The uterus resembles a flattened pear in shape and consists of two major but unequal parts: an upper triangular shaped portion referred to as the *body* or *corpus* and a lower fusiform or cylindrical portion, the *cervix*. The demarcation line of these two portions is known as the *isthmus*. The anterior surface of the uterus is practically flat while the posterior surface is distinctly convex. The fallopian tubes emerge from the *cornua* of the uterus at the junction of the superior and lateral margins. The visible openings of the fallopian tubes are referred to as *ostia*. The upper or "top" portion of the uterus between the points of insertion of the fallopian tubes is called the *uterine fundus*. The cervical canal openings are called the *external os* and the *internal os*. The external os protrudes into the vaginal vault. The internal os is an important anatomic landmark during hysteroscopy because it marks the boundary between the uterine cavity and the endocervical canal, the location at which the main blood supply, the *uterine arteries and veins*, enters the uterus. Manipulation of the scope during hysteroscopy should cease when this landmark is reached. Vigorous operative procedures, including an unsuspected perforation during cervical dilation, in this area may result in excessive bleeding.

The wall of the body of the uterus is composed of three layers: (1) the outermost layer, the *serosa*, (2) the middle and thickest layer, the *myometrium*, and (3) the innermost portion, which lines the entire uterine cavity, the *endometrium*. The endometrium is a thin, pale pink, velvet-like membrane normally measuring in thickness from 0.5 mm to 5 mm, depending on cyclic changes that occur throughout the reproductive life of a woman. The endometrium is perforated by a large number of tiny openings, referred to as *uterine gland ostia*, which are easily visualized during a hysteroscopy.

Hysteroscopic findings should be described schematically, mentioning both negative and positive findings at the different levels of anatomy of the uterine cavity: cornua and tubal ostia, fundus, isthmus, internal cervical os, and the endocervical canal. A description of the appearance of the endometrium and endocervical mucosa should also be included.

INDICATIONS

- Unexplained abnormal uterine bleeding (pre- or postmenopausal)
  - Endometrial polyps
  - Submucous leiomyoma
  - Hyperplasia/malignancies
  - Endometritis
  - Adenomyosis
- Evaluation of selected infertility cases
  - Abnormal hysterosalpinogram (HSG)
  - Foreign body (e.g., lost intrauterine device [IUD])
  - Uterine adhesions (Asherman's syndrome)
  - Occluded tubal ostia
- Repeated pregnancy loss
  - Recurrent miscarriage
  - Abnormal uterine cavity (i.e., septum or other uterine anomaly)
  - Retained products of conception
- Preprocedural evaluation of uterine cavity (i.e., endometrial ablation [any method])
- Visually directed insertion of tubal occlusion contraceptive device
- Essure microinsert hysteroscopic sterilization procedure (see Chapter 148, Insertion of Essure [Hysteroscopically Assisted Female Sterilization])
- Adiana permanent contraceptive system (see Chapter 148, Insertion of Essure [Hysteroscopically Assisted Female Sterilization])
- Localization of lost intrauterine device

CONTRAINDICATIONS

Absolute

- Cardiac or pulmonary instability
- Acute pelvic infection

Relative

- Pregnancy
- Coagulopathies: idiopathic thrombocytopenic purpura (ITP), von Willebrand's disease
- Previous uterine perforation or recent surgery or synechiae
- Known cervical or uterine carcinoma
- Morbidly obese patients
- Acute uterine bleeding

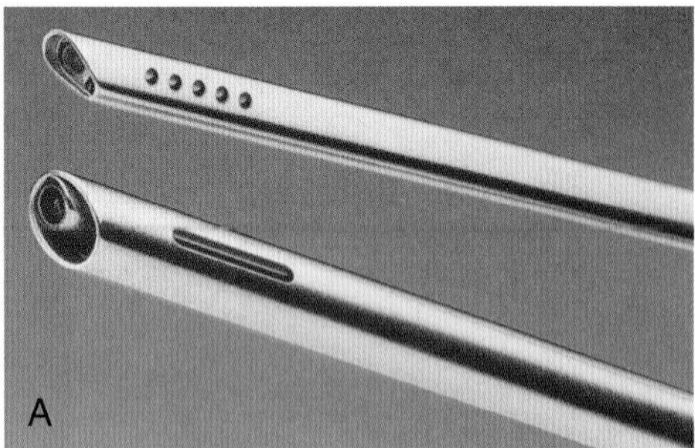

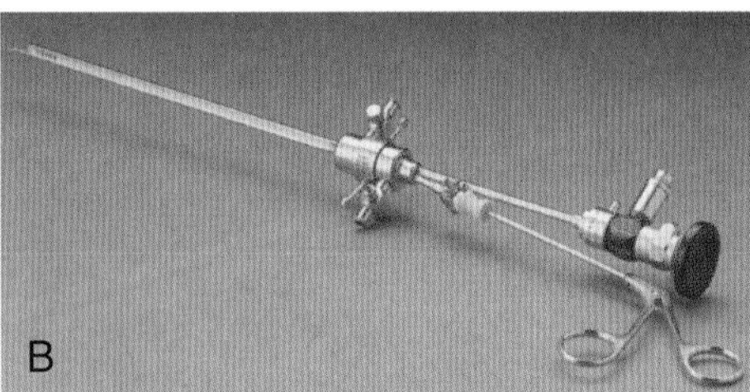

Figure 140-1 **A,** Diagnostic hysteroscopes with continuous-flow outer sheaths. The fenestrations on the distal tip of the sheath improve circulation of the liquid distention media. When using CO_2 distention, a single-flow sheath may be preferable. **B,** Example of a diagnostic rigid hysteroscope and continuous-flow operating sheath with an operating channel used to pass a biopsy forceps or other instrumentation.

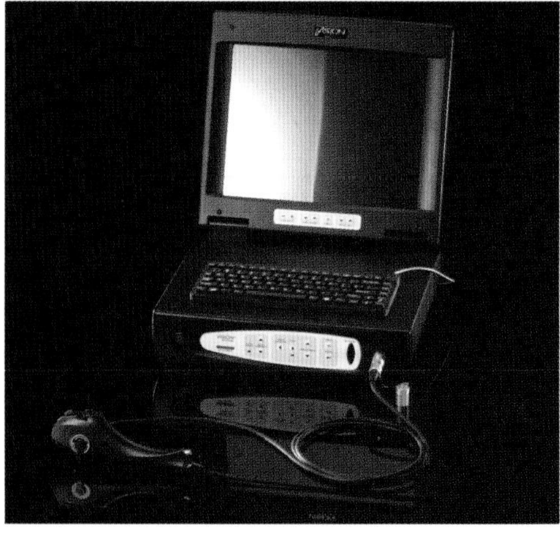

Figure 140-3 Technologic advances in electronics and hysteroscope designs have produced "all-in-one" systems that contain a camera controller, light source, documentation digital photo/video recorder, and, in this example, a flexible hysteroscope. These systems are portable and have a small "footprint," allowing them to fit easily on a countertop. (Courtesy of VisionSciences, Inc.)

Equipment

In order to perform hysteroscopy safely the mind set of the physician should be the same, whether the procedure is performed in the office or in an operating room. The choice of equipment is important, especially if the physician plans to perform "operative procedures" after gaining proficiency with simple diagnostic hysteroscopies.

The *basic* hysteroscope is a simple rigid (solid rod lens) device (Fig. 140-1). The diameter of the scope preferably is no greater than 5 to 5.5 mm when the introducing sheath is over the scope (used to protect the scope from breaking and provides a channel for continuous flow for fluid distention or an instrument). Size is important because the smaller the diameter of the scope, the less cervical dilation is required, and the more comfortable the procedure is for the patient. The angle of view for the scope is commonly 0 degrees, which provides a panoramic view once inside the uterine cavity and is an ideal all-around hysteroscope. Some surgeons prefer a 30-degree view with a more limiting, downward-looking vista.

Currently the most common device used is the *flexible* hysteroscope (Fig. 140-2). The flexible distal tip can improve maneuverability once inside the uterine cavity because of the ability to deflect the distal tip from 90 degrees to over 120 degrees. These flexible scopes are small in diameter (3.5 to 5 mm), do not require an outer sheath, and possess an operating channel, and the latest generations have moved from fiberoptic bundle technology to digital chip-on-the-tip camera sensors (Fig. 140-3).

All newer flexible hysteroscopes are designed to accommodate instrumentation for office procedures such as the Essure sterilization. These flexible scopes are more costly than a rigid system. The high initial cost may be offset by the increased reimbursement achieved with the variety of procedures that can be performed with the flexible scope.

A *light source* ranging from 100 to 300 watts is needed. A halogen light is acceptable, but a xenon light source is preferred because it emulates natural daylight and provides superior illumination of the uterine cavity.

In addition, a *simple grasping forceps*, *biopsy forceps*, and *scissors* will round out the special instrumentation necessary to perform simple operative procedures such as endometrial biopsy, polyp removal, and removal of retained IUDs.

An optional piece of equipment is a *video endoscope* (Fig. 140-4). A camera eliminates the need to look through the eyepiece of the hysteroscope and improves the working position, comfort, and visualization. It also allows the patient to partake in the procedure by watching simultaneously as the hysteroscopic evaluation is performed. Some vendors now produce systems with all these components in one stand-alone unit (Fig. 140-5).

Additional video equipment provides the ability to record and document the procedure so that photographic documentation of findings can be included in the patient's operative report. It also allows a physician to send detailed information back to a referring

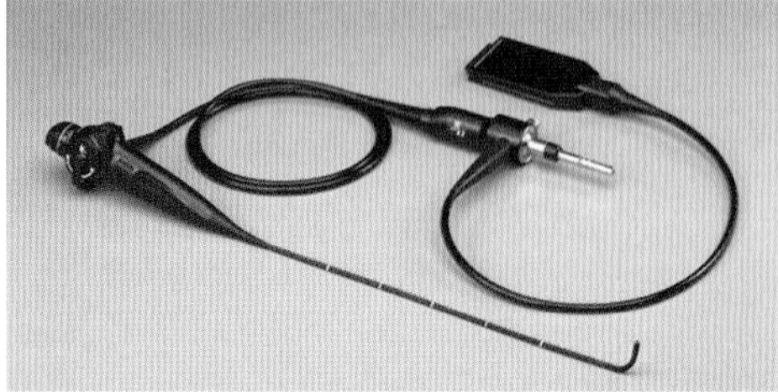

Figure 140-2 Flexible small-diameter hysteroscopes are easy to manipulate and are comfortable for patients but may lack a large-diameter operating channel for the passage of biopsy instruments, tubal sterilization inserts, or other procedure instrumentation. (Courtesy of Olympus Surgical America.)

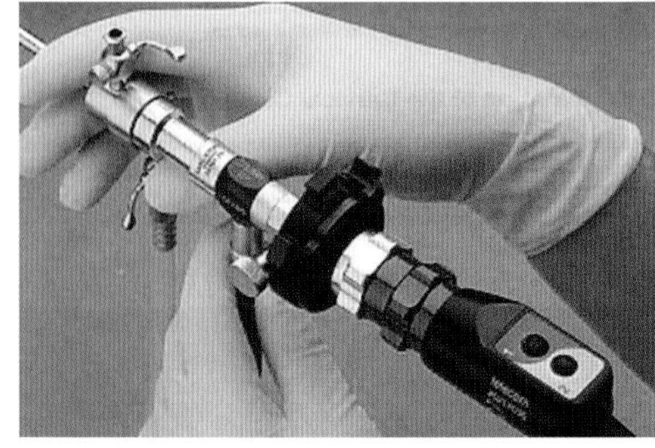

Figure 140-4 Video cameras can directly attach to the eyepiece of the hysteroscope, dramatically improving visualization of the uterine cavity.

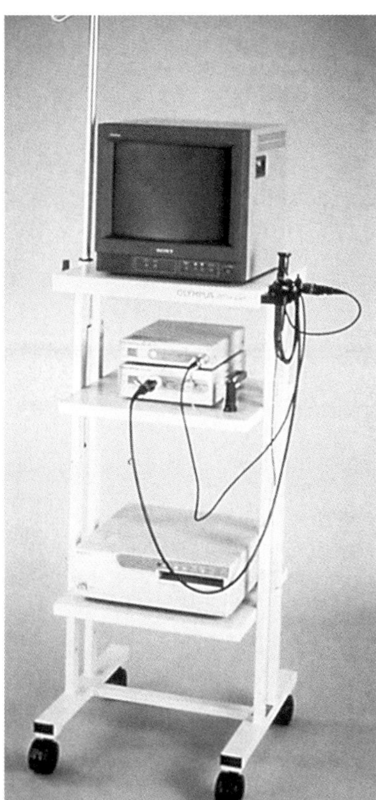

Figure 140-5 New electronic equipment designs for office hysteroscopy have resulted in systems that allow the hysteroscope (in this case a flexible design) to connect directly to one unit, which contains the camera controller, light source, documentation recorder, and LCD monitor.

colleague. These pictures should be maintained as an integral part of the patient's chart.

Choose a *distention medium*. Uterine distention is crucial to the success of any hysteroscopic procedure. Most office hysteroscopic procedures are performed with saline. CO_2 distention is mainly used for diagnostic hysteroscopy. Hyskon is difficult and "messy." CO_2 is more difficult for the novice because of the tendency for troublesome gas bubbles to form, and it cannot be used if any bleeding occurs. Sorbitol and glycerine are for electrical (bipolar) operative procedures. *Saline, then, is the "consensus gold standard" for office hysteroscopy*. It is safe, physiologic, and inexpensive. A *gravity flow system* can be used for the majority of diagnostic procedures, providing more than adequate uterine distention (Fig. 140-6). A method for monitoring the amount of fluid used to distend the uterus is needed. It is uncommon to have fluid and electrolyte complications if less than 1 L of fluid is used during the procedure. Commercial systems are available to control the flow and accurately record the fluid deficit during hysteroscopy. For short diagnostic procedures, the amount of fluid used to distend the uterus to 500 mL or less is sufficient. For slightly larger volumes, monitoring the amount of fluid used to distend the uterus and collecting the residual fluid in a pouched drape for subsequent measurement is an option. *Carbon dioxide* is also commonly used with few complications and low risks of complications (Fig. 140-7). Instructions on the use of both normal saline and carbon dioxide are noted later.

A standard tray for hysteroscopy includes instruments for anesthesia and cervical dilation (Fig. 140-8A and B):

- Antiseptic solution (e.g., povidine–iodine)
- Large cotton-tipped swabs
- Vaginal speculum (unhinged one side, open-sided Graves, or disposable illuminated types) (Fig. 140-8C)
- Cervical tenaculum
- Ring forceps
- Uterine sound
- Cervical dilators (see Chapter 136, Cervical Stenosis and Cervical Dilation)
- Topical 2% benzocaine
- Lidocaine without epinephrine 1% to 2% (optional but helpful); anesthesia can be accomplished with topical and local anesthetic
- 10-mL syringe with 4-inch needle extender and 25- to 27-gauge needle, or a dental syringe, if anesthetic is to be given into the cervix (see Chapter 149, Loop Electrosurgical Excision Procedure for Treating Cervical Intraepithelial Neoplasia, and Chapter 173, Paracervical Block)
- Endocervical curette

PRECAUTIONS

Poor visualization increases the risk of complications. Larger uteri may take a bit longer to achieve adequate distention. Plan on

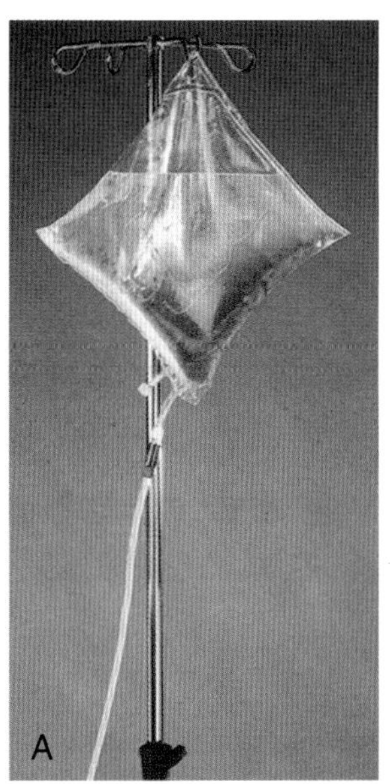

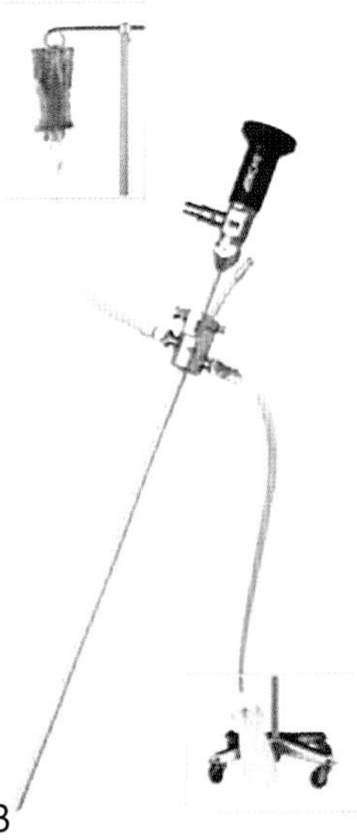

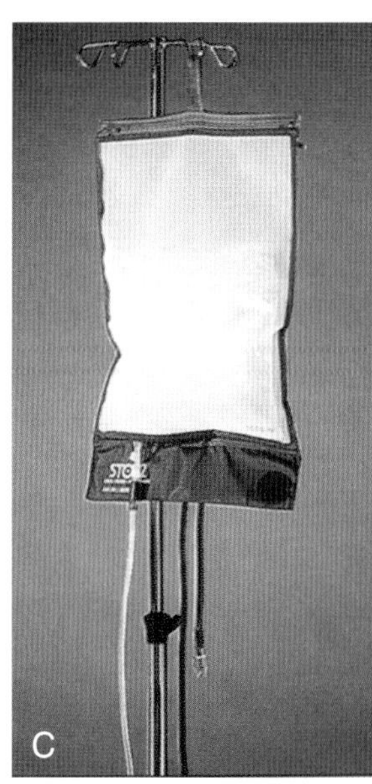

Figure 140-6 Systems used to achieve distention of the uterine cavity during diagnostic hysteroscopy. **A,** A 1000-mL bag of saline with large-bore tubing used for gravity flow distention. **B,** A closed system designed to capture the outflow distention fluid. **C,** A simple pressure cuff used to increase flow of distention medium; it offers no control of intrauterine pressure. (**B,** Courtesy of Gynex.)

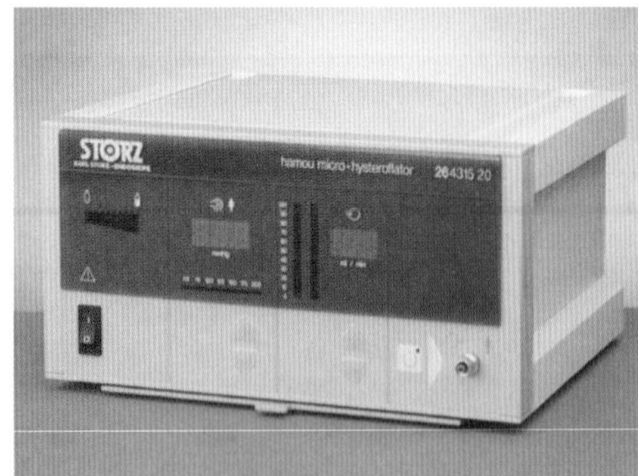

Figure 140-7 Use of CO_2 as a distention medium for diagnostic hysteroscopy mandates an appropriate device for instillation of the CO_2 gas. Intrauterine pressure must be precisely maintained to avoid passage of distention media into the fallopian tubes and subsequently into the abdominal cavity. (Courtesy of Karl Storz.)

spending the amount of time needed with each patient to ensure adequate distention and visualization.

- Be aware that not all insufflators, light sources, and scopes are interchangeable. Mixing and matching may be dangerous. Check compatibility issues with your suppliers.
- A pregnancy test is advised in all reproductive-age patients prior to the procedure.
- Cervical cultures should be obtained for patients at high risk for pelvic infections before hysteroscopy is performed.
- Avoid hysteroscopy during menses or heavy bleeding if possible—it is more difficult to see uterine contents and landmarks.
- As with any in-office invasive procedure, proper emergency resuscitation equipment and action plan should be readily available (see discussion of the Banyan kit in Chapter 220, Anaphylaxis).

Preprocedure Preparation

- The patient is best served if provided a *patient education* handout or pamphlet prior to the procedure.
- A *consent* form for diagnostic hysteroscopy with or without endometrial biopsies should be obtained.
- Document the last menstrual period, contraceptive method, and pregnancy test (if indicated) results on every patient.
- Preprocedure antibiotics are not required.
- *Nonsteroidal anti-inflammatory drugs* (NSAIDs) (e.g., ibuprofen 800 mg) administered 30 minutes before the procedure can significantly diminish the discomfort of the procedure.

Procedure

There are multiple variations of how to perform a hysteroscopy. The steps listed here are one such method.

1. Throughout the procedure, attempt to maintain a sterile environment, especially with equipment and instrumentation that are inserted into the uterus. The vaginal component of the procedure is considered a "clean" field, but it is a good habit to maintain sterile technique throughout the entire procedure.
2. With the patient in dorsal lithotomy position and preferably on an electric-powered examination table, *perform a bimanual pelvic examination* to ascertain the size, shape, and position of the uterus. Failure to do this may result in a uterine perforation during cervical dilation or initial insertion of the hysteroscope.
3. Insert a disposable illuminated vaginal speculum or a reusable open-sided Graves speculum.
4. Prep the cervix and vagina with antiseptic solution.
5. Insert a large cotton applicator under the cervix and *spray a small amount of topical 2% benzocaine* oral anesthetic on the cervix. The cotton applicator will absorb the anesthetic. Allow the applicator to remain in contact with the cervix as you talk to the patient and prepare your instruments. Remove the applicator.
6. *Anesthetize the cervix.* Using a dental-style cartridge syringe with ampules of 2% lidocaine (or other anesthetic) and a 25- to 27-gauge dental needle, place a minimum of 1 mL (maximum amount per quadrant is up to 2 mL) of anesthetic at the 3, 6, 9, and 12 o'clock positions of the cervix into the subserosal layer. (For detailed instructions, see chapters noted earlier.)
7. Grasp the anterior (or posterior, depending on uterine position) *lip of the cervix* with a tenaculum.
8. Perform an *endocervical curettage* (ECC) if indicated.
9. *Sound the uterus* to determine depth and direction of the central uterine axis.
10. *Dilate the cervical canal.* Using a set of silastic or metal graduated dilators, insert the os finder or a 3 mm dilator into the cervix, and, feeling for resistance, pass this through to the internal os, if possible. Continue progressive dilation up to a size 1 mm over the diameter of the hysteroscope. Dilation should be done slowly with a constant gentle pressure, especially in the nulligravid patient. Multiparous patients are generally easier to dilate. You may leave this dilator in the cervix to maintain patency as you reach for the hysteroscope. For stenotic patients, see Chapter 136, Cervical Stenosis and Cervical Dilation.
11. Remove the dilator.
12. The *saline is suspended 60 cm above the uterus* and will enter the cavity with a pressure of 45 mm Hg (see Fig. 140-6). The maximum uterine pressure via any distention method should

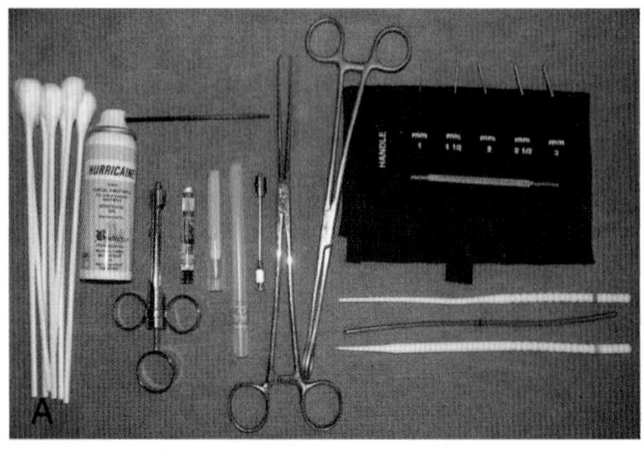

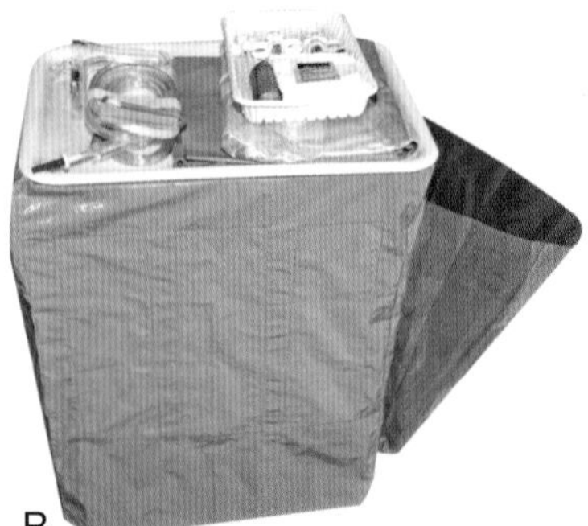

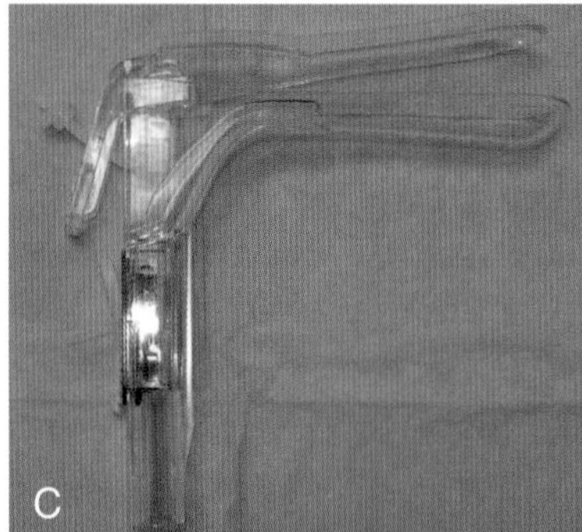

Figure 140-8 **A,** Typical instrument setup for office diagnostic hysteroscopy. **B,** Disposable office packs make procedure setup and clean-up simple. These packs contain all the necessary items required to perform an office hysteroscopy. **C,** Example of a disposable, self-illuminating LED, open-sided speculum. (**B** and **C,** Courtesy of OBP Medical, Inc.)

not exceed 70 mm Hg, which is below the capillary pressure of 100 mm Hg. Varying the height of the saline bag will alter this infusion pressure. If a pressure sleeve is placed around the bag of saline, additional pressure required to increase flow rate of the distention medium can be achieved by inflating the sleeve as needed. This is a useful technique in patients with a larger uterus or when a faster flow of distention medium is required to "clear" the field of view (see Fig. 140-6C).

If *carbon dioxide* is used, begin insufflation once the scope engages the external os. Use the instillation port on the scope at an initial rate of 30 mL/min. As the hysteroscope traverses the endocervical canal, the carbon dioxide will create a visual space ahead of the scope. Advance the scope only if the view is clear. The internal os is seen as a narrow constriction at the upper portion of the endocervical canal. Increase the carbon dioxide insufflation rate to 40 to 60 mL/min when the isthmus of the uterus is entered. The carbon dioxide insufflation must be critically controlled during the procedure. If the gas is instilled too quickly, obstructive bubbles of carbon dioxide will form. The maximum flow rate should not exceed 100 mL/min and a maximum pressure of 100 mm Hg. The risk of gas embolism is proportional to the flow rate of the infused gas. Embolization of small amounts of CO_2 is not dangerous, and over 50% of CO_2 hysteroscopies have some amount of carbon dioxide embolized.

If *saline* is used, the hysteroscope is inserted under direct visualization, advancing the scope slightly into the endocervical canal. Start the distention fluid (e.g., normal saline) flowing and continue to gently advance the scope until you feel a slight resistance. You are now at the uterine fundus. Pause to confirm that the distention fluid is flowing into the cavity. Using a continuous flow hysteroscope and a bag of saline hanging from an intravenous (IV) pole approximately 60 cm above the patient, the distention fluid flow rate will range between 125 and 200 mL/min with an average intrauterine pressure of approximately 45 mm Hg; this rate creates no problems. This flow rate may vary based on parameters such as the diameter of the tubing used, exact height of the IV pole, if suction aspiration is used on the outflow side of the hysteroscope, and if a pressure cuff is employed around the saline bag.

13. Withdraw the scope ever so slightly from the fundus and wait. As the distention fluid clears, the fundus will come into view. If you have successfully reached this point, the hysteroscopy is 75% complete and all that remains is the visual inspection of the cavity. Remember, failure to achieve adequate distention and repeated attempts to do so increase the risk of procedure failure and complications. If the uterus cannot be easily distended, consider stopping the procedure. It is important to recognize when to stop!
14. *Inspect the uterine cavity*. Withdraw the scope slightly and look at the fundus. Move the hysteroscope to the patient's right, then left. You can move the scope in or out, up or down, and rotate it to achieve the best views (Figs. 140-9 and 140-10). The central point of müllerian duct fusion projects down from the fundus. The cornua are located on both sides of this fused tissue. Evaluate the tubal ostia. Continue to withdraw the hysteroscope down into the lower segment of the uterine cavity. Visualize the anterior, posterior, and lateral walls of the cavity, maneuvering the scope ever so slightly when needed. Document any findings with photo or video recording as the procedure is performed. Continue to withdraw the scope until a "ring" appears over the scope. This is the level of the internal os of the cervix and the start of the endocervical canal. It is an important landmark to document and confirm the completion of the uterine cavity inspection (Figs. 140-11 and 140-12).

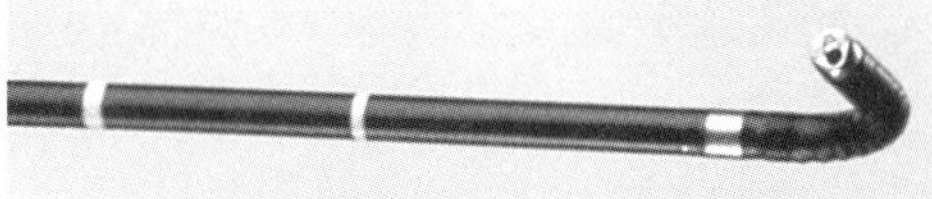

Figure 140-9 Mobile tip at the end of the hysteroscope. (Courtesy of Olympus Corp., Melville, NY.)

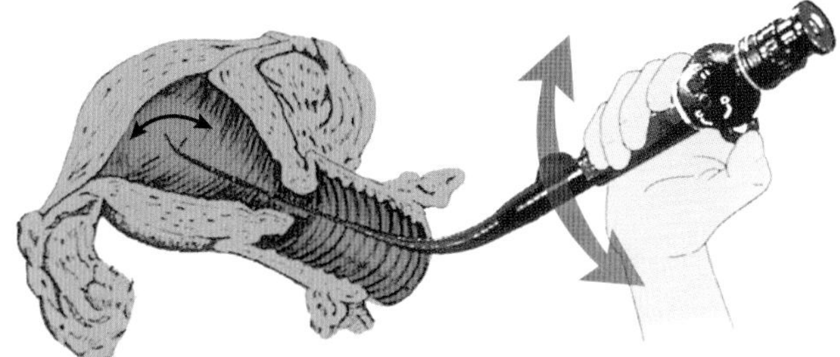

Figure 140-10 Hysteroscopic examination of the uterine cavity.

15. *Biopsy any suspicious areas*. Remove stalked endometrial polyps with grasping forceps. Generally, any bleeding will stop on its own and no cautery or chemicals are needed. All biopsies are taken after a complete inspection of the uterine cavity and prior to terminating hysteroscopy. Bleeding from the biopsies, even minimal, may decrease visualization regardless of the distention medium selected. With CO_2, this will decrease the view and may not allow re-entry into the cavity and require terminating any further observation. With saline, the clouding will dissipate as fluid continues to flow through the uterine cavity. The field generally clears, allowing the procedure to continue if necessary, but this may not always be the case.
16. *Continue to withdraw the scope* through the endocervical canal, observing and documenting when necessary. You have now completed what is referred to as a retrograde diagnostic hysteroscopy. Shut off the distention flow and remove the scope from the vagina. Remove the tenaculum and observe for any bleeding. Remove all other instrumentation and the procedure is complete.
17. Clean the scope.
18. Dictate an operative report.

Sample Operative Report

Preoperative diagnosis:	Abnormal uterine bleeding
Procedure performed:	Diagnostic hysteroscopy with endometrial biopsies; endocervical curettage
Postoperative diagnosis:	Endometrial polyps, hypertrophic endometrium
Surgeon:	Dr. ________________
Assistant:	________________ (Dr.'s name, assistant's name, or none)
Estimated blood loss:	Nil
Complications:	None
Findings:	________________
Total distention fluid instilled:	Approx. 350 mL of normal saline
Total fluid recovered:	Approx. 300 mL

With the patient on the procedure table in dorsal lithotomy position and in Allen stirrups, the patient was prepped and draped for hysteroscopy. Bimanual examination revealed a normal size, anteverted uterus and no significantly palpable adnexal masses.

An illuminated speculum was inserted into the vagina and the cervix was cleansed with a Betadine solution. Topical bupivicaine (Hurricaine solution) was applied to the cervix and the run-off collected by a sponge stick. After waiting a few minutes for the topical

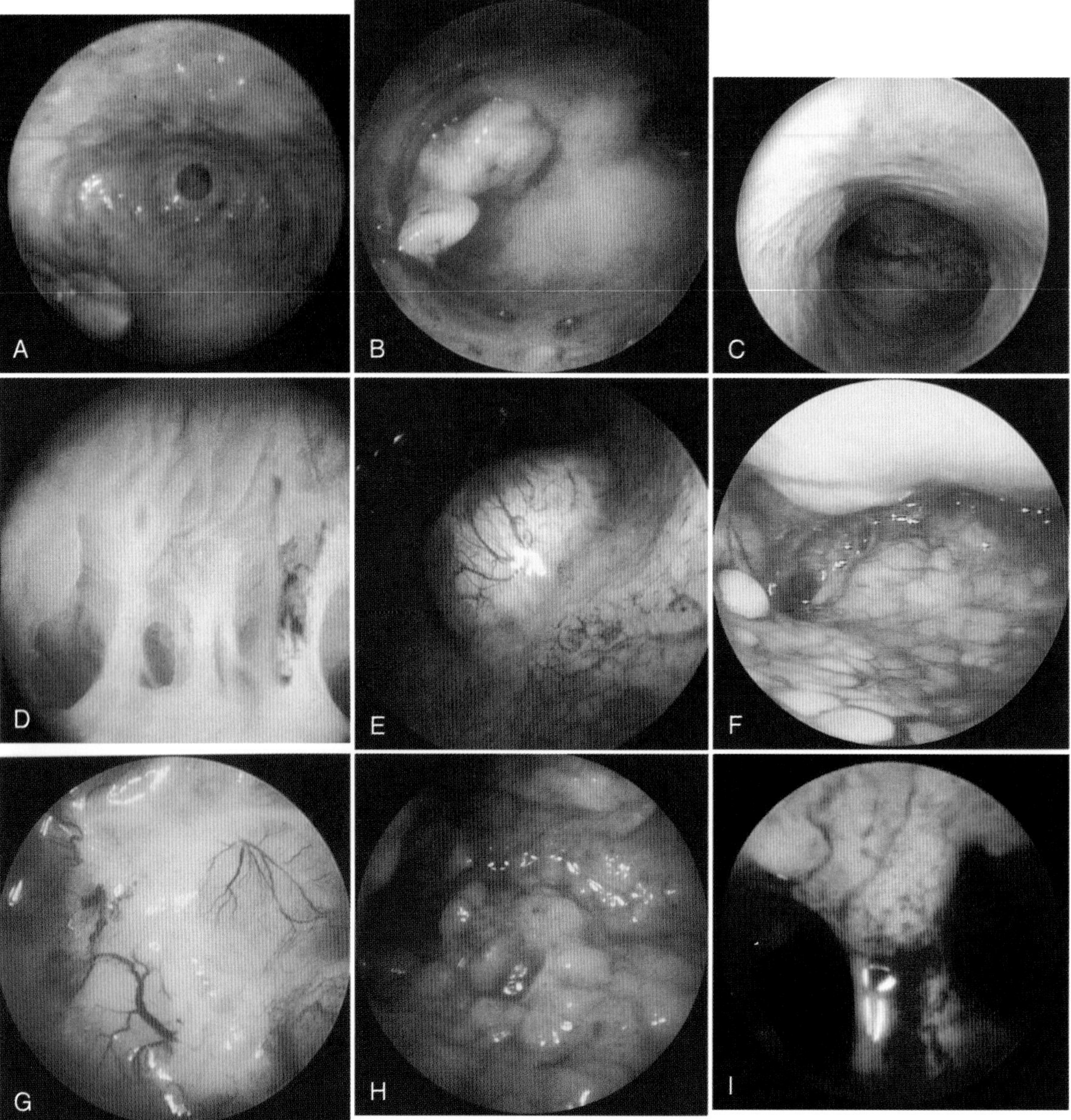

Figure 140-11 Typical uterine anatomy and pathology seen during diagnostic hysteroscopy: Tubal ostium (normal) (**A**); benign polyp in right cornua of uterine cavity (**B**); atrophic endometrium (**C**); uterine adhesions (synechiae) (**D**); submucosal fibroid (**E**); benign endometrial hyperplasia (cystic) (**F**); endometrial hyperplasia (high risk) (**G**); endometrial cancer (**H**); uterine septum (side-by-side double-barrel shotgun appearance) (**I**).

anesthetic to take effect, an intrastromal cervical block was performed. Approximately 1.8 mL of 2% lidocaine without epinephrine per quadrant was instilled at 12, 3, 6, and 9 o'clock positions on the cervix with a 27-gauge needle and Tubex syringe. The anterior lip of the cervix was grasped with a single-tooth tenaculum and an endocervical curettage was performed, followed by uterine sounding. Progressive dilation of the cervix with graduated dilators was carried out up to 6 mm. The uterus sounded to 10 cm. Thereafter, a 30-degree hysteroscope with diagnostic/operating sheath was inserted into the uterus under direct visualization and gently brought to bear against the fundus of the uterus. Using a gravity flow saline distention, the uterine cavity was distended until a clear image was achieved. (*Optional to mention*: video footage or digital photos were taken.) The hysteroscope was withdrawn farther away from the fundus until both tubal ostia could be visualized; both appeared normal. As the hysteroscope was withdrawn farther down into the uterine cavity, the entire fundus and upper portion of the cavity were visualized. Inspection of the cavity did not reveal the presence of any adhesions, submucous fibroids, or abnormal configuration. Of note were areas with visible large vessels coursing superficially beneath the thickened, hypertrophic endometrium. Multiple biopsies were taken with the biopsy forceps via the operating channel and individually marked according to their location. As the hysteroscope was withdrawn further, the level of the internal os was clearly identified. Three small endometrial polyps, the largest measuring approximately 0.5 cm, were seen. (Mention that a photograph or video was taken.) The hysteroscope continued to be withdrawn in a retrograde fashion under direct visualization through the endocervical canal, which was unremarkable. The hysteroscope was then removed from the vagina and the saline distention discontinued. Any residual fluid was evacuated from the vagina and the cervical tenaculum removed. No bleeding was noted from the cervix. Remainder of the instrumentation was removed from the vagina. The procedure was complete. Patient tolerated the procedure well and after a 15-minute recovery left the office feeling well and in good condition.

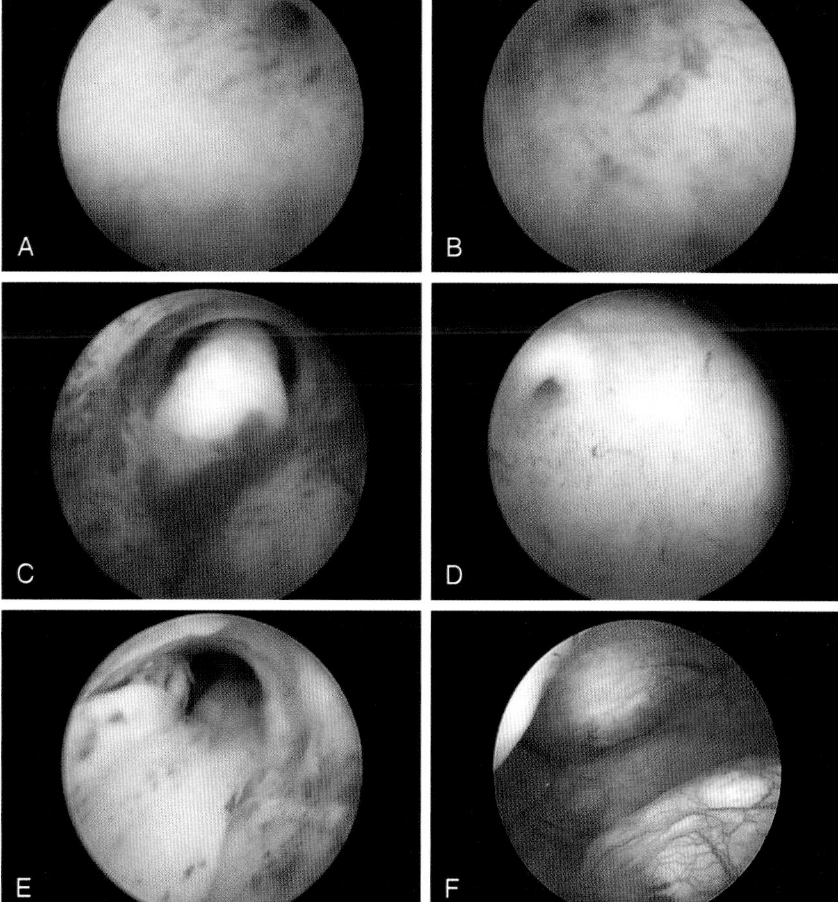

Figure 140-12 **A** and **B,** Fallopian tube. **C,** Endometrial polyp arising from fundus (seen on entrance into uterus). **D,** Fallopian tube. **E,** Attachment site of endometrial polyp at fallopian tube. **F,** Uterine fibroids.

Common Errors

- Attempting procedure with inadequate distention of the uterus.
- Performing the procedure under poor visualization. If the distention fluid is murky or bloody, stop until the field clears. Then proceed slowly. If the field is still cloudy, check your distention connection tubing and bag of fluid. If this problem continues, stop the procedure and reschedule the patient. You do not want to perforate!
- If you suspect a perforation, just stop. Remove all instruments. Place the patient in a semi-upright position and observe her for changes in vital signs, pallor, complaint of pain, or vaginal bleeding. Be prepared to consider a diagnostic laparoscopy. Most perforations are uneventful and the puncture closes readily, but always err on the side of caution. Repeat hysteroscopy can be performed in 6 weeks.
- Performing a biopsy prior to completing inspection of the entire uterine cavity may cause bleeding, thus clouding the visual field and resulting in the inability to complete the uterine cavity evaluation.

Complications

- Cervical laceration secondary to forceful dilatation.
- Uterine perforation.
- Infection.
- Fluid overload (usually not a concern with diagnostic hysteroscopies since most require only 250 to 350 mL of distention medium).
- Complications related to carbon dioxide insufflation (if used) are rare with the use of a constant-flow insufflator. Acidosis and hypercarbia are rare events. Patients can experience shoulder pain secondary to irritation of the diaphragm from the CO_2 in 2% to 5% of the cases. If the patient complains of shoulder pain, keep her lying flat and ask her to breathe deeply. The pain may last up to 20 minutes before dissipating.
- Inability to perform the procedure secondary to cervical stenosis
- Vasovagal reactions occur in less than 1% of patients, but physicians should be prepared to manage these reactions and symptomatic bradycardia.

Postprocedure Management

- Keep the patient in a semi-upright position for about 15 minutes.
- Observe for any watery discharge or excessive bleeding.
- Suggest NSAIDs as needed for any postprocedure discomfort.
- Patient resumes normal activity within 4 to 6 hours.

Postprocedure Patient Education

- Patients may notice mild cramping after the procedure. Reassure them that it is transitory and to use NSAIDs for relief.
- Some watery or blood-tinged discharge is normal for up to 2 to 3 hours. Instruct the patient to use a sanitary pad and to report any prolonged episodes of vaginal discharge, bright red bleeding, fever, or excessive abdominal pain.
- Instruct patients to avoid inserting anything in the vagina for 24 hours. They may resume intercourse after 24 hours.
- Patients generally will return to their daily lifestyle activities within 8 hours after the procedure with no restrictions on physical activity.
- Patients should call if there is any foul odor or discharge, which could signal an infection.

Interpretation of Findings

- *Abnormal uterine bleeding* (AUB) is probably the most common symptom investigated by hysteroscopy. Endometrial biopsy or D&C can be carried out at the end of the hysteroscopic examination. The main causes of AUB are submucous myomas, endometrial polyps, endometrial atrophy, and postpregnancy metrorrhagia.
- *Submucous myomas* can vary in appearance. At times they have a regular, smooth surface covered by a homogeneous endometrium similar to that of the remainder of the uterine cavity. If there is extensive intracavitary progression, then the ensuing compressed endometrium may give rise to ulceration and necrosis near the apex of new growth. At times, the surface of the myoma appears lobulated, pearly white in color, and grooved with one or more large blood vessels (see Fig. 140-11E).
- *Endometrial polyps* are exophytic, usually sessile mucous lesions varying in shape, number, size, and appearance. Their surface is similar to that of the surrounding endometrium and soft in consistency upon contact with biopsy forceps or a hysteroscope. Pedunculated polyps have a variable length to their pedicle consisting of vascularized connective tissue. These lesions have cubic, short, cylindrical epithelium interspersed with hypertrophic blood vessels. Polyps can be associated with glandular endometrial hyperplasia and can remain latent for long periods (see Fig. 140-11B).
- *Endometrial atrophy* is a postmenopausal physiologic change that may cause bleeding. The hysteroscopic image is quite characteristic: since the endometrial mucosa is quite thin, it often appears transparent, revealing the underlying vascular structures. The presence of hemorrhagic petechiae is very typical. In severe endometrial atrophy the epithelium is smooth and pale, nearly white (see Fig. 140-11C).
- *Postpregnancy metrorrhagia*. In patients with postpartum or postabortal bleeding, hysteroscopy may be used to confirm evacuation or removal of all abortive debris from the uterine cavity. The overall appearance is that of an atrophic endometrium infused with hemorrhagic areas and petechiae along with dangling pedicles and fragments of benign, shredded endometrium.
- *Intrauterine adhesions*. Hysteroscopically, synechiae may be centrally or marginally located and may be classified as endometrial, myometrial, or connective fiber synechiae. Endometrial synechiae often grow from abortive tissue and create filmy adhesions, which are easy to remove. Myometrial synechiae appear "buttress"-like, usually marginally located throughout the cavity, and as distinct "organized" structures, and connective fiber adhesions often change the normal morphology and structure of the uterine cavity (see Fig. 140-11D).
- *Uterine cavity septum* appears as either arcuate (involves the fundus) or as an incomplete or complete septum. The latter two are generally discovered upon entry into the uterine cavity just past the internal os. The appearance is likened to looking at a double barrel shotgun head-on or a "pig's snout." The septum generally has the same appearance as the surrounding endometrium. The arcuate type is usually visualized as a bulge in the top of the fundus protruding downward into the uterine cavity. The surface area may appear more "atrophic" than the rest of the uterine cavity endometrium (see Fig. 140-11I).
- *Endometrial carcinoma and precursors*. Abnormal uterine bleeding is the first symptom in over 90% of cases, so early detection is relatively straightforward if proper procedures are performed. In fact, 75% of endometrial cancers are diagnosed as stage I.

  Hysteroscopic findings include the following:

- Endometrial hyperplasia is a precursor of endometrial cancer. The hysteroscopic appearance generally resembles normal glandular epithelium, and the thickness of the mucosa can be determined by pressing with the hysteroscope (see Fig. 140-11F).
- Low-risk endometrial hyperplasia (EH) often shows a specific pattern of widened glandular ostia with cystic-glandular formations about 1 mm in diameter. The same formation can be found in an endometrium of reduced thickness, where they indicate cystic atrophy. Aside from the cystic form, EH is characterized by a variety of other hysteroscopic changes such as increased endometrial thickness, nonhomogeneous endometrial regeneration, increased vascularization, presence of ciliated epithelium, cystic dilation, polypoid formations, irregularly arranged glandular orifices, and necrotic areas. If one or more of these elements are found, hyperplasia must be suspected and endometrial biopsies should be performed.
- High-risk endometrial hyperplasia (EIN) presents a varied hysteroscopic image with polypoid appearance and vascularization clearly evident. This vascularization takes on an arborescent appearance, sometimes described like a "corkscrew" in that it surrounds groups of glandular ostia. The appearance of the mucosa could be described as "cerebroid" due to the abnormal growth and vascularization, similar to the irregular surface of brain tissue (see Fig. 140-11G).
- Endometrial neoplasia. Hysteroscopy is an extremely reliable technique for the diagnosis of endometrial neoplasia. The hysteroscopic images are clear and so obvious that they are rarely confused with other lesions. In its initial stage, adenocarcinoma presents a germinative scenario, with irregular, polylobular, delicate excrescences, which may be bleeding or necrotic; vascularization is irregular or anarchic. In some instances, the involved area may be clearly demarcated from the normal endometrium. In other cases, it may be possible to see focal lesions, sometimes on the tubal cornua or sporadic implants throughout the uterine cavity (see Fig. 140-11H).

CPT Billing Codes

57505	Endocervical curettage, not with D&C
57800	Dilation; cervical canal, instrumental
58555	Hysteroscopy, diagnostic
58558	Hysteroscopy with biopsy of endometrium or polypectomy with or without D&C.
58559	With lysis of intrauterine adhesions
58560	With division or resection of intrauterine septum
58561	With removal of leiomyomas
58562	With removal of impacted foreign body
58563	With endometrial ablation, any method
58565	Hysteroscopic sterilization (Essure, Adiana)

ICD-9-CM Diagnostic Codes

182.0	Malignancy, corpus uteri except isthmus
182.1	Malignancy, isthmus of uterus
218.0	Submucous leiomyomas, uterus
218.1	Intramural leiomyoma
219.1	Uterine neoplasm, benign
233.2	Carcinoma in situ, unspecified part of uterus
621.0	Polyps, uterine
621.3	Hyperplasia of endometrium, unspecified
621.5	Adhesions, intrauterine (synechiae)
622.4	Stricture and stenosis of cervix
622.7	Mucous polyp of cervix
625.3	Dysmenorrhea
626.0	Absence of menstruation
626.2	Excessive or frequent menstruation
626.4	Irregular menstrual cycle
626.6	Metrorrhagia
627.0	Premenopausal menorrhagia
627.1	Postmenopausal bleeding

SUPPLIERS

Full contact information is available online at www.expertconsult.com.

Conventional rigid and flexible hysteroscopes, graspers, biopsy forceps and scissors, endoscopic cameras, light sources and video monitors, and recording systems:
CooperSurgical
Karl Storz Endoscopy-America, Inc.
Olympus America, Inc.
Pentax Precision Instruments Corporation
Richard Wolf Medical Instruments Company

Disposable endoscopes and hysteroscopes:
Micro-Imaging Solutions, Inc.

Disposable side-opening speculum with built-in LED light source, office "all-in-one" pack/procedure kits for office hysteroscopy (includes custom mayo drape with built-in instrument pockets and trash container, disposable side-opening speculum with built-in LED light, 1.2-mm endoscopic double sealing seal, inflow and outflow tubing with Luer-Lok adapters, under buttocks drape with graded drain bag, and a drawstring for easy postprocedure disposal):
OBP Medical, Inc.

Flexible fiber or digital hysteroscopes, special designed office hysteroscopes, EndoSheath sterile, disposable single-use sheaths (diagnostic and therapeutic designs), video processor (light source) with built in LCD screen:
Vision-Sciences, Inc.

IV saline bags, TURP tubing, Gyn applicators, topical anesthetics, gauze, disinfectant solutions, Welch Allyn Kleenspec disposable vaginal speculum, power examination tables, mayo stands, and vital signs monitors:
Moore Medical

Special open-sided speculum, large speculum, cervical dilators and os finders, dental syringe and supplies, needle extenders and topical anesthetics, drapes, tenaculum, long forceps, sponge sticks and specialized fluid collection devices:
Gynex

ONLINE RESOURCES

Patient Education Information and Brochures

Hysteroscopy Patient Education/Brochure, available online at American College of Obstetricians and Gynecologists: http://acog.org/publications/patient_education/bp084.cfm. To order pamphlets: 800-762-2264.

Hysteroscopy Patient Information, available at American Association of Gynecologic Laparoscopists: http://www.aagl.org/topics, Select Treatments then Hysteroscopy.

Krames Online, Hysteroscopy:
www.geisinger.kramesonline.com/HealthSheets/3,S,82976.

Hysteroscopy "How to" and Procedure Videos

American Association of Gynecologic Laparoscopists website: www.aagl.org.

Conceptus website for physicians: www.essuremd.com.

Karl Storz: www.karlstorz.de/cps/rde/xchg/SID-388011F6-05A9997C/karl-storz-en/hs.xsl/7239.htm.

Office Hysteroscopy Procedure Videos: contact SA Grochmal via email address: endoreprogyne@aol.com.

Richard Wolf USA: www.richardwolfusa.com/specialties/gynecology/office-hysteroscopy.html.

BIBLIOGRAPHY

AAGL Practice Report: Practice Guidelines for Management of Intrauterine Synechiae. J Minimal Invasive Gynecol 17:1–7, 2010.

American College of Obstetricians and Gynecologists: Antibiotic prophylaxis for gynecologic procedures. ACOG Practice Bull. No. 104, Washington, DC, May 2009.

American College of Obstetricians and Gynecologists: ACOG Committee opinion no. 450: Increasing use of contraceptive implants and intrauterine devices to reduce unintended pregnancy. Obstet Gynecol 114:1434–1438, 2009.

Bettocchi S, Nappi L, Ceci O, Selvaggi L: In-office hysteroscopy is feasible. Women's Health Law Weekly 5:1–3, 2004.

Bradley LD: Assessment of abnormal uterine bleeding: Three office-based tools. J Fam Pract 15:1–11, 2004.

Bradley LD: Instrumentation in office hysteroscopy: Flexible hysteroscopy. In Bradley LD, Falcone T (eds): Hysteroscopy. Philadelphia, Mosby, 2009, pp 7–18.

Bradner P, Neis KJ, Ehmer C: The etiology, frequency, and prevention of gas embolism during hysteroscopy. J Am Gynecol Endosc 6:421–428, 1999.

Brooks PG: In the management of abnormal uterine bleeding, is office hysteroscopy preferable to sonography? The case for hysteroscopy. J Minimal Invasive Gynecol 14:12–15, 2007.

Buchanan EM, Weinstein LC, Hillson C: Endometrial cancer. Am Fam Physician 80:1075–1080, 2009.

de Jong P, Doel F, Falconer A: Outpatient diagnostic hysteroscopy. Br J Obstet Gynecol 97:299–303, 1990.

Di Spiezio A, Bettocchi S, Guida AM, et al: "See and treat" hysteroscopy in daily practice. J Minimal Invasive Gynecol 15:41–43, 2008.

Garbin O, Kutnahorsky R, Gollner JL, et al: Vaginoscopic versus conventional approaches to outpatient diagnostic hysteroscopy: A two-centre randomized prospective study. Hum Reprod 21:2996–3000, 2006.

Garratt D, Grochmal SA: A survey of patient response to office surgery. J Am Assoc Gynecol Laparosc 3(4 suppl):S14, 1996.

Garry R: Uterine distention methods and fluid management in operative hysteroscopy. In Grochmal SA (ed): Minimal Access Gynecology. Oxford, Radcliffe Medical Press, 1995, pp 301–315.

Gimpleson R, Rappold HO: A comparative study between panoramic hysteroscopy with directed biopsies and dilatation and curettage. A review of 276 cases. Am J Obstet Gynecol 158(pt 1):489–492, 1988.

Grochmal SA: Office hysteroscopy: The time has come. Female Patient 32:15, 2007.

Hill D, Maher P, Wood C, et al: Complications of operative hysteroscopy. Gynaecol Endosc 1:185–189, 1992.

Hill DA: Abnormal uterine bleeding: Avoid the rush to hysterectomy. J Fam Pract 58:136–142, 2009.

Hulf JA: Blood carbon dioxide changes during hysteroscopy. Fertil Steril 32:193–196, 1979.

Issacson K: Office hysteroscopy: A valuable but under-utilized technique. Curr Opin Obstet Gynecol 2002;14:381–385.

Itzkowic DJ, Laverty CR: Office hysteroscopy and curettage—A safe diagnostic procedure. Aust NZ J Obstet Gynecol 30:150–153, 1990.

Lethaby A, Shepperd S, Cooke I, Farquhar C: Endometrial resection and ablation versus hysterectomy for heavy menstrual bleeding. Cochrane Database Syst Rev:CD000329, 2000.

Levie MD, Chudnoff SG: Prospective analysis of office-based hysteroscopic sterilization. J Minimal Invasive Gynecol 13:98–101, 2006.

Loffer FD: Complications of hysteroscopy—Their cause, prevention and correction. J Am Assoc Gynecol Laparosc 3:11–26, 1995.

Loffer FD, Bradley LD, Brill AI, et al: Hysteroscopic training guides. J Am Assoc Gynecol Laparosc 7:165, 2000.

Nagele F, O'Connor H, Baskett TF, et al: Hysteroscopy in women with abnormal uterine bleeding on hormone replacement therapy: A comparison with postmenopausal bleeding. Fertil Steril 65:1145–1150, 1996.

Nichols M, Carter JF, Fylstra DL, Childers M, for the Essure System U.S. Post-Approval Study Group: A comparative study of hysteroscopic sterilization performed in-office versus a hospital operating room. J Minimal Invasive Gynecol 13:447–450, 2006.

Oehler MK, Rees MC: Menorrhagia: An update. Acta Obstet Gynecol Scand 82:405–422, 2003.

Presthus JB: Office-based hysteroscopy: Getting started now. Contemp Obstet Gynecol 15:1–6, 2006.

Raimondo G, Raimondo D, D'Aniello G, et al: A randomized controlled study comparing carbon dioxide versus normal saline as distension media in diagnostic office hysteroscopy: Is the distension with carbon dioxide a problem? Fertil Steril Jan 14, 2010. [Epub ahead of print.]

Rogerson L, Duffy S: A national survey of office hysteroscopy. Gynecol Endosc 10:343–347, 2001.

Sagiv R, Sadan O, Boaz M, et al: A new approach to office hysteroscopy compared with traditional hysteroscopy: A randomized controlled trial. Obstet Gynecol 108:387–392, 2006.

Shah J: Endoscopy through the ages. BJU Int 89:645–652, 2002.

Tidwell C, Soll D, Snyder D: In-Office Procedures: Emerging Trends and Practical Views. OBG Mgmt Suppl:S1–S12, 2007, available online at: www.obgmanagement.com.

Uenol J, Ikeda F, Carvalho FM, et al: Routine hysteroscopy with endometrial biopsy in an infertility clinic. J Minimal Invasive Gynecol 16:118–120, 2009.

Vilos GA, Edris F, Abu-Rafea B, et al: Miscellaneous uterine malignant neoplasms detected during hysteroscopic surgery. J Minimal Invasive Gynecol 16:318–325, 2009.

Wang JH, Zhao J, Lin J: Opportunities and risk factors for premalignant and malignant transformation of endometrial polyps: Management strategies. J Minimal Invasive Gynecol 17:53–58, 2010.

Weekes A, Voss E: Complications of office hysteroscopy. In Grochmal SA (ed): Minimal Access Gynaecology. Oxford, UK, Radcliffe Medical Press, 1995, pp 370–381.

CHAPTER 141

Dilation and Curettage

Verneeta L. Williams • Sheila Thomas

Dilation and curettage (D&C) is a valuable diagnostic and therapeutic tool in the management of abnormal uterine bleeding (AUB) and pregnancy-related disorders. Endometrial biopsy techniques have replaced D&C in most diagnostic situations, and hysteroscopy (see Chapter 140, Hysteroscopy) is now often performed in place of the "blind" D&C when initial diagnostic and therapeutic interventions fail. When the operator is experienced and the proper ancillary personnel are available, the office D&C proves to be a very cost-effective and safe procedure for the patient. Otherwise, the procedure can be performed in the operating room. In many instances of abnormal bleeding, diagnosis is facilitated if the sampling is done just before an anticipated period (e.g., for anovulatory bleeding). Unless the procedure is pregnancy related, the clinician should ensure that the patient is not pregnant and should know the status of the Papanicolaou (Pap) smear before the surgery. In addition to this chapter, it would be helpful for the clinician to review Chapter 143, Endometrial Biopsy.

On reaching menopause all women should be informed about the risks and symptoms of endometrial cancer and strongly encouraged to report any unexpected bleeding or spotting to their physician.

Indications

Diagnostic

- To determine the cause of abnormal premenopausal bleeding that has not been corrected by medical management
- To determine the cause of abnormal premenopausal bleeding that occurs in women older than 40 years of age with inadequate endometrial biopsies
- To determine the cause of postmenopausal bleeding when endometrial aspiration is nondiagnostic
- To rule out cancer and adenomatous hyperplasia with atypia when complex hyperplasia (adenomatous hyperplasia) is found on endometrial biopsy
- When the endometrial lining (stripe) measures more than 5 mm on ultrasonography
- To determine the cause of significant uterine bleeding that is too excessive for an endometrial biopsy
- When a reliable pelvic examination is required but cannot be obtained to evaluate the internal organs before endometrial biopsy, and thus anesthesia would be helpful
- For a debilitated or apprehensive patient when endometrial biopsy cannot be performed
- When cervical stenosis cannot be resolved and prevents an office procedure
- When pregnancy-related causes are suspected for AUB
- When atypical glandular cells are reliably found and confirmed on Pap smear, but no cause is found in a less invasive work-up

Therapeutic

- For removal of suspected endometrial polyp
- For removal of retained products of conception associated with postpartum infection or hemorrhage
- For removal of retained products of conception after an incomplete abortion
- For therapy of excessive hemorrhaging
- For use in combination with hysteroscopy

NOTE: Performing a D&C to resolve hormonally related AUB has been found to be ineffective.

Other

Elective termination of pregnancy (see Chapter 127, Pregnancy Termination: First-Trimester Suction Aspiration) is another indication for D&C.

Contraindications

Absolute

- Existence of comorbid medical conditions that are unstable (e.g., renal failure, active cardiac compromise)
- Desired viable intrauterine pregnancy

Relative

- The presence of an active pelvic infection
- Signs of a systemic coagulopathy (i.e., diffuse intravascular coagulation or unknown anticoagulation status)
- Uncertainty concerning the viability of an intrauterine pregnancy
- Patient's preference to defer procedure in anticipation of a spontaneous resolution of a miscarriage
- Prior history of uterine procedures and the development of Asherman's syndrome (i.e., endometrial synechiae)

NOTE: A D&C should be performed in the office only with a cooperative patient who has no other significant health risk factors and only if adequate resuscitation equipment is available.

Equipment

See Figure 141-1.

- Sterile gowns (optional)
- Sterile gloves
- Sterile drapes
- Sterile sponge gauze
- Formalin bottles

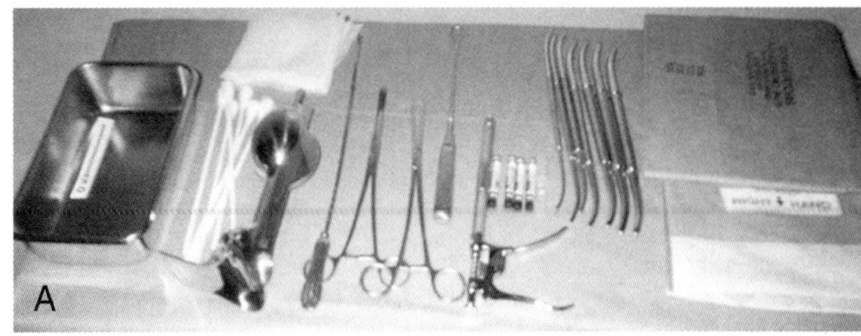

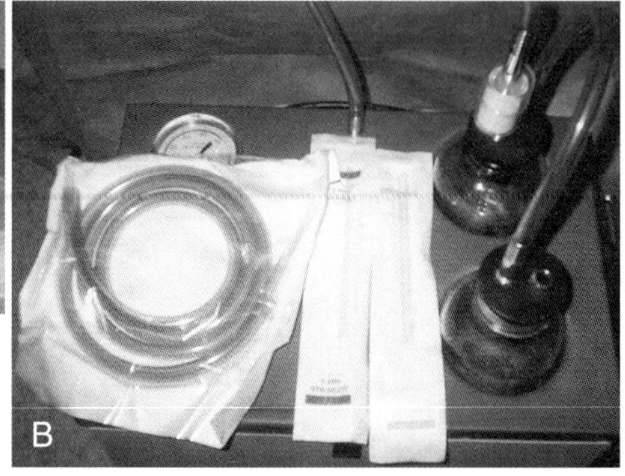

Figure 141-1 **A,** Equipment used for dilation and curettage *(left to right)*: sterile basin, 4 × 4 sterile sponge gauze, large obstetrics/gynecology applicators, weighted speculum, uterine sound, ring forceps, single-tooth tenaculum, curette, dental anesthetizing gun, 1.8 mL of 2% lidocaine with epinephrine, uterine dilators, leggings, and sterile covering. **B,** Suction device and tubing.

- Lens paper or Telfa pads for endocervical curettage and uterine curettage tissue
- Antiseptic cleansing solution
- Sterile bowl
- Suction hosing and apparatus with pump (for some situations, especially if significant bleeding or pregnancy related)
- Ring forceps
- Uterine sound
- Graves or weighted (Auvard) speculum
- Polyp (Stone) forceps
- Cervical dilators
- Kevorkian endocervical curette for endocervical curettage
- Curved and straight suction catheters (size 8 to 12 mm) when applicable
- Sharp uterine curette
- Intravenous (IV) needle, catheter, and tubing
- IV fluids (optional)
- A 20-gauge spinal needle and syringe, dental anesthetizing gun, or needle extender when local anesthesia (submucosal block) will be used
- Lidocaine 5 mL (2%) with epinephrine for submucosal block or 10 mL of lidocaine without epinephrine for paracervical block or equivalent

NOTE: Review Chapter 149, Loop Electrosurgical Excision Procedure for Treating Cervical Intraepithelial Neoplasia, for information regarding local anesthetic use (it is not needed if general anesthesia is given).

- Tenaculum
- Ultrasonography (optional)
- Pulse oximeter if IV sedation is given

Preprocedure Patient Education

Each patient should be comfortable with the decision to perform a D&C. All questions regarding the procedure, alternatives, and risks should be explained carefully so the patient can give informed consent (see the sample patient consent form online at www.expertconsult.com). If performed in the office with sedation, appropriate knowledge and equipment must be available for possible complications and resuscitation. A nurse should be available throughout the procedure to aid with preparing the patient for the procedure, injecting IV medications, and handling equipment, and to provide assistance during the postoperative and recovery periods. The patient's vital signs must be stable for the clinician to perform an office D&C. If bleeding has been prolonged or heavy, a hemoglobin or hematocrit should be obtained. The ability to obtain IV access is also important should the need arise to correct hemodynamic instability.

Anesthesia and Analgesia

In the outpatient setting, anesthetic and analgesic choice is somewhat limited. For D&C procedures performed in the hospital, the choice of sedation is much wider. No matter which drug regimen is selected, it is important that personnel and equipment for resuscitation be available should anaphylaxis, bleeding, or oversedation occur.

When making anesthetic and analgesic choices for D&C, the clinician should consider the following:

- A paracervical block is useful before placement of a tenaculum onto the cervix and before cervical dilation, unless a general anesthetic is used (see Chapter 173, Paracervical Block).
- Alternatively, a submucosal cervical local block is generally sufficient and easier to perform (see Chapter 149, Loop Electrosurgical Excision Procedure for Treating Cervical Intraepithelial Neoplasia).
- Consider a nonsteroidal anti-inflammatory drug (NSAID) 1 hour before the procedure for office procedures to reduce cramping and decrease uterine bleeding. Diazepam (Valium) 10 mg orally 1 hour before the procedure combined with a maximum-dose NSAID and local lidocaine are generally sufficient to accomplish a D&C.
- IV medication can be used for sedation if needed (see Chapter 2, Procedural Sedation and Analgesia).

Technique

1. A hematocrit and hemoglobin, Rh, blood type, and screen should be considered if the patient's problem is pregnancy related. Platelet count, prothrombin time, partial thromboplastin time, and fibrin split products may be indicated in some situations. If uncertain of pregnancy status, obtain a pregnancy test.
2. Start an IV line and administer fluids. Sedate the patient if needed.
3. Prophylactic antibiotics, including subacute bacterial endocarditis prophylaxis, are not indicated in routine D&Cs.
4. Place the patient in the dorsal lithotomy position.
5. Determine the position of the uterine fundus by performing a bimanual examination or using ultrasonographic guidance, if skilled in its use.
6. Expose the cervix using a Graves or Auvard speculum and cleanse the vagina, cervix, and posterior fornix with an antiseptic solution (e.g., povidone–iodine, cyproheptadine).
7. Put on a sterile gown and gloves.
8. Place sterile drapes around the perineum.
9. Empty the bladder (if full) with an in-and-out catheter. Alternatively, ask the patient to void just before the procedure.

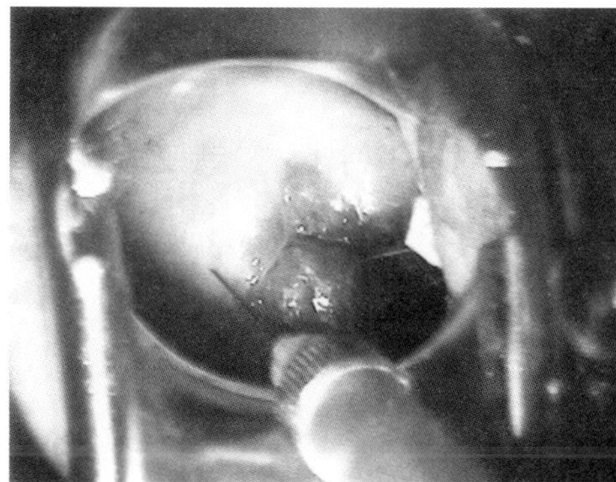

Figure 141-2 Dental anesthetizing gun used for submucosal block.

10. Perform a paracervical block (see Chapter 173, Paracervical Block) or submucosal block (Fig. 141-2). This can be omitted if the patient has general anesthesia.
11. Grasp the cervix at the 12 o'clock position and elevate it using a tenaculum (Fig. 141-3).
12. Perform an endocervical curettage unless the problem is pregnancy related or if one has been performed during a recent evaluation (see Chapter 137, Colposcopic Examination). This is called a *fractional curettage* because the endocervical canal is being evaluated separately from the uterine cavity.
13. Use short, firm, in-and-out strokes from the internal os to the external os, curetting in a full 360-degree circle, twice.
14. Place the collected tissue on a Telfa pad or common lens paper and send this specimen in a separate formalin container to the pathology laboratory.
15. Insert a uterine sound into the os to determine the axis of the cervix and uterine cavity, as well as the depth of the uterus. Greater than 10 cm is abnormal in a premenopausal woman. Most postmenopausal uteri sound less than 8 cm. (For information regarding steps to take when either external or internal os stenosis is encountered, see Chapter 136, Cervical Stenosis and Cervical Dilation).
16. Dilate the os to 8 to 12 mm using dilators.
17. If using a suction method, insert the largest suction curette that can easily pass through the os and attach the other end to the suction hosing.
18. Make sure the suction hosing has a tissue trap.
19. Place the curette in the center of the uterus, turn on the suction machine, and close the suction valve on the handle of the curette. A pressure of 60 mm Hg is needed to obtain adequate suction. Use a rotary, slightly in-and-out motion, until an increased resistance to rotation is achieved.

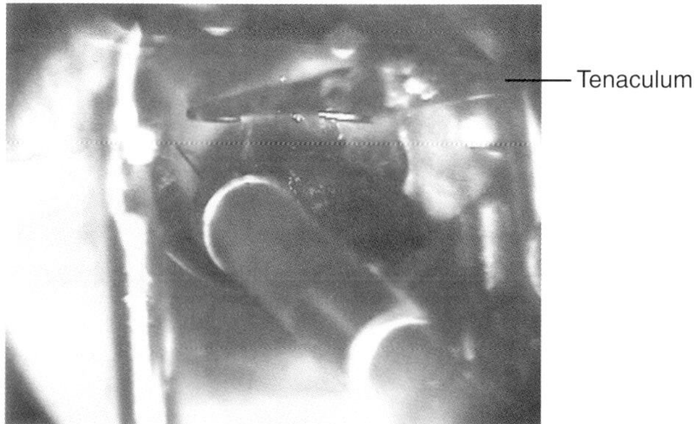

Figure 141-3 Dental anesthetizing gun used for a paracervical block at fornix. The single-tooth tenaculum has been placed on the anterior tip of the cervix.

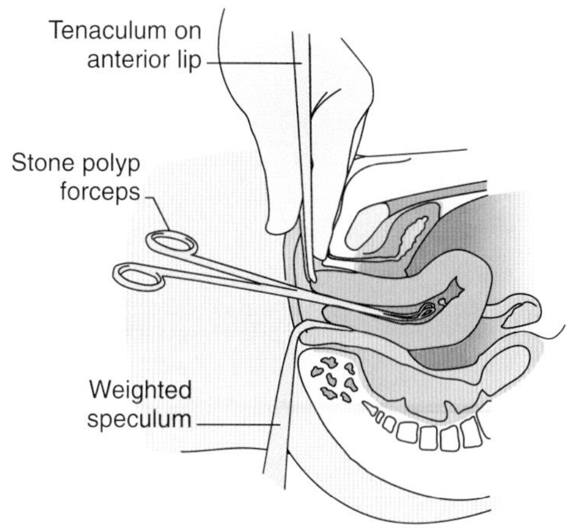

Figure 141-4 Stone polyp forceps used to remove polyp from uterine cavity. (Redrawn from Junnila RD: Dilation and curettage. In Benjamin RB [ed]: Atlas of Outpatient and Office Surgery, 2nd ed. Philadelphia, Lea & Febiger, 1994.)

20. Curette the entire endometrial lining using a to-and-fro motion. Do not pull the curette past the internal os lest suction be lost. Continue to suction until the entire cavity is sampled and there is no further return of tissue. Turn off the suction and remove the curette.
21. Place a Telfa pad or large sheet of lens paper into the posterior vaginal vault.
22. Insert a sharp uterine curette and lightly scrape all sides of the uterine cavity. Collect the materials on the Telfa pad or lens paper and send in separate laboratory container.
23. Using the Stone forceps, explore the uterine cavity for polyps by systematically opening and closing the forceps while moving across the dome and anterior and posterior walls of the uterus (Fig. 141-4). Remove any tissue grasped with the forceps with gentle pressure or twisting.
24. Reinsert the curette and suction out any remaining tissue (optional).

Optional Methods

- The entire procedure can be performed under ultrasonographic guidance (Fig. 141-5).
- Laminaria can be placed in the os the night before the procedure for dilation of the cervix (Chapter 136, Cervical Stenosis and Cervical Dilation).
- A sharp curette alone can be used instead of a suction curette to remove endometrial tissue.
- A curved suction curette is used if the uterus is anteflexed or retroflexed. A straight suction curette is used if the uterus is in midposition.

Complications

- *Hemorrhage*: This is very rare (<1%) unless the problem is pregnancy related. Most women will have some spotting for a few weeks afterward.
- *Infection*: This is extremely rare; it is treatable with a broad-spectrum antibiotic covering anaerobes.
- *Perforated uterus*: This is more likely to occur in the presence of uterine infection; with a stenotic cervical os (especially in elderly postmenopausal women); in cases in which a sharp (as opposed to vacuum) curette is used; if there is unrecognized marked anterior or posterior flexion; and in patients who are less than 8 weeks postpartum.

  With lateral perforation, injury to the uterine artery is possible. Anteroposterior perforation is usually not serious if a small curette is used.

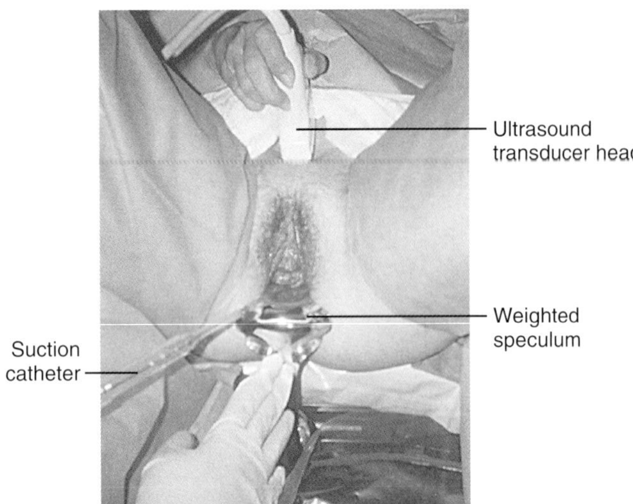

Figure 141-5 Weighted speculum and suction equipment used in dilation and curettage. Ultrasonography is used to guide the physician during the procedure.

- Perforation with a blunt object (usually the uterine sound) is generally uncomplicated.
- Perforation with a sharp object is more significant.
- In most cases, treatment for perforation is simple observation. Perforation should be suspected if the uterine sound or curette passes beyond 9 to 10 cm in the postmenopausal or beyond 12 cm in menstruating women (unless the uterus is actually this large on palpation). If perforation occurs, the procedure should be terminated. Before discharging the patient, the clinician should look for unstable vital signs and significant pelvic pain or bleeding. Some physicians provide antibiotic coverage, although this is not generally done. The patient should report any fever, pelvic pain, or discharge. The risk of perforation is reduced if the D&C is carried out under ultrasonographic guidance.

- Asherman's intrauterine adhesions may cause secondary amenorrhea, infertility, recurrent abortion, or other menstrual irregularities. Postoperative adhesions are more common when the D&C is performed on the puerperal uterus.
- Disease may be missed. In even vigorous D&Cs, studies show only 50% to 60% of the endometrial cavity is actually curetted. The patient and physician must understand that if symptoms persist, a further or repeat diagnostic test may be needed.

Postprocedure Management

Immediately after the Procedure

- After completing the D&C, observe the vital signs for any indication of deleterious effects (i.e., lowered blood pressure, elevated pulse rate, decreased oxygen saturation).
- If continued vaginal bleeding is evident after the procedure, give 10 to 20 U of IV oxytocin (Pitocin) in 1 L of lactated Ringer's solution, and methylergonovine maleate (Methergine) 0.2 mg intramuscularly. This is especially helpful in pregnancy-related procedures.
- If bleeding does not stop, the clinician should inspect for lacerations and use ultrasonography to visualize intrauterine contents to rule out an incomplete evacuation.
- If a significant decrease in blood volume has occurred, it may be necessary to replenish body fluids intravenously using normal saline or lactated Ringer's solution.
- Provide RhoGAM if the patient is Rh negative and the procedure is pregnancy related.

Before Discharge

- The patient should be alert and ambulatory and should have stable vital signs before discharge.
- Consider NSAIDs for pain.
- If the patient is at risk for vaginal infection, consider doxycycline 100 mg twice daily for 7 to 10 days.
- Ergonovine 0.2 mg every 4 hours for 1 to 2 days can be given to decrease bleeding in pregnant patients.

After discharge, consider a postoperative check in 1 to 2 weeks to discuss pathologic tissue findings and assess the patient's well-being.

Postprocedure Patient Education

- Instruct the patient to insert nothing in vagina for 2 weeks. This includes sexual activity.
- The patient is to call the office if bleeding is greater than one sanitary napkin per hour or if there is fever, purulent discharge, or unrelieved abdominal pain.

Interpretation of Results

Normal Findings

- Proliferative endometrium
- Secretory endometrium
- Atrophic endometrium
- Products of conception

Abnormal Findings

- Endometrial polyp
- Chronic endometritis
- Intrauterine synechiae
- Submucous leiomyoma
- Intramural leiomyoma
- Uterine enlargement
- Vaginal bleeding
- Premenopausal menorrhagia
- Postmenopausal bleeding
- Personal history of cancer uterus
- Endometrial hyperplasia (adenomatous, cystic, glandular)
- Simple endometrial hyperplasia without atypia
- Complex endometrial hyperplasia without atypia
- Complex endometrial hyperplasia with atypia
- Adenocarcinoma in situ
- Endometrial carcinoma (i.e., adenocarcinoma)
- Hydatidiform mole (i.e., trophoblastic disease)
- Malignant hydatidiform mole
- Variations of cervical dysplasia (from endocervical curettage)
  - Cervical intraepithelial neoplasia (CIN) I
  - CIN II
  - CIN III

Patient Education Guides

See sample patient education and consent forms online at www.expertconsult.com.

CPT/Billing Codes

00946 Paracervical block
36000 Starting an IV
36415 Venipuncture

57505	Endocervical curettage*
58120	D&C (diagnostic or therapeutic but nonobstetric)
59160	D&C (postpartum)
76856	Ultrasound, pelvic (nonobstetric)
76857	Ultrasound, pelvic, limited or for follow-up
78630	Transvaginal ultrasound

ICD-9-CM Diagnostic Codes

Adenocarcinoma in situ	233.2
Chronic endometritis	615.1
Complex endometrial hyperplasia w/o atypia	621.32
Complex endometrial hyperplasia with atypia	621.33
Endometrial carcinoma (i.e., adenocarcinoma)	182.0
Endometrial hyperplasia (adenomatous, cystic, glandular)	621.3
Endometrial polyp	621.0
Hydatidiform mole (i.e., trophoblastic disease)	630.0
Hydatidiform mole, malignant	236.1
Intramural leiomyoma	218.1
Intrauterine synechiae	621.5
Personal history of cancer of the uterus	V10.4
Postmenopausal bleeding	627.1
Premenopausal menorrhagia	627.0
Simple endometrial hyperplasia w/o atypia	621.31
Submucous leiomyoma	218.0
Uterine enlargement	621.2
Vaginal bleeding	623.8
Variations of cervical dysplasia (from endocervical curettage)	
CIN I	622.11
CIN II	622.12
CIN III	233.1

*The endocervical curettage is now "bundled" with a D&C and cannot be charged separately (unless it is not performed as part of D&C)

BIBLIOGRAPHY

American College of Obstetricians and Gynecologists: Antibiotic prophylaxis for gynecologic procedures. ACOG Practice Bulletin No. 104. Washington DC, ACOG, May 2009.

Buchanan EM, Weinstein LC, Hilson C: Endometrial cancer. Am Fam Physician 80:1075–1080, 2009.

Canavan TP, Doshi NR: Endometrial cancer. Am Fam Physician 59: 3069–3077, 1999.

Feldman S, Berkowitz RS, Tosteson AN: Cost-effectiveness of strategies to evaluate postmenopausal bleeding. Obstet Gynecol 81:968–975, 1993.

Grimes DA: Diagnostic dilation and curettage: A reappraisal. Am J Obstet Gynecol 142:1–6, 1982.

Hacker N, Moore JG, Gambone J (eds): Essentials of Obstetrics and Gynecology, 4th ed. Philadelphia, Saunders, 2004.

Johnson BE, Johnson CA, Murray JL, Apgar BS: Women's Health Care Handbook, 2nd ed. Philadelphia, Hanley & Belfus, 2000.

Junnila RD: Dilation and curettage. In Benjamin RB (ed): Atlas of Outpatient and Office Surgery, 2nd ed. Philadelphia, Lea & Febiger, 1994.

Oriel KA, Schrager S: Abnormal uterine bleeding. Am Fam Physician 60:1371–1380, 1999.

Smith RA, Cokkinides V, Eyre HJ: American Cancer Society guidelines for the early detection of cancer, 2006. CA Cancer J Clin 56:11–25, 2006.

CHAPTER 142

Human Papillomavirus DNA Typing

Gary R. Newkirk

Papanicolaou cervical screening (Pap test) has dramatically reduced the incidence of cervical cancer in developed countries. For nearly 20 years a relationship between human papillomavirus (HPV) infection and cervical cancer has been recognized. HPV is a sexually transmitted DNA virus that causes over 99% of cervical cancer. Of the 120 HPV types, at least 40 are known to infect the anogenital tract causing genital warts or dysplasia (Table 142-1). HPV types have unique biologic potential and often prefer specific sites of infection (hands, feet, and genitals). Among the types that infect a given target tissue, such as the cervix, specific types are more likely to predispose to cancer. HPV types that infect the genitalia can be categorized as high, low, and intermediate risk based on their predilection for causing severe dysplasia.

Other cancers have also been linked to the high-risk HPV viruses, including anorectal, vulvar, vaginal, oropharyngeal, bladder, and nonmelanoma skin cancers, among others. Sophisticated new tests for the detection of HPV hold great promise for improving both the sensitivity and specificity of cervical cancer screening. These new tests have also supported the development of triage mechanisms to help identify women who are at greatest risk for the development of high-grade cervical intraepithelial neoplasia (CIN) or recurrence of disease after treatment for CIN.

Testing for HPV relies on the detection of viral DNA. The only test currently approved by the U.S. Food and Drug Administration (FDA) for the detection of HPV DNA is Hybrid Capture 2 (HC2) system (Digene Corporation, Gaithersburg, MD). This commercially available test uses a liquid hybridization format to detect 13 high-risk HPV types (HR HPV) (genotypes 16, 18, 31, 33, 35, 39, 45, 51, 52, 56, 58, 59, and 68). This test does not distinguish individual HPV types but, rather, identifies "the group." Recently, a standardized polymerase chain reaction (PCR)-based technique (AMPLICOR HPV test, Roche Molecular Systems) for the detection of the 13 HR HPV genotypes has been commercialized. This test is available for clinical diagnostic laboratories, but few data are available on its performance in clinical settings. This discussion will focus on use of the HC2 HPV test. HC2 testing can be performed as both a stand-alone test or combined with Pap testing when a liquid-based Pap test is used (see Chapter 151, Pap Smear and Related Techniques for Cervical Cancer Screening). "Reflex" HPV testing refers to an automatic HPV DNA analysis on a liquid-based Pap test based on the cytologic diagnosis, such as atypical squamous cells of undetermined significance (ASCUS). In this setting, because the same sample aliquot is used, the patient need not return for a separate HPV sample collection examination.

HPV is very common among sexually active women. Nearly 75% of women are infected by age 30. Because most HPV infections are transient and do not progress to severe dysplasia or cancer, the isolated finding of HPV by current technology does not offer sufficient predictive value to replace current cytologic Pap screening. Accordingly, the FDA has not approved currently available HPV DNA tests as a sole primary method for cervical cancer screening. At present, testing for HPV should be reserved mainly for triage of patients with ASCUS (see Chapter 151, Pap Smear and Related Techniques for Cervical Cancer Screening, Box 151-2, Terminology and Definitions, and Appendix K: Management Guidelines for Abnormal Cervical Cancer Screening Tests and Histologic Findings), screening otherwise healthy women over age 30, and post-treatment or postcolposcopy follow-up. Use of HC2 HPV has clearly been shown to be a useful tool in screening women with ASCUS cytologic features, especially if performed as a "reflex" test after liquid-based Pap smears. HC2 HR HPV detects over 90% of high-grade CIN; a negative test greatly reduces unnecessary colposcopy and treatment. Evidence supports lengthening the screening interval for women over age 30 to 3 years when both Pap and HPV tests are normal. Combined cytologic and HPV DNA testing in women aged 30 years and older is highly sensitive and cost-effective, reducing overall costs by 30%. HPV testing also can be used for postcolposcopy and post-treatment follow-up. Patients with an ASCUS, atypical squamous cells (cannot exclude high-grade squamous intraepithelial lesion [ASC-H]), or LSIL (low-grade squamous intraepithelial lesion) Pap test result who are diagnosed with CIN 1 after colposcopy can be screened either by repeat cytology at 6 and 12 months or with a single HPV test at 12 months. Likewise, women who are treated for CIN 2/3 can be followed by a repeat Pap test with HPV testing at 6 months. If these tests are both negative, the patient can safely return to routine screening. An abnormal HPV or Pap test result necessitates follow-up colposcopy. Of note, HPV testing can be performed on tissue samples (in situ sampling) to help correlate histologic finding with the presence of HPV. Currently, testing for low-risk types of HPV is not recommended. HPV testing is not approved for males.

The American Society for Colposcopy and Cervical Pathology (ASCCP) 2006 Consensus Guidelines for the management of both cytologic and histologic cervical abnormalities are presented as algorithms in Appendix K: Management Guidelines for Abnormal Cervical Cancer Screening Tests and Histologic Findings.

Anatomy

Cervical testing requires sampling the same area targeted by the Pap smear, namely, the active transformation zone (see Chapter 151, Pap Smear and Related Techniques for Cervical Cancer Screening, Figs. 151-3 and 151-4, and Chapter 137, Colposcopic Examination).

Indications

- Adjunct to triage of ASCUS cytologic finding
- In combination with Pap testing for women over age 30 years

TABLE 142-1 Human Papillomavirus (HPV) Types Associated with Various Lesions

Lesion	HPV Type
Common wart	2
Planar	4
Butcher's	7
Flat	3
Plantar	1
Epidermodysplasia verruciformis	3, 5, 8, 9, 10, 12, 14, 15, 17, 19, 26, 27
Respiratory	11, 16, 30, and others
Genital	
Low-risk	6, 11, 42, 43, 44
High-risk	16, 18, 31, 33, 35, 39, 45, 51, 52, 56, 58, 59, 68

- For follow-up of women who have colposcopic/histologic findings consistent with CIN 1 without treatment
- For follow-up of women who have had treatment of the cervix for CIN 2/3
- To evaluate the presence of HPV-related abnormal histologic findings (in situ testing)

HPV testing potentially could be useful for evaluation of persistent low-grade cytologic changes in the postmenopausal patient, potential cases of child abuse, and cases of anal-canal disease.

There are no indications at present for testing noncervical lesions for HPV. Some men who have sex with men are now being screened with Pap smears of the anal canal, and HPV testing may become an adjunctive test.

Contraindications

There are no absolute contraindications. As this procedure is frequently performed at the time of Pap smear, see Chapter 151, Pap Smear and Related Techniques for Cervical Cancer Screening, for contraindications to collection of the sample.

Equipment and Supplies

The only test currently approved by the FDA for the detection of HPV DNA is the HC2 system. At the present time the HC2 collection and specimen transport medium (STM) kit is the only HPV DNA testing assay used by clinical reference laboratories. When used in combination with the Pap smear, both the cervical sampling and HPV DNA testing sample can be obtained with the same sampling device. Either a brush type or broom type sampler may be used. ThinPrep is the only liquid-based Pap smear system that is FDA approved for reflex HPV testing. The SurePath collection system is the only other liquid-based Pap system used in the United States.

- Digene HC2 cervical sampling kit with brush, transport tube, and medium is used for stand-alone HPV DNA testing when a liquid-based Pap is not performed.
- Cervical biopsies (or other genital biopsies) are taken with the usual biopsy equipment and placed in the tube with the STM.
- Tissue biopsies from lesions located anywhere on the body can also be placed in standard formalin for transport, although the STM is preferred.
- Pap smear specimens can be collected with either broom or brush devices and placed in the Cytyc PreservCyt solution (Cytyc Corporation, Boxborough, MA).

Procedure

Cervical Sample without Pap Smear Collection

1. The cervix is placed in view as for collecting a Pap specimen (see Chapter 151, Pap Smear and Related Techniques for Cervical Cancer Screening, Fig. 151-3).
2. Blot and gently remove excess cervical mucus.
3. The special cervical conical brush supplied by the Digene Specimen Collection Kit is inserted into the cervical os until the outer or widest bristles make contact with the cervix or reasonable resistance is encountered for further advancement (Fig. 142-1).
4. There is no need to advance the brush farther than 10 to 15 mm.
5. Rotate the brush three full turns in a counterclockwise direction.
6. Insert the brush into the bottom of the transport tube, snap off the shaft at the scored line, and cap securely.

Cervical Sample at the Time of Liquid-Based Pap Testing

1. The cervix is sampled with the broom or brush (see Chapter 151, Pap Smear and Related Techniques for Cervical Cancer Screening, Fig. 151-4) and rinsed thoroughly in Cytyc PreservCyt solution for use in transporting material for the ThinPrep Pap process.
2. The ThinPrep Pap preparation renders a slide for cytologic evaluation. The remaining supernatant must be at least 4 mL and is processed with the Digene HC2 protocol.
3. If the Digene sampling kit is used for HPV sampling at the time of a Pap smear (i.e., either in addition to the liquid-based Pap or with conventional Pap testing), the HPV DNA sample should be taken *after* the Pap sample is taken.
4. If HPV DNA sampling is performed at the time of colposcopy, the HPV sample should be collected *before* the use of any applied solutions such as saline, acetic acid, or Monsel's solutions and prior to cervical biopsies.

Biopsy Testing for Human Papillomavirus

1. Biopsies may be taken from the cervix, vagina, rectum, vulva, or any other anatomic location and placed in the Digene Specimen Transport Medium. Because there is no other preservative, this sample must be frozen immediately.

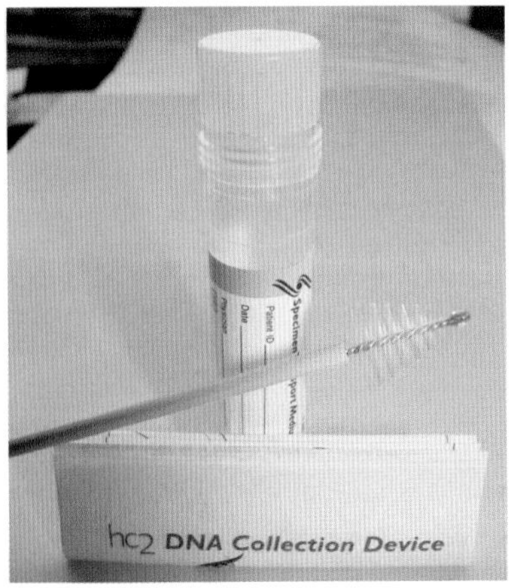

Figure 142-1 The Digene Hybrid Capture 2 (HC2) human papillomavirus (HPV) DNA kit (Qiagen, Inc., Valencia, CA) tests for the 13 most common HPV types known to be associated with high-grade cervical dysplasia and cervical cancer. The kit includes a transport vial with fluid medium and a special conical sampling brush, which is rotated three times in the cervical os and then placed in the transport tube, snapped off, and sealed.

2. Biopsy specimens can be tested for in situ hybridization in formalin-preserved and paraffin-prepared histologic blocks.
3. Clinicians should check with their reference laboratory regarding the sampling, preparation, and handling of biopsy samples. Opinion differs on the ideal manner to handle this tissue for the somewhat rare in situ hybridization protocols.

Complications

None have been reported. Minor spotting as per routine Pap testing is normal.

Postprocedure Management

The ASCCP guidelines suggest management based on the results of the HPV testing. These guidelines will be appropriate for most patients but are not a substitute for clinical judgment in the management of cervical dysplasia.

NOTE: Operative report, complications, and postprocedure management are identical to Pap smear protocol (see Chapter 151, Pap Smear and Related Techniques for Cervical Cancer Screening).

Interpretation of Results

The HC2 HPV test will be reported as "positive" or "negative." A positive test indicates the presence of one or more of the 13 high-risk HPV viral types in the test. The overwhelmingly most common type causing a positive result is type 16. A negative test indicates either absence of these types or an amount of viral DNA deemed clinically irrelevant. Appendix K, Management Guidelines for Abnormal Cervical Cancer Screening Tests and Histologic Findings, presents the ASCCP 2006 Consensus guideline algorithms, which offer suggested evidence-based management interventions based upon a positive HPV test.

CPT/Billing Code

87621 HPV amplified probe technology interpretation

There is no specific code for collection of the specimen.

Supplier

Full contact information is available online at www.expertconsult.com.

Digene HC2 HPV DNA Kit
Qiagen, Inc.

Online Resource

Digene hosts a patient education site at www.thehpvtest.com/.

Bibliography

ACOG Practice Bulletin on Clinical Management Guidelines for Obstetricians-Gynecologists: Cervical cytology screening. In ACOG Women's Health Care Physician's Compendium of Selected Publications, Practice Bulletin No. 45, Aug. 2003. Washington, DC, ACOG Distribution Center, 2006, pp 398–408.

ACOG Practice Bulletin on Clinical Management Guidelines for Obstetricians-Gynecologists: Management of abnormal cervical cytology and histology. In ACOG Women's Health Care Physician's Compendium of Selected Publications, Practice Bulletin No. 66, Sept. 2005. Washington, DC, ACOG Distribution Center, 2006, pp 603–622.

Apgar BS, Brotzman GL, Spitzer M: Colposcopy: Principles and Practice, 2nd ed. Philadelphia, Saunders, 2008.

ASCUS-LSIL Triage Study Group (ALTS): Results of a randomized trial on the management of cytology interpretations of atypical squamous cells of undetermined significance. Am J Obstet Gynecol 188:1383–1392, 2003.

Wright TC, Massad LS, Dunton CH, et al: 2006 consensus guidelines for the management of women with abnormal cervical cancer screening tests. Am J Obstet Gynecol 197:340–345, 2007.

Wright TC, Massad LS, Dunton CH, et al: 2006 consensus guidelines for the management of women with cervical intraepithelial neoplasia or adenocarcinoma in situ. Am J Obstet Gynecol 197:346–355, 2007.

CHAPTER 143

Endometrial Biopsy

Beth A. Choby

Endometrial biopsy (EMB) is a safe and cost-effective diagnostic method of evaluating the endometrium. EMB is an office-based procedure most commonly used in perimenopausal and postmenopausal women to investigate abnormal uterine bleeding (AUB) and to rule out endometrial cancer. Endometrial cancer is the most common invasive gynecologic malignancy, and endometrial hyperplasia is sometimes a precursor. EMB may be considered in any woman with risk factors for endometrial hyperplasia or cancer (Box 143-1).

Although EMB is sensitive enough to diagnose hyperplasia or cancer, it is less useful for detecting abnormalities such as endometrial polyps or the changes of endometrial atrophy. The false-negative rate for EMB is 5% to 15%. Although EMB was the preferred initial procedure for evaluating AUB and had mostly replaced dilation and curettage (D&C), it is now more often used in conjunction with other procedures. Hysteroscopy, transvaginal ultrasonography for endometrial thickness, and sonohysteroscopy are often combined with or done in lieu of EMB (see Chapter 140, Hysteroscopy). Because EMB is cost effective, efficient, and readily available in the outpatient setting, it continues to be an important diagnostic tool.

Anatomy

The EMB involves transcervical sampling of the endometrial lining. An endocervical curettage of the cervical canal is performed as part of the EMB.

Indications

- Evaluation of premenopausal and postmenopausal AUB
- Work-up of infertility, especially short luteal phase or anovulation
- Assessment of the effects of hormone therapy
- Investigation of atypical glandular cells or endometrial cells on Papanicolaou (Pap) smear in women older than 40 years of age
- Failure to respond to medical treatment of AUB
- Evaluation of abnormal endometrial thickness on transvaginal ultrasonography
- Surveillance in women previously diagnosed with endometrial hyperplasia
- AUB in women with risk factors for endometrial cancer (see Box 143-1)
- Women with an intact uterus receiving unopposed estrogen therapy
- Evaluation for endometrial carcinoma or precancerous changes
- Identification of causes of dysfunctional uterine bleeding
- Evaluation of uterine enlargement in conjunction with ultrasonography
- Screening in hereditary nonpolyposis colon cancer syndrome (HNPCC). The lifetime risk of endometrial cancer in women with HNPCC ranges between 32% and 60%. Annual or biennial endometrial biopsy or transvaginal ultrasonography is recommended in women with HNPCC beginning at 30 to 35 years of age. Recommendations are based on expert opinion because the effectiveness of gynecologic surveillance is not definitive. Diagnosis of HNPCC requires histologically confirmed colorectal cancer in three relatives, at least one of whom must be a first-degree relative. Two successive generations must be affected and one case has to be diagnosed before 50 years of age. Screening is appropriate in known carriers of this autosomal dominant gene or in cases where there is strong suspicion of HNPCC.

Contraindications

Absolute

- Pregnancy
- Bleeding diathesis/coagulopathy

Relative

- Use of anticoagulant therapy
- Active vaginal, cervical, uterine, or pelvic infection
- Cervical stenosis
- Morbid obesity
- Significant pelvic relaxation with uterine prolapse

Equipment

A variety of instruments are available for EMB. The more popular methods are described for comparison. Equipment common to all methods is listed here; additional items required with specific aspirators are listed in the aspirator descriptions.

- Large Graves vaginal speculum
- Povidone–iodine solution in nonallergic patients
- Cotton balls
- Ring forceps
- Uterine sound
- Single-tooth tenaculum
- Endocervical curette without basket (e.g., Kevorkian curette)
- Buffered formalin specimen containers with patient identification labels (two)*
- Endometrial sampler (special equipment requirements by method)
  - Disposable flexible plastic endometrial aspirator (e.g., Pipelle, Pipet Curet, Endocell)
  - Scissors
  - Reusable stainless steel curette (Novak or Randall)
  - 20-mL syringe
  - Disposable endometrial aspirators with syringe suction (Cannula Curette, Uterine Explora, Explora II)

*The Tao Brush uses CytoRich Red solution instead of buffered formalin for specimen preservation.

Box 143-1. Risk Factors for Endometrial Hyperplasia and Cancer

Age >50 years
Atypical endometrial hyperplasia
Chronic anovulation
Diabetes
Infertility
Menopause after 55 years of age
Nulliparity Chronic anovulation
Obesity*
Tamoxifen
Unopposed estrogen therapy

*21 to 50 pounds overweight carries relative risk three times less than >50 pounds overweight.

- A Tis-U-Trap endometrial curette or a Vabra aspirator (disposable)
- External suction pump
- Brush sampler (Tao Brush)

Cervical dilators should be kept available (see Chapter 136, Cervical Stenosis and Cervical Dilation).

Precautions

- The previous Pap smear should be reviewed before the procedure. If no recent smear report is available and it is indicated, obtain one before proceeding with the endometrial biopsy (EMB).
- A bimanual examination identifies extreme uterine anteversion or retroflexion. There is an increased risk of uterine perforation when sounding the uterus or collecting the EMB if significant angulation is present between the cervical neck and uterus.
- The use of small cervical dilators is often necessary in women found to have cervical stenosis, so they should be available. Methods for managing cervical stenosis are described in Chapter 136, Cervical Stenosis and Cervical Dilation.

Preprocedure Patient Education and Forms

- Obtain a thorough history and review pertinent clinical records (see encounter form online at www.expertconsult.com). Explain to the patient the indications for the procedure, the process itself, side effects, and potential complications so that she may provide informed consent. See the sample patient education handout and the sample patient consent for "Endometrial Biopsy" available online at www.expertconsult.com.
- Nonsteroidal anti-inflammatory drugs (NSAIDs) effectively decrease uterine cramping during EMB. Patients can be instructed to take 600 to 800 mg of ibuprofen orally 30 to 60 minutes before the procedure unless they are allergic to aspirin or NSAIDs. Other NSAIDs have similar efficacy.
- In extremely anxious patients, premedication with an oral anxiolytic such as 10 mg of diazepam (Valium) 1 hour before the EMB is an option. Patients receiving these medications should be counseled to bring a family member to drive them home.
- The American Heart Association does not recommend antibiotic prophylaxis against bacterial endocarditis before EMB because the procedure is unlikely to cause bacteremia. No current studies specifically stratify this risk.
- Postmenopausal women can be scheduled for EMB at any time, although significant bleeding episodes are best avoided to optimize sample size.
- EMB in reproductive-age women is best performed on day 22 or 23 after the first day of the last menstrual period. The presence of secretory glands confirms that ovulation has occurred. Avoid EMB during menses because stromal breakdown can be misinterpreted as cell fragmentation and hemorrhage due to malignancy.

Procedure

The initial steps for endometrial biopsy are similar for the various methods. These are listed first (steps 1 through 8) and followed by descriptions of individual endometrial aspirators and specific instructions for their use. *Confirm that the patient is not pregnant, if appropriate, before beginning the procedure.*

1. The patient is placed in stirrups in dorsal lithotomy position (after the Pap smear is obtained, if indicated) and a *bimanual examination* is performed to determine the size and position of the uterus. The provider wears nonsterile gloves for this portion of the procedure.
2. *Insert a large Graves speculum* vaginally. Visualize the cervix and remove any mucus or debris.
3. Change into sterile gloves.
4. *Prepare the cervix and vagina with povidone–iodine*–soaked cotton balls using the ring forceps.
5. *Perform an endocervical curettage* in cases where neoplasm is suspected (see Chapter 137, Colposcopic Examination). Insert a Kevorkian curette without basket or a disposable curette into the endocervical canal. Manipulate the curette 360 degrees circumferentially around the entire canal, scraping in and out for two full rotations. Warn the patient about cramping. Collect all of the available material. Use ring forceps to collect any blood or secretions draining from the os. Place all the material on lens paper and then place it in formalin.
6. *If insertion of the curette is difficult*, use a single-tooth tenaculum to grasp the cervix at 12 o'clock. Traction on the tenaculum straightens the cervical neck and allows for easier endocervical curettage. Avoid grasping the 3 and 9 o'clock positions because of the presence of arteries at these points. Topical benzocaine gel (20%) or benzocaine spray (Hurricaine) may be applied to the tenaculum site to decrease pain. If used, the anesthetic needs to be in place several minutes before it has an effect. A submucosal injection of lidocaine works well (see explanation in Chapter 149, Loop Electrosurgical Excision Procedure for Treating Cervical Intraepithelial Neoplasia).
7. Once a gritty sensation is noted, remove the curette. *Collect all tissue* obtained and place it in formalin.
8. *Proceed with EMB* using one of the following techniques. With all endometrial biopsy techniques, insert the sterile sampling device through the cervical os without touching the vulva or vaginal walls. Do not touch or contaminate the part of the sampler that is placed into the uterus. Sterile gloves and speculum are not necessary if a "no-touch" technique is used.

Plastic Endometrial Aspirators (Pipelle or Endocell Endometrial Aspirator)

Disposable flexible endometrial sampling devices are the most popular method for EMB (Fig. 143-1A and B). The device is made of a clear, flexible polypropylene tube with an inner plunger. This functions as a piston and creates negative pressure when retracted quickly. A 2.4-mm distal side port allows for tissue sampling. The stiffer-tipped aspirators are more useful when cervical stenosis is present. More flexible types may be "stiffened" by placing them in a freezer for 10 to 15 minutes.

The Pipelle samples 5% to 15% of the endometrial surface. Several types are calibrated and can be used to sound the uterus (6.5 to 10 cm is normal). Seventy-seven to 99% of specimens obtained using the Pipelle are adequate for histopathologic diagnosis.

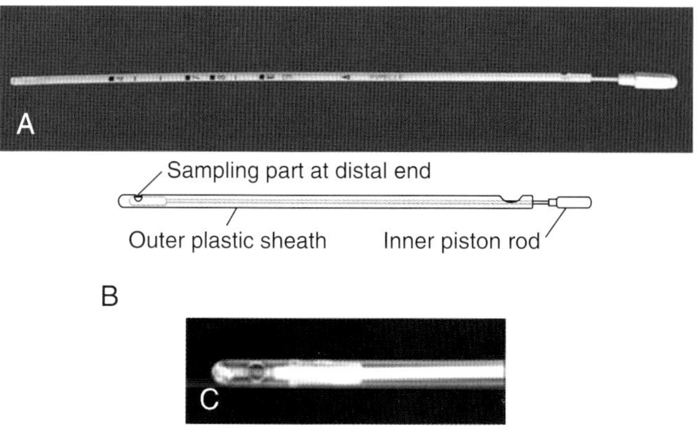

Figure 143-1 **A,** Pipelle endometrial sampler. **B,** Depiction of Pipelle sheath and piston. **C,** The opening at the end of the Pipelle. (Courtesy of CooperSurgical, Inc., Trumbull, Conn, with permission.)

The procedure for flexible endometrial aspirators follows, continued from previous steps 1 through 8.

9. *Sound the uterus* using either a calibrated flexible aspirator with the piston fully inserted or a metal sound (when using an uncalibrated product). Document the depth of the endometrial cavity (usually 6.5 to 10 cm). If the sound cannot be inserted, use a tenaculum to grasp the cervix at 12 o'clock. Outward traction straightens the cervical neck and allows the sound to pass through the cervical os. If the sound still will not pass, cervical dilation may be necessary (see Chapter 136, Cervical Stenosis and Cervical Dilation).
10. *Introduce the aspirator*, with internal piston fully inserted, into the endocervix. Pass it through the cervix and into the uterine cavity. Stop once the fundus is reached or resistance is encountered (Fig. 143-2A).
11. Stabilize the sheath with one hand while the *piston is drawn back* with the other hand. Negative pressure builds up in the lumen of the tube (Fig. 143-2B).
12. *Rotate the sheath 360 degrees* between the thumb and index finger. At the same time, *withdraw the aspirator going from the fundus to the internal os*. Most of the endometrial cavity can be sampled with a minimum of four complete in-and-out circumferential passes. As the aspirator completes a helical arc against the uterine walls, negative pressure within the sheath draws the sheared-off endometrial tissue through the distal port and into the lumen. The aspirator must be kept within the cervix or suction is lost (Fig. 143-2C).
13. *Withdraw the entire device from the uterus*, with the piston pulled back the full distance. Avoid contaminating the tip. *Do not* push the piston back into the sheath before removal because the tissue sample will be lost.
14. *Expel the sample into formalin* by advancing the piston into the sheath (Fig. 143-2D–F). *If insufficient tissue is obtained or if the aspirator fills with blood or other material* before four complete passes have been made, a second insertion may be attempted using the same catheter as long as it has not touched the formalin or vaginal sidewalls. The manufacturers often recommend that the tip of the catheter be cut off using scissors before the sample is expelled into formalin, although this is unnecessary. Additional sampling would then require an additional unused aspirator.
15. *Remove the speculum from the vagina.*

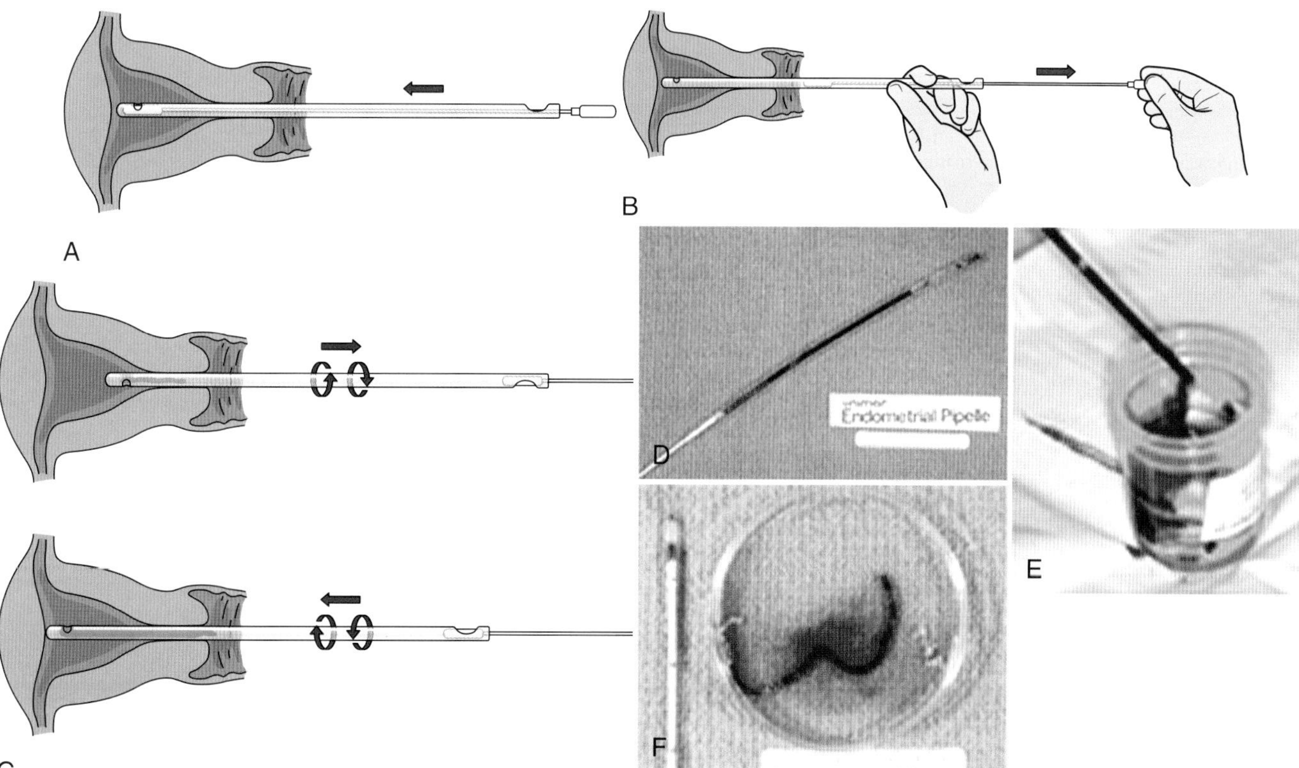

Figure 143-2 **A,** With the piston fully advanced in the sheath, insert the aspirator transcervically into the endometrial cavity. **B,** Hold the outer sheath with one hand while simultaneously pulling back the piston to create negative pressure. **C,** Roll the sheath between the fingers while simultaneously moving the sheath in and out from the fundus to the internal os. Complete a minimum of four passes. **D,** Appearance of tissue in the sampler. **E,** Expressing the tissue into the formalin bottle. **F,** The sample as it appears in the formalin container.

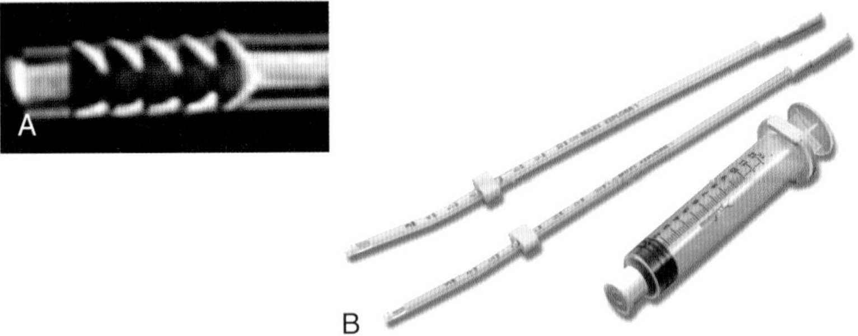

Figure 143-3 **A,** Close-up of the end of the Novak stainless steel curette. **B,** Uterine Explora and Explora II endometrial aspirators. (Courtesy of CooperSurgical, Inc., Trumbull, Conn, with permission.)

Reusable Stainless Steel Curette (Novak or Randall) and Disposable Endometrial Aspirators with Syringe Suction (Cannula Curette, Uterine Explora, Explora II)

The Novak curette is made of *stainless steel* and has been available for over 50 years (Fig. 143-3A). The cannula is rigid and is attached to a 10- to 20-mL disposable plastic syringe. When the syringe plunger is pulled, the negative pressure generated draws endometrial tissue into the cannula. Both the Novak and Randall curettes are reusable after sterilization. A disadvantage of this method is that patients complain of greater pain than with flexible plastic aspirators.

Several *disposable methods* allow easier use of suction by connecting a locking syringe to the end of the plastic aspirator. The Cannula Curette, Uterine Explora, and Explora II combine the benefits of a rigid cannula with disposability. Both Explora models are nylon with a sharp Randall-type cutting edge (Fig. 143-3B and C). The Explora has one distal port, whereas the Explora II has two distal ports on opposing sides of the aspirator. Tissue is obtained with suction using a scraping and peeling action. In women with large endocervical canals, the Cannula Curette may be a better option (Fig. 143-4). It comes in sizes ranging from 3 to 7 mm, whereas the Explora and Explora II are available only in 3- and 4-mm sizes. When AUB is present, the larger-diameter Cannula Curette is less likely to clog than the smaller curettes. Sensitivity and specificity of these types of endometrial samplers are similar to those for the flexible plastic endometrial aspirators.

After completing previous steps 1 through 8, the procedure for the reusable stainless steel curette (Novak or Randall) and disposable endometrial aspirators with syringe suction (Cannula Curette, Uterine Explora, Explora II) is as follows:

9. *Apply a tenaculum* to the anterior or posterior tip of the cervix, depending on the direction of flexion of the uterus. Grasp the cervix with the tenaculum teeth in the horizontal position. Grasping the cervix at the 3 or 9 o'clock position with the tenaculum in the vertical plane decreases the diameter of the external os. Local anesthesia (2 mL 2% lidocaine solution or spray) where the tenaculum teeth are applied decreases patient discomfort (*optional*).
10. *Insert a uterine sound* into the cervix while applying gentle traction to the tenaculum. Halt when the fundus is reached and note the insertion measurement in centimeters. Remove the sound from the patient. If stenosis is present, cervical dilation may be necessary (see Chapter 136, Cervical Stenosis and Cervical Dilation).
11. Gently *insert the curette* into the endometrial cavity while applying traction with the tenaculum. Stop insertion once the curette is at the depth that was sounded.
12. Before attaching the curette, *draw up 1 to 2 cm of air into the syringe*. This will be used to evacuate the curette when the procedure is completed.
13. *Attach a 20-mL syringe to the curette hub*. Pull the syringe back to the 10- to 15-mL mark to create suction. The Explora models recommend pulling the syringe back to 1 or 2 mL to avoid discomfort.
14. Apply pressure against the uterine sidewalls and *perform four to six single-strip curettages*. Sample from the fundus to the lower uterine segment and obtain at least one sample from each quadrant. More sampling can be done if the patient is tolerating the procedure well.
15. *Release the pressure on the syringe, withdraw the curette from the uterus, and express the sample into the formalin* bottle by pushing the plunger of the syringe toward the curette. Label the formalin bottle.
16. *Remove the speculum* from the vagina.

Tis-U-Trap and Vabra Aspirator

The sterile and disposable Tis-U-Trap is a clear *plastic* tissue collection chamber (Fig. 143-5). It comes with a funnel, two sealing caps, a resealable bag, and either a flat or cone-shaped tissue trap. The Tis-U-Trap is used with one of several types of endometrial curettes. The trap is attached to an external suction source such as a pump

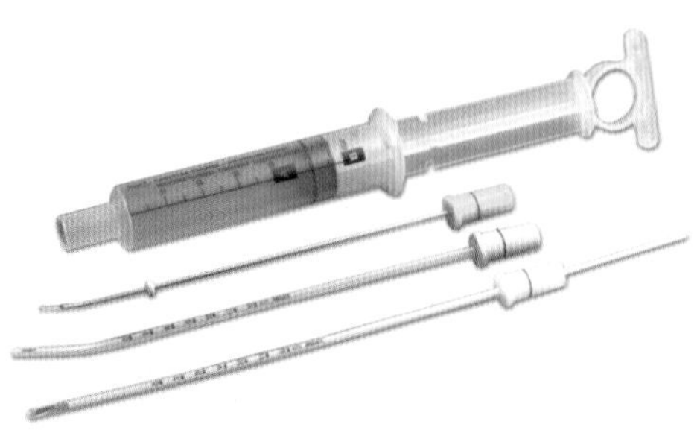

Figure 143-4 Cannula curette endometrial aspirator. (Courtesy of CooperSurgical, Inc., Trumbull, Conn, with permission.)

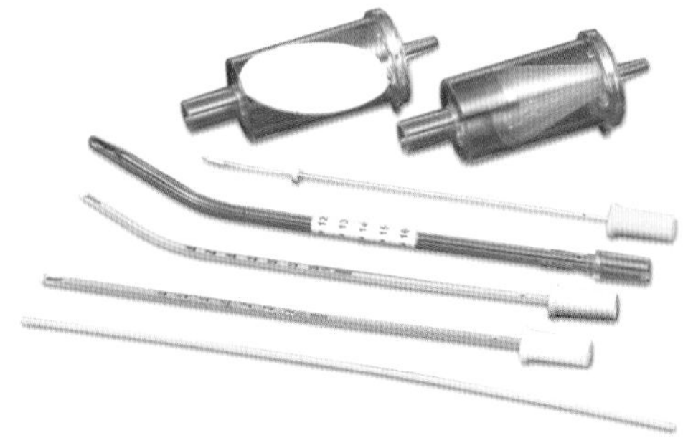

Figure 143-5 Tis-U-Trap plastic disposable aspirator, including flat and cone-shaped collection chamber, sound, and endometrial curettes. (Courtesy of CooperSurgical, Inc., Trumbull, Conn, with permission.)

or wall suction. Endometrial tissue is aspirated directly into the collection chamber, eliminating the need to transfer the tissue sample into another container. The design of the collection chamber permits easy visualization of the tissue collected and simplifies routine tissue handling for pathology.

The Vabra aspirator uses a 4-mm disposable curette or 2- to 3-mm stainless steel curette with an external vacuum pump. The vacuum pump is noisy, and this method is less commonly used than those listed previously. Tissue collected is gathered from a trap and placed in formalin. An advantage of the Vabra aspirator is the large tissue sample obtained, although the larger, rigid cannula is more uncomfortable for the patient.

After completing previous steps 1 through 8, follow these steps for using the Tis-U-Trap or Vabra aspirator:

9. *Apply a tenaculum* to the anterior or posterior lip of the cervix.
10. Using a metal sound, carefully *measure the depth of the endometrial cavity*. Measurements usually range between 6.5 and 10 cm. If stenosis is present, cervical dilation may be necessary (see Chapter 136, Cervical Stenosis and Cervical Dilation).
11. *Attach the device to the external suction pump*.
12. *Insert the curette* through the cervical os and gently advance until the fundus is reached. The depth should coincide with the uterine sound measurement.
13. *Activate the pump to 55 cm H_2O*.
14. *Initiate suction* by covering the suction hole with a finger (Fig. 143-6A).
15. Carefully *curette the entire endometrium* using a circumferential in-and-out movement. Keep the curette within the uterine cavity. The tissue passes through the curette and into the trap, where it collects on the grid.
16. When sufficient tissue accumulates in the trap, *halt suction* and then remove the curette from the uterus.

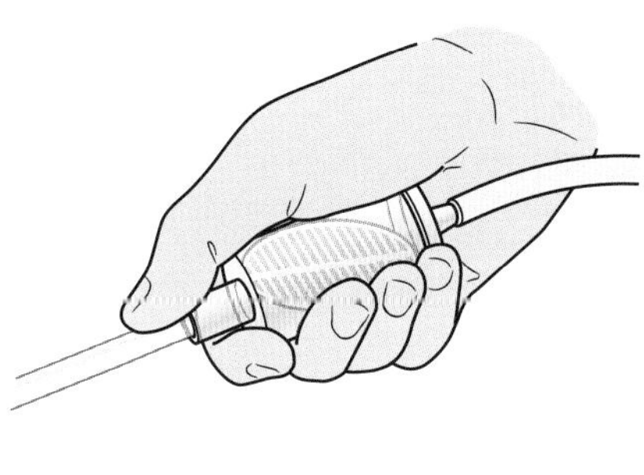

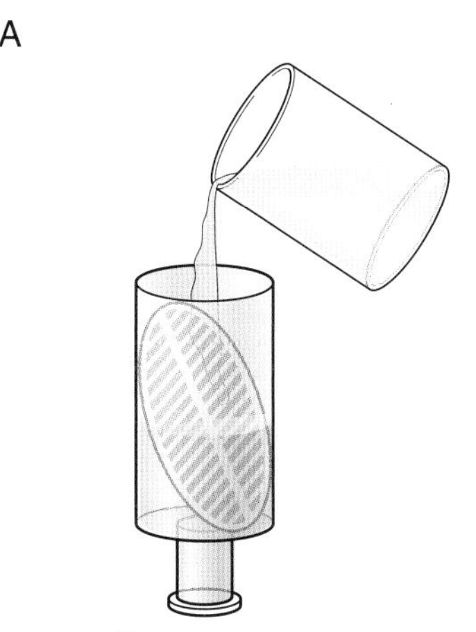

Figure 143-6 **A,** Initiate suction by covering the hole on the curette. **B,** Remove the curette from the trap and cap the outlet. Pour formalin into the trap to cover all tissue and then seal.

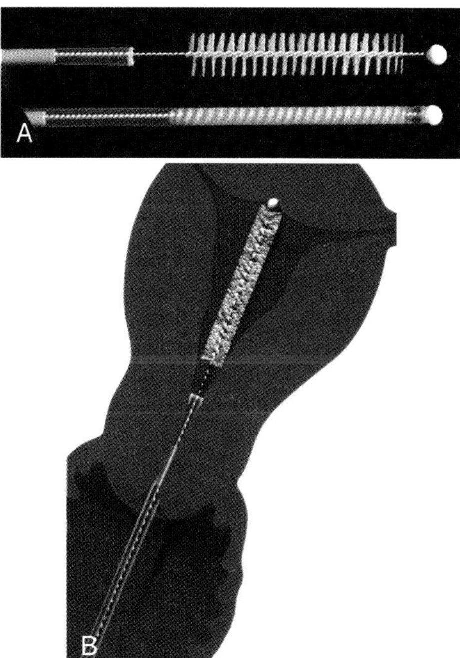

Figure 143-7 Tao Brush. **A,** Endometrial sampler with sheath. **B,** Brush inserted in the endometrial cavity with sheath retracted to allow for sampling. (Courtesy of Cook Women's Health, Spencer, Ind, with permission.)

17. *Turn the suction pump* off and disconnect the curette from the trap.
18. *Add formalin* to the trap and ensure that all tissue is exposed. Cap and label the trap for submission to pathology (Fig. 143-6B).
19. *Remove the speculum* from the vagina.

Tao Brush

The Tao Brush sampler consists of a tube with a distal brush (Fig. 143-7A). The brush is covered by a 26-cm, 9.0-Fr vinyl sheath. By keeping the brush covered during insertion, the sheath allows for sampling of endometrial cells only, without contamination from the vagina or cervix, because the brush is uncovered only once it is in the uterine cavity. The brush obtains an adequate sampling from the entire endometrium. It is supplied in a sterile package and intended for one-time use only. The Tao Brush may be used alone or before or after use of a plastic aspirator.

After following previous steps 1 through 8, the Tao Brush procedure is as follows:

9. *Sound the uterus* (up to 10 cm is normal). If stenosis is present, cervical dilation may be necessary (see Chapter 136, Cervical Stenosis and Cervical Dilation).
10. *Insert the Tao Brush* with the outer sheath covering the brush. Gently advance it until the fundus is reached, based on the initial sounding depth.
11. *Slide back the outer sheath* to expose the plastic bristles and rotate 360 degrees 10 times against the uterine walls (Fig. 143-7B).
12. Slide the sheath back in to cover the brush and then remove the Tao Brush and speculum.
13. Place the brush into the supplied CytoRich Red. Pull the sheath back and forth 10 times to dislodge the endometrial tissue. CytoRich Red hemolyzes blood and allows the pathologist to prepare a "thin-layer" sample (liquid-based cytology).

Sample Operative Report

See the sample encounter form online at www.expertconsult.com.

Common Errors

- *Inability to develop suction with a Pipelle or Novak/Randall-type endometrial aspirator.* If the endocervical canal is large, change to a larger-diameter cannula and reattempt aspiration.
- *Loss of suction during the biopsy.* If the distal port of the Pipelle or syringe suction aspirator is pulled too far outside the endocervix, suction is lost as air is pulled in. Keep the aspirator within the uterine cavity and endocervix until the sample is obtained.
- *Use of a small-diameter cannula in the setting of significant uterine bleeding.* Large clots clog the cannula and make obtaining an adequate sample (rather than just blood) challenging. Switch to a larger-diameter cannula and reattempt aspiration.

Complications

- *Uterine perforation* occurs in 0.1% to 1.3% of EMBs. Perforation most often occurs with the use of rigid devices, while sounding the uterus, or when the cervix is stenotic. If the uterine sound passes more than 12 cm in a uterus that does seem that large on palpation, perforation is suspected. Stop the procedure and withdraw all instruments. Observe the patient closely for bleeding. No other intervention is indicated unless symptoms develop. Patients may be discharged home with close follow-up if bleeding is minimal and vital signs are stable after 30 minutes of observation. Precautions regarding infection and bleeding should be discussed before release. Repeat biopsy can be attempted in 6 to 8 weeks.
- *Excessive uterine bleeding* is possible, especially in patients with undiagnosed coagulation disorders or perforation.
- *Missed pathology* is possible because only a small area of the endometrium is sampled. Although the sensitivity of EMB is estimated to be high as 96%, it may miss up to 18% of focal lesions. Fibroids and polyps will also not be identified.
- A *vasovagal response* occurs in an estimated 10% of patients after EMB.
- Although most women experience *cramping during* the endocervical curettage, *pain after* the procedure is usually minimal. Pain lasting longer than 24 hours should be reported to the provider.
- *Bacteremia, septicemia, and endocarditis* have been reported after EMB, although they are exceedingly rare. The patient should report any fever or foul discharge.

Postprocedure Management

- Patients should remain semirecumbent for 10 minutes after the EMB has been taken. Assess for vasovagal reaction.
- Painful uterine cramps (if present) usually subside rapidly or are relieved with NSAIDs.
- Patients with minimal cramping and bleeding may be discharged home.
- Although a follow-up visit is usually not necessary, it may be needed to discuss pathology findings. *If AUB persists,* further evaluation with a repeat EMB, D&C, hysteroscopy, or pelvic ultrasonography is indicated.

Postprocedure Patient Education

Bleeding and cramping usually resolve within 24 to 48 hours. Fever, cramping lasting longer than 48 hours, or bleeding heavier than a normal period should be reported. NSAIDs can be used for pain or cramping. Sexual relations may be resumed after bleeding has stopped.

Interpretation of Results

1. When submitting an endometrial biopsy, *conveying adequate clinical history to the pathologist* is essential. The patient's age, clinical indication for biopsy, menopausal status, and date/length of last menstrual period in premenopausal women are important. Exogenous hormones, hormonal contraceptives, and drugs like tamoxifen can alter the morphology of the endometrium and cause false-positive or false-negative results (Fig. 143-8).
2. Biopsy interpretation is based on the status of the functionalis layer located in the upper two thirds of the endometrium. The basalis layer usually shows minimal change. Atrophic, denuded, or scarred endometrium may not yield sufficient tissue for diagnosis. *Inadequate samples* are possible in biopsies immediately after menses, with hypoestrogenism, with prolonged bleeding, or with intrauterine adhesions/synechiae. Menopausal status has a greater effect on specimen adequacy than the type of instrument used (Box 143-2).
3. The *classification of endometrial hyperplasia* is made according to guidelines from either the International Society of Gynecological Pathologists or the World Health Organization (Box 143-3). Endometrial hyperplasia covers a spectrum of alterations in the stroma and glands of the endometrium. Changes range from hyperplasia to atypical hyperplasia to carcinoma. Both hyperplasia and atypical hyperplasia are further categorized as either simple or complex:
   - *Simple hyperplasia* describes an increased glandular-to-stromal ratio without evidence of glandular crowding or cellular atypia. *Cystic hyperplasia* is an older term that is no longer used. There is no clinical significance to this finding and no treatment is needed.
   - In *complex hyperplasia*, infolding and budding of the glands is noted. Glands are crowded in comparison to simple hyperplasia, but no atypia is noted. The older term *adenomatous hyperplasia* is no longer in use.
   - In *atypical hyperplasia*, cytologic atypia is divided into simple or complex categories depending on the glandular architecture. Large nuclei of varying shape and size, increased nuclear-to-cytoplasm ratio, and prominent nucleoli are commonly described.
4. *Endometrial hyperplasia without cytologic atypia is usually managed with progestins;* 20 mg medroxyprogesterone acetate given twice daily is prescribed for 3 to 6 months. EMB is repeated after therapy, and complete reversal of lesions is often noted. If hyperplasia *without atypia* is again confirmed, a repeat course of progestin with follow-up EMB or hysteroscopy can be performed. Some patients may opt for a hysterectomy at this point.
5. *Hyperplasia with cytologic atypia* is best managed with a hysterectomy because of the risk of progression to adenocarcinoma. Approximately 10% of women with postmenopausal bleeding have endometrial cancer.
6. Histology determines management. Severity of endometrial hyperplasia and the probability of cancer *cannot* be determined by the amount of bleeding, at what point during the menstrual cycle the bleeding occurs, the gross appearance of the sample, or the tissue volume obtained by biopsy. Histopathology must be determined. Transvaginal endometrial thickness measurement is never a substitute for histologic tissue assessment in symptomatic women.

Patient Education Guides

See the patient education and consent forms online at www.expertconsult.com.

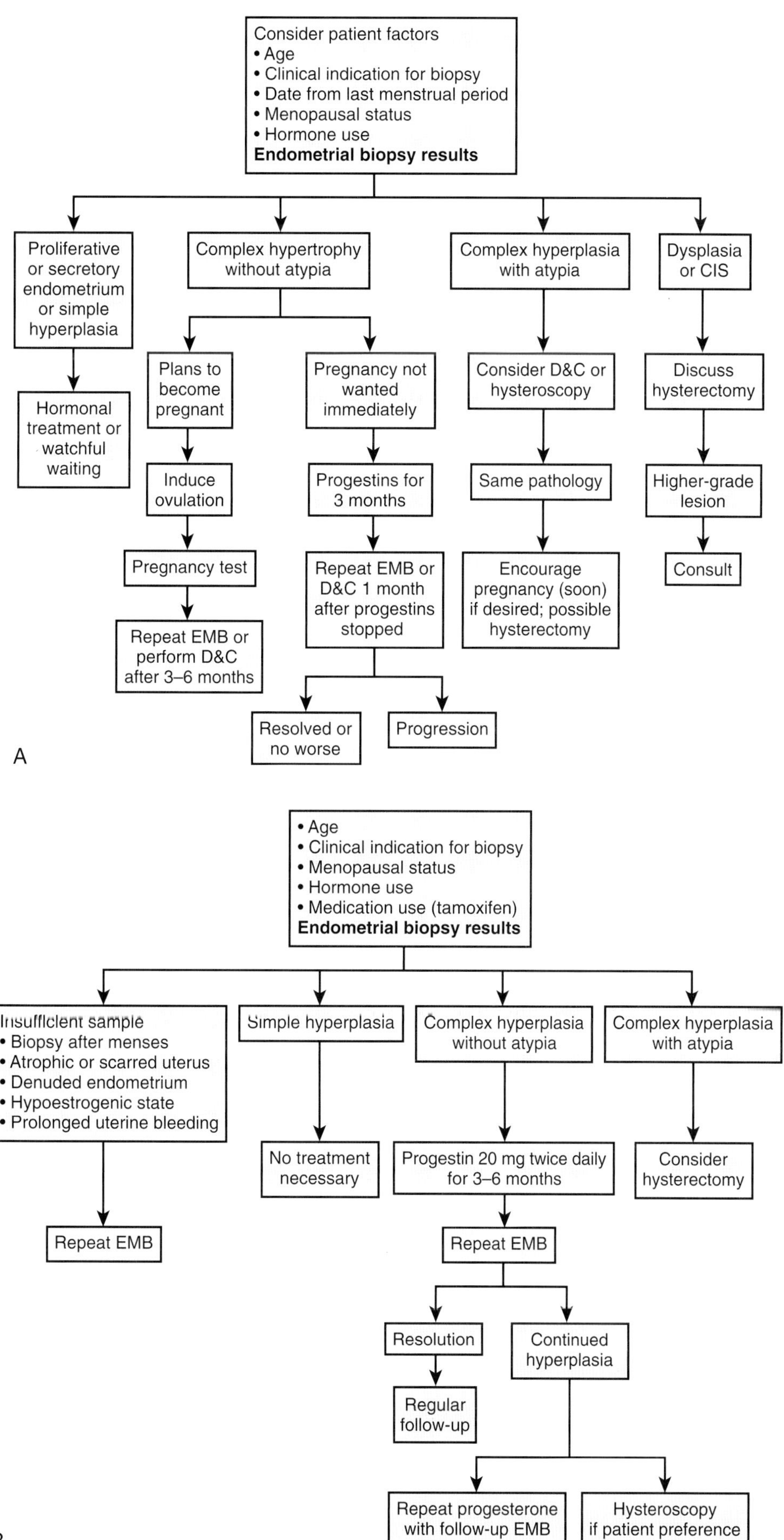

Figure 143-8 Management options after endometrial biopsy in premenopausal (**A**) and postmenopausal (**B**) women. CIS, carcinoma in situ; D&C, dilation and curettage; EMB, endometrial biopsy.

Box 143-2. Findings on Endometrial Biopsy Sampling

Insufficient Tissue

Follow-up depends on clinical situation; may need to repeat or use other diagnostic techniques

Normal

Proliferative endometrium
Secretory endometrium
Atrophic endometrium

Pregnancy Related

Retained products of conception
Decidua (consider an ectopic or missed abortion)

Infectious Etiology

Endometritis, treat as indicated

Abnormal

Rarely, endometrial polyp
Simple (cystic) hyperplasia
- Risk for progression to cancer extremely small; little need for follow-up unless symptoms present.

Complex (adenomatous) hyperplasia
- Low but some risk for progression to cancer.
- Treat with progestational agents and follow up with tissue sampling in 6 months.

Atypical hyperplasia (simple and complex)
- Significant risk for progression to cancer.
- Consider hysterectomy because of significant risk of progression to invasion and need for long-term follow-up to detect progression. If childbearing not complete, treat with progestational agents and follow with frequent biopsies. Referral and consultation should be strongly considered.

Adenocarcinoma
- Referral indicated for appropriate work-up and treatment.

If the endocervical curettage is positive for dysplasia, a conization is indicated. If symptoms persist in spite of treatment, regardless of biopsy results, further evaluation is indicated.

CPT/Billing Codes

57505 Endocervical curettage not done as part of dilation and curettage
57800 Dilatation of cervical canal, instrumental
58100 Endometrial sampling (biopsy) with or without endocervical sampling, without cervical dilation, any method
59200 Insertion of cervical dilator (e.g., laminaria)

Box 143-3. International Society of Gynecological Pathologists Classification for Endometrial Hyperplasia

Endometrial hyperplasia
- Simple
- Complex

Endometrial hyperplasia with atypia
- Simple
- Complex

ICD-9-CM Diagnostic Codes

182.0 Ca uterus
219.9 Benign neoplasm of uterus
233.2 Ca in situ, uterus
236.3 Neoplasm of uncertain behavior, uterus
621.0 Polyp of endometrium
621.2 Hypertrophy of uterus; bulky or enlarged uterus
621.30 Endometrial hyperplasia unspecified
621.31 Endometrial hyperplasia without atypia
621.32 Complex hyperplasia without atypia
621.33 Endometrial hyperplasia with atypia
622.1 Atypical glandular cells
625 Pain associated with female genital organs (requires a fourth digit and must be as specific as possible)
625.9 Unspecified symptoms associated with female genital organs
626.5 Ovulation bleeding (regular intermenstrual bleeding)
626.6 Metrorrhagia (bleeding unrelated to menstrual cycle; irregular intermenstrual bleeding)
626.8 Dysfunctional uterine bleeding
626.9 Unspecified uterine bleeding
627.0 Premenopausal menorrhagia
627.1 Postmenopausal bleeding
V07.4 Postmenopausal HRT
V10.40 Personal history of cancer of female genital organ, unspecified
V10.41 Personal history of cancer of cervix, uteri

Acknowledgment

The editors wish to recognize the contributions by Barbara S. Apgar, MD, and John L. Pfenninger, MD, to this chapter in the previous two editions of this text.

Suppliers

(See contact information online at www.expertconsult.com.)

Endocell endometrial sampler
Wallach Surgical
Plastic endometrial aspirator
Cannula Curette with 60-cc Handyvak Locking Syringe
Milex Products, Inc. (Division of CooperSurgical, Inc.)
Endocervical curette with Vac-Loc syringe
Pipelle de Cornier endometrial suction curette
CooperSurgical, Inc.
Uterine Explora Models 1 and 2
Tao Brush
Cook Women's Health
Tis-U-Trap Sampler Device, endometrial suction curette (flat trap and cone trap)
Milex Products, Inc. (Division of CooperSurgical, Inc.)
Vabra aspirator
Berkeley Medevices

Online Resource

National Cancer Institute: Endometrial cancer. Available at www.cancer.gov/cancertopics/types/endometrial.

Bibliography

Albers J, Hull S, Wesley R: Abnormal uterine bleeding. Am Fam Physician 69:1915–1926, 1931–1932, 2004.

American College of Obstetricians and Gynecologists: Antibiotic prophylaxis for gynecologic procedures. Practice Bulletin no. 104. Obstet Gynecol 113:1180–1189, 2009.

American College of Obstetricians and Gynecologists: The role of transvaginal ultrasonography in the evaluation of postmenopausal bleeding. Committee Opinion no. 426. Obstet Gynecol 113:462–464, 2009.

Buchanan EM, Weinstein LC, Hillson C: Endometrial cancer. Am Fam Physician 80:1075–1080, 2009.

Dunn TS, Stamm CA, Delroit M, Goldberg G: Clinical pathway for evaluating women with abnormal uterine bleeding. J Reprod Med 46:831–834, 2001.

Hill DA: Abnormal uterine bleeding: Avoid the rush to hysterectomy. J Fam Pract 58:136–142, 2009.

McCluggage W: My approach to the interpretation of endometrial biopsies and curettings. J Clin Pathol 59:801–812, 2006.

Mounsey A: Postmenopausal bleeding: Evaluation and management. Clin Fam Practice 4:173–192, 2002.

Renkonen-Sinisalo L, Butzow R, Leminen A, et al: Surveillance for endometrial cancer in hereditary nonpolyposis colorectal cancer syndrome. Int J Cancer 120:821–824, 2006.

Sierecki AR, Gudipudi DK, Montemarano N, Del Priore G: Comparison of endometrial aspiration biopsy techniques: Specimen adequacy. J Reprod Med 53:760–764, 2008.

Smith R, Cokkinides V, Eyre HJ: American Cancer Society Guidelines for early detection of cancer, 2006. CA Cancer J Clin 56:11–25, 2006.

Tanriverdi H, Barut A, Gün B, Kaya E: Is Pipelle biopsy really adequate for diagnosing endometrial disease? Med Sci Monit 10:CR271–CR274, 2004.

Tuggy M, Garcia J: Procedures Consult. Available at www.proceduresconsult.com.

CHAPTER 144

HYSTEROSALPINGOGRAPHY AND SONOHYSTEROGRAPHY

Steven Fettinger • Linda Fanelli

Hysterosalpingography (HSG) is a radiologic examination of the female genital tract. It allows for the evaluation of the cervical canal, endometrial cavity, tubal lumen, and the periadnexal area. The *basic infertility work-up* includes HSG, although some physicians feel that it has been superseded by laparoscopy with hysteroscopy. However, it remains an integral part of many other diagnostic work-ups. HSG is a relatively easy procedure, requires no anesthesia, and has a low complication risk. Its use as a *therapeutic* procedure for enhancing fertility is promoted by some clinicians. The addition of selective cannulation of the cornual ostia has eliminated many false positives (or blockage) and opened new therapeutic options. These additions, however, require special training and currently limit the use of HSG in this manner to an infertility specialist or an interventional radiologist. The radiation exposure is usually minimal, in the 50 to 500 mrem ranges.

Saline infusion sonohysterography (SIS) is a technique for visualization of the reproductive tract using ultrasound and the injection of sterile normal saline as an ultrasonic contrast medium. The ease of this procedure and the availability of ultrasound in the office have been responsible for its rapid growth. The discomfort involved is usually less than that of HSG, but the complications and contraindications are similar. A vaginal probe ultrasound and catheter-injected normal saline (or ultrasonic contrast medium, not yet FDA [Food and Drug Administration] approved for gynecology) are used for imaging of the anatomy. The procedure itself is simple, but the expertise and experience needed for interpretation require specialized training. The decreased accuracy in visualizing the fallopian tubes limits its use for this purpose. However, these limitations are compensated for by the ability to identify endometrial pathologic changes and to define uterine anomalies.

Many clinicians start their *work-up of a patient with abnormal uterine bleeding* with a transvaginal ultrasonic measurement of the thickness of the endometrial stripe to rule out endometrial cancer. Ultrasonic evaluation of the endometrial stripe thickness in the work-up of abnormal uterine bleeding has been enhanced greatly by using SIS in combination. Endometrial thickness of 5 mm or less is thought to represent dysfunctional uterine bleeding. However, ethnic variations exist and cancer has been found in Japanese women with stripes only 3 to 4 mm thick. SIS is performed in patients with double layer endometrium thicker than 5 mm. Single layer endometrium of 3 mm or less, with no focal abnormalities on SIS, is also treated as dysfunctional uterine bleeding (Fig. 144-1). Symmetrical thickening of the single layer endometrium greater than 3 mm, with no focal lesions, is evaluated by an office endometrial biopsy. A newly available SIS catheter allows an immediate endometrial biopsy, if indicated, through the same catheter. Endometrium with focal lesions or asymmetry requires hysteroscopy and directed biopsy (Fig. 144-2). Hormone replacement and the use of tamoxifen also affect uterine lining, requiring the use of different discrimination thicknesses.

INDICATIONS

- Infertility (uterine)
  - Endometrial adhesions (Asherman's syndrome)
  - Submucosal polyps
  - Pedunculated endometrial leiomyomas
  - Uterine anomalies
  - Diethylstilbestrol (DES): T-shaped uterus
- Infertility (tubal)
  - Assessment of tubal patency
  - Salpingitis isthmica nodosa
  - Periadnexal adhesive disease
  - Tubal cannulation procedures
  - Follow-up after a medically or a surgically treated ectopic pregnancy
- Habitual abortions
  - Asherman's syndrome
  - Uterine anomaly
  - DES changes
  - Leiomyomas
- Cervical incompetency (controversial indication)
- Preoperative and postoperative evaluation
  - Tubal reanastomosis/reimplantation, tuboplasty
  - Confirmation of tubal occlusion after Essure contraceptive coil insertion (Fig. 144-3)
  - Uterine septal resection, metroplasty
  - Myomectomy
- Localization of lost intrauterine contraceptive device (IUD); ultrasound alone is the procedure of choice
- Abnormal uterine bleeding (SIS)

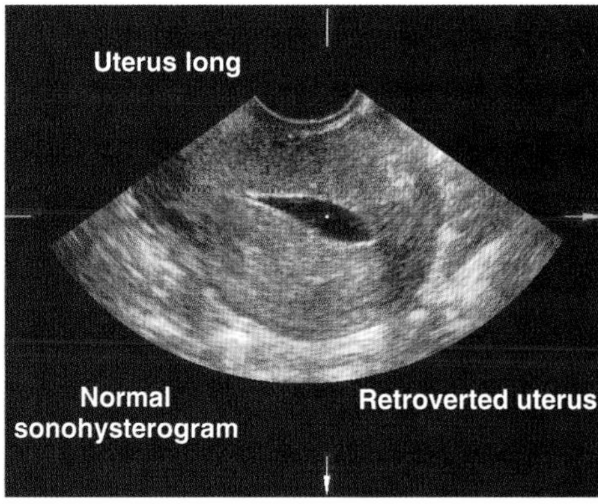

Figure 144-1 Normal saline infusion sonohysterogram with normal thin endometrial stripe. Longitudinal view (uterus long) with fundus to the right and posterior position inferior.

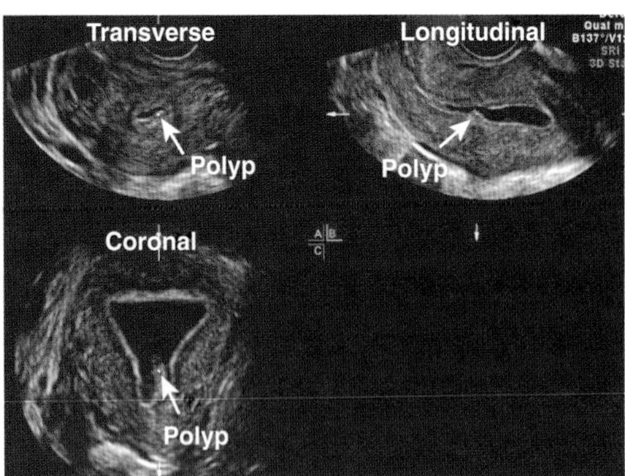

Figure 144-2 Abnormal saline infusion sonohysterogram with thin normal endometrial stripe and a focal lesion (endometrial polyp) in three planes of view.

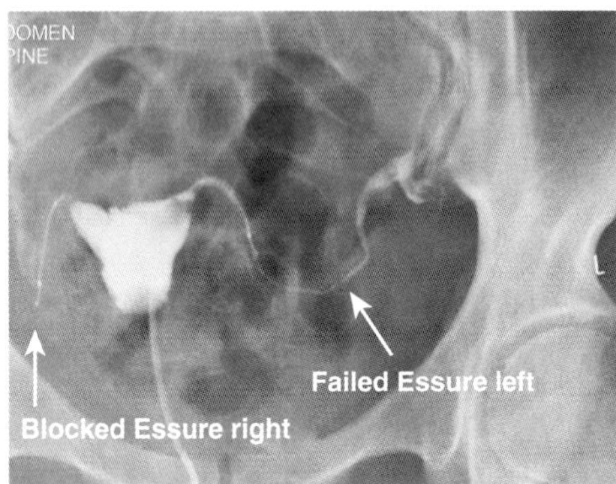

Figure 144-3 Hysterosalpingography after an Essure cornual occlusion procedure.

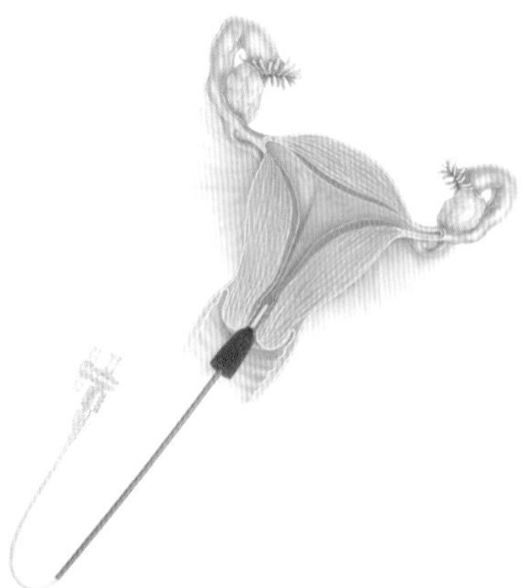

Figure 144-4 Saline infusion sonohysterography using EZ-HSG. (Courtesy of CooperSurgical, Trumball, CT.)

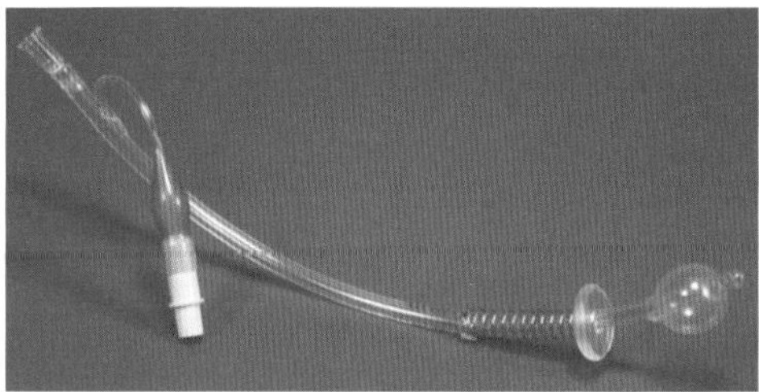

Figure 144-5 HUI catheter. (Courtesy of CooperSurgical, Trumball, CT.)

Contraindications

Absolute

- Active salpingitis
- Pregnancy

Relative

- Recent dilation and curettage
- Allergy to contrast medium
- Untreated sexually transmitted disease (STD)

Equipment and Supplies

- Cannulas

Many types of HSG cannulation devices are available. The choice of catheters used may depend on procedure indication and physician preference. Three general types are in common use, with multiple modifications (the flexible balloon cannulas are also used for SIS):

1. *Olive-tipped cannulas*. A small cannula traverses the cervical canal, and an olive- or cone-shaped seat is held against the cervix os to seal it (Fig. 144-4).
2. *Suction cannulas*. A small cannula is held in place and sealed by a suction cup on the ectocervix.
3. *Balloon cannulas*. One or two balloons are used to fix and seal the cervix. A primary intrauterine balloon is pulled down against the internal cervical os by a second balloon, a spring-loaded platform, or manual traction. The balloon catheters (including pediatric Foley catheters) obscure the lower uterine anatomy; however, the balloon can be deflated near the end of the procedure, and additional contrast dye can be injected to evaluate this area (Figs. 144-5 and 144-6).

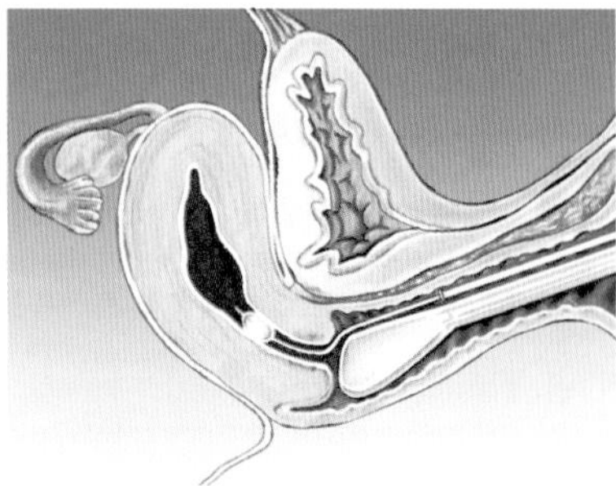

Figure 144-6 Saline infusion sonohysterography using H/S Elliptosphere catheter. (Courtesy of CooperSurgical, Trumball, CT.)

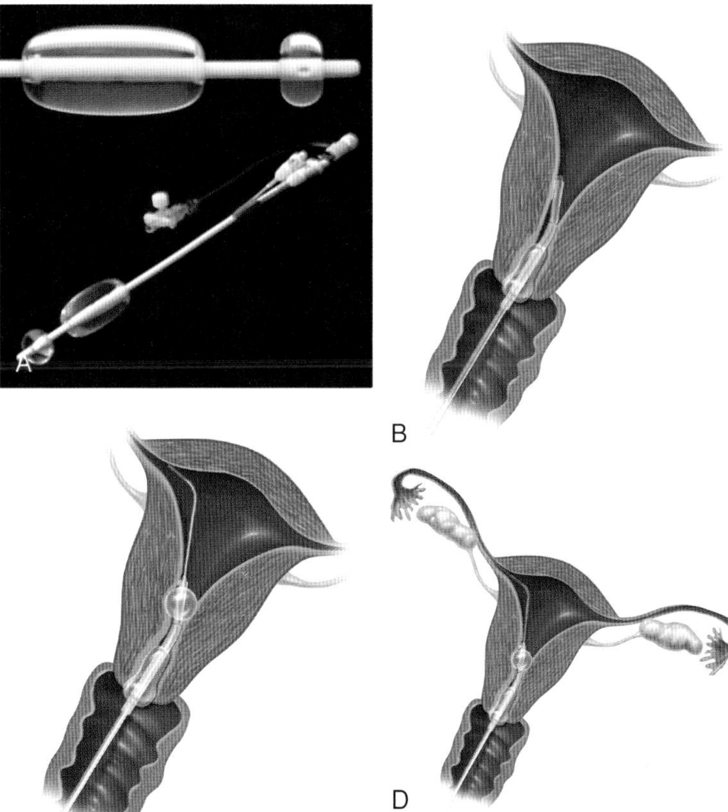

Figure 144-7 Selective cannulation of the fallopian tube. **A,** Preassembled Mencini double balloon catheter. **B,** Balloon cervical cannula (BCC) in uterus. **C,** Selective salpingography catheter (SSC) passes through BCC. **D,** Inner catheter through SSC. (Courtesy of Cook Ob/Gyn, Spencer, IN.)

Special selective cannulation catheterization systems are available from Cook Medical (see the "Suppliers" section). These catheters are used to selectively cannulate and evaluate a fallopian tube in special circumstances (e.g., unilateral or bilateral nonvisualization, salpingitis isthmica nodosa, or prior ectopic pregnancy). They may also be used therapeutically in some patients to open a blockage in the proximal tubes (Fig. 144-7).

SIS catheters with and without cervical sealing balloons and sponges are used for these procedures. In addition, an infusion/endometrial biopsy catheter makes it possible to biopsy at the same time (Box 144-1).

Box 144-1. Common Cannulas by Brand Names

EZ-HSG (CooperSurgical) (see Fig. 144-4)
Goldstein sonohysterography catheter (CookMedical) (Fig. 144-8)
Goldstein sonobiopsy catheter (Cook Medical) (Fig. 144-9)
H/S Elliptosphere catheter set (Ackrad/CooperSurgical)
HUI catheter (CooperSurgical) (see Fig. 144-5)
HUI Mini-Flex catheter (CooperSurgical)
Hysterocath (CookMedical)
Mencini double balloon hysterosalpingography catheter (CookMedical) (see Fig. 144-7)
Jaco or Kuhn catheter (nondisposable)
Thurmond-Rosch movable cup hysterocath (CookMedical) (Fig. 144-10)
ZUMI 2.0/4.0/4.5 catheter (CooperSurgical/Zinnanti) (Fig. 144-11)
Pediatric Foley catheter

- Contrast medium
  - HSG contrast
    - Water-soluble: Salpix (Ortho Pharmaceutical), Sinografin (Squibb)
    - Conray 60 (Mallinckrodt Pharmaceutical)
    - Oil-based (Lipiodal or Ethiodol)
    - Nonionic water-soluble: Hypaque-60 (Winthrop-Breon Pharmaceutical)
  - SHSG contrast
    - Normal saline
    - Echovist (Schering-Berlin Pharmaceutical)
    - Albunex (Mallinckrodt Pharmaceutical)

Most centers currently use water-soluble dye. There has been continued controversy regarding the use of water-soluble versus oil-based media (Table 144-1). The question of ionic or nonionic water-soluble dye depends on the preference of the radiologist. The majority of centers are using the less expensive ionic dyes, except

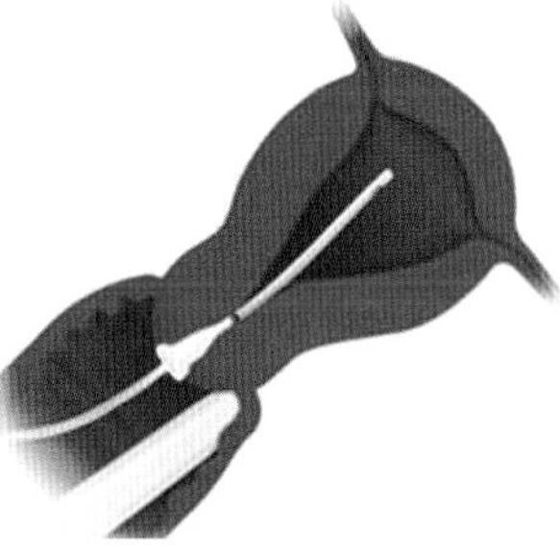

Figure 144-8 Goldstein sonohysterography catheter. (Courtesy of Cook Medical, Bloomington, IN.)

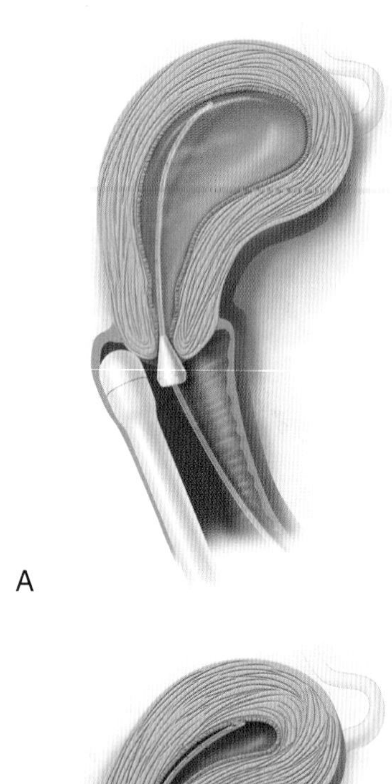

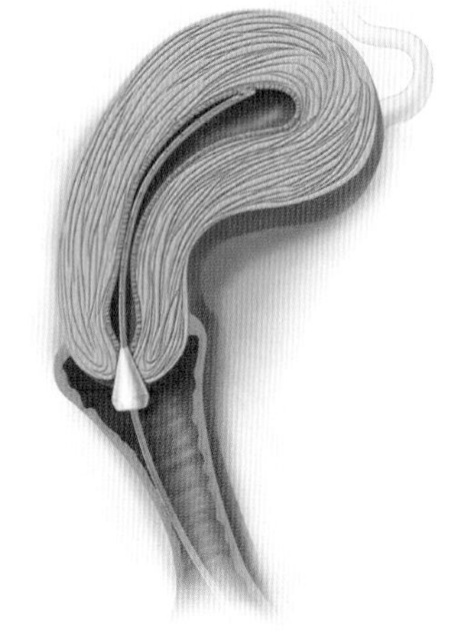

Figure 144-9 Goldstein sonobiopsy catheters. **A**, Saline infusion sonohysterography catheter. **B**, Endometrial biopsy catheter. (Courtesy of Cook Medical, Bloomington, IN.)

in patients with a history of an iodine allergy. Preprocedural administration of antihistamines and steroids may reduce this risk in allergic patients. Alternatively, gadolinium radiologic contrast agent can be used in iodine-allergic patients without renal failure.

- Prep tray, including 4 × 4 inch gauze pads, ring forceps, povidone–iodine solution, medicine cups, lubricating jelly, and a plastic speculum (prep trays with catheters included are available)

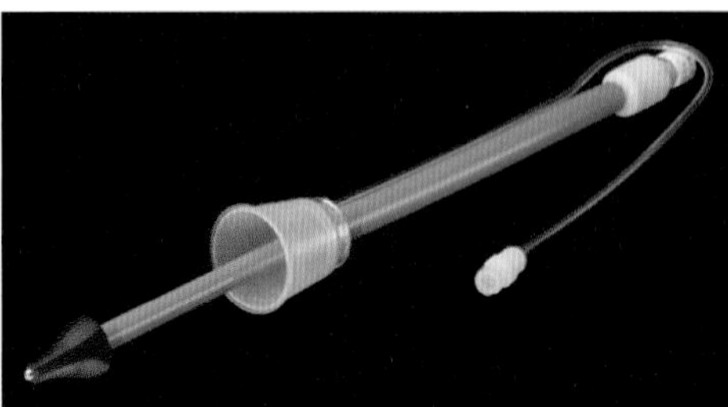

Figure 144-10 Thurmond-Rosch movable cup hysterocath. (Courtesy of Cook Medical, Bloomington, IN.)

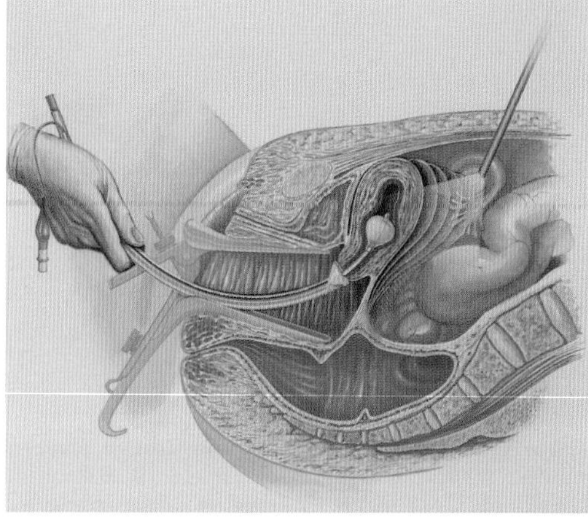

Figure 144-11 ZUMI (Zinnanti) catheter inserted for hysterosalpingography at the time of laparoscopy.

- Vaginal speculum
  - One-armed Graves speculum (removable after placement of cannula)
  - Plastic nonradiopaque (disposable)
- Tenaculum (if needed to fixate cervix for cannula placement)
- Syringe, 10 or 20 mL

Precautions

- HSG *should be performed in the preovulatory phase of the menstrual cycle* to avoid exposing an embryo to radiation and to decrease the risk of infection (infection rates are higher if the procedure is performed during the secretory phase). SIS is performed as soon as possible after menstruation ends to minimize endometrial growth/thickness. HSG/SIS during the preovulatory phase will also avoid the possibility of dislodging a preimplantation conception, and thereby theoretically prevent an ectopic pregnancy.
- Patients with a *history of salpingitis require negative cultures* for sexually transmitted disease and a nontender preprocedure pelvic examination. Some practitioners require a normal sedimentation rate as well.
- Patients with a *history of pelvic inflammatory disease or prior tuboplasty* should be treated with *prophylactic antibiotics*. One option shown to be effective is doxycycline 200 mg the morning of the procedure and 100 mg twice a day for 5 days following the procedure. Antibiotic prophylaxis is controversial for patients without a history of pelvic inflammatory disease or prior tuboplasty. Many physicians now use prophylaxis with all patients undergoing HSG, despite the lack of evidence of its usefulness in low-risk patients. The use of prophylactic antibiotics for SIS is even less well studied, but they are used by some sonographers.

TABLE 144-1 Selection of Contrast Medium

Medium	Advantages	Disadvantages
Water-soluble	Rapidly absorbed Less need for delayed films Improved visualization of details Extravasation tolerated	No enhancement of fertility
Oil-based	Possible fertility enhancement	Delayed films may be needed Granuloma formation possible Embolism if extravasation occurs

- *Preoperative medications* may include a nonsteroidal anti-inflammatory agent, such as ibuprofen 600 mg, given 1 to 2 hours preoperatively, to decrease pain and cramping. The effectiveness of this premedication, however, is limited at best. Diazepam 10 to 20 mg 1 to 2 hours preoperatively may be given for extreme apprehension.

Preprocedure Patient Education

- Discuss the procedure, the typical findings, and alternatives to, risks of, and possible complications of the procedure with the patient (obtain informed consent).
- Explain to the patient that mild discomfort will be experienced during the procedure and that spotting for up to a few days after the procedure is expected.
- Educate the patient about the warning signs of complications (e.g., increasing pain, heavy bleeding, and fever).

Procedure

Hysterosalpingography

1. Check all equipment to ensure that the setup is complete and in proper working condition.
2. Draw up the contrast material and preload the cannula (bubbles may obscure intrauterine disease or be confused with intrauterine polyps).
3. Position the patient on a high-resolution image-intensifier fluoroscopy table in the dorsal lithotomy position. An adequate light should be available.
4. Perform a bimanual pelvic examination to assess the degree of flexion or retroflexion of the uterus and to exclude pelvic tenderness (the latter is a contraindication to HSG if there is suspected inflammation).
5. Insert the vaginal speculum.
6. Cleanse the cervix and upper vagina with antiseptic.
7. If indicated by the cannula choice, grasp the anterior lip of the cervix with the tenaculum (slowly, to minimize pain).
8. Insert the cannula and seat it as indicated by the specific cannula:
   - Inflate the upper balloon, then the lower balloon—Mencini Double Balloon Hysterosalpingography Catheter (Cook-Medical) (see Fig. 144-7).
   - Inflate the upper balloon and set the spring platform—HUI/Zinnanti (CooperSurgical) (see Figs. 144-5 and 144-11).
   - Inflate the balloon and pull down—pediatric Foley and H/S Elliptosphere (CooperSurgical) (see Fig. 144-6).
   - Insert the cannula and set spring to tenaculum (Jaco).
   - Insert the cannula and seat suction cup onto the cervix, then apply suction to the cup—Thurmond-Rosch movable cup Hysterocath (CookMedical) (see Fig. 144-10).
9. Remove the speculum (nonradiopaque plastic speculum may be left in place).
10. Place the patient in the recumbent position for fluoroscopy.
11. Inject the contrast slowly. Between 1 and 3 mL may be sufficient to show intrauterine detail; greater volumes may obscure small polyps or adhesions. The injection should be viewed concurrently, and a single spot film taken. Upward or downward movement of the tenaculum will often change the degree of flexion to obtain a better view. Warming the dye preprocedurally may decrease associated cramps.
12. Continue to inject dye until the tubes start to fill. A spot film at this point may show tubal detail that will be obscured after dye spills.
13. Continue to inject dye until intra-abdominal spill of dye is seen bilaterally. A spot film at this point will sometimes show peritubal detail. A delayed film may be needed to confirm location of dye in peritubal adhesions.
14. Rolling the patient from side to side during the procedure sometimes helps the clinician to visualize lesions but increases the radiation exposure.
15. If visualization of one tube cannot be accomplished initially, try relaxing tubal spasm by relieving the pressure on the syringe and waiting 1 to 2 minutes.
16. Remove the instruments.
17. Observe the patient for 30 minutes for allergic reactions and heavy bleeding.
18. Selective cannulation of the ostium is briefly done as follows (see Fig. 144-7):
    - Preassemble coaxial catheter portions to be used or add portions as indicated, for the given patient.
    - Place the cervical access catheter (CAC) as previously discussed (catheter type must match the system used).
    - Introduce the uterine ostial access catheter (UOAC) through the CAC under radiologic guidance until the tip reaches the tubal ostium (this may be aided by the injection of a small amount of a contrast agent).
    - Pass the uterine cornual access catheter (UCAC) through the UOAC until the ostium is reached.
    - Advance the guidewire into the tube for a short distance, advance the UCAC over the wire, and then repeat the process until the UCAC is well within the tubal lumen.
    - While holding the UCAC in place, remove the wire.
    - Confirm placement by injecting contrast material into the UCAC.

Sonohysterography

1. Using the infusion port of the catheter, fill the catheter with sterile normal saline, purging all air. Even a few tiny air bubbles can create difficulties when evaluating the images.
2. A brief transvaginal ultrasound should be done prior to the SIS to establish the angle of the uterus and to measure the endometrial stripe. If other than a thin endometrial stripe is noted, a pregnancy test should be ordered prior to insertion of the catheter. Tenderness noted at this point should prompt the question of inflammation and may be a contraindication to continuation with the SIS.
3. Position the patient in the lithotomy position and insert a speculum (one-armed Graves speculum is preferred because it will be removed after placement of the catheter and before the reintroduction of the vaginal ultrasound probe).
4. Prep the vagina and cervix with antiseptic.
5. Insert the SIS catheter of choice and inflate the balloon. If the patient has not had a vaginal delivery, the balloon can frequently be inflated in the endocervix instead of in the endometrial cavity, enhancing the evaluation of the lower uterine segment and decreasing the discomfort.
6. Remove the speculum and insert the transvaginal ultrasound transducer into position, taking care not to displace the cannula (see Fig. 144-6).
7. While imaging the uterus, slowly inject 5 to 10 mL of contrast agent. In some cases up to 20 mL of normal saline is necessary.
8. The uterine distention allows evaluation of the cavity for polyps or other disease.
9. Continued injection (especially if Albunex is used) fills the tubes for study; if spillage into the abdomen occurs, patency of at least one fallopian tube is verified.
10. If an endometrial biopsy is indicated and a Sonobiopsy Catheter is used, the biopsy is performed without removing the catheter. The saline is removed and suction applied to the catheter while it is moved in and out and rotated at the same time to obtain an endometrial sample (see Fig. 144-9).

Complications

- Infection rates may be as high as 3% in patients with a prior history of pelvic infection. Antibiotic prophylaxis is indicated in select patients (as mentioned previously) to decrease this risk.
- Tenaculum site bleeding is rare but may require suturing.
- Extravasation of dye into the intravascular space warrants discontinuation of the procedure, especially if an oil-based dye is used (there is a risk of oil pulmonary embolus).
- Granuloma formation after use of an oil-based dye is a rare late complication.
- Perforation of the uterus (or tube with selective cannulization) should prompt discontinuation.
- Rupture of a hydrosalpinx can occur.

Interpretation of Results

Interpretation of results is not reviewed in this chapter, but a few points may be helpful.

- The normal HSG should show (1) a smooth triangular endometrial cavity, (2) a narrow smooth isthmic tube, (3) a progressively enlarging, increasingly convoluted ampullary tube with internal mucosal folds, and (4) spillage into the peritoneal cavity with dispersion between bowel loops.
- The correlation of HSG and laparoscopy may be as poor as 25% false positives and false negatives (the use of selective cannulation may decrease this). *Therefore, absolute statements regarding tubal patency and chances for conception should be avoided.*
- Uterine anomalies are classified according to Buttram and Gibbons, and may also require SIS or laparoscopy to fully define the abnormality. SIS has the advantage over HSG in classifying uterine anomalies, because it can evaluate the myometrium, as well as the endometrial cavity, without the risk of anesthesia or surgery. Ultrasound of the late menstrual endometrium with three-dimensional (3-D) sonography allows better delineation of these uteri (Fig. 144-12).
- The association of renal with uterine developmental anomalies may be as high as 20%; therefore, renal evaluation may be indicated.

The benefits of HSG over SIS are as follows:

- HSG establishes patency of both fallopian tubes.
- HSG can give the appearance of pelvic adhesions if loculations of dye occur in the adnexa.
- HSG can be "therapeutic" and increase pregnancy rates for unknown reasons if oil-based contrast agent is used (see Table 144-1).

The benefits of SIS over HSG are as follows:

- SIS enables visualization of the entire uterus, including the myometrium as well as the endometrial cavity. It is becoming the gold standard for evaluation of uterine anomalies, and can more accurately differentiate between a bicornuate and a septate uterus, for example (see Fig. 144-12). Adding 3-D ultrasound enables further evaluation, as one can reconstruct and rotate the 3-D uterus for additional views (see Fig. 144-12).
- For patients with abnormal uterine bleeding, SIS will reveal global or focal thickening. If there is focal thickening, from a polyp, for example, it can determine anatomic location and size (Fig. 144-13; and see Fig. 144-2).
- SIS is helpful for evaluating fibroids, particularly if they are submucosal or intracavitary. The degree to which a fibroid extends into the endometrial cavity can be established and help to determine if hysteroscopic removal is feasible.

Suppliers

Full contact information is available online at www.expertconsult.com.

Cook Medical, Inc.
CooperSurgical (Ackrad)

CPT/Billing Code

58340 Catheterization and introduction of saline or contrast medium for the HSG or SIS
58345 Transcervical introduction of fallopian tube catheter for diagnosis or re-establishing patency (selective catheterization)
74740 Hysterosalpingography, with radiologic supervision and interpretation
74742 Transcervical introduction of fallopian tube catheter for diagnosis or treatment, radiologic supervision, and interpretation
76830 Transvaginal ultrasound, nonobstetric (with radiologic interpretation)
76831 Saline infustion sonohysterography (SIS) (with radiologic interpretation)
99070 Supplies and materials

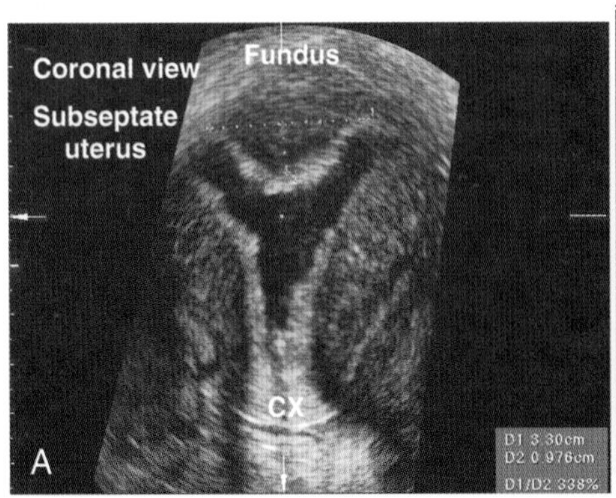

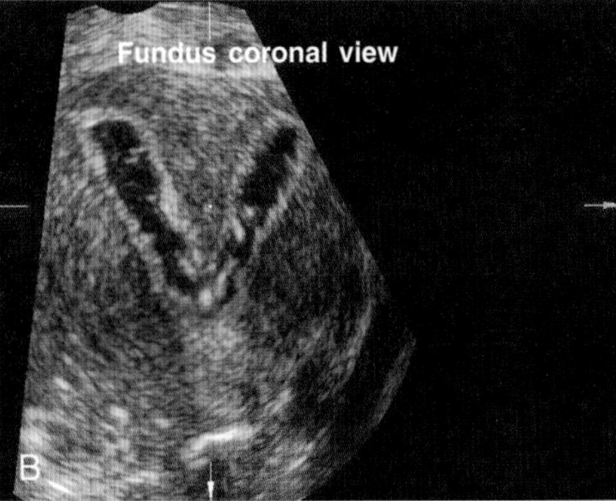

Figure 144-12 Septate uterus diagnosed by saline infusion sonohysterography. **A**, Subseptate uterus. **B**, Large septum. Notice the fundus is intact, not bicornuate, and the septum does not reach the cervix.

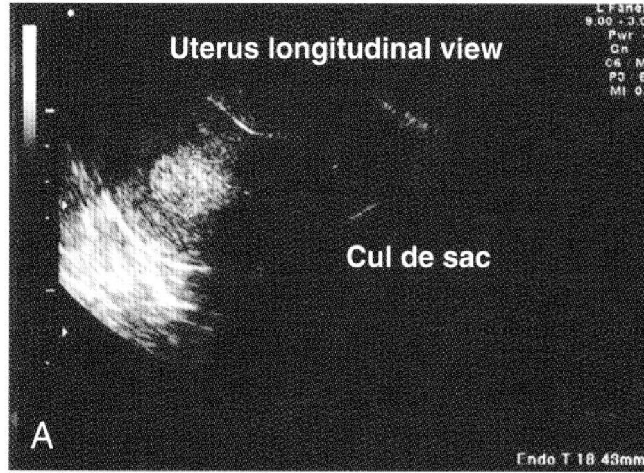

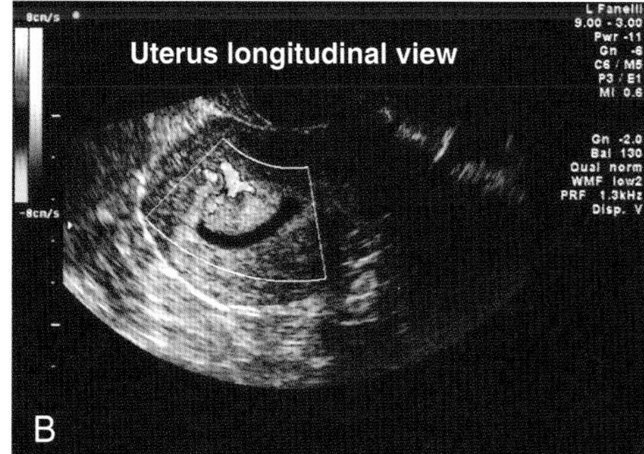

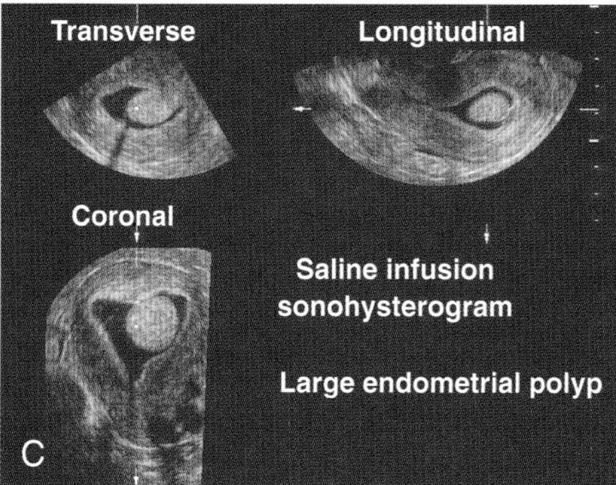

Figure 144-13 Example of a large endometrial polyp. **A**, Transvaginal ultrasound shows a thickened endometrium. **B**, Saline infusion sonohysterography (SIS) with Doppler shows a large polyp with its blood supply. **C**, Three-dimensional reconstruction of this SIS polyp in three orthogonal planes.

ICD-9-CM Diagnostic Codes

V26.21	Fertility testing, fallopian insufflation
V26.22	Aftercare following sterilization reversal
V26.29	Other investigation and testing for procreative management
V26.51	Tubal ligation status
218.9	Uterine leiomyoma, unspecified
621.0	Endometrial polyp
622.5	Incompetence of cervix
626.2	Menorrhagia or menometrorrhagia
626.6	Metrorrhagia
626.7	Postcoital bleeding
626.8	Other abnormal uterine bleeding
627.1	Postmenopausal bleeding
629.81	Habitual aborter without current pregnancy
752.XX*	Congenital anomaly of genital organs

*See ICD-9 code book for more specific codes.

BIBLIOGRAPHY

Alborzi S, Dehbashi S, Khodaee R: Sonohysterosalpingographic screening for infertile patients. Int J Gynaecol Obstet (Ireland) 82:57–62, 2003.

American College of Obstetricians and Gynecologists: Antibiotic prophylaxis for gynecologic procedures. ACOG Practice Bull. No. 104. Obstet Gynecol 113:1180–1189, 2009.

American College of Obstetricians and Gynecologists: Cervical insufficiency. Bull. No. 48. Obstet Gynecol 102:1091–1099, 2003.

American College of Obstetricians and Gynecologists: Management of recurrent early pregnancy loss. Bull. No. 24. Obstet Gynecol 97(2), 2001.

American College of Obstetricians and Gynecologists: Technology assessment in obstetrics and gynecology, No. 3. Saline Infusion Sonohysterography. Obstet Gynecol 102:659–662, 2003.

Buchanan EM, Weinstein LC, Hillson C: Endometrial cancer. Am Fam Physician 80:1075–1080, 2009.

Buttram VC Jr, Gibbons WE: Mullerian anomalies: A proposed classification. Fertil Steril 32:40–46, 1979.

Carson S, Heard MJ: Hysterosalpingography. Female Patient 26:29–34, 2001.

deKroon CD, Jansen FW: Saline infusion sonography in women with abnormal uterine bleeding; an update of recent findings. Curr Opin Obstet Gynecol 18:653–657, 2006.

Hill DA: Abnormal uterine bleeding: Avoid the rush to hysterectomy. J Fam Pract 58:136–142, 2009.

Jansen FW, deKroon DC, van Dongen H, et al: Diagnostic hysteroscopy and saline infusion sonography; prediction of intrauterine polyps and myomas. J Minimal Invasive Gynecol 13:320–324, 2006.

Kempers RD, Cohen J, Haney AF, Younger JB: Fertility and Reproductive Medicine. New York, Elsevier Science, 1998.

Lee C, Salim R, Ofili-Yebovi D, et al: Reproducibility of the measurement of submucous fibroid protrusion into the uterine cavity using three-dimensional saline contrast sonohysterography. Ultrasound Obstet Gynecol 28:837–841, 2006.

Lin PC: Reproductive outcomes in women with uterine anomalies. J Women's Health (Larchmt) 13:33–39, 2004.

Mishell DR Jr: Infertility, Contraception and Reproductive Endocrinology, 3rd ed. Montvale, NJ, Medical Economics Company, 1991.

Noorhasan D, Heard MJ: Gadolinium radiologic contrast is a useful alternative for hysterosalpingography in patients with iodine allergy. Fertil Steril 84:1744, 2005.

Oriel K, Schrager S: Abnormal uterine bleeding, Am Fam Physician 60:1371, 1999.

Rantala M, Makinen J: Tubal patency and fertility outcome after expectant management of ectopic pregnancy. Fertil Steril 68:1043–1046, 1997.

Salim R, Woelfer B, Backos M, et al: Reproducibility of three-dimensional ultrasound diagnosis of congenital uterine anomalies. Ultrasound Obstet Gynecol 21:578–582, 2003.

Simpson WL, Beitia LG, Mester J: Hysterosalpingography: A reemerging study. Radiographics 26:419–431, 2006.

Smith-Bindman R, Kerlikowske K, Feldstein VA, et al: Endovaginal ultrasound to exclude endometrial cancer and other endometrial abnormalities. JAMA 280:1510–1517, 1998.

Soares SR, Barbosa dos Reis MM, Camargos AF: Diagnostic accuracy of sonohysterography, transvaginal sonography, and hysterosalpingography in patients with uterine cavity diseases. Fertil Steril 73:406–411, 2000.

Steiner AZ, Meyer WR, Clark RL, Hartmann KE: Oil-soluble contrast during hysterosalpingography in women with proven tubal patency. Obstet Gynecol 101:109–113, 2003.

Stovall DW: The role of hysterosalpingography in the evaluation of fertility. Am Fam Physician 55:621–628, 1997.

Swart P, Mol BW, van der Veen F, et al: The accuracy of hysterosalpingography in the diagnosis of tubal pathology: A meta-analysis. Fertil Steril 64:486–491, 1995.

Timor-Tritsch IE, Goldstein SR: Ultrasound in Gynecology, 2nd ed. Philadelphia, Elsevier, 2007.

Tsuda H, Kawabata M, Kawabata K, et al: Differences between Occidental and Oriental postmenopausal women in cutoff level of endometrial thickness for endometrial cancer screening by vaginal scan. Am J Obstet 172:1494–1495, 1995.

Watson A, Vanderkerckhove P, Lilford R, et al: A meta-analysis of the therapeutic role of oil soluble contrast media at hysterosalpingography: A surprising result? Fertil Steril 61:470–477, 1994.

Wittmer MH, Famuyide AO, Creedon DJ, Hartman RP: Hysterosalpingography for assessing efficacy of Essure microinsert permanent birth control device. Am J Roentgenol 187:955–958, 2006.

CHAPTER 145

Intrauterine Device Insertion

Ashley Christiani

The intrauterine contraceptive device (IUD) has been in use for over five decades and is the most commonly used method of reversible birth control, with current use estimated at over 160 million women worldwide. In the United States, two types of IUDs are available: the *ParaGard T380A*, a copper IUD containing no hormones that may be left in place for 10 years; and the *Mirena Levonorgestrel Intrauterine System (LNG IUS)*, a progesterone-secreting device that is effective for 5 years. The primary mode of action for IUDs is through inhibition of sperm function (thus preventing ova fertilization) through release of endometrial prostaglandins and leukocytes, enzymes, and copper ions. As a secondary effect, the endometrium is typically rendered inhospitable to embryonic implantation. The LNG IUS has additional effects related to hormonal suppression of the endometrium, thickening of cervical mucus, and inhibition of ovulation.

Although IUDs fell out of favor in the United States many years ago after a reported increase in the incidence of pelvic inflammatory disease (PID) and the highly publicized Dalkon Shield lawsuits, contemporary IUDs have reemerged as an excellent option for reversible, long-term birth control owing to their well-demonstrated safety and potential therapeutic effects (Tables 145-1 and 145-2). Numerous studies demonstrate that the risk of PID and upper genital tract infection is low in properly selected patients. *Features that make the IUD an attractive form of birth control* for many women are an efficacy rate that rivals sterilization, favorable safety profile, ease of use once inserted, and relative lack of systemic effects. *Disadvantages* include altered bleeding patterns (especially in the first few months after IUD placement), the need for a procedure to place and remove the device, cramping and pain at time of insertion (as well as possibility of increased dysmenorrhea with copper IUDs), risk of expulsion of the device (2% to 10% in first year), and the risk of uterine perforation at the time of the procedure (risk is 1 per 1000 in experienced hands).

Indications

- The *ideal* candidate for an IUD is a parous woman in a stable, mutually monogamous relationship, with no sexually transmitted infection (STI) risk factors who is looking for long-term but reversible birth control. The patient should be willing to check for the presence of IUD threads on a monthly basis.
- The IUD is especially appropriate for women who have difficulty remembering to take oral contraceptives or are intolerant to them, who wish to maintain fertility, and who want to avoid systemic hormones.
- Women older than 35 years of age who are smokers and others with increased risk of thromboembolic events, cardiac disease, hypertension, or other contraindications to hormonal therapy are also good candidates.
- Although not listed as an indication by the company, the LNG IUS may be a preferred contraceptive method in women with endometriosis, dysmenorrhea, hypermenorrhea, or significant anemia given that menstrual bleeding and cramping generally decrease significantly within 3 to 6 months. Overall blood loss drops approximately 90% and some 20% of women experience absence of bleeding because of the localized progestin effect. Other possible off-label uses of the LNG IUS are to treat endometrial hyperplasia and for postmenopausal women on hormone replacement who are intolerant to oral progestins. The progesterone component provides endometrial lining suppression, decreasing the risk of endometrial hyperplasia and uterine cancer.
- The IUD is also acceptable for women who were once considered poor candidates for the device, including adolescents, nulliparous women, women in nonmonogamous relationships, and those with a history of PID or ectopic pregnancy. Use of the IUD in these populations is reasonable in the context of appropriate screening and counseling regarding side effects and STI prevention (Table 145-3).
- Emergency contraception may be provided with the copper IUD only.

Contraindications

The World Health Organization (WHO) Medical Eligibility Criteria provide guidance in risk assessment for the IUD and LNG IUS. The full-eligibility screening tool is available online at www.who.int/reproductive-health/publications/mec/iuds.html. Category 4 indicates unacceptable health risk, Category 3 indicates that the risks generally outweigh the benefits, Category 2 indicates the benefits generally outweigh the risks, and Category 1 indicates no restrictions.

World Health Organization Category 4 (Unacceptable Health Risk)

For All IUDs

- Congenital or acquired uterine cavity malformations that would distort the uterine cavity, making it incompatible with IUD insertion. Includes large fibroids, bicornate uterus, abnormally large or small uterine cavity (axial length <6 cm or >9 cm).
- Pregnancy or suspicion of pregnancy (except in the setting of emergency contraception).
- Immediate postseptic abortion or puerperal sepsis.
- Postpartum endometritis or infected abortion within the past 3 months.
- Current or recent STI (within past 3 months).
- Current or recent PID (within past 3 months).
- Known *pelvic* tuberculosis (insertion of IUD may substantially worsen the disease).
- Genital bleeding of unknown cause.
- Known or suspected uterine or cervical neoplasia (awaiting treatment).
- Malignant gestational trophoblastic disease.

TABLE 145-1 Rate of Continuation of Contraceptive Method at 1 Year

Method	Continuing Method after 1 Year
Mirena intrauterine device (IUD)	81%
ParaGard Copper IUD	78%
Oral contraceptive pill	68%
Depo-Provera	56%
Condom	53%
Diaphragm	57%
Spermicide	42%

Data adapted from Trussell J, Kowal D: The essentials of contraception: Efficacy, safety and personal considerations. In Hatcher RA, Trussell J, Stewart F, et al (eds): Contraceptive Technology. New York, Ardent Media, 1998, pp 211–247.

For LNG IUS Only

- Breast cancer (Category 1 for copper IUD).

World Health Organization Category 3 (Risks Generally Outweigh Benefits)

For All IUDs

- Acquired immunodeficiency syndrome (AIDS) or human immunodeficiency virus (HIV) positive. Some studies suggest it is safe to use IUDs in patients with well-controlled HIV infection, but caution is advised.

TABLE 145-2 Annual Failure Rates for Birth Control Methods

Method	"Typical Use" Failure	"Ideal Use" Failure
Sterilization		
Male sterilization	0.15%	0.1%
Female sterilization	0.5%	0.5%
Hormonal Methods		
Implanon	<0.1%	<0.1%
Hormone shot (Depo-Provera)	3%	0.3%
Combined pill (estrogen/progestin) and minipill	8%	0.3%
Intrauterine Devices		
Copper T	0.8%	0.6%
LNG 20	0.1%	0.1%
Barrier Methods		
Male latex condom*	15%	2%
Diaphragm†	16%	6%
Vaginal sponge (no previous births)‡	16%	9%
Vaginal sponge (previous births)‡	32%	26%
Cervical cap (no previous births)†	16%	9%
Cervical cap (previous births)†	32%	26%
Female condom	21%	5%
Spermicide (Gel, Foam, Suppository, Film)	29%	18%
Natural Methods		
Withdrawal	27%	4%
Natural family planning (e.g., calendar, temperature, cervical mucus)	25%	1%–9%
No Method	85%	85%

*Used without spermicide.
†Used with spermicide.
‡Contains spermicide.
Data adapted from Trussell J, Kowal D: The essentials of contraception: Efficacy, safety and personal considerations. In Hatcher RA, Trussell J, Stewart F, et al (eds): Contraceptive Technology. New York, Ardent Media, 1998, pp 211–247.

- Fewer than 4 weeks postpartum (although <48 hours is Category 2 for copper IUDs).
- Multiple current sexual partners, a partner who is not monogamous or is otherwise at increased risk for STIs, including HIV.
- Benign gestational trophoblastic disease.
- Ovarian cancer (contraindication to IUD insertion, but existing IUD may remain in place until time of treatment if contraception needed).

For LNG IUS Only

- Active viral hepatitis (Category 1 for copper IUDs), related to concerns regarding impact of hormonal effect on viral load.
- Active liver disease, including severe decompensated cirrhosis, liver adenoma, or hepatoma (Category 1 for copper IUDs).
- Current deep vein thrombosis (DVT) or pulmonary embolism (Category 1 for copper IUDs).
- History of breast cancer, disease free for 5 years (but Category 1 for copper IUDs).
- Migraines with focal neurologic symptoms for LNG IUS (Category 1 for copper IUDs).

World Health Organization Category 2 (Benefits Generally Outweigh Risks)

- Nulliparity (or, more specifically, nulligravidity). Although the manufacturers list nulliparity as a contraindication to an IUD, many authorities state that any nulliparous woman who feels confident she can avoid STIs should be considered a possible candidate for an IUD. These women should be warned of the risk of PID and of the slightly elevated risk of IUD expulsion. These women may benefit from cervical priming with misoprostol 400 μg or osmotic laminaria before insertion.
- Recent second-trimester abortion (increased risk of expulsion).
- Heavy or prolonged uterine bleeding (includes regular and irregular patterns).
- Minor anatomic anomalies such as cervical stenosis or laceration or small uterine fibroids that do not distort the uterine cavity or significantly interfere with IUD insertion.
- History of PID without current risk factors for STIs but without subsequent pregnancy (note that if patient has had subsequent pregnancy, risk is reduced to Category 1).
- Vaginitis without cervicitis.
- Complicated valvular heart disease.*
- Postpartum less than 48 hours for copper IUD (Category 3 for LNG IUS).

For Copper IUDs Only

- Endometriosis or severe dysmenorrhea, which may worsen symptoms (Category 1 for LNG IUS).
- Thalassemia (Category 1 for LNG IUS).
- Sickle cell disease (Category 1 for LNG IUS).
- Iron-deficiency anemia (Category 1 for LNG IUS).

For LNG IUS Only

- Diabetes (Category 1 for copper IUDs).
- Gallbladder disease (Category 1 for copper IUDs).
- Mild compensated cirrhosis (Category 1 for copper IUDs).
- Obesity (BMI ≥30) (Category 1 for copper IUDs).
- Cardiac risk factors (e.g., smoking, diabetes, advanced age, hypertension, hyperlipidemia, known ischemic heart or vascular disease; Category 1 for copper IUDs).
- History of stroke for LNG IUS (but Category 1 for copper IUDs).
- Recent major surgery with prolonged immobilization (due to DVT risk; Category 1 for copper IUDs).

*Prophylactic antibiotics may be advised for insertion (see Chapter 221, Antibiotic Prophylaxis).

TABLE 145-3 Special Populations and Considerations

Population	Considerations
Adolescents	Despite increased risk of pregnancy, expulsion, and removal for bleeding or pain, the IUD is still more effective than other forms of reversible contraception in this age group, and age should not be the primary determinant of candidacy for the device. Rates of infection are similar to those in adults.
Nulliparous women	Nulliparous women have similar rates of infection and efficacy with IUD use compared to multiparous women; however, higher rates of expulsion and discomfort can limit tolerance for the device.
Fertility	Most women, including nulliparous patients, can expect a rapid return to fertility after discontinuing copper or hormone-releasing IUDs. Contrary to common belief, use of a copper IUD does not appear to increase the risk of tubal infertility in nulligravid women in the absence of chlamydial infection.
Prior ectopic pregnancy	The IUD is *protective* against ectopic pregnancy and is appropriate for women with a history of an ectopic pregnancy.
Insertion after abortion	IUD insertion is safe immediately after spontaneous or induced abortion and is not associated with an increased risk of perforation or infection. Expulsion rates are higher when inserted immediately after second-trimester abortion.
Insertion postpartum	Postpartum insertion appears to have a higher rate of expulsion, but no increase in perforation or infection. Expulsion is less likely when insertion is performed within 10 minutes of delivery of the placenta compared to 1 to 2 days postpartum. If immediate postpartum insertion is not done, then waiting 4 to 6 weeks is advisable. Only the Paragard Cu380A has approval for immediate postpartum insertion. The LNG IUS can be inserted at the 6-week postpartum visit. Breast-feeding women can safely use either device.
Use for emergency contraception	The ParaGard IUD can be inserted within 120 hours of unprotected intercourse for emergency contraception with an efficacy of 98.1% in parous women and 92.4% in nulliparous women.
Valvular heart disease	There is no contraindication to use of the IUD in women with uncomplicated valvular heart disease (including mitral valve prolapse and aortic stenosis). Even in women with complicated valvular heart disease, the benefits an IUD generally outweigh risks. Advantages include avoidance of pregnancy risks and those associated with estrogen-containing contraceptives. Prophylactic antibiotics are recommended at the time of insertion to prevent infective endocarditis in those with high-risk valvular heart disease.
Coexistent gynecologic conditions	There is no contraindication to use of the IUD in women with irregular menses, vaginitis, cervical dysplasia or cervical ectropion, a history of benign ovarian cysts, past PID with a subsequent pregnancy, or prior cesarean delivery. In some situations, such as menorrhagia, use of the LNG IUS is therapeutic. The cause of any abnormal bleeding should be defined prior to insertion. It is best to evaluate significant abnormal Pap smears prior to insertion since performing a LEEP procedure can be difficult if not impossible to do with the strings in place.
Coexistent chronic medical conditions	There is no contraindication to use of the copper IUD in women with diabetes mellitus, cardiovascular disease, migraine headaches, breast cancer or benign breast disease, smoking, obesity, epilepsy, or liver, gallbladder, or thyroid disease. There is no increased risk of pelvic infection in women with diabetes mellitus. Neither the copper IUD nor LNG IUS adversely affects glycemic control in diabetic patients.
Immunocompromise	IUD use does not enhance the risk of HIV acquisition over that in users of other contraceptives. Limited data suggest no increased risk of PID in HIV-positive IUD users. In conjunction with appropriate condom use, the IUD may be safely used in women with or at risk for HIV infection. However, for women at risk of HIV and other sexually transmitted infections, hormonal contraception may be preferable due to protection against ascending infections.
Cancer	The copper IUD use has been associated with lower risks of endometrial and cervical cancer. The LNG IUS likely reduces the risk of endometrial cancer but may increase risk of breast cancer.
Menopausal women	An IUD inserted for contraception should be removed one year after the last menstrual period in menopausal women.

HIV, human immunodeficiency virus; LEEP, loop electrosurgical excision procedure; PID, pelvic inflammatory disease.

- Migraines (Category 1 for copper IUDs).
- Cervical intraepithelial neoplasia (Category 1 for copper IUDs).

Other Contraindications

- Allergy to copper (for ParaGard); hypersensitivity to any component of the IUD, including levonorgestrel, silicone, or polyethylene; or any past history of IUD intolerance.
- Wilson's disease (for ParaGard).
- Desire for short-term contraceptive use (may be more cost effective to use any other method).

Equipment

- The desired prepackaged IUD (ParaGard, LNG IUS; Fig. 145-1)
- Speculum
- Sterile basin with cotton balls moistened with a water-based antiseptic, such as povidone–iodine (Betadine) or chlorhexidine gluconate
- Ring forceps
- Cervical tenaculum
- Uterine sound

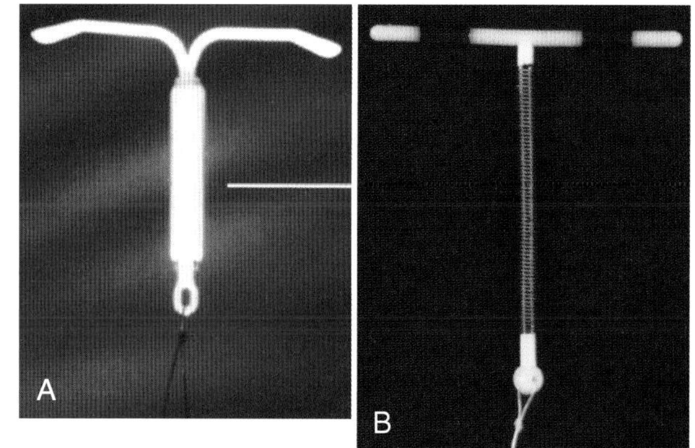

Figure 145-1 Available intrauterine devices. **A,** Mirena LNG IUS. **B,** ParaGard T380A. (A, Courtesy of Berlex Laboratories, Wayne, NJ. **B,** Courtesy of Ortho-McNeil Pharmaceutical, Inc., Raritan, NJ.)

- Nonsterile gloves (for bimanual examination before insertion procedure)
- Sterile gloves (for IUD insertion phase)
- Sterile towel to cover tray
- Long suture scissors (to cut IUD threads after insertion)

Optional Equipment

- Nonsteroidal anti-inflammatory drug (NSAID), to be taken before procedure (e.g., 800 mg ibuprofen).
- Although not generally necessary, local anesthetic may be helpful in some patients. Lidocaine 2% without epinephrine may be used to perform a paracervical or submucosal block (additional equipment includes 10-mL syringe, needle extender with a 22-gauge long needle, Monsel's solution, and cotton-tipped swabs; see Chapter 149, Loop Electrosurgical Excision Procedure for Treating Cervical Intraepithelial Neoplasia, and Chapter 173, Paracervical Block, for submucosal injection technique).
- Cervical dilators (see Chapter 136, Cervical Stenosis and Cervical Dilation).

Preprocedure Patient Preparation

A separate office visit for patient counseling, consent, and preparation is advised before the IUD insertion visit. However, current guidelines suggest that the patient may be counseled, evaluated, and have the IUD inserted, if appropriate, on the first visit. A separate visit allows the patient the opportunity to review the material, consider her contraceptive options, ask questions, examine sample IUDs, and plan for the procedure. This visit also provides the clinician with the opportunity to assess potential risks and benefits of IUD insertion, provide counseling, address common myths and misconceptions regarding the device (Table 145-4), and perform the screening evaluation. An insertion date is more easily planned and scheduled at another time.

Patient Counseling and Consent

Federal guidelines require that patients be given an IUD patient information brochure as part of the consent process before IUD insertion. Brochures are provided through the manufacturers of ParaGard and the Mirena LNG IUS (see the "Suppliers" section). These brochures are excellent resources and can serve as consent documents when the patient reviews the checklists and signs the forms. The clinician should confirm that the patient understands her *risks, benefits, and alternatives* to IUD placement and the common side effects experienced with this form of contraception. The clinician should advise of the *cramping and discomfort* associated with IUD insertion as well as removal and the potential for *transient nausea, dizziness, or faintness during and immediately after the procedure*.

It is common to have *mild spotting and cramping* for a few days after the procedure and up to 8 weeks after insertion of IUDs, but if these symptoms are severe or the discomfort is not alleviated with over-the-counter analgesics, the patient will need medical evaluation.

Patients must be willing to *check for the presence of IUD threads* after the first menstrual period and each month thereafter. If the threads cannot be found or seem to be migrating upward, the patient must notify her physician. Although patients may expect reliable birth control immediately after IUD insertion, some authorities recommend *1 to 2 weeks of pelvic rest* after the procedure to minimize risk of infection and other complications. The importance of a mutually monogamous relationship should be emphasized with the explanation that *any new partners will increase the risk of PID* while the IUD is in place. Although the IUD has *not* been shown to increase risk of cervical dysplasia, women using this form of contraception may be less likely to present for routine gynecologic examinations and should be specifically instructed to *continue regularly scheduled pelvic examinations and Pap smears*. After insertion, the patient should be given an identification card or form with the name and design of her IUD, the date of insertion and recommended date for removal, and the date of her follow-up appointment.

Screening Evaluation

Before IUD insertion, a Pap smear (within 6 months) and pelvic examination along with any appropriate STI screening should be performed and the results documented as negative. The pelvic examination should include assessment of uterine size and position, examination for signs of cervicitis or vaginitis, and evaluation of the general morphology of the cervix and os, including signs of cervical stenosis.

Timing of Procedure

Because of higher risk of expulsion during menses (5% risk of expulsion with insertion during the first 5 days of the menstrual cycle, compared with 2% risk with luteal-phase insertions), and slightly higher risk of postinsertion pain or bleeding with luteal-phase insertions, the optimal timing is the late follicular phase (day 5 to 10 of cycle). However, the IUD may be inserted at any time provided the patient is consistently using a reliable method of contraception, has been abstinent since the last menses, or is within 5 days of a single act of unprotected intercourse and desires emergency contraception with a copper IUD.

Pretreatment

Patients should consider taking ibuprofen (600 to 800 mg) or other NSAID 45 to 60 minutes before IUD insertion to minimize cramping and discomfort during the procedure. Local anesthetic is usually

TABLE 145-4 Myths and Misconceptions about IUDs

Myth	Fact
IUDs are abortifacients.	IUDs prevent fertilization and thus are true contraceptives.
IUDs increase the risk of ectopic pregnancy.	IUDs significantly reduce a woman's risk of an ectopic pregnancy because the IUD prevents all types of pregnancies. Should a pregnancy occur with an IUD in place, the ratio of ectopic to intrauterine pregnancies may be increased.
IUDs expose the provider to medoicolegal risk.	In past decades, product liability suits against manufacturers alleged inherently unsafe products or failure to warn of risks. Today, IUDs have been judged safe by the U.S. Food and Drug Administration. Package inserts and patient brochures provide extensive information about risks and benefits. Hence, litigation related to IUDs has virtually disappeared.
IUDs increase the risk of PID.	The IUD itself appears to have no effect on the risk of upper genital tract infection. Rather, the insertion process carries a small, transient risk in some women. The risk of PID in appropriately selected IUD candidates is so small that prophylactic antibiotics are not warranted.

PID, pelvic inflammatory disease.

From Stewart F, Gary K: Intrauterine devices (IUDs). Hatcher RA, Trussell J, Stewart F, et al (eds): Contraceptive Technology. New York, Ardent Media, 1998, pp 511–543.

not necessary but may be helpful in the apprehensive patient, particularly those at risk for significant discomfort (nulliparas, those requiring cervical dilation, those with history of pain with prior cervical procedures) or vasovagal reaction. If desired, use lidocaine 1% to 2% without epinephrine to perform a paracervical or submucosal block (see Chapter 149, Loop Electrosurgical Excision Procedure for Treating Cervical Intraepithelial Neoplasia, and Chapter 173, Paracervical Block, for the submucosal injection technique). Some clinicians advocate the use of topical benzocaine spray (e.g., Hurricaine); however, studies with patients undergoing endometrial biopsy failed to demonstrate a pain control benefit compared with placebo. Per current American College of Obstetricians and Gynecologists (ACOG) and American Heart Association (AHA) guidelines, routine antibiotic prophylaxis for PID prevention and for bacterial endocarditis is not recommended (see Chapter 221, Antibiotic Prophylaxis).

Technique

The IUD insertion technique described here provides general guidelines for the procedure. For further details, the clinician should refer to the physician insert provided by each manufacturer in the respective packaging.

Initial Steps (Both IUDs)

1. Ensure that the patient understands the method of and alternatives to IUD placement and that the consent form has been signed. Confirm that the patient is still a candidate for the IUD (i.e., is in a stable, monogamous relationship and has not developed any contraindications as listed previously). Confirm a negative Pap smear result.
2. Confirm a negative pregnancy test if there is any question of pregnancy.
3. Reassess the need for an NSAID, antibiotic prophylaxis (not routinely recommended), heating pad (low to medium heat) for the patient's abdomen, or other special accommodations.
4. Perform a bimanual pelvic examination to reconfirm the size, position, consistency, and mobility of the uterus and to screen for the presence of any signs or symptoms of acute pelvic infection. A speculum examination may be repeated at this time if desired.
5. Change to sterile gloves and observe sterile technique from this point on in the procedure.
6. Prepare a sterile field containing the supplies discussed previously. Request an assistant, if desired.
7. With the patient in the lithotomy position, insert a warm, sterile speculum into the vagina. The cervix should be well visualized and the os centered in the midline.
8. Using the ring forceps, cleanse the cervix with the antiseptic-soaked cotton balls.
9. Perform a paracervical (see Chapter 173, Paracervical Block) or submucosal block if desired.
10. Clamp a single-tooth tenaculum to the anterior lip of the cervix. It may be helpful to ask the patient to cough as you apply the device or to inject 1 to 2 mL of lidocaine into the tenaculum site before placement. Apply gentle downward traction on the tenaculum to correct for any angulation and to stabilize the cervix.
11. Gently and slowly sound the uterus. Careful technique will decrease the patient's discomfort and the risk of perforation, laceration, and other complications. The uterine depth should be between 6.5 and 8.5 cm. Do not place an IUD if the depth is outside the normal range (there is an increased risk of

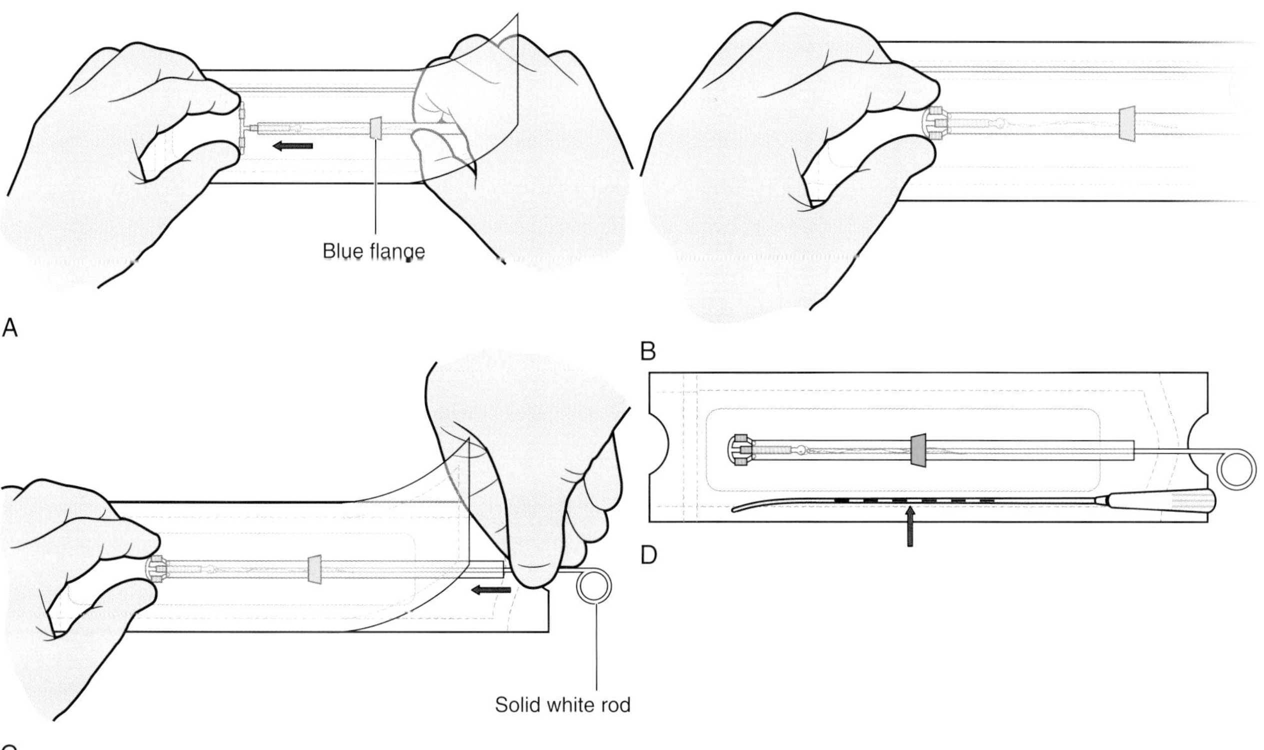

Figure 145-2 Loading the ParaGard intrauterine device (IUD) using the "no-touch" technique just before insertion. **A,** After the bimanual examination and antiseptic solution preparation and after the uterus has been sounded, the IUD is inserted into the hollow inserter tube. **B,** The arms are bent down and inserted just far enough to retain them in the tube. **C,** The solid white inserter rod is placed into the hollow insertion tube from the other end so that it just touches the bottom of the vertical arm of the IUD. **D,** The blue flange is set so that the distance from the tip of the IUD to the flange is the same distance as the depth of the uterus (as determined by the uterine sound; *red arrow*). (Redrawn from Pfenninger JL: Techniques for inserting an IUD. Fam Pract Recertification 14:131–138, 1992.)

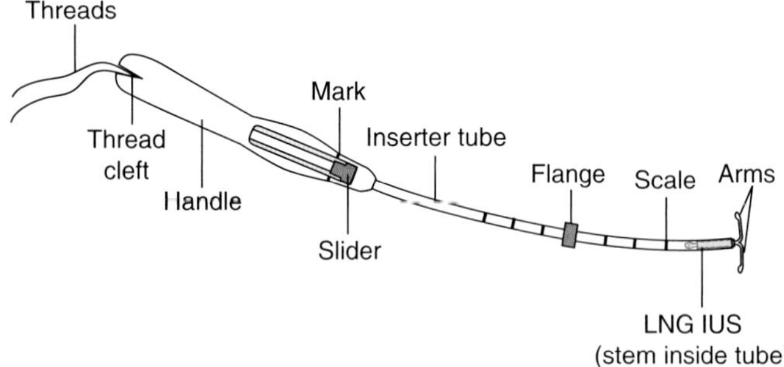

Figure 145-3 Mirena Levonorgestrel Intrauterine System (LNG IUS) and inserter. (Redrawn from Berlex Laboratories, Wayne, NJ.)

complications in this setting). If the sound cannot be inserted because of stenosis, dilate the cervix (see Chapter 136, Cervical Stenosis and Cervical Dilation).

12. Prepare the IUD/IUS for insertion. The two units are totally different. The *inserter tube* refers to the hollow cylinder in which the IUD fits. It may be possible to load the ParaGard IUD into the inserter while it is still in the original packaging. This is referred to as the "no-touch technique" and is described in the packaging information of IUDs that provide this loading option (Fig. 145-2). Alternatively, sterile gloves are used to "load" the unit by folding the arms down and inserting them in the inserter tube. The inserter "rod" for the ParaGard refers to the solid trocar that fits inside the inserter tube. Figure 145-3 is a graphic depiction of the Mirena IUS. Loading this system is quite different and will be shown as part of the procedure in Figure 145-5.
13. Insert the chosen IUD, using the appropriate technique for the ParaGard or LNG IUS.

ParaGard Insertion

After following the previous initial steps, insert the ParaGard IUD as follows (Fig. 145-4):

1. Make certain that the horizontal arms of the IUD are parallel to the horizontal orientation of the blue flange to ensure proper placement in the uterus. Slide the blue flange so it is the same distance from the tip of the inserter tube as the depth the uterus sounded, maintaining the horizontal orientation.
2. Grasping with the single-tooth tenaculum, insert the IUD inserter unit into the cervical canal up to the flange (see Fig. 145-4A). You may wish to have an assistant hold the tenaculum. With the solid white rod in your dominant hand, use the other hand to *withdraw* the clear plastic inserter tube toward you approximately 2 cm *as the white rod is held in place* (see Fig. 145-4B). This maneuver will allow the IUD to "fall" into place. Pushing in on the solid rod could cause a perforation. A small "pop" can often be felt as the IUD unfolds.
3. Now, *while holding the white rod stable*, gently and slowly *push the hollow tube inserter toward the fundus* until resistance is felt to allow "high placement" of the IUD (see Fig. 145-4C[1]). Fundal placement of the IUD decreases the risk of expulsion, accidental pregnancy, and other complications. *Withdraw the solid rod only* (see Fig. 145-4C[2]). *Do not* withdraw the tube before removing the rod first. The strings are inside the tube and compressed against the tube by the rod. Pulling both out at the same time could immediately pull out the IUD.
4. Withdraw the insertion tube (see Fig. 145-4D).
5. Complete the procedure as noted in the "Completion of Procedure" section.

LNG IUS Insertion

After following the initial steps provided previously, insert the LNG IUS (Mirena) as follows (Fig. 145-5):

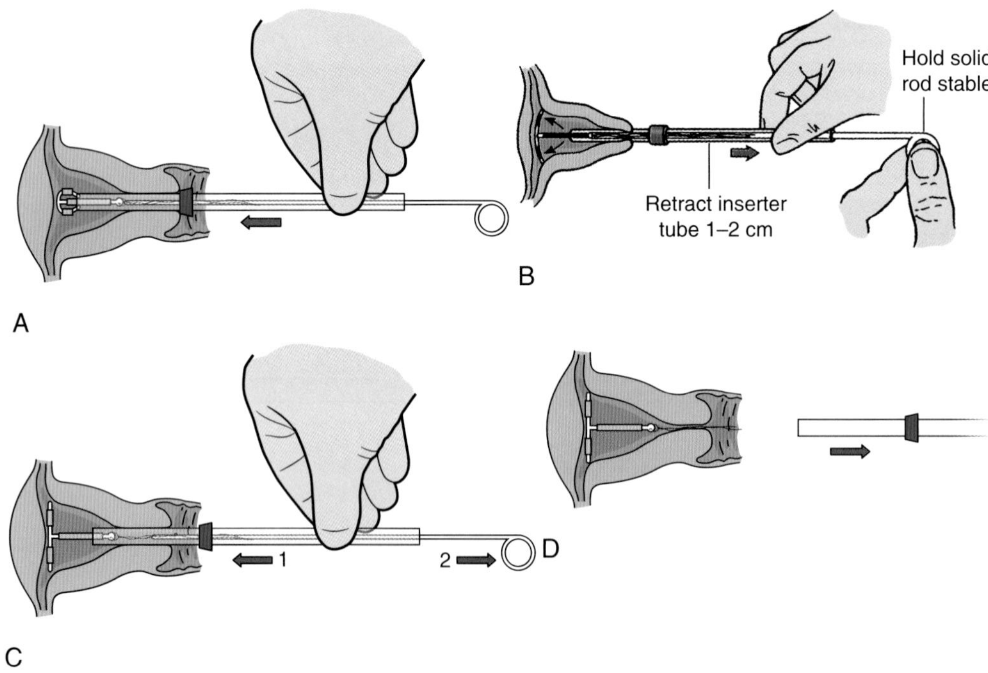

Figure 145-4 Inserting the ParaGard intrauterine device (IUD). **A,** The single-tooth tenaculum is applied to stabilize the cervix, and the IUD–inserter unit is placed into the cervical canal up to the flange. **B,** While an assistant holds the tenaculum, the clinician holds the solid white rod stable in the dominant hand and withdraws the insertion tube approximately 2 cm. **C,** *1,* The inserting tube (with the rod held stable and still in place) is gently advanced to ensure high placement of IUD; 2, the *solid inserting rod* is withdrawn while holding the *tube* steady. **D,** The insertion tube is withdrawn and the threads are cut, ensuring adequate length. (Redrawn from Pfenninger JL: Techniques for inserting an IUD. Fam Pract Recertification 14:131–138, 1992.)

Figure 145-5 Loading and inserting the Mirena Levonorgestrel Intrauterine System (LNG IUS) using sterile glove technique. **A** and **B,** The package is opened. The LNG IUS is prepared for insertion. **C,** The upper end of the flange is set at the uterine depth found with sounding. **D,** The LNG IUS is inserted with the flange 1.5 to 2 cm from the ectocervix. **E,** The arms are released by pulling the slider back to the mark. **F,** For fundal positioning, the clinician holds the slider in position at the mark and pushes the inserter gently inward until the flange touches the cervix. The LNG IUS should now be in the fundal position. **G,** Finally, the LNG IUS is released by pulling the slider all the way back, which releases the strings. The insertion tube is then removed. Cut the strings to leave 2 to 3 cm visible outside the cervix. (Courtesy of the Association of Reproductive Health Professionals, Ithaca, NY, copyright 2000, used by permission. B *(center)*, Redrawn from Association of Reproductive Health Professionals, Ithaca, NY.)

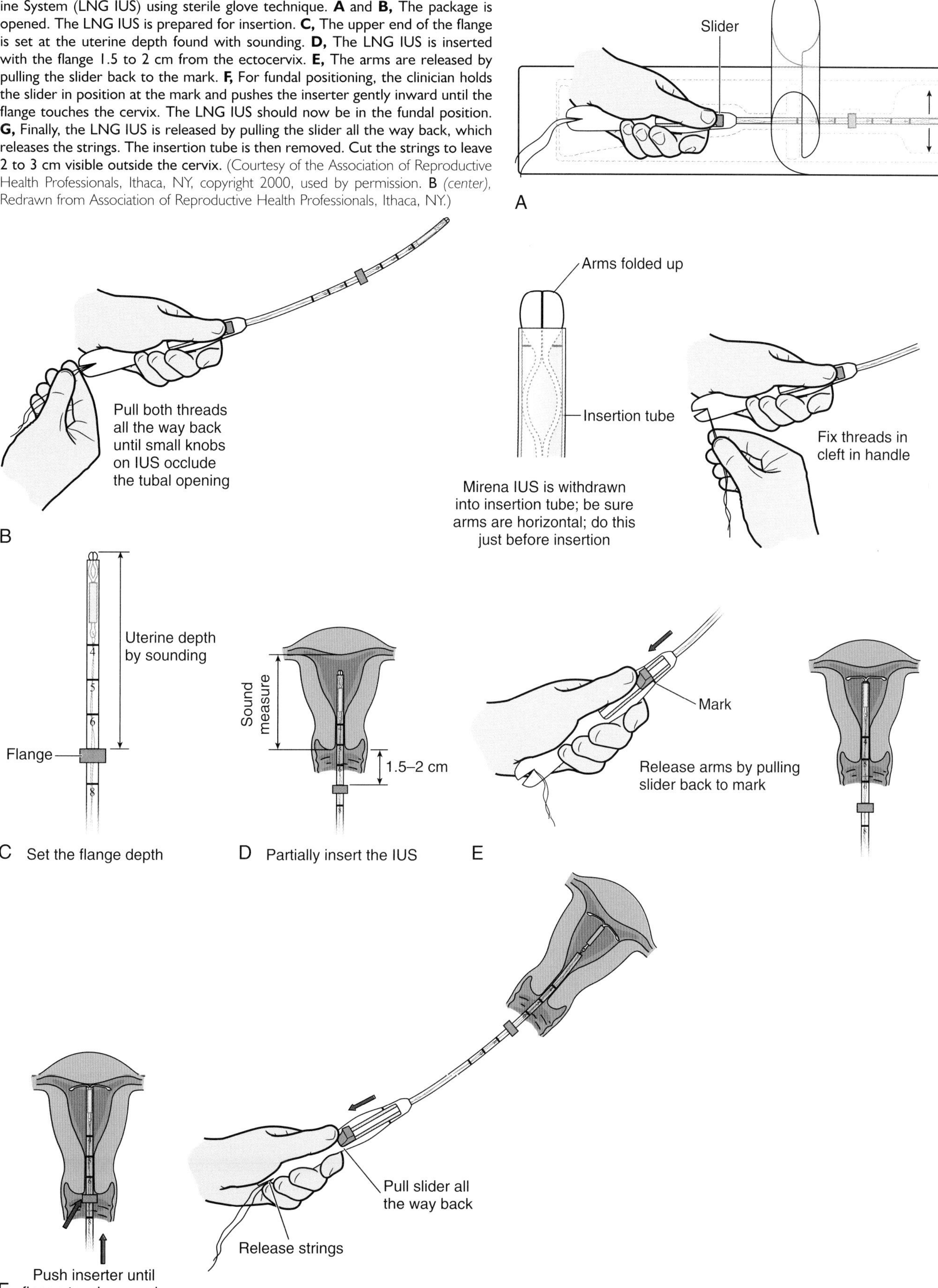

1. After opening the sterile package, release the threads, making sure the slider is in furthest position from you. Use the sterile packaging to rotate the arms of the system to be horizontal when the lettering on the handle is facing upward (see Fig. 145-5A).
2. Load the LNG IUS for insertion. Pull on both threads to draw the LNG IUS into the insertion tube. The arms will fold upward (the ParaGard arms fold down). The knobs at the ends of the arms should occlude the open end of the inserter. Fix the threads tightly in the cleft at the near end of the inserter shaft (see Fig. 145-5B).
3. Set the upper end of the flange at the uterine depth measured previously (see Fig. 145-5C).
4. Hold the slider firmly with the forefinger or thumb in the furthermost position, and advance the inserter into the cervical canal until the flange is about *1.5 to 2 cm from the cervix. This is a significant difference from the method of inserting the ParaGard.* Keeping the flange 1.5 to 2 cm away from the cervical os allows sufficient space for the arms to open within the uterus (see Fig. 145-5D).
5. While holding the inserter steady, release the arms of the LNG IUS by pulling the slider back until it reaches the mark (i.e., raised horizontal line; see Fig. 145-5E).
6. Stabilize the slider in the current position and push the inserter gently inward until the flange now touches the cervix. The LNG IUS should now be in the fundal position (see Fig. 145-5F).
7. Holding the inserter rod steady, release the LNG IUS by pulling the slider all the way back. The threads will be released automatically (see Fig. 145-5G). Remove the inserter carefully from the uterus.
8. Complete the procedure as noted in the next section.

Completion of Procedure

1. After insertion, the IUD should remain within the uterine cavity. If any portion of the device is visible or protruding from the endocervical canal, the device should be removed by pulling the string, and then a sterile device from a new package should be used.
2. After the inserter is removed from the uterus, cut the IUD threads to a length of 2 to 3 cm beyond the os (Fig. 145-6). It is better to leave the threads too long than too short because they can be shortened on subsequent visits if necessary and short threads may be irritating or painful for a male partner.
3. Remove the tenaculum and observe the site for bleeding. If bleeding is seen, apply pressure or Monsel's solution to achieve hemostasis.
4. Remove the speculum.
5. Provide postprocedure counseling to the patient and arrange a follow-up appointment for an IUD and symptom check after the first postinsertion menses.
6. Complete the encounter form (Fig. 145-7) or dictate a complete note.

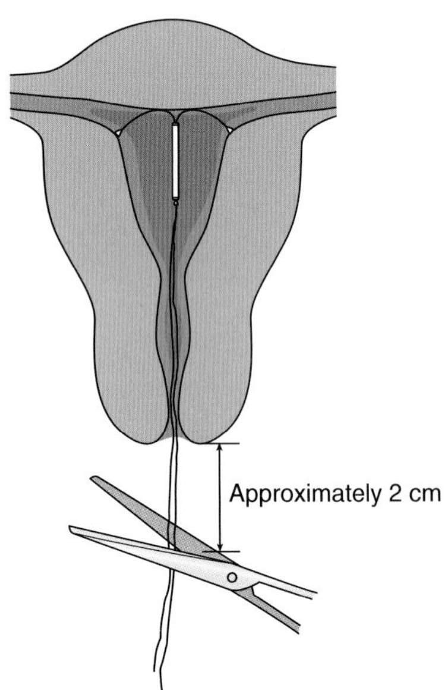

Figure 145-6 Threads are cut (leaving about 2 to 3 cm visible outside the cervix). (Redrawn from Berlex Laboratories, Wayne, NJ.)

Common Errors

- Cutting the strings too short
- Device slips back out during the insertion process
- Contaminating the IUD
- Not doing a pelvic examination and determining the uterine position
- Not using a tenaculum to straighten the cervical angle
- The last common error that can cause a significant problem is pushing in on the inserter rod (for the ParaGard) instead of pulling back on the inserter tube (see Fig. 145-4B) to "release" the IUD. Pushing in on the rod could cause a perforation.

Short Strings

It is better to cut the strings too long than to risk cutting them too short. Short strings may make it difficult for the patient to check her strings and can cause discomfort to her partner (see later). If the strings are accidentally cut too short (<2 cm), the clinician should consider inserting a new device. If the patient is able to reach the strings and prefers to keep the IUD in place, she can be monitored with instructions to return for any difficulty or complications.

Contamination of the IUD

Contamination of the device most commonly occurs when the IUD or the distal tip of the insertion tube is touched with a nonsterile hand during the preparation or insertion process. If this occurs, a new package must be opened and the procedure repeated with a sterile device. The contaminated IUDs may be returned to the manufacturer for refund.

Complications

Placement of an IUD is a relatively safe procedure with significantly less morbidity and mortality than pregnancy and delivery. The IUD itself is generally well tolerated, as demonstrated by the 1-year continuation rate for this birth control method compared with other methods. Nonetheless, it is important to counsel patients on the risk of complications and common side effects of the IUD, which are discussed in the following sections.

Vasovagal Reaction

Some women experience vasovagal reactions with instrumentation of the cervix or immediately after insertion. Such reactions may include lightheadedness, hypotension, bradycardia, nausea, or even syncope. If such symptoms occur, the patient should be kept in the supine position and given supportive care until the reaction resolves. Rarely do such symptoms persist. In severe cases a paracervical block may be done (or repeated) or atropine (0.4 to 0.6) can be given intramuscularly or intravenously. Occasionally the IUD may need to be removed.

IUD ENCOUNTER FORM

Patient to fill out:

Name ____________________ Date ________________

Birth date ____________________ Age ________________

Number of pregnancies ____________ Miscarriages or abortions ________

Current contraceptive method ________________________

Have you had:

A pregnancy in your tubes?	Y N	Are you allergic to copper?	Y N
Infection in your tubes?	Y N	How long is your usual period?	______ days
Any venereal disease?	Y N	Have you ever had a low blood count?	Y N
An IUD before?	Y N	Number of lifetime sexual partners? ________	
Leukemia, AIDS, heart murmur?	Y N	Current number of sexual partners? ________	
Rheumatic fever, diabetes?	Y N	Last Pap smear: Date ______ Result ______	
Are you on steroids?	Y N	Did you read and understand the company handout?	Y N

For the doctor:

Company handout explained? Y N

Impression ____________

Plan ____________

PMH: PMI: ____________

All: ____________

Meds: ____________

Surgeries: ____________

Procedure/(Insertion): Date ____________

LMP ____________

Pap: Y N

Type of IUD: ParaGard T380A

Mirena IUS

Bimanual: uterus: adnexa:

Prep with tenaculum Y N

Sound cm

Insertion:

Patient tolerance:

Complications:

Reinforce: bleeding, pregnancy, infection, pain, expulsion

Remove on: ____________

Given new company handout? Y N

Given card? Y N

Follow-up: ____________

____

Physician Signature

cc: ____________________

Figure 145-7 Sample intrauterine device encounter form. (From The Medical Procedures Center, PC, Midland, Mich.)

Perforation

Perforation of the uterus or cervix is extremely rare (<0.1%). It generally occurs at the time of uterine sounding or occasionally with insertion. Perforation should be suspected if the sound enters the uterine cavity more than 12 cm and uterine palpation has indicated a normal size. The perforation itself is usually painless and often occurs in the setting of forceful pressure through a tight cervical os. Should perforation be suspected, the clinician should pull out the IUD (if already inserted) and observe the patient for 30 minutes. If stable, the patient can be discharged and told to report any signs of infection, abdominal pain, rapid pulse, or shortness of breath. Usually there is an uncomplicated resolution, and insertion can be attempted again in 6 to 8 weeks (no prophylactic antibiotics are indicated). Unstable patients may require immediate surgical consultation.

Uterine Bleeding and Cramping

Intrauterine devices may cause abdominal or low back pain and cramping, as well as irregular uterine bleeding, particularly in the first 3 months of use. Some women will have heavier bleeding and increased dysmenorrhea with the IUD, particularly when using the ParaGard. Conversely, approximately 20% of women using the Mirena LNG IUS will cease having periods after 3 to 6 months. Menstruation returns rapidly once the device is removed.

Spontaneous Expulsion

Although uncommon, most IUD expulsions occur within the first 6 months after insertion. The patient may experience cramping, pain, vaginal discharge, abnormal vaginal spotting, dyspareunia, or lengthening of the IUD strings. However, expulsion may be asymptomatic. For this reason the patient should be instructed to check for IUD strings each month after menstruation. Occasionally the IUD will become lodged in the cervical os, which may cause cramping and discomfort. In this case, the IUD should be removed and a new one may be placed if desired. If an IUD is spontaneously passed, is removed because of a complication, or becomes contaminated during the insertion process, it may be returned to the company for a free replacement.

Embedded or Lost Intrauterine Device String

Missing strings may indicate unsuspected perforation or spontaneous expulsion (see previous section), or migration of the IUD into the endometrial cavity. If the strings are not visible in the os, the clinician should first rule out pregnancy. Ultrasonography may quickly confirm intrauterine location. If the IUD is in place, nothing needs to be done. If the patient desires removal of an IUD whose strings are not visible in the os, special procedures may assist in recovering the IUD (see Chapter 146, Intrauterine Device Removal). Occasionally the IUD may become embedded in the uterine lining, which complicates removal and may necessitate cervical dilation and instrumentation to remove the device.

Partner Discomfort (due to IUD Strings)

The IUD strings should be cut to a length of 2 to 3 cm from the external os. It is preferable to leave the strings slightly too long than to risk trimming them too short, which may cause irritation to the partner during intercourse. If the partner complains of penile discomfort (a barblike sensation), the strings can be trimmed further, or the device may need to be replaced. Strings that are too long may be trimmed. Strings that lengthen over time may be a sign of impending expulsion.

Contraception Failure

Although rare (<1%), pregnancy is possible, even with the IUD in place. In this event, the patient must immediately be assessed for ectopic pregnancy. Although patients with IUDs do not have a higher ectopic pregnancy rate (the risk is actually lower), if pregnancy does occur, nearly 50% will be extrauterine. The IUD should be promptly removed if the woman is in the early stages of pregnancy regardless of whether she desires to continue the pregnancy. Although there is a risk of inducing abortion with removal of an IUD, if it is left in place there is a significant risk of premature labor, sepsis, and spontaneous abortion. Whether the IUD is removed or left in place, there is no increased risk of fetal anomalies.

Pelvic Inflammatory Disease

The risk of PID is elevated only the first 20 days after IUD insertion or in the setting of exposure to a new sexual partner. If the clinician suspects PID, it should be promptly treated according to Centers for Disease Control and Prevention (CDC) guidelines, with initiation of antibiotics before IUD removal.* A new IUD may be placed 3 months after resolution of the infection. However, because of the risk of recurrent STIs and PID, other contraceptive options should be strongly considered.

Actinomyces

Actinomyces is an anaerobic, gram-positive bacterium. It is more frequently found in IUD users (on routine Pap smear) and is generally asymptomatic. Most authorities recommend removal of the device and antibiotic treatment only in the presence of clinical symptoms. Rarely do the bacteria cause a systemic problem in healthy individuals, but if present or past infection is known, it is best not to insert the IUD because *Actinomyces* preferentially grows on foreign bodies.

Ovarian Cysts

Ovarian cysts may develop in patients using the Mirena LNG IUS because of hormonal stimulation. Enlarged follicles are seen in about 12% of LNG IUS users. Most of the cysts are asymptomatic and self-limiting, but on occasion they may cause pelvic pain or dyspareunia.

Hormonal Side Effects and Use during Lactation

Hormone-containing IUDs, such as the LNG IUS, may have side effects such as mood changes, acne, headache, breast tenderness, dysmenorrhea, nervousness, vaginitis, hypertension, and nausea. Weight gain is usually not a problem. Other forms of contraception may be preferable for lactating women.

Pap Smears and Cervical Dysplasia

Although no known association has been shown between cervical dysplasia and use of the IUD, it is essential that the Pap smear be normal before insertion. Should the patient present with abnormality on her Pap smear, the IUD may complicate the process of cervical and endocervical sampling and procedures such as the loop electrosurgical excision procedure or conization. Because patients using IUDs do not require annual renewal of their contraception, they are at greater risk of neglecting their regular Pap smears. When treating these patients, the clinician should emphasize that they must return for their routine Pap smear and pelvic examinations.

POSTPROCEDURE PATIENT EDUCATION

- Give the patient a copy of the IUD handout provided by the manufacturer, including the name and design, the date of insertion, and recommended date for removal. Discuss the following:
  - The patient should check for the presence of IUD strings after each menstruation.
  - The patient should be clear on the signs and symptoms of IUD expulsion, infection, and other possible complications. Instruct her to return for fever, worsening pelvic or abdominal pain, foul-smelling or abnormal vaginal discharge, excessive bleeding (other than spotting for a few months), pain with intercourse, prolonged amenorrhea, any type of genital lesions, or signs of STI or pregnancy.

*WHO guidelines state that in resource-poor settings, it is an option to treat mild to moderate PID without removal of the device.

- Reiterate that the IUD will not protect her from infection from HIV, herpes simplex virus, human papillomavirus, *Chlamydia*, gonorrhea, or any other STI and she must take precautions to avoid these infections.
- A routine follow-up examination to check for strings and review symptoms is scheduled for 1 to 3 months. The IUD is removed when the patient desires pregnancy or as indicated by the manufacturer. The ParaGard IUD should be replaced after 10 years and the Mirena LNG IUS should be replaced after 5 years.

CONCLUSION

The safety issues and misconceptions that plagued IUDs in the past have largely been resolved, offering patients an excellent option for long-term, reversible contraception. IUDs have high efficacy; require little maintenance; provide long-term, yet reversible, contraception; and are cheaper than birth control pills over a 5-year period. The LNG IUS offers the benefit of decreased vaginal bleeding and may be used in hormone replacement to protect against uterine malignancy and hyperplasia. Conversely, the copper IUD offers the potential advantage of being hormone free.

CPT/BILLING CODES

58300 Insertion of intrauterine device (IUD), not including device
58301 Removal of IUD
J7300 Charge for cost of copper IUD (ParaGard T380A)
J7302 Charge cost Levonorgestrel-Releasing Intrauterine System (Mirena)

ICD-9-CM DIAGNOSTIC CODES

V25.1 Encounter of contraceptive management; insertion of intrauterine contraceptive device
V25.42 Intrauterine contraceptive device; checking, reinsertion, or removal of intrauterine device

SUPPLIERS

(See contact information online at www.expertconsult.com.)

NOTE: Most companies will provide videotapes and training models for their devices.

Mirena
Bayer Healthcare Pharmaceuticals, Inc.

ParaGard T380A
Duramed Pharmaceuticals, Inc.

BIBLIOGRAPHY

American College of Obstetricians and Gynecologists: Antibiotic prophylaxis for gynecologic procedures. Practice Bulletin no. 104. Obstet Gynecol 113:1180–1189, 2009.

Boutet G: Levonorgestrel-releasing intrauterine device (Mirena) and breast cancer: What do we learn from literature for clinical practice? [in French]. Gynecol Obstet Fertil 34:1015–1023, 2006.

Darney PD: Time to pardon the IUD? N Engl J Med 345:608–610, 2001.

Einarsson JI, Henao G, Young AE: Topical analgesia for endometrial biopsy: A randomized controlled trial. Obstet Gynecol 106:128–130, 2005.

Fortney JA, Feldblum PJ, Raymond EG: Intrauterine devices: The best long-term contraceptive method? J Reprod Med 44:269–274, 1999.

Hatcher RA, Trussell J, Stewart F, et al. (eds): Contraceptive Technology, 18th rev ed. New York, Ardent Media, 2004.

Hill DA: Abnormal uterine bleeding: Avoid the rush to hysterectomy. J Fam Pract 58:136–142, 2009.

Hov GG, Skjeldestad FE, Hilstad T: Use of IUD and subsequent fertility: Follow-up after participation in a randomized clinical trial. Contraception 75:88–92, 2007.

Hubacher D, Lara-Ricalde R, Taylor DJ, et al: Use of copper intrauterine devices and the risk of tubal infertility among nulliparous women. N Engl J Med 345:561–567, 2001.

Johnson BA: Insertion and removal of intrauterine devices. Am Fam Physician 71:95–102, 2005.

Mirena Package Insert. Montville, NJ, Berlex Laboratories, 2003.

Nelson AL: The intrauterine contraceptive device. Obstet Gynecol Clin North Am 27:723–740, 2000.

Paladine HL, Blenning CE, Judkins DZ, Mittal S: Clinical inquiries: What are contraindications to IUDs? J Fam Pract 55:726–729, 2006.

ParaGard Package Insert. Tonawanda, NY, FEI Products, 2003.

Stanford JB, Mikolajczyk RT: Mechanisms of action of intrauterine devices: Update and estimation of postfertilization effects. Am J Obstet Gynecol 187:1699–1708, 2002.

Tuggy M, Garcia J: Procedures Consult. Available at www.proceduresconsult.com.

Usatine RP: The Color Atlas of Family Medicine. New York, McGraw-Hill, 2009.

Walsh T, Grimes D, Frezieres R, et al: Randomised controlled trial of prophylactic antibiotics before insertion of intrauterine devices. IUD Study Group. Lancet 351:1005–1008, 1998.

World Health Organization: Medical Eligibility Criteria for Contraceptive Use, 3rd ed. Intrauterine devices (IUDs). 2004. Available at www.who.int/reproductive-health/publications/mec/iuds.html.

Zieman M, Kanal E: Copper T 380A IUD and magnetic resonance imaging. Contraception 75:93–95, 2007.

CHAPTER 146

Intrauterine Device Removal

Ashley Christiani

Generally, intrauterine contraceptive device (IUD) removal is a simple and uncomplicated procedure that takes only a few minutes. The rare case in which the IUD string is not visible ("lost" IUD) presents a more challenging situation.

Indications

- Desire for pregnancy
- Postmenopause (no need for contraception)
- Pregnancy confirmed (early)
- Pelvic infection
- Before loop electrosurgical excision procedure (LEEP)/conization (but with careful precautions, a LEEP can be performed without cutting the string)
- Patient intolerance: pain, bleeding, other
- Manufacturer recommendations
  - ParaGard T380: 10 years
  - Mirena: 5 years
- Inability to identify the strings

Contraindications

- Advanced pregnancy (second or third trimester; generally contraindicated because of risk of spontaneous abortion)
- Suspected extrauterine location

Preprocedure Patient Preparation

Patient Counseling and Consent

Although typically a straightforward and simple procedure, as with any other procedure, patients should receive counseling on the risks, benefits, and alternatives to IUD removal and provided a general overview of what to expect during the process. Depending on the reason for IUD removal, appropriate discussion of contraceptive options, preconception counseling, or management of menopause should be discussed. The clinician should advise of possible cramping and discomfort associated with IUD removal as well as the potential for transient nausea, dizziness, or faintness during and immediately after the procedure. Mild spotting and cramping may occur.

Pretreatment

Patients may consider taking ibuprofen (600 to 800 mg) or other nonsteroidal anti-inflammatory drug 45 to 60 minutes before IUD removal to minimize cramping and discomfort during the procedure. Local anesthetic is usually not necessary, but may be helpful in the case of a complicated removal, particularly in those at risk for significant discomfort (nulliparas, those requiring cervical dilation, those with history of pain with prior cervical procedures) or vasovagal reaction. In this case, lidocaine 1% to 2% without epinephrine may be used to perform a paracervical or submucosal block (see Chapter 149, Loop Electrosurgical Excision Procedure for Treating Cervical Intraepithelial Neoplasia, and Chapter 173, Paracervical Block, for the submucosal injection technique).

Technique

Removal with Visible IUD Strings

The usual IUD removal is straightforward, and there is no need for sterile technique. Insert the speculum and visualize the IUD strings. Using ring forceps, grasp the strings and pull toward the introitus in a firm and deliberate motion until the IUD is delivered. The patient will likely experience momentary discomfort, which may be prevented somewhat by premedicating with 800 mg of ibuprofen. Remove the speculum and send the patient home. Some minor spotting may be expected for a few days. There is no need to culture the IUD unless infection is suspected.

Removal when IUD Strings Are Not Visible

If the speculum is inserted and IUD strings cannot be visualized after a diligent search, one of several approaches may be used. *First,* try using a Cytobrush or similar instrument and insert the brush portion the full depth into the cervical canal (approximately 2 cm). After insertion, rotate and extract the brush in a continuous motion. Repeat several times if needed. In one study, 24 of 27 lost strings were retrieved in this maneuver when other methods had failed.

If this fails, try a *second* method. Insert a long-handled alligator forceps or other hemostat-like instrument such as a uterine packing forceps into the os, with the instrument opened as much as the os will allow. Close the jaws in a blind attempt to catch any strings that may be present. If the strings are indeed grasped, resistance will be felt when the instrument is removed. Carry out this maneuver four or five times in an attempt to grasp the strings. If unsuccessful, or if the os is too small, other methods will be needed to find the strings.

A *third* approach uses an endocervical speculum along with a colposcope to identify the strings. Frequently, the end of the string is just within the os. Once visualized, it is much more easily grasped with forceps and removed.

Should these techniques fail, proceed with a more invasive *fourth option* (see Chapter 136, Cervical Stenosis and Cervical Dilation, for the instrumentation to be used). Perform a bimanual examination to identify the position of the uterus. Prepare the area with an antiseptic solution. Grasp the anterior lip with a single-toothed cervical tenaculum and apply slight traction to straighten the uterus. A uterine sound may be used to dilate the internal os if needed. An IUD remover is then used to enter the intrauterine cavity (Fig. 146-1). Using the larger-sized instruments will prevent or minimize the potential for perforation of the uterus. The double IUD extractor and flexible IUD hook are commonly used. The *double IUD extractor* resembles a crochet hook that "hooks" the IUC (Fig. 146-2). Use a twist-and-pull motion to "catch" the IUD.

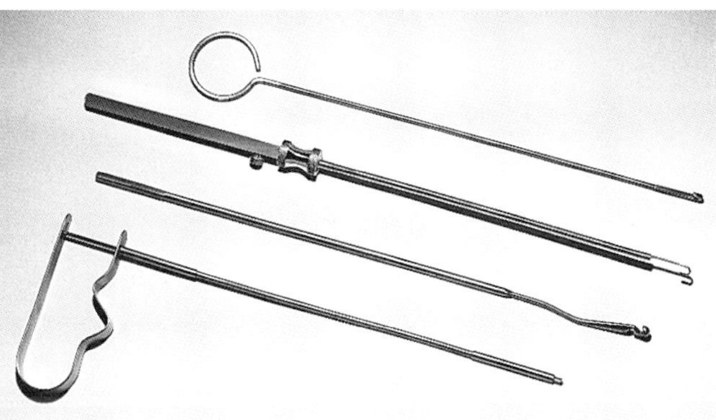

Figure 146-1 Intrauterine device (IUD) removal instruments. From top to bottom: simple IUD hook, universal IUD hook, double IUD extractor, and flexible IUD hook.

Frequent, repeated passes are often needed. The *flexible IUD hook* is actually a forceps. Insert the stem into the uterus and compress the handle to open the jaws. When the handle is released, the jaws grasp the IUD as they close. Then withdraw the unit. With either instrument, if the string or the IUD is grasped, resistance will be felt.

Embedded IUDs

If the IUD has been in place for a significant length of time, it may have become embedded in the endometrium and significant force will be required to remove it. Firm pressure rarely if ever breaks the strings. If the force seems to be extreme, there is excessive pain, or there is any question whether the IUD is still in place, it may be best to defer removal. Although a flat-plate radiograph of the abdomen will identify whether the IUD is present (IUDs are radiopaque), the x-ray film will not indicate whether the IUD *is intrauterine*. A pelvic ultrasonographic examination, on the other hand, will confirm whether it is present *and* whether it is intrauterine. If the IUD has moved to an extrauterine position, surgery will be required.

If an intrauterine IUD is confirmed by ultrasonography, the patient must return for a visit when further, more aggressive attempts can be made to remove it. If all else fails, the patient may require a dilation and curettage procedure, with the IUD removed under anesthesia or with the aid of a hysteroscope.

No prophylactic antibiotics are needed.

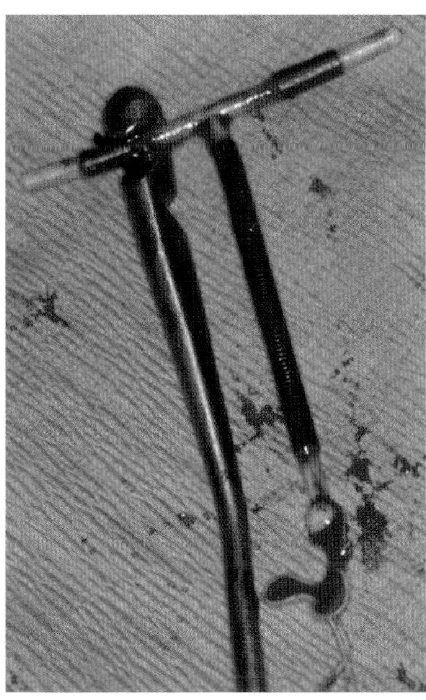

Figure 146-2 Double intrauterine device (IUD) extractor after retrieving a "lost" IUD (ParaGard T380).

Complications

Other than slight discomfort and the possibility of vasovagal reactions, there are no significant complications from routine IUD removal. If other instrumentation is required because of lost strings, rare complications include perforation, infection, and bleeding. If the IUD is being removed in the context of pregnancy, there is significant risk of miscarriage, with rates as high as 50% to 60% in some studies.

Postprocedure Patient Education

Provide contraception, preconception counseling, or hormone replacement and menopause counseling as appropriate. If the patient desires to continue IUD use, there is no need to delay insertion. An IUD may be removed and a new IUD (same or different type) can be inserted at the same visit (see Chapter 145, Intrauterine Device Insertion).

CPT/Billing Codes

58300 IUD insertion
58301 IUD removal

ICD-9-CM Diagnostic Codes

Contraceptive Device

996.32 Complications (lost IUD)
996.76 Causing menorrhagia
V25.1 Insertion
V25.42 Reinsertion
V25.42 Removal
V25.42 Maintenance/surveillance/checking IUD

Suppliers

(See contact information online at www.expertconsult.com.)

The various IUD removal instruments should be available from most medical supply firms. Those shown in Figure 146-1 are from CooperSurgical, Inc.

Bibliography

Ben-Rafael Z, Bider D: A new procedure for removal of a "lost" intrauterine device. Obstet Gynecol 87:785–786, 1996.

Bounds W, Hutt S, Kubba A, et al: Randomised comparative study in 217 women of three disposable plastic IUCD thread retrievers. Br J Obstet Gynaecol 99:915–919, 1992.

Hatcher RA, Trussell J, Stewart F, et al (eds): Contraceptive Technology, 18th rev ed. New York, Ardent Media, 2004.

Tuggy M, Garcia J: Procedures Consult. Available at www.proceduresconsult.com.

CHAPTER 147

INSERTION AND REMOVAL OF IMPLANON

Stephen A. Grochmal • Dale A. Patterson

Implanon is an implantable contraceptive device that functions like other progestin-based contraceptives by developing a thick, hostile cervical mucus and eventual atrophy of the uterine endometrium. Compared to the original Norplant System, Implanon appears to cause a greater inhibition of ovulation in patients. Implanon is designed as a single implant measuring 4 cm long with a diameter of 2 mm and an outer structural membrane composed of ethylene vinyl acetate (EVA) copolymer (Fig. 147-1). This copolymer outer membrane may not react with the surrounding tissue as much as Norplant did, leading to less tissue fibrosis; thus permitting easier extraction when its content is exhausted. The implant core contains 68 mg of etonogestrel in EVA. The progestin is released initially at the rate of 60 µg/day in weeks 5 to 6 of use and then decreases to 35 to 45 µg/day at the end of the first year. The released amount of etonogestrel continues to decrease to 30 to 40 µg/day and 25 to 30 µg/day at 2 and 3 years of use, respectively. Implanon is effective for 3 years and has a shelf life of 5 years. The implant is placed in the subcutaneous tissue of the upper arm with a 19-gauge disposable, preloaded inserter. The insertion is a minor surgical procedure performed in the office. Implanon was approved in July 2006 by the U.S. Food and Drug Administration (FDA).

INDICATIONS

Implanon is used for contraception.

CONTRAINDICATIONS

Absolute

Pregnancy is an absolute contraindication.

Relative

- Thromboembolism
- Breast cancer
- Hepatic disorders
- Unexplained abnormal vaginal bleeding
- Hypersensitivity to the components of the product

A detailed discussion of relative risks is available in the complete prescribing information at: www.implanon-usa.com/hcp.

EQUIPMENT

- Examination table
- Sterile surgical drapes and gloves, antiseptic solution, sterile skin marker
- Local anesthetic (1% lidocaine without epinephrine), syringes (3 mL), and needles (25 to 27½ g)
- Sterile gauze, adhesive bandage (self-adhesive wrap like Coban), pressure bandage
- Implanon product kit (Fig. 147-2) (no. 11 blade, straight and curved mosquito clamps, and forceps are needed for removal)

PRECAUTIONS

Although progestin-containing contraceptives have not been shown to cause birth defects, it is imperative to ensure that a patient is not pregnant prior to inserting Implanon. If a patient is found to be pregnant or becomes pregnant after insertion, the device should be removed.

Caution is also advised in patients with bleeding disorders and patients taking anticoagulants. Implanon may be an appropriate contraceptive for these patients, but precautions should be taken to minimize bleeding.

PREPROCEDURE PATIENT EDUCATION

Implanon is more than 99% effective, and when the device is inserted correctly risk of pregnancy is less than 1 per 100 women who use it. Approximately 82% of women continue to use Implanon for 2 or more years. Implanon may be less effective in women who are overweight or are taking certain types of medications. Contraception with progestins is very useful in patients with known hepatic disease, hypertension, psychosis, mental retardation, or a history of thromboembolism. It should be noted that the manufacturer lists thromboembolism, hepatic disorders, and breast cancer as contraindications to the use of Implanon but that clinical practice has shown that progestin-based contraceptives are safe in these patients and preferred over estrogen-containing products.

The implant must be removed after all the progestin is released, generally by the end of the third year. Women should be informed that Implanon does not protect against human immunodeficiency virus (HIV) or other sexually transmitted diseases. A detailed patient consent form is available from the manufacturer's website and online at www.expertconsult.com.

ADVANTAGES

- *Menstrual*: Menstrual and ovulatory discomfort and cramping are decreased. There is less bleeding as compared to other implant devices, with more consistent amenorrhea reported (20% at 1 year). In Implanon users, uterine pain was reduced or eliminated in 88% of women previously experiencing dysmenorrhea.
- *Sexual and psychological*: Sexual intercourse may be more pleasurable because fear of pregnancy is reduced, allowing for more spontaneity.
- *Risk of cancer*: None known.

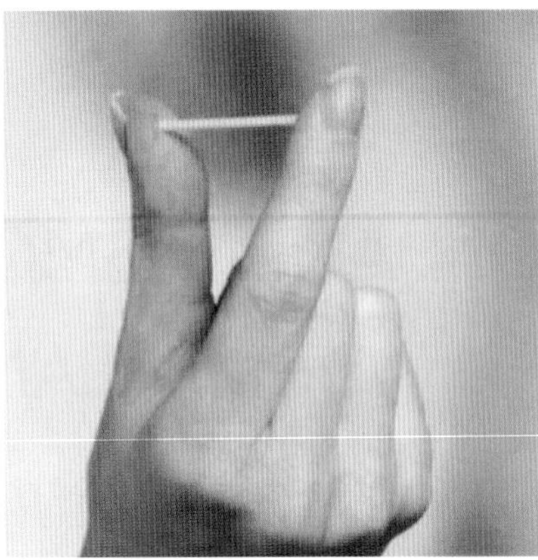

Figure 147-1 Implanon device. (Courtesy of Schering-Plough Corp., Kenilworth, NJ.)

- *Additional factors*: There was a high continuation rate reported in the clinical trials, and asymptomatic follicular cysts were less common than with users of Mirena or Norplant. The single implant permits quick removal.

Disadvantages

- *Menstrual*: Amenorrhea and oligomenorrhea are commonly reported. A more common patient complaint is persistent irregular and less predictable menstrual bleeding.
- *Sexual and psychological*: The irregular bleeding may become disconcerting and possibly discourage sexual intercourse.
- *Headache* and *acne* are commonly reported side effects.
- *Interactions with other medications* may make Implanon less effective. These medications include barbiturates, griseofulvin, rifampin, phenylbutazone, carbamazepine, felbamate, oxcarbazepine, topiramate, and modafinil. Herbal remedies such as St. John's wort may also reduce effectiveness. In these situations, a secondary nonhormonal method of birth control should be considered.

Patient Selection

The Implanon implant is particularly useful for women with contraindications to or severe side effects from estrogen. As previously mentioned, Implanon candidates would include those patients with a personal history of thrombosis, coronary artery disease, cerebrovascular disease, hypertension, or hepatic disorders. Included in this list are those patients who suffer from other related estrogen side effects including migraine headaches, previous history of drug-induced chloasma, and hypertriglyceridemia, and those women who are recently postpartum, breastfeeding, over the age of 35 years, or smokers. The published prescribing precautions are the same as for other progestin-only pills. Patients concerned about their fertility after discontinuation of Implanon should be counseled that they will experience a rapid return to baseline fertility, with over 94% of patients demonstrating ovulation within 3 to 6 weeks after removal of the implant. It is important to inform patients that irregular bleeding may be expected and might persist while the implant rod is in place. If the pattern of bleeding becomes intolerable, additional treatments can be employed to make the bleeding pattern more acceptable.

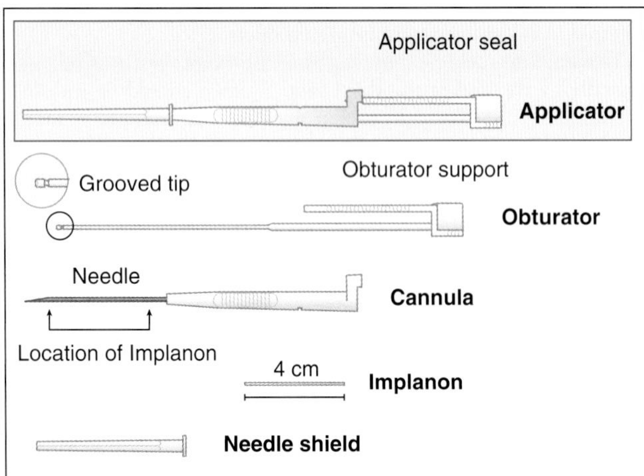

Figure 147-2 Implanon kit (see text for details). (Courtesy of Schering-Plough Corp., Kenilworth, NJ.)

Procedure

Ideally, the insertion should be scheduled within the first few days of a regular menstrual bleed, and the use of a "backup" method of birth control (i.e., condoms) should be recommended for 7 days after insertion.

The insertion procedure for Implanon is somewhat opposite that of an injection. The manufacturer has specific training seminars and onsite support available for health care providers wishing to offer this device to their patients. A provider must complete the manufacturer's course before being able to order Implanon and perform the procedure. This procedure is performed in the office setting. The Implanon rod and inserter should remain sterile throughout the procedure. If at any time sterility is compromised, a new device should be used.

Insertion Technique

A video can be reviewed on the Implanon website, www.implanon-usa.com.

1. Have the patient lie on her back on the examination table with her nondominant arm flexed at the elbow and externally rotated. Her hand should be next to her head (Fig. 147-3A).
2. Mark a site for insertion 6 to 8 cm above the elbow crease on the nondominant arm. The site should be on the medial aspect of the arm, between the biceps and triceps. A second mark should be made on the same arm 6 to 8 cm *proximal* (farther up the arm) to the first mark (Fig. 147-3B).
3. Prep the insertion site with the antiseptic of choice.
4. Anesthetize the area locally with 1 to 3 mL of 1% to 2% lidocaine with or without epinephrine (see Chapter 4, Local Anesthesia).
5. Remove the inserter device (without the contraceptive rod in the needle/cannula) from the packaging.
6. Keeping the shield on the needle, identify the white rod inside the needle tip.
7. If not visible, tap the side of the device, with needle pointing down, to slide the rod into the needle tip.
8. Turn the needle up and shake or tap the rod back into the needle tip and remove the shield.
9. It is now possible for the rod to fall out of the needle. Keep the applicator in the upright position until insertion to minimize this risk.
10. While applying countertraction to the skin (Fig. 147-3C), insert the tip of the needle bevel up into the skin. The angle of insertion should be less than 20 degrees (Fig. 147-3D).
11. Put the applicator in a position horizontal to the skin and lift the skin up with the tip of the needle keeping the needle subdermal (Fig. 147-3E).
12. Tent the skin and insert the needle fully into the subdermal tissue, aiming for the second mark made earlier on the arm (Fig. 147-3F).

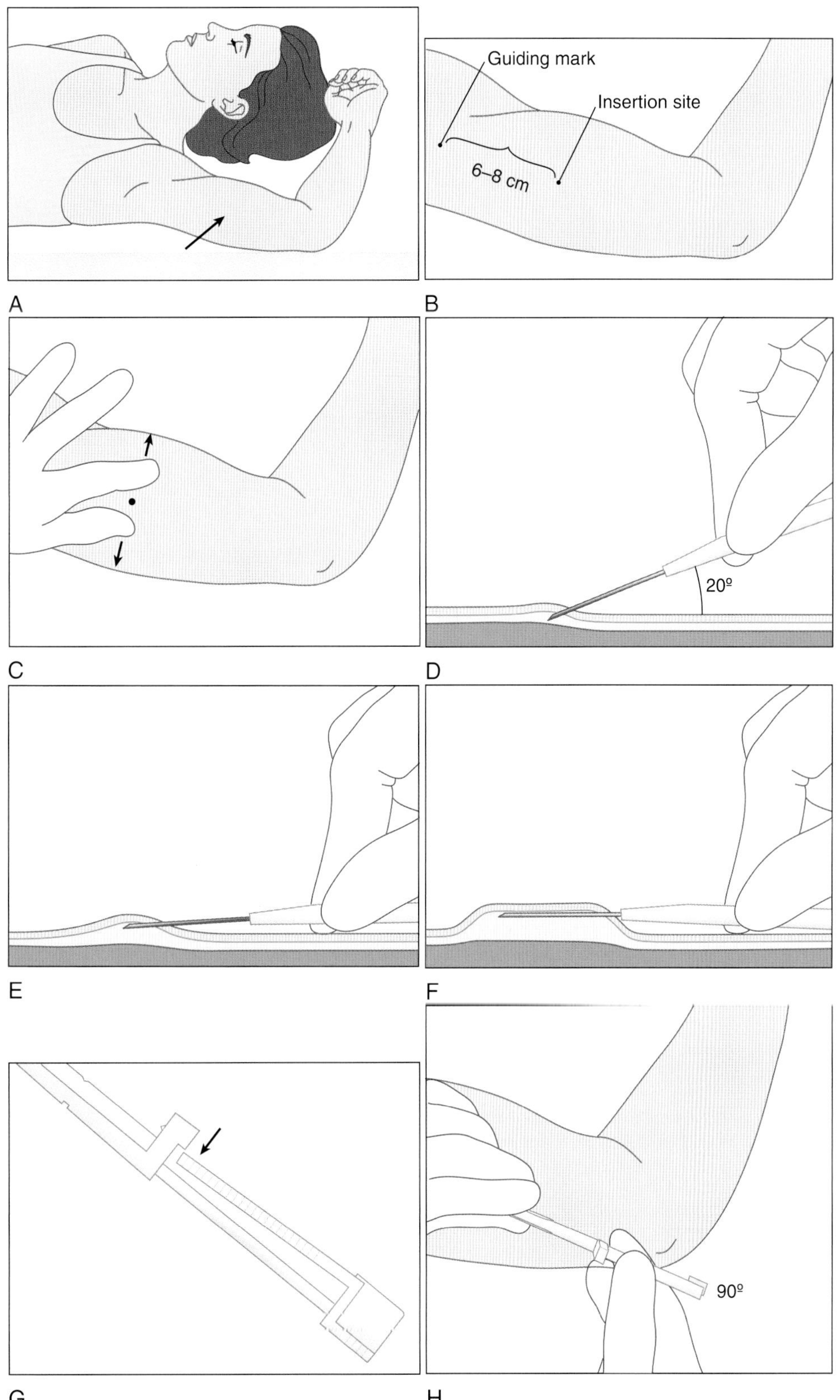

Figure 147-3 **A–J,** Insertion procedure (see text for details). (Courtesy of Schering-Plough Corp., Kenilworth, NJ.)

Figure continues on following page.

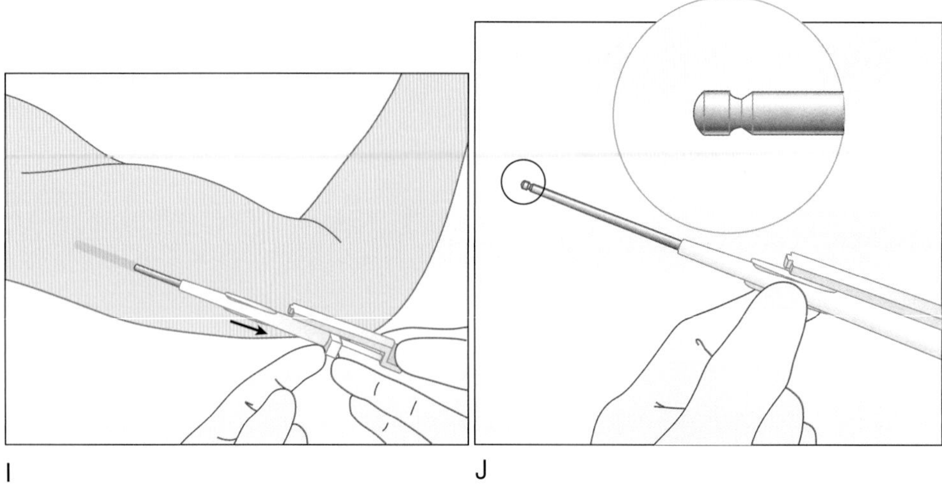

Figure 147-3, cont.

13. Break the applicator seal by pressing the support for the obturator. Turn the obturator 90 degrees in either direction (Fig. 147-3G and H).
14. Hold the obturator in place on the arm and retract the cannula. Do not push or pull on the obturator. Slide the cannula off the device, allowing the insert to "fall in place" and be implanted in the patient (Fig. 147-3I).
15. Confirm placement of the device. Check the needle to make sure the device is not in it. The grooved tip of the applicator should now be visible (Fig. 147-3J). Palpate the skin to feel the device in the proper location. If a rod cannot be palpated, it can be seen on ultrasound or magnetic resonance imaging (MRI). The rod *cannot* be seen on plain x-ray. An alternative form of contraception must be used until correct placement is verified.
16. The wound can be dressed with an adhesive bandage and pressure dressing.
17. A card is provided to give to the patient with details of the device implanted.

Removal Technique

A video can be viewed on the Implanon website, www.implanon-usa.com.

1. Removal is performed with the patient in a position similar to that for insertion. The rod should be palpated or located with ultrasound prior to removal. The removal site should also be prepared with antiseptic solution.
2. Locally anesthetize the area for removal, including the area under the rod (see Chapter 4, Local Anesthesia).
3. Make a 2- to 3-mm incision longitudinally at the end of the rod closest to the elbow using a no. 11 blade.
4. Push the rod toward the incision until it is visible. It may be necessary to further dissect the tissue to visualize the device.
5. Grasp the device with a hemostat and remove (Fig. 147-4A).
6. If unable to see the device, it may be grasped with one fine hemostat through the skin and further dissected with a second fine hemostat to facilitate removal (Fig. 147-4B). The fascia over the capsule may need to be incised with scissors or the no. 11 blade (Fig. 147-4C).
7. Ensure that the entire device has been removed by measuring it (length is 4 cm).
8. A new device may be inserted into the same incision or the opposite arm if desired.
9. Dress the wound with an adhesive bandage and pressure dressing.

Sample Operative Report

Preoperative diagnosis: Elective contraception with implantable device
Postoperative diagnosis: Same
Procedure performed: Insertion of Implanon contraceptive device
Surgeon: Dr. ______________
Blood loss: None
Complications: None

Procedure: The patient was placed in the supine position with her left arm up above her head exposing the medial (inside) portion of the upper left arm. The region above the antecubital space was prepped and draped. Local infiltration of the skin with 2 to 4 mL of 1% lidocaine with epinephrine was accomplished along a 3- to 4-cm line approximately 2 fingerbreadths from the antecubital space using a 27-gauge needle, and satisfactory anesthetic effect was achieved. A small vertical incision was made into the skin. The 19-gauge preloaded insertion cannula was directed at a 20-degree angle, beveled side up, through the incision and into the subcutaneous tissue, tenting up the skin to keep the needle just under the skin. The inserter cannula was stabilized and the Implanon implant passed down the cannula sleeve and deposited into the subcutaneous space. The inserter cannula was removed after the terminal ends of the deposited implant were palpated to confirm accurate placement within the designated tissue space. The skin incision was then closed with Steri-Strips (or adhesive bandage) and a small sterile pressure dressing was applied. Patient tolerated the insertion procedure well and will return to the office for follow-up in 3 days.

Common Errors

- Shallow insertion, causing the implant to be clearly visible directly under the skin surface.
- More commonly, the implant is inserted too deeply, which will make it difficult to palpate and complicate the removal process.
- Inadvertent removal of the obturator portion of the cannula results in the inability to advance the implant device.
- Inability to confirm proper placement of the Implanon device by digital palpation after the procedure may be due to placing the rod too deep in the fatty tissue (as noted earlier). Confirmation of correct placement should be attained by ultrasound or MRI. The patient must use a barrier method of contraception until proper placement is confirmed. Document this activity at the end of the operative report and in the patient's chart.

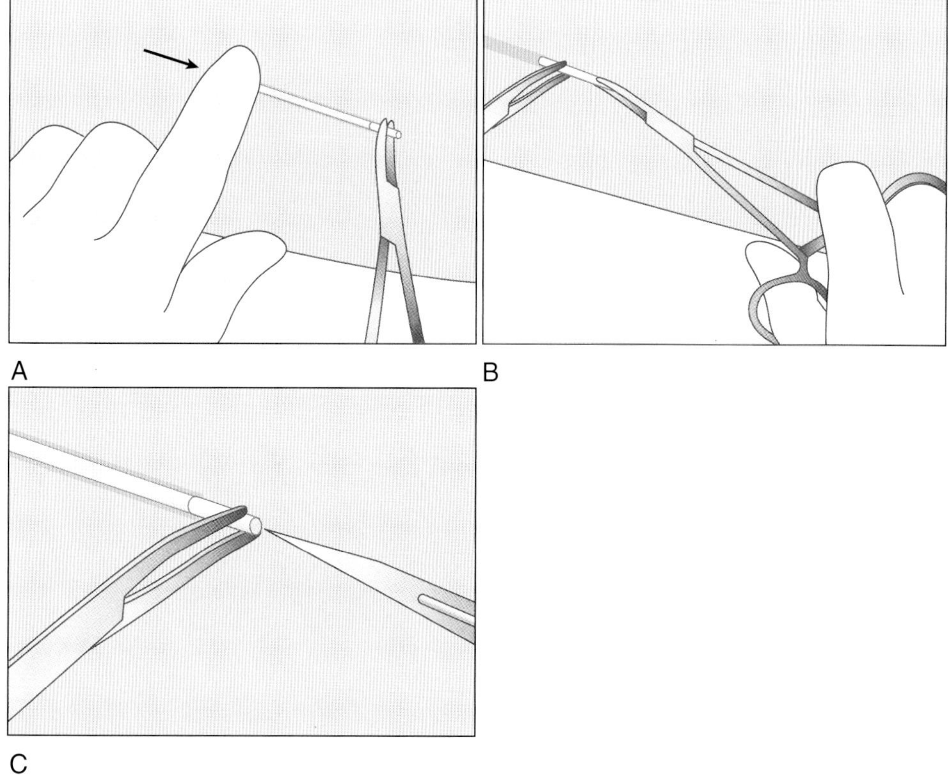

Figure 147-4 **A–C,** Removal procedure (see text for details). (Courtesy of Schering-Plough Corp., Kenilworth, NJ.)

Complications

- Postprocedure pain (insertion area of arm)
  - Determine if there is evidence of local nerve damage (extremely rare and unlikely).
  - Ecchymosis: confirm bandage is not applied too tightly. Apply ice packs for 24 hours.
  - Recommend NSAIDs or acetaminophen as needed.
- Infection in the insertion area
  - *No abscess present.* Suspect a localized cellulitis. Do not remove the rod. Clean the infected area with antiseptic solution and begin an oral antibiotic for 7 days. Evaluate in 24 hours and again after course of antibiotics is concluded.
  - *Abscess is present.* Begin course of antibiotics for 7 to 10 days. Prepare infected area, incise and drain any purulent material, and remove the rod. Drain and dress the wound and continue antibiotic therapy and wound care until resolved.

Postprocedure Management

- After insertion, apply a pressure dressing on the insertion site for 24 hours; thereafter, apply just a small bandage for approximately 3 to 5 days.
- After removal, Steri-Strips should be left in place until they "fall off." The wound should be treated as a simple laceration.

Postprocedure Patient Education

The process of wound healing should be discussed with the patient, and she should be reminded that the device does not protect against sexually transmitted diseases. The Implanon website has downloadable patient education materials available (www.implanon-usa.com).

CPT/Billing Codes

11981 Insertion, nonbiodegradable drug delivery implant (11975, 11976, 11977, 11980 used for other implant types)
11982 Removal, nonbiodegradable drug delivery implant
11983 Removal with reinsertion, nonbiodegradable drug delivery implant

ICD-9-CM Diagnostic Codes

V25.5 Insertion of implantable subdermal contraceptive
V25.43 Surveillance of subdermal implantable contraceptive
V45.52 Other postprocedural states, presence of contraceptive device, subdermal contraceptive implant

HCPCS

J7307 Etonogestrel (contraceptive) implant system, including implant and supplies (It is necessary to include this code on CMS form 1500 to be reimbursed for the cost of the device.)

Supplier

Full contact information available online at www.expertconsult.com.

Implanon
Schering-Plough Corporation

Editor's Note: The company's website is excellent and comprehensive. It includes videos on insertion and removal as well as patient education materials.

ONLINE RESOURCES

Implanon Insertion/Removal form online at www.expertconsult.com.

Implanon patient support. Schering-Plough Corp. Kenilworth, NJ 07033. Available at implanon-usa.com/hcp.

Implanon website for health care professionals, accessed May 2010: http//:www.spfiles.com/piimplanon.pd.pdf.

BIBLIOGRAPHY

American College of Obstetricians and Gynecologists: Increasing use of contraceptive implants and intrauterine devices to reduce unintended pregnancy. Opinion no. 450. Obstet Gynecol 114:1434–1438, 2009.

Chrousos GP: Contraceptive steroids. In Katzung BG (ed): Basic and Clinical Pharmacology, 10th ed. New York, McGraw Hill Lange, 2007, pp 666–670.

Grenwal M, Burkman RT: Contraception and family planning. In DeCherney AH, Nathan L (eds): Current Obstetric and Gynecology Diagnosis and Treatment, 9th ed. New York, Lange Medical Books/McGraw Hill, 2004, pp 639–641.

Hatcher RA, Zieman M, Cwiak C, et al: Progestin-only contraceptives. In Managing Contraception, 8th ed. Tiger GA, Bridging the Gap Foundation, 2005–2007, pp 124–139.

Nakajima ST: Future methods and areas of investigation: Implants—progestin based. In Contemporary Guide to Contraception, 2nd ed. Newton, PA, Handbooks in Health Care Co., 2006, pp 189–191.

Usatine RP: The Color Atlas of Family Medicine. New York, McGraw-Hill, 2009.

CHAPTER 148

INSERTION OF ESSURE (HYSTEROSCOPICALLY ASSISTED FEMALE STERILIZATION)

Stephen A. Grochmal • Lydia A. Watson • Dale A. Patterson

Female tubal sterilization remains the most widely utilized method of permanent contraception worldwide. Approximately 700,000 female sterilizations are performed annually, and about of half of these are completed within 48 hours post partum. The remaining 345,000 sterilizations are "interval" procedures, meaning they do not occur immediately following pregnancy. Until recently, the majority of interval sterilization procedures in the United States were performed laparoscopically, under general anesthesia or intravenous (IV) conscious sedation, in either the hospital or an out-patient surgery setting. Although the laparoscopic approach is considered safe and effective, it is not without complications, including infection, anesthesia complications, vascular damage, failure, and injury to internal organs; and occasionally, as a result of a failed laparoscopic attempt, an unintended laparotomy may occur. Annually, an average of 14 women die in the United States from complications of tubal ligation surgery, and there is a reported 1/200 failure rate. Sterilization rates have remained the same for men and women over the past 45 years; however, the types of surgical procedures utilized have changed, influenced by improvements in medical device technologies and anesthesia.

Historically, the concept of hysteroscopic or transcervical occlusion of the fallopian tubes (using electrocoagulation) was first described by Schroeder in 1927. Unfortunately, there was sporadic interest in this hysteroscopic "scarless" tubal ligation procedure and further progress to find an acceptable method was plagued by numerous attempts and failures. An innovative technology was approved by the Food and Drug Administration (FDA) in November 2002 as the first hysteroscopic tubal occlusion device for permanent female sterilization in the United States. Now in its third generation, the Essure (ESS305, Conceptus, Inc., Mountain View, CA) is a less invasive, incisionless alternative to tubal ligation that provides significant advantages, such as decreased morbidity, rapid patient recovery, ability to detect failures, decreased expense, and a high level of patient satisfaction, when compared to tubal ligation.

Transcervical sterilization lends itself nicely to the office setting because it can be performed with little to no anesthesia or sedation in a standard gynecologic examination room. Patients describe only minimal postoperative discomfort and have a high tolerance for the procedure. A recent survey reported that more than 97% of patients who underwent the procedure would recommend it to a friend. Now, more than 8 years after its introduction, transcervical hysteroscopic sterilization (Essure) has proven to be an enduring technology, making hysteroscopic tubal occlusion increasingly popular as the option of choice for permanent interval female sterilization.

An investigation of the trends in female sterilization between January 1, 2002, and December 31, 2007, at the Detroit Medical Center, Michigan, revealed a significant decrease in the percentage of interval laparoscopic sterilizations and postpartum tubal ligations performed after vaginal delivery. Of the interval sterilizations performed, the percentage of hysteroscopic sterilizations (Essure) increased significantly from 0% to 51.3% of all procedures performed. Although not indicative of a universal shift in trends across the United States, this study suggests that a minimally invasive, incisionless procedure is an appealing alternative choice for many patients.

The transcervical hysteroscopic sterilization procedure (Essure) entails one office visit, followed by a postprocedure low-pressure hysterosalpingogram (HSG) 3 months later. (See sample Essure confirmation test checklist online at www.expertconsult.com.) The placement of the Essure microinserts can be accomplished in about 9 minutes with a 97% to 99% successful bilateral placement rate with little to no patient discomfort and downtime.

If the physician is proficient with basic diagnostic office hysteroscopy, then performing the Essure procedure (after attending a certified device user course) would be a logical "next step" office procedure. Presently, many gynecologists and a few primary care physicians perform hysteroscopic sterilizations. Increased awareness and available training for hysteroscopic sterilization for "seasoned" practitioners or recent residency graduates will increase the popularity and availability of this permanent contraception option to patients.

A second method of transcervical sterilization has also become available. In July 2009, the Adiana Permanent Contraception System (Hologic, Inc., Bedford, MA) received FDA approval in the United States. Under hysteroscopic guidance, a catheter is introduced into the tubal ostium. Once correct placement inside the intramural portion of the fallopian tube is confirmed, a radiofrequency (RF) energy burst lasting for 1 minute produces a 5-mm lesion within the fallopian tube. Following this thermal injury, a 3.5-mm silicone matrix "plug" is deployed into this thermal lesion. During the next several weeks after the procedure, tubal occlusion occurs from in-growth of fibroblasts within the matrix, which acts like a permanent scaffolding permitting a "space-filling" effect to develop. Like the Essure procedure, confirmed tubal occlusion must be assessed by hysterosalpingogram in 3 months after the device has been placed.

Presently, experience with the Adiana system in the United States is limited. The cumulative available worldwide data cover up to 3 years; however, the data from the pivotal trial provide important clinical information. Additional information for the reader can be found at the end of this chapter. Although appropriate to highlight new, emerging technologies and treatment

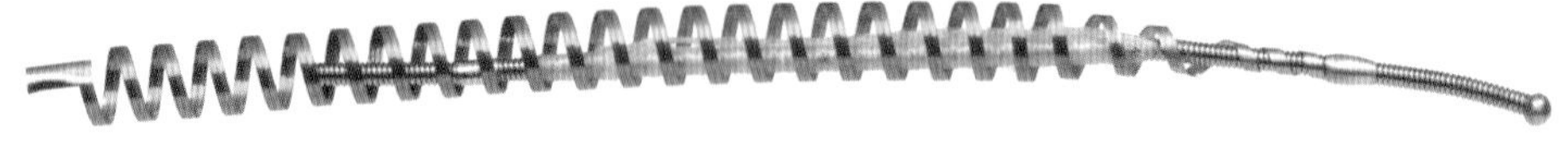

Figure 148-1 Essure microinsert. (Courtesy of Conceptus, Inc., Mountain View, CA.)

options, our discussion in this chapter will focus only on the Essure procedure.

Anatomy

The anatomy relevant to Essure placement is identical to that described in Chapter 140, Hysteroscopy.

Indication

Hysteroscopic sterilization is indicated for any woman who desires permanent elective sterilization.

Contraindications

Absolute

- Pregnancy or suspected pregnancy
- Less than 6 weeks after delivery or abortion
- Inability to observe both tubal ostia during hysteroscopy
- Patients who have previously undergone a tubal ligation
- Nickel allergy (documented by skin testing)

Relative

- Radiologic contrast allergy
- Active or recent pelvic infection
- Uterine anomalies
- Immunosuppressive therapy

Equipment and Supplies

- Materials for a paracervical block (see Chapter 173, Paracervical Block)
- Powered examination table
- The standard hysteroscopic equipment already available in the physician's office (see Chapter 140, Hysteroscopy)

The *third generation Essure system* (ESS305) consists of two Essure microinserts (Fig. 148-1) (one insert per disposable delivery catheter) and two disposable introducers (Fig. 148-2). A standard hysteroscope with a 5 French operating channel, preferably with continuous flow and an angle of view between 12 and 30 degrees is required equipment necessary for this procedure. The only uterine distention medium recommended for hysteroscopic sterilization is normal saline using a gravity flow system (see Chapter 140, Hysteroscopy).

The *Essure microinsert* (see Fig. 148-1) consists of two coils composed of a flexible stainless steel inner coil and an outer coil made of nickel-titanium alloy (nitinol) and polyethylene terephthalate (PET) fibers. The insert measures 3.85 cm in length and 0.8 mm in diameter in the "wound down" or contracted configuration. The microinserts do not contain or release hormones. Once inserted, the PET fibers stimulate a local, benign tissue growth that surrounds and infiltrates the device over the course of several weeks, leading to occlusion of the tubal lumen.

The disposable *delivery device handle* contains a delivery wire, release catheter, and delivery catheter housing the microinsert. An ergonomic, single-use handle provides effortless control of the microinsert deployment via a button-thumbwheel combination built in to the handle (see Fig. 148-2). The valved, DryFlow introducer permits passage of the Essure introducer catheter into the operating channel without any valve manipulation on the hysteroscope, thus preventing backflow of fluid. The ESS305 has a new gold band where the notch used to be on the previous version, making it easier to visualize and correctly place the device into the tubal ostia. The release catheter has a contrasting green color to improve visibility. Also, the device has an automatic release mechanism on the handle that eliminates the need, as was required with the previous generation, for counterclockwise rotations to disconnect the introducer catheter from the actual implanted insert (Fig. 148-3).

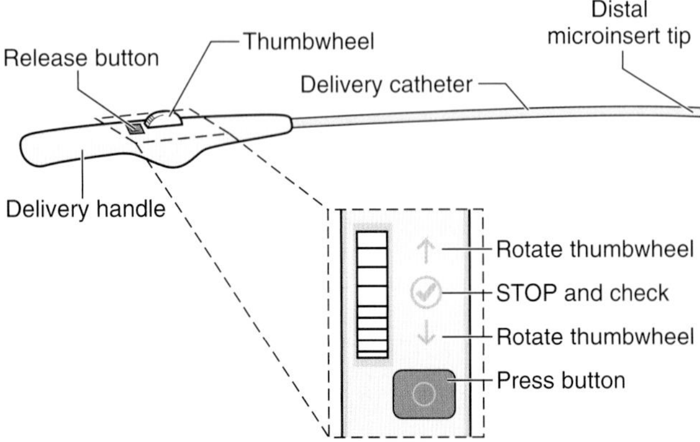

Figure 148-2 Delivery system. (Redrawn from images courtesy of Conceptus, Inc., Mountain View, CA.)

Precautions

- Patient must use an alternative form of contraception until an HSG is done to confirm both placement and tubal occlusion.
- Essure does not prevent sexually transmitted diseases.
- Essure is considered permanent and irreversible.
- Caution should be used when performing surgeries with electrosurgical or radiofrequency devices in the pelvis because Essure microinserts may conduct energy and potentially injure the patient.
- If both tubal ostia cannot be visualized, the procedure cannot be performed.
- If patient has a known prior history of intrauterine disease, previous surgical procedure, or uterine anomaly, consideration should be given to performing a "presterilization" diagnostic hysteroscopy to rule out any abnormal uterine conditions prior to the day of the planned hysteroscopic sterilization.
- The presence of an intracavitary lesion may obstruct the view of the tubal ostia and the Essure procedure may be technically difficult to perform. Removal of the lesion (e.g., submucous fibroid, endometrial polyp) may be necessary before the Essure microinserts can be placed.

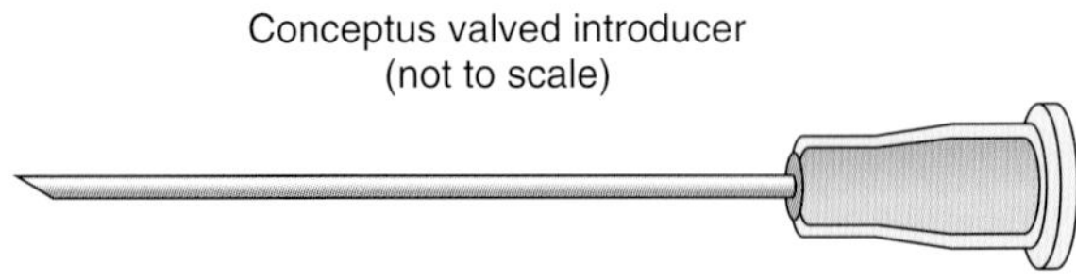

Figure 148-3 Valved DryFlow introducer for the Essure ESS305. (Redrawn from images courtesy of Conceptus, Inc., Mountain View, CA.)

Preprocedure Patient Education

Presurgical counseling is important. The patient should understand that she is contemplating a permanent procedure. This is particularly important in young patients, who may later regret their decision to be sterilized. A history of nickel allergy should be elicited in preprocedure discussion. Patients with a possible nickel allergy must undergo specific allergy testing prior to the procedure. Patients should also be queried about an allergy to contrast dye because the HSG is still required postprocedurally by the FDA protocol. If an allergy exists to dye, ultrasound is a useful alternative and is equally effective at confirming tubal occlusion; however, the patient must be told that the postprocedure evaluation of her fallopian tubes will be a deviation from the recommended FDA protocol.

It is important to schedule the patient during the early proliferative phase of her cycle. If needed, medical preparation of the endometrium with low-dose oral contraceptives or norethindrone (5 mg) or medroxyprogesterone (10 mg) can begin around day 4 or 5 of the cycle and continue until the procedure date. This helps prevent menstruation and produces a temporary atrophy of the uterine endometrium, which aids in improving visualization and manipulation within the uterine cavity during the hysteroscopic procedure. Hysteroscopic sterilization may be successfully performed in patients with a Mirena IUD in place within the uterine cavity. The IUD's presence may be advantageous by allowing more flexibility in the timing of the Essure procedure, providing continuous contraceptive effect until confirmation of tubal occlusion at 12 weeks.

The risks of hysteroscopy (see Chapter 140, Hysteroscopy), including an unlikely but small risk of tubal perforation, should also be discussed with the patient. The sterilization procedure is 99.74% effective in preventing pregnancy after 5 years of follow-up. It should again be emphasized that a backup birth control method must be used until bilateral tubal occlusion and correct placement are confirmed by HSG. (See sample consent form online at www.expertconsult.com.)

Procedure

Figure 148-4 illustrates the insertion procedure. Because the procedure is short, there is no need for conscious sedation or general anesthesia. A paracervical block (see Chapter 173, Paracervical Block) along with nonsteroidal premedication (recommended to prevent tubal spasm) is all that is needed to keep the patient comfortable during the procedure. The average office visit time "start to finish" is approximately 30 minutes with just about 9 to 10 minutes of actual hysteroscopy time to place the microinserts.

1–8. The procedure begins with insertion of the hysteroscope (steps 1–8 are identical to the procedure described in Chapter 140, Hysteroscopy). Once both tubal ostia have been identified, the insertion procedure begins as outlined in Figure 148-4.

9. Identify both tubal ostia and ensure that they are normal in appearance.

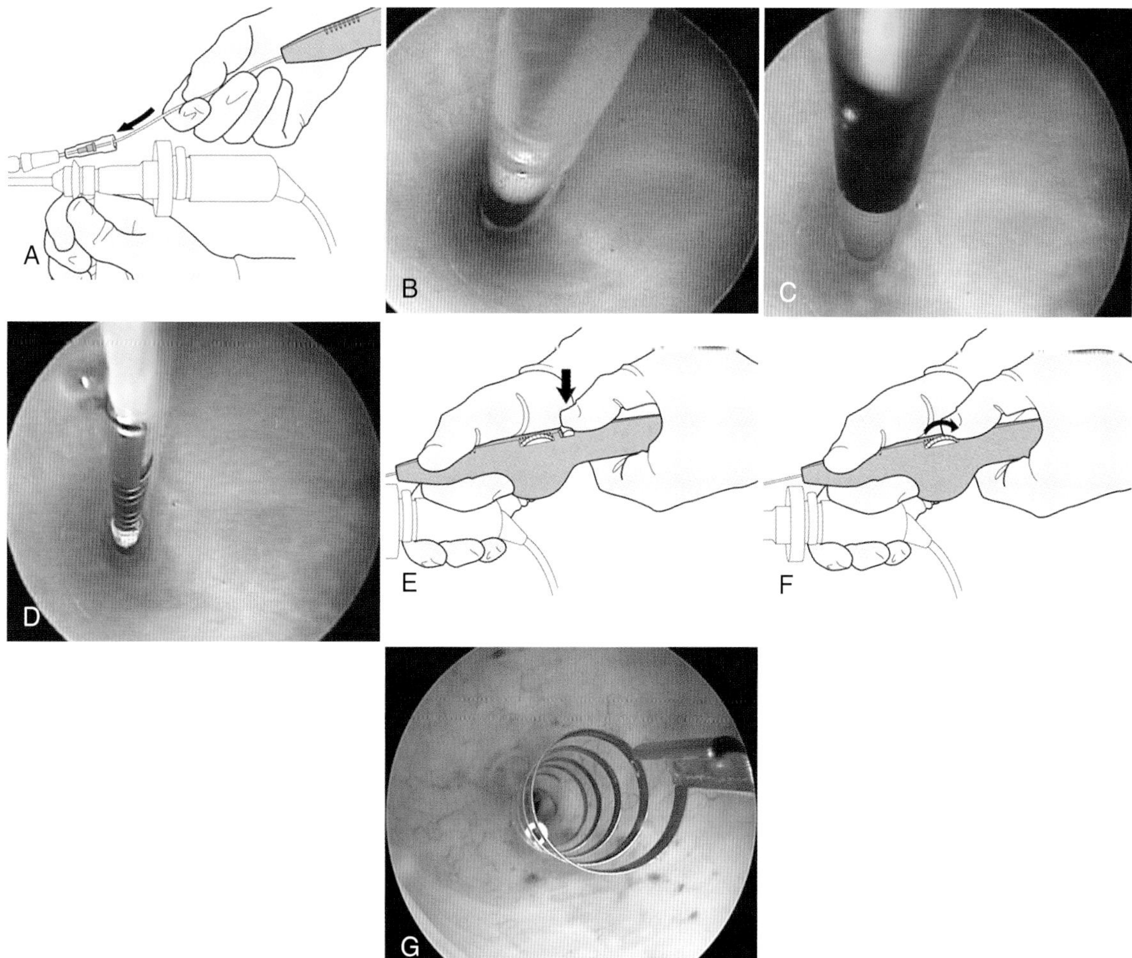

Figure 148-4 **A–G,** Essure placement steps for procedure. See text for details. Note especially how the inserter device is stabilized with the hand on the hysteroscope.

10. Insert the introducer through the working channel of the hysteroscope (see Fig. 148-4A).
11. Advance the catheter through the introducer to the tubal ostium on one side. There is a black marker on the introducer to signify the correct location of the catheter at the ostium (see Fig. 148-4B).
12. Stabilize the device handle on the hysteroscope.
13. Roll the thumbwheel on the inserter handle back so that the black positioning marker on the catheter moves toward you until reaching a hard stop. The handle is marked with a "1" and an arrow at this location (see Fig. 148-4C).
14. Check the placement of the microinsert by locating the gold band, which should be just outside the ostium with the green release catheter in view (see Fig. 148-4D).
15. Deploy the insert by pressing the button on the handle. The microinsert will not yet expand, allowing for any final positioning adjustments for the insert at this time (see Fig. 148-4E).
16. Expand and detach the microinsert by rolling the thumbwheel back to a second hard stop (see Fig. 148-4F).
17. Document visualization of the coils at the ostium to show proper placement (see Fig. 148-4G).
18. Withdraw the catheter, leaving the introducer in place.
19. Insert another catheter into the hysteroscope and repeat steps 11 to 18 on the other tubal ostium.
20. Remove the introducer. Then remove the hysteroscope from the uterine cavity under direct visualization.

When inserted, the device is placed in the proximal fallopian tube in the contracted state (Fig. 148-5A) and then deployed to an expanded state once correctly positioned in the interstitial portion of the tubal lumen. After release, the outer coil expands to 1.5 to 2.0 mm in diameter, anchoring and embedding the microinsert in each fallopian tube (Fig. 148-5B).

The trailing coils of the microinsert are easily visualized at each tubal ostium, ensuring "on-site" confirmation of proper placement within the fallopian tubes. Once the inserts are in place, the PET fibers elicit tissue in-growth. The PET fiber mesh and the microinsert act as scaffolding into which the tissue grows, further embedding the microinsert within the proximal uterotubal junction, thus resulting in sterilization (Fig. 148-5C). Correct placement of the radiopaque microinserts and tubal occlusion is confirmed by HSG 12 weeks following the procedure (Fig. 148-5D).

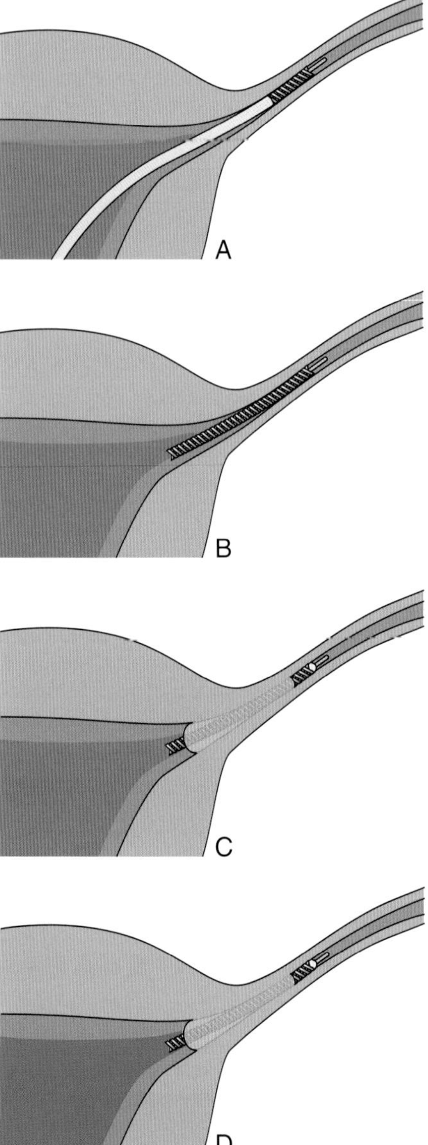

Figure 148-5 Essure procedure for permanent birth control. **A,** Using a hysteroscope, the Essure microinsert is inserted into the fallopian tube using a small catheter. **B,** Once deployed, the Essure microinserts expand to fit the fallopian tube, which anchors them in place. **C,** After approximately 12 weeks after procedure, tissue grows into the Essure microinserts, forming a permanent natural barrier, which occludes the fallopian tube. **D,** At 3 months, low-pressure hysterosalpingography is performed. The radiologic study documents that injected dye remains in the uterine cavity and does not pass through the fallopian tubes, confirming tubal occlusion. (Courtesy of Conceptus, Inc., Mountain View, CA.)

Sample Operative Report

Identifying data: Patient is a 36-year-old white G2P2 who requests sterilization by Essure micoinserts

Preoperative diagnosis: Elective permanent sterilization

Postoperative diagnosis: Bilateral Essure insertion

Estimated blood loss: None

Complications: None

Operation performed: Hysteroscopically guided bilateral tubal sterilization with Essure microinserts

Surgeon: Dr. ____________

Anesthesia: Paracervical block

Procedure: The patient's preoperative examination and consent were obtained with a prior office visit. A negative urine pregnancy test was confirmed prior to starting the procedure. The patient was placed in the dorsolithotomy position and a bimanual examination demonstrated a normal-sized, mobile uterus without abnormality. An open-sided self-illuminating speculum was inserted into the vagina and the cervix identified and prepped with antiseptic solution. A paracervical block was performed with approximately 5 mL of 1% lidocaine. The anterior lip of the cervix was grasped with a single-tooth tenaculum. The cervix was progressively dilated to approximately 6 mm. The hysteroscope was inserted under direct visualization into the uterine cavity. The uterine cavity was distended with normal saline via a gravity flow system. The uterine fundus was well visualized. Both tubal ostia were identified and appeared normal. The tip of the hysteroscope was brought within close proximity of the patient's left tubal ostium. The Essure microinsert was advanced through the operating channel of the hysteroscope and maneuvered easily into the left fallopian tube. Under direct visualization, the microinsert was deployed without difficulty. After release, the trailing coils of the microinsert were easily visualized at the tubal ostium. The preceding technique was repeated, resulting in a successful, confirmed placement of a microinsert into the patient's right fallopian tube. The hysteroscope was withdrawn under direct visualization. All instrumentation was removed from the vagina. The patient tolerated the procedure well.

Common Errors

- Performing sterilization on a patient who is uncertain about future childbearing. Be certain to discuss the permanent nature of the procedure.
- Failure to obtain HSG 12 weeks after the procedure. Be certain to arrange follow-up for this portion of the procedure to ensure efficacy and proper placement. Alternatively, ultrasonography (two or three dimensional) can be utilized to determine successful bilateral placement because the microinserts are highly echogenic on pelvic ultrasound.
- Failure of physician to properly reinforce patient compliance regarding the importance of back-up contraception until the HSG confirms both correct placement and tubal occlusion. Should the HSG be inconclusive, the patient must continue back-up contraception until a final determination is reached.
- Microinsert removal should not be attempted hysteroscopically once the microinsert has been placed and detached from the delivery wire. Attempted removal of a microinsert having less than 18 coils trailing into the uterine cavity may result in tubal perforation or other patient injury. Consult product Information for Users guide (IFU) for complete details and exceptions.

Complications

Failure rates. Evaluation of all available clinical data from 2001 to 2009 reveals 503 reported pregnancies with 372,112 Essure systems sold commercially. Most pregnancies are avoidable and occur as a result of physician/patient noncompliance with recommended follow-up or misinterpreted confirmation test.

Although no major complications are associated with transcervical sterilization, *short-term complications* reported in the IFU or recent clinical studies include the following:

- Inability to place two microinserts in the first procedure, ~3.1% (Levie, 2009).
- An initial tubal patentcy rate of 3.5% at 3 months and 0% at 6 months.
- Expulsion rate of 2.9%.
- Unsatisfactory device location, 0.6%.
- Risks related to the insertion procedure itself include cramping (29.6%) and pain (12.9%) on the day of the procedure, dizziness (8.8%), bleeding or spotting (6.8%), vasovagal response/fainting (1.3%). The majority of patients actually consider the procedure painless or scarcely painful. Cramping pain during the procedure was reported comparable to or less than menses.
- Tubal perforation rate of 1.1%. Tubal perforation may often go undiagnosed during the procedure or even at the HSG 3 months after the sterilization. The microinsert may perforate into the peritoneal cavity and be entrapped by the omentum causing chronic pain or can lead to complications such as hemorrhage, infection, or bowel injuries and compromise the contraceptive efficiency of Essure (Fig. 148-6). Therefore, in the case of a suspected perforation into the abdominal cavity, the prudent option is to investigate sooner rather than later. The possible need for a laparoscopic evaluation (carried out elsewhere if procedure is office-based) should always be discussed prior to the procedure as part of the informed consent. Alternatively, the use of fluoroscopy and two- or three-dimensional ultrasound have been suggested as useful tools in locating microinserts dislodged into the abdominal cavity

Postprocedure Management

- Patients return to work in 1 day and most resume their daily activities the same day as the procedure.
- Patients should be counseled to use an alternative form of contraception until HSG confirmation of placement and occlusion of tubal lumen.

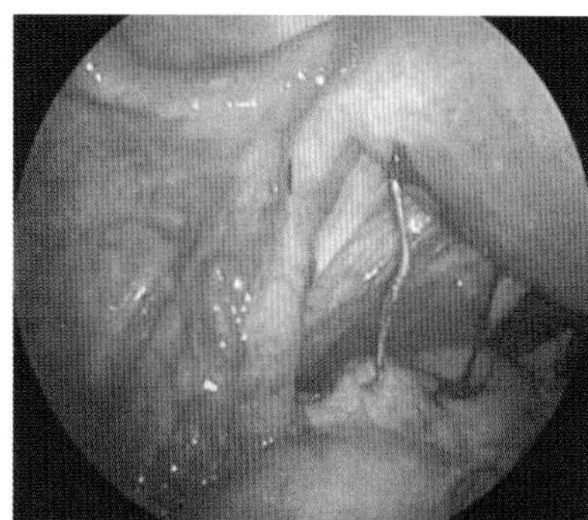

Figure 148-6 Perforation by Essure microinsert of left side of the proximal tube. The microinsert remains attached to the tube by its distal portion while the proximal end rests on the fatty tissue of the sigmoid colon. (Courtesy of V. Thoma, MD.)

- Patients should be educated to inform their health care providers of the presence of Essure microinserts prior to undergoing any future medical or surgical procedure.

Concomitant Hysteroscopic Sterilization and Global Endometrial Ablation

Initially, FDA approval was granted for a Thermachoice endometrial ablation (see Chapter 156, Endometrial Ablation) to be performed concomitantly on those women who had a transcervical microinsert hysteroscopic sterilization. After evaluation of postapproval study data, the FDA later recommended a modification to the microinsert procedure label stating that the Thermachoice treatment should not be performed until after the completion of the 3-month HSG.

Until recently, little was known about concomitant use of global endometrial ablation (GEA) methods for endometrial ablation (e.g., balloon, cryoablation, hydrothermablation [HTA] microwave or RF energy) and hysteroscopic sterilization with microinserts. Studies assessing Thermachoice and Essure in a perihysterectomy setting demonstrated no interference with achieving a uniform ablation effect and no conduction of heat via the Essure microinsert to the serosal surface of either fallopian tube or cornua. Another retrospective study of concomitant use of Thermachoice, NovaSure, and HTA demonstrated an 85% patient satisfaction rate and no adverse events leading to the conclusion that performance of combined GEA and hysteroscopic sterilization is effective in the treatment of menometrorrhagia.

Although current data support that it is feasible and effective to perform GEA and hysteroscopic sterilization at the same session, long-term data are still needed. Either the Essure or ablation can be performed first, depending on the topography of the uterine cavity, surgeon's expertise, and the type of energy utilized for the ablation.

- Remember that, if a concomitant procedure is planned, you must inform the patient that this is an off-label, non-FDA approved use of these combined technologies.
- It would be prudent that, taking into consideration all of the preceding information, until a level of proficiency is reached with office hysteroscopic sterilization, any endeavor to perform a concomitant procedure should be carried out with particular caution.

CPT/Billing Codes

Physician reimbursement for this procedure is substantially greater if the procedure is performed in the office rather than the hospital.

58340 Catheterization and introduction of saline or contrast material for saline infusion sonohysterography or hysterosalpingography
58565 Hysteroscopy, with bilateral fallopian tube cannulation to induce occulsion by placement of permanent implants

ICD-9-CM Codes

V25.09 Family planning advice
V25.2 Sterilization, admission for interruption of fallopian tubes/vas deferens
V25.40 Contraceptive surveillance, unspecified

Acknowledgment

The authors wish to thank Jeanne Ballard, MD, for her assistance with this chapter.

Suppliers

Full contact information is available online at www.expertconsult.com.

Adiana Permanent Contraceptive System, patient information, physician education, and instructional videos
Hologic, Inc., Bedford, MA
www.adiana.com

Essure ESS305 microinsert device, patient education, physician information, procedure videos, and training/credentialing information
Conceptus, Inc.
http://essuremd.com/

Hysteroscopy equipment, disposable illuminated vaginal speculums, distention media, miscellaneous supplies
See Chapter 140, Hysteroscopy.

BIBLIOGRAPHY

American College of Obstetrics and Gynecology: Use of hysterosalpingography after tubal sterilization. Committee Opinion No. 458. Obstet Gynecol 115:1343–1345, 2010.

Arjona JE, Mino M, Cordon J, et al: Satisfaction and tolerance with office hysteroscopic tubal sterilization. Fertil Steril 90:1182–1186, 2008.

Connor VF: Essure: A review six years later. J Minimal Invasive Gynecol 16:282–290, 2009.

Essure® Information For Use (IFU). Conceptus, Inc., Mountain View, CA, revised 09/09/2009, pp 1–6.

Guiahi M, Goldman KN, McElhinney MM, Olson CG: Improving hysterosalpingogram confirmatory test follow-up after Essure hysteroscopic sterilization. Contraception 81:520–524, 2010.

Levie M, Chudnoff S: Office hysteroscopic sterilization compared with laparoscopic sterilization: A critical cost analysis. J Minimal Invasive Gynecol 12:318–322, 2005.

Levie MD, Chudnoff SG: Prospective analysis of office-based hysteroscopic sterilization. J Minimal Invasive Gynecol 13:98–101, 2006.

Levie M, Weiss G, Kaiser B, et al: Analysis of pain and satisfaction with office-based hysteroscopic sterilization. Fertil Steril 2009 (in press). Epub: http://www.fertstert.org/article/S0015-0282(09)02490-X/abstract.

Mino M, Arjona JE, Cordon J, et al: Success rate and satisfaction with Essure sterilization in an outpatient setting: A prospective study of 857 women. Br J Obstet Gynecol 114:763–766, 2007.

Nichols M, Carter JF, Fylstra DL, et al: A comparative study of hysteroscopic sterilization performed in-office versus a hospital operating room. J Minimal Invasive Gynecol 13:447–450, 2006.

Ory EM, Hines RS, Cleland WH, Rehberg JF: Pregnancy after microinsert sterilization with tubal occlusion confirmed by hysterosalpingogram. Obstet Gynecol 111:508–510, 2008.

Palmer SN, Greenberg JA: Transcervical sterilization: A comparison of Essure® Permanent Birth Control System and Adiana® Permanent Contraception System. Rev Obstet Gynecol 2:84–89, 2009.

Peterson HB: Sterilization. Obstet Gynecol 111:189–203, 2008.

Shavell VI, Abdallah ME, Shade GH, et al: Trends in sterilization since the introduction of Essure hysteroscopic sterilization. J Minimal Invasive Gynecol 16:22–27, 2009.

Syed R, Levy J, Childers ME: Pain associated with hysteroscopic sterilization. JSLS 11:63–65, 2007.

Tatalovich JM, Anderson TL: Hysteroscopic sterilization in patients with a Mirena intrauterine device: Transition from interval to permanent contraception. J Minimal Invasive Gynecol 17:228–231, 2010.

Thoma V, Chua I, Garbin O, et al: Tubal perforation by Essure microinsert. J Minimal Invasive Gynecol 13:161–163, 2006.

Valle RF: Tubal perforation by Essure microinsert: Clearly not a tubal perforation but a cornual-uterine perforation. J Minimal Invasive Gynecol 13:487–488, 2006.

Vancaillie TG, Anderson TL, Johns DA: A 12-month prospective evaluation of transcervical sterilization using implantable polymer matrices (EASE study). Obstet Gynecol 112:1270–1277, 2008.

Veersema S, Vleugels MP, Timmermans A, Brölmann HA: Follow-up of successful bilateral placement of Essure microinserts with ultrasound. Fertil Steril 84:1733–1736, 2005.

CHAPTER 149

Loop Electrosurgical Excision Procedure for Treating Cervical Intraepithelial Neoplasia

Thomas C. Wright, Jr.

A variety of techniques can be used to treat cervical intraepithelial neoplasia (CIN). The appropriateness of a particular technique to treat a particular lesion depends on a number of factors, including lesion size, location, and extension into the endocervical canal. Many clinicians now use the loop electrosurgical excision procedure (LEEP) to treat most women with biopsy-confirmed CIN 2 or CIN 3. With LEEP, thin wire loop electrodes are used to excise the entire cervical transformation zone. This procedure is referred to by a number of different names, including loop electrosurgical excision procedure (LEEP), large loop excision of the transformation zone (LLETZ), and loop excision. Many clinicians subdivide LEEP into two procedures: (1) routine LEEP, which is used to excise lesions confined to the exocervix (or visible portion of the cervix), and (2) LEEP conization, which is used when lesions extend into the endocervical canal. LEEP has a number of advantages over other treatment modalities for CIN, including the following:

- The equipment is less expensive than laser equipment.
- The entire lesion is excised and can be assessed histologically to rule out invasive cancer.
- Patients can be diagnosed and treated in a single office visit.
- It allows cervical conization to be performed in the office at a significantly reduced cost (LEEP conization).
- Complications are few for the procedure itself, but it can affect future pregnancies.

Anatomy

The anatomy relevant to the LEEP is reviewed in detail in Chapter 137, Colposcopic Examination. As the procedure involves complete removal of the transformation zone, it is important to understand the anatomy of the cervix, including normal and abnormal appearances. In most circumstances, a colposcopy will be completed prior to the LEEP to define the anatomy of the cervix.

Indications

The following indications are based on the 2006 American Society for Colposcopy and Cervical Pathology (ASCCP) guidelines that are reproduced in Appendix K, Management Guidelines for Abnormal Cervical Cancer Screening Tests and Histologic Findings. Several options are given for treatment of most of these indications. This chapter presents the possible indications for the LEEP.

Routine LEEP

- Biopsy-confirmed CIN 2 or CIN 3 and a satisfactory colposcopy
- High-grade squamous intraepithelial lesion (HSIL) on referral cytologic examination that is immediately treated in a patient over age 20 ("screen and treat")
- Persistent HSIL on screening for 6 to 12 months (without CIN 2 or 3 documented by biopsy)
- CIN 1 on biopsy after screening result of HSIL or atypical glandular cells–not otherwise specified (AGC-NOS)

When several treatment options exist with the treatment guidelines, LEEP is preferred over ablative therapies such as cryotherapy in the following conditions:

- High-grade lesion involving three or more quadrants
- Complex-appearing CIN 2 or 3 with prominent abnormal vessels
- Lesion is not covered by cryoprobe
- Ectocervix is irregular
- Patients have recurrent CIN after previous therapy (e.g., cone biopsy, LEEP, cryotherapy)

LEEP Conization

- Unsatisfactory colposcopy in women with biopsy-confirmed CIN of any grade (e.g., cannot see entire lesion, squamocolumnar junction [SCJ], or transformation zone [TZ])
- HSIL on referral cytologic examination and unsatisfactory colposcopy
- HSIL on referral cytologic examination with satisfactory colposcopy and either no CIN or only CIN 1 identified ("lack of correlation principle")
- Positive endocervical sampling (e.g., neoplasia of any grade present)
- Microinvasive lesions on cervical biopsy

Contraindications

Relative

- Bleeding diathesis
- Patient exposed in utero to diethylstilbestrol
- Patient fewer than 12 weeks after delivery
- Equivocal cervical abnormalities
- Heavy menses

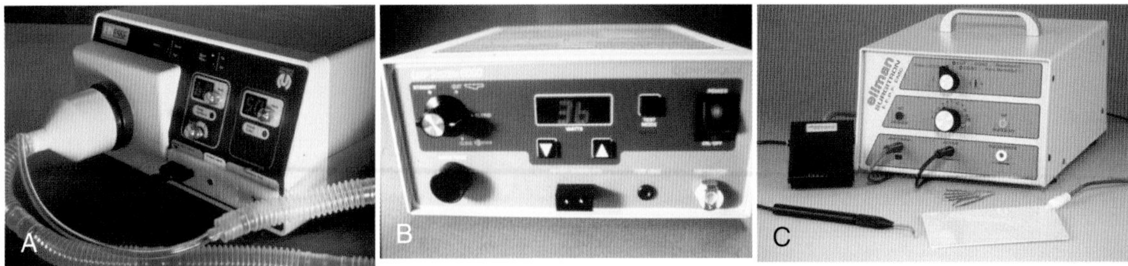

Figure 149-1 Electrosurgical units used for loop electrosurgical excision procedure (LEEP). **A,** Utah Medical electrosurgical unit. The smoke evacuator is included in the basic unit. **B,** CooperSurgical LEEP unit. **C,** Ellman Surgitron with handpiece, electrodes, antenna plate, and foot pedal. (**A,** Courtesy of Utah Medical Products, Inc., Midvale, UT. **B,** Courtesy of CooperSurgical, Trumbull, CT. **C,** Courtesy of Ellman International, Hewlett, NY.)

- A preexisting short cervix (clinician should consider referral)
- Patients with pacemakers (special precaution necessary)
- Severe cervicitis

Absolute

- Pregnancy
- Clinically apparent invasive carcinoma of the cervix
- Lack of expertise to control potential severe cervical bleeding

Equipment and Supplies

- Electrosurgical generator or unit (ESU) (Fig. 149-1) with the following features:
  - Minimum output capability of 50 watts in both cutting and coagulation modes
  - Rapid-start features
  - Patient grounding pad monitor (beneficial if the patient is under anesthesia)
  - Isolated circuitry

EDITOR'S NOTE: Although the Ellman Surgitron does not meet some of these qualifications, it has been used extensively for the LEEP.

- Loop electrodes of the appropriate size and a ball electrode for fulguration (Fig. 149-2). (These electrodes can be either of the disposable or of the reusable variety.)

  It is recommended that clinicians use only the shallow loop electrodes (i.e., either 0.8 or 1.0 cm deep) for routine LEEP. Larger electrodes can be used with large cervices or when lesions extend into the endocervical canal (e.g., LEEP conization). A variation is the Fischer electrode, which provides a true "cone" specimen.
- Electrode handle and a patient return electrode (grounding pad or antenna).
- Nonconductive speculum (either coated with a nonconductive material or made of plastic) capable of being used in conjunction with a smoke evacuator (Fig. 149-3).
- Smoke evacuator equipped with an adequate viral and odor filter.
- Colposcope capable of low magnification (4× to 7.5×).
- Nonsterile gloves.
- Acetic acid (5%).
- Full-strength aqueous Lugol's solution.
- Cotton balls and large OB-GYN applicators.
- Ring forceps.
- Syringe (5 mL) with 4-inch needle extender and 1½-inch, 25-gauge needle as well as 5 mL of 2% lidocaine with epinephrine, or dental type of syringe equipped with a 25- to 27-gauge needle at least 1½ inches long with two 1.8-mL ampules of 2% lidocaine with 1:100,000 epinephrine (Fig. 149-4).
- Coated vaginal sidewall retractor (*arrow*, see Fig. 149-3).
- Kevorkian endocervical curette.
- Monsel's paste, which is made by allowing Monsel's solution to evaporate until it forms a thick yellow paste.
- Containers of histologic fixative (usually 10% formalin).
- A 12-inch needle holder and 2-0 Vicryl suture material together with a vaginal pack in the event that large-vessel bleeding occurs.
- Power examination table with adjustable height (recommended).

Precautions

It is imperative that the LEEP not be used to excise the TZ indiscriminately in women with atypical Papanicolaou (Pap) smears. The procedure should be reserved to treat advanced lesions as per the established indications, not just atypical Pap smears or CIN 1. CIN 1 has a high rate of regression and should usually be observed or

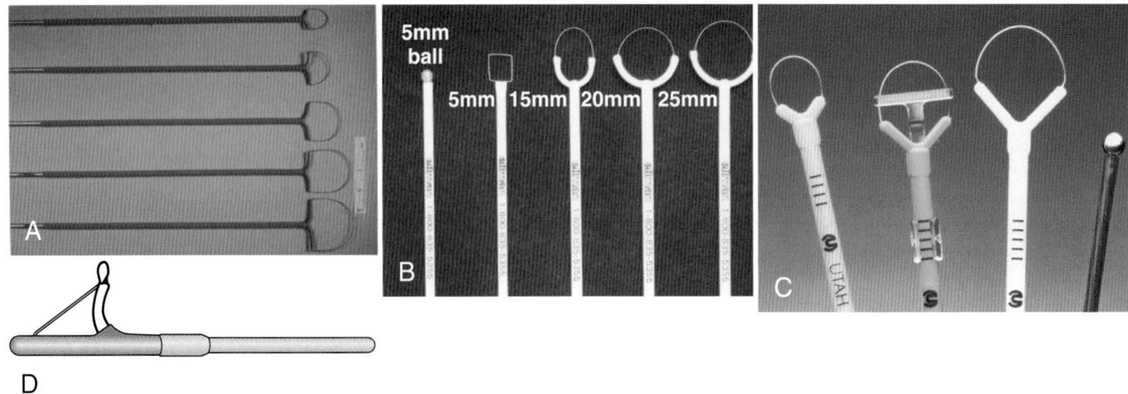

Figure 149-2 Wire loop electrodes for loop electrosurgical excision procedure (LEEP). **A,** Loop electrodes come in a variety of sizes and shapes. **B,** Ellman electrodes. **C,** Utah Medical electrodes with an optional adjustable stop to limit depth (*middle*, green-handled loop). **D,** Fischer electrode, which removes more of a conical piece. (**A–C,** Courtesy of The Medical Procedures Center, PC, John L. Pfenninger, MD.)

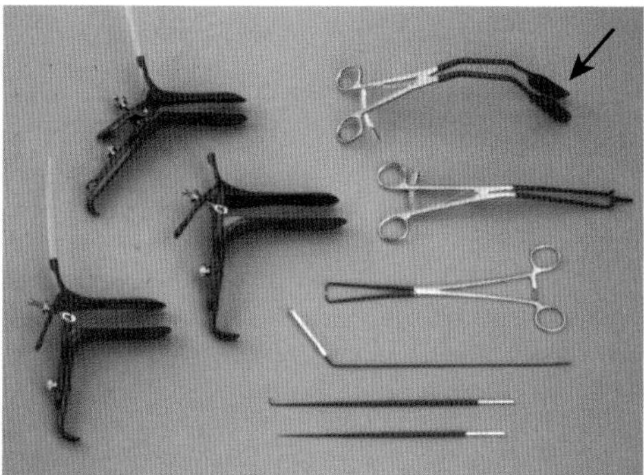

Figure 149-3 Coated instruments to prevent electrical shocks. Vaginal sidewall retractors (*arrow*) are essential in many cases to avoid lacerating the vaginal walls. Three different vaginal speculums are on the left, each with a vented tube to attach to the smoke evacuator tubing.

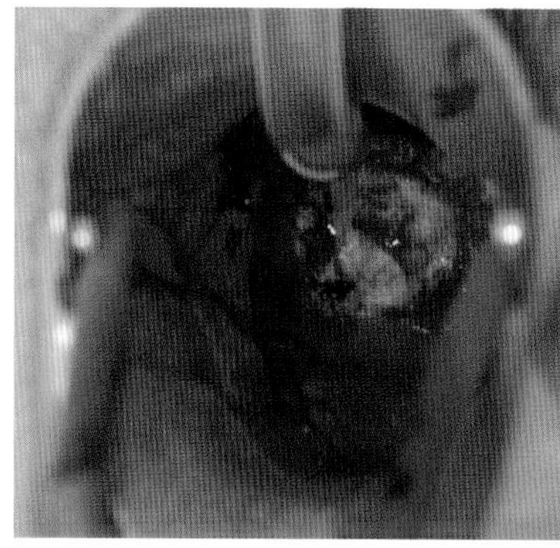

Figure 149-5 The cervix as seen through a coated vaginal speculum with coated, nonconductive sidewall retractors in place.

treated with less invasive options. Cryotherapy is less expensive, has fewer complications, and has equal outcomes in properly selected patients (while at the same time removing less tissue) (see Chapter 138, Cryotherapy of the Cervix). Cold-knife conization is preferred when conization is being performed for a glandular abnormality.

Preprocedure Patient Education

- Provide a patient education handout (see the sample patient education handout online at www.expertconsult.com).
- Instruct the patient to take 600 to 800 mg of ibuprofen or a preferred nonsteriodal anti-inflammatory drug 1 to 2 hours before the procedure.
- Obtain informed consent.

Procedure

The procedure is best performed immediately after menses so that any vaginal bleeding is not confused with menses.

1. Have the patient undress from the waist down and lie on the gynecologic examination table. It is important that the patient not move, cough, or change position once the excision is started. Thus, a cooperative patient is essential.
2. Attach the patient return electrode grounding pad to the patient's thigh and connect the grounding pad to the ESU (or place the "antenna plate" under the hip).
3. Insert a nonconductive speculum with the smoke evacuator attachment into the vagina and connect it to the smoke evacuator. It is important that the speculum be large enough to allow complete, unobstructed visualization of the cervix. If the vaginal sidewalls remain in the way, use a vaginal sidewall retractor (Fig. 149-5, and see Fig. 149-3).
4. Apply the acetic acid solution, examine the cervix colposcopically, and identify all lesions and the TZ.
5. Apply full-strength Lugol's solution to the cervix (this lasts longer than acetic acid). Use cotton balls or a large OB-GYN applicator.

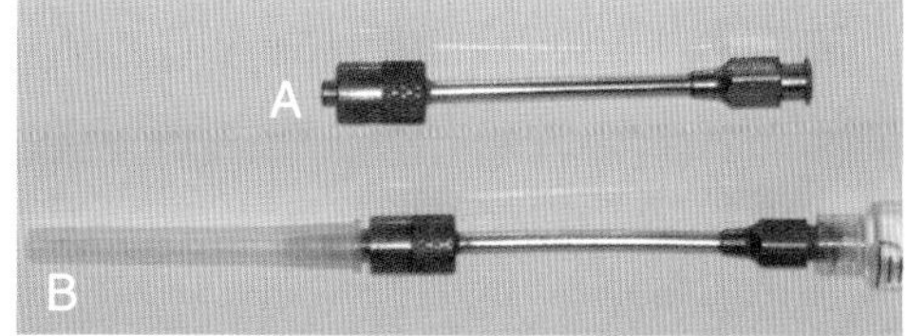

Figure 149-4 **A,** Needle extender (5 inch). **B,** Needle extender placed on the end of a 5-mL syringe with 25-gauge, 1½-inch needle attached. (Courtesy of The Medical Procedures Center, PC, John L. Pfenninger, MD.)

6. Inject approximately 0.5 to 1.5 mL of 2% lidocaine with epinephrine 1 : 100,000 intracervically (submucosally) at each of the 12, 3, 6, and 9 o'clock positions (to a total of 2 to 6 mL), usually just outside the TZ. Take care to inject the cervix superficially, only 3 to 5 mm deep. Additional injections may be needed at intervals between those noted previously, depending on the size of the cervix.
7. Although loops of many different sizes are available from various manufacturers, a round loop 2 cm wide by 0.8 cm deep (R2008) is most frequently used for CIN lesions confined to the portio. For a small, nulliparous cervix, use a 1.5 × 0.7 cm loop (R1507). For LEEP conizations when lesions extend into the endocervical canal, a 1 × 1 cm loop electrode can be used to excise the endocervical canal itself. This can be performed after the ectocervical excision has been completed to perform a "cowboy hat" type of procedure (see Fig. 149-7C).

   The power required will depend on the ESU used and the diameter of the loop. In general, a 2.0 × 0.8 cm loop will require between 35 and 45 watts of power, whereas a 1 × 1 cm loop will require only 20 to 30 watts of power. For LEEP, the use of a blended (cut and coagulate) current provides the combination of minimal tissue artifact and minimal amounts of bleeding. However, many use a *pure cutting* setting, which provides even less burn artifact for the pathologist while still controlling bleeding. It also allows for the use of less power so less tissue is damaged.

   Three different types of cervical LEEP excisions can be performed, depending on the size and location of the CIN lesion: (1) LEEP for small lesions confined to the exocervix, (2) LEEP for large lesions confined to the ectocervix, and (3) LEEP conization for lesions extending into the endocervix.

   For small lesions confined to the ectocervix, the following is suggested:
   - Select a loop electrode 1.5 to 2.0 cm wide and 0.8 cm deep. Place the loop several millimeters lateral to the edge of the CIN lesion and make a test pass over the lesion to ensure that the path is clear.
   - Hold the loop just above the surface, activate the loop, and then push it perpendicularly, gradually, into the tissue to a depth of about 4 mm.
   - While pushing the loop deeper into the cervical stroma to the full depth of 8 mm, draw it laterally and through the endocervical canal. Pull it to the other side several millimeters past a lesion or several millimeters beyond the TZ, whichever is more lateral, before removing it (Fig. 149-6).

NOTE: In most instances the entire CIN lesion and the TZ can be removed in a single pass. This produces a donut-shaped specimen with the endocervical canal in the center.

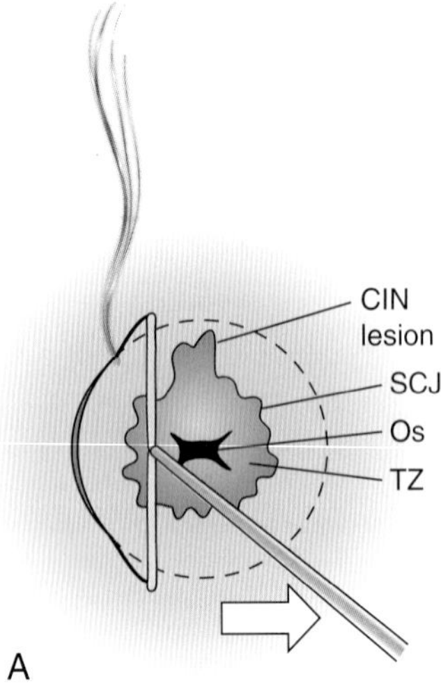

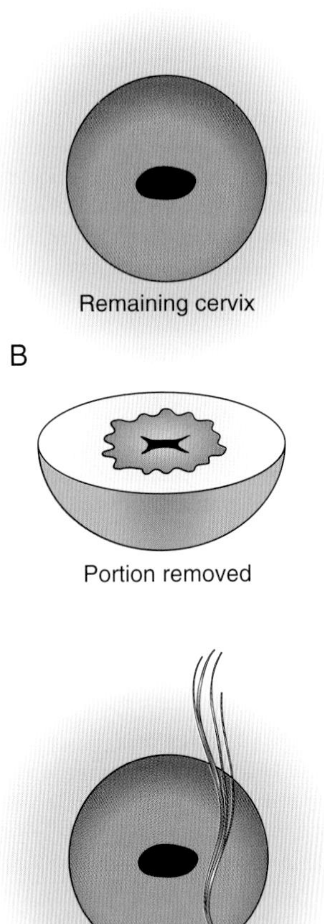

Figure 149-6 Standard loop electrosurgical excision procedure (LEEP) for cervical intraepithelial lesions that can be removed in a single pass. After painting the cervix with Lugol's solution and injecting lidocaine, the clinician uses an ectocervical loop (2 cm wide and 0.8 cm deep) to resect the entire lesion (**A** and **B**). Then the crater base is coagulated using a 5-mm ball electrode followed by the application of Monsel's paste (**C**). CIN, cervical intraepithelial neoplasia; SCJ, squamocolumnar junction; TZ, transformation zone.

For larger lesions confined to the ectocervix, the following technique is advised:

- In some instances, CIN lesions may be too extensive to be removed in a single pass. In this event, remove the central portion of the lesion using a 2-cm wide loop electrode, as previously described.
- Then, excise the remaining CIN and TZ with additional, more superficial passes using the same loop electrode. Alternatively, the remaining tissue can be ablated using electrocoagulation with a ball electrode (Fig. 149-7).

For CIN extending into the endocervical canal, LEEP conizations are performed and lesions are removed in a two-step procedure that uses a 2-cm wide exocervical electrode in conjunction with a 1 × 1 cm loop or square endocervical electrode to produce a cowboy-hat type of excision. For this procedure, one of two methods can be used:

- The *first method* involves excising the endocervical portion of the lesion first using the 1 × 1 cm endocervical electrode. Once the endocervical portion of the lesion is excised, the exocervical portion is excised using a standard 2.0 × 0.8 cm loop electrode (Fig. 149-8A).

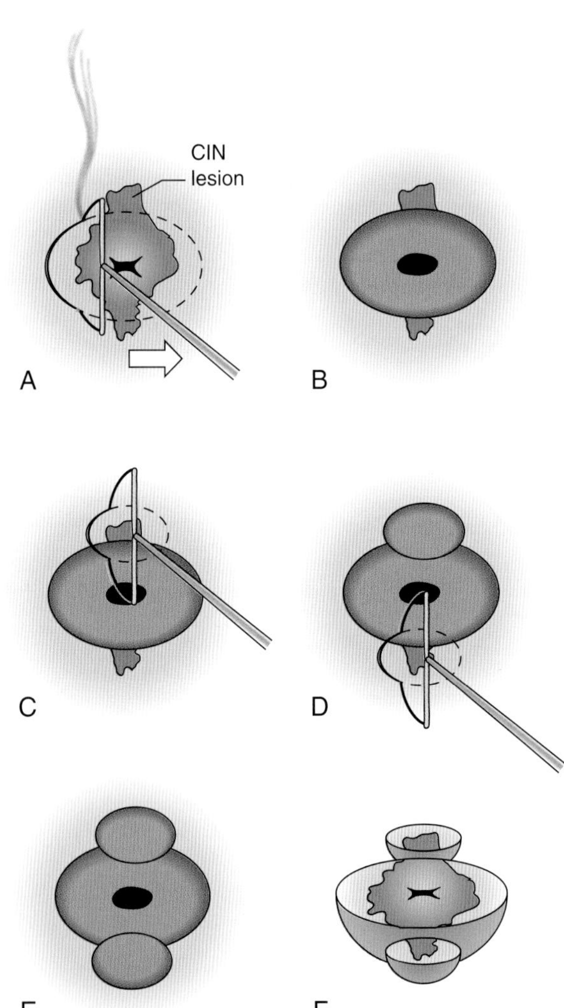

Figure 149-7 For lesions too large to be removed in a single pass, the clinician uses a 2 × 0.8 cm loop electrode to resect the central portion of the lesion (**A** and **B**). Then, the remaining tissue is resected with additional passes using the same electrode (**C–E**). Tissue specimens (**F**) are placed in the same bottle of formalin. CIN, cervical intraepithelial neoplasia.

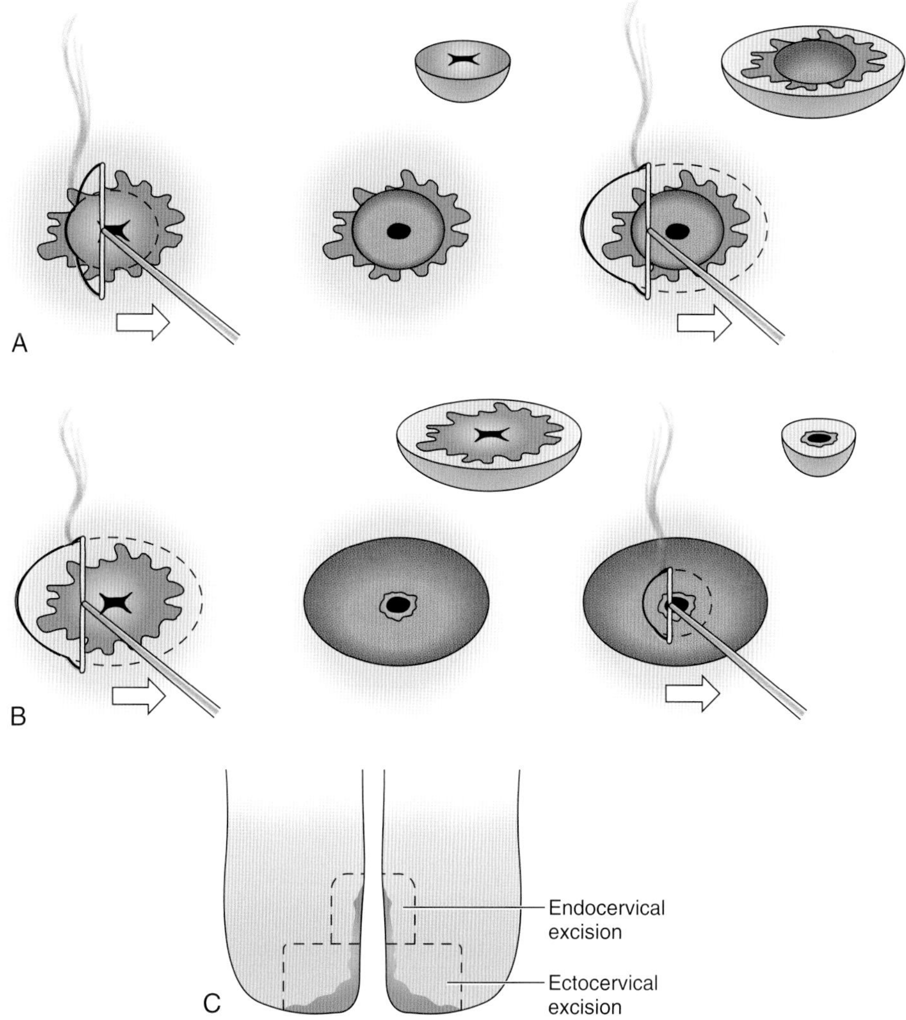

Figure 149-8 Two methods for obtaining an endocervical sample with the loop electrosurgical excision procedure: **A,** The clinician resects the endocervical portion of the lesion using a 1 × 1 cm loop. Then a 2.0 × 0.8 cm loop is used to resect additional cervical intraepithelial neoplasia extending onto the portio. **B,** In some cases it may be necessary to excise the ectocervical portion first. Excising to a depth greater than 1.5 cm into the canal increases the chances of significant bleeding. **C,** Longitudinal section showing the "cowboy-hat" procedure.

In the *second method,* the large ectocervical portion is excised first, followed by the smaller endocervical portion (Fig. 149-8B). Care should be taken not to excise the endocervical canal too deeply. Both approaches leave a cowboy-hat shaped excision on the cervix (Fig. 149-8C). The endocervical and exocervical excisional specimens should be submitted for pathologic assessment in separate containers.

Some pathologists prefer that after the specimen is excised, it be removed from the cervix using forceps, opened along one side, and placed in a plastic holder to allow it to fix in formalin in the proper orientation. Other pathologists prefer the specimen to be tagged at a certain location. Clinicians should check with the particular pathologist to determine preferences. Generally "tagging" the tissue to provide location provides little practical information. Although some clinicians want to know whether or not the endocervical margin of the specimen is involved with CIN, this can be difficult to evaluate because of tissue orientation on the histology slide and thermal damage. An endocervical curettage (ECC) taken immediately after the LEEP can also be used to evaluate whether the CIN lesion has been removed in its entirety. In most instances when the margin or post-LEEP ECC is positive, the patient should simply be followed up 4 to 6 months later with cytologic examination and a repeat ECC (see Complications).

8. Inspect the ectocervix and the endocervical canal to ensure that all nonstained (iodine negative) ectocervix and all acetowhite epithelium (AWE) in the canal have been excised. (More acetic acid may need to be applied with a Q-Tip to the canal.) If AWE remains in the canal (often identified by a thin rim of white along the margin of the os), another excision should be carried out and the process repeated until there is no AWE remaining. Care should be taken not to interpret thermal cautery effect in the endocervical canal as residual neoplasia.
9. Perform an ECC above the excisional base. This helps confirm there was no dysplasia above the excision.
10. Fulgurate any bleeding points at the base of the excision using a ball electrode with the "coagulation" setting on the ESU. For 5-mm ball electrodes, power settings of 40 to 55 watts are usually required to obtain adequate arcing between the electrode and the tissue. (Excessive bleeding is more frequent in patients with severe cervicitis and in those less than 12 weeks after delivery.) Frequently the entire base of the excision is lightly coagulated. Perform the coagulation up to the endocervical canal, but take care not to insert the electrode into the

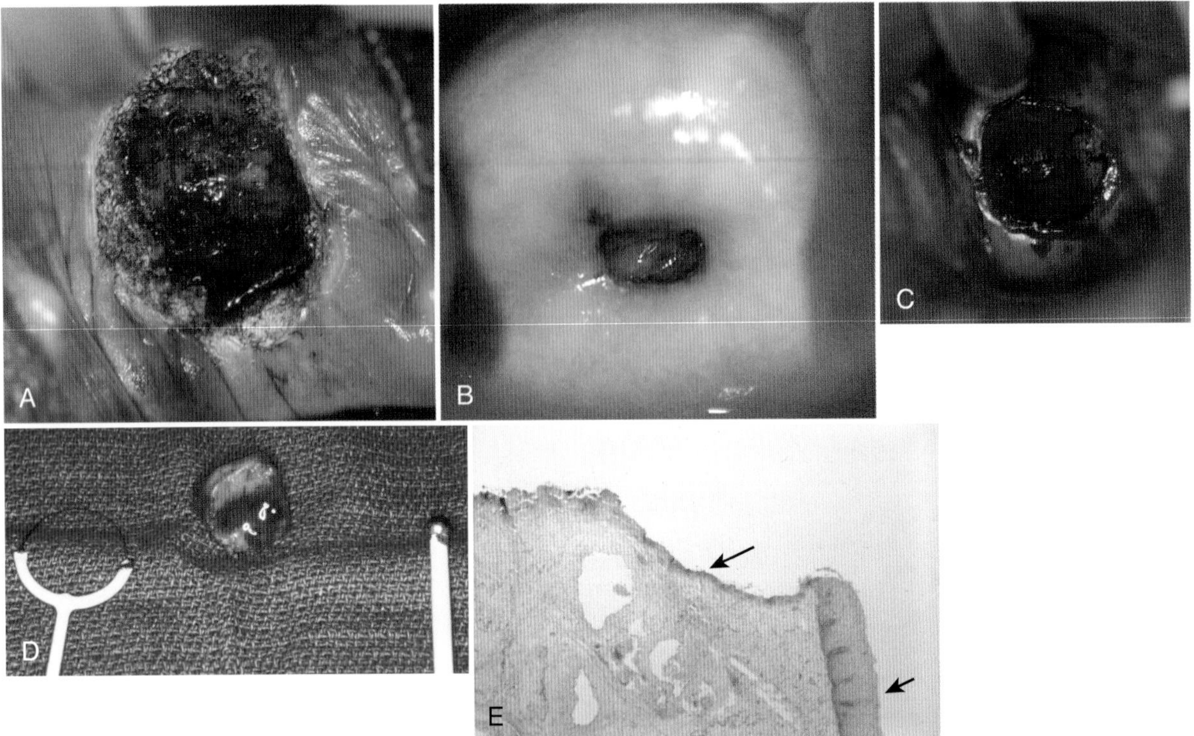

Figure 149-9 **A,** Appearance of the cervix as seen through a nonconductive speculum immediately after the loop electrosurgical excision procedure (LEEP). **B,** Appearance of cervix 4 months after LEEP. Note the absence of an ectocervical transformation zone. **C,** Appearance of cervix immediately after the "cowboy-hat" LEEP procedure (ectocervical and endocervical excision). Coated speculum and smoke evacuator tubing are in place. **D,** Tissue specimen from a single-pass LEEP procedure. **E,** Microscopic view of the removed tissue. Note the minimal tissue damage on the resected edge (*arrows*). (Courtesy of The Medical Procedures Center, PC, John L. Pfenninger, MD.)

canal. Excessive coagulation is not warranted and may be detrimental to optimal healing.

11. Apply Monsel's paste to the entire area. Figure 149-9A to E shows the typical cervix upon completion of the procedure with Monsel's applied (A) and 4 months after the procedure (B). Part C shows another cervix after the "cowboy hat" procedure as seen through a coated vaginal speculum. Part D shows the average tissue specimen from the LEEP. Part E is a microphotograph showing the minimal amount of thermal tissue damage from the LEEP.

Sample Operative Report

Preoperative diagnosis: CIN 3
Postoperative diagnosis: CIN 3
Surgeon: Dr. ____________
Anesthesia: Local, 1% lidocaine with epinephrine, 5 mL
Procedure: LEEP
Indications: The patient is a 35-year-old female with a history of several abnormal Pap smears including the most recent with HSIL. She underwent colposcopy with biopsy revealing a large CIN 3 lesion. After discussion of the options for treatment, the patient prefers LEEP.
Procedure: Informed consent was obtained and prior colposcopic findings were reviewed. The patient was placed in the dorsal lithotomy position and an insulated vaginal speculum was introduced with good visualization of the cervix. Acetic acid was applied and the previously noted lesion at 3 o'clock was again visualized under colposcopic magnification as was the entire squamocolumnar junction. No other abnormalities were noted. Lugol's solution was applied and the cervix again visualized with the colposcope. Anesthesia was provided with injections of 1% lidocaine with epinephrine at 3, 6, 9, and 12 o'clock just peripheral to the transformation zone. Approximately 5 mL was used in total. After adequate anesthesia was confirmed, a round 2.0 cm by 0.8 cm loop electrode was used on a pure cutting setting at 35 watts to remove the entire transformation zone in one pass. The edges of the lesion were visualized and included in the excision. There was minimal bleeding, which was controlled with coagulation using a ball electrode. Monsel's solution was applied prior to removing the speculum. Patient tolerated the procedure with minimal discomfort.
Estimated blood loss: Negligible
Specimen removed: One cervical specimen removed and sent to pathology
Complications: None

Common Errors

- The patient experiences an electric shock. Using a coated, nonconductive speculum prevents electric shock, which is caused by touching the speculum with the electrode during the procedure. An "electric shock" sensation can make the patient jump, causing significant injury.
- The loop electrode "stalls" as it is going through the tissue. Possible causes include the following:
  - If using a reusable loop, it must be free of carbon. Use a piece of fine sandpaper to shine the loops before the procedure. When using disposable loops, this will not be a problem.
  - The operator is moving the loop too quickly through the tissue. Go fast enough to prevent excessive tissue damage but slow enough to maintain a cutting function.
  - The cutting power is too low on the unit. Often, a pure cutting current will be easier to use than the "cut and coag" mode.

The unit has an automatic shut-off and the patient is not grounded. Check that the grounding pad is securely inserted to the main unit and attached to the patient.

If a stall occurs for any reason, withdraw the electrode and either try passing it through the same tissue again after the problem has been corrected or approach from the other side.

- The electrode won't "cut" when touching the cervix. The electrode has not been activated before touching the patient or the tissue is too dry. In order for the electrode to cut, the tissue must be moist. Apply some acetic acid. Always activate the unit before touching the tissue with the loop.
- Pathologist reports excessive thermal damage on the tissue. Turn down the power on the unit or switch to the pure cutting mode for future procedures.

Complications

- Significant *intraoperative bleeding* is an uncommon but potentially serious complication. It sometimes occurs when the electrode is inserted too deeply into the tissue at the 3 and 9 o'clock positions (where the cervical branches of the uterine artery are located) or when the patient has severe cervicitis. The most effective way to control bleeding is to first apply pressure directly to the bleeding site using a large cotton-tipped applicator. Once the bleeding has slowed, the ball electrode is then placed in direct contact with the bleeding site and tissue is "desiccated" using coagulation current. If the bleeding is not controlled with pressure, the clinician should inject 1 to 2 mL of 2% lidocaine *with epinephrine* into the bleeding site. With the bleeding slowed or stopped, the ball electrode may then be effective. For rare cases of persistent bleeding a "figure of eight" hemostatic stitch can be placed or the vagina and cervix can be packed tightly with 4 × 4 gauze and the patient transported to the emergency room.
- *Postoperative bleeding* occurs in less than 5% of patients. These patients experience a modest amount of bleeding 4 to 10 days after LEEP. It can usually be managed by electrofulguration or by packing the crater base with Monsel's paste. Minimal spotting is to be expected up to 14 days after the procedure and after initial intercourse.
- Post-treatment *cervical stenosis* (Fig. 149-10) is an uncommon complication (<1%) and occurs more commonly in postmenopausal women and those lacking estrogen stimulation (postmenopausal women, Implanon and Depo-Provera users; lactating women). For postmenopausal patients and hypoestrogenic states, consider replacement estrogen for 2 to 3 weeks after the procedure (one applicator of estrogen cream in the vagina every night).
- *Inadvertent burns or lacerations* to the lateral vaginal wall or other sites can occur but are rare. The clinician should instruct the patient not to move. Ureters, bowel, and bladder are only millimeters away from the vaginal sidewalls.
- *Pain and discomfort* are minimal and generally can be controlled with nonsteroidal anti-inflammatory drugs (NSAIDs).
- *Infection* is rare. Metronidazole or doxycycline can be used.
- *Recurrence or persistence* of disease occurs in 5% to 10% of cases.
- *Cervical incompetence.* Although it is generally recognized that cold-knife conization is associated with adverse obstetric outcomes, most of the studies published in the early 1990s showed little impact of LEEP on obstetric outcomes. Recently larger studies have been published and these newer studies indicate that all forms of excisional procedures used to treat CIN produce similar obstetric risks. A meta-analysis of these published trials found that LEEP has a significant association with preterm delivery (11% risk in treated women versus 7% risk in untreated women), low-birth-weight infants (8% in treated women versus 4% in untreated women), and premature rupture of membranes (5% in treated women versus 2% in untreated women). Therefore, when treating women likely to become pregnant in the future, consideration should be given to using an ablative method such cryotherapy rather than LEEP, provided the colposcopy is satisfactory and there is no suspicion of occult invasive cancer.

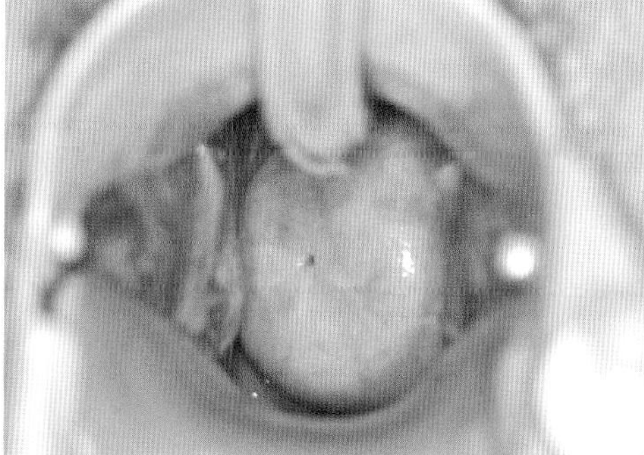

Figure 149-10 Cervical stenosis following a loop electrosurgical excision procedure. (Courtesy of The Medical Procedures Center, PC, John L. Pfenninger, MD.)

Postprocedure Management

Patients are seen 4 to 6 weeks after the procedure for a review of the pathology report and for a brief postoperative check. This visit helps reassure the patients and decreases their anxiety about how well they have healed. It also provides an opportunity to reinforce prevention methods, such as not smoking. It is important to check for cervical stenosis. The os is easier to dilate early rather than waiting for a more mature scar (see Chapter 136, Cervical Stenosis and Cervical Dilation).

The clinician should then reevaluate the patient using either a program of repeat cytologic examination at 6 and 12 months, a single HPV DNA test for high-risk types of HPV at 6 to 12 months, or a combination of cytologic examination and colposcopy at 6 and 12 months. If a program of repeat cytologic examination is used for follow-up, patients with a cytologic result of atypical squamous cells or higher classification should be referred for colposcopy. If HPV DNA testing at 6 to 12 months is used, patients with high-risk types of HPV identified should be referred for colposcopy.

Postprocedure Patient Education

See the sample patient education handout online at www.expertconsult.com.

- The clinician should instruct the patient to avoid vaginal intercourse, douching, use of tampons, and heavy exercise (especially weight lifting) for 3 weeks.
- If significant bleeding persists for more than 2 weeks (if the volume is comparable to that of a normal period or greater), if the patient begins passing large blood clots, if the vaginal discharge becomes foul smelling, or if there is significant pelvic pain (especially if it is associated with a fever), the patient should call the physician or return to the clinic.

Interpretation of Results

The specimen removed during LEEP should be sent to pathology as previously discussed. The pathologic diagnosis should confirm the prior biopsy and examination findings. The extent of dysplasia and involvement of the margins of resection will be reported. If invasive carcinoma is present, immediate reevaluation and follow-up are essential and the patient is generally referred to a gynecologic oncologist. Ideally, the lesion should be completely excised and the margins should be clear of any abnormal findings. If the ectocervical or endocervical excisional margins are "positive" on histologic examination or if the ECC is positive for neoplasia, the patient is at higher risk for recurrence. However, even in these situations, less than one third of lesions will persist. The cautery and inflammatory response appears to resolve most of these. In these cases it is prudent to perform colposcopy with endocervical curettage and repeat cytologic examination approximately 3 to 4 months after the initial LEEP. In some instances, especially high-risk and postmenopausal patients, consideration should be given to performing a repeat diagnostic conization procedure (e.g., either a cold-knife or LEEP conization) once the cervix has healed.

CPT/Billing Codes

57460 Colposcopy with loop electrode excision or excisions of the cervix (LEEP)
57461 Colposcopy with loop electrode conization of cervix (LEEP cone)
57500 Cervical biopsy
57505 Endocervical curettage
57520 Cervical conization, with or without fulguration (cold knife or laser)
57522 Cervical conization using loop electrode technique (LEEP cone)
99070 Supplies and materials for kits and electrodes (a surgical tray charge is generally allowed for an office LEEP)

ICD-9-CM Diagnostic Codes

180.9 Cervical cancer
233.1 CIN 3 (severe dysplasia, carcinoma in situ)
622.11 CIN 1
622.12 CIN 2
795.04 HSIL
795.00 Atypical glandular/endocervical cells

Suppliers

Full contact information is available online at www.expertconsult.com.

Equipment

Bovie Medical Corporation
ConMed
CooperSurgical
Ellman International, Inc.
ERBE USA, Inc.
MedGyn Products, Inc.
Premier Medical Products
Utah Medical Products, Inc.
Valleylab, Inc.
Wallach Surgical Devices, Inc.
Welch Allyn

Patient Education Guides

See the sample patient education handout online at www.expertconsult.com.

BOOKLETS ON PATIENT EDUCATION

American College of Obstetrics and Gynecology (ACOG)
American Society of Colposcopy and Cervical Pathology (ASCCP)
Krames Communications

BIBLIOGRAPHY

American College of Obstetricians and Gynecologists: Role of loop electrosurgical excision procedure in the evaluation of abnormal Pap test results. Committee Opinion No. 195. Int J Gynaecol Obstet 61:203, 1998.

American College of Obstetricians and Gynecologists: Evaluation and management of abnormal cervical cytology and histology in the adolescent. Committee Opinion No. 330. Obstet Gynecol 107:963, 2006.

American College of Obstetricians and Gynecologists: Management of abnormal cervical cytology and histology. Practice Bulletin No. 99. Obstet Gynecol 112:1419, 2008.

Apgar B, Brotzman G, Spitzer M: Colposcopy: Principles and Practice. St. Louis, Elsevier, 2008.

Apgar BS, Wright TC Jr, Pfenninger JL: Loop electrosurgical excision procedure for CIN. Am Family Physician 46:505, 1992.

Brockmeyer AD, Wright JD, Gao F, et al: Persistent and recurrent cervical dysplasia after loop electrosurgical excision procedure. Am J Obstet Gynecol 192:1379, 2005.

Crane JM: Pregnancy outcome after loop electrosurgical excision procedure: A systematic review. Obstet Gynecol 102:1058, 2003.

Dunn TS, Bajaj JE, Stamm CA, et al: Management of the minimally abnormal Papanicolaou smear in pregnancy. J Low Genit Tract Dis 5:133, 2001.

Kyrgiou M, Koliopoulos G, Martin-Hirsch P, et al: Obstetric outcomes after conservative treatment for intraepithelial or early invasive cervical lesions: Systematic review and meta-analysis. Lancet 367:489, 2006.

Kyrgiou M, Tsoumpou I, Vrekoussis T, et al: The up-to-date evidence on colposcopy practice and treatment of cervical intraepithelial neoplasia: The Cochrane colposcopy and cervical cytopathology collaborative group (C5 group) approach. Cancer Treat Rev 32:516, 2006.

Lindeque BG: Management of cervical premalignant lesions. Best Pract Res Clin Obstet Gynaecol 19:545, 2005.

Lozeau AM, Schrager S, Lowrie R, et al: Clinical inquiries. What's the best treatment for CIN 2 or 3? J Family Pract 56:650, 2007.

Mossa MA, Carter PG, Abdu S, et al: A comparative study of two methods of large loop excision of the transformation zone. Br J Obstet Gynaecol 112:490, 2005.

Paraskevaidis E, Arbyn M, Sotiriadis A, et al: The role of HPV DNA testing in the follow-up period after treatment for CIN: A systematic review of the literature. Cancer Treat Rev 30:205, 2004.

Paraskevaidis E, Kalantaridou SN, Paschopoulos M, et al: Factors affecting outcome after incomplete excision of cervical intraepithelial neoplasia. Eur J Gynaecol Oncol 24:541, 2003.

Pfenninger JL: Colposcopy, LEEP, and other procedures: The role for family physicians. Family Med 28:505, 1996.

Pfenninger JL: Good things still come in old packages: Cryosurgery vs. loop electrosurgical excision procedure. J Am Board Family Pract 12:416, 1999.

Prendiville W: Large loop excision of the transformation zone. Baillières Clin Obstet Gynaecol 9:189, 1995.

Spitzer M, Brotzmon GL, Apgar BS: Practical therapeutic options for treatment of cervical intraepithelial neoplasia. In Apgar BS, Brotzman GL, Spitzer M (eds): Colposcopy Principles and Practice, 2nd ed. Philadelphia, Saunders, 2008, pp 505–509.

Tuggy M, Garcia J: Procedures Consult. Available at www.proceduresconsult.com, and as an app at www.apple.com/iTunes.

Wright TC Jr, Massad LS, Dunton CJ, et al: 2006 consensus guidelines for the management of women with cervical intraepithelial neoplasia or adenocarcinoma in situ. Am J Obstet Gynecol 197:340, 2007.

Wright TC, Richart RM, Ferenczy AF: Electrosurgery for HPV-Related Lesions of the Anogenital Tract. New City, NY, Arthur Vision, 1992.

CHAPTER 150

Fertility Awareness–Based Methods of Contraception (Natural Family Planning)

William Ellert

Fertility awareness–based (FAB) methods of contraception are frequently referred to as *natural family planning* (NFP). FAB methods are an approach to contraception that identifies the days of the menstrual cycle when couples should avoid unprotected intercourse as determined by the normal physiology of the menstrual cycle and the life expectancy of a sperm and ovum. Studies in multiple countries have shown that couples choose this method of contraception for a variety reasons, the most common of which are health issues and concerns about side effects of other methods. Other reasons include financial concerns, religious beliefs, and a belief that "natural" is better.

Currently, six major methods are discussed when referring to FAB methods of contraception. Two are considered "historical methods," and four methods are currently considered more practical for clinical use.

The historical methods are

- Calendar rhythm
- Basal body temperature (BBT)

The current FAB methods are

- Standard Days method
- Ovulation method
- TwoDay method
- Symptothermal method

Physiology

The physiologic basis of the Standard Days method is based on hormonal studies indicating that a woman is generally fertile 5 days before ovulation and 24 hours after ovulation. This conclusion is based on the viability of the sperm after sexual intercourse being no more than 5 days and the viability of the egg after ovulation being less than 24 hours. Based on these studies, the probability of pregnancy from unprotected intercourse is as follows:

- 4% 5 days before ovulation
- 25% to 28% for the 2 days before ovulation
- 8% to 10% for the 24 hours after ovulation
- 0% for the remainder of the cycle

The remaining three methods for current FAB contraception rely on interpretation of the physiologic signs of fertility. Before ovulation, estradiol levels increase and cause the production of characteristic cervical secretions. The environment created by estradiol production is conducive to the transportation of sperm to the ovum. After ovulation, progesterone produced by the corpus luteum causes a distinct change in the secretions. There is a typical obvious pattern to the secretions. No noticeable vaginal secretions are present for approximately 3 to 4 days after menstruation. After this, there is a distinctly sticky and elastic secretion that lasts for approximately 3 to 4 days. After this, the secretions turn clear and wet for approximately 3 to 4 days. Then, there is again an absence of secretions for approximately 11 to 14 days before the next menstrual cycle. This pattern is seen in the typical menstrual cycle lasting 26 to 32 days (Fig. 150-1).

Indications

Fertility awareness–based methods of preventing pregnancy are indicated for those couples who wish to avoid hormone-based and operative-based methods of contraception; who wish to minimize the use of barrier methods of contraception; and who are able to avoid unprotected intercourse on fertile days. These methods require the active participation of both partners and a willingness to assess the signs of fertility daily. The ability to use modern methods of FAB contraception relies ultimately on the acceptance of the technique(s) by physicians and other health care providers as legitimate and effective methods of family planning. The availability of trained instructors and other resources that readily convey the needed information is also crucial. These methods of fertility awareness are also very helpful for couples who desire pregnancy.

Contraindications

There are no absolute contraindications to these methods of contraception. Relative contraindications are related to an unreliable hormone status and include the following:

- Breast-feeding
- Recent menarche
- Recent childbirth
- Recent discontinuation of some hormonal contraceptives
- Perimenopausal
- Menstrual cycles that are frequently shorter than 26 days or longer than 32 days (for the Standard Days method)
- Persistent reproductive tract infections that affect the signs of fertility
- An inability to interpret the signs of fertility correctly

Most of these relative contraindications can be overcome through more extensive counseling and follow-up.

		Fertile period			
Folicular phase					Luteal phase
Menstruation	No secretions (3–4 days)	Sticky and elastic secretions (3–4 days)	Wet secretions (3–4 days)	Ovulation	No secretions
1 2 3 4	5 6 7	8 9 10	11 12 13	14	15 16 17 18 19 20 21 22 23 24 25 26 27 28

Figure 150-1 Physical signs associated with days of the typical 28-day menstrual cycle.

Methods

Historical Methods

The calendar rhythm method and the basal body temperature method are rarely used by practitioners familiar with more current FAB methods of contraception. The *calendar rhythm method* consists of recording the length of six cycles. Eighteen days are subtracted for the number of days in the shortest cycle and 11 days are subtracted from the number of days in the longest cycle. This determines the period in which sexual intercourse should be avoided. For example, if the shortest cycle is 23 days and the longest cycle is 31 days, then the fertile period is from day 5 until day 20.

The *basal body temperature method* is based on the fact that in a normal cycle, the basal body temperature is approximately 0.5° F (0.3° C) higher in the luteal phase than in the follicular phase. This method requires avoiding unprotected sexual intercourse from the beginning of the cycle until 3 days of elevated temperatures have occurred. This method requires the daily monitoring of temperature before any activity or food consumption.

Current Methods

Standard Days Method

- Screening: The Standard Days method is appropriate for women whose cycles are usually between 26 to 32 days long. Women who have more than one cycle outside of the 26- to 32-day range in a 12-month period should be encouraged to use another method.
- Instructions: Avoid unprotected intercourse from day 8 of the cycle through day 19. Day 1 is defined as the first day of menstrual bleeding.

Ovulation Method

- Screening: This method is appropriate for women regardless of their cycle length. Women who are breast-feeding, have recently used hormonal contraception, or who are perimenopausal require more detailed counseling and instructions.
- Instructions: This method requires women to observe, record, and interpret their cervical secretions at the vulva several times each day, generally before each urination. Women are taught to chart the days of their menses, the days with secretions (including the characteristics of secretions), and the days when pregnancy is likely. Unprotected intercourse is to be avoided at the following times:
  - During menses (because menstrual bleeding could obscure the presence of secretions).
  - On preovulatory days after days with intercourse (because of the possible confusion with semen).
  - On all days with fertile secretions (see description under "Physiology").

TwoDay Method

- Screening: The screening criteria for this method are identical to those for the ovulation method.
- Instructions: This method is very similar to the ovulation method, but is much simpler. The TwoDay method also requires women to determine the presence or absence of cervical secretions. Two questions are then asked: "Were there any secretions today?" and "Were there any secretions yesterday?" If the patient notes 2 consecutive days without secretions she is deemed to be in a nonfertile period. If the answer to either of those questions is "yes," she is potentially fertile on that day.

Symptothermal Method

- Screening: The screening criteria for this method are identical to those for the ovulation method.
- Instructions: The symptothermal method allows for several different "rules" for avoiding pregnancy. Each rule recognizes the appearance of cervical mucus at the vulva or vagina as the first sign of fertility. In determining the end of the fertile window, couples may choose to emphasize mucus observations over temperature observations (and vice versa). The most conservative rule recognizes both observations equally. For example, postovulatory infertility commences after the third day (or more) of a thermal shift (>0.4° F), cross-checked by 4 or more days of "drying up" of the cervical mucus. This allows the couple to personalize their method and focus on a marker they prefer, while still using an alternative to "back-up" their primary marker.

Efficacy

The effectiveness of FAB methods of contraception, when taught and used correctly (i.e., method effectiveness), ranges from 97% to 100% in all published studies. It must be emphasized, however, that these methods rely on the ability of the couple to abstain from genital contact during periods of fertility, and the "use effectiveness" rate typically approaches about 80%.

Conclusion

Fertility awareness–based methods of avoiding pregnancy (or facilitating pregnancy) are very useful tools for women to become more aware of and knowledgeable about the physiologic changes that occur during their menstrual cycle. Frequently this can be used to facilitate communication between partners regarding mutual reproductive responsibility. The personal choice of a couple to choose this method of contraception should be supported by primary care providers in a responsible and informed manner.

ICD-9-CM Diagnostic Codes

623.5 Vaginal discharge
626.4 Irregular menses
V25.04 Counseling and instruction in natural family planning to avoid pregnancy
V25.09 Family planning advice
V25.40 Contraception, maintenance/examination

V25.49 Unspecified contraceptive management
V26.41 Procreative counseling and advice using natural family planning

RESOURCES

Billings Ovulation Method—USA (BOMA)
P.O. Box 16206
St. Paul, Minn 55116
Phone: 1-800-637-6371
www.boma-usa.org

Institute of Reproductive Health
Georgetown University
Washington, DC
www.irh.org/

Pope Paul VI Institute
6901 Mercy Road
Omaha, Neb 68106-2604
Phone: 1-402-390-6600
www.popepaulvi.com

BIBLIOGRAPHY

Alliende ME, Cabezon C, Figueroa H, Kottmann C: Cervicovaginal fluid changes to detect ovulation accurately. Am J Obstet Gynecol 193:71–75, 2005.

Arevalo M, Jennings V, Nikula M, Sinai I: Efficacy of the new TwoDay method of family planning. Reprod Endocrinol 82:885–891, 2004.

Febring R, Kitchen S, Shivanandan M: An Introduction to Natural Family Planning [booklet]. Washington, DC, Diocesan Development Program for Natural Family Planning, National Conference of Catholic Bishops, 1999.

Geerling JH: Natural family planning. Am Fam Physician 52:1749–1756, 1995.

Guida M, Tommaselli GA, Pellicano M, et al: An overview on the effectiveness of natural family planning. Gynecol Endocrinol 11:203–219, 1977.

Howard M, Stanford J: Pregnancy probabilities during use of the Creighton Model Fertility Care System. Arch Fam Med 8:391–402, 1999.

Jennings V: Fertility awareness-based methods of pregnancy prevention. In Rose BD (ed): UpToDate. Waltham, Mass, UpToDate, 2007. Available at www.uptodate.com.

Pallone SR, Bergus GR: Fertility awareness-based methods: Another option for family planning. J Am Board Fam Med 22:147–157, 2009.

Sinai I, Jennings V, Arevalo M: The importance of screening and monitoring: The Standard Days method and cycle regularity. Contraception 69:201–206, 2004.

PAP SMEAR AND RELATED TECHNIQUES FOR CERVICAL CANCER SCREENING

Gary R. Newkirk

Despite the controversies surrounding cervical Papanicolaou (Pap) smear testing, it remains an effective tool for cancer prevention and detection. Numerous studies have documented a statistically valid drop in the incidence and mortality rates of invasive cervical carcinomas since the introduction of the Pap smear. Unfortunately, cervical cancer screening has not eradicated this potentially preventable disease. The current cervical cancer detection system relies on a complex system of clinical and laboratory procedures that have potential for error at numerous points. Koss' (1989) landmark discussion summarizes major sources of error, including (1) problems with the initial clinical examination, (2) inappropriate smear collection technique, (3) laboratory errors in sample preparation and interpretation, (4) errors in report interpretation, (5) failure of the clinician to understand or appropriately respond to Pap smear–generated data, and (6) failure of the patient to follow the clinician's recommendations.

Compelling data link cervical intraepithelial neoplasia (CIN) with human papillomavirus (HPV) infection. Epidemiologic data further document the epidemic proportions of new genital HPV infections. Box 151-1 summarizes these risk factors for cervical dysplasia. Most women who are exposed to HPV have transient infections and do not develop cervical cancer. Current evidence indicates that patients with the *persistence of HPV* as detected by either abnormal cytologic features (Pap) with or without positive high-risk HPV DNA testing (see Chapter 142, Human Papillomavirus DNA Typing) are the subgroup of women who remain at greatest risk for developing cervical cancer. Despite the success of Pap smear screening methodology, numerous studies indicate that there remains between a 20% and 50% false-negative rate for a single Pap smear in identifying patients with cervical dysplasia, and this includes even the latest ThinPrep method. Accordingly, the clinician should be aware that Pap smear screening guidelines are evolving to take in consideration not only the enhanced sensitivity of screening, but also the enhanced specificity of combining cytologic findings with high-risk HPV DNA results.

Furthermore, the sampling devices, method of preparation, and transport systems for Pap samples are evolving as well. Liquid-based Pap systems such as ThinPrep and SurePath are currently approved by the U.S. Food and Drug Administration (FDA) as alternatives to conventional slide smear techniques for Pap sample preparation. Liquid-based Pap smear cytologic examination also allows simultaneous collection of material that can be submitted for HPV DNA testing at the request of the clinician or as a "reflex" test dependent on the cytologic interpretation (see Chapter 142, Human Papillomavirus DNA Typing and the ASCCP Guidelines in Appendix K). *Reflex testing* means the DNA testing is automatically performed if an ASC-US (atypical squamous cells of undetermined significance) Pap smear is found. As a result of these advancements and a better understanding of HPV screening, cervical cancer screening guidelines have become more complicated.

Clinicians are advised to keep current regarding the seemingly ever-changing cervical cancer screening recommendations because these guidelines will continue to evolve as new evidence-based and outcome data become available. At the present time, clinicians can continue to make significant contributions to cancer prevention in women by refining their method of Pap smear sampling, enhancing their understanding of Pap smear report interpretation, clarifying their recommendations for patient management, and making sure that their efforts are implemented by an effective follow-up and intervention system. Clearly, efforts to prevent cervical cancer are inconsequential if mechanisms for follow-up and quality assurance are not developed. Unfortunately, nearly 70 years after the advent of Dr. Papanicolaou's revolution with cervical cancer prevention, nearly 50% of the women who develop cervical cancer in the United States have either never had a single Pap test or have not had a Pap smear for 10 years prior to their diagnosis! This is unacceptable in this modern age of medical care.

This chapter focuses on a contemporary approach to Pap smear screening; it is assumed that basic pelvic examination skills have been mastered. Box 151-2 offers a brief summary of the terminology used throughout this discussion.

Box 151-1. Risk Factors and Historical Characteristics Correlated with Abnormalities on Pap Smear

- Diethylstilbestrol (DES) exposure (should be extremely rare now)
- Early age at first intercourse (before age 16 years)
- History of abnormal Pap smear, cervical dysplasia, or cervical cancer
- History of genital or anal condyloma
- History of sexual abuse
- History of vulvar dysplasia
- Illicit drug use (intravenous or oral)
- Immunocompromised patient, including HIV-positive status
- Multiple sexual partners (more than three)
- Other sexually transmitted disease history
- Sexual partner with condyloma or history of intercourse with a woman with cervical dysplasia or cancer
- Sexual partner with more than three previous sexual partners
- Tobacco smoking

HIV, human immunodeficiency virus; Pap, Papanicolaou.

Box 151-2. Terminology and Definitions

Atypical glandular cells (AGC): In the past these were called "AGC-US" (atypical glandular cells of undetermined significance), but because the incidence of significant pathology is so high with this finding (10% cancers and 25% high-grade lesions), the "US" has been dropped by Bethesda-2001. All AGC reports need further investigation.

Atypical squamous cells (ASC): Bethesda-2001 divides these into ASC-US (atypical squamous cells of undetermined significance) and ASC-H (atypical squamous cells, cannot exclude HSIL).

Carcinoma in situ (CIS): Dysplasia involves the entire squamous epithelium but does *not* penetrate the basement membrane. Included in CIN 3 and HGSIL designations.

Cervical intraepithelial neoplasia (CIN): See "Dysplasia." *CIN 1* refers to mild dysplasia, *CIN 2* to moderate dysplasia, and *CIN 3* to severe dysplasia, including carcinoma in situ (CIS).

Columnar epithelium: Single-layer, mucin-secreting epithelium on the surface of the endocervix. It can often be seen on the ectocervix and is proximal to the SCJ.

Dysplasia: Premalignant change in the cervical epithelium displaying proliferation of parabasal cells with disordered polarity, loss of cellular junctions, coarse nuclear chromatin clumping, abnormal nuclear cytoplasmic ratio, and high mitotic index. Reported as *mild, moderate*, and *severe* dysplasia. Usually refers to histologic features.

Ectocervix (also called exocervix): The flat portion of the cervix that is readily visible. The cervical os is located centrally.

Endocervical cells: Glandular, columnar-shaped cells obtained from the endocervical (columnar) epithelium in the endocervical canal.

Endocervix: The area within the endocervical canal.

Exocervix: See "Ectocervix."

Frankly invasive squamous cell carcinoma of the cervix: Invasion greater than 3 mm (or 5 mm, depending on classification used) below the basement membrane.

Koilocytotic or koilocytic: Equivalent terms include condylomatous atypia and human papillomavirus (HPV) effect; these terms describe cells that have perinuclear halos or vacuoles that vary in shape and configuration, and that show a distinct zone of clearing between the nucleus and cytoplasmic membrane. The abnormal nuclei are characterized by wrinkling, variation in size and shape, binucleate forms, and hyperchromasia. Usually indicative of HPV infection.

Microinvasive cervical cancer: Invasion 3 mm or less below the basement membrane. Some terminologies allow 5 mm of invasion and include other descriptive factors.

Reflex DNA testing: Automatically obtaining HPV DNA test for patients that have an ASC-US report.

Squamocolumnar junction (SCJ): The line where the squamous epithelium of the ectocervix joins the mucus-secreting columnar epithelium of the endocervix.

Squamous cells: Epithelial cells on the surface of the ectocervix. These cells appear smooth and pink on the cervix.

Squamous intraepithelial lesion (SIL): Reported as either low-grade (LGSIL, LSIL) or high-grade (HGSIL, HSIL), corresponding to increasing severity of dysplasia (Bethesda terminology). Originally referred to cytologic diagnosis, but now often used to describe histologic findings as well.

Squamous metaplasia: A type of tissue present where the columnar epithelium is being replaced (transformed) by squamous epithelium. This normal tissue occurs within the cervical transformation zone, and the transformation of columnar to squamous epithelium is a totally normal process.

Transformation zone (TZ): Area of transformation or replacement of the cervical columnar epithelium by squamous epithelium through a process called metaplastic change. The *active* TZ goes from the outermost gland to the SCJ. The TZ is the principal site of origin for precancerous and invasive squamous cell carcinomas of the cervix.

See Figures 151-1 and 151-2, and Chapter 137, Colposcopic Examination.

ANATOMY

Figure 151-1 depicts the anatomy involved. Successful Pap smear technique requires sampling from the active transformation zone in women with an intact cervix or from the vaginal cuff for those who have undergone hysterectomy. Figure 151-2 provides a graphic representation of the changes involved with preinvasive and invasive disease of the cervix as well as a depiction of histologic and cytologic correlates. (Refer to Chapter 137, Colposcopic Examination, for further discussion of anatomy.)

INDICATIONS

The Pap smear is a screening test only; it is not diagnostic. Thus, if an abnormality is seen or palpated at the time of the pelvic examination, it should be examined with a colposcope and a directed biopsy performed. *The physician cannot rely on the Pap smear alone to be diagnostic for an observed lesion.*

- *Screening*: Current cervical cancer screening guidelines are summarized in Box 151-3. These guidelines also consider recommendations concerning the use of liquid-based cytologic and HPV testing. Clinicians are advised to consider these guidelines in relation to the patient population they serve and their practice and patient resources.
- *Follow-up after treatment for cervical dysplasia, malignancy*: See the ASCCP Guidelines in Appendix K. All women with a history of cervical dysplasia remain at significant risk for disease recurrence and should undergo Pap smear testing at least annually for life. There are numerous schemes for follow-up after treatment for cervical dysplasia and carcinoma. All involve increased frequency of Pap smear testing or HPV testing for a period of time. Repeat colposcopic examination is often performed with endocervical curettage or cervical biopsy in circumstances where the clinician is concerned about the recurrence of cervical dysplasia or cancer.
- *Diethylstilbestrol (DES)-exposed offspring*: DES-exposed offspring require colposcopic evaluation (and repeat colposcopy with biopsy as necessary). Modified Pap smear and colposcopy protocols have been developed. The appropriate Pap smear follow-up usually requires modified routines determined by coordinated exchange of expert opinion between the clinician, pathologist,

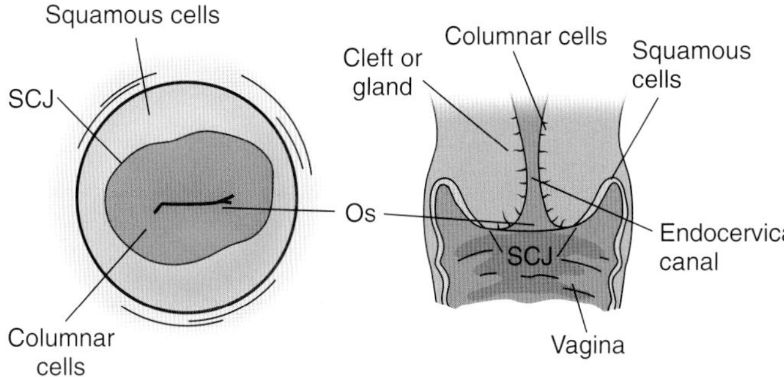

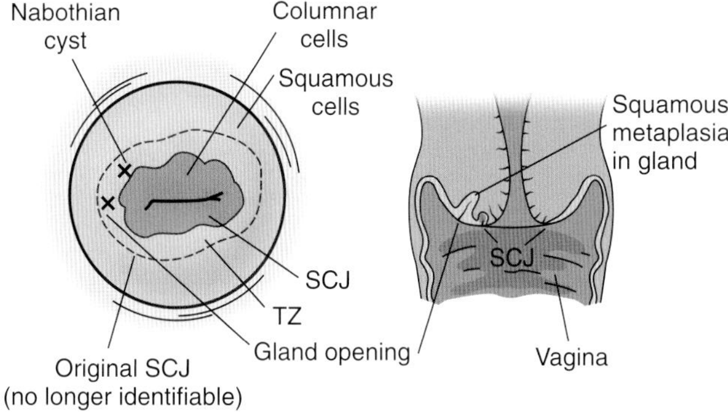

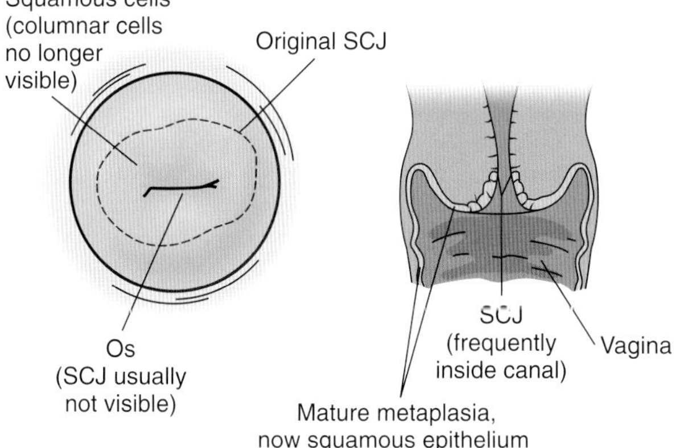

Figure 151-1 Appearance of cervix in various age groups. The area most at risk in all age groups is the transformation zone (TZ), including the squamocolumnar junction (SCJ). Note how location varies with age. The SCJ and TZ are readily visible in younger women and may be quite large. The SCJ migrates inward with aging, and by menopause, it is usually within the canal and is not visible. The entire TZ must be sampled to maximize efficacy of the Papanicolaou smear. Also see Figure 137-2 (Chapter 137, Colposcopic Examination) for cervical photographs showing these findings and developmental changes.

and, quite often, a gynecologist familiar with this small subgroup of women. The vagina must also be observed closely, because it has a much higher risk for dysplasia and cancer.

- *Any visible or palpable lesion of the cervix*: Follow the precaution that the Pap smear is not diagnostic and further assessment is usually done with a biopsy directed by the colposcope.
- *Any abnormal vaginal bleeding or discharge*.
- *Following hysterectomy for benign disease*: Discontinue Pap smears if for benign reasons and no prior history of high-grade CIN. Exceptions include immunocompromised women or women who have a history of prenatal exposure to DES.
- *Following hysterectomy for dysplasia, carcinoma*: Continue Pap smears annually after three or four normal Pap smears at 4- to 6-month intervals.
- *Supracervical (subtotal) hysterectomy*: Routine recommendations should be followed.
- *Victims of rape, incest, abuse*: Pap smear is part of the initial work-up. Evaluations in these circumstances require expertise and strict adherence to medical/legal chain of evidence. (See Chapters 157, Treatment of the Adult Victim of Sexual Assault, and 158, Management of the Young Female as Possible Victim of Sexual Abuse.)

Contraindications

Absolute

There are no absolute contraindications to obtaining a Pap smear.

Relative

Relative contraindications include clinical circumstances in which sample collection is difficult to obtain or difficult to interpret (e.g., active vaginitis or cervicitis, pelvic inflammatory disease [PID], or menses). The clinician must weigh the benefits versus the risk of obtaining the screening Pap smear under these circumstances. For instance, if a woman presents with abnormal vaginal bleeding, a Pap smear is advised, despite the presence of blood. This contrasts with a patient who comes in for a routine Pap smear screening and has begun to menstruate. In the latter instance, the Pap smear can be deferred to a more favorable time. See the sample patient education handout available online at www.expertconsult.com, which includes advice on what women can do to optimize Pap smear results.

Equipment

- Examination table appropriate for placing the patient in the lithotomy position
- A warm, well-lit examination room
- Various-sized speculums: Graves (metal); Pederson (metal); plastic, disposable (Welch Allyn, Inc; Durr-Fillauer Medical, Inc.)
- Water-soluble lubricant (e.g., K-Y Jelly)
- Nonsterile examination gloves
- Large swabs for gently blotting excess discharge
- Cotton swabs
- Method for warming the speculum (warm water or speculum drawer warmer [light bulb])
- Sampling devices (see Fig. 151-5)
  - Wooden spatulas (Cervical Scraper No. 7, Hardwood Products Co.) or plastic spatula (Cervical Scraper [8½ inch], Milex Products) for ectocervical sample
  - Cytobrush Plus for endocervical sample (Medscand)
  - As an alternative to taking two samples, a "broom" device can be used for both the ectocervical and endocervical samples (Cervex-Brush, CooperSurgical, Inc.; Papette, Wallach Surgical Devices, Inc.)
- Microscope slides, fixative (consult with reference laboratory performing cytologic evaluation for its preference), or medium for liquid-based testing
- Appropriate patient identification, history forms to accompany Pap smear and other tests
- Culture or transport media and swabs as necessary for detection of gonorrhea, chlamydia, herpes, and fungal infection, and KOH/wet mount
- Cervical tenaculum or cervical hook (rarely needed)
- Ring forceps

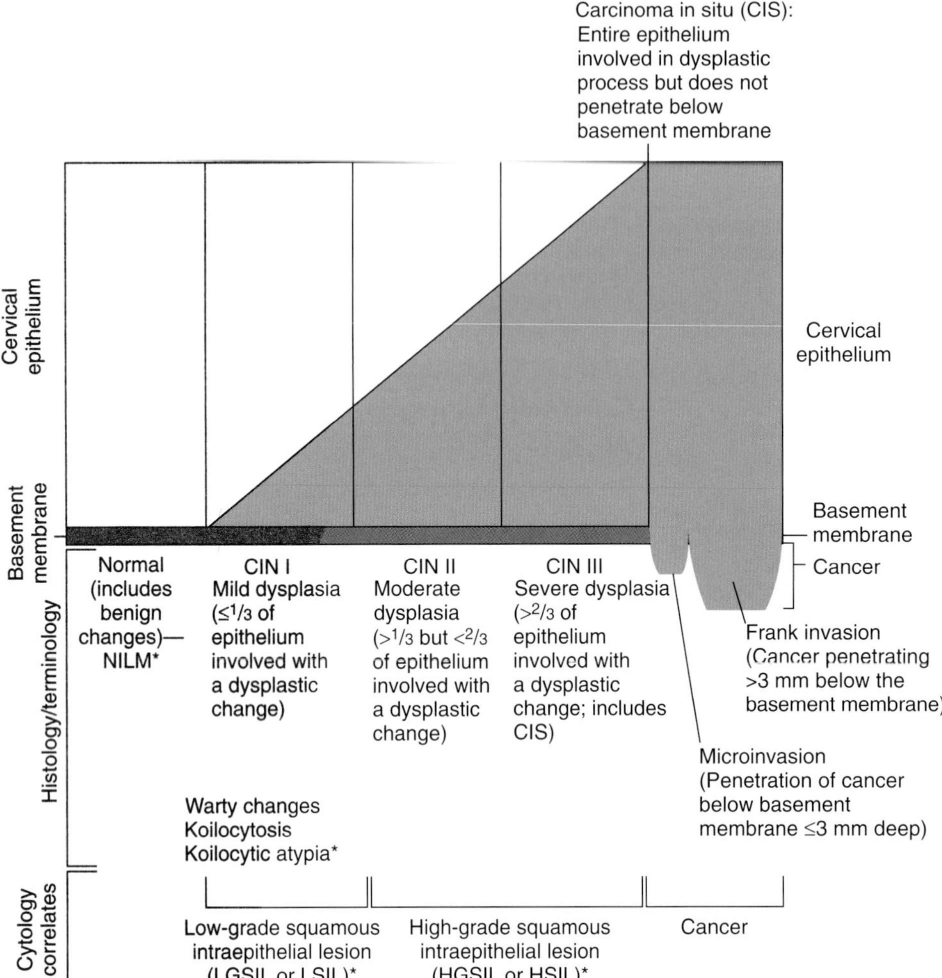

Figure 151-2 Histologic and cytologic correlations of various terms used to describe preinvasive and invasive squamous cell disease of the cervix. Also see Box 151-2 for further description of the terms. The degree of epithelial involvement correlates with the severity of cytologic findings as well as the total degree of involvement of the dysplastic tissue in relation to the thickness of the cervical squamous epithelium. On histologic examination, involvement below the basement membrane supports a diagnosis of invasive cancer. NILM, negative for intraepithelial lesion or malignancy. *Atypical squamous cells (ASC), atypical squamous cells of undetermined significance (ASC-US), and atypical squamous cells that cannot exclude HSIL (ASC-H) are not depicted here because they include a variety of histologic diagnoses. Note, too, that glandular cell abnormalities include atypical glandular cells (AGC), endocervical adenocarcinoma in situ (AIS), and adenocarcinoma, and are also not depicted in this graph.

- Materials and solutions for liquid-based Pap smears (e.g., ThinPrep)

Sampling Devices

Concern over the frequency and occurrence of false-negative Pap smears has led to the development of newer Pap smear sampling, preparation, and processing techniques. Despite the higher costs for the newer sampling devices (nominally \$0.40 to \$0.80 each), the increased quality of smears, the improved detection rates, and, ultimately, the fewer patients who must return for "inadequate" repeat smears more than justify this added expense. The routine use of the Cytobrush, Cervex-Brush, Papette, or similar devices is recommended (see later discussion of liquid-based technologies). *A Pap smear consists of sampling the endocervical canal and the entire transformation zone* (Figs. 151-3 and 151-4). At times, the broom device will not be wide enough to sample the entire area at risk (the transformation zone). Additional sampling of the missed area is then required. Clinicians should not be locked into using a single method of transformation zone sampling. A good strategy for obtaining ideal Pap smears is to have several types of sampling devices such as the brush and broom available. "One size fits all" strategies are less effective than using the sampling device that matches the patient's particular cervical anatomy.

The Pap smear test samples "exfoliated" cells. As such, the transformation zone need not be denuded of its mucosa to obtain an adequate sample! There are enough cells from one Cytobrush and a wooden spatula sample, for instance, to provide material for cytologic interpretation for five slides! Sharp, fine-edged plastic devices are advocated by some physicians; however, wood works fine for sampling of the ectocervix. Both should be accompanied by brush sampling of the endocervical canal. A bloody Pap smear sample decreases detection rates. Figure 151-5 illustrates several of the common sampling devices that achieve satisfactory sampling.

Liquid-Based Pap Smears

In the United States there are two FDA-approved *liquid-based Pap smear systems* available. Both rely on a method of sampling the cervix that is similar or identical to conventional slide prepared smears, but they differ in the transport media and the technical methods of cytologic preparation. With liquid-based Pap smears, the same principles apply regarding collection of cells. The sample, however, instead of being spread on a glass slide, is "swished" in a vial of liquid that is subsequently processed to eliminate blood and other debris.

Prior study suggested that liquid-based Pap testing is more sensitive and specific than conventional slide methods; however, a recent systematic review and meta-analysis indicated that *liquid-based Pap smear testing is neither more sensitive nor more specific for high-grade CIN when compared with the conventional Pap test*. A clearer advantage of the liquid-based technique is that the residual cytologic material left over after the cytologic examination is completed in the laboratory can be used for HPV DNA testing. (Refer to Chapter 142, Human Papillomavirus DNA Typing, and Appendix K to guide when HPV testing may be useful.) In particular, the data

Box 151-3. American Cancer Society Guidelines for the Early Detection of Cervical Neoplasia and Cancer, 2003–2009

1. When to start screening
   - Begin approximately 3 years after the onset of vaginal intercourse but no later than 21 years of age.
   - Adolescents who may not need a Pap smear should still obtain appropriate preventive health care, including contraception and education, other screening, and treatment of sexually transmitted diseases.
2. When to discontinue screening
   - Women who are age 70 and older with an intact cervix and who have had three or more documented consecutive technically satisfactory, normal/negative cervical cytologic tests and no abnormal/positive cytologic tests within a 10-year period before age 70 may elect to cease cervical cancer screening.
   - When comorbid or life-threatening illnesses are present, Pap smears are not needed.
   - Screening should be continued for women older than 70 years:
     If they have not been previously screened
     When previous Pap smear screening information is unavailable
     If there was in utero exposure to diethylstilbestrol (DES)
     For immunocompromised women (including those with HIV-seropositive status)
     For women older than 70 years who have tested positive for HPV DNA
3. Screening after hysterectomy
   - After a total hysterectomy with removal of the entire cervix for benign lesions, Pap smears using vaginal cytologic samples are not indicated.
   - The presence of CIN 2/3 is not considered a "benign lesion," so continued screening would be indicated.
   - Women who have had a subtotal hysterectomy (the cervix remains) should continue cervical cancer screening.
   - With history of CIN 2/3, or if it is not possible to document the absence of the same prior to the hysterectomy, three documented consecutive technically satisfactory normal/negative cervical cytologic tests should be obtained before ceasing screening. In addition, there should have been no abnormal tests within the previous 10-year period.
   - Women with DES exposure or history of cervical carcinoma should continue screening after hysterectomy as long as they are in reasonably good health and do not have a life-limiting chronic condition.
4. Screening interval
   - Perform annually with conventional cervical cytology smears *or* every 2 years using liquid-based cytologic test. At or after age 30 years, women who have had three consecutive technically satisfactory normal/negative cytologic results may be screened every 2 to 3 years (unless they have a history of in utero DES exposure, are HIV-seropositive, or are immunocompromised).
5. New technologies
   - The panel did not issue a statement on new technologies that are under development. These include aided visualization (i.e., speculoscopy), cervicography, computer-assisted screening devices, optical probe devices, self-collected vaginal samples for HPV DNA testing, and spectroscopy/electronic detection devices.
   - Liquid-based Pap technology: As an alternative to conventional cervical cytologic smears, conventional screening may be performed every 2 years using liquid-based cytologic test; at or after age 30, women who have had three consecutive, technically satisfactory normal/negative cytologic results may be screened every 2 to 3 years (unless they have a history of in utero DES exposure, are HPV positive, or are immunocompromised).
   - HPV/DNA testing with cytologic test: Primary cervical cancer screening has not been approved by the FDA. Should the FDA approve HPV DNA testing for primary screening, it would be reasonable to consider it for women age 30 and over, as an alternative to cervical cytologic testing alone. Cervical screening may be performed every 3 years using conventional or liquid-based cytologic test combined with a test for DNA for high-risk HPV types.
6. Additional recommendations
   - Patients need to be educated (especially teens) that a pelvic examination does not equate with a cytologic (Pap) test. They still need regular health care visits.
   - No recommendation was made regarding pelvic and rectal examinations. They are not effective in detecting cervical cancer early enough, but there are other reasons to consider them. These should be discussed on an individual basis with the primary care physician.
   - Referrals of women with low-grade lesions for colposcopy may be less necessary for adolescents given the self-limited nature of many low-grade squamous intraepithelial lesions (LSILs) in this age group. Detection and treatment of high-grade squamous intraepithelial lesions (HSILs) should be the goal of adolescent screening and referral.
   - Health insurance payers should not exclude adolescents or women of any age from coverage for cervical health on the basis of false positive cytologic results and/or mild abnormalities on cervical cytologic test.
   - Health insurance coverage for new cervical screening technology is not uniform. Patients should be advised of this by their primary care provider.
   - There is considerable clinical evidence with the use of the cytobrush in pregnant women with no apparent complications.
   - Cervical broom instruments and other single sampling instruments are comparable to the spatula and brush.
   - An endocervical swab is less sensitive than an endocervical brush and its use is discouraged. It may be considered for pregnant women.

CIN, cervical intraepithelial neoplasia; DES, diethylstilbestrol; FDA, Food and Drug Administration; HIV, human immunodeficiency virus; HPV, human papillomavirus; Pap, Papanicolaou.
Adapted from Smith RA, Cokkinides V, Brawley OW: Cancer screening in the United States, 2009: A review of current American Cancer Society guidelines and issues in cancer screening. CA Cancer J Clin 59:27–41, 2009.

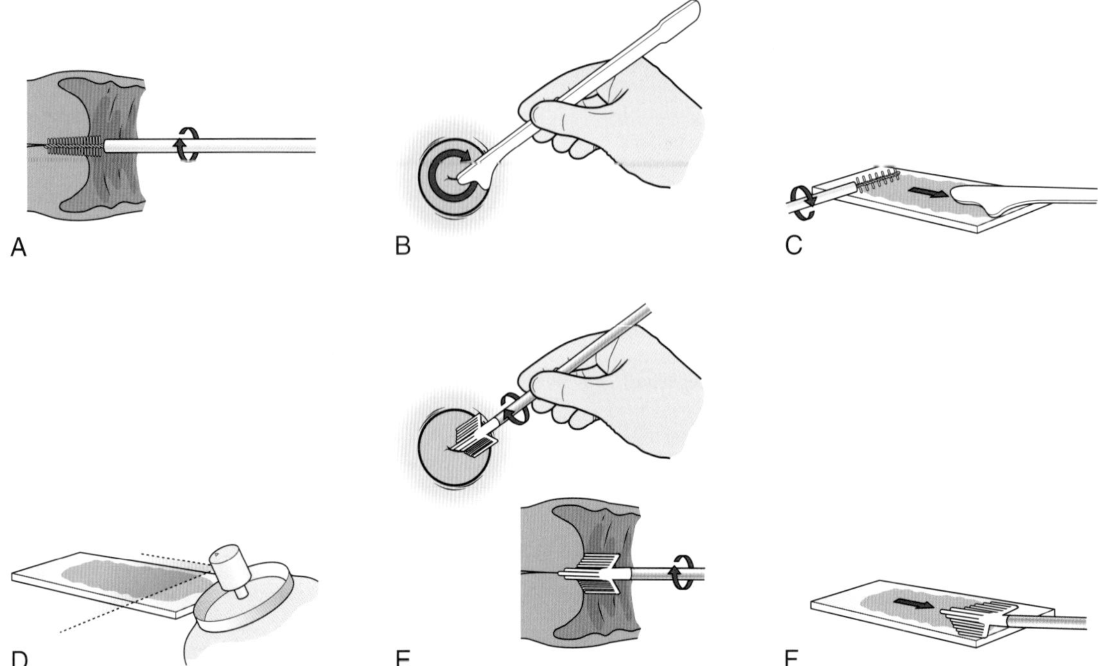

Figure 151-3 Obtaining the Papanicolaou smear. **A,** Endocervical sample with Cytobrush; rotate 90 to 180 degrees. **B,** Ectocervical sample obtained with a wooden or plastic spatula. **C,** A single-slide technique is preferred. First, the spatula sample is spread, which is then followed by "unrolling" of the brush sample directly over the first sample. **D,** Immediate fixation of the slide with cytologic fixative. **E,** Alternatively, a single sampling device may be used (Papette, Cervex-Brush, or "broom") to obtain both ectocervical and endocervical samples at the same time. Rotate 360 degrees five times. **F,** Spreading the sample from broom device onto slide.

support that reflex HPV testing will enhance management of women with ASC-US cytologic findings, separating those who need colposcopy (HPV DNA high-risk positive) from those who can be returned to standard screening (HPV DNA negative). If the HPV testing is performed automatically (reflex) based upon an ASC-US cytologic findings, the patient need not return for a separate HPV screening visit. Data support the cost effectiveness of this strategy. Furthermore, the combined use of liquid-based cytologic examination and same-time HPV testing has immediate advantage for management of women over age 30 and women in certain post-treatment categories (see Chapter 142, Human Papillomavirus DNA Sampling, and the ASCCP Guidelines in Appendix K).

In addition to the reflex HPV testing potential, liquid-based Pap techniques are also directly adaptable to computer-based automated screening devices. Development of automated screening devices has been driven more by the need to reduce labor costs than the need for accuracy. It is not clear that they will improve traditional human review of light microscopy samples. Currently these computer systems are utilized for either repeat evaluation of previously read Pap smears or for selecting certain cells for technicians to view. Computers can interpret only liquid-based preparations at the present time.

Preprocedure Patient Preparation

The patient should understand the reason for performing the Pap smear. The Pap smear is best performed during midcycle. The patient should avoid douching, vaginal medications, and intercourse for 24 hours prior to the procedure. In most instances the examination should be rescheduled if the patient is actively menstruating. The patient should void before undressing for the examination. Make sure the room is warm enough and the speculum is warmed as well. Question the patient regarding her concerns. Not infrequently, women are hesitant to discuss symptoms related to the genitals, such as vaginal dryness, itchiness, or discharge, unless the clinician asks. The clinician should explain each step of the pelvic examination prior to proceeding. Inform the patient of the mechanisms that you use to follow up on test results (Pap smear, cultures, etc.). (See the sample patient education handout online at www.expertconsult.com.)

Technique

1. *Obtain history* (especially sexual aspects of age at first intercourse, number of sexual partners, and history of sexual abuse or rape), perform review of systems, and answer questions. Clarify the patient's risk factors for cervical dysplasia. Review past Pap results if available.
2. *Proceed with the general medical and breast examination*, leaving the pelvic examination for last.
3. Label the frosted end of the glass slide or the liquid Pap vial with the patient's name and other identifying data prior to applying the sample.
4. *Place the patient in the lithotomy position*, and begin the examination. Wear nonsterile gloves. Inspect the vulva, and assess hair pattern, anatomy, estrogen effect, discharge, and any abnormal areas. Ask the patient if she has any concerns.
5. *Place a small amount of water-soluble lubricant on the warmed speculum and insert it*. Carefully advance the speculum, applying gentle pressure posteriorly. In patients whose vaginal walls prolapse and obstruct view, consider using a vaginal "stent." This can be fashioned by cutting off both ends of a single finger of a latex rubber glove and placing it over the blades of the speculum (Fig. 151-6). For those who are very obese or have excessively deep vaginas, a special, long *"Snowman" speculum* is available from CooperSurgical, Inc.
6. Adjust the speculum to obtain adequate visualization of the cervix, and tighten the screw or lock the speculum open.
7. Determine whether the vagina or cervix appears inflamed or infected. Avoid rubbing or otherwise traumatizing the cervix.

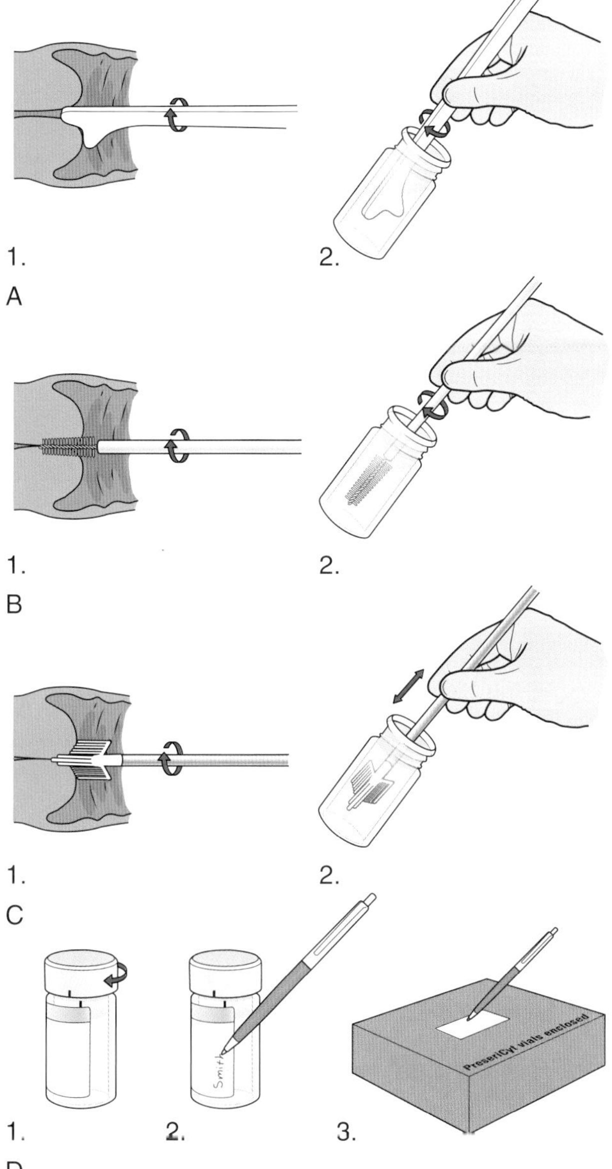

Figure 151-4 Liquid-based (ThinPrep) methods using plastic spatula (**A**), endocervical brush (**B**), or broom-like device (**C**). **D** shows the final three steps for each method. **A,** 1. Obtain an adequate sampling from the ectocervix using a plastic spatula. 2. Rinse the spatula as quickly as possible into the PreservCyt Solution vial by swirling the spatula vigorously in the vial 10 times. Discard the spatula. **B,** 1. Obtain an adequate sampling from the endocervix using an endocervical brush device. Insert the brush into the cervix until only the bottom-most fibers are exposed. Slowly rotate 1/4 or 1/2 turn in one direction. *Do not over-rotate*. 2. Rinse the brush as quickly as possible into the PreservCyt Solution by rotating the device in the solution 10 times while pushing against the PreservCyt vial wall. Swirl the brush vigorously to further release material. Discard the brush. **C,** 1. Obtain an adequate sampling from the cervix using a broom-like device. Insert the central bristles of the broom into the endocervical canal deep enough to allow the shorter bristles to fully contact the ectocervix. Push gently, and rotate the broom in a clockwise direction five times. 2. Rinse the broom as quickly as possible into the PreservCyt Solution vial by pushing the broom into the bottom of the vial 10 times, forcing the bristles apart. As a final step, swirl the broom vigorously to further release material. Discard the collection device. Be sure entire transformation zone has been sampled. **D,** 1. Tighten the cap so that the torque line on the cap passes the torque line on the vial. 2. Record the patient's name and ID number on the vial, and record the patient information and medical history on the cytology requisition form. 3. Place the vial and requisition in a specimen bag for transport to the laboratory. (Courtesy of CYTYC Corp., Boxborough, MA.)

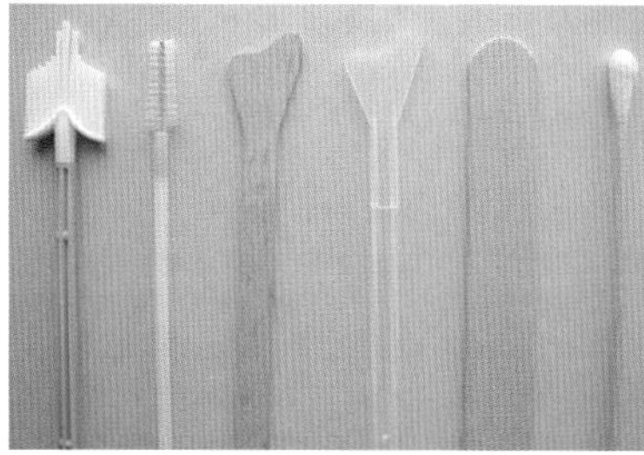

Figure 151-5 Papanicolaou sampling devices. *Left to right*: Cervex-Brush, Cytobrush, wooden spatula, plastic spatula, tongue blade, and cotton swab. Use of the swab and tongue blade is discouraged.

8. *Identify cervical landmarks*, including the transformation zone with its squamocolumnar junction. Note the nature of the cervical mucus. Markedly excessive mucus or discharge may be gently blotted, not rubbed, from view. However, mucus may actually contain the exfoliated cells needed for the microscopic examination. So, unless truly necessary, do not remove this mucus; include it in the sample. Note any gross cervical lesions, such as erosions (ulcerations), leukoplakia (white areas), nabothian cysts, or condylomas. Examine the vaginal fornices for obvious abnormalities.
9. *Obtain the Pap smear* by using an endocervical sampling device (Cytobrush, Papette, or Cervex-Brush). Q-Tips are not to be used. If the Cytobrush is used, first insert the Cytobrush into the canal and *rotate it 90 to 180 degrees*. Do not rotate it more than this, since that may cause bleeding, which can wash away or obscure abnormal cells. Follow this by a gentle sampling of the entire transformation zone using a spatula device, rotating *it 360 degrees*. If broom devices (Papette, Cervex-Brush) are used, insert and rotate them *360 degrees five times*. The broom will obtain both endocervical and ectocervical samples at the same time but must be rotated multiple times to collect an adequate number of cells.

   Sampling the vaginal pool has little advantage during Pap smear screening unless the patient has had a hysterectomy. In this instance, be sure to sample the vaginal cuff itself. If vaginal abnormalities are seen, another Pap smear of these areas (using a spatula) may be submitted on a separate slide. Areas that appear abnormal on visualization will ultimately require colposcopy and biopsy.
10. Glass slide method
    - If a *one-slide smear technique* is suggested by your reference laboratory (check with your pathologist), withhold smearing the endocervical Cytobrush sample on the slide until the ectocervical spatula sample is smeared on the slide first. Once this is done, then quickly roll out the Cytobrush sample (which is less subject to drying artifact) right over the spatula smear material and spray immediately with cytofixative.

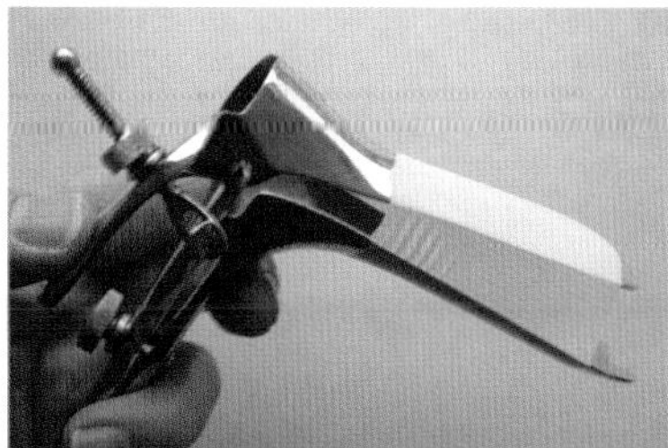

Figure 151-6 Vaginal speculum stent. To aid in the visualization of the cervix, a single finger of a latex examination glove can be cut off and placed over the blades of a standard vaginal speculum. This is helpful if there is redundant vaginal mucosa, as seen with pregnancy, obesity, or multiparity.

- If a *two-slide smear technique* is used, each sample (ectocervical and endocervical) is evenly applied to different slides immediately after sampling, and then the slide is sprayed or dipped in preservative within 5 seconds. (The broom devices will provide only a single slide because they sample both the ectocervical and endocervical areas at the same time.)

11. If a *thin-layer liquid-based technology Pap smear method* is utilized, follow the instructions of the manufacturer, which usually require rinsing the Pap sample (collected on the brush, broom, or spatula) directly into a vial of transport liquid rather than smearing the sample on glass slides. (See later discussion under "ThinPrep Pap Smears.")
12. *Perform the appropriate cervical cultures* after cytologic sampling, if indicated. (The Centers for Disease Control [CDC] recommends that all sexually active females under age 25 be routinely screened for chlamydia and rechecked after treatment is completed.)
13. *Examine the vagina* by slowly withdrawing the speculum, which is held slightly open, allowing the vagina to collapse over the blades. Note abnormalities.
14. Lubricate the gloved hand as necessary and *proceed with the bimanual examination*. Pay particular attention to palpated abnormalities of the introitus, vagina, fornices, and cervix. Palpate the areas of Skene's and Bartholin's glands. Ask your patient to bear down, and observe for uterine or pelvic floor prolapse and for leaking of urine. Having her cough facilitates assessment of pelvic support.
15. Complete the remainder of the bimanual examination, noting the size, contour, tenderness, and mobility of the uterus and adnexal structures.
16. Perform a rectal examination on women with rectal complaints, or who are over age 40. Be sure to put on a new glove before the rectal examination, which may prevent the spread of HPV or other infectious agents to the anus. For women who have had abnormal high-grade Pap or biopsy results, a rectal examination may be indicated at any age because high-risk HPV viruses also cause anal cancers.
17. Allow the patient to dress.
18. Make sure the Pap smear requisition form includes all pertinent data regarding your patient. Include clinical findings, patient risk factors, or your concerns as part of this "referral" (Bethesda recommendation).

ThinPrep Pap Smears

1. Use a nonwooden spatula or supplied sampling device.
2. The Cytobrush should not be rotated more than 180 degrees, and only in one direction.
3. The collecting devices are then swished along the inner surface of the fluid container at least 20 times around.

SurePath Pap Smears

1. A cervical broom is provided with the transport fluid and vial.
2. Insert the central or longest bristles into the cervical canal.
3. Apply gentle pressure to allow the outer bristles to contact the cervix.
4. Rotate the broom five full turns in one direction making sure it samples the entire transformation zone.
5. Pop the broom head off into the transport vial.

Pap Smears during Pregnancy

During pregnancy, the cervix progressively enlarges, the squamocolumnar junction displaces outward, the mucus becomes thicker and more abundant, and the cervix becomes much more vascular. Extra care must be used to gently blot off excess mucus and when applying the Pap sampling device to collect the sample, especially after 20 weeks' gestation. Despite these changes, the Pap smear in a pregnant woman maintains a similar sensitive and specific profile when compared to the nonpregnant state. Pregnancy itself does not accelerate or worsen cervical dysplasia. In most women, the first trimester cervix appears very similar to the nonpregnant cervix. The active transformation zone everts, or externalizes, progressively with advancing gestation, so there is little need to probe or sample the cervical canal, especially with wire tip brush devices. (In the author's opinion, broom or spatula devices are preferred in pregnancy, and the brush is avoided to reduce the risk of bleeding.)

1. Ideally, obtain the Pap smear as early in pregnancy as possible to avoid exaggerated spotting. Patients are also more uncomfortable in the lithotomy position with an advanced gestation.
2. Although there is controversy with using brush devices in pregnancy, the broom or spatula devices make excellent sampling devices and are preferred.
3. Be gentle while rotating the brush because bleeding is more common in pregnancy.

Sample Procedure Note

This 32-year-old G3P3 white female is here for a screening Pap smear. She had a tubal ligation 4 years ago. Last Pap smear was 2 years ago. Prior Pap testing has been reviewed and is normal. With chaperone present and the patient in the lithotomy position, the external genitalia were inspected and found to be free of abnormality. A standard metal Graves speculum was warmed, lightly lubricated, and gently inserted. The cervix was manipulated into view and found to be free of inflammation, infection, and abnormal discharge. The squamocolumnar junction was seen in its entirety and was about 10 mm in diameter. A Cytobrush sample and spatula sample were obtained, sampling the entire visible transformation zone, and quickly smeared and fixed on a single identified glass slide. Cultures were not deemed necessary by history and examination. Bimanual examination revealed a smooth, midline, freely mobile, nontender uterus that was not enlarged. Ovaries and adnexal structures were of normal size and position and were not painful. No pelvic masses were identified. The vagina and cervix were normal on palpation.

Common Errors

1. Lack of understanding of the basic anatomy of the cervix, including the squamocolumnar junction and the transformation zone can lead to incorrect sampling.
2. Inadequate exposure of the cervix with the speculum can lead to incomplete sampling of the transformation zone.
3. Failure to review the patient's history for prior abnormal Pap smears or cervical treatment. The patient may require colposcopy (see the ASCCP Guidelines in Appendix K).
4. Failure to inform or follow up with patients with Pap results, especially if abnormal.
5. Not obtaining recent contact information from the patient, confounding attempts to notify the patient of Pap smear results.
6. An aggressive approach to Pap smear sampling can lead to unnecessary bleeding, patient concern, and potentially less than satisfactory sample.
7. Obtaining cervical cultures or DNA probes for sexually transmittable infections prior to the Pap smear may cause bleeding or remove valuable cytologic material from the Pap smear sample.
8. Relying on the Pap smear result even when the cervix appears abnormal. An abnormal-appearing cervix warrants colposcopy regardless of the Pap smear result.
9. Interpretative confusion on the part of the clinician regarding the recommended follow-up of cytologic examination indicating atypical glandular cells versus atypical squamous cells (AGC vs. ASC-US, Bethesda-2001).

10. Inappropriately ordering DNA testing in women younger than 30 years of age for routine screening.

Complications

The Pap smear is only a *screening test*. False-negative rates are high (20% to 50%, with an average of 25%), and significant disease can be missed or underestimated. More frequent Pap smear screening or colposcopy may be indicated, depending on patient history and risks of having or developing genital malignancy. Minor spotting and occasional uterine cramps can commonly follow Pap smear sampling. Many of the shortfalls of Pap smear screening can be addressed by adhering to the following "golden rules":

- Identify cervical landmarks and gross abnormalities, and sample both the endocervical canal and the entire transformation zone. Choose a transformation zone sampler that fits your patient.
- All Pap smears reported as abnormal require some form of intervention. A report of dysplasia warrants colposcopy. Many clinicians also recommend colposcopy for reports of ASC, especially in patients with numerous risk factors. At the least, repeat Pap smear is indicated, or DNA typing is needed to determine which ASC Pap sample has high-risk HPV. Atypical glandular cells (AGCs) definitely need further evaluation. (See Chapter 137, Colposcopic Examination, and Appendix K, Management Guidelines for Abnormal Cervical Cancer Screening Tests and Histologic Findings.)
- Clarify your patient's risk factors for having HPV infection and cervical dysplasia as part of the routine examination. Anyone with substantial risks requires at least annual Pap smears.
- An observed abnormality on the cervix that cannot be readily explained by normal variants (e.g., nabothian cysts) warrants colposcopic examination. A normal Pap smear report in the face of an observed abnormal cervix should *not* dissuade the clinician from performing colposcopy and biopsy.
- Know your cytopathologist. Interpretive problems should be discussed directly with the pathologist, who can address your questions, including the option to review the cytologic findings at issue.
- The optimal way to reduce morbidity and mortality rates from cervical cancer may not be new technology, but rather convincing women who have not been screened for large intervals, or at all, to have a Pap smear.

Postprocedure Management

Most of the postprocedure management issues with the pelvic examination including Pap smear sampling can be addressed by environmental issues and having an informed patient. Inform the patient to expect minor spotting or cramping. This is especially important for Pap smears during pregnancy, when these symptoms can be very concerning. Make sure that you have accurate follow-up contact information and patient preferences for contact methods. Take time to explain when you feel the next Pap smear is due. With the new Pap smear screening recommendations, which may include HPV testing, patients and clinicians alike are often confused regarding what is recommended. Clearly document your recommendation.

Interpretation of Results

Adequacy

The Pap smear report should indicate whether the smear was adequate. Unless the patient has had a hysterectomy, the report should include cytologic evidence that the transformation zone was sampled. Ordinarily, the reporting of endocervical cells along with squamous cells implies adequate sampling. Many cytologists attribute the same significance to "squamous metaplasia" as the reporting of "endocervical cells present." Either is considered objective evidence that the transformation zone was sampled, which implies an adequate sample. Many reports will in some way use or check the word "adequate" on a form. Bethesda-2001 further delineates adequacy.

Interpretation System

The "Bethesda system," named after the national consensus conference for Pap smear interpretation, has provided a uniform nomenclature for Pap smear cytologic interpretation and attempts to address much of the confusion regarding Pap smear terminology. In September 2001, the Bethesda consensus conference convened for the third time and provided revisions of the reporting system, with general recommendations as follows:

- The Pap smear report should use terminology that is understood by the clinician.
- The clinician should be able to discuss the Pap smear report with the cytopathologist if questions arise.
- All abnormal Pap smears require some form of intervention in addition to the routine yearly screening interval.
- See the discussion in the following section regarding findings in postmenopausal women.

Follow-up Recommendations

A consensus group hosted by the American Society of Colposcopy and Cervical Pathology (ASCCP) convened in 2006 in Bethesda, Maryland, and developed guidelines for the management of abnormal cervical cytologic findings. These recommendations use the terminology of the 2001 Bethesda interpretation system and are applicable to clinical circumstances. (See also Chapter 137, Colposcopic Examination.) The ASCCP guidelines are summarized with algorithms that can be found in Appendix K. These algorithms can guide clinicians through evidence-based recommendations for the majority of abnormal Pap smear scenarios. General "new" tenets of these guidelines include the following:

1. Less aggressive management of adolescents with abnormal Pap smears.
2. A recommendation to avoid HPV screening in adolescents and those under 30 years of age.
3. Options to use HPV testing for follow-up of ASC-US cytologic findings with reflex testing preferred if liquid-based Pap techniques are already used for cytologic evaluation.
4. Specific suggestion for management of pregnant women with abnormal cytologic features.
5. Preferred recommendations for follow-up of both adolescent and nonadolescent women with low-grade squamous intraepithelial lesion (LSIL).
6. Suggested work-up of women with initial and subsequent atypical glandular cells.
7. Use of HPV testing for screening and management of results in women age 30 years and older.
8. Reconfirmation that all women with high-grade squamous intraepithelial lesion (HSIL) will require colposcopy. However, follow-up for high-grade dysplasias may differ for adolescent and nonadolescent women.
9. A statement that although these guidelines are based upon available evidence, they remain only guidelines and clinicians are advised to utilize them as they may apply to a specific patient and are encouraged to consider alternative management or follow-up strategies based upon the social, economic, risk stratification, and other factors that may influence management decisions.

A report describing *glandular* or *adenomatous atypia* (also called *atypical glandular cells [AGC]*, and previously termed *atypical glandular cells of uncertain significance [AGCUS]*, which is to be differentiated from squamous atypia) warrants immediate colposcopy with endocervical curettage to rule out a high-grade lesion and cervical adenocarcinoma. Furthermore, *endometrial carcinoma* may be suggested by abnormal cytologic findings detected by a Pap smear. In such instances, formal endometrial sampling is mandated in patients over 40 years of age if no cervical abnormality is found. In *postmenopausal women* who are *not* on estrogen replacement, a report of *estrogen effect or endometrial cells* on the Pap smear is *not* normal. Evaluate the ovaries and uterus. If the findings of adenomatous atypia, or of estrogen effect/endometrial cells (in a postmenopausal woman not on estrogen) are definite, conization, pelvic ultrasound, and even laparoscopy may be indicated.

Patients who are *immunocompromised* (chronic immunosuppression after transplant, HIV positive, etc.) may require different, and in general more aggressive, follow-up and management strategies. Colposcopy is recommended for circumstance when there remains concern regarding potential severe or malignant changes.

From the 2006 ASCCP Guidelines, colposcopy is used for follow-up of the following Pap smear and pelvic examination findings:

1. Women with ASC-US
2. Adolescent women with HSIL or persistent ASC or LSIL
3. Women with LSIL
4. Nonadolescent women with LSIL or greater
5. Women with HSIL, both adolescent and nonadolescent
6. Initial work-up of women with AGCs
7. Women over age 30 with either persistent abnormal cytologic features or positive HPV testing
8. Pelvic examination findings of
   - Abnormal-appearing cervix
   - Abnormal-feeling cervix or vagina

Other indications for colposcopy:

- DES offspring
- History of sexual abuse or rape
- Other sexually transmissible disease (relative)

CPT/Billing Codes

Q0091	Screening Papanicolaou smear; obtaining, preparing, and conveyance of cervical or vaginal smear to laboratory*
57500	Biopsy of cervix†
57505	Endocervical curettage†
88150	Pap smear interpretation‡
99201–99215	For a Pap smear, use office visit codes

ICD-9-CM Diagnostic Codes

180.9	Malignant neoplasm of the cervix, unspecified
219.0	Neoplasm of the cervix, benign
233.1	Cervical carcinoma in situ, severe dysplasia of cervix
622.0	Cervical ulcer
622.2	Cervical leukoplakia
622.7	Cervical polyp
622.8	Cervical atrophy
622.10	Cervical dysplasia, unspecified
622.11	Mild dysplasia of cervix
622.12	Moderate dysplasia of cervix
623.8	Abnormal vaginal bleeding
626.8	Uterine bleeding
795.0	Abnormal Pap smear (some insurances will not reimburse for this code)
V15.89	Other specified personal history presenting hazards to health; other (for high-risk patients)
V76.2	Special screening for malignant neoplasms; cervix
V76.47	Special screening for malignant neoplasms; vagina

*One Pap test is covered by Medicare every 2 years for low-risk patients and every 1 year for high-risk patients. Q0091 can be reported with a separate E&M code for Medicare patients.

†The majority of cervical biopsies and the endocervical curettage (ECC) will be performed as part of the formal colposcopic examination. Please refer to Chapter 137, Colposcopic Examination, for appropriate billing information.

‡This code is used by the cytopathologist for billing. Very few clinicians (i.e., nonpathologists) interpret their patients' cytologic findings.

Patient Education Guides

See the sample patient education handout available online at www.expertconsult.com.

Suppliers

Full contact information is available online at www.expertconsult.com.

BD Diagnostics (SurePath)
CooperSurgical, Inc.
CYTYC Corp. (ThinPrep)
Hardwood Products Co. (Cervix Brush, spatulas)
Milex Products
Wallach Surgical Devices, Inc. (Brush device, spatulas)

Online Resources

American Cancer Society recommendations: http://caonline.amcancersoc.org/cgi/content/full/52/6/342.

American Society for Colposcopy and Cervical Pathology: Consensus guidelines for abnormal cytology: www.ASCCP.org.

Tuggy M, Garcia J: Procedures Consult: www.proceduresconsult.com; also available as an application at www.apple.com/iTunes.

USPSTF recommendations: www.ahcpr.gov/clinic/uspstf/uspscerv.htm.

Bibliography

American College of Obstetricians and Gynecologists: Clinical Management Guidelines for Obstetricians-Gynecologists. Cervical cytology screening. In ACOG Women's Health Care Physician's Compendium of Selected Publications, Practice Bulletin No. 45, Aug. 2003. Washington, DC, ACOG Distribution Center, 2006, pp 398–408.

Apgar BS, Brotzman GL, Spitzer M: Colposcopy: Principles and Practice, 2nd ed. Philadelphia, Saunders, 2008.

Arbyn M, Bergeron C, Klinkhamer P, et al: Liquid compared with conventional cervical cytology. Obstet Gynecol 111:167–177, 2008.

Koss LG: The Papanicolaou test for cervical cancer detection: A triumph and a tragedy. JAMA 261:737–743, 1989.

Solomon D, Davey D, Kurman R, et al: The 2001 Bethesda System: Terminology for reporting results of cervical cytology. JAMA 287:2114–2119, 2002.

Tuggy M, Garcia J: Procedures Consult. Available at www.procedurescounsult.com.

Wright TC, Massad LS, Dunton CH, et al: 2006 consensus guidelines for the management of women with abnormal cervical cancer screening tests. Am J Obstet Gynecol 197:340–345, 2007.

Wright TC, Massad LS, Dunton CH, et al: 2006 consensus guidelines for the management of women with cervical intraepithelial neoplasia or adenocarcinoma in situ. Am J Obstet Gynecol 197:346–355, 2007.

CHAPTER 152

Permanent Female Sterilization (Tubal Ligation)

Gary R. Newkirk

In the United States, voluntary sterilization remains one of the most widely used contraceptive methods, chosen by nearly 20% of married women. Family physicians skilled with basic surgical technique are in an ideal position to discuss and perform permanent sterilization procedures for both men and women. Approximately 600,000 tubal ligations are performed each year in the United States. A similar number of vasectomies are carried out. No man has ever died from the vasectomy procedure itself. Between 10 and 14 women die each year (in the United States) from tubal ligation. The failure rate for vasectomy is 1 in 1200 in the United States, whereas tubal ligation failures occur in 1 in 200 procedures within the first year and may increase in frequency over time. Although vasectomy allows detection of failures, no simple technique allows the surgeon to find tubal ligation failures. The cost of a tubal ligation is five to six times that of an office vasectomy. When a patient asks about permanent contraception, it behooves the primary care physician to point out the benefits of vasectomy over a tubal ligation. Even the American College of Obstetricians and Gynecologists (ACOG) agrees that, all things considered, a vasectomy is the procedure of choice. Nevertheless, when vasectomy is inappropriate for any reason, tubal ligation remains an excellent choice for permanent surgical contraception.

Despite numerous variations, female sterilization consists of two basic steps: (1) exposing the fallopian tubes, and (2) partially resecting or occluding the tubes to prevent conception. This chapter discusses the minilaparotomy approach to permanent female sterilization, both as an interval and as a postpartum procedure.

Box 152-1 outlines basic terminology related to permanent female sterilization methodology. Minilaparotomy and laparoscopy are abdominal surgical approaches that are considered safe, quick, and readily available.

Table 152-1 shows advantages and disadvantages of the minilaparotomy and the laparoscopic techniques. Despite the recognized advantages of laparoscopy for certain situations, minilaparotomy—because of its reliance on readily available surgical equipment, fewer technical demands, and applicability to both interval and postpartum periods—is the method of choice for many primary care physicians. Box 152-2 summarizes the more common methods for ligating the tubes.

This chapter outlines the minilaparotomy approach and the modified Pomeroy or "Parkland" method for ligation (Figs. 152-1 and 152-2). The ideal method is still under debate; however, the modified Pomeroy and Parkland methods (with their variations) remain popular in the United States. Prudent physicians should identify patients who may benefit by referral, either for alternative methods that the referring physician cannot offer because of a lack of skill, training, equipment, or facility or because of the patient's clinical condition.

Anatomy

Figure 152-3 demonstrates the anatomy relevant to a tubal ligation.

Indications

- Desire for permanent sterilization
- Medical conditions that place the patient at significant risk for irreversible morbidity or death if she should become pregnant
- Known severe inheritable genetic disease (that makes childbearing undesirable)

Contraindications

Absolute

- Active peritoneal infections
- Severe chronic heart, lung, or metabolic disease (abdominal insufflation [laparoscopy] and the head-down [Trendelenburg] position can cause acute cardiopulmonary decompensation)
- Any unstable medical condition (including unstable postpartum condition)
- Lack of informed consent
- Inability to tolerate necessary anesthesia
- Patient unsure of desire for permanent sterilization

Relative

- Prior significant pelvic or abdominal infection: minilaparotomy or laparoscopy may be more difficult. (Laparotomy may be necessary.)
- Severe obesity, especially with a history of pelvic or abdominal infection.
- Chronic heart disease, irregular pulse, uncontrolled hypertension, pelvic masses, uncontrolled diabetes, bleeding disorders, severe nutritional deficiencies, severe anemia, and umbilical or hiatal hernia. (The risks of future pregnancies must be weighed against the risks of permanent sterilization procedures.)

Equipment

- A laparotomy pack contains most of the instruments necessary for basic abdominal surgery and is available in most hospital outpatient and inpatient surgical suites.
- Suction catheter: Generally, suction is not used during a routine minilaparotomy tubal ligation. Suction is available on demand at most surgical suites; it is mandatory if complications such as bleeding develop.

Box 152-1. Female Sterilization Terminology

Colpotomy: A vaginal approach to tubal ligation through the posterior vaginal fornix.

Interval tubal ligation: Tubal ligation performed at times other than during the immediate postpartum period—generally 6 weeks or more after delivery.

Laparoscopy: Involves inserting an illuminated telescope-like instrument into the abdomen that allows visualization of the fallopian tubes in order to accomplish electrocoagulation or application of clips or rings. For *open* laparoscopy, a small incision is made within or just below the umbilicus to allow passage of a special cannula, around which the skin makes an airtight seal. The cannula allows for insufflation of the abdomen, passage of the laparoscope and instruments, and occlusion of the tubes. Open laparoscopy is considered safer than traditional *closed* laparoscopy, especially in women with prior pelvic or abdominal surgery or infection. With the *closed* laparoscopic procedure, the laparoscope is inserted blindly through the abdominal wall.

Laparotomy: A relatively large abdominal incision performed to optimize surgical exposure for a variety of intra-abdominal surgeries.

Minilaparotomy: Sometimes referred to as a *minilap*; involves a small abdominal incision, usually less than 5 cm (2 inches).

Postpartum tubal ligation: Tubal ligation performed within 72 hours of delivery.

Technical failure: Inability to complete the planned sterilization during the operation, which results in a change of method or failure to perform the sterilization.

TABLE 152-1 Advantages and Disadvantages of Minilaparotomy and Laparoscopy

	Advantages	Disadvantages
Minilaparotomy	Easy to learn Basic surgical training and skill Inexpensive instruments Complications are usually minor Can be performed as a postpartum or interval	Takes longer than laparoscopy Difficult to perform on patients who are obese or who have pelvic scarring or adhesions Scar slightly larger More pain from the abdominal incision Higher infection rate than laparoscopy procedure
Laparoscopy	Very low complication rate Quick procedure (10–15 min) Very small incision Useful for other diagnostic and therapeutic purposes Less painful	Complications may be serious Requires abdominal insufflation, with its added risk More difficult to learn; requires specialized training for physician and staff Equipment is more expensive and requires more maintenance and repair Not recommended as a postpartum procedure

Box 152-2. Common Tubal Ligation Methods

Minilaparotomy ("Open" Procedure)

Electrocoagulation: A bipolar probe is passed through a small segment of tube to cauterize and obstruct the lumen.

Fimbriectomy: This method is accomplished by the complete removal of the fimbriated end of the tube. The procedure appears to have a higher pregnancy failure rate, and reversal is unlikely.

Irving technique: An extremely effective, though more difficult, method that cannot be reversed easily. The tube is cut and the uterine end buried beneath the peritoneum within the wall of the uterus. The remaining end is buried within the mesosalpinx.

Laparoscopy clips: Under laparoscopic guidance, clips are applied to occlude the tubal lumen. Hulka (spring-loaded) and Filshie clips (titanium and silicone rubber) are commonly used. Clips destroy less than 1 cm of tissue, and reversals are considered much easier.

Parkland technique: A small length of tube is separated from the mesosalpinx and ligated at each end, about 2 cm apart; the free segment between the ligatures is removed (see Fig. 152-3).

Pomeroy technique: The most common procedure performed for both interval and postpartum tubal ligations. Absorbable catgut sutures are used to tie the base of a loop of midportion (ampullary) tube. The ligated loop of tube is then removed. As the suture absorbs, the ends pull apart and are obstructed by the healing and scarring process. From 3 to 6 cm of the tube is destroyed (see Fig. 152-2).

Tubal ring: A small Silastic ring is stretched and placed over a loop of fallopian tube and then released. The tube is blocked by compression. Usually a 2- to 3-cm segment of the tube is involved. Reversal is more successful than with the electrocauterization, Irving, or Uchida techniques.

Uchida technique: A technically demanding, yet extremely effective, method that is becoming more popular in the United States. The tube is severed and the uterine end is buried within the mesosalpinx.

Vaginal Approaches

Ligation, clips, and electrocoagulation rings: Two varieties have been used.

1. *Colpotomy*, which involves a surgical incision in the posterior vaginal fornix through which the tube is delivered and occluded by ligation, clips, or rings.
2. *Culdoscopy*, in which a culdoscope is passed through a smaller colpotomy incision to allow identification of the tubes and application of the electroprobe, clips, or rings.

Both of these less popular methods share higher complication and failure rates. They are not postpartum methods.

Transcervical Approaches

Essure: In the fall of 2002, the Food and Drug Administration approved a new method, called Essure, whereby a device with a small stainless steel inner coil and superelastic outer coil (4 cm × 0.8 mm, after release 4 cm × 1.5–2 mm) is inserted hysteroscopically into the fallopian tubes for permanent sterilization. (See Chapter 148, Insertion of Essure [Hysteroscopically Assisted Female Sterilization].)

Others: Still considered experimental procedures, these methods of blocking the tubes from a transcervical-intrauterine approach continue to evoke interest. One method is to use Silastic "plugs" placed under hysteroscopic guidance. Various techniques are under development to provide a reversible sterilization by "pulling the plugs" when a pregnancy is desired.

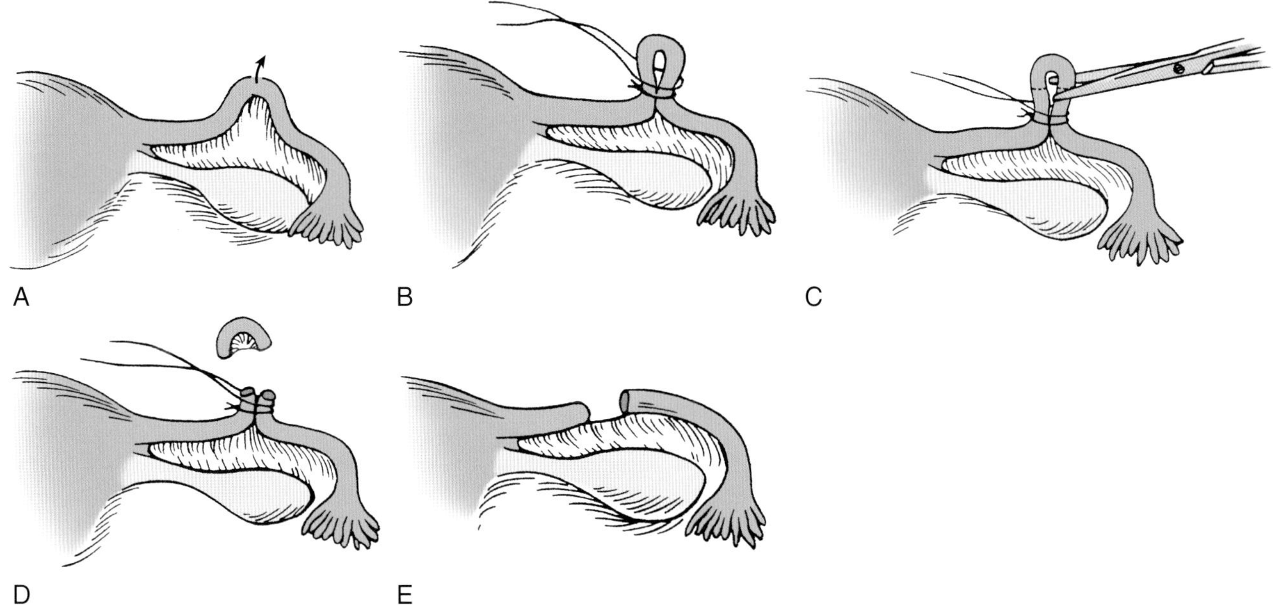

Figure 152-1 Modified Pomeroy technique. **A,** Lift loop. **B,** Double ligation 0 or 2-0 plain gut suture, no crushing. **C,** Each limb of tubal loop is cut separately. **D,** Loop is cut off. **E,** Later results.

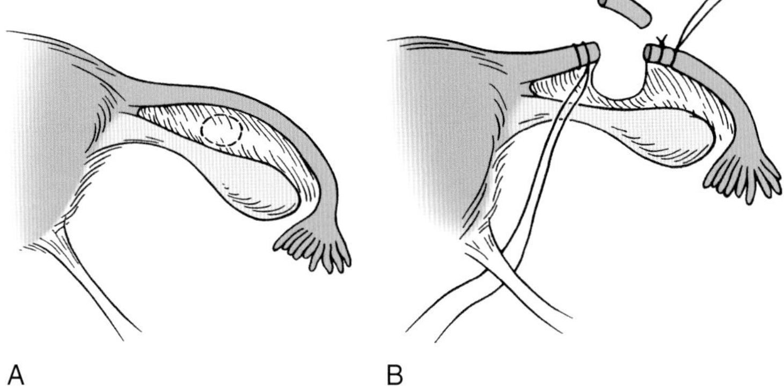

Figure 152-2 Parkland method of tubal ligation. **A,** A relatively avascular area of the mesosalpinx is identified within the isthmic portion of the tube. **B,** A segment of tube is isolated and removed after double ligation with chromic suture.

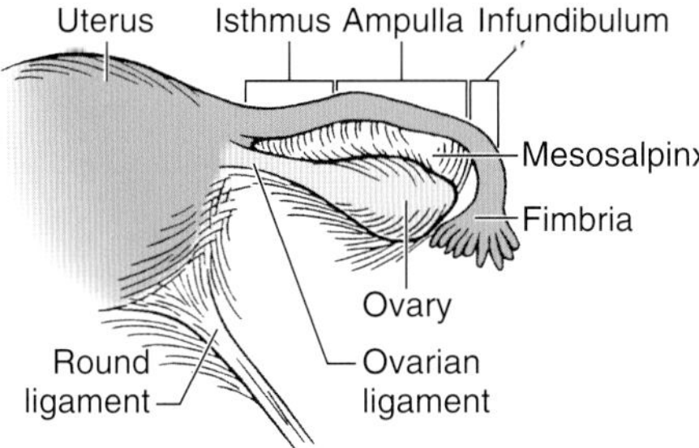

Figure 152-3 Basic anatomy of the parauterine structures.

- Coagulation device: Most operative suites have a Bovie or similar coagulation device available. Some surgeons prefer to have this available for all cases; others use this electively, or when complications develop. Because a Bovie requires grounding, it should be set up in advance. A ground plate can be attached before the patient is draped and scrubbed.
- Sutures

Anatomic Site	Suture
Tubal ligation	0 Plain or chromic
Peritoneum	2-0 Chromic
Fascia	0 Dexon
Scarpa's fascia	2-0 Chromic
Skin	Metal clips, 4-0 Dexon

- 8-inch Babcock forceps to separate and retract fallopian tube (Fig 152-4A)
- Ring sponge (a ring forceps holding a tightly folded gauze pad)
- Small Richardson or Army-Navy retractors for holding the incision open (Fig. 152-4B)
- Adson tissue forceps with teeth for skin manipulation (Fig. 152-4C)
- Metzenbaum scissors for general tissue blunt dissection and incision (Fig. 152-4D)
- Kelly clamps for blunt dissection, and for grasping and tagging suture, bleeders, or tissue planes (fascia, peritoneum)
- Uterine manipulators for use with the cervical tenaculum or the newer uterine manipulators (Fig. 152-4E)
- 5-mL, 0.5% bupivacaine (Marcaine) (optional)

Precautions

Tubal ligation is elective surgery and should be performed when optimal preparation of both the patient and surgical environment are at hand. Patients must be competent to offer informed consent or the appropriate arrangements (legal guardianship for health care decisions) made to assure legal basis to proceed with permanent sterilization. As with all elective surgeries, the patient's medical condition should be optimized for the stress of regional or general anesthesia to allow for this intra-abdominal surgery. It is not uncommon to postpone a postpartum tubal ligation, which was planned

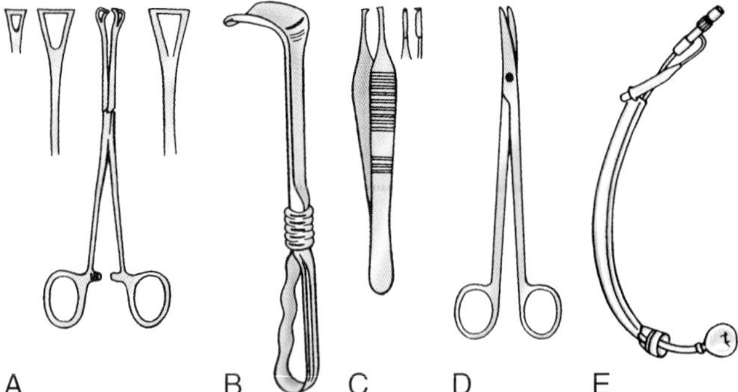

Figure 152-4 Instruments for tubal ligation. **A,** Babcock forceps; **B,** small Richardson retractor; **C,** Adson tissue forceps; **D,** Metzenbaum scissors; **E,** uterine manipulator. (Also see Chapter 144, Hysterosalpingography and Sonohysterography.)

well in advance, because of intrapartum complications such as unexpected blood loss or unstable condition of the newborn. In these instances, delaying a postpartum tubal ligation as well as reevaluation for other contraceptive options may be prudent and appropriate.

Preprocedure Patient Preparation

Preprocedure Visits

Preprocedure evaluation and counseling for women who want permanent sterilization warrant focused attention. A special visit should be scheduled to discuss contraceptive options, risks, technique, and follow-up demands of sterilization surgery. (See the sample patient education form online at www.expertconsult.com.) In addition, many insurance companies require preauthorization, which should be obtained at this visit. The counseling session should not be hurried or added to the end of a visit for an acute illness. Written materials should be given to the patient at this time. Federal payment programs require that counseling precede surgery by at least 30 days and not more than 180 days. Special forms need to be signed, and the patient must be at least 21 years of age. If the patient is involved in a monogamous relationship, it is wise to have the partner present during the consultation to address any concerns. Partner written consent is not mandatory, but if there is disagreement with this decision, it should be discussed and the reasons explored. It is also important to address the issues and benefits of vasectomy (refer to the opening paragraph of this chapter).

A *preprocedure examination*, which requires a reasonable amount of time, should occur within 10 days (some hospitals require less than 5 days) of anticipated surgery. Review the patient's complete medical history, paying particular attention to prior pelvic or abdominal surgery and infection. Are there drug allergies or drug intolerances? Are there medications (such as aspirin) that should be stopped? Is the patient on chronic anticoagulants? Is there a history of heart disease, diabetes, bleeding disorder, endometriosis, or dysfunctional uterine bleeding? Is other concomitant surgery necessary (e.g., dilation and curettage [D & C], breast biopsy, or procedure for urinary incontinence)? Is the Pap smear normal? Discuss the method of anesthesia that is to be used. Carefully review anticipated postprocedure morbidities (e.g., pain, the necessity of limited lifting). Remain mindful of the risk factors for regret (see later discussion under General Information). Review current contraceptive methods. Is pregnancy a possibility at the time of surgery? If the patient smokes, can she quit before surgery?

Preprocedure examination should be thorough. Focus on the heart, lung, breast, and abdominal examinations. During the pelvic examination, assess for the presence of vulvar, vaginal, or cervical disease. Obtain specimens for culture (e.g., gonorrhea, chlamydia) as necessary. Assess the degree of uterine prolapse and urinary incontinence; have the patient bear down and cough. Perform a bimanual examination to assess uterine size, shape, and tenderness. Palpate the ovaries for enlargement. Pay particular attention to uterine mobility. Can the uterus be brought out of the pelvis easily, or is it frozen in a particular direction? Estimate the degree of abdominal wall obesity. Show the patient the location and size of the anticipated abdominal incision and eventual scarring.

Perform laboratory tests as necessary. Typically, hospitals require *hemoglobin* levels and a *urinalysis* as the minimum prerequisites for general anesthesia. Perform a *pregnancy test* if there is any question of pregnancy. If there is clinical evidence of cervicitis or pelvic inflammation, obtain specimens for culture, and treat the condition accordingly. In this case, schedule the surgery only when treatment and clinical response have been adequate.

Many same-day and outpatient surgery services offer *preanesthesia counseling*. The patient can meet with the anesthesia clinician to discuss anesthesia, risks, time to arrive at the hospital, how long to fast before surgery, and other issues. This counseling should be used whenever it is available; for many hospitals, it is a requirement.

Call the hospital surgery personnel with any special requests for the anticipated surgery. Will a D & C be performed? (If so, it should be done *after* minilaparotomy.) Is a uterine manipulator necessary, and what type will be used?

General Information

- *Minilaparotomy is the safest sterilization method in the postpartum period*, with a complication rate approaching that of interval sterilization, which is usually less than 3%. Laparoscopy is not as safe during the immediate postpartum period as at other times.
- Average *rates for tubal sterilization failures* are 1 in 250 at 1 year.
- Postpartum and postabortion sterilization appears to be somewhat less effective than interval sterilization.
- Of the women who have tubal sterilization, *1% to 2% seek reversal*; however, sterility is not easily reversed. Only 30% to 70% of these women are candidates for reversal surgery (this broad range for reversal success is related to the original method of the tubal ligations), and pregnancy occurs in about 50% of those who do undergo reversal procedures. Reversal is most successful if less than 3 cm of the tubes was originally damaged or removed. The most "reversible" techniques include those that do not involve electrocautery and those in which the smallest segment is removed from within the isthmic portion of the tube. Women with the following *risk factors for regret* should not necessarily be denied surgery; however, the prudent physician should counsel these patients before performing sterilization.
  - *Marital disharmony* at the time of sterilization. (Remarriage is the reason 90% of women request reversal.)
  - *Age less than 30 years* at the time of sterilization. (Some clinicians debate whether this is a significant risk factor.)
  - Religious, socioeconomic, and educational backgrounds show much less correlation with regret. Low parity or number of live children is also less well correlated.
  - Regret may be slightly more prevalent after postpartum sterilization procedures; however, as a risk factor, this is less well defined.
  - Regret is more likely when sterilization is chosen because of financial difficulties, health, or emotional problems.

Procedure

Figure 152-5 illustrates the procedure for tubal ligation. According to the latest ACOG and American Heart Association guidelines, prophylactic antibiotics are not indicated for laparoscopy or laparotomy sterilization procedures.

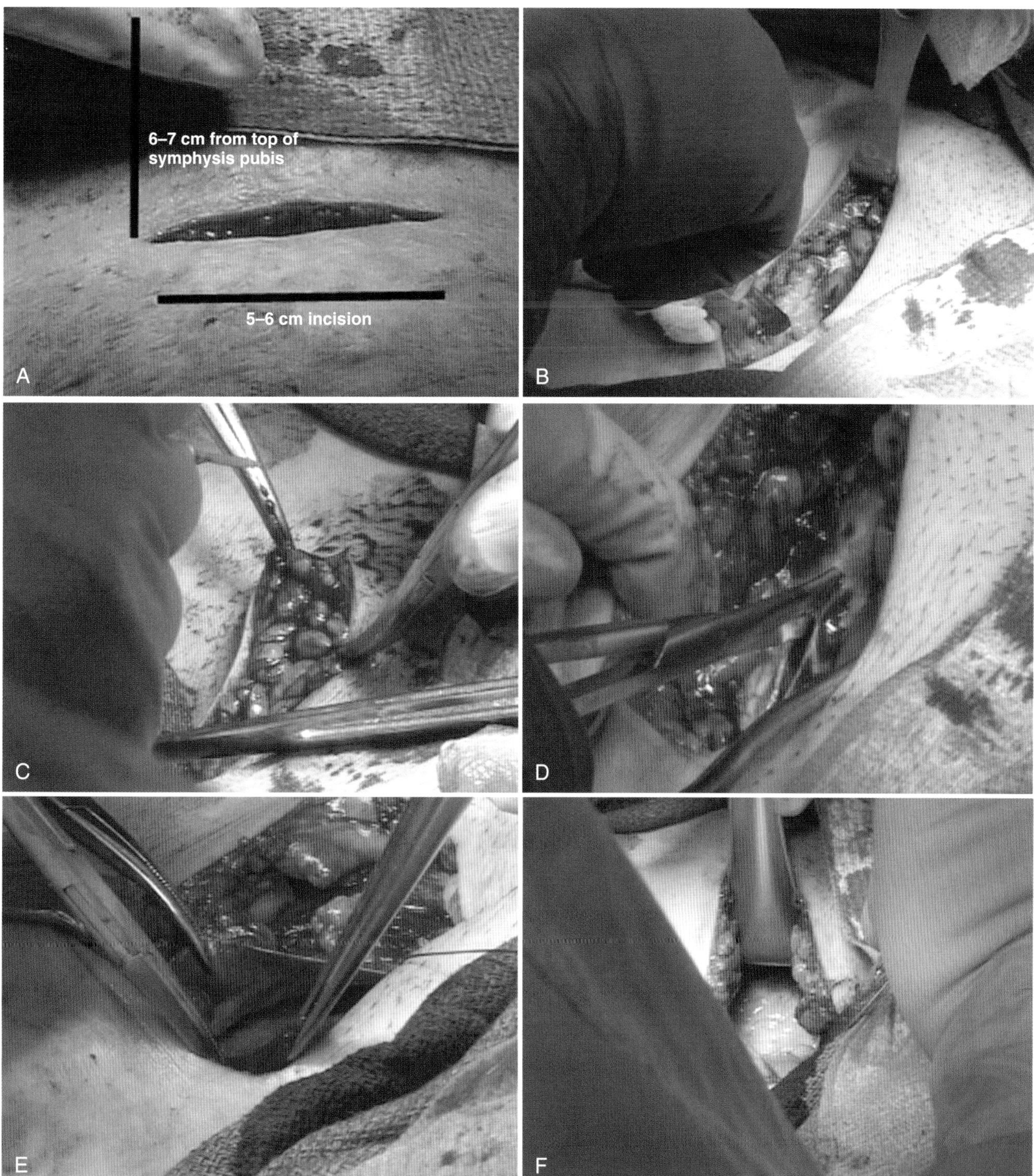

Figure 152-5 Procedure for tubal ligation. **A,** A transverse abdominal incision is made about 6 cm above the top of the symphysis pubis and about 5 cm wide. **B,** A small retractor is used to part the incised tissue and improve exposure as the incision is carried through the abdominal wall. **C,** Small bleeders encountered can be grasped with a hemostat and coagulated by touching the electrosurgical coagulator to the hemostat. **D,** As the fascia is encountered, it is carefully divided transversely and the incision is carried down to the peritoneum. **E,** The peritoneum is identified by its thin, translucent quality and is divided entering the abdominal cavity. **F,** A small Richardson retractor with counter-retraction by the surgeon's fingers improves visual access to the abdominal contents.

Figure continues on following page

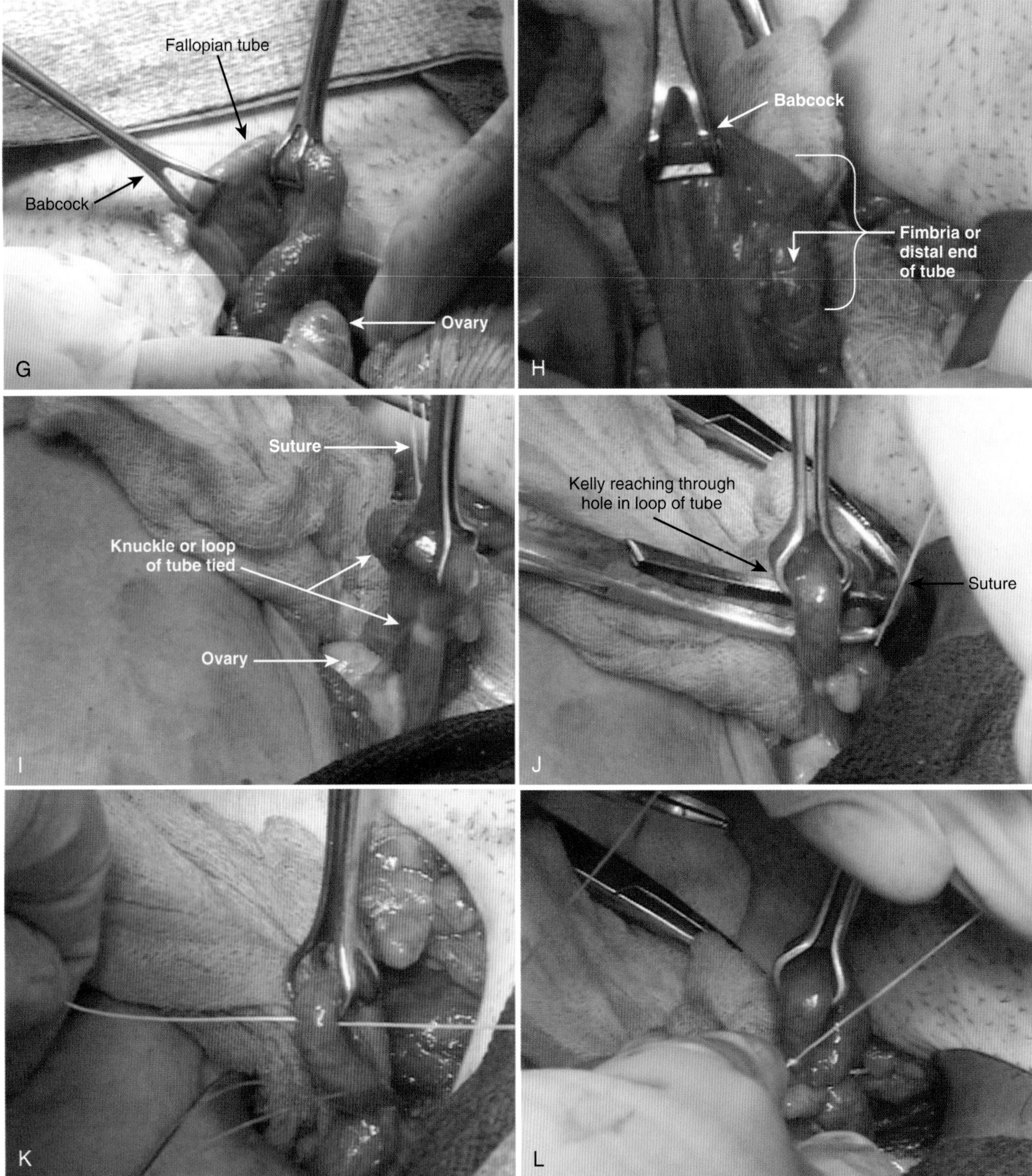

Figure 152-5, cont. **G,** The Babcock clamps are used in pairs to carefully retrieve the fallopian tube and follow it to the fimbriated end and ovary confirming its identification. **H,** Here a single Babcock clamp retracts the tube and demonstrates the widened fimbriated end. **I,** A loop of suture on a reel is used to tie off a loop of fallopian tube in the simple Pomeroy procedure. With the modified Pomeroy technique, a hemostat is passed through the center of the tied-off loop of fallopian tube and is used to guide suture material to individually tie off each side of the fallopian loop. **J–L,** Scissors are used to cut through the fallopian tube just above where the prior ties were seated. The incision is made at the crush mark left by the hemostats that were used to cross-clamp the tube.

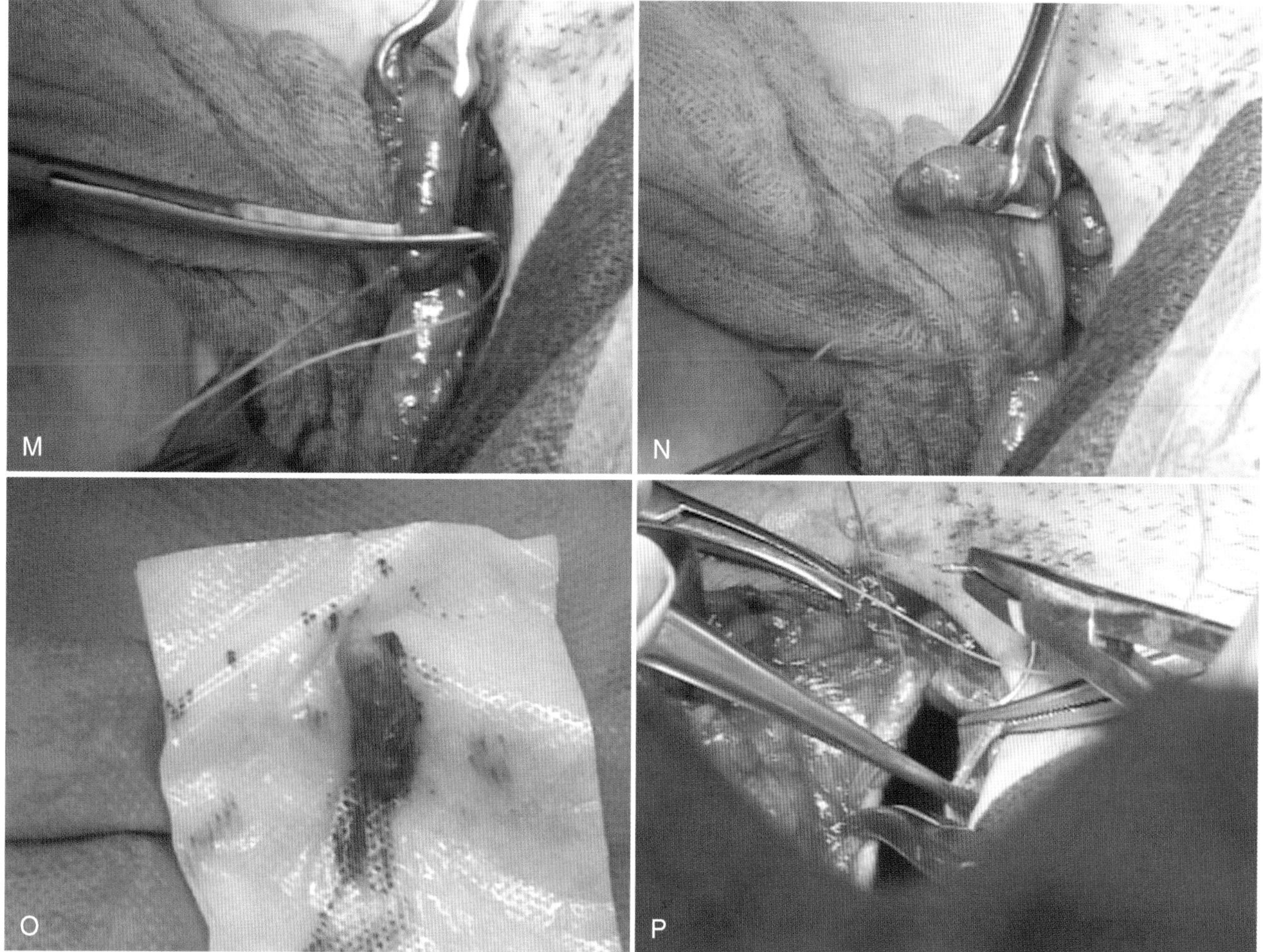

Figure 152-5, cont. **M–O,** The severed end is retracted and the opposite side of the loop is cut, freeing a 2- to 3-cm section of fallopian tube. **P,** It is critical to completely close the fascial layers identified by their white, thick, and tough nature.

Check in with the preoperative holding area. Is the patient's chart complete and informed consent form available and signed? Are the laboratory values within normal range? Does your patient have any questions? Is the family in the waiting room?

Tell the operating room scrub or float nurse what equipment and sutures you will need. Clarify the position that the patient will be placed in for the surgery (e.g., lithotomy, frog-legged, or standard supine position). Request a specific cleansing agent for patients who are allergic to iodine.

1. *Cleanse the vulva and vagina.* A vaginal prep is necessary if the bladder is to be catheterized or a uterine manipulator is to be applied.
2. *Drain the bladder.* Perform a quick, gentle, straight catheterization to decompress a distended bladder from the operative field. Catheterization of the bladder is not universally performed. This is particularly true for patients under local anesthesia who can void sufficiently just before anesthesia. However, when the surgeon is new to this technique or when delay is anticipated in completing the abdominal entry (obesity, prior pelvic surgery, or infection), bladder injury is more likely. Draining the bladder helps reduce this risk. "Fluid blousing" at the time of general anesthesia induction is common, and the bladder can fill quickly.
3. *Apply the uterine manipulator* (for interval minilaparotomy) as deemed necessary. Traditional devices include acorn or Hulka devices. Adaptations, such as CooperSurgical's uterine manipulator (Fig. 152-4E), are easy to apply and are rarely traumatic. Many clinicians use manipulators routinely; others reserve them for anticipated problems with adequate exposure (abdominal obesity, prior pelvic surgery or infection, or retroversion or flexion of the uterus). Less-experienced surgeons will find them helpful. The patient must be in either the lithotomy or the frog-leg position, and general anesthesia is required.
4. *Sterile gloves* may be used without formal *gowning* for insertion of the uterine manipulator or for straight catheterization of the urinary bladder. In fact, it is advisable for the surgeon not to perform these procedures with the same formal gowning and gloving worn for the minilaparotomy, because contamination is likely when the patient is in the lithotomy position.
5. *Prepare and scrub the abdomen.* Minilaparotomy should not be performed through pubic hair. Depending on patient pubic hair distribution, shaving a small strip of pubic hair over the operative site may be necessary.
6. After *thorough surgical scrub and gowning,* perform the procedure.
7. *Apply surgical drapes* as for abdominal surgery.
8. *Locate the site for the incision.* Palpate *three fingerbreadths above the symphysis pubis.* With one hand on the abdomen above the symphysis, move the uterine manipulator. Often the uterus can be felt with the abdominal hand, which offers reassurance that the incision will provide ready access to the uterus and adnexa. Using the skin scalpel with a no. 10 blade, *make a transverse incision.* There is no need to arc this incision. Often the linea nigra, the faint line demarcating the midline, can be visualized.

The incision should be no more than 5 *cm long*, and often a smaller incision will suffice (see Fig. 152-5A).

9. *Switch to the deep knife (new no. 10 blade) and progress through Scarpa's fascia* (within the fat) until the rectus sheath is encountered (see Fig 152-5B). Often, once Scarpa's fascia is divided, the sub-Scarpa's fat can be brushed away with a sponge, using a wiping motion. *Bleeders can be cauterized* using the electrocoagulator. Do not tunnel the incision, especially in the obese abdomen; this can be prevented by ensuring that the subcutaneous fat has been divided all the way to both edges of the skin incision. The subcutaneous fat presents an excellent opportunity to test the power on the Bovie before entering the abdomen. The Bovie device should never be used for the first time on intra-abdominal tissue, in case the power is set dangerously high (see Fig. 152-5C).
10. Once the rectus fascia is identified by its dense, white fibrous appearance, *make a small transverse incision on each side of the linea alba*. Using a Metzenbaum scissors, carefully extend the fascial incision to the lateral margin of the skin incision and across the midline (see Fig. 152-5D). Place two Kelly clamps on the incised lower fascial edge and gently retract and elevate the fascia. Gently place the index finger (preferably) or the blunt end of the scalpel along the midline under the incised fascial edge, and gently roll it toward the lateral margins, freeing the sheath from the underlying rectus muscle. In the midline, the pyramidalis remains adherent; use the Metzenbaum scissors to carefully cut along the inferior linea alba, freeing the muscle and making more room. Apply Kelly clamps to the upper segment of the anterior rectus sheath, and free the underlying muscles in a similar fashion. You do not need to roll the index finger under the rectus sheath any further than the skin incision. Perforating vessels arise more laterally and can be ruptured. Carefully use cautery to control bleeding.
11. Using blunt dissection with the index finger or the blunt end of the knife, *separate the rectus muscles from the transversalis fascia and peritoneum in the midline*. A gentle rolling action of the index finger (or the blunt end of the scalpel) under each lateral band of rectus muscles ensures adequate room.
12. Using two Kelly clamps or pickups, opposing each other, *lift the transversalis and peritoneum, thereby tenting these layers away from underlying abdominal structures*. Using either the scalpel or Metzenbaum scissors, make a small buttonhole incision between the two clamps. This incision should be well above the symphysis pubis, favoring the cephalad (toward the umbilicus) portion of the wound to avoid the bladder. At this point, use a Kelly clamp to enter the small incision, and with a combination of blunt dissection and retraction of tissues, enter the abdomen. *The key maneuver is to maintain this elevation of the incision edges to expose abdominal viscera*. The obese abdomen may contain a significant amount of fat below the peritoneum, which requires special care when dissecting. It may be difficult to distinguish this tissue from omentum or mesenteric fat that may be adherent in the lower pelvis, especially in women with a history of abdominal surgery or infection. The peritoneal incision may be extended either transversely (preferred) or vertically. The edges of the incised peritoneum are grasped and elevated and the incision inspected to ensure the abdominal cavity has been entered (see Fig. 152-5E).
13. Place the small Richardson retractors, and with gently opposed and elevating retraction, lift *the abdominal wall and inspect the abdominal cavity* (see Fig. 152-5F). If the small intestine obscures the view, place the patient in the reverse Trendelenburg position (head down) to allow the bowel to gravitate cephalad out of view. Use a gauze pad rolled tightly on a ring clamp to brush the bowel and adnexal structures aside if they are obstructing the view. Using Babcock forceps, identify the adnexal structures. Once the fallopian tube is identified, use Babcock forceps to gently retract the tube until the ovary and fimbriated end are clearly identified (see Fig. 152-5G). Apply further slight traction on the Babcock to deliver the tube through the incision. Note the glistening white ovary, which assures the surgeon that the fallopian is being grasped (see Fig. 152-5H). Gentle traction is always advised because the tube can be adherent to vascular structures, which may bleed if torn. Use the uterine manipulator to help with visualization and exposure.
14. For the traditional Pomeroy tubal ligation technique, the Babcock forceps delivers a knuckle of tube, which is tied off with the 2-0 chromic suture. A second suture around this isolation knuckle of tube is often applied to achieve a tight, hemostatic construction before the knuckle of tube is excised (see Fig. 152-5I).
15. For the *modified Pomeroy tubal ligation procedure*, carefully elevate the fallopian tube and identify a relatively avascular area of the mesosalpinx. Using a Kelly clamp to gently penetrate or the Bovie on "coag" (*not* "cutting") to avoid making too large of a hole, make a small hole through the mesosalpinx (see Fig. 152-5J). Then clamp the tube with a Kelly, placing one jaw through this hole and the other across the tube. Place another Kelly clamp 2 cm distal to the first one, isolating a segment of tube. Using a 2-0 chromic suture on a needle, place a stick-tie on the uterine side of the tube so that the suture encircles the tube next to the portion of the tube that connects to the uterus Kelly clamp (see Fig. 152-5K). Tag this tie (Kelly is placed on the suture to maintain control). Most surgeons place a second tie on the same side and cut (see Fig. 152-5L). Place a similar tie on the fimbriated side of the tube. Remove the Kelly clamps. Incise through each of the two crush marks made by the Kelly clamps that lie on the side of the encircling suture toward the excised piece of tube; remove the segment of the tube (see Figs. 152-5M and N). Place the cut segment of tube on a piece of Telfa, note right or left side, and submit for pathologic evaluation when the sugery is completed (see Fig 152-5O). Lightly cauterize the exposed mesosalpinx if bleeding is observed. Cut the tags and repeat this procedure on the other tube. Current evidence supports the use of preemptive analgesia using infiltration of the incised skin and uterine tubes at cut ends with 0.5% bupivacaine. Postoperative pain, nausea, vomiting, and cramping were significantly lessened by this practice.
16. Perform a *sponge count* and, if it is correct, close the abdomen.
17. Identify and hold the edges of the *peritoneum* with Kelly clamps or pickups (see Fig. 152-5E). Use a running 3-0 chromic suture to *reapproximate* the cut edges. Identify and tag the fascial sheath edges with Kelly clamps. Close this sheath with a running 0 Dexon suture (see Fig. 152-5P). Palpate the closure to make sure there are no buttonhole defects in the fascial repair that could later manifest as incisional hernias. If there is more than 1 cm of subcutaneous fat, close Scarpa's fascia with interrupted 2-0 chromic sutures. The skin may be closed with staples or by running a subcuticular stitch of 3-0 chromic suture on a Keith needle.
18. Cleanse the surgical site with normal saline and apply a gauze dressing.
19. Take the patient to the recovery room. She may be discharged when she is awake, is tolerating oral liquids, and is ambulatory. Send the tubal segments for routine pathologic examination; place them in separate bottles marked "right" and "left." Write a brief operative note in the chart. State any complications, blood loss, and other findings. Dictate a complete operative report immediately after surgery. The patient is generally seen in the office within 7 to 14 days or at any time a complication develops. Review the tubal histologic report.

Postpartum Tubal Ligation

Postpartum tubal ligation (PTL) has many similarities to interval tubal ligation, but there are also major differences. Despite the convenience, cost savings, and ultimate desires of the patient, PTL remains an elective surgery. Numerous *contraindications* include maternal fever, pregnancy-related hypertension, uncontrolled diabetes mellitus, and excessive blood loss. Concerns regarding the viability and health of the newborn must be considered as well. Women who must postpone their postpartum sterilization should be reassured that interval tubal ligation as early as 6 weeks after delivery is also an excellent method of sterilization surgery. PTL can readily be performed during cesarean section; however, never assume that PTL remains the patient's desire if the cesarean section was performed because of concern over the condition of the fetus. (See the sample patient education form online at www.expertconsult.com.)

Technique

Review the technique described earlier for interval tubal ligation.

1. PTL can often be performed with the same block (epidural, caudal) that was used during labor. If this is not desirable or possible, there are many advantages to allowing the patient to rest and recover from labor and to schedule the PTL procedure for the next morning. A repeat hemoglobin determination will be much more meaningful after equilibration of fluid, especially if there is concern over blood loss during delivery. This delay also allows more time to observe the condition of the newborn.
2. The bladder should be drained either by having the patient void immediately before surgery or by straight catheterization (preferred method). Prepare the abdomen in the immediate umbilical area. Surgical scrub and draping are required.
3. Make a curved infraumbilical incision in the abdomen with the skin knife (no. 10 blade) (Fig. 152-6). Gentle inferior retraction on the abdominal skin at the time of this incision ensures that the scar will be close to or within the umbilical crater.
4. Carry the incision deeper with the deep knife (no. 10 blade). Once the skin and subcutaneous fat have been divided, enter the abdomen by favoring the inferior portion of the wound. (Dissecting through the substance of the umbilicus can be frustrating because tissue planes are not well defined.) Blunt dissection with Kelly clamps, which can probe and spread, is the preferred method for exploring and defining the portal of entry into the abdominal cavity. Some surgeons prefer to grasp each lateral side of the incision with towel clamps and elevate the entire incision away from underlying structures, such as the bowel and the uterus, when entering the peritoneum. Once the abdominal cavity is identified, the incision through the fascia and peritoneum can be extended, but it rarely needs to be longer than 4 to 5 cm.
5. Push the uterus gently to one side to rotate the adnexal structures into view. Use Babcock clamps to identify the fallopian tube, which in the postpartum period is typically swollen and engorged compared with the nonpregnant state. Follow each tube until the fimbriated ends and ovaries are identified. Extremely gentle traction is warranted because vessels within the mesosalpinx can be huge and easily damaged by traction. Tears in these vessels can cause profound bleeding.
6. Once the tube has been identified clearly, perform a tubal ligation as described previously for the interval sterilization technique. If the mesosalpinx is extremely fragile, many clinicians prefer the more traditional modified Pomeroy technique. The loop, tie, and cut features of the Pomeroy render a quick hemostatic procedure that can minimize the traction injuries or raw cut edges of the mesosalpinx produced by other procedures. Remember that if the tube cannot be delivered through the incision for a tubal ligation procedure, clips may be applied to the correctly identified fallopian tube.
7. Close the abdomen in a layered fashion as previously described. With periumbilical incisions, it is sometimes difficult to clearly redefine the peritoneal edges for closure. However, closure of the fascia is crucial and time should be spent clearly identifying the edges of this layer for definitive suturing.
8. The patient is generally seen within 2 weeks of PTL. At this time, the histology report should be reviewed.

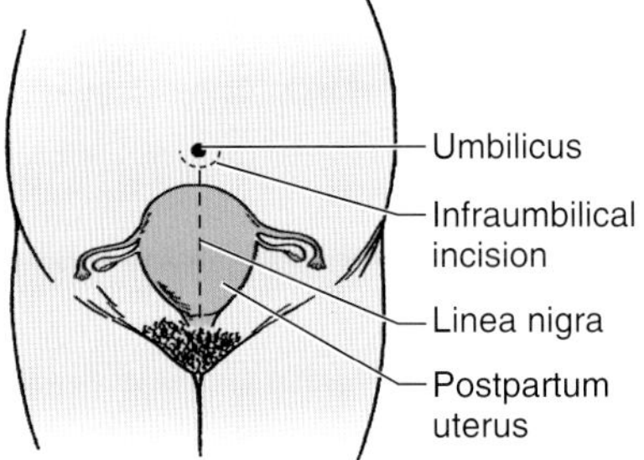

Figure 152-6 Postpartum tubal ligation by minilaparotomy requires a small transverse infraumbilical incision.

Sample Operative Report

Identifying data: Patient is a 36–year-old white G2P2 who requests sterilization
Procedure performed: Minilaparotomy tubal ligation
Preoperative diagnosis: Elective permanent sterilization
Postoperative diagnosis: Bilateral tubal ligation
Estimated blood loss: Less than 5 mL
Complications: None
Operation performed: Modified Parkland excision of tubal segments
Surgeon: Dr. ________________________
Assistant: Dr. ________________________
Anesthesia: General with intubation
Procedure: The patient's preoperative examination and consent were obtained with prior office visit. The preoperative hematocrit and urinalysis are normal and the pregnancy test negative. The patient was identified by me prior to surgery. The patient was placed in the lithotomy position and a bimanual examination demonstrated a normal-sized, mobile uterus without abnormality. A Foley catheter was placed. The vulva and vagina were cleansed with Betadine, the cervix identified, and a Hulka intrauterine manipulator applied. The patient was then prepped and draped in the usual fashion. An incision site was identified three fingerbreadths above the pubic symphysis. A 4-cm transverse incision was performed and advanced, layer by layer, into the abdomen. Richardson retractors were used for exposure. The uterine manipulator was used to help identify the right tube. The tube was confirmed by inspecting its length distally to the right ovary. Babcock forceps were used to gently deliver a loop of tube through the abdominal incision. A relatively avascular window in the mesosalpinx was identified, the tube was cross-clamped on each side of this window. Stick-ties with 2-0 chromic suture were placed on each side of the clamps encircling the tube. Double ties were placed on the uterine side. A 2-cm section of the tube was removed and sent for pathologic evaluation. Minor bleeding was controlled with minimal coagulation. A similar procedure was performed for the left tube. The instrument and sponge count was correct and the incision was closed layer by layer with 2-0 chromic on the peritoneum, 0 Dexon suture on the fascia, 2-0 chromic on Scarpa's fascia, and a 3-0 chromic running subcuticular suture on the skin. The urine was noted to remain clear during and after the procedure. The Foley catheter and uterine manipulator were removed. The patient was extubated and taken to the recovery room in stable condition.

Common Errors

1. *Incomplete preoperative assessment* overlooking medications (e.g., aspirin), prior pelvic surgeries (e.g., appendectomy), medical morbidities (e.g., poorly controlled diabetes).
2. *Failure to have a contraception plan to prevent pregnancy prior to the tubal ligation.*
3. Performing procedure when the patient's *ability to make the decision for permanent sterilization is questioned* (e.g., mentally challenged, unstable emotional or psychiatric status, consider legal and/or psychiatric consultation).
4. Attempting interval tubal ligation by minilaparotomy in women with significant abdominal obesity.
5. *Failing to discuss alternatives* to permanent sterilization.
6. *Failing to review the postprocedure pathology report.* Are there two segments of tube resected?

Complications

Minilaparotomy and laparoscopy have similar complication rates.

Major

- Major factors related to the development of complications include clinician inexperience, patient obesity, prior pelvic or abdominal surgery, and other medical problems such as diabetes mellitus, heart disease, asthma, bronchitis, and emphysema.
- Major complications occur in less than 2% of all procedures and may require prolonged hospitalization (0.3% requiring three or more nights in the hospital) or laparotomy (0.02% to 1.2% in large studies) to resolve complications.
- Delayed complications requiring readmission to the hospital occur after less than 1% of procedures.
- Female sterilization causes very few deaths (10 to 15 deaths per 500,000 procedures per year in the United States), and most are related to anesthetic complications (overdose or drug reaction), infection, and hemorrhage. Mortality rates from sterilization are far lower than with childbirth.
- Rare complications of tubal litigations include pregnancy (intrauterine and ectopic) and luteal phase pregnancy.

Minor

- Minilaparotomy appears to have a higher rate of minor complications (12% versus 7%) and a longer average operating time when compared with laparoscopy. Minilaparotomy convalescence appears to be slightly longer and more painful. Higher complication rates have been reported when laparoscopy is performed by inexperienced physicians.
- Minor minilaparotomy complications include wound infections, slight blood loss, uterine perforation by uterine manipulation instruments, and bladder injury. Most minor injury complications are immediately recognized and managed intraoperatively.
- Laparoscopy complications include those of minilaparotomy, as well as unique problems related to insertion of the instrument and gas insufflation of the abdomen. These complications include gas embolism, subcutaneous emphysema, and cardiac arrest. Vessel or organ laceration may occur. Open laparoscopy may make some of these complications less likely.
- Pain occurs after both minilaparotomy and laparoscopy. Chest and shoulder pain is common after laparoscopy and is caused by trapped gas under the diaphragm after insufflation of the abdomen. Most postprocedure and recovery pain can be managed with oral drug therapy, and narcotics are rarely necessary after the third postprocedural day.
- There is no compelling evidence that female sterilization causes menstrual cycles to change significantly; but abnormalities may persist if they existed before surgery. Among women who do experience menstrual changes, about half observe improvements and half experience irregular cycles or increased bleeding.
- Sterilized women do not appear to have different rates of pelvic inflammatory disease, cervicitis, hysterectomy, or D & C. Ovarian cancer may be diminished.
- Sterilized women are no more likely to experience severe psychiatric problems than unsterilized women.

Postprocedure Management

The surgeon is advised to check in on the recovery of the patient prior to leaving the hospital. Speak with family members in the waiting room, if available. Postoperative instructions can often be reviewed at this time. In most circumstances, patients can resume normal activities within 5 days following tubal ligation. Until then, heavy lifting and vigorous activities, such as jogging or weight training, should be postponed for about 5 days or until comfortable. Baths or hot tubs should be avoided for 10 days. Showers are recommended. A postoperative visit in the office in 7 to 10 days is advised. At this time, recovery experience, tubal pathology report, and other questions can be explored.

Postprocedure Patient Education

Give the patient postprocedure instructions and inform the family of any follow-up instructions. (See the sample patient education form online at www.expertconsult.com.)

Interpretation of Pathology Results

The surgeon must review the pathology report, which is generally available within 7 to 14 days following the procedure. Two segments of fallopian tube with evidence of complete resection of their diameter should be obtained. Failure to document two segments requires that the patient be informed and appropriate steps be initiated to prevent pregnancy and allow time for evaluation. In most instances, waiting 8 weeks to allow for internal healing and performance of a hysterosalpingogram will help assess whether or not both tubes are indeed blocked or, in fact, whether the wrong structures, such as the round or ovarian ligaments, were removed. Avoid performing the hysterosalpingogram prior to 8 weeks to allow for adequate healing. Each patient requires individual management in this circumstance. Some may opt for repeat procedures while others will reconsider other options of contraception.

CPT/Billing Codes

58600 Interval tubal ligation
58605 Postpartum tubal ligation
58670 Laparoscopic tubal ligation

ICD-9-CM Diagnostic Codes

V25.09 General counseling and family planning advice
V25.2 Sterilization; admission for interruption of fallopian tubes or vas deferens

Patient Education Guides

See the sample patient education form online at www.expertconsult.com.

Supplier

Full contact information is available online at www.expertconsult.com.

HUMI Intrauterine Manipulators
CooperSurgical, Inc.

BIBLIOGRAPHY

American College of Obstetricians and Gynecologists: Antibiotic prophylaxis for gynecologic procedures. ACOG Practice Bulletin No. 104. Obstet Gynecol 113:1180–1189, 2009.

Hillis SD, Marchbanks PA, Tylor LR, Peterson HB: Poststerilization regret: Findings from the United States Collaborative Review of Sterilization. Obstet Gynecol 93:889–895, 1999.

Kuilier R, Boulvain M, Walker D, et al: Minilaparotomy and endoscopic techniques for tubal sterilization. Cochrane Database Syst Rev CD001328, 2004.

Peterson HB: Sterilization. Obstet Gynecol 111:189–203, 2008.

Peterson HB, Xia Z, Hughes JM, et al: The risk of pregnancy after tubal sterilization: Findings from the U.S. Collaborative Review of Sterilization. Am J Obstet Gynecol 174:1161–1168, 1996.

Peterson HB, Xia Z, Hughes JM, et al: The risk of ectopic pregnancy after tubal sterilization: U.S. Collaborative Review of Sterilization Working Group. N Engl J Med 336:762–767, 1997.

Rulin MC, Davidson AR, Philliber SG, et al: Long-term effect of tubal sterization on menstrual indices and pelvic pain. Obstet Gynecol 82:118–121, 1993.

Speroff L, Darney PD: Sterilization. In Speroff L, Darney PD (eds): A Clinical Guide for Contraception, 4th ed. Philadelphia, Lippincott Williams & Wilkins, 2005, Chap. 12.

CHAPTER 153

Pessaries

Sandra M. Sulik

Historically, pessaries have been used to correct pelvic floor deformities and dysfunctions and symptoms associated with genital prolapse, uterine retrodisplacement, and cervical incompetence in women. In addition to hanging women by their heels, physicians as early as Hippocrates reported the use of half a pomegranate soaked in vinegar in the vagina for women with prolapse! In 1860, Hugh Lenox Hodge, Professor of Gynecology at the University of Pennsylvania, designed a pessary using Goodyear's newly patented vulcanized rubber. Since that time, technological advances in composition and a wide variety of sizes and shapes now make fitting pessaries an art (Fig. 153-1).

Indications

- Stress urinary incontinence (including athletic stress urinary incontinence)
- Uterine prolapse
- Vaginal vault prolapse
- Uterine retrodisplacement
- Pelvic relaxation
- Cystocele
- Enterocele
- Rectocele
- Poor surgical candidates with significant symptoms
- Prophylactic, postoperatively
- Preoperative diagnostic aid while awaiting surgery
- Cervical incompetence (proposed indication)

Indications for pessary use include reduction of pelvic organ prolapse and stress urinary incontinence. Preoperative use of pessaries as a diagnostic tool for any of the preceding indications can be helpful to estimate the amount of normal function that may be restored after surgery. A pessary can also help determine if the patient will develop incontinence once the prolapse is surgically corrected. Although surgery generally produces a more permanent cure, a pessary may be the treatment of choice for women who are poor surgical candidates, who want to postpone surgery indefinitely, or who prefer a nonsurgical treatment option. Pessaries may also be used postoperatively in women at risk for recurrent prolapse. Use of the pessary has been proposed as an alternative to cerclage to prevent preterm delivery. Only limited data support this indication, and it has not achieved widespread use.

Contraindications

- Noncompliant patient
- Impaired mental capacity leading to inability to follow up
- Persistant vaginal ulceration/erosions (relative)
- Active vaginitis (relative)
- Any pelvic infections or lacerations (relative)
- Severe atrophic changes (relative)
- Lack of manual dexterity

Active vaginitis including atrophic changes and vaginal ulcerations should be treated and resolved before pessary use. Although ulcerations are generally considered a contraindication, when they are a direct result of an exteriorized prolapse, a pessary may prevent further injury and promote healing. Severe atrophic changes are a contraindication to immediate pessary use; however, once the vagina is re-estrogenized, the pessary may be used. The woman using a pessary must be mentally and physically capable of using the device as recommended and able to return for appropriate follow-up.

Equipment and Supplies

Approximately 75% of women with prolapse can be successfully fitted with a pessary. Unsuccessful fitting is more likely with a shorter vagina (<7 cm) or a wide introitus (>4 fingerbreadths), higher parity, and previous hysterectomy. Most women with pessaries are satisfied and experience improvement in their symptoms.

There are *two major types of pessaries: support and space filling.* Most pessaries are made of silicone, some from rubber (avoid in latex allergic patients), and a few from plastic. Silicone has the advantage of being nonallergenic, and it does not absorb odors or secretions and is pliable and soft, so it is well tolerated.

A properly fitted pessary should be comfortable for the patient; it should remain in place while walking and standing, and during provocative maneuvers (e.g., coughing, standing, Valsalva's maneuver); and it should not interfere with bladder and bowel function. The pessary should fill the vagina, but should easily admit the examiner's finger between the pessary and the vaginal wall.

Pessary Selection

Pessaries are available in a wide range of sizes and shapes, each with a specific indication and function. *Selection depends on anatomy, symptomatology, and the overall goal of treatment.* Identifying the best choice is often a trial-and-error process; clinicians and patients should not be discouraged if the first selection is unsuccessful. *The most commonly prescribed pessaries are the ring, the Gellhorn and the donut.* For the novice starting to fit pessaries for the first time, obtaining fitting kits and samples of the most commonly used pessaries from the various companies may lessen the difficulty of pessary fitting.

Pessaries are made with several modifications on the same theme. For example, the ring pessary has a version "with support," which has a silicone web across the central opening. This "supports" the bladder, effectively reducing a mild to moderate cystocele. The "ring

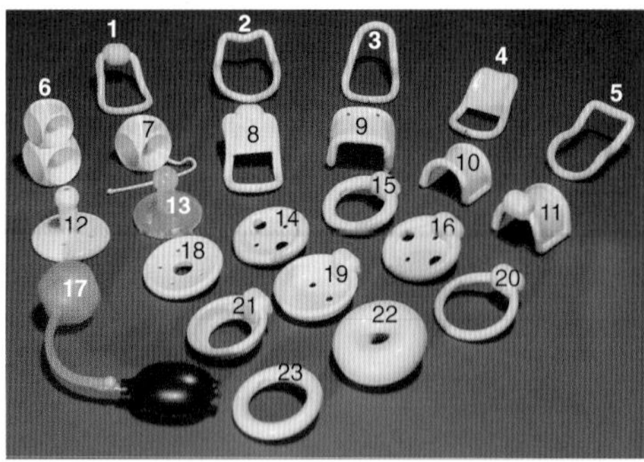

Figure 153-1 Various type of pessaries. 1, Hodge with knob; 2, Risser; 3, Smith; 4, Hodge with support; 5, Hodge; 6, tandem cube; 7, cube; 8, Hodge with support and knob; 9, Regula; 10, Gehrung; 11, Gehrung with knob; 12, Gellhorn flexible; 13, Gellhorn rigid (acrylic silicone); 14, ring with support; 15, ring with knob; 16, ring with knob and support; 17, Inflatoball; 18, Shaatz; 19, incontinence dish with support; 20, incontinence ring; 21, incontinence dish; 22, donut; 23, ring. (Courtesy of CooperSurgical, Inc., Trumbull, CT.)

with knob" has a bulbous portion that is placed retropubically (at the pubic notch) to restore the urethral-vesical (U-V) angle and increase urethral closing pressure. The addition of the "knob" is for stress urinary incontinence from a hypermobile U-V angle. Some devices have both modifications.

Pessary Types by Indication

- *Stress incontinence:* ring with knob, Hodge, Hodge with knob, Smith, Risser, incontinence ring, incontinence dish, Mar-Land, Gehrung with knob (Fig. 153-2)
- *Preoperative evaluation for Burch procedure for stress incontinence:* Hodge, Risser, and Hodge with support
- *Uterine retrodisplacement:* Smith, Risser, and Hodge
- *Uterine prolapse, first or second degree:* ring, ring with support, Shaatz, Regula, Oval, Smith, Risser, Hodge
- *Uterine or vaginal vault prolapse, third or fourth degree:* donut, Inflatoball, cube, tandem cube, Gellhorn (not well suited for severe vaginal prolapse)
- *Stress incontinence with cystocele, first or second degree:* ring with support (with or without knob) incontinence dish with support, Gehrung with knob, and Hodge (with/without support, with/without knob), Mar-Land with support (Fig. 153-3)

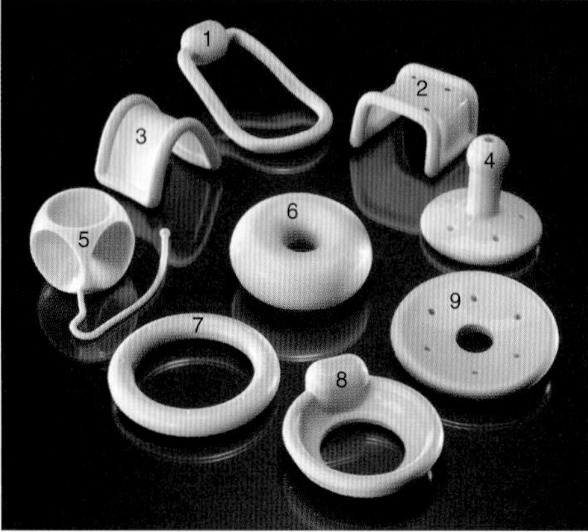

Figure 153-2 Stress urinary incontinence pessaries (made with silicone). 1, Hodge with knob; 2, Regula; 3, Gehrung; 4, Gelhorn flexible; 5, tandem cube; 6, donut; 7, ring; 8, incontinence dish; 9, Shaatz. (Courtesy of CooperSurgical, Inc., Trumbull, CT.)

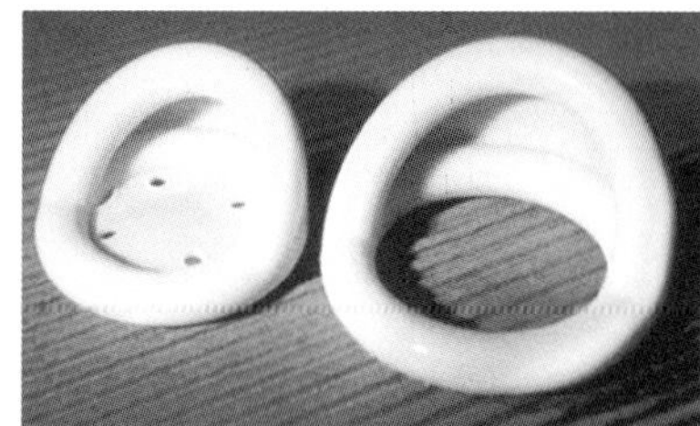

Figure 153-3 Mar-Land pessaries with (*left*) and without (*right*) support. (Courtesy of Coloplast Corporation [formerly Mentor Corporation], Minneapolis, MN.)

- *Stress incontinence with uterine prolapse, first or second degree:* ring, incontinence ring, ring with support and knob, incontinence dish (with/without support), Mar-Land, Mar-Land with support, Hodge (with/without support, with/without knob and support)
- *Cystocele:* Gehrung, Gehrung with knob, ring with support, Gellhorn, donut, Inflatoball, cube, and tandem cube
- *Enterocele:* Gellhorn, Gehrung, donut, Inflatoball, cube, tandem cube
- *Rectocele:* Gellhorn, Gehrung, donut, Inflatoball, cube, tandem cube
- *Incompetent cervix:* Hodge

Procedure

Fitting Pessaries

Pessaries are fit by trial and error. Proper fitting often requires multiple sizes and or styles. Fitting pessaries can be done from fitting kits obtained from the manufacturer or by stocking multiple sizes and fitting the pessary from stock. Fitting kits are available from the two largest manufacturers of pessaries in the United States: Milex and Coloplast Corporation. Milex has kits for the ring, the Gellhorn, the cube, and the Gehrung pessaries. The Coloplast Corporation has a kit for fitting the ring pessary with a conversion chart for converting the size of the ring pessary to other types it manufactures. Conversions of pessary sizes are difficult, however. The totally different shape of each pessary and whether the pessary fits in front of the cervix (e.g., the Gellhorn, donut, or cube), behind the cervix (e.g., the lever pessaries), or over the cervix (e.g., the Gehrung) precludes simple conversions. The manufacturer should be contacted for product information and obtaining pessary fitting kits.

When fitting a pessary for *incontinence*, it is best for the patient to have a full bladder. If fitting for *prolapse*, the patient should empty her bladder before the fitting process. Once the correct pessary has been determined, the patient should be able to void comfortably with the pessary in place before she leaves the office. Ideally, the patient should insert and remove the pessary on a daily basis. Women can remove the pessary at bedtime, wash it with soap and water, and then replace it in the morning. If daily changing is too cumbersome, a schedule of twice weekly can be used. In this setting, an early follow-up should be arranged to assess the vaginal walls and ensure no erosions are developing. If the patient is unable to remove her pessary regularly, most pessaries can be left in place and removed on a monthly basis, cleaned, and reinserted by the clinician. On the other hand, the cube and Inflatoball pessaries *must be* removed daily. An applicatorful of an acidifying gel such as Trimo-San inserted into the vagina two or three times per week should be recommended to help decrease the amount and odor of vaginal discharge.

Prior to fitting the pessary, the vagina should be inspected for estrogen status, erythema, erosions, and ulcerations. A Papanicolaou (Pap) smear should be obtained if indicated. *Determining pessary size for all round pessaries is similar to fitting a contraceptive diaphragm* (see Chapter 130, Barrier Contraceptives: Cervical Caps, Condoms, and

Diaphragms). A rough estimate of length of the vagina is determined by measuring the distance from the posterior fornix or vaginal apex to the symphysis pubis. The second and third fingers are placed in the vagina with the third finger in the posterior fornix. The depth of insertion is marked on the second finger. The distance between the tip of the third finger and the mark on the second finger approximates vaginal depth (see Figure 130-5 in Chapter 130, Barrier Contraceptives: Cervical Caps, Condoms, and Diaphragms). This is also a good opportunity to evaluate pelvic floor strength and teach the patient how to do Kegel exercises. Several pessary sizes can be tried to find the proper fit.

Once the appropriate pessary is found, the patient should be reexamined after performing provocative maneuvers. Provocative maneuvers include coughing, standing, sitting, walking, squatting, and Valsalva's maneuver. Then the patient should try to void. If the patient is unable to void comfortably or if discomfort is noted during these maneuvers, the next smaller size of pessary should be tried. If the pessary has shifted position or falls out after these maneuvers, a larger size or different pessary should be tried.

USE OF SPECIFIC PESSARIES

Uses for specific pessaries are listed in Table 153-1.

COMPLICATIONS

- Vaginitis
- Vaginal erosion or ulceration
- Discomfort
- Obstructed defecation and/or urination
- Impaction of the pessary

It is normal for the patient to experience an increase in vaginal discharge. However, odor, itching, change in color of discharge, or bleeding should be reported to the health care provider. Use of vaginal estrogen with pessaries generally prevents vaginal erosion and ulceration. Many health care providers overlook the importance of estrogen in maintaining the acid pH balance necessary to prevent vaginitis. The vagina should be re-estrogenized by using vaginal estrogen cream, 1 g every other night for 1 month, then two to three times per week thereafter. Alternating a pH-adjusted vaginal gel (e.g., Trimo-San gel, half applicator, two or three times per week) with the estrogen cream is beneficial as well if the pessary is left in place and not removed nightly. In addition to atrophic changes, ulcerations may be associated with a device that is too large or not removed on a regular basis. Discomfort is usually associated with anterior displacement during Valsalva's maneuver or a device that is too large. If anterior displacement is noted, the patient should push the pessary further into the vagina. If that does not alleviate the discomfort, a smaller size should be tried. Obstruction of defecation should be promptly reported to the provider. Removal of the pessary should resolve the problem, and delay in removal may lead to obstipation. Obstruction of urination should be uncommon if voiding was performed in the office with the device in place. A smaller pessary should resolve the problem. Impaction of the device is rare and typically associated with "forgotten pessaries." A reminder system such as a tickler file will help to alleviate this problem and ensure appropriate follow-up.

POSTPROCEDURE MANAGEMENT

Pessary Care

Patients should remove the pessary and wash it with warm, soapy water. Soap with deodorants, perfumes, or detergents should not be used. Autoclaving (15 lb pressure for 15 minutes) is the recommended method of sterilization for pessaries from the fitting sets between fittings.

Follow-up Care

Ideally, the pessary should be removed nightly, and cleaned and replaced the next morning. Realistically, women are reluctant to comply with such frequency. In many cases, pessaries have been left in the vagina for months at a time without complication. (The cube and tandem cube and Inflatoball must be removed nightly because there are no holes for drainage.) The final decision is left to the health care provider and the patient and should be based on several factors: the patient's mental and physical capacity to insert and remove the device and willingness to do so on a regular basis; the health of the vaginal mucosa; the potential for complications; how well the device fits; and the patient's ability to comply with follow-up visits.

In general, reevaluate the patient 1 week after the initial fitting, and then at 1 month and 3 months later. At a minimum, the patient should be seen every 6 months thereafter. Patients unable to care for the device themselves should be seen at least every 2 to 3 months. At each visit the patient should be questioned about bowel and bladder function, symptoms associated with vaginitis, vaginal bleeding, and problems with insertion and removal. The device should be removed and the vaginal mucosa should be inspected for erythema, ulceration, laceration, and estrogen status. The device may be cleaned and reinserted if there are no complications. The pessary is a foreign body in the vagina. Inspection of the vaginal vault at regular intervals seems prudent and warranted.

TIPS

The following are anecdotal helpful hints and not manufacturers' recommendations.

- *Diaphragms:* A diaphragm can be very effective for mild degrees of prolapse or incontinence.
- *Stay relaxed for device removal:* The patient should keep the pelvic floor muscles relaxed and even perform a gentle Valsalva maneuver to assist with removal.
- *Estrogen:* Regular use of vaginal estrogen cream should be strongly encouraged. The Estring may also be used with several of the pessaries.
- *Double pessaries:* A small donut coupled with a Gellhorn pessary may be useful for patients with excessive redundant tissue. The donut is placed closest to the cervix with the Gellhorn facing out into the vagina. The stem of the Gellhorn does not fit through the hole in the donut (Fig. 153-4).
- *Pelvic floor muscle exercises/Kegel exercises:* Ongoing performance of Kegel exercises is important to maintain and improve pelvic floor tone and should be encouraged with all follow-up visits. If a patient is unable to perform Kegel exercises on her own, useful patient devices include *Kegel Kones* (a set of six weighted devices, which get progressively smaller and heavier). The *Kegel Exersizer* is an intravaginal device that measures intravaginal pressure. The cone-shaped device has an approximately 2-foot flexible hose to transmit the pressure to a gauge to give the patient positive feedback with a proper perineal (Kegel) contraction. Some physical therapy departments have assisted patients with proper technique for Kegel exercises by using this type of device.
- *A woman with very little or no vaginal muscle tonicity or marked vaginal wall prolapse* may have difficulty even retaining a donut or a Gellhorn pessary. In such cases the cube pessary is indicated.
- *Sexual activity:* Some pessaries can be left in place during intercourse. Most often, women remove the pessary prior to engaging in sexual activity. A ring pessary is an effective device for women who leak urine with orgasm.
- *Pessaries and x-rays:* Some pessaries contain wire coils; these pessaries must be removed before an x-ray or magnetic resonance imaging. The face page of each pessary instructional brochure indicates whether the pessary contains metal. An instructional brochure is enclosed with each pessary.

TABLE 153-1 Use of Pessaries

Condition	Pessary	Common Sizes	Features	Company	Insertion	Removal	Other Pessaries to Try
First-degree and Second-degree prolapse	Ring	0–13, 2–7 most common	One of the easiest to use, requires a well-defined pubic notch for pessary to rest	Milex, EvaCare	The device is hinged and will fold in only one direction; once inserted rotate 90 degrees to decrease chance of expulsion with Valsalva.	Insert the index finger into the notch and rotate the hinge anteriorly; pull down and out.	Gelhorn, donut, Gehrung, Shaatz, oval, Inflatoball, Regula
	Ring with support	0–13, 3–5 most common	Supports mild cystocele as well	Milex, EvaCare	Insert same as ring	Same as for ring	Same as for ring
	Shaatz	1 ½ inches to 3 ½ inches, most common 2 ¼ inches to 3 inches	Utilizes levators for support, especially effective in patients where ring pessary does not stay in place	Milex, EvaCare	Compress the sides and turn the device parallel to the introitus, advance until it rests against cervix; insert with concave surface facing up.	Hook the index finger in the center hole; bring device down to introitus; pull down and out.	Gellhorn, Gehrung, ring with support, oval, donut
	Regula	Most common 2–8	The pressure exerted by the prolapsed uterus/cervix on the flexible anatomically adjusting arch or bridge of the regula automatically spreads the heels outward, thereby helping to prevent the expulsion of the pessary. The patient should be forewarned that it may be necessary for her to be refit several times.	Milex	The flexibility of the bridge, which alters the support dimensions of the pessary, must be balanced with the size of the patient's vaginal vault and the degree of uterine prolapse.	Reach in, grasp pessary and pull down toward introitus.	Gelhorn, donut, Gehrung, Shaatz, oval, Inflatoball
	Oval	Most common 1–9	Designed specifically to fit a narrow vaginal vault. Works extremely well in women with a prior history of vaginal surgery that resulted in scarring, and in some cases palpable sutures from anterior repair or bladder suspension procedures.	EvaCare	Fold pessary at flexible joint; insert and rotate to fit.	Reach in, grasp pessary and pull down toward introitus.	
Third-degree prolapse	Donut	2 inches to 3 ¾ inches most common, also 2 ½ to 3 ¼ inches	The most commonly used pessary. A space-occupying device that is useful in patients with excessive redundant tissue; works well in a vaginal vault with little or no support; most commonly used in older, postmenopausal women; works well for vaginal prolapse also.	Milex, EvaCare	Turn the device parallel to the introitus; exert pressure posteriorly, and advance until it is fully intravaginal; then rotate until the pessary is transverse and up against the cervix.	Hook the index finger in the center hole, bring device down to introitus; pull down and out.	Gellhorn, Inflatoball, Gehrung

TABLE 153-1 Use of Pessaries—cont.

Condition	Pessary	Common Sizes	Features	Company	Insertion	Removal	Other Pessaries to Try
Third-degree prolapse—cont.	Gellhorn	1 ½ to 3 ½ inches, most common 2 ¼ to 3 inches	Requires a relatively capacious vaginal vault so that the base is broad enough to rest above the levators. The stem functions to stabilize the device in the vagina and facilitates removal. A shorter stem is available by special order. Can be ordered as rigid silicone or acrylic for severe prolapse. Not well suited for severe vaginal prolapse because the walls can prolapse around the pessary.	Milex, EvaCare	Fold the knob of the device; position the disk portion parallell to the introitus, angling downward to avoid pressure on the urethra; push posteriorly until the entire disk is within the vagina; then turn and push the knob upwards toward the cervix.	Insert finger up to the disk and release the suction; pull disk towards introitus and remove. Can use a barber pole action. Can inject a small amount of water or saline into the hole in the knob to help release the suction.	Donut, Inflatoball, or Gehrung
	Cube	0–7, most common 2–5	May be used in women with either a small or a large introitus because of its malleability. Has no area for drainage, must be removed nightly. Support is achieved by creating negative presssure on the vaginal walls. Atrophic changes increase the risk of ulceration and erosion.	Milex, EvaCare	Compress the cube and insert it high into the vagina.	The string is used to help locate the pessary; it should not be used to pull on to remove the pessary. The suction should be released by squeezing the walls of the cube and then pulling the device in a downward fashion. The pessary must be removed and cleaned daily. Regular use of estrogen cream in postmenopausal women is recommended.	Tandem cube, Gellhorn, Inflatoball, donut
	Tandem cube	The larger cube is 2 sizes bigger than the small one. 2/0–7/5, most common 4/2–7/5.	Try if single cube does not work. Can be used in young women who experience stress incontinence with vigorous exercise when other pessaries are ineffective.	Milex	Insert with larger cube towards cervix.	Same as for cube	Gellhorn, Inflatoball
	Inflatoball	Small (2 inches), medium (2 ¼ inches), large (2 ½ inches), extra large (2 ¾ inches); medium and large are the most common sizes	Can be used for mild cystocele or rectocele associated with a procidentia/prolapse. The unique design permits individualized fitting and adjustments by varying the amount of air pressure within the pessary. The fully deflated pessary is easy to insert or remove, even with a narrow introitus. Inflatoball is sometimes the only pessary the patient can tolerate. Manual dexterity is needed for use of this pessary. This is a latex rubber pessary. Must be removed daily.	Milex	Compress all the air out of the ball, insert into vagina, and position high. Inflate to the desired pressure, remove the pump, push the small ball up to keep the pessary inflated, then tuck the tube into the vagina.	Deflate by pushing the small ball down to release the air; reach into the vagina, grab the pessary, pull towards the introitus, and remove.	Gellhorn, Gehrung, donut

Table continued on following page

TABLE 153-1 Use of Pessaries—cont.

Condition	Pessary	Common Sizes	Features	Company	Insertion	Removal	Other Pessaries to Try
Incontinence pessaries	Incontinence ring (ring with knob)	0–10, 2–7 most common sizes	The device stabilizes the bladder base and increases urethral functional length and closure pressure.	Milex	Compress the ring and insert with the knob in the anterior direction; knob fits just below pubic notch.	Grasp, and pull in a downward fashion.	Incontinence dish, ring with support and knob, Gehrung with/without knob, Hodge, Smith, Risser, Mar-Land
	Incontinence dish with/without support	55–85 mm, most common 60–75 mm (Milex brand), 0–7 (EvaCare brand)	Continence is restored by stablizing the bladder base, increasing urethral closure pressure, and lengthening the functional urethra. It also offers support to an accompanying mild prolapse.	Milex, EvaCare	Compress the device and turn it parallel to the introitus. Rotate the device once it is intravaginal so that the heel is posterior to the cervix and the knob is retropubic.	Hook the index finger and pull down and out *or* Insert index finger between the device and the symphysis; grasp between the finger and thumb, and pull down and out.	Hodge with/without support, Mar-Land with support
	Mar-Land with/without support	2–8, most common 2–5	An adaptation of the ring pessary; has a round Silastic base with a half-moon support that fits retropubically	EvaCare	Compress the device and turn it parallel to the introitus. Rotate the device once it is intravaginal so that the heel is in the vault or posterior fornix and the arch is positioned retropubically. May also be inserted by folding the pessary in half so that the back ring collapses the supportive sling. The folded pessary should be in a crescent shape and inserted by directing the cresecent shape downward; advance it until the device is fully intravaginal and the supportive sling is retropubic.	Hook the device with the index finger and rotate parallel while pulling down and out.	Hodge with/without support, incontinence ring, incontinence dish.
	Gehrung with/without knob	0–9, most common sizes 2–5	"Saddle pessary"; manually shapeable, which allows for fit in most women. Support derived from the lateral remnants of the elevator sling. Gehrung with knob useful for cystocele coupled with stress incontinence.	Milex	Compress the sides of the device and turn it parallel to the introitus. Insert the left heel and advance until the device is fully intravaginal; rotate the anterior arch forward so that the cystocele rests on the bridge. The heels of the pessary rest on the vaginal floor.	Push the anterior arch posteriorly toward the rectum; grasp the lateral heel and fold to remove.	Hodge with/without support, incontinence ring, incontinence dish with/without support

TABLE 153-1 Use of Pessaries—cont.

Condition	Pessary	Common Sizes	Features	Company	Insertion	Removal	Other Pessaries to Try
Incontinence pessaries—cont.	Hodge with/without knob Hodge with/without support	0–9, most common size 2–5	Originally designed for uterine retrodisplacement, Hodge with knob restores continence by stabilizing the bladder base and increasing urethral closure pressure and functional urethral length. Designed for patients with a shallow pubic notch. Can be used for patients with stress incontinence associated with urethral hypermobility, first- and second-degree prolapse, and uterine retrodisplacement. The Hodge can be used as a test of effectiveness of the Burch procedure for stress incontinence. Has also been used for treatment of incompetent cervix with or without cerclage.	Milex	Compress the sides and insert the rounded end into the vagina; direct the heel into the vault or posterior fornix and position the anterior portion retropubically. The device should fit snugly, should not rotate, and should remain retropubic.	Hook the device with the index finger to fold it, and pull the device down and out.	Incontinence ring, incontinence dish, or Mar-Land
Uterine retrodisplacement	Smith (designed for a patient with a well-defined pubic notch) Risser (designed for a patient with a shallow pubic notch; has a larger weight-bearing zone to support the vaginal aspect of the pubis)	Smith: 0–8, 2–5 most common Risser: 0–9, 2–5 most common	Can be used for a number of other conditions, including dysmenorrhea when no other cause except uterine retroversion is noted, infertility if retroversion is considered the cause, and backache if attributed to uterine retroversion.	Milex	Insertion same as for Hodge	Same as for Hodge	Hodge with/without support/knob, Mar-Land, incontinence ring, or incontinence dish

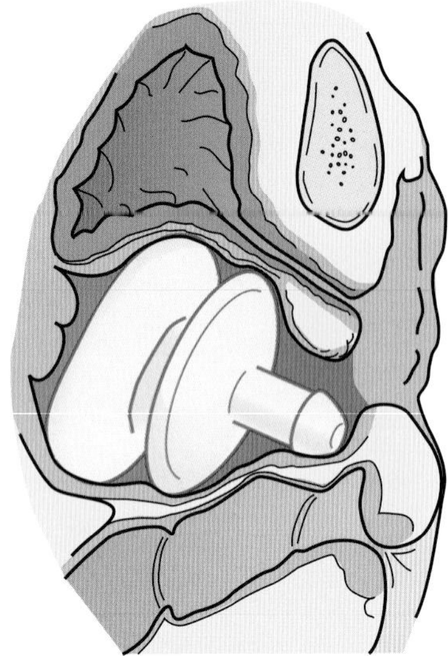

Figure 153-4 Double pessaries in place. The donut pessary is inserted first, and the Gellhorn pessary (stem out) is inserted second. (Redrawn from Myers DL, Lasala CA, Murphy JA: Instruments and methods: Double pessary used in grade 4 uterine and vaginal prolapse. Obstet Gynecol 91:1019, 1998.)

CONCLUSION

Although surgical repair remains the treatment of choice for many urogynecologic dysfunctions, pessaries are a viable option for a variety of situations. Pessaries are useful for both the rising elderly population but also for younger active women who wish to maintain their activities without the discomfort of prolapse or leaking of urine.

CPT/BILLING CODES

The pessary cost is considered a supply. It should be billed to the local Medicare Part B carrier or the patient's insurance company.

57160 Pessary fitting and insertion

An E/M code may also be billed with a -25 modifier depending on documented examination and decision-making complexity. Only the E/M code is to be used when the patient comes in for removal and cleaning and reinsertion.

A4561 Rubber pessaries or intravaginal devices
A4562 Nonrubber pessaries or intravaginal devices

In some areas, the alternative for Part B providers is to write a prescription for the device, have the patient fill the prescription at a local pharmacy or medical supply store, and return with the pessary for insertion. Place of service is the home of the patient.

ICD-9-CM DIAGNOSTIC CODES

618.00 Vaginal wall prolapse, unspecified (w/o uterine prolapse)
618.01 Cystocele midline or lateral (w/o prolapse)
618.04 Rectocele (w/o uterine prolapse)
618.1 Uterine prolapse (w/o vaginal wall prolapse)
618.2 Uterovaginal prolapse, incomplete
618.3 Uterovaginal prolapse, complete
618.4 Uterovaginal prolapse, unspecified
618.5 Posthysterectomy vault prolapse
618.6 Enterocele, vaginal
618.9 Unspecified genital prolapse
618.81 Incompetence or weakening of pubocervical tissue
618.82 Incompetence or weakening of rectovaginal tissue
618.83 Pelvic muscle wasting
621.6 Retroflexed uterus, symptomatic
625.6 Incontinence, stress
654.5 Cervical incompetence in pregnancy

ACKNOWLEDGMENT

The editors wish to recognize the contributions by Edward J. Mayeaux, Jr., MD, to this chapter in the previous edition of this text.

SUPPLIERS

Full contact information is available online at www.expertconsult.com.

Estring
Pharmacia and Upjohn Company
Pessaries, Kegel Kones, Kegel Exersizer
Coloplast (formerly Mentor Corporation) Corporation (EvaCare Pessaries)
Milex Products, Inc.

ONLINE RESOURCES

www.webmd.com/urinary-incontinence.../vaginal-pessaries
See the sample patient education form online at www.expertconsult.com.

BIBLIOGRAPHY

Adams E, Thomson A, Maher C, Hagen S: Mechanical devices for pelvic organ prolapse in women. Cochrane Database Syst Rev 2:CD004010, 2004.

American College of Obstetricians and Gynecologists: Pelvic Organ Prolapse. ACOG Practice Bulletin No. 85. Obstet Gynecol 110:717, 2007.

Anders K: Devices for continence and prolapse. Br J Obstet Gynaecol 111:Suppl 1:61, 2004.

Bernier F, Harris L: Treating stress incontinence with the bladder neck support prosthesis. Urol Nurs 16:1, 1995.

Bernier F, Jenkins P: The role of vaginal estrogen in the treatment of urogenital dysfunction in postmenopausal women. Urol Nurs 17:3, 1997.

Deger R, Menzin A, Mikuta J: The vaginal pessary: Past and present. Postgrad Obstet Gynecol 13:18, 1993.

Fernando R, Thakar R, Sultan A, Shah S: Effect of vaginal pessaries on symptoms associated with pelvic organ prolapse. Obstet Gynecol 108:1, 2006.

Myers DL, LaSala CA, Murphy JA: Instruments and methods: Double pessary use in grade 4 uterine and vaginal prolapse. Am Coll Obstet Gynecol 91:6, 1998.

Newcomer J: Pessaries for the treatment of incompetent cervix and premature delivery. Obstet Gynecol Surv 55:443, 2000.

Shaikh S, Ong EK, Glavind K, Cook J, N'Dow JMO: Mechanical devices for urinary incontinence in women. Cochrane Database Syst Rev 3:CD001756, 2006.

Sulak R, Kuehl T, Shull B: Vaginal pessaries and their use in pelvic relaxation. J Reprod Med 38:12, 1993.

Sultana C: Pessaries for pelvic organ prolapse. Female Patient 28:59, 2003.

Viera AJ, Larkins-Pettigrew M: Practical use of the pessary. Am Fam Physician 61:2719, 2000.

Weber A, Richter H: Pelvic organ prolapse. Obstet Gynecol 106:3, 2005.

Wu V, Farrell S, Baskett T, Flowerdew G: A simplified protocol for pessary management. Obstet Gynecol 90:6, 1997.

Zeitlin MP, Lebherz TB: Pessaries in the geriatric patient. J Am Geriatr Soc 40:6, 1992.

CHAPTER 154

Postcoital Test (Sims-Huhner Test)

Julie M. Sicilia

The postcoital test (PCT) is an evaluation of the survival and motility of sperm in the cervical mucus. The PCT is a way of detecting if sperm are present in the ejaculate and cervical mucus; it is not a diagnostic test for cervical factor infertility. The PCT should be used in conjunction with semen analysis, not as a substitute for it. Result validity has been questioned because of the lack of reproducibility and universal standards for obtaining and interpreting samples with the PCT. The PCT was previously a routine test in the infertility evaluation. A 1998 randomized controlled trial concluded that routine PCT for infertile couples increased the amount of testing but did not increase the pregnancy rate for the couples. Currently, the PCT is used only for guiding treatment decisions for couples with certain indications.

Indications

- Investigation of the sperm and cervical mucus interaction
- Monitoring the cervical mucus during the first ovulatory cycle of treatment with clomiphene citrate for couples planning timed intercourse infertility treatment
- To assist in deciding if a couple is a candidate for expectant management versus aggressive therapy (intrauterine insemination [IUI] or in vitro fertilization [IVF]) with suspected cervical factor infertility

Contraindications

- Any condition that would preclude unprotected sexual intercourse followed by examination and sampling of the cervix
- Active vaginal infection

Equipment

- Nonsterile examination gloves
- Vaginal speculum (no lubricant) and swabs
- Tuberculin syringe with cap
- Ring forceps
- Microscope, slides, and coverslips
- Plastic endometrial aspirator (optional)

Preprocedure Patient Education

- One month prior to PCT, have patient start measuring basal body temperature (BBT) or urinary luteinizing hormone (LH) ovulation testing. Review the BBT or LH graphs to determine the proper timing of intercourse. Have the patient watch for clear cervical mucus (more estrogenic). (See Chapter 150, Fertility Awareness–Based Methods of Contraception [Natural Family Planning].) The PCT should be performed as near as possible to ovulation. The test is usually performed on day 12 to 14 of an ideal 28-day cycle.
- Instruct the couple to abstain from intercourse or masturbation for 48 hours before the test. Before performing the PCT, determine that the BBT is in accord with the proper timing of the menstrual cycle for the performance of the test. Nothing (lubricants, medications, douches, etc.) should be placed in the vagina for 24 hours prior to the test and up to the time of the PCT.
- Instruct the patient to come to the office 6 to 10 hours after intercourse.

Procedure

1. Place the patient in the dorsal lithotomy position. Insert a vaginal speculum (without lubricant) and visualize the cervix. Gently wipe the cervix with a vaginal swab.
2. Insert a tuberculin syringe (without the needle) into the endocervical canal and retract the plunger to draw the mucus into the syringe (collect at least 0.2 mL of mucus). An endometrial aspirator may make this collection easier in some patients. Place the syringe cap over the hub of the syringe once the sample is obtained so that the mucus will be stored in an airtight container until it is ready for processing.
3. Record the amount and clarity of the mucus.
4. Record the degree of stretchability (i.e., spinnbarkeit) of the mucus. A ring forceps may be used to grasp the mucus at the cervical os to measure the mucus stretch as the forceps is removed from the vagina. The mucus can also be placed between the index finger and thumb with the stretch determined as the fingers are drawn apart. A normal mucus stretch greater than 5 to 10 cm is indicative of a high estrogenic state. A spinnbarkeit of less than 3 cm indicates a low likelihood that sperm could penetrate through the mucus and indicates an unfavorable situation for fertilization.
5. Place a drop of the mucus from the syringe on a glass slide and immediately place a coverslip over the sample. Examine the cervical mucus under low power for the presence of sperm and other components, such as trichomonads, leukocytes, squamous cells, or *Candida*. Make a note of the number of sperm. Examine the specimen under high power. The number of sperm in at least five different fields should be averaged. Record an average number or range of numbers of sperm present. Note whether the sperm are mobile, whether they have normal or abnormal morphology, and, if possible, whether they exhibit forward progression. For a normal study, if specimens are examined 6 to 10 hours after intercourse, *there should be an average of at least 5 to 10 actively motile sperm per high-power field*. Actively moving sperm are facilitated by the presence of optimal cervical mucus. A decrease in the quality of the cervical mucus and an increase in viscosity and cellularity caused by rising progesterone levels after ovulation impair sperm survival. The presence of ferning, increased elasticity, and decreased viscosity of the cervical mucus is an indirect indication of estrogen production and ovulation.

Common Errors

The primary cause of an inconclusive or abnormal PCT is failure to accurately time the test. PCTs are also usually abnormal in anovulatory cycles. If the initial PCT yields poor results, a second test should be performed 1 to 3 hours after intercourse in the next menstrual cycle month.

Complications

Falsely abnormal results can result from poor timing of the menstrual cycle, poor mucus quality because of infection, coital positions not favoring vaginal sperm retention, and low semen volume or low numbers of sperm. Although a normal PCT is encouraging, an inadequate test does not necessarily preclude fertilization.

Postprocedure Patient Education

If the test is inconclusive or abnormal, the PCT may be repeated. IUI or IVF, although expensive, are readily available in the United States. IUI and IVF bypass cervical mucus/sperm interaction abnormalities and should be offered to couples as a treatment option when indicated, especially in couples wanting multiple pregnancies or older couples (>35 years old).

Interpretation of Results

A normal result is 5 or more motile sperm per high power field. The mucus should also be thin, clear, and have a stretch of more than 5 cm.

CPT/Billing Code

89300 Semen analysis; presence or motility (or both) of sperm, including Huhner test

ICD-9-CM Diagnostic Codes

606.0 Infertility, male (due to azoospermia)
606.1 Oligospermia
606.9 Infertility, male, unspecified
628.4 Infertility, female (due to cervical origin)
628.9 Infertility, female (of unspecified origin)

Acknowledgment

The editors wish to recognize the contributions by Barbara Apgar, MD, to this chapter in the previous edition of this text.

BIBLIOGRAPHY

American Society for Reproductive Medicine: Optimal evaluation of the infertile female. A practice committee report. Fertil Steril 86(5 suppl):S264–S267, 2006 (www.asrm.org).

Carson SA, Kovanci E: Female infertility and evaluation of the infertile couple. In Bieber EJ, Sanfilippo JS, Horowitz IR (eds): Clinical Gynecology. Philadelphia, Churchill Livingstone, 2006, pp 751–766.

Glazener CM, Ford WC, Hull MG: The prognostic power of the postcoital test for natural conception depends on duration of infertility. Hum Reprod 15:1953–1957, 2000.

Griffith CS, Grimes DA: The validity of the postcoital test. Am J Obstet Gynecol 162:615–620, 1990.

Oei SG, Helmerhorst FM, Bloemenkamp KW, et al: Effectiveness of the postcoital test: Randomized controlled trial. BMJ 317:502–505, 1998.

Speroff L, Fritz M: Female infertility. In Speroff L, Fritz M (eds): Clinical Gynecologic Endocrinology and Infertility. Philadelphia, Lippincott Williams & Wilkins, 2005.

Treatment of Noncervical Condylomata Acuminata

Harris Mones

The increased incidence of human papillomavirus (HPV) infection combined with increased public awareness of the association of HPV with cervical carcinoma has led to a greater number of patients seeking counseling and treatment for condylomata (genital warts). Over 5 million new infections occur every year in the United States, and 74% are in those 15 to 24 years of age. Although there is some evidence that treatment reduces infectivity, there is no evidence supporting the concept that treatment of condylomata (the warty lesions themselves) reduces the incidence of cervical or genital neoplasia. In the majority of cases, genital HPV infection is subclinical and resolves on its own (Fig. 155-1). Treatment of subclinical asymptomatic genital HPV infection, regardless of its mechanism of detection (e.g., colposcopy, biopsy, acetic acid application, laboratory testing), is not recommended. The purpose and goal of treatment are to eliminate visible warts or symptomatic infection, to identify and resolve any associated dysplasia, and to educate the patient and any partners about the disease.

HPV is a multicentric infection. Coexisting external and internal lesions, or multiple lesions involving the entire lower genital system of both men and women, may be present. They can present as totally flat or 1- to 2-mm papular lesions, or as large, 1- to 2-cm cauliflower-like growths (see Chapter 118, Androscopy, Figs. 118-1 and 118-5). Some may be detected only with magnification (e.g., a colposcope), whereas others will be detected by a white discoloration after application of acetic acid (white epithelium). Some are flesh colored, whereas others are pigmented (see Chapter 118, Androscopy, Fig. 118-4; for a differential diagnosis, see Box 118-1). Warts may be found in and around the anus and inside the mouth. *Because of the risk of neoplastic transformation, a biopsy should be obtained if the clinician is uncertain about the diagnosis, lesions fail to respond or worsen during therapy, the patient is immunocompromised, or the lesion has an atypical, suspect appearance including pigmentation, bleeding, or ulceration.*

Biopsy of suspect lesions should be performed before treatment is initiated. If biopsy is performed after treatment, it is important to communicate to the pathologist the type and amount of preceding treatment.

The clinician must decide which treatment modality is best based on clinical skill, extent of disease, cost, patient preferences, and overall chance of success. The 2006 Centers for Disease Control and Prevention Treatment Guidelines point out that there is no definite evidence suggesting any of the available treatments are better than the others or ideal for all patients. Spontaneous resolution is a possibility, and therefore observation alone without specific treatment may be a reasonable alternative for some patients. Because there is no specific "cure" for HPV infection itself, the goal of treating HPV infection is the elimination of obvious visible or troublesome lesions (the disease caused by the virus). Treatment of HPV infection is analogous to the treatment of herpes virus infection. The virus will not be eliminated, but symptoms can be controlled.

Some infections may not be grossly visible, yet still cause anogenital pruritus, burning, vaginal discharge, or bleeding. Conversely, the treatment of asymptomatic intraurethral, intravaginal, or cervical condylomata (without dysplasia) exposes the patient to treatment risk without obvious benefit.

The patient may harbor HPV DNA for life; therefore, patient education is important to prevent unreasonable expectations. Treating male sexual partners with HPV infection has not appeared to change the post-treatment failure rate in women with cervical dysplasia. These findings should not deter the clinician from appropriately counseling, examining, and treating HPV-infected men (see Chapter 118, Androscopy). All methods of treating HPV have significant failure and recurrence rates. Common modalities for treatment are noted in Table 155-1; additional information is presented in Chapter 14, Cryosurgery; Chapter 30, Radiofrequency Surgery (Modern Electrosurgery); Chapter 118, Androscopy; Chapter 137, Colposcopic Examination; and Chapter 142, Human Papillomavirus DNA Typing.

The latest in the "treatment" of HPV infection is prevention. A quadrivalent vaccine (Gardasil) is available and approved by the U.S. Food and Drug Administration (FDA) for women between the ages of 9 and 26 years. It protects against HPV types 6, 11, 16, and 18; 95% to 99% of condylomata are due to an infection with HPV 6 or 11, and 75% of cervical cancers are caused by HPV 16 and 18. Theoretically, a series of three injections effectively prevents nearly all genital warts. The vaccine has no effect on treating an infection once it is present. In October 2009, the FDA approved Gardasil for use in males ages 9 to 26 for prevention of genital warts. At the same time, the FDA also approved another HPV vaccine, Cervarix (types 16 and 18), a GlaxoSmithKline product.

Indications for Treatment of Human Papillomavirus Infection

- Visible, acuminate condylomata
- Symptomatic condylomata

Contraindications to Treatment of Human Papillomavirus Infection

Relative

- Any known adverse reactions to the selected treatment modality.
- Any lesion that is possibly cancerous. (These lesions should be sampled for biopsy before treatment.)

Preprocedure Patient Education

Explain the procedure along with the *risks* and *benefits* to the patient. If an investigational drug is to be used, such as 5-fluorouracil ([5-FU]

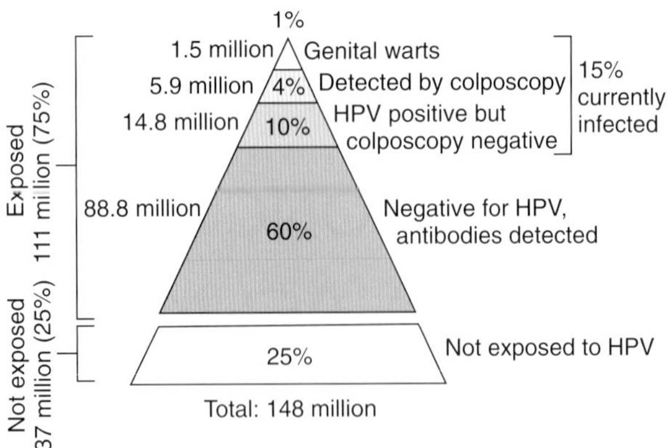

Figure 155-1 Hierarchy of clinically apparent and subclinical human papillomavirus infections: 15 to 49 years of age, United States, 2004. HPV, human papillomavirus. (From U.S. Census estimates of population as of July 1, 2004. Adapted from Koutsky L.)

Efudex; Valeant Pharmaceuticals, Aliso Viejo, Calif), review the non–FDA-approved status and why it is still being used. *Counseling* and *education* are key components in the comprehensive management of HPV-infected individuals. It is imperative that appropriate time be taken by physicians and staff to counsel patients and answer questions. Educational materials include pamphlets, printouts, videotapes, hotlines, and Internet sites (e.g., www.cdc.gov/std/hpv). Advise patients and sexual partners that although HPV infection itself has been associated with carcinoma, it is very common among sexually active adults and usually remains a benign disease that resolves on its own. Most sexually active adults will be exposed to the virus at some point in their lives. Penile penetration of the vagina is the most common mode of transmissions, but HPV can also be spread through nonpenetrative contact. Most sex partners are infected by the time the patient's diagnosis has been made, even though they may not have any clinical evidence of infection. HPV DNA testing is currently not indicated for partners of patients with genital warts. In female patients, if not already immunized, HPV recombinant vaccine should be administered to protect against types 6, 11, 16, and 18. Prior infection with HPV is not a reason to withhold the vaccine because it may prevent infection from HPV types other than the one(s) causing the current situation. In the past, condoms were not thought to be of much benefit in providing protection, but a 2006 study by Winer and colleagues suggests a 70% decrease in risk of new infection with consistent use.

Women who develop signs of HPV infection or who are sexually active with a partner who has HPV must be advised to obtain regular Pap smears because they are at higher risk for development of dysplasia.

CRYOSURGERY

See Chapter 14, Cryosurgery, and Chapter 138, Cryotherapy of the Cervix.

Equipment

Cryosurgery may be carried out with a variety of methods:

- Cryogun with nitrous oxide tank and small dermal tips
- Liquid nitrogen and cotton-tipped applicators
- Liquid nitrogen pressurized sprayer (Wallach Ultrafreezer, Brymill Cry-Ac)
- Canister gases (Verruca-Freeze, Ellman Medi-Frig)

Techniques

General Techniques for All Methods

1. No anesthetic is required for cryotherapy, although if there are large or multiple lesions, patients may prefer it (see Chapter 10, Topical Anesthesia).

TABLE 155-1 Therapies Currently Available for the Treatment of Genital Warts*

Treatment Modality	Average No. of Treatments	Success Rate†	Recurrence <6 Months	Average Length of Study Follow-up	Total Cost to Patient‡
Ablative Therapy					
CO_2 laser	1.3	89%	8%	13.9 mo	$$
Cryotherapy	1.9	83%	28%	2.7 mo	$$
Electrocautery	1.4	93%	24%	3 mo	$$
Infrared coagulator	1.5	80%	20%	6 mo	$$
Chemical–Ablative Therapy					
Topical 5-fluorouracil (Eudex)	Patient applied	71%	13%	10.9 mo	$$
85% Trichloroacetic acid	4	81%	36%	2 mo	$$$
Podophyllin	4.2	65%	39%	6 mo	$$$
Podophyllotoxin (Condylox)	10.5 (patient applied)	61%	34%	3.2 mo	$$
Chemical–Immune Enhancer Therapy					
Imiquimod (Aldara)	30 (patient applied)	56%	—§	7 mo	$$$
Interferon (local injection)	11	52%	25%	7.8 mo	$$$$
Other					
Sinecatechins	300 (patient applied)	55%	6%	4.0 mo	$$$$
Excisional Therapy					
Blade/scissors	1.1	93%	24%	8.3 mo	$$
Radiofrequency (loop)	1	90%	—§	8 mo	$$

*Based on an estimate from the previous edition's author (Edward J. Mayeaux, Jr.) as compiled from available English-language literature. Very small studies, study results that fell 2 standard deviations beyond the means, and very poorly designed studies were excluded.

†Defined as clearance of all condylomata at end of therapy or healing from therapy.

‡Relative cost based in office visits and cost of treatment for each method. $, low cost; $$, low-moderate cost; $$$, high-moderate cost; $$$$, high cost.

§No data or not recorded.

2. Place the patient in the lithotomy position and examine the vulva, perineum, and rectum (or scrotum and penis). If the lesions cover a large area, it may be prudent to treat subsections at separate visits to prevent excessive post-treatment discomfort. Treatment should be directed at the acuminate warts rather than at subclinical condylomata that cannot be seen with the naked eye. Staining with dilute acetic acid may make smaller acuminate lesions more prominent.

Nitrous Oxide

1. Select the proper size of cryotip based on the size of the lesion. The tip should cover small lesions; larger lesions may be frozen in sections or clusters.
2. Moisten the lesion with water-soluble gel before positioning the probe to improve tip-to-tissue adhesion. With the cryotip at ambient temperature, place the tip on an individual lesion. Activate the cryogun to initiate the flow of gas within the probe, which begins the freezing process. Apply gentle traction on the lesion to lift the skin away from underlying tissue as soon as ice appears on the tissue (this is especially important on the penile shaft). This traction isolates the lesion from the surrounding tissue, minimizes discomfort, and ensures cold transfer. Clumped lesions may be frozen in clusters but will require longer freezing times. Clusters also require the freeze–thaw–refreeze technique to produce the necessary cryonecrosis. (The tissue is frozen until it appears solid white, then thawed until it turns pink again, and then frozen a second time.) Stop freezing as soon as the ice extends just 2 to 3 mm beyond each lesion's border. This generally takes only 15 to 30 seconds. Some practitioners prefer a second application after the initial thaw in all cases.
3. Explain to the patient that a tingling or burning sensation is normal, especially with thawing.

Liquid Nitrogen (Cotton-Tipped Applicator and Spray)

1. Standard or large cotton-tipped applicators may be used to apply liquid nitrogen. Standard applicators (Q-Tips) work better if wisps of cotton are pulled from a cotton ball and twirled to add bulk to the end of the applicator. Pour liquid nitrogen into a Styrofoam cup. Dip the cotton-tipped applicator into the liquid nitrogen and apply immediately to the lesion. Reapply until the lesion turns white. Avoid freezing more than 2 to 3 mm beyond the border of the lesion. Thaw time should take at least 1 minute.
2. With the thermos-type containers (Brymill Cry-Ac and Wallach Ultrafreezer), spray a jet of liquid nitrogen on the lesions. Select an orifice large enough to have the site of the spray cover the lesion, but do not overspray. (This is a quick and economical use of liquid nitrogen.) Apply the liquid nitrogen until the lesion turns white. Avoid freezing more than 2 to 3 mm beyond the lesion. It generally takes only 5 to 10 seconds, depending on the size of the lesion. Thaw time should take at least 1 minute. A spray guard is available to protect surrounding skin. Alternatively, the physician can place an ear speculum around the lesion to limit overspray.

Gases (Verruca-Freeze and Medi-Frig)

Verruca-Freeze and Medi-Frig work similarly to liquid nitrogen. Compressed gas in a can is sprayed into an ear speculum that should just cover the lesion. The compressed gas liquefies with spraying, and rapid evaporation results in freezing of the lesion. Use of this agent obviates the need for storing large amounts of liquid nitrogen. The speculum must be positioned so that it is perpendicular to the lesion; in this way it acts like a funnel. This position requirement may be impractical on the genitalia. Once the material is sprayed into the speculum, it is held in place until the bubbling stops. Care must be taken that the liquid does not leak out from under the speculum and freeze normal tissue. One application may suffice on small lesions. If the lesions are large, a second application may be necessary after thawing. There are also cotton-tipped applicator–like attachments that allow this device to be used in a manner similar to liquid nitrogen.

Postprocedure Patient Education

- Usually no postprocedure medication is needed. Topical anesthetic ointments may be used to minimize discomfort (e.g., lidocaine 5% ointment). Sitz baths may aid resolution when large areas are treated. Silver sulfadiazine (Silvadene) ointment or other over-the-counter antibiotic ointments (Polysporin, Bacitracin) may not only be soothing but may reduce the possibility of superficial infection. They also help keep the denuded tissue from sticking to underclothing. No dressing is required, but some patients may request a sanitary napkin.
- Lesions that are cryonecrosed progress from erythema to edema and then turn black. They may also blister. The blister may be left intact or removed. The lesions disappear within a few days, and healing should be complete in 7 to 8 days.
- The patient should be advised to report any signs of infection or excessive discomfort.
- Treated areas should be washed with mild soap and water several times each day. Postcryotherapy management is similar to that for a second-degree burn.

Complications

- If the area treated at one visit is too large, extensive necrosis and pain may occur. It is prudent to treat large areas over multiple visits. Infection may occur at the treatment site if the area is not kept clean by normal hygienic measures.
- Recurrence or persistence of lesions is common.
- Cryotherapy is probably the safest therapy for treating HPV lesions during pregnancy.
- Nitrous oxide cryoguns are associated with a higher risk of perforation and fistula formation inside the vagina compared with the cotton-tipped applicator method.

Suppliers

See Chapter 14, Cryosurgery.

Chemical Cautery

Equipment

- Bichloracetic acid (BCA), 85% trichloroacetic acid (TCA), or 0.5% podofilox (Condylox)
- Cotton-tipped applicators or toothpicks

Technique

1. For BCA, TCA, or podophyllin, identify the lesions to be treated. For small lesions, use the wooden end of the cotton-tipped applicator or a toothpick to apply the solution directly on the lesion. Avoid getting the solution on normal skin. However, the wart virus is often present 3 mm beyond the obvious lesion. *Do not* apply petrolatum or other ointments around the lesions, as may have been the custom in the past. Besides being time consuming, it often covers the lesion itself and protects exactly what is meant to be treated. For larger lesions, use the cotton-tipped end of the applicator to apply the solution, again being careful to avoid getting the solution on normal skin. Continue in the same manner until all the lesions are treated. With high-strength acid application, the warty tissue rapidly turns white (see Chapter 118, Androscopy, Fig. 118-7A and B). Although in the vast majority of patients this treatment method is extremely well tolerated, patients treated with acids do experience intense, burning-like pain that subsides in about 5 minutes. In 1 to 2 days

the skin will slough. Patients may need retreatment every 1 to 3 weeks until the lesions resolve. The acids can be used in pregnancy and on mucous membranes.

2. Patients may apply topical 0.5% podofilox solution or gel themselves at home. Podofilox is a pure standardized compound of the active ingredient in podophyllin. Podofilox is indicated for topical treatment of external genital warts, but it is not indicated for the treatment of mucous membrane (urethra, rectum, vagina) condylomata. Podofilox is applied to the warts with a cotton-tipped applicator supplied with the medication. Treatment should be limited to an area less than 10 cm^2, and no more than 0.5 mL of the solution should be used each day. The solution is applied in the morning and evening for 3 consecutive days; then a 4-day waiting period is observed, during which the solution is not applied. This 1-week treatment cycle may be repeated up to four times, until there is no visible wart tissue. Remember the "2-3-4-4 Rule": twice a day for 3 days, off for 4 days, used for up to 4 weeks. Later, the entire treatment can be repeated if needed. Podofilox should not be used in pregnant women, young children, and nursing mothers.

Complications

- Treatment with too much solution can lead to excessive tissue damage and prolonged healing.
- Persistence and recurrence of the warts are not uncommon.
- Systemic reactions with extensive exposure to podophyllin may include nausea, vomiting, fever, confusion, coma, renal failure, ileus, and leukopenia. Local reactions include erosions, ulcerations, scarring, balanitis, and phimosis.
- Seizures and death have occurred with application of podophyllin to occluded mucous membranes.

Postprocedure Patient Education

- For lesions that are cauterized chemically, the healing process is usually less than 1 week but may take longer.
- Patient education sheets are supplied by the manufacturer of podofilox.

Interferon Therapy

Indication

Interferon therapy is indicated for recalcitrant condylomata unresponsive to other modalities.

Contraindication

Pregnancy is the only contraindication.

Equipment

- Recombinant interferon alfa-2b
- 27- to 30-gauge needle and a 1-mL syringe

Technique

1. The manufacturer recommends that only five warts be treated at one time, making this treatment time consuming and expensive. It is rarely used.
2. The standard dose is 1 million U of interferon (0.1 mL) intralesionally three times a week for 3 weeks (total of nine injections).
3. Use a 27- to 30-gauge needle to inject the interferon directly into the center of the wart's base (intralesional).
4. Maximum response should occur within 4 to 6 weeks. If there is no clinical response after 16 weeks, a second 3-week course should be completed.

Complications

- Flulike symptoms such as myalgias, fatigue, headache, chills, and fever may occur.
- May cause menstrual problems in adolescents.
- Treatment beyond 3 weeks may cause reversible leukopenia and liver enzyme elevations.

Postprocedure Patient Education

- The patient may take an analgesic if flulike symptoms develop.

Electrosurgery or Laser Therapy

Treatment of warts with electrosurgery can be ablative or excisional (see later). Lesions that are small or few in number can be cauterized easily with a ball or needle electrode. Place the electrosurgical unit on coagulation (or hemostasis) with just enough power to "cook" the wart. Wipe away the debris. If viable tissue remains, touch the wart again with the electrode. Condylomata are epidermal, and there is little need to go deep. With "just enough" current there will be little scarring. An alternative approach is laser ablation, but this treatment is expensive. Its use is more commonly reserved for when there are extensive condylomata on the vulva or when the vagina or cervix also needs treatment (Fig. 155-2).

Infrared Coagulation

Infrared coagulation can also be used to ablate warts on the external genitals as well as mucous membranes. Its advantages are that it is quick and the depth of destruction is readily controlled by the automatic timer (see Chapter 106, Office Treatment of Hemorrhoids). Destruction occurs when infrared light travels down the light guide and concentrates on the lesion. There is no electrical current involved.

Technique

1. Anesthetize lesions.
2. Set timer on 1 to 1.25 seconds for the average lesion. If the lesion is quite thick, the unit can be set up to 3 seconds. The depth of penetration will be roughly 1 mm/sec.
3. Apply the Teflon-coated tip inside the disposable sheath to the lesion using slight pressure.
4. Pull the trigger and hold it in place until it automatically turns off. The light will not harm the eyes, although it is bright and uncomfortable if directly viewed.
5. Wiping the tip and allowing the tip to cool for a few seconds between applications is recommended.
6. If the lesion is large, reapplication is carried out with slight overlapping.
7. Wipe away the ablated tissue with moistened gauze and determine if depth is adequate.
8. Treat the next lesion.
9. Postoperative treatment is the same as noted for other ablative treatments with electrocautery and acids.
10. Reexamine and retreat if necessary in 3 to 4 weeks. Expect slight denuding of the epithelium and mild ulceration as seen with topical acid treatments. There usually is little residual scarring.

Surgical Removal

Condylomata can be excised surgically with sharp iris scissors (see Chapter 118, Androscopy, Fig. 118-6) or a knife blade after appropriate anesthesia. However, the penile and vulvar skin is thin; it is easy to resect too deeply, which may result in scarring. Sharp disposable curettes offer a good alternative. Warty lesions also tend to be vascular and bleed easily. Although this can be controlled with

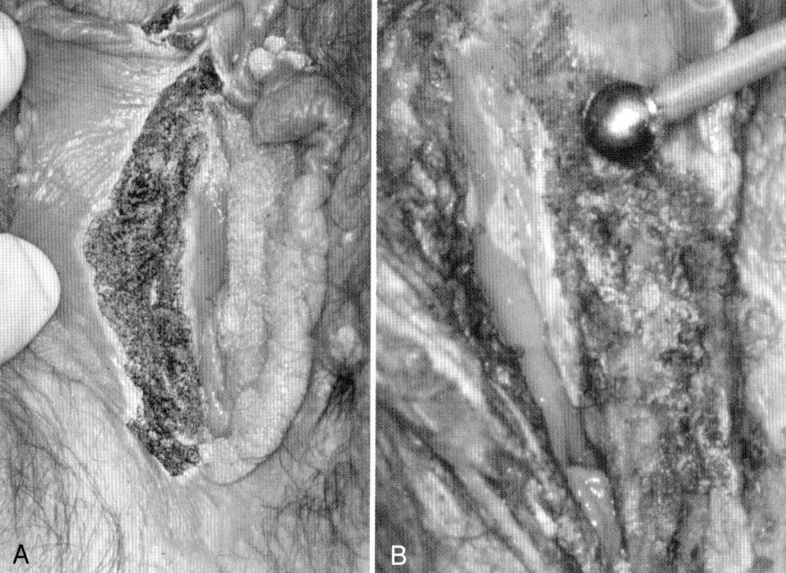

Figure 155-2 Treatment of condyloma with laser (**A**) and ball electrocautery (**B**). (From Ferenczy A, Behelak Y, Wright TC, et al: Treating vaginal and external anogenital condylomas with electrosurgery vs CO_2 laser ablation. J Gynecol Surg 11:41–50, 1995.)

Monsel's solution, it is often easier to use radiofrequency (loop) excisional surgery, especially for bigger lesions (see later discussion, as well as Chapter 30, Radiofrequency Surgery [Modern Electrosurgery]). For small pedunculated growths, scissor excision may be ideal. Flatter papular lesions can usually be easily curetted with a sharp, disposable 2- to 4-mm dermal curette.

Loop Radiofrequency Electrosurgical Excision

This technique is especially useful for large condylomata, in which any type of excisional process can create excessive bleeding. Use of the radiofrequency (a type of electrosurgery) unit can readily control this excess. Using a pure cutting setting minimizes any scarring, and there is still at least a 10% coagulation current. Thus, removal is carried out quickly with minimal residual tissue destruction. Complete details of this technique are found in Chapter 30, Radiofrequency Surgery [Modern Electrosurgery].

Equipment

- Square or round/oval loop electrodes (Usually the larger oval loops work best. Use dermatology electrodes with shorter shafts rather than the longer ones used to carry out the loop electrosurgical excision procedure [LEEP]. The shorter shafts allow better control of depth, and the operator's hand can be stabilized against surrounding tissue.)
- Electrosurgical generator
- Colposcope or 3× to 5× magnification lens (helps to keep the loop superficial, avoiding deep excisions as well as ensuring that all the lesion has been removed)
- Grounding pad or antenna
- Smoke evacuator
- 2% lidocaine with or without epinephrine (epinephrine is generally not used on the penis)
- Syringe with 30-gauge needle
- Ball electrodes (5 mm) to cauterize any bleeders
- Antibiotic ointment (over-the-counter preparations Bacitracin and Polysporin work well)
- Virus-filtering (submicron) mask and nonsterile gloves
- 4 × 4 sterile gauze pads
- Acetic acid
- Monsel's solution
- Formalin bottles
- 5% lidocaine ointment to apply after excisions completed

Suppliers

See the list of companies for radiofrequency units in Chapter 30, Radiofrequency Surgery [Modern Electrosurgery], and Chapter 149, Loop Electrosurgical Excision Procedure for Treating Cervical Intraepithelial Neoplasia.

Preprocedure Patient Preparation

Explain the procedure to the patient and obtain informed consent. The major risks are pain, bleeding, infection, recurrence, and scarring.

Technique

See Figures 155-3 and 155-4.

1. Apply 5% acetic acid (or white vinegar) to the warts. Keep the tissue moist by repeated acetic acid application.
2. Turn on the electrosurgical generator power supply. Check the manufacturer's guidelines for proper power settings (usually around 15 to 20 W or, if using the Ellman unit, level 2).
3. Select the cutting (preferred) or blend mode on the electrosurgical generator.
4. Place the grounding pad or antenna on the patient's thigh or buttocks.
5. With a 27- to 30-gauge needle, inject 2% lidocaine under the base of the wart(s) to make a wheal that extends beyond the margin of the wart.
6. Activate the smoke evacuator and place the hose close to the excisional site.
7. Using a method of magnification allows more precise removal and assurance that small lesions are not missed. The loop should not excise deeper than 1 mm to the dermal–epidermal junction (looks like chamois cloth). Often it is best just to "debulk" the wart on the first pass. Then make fine, superficial "feathering" strokes to remove the remaining tissue. Significant bleeding may be a sign that the excision is too deep or, paradoxically, that there is residual wart tissue. To control the depth of

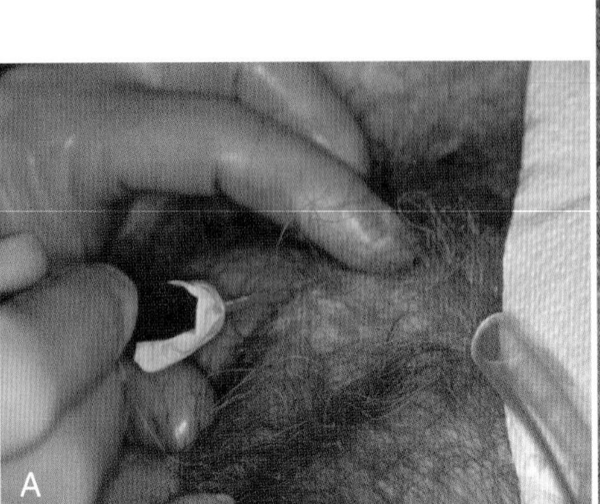

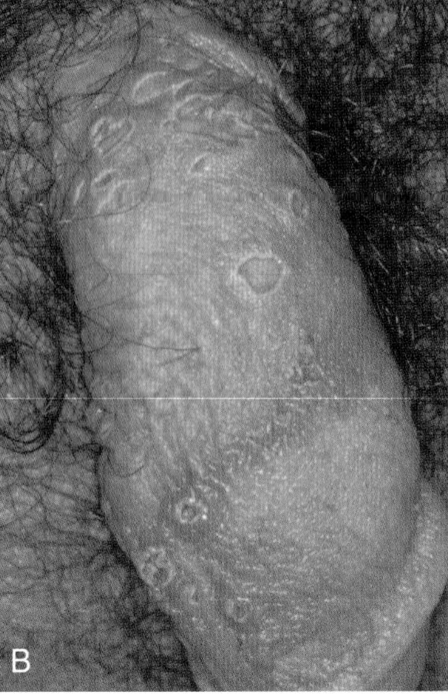

Figure 155-3 Treatment of condyloma using radiofrequency loop excision. During (**A**) and immediately after (**B**) removal. Note lack of bleeding. (Courtesy of The Medical Procedures Center, PC, Midland, Mich/John L. Pfenninger, MD.)

excision and stabilize the loop, place the fifth finger of the hand holding the electrode in the pencil wand on the patient. Should the patient jump or move, the operating hand will move too, avoiding a deep cut. Hold the pencil wand close to where the electrode inserts into the wand. Use caution because the loops cut very quickly. Be especially cautious over the penis.

8. After the loop electrode has been used to excise the wart, the ball electrode may be used to coagulate any bleeders or residual tissue, although this is rarely necessary.
9. Remove the coagulated remnants with gauze sponges soaked with acetic acid (5%).
10. On completion, inspect the excised area with the colposcope to ensure that the entire wart has been removed and that no coagulated remnants are left at the base of the excised lesion. Also be sure no small lesions have been missed.
11. Apply an antibiotic ointment and/or lidocaine ointment to the excision area and use gauze pads to cover the excision sites.
12. Although not mandatory, consider sending all tissue that was removed for histologic evaluation. Many lesions that appear totally benign and clinically are condylomata can be dysplastic or, albeit rarely, verrucous carcinoma.

NOTE: Many patients prefer this modality over chemical cautery methods because healing is often more rapid and less painful.

Complications

- Hypopigmentation may rarely occur at the excision site.
- If Monsel's is used to control bleeding, there may be some residual ferrous pigmentation for several months. This gradually fades.
- Keloids may form on skin that has a tendency toward keloid formation.
- Postprocedure bleeding and wound infection are extremely rare.
- According to Ferenczy (1990), the treatment failure rate at 8 months (average two treatments) is 19%.
- If the procedure is performed correctly, scarring is minimal and comparable to that with laser ablation.

Postprocedure Patient Education

- Provide the patient with the sample patient education handout available online at www.expertconsult.com. Instruct the patient that some postprocedure discomfort may last for up to 2 weeks. However, initial discomfort should resolve in 24 to 48 hours and is well controlled with nonsteroidal anti-inflammatory drugs. When large areas have been treated, sitz baths may be taken two to three times a day during the initial recovery period. At a minimum, the area should be washed three to four times per day, followed by application of an antibiotic ointment. This is

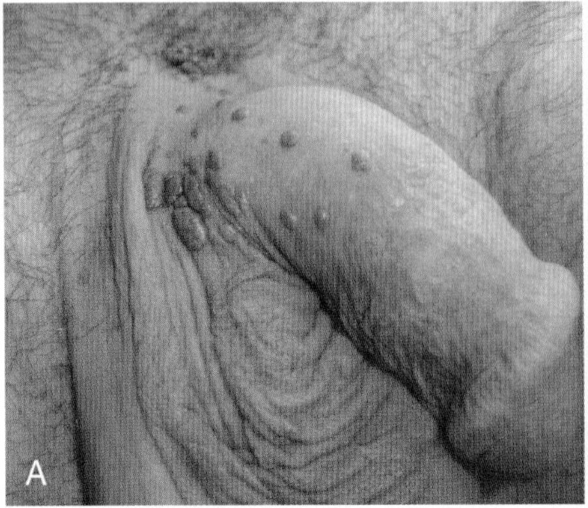

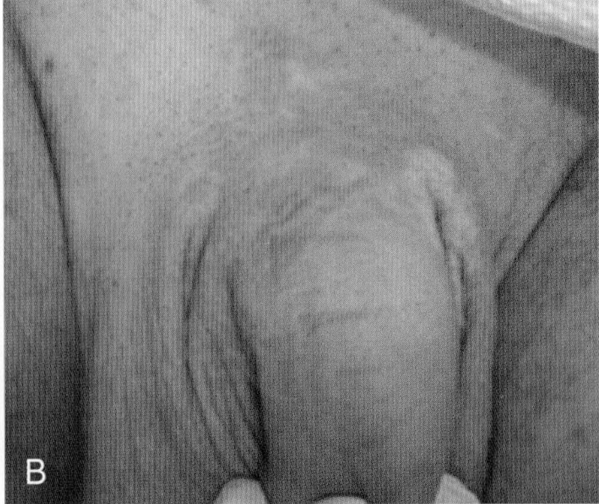

Figure 155-4 Treatment of condyloma using radiofrequency loop excision. Appearance before (**A**) and 1 month after (**B**) removal. (Courtesy of The Medical Procedures Center, PC, Midland, Mich/John L. Pfenninger, MD.)

continued for 5 to 7 days until reepithelialization has taken place. Ice packs may also be used initially. For those patients who have perianal removals, stool softeners (docusate sodium) are important throughout the entire recovery period.

- If acute discomfort persists beyond 48 hours, instruct the patient to contact the physician. Rarely, a mixture of equal parts of 20% benzocaine (Hurricaine) ointment and topical antibiotics may be used. Lidocaine ointment 5% provides excellent relief and also keeps the tissues moist.
- Instruct the patient to return to the office in 4 to 6 weeks and to call if fever, chills, or purulent discharge develops.

Imiquimod Cream (Aldara)

Use of imiquimod (Aldara) cream is a unique approach to HPV treatment. It acts as an immune stimulator by inducing multiple subtypes of interferon-α. This causes induction of several cytokines, including tumor necrosis factor and interleukins. These in turn activate natural killer cells, T cells, polymorphonuclear neutrophil leukocytes, and macrophages, thus increasing antitumor activity. The drug has almost no systemic side effects. Use of this drug is not indicated in children younger than 12 years of age. It can be used primarily or after other treatments to reduce recurrences. In randomized, placebo-controlled trials, 37% to 54% of treated patients showed clearance after 16 weeks. Although it is an off-label indication, imiquimod has been used with excellent results to treat extensive intravaginal condylomata.

Indications

It can be used on all external HPV-infected sites.

Contraindications

- It is a pregnancy class C drug.
- It is not approved for use on occluded mucous membranes or on the uterine cervix. However, an off-label use for extensive intravaginal lesions is to use one packet of the cream at bedtime, once a week, for 4 to 6 weeks. It is very efficacious but may cause irritation.
- It is not recommended for use with condoms or diaphragms because of possible latex damage.

Technique

The cream comes in small packets (box of 12 or 24) and is applied to the lesions three times a week for up to 16 weeks. The cream may be applied to the affected area, not strictly to the lesion itself. For best results it must be rubbed in well, not just lightly applied to the involved areas.

Complications

- Side effects can include pain, pigmentary changes at application site, erythema, erosion, itching, skin flaking, and edema. Therapy may be temporarily halted if symptoms become problematic. Systemic symptoms have been reported but are extremely rare.

5-Fluorouracil

Treatment with 5-FU should be considered only for extensive, intractable condylomata resistant to other modalities or for the treatment of vaginal intraepithelial neoplasia (VAIN). The FDA has not approved labeling of 5-FU for treatment of these diseases, and the patient should be advised that this is technically an investigational use. Because of the reported teratogenic potential, 5-FU should be used with extreme caution—if at all—in nonsterile women of reproductive age. If used, a signed consent form is advised indicating the patient will not become pregnant. Although commonly used historically, 5-FU use has fallen into disfavor for HPV treatment because of complications of vaginal scarring and the development of other, more acceptable methods. It is still one of the easiest-to-use and most effective treatments for male urethral/meatal lesions.

Indications

- Extensive vulvar, perianal, penile, or vaginal condylomata
- VAIN
- Vulvar intraepithelial neoplasia
- Urethral meatus lesions
- Bowenoid carcinoma in situ of the penis (erythroplasia of Queyrat)

CAUTION: Patients with blond or red hair, or with very light complexions, may be more sensitive to 5-FU. Also use cautiously in patients with known skin sensitivities such as atopic dermatitis. Mucosal areas are much more sensitive than keratinized skin.

Contraindications

- Pregnancy
- Lack of birth control method (relative contraindication)
- Lack of informed consent with regard to absence of FDA approval

Equipment

- 5% 5-FU (Efudex, Fluoroplex) cream
- Vaginal applicator marked with dosage lines

Preprocedure Patient Preparation

- Obtain informed consent before initiating treatment.
- Advise the patient of alternative methods of treatment. Frequently when 5-FU is being considered, laser ablation or LEEP therapy is also an option.
- The patient should know that the inflammatory response is delayed by 3 to 4 days. The patient may believe the medication is not working and so apply it more frequently, leading to complications.
- Use of 5-FU should be limited to clinicians experienced with managing side effects, which are similar to those experienced when treating the face for actinic changes (e.g., chemical burns). See the sample patient education form online at www.expertconsult.com.

Technique

For the Vagina

1. Instruct the patient to use 1.5 g of 5-FU per week for 10 weeks. A standard Ortho vaginal applicator will hold 10 mL of cream (5 g of 5-FU). Patients should then use only one third of an applicator of cream for each treatment. The 5-FU should be inserted intravaginally or applied directly to any external lesions at bedtime (e.g., for perianal lesions).
2. Instruct the patient to apply zinc oxide to the vulva (where treatment is not necessary) to protect it in the event that intravaginal, perineal, or perianal 5-FU should leak out or come into contact with the vulva. This is not necessary if external condylomata exist in this area.
3. The patient may insert a small tampon into the vagina to keep the 5-FU within the introitus.
4. If there is no inflammatory response after 3 weeks, the patient may increase the frequency of application to every 5 days.

For the Urethral Meatus

Use a cotton-tipped applicator and apply a small amount of 5-FU cream into the meatus for a distance of 5 to 6 mm. Apply after voiding at bedtime and again after voiding and showering in the morning. Repeat for 7 days. Lesions will generally resolve. If not, repeat for another 7 days. Allow any inflammation to resolve before reapplication.

For the Penis (Carcinoma in Situ, Erythroplasia of Queyrat)

This lesion usually occurs under the foreskin. Because of occlusion, the effects are magnified. Although quite efficacious, the treatment can be quite painful, especially if the medication is overused. Also, these lesions generally occur in older men, so compliance can be difficult. Cream will often drip out on the scrotum, so it must be protected. A small amount of cream is applied once a week to the affected area for 6 weeks. If there is little reaction after the first week, the schedule can be increased to every 5 days for two periods. If there is still minimal response, the cream can be tried every 3 to 4 days, but must be monitored closely. Treatment for 6 weeks usually resolves the dysplasia, but longer treatment may be needed. Recheck 6 weeks after completing treatment to be sure the abnormality has resolved. Small residual spots may be treated with excision or electrocautery, or even more 5-FU.

Complications

- Pain.
- Bleeding.
- Persistence of disease.
- Persistent vaginal ulcers may develop in patients who are extremely sensitive to 5-FU or in patients who overuse the medication. For some patients, the vaginal ulcers may fail to heal with time, and the patient may have persistent vaginal discharge and bleeding (rare). Patients who fail to heal may require surgical excision of the ulcer and primary closure of the defect.
- Vaginal stenosis (rare).
- If 5-FU is to be used after cryotherapy of the cervix, wait at least 4 weeks before initiating 5-FU therapy to avoid cervical stenosis.
- Inflammation of the scrotum, if not properly protected, when treating Bowen's disease (squamous cell carcinoma in situ).
- Foreskin adhesions.

Postprocedure Patient Education

Instruct the patient to contact the physician if severe inflammation or any hypersensitivity reaction occurs. Intravaginal estrogens or steroid creams may be used to decrease the inflammatory reaction. See the sample patient education handout online at www.expertconsult.com.

SINECATECHINS

Sinecatechins, a green tea extract, is approved by the FDA for the treatment of genital and perianal warts. It is a 15% ointment, produced by Bradley Pharmaceuticals (Fairfield Township, NJ), and marketed as Veregen. It is approved for use in immunocompetent patients 18 years of age or older. The recommended initial dose of the Veregen is a 0.5-cm strand applied in a thin layer over all external and perianal warts, three times a day.

In clinical trials patients applied 10% or 15% ointment three times daily for a maximum of 16 weeks or until complete resolution of the warts occurred. Complete clearance of warts was seen in 56.3% and 57.2% of patients, respectively. Partial clearance rates of at least 50% were reported for 74% and 78.4% of patients.

GUIDELINES FOR TREATING PERIANAL AND INTRA-ANAL LESIONS

Treatment of perianal and intra-anal lesions is similar to treatment for vaginal condylomata. Additional guidelines are as follows:

- Podofilox and imiquimod should not be used on mucous membranes (i.e., inside the anus). TCA, excisional therapy, electrocautery, and infrared coagulation may be used intra-anally.
- Anoscopy should be performed on all patients with perianal lesions to rule out more proximal lesions. This is often done after resolution of the external lesions to avoid possible trauma and potential spread of the virus proximally.
- The risk of rectal carcinoma is increased 50 times in receptive homosexual men, and HPV appears to be involved in the process. Some suggest Pap smears of the dentate line of the anus to detect early dysplastic lesions just as with the cervix, followed by staining and biopsy (see Chapter 99, High-Resolution Anoscopy).

GUIDELINES FOR TREATING CONDYLOMATA IN PREGNANCY

Condylomata may grow rapidly and multiply quickly during the second-trimester immune suppression. After delivery, they may, and often do, resolve spontaneously. Women who have warts in the perineum with subsequent tears or episiotomies have a higher risk of wound dehiscence. Most physicians recommend treatment of perineal condylomata during the third trimester. Safe modalities include cryotherapy, 85% TCA, electrocautery, laser therapy, infrared coagulation, and radiofrequency (loop) or sharp tissue scissor excision. Although cryotherapy may be used, there is often more swelling and discomfort.

It appears that HPV is in the amniotic fluid of infected mothers, so there is no indication for cesarean section unless the lesions are so large that they inhibit normal delivery.

OTHER METHODS FOR TREATING CONDYLOMATA ACUMINATA

Although *Candida* antigen injection is used for verrucae, there have been no published reports of its use in treating condylomata. There is theoretically no contraindication to its use, and it has been tried to some degree of success (editor's experience).

GENERAL CONSIDERATIONS FOR ALL METHODS

See Box 155-1 for a summary of treatment options for various locations. See Figure 155-5 for an algorithm on treatment protocol selection.

- HPV is associated with cervical cancer, and women must be followed closely with Pap smears, HPV DNA typing, or colposcopy.
- The patient and partner must not smoke. Even passive smokers have been found to have lower folate levels—a known risk for HPV. Reducing smoking leads to a reduction in cervical dysplasia, whereas continuing to smoke encourages progression.
- The patient should consume a diet with at least five helpings of fruits and vegetables daily.
- Patients must be informed that they can spread the disease at any time and that monogamy is most prudent.

Box 155-1. Preferred Methods of Treatment for Condylomata in Various Locations and during Pregnancy*

External Genital and Perianal
Cryotherapy
Electrocautery
Electrofrequency/radiofrequency excision
Imiquimod (Aldara)
Laser
Podofilox (Condylox)
Sinecatechins (Veregen)
85% TCA

Cervical
Must rule out dysplasia before treatment (perform colposcopy), then the following:
Cryotherapy
Electrocautery
Excision with radiofrequency or multiple biopsies
85% TCA

Vaginal
Cryotherapy
Electrocautery
5-FU (extensive disease)—not FDA approved
Imiquimod (Aldara)—not FDA approved
Laser
85% TCA

Urethral Meatus
Cryotherapy
Electrocautery
Excision
5-FU
85% TCA

Penis or Bowen's Disease
Electrocautery
5-FU
Frank excision of lesion

Intra-anal
Cryotherapy
Electrocautery
Surgical
85% TCA

Oral
Cryotherapy
Electrocautery
Excision

Pregnancy
Cryotherapy
Electrocautery/excision
85% TCA

*See text for details.
FDA, Food and Drug Administration; 5-FU, 5-fluorouracil; TCA, trichloroacetic acid.

- Condoms are not needed with current partners if there has been unprotected intercourse because they already have the virus; theoretically, once infected, the patient will always harbor the virus. Condoms may protect against transmission with new partners and against other sexually transmitted infections.

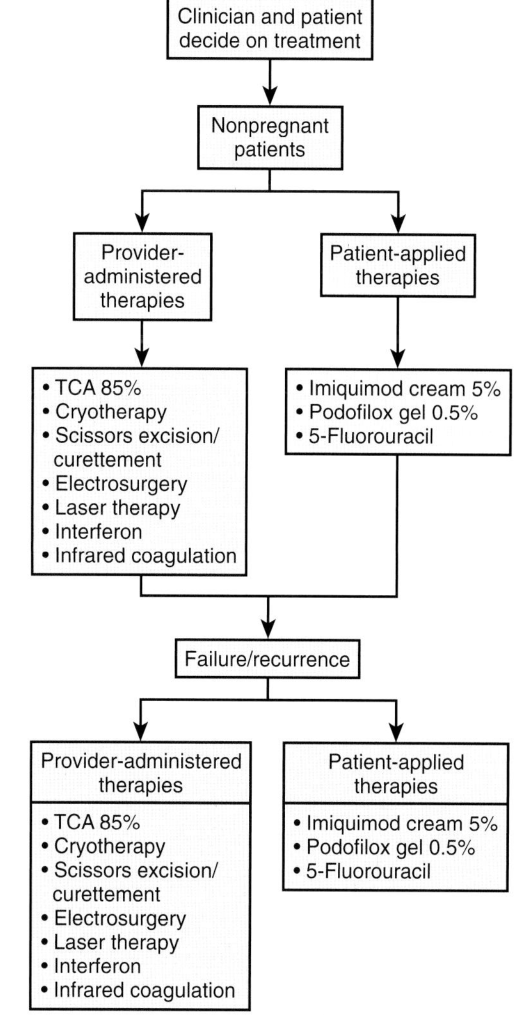

Figure 155-5 Algorithm for treatment protocol selection for condyloma. TCA, trichloroacetic acid. (From Ferenczy A: External anogenital warts: Old and new therapies. J SOGC December:1305–1313, 1999.)

CPT/Billing Codes

11900 Injection, intralesional; up to and including seven lesions (interferon)
11901 Injection intralesional; more than seven lesions

For destruction codes, if it takes less than 15 minutes, use "simple" codes. If treatment takes longer than 15 minutes, requires use of the colposcope and an extensive examination, or is particularly complicated because of the size or extent of the condylomata, use the "extensive" codes.

46900 Destruction of lesion(s); anus (e.g., condyloma), simple; chemical
46910 Destruction of lesion(s); anus electrodesiccation, simple
46916 Destruction of lesion(s); anus cryosurgery, simple
46917 Destruction of lesion(s); anus laser surgery, simple
46922 Destruction of lesion(s); anus surgical excision, simple
46924 Destruction of lesion(s); anus, extensive; any method
54050 Destruction of lesion(s); penis (e.g., condyloma), simple; chemical
54055 Destruction of lesion(s); penis electrodesiccation, simple
54056 Destruction of lesion(s); penis cryosurgery, simple
54057 Destruction of lesion(s); penis laser surgery, simple
54060 Destruction of lesion(s); penis surgical excision, simple

54065 Destruction of lesion(s); penis, extensive, any method
54100 Biopsy, cutaneous, penis
56501 Destruction of lesion(s); vulva, simple; any method
56515 Destruction of lesion(s); vulva, extensive, any method
56605 Biopsy, vulva introitus
57061 Destruction of lesion(s); vagina, simple; any method
57065 Destruction of lesion(s); vagina, extensive; any method
57100 Biopsy, vagina

ICD-9-CM Diagnostic Codes

078.10 Viral warts, unspecified
078.11 Condyloma acuminatum

Acknowledgment

The editors wish to recognize the many contributions by Edward J. Mayeaux, Jr., MD, to this chapter in a previous edition of this text.

ADDITIONAL RESOURCES

The following videotapes are available from Creative Health Communications, distributed through The National Procedures Institute, Midland, Michigan (www.npinstitute.com).

Physician Education

Pfenninger JL: Removal of condyloma with radiofrequency (33 minutes)

Patient Education

Pfenninger JL: Genital warts and cancer: The man's side (21 minutes)
Pfenninger JL. Genital warts and cancer: The woman's side (35 minutes)

BIBLIOGRAPHY

Baker DA, Douglas JM Jr, Buntin DM, et al: Topical podofilox for the treatment of condylomata acuminata in women. Obstet Gynecol 76:656–659, 1990.

Bekassy Z, Westrom L: Infrared coagulation in the treatment of condyloma acuminata in the female genital tract. Sex Transm Dis 14:209–212, 1987.

Bergman A, Bhatia NN, Broen EM: Cryotherapy for the treatment of genital condylomata during pregnancy. J Reprod Med 29:432–435, 1984.

Centers for Disease Control and Prevention: Sexually transmitted disease treatment guidelines, 2006: Genital warts. Available at www.cdc.gov/std/treatment/2006/genital-warts.htm#warts1.

CenterWatch: Drug information: Veregen (kunecatechins). Available at www.centerwatch.com/patient/drugs/dru938.html. Accessed January 21, 2010.

Doorbar J: The papillomavirus life cycle. J Clin Virol 32(Suppl 1):S7–S15, 2005.

Edwards L, Ferenczy A, Eron L, et al: Self-administered topical 5% imiquimod cream for external anogenital warts. Arch Dermatol 134:25–30, 1998.

Ferenczy A: Diagnosis and treatment of anogenital warts in the male patient. Prim Care 10:11, 1990.

Ferenczy A: External genital condyloma. In Apgar BS, Brotzman GL, Spitzer M (eds): Colposcopy: Principles and Practice, 2nd ed. Philadelphia, Saunders, 2008, pp 381–400.

Fletcher JL: Perinatal transmission of human papillomavirus. Am Fam Physician 43:143–148, 1991.

Friedman-Kien AE, Eron LJ, Conant M, et al: Natural interferon alfa for treatment of condylomata acuminata. JAMA 259:533–538, 1988.

Frisch M, Fenger C, van den Brule AJ, et al: Variants of squamous cell carcinoma of the anal canal and perianal skin and their relation to human papillomaviruses. Cancer Res 59:753–757, 1999.

Kodner C, Nasarty S: Management of genital warts. Am Fam Physician 70:2335–2342, 2345–2346, 2004.

Krebs HB, Helmkamp BF: Treatment failure of genital condylomata in women: Role of the male sexual partner. Obstet Gynecol 165:337–339, 1991.

Maw RD: Treatment of anogenital warts, Dermatol Clin 16: 829, 1998.

Mayeaux EJ Jr: External genital warts: An update. The Female Patient, December 2007. Available at http://www.femalepatient.com/html/cme/articles/032_12_038.asp.

Mayeaux EJ Jr, Dunton C: Modern management of external genital warts. J Low Genit Tract Dis 12:185–192, 2008.

Pfenninger JL: Androscopy: Examination of the male partner. In Apgar BS, Brotzman GL, Spitzer M (eds): Colposcopy: Principles and Practice, 2nd ed. Philadelphia, Saunders, 2008, pp 483–496.

Richart R: Ways of using LEEP for external lesions. Contemp Obstet Gynecol 5:138–152, 1992.

Slattery ML, Robison LM, Schuman KL, et al: Cigarette smoking and exposure to passive smoke are risk factors for cervical cancer. JAMA 261:1593–1598, 1989.

Swinehart JM, Sperling M, Phillips S, et al: Intralesional fluorouracil/epinephrine injectable gel for treatment of condylomata acuminata: A phase 3 clinical study. Arch Dermatol 133:67–73, 1997.

Szarewski A, Jarvis MJ, Sasieni P, et al: Effect of smoking cessation on cervical lesion size. Lancet 347:941–943, 1996.

Tatti S, Swinehart JM, Thielert C, et al: Sinecatechins, a defined green tea extract, in the treatment of external anogenital warts: A randomized controlled trial. Obstet Gynecol 111:1371–1379, 2008.

Tyring SK, Friedman-Kien AE, Kent HL, et al: Alpha interferon in the management of genital warts. Female Patient 18:33–39, 1993.

Usatine RP, Smith MA, Mayeaux EJ Jr, et al: The Color Atlas of Family Medicine. New York, McGraw-Hill, 2008.

Villa LL, Costa RL, Petta CA, et al: High sustained efficiency of a prophylactic quadrivalent human papilloma virus types 6/11/16/18 L1 virus-like particle vaccine through 5 years of follow up. Br J Cancer 95:1459–1466, 2006.

Winer RL, Hughes JP, Feng Q, et al: Condom use and the risk of genital human papillomavirus infection in young women. N Engl J Med 354:2645–2654, 2006.

CHAPTER 156

Endometrial Ablation

Thomas A. Kintanar

For over a century, physicians have attempted a variety of methods to control abnormal uterine bleeding as an alternative to hysterectomy. It is estimated that nearly 50% of women will have significant, heavy menstrual bleeding during their lifetime, particularly during the fifth and sixth decades of life. In the late 1880s there was a report of a physician placing a uterine sound into the endometrial cavity of patients and attaching the sound to a series of batteries. It was noted that women who did not have uterine fibroids had significant improvement in their heavy bleeding. However, because of the lack of suitable equipment and delivery systems, interest in endometrial ablation for the treatment of abnormal bleeding was essentially nonexistent. The technique of dilation and curettage (D&C) was introduced and became the gold standard for the treatment of abnormal bleeding, even though this procedure continues to be ineffective in controlling abnormal uterine bleeding. More recently, different methods of hormone manipulation have been used with limited success.

Modern methods of achieving endometrial coagulation by heat had their beginning when Goldrath successfully used the neodymium-doped yttrium-aluminum garnet (Nd:YAG) laser in the early 1980s. His technique was quickly followed by other methods in which a urologic resectoscope was used to remove the endometrial lining. Resection was soon followed by rollerball endometrial ablation, in which the lining is not removed, but is destroyed by cauterization. For the past decade, the Nd:YAG laser, uterine resection, and rollerball ablation have been the primary methods used to control abnormal bleeding when hysterectomy was not desired and hormones were ineffective.

Endometrial ablation is safe, effective, efficient, and readily learned. It allows patients to address problematic vaginal bleeding from the endometrium while allowing them to keep their uterus. Methodologies that use hysteroscopy for visualization of the uterus are considered invasive. The newer techniques that do not require the use of hysteroscopy are termed *minimally invasive nonhysteroscopic methods for endometrial ablation*. This chapter covers the more contemporary approaches to endometrial ablation with a brief historical discussion of the classic techniques of rollerball, hysteroscopic methods of resection, and laser. At the end of the discussion, a table highlighting the U.S. Food and Drug Administration (FDA) comparative data on the five second-generation approaches is provided (Table 156-1). These data reflect the FDA Manufacturer and User Facility Device Experience (MAUDE) database review.

Advantages

- Minimal anesthesia (cryoablation)
- Short operating time
- Performed in outpatient facility (rollerball and thermal balloon ablation) or office (cryoablation)
- Few complications
- Rapid postoperative recovery and return to normal activity
- Highly effective in controlling bleeding (95% success rate)
- Highly effective in controlling or eliminating associated symptoms (e.g., premenstrual syndrome, dysmenorrhea, moodiness)
- Easily mastered (cryoablation)

Indications

The ideal candidate for endometrial ablation meets all of the following criteria. However, there are differences in indications and contraindications depending on which technique is used.

- Menorrhagia or heavy menstrual bleeding (defined as blood loss >80 mL/cycle; bleeding for longer than 8 days; blood loss or symptoms that interfere with normal activities; or blood loss sufficient to cause anemia)
- Pharmaceutical treatment contraindicated, failed, refused, or created adverse effects
- Desire to avoid hysterectomy, especially in those with significant medical problems and surgical risks

Prerequisite Conditions

- Absence of any precancerous or cancerous lesions of the endometrium or cervix; normal Papanicolaou (Pap) smear and negative endometrial biopsy or hysteroscopy.
- Uterine size less than 12 weeks of gestation and uterine cavity less than 12 cm in length (with the cryoablation technique, large uterine size does not preclude performing the procedure).
- Other potential causes of excessive menstrual bleeding that could be treated medically or by other alternative forms of surgery have been excluded.
- No underlying uterine lesions requiring surgery.
- Childbearing has been completed.
- No active pelvic infection.

Contraindications

Absolute

- Current or planned pregnancy
- Presence of cervical or endometrial cancer or precancer
- Myomas in uterus larger than 4 cm
- Previous uterine surgeries such as myomectomy, classic cesarean section (excluding low transverse cesarean section), or any uterine surgery that would render the myometrium thin (e.g., deep myomectomy)
- Clotting or bleeding disorders
- Adnexal masses

TABLE 156-1 Comparative Data from 2001 U.S. Food and Drug Administration Trial of Five Second-Generation Endometrial Ablation Devices

Device Characteristic	Balloon	Cryotherapy	Radiofrequency	Hydrothermal	Microwave
Operating principle	Balloon filled with fluid (5% dextrose in water) at 87° C	Probe with transfer media creates ice ball at −100° C to −120° C	Bipolar, radiofrequency ablation at 180 W	Hydrothermal circulation of saline at 90° C	Controlled microwave tissue ablation delivered through hand-held applicator
Average treatment time	8 min	10–18 min	90 sec	10 min	3.5 min
Average procedure time	20 min	30 min	4.2 min	30 min	Not reported (~11 min including hysteroscopy)
Direct visualization	None; done before procedure	Ultrasonography	None required; visualization before and after procedure	Hysteroscopy	Done before procedure; continuous temperature readings taken during procedure
Pretreatment	3-min suction curettage	Leuprolide acetate	None required	In FDA trial, patients received a 7.5-mg dose of leuprolide acetate administered 3 wk before ablation; other trials used 3.75-mg dosages. Treatment occurred on days 19–27 after injection.	Leuprolide acetate (3.75 mg)
Safety features	Pressure shut-off at >210 mm Hg or <45 mm Hg; terminates if temperature >95° C or <75° C	Ultrasonographic visualization provides guidance for ice ball progression	Tests for perforations; terminates procedure at proper tissue impedance	Automatic shut-off at fluid loss of 10 mL or increase of 20 mL	Tests for abnormal temperature rise; terminates procedure
Patients enrolled in FDA trial: selected inclusion criteria	Uterine sound measurement of 4–10 cm	Uterine sound measurement of <10 cm Uterine volumetric measurement <300 mL	Uterine sound measurement of 6–10 cm Polyps <2 cm Submucous fibroids that did not distort the uterine cavity	Endometrial cavity measuring <10.5 cm	Uterine sound measurement of 6–14 cm Polyps or submucous fibroids allowing distortions up to 3 cm
Patients enrolled in FDA trial: selected exclusion criteria	Cavity >10 cm Submucous fibroids Polyps Septate uterus Previous endometrial ablation procedure Classical cesarean section	Intramural myomas >2-cm diameter Intrauterine polyps Pedunculated fibroids Septate uterus	Abnormal/obstructed uterine cavity as confirmed by hysteroscopy, saline-infused sonogram, or hysterosalpingogram Specifically, septate or bicornuate uterus, pedunculated submucosal leiomyomata, or polyps (>2 cm) likely to cause menorrhagia Previous uterine surgery interrupting integrity of uterine wall	Intramural fibroids >4 cm on sonography contributing to menorrhagia Uterine anatomic anomaly Previous endometrial ablation procedure Classical cesarean section	Previous uterine surgery or other condition that interrupts integrity of myometrial wall

Data from Sanfilippo JS (ed): Options in Endometrial Ablation. Supplement to OBG Management, December 2005. Available at www.obgmanagement.com/medediibr/PDFs/1205Suppl_EA.pdf.

Relative

- Uterine size greater than 12 cm (this may vary depending on the procedural approach of the surgeon).
- Total cervical stenosis.
- Previous endometrial ablation.
- Unusual anatomic variation that may preclude adequate ablation, such as congenital uterine abnormalities. If there is a septate or bicornuate uterus, both cavities must be ablated separately; in the case of hydrothermablation, this may constitute a relative contraindication. Clinical consideration and procedural approach must be taken into account before proceeding with the ablation procedure of choice.

EQUIPMENT AND SUPPLIES

Because there are different systems that use supplies specific to the particular procedure, the following equipment/supply list provides the most often required supplies to perform the majority of the procedures. A list of equipment/supplies germane to each procedure is listed with each particular section.

- For hysteroscopy-based ablation, a rigid (0-, 12-, or 30-degree viewing angle) hysteroscopic resectoscope (Fig. 156-1)
- Uterine sound
- Hegar cervical dilators
- Tenaculum

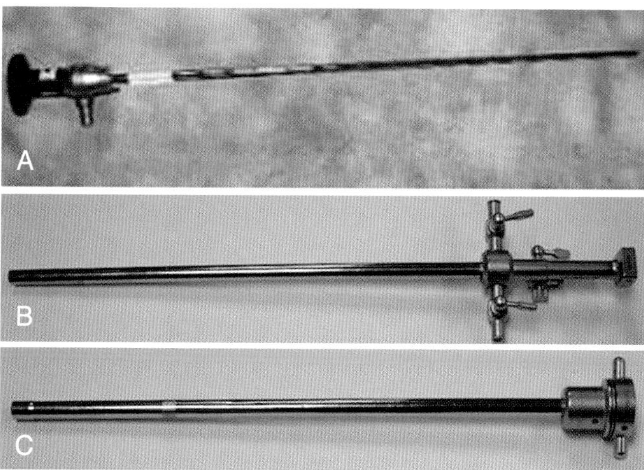

Figure 156-1 Full resectoscope kit. **A,** Hysteroscope. **B,** Operating sheath. **C,** Continuous-flow sheath.

- Vaginal bivalve speculum
- Antiseptic solution
- Lidocaine 1% with 10-mL syringe and 4-inch needle extender, 25-gauge needles *(optional)*
- Light source
- Uterine distention system (CO_2 or fluid) for hysteroscopy-based systems (see Chapter 140, Hysteroscopy)
- Energy source and ablative attachments (laser or cautery, thermal balloon, and cryosurgical ablation techniques do not require these components)
- Video camera and display monitor for hysteroscopy-based systems

Precautions

Endometrial ablation does not exclude the possible future development of endometrial cancer or pregnancy. Although the risks of these are low, patients should be made aware of this before undergoing the procedure. If a patient is on estrogen therapy after endometrial ablation, progestin supplementation is still necessary to prevent the development of atypical endometrium.

If the patient is still of childbearing age and pregnancy is a distinct although distant possibility, contraceptive measures should be taken to ensure pregnancy is prevented.

Preprocedure Patient Education and Forms

Endometrial ablation is such a life-altering procedure that it is the surgeon's obligation to provide the patient with all of the information needed to understand all of the possible outcomes (see the example patient education form online at www.expertconsult.com). Some key elements of discussion are to emphasize that ablation *may* induce sterility but does not guarantee that pregnancy will not occur. Another element is that sexual desire should not be affected by the procedure. Because the endometrium is the only focus of treatment, and not the ovaries, hormonal cycles will continue if the patient is premenopausal.

Preprocedure Patient Preparation

- In most instances, the patient will have already had *endometrial sampling* performed in the investigation of her abnormal bleeding. If this has not been done, endometrial sampling should be performed in advance of the procedure to verify the absence of malignant or premalignant lesions.
- Screening for cervical cancer *(Pap smear)* should also be up to date.
- *Pregnancy should be excluded* at the time of the procedure.
- Preoperative *ultrasonography* is helpful to ascertain the endometrial thickness and assess the uterine anatomy. *The ideal thickness of the endometrium for ablation is less than 3 to 4 mm.* There are several ways to reach this goal:
  - *Physiologically, the late menstrual or early proliferative phase of the* cycle will provide the ideal setting for proceeding without the use of pharmacologic agents.
  - Another simple approach would be to perform the ablation immediately after curettage.
  - To produce an atrophic, thin endometrium before the surgery, pharmacologic agents may be used. This will allow for more efficient ablation and lessen bleeding to decrease postoperative anemia. Agents available are either antiestrogenics such as danazol (600 to 800 mg daily for 3 to 12 weeks) or gonadotropin-releasing hormone (GnRH) agonists such as leuprolide acetate (two 3.75-mg intramuscular injections administered 3 to 4 weeks before surgery) or goserelin (3.6 mg injected subcutaneously 3 to 4 weeks before surgery). Pharmacologic preparation is not required with use of the NovaSure.
- Laminaria tent placement the day before the procedure will enhance cervical dilation. However, care must be taken to limit cervical dilation owing to concerns regarding the seal that the cervix can provide during the procedure, as in the case of the hydrothermablation procedure or the NovaSure.
- Antibiotic prophylaxis is unnecessary in most cases.

Preoperative preparation in this manner can decrease surgical time, lessen fluid absorption, and improve safety and surgical outcome for the patient.

Appropriate anesthesia for these procedures varies with the procedure, patient, physician, and clinical setting. Paracervical block, sedation, regional anesthesia, general anesthesia, or a combination of these should be considered.

Procedure

The following descriptions summarize the procedures in the most succinct manner. However, the focus is on the more contemporary techniques, with as much detail as possible. Inclusion of the rollerball and laser ablation is of more historical rather than practical value given the advent of the more contemporary ablative techniques. Some of the new-generation techniques for endometrial ablation do not require the use of the hysteroscope and are termed *minimally invasive nonhysteroscopic methods for endometrial ablation*. Discussion of long-term success rates regarding issues such as amenorrhea, patient satisfaction, and the eventual need for hysterectomy is well covered in the references provided in the Bibliography.

Anesthesia

The anesthesia provided for the rollerball and laser procedures is usually general anesthesia, but with the new procedural approaches, paracervical block along with oral analgesics may be all that is required to effect adequate clinical comfort. The paracervical block is used in several of the new techniques (see Chapter 173, Paracervical Block).

Technique of Hysteroscopic Endometrial Ablation with Rollerball

A rigid (0-, 12-, or 30-degree viewing angle) hysteroscopic resectoscope (see Fig. 156-1) is necessary for this procedure.

The objective of this procedure is to ablate the basal layer of the endometrium as well as the first few millimeters of the myometrium in order to ensure endometrial destruction. The first pass of the rollerball ablates to a depth of approximately 3 mm, exposing the base of the endometrial glands. The second pass ablates 2 to 3 mm of myometrium.

For the surgeon to adequately visualize the entire uterine cavity, it must be distended with liquid. Operative hysteroscopy usually uses a low-viscosity medium that continuously flows into and out of the uterus, clearing out surgical debris and blood and improving the surgeon's field of view. An inflow pressure of 80 to 110 mm Hg ensures optimal distention and continuous irrigation. An automated irrigation delivery system may be used, or a bag of distending medium is hung 1 m above the patient and produces distention through gravity. Distention media used during endometrial ablation include hypotonic agents such as glycine (1.5%), sorbitol (3%), or mannitol; isotonic agents such as normal saline; or the high-viscosity agent, dextran 70 (a viscous solution of 32% dextrose). Infused and collected fluid volumes are measured every 5 minutes, and consideration should be given to terminating the procedure if the fluid accumulation exceeds 1 to 1.5 L.

Procedure

Under sterile conditions, perform a standard bimanual pelvic examination to ascertain uterine position.

1. Insert bivalve speculum to expose the the cervix. Another alternative would be to place a weighted speculum in the posterior vaginal cavity and use an anterior retractor to expose the cervix, thus maximizing exposure of the cervix.
2. Grasp anterior lip of cervix with fine-tooth tenaculum.
3. Gently sound the uterus with a uterine sound. The tenaculum can be used to provide uterine stability.
4. Use Hegar dilators to gradually dilate the cervix (usually 8 to 12 mm to provide enough width to advance the resectoscope component of the hysteroscope). Also be careful to not overdilate the cervix because this may induce leakage of distention media, thus limiting the view. If this does occur, a fine-tooth tenaculum may be used to approximate the loose cervical edges.
5. Assemble the resectoscope, making sure the advance and retraction capability is in order. (There is a paradoxical mechanism in all resectoscopes. Pulling the trigger advances the rollerball and gently relaxing pressure retracts the rollerball. The pushing and pulling of the trigger creates the extension/retraction of the rollerball, which effects the rowlike destruction of the endometrium. The rollerball is a spherical or barrel-shaped electrode that rolls over the endometrium at a speed of 10 to 15 mm/sec [Fig. 156-2]).
6. Insert the resectoscope by gentle advancement under direct visualization, following the lumen, with the irrigating fluid flowing (very similar to advancing a rigid sigmoidoscope).
7. Identify landmarks (bilateral tubal ostia and fundal area; see Chapter 140, Hysteroscopy).
8. Gently advance the rollerball by pulling the trigger until it approximates the proximal segment of the internal os. About 1.5 cm below (distal to) the internal os, set the end-point line of demarcation for ablation. Cauterize the entire circumference of this area by placing the rollerball directly on the segment by gently maneuvering the resectoscope. This creates a ringlike area of destruction that marks the eventual end point for the rollerball retraction.
9. Activate the cautery source by the foot pedal, set to a coagulating power of 50 to 80 W. There are differing viewpoints on the average power. Some operators use up to 200 W. There are also recommendations to start at 60 W to destroy the endometrial tissue for the first layer of endometrial destruction, followed by an increase to 80 to 100 W for subsequent passes. Visualize the entire distended uterine fundus and then start ablating the fundus by contacting the rollerball with the fundal tissue in a right-to-left manner. When performing ablation on the fundus, the rollerball is extended to near its maximum. The rollerball "paints" the fundus in a right-to-left manner in rows until the fundal area is entirely ablated. The ostia are handled in a similar fashion. However, because the ostial area is spherical, the rollerball must be rotated within the resectoscope to contact the tissue, consistent with the anatomy being ablated. After the line of demarcation has been established at the internal os, the corpus is ablated with the rollerball fully extended, starting at the fundus at around 6 o'clock. Advance the rollerball to the fundus to ablate the entire fundal and periostial area. Gently advance the rollerball to full or nearly full extension to the fundus, then retract in a linear fashion while activating the energy source to destroy the endometrium. A count of "one thousand one, one thousand two, one thousand three" should be used to effect a subjective but fairly accurate time for contact of the rollerball with the tissue during the ablation process. Continue this in a row-by-row fashion, destroying 360 degrees around the entire endometrial cavity two to three times, ending once again at 6 o'clock position.
10. On completion of the procedure, check the fluid balance to confirm minimal risk of postoperative fluid overload.
11. Remove all instruments and transport the patient to recovery.

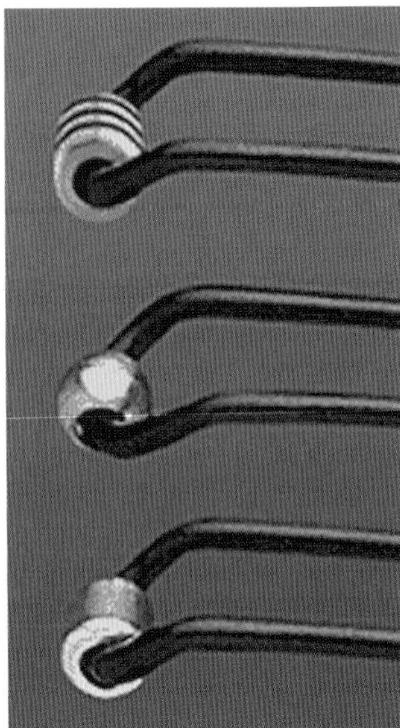

Figure 156-2 Examples of rollerball ablation probes.

Common Errors

- Equipment malfunction or poor assemblage of the equipment
- Poor endometrial preparation resulting in less than optimal long-term outcomes
- Fluid leakage resulting in inaccurate fluid balance estimation

Complications

The media used to distend the uterine cavity during hysteroscopy can cause fluid overload, allergic reactions, and other toxic reactions. Fluid overload is associated with prolonged operating times and the use of high distending pressures.

- Absorption of excess amounts of hypotonic distending solution results in increased central venous pressure and hyponatremia that, if untreated, lead to pulmonary edema, hypotension, cerebral edema, and potentially fatal cardiovascular collapse. To avoid these complications, intraoperative fluid use must be strictly monitored during the procedure and the patient observed for signs and symptoms of fluid overload. Most physicians will stop a hysteroscopic procedure at a 1- to 1.5-L fluid deficit when using glycine, sorbitol, or mannitol to avoid hyponatremic hypovolemia. A lower threshold may be required for older patients or those with preexisting cardiovascular problems. Dextran 70 has been associated with fluid overload, pulmonary edema, intravascular coagulopathy, renal insufficiency or failure, rhabdomyolysis, and anaphylactoid reactions. Glycine can result in hyperammonemic encephalopathy and transient blurred vision and blindness.

- Mechanical complications include air embolism, cervical laceration, perforation of the uterus, and severe hemorrhage.
- Thermal damage to the bowel, although rare, may occur with rollerball or laser ablation.
- Endometrial cancer may persist if occult presence is not diagnosed before the ablation, making diagnosis afterward very difficult.
- Pregnancy, although rare, is possible. With a very thin posttreatment endometrium, there is a higher risk of ectopic pregnancy as well as poorly sustained placenta and embryonic implantation.
- Infection.

Postprocedure Management

Consideration should be given to the use of postoperative antiemetics and pain medication. Options for pain control include nonsteroidal anti-inflammatory drugs (NSAIDs), opiates, and acetaminophen. The patient should be instructed to have a return appointment at the surgeon's office within 1 to 2 weeks and be apprised of possible postoperative complications such as prolonged bleeding, vaginal discharge, infection, and abdominal discomfort.

Endometrial Laser Ablation

A resective hysteroscope with Nd:YAG laser attachment is necessary for this procedure.

Endometrial laser ablation is performed as an inpatient or outpatient procedure under general or regional anesthesia. A distention medium, usually normal saline, is delivered into the uterus by peristaltic pump, sphygmomanometer, or gravity, and uterine pressure is maintained between 80 and 100 mm Hg. The amount of medium is measured so that the development of fluid overload can be monitored. The Nd:YAG 600-μm fiber can produce 17,000 W/cm^2 at 60-W power when maximally focused. Characteristic front-scatter, coagulation, and bubbling occur during the process. A 1200-mm microfiber at same power will produce 4200 W/cm^2.

Procedure

1. Repeat steps 1 to 7 from the hysteroscopic rollerball ablation section, earlier.
2. The rigid hysteroscope is placed, and the endometrium is visualized. The laser attachment is placed through the operating channel of the hysteroscope and activated at a power level of approximately 60 to 80 W delivered by a 600-μm bare quartz fiber.
3. There are two techniques used for endometrial laser ablation, the touch or drag technique and the nontouch or blanching technique. During the *touch technique*, the laser tip is lightly applied to the endometrial surface and gently swept across the uterine cavity. For the *nontouch technique*, the laser tip is brought within 1 to 5 mm of the endometrial surface but does not touch it. Compared with the touch technique, this technique reduces the potential for fluid absorption because the blood and lymphatic vessels are coagulated as opposed to being cut open. Some physicians use a combination of the two techniques. Ablation begins at the cornual and fundal areas with the delivery of short, 5- to 10-second bursts of laser energy. The anterior wall is ablated to the level of the cervical os, followed by ablation of the lateral and posterior walls.
4. The Nd:YAG laser coagulates and denatures the endometrium to a depth of approximately 4 to 6 mm. As coagulation proceeds, tissue damage is minimized because the laser energy absorbed decreases and the amount reflected increases. Fluid balance is calculated every 5 minutes and intravenous (IV) furosemide is given if the fluid absorption exceeds 1500 mL. Endometrial laser ablation takes approximately 30 to 180 minutes. If the procedure is successful, postablation histologic study months later will reveal a single layer of simple cuboidal epithelium devoid of endometrial glands.
5. Remove all of the instruments and transport patient to recovery.

Common Errors

Potential errors are the same as for the rollerball technique.

Complications

Complications are the same as for the rollerball technique.

Postprocedure Management

Postprocedure management is the same as for the rollerball technique.

Thermal Balloon Ablation of the Endometrium

A 30-mL syringe, ThermaChoice III disposable kit, and generator are necessary for this procedure.

The ThermaChoice (Gynecare, Inc., Menlo Park, Calif) kit consists of a disposable balloon catheter with an outside diameter of 5 mm and a plastic catheter that connects the balloon catheter to the fluid line and the umbilical cable. The controller unit displays the temperature, pressure, and clock (time) as well as providing the base of connections for power and the umbilical cord to the catheter (Fig. 156-3). An excellent educational module is available that covers all aspects of the procedure in detail (available at www.interact3d.com/modules/).

Procedure

This procedure does not require the use of a hysteroscope as in the previously described techniques. This approach was the first of the newer minimally invasive nonhysteroscopic methods for endometrial ablation.

1. *Priming the catheter* with 15 mL of D_5W is the first step in the procedure. Fill the catheter with the balloon tip facing downward, keeping the catheter vertical until priming is complete and the catheter is full. Once the priming is finished, attach the syringe with D_5W to the catheter and inflate the balloon with 10 mL of D_5W to ensure its patency. Withdraw air bubbles and D_5W through the syringe until a negative pressure of 150 to 200 mm Hg is attained as noted on the monitor.
2. Repeat steps 1 to 3 from the hysteroscopic rollerball ablation section. The ThermaChoice is approved in the United States for ablation in uteri sounding from 4 to 10 cm, although it may be used in uteri sounding up to 12 cm.
3. A *paracervical block* is administered along with preoperative provision of long-acting NSAIDs to minimize patient discomfort. This procedure is routinely performed in the office setting, but it may also be performed in an operating suite. The choice of anesthesia will depend on patient–physician interaction.
4. *Sound the uterus, then insert the balloon catheter* into the cervix. The outer sheath measures 5 mm, which makes insertion relatively easy and usually obviates the need for cervical dilation.
5. *The catheter is filled with a small volume of sterile D_5W (usually 15 to 30 mL)* to conform to the shape of the uterus and until a balloon pressure of 160 to 180 mm Hg is identified on the ThermaChoice generator. Titration of the fluid volume will achieve the proper therapeutic pressures. Pressing the valve control button on the catheter adds or removes fluid to titrate the pressure. As the balloon enlarges, the endometrial cavity will relax

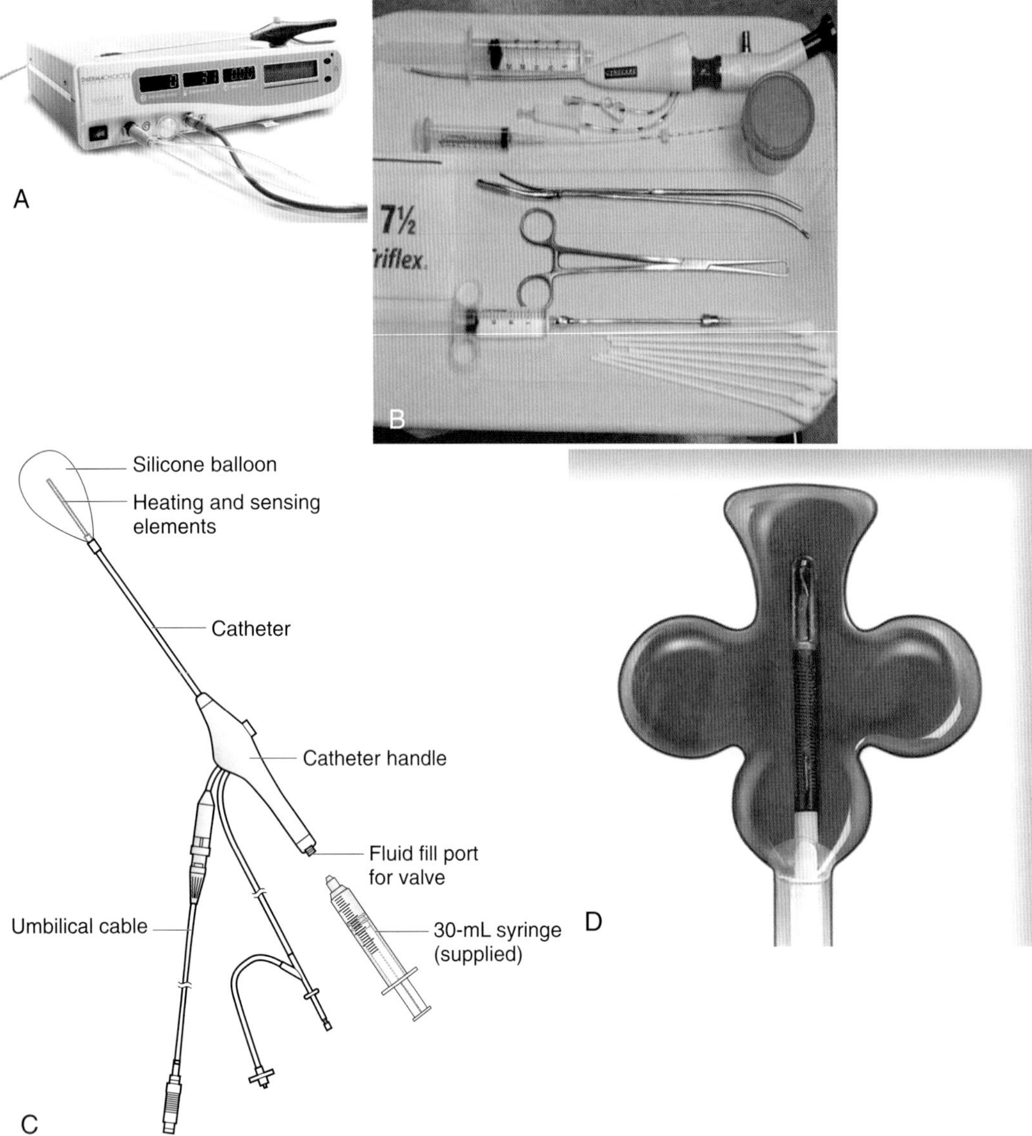

Figure 156-3 Gynecare ThermaChoice III Uterine Balloon Therapy System for performing thermal balloon ablation, with element tray and demonstration of balloon insufflation in a model uterine cavity. **A,** ThermaChoice III module. **B,** ThermaChoice surgical tray. **C,** ThermaChoice III device elements. **D,** ThermaChoice III device inflated in uterine model with abnormal cavity. (Courtesy of Ethicon, Inc., Somerville, NJ. Reproduced with permission.)

to accommodate the volume, causing a pressure reduction. Judicious addition of D_5W in small increments will likely be necessary to maintain proper balloon pressure.

6. After titration of pressure, *allow approximately 1 minute to pass before activating the ablation process by pressing the "Start" button*. There are integrated safeguards on the generator that assist the surgeon in avoiding or detecting some potential problems. If uterine *perforation* occurs during the balloon insufflation process, the pressure does not stabilize, thus rendering the start process inactive. Another cause of unstable pressure readings is a *leak* in the catheter, which should prompt the surgeon to reevaluate the integrity of the connections and the stability of the uterus. If the surgeon insufflates the balloon to a *pressure greater than 220 mm Hg*, the balloon may become damaged and rendered unusable by bursting a safety valve. The patient's safety is ensured with the ThermaChoice system in that there is no override process incorporated in the generator if there is any inclination to add more D_5W during the process or start the process without all of the elements for ignition in place.
7. After the start button has been activated safely, a *heating element located inside the balloon raises the temperature of the fluid to 87° C*. The time to reach the required temperature takes anywhere from 15 seconds to 4 minutes, but averages around 40 seconds. Once the balloon reaches the required temperature, thermal coagulation of 3 to 5 mm of the endometrium by heat transfer through the balloon occurs. It is important that the surgeon hold the catheter steady and in the center of the uterus during the 8-minute ablation process. A variance in uterine pressure is a not uncommon occurrence because of uterine relaxation. The controller connected to the catheter monitors and displays catheter pressure, regulates temperature, and controls therapy time until the process has been completed. It then *automatically shuts the unit off*. The balloon is then deflated and withdrawn from the uterus after a 1-minute cooling period. Very detailed demonstrations are available at the ThermaChoice website (www.interact3d.com/modules/).
8. Withdraw the tenaculum and speculum and disconnect all cords connected to the catheter. The entire procedure can be

performed in less than 1 hour on an outpatient basis if local anesthesia and IV sedation are used. Mild to moderate uterine cramping may occur during the first day postablation. Otherwise, recovery is usually uncomplicated. Vaginal discharge or spotting may occur during the first week. Patients generally resume normal activities within 24 hours of treatment.

Common Errors

- Improper assembly of unit and components
- Incomplete preoperative work-up
- Attempting to exceed the recommended 60 mL of fluid in the balloon
- Attempting to perform ThermaChoice ablation on a uterus sounding greater than the recommended 12 cm

Complications

Complications are rare and less common than with traditional endometrial ablative techniques. Possible adverse events include uterine perforation, fluid overload in the balloon, perforation of the balloon (rare), and the balloon compromising cervical integrity (cervical overload).

Postprocedure Management

Postoperative pain medications should be administered as needed, including NSAIDs, opiates, or acetaminophen. The patient should make a return appointment within 1 to 2 weeks and call if there are signs of fever, pain or infection, prolonged vaginal discharge, or bleeding. Normal activities can generally resume immediately; intercourse should be avoided for 2 weeks.

Radiofrequency (NovaSure) Ablation of the Endometrium

Equipment and Supplies

- NovaSure endometrial ablation device and radiofrequency controller
- Miller speculum (open sided)
- Hegar dilators in sizes up to 9 mm
- Dressing forceps
- Two single-tooth tenacula
- Uterine sound
- Paracervical block supplies (see Chapter 173, Paracervical Block)
- Optional instrumentation: 5.5-mm diagnostic hysteroscope, weighted speculum, Simms retractor, small Deaver retractor, 16-Fr straight catheter

Appropriate resuscitative equipment is necessary and varies depending on the setting and type of anesthesia administered.

Use of the NovaSure radiofrequency device (Cytyc Corporation, Marlborough, Mass) involves inserting a slender wand through the cervix (Figs. 156-4 to 156-6). A triangular, meshlike device (the electrode array) is then passed through the wand and expands to fit the uterus. Radiofrequency electrical energy is passed through it for about 90 seconds and the mesh and wand are then withdrawn. As with many other second-generation ablation techniques, it is quick and effective and does not require pretreatment to expand the uterus. The following description is as detailed as the procedural instructions given by the manufacturer. However, the manufacturer's website animation provides a superb simulation of the actual procedure (www.novasure.com/novasure-procedure/procedure-animation.cfm).

Procedure

1. Repeat steps 1 to 3 from the hysteroscopic rollerball ablation section.
2. Anesthetic administration is similar to that for the other second-generation techniques. It can be performed in the operating room under general anesthesia or with IV sedation with paracervical block. It can also be performed in the office with NSAIDs and a paracervical block.
3. Insert the untapered Hegar dilator until resistance is met at the internal os to measure *endocervical canal length.* Subtract this length from the original uterine sound length to obtain uterine cavity length. *This is a very crucial measurement.*
4. Diagnostic hysteroscopy is optional.
5. Squeeze the handles of the sterile NovaSure device into the locked position to open the mesh electrode array before inserting it into uterus to ensure that it deploys. Verify that the cornual width gauge found on the instrument is greater than 4 cm. On deployment of the device, the electrode array indicator light should no longer illuminate.
6. Unlock the device and retract the array into the protective sheath by pulling back the handle using the "bow and arrow" technique.
7. Adjust the cavity length (the total uterine cavity length on uterine sounding minus the cervical cavity length) using the length-adjusting feature on the handle of the device.
8. Dilate the cervix to 8 mm with tapered Hegar dilators.
9. Slide the cervical collar onto the sheath in its entirety. Insert the device into the cervix while holding the handle until the distal sheath reaches the fundus.
10. *Tap the fundus with the array* while slowly squeezing the handles, which deploys the electrode array inside the uterine cavity.
11. *Seat the device* by maneuvering it laterally, medially, anteriorly, and posteriorly, rotating it clockwise and counterclockwise. Pull the device backward until a decrease in value is noted on the cornual width gauge. Advance toward the fundus at this point. Repeat until maximum width is gained as demonstrated on the cornual width gauge. Input the width and length measurements

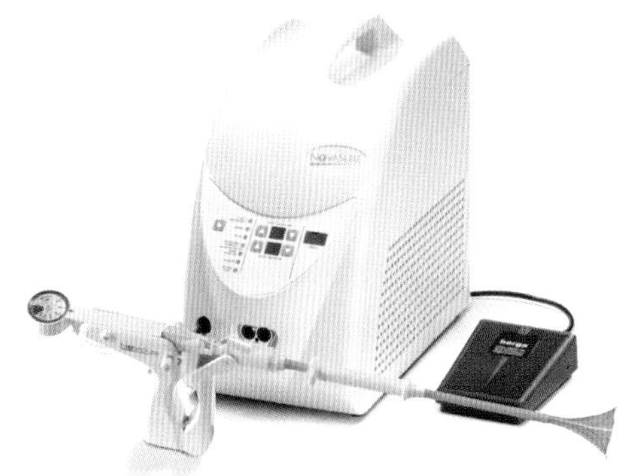

Figure 156-4 The NovaSure Controller. (Courtesy of Hologic, Inc., and affiliates, Marlborough, Mass.)

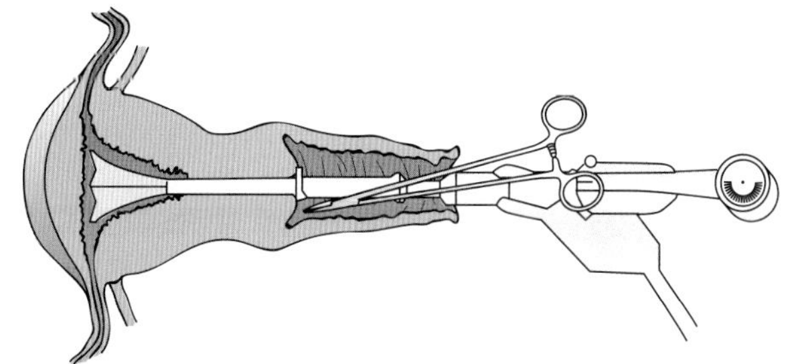

Figure 156-5 Fully expanded NovaSure device in vaginal cavity with fully expanded bipolar electrode in the uterine cavity. (Redrawn from Hologic, Inc., and affiliates, Marlborough, Mass.)

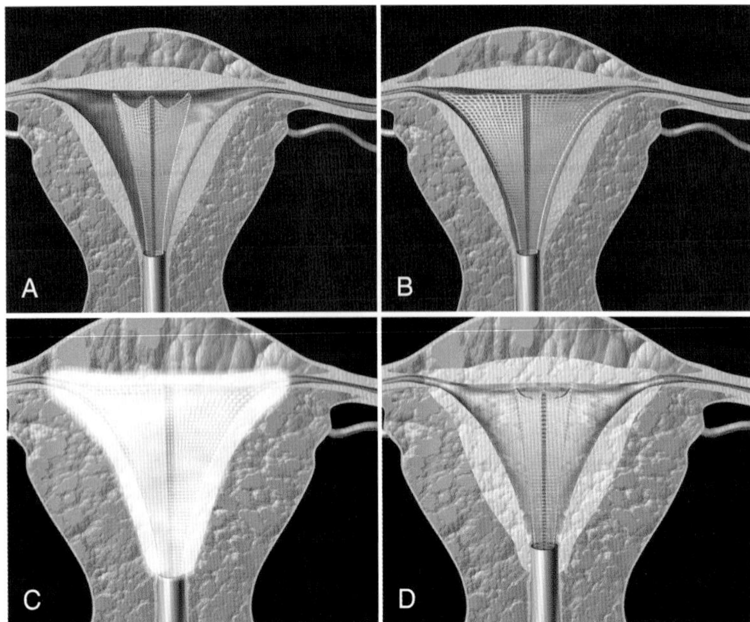

Figure 156-6 NovaSure procedure. **A,** Step 1: The NovaSure bipolar electrode expands from the slender sheath to conform to the contours of the uterine cavity. **B,** Step 2: The system insufflates the uterine cavity with CO_2 to perform the cavity integrity assessment. **C,** Step 3: NovaSure delivers bipolar radiofrequency energy for a complete and contoured ablation in approximately 90 seconds. **D,** Step 4: The electrode array is retracted into the sheath for easy removal, leaving the uterine lining desiccated down to the superficial myometrium. (Courtesy of Hologic, Inc., and affiliates, Marlborough, Mass.)

into the controller (the length is the total uterine cavity length on uterine sounding minus the cervical cavity length).

12. Use one hand to *stabilize the cervix* with the tenaculum while holding the device. Slide the cervical collar forward to create a seal.
13. *Assess the cavity integrity* by stabilizing the cervical collar, then stepping on the footswitch once to activate this function on the controller. Carbon dioxide is insufflated into the uterine cavity. When the uterine cavity is insufflated to 50 mm Hg for approximately 4 seconds, the control unit must recognize no evidence of perforation. The procedure cannot proceed if perforation is evident; there is no way to override the device.
14. Once the cavity integrity is established, the controller will signal that the ablation process is enabled. The operator then steps on the footswitch once to *activate the ablation cycle*. The cycle using radiofrequency power lasts at least 90 seconds and not over 2 minutes. The controller signals when the cycle is complete.
15. Remove the cervical sheath and retract the array carefully.
16. Remove all instruments and transport the patient to recovery.

Common Errors

- Deployment problems with the device due to improper patient selection
- Errors in connecting and setting up the equipment properly
- Improper interpretation of measurement data, thus prolonging procedural time

Complications

Perforation, thermal burns to adjacent tissue, prolonged bleeding, infection, prolonged pain (beyond the usual expected postoperative discomfort), pregnancy, and prolonged discharge are some of the most common complications encountered.

Postprocedure Management

The usual analgesics of the surgeon's choice should be used. These include NSAIDs, opiates, and acetaminophen. There will be a vaginal discharge for 3 to 6 weeks. Uterine cramping will likely occur. The patient should return for a reevaluation appointment in 2 weeks and for possible complications such as prolonged bleeding, pain, fever, or septic symptoms such as fever and tachycardia.

Cryoablation of the Endometrium

The Her Option Cryoablation System (American Medical Systems, Inc., Minnetonka, Minn) is another minimally invasive nonhysteroscopic method for endometrial ablation.

Cryoablation of the endometrium destroys tissue by the application of extreme cold through the use of the gas-cooled cryoprobe. Its operation is based on the Joule-Thomson principle, in which pressurized gas is expanded through a small orifice to produce cooling. Temperatures of −100° C to −120° C are achieved at the tip, producing an ice ball. As this ice ball grows, tissue that comes into contact with the portion of the ice ball that is −20° C or colder is destroyed. Activation of the cooling process initiates efflux of gas through the cryoprobe; it expands at low pressure at the tip of the cryoprobe, causing an abrupt drop in temperature and freezing of the endometrium. The gas then is transported back to the compressor for recirculation.

A recently completed study directed by the FDA demonstrated the safety and effectiveness of the cryoablation system in controlling abnormal uterine bleeding. Cryoablation was found to be as effective as rollerball ablation, but is much easier to learn and causes less significant side effects. It is safer than rollerball ablation because it does not require distention of the uterus or the use of large amounts of fluid necessary with operative hysteroscopy. Moreover, cryoablation requires minimal anesthesia and can be performed in a physician's office, although the surgical suite is still an option if dictated by clinical circumstances.

The work-up and preparation of a patient for a cryoablation procedure is similar to that for rollerball ablation, except that all patients *must have an ultrasonographic examination* performed to determine whether they have endometrial polyps or myomas. If submucous fibroids or polyps are found in the uterine cavity, the tissue should be sampled to rule out a premalignant or malignant process. This is accomplished by hysteroscopy and D&C. If the submucous myomas are greater than 3 cm in diameter or extend over halfway into the uterine cavity, the patient is not a good candidate for cryoablation. This is because the depth of tissue destruction is characteristically 9 to 15 mm. In this case, the resectoscope should be considered to remove the myomas before ablation. Pretreatment with a GnRH agonist is not necessary. Tutorial materials and an excellent training video can be accessed online at www.heroption.com.

Equipment and Supplies

The Her Option self-contained control console comes with an attached, slim 5-mm disposable cryoprobe with two-button control (Control Unit [CU]). The console also provides an audio-guided, step-by-step tutorial. A 3-L bag of 0.9% saline, a catheter that inserts into the machine, and a portable ultrasonography unit are also required.

Procedure

1. Repeat steps 1 to 3 from the hysteroscopic rollerball ablation section.
2. Provide the appropriate anesthetic. (This procedure may involve less pain because of the cryoanesthesia conferred by the instrument and procedure.)
3. Once the anesthetic is administered, a Foley catheter is inserted to *instill 300 to 400 mL of saline into the bladder* to facilitate ultrasonographic visualization of the uterus during the procedure.
4. *Place the disposable CU over the cryoprobe.* It is provided sterile, for single use only. A fuse in the disposable CU prevents function of the system if reuse is attempted. The "heat" button is used at the end of the each freeze cycle to thaw the probe away from the tissue for the next freeze cycle.
5. Dilate the cervix to 5.5 mm to accept the cryoprobe.
6. Gently insert the cryoprobe into the uterine cavity (Fig. 156-7). The probe is provided with measurement markers enabling the surgeon to measure the uterine cavity. Confirm successful cannulation with ultrasonography.
7. Aim the CU toward one of the cornua and *inject 5 mL of saline into the uterus* through the accessory port on the cryoprobe. This will help to effect optimal tissue adherence to the cryoprobe during the freezing process.
8. *Active freezing* is initiated by pressing the "freeze" button on the CU (Fig. 156-8). Freezing continues until the user presses the freeze button again to pause freezing (freeze time will stop counting and resume when the user presses the freeze button again) or presses the heat button to begin heating, or until the safety time limit of 10 minutes is reached. The user presses the heat button to terminate the freeze. The heater cycles automatically to maintain a temperature of 37° C on the probe surface until the user pushes the freeze button again to complete a second freeze cycle.
9. The cornua are subjected to cryoablation first, with the process taking 4 to 6 minutes for each (Fig. 156-9). *After the first cornu is finished, ultrasonography may be used to ascertain the depth of cryoablation.* Ideally, the cryoablation process stops before the edge of the ice ball reaches the serosa. Ultrasonography also helps to assess the progress of the procedure and will help determine the number of passes required to effect successful ablation. Uterine size also determines the number of passes required. When the tip of the cryoprobe cools to a temperature of less than −90° C, an ice ball ellipse 3.5 to 5 cm in size forms around the probe. The edge of the ice ball is approximately 0° C and is nonlethal to the endometrial tissue. The lethal temperature for the tissue is −20° C and is found approximately 1.5 cm from the edge of the ice ball. Again, ultrasonography can be used to assess the characteristic changes in the tissue that denote adequate destruction. After satisfactory destruction of the tissue of the second cornu is completed, the heat button is pressed to pull the CU away from the destroyed endometrium. *The CU is then reactivated at the midline in the uterus in the same manner as for the cornua.* The ice ball is monitored by ultrasonography to assess destruction. Again, the procedure takes from 4 to 6 minutes, depending on the depth of destruction. Because there is no distention medium and saline is injected to effect maximal contact, both anterior and posterior components of the uterine cavity may be destroyed simultaneously. Examples of the varied options for passes made with the CU include (1) one freeze for 6 minutes in both cornua and one freeze for 6 minutes in the midline; (2) two freezes in both cornua for 6 minutes; (3) two freezes in both cornua for 6 minutes and two freezes in the midline for 4 minutes; and (4) one freeze in the midline for 4 minutes and two freezes in both cornua for 6 minutes. The number of variations depends on the anatomy and desired clinical outcome as defined by the surgeon and the ultrasonographic findings.
10. Once adequate tissue destruction is achieved, remove all instruments and transport the patient to recovery or allow recovery in the procedure suite.

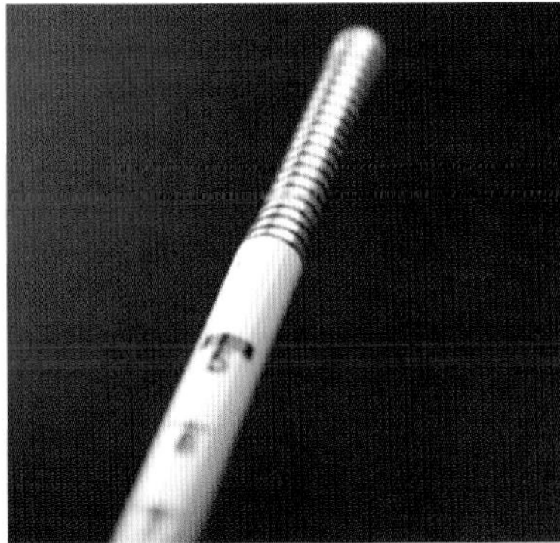

Figure 156-7 Her Option cryoprobe tip. (Courtesy of CooperSurgical, Inc., Trumball, Conn.)

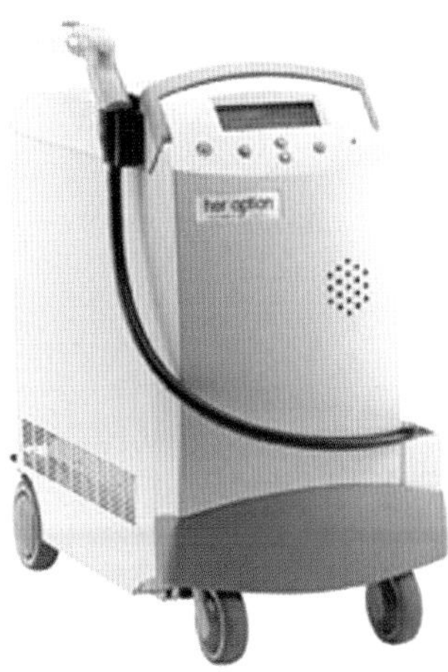

Figure 156-8 Her Option P30 module. (Courtesy of CooperSurgical, Inc., Trumball, Conn.)

Common Errors

- Inadequate assembly of equipment, thus delaying procedural start
- Operator error causing failure of equipment to perform as expected
- Insufficient freeze time to provide adequate cryoablation
- Inadequate destruction of fibroid tumors

Complications

Potential complications include adjacent tissue damage, perforation, prolonged bleeding, prolonged pain, and infection.

Postprocedure Management

Cryoablation usually does not cause a great deal of pain because of the nature of the destruction. However, if postoperative pain does present, the usual pain medications of the surgeon's choice should

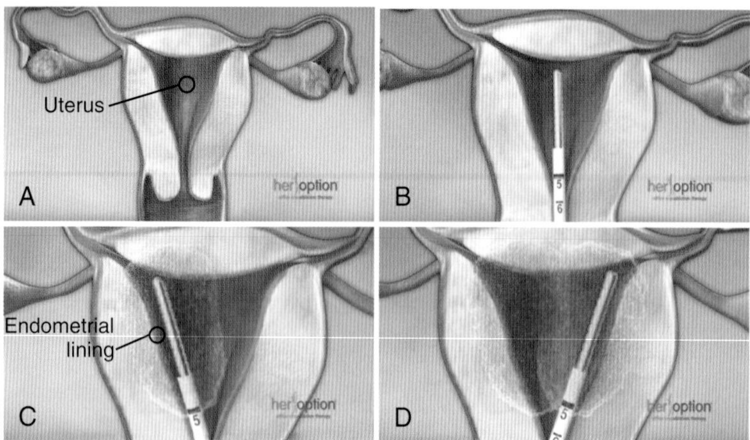

Figure 156-9 Stages of cryoablation. **A,** Uterus before cryoablation. **B,** Insertion of cryoprobe. **C,** Cryoablation of right cornua. **D,** Cryoablation of left cornua. (Courtesy of CooperSurgical, Inc., Trumball, Conn.)

be used. An NSAID, opiate, or acetaminophen is appropriate. A follow-up appointment should be scheduled for 1 to 2 weeks. The patient should be instructed to call in the event of prolonged postoperative bleeding, pain, fever, or infection.

Hydrothermablation

Equipment and Supplies

- *Hydrothermablation (HTA) control unit.* The control unit has a microprocessor that relays a series of instructions noted on the monitor for system setup as well as providing leakage alerts. The microprocessor also monitors fluid loss and alerts the operator if a loss of 10 mL is detected at any time during the setup or ablation procedure. The control unit uses room-temperature saline to purge air from the delivery system.
- *A 3-L bag of sterile 0.9% saline* is suspended from an IV pole connected to the control unit (ideally 115 cm above the uterus to ensure good outflow pressure).
- *A sterile procedure kit and an unsterile fluid management reservoir.* The one-use sterile procedure kit consists of a cassette assembly, heater canister, a disposable HTA sheath that connects to the hysteroscope, and fluid tubing. Some institutions use the heater canister 10 times, repackaging and resterilizing the unit and marking the number of sterilizations before each use and subsequent disposal.
- *A rigid hysteroscope* of the surgeon's choice is also needed (the 12-degree scope is the most versatile). If one uses the 30-degree scope, care must be taken to avoid aiming the end of the scope toward the wall of the uterine cavity so as not to traumatize the area.
- A silicone tip that creates the closed-loop circulation system when attached to the HTA sheath is also needed.

Procedure

1. Repeat steps 1 to 3 from the hysteroscopic rollerball ablation section.
2. With HTA, *it is essential that the cervix* **not** *be dilated greater than 8 mm.* It is also important *not* to use cervical dilating agents such as laminaria tents. If the cervix is dilated greater than 8 mm, the seal of the cervix around the sheath may be compromised, resulting in leakage. This may lead to thermal burns, which is a potential complication of this procedure.
3. Proceed with *paracervical block* (see Chapter 173, Paracervical Block).
4. *Remove the HTA sterile sheath from its pouch and connect it using appropriate adapters* (if needed) to the hysteroscope of choice. Be sure to use a hysteroscope with a diameter of less than 3 mm. This will ensure proper flow of the heated fluid from the HTA sheath.
5. Place the silicone tip attachment over the end of the sheath. This is crucial in maintaining the closed loop for circulating the heated fluid in and out of the uterus during the procedure.
6. Have an assistant *connect the inflow and outflow tubes to the pump mechanism* on the machine. Tips are color coded to ensure correct placement.
7. Press the start button. This commences the procedure, and the unit circulates saline through all of the tubing, eliminating any residual air. This takes approximately 1 minute; the main unit displays a counter until this portion of the process is complete.
8. During the countdown phase, *all tubing connections and the sheath should be checked* for leaks, and the light source and hysteroscope unit can be assembled in their entirety.
9. The circulation of the proper amount of saline at the proper pressure is ensured by *placing the bag of saline 115 cm (45 inches) above the patient's pelvic region.* This provides approximately 50 to 55 mg Hg intrauterine pressure, ample circulating pressure but below the tubal ostia opening pressure of 70 mm Hg. The circulating function begins with the pressure created by the height of the saline bag. The sheath functions as the circulating conduit for the saline. The HTA control unit functions as an aspiration pump, returning saline from the uterus to the reservoir and heater canister on the control unit for heating and reheating.
10. *Gently insert the hysteroscope sheath unit under direct visualization and with saline flowing into the intrauterine cavity.* This procedure requires an assistant to observe the ablation process and operate the ablation control unit. The intrauterine cavity is inspected at this point.
11. Once the cavity has been evaluated, *the hysteroscope–sheath unit is withdrawn to the level of the internal os to ensure the ablation treatment area remains in the uterine cavity and does not extend into the cervix.* A tight uterine seal is essential to avoid the potential complication of vaginal burns from leakage of fluid onto the vaginal mucosa. This can be effected by adding one or two tenacula to the cervix to tighten the seal.
12. *Commence the ablation process by starting the fluid warming cycle.* Once the fluid reaches 90° C (194° F; Fig. 156-10A), the ablation cycle begins as the microprocessor on the main unit is triggered. Ablation is performed under the surgeon's direct visualization until the approximately 10-minute cycle is completed. Tissue necrosis is usually appreciated to a depth of 2 to 4 mm after 10 minutes.
13. *After the ablation cycle has ended, the control unit triggers a 1-minute cooling cycle* to evacuate the superheated saline from the delivery system tubing. *This must be completed* before removing the hysteroscope–sheath unit from the cervix (Fig. 156-10B). Room-temperature saline flows into the uterus, which circulates the heated saline into the collection bag. When the cooling cycle

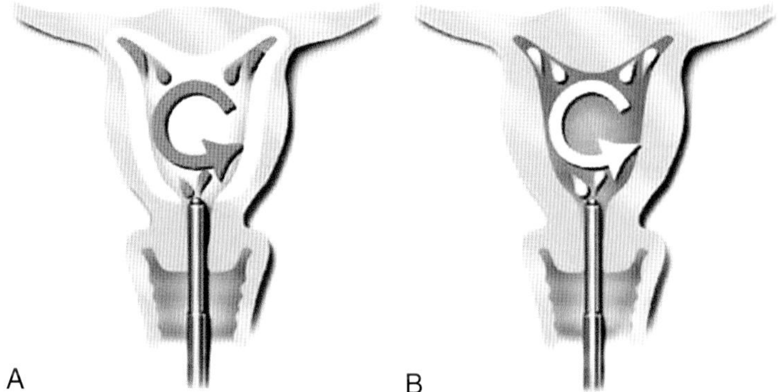

Figure 156-10 Hydrothermablation. **A,** Heating component of the ablative procedure. **B,** Cooling component of the ablative procedure, showing circulation of saline.

is complete, the control unit displays a message indicating safe conditions exist for removal of the sheath from the uterus and cervix. Again, this prevents efflux of superheated saline into the vaginal cavity with subsequent burns to the area.

14. Before disassembling the unit, the team must *wait for the entire system to cool down*. This includes the canister, tubing, cassette, heater, and reservoir. This is indicated by a message in the control unit when the temperature in the heater canister falls below 45° C.

Common Errors

- Improper assembly or construction of the system
- Inefficient dilation of the cervix
- Improper placement of IV tubing into the unit, thus decreasing saline pressure for HTA
- Hysteroscopy malfunction
- Improper cervical seal
- Removing the unit prematurely from the cervix before the cooling process is complete

Complications

Potential complications include thermal burns from leakage of fluid into the peritoneal or vaginal cavity, perforation, postoperative infection, vaginal discharge (greater than expected), and abdominal cramping longer than expected.

Postprocedure Management

Postprocedure management is the same as for thermal balloon ablation of the endometrium.

Microwave Endometrial Ablation

The Microsulis (Denmead, United Kingdom) microwave endometrial ablation (MEA) device was approved for use in the United States in 2003. It uses microwave energy at a frequency of 9.2 GHz, at which the microwave tissue-heating effect penetrates to less than 3 mm. Heat may be thermally conducted another 2 to 3 mm, creating a total depth of tissue destruction of 5 to 6 mm. The chosen frequency for MEA ablates the endometrium to the basal layer. Treatment of the entire uterine cavity is achieved by sweeping the applicator tip across the endometrial lining of the uterus. Microwaves are emitted from the distal end of the MEA applicator tip, providing controlled heat to the adjacent tissue. The process creates a hemispherical pattern of destruction at the applicator tip; because uterine tissue has a robust water content, this results in the reduction of the microwave field amplitude by approximately 90% 3 cm from the applicator tip. Destruction beyond this point of high-intensity heat still occurs by thermal conduction. Thus, endometrial destruction is achieved by direct and conductive heating effects. MEA treatment is fully adaptable to most sizes, shapes, and conditions of the uterine cavity. The thermocouple at the tip of the MEA applicator allows the operator to monitor and control localized temperatures, giving the most effective and maximal dispersion of microwave energy throughout the uterine cavity to achieve a complete ablation.

Prerequisites that need to be considered before proceeding with MEA include uterine cavity length less than 12 cm and uterine wall thickness greater than 12 mm. If present, fibroids in the uterine cavity should be less than 5 cm in diameter and must not obstruct the progress of the transcervical applicator. Repeat procedures are not recommended. Irregular cavities can be considered for treatment.

Equipment and Supplies

The Microsulis device is equipped with a disposable transcervical applicator connected to an ergonomic handle designed specifically for a "sweeping" technique. The controller system permits real-time information monitoring of localized temperatures from the thermocouple at the tip of applicator. A diagnostic hysteroscope of the surgeon's choice, with all of its attachments, is necessary.

Procedure

1. Repeat steps 1 to 4 of the hysteroscopic rollerball ablation section.
2. Proceed with *hysteroscopy* to ascertain/confirm positive or negative preoperative ultrasonographic findings. This will also help to ensure there are no perforations or anatomic obstructions that will obstruct probe placement in the uterine cavity.
3. *Insert the applicator to the midline of the fundus*. The applicator has centimeter markings on its side, enabling the surgeon to make sure the original uterine sounding measurement is the same as observed with the applicator. The microwave generator is activated by depressing the footswitch.
4. *Once the temperature reaches 70° C to 80° C, begin the sweeping motion* in the fundal region, starting in one cornu then moving to the opposite cornu. Then move the applicator downward through the rest of the uterine cavity. The ablative process is effected by microwave energy emitted from the tip of the device, where a thermocouple allows real-time temperature monitoring during the treatment process. A second sensor located at the base of the applicator provides a temperature gradient. The intraoperative temperature is displayed digitally on the control unit, which has a graphic band highlighting the 70° C to 80° C level. This enables the surgeon to monitor the process of effective ablation and prompts him or her to maneuver the applicator to maintain the temperature within the therapeutic band. It must be understood that endometrial destruction takes place even when temperatures are not ideal. The ideal 5- to 6-mm depth of destruction is not achieved with temperatures less than the indicated 70° C to 80° C range. The device is moved back and forth and gradually downward in a sweeping manner, as described. The temperature is observed on the system monitor. As the applicator is retracted further, a yellow marker 4 cm from the tip of the applicator wand helps to prevent treatment of the endocervical

canal, which could result in cervical stenosis. The usual time for the procedure is approximately 2 to 4 minutes and depends on uterine length and thickness.
5. The applicator is then withdrawn gradually from the uterine cavity.

Common Errors

Most errors are user related. Some of the more common issues include the following:

- Improper connection of the system parts
- Poor preoperative dilation of the cervix
- Triggering the procedure before the applicator is fully deployed
- Continuing with ablation past the yellow marker on retraction of the applicator, thus damaging the endocervical canal

Complications

The most common complications have been uterine perforation, serosal thermal injury to adjacent organs, and escape of thermal energy outside of the cervical canal. One of the best general preventive measures is to perform hysteroscopy before the procedure. This alerts the surgeon to any anatomic differences or anomalies that may increase the risk of complications during the ablation procedure.

The MEA system has safety mechanisms that help to prevent complications before the procedure starts. The system will prevent initiation of the procedure if the applicator insertion depth is greater than the original sounding measurement. An increase in the measured length of the applicator raises the concern of possible misplacement of the applicator in a perforation or commencement of the procedure before full insertion of the applicator in the uterine cavity.

The system also has a temperature alarm when the surface temperature of the applicator reaches 85° C. The system automatically shuts down if the temperature reaches 90° C.

Postprocedure Management

Postprocedure management is the same as for thermal balloon ablation of the endometrium.

Final Comments

Table 156-1 summarizes and compares the different second-generation techniques of endometrial ablation.

The procedure of endometrial ablation enables physicians to serve patients who have abnormal endometrial bleeding. It has evolved from a surgical suite procedure with the hysteroscope into a potentially office-based service that provides convenience, safety, and the avoidance of hysterectomy. The particular approach depends on the physician performing the procedure and his or her training, level of expertise, and comfort level with the service performed. Although the results from the newer procedures are similar to those with the traditional ablative techniques, complications are fewer and recovery is quicker with the newer methods.

Patient and Physician Education Guides

Each company listed in this chapter has its own brochure for physicians and patients. In addition, there may be descriptive instructional videos available. The company websites should be reviewed for examples.

CPT/Billing Codes

57800 Dilation of the cervical canal, instrumental (separate procedure)
58353 Endometrial ablation, thermal, without hysteroscopic guidance
58356 Endometrial cryoablation with ultrasonic guidance, including endometrial curettage, when performed
58555 Hysteroscopy, diagnostic (separate procedure)
58558 Hysteroscopy, surgical with sampling, with or without D&C
58561 Hysteroscopy with removal of leiomyomata
58563 Hysteroscopy, surgical; with endometrial ablation (e.g., endometrial resection or electrosurgical ablation or thermoablation)
59200 Laminaria insertion

ICD-9-CM Diagnostic Codes

626.2 Excessive or frequent menstruation, menometrorrhagia, menorrhagia
626.8 Dysfunctional uterine bleeding

Acknowledgment

The editors wish to recognize the many contributions by Duane E. Townsend, MD, to this chapter in the previous edition of this text.

Suppliers

(See contact information online at www.expertconsult.com.)

Bipolar cautery equipment/mesh
Cytyc Corporation (NovaSure)
Cryoablation
American Medical Systems
Hydrothermablation
Boston Scientific Corporate Headquarters
Microwave endometrial ablation
Microsulis
Rollerball endometrial ablation: The equipment required for rollerball endometrial ablation includes a standard urologic resectoscope, a video system, and an electrocautery system. The following companies manufacture these systems:
ACMI Circon
CooperSurgical
Karl Storz Endoscopy-America, Inc.
Olympus America Inc.
Richard Wolfe Medical Instruments Corp.
Thermal balloon
Gynecare, Inc. (Division of Ethicon, Inc.)

Bibliography

Agency for Health Care Policy and Research (AHCPR): Common Uterine Conditions: Options for Treatment. AHCPR publication no. 98-0003. Rockville, Md, U.S. Department of Health and Human Services, Public Health Service, Agency for Health Care Policy and Research, 1997.

American College of Obstetricians and Gynecologists (ACOG): Endometrial ablation: ACOG Practice Bulletin No. 81. Obstet Gynecol 109: 1233–1248, 2007.

Baggish MS, Valle RF, Guedj H: Hysteroscopy: Visual Perspectives of Uterine Anatomy, Physiology and Pathology. Philadelphia, Lippincott Williams & Wilkins, 2007.

Bongers MY, Bourdrez P, Willem B, et al: A prospective, double-blind, randomized, and controlled trial of two second-generation ablation devices, NovaSure GEA and ThermaChoice. J Am Assoc Gynecol Laparosc 8(3 Suppl): S5–S6, 2001.

Gurtcheff SE, Sharp HT: Complications associated with global endometrial ablation: The utility of the MAUDE Database. Obstet Gynecol 102:1278–1282, 2003.

Health Technology Advisory Committee—Minnesota: Surgical alternatives to hysterectomy for vaginal bleeding. Bethesda, Md, National Library of Medicine (US), National Center for Biotechnology Information, June 2000. Available at www.ncbi.nlm.nih.gov/bookshelf/br.fcgi?book=hsarchive&part=A3397.

Hill DA: Abnormal uterine bleeding: Avoid the rush to hysterectomy. J Fam Pract 58:136–142, 2009.
Lethaby A, Hickey M, Garry R, Penninx J: Endometrial resection/ablation techniques for heavy menstrual bleeding. Cochrane Database Syst Rev 4:CD001501, 2009.
Pasic R, Levine RL: A Practical Manual of Hysteroscopy and Endometrial Ablation Techniques. London, Taylor and Francis, 2004.
Sanfilippo JS (ed): Options in Endometrial Ablation. Supplement to OBG Management, December 2005. Available at www.obgmanagement.com/mededlibr/PDFs/1205Suppl_EA.pdf.
United States Food and Drug Administration: MAUDE: Manufacturer and user facility device experience. Available at http://www.accessdata.fda.gov/scripts/cdrh/cfdocs/cfMAUDE/TextSearch.cfm.
Weber AM: Endometrial ablation. Obstet Gynecol 99:969–970, 2002.

CHAPTER 157

Treatment of the Adult Victim of Sexual Assault

Olasunkanmi W. Adeyinka

Current statistics indicate that a sexual assault occurs every 4 seconds in this country. One in every four women will be sexually assaulted in her lifetime. But not only women are affected: almost 10% of assault victims are male. Sexual assault is the fastest-growing, most frequently committed, and most under-reported violent crime in the United States.

Sexual assault is under-reported for many reasons, including societal misconceptions about the victims of sexual assault, feelings invoked by such an assault, and the burden of reporting an assault. Misconceptions persist, despite enhanced public education, that individuals who are assaulted may have encouraged the act by their behavior, dress, lack of resistance, or previous promiscuity. Complex law enforcement and health care systems are often perceived as being impersonal and nonsupportive. An estimated 75% of victims know their perpetrators, possibly enhancing feelings of embarrassment, guilt, and fear of retribution. These feelings and misconceptions combined with inadequate support systems often prevent a victim from reporting a sexual assault.

The purpose of the medical evaluation after sexual assault is to assess the patient for physical injuries or possible disease, to document injuries, and to collect the necessary evidence. The remainder of the encounter should be used to treat any injuries, to prevent pregnancy and disease, and to find the proper support services for the victim. The examination and treatment should be completed as soon as possible after the assault, especially the collection of evidence. Although an evaluation within 48 hours is preferred, victims are encouraged to see a clinician even if more than 72 hours have elapsed (this still allows a clinician to treat and prevent many problems).

Collaboration between hospitals, community services, and local law enforcement agencies for the establishment of protocols is very helpful, and such protocols will ease victims' pain and suffering. Primary care clinicians can be instrumental in ensuring that this collaboration takes place. Such collaboration is effective at not only streamlining the evaluation process but for easing the burden of reporting. Some institutions offer 24-hour availability of specially trained and experienced volunteers, such as a nurse on every shift. These volunteers can provide the victim continuous support during the cumbersome process of answering questions and the examination. They can also act as witnesses for the chain of evidence. A supportive volunteer system can offer such simple things as a change of clothing (victims often need to leave their clothing as evidence), which are hugely appreciated by victims.

Indication

Sexual assault requires treatment.

NOTE: Sexual assault is any form of nonconsenting sexual activity. It encompasses all unwanted sexual acts, from fondling to forcible penetration.

Contraindication

A lack of patient consent contraindicates treatment.

Equipment and Supplies

- Camera and film
- Wood's light or other high wavelength light
- Sexual assault kit: Most emergency departments have a standard kit that contains a protocol for care and all the necessary specimen containers. These should be in compliance with and fulfill state laws for sexual assault (Table 157-1). In general, kits should contain the following:
  - Information for the victim
  - Consent form for the examination
  - Instructions, checklist, and chain of custody form
  - History and physical examination forms
  - Diagrams for use in documentation of injuries (Fig. 157-1)
  - Specimen containers, equipment, and labels
- Colposcope *(optional)*

Preprocedure Patient Education

If a patient calls before presenting to the emergency department, first make sure that the patient is safe. If not, encourage the patient to call the police. Next, encourage the patient not to take a bath or remove the clothing worn during the assault. If possible, they should postpone urinating, defecating, brushing their teeth, or drinking anything until samples are collected. Also, ask them to bring a change of clothing. Patients should sign for informed consent before starting the evaluation (see the patient consent form available online at www.expertconsult.com).

Explain the process of the evaluation to patients. Let them know that you will explain every step of the examination before performing it. Even if they may not want to report the assault, a very thorough examination is necessary in case of a later change of mind. Continue to reassure patients that they are safe and that someone else will always be in the room to comfort them during the evaluation.

Procedure

1. Open the sexual assault kit. Once the kit is opened, the chain of evidence must be maintained and evidence must not be left unattended. Signatures of those in attendance must be documented on the form for any and all evidence collected. (See Chapter 158, Management of the Young Female as a Possible Victim of Sexual Abuse, Fig. 158-8, for a sample chain of evidence form.) The kit should be labeled as a biohazard. After the patient has signed the consent form, proceed with taking the history.

TABLE 157-1 Sexual Assault Kit Equipment*

Contents	Purpose
Two urine containers	Urine for microscopic urinalysis, pregnancy test, and drug screen
Fingernail clippers, file, and envelope	Fingernail clippings and scrapings
Forceps, scissors, two envelopes	Pubic hair trimming in one envelope, head hair trimming in other envelope
Plastic comb, large paper towel, two envelopes	Pubic hair combing in one envelope, head hair combing in other envelope
Vaginal speculum, aspiration pipette, red-topped test tube and stopper	Aspiration of vaginal contents
Four cotton-tipped swabs and a test tube or envelope, one slide	Vaginal (or penile) swabbing, and smear (same for rectal swabbing and smear if indicated)
Saline, 10 mL; two aspiration pipettes and bulbs; two test tubes, two slides	Vaginal washing (and rectal if indicated using second pipette and test tube)
Cervical scraper, brush, slides, Pap smear fixative	Pap smear
Thayer-Martin plates and *Chlamydia* cultures and/or sample tubes for gonorrhea/*Chlamydia* enzymatic probes	Gonorrhea and *Chlamydia* evaluation (positive cultures are the gold standard for court, but probes have greater sensitivity)
Four cotton-tipped swabs and a test tube or envelope, one slide	Oral swabs and smear
Two cotton-tipped swabs and a test tube or envelope	Saliva collection for secretor status
Three red-topped test tubes and stoppers, tourniquet, nonalcohol swab to prepare skin, syringe and needle	Blood samples
Labeled paper bags	Collection of clothing and dried body fluids
Necessary and helpful forms Patient education handout Consent form History and physical examination form Diagrams for documentation of injuries Chain of custody form Any necessary instructions Checklist	Information, consent, and documentation

*Contents should be refrigerated after collection.

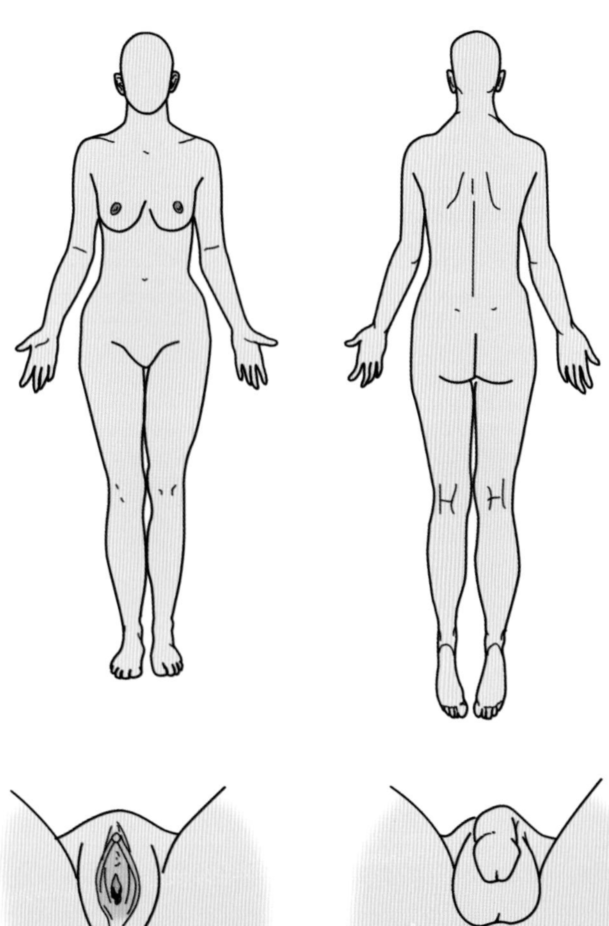

Figure 157-1 **Traumagram. Mark and label locations where there is evidence of trauma.** (From Botasch AS, Braen GR, Gilchrist VJ: Acute care for sexual assault victims. Patient Care 28:112–137, 1994. Copyright Marcia Hartsock, Artist.)

History

2. The history should be taken in a quiet room, with a witness present, after the patient has been assured that she or he is safe. Be cautious about the terms used in stating patient complaints. Avoid use of the word "rape" because this is a legal term. Instead, state the patient complaint as being a "sexual assault." Also, try to avoid the phrases "why didn't you ..." or "you shouldn't have ..." or "Did you do anything to lead them on?" In fact, try to avoid the words "why" and "alleged" altogether; "why" implies blame and "alleged" implies disbelief.

   Questions should be directed to the victim in a nonjudgmental way, and the patient should be allowed to talk about the assault at a comfortable pace, using her or his own words. It is important to observe nonverbal communication that may indicate a need for further questioning. Supportive terms worth using include "I'm glad you're alive," "You did what you needed to survive," "I'm sorry this happened to you," and "It was not your fault." Allow the victim to express her or his feelings. To build rapport, it may be worth obtaining the medical and sexual history before obtaining the assault history.

NOTE: If you have a long-term relationship with the patient, the patient may prefer to be examined in your office. However, in many jurisdictions, legally admissible evidence of a sexual assault cannot be collected without using the kit and other resources that are often available only in the emergency department. It is important for practitioners to know the assault and rape laws in their state so that they can comply with any legal requirements.

Medical and Sexual History (Gynecologic History for Women)

- Medical disease, if present, should be documented.
- Last voluntary sexual encounter up to 1 week before the assault and the race of that individual should be documented. If the encounter is less than 48 hours ago, blood and fluid samples may be requested from that individual at a later date.
- The victim's alcohol and drug intake should be documented.
- For women, the date of the victim's last menstrual period, her contraceptive use, pregnancy history, use of tampons, and any previous episode of gynecologic infection or pelvic surgery should be documented.

Assault History

An accurate but brief description of the assault is crucial for proper collection and analysis of the physical evidence. This includes documenting the following:

- Age and identifying information for victim, and assailant(s), if available.
- Date, time, and location of the alleged assault.
- Details of sexual contact, such as actual or attempted oral, rectal, or vaginal penetration of the victim. Attempt to determine whether there was an ejaculation, digital penetration, or penetration with foreign objects. It should be documented whether a tampon was present, or if a lubricant, contraceptive foam, a spermicide, or a condom was used. If any of these are unknown, that should be documented.
- Type of physical restraints used, if any, and whether there were any threats, weapons, drugs, or alcohol involved. Was the assailant injured during the assault?
- Activities of the victim after the assault, such as changing clothes, wiping, washing, bathing, douching, dental hygiene, urination, vomiting, smoking, eating, drinking, or defecation.

Physical Examination

3. Having a trained, experienced volunteer in the room in addition to the nurse may help distract the victim from her or his emotional and physical pain during the examination. The physical examination and collection of evidence are performed congruently. Carefully examine the entire body and photograph or make drawings of the injured areas (see Fig. 157-1). The clinician should search for bruises, abrasions, or lacerations about the head, neck, back, buttocks, and extremities. A victim who was choked may have petechiae on the face and conjunctiva. Physical trauma may be greater in sexually assaulted men, perhaps because only those who have been more seriously injured are likely to report the crime.
4. Examine the oral cavity. Broken teeth, a torn frenulum of the tongue or lip, or pharyngeal trauma may indicate that the mouth was forced open. Using two swabs simultaneously, swab the oral cavity and along the teeth for evidence of semen. Do not moisten the swabs before sample collection.

   Repeat with two additional swabs. Prepare one smear on the slide by gently smearing the swabs over the surface. Allow the swabs and smear to air dry. Place swabs in envelope or test tube provided.
5. The victim's clothing should be collected and placed in a paper bag that is sealed and signed. Allow any wet clothing to air dry before packaging. If additional bags are needed, use only new paper (grocery-type) bags.

   It may be helpful to photograph the patient before she or he disrobes. Semen may appear as flaking, crusty stains on clothing and will fluoresce under a high wavelength light. Have the patient disrobe while standing on paper from the examination table. Each item of clothing should be placed in a separate paper bag. Do not use plastic bags for clothing collection because they promote bacterial growth on blood or semen. Use gloves when touching the victim's clothes to avoid contaminating the evidence with your DNA or blood type from sweat.
6. For women, a pelvic examination should be performed to complete the physical examination. Lesions around the vulva or rectum may be present because of trauma from a hand, penis, or other foreign body. Superficial or extensive lacerations of the hymen and vagina, injury of the urethra, and, occasionally, rupture of the vaginal wall may be present. Swab and preserve any semen for later DNA analysis. Although historically recommended and still used in many locations, a Wood's lamp does not cause semen to fluoresce more than other commonly found substances. Alternative light sources with a higher wavelength may be more effective than the traditional Wood's lamp. The procedure is as follows:
   - Lubricate the speculum with water. Standard lubricants may adversely affect the results of the acid phosphatase test and alter sperm motility. Examine the vaginal wall and cervix for abrasions, ecchymoses, and lacerations. A colposcope may be helpful to document any microtrauma to the cervix or vagina. It can also be used to take photographs. The cervix should be swabbed and cultures and probes sent for gonorrhea and chlamydial infection. Four swabs should be used and a smear prepared in a manner similar to the oral swabs. The swabs should be allowed to air dry before sealing.
   - A Pap smear should be performed. Intact spermatozoa may be seen several days later on a Pap smear.
   - Any fluid from the posterior fornix should be aspirated and examined under the microscope. A sample of the aspirated fluid should be saved for DNA testing, as well as for testing for acid phosphatase and blood group antigens.
   - If no secretions are visible, a small amount of saline (about 5 mL) may be used to lavage the cervix and posterior fornix. Aspirate this fluid and save while using some to prepare slides. Examine the slides under the microscope for spermatozoa. Lavage with normal saline may enhance motility of spermatozoa for up to 2 hours. Motile sperm from the vagina imply intercourse within the past 6 hours (rarely within the past 12 hours) and their presence should be documented.

Immotile sperm imply intercourse within the past 12 to 18 hours (in rare cases, up to 24 hours). In addition to examining for spermatozoa with a wet smear, the slide should be examined for *Trichomonas*, bacterial vaginosis, and the presence of any *Candida* species.

7. The victim's pubic hair should be combed to detect foreign bodies, as well as for perpetrator pubic hair samples. If present, 15 to 20 perpetrator hairs should be collected as part of the evidence. In a separate container, 15 to 20 of the victim's trimmed pubic hairs should be saved. This process should be repeated for head hair, using separate specimen containers.
8. Bimanual and rectal examinations should be performed. Anal assault is more common in men. Look for erythema, edema, bleeding, mucosal tears, fissures, a hematoma, or sphincter laxity or spasm. The digital rectal examination is usually sufficient if nothing suspect is palpated and bleeding is absent or insignificant.
9. Anoscopy or proctoscopy are difficult for the patient, but may be required if you suspect a tear. The rectal area should be swabbed for *Chlamydia*. If anal intercourse is known to have occurred, four anal swabs should be used and a smear prepared in a manner similar to the oral swabs. Anal swabs can be moistened with sterile normal saline before using, if necessary. They should be allowed to air dry before sealing. (Penile swabs and smears can be performed in the same manner by swabbing the outside of the penile shaft.)

   Next, wash the rectal vault with 5 to 10 mL of normal saline introduced through the anus with the hub of a syringe. Allow the saline to stand for 5 to 10 minutes, then aspirate and preserve as evidence. These samples can be examined for motile sperm, immotile sperm, and acid phosphatase. Fecal contamination precludes their use for blood group antigen analysis.

NOTE: Pelvic, rectal, and proctoscopic examinations should be done gently and with careful explanation because the victim not only may experience severe discomfort because of the local trauma but may experience flashbacks.

Laboratory Tests

10. Obtain fingernail clippings and scrapings. These may harbor bits of the assailant's blood, skin, or hair. Photographs of bite marks may also be used to match dental records.
11. Saliva samples should be taken. The victim should not be allowed to smoke or eat for 30 minutes before taking a sample. If there is trauma to the mouth, this procedure should be delayed until the wound is healed. The swabs should be allowed to air dry before sealing. They should not be removed from the victim's mouth by anyone other then the victim or the examiner.
12. Guided by the history of the assault, the victim's symptoms, and any local protocol, determine which laboratory tests are appropriate. Recommended laboratory tests in all cases of sexual assault include the following:
    - A Venereal Disease Research Laboratory (VDRL) test for syphilis or rapid plasma reagin (RPR) test should be obtained at the initial visit and repeated at 6 weeks, 3 months, and 6 months.
    - Hepatitis B serology should be checked (hepatitis B surface antigen and antibody and the hepatitis B core antibody).
    - Serology for human immunodeficiency virus (HIV) should be obtained at the initial visit and repeated at 6 weeks, 3 months, and 6 months after exposure, after proper patient counseling.
    - The patient's blood type should be determined from blood or saliva swabs.
    - For women, a urine or serum β-human chorionic gonadotropin (hCG) pregnancy test at the initial examination is needed to rule out existing pregnancy.

Treatment

13. Treatment of major or life-threatening injuries should occur before initiating the evaluation. After the patient is stable, treatment of other physical injuries should depend on the type sustained.
14. Sexually transmitted infection (STI) prevention
    - Antibiotic prophylaxis: The current recommendation for the treatment of trichomoniasis, bacterial vaginosis, gonorrhea, and chlamydial infection is 250 mg of ceftriaxone intramuscularly and 2 g of metronidazole orally and either 100 mg of doxycycline twice daily for 7 days or 1 g of azithromycin once. Doxycycline should not be prescribed for pregnant patients.

      This regimen will probably treat incubating syphilis. Although the overall risk of acquiring an STI from a single sexual encounter is only 5% to 10%, the aforementioned treatment should be prescribed for all victims of sexual assault.
    - Hepatitis B prophylaxis: If the patient has not been immunized, hepatitis B virus vaccine should be given at the initial visit, then repeated at 1 and 6 months. Hepatitis B immunoglobulin (HBIG) 0.06 mL intramuscularly should be offered if the assailant is thought to be in a high-risk group for hepatitis B and the victim has experienced vaginal or anal bleeding from the assault. The same dose can be repeated in 1 month if the victim's serology is negative.
    - HIV prophylaxis is not universally recommended. However, it should be understood that if the assailant cannot be apprehended and tested (most cases), the victim's infection status may not be known for 6 months. Treatment should be tailored to the patient's needs after counseling for medication costs and potential toxicity.
    - Tetanus prophylaxis is indicated for anyone not immunized in the past 5 years.
15. For women, if the pregnancy test is negative, pregnancy prevention should be offered. See Chapter 129, Emergency Contraception, for available methods and dosing. These treatments are most effective for prevention of pregnancy if used within 72 hours of intercourse.

NOTE: Because up to half of all victims do not report for their follow-up visits, it is very important to perform adequate prophylaxis on patients during the initial visit.

Follow-up

16. The patient should have a follow-up visit with a clinician within 72 hours to again document bruising and to evaluate the results of cultures if prophylactic antibiotics were not given. HIV and syphilis testing should be repeated at 6 weeks, 3 months, and 6 months. Follow-up counseling referrals should be made at the first visit. An additional follow-up visit should be made at 1 to 2 weeks to monitor patient progress (and to evaluate for pregnancy in women) as a result of the assault. If the patient did not receive prophylaxis for infection, STI testing should be repeated at this 1- to 2-week follow-up visit. If the patient received prophylaxis, repeat testing is indicated only if the patient is symptomatic. For women who are pregnant, counseling can be initiated and appropriate options for care can be discussed.

Postprocedure Patient Education

Sexual assault is associated with major emotional and psychologic sequelae. Most women go through the three stages of rape trauma syndrome: (1) trauma (e.g., fear of being alone, fear of men, sexual problems, depression); (2) denial (not wanting to talk about it); and

(3) resolution (dealing with fears and feelings, regaining a sense of control over life). During the first two stages, patients may experience flashbacks, numbness or constriction of feeling, or hypervigilance. Mood swings, irritability, and anger are common and may indicate signs of healing. Insomnia, tension headaches, anorexia, fatigue, nausea, abdominal pain, and genitourinary symptoms are not uncommon. The last stage may take years to reach. The patient should be aware that should the case go to court, it may be necessary to gather additional evidence at a later time. Adequate follow-up and a counseling referral are an essential component of management. Men go through similar stages and need similar counseling.

Patients should receive a written outline of what was performed with the initial evaluation and what treatments were provided. They should also be given a written list of specific instructions and follow-up appointments. It should be written because most assault victims will not remember the evaluation and treatment they received, much less the instructions they were given after the treatment. Many communities have sexual assault centers that will provide advocates and support personnel for the victims during medical visits and for follow-up appointments. If this is not available or feasible, after obtaining the victim's permission, a trained counselor should be consulted. The most important contributing factor to the patient's recovery is contact with a trained advocate or counselor within the first 72 hours of a sexual assault.

The Rape, Assault and Incest National Network (RAINN; phone: 1-800-656-HOPE; website: www.rainn.org) can assist with finding local agencies and counselors trained to assist sexual assault victims.

Additional Resources

See the patient education and consent forms available online at www.expertconsult.com.

CPT/Billing Code

Use E/M codes for established or new patients for the noncolposcopic portion of the examination.

57452 Colposcopy

In some states, the law enforcement agency is required to pay for the evidence collection examination in the case of a reported sexual assault. The patient should sign a consent form to allow the law enforcement agency to be billed.

ICD-9-CM Diagnostic Codes

878.4 Open wound, vulva, without mention of complication
878.5 Open wound, vulva, complicated
878.6 Open wound, vagina, without mention of complication
878.7 Open wound, vagina, complicated
995.83 Adult sexual abuse
V71.5 Rape, alleged, observation or examination, victim or culprit
V71.81 Observation for adult abuse and neglect
V72.31 Gynecologic examination, Papanicolaou smear as part of general gynecologic examination, pelvic examination (annual) (periodic)

Suppliers

(See contact information online at www.expertconsult.com.)

Sexual assault evidence collection kit

Gieserlab Equipment and Supply
MedTech International
Sirchie Fingerprint Laboratories, Inc. (standardized kit available that fulfills laws for many western states)

ONLINE RESOURCE

Centers for Disease Control and Prevention: Sexual assault and STDs. Available at www.cdc.gov/std/treatment/2006/sexual-assault.htm.

BIBLIOGRAPHY

Anderson A: "Don't scream, Miss Annie. Don't scream." Am Fam Physician 59:213–214, 1999.
Centers for Disease Control and Prevention: Sexually transmitted diseases treatment guidelines 2006. MMWR Recomm Rep 55(RR-11):1–94, 2006.
Dunn S: Lavage fluid in sexual assault examination. CMAJ 138:400, 1988.
Holmes MM, Resnick HS, Frampton D: Follow-up of sexual assault victims. Am J Obstet Gynecol 179:336–342, 1998.
Lenahan LC, Ernst A, Johnson B: Colposcopy in evaluation of the adult sexual assault victim. Am J Emerg Med 16:183–184, 1998.
Luce H, Schrager S, Gilchrist V: Sexual assault of women. Am Fam Physician 81:489–495, 2010.
Nelson DG, Santucci KA: An alternate light source to detect semen. Acad Emerg Med 9:1045–1048, 2002.
Usatine RP: The Color Atlas of Family Medicine. New York, McGraw-Hill, 2009.
Young WW, Bracken AC, Goddard MA, Matheson S: Sexual assault: Review of a national model protocol for forensic and medical evaluation. Obstet Gynecol 80:878–883, 1992.

CHAPTER 158

Management of the Young Female as a Possible Victim of Sexual Abuse

David B. Bosscher

Sexual abuse is so common that primary care clinicians should consider it as a possibility even during routine office visits. The prevalence is estimated to be 22.3% for girls and 8.5% for boys. Although child advocacy centers are increasingly available in many regions and communities, the generalist clinician is often the critical first line of evaluation.

In young females, common initial complaints include itching, redness, burning, irritation, discharge, or bleeding at the vagina. The abuse may be disclosed initially or discovered later. Occasionally, the abuse will be discovered when a parent wants a child examined after their use of sexually explicit language, demonstration of a sexual act on their doll, or other overtly sexual behavior. Because children may be exposed to sexually explicit media, the examiner must carefully sift through such allegations and concerns. Often the complaints are nonspecific and parents hope that a medical test can prove or disprove abuse. Unfortunately, in the majority of cases, children are seen long after the incident may have occurred. If, however, the alleged incident took place within 72 hours of complaint, immediate examination using a carefully structured protocol (e.g., a rape kit; see Chapter 157, Treatment of the Adult Victim of Sexual Assault) is mandatory.

A careful physical examination for children with allegations of sexual abuse is imperative, either in the clinician's office or through a regional child advocacy center. Nonetheless, only about 4% of physical examinations result in positive findings. A negative finding does not negate the claim of abuse, but does make interviews with social workers and other trained interviewers critically important to sort out allegations.

Although this chapter focuses on females, it is not meant to deny the possibility of abuse in males. If abuse is suspected in a young male, many of the same principles apply. It is important to know local laws regarding collection of evidence because they vary by location. The examiner should be certain to follow local standards for collection of forensic specimens.

Indications

- Suspicion of sexual abuse after initial questioning or preliminary physical examination
- Referral from teacher, parent, or other responsible person alleging sexual abuse

Contraindications

- Lack of the instruments or supplies needed to carry out the examination
- Lack of forms to preserve the chain of evidence
- Lack of a witness for the examination to preserve the chain of evidence
- Lack of consent to examine or treat a minor if a parent or guardian is not present

Equipment

- Either a hand-held lens with an adequate examination light or a colposcope to examine details. One major benefit of a colposcope is that it allows the clinician to use both hands for the examination. If a hand-held lens is used, an assistant will be needed.
- Camera (helpful but not mandatory).
- A rape kit should be available in case it is necessary to document rape. If alleged sexual contact was within the past 72 hours, consider using the rape kit to collect evidence in an organized manner (see Chapter 157, Treatment of the Adult Victim of Sexual Assault).

Equipment on a Mayo Stand

- Room-temperature culture media for gonorrhea or culture transport media from your reference laboratory
- *Chlamydia* and herpes culture media or culture transport media from your reference laboratory
- Materials for wet prep and potassium hydroxide (KOH) prep
- Cotton swabs, calcium alginate swabs (Calgiswab) or equivalent

NOTE: Do not use current available DNA probes for sexually transmitted infection (STI) testing in examinations for sexual abuse. As of October 2009, the package insert specifically states: "Do not use for medicolegal purposes or in sexual abuse cases." Although the technology may be better, and the DNA probes may be the standard of the future, they should not be used in these cases at present.

Preprocedure Patient Preparation

Explain the entire procedure to the caregiver and the child at a language level that both will understand. The child needs to know that she will be asked a lot of questions and that some may seem "silly." Explain that after the questions, the child will be examined.

It is often helpful to allow a young girl to maintain her sense of control over the process. After establishing rapport with the child, assure her that she will be allowed to be as active a participant as possible. If possible, she should know that she will be asked for permission before proceeding with any part of the examination.

Issues of privacy and confidentiality are important when examining older children. Although most young girls will prefer to have a parent, usually the mother, in the room at all times, in some cases it will be helpful to later spend time alone with the child. When alone with an examiner, a child may disclose abuse or other concerns. Letting her and the parent(s) know ahead of time (before the examination) that the clinician will be spending time alone with her may increase her comfort. Allowing that time alone may give her a greater sense of control and a feeling of responsibility for her own health. Consideration should be given to having a second person in the room with the patient and examiner at all times to serve as an assistant, chaperone, and witness. If the examiner is male, having a female assistant in the room may make the patient more comfortable.

Parents should be reassured that the child's hymen will not be altered in any way by the examination. Anatomic diagrams may be helpful for demonstration.

TECHNIQUE

Taking the History

1. Assuming that a social worker or trained interviewer is responsible for taking a detailed history, the primary care clinician should take sufficient history to perform all pertinent portions of the examination. If no trained interviewer is available, a complete history should be taken in an unhurried and comfortable setting. Consider setting aside separate visits for the history and the physical examination.
2. Take some time to establish rapport. Ask about the current family structure, recent life changes, and which activities she enjoys, as well as about school and friends. Take notes while obtaining the history. It is often complicated. Obtain the names of persons potentially involved.
3. Document the descriptions of any potential sexual abuse in the child's own words. When the meaning of a word is unclear, ask clarifying questions. Document the meaning of the word in her terms. For example, if the child mentions sex, ask her what that means (e.g., because of depictions on television, children often think that sex means just being naked and in bed with another person).
4. Do not be any more leading in questioning than is absolutely necessary. Begin with very general questions and go to more specific ones if the child does not offer sufficient information. For example, ask "Has anyone touched you in a way that made you feel funny or bad?" before asking "Has anyone touched your bottom?" Leading questions can not only misdirect the child and, subsequently, the examiner, they can also be neutralized by a defense attorney.
5. Do not allow the caregiver(s) to adopt a coaching role. Such a role may negate the clinician's testimony as well as the child's.
6. Young children have an incomplete concept of numbers and time. They often cannot tell how many times something occurred, but can often specify in general terms: "a lot," "once in a while," or "one time." Likewise, regarding time, small children do not understand the difference between "3 months ago" and "8 months ago."

Preparing for the Vaginal Examination

1. Again, take time to establish a comfortable setting. A child-friendly, compassionate medical assistant or nurse can be very helpful in using a toy, book, or stuffed animal to distract the child during the examination.
2. Explain the examination to the caregiver and the child at a language level they will comprehend. This is an important step toward reinforcing the child's sense of control over the examination. Begin by describing familiar portions of the examination ("I'm going to listen to your heart and then feel your tummy"). Then simply state that you are going to examine her genitalia ("Then I'm going to look at your bottom").
3. Explain to the child that the most important part of the examination is when the examiner merely "looks" around and that it is important for her to communicate with the examiner during the examination. Reassure the child that the examination should not hurt.
4. Perform the physical examination except for the vaginal–rectal portion. The examination should proceed from the least to the most intrusive while gaining the confidence of the child with each step.
5. Before performing the vaginal examination, it is helpful to recall normal anatomy (Fig. 158-1).

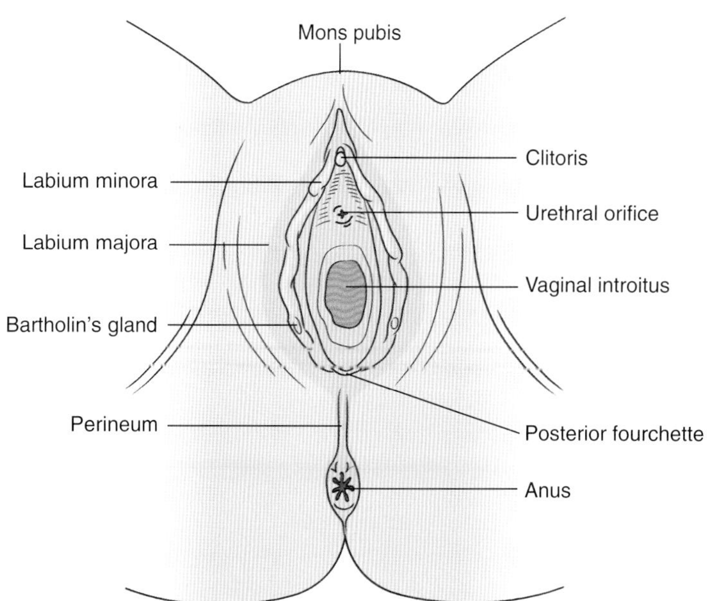

Figure 158-1 Anatomy of genitalia in prepubertal girl. (From Dieckmann RA, Fiser DH, Selbst SM [eds]: Illustrated Textbook of Pediatric Emergency and Critical Care Procedures. St. Louis, Mosby, 1997.)

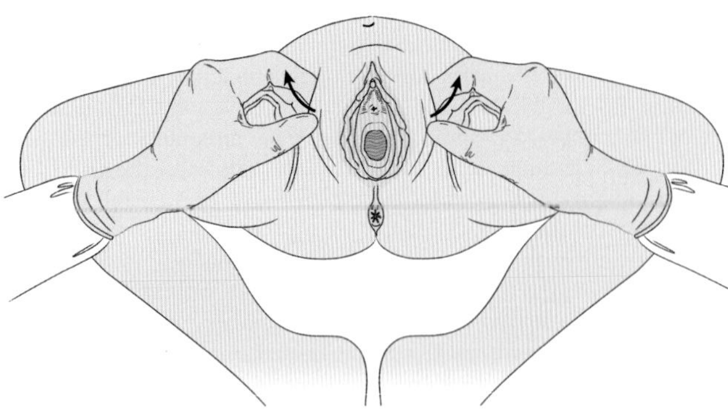

Figure 158-2 **Frog-leg position for examining labia. Note gentle traction on posterior labia to enhance visualization.** (From Dieckmann RA, Fiser DH, Selbst SM [eds]: Illustrated Textbook of Pediatric Emergency and Critical Care Procedures. St. Louis, Mosby, 1997.)

Performing the Vaginal Examination

1. Talk constantly ("verbal anesthesia"). A calm, quiet, confident voice can be reassuring. A relaxed and unhurried approach may decrease the child's anxiety. Having the parent sit close by or hold the child's hand may also provide comfort. If the child is provided a hand mirror, it may distract her, promote education, and allow her to participate more actively in the process.
2. Tell the child that it is acceptable to undress because she is in a clinician's office.
3. Frog-leg examination
   - Begin with the frog-leg examination. The child is supine with knees apart and feet touching in the midline with buttocks at the end of the table (Fig. 158-2). Alternatively, the mother may assist with the frog-leg position (Fig. 158-3). Older children may be placed in adjustable stirrups (Fig. 158-4).
   - Inspect the vulva and areas lateral to it. Use the colposcope or a hand lens with adequate lighting to best visualize the introitus.
   - Gently open the labia by applying gentle lateral and posterior traction just lateral to the vulva at the level of the posterior introitus. Do not force the labia open; they will usually open with persistent gentle traction or the child may assist by holding her labia apart.
   - Examine carefully the entire circumference of the introitus and hymen. Normal hymenal variants are illustrated in Figure 158-5. Look carefully for asymmetry, for notching in the posterior hymen, and for posterior hymenal attenuation (thinning; Fig. 158-6). These findings are usually caused by sexual abuse, and rarely by accidental trauma. The significance of the diameter of the hymenal orifice is controversial; do not worry about measurements. If the hymen cannot be fully visualized, ask the child to cough or take a deep breath. Pull the labia gently forward and down or laterally. A colposcope is helpful at this stage. A hand lens can also be used if an assistant can help with the examination.
   - Acute trauma from sexual abuse is evidenced by the presence of hematomas, abrasions, lacerations, hymenal transections, or vulvar erythema. These conditions usually resolve within 10 to 14 days.
   - Cultures can be taken at this time (assuming the child is comfortable) or after the knee–chest examination.
4. Knee–chest examination (for children older than 2 years)
   - Most young children readily adopt this position with a little encouragement. Buttocks should be higher than the back, with knees approximately 25 cm (12 inches) apart. The child can rest her head to one side on her folded arms or pillow (Fig. 158-7).
   - Gentle traction laterally will often open up the labia. Ask the patient to take 10 slow, deep breaths because this will also relax the perineal structures.
   - Use the colposcope (or hand lens with an assistant) to look at the posterior hymen. The knee–chest position is the preferred position for detecting small but significant abnormalities of the hymen. Again, look for asymmetries, notching, or attenuation. Take photographs or carefully document if abnormalities are seen.
   - The lower vagina may be visualized in this position, and the upper vagina and cervix in 80% to 90% of prepubertal girls. Also, examine the rectum in this position.
5. Resume the frog-leg position if cultures are needed. Perform the following *only* if vaginal discharge or pain is noted, if there is genital itching or odor or urinary symptoms, or if there are genital ulcers or lesions. Consider cultures if the prevalence of STIs in the community is high, if a sibling or another child or adult in the household has an STI, or a known assailant has an STI or is at high risk.
   - Culture for *Chlamydia*. Collect the specimen as deeply in the posterior vagina as you can. Use a cotton or calcium alginate swab. If possible, it should be moistened with nonbacteriostatic saline to minimize the discomfort. Before inserting, allow the child to feel a similar swab on her skin. Avoid touching the hymen when obtaining the culture. It may also be helpful to ask the child to cough in order to distract her and open the hymen. A male urethral swab may also be used to gently scrape the vaginal wall.
   - Alternatively, a vaginal wash and aspiration can be obtained. Using a small feeding tube attached to a small syringe, insert the tube into the vagina and inject and aspirate 0.5 to 1 mL of sterile saline. A soft plastic or glass eyedropper with 4 to 5 cm of intravenous plastic tubing attached can also be used in the same manner. Insert the catheter into the vagina and inject and then aspirate the saline.
   - For gonorrhea (gonococci), use a cotton or calcium alginate swab to obtain samples from the following: throat, deep in the posterior vagina, and rectum. Place them on a single plate partitioned into thirds (this is done to reduce the number of cultures needed). If any area of the plate is actually positive, you will need to reculture each area separately to confirm the

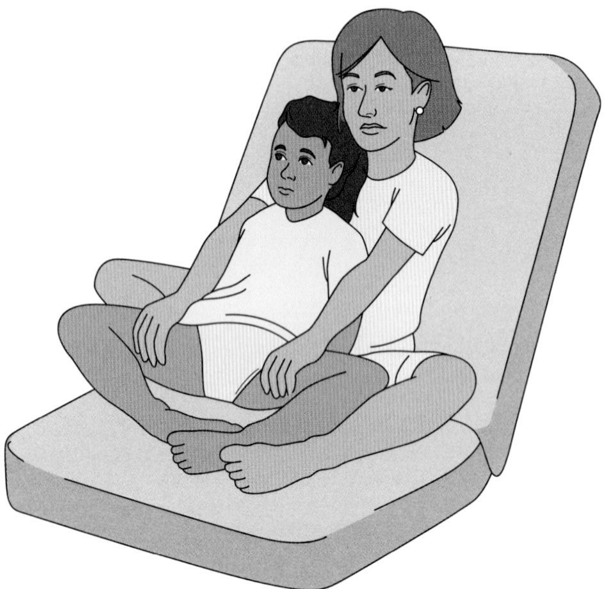

Figure 158-3 **Frog-leg position with mother's assistance.** (Modified from Khan JA, Emans SJ: Gynecologic management of rape in adolescent girls. Patient Care 33:71, 1999.)

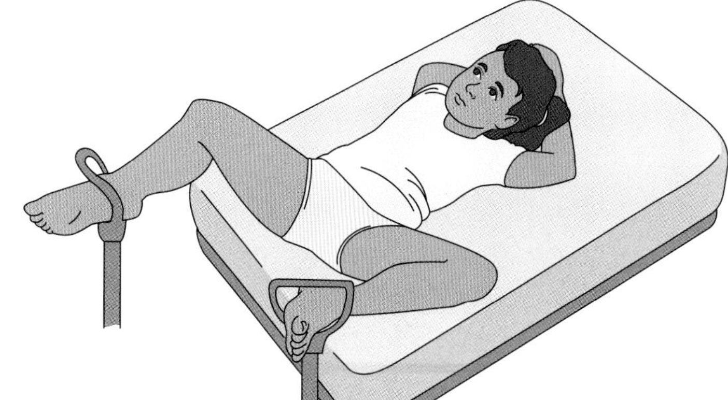

Figure 158-4 Lithotomy position with use of stirrups. (Modified from Khan JA, Emans SJ: Gynecologic management of rape in adolescent girls. Patient Care 33:71, 1999.)

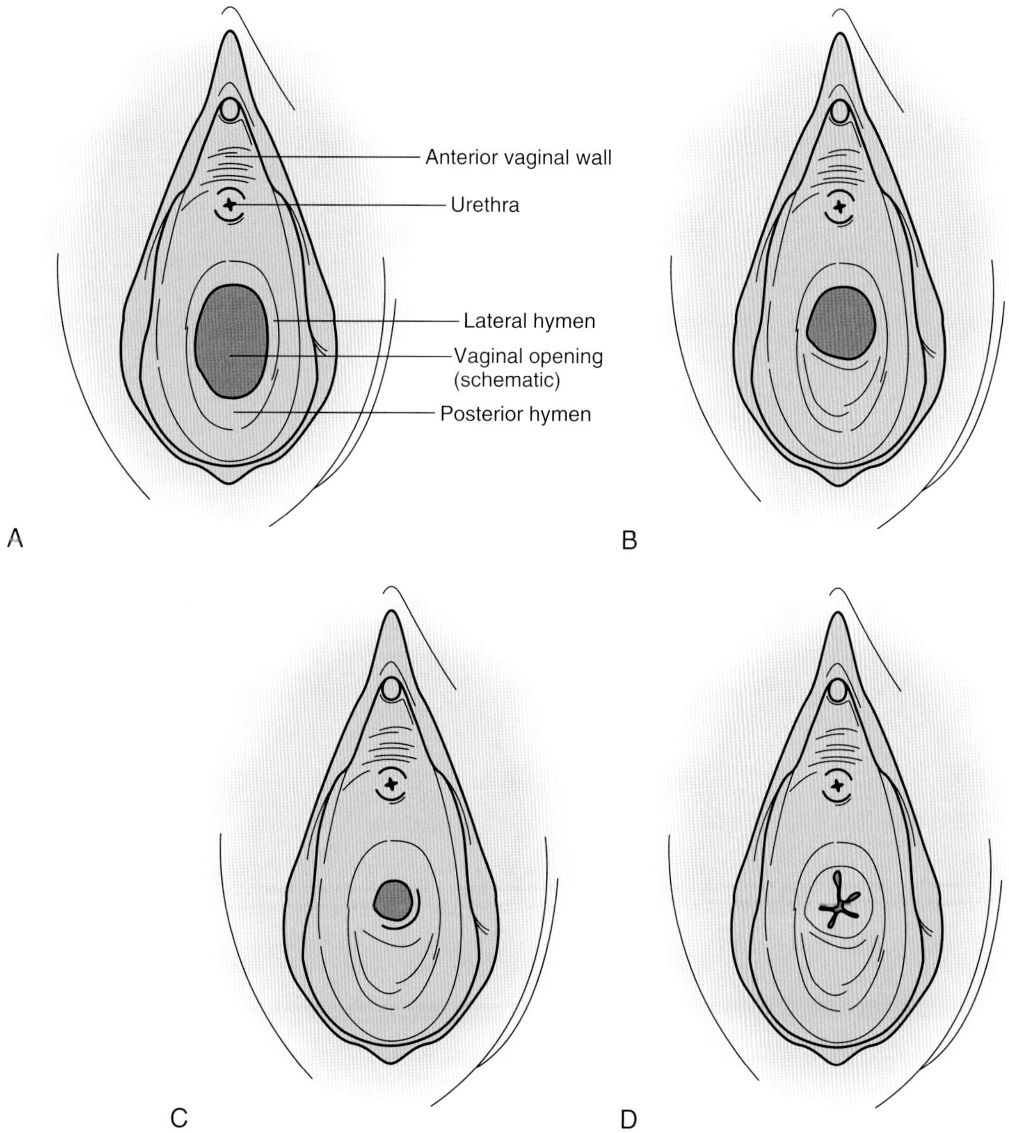

Figure 158-5 Variants of normal hymen. **A,** Normal hymen. **B,** Posterior rim or crescentic hymen. **C,** Circumferential or annular hymen. **D,** Fimbriated or redundant hymen. (Modified from Khan JA, Emans SJ: Gynecologic management of rape in adolescent girls. Patient Care 33:71, 1999.)

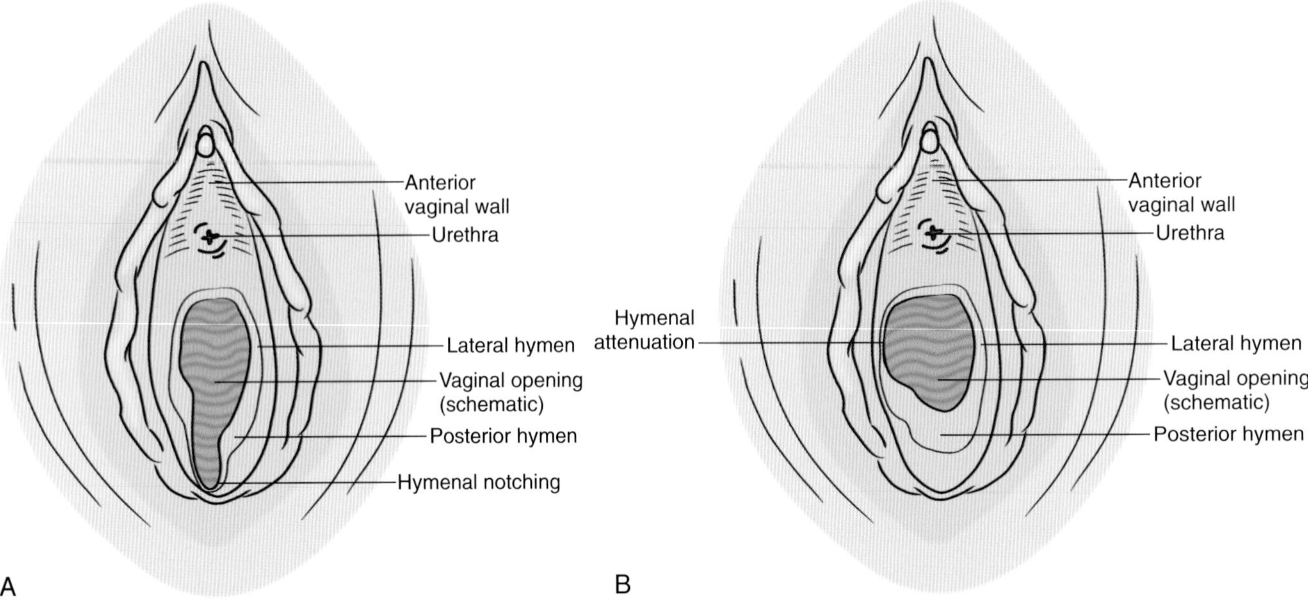

Figure 158-6 **A,** Hymenal notching. **B,** Hymenal attenuation.

location. A false-positive chlamydial or gonococcal culture is very rare, so it should be investigated.

- Obtain a herpes culture if it is suspected.
- Cultures for other organisms can be obtained by placing the calcium alginate swab into a transport Culturette II (contains medium) or by sending the aspirated fluid to your local hospital laboratory for direct plating.
- Obtain a wet prep or KOH prep if indicated.
- Note and document the presence of any condylomata.

NOTE: Cultures are the standard for forensic evidence. DNA probe specimens may, however, be helpful in some instances as an adjunct to cultures.

6. In addition to the aforementioned studies, consider a urine culture, syphilis serology, and hepatitis B and human immunodeficiency virus testing on all patients because of the paucity of clinical findings with these diseases. Parents may also be reassured by doing these studies.

NOTE: Foreign bodies are often found as the cause of a discharge. Removal may be possible with a cotton-tipped applicator or by lavaging the vagina with saline or warm water. Viscous lidocaine may be useful for anesthesia at the introitus.

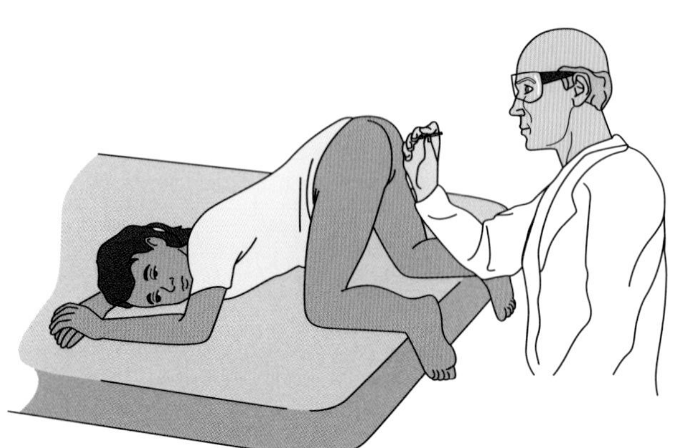

Figure 158-7 **Knee–chest position.** (Modified from Khan JA, Emans SJ: Gynecologic management of rape in adolescent girls. Patient Care 33:71, 1999.)

7. Send all cultures to the laboratory, using *chain of evidence* form and precautions (Fig. 158-8).
8. After the examination, congratulate the child for her cooperation. Discuss the results and the diagnosis and management plan with the child and her parent(s) after she is dressed. Because the results of the examination are often inconclusive, help the parent(s) to understand that a careful and complete investigation includes protective services or law enforcement officials, or both.
9. Implications of positive laboratory findings are set out in Table 158-1. Table 158-2 contains guidelines for making reporting decisions.

Uncooperative Patients

The uncooperative patient calls for patience and artistry on the part of the examiner. Often (but not always), proceeding through the examination slowly will result in a satisfactory examination. Leaving the room and returning when she is ready often allows a child to regain control.

Nasally administered midazolam (Versed), a short-acting benzodiazepine (dosage 0.2 to 0.4 mg/kg of the *injectable* solution) can enhance cooperativeness. When administered by this route (use a tuberculin syringe without a needle), the drug will be effective within 15 minutes. Side effects are rare. Versed syrup is available as another option, but therapeutic onset is longer. The child must be observed by a knowledgeable parent or by your staff for about 1 to 2 hours after the drug is given. This anxiolytic technique requires no intensive monitoring (see Chapter 7, Pediatric Sedation and Analgesia).

Antibiotics are rarely indicated. Usually, the alleged abuse occurred long ago.

Patient Education Guides

See the patient education form available online at www.expertconsult.com. To find a regional child advocacy center, consult the National Children's Alliance website at www.nca-online.org.

Chain of Evidence Form

* *PLEASE COMPLETE* CAREFULLY—*THIS FORM IS REQUIRED FOR LEGAL PURPOSES*

1. Use this LOG to document specimen transfer so that "chain of evidence" can be preserved.
2. Each time the specimen changes hands, the new carrier-technologist must place his or her initials on the form in the appropriate location and must mark the date and time.
3. When the final laboratory report is prepared, staple securely to the LOG before sending the report to the ordering clinician.
4. Please use separate forms if specimens of different types are submitted (e.g., blood specimen and GC culture) or if specimens are sent to different labs.
5. If you perform the laboratory test in your office, have each staff member who handles the specimen initial the form. Anyone in attendance during the history and examination should sign as a witness at the bottom of the form.
6. If you have questions, call the ordering clinician.

Patient's name: ______________________ Date: __________

Laboratory test(s) ordered (circle): RPR Urine culture Culture for GC/Chlamydia HIV

Other: ______________________

Patient's medical record number: ______________ Date of birth: __________

Ordering clinician: ______________________

Each person handling the specimen should *place initials in the first column, then mark the time and date.*

1. Specimen collected by ______	1. Date ________	Time ________
2. Delivered to lab by ______	2. Date ________	Time ________
3. Received in lab by ______	3. Date ________	Time ________
4. Processed by ______	4. Date ________	Time ________
5. Processed by ______	5. Date ________	Time ________
6. Final report prepared by ______	6. Date ________	Time ________

Witnesses to examination:

1. ______________	1. Date ________	Time ________
2. ______________	2. Date ________	Time ________
3. ______________	3. Date ________	Time ________
4. ______________	4. Date ________	Time ________
5. ______________	5. Date ________	Time ________
6. ______________	6. Date ________	Time ________

Figure 158-8 Chain of evidence form.

TABLE 158-1 Implications of Commonly Encountered STIs in Prepubertal Children

STD Confirmed	Sexual Abuse	Suggested Action
Gonorrhea	Certain	Report
Syphilis	Certain	Report
Chlamydial infection	Probable	Report
Condylomata	Probable	Report
Trichomoniasis	Probable	Report
Herpes simplex type 1 (on genitals)	Possible	Report
Herpes simplex type 2	Probable	Report
Bacterial vaginosis	Uncertain	Medical follow-up
Candida infection	Unlikely	Medical follow-up

STD, sexually transmitted disease; STI, sexually transmitted infection.
Adapted from American Academy of Pediatrics Committee on Child Abuse and Neglect: Guidelines for the evaluation of sexual abuse of children. Pediatrics 87:254–260, 1991.

CPT/Billing Code

Use E/M codes for the noncolposcopic portion of the examination.

57452 Colposcopy

ICD-9-CM Diagnostic Codes

V71.5 Rape, alleged, observation or examination, victim or culprit
878.4 Open wound, vulva, without mention of complication
878.5 Injury to vulva, complicated
878.6 Open wound, vagina, without mention of complication
878.7 Injury to vagina, complicated
995.53 Child sexual abuse

TABLE 158-2 Guidelines for Making the Decision to Report Sexual Abuse of Children

History	Physical Examination	Laboratory Abnormality	Level of Concern about Sexual Abuse	Action
None	Normal	None	None	None
Behavioral changes	Normal	None	Low	±Report, follow closely
None	Nonspecific	None	Low	±Report, follow closely
Nonspecific history by child or history by parent only	Nonspecific	None	Possible	±Report, follow closely
None	Specific findings	None	Probable	Report
Child's clear statement	Specific findings	None	Probable	Report
None	Normal, nonspecific, or specific findings	Positive culture for gonococci, *Chlamydia*, or *Trichomonas*, +RPR, presence of sperm	Definite	Report
Behavioral changes	Nonspecific changes	Other sexually transmitted infections	Probable	Report

RPR, rapid plasma reagin test.

Adapted from American Academy of Pediatrics Committee on Child Abuse and Neglect: Guidelines for the evaluation of sexual abuse of children. Pediatrics 87:254–260, 1991.

BIBLIOGRAPHY

American College of Emergency Physicians: Evaluation and Management of the Sexually Assaulted or Sexually Abused Patient. 1999. Available at http://www.acep.org/WorkArea/DownloadAsset.aspx?id=8984.

Berkoff MC, Zolotor AJ, Makoroff KL, et al: Has this prepubertal girl been sexually assaulted? JAMA 300:2779–2792, 2008.

Centers for Disease Control and Prevention: Sexually transmitted diseases treatment guidelines 2006. MMWR Recomm Rep 55(RR-11):1–94, 2006.

Kellogg N, for the American Academy of Pediatrics Committee on Child Abuse and Neglect: The evaluation of sexual abuse in children. Pediatrics 116:506–512, 2005. Also available online at http://aappolicy.aappublications.org/cgi/content/full/pediatrics;116/2/506.

McDonald KC: Child abuse: Approach and management. Am Fam Physician 75:221–228, 2007.

O'Connell BJ: Evaluation of the sexually abused child, including the role of colposcopy. J Low Genit Tract Dis 5:87–93, 2001.

Usatine RP, Smith MA, Mayeaux EJ Jr, et al: The Color Atlas of Family Medicine. New York, McGraw-Hill, 2009.

CHAPTER 159

VULVAR BIOPSY

Gregory L. Brotzman

Evaluation of the vulva is an important component of a routine gynecologic examination. Although most lesions found are benign, such as skin tags, condylomata, and simple nevi, biopsy is occasionally needed to obtain a clearer understanding of the lesion present. This is especially true in older women and in those who smoke, because they have a significantly increased risk of developing vulvar intraepithelial neoplasia (VIN) or cancer.

Depth of biopsy is an important consideration. Disease of the *non–hair-bearing areas* of the vulva (labia minora, fourchette, interior aspect of the labia majora) is usually only 1 to 2 mm in depth. In contrast, *hair-bearing areas* (outer aspect of labia majora) may have disease that follows the hair shaft and may be several millimeters in depth. Deep biopsies are not necessary for non–hair-bearing vulvar skin areas, but biopsies should go down full depth to adipose tissue where hair is present. An elevated lesion can be shaved off (see Chapter 32, Skin Biopsy) if it is certain not to be a melanoma (e.g., seborrheic keratosis, condyloma, or benign nevus).

Examination of the vulva is aided by the use of a colposcope (low-power setting, 5×) or a magnifying glass after soaking the skin with 3% to 5% acetic acid (vinegar) using a spray bottle or large cotton applicators. Use of vinegar helps delineate dysplastic tissue and warty changes by turning them white (acetowhite epithelium).

Vulvar biopsy is a straightforward, easy-to-perform office skill that allows the practitioner to differentiate benign from neoplastic lesions, often being curative when the entire lesion is encompassed by the biopsy.

In addition to this chapter, see Chapters 22 to 25 on excision of lesions and follow-up repair; Chapter 32, Skin Biopsy; and Chapter 155, Treatment of Noncervical Condylomata Acuminata.

ANATOMY

Figure 159-1 shows basic vulvar anatomy as well as the orientation of lines of skin tension. Skin tension lines are important in considering excisional or punch biopsies of the vulva. With the index finger and thumb of the nondominant hand, the skin should be stretched in the opposite direction of (perpendicular to) the tension lines, so that the excision margins form an ellipse after release. This allows an easier closure if sutures are used.

INDICATIONS

- Pigmented lesions
- Vulvar ulceration of uncertain etiology or a nonhealing ulcer
- White epithelium (skin that turns white after the application of 5% acetic acid)
- Leukoplakia (white skin before the application of acetic acid)
- Presumed condylomata that do not readily respond to conventional therapy (if not resolved or significantly improving after two treatment attempts of any kind)
- Any skin abnormality that needs definitive diagnosis

CONTRAINDICATIONS

Absolute

An allergy to local anesthetic/preservatives is the only absolute contraindication.

Relative

- Bleeding diathesis
- Recent (<3 weeks) chemical destruction attempts. These may result in false-positive histologic findings owing to reparative changes. It is best to wait until healing has occurred after any treatment before attempting a biopsy of such lesions.

EQUIPMENT

- 3-mm Keyes punch biopsy (4 and 5 mm also acceptable but may require suturing, whereas 3 mm does not; Fig. 159-2A), a cervical punch biopsy forceps (Fig. 159-2B), or sharp tissue scissors (Fig. 159-2C) or a no. 15 blade for elevated or non–hair-bearing areas ("shave biopsy")
- No. 15 scalpel blade for excision
- 1% lidocaine (Xylocaine) with or without epinephrine (can mix 1:10 with sodium bicarbonate solution to decrease discomfort)
- 30-gauge, ½-inch needles
- 1- to 5-mL syringe
- Nonsterile gloves (sterile gloves needed if placing sutures)
- Formalin containers
- Iris scissors (see Fig. 159-2C)
- Pickups (Fig. 159-2D)
- Povidone–iodine or alcohol swabs
- Monsel's solution (thickened ferric subsulfate solution) or aluminum chloride solution (Drysol)
- Small cotton-tipped applicators
- Antibiotic ointment
- 3 mm disposable (sharp) dermal curette

PREPROCEDURE PATIENT EDUCATION

If there are no contraindications, have the patient take 600 mg of ibuprofen 1 hour before the procedure to help with postprocedure discomfort.

PROCEDURE

There are four ways to perform a biopsy of the vulva:

1. Punch biopsy (with a Keyes punch or cervical biopsy forceps)
2. Excisional biopsy (using a no. 15 scalpel blade)
3. Shave excision (using tissue scissors or a blade)
4. Curettement using a 3-mm disposable (sharp) dermal curette

Deciding which type of biopsy technique to use depends on the size and location of the lesion (see earlier discussion). A large or

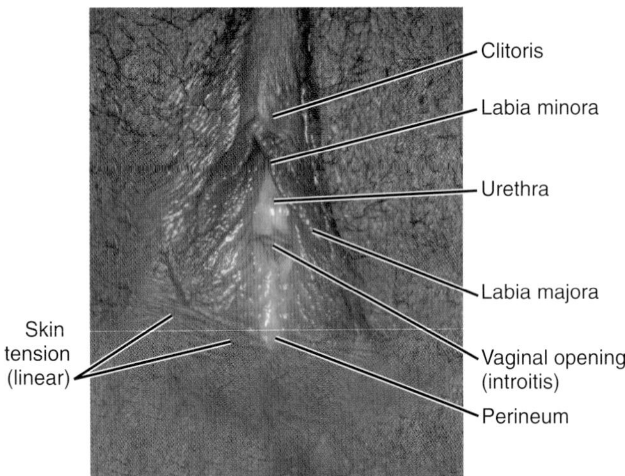

Figure 159-1 Vulvar anatomy. The vertical and horizontal lines demonstrate the lines of skin tension. When a biopsy is being performed, stretch the skin in the direction opposite to the skin tension lines so that after the biopsy is done, the skin will form an ellipse when relaxed, making it easier to close if sutures are needed.

deep lesion would likely require punch biopsies to sample it, or it may be possible to excise it in its entirety with an excisional biopsy technique. Frequently, small lesions can be excised completely with a punch or shave biopsy. Most punch biopsies do not require suturing, whereas excisional biopsies do. The curette technique can be used to sample a large lesion or to remove small, especially papular, lesions.

General Technique

1. Draw up 1 to 5 mL lidocaine with or without epinephrine, mixed with a 10 : 1 ratio of lidocaine to bicarbonate solution, 1 mEq/mL (avoid use of epinephrine around the clitoral area). One may also use a small amount of a topical anesthetic such as 5% lidocaine cream (LMX5) applied with a cotton-tipped applicator to the area to be sampled. This is left on for 5 minutes before local anesthetic infiltration.
2. Identify the lesion.
3. Prepare the skin with a povidone–iodine swab or alcohol.
4. Inject around and under lesion with local anesthetic to raise the lesion (Fig. 159-3A).
5. Test skin with needle to be sure anesthesia is adequate (should be immediately effective).
6. Stretch the skin in direction opposite of skin tension lines in the vulvar area (i.e., stretch horizontally for a labial biopsy and stretch vertically for a perineal biopsy).
7. If using a blade, curette, or scissors to remove lesion, stay more superficial in non–hair-bearing areas.

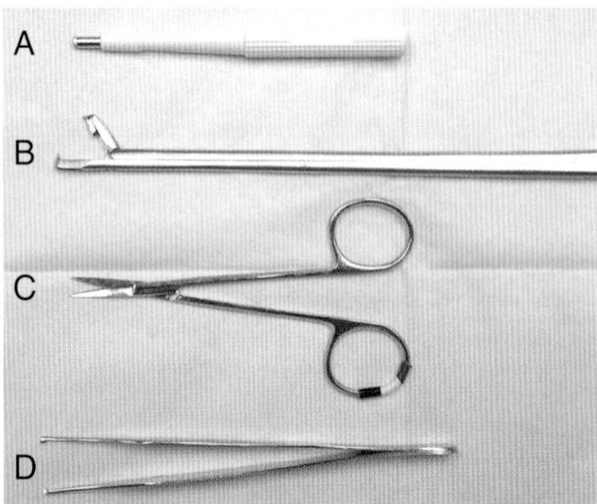

Figure 159-2 **A,** Keyes punch biopsy. **B,** Cervical punch biopsy forceps. **C,** Iris scissors. **D,** Tissue forceps.

Technique for a Keyes Punch

1. To obtain deeper samples (e.g., hair-bearing areas), place punch over lesion perpendicular to the surface and slowly twist with minimal pressure on the punch instrument (let the cutting occur with the instrument; Fig. 159-3B).
2. Continue until you feel a "give" and the punch is loose from the surrounding tissues.
3. Gently grasp the edge of the lesion or the subcutaneous portion of the biopsy with the tissue forceps and lift up (avoid grasping the central portion of the lesion because this may cause crush artifact to the specimen).
4. Snip the base of the specimen with iris scissors and remove the biopsy sample (if multiple biopsies of the same lesion are obtained, each sample should be placed in its own container; Fig. 159-3C).
5. Apply a small amount of Monsel's solution or aluminum chloride solution to the biopsy crater, using a small cotton-tipped applicator.
6. More resistant bleeding may be treated with a small piece of Gelfoam, electrocautery, or an absorbable suture.
7. Wipe away any excess hemostatic agent or blood with saline-moistened gauze.

NOTE: After either a punch biopsy or an excisional biopsy, apply a small amount of antibacterial ointment to the biopsy site.

Technique for Using Cervical Punch Biopsy Forceps

1. Place the forceps jaws perpendicular to the surface of the lesion and grasp the skin. This will cause tenting of the skin (Fig. 159-3D).
2. Close the biopsy forceps to obtain the biopsy. The goal is to obtain approximately a 3-mm-wide and -deep biopsy.
3. Apply a small amount of Monsel's solution or aluminum chloride solution to the biopsy crater, using a small cotton-tipped applicator.
4. Wipe away any excess hemostatic agent or blood with saline-moistened gauze.

Technique for an Excisional Biopsy

Figure 159-4 illustrates an excisional biopsy. See Chapter 32, Skin Biopsy, for further details on performing an excisional biopsy with repair.

Common Errors

- Not sampling the most advanced part of the lesion. If uncertain, take multiple biopsies for large lesions. An area that is more darkly pigmented and raised, or an area of leukoplakia, is usually more advanced.
- Taking too deep of a sample. Use careful technique to take only the depth of specimen necessary.

Complications

The following complications are extremely rare:

- Infection
- Bleeding, hematoma, ecchymosis

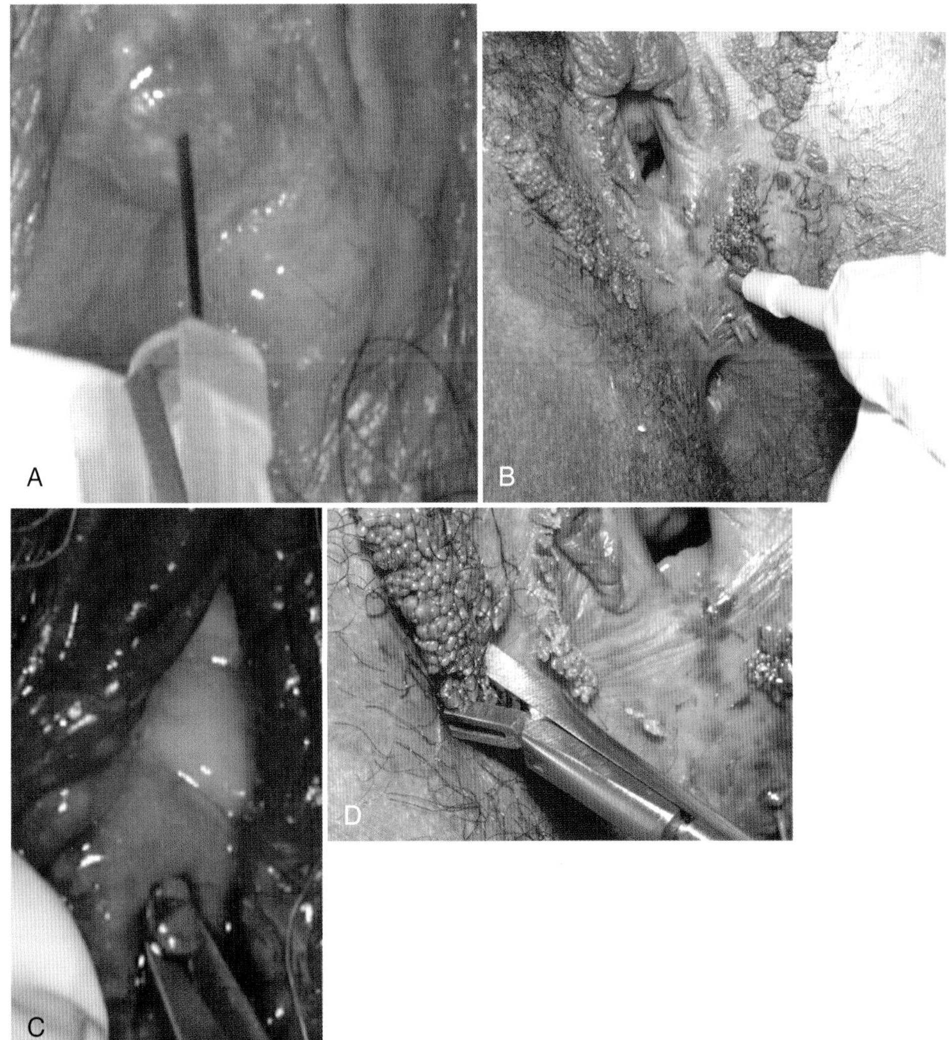

Figure 159-3 Example of punch biopsy. **A,** The lesion is anesthetized. **B,** Biopsy is performed with a Keyes punch. **C,** If a Keyes punch is used, once the skin is free from surrounding tissues, snip base with iris scissors. **D,** Alternatively, biopsy is performed with a cervical biopsy forceps. (**B** and **D,** Courtesy of Hope Haefner, MD.)

- Hypopigmentation
- Pain
- Scar
- Recurrence
- Hyperpigmentation from Monsel's solution (usually temporary)

Postprocedure Patient Education

Instruct the patient to perform the following after the procedure:

- Wash the area twice a day with soap and water.
- Apply antibiotic ointment after each cleansing.
- Use acetaminophen or ibuprofen for discomfort (first determine any contraindications to the use of these medications in the patient).
- Take sitz baths as needed for discomfort if extensive removals are performed.
- Use ice packs as needed.
- For more recalcitrant pain, use over-the-counter benzocaine gel (toothache-type pain reliever) as needed.
- Call if there is persistent pain, redness, or swelling.
- Avoid intercourse until discomfort is gone (usually 3 to 5 days).
- Arrange a follow-up appointment or phone call to discuss biopsy results.

Patient Education Guides

See patient education and patient consent forms available online at www.expertconsult.com.

CPT/Billing Codes

56501 Destruction benign lesion vulva, single
56515 Destruction benign lesion vulva, extensive
56605 Biopsy of vulva or perineum (one lesion)
56606 Biopsy of each additional vulvar or perineal lesion

For complete excisional removals, also see excision codes.

ICD-9-CM Diagnostic Codes

078.11 Condyloma acuminatum
221.2 Benign vulvar neoplasm
233.32 VIN III
616.10 Vulvitis
624.01 Vulvar intraepithelial neoplasia I (VIN I)
624.02 VIN II
624.9 Unspecified noninflammatory disorder of vulva and perineum
701.9 Skin tag

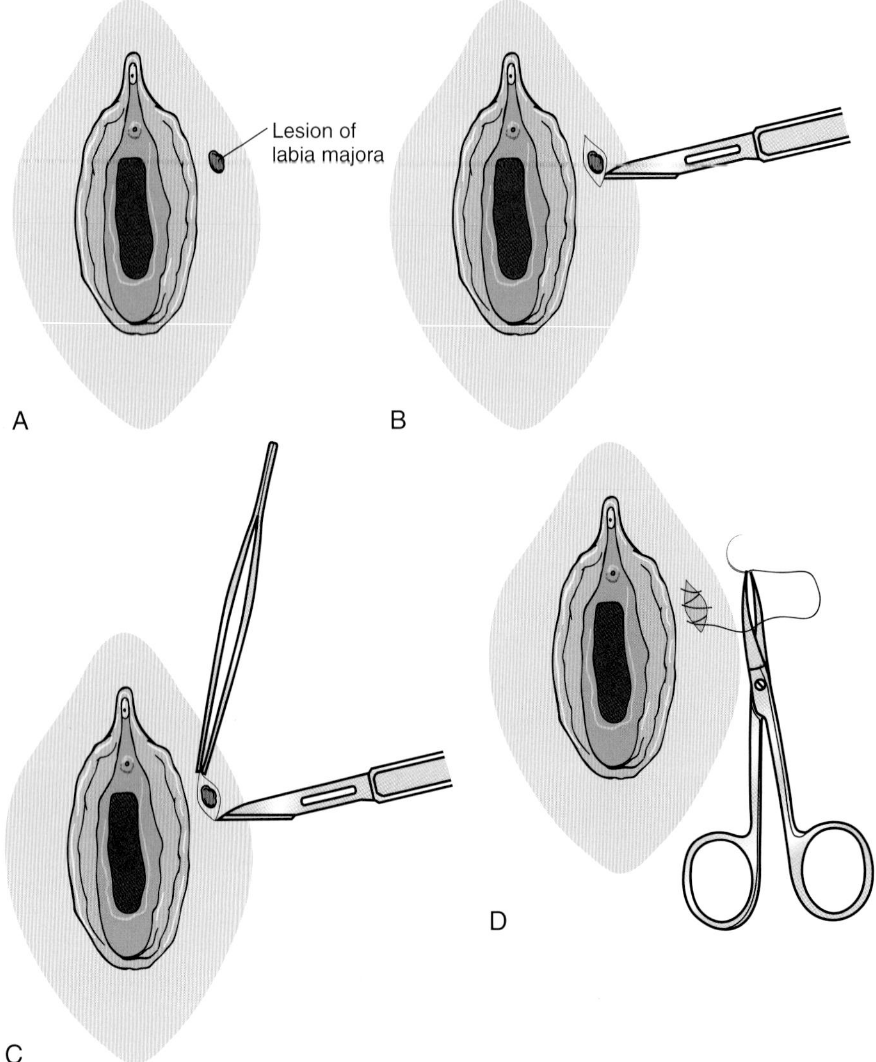

Figure 159-4 Example of excisional biopsy. **A,** Lesion of labia majora. **B,** After anesthesia, an elliptical incision is made along skin tension lines. **C,** Scalpel is used to free base from apex toward center of excised area. **D,** Skin is closed with subcuticular running absorbable suture.

BIBLIOGRAPHY

Apgar BS, Brotzman GL, Spitzer M (eds): Colposcopy: Principles and Practice, 2nd ed. Philadelphia, Saunders, 2008.

Apgar BS, Cox JT: Differentiating normal and abnormal finding of the vulva. Am Family Physician 53:1171–1180, 1996.

Berek J (ed): Novak's Gynecology, 13th ed. Philadelphia, Lippincott Williams & Wilkins, 2002.

Clarke-Pearson DL, Dawood MY (eds): Green's Gynecology: Essentials of Clinical Practice, 4th ed. Boston, Little, Brown, 1990.

DiSaia P, Creasman W (eds): Clinical Gynecologic Oncology, 7th ed. St. Louis, Mosby, 2007.

Gibbs R, Karlan B, Haney A, Nygaard I (eds): Danforth's Obstetrics and Gynecology, 10th ed. Philadelphia, Lippincott Williams & Wilkins, 2008.

Kurman R (ed): Blaustein's Pathology of the Female Genital Tract, 5th ed. New York, Springer-Verlag, 2002.

Ostergard D, Berman M, Yee B (eds): Atlas of Gynecologic Surgery. Philadelphia, WB Saunders, 2000.

Rock J, Jones H III (eds): Te Linde's Operative Gynecology, 10th ed. Philadelphia, Lippincott Williams & Wilkins, 2009.

Tuggy M, Garcia J: Procedures Consult. Available at www.proceduresconsult.com.

Wheeless C Jr, Roenneburg M: Atlas of Pelvic Surgery: On-Line Edition. Available at www.atlasofpelvicsurgery.com/home.html.

CHAPTER 160

Wet Smear and KOH Preparation

Gary R. Newkirk

Abnormal vaginal discharge is a common complaint. In fact, vaginitis is the most common gynecologic diagnosis in primary care. Vulvovaginal candidiasis (VVC), bacterial vaginosis (BV), and trichomoniasis (trich) account for over 90% of abnormal vulvovaginal symptoms and discharge. Frequently, several pathogens may coexist. Office-based wet smear, potassium hydroxide (KOH) preparation, and vaginal secretion pH should be used to ensure a more accurate diagnosis and effective treatment of vaginitis. Empiric treatment for vulvovaginal symptoms including vaginal discharge should be avoided until appropriate testing is performed making a specific diagnosis.

Anatomy

Obtaining vaginal or vulvar samples to determine the cause of vulvovaginal symptoms and discharge requires familiarization with lower female genital anatomy and the basic skills of pelvic examination. Chapter 137, Colposcopic Examination, and Chapter 151, Pap Smear and Related Techniques for Cervical Cancer Screening, review the anatomy and basic steps of the pelvic examination.

Indications

- Abnormal vaginal discharge
- Vulvar or vaginal itching, burning, or pain
- Discomfort with intercourse

Contraindictions

- Active menses (clinician should not postpone evaluation for significant discharge or vulvovaginitis during menses)
- Recent douching (relative contraindication)
- Recent application of vaginal creams or lubricants (relative contraindication)

Equipment and Supplies

- Vaginal speculum
- Small cotton-tipped applicators
- Small test tubes
- Normal saline
- 10% potassium hydroxide solution
- Glass slides and coverslips
- pH test tape (narrow range needed: Micro Essential laboratory; pH paper on a stick: Imagyn Gynecology)
- Microscope

Precautions

- In some instances, women with extremely inflamed vulvovaginitis cannot tolerate speculum insertion. The clinician should be prepared to perform a limited examination by obtaining samples from the distal vagina or vulva.
- The clinician should maintain a high index of suspicion for a primary cervical infection with either *Chlamydia trachomatis* or *Neisseria gonorrhoeae* in patients at risk or for those who have an observed mucopurulent cervicitis.

Preprocedure Patient Preparation

- Discuss the need for pelvic (speculum) examination and testing requirements that may incur additional costs.
- Written consent is not required, although women should be informed if testing for gonorrhea or *Chlamydia* is performed.
- Educate women during annual pelvic examinations regarding avoidance of douching, creams, and lubricants prior to the evaluation of abnormal discharge.

Procedure

1. With the patient in the lithotomy position begin with careful examination of the vulva for inflammation, ulcers, lesions, and discharge.
2. Insert a warm lubricated speculum and expose the cervix.
3. Inspect the cervix, vaginal walls, and fornices. Perform cervical sampling for gonorrhea, *Chlamydia*, or herpes as deemed appropriate. Consult with your laboratory on the detection methodology (culture, DNA testing) and technique for sample collection, preparation, and transport.
4. Collect secretions from both the vaginal fornices and lateral vaginal walls by gently rubbing with a cotton-tipped applicator. Place the cotton-tipped applicator with sample in a patient identified small test tube that contains 1 mL of 0.9% (normal) saline. Leave the applicator in the test tube until the wet smear is performed in the laboratory. Remove the speculum from the vagina.
5. To properly prepare the slide for review, vigorously mix the swab in the saline solution. Remove the swab from the tube and depress it on the slide to express a small amount of fluid. Apply a coverslip over the sample. The slide ("wet prep" or "wet smear") is then immediately examined with the microscope under low power (10×) for vaginal squamous cells, white blood cells, lactobacilli, clue cells, and trichomonads. Examine under low and high power (40×). If a KOH slide is needed, prepare another slide exactly as previously described. Before placing the coverslip, put one drop of a 10% KOH solution on the sample. Apply a coverslip. Allow to air- or flame-dry and examine under low power for hyphae, mycelial tangles, or spores. The "whiff test" is performed when KOH is applied to the sample (see later discussion).
6. A pH test of vaginal secretions can improve diagnostic specificity. A vaginal secretion pH of 3.8 to 4.5 is considered normal in premenopausal women. A piece of the pH test tape may be directly applied to the moist vaginal wall or to the vaginal secretions adhering to the speculum when it is removed from the vagina. Standard nitrazine paper is not accurate and narrower pH range test method should be used (narrow range test paper: Micro Essential Laboratory; pH paper on a stick: Imagyn Medical

Technologies, Inc.). Cervical mucus, semen, douche solutions, and blood are alkaline and can interfere with pH testing.

7. Cultures of vaginal secretions can be obtained for *Candida* and non-*Candida* yeast, aerobic vaginitis, or trichomonas. DNA testing is available for candidiasis or trichomoniasis. Cultures are recommended when microscopy and pH testing fail to document a cause for recurrent vaginitis.

Common Errors

- Not obtaining cervical cultures for gonorrhea, *Chlamydia*, or herpes in settings where this may be probable. These infections often cause vaginal discharge as well.
- Not obtaining samples from the vaginal wall as well as the cervical fornices.
- Not performing a careful history of patient-directed treatment, such as douching or over-the-counter treatments that can interfere with testing, prior to examination.
- Failure to consider the contribution of chronic douching, spermicidal compounds, or condom-related latex allergy as contributors of vaginal irritation and discharge.

Complications

The most common complication is allowing confusing or conflicting results to lead to misguided or "shotgun" treatment.

Postprocedure Management

- Offer general education regarding the relationship of vulvovaginitis to self-treatment, douching, use of female "deodorant" or cleansing, latex, or spermicidal products.
- Offer specific instructions regarding the treatment modalities recommended such as intravaginal creams with applicator, oral medications, and side effects (e.g., metronidazole for BV).

Interpretation of Results

At least five different microscopic fields should be surveyed to observe an adequate number of representative fields. Initially low (10×) and high (40×) power should be used.

Findings: Saline Examination ("Wet Prep" or "Wet Smear")

- *Lactobacillus* species are normal vaginal flora. Lactobacilli are large, long bacillary rods. Their absence or decrease, coupled with an abundance of clue cells and a vaginal pH greater than 4.7, may be consistent with the clinical findings observed in bacterial vaginosis (Fig. 160-1).

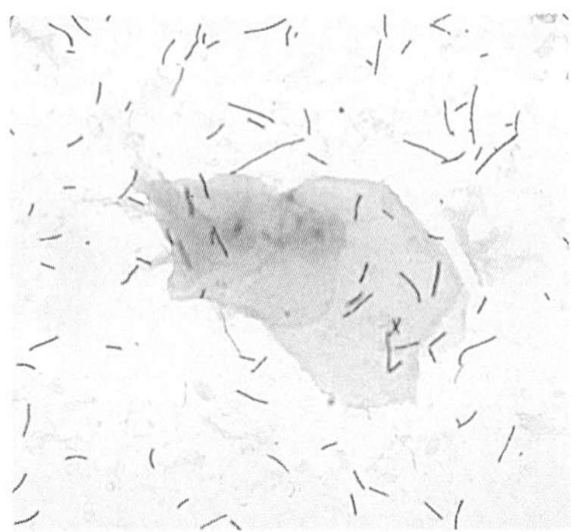

Figure 160-1 *Lactobacillus* species. (From Morse SA, Moreland A, Holmes K: Atlas of Sexually Transmitted Diseases and AIDS, 2nd ed. London, Gower Medical, 1996.)

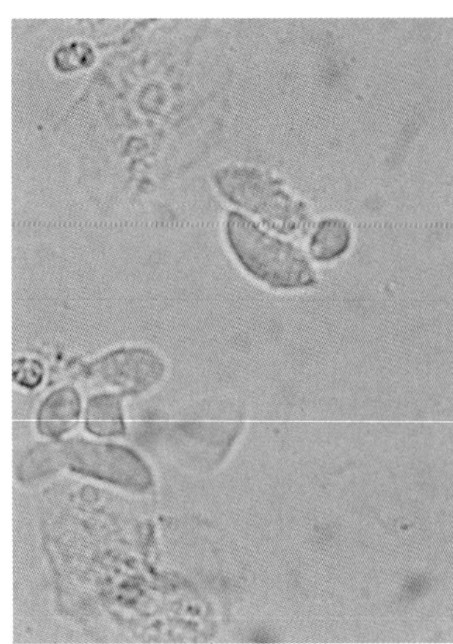

Figure 160-2 Microscopic examination of a wet mount reveals multiple motile trichomonads. (From Zitelli BJ, Davis HW: Atlas of Pediatric Physical Diagnosis, 4th ed. St Louis, Mosby, 2002.)

- Leukocytes at a concentration of more than 5 to 10 cells per high power field (HPF) may indicate infection. If the number of leukocytes exceeds the number of squamous cells, an inflammatory process should be suspected.
- Parabasal cells may indicate low estrogenic state.
- Trichomonads (*Trichomonas vaginalis*) distinctively appear as actively motile protozoans with whipping flagella (Fig. 160-2).
- Clue cells are epithelial cells with indistinct borders often described as "fuzzy" or "dirty" caused by abundant adherent multiple coccobacilli organisms. Clue cells are indicative of bacterial vaginosis (see Figs. 160-1 and 160-2).

Findings: KOH Examination

Hyphae or buds suggest candidiasis (Figs. 160-3 and 160-4). The absence of hyphae but presence of budding spores suggests infection with a non-*albicans* type of *Candida*, such as *C. glabrata* (Fig. 160-5).

pH Test

The range of values will be determined by the color of the tape.

Normal flora	pH 4.5
Candidiasis	pH 3.8 to 4.5
Bacterial vaginosis	pH 4.7
Trichomonas	pH above 4.5

NOTE: Combined infections such as yeast and BV can produce variable pH results.

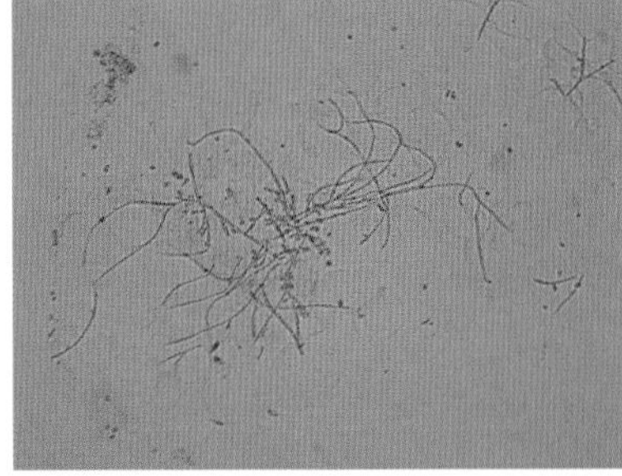

Figure 160-3 Low power of KOH preparation, which shows the ghost-like appearance of disintegrating epithelial cells from the KOH and the fungal mycelia and spore forms becoming evident. (Courtesy of Gary R. Newkirk, MD.)

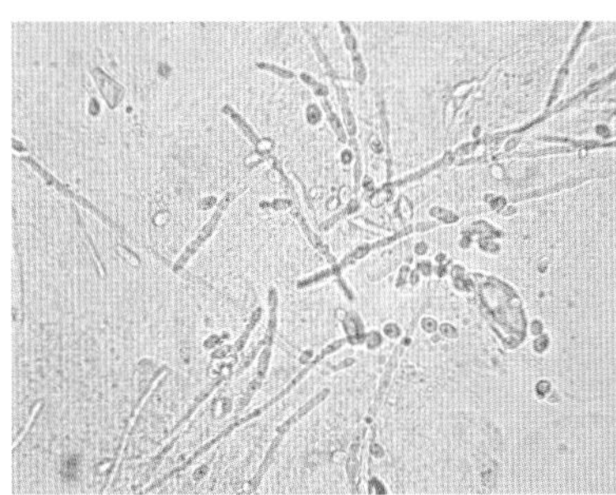

Figure 160-4 Higher power (40×) of mycelia, budding yeast, and spores supporting the diagnosis of yeast vaginitis. (Courtesy of Gary R. Newkirk, MD.)

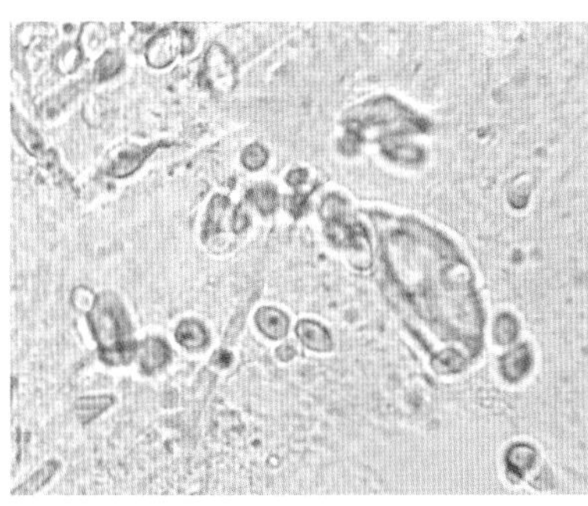

Figure 160-5 High power of KOH preparation with predominately spore forms suggesting Candida glabrata yeast vaginitis. (Courtesy of Gary R. Newkirk, MD.)

Whiff Test

The presence of a strong amine or "fishy" odor after application of 10% KOH implicates BV. A positive whiff test was predictive of positive culture results for anaerobic flora such as *Bacteroides* species with 67% sensitivity, 94% specificity, and a positive predictive value of 95%.

CPT/Billing Codes

58999 Unlisted procedure, female genital system (wet smear and KOH preparation)
87220 Tissue examination by KOH slide from skin, hair, or nails

ICD-9-CM Diagnostic Codes

112.1 Monilial vulvovaginitis (candidiasis)
131.01 Trichomonal vaginitis
616.10 Vaginitis and vulvovaginitis, unspecified (includes bacterial vaginosis)
623.5 Vaginal discharge
625.9 Unspecified symptom associated with female genital organs
627.3 Atrophic vaginitis

Acknowledgment

The editors wish to recognize the many contributions by Barbara Apgar, MD, to this chapter in a previous edition of this text.

ONLINE RESOURCE

Center for Disease Control: Diagnosis and treatment of vaginitis, at http://www.cdc.gov/std/treatment/2006/vaginal-discharge.htm.

BIBLIOGRAPHY

French L, Horton J, Matousek M: Abnormal vaginal discharge: Using office diagnostic testing more effectively. J Fam Practice 53:805–814, 2004.
Sobel JD: Vaginitis. N Engl J Med 337:1896–1903, 1997.
Usatine RP: The Color Atlas of Family Medicine. New York, McGraw-Hill, 2009.
Wiesenfeld HC, Macio I: The infrequent use of office-based diagnostic tests for vaginitis. Am J Obstet Gynecol 181:39–41, 1999.

SECTION 10

Obstetrics

Section Editor: DALE A. PATTERSON

CHAPTER 161

Amniocentesis

Dale A. Patterson • John J. Andazola

Amniocentesis is very helpful for evaluating an inaccessible in utero patient. Although genetic studies were first performed on amniotic fluid in the 1950s, before the 1970s the primary indication for amniocentesis was the Rh-immunized patient. Since that time, the indications have expanded to include evaluation of fetal lung maturity, fetal genetics, rupture or infection of the amniotic membranes or fluid, and other factors related to fetal health. In some centers caring for high-risk patients, amniocentesis is a routine procedure in approximately 15% of pregnancies. However, the overall frequency of amniocentesis has decreased every year since 1989—down to 1.7% of pregnancies in 2003. It is important to remember that complications from amniocentesis can be serious and occasionally lethal.

Indications

Prenatal Diagnosis (First and Second Trimester)

- *Chromosomal studies*. This is the most common reason for amniocentesis in the United States. Amniotic fluid contains fetal and amniotic cells. The fetal cells include desquamated squamous cells and cells from the gastrointestinal tract, respiratory tract, and urinary system. Although it requires 2 to 3 weeks for results, culture of these cells allows accurate fetal chromosome analysis for chromosomal, sex-linked, and metabolic disorders. For chromosomal analysis, amniocentesis is usually performed at 15 to 17 weeks, when there are sufficient numbers of desquamated fetal cells to allow successful culture. Although early amniocentesis (i.e., 10 to 14 weeks gestation) can be performed, chorionic villus sampling can also be performed around this time for similar indications. The risks and benefits of these procedures are similar but vary slightly by location and indication. Local availability and standards may influence the choice of procedure. Indications for early amniocentesis include the following:
  - Advanced maternal age (35 years of age or older)
  - Parent who is a carrier of a genetic disease that can be diagnosed by amniocentesis
  - Mother who is a carrier of an X-linked disorder
  - History of a child with a chromosomal disorder, neural tube defect, inherited biochemical disorder, or multiple anomalies
  - Mother with a history of three or more spontaneous abortions

NOTE: Some experts recommend that mothers be referred to specialized medical centers that perform 50 or more procedures per year for first-trimester or early second-trimester amniocentesis and genetic studies. Less fluid is available at this stage, and there may be less risk of complications with more operator experience. This is particularly important if the procedure must be performed *through* the placenta. A cell culture is also very fragile, and proper transport and assurance against loss or mix-up are essential. It may be best to perform the study at the institution where the cells will be cultured.

- *Abnormal prenatal testing results*. Triple screen, quad screen, and combined first-trimester screening are examples of frequently used prenatal tests for birth defects. Careful sonographic fetal evaluation in patients with abnormal prenatal testing results may diagnose (or exclude) an open neural tube defect or Down syndrome. Occasionally, amniocentesis may be required for clarification.
- *Evaluation for amnionitis*. In a patient with ruptured membranes and clinical signs of amnionitis, Gram's stain and culture of amniotic fluid may be performed before initiation of treatment (i.e., antibiotics and prompt delivery of the infant).

Evaluating Fetal Health (Late Second or Third Trimester)

Bilirubin levels, measured spectrophotometrically as ΔOD450, are no longer the standard of care for following the Rh or other blood group isoimmunized pregnancy. This has been replaced by Doppler ultrasonographic measurement of the peak velocity of systolic blood flow in the middle cerebral artery. The sensitivity and specificity of Doppler ultrasonography have been shown to be superior to those of measurement of the amniotic fluid ΔOD450. Doppler ultrasonography is noninvasive and thus does not carry the risk associated with amniocentesis. It is recommended that patients with Rh alloimmunization be referred to a center where Doppler ultrasonography of the middle cerebral artery is performed.

Evaluating Fetal Maturity (Third Trimester)

Another common reason for performing amniocentesis is to assess fetal lung maturity. Lecithin (L), sphingomyelin (S), and phosphatidylglycerol (PG) are phospholipids in the newborn lung that act as surfactants and lower the surface tension in the alveoli. Using amniocentesis to determine the L/S ratio, the presence of PG, or both, may minimize the risk of delivering an infant who will develop respiratory distress syndrome (RDS). Other methods to help determine fetal lung maturity include the foam stability index, fluorescence polarization, and lamellar body counts (Table 161-1). Kits are commercially available to help determine these measurements, or variations on them, and are therefore useful for predicting fetal lung maturity.

Therapeutic Interventions

- Relief of symptomatic polyhydramnios, although this is temporary because the fluid rapidly reaccumulates
- Intrauterine transfusion for Rh-hemolytic disease

Contraindications

Absolute

- Infected lesions of the abdominal wall where amniocentesis must be performed
- Patient refusal
- When the results of tests will not change the clinical course

TABLE 161-1 Commonly Used Direct Tests of Fetal Lung Maturity

Test*	Technique	Time and Ease of Testing†	Threshold	Typical Predictive Value (%): Mature — Negative Predictive Value	Typical Predictive Value (%): Immature — Positive‡ Predictive Value	Blood Contamination Affects Results	Meconium Contamination Affects Results	Vaginal Pool Sample
Fluorescence polarization	Fluorescence polarization with TDx-FLM II	1+	≥55 mg/g of albumin§	96–100	47–61	Yes	Yes	Yes
Lecithin/sphingomyelin ratio	Thin-layer chromatography	4+	2–3.5	95–100	33–50	Yes	Yes	No
Phosphatidylglycerol	Thin-layer chromatography	4+	Present (usually >3% of total phospholipids)	95–100	23–53	No	No	Yes
	Antisera with AminoStat-FLM	1+	0.5 = low positive 2 = high positive	95–100	23–53	No	No	Yes
Lamellar body counts	Counts using commercial hematology counter	2+	30,000–40,000 (still investigational)	97–98	29–35	Yes	No	Not available
Optical density at 650 nm	Spectrophotometric reading	1+	Optical density of ≥0.15	98	13	Not available	Not available	Not available
Foam stability index	Ethanol added to amniotic fluid, solution shaken, presence of stable bubbles at meniscus noted	2+	≥47–48	95	51	Yes	Yes	No

*Commercial versions are available for all tests except optical density and lamellar body counts.
†Range in complexity: 1+ indicates procedure is simple, procedure is available all the time, procedure time is short, and personnel effort is not intensive; 4+ indicates procedure is complex or difficult, time consuming, and, therefore, frequently not available at all times.
‡Positive predictive value is the probability of neonatal respiratory distress syndrome when the fetal lung maturity test result is immature.
§The manufacturer has reformulated the product and revised the testing procedure. Currently, the threshold for maturity is 55; with the original assay, it was 70.

Relative

- Maternal coagulopathy
- Placental abruption
- Problems not diagnosable by evaluation of the amniotic fluid (e.g., teratogen exposure, radiation exposure, drug use early in pregnancy, history of genetic disorders not diagnosable by amniocentesis)

EQUIPMENT AND SUPPLIES

- Real-time diagnostic ultrasonography unit
- Commercial amniocentesis tray or sterile tray containing at least three plain sterile specimen tubes (5 to 10 mL each) with caps; standard-length 20- or 22-gauge spinal needle (no larger than 20 gauge should be used); 20-mL syringe; 5-mL syringe; 1½-inch, 22- or 23-gauge needle; sterile 4 × 4 gauze pads; sterile Band-Aids; and sterile towels for drapes
- Skin antiseptic (e.g., povidone–iodine, chlorhexidine gluconate)
- Fetal heart rate monitor
- Sterile gloves
- Local anesthetic solution (e.g., 1% or 2% lidocaine, *without* epinephrine) *(optional)*

NOTE: To obtain disposable amniocentesis trays, the clinician should check with a local surgical supplier.

PREPROCEDURE PATIENT EDUCATION AND FORMS

The clinician should discuss the procedure with the patient (and the patient's partner, if available) beforehand. Both people should be informed of the risks and the benefits of having an amniocentesis. In addition, the clinician should describe alternative modes of evaluation or treatment (if any) and obtain signed informed consent. (See the sample patient education and consent forms available online at www.expertconsult.com.)

TECHNIQUE

1. Have the patient lie on the examining table or bed with the head elevated 20 to 30 degrees. Alternatively, perform the procedure with the patient in the slight (15 degrees) left lateral decubitus position. Monitor the fetal heart rate for 20 minutes to establish a baseline.
2. Locate a pocket of fluid with real-time ultrasonography (Fig. 161-1). Try to find a pocket that the needle will be able to reach without going through the placenta or near the fetal face. The best locations (associated with low risk of cord puncture) are usually in the area of the fetal extremities. Use the ultrasound *electronic* calipers to measure the depth from the skin that the needle must penetrate to enter the pocket. Note the desired longitudinal angle for the needle. If not perpendicular to the abdomen, note the lateral angle of the probe used to locate the pocket. The needle should be directed at the same lateral angle. Mark the location of the puncture site on the skin using pressure from a needle hub.
3. Prepare the abdomen with antiseptic solution.
4. The use of local anesthetic is optional. If desired, wearing sterile gloves, raise a skin wheal with the anesthetic at the puncture site, then continue to anesthetize along the course of the needle track to the parietal peritoneum and serosal surface of the uterus (requires 4 to 5 mL of anesthetic solution). Remove the needle.
5. With the stylet in place and with concurrent real-time ultrasonographic guidance (transducer in sterile plastic bag, glove, or cover), insert the 20- or 22-gauge spinal needle along the selected track (at the correct angles) to the previously measured depth. The clinician should feel a little "pop" as the needle moves through the fascia. When it penetrates the amniotic membrane, there is sudden free movement.
6. Remove the stylet. In most cases the amniotic fluid will flow through the needle. If not, rotate the needle (this may move the tip away from membranes, fetal parts, etc.). If there is no flow of fluid, attach the empty 5-mL anesthetic syringe to the needle hub and apply gentle suction. If there is still no fluid, replace the stylet and advance the needle another 0.5 to 1 cm or until resistance

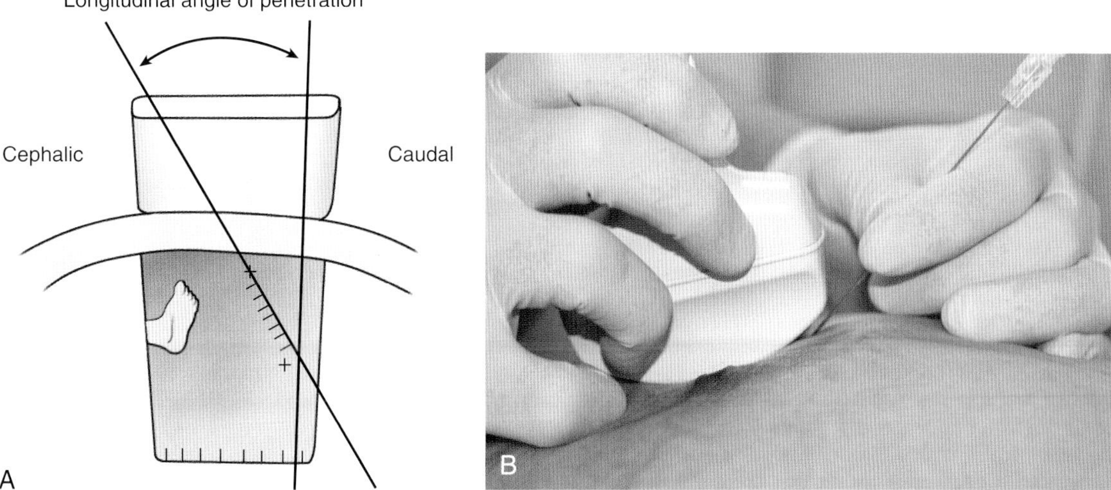

Figure 161-1 Proper insertion of needle. **A,** Graphical depiction. Note measurements with calipers; the needle direction is also determined. **B,** Photograph. Needle is inserted to previously measured depth at the proper angle.

is felt. Again, remove the stylet. If there is no fluid, reattach the small syringe and withdraw the needle slowly with gentle suction, rotating it as it is withdrawn.

7. Once the fluid pocket is located, withdraw 2 or 3 mL of fluid in the small syringe and then discard it. This minimizes the amount of blood in the remaining fluid sample (blood can affect laboratory results). Next, withdraw 15 to 25 mL of fluid (or the volume needed for the tests planned). Remove the needle, clean the excess antiseptic from the abdominal wall, and cover the puncture wound with a Band-Aid. If the patient is unsensitized Rh-negative, administer 300 mg of Rh-immune globulin.
8. If no amniotic fluid is obtained, repeat the ultrasonographic examination and again localize the fluid pocket, its angle, and its distance from the skin; prepare the skin with antiseptic and repeat the tap (again under continuous ultrasonographic guidance). It is recommended that no more than two attempts be made because repeated attempts increase the risk of significant fetal injury or induction of labor. It is also important not to use a needle larger than 20 gauge because the incidence of complications rises with needle gauge.

Sample Operative Report

The patient was placed in low semi-Fowler's position and the fetal heart tones were monitored for 20 minutes. Real-time ultrasonography was used to locate a collection of amniotic fluid in the area of the fetal extremities at a depth of 5 cm. No loops of cord were noted. The overlying skin was marked, prepped with povidone–iodine solution, and draped with sterile towels. After local anesthesia with 1% lidocaine (if used), a 20-gauge spinal needle was inserted into the fluid pocket under continuous ultrasound guidance. A total of 15 mL of clear (or "meconium stained," "slightly blood tinged," "grossly bloody") amniotic fluid was removed without (with) difficulty. A sterile dressing was applied to the puncture site, and the fetal heart tones were monitored for another 20 minutes; these remained reassuring. The patient felt well and was discharged with warnings and instructions for follow-up.

Complications

A wide variety of complications have been reported, including injuries and even fetal death. However, serious complications are uncommon and the procedure is considered relatively safe in experienced hands. Complications from amniocentesis include the following:

- Pain, bruising, or infection at the puncture site
- Abdominal visceral injury
- Uterine contractions, occasionally progressing to labor but usually self-limited
- Occasional (0.8% to 1.1% risk) spontaneous abortion after late first-trimester or midtrimester amniocentesis
- Premature rupture of membranes
- Placental separation or abruption
- Fetal injury, such as skin scars, dimpling, eye injury, genital injury (risk increases with oligohydramnios)
- Orthopedic deformities of the newborn
- Cord or placental blood vessel injury with resultant fetal hemorrhage
- Rh-factor isoimmunization
- Uterine or amniotic fluid infection
- Fluid leak with resultant oligohydramnios *(rare)*

Postprocedure Management

After a normal successful amniocentesis, monitor the fetal heart rate and the mother's response for 20 to 30 minutes, after which the patient may leave. Prolonged monitoring for 1 to 2 hours may be indicated if there are frequent uterine contractions or if the sample was grossly bloody. Often, placental bleeding can be seen on ultrasonography and monitored visually.

Postprocedure Patient Education

Printed instructions help patients remember what they are told. The clinician should give the patient an instruction sheet to use after amniocentesis.

Interpretation of Results

1. PG by itself can be used as an indicator of fetal lung maturity. Blood, meconium, or vaginal secretions (as contaminants) in the amniotic fluid do not affect PG. PG does not appear until 35 weeks' gestation; therefore, although it is not an absolute guarantee, the presence of PG provides considerable reassurance against the occurrence of RDS. Also important, the absence of PG is not necessarily a strong predictor of RDS after delivery. Although commercially available kits can be used to document PG presence rapidly and with considerable accuracy, it still usually takes several hours to obtain the results. That is why L/S studies are usually more convenient and still considered the gold standard for fetal lung maturity.
2. At about 33 weeks' gestation, the concentration of L relative to S begins to rise, and both can be measured directly. It has been

frequently reported that the risk of RDS is very slight when the L/S ratio is greater than 2, and there is an increased risk of RDS when the ratio is below 2. It should be noted that with some complications of pregnancy, such as maternal diabetes, RDS may occur despite a mature L/S ratio. As a result, some clinicians require the presence of PG before an elective delivery of a diabetic mother. In addition, the presence of blood has been reported to both increase and decrease the ratio, and the presence of meconium can produce falsely mature results.

3. The "shake test" is a rapid screening test for L/S ratio in which varying dilutions of amniotic fluid are shaken with ethanol. Ethanol is a nonfoaming, competitive surfactant that eliminates the contributions of protein, bile salts, and salts of free fatty acids to the formation of a stable foam. At an ethanol concentration of 47.5%, stable bubbles that foam after shaking are due entirely to lecithin in the amniotic fluid. Positive tests, a complete ring of bubbles at the meniscus with a 1 : 2 dilution of amniotic fluid, are rarely associated with RDS. The shake test is moderately good, but not excellent, at predicting RDS, and it should therefore be regarded as a screening procedure.

   To perform the shake test, the clinician should mix 1 mL of amniotic fluid with 1 mL of 95% ethanol. This vial should be compared with a second vial of 1 mL of amniotic fluid mixed with 0.5 mL of 95% ethanol and 0.5 mL of normal saline. After 30 seconds of vigorous shaking, a ring of bubbles in the second vial indicates an L/S ratio of 2 or greater. Bubbles in the 1 : 1 mix, but not in the second vial, indicate that the fetus is in a bordering stage of development but not yet mature.
4. The foam stability index (FSI) is a commercially available variation of the shake test. The kit has test wells built into it containing predispensed amounts of ethanol. Amniotic fluid (0.5 mL) is added to each well and shaken. A "control" demonstrates an example of the stable foam end point. The FSI is read as the highest reading corresponding to a well in which a ring of stable foam persists. This test appears to be a reliable predictor of fetal lung maturity if the FSI is 47 or higher; however, this test is unreliable if the amniotic fluid is contaminated with blood.
5. Although results are not available as rapidly as with the shake test, the fluorescence polarization test, or fetal lung maturity (FLM) assay, usually provides results faster than a PG assay. The FLM assesses overall surfactant activity, using polarized light to quantify the competitive binding of a probe to albumin and surfactant in amniotic fluid. An FLM result greater than 55 mg of surfactant per gram of albumin indicates maturity, from 35 to 55 indicates borderline maturity, and less than 35 indicates immaturity.
6. Lamellar counts on the amniotic fluid are also quite reliable if they show fetal lung maturity. They are quick, inexpensive, and readily available anywhere that platelet counts are done. Clinicians experienced with lamellar counts often use them as a quick screen to decide who needs the full L/S or PG evaluation. Values of 50,000/μL or greater are consistent with fetal lung maturity.

Patient Education Guides

See patient education and consent forms available online at www.expertconsult.com.

CPT/Billing Codes

The clinician should include a picture of the amniotic fluid pocket from the ultrasonographic examination (when possible; Fig. 161-2) and a procedure note in the documentation.

59000 Amniocentesis, diagnostic
59001 Amniocentesis, therapeutic amniotic fluid reduction (includes ultrasound guidance)
76946 Ultrasonic guidance for amniocentesis, imaging supervision and interpretation

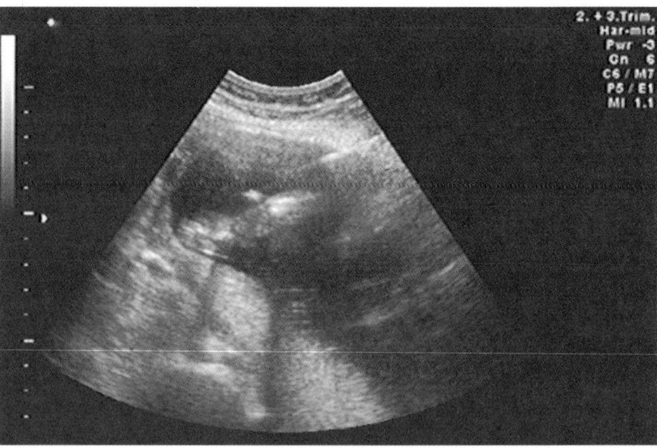

Figure 161-2 Example of an ultrasonographic image to be photographed for documenting the site chosen for amniocentesis. Note the large pocket of fluid and the absence of the cord. Also note the visualization of the needle.

ICD-9-CM Diagnostic Codes

These are illustrative codes for conditions commonly associated with amniocentesis. A fifth digit (represented by an asterisk) is used in codes 640 to 648 and 651 to 659. Following are the fifth digits used and the episodes of care they represent:

0 Unspecified
1 Delivered, with or without mention of antepartum condition
2 Delivered, with mention of postpartum complication
3 Antepartum condition or complication
4 Postpartum condition or complication
642.5* Severe preeclampsia
644.0* Threatened premature labor (after 22 weeks)
645.2* Prolonged pregnancy
646.3* Habitual aborter
654.2* Previous cesarean delivery, NOS
655.1* Chromosomal abnormality in fetus
655.2* Hereditary disease in family, possibly affecting fetus
655.8* Other known or suspected fetal abnormality, not elsewhere classified
656.1* Rh isoimmunization
656.3* Fetal distress
657.0* Polyhydramnios
658.1* Premature rupture of membranes
658.4* Chorioamnionitis
659.6* Advanced maternal age, primiparous or multiparous

Acknowledgment

The editors wish to recognize the contributions by Clark B. Smith, MD, to this chapter in the previous two editions of this text.

BIBLIOGRAPHY

Caughey AB, Hopkins LM, Norton ME: Chorionic villus sampling compared with amniocentesis and the difference in the rate of pregnancy loss. Obstet Gynecol 108:612–616, 2006.

Oepkes D, Seaward PG, Vandenbussche FP, et al: Doppler ultrasonography versus amniocentesis to predict fetal anemia. N Engl J Med 355:156–164, 2006.

Reece EA: Early and midtrimester genetic amniocentesis: Safety and outcomes. Obstet Gynecol Clin North Am 24:71–81, 1997.

Seeds JW: Diagnostic mid trimester amniocentesis: How safe? Am J Obstet Gynecol 191:608–616, 2004.

Silver RK, Russell TL, Kambich MP, et al: Midtrimester amniocentesis: Influence of operator caseload on sampling efficiency. J Reprod Med 43:191–195, 1998.

CHAPTER 162

CESAREAN SECTION

Lee I. Blecher • Benjamin Mailloux

Cesarean section is the operative delivery of an infant and is usually performed to decrease risk of perinatal morbidity and mortality. The term *cesarean* is considered to have been derived from the Latin verb *caedere*, "to cut." The first reported case series of cesarean sections was published in 1591 by Rouseto and Casparo. In the United States, the rate of cesarean deliveries has been increasing every year since 1996, and in 2005 cesarean sections made up approximately 30% of all deliveries. For many years before 1960, the cesarean rate was closer to 5%.

Among family physicians in the United States, 23% actively perform vaginal deliveries and about 7% perform cesarean deliveries. These family physicians are found in a wide variety of practice settings ranging from urban teaching institutions to isolated rural practices. Several family medicine obstetrics fellowships exist to offer additional training for family physicians to perform cesarean sections.

This chapter discusses one standard technique for performing an uncomplicated low transverse cesarean section. It does not attempt to discuss all of the possible techniques or medical situations in which a cesarean section may be necessary. For a more exhaustive review of how to handle complications or more complex surgical deliveries, references are listed in the bibliography.

INDICATIONS

Maternal Indications

- Repeat cesarean when mother declines or fails a trial of labor
- Repeat cesarean when a trial of labor is not indicated (e.g., prior classical uterine incision)
- Antepartum hemorrhage
- Obstructive pelvic, vaginal, or vulvar tumors or condylomata
- Cervical cancer
- Severe hypertension or severe preeclampsia
- Contracted pelvis (cephalopelvic disproportion)
- Labor intolerance resulting from medical disease
- Uterine rupture
- Maternal thrombocytopenia
- Active maternal herpes simplex genital infection
- Maternal exhaustion or arrest of labor
- Failed postdates induction
- Placenta previa
- Placental abruption

Fetal Indications

- Malpresentation (e.g., brow or face presentation, transverse or breech lie)
- Failed trial of forceps or vacuum
- Arrest of the active stage, including deep transverse arrest
- Nonreassuring fetal heart rate (e.g., recurrent late decelerations, bradycardia, lack of heart rate variability)
- Fetal anomalies
- Cord prolapse
- Shoulder dystocia
- Very low birth-weight infant (<1500 g)
- Multiple gestation or twins with first being nonvertex
- Perimortem
- Macrosomia (controversial; estimated fetal weight >4500 g or >4000 g in diabetic mother)
- Maternal human immunodeficiency virus infection

CONTRAINDICATIONS

Because cesarean section is considered a life-saving procedure in many instances, there are no absolute contraindications other than patient refusal after the consequences have been explained clearly and accepted by the mother.

EQUIPMENT

- Intravenous antibiotic such as cefoxitin 1 g, or for penicillin-allergic patient, clindamycin 600 mg
- Terbutaline
- Standard operating room cesarean section package to include the following:

Quantity Needed	Instrument
2	Babcock clamps (if tubal ligation planned)
6	Allis clamps
4	Pennington clamps (8 inch)
2	Tissue forceps (toothed; 6 and 8 inch)
2	Dressing forceps (smooth; 6 and 8 inch)
2	Russian forceps (6 and 8 inch)
4	Sponge forceps
2	Adson forceps with teeth
2	No. 20 blade scalpels
1	No. 10 blade scalpel
6	Curved hemostats (5½ inch)
6	Curved Kelly clamps
2	Needle holders
4	Kocher or Ochsner clamps (7½ inch)
2	Army-Navy retractors
1	DeLee, Fritsch, or Rochard universal retractor
3	Richardson retractors (small, medium, and large)
1	Bandage scissors (7¼ inch)
1	Metzenbaum scissors (7 inch)
1	Curved Mayo scissors (6½ inch)
1	Suture scissors
1	Straight Mayo scissors (6½ inch)
1	Poole suction tip
1	Yankauer tonsil suction tip
4	Packages of suture (two packages each of 0 chromic and 1-0 Vicryl; 2-0 and 3-0 chromic, optional)
20	Lap sponges
1	Surgical stapler
1	Bovie cautery device
1	Cervical dilators set

Box 162-1. Typical Preoperative Orders for Cesarean Section

CBC without diff, urinalysis
Type and hold 2 units PRBCs
Foley to gravity
Anesthesia pre-op for epidural, spinal, or general anesthesia
NPO
IV lactated Ringer's at 125 mL/hr
Prep abdomen per MD preference

PRECAUTIONS

There are several conditions that increase the risks associated with performing a cesarean section that should be known, prepared for, and managed where possible.

- Grand multiparity
- Preterm delivery
- Placenta previa
- Placenta accreta
- Morbid maternal obesity
- Transverse lie
- Maternal coagulopathy
- Large uterine fibroids
- Multiple gestation
- Repeat cesarean on patient with extensive adhesions

PREPROCEDURE PATIENT EDUCATION

Informed consent should be obtained, the patient's questions should be answered, and a consent form signed. A standard hospital consent form can be used, emphasizing the following risks to the patient and infant undergoing cesarean section:

- Complications due to anesthesia
- Injury to the bladder or ureters
- Injury to the bowel
- Need for hysterectomy
- Hemorrhage requiring transfusion
- Infection
- Injury to the fetus (rare)
- Rupture of the uterus during future labors

A consent for use of blood products in the event of hemorrhage should also be obtained. Box 162-1 shows typical preoperative orders for a cesarean section.

TECHNIQUE

There are three choices of uterine incision when performing a cesarean section: low transverse (Kerr), low vertical (Krönig), and classic. These are outlined in Table 162-1. The most popular technique, the low transverse (Kerr), is described here.

1. Create a left tilt by either tilting the operating table or placing a wedge under the patient when regional anesthesia is used. (This displaces the uterus to the left, which permits better venous return and improves fetal oxygenation.)
2. After anesthesia is induced by a regional (epidural), spinal, or general anesthetic, test for anesthesia of the abdominal skin with the Allis clamp.
3. When anesthesia is deemed adequate, perform a Pfannenstiel skin incision by incising the abdominal skin to a width of approximately 13 to 15 cm, two fingerbreadths above the symphysis pubis, using a no. 10 blade (Fig. 162-1). Maintain hemostasis from dermal bleeding with Bovie cautery.
4. Carry the incision down through the subcutaneous fat to the fascia with the no. 20 blade. In the midline, make a 2-cm horizontal incision in the fascia with the scalpel. Lift the fascia and extend the cut edges laterally and superiorly in a curvilinear fashion with the curved Mayo scissors (Fig. 162-2).
5. Grasp the superior edge of the fascia with two Kocher clamps to elevate the fascia off of the underlying muscle, and bluntly dissect the fascia and the heavier fibers of the linea alba away from the muscle with fingers, staying in the midline (Figs. 162-3 and 162-4). This may be more difficult in a repeat case because of adhesive scar formation. In such cases, use the Mayo scissors to cut the adhesions. Then use the Mayo scissors again to cut through the midline fibers of the linea alba. Be careful not to cut the muscle tissue or to cut a "buttonhole" through the fascia. Repeat this dissection on the inferior edge of the fascia, bluntly and sharply dissecting the fascia away from the muscular tissue.
6. Bluntly separate the rectus muscle in the midline in a vertical fashion to expose the peritoneum. Grasp the peritoneum superiorly with two hemostats, tent it away from the underlying viscera, and incise with the no. 20 blade (Fig. 162-5). Keep this incision above the urachus (if visualized) to ensure you are above the bladder. Bluntly extend this incision vertically, slightly, being careful not to extend to the bladder inferiorly.
7. Place the DeLee bladder blade to retract and identify the bladder.
8. Develop the bladder flap (Fig. 162-6) by picking up the peritoneum over the lower uterine segment with tissue forceps and incising it laterally to make a flap approximately 12 cm long

TABLE 162-1 Types of Uterine Incisions

Incision	Advantages	Disadvantages
Low transverse	Lower uterine segment is thin and less vascular Incision heals well, less risk of subsequent dehiscence Most popular, >90% of all cesarean births	Risk of lateral extension into the uterine vessels
Low vertical	Useful if lower uterine segment is thick or has fibroids For transverse lie with back down For fetal anomalies such as hydrocephalus	Need for greater separation of the bladder from lower uterine segment Need for repeat cesarean section if upper segment entered
Classic incision	Suitable for emergent cases, easiest and fastest access to the infant Better exposure Ability to develop a larger opening for delivery	Increased blood loss Difficult repair (three-layer) Increased risk of rupture in subsequent pregnancies Adhesion formation between incision and abdominal organs Eight times greater risk of dehiscence than transverse incision

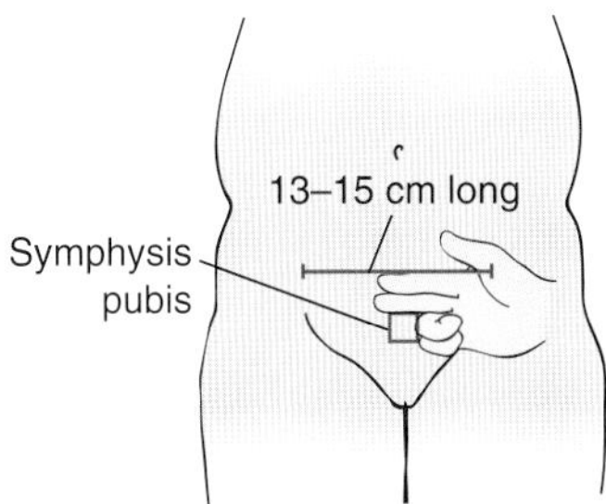

Figure 162-1 Pfannenstiel skin incision. The horizontal incision is carried out two fingerbreadths above the symphysis pubis.

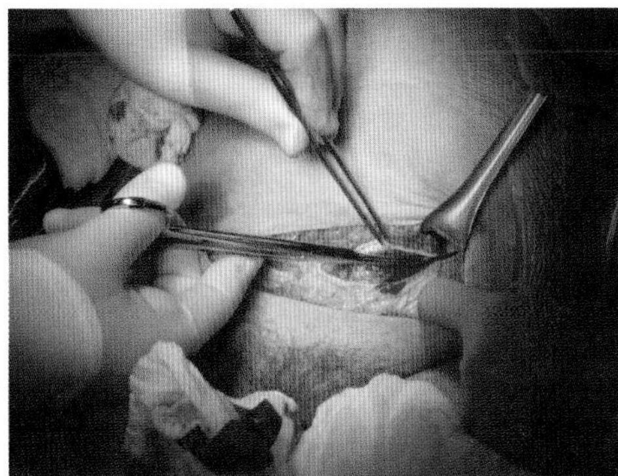

Figure 162-2 Extending the fascia incision using curved Mayo scissors.

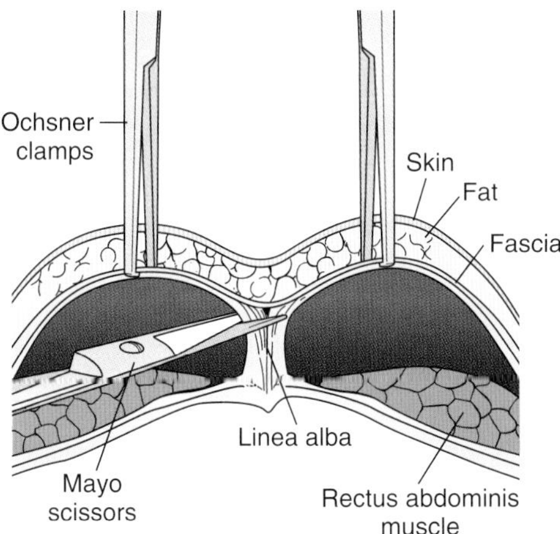

Figure 162-3 Dissection of the linea alba.

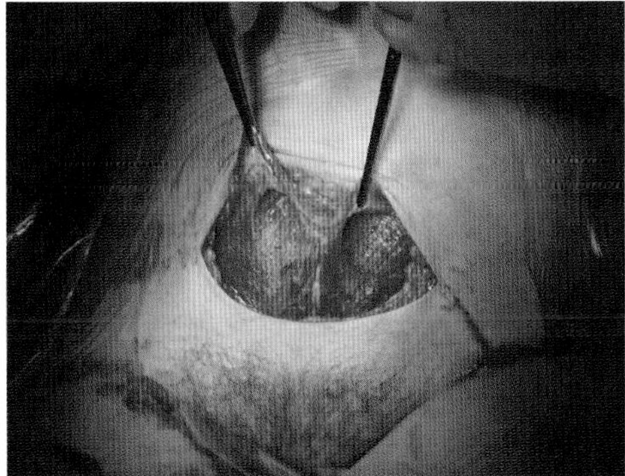

Figure 162-4 Elevating the fascia off the underlying muscle by gripping the superior edge using two Kocher clamps.

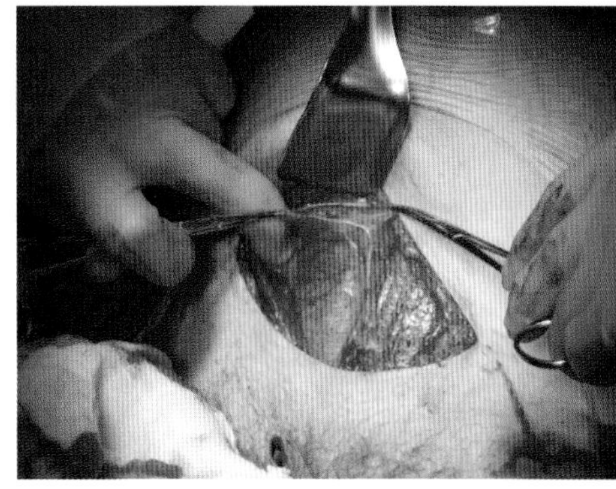

Figure 162-5 After tenting the exposed peritoneum with two hemostats, a small incision is made before bluntly extending it.

(Figs. 162-7 and 162-8). Dissect the peritoneum off of the uterus bluntly with the fingers. Reapply the DeLee bladder blade to include the inferior bladder flap just created.

9. Determine the position of the lateral uterine vessels as well as the orientation of the uterus. Next, incise the lower uterine segment over the fetal head, known as *scoring the uterus* (Fig. 162-9). Announce "uterine incision" so that the anesthesiologist and nursery attendant can prepare for imminent delivery. It is best to use a no. 20 blade and a 2- to 3-cm incision, proceeding millimeter by millimeter in depth to avoid injuring the presenting fetal part below (Fig. 162-10).
10. Extend the uterine incision bluntly with fingers. A bandage scissors may then be used to extend (protecting the fetal parts with two fingers inside the opening) the incision in a superior and lateral direction through the lower uterine segment for a total incision of approximately 10 to 11 cm (Fig. 162-11). However, this carries the added risk of extending the incision into the uterine arteries, so proceed with caution.
11. Rupture the membranes with the Allis clamp.
12. Deliver the fetal head by inserting a cupped hand over the head and occiput, keeping the wrist straight. Gently lift upward without flexing the wrist, bringing the head out of the incision along with your hand (Fig. 162-12). It may be necessary for the assistant to exert gentle fundal pressure after the occiput has cleared the incision.

NOTE: If the head is flexed tightly or stuck from excessive pushing before the procedure, as is common in arrest of descent cases or true cephalopelvic disproportion, have an assistant push

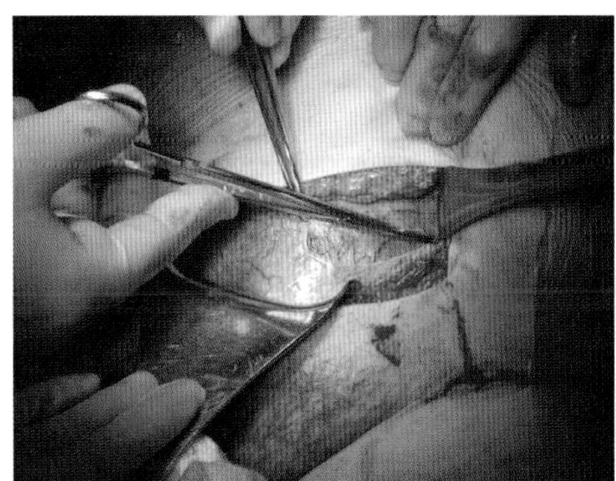

Figure 162-6 Developing the bladder flap.

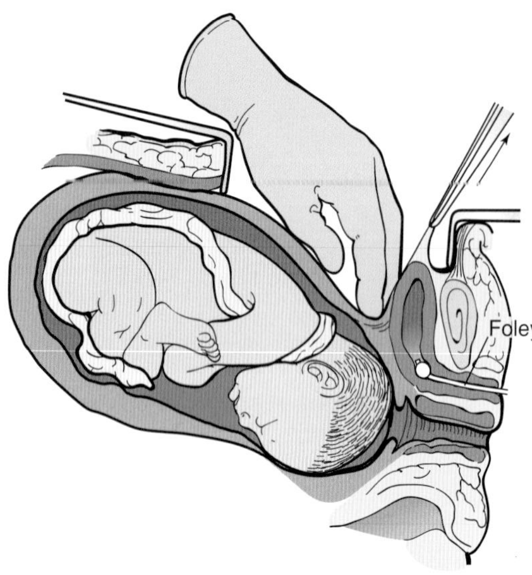

Figure 162-7 Dissection of the bladder away from the uterus.

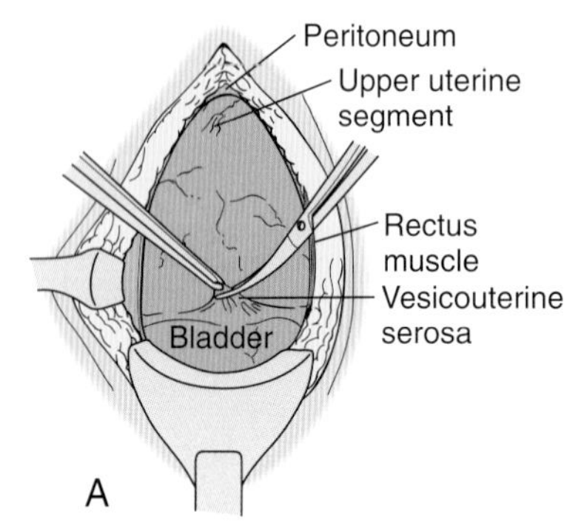

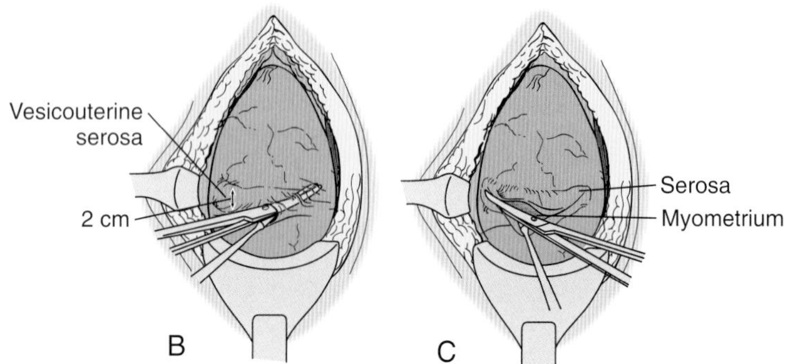

Figure 162-8 Development of the bladder flap. **A,** Tenting of the peritoneum. **B,** Undermining the peritoneum. **C,** Incising the peritoneum. (Redrawn from Cunningham FG, MacDonald P, Gant NF, et al [eds]: Williams Obstetrics, 19th ed. Norwalk, Conn, Appleton & Lange, 1993, pp 591–613.)

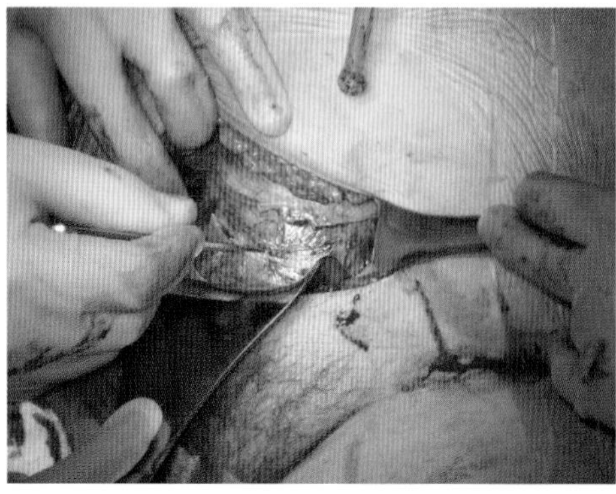

Figure 162-9 Scoring the uterus.

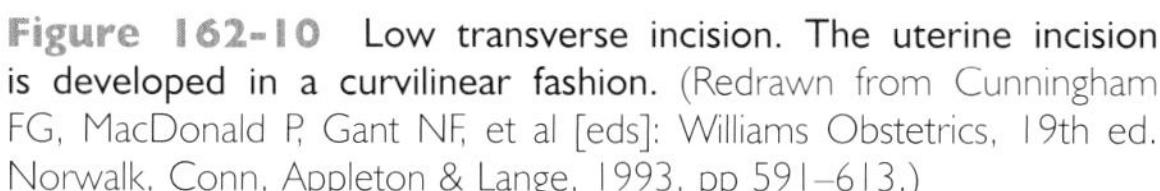

Figure 162-10 Low transverse incision. The uterine incision is developed in a curvilinear fashion. (Redrawn from Cunningham FG, MacDonald P, Gant NF, et al [eds]: Williams Obstetrics, 19th ed. Norwalk, Conn, Appleton & Lange, 1993, pp 591–613.)

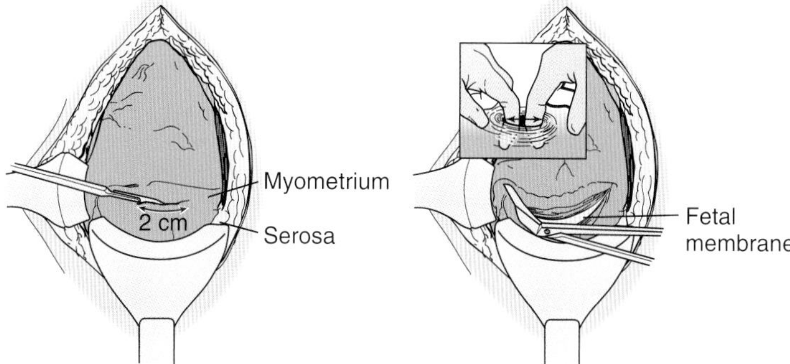

the head inward and upward from below (Fig. 162-13). Occasionally it may be necessary to inject 0.25 mg terbutaline subcutaneously or intravenously (IV) to relax the uterus in order to move the infant upward far enough to allow for delivery. Note that use of terbutaline can increase blood loss from uterine atony.

13. Suction the infant's mouth and nose; deliver the anterior shoulder, the posterior shoulder, and then the rest of the infant as in a vaginal delivery. Clamp and cut the cord and hand the infant to the nurse in attendance. Obtain cord blood if necessary, and then manually extract the placenta bluntly with the fingers (Fig. 162-14). Remove the last adherent membranes with the aid of ring forceps.
14. Give one dose of perioperative antibiotics after the cord is clamped. This has been proved to reduce postoperative wound infection by 50%. A broad-spectrum cephalosporin, such as cefoxitin 1 g IV, can be used. In penicillin-allergic patients, use clindamycin 600 mg IV in one dose.
15. You may choose to externalize the uterus for improved visualization and access, but this is optional. To control blood loss, place two Pennington clamps at the edges of the incision where bleeding is most vigorous. Wrap the uterine fundus in a clean, moist lap sponge as you massage the uterus; gently clean the inner endometrium with moist lap sponges so that it is free of any clots, membranes, and debris. Should the cervix be closed, dilate it with cervical dilators at this point.
16. Now close the hysterotomy incision with a running locked stitch of 0 chromic (Figs. 162-15 and 162-16). Should bleeding or oozing continue after a one-layer closure, imbricate with another layer of 0 chromic. Do not include the endometrial layer in the closure of the myometrium. Should an extension of the incision occur (typically inferiorly toward the cervix), repair the extension first, and then repair the hysterotomy incision. Occasionally, one small area of the hysterotomy incision may bleed and can be repaired with a figure-of-8 stitch for hemostasis.
17. Inspect the uterus, tubes, and ovaries. If a bilateral tubal ligation is desired, this is the time to do it.
18. Irrigate and suction the pouch of Douglas of clots and debris using warm saline and a tonsil suction tip, and then return the uterus to the abdominal cavity.
19. Irrigate and suction the abdominal cavity of clots and debris using warm saline and a tonsil suction tip. Palpate the right and left colic gutters for abnormal structures, and inspect the appendix and gallbladder.
    Optional: Close the bladder flap/parietal peritoneum with 2-0 chromic. However, most experts do not recommend closing the peritoneum because it will reapproximate on its own without suturing.
20. Close the two-layered fascia in a running stitch with 1-0 Vicryl or any other strong monofilament suture. Make sure that the sutures are placed equally across the incision and no more than 1 cm apart (Fig. 162-17).
21. Irrigate the subcutaneous fat and stop any bleeding with Bovie cautery (Fig. 162-18).
    Optional: Close the subcutaneous dead space. This is necessary only for patients with a very large pannus in which it is difficult to reapproximate the skin without this step. Remember that every suture placed is a nidus for possible infection,

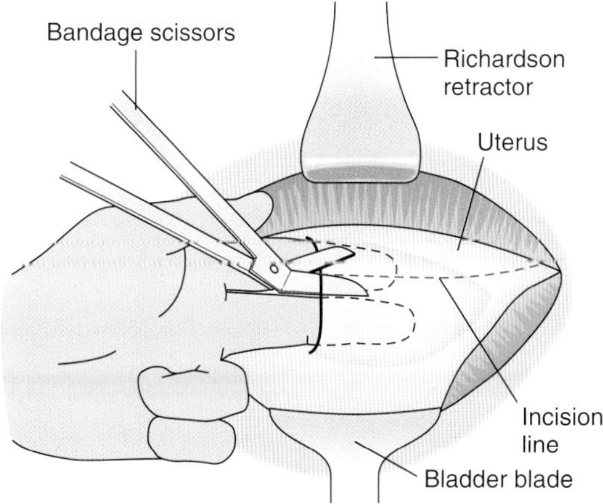

Figure 162-11 Protecting the fetal head from the bandage scissors when incising the uterus. Two fingers are placed under the incision to protect the infant from the bandage scissors.

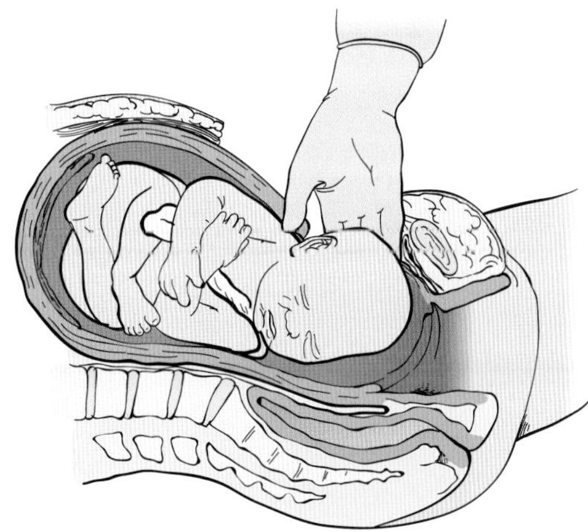

Figure 162-12 Lifting the fetal head out of the uterus. Keep the wrist straight to avoid using the uterus as a fulcrum.

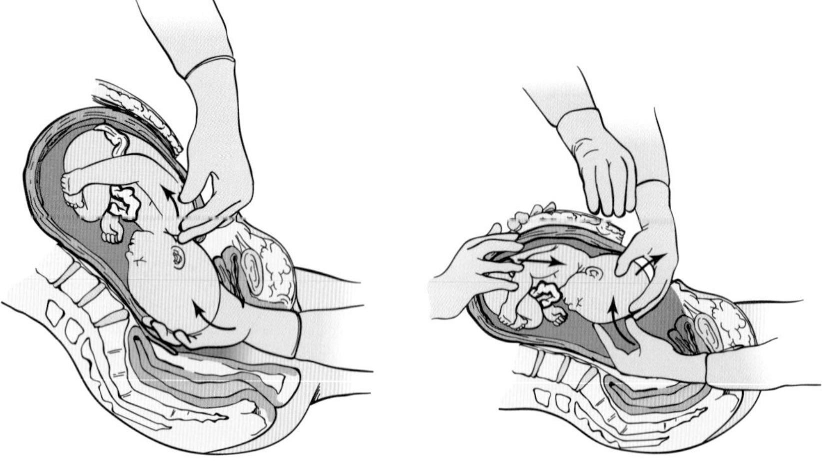

Figure 162-13 Technique to extract an impacted fetal head. An assistant exerts gentle upward force on the head from the vagina as the operator exerts steady upward pressure on the head and shoulders. (Redrawn from Plauché WC, Morrison JC, O'Sullivan MJ [eds]: Surgical Obstetrics. Philadelphia, WB Saunders, 1992, pp 431–436.)

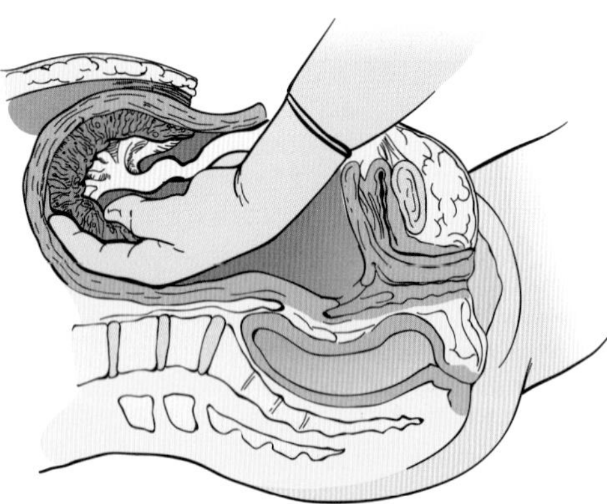

Figure 162-14 Manual extraction of the placenta.

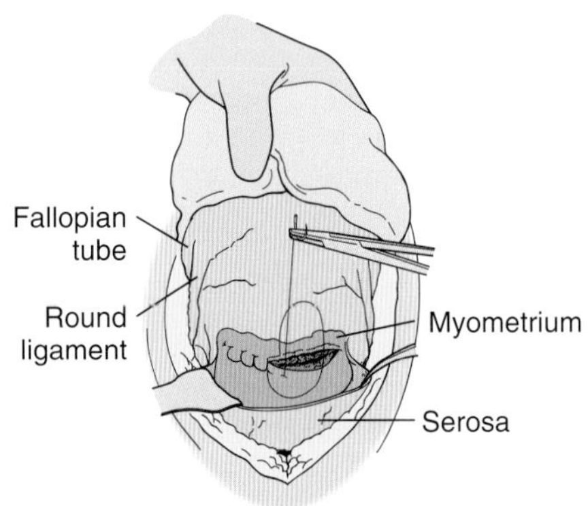

Figure 162-15 Uterine closure with a running locked stitch of 0 chromic catgut suture. (Redrawn from Cunningham FG, MacDonald P, Gant NF, et al [eds]: Williams Obstetrics, 19th ed. Norwalk, Conn, Appleton & Lange, 1993, pp 591–613.)

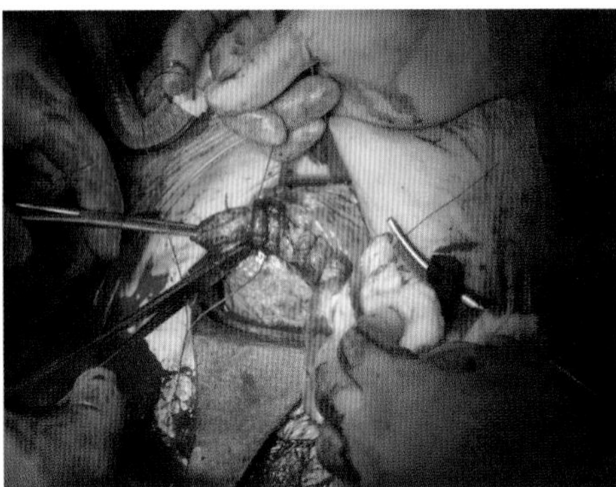

Figure 162-16 Closing the uterus using running locked stitch.

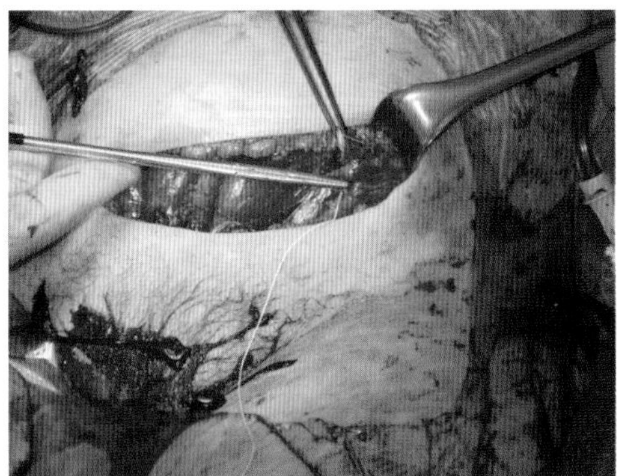

Figure 162-17 Closing the fascia.

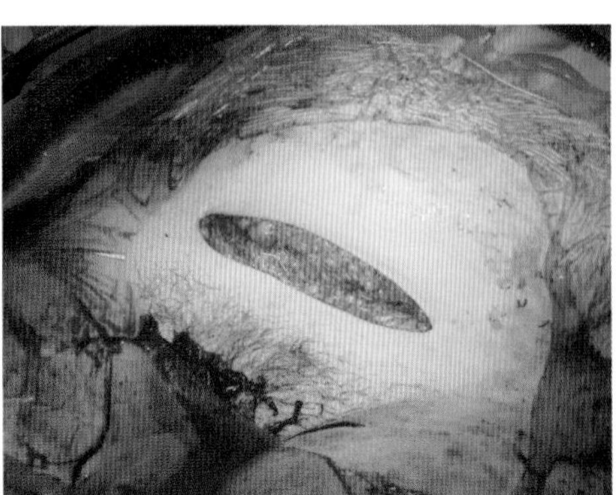

Figure 162-18 The subcutaneous fat after closure.

so keep the amount of suturing to the required steps only. If suturing is required for closure, use interrupted sutures with absorbable suture material, such as 3-0 chromic gut.

22. Close the skin. Most surgeons prefer the skin stapler, which does an excellent job when staples are placed 1 cm apart. However, a plastic skin closure with deep buried sutures and a final subcuticular stitch is certainly acceptable if time permits.

Sample Operative Report

The sample operative report, available online at www.expertconsult.com, shows an example of an ordinary, uncomplicated case. Any complications should be added and noted in the dictation.

Complications

- From anesthesia
- Injury to the bladder or ureters
- Injury to the bowel
- Uterine hemorrhage
- Infection: endometritis, urinary tract infection, respiratory infection, atelectasis, wound infection, septic pelvic thrombophlebitis
- Pulmonary embolism
- Risk of rupture in future deliveries
- Injury to the child

Postoperative Orders

Box 162-2 shows typical postoperative orders for cesarean section.

Box 162-2. Typical Postoperative Orders for Cesarean Section

1. Admit to the service of ____________________.
2. Admit to recovery room, then to floor as per PACU protocol.
3. Monitor vital signs every 15 minutes until stable, then every 30 minutes until anesthesia wears off, then every 4 hours on the floor × 24 hours, then per routine.
4. IV lactated Ringer's with 20 units of oxytocin at 125 mL/hr × 1 liter (started in OR).
5. After first liter, follow with IV lactated Ringer's at 125 mL/hr.
6. Activity: out of bed as tolerated with assistance first time and PRN thereafter.
7. Diet: Clear liquids, advance as tolerated.
8. Labs: CBC in AM first postpartum day.
9. Foley to gravity drainage. Discontinue after 24 hours if urine is clear and patient ambulating.
10. Strict intake and output every shift. Discontinue after patient voids at least 250 mL × 2, is tolerating oral intake, and IV fluids are discontinued.
11. K-Pad as needed to abdominal incision after 24 hours.
12. Call clinician for the following:
    - Temperature over 100.4° F
    - Pulse over 110
    - Increasing uterine tenderness
    - Foul-smelling lochia
    - Excessive vaginal bleeding
13. Pain medication
    - PCA pump if available × 24 hours.
    - If not tolerating PO—morphine 2 mg IV q6h PRN.
    - If tolerating PO—Percocet 1–2 tabs PO q4h PRN pain or Dilaudid 2 mg PO q4h PRN pain.
14. Other medications to consider
    - Promethazine 6.25–12.5 mg IV q4h PRN nausea.
    - Ondansetron 4 mg IV × 1 PRN nausea.
    - Diphenhydramine 25 mg PO/IV q6h PRN itching or as sleep aid.
    - Simethicone 80 mg 1–2 tablets PO after meals and QHS PRN gas.
    - Bisacodyl 10 mg PR × 1 PRN severe gas/constipation.
    - Methylergonovine 0.2 mg PO/IM q6h PRN excessive vaginal bleeding.
15. Breast care and lactation consult PRN.
16. Sitz bath 3–4 times daily PRN hemorrhoids and/or perineal discomfort.
17. Patient self-administered medications to bedside
    - Sennosides 8.6 mg and docusate 50 mg 2 capsules PO QHS PRN constipation.
    - Perineal spray to perineum PRN pain.
    - Witch hazel pads. Apply 1 pad to perineum/hemorrhoids PRN discomfort.
    - Anusol-HC ointment to hemorrhoids 3 times daily PRN discomfort.
18. Provide RhoGAM if indicated.

Postprocedure Patient Education

First 24 Hours

The patient should be told what to expect, such as pain control issues (e.g., patient-controlled analgesia [PCA] pump versus IV narcotic analgesia). She will experience some uterine cramping and receive fundal massage by the nurses. Her Foley catheter remains in place. She may have the infant with her as early as possible to start breast-feeding and bonding. Most patients stay in the hospital 3 to 5 days after a cesarean section.

First Postoperative Day

The patient should ambulate to prevent atelectasis and pneumonia. If bowel sounds are present, diet should be advanced to clear liquids and then to full liquids as tolerated. If she is ambulating well, the Foley catheter can be removed and she can walk to the bathroom. The IV line should be changed to a heparin lock. Oral narcotic analgesia can replace a PCA pump, or IV or intramuscular narcotics. She should note some flatus, and urination should increase from postpartum diuresis.

Second Postoperative Day

The criteria for discharge may include a bowel movement, ability to tolerate a regular diet, lack of fever, and full ambulation on oral pain medication only. Many patients can be discharged 36 hours after a cesarean section. *If the skin is closed*, staples can be removed and replaced with Steri-Strips. If not, this can be done at postoperative day 5 on an outpatient basis.

Discharge Instructions

- No driving for 10 days.
- Refrain from intercourse for 4 to 6 weeks.
- Care of the surgical incision is relatively simple. Water can wash over the wound as long as there is no direct impact of water onto the wound. Keeping the wound clean and dry is important for adequate healing. This includes avoiding coverage by skin folds, which can lead to excessive moisture and infection.
- Notify the physician's office for the following problems: pus seeping out of the wound, fever, painful urination, difficulty breathing, shortness of breath, or increasing pain.
- Follow-up in the office for a wound check in 1 week.
- Limit activity to walking for the first week, back to full activity by 6 weeks.

CPT/Billing Codes

59510 Routine obstetric care including antepartum care, cesarean delivery, and postpartum care
59514 Cesarean delivery only
59515 Cesarean delivery only, including postpartum care
59618 Routine obstetric care including antepartum care, cesarean delivery, and postpartum care, following attempted vaginal delivery after previous cesarean delivery
59620 Cesarean delivery only, following attempted vaginal delivery after previous cesarean delivery
59622 Cesarean delivery only, following attempted vaginal delivery after previous cesarean delivery, including postpartum care

ICD-9-CM Diagnostic Codes

641.01 Placenta previa without hemorrhage, delivered, with or without mention of antepartum complication
641.21 Premature separation of placenta (e.g., abruptio placentae), delivered, with or without mention of antepartum complication
641.31 Antepartum hemorrhage associated with coagulation defects, delivered, with or without mention of antepartum complication
642.51 Severe preeclampsia, delivered, with or without mention of antepartum complication
645.11 Prolonged pregnancy, beyond 42 completed weeks of gestation, delivered, with or without mention of antepartum complication
647.81 Other viral diseases complicating pregnancy, childbirth, the puerperium, delivered, with or without mention of antepartum complication
652.21 Breech presentation, without mention of version, delivered, with or without mention of antepartum complication
652.31 Transverse or oblique presentation, delivered, with or without mention of antepartum complication
652.41 Face or brow presentation, delivered, with or without mention of antepartum complication
652.61 Multiple gestation with malpresentation of one fetus or more, delivered, with or without mention of antepartum complication
653.51 Unusually large fetus causing disproportion, delivered, with or without mention of antepartum complication
654.21 Previous cesarean delivery, delivered, with or without mention of antepartum complication
656.31 Fetal distress, delivered, with or without mention of antepartum complication
659.11 Failed medical or unspecified induction, delivered, with or without mention of antepartum complication
660.03 Obstructed labor, caused by malposition of fetus at onset of labor, delivered, with or without mention of antepartum complication
660.11 Obstructed labor, caused by bony pelvis, delivered, with or without mention of antepartum complication
660.31 Obstructed labor, caused by deep transverse arrest and persistent occipitoposterior position, delivered, with or without mention of antepartum complication
660.41 Shoulder dystocia, delivered, with or without mention of antepartum complication
660.61 Failed trial of labor, unspecified, delivered, with or without mention of antepartum complication
660.71 Failed forceps or vacuum extractor, unspecified, delivered, with or without mention of antepartum complication
661.01 Abnormality of forces of labor, primary uterine inertia, failure of cervical dilation, primary hypotonic uterine dysfunction, delivered, with or without mention of antepartum complication
661.11 Abnormality of forces of labor, secondary uterine inertia, arrested active phase of labor or secondary hypotonic uterine dysfunction, delivered, with or without mention of antepartum complication
662.01 Prolonged labor, first stage, delivered, with or without mention of antepartum complication
662.21 Prolonged labor, second stage, delivered, with or without mention of antepartum complication
663.03 Prolapse of cord, delivered, with or without mention of antepartum complication
665.1 Rupture of uterus during labor

Acknowledgment

The editors wish to recognize the contributions by Rebecca H. Gladu, MD, to this chapter in a previous edition of this text.

BIBLIOGRAPHY

Abuhamad A, O'Sullivan MJ: Operative techniques for cesarean section. In Plauché WC, Morrison JC, Sullivan MJ (eds): Surgical Obstetrics. Philadelphia, WB Saunders, 1992, pp 417–429.

American Academy of Family Physicians: Cesarean Delivery in Family Medicine (Position Paper). Available at www.aafp.org/online/en/home/policy/policies/c/cesarean.printview.html. Accessed June 14, 2009.

American Academy of Family Physicians: Facts about Family Medicine. Table 41: Performance of OB-cesarean sections in hospital practices of family physicians by census division, July 2008. Available at www.aafp.org/online/en/home/aboutus/specialty/facts/41.html. Accessed June 14, 2009.

Centers for Disease Control and Prevention: Morbidity and Mortality Weekly Report QuickStats: Total and primary cesarean rate and vaginal birth after previous cesarean (VBAC) rate—United States, 1989–2003. Available at www.cdc.gov/mmwr/preview/mmwrhtml/mm5402a5.htm. Accessed June 14, 2009.

Damos J, Deutchman M, Ratcliffe S, Sakornbut E: Intrapartum procedures. Section G: Cesarean section. In Ratcliffe S, Sakornbut E, Byrd J (eds): Handbook of Pregnancy and Perinatal Care in Family Practice. Philadelphia, Hanley & Belfus, 1996, pp 360–395.

Gordon J, Rydfors J, Druzin M, Tadir Y: Obstetrics, Gynecology and Infertility: Handbook for Clinicians, 5th ed. Arlington, Va, Scrub Hill Press, 2001.

Hankins GDV, Gilstrap L, Cunningham EG, Clark SL (eds): Operative Obstetrics. East Norwalk, Conn, Appleton & Lange, 1995.

Raimer KA, O'Sullivan MJ: Cesarean section: History, incidence, and indications. In Plauché WC, Morrison JC, O'Sullivan MJ (eds): Surgical Obstetrics. Philadelphia, WB Saunders, 1992, pp 405–416.

Tuggy M, Garcia J: Procedures Consult. Available at www.proceduresconsult.com.

Yasin SY, Walton DL, O'Sullivan MJ: Problems encountered during cesarean delivery. In Plauché WC, Morrison JC, O'Sullivan MJ (eds): Surgical Obstetrics. Philadelphia, WB Saunders, 1992, pp 431–446.

CHAPTER 163

Induction of Labor

Scott T. Henderson

Although labor usually begins spontaneously, the induction of labor is one of the most common procedures in obstetrics. It is indicated for both maternal and fetal reasons as well as for elective and social reasons. The frequency at which patients undergo induction of labor has risen from 9% in 1989 to over 20% today. To induce labor, it may also be necessary to manipulate the cervical connective tissue. Therefore, induction can be viewed in two phases, cervical ripening followed by induction of contractions by artificial stimulation of the uterus.

The status of the cervix plays a vital role in the success or failure of an induction. The Bishop Scoring System is a tool that has been used for many years to help quantify the readiness of the cervix for labor (Table 163-1). The maximum score is 13. When the score exceeds 8, the likelihood of a successful vaginal delivery with use of oxytocin approaches that of spontaneous labor. A Bishop score of less than 6 correlates with a prolonged labor or failed induction. For research purposes, there is slight variation in the definition of an unfavorable cervix, with a Bishop score ranging from 4 to 6.

When a cervix is assessed as not favorable, ripening methods should be considered. Historically, nonpharmacologic methods such as breast stimulation, acupuncture, stripping (sweeping) of membranes, and placement of a Foley catheter or laminaria in the cervical os have been used. With the development of artificial prostaglandins (dinoprostone [prostaglandin E_2; PGE_2] and misoprostol [PGE_1]), use of pharmacologic methods has surpassed these other methods. If a cervix is favorable or ripening techniques have been used, it is reasonable to use oxytocin or amniotomy (see Chapter 164, Amniotomy) to stimulate the uterus to have regular and rhythmic contractions.

Providers and nursing staff should develop protocols, as a team, for management of labor induction, including possible complications. These policies should be in written form and followed to maximize safety for the mother and infant and to reduce liability for the providers and institution. Protocols should outline not only the procedural technique but the indications and contraindications. Special attention should be given to the protocols for elective inductions and for induction in women with a previous cesarean section.

Anatomy

The uterus is normally spontaneously contractile. During gestation, various physiologic mechanisms maintain it in an inactive state. Retention of the fetus is also aided by the cervix, a tight sphincter composed mainly of connective tissue, which maintains the pregnancy's integrity. During the final 4 to 5 weeks of pregnancy, the cervix normally undergoes a "ripening" process. Hormone-mediated changes alter the cervix in both composition and structural organization. It becomes softer and more pliable, and dilates. Endogenous prostaglandins play an important role in this process and also sensitize the uterus to prepare for labor.

Indications

Induction is indicated when the benefits of delivery to the mother or fetus outweigh the potential risks of continuing the pregnancy. Pregnancy-induced hypertension and prolonged or post-term pregnancies are among the most common indications, accounting for more than 80% of reported inductions. Indications include the following:

- Pregnancy-induced hypertension, preeclampsia, or eclampsia
- Prolonged or post-term pregnancy
- Abruptio placentae
- Abnormal antepartum testing results and delivery indicated
- Chorioamnionitis
- Suspected fetal compromise (e.g., severe fetal growth restriction, isoimmunization)
- Fetal demise
- Premature rupture of membranes
- Maternal medical complications (e.g., diabetes mellitus, renal disease, chronic pulmonary disease, chronic hypertension)

Elective (without medical or obstetric indications) induction of labor is generally not recommended. However, logistic factors such as distance from the hospital, a history of rapid labor and delivery, or psychosocial issues may be reasonable indications for elective induction.

Contraindications

Absolute

Absolute contradictions are the same as those for spontaneous labor or delivery, including the following:

- Placenta previa
- Vasa previa
- Transverse fetal lie
- Severe hydrocephalus
- Prolapsed umbilical cord
- Previous classic cesarean incision or other longitudinal uterine scar
- Small maternal size or distorted pelvic anatomy
- Active genital herpes infection
- Invasive cervical carcinoma
- Nonreassuring fetal status
- Known hypersensitivity to prostaglandins (dinoprostone [PGE_2] or misoprostol [PGE_1])
- Previous asthma, glaucoma, or myocardial infarction (dinoprostone)

Relative

- Multiple gestation
- Polyhydramnios

TABLE 163-1 Bishop Scoring System

Assessment Score	Dilation (cm)	Effacement (%)	Station	Consistency	Position of Cervix
0	Closed	0–30	−3 (engaged)	Firm	Posterior
1	1–2	40–50	−2	Moderate	Mid
2	3–4	60–70	−1/0	Soft	Anterior
3	≥5	≥80	+1/+2		

Add the score for each of the clinical assessments. If the total score is greater than 8, the success of induction approaches that of spontaneous labor.

- Appreciable macrosomia
- Maternal cardiac disease
- Grand multiparity
- Previous cesarean delivery
- Breech presentation
- Malpresentations
- Presenting part above pelvic inlet
- Unexplained vaginal bleeding during pregnancy
- Prematurity
- Ruptured membranes

Equipment and Supplies

- External device for monitoring fetal heart rate (FHR) and uterine activity.
- Sterile gloves.
- Sterile speculum (if membranes ruptured or using dinoprostone gel).
- Intravenous (IV) access (e.g., heparin lock, lactated Ringer's, normal saline).
- Pharmacologic induction supplies: dinoprostone (PGE_2) gel 0.5 mg in 2.5 mL (Prepidil) or insert 10 mg (Cervidil); misoprostol (PGE_1) 100-μg tablet; or oxytocin 10 U/mL (Pitocin).

  NOTE: Dinoprostone should be stored between −20° C and −10° C. Because misoprostol is available only in a 100-μg dosage, it is recommended to have the pharmacist cut the tablet into quarters to ensure the correct dose.

  EDITOR'S NOTE: A meta-analysis of randomized, controlled trials comparing dinoprostone with misoprostol for cervical ripening and induction of labor found the time to delivery was shorter and the rate of cesarean delivery was lower in the misoprostol group.

- Oxytocin, usually 10,000 to 20,000 mU is diluted in 1 L of lactated Ringer's or normal saline to provide a 10 to 20 mU/mL mixture.
- Infusion pump, if oxytocin is to be used.
- Mechanical induction device (16- to 26-Fr Foley catheter or laminaria [from the brown, cold-water seaweed *Laminaria digitata* or *japonica*], available in small, medium, and large sizes) and povidone–iodine solution, sterile 4 × 4 gauze sponges, sponge or uterine packing forceps. One author (Freedman, 2002) suggests use of a blunt-tipped stylet (urologic sound) to help with insertion of the Foley.
- Terbutaline 0.25 mg (at least two doses should be readily available before initiating use of dinoprostone or misoprostol).

Precautions

Before proceeding with an elective induction, the provider should review and confirm the dating of pregnancy by at least one of the following:

1. Fetal heart tones present for 30 weeks by fetal Doppler or 20 weeks by nonelectronic fetoscope
2. Thirty-six weeks since a positive β-human chorionic gonadotropin
3. A crown–rump length obtained at 6 to 12 weeks that supports a gestational age of at least 39 weeks
4. An ultrasonographic study obtained at 13 to 20 weeks that confirms the gestational age of at least 39 weeks
5. Documented fetal lung maturity by amniocentesis (see Chapter 161, Amniocentesis)

Before proceeding with induction in a patient who has had a previous caesarean section, the provider must consider the fact that these patients have an increased rate of uterine rupture, especially those with a failed trial of labor. Although labor induction may be a reasonable option for patients attempting vaginal birth after a cesarean delivery (VBAC), the risk of uterine rupture should be discussed with the patient and documented in the medical record.

EDITOR'S NOTE: At many institutions, documented informed consent is required before induction of labor or VBAC.

Caution should be exercised with the use of dinoprostone in patients with ruptured membranes and in patients with a history of previous uterine hypertonia, glaucoma, myocardial infarction, or childhood asthma (even if there have been no asthma attacks in adulthood).

Preprocedure Patient Education and Forms

All patients should be counseled regarding the indications for induction, the expected results, the alternatives, and the possible adverse effects, including the increased risks for cesarean section, uterine hyperstimulation, and fetal distress. The U.S. Food and Drug Administration (FDA) has approved only oxytocin and dinoprostone for labor induction. Review the possible complications with the patient (and family, if present). The clinician should be familiar with the package insert information. With use of prostaglandins, vomiting, diarrhea, or fever may occur, but a recent review of the literature indicated no difference between treatment and control for use of prostaglandins for cervical ripening. Laminaria are made from brown seaweed and act by drawing water from the cervix and swelling, which softens and then dilates the cervix. If a laminaria is inserted, some clinicians will let the patient go home; however, there is a slight increased risk of infection. Anaphylaxis has also been reported. With either laminaria or Foley catheter, the patient will typically experience cramping as the cervix dilates.

Misoprostol is *not* approved by the FDA for this use. There is a "black box warning" against the use of misoprostol during pregnancy. Patients should be informed of the off-label use and possible complications of any prostaglandin, as listed later. It may be helpful to remind the patient that clinicians frequently use medications off-label (e.g., most of the common medications used to halt preterm labor are off-label). Furthermore, misoprostol is contraindicated in patients who have had a previous cesarean delivery.

Technique

Before initiating any method of labor induction, the provider should perform a cervical assessment and calculate a Bishop score. In addition, the patient should have a nonstress test (NST) and be assessed for regular uterine contractions (see Chapter 165, Antepartum Fetal Monitoring). If the NST is nonreactive or a normal uterine contraction pattern is noted, the provider should not proceed with the insertion of any labor induction medication at that time.

Mechanical

Foley Catheter

1. Using sterile technique, cut off the tip (the portion beyond the balloon) of the 16- to 26-Fr Foley catheter. After cleansing the cervix with a povidone–iodine soaked gauze sponge or swab, the Foley is introduced into the endocervix by direct visualization. (One author [Freedman, 2002] uses a 16-Fr Foley to ensure adequate diameter for inserting a stylet; this keeps the Foley stiff when inserting. Make sure the stylet does not protrude beyond the tip of catheter, where it might rupture membranes). The Foley is then guided through the endocervix and into the potential space between the amniotic membrane and the lower uterine segment.
2. The balloon reservoir is inflated with 30 to 50 mL of normal saline.
3. The balloon is then retracted so that it rests on the internal os.

The following additional steps may be taken:

4. Pressure, either constant or intermittent, may be applied by adding weights to the catheter end. Constant pressure can be achieved by attaching 1 L of IV fluid to the catheter end and suspending it from the end of the bed. Intermittent pressure can be obtained by a gentle tug on the catheter end two to four times per hour.
5. Remove the catheter 6 hours later, at the time of spontaneous expulsion, or rupture of membranes (whichever occurs first).

Laminaria

1. After cleansing the cervix with a povidone–iodine soaked swab, the anterior aspect is grasped with a tenaculum.
2. Using a sponge or uterine packing forceps, a laminaria of appropriate size is then inserted so that the tip will rest against the internal os. The laminaria will increase in diameter by three- to fourfold.
3. After 4 to 6 hours, remove the laminaria and reevaluate the cervix. If the cervix remains unfavorable, the procedure may be repeated with a second laminaria of larger diameter.

Pharmacologic

Dinoprostone Gel

1. Obtain IV access *(optional)*.
2. Connect the appropriate shielded catheter (20 mm in length if no cervical effacement is present or 10 mm if greater than 50% effacement) to the filled syringe.
3. For proper gel administration, the patient should be in a dorsal position. To help ensure proper placement of the gel, a speculum can be used to visualize the cervix.
4. Under sterile conditions, insert the catheter into the vagina. Use a gentle expulsion technique to express the contents of one syringe (0.5 mg) into the cervical canal just below the level of the internal os (Fig. 163-1). If the tube becomes disconnected, spread the remaining contents of the syringe onto the cervix with your fingers. Use the contents of one syringe for one patient only. After injection, do *not* attempt to administer the small amount of gel remaining in the catheter. Discard the syringe, catheter, and any unused package contents after use.
5. The patient should remain supine for at least 15 to 30 minutes to minimize leakage from the cervical canal. Maintain external fetal monitoring of FHR and uterine activity for 2 hours after the installation. Monitoring may be discontinued after 2 hours if there is no uterine activity or FHR abnormality.

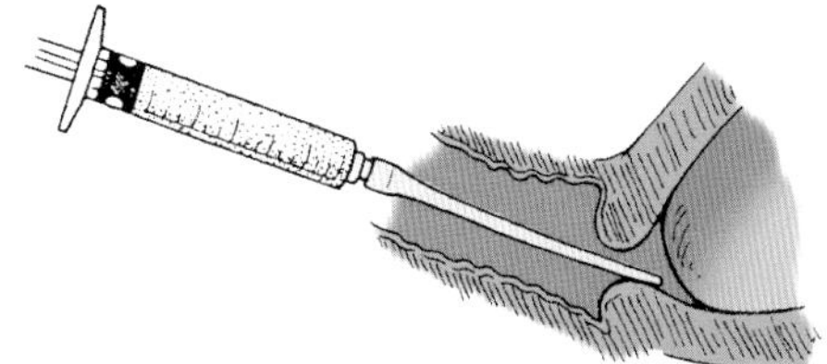

Figure 163-1 Application of dinoprostone (PGE_2) gel.

6. Reevaluate the cervix after 6 hours. If there is minimal change, the procedure may be repeated with a second dose. If needed, a third dose may be administered after 6 more hours. The maximum recommended cumulative dose for a 24-hour period is 1.5 mg of dinoprostone.
7. The package insert recommends an interval of 6 to 12 hours between the use of dinoprostone gel and oxytocin. However, some clinicians will initiate oxytocin in 4 hours if there is no uterine hyperactivity.

Dinoprostone Insert

1. Obtain IV access *(optional)*.
2. Cervidil is supplied in an individually wrapped aluminum/polyethylene package with a tear mark on one side of the package. The package should be opened only by tearing the aluminum package along the tear mark. The package should *never* be opened with scissors or other sharp objects, which may compromise or cut the knitted polyester pouch that serves as the retrieval system for the polymeric slab.
3. On bimanual examination, insert the dinoprostone 10 mg insert and then place it transversely in the posterior fornix of the vagina (Fig. 163-2). A minimal amount of water-soluble lubricant can be used to assist with insertion. The vaginal insert must not be used without its retrieval system.
4. The patient should remain supine for at least 2 hours after insertion but thereafter may be ambulatory. Maintain external fetal monitoring for 2 hours after the installation. Monitoring may be discontinued after 2 hours if there is no uterine activity or FHR abnormality.
5. The insert should be removed on onset of labor or 12 hours after insertion. Reevaluate the cervix at that time. On removal of the insert, it is essential to confirm that the slab has been removed by visualizing the knitted polyester retrieval system and confirming that it contains the slab. In the rare event that the slab is not contained within the polyester retrieval system, a vaginal examination should be performed to remove the slab and prevent the continuing delivery of the active ingredient.
6. The insert should be removed at least 30 minutes before oxytocin administration, if uterine hyperstimulation is encountered, or before amniotomy.

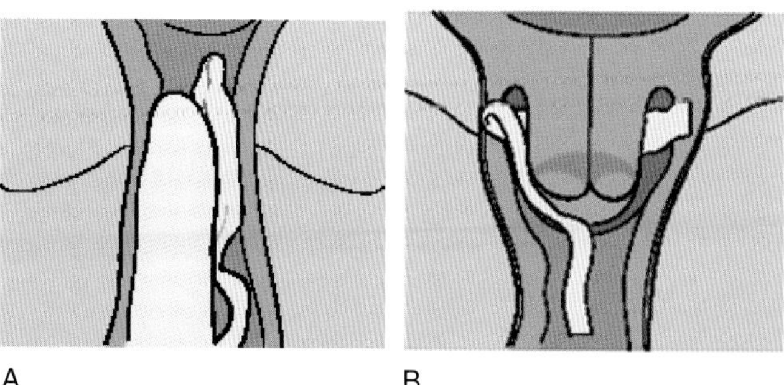

Figure 163-2 Application of dinoprostone (PGE_2) insert. **A,** Insertion, **B,** Final placement. (Redrawn from Cervidil insert, Forest Pharmaceuticals, Inc., St. Louis.)

Misoprostol

1. Obtain IV access *(optional)*.
2. On bimanual examination, insert 25 μg of misoprostol (one quarter of 100-μg tablet) into the vaginal fornix (Fig. 163-3). Certain protocols recommend continuous uterine and fetal monitoring after insertion. At a minimum, maintain external fetal monitoring for 2 hours after the installation.
3. Reevaluate the cervix after 4 hours. If there is minimal change, the procedure may be repeated with a second dose.
4. Misoprostol should be held if two or more contractions occur in 10 minutes, a Bishop score of 8/13 has been achieved, active labor begins, or the FHR pattern is nonreassuring. Oxytocin should not be administered sooner than 2 hours after the last dose of misoprostol.
5. Misoprostol is not recommended for use in this manner for more than 24 hours.

Studies have been done on higher doses and shorter dosing intervals of misoprostol. However, both are associated with a greater incidence of side effects such as hyperstimulation and FHR abnormalities. Studies have also been done on the use of oral misoprostol. It appears that oral misoprostol, 100 mg every 3 to 4 hours, is safe and effective for cervical ripening.

Oxytocin

Oxytocin is the preferred pharmacologic agent for inducing labor when the cervix is favorable or ripe. It is administered as a dilute IV solution, with the flow rate precisely regulated by an infusion pump. Protocols vary on the number of units of oxytocin per liter of fluid (typically lactated Ringer's or normal saline). Providers can speak with their hospital's pharmacy to determine which concentrations are typically used at their institution.

As with other pharmacologic means of induction, fetal monitoring is indicated before beginning the infusion. Monitoring of FHR and uterine activity should continue throughout the administration of oxytocin. If higher doses are used, strong consideration should be given to the use of an internal fetal monitor and an intrauterine pressure catheter (see Chapter 171, Intrauterine Pressure Catheter Insertion).

Multiple protocols have been established regarding the initial dose of oxytocin and the amount and frequency of dosage increases (Table 163-2). Starting doses typically range from lower doses of 0.5 to 2 mU/min to as much as 6 mU/min. The increment of dosage increase has ranged from as low as 1 to 2 mU/min to as much as 6 mU/min, with adjustments for uterine hyperstimulation. Time intervals between dosage increases in protocols usually range from 15 to 40 minutes. The goal of any protocol is to obtain an adequate labor pattern with contractions 2 to 3 minutes apart, of 45- to 60-second durations, with 50- to 75-mm Hg intensity, and a normal resting tone between contractions. The higher initial doses and more frequent increases in dosing appear to decrease the risk of cesarean section for uterine dystocia, especially for nulliparas. This has resulted in the development of Active Management of Labor

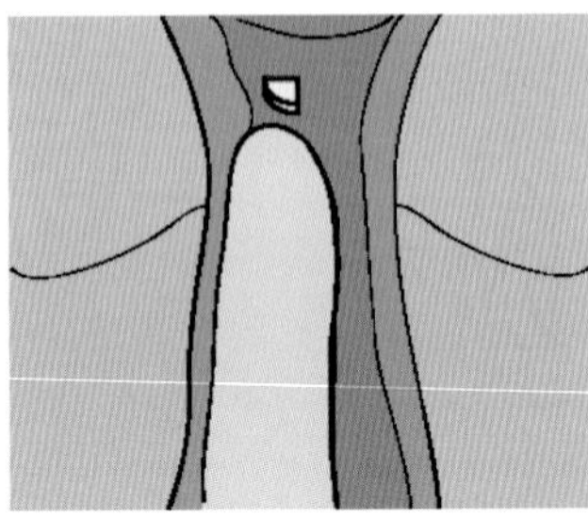

Figure 163-3 Insertion of ¼ tablet of misoprostol (PGE_1).

TABLE 163-2 Oxytocin Protocols

Regimen	Starting Dose (mU/min)	Incremental Increase (mU/min)	Frequency of Increasing Dosage (min)
Low dose	0.5–1	1	30–40
Alternative low dose	1–2	2	15
High dose	6	6 (max. 40 mU/ min)	15
Alternative high dose	4	4 (max. 32 mU/ min)	15

protocols that seem to reduce the risk of cesarean section in nulliparas. Regardless of protocol, approximately 90% of patients typically respond to 16 mU/min or less, whereas it is most unusual for a patient to require more than 20 to 40 mU/min to obtain an adequate labor pattern. In fact, higher doses may predict failure. In a study of 1151 consecutive nulliparous patients (Wen and colleagues, 2001), the likelihood of progressing to a vaginal delivery decreased at or beyond an oxytocin dose of 36 mU/min. However, at a dose of 72 mU/min, half of nulliparas delivered vaginally. This must be weighed against the fact that if the FHR is reassuring and labor has arrested (i.e., contractions not adequate [<200 Montevideo units]), there are no apparent risks to oxytocin doses greater than 48 mU/min. It should be kept in mind that oxytocin is a homolog to vasopressin; therefore, it has significant antidiuretic properties and when infused at doses greater than 20 mU/min may result in renal retention of free water. Infusion of oxytocin in aqueous fluid in appreciable amounts can result in water intoxication and hyponatremia, which can lead to coma, convulsions, and even death.

COMMON ERRORS

The provider must be prepared to handle both maternal and fetal complications before an induction is initiated. Once applied (except for the dinoprostone insert, which can be removed by using its retrieval system) prostaglandins cannot be removed or reduced like oxytocin. For practical purposes, all of these ripening techniques can be performed in the evening and overnight, with planned oxytocin administration or amniotomy the following morning. The provider must also ensure that the resources are available to perform an immediate delivery (either vaginally or by cesarean section) and newborn resuscitation, if necessary.

COMPLICATIONS

- Uterine hyperstimulation (defined as stimulated uterine contractions of moderate to strong intensity in >50% of contractions in a 10-minute segment) and possible premature separation of placenta
- Failed induction with increased risk of cesarean delivery
- Abnormalities or changes in FHR pattern
- Premature infant if dates calculated incorrectly
- Fetal acidosis
- Fetal distress
- Infant with low Apgar scores
- Precipitous delivery
- Prolapsed umbilical cord
- Maternal or newborn infection
- Uterine rupture

POSTPROCEDURE MANAGEMENT

The goal of an induction is an otherwise normal vaginal delivery. However, the provider must be prepared to manage all situations that can occur during induction and delivery. Should hyperstimulation occur, the FHR pattern should be assessed immediately. If at that time, or any other time, the FHR pattern is not reassuring, immediate intrauterine resuscitation should be initiated. This includes an IV fluid bolus of 1000 mL, lateral positioning of the mother, and oxygen administration at 10 L/min through a nonrebreather face mask to increase fetal oxygenation. If hyperstimulation occurs and a dinoprostone insert is being used, it should be removed; if oxytocin is being used it should be stopped. Likewise, an oxytocin infusion should be halted if a nonreassuring FHR occurs. Some protocols suggest oxytocin can be restarted when indicated (hyperstimulation resolved and FHR reassuring) at half the dose used when stopped. If other pharmacologic methods are being used, they cannot be removed, so terbutaline 0.25 mg as a subcutaneous injection can be administered and repeated as necessary. If the FHR pattern does not respond in a satisfactory manner, the provider should proceed to an immediate operative delivery. If the FHR pattern is reassuring despite the uterine hyperactivity, the oxytocin should be titrated down until the uterine response is acceptable.

CPT/Billing Codes

No specific CPT codes exist for labor induction. According to the CPT manual, labor that is preterm, post-term, induced, augmented or otherwise complicated is not routine and requires additional time and resources. The clinician should code these situations with hospital Evaluation and Management codes.

99356 Prolonged physician service in the inpatient setting, requiring direct (face-to-face) patient contact beyond the usual service (e.g., maternal fetal monitoring for high-risk delivery or other physiological monitoring); first hour (list separately in addition to code for inpatient Evaluation and Management service).

99357 Each additional 30 minutes (list separately in addition to code for prolonged physician service).

And, if prolonged, but not face-to-face, care

99358 Prolonged Evaluation and Management service before and/or after direct (face-to-face) patient care (e.g., review of extensive records and tests, communication with other professionals and/or the patient/family); first hour (List separately in addition to code[s] for other physician service[s] and/or inpatient or outpatient Evaluation and Management service).

ICD-9-CM Diagnostic Codes

Multiple possible diagnostic codes exist to support the induction of labor. The fifth digit (X) is required for codes 640 to 648 and 651 to 659 to denote the following common codes:

0 Unspecified
1 Delivered, with or without mention of antepartum condition
2 Delivered, with mention of postpartum complication
3 Antepartum condition or complication
4 Postpartum condition or complication

641.2X Premature separation of placenta
642.0X Benign essential hypertension complicating pregnancy, childbirth, and the puerperium
642.1X Hypertension secondary to renal disease complicating pregnancy, childbirth, and the puerperium
642.4X Mild or unspecified preeclampsia
642.5X Severe preeclampsia
642.6X Eclampsia
642.7X Preeclampsia or eclampsia superimposed on preexisting hypertension
645.1X Post-term pregnancy, 40 to 42 weeks' gestation, delivered with or without antepartum condition
645.2X Prolonged pregnancy, beyond 42 weeks' gestation, delivered with or without antepartum condition
646.2X Unspecified renal disease, without mention of hypertension
648.0X Diabetes mellitus
648.8X Gestational diabetes
656.1X Rh isoimmunization
656.2X Isoimmunization from other and unspecified blood-group incompatibility
656.3X Fetal distress
656.4X Intrauterine fetal death
656.5X Intrauterine growth retardation
658.1X Premature rupture of membranes (membranes ruptured <24 hours before onset of labor)
658.2X Delayed delivery after spontaneous or unspecified rupture of membranes (ruptured >24 hours before onset or prolonged rupture of membranes)
658.4X Infection of amniotic cavity
659.0X Failed mechanical induction
659.1X Failed medical or unspecified induction
659.7X Abnormality in fetal heart rate or rhythm

BIBLIOGRAPHY

American College of Obstetricians and Gynecologists: Induction of labor. ACOG Practice Bulletin No. 10. Washington, DC, American College of Obstetricians and Gynecologists, 1999.

Archie CL: The course and conduct of normal labor and delivery. In DeCherney AH, Nathan L, Goodwin TM, Laufer N (eds): Current Diagnosis and Treatment in Obstetrics and Gynecology, 10th ed. New York, McGraw-Hill, 2007, pp 203–211.

Cunningham FG, Leveno KJ, Bloom SL, et al: Labor induction. In Cunningham FG, Leveno KJ, Bloom SL, et al (eds): Williams Obstetrics, 22nd ed. New York, McGraw-Hill, 2005, pp 500–510.

Freedman LJ: Simplified Foley insertion for cervical ripening. OBG Management 14(10), 2002. Available at www.obgmanagement.com/article_pages.asp?AID=3003&UID. Accessed July 8, 2009.

Merovitz L, Whittle W, Farine D: Should labour be induced using a non-pharmacologic approach? Can J Clin Pharmacol 12:e1–e3, 2005.

Sanchez-Ramos L: Induction of labor. Obstet Gynecol Clin North Am 32:181–200, 2005.

Tenore JL: Methods of cervical ripening and induction of labor. Am Fam Physician 67:2123–2128, 2003.

Wen T, Beceir A, Xenakis E, et al: Is there a maximum effective dose of Pitocin? Am J Obstet Gynecol 185:S212, 2001.

CHAPTER 164

AMNIOTOMY

Rebecca H. Gladu

Amniotomy, or artificial rupture of the membranes, is often used in the management of laboring patients. This procedure is used to prepare for insertion of an intrauterine pressure catheter monitor or a fetal scalp electrode, to stimulate labor progress in active management protocols, to check the volume of amniotic fluid, to check for the presence of meconium where the fetal tracing may indicate difficulty, and to produce a presumably more rapid labor. Many studies and reports suggest that with artificial rupture of membranes labor is shortened slightly, but there is no evidence that a shorter labor in any way benefits the mother or fetus. If amniotomy is performed, an aseptic technique should be used. The clinician should be careful during amniotomy to avoid dislodging the fetal head and to avoid cord prolapse (if the head is not fully engaged when amniotomy is performed, it increases the risk of prolapse). Overall, amniotomy is a simple and relatively safe procedure that may be beneficial to the management of some women in labor.

EDITOR'S NOTE: Amniotomy should not be performed routinely. Some experts perform it only if there is a strong indication; in most cases, nature will run its course without an intervention. Depending on the station of the fetal head, any attempt to rotate it and change the position (e.g., from occiput posterior to occiput anterior) should probably be made before amniotomy.

INDICATIONS

- Necessity of internal uterine or fetal monitoring when membranes are intact
- Active management of labor protocol
- Questionable meconium
- Induction of labor
- Hastening labor

NOTE: Although a fetal scalp electrode can be applied through the amniotic membranes, performing an amniotomy first will usually simplify that procedure (see Chapter 168, Fetal Scalp Electrode Application). Although a fetal scalp electrode can be applied through the membranes to create a "slow leak" of fluid, perhaps enhancing engagement (as opposed to an "abrupt" amniotomy), there is no evidence to support the use of a fetal scalp electrode in this manner.

CONTRAINDICATIONS

Absolute

- Malpresentation
- Cord palpable below or near fetal head
- Unstable lie
- Suspected velamentous insertion of umbilical cord

Relative

- Presentation unknown or not fully engaged—if head not fully engaged, it increases risk of prolapse
- Cervix dilated less than 3 cm, or patient not in active labor
- Patient refusal

EQUIPMENT AND SUPPLIES

- Amniotomy hook (Fig. 164-1) *or* amniotomy glove (Fig. 164-2).
- Sterile gloves and lubricant.
- Absorbent pads and towels to be placed under the patient.
- Fetal monitor.
- Tocolytics should be available, especially if the patient is being augmented.
- Equipment necessary for the clinician to observe universal blood and body fluid precautions.

PRECAUTIONS

Risks to the patient (and infant) include the following:

- Infection such as chorioamnionitis (especially if labor is prolonged)
- Need for antibiotics (especially if labor is prolonged)
- Bleeding
- Cord prolapse
- Uterine tetany
- Fetal scalp scratch or laceration

PREPROCEDURE PATIENT EDUCATION AND FORMS

The procedure should be explained to the patient as well as its possible benefits, risks, and any alternatives (see patient consent form available online at www.expertconsult.com). The patient should be informed about the risk of cord prolapse and the precautions the clinician will take to avoid this as well as all possible complications. If the procedure is being used to stimulate labor progression, it should be clear to the patient that sometimes this procedure alone does not reduce the length of labor. On the other hand, the contractions may become more frequent and very strong, even requiring a medication to block them. The possible increased risk of infection (and need for antibiotics) and bleeding should be explained. Rupture of membranes commits the patient to delivery, usually within 24 hours. After 24 hours, the risk of chorioamnionitis increases significantly, so cesarean delivery may be indicated or necessary. There is a rare chance that the infant's head could be scratched or cut.

TECHNIQUE

Amniotomy Hook

1. The patient should attempt to relax in the recumbent position with feet together and hips externally rotated (i.e., frog-legged) or in stirrups. Observe universal blood and body fluid precautions when performing this procedure. The fetal heart rate should be

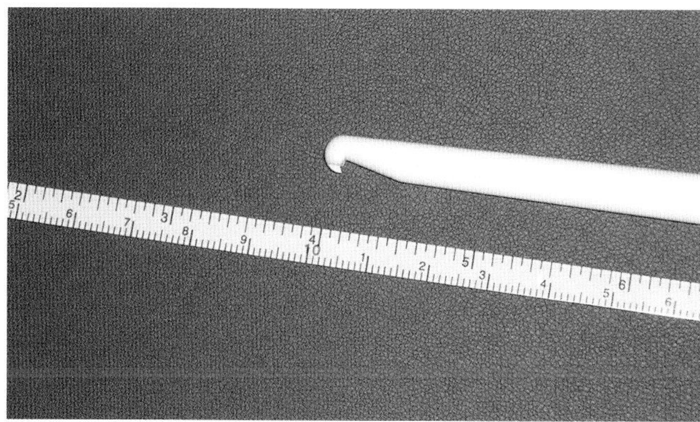

Figure 164-1 Amniotomy hook.

recorded before, during, and after amniotomy. Perform a cervical examination to confirm that the membranes are intact, with at least 3 cm dilation, and that the head is well applied. The presence of an umbilical cord should be excluded.

2. Introduce the second and third digits (index and middle fingers) of the nondominant hand, palmar side up, into the vagina. Insert the fingertips past the cervical lip, into the uterus, and against the membranes. *Make sure that the fingers are truly against the membranes and not against a thin cervical lip.*
3. Grasping the amniotomy hook with your dominant hand, introduce the tip into the vagina and into a position between the two fingers on the nondominant hand already applied against the membranes (Fig. 164-3). The hook should be pointed downward (away from the membranes). Ask an assistant to apply fundal and suprapubic pressure to reduce the risk of cord prolapse. This maneuver may also increase the amount of fluid bulging between the membranes and the head. This bulge should mimic a bag, hence the description of the mother's "bag of water." Avoid compressing the membranes too tightly against the infant's head with the nondominant hand; this may make it more difficult to hook the bag.
4. Invert the hook upward (i.e., rotate it 180 degrees), apply pressure to the bag with the hook, and rupture the bag with a single motion of the sharp hook. If successful, fluid should run from the vagina. If no fluid appears, this step may be repeated two or three times until fluid is noted to flow from the vagina. If these attempts are unsuccessful, and the bag is still palpable, relax the fingertips away from the membranes and move them slightly. This will allow you to attempt hooking the bag from a different direction. Make sure the fingers of your nondominant hand are against the membranes (and not the cervix) and again attempt to rupture the bag with a single motion of the hook. The bag may be quite slippery, so it may take several attempts, redirecting several times, before the amniotomy is successful. Apply varying amounts of pressure against the membranes with the nondominant hand with each attempt. If unsuccessful at this point, request a new hook because the hook may be defective. If there is little fluid palpable (no bag) at the beginning of the procedure, instead of rupturing the membranes or "breaking the bag of water" with the hook, the clinician should attempt to grasp and tear the membranes with the hook. If successful, even though fluid was not apparent as a bag before amniotomy, it may still run out of the vagina. Without a full bag, the sensation of performing amniotomy is quite different; the clinician may have the sensation of merely scratching the fetal scalp with the hook. As long as the clinician is sure that the presentation is vertex and only gentle attempts are made at hooking the bag, it should minimize the risk of actually scratching or lacerating the infant's scalp.

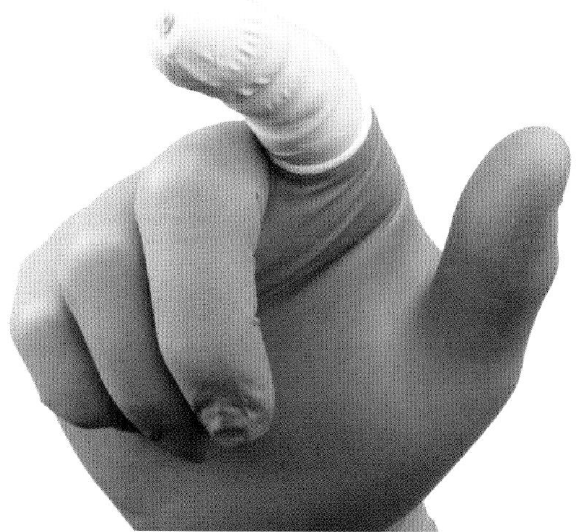

Figure 164-2 Amniotomy glove: AROM-COT. (Courtesy of Utah Medical Products, printed with permission.)

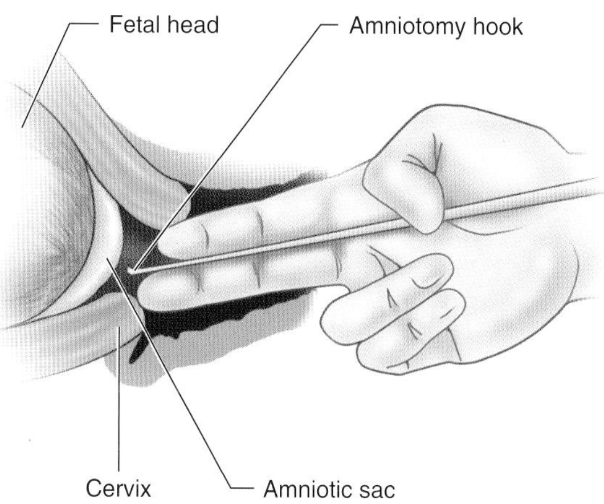

Figure 164-3 Proper insertion of amniotomy hook.

5. After successful amniotomy, remove the hook. Note the volume of fluid that has drained. If very little fluid has drained, no prior ultrasonography was performed, and the membranes were thought to be previously intact, the diagnosis of oligohydramnios should be considered. If so, be prepared for additional resuscitative needs for the infant, especially if it is a small infant. (Also, don't forget to check for a second infant!)
6. Keep the fingers of the nondominant hand applied against the fetal head as fluid is allowed to leak out, noting the color of the fluid (clear or meconium stained). Be sure to confirm that the umbilical cord is not prolapsing.
7. Remove the fingers and observe the fetal monitor for any signs of distress, such as fetal bradycardia or tachycardia.

Amniotomy Glove

Steps 1 and possibly 2 are the same as with the amniotomy hook except that the finger cot is placed on the index finger with the hook pointing toward the palm of the hand, and then against the amnion to rupture it. This simplifies the procedure and prevents the clinician from having to use an instrument blindly. Clinician preference dictates whether the cot is placed on the dominant hand or the nondominant hand. No matter which hand is used for the cot, the other hand can be inserted behind the cervix and against the membranes, as with the amniotomy hook. It can then be used after amniotomy to stabilize the head. Alternatively, because only one hand needs to be inserted into the vagina to perform the amniotomy, the other hand can be used to apply fundal or suprapubic pressure, which can then be released after successful amniotomy. Universal blood and body fluid precautions should be observed when performing this procedure.

3. Use the finger cot to apply pressure to the membranes with the sharp device. This step may be repeated until fluid is noted to flow from the vagina.
4. See steps 4 through 7 from the Amniotomy Hook section.

Sample Operative Report

See the sample operative report online at www.expertconsult.com.

Common Errors

- Failure to fully rupture the amnion. Should this error occur, reposition the hand and repeat the procedure. Occasionally, only a partial amniotic tear is accomplished or only one layer is ruptured, requiring repetition of the procedure ("the double bag").
- Mistaking a thinned cervical lip for the amnion. This mistake can cause the patient some discomfort if she is not under some type of anesthesia.

Complications

- Fetal distress
- Failure to induce or augment labor
- Increase in pain sensation with labor
- Prolapsed cord
- Infection due to prolonged rupture of membranes
- Possibly increased risk of cesarean delivery

Postprocedure Management

Observe the patient and fetus for signs of distress, such as fetal heart rate decelerations on the fetal monitor. Ensure that the cord did not prolapse and that the amniotomy hook did not lacerate the cervix or infant.

Postprocedure Patient Education

The patient should be instructed to expect the leakage of fluid. Should she develop any pain or bleeding after the procedure, she should notify the clinician immediately. In general, most patients are not given a handout about the procedure for postprocedure education.

CPT/Billing Codes

Amniotomy is not a separate billable procedure. It is considered part of labor management.

ICD-9-CM Diagnostic Codes

656.83 Meconium-stained fluid, affecting management of pregnancy or delivery, antepartum complication
656.83 Fetal distress, NOS, affecting management of pregnancy or delivery, antepartum complication
657.03 Polyhydramnios, antepartum condition or complication
661.11 Secondary uterine inertia, arrested active phase of labor or hypotonic uterine dysfunction, delivered with or without mention of antepartum condition
662.01 Prolonged labor, first stage, delivered with or without mention of antepartum condition
662.21 Prolonged labor, second stage, delivered with or without mention of antepartum condition

Suppliers

(See contact information online at www.expertconsult.com.)

Amniotomy hook
Advanced Surgi-Pharm, Inc.
Amniotomy glove (AROM-COT)
Utah Medical Products

BIBLIOGRAPHY

Archie CL: The course and conduct of normal labor and delivery. In DeCherney AH, Nathan L, Goodwin TM, Laufer N (eds): Current Diagnosis and Treatment in Obstetrics and Gynecology, 10th ed. New York, McGraw-Hill, 2007, pp 203–211.

Bricker L, Luckas M: Amniotomy alone for induction of labour. Cochrane Database Syst Rev 4:CD002862, 2000.

Neilson JP: Amniotomy for shortening spontaneous labour. Obstet Gynecol 111:204–205, 2008.

Smyth RMD, Alldred SK, Markham C: Amniotomy for shortening spontaneous labour. Cochrane Database Syst Rev 4:CD006167, 2007.

Tuggy M, Garcia J: Procedures Consult. Available at www.proceduresconsult.com.

CHAPTER 165

Antepartum Fetal Monitoring

Stephen D. Ratcliffe

Since the 1960s, certain fetal heart rate patterns have been associated with poor outcomes. Subsequently, several techniques for evaluating fetal well-being and uteroplacental function have evolved. Although there is currently no "best test," largely because of a lack of randomized clinical trials (RCTs), the majority of centers use a combination of fetal movement counting (FMC), the nonstress test (NST), the biophysical profile (BPP), the modified BPP, and the contraction stress test (CST). Some also use arterial Doppler velocitometry. FMC, NST, modified BPP, and CST are covered in this chapter, Doppler velocitometry will be discussed, and the BPP is discussed in Chapter 172, Obstetric Ultrasonography.

Whether NST, CST, modified BPP, or BPP is used, a negative test is very reassuring, with negative predictive values (no fetal death within a week of the test) of 99.8% or higher. Unfortunately, positive predictive values are quite low, ranging from 10% to 40%, which can be problematic for the clinician. Additional challenges include deciding when to start and the frequency of testing. Most experts start testing high-risk pregnancies at 32 to 34 weeks. Pregnancies with severe complications may need testing as early as 26 to 28 weeks.

Doppler Velocitometry

Real-time ultrasonography machines equipped with Doppler technology can assess arterial velocity and flow. Fetal Doppler studies were initially used to evaluate the placenta by measuring umbilical artery outflow. However, with improved technology, multivessel evaluation became possible. Subsequently, this antenatal test has been the subject of more RCTs than any other antenatal test. The current position of the American College of Obstetricians and Gynecologists (ACOG) on umbilical artery velocitometry is that there is no benefit other than in pregnancies with suspected growth restriction. Its use may alert the clinician to the need for an additional study such as a BPP, continuous fetal monitoring, or delivery.

Fetal Movement Counting

Both human and animal studies indicate that a fetus in trouble (having hypoxemia) will reduce its oxygen requirements by reducing its activity. As a result, FMC is a potentially useful tool for monitoring the fetus during the third trimester of pregnancy. FMC is commonly used to monitor high-risk pregnancies, although there is no RCT evidence to support its use.

Studies of women presenting with decreased fetal movement have produced variable results, ranging from no increase in adverse outcomes to a 3.8% perinatal mortality rate in a cohort of 599 low-risk pregnancies. Grant and colleagues (1989) performed the largest RCT (N = 68,000), which demonstrated that the routine use of FMC in low-risk pregnancies did not improve perinatal outcomes. Although the study authors did not find improved outcomes with FMC, they did conclude that maternal perceptions of decreased fetal movement were as good as formally counted and recorded fetal movement.

Indications

The clinician needs to decide when to use FMC.

- All pregnancies as a routine practice: The evidence does not support daily FMC in all pregnancies (Mangesi and Hofmeyr, 2007). It does support being on the alert for overall decreased fetal movement. Patients who report decreased fetal movement should be instructed to contact their clinicians or to report to labor and delivery.
- High-risk pregnancies: RCTs have not been performed to study the use of FMC in these patients. However, it is a common practice to recommend FMC as a secondary method of fetal surveillance in these pregnancies.

Contraindications

- Impaired mental status or significant linguistic or cultural barrier—any barrier preventing adequate communication or the proper use of FMC could cause screening errors or failures.
- Mother unable to sense fetal movements—there are cases where the clinician can actually see the fetus moving (e.g., during a routine visit, while measuring the fundal height, or otherwise observing the anterior abdomen), yet the patient cannot sense the movement. It may not be possible to use FMC with these patients.

Technique

1. The patient should be instructed in the count-to-ten method of FMC (see patient education handout online at www.expertconsult.com). The "Cardiff" count-to-ten method has been studied and compared with the Sadovsky method (three 30- to 60-minute counts at preset times each day) and the Rayburn method (FMC for 60 minutes, once a day). There is a higher patient compliance rate with the count-to-ten method. Instruct the patient to count 10 fetal movements (e.g., swishes, rolls, kicks). The test is complete and considered to be "reassuring" when 10 movements are counted in less than 2 hours. Tests are usually performed in the evening and are often completed within 20 minutes.
2. The patient is instructed to report to labor and delivery or to notify her clinician if 10 movements are not recorded within a 2-hour period. Such a result is a "nonreassuring" screening test.

Complications

Unfortunately, FMC produces frequent false-positive results. A nonreassuring FMC may be further complicated by false-positive follow-up antenatal testing results. These abnormal findings often result in the decision to induce labor, thereby unnecessarily exposing the mother and child to the risks of induction.

Interpretation of Results

A reassuring test is described in the earlier section on Technique. Patients arriving at labor and delivery with a complaint of decreased fetal movement usually undergo an NST. A normal or reactive NST is sufficient to assess fetal well-being. If the NST is not reassuring, then additional antenatal fetal testing will be necessary, such as a BPP or a CST.

NONSTRESS TEST

The NST was introduced in the United States in the early 1970s. Despite the lack of RCT evidence to support its use, the NST is the workhorse of antenatal fetal surveillance. It is usually the first-line test to evaluate high-risk pregnancies and fetal well-being. The NST uses fetal monitoring to document fetal heart rate accelerations that occur in conjunction with fetal movements. Extensive clinical observations have shown a strong correlation between *absent* or *less frequent* fetal heart rate accelerations and *progressive fetal hypoxia*. Conversely, the *presence* of fetal heart rate accelerations associated with fetal movement (reactive NST) is a reassuring indicator of *good fetal health*. Although this is not a complex procedure, the clinician must be adept at the proper interpretation of the NST. Important considerations include the indication for testing, gestational age, and any known congenital anomalies or maternal medical conditions. The clinician should also know whether the patient has taken any medications (e.g., narcotics, barbiturates) that might affect the reactivity of the fetal tracing.

Indications

The NST is used to monitor high-risk pregnancies as early as 32 weeks' gestation. Some of these high-risk conditions include the following:

- Suspected or confirmed intrauterine growth restriction (IUGR; may also use umbilical artery Doppler velocitometry)
- Maternal or gestational diabetes
- Hypertensive disorders of pregnancy
- Prolonged or post-term pregnancy
- Decreased fetal movement
- Maternal trauma
- Other maternal or fetal condition posing risk to the fetus (e.g., renal disease, multiple gestation, substance abuse, prior fetal demise, trauma)

Some clinicians use the NST as early as 26 weeks' gestation. Different criteria are used to define a reactive or reassuring fetal heart rate tracing before 32 weeks (see Interpretation of Results section). As experience has evolved with the NST, the interval between testing has shortened. Originally set rather arbitrarily at 7 days, more frequent testing is advocated for women with prolonged or post-term pregnancy, type 1 diabetes mellitus, IUGR, or gestational hypertension. In these circumstances, many experts perform twice-weekly NSTs, with more frequent testing for maternal or fetal deterioration. Some even perform NSTs daily, or more frequently, especially for severe preeclampsia remote from term.

Contraindications

There are no specific contraindications to performing an NST, although the test should be aborted if the mother goes into labor and there is marked fetal intolerance of labor.

Equipment

- Fetal heart rate and uterine pressure monitor (Fig. 165-1)
- Blood pressure cuff
- Fetal stimulation device (vibroacoustic stimulator [VAS], such as an artificial larynx)
- Ultrasonic gel for monitor
- Bed or comfortable reclining chair

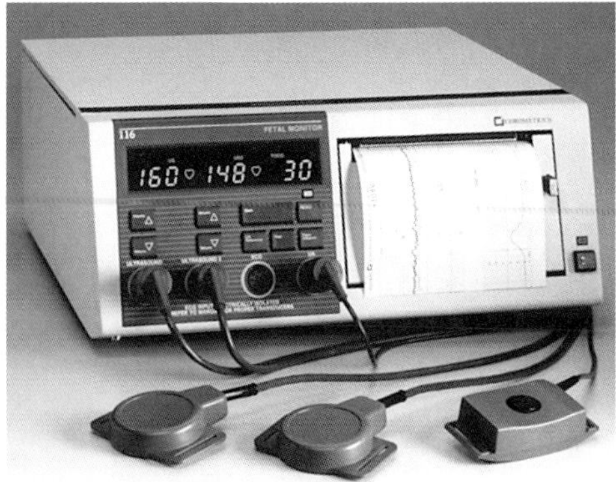

Figure 165-1 Intrapartum fetal and uterus monitor. (Courtesy of GE Medical Systems.)

Preprocedure Patient Education

Before the NST is performed, the patient should be given a handout outlining the procedure and the steps to follow (see sample patient education handout online at www.expertconsult.com). Many testing centers use standardized protocols in an attempt to minimize confounding environmental variables. These protocols encourage the patient to eat about 2 hours before the NST, to *not* smoke or take sedative drugs before the test, and to remain sedentary during the hour before testing.

Technique

1. Place the patient in a semirecumbent (semi-Fowler's) position, tilted slightly to her left or with slight left lateral hip displacement. She can also be seated in a reclining chair at a 30- to 45-degree angle.
2. Apply external uterine and fetal monitors (tocodynamometer and Doppler) to record any uterine contractions and the fetal heart rate. Record the patient's blood pressure before the test to make sure she does not have supine hypotension, which could cause a falsely abnormal test result. Check the blood pressure every 10 to 15 minutes during the test.
3. Ask the patient to report or record any fetal movements.
4. Monitor the patient for a 30-minute baseline period. Two additional 30-minute monitoring periods should be considered if the tracing is nonreactive.
5. If there is insufficient fetal movement in the first or second 30-minute observation period, there is strong evidence (based on multiple RCTs) supporting the use of a fetal stimulation device such as a VAS to induce fetal movements. According to ACOG, this can be used for 3 seconds and repeated up to three times. Use of a VAS does not decrease the sensitivity of the NST or result in an increase of falsely reassuring tests. One investigator found that using the VAS with every NST shortened the average time for the NST from 24 to 15 minutes.

Complications

False-positive results can occur. Such results may lead to premature interventions that could lead to iatrogenic perinatal complications, such as an unnecessary cesarean intervention with its associated complications.

Interpretation of Results

A fetal tracing is considered reactive if there are two or more accelerations of more than 15 beats per minute (bpm) lasting for at least 15 seconds but not more than 2 minutes (Fig. 165-2A). ACOG considers accelerations occurring without fetal movement to also be reactive.

Because the premature fetus has less pronounced heart rate accelerations than the more mature fetus, the National Institute of Child Health and Human Development (1997) defines a 10-bpm acceleration lasting for 10 seconds to be a reassuring or reactive NST for fetuses before 32 weeks' gestation.

In a low-risk pregnancy, nonreactivity (Fig. 165-2B) usually indicates the infant is sleeping. The clinician should extend the observation period for as long as 90 minutes total to decrease the likelihood of a false-positive test result. Alternatively, the clinician may safely use VAS to induce fetal movements. In addition, make sure that the patient undergoing an NST is in a semirecumbent position to avoid supine hypotension and a false positive (nonreactive) NST.

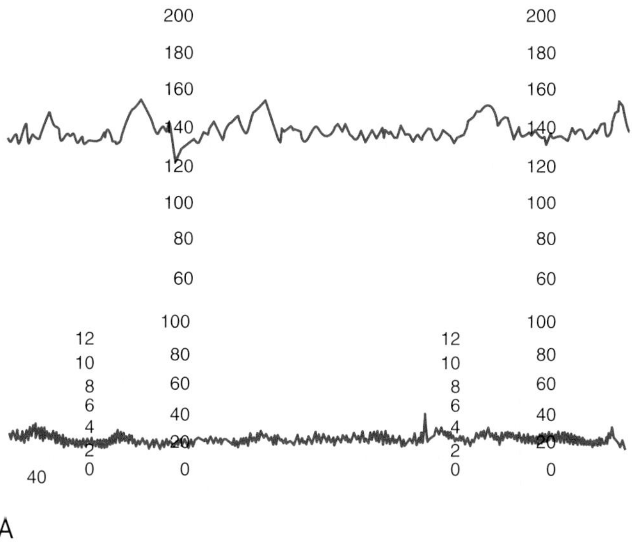

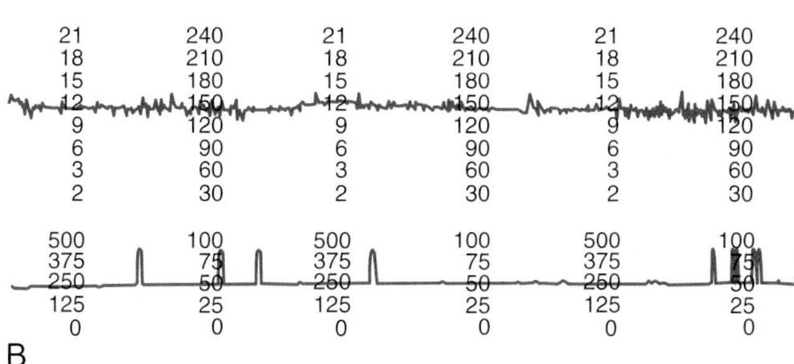

Figure 165-2 **A,** Reactive (normal) nonstress test (NST), with two or more accelerations of 15 beats per minute lasting for at least 15 seconds but not more than 2 minutes. Note the fetal heart rate in the upper tracing accelerates with fetal movement, which is noted by the vertical marks on the lower tracing. The vertical marks are made when the mother presses the button as she perceives fetal movement. **B,** Nonreactive (abnormal) NST. Although the mother perceives fetal movement, as noted by the vertical marks on the lower tracing, there are no fetal heart rate accelerations. (**A,** From Biophysical profile scoring. In Rumack CM, Wilson SR, Charboneau JW, Johnson J-A [eds]: Diagnostic Ultrasound, 3rd ed. Philadelphia, Mosby, 2005, Fig. 46-2; **B,** From Antepartum fetal evaluation. In Gabbe SG, Niebyl JR, Simpson JL, et al [eds]: Obstetrics: Normal and Problem Pregnancies, 5th ed. New York, Churchill Livingstone, 2007, Fig. 11-7.)

The clinician must take into account the risk status of the patient and the indication for ordering an NST when interpreting a nonreactive NST and before proceeding with further interventions. The positive predictive value of an abnormal NST ranges from 15% for evaluating a post-term pregnancy to 69% for evaluating IUGR. Hence, false-positive tests are common.

Reactive NSTs that have no other abnormalities on the tracing (e.g., variable decelerations) have a very low false-negative rate (2 in 1000). Combining an NST with an amniotic fluid index (AFI; see Chapter 172, Obstetric Ultrasonography, for a more complete discussion of evaluating amniotic fluid volume) produces a "modified BPP" and results in an even more sensitive test, with a false-negative rate of 0.8 per 1000.

In addition to obtaining a modified BBP, options available for the clinician to evaluate a fetus with a persistently nonreactive NST include BPP, CST, or proceeding with induction when the infant is mature and the mother has a favorable cervix. A sample flowchart for the management of an NST is shown in Figure 165-3. In settings that do not routinely perform modified BPPs, the occurrence of repetitive variable decelerations in an otherwise reactive NST should prompt a measurement of the AFI. This subgroup of fetuses is at increased risk of cord compromise during labor.

Postprocedure Patient Education

It is essential that patients receive a detailed explanation of the results of the NST and the specific signs and symptoms (e.g., decreased fetal movement, vaginal bleeding, leakage of fluid) for which they should watch. Patients should receive explicit instructions regarding follow-up appointments and when to go to labor and delivery.

Modified Biophysical Profile

Although a normal weekly BPP result can somewhat ensure fetal well-being, this is a labor-intensive process and requires a high level of expertise—a sonographer or clinician trained to perform and interpret ultrasonography scans. Therefore, the modified BPP (NST combined with an AFI) was developed in the late 1980s. An AFI less than 5 cm, or oligohydramnios, is suspected to be due to decreased urine production, in turn due to decreased fetal renal blood flow, which suggests uteroplacental insufficiency. One of the early studies reported that it took only about 10 minutes to perform a modified BPP when a VAS is used for the NST; if nursing staff are trained to perform an AFI, they can perform the entire modified BPP. In centers using modified BPPs for surveillance, most perform it twice weekly. In 1996, Miller and colleagues reported results from more than 54,000 modified BPPs in 15,400 high-risk pregnancies and described a false-negative rate of 0.8 per 1000 and a false-positive rate of 1.5%. Subsequently, ACOG endorsed the modified BPP as an acceptable means of antepartum monitoring.

Indications

- High-risk pregnancy, especially a prolonged or a post-term pregnancy
- A follow-up evaluation of a suspect or abnormal NST

Equipment

- Real-time ultrasonography machine with a 3-MHz or higher transducer. Among state-of-the-art machines, differences between different manufacturers are primarily subjective. (See the Suppliers section of Chapter 172, Obstetric Ultrasonography.)
- Bed
- Ultrasonic gel
- Towels to remove gel when study completed
- Appropriate forms for documentation

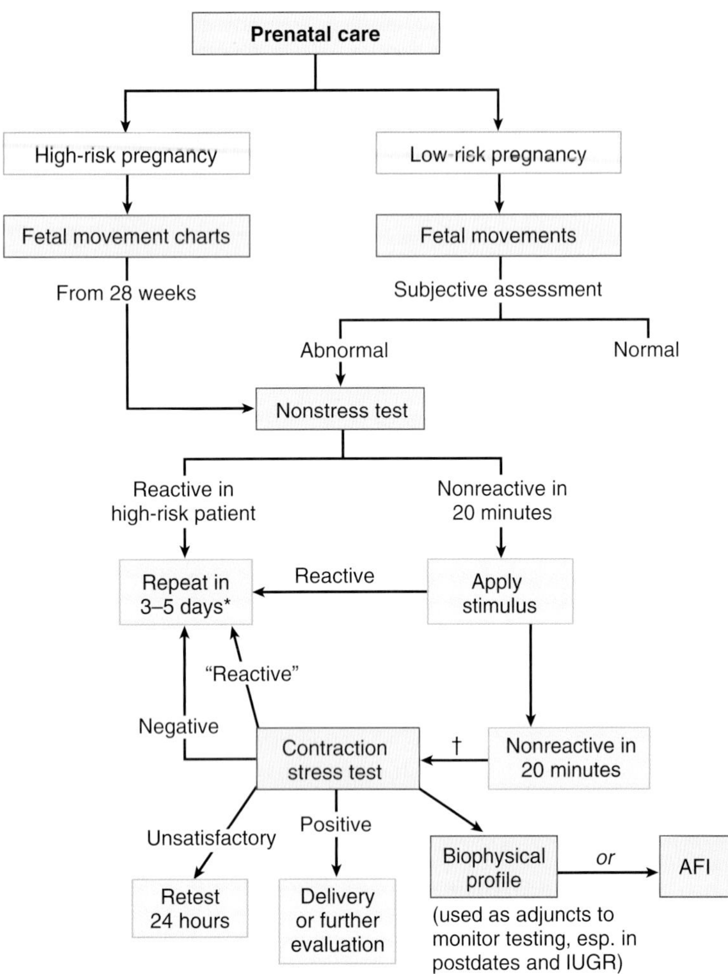

Figure 165-3 Sample flowchart for management of the nonstress test (NST) and modified biophysical profile. AFI, amniotic fluid index; IUGR, intrauterine growth retardation. *"Twice weekly" NSTs recommended. †"Prolonged" NST may be repeated in 2 to 3 hours. (Courtesy of Kent Petrie, MD, Vail, Colo.)

Preprocedure Patient Education

Before the modified BPP is performed, the patient should be given a handout outlining the procedure and the steps to follow (see sample patient education handout online at www.expertconsult.com). Unlike in nongravid pelvic ultrasonography, the patient will not need a full bladder. The patient should also be aware that although the sonogram will demonstrate a fetus and probably fetal activity, it will be used only to evaluate the amount of amniotic fluid. See Chapter 172, Obstetric Ultrasonography, for more Preprocedure Patient Education.

Technique

1. After the NST has been completed, place the patient in the recumbent or a semirecumbent (semi-Fowler's) position, tilted slightly to her left or with slight left lateral hip displacement.
2. The uterus is divided into four quadrants. The ultrasound transducer is then held in a vertical and sagittal alignment (marker dot on the probe turned toward the mother's head [cephalad]). With the patient supine, the transducer is held perpendicular to the plane of the floor and aligned longitudinally with the mother's spine. Starting in one quadrant, the pocket of fluid with the largest vertical dimension is identified, measured, and recorded. Care must be taken not to include segments of the umbilical cord in the measurement. Coiled cord can fill the space and appear to be fluid.
3. This procedure is repeated in each quadrant and the values summed. If the sum (AFI) is less than 8 cm, perform the four-quadrant evaluation three times and average the values.

Interpretation of Results

Most published results considered a nonreactive NST or an AFI less than 5 cm to be abnormal, and abnormal modified BPP results are usually followed up with a BPP, a CST, or delivery if the fetus is mature and the cervix favorable (see Fig. 165-3). At least one study (Nageotte and colleagues, 1994) found that when patients with an abnormal modified BPP were randomized to either BPP or CST, the CST resulted in a higher false-positive rate.

NOTE: On noting an abnormal AFI, most clinicians will either immediately perform a BPP or call a clinician capable of performing a BPP.

Contraction Stress Test

The CST was one of the earliest antepartum fetal surveillance tests, and it is used infrequently today. It is designed to identify fetuses at risk from uteroplacental insufficiency and is usually performed in a hospital setting. A CST is usually a secondary antenatal test used when an NST, modified BPP, or BPP does not provide the reassurance needed to continue an expectant course of pregnancy management. The basis of the test is to determine whether uterine contractions cause late decelerations in the fetal heart tracing. A secondary use of the CST is to determine if regular uterine contractions provoke recurrent variable decelerations suggestive of umbilical cord compression.

In the setting of uteroplacental insufficiency, fetal oxygen reserves are diminished. As a result, a brief hypoxic episode from a uterine contraction can cause a vagally mediated fetal bradycardia that in turn produces a late deceleration. Hypoxia can also directly affect the fetal myocardium and trigger a late deceleration.

Research in the mid-1960s demonstrated that late decelerations were associated with adverse perinatal outcomes such as an increased stillbirth rate and low Apgar scores. Ray and colleagues (1972) instituted the *oxytocin challenge test* because it relied on an infusion of synthetic oxytocin. Clinicians may choose to use spontaneous contractions or those induced by breast stimulation in place of oxytocin administration. This simplification of the procedure has also resulted in the procedure being called the CST.

In case series, the CST has been shown to be the most sensitive test for antenatal fetal surveillance, with a fetal loss rate of 0.03% within 1 week of a negative or normal CST, compared with a 0.08% loss rate for BPP and modified BPPs, and a 0.18% loss rate for a normal or reassuring NST. Disadvantages to the CST include the length of time required for testing (an average of 90 minutes in one study) and the need to have intravenous access if oxytocin is used.

Indications

- Suspected fetal compromise in a high-risk pregnancy
- Follow-up evaluation of a suspect or abnormal NST, modified BPP, or BPP

Contraindications

Absolute

If labor is contraindicated, the CST is contraindicated (e.g., prior premature labor and considerable cervical dilation and effacement have already occurred, incompetent cervix with nonmature fetus, placenta previa, classic cesarean scar).

Relative

A breech or other fetal indication for cesarean is a relative contraindication.

Equipment

- Fetal heart rate and uterine pressure monitors (see Fig. 165-1)
- Ultrasonic gel for monitors
- Blood pressure cuff
- Intravenous setup
- Terbutaline
- Bed or comfortable reclining chair

Preprocedure Patient Education

Give the patient a teaching guide explaining the CST and answer any questions she may have. Risks, benefits, and alternatives should be explained and informed consent obtained.

Technique

1. Place the patient in a semirecumbent (semi-Fowler's) position, tilted slightly to her left, or with slight left lateral hip displacement. She can also be sitting in a reclining chair at a 30- to 45-degree angle. Attach fetal and uterine monitors.
2. Take a baseline blood pressure to ensure that supine hypotension, which could cause a false-positive CST result, does not exist. Repeat every 10 to 15 minutes during the test.
3. Record a baseline fetal heart rate tracing for 20 to 30 minutes to assess for reactivity. Concurrently, the uterus should be monitored to determine whether there are spontaneous uterine contractions. Subcutaneous terbutaline, which relaxes uterine muscle in the event of serious uterine hyperstimulation and hypertonic contractions, should be readily available. If there are adequate spontaneous contractions (three or more per 10 minutes, lasting 40 seconds or longer), monitor the fetal heart rate during these contractions, and the study is completed.
4. If there are not enough adequate spontaneous contractions, after obtaining the baseline NST ask the patient to stimulate one nipple by massaging it through her clothing for about 2 minutes (or less if a contraction starts). She can restart the stimulation in 5 minutes if three contractions do not occur in 10 minutes. If no contraction is induced after 2 minutes, have her stop the stimulation for 2 minutes before repeating the process on the other side. If intermittent stimulation does not achieve the desired uterine contractions, bilateral stimulation should be performed for about 10 minutes.
5. Once an adequate contraction pattern is achieved, the breast stimulation should be stopped. Uterine hyperstimulation patterns (more than five contractions per 10 minutes or contractions lasting 90 seconds or more) occur in 3% to 4% of CSTs using breast stimulation. Provide continuous fetal and uterine monitoring.

   NOTE: The nipple-stimulation CST is frequently used because it bypasses the need for placing an intravenous line. If successful, it also reduces the testing time.
6. If nipple stimulation does not produce an adequate contraction pattern, oxytocin can be administered. Initiate the intravenous infusion of oxytocin at 0.5 to 1.0 mU/min. This rate may be increased every 15 minutes by increments of 0.5 to 1.0 mU/ min until regular uterine contractions are achieved. (Another published protocol doubles the infusion rate every 20 minutes.) An adequate CST has been achieved when there are three contractions lasting 40 seconds or longer within a 10-minute period. If oxytocin is used, the majority of patients will achieve this contraction pattern by the time they reach an infusion level of 4 to 8 mU/min. Uterine hyperstimulation occurs during oxytocin challenge testing in about 1% of patients and generally responds to stopping the oxytocin infusion. If the contractions do not decrease rapidly after stopping the oxytocin, administer subcutaneous terbutaline, 0.25 to 0.5 mg.

Complications

- Uterine hyperstimulation often provides a false-positive CST that may lead to improper management if not correctly identified.
- Fetal distress requiring an emergency intervention is a rare complication of uterine hyperstimulation. Uterine hyperstimulation almost always resolves if the oxytocin infusion or breast stimulation is stopped. If this is not sufficient, subcutaneous terbutaline may be used as described previously.

Interpretation of Results

"Negative" test results are reassuring. "Positive" or "suspect" results are causes for concern. A CST is positive if more than 50% of the contractions are accompanied by late decelerations in the absence of uterine hyperstimulation. The reactivity of the fetal tracing is an important factor to weigh when evaluating a positive CST. A *reactive*, positive CST is associated with a high incidence of false-positive results, whereas a *nonreactive*, positive CST has a much higher predictive value for identifying a compromised fetus (Fig. 165-4).

A suspect or equivocal CST is one in which less than 50% of the contractions result in late decelerations. The result is also considered equivocal if the decelerations occur during hyperstimulation because it cannot be determined whether the CST is negative or positive.

A negative CST is one in which no late decelerations occur when the contraction frequency is at least three per 10 minutes. In addition, no significant variable decelerations should occur. A

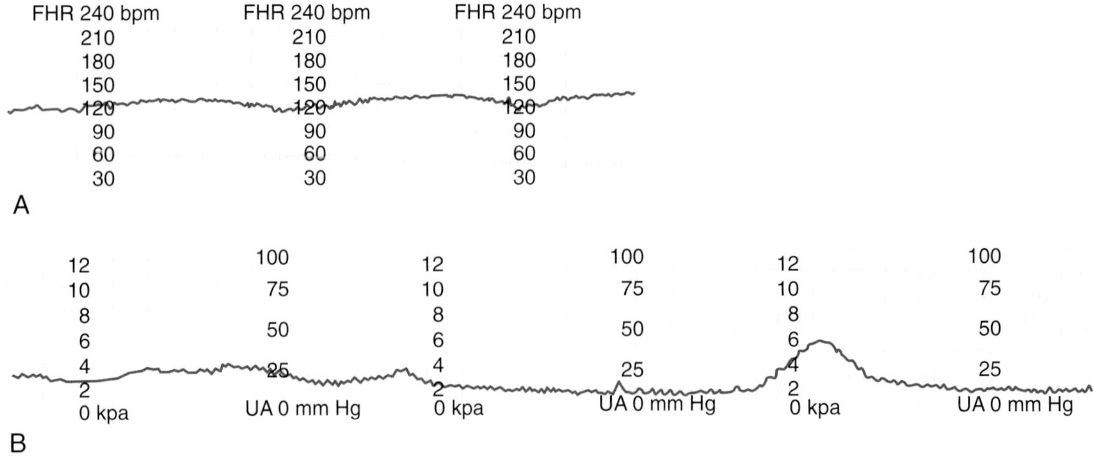

Figure 165-4 Nonreactive positive contraction stress test. **A,** Fetal heart rate (FHR). **B,** Uterine activity (UA; i.e., contractions).

negative CST that is *nonreactive* is uncommon. This test result deserves further scrutiny to determine if the cause is a medication (e.g., narcotics, phenobarbital), a fetal central nervous system defect, subtle fetal distress, or a premature infant.

A positive or suspect CST result should be given careful consideration. Maternal factors that affect placental function such as dehydration or hypotension should be addressed. If improvement in the fetal heart rate tracing cannot be attained, and if fetal pulmonary maturity has been confirmed, labor is often induced.

Postprocedure Education

A CST must be interpreted in the context of the patient's overall clinical condition. Because CSTs are usually reserved for high-risk patients, clear postprocedure instructions for these patients are essential. Even patients with negative CSTs require explicit instructions for follow-up antenatal testing, clinician visits, and any signs and symptoms for which they should be watching. The fetal deaths that have been reported after negative CSTs are often attributed to congenital malformations, placental abruption, and poor glucose control in women with diabetes; counseling for patients at risk should be appropriate.

Patient Education Guides

See patient education and consent forms available online at www.expertconsult.com.

CPT/Billing Codes

59020 Fetal contraction stress test
59025 Fetal nonstress test

If the patient has a diagnosis in addition to normal pregnancy, counseling for FMC is coded with an E/M code. If there is no additional diagnosis (normal pregnancy), preventive medicine codes should be used.

ICD-9-CM Diagnostic Codes

V22.0 Supervision of normal first pregnancy
V22.1 Supervision of other normal pregnancy
642.03 Benign, essential hypertension complicating pregnancy, antepartum
642.43 Mild or unspecified preeclampsia, antepartum
642.53 Severe preeclampsia, antepartum
642.63 Eclampsia, antepartum
642.73 Preeclampsia or eclampsia superimposed on preexisting hypertension, antepartum
645.13 Post-term pregnancy, pregnancy over 40 completed weeks to 42 completed weeks, antepartum
645.23 Prolonged pregnancy, pregnancy which has advanced beyond 42 completed weeks, antepartum
646.23 Unspecified renal disease, without mention of hypertension, antepartum
646.33 Habitual aborter, antepartum
648.03 Diabetes mellitus, preexisting, antepartum
648.83 Abnormal glucose tolerance (i.e., gestational diabetes), antepartum
656.43 Fetal demise, antepartum
656.53 Intrauterine growth restriction, antepartum
760.5 Maternal injury, fetus or newborn affected by maternal conditions

Suppliers

(See contact information online at www.expertconsult.com.)

Philips Medical Systems

Corometrics
General Electric Healthcare

For real-time ultrasonography equipment, see the Suppliers section of Chapter 172, Obstetric Ultrasonography.

BIBLIOGRAPHY

American College of Obstetricians and Gynecologists: Antepartum fetal surveillance. ACOG Practice Bulletin No. 9. Obstet Gynecol 94(4), 1999.

American College of Obstetricians and Gynecologists: Intrauterine growth restriction. ACOG Practice Bulletin No. 12. Obstet Gynecol 95(1), 2000.

American College of Obstetricians and Gynecologists: Special tests for monitoring fetal health. Patient Education Pamphlet. Washington, DC, American College of Obstetricians and Gynecologists, 2006.

Antepartum assessment. In Cunningham FG, Leveno KJ, Bloom SL, et al (eds): Williams Obstetrics, 22nd ed. New York, McGraw-Hill, 2005.

Castillo RA, Devoe LD, Arthur AM, et al: The preterm nonstress test: Effects of gestational age and length of study. Am J Obstet Gynecol 160:172–175, 1989.

Devoe LD: The nonstress test. Obstet Gynecol Clin North Am 17:111–128, 1990.

Dubiel M, Gudmundsson S, Thuring-Jonsson A, et al: Doppler velocimetry and nonstress test for predicting outcome of pregnancies with decreased fetal movements. Am J Perinatol 14:139–144, 1997.

Grant A, Elbourne ED, Valentin L, Alexander S: Routine formal fetal movement counting and risk of antepartum late death in normally formed singletons. Lancet 2:345–349, 1989.

Harrington K, Thompson O, Jordan L, et al: Obstetric outcome in women who present with a reduction in the fetal movements in the third trimester of pregnancy. J Perinat Med 26:77–82, 1998.

Lagrew D: The contraction stress test. Clin Obstet Gynecol 38:11–25, 1995.

Mangesi L, Hofmeyr GJ: Fetal movement counting for assessment of fetal well-being. Cochrane Database Syst Rev 1:CD004909, 2007.

Miller DA, Rabello Y, Paul R: The modified biophysical profile: Antepartum testing in the 1990s. Am J Obstet Gynecol 174:812–817, 1996.

Moore TR, Piacquadio K: A prospective evaluation of fetal-movement screening to reduce the incidence of antepartum fetal death. Am J Obstet Gynecol 160:1075–1080, 1989.

Nageotte MP, Towers CV, Asrat T, Freeman RK: Perinatal outcome with the modified biophysical profile. Am J Obstet Gynecol 170:1672–1676, 1994.

National Institute of Child Health and Human Development Research Planning Workshop: Electronic fetal heart rate monitoring: Research guidelines for interpretation. Am J Obstet Gynecol 177:1385–1390, 1997.

Pattison N, McCowan L: Cardiotocography for antepartum assessment. Cochrane Database Syst Rev 2:CD001068, 2000.

Ray M, Freeman R, Pine S, Hesselgesser R: Clinical experience with the oxytocin challenge test. Am J Obstet Gynecol 114:1–9, 1972.

Rosenzweig B, Levy J, Schipiour P, Blumenthal PD: Comparison of nipple stimulation and exogenous oxytocin contraction stress tests: A randomized, prospective study. J Reprod Med 34:950–954, 1989.

Smith CV, Davis SA, Rayburn WF: Patients' acceptance of monitoring fetal movement: A randomized comparison of charting techniques. J Reprod Med 37:144–146, 1992.

Tan K, Smyth R: Fetal vibroacoustic stimulation for facilitation of tests of fetal well-being. Cochrane Database Syst Rev 1:CD002963, 2001.

Willis D, Blanco J, Hamblen K, Stovall DW: The nonstress test: Criteria for the duration of fetal heart rate acceleration. J Reprod Med 35:901–903, 1990.

CHAPTER 166

EPISIOTOMY AND REPAIR OF THE PERINEUM

Montiel T. Rosenthal

Episiotomy is an intentional incision in the perineum used to facilitate the second stage of labor. Today, it is performed much less often in the United States than in previous years, when routine episiotomy was common. However, clinicians in Europe use it even less often, affirming that vaginal delivery is a natural process that does not necessarily benefit from intervention. Although use of an episiotomy may slightly decrease the risk for labial and anterior vaginal lacerations, *avoidance* of episiotomy leads to *less* maternal blood loss, *less* overall perineal trauma, *less* risk of disruption of the anal sphincter (third-degree extension) or rectal mucosa (fourth-degree extension), and *less* delay in the patient's resumption of sexual activity. Avoidance may also decrease risk of spontaneous lacerations with future deliveries. Eight studies that compared a restrictive policy of episiotomy with a policy of its routine use were reviewed for the Cochrane Database and found less posterior vaginal or perineal trauma with a restrictive policy and less overall need for suturing. Episiotomy therefore falls into the Cochrane category of "Forms of Care Likely to be Ineffective or Harmful," and it should not be performed routinely. However, for certain situations or indications, episiotomy may be unavoidable or extremely useful.

An episiotomy is performed to enlarge the vaginal outlet to facilitate delivery. Clinicians should be familiar with the anatomy of the vagina, introitus, and perineum (Fig. 166-1) before performing an episiotomy. In a midline or median episiotomy, the incision is made in a direct line posteriorly from the vagina, through the attachments of the bulbospongiosus muscle and the tendinous perineal body, and toward the anus. Mediolateral episiotomy directs the incision 45 degrees laterally from the midline at the base of the introitus (Fig. 166-2). Although performed more commonly in Europe, mediolateral episiotomy is rarely performed in the United States and is associated with more bleeding, a more difficult surgical repair, complicated healing, and a higher risk of postoperative pain, including dyspareunia. The only benefit to mediolateral episiotomy is a decreased risk of extension to a third- or fourth-degree tear. This chapter focuses on the midline or median episiotomy, although a modified "hockey stick" version of the midline and the mediolateral episiotomy is also discussed. In addition to the general risk factors for midline episiotomy, risk factors for third- or fourth-degree extensions include nulliparity, arrest of second-stage labor, persistent occiput posterior position, very short perineum, use of mid- or low-outlet forceps, and use of local anesthetics.

INDICATIONS

Any situation that prolongs the second stage of labor and thereby significantly endangers the life of the mother, the integrity of her perineum, or fetal well being could warrant episiotomy. The fact that episiotomy is a surgical procedure with attendant risks and potentially fatal complications has to be weighed against the need to shorten the second stage of labor by a few minutes. Current obstetric literature suggests that episiotomy may be indicated when vaginal delivery is anticipated and one of the following maternal or fetal indications exists.

Maternal Indications

- Significant cardiac disease (e.g., mitral stenosis)
- Risk of significant perineal trauma (e.g., large infant, use of forceps or vacuum, imminent perineal rupture)

Fetal Indications

- Significant fetal distress in second stage
- Prematurity
- Breech or face presentation
- Shoulder dystocia
- Occiput posterior position (possible benefit)

Precipitous deliveries are associated with more perineal and pelvic injuries; therefore, a timely episiotomy is critical in this situation. For all other deliveries, less invasive maneuvers (e.g., perineal massage, warm perineal compresses, sitting for delivery, breathing, hands off until crowning, and slowing delivery of fetal head—delivering head between contractions and avoiding maternal pushing while the head is being delivered) may be helpful in alleviating second-stage complications or in reducing trauma. Again, recent evidence has suggested that episiotomy use should be restricted to instances where it is clearly indicated.

CONTRAINDICATIONS

Absolute

The only absolute contraindication is patient refusal.

Relative

- Prior fourth-degree laceration or fourth-degree repair breakdown
- Severe scarring or malformation of perineum
- Extensive or large condylomata that may lead to frank hemorrhage if incised
- Prior or concurrent fistula
- Maternal disorders that impair healing such as autoimmune disorders, diabetes, or human immunodeficiency virus infection

EQUIPMENT

- Sterile gown, gloves, drapes and any other equipment necessary for the clinician to follow universal blood and body fluid precautions.

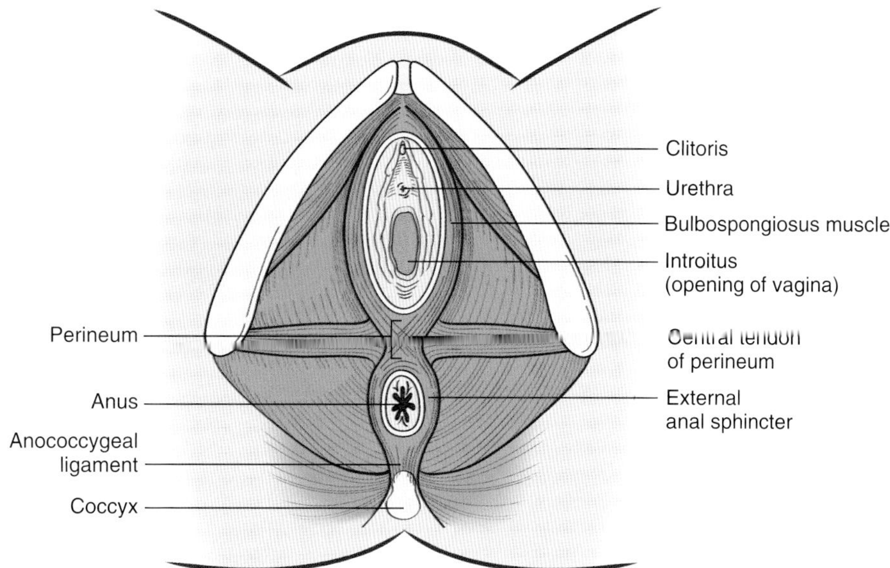

Figure 166-1 Anatomy of the vagina, introitus, and perineum.

- Povidone–iodine solution (or chlorhexidine if patient allergic to iodine).
- Blunt-tipped straight surgical scissors (e.g., Mayo scissors; a scalpel may also be used but the editors do not recommend this because it can cause significant injury to the mother, fetus, or clinician).
- Needle holder.
- Nontraumatic forceps.
- Vaginal retractor(s).
- Ring forceps.
- 4 × 4 sterile gauze sponges.
- 2-0 or 3-0 polyglycolic braided absorbable sutures (e.g., Vicryl, Dexon, Polysorb; preferred over chromic, which is associated with an increased risk of episiotomy breakdown and more discomfort during the first 3 days of healing; however, polyglycolic sutures may more frequently cause local irritation and work themselves to the skin surface or fail to heal and have to be removed weeks later) on a large, curved cutting or tapered-point needle. Rapidly absorbable versions of polyglycolic sutures are now also available and may decrease the need for suture removal within the first 3 months after episiotomy repair.
- Allis clamps (especially for third- and fourth-degree extension repairs).
- 4-0 or 5-0 polyglycolic suture on smaller curved needle (for fourth-degree extension repairs).

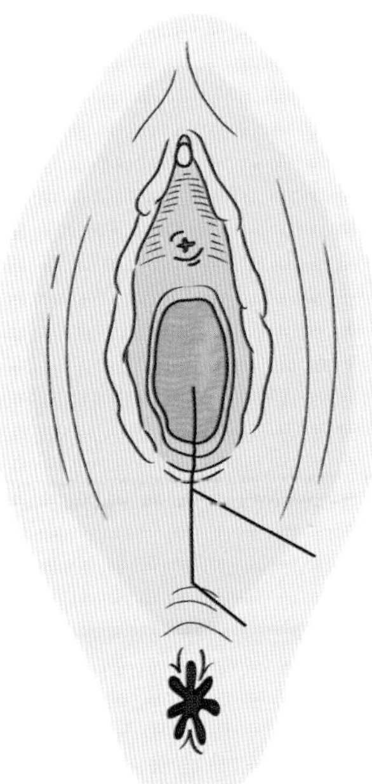

Figure 166-2 "Hockey stick" extension of midline episiotomy versus mediolateral episiotomy.

NOTE: If effective regional (e.g., epidural, pudendal) anesthesia is not in place, a 10-mL syringe with a 1½-inch, 27-gauge needle should be available to locally infiltrate the anesthetic of preference (usually 10 mL 1% lidocaine *without* epinephrine; use ≤30 mL lidocaine).

Preprocedure Patient Education

Discuss potential risks and possible benefits of an episiotomy with the patient (and partner) during prenatal care, *before* an emergent moment of need when neither the clinician nor the patient is in an optimal situation for exchange of information. Ideally, the patient's desires are part of a birth plan, and this should be discussed and written well before the pregnancy is at term. (See also Chapter 3, Epidural Anesthesia and Analgesia, Chapter 174, Pudendal Anesthesia, and Chapter 177, Vaginal Delivery, for examples.)

Technique

In the second stage of labor, as the fetal cranium begins to distend the maternal perineum, if time permits, effort should be directed toward assisting with the natural thinning of the perineum and dilation of the introitus (Fig. 166-3). These efforts should include applying warm compresses and placing tension on the perineum and gently stretching it from inside the introitus with the index and middle fingers. Labeling posterior as the 6 o'clock direction, rotate these fingers, under gentle tension (directed outwardly), from about the 4 o'clock to the 8 o'clock positions. Gentle exterior massage with the thumb or other hand at the same time, in this same location, may also help with thinning of the perineum.

The decision for episiotomy is usually made after the fetal cranium (not just the caput) distends the introitus. Waiting until

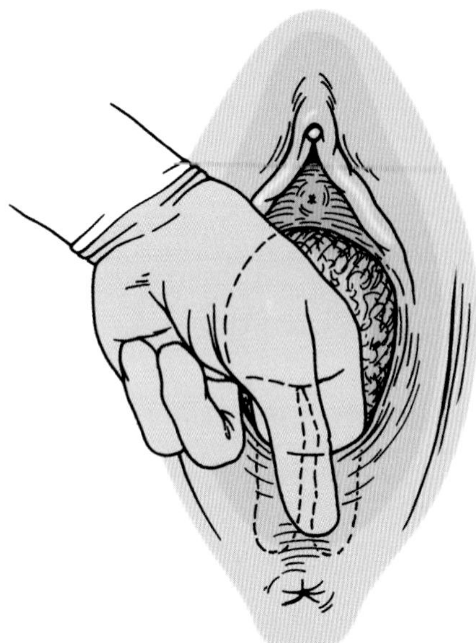

Figure 166-3 Palpating and attempting to stretch and thin the perineum before episiotomy.

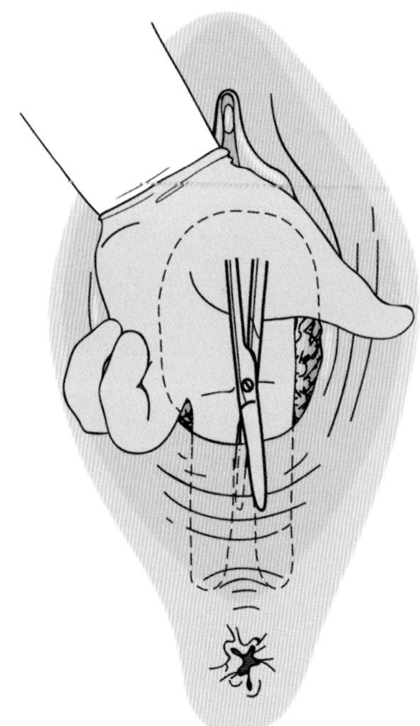

Figure 166-4 Performing the midline episiotomy.

a minimum of 3 to 4 cm of the fetal scalp diameter is visible and delivery is imminent will prevent excessive blood loss. If the indication for episiotomy is for a forceps or vacuum delivery, most clinicians perform the episiotomy after application of the blades or vacuum device. Until this time, massaging the perineum, as described previously, may not only minimize bleeding but may provide some anesthesia by placing pressure on the local nerve endings. As the head further distends the introitus, an episiotomy may be needed if it appears that the head will not be deliverable without an episiotomy or that there will be so much tension on the perineum that it will tear (i.e., imminent rupture). An episiotomy may also be necessary for one of the other indications. If the patient is in stirrups, make sure the legs are not separated too widely or one leg placed higher than the other; this may produce excess tension on the perineum, resulting in an extension of the episiotomy into a third- or fourth-degree laceration. When performing this procedure, the clinician should follow universal blood and body fluid precautions.

1. With the palm of the clinician's nondominant hand facing outward, the index and middle fingers are inserted between the fetal scalp (or presenting part) and the maternal perineum, directed toward the maternal anus (toward the 6 o'clock position). The thumb should be placed on the exterior perineum. The thumb and fingers serve two functions: to protect the fetus and to palpate the anal sphincter as a reminder of its location for the clinician. The thumb defines the bottom of the episiotomy (see Fig. 166-3).
2. Check for adequate anesthesia by gently scratching the perineum with tissue forceps. If there is no anal "wink" reflex (i.e., sphincter contraction) with this scratching, it suggests adequate anesthesia. Further confirm anesthesia by gently pinching the perineum with the tissue forceps or an Allis clamp. Even epidural anesthesia or a pudendal block is not always effective, so be prepared to locally anesthetize the midline of both the perineum (for a median episiotomy) and the floor of the vagina. The middle and index fingers should be in place between the fetus and the perineum/floor of the vagina to avoid fetal injection with anesthetic.
3. Insert the blunt blade of the scissors inside the introitus to cut parallel to and between the fingers. Make the incision downward after bringing the other blade of the scissors flat against the skin on the outside of the perineum (Fig. 166-4). Again, take care to protect the fetal presenting part. After the incision has passed the fetus, avoid cutting the external sphincter of the anus by keeping pressure posteriorly just above the fullness of the anus. Under direct visualization, extend the incision up the vaginal mucosa an additional 2 to 4 cm, through the hymenal ring, to release tension and prevent tearing. The introitus should readily open after making the episiotomy and delivery should proceed expeditiously to minimize blood loss.

In the patient with a very short perineum (especially if nulliparous or with prolonged second stage of labor, or the fetus is in the occiput posterior position), consider performing a variant of the median episiotomy, the "hockey stick" episiotomy (see Fig. 166-2). To form the hockey stick, as the midline incision is being made and before it reaches the anus, extend it laterally 1 to 2 cm. That way, if the incision extends further by tearing, it should naturally follow the "L" shape and avoid the anal sphincter. Another option is a mediolateral episiotomy (see Fig. 166-2). The incision is directed at a 45-degree angle to the midline of the posterior fourchette, from the hymenal ring toward the ischial tuberosity. The mediolateral episiotomy is usually made on the same side of the patient as the handedness of the clinician (e.g., right side of patient at about the 7 o'clock position for a right-handed clinician). The length of the incision is not as critical for a midline incision; however, the longer the incision, the more extensive the repair.

Repair

1. Repair the episiotomy *after* the third stage of labor. This avoids disturbing the episiotomy repair with the delivery of the placenta. (If the episiotomy repair has already been completed, the sutures could become disrupted with delivery of the placenta, especially if a manual extraction is necessary. If the episiotomy is in the process of being repaired, delivery of the placenta often obscures the field with blood.) Again, the clinician should follow universal blood and body fluid precautions.
2. Check again for adequate anesthesia by gently scratching the perineum, and if there is no anal "wink" reflex, by gently pinching the perineum with tissue forceps. If not already done, a pudendal block (see Chapter 174, Pudendal Anesthesia) can

again be considered, especially if a third- or fourth-degree extension needs to be repaired. Check patients with an epidural in the same manner; additional local anesthesia may be helpful during repair.

3. A digital rectal examination should be performed after every delivery. After donning a clean glove and lubricating a finger with antiseptic solution, palpate the distal 6 cm of the rectal mucosa. The gloved finger should not be visible in the vaginal wound. Such a tear or "buttonhole," usually located superior to the sphincter, could later produce a rectovaginal fistula if left unrepaired. Determine whether the sphincter has sufficient "bulk" remaining (i.e., produces the sensation of a small doughnut being palpated). In the absence of this sensation, evaluate closely for a third-degree extension. Carefully examine the remainder of the lower urogenital tract for lacerations not contiguous with the episiotomy, repairing those that need it.

Repair of Third- and Fourth-Degree Extensions (Tears)

1. If the rectal mucosa is no longer intact (fourth-degree extension), it must be repaired to prevent fistula formation. Reapproximate the submucosa and muscularis with 4-0 or 5-0 polyglycolic stitches (Fig. 166-5A). Use running or interrupted stitches placed 3 to 5 mm apart. (These are basically subcuticular stitches, but unlike subcuticular stitches placed in skin, these are placed from the other side—the back side—of the mucosa.) Reapproximating the submucosa and muscularis in this manner should invert the mucosa back into the lumen (Fig. 166-5B). Doing so will eliminate the risk of sequestering rectal mucosa in overlying tissue. Sutures should begin just above the apex of the laceration and proceed distally.

   NOTE: If the apex of the laceration is not visible, an interrupted suture can be placed as close as possible to the apex and used to apply gentle traction toward the clinician, bringing the apex of the wound into view. This suture can later be removed. (A similar technique can be applied to *any* vaginal or even a cervical laceration when there is difficulty visualizing the apex.)

   The musculature of the anal canal, including the anal sphincters, basically consists of two tubes, one inside the other. The inner cylinder, closest to the rectal mucosa, contains the internal anal sphincter, which consists of smooth muscle under involuntary control and provides the resting tone noted when performing a digital rectal examination. This cylinder, in turn, is surrounded by the thicker cylinder containing the external anal sphincter, which consists of skeletal muscle under voluntary control and can be used to squeeze the clinician's finger when a digital rectal examination is being performed.

2. After reapproximation of the mucosa, a second layer of running or interrupted 3-0 polyglycolic sutures should be placed to provide a reinforcing layer of fascia over the stitches in the submucosa. This layer should also close the torn ends of the internal anal sphincter, a roughly 2.5-cm-long (the most distal 2.5 cm of the anal canal) fibrous layer lying between the rectal mucosa and the external anal sphincter. It is identified as a white, glistening, fibrous structure that may have retracted laterally and need to be retrieved with an Allis clamp for repair. These sutures should give the wound additional strength, again decreasing the chance for fistula formation.
3. The external anal sphincter (third-degree extension) is then repaired by using three or four interrupted stitches. Suturing the sphincter muscle alone will not provide sufficient strength to hold until healing is complete, so the fibrous sphincter sheath (fascia) must also be reapproximated. It is identified as a tenacious white sheath, often retracted further laterally than the muscle edges. Search for the sheath on the posterior, inferior (caudal), superior (cephalic), and anterior aspects of the muscle. Again, lateral probing and fixation with an Allis clamp may be necessary.
4. Several techniques are described in the literature for external anal sphincter repair. Four simple sutures (Fig. 166-5C–I) can be placed in the posterior, superior (cephalic), inferior (caudal), and anterior portions of the muscle and the adjacent aspects of the torn sphincter sheath for an end-to-end repair. (Some experts place the posterior and caudal sutures first and then tie them last.)

   Alternatively, the ends of the sphincter may be pulled to overlap and sutured with three sutures. (Although the overlapping-type repair was initially thought to provide superior results, randomized trials comparing it with traditional end-to-end repair have failed to demonstrate superior anatomic or functional results.) Another method of end-to-end repair is to merely place two large transfixion sutures in the posterior and anterior aspects of the external sphincter. Usually it is easier to place the posterior transfixion suture first, followed by the anterior suture. These large transfixion sutures should also traverse the superior (cephalic) and inferior (caudal) sheaths in both locations (Fig. 166-5J).
5. On completion, a repeat rectal examination should confirm adequate sphincter reapproximation and adequate "bulk"/support. Examination glove should be discarded after rectal examination.

Repair of the Episiotomy

1. After any injury to the rectal mucosa and anal sphincters has been repaired, carefully examine the wound. Use 2-0 or 3-0 polyglycolic suture to place a stitch above the apex on the vaginal incision. Tie there, and then run it down to the introitus and reapproximate the hymenal ring (Fig. 166-6). It is critical that these stitches provide hemostasis, close all dead space, and not enter the rectum. Although some clinicians use a subcuticular running stitch for this reapproximation, it seems that simple stitches would be more effective at providing hemostasis and closing the dead space. One way to avoid entering the rectum is to take wide bites laterally on each side and then to bring the needle out at the base of the incision, ensuring that it does not go as deep as the rectum (merely piercing the rectum with a needle increases the risk of rectovaginal fistula). Either locked or unlocked sutures may be used, although the literature suggests that unlocked sutures are associated with less pain. If locked sutures are used, take care to avoid too much tension, which might cause tissue ischemia and necrosis.
2. At this point, two techniques are available, either continuing with the current suture to close the perineum for the one-suture technique (Fig. 166-7), or using an additional suture for the two-suture technique (Fig. 166-8). If the one-suture technique is chosen, after approximating the hymenal ring, the needle is buried beneath the hymenal ring to exit at the apex/top of the perineal wound. From there, running stitches are placed in the deep perineal tissue, roughly approximating the perineum (or at least taking the tension off the eventual subcuticular stitch) while proceeding to the most posterior aspect/bottom of the wound. After the deep perineal tissue has been reapproximated and the posterior aspect of the wound reached, the suture is redirected to become a running subcuticular stitch and used to close the skin of the perineum. The suture is run back up the perineum, and then the needle is again buried beneath the hymenal ring to exit through the already sutured incision in the vaginal mucosa. One final stitch is placed beneath the incision in the vaginal mucosa, to hide or invert it, a knot tied, and any remaining suture cut.

   NOTE: Deep placement of the perineal subcuticular stitches (but leaving the perineal wound gaping only 2 to 3 mm) significantly decreases itching during healing with no loss of cosmesis or function. Also, avoid interrupted transcutaneous sutures when closing the perineum because they are associated with more pain in the immediate postpartum period compared with continuous subcuticular sutures.

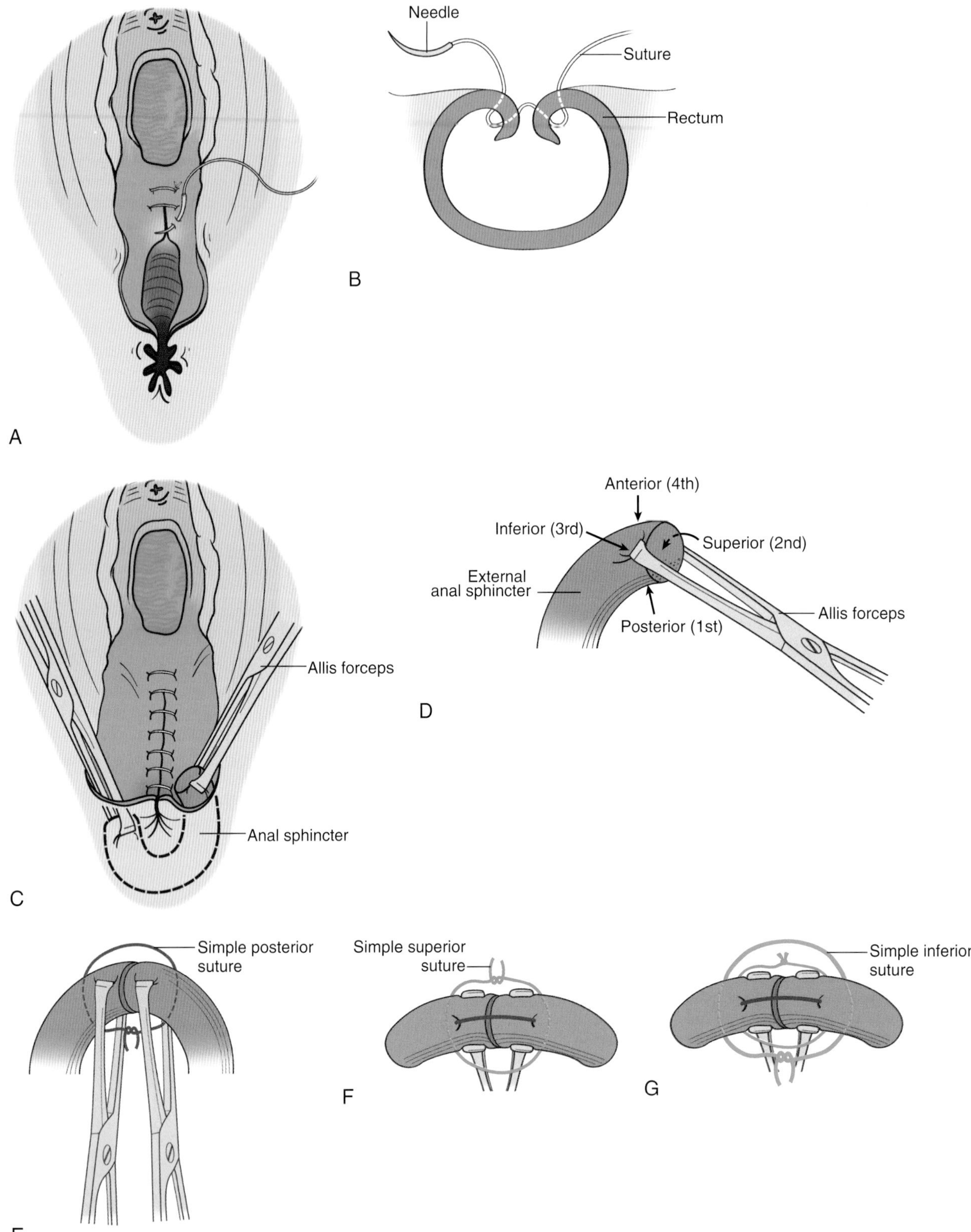

Figure 166-5 Repair of fourth-degree extension of a midline episiotomy. **A,** The rectal mucosa is repaired using interrupted submucosal stitches. **B,** Cross-sectional view of rectal laceration closure, inverting mucosa. **C,** The sphincter is retrieved with Allis forceps. **D,** Right edge of external anal sphincter from perineal view with order of placement of sutures. **E,** Placement of simple posterior suture, perineal view. **F,** Placement of simple superior (cephalic) suture, anterior view. **G,** Placement of simple inferior (caudal) suture, anterior view.

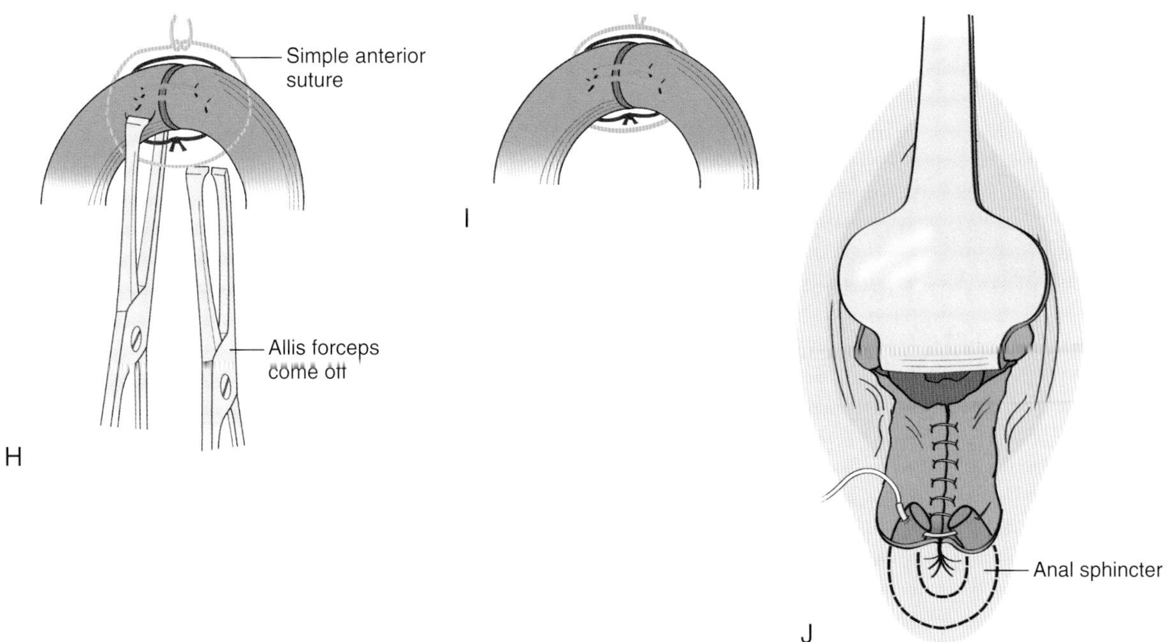

Figure 166-5, cont. **H,** Placement of simple anterior suture with removal of Allis clamps (perineal view). **I,** Complete closure of external anal sphincter (perineal view). **J,** Alternative technique of reapproximating external anal sphincter using two large transfixion sutures.

3. If the two-suture technique is used, after the hymenal ring is approximated with the first suture, the needle is buried beneath the hymenal ring to exit into the perineal wound. The needle is then laid aside or tagged with a hemostat to keep it out of the wound and ready for later use. With the second suture, a crown stitch is placed to carefully reapproximate the perineum where the bilateral bulbospongiosus (formerly known as bulbocavernosus) muscles merge (see Fig. 166-6B). Then, either interrupted or running sutures can be placed to close the perineum from the apex/top to the posterior/bottom of the wound. If a running suture is used, after the deep perineal tissue has been reapproximated, the suture can then be redirected as a subcuticular stitch and run back up to close the skin of the perineum. At that point, when the first suture is reached, both needles are removed and the sutures tied together into an inverted knot. Alternatively, if interrupted sutures are used to repair the deep perineal tissue (see Fig. 166-8), the suture tagged after reapproximating the hymenal ring can then be used for a running subcuticular stitch to close the skin of the perineum.
4. To repair a hockey stick extension, merely follow the incision with the subcuticular suture. Figure 166-9 diagrams the repair of a mediolateral episiotomy.
5. Once repair is complete, perform a final rectovaginal examination. Verify again that the rectal mucosa is intact and is not obstructed by suture, and that no gauze sponges or instruments remain in either the rectum or the vagina. Immediate correction, by removal of the existing repair and repeating the procedure with care, is imperative to minimize the risk of infection and fistula formation.

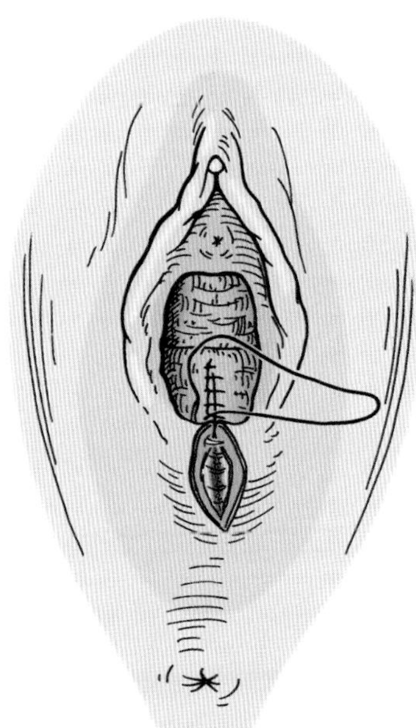

Figure 166-6 Closure of the vaginal mucosa. The first stitch is placed *above* the apex of the wound and tied. This stitch is then usually continued as a simple or locked running stitch down to the introitus. The hymenal ring has been reapproximated and the needle is then taken to the depth of the perineum.

Figure 166-10 provides a flowchart that summarizes the episiotomy and repair technique.

Complications

- Blood volume loss is reported to be approximately 300 mL from an uncomplicated median episiotomy, but easily may be more if there is an unexpected delay in delivery or repair. Observe the patient carefully and treat proactively, especially if other conditions threaten to compromise the patient's blood volume (e.g., intravascular hypovolemia resulting from other blood loss or preeclampsia).
- Hematoma formation with acute swelling and pain is unusual but not rare. In addition to large vulvar hematomas, paravaginal and ischiorectal hematomas can occur. If present, a hematoma may need to be opened immediately. The bleeding must then be arrested and the space either closed or drained to prevent recurrence.
- Infection is probably the most serious threat to episiotomy recovery. A range of wound infections is possible, from a minor

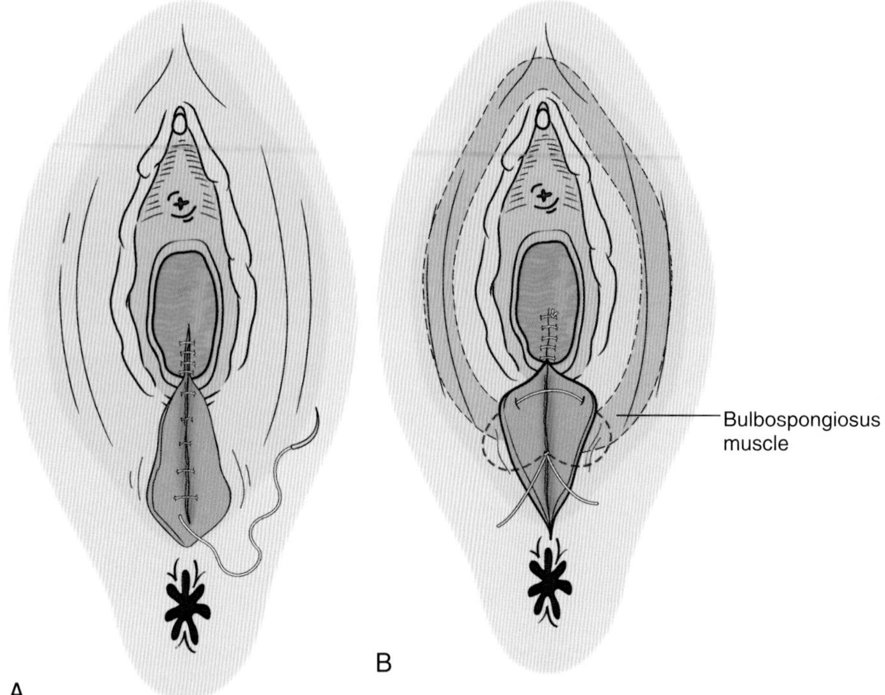

Figure 166-7 **A,** Repair of the vaginal mucosa has been completed with locked stitches. The hymenal ring and perineal body have been reapproximated and a deep running layer of perineal sutures has been placed, using the same suture. Finishing the perineal closure would entail running the subcuticular stitches back to the introitus. **B,** Alternative closure of deep perineum after running vaginal suture. The crown stitch approximates the perineal body, where the fibers of the bulbospongiosus muscles join from either side. (*Dotted line* indicates placement of suture out of view of the person doing the repair.)

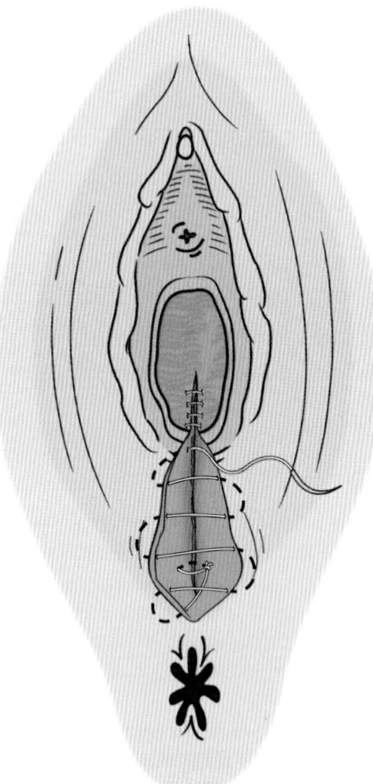

Figure 166-8 Two-suture technique of closing the deep perineal space. The second suture is used for deep interrupted stitches. The perineal skin is closed with a subcuticular stitch using either the second suture or the remaining first suture from the vaginal repair. (*Dotted line* indicates placement of subcuticular suture.)

superficial exudative wound infection to a life-threatening septic hematoma or necrotizing fasciitis. Maternal fever and unusual pain or swelling in the perineum must be evaluated thoroughly to rule out serious infection.

- Incontinence of stool or urine and flatus are possible complications of episiotomy, especially when associated with extensions.
- Rectovaginal and urogenital fistulas (vesicovaginal, vesicocervicovaginal, urethrovaginal, and ureterovaginal) may occur from either direct trauma (hence the importance of careful examination of the entire lower genital tract) or from infection or necrosis associated with suturing. Incontinence of either feces or urine starting 10 or more days after delivery should alert the clinician to the possibility of these complications.
- Pelvic relaxation and poor perineal tone, once thought to be minimized by performing an episiotomy, may actually be exacerbated by the procedure. Although not life-threatening, they may lead to a lifetime of misery and disability.
- Local pain or wound breakdown and dyspareunia are usually self-limited complications. Bartholin's duct cysts, inclusion cysts, and endometriosis at the wound site are rarely encountered but may require surgical repair.
- In addition to maternal complications, episiotomies place a nearby patient in jeopardy: the fetus. Fetal complications may range from injecting the scalp with anesthetic, producing lidocaine toxicity, to minimal abrasions, to rare but significant lacerations on the presenting part (e.g., eyelid lacerations and even castration of a male breech infant).

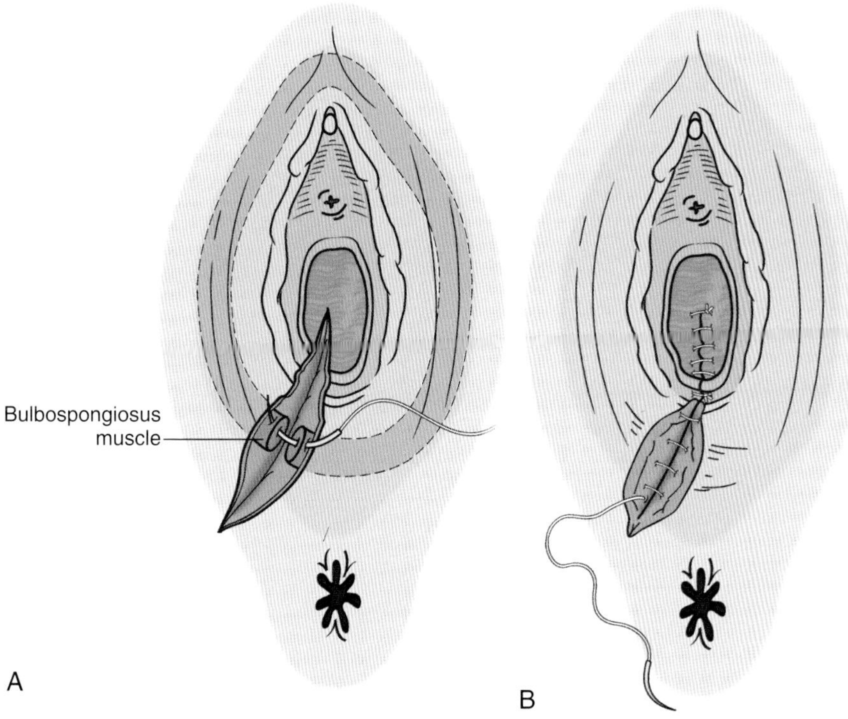

Figure 166-9 Repair of a mediolateral episiotomy. **A**, Similar to placing a crown stitch, the bulbospongiosus muscle is first approximated. **B**, The remainder of the episiotomy is repaired in a manner similar to a midline episiotomy, using either a one- or two-suture technique.

Postprocedure Management and Patient Education

After delivery, patients with sutures are less comfortable than patients without sutures, and women with episiotomies may experience more pain than women with minor lacerations. Many women will desire analgesia, and nonsteroidal anti-inflammatory drugs (e.g., ibuprofen) are increasingly used instead of acetaminophen with codeine. Codeine can be constipating, which is especially problematic among women after a third- or fourth-degree repair. Stool softeners may decrease pain with defecation as well as the risk of episiotomy disruption, especially after third- or fourth-degree extensions. The application of ice packs to the perineum the first 24 hours after delivery is efficacious for reducing swelling and postpartum pain, whereas warm sitz baths can provide comfort beyond the immediate postpartum period. Alternatively, adding ice cubes to a lukewarm sitz bath and soaking for 20 to 30 minutes may be preferred by some patients for pain relief. Potential complications must be discussed so that she is aware of the signs and symptoms for which she must immediately contact the clinician, especially bleeding, fever, or severe or persistent pain. Patients should also know that if a suture works its way to the surface, they can return to the clinician for removal.

CPT/Billing Codes

59300 Episiotomy or vaginal repair by other than the attending physician
59400 Routine obstetric care, including antepartum care, vaginal delivery (with or without episiotomy, and/or forceps) and postpartum care
59409 Vaginal delivery only (with or without episiotomy and/or forceps)

ICD-9-CM Diagnostic Codes

650 Normal delivery, requiring minimal or no assistance, with or without episiotomy, without fetal manipulation or instrumentation (forceps) of a spontaneous, cephalic, vaginal, full-term, single, live-born infant

The fifth digit (X) is required for codes 660 to 669 to denote the following:

0 Unspecified
1 Delivered, with or without mention of antepartum condition
2 Delivered, with mention of postpartum complication
3 Antepartum condition or complication
4 Postpartum condition or complication

The following codes are related to deliveries with forceps or vacuum:

659.7X Abnormality in fetal heart rate or rhythm
662.2X Prolonged second stage of labor

The following codes are related to episiotomy and episiotomy repair, and for repair of low vaginal lacerations:

664.0X First-degree perineal laceration
664.1X Second-degree perineal laceration
664.2X Third-degree perineal laceration
664.3X Fourth-degree perineal laceration
664.4X Unspecified perineal laceration

Acknowledgment

The editors wish to recognize the many contributions by Donald N. Marquardt, MD, PhD, to this chapter in the previous two editions of this text.

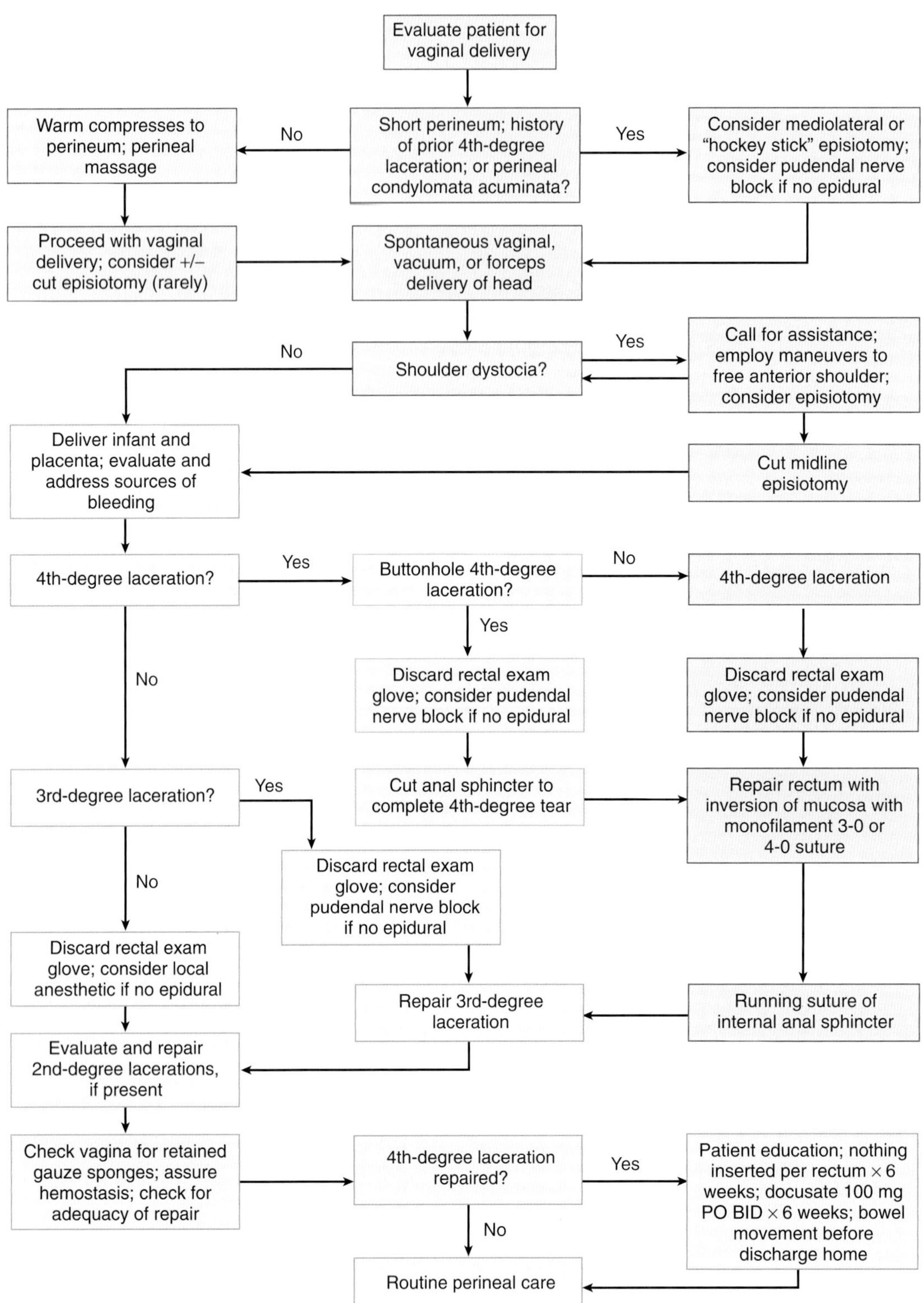

Figure 166-10 Flow diagram for episiotomy and repair.

ONLINE RESOURCE

The Cochrane Collaboration: Cochrane abstracts. Available at www.cochrane.org.

BIBLIOGRAPHY

Albers LL, Sedler KD, Bedrick EJ, et al: Midwifery care measures in the second stage of labor and reduction of genital tract trauma at birth: A randomized trial. J Midwifery Womens Health 50:365–372, 2005.

Carroli G, Belizan J: Episiotomy for vaginal birth. Cochrane Database Syst Rev 2:CD000081, 2000.

Forghani A, Hendricks SK: Episiotomy. In Reichman EF, Simon RR (eds): Emergency Medicine Procedures. New York, McGraw-Hill, 2004, pp 1033–1042.

Kettle C, Johanson RB: Continuous versus interrupted sutures for perineal repair. Cochrane Database Syst Rev 2:CD000947, 2000.

Power D, Fitzpatrick M, O'Herlihy C: Obstetric anal sphincter injury: How to avoid, how to repair: A literature review. J Fam Pract 55:193–200, 2006.

Tuggy M, Garcia J: Procedures Consult. Available at www.proceduresconsult.com.

Williams FL, Florey CV, Ogston SA, et al: UK study of intrapartum care for low risk primigravidas: A study of interventions. J Epidemiol Community Health 52:494–500, 1998.

CHAPTER 167

EXTERNAL CEPHALIC VERSION

Andrew S. Coco

In about 4% of term pregnancies, the fetus is in the breech position. Because the risk of complications with vaginal breech delivery is generally considered high, almost 90% of these fetuses are delivered by cesarean section without a trial of labor. Practiced since the time of Aristotle, external cephalic version (ECV) is a procedure that externally rotates the fetus from a breech presentation to a vertex presentation. Trials of ECV conducted over the past 25 years demonstrate an extremely strong safety record, a success rate of about 60%, and factors predictive of success and failure (Box 167-1). As a result of these studies, as well as the widespread availability of ultrasonography, electronic fetal monitoring, and effective tocolytic agents, ECV has made a resurgence. In addition to reducing cost and being safe and effective, the manual skills to perform ECV are easily acquired. Despite these favorable features, ECV is still underused. In fact, breech presentation is the third most frequent indication for cesarean section (after labor dystocia and repeat cesarean), and it accounts for 12% of the cesarean sections in the United States. Routine use of ECV could substantially reduce the rate of cesarean section, even in patients undergoing vaginal birth after cesarean (VBAC; however, see section on Relative Contraindications). ECV can be performed in basically any setting that has an ultrasonography machine and an experienced clinician (comfortable with ultrasonography and ECV). Clinicians must also be equipped and prepared for cesarean section if the need for an immediate delivery arises.

INDICATIONS

- Low-risk gestation at 36 weeks or more, by good dating criteria (at 36 weeks, likelihood of spontaneous version is low; alternatively, at 36 weeks, complications of immediate, iatrogenic, even preterm delivery are not severe).
- The type of breech (e.g., frank, complete, footling) is not a factor in determining suitability. Women with a fetus in transverse lie are also excellent candidates, as are those who are attempting VBAC (however, see section on Relative Contraindications).

NOTE: To perform ECV, it is preferable that the diagnosis of breech be made before the patient is in active labor! The further the breech is engaged in the pelvis, the more difficult the ECV; therefore the clinician should screen for breech, at least with Leopold's maneuvers, in every pregnancy near term.

CONTRAINDICATIONS

Absolute

- Indications for cesarean delivery aside from fetal presentation (e.g., placenta previa)
- Major uterine or fetal anomaly
- Nonreassuring fetal monitoring pattern
- Multiple gestation
- Abruptio placentae
- Ruptured membranes

Relative

- Suspected intrauterine growth restriction
- Decreased amniotic fluid volume
- Maternal cardiac disease
- Maternal hypertension
- Previous cesarean delivery (in small studies, ECV was not associated with uterine rupture in patients with previous cesarean or VBAC; however, repeat cesarean is generally a safe operation)
- Maternal obesity

EQUIPMENT AND SUPPLIES

- Intravenous catheter with heparin lock
- Blood-drawing equipment for a complete blood count and blood type and screen
- Syringe with 0.25 mg of terbutaline (Brethine)

Box 167-1. Factors Predictive of Successful and Failed External Cephalic Version

Factors Predictive of Successful Version

Increasing parity (most consistent factor in studies)
Normal amount of amniotic fluid (may be linear correlation between success rate of ECV and AFI, i.e., higher success rate with increasing AFI)
Fetal presentation (success rate with transverse lie approaches 90%)
Unengaged fetal part
Earlier attempts at ECV (increase success rate, but also increase risk of spontaneous reversion to breech)

Factors Predictive of Failed Version

Engaged fetal presenting part*
Difficulty palpating the fetal head*
Uterus tense to palpation*
Maternal obesity
Cervical dilation
Anterior placenta
Anterior or posterior positioning of fetal spine
Descent of breech into pelvis
Decreased AFI

AFI, amniotic fluid index; ECV, external cephalic version.
*The success rate is >90% if none of the factors marked by an asterisk is present and <20% if two of these factors are present. There have been no successful ECVs when all three factors are present.

- Fetal heart rate monitor
- Examination table with Trendelenburg's position
- Ultrasonography machine
- Ultrasonic gel
- Towels
- Sterile gloves and lubricant (if vaginal examination is required)
- Syringe of Rh_0 (D) immune globulin (RhoGAM) for Rh-negative patients

Preprocedure Patient Education

Usually the patient is examined and counseled in one clinic visit about risks, benefits, and alternatives to ECV (see the sample patient education form online at www.expertconsult.com) and returns for ECV at another visit. This delineation allows time for both the patient and her partner to make an informed decision about ECV. At the ECV visit, the patient should bring a signed consent form (see the sample patient education form online at www.expertconsult.com). The procedure should be scheduled as close to (but not before) 36 weeks' gestational age as possible to maximize the chances of success while, it is hoped, avoiding a preterm birth. Before 36 weeks, although there is a high success rate for ECV, fetuses are more likely to spontaneously revert to breech. The patient should be instructed not to eat a heavy meal during the 3 hours before ECV. The clinician should also reassure the patient that ECV causes only minimal discomfort. The results of studies are mixed regarding use of conduction analgesia. Some studies show an increased success rate with epidural analgesia, whereas other studies showed no benefit with use of spinal analgesia. This has led the American College of Obstetricians and Gynecologists (2000) to conclude that there is insignificant evidence to recommend routine use of conduction analgesia with ECV.

Technique

1. Perform an ultrasonographic examination to confirm a singleton in breech or transverse presentation, determine the amniotic fluid index, note the placental location, and rule out uterine malformations or congenital anomalies. The patient should empty her bladder after the ultrasonographic examination.
2. Perform a nonstress test to confirm a reassuring fetal heart rate tracing.
3. Draw blood for a complete blood count; type and screen. Establish intravenous access.
4. Administer a tocolytic agent, such as terbutaline (Brethine), subcutaneously about 15 minutes before the procedure. (This is optional because studies show conflicting efficacy. However, some type of relaxation technique should be used. One study in the literature demonstrates efficacy of hypnosis for spontaneous version.)
5. Place the patient in slight Trendelenburg's position to facilitate disengagement and mobility of the breech. Liberally coat the abdomen with ultrasonic gel to decrease friction and lessen the chances of an overly vigorous manipulation.
6. One or two persons may perform ECV. Determine the degree of pelvic engagement of the breech and perform gentle disengagement, if possible. Sometimes this requires a second operator to attempt vaginal disengagement. Successful disengagement is usually the key factor in achieving success. After the buttocks are elevated out of the pelvis and displaced laterally, the clinician(s) grasps each fetal pole in a hand.

   NOTE: The breech (i.e., buttocks) is what is actually manipulated during the maneuver. The head is merely guided gently toward the pelvis while the breech is actively moved cephalad.

7. Attempt either the classic forward roll or the back flip. Most clinicians tend to try the forward roll first (Fig. 167-1). However, some base their preference on whether the fetus is mostly on one side of the uterus (e.g., fetal head and spine are on the same side of the maternal midline) or not. A forward roll is chosen if the fetal head and spine are on different sides of the maternal midline, and a back flip (Fig. 167-2) is chosen if they are on the same side. Emphasis should be on gentle persuasion of the fetus, as opposed to forceful movements.
8. In most cases, if it is going to occur at all, success is attained quite easily. If the first attempt is unsuccessful, a second attempt is made in the opposite direction. An attempted version should be discontinued for significant maternal discomfort or a persistently abnormal fetal heart rate. After two failed attempts, if another attempt is to be made, it should be rescheduled.
9. It is important to monitor the fetal heart rate with the ultrasonography probe for fetal distress (e.g., bradycardia) immediately after all attempts. If persistent fetal bradycardia is noted after a successful version, return the infant to its previous breech presentation in hopes of reducing umbilical cord compression. Ultrasonography is also used after all attempts to confirm success or failure.
10. Regardless of success or failure, perform a nonstress test after the procedure to exclude fetal heart rate abnormalities.
11. Administer RhoGAM after the procedure to all Rh-negative patients because of a 4.1% risk of fetomaternal blood exchange.

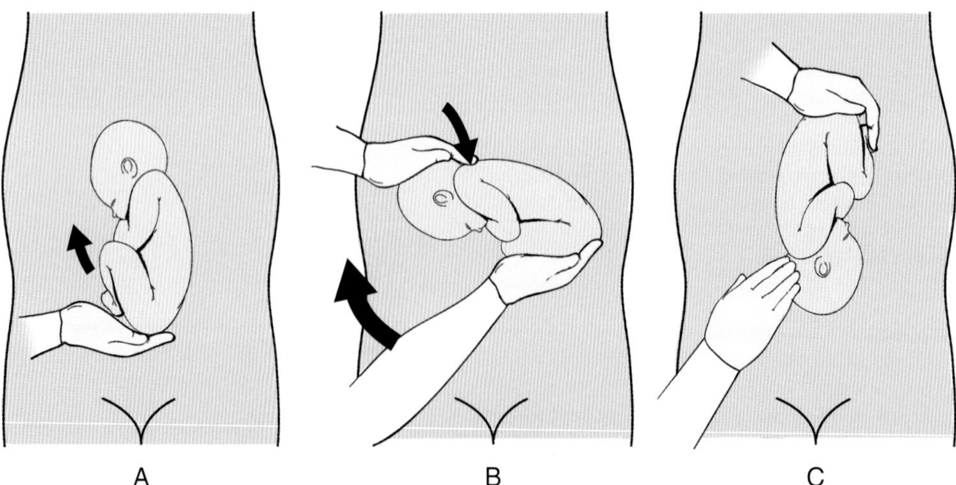

Figure 167-1 External cephalic version using the classic forward roll. **A,** The breech is mobilized. A second person is sometimes needed to vaginally disengage the fetus. **B** and **C,** At the same time, the breech is gently pushed upward while the head is directed into the pelvis.

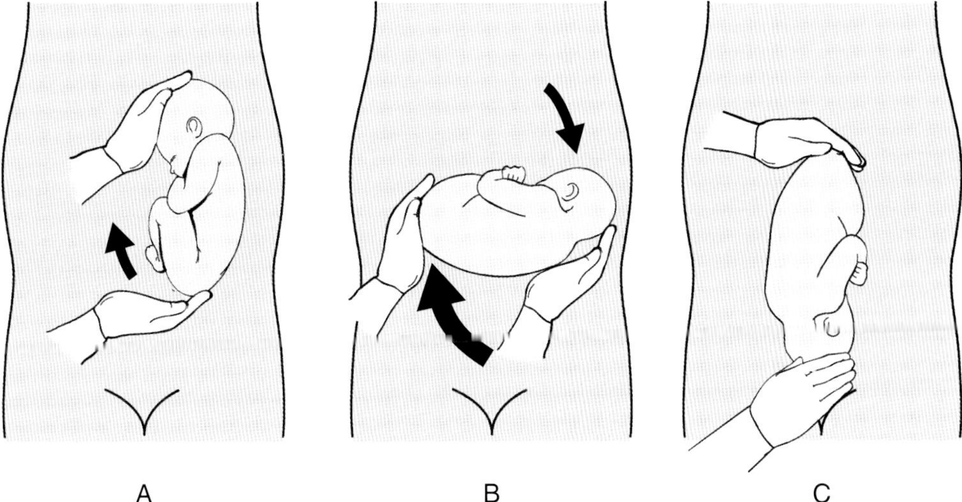

Figure 167-2 External cephalic version using the back flip. **A,** As with the forward roll, the breech is mobilized, possibly using a second person to vaginally disengage the fetus. **B** and **C,** At the same time, the breech is gently pushed upward while the head is directed into the pelvis.

12. If an attempt is unsuccessful and no evidence of fetal compromise is found, it is safe and cost effective to repeat ECV several days to 1 week later.

NOTE: ECV is easier to perform with multiparous mothers and when there is plenty of amniotic fluid. ECV may be worth considering, even in early labor, in multiparous women while en route to cesarean. It should never be performed under anesthesia unless the clinician is very experienced or is preparing for cesarean section. The technique should never be so forceful as to cause so much discomfort that anesthesia is necessary.

Sample Operative Report

See sample operative report online at www.expertconsult.com.

Common Error

Attempting to turn the fetus before mobilizing the breech from the pelvis is the most common error.

Complications

In general, ECV is very safe. When a protocol is used that includes fetal heart rate monitoring, ultrasonography, and ready access to operative delivery, the complication rate has ranged from about 1% to 2% since 1979. Most important, the literature provides overwhelmingly reassuring evidence against the risk of fetal death. Since 1980, only two fetal deaths have been reported with ECV. Both occurred when ECV was performed without the use of fetal heart rate monitoring or ultrasonography in preterm infants in Zimbabwe. In other words, there are no reports of fetal death when a protocol has been used similar to that outlined in this chapter.

- The risk of spontaneous reversion to a breech presentation after successful version is about 7%.
- Occasionally, the procedure needs to be discontinued because of significant or excessive maternal discomfort.
- There is a small risk of premature rupture of membranes or active labor within several days after the procedure. If the ECV was unsuccessful, either of these events could lead to a cesarean section for breech presentation, depending on patient and provider interest in an attempt at vaginal breech delivery.
- Transient, benign changes in fetal heart rate tracings are common (up to 39% in one study). There is a small risk of more worrisome changes, such as severe variable decelerations, late decelerations, or persistent bradycardia. These changes could signify placental abruption or umbilical cord entanglement and therefore necessitate an urgent cesarean section.
- Nonfatal fetomaternal hemorrhage occurs in about 4% of cases. A case of fetal brachial plexus injury has been reported.
- One maternal death has been reported due to amniotic fluid embolism. There is also risk of uterine rupture.
- After successful ECV, several reports suggest that the risk of cesarean delivery does not revert to institutional risk for vertex presentations. Dystocia, malpresentation, and nonreassuring heart rate patterns may be slightly more common after ECV.
- Authors of a systematic review of 44 studies involving 7377 patients from 1990 until 2002 concluded in 2004 that ECV is a safe procedure for both the mother and fetus.

Postprocedure Management

Follow-up visits and plans for a repeat attempt at ECV (in the event of an unsuccessful attempt), or a cesarean section when labor ensues are important to discuss with the patient.

Postprocedure Patient Education

- The clinician should discuss the postprocedure information on the sample patient education handout (see the sample patient education handout online at www.expertconsult.com), reemphasizing the major concerns.
- Clinicians should teach women who have undergone a successful ECV how to check their abdomen for reversion to breech, and women should do so daily. If the fetus has reverted, they should call or return to the clinic. One study has shown that training women to make regular self-assessments of the presenting part after successful ECV could improve the ultimate rate of vaginal delivery through the use of prompt, repeat ECV when reversion is detected before labor.
- Patients should call for any signs of premature rupture of membranes or labor. They should be instructed about the symptoms of both.

Patient Education Guides

See patient education and patient consent forms available online at www.expertconsult.com.

CPT/Billing Code

59412 External cephalic version (ECV), with or without tocolysis

ICD-9-CM Diagnostic Codes

652.23 Breech presentation without version, antepartum
652.33 Transverse or oblique fetal presentation, antepartum
761.7 External version before labor, malpresentation before labor

ONLINE RESOURCES

The Cochrane Collaboration. Available at www.cochrane.org (for updates on most obstetric issues).

Familydoctor.org: Breech babies: What can I do if my baby is breech? Available at familydoctor.org/handouts/310.html.

OBFOCUS: High-Risk Pregnancy Directory. Available at www.obfocus.com/resources/breech.htm (information on breech deliveries).

The WHO Reproductive Health Library: External cephalic version for the management of breech presentation (includes access to a video, "External cephalic version: Why and how?"). 2006. Available at http://apps.who.int/rhl/pregnancy_childbirth/childbirth/breech/rlcom/en/index.html.

BIBLIOGRAPHY

American College of Obstetricians and Gynecologists: Mode of singleton breech delivery. ACOG Committee Opinion No. 265. Int J Gynaecol Obstet 77:65–66, 2002.

American College of Obstetricians and Gynecologists: External cephalic version. ACOG Practice Bulletin No. 13. Washington, DC, 2000.

Breech presentation and delivery. In Cunningham FG, Leveno KJ, Bloom SL, et al (eds): Williams Obstetrics, 22nd ed. New York, McGraw-Hill, 2005, pp 565–586.

Coco AS, Silverman SD: External cephalic version. Am Fam Physician 58:731–738, 742–744, 1998.

Collaris RJ, Oei SG: External cephalic version: A safe procedure? A systematic review of version-related risks. Acta Obstet Gynecol Scand 83:511–518, 2004.

Hannah ME, Hannah WJ, Hewson SA, et al: Planned caesarean section versus planned vaginal birth for breech presentation at term: A randomised multicentre trial. Term Breech Trial Collaborative Group. Lancet 356:1375–1383, 2000.

Hofmeyr GJ: External cephalic version facilitation for breech presentation at term. Cochrane Database Syst Rev 4:CD000184, 2001.

Hutton EK, Hofmeyr GJ: External cephalic version for breech presentation before term. Cochrane Database Syst Rev 1:CD000084, 2006.

CHAPTER 168

Fetal Scalp Electrode Application

Beth A. Choby

Fetal heart rate monitoring is the most common obstetric procedure in the United States, with approximately 85% of fetuses being assessed with internal or external monitoring during labor. Electronic fetal monitoring (EFM) became possible in the 1950s with Edward Hon's design of an electrode that directly attached to the fetus. EFM entered widespread clinical use in the late 1960s despite the fact that evidence supporting its benefit was nominal (i.e., limited to case reports and retrospective studies).

Intermittent auscultation and continuous EFM are both available for assessing fetal heart rate trends. To perform intermittent auscultation, a hand-held Doppler ultrasonography transducer is used at specific intervals during labor. However, this requires a one-to-one nurse-to-patient ratio and an explicit auscultation schedule; therefore, intermittent auscultation is both difficult and expensive to perform. Although the majority of professional maternity care societies believe that some type of fetal monitoring is needed during labor, no randomized, controlled trials have compared either intermittent auscultation or continuous EFM with no monitoring. Because continuous EFM is simpler and less expensive and provides more data, it has become the default method of monitoring on most labor units, especially in the United States.

Continuous EFM is available either through external or internal monitoring. With external monitoring, a cardiotocometer measuring fetal heart rate is attached across the maternal abdomen using a belt. Internal EFM technology makes use of a bipolar spiral electrode that attaches directly to the fetal scalp. An electrical circuit is created between the wire electrode that twists into the fetal scalp and the metal wing on the electrode. Vaginal fluids create a saline electrical bridge and close the circuit. The resulting voltage difference (fetal cardiac signal) is amplified and transferred to a cardiotocometer that calculates heart rate. The bipolar wires also connect to a reference electrode on the maternal thigh to minimize electrical interference.

Both internal and external EFM are hindered by poor intraobserver consistency and a high false-positive rate. Continuous EFM is usually performed with the patient in dorsal lithotomy position and likely contributes to dysfunctional labor. Widespread use of EFM is associated with higher rates of cesarean delivery, operative vaginal delivery, and litigation. Continuous EFM has limited ability to identify a truly hypoxic–ischemic fetus and fails to decrease rates of cerebral palsy. In a recent meta-analysis of 13 randomized, controlled trials, the only clinically significant benefit for routine continuous EFM was the prevention of neonatal seizures.

With older EFM technology, internal scalp electrodes provided more accurate information on fetal heart rate trends than external monitoring. Newer-generation equipment allows for better evaluation of beat-to-beat variability (short-term variability) using the external monitor. Scalp electrodes are less frequently used as a result of these improvements in technology. Because certain situations still necessitate the use of an internal monitor, understanding both the application and use of the fetal scalp electrode is important for maternity care providers.

NOTE: Discussion of the subtleties of the abnormal fetal heart rate tracing is beyond the scope of this chapter. The practitioner of maternal and fetal care is referred to any recent comprehensive obstetrics textbook for this information. The entire clinical picture, including stage of labor, concurrent medical problems, current medications, and availability of a physician to perform an operative delivery, should be considered when making management decisions.

Indications

Most healthy, low-risk pregnancies are safely monitored with intermittent auscultation or continuous external monitoring. Higher-risk pregnancies affected by maternal or fetal medical complications often require continuous monitoring. Although continuous external monitoring is usually adequate, the following situations warrant consideration of internal monitoring with a fetal scalp electrode (FSE):

- Ineffective external monitoring or inadequate fetal tracing as a result of
  - Maternal body habitus
  - Excessive maternal movement
  - Excessive fetal movement
- Inadequate staffing for provision of intermittent auscultation
- Nonreassuring fetal heart rate patterns
  - Persistent fetal bradycardia (fetal heart rate [FHR] < 110 beats per minute [bpm])
  - Persistent fetal tachycardia (FHR > 160 bpm)
  - Decreased beat-to-beat variability on external monitoring
  - Lack of FHR accelerations
  - Moderate to severe variable decelerations
  - Repetitive late decelerations

Contraindications

Absolute

- Nonreassuring fetal status mandating emergent delivery
- Nonvertex presentation
- Patient refusal/uncooperative patient
- Active maternal hepatitis C, human immunodeficiency virus (HIV), or transmissible blood infection
- Placenta previa
- Vasa previa

- Head not fully engaged in maternal pelvis (membranes may rupture when applying FSE; possibility of prolapsed cord cannot be excluded)
- Inadequate cervical dilation to allow safe placement of FSE

Relative

- Untreated group B *Streptococcus* (GBS) infection
- Imminent delivery (relative)

Equipment and Supplies

- Scalp electrode (FSE; Fig. 168-1)
- Fetal monitor
- Sterile gloves
- Connecting wires between FSE and electronic monitor
- Surgical lubricant or povidone–iodine solution

Scalp electrodes and fetal monitoring equipment are available on all labor units. Familiarity with locally available equipment is suggested.

Precautions

- Vertex presentation
- Cervical dilation greater than 2 cm
- Ruptured membranes
- Head well engaged in maternal pelvis to decrease the risk of cord prolapse during FSE application

The fetal presentation, station, and position are determined from a sterile vaginal examination. If the placental location is unknown, bedside ultrasonography is helpful to rule out placenta previa and confirm vertex presentation. Rupturing the membranes (see Chapter 164, Amniotomy) makes applying an FSE easier, although it can be applied through the amniotic sac to create a "slow leak" of amniotic fluid. Rupturing membranes when the head is not fully engaged (i.e., "floating" in uterus) can result in cord prolapse. When meconium-stained fluid is encountered, fetal well-being should be closely assessed using continuous monitoring or a biophysical profile.

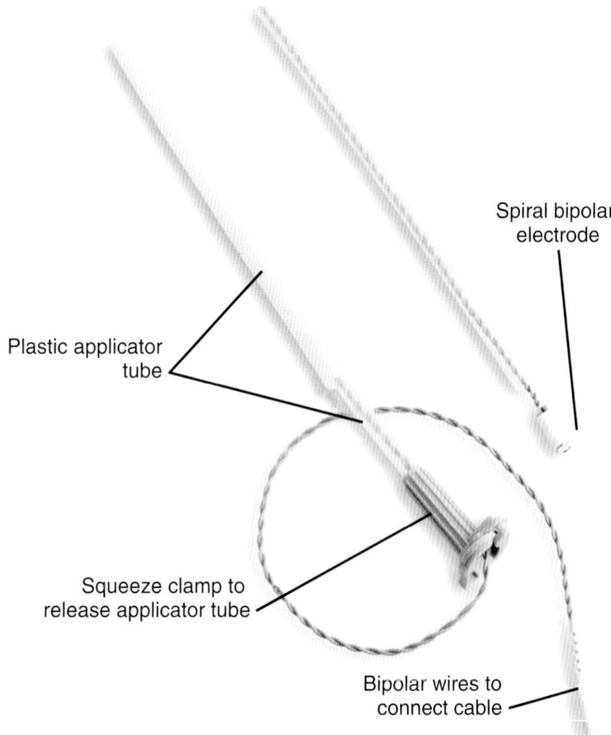

Figure 168-1 **Fetal scalp electrode with applicator tube.** (Courtesy of GE Healthcare, Waukesha, Wisc.)

Preprocedure Patient Education and Forms

Indications for FSE placement are discussed with the patient. Patient discomfort is generally minimal, and the procedure usually takes only a few minutes. Pain to the fetus is thought to be minimal. Showing the patient an FSE may help allay her concerns.

The patient lies in dorsal lithotomy position and the FSE is placed after a cervical examination to confirm fetal presentation. Fundal pressure from an assistant is helpful to reduce the risk of cord prolapse. Most hospitals do not require patients to sign specific operative consents for this procedure; obtaining verbal informed consent from the patient is prudent.

Technique

The following steps are performed when applying an FSE:

1. Read the package insert accompanying the FSE.
2. Put sterile gloves on both hands.
3. Confirm vertex presentation and assess for adequate cervical dilation (>2 cm).
4. Perform an amniotomy if membranes are intact and there are no contraindications (see Chapter 164, Amniotomy).
5. Ask an assistant to apply the adhesive pad (reference electrode) to the maternal thigh and connect the leads to the fetal electrocardiographic (ECG) monitor.
6. Holding the scalp electrode, free the tail wire to permit clockwise rotation of the electrode in the applicator tube.
7. Place the tip of applicator tube between the pads of the index and middle fingers of the hand used for vaginal examination.
8. Insert the fingers and applicator into the vagina and slide them toward the fetal vertex.

   NOTE: Be careful to avoid the fetal fontanelles. The electrode should not be placed on or near the anterior or posterior fontanelle.

9. Place the electrode against the fetal skull. Turn the outer portion of the FSE clockwise approximately two times until a "pop" is felt. Applying the electrode during a contraction or with fundal pressure from an assistant makes placement easier and decreases the risk of cord prolapse.
10. Ensure that the scalp electrode tip is well anchored by applying gentle, external/outward traction on the electrode applicator (which is still attached to the wires of the FSE). If the FSE holds in place with this maneuver, it is likely well anchored. If the FSE pulls loose with this maneuver, a second attempt should be made to implant the FSE nearby. Before attempting to reimplant, the FSE should be turned counterclockwise twice in the applicator (i.e., to untwist the wires). Then, while applying the FSE with slightly more pressure against the fetal skull than last time, a reassuring "pop" should be felt with two more clockwise turns of the tip. If the clinician is unable to anchor the electrode after a second attempt, the next attempt should be made with a new FSE.
11. Palpate the area around the scalp electrode to check that it is not applied to the maternal cervix or vaginal walls. Also ensure that it is not connected on or around the anterior or posterior fontanelle.
12. Unwind the wires from the clamp located on the exterior end of the scalp electrode.

13. Gently squeeze the clamp and allow the applicator to slide over the wires and out of the vagina. If the FSE pulls loose with this maneuver, it was not well anchored and should be removed. The next attempt should be made with a new FSE.
14. Have the assistant connect the red and green FSE wires to the cable that attaches to the fetal monitor.
15. Switch the fetal monitor setup from Doppler to ECG.
16. Review the ECG tracing for nonreassuring signs, including persistent tachycardia/bradycardia, decreased variability, or decelerations (discussed in Chapter 165, Antepartum Fetal Monitoring). If severe decelerations are noted, check for umbilical cord prolapse immediately. If cord prolapse is noted, the vertex should be pushed up into the uterus while an emergent cesarean delivery is arranged.
17. Consider whether placing an intrauterine pressure catheter is necessary (see Chapter 171, Intrauterine Pressure Catheter Insertion).

Sample Operative Report

A formal note detailing the indications for FSE placement and specifics of the procedure should be documented in the chart.

Procedure: Fetal Scalp Electrode placement for internal EFM
Indication: Inability to perform external monitoring due to (circle one):
  Maternal body habitus
  Maternal activity
  Fetal movement
  Poor external tracing
  Other: __________
Procedure: Risks, benefits, and alternative options were discussed with the patient/family. The patient provided informed consent and agreed to proceed. A sterile vaginal exam was performed demonstrating vertex presentation, cervical dilation of ____ cm, and a well-engaged fetal head. The membranes were/were not artificially ruptured. The FSE was applied to the fetal scalp, avoiding the fetal fontanelles. The patient and fetus tolerated the procedure well and a reassuring tracing was noted after FSE placement.

Common Errors

- Incorrect placement of the FSE onto maternal tissue
- Placement of the FSE close to the maternal cervix
- Entanglement of the FSE in fetal hair without fetal scalp attachment
- FSE attachment on or close to the fetal fontanelles
- Puncture injury to operator's finger from an extended bipolar wire

Scalp electrodes inadvertently attached to the maternal cervix or vagina do not provide an ECG tracing when connected to the monitor. FSEs placed close to the maternal cervix create pronounced vertical spikes on the tracing secondary to "bumping" against the cervix. No ECG tracing is apparent if the electrode is tangled in the fetal hair. Scalp electrodes attached on or near a fontanelle or on locations other than the fetal scalp should be removed immediately. Keeping the electrode sheathed in the applicator until the fetal skull is palpated helps avoid an unintentional puncture injury to the person applying the FSE.

Complications

- Fetal scalp abscess
- Meningitis, cerebrospinal fluid leak, or infection if an FSE is applied on a fontanelle
- Cephalohematoma or subcutaneous scalp emphysema if vacuum extraction is performed. The FSE should be removed before vacuum application. Depending on clinician experience, forceps may be preferred over vacuum-assisted delivery after FSE placement.
- Fetal trauma if FSE is incorrectly placed or applied in nonvertex positions: ocular injury in face presentation; scrotal, labial, or buttock lacerations with breech presentation
- Umbilical cord prolapse
- Increased risk of neonatal GBS sepsis if intrapartum antibiotic treatment is not given to mothers with GBS infection
- Puncture injury to the clinician applying the FSE

Postprocedure Management and Patient Education

Patients should be warned not to make sudden position changes or attempt to get out of bed without the hospital staff disconnecting the wire leads for the FSE. Internal monitoring generally limits patient mobility, although women may elect to sit in a rocking chair or on a birthing ball if close attention is paid to the wire leads.

Removing the Fetal Scalp Electrode

Indications

- Impending delivery (fetal head crowning)
- Application of vacuum-assisted device
- Cesarean delivery
- Inadvertent electrode placement on maternal tissue or nonscalp fetal parts
- Signal interference because of proximity of electrode to cervix

Technique

1. Remove the electrode when the fetal skull is visible between contractions with the head on the perineum.
2. Cut the wire leads with scissors approximately 2 inches from the perineum.
3. Manually untwist the wires until they can be easily unwound.
4. The electrode tip spins counterclockwise and unscrews from the fetal scalp. This usually happens as the wires are being untwisted.
5. Electrodes occasionally become tangled in the fetal hair. In this situation scissors are helpful for FSE removal.
6. During precipitous deliveries, cut the wire leads close to the perineum to prevent the electrode from catching and pulling on the fetal scalp. The electrode is easily removed after delivery.

CPT/Billing Codes

A specific code does not exist for FSE placement.

59050 Fetal monitoring during labor by consulting physician (not attending physician) with written report; supervision and interpretation
59051 Fetal monitoring during labor by consulting physician (not attending physician) with written report; interpretation only
59400 Routine obstetric care including antepartum care, vaginal delivery with or without episiotomy, forceps, or both, and postpartum care
59409 Vaginal delivery only (with or without episiotomy, forceps, or both)
59410 Vaginal delivery including postpartum care (excluding antepartum care)
59610 Successful vaginal birth after previous cesarean (VBAC)

ICD-9-CM Diagnostic Codes

656.33 Fetal distress, acid-base imbalance, affecting management of pregnancy or delivery, antepartum complication
656.53 Placental insufficiency affecting management of mother, antepartum complication
656.83 Meconium-stained fluid, affecting management of pregnancy or delivery, antepartum complication
656.83 Fetal distress, NOS, affecting management of pregnancy or delivery, antepartum complication
663.00 Umbilical cord prolapsed, antepartum
762.2 Placental insufficiency, affecting fetus or newborn
767.19 Cephalohematoma, because of birth injury
768.3 Fetal distress, liveborn, during labor and delivery
792.3 Meconium-stained amniotic fluid

Acknowledgment

The editors wish to recognize the many contributions by Timothy J. Downs, MD, to this chapter in a previous edition of this text.

Supplier

(See contact information online at www.expertconsult.com.)

Qwik Connect Plus fetal scalp electrodes and Abcorp belts
Utah Medical Products, Inc. (United States and Europe)

Online Resources

American College of Obstetricians and Gynecologists: Fetal heart rate monitoring during labor. ACOG Patient Education Pamphlet, 2001. Available at www.acog.org/publications/patient_education/bp015.cfm.

U.S. National Library of Medicine, Medline Plus Encyclopedia: Fetal heart monitoring. Available at www.nlm.nih.gov/medlineplus/ency/article/003405.htm.

Bibliography

Graham E, Peterson S, Christo D, et al: Intrapartum electronic fetal heart rate monitoring and the prevention of perinatal brain injury. Obstet Gynecol 108:656–666, 2006.

Hofmyer G: Evidence-based intrapartum care. Best Pract Res Clin Obstet Gynaecol 19:103–115, 2005.

Miyashiro M, Mintz-Hunter H: Penetrating ocular injury with a fetal scalp monitoring spiral electrode. Am J Ophthalmol 128:526–528, 1999.

Thacker S, Stroup D, Chang M: Continuous electronic fetal monitoring for fetal assessment during labor. Cochrane Database Syst Rev 3:CD000063, 2007.

Tuggy M, Garcia J: Procedures Consult. Available at www.proceduresconsult.com.

CHAPTER 169

FORCEPS- AND VACUUM-ASSISTED DELIVERIES

Carol Osborn • Jennifer Bell • Dale A. Patterson

Knowledge and experience with instrument-assisted (forceps or vacuum) delivery are important for all obstetrics providers managing the second stage of labor, particularly if there is an emergency, such as severe fetal or maternal compromise. In unexpected situations the knowledgeable use of an assisted delivery may be lifesaving and help reduce morbidity. Assisted deliveries are also a safe alternative to an operative delivery, as long as criteria and indications are followed. The incidence of assisted delivery is decreasing (especially forceps deliveries), in part because the incidence of cesarean delivery is increasing. Only 6% of all vaginal deliveries were assisted deliveries in the United States in 2002. The safe use of these procedures depends on understanding and clinically establishing the station and position of the vertex. A Cochrane review comparing forceps with vacuum found slightly more deliveries with vacuum, and fewer cesarean sections, less maternal trauma, and less general and regional anesthesia use with vacuum. However, the vacuum extractor was associated with an increase in neonatal cephalhematoma and retinal hemorrhages. Serious neonatal injury was uncommon with either form of assisted delivery or instrument.

CLASSIFICATION

Because of difficulties in estimating engagement and in defining different stations, the American College of Obstetrics and Gynecology (ACOG) defined and reclassified instrumented deliveries. The intention of this reclassification is to improve the safety of assisted deliveries and is discussed in the following sections.

Outlet Forceps or Vacuum

- Fetal skull has reached the pelvic floor.
- Fetal scalp is visible between contractions.
- Sagittal suture is in an anteroposterior diameter (i.e., occipitoanterior [OA], right occipitoanterior [ROA], left occipitoanterior [LOA], occipitoposterior [OP], right occipitoposterior [ROP], or left occipitoposterior [LOP]) that is less than 45 degrees from the midline.

Low Forceps or Vacuum

- Leading edge of the vertex is at +2 or greater station.
- Fetal head at this station fills the hollow of the sacrum.
- Head is not on the pelvic floor.
- Rotations are less than 45 degrees.

Midforceps or Vacuum

- Head is engaged.
- Vertex is higher than +2 station.
- Advisable only in emergency situations.

With the classification change, the term *high forceps* has been eliminated. High forceps describes application of the forceps before engagement of the vertex. This procedure has no place in modern obstetrics because of unacceptably high morbidity rates. Mid-instrumentation is reserved for providers who are experienced with this application. If an obstetrics provider is uncomfortable with the evaluation or application of forceps, a cesarean section is likely a safer route of delivery.

Before any forceps or vacuum application proceeds, the position and station of the vertex presentation must be determined. First, fetal engagement is verified. By definition, engagement indicates the biparietal diameter has passed the plane of the inlet. Clinically the fetal skull is at or below the ischial spines (i.e., 0 station). Checking the amount of space between the fetal head and the symphysis gives an additional measurement of station (Fig. 169-1).

Two things that complicate the clinician's ability to ensure complete engagement and assess descent are (1) molding, which leads to overestimation of descent or station, and (2) asynclitism or OP presentation, which also leads to overestimation of station. To avoid this miscalculation, the clinician should always confirm that the fetal head fills the sacral hollow. When the vertex fills the sacral hollow there should not be room to admit the fingers of the examining hand.

Position can be difficult to determine, especially if the head has marked caput. The following method helps determine position:

- Anterior fontanelle is shaped like a cross or plus (+) and is usually larger than the posterior fontanelle.
- Posterior fontanelle is shaped like a Y.
- When in doubt, the clinician should find the fetal ears to determine position.

If the position and descent meet criteria for an outlet or low instrumentation, then the provider needs to consider whether to use forceps or a vacuum to assist the delivery. The pros and cons of forceps versus vacuum extraction are described in Box 169-1.

INDICATIONS

Conditions Required for Instrumentation

- Vertex presentation (As noted previously, instrumentation may also be required to deliver the head in breech presentation. However, vertex presentation is required for the usual suction and outlet or low forceps applications.)
- Complete cervical dilatation
- Ruptured membranes
- No known severe cephalopelvic disproportion
- If unsuccessful, willingness to abandon procedure and proceed to cesarean section
- Adequate anesthesia is established

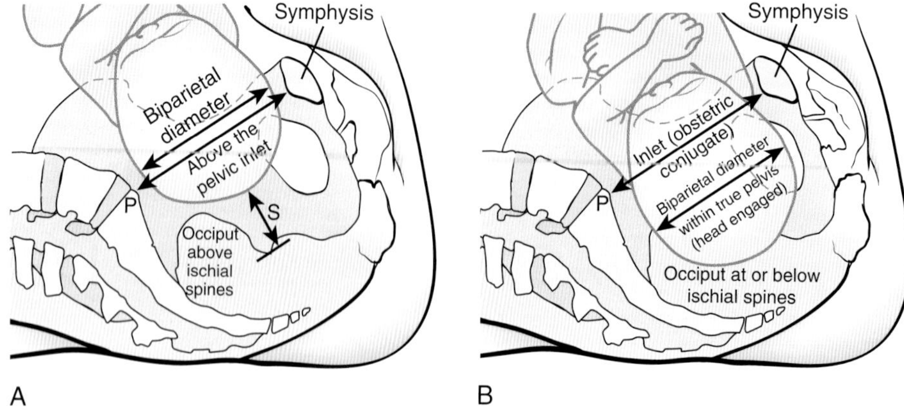

Figure 169-1 **A,** When the lowermost portion of the fetal head is above the ischial spines, the biparietal diameter of the head is not likely to have passed through the pelvic inlet and therefore is not engaged. **B,** When the lowermost portion of the fetal head is at or below the ischial spines, it is usually engaged. Exceptions occur when there is considerable molding, caput formation, or both. P, sacral promontory; S, ischial spine. (Modified from Cunningham FG, MacDonald P, Gant N, et al [eds]: William's Obstetrics, 19th ed. East Norwalk, Conn., Appleton & Lange, 1993.)

Maternal Indications for Instrument Delivery

- *Maternal exhaustion*. This is associated with prolonged second-stage pushing. Maternal exhaustion is especially common in the nulliparous labor. The lack of a trained labor companion during the second stage is associated with a longer labor and increased use of instrumentation.
- *Lack of maternal cooperation*.
- *Prolonged second stage or failure to progress*. The average second stage is 50 minutes for primiparous patients and 20 minutes for multiparous patients. Regional anesthesia prolongs the second stage by inhibiting the maternal urge to push (Table 169-1).
- *Medical conditions for which the strain of the second stage of labor would be deleterious*. Examples include cardiac valvular disease, respiratory disease (e.g., active asthma), cerebrovascular disease, toxemia, and chronic hypertension.

Maternal and Fetal Indications for Instrument Delivery

- Relative cephalopelvic disproportion.
- Malposition (OP or OT).
- Malpresentation (face or breech); use forceps only. For breech deliveries, forceps are often needed for the aftercoming head once the body has been delivered.
- Hemorrhage.
- Intrapartum infection.

Fetal Indications for Instrument Delivery

- Nonreassuring fetal heart tracing
- Rapid deterioration of the tracing or any condition that makes it unsafe for the fetus
- Premature placental separation

CONTRAINDICATIONS

Absolute

- Fetal head not engaged
- Position of the head not determined (forceps)

Relative

- History of a failed forceps or vacuum delivery with a macrosomic fetus

Box 169-1. Forceps versus Vacuum Extraction

Forceps	*Vacuum*
Pros	*Pros*
Higher rate of successful vaginal delivery	Easy to apply
Usually a more rapid delivery (e.g., for fetal distress)	Teaches the clinician to follow the pelvic curve
Useful in breech (for the aftercoming head) and face presentations	Allows autorotation from occipitoposterior and occipitotransverse positions
Useful for rotations if clinician is experienced with these	Less force applied to the head
Cons	Requires less anesthesia
Requires significant experience	Results in fewer cervical, vaginal, and perineal lacerations
Increased risk of neonatal craniofacial injuries	Easier to learn
Increased risk of intracranial hemorrhage	Clinician can use if not completely sure of head position
Requires more maternal anesthesia	*Cons*
Associated with more cervical, vaginal, and perineal lacerations	Difficult to maintain vacuum if head is molded or infant has full head of hair
	Pull only with contractions, which increases time needed for successful delivery
	Associated with intracranial hemorrhage at a greater rate than spontaneous deliveries
	Only useful in vertex presentations
	Increased incidence of cephalhematomas and retinal hemorrhage

TABLE 169-1 Limits of the Duration of the Second Stage of Labor before Intervention

Parity	Without Regional Anesthetic	With Regional Anesthetic
Nullipara	2 hr	3 hr
Multipara	1 hr	2 hr

- Suspected fetal coagulation defect
- Incomplete cervical dilatation (only exceptions are the urgent delivery of a second twin and a severely abnormal tracing without immediately available cesarean section)
- Delivery requiring excessive traction
- Prematurity (vacuum not recommended before 34 weeks' gestation because of increased risk of intracranial hemorrhage)
- Malpresentation (e.g., breech, face, brow, transverse lie)
- Prior scalp sampling (vacuum)
- Position of fetal head not precisely determined in vertex presentation (vacuum)

EQUIPMENT

Include all equipment listed for normal vaginal delivery (see Chapter 177, Vaginal Delivery). Modern vacuum extractors are available from numerous suppliers. Both rigid and soft cups are available; each has advantages over the other. Rigid cups more often result in a successful assisted delivery, but they are also more likely to be associated with complications. The operator should be familiar with the models available at the institution and should be trained in their proper use. Any associated tubing or pumps must also be available. The Mityvac is one example of a vacuum apparatus (Fig. 169-2). Tucker-McLean (Fig. 169-3) and Simpson (Fig. 169-4) forceps are commonly used forceps with vertex presentation of term infants. Again, local availability and user training should determine the type of forceps employed. Both forceps and vacuum equipment should be readily available on all labor floors.

PRECAUTIONS

The Food and Drug Administration (FDA) published a public advisory in 1998 concerning complications resulting from vacuum deliveries. The FDA found a fivefold increase in death and serious injury after vacuum deliveries. Although part of this increase may be due to the increased use of this procedure, the blame may also lie in failing to follow established protocols. The most concerning complication is a life-threatening subgaleal hematoma. The length of application of the vacuum may also be an important factor in the development of complications. It is not recommended to apply a vacuum for more than 20 minutes.

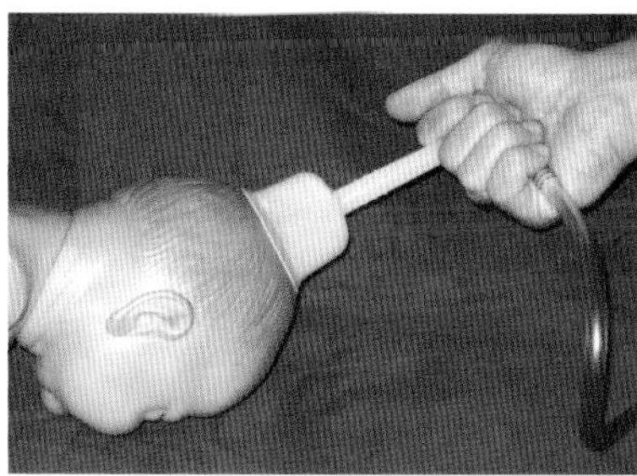

Figure 169-2 Mityvac extractor.

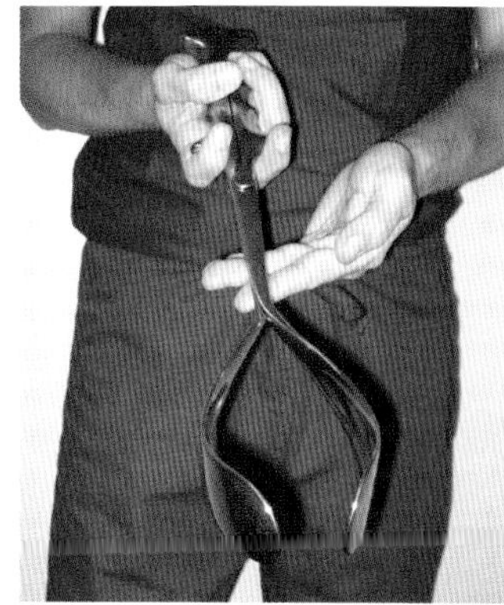

Figure 169-3 Tucker-McLean forceps.

PREPROCEDURE PATIENT EDUCATION

Assisted delivery is a procedure that most women would choose to avoid during their labor. It is optimal to discuss the possibility of the need for vacuum or forceps delivery before a patient is in labor, but this is not always possible. Nonetheless, the risks and benefits of the procedure must be explained to the patient in as much detail as possible prior to attempting an assisted vaginal delivery. Consent for the procedure should be obtained.

TECHNIQUE

Forceps Delivery

The forceps have interlocking parts with a right and a left side that correspond to the side of the maternal pelvis in which they lie when applied. Each side has a handle, shank, and blade. The Simpson forceps is most commonly used for low and outlet deliveries.

Initially developed by Dr. J. Bachman, the acronym *ABCDEFGHIJ* has become part of the Advance Life Support in Obstetrics (ALSO) curriculum; it is useful when training for forceps- and vacuum-assisted deliveries. Except for *F*, *G*, and *H*, the acronym is essentially the same for both procedures:

A: Is the *anesthesia* adequate? Consider a local or pudendal block or both. *Ask* for help.
B: Is the *bladder* empty? Straight catheterize if needed.
C: Is the *cervix* completely dilated?
D: *Determine* the position of the fetal head. Consider shoulder *dystocia* (i.e., why is there a delay?).
- Anterior fontanelle is larger and forms a cross.
- Posterior fontanelle is smaller and forms a Y.
- Find the ear, feeling which way it bends.
- The descent should be to a +2 station, with the vertex filling the sacrum.

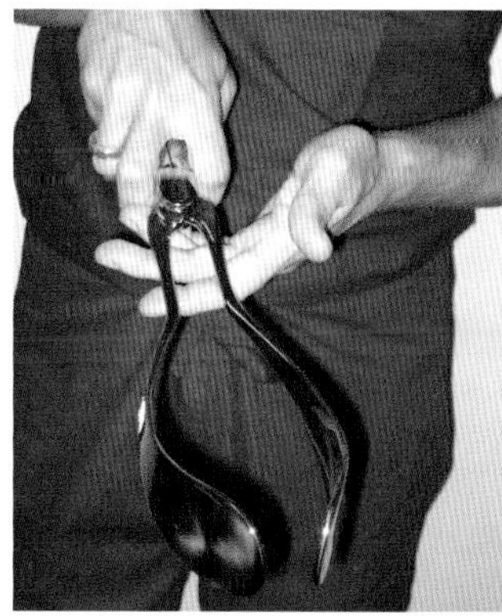

Figure 169-4 Simpson forceps.

E: Is the *equipment* ready (e.g., infant suction bulb, cord clamp, instrument table)?
F: Are the *forceps* ready for application?
1. Articulate the forceps to ensure a proper fit.
2. Disarticulate the handles and take the left handle in your left hand (holding it like a pencil with concave cephalic curve toward the vulva and the shank directed upward, perpendicular to the floor).
3. Begin to ease the forceps along the left side of the fetal head (OA); use your right hand to protect the maternal sidewalls and guide the blade into position. (The right thumb is placed on the heel of the blade and gently inserted.)
4. Right forceps handle is then held in your right hand.
5. Insertion is along the right side of the fetal head, with the left hand protecting the maternal right pelvis and guiding the blade into place.
6. If correctly applied, the handles should fit together easily and lock easily.
7. Check the application position for safety (posterior fontanelle, fenestration, sagittal suture).
   - Posterior fontanelle should be midway between the shanks and 1 cm above the plane of the shanks.
   - Fenestrations of the forceps should admit no more than one fingertip.
   - Sagittal suture should be midline and midway between the shanks. (For OP deliveries, the blades should be equidistant from the midline of the face and brow.)

G: Use *gentle* traction (i.e., Pajot's maneuver) (Fig. 169-5).
1. The pelvic curve from the inlet through the outlet is described as a J-shaped curve.

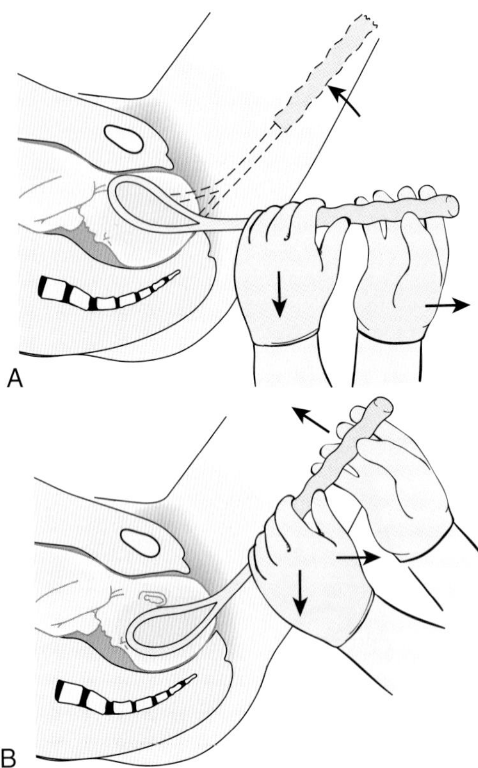

Figure 169-5 Occiput anterior delivery by outlet forceps (Simpson). The direction of gentle traction for delivery of the head is indicated. Initially, the forceps are horizontal (**A**) and they are gradually rotated forward (**B**). Forces are as noted.

2. Initially, one hand pulls the forceps handles in the same direction that the handles extend (an approximately horizontal vector, outward and away from the mother).
3. The other hand is placed on the shaft close to the perineum and pushes in a downward vector.
4. The summation of these two vectors creates an outward-and-downward force.
5. As the crown of the head moves from under the symphysis, the traction should begin upward. (For OP deliveries, the horizontal traction continues until the base of the infant's nose passes under the symphysis.)

H: The *handle* is elevated to follow the J-shaped pelvic curve (see Fig. 169-5B).
I: Evaluate for the need for an episiotomy *incision*. The amount of distention of the perineum will dictate the need. (For OP deliveries, there will be greater distention of the vulva, and a large episiotomy may be needed.)
J: The forceps are removed when the *jaw* of the infant is reachable.

Vacuum Delivery

A: Is the *anesthesia* adequate? *Ask* for help.
B: Is the *bladder* empty?
C: Is the *cervix* completely dilated?
D: *Determine* the position of the fetal head. Consider shoulder *dystocia* (i.e., why is there a delay?).
   - Anterior fontanelle is larger and forms a cross.
   - Posterior fontanelle is smaller and forms a Y.
   - Find the ear, feeling which way it bends.
   - Descent should be to a +2 station, with the vertex filling the sacrum.

E: *Equipment* and *extractor* ready (infant suction bulb, cord clamp, instrument table, etc.)?
F: Insert and apply the cup over the posterior *fontanelle*.
   - Wipe vertex clean of blood and fluid.
   - Spread the labia.
   - Compress and insert the cup.
   - Place the cup over the posterior fontanelle (or over the sagittal suture up to 3 cm in front of the posterior fontanelle, toward the face).
   - Sweep the finger around the cup to check for trapped maternal tissue.
   - Calibrate the vacuum dials, noting that yellow (10 mm Hg) is the resting suction and that red (50 mm Hg) is the suction pressure required for traction during contractions.

G: Use *gentle* traction (Fig. 169-6).
1. Apply traction at right angles to the plane of the applied surface of the cup.

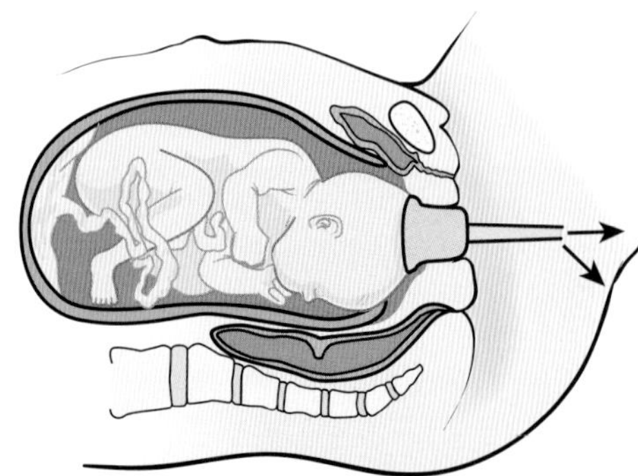

Figure 169-6 Correct position of the vacuum cup and the correct direction of traction before the vertex clears the symphysis pubis. (Modified from Epperly T, Breitinger R: Vacuum extraction. Am Fam Physician 38:205, 1988.)

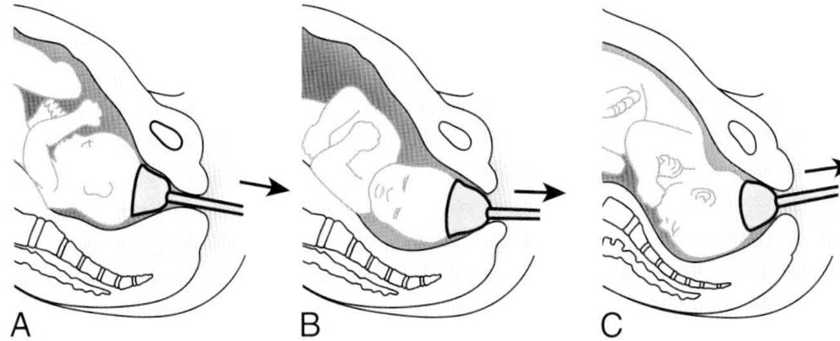

Figure 169-7 Occipitoposterior application (**A**), rotation (**B**), and delivery (**C**) using vacuum extractor. (Modified from Lowdermilk DL, Perry SE, Bobak IM: Maternity and Women's Health Care, 7th ed. St. Louis, Mosby, 2000.)

2. Do not rock or torque the cup or handle. Only use gentle, steady traction.
3. As the fetal head moves around the symphysis and extends, the vacuum handle will rise from a horizontal to a nearly vertical position. (The angles and traction are more difficult for OP deliveries, with the handle often pointing toward the floor.)
4. If the cup detaches, consider the following problems: inadequate vacuum suction, trapped maternal tissue, a fetal scalp electrode in the way, incorrect application of the extractor (not over the flexion point), or bending or rotation of the shaft.

H: *Halt* traction when the contraction is over.
1. Reduce the vacuum to 10 mm Hg between contractions.
2. Repeat the gentle-traction cycle with the next contraction.
3. *Halt* the procedure if the cup disengages more than three times, if no progress is noted after three consecutive pulls, or if a delivery does not occur after 20 minutes of intermittent traction.
4. Use caution when attempting a forceps delivery after a failed vacuum extraction (only if the vertex is right on the perineum). A cesarean section may be a better choice (intracranial hemorrhage is more common after a failed vacuum extraction followed by a forceps delivery).

I: Make an *incision* for episiotomy, if necessary. A midline episiotomy may be associated with increased risk of third- and fourth-degree perineal lacerations.

J: Remove the vacuum cup when *jaw* of the infant can be reached or is delivered.

A suction application can also be used to rotate the head from an OP to an OA position before delivery (Fig. 169-7).

Sample Operative Report

The operative report from an assisted vaginal delivery should be included in the delivery note. The actual note will vary greatly depending on the individual labor and local custom. Following is an outline of suggested topics to include in this note:

- Preoperative diagnosis (note indication for the assistance, such as maternal exhaustion)
- Postoperative diagnosis (note preoperative diagnosis and result of the procedure [e.g., vaginal delivery, term infant, weight, Apgar score, cord pH])
- Operation (note outlet forceps or vacuum extraction)
- Instrument (e.g., Simpson forceps)
- First stage (note length, interventions, any complication)
- Second stage (same information as in first stage, including type of fetal monitoring)
- Third stage (type of placenta delivery, description of placenta)
- Repairs
- Bladder
- Estimated blood loss
- Anesthesia

Common Errors

- Starting the procedure too soon: Be sure that head is engaged and position is clear prior to attempting assisted vaginal delivery.
- Incorrectly positioning the instrument: Ensure proper placement of vacuum or forceps prior to pulling.
- Including vaginal tissue in the vacuum application: Circle finger around cup to ensure no tissue has been trapped between the cup and the head.
- Continuing with assisted vaginal delivery when success is unlikely: Be prepared to stop and proceed to a cesarean section if unable to deliver within 20 minutes or if vacuum "pops off" three times.

Complications

- Cervical, vaginal, or perineal lacerations
- Postpartum hemorrhage from the lacerations
- Fetal birth trauma (e.g., fractured clavicle, cephalhematoma, lacerations, abrasions, facial nerve palsy, intracranial and retinal hemorrhage)
- Subgaleal hematoma
- Shoulder dystocia
- Neonatal scalp emphysema
- Cephalhematoma
- Hyperbilirubinemia
- Fetal cervical trauma
- Maternal discomfort at delivery
- Maternal urinary retention

Postprocedure Patient Education

Instrument-assisted deliveries increase the level of maternal concern for the infant. The provider should discuss the need for the instrument delivery and maternal perceptions regarding the delivery on the first postpartum day. After the procedure, the patient should be advised to monitor the following and report any changes to the practitioner:

- Bleeding
- Fever
- Dysuria and urinary retention
- Pelvic pain (could indicate hematoma)

CPT/Billing Codes

59400 Global vaginal delivery (antepartum, vaginal delivery with or without episiotomy and/or forceps or vacuum) and postpartum care
59409 Vaginal delivery *only* (with or without episiotomy and/or forceps or vacuum)
59410 Vaginal delivery *only* (with or without episiotomy and/or forceps or vacuum) including postpartum care
59610 VBAC (global)
59899 Unlisted procedure, maternity care and delivery (induction)

ICD-9-CM Diagnostic Code

669.51 Forceps or vacuum delivery, without mention of indication

BIBLIOGRAPHY

American College of Obstetricians and Gynecologists: Operative vaginal delivery. Practice Bulletin No. 17. Washington, DC, American College of Obstetricians and Gynecologists, June 2000.

Bachman J: Forceps delivery (letter). J Fam Pract 29:360, 1989.

Damos J: ALSO Curriculum. Leawood, KS, American Academy of Family Physicians, 2000.

Forceps delivery and vacuum extraction. In Cunningham FG, Hauth JC, Leveno KJ, et al (eds): William's Obstetrics, 22nd ed. New York, McGraw-Hill, 2005.

Hook CD, Damos RJ: Vacuum-assisted vaginal delivery. Am Fam Physician 78:953–960, 2008.

Johanson RB, Menon BK: Vacuum extraction versus forceps for assisted vaginal delivery. Cochrane Database Syst Rev 2:CD000224, 2000.

Putta LV, Spencer JP: Assisted vaginal delivery using the vacuum extractor. Am Fam Physician 62:1316–1320, 2000.

Ratcliffe S, Byrd J, Sakornbut E: Pregnancy and Perinatal Care in Family Practice. Philadelphia, Hanley & Belfus, 1996.

Society of Obstetricians and Gynaecologists of Canada: Guidelines for operative vaginal birth. Int J Gynaecol Obstet 88:229–236, 2005.

Tuggy M, Garcia J: Procedures consult. Available at www.proceduresconsult.com, and as an application at www.apple.com/iTunes.

CHAPTER 170

Intrathecal Analgesia in Labor

Thomas E. Howard • Renae Rasmussen

Intrathecal analgesia uses the subarachnoid (dural) space for the injection of analgesic narcotics and anesthetics. This space is filled with cerebrospinal fluid (CSF) and is the same space used for a spinal or saddle block (see Chapter 175, Saddle Block Anesthesia). Analgesics injected into this space diffuse through the CSF to coat the visceral pain receptors in the dorsal horn of the spinal cord (T10–L1). Although it does not provide complete pain relief, this technique provides considerably more pain relief than the parenteral or intravenous (IV) route. In addition, pain relief is more rapid than with epidural analgesia. In comparison to spinal or saddle block anesthesia, which often uses hyperbaric anesthetic solutions (i.e., solutions more dense than CSF so they drift caudally), the dose with intrathecal analgesia is significantly less. Overall, intrathecal analgesia allows for profound analgesia without clinically significant motor or autonomic blockade (i.e., minimal anesthesia).

This procedure is not technically difficult to perform and does not adversely affect the infant or the progress of labor. Clinicians comfortable with performing lumbar puncture can easily learn this procedure and perform it without an anesthesiologist. It is useful in many clinical settings, especially where epidural analgesia is not readily available or when complete anesthesia is not necessary (Box 170-1). It is also used in combination with epidural analgesia (combined spinal-epidural [CSE]).

Often performed with a needle-through-needle technique, CSE provides faster onset of analgesia with a smaller dose of anesthetic than epidural alone. Although it was thought, at one time, that a smaller dose of anesthetic would result in less motor block and maternal leg numbness and therefore improved mobility, it turns out this may not be the case. A recent Cochrane Review comparing CSE with epidural alone concluded that although there was no difference in postdural puncture headache (PDPH), progress of labor, incidence of instrumented deliveries or cesareans, or adverse effects on the infant, there was also no difference in maternal mobility during labor. Although analgesia was faster in onset with CSE, more women had pruritus than with epidural alone. Consequently, there was no difference in patient satisfaction in the CSE group compared with epidural alone.

Intrathecal analgesia is ideally suited for patients in the first stage of labor who are anticipated to deliver vaginally (if cesarean is anticipated, epidural or CSE may be preferred). The pain in this stage is primarily due to uterine contractions and cervical dilation. Pain in the second stage of labor is due to both uterine contractions and fetal descent through the birth canal. Because fetal descent stimulates the pudendal nerve (S2–S4), intrathecal analgesia is less effective; however, it does continue to provide analgesia for the uterine contractions. The real overall benefit for intrathecal analgesia is improved tolerance of the contractions, thereby resulting in a more rested mother for the second stage of labor. This in turn should enhance the overall birthing experience.

Because the duration of intrathecal analgesia is limited, it should be used as the sole method for pain control only when the remaining duration of the first stage of labor is expected to be less than 6 hours. Although the procedure can be repeated later in labor, each additional dural puncture increases the risk of PDPH. If a cesarean section becomes necessary, general, spinal, or epidural analgesia may be used after intrathecal analgesia.

Anatomy

Intrathecal analgesia is produced when medications are injected directly into the thecal sac. Unlike an epidural injection, the intrathecal injection penetrates the dura and enters the space occupied by the CSF. The anatomy is identical to that for an adult lumbar puncture and this is described in detail in Chapter 206, Lumbar Puncture. The anatomy is also identical to that for saddle block anesthesia, as described in Chapter 175, Saddle Block Anesthesia.

Indications

- Active first stage of labor with anticipated vaginal delivery
- Epidural analgesia not available (many rural and community hospitals), not needed, or not desired

Contraindications

Absolute

- Allergy to selected narcotics
- Patient refusal or uncooperative patient
- Patient with known coagulopathy
- Use of once-daily–dose low–molecular weight heparin within 12 hours
- Refractory maternal hypotension

Box 170-1. Advantages and Disadvantages of Intrathecal Narcotics in Labor

Advantages

Prolonged, superior analgesia compared with intravenous administration
No effect on expulsive forces in labor
Rapid onset of analgesia
Technique similar to lumbar puncture
Low incidence of serious side effects
Cost advantages compared with epidural anesthesia

Disadvantages

Analgesia is usually inadequate for second stage of labor
No anesthesia for instrumented delivery or episiotomy
Does not provide surgical anesthesia
Risk of respiratory depression
High incidence of mild side effects
May require a repeat injection, which increases the risk of postdural puncture headache

TABLE 170-1 Duration and Onset of Action for Intrathecal Narcotics

Medication	Dosage	Onset of Action (min)	Duration of Action (hr)
Fentanyl	10–25 μg (usual dose 15 μg)	5	1.4–3.5
Sufentanil*	2.5 μg	5–10	1–3
Morphine†	0.1–1.0 mg‡ (usual dose 0.15 mg)	15–60	2–6

*Although fetal outcomes were the same, bradycardia has been associated with higher doses of sufentanil; therefore, at Parkland Hospital, fentanyl or this dose of sufentanil are preferred.

†Astramorph and Duramorph are commercially available, preservative-free morphine preparations. It is important to use preservative-free medications to avoid the complication of arachnoiditis from the preservative.

‡Morphine at doses of 0.5–1.0 mg can have duration of action up to 12 hours but with a higher rate of side effects; it is therefore not recommended.

- Active infection at the site of puncture
- Increased intracranial pressure
- Supratentorial mass lesion
- Untreated maternal bacteremia

Relative

- Spinal abnormalities, such as marked scoliosis, making the procedure technically difficult
- Treated active systemic infection, such as that resulting in maternal bacteremia
- Cutaneous lesion/skin compromise of the lower back, such as cellulitis or dermatitis

Equipment and Supplies

- Spinal anesthesia kit, which includes sterile preparation materials, local anesthetic, a 25-gauge or smaller atraumatic spinal anesthesia needle, and an 18- or 19-gauge introducer

  NOTE: Thin, atraumatic spinal needles (Sprotte or Whitacre needles, with rounded or pencil-point, conical ends) have been proven to decrease the risk of PDPH.

- Syringe with filter-tip needle for drawing up narcotic for injection
- Narcotic for injection (Table 170-1)
- Bupivacaine 0.5% to 0.75% suitable for spinal injection, 2.5 mg total
- Ephedrine for injection
- Naltrexone, 25-mg tablet
- Naloxone ampules, 0.4 mg
- Continuous fetal monitoring (internal or external)
- Sterile gloves
- Personnel to monitor for side effects, including monitoring blood pressure
- Pulse oximeter

Precautions

Intrathecal analgesia is a fairly safe procedure in the right clinical setting. Nonetheless, it should be approached with caution. The procedure should not be performed too early in labor unless another form of analgesia or repeat injection is planned. The injection should also not be performed too late in labor because the medication is primarily given to ease the discomfort of contractions; it is not as effective in the second stage of labor where much of the discomfort is due to descent of the fetus. Care should be taken to minimize the side effects, particularly the itching seen in many patients. Finally, the provider should remember to avoid the possibility of introducing infection to the central nervous system by following aseptic technique and avoiding injection through an area that may be infected or compromised.

Preprocedure Patient Education

The patient should be informed of available analgesia and anesthesia options during the prenatal period to aid in giving informed consent (see the sample patient consent form online at www.expertconsult.com). Preferably, desired analgesia or anesthesia should be determined as part of a written birthing plan. Staff providing prenatal education should be knowledgeable about this technique and offer information to their clients. An educational handout can be given to them to read before the onset of labor (see patient education form online at www.expertconsult.com). It should be explained to the mother that any analgesia/anesthesia during labor is optional and does have certain risks. It is not necessary to have any procedure for analgesia/anesthesia in order to have a healthy baby. However, excessive fatigue due to discomfort during labor is also unnecessary; it may affect not only the quality of labor but the ability to complete labor.

During labor, the clinician should review the benefits and risks with the patient and obtain informed consent. Ideally, because the pain of labor might impair the mother's understanding of this information, the counseling should be done in the presence of the mother's labor coach.

Technique

1. Ensure continuous fetal monitoring is in place and check for contraindications to intrathecal analgesia.
2. Obtain informed consent.
3. Establish IV access and, if possible, give a 500-mL bolus of fluid to help prevent the rare side effect of maternal hypotension (give this bolus very slowly for women with pregnancy-induced hypertension).
4. Place the patient in the desired position for dural puncture (sitting or lying on left side) and locate the L3-4 interspace (Fig. 170-1).

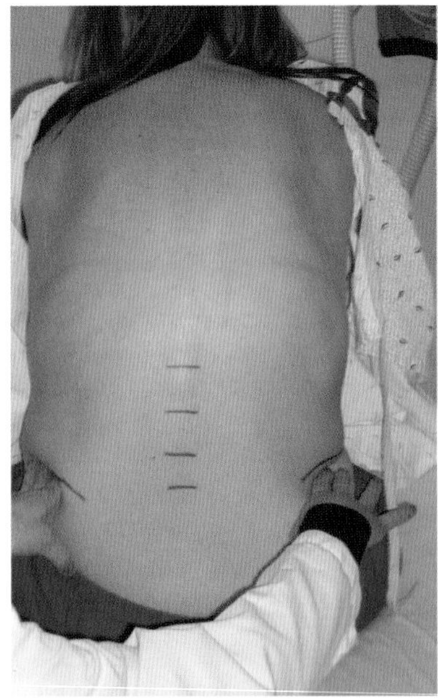

Figure 170-1 To locate the L3-4 interspace, the iliac crests are palpated. The line between the crests intersects the L4 spinous process. The L3-4 interspace is found slightly above (cephalic to) the L4 spinous process.

5. Perform sterile preparation and draping. Administer the local skin anesthetic as you would for a lumbar puncture.
6. Insert the introducer needle through the anesthetized skin and into the supraspinous ligament. It is especially important to use an introducer in larger patients because the spinal needle is otherwise difficult to direct. Spinal anesthetic needles used for this procedure are thinner and less rigid than the needles most clinicians use for lumbar puncture. The advantage of the narrower-gauge, atraumatic needles is that they lower the risk of PDPH.
7. Draw up selected rapid-onset narcotic (fentanyl or sufentanil) in a syringe with a filter-tip needle (filter prevents drawing up tiny glass particles).
8. If desired, also draw up preservative-free morphine into the same syringe with the filter-tip needle. The decision to add morphine in part depends on the anticipated length of time needed for analgesia; adding morphine prolongs the duration (see Table 170-1). Use of morphine has also been shown to decrease the need for postpartum pain medications and to enhance the pain relief with subsequent epidural analgesia.
9. In the same syringe, draw up 2.5 mg of bupivacaine. Ensure that the bupivacaine is suitable for spinal anesthesia. Bupivacaine at much higher doses is commonly used to obtain complete surgical anesthesia. This small dose of bupivacaine increases the duration while decreasing the time to onset of analgesia compared with using a narcotic alone. Its use also reduces the incidence of pruritus.
10. Insert a narrow-gauge, bullet-type or pencil-point atraumatic anesthetic needle (25 to 27 gauge) through the introducer into the intrathecal space. You will detect a distinct pop or snap when passing through the ligamentum flavum (this pop may be less pronounced with atraumatic needles). Whereas minimal or no fluid returns when passing through the epidural space, CSF returns when the intrathecal space has been entered (just as with a lumbar puncture). Remove the trocar from the anesthesia needle and confirm that CSF is flowing into the hub of the needle.
11. Place the syringe with the narcotic and anesthetic agents onto the spinal needle. Aspirate a small amount of CSF (0.25 to 0.5 mL) into the syringe, allowing it to mix with the medications in the syringe, and then inject the contents of the syringe back through the needle over 5 to 10 seconds. Aspiration and injection should be performed between contractions.
12. Remove the spinal needle, introducer, and syringe as a unit and place the patient on her left side for uterine displacement. Monitor her pulse and blood pressure every 5 minutes for 15 minutes; if stable, she can then move to a more comfortable position. Maternal hypotension (rare) occurs soon after the medication is given, if it is going to happen. If this occurs, it should be treated with another IV fluid bolus and with ephedrine 5 to 10 mg IV push. This ephedrine dose can be repeated every 5 minutes as necessary.
13. If pain relief diminishes before delivery, there are four options:
    - Intrathecal narcotic and bupivacaine can be repeated, especially if the patient is still in the first stage of labor.
    - A supplemental parenteral narcotic injection can be given. However, it is important to give this at half the usual dose to avoid the side effect of respiratory depression.
    - Epidural analgesia can be administered.
    - Some anesthesiologists perform CSE. To do this, an epidural catheter is placed at the time of the intrathecal injection and can be used later if operative delivery is necessary, or if added pain relief is desired.

Sample Operative Report

See a sample operative report online at www.expertconsult.com.

Common Errors

- *Incorrect dosing of medications*: Be certain that medications are properly labeled and dosed. The use of multiple medications with different dosing scales can lead to confusion and medication errors.
- *Failure to monitor patient*: The peak of respiratory depression that may develop after injection usually occurs after delivery of the infant. Patients who receive intrathecal injections should be monitored in the postpartum area for signs of respiratory depression for at least 12 hours after the injection.
- *Insufficient pain relief*: Intrathecal injection works well in most instances, but may not be effective for all patients. Dosing may need to be repeated or alternative forms of analgesia used. If multiple doses or multiple routes of analgesic administration are used, be certain to monitor closely for deleterious effects of the medications.

Complications

Although serious complications with intrathecal analgesia are rare, the incidence of less severe side effects is relatively high (Table 170-2). Pruritus, although seldom severe, is quite common. However, only about one third of patients request treatment for pruritus. It responds to naloxone at the doses listed. However, the analgesic effect may be affected by naloxone. Nalbuphine (Nubain) is an opioid agonist–antagonist that can be used for pruritus alone. Another option is diphenhydramine (Benadryl). Nausea and vomiting are treated symptomatically. For PDPH, oral or IV caffeine or use of an autologous blood patch may be helpful. See Chapter 206, Lumbar Puncture, for these treatments.

There are no adverse fetal outcomes expected from this procedure. Rarely (<10% of cases), fetal heart rate decelerations are seen and these are generally transient. Fetal heart rate monitoring is recommended according to institutional protocols. There is no effect on the normal course of labor at the suggested doses of agents.

TABLE 170-2 Side Effects and Their Management for Intrathecal Analgesia in Labor

Side Effects	Incidence	Treatment
Pruritus (usually mild)	≥50%	May not be related to histamine release, but can try diphenhydramine (Benadryl) 20–50 mg orally, IM, or IV every 6 hr as necessary or naloxone (Narcan) 0.2–0.4 mg IV.
Nausea and vomiting	30%–50%	Metoclopramide (Reglan) 10 mg orally or IV every 6 hr or promethazine (Phenergan) 25 mg IM every 6 hr.
Urinary retention	4%–20%	In-and-out catheterization as necessary.
Postdural puncture headaches	1%–6%	Usually no treatment is necessary. Blood patch if not resolved with conservative management (rest, fluids, analgesics, caffeine).
Maternal hypotension	Up to 15%	Generally transient. If systolic blood pressure <90 mm Hg or any fetal distress, use IV fluid bolus, uterine displacement, and/or ephedrine (5–10 mg IV push). Repeat every 5 min as necessary.
Respiratory depression	0.2%–0.4%	Naloxone (Narcan) 0.2–0.4 mg IV. Consider oxygen with decreased SaO_2.

TABLE 170-3 Sedation Scale to Monitor for Respiratory Depression from Intrathecal Narcotics

Sedation Level	Assessment
None	Awake and alert
Minimal	Drowsy or sleeping but easily aroused
Moderate	Drowsy or sleeping but not easily arousable
Somnolent	Drowsy or sleeping and cannot be fully aroused

Postprocedure Management

Vital signs (respiratory rate, heart rate, and blood pressure) are monitored every 30 minutes for the duration of labor. Increased monitoring should be maintained after delivery until the analgesic is metabolized. Nursing staff should assess for sedation and arousability (Table 170-3).

If moderate or somnolent sedation is noted by nursing staff, the clinician should be notified and the patient's oxygen saturation (SaO_2) checked. Use naloxone for treatment of respiratory depression at doses of 0.2 to 0.4 mg IV. This can be repeated every 3 minutes until the respiratory depression or sedation is reversed. Administer oxygen if the SaO_2 is diminished. Naloxone can also be given by a continuous IV infusion at 0.4 mg/hr if necessary. Although the exact mechanism is unknown, respiratory depression may be caused by ascending spread of the analgesic agent. In theory, if the narcotic spreads too far cephalad, it can suppress the respiratory centers in the fourth ventricle of the brain. The incidence of respiratory depression peaks at between 4 and 9 hours, but it has been noted as late as 12 hours after administration of intrathecal narcotics. The time of highest risk for the mother is after delivery, when her respiratory drive may be decreased. Unfortunately, this is also a time when mothers are monitored less frequently. Some protocols call for postpartum continuous pulse oximetry or frequent hands-on measurement of vital signs and mental status.

Oral naltrexone 12.5 to 25 mg is given within 30 minutes after the delivery. This is a long-acting narcotic antagonist that reduces the side effects of the intrathecal narcotic, including the risk of respiratory depression, and is generally free of side effects at these dosages.

Patient Education Guides

See examples of patient education and consent forms online at www.expertconsult.com.

CPT/ Billing Codes

62273 Injection, lumbar epidural, of blood or clot patch
62311 Injection, single (not via indwelling catheter), not including neurolytic substances, with or without contrast, of diagnostic or therapeutic substance(s) (including anesthetic, antispasmodic, opioid, steroid, other solution), epidural or subarachnoid; lumbar, sacral (caudal)

ICD-9-CM Diagnostic Codes

V22.2 Pregnant state, NOS
650 Normal delivery

The fifth digit (X) is required for codes 640–648, 651–659, and 660–669 to denote the current episode of care:

0 Unspecified
1 Delivered, with or without mention of antepartum condition
2 Delivered, with mention of postpartum complication
3 Antepartum condition or complication
4 Postpartum condition or complication

644.23 Premature labor with delivery (<37 weeks)
646.83 Other specified condition of labor (pain)
652.23 Breech presentation
653.53 Unusually large fetus causing disproportion

Codes Related to Deliveries with Forceps or Vacuum

662.03 Prolonged first stage of labor
662.23 Prolonged second stage of labor
659.73 Abnormality in fetal heart rate or rhythm or fetal distress

Suppliers

(See contact information online at www.expertconsult.com.)

Covidien
Kendall Company
Disposable trays, needles
B. Braun Medical, Inc.
Baxter Healthcare Corporation
Becton, Dickinson and Co.
Teleflex
Rusch, Inc.

BIBLIOGRAPHY

American College of Obstetricians and Gynecologists: Obstetric analgesia and anesthesia. ACOG Practice Bulletin No. 36. Obstet Gynecol 100:177–191, 2002.

American College of Obstetricians and Gynecologists Committee on Obstetric Practice: Optimal goals for anesthesia care in obstetrics. ACOG Committee Opinion No. 433. Obstet Gynecol 113:1197–1199, 2009.

American Society of Anesthesiologists Practice Guidelines for Obstetric Anesthesia: An Updated Report by The American Society of Anesthesiologists Task Force on Obstetric Anesthesia. Last amended October 18, 2006. Available at www.asahq.org/publicationsAndServices/practiceparam.htm#ob. Accessed August 20, 2009.

Asokumar B, Newman LM, McCarthy RJ, et al: Intrathecal bupivacaine reduces pruritus and prolongs duration of fentanyl analgesia during labor: A prospective, randomized controlled trial. Anesth Analg 87:1309–1315, 1998.

Fontaine P, Adam P, Svendsen KH: Should intrathecal narcotics be used as a sole labor analgesic? A prospective comparison of spinal opioids and epidural bupivacaine. J Fam Pract 51:630–635, 2002.

Hawkins JL: Obstetric analgesia and anesthesia. In Gibbs RS, Karlan BY, Haney AF, Nygaard IE (eds): Danforth's Obstetrics and Gynecology, 10th ed. Philadelphia, Lippincott Williams & Wilkins, 2008.

Herman NL, Choi KC, Affleck PJ, et al: Analgesia, pruritus, and ventilation exhibit a dose-response relationship in parturients receiving intrathecal fentanyl during labor. Anesth Analg 89:378–383, 1999.

Hess PE, Vasudevan A, Snowman C, Pratt SD: Small dose bupivacaine–fentanyl spinal analgesia combined with morphine for labor. Anesth Analg 97:247–252, 2003.

Palmer CM, Cork RC, Hays R, et al: The dose-response relation of intrathecal fentanyl for labor analgesia. Anesthesiology 88:355–361, 1998.

Palmer CM, Van Maren G, Nogami WM, Alves D: Bupivacaine augments intrathecal fentanyl for labor analgesia. Anesthesiology 91:84–89, 1999.

Regional analgesia. In Cunningham FG, Leveno KJ, Bloom SL, et al (eds): Williams Obstetrics, 22nd ed. New York, McGraw-Hill, 2005.

Rust LA, Waring RW, Hall GL, Nelson EI: Intrathecal narcotics for obstetric analgesia in the community hospital. Am J Obstet Gynecol 170:1643–1646, 1997.

Simmons SW, Cyna AM, Dennis AT, Hughes D: Combined spinal-epidural versus epidural analgesia in labour. Cochrane Database Syst Rev 2:CD003401, 2007.

Stephens MB, Ford RE: Intrathecal narcotics for labor analgesia. Am Fam Physician 56:463–470, 1997.

Wong CA, Scavone BM, Loffredi M, et al: The dose-response of intrathecal sufentanil added to bupivacaine for labor analgesia. Anesthesiology 92:1553–1558, 2000.

Yeh HM, Chen LK, Shyu MK, et al: The addition of morphine prolongs fentanyl-bupivacaine spinal analgesia for the relief of labor pain. Anesth Analg 92:665–668, 2001.

CHAPTER 171

Intrauterine Pressure Catheter Insertion

Beth A. Choby

The intrauterine pressure catheter (IUPC) allows for direct intrauterine monitoring of contraction strength and frequency when external tocodynamometry is ineffective. Approximately 20% of laboring patients in the United States are monitored using an IUPC. IUPC placement is appropriate for specific intrapartum indications. Maternal indications include excessive movement or elevated body mass index. IUPC use is common with protracted/dysfunctional labor and increasingly used during trial of labor after cesarean (TOLAC). When meconium or significant variable decelerations are present, IUPC placement allows for amnioinfusion.

Intrauterine pressure monitoring was first developed in the 1860s using intrauterine balloons placed transabdominally to determine contraction strength. The current transcervical route for IUPC placement was developed in the late 1960s, when one clinical monitoring unit became available that concurrently monitored fetal heart rate and contractions. Early IUPC technology determined intrauterine pressure using a column of water, although this was later replaced by an electronic microtip pressure sensor.

Today's IUPC technology uses either electronic pressure transducer-tip catheters or air-coupled flexible balloon catheters. Both types graphically represent intrauterine pressure through measurements of the frequency, duration, and amplitude of contractions. In women with arrest of labor, internal monitoring allows for an assessment of contraction strength with Montevideo units (MvU). Montevideo units are calculated as the product of contraction intensity multiplied by frequency (i.e., number of contractions in a 10-minute period multiplied by the mean amplitude of contractions during this time). During active labor, individual contraction amplitude ranges from 30 to 80 mm Hg; calculated Montevideo units between 180 and 220 are considered adequate. Demonstrating a pattern of 200 MvU for at least 2 hours during active labor is a reasonable criterion for making the diagnosis of failure to progress (Miles and colleagues, 2001).

Whether women with a previously scarred uterus attempting TOLAC benefit from IUPC monitoring is uncertain. An elevated uterine resting tone or abnormalities in the contraction pattern may suggest uterine rupture, although the best predictor seems to be an abnormal fetal heart tracing (variable or late decelerations). Fetal indications for an IUPC include amniotic fluid sampling and meconium dilution through amnioinfusion (discussed in Chapter 176, Transcervical Amnioinfusion).

Indications

Eighty-five percent of patients in labor in the United States are managed using continuous fetal monitoring. Surveillance with external monitoring for fetal heart rate and contractions is most frequently used. When external monitoring is not possible, internal monitoring with a fetal scalp electrode and IUPC is sometimes necessary. Indications for an IUPC include the following:

- Inadequate contraction pattern
- Failure to progress/descend
- Arrest of labor
- TOLAC
- Ineffective use of external monitoring secondary to maternal motion or body habitus
- Need for amnioinfusion
  - Amniotic fluid sampling
  - Meconium dilution
  - Oligohydramnios with variable decelerations

Contraindications

Absolute

- Intact fetal membranes (absolute unless rupture acceptable; see Chapter 164, Amniotomy)
- Complete placenta previa

Relative

- Inadequately dilated cervix
- Partial placenta previa
- Vasa previa
- Uterine bleeding of undetermined etiology
- Nonreassuring fetal status
- Fetal anomalies (e.g., gastroschisis)

Equipment and Supplies

- Sterile gloves
- Amniotomy hook if membranes are not ruptured
- Intrauterine pressure catheter (sterile; Fig. 171-1)
- Cable to join IUPC with fetal monitor (nonsterile)
- Fetal monitor
- Intravenous tubing, pole, and fluid if amnioinfusion is planned (see Chapter 176, Transcervical Amnioinfusion)

Precautions

- Ascertain fetal presentation to avoid traumatizing fetus.
- Ascertain placental location to avoid traumatizing the placenta.

Preprocedure Patient Education and Forms

The patient's medical record and progress in labor are reviewed. If the placental location is unknown, bedside ultrasonography confirms whether a partial or complete placenta previa is present.

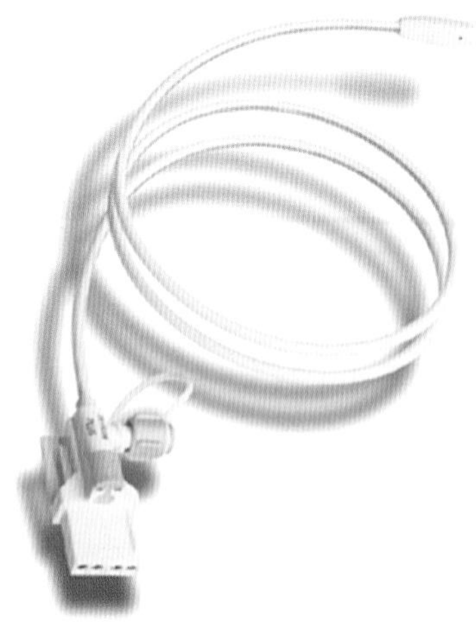

Figure 171-1 Intrauterine pressure catheter. (Courtesy of Utah Medical Products, Inc., Midvale, Utah.)

Indications for IUPC placement and risks and benefits of the procedure are discussed with the patient in a manner consistent with providing informed consent.

The patient is placed in dorsal lithotomy position. A cervical examination is necessary to determine cervical dilation and fetal presentation. If the membranes are unruptured, artificial rupture may be performed during the cervical examination if appropriate. IUPC placement is not usually painful, although some women experience mild discomfort during the procedure.

Technique

1. Read the package insert to ensure familiarity with the equipment.
2. Ensure that all necessary supplies are present. Prepare a sterile field on the delivery bed or table.
3. Turn on the fetal monitor. Connect the interface cable (nonsterile) to the fetal monitor. Switch the fetal monitor from the external tocometer setting to the IUPC setting.
4. Open the IUPC package. Don sterile gloves. Remove the IUPC and plastic introducer (guide) from the package and observe the double hatch marks at 45 cm. Hand the end of the IUPC that connects to the interface cable to an assistant.
5. Establish a "0" baseline for the monitor as described by the manufacturer.
6. Perform a sterile vaginal examination to assess cervical dilation and confirm that the membranes are ruptured. Place the index and third fingers posteriorly between the fetal vertex and cervix. Position the fingers away from the area above which the placenta is located.
7. Use the opposite hand to slide the IUPC/plastic introducer into the vagina over the palmar aspect of the intravaginal hand. Pass the catheter through the vagina and into the cervical os. Stop advancement of the IUPC/introducer when the tip of the IUPC rests between the fingers of the examining hand.
8. Hold the plastic introducer with the intracervical fingers and push the external (outside) part of the IUPC with the opposite hand to advance it through the introducer. The IUPC should pass the fetal vertex with minimal resistance and advance into the amniotic sac.
9. Stop advancing the IUPC when the double hatch marks (45 cm) reach the maternal introitus or when resistance is felt. IUPC advancement should proceed smoothly and without resistance. If resistance is encountered, change the direction of the catheter until insertion proceeds easily. Do not force the catheter because this increases the risk for placental, uterine, or fetal damage. Planning for insertion in an area remote from the placenta decreases risk for iatrogenic abruption. The double hatch marks correlate with normal placement of the IUPC. Checking for a flash of amniotic fluid in the IUPC channel during insertion is recommended to guard against extramembranous placement.
10. With the IUPC properly positioned, hold the external IUPC with the external hand. Remove the intravaginal hand and use it to "peel" the introducer away from the IUPC as the introducer is simultaneously pulled out of the vagina. Take care not to remove the IUPC when the introducer is being removed.
11. Connect the distal end of the IUPC to the interface cable. Secure the IUPC to the patient's thigh using the belt or adhesive pad provided. Leave some slack between the introitus and the belt to prevent inadvertent IUPC expulsion with patient repositioning or movement. Proper IUPC placement is again confirmed by checking that the double hatch marks are at the introitus.
12. Confirm that connections between the IUPC and the reusable monitor cable and from the monitor cable to the monitor are all secure.
13. Have the patient cough or perform a Valsalva maneuver to check for proper IUPC functioning. Palpable contractions should correlate with increased intrauterine pressure on the monitor.
14. Write a brief procedural note in the chart. When amnioinfusion is indicated, please refer to Chapter 176, Transcervical Amnioinfusion.

Intrauterine Pressure Catheter Removal

Removal of the IUPC is straightforward and usually performed before delivery. Apply traction to the IUPC between contractions. The IUPC should come out easily. If resistance is encountered, stop and redirect the catheter until it can be removed with minimal resistance.

Sample Operative Report

See a sample operative report online at www.expertconsult.com.

Common Errors

- Extramembranous placement. This problem occurs when the IUPC is positioned between the uterine wall and the amniotic/chorionic membranes. Complications include placental perforation, uterine perforation, and abruptio placentae. Estimates of the frequency of incorrect IUPC placement range from 14% to 38% (Lind, 1999). The percentage of intra-amniotic placements increases if the clinician watches for a flash of amniotic fluid each time an IUPC is being inserted.
- Inability to thread the IUPC into the amniotic cavity. Redirect the IUPC tip and gently reintroduce. As the fetal head descends, placement becomes more challenging.
- The baseline tone on the uterine monitor is above zero. Re-zero the IUPC using the slide switch on the base of the IUPC.
- No contraction pattern is evident after the IUPC is zeroed. Suspect extramembranous placement. Withdraw the IUPC and check for blood in the IUPC tip.

Complications

- Extramembranous (extraovular) placement of the IUPC
- Inaccurate pressure tracings
- Placental perforation

- Uterine perforation
- Fetal vessel laceration
- Fetal trauma
- Amnionitis
- Disseminated intravascular coagulation (rare)
- Maternal cardiac failure secondary to amniotic fluid embolus (rare)

Postprocedure Management and Patient Education

The fetal heart rate and contraction pattern are monitored closely to ensure fetal and maternal well-being. Vaginal bleeding should be reported. Counsel the patient that mobility is limited with an IUPC. The patient can be disconnected from the monitor but should ask for assistance when she needs to get out of bed. Some providers prefer placing Foley catheters in women who have internal monitors.

CPT/Billing Codes

Although there is no CPT code for IUPC insertion, labor that is post-term, augmented/induced, or complicated can be billed in addition to a routine delivery charge. Code this increased acuity of care using hospital evaluation and management (E/M) codes. Obstetric care and delivery charges should be submitted in addition to these codes.

99356 Prolonged physician service in the inpatient setting, requiring direct (face-to-face) patient contact beyond the usual service first hour*
99357 Each additional 30 minutes*
99358 Prolonged evaluation and management service before and/or after direct (face-to-face) patient care (e.g., review of extensive records and tests, communication with other professionals and/or patient/family); not face-to-face care; first hour*
99359 Each additional 30 minutes*

*This is an add-on code and is designed to be used in addition to the E/M code.

ICD-9-CM Diagnostic Codes

658.0X Oligohydramnios
658.4X Infection of amniotic cavity
661.0X Abnormality of forces of labor
662.1X Prolonged labor
665.1X Rupture of uterus during labor
792.3 Nonspecific abnormal findings in fluid surrounding fetus

"X" indicates the need for a fifth digit for complete coding: 0, unspecified as to episode of care; 1, delivered; 3, antepartum condition.

Acknowledgment

The editors wish to recognize the many contributions by Christian Raigosa, MD, to this chapter in a previous edition of this text.

Suppliers

(See contact information online at www.expertconsult.com.)

Intran Plus IUP-400 (An electronic pressure transducer-tip catheter)
Utah Medical Products, Inc. (United States and Europe)
Koala IUPC (Air-coupled flexible balloon catheter)
Clinical Innovations, Inc.

Online Resources

Clinical Innovations: Koala: Essentials in IUP monitoring. Available at www.clinicalinnovations.com/koala_video.htm.
Utah Medical Products, Inc.: Intran Plus intrauterine pressure catheters. Available at www.utahmed.com/intran.htm.

Bibliography

Dowdle M: Comparison of two intrauterine pressure catheters. J Reprod Med 48:501–505, 2003.
Lind B: Complications caused by extramembranous placement of intrauterine pressure catheters. Am J Obstet Gynecol 180:1034–1035, 1999.
Macones G, Cahill A, Pare E, et al: Obstetric outcomes in women with two prior cesarean deliveries: Is vaginal birth after cesarean delivery a viable option? Am J Obstet Gynecol 192:1223–1229, 2005.
Miles A, Monga M, Richeson K: Correlation of external and internal monitoring of uterine activity in a cohort of term patients. Am J Perinatol 18:137–140, 2001.
Wilmink FA, Wilms FF, Heydanus R, et al: Fetal complications after placement of an intrauterine pressure catheter: A report of two cases and review of the literature. J Matern Fetal Neonatal Med 21:880–883, 2008.

CHAPTER 172

OBSTETRIC ULTRASONOGRAPHY

Thomas A. Kintanar

Ultrasound is defined as the range of sound waves with frequencies greater than 20,000 cycles per second (Hz), and they are undetectable by the human ear. Most ultrasound scanners use frequencies of from 1 to 10 MHz; 3 to 5 MHz are the most common for obstetric transabdominal examinations, although 2 to 2.25 MHz may be needed for obese patients. According to natality data, ultrasonography is being used more commonly in the United States. In 2002, 67% of mothers who had live births underwent ultrasonographic scanning during pregnancy, compared with 48% in 1989.

To evaluate the use of ultrasonography as a routine screening procedure during pregnancy, the National Institutes of Health (NIH) sponsored a landmark Consensus Development Conference in 1984. The consensus was that routine screening was not justified and that ultrasonography should be used only for specific indications. Those indications have remained fairly constant and are similar to those listed in the Indications section. This consensus was further supported by evidence from the large RADIUS study (N = 15,151), published in 1993 (Ewigman and colleagues), although there continues to be controversy regarding this study, specifically over whether the study population is generalizable (e.g., 93% of women in the study were white, 71% had at least some college education). The current position of the American College of Obstetrics and Gynecology (ACOG) allows the clinician and patient to opt for screening, but does not recommend routine use. As it turns out, the majority of women will develop one of the indications listed by the Consensus Development Conference during pregnancy.

The U.S. consensus regarding screening is not a worldwide consensus. The Royal College of Obstetricians and Gynecologists and the European Committee for Ultrasound Radiation Safety endorse routine prenatal ultrasonographic examinations. Ultrasonography is routinely used in several European countries, including Sweden and Germany. The Canadian Task Force on Preventive Health Care finds fair evidence for routine ultrasonographic screening in the second trimester, even in women without clinical indications. Many U.S. insurers, including managed care organizations, now reimburse for routine obstetric ultrasonographic screening. The advent of three- (3D) and four-dimensional (4D) ultrasonography (3D imaging is three-dimensional in appearance; 4D is 3D imaging in real time) has conferred some proprietary advantages in terms of the quality of fetal features appreciated (recent literature cites improved diagnosis of facial anomalies, skeletal malformations, and neural tube defects with 3D and 4D ultrasonography).

EDITOR'S NOTE: Routine first-trimester scanning in a high-risk population to confirm gestational age is very helpful (investigators have proven it more accurate than last menstrual period), especially when later managing intrauterine growth retardation (IUGR) or postdate pregnancies (in two studies, postdate deliveries and inductions were reduced by more than 50%). Such accurate dating may also alter the method of pregnancy termination; conversely, its use may improve maternal bonding.

Obstetric ultrasonography can be performed transabdominally, transvaginally, or transperineally (or a combination), with transabdominal and transvaginal scanning being used much more frequently than transperineal. Transvaginal scanning is performed predominantly in the first trimester and usually facilitates visualization of fetal structures 1 week earlier than with transabdominal scanning. Transvaginal and transperineal scanning may also be useful during the second and third trimesters for scanning the cervix and endocervical areas in cases of preterm labor, incompetent cervix, and placenta previa.

Ultrasonography can detect 35% to 50% of major fetal malformations, but its sensitivity is very technician or clinician dependent. It is important for the clinician performing the examination to have adequate training and equipment and a willingness to seek appropriate consultation for complicated cases. Although a complete survey of fetal anatomy can often be performed by the end of the first trimester, the American Institute of Ultrasound in Medicine (AIUM) suggests that such a survey is best if performed after 18 weeks.

Obstetric ultrasonographic studies are classified in three different ways: for billing purposes, radiologically, and by training requirements. For billing purposes, a *standard* (survey), a *limited* (e.g., in emergencies, to evaluate a single organ, to guide a procedure, to answer a clinical question [e.g., "Is there fetal heart activity," or "Is there a placenta previa?"]), or a *follow-up* (to a standard scan) scan has been performed. Radiologically, a *standard* (also termed *basic*), a *limited*, or a *specialized (targeted)* scan is performed (the terms *level I* and *level II* scans are outdated). A limited scan is a goal-directed search for a problem or finding, and in most cases is appropriate only when a prior standard scan is already in the medical record (exceptions include women with no prenatal care). A specialized evaluation is done to identify, characterize, or exclude fetal anomalies, often based on an abnormal history, maternal serum screening results, or an abnormal standard scan, and is usually performed by individuals with special expertise. The American Academy of Family Physicians, the Advanced Life Support in Obstetrics (ALSO) advisory board, and others classify ultrasonographic applications as either *basic* or *extended*. With basic applications (e.g., most of the intrapartum indications), practicing clinicians with a base of knowledge in maternal–fetal anatomy and physiology can usually master scanning in a 1-day workshop. For extended applications, significant additional study and supervised practice are needed such as can be obtained in residency or other training programs. More advanced applications, such as measurement of Doppler velocimetry, require specialized training and are beyond the scope of this chapter.

DOCUMENTATION

Adequate documentation for every ultrasonographic study is essential. This should include a permanent written report, complete with the ultrasonographic images incorporating measurement parameters and anatomic findings. Figure 172-1 is an example of an ultrasonography report form. Suggested documentation (adapted from the

OBSTETRIC ULTRASOUND						PATIENT IDENTIFICATION Name Age DOB PMD LMP EDC				
Age	Gravidity	Term	Preterm	Abortion	Living	Parameter	Measurement	Gestational age	Indices	
Reason for examination						GEST SAC			CI	
Requested by						CRL			HC/ AC	
Estimated gestational age at examination						BPD			FL/ AC	
Number of fetuses			Presentation			OFD			FL/ BPD	
Placental location			Placental grade			HC			AC/ BPD	
AFI=			☐ Septum cavum pellucidum ☐ Cisterna magna ☐ Lateral ventricle ☐ Extremities ☐ 4 Chamber heart ☐ Stomach ☐ Fetal kidneys ☐ Fetal bladder ☐ Normal abd. wall ☐ Normal spine ☐ 3-Vessel cord ☐ Normal diaphragm			AC			Distal femoral epiph?	
Biophysical profile score= Movement Breathing Tone Fluid NST TOTAL						FL			Proximal humeral epiph?	
						OTHER			Proximal tibial epiph?	
						Estimated fetal age			Other	
						Estimated fetal weight	EFW	Percentile		
Birth weight (grams) chart: 5000, 4500, 4000, 3500, 3000, 2500, 2000, 1500, 1000, 500; 97%, 90%, 50%, 10%, 3%; 0 22 24 26 28 30 32 34 36 38 40 42 44 46 48 50 Weeks gestation completed						*Impressions/recommendations:* Uterus Adnexa				
Prepared by: (Signature and title)						*Date of examination:*				

Figure 172-1 Sample obstetric ultrasonography report form.

AIUM guidelines) for first-trimester, second- and third-trimester, and intrapartum scans is discussed in the following sections. Only standard obstetric ultrasonographic studies are discussed here, and they should include the elements described in the following sections.

First-Trimester Standard Scan Documentation

1. Document the location of the gestational sac. If visible, the embryo should be identified and the crown–rump length (CRL) measured and recorded. If an embryo is not visible, the mean gestational sac diameter should be recorded and can be used for estimating gestational age (Box 172-1).
2. Report the presence or absence of fetal life (e.g., cardiac or somatic activity). With transvaginal scanning, cardiac activity is usually observed when the embryo is 5 mm or greater in length; if not, a later scan may be needed to document cardiac activity.
3. Document fetal number.

Box 172-1. Indicated Dating Parameters Based on Gestational Age

1. From 7–10 wk: use an average of GS and CRL
2. From 11–14 wk: use an average of CRL, BPD, and FL, although CRL most accurate
3. From 15–28 wk: use an average of BPD, HC, FL, and AC; BPD most accurate, AC least accurate
4. After 28 wk: use an average of BPD (with CI), HC, FL, and AC; discard any that are significantly different from others

AC, abdominal circumference; BPD, biparietal diameter; CI, cephalic index; CRL, crown–rump length; FL, femur length; GS, gestational sac; HC, head circumference.

4. Assess embryonic/fetal anatomy to ascertain that it is appropriate for the first trimester.
5. Perform an evaluation of the uterus (including the cervix), adnexal structures, and the cul de sac for any abnormalities.
6. Fetal nuchal translucency should be measured between 11 and 14 weeks.

Second- and Third-Trimester Standard Scan Documentation

1. Document fetal life, number, presentation, and activity.
2. Report a quantitative and qualitative estimate of the amount of amniotic fluid (increased, decreased, normal; amniotic fluid index [AFI], single deepest vertical pocket, 2-diameter pocket).
3. Record the placental location and determine its relationship to the internal cervical os. The umbilical cord should be imaged and the number of vessels evaluated, when possible.
4. Assess gestational age using a combination of biparietal diameter (BPD; or head circumference) and femur length. Abdominal circumference can also be used to assess gestational age (see Box 172-1).
5. Assess fetal growth with the abdominal circumference measurements. If previous studies have been performed, give an estimate of the appropriateness of the interval growth. Fetal weight should be estimated in late second- and all third-trimester scans. It can be estimated from BPD, head circumference, abdominal circumference, and femoral diaphysis length. Significant discrepancies between gestational age and fetal weight may suggest the possibility of fetal growth abnormality, intrauterine growth restriction, or macrosomia.
6. Perform an evaluation of the uterus, cervix, and adnexal structures.
7. The study should include, but not necessarily be limited to, the following fetal anatomy: head and neck, lateral cerebral ventricles, midline falx, cavum septum pellucidum, choroid plexus, cisterna magna, cerebellum, four-chamber view of heart, spine (cervical, thoracic, lumbar, and sacral), stomach (presence, size, and site), diaphragm, kidneys, urinary bladder, umbilical cord insertion site, number of umbilical vessels, extremities (presence and number), intactness of the anterior abdominal wall, and sex (medically indicated only in low-risk pregnancy with multiple gestations to possibly determine number of chorions).

Intrapartum Standard Scan Documentation

1. Document fetal life, number, and presentation.
2. Report an estimate of the amount of amniotic fluid.
3. Record the placental location and determine its relationship to the internal cervical os.

Indications

- Confirmation of pregnancy
- Vaginal bleeding of undetermined etiology during pregnancy
- Determination of fetal presentation/presenting part
- Suspected multiple gestations
- Estimation of gestational age
- Evaluation of fetal growth, including multiple gestations
- Significant uterine size/dates discrepancy
- Pelvic mass/pain
- Suspected hydatidiform mole
- Suspected ectopic pregnancy
- Suspected fetal death (see Chapter 225, Emergency Department, Hospitalist, and Office Ultrasonography [Clinical Ultrasonography])
- Suspected uterine abnormality
- Intrauterine contraceptive device localization (see Chapter 225, Emergency Department, Hospitalist, and Office Ultrasonography [Clinical Ultrasonography])
- Ovarian follicle development surveillance for infertility
- Biophysical profile (BPP) or modified BPP (nonstress test combined with AFI)
- Suspected polyhydramnios or oligohydramnios
- Follow-up evaluation of placental location for identified placenta previa
- Suspected placental abruption
- Premature rupture of membranes or preterm labor (e.g., estimation of fetal weight and/or presentation and/or cervical dilation)
- Evaluate need for cervical cerclage placement
- Evaluation of fetal condition in late registrants for prenatal care
- Observation of intrapartum events
  - Management of second twin
  - Manual removal of placenta
- Adjunct to special procedure
  - Amniocentesis
  - External cephalic version
  - In vitro fertilization/embryo transfer
  - Chorionic villous sampling
- Measure nuchal translucency as part of a screening program for fetal aneuploidy
- Follow-up observation of identified anomaly*
- History of previous infant with congenital anomaly*
- Abnormal maternal serum markers for aneuploidy or neural tube defects (screening for anomalies)*
- Evaluation of fetal well-being by Doppler flow velocities in suspected IUGR*

Contraindication

Maternal refusal is the only contraindication.

Equipment

- Real-time ultrasonography machine with either a 3-MHz or higher transducer for transabdominal or transperineal scans (2 to 2.25 MHz may be needed for obese patients) or a 5-MHz or higher transducer for transvaginal scans (Among state-of-the-art machines, differences between manufacturers are primarily subjective [see the Suppliers section].)
- Ultrasonic gel
- Towels to remove gel when study completed
- Sheaths, probe covers, or a glove for transvaginal or transperineal scanning
- Appropriate forms for documentation

Preprocedure Patient Preparation

If the pregnancy is more than 20 weeks along, the bladder should be empty if performing transabdominal scanning. The patient's bladder should be empty or only slightly full for transvaginal or transperineal scanning. Patients should know about the necessary position (recumbent or semirecumbent for transabdominal or transperineal; dorsal lithotomy for transvaginal or optionally for transperineal scanning), and to expect the insertion of a probe for transvaginal scanning.

Issues to be discussed with patients who undergo obstetric ultrasonography include the following:

- Safety
- Purpose of the examination
- Detection of birth defects
- Accuracy of measurements
  - Dating
  - Estimated fetal weight

---

*Usually a targeted examination performed by individuals experienced in this area.

After many years, no study of safety has ever indicated more than a theoretical risk to the fetus from routine ultrasonographic scanning (see the Complications section). AIUM is a not-for-profit national professional organization that continues to monitor ultrasonography safety. They have never noted any safety problems (for mother or child) with ultrasonography. However, the clinician should comment that ultrasonographic examinations are generally performed in the United States only for indications and that the least amount of ultrasound that is necessary will be used to obtain the needed information.

When asked why they think an ultrasonographic examination is being performed, patients commonly state "to make sure the baby is okay." It may be important to explain that the examination is being performed to answer a particular clinical question, not for general screening. They should be aware, especially if a limited study is being performed, that no ultrasonographic study can ensure a perfect infant. Patients also frequently request ultrasonography to determine the sex of the infant. They should be informed that national guidelines (NIH or otherwise) do not list this as an indication for ultrasonography. After providing this information, it is the clinician's choice as to whether to attempt to determine the sex of the infant.

A handout for the patient to review before scanning can be quite helpful (see the sample patient education form available online at www.expertconsult.com). After scanning, giving the patient a picture of the fetal hand profile, the facial profile, or even the genitalia should enhance bonding with minimal legal hazard.

Technique

1. For transabdominal scanning, the mother is usually most comfortable in the recumbent or semirecumbent position, tilted slightly to her left or with slight left lateral hip displacement. An adequate amount of gel should be applied to the abdomen. This position can also be used for transperineal scanning if the legs are flexed and wide apart. For transvaginal (and often for transperineal scanning), the mother is placed in the dorsal lithotomy position. An adequate amount of gel should be applied to the tip of the transducer before it is inserted into the sheath or glove for transvaginal or transperineal scanning.
2. By convention, transabdominal scanning is performed with the clinician on the right side of the bed, and the transducer position and image orientation are described relative to the mother (not the body of the fetus). When the marker dot of the transducer is located toward the mother's head, a longitudinal (sagittal) scan is performed; the mother's head will be located beyond the left side of the image (cranial direction) and her feet beyond the right side (caudal direction). When the marker dot is placed on the mother's right side, a transverse image is produced; the mother's right side will be located on the left side of the image and vice versa. (See Chapter 225, Emergency Department, Hospitalist, and Office Ultrasonography [Clinical Ultrasonography], for a more complete discussion of orientation.) By convention, transvaginal and transperineal scanning follow the same orientation for images.
3. For transvaginal scanning, additional gel is applied to the outside of the sheath and the transvaginal transducer is introduced into the vagina. Scanning starts as soon as the transducer is inserted; avoid inserting the transducer too far, which can cause the clinician to miss the cervix and lower uterine segment. The transducer handle is moved to the opposite side of the vaginal opening to evaluate the adnexa (e.g., the transducer handle is moved to the mother's right side to evaluate her left adnexum).
4. For transperineal scanning, use the same transducer as for abdominal scanning. Additional gel is applied to the outside of the sheath or glove covering the transducer and the transducer is then placed against the introitus, labia, and perineum. During transperineal scanning, the vagina appears as a bright line usually meeting the cervix at a 90-degree angle. The distance from the perineum to the cervix usually places the cervix at an ideal distance for (and within) the focal zone of the transducer. Bowel gas in the rectum can sometimes obscure the external os. The image is sometimes improved if the patient is placed in the left-side-down decubitus position.
5. Follow a routine when performing a standard scan of an apparently normal pregnancy. However, even with a normal pregnancy you should have a low threshold for varying from the routine. For example, if you see an excellent sonographic view of something that will later need to be documented (e.g., placenta), freeze it and record an image. (You may not get another chance.) If an abnormality is noted, document it but do not forget to complete the routine scan.
6. First, briefly sweep the entire uterus to check for fetal viability and gross pathology as well as to determine the direction in which the fetus is lying. For first-trimester scans, it is important to methodically sweep the entire uterus to exclude multiple gestations. After gross pathology is excluded, it may enhance bonding to allow the patient and family to watch the images during scanning.
7. Next, with second- and third-trimester scanning, evaluate the lower uterine segment before the bladder fills and distorts the cervical length or its relationship to the placenta.
8. To maintain orientation, evaluate the long axis and transverse views of the spine if the fetus is in a convenient position. After getting oriented to the fetal spine, you will be three-dimensionally oriented to how the fetus is lying (e.g., on all fours). Transverse views of various organs will then be easier to obtain and will make more sense.
9. Evaluate the fetus in transverse views from head to pelvis. In particular, transverse views of the brain, spine, chest, heart, diaphragm, abdomen, stomach, kidneys, and bladder should be obtained. The cord insertion site should be imaged. Record appropriate images for documentation.
10. Longitudinal views of the spine, diaphragm, stomach, kidneys, and bladder should also be visualized. Record appropriate images for documentation.
11. Next, evaluate the extremities. The clinician should visualize all four extremities. Record an image of a femur for measurements.
12. A final sweep should be made through the entire fetus and at least an informal BPP performed for late-trimester pregnancies.
13. Finally, the placental site and amniotic fluid volume should be evaluated. For transabdominal scanning, if the placenta has not already been visualized during the previous scanning, it is usually located posteriorly. If there has been difficulty imaging the fetus, the amount of amniotic fluid is probably reduced.
14. While scanning, the necessary measurements listed in the next section should be obtained. Techniques and formulas for obtaining specific measurements are also discussed in the following sections. Use the appropriate sections when attempting to answer particular clinical questions or for certain situations as needed.

Measurements

NOTE: Newer ultrasonography machines calculate many of these values for the sonographer based on the formulas given in the text. Many also use nomograms for making estimates; estimates on age or weight are most accurate when multiple parameters are used and the nomograms have been derived from fetuses of the same ethnic or racial background living at similar altitude.

The BPD, abdominal circumference, and femur length are measured as the basis of most obstetric ultrasonographic evaluations. Early in pregnancy, CRL and gestational sac measurements are also important. Certain early developmental landmarks, if noted, may

TABLE 172-1 Developmental Landmarks According to Abdominal Ultrasonography*

Landmark	Fetal Age (from LMP)
Visualization of gestational sac	5–6 wk
Embryonic pole	6–7 wk
Fetal heart motion	7–8 wk
Fetal movement	8–9 wk
Biparietal diameter measurable	12–13 wk

LMP, last menstrual period.
*Many of these may be visualized up to a week earlier with transvaginal scanning.

also provide worthwhile information for estimating gestational age (Table 172-1).

1. CRL
   - The formula is as follows:

     $$\text{Gestational age (weeks)} = (\text{CRL [mm]} + 65)/10$$

   - The CRL is the longest length of the fetus in the sagittal plane and excludes the fetal limb buds and the yolk sac. One should average crown–rump measurements from three satisfactory images.
   - Transabdominally, CRL is most accurate between 9 and 11 weeks. Even more accurate is CRL by transvaginal scanning between 7 and 9 weeks. The greatest problem with measuring CRL transabdominally earlier than 9 weeks is that the fetus is very small and the borders may be unclear. As a result, it may be very difficult to obtain the maximum longitudinal diameter (CRL) of the fetus. After 11 or 12 weeks, the fetus flexes and extends so much that it may be difficult to obtain the true maximal diameter (Fig. 172-2).
2. Gestational sac (GS) diameter
   - The formula is as follows:

     $$\text{Gestational age (weeks)} = (\text{Avg GS [mm]} + 25.43)/7.02$$

   - The gestational sac measurement is not the best value to use for estimating gestational age, and it should be used only if other dating parameters are *not* available.
   - The gestational sac consists of a hypoechogenic area, which corresponds to the chorionic vesicle, and an echogenic rim or ring, which corresponds to the trophoblast. The gestational sac of a normal pregnancy also may be characterized by a *double echogenic ring*. The inner ring is the decidua capsularis plus the chorion laeve. The outer ring is the decidua vera. At the implantation site, the hyperechoic rim is thicker, and it comprises the decidua basalis and chorion frondosum (Fig. 172-3).
   - The in utero presence of a normal gestational sac, complete with contents (Fig. 172-4), usually confirms an intrauterine pregnancy and indirectly excludes ectopic gestation. In some cases, however, it may be difficult to differentiate between the gestational sac seen with an early intrauterine pregnancy and the *pseudogestational sac* sometimes seen with an ectopic pregnancy (see the First-Trimester Standard Scan Documentation section, and Chapter 225, Emergency Department, Hospitalist, and Office Ultrasonography [Clinical Ultrasonography]).

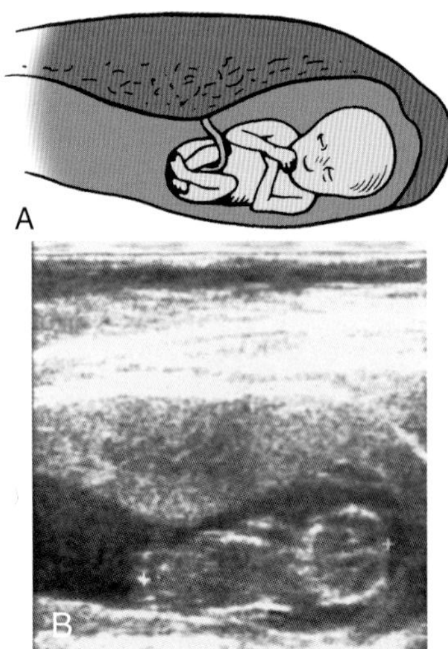

Figure 172-2 Measurement of the crown–rump length. **A,** Fetus at 12 to 13 weeks. **B,** Sonogram showing the longest length of a 12-week fetus. Measurement should be made from the top of the crown (head) to the bottom of the rump.

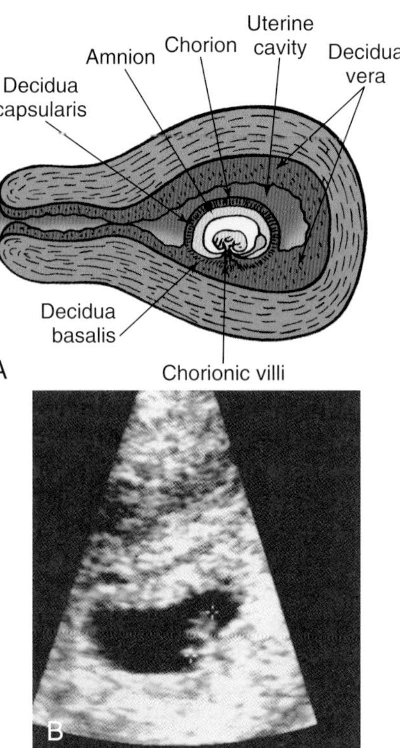

Figure 172-3 **A,** Illustration accompanying a transvaginal photograph detailing an early gestation. The decidua capsularis and the decidua vera form the double echogenic ring. **B,** The sonogram contains a fetal pole with 7-mm crown–rump length, which corresponds to a 6-week gestation. Pregnancies earlier than 5 weeks by transvaginal scanning and earlier than 6 weeks by transabdominal scanning generally do not show a fetal pole. Usually, only a hypoechogenic area corresponding to the chorionic vesicle is seen at this age.

NOTE: This method of exclusion of ectopic pregnancy may not be helpful for patients taking ovulation induction medications for fertility (see the First-Trimester Standard Scan Documentation section).

   - The gestational sac is measured inside the hyperechoic rim, including only the anechoic (dark or fluid-filled) space. If the sac is round, only one dimension is needed; if ovoid, three measurements are taken and an average diameter calculated (Avg GS).
3. BPD
   - The BPD is measured ideally when the fetus is lying in the occiput transverse position. In this position, BPD is the distance measured between the outer table of the proximal

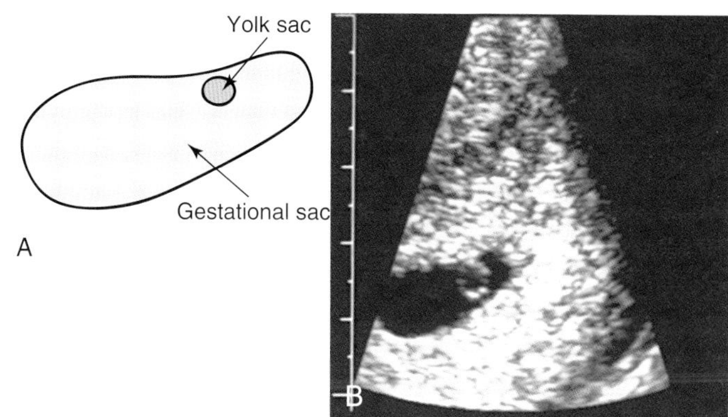

Figure 172-4 Gestational sac with yolk sac on transvaginal ultrasonography. **A,** Yolk sac is generally first seen at about 5 weeks' gestation by transvaginal scanning and at 6 to 7 weeks' gestation by transabdominal scanning. Its presence confirms an intrauterine gestation but does not rule out a rare concomitant ectopic pregnancy (see text). **B,** Sonogram of gestational sac with yolk sac demonstrated.

fetal skull and the inner table of the contralateral side of the skull.

NOTE: The BPD is one of the only outer-to-inner diameter measurements used in all of sonography. Inner diameter is used because the posterior calvarium causes a lot of artifact and tends to distort outer-to-outer diameter measurements (Fig. 172-5).

- The most commonly accepted reference plane for BPD is a cross-section parallel to the canthomeatal line and slightly above it. This cross-sectional plane cuts through the falx cerebri, the thalamus, the cavum septi pellucidi, and the medial cerebral artery. The head shape should be oval at this plane.

4. Head circumference (HC)
   - The formula is as follows:

$$HC = 1.57\,(BPD + \text{occipital–frontal diameter [OFD]}).$$

NOTE: Some clinicians use HC = 1.57 (BPD + 0.3 cm + OFD) because of the manner in which BPD is measured.

- The OFD is measured in the same plane as the BPD. The OFD diameter measurement should be made from the skull's outer-to-outer aspect.

5. Cephalic index (CI)
   - The formula is as follows:

$$CI = BPD/OFD$$

- Prenatal molding of the fetal skull is common and may result in an inaccurate determination of the BPD. The CI (the ratio of the BPD to the OFD) can be used to screen for cranial shape abnormalities. The CI is a constant throughout pregnancy. The normal value is 78.3% ± 8% (±2 standard deviations [SD]). Values below this normal range indicate a dolichocephalic head (an ellipse with a BPD that is shorter than expected, or "too flat"). Values above this normal range indicate a brachycephalic head (an ellipse with a BPD that is wider than expected, or "too round").
- If the CI is significantly above or below the normal range, the BPD may not be a reliable estimation of gestational age. Instead, the HC should be used for estimating gestational age.

6. Abdominal circumference (AC)
   - The formula is as follows:

$$AC = 1.57\,(D_1 + D_2)$$

- Two diameters (D_1 and D_2), the anteroposterior abdominal diameter and the transverse abdominal diameter, are taken at the level of the stomach, the liver (if kidneys or ribs are visualized, the level is too high), and the junction of the umbilical vein and the left portal vein. This junction appears as an echolucent structure shaped like a hockey stick. These diameters should be at right angles to one another, and the plane in which they are taken should be at a right angle to the fetal spine. These measurements should also be outer-to-outer diameter measurements.
- For estimating gestational age, the AC is useful only when there is no clinically apparent maternal or fetal condition that would modify liver growth. Because it relies on measurement of soft tissues, the AC is the least accurate of these methods for estimating gestational age. That said, it is most useful for estimating gestational age in midgestation and late pregnancies (Fig. 172-6).

7. *Femur length (FL).* The central diaphysis of the shaft of the femur should be measured (not including the epiphysis), and the beam should be as perpendicular to the shaft as possible (Fig. 172-7).

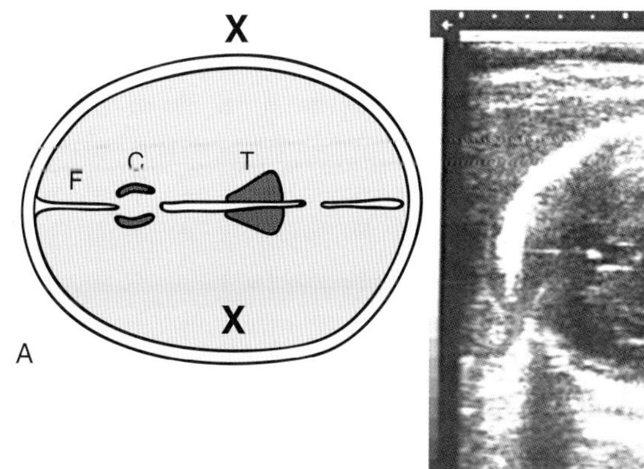

Figure 172-5 **A,** Biparietal diameter (BPD) is measured from outer to inner aspects of the skull. C, cavum septi pellucidi; F, falx cerebri; T, thalami. **B,** Sonogram of the fetal cranium at the proper level for a BPD, the level of the cavum septi pellucidi and thalamus. Note artifact behind posterior skull table.

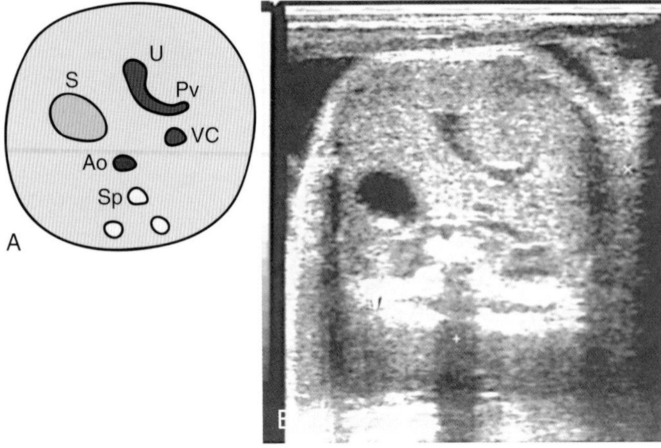

Figure 172-6 Abdominal circumference. **A,** This third-trimester cross-section of the fetal abdomen shows the junction of the umbilical vein and left portal vein. The stomach is seen on the left side of the fetus. **B,** Cross-sectional sonogram of fetal abdomen. Ao, aorta; Pv, portal vein; S, stomach; Sp, spine; U, umbilical vein; VC, vena cava.

This is not necessarily the largest or longest measurement that can be obtained. (The longest measurement may include the femoral neck, which, if included, would overestimate the true value.)

Fetal Body Ratios

1. *Cephalic index.* (See previous discussion.)
2. *Head circumference/abdominal circumference.* This ratio has a positive predictive value of 62% for detecting asymmetric IUGR and a negative predictive value of 98%. The HC/AC is normally about 1.2 at 20 weeks' gestation and drops linearly to about 1 at 36 to 38 weeks' gestation. From that time, it remains about 1 or below until delivery. Screening for an HC/AC greater than 1 after 36 weeks detects 85% of IUGRs. This method fails to detect symmetric IUGR.
3. *Femur length/abdominal circumference.* The FL/AC ratio will not detect symmetric IUGR, but it is sensitive for asymmetric IUGR. This ratio has the further advantage of having normal-range values that do not change with time after 20 weeks. The normal value for this ratio expressed as a percentage is 22% ± 2% (±2 SD). A value greater than 24% indicates IUGR. A value less than 20.5% is suggestive of macrosomia. However, even though the negative predictive value is 92% to 93%, the positive predictive value is only 18% to 20%.
4. *Femur length/biparietal diameter.* After 22 weeks' gestational age, the FL/BPD ratio is almost constant, with a normal range of 79% ± 8% (±2 SD) from 22 to 40 weeks. The predictive values of this ratio are similar to those for FL/AC. The FL/BPD has three important uses: (1) evaluation of the ultrasonographic examination for measurement error, (2) detection of diseases of the fetal head and limbs, and (3) classification of IUGR.

Ultrasonographic Dating

1. Because of biologic variability, traditional clinical methods can estimate gestational age with 90% certainty only to within 2 weeks. This is the limit when even the best clinical methods are applied (using last menstrual period, date when uterus reaches umbilicus, first heard fetal heart tones, fundal height, and quickening). In part, this is because 25% to 45% of women are unable to provide an accurate menstrual history. For this and other reasons, the estimated date of confinement derived from the last menstrual period differs by more than 2 weeks from the actual date of birth in nearly one fourth of pregnancies. Ultrasonographic dating early in pregnancy is more accurate and can be helpful for correcting the estimated date of confinement.
2. Ultrasonographically determined size of certain body parts correlates with gestational age. In general, growth is quite uniform in the first 20 weeks of gestation. Thereafter, the progressive increase in variability makes estimation of gestational age difficult and less accurate (Table 172-2).
3. When reporting ultrasonographic estimates of age, it is very important to understand and report the associated uncertainties. The uncertainty or variability is usually expressed as plus or minus two standard deviations (±2 SD), which should be applicable to 95% of fetuses in a normal population. Reporting a single age estimate for a given fetal measurement gives a false impression about the accuracy of the method. Thus, the variability of the estimate (in SD) should be given as well.

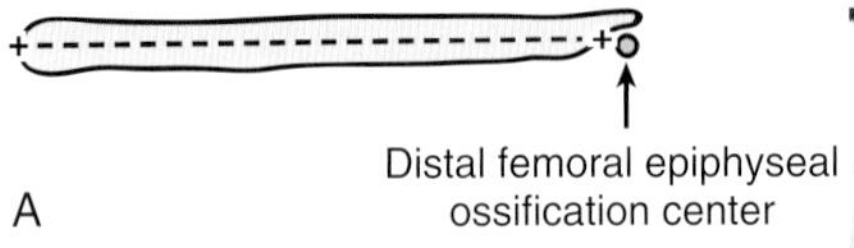

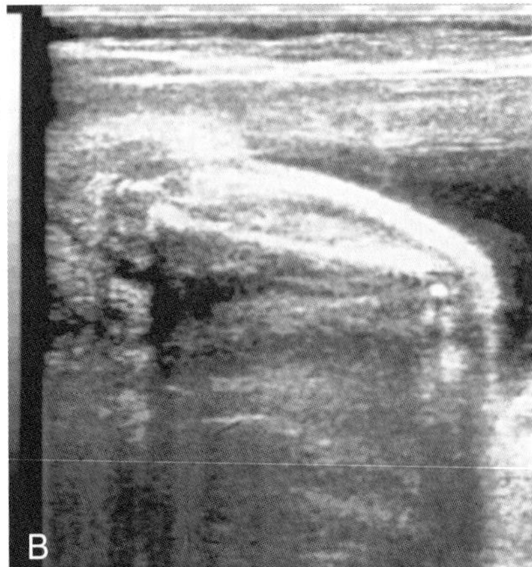

Figure 172-7 **A,** Third-trimester femur is measured along the central shaft of the diaphysis. **B,** Sonogram demonstrating the echogenic distal femoral epiphyseal ossification center on the right, which indicates a gestational age of 33 weeks or more.

TABLE 172-2 Outline of Ultrasonographic Dating of Pregnancy

Weeks of Gestation	Recommended Dating Measurement	Accuracy
3–5	None	
5–6	GS	±1 wk
6–12	CRL	±3–5 days
12–20	1. BPD 2. FL	±1 wk ±1 wk
20–30	1. BPD 2. FL 3. AC	±2 wk ±2 wk ±3 wk
30–40	1. BPD 2. FL 3. AC	±3 wk ±3 wk ±3.5 wk

AC, Abdominal circumference; BPD, biparietal diameter; CRL, crown–rump length; FL, femur length; GS, gestational sac.

4. Pregnancy dating often uses an average of estimates of age from several methods; see Box 172-1 for suggestions as to which parameters to use with each stage of pregnancy. Any of the measurements may be technically incorrect, especially by the third trimester. However, it is unlikely that several measurements will be incorrect in the same direction. Therefore, when averages are used, measurement errors tend to be self-canceling and a more accurate overall estimate of gestational age is made. However, each measurement should be assessed individually; if one measurement is significantly different from the others, it can be excluded from the calculation.
5. When using the multiple-parameter dating approach, or an averaged estimate of age, it is also critical to avoid using any measurements that might have been affected by a pathologic process in the fetus (e.g., hydrocephaly, microcephaly, macrosomia, IUGR, or fetal dwarfism). After 22 weeks' gestational age, potential errors can be minimized by making certain that the fetal body ratios are within normal limits (see the Fetal Body Ratios section). If the CI indicates a normally shaped head, the FL/BPD ratio can be calculated. If the FL/BPD ratio is below 70%, the FL should be eliminated; if the ratio is above 86%, the fetal head measurements should be discarded. If the FL/BPD ratio is normal, the FL/AC ratio can be calculated. If the FL/AC ratio is less than 20%, the AC should not be used because of possible macrosomia; if the ratio is above 24%, the AC should not be used because of possible IUGR.
6. The presence of certain fetal epiphyseal ossification centers may be helpful when estimating gestational age for pregnancies beyond 30 weeks. This is especially useful at this stage of pregnancy because we know dating by other ultrasonographic parameters has limited reliability (see Table 172-2). A visible distal femoral epiphysis (see Fig. 172-7) indicates a menstrual age of at least 33 weeks, a visible proximal tibial epiphysis indicates a menstrual age of at least 35 weeks, and a visible proximal humeral epiphysis indicates a gestational age of at least 38 weeks.

Organ Survey

1. Fetal organs should be categorized as anatomically normal, abnormal, or not visualized. Among all anomalies, cardiac defects are the most common; central nervous system defects are almost as common, especially neural tube defects. Deviations from normal anatomy require a specialized scan.
2. The brain should be surveyed in three transverse (axial) views. The transthalamic view is used to measure BPD and HC and is at the level of the thalamus and cavum septi pellucidi. Moving slightly superiorly, with the transventricular view, the lateral ventricles and their atria are visualized, and this is where the echogenic choroid plexus is noted. (The atria are the confluens of the lateral and occipital horns.) The diameter of an atrium is normally between 5 to 10 mm from 15 weeks to term; ventriculomegaly is quantified by amount of dilation (>10 mm but <15 mm, mild; >15 mm, moderate to severe). Angling posteriorly through the posterior fossa produces the transcerebellar view. The cisterna magna and cerebellum are usually measured, with the cerebellar diameter in millimeters being roughly equivalent to the gestational age in weeks for up to 20 weeks (accurate enough to help establish gestational age in late registrants; tables are available for after 20 weeks).
3. The spine should be surveyed in its entire length in both longitudinal and transverse views. Neural tube defects result from incomplete closure by 6 weeks. In 90% of cases of spina bifida, not only is there an opening in the vertebrae through which the meninges protrude (meningocele), but the sac also contains neural elements (meningomyelocele). One or more additional defects are classically associated with spina bifida (e.g., small BPD, ventriculomegaly, frontal bone scalloping, elongation and downward displacement of the cerebellum, effacement or obliteration of the cisterna magnum).
4. The lungs are best visualized from 20 to 25 weeks, and they should be homogeneous. Cystic or solid lesions may need further evaluation with a specialized scan. Ninety percent of diaphragmatic hernias are located on the left side and posteriorly, and almost half are associated with other major anomalies or aneuploidy. The heart may be pushed to the middle or right side of the thorax, the stomach bubble may be missing from the abdomen, and the AC may be decreased.
5. The basic survey of the heart should include a four-chamber view, rate, and rhythm. The four-chamber view is obtained with a transverse view immediately above the diaphragm. The two atria should be about the same size, and likewise the two ventricles, respectively. The apex of the heart should form a 45-degree angle with the left anterior chest wall; abnormalities of axis should be followed with a specialized scan. Thirty to 40% of cardiac defects are associated with chromosomal abnormalities. An attempt should be made to evaluate the left and right ventricular outflow tracts.
6. The stomach is visible in 98% of fetuses after 14 weeks. Nonvisualization could be the result of various abnormalities (e.g., esophageal atresia, abdominal wall defects, diaphragmatic hernia), so ultrasonography should be repeated in a week, possibly with a specialized scan. The liver, spleen, gallbladder, and intestine are visible in many second- and third-trimester scans. After visualizing the stomach, the abdominal wall should be scanned because defects are quite common. Gastroschisis is typically located to the right of the umbilical cord insertion, and bowel herniates into the amniotic cavity. In over half of cases, an omphalocele is associated with other major anomalies or aneuploidy.
7. The kidneys and urinary tract should be scanned, with kidneys visualized as early as 14 weeks and almost always by 18 weeks. Renal agenesis or cysts in the kidneys (infantile polycystic kidney disease, multicystic dysplastic kidney disease) should be noted. After 16 to 20 weeks, most of the amniotic fluid is produced by the kidneys, so oligohydramnios suggests a need to carefully scan the kidneys. Conversely, a normal AFI indicates at least one urinary tract is patent and functioning. A normal renal pelvis diameter is less than 4 mm before 20 weeks; if it is enlarged, ultrasonography should be repeated at 34 weeks, and if it is greater than 7 mm at that point, neonatology should be consulted. Pyelectasis is dilation at the level of the renal pelvis, and two thirds of infants with pyelectasis greater than 7 mm will have a renal abnormality. Duplicate collecting ducts occur in 4% of the population, and the classic finding is pyelectasis of the upper pole. Reflux of the lower pole is common, so antimicrobial therapy from birth onward may reduce the incidence of urinary

tract infections. Posterior urethral valves in a male fetus will result in dilation of the bladder and proximal urethra; associated oligohydramnios portends a poor prognosis because of pulmonary hypoplasia.

Placental Imaging

1. Maturational changes of the placenta occur in its three basic anatomic areas (the amniochorionic plate, the placental body, and the basal layer) and form the basis for the following grading system of placental maturity (Fig. 172-8):
   Grade 0: Placenta has a chorionic plate that is very smooth. The placental substance is homogeneous and without calcifications.
   Grade I: There is some undulation and some indentations in the chorionic plate. There are also scattered echogenic areas, which represent calcifications in the placental substance.
   Grade II: The chorionic plate has more indentations, but they do not reach the basal plate. The grade II placenta is characterized by a straight line of echoes with calcifications present along the axis of the basal plate. These echoes are high-amplitude, bright, white, and linear or comma-shaped.
   Grade III: The chorionic plate indentations reach the basal plate. There is complete compartmentalization of the placenta with extensive echogenic areas representing calcifications. They may cast shadows.

NOTE: In a third-trimester transabdominal scan, if the placenta has not been located by the time the other parameters have been obtained, it is usually located posteriorly, having been obscured by infant body parts.

2. Grade 0 is most common in the first trimester; grade I appears after 14 weeks' gestation and is most common until around 34 weeks. Grade II may appear after 26 weeks' gestation and is most common at around 36 weeks. Grade III most commonly appears after 35 weeks' gestation. Even with a grade III placenta, there is a 4% chance of fetal pulmonary immaturity.
3. A grade II placenta before 26 weeks or a grade III placenta before 35 weeks is abnormal.
4. IUGR, oligohydramnios, and hypertension are associated with accelerated placental maturation. Diabetes mellitus and Rh sensitization are associated with delayed maturation. Preeclampsia and pregnancy-induced hypertension do not affect placental maturation.
5. The principal purposes of the ultrasonographic examination for bleeding in the second and third trimesters are to delineate the placental implantation site, to exclude placenta previa, and to attempt to determine whether there has been an abruption. Scanning transvaginally or transperineally may improve visualization of these abnormalities in the second and third trimester and during labor.

NOTE: In the proper scenario, unless a large abruptio placentae is clearly confirmed on ultrasonography, the possibility should be managed clinically (as if there is an abruptio placentae). With ultrasonography, there is a risk of false-negative findings; most placental abruptions are small and easy to miss. There is also the risk of a false-positive result; venous lakes can appear very similar to abruptio placentae.

Amniotic Fluid Volume

1. Estimation and documentation of amniotic fluid volume (AFV) is the standard of care during routine ultrasonographic examinations. Although there is no precise method of determining AFV, there are several indirect methods of estimation.
   - *Subjective assessment*: Although simple and rapid, if used alone a subjective assessment (e.g., increased, decreased, normal fluid volume) requires an experienced sonographer. Because the result lacks a numeric value, it is difficult to follow trends; therefore most centers prefer an AFI over subjective assessment for estimating AFV. That said, even if a maximal vertical pocket or AFI will be measured, clinicians should practice making a subjective assessment and record it.
   - *Maximum vertical pocket or 2-diameter*: The maximal vertical pocket technique involves measuring the single deepest vertical pocket of amniotic fluid, not including segments of the umbilical cord. *Oligohydramnios* is defined as the absence of a pocket of fluid at least 2 cm in depth, and *polyhydramnios* is diagnosed when any pocket exceeds 8 cm. This technique is most helpful for quantitating fluid with a multiple-gestation pregnancy or in the assessment of polyhydramnios. The 2-diameter method has been used in BPPs. Excluding

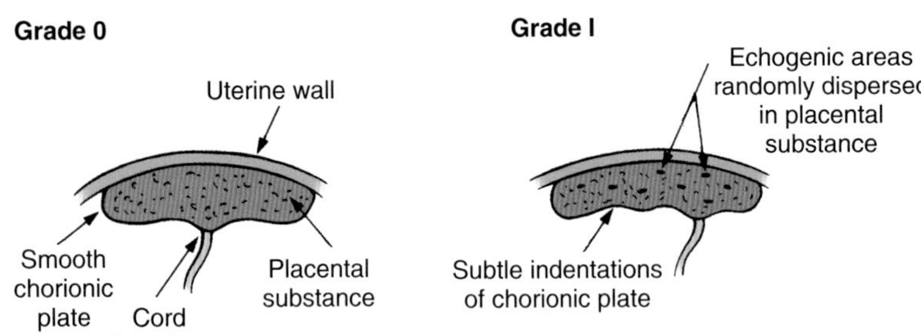

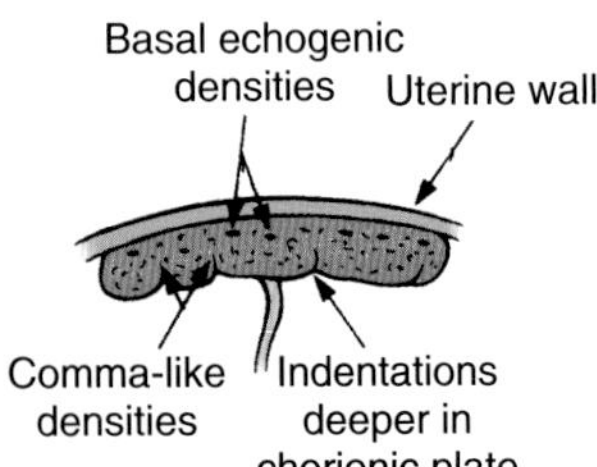

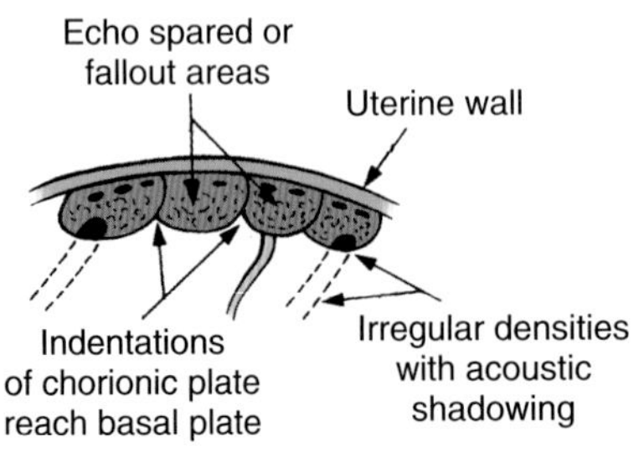

Figure 172-8 Four grades of placental maturity. (Redrawn from Grannum P, Berkowitz R, Hobbins J: The ultrasonic changes in the maturing placenta and their relation to fetal pulmonic maturity. Am J Obstet Gynecol 133:915–922, 1979.)

umbilical cord, there should be at least one pocket of amniotic fluid measuring 2 cm in both the horizontal and vertical planes (i.e., 2 × 2 cm), which results in a score of 2. Failure to identify a fluid pocket of at least this size results in a score of 0.
- *Amniotic fluid index*: This is the quantitative approach to estimating the AFV used by most centers. The uterus is divided into four quadrants. The ultrasound transducer is then held in a vertical and sagittal alignment (marker dot on the probe turned toward the mother's head/cephalad). With the patient supine, the transducer is held perpendicular to the plane of the floor and aligned longitudinally with the mother's spine. Starting in one quadrant, the pocket of fluid with the largest vertical dimension is identified, measured, and recorded. Care must be taken not to include segments of the umbilical cord in the measurement. Coiled cord can fill the space and appear to be fluid (color Doppler can be used to identify the cord). This procedure is repeated in each quadrant and the values summed. If the sum (AFI) is less than 8 cm, perform the four-quadrant evaluation three times and average the values. From 16 weeks onward, the majority of normal pregnancies have an AFI between 8 and 24 cm.

2. Polyhydramnios
   - In nondiabetic women, polyhydramnios is defined as an AFI of 24 cm or more.
   - The most likely etiology is idiopathic (34.6%), followed by diabetes mellitus (24.6%), congenital anomalies (20.1%), erythroblastosis fetalis (11.5%), and multiple gestation (9.2%).
   - Once identified, a patient with an AFI of 24 cm or more should have a detailed or targeted ultrasonographic examination to rule out fetal anomalies.
   - Abnormal fetal lie, operative delivery, and placental abruption all occur more frequently during labor in patients with polyhydramnios.
3. Oligohydramnios
   - Significant oligohydramnios is defined as an AFI of less than 5 cm.
   - Excluding patients with premature rupture of membranes, approximately 83% of patients with oligohydramnios will have fetal IUGR; however, only 16% of patients with fetal IUGR will have oligohydramnios.
   - Fetal weight should be estimated whenever oligohydramnios is present.
   - Premature rupture of membranes can cause severe oligohydramnios or anhydramnios.
   - Fetal causes of oligohydramnios are usually related to urinary tract anomalies.
   - Fetal heart rate abnormalities, depressed Apgar scores, and passage of meconium all occur more frequently during labor in patients with oligohydramnios.
   - In most cases, oligohydramnios in a term infant is an indication for delivery.

Fetal Assessment (Biophysical Profile)

1. A combination of biophysical variables (the BPP) was first introduced by Manning in 1980. The most important aspect in the sensitivity of this test is that it combines both acute and chronic markers of the fetal and placental condition (Table 172-3). Documenting the acute markers (fetal heart rate reactivity [FR; normal is reactive on nonstress test], fetal movement [FM; normal is three or more significant body or limb movements in 30 minutes], fetal breathing movement [FBM; normal is 30 seconds or more of breathing movements in 30 minutes], and fetal tone [FT; normal is extension/flexion of an extremity or spine and then return to normal position]) is very similar to performing an in utero neurologic examination of the infant. It can demonstrate acute oxygenation of various parts of the neurologic system. Normal acute markers result in a score of 2 each; abnormal, a score of 0. Documenting the chronic marker (AFI) is similar to obtaining a "hemoglobin A_{1C}" of fetal oxygenation; it demonstrates how well the fetus has been oxygenated over the past few days, weeks, or maybe even a month. Normal AFI, maximal vertical pocket, or a 2-diameter pocket results in a score of 2. Failure to identify a 2-diameter fluid pocket (one at least 2 × 2 cm in diameter) results in a score of 0. Conversely, even if there is oligohydramnios using an AFI (i.e., AFI <5 cm), if there is a 2 × 2-cm diameter pocket, the score for BPP is 2. Adding the acute and chronic markers, the highest possible score for a normal fetus is 10.
2. A normal BPP is indirect evidence that each of the portions of the central nervous system that control particular activities is functioning and, therefore, oxygenated. When all of the various portions of the central nervous system are active, it indicates that overall the fetus is well oxygenated at that time. The absence of a given BPP activity, however, is difficult to interpret because it may reflect either pathologic depression or normal periodicity.
3. In chronic sustained fetal hypoxia, a protective redistribution of fetal cardiac output may occur, with blood being directed away from nonvital fetal organs (kidneys or lung) toward vital fetal

TABLE 172-3 Fetal Biophysical Profile (BPP) Scoring

Variable	Score 2	Score 0
Fetal breathing movement (FBM)	The presence of at least 30 sec of sustained FBM in 30 min of observation	<30 sec of FBM in 30 min
Fetal movement	Three or more gross body movements in 30 min of observation; simultaneous limb and trunk movements are counted as a single movement	Two or fewer gross body movements in 30 min of observation
Fetal tone	At least one episode of motion of a limb from a position of flexion to extension and a rapid return to flexion	Fetus in a position of semi- or full limb extension with no return to flexion with movement; absence of fetal movement is counted as absent tone
Fetal reactivity*	The presence of two or more fetal heart rate accelerations of at least 15 bpm and lasting at least 15 sec and associated with fetal movement	No acceleration or less than two accelerations of the fetal heart rate during observation (see Chapter 165, Antepartum Fetal Monitoring)
Qualitative amniotic fluid volume†	A pocket of amniotic fluid that measures at least 2 cm in two perpendicular planes	Largest pocket of amniotic fluid measures <2 cm in two perpendicular planes
Maximal score	10	—
Minimal score	—	0

*Most centers perform a nonstress test.
†Most centers usually determine an amniotic fluid index.
Updated from Manning FA, Platt LD, Sipos L: Antepartum fetal evaluation: Development of a fetal biophysical profile. Am J Obstet Gynecol 136:787–795, 1980.

organs (heart, brain, and adrenals). This redistribution leads to decreased renal perfusion and urine production, oligohydramnios, and a low AFI. A low AFI may be the earliest marker of placental insufficiency.

4. A fetal BPP score of 8 or more is reassuring of fetal well-being; a BPP of less than 8 is nonreassuring, and repeated testing or delivery is indicated (see Table 172-3). The presence of oligohydramnios constitutes an abnormal biophysical assessment regardless of the overall score.

Fetal Size

1. Many formulas and tables are available for prediction of fetal weight. These formulas are based on a variety of combinations of BPD, HC, AC, and FL. The predictive accuracy of these formulas ranges from ±14.8% to ±20.2% (±2 SD). Formulas are often compared against a commonly used table (Shepard and colleagues, 1987).
2. On clinical examination, a discordance between size and dates should arouse suspicion of specific disorders, depending on gestational age. In early pregnancy, suspect multiple gestation, a hydatidiform mole, incorrect menstrual history, and genetic or developmental defects. Later in pregnancy, fetal malposition, IUGR, fetal dysmaturity, genetic or developmental defects, multiple gestation, fetal macrosomia, and abnormal AFV are causes to consider. Many of these possibilities can be further evaluated with ultrasonography.

Intrauterine Growth Retardation

1. Clinical signs of IUGR include poor increase in fundal height (>4 cm difference from expected fundal height) or maternal weight gain (<100 to 200 g [3.5 to 7 oz] per week in third trimester), or both. However, diagnosis of IUGR by clinical means is possible in only about 33% of pregnancies.
2. By comparison, a diagnosis of IUGR by ultrasonography is much more accurate, especially if dating is accurate (e.g., from transabdominal ultrasonography at 9 to 11 weeks). However, even with ultrasonography, sensitivities and specificities are variable, so ultrasonographic information should be correlated with clinical data. This combination of information will significantly improve a clinician's ability to diagnose IUGR.
3. The following are important ultrasonographic parameters for evaluating potential IUGR.
   - Oligohydramnios
     For the general population, the sensitivity of oligohydramnios in the diagnosis of IUGR is approximately 16%.
     For high-risk populations, the predictive value and sensitivity of oligohydramnios are enhanced (sensitivity can exceed 85%). If oligohydramnios is present and there is no evidence of premature rupture of membranes or congenital anomalies, IUGR is the likely cause. The combination of oligohydramnios and IUGR portends a less favorable outcome, and early delivery should be considered. Generally, if the pregnancy is at 36 weeks or more, the high risk of intrauterine loss may mandate delivery.
   - Biparietal diameter. BPD alone is not a very helpful parameter when diagnosing IUGR; however, it is useful for ratios. With symmetric IUGR, both head and body measurements fall off the growth curve together and result in an erroneous estimate of gestational age. Even with asymmetric IUGR, the BPD remains normal until late in the course.
   - Head circumference. The HC is a more shape-independent measurement of fetal head size than the BPD. In cases of cranial shape abnormalities, its inclusion in the growth profile will significantly decrease the high number of false-positive results seen when BPD is used. However, because IUGR may not selectively affect brain and head growth, or is "relatively head-sparing," HC alone is also not a very useful measurement. The HC is most useful when it is used with another measurement as a ratio.
   - Femur length. The FL can also be misleading when trying to diagnose IUGR. In asymmetric IUGR, FL usually parallels the gestational age as calculated from the last normal menstrual period. Therefore, for asymmetric IUGR, FL may not be helpful. In symmetric IUGR, all measurements will be small and result in an erroneously early gestational age estimate, so again FL is not helpful. Similar to HC, FL is most useful for prediction of IUGR when it is used in a ratio.
   - Abdominal circumference. The AC is useful for assessing fetal nutritional status. The AC involves measurement of the liver, which is smaller in chronic hypoxia. With inadequate oxygen or nutrition, the liver cannot produce substrate (glycogen); thus the AC is the best single predictor of IUGR.
   - Calculation of fetal body ratios (see the Fetal Body Ratios section).
   - Placental grade. When fetal growth pattern and estimated weight suggest a small fetus, the finding of a prematurely grade III (before 35 weeks) placenta is further evidence of IUGR.
   - Use of fetal epiphyseal ossification centers (see the Ultrasonographic Dating section).
4. Suspect IUGR by ultrasonography if the following occur:
   - AC falls in the lower 15th percentile. (Sensitivity of ultrasonography is >95% if AC <2.5th percentile.)
   - Weight falls in the lower 15th percentile.
   - HC/AC ≥0.95 (HC/AC >1.0 after 36 weeks detects 85% of IUGR).
   - FL/AC ≥23.5%.
5. In the absence of an accurate gestational age, the assessment of risk for IUGR relies predominantly on fetal disproportionality and asymmetry. This may lead to the diagnosis of asymmetric IUGR. However, to diagnose symmetric IUGR, unless dates are very accurate, serial ultrasonographic studies must be performed to assess fetal growth. Some experts recommend serial scans at 2- or 3-week intervals to identify IUGR in the absence of reliable dating. Therefore, for those at risk, liberalizing the use of early ultrasonography for establishing gestational age may be the best way to diagnose symmetric IUGR.
6. Newer techniques to identify IUGR are being evaluated, including Doppler velocimetry of the umbilical artery or other placental vessels and M-mode echocardiography of the fetal heart. Abnormal placental vessel Doppler velocimetry may alert the clinician to the need for an additional study such as a BPP, continuous fetal monitoring, or delivery.

Macrosomia

1. Fetal macrosomia is defined in absolute terms as a fetal weight of greater than 4000 g, regardless of gestational age. However, macrosomia is also considered when a fetal weight falls in the upper 90th percentile for any gestational age at any point during the pregnancy.
2. Symmetric macrosomia occurs when the excessive fetal weight is the result of proportionate growth of all fetal parameters. For example, the weight, length, and head size may all be above the 90th percentile for age. Symmetric macrosomia is usually the result of a prolonged gestation or genetics (i.e., large parents). The HC/AC and the FL/AC ratios are usually within the normal range for age.
3. Asymmetric macrosomia generally occurs in patients with class A to C gestational diabetes mellitus. Although the values of HC and FL are higher than average, they usually fall below the 90th percentile for age. The excessive weight results from profound increases in soft tissue mass that are reflected by an AC and an estimated fetal weight above the 90th percentile. The HC/AC and the FL/AC ratios usually fall below the 10th percentile for age.

NOTE: Sonographic diagnosis of macrosomia does *not* predict prognosis for vaginal delivery, largely because the positive predictive rate for macrosomia in postdates pregnancies is only about 50%. In fact, for suspected macrosomia, the accuracy of estimated fetal weight by ultrasonography is no better than that obtained with clinical palpation (Leopold's maneuvers). As a result, ACOG guidelines (November 2000) state that suspected macrosomia is not a contraindication to attempted vaginal birth. However, they do state that prophylactic cesarean delivery may be considered with estimated fetal weights of more than 5000 g in women without diabetes and more than 4500 g in diabetic women.

Preterm Labor

1. Preterm labor is defined as onset of labor before a gestational age of 37 weeks. Preterm labor affects 10% of pregnancies and accounts for 75% of perinatal morbidity and mortality.
2. Ultrasonographic parameters that are important when evaluating the patient in preterm labor include the following:
   - Fetal number. Multiple gestations have an increased risk of preterm labor.
   - Estimated fetal weight. Preterm labor is associated with IUGR.
   - Amniotic fluid index. Preterm labor is associated with both oligohydramnios and polyhydramnios.
   - BPP score. A low BPP score may contraindicate tocolysis.
   - Other possible contraindications to tocolysis
     - Fetal malformations.
     - Evidence of concealed placental abruption.
   - Ultrasonographic cervical evaluation
     - Cervical shortening (present if the distance from internal os to external os [or the leading edge of the portio vaginalis] is <3 cm). Transperineal and transvaginal scanning appear to be equally accurate for making this measurement. Transvaginal scanning does not seem to increase the risk of infection in women with preterm premature rupture of membranes. A cervical length of less than 2 cm or funneling (dilation and shortening of the upper half of the cervix) has been associated with a short time-interval between rupture of membranes and delivery.
     - Dilation of the endocervical canal (present if the maximal diameter of the endocervical canal exceeds 1 cm).
     - Bulging of the fetal membranes into the endocervical canal (conical or funnel-shaped rather than flat or slightly rounded shape of the internal os).
     - Thinning of the lower uterine segment (anterior wall thickness <0.6 cm).
3. Although studies have shown variable results with the use of cervical cerclage for cervical incompetence, at least one large prospective study found that fewer women delivered before 32 weeks if a cerclage was placed in those with a cervical length of 15 mm or less at 23 weeks.

Postdates Pregnancy

1. Expected date of confinement is defined as 40 weeks (280 days) from the first day of the last normal menstrual period, or 266 days after ovulation, provided cycles are regular and occur at 28-day intervals. Normal term ranges from 38 to 42 weeks.
2. A postdates pregnancy is one with a duration that has exceeded 42 weeks (294 days) from the last normal menstrual period, assuming a 28-day cycle.
3. One study showed that the incidence of postdates pregnancy was overestimated by 7.5% when gestational age was determined using just the menstrual history, but it fell to 2.6% with early ultrasonographic examination, and to 1.1% when both menstrual history and early ultrasonographic measurements were used.
4. Complications detectable by ultrasonography include the following:
   - Physiologic oligohydramnios (these are detectable by AFV determination).
   - Macrosomia (this is detectable by calculation of estimated fetal weight).
   - Dysmaturity resulting from chronic uteroplacental insufficiency (this is detectable by evidence of asymmetric IUGR).
   - Congenital anomalies (these are detectable by anatomic survey).
   - Inaccurate dating (e.g., a preterm delivery could be prevented by having good estimates of gestational age).
5. The contraction stress test (CST) is still regarded as the most reliable method of antenatal surveillance for a postdates pregnancy. However, it has basically been replaced by the modified BPP (nonstress test [NST] combined with an AFI) or the BPP (which usually includes an NST). Studies comparing the use of twice-weekly modified BPP or BPP with a CST do not show a significant difference between the tests (see Chapter 165, Antepartum Fetal Monitoring). All are characterized by minimal morbidity and mortality but unfortunately high intervention and cesarean section rates. The benefits of obtaining twice-weekly modified BPP over the other techniques include the fact that a sonographer or physician is not required to perform a modified BPP. Specially trained personnel (nursing) are certainly capable of performing these two evaluations.

First-Trimester Scanning

See Chapter 225, Emergency Department, Hospitalist, and Office Ultrasonography [Clinical Ultrasonography], for a detailed description.

1. Caution should be used in making the presumptive diagnosis of a gestational sac in the absence of a yolk sac or a definite embryo. Therefore, this portion of the study deserves special attention. It is very easy to overlook a second or third gestational sac in first-trimester scans, and this is the most common time that one is overlooked. This is also the best time to determine the number of chorions for multiple gestations (monochorionic twins are at higher risk for complications such as cord entanglement).
2. First-trimester scanning is the best opportunity to evaluate the uterus (including the cervix), adnexa, and cul de sac for abnormalities.
3. The most common causes of bleeding in the first trimester include the following:
   - Unknown causes
   - Embryonic resorption/ blighted ovum
   - Threatened, missed, incomplete, or complete abortion
   - Ectopic pregnancy
   - Abortion of one member of a multiple gestation
   - Hydatidiform mole
4. Transvaginal scanning is preferred at this gestational age; color flow and Doppler should generally be avoided (there are few clinical uses and the ultrasonic "dose" is higher). When evaluating for ectopic pregnancy by transabdominal scanning, an extrauterine gestational sac is seen in less than 10% of cases (rates are higher with transvaginal scanning). Ultrasonography is more helpful for excluding ectopic pregnancy by demonstrating an intrauterine gestation. When an intrauterine gestation is clearly demonstrated, the likelihood of simultaneous extrauterine and intrauterine gestations (i.e., a combination pregnancy) is only 1 in every 7000 to 8000 cases or 1 in 30,000 low-risk pregnancies. If a patient has had infertility treatment, the risk of a heterotopic pregnancy increases and must be considered.

   An ectopic pregnancy becomes almost certain with transvaginal scanning if (a) there is no intrauterine pregnancy, (b) the patient has no vaginal bleeding, and (c) the quantitative human chorionic gonadotropin (hCG) is more than 2000 IU.

5. The sonographic appearance of a gestational sac can be simulated by the exfoliation of hyperplastic endometrium associated with an ectopic pregnancy. This sonographic finding, known as a *pseudogestational sac*, can appear very similar to a gestational sac. A pseudogestational sac occurs in 10% to 20% of ectopic pregnancies. Thus, the unequivocal diagnosis of an intrauterine pregnancy should not be made until the gestational sac contains two concentric rims, a fetal pole, and a yolk sac, or fetal heart activity can be identified within the sac.
6. In a normal pregnancy, the mean serum hCG doubling time is 1.98 days. If serial hCG titers show a plateau or fall, an abnormal (ectopic) or nonviable pregnancy is likely.
7. There are many reasons variations can exist between institutions when measuring hCG. Purity differences among test kits (different manufacturers) can contribute to variations in measurement. Variations can even exist in the same laboratory in different runs, or occasionally in the same run. With this much variation, even using a given standard, it is important to be aware which test kit is being used when correlating the sonographic findings with the quantitative hCG levels.
8. Optimally, each institution should correlate its ultrasonography equipment and sonographers' skill with quantitative hCG levels obtained from its own reference laboratory. When this is accomplished, externally published quantitative hCG reference levels and expected ultrasonographic findings should be used only as rough guidelines. Current published quantitative hCG levels and ultrasonographic correlations are outlined in Table 172-4.
9. If a gestational sac is absent at an hCG value above the institution's threshold, ectopic pregnancy, recent spontaneous abortion, and early hydatidiform degeneration should be considered. Suspicion of an ectopic pregnancy should be even higher if there is significant fluid in the cul de sac.
10. Ultrasonographic examination can be very helpful for evaluating whether tissue is remaining after a spontaneous abortion, for diagnosing the vanishing twin syndrome (abortion of one member of a multiple gestation), and for establishing fetal viability in threatened abortion. It is the procedure of choice for evaluation of gestational trophoblastic disease.
11. With ultrasonographic examination alone, a normal gestational sac can often be distinguished from an abnormal sac doomed to miscarriage, even before the embryo is visible. The size and appearance of the gestational sac should be evaluated according to major and minor criteria for normality. A gestational sac of abnormal size or appearance correlates highly with an abnormal outcome.
    - Major criteria for a normal-appearing gestational sac
      A sac of 25 mm or more in diameter must reveal an embryo within it (17 mm in diameter for transvaginal scanning).
      The sac must be round.
    - Minor criteria for a normal-appearing gestational sac
      The gestational sac is located in the fundus of the uterus.
      A thick, echogenic decidual ring surrounds the gestational sac.
      There is evidence of the double-ring sign.
12. When a gestational sac with a mean diameter greater than 25 mm (17 mm for transvaginal scanning) lacks an embryo or when the gestational sac is grossly distorted, abnormal pregnancy is almost certain. Using these criteria, 76% of abnormal pregnancies and 93% of normal pregnancies will be correctly classified by only one ultrasonographic scan. Failure to meet any single major criterion or all three minor criteria will identify 53% of abnormal pregnancies but will be 100% specific in predicting spontaneous abortion.
13. Once embryonic cardiac motion is seen on ultrasonography, the likelihood of spontaneous abortion is very low (<16% for pregnancies less than 8 weeks; <2% to 4% after 12 weeks).
14. Nuchal translucency is the maximum thickness of the subcutaneous translucent area between the skin and soft tissue that overlies the fetal spine in the sagittal plane at the neck. It can be accurately measured between 11 and 14 weeks; with several large studies (e.g., N >8500, N >33,000) detecting 85% of cases of Down syndrome by ultrasonography combined with serum markers, ACOG has recognized it as an acceptable option to screen for trisomy 18 and 21.

Intrapartum Scanning

1. Limited scans can usually be performed by individuals with minimal training in ultrasonography to document fetal life, number, and presentation, to estimate the amount of amniotic fluid, and to record the placental location and determine its relationship to the internal cervical os. However, several factors unique to late pregnancy and labor may make such scanning more difficult (e.g., physical crowding due to advanced gestational age, the low station during labor, loss of the acoustic window due to fluid loss after rupture of membranes). That said, fetal life is usually documented by observing fetal cardiac motion. It can also be documented on a still image by performing an M-mode tracing. Diagnosis of fetal demise is discussed in detail in Chapter 225, Emergency Department, Hospitalist, and Office Ultrasonography [Clinical Ultrasonography]. Fetal lie is defined by the orientation of the fetal spine to the maternal spine (longitudinal, transverse, oblique). After several sweeps of the uterus with ultrasonography, the fetal lie and presentation are usually apparent. If the fetal lie is transverse, it is helpful to know if the fetal spine is up or down in relation to the lower uterine segment because the choice of uterine incision for cesarean may be affected (risk of cord prolapse increases if the spine is up). Methods of estimating AFV are discussed elsewhere. Often the placenta is located when

TABLE 172-4 Possible Outcomes Based on Ultrasonography and Quantitative Human Chorionic Gonadotropin Correlations

hCG Level (mIU/mL)*	Presence/Absence of GS on TAUS	Significance
>1800	+GS	Intrauterine pregnancy; if fetal pole or yolk sac is identified, no further ultrasound is required. Ectopic pregnancy is basically ruled out. (<1 : 7000 risk unless patient taking fertility ovulation induction medications; see text).
<1800	+GS	Failed intrauterine pregnancy or absorbed pregnancy; ectopic pregnancy with pseudogestational sac; or very rarely, an early pregnancy that may continue.
>1800	–GS	Suspect ectopic pregnancy.
<1800	–GS	Indeterminate. May be result of an early intrauterine pregnancy, or ectopic or failed pregnancy. Follow hCG titer every 2 to 4 days; for normal pregnancies, hCG should double. However, normal hCG trends occur in 15% of ectopic pregnancies. Thus, as soon as the level crosses the threshold for the practitioner's facility, repeat the ultrasonographic examination.

GS, gestational sac; TAUS, transabdominal ultrasonography.
*Actual values will vary from institution to institution based on particular assay used, quality of TAUS machine, and the skill of the ultrasonographer.

performing other parts of an intrapartum scan. If not, it is probably posterior; however, uterine contractions can alter the apparent location, thickness, and appearance of the placenta. A more thorough evaluation of the placenta usually requires more comprehensive training.

2. Extended applications (require more training) of intrapartum scanning include examination for placenta previa or abruptio placentae (see section on Placental Imaging), evaluation of the cervix in preterm labor or for incompetent cervix (see section on Preterm Labor), evaluation for procedural guidance (see appropriate chapters), and evaluation for intrapartum twin management. Such applications may also include organ survey and biometry for fetal age and weight (see sections on Ultrasonographic Dating, Organ Survey, Fetal Size, and Postdates Pregnancy). When evaluating for placenta previa, make sure the maternal bladder is not overdistended, which can compress the lower uterine segment and cause the appearance of a placenta previa. Such scanning is probably best performed with the bladder partially full and then with an empty bladder. It should also be performed between contractions, if at all possible.
3. When managing intrapartum twins, the initial presentation and lie of the fetuses should be determined. After delivery of the first twin, the cardiac rate and rhythm of the second twin should be observed. Using a technique similar to external cephalic version (see Chapter 167, External Cephalic Version), guide the second twin into the cephalic presentation for delivery.

Complications

Although there are theoretical risks of ultrasound damaging human fetuses, no proven harm has been documented to any human fetus or mother. The only other possible complications from obstetric ultrasonography are failure to diagnose an anomaly or condition, an inaccurate estimate of gestational age or weight, inappropriate reassurance of a perfect infant, or inaccurate determination of the sex of the infant. Because fetal anomalies can remain undetected even by the best sonographer with the best equipment, the patient should never be unequivocally assured that the fetus is "fine." However, the patient can be reassured with answers to certain specific questions provided by the scan.

Postprocedure Patient Education

If follow-up scans or other management will be needed, the patient must know when and where to go for them.

Patient Education Guides

See the patient education and patient consent form available online at www.expertconsult.com.

CPT/Billing Codes

76801 Ultrasound, pregnant uterus, real time with image documentation, fetal and maternal evaluation, first trimester (<14 weeks 0 days), transabdominal approach; single or first gestation
76802 Each additional gestation (List separately in addition to code for primary procedure. List 76802 in conjunction with 76801.)
76805 Ultrasound, pregnant uterus, real time with image documentation, fetal and maternal evaluation, after first trimester, transabdominal approach, single or first gestation
76810 Each additional gestation (List separately in addition to code for primary procedure. List 76810 in conjunction with 76805.)
76813 Nuchal translucency, single or first gestation
76814 Nuchal translucency, each additional gestation
76815 Limited (e.g., fetal heart beat, placental location, fetal position, and/or qualitative amniotic fluid volume)
76816 Follow-up or repeat of 76815
76817 Ultrasound, pregnant uterus, transvaginal
76818 Fetal biophysical profile; with nonstress testing
76819 Fetal biophysical profile; without nonstress testing

ICD-9-CM Diagnostic Codes

623.8 Vaginal bleeding, nonpregnant
630 Hydatidiform mole
631 Blighted ovum
632 Missed abortion
633.9 Ectopic pregnancy, unspecified
634.91 Abortion or miscarriage, incomplete, without complications
634.92 Abortion or miscarriage, complete, without complications
640.03 Threatened abortion, antepartum
640.93 Unspecified hemorrhage in early pregnancy, antepartum
641.03 Placenta previa without hemorrhage, antepartum
641.13 Placenta previa with hemorrhage, antepartum
641.21 Placental abruption, delivered
641.23 Placental abruption, antepartum
642.03 Benign essential hypertension complicating pregnancy, antepartum
642.43 Mild or unspecified preeclampsia, antepartum
642.53 Severe preeclampsia, antepartum
642.73 Preeclampsia or eclampsia superimposed on preexisting hypertension, antepartum
644.21 Preterm labor, delivered
644.23 Preterm labor, antepartum
645.13 Post-term pregnancy (40 to 42 weeks), antepartum
645.23 Prolonged pregnancy (>42 weeks), antepartum
646.83 Uterine size–date discrepancy, antepartum
648.03 Diabetes mellitus, preexisting, antepartum
648.83 Abnormal glucose tolerance (gestational diabetes)
651.03 Multiple gestation, twins, antepartum
651.93 Multiple gestation, unspecified, antepartum
656.43 Fetal demise, antepartum
656.53 Intrauterine growth retardation, antepartum
656.63 Fetal macrosomia, antepartum
657.3 Polyhydramnios, antepartum
658.3 Oligohydramnios, antepartum
760.5 Maternal injury, fetus or newborn affected by maternal conditions

Acknowledgment

The editors wish to recognize the contributions by Richard E.A. Brunader, MD, to this chapter in the previous two editions of this text.

Suppliers

(See contact information online at www.expertconsult.com.)

Note that ultrasonography machine technology has evolved substantially. However, the variance in pricing for the most basic equipment can be substantial.

Acuson (owned by Siemens)
Agilent Technology (formerly Hewlett-Packard)
Aloka
Biosound Esaote, Inc.
General Electric Medical Systems
Hitachi Medical Corp.
Medison America, Inc.
Philips
Toshiba America Medical Systems

BIBLIOGRAPHY

American College of Obstetricians and Gynecologists: Fetal Macrosomia. ACOG Practice Bulletin no. 22. Washington, DC, ACOG, 2000.

American College of Obstetricians and Gynecologists: Ultrasonography in Pregnancy. ACOG Practice Bulletin no. 58. Washington, DC, ACOG, 2004.

American Institute of Ultrasound Medicine: AIUM Practice Guidelines: Obstetric Ultrasound. Laurel, Md, AIUM, 2007.

Benacerraf BR, Benson CB, Abuhamad AZ, et al: Three- and 4-dimensional ultrasound in obstetrics and gynecology: Proceedings of the American Institute of Ultrasound in Medicine Consensus Conference. J Ultrasound Med 24:1587–1597, 2005.

Brunader R: Accuracy of prenatal sonography performed by family practice residents. Fam Med 28:407–410, 1996.

Callen PW (ed): Ultrasonography in Obstetrics and Gynecology, 4th ed. Philadelphia, WB Saunders, 2000.

Canadian Task Force on Preventive Health Care: Routine prenatal ultrasound screening. In Canadian Guide to Clinical Preventive Health Care. Ottawa, Health Canada, 1994 (rev 1998).

Deutchman M, Sakornbut E: Diagnostic ultrasound in labor and delivery. In Syllabus for Advanced Life Support in Obstetrics. Kansas City, Mo, American Academy of Family Physicians, 2001.

Ewigman BG, Crane JP, Frigoletto FD, et al: Effect of prenatal ultrasound screening on perinatal outcome: RADIUS Study Group. N Engl J Med 329:821–827, 1993.

Gonçalves LF, Lee W, Espinoza J, Romero R: Three- and 4-dimensional ultrasound in obstetric practice: Does it help? J Ultrasound Med 24: 1599–1624, 2005.

Keith R, Frisch L: Fetal biometry: A comparison of family physicians and radiologists. Fam Med 33:111–114, 2001.

Manning FA, Platt LD, Sipos L: Antepartum fetal evaluation: Development of a fetal biophysical profile. Am J Obstet Gynecol 136:787–795, 1980.

Sabbagha RE (ed): Diagnostic Ultrasound Applied to Obstetrics and Gynecology, 3rd ed. Philadelphia, JB Lippincott, 1994.

Sanders RC, Winter TC (eds): Clinical Sonography: A Practical Guide, 4th ed. Philadelphia, Lippincott Williams & Wilkins, 2007.

Shepard MJ, Richards VA, Berkowitz RL, et al: An evaluation of two equations for predicting fetal weight by ultrasound. Am J Obstet Gynecol 156:80, 1987.

Timor-Tritsch IE, Rottem S (eds): Transvaginal Sonography, 3rd ed. New York, Elsevier, 1997.

Tuggy M, Garcia J: Procedures Consult. Available at www.proceduresconsult.com.

Usatine RP: The Color Atlas of Family Medicine. New York, McGraw-Hill, 2009.

CHAPTER 173

PARACERVICAL BLOCK

Scott T. Henderson

A paracervical block anesthetizes the paracervical (Frankenhäuser's) ganglion. By injecting local anesthetic submucosally into the fornix of the vagina (i.e., cervicovaginal junction), anesthesia during the first stage of labor can be attained. Although a paracervical block should enhance the experience, the pudendal nerves are not blocked. Therefore, additional anesthesia may be required for delivery. These anesthetics are also fairly short acting, so the procedure may need to be repeated during labor. This procedure is rarely used because of the availability of other techniques for regional analgesia during the first stage of labor and the potential for postparacervical block fetal bradycardia. A paracervical block can also be used for anesthesia for other procedures involving the cervix (e.g., cryosurgery, ablation, conization, loop electrosurgical excision procedure [LEEP], dilation and curettage).

ANATOMY

During the first stage of labor, pain is due to increased intrauterine pressure and cervical dilation. The pain arises from the visceral sensory nerve fibers of the uterus, cervix, and upper vagina, passes through the paracervical ganglion to the hypogastric and then the preaortic plexuses, and then enters the spinal cord at T10-T12 and L1. These same fibers carry pain during a cervical procedure in the nongravid patient.

INDICATIONS

- First stage of labor
- Cervical ablation or conization procedures
- Dilation and curettage
- Possibly with endometrial biopsy and intrauterine device insertion

CONTRAINDICATIONS

Absolute

- Uteroplacental insufficiency
- Preexisting fetal distress
- Nonreassuring fetal heart tracing
- Delivery appears imminent
- Allergy to anesthetic agent
- Presence of local infection

Relative

- Known coagulopathy or anticoagulant therapy (e.g., heparin or its analogs, warfarin, clopidogrel [Plavix])

EQUIPMENT AND SUPPLIES

- 10-mL syringe (with finger rings if available; otherwise a plain syringe can be used)
- Iowa trumpet with a 6-inch, 20-gauge needle (a must during labor; or a 3-inch needle extender on the end of a syringe with a 1½-inch, 22-gauge needle
- Anesthesia
  - Gravid: lidocaine (Xylocaine or generic) 1% (10 mg/mL) *without* epinephrine, or chloroprocaine (Nesacaine or generic) 1% (10 mg/mL). (Note with lidocaine that toxicity may occur with doses >1 mg/kg [70 mg or 7 mL in a 70-kg patient].) With lidocaine or chloroprocaine, toxicity can occur with rapid absorption or with intravascular administration. With lidocaine, maximum dosage should not exceed 4.5 mg/kg or a maximum of 30 mL of a 1% solution (300 mg), and maximum dose should not be repeated in less than 2 hours. With chloroprocaine, maximum recommended dose is 120 mg, and it should not be repeated in less than 1 hour.
  - Nongravid: up to 2% lidocaine or chloroprocaine can be used, with maximum recommended dose of 300 mg lidocaine or 120 mg chloroprocaine.
  - Gravid or nongravid: bupivacaine (Marcaine or generic) is contraindicated because of an increased risk of cardiotoxicity.
- Sterile gloves
- Antibacterial solution and sterile gauze pads
- Sterile ringed forceps
- Sterile speculum
- Sterile tenaculum for nongravid cervix
- Fetal heart monitor (for gravid patient)

PREPROCEDURE PATIENT EDUCATION

Obtain informed consent and outline the possible complications, risks, benefits, and alternatives to anesthesia. (See the sample patient education and patient consent forms online at www.expertconsult.com.)

TECHNIQUE

1. Place the patient in the lithotomy position. Observe universal blood and body fluid precautions during this procedure.
2. In the gravid patient, assess the cervix and proceed if dilation is 5 to 9 cm. If the cervix is dilated greater than 7 or 8 cm, proceed with caution to preclude injecting the fetal scalp.
3. Some clinicians swab the injection sites in the vaginal fornix with antibacterial solution–soaked sterile gauze pads, held in ringed forceps, before the procedure. For a conization procedure, some clinicians prepare the entire perineal area with an

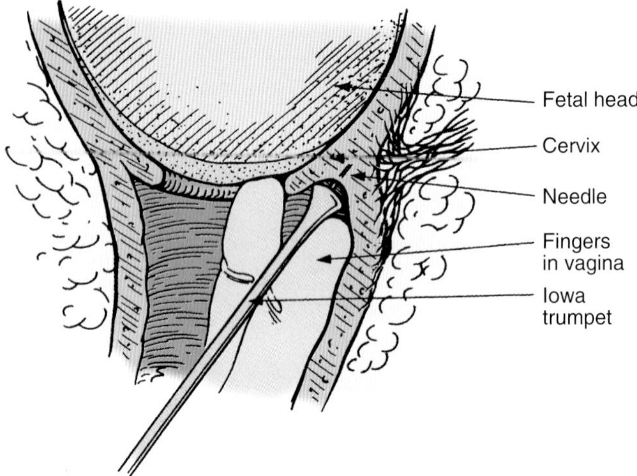

Figure 173-1 Technique of administering a paracervical block during labor using an Iowa trumpet.

antibacterial solution, as for gynecologic surgery, and then swab the injection sites in the fornix with antibacterial solution–soaked sterile gauze pads held in ringed forceps.

4. Using your sterile-gloved, lubricated index and middle fingers as a guide, lay the trumpet against them and insert it into the vagina (Fig. 173-1). For a nongravid cervix, paracervical block is usually performed under direct visualization, using the sterile speculum and a tenaculum placed on the anterior lip of the cervix (Fig. 173-2).
5. Place the 20-gauge needle within the trumpet (or 1½-inch needle on an extender) through the mucosa at the *cervicovaginal junction* at the 3 o'clock position. Take great care not to inject yourself. Also take care not to insert the needle deeper than 0.5 cm into the tissue (see Fig. 173-1). Note that in the nongravid cervix and in early labor, the nerves are located at the 4 and 8 o'clock positions, respectively (see Fig. 173-2). As labor progresses, the position of the paracervical nerves "migrates" anteriorly during progressive dilation.
6. After aspirating for blood (to avoid intravascular injection), inject 5 to 10 mL of the chosen local anesthetic for the gravid cervix. (Alternatively, 2 to 3 mL may be placed in two or three locations around the probable location of the nerve.) After aspirating for blood in the nongravid cervix, some clinicians inject at four locations, at the 3, 6, 9, and 12 o'clock positions. Because there is no risk to a fetus, they inject 10 to 15 mL of a 2% solution in each site. Others inject in multiple locations in a cufflike fashion around the cervix.
7. For the gravid patient, monitor the fetal heart rate for approximately 5 minutes. If the tracing is reassuring (e.g., no apparent bradycardia), inject on the contralateral side at the 9 o'clock position (or the 8 o'clock position in early labor). Then monitor the fetal heart rate for 20 to 30 minutes, along with maternal blood pressure and pulse. In the nongravid patient, if there is no untoward reaction to the first injection, repeat the injection in the previously indicated location(s).

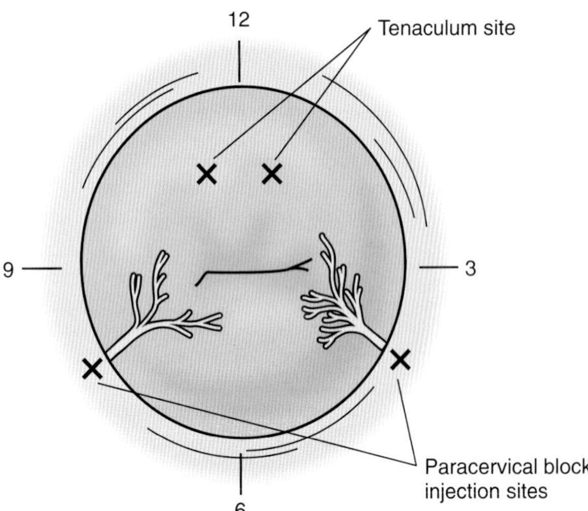

Figure 173-2 Paracervical block location in nongravid or early-labor patient and where to place the tenaculum in the nongravid cervix.

Common Error

Failure to inject at proper locations, and therefore not gaining maximum effect, is the most common error.

Complications

- Intrafetal injection.
- Postparacervical block fetal bradycardia. This may occur in 10% to 20% of blocks. This usually occurs within 10 minutes and may last up to 30 minutes. Most studies report only a small to moderate decrease in fetal heart rate of short duration (<10 minutes). Some investigators suggest that the fetal bradycardia associated with this procedure is not a sign of fetal asphyxia because it is almost always transient and the infants are usually vigorous at birth. However, there have been occasional reports of profound bradycardia, low fetal scalp pH, depressed Apgar scores, and other adverse outcomes, including fetal demise.
- Subgluteal, paracervical, parametrial, or retropsoas hematoma or infection.
- Neuropathy resulting from hematoma formation or direct sacral plexus trauma.
- Cardiotoxicity or neurotoxicity resulting from intravascular injection.
- Allergic reactions (rare).

Postprocedure Management

Continue to monitor the fetal heart rate after placing the block. It may be necessary to repeat the entire procedure, depending on the duration of activity of the anesthetic agent. A good response is generally maintained for 45 to 75 minutes. However, the effect may last only 30 minutes, or it can last as long as 90 minutes.

The patient should know to report any significant signs or symptoms of a complication after the procedure. Major late complications include a hematoma or infection, so the patient should report any fever, areas of numbness, vaginal bleeding, or abdominal, vaginal, or pelvic pain in the weeks after the procedure.

Patient Education Guides

See patient education and patient consent forms available online at www.expertconsult.com.

CPT/Billing Codes

64435 Injection, anesthetic agent; paracervical (uterine) nerve

ICD-9-CM Diagnostic Codes

Please see the Diagnostic Codes sections in Chapters 127, Pregnancy Termination: First-Trimester Suction Aspiration; 141, Dilation and Curettage; 143, Endometrial Biopsy; 145, Intrauterine Device Insertion; 149, Loop Electrosurgical Excision Procedure for

Treating Cervical Intraepithelial Neoplasia; and 177, Vaginal Delivery.

EDITOR'S NOTE: For colposcopy, the patient does not need a paracervical block, but all the rest of the cervical procedures require one.

BIBLIOGRAPHY

Althaus J, Wax J: Analgesia and anesthesia in labor. Obstet Gynecol Clin North Am 32:231–244, 2005.

American College of Obstetricians and Gynecologists: Optimal goals for anesthesia care in obstetrics. Committee opinion no. 433. Obstet Gynecol 113:1197–1199, 2009.

Cunningham FG, Leveno KJ, Bloom SL, et al (eds): Obstetrical Anesthesia. In Williams Obstetrics, 23rd ed., chapter 19. Available at http://www.accessmedicine.com.proxy.lib.uiowa.edu/content.aspx?aID=602481.

Eberle RL, Norris MC: Labour analgesia: A risk-benefit analysis. Drug Saf 14:239–251, 1996.

Leeman L, Fontaine P, King V, et al: The nature and management of labor pain: Part II. Pharmacologic pain relief. Am Fam Physician 68:1115–1120, 2003.

Levy BT, Bergus GR, Hartz A, et al: Is paracervical block safe and effective? A prospective study of its association with neonatal umbilical artery pH values. J Fam Pract 48:778–784, 1999.

Rosen MA: Paracervical block for labor analgesia: A brief historic review. Am J Obstet Gynecol 186(5 Suppl):S127–S130, 2002.

Salam GA: Regional anesthesia for office procedures: Part II. Extremity and inguinal area surgeries. Am Fam Physician 69:896–900, 2004.

Tuggy M, Garcia J: Procedures Consult. Available at www.proceduresconsult.com.

CHAPTER 174

Pudendal Anesthesia

John J. Andazola • Dolores M. Gomez

Pudendal nerve anesthesia is a common nerve block technique used in obstetrics and minor gynecologic surgery. Its advantages include its safety, ease of administration, and rapidity of onset. Pudendal nerve block can be used to provide analgesia during the second stage of labor and to facilitate pelvic floor relaxation when using low forceps and vacuum extraction. It also provides anesthesia for the perineum in order to create or repair an episiotomy. Pudendal nerve anesthesia can be used for minor surgery of the lower vagina and perineum. Epidural anesthesia has largely supplanted the use of pudendal nerve anesthesia, but pudendal blocks are an alternative when neuraxial blockade is not feasible, not effective, or contraindicated. Although both transperineal and transvaginal approaches for pudendal blockade are options, the transvaginal approach is more practical and used most often. Therefore, only the transvaginal approach is discussed here.

Anatomy

The pudendal nerve supplies both sensory and motor innervation to the perineum. It is composed of parts of the second, third, and fourth sacral nerves and has three branches. In a woman, these branches supply the following structures:

1. The dorsal nerve of the clitoris, which innervates the clitoris and its erectile tissues
2. The perineal nerve, which innervates the muscles of the perineum and the skin of the labia minora, labia majora, and vestibule
3. The inferior hemorrhoidal nerve, which innervates the external sphincter of the anus and perianal skin (responsible for the anal "wink" reflex)

Pudendal anesthesia attempts to block the nerve as it enters the lesser sciatic foramen, usually inferior and medial to the insertion of the sacrospinous ligament on the ischial spine. The pudendal vessels lie lateral to the nerve at this location, so care must be taken to avoid intravascular injection. Although total block of the pudendal nerve should abolish pain and sensation over this entire area, there are other nerves that may also supply the sensory innervation to the perineum. Thus "skip" areas of analgesia may be noted, and complete nerve blockade can be ineffective on one or both sides as frequently as 50% of the time.

Indications

- Obstetric anesthesia for spontaneous vaginal delivery, episiotomy and episiotomy repair, repair of low vaginal lacerations, and low (outlet) forceps or vacuum-assisted delivery
- When epidural anesthesia is incomplete or inadequate
- For minor surgery of the lower vagina and perineum

NOTE: Because the upper vagina, cervix, and uterus receive separate innervation from the lower thoracic nerves, pudendal anesthesia alone is insufficient for midforceps application or for high vaginal, cervical, or uterine manipulation or repair.

Contraindications

Absolute

- Patient refusal
- Allergy to local anesthetic agents
- Current infection in the ischiorectal space or neighboring structures, including the vagina and perineum

Relative

Coagulopathy or anticoagulant therapy (e.g., warfarin, heparin or its analogs) or antiplatelet therapy (clopidogrel [Plavix]) is a relative contraindication for this procedure.

Equipment and Supplies

- Local anesthetic: 1% lidocaine (Xylocaine or generic) without epinephrine or 1% or 2% chloroprocaine (Nesacaine or generic; this may have lower toxicity than lidocaine but does not last as long)
- Iowa trumpet (Fig. 174-1A) or similar guide to facilitate placement of the needle
- 10-mL syringe with finger ring (Fig. 174-1B)
- Needle, usually 6-inch, 22-gauge (see Fig. 174-1B) (The operator should check, before the procedure, that the needle is longer than the guiding device and equipped with a "stop" to prevent penetration of tissue deeper than 10 to 15 mm.)
- Sterile gloves

Precautions

Care must be taken to avoid intravascular injection because the pudendal vessels lie lateral to the pudendal nerve. Toxicity may occur with 1% lidocaine *without* epinephrine (10 mg/mL) above 1 mg/kg (70 mg or 7 mL in a 70-kg patient) with intravascular administration. Maximum dosage should not exceed 4.5 mg/kg or a maximum of 30 mL of 1% solution (300 mg), and the maximum dose should not be repeated in less than 2 hours (see Chapter 4, Local Anesthesia, for maximum dosages). A successful pudendal block may impair some reflexive maternal pushing, which may prolong the second stage of labor in women who are ineffective at pushing.

Preprocedure Patient Preparation

Explain the potential risks (see the Contraindications and Complications sections) and the potential benefits to the patient so she may make an informed decision. This discussion should include alternatives and occur before the moment of greatest anesthetic need, when neither the patient nor the clinician can communicate optimally. Ideally, anesthesia should be decided as part of a birth plan, and this should be discussed and written well before the pregnancy is at term.

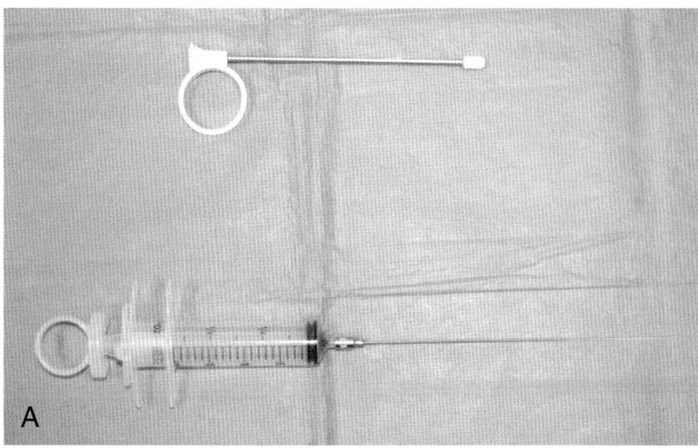

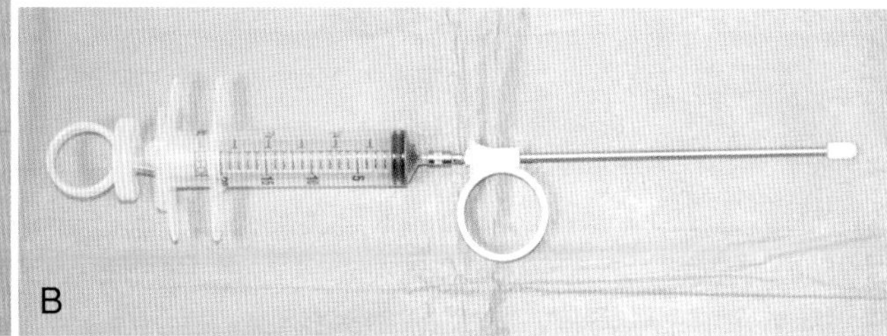

Figure 174-1 **A,** Iowa trumpet and syringe with finger rings separated. **B,** Iowa trumpet and syringe with finger rings together.

TECHNIQUE

Because a fairly large volume of anesthetic agent is given, appropriate monitoring of the patient (and, in obstetric cases, the fetus) should be considered. See the Complications section, or Chapter 5, Local and Topical Anesthetic Complications, for symptoms of adverse reactions.

1. Timing is important for pudendal anesthesia. Approximately 5 to 10 minutes must be allowed for the anesthetic to infiltrate the nerve and cause its effect. However, for obstetric indications, the anesthetic should be administered neither so early that it blocks effective reflex pushing, nor so late that it wears off before delivery. In nulliparous women, it is usually administered after the cervix has completely dilated and the head has descended to a +2 to +3 station. In multiparous women, the pudendal block may be administered earlier when rapid delivery is expected but should be avoided before the cervix has dilated to 5 cm because it may slow or arrest labor. The resultant anesthetic effect may last for 20 to 60 minutes.
2. Place the patient in the dorsal lithotomy position; usually no vaginal preparation is done. In obstetric procedures, (a) the length of time the patient is flat should be minimized, and (b) *the fetus must be carefully monitored* throughout the procedure and after anesthesia. Universal blood and body fluid precautions should be observed during any obstetric or anesthetic procedure.
3. Grasp the Iowa trumpet or needle guide with your sterile-gloved, nondominant hand. The wrist should be pronated, with the thumb through the ring and the shaft between the index and middle fingers. Adequately lubricate the index and middle fingers and use them to protect the vaginal mucosa (and, in obstetric cases, the fetal head). Insert the fingers into the vagina and direct the tip of the guide to the patient's ipsilateral ischial spine (i.e., the left hand of the right-handed operator is used to direct the guide to the patient's left ischial spine). Maintain the guide at an angle nearly parallel to the patient's back (Fig. 174-2).
4. Carefully define the anatomy to increase the likelihood of a successful procedure. Attempt to delineate the ischial spine. Slightly below the spine, on its inferoposterior surface, the sacrospinous ligament is attached. Next, attempt to palpate the pudendal artery laterally. Locating these landmarks helps prevent injection of the anesthetic directly into the vessels. It also helps to define the location of the nerve, which is medial to the vessels. If the anatomy is particularly difficult to define, injection just below the ischial spine should be sufficient (but only after aspirating to be certain the needle is not in a vessel).
5. With your nondominant hand grasping the syringe, use your dominant hand to direct the needle through the guide, and insert it to the appropriate depth at the desired injection site(s).

   NOTE: *Aspirate for blood with the syringe before injecting anesthetic each time the needle placement is changed.* If blood is aspirated, intravascular injection is likely; withdraw the needle and redirect medially, away from the vessels.
6. Inject the desired sites. Usually two to three sites are injected on each side in a fanlike fashion, with a total of 10 mL of local anesthetic injected per side. For the sacrospinous ligament (below/inferior/posterior to spine), some clinicians raise a mucosal wheal at this site with 1 mL of anesthetic and then insert the needle through the wheal until it contacts the ligament. After infiltrating the ligament with 2 to 4 mL of anesthetic, the needle is advanced through the ligament. The clinician will know that the ligament has been traversed when resistance to the plunger decreases. Another 2 to 4 mL of anesthetic can then be easily injected into the loose areolar tissue behind the ligament; another 2 to 4 mL can be injected above/superior/anterior to the ischial spine; and another 2 to 4 mL can be injected medial to the tip of the spine.

   NOTE: At each site (except when raising the mucosal wheal below the ischial spine), the needle should be inserted at least 10 mm but not more than 15 mm beyond the needle guide. Each time the needle is redirected, the tip should be drawn back into the guide, the guide redirected, and then the needle advanced to the desired depth.
7. Withdraw the needle, refill the syringe, and inject into the opposite side if bilateral anesthesia is desired. Most clinicians prefer to use the same hand for the guide; however, some claim switching hands for the opposite side is more effective. If switching hands, make sure the needle tip is withdrawn to protect yourself from a puncture wound.
8. After 5 minutes, check anesthesia on *each* side. Using an Allis forceps, gently scratch over the perineum and watch for the anal "wink" reflex. If there is no reflex to mild stimulus, confirm that the anesthesia is complete with a pinch on each side.
9. A smaller repeat dose on a side not demonstrating adequate anesthesia may be used, but care must be taken to avoid doses at which, even with slow absorption from the tissues, toxic serum levels could be reached. Local anesthesia may be used on the perineum to augment the effect, if necessary (when the pudendal block is not completely effective or if it has not had time to take full effect). For example, in the pregnant patient, if the head is descending rapidly, local anesthetic can also be infiltrated into the area where an episiotomy will be made. After the head has been delivered, the pudendal block should have had time to take effect and will usually provide anesthesia for the episiotomy repair.
10. As discussed earlier, a pudendal block usually does not provide anesthesia for the upper vagina or cervix. This is important to

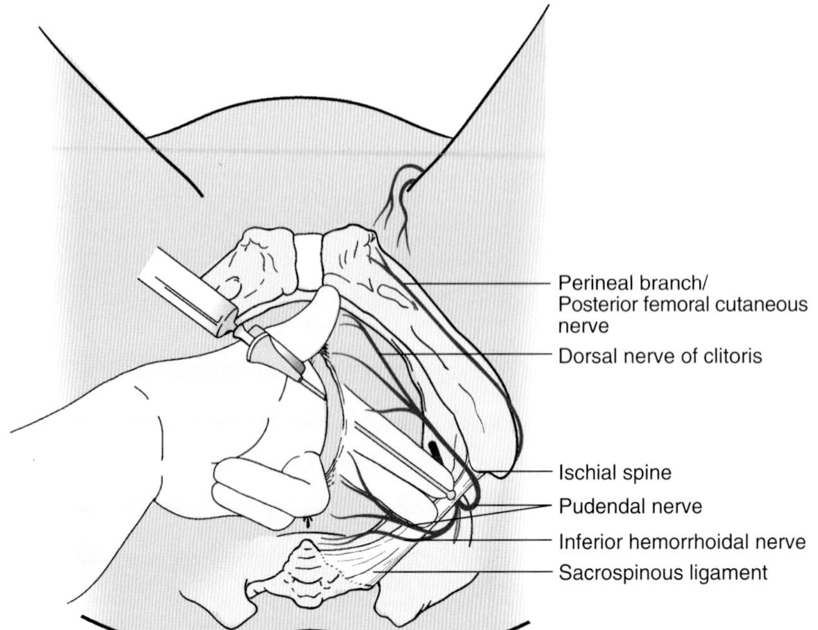

Figure 174-2 Practitioner's left hand is directing guide and needle toward the patient's left pudendal nerve.

remember after delivery when attempting to visualize the entire cervix and upper vagina. If manual exploration of the uterus is necessary, the addition of an intravenous narcotic analgesic may be helpful and appreciated.

Complications

- Systemic anesthetic toxicity is rare and usually results from intravascular administration or an inappropriately high dose. Toxicity may initially cause palpitations, tinnitus, dysarthria, or drowsiness. It may progress to confusion, loss of consciousness, convulsions, hypotension, and bradycardia. Although complications are usually transient, support of the patient's oxygenation and blood pressure is essential (especially to minimize fetal complications in obstetric cases). See Chapter 5, Local and Topical Anesthetic Complications, for management of complications.
- The most frequent complication with pudendal anesthesia is failure to provide adequate anesthesia. Local or regional (e.g., saddle block or epidural) anesthesia should be offered if available.
- Hematomas and infections have been reported but are rare. Infection may spread into the hip joint, the gluteal musculature, or the retropsoas space. Infections may be life-threatening and must be suspected when there is severe pain in the pelvis, back, or hip, limitation of motion, and increasing fever.
- Despite the fact that the anesthetic reaches the neonatal bloodstream after regional anesthesia, studies have failed to demonstrate neonatal neurobehavioral effects or other adverse effects.

Postprocedure Management and Patient Education

There is little need for specific postanesthesia instruction. Remind the patient of the rare but possible complications so that she will report to her clinician if any symptoms develop, especially pelvic, back, or hip pain, limited range of motion, or fever.

CPT/Billing Code

64430 Injection, anesthetic agent, pudendal nerve

ICD-9-CM Diagnostic Codes

650 Normal delivery

The fifth digit (X) is required for codes 651–659 and 660–669 to denote the following:

0 Unspecified
1 Delivered, with or without mention of antepartum condition
2 Delivered, with mention of postpartum complication
3 Antepartum condition or complication
4 Postpartum condition or complication

Codes related to deliveries with forceps or vacuum

659.7X Abnormality in fetal heart rate or rhythm
662.2X Prolonged second stage of labor

Codes related to episiotomy and episiotomy repair, and for repair of low vaginal lacerations

664.0X First-degree perineal laceration
664.1X Second-degree perineal laceration
664.2X Third-degree perineal laceration
664.3X Fourth-degree perineal laceration
664.4X Unspecified perineal laceration

Acknowledgment

The editors wish to recognize the contributions by Donald N. Marquardt, MD, PhD, to this chapter in the previous two editions of this text.

Bibliography

American College of Obstetricians and Gynecologists: Optimal goals for anesthesia care in obstetrics. Committee opinion no. 433. Obstet Gynecol 113:1197–1199, 2009.

Cunningham FG, Leveno KJ, Bloom SL, et al (eds): Obstetrical Anesthesia. In Williams Obstetrics, 23rd ed., chapter 19. Available at http://www.accessmedicine.com.proxy.lib.uiowa.edu/content.aspx?aID=602481.

Hawkins JL: Obstetric analgesia and anesthesia. In Gibbs RS, Karlan BY, Haney AF, Nygaard IE (eds): Danforth's Obstetrics and Gynecology, 10th ed. Philadelphia, Lippincott Williams & Wilkins, 2008, pp 43–59.

Svancarek W, Chirino O, Schaefer G Jr, Blythe JG: Retropsoas and subgluteal abscesses following paracervical and pudendal anesthesia. JAMA 237:892–894, 1977.

CHAPTER 175

Saddle Block Anesthesia

Peter W. Grigg

Saddle block anesthesia provides pain relief in the area of the perineum, buttocks, and inner thigh by using an intrathecal (spinal) injection of local anesthetic. A saddle block may be confused with a caudal block (injection of local anesthetic into the sacral canal through the sacral hiatus) because the resultant anesthesia may be similar, but the technique is different. This chapter describes the low-spinal saddle block technique. An ideal "saddle block" anesthetizes the area that would touch a saddle if the patient were riding a horse.

With the advent of more complex techniques for producing analgesia and anesthesia, including single-dose intrathecal opiates and combined spinal epidural and continuous spinal infusions, traditional saddle block (low spinal) is used less often.

Saddle block anesthesia has been used for many years for both surgical procedures and obstetric deliveries. Past problems with profound motor paralysis can be avoided by using lower doses of bupivacaine (e.g., 1 to 2 mL 0.25% bupivacaine [Sensorcaine-MPF] with or without a narcotic). Therefore, variations of saddle block anesthesia can be used midlabor or near delivery.

Clinicians administering saddle block anesthesia must have a good understanding of the anatomy, needle placement techniques, pharmacology, and physiology involved, particularly with regard to the obstetric patient. They must be familiar and experienced with the diagnosis and management of possible complications. A review of the updated American Society of Anesthesiologists (ASA) Guidelines for Obstetric Anesthesia (2006) and the ASA Difficult Airway Algorithms is highly recommended for medical professionals anesthetizing obstetric patients.

Saddle blocks should be performed only in hospitals, surgical centers, or facilities where drugs, equipment, and adequately trained personnel are available to manage any and all possible complications. The equipment available should be comparable with that of the main operating rooms.

Indications

- For use in obstetrics when time or other circumstances do not allow the use of continuous catheter spinal or epidural anesthetic techniques (e.g., routine delivery, assisted delivery [forceps, vacuum], episiotomy or perineal repair, or other obstetric procedures).
- To provide quick relief so that a laboring patient can remain stationary for epidural catheter placement.
- Genital surgery (e.g., dilation and curettage, hysteroscopy, vaginal surgery, adult circumcision, orchiectomy, or complicated vasectomy).
- Anorectal surgery (e.g., hemorrhoidectomy, fistulectomy, or rectal-anal biopsy).
- As part of a combined spinal epidural technique, when the spinal needle is placed through an epidural needle that is in the epidural space.

Contraindications

Absolute

- Patient declines.
- Lack of proper resuscitative equipment, skills, or trained staff.
- Allergy to specific local anesthetics.
- Active systemic infection.
- Moderate to severe hypovolemia.
- Blood dyscrasias; coagulopathy; prolonged international normalized ratio, prothrombin time, or activated partial thromboplastin time; thrombocytopenia.
- Anticoagulant therapy (e.g., heparin, warfarin, enoxaparin [Lovenox], clopidogrel [Plavix]).

Relative

- Cutaneous lesions of the lower back.
- Spinal abnormalities, including scoliosis and other structural abnormalities.
- Preexisting neurologic diseases (amyotrophic lateral sclerosis, other degenerative nerve diseases, poliomyelitis).
- Preoperative headache.

Equipment and Supplies

- Disposable sterile gloves
- Equipment for the clinician to observe universal blood and body fluid precautions
- Disposable spinal tray containing the following
  - Appropriate prep solutions, swabs, and sterile 4 × 4 gauze pads
  - Disposable drapes
  - Syringes
    - 3-mL plastic Luer-Lok for local infiltration of lidocaine 1%
    - 5-mL procedural syringe for administration of intrathecal agent
  - Needles
    - 3½-inch, 25-gauge spinal needle (pencil point instead of cutting bevel)
    - 20-gauge introducer needle
    - 19-gauge filter needle for drawing solutions into the syringes
    - 25- or 27-gauge skin wheal needle
  - Medications
    - Lidocaine 1% (available in 5-mL vial) for local infiltration
    - Hyperbaric anesthetic
      - Lidocaine 5% (preservative free) in 7.5% dextrose for intrathecal administration (2-mL vial), *or*
      - Tetracaine 1% (2-mL vial) mixed at the time of use with an equal volume of dextrose 10% (5-mL vial) to make the solution hyperbaric, *or*
      - Bupivacaine 0.75% in 8.25% dextrose (2-mL vial)

Bupivacaine 0.25% methyl paraben free (MPF; for epidural use) plain

Epinephrine 1:1000 (1-mL vial); addition of 0.2 to 0.3 mg (0.2 to 0.3 mL of 1 : 1000) epinephrine to tetracaine will produce vasoconstriction and prolong the duration of anesthesia by about 50%

Ephedrine 5% (1-mL) in case hypotension develops (the usual dose to treat hypotension is 10 mg [0.2 mL] intravenously [IV])

Fentanyl 50 μg/mL for injection

NOTE: A 1% solution equals 10 mg/mL.

- IV fluids (Ringer's lactate, normal saline)
- Continuous fetal monitoring equipment if used for labor and delivery
- Patient monitoring equipment, including automated blood pressure (BP) device, continuous electrocardiograph (ECG), and pulse oximeter
- Emergency and resuscitative equipment, including suction, positive-pressure breathing device (Ambu-Bag), oxygen, and defibrillator (Having general anesthesia equipment available may be useful [e.g., endotracheal tubes, laryngoscope].)
- Emergency and other drugs not included in the spinal kit
  - Atropine
  - Diphenhydramine (Benadryl)
  - Ephedrine (not included in all commercial spinal kits)
  - Lidocaine for IV injection
  - Metoclopramide (Reglan)
  - Neo-Synephrine
  - Epinephrine
  - Phenylephrine
  - Succinylcholine
  - Propofol, thiopental, and midazolam

Anesthetic Agents and Doses

For saddle block, the three commonly used local anesthetics are lidocaine, tetracaine, and bupivacaine. Lidocaine produces a more rapid onset of anesthesia than tetracaine or bupivacaine; however, it is the shortest acting of the three. Lidocaine generally produces adequate surgical analgesia for 45 to 90 minutes, whereas tetracaine and bupivacaine will last 1½ to 3 hours.

Recently, reports of neurologic sequelae (transient radicular irritation) have raised concerns about the use of lidocaine for intrathecal anesthesia. The risk appears to be reduced if the lidocaine solution is diluted before injection with an equal volume of cerebrospinal fluid (CSF). Tetracaine and bupivacaine are excellent alternatives to lidocaine; however, their increased duration of action requires a longer recovery period.

NOTE: For a rapidly progressing obstetric patient, lidocaine may be the only option that will work quickly enough.

Hyperbaric solutions (solutions more dense than CSF) are used for saddle block anesthesia so that in the sitting position the anesthetic solution travels caudad, affecting only the lower levels of the spinal cord. It is important to remember that during pregnancy, inferior vena cava compression will cause engorgement and distention of the vertebral venous system. As a result, there is a decrease in the CSF capacity of the subarachnoid space; therefore, the dose requirements are generally reduced in the pregnant patient.

Near delivery, the usual dose of lidocaine for a saddle block is 25 to 50 mg of 5% lidocaine in 7.5% dextrose (0.5 to 1.0 mL). It should be mixed with equal amounts of CSF before injecting. The equivalent dose of 1% tetracaine is 4 to 6 mg (0.4 to 0.6 mL) plus an equal volume of 10% dextrose solution. For bupivacaine, 5 to 6 mg (0.66 to 0.8 mL of the 0.75% bupivacaine in 8.25% dextrose) should be used. Epidural bupivacaine 0.25% MPF 1 mL (2.5 mg) with 25 μg fentanyl provides less motor block. In surgical procedures for the nonpregnant patient, the doses should be increased.

Confining the anesthetic to a saddle block distribution depends on the dosage and the time that the patient remains in the sitting position after administration of the anesthetic. Too little time in the sitting position (lying down too soon) may produce a higher level of anesthesia than desired, placing the patient at higher risk of hypotension and a higher level of block.

NOTE: From an anesthetic perspective, the *level* of anesthesia refers to an anatomic level or segment of effect (e.g., up to the level of the umbilicus [T10], the lower border of the ribs [T8], or the level of the xiphoid [T6]), whereas *depth* refers to the amount of remaining sensation. With saddle block, both motor and sensation are blocked; however, the level of the sensory block is usually two segments above the motor block.

Precautions

In addition to a physical examination, a focused history (general maternal health, anesthetic history, allergies, relevant obstetric history, current medications, and NPO status) should be performed with special attention to the airway, vital signs, heart, lungs, and back. Look for contraindications to performing the block.

Expert witnesses in medical liability cases often note a lack of preblock examinations by the anesthesiologist. Laboratory studies are obtained on an individualized basis. Patients should be informed of the risks, benefits, and alternatives to analgesia and anesthesia.

Preprocedure Patient Education and Forms

A fact sheet should be given to the patient to read preoperatively or before the onset of labor (see patient education form available online at www.expertconsult.com). Preferably, the fact sheet should be given to the patient as part of her preoperative assessment or as part of her prenatal care. Shortly before labor, before surgery, or during early labor, the clinician should review the options again with the patient and obtain a signed informed consent (if not done previously).

Desired anesthesia or analgesia should be included in the patient's birth plan. Early and ongoing contact between the obstetrician and anesthesiologist is vital, particularly when significant anesthetic and obstetric risk factors are elucidated.

Technique

1. Consider giving nonparticulate antacids (Bicitra 30 mL), histamine type 2 blocker (e.g., ranitidine 150 mg), and metoclopramide (Reglan 10 mg) 30 minutes before the saddle block, especially before a cesarean delivery or postpartum tubal ligation. Some clinicians withhold Bicitra because they believe it causes vomiting. ASA Guidelines for Obstetric Anesthesia (2006) permit clear liquids up to 2 hours before saddle block, even in uncomplicated patients undergoing an elective cesarean section.
2. Confirm that informed consent and permission forms are signed and in order.
3. Establish IV access with a 20-gauge or larger catheter and give a bolus of 500 to 1000 mL of IV fluids. The patient should be well hydrated before the procedure to minimize the risk of developing hypotension.

   NOTE: Administer IV fluids slowly in women with pregnancy-induced hypertension.

4. For patients in labor, fetal monitoring should be used. For all patients, secure the continuous BP, ECG, and pulse oximetry

monitors and record the initial values. Thereafter, monitor carefully for hypotension by cycling the BP monitor to take measurements at least every 2.5 minutes. Vital signs should be recorded on the anesthesia chart at least every 5 minutes.

5. Open the disposable spinal kit and mix the appropriate solutions. Use the filtered needle to draw up any solutions that will be administered intrathecally.
6. Place the patient in the sitting position with the back and neck flexed and the spine straight and not rotated. An assistant should stand in front of the patient during the procedure, helping the patient to maintain the proper position.
7. Locate the L2-3, L3-4, or L4-5 interspace. Perform the sterile preparations and drape the area.
8. Administer the local anesthesia (lidocaine 1%) to the interspace area by first making a skin wheal, then injecting into the deeper tissues in the same direction that the spinal needle will be advanced.
9. Insert the introducer needle into the supraspinous ligament at the proper angle to later direct the spinal needle into the subdural space.

   NOTE: The proper angle depends on which interspace is used. At the L4-5 interspace, the proper direction for the needle tip is basically perpendicular (90 degrees) to slightly cranial, whereas it decreases to about 70 degrees (and aimed cranial) at the L2-3 interspace. The proper location is usually just below the inferior edge of the spinous process or slightly below that level (Fig. 175-1). For saddle block anesthesia, insertion angle and location are identical to those used for epidural anesthesia; however, the depth of insertion is unique to each procedure.

10. Insert the 3½-inch, 25-gauge spinal needle into the introducer. Next, advance the spinal needle into the intrathecal space. A "pop" is usually felt when the needle passes through the ligamentum flavum and into the space. Confirmation is obtained when CSF flows from the hub of the spinal needle and continues to do so after the needle is rotated 360 degrees. Rotating the needle ensures that there is no tissue right at the tip of the needle that could later cause an obstruction and prevent injection (Fig. 175-2).

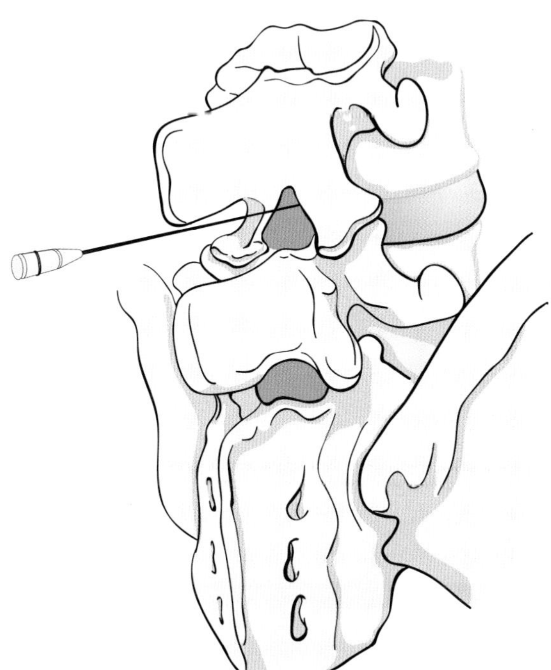

Figure 175-1 Spinal needle introduced through the L4-5 interspace. Note that the needle is introduced just below the inferior border of the L4 spinous process. The tip is directed at 90 degrees to the spine or slightly cranial.

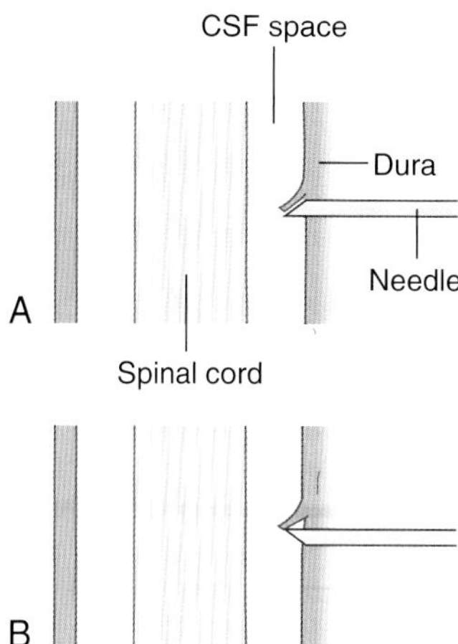

Figure 175-2 **A,** Bevel of spinal needle occluded by a dural flap after puncture. The flap prevents free flow of cerebrospinal fluid (CSF) through the spinal needle. **B,** Rotating the needle 180 degrees separates the dural flap from the bevel, allowing free flow of CSF through the needle.

11. With the anesthetic solution syringe connected to the hub of the spinal needle, aspirate a small amount of CSF to confirm the placement of the needle. Next, if using lidocaine, withdraw an amount of CSF (0.5 to 1 mL) equal to the amount of lidocaine already in the syringe. Reinject the lidocaine/CSF mixed solution through the spinal needle, slowly, over a period of 5 to 10 seconds. Tetracaine or bupivacaine should also be injected slowly. Do not aspirate or inject during a uterine contraction.
12. Remove the spinal needle, syringe, and introducer as a unit. Have the patient remain in the sitting position for 2 to 5 minutes to allow the anesthetic to "set" while it drifts downward into the spinal canal. Allowing the patient to become recumbent or lie in the lithotomy position too soon can result in a higher level of anesthesia than desired. However, if the patient becomes hypotensive, he or she should be returned to the recumbent position immediately and treatment initiated. Otherwise, at the end of the sitting period, place the patient in the lithotomy position. For pregnant women, left uterine displacement should be performed by lifting the uterus slightly and manually pushing or pulling it toward the patient's left side. An assistant should perform this maneuver. This may be facilitated by having the patient turn slightly toward her left side. Left uterine displacement helps minimize or avoid vena caval compression syndrome (decreased venous return to the heart combined with venous congestion around the spinal cord). In a late-trimester pregnancy, this syndrome can lead to prolonged hypotension.
13. Check sensation to sharp objects (e.g., a needle) and record the level of anesthesia on the anesthesia record. Once adequate anesthesia has been established, the patient is prepared for delivery.

NOTE: The factors affecting the level of anesthesia include (1) the lumbar puncture site, (2) the volume of solution used, (3) the rate of injection, (4) the specific gravity of the solution used, and (5) the position of the patient.

Complications

Intraoperative and postoperative complications of saddle block anesthesia are essentially the same as for higher levels of spinal anesthesia.

Intraoperative Complications

- Hypotension may occur at any time, particularly during and shortly after administration of the anesthetic. It must be corrected rapidly by (1) placing the patient in a recumbent position, (2) infusing a rapid bolus of IV fluids (500 mL), (3) rapidly administering ephedrine 10 mg (IV), and (4) relieving pressure on the vena cava from the pregnant uterus by left uterine displacement. If bradycardia and hypotension occur (from block of cardiac accelerator nerves) give epinephrine quickly. If hypotension and maternal tachycardia are present, then phenylephrine in a 0.1- to 0.5-mg IV bolus dose is acceptable.
- High spinal block with respiratory insufficiency or total spinal block with total respiratory arrest must be treated immediately with respiratory assistance and continued as needed for the duration of the block. Hypotension commonly occurs concurrently.
- Nausea and vomiting may occur concurrently with a drop in blood pressure and usually are relieved with correction of the hypotension by ephedrine (10 mg IV). If accompanied by bradycardia, the nausea and vomiting may regress after treatment with atropine (0.4 to 0.6 mg IV). Nausea and vomiting in the absence of other symptoms may be treated with metoclopramide (10 mg IV).
- Allergic reactions: use diphenhydramine 25 to 50 mg IV.
- Systemic reactions, including cardiac arrhythmia/arrest, are rare. To treat this, routine advanced cardiac life support protocols should be followed.

Postoperative Complications

- Headache may occur, with an incidence as high as 5%. Most postspinal puncture headaches can be treated conservatively (oral analgesics, fluids, rest), but some require more aggressive treatment, including a blood patch (see Chapter 206, Lumbar Puncture, for instructions on performing a blood patch).
- Urinary retention sometimes occurs, requiring catheterization.
- Neurologic sequelae (rare), including arachnoiditis, meningitis, palsies, and paralysis.

Patient Education Guides

See the sample patient education form available online at www.expertconsult.com.

CPT/Billing Codes

62273 Injection, lumbar epidural, of blood or clot patch
62311 Injection, single (not via indwelling catheter), not including neurolytic substances, with or without contrast, of diagnostic or therapeutic substance(s) (including anesthetic, antispasmodic, opioid, steroid, other solution), epidural or subarachnoid; lumbar, sacral (caudal)

ICD-9-CM Diagnostic Codes

For other than pregnancy codes, see the appropriate procedure chapter for ICD-9-CM codes.

650 Normal delivery
V22.2 Pregnant state, NOS

The fifth digit (X) is required for codes 640–648, 651–659, and 660–669 to denote the current episode of care.

0 Unspecified
1 Delivered, with or without mention of antepartum condition
2 Delivered, with mention of postpartum complication
3 Antepartum condition or complication
4 Postpartum condition or complication
644.2X Premature labor with delivery (<37 weeks)
652.2X Breech presentation
653.5X Unusually large fetus causing disproportion

Codes related to deliveries with forceps or vacuum

659.7X Abnormality in fetal heart rate or rhythm or fetal distress
662.2X Prolonged second stage of labor

Codes related to episiotomy and episiotomy repair and codes for repair of low vaginal lacerations

664.0X First-degree perineal laceration
664.1X Second-degree perineal laceration
664.2X Third-degree perineal laceration
664.3X Fourth-degree perineal laceration
664.4X Unspecified perineal laceration

Acknowledgment

The editors wish to recognize the contributions of Thomas H. Corbett, MD, MPH, to this chapter in the previous edition of this text.

Suppliers

(See contact information online at www.expertconsult.com.)

Disposable trays, infusion pumps, and needles
B. Braun Medical Inc.
Baxter Healthcare Corporation
Becton, Dickinson and Co.
Rusch Inc. (Teleflex)
Smiths Medical USA
Epidural and saddle block needles
The Kendall Company (Covidien)

BIBLIOGRAPHY

American College of Obstetricians and Gynecologists: Optimal goals for anesthesia care in obstetrics. Committee opinion no. 433. Obstet Gynecol 113:1197–1199, 2009.

American College of Obstetricians and Gynecologists Committee on Obstetric Practice: Analgesia and cesarean delivery rates. Committee opinion no. 339. Obstet Gynecol 107:1487–1488, 2006.

American Society of Anesthesiologists: Practice Guidelines for Obstetric Anesthesia (last amended on October 18th, 2006). An updated report by the American Society of Anesthesiologists Task Force on Obstetric Anesthesia. Available at www.asahq.org/publicationsAndServices/practiceparam.htm#ob. Accessed July 20, 2008.

American Society of Anesthesiologists Task Force on Management of the Difficult Airway: Practice guidelines for the management of the difficult airway: An updated report by the American Society of Anesthesiologists Task Force on Management of the Difficult Airway. Anesthesiology 98:1269–1277, 2003.

Gerancher JC: Cauda equina syndrome following a single spinal administration of 5% hyperbaric lidocaine through a 25-gauge Whitacre needle. Anesthesiology 87:687–689, 1997.

Johnson ME: Potential neurotoxicity of spinal anesthesia with lidocaine. Mayo Clin Proc 75:921–932, 2000.

CHAPTER 176

TRANSCERVICAL AMNIOINFUSION

David G. Weismiller

Amnioinfusion is an inexpensive, minimally invasive, proven therapeutic measure used since 1983 to restore or replace amniotic fluid during labor. It is performed by infusing normal saline or lactated Ringer's transcervically through a catheter. There are two common applications: (1) to assist with the management of variable or prolonged (e.g., lasting as long as the contraction) fetal heart rate decelerations; and (2), until recently, to dilute thick meconium fluid. Overall, the procedure appears to pose little risk while offering considerable benefit in properly selected patients. A survey of 186 teaching hospitals in the United States found that 96% use amnioinfusion, and an estimated 3% to 4% of women in labor receive such an infusion.

In theory, artificially increasing the amniotic fluid volume should protect the umbilical cord from compression, thus reducing the number and severity of variable decelerations. If decelerations become severe, persistent, or prolonged, it is possible for the fetus to become distressed and even require emergency operative delivery. A recent meta-analysis of nine randomized trials provides supportive evidence for amnioinfusion for variable decelerations. Another summary of 12 published randomized trials suggests that using amnioinfusion for infants at risk of cord compression (e.g., repetitive variable decelerations, especially in the presence of oligohydramnios or amniotomy) decreases not only the occurrence of variable decelerations but the number of cesarean sections. Interestingly, amnioinfusion is also associated with a reduction in postpartum endometritis for women at risk.

Previous randomized, controlled trials had suggested that the *prophylactic* use of amnioinfusion for oligohydramnios might reduce the incidence of fetal distress and cesarean intervention. However, recent comparison studies found no advantage to prophylactic amnioinfusion as opposed to using amnioinfusion only when fetal heart rate decelerations occur.

Amnioinfusion has been advocated as a technique to reduce the incidence of meconium aspiration and to improve neonatal outcome. Meta-analyses had suggested that amnioinfusion for moderate to thick meconium reduced the frequency of meconium being found below the infant vocal cords, the incidence of meconium aspiration syndrome, and the cesarean delivery rate. However, a large proportion of infants have already aspirated meconium before meconium-stained amniotic fluid is noted and before amnioinfusion can be performed; meconium passage may predate labor. Meconium passage occurs in three distinct situations: (1) as a physiologic or maturational event, (2) as a response to acute hypoxic events, and (3) as a response to chronic intrauterine hypoxia. It has long been known that the risk of meconium aspiration is high in infants of mothers with thick meconium, particularly if associated with an episode of fetal hypoxia. In contrast, thin meconium is not associated with an increased perinatal mortality rate or incidence of meconium aspiration syndrome. Therefore, diluting meconium in the already potentially compromised fetus is postulated to have a positive effect on neonatal outcome.

Based on current literature (e.g., evidence from a well-designed, randomized, multicenter, prospective trial of 1998 women [Fraser and colleagues, 2005]), routine prophylactic amnioinfusion for the dilution of meconium-stained amniotic fluid is not recommended. For women in labor who have thick meconium staining of the amniotic fluid, amnioinfusion does not reduce the risk of moderate or severe meconium aspiration syndrome, perinatal death, or other major maternal or neonatal disorders. Prophylactic use of amnioinfusion for meconium-stained amniotic fluid should be done only in the setting of additional clinical trials. Data are not available to determine whether amnioinfusion for fetal heart rate decelerations in the presence of meconium-stained amniotic fluid decreases meconium aspiration syndrome or other meconium-related morbidities.

Different protocols for amnioinfusion are used. However, they all appear to be safe, easy to perform, and associated with few complications.

INDICATION

Repeated severe or prolonged (e.g., lasting longer than the contraction) variable fetal heart rate decelerations that are unresponsive to conventional therapy (e.g., left-sided labor, intravenous hydration, oxygen therapy), regardless of amniotic fluid meconium status, are the indication for amnioinfusion.

EDITOR'S NOTE: Obviously, amnioinfusion might be a consideration during labor in *many* pregnancies because variable decelerations are very common. In reality, experienced clinicians use amnioinfusion in certain selected situations. An example is the multiparous patient who has only an hour or so remaining before the second stage of labor, yet the fetal strip shows very deep, severe variables that last a long time (perhaps as long as the contraction). We have all nervously watched such a labor fearing that these deep variables may exhaust the fetus. It is reassuring to have amnioinfusion available as a possible preventive measure. A similar situation may be seen with oligohydramnios, or even borderline oligohydramnios. Often these infants endure a stormy labor with deep variables early in labor. Amnioinfusion may be an option in these situations.

CONTRAINDICATIONS

- Amnionitis
- Polyhydramnios
- Uterine hypertonus
- Multiple gestation
- Known fetal anomaly
- Known uterine anomaly
- Severe fetal distress
- Nonvertex presentation
- Fetal scalp pH <7.20
- Placental abruption or placenta previa (known or suspected)
- Patient refusal or uncooperative patient

EQUIPMENT

- Intrauterine pressure catheter (see Chapter 171, Intrauterine Pressure Catheter Insertion)
- Normal saline or lactated Ringer's at room temperature
- Fetal monitor
- Intravenous tubing
- Intravenous pump
- Fetal scalp electrode*
- Sterile gloves (for insertion)
- Vaginal lubricant (for insertion)
- Fluid warmer (if the fluid is to be infused at a rate >15 mL/min)

PREPROCEDURE PATIENT PREPARATION

Before performing the procedure, discuss it with the patient (and family, if present). Inform her of the risks and explain why amnioinfusion should be beneficial. (For severe repetitive or prolonged variable decelerations, amnioinfusion decreases the number of variable decelerations and cesarean sections and possibly the risk of postpartum endometritis.) Describe alternative modes of intervention (if applicable) and obtain informed consent. Answer any questions that the patient (or family) may have.

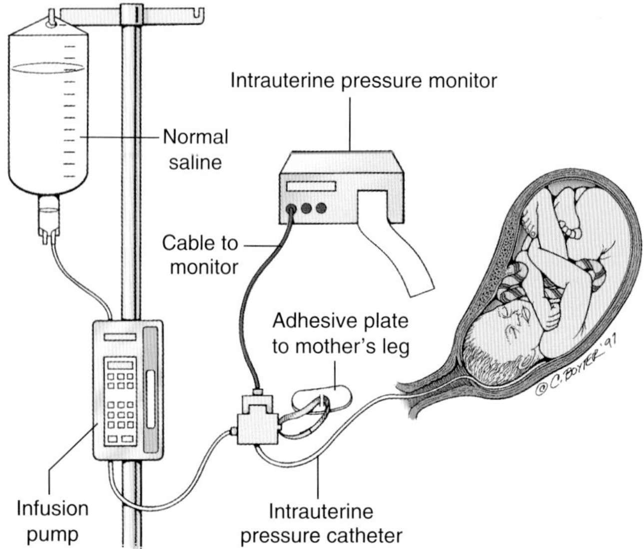

Figure 176-1 **Procedure for amnioinfusion.** (From Weismiller DG: Transcervical amnioinfusion. Am Fam Physician 57:504–510, 1998.)

TECHNIQUE

1. Perform a sterile vaginal examination to confirm cephalic presentation and that the membranes are ruptured (see Chapter 164, Amniotomy), determine the degree of dilation, and exclude a cord prolapse.
2. Place a fetal scalp electrode (recommended, not required; see Chapter 168, Fetal Scalp Electrode Application) or ensure adequate fetal monitoring.
3. Insert an intrauterine pressure catheter (see Chapter 171, Intrauterine Pressure Catheter Insertion) and document the resting tone. The resting tone should be less than 15 mm Hg.
4. Link room-temperature normal saline (or lactated Ringer's) to the intravenous tubing. Prime the tubing as would be done for intravenous use.
5. Attach the tubing to the infusion port of the intrauterine pressure catheter (Fig. 176-1).
6. For patients with repetitive severe or prolonged variable decelerations
   - Start the infusion with an initial bolus of 250 to 500 mL of fluid over 20 to 30 minutes.
   - Next, adjust the rate of infusion according to the severity of decelerations. The usual infusion rate is 10 to 20 mL/min up to a total of 600 to 800 mL infused or until resolution of the variable decelerations, if that occurs first. (Other experts start with a bolus of 500 mL of room-temperature fluid followed by a continuous infusion of 3 mL/min.)
   - With resolution, continue the infusion for an additional 250 mL beyond the volume at which the decelerations resolved.
   - Terminate the infusion if 800 to 1000 mL of saline does not resolve the decelerations. However, if decelerations do not resolve completely, yet there is an increase in frequency and severity when the fluid is discontinued, it may be prudent to resume the infusion.
7. Warm the fluid to body temperature if it is administered at a rate greater than 15 mL/min.
8. Monitor fetal heart rate and resting uterine tone continuously during the intervention; monitor intrauterine pressure using the same intrauterine pressure catheter, a second one, or a double-lumen catheter.
9. Discontinue the infusion if uterine tone becomes persistently elevated or if the flow of fluid from the vagina stops. Allow the uterine pressure to equilibrate over 5 minutes and reassess the resting uterine tone. Discontinue the infusion if the new resting tone is 15 mm Hg above the baseline resting tone or 30 mm Hg maximum.
10. After the initial bolus, it is extremely important to verify that fluid is flowing from the vagina and that volume overload is not occurring.

COMPLICATIONS

There are occasional amnioinfusion failures. The possible causes for failure include inadequate infusion volume or rate, rapid progression to second stage of labor, or cord complications; however, the cause of the majority of failures is unknown.

In another teaching hospital survey intended to determine how, when, and with what results amnioinfusion is being performed in the United States, it was found that neither the method used nor the number of infusions performed appears to significantly increase the risk for complications. The fact that the mean number of amnioinfusions performed per year is similar between centers that did and centers that did not report complications suggests that complications are generally infrequent or, perhaps, that the risk of complication decreases as clinician experience increases. (It also might indicate a reporting problem!)

- Isolated cases of umbilical cord prolapse have been reported, but they are well within the usual occurrence rate of prolapse in pregnancies with vertex presentation, even when amnioinfusion is not used.
- Uterine tone may increase and hypertonus has been reported; thus monitoring intrauterine pressure, the total volume infused, and the continuous flow of fluid from the vagina is important. In one study, this was the most common complication.
- Abnormal fetal heart rate tracings were the second most common complication in one study.
- Prolonged fetal bradycardia has been reported after rapid administration (50 mL/min) of unwarmed fluid.
- Prophylactic amnioinfusion (although not recommended) was associated with increased intrapartum fever.

*Recommended, not required.

- Other reported rare complications
  - Uterine scar disruption (one reported case)
  - Iatrogenic polyhydramnios and elevated intrauterine pressure resulting in fetal bradycardia (one reported case)
  - Amniotic fluid embolism (five reported cases, all associated with previously reported risk factors for amniotic fluid embolism)
- Rare complications associated with placement of an intrauterine pressure catheter
  - Uterine perforation
  - Umbilical cord trauma
  - Placental abruption
  - Fetal trauma
- Amnionitis is a possible complication. Prolonged use of an intrauterine pressure catheter is also associated with an increased risk of amnionitis and perinatal infection.

NOTE: Most trials reviewed have been too small to address the possibility of rare but serious adverse maternal effects of amnioinfusion.

Patient Education Guides

See patient education and patient consent forms available online at www.expertconsult.com.

CPT/Billing Code

59899 Unlisted procedure, maternity care and delivery

ICD-9-CM Diagnostic Codes

656.33 Fetal distress, antepartum
659.73 Abnormality in fetal heart rate or rhythm, antepartum
663.2 Cord compression

Online Resource

Birthsource.com: Amnioinfusion. Available at www.birthsource.com/scripts/article.asp?articleid=42. Accessed July 31, 2008.

Bibliography

American College of Obstetricians and Gynecologists: Amnioinfusion does not prevent meconium aspiration syndrome. Committee opinion no. 346. Washington, DC, American College of Obstetricians and Gynecologists, 2006.

Fraser WD, Hofmeyr GJ, Lede R, et al: Amnioinfusion for the prevention of meconium aspiration syndrome. N Engl J Med 353:909–917, 2005.

Hofmeyr GJ: Amnioinfusion for meconium-stained liquor in labour. Cochrane Database Syst Rev 1:CD000014, 2002.

Hofmeyr GJ: Amnioinfusion for potential or suspected umbilical cord compression in labour. Cochrane Database Syst Rev 2:CD001182, 2005.

Xu H, Hofmeyr J, Roy C, Fraser WD: Intrapartum amnioinfusion for meconium-stained amniotic fluid: A systematic review of randomized controlled trials. Br J Obstet Gynaecol 114:383–390, 2007.

CHAPTER 177

VAGINAL DELIVERY

Dale A. Patterson • Coral D. Matus • Jacob Curtis

Vaginal delivery is a natural process that has gradually become a medical procedure. Although early medical efforts were successful at decreasing the maternal and fetal death rates, more recent and advanced interventions have not been shown to be as successful. Despite routine use in numerous settings, interventions such as electronic fetal monitoring, routine amniotomy, and fetal pulse oximetry have not been shown to improve outcomes. A few medical interventions, including routine episiotomy, have actually been shown to be harmful to the mother or the baby. As in all aspects of modern medicine, new information is available on a regular basis, and it is prudent to stay up to date with this information if attending deliveries.

Even though it is a natural process, labor and delivery is also very complex and varies among patients. Labor can last as little as an hour or less in some patients and take several days in others. The underlying hormonal changes associated with labor are only superficially understood. It is beyond the scope of this text to explore all of the possible variables and complications that could occur during a vaginal delivery. The focus of this chapter is on the uncomplicated vaginal delivery of a single newborn in the vertex position. When available, evidence-based recommendations will be made regarding the delivery technique.

Women in labor frequently undergo procedures related to vaginal delivery. Many of these are described in Section 10, Obstetrics, Chapters 161–177.

ANATOMY

Vaginal delivery begins with the onset of true labor, which is defined by the onset of contractions that are regular, are of increasing intensity, and cause progressive dilation and effacement of the cervix with descent of the fetal presenting part.

Labor is divided into three progressive stages: *first stage*, from onset of labor until complete cervical dilation; *second stage*, from complete dilation to delivery of the infant; and *third stage*, from delivery of the infant to delivery of the placenta.

The average time of each stage is different for nulliparas than for multiparas (Table 177-1). The cervix should dilate 1 cm/hour or more in nulliparas and 1.2 cm/hour or more in multiparas, once active labor begins. Descent should occur at 1 cm/hour or more in nulliparas and at least 2 cm/hour in multiparas. Protraction disorders are defined by a rate of either dilation or descent slower than these minimums.

The first stage of labor may be subdivided into two phases: latent and active. Latent phase labor may occur prior to the onset of the active phase. Latent labor is characterized by mild, irregular uterine contractions that cause softening, effacement, and slow dilation of the cervix. A prolonged latent phase is defined as more than 25 hours for nulliparas and 14 hours for multiparas. Progression at a rate below those defined numbers may warrant intervention, especially in a post-term or prolonged pregnancy (see Chapter 163, Induction of Labor).

As the cervix dilates, the fetus starts its descent through the birth canal. Using the force of each contraction, the fetal head negotiates incrementally through the angles of the maternal pelvis, following a standard pattern known as the cardinal movements of labor:

1. Engagement
   - Defined by descent of the biparietal diameter of the fetus to a level below the maternal pelvic inlet. The borders of the pelvic inlet are formed by the sacral promontory posteriorly and the inner pubic arch anteriorly; this diameter is also referred to as the "obstetric conjugate." In most cases, the anteroposterior diameter of the pelvic inlet is the smallest dimension. Thus, the smallest diameter of the fetal head (biparietal diameter) must align with the anteroposterior diameter of the pelvic inlet.
   - Suggested clinically when the lowest portion of the occiput (not caput) is palpated at or below the maternal ischial spines (0 station).
   - In most cases, it indicates the maternal pelvic inlet is sufficient to allow descent of the head.
   - Often occurs before the onset of labor, especially in nulliparas.
   - Verification may be difficult if the fetal head is molded or in the occipitoposterior (OP) presentation.
2. Descent (Fig. 177-1)
   - Slow, progressive process.
   - Measured by station (level of presenting part) and quantified by number of centimeters the presenting part is above (e.g., −2, −1) or below (e.g., +1, +2) the ischial spines.
3. Flexion
   - The force of contractions against the cervix and maternal tissue eventually pushes the head into a flexed position so that the smallest diameter of the fetal head presents primarily, further aiding in descent of the presenting part (Fig. 177-2A). It remains in this position until the head has descended to the level of the vulva.

TABLE 177-1 Average Lengths and Upper Limits of Normal for Stages of Labor in Primiparous and Multiparous Women

	Lengths	
Stage of Labor	**Primiparous Women**	**Multiparous Women**
First (latent phase)	5.9 to 6.4 (25.1*) hrs	4.8 (13.6*) hrs
First (active phase)	3.3 to 7.7 (17.5*) hrs	3 to 7 (13.8*) hrs
Second	33 to 54 (146*) mins	8.5 to 18 (64*) mins
Third	5 (30*) mins	5 (30*) mins

*Upper limit of normal.
From Patterson DA, Winslow M, Matus CD: Spontaneous vaginal delivery. Am Fam Physician 78:336–341, 343–344, 2008.

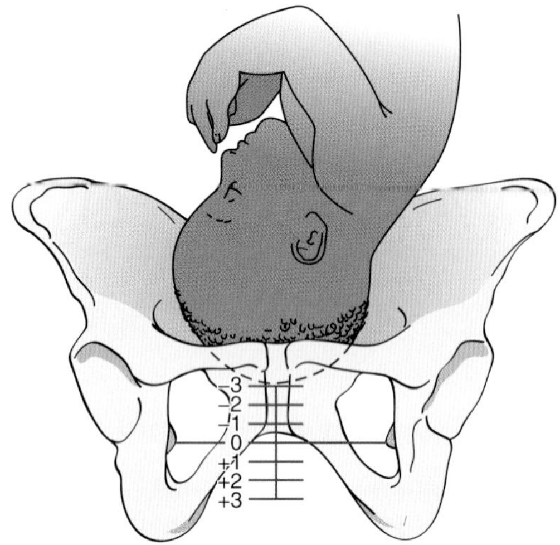

Figure 177-1 Descent of fetal head into the pelvis. Zero station is diagnosed when the fetal vertex has reached the level of the ischial spines. (Redrawn from Niswander K: Obstetrics: Essentials of Clinical Practice, 2nd ed. Boston, Little, Brown, 1981.)

- Normally, the posterior fontanelle is in the center of the dilating cervix, allowing for optimal "molding" of the fetal cranial bones and sutures.
- Infants in an OP position often assume a more "deflexed" position due to their orientation in the maternal pelvis. This causes a less favorable alignment between the fetal head (passenger) and the maternal pelvis (passageway).

4. Internal rotation
   - As the fetal head continues to descend, the biparietal diameter of the fetus rotates to align with the lateral diameter (intertuberous diameter, or the distance between the ischial tuberosities) of the maternal pelvic outlet. Typically this intertuberous diameter constitutes the smallest dimension of the pelvic outlet. The borders of the pelvic outlet are formed by the ischial tuberosities laterally, and the angle of the pubic symphysis anteriorly.
   - The final position of the vertex is usually left occipitoanterior (LOA) (Fig. 177-2B), occipitoanterior (OA) (Fig. 177-2C), or right occipitoanterior (ROA); however, in about 5 to 10 percent of cases, the vertex presents in an OP position.
5. Extension
   - The force of contractions from above meets the force of resistance from the pelvic muscles below and interacts to use the pubic symphysis as a fulcrum. This combination of forces and a fulcrum pushes the head around the pubic bone (Fig. 177-2D).
   - The head becomes extended with delivery as a result of these forces.
   - Extension occurs fairly rapidly and is observed clinically when the perineum distends.
6. External rotation and restitution
   - After delivery, the head rotates back to a transverse position and the shoulders rotate into an anteroposterior (AP) position, before they are delivered (Fig. 177-2E).

Although dilation and descent may occur predictably, more often the pattern of labor is irregular and erratic. The original labor curves plotted by Friedman in the 1950s have since been adjusted to fit a slower average progression of labor as seen in many patients with epidural analgesia (see Table 177-1). Common pitfalls of early labor management include admission to the hospital too early during latent phase labor. Women admitted in latent labor tend to spend more time in the labor unit and have more interventions than those in whom admission is delayed until active labor is confirmed.

In an attempt to reduce prolonged labor in nulliparas, the active management of labor (AML) protocol was created and studied at the National Maternity Hospital in Dublin, Ireland. AML refers to active control, rather than passive observation, by the obstetric provider during the active phase of the first stage of labor. Initially, this protocol demonstrated a shortened labor and a decrease in the cesarean delivery rate. Subsequent studies in the United States did

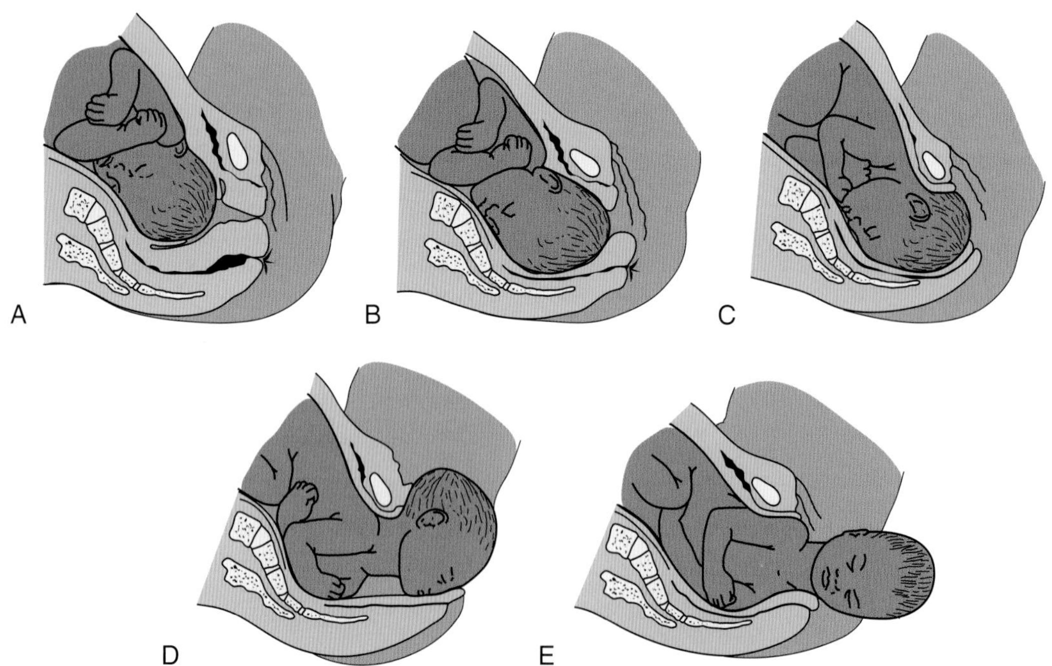

Figure 177-2 **A,** Engagement of flexed head. **B,** Left occipitoanterior (LOA) position. **C,** Internal, anterior rotation of head to occipitoanterior (OA) position. **D,** Extension of head. **E,** External rotation of head. (Redrawn from Pernoll M: Benson and Pernoll's Handbook of Obstetrics and Gynecology, 9th ed. New York, McGraw-Hill, 2001.)

not confirm the decrease in cesarean deliveries. This protocol has generated much controversy and there is no clear consensus that it should be universally adopted. However, it may be appropriate for some patients. The AML protocol for nulliparas has four underlying tenets.

1. Extensive prenatal education
   - Women are educated about the signs of true labor and reasonable expectations during active labor. They are also assured that they will have continuous support during labor. Continuous support by an experienced (parous) laywoman or doula and emotional support early in labor may be more critical than support given to a woman after she is admitted to the hospital and may have already chosen an epidural.
2. A specific definition of labor, which includes not only the presence of painful uterine contractions, but also *one* of the following:
   - Presence of bloody show (blood-stained mucus)
   - Complete cervical effacement, regardless of dilation
   - Rupture of the membranes

   NOTE: The correct diagnosis of labor is considered to be the single most important factor in AML because an incorrect diagnosis may lead to inappropriate or ineffective interventions.
3. Close monitoring of labor progress, every 1 hour for the first 3 hours after diagnosis of labor and admission to the labor ward. Subsequently, examinations are performed at no longer than 2-hour intervals. If cervical dilation is not progressing at a rate of at least 1 cm/hour, intervention is indicated.
4. Intervention if progress does not proceed as expected
   - Early amniotomy (1 hour after admission, see Chapter 164, Amniotomy) to allow assessment of amniotic fluid was a component of the original AML protocol, although it has not been shown to significantly reduce the duration of labor.
   - High-dose oxytocin (start with 6 mU/min and increase every 15 minutes) was also a component of the original AML protocol. Subsequent studies have questioned the safety of such high-dose protocols, citing complications such as maternal water intoxication and uterine hyperstimulation.

INDICATIONS

- Vertex presentation, active labor, vulva distended, and deliverable baby
- Fetal distress in a deliverable baby

CONTRAINDICATIONS

Absolute

- Cord prolapse
- Complete placenta previa or vasa previa
- Abnormal fetal lie (e.g., footling breech, transverse lie, persistent brow presentation)
- Prior classical cesarean section or transfundal uterine surgery
- Herpes simplex infection with active genital lesions or prodromal symptoms
- Untreated human immunodeficiency virus (HIV) infection

Relative

- Pelvic deformities
- Congenital deformities (hydrocephalus)
- Invasive cervical carcinoma
- Treated HIV infection
- Macrosomia
- Malpresentation (including breech)
- Previous low transverse cesarean deliveries
- Multiple gestation

EQUIPMENT AND SUPPLIES

Although equipment setups vary, depending on the hospital or the staff, the following list is found in a standard *birthing room*. In addition to what is listed, deliveries in an *operating room* require a full gown, a mask, and foot and head covers.

- Oxygen with flowmeter (one setup for mother and another for infant)
- Delivery bed (should be able to break down into a modified lithotomy position and have adjustable height)
- Setups for uterine contraction and fetal monitoring (optional, see Chapter 168, Fetal Scalp Electrode Application)
- Setup for infant (infant warmer, oxygen with bag and mask, suction with DeLee, infant laryngoscope, intubation equipment, umbilical catheter, medications, and monitoring equipment for resuscitation [see Chapter 180, Neonatal Resuscitation])
- Sterile equipment tray or table containing the following (Fig. 177-3)
  - 10-mL tube for cord blood
  - Two pairs of scissors (blunt Mayo-Noble straight scissors for cutting the cord and episiotomy and sharp scissors for cutting suture and dressings)
  - Bulb syringe
  - One plastic cord clamp (may use curved artery Kocher clamp for the other; some clinicians use three plastic cord clamps if cord blood is routinely sent for gases)
  - Two curved artery Kocher clamps (some clinicians like to have four of these clamps, especially if cord blood gases are to be sent)
  - Needle holder
  - Two ring forceps clamps (also called a sponge stick or placenta forceps)
  - Drapes and towels (including under buttocks drape with fluid pouch)
  - Placenta basin
  - Gown (optional) and sterile gloves (latex-free recommended)
- Optional equipment for sterile tray or table (also see Chapter 166, Episiotomy and Repair of the Perineum)
  - Additional pair needle holder
  - Two Allis clamps (for third- or fourth-degree repair)
  - Two thumb tissue forceps (one with teeth and one without teeth)
  - Gelpi retractor (for added visualization during a third- or fourth-degree repair)

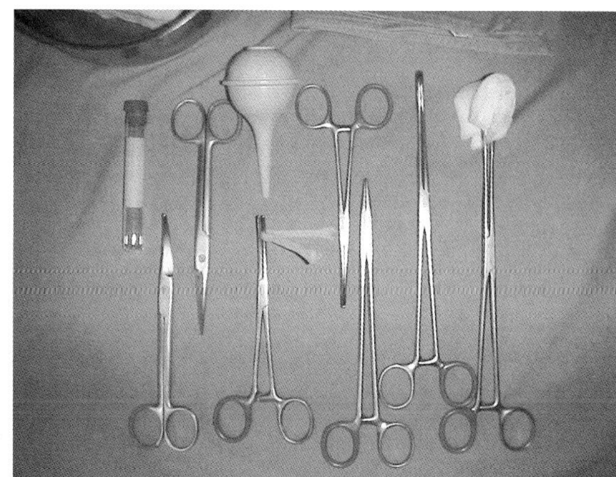

Figure 177-3 Instruments for vaginal delivery. *Left to right:* Cord blood tube, two scissors (blunt and sharp edge), bulb syringe, plastic cord clamp, two curved artery Kocher clamps (one is holding plastic cord clamp), needle holder, two ring forceps (one grasping folded 4 × 4 gauze is called sponge stick).

- Weighted speculum (offers greater visualization of the vaginal wall and cervix)
- 10-mL syringe
- 22-gauge, 1½-inch needle (for local anesthesia)
- 1% lidocaine, without epinephrine
- Two 3-0 absorbable synthetic sutures with tapered needles
- Gauze pads (4 × 4 inch)
- Sterile speculum
- Red rubber, straight, in and out catheter— povidone–iodine, chlorhexidine, or surgical soap or solution for preparation
- Emergency kit (for precipitous deliveries)
  - Sterile gloves (large size)
  - Two sterile towels
  - One pair of blunt-ended scissors
  - One plastic cord clamp
  - Two curved artery Kocher clamps
  - Gauze pads (4 × 4 inch)
  - Bulb syringe
  - Placenta basin

Precautions

All women with prior history of cesarean delivery for any indication should be cautioned about the options for mode of delivery in subsequent pregnancies and the risks and benefits of each option. Certain patients (those with prior "classical" or "T" type uterine incision) should be cautioned against laboring. Those with a single prior low transverse uterine incision should be allowed to consider a trial of labor with informed consent. It is imperative that these patients understand the risk of uterine rupture with vaginal delivery and the risks of repeat surgical delivery. Selecting women most likely to give birth vaginally (e.g., those with prior vaginal birth or those with indication for prior cesarean delivery other than dystocia) and avoiding the use of prostaglandins or misoprostol offer the lowest risk of complication. Many institutions have strict criteria for allowing women with prior cesarean delivery to attempt a vaginal birth after cesarean delivery (VBAC). It is prudent to ensure that facilities are able to provide immediate repeat cesarean delivery in case of emergency and that close monitoring by trained personnel is available.

Group B streptococcus (GBS) colonization occurs in 10% to 30% of women. The incidence of early onset neonatal infection with GBS, the most common serious infection of the newborn period, can be reduced with intrapartum chemoprophylaxis of women who test positive for GBS. The Centers for Disease Control and Prevention recommends routine screening for GBS in all pregnant women at 35 to 37 weeks' gestation with rectal and vaginal swab. If positive, treatment with penicillin (5 million units) at least 4 hours prior to delivery and repeat doses every 4 hours (2.5 million units) is first-line therapy. If unable to use penicillin, options for GBS prophylaxis during labor include ampicillin, cefazolin, clindamycin, erythromycin, and vancomycin. Other indications for intrapartum prophylaxis are GBS bacteriuria during pregnancy and previous neonatal infection with GBS. Women with these risks should not be screened at 35 to 37 weeks; they should just be treated (regardless of results).

Other maternal conditions that warrant preprocedure evaluation and counseling include maternal cardiovascular conditions, coagulopathies, diabetes, and other chronic medical conditions. Discussion of each of these is beyond the scope of this text, but each patient with potential complications should have an appropriate management plan prior to the onset of labor and a labor and birth plan accounting for the risks formulated.

Preprocedure Patient Education

One focus of prenatal care is education. In an ideal situation, the patient will have several months to prepare and numerous encounters with her provider prior to a vaginal delivery. The breadth of prenatal education is beyond the scope of this text. There are many resources available to guide education and many prenatal record keeping products incorporate education into their program. See the resources listed under "Useful Continuing Education" later in this chapter.

In general, a pregnant patient should be educated about the process of pregnancy and behaviors that increase her chances of an uncomplicated delivery with a healthy newborn. Topics that should be addressed in pregnancy include whether to continue exercise and for how long; avoiding tobacco, alcohol, and other drugs; and eating a healthy diet.

The birth process is intimidating for many women, especially first-time mothers. Education about the normal birth process can greatly relieve these fears and improve a women's experience of labor. Some form of a birth plan is helpful for the patient and the provider (Fig. 177-4). Topics to discuss include pain control, the uncertainty of labor, and the possibility of interventions, including episiotomy and cesarean delivery. The patient should be encouraged to ask questions so that her concerns are adequately addressed.

As the rate of operative deliveries in the United States continues to increase, more patients may express a desire for an elective cesarean delivery or a repeat cesarean delivery. The question of whether a patient should be allowed to choose an elective primary cesarean delivery is an ethical debate. Despite advances in anesthesia and surgical care, a vaginal delivery is a safer procedure than a cesarean delivery. Vaginal birth after cesarean delivery can also be a safe procedure in the appropriate setting. See earlier discussion under "Precautions."

Overall, patients should be educated about the normal birth process and the risks and benefits of the multiple options they may encounter during labor. Because vaginal delivery is the safest method of delivery, it should be encouraged. The provider should be aware of local standards of care and communicate these to the patient prior to the onset of labor when they may affect the management of her labor.

Technique

First Stage

Management of the first stage of labor should be passive during the latent phase. Once the active phase has begun, labor should be monitored for progression and intervention considered if adequate progress toward delivery is not achieved. AML can be considered by the patient and maternity care provider. Arrest of labor is defined as no change in dilation with adequate contractions for 2 hours. Adequacy of contractions can be assessed by inserting an intrauterine pressure catheter (IUPC; see Chapter 171, Intrauterine Pressure Catheter Insertion). Although there is no definitive time to mandate cesarean delivery, it should be considered after 2 to 4 hours of oxytocin augmentation of labor without cervical change.

Second Stage

Typically, as the cervix nears complete dilation, the intensity of the contractions increases and the patient starts to feel the urge to push. Even if the patient has regional anesthesia, she will usually feel pressure as the fetus begins to descend more rapidly. When the cervix is completely dilated, the second stage of labor has begun and the patient may begin to push. It is contraindicated to push prior to complete dilation of the cervix as soft tissue injury and maternal exhaustion are likely.

After the second stage of labor has begun, the length of time until delivery varies (see Table 177-1). Two or three explosive pushes may be enough to deliver a multipara, whereas a nullipara with regional anesthesia may push for more than an hour. If labor stalls during this stage, oxytocin augmentation should be considered. To prevent maternal exhaustion, if the infant is stable, alternating periods of rest and pushing is recommended. If the mother is comfortable and the infant appears to be tolerating the labor process, it

Anticipatory Guidance and Patient Preferences for Birthing Plan (Checklist Completed by Clinician)

Patient name: ______________________________

Date: ______________ **Clinician:** ______________________

Answers to the following will help determine the patient's individual preferences and amount of preparation during prenatal care, labor, and postpartum care:

Is prenatal birth education (Lamaze) planned? ☐ Yes ☐ No

Who will attend Lamaze? ______________________

If no rupture of membranes has occurred (ROM), is an enema desired? ☐ Yes ☐ No

Diet preferences: ☐ Clear liquids ☐ Ice chips ☐ Nothing

IV access preferences: ☐ Hep-Lock ☐ None ☐ IV with lactated Ringer's at 100 mL/hr

Fetal assessment (low-risk patient):

- ☐ Continuous electronic fetal monitoring for 20 minutes (baseline strip); then, if baseline is reassuring, periodic auscultation every 30 minutes in first stage, then every 15 minutes in second stage (auscultation done during contraction and for 30 seconds following).
- ☐ Continuous electronic fetal monitoring.
- ☐ Scalp clip okay.

Preferences for maximizing comfort during labor (anesthesia?): ____________ Position ____________

Father to be present during labor? ☐ Yes ☐ No

Female support person (doula) to be present? ☐ Yes ☐ No

Patient attitude toward episiotomy? ______ (desired) ______ (only if necessary)

Infant feeding preferences? ☐ Breast-feeding ☐ Bottle feeding

For male infant, is circumcision desired? ☐ Yes ☐ No

Preferred clinician for baby: ______________________

Rooming-in with baby? ☐ Yes ☐ No

Postpartum contraception preference: ______________________

Baby's name? ______________________

Hospital preregistration? ☐ Yes ☐ No

Mother has visited labor and delivery? ☐ Yes ☐ No

Encouraged intrapartum ambulation, frequent position changes? ☐ Yes ☐ No

Practiced positions for emergencies (e.g., knee chest, rolling onto hands/knees)? ☐ Yes ☐ No

If the clinician provides anticipatory guidance, it may not only improve the outcomes, but it may also give mother a greater sense of security. The results of this questionnaire should be dictated or copied, signed by the patient, and a copy given to the patient. She should bring it to labor and delivery when admitted.

Figure 177-4 Sample birthing plan.

is reasonable to delay pushing until the vertex is at the introitus or the mother feels a strong urge to push. If the vertex is at +2 or greater station, forceps or vacuum-assisted delivery may be considered after 1 hour of pushing in a multipara or 2 hours in a primipara (after 2 hours in a multipara or 3 hours in a nullipara if a regional anesthetic is being used; see also Chapter 169, Forceps- and Vacuum-Assisted Deliveries).

One of the most common reasons for a prolonged second stage of labor is persistent OP position. On average, the OP position will prolong labor by 1 hour in multiparas and 2 hours in nulliparas. Consider the possibility of OP position if labor is predominantly felt in the back. A persistent anterior cervical lip or an easily palpable anterior fontanelle may also be associated with the OP position. To confirm the OP position by examination, the infant's skull sutures should be followed until the posterior fontanelle can be palpated. (Recall that the anterior fontanelle is shaped like a cross or plus (+) and is usually larger than the posterior fontanelle; the posterior fontanelle is shaped like a Y.) If an ear is palpable, the direction that the ear is facing will also help determine which direction the baby is facing.

To rotate the fetus from the OP position, any maternal position that causes her to curl forward from the hips is felt to be helpful. Various positions and activities can be tried, such as squatting or ambulating, or placing mother on her hands and knees, on her side, or with her back arched. The theory is that with most of these positions, the infant will become uncomfortable and be encouraged to turn itself. If the various positions fail to cause rotation, manual rotation can be attempted. Place the mother in the lithotomy, lateral Sims', or hands and knees position. With a hand in the posterior pelvis behind the occiput, attempt to rotate and flex the head, during a contraction, while the mother is pushing. If the fetus is straight OP, the clinician's dominant hand should be used. If the fetus is partially rotated, use whichever hand is easiest to rotate it in the direction of the shortest distance to OA. (If a vacuum-assisted delivery is to be performed, the vacuum device can sometimes help rotate the infant from OP to OA; see Chapter 169, Forceps- and Vacuum-Assisted Deliveries.)

Preparation for delivery should begin at the onset of the second stage for the multipara and as the vertex reaches the pelvic floor in the nullipara.

Preparation

1. Put on sterile gloves and consider a gown. Remember to observe universal blood and body fluid precautions.
2. Prepare the delivery tray.
3. Turn on the warmer for the bassinette and notify the nursery staff for meconium-staining or fetal distress. Make sure that all necessary equipment is available for a neonatal resuscitation (see Chapter 180, Neonatal Resuscitation).
4. Verify that all needed equipment is on the sterile tray or table and within reaching distance. Empty the mother's bladder (usually requires using a catheter with aseptic technique if she has had an epidural).
5. Make an attempt to rotate a persistent OP vertex to an OA position if necessary.
6. Wash the perineal area with a surgical soap or solution (*optional*). There is no evidence to support shaving the perineum or enemas at this stage of delivery.

Position of the Woman

Allow the patient to find a comfortable position for pushing and resting (Fig. 177-5). The rationale for each position is noted here, as well as possible inconveniences or complications for each position:

1. Modified dorsal
   - Semisitting position with knees flexed and legs widely separated; the mother can grip below her knees for leverage when pushing
   - Good position for multipara deliveries
2. Squatting, kneeling (see Fig. 177-5A)
   - More physiologic for pushing
   - Less discomfort with pushing
   - Fewer perineal tears
   - Increased incidence of hemorrhage
3. Lithotomy (see Fig. 177-5B)
   - Better access for the provider, so this position is often used for instrumentation
   - Difficult position for pushing
   - Increased risk for maternal aspiration
4. Left lateral (see Fig. 177-5C)
   - Left side with knees flexed and separated
   - Offers better clinician access for head control
   - Need an assistant to hold upper leg

Anesthesia (Optional)

- Regional anesthesia (see Chapter 3, Epidural Anesthesia and Analgesia; Chapter 170, Intrathecal Analgesia in Labor; and Chapter 175, Saddle Block Anesthesia)
- Paracervical block, for first stage of labor to decrease the discomfort with contractions (see Chapter 173, Paracervical Block)
- Pudendal block, for perineal pain (see Chapter 174, Pudendal Anesthesia)
- Local infiltration of lidocaine if episiotomy is required (routine episiotomy is contraindicated; see Chapter 166, Episiotomy and Repair of the Perineum)

Delivery

There are many variations in technique for vaginal delivery. There is not one "right" way to deliver a vertex infant. Two commonly debated techniques are the "hands on" and "hands poised" techniques. Essentially, the "hands on" technique is a process by which the provider puts pressure on the baby's head and supports the mother's perineum throughout the delivery process. The "hands poised" technique requires the provider to allow spontaneous

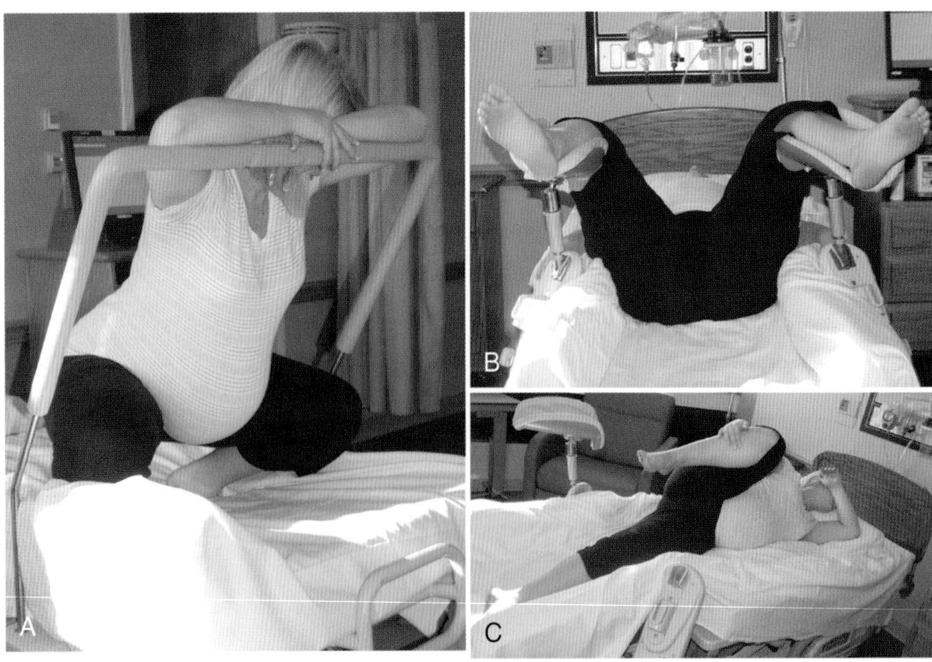

Figure 177-5 Maternal birthing positions. **A,** Squatting; **B,** lithotomy; **C,** left lateral.

delivery of the head prior to any intervention. No significant differences in outcomes have been shown between the two methods and either is acceptable practice. This section will describe the "hands on" technique. The "hands poised" method is similar after delivery of the infant's head.

1. Observe the perineum for distention due to the fetal head. When the head is visible ("crowning"), it is appropriate to apply pressure to the infant's head to control the force of delivery and to support the perineum with gentle pressure. Either hand may be used.
2. If an episiotomy is to be performed, the best time to perform it is when the opening is 5 to 6 cm (see Chapter 166, Episiotomy and Repair of the Perineum). This procedure is clearly *not* indicated as a routine part of every vaginal delivery. It is usually performed only if it is unsafe for the mother to push (cardiac disease or prolonged second stage), for significant fetal distress (to expedite delivery), before reducing a shoulder dystocia, if an infant is premature or breech, or to make room if there is risk of perineal trauma (e.g., large infant or use of forceps or vacuum). Many episiotomies are appropriately cut at the time an indication presents and may not be performed at this "ideal" time.
3. As the head advances, make sure to control its progress. Maintain flexion of the head with pressure applied through a towel placed on the perineum. The head should be delivered slowly, in a controlled manner, as it edges forward with each contraction. Between contractions the head will gradually extend. Recall that as the head extends, it will increase in diameter. Therefore, do not allow the head to extend too rapidly or the chin may tear the perineum. In other words, palpate the chin (through the towel over the perineum), and prevent it from "popping" (suddenly extending) and tearing the perineum.
4. If a rapid delivery is necessary (e.g., fetal distress) or assistance is needed (e.g., inadequate pushing because of regional anesthesia or maternal exhaustion), a modified Ritgen maneuver can be used. The Ritgen maneuver merely assists or exacerbates the extension of the fetal head. To perform it, while palpating the infant's chin (through the towel on the perineum), pull outward on the chin and then press it upward to extend the head. Again, this effort should be weighed against the possibility of the chin "popping" through the perineum and tearing it. In most cases, the chin can be controlled and extended enough for delivery without "popping" the perineum.
5. For an OP delivery, the head is usually delivered more readily by applying flexion, not extension. The tension on the perineum can be very high, resulting in a third- or fourth-degree laceration. Again, assisting and controlling the amount of flexion with a hand, through the towel on the perineum, may minimize the risk of lacerations.
6. As the head is slowly delivered, reach around the neck to check for and reduce a nuchal cord (occurs in 20% of deliveries). Reduction is accomplished by pulling the cord over the delivered head. If the nuchal cord cannot be reduced, it can be doubly clamped and cut at the perineum. (At that point, the infant should be delivered without delay because the infant's blood supply and oxygenation are interrupted until fully delivered.) After the head is delivered, in most cases the mother should be instructed to stop pushing. Wipe the mucus off the infant's nose and mouth while suctioning both orifices with a bulb syringe. The head has now rotated to allow the shoulders to assume an AP position.
7. Delivery of the shoulders should be performed with slow and deliberate motions and without exerting excessive traction. Gently depress the head toward the maternal coccyx (Fig. 177-6A), and when the anterior shoulder has passed the symphysis (downward traction becomes much easier and a "pop" may be felt), lift the fetal head upward (Fig. 177-6B). Lifting the head in this way allows for delivery of the posterior shoulder. It is important to protect the perineum again with one hand through a sterile towel. As the posterior shoulder is delivered, it should also be prevented from "popping" through the perineum and tearing a third- or fourth-degree laceration. If shoulder dystocia is a concern, attempt to deliver the head and shoulders in one continuous motion, which may prevent the anterior shoulder from lodging or becoming impacted against the symphysis.

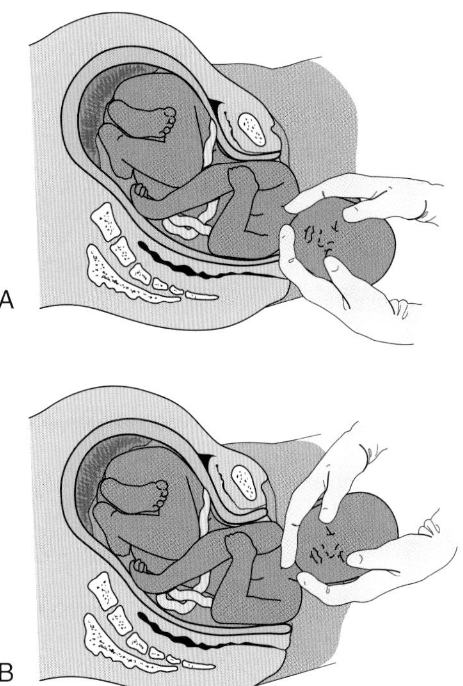

Figure 177-6 **A,** Gentle downward traction to bring about descent of anterior shoulder. **B,** With delivery of the anterior shoulder completed, applying gentle upward traction delivers the posterior shoulder. (Redrawn from Ratcliffe S, Baxley EG, Byrd J, Sakornbut E: Family Practice Obstetrics, 2nd ed. Philadelphia, Hanley & Belfus, 2001.)

EDITOR'S NOTE: Although management of shoulder dystocia is beyond the scope of this chapter (see "Useful Continuing Education" section), one or two of the maneuvers used in that situation, known as the Rubin II or Woods' screw maneuvers, can be used for all large babies (or small pelves), even in the absence of dystocia. It is the editor's opinion that by using such maneuvers with all large babies, it may minimize the number of tears and the amount of local trauma. Having practiced these maneuvers during routine deliveries may also be beneficial when a shoulder dystocia finally occurs. To perform the Rubin II maneuver, enter the vagina with your hand and apply two fingers to the back of the anterior shoulder of the infant. Apply pressure to rotate it toward the front of the infant and in effect "shrug" the baby's shoulders (adduct them). This will decrease their AP diameter. At the same time, the clinician's other hand can be applied to the infant's posterior shoulder from the front of the infant. Applying pressure here will abduct this shoulder, and rotate it toward the back of the infant. With both maneuvers applied at the same time, the infant's shoulders turning together approximates the turning of a threaded screw (Woods' screw).

8. Next, hold the baby's neck and place a finger in the infant's axilla to maintain lateral flexion of the trunk. The trunk is easily delivered with gentle, continuous traction. Support the trunk with the hand not supporting the neck. Many clinicians feel that the infant should be held just below the level of the introitus with the head down to be suctioned. The cord should then be clamped.

In vitro data support that this is the proper level and time for optimal placental–fetal transfusion. However, no outcome studies support this assertion. In an attempt to increase bonding, some clinicians place the newborn on the mother's chest or abdomen while clamping the cord. The infant should be dried rapidly with towels while assessing it.

Third Stage

Active management of the third stage of labor has been shown to decrease maternal blood loss, postpartum hemorrhage, length of the third stage, and the need for maternal blood transfusion. Despite an increase in maternal nausea and vomiting, active management of the third stage of labor is highly encouraged.

1. Once the anterior shoulder has been delivered, administer an oxytocic agent. Twenty to 40 units of oxytocin added to a liter of intravenous (IV) fluid is a common choice.
2. When clamping the cord soon after delivery, the plastic clamp should be placed about 3 to 4 cm from the umbilicus. A curved artery Kocher clamp should then be placed about 3 to 5 cm distally. Cut the cord between the clamps and, as clinically indicated, pass the infant to the mother, nurse, or nursery personnel. (If the collection of cord blood gases is desired, two additional plastic or Kocher clamps should be applied to the cord 10 to 20 cm distal to the curved artery clamp [closer to the introitus]. The cord can be cut again between the most distal clamps and the interval portion of cord sent to the laboratory doubly clamped. Alternatively, the blood for gases can be collected on-site. Samples should be obtained from the umbilical vein, as well as from one of the umbilical arteries, by drawing blood into a 1- or 2-mL syringe flushed with heparin; the samples should be labeled and transported on ice to the laboratory immediately. A delay in clamping or collection can cause inaccurate results.)
3. Release the clamp on the cord still attached to the placenta to collect 7 to 10 mL of cord blood while verifying that the cord has two arteries and a vein. Fetal anomalies are associated with cords having fewer than three vessels. After the cord blood is collected, the clamp may be reapplied or left off to allow the placenta to drain. Allowing cord blood to drain will decrease the length of the third stage.
4. While waiting to deliver the placenta, place one hand (on a sterile drape) over the fundus and palpate it. Use the other hand to apply firm traction on the cord. Avoid overaggressive traction, however, which may detach the placenta from the cord and cause hemorrhage. Monitor the uterus for atony and uterine inversion (see "Complications" section) by continuous palpation.
5. As the uterus becomes more rounded, the cord will usually lengthen, and a gush of vaginal blood indicates placental separation. Usually the placenta separates within 5 minutes of the delivery but it can take as long as 30 minutes. Once the separation occurs, have the mother bear down gently. This is normally enough pressure to expel the placenta. If not, "milk" the placenta out of the birth canal by placing one hand on the fundus and using it to exert a slight to moderate amount of pressure. This should propel the placenta into the vagina (Fig. 177-7). Most clinicians deliver the placenta with gentle twisting traction to help remove membranes. After the placenta has passed through the introitus, gently remove any remaining or attached membranes with a ring forceps. This removal prevents tearing the membranes and decreases the chance of any being left behind.

If the placenta has not delivered within 30 minutes, it may be trapped by a contracted cervical ring. This diagnosis is likely if the uterus has already contracted, the gush of vaginal blood occurred, and the cord lengthened. The Brandt maneuver will often deliver the placenta: apply firm pressure suprapubically to hold the uterus in place, apply firm traction on the umbilical cord, and attempt to deliver the placenta.

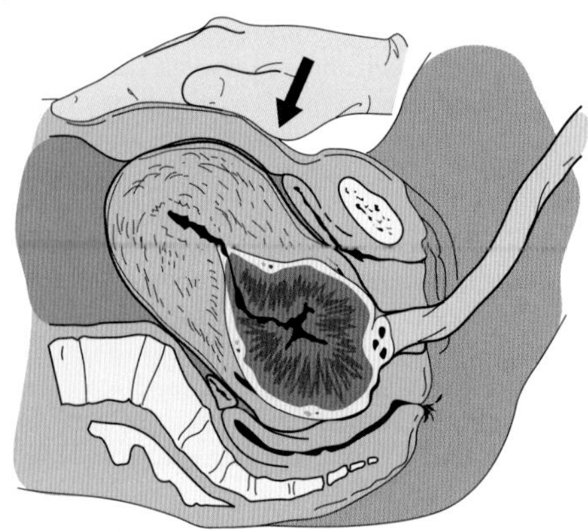

Figure 177-7 Expression of placenta. Note that the hand is *not* trying to push the fundus of the uterus through the birth canal! As the placenta leaves the uterus and enters the vagina, the uterus is elevated (fundus pushed upward and posteriorly) by the hand on the abdomen (*arrow*) while the cord is held in position. The mother can aid in the delivery of the placenta by bearing down. As the placenta reaches the perineum, the cord is lifted, which in turn lifts the placenta out of the vagina. Adherent membranes are eased away from thin attachments to prevent their being torn off and retained in the birth canal. (Redrawn from Cunningham FG, Gant NF, Leveno KJ, et al (eds): Williams' Obstetrics, 18th ed. East Norwalk, Conn, Appleton & Lange, 1989.)

Manual Delivery of the Placenta

Manual removal of the placenta is indicated (3% of vaginal deliveries) if the placenta does not deliver within 30 minutes or if significant bleeding occurs and the uterus does not contract. For failure of the uterus to contract, the injection of oxytocin (2 mL/20 IU in 20 mL of normal saline) into the placental side of the clamped cord may be helpful. It will occasionally result in contraction of the uterus and delivery of the placenta.

For manual removal, change gloves and enter the vagina with the dominant hand, palpating for lacerations. Next, find the cervix and enter the uterus. With two or three fingers, and then the whole hand if necessary, find the plane between the placenta and the uterine wall. Gently follow this plane and use the hand to separate the placenta from the uterine wall. After complete separation, hold onto the placenta with the dominant hand, and slowly withdraw the hand with the placenta. If the cleavage plane cannot be separated or parts of the plane cannot be developed completely, prepare for surgical removal of the placenta.

After the third stage, always examine the placenta to see if it is complete while it is in the basin or on the table. If a portion is missing, re-enter the vagina and uterus manually to perform this same maneuver to retrieve any fragments. Covering the sterile glove on the inserted hand with one 4 × 4 gauze pad may give additional traction when sweeping the uterus. Such sweeps may also be useful in patients after VBAC, for those bleeding excessively, or for premature deliveries. When the placenta is being examined for completeness, this is another chance to confirm (if you have not already done so) that the cord has three vessels.

If it has not already been given, IV oxytocin should be administered and gentle uterine massage performed to prevent atony. Currently, in the United States, it is the clinician's choice as to whether to give oxytocin with the delivery of the shoulders or after the placenta is expelled. The evidence suggests that giving the oxytocic agent immediately after delivery of the anterior shoulder is beneficial to the patient. Usually this is given intravenously (20 to 40 units in 1 L of isotonic solution over 8 hours). If atony and bleeding persist, intramuscular (IM) methylergonovine (2 mg IM [normotensive patients only]) or 15-methyl prostaglandin (250 μg IM) can be given. After the uterus is firm, begin any necessary repair.

Sample Operative Report

Patient is a 28-year-old female G2P1 at 39 weeks' gestation, admitted for rupture of membranes and contractions. She was 3 cm dilated at admission and progressed to complete without intervention. Fetal heart monitoring remained reassuring throughout labor. Epidural anesthesia was provided. Patient delivered a viable female infant over intact perineum via normal spontaneous vaginal delivery (NSVD) at 08:35. Amniotic fluid was clear. Nuchal cord × 1 easily reduced. Anterior shoulder delivered with gentle traction. Infant was bulb suctioned at perineum. Infant was vigorous, with Apgar scores of 8 and 9 at 1 and 5 minutes. Cord was clamped and cut immediately after delivery and infant was placed on maternal abdomen. Cord blood sent for analysis. Blood gas with pH 7.28. Oxytocin 40 units in 1 L of normal saline started IV at delivery of the anterior shoulder. Placenta delivered intact with three-vessel cord via active management at 08:42. Cervix, vagina, and perineum explored and intact. Estimated blood loss 300 mL. Mother and newborn were stable and remained in the delivery room.

If vacuum or forceps are applied, be sure to include in the delivery note indication, consent, position, station, number of applications, and time of application.

Common Errors

- Admitting patient to the labor ward prior to the onset of active labor. Being certain of the diagnosis of active labor and delaying admission to the hospital until active labor is confirmed have been shown to decrease the number of interventions a woman undergoes prior to delivery.
- Failure to diagnose breech presentation (or other malpresentation). If not completely certain of the position of the baby after performing Leopold's maneuvers, intrapartum ultrasound confirmation of lie should be considered (see Chapter 172, Obstetric Ultrasonography).
- Failure to recognize nonreassuring fetal tracing. A team approach involving the nurses and delivering providers enhances the ability to detect abnormalities in the fetal heart tracing. As with all skills, continuing education is essential for all caregivers interpreting strips.
- Failure to actively manage the third stage of labor. Good evidence shows that this protocol will decrease postpartum hemorrhage, but it has been slow to be adopted in some settings.
- Performing unnecessary episiotomy. Routine episiotomy should not be performed.
- Poor documentation of labor and delivery. It is essential to document the provider's presence and involvement in the delivery process. As with all care, any intervention needs to be documented in the medical record.

Complications

Maternal Complications

- Perineal pain and dyspareunia are common complications of vaginal delivery, especially those involving perineal or vaginal trauma. Restrictive use of episiotomy has been shown to reduce the risk of more severe tears and postpartum perineal pain. When perineal repair is required, a continuous, knotless suturing technique with absorbable synthetic suture decreases postpartum analgesia use as well as dyspareunia at 12 months.
- Postpartum hemorrhage occurs in 4% of all vaginal deliveries, and is defined as greater than 500 mL of blood loss in the first 24 hours. It may also be defined as blood loss significant enough to cause hemodynamic instability. The causes of postpartum hemorrhages may be broken down into four categories:
  1. Tone: Tone refers to uterine atony, and is responsible for 70% of postpartum hemorrhages. Uterine massage, and the use of agents such as oxytocin, methylergonovine, and carboprost should be considered to stimulate uterine contractions.
  2. Trauma: Perineal, cervical, and vaginal lacerations, as well as uterine rupture or inversion, should be sought as a source of bleeding. These sources account for 20% of cases of postpartum hemorrhages.
  3. Tissue: Retained tissue or, less commonly, invasive placenta causes up to 10% of postpartum hemorrhages. In some cases, manual removal of the placenta is required, and in the case of invasive placenta (placenta accreta, increta, or percreta), surgical consultation and intervention are required.
  4. Thrombin: Coagulation disorders are rare causes (<1%) of postpartum hemorrhages, as most of these are identified previously, allowing for planning and management prior to vaginal delivery. Management of postpartum hemorrhage includes early recognition, immediate fluid resuscitation, and identification and treatment of the underlying cause.
- Endometritis can occur after an uncomplicated vaginal delivery. It is more common if uterine manipulation, instrumentation, or prolonged labor and rupture of membranes have occurred. Retained products of conception (placenta or membranes) also increase the risk of infection.
- Uterine inversion is an infrequent complication of vaginal delivery. Uterine inversion is associated with fundal placentas, uterine atony, and congenital weakness of the uterus. Management begins with calling for assistance, including general anesthesia, and immediately attempting to replace the uterus. If possible, it should be replaced without removing the placenta. If the uterus is not replaceable immediately, there is an 85% to 90% success rate of replacing the uterus with tocolysis. (Oxytocin should be discontinued and the uterus relaxed with IV beta-mimetic medications or magnesium sulfate [preferred].) The remaining 15% to 20% of patients will require general anesthesia for the abdominal relaxation needed for uterine replacement. After replacement, oxytocin should be restarted and the postpartum hemorrhage managed appropriately.
- A rare complication of vaginal delivery is amniotic fluid embolism (AFE), occurring in 1 of 20,000 pregnancies, with a mortality rate as high as 85%. AFE presents with rapid, unexpected respiratory distress and cardiovascular collapse, leading to disseminated intravascular coagulopathy (DIC), coma, and death. Rapid clinical diagnosis and aggressive intensive care unit (ICU) management can reduce mortality risk, but progression can be very rapid and difficult to reverse.

Fetal Complications

The main risks to a fetus through the delivery process are trauma and hypoxia. Numerous problems can occur during the process, but most newborns survive delivery without complication. Following is a partial list of possible fetal complications:

- Respiratory distress
- Hemodynamic instability
- Neonatal sepsis
- Intracranial hemorrhage
- Brachial plexus damage
- Fractures (humerus and clavicle common)
- Asphyxia and associated problems

Management of these complications is beyond the scope of this chapter. Chapter 180, Neonatal Resuscitation, gives an overview of the acute treatment of emergent complications.

Postprocedure Management

Unless delivered in a labor-delivery-recovery-postpartum (LDRP) room, the patient is transferred to a postpartum room approximately

2 hours after a normal spontaneous delivery. She remains there until discharged home approximately 2 days later.

While in the recovery stage, the patient should be regularly assessed for postpartum hemorrhage. This can be best evaluated with observation of the perineum, which should be absent of continuous blood flow. The uterine fundus should be firm and below the umbilicus. The patient should remain hemodynamically stable with normal vital signs before transfer. If concern for postpartum hemorrhage or other complication exists, transfer to the postpartum floor should be delayed.

After being taken to the postpartum room the patient should be assessed at least daily by a clinician. The assessment should include evaluation for vaginal bleeding or infection. The patient should be instructed regarding the normal amount of vaginal bleeding after delivery (lochia rubra) and return to normal function. She should also be monitored for signs and symptoms of postpartum blues and depression, mastitis, venous thromboembolism, constipation, and sleep disturbance. Pain control is generally obtained with any of the following: acetaminophen, ibuprofen, naproxen, and acetaminophen with codeine. For constipation, Milk of Magnesia, docusate sodium, Dulcolax suppository, or psyllium may be helpful. Routine blood count measurements are generally not indicated following an uncomplicated vaginal delivery. Prior to discharge, birth control measures should be discussed and instructions given.

Postprocedure Patient Education

On discharge from the hospital, patients should be given specific instructions about their medications and other postpartum care. Any and all questions should be answered. Whether patients are breast-feeding or not, new mothers will require instructions for breast care. They should also be instructed about sitz baths, Peri-Pads, and other perineal care. Inform them about when to call the clinician. Pelvic rest should be maintained for at least 1 month. The follow-up appointment should be 4 to 6 weeks after the delivery.

Interpretation of Results

The most objective way to assess for fetal acidosis at birth is by analysis of umbilical cord blood at delivery. This information can be useful in differentiating those newborns who are "depressed" (have low Apgar scores) from those who are truly acidotic at delivery. The pH, PCO_2, PO_2, CO_2, hemoglobin, and oxygen content of the blood can be measured, and the bicarbonate concentration, oxygen saturation, and base excess/deficit can be calculated from these measurements. Table 177-2 shows normal values for these measurements.

The most useful value for assessing fetal condition is pH. Fetal pH is typically 0.1 unit lower than maternal pH. The mean arterial fetal pH is 7.28, with the 5th and 95th percentiles at 7.14 and 7.40, respectively. The risk of neonatal morbidity is inversely related to pH, with the highest risk for those with pH less than 6.9. In several studies, umbilical artery pH lower than 7 was predictive of neonatal morbidity (e.g., seizures). However, it should be noted that the majority of newborns with pH less than 7 were admitted to the regular newborn nursery and had an uncomplicated neonatal course. Umbilical artery PO_2 is not predictive of any adverse neonatal outcome.

TABLE 177-2 Normal Ranges for Cord Blood Gas Analysis

pH	7.27 to 7.28
PCO_2 (mm Hg)	49.2 to 50.3
HCO_3^- (mEq/L)	22 to 23.1
Base excess (mEq/L)	−2.7 to −3.6

The calculated base deficit or excess is also useful, because metabolic acidosis leads to excess production of acid, or a negative base excess (base deficit). A base deficit greater than 12 mmol/L is predictive of neonatal complications. Fetal blood gas analysis does not distinguish between potential causes of fetal acidosis; fetal, placental, and maternal factors could all play a role.

CPT/Billing and Coding

59400 Global vaginal delivery (routine obstetric care, including antepartum care, vaginal delivery [with or without episiotomy, and/or forceps] and postpartum care)
59409 Vaginal delivery *only* (with or without episiotomy, and/or forceps)
59410 Vaginal delivery *only* (with or without episiotomy, and/or forceps) and postpartum care (no antepartum care)
59430 Postpartum care only
59610 Global VBAC delivery (routine obstetric care including antepartum care, vaginal delivery [with or without episiotomy and/or forceps] and postpartum care after previous cesarean delivery)
59612 Vaginal delivery only, after previous cesarean delivery
59614 Vaginal delivery only, after previous cesarean delivery including postpartum care
59899 Unlisted procedure maternity care and delivery (induction, etc.)

NOTE: A patient who is admitted for labor that is post-term, induced, augmented, or otherwise complicated (blood pressure problems, arrest of labor, fetal distress, etc.) is not included in a routine delivery. These types of deliveries should be coded with routine inpatient or outpatient evaluation and management codes (e.g., 99221 to 99223).

99291 Critical care, evaluation of the critically ill or critically injured patient, first 30 to 74 minutes (e.g., preeclampsia, placenta previa or abruptio, postpartum hemorrhage, pulmonary or amniotic fluid embolism)
99292 Each additional 30 minutes
99356 Prolonged physician service in the inpatient setting, requiring direct (face-to-face) patient contact beyond the usual routine service, but not in critical care unit (e.g., maternity fetal monitoring for high-risk delivery or other physiologic monitoring); first hour
99357 Each additional 30 minutes
99358 Prolonged evaluation and management service before and/or after direct face-to-face patient care (e.g., review of extensive records and tests, communication with other professionals and/or patient/family); first hour
99359 Each additional 30 minutes

NOTE: A good reference for coding is provided by the American Academy of Family Physicians at http://www.aafp.org/online/en/home/practicemgt/codingresources/codingob.html.

ICD-9-CM Diagnostic Codes

Codes 630 to 677 cover the "Complications of Pregnancy, Childbirth and Puerperium." Commonly used codes at the time of delivery are shown in the following list. The fifth digit is required for codes 640 to 676. For these codes the following applies:

0 indicates unspecified as to episode of care
1 indicates delivered with or without mention of antepartum condition
2 indicates delivered, with mention of postpartum condition
3 indicates antepartum condition or complication
4 indicates postpartum condition or complication

645.1 Post-term pregnancy (40–42 weeks)
645.2 Prolonged pregnancy (>42 weeks)
649.1 Obesity complicating pregnancy, childbirth, or the puerperium
650 Normal delivery (not to be used with any other code in 630 to 676, fourth and fifth digits not required)
654.2 Previous cesarean section
656.3 Fetal distress
658.0 Oligohydramnios
658.1 Premature rupture of membranes
659.2 Pyrexia in labor
659.4 Grand multiparity
659.7 Abnormality in fetal heart rate or rhythm (e.g., fetal bradycardia or tachycardia)
662.0 Prolonged first stage of labor
662.2 Prolonged second stage of labor
663.0 Prolapse of cord
663.1 Cord around neck, with compression
664.1 Perineal laceration, second degree
664.2 Perineal laceration, third degree
664.3 Perneal laceration, fourth degree
666.12 Postpartum hemorrhage
667.12 Retained placenta/membranes
792.3 Meconium staining

ACKNOWLEDGMENT

The editors wish to recognize the many contributions by Carol Osborn, MD, to this chapter in a previous edition of this text.

ONLINE RESOURCES

AAFP coding resources: http://www.aafp.org/online/en/home/practicemgt/codingresources/codingob.html.

The Cochrane Collaboration: www.cochrane.org.

Patient Education from the U.S. government: http://www.4women.gov/pregnancy/.

Tuggy M, Garcia J: Procedures Consult. Available at www.proceduresconsult.com, and as an application at www.apple.com/iTunes.

See the sample patient education and consent forms online at www.expertconsult.com.

USEFUL CONTINUING EDUCATION

Advanced Life Support in Obstetrics (ALSO)

This course provides practice for both the cognitive and the manual skills for simple or complicated deliveries. Lifelike pelvic and infant mannequins allow the learner to practice in a calm environment, even using forceps or vacuum-assisted delivery equipment. Courses are taught throughout the United States as well as internationally. More information can be found at www.aafp.org/also.

Family-Centered Maternity Care Conference

This course is designed to provide state-of-the-art, evidence-based education in the knowledge, training, and skills of caring for patients and their families during pregnancy and the birth process. It is organized by the American Academy of Family Physicians (AAFP). More information is available at http://www.aafp.org/.

BIBLIOGRAPHY

Akoury HA, MacDonald FJ, Brodie G, et al: Oxytocin augmentation of labor and perinatal outcome in nulliparas. Obstet Gynecol 78:227–230, 1991.

Albers LL: The duration of labor in healthy women. J Perinatol 19:114–119, 1999.

American Academy of Family Physicians (AAFP): Advanced Life Support in Obstetrics (ALSO) Provider Course Syllabus, 4th ed. Kansas City, AAFP, 2000.

American Academy of Pediatrics, American College of Obstetricians and Gynecologists: Neonatal encephalopathy and cerebral palsy: Defining the pathogenesis and pathophysiology. Elk Grove Village, IL, AAP; Washington, DC, ACOG; 2003.

American College of Obstetricians and Gynecologists: Induction of labor for vaginal birth after cesarean delivery. Committee on Obstetric Practice Opinion No. 342. Obstet Gynecol 108:465–468, 2006.

American College of Obstetricians and Gynecologists: Optimal goals for anesthesia care in obstetrics. ACOG Committee on Obstetric Practice Opinion No. 433. Obstet Gynecol 113:1197–1199, 2009.

American College of Obstetricians and Gynecologists: Scheduled cesarean delivery and the prevention of vertical transmission of HIV infection. Committee Opinion No. 234. Int J Gynaecol Obstet 73:279–281, 2001.

American College of Obstetricians and Gynecologists: Umbilical cord blood gas and acid-base analysis. Committee Opinion No. 348. Obstet Gynecol 108:1319–1322, 2006.

American College of Obstetricians and Gynecologists: Vaginal birth after previous cesarean. Practice Bulletin No. 54. Obstet Gynecol 104:203–212, 2004.

Andres RL, Saade G, Gilstrap LC, Wilkins I: Association between umbilical blood gas parameters and neonatal morbidity and death in neonates with pathologic fetal acidemia. Am J Obstet Gynecol 181:867–871, 1999.

Brown D, Hendricks SK, Waechter A: Normal spontaneous vaginal delivery. In Reichman EF, Simon RR (eds): Emergency Medicine Procedures. New York, McGraw-Hill, 2004.

Duignan NM, Studd JW, Hughes AO: Characteristics of normal labour in different racial groups. Br J Obstet Gynaecol 82:593–601, 1975.

Fraser WD, Turcot L, Krauss I, Brisson-Carrol G: Amniotomy for shortening spontaneous labour. Cochrane Database Syst Rev 2:CD000015, 2000.

Friedman EA: Labor: Clinical Evaluation and Management, 2nd ed. New York, Appleton-Century-Crofts, 1978, p 49.

Frigoletto FD Jr, Lieberman E, Lang JM, et al: A clinical trial of active management of labor. N Engl J Med 333:745–750, 1995.

Lauzon L, Hodnett E: Labour assessment programs to delay admission to labour wards. Cochrane Database Syst Rev 3:CD000936, 2001.

Lopez-Zeno JA, Peaceman AM, Adashek JA, Socol ML: A controlled trial of a program for the active management of labor. N Engl J Med 326:450–454, 1992.

Patterson DA, Winslow M, Matus CD: Spontaneous vaginal delivery. Am Fam Physician 78:336–341, 343–344, 2008.

Pattinson RC, Howarth GR, Mdluli W, et al: Aggressive or expectant management of labour: A randomised clinical trial. Br J Obstet Gynaecol 110:457–461, 2003.

Pitkin RM, Scott JR: Active management of labor: The American experience. Clin Obstet Gynecol 40:510, 1997.

Prendiville WJ, Elbourne D, McDonald S: Active versus expectant management in the third stage of labour. Cochrane Database Syst Rev 2:CD000007, 2000.

Public Health Service Task Force, Perinatal HIV-1 Guidelines Working Group: Recommendations for use of antiretroviral drugs in pregnant HIV-1-infected women for maternal health and interventions to reduce perinatal HIV-1 transmission in the United States. October 12, 2006; http://www.ucsf.edu/hivcntr/Perinatal/PerinatalGL.pdf. Accessed Feb. 13, 2008.

Smyth R, Alldred S, Markham C: Amniotomy for shortening spontaneous labour. Cochrane Database Syst Rev 4:CD006167, 2007.

Zhang J, Troendle JF, Yancey MK: Reassessing the labor curve in nulliparous women. Am J Obstet Gynecol 187:824–828, 2002.

SECTION 11

Pediatrics

Section Editor: DALE A. PATTERSON

CHAPTER 178

DeLee Suctioning

David B. Bosscher

Suctioning with a DeLee suction device may clear the upper airway of the neonate. Meconium is present in the amniotic fluid in 9% to 20% of deliveries. For many years, it was thought that DeLee suctioning of the oropharynx and stomach carried out before delivery of the neonate's chest would prevent meconium aspiration syndrome, and there were studies to support this practice. It is now known that some infants aspirate before delivery and therefore no intrapartum intervention can prevent all meconium aspiration. Although DeLee suctioning after delivery of the anterior shoulder and before delivery of the chest (i.e., intrapartum suctioning, before the neonate's first breath) may prevent further meconium aspiration with the first breath, it is no longer part of neonatal resuscitation guidelines (published in 2005; see Chapter 180, Neonatal Resuscitation). This change is because one large, randomized multicenter trial (Vain and colleagues, 2004) found no benefit to performing such an intrapartum procedure. That said, many experts in both obstetrics and pediatrics still recommend suctioning the oropharynx or nasopharynx if the amniotic fluid or infant is meconium stained. Most agree that nothing more needs to be done if the infant is vigorous (defined by strong respiratory efforts, a heart rate >100 beats per minute, and good muscle tone), and this is supported by randomized, controlled trials. Most also agree that further intervention, such as endotracheal intubation and direct suctioning of the trachea (usually with a meconium aspirator applied to the endotracheal tube as the endotracheal tube is withdrawn) is indicated in those infants who are not vigorous, especially premature infants. (This assumes that the equipment and expertise are available and that, if so, and if at all possible, endotracheal suctioning should occur before stimulating these infants.)

Indications

- To help clear secretions in the newborn, including meconium-stained secretions, before stimulation (however, this should not delay more definitive endotracheal suctioning in the nonvigorous infant)
- To help relieve respiratory distress in the newborn when the stomach is full or when regurgitated stomach contents partially occlude the airway (again, this should not delay more definitive endotracheal suctioning in the nonvigorous infant)
- To assist in the diagnosis of choanal atresia
- To help exclude certain types of tracheoesophageal fistula

NOTE: In some tertiary care hospitals, DeLee suctioning is performed by the nursing staff before stimulation, while the infant is under the warmer and awaiting the neonatal resuscitation team. In such a setting, hospital bylaws may require the presence of a resuscitation team whenever there is meconium staining.

Contraindications

Absolute

- A neonate with known choanal atresia should not receive DeLee suctioning by the *nasal* route.
- As mentioned previously, DeLee suctioning should not delay more definitive resuscitative efforts such as direct endotracheal suctioning; however, equipment and expertise for this are not always immediately available.

Relative

Thick particulate meconium cannot be adequately suctioned with a DeLee suction device alone.

Equipment and Supplies

- A DeLee or similar suction device, 8 to 10 Fr (Fig. 178-1)
- A bulb syringe to clear the mouth and nasal openings
- Gloves, facial coverings, and other necessary items for the clinician to observe universal blood and body fluid precautions
- Mechanical or wall vacuum or suction

NOTE: Newborns have a high degree of vagal tone and the pharynx is heavily innervated by the vagus nerve. Excessive vagal stimulation in a newborn, such as from overstimulation of the pharynx, can result in secondary apnea, bradycardia, or distress.

Technique

1. Prepare the equipment. First make certain that the large-diameter end of the DeLee device, the end that will be attached to the external vacuum or suction source, is functioning. This can be done by handing this end to an assistant, who should then attach it to the external vacuum source. Cover the thumb opening/occluder and listen for a change in the noise from the vacuum. This also ensures that the vacuum source is functioning. Human-powered suctioning is no longer recommended.
2. Quickly clear the mouth and nose of the neonate with a bulb syringe.
3. Use your index finger to open the infant's mouth and to depress the back of the tongue. Using your other hand, gently unroll and insert the much smaller-diameter mouth end of the DeLee device into the mouth of the neonate. Attempts should be made to keep this end as sterile as possible.
4. Slowly advance the catheter into the oropharynx, then direct it down into the esophagus (hypopharynx) with your finger.

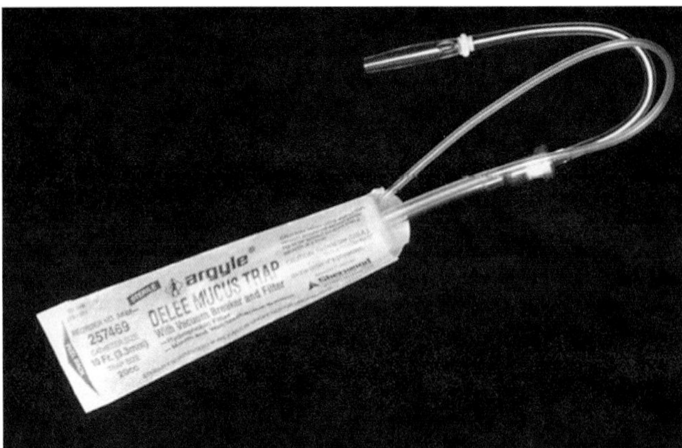

Figure 178-1 DeLee suction device.

5. Continue to advance the catheter until approximately 5 cm of its length remains outside the infant's mouth. The distal end is now in the infant's stomach.
6. Using a vacuum source that does not exceed 100 mm Hg, again apply vacuum to the suction end of the DeLee device by covering the thumb opening/occluder. After applying vacuum for a few seconds, slowly withdraw the catheter while continuously maintaining a vacuum. If time allows, use the same technique to suction the infant's nose.
7. After suctioning, check for any respiratory distress. Treat minor degrees of distress with proper positioning and oxygen administration, if necessary (see Chapter 180, Neonatal Resuscitation).
8. As part of documenting the care of the newborn in the postdelivery period, always mention that DeLee suctioning was performed. Document any complications.

Complications

- Stimulation of the neonatal pharynx with any suction device during the first few minutes after delivery can evoke a vagal response and induce apnea, bradycardia, or fetal distress.
- Vigorous DeLee suctioning could cause trauma to the upper airways, the esophagus, and the stomach.
- In a neonate with a tracheoesophageal fistula, the DeLee suction device could enter the airway below the larynx, causing respiratory distress.
- Older DeLee suction devices, and even some of the newer ones that use human-powered suction, allow aspirated neonatal stomach contents to enter the mouth of the person applying suction. This method has the potential for spreading infectious diseases. A human mouth should not be used to apply suction on a DeLee. Newer models use mechanical or wall vacuum suction and are safer for the clinician; however, they are more cumbersome and difficult to use in a sterile field.

CPT/Billing Codes

99431 History and examination of the normal newborn infant, initiation of diagnostic and treatment programs and preparation of hospital records
99436 Attendance at delivery (when requested by the delivering physician) and stabilization of newborn
99440 Newborn resuscitation; provision of positive-pressure ventilation and/or chest compressions in the presence of acute inadequate ventilation and/or cardiac output

99436 may be reported in addition to 99431 but may *not* be reported in addition to 99440.

ICD-9-CM Diagnostic Codes

656.83 Meconium passage during delivery
656.84 Meconium passage after delivery
763.84 Meconium passage during delivery, affecting newborn, excludes 770.11, 77.12, 779.84
768.6 Asphyxia, newborn, mild/moderate at birth
770.18 Newborn aspiration, 2000 to 2499 grams
770.19 Newborn aspiration, >2500 grams
770.11 Meconium aspiration, newborn, without respiratory symptoms
770.12 Meconium aspiration, newborn, with respiratory symptoms
770.84 Respiratory failure, newborn
770.85 Aspiration of postnatal stomach contents, newborn, without respiratory symptoms
770.86 Aspiration of postnatal stomach contents, newborn, with respiratory symptoms
770.87 Respiratory arrest, newborn
770.88 Hypoxemia of newborn
770.89 Other respiratory problems after birth
779.81 Bradycardia, newborn
779.84 Meconium staining, newborn
779.85 Cardiac arrest, newborn
792.3 Amniotic fluid, nonspecific abnormal finding

Online Resource

Agency for Healthcare Research and Quality (AHRQ) National Guideline Clearinghouse: Brief Summary: Neonatal resuscitation: 2005 International Consensus Conference on Cardiopulmonary Resuscitation and Emergency Cardiovascular Care Science with Treatment Recommendations. Available at www.guidelines.gov/summary/summary.aspx?doc_id=8485&nbr=004736&string=neonatal+AND+resuscitation. Accessed February 2, 2010.

Bibliography

American Academy of Pediatrics and American Heart Association: Textbook of Neonatal Resuscitation, 5th ed. Elk Grove Village, Ill, American Academy of Pediatrics, 2005.

American Heart Association: 2005 American Heart Association Guidelines for Cardiopulmonary Resuscitation and Emergency Cardiovascular Care: Part 13. Neonatal resuscitation guidelines. Circulation 112: IV-188–IV-195, 2005.

American Heart Association and American Academy of Pediatrics: American Heart Association (AHA) guidelines for cardiopulmonary resuscitation (CPR) and emergency cardiovascular care (ECC) of pediatric and neonatal patients: Neonatal resuscitation guidelines. Pediatrics 117:e1029–e1038, 2006.

Halliday HL: Endotracheal intubation at birth for preventing morbidity and mortality in vigorous, meconium-stained infants at term. Cochrane Database Syst Rev 2:CD000500, 2000.

Raab EL: Essentials of normal newborn assessment and care. In DeCherney AH, Nathan L, Goodwin TM, Laufer N (eds): Current Diagnosis and Treatment in Obstetrics and Gynecology, 10th ed. New York, Lange McGraw-Hill, 2007, pp 212–221.

Thilo EH, Rosenberg AA: The newborn infant. In Hay WW, Levin MJ, Sondheimer JM, Deterding RR (eds): Current Diagnosis and Treatment in Pediatrics, 18th ed. New York, Lange McGraw-Hill, 2007, pp 1–64.

Vain NE, Szyld EG, Prudent LM, et al: Oropharyngeal and nasopharyngeal suctioning of meconium-stained neonates before delivery of their shoulders: Multicentre, randomised controlled trial. Lancet 364:597–602, 2004.

Subcutaneous Ring and Dorsal Penile Block for Newborn Circumcision

Grant C. Fowler

The American Academy of Pediatrics has recommended routine use of analgesia for circumcision since 1999. A recent survey of residency program directors found that 97% of pediatric, family medicine, and obstetrics and gynecology programs that teach circumcision teach the administration of an anesthetic, either locally or topically. Therefore, the controversy about whether or not infants should receive analgesia or anesthesia for circumcision has ended. Previously, the controversy weighed whether the incompletely developed neonatal nervous system was capable of experiencing pain against the risk of anesthesia. Many clinicians chose not to use circumcision anesthesia, in part because of this controversy, but also owing to their lack of training or experience in the techniques available, the additional steps (and time) required to perform the procedure, and the time required for the anesthesia to take effect. However, with proper planning, the number of steps and the time required are minimal. In addition, studies have documented the safety of anesthesia as well as the improved outcomes in neonates.

Common analgesic and anesthetic techniques for circumcision include subcutaneous ring block, dorsal penile nerve block (DPNB), topical anesthesia (see Chapter 10, Topical Anesthesia), and precircumcision oral analgesics. Several studies have reported that the subcutaneous ring block is the most effective, and it has therefore basically replaced DPNB as the anesthetic technique of choice. (This is different in adults, where the most effective anesthesia for office circumcision is probably a combination of all three.) This chapter discusses subcutaneous ring block, DPNB, and an alternative technique of DPNB using a single injection. All three techniques appear to be more effective than topical or oral anesthesia, and no major complications have been reported with any of these methods. Studies have found that anesthetized infants show less crying, tachycardia, and irritability and exhibit fewer behavior changes for the 24 hours after circumcision. They also have less variability in oxygen saturation and blood pressure during the procedure and lower serum cortisol levels after the procedure. One small study in children found that lidocaine–prilocaine (eutectic mixture of local anesthetics, or EMLA) cream applied an hour before the ring block reduced the pain of needle puncture. However, because most clinicians are not able to prepare a newborn an hour before its circumcision, they would probably rely on the nursing staff to apply the cream. Conversely, in adults and children who are about to undergo office circumcision under local anesthesia, waiting an hour for the lidocaine–prilocaine cream to take effect may be very worthwhile.

Indication

Parental desire (however, parents should be encouraged to consent to this procedure in any healthy newborn undergoing circumcision).

Contraindications

- Known hypersensitivity to anesthetic
- A known bleeding disorder *(relative contraindication)*

Equipment

- 1% lidocaine without epinephrine
- 1-mL syringe with 27-gauge needle (some tuberculin syringes come with this combination). If the needle is removable, using a 30-gauge needle to administer the anesthetic may minimize bleeding and discomfort.
- Alcohol wipe
- Infant restrainer (papoose board or Circumstraint) if assistant not available to hold infant
- Lidocaine–prilocaine (EMLA) cream *(optional)*

NOTE: There is a risk of methemoglobinemia after use of EMLA cream in certain situations. However, this risk is minimized with circumcision because it is used only once on intact skin and not with other drugs known to cause methemoglobinemia (e.g., nitric oxide).

Preprocedure Patient Preparation

Discuss the risks, benefits, and alternatives with the parents, and obtain informed consent. Most clinicians combine this consent with the circumcision consent form.

Technique

Before the procedure, note the anatomy as shown in Figure 179-1. Consider giving the infant a few swallows of glucose water or a sugar-coated pacifier to minimize distress. In a warm room, have an assistant hold the infant or place the infant's legs in restraints. Fold back the diaper to expose the penis.

NOTE: As the clinician becomes more comfortable performing ring block or DPNB, time may be saved by performing the procedure

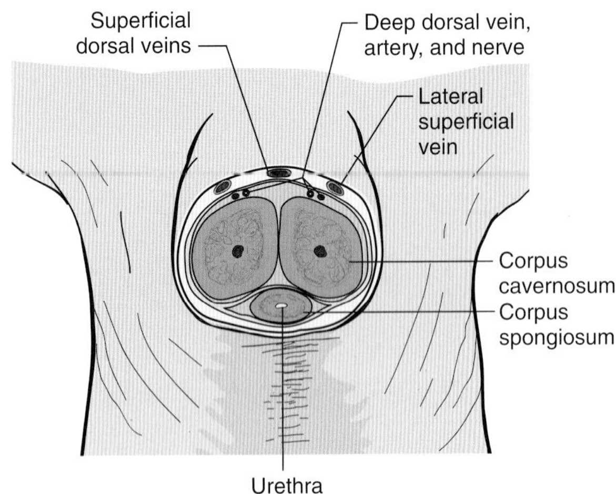

Figure 179-1 Anatomy of the penile root (cross-section).

before the infant is surgically prepared. This allows time for the anesthetic to take effect while other preparations are being made.

Subcutaneous Ring Block

1. Prepare the skin both at the base of the penis as well as around the penis with an alcohol pad. Using aseptic technique and stabilizing the penis by gentle, slightly downward or ventral traction, insert the needle into the lateral side of the penis at the base (Fig. 179-2). Staying superficial to Buck's fascia, place a subcutaneous bleb of lidocaine. Then advance the needle circumferentially around the base of the penis while injecting. A couple of punctures may be necessary to accomplish this.
2. After completing a 180-degree half-circle, the same procedure is followed on the opposite side of the penis. A maximum of 1 mL of lidocaine should be used to complete the 360-degree circumferential ring. Intravascular injection can be avoided by frequently aspirating with the syringe to check for any blood return prior to each ¼ mL injected.

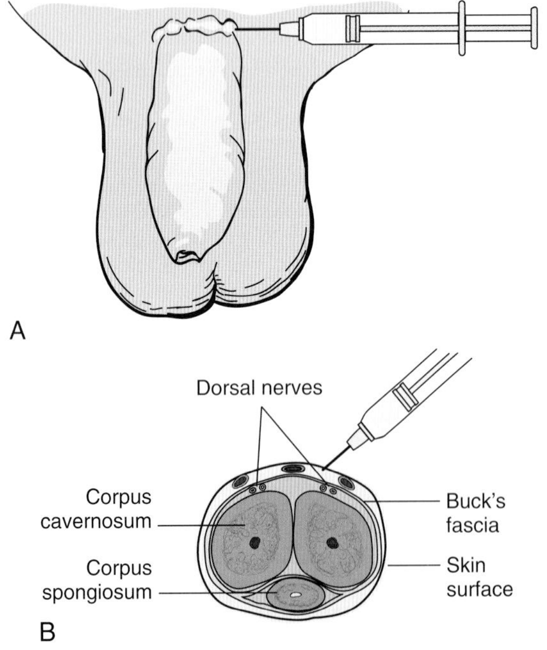

Figure 179-2 Subcutaneous ring block. **A,** Needle is inserted at base of penis and a subcutaneous bleb of lidocaine is placed. A 360-degree ring of anesthesia is completed around the penis. **B,** Cross-section of penis at base showing paired dorsal nerves deep to Buck's fascia.

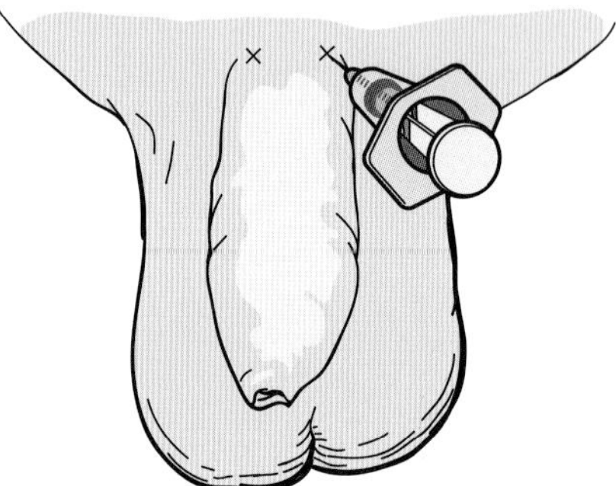

Figure 179-3 Injection sites and direction of needle for administering dorsal penile nerve block.

Dorsal Penile Nerve Block (Two Techniques)

Standard Technique

1. Using an index finger, palpate the lateral side of the penis to determine the depth of the root of the penis, which is usually about 0.75 to 1 cm beneath the skin surface. Often it is about the size, shape, and consistency of a large blueberry and is located just under the symphysis pubis.
2. Prepare the skin at the base of the penis with an alcohol pad. Using aseptic technique and stabilizing the penis by gentle, slightly downward or ventral traction, insert the needle at the 1 o'clock position (the dorsal or cranial direction being the 12 o'clock position, and the ventral direction being the 6 o'clock position) and direct it posteromedially (Fig. 179-3). Insert to a depth of 0.3 to 0.5 cm, which corresponds to 0.5 to 0.7 cm distal to the penile root, and this is slightly proximal to where the dorsal nerves branch (Fig. 179-4). The tip of the needle should be freely movable, indicating that it is in loose connective tissue, and this should prevent injection into the corpus cavernosum. Taking care not to inject into a blood vessel (check by aspirating), inject 0.4 mL of lidocaine. Repeat the injection at the 11 o'clock position with another 0.4 mL of lidocaine. (Avoid exceeding a total of 0.8 mL of lidocaine.)
3. In the infant whose penile root is not palpable because it is embedded in pubic fat, the anesthetic can be injected at the same locations, depths, and directions but about 0.3 to 0.5 cm inferolateral to the penile–suprapubic skin junction (Fig. 179-5).

Alternative Technique Using Single Injection Site

1. Instead of making two skin punctures (at the 11 and 1 o'clock positions), an alternative is to insert the needle at the 12 o'clock

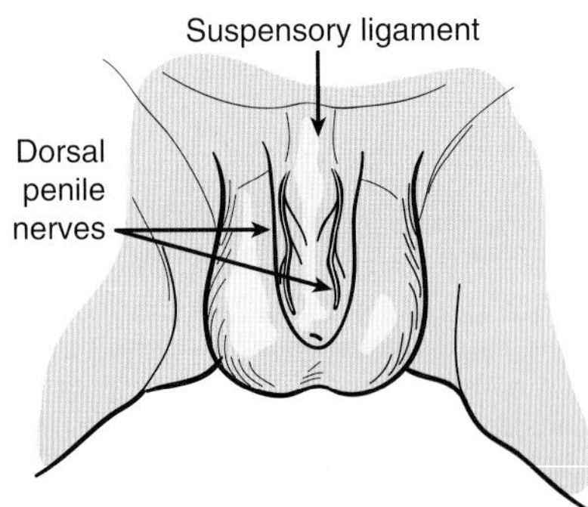

Figure 179-4 Location of dorsal penile nerves. Note branching begins after emergence from the suspensory ligament of the penis.

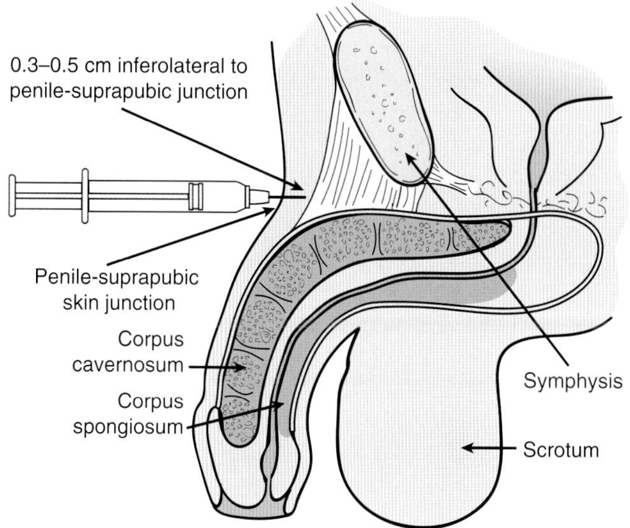

Figure 179-5 Sagittal view through the perineum showing anesthetic injection in a posteromedial direction at a depth of 0.3 to 0.5 mm.

position and angle the needle toward the 11 and 1 o'clock positions. In other words, if the 12 o'clock position is where the dorsal skin of the penis reflects onto the abdomen (penile–suprapubic skin junction), insert the needle here and angle it toward the 1 o'clock position to a depth of about 0.5 cm. The tip of the needle should be freely movable, indicating that it is in loose connective tissue, and this should prevent injection into the corpus cavernosum. After aspirating to ensure the needle is not in a blood vessel, inject 0.4 mL of lidocaine.

2. Withdraw the needle until the tip is just below the skin surface, and then advance it again toward the 11 o'clock position (Fig. 179-6). The second injection can then be made, taking care not to exceed a total of 0.8 mL of lidocaine.

NOTE: A combination of ring block and DPNB has been demonstrated to be effective in adults undergoing office circumcision. Obviously, larger doses of lidocaine are used in adults.

Notes Regarding Optimal Effects

- One study in adults has found that using slower injection rates (i.e., longer injection times, such as 100 to 150 seconds) caused less pain than shorter injection times (40 to 80 seconds). Using a 30-gauge needle will not only slow the injection rate, it will increase overall patient comfort and cause less bleeding.

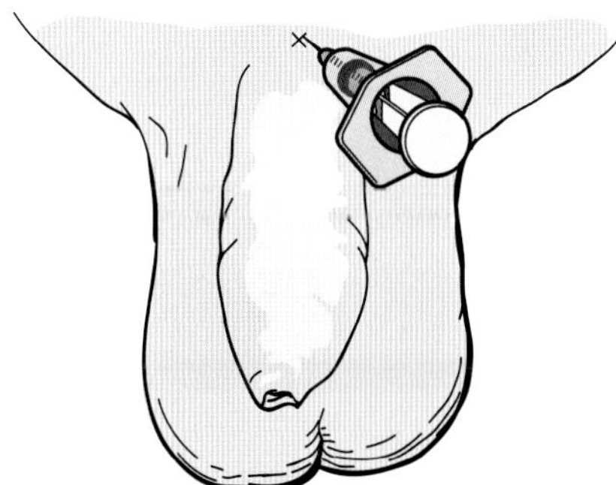

Figure 179-6 Dorsal penile nerve block using a single injection site at the 12 o'clock position.

- Another study comparing plain and buffered lidocaine in newborns failed to demonstrate a difference in oxygen saturations, crying, heart rate, or any other measure of distress.
- Although some anesthesia will take effect in as little as 2 to 3 minutes, ideally 3 to 5 minutes should be allowed for the full effect of the anesthesia before performing circumcision. Conveniently, this is about the amount of time it takes to prepare and drape the infant and appropriately arrange the instruments.
- Avoid injecting air, which can cause pain.

Common Errors

- Insufficient time allowed for anesthetic to take effect
- Lidocaine injected in the wrong location

Complications

- Inadequate anesthesia
- Localized edema, bleeding, or hematoma at the injection site
- Local skin infection or necrosis
- Allergic reaction to lidocaine
- Systemic reaction to intravascular lidocaine
- Erythema and mild skin pallor observed with use of EMLA
- Penile necrosis (This is theoretical, because it has not been reported. Only lidocaine *without* epinephrine should be used because epinephrine can cause vasospasm of the penile arteries.)

CPT/Billing Code

64450-47 Nerve block, diagnostic or therapeutic, other peripheral nerve, anesthesia by surgeon

(A few insurers will pay for this as a separate procedure from the circumcision.)

ICD-9-CM Diagnostic Code

V50.2 Routine or ritual circumcision, in absence of significant medical indication

Supplier

(See contact information online at www.expertconsult.com.)

Circumstraint
Olympic Medical Corp. (Natus)

Bibliography

American Academy of Pediatrics: Committee statements: Report of the task force on circumcision. Pediatrics 103:686–693, 1999.

American Academy of Pediatrics, Committee on Fetus and Newborn and Section on Surgery, Canadian Paediatric Society, and Fetus and Newborn Committee: Prevention and management of pain in the neonate: An update. Pediatrics 118:2231–2241, 2006.

Anesthesia for circumcision. In Cunningham FG, Leveno KJ, Bloom SL, et al (eds): Williams Obstetrics, 22nd ed. New York, McGraw-Hill, 2005.

Brady-Fryer B, Wiebe N, Lander JA: Pain relief for neonatal circumcision. Cochrane Database Syst Rev 4:CD004217, 2004.

Lander J, Brady-Fryer B, Metcalfe JB, et al: Comparison of ring block, dorsal penile nerve block, and topical anesthesia for neonatal circumcision: A randomized controlled trial. JAMA 278:2157–2162, 1997.

Serour F, Mandelberg A, Mori J: Slow injection of local anesthetic will decrease pain during dorsal penile nerve block. Acta Anaesthesiol Scand 42:926–928, 1998.

Stellwagen L, Wang M: Local anesthesia for neonatal circumcision video. American Academy of Pediatrics, 2000. Available for purchase at www.aap.org/bst/showdetl.cfm?&DID=15&Product_ID=2370.

CHAPTER 180

Neonatal Resuscitation

Eric M. Hughes

The first few moments of a newborn's life can be the most critical. If needed, effective emergency care during this transition can prevent lifelong consequences. Proper resuscitation requires essential equipment and knowledge of necessary protocols before delivery. Prior knowledge of the gestational age of the newborn is helpful in anticipating the need for resuscitation. Low birth weight and premature delivery predispose infants to the need for resuscitative efforts.

Indications

Neonate with the following:

- Inadequate or ineffective respirations
- Inadequate heart rate
- Central cyanosis
- Other evidence of cardiorespiratory distress

Equipment

- Suction equipment, including a bulb syringe, mechanical suction device, suction catheters (6, 8, 10 French), pediatric feeding tube (8 French), and meconium aspirator (Fig. 180-1)
- Oxygen source with flowmeter, infant resuscitation bag (750 mL) with appropriately sized face masks, laryngoscope with no. 0 and no. 1 straight blades, and sterile newborn endotracheal tubes (2.5, 3, 3.5, and 4 mm), CO_2 monitor
- Drugs, including epinephrine 1:10,000 (0.1 mg/mL), naloxone (0.04 mg/mL), volume expanders (crystalloid or blood), and normal saline for injection
- Miscellaneous items, including a radiant warmer, pediatric stethoscope, needles (25, 21, and 18 gauge), syringes (1, 3, 10, 20 mL), adhesive tape (½-inch width), an umbilical catheter (3.5 or 5 French), and food grade heat-resistant plastic wrap

Technique

As with all medical procedures, universal precautions against exposure to blood and other body fluids should be followed during this procedure. Initial measures, including proper positioning, drying, suctioning, and stimulation, should be provided to all newborns. Figure 180-2 is a flow diagram of the protocol for neonatal resuscitation that is explained in the following sections.

Positioning, Suction, and Stimulation

1. Prevent heat loss by placing the infant under a radiant heat source, then quickly drying him or her and removing the wet linen. (Recovery from acidosis is delayed by hypothermia.) Infants of low birth weight (<1500 g) need extra equipment and effort to keep them warm because the traditional radiant warmer and blankets are insufficient. The body, *but not the head*, of the neonate may be covered with food grade heat-resistant plastic wrap in addition to providing radiant heat. Use of this technique requires constant monitoring to assure overheating does not occur.
2. Open the airway by positioning the infant on its back with the neck slightly extended. Avoid extreme hyperextension or flexion of the infant's neck, which may diminish airflow.
3. Clear the airway by suctioning the mouth, then the nose, with a bulb syringe or mechanical device (suction catheter; see Chapter 178, Delee Suctioning). If mechanical suction is used, pressure should not exceed 100 mm Hg. Deep suctioning of the oropharynx may produce a vagal response and cause bradycardia and apnea. Infants with meconium-stained amniotic fluid should no longer be suctioned with mechanical devices after the head is delivered and prior to the body being delivered. Direct tracheal suctioning should be carried out only if the newborn has absent or depressed respirations, a heart rate below 100 bpm, or poor muscle tone. A meconium aspirator is very helpful in performing this procedure (see Fig. 180-1). This unique piece of equipment is used only for neonates. One end of the device is for a neonatal endotracheal tube, the other end is for suction, and the top hole is for the operator's thumb.
4. Promote respiratory activity by providing tactile stimulation (e.g., slap the sole of the foot or gently rub the back).

Initial Assessment

1. Assess the infant's respiratory status, heart rate, and color.
2. Infants with adequate respiratory and cardiac function (good ventilation and heart rate >100 bpm) and with no evidence of central cyanosis can be merely observed.
3. Infants with depressed respiratory function (shallow, slow, or absent respirations), an abnormal heart rate, or central cyanosis should undergo further resuscitation.

General Guidelines of Resuscitation

As with all resuscitations, the order of importance is **a**irway, **b**reathing, and **c**irculation. The three cardinal indicators in neonatal resuscitation are **r**espirations, **h**eart **r**ate, and **c**olor. In general, the initial assessment should take no more than 30 seconds; should the need for further resuscitation occur, reassessment of interventions should occur every 30 seconds. Apgar scores should be determined and recorded at appropriate intervals. Special circumstances may arise and may be treated with procedures used in general pediatric resuscitation (e.g., chest tube for pneumothorax).

Ventilation

1. Ventilatory insufficiency produces the majority of respiratory and circulatory abnormalities during the newborn period. *Rapid* institution of ventilatory support in newborns with abnormalities of respiratory function or heart rate or central cyanosis maximizes the chances of a successful outcome.

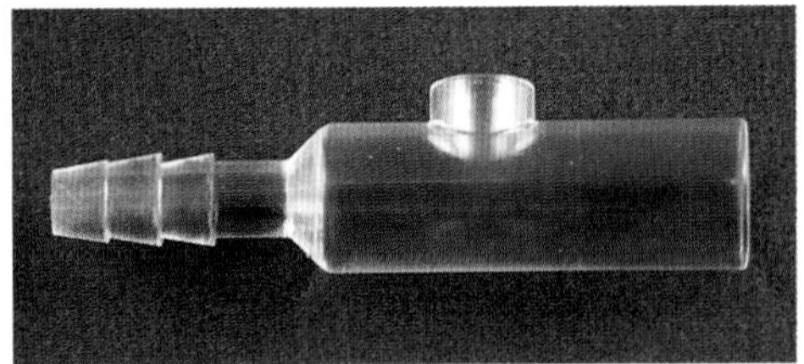

Figure 180-1 Meconium aspirator.

TABLE 180-1 Endotracheal Tube Selection

Infant Weight (g)	Gestation Age (wk)	Endotracheal Tube Size (mm)
<1000	<28	2.5
1000–2000	28 34	3
2000–3000	34–38	3.5
>3000	>38	3.5–4

2. Positive pressure ventilation (PPV) with 100% oxygen is indicated for infants with inadequate respiratory effort or a heart rate less than 100 bpm. Free-flow oxygen administration may be adequate for the infant with central cyanosis if respiratory function is adequate and the heart rate is over 100 bpm. (The cause for cyanosis should be sought.) If central cyanosis persists despite oxygen administration, PPV should be applied.
3. PPV is usually accomplished with a bag and mask, using either a self-inflating bag or an anesthesia bag. A good seal should be maintained by using an appropriately sized face mask with a cushioned rim. A pressure gauge or pop-off valve should be used to ensure adequate ventilatory pressures.
4. Ventilate the infant at a rate of 40 to 60 breaths per minute with a tidal volume of 6 to 8 mL/kg. Adequate ventilation is verified clinically by observing bilateral symmetrical chest expansion and the presence of bilateral breath sounds. Inadequate ventilation may indicate an inadequate face mask seal, a blocked airway, or inadequate ventilation pressure. After initial ventilations, pressures of less than 30 to 40 cm H_2O (20 to 25 cm H_2O for preterm infants) should be adequate.
5. Perform an endotracheal intubation when prolonged PPV is required, bag and mask ventilation is ineffective, chest compressions are used, endotracheal delivery of medication is necessary, or diaphragmatic hernia is suspected. Select an endotracheal tube of appropriate size (Table 180-1) and insert it under direct visualization using the laryngoscope. The tip should rest above the tracheal bifurcation. Appropriate endotracheal tube location is verified clinically by the presence of bilaterally symmetrical breath sounds and confirmation of expired CO_2. Most clinicians also confirm endotracheal tube placement with a chest radiograph.
6. Oral airways are rarely required during neonatal resuscitation but are indicated for bilateral choanal atresia, Pierre Robin syndrome, and when necessary for adequate ventilation.
7. Use of a laryngeal mask airway (LMA) (Fig. 180-3) can be an acceptable alternative when bag-mask ventilation and endotracheal intubation have failed. (The LMA is a substitute in certain cases for traditional endotracheal intubation.) The LMA should be used only by properly trained personnel and is not considered a routine substitute for endotracheal intubation.
8. Gastric catheter placement (8 French) is indicated in prolonged resuscitation efforts to prevent stomach distention, a frequent problem in newborns who are being ventilated by mask.

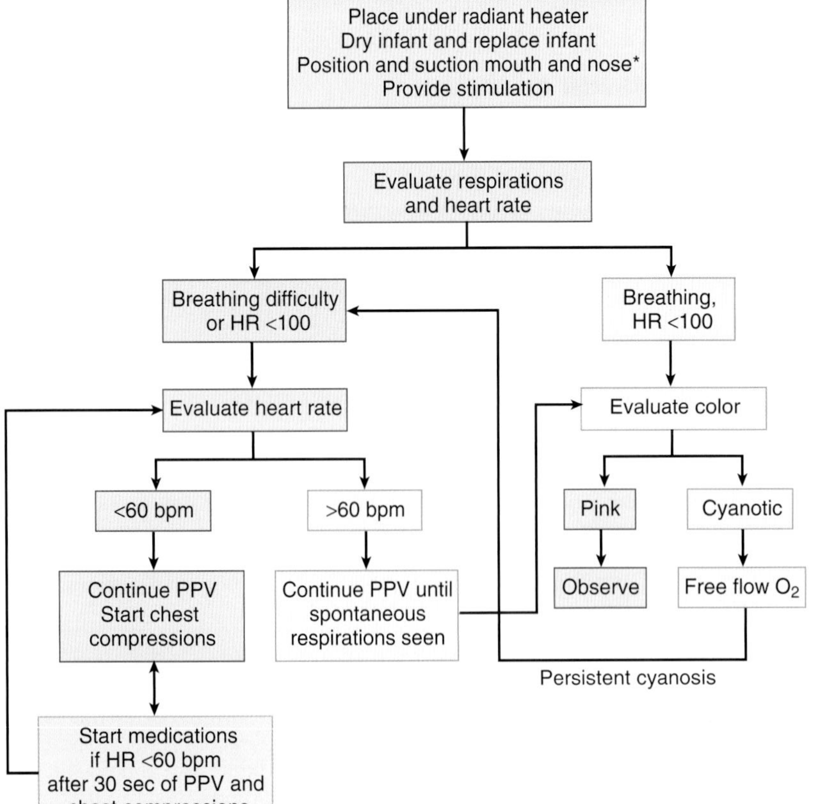

Figure 180-2 Resuscitation flowchart. bpm, beats per minute; HR, heart rate; PPV, positive pressure ventilation. *Consider endotracheal intubation if meconium present and infant not vigorous.

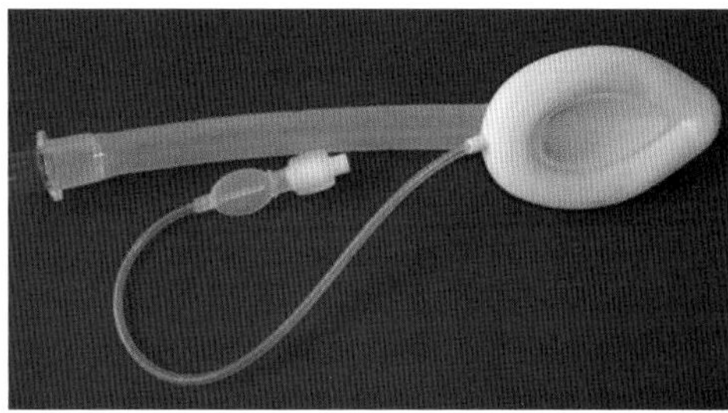

Figure 180-3 Laryngeal mask airway. (Courtesy of Legend Medical Devices, Inc.)

Chest Compressions

1. Administer chest compressions if the infant's heart rate is less than 60 bpm after adequate PPV for 30 seconds. Chest compressions can be accomplished with the thumbs placed on the sternum and the hands encircling the chest (preferred method), or with the tips of the middle and index fingers (Fig. 180-4). Chest compressions should be applied to the lower third of the sternum. The sternum should be depressed one third of the anteroposterior dimension of the chest, rather than an exact depth of compression. The compression depth must be adequate to produce a palpable pulse.
2. Chest compressions should be administered at a ratio of 3:1 with PPV, at a rate of 90 compressions and 30 ventilations every minute. Reassess the pulse every 30 seconds. The umbilical cord stump is a convenient location to palpate the pulse.
3. Continue chest compressions until the spontaneous heart rate is 60 bpm or higher (see Fig. 180-2).

Medications

Table 180-2 summarizes the medications used in neonatal resuscitation. Administer medications for asystole or if the heart rate remains less than 60 bpm after adequate PPV and chest compressions for a minimum of 30 seconds. Medications may be administered through the umbilical vein with a 3.5- or 5-French umbilical catheter placed just below the skin level. (See Chapter 184, Umbilical Vessel Catheterization.) Alternative access can be obtained through a peripheral vein or, in the event that no other access is available, by intraosseous access (see Chapter 198, Intraosseous Vascular Access). Intraosseous access can be very difficult to obtain in premature infants. Alternative routes of administration (endotracheal, intramuscular, or subcutaneous) are available for some medications.

Termination of Resuscitation

Discontinuation of resuscitative efforts may be appropriate if resuscitation of an infant with cardiorespiratory arrest does not produce spontaneous circulation within 10 minutes. Resuscitation of newly born infants after 10 minutes of asystole is also very unlikely to result in survival or survival without severe disability. Those involved in neonatal resuscitation should pursue local discussions to formulate guidelines consistent with local resources and outcome data.

Postprocedure Patient Management

- Maintain careful monitoring in an appropriately staffed intensive care unit (or arrange transfer to such a facility).
- Continue evaluation with serial arterial blood gases, frequent determination of fluid and electrolyte status, chest radiographs, and other modalities as indicated by clinical findings.
- Completely document the resuscitation effort in the medical record.
- Discuss situation with parents.

Complications

Suction

- Vagal response (bradycardia or apnea)
- Hypoxia

Ventilation

- Pneumothorax
- Hypoxia resulting from inadequate ventilation

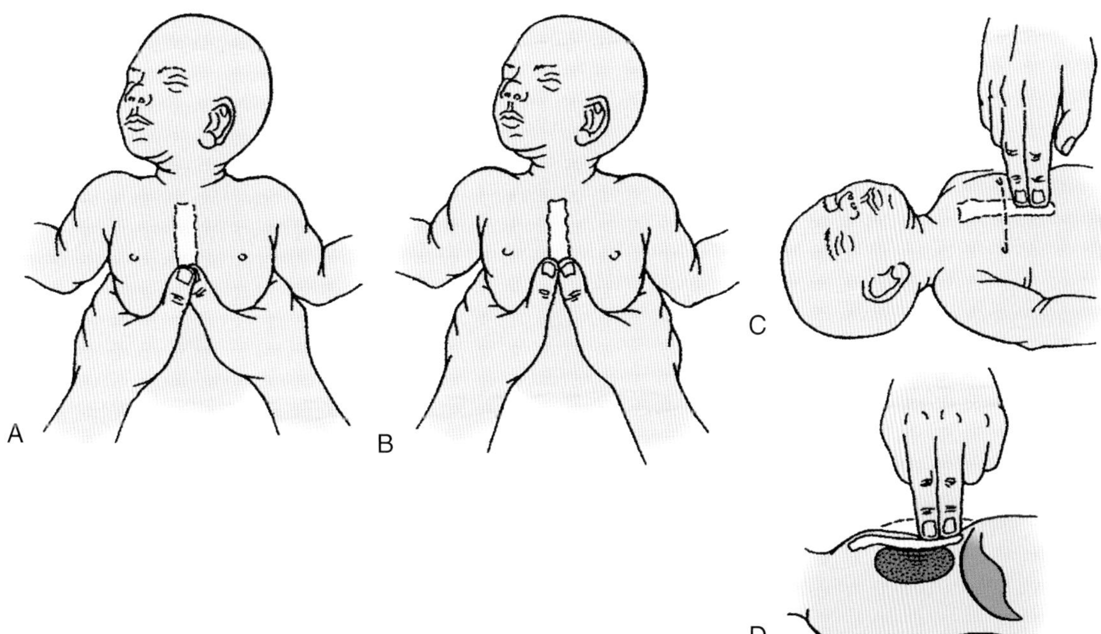

Figure 180-4 Chest compression. Two-thumb technique with, **A,** thumb over thumb and, **B,** thumbs side by side. **C,** Two-finger technique. **D,** Chest compression depth is one third to one half of the anteroposterior diameter of the chest or one third of the depth of the chest.

TABLE 180-2 Medications Used for Neonatal Resuscitation

Medication	Indication	Dose	Route of Administration
Epinephrine	Asystole or HR <60, despite adequate PPV and chest compressions for 30 sec	0.1–0.3 mL/kg of a 1 : 10,000 solution *or* 0.01–0.03 mg/kg	IV (preferred) or ET; can repeat every 3–5 min
Volume expander (crystalloid or blood)	Evidence of acute blood loss with signs of hypovolemia, or failure to respond to resuscitation or signs of shock	10 mL/kg	IV over 5–10 min
Naloxone	History of maternal narcotic administration within 4 hr of delivery; not recommended for initial efforts, heart rate and color should be restored by supporting ventilation first	0.1 mg/kg	IV preferred, IM

ET, endotracheal; HR, heart rate; IM, intramuscular; IV, intravenous; PPV, positive pressure ventilation.

- Complications from intubation (see Chapter 213, Tracheal Intubation)

CPT/Billing Codes

99431 History and examination of the normal newborn infant, initiation of diagnostic and treatment programs, and preparation of hospital records

99436 Attendance at delivery (when requested by delivering physician) and initial stabilization of newborn

99440 Newborn resuscitation: provision of positive pressure ventilation and/or chest compressions in the presence of acute inadequate ventilation and/or cardiac output

NOTE: 99436 *may* be reported in addition to 99431; 99436 *may not* be reported in addition to 99440

ICD-9-CM Diagnostic Codes

427.5 Cardiorespiratory arrest
768.5 Asphyxia, newborn, severe
768.6 Asphyxia, newborn, mild/moderate
770.12 Meconium aspiration, with respiratory symptoms
770.84 Respiratory failure, newborn
770.87 Respiratory arrest, newborn
770.88 Hypoxemia of newborn
770.89 Other respiratory problems after birth
779.81 Bradycardia, newborn
779.85 Cardiac arrest, newborn

Acknowledgment

The editors wish to recognize the many contributions by Marvin A. Dewar, MD, JD, to this chapter in the first edition of this text.

BIBLIOGRAPHY

American Heart Association: 2005 American Heart Association (AHA) guidelines for cardiopulmonary resuscitation (CPR) and emergency cardiovascular care (ECC) of pediatric and neonatal patients: Neonatal resuscitation guidelines. Pediatrics 117:e1029–e1038, 2006.

International Liaison Committee on Resuscitation (ILCOR) Consensus on Science with Treatment Recommendations for Pediatric and Neonatal Patients: Pediatric basic and advanced life support. Pediatrics 117: e955–e977, 2006.

CHAPTER 181

NEWBORN CIRCUMCISION AND OFFICE MEATOTOMY

Ronald D. Reynolds • Grant C. Fowler

Newborn circumcision is the most common surgical procedure performed in the United States, yet controversy exists over the need for the procedure. Studies have shown a lower incidence of urinary tract infection (UTI), phimosis, paraphimosis, balanoposthitis, and some sexually transmitted infections (STIs), including human immunodeficiency virus (HIV), in circumcised men. Circumcision clearly helps prevents penile cancer and may decrease the risk of cervical cancer in the sexual partner. However, some of these problems (i.e., penile cancer, UTIs, foreskin problems, and HIV infection) are rare even in uncircumcised men.

In developed countries where it is much less common for males to be circumcised, there is a low incidence of foreskin problems later in life. Behavioral factors also appear to be far more important than circumcision status in regards to the acquisition of STIs and HIV infection. Therefore, the decision to circumcise is not currently based on scientific evidence. Rather, this decision is generally made based on cultural, familial, or ethnic preference.

There is controversy in the literature regarding the cost effectiveness of newborn circumcision. Authors of a retrospective cost–benefit analysis of almost 15,000 newborn boys born in 1996 and insured by Kaiser Permanente Northern California (a large health maintenance organization) concluded that neonatal circumcision can be achieved at basically no cost. When total costs of newborn circumcision were weighed against total medical costs of not having it, the costs were basically equal. This was largely because postneonatal circumcision costs were about 10 times more than neonatal circumcision costs ($1921 per child versus $165 per newborn), and circumcision was eventually medically indicated in 9.6% of uncircumcised boys. However, other cost–benefit analysis studies have reached opposite conclusions. Also, there is controversy in the literature as to whether the percentage of newborns undergoing circumcision is increasing. If that is the case, it may start becoming more of a norm.

Clinicians performing circumcision are encouraged to remain current with guidelines and the scientific evidence. The American Academy of Pediatrics (AAP) circumcision position from March 1999, endorsed by the American College of Obstetricians and Gynecologists (ACOG) in 2001, and reaffirmed in 2005, reads as follows:

> Existing scientific evidence demonstrates potential medical benefits of newborn male circumcision; however, these data are not sufficient to recommend routine neonatal circumcision. In circumstances in which there are potential benefits and risks, yet the procedure is not essential to the child's current well-being, parents should determine what is in the best interest of the child. To make an informed choice, parents of all male infants should be given accurate and unbiased information and be provided the opportunity to discuss this decision. If a decision for circumcision is made, procedural analgesia should be provided.

Of note, 97% of pediatric, family medicine, and obstetrics and gynecology residency programs that teach circumcision teach the administration of an anesthetic, either locally or topically. Common methods of analgesia administration include subcutaneous ring block, dorsal penile nerve block (DPNB; see Chapter 179, Subcutaneous Ring and Dorsal Penile Block for Newborn Circumcision), topical anesthesia such as lidocaine–prilocaine cream (also known as eutectic mixture of local anesthetic, or EMLA; see Chapter 10, Topical Anesthesia), and precircumcision oral analgesics. Although studies have shown lidocaine–prilocaine cream to be helpful, injected blocks appear to be more effective, and the ring block is more effective than a DPNB. Studies have shown that infants anesthetized with a block cry less, are less likely to have tachycardia, are less irritable, and have fewer behavior changes during the 24 hours after the procedure. They also have less variability in oxygen saturation and blood pressure during, and lower serum cortisol levels after, the procedure.

Three techniques of newborn circumcision are common in the United States: Mogen, Gomco, and Plastibell. Most clinicians continue to use the technique they were taught in their training. Both Gomco and Plastibell require a dorsal slit and considerable manipulation to prepare the foreskin for excision, and result in removal of a cylindrical sleeve of tissue. Both techniques carry the risk of removing too much tissue from the ventral side. In addition, Plastibell leaves behind a foreign body that may contribute to infection. One study comparing Gomco with Plastibell indicated that there was not only a higher rate of infection with Plastibell but also a slightly higher rate of bleeding.

Most clinicians who learn to use the Mogen clamp tend to prefer this technique because it is quicker and simpler, and it follows the angle of the corona so as to avoid removing excess tissue ventrally. At least two studies (Kurtis and colleagues, 1999; Kaufman and colleagues, 2002) comparing the use of the Mogen with the Gomco technique found that the Mogen procedure took about half the time and seemed to cause less discomfort (however, discomfort may be a moot point when anesthesia is used). Contrary to popular belief, the Mogen clamp is not a guillotine. It is simply a crushing device with a narrow slot that, when used appropriately, does not allow entry of the glans into the slot.

One apparent complication of circumcision is meatal stenosis (i.e., it is very rare in uncircumcised boys). Whether circumcision or a chronic inflammatory process due to superabsorbent disposable diapers, ammonia dermatitis, or inadequate parental postprocedure care is to blame is yet to be determined. In the last edition of this text, a technique for newborn meatotomy was included; however, there are few data suggesting that such a procedure might decrease the later incidence of meatal stenosis. (And it must be very rare or it would be more common in uncircumcised men.) This scarcity of data is partially because it is difficult to define meatal stenosis in a newborn. It is usually diagnosed later in life, at the time of toilet training or even later, because of its complications (e.g., painful urination that may require straining or standing, difficulty aiming stream, blood spotting in underwear). To make the diagnosis may require observed voiding (i.e., pinpoint meatus and a dorsally deflected, very fine caliber, forceful urine stream with a long voiding distance) because the appearance of the glans may be somewhat normal and thereby misleading. However, newborn meatotomy is included again in this edition because the risk of such a procedure is minimal compared with potential benefits (e.g., repair in an older male patient can be somewhat psychologically traumatic). Also, in certain situations, newborn meatal stenosis is obvious and because the infant is already anesthetized for circumcision, it would seem prudent to repair it at that time.

After toilet training, a popular method of defining meatal stenosis is by what size feeding tube or pediatric urethral catheter can be easily inserted. Because meatal stenosis is a possible complication of newborn circumcision, it seems appropriate to also include a technique for later repair (i.e., office meatotomy) in this chapter. Although it might seem somewhat psychologically traumatic to repair meatal stenosis under mere topical anesthesia, boys having difficulty with urination may be very motivated to cooperate, especially if assured of the adequacy of topical anesthesia. Pediatric sedation may also be useful (see Chapter 7, Pediatric Sedation and Analgesia).

Anatomy

The neonatal foreskin is composed of three layers: skin, loose subcutaneous tissue, and mucosa. At birth, the foreskin mucosa is adherent to the glans penis, with just a small distal opening to allow for urination. The ventral side of the mucosal surface has the highest density of nerve endings. A band of tissue called the *frenulum* attaches the foreskin along the ventral side of the penis and ends distally near the urethral meatus. The frenulum contains a small artery.

Circumcision

Indication

Parental desire is the only necessary indication for circumcision.

Contraindications

Absolute

- Hypospadias, epispadias, or megaurethra (the foreskin is used for later repair)
- Unusual-appearing genitalia
- Inability to determine the sexual phenotype of the child (ambiguous genitalia)

Relative

- Age younger than 12 hours (physiologic adaptation requires 12 to 24 hours)
- Age greater than 6 to 8 weeks
- Severe illness
- Prematurity (until the child is ready for discharge from the hospital)

Precautions

If there is a family history of bleeding problems, appropriate laboratory studies should be performed before the procedure. If the mother is thrombocytopenic, the infant's platelet count should be checked.

By the age of 6 to 8 weeks, maternal clotting factors have been metabolized, possibly predisposing the infant to increased blood loss. The foreskin may also develop significant edema after defining the plane and breaking up adhesions between the glans and the foreskin, making it difficult to use the Gomco clamp or Plastibell.

Preprocedure Patient and Parent Preparation

Discuss the risks and benefits of the procedure with the parents. Informed consent is obtained and a patient teaching guide is given to the parents. (See patient education and patient consent forms available online at www.expertconsult.com.) The AAP has two brochures that may be used: (1) *Circumcision: Information for Parents* and (2) *Care of the Uncircumcised Penis* (see the Suppliers section). The parents are usually asked to leave the room during the procedure. If they desire to stay, they should be given the option to look away while the procedure is being performed because it can be disconcerting to some.

Because of the risks of regurgitation and aspiration, infants being circumcised should be at least 1 hour postprandial. Confirm that the infant has had at least one void since birth.

Equipment

Equipment Common to All Techniques

- Assistant for holding infant, infant restraint or papoose board (Circumstraint) with leg straps (e.g., Circumstraint), or circumcision chair (e.g., Stang)
- Anesthetic supplies: gloves, alcohol wipes, 1% plain lidocaine, 1-mL syringe, 30-gauge needle
- Sterile gloves
- Antiseptic solution (e.g., alcohol wipes, povidone–iodine, chlorhexidine) or swabsticks
- Sterile drape with 1-inch fenestration
- Sterile 2 × 2 or 4 × 4 gauze pads
- Three straight mosquito hemostats
- White petrolatum ointment (e.g., Vaseline)
- Disposable diaper
- Adequate light source
- Glucose water or sugar-coated pacifier *(optional)*
- Skin marking pen *(optional)*
- Flexible blunt probe *(optional)*
- Acetaminophen drops or solution (10 to 15 mg/kg) *(optional)*

Equipment for the Mogen Technique

- Mogen clamp, neonatal size (2.5-mm slot)

  NOTE: The larger adult size is dangerous to use on a newborn because the glans can become trapped in the larger slot. The clinician should confirm that the neonatal size does not open more than 2.5 mm.

- No. 10 blade scalpel

Equipment for the Gomco Technique

- Straight scissors with one blunt tip
- Gomco circumcision clamps (1.1-, 1.3-, and 1.45-cm sizes)

  NOTE: The most commonly used size is 1.3 cm. The 1.1-cm size is used for a very small infant, whereas the 1.45-cm clamp usually fits a large infant. Even larger sizes are available for children and adults.

- No. 10 blade scalpel
- Sterile safety pin *(optional)*

Equipment for the Plastibell Technique

- Straight scissors with one blunt tip
- Plastibell device (1.1-, 1.2-, 1.3-, and 1.4-cm sizes)

  NOTE: Similar to the Gomco technique, 1.3 cm is the most commonly used Plastibell size.

- Iris scissors

Equipment for Bleeding Complications in All Three Techniques

- Topical epinephrine
- Topical hemostatic agent of choice (e.g., Gelfoam, Surgicel, silver nitrate; see Chapter 40, Topical Hemostatic Agents)
- 5-0 absorbable suture (chromic or catgut) on a taper-point needle
- Needle holder and suture scissors

Mogen Technique

1. Consider using a skin marker to mark the coronal edge. Inspect the penis for abnormalities and for the location of the meatus on the glans. If epispadias or hypospadias is found, terminate the procedure because the foreskin may be used for later repair by a urologist.
2. The clinician should follow universal blood and body fluid precautions. If penile anatomy is normal, anesthetize the penis with a subcutaneous ring block (see Chapter 179, Subcutaneous Ring and Dorsal Penile Block for Newborn Circumcision). Consider doing the block with the infant still in his crib to allow time for the block to take effect while the rest of the surgical preparations are made. Position the infant appropriately in a warm room. An infant may experience discomfort when you extend his legs on an infant restraint board. As a result, special circumcision chairs have been developed for exposure of the penis without extension of the legs. If such a chair is not available, an assistant can hold the infant on a pillow with the knees flexed and legs abducted for adequate exposure. Most often, though, an infant restraining board is used. Leave the infant's arms free to minimize distress. Offer him a swallow or two of glucose water or a sugar-coated pacifier to calm him.
3. Using antiseptic solution or swabsticks, prepare the entire penis and a 1-inch area surrounding the penis. Wear sterile gloves when placing the fenestrated drape.
4. Grasp the very edge of the foreskin with hemostats at the 2 and 10 o'clock positions, taking care not to grasp the glans. (When describing the penis, use the dorsal midline as the 12 o'clock position. To identify the true dorsal midline, identify the ventral raphe at the frenulum, which is the 6 o'clock position, and consider the foreskin 180 degrees opposite it to be the 12 o'clock position [Fig. 181-1]. This orientation technique is important in case the penile shaft gets rotated.)
5. Place gentle traction on the foreskin by holding the two hemostats side by side in your nondominant hand. Gently insert the third hemostat with your dominant hand, closed and from below the grasping hemostats, at the 12 o'clock position between the foreskin and the glans. Advance to the depth of the coronal sulcus (Fig. 181-2). To ensure that the meatus is not entered, keep the foreskin tented up as this hemostat is advanced. Open this hemostat and sweep it clockwise and counterclockwise to free the foreskin off the glans. This may take a number of open–close cycles starting at different places around the corona. Do not free the area from the 5 to 7 o'clock positions (the frenulum) because it contains an artery. Do not dissect beyond the depth of the coronal sulcus. As an alternative to opening and closing a hemostat, a blunt probe may be used to free the foreskin off of the glans.
6. Tent the foreskin away from the glans by gently lifting the grasping hemostats. Ensure that no part of the glans is in the way. Advance the lower blade of the third hemostat between the glans and foreskin at the 12 o'clock position to a position no less than 5 mm distal to the coronal sulcus (Fig. 181-3). Do not apply traction to the grasping hemostats as this dorsal hemostat is applied or you will remove too much foreskin. Close and lock the hemostat in place.
7. Remove the two foreskin edge–grasping hemostats.
8. Using the thumb and index finger of your nondominant hand, pinch the free foreskin underneath the dorsal hemostat while curling your other fingers of the same hand around the handles of the hemostat. This pushes the glans back out of the way of the Mogen clamp. Release any traction on the hemostat and foreskin because traction on the frenulum can dorsally rotate the glans and bring the meatus into the path of the Mogen clamp. Maintain the pinch while the Mogen clamp is placed. The tips of the pinching fingers should be slightly proximal to the tip of the grasping hemostat.
9. Inspect the Mogen clamp to be sure that its joint is not loose and that it opens only 2.5 mm, then open it fully. Hold it so

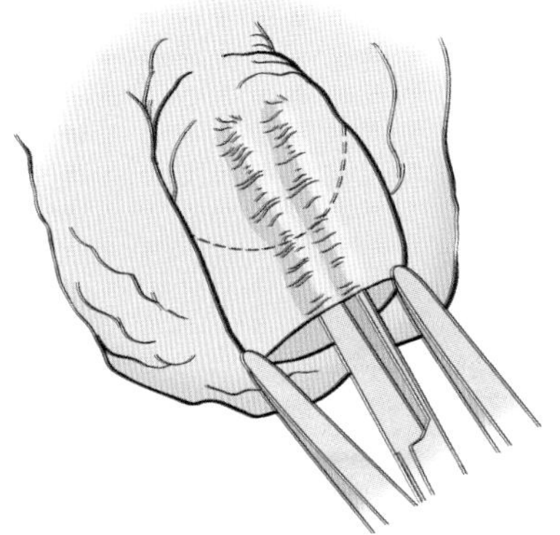

Figure 181-2 Insert the third hemostat between the foreskin and the glans, tenting the foreskin as it is advanced. Here the surgeon is just beginning to open the hemostat to free the foreskin off the glans.

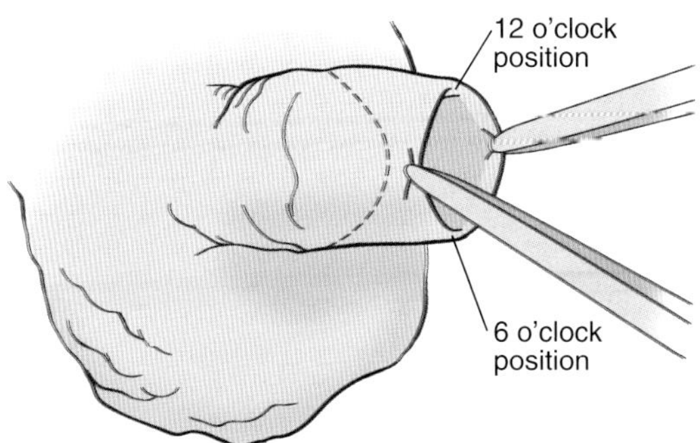

Figure 181-1 Using 6 o'clock as the ventral position of the frenulum, 12 o'clock is the dorsal midline position.

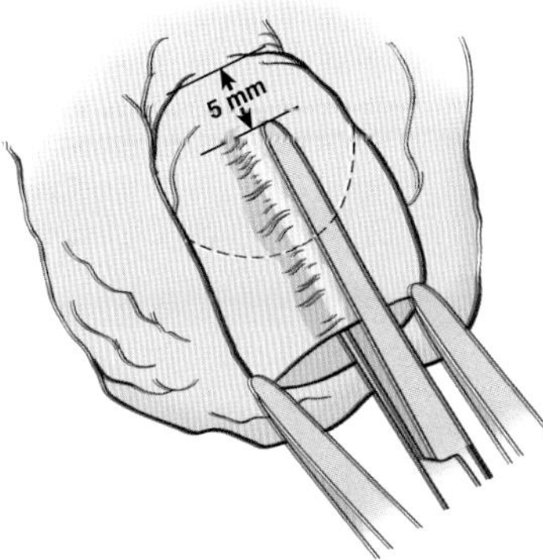

Figure 181-3 Place a dorsal hemostat with its tip 5 mm from the corona.

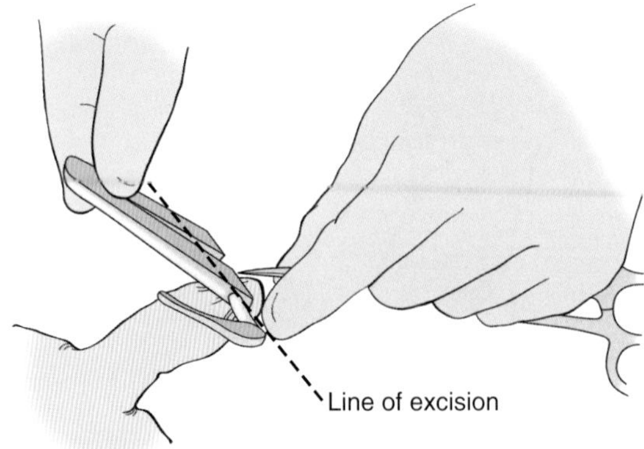

Figure 181-4 Pinch the foreskin to push the glans back while advancing the Mogen clamp vertically along the angle of the corona.

that the open end of the slot is down and the flat surface faces you. With your dominant hand, advance the Mogen slot across the foreskin, starting immediately behind the tip of the dorsal hemostat (Fig. 181-4). Angle the Mogen's advancement to remove more foreskin dorsally than ventrally, following along the angle of the corona (dorsum of the glans). Slide the clamp across the foreskin as far as it will go easily. At this point, the use of previous skin markings can ensure that an adequate, but not excessive, amount of foreskin is removed.

10. Before locking the Mogen clamp, drop the foreskin pinch and attempt to move the glans beneath the slot. You should be able to move the glans freely for a few millimeters up and down and side to side. If the glans is not free, *do not* lock the Mogen clamp.
11. Lock the Mogen clamp by moving the bar across the slot and closing the cam lever fully.
12. Use the scalpel to cut the foreskin off flush with the flat surface of the Mogen clamp (Fig. 181-5). Discard the foreskin in a biohazard waste container.
13. Unlock and remove the Mogen clamp. There is no medical rationale for leaving the clamp on for any specific length of time.
14. Gently separate the crushed edges of the foreskin to liberate the glans. Grasp the penile shaft skin at the 3 and 9 o'clock positions to pull the crush line apart (Fig. 181-6). Be sure to separate fully to avoid the possibility of causing a paraphimosis. It is not unusual to have a few remaining attachments between the glans and the mucosal surface of the remaining foreskin next to the corona. The easiest way to divide these is to use the tip of a closed and locked hemostat to follow the coronal sulcus, but a blunt probe can also be used. Do not be too vigorous or try to free the frenular area because this will cause bleeding.

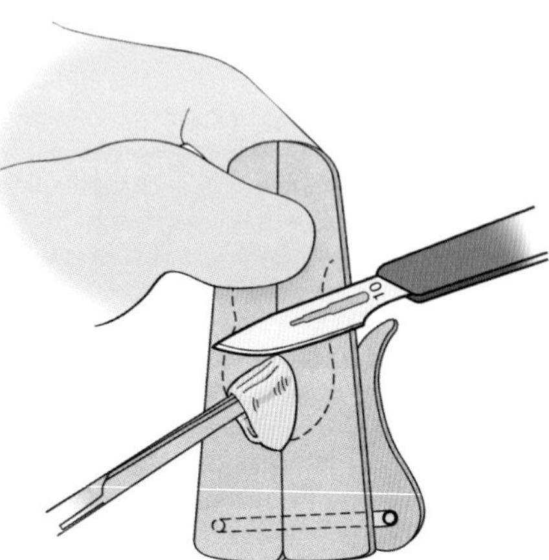

Figure 181-5 Excise the foreskin.

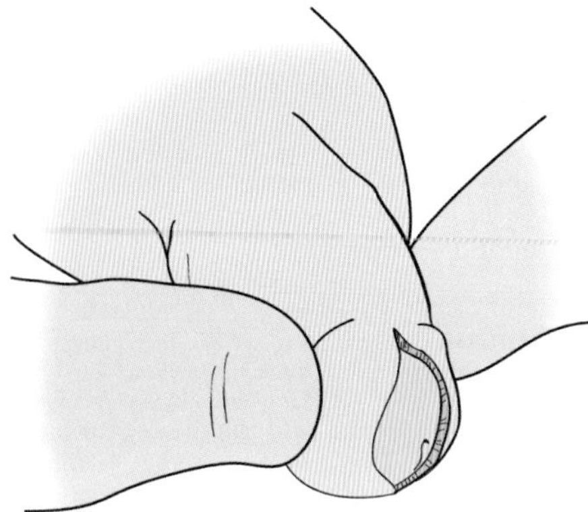

Figure 181-6 Liberate the glans with thumb pressure.

15. Check for hemostasis. To control any bleeding, apply pressure or topical epinephrine to the specific source. In rare cases of persistent bleeding, topical hemostatic agents can be applied with pressure to hasten clotting. Rarely will bleeding require suturing. In the event that it does, use an absorbable suture at the site of the bleeding, which is usually an arteriole. Persistent bleeding after circumcision is a common presenting sign for a factor-deficient bleeding disorder, such as hemophilia. If bleeding persists after following these described measures, obtain clotting studies and consider a hematology consultation.
16. Cover the glans with white petrolatum ointment, and reapply the diaper.
17. Administer an oral dose of acetaminophen (10 to 15 mg/kg) *(optional)*.
18. Document the procedure and time in the chart. To ensure continued hemostasis, do not discharge the infant for about an hour after the procedure. The infant should also have urinated before discharge.

Gomco Technique

1. Choose an appropriate-size Gomco clamp, which is 1.3 cm for most newborns. (The bell diameter should be slightly larger than the diameter of the glans; although the bell should cover the glans completely, it should just barely cover it.) Carefully inspect the clamp. If the clamp was packaged disassembled, reassemble it in the sterile field. Because there is more than one manufacturer for Gomco clamps, make sure the reassembled clamp parts fit together properly. (Reassembled parts may be from different manufacturers.) Make sure the bell is the correct size for the clamp and that there are no defects. Lightly tighten the clamp with the bell in place. Make sure that no light can be seen around the bell where it meets the clamp at the base plate. This ensures a complete circumferential crush for optimal hemostasis. Next, verify that the top surface of the base plate is flat (it can become warped over time). Last, there should be at least 2 mm between the back of the lever arm and the base plate beneath the nut before tightening. This also ensures adequate clamping.
2. As in steps 1 through 5 of the Mogen Technique section, inspect the penis for abnormalities, consider marking the coronal edge, administer a penile subcutaneous ring block, position the infant (restrain if necessary), apply antiseptic and drapes, and free the foreskin from the glans.
3. As in step 6 of the Mogen Technique section, place a crushing dorsal hemostat at the 12 o'clock position, but apply it only to the distal third or half of the length of the foreskin (the total

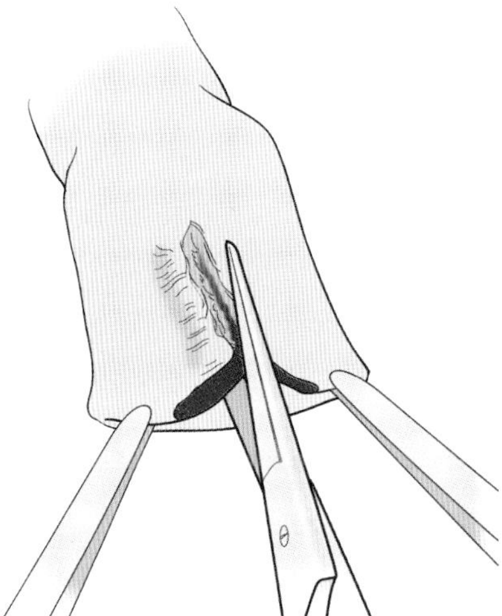

Figure 181-7 Incise the dorsal slit.

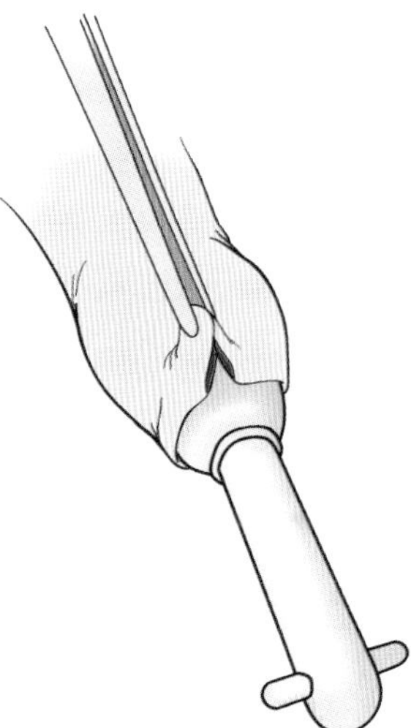

Figure 181-8 Reapproximate the dorsal slit around the Gomco bell.

length of the foreskin extends from the foreskin edge to the coronal sulcus). This hemostat is not applied more proximal than 1 cm from the coronal sulcus. Make sure that the crushing hemostat contains both the mucosal and skin layers of the foreskin.

4. The hemostat can be removed immediately after crushing. Removal reveals a crushed straight line down the dorsal aspect of the foreskin; this crushed tissue has been devitalized and therefore will not bleed when cut. Insert the blunt blade of the scissors between the foreskin and the glans, underneath the crush line, and tent the foreskin with the two edge hemostats and this blade of the scissors. The crushed dorsal line should be thin enough to somewhat visualize the blunt blade through it when it is tented up. With the scissors placed in this manner, cut a dorsal slit down the center of the crush line (Fig. 181-7). Be careful to cut only in the crush line; do not extend laterally or past the apex of the crush line. Venturing beyond or outside the crush line will often result in unnecessary bleeding.
5. Separate the cut edges of the foreskin; this should then allow you to retract the foreskin back from around the glans. If, at this point, you cannot fully retract the foreskin, and it is due to an inadequate incision (and not due to adhesions), recrush a bit further dorsally on the foreskin and extend the dorsal slit. Lyse any remaining adherence between the foreskin and glans with the closed tips of a locked hemostat or the blunt probe. You should be able to fully reveal the sulcus behind the corona. Be very careful when dissecting between the 5 and 7 o'clock positions to avoid the frenulum and its artery.

   NOTE: If the clinician notices hypospadias or epispadias after the dorsal slit has been made, terminate the procedure. After termination, if there is bleeding from the dorsal slit, whipstitch the edges or close the dorsal slit using fine chromic suture. Repair of penile congenital anomalies by a urologist may require foreskin tissue; do not remove any, if possible.

6. Place the bell of an appropriate-size Gomco clamp over the exposed glans. (If the bell and Gomco are not in the same package, another package may need to be opened by an assistant and handed to you in a sterile manner.)
7. Use the two still-attached edge hemostats to reapproximate the foreskin around the outside of the bell while applying gentle downward pressure on the bell's stem. Make sure that both mucosal and skin layers of the foreskin are reapproximated. The bell should occupy the space between the glans and the foreskin and sit against the coronal edge.
8. Once the Gomco bell is appropriately placed, grasp both sides of the dorsal slit near the middle of the incision with the tips of a third hemostat. This reapproximates the foreskin around the stem (Fig. 181-8). The approach with the hemostat is from above at a low angle, with handles up near the infant's umbilicus. This will ease the next step. (Some clinicians use a safety pin to hold the dorsal slit edges together in this step, but this unnecessarily increases the risk of a puncture injury to the clinician.)
9. Remove the two foreskin edge hemostats.
10. Place the end of the stem through the hole in the Gomco baseplate as far as it will go without dislodging the foreskin.
11. Reaching through the baseplate hole with a hemostat, grasp across the foreskin's dorsal slit just above the tips of the lower hemostat (Fig. 181-9). Remove the lower hemostat. Pull the stem and surrounding foreskin fully up through the baseplate hole. (If using a safety pin, pull the entire pin along with the bell through the baseplate hole. The safety pin will need to be turned parallel to the stem of the bell to pull it through the hole. The safety pin can then remain in place throughout the remainder of the procedure to avoid exposing its sharp tip.)
12. Assemble the Gomco clamp by grasping the wings of the bell's stem in the rocker arm's end, placing the rocker arm in its fulcrum slot, and loosely placing the nut on its screw.

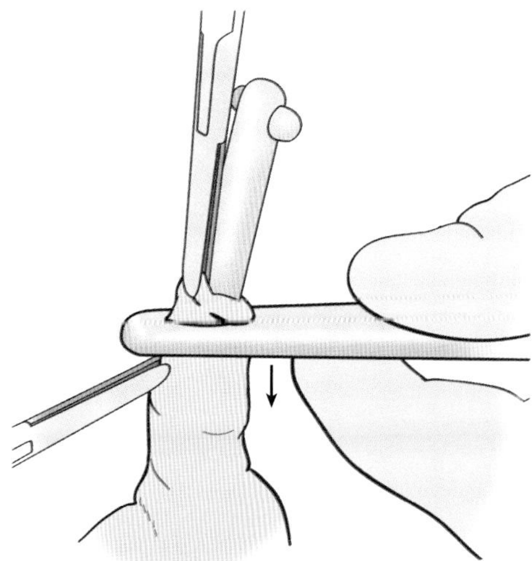

Figure 181-9 Bring the bell's stem and foreskin through the ring by exchanging hemostats.

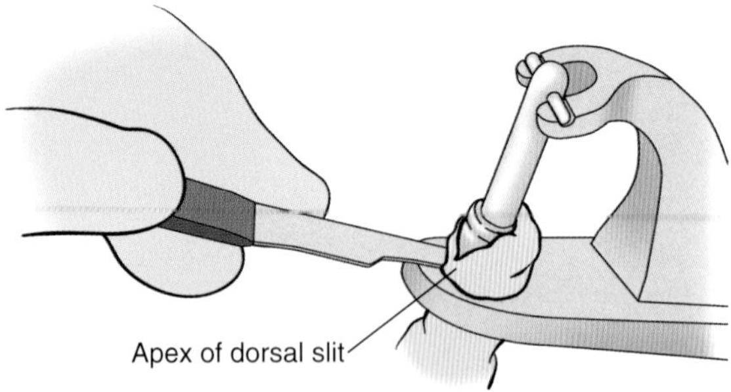

Figure 181-10 Excise the foreskin. The apex of the dorsal slit should be visible above the baseplate.

13. Make sure that the foreskin has been drawn through the hole in the Gomco clamp evenly from all sides. The apex of the dorsal slit must be above the baseplate. Using a hemostat or forceps, pull on the mucosal edge of the dorsal slit to be sure that the mucosal apex of the dorsal slit is also above the baseplate. Prior marking of the coronal edge position on the foreskin with a skin marker can be helpful at this point. When you are sure that the foreskin is evenly pulled through the Gomco clamp and the apex of the dorsal slit is visible above the baseplate, firmly tighten the clamp.
14. On the top side of the baseplate, the scalpel can be used to immediately excise the foreskin. It should be excised circumferentially and completely, on the top side, at the junction of the baseplate and the bell (Fig. 181-10). The top side of the baseplate is on the same side as the stem of the bell. Make sure that all skin and mucosal layers are removed. Any remaining tissue above the clamp will become necrotic and a possible source of infection. The excised ring of foreskin should be removed from the bell (it may be slid over the stem or cut away from the stem with scissors) and discarded in a biohazard waste container. Alternatively, the excised foreskin may be left on the stem until the device is disassembled.
15. Loosen and disassemble the Gomco clamp. There is no medical rationale for leaving the clamp on for any specific length of time.
16. To remove the adherent foreskin edge from the bell, gently tease it away using a piece of gauze (Fig. 181-11).

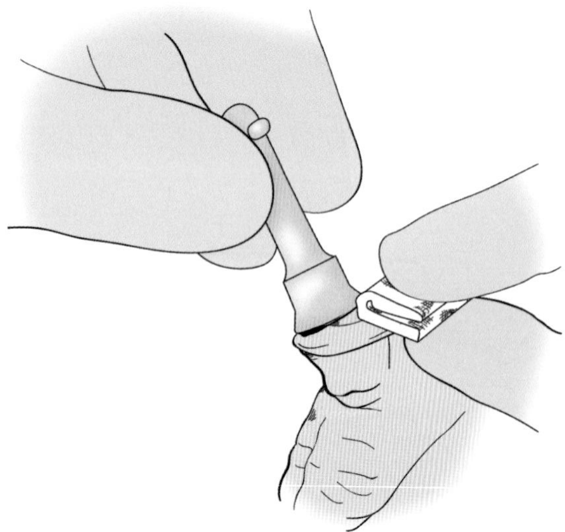

Figure 181-11 Tease the adherent tissue off the bell edge with gauze.

17. Follow steps 15 through 18 of the Mogen Technique section to check hemostasis, dress the wound, and document the procedure.

NOTE: A rare complication of using a Gomco clamp that is too large, or from pulling too much foreskin through the baseplate hole, is degloving of the penile shaft skin. In this situation, after the clamp and bell are removed, the shaft skin will retract too far and expose the underlying tissue proximal to the coronal sulcus. Attempts to control bleeding in the usual manner often fail. If bleeding is not controlled, a primary closure with four absorbable (5-0 chromic) sutures should be made. Sutures are placed circumferentially to reposition the retracted shaft skin to a point just proximal to the corona. Care must be taken in the ventral area to avoid the urethra. Some clinicians catheterize the infant with a 5-Fr feeding tube before performing the repair. Otherwise, no special aftercare is needed. If bleeding is controlled, degloving does not need to be repaired.

Plastibell Technique

1. Choose an appropriate-size Plastibell, which is 1.3 cm for most normal newborns. (The Plastibell should fit like an appropriate-size Gomco bell.) Drop the device into the sterile field.
2. As in steps 1 through 5 of the Mogen Technique section, inspect the penis for abnormalities, consider marking the foreskin at the coronal edge, administer a penile subcutaneous ring block, position the infant (restrain if necessary), apply antiseptic, drape, and free the foreskin from the glans.
3. As in steps 3 through 5 of the Gomco Technique section, place a dorsal crushing clamp and remove it, cut a dorsal slit, and retract and fully free the foreskin. Leave the two foreskin edge hemostats in place.
4. Place the Plastibell string loosely around the base of the penis and put two twists in the string to start a surgeon's knot.
5. Place the Plastibell over the glans (Fig. 181-12) with its "wishbone" vertical (along the 12 to 6 o'clock axis). The edge of the Plastibell should just touch the coronal edge. Exchange the Plastibell for one of an appropriate size if this is not the case. It is particularly dangerous to use too large a Plastibell because the glans can push through its center and cause a paraphimosis, with resultant necrosis of the glans. If the size is correct, pull the foreskin over the device by manipulating the two grasping hemostats.
6. Once the Plastibell is appropriately placed, use a third hemostat to grasp both sides of the dorsal slit with the hemostat tips at about the middle of the incision. This will reapproximate the foreskin around the device and hold it in place (Fig. 181-13).

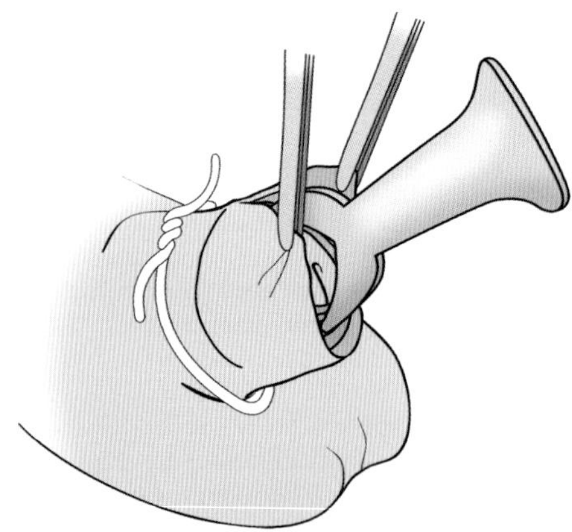

Figure 181-12 Place the Plastibell on the glans and check for proper size.

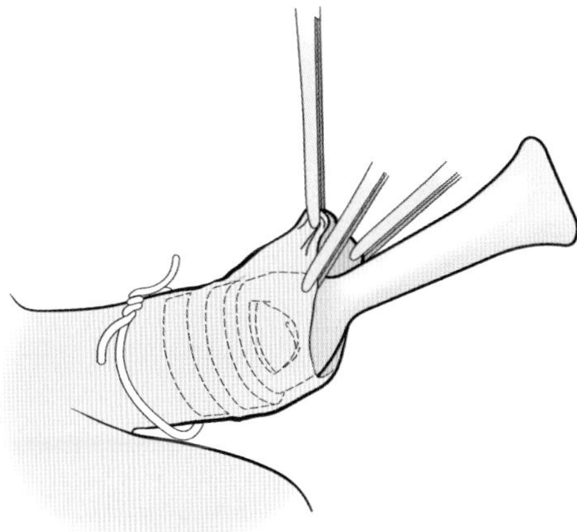

Figure 181-13 Reapproximate the foreskin around the Plastibell and hold it in place with a hemostat.

7. Ensure that the string groove of the Plastibell is below the apex of the dorsal slit and at the appropriate place on the foreskin. Adjust the grasping hemostat if necessary. When certain of Plastibell placement, remove the two foreskin edge hemostats.
8. Place the string over the groove in the Plastibell and tighten the string just until it remains in place.
9. Check the placement of the string and bell again, making sure that the apex of the foreskin incision is distal to the string. Be sure that you are not removing too much foreskin and that the Plastibell can move freely on the glans.
10. Tighten the string as much as possible and hold at this tension for a few seconds. Complete the surgeon's knot in the string and trim the excess string to ¼ inch in length (Fig. 181-14).
11. Remove the hemostat that has been approximating the dorsal slit.
12. Using iris scissors, cut the foreskin away to within 3 mm of the string. Be careful not to cut the string (Fig. 181-15). Discard the foreskin in a biohazard waste container.
13. Holding the body of the Plastibell between the index finger and thumb of one hand, bend the wishbone with the other hand until it snaps at its junction with the bell (Fig. 181-16).
14. Verify again that the Plastibell can move up and down on the glans and that the meatus is not occluded.
15. As in steps 15 through 18 of the Mogen Technique section, check for bleeding, cover with white petrolatum, reapply the diaper, and record the procedure in the chart.

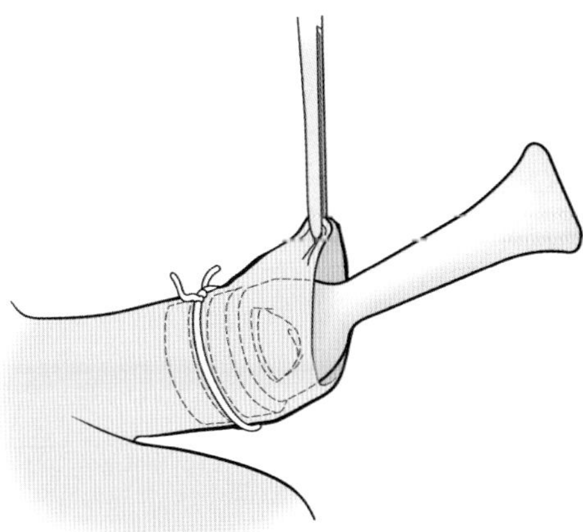

Figure 181-14 String in the groove of the Plastibell with knot trimmed.

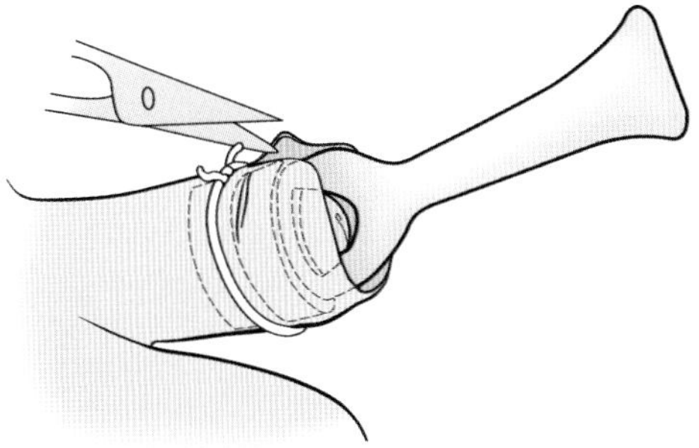

Figure 181-15 Trim the excess foreskin with iris scissors.

Postprocedure Management and Parent Education

All Techniques

Parents should report any bleeding or signs of infection. It is normal to have a red, angry-looking glans, often with a yellowish crust that may last for a week. Acetaminophen (10 to 15 mg/kg every 6 to 8 hours) is given for any apparent pain or irritability. Rarely is any analgesic needed beyond 24 hours. The patient education handout includes postprocedure instructions for parents. (See the sample handout titled "Newborn Circumcision" available online at www.expertconsult.com.)

After a Mogen or Gomco procedure, parents are told to retract the penile shaft skin back from the corona and to apply white petrolatum to the area at each diaper change. After the Plastibell falls off, this same procedure is followed. This should continue for a week to prevent adhesions from forming. To prevent the glans from sticking to the diaper, parents should apply a smear of white petrolatum to the front of the diaper for the first week. They can wash the penis with soap and water the day after surgery.

Parents are instructed to watch for meatal stenosis. Meatal stenosis appears as a pinhole urethra causing a narrow or angulated urinary stream. This can be associated with enuresis or incontinence. Meatotomy is a simple office procedure and will usually correct the problem.

Plastibell Technique

In addition to following all of the same basic instructions for patients who undergo circumcision using the Mogen or Gomco clamp, parents need to know what to expect with a Plastibell. They should know that the foreskin remaining beyond the string will turn black and necrotic and fall off along with the Plastibell within 1 week. Each Plastibell device comes with a postoperative education card that is given to the parents.

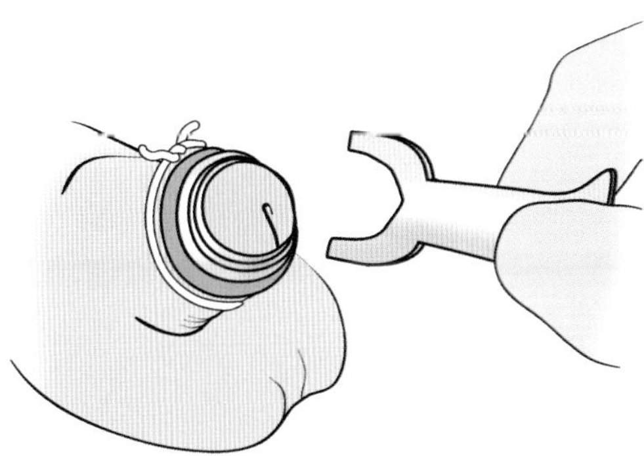

Figure 181-16 Snap the Plastibell at the junction of the ring and the wishbone.

Complications

- Bleeding.
- Infection (most common with Plastibell because of the retained tissue and the presence of a foreign body).
- Trauma to the glans or urethra.
- Poor cosmetic result due to remaining adherence of mucosa to glans, removal of too much or too little foreskin, or uneven removal of foreskin. Most cosmetic problems resolve as the infant grows and the wound heals. Secondary intervention is very infrequently necessary.
- Paraphimosis from inadequate opening of the Mogen crush line after the procedure is completed or from the use of Plastibell that is too large. A Plastibell may be removed with orthopedic bone-cutting forceps.
- Degloving of penile shaft skin (Gomco only; see the Gomco Technique section).
- Meatal stenosis: rare, but a possible late complication.

Meatotomy (Newborn and Office)

Indications

- Newborn (following circumcision): width of meatus less than 2 mm or less than 25% to 30% of diameter of glans
- Male infant younger than 1 year of age: symptoms of meatal stenosis and unable to easily insert 5-Fr feeding tube
- Male child older than 1 year and younger than 6 years of age: symptoms of meatal stenosis and unable to easily insert 8-Fr feeding tube

Contraindications

The contraindications are the same as for circumcision, except the child can be older than newborn for office meatotomy.

Preprocedure Patient Preparation

If there is a possibility that newborn meatotomy may be performed, the procedure, its alternatives, and its risks and benefits should be explained. Meatotomy is often added to the informed consent for circumcision. If office meatotomy is to be performed in an older male child, similar explanations should be made and informed consent obtained.

Equipment

- Antiseptic solution (e.g., povidone–iodine, chlorhexidine)
- Antibiotic ointment
- Fenestrated drape
- Straight mosquito hemostat
- Straight iris scissors
- Lidocaine–prilocaine cream or gauze soaked with 2% lidocaine (office meatotomy)
- 30-gauge needle with 1-mL syringe and 1% lidocaine without epinephrine (office meatotomy, *alternative for anesthesia*)

Technique

1. Anesthesia is usually already adequate for a newborn having just undergone circumcision. For office meatotomy, lidocaine–prilocaine cream should be smeared liberally over the entire glans, especially the ventral portion and the meatal opening. It should be secured in place with occlusive dressing and left for at least an hour of contact time before the procedure. Alternatively, a small amount of lidocaine can be injected directly into the meatal skin. For very anxious children (for 2 of 58 children in one study, ages 30 months to 10 years, a preoperative anxiolytic was used), it may be useful to use pediatric sedation (see Chapter 7, Pediatric Sedation and Analgesia).
2. Apply antiseptic solution to the penis and place a fenestrated drape.
3. Place one tip of the straight mosquito hemostat, lubricated with antiseptic solution, inside the meatus at the 6 o'clock position. The tip should be several millimeters inside the meatus, the distance being judged by the severity of stenosis and patient age. In the newborn, the other tip should be no farther than the frenulum.
4. Close the hemostat to obtain a crush line of hemostasis on the inferior side of the meatus. Frequently the majority of the crush line will be located on the thin, sometimes translucent, inflammatory membrane that has caused the meatal obstruction.
5. Using the fine iris scissors, cut through the center of the crush line (Fig. 181-17). Be careful to cut only in the crush line; if you extend laterally or past the crush line, bleeding may occur.
6. A closed hemostat can then be inserted into the urethra to gently and blindly palpate for distal urethral webs. If webs are noted, urologic referral is indicated.
7. A small amount of antibiotic ointment is then placed on the incision.

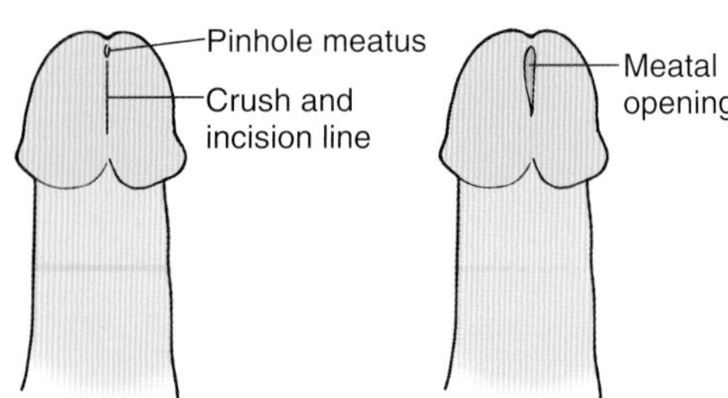

Figure 181-17 **A,** Meatal stenosis and location of crush line. **B,** Meatus after meatotomy.

Postprocedure Management and Parent Education

The meatotomy site should be shown to parents, and they can then be given instructions for care. Parents are instructed to insert a small dilator into the meatus daily for 2 weeks to prevent recurrence of the stenosis. Use either a small eyedropper or the tip of a tube of ophthalmic antibiotic ointment as the dilator. White petrolatum ointment can be used as a lubricant.

Sample Operative Report

After most neonatal circumcisions (or meatotomies) in the United States, only a cursory operative note is made in the chart—for example, "1% lido ring block, Mogen circ without complication, infant tolerated well, parents given instructions for care." This chart is signed by the clinician, and the date and time are noted.

Patient Education Guides

See patient education form available online at www.expertconsult.com.

CPT/Billing Codes

53025 Meatotomy, infant
54150 Circumcision by clamp or other device with regional dorsal penile or ring block, regardless of age
54150-52 Circumcision using clamp or other device without regional dorsal penile or ring block, regardless of age (reduced services)
64450-47 Nerve block, diagnostic or therapeutic, other peripheral nerve, anesthesia by surgeon (A few insurers will pay for this as a separate procedure from the circumcision)

ICD-9-CM Diagnostic Codes

V50.2 Circumcision, routine or ritual (in the absence of significant medical indication)
599.6 Urethral obstruction, unspecified

Acknowledgment

The editors wish to recognize the many contributions by S. Shevaun Duiker, MD, to this chapter in a previous edition of this text.

Suppliers

(See contact information online at www.expertconsult.com.)

Brochures
American Academy of Pediatrics
Circumstraint
Natus Medical Incorporated
Gomco circumcision clamps (1.1-, 1.3-, and 1.45-cm sizes)
Allied Healthcare Products, Inc. (Gomco Division)
Mogen clamp
Mogen Instrument Co.
Plastibell device (1.1-, 1.2-, 1.3-, 1.4-, 1.5-, and 1.7-cm sizes)
Briggs Corporation (Hollister Global)
Stang Circumcision Chair
Pedicraft

Online Resource

U.S. Food and Drug Administration: Potential for injury from circumcision clamps. August 29, 2000. Available at www.fda.gov/MedicalDevices/Safety/AlertsandNotices/PublicHealthNotifications/ucm062279.htm.

Bibliography

American Academy of Pediatrics Task Force on Circumcision: Circumcision policy statement. Pediatrics 103:686–693, 1999. Available online at http://aappolicy.aappublications.org/cgi/reprint/pediatrics;103/3/686.pdf. Accessed February 2, 2010.
Brown MR, Cartwright PC, Snow BW: Common office problems in pediatric urology and gynecology. Pediatr Clin North Am 44:1091–1115, 1997.
Cartwright PC, Snow BW, McNees DC: Urethral meatotomy in the office using topical EMLA cream for anesthesia. J Urol 156:857–858; discussion 858–859, 1996.
Castellsagué X, Bosch FX, Muñoz N, et al: Male circumcision, penile human papillomavirus infection, and cervical cancer in female partners. N Engl J Med 346:1105–1112, 2002.
Haouari N, Wood C, Griffiths G, Levene M: The analgesic effect of sucrose in full term infants: A randomized controlled trial. BMJ 310:1498–1500, 1995.
Kaufman GE, Cimo S, Miller LW, Blass EM: An evaluation of the effects of sucrose on neonatal pain with 2 commonly used circumcision methods. Am J Obstet Gynecol 186:564–568, 2002.
Kunz HV: Circumcision and meatotomy. Prim Care 13:513–525, 1986.
Kurtis PS, DeSilva HN, Bernstein BA, et al: A comparison of the Mogen and Gomco clamps in combination with dorsal penile nerve block in minimizing the pain of neonatal circumcision. Pediatrics 103:E23, 1999.
Laumann EO, Masi CM, Zuckerman EW: Circumcision in the United States: Prevalence, prophylactic effects, and sexual practice. JAMA 227:1052–1057, 1997.
Peleg D, Steiner A: The Gomco circumcision: Common problems and solutions. Am Fam Physician 58:891–898, 1998.
Reynolds RD: Use of the Mogen clamp for neonatal circumcision. Am Fam Physician 54:177–182, 1996.
Schoen EJ: The increasing incidence of newborn circumcision: Data from the nationwide inpatient sample. J Urol 175:394–395, 2006.
Schoen EJ, Colby CJ, To TT: Cost analysis of neonatal circumcision in a large health maintenance organization. J Urol 175:1111–1115, 2006.
Spach DH, Stapleton AE, Stamm WE: Lack of circumcision increases the risk of urinary tract infection in young men. JAMA 267:679–681, 1992.

CHAPTER 182

Pediatric Arterial Puncture and Venous Minicutdown

John J. Andazola • Karyn B. Kolman

Arterial Puncture

Arterial blood may be needed for blood gas analysis or for routine laboratory analysis. In the infant or child, the radial artery is the most appropriate and most commonly selected site for arterial puncture. The posterior tibial and dorsalis pedis arteries are optional sites, but each has its own risk of complications. Because of the risk of thrombosis, use of the femoral artery for arterial puncture in the infant or child should be reserved for emergencies. Likewise, because of the risk of median nerve damage and the fact that the brachial artery has minimal collateral circulation, the brachial artery should be reserved as a last resort in emergencies. The temporal artery should probably not be used because of the high risk of neurologic complications.

The radial artery is located just medial to the styloid process of the radius. It is palpable between the radius and the tendon of the flexor carpi radialis (see Chapter 208, Arterial Puncture and Percutaneous Arterial Line Placement).

Indications

- To obtain arterial blood from the pediatric patient in respiratory distress or for other studies that require arterial blood
- To guide the management of the pediatric patient receiving ventilatory support or undergoing intensive respiratory therapy (e.g., to confirm hypoxia or hypercapnia when pulse oxymetry [SaO_2] or end-tidal CO_2 [$ETCO_2$] monitoring, respectively, indicates it)
- To obtain blood for routine laboratory analysis when venous blood cannot be obtained

NOTE: The last indication is controversial. The benefit must outweigh the higher risk of obtaining an arterial sample.

Contraindications

Infection, burns, local skin damage, trauma, or severely disturbed anatomy at the site of the intended puncture are all contraindications. They are considered *relative* contraindications in a life-threatening situation.

Equipment and Supplies

- Commercially available heparinized arterial blood gas (ABG) syringe or 1-mL (tuberculin syringe) to 3-mL syringe (to be flushed with heparin)
- Rubber stopper or syringe plug to seal blood sample
- 23- to 27-gauge butterfly scalp vein needle or standard 23- to 27-gauge needle (the smaller the needle, the lower the risk of complications)
- Antiseptic skin preparation, such as povidone–iodine or chlorhexidine, and 70% isopropyl alcohol
- Container of crushed ice for sample transport
- Sterile 4 × 4 gauze pads
- Sterile gloves
- Goggles or eye protection
- Bright light source (e.g., bright penlight, otoscope) for transillumination *(optional)*
- 1 or 2 mL heparin, 1000 U/mL *(optional, for use in nonheparinized syringe)*
- In the alert patient *(optional)*, 1% or 2% lidocaine *without* epinephrine and a 1- or 3-mL syringe with 25- or 27-gauge, ⅝-inch (1.6-cm) needle
- Arm or leg board *(optional)*

Precautions

The modified Allen test is performed to ensure patency of the ulnar artery before an arterial puncture or the placement of an indwelling arterial catheter. Verifying adequate collateral circulation may reduce the risk of ischemic complications if thrombosis of the radial artery occurs. (See Chapter 208, Arterial Puncture and Percutaneous Arterial Line Placement, for a description of the modified Allen test as well as other techniques available to test for collateral circulation.)

Technique

1. Always perform a modified Allen test (or equivalent) to confirm adequate collateral circulation.
2. Attach a butterfly needle (preferred for infants and neonates) or a standard 23- to 27-gauge needle to a heparinized ABG syringe. Alternatively, draw a small amount of heparin into the syringe and eject the heparin. The heparin remaining in the syringe will prevent the sample from clotting as well as decrease the dead space in the syringe. Heparin has a very low pH, so avoid using excessive heparin, which could result in falsely abnormal ABG results. If the sample will be used for another laboratory test, do not use heparin.
3. Immobilize the upper extremity by taping it to an arm board or by having an assistant manually stabilize it.
4. Grasp the wrist with the nondominant hand and identify the radial artery by dorsiflexing and slightly externally rotating the wrist and palpating over the distal volar (palmar) radius. Using a bright light source for transillumination may help locate the artery, especially in newborns. Cleanse the site of intended puncture with an antiseptic solution, which can be wiped off with alcohol swab. If the patient is alert, the area can also be infiltrated with 1% to 2% lidocaine without epinephrine.
5. Universal blood and body fluid precautions should be followed. Insert the needle with the bevel up, at the point of maximum

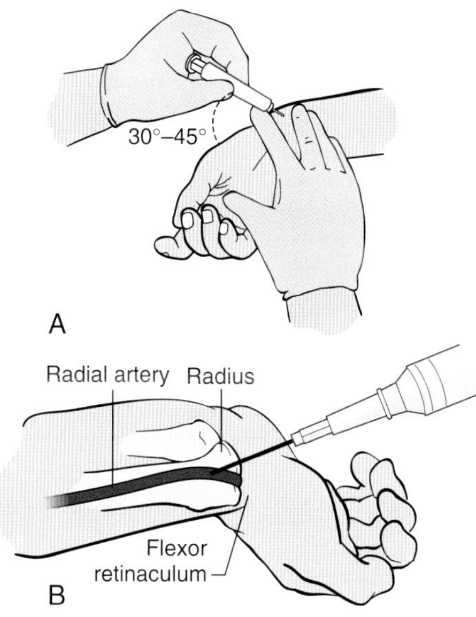

Figure 182-1 Pediatric arterial puncture. **A,** Anatomic location of the radial artery with immobilization of the wrist in hyperextension. **B,** The artery is entered with the bevel up and the needle at 30 to 45 degrees from horizontal.

pulsation, at a 30- to 45-degree angle (Fig. 182-1) to the distal skin. Usually little aspiration is needed to fill the syringe when the artery is pierced. If the syringe does not flash blood immediately, continuous gentle suction can be applied with the plunger of the syringe as the needle is removed or on the next attempt. Be aware that arterial blood may not flash into the syringe as vigorously in a child as in the adult patient. If using the butterfly needle, have an assistant maintain gentle suction while the needle is advanced.

6. If resistance is encountered, most likely the needle has made contact with underlying bone (radius). At this point, withdraw the needle very slowly while maintaining gentle suction on the plunger until there is blood return. If there is no blood return and the tip of the needle has been withdrawn to a point just beneath the skin, readvance the needle toward the point of maximal pulsation before withdrawing it from the skin. Although the risk of complications increases with the number of attempts, several attempts can be made in this manner causing minimal trauma to the infant before choosing another site.
7. When arterial blood is encountered, withdraw 0.3 to 0.5 mL into the syringe before removing the needle. Leave the butterfly needle in place (with its extension tubing) if more blood is needed for other analyses. This will facilitate changing the syringe. For blood gas analysis, remove any bubbles from the syringe and then seal it. Place it on ice and immediately transport to the laboratory.

   NOTE: The total blood volume in a neonate is usually about 80 mL/kg, and the volume of blood withdrawn should not exceed 3% to 5% of this total blood volume. As an example, 8 mL is 5% of the total blood volume in a 2-kg infant.

8. After removing the needle, always maintain manual compression at the arterial puncture site for a minimum of 5 minutes to prevent the formation of a hematoma. Apply firm, but not occlusive pressure.

Sample Operative Report

See the sample operative report online at www.expertconsult.com.

Complications

- Bleeding and hematoma formation (to minimize this risk, use the smallest needle possible)
- Arterial spasm, thrombosis, and embolism (risk increases with repeated punctures in the same location; however, arterial spasm will usually resolve spontaneously, and the artery will usually recanalize over time after thrombosis)
- Nerve injury
- Infection
- Spurious laboratory results (see Chapter 208, Arterial Puncture and Percutaneous Arterial Line Placement, for a discussion)

NOTE: Because the radial artery is not close to a nerve or vein, its puncture usually results in fewer complications than puncture of the posterior tibial or dorsalis pedis artery. Repeated puncture at the same site increases the chance of complications but may be unavoidable.

Interpretation of Results

See Table 182-1.

VENOUS MINICUTDOWN

Obtaining percutaneous venous access in infants or in hypovolemic children can be a challenge. In an emergent situation, when percutaneous venous access in not easily obtainable, intraosseous line placement is the preferred alternative (see Chapter 198, Intraosseous Vascular Access). If intraosseous line placement is not possible, venous cutdown can be used to gain vascular access. Venous cutdown can often be performed rapidly, usually in a matter of minutes. Chapter 209, Venous Cutdown, offers technical advice on the overall mechanics of venous cutdown. This chapter offers an abbreviated and clinically easier method for pediatric patients in emergencies: the minicutdown. Although standard venous cutdown takes 5 to 15 minutes, even in the hands of a skilled clinician, minicutdown is less complicated and can usually be performed in less than 5 minutes.

The saphenous vein is a consistent anatomic structure and is located a fingerbreadth (1 cm) anterior to and a fingerbreadth (1 cm) superior to the medial malleolus at the ankle in infants and 2 cm anterior and superior in older children (Fig. 182-2). Because of its superficial and consistent location, the saphenous vein is the most common site for cutdown in the pediatric patient. The saphenous nerve travels with the saphenous vein and is often transected when isolating the saphenous vein at the ankle, but fortunately it is of minimal clinical significance. In this location, there is very little subcutaneous tissue, and other than the saphenous vein and nerve, there are few other structures between the dermis and the tibial periosteum.

Indications

In an emergency, the inability to obtain needed percutaneous intravenous (IV) or intraosseous vascular access in a matter of minutes

TABLE 182-1 Normal Values for Arterial Blood Gases Based on Age

Age	pH	Pa_{O_2} (mm Hg)	Pa_{CO_2} (mm Hg)	HCO_3 (mEq/L)
Birth	7.26–7.29	60	55	19
Birth–1 yr	7.37	70	33	20
1–2 yr	7.40	90	34	20
7–19 yr	7.39	96	37	22
>19 yr	7.35–7.45	90–110	35–45	22–26

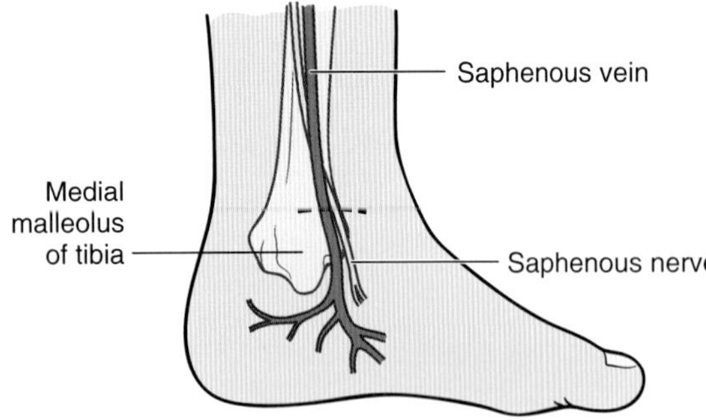

Figure 182-2 Path of the saphenous vein as it courses anterior to the medial malleolus of the tibia. An incision (about 1 to 2 cm in length) through the skin is made perpendicular to the long axis of the tibia. (Redrawn and modified from Bailey P: Vascular access for pediatric resuscitation and other pediatric emergencies. In Rose BD [ed]: UpToDate. Waltham, Mass, UpToDate, 2007.)

or the inability to maintain a peripheral IV line indicates the need venous minicutdown.

Contraindications

- Vascular injury or long bone fracture proximal to the site of the intended cutdown *(proximal venous flow or vascular access may be obstructed, so this is a relative contraindication because the minicutdown may not work)*
- Infection, burn, trauma, or severely disturbed anatomy at the site of the intended cutdown *(relative contraindication in life-threatening situation)*
- Anticoagulation from bleeding disorders or anticoagulant therapy *(relative contraindication in life-threatening situation)*

Equipment and Supplies

- Mounted no. 15 blade scalpel
- Mosquito hemostat
- Antiseptic skin preparation, such as povidone–iodine or chlorhexidine, and 70% isopropyl alcohol
- 4-0 silk suture, 4-0 nylon skin suture
- Sterile 4 × 4 gauze pads
- Sterile gloves
- Goggles or eye protection
- 16- to 20-gauge standard over-the-needle IV catheter
- Skin retractors *(optional)*
- Leg board *(optional)*
- In the alert patient *(optional)*, 1% or 2% lidocaine *without* epinephrine and a 1- or 3-mL syringe with 25- or 27-gauge, ⅝-inch (1.6-cm) needle

Technique

1. Immobilize the lower extremity by securing it to a board or by having an assistant manually hold the patient. The lower extremity should be extended and slightly externally rotated.
2. Cleanse this area with an antiseptic solution. If time allows, wipe the antiseptic solution off with an alcohol pad. Follow universal blood and body fluid precautions. If time allows and the patient is alert, anesthetize the area with lidocaine.
3. Locate the medial malleolus, and at the appropriate location anterior (one to two fingerbreadths [1 to 2 cm], depending on age) and superior (1 to 2 cm, depending on age) to it, make a 1- to 2-cm transverse (perpendicular to the vein and the tibia) incision through the dermis, exposing the underlying subcutaneous tissue. (In other words, the incision should be made in the anteroposterior direction.)

   NOTE: The incision should be very superficial, limited to the skin and only exposing the subcutaneous tissue. Incising into the subcutaneous tissue may result in transection of the vein with subsequent bleeding into the surgical field, obscuring the vein.
4. Exposure of the vein is accomplished with traction on either side of the incision with the nondominant hand (or skin retractors) and blunt dissection with a mosquito hemostat. Most clinicians insert the hemostat with the tips down against the posterior tibia, down to the periosteum, and aim it in the direction of the incision (transverse to the vein). The tips are then advanced across the tibia, with downward pressure so that they slide across the periosteum, until they reach the anterior border of the tibia (the tips will slide beneath the saphenous vein). The tips are then rotated 180 degrees (until they are facing upward), and all of the tissue between the skin and the tibial periosteum should be on top of the hemostat. When the hemostat is opened widely, the saphenous vein should be visualized in this tissue (usually a scant amount of subcutaneous tissue). Frequently, in older children, the saphenous nerve can also be visualized and avoided.

   Alternatively, the clinician can attempt to visualize the vein by bluntly spreading the subcutaneous tissue with the hemostat tips, staying parallel to the course of the vein (perpendicular to the incision; Fig. 182-3A). However, some experts consider this technique to take longer because it may be difficult to find the vein against the white background of the periosteum.

   With either technique, if there is difficulty visualizing the vein, the foot can be squeezed to backfill the vein. This should improve localization of the vein.
5. When the saphenous vein is identified, pass a 4-0 silk suture beneath the vessel and clamp both ends of the suture with a hemostat (Fig. 182-3B).
6. Using upward traction on the vein with the suture to stabilize it, cannulate the vessel with an IV catheter under direct visualization (Fig. 182-3C). Advance the catheter in the usual fashion, then attach IV tubing and begin infusing fluid. As with percutaneous line placement, steady fluid flow indicates successful cannulation.
7. Suture the catheter in place. (With the minicutdown technique, the vein is not ligated after cannulation.)
8. The incision site is then sutured with nylon suture and a sterile occlusive dressing applied. Because the minicutdown technique does not destroy the vein, standard cutdown can still be performed if needed.

Sample Operative Report

See the sample operative report online at www.expertconsult.com.

Complications

- Wound infection
- Local hematoma
- Phlebitis
- Sensory nerve damage
- Damage to adjacent structures from incision and dissection

NOTE: Because this is only a temporary procedure, the risk of these complications is minimal.

Postprocedure Management

A sterile occlusive dressing should be placed immediately and routine wound care provided. Once other means of vascular access are obtained, the venous minicutdown catheter should be removed and the incision repaired with appropriate suture material.

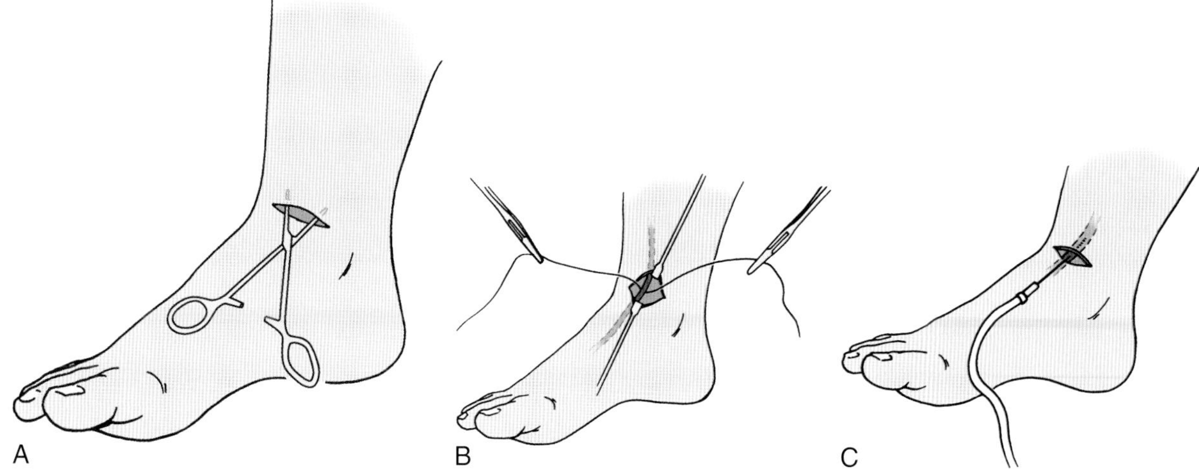

Figure 182-3 Venous minicutdown. **A,** Blunt dissection after making a transverse incision. **B,** Localization of the vein. **C,** Cannulating the vein.

CPT/Billing Codes

36420 Venipuncture, cutdown; younger than age 1 year
36425 Venipuncture, cutdown; age 1 or over
36600 Arterial puncture, withdrawal of blood for diagnosis
36625 Arterial cutdown

ICD-9-CM Diagnostic Codes

Pediatric Arterial Puncture

250.1 Diabetic ketoacidosis
276.2 Acidosis
276.3 Alkalosis
276.4 Acid–base mixed disorder
427.5 Cardiac or cardiorespiratory arrest
428.1 Pulmonary edema (left heart failure)
493.00 Asthma, extrinsic, unspecified
493.01 Asthma, extrinsic, with status asthmaticus
493.9 Dyspnea, asthma; or asthma, unspecified
518.5 Pulmonary insufficiency following shock, trauma, or surgery
518.81 Respiratory failure, acute, NOS
518.82 Respiratory distress or failure, acute
518.83 Respiratory failure, chronic
518.84 Respiratory failure, acute and chronic
769 Respiratory distress syndrome of newborn
770.12 Meconium aspiration syndrome
780.01 Coma
785.50 Shock, unspecified, without mention of trauma
785.51 Shock, cardiogenic
785.52 Shock, septic
785.59 Shock, other (hypovolemic, septic)
786.05 Shortness of breath
786.06 Tachypnea
786.09 Respiratory distress or insufficiency, NOS
799.01 Asphyxia
799.02 Hypoxemia
799.1 Respiratory arrest
986 Carbon monoxide, toxic effect

Venous Minicutdown

459.0 Hemorrhage, unspecified
459.89 Venofibrosis
772.9 Hemorrhage, in newborn, NOS
958.4 Hemorrhagic shock due to trauma

Acknowledgment

The editors wish to recognize the contributions by Gregg K. Phillips, MD, and Rebecca H. Gladu, MD, to this chapter in the previous two editions of this text.

BIBLIOGRAPHY

Gomella TL, Cunningham MD, Eyal FG, Zenk KE: Arterial access. In Neonatology: Management, Procedures, On-Call Problems, Diseases, and Drugs, 5th ed. New York, Lange McGraw-Hill, 2004, pp 157–164.
Johns Hopkins Hospital; Robertson J, Shilkofski N (eds): The Harriet Lane Handbook: A Manual for Pediatric House Officers, 17th ed. St. Louis, Mosby, 2005.
Klofas E: A quicker saphenous vein cutdown and a better way to teach it. J Trauma 43:985–987, 1997.
Nobay F: Peripheral venous cutdown. In Reichman EF, Simon RR (eds): Emergency Medicine Procedures. New York, McGraw-Hill, 2004, pp 367–382.
Sweeney MN: Vascular access in trauma: Options, risks, benefits, and complications. Anesthesiol Clin North Am 17:97–106, 1999.

CHAPTER 183

Pediatric Suprapubic Bladder Aspiration

Carlos A. Moreno

Suprapubic bladder aspiration is a method of obtaining a sterile urine specimen in a young infant when other methods are unsatisfactory. This procedure is most successful in an infant younger than 2 years of age because at that age the bladder is an abdominal organ. After 2 years, as the child grows, the bladder moves into the pelvis, increasing both the difficulty of the procedure and the risk of complications. (See Chapter 225, Emergency Department, Hospitalist, and Office Ultrasonography [Clinical Ultrasonography], for a method of confirming a full bladder and determining where to direct the needle.)

Indications

- To obtain sterile urine for culture in an infant or child younger than 2 years of age (e.g., suspected urinary tract infection [UTI] or sepsis)
- To decompress the urinary bladder when there is urethral obstruction (after decompression, a referral should be made to pediatric urology)

Contraindications

Absolute

There are no absolute contraindications.

NOTE: Some experts now consider "blind" aspiration to be an absolute contraindication. They suggest that the bladder location should be confirmed by palpation, percussion, or transillumination or visualized with ultrasonography.

Relative

- Bleeding abnormality or coagulopathy
- Infection or loss of integrity of skin or fascia at the site of needle insertion (e.g., burn, cellulitis)
- Anatomic genitourinary tract anomalies
- Bowel distention (e.g., ileus, obstruction)
- Scars from previous lower abdominal surgery that might cause adhesions

NOTE: With ultrasonography-directed aspiration, the last three contraindications may be overcome (see Chapter 225, Emergency Department, Hospitalist, and Office Ultrasonography [Clinical Ultrasonography]).

Equipment and Supplies

- Povidone–iodine solution
- 70% isopropyl alcohol
- Sterile 4 × 4 gauze pads
- Sterile gloves
- 3-mL sterile syringe with 1- or 1½-inch, 22- or 23-gauge needle
- Sterile urine specimen container
- Adhesive bandage
- 1% lidocaine in a tuberculin syringe with ½-inch, 27-gauge needle *(optional)*
- High-frequency ultrasound (5- to 10-MHz) probe and acoustic gel *(optional)*

Preprocedure Patient Preparation

The parent(s) should be informed about the indication(s) for suprapubic aspiration, as well as alternatives and possible complications. In nonemergent situations, informed consent should be obtained. The parent(s) should be given the option to leave the room or to look away as the procedure is being performed because it can be disconcerting to some parents.

Procedure

1. Before bladder aspiration, the infant's diaper should be dry and urination should not have occurred within the previous hour. Often the full bladder can be palpated, percussed, or transilluminated to ensure a full bladder. An alternative is to perform a quick ultrasonographic examination to confirm a full bladder.
2. Hold the infant in the supine, frog-leg position. Observe universal blood and body fluid precautions.
3. Urination can be prevented by gently pinching the penis or by applying manual pressure in the area of the anterior rectum or urethral meatus in a female infant.
4. Cleanse the lower abdomen with povidone–iodine and then remove the iodine with 70% isopropyl alcohol.

   NOTE: At this point, some clinicians inject a small amount (<1 mL) of a local anesthetic, such as 1% lidocaine, to raise a subcutaneous wheal in the area of the intended puncture site. However, this is considered optional by many clinicians because the discomfort caused by the lidocaine is similar to that caused by the puncture for bladder aspiration.

5. With the needle attached to a 3-mL sterile syringe, direct the needle into the midline of the abdomen at a point 1 cm above the symphysis pubis (there is usually a transverse suprapubic crease at this location). Hold the needle perpendicular to the abdomen or direct it slightly caudal (Fig. 183-1).
6. Aspirate gently with the syringe while advancing the needle. To avoid puncturing the posterior bladder wall or retroperitoneal structures, do not advance the needle after urine begins to enter the syringe. If the bladder is full, urine is usually obtained before the needle is inserted to its full depth.

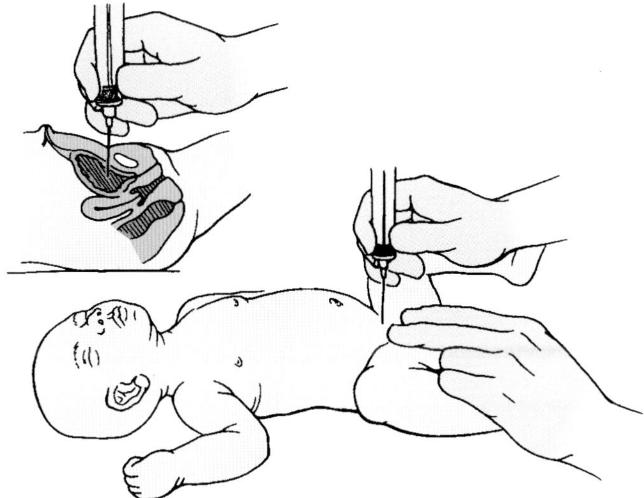

Figure 183-1 Proper technique for suprapubic bladder aspiration.

7. If no urine is obtained, withdraw the needle without removing it from the skin and attempt bladder puncture again, angling 20 degrees more caudal. If three attempts are unsuccessful, the bladder is considered empty. The procedure can be repeated in an hour if the patient is stable. Some urine should have accumulated over this time.

   NOTE: An alternative is to catheterize the infant, especially if he or she is too unstable to wait an hour. If ultrasonography is available, it can be helpful to confirm the presence of urine before subjecting the infant to catheterization and risk of iatrogenic UTI.

8. After withdrawing the needle, immediately apply pressure to the puncture site until it can be covered with a sterile gauze dressing. Next, apply mild pressure to the dressing for a minute. After a minute, if there is adequate hemostasis and no urine draining from the puncture site, pressure can be discontinued and the bandage applied.
9. Transfer the aspirated urine to a sterile container and transport to the laboratory for analysis, culture, and sensitivity.

Complications

- Microscopic hematuria (typically transient, resolving without specific treatment)
- Iatrogenic UTI (risk is minimized by the use of sterile technique)
- Perforation of the bowel (rare and may be managed by close observation and, if necessary, antibiotic administration)
- Retroperitoneal hematoma or damage to retroperitoneal structures (very rare)
- Infection of the abdominal wall

Postprocedure Patient Education

The parent(s) should be given instructions to keep the site clean and to seek medical care for fever, nausea, vomiting, or infection at the puncture site.

CPT/Billing Codes

51000 Aspiration of bladder by needle
76942 Ultrasonic guidance for needle placement, imaging supervision, and interpretation

ICD-9-CM Diagnostic Codes

595.0 Acute cystitis
771.81 Septicemia (sepsis) of the newborn
771.82 Neonatal urinary tract infection
771.83 Bacteremia of the newborn
788.20 Urinary retention, unspecified
788.21 Incomplete bladder emptying

Acknowledgment

The editors wish to recognize the many contributions by Marvin A. Dewar, MD, JD, to this chapter in the first edition of this text.

Bibliography

Hoekelman RA (ed): Primary Pediatric Care, 4th ed. St. Louis, Mosby, 2001.

James DM: Suprapubic bladder aspiration and placement of a suprapubic catheter. In James DM (ed): Field Guide to Urgent and Ambulatory Care Procedures. Philadelphia, Lippincott Williams & Wilkins, 2001, pp 189–193.

Johns Hopkins Hospital; Robertson J, Shilkofski N (eds): The Harriet Lane Handbook: A Manual for Pediatric House Officers, 17th ed. St. Louis, Mosby, 2005.

Stokes S, Kulkarni A: Suprapubic bladder aspiration. In Reichman EF, Simon RR (eds): Emergency Medicine Procedures. New York, McGraw-Hill, 2004, pp 1128–1133.

CHAPTER 184

Umbilical Vessel Catheterization

Carman H. Whiting

Being able to quickly assess and rapidly intervene in a severely ill infant is essential. Because the umbilical vessels are easily visualized, they are an excellent route for catheterization to provide central vascular access. Whereas umbilical artery catheterization allows for accurate monitoring of central arterial pressure directly through the aorta, umbilical vein catheterization allows for central venous pressure (CVP) monitoring through the inferior vena cava. Umbilical vein catheterization also provides access for rapid infusion of life-sustaining therapies (Fig. 184-1).

Primary care clinicians may need to perform umbilical vessel catheterization in the delivery room for a newborn resuscitation or in the emergency department for a newborn or infant in distress. They may also need to perform it in the nursery or neonatal intensive care unit (NICU) for an infant requiring continuous monitoring or frequent infusions of medications or fluids. In fact, both vessels are frequently catheterized in the NICU for premature infants requiring prolonged vascular access or monitoring.

Compared with the vein, the umbilical artery is a more durable vessel with higher-velocity blood flow; therefore it is easier to visualize and there is a slightly lower risk of complications when it is catheterized. Inserting an umbilical artery catheter (UAC) or an umbilical vein catheter (UVC) is easier if performed in the first 30 to 60 minutes of the infant's life. However, a UAC may be inserted up to the 7th day of life and a UVC at up to 2 weeks of age. Despite the fact that the vessels are easily accessible, placing a UAC can be a time-consuming procedure and requires skill and experience. Contraindications or difficulty obtaining a UAC insertion may necessitate the need for a UVC for infusions because a UVC insertion is easier to perform. A UVC is also an option if peripheral intravenous access is difficult to obtain, which is likely the case in very premature infants. After the first day of life, there are few data supporting any benefit of a UAC over a UVC for infusion, although an attempt should always be made to obtain peripheral venous access before either of these is inserted, except in infants of very low birth weight.

Indications

Umbilical Artery Catheterization

- Newborn resuscitation requiring monitoring for cardiorespiratory distress (e.g., arterial pressure monitoring, frequent arterial sampling)
- Newborn or infant in a NICU requiring
  - Mechanical ventilation for respiratory distress (i.e., frequent arterial sampling)
  - Oxygen hood and greater than 40% oxygen (FIO_2 >0.4) requirement with an abnormal chest radiograph (i.e., frequent arterial sampling)
  - Exchange transfusion that can be performed through a UAC (e.g., newborn weighing <1800 g)

Umbilical Vein Catheterization

- Newborn resuscitation requiring
  - Administration of drugs, blood, blood expanders, or fluids
  - Monitoring for possible cardiorespiratory distress (e.g., CVP monitoring)
- Newborn or infant in the NICU requiring
  - Greater than 12.5% dextrose to maintain blood glucose while taking nothing by mouth (NPO)
  - Pressor drips, total parenteral nutrition (TPN) solution, or hypertonic medications (e.g., newborn weighing <1000 g or who is critically ill)
  - Exchange transfusion or partial exchange transfusions that can be performed through a UVC (e.g., newborn weighing <1800 g)

NOTE: By convention, a newborn is defined as an infant younger than 1 month of age.

Contraindications

- There are no contraindications during the first hours of life if the newborn has normal anatomy and no local skin infections.
- Vascular insufficiency of a lower extremity is a contraindication to UAC.
- Local infection (e.g., omphalitis, impetigo) and abdominal distention (possibly caused by intestinal hypoperfusion or necrotizing enterocolitis) are contraindications that can develop after the first few hours of life.

Equipment

- Sterile measuring tape
- 3.5- to 5.0-Fr umbilical catheter for UAC; up to 8-Fr umbilical catheter for UVC
- Surgical cap and mask; sterile gown and gloves
- Eye protection for clinician
- Povidone–iodine or antiseptic scrub solution
- Three-way stopcock (sterile); locking connectors
- Heparin for flush (1 to 2 U heparin/mL of 0.25 normal saline [NS])
- Sterile instrument tray with small hemostats, forceps (iris curved), scissors, needle holder, straight forceps, mounted no. 11 scalpel blade, and drapes
- Antibiotic ointment
- 4-0 or 5-0 silk suture with a small needle or a catheter stabilizer

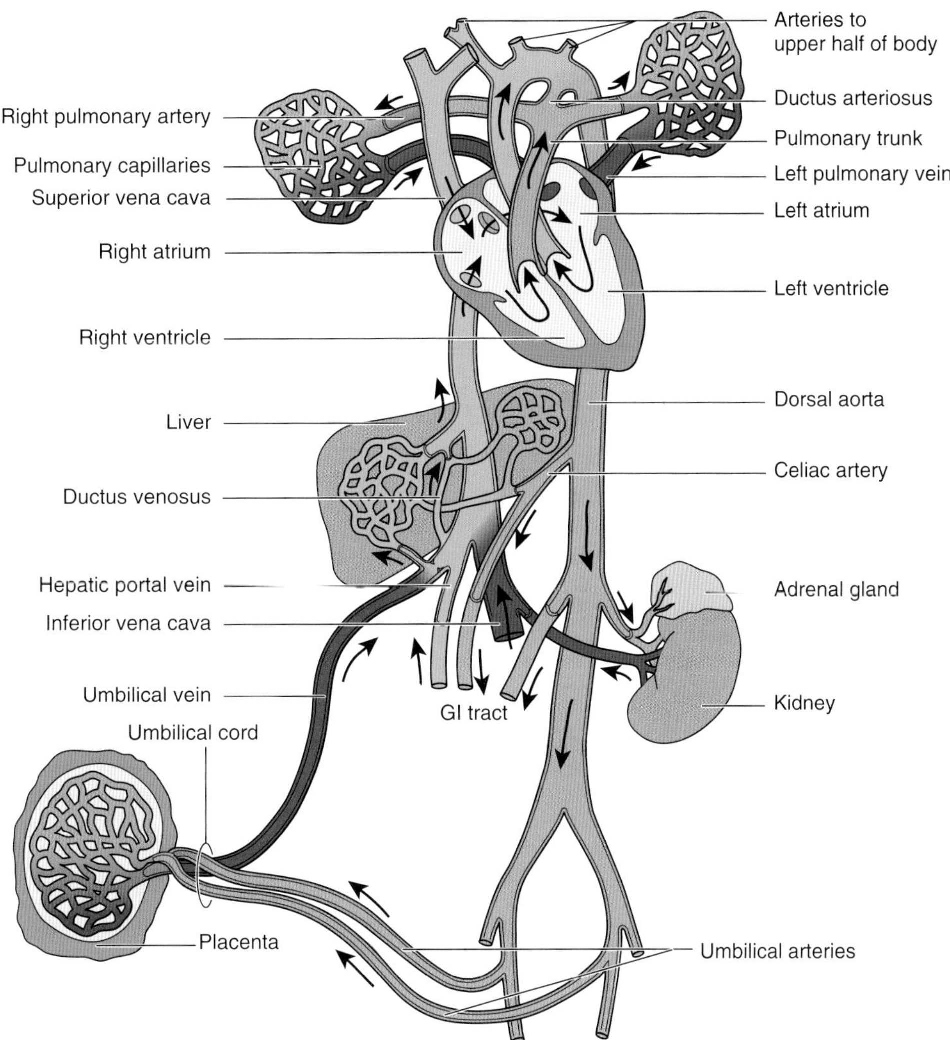

Figure 184-1 Fetal circulation at term. (Modified from Carlson B: Human Embryology and Developmental Biology, 2nd ed. St. Louis, Mosby, 1999.)

- Sterile umbilical tape
- Infant radiant warmer, means of restraint, cardiac and oxygen saturation monitors, supplemental oxygen
- 5% or 10% dextrose in water or NS infusion setup (use heparin 1 U/mL, unless medications are to be administered that are incompatible with heparin) with fluid chamber, 0.22-μg filter, and infusion pump
- Adhesive tape

A rule of thumb for selecting UAC size is to use a 5-Fr catheter for infants weighing more than 2000 g and a 3.5- to 4-Fr catheter for infants weighing less. Because the lumen of the vein is larger, a 5- to 8-Fr catheter can be used for UVC in term infants (>1800 g), especially infants requiring exchange transfusion. The catheter may be composed of any U.S. Food and Drug Administration–approved material; double-lumen catheters are also available.

Preprocedure Patient Preparation

The newborn needing umbilical catheterization typically demonstrates signs and symptoms of cardiorespiratory distress shortly, if not immediately, after birth. If performed as an emergency procedure, implied consent and the indications should be documented in the chart. Explain the need for the procedure to the parent(s) when there is time. For less urgent insertions, obtain informed consent from the parent(s) after discussing the alternatives, risks, and potential benefits of the procedure.

Technique

When the infant arrives at the nursery, if umbilical catheterization is probable, the umbilical stump should be left at least 4 cm long. The two thick-walled arteries and the single vein should be easily identifiable. Place the infant under an infant warmer and restrain, if possible. The cardiac rate should be monitored and adequate oxygenation should be provided throughout the procedure.

1. Set up the tubing, fluids, fluid chamber, 0.22-μg filter, and infusion pump. Flush and fill the tubing with heparin flush to remove air from the system.
2. Prepare the entire abdomen from xiphoid to pubis with sterile povidone–iodine or antiseptic scrub solution. Scrub the umbilical stump and apply sterile drapes. Observe universal blood and body fluid precautions when performing the procedure.
3. Calculate the insertion length of the catheter for proper placement.
   - UAC. There are two commonly used, standard insertion depths for UAC. One results in "high" placement of the catheter tip, which is above the diaphragm at the level of the thoracic aorta (spinal level T6–T9). This site places the tip

between the ductus arteriosus and the origin of the celiac axis. The second site results in "low" placement of the catheter tip (spinal level L3–L5), which is below the diaphragm. This site places the tip between the inferior mesenteric artery and the bifurcation of the aorta.

For high placement: (a) measure the axial or longitudinal distance from the level of the umbilicus to the level of the shoulder or clavicle (shoulder–umbilicus length). Then use the nomogram shown in Figure 184-2A; or (b) calculate the length based on birth weight (BW): length (cm) = (3 × BW [kg]) + 9.

When a nomogram or the birth weight is not available or the situation is urgent, if the shoulder–umbilicus length is greater than 13 cm, simply add 1 cm to the shoulder–umbilicus length. This results in a reasonable estimate for the catheter insertion depth. When the shoulder–umbilicus length is less than 13 cm, insert the catheter 2 cm further than the shoulder–umbilicus length.

For low placement: (a) use the nomogram (see Fig. 184-2A) with the shoulder–umbilicus length, or (b) calculate the length based on birth weight: length (cm) = BW (kg) + 7.

If a nomogram or the birth weight is unavailable or the situation is urgent, insert the catheter until blood is first encountered and then advance it 1 additional centimeter.

NOTE: One meta-analysis study found that high-placement UACs (compared with low placement) have fewer acute vascular complications and no increase in permanent vascular sequelae.

- UVC. For CVP readings, place the catheter tip 0.5 to 1 cm above the diaphragm. The insertion depth can be estimated with a nomogram (Fig. 184-2B) or with one of two formulas: (a) length (cm) = shoulder–umbilicus length (cm) × 0.6, or (b) length (cm) = (UAC insertion length [cm] × 0.5) + 1. If a nomogram or the birth weight is not available or the situation is urgent, a second option is to insert the UVC gently for 4 to 5 cm until blood return is noted. *Never insert the UVC more than 5 cm without radiographically checking the placement because the tip may be in the portal vein*. If the catheter is being placed for a single exchange transfusion, it may be inserted to just beneath the skin (3 to 5 cm), as long as good blood flow is noted and there is no leakage around the catheter.

4. Loosely tie the sterile umbilical tape around the proximal stump. It should be tight enough to control bleeding but loose enough to allow later passage of the catheter. A silk suture can be used as a pursestring ligation in the same manner.
5. Holding the cord with straight forceps, transect it with the scalpel approximately 1 cm above the umbilical tape (Fig. 184-3A). Correctly identify the arteries and the vein. Because the vein is the single vessel and has the largest lumen, it is usually the easiest to identify. It can then be distinguished from the thicker-walled arteries that are usually lateral to the vein.
6. The cord stump should be grasped with one or two hemostats (on opposite sides of the umbilicus) and the cut edge everted. Gently dilate the desired vessel with small curved forceps (Fig. 184-3B). To do so, insert one prong, then both prongs of the iris forceps, then open the forceps prongs slightly to dilate the lumen to a depth of about 1 cm. Next, grasp the catheter approximately 1 cm from the tip with your thumb and forefinger or with the forceps. Gently insert the catheter through the vessel lumen to the length previously measured (Fig. 184-3C).
7. Insertion
   - UAC. Placing traction on the cord stump in a cranial direction usually facilitates directing the catheter caudally. With insertion, use gentle, constant pressure to overcome any resistance. Resistance is usually encountered at a depth of about 1 to 2 cm as the vessel turns caudad. Slight resistance may again occur when the catheter enters the internal iliac artery at approximately 5 to 6 cm. At this depth, the

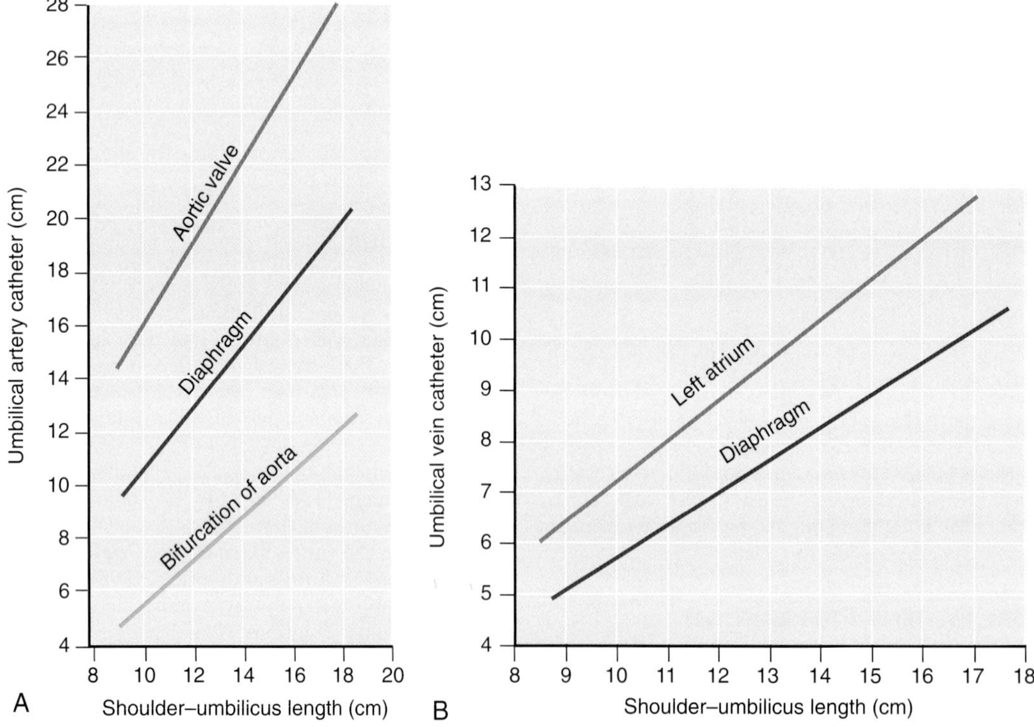

Figure 184-2 Approximate distances for catheter insertion, with radiographic confirmation of proper placement after insertion. **A,** Umbilical artery catheter (avoid inserting to level of aortic valve). **B,** Umbilical vein catheter. (From Johns Hopkins Hospital; Siberry G, Iannone R [eds]: The Harriet Lane Handbook: A Manual for Pediatric House Officers, 15th ed. St. Louis, Mosby, 2000.)

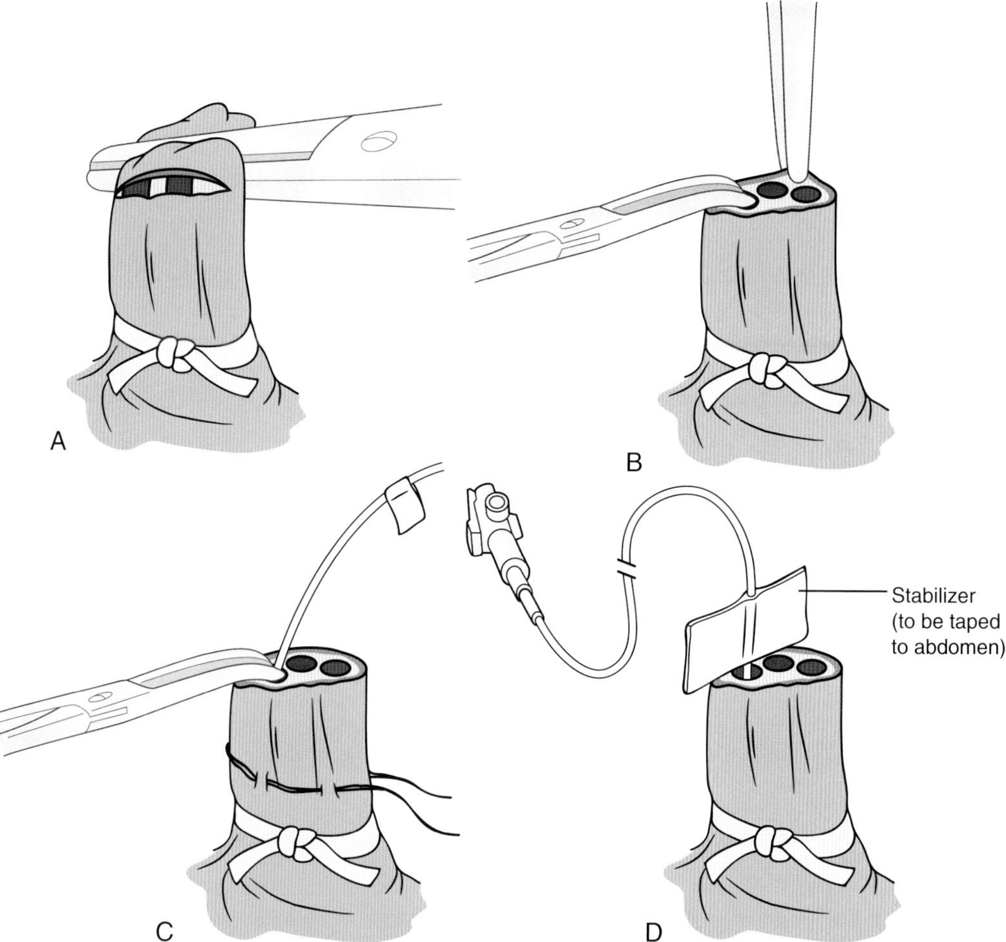

Figure 184-3 Umbilical artery catheter placement. **A,** The cord is transected approximately 1 cm above the umbilical tape. **B,** The desired artery is dilated with small curved forceps. **C,** The catheter is inserted through the vessel lumen to the length previously measured and secured with a silk pursestring suture. **D,** Alternatively, the catheter can be secured by a stabilizer taped to the abdomen.

catheter must turn cephalad. Twisting the catheter slightly may also help overcome resistance. Occasionally, resistance from vasospasm may be overcome by applying constant gentle pressure for 30 to 60 seconds, causing the spasm to subside. Another technique for relieving vasospasm is to fill the tip of the catheter with 2% lidocaine and then to flush some of it at the level where the resistance is noted. After waiting 1 to 2 minutes, attempt to advance the catheter again. Do *not* advance against significant resistance, especially at a depth of 4 to 5 cm. Resistance at this depth generally indicates that a false tract has been created. Rather than continuing to advance the catheter, withdraw it and attempt to cannulate the other artery.

UVC. Insert in the same manner as a UAC. At the insertion depth previously determined, CVP can be measured, hyperalimentation solutions can be administered, and medications can be infused. If an obstruction is encountered at a depth of 5 to 10 cm, the catheter has probably entered a branch of the portal vein of the liver and should be withdrawn.

8. Secure the catheter with the umbilical tape. Also use a silk suture in a pursestring fashion (see Fig. 184-3C), *or with a stabilizer* (Fig. 184-3D). *Once the sterile field is taken away, the catheter may not be advanced.* For that reason, it is often more convenient to insert the catheter slightly further than necessary. (For a UAC, *never* exceed the distance to the aortic valve [see Fig. 184-2].) Then it can be withdrawn slightly after radiographic confirmation of the location of the tip.

NOTE: Occasionally a persistent urachus in the umbilical stump is mistaken for the umbilical vein. Catheterization of the urachus results in the return of urine instead of blood and is easily identified and corrected.

9. Apply sterile gauze over the antibiotic ointment and tape the catheter to the abdomen.
10. Obtain radiographic confirmation of proper placement. Again, the ideal location of the UAC tip is either high placement at T6–T9 (above the diaphragm and the celiac axis but below the ductus arteriosus) or low placement at L3–L5 (above the aortic bifurcation but below the inferior mesenteric artery). If radiographic confirmation is not possible, a UVC should be used instead of a UAC and should be inserted only 3 to 5 cm or until prompt return of blood is noted.
11. Check the catheter frequently for patency and the infant for signs of infection. If signs of infection are noted, take cultures from the catheter.
12. As soon as the catheter is no longer needed, it should be removed. In addition, remove the catheter in the face of complications. When the catheter is no longer needed for arterial sampling or for CVP monitoring, in some NICUs it is simply pulled out enough to leave the tip in the midline. This maintains peripheral access if it is extremely critical or has been difficult to obtain. At that level, it then can be used for infusions.
13. If vasospasm occurs while the UAC is in place, causing ischemia of one buttock or leg, apply warm compresses to the

contralateral limb in an attempt to trigger reflex vasodilation in the affected limb. If no improvement in limb color or pulse is observed in 15 minutes, the catheter should be withdrawn. An attempt can also be made to relieve vasospasm by repositioning the catheter. Withdraw it a short distance or rotate it, while observing limb color. If successful, obtain radiographic confirmation of proper placement. Other options include withdrawing the line completely and catheterizing the other artery or using a smaller catheter in the same artery.

14. For catheter removal, the stopcock should be turned off. Umbilical tape should be tied loosely around the stump. The catheter should then be gradually withdrawn over 3 to 5 minutes. If there is bleeding, tighten the umbilical tape or grasp the vessel with forceps and apply pressure until it stops.

Complications

- Air embolization (use a three-way stopcock and flush all tubing before connecting)
- Necrotizing enterocolitis
- Bladder rupture
- Pelvic exsanguination
- Exsanguination from disconnected tubing (use locking connectors on tubing, secure the line)
- Bacteremia or sepsis (to minimize risk, remove the catheter once the infant is stabilized or within 5 days)
- Vascular perforation or malformation
- Congestive heart failure
- Fluid around the umbilicus, if the catheter is placed too low or withdrawn too far
- Silent thrombus (difficult to diagnose without contrast studies)
- UAC complications (risk of complications is as high as 10%)
  - Ischemia to bowel, liver or other intraabdominal organ, or lower extremity
  - Systemic hypertension as a result of renovascular stenosis or thrombosis
  - Embolization of clots causing loss of digits, organ infarcts, or skin ulceration
  - Hypoglycemia
- UVC complications (risk of complications is as high as 20%)
  - Portal hypertension
  - Pericardial perforation (if placed in the right atrium for central monitoring)
  - Arrhythmias
  - Hepatic abscess or necrosis
  - Pulmonary embolism

Postprocedure Patient Education

If the procedure is successful, this should be explained to the family. If there were any complications, this should also be explained, as well as what will be done about them. Any questions regarding the umbilical catheter should be answered. The family should be informed of the need for and value of having the catheter in place, and reassured that it will be monitored continuously for any signs of complications. They should be aware that it will be withdrawn to a safer level or removed as soon as it is no longer needed. It will also be removed at the first signs of a complication. Families also usually appreciate any other reassurances and guidance provided when they have a critically ill loved one in an intensive care setting, especially an infant.

CPT/Billing Codes

36510 Catheterization, umbilical vein, for diagnosis or therapy; newborn
36660 Catheterization, umbilical artery, for diagnosis or therapy; newborn

ICD-9-CM Diagnostic Codes

459.0 Hemorrhage, unspecified
769 Respiratory distress syndrome of newborn
770.12 Meconium aspiration syndrome
770.89 Other respiratory problems after birth (e.g., perinatal apnea, newborn bradycardia)
771.81 Neonatal sepsis
772.3 Hemorrhage, in newborn, umbilical
772.9 Hemorrhage, in newborn, NOS
773.0 Newborn hemolytic disease caused by Rh isoimmunization
775.4 Hypocalcemia and hypomagnesemia of newborn
775.6 Neonatal hypoglycemia
779.3 Feeding problems in newborn
785.59 Hypovolemic shock, necrotizing enterocolitis
958.4 Hemorrhagic shock as a result of trauma

Acknowledgment

The editors wish to recognize the many contributions by James A. Sterling, MD, and Susan E. Murphey, MD, to this chapter in the previous two editions of this text.

BIBLIOGRAPHY

Advanced Life Support Group: Advanced Paediatric Life Support: The Practical Approach, 3rd ed. London, BMJ Books, 2001.

Barrington KJ: Umbilical artery catheters in the newborn: Effects of position of the catheter tip. Cochrane Database Syst Rev 1:CD000505, 1999.

Carlson B: Human Embryology and Developmental Biology, 2nd ed. St. Louis, Mosby, 1999.

Fanaroff A, Martin R, Walsh M (eds): Neonatal-Perinatal Medicine: Diseases of the Fetus and Infant, 8th ed. St. Louis, Mosby, 2005.

Gomella TL, Cunningham MD: Neonatology: Management, Procedures, On-Call Problems, Diseases, and Drugs, 5th ed. New York, McGraw-Hill, 2004.

Johns Hopkins Hospital; Robertson J, Shilkofski N (eds): The Harriet Lane Handbook: A Manual for Pediatric House Officers, 17th ed. St. Louis, Mosby, 2005.

Kang I, Reichman EF: Umbilical vessel catheterization. In Reichman EF, Simon RR (eds): Emergency Medicine Procedures. New York, McGraw-Hill, 2004, pp 390–397.

Spitzer AR: Intensive Care of the Fetus and Neonate, 2nd ed. St. Louis, Mosby, 2005.

SECTION 12

Orthopedics

Section Editor: MIKE PETRIZZI

CHAPTER 185

MUSCULOSKELETAL ULTRASONOGRAPHY

John Hill • Mark Lavallee • Grant C. Fowler

Ultrasonography has been used to assess the musculoskeletal system since the 1980s. The diagnostic and interventional aspects of this imaging modality were once the sole province of radiologists, and it was used primarily in Europe (especially the United Kingdom) and Canada for these applications. This technology was not largely embraced by radiologists in the United States because it was overshadowed by the growth of computed tomography (CT) and magnetic resonance imaging (MRI). However, additional innovations in instrumentation, advances in clinical applications, and availability of clinician training programs have led us out of the infancy of musculoskeletal ultrasonography (MSK US). These technologic improvements, combined with increasing recognition of the benefits over traditional CT and MRI (e.g., less cost, higher patient satisfaction, ease of use, dynamic capabilities including guiding interventions), have led to a resurgence of interest. Primary care clinicians, particularly those skilled in sports medicine, are applying their knowledge of anatomy and pathophysiology to use this diagnostic tool as an extension of the history and physical examination. The diagnostic applications for MSK US in the upper and lower extremities and for special populations, including pediatric patients, are immense. There are also a significant number of procedural applications. To cover every joint and procedural application of MSK US would be beyond the scope of this book; therefore, this chapter addresses some of the more common clinical uses.

TECHNOLOGY AND TERMINOLOGY

Various terms are used to describe ultrasonographic equipment and images. *B-mode US* refers to brightness mode, and it allows real-time imaging. B-mode US is the precursor to gray-scale US and is somewhat limited beyond differentiating fluid from solid; consequently, it has largely been replaced by *gray-scale US*. Gray-scale US differentiates between intensities of echoes and displays them in black, white, and various shades of gray, which improves not only the resolution of the images but the ability to distinguish between different types of tissue. However, even gray-scale US cannot differentiate between fibrous synovial tissue and active synovitis; such a differentiation requires characterization of blood flow. *Color Doppler US* uses the principle that sound waves *increase* in frequency when they reflect from objects moving *toward* the transducer and *decrease* when they reflect from objects moving *away*. This is combined with real-time imaging to indicate the presence and direction of blood flow. Red signals indicate flow toward the transducer and blue signals indicate blood flow away from the probe. *Power Doppler US* has increased sensitivity for imaging small vessels and slow blood flow, which better demonstrates hyperemia and can help differentiate between inflammatory (hyperemic) and scar tissue. Power Doppler US may help visualize neovascularization or angiogenesis in inflamed or otherwise affected tissues (e.g., chronic tendinosis). Both color and power Doppler US allow one to clearly differentiate cystic lesions from vessels. (See also Chapter 225, Emergency Department, Hospitalist, and Office Ultrasonography [Clinical Ultrasonography], for discussions of principles of ultrasound and beginner scanning. Quality assurance, credentialing, and liability are also discussed.)

MSK US should be performed with a high-resolution linear-array transducer with frequencies between 7.5 and 20 MHz. The lower frequencies allow visualization of the deeper structures (e.g., hip joint), whereas the higher frequencies are better for superficial structures (e.g., finger joints). In addition to gray-scale US, machines with *tissue harmonic* imaging or *compound* imaging are useful for musculoskeletal applications. Advances in ultrasonographic equipment mirror changes in computer technology, and the actual machine used does not have to be the latest version. Although the newer machines have more features and are more portable, they are more expensive. To reduce startup costs, instead of purchasing a new machine, it may be possible to purchase a high-frequency linear-array transducer for a machine already owned or to purchase a used machine when someone else upgrades his or her equipment. Standoff probe attachments are available to enhance resolution in certain older equipment; they are also useful with most equipment when scanning very superficial structures.

ORIENTATION AND ANATOMY

Ultrasonographic scans are defined by two views oriented perpendicular to one another, the *transverse/axial/short-axis view* and the *longitudinal/long-axis view* (Fig. 185-1). Long-axis images are further defined as *sagittal* or *coronal*. Understanding anatomy as viewed by ultrasonography is a "learned skill" that takes both patience and practice to acquire. One must keep two principles in mind. First, three-dimensional structures are seen on a screen in only two dimensions. Second, a 90-degree turn of the probe will change the orientation of a two-dimensional view from axial (short axis) to longitudinal (long axis) or vice versa

SCANNING

The position of the probe in the practitioner's hand is variable; many hold it as a large pencil or like a computer mouse (Fig. 185-2). Artifact is minimized by keeping the probe as perpendicular as possible to the tissue being scanned. By convention, solid or echogenic tissue or structures are whiter on the image, whereas fluid or fluid-filled tissue or structures are darker, hypoechoic, or echolucent. Table 185-1 shows some common superficial anatomic structures seen with MSK US as well as the common views used to scan these structures.

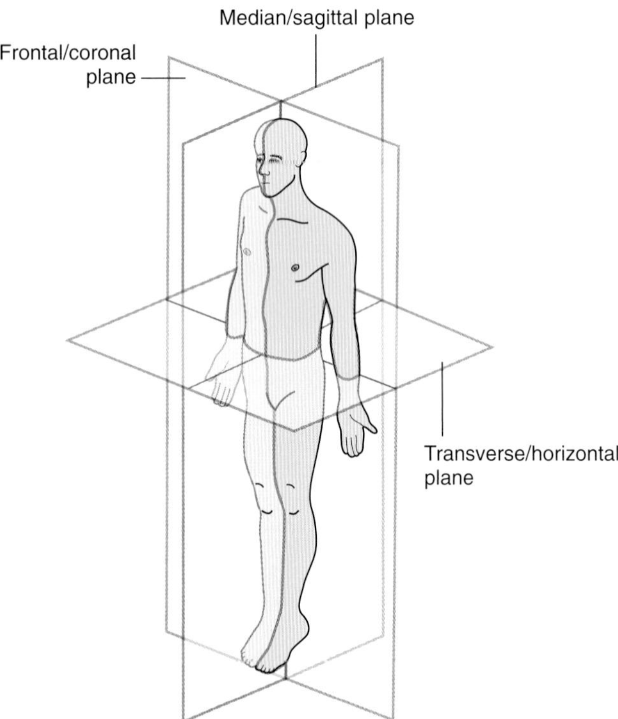

Figure 185-1 Short-axis (transverse/axial) and long-axis (longitudinal/sagittal/coronal) views in ultrasonographic scanning.

Indications

See Table 185-2.

Precautions and Contraindications

Diagnostic MSK US is a safe imaging modality with no exposure to radiation, no risks of a large magnet disrupting vascular clips, and no issues related to claustrophobia. The fact that ultrasonography has been used for years in maternal-fetal medicine with no documented ill effects speaks to its safety. Therefore, the major precaution is related to the imaging abilities; this procedure is highly operator and interpreter dependent. The sensitivity and specificity are related to the ability to visualize the individual structures and, once these are seen, to distinguish normal from abnormal anatomy. It is quite easy to visualize and diagnose an inflamed biceps tendon; however, it can be quite difficult to differentiate between chronic hamstring inflammation and a high hamstring injury. Clinicians must know their limitations and caution must be used to avoid scanning, diagnosing, or performing procedures beyond their skills.

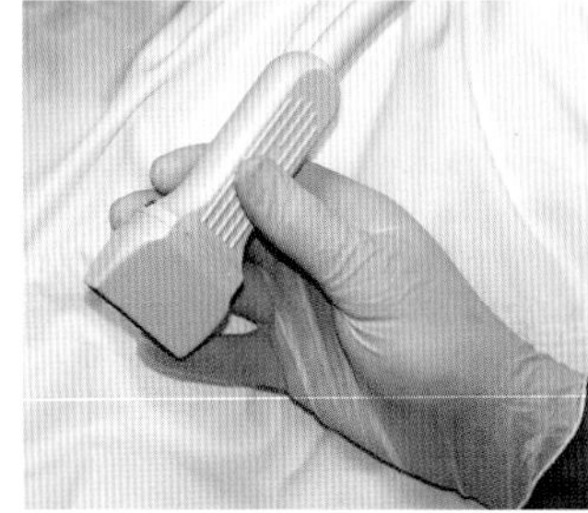

Figure 185-2 Hand and probe position.

Although procedures performed using ultrasonographic guidance are safer than blindly performing injections and aspirations, whenever a needle enters the skin, there are inherent risks of pain, bleeding, infection, and damage to underlying or surrounding tissues. No absolute contraindications to MSK US exist, but similar to all procedures, using good judgment and proper techniques will protect you and your patient.

Equipment

- Ultrasonography machine with a high-frequency (7.5 to 20 MHz), high-resolution, linear-array transducer able to capture images (see Suppliers section). Standoff disks are available to artificially increase the transducer frequency.
- Printer paper for images.
- Ultrasonic gel.
- Towels to drape the area and for cleanup afterward.
- Equipment necessary to perform procedure such as sterilizing solution (alcohol, povidone–iodine [Betadine], chlorhexidine [Hibiclens]), sterile needles, local anesthetic, or any necessary instruments.

NOTE: Linear-array transducers do have one significant limitation: they accentuate anisotropy. This hypoechogenic artifact of the tendon insertions can look like a tendon tear (Fig. 185-3); it is due to the lack of divergent beam geometry.

Preprocedure Patient Education and Preparation

Diagnostic ultrasonography, and any possible ultrasonography-guided procedure, should be briefly explained to the patient (or representative) before obtaining consent verbally and often in writing. The approximate length of time to accomplish the procedure, the few risks involved (e.g., irritation from ultrasonic gel, having to remain still during the examination, missed diagnosis), the amount of discomfort to expect from an ultrasonography-directed procedure, the benefits of having this procedure, and any alternatives should be explained. For an ultrasonography-guided procedure, any additional risks should be explained (e.g., risks of infection, injury to a nearby structure such as a vessel or nerve, scar formation, tendon rupture, hematoma) as well as any alternatives. Any other aspects should be addressed, depending on the practitioner's personal style (e.g., some clinicians curtail use of nonsteroidal anti-inflammatory drugs [NSAIDs] or aspirin before certain procedures [e.g., dry-needling tendon]; other clinicians use topical ethyl chloride "cold" spray before needling instead of injecting an anesthetic). The cost should also be explained, especially for Medicare patients; a Medicare waiver should be signed. There may be benefit to discussing postprocedure expectations at this point, especially those regarding activity, physical therapy, and restrictions. The patient should know that the room lights may be dimmed to improve visualization of the screen. (See the sample forms online at www.expertconsult.com for checklists for diagnostic and ultrasonography-guided procedures.)

Technique

Overall

1. There are several prerequisites essential to performing adequate MSK US; these should be ensured before scanning. Enough time should have been allocated to provide the imaging and perform the procedure (10 to 60 minutes). There must be adequate support staff, and they can help prepare the patient (e.g., obtain informed consent, appropriately uncover the body part to be

TABLE 185-1 Common Superficial Anatomic Structures Seen with Musculoskeletal Ultrasound

Structure	Probe/Setting	Best Views	Example
Skin/integument (dermis and epidermis at *large arrow*)	Linear/High resolution/2D and Doppler	Transverse and longitudinal	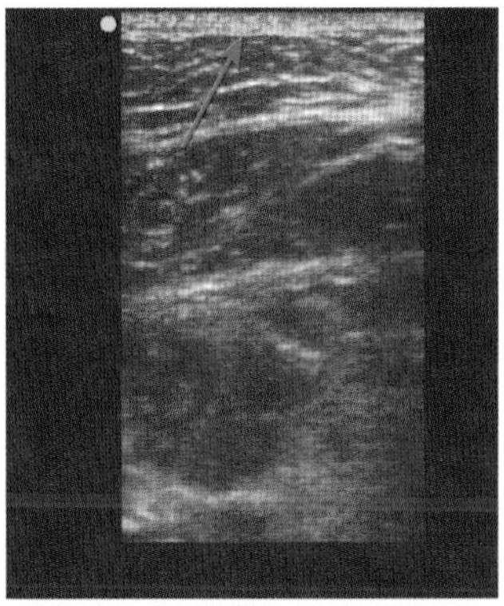
Patellar tendon (*large arrow*)	Linear/Midresolution/2D	Transverse and longitudinal	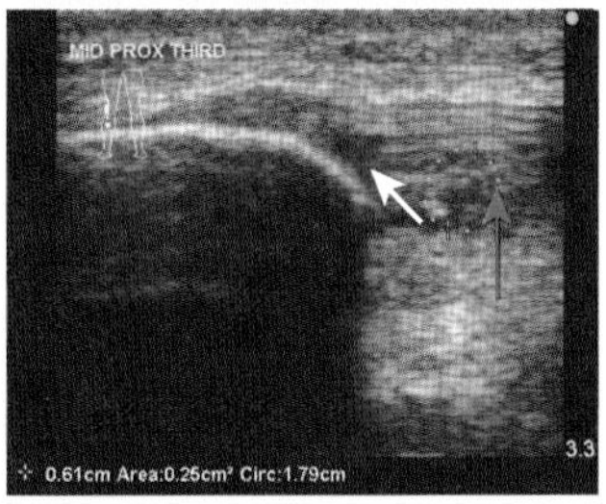
Achilles tendon (*large arrow*)	Linear/Midresolution/2D	Transverse and longitudinal	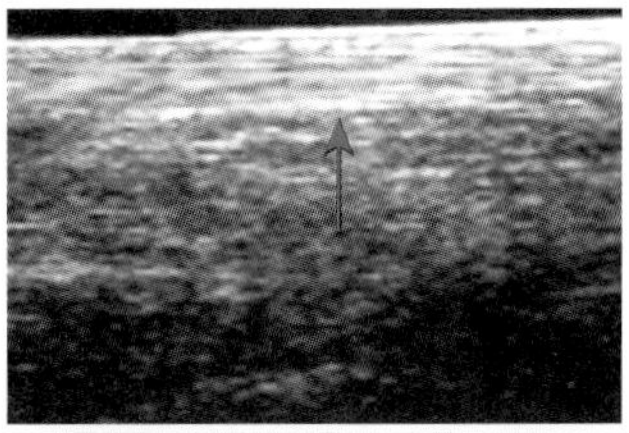
Vasculature, femoral artery in right groin (*large arrow*)	Linear/High resolution/Doppler	Transverse and longitudinal	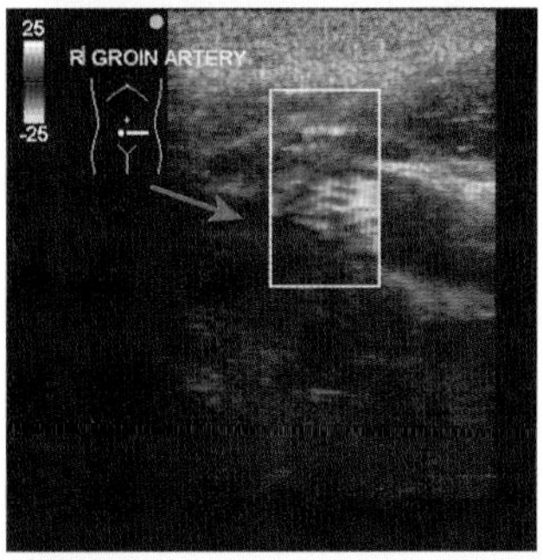
Supraspinatus tendon, longitudinal view (*large arrow*)	Linear/Low resolution/2D	Transverse and longitudinal	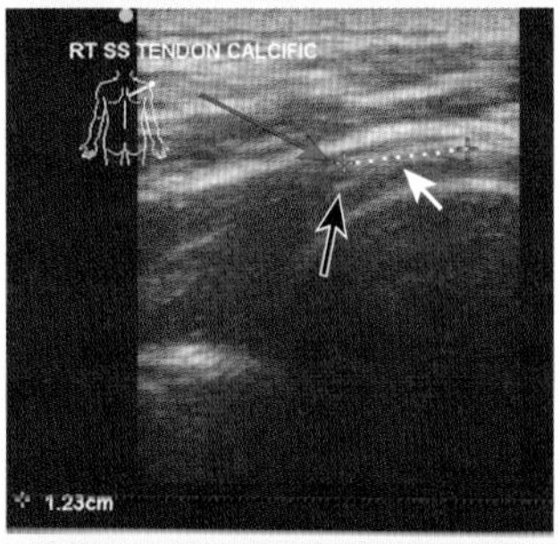
Biceps tendon, axial view (*large arrow*)	Linear/Midresolution/2D	Transverse and longitudinal	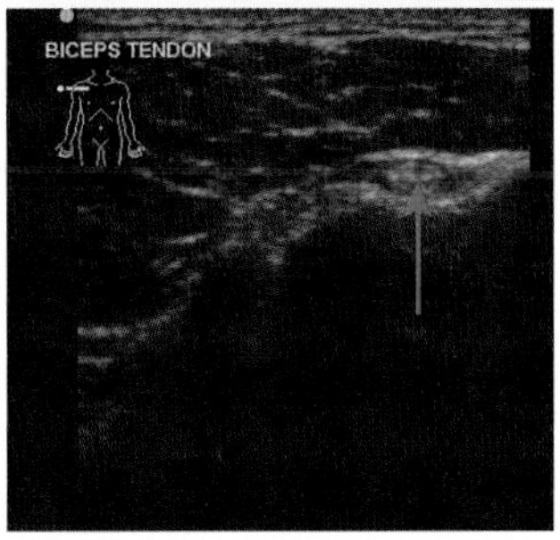

Table continues on following page.

TABLE 185-1 Common Superficial Anatomic Structures Seen with Musculoskeletal Ultrasound—cont.

Structure	Probe/Setting	Best Views	Example
Biceps tendinopathy, hypoechoic fluid surrounding thickened tendon (*large arrow*)		Longitudinal and axial	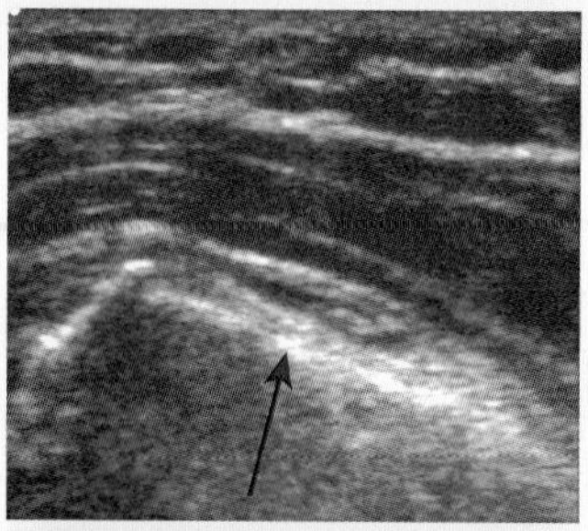
Bursa, right subacromial (*large arrow*)	Linear/High resolution/2D	Transverse and longitudinal	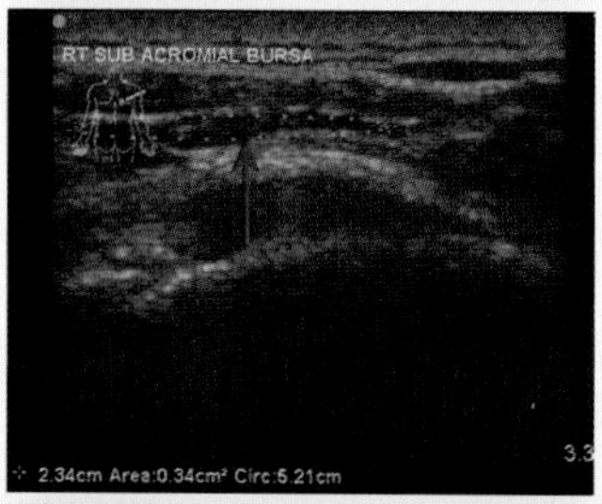
Muscle, pectoralis major (relaxed)	Linear/Mid–low resolution/2D	Longitudinal defect in pectoralis major	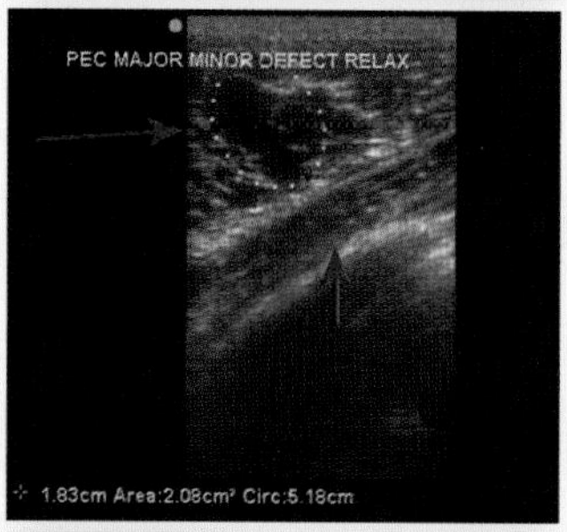
Muscle, pectoralis major (contracted)	Linear/Mid–low resolution/2D	Longitudinal	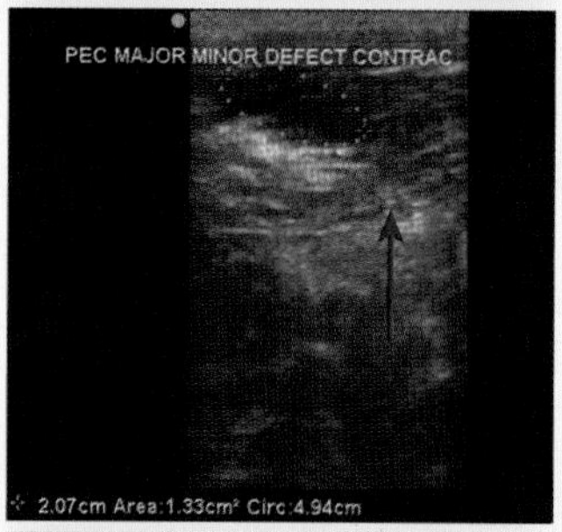
Joint capsule/Synovial fluid Acromioclavicular joint	Linear/High resolution/2D	Transverse and longitudinal	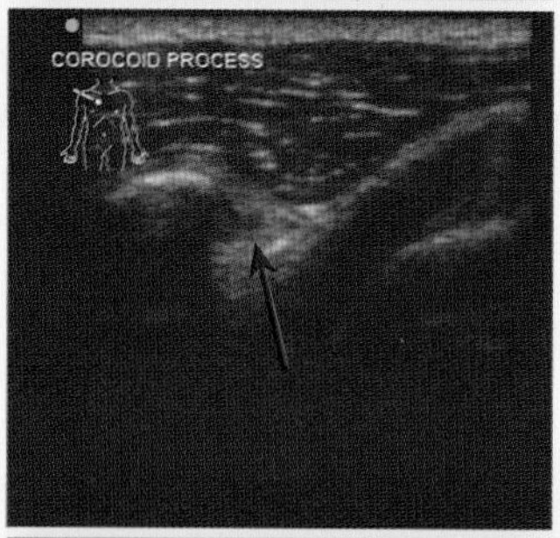
Nerves, carpal tunnel	Linear/High resolution/2D	Transverse/axial or longitudinal	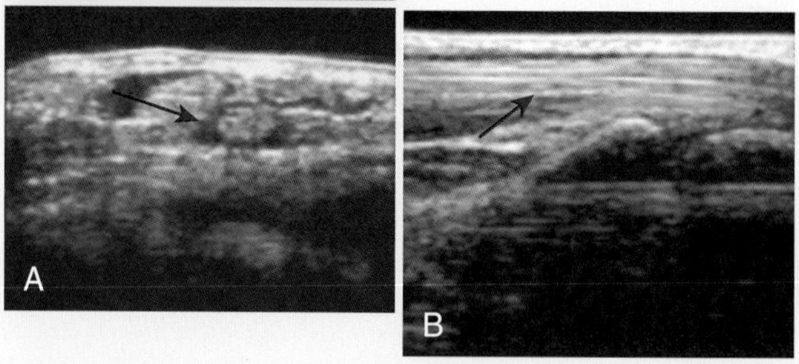

TABLE 185-2 Summary of Musculoskeletal Ultrasonography Uses

Indications, Examples, and Interventional Uses of Musculoskeletal Ultrasound		
General Indications	**Specific Applications**	**Ultrasound-Guided Interventional Technique**
Traumatic ligament tears	UCL sprain (skier's thumb)	Stress testing
Chronic tendon injury	Partial- vs. full-thickness rotator cuff tear	Motion testing
Calcific tendinopathy	Calcific supraspinatous	Steroid injection or needle débridement
Chronic tendinopathy	Proximal hamstring overuse	Dry needling, ABI, or PRPI
Bursitis	Trochanteric bursitis	Steroid injection
Effusion/Infection	Hip effusion/Septic joint	Aspiration/Arthrocentesis/Viscous supplementation
Cysts and masses	Popliteal cyst	Aspiration (avoiding popliteal aneurysm)
Wound/Abscess management	Abscess vs. cellulitis	Abscess aspiration
Elbow pain	Lateral epicondylitis	Dry needling, ABI, or PRPI
Muscle tear versus hematoma	Quadriceps muscle tear	Hematoma aspiration
Neuropathy	Carpal tunnel syndrome	Steroid injection (avoiding nerve)
Foot/Heel pain	Plantar fasciitis	Needle tenotomy/Injection

Specific Indications by Joint, Abnormality, or Procedure	
Joint	**Indication**
Shoulder	Shoulder pain or dysfunction
Elbow, wrist and hand, hip, knee, ankle and foot	Soft tissue injury, tendon or ligament pathology, arthritis, loose intra-articular body, soft tissue mass, nerve entrapment, joint effusion, foreign body, bone injury
Prosthetic hip	Joint effusion and extra-articular fluid collection (often for ultrasound-guided aspiration)
Foot	Morton's neuroma, plantar fasciitis
Peripheral nerves	Compression neuropathies, neuritis, nerve mass, nerve trauma, nerve subluxation
Soft tissue mass	Differentiating cystic from solid mass; determining size, vascularity, margins, and relationship to adjacent structures
Soft tissue foreign body	Detection and localization of foreign body, especially nonradiopaque foreign body from wood, plastic, or certain types of glass
Interventional ultrasound/Ultrasound-guided procedures	Aspiration of cysts, fluid collection or abscess; arthrocentesis or insertion of drain; injection of medication, ABI, PRPI, or contrast; ultrasound-guided biopsy or foreign body removal; lavage or aspiration of tendon calcification

ABI, autologous blood injection; PRPI, platelet-rich plasma injection; UCL, ulnocollateral ligament.

imaged), turn on the machine, and record the patient's demographic information. Often an assistant is needed to operate the machine during a procedure because the clinician's hands may be occupied with the probe and needle. Both the patient and clinician should be positioned in a manner that will be comfortable for the duration of the procedure. Any additional questions should be answered before starting the procedure.

2. Apply ultrasonic gel to the patient's skin. If planning an ultrasonography-guided percutaneous procedure, certain additional steps should be taken.
   - Apply a sterile cover over the probe/transducer (a sterile glove can be used). Some clinicians apply a small ribbon of gel to the probe before applying the sterile cover.
   - Cleanse the area of skin with antiseptic solution.

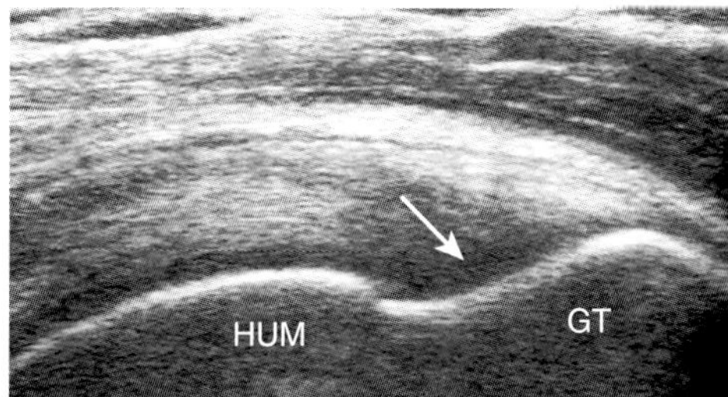

Figure 185-3 Anisotropy (*arrow*) of supraspinatus insertion on greater tuberosity (GT). HUM, humerus.

   - Apply to the area any of the following:
     - Sterile ultrasonic gel
     - Packet of sterile KY Jelly
     - Betadine-impregnated gel (if you are not using a disposable probe cover, this will stain the transducer)
   - Apply sterile probe to site.

NOTE: Preferably a sterile probe cover should be over the probe.

3. Capture basic images (Table 185-3 shows some common sonographic pathologic findings):
   - Identify large and obvious structures first.
   - Get into the habit of viewing most structures in both transverse and longitudinal planes.
   - When needed, capture images of the area in question in both static and dynamic positions (i.e., relaxed and contracted or flexed and extended).
   - Consider using color or power Doppler to look for blood flow in low- to high-flow states to assess for inflammation or neovascularization, or to differentiate between a cyst and a vessel.
   - When performing percutaneous needling (aspiration/injection or dry needling), try to obtain and document images. Because the clinician's hands will be occupied with the probe and syringe (Fig. 185-4), an assistant may be needed to run the machine.
4. Postprocedure: Once the procedure is completed, wipe the ultrasonic gel off of the patient and the probe.
   - It is important to remove the gel before it dries.
   - If a percutaneous procedure has been performed, remove and discard the sterile cover. Clean the probe head with manufacturer's approved cleaning solution.

TABLE 185-3 Common Sonographic Pathologic Findings

Diagnosis	Views Needed	Characteristics	Example
Full-thickness supraspinatus tear	Coronal, adduction, and abduction	Retraction of supraspinatus muscle, disrupted tendon	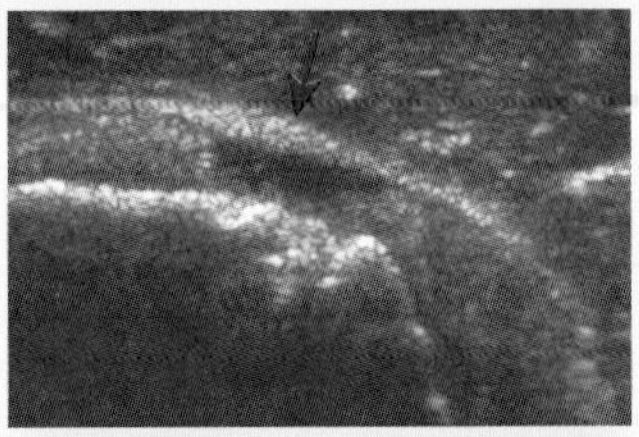
Calcific tendinopathy of supraspinatus	Longitudinal and axial	Intense echogenic mass within tendon; shadowing below mass similar to bone shadows	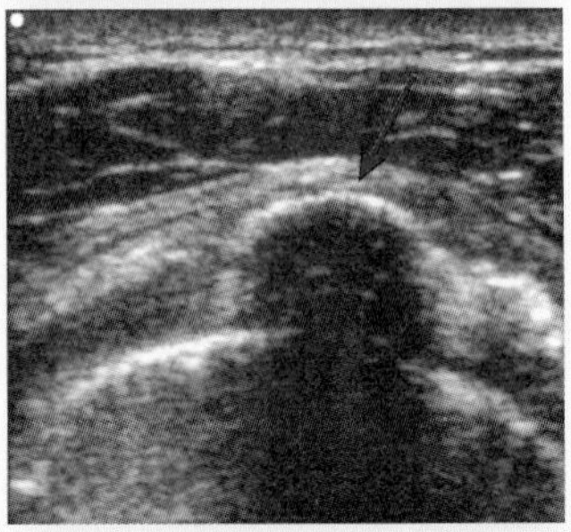
Chronic, partial-thickness supraspinatus tear	Coronal, adduction, and abduction	Hypoechoic defect within supraspinatus tendon, but no complete disruption	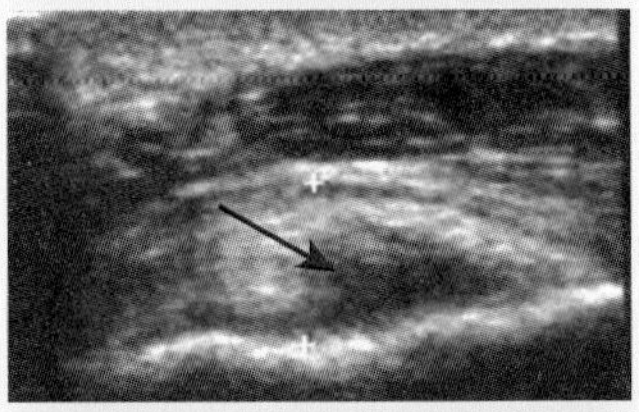
Lateral epicondylitis (tennis elbow)	Longitudinal and axial	Hypoechoic (edema) and thickening within normal tendon	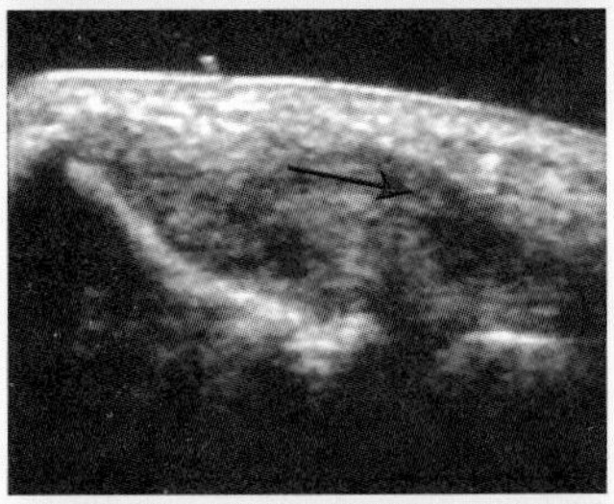
Thumb, UCL partial-thickness tear (skier's thumb)	Longitudinal and stress	Hypoechoic thickened tendon with joint laxity on stress	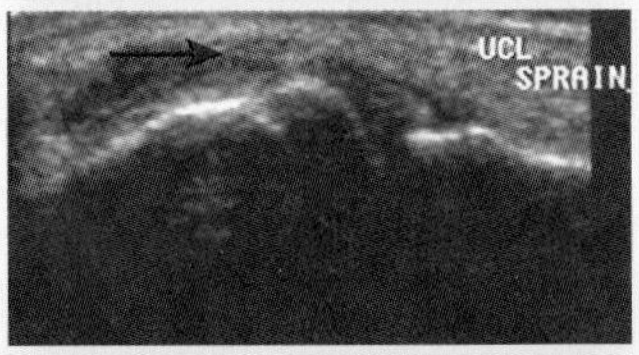 UCL SPRAIN
Soft tissue abscess	Longitudinal and axial	Hypoechoic cystic structure with bright internal echoes	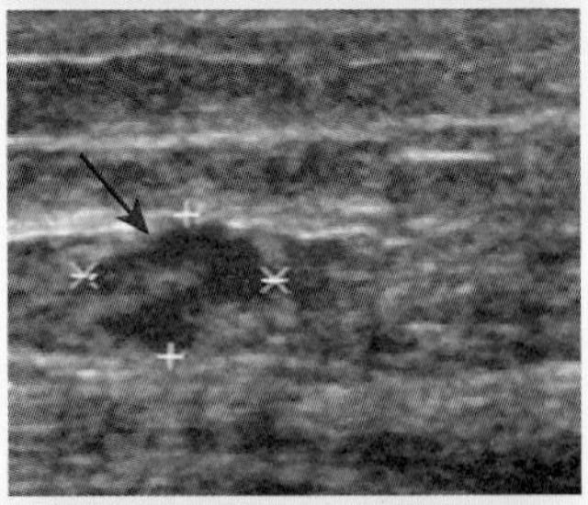
Long head of biceps tendon rupture (*large arrow*)	Longitudinal and axial	Tendon disrupted and hypoechoic fluid replacement within tendon sheath	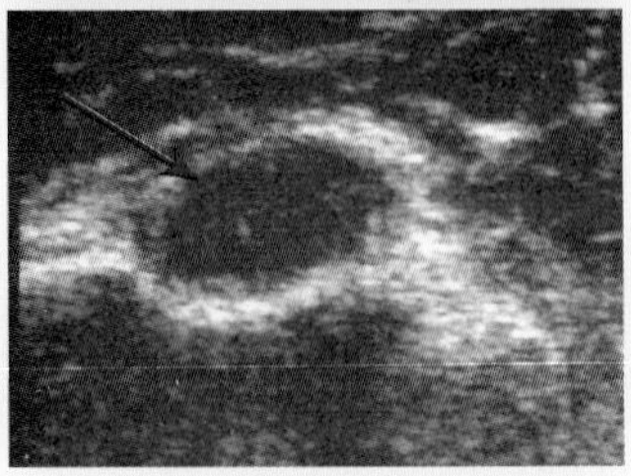

TABLE 185-3 Common Sonographic Pathologic Findings—cont.

Diagnosis	Views Needed	Characteristics	Example
Achilles tendinosis (*large arrow*)	Longitudinal and axial	Thickened, mixed echogenicity of focal site within tendon	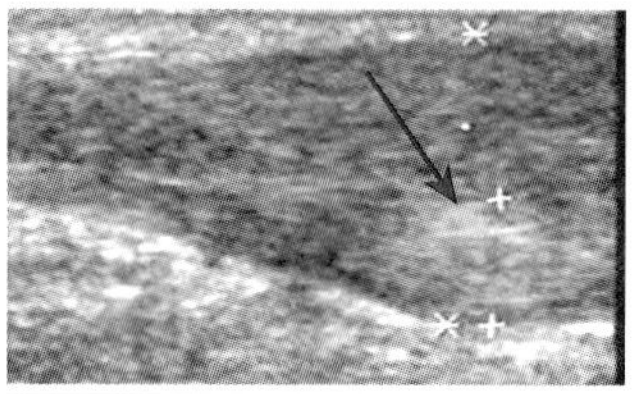
Hematoma in muscle (*large arrows*)	Longitudinal and axial	Hypoechoic fluid-filled pocket within muscle	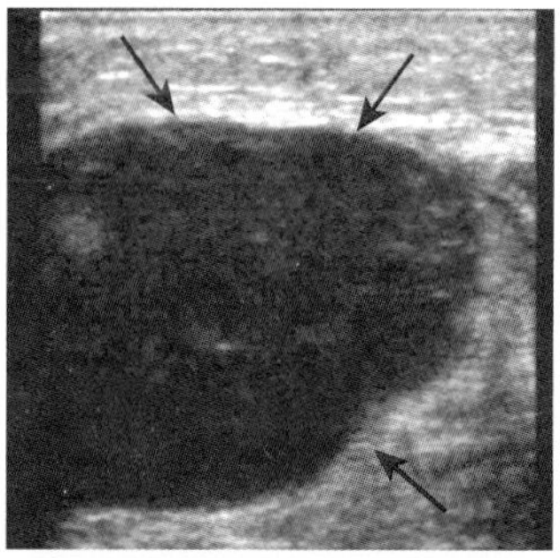
Fracture of distal radius (*large arrow*)	Longitudinal	Defect in appearance of cortex +/– angulation	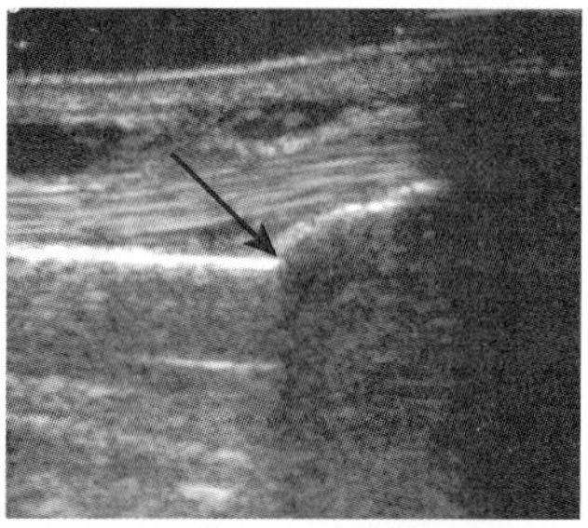
Ganglion cyst (*large arrow*)	Longitudinal and axial	Complex, multiloculated cystic structure	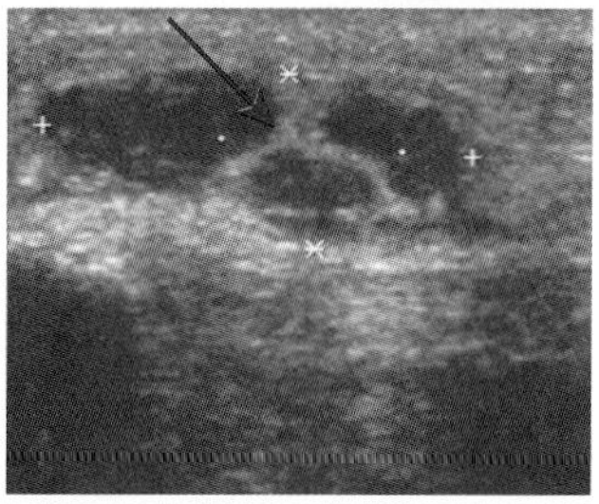
Vasculature	Transverse and longitudinal	Radial artery next to ganglion cyst	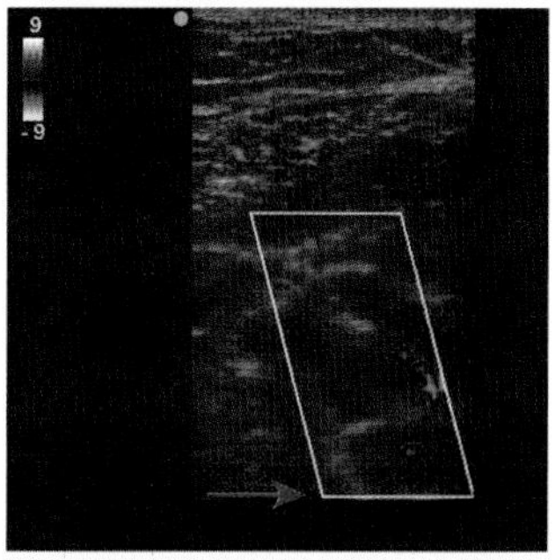
Finger/hand	Longitudinal	Hematoma on dorsum of hand	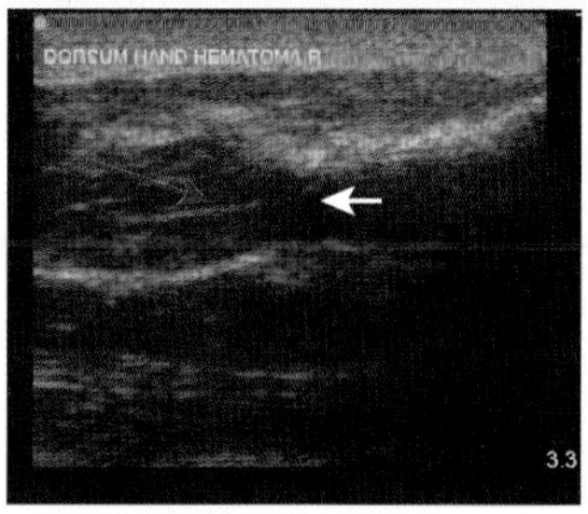

Table continues on following page.

TABLE 185-3 Common Sonographic Pathologic Findings—cont.

Diagnosis	Views Needed	Characteristics	Example
Joint space, acromioclavicular joint	Transverse and longitudinal	Cyst A/C joint	
Ligaments, lateral collateral	Longitudinal	Lateral collateral ligament disruption	

UCL, ulnocollateral ligament.

- If blood, body fluids, or Betadine somehow gets onto the probe surface, wash it with soap and water and then follow the manufacturer's recommendation to disinfect the probe.

NOTE: Povidone–iodine, if allowed to stay on the probe even for a short length of time, will discolor the probe and may shorten its working life.

- Complete and save any documentation on the ultrasonography unit and in the patient's chart.

Specific

Shoulder

1. To examine the biceps tendon, the patient's hand should be in the supine position and resting on the thigh or a pillow on the examination table with the arm slightly rotated externally. To localize the tendon, it can be scanned transversely, from where it emerges under the acromion, and followed distally to where it inserts. The tendon should then be scanned longitudinally. While scanning, determine whether the tendon is properly located in the bicipital groove, or if it can be subluxated or dislocated. Also, attempt to determine whether it is torn or disrupted.

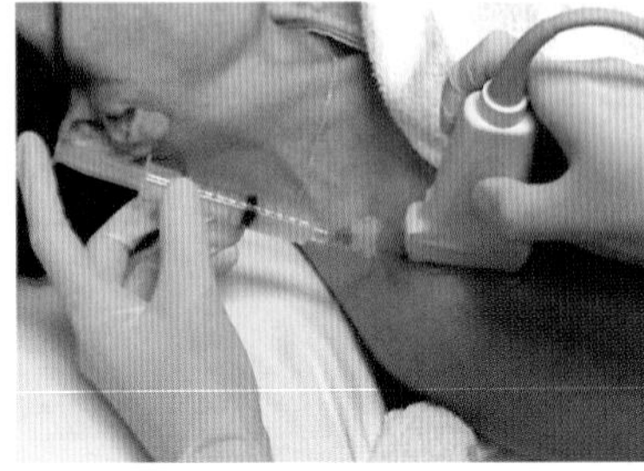

Figure 185-4 Example of positioning for an ultrasonography-guided injection.

2. To scan the subscapularis tendon, the patient's elbow should be by the side and the arm externally rotated. The tendon should be scanned transversely and then longitudinally. It may be helpful to observe the tendon as the patient moves the arm from externally to internally rotated.
3. To scan the supraspinatus tendon, ask the patient to place the hand in his or her back pocket on the same side. In this position, the elbow will be flexed, the arm extended posteriorly, and the palm of the hand placed against the posterior pelvis (iliac wing). The tendon should be scanned longitudinally and then transversely. The infraspinatus tendon can be scanned with the arm in the same location. The probe can be placed anteriorly and posteriorly to get longitudinal scans of both tendons, and will usually need to be angled 45 degrees to the sagittal plane, or in between the sagittal and coronal planes, to obtain good views. Transverse images are then obtained by rotating the probe 90 degrees. Sweep the transducer over the tendons laterally from the acromion to their insertion on the greater tuberosity of the humerus.
4. The arm is then returned to rest supinated on the thigh. In this position, the most posterior aspect of the infraspinatus tendon can be scanned as well as the posterior teres minor tendon. Internal and external rotation of the arm will help identify the infraspinatus tendon. The probe will usually need to be directed inferiorly to evaluate the entire teres minor tendon.
5. Scan also the posterior aspect of the glenohumeral joint below the scapular spine, perhaps while internally and externally rotating the arm. Small joint effusions may be noted with the transducer in this position.
6. When scanning the rotator cuff tendons, comparison with the contralateral side may be useful. Also, be on the alert for tendon calcification, bursal thickening, or loose bodies. Compression of the cuff may help identify nonretracting tears.

Elbow

1. For scanning, the elbow is divided into anterior, posterior, medial, and lateral quadrants. The patient should be sitting or lying with the hand supine and the arm extended.

2. To scan the anterior elbow, the bicipital tendon can first be followed down to its insertion on the radial bicipital tuberosity. Next, assess the articular cartilage and cortical bone while scanning the anterior humeroradial and humeroulnar joints and the coronoid and radial fossae, both longitudinally and transversely. Also look for joint effusions, synovial thickening, or loose bodies. Note the brachialis muscle, the adjacent radial and brachial nerves and vessels, as well as the median nerve. While the patient is supinating and pronating the forearm, scan the annular recess of the neck of the radius.
3. To scan the lateral elbow, have the patient put both palms together if sitting; if lying, have him or her place the forearm across the abdomen. Scan the lateral epicondyle and the attachments of the common extensor tendon, extensor carpi radialis longus, and brachioradialis. The radial collateral ligament is then scanned by having the patient pronate the hand while the transducer is on the posterolateral aspect of the elbow.
4. The medial elbow is scanned with the hand in the supine position. The medial epicondyle, common flexor tendon, and ulnar collateral ligaments should be scanned in longitudinal and transverse planes. While scanning, the integrity of the ulnar collateral ligament can be tested by applying valgus stress with the elbow slightly flexed. Scan the ulnar nerve in the cubital tunnel between the olecranon process and the medial epicondyle. Test for ulnar nerve subluxation by scanning while the patient flexes and extends the elbow.
5. Scan the posterior elbow by placing the palm down on the examination table (if the patient is sitting) or by placing the forearm across the abdomen with the elbow flexed 90 degrees (if the patient is lying). Scan the posterior joint space, the triceps tendon, the olecranon process, and the olecranon bursa in both longitudinal and transverse planes.

Wrist

1. The wrist is scanned from volar, ulnar, and dorsal locations.
2. To scan the volar wrist, the hand is placed on the examination table (if the patient is sitting) or pillow (if the patient is lying) with the palm up. Slight dorsiflexion may facilitate scanning. Scan from the wrist crease distally to the thenar muscles in both longitudinal and transverse planes. Within the carpal tunnel, the flexor retinaculum, the flexor digitorum profundus, and superficialis tendons, and the adjacent flexor pollicis longus tendons, should be identified. The median nerve lies superficial to these tendons but deep to the retinaculum. Flexion and extension of the fingers will demonstrate normal motion of these tendons and, to a lesser degree, the median nerve. Superficial to the retinaculum is the palmaris longus tendon. On the ulnar side of the wrist, branches of the ulnar nerve and artery lie within Guyon's canal. The flexor carpi ulnaris tendon borders the ulnar aspect of Guyon's canal. On the radial side of the wrist, the flexor carpi radialis longus tendon lies in its own canal. Whichever tendon is clinically indicated should be scanned for integrity, both longitudinally and transversely, to its site of insertion. Occult ganglion cysts can occasionally be noted originating from the radiocarpal joint capsule.
3. On the ulnar side, the triangular fibrocartilage can be scanned in its long axis by placing the transducer in a transverse position and scanning distal to the ulnar styloid. Rotating it 90 degrees allows for scanning the cartilage in short axis. The meniscus homolog lies distal to the triangular fibrocartilage and deep to the extensor carpi ulnaris longus tendon. This tendon should also be scanned for subluxation by pronating and supinating the wrist.
4. Dorsal scanning may be facilitated by placing the wrist in slight volar flexion. Structures on the dorsal wrist are very superficial, and the extensor retinaculum divides the dorsal wrist into six compartments. These compartments contain nine tendons that should be scanned longitudinally and transversely, at rest and in motion, to their point of insertion, as clinically indicated. With the transducer turned transversely, the scapholunate ligament can be scanned distal to Lister's tubercle. This is a common site for ganglion cysts and ligamentous tears. Otherwise, the remaining intercarpal ligaments are not routinely assessed. With an inflammatory arthritis, the metacarpophalangeal joints and, if symptomatic, the proximal interphalangeal joints can be scanned, both longitudinally and transversely. The clinician should look for effusions, synovial hypertrophy, or bony erosion. Color and power Doppler may be useful for detecting synovial hyperemia. Because the structures on the dorsal wrist are very superficial, a standoff pad may be helpful.

Hip

1. The hip can be scanned from anterior, posterior, medial, or lateral locations. In adults, a lower-frequency probe may be necessary for adequate tissue penetration; however, use the highest-frequency probe that will allow visualization of the deeper structures.
2. To scan from the anterior location, the patient should be supine with the hip rotated slightly externally. Scan longitudinally along the femoral head and neck. Evaluate the joint for any signs of an effusion, and then evaluate the labrum, the iliopsoas tendon and bursa, and the sartorius and rectus femoris muscles. These structures should also be scanned in short-axis views. The femoral vessels can be scanned. An anterior "snapping hip" is sometimes caused by the iliopsoas muscle tendon where it passes over the superior pubic bone.
3. To scan from the lateral location, rotate the patient to the lateral decubitus position with the symptomatic side up. Scan the greater trochanter, the greater trochanteric bursa, the tensor fascia lata, and the glutei medii, maximi, and minimi, all longitudinally and then transversely. Another type of snapping hip can be diagnosed when scanning from this position if the iliotibial tract snaps when passing over the greater trochanter while the hip is being moved from extension to flexion, or vice versa.
4. To scan from the medial location, the hip is placed in the frog-leg position (externally rotated with 45 degrees of knee flexion). The abductor muscles can be scanned longitudinally, as well as the distal iliopsoas tendon, and then in their short-axis plane. The pubic bone and symphysis as well as the distal insertion of the rectus abdominis on the pubic bone should be scanned from this position.
5. To scan from the posterior position, the patient should be turned to the prone position with the leg extended slightly. The glutei, hamstrings, and sciatic nerve can be scanned longitudinally and then transversely. The glutei can be scanned from origin to insertion on the greater trochanter (minimus and medius) or linea aspera (maximus). The sciatic nerve can be followed from its exit under the greater sciatic foramen, deep to the gluteus maximus muscle, and then distally to where it lies superficial to the quadratus femoris muscle. Along its course, it lies midway between the ischial tuberosity and the greater trochanter. It should be scanned both longitudinally and transversely.
6. The prosthetic hip is typically scanned for the presence of an effusion or extra-articular fluid collection. It is usually scanned from the anterior or lateral location, as described previously, and effusions are usually located at the prosthesis–bone junction. Any effusions should be measured and documented. The greater trochanteric and iliopsoas bursae should also be scanned for the presence of fluid.

Knee

1. The knee is also divided into anterior, medial, lateral, and posterior quadrants when scanning.
2. To scan the anterior knee, the patient is usually supine with the knee flexed 30 degrees. Longitudinal and transverse scans are

obtained of the quadriceps and patellar tendons, the patellar retinacula, and the suprapatellar recess. The prepatellar, superficial, and infrapatellar bursae should also be evaluated. The patella can be scanned for occult injury if clinically indicated. With the knee in maximal flexion and the transducer in the transverse plane, the suprapatellar recess can be scanned and the distal femoral cartilage assessed. This cartilage can also be assessed using longitudinal scans over the medial and lateral condyles, if indicated. While maintaining the knee in maximal flexion, the distal anterior cruciate ligament can be followed longitudinally with the probe to its insertion into the anteromedial tibial plateau.

3. To scan the medial knee, the patient remains supine with the knee slightly flexed and the hip slightly externally rotated. Alternatively, the patient can be in the lateral decubitus position with the affected knee located inferiorly. Scan the medial joint space in both longitudinal and transverse planes. The medial collateral ligament, the pes anserine tendons and bursa, and the medial patellar retinaculum should be evaluated. The anterior body and horn of the medial meniscus can be scanned from this position, possibly facilitated by the application of some valgus stress.
4. To scan the lateral knee, the patient may remain supine with the ipsilateral leg internally rotated or in the lateral decubitus position with the affected knee located superiorly. Placing a pillow between the knees may increase patient comfort. Scanning longitudinally and transversely, and moving from posterior to anterior, the popliteus tendon, fibular collateral ligament, iliotibial band, and bursa should be evaluated. The lateral patellar retinaculum can also be assessed from this location. The lateral meniscus can be evaluated by scanning in the joint line.
5. The posterior knee is scanned with the patient lying prone and the leg slightly extended. Scanning both longitudinally and transversely, the popliteal fossa and the semimembranosus and medial and lateral gastrocnemius muscles, tendons, and bursae can be assessed. The posterior horns of both menisci can be assessed by scanning transversely from this location, and the posterior cruciate ligament can be followed longitudinally. The superior aspect of the anterior cruciate ligament can be assessed somewhat when scanning transversely in the intercondylar region. To confirm a popliteal cyst, it should be demonstrated to originate from the posterior joint capsule between the medial head of the gastrocnemius tendon and the semimembranosus tendon when scanning transversely.

Ankle

1. The ankle is divided into the anterior, medial, lateral, and posterior quadrants.
2. To scan the anterior quadrant, the patient lies supine with the knee flexed and the foot flat on the examination table. From medial to lateral, the tibialis anterior, extensor hallucis longus, extensor digitorum longus, and peroneus tertius (occasionally congenitally absent) tendons are scanned in longitudinal and transverse planes. They should be followed from their musculotendinous origins to their distal insertions. The anterior joint recess is scanned for effusions, loose bodies, and synovial thickening. It may need to be compared with the contralateral side joint recess. The anterior joint capsule is attached to the anterior tibial margin, superiorly, and the neck of the talus, inferiorly. The cartilage of the talus appears as a thin, hypoechoic line. Assess the anterior tibiofibular ligament by moving the transducer over the distal tibia and fibula, superior and medial to the lateral malleolus, and scanning in an oblique transverse plane.
3. The medial ankle can be scanned with the patient in the same position. Scanning from anterior to posterior with the transducer in the transverse position, the posterior tibial, flexor digitorum longus, and flexor hallucis longus tendons can be located proximal to the medial malleolus. They can then be scanned transversely and longitudinally from their muscle of origin above the malleolus to their distal insertions. The probe angle may need to be varied to follow the tendon around the medial malleolus. The tibial nerve can then be identified at the level of the malleolus where it travels between the tendons of the flexor digitorum, anteriorly, and flexor hallucis longus, posterior to it. The nerve can be followed proximally and distally. The flexor hallucis longus can also be scanned in the posterior position where it lies medial to the Achilles tendon. The deltoid ligament is then scanned longitudinally from the medial malleolus to its attachments on the navicular, talus, and calcaneus bones.
4. The ankle is scanned from the lateral location with the patient in the same position. Slight inversion of the foot may facilitate scanning. Scanning transversely, proximal to the lateral malleolus, the peroneus brevis and longus tendons are usually easy to identify. They can then be scanned transversely and longitudinally from their proximal muscle of origin to their distal insertion. The peroneus longus tendon can be followed to the cuboid groove, where it turns to course medially along the plantar aspect of the foot to insert at the base of the first metatarsal and medial cuneiform. The peroneus brevis tendon is followed to its insertion on the base of the fifth metatarsal. These tendons should be assessed for subluxation by scanning while dorsiflexing and everting the foot. The lateral ligament complex is then assessed by placing the transducer on the tip of the lateral malleolus. From this position, the transducer will need to be turned out of the strict sagittal plane to scan and follow the anterior and posterior talofibular and calcaneofibular ligaments longitudinally.
5. The posterior ankle is scanned with the patient supine and the foot extended over the end of the examination table. Scan the Achilles tendon longitudinally and transversely from its origin, the medial and lateral heads of the gastrocnemius and soleus muscles, to its insertion on the posterior surface of the calcaneus. Plantar flexion and dorsiflexion of the foot while scanning may assist in the diagnosis of a tear. Along the medial aspect of the Achilles, the plantaris tendon may be noted to insert on the posteromedial calcaneus. Although absence of this tendon may be a normal variant, it often remains intact despite a full-thickness Achilles tendon tear. The retrocalcaneal bursa deep to the Achilles tendon can also be scanned. The plantar fascia should be scanned transversely and longitudinally from its origin on the medial calcaneal tubercle to where it divides distally and merges with soft tissue.

Foot

1. Similar to the hand, in patients with inflammatory arthritis, the metatarsophalangeal joints can be scanned, as well as the proximal interphalangeal joints if symptomatic, looking for effusions, synovial hypertrophy or hyperemia, or bony erosions. These joints, as well as any other symptomatic joints in the foot, should be scanned longitudinally and transversely. They can be scanned from dorsal or plantar locations.
2. The interdigital spaces of the foot can be scanned from either dorsal or plantar locations. Starting at the level of the first interdigital space, with the transducer in the longitudinal orientation, the interdigital spaces are scanned while moving the transducer laterally. The same areas should also be scanned transversely. The intermetatarsal bursa lies on the dorsal aspect of the interdigital nerve, so care must be taken to differentiate it from a Morton's neuroma. Pressure can be applied to reproduce the symptoms with a Morton's neuroma.

Peripheral Nerves

1. Common peripheral nerve problems include entrapment and subluxation. The most common locations for entrapment are within fibro-osseous tunnels such as the cubital or Guyon's tunnel for the ulnar nerve, the carpal tunnel for the median nerve, the tarsal tunnel for the tibial nerve, or the tunnel formed by the fibular neck and the common peroneal nerve. The most

common subluxating nerve is the ulnar nerve in the cubital tunnel.
2. Nerves course adjacent to tendons and vessels, and Doppler ultrasonography can be used to distinguish them from vessels. Tendons can be distinguished by the fact that they move much more readily than nerves with flexion or extension of the nearest joint. Surrounded longitudinally by hyperechoic fascicles, nerves are usually hypoechoic and may be interspersed with hyperechoic endoneurium or further surrounded by hyperechoic epineurium. It may be easier to follow the course of a nerve and to differentiate it from nearby tendons by scanning transversely, at first, and then scanning longitudinally.
3. For an entrapment neuropathy, after locating the nerve in the tunnel, nearby tissues (e.g., tendons, soft tissue, bones) should be scanned in an attempt to identify the source of entrapment.
4. A statically dislocated nerve is usually readily identified with ultrasonography; however, an intermittently subluxating nerve may need to be imaged during flexion or extension of a nearby joint.

Soft Tissue Masses

A soft tissue mass should be scanned longitudinally and transversely, and diameters measured in three planes. Cysts should be differentiated from solid masses, and nearby structures should be determined, particularly neurovascular bundles, bones, tendons, and joints. Compressibility of the mass should be determined. Vascularity can be evaluated using Doppler.

Foreign Bodies

When scanning a foreign body, the approximate size, location, and nearby structures should be determined. Most foreign bodies larger than a certain diameter (depending on the frequency and quality of the probe) will cast an acoustic shadow or a comet tail artifact. A standoff pad may be needed for the probe to scan very superficial foreign bodies in subcutaneous tissues. (See also Chapter 225, Emergency Department, Hospitalist, and Office Ultrasonography [Clinical Ultrasonography].)

Interventional Ultrasonography

1. Ultrasonography provides direct visualization of the needle pathway, and if the probe is equipped with a needle guide, it may provide direct visualization of the needle and show the position of the needle as it enters the target area.
2. Nearby structures should be evaluated, in an attempt to avoid them, and the shortest pathway to the interventional site is usually determined. For ultrasonography-guided biopsy, focal areas of vascularity may indicate viable tissue.
3. Ultrasonography-guided procedures can be performed either statically or in real time. For statically guided interventions, the insertion site, angle, and depth are initially identified with ultrasonography and then the probe is laid aside while the procedure is performed. For real-time guidance, the procedure is performed with simultaneous ultrasonographic imaging. Either a one-person or two-person technique can be used for ultrasonography-guided procedures. (See also Chapter 225, Emergency Department, Hospitalist, and Office Ultrasonography [Clinical Ultrasonography].)

Sample Operative Report

Diagnostic: Patient (or patient's proxy) was informed about the protocol and the risks of having a diagnostic ultrasound. Written informed consent was obtained. Longitudinal and axial views were captured, reviewed, measured, and archived. Doppler ultrasound views were also obtained and the following vascular structures were identified. The following anatomic structures were seen via ultrasound, and noted caliper measurements were archived. Images of the area in question were viewed both in a relaxed (or static) phase and also in a contracted (or dynamic) phase, captured and archived. No complications were noted from this scan, and the patient tolerated the procedure well. Results were explained to the patient before discharge from the office. [Finally, the impression should state a defined diagnosis and the plan should include any pertinent instructions.]

Percutaneous needling: Patient (or patient's proxy) was informed verbally about the protocol and the risks of having this procedure performed as well as having a diagnostic ultrasound. Written informed consent was obtained. Topical ethyl fluoride or local lidocaine was used for anesthesia. Normal sterile preparation of both patient and equipment was done using antiseptic solutions and sterile barrier devices. Pre- and postpercutaneous images were reviewed, measured, and archived. Images of the needle in the appropriate location were viewed and documented (Table 185-4).

TABLE 185-4 Additional Documentation Needed for Percutaneous Needling Procedure

Aspiration	Cortisone	PRP/Autolog Blood	Dry Needling
Anesthetic and amount	Anesthetic and amount	Anesthetic and amount	Anesthetic and amount
Gauge needle	Gauge needle	Gauge needle	Gauge needle
Amount of fluid removed	Amount/Type of steroid	Location of blood/Plasma	Amount of needling
Description of fluid		Amount injected	
Fluid sent for analysis?		Amount of needling	

PRP, platelet-rich plasma.

There were no complications, adverse reactions, or premature termination of this procedure. [Finally, the impression should state a defined diagnosis and the result of the procedure, and the plan should include any pertinent instructions.]

NOTE: Images should be saved when billing for an ultrasonography-guided procedure.

Common Errors

Musculoskeletal ultrasonography is often considered the most operator-dependent imaging technique available. In other words, the most common errors in using this tool are using it incorrectly and incorrectly interpreting the images. In Europe, standardized training courses are available, taught by experienced sonographers, and a set preceptorship period is established after the introductory course. At the conclusion of training, individuals are assessed on their ability to make ultrasonographic diagnoses; thus, interoperator variability is minimized. Standardized teaching methods are lacking in the United States. The American Institute of Ultrasound in Medicine (AIUM) has a set of practice guidelines for the performance of MSK US. These guidelines have been developed to provide practitioners with the minimum requirements for performing diagnostic procedures. Although it is not possible to detect every abnormality, by using a standardized approach one can maximize the ability to detect most problems. These guidelines specifically address examinations of the shoulder, elbow, wrist, hand, hip, knee, ankle, foot, peripheral nerves, and soft tissue masses, as well as the performance of interventional MSK US.

To avoid obvious errors, general scanning principles should be followed that require axial/transverse and longitudinal views of each structure. In an axial scan, one might see a structure that looks like a fluid-filled cyst; however, in the longitudinal image it will be obvious that the structure is in fact a vessel. A full understanding of the underlying anatomy and common abnormalities that might be relevant will increase the operator's scanning sensitivity and accuracy.

Complications

Ultrasonography is generally a safe procedure; the main complication is misdiagnosis. If, when evaluating a shoulder injury, an acute full-thickness supraspinatus tendon tear is missed, surgery could be delayed, which could ultimately lead to a less-than-ideal outcome. If performing an ultrasonography-guided injection, one must follow the usual standards for all interventional procedures: appropriate consent, sterile technique, and, to avoid damage to nerves and vessels, proper positioning of the needle.

Postprocedure Management and Patient Education

The patient should be repositioned into a comfortable position and the results of the ultrasonographic examination explained. At this point, some clinicians review the images with their patients. Future patient care management should also be discussed based on the results.

If an ultrasonography-guided procedure was performed, the postprocedure plan should be reviewed with the patient. The patient should know to watch for signs of infection, increasing pain or swelling, or fever, and know how to reaccess medical personnel if necessary. After aspiration, the patient should know to watch for reaccumulation of aspirated fluid. A pressure dressing for 1 to 3 days may prevent this. Depending on the clinician, restrictive dressings, bracing, immobilizers, sterile bandages, and limits on bathing or activity may be recommended. These are best communicated in writing and shared with the patient and his or her responsible friend or family member. Certain procedures may benefit from a 24 to 48 hours' postprocedure check in the office to assess for pain control, development of a hematoma, or signs of infection. As with many procedures in musculoskeletal medicine, certain home exercises and formal physical therapy protocols may be initiated depending on the clinician's personal protocol. Discuss with patients how to control their pain and give them appropriate medications. Many clinicians now avoid NSAIDs or aspirin in the postprocedure phase because of their antiplatelet effects and inhibition of the normal physiologic inflammatory cycle.

Specific instructions may be warranted with certain procedures:

Injection: Look for local reaction to the injected substance (e.g., cortisone, lidocaine, autologous blood, platelet-rich plasma) or development of a hematoma. A pressure dressing for 1 to 3 days may prevent this. Restrictions and expectations should be discussed.

Dry needling and tenotomy: Look for excessive swelling or new-onset hematoma. A pressure dressing for 1 to 3 days may prevent this. Sometimes elevation of the limb, compression dressing, and ice may be needed postprocedure. Limited, short-term extremity immobilization is often recommended when extensive needling is done to protect against tendon/ligament rupture. The role of physical therapy is crucial when dealing with long-standing injuries that have had needling. Restrictions and expectations should be discussed.

Interpretation and Results

See Table 185-3.

CPT/Billing Codes

20550 Injection, single tendon sheath, or ligament
20551 Injection, single tendon origin/insertion
20552 Injection(s), single or multiple trigger point(s), one or two muscles
20553 Injection(s), single or multiple trigger point(s), three or more muscles
27096 Injection into sacroiliac joint
76880 Diagnostic ultrasound examination of extremity, nonvascular, including image documentation
76942 Ultrasound-guided biopsy, aspiration, injection, localization device
93922 Color or spectral waveform Doppler of upper or lower extremity arteries, single level

Modifiers

25 To be used with separate E&M code
50 Bilateral procedures
51 Multiple procedures

Coding Example

If a patient is referred from another clinician for consultation on shoulder pain and you perform a diagnostic MSK US, you can code (99243) for the consultation, use a (25) modifier, and perform a diagnostic MSK US (76880). If you determine the patient has a long head of the biceps tendinopathy and would benefit from an ultrasonography-guided injection of the tendon sheath, then you can add 76942 and 20550 to your procedures.

ICD-9-CM Diagnostic Codes

354.0 Carpal tunnel syndrome
354.2 Cubital tunnel syndrome
355.5 Tarsal tunnel syndrome
355.6 Morton's neuroma
355.9 Mononeuritis of unspecified site (e.g., compression neuropathy)
682.9 Other cellulitis and abscess, unspecified site
718.00 Articular cartilage disorder, site unspecified
718.10 Loose body in joint, site unspecified
719.00 Effusion of joint, site unspecified
719.40 Pain in joint, site unspecified
719.60 Other symptoms referable to joint, site unspecified (e.g., snapping hip)
726.4 Enthesopathy of wrist and carpus
726.5 Enthesopathy of hip
726.6 Enthesopathy of knee
726.10 Disorders of bursae and tendons in shoulder region, unspecified
726.30 Enthesopathy of elbow, unspecified
726.33 Olecranon bursitis
726.65 Prepatellar bursitis
726.70 Enthesopathy of ankle and tarsus, unspecified
727.41 Ganglion of joint
727.42 Ganglion of tendon sheath
727.51 Baker's cyst
727.60 Nontraumatic rupture of unspecified tendon
727.61 Complete rupture of rotator cuff
727.62 Rupture of tendon of biceps
727.63 Rupture of extensor tendons of hand and wrist
727.64 Rupture of flexor tendons of hand and wrist
727.65 Rupture of quadriceps tendon
727.66 Rupture of patellar tendon
727.67 Rupture of Achilles tendon
727.81 Contracture of tendon or tendon sheath
727.82 Calcium deposits in tendon and bursa
728.4 Laxity of ligament
728.5 Hypermobility syndrome
728.83 Rupture of muscle, nontraumatic
729.6 Residual foreign body in soft tissue
729.81 Swelling of limb

SUPPLIERS

(See contact information online at www.expertconsult.com.)

General Electric Medical Systems
Mindray Medical International (Mindray DP-6600)
MySono/Medison/Sonoace America
Siemens/Acuson
SonoSite
Sonoscape USA
Toshiba America

ONLINE RESOURCE

American Institute of Ultrasound in Medicine: Available at www.aium.org.

BIBLIOGRAPHY

Bianchi S, Martinoli C: Ultrasound of the Musculoskeletal System. New York, Springer, 2007.

Bryun GAW: Musculoskeletal ultrasonography: Nomenclature, technical considerations, validation, and standardization. In Rose BD (ed): UpToDate. Waltham, Mass, UpToDate, May 10, 2007. Available at www.uptodate.com.

Jacobson JA: Fundamentals of Musculoskeletal Ultrasound. Philadelphia, Saunders, 2007.

McNally EG: Practical Musculoskeletal Ultrasound. Philadelphia, Churchill Livingstone, 2005.

Nazarian L, Jacobson JA, Smith J, et al: AIUM Practice Guideline for the Performance of the Musculoskeletal Ultrasound Examination. American Institute of Ultrasound in Medicine, 2007. Available at www.aium.org/publications/guidelines/musculoskeletal.pdf.

CHAPTER 186

Ankle and Foot Splinting, Casting, and Taping

Gregory A. Marolf

Primary care clinicians encounter a wide variety of acute and chronic foot and lower leg injuries that may benefit from immobilization. The value of immobilization as an initial means of therapy has been known for centuries. Treatment of foot and ankle injuries involves an accurate clinical evaluation and, when indicated, radiographic assessment of potential fractures, avulsions, or instability. Casting and cast splinting are commonly used in acute situations and fractures (see Chapter 190, Fracture Care), whereas splinting and taping are probably best used to control chronic instabilities and as adjuncts in rehabilitation. PRICES (**p**rotect, **r**est, **i**ce, **c**ompression, **e**levation, **s**plint) is the mnemonic often utilized when acute immobilization is indicated. *It should also be noted that rapid remobilization is an important part of the rehabilitation for most soft tissue injuries to the ankle.*

Indications

Soft Tissue Injuries

- Ankle sprains: Treatment options include use of a sugar-tong splint, taping, and braces (stirrup or lace-up type) for support as the patient returns to weight bearing.
- Plantar fasciitis: Immobilization can be achieved with a nocturnal posterior leg splint, which provides a constant stretch to the plantar fascia. (See Chapter 195, Podiatric Procedures, for other treatments, including customized orthotics.)

Fractures

- Tibial or fibular: Stable distal tibial or fibular fractures, including malleolar fractures, can be immobilized with a splint or short-leg walking cast (see Chapter 190, Fracture Care).
- Fifth metatarsal: Immobilize avulsion fractures with a postoperative shoe, posterior splint, or short-leg cast (see Chapter 190, Fracture Care).
- Other: Primary care clinicians may also encounter fractures of the tarsals, or first through fourth metatarsals. When these fractures are nondisplaced and stable, immobilization alone may be appropriate; otherwise, surgical referral may be necessary (see Chapter 190, Fracture Care).

Prophylaxis against Injuries

Ankle taping or bracing may be used as prophylaxis against injury in ankles that need additional stabilization and improved proprioception.

Contraindications

- Early (premature) casting: Casting before maximal swelling has occurred can cause necrosis and compartment syndrome.
- Open wound: Never place a cast over an open wound because of the potential for infection. If the wound is not too large, a window may be cut in the cast to monitor it.
- Unstable fractures: These fractures need surgical repair; splint only until definitive treatment can be provided.

Benefits of Different Types of Immobilization

The type of immobilization used may vary with the location and severity of the injury, patient or clinician preference, and the plan of treatment. The following list of benefits for each option may help when making decisions.

Splinting

- Stability for soft tissue injuries
- Pain relief
- Easily removable to apply ice massage, etc.
- Provides temporary support for patients needing surgery

Casting

- Marked stability
- Significant pain relief
- Immobilization for hard-to-treat soft tissue injuries as well as fractures

Taping

- Supports acutely injured ankles
- Supports chronically weak ankles or a chronically injured plantar fascia
- Enhances proprioception
- Prophylaxis against injury

Equipment

Casting

Figure 186-1 illustrates the materials needed for casting.

- Stockinette: 4-inch stockinette is appropriate for most patients, but 3-inch stockinette may be needed for smaller patients
- Cast padding: 3- or 4-inch rolls (depending on patient size), soft cotton (e.g., Webril) or synthetic (e.g., polyester)
- Synthetic waterproof cast liner (e.g., Gore Procel, Scotchcast Wet or Dry, Delta-Dry, Waterpruf) (*optional*)
- Cast material: 3- or 4-inch rolls, depending on patient size, plaster or synthetic (e.g., fiberglass)

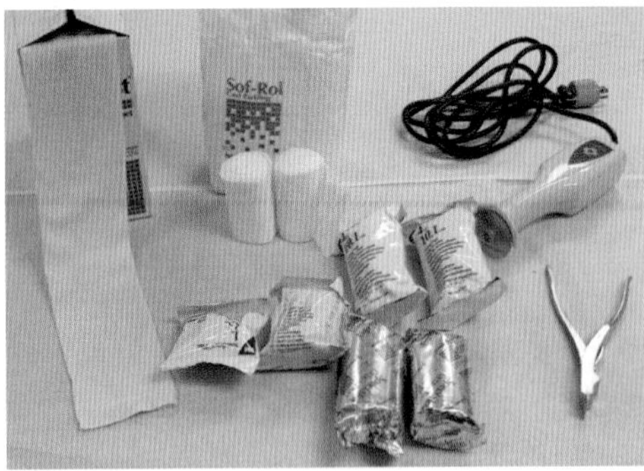

Figure 186-1 Materials needed for casting: cast padding, casting material, cast spreader, cast cutter, and stockinette.

- Rubber heels (for walking cast, but may not be needed for fiberglass cast)
- Gloves, nonsterile
- Gown and shoe covers for the clinician
- Patient towels or drapes
- Water bucket with tepid water (if using plaster, should have traps in drains)
- Chinese finger traps
- Foot stand (*optional*)
- Scissors
- Cast cutter
- Cast spreader
- See Chapter 187, Cast Immobilization and Upper Extremity Splinting, if cast removal protective strips (e.g., De-Flex) indicated or desired to protect skin from cast saw during removal

Splinting

- Most of foregoing supplies for casting *or* premade splint material (plaster or synthetic)
- Compression wrap elastic bandage (Ace bandage)

Taping for Ankle

- Skin preparation (benzoin)
- Lubricant (*optional*)

NOTE: The lubricant may be applied to the skin at sites of potential friction or irritation.

- Underwrap
- 1½- or 2-inch athletic tape
- Pressure pads or moleskin

Taping for Plantar Fasciitis

Equipment is similar to that used for the McConnell method of taping for patellofemoral knee pain:

- 2-inch dressing retention sheet (skin tape, white)
- 1½-inch patellofemoral adhesive tape (high-tensile strength tape, brown; some of the original work with McConnell taping was rumored to have used duct tape!)
- Alcohol swabs
- Commercial adhesive remover

Preprocedure Patient Preparation

Obtain verbal or written consent. Possible complications should be explained to the patient. For example, the patient should be aware that there will be a temporary loss of flexibility following immobilization, especially in the foot. In some cases, a partial loss of flexibility can become permanent. Place the patient in a seated or supine position. Some clinicians prefer a prone position with the knee flexed 90 degrees.

Technique

Splinting

Most clinicians have access to premade splinting materials that are fixed or inflatable (e.g., Aircast). However, inexpensive splints can be made from a plaster cast roll and cast padding:

1. Estimate the length of the splint you plan to use.
2. Unroll cast material into layers, making 11 to 13 layers.
3. In a similar fashion, unroll cast padding into layers, making 6 to 8 layers.
4. Unroll a single layer of cast padding for the outside of the splint.
5. The plaster cast material will be placed between the inner and outer layers of cast padding. The inner layers (6 to 8 layers) are placed between the splint and the skin, while the single outer layer of cast padding is placed on the outside of the splint. The latter is used to prevent the Ace bandage from adhering to the plaster.

Generally, when making a splint from casting materials, plaster is used. With this type of splint, the padding will not be wet. The casting material is immersed in water separately. Premade splints may be plaster or fiberglass. With premade materials, the padding will be wet. Premade splint material can also be simulated by rolling a stockinette over the outside of the 11 to 13 layers of cast materials. Fold over the ends of the stockinette and tape them to keep the splint neat. Both the stockinette and the casting materials are then immersed in water together. Both will be wet when applying. Several layers of cast padding are then placed between the patient's skin and this splint to prevent skin breakdown.

Two types of ankle splints will be discussed: sugar tong and posterior. Application depends on the indication and degree of stabilization desired. The sugar-tong (stirrup) splint may be used in ankle sprains to prevent inversion or eversion.

Sugar-Tong (Stirrup) Splint

1. Measure from the fibular head (at the knee) to the calcaneus, double that measurement, and cut the splint material and padding to size.
2. Wet the splint material and remove excess water by applying gentle pressure across the width of the splint material.
3. Place the padding against the patient's skin and have the patient or an assistant hold it in place.
4. Apply the splint material against the lateral aspect of the leg, starting just distal to the fibular head (2 fingerbreadths below). Wrap the splint under the heel, and return it up the medial side of the leg to just below the knee (Fig. 186-2). (It is U-shaped like a long sugar tong; the anterior and posterior aspects are open.)
5. Mold the splint material to support the ankle and heel.
6. Place a layer of padding over the splint.
7. Wrap the splint material to hold it in place with an elastic bandage or a roll of cast padding (Fig. 186-3).

Posterior Splint

The posterior splint may be used with stable tibial or fibular fractures and plantar fasciitis to restrict dorsiflexion or plantar flexion of the foot and ankle complex.

1. Measure from the metatarsal heads to just distal to the popliteal fossa (2 fingerbreaths above), and cut the splint material and padding to size.
2. Wet the splint material and remove excess water.
3. Place the padding against the patient's skin and have the patient or an assistant hold it in place.

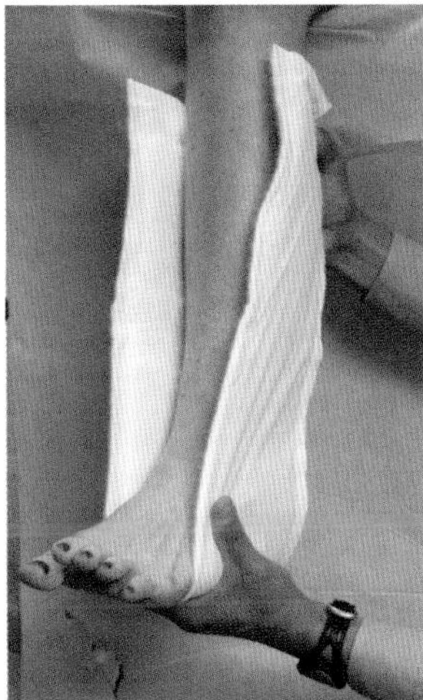

Figure 186-2 Splint material in the shape of a U (sugar tong). The splint allows for swelling while providing medial and lateral support.

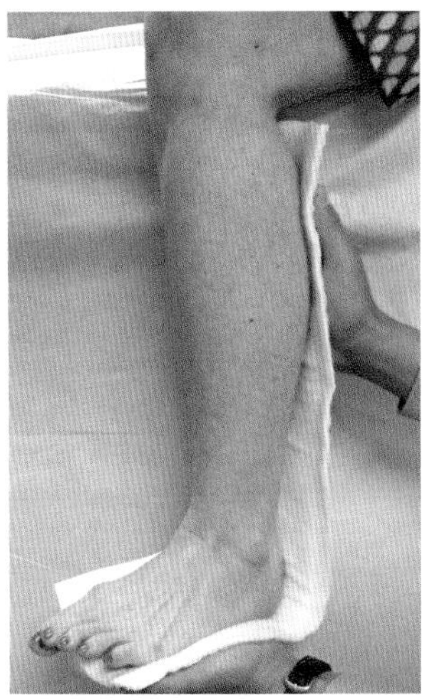

Figure 186-4 Cast material runs along the posterior aspect of the lower leg and the plantar surface, providing immobilization for ankle dorsiflexion and plantar flexion.

4. Apply the splint material over the padding and against the plantar aspect of the foot and along the posterior aspect of the leg. Extend the splint from the metatarsal heads to just distal to the popliteal fossa (Fig. 186-4).
5. Mold the splint material to support the ankle and heel.
6. Place a layer of padding over the outside of the splint.
7. Wrap the splint material to hold it in place with an elastic bandage or a roll of cast padding (Fig. 186-5).

Casting

Short-Leg Cast

A short-leg cast may be used for stable tibial or fibular fractures, fifth metatarsal fractures, or severe ankle sprains (after acute swelling subsides).

1. Measure from the metatarsal heads to the knee and cut the stockinette to length. Be sure to allow extra stockinette to fold over the ends of the cast.
2. Slide stockinette on and smooth all wrinkles or folds. The crease that will be formed at the anterior ankle should be trimmed away (Fig. 186-6).
3. Place the ankle in neutral position (90 degrees). Failure to flex it to 90 degrees may lead to difficulty in ambulating and to Achilles tendon shortening. A foot stand may be useful to support the foot.
4. Wrap the cast padding over the stockinette, starting at the foot. The padding should overlap 50% with each consecutive wrap. The padding should extend from the metatarsal heads to just distal to the fibular head. Care should be taken to provide adequate padding around the heel, the malleoli, the metatarsal heads, the proximal fibula, and the anterior tibia (Fig. 186-7).
5. Wet the cast material. Wrap the foot and ankle with the cast material in a manner similar to that already done with the cast padding. It should be wrapped over the cast padding. Maintain moderate tension, and overlap the rolls by 50% (Fig. 186-8).
6. Mold the cast to ensure neutral position of the ankle at 90 degrees.
7. Fold the stockinette over the ends of the cast to provide a smooth edge (Fig. 186-9).
8. Apply a final layer of cast material over the initial layer and the folded-down edge of the stockinette at the ends (Fig. 186-10). For a walking cast, 6 to 8 layers of reinforcing strips may be placed under the heel and foot prior to the final cast layer.

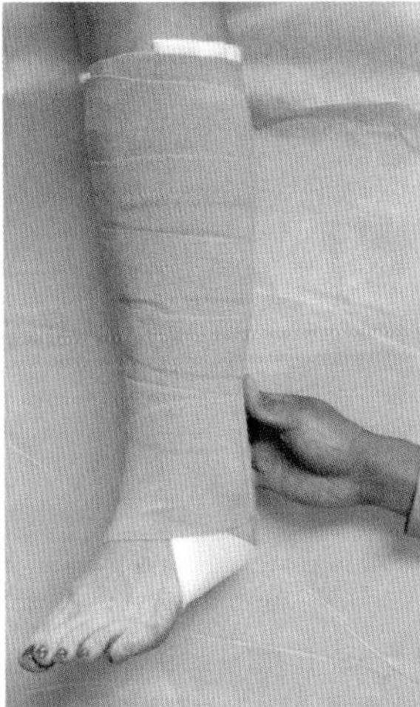

Figure 186-3 Finished sugar-tong splint held in place with a compression wrap.

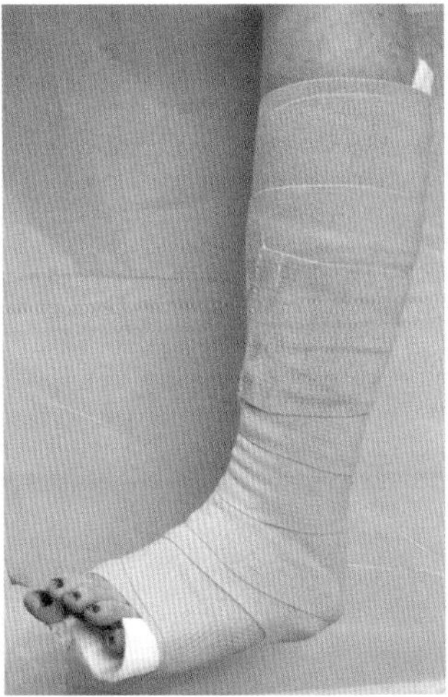

Figure 186-5 Finished posterior splint held in place with a compression wrap.

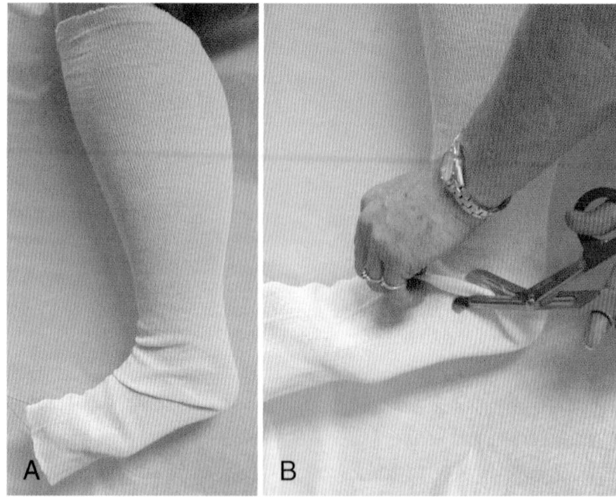

Figure 186-6 **A,** Stockinette is placed on the lower leg from the knee to the toes. **B,** The transverse crease formed at the ankle should be removed.

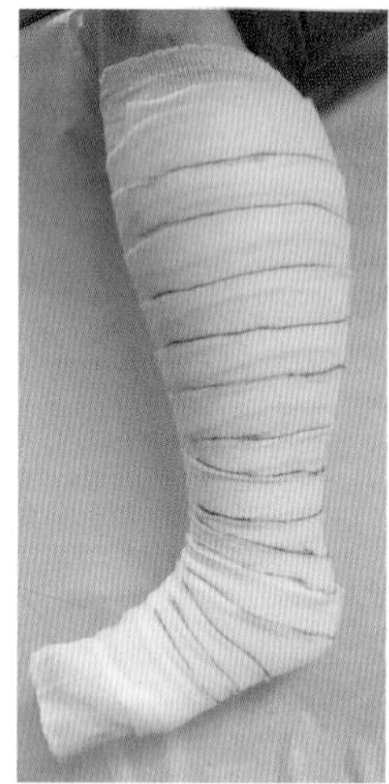

Figure 186-7 Cast padding is applied with 50% overlap on each turn.

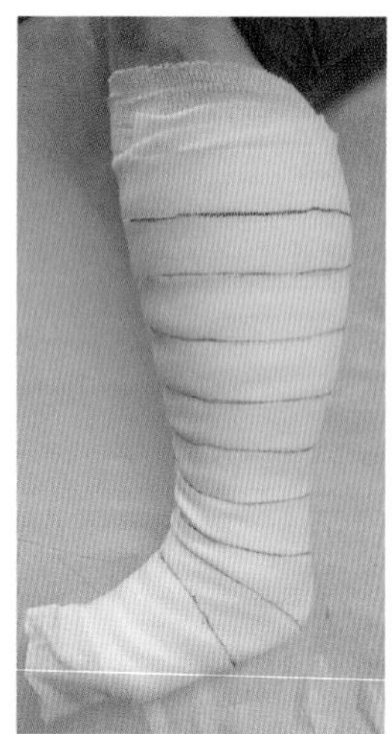

Figure 186-8 Application of cast material with 50% overlap on each turn.

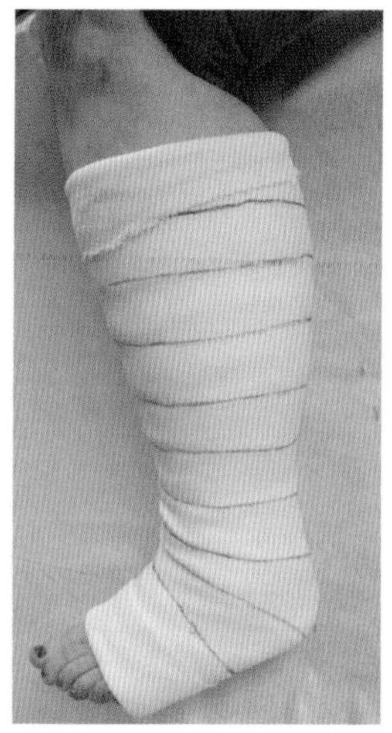

Figure 186-9 After the first roll of cast material is placed, the stockinette is folded back over the ends.

These are shaped like an L and go from the metatarsal heads to the midcalf to provide additional support.

9. Allow 10 minutes for the cast to set, and instruct the patient not to bear weight for at least 24 hours. Provide crutches for ambulation.
10. A walking boot may be fitted to ease ambulation. Again, wait 24 hours for the cast to set before allowing weight bearing. A cast check by the clinician the next day can assure a proper fit.

NOTE: A walking heel is unnecessary for a fiberglass cast.

Cast Removal or Bivalving

1. When splitting the cast, both the medial and lateral sides should be cut.
2. Starting at the top of the cast, make straight cuts that run posterior to the malleoli. Use a finger to stabilize the saw against the cast and to control the depth of the cut.

   NOTE: When using a cast saw, make plunging cuts along the length of the cut. Do not attempt to steadily drag the saw along the length of the cut, as this will cause the blade to heat up, and may burn the patient.
3. Next, make cuts along the medial and lateral sides of the foot that intersect with the initial cuts. Take care to avoid cutting over bony prominences (Fig. 186-11).

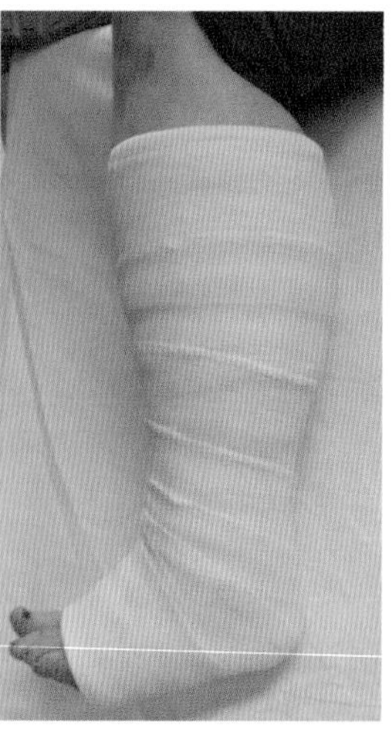

Figure 186-10 Finished short-leg cast.

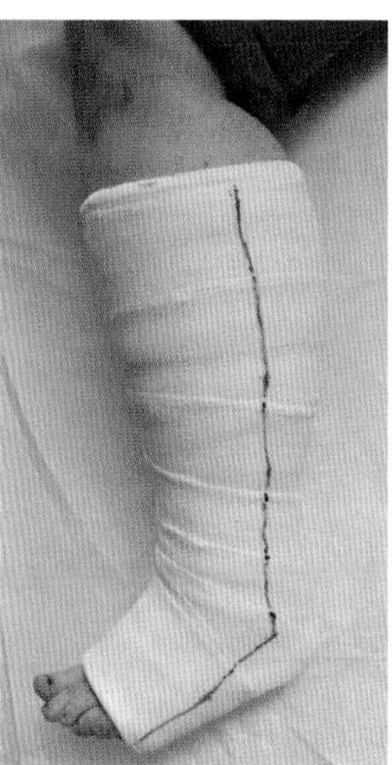

Figure 186-11 When a cast is being removed, medial and lateral cuts are made posterior to the malleoli.

4. After the cuts are complete, a cast spreader is inserted into the cut and spread to widen the cut.
5. The cast padding and stockinette are then cut with blunt-tipped scissors.
6. The cast may then be opened and removed, or wrapped with a compression bandage to serve as a splint.

NOTE: When wrapped with a compression bandage, the resultant splint provides almost as much support as a cast; therefore a clinician should have a low threshold for bivalving a cast to minimize complications. The same saws can be used for both plaster and fiberglass.

Bracing

Ankle bracing may be used prophylactically (to prevent injury), therapeutically, after an acute injury, or after injury to prevent reinjury. Commercial premade braces come in several styles. All styles may be used for any of these indications. Consider patient comfort and stability in choosing a brace. If the patient does not tolerate one style, consider a different one. Available styles include a lace-up, stirrup, or hinged brace.

Taping

Plantar Fasciitis

For this procedure, two pieces of skin tape will be applied followed by two pieces of high-tensile adhesive tape placed over them. The first three pieces of tape are simply applied smoothly and without wrinkles or any tension; the last piece of tape is the only one applied under tension.

SKIN PREPARATION. With the patient sitting on an examination table, skin oils and other debris should be cleansed from the plantar aspect of the affected foot with alcohol. While the alcohol is allowed to dry, palpate the dorsalis pedis pulse. Document the presence or absence of the pulse.

APPLICATION

1. Place the foot in a neutral position (90 degrees), approximately the same position as if the patient were standing on it. From this position, it should be slightly inverted or "turned in" (sole of the foot facing slightly medially).
2. Apply skin tape (white tape) from the ball of the foot (Fig. 186-12A) to the middle of the heel (Fig. 186-12B). The upper edge of the tape will extend slightly up the medial side of the foot, but it should not be higher than one third of the way up to the medial malleolus. In fact, keeping it low on the foot and simply taping around the posterior calcaneus may minimize any friction on the Achilles tendon. Smooth the wrinkles and bubbles; there should be no tension applied to this piece of tape.
3. Locate the navicular bone. It causes the bony projection about 1 inch anterior to the medial malleolus. Apply skin tape (white tape), under no tension, from the heel (Fig. 186-12C) up the medial aspect of the foot to end on top of the foot (Fig. 186-12D). This tape should cover and include the navicular bone and extend past the midline of the dorsum of the foot.
4. Apply tensile tape (brown tape) of the same length in the same location and manner as the first piece of skin tape, simply covering that skin tape. Smooth any wrinkles or bubbles, but do not apply any tension.
5. Apply a second piece of tensile tape (brown tape) over the second piece of skin tape. This tape should be applied under tension, but not so much as to occlude the dorsalis pedis pulse.
6. When the patient stands, he or she should be almost symptom free because the tape bears the weight of the plantar fascia. For severe cases of plantar fasciitis, adding a slight degree of plantar

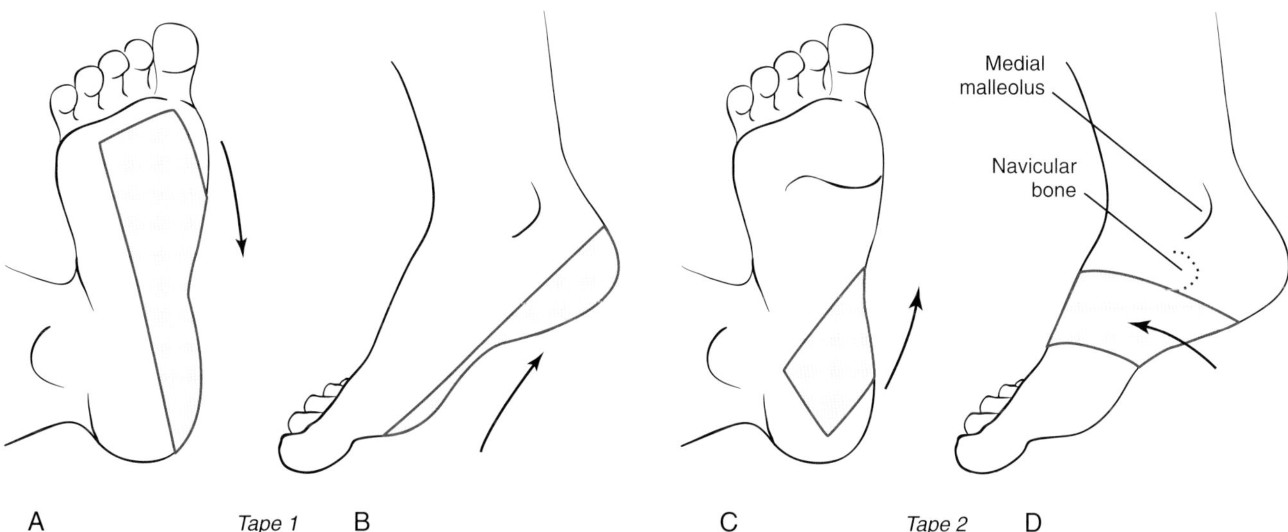

Figure 186-12 Skin tape 1 (white tape) is applied from the ball of the foot (**A**) to the middle of the heel (**B**). Skin tape 2 (white tape) is applied from the heel (**C**) up the medial aspect of the foot to end on top of the foot (**D**). Tensile tape pieces 1 and 2 are applied in the same locations and directions. They should be the same lengths as the skin tape.

flexion to the foot prior to taping, in addition to the slight inversion, will take the weight off the fascia even more.

7. Because it loses strength with weight bearing, the tape should be removed and reapplied daily for 4 to 6 weeks. Outlining the outside edges of the tape with a permanent marker may be helpful for patient education purposes. This outline may help them when reapplying the tape the next day. They may want to outline it each day or use a copy of Figure 186-12 to remind them of how to reapply the tape. When the tape is being changed, the foot should be massaged and put through range-of-motion exercises. Using a commercial adhesive remover will help remove the debris from the prior day's skin tape.
8. For more severe cases, if the patient is symptomatic when bearing weight following taping, gradually more degrees of plantar flexion should be applied with each day of subsequent taping. The goal should be to bear weight with almost no symptoms for 4 to 6 weeks. This allows the fascia to heal.
9. Following resolution of symptoms and completion of the taping regimen, the foot should be rehabilitated aggressively with stretching and range-of-motion exercises.

NOTE: One of the success stories of the physical therapists that first utilized this technique was a woman who had had plantar fasciitis for 7 years!

Ankle

SKIN PREPARATION. Ankle taping provides the greatest support when applied directly against the skin. Daily application, however, will likely cause skin irritation. The use of underwrap material can prevent this. Shave the foot and ankle. Apply a coating of skin preparation, usually benzoin, to protect the skin and provide better adhesion. Avoid the use of skin preparation in patients with a history of sensitivity or allergy to these products (underwrap is recommended in these patients [Fig. 186-13A]). Lubrication or padding may be applied to the skin at sites of potential friction or irritation (Fig. 186-13B).

APPLICATION. Several methods can be used for taping the ankle. The most commonly used is the *closed basket-weave technique*, also known as the Gibney technique, which provides strong tape support (see Fig. 186-13). This extra support may be needed in either recently sprained or chronically weak ankles.

1. An anchor strip is placed around the ankle 5 to 6 inches above the malleoli (Fig. 186-13C).
2. A second anchor strip is placed around the instep.
3. A stirrup strip is placed posterior to the malleoli (Fig. 186-13D). For an inversion injury, hold the foot in *eversion* when applying the stirrup strips. Conversely, hold the foot in *inversion* for an eversion injury.
4. The first horizontal (Gibney) strip is placed under the malleoli, and attached to the foot anchor (Fig. 186-13D).
5. A second stirrup is placed overlapping the first by 50%, followed by a second Gibney strip, also overlapping the first by 50%. A third stirrup and Gibney are then placed in similar fashion (Fig. 186-13E).
6. Placement of the Gibney strips is then continued up the ankle to the anchor strip (Fig. 186-13F).
7. Two or three strips are placed around the arch for added support (Fig. 186-13G).
8. Lastly, heel locks are applied as a final support. Starting high on the instep, wrap the tape posteriorly across the Achilles tendon, downward, hooking the heel. It should then lead under the arch and up the opposite side to finish at the starting point. The heel lock is completed by repeating the wrap in the opposite direction (Fig. 186-13H).

An alternative method, the *open basket-weave technique*, allows for some degree of dorsiflexion and plantar flexion. This technique accommodates swelling and may be used after acute injury. The procedure for the open basket weave is the same as for the closed basket weave, with the notable exception of the Gibney strip placement. The Gibney strips are placed with a gap anteriorly. After the Gibney strips are placed, the gap is closed and the ends are locked by two to four strips running down the instep.

COMPLICATIONS

- *Nerve entrapment:* When casting, compression of the common peroneal nerve at the fibular head may lead to foot drop. Correct placement of the proximal end of the cast is essential.
- *Compartment syndrome:* This may be seen in patients with injuries due to high-velocity forces (e.g., motor vehicle accidents) or by applying the cast before swelling has reached its maximum. If the patient notes any pain caused by the cast, pain out of proportion to the injury, pain not controlled with oral analgesics, or progressively increasing pain, the cast should be bivalved or removed immediately to check compartment pressures (see Chapter 188, Compartment Syndrome Evaluation) and to evaluate for any neurovascular compromise. Treatment of the fracture or maintenance of reduction of the fracture is always a second priority to preserving the blood supply to the soft tissue and bone.

  NOTE: One of the earliest signs of an impending compartment syndrome is pain on resisted plantar flexion of the great toe. Have the patient dorsiflex his or her toe, and if pain radiates into the leg when the clinician attempts to plantarflex the toe, the cast should be bivalved or removed immediately.

- *Loosening of the cast:* Application of a cast when swelling is present may lead to cast looseness when the swelling abates. A loose cast will no longer provide adequate stability and immobilization.
- *Skin necrosis:* Skin necrosis may be caused by pressure over bony prominences. This is best prevented by placing extra padding at potential pressure points (Fig. 186-14). If necessary, a window may be cut in the cast to remove the source of irritation. A window should not be cut, however, in areas that have acute swelling. In that case, a different form of immobilization should be employed.
- *Delayed union, nonunion, atrophic or hypertrophic union, or malunion:* All are possible complications of fractures. Inadequate assessment of the initial radiographs, improper management of the fracture (including incomplete reduction), poor patient adherence and compliance, increased age, medications, and presence of osteopenia or osteoporosis are all possibly causes of these complications. Smoking or taking anti-inflammatory medications delays the healing time and increases the risk for improper fracture healing, especially in weight-bearing bones such as the ankle, foot, or calcaneous. If the patient smokes, the fracture healing time in the ankle is doubled compared to a nonsmoker.
- *Joint stiffness:* Patients often suffer from joint stiffness as a result of immobilization. This is best prevented by not immobilizing joints any longer than what is needed for fracture healing.

POSTPROCEDURE PATIENT EDUCATION

In an acute injury, after immobilization the patient should elevate the leg for 48 to 72 hours to prevent swelling. Ice can be used, in a sealed container, over the cast or splint to help alleviate pain. If a non-waterproof cast or splint is used, every effort should be made to keep the cast or splint dry. Patients should remove or cover it when bathing. If a non-waterproof cast or splint does become wet, patients may dry it with a hair dryer set on the cool setting.

Nothing should be inserted between a cast and the skin. This may cause abrasions and undetected infections. With a cast, patients should call immediately if they notice pain, fever, tightness or irritation, numbness, or discolored or cool toes.

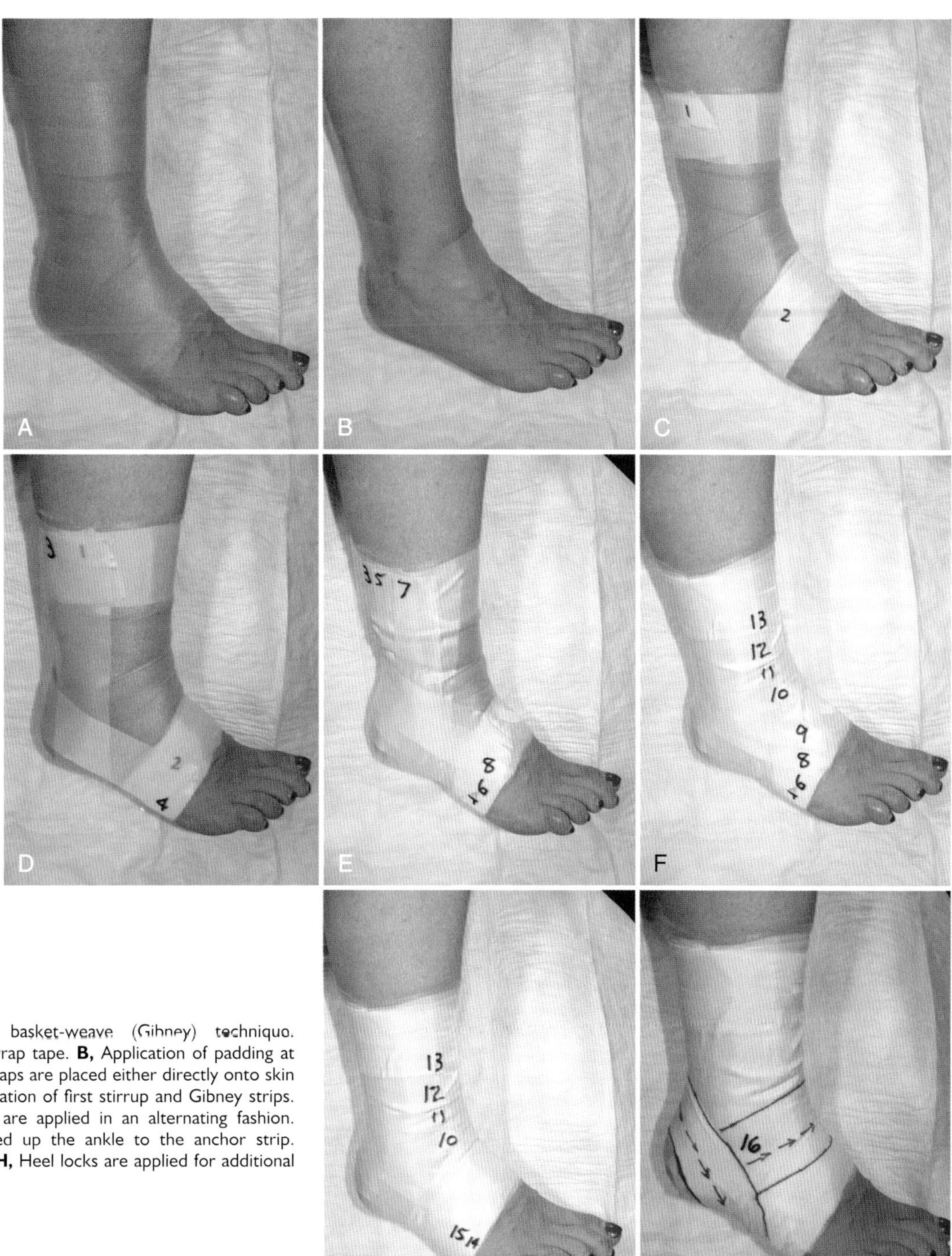

Figure 186-13 Closed basket-weave (Gibney) technique. **A,** Application of thin underwrap tape. **B,** Application of padding at pressure points. **C,** Anchor straps are placed either directly onto skin or over underwrap. **D,** Application of first stirrup and Gibney strips. **E,** Stirrup and Gibney strips are applied in an alternating fashion. **F,** Gibney strips are continued up the ankle to the anchor strip. **G,** Application of arch strips. **H,** Heel locks are applied for additional support.

CPT/Billing Codes

Fracture Management

Fracture care CPT codes include initial management of fractures, along with initial splint or cast application. These codes include subsequent routine cast care and removal.

Codes for closed treatment *without* manipulation include the following:

27750 Tibial shaft fracture
27760 Medial malleolus fracture
27780 Proximal fibula or fibular shaft fracture
27786 Distal fibular (lateral malleolus) fracture

Codes for closed treatment *with* manipulation include the following:

27752 Tibial shaft fracture
27762 Medial malleolus fracture
27781 Proximal fibula or fibular shaft fracture
27788 Distal fibular (lateral malleolus) fracture

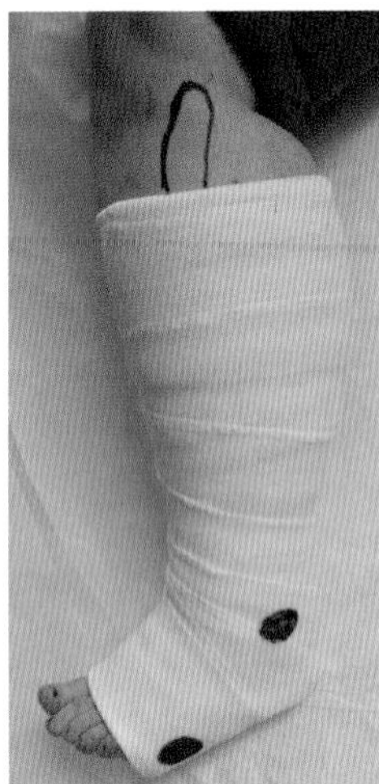

Figure 186-14 Common locations for pressure sores are noted on the cast. Note the outline of the fibular head above the cast. This is the site of possible peroneal nerve entrapment.

Cast or Splint Application

The following codes can be used when not part of comprehensive fracture management, or when used for soft tissue injuries. If a cast needs replacement, these codes can also be used.

29405 Application of short-leg cast (below knee to toes)
29425 Walking or ambulatory type
29440 Adding walker to previously applied cast
29515 Application of short-leg splint (calf to foot)
29540 Strapping; ankle and/or foot
29700 Removal or bivalving of short-leg cast applied by another physician
29705 Removal or bivalving of full-leg cast applied by another physician
29730 Windowing of cast applied by another physician
29740 Wedging of cast applied by another physician
29799 Unlisted procedure, casting or strapping

Supplies

A4565 Sling
A4570 Splint material
A4580 Plaster cast supplies
A4590 Special cast supplies (fiberglass)
99070 Miscellaneous supplies/materials provided over and above other services rendered

ICD-9-CM Diagnostic Codes

728.71 Plantar fasciitis
733.94 Stress fracture of the metatarsal (march)
823.00 Tibial fracture, upper end, closed
823.01 Fibular fracture, upper end, closed
823.02 Tibial and fibular fracture, upper end, closed
823.20 Tibial shaft fracture, closed
823.21 Fibular shaft fracture, closed
823.22 Tibial and fibular shaft fracture, closed
824.0 Medial malleolus fracture, closed
824.2 Lateral malleolus fracture, closed
824.4 Bimalleolar fracture, closed
824.6 Trimalleolar fracture, closed
825.0 Calcaneal fracture, closed
825.21 Talar fracture, closed
825.22 Navicular fracture of foot, closed
825.23 Cuboid fracture, closed
825.24 Cuneiform fracture, closed
825.25 Metatarsal fracture, closed
845.0 Ankle sprain and strain

Suppliers

Full contact information is available online at www.expertconsult.com.

Braces
Swede-O, Inc.
Casting and splinting materials
Johnson & Johnson Professional, Inc. (extra-fast setting casting splints available)
3M Health Care
Casting and splinting materials, accessories, braces
M-Pact (now owned by Jobst/BSN Medical)
Dressing retention sheet (skin tape)
Hypafix
Smith & Nephew, Inc.
High-tensile strength adhesive tape
FLA Orthopedics
Jobst/BSN Medical
Leukotape-P (this brand was specifically developed for use with McConnell taping)
Nocturnal splints
AliMed, Inc.
Freedom PF Night Splint II
Splints and braces
Aircast, Inc., and DonJoy are now owned by DJO

BIBLIOGRAPHY

Batt ME, Tanji JL, Skattum N: Plantar fasciitis, a prospective randomized clinical trial of the tension night splint. Clin J Sport Med 6:158–162, 1996.

Black WS, Becker JA: Common forearm fractures in adults. Am Fam Physician 80:1096–1102, 2009.

Boyd AS, Benjamin HJ, Asplund C: Principles of casting and splinting. Am Fam Physician 79:16–22, 23–24, 2009.

Eiff MP, Hatch RL, Calmbach WL: Fracture Management for Primary Care, 2nd ed. Philadelphia, Elsevier, 2003.

Hutson AM, Rovinsky D: Casts and splints. In Reichman EF, Simon RR (eds): Emergency Medicine Procedures. New York, McGraw-Hill, 2004.

Mellion MB, Walsh WM, Madden C, et al: The Team Physician's Handbook, 3rd ed. Philadelphia, Hanley & Belfus, 2001.

Petrizzi MJ, Petrizzi MG (eds): Casting and splinting of soft-tissue injuries and fractures, vol. 5, no. 3. In: The Clinics Atlas of Office Procedures. Philadelphia, Saunders, 2002.

Petrizzi MJ, Petrizzi MG, Miller A: A "three-way" ankle splint for acute ankle injury. Phys Sportsmed 28:99–100, 2000.

Petrizzi MJ, Petrizzi MG, Roos RJ: Making a tension night splint for plantar fasciitis. Phys Sportsmed 26:113–114, 1998.

Pfeffer G, Bacchetti P, Deland J, et al: Comparison of custom and prefabricated orthoses in the initial treatment of proximal plantar fasciitis. Foot Ankle Int 20:214–221, 1999.

Prentice W, Arnheim D: Principles of Athletic Training, 9th ed. Madison, WI, Brown & Benchmark, 1996.

Shahady E (ed): Primary Care of Musculoskeletal Problems in the Outpatient Setting. Cambridge, Blackwell Science, 2006.

Strayer SM, Reece SG, Petrizzi MJ: Fractures of the proximal fifth metatarsal. Am Fam Physician 59:2516–2522, 1999.

CHAPTER 187

Cast Immobilization and Upper Extremity Splinting

Scott W. Eathorne • Todd M. Sheperd

Cast immobilization is a technique used to treat a variety of medical conditions encountered by the primary care clinician. Although newer technologies have led to an evolution in casting materials, the general principles of this valuable technique have stood the test of time. By having knowledge of the materials available and an understanding of the indications and fundamental precepts of cast immobilization, and by developing the necessary manual or dexterity skills, the primary care clinician can easily treat the patient who has an injury amenable to such therapy.

In the upper extremity, splints made from casting material (e.g., thumb spica, sugar-tong) are occasionally used in place of circumferential casts. Some of these will be covered in this chapter. Please note that splinting and casting in the lower extremity are also discussed in Chapter 186, Ankle and Foot Splinting, Casting, and Taping.

History

The use of immobilization to treat acute fractures dates back to the era of the Fifth Dynasty of Egypt (2498–2345 BCE) when bark was used to splint fractures of the forearm. Gypsum, from which plaster of Paris is derived, was initially used around the sixteenth century in parts of the Ottoman Empire. With the development, in 1927, of the hard-coated plaster of Paris rolls, a binder was incorporated that improved the adherence of the plaster to the cloth. Since then, various additives have been used to either accelerate (salicylic acid, zinc, or aluminum) or slow down (gums or glue) the setting process.

Currently, fiberglass is the most common material used in casting. It has the advantages of being stronger and lighter (approximately two to three times stronger for any given thickness) than plaster, and it creates less heat during application. However, it is more difficult to mold. The cost of fiberglass continues to be more than that of plaster, but in recent years this difference has decreased significantly. In addition to newer casting materials, the development of synthetic padding (Gore-Tex) has allowed most casts to survive significant exposure to water without damage.

Indications

- A variety of stable, acute fractures
- Dislocations that have been reduced
- Injuries to the soft tissues, including muscle, tendon, and ligament
- Congenital and acquired deformities (e.g., correction of talipes equinovarus, congenital clubfoot)
- For the stabilization and protection of vascular, tendon, and nerve injuries following surgical repair

The most common diagnosis for which the primary care clinician uses cast immobilization is the stable, nondisplaced, closed fracture of a long bone. The primary care clinician often treats fractures involving the radius or ulna, phalanges, metacarpals, metatarsals, and malleoli. (See Chapter 190, Fracture Care.) Other conditions include certain grade III ligament sprains (e.g., ankle), Achilles tendon disruptions, and tendonitis refractory to other forms of therapy.

Cast Application Equipment

- Rubber gloves
- Gown and shoe covers for the clinician
- Patient towels or drapes
- Stockinette (2-, 3-, and 4-inch widths)
- Felt padding, soft cotton (e.g., Webril), or synthetic (e.g., polyester) bandages (2-, 3-, 4-, and 6-inch widths)
- Synthetic waterproof cast liner (e.g., Gore Procel, Scotchcast Wet or Dry, Delta-Dry, Waterpruf)
- Rubber heels (walking cast)
- Cast removal protective strip (e.g., De-Flex) to eventually protect skin from cast saw
- Casting material (Fig. 187-1)
  - Plaster (e.g., plaster of Paris, avoid thicker than 10 ply, which can cause thermal injury to patient)
  - Synthetic (e.g., fiberglass)
- Water source (if using plaster, should have traps in drains and water temperature less than 24° C/75° F)
- Elastic (e.g., Ace) bandages (2-, 3-, 4-, and 6-inch widths)
- Slings
- Scissors
- Chinese finger traps
- Leg stand

When water is added to the plaster, the water molecules are incorporated into the calcium sulfate hemihydrate (i.e., plaster of Paris) molecules with a resultant exothermic reaction. The powdery white substance is converted into a solid, rock-hard material, and a significant amount of heat is generated. A curing process then follows over the next few days, characterized by continued water evaporation; this process is accelerated by low humidity, high ambient temperature, and increased air circulation.

Synthetic materials require immersion in water to activate the curing process, with generally less heat generated than plaster. *Attention to water temperature in this process is especially important,* because water that is too warm (>24° C/75° F) can lead to rapid curing and significant difficulty in application. Water at higher than these temperatures or plaster of Paris thicker than 10 ply can also result in thermal injury to the patient.

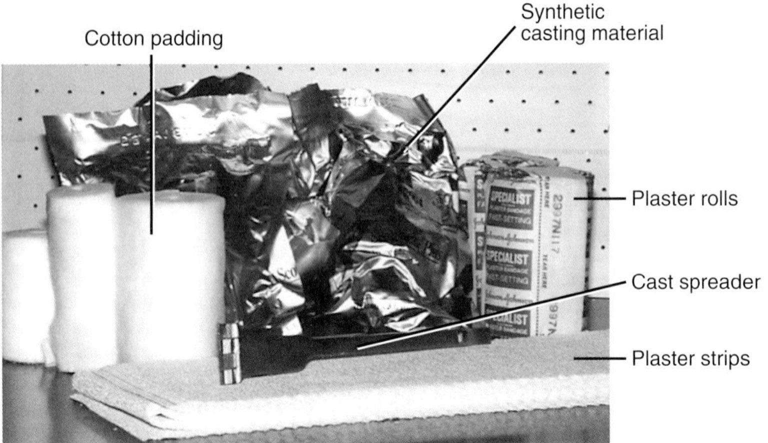

Figure 187-1 Materials needed for casting: cotton padding, synthetic casting material or plaster rolls, cast spreader, cast cutter (not shown), and plaster strips.

Advantages of plaster casts over fiberglass include low cost, ease of molding, long shelf-life, and low allergenicity. Synthetic cast material is more expensive, but this margin has narrowed in the years since fiberglass was introduced. Fiberglass has also improved in its ease of application and continues to be superior in strength, durability, weight, water resistance, and drying time. Both materials are available in multiple sizes, ranging from 2 to 5 inches in width for general, circumferential cast use.

Ideally, a single room or area in the clinic, emergency department, or hospital should be dedicated to the application of casts and splints. This room should have a plaster trap in the sink, and all materials should be easily available. Rubber gloves, gowns, shoe covers, and towels or drapes should be available to protect both the clinician and patient from the inevitable exposure to casting materials. An easily cleaned examination table, stool, and leg stand can greatly facilitate the process of cast application.

Common Cast Types

See Chapter 190, Fracture Care.

Short-Arm Casts

Short-arm casts are generally indicated in the treatment of stable sprains of the wrist, as well as some stable fractures of the distal radius, ulna, carpal bones, and metacarpals. Clinicians performing cast immobilization should be aware of those fractures requiring orthopedic evaluation for possible open reduction and internal fixation. Materials required for short-arm cast applications include a 3-inch stockinette, two rolls of 3-inch cast padding (the waterproof liner replaces the need for both stockinette and padding), and two to four rolls of either 3- or 4-inch plaster bandage (or 2- or 3-inch fiberglass bandage). In general, adult males will require 4-inch plaster (3-inch fiberglass) and children will require 3-inch plaster (2-inch fiberglass). Adolescents and females may require either size depending on preference and size of extremity. The patient should be supine or seated, with the arm abducted 90 degrees and the elbow flexed 90 degrees. The wrist should be slightly extended and in a position of function (Fig. 187-2). Chinese finger traps attached to the patient and suspended from above can support the arm and assist in maintaining the position of function. The cast extends from the proximal forearm (approximately 1 inch distal to the flexion crease of the elbow) distally to include the palm and dorsum of the hand, completely covering the forearm. The metacarpal-phalangeal (MCP) joints are allowed complete motion, with the cast stopping just proximal to the distal palmar crease (Fig. 187-3). Extra padding should be applied over the ulnar styloid. Short-arm casts only partially immobilize the wrist joint and allow movement of the thumb, including opposition with the fifth digit. In addition, they allow for supination and pronation to occur because the elbow is not included. An adaptation of the short-arm cast is the *short-arm thumb spica,* in which the thumb is included to the level of the interphalangeal (IP) joint (Fig. 187-4). This type of cast may be used for injuries to the scaphoid, trapezium, or first metacarpal, or for any injury requiring wrist and thumb immobilization.

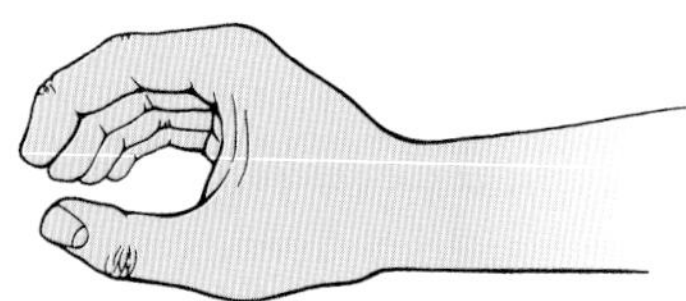

Figure 187-2 Position of the wrist in the application of arm casts.

Long-Arm Casts

Long-arm casts can be fashioned by extending a short-arm cast proximally, with the elbow maintained in 90 degrees of flexion. The padding and plaster should be extended to the proximal humerus, ending 2 to 3 fingerbreadths below the axilla. Be careful to provide extra padding over the pressure point at the olecranon. Plenty of padding should also be placed over the proximal end of the cast or the patient will complain of the sharp edges.

Short-Leg Casts

Short-leg casts are generally indicated in the treatment of some stable ligamentous injuries to the ankle, and stable fractures of the ankle, calcaneus, tarsals, and metatarsals. Materials include a 4-inch stockinette and three rolls of 4-inch cast padding (or waterproof liner). Use of fiberglass is generally preferred in these casts because of its increased durability. With fiberglass casts, three rolls of 4-inch fiberglass bandage are generally needed. An extra reinforcing strip of heavy-duty fiberglass can also be used posteriorly along

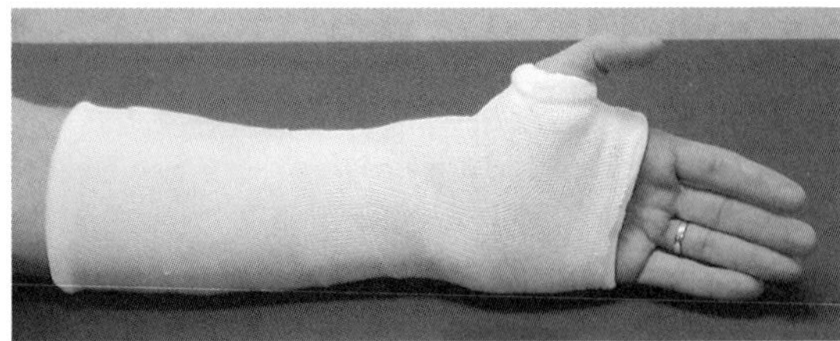

Figure 187-3 Appearance of a completed short-arm cast. Note that the thumb and fingers are free to move.

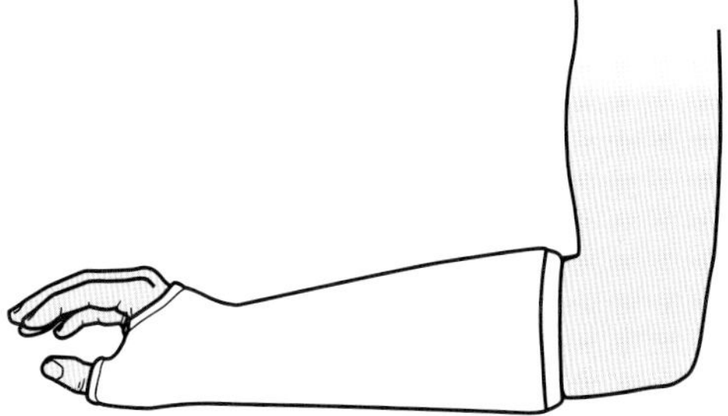

Figure 187-4 Short-arm cast with thumb spica.

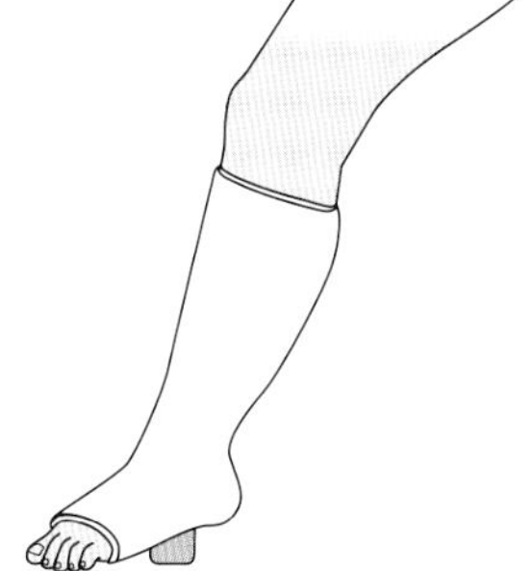

Figure 187-6 Short-leg cast with walker.

the bottom of the foot up the back of the leg. For plaster casts (used less often), materials vary widely based on personal preference, but they usually include two to three rolls of 6-inch plaster bandage and an adequate number of plaster splint strips (again for posterior and foot reinforcement), with size based on patient limb size. Application of the short-leg cast is achieved either in the sitting position, with the leg hanging over the table, or prone, with the knee flexed to 90 degrees to help relax the gastrocnemius muscle. The ankle is usually held at a 90-degree angle to the leg, but this angle may be altered depending on the type of injury. A foot-stand or assistant can provide support to the foot. The cast extends from just below the knee joint, usually including the fibular head, distally to the base of the toes, including the metatarsal heads (Fig. 187-5). Again, the ankle joint is only partially immobilized, since the cast does not involve both the joint above and below. For *walking short-leg casts* (Fig. 187-6), a posterior reinforcing strip is placed and molded after application of the second roll of fiberglass bandage and before placing the final roll. The walker can be applied the same day or at a later time. If applied initially, patients have a tendency to walk on it before the primary cast is dry enough, leading to breakdown of the cast.

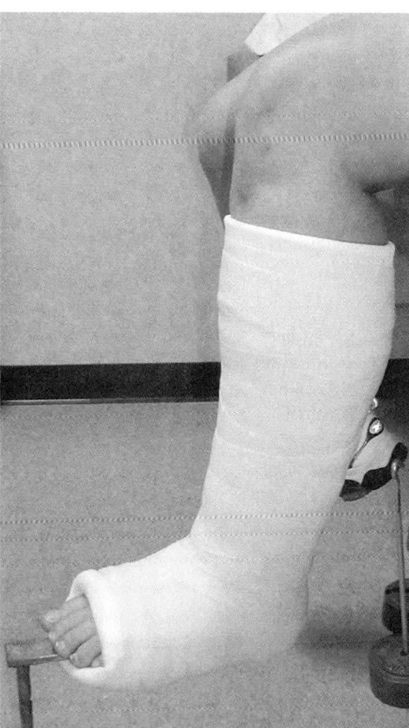

Figure 187-5 Appearance of a completed short-leg cast. The cast should hold the ankle at 90 degrees. In addition, the proximal end of the cast should be far enough from the knee to eliminate the possibility of skin irritation with knee flexion.

Long-Leg Casts

Long-leg casts can be fashioned by extending a short-leg cast proximally up to the groin. The padding and plaster should be extended to the proximal femur, ending several fingerbreadths below the groin. The knee is in slight flexion and the foot is at 90 degrees. There should be no internal or external rotation of the foot. The knee should be supported in this slight flexion while the cast sets. To maintain strength, make sure there is adequate overlap of the casting material when extending proximally from the knee. In addition, make sure extra padding is provided over the pressure point at the anterior patella. Plenty of padding should also be placed over the proximal end of the cast or the patient will complain of the sharp edges.

Other Casts and Splints

Other types of common casts and splints are shown in Figure 187-7. Even with splints, where casting materials do not totally surround the extremity, there is generally a layer of stockinette around the entire area followed by the padding, then the casting material. The casting material is held in place with an Ace wrap or similar material.

Preprocedure Patient Preparation

After diagnosing an injury requiring cast immobilization, and before application of the cast, the indications for casting, estimated duration of immobilization, and potential impact on activities of daily living should be discussed with the patient. Typically, discussion of common problems and potential complications from casting occur following application. Online references for patient education handouts can be found at the end of this chapter (www.expertconsult.com). If there is a chance that the cost of synthetic material will not be covered by the patient's insurance, this should be discussed prior to its use.

Technique

Casts are generally applied to immobilize and protect an injured part of the body in a position that will facilitate healing. Three-point contact and stabilization are necessary to maintain most closed reductions. The following simple principles direct the fundamentals of cast immobilization. First, to best approach complete immobilization, *a cast must conform precisely to the anatomy of the region being immobilized*. Failure to accomplish this can lead to unacceptable movement of the injured area, leading to potential loss of reduction, malalignment of a reduced dislocation, or persistent inflammation in a refractory tendonitis. Second, *effective immobilization is achieved only by including a sufficient amount of injured area in the cast*. Ideally, this is accomplished by including the joint above and below the area of injury. However, exceptions to this rule are made based on the nature of the injury. Achieving adequate immobilization requires attention to these fundamentals before application of the cast. If

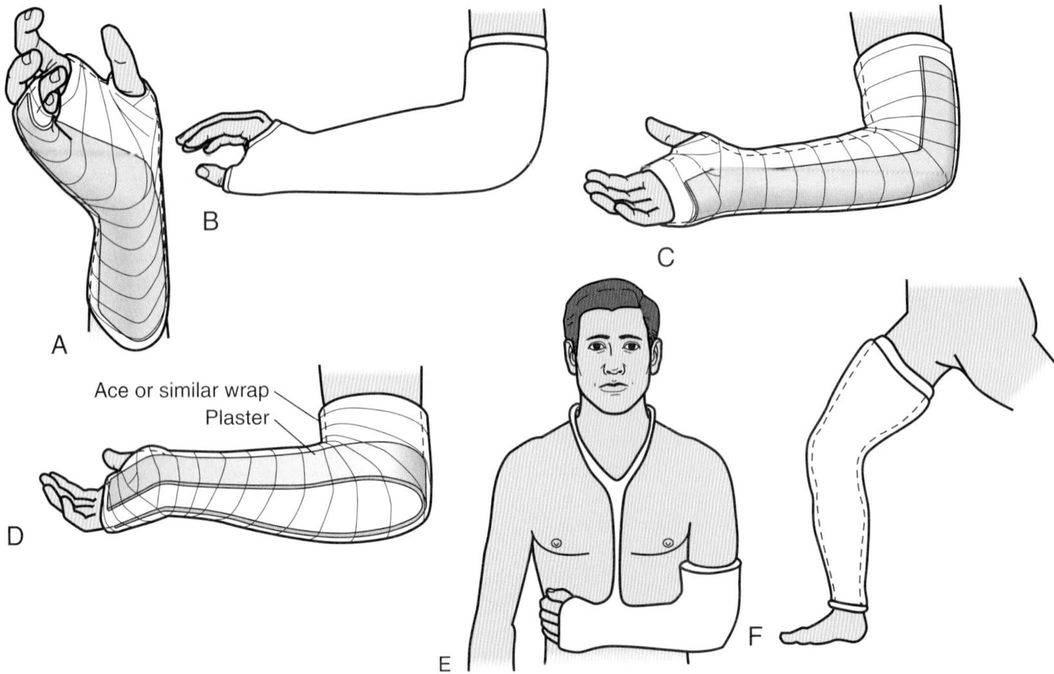

Figure 187-7 Common casts and splints. **A,** Ulnar gutter splint is used to immobilize fractures and serious soft tissue injuries of the ring and little fingers and fractures of the neck, shaft, and base of the fourth and fifth metacarpals. **B,** Long-arm cast with thumb spica is used to treat navicular fractures, complicated Colles' fractures, and nondisplaced radius and ulnar shaft fractures. **C,** Long-arm posterior splint is used for severe lateral epicondylitis and elbow dislocation. **D,** Sugar-tong splint is used for fractures of the distal radius and ulna. **E,** Long-arm hanging cast. **F,** Long-leg cast is used for fractures such as patellar, uncomplicated tibial plateau, and minimally displaced tibial/fibular shaft fractures as well as for medial collateral ligament or lateral collateral ligament avulsion and nondisplaced osteochondritis.

these goals cannot be met, the injury may best be served by another means of immobilization.

1. Before application of any casting materials, cleanse, dry, and thoroughly inspect the skin to be included in the cast for any lesions such as lacerations, abrasions, and ulcers. If present, they should be noted and, if significant, may contraindicate inclusion in the cast or may require special "window" techniques. Depending on the acuity of the injury and degree of soft tissue swelling, immobilization using circumferential casting may be contraindicated. In this situation, the injury may require the use of a splint for immobilization until the swelling has diminished.
2. After this assessment is completed, position the patient so that the injured area can be held most easily in the desired position throughout the application process. This positioning often requires the use of an assistant or assistive device (e.g., leg stand, finger traps).

NOTE: Cast application is performed in a step-wise manner, and development of a systematic approach will help ensure consistency and minimize the potential for error.

3. The *first layer* generally applied in casting is the *stockinette*. A poorly fitting stockinette can contribute to skin breakdown, so it must be applied carefully. Use a 3-inch-wide stockinette for adult arm casts, and a 4-inch-wide for legs, with exceptions based on the extremes of limb size. The material should go well past the toes or fingertips and 4 to 5 inches above the elbow or knee (Fig. 187-8A). (Cutting the stockinette too short is a common problem among those learning the procedure.) Some of this "extra" material is ultimately incorporated into the cast or, eventually, cut off.
4. Remove all transverse wrinkles; they become pressure points after cast application and can cause skin breakdown. This can be achieved by cutting the redundant material, which is usually at a joint. Figure 187-8B shows a short-leg stockinette that has been cut and then overlaid at the anterior ankle to reduce wrinkles.
5. After ensuring that the stockinette overlying the area is smooth and free of wrinkles, apply the second layer. The *second layer consists of soft cast padding material (Webril)*, which comes in rolls and is applied in a circular manner. Start at one end (usually distal) and work toward the other; on the first turn around the extremity, roll the padding over itself to create an anchor. After this, each subsequent turn will overlap itself by 50% (Fig. 187-9).

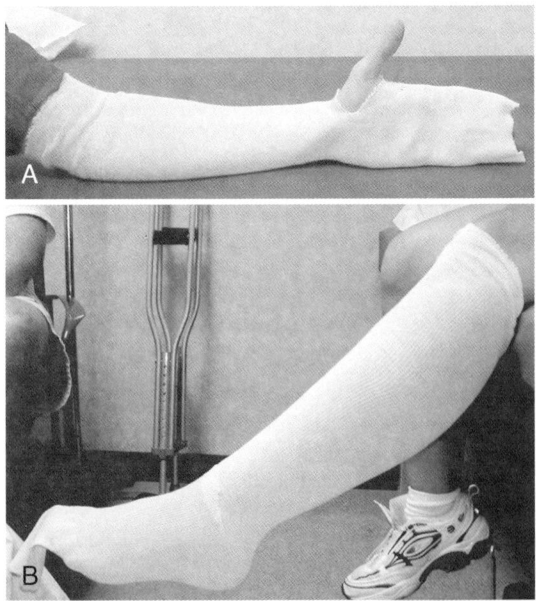

Figure 187-8 **A,** Demonstration of proper stockinette application for short-arm cast. Enough excess is present to allow a cuff to be created below the final layer of casting material. **B,** Application of stockinette for a short-leg cast, demonstrating the technique to eliminate transverse wrinkle at ankle. Note the length of the stockinette for a short-leg cast.

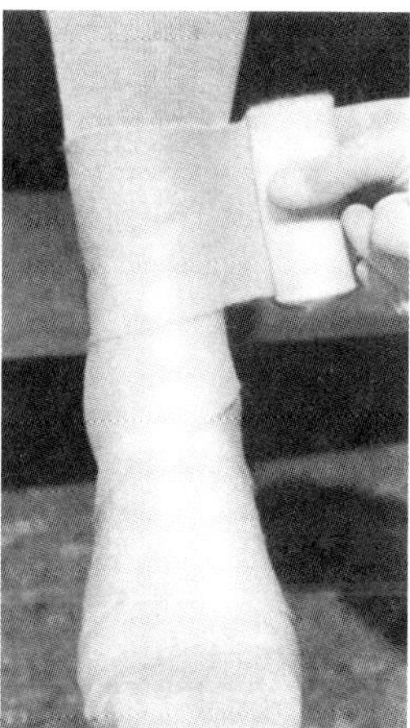

Figure 187-9 Application of soft cast padding. Beginning at one end, cast padding is added while overlapping each turn by half. (From Mercier LR: Practical Orthopedics, 5th ed. St Louis, Mosby, 2000.)

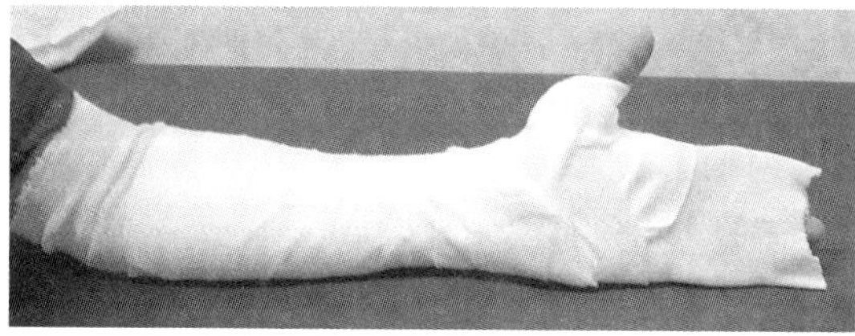

Figure 187-10 Short-arm cast after application of cast padding and before addition of casting material.

Two layers of cast padding can be applied, but care should be taken not to pad too much because this can lead to a loose cast. The goal with padding, as with the stockinette, is to avoid wrinkles, which may contribute to pressure points. Stretch or tear the advancing edge that is to encircle a larger portion of the extremity in order to avoid wrinkles. Keeping in mind the local anatomy, apply additional padding to bony prominences and likely areas of increased local pressure (e.g., flexion creases; fulcrum points such as the proximal anterior tibia where short-leg walking casts may rub; and common areas of nerve compression or pressure necrosis, such as over the proximal fibula). Felt pads appropriately fashioned can prevent common complications and improve comfort. Figure 187-10 shows a short-arm cast after cast padding application and before application of cast material. Although padding is important, excess padding over bony prominences can also lead to excess pressure; therefore, it should be avoided.

6. When using the *waterproof cast liner*, it is applied in a manner identical to the application of cast padding and eliminates the need for stockinette use. By using this material, only two total layers of material are needed (cast liner and cast material). To apply, start unrolling onto the extremity from either the distal or proximal end. Remember to keep the adhesive side of the cast liner *away* from the patient's skin. The material is applied until the opposite end of the desired endpoint is reached and is extended 4 to 5 cm beyond the desired length of the cast. The excess will allow the ends to be folded back at the margins before casting material application (Fig. 187-11A). Apply additional material to bony prominences to prevent pressure-related complications. Unlike traditional cast padding, the waterproof cast liner must be cut to achieve proper sizing because it does not tear (Fig. 187-11B and C). In addition, because fewer layers of padding are used, waterproof cast liner requires the use of a protective strip below the cast material (Fig. 187-11D) to protect from the cast saw.
7. A protective strip can be placed under any cast to minimize the risk of thermal injury or damage to the skin with later use of the cast saw to remove the cast. Many experts will extend the strip an inch or so beyond the anticipated margin of the cast, far enough to enfold it into the end or cuff of the cast, right over the stockinette. This simplifies locating and following the strip

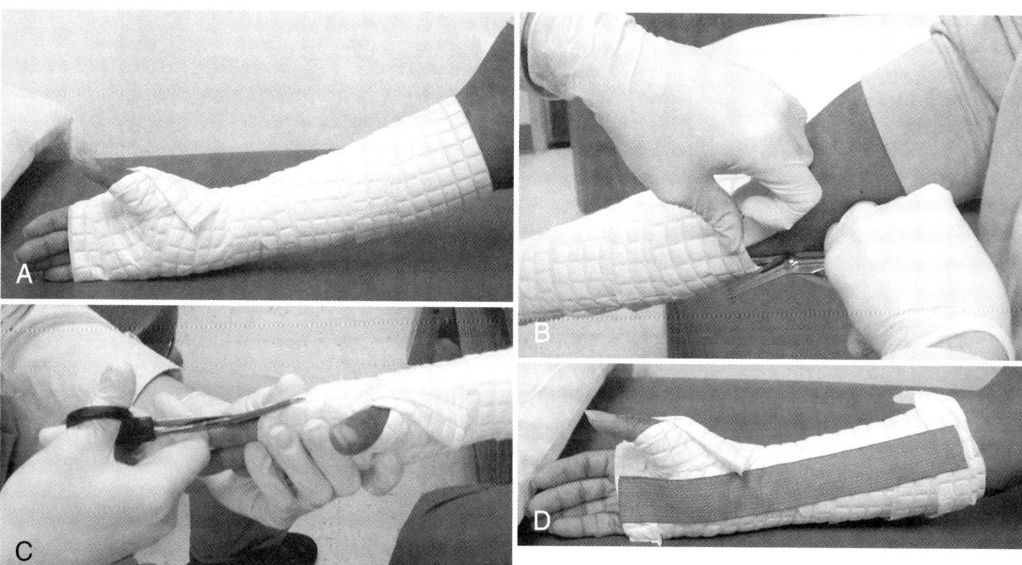

Figure 187-11 Gore-Tex application. **A,** Gore-Tex liner applied 4 to 5 cm beyond desired cast length. **B** and **C,** Using scissors to cut material and allow liner to be folded. **D,** Protective strip applied before application of cast materials. Extend the strip beyond the anticipated margin of the casting material.

when later using the cast saw, especially if the strip is extended into both the proximal and distal cuffs of the cast. The resistance of the strip to being cut by the saw is compromised over hard, bony surfaces; therefore, use over bony prominences should be avoided.

8. Apply the *third layer* (or second layer if cast liner was used), *which consists of the cast material itself*. The type of material used (plaster versus synthetic) dictates how the next step will be completed. Although application is quite similar, a few significant differences are worth noting. When using *plaster-impregnated rolls*, place each roll individually in water at room temperature and submerse until the bubbling stops. Cold water slows the setting process, whereas warmer water speeds it. A faster setting may be desirable when immobilizing a recently reduced dislocation. After removing from the water, gently squeeze and twist the roll to eliminate excess water and begin the application (Fig. 187-12A). Placement of the plaster rolls should follow the direction of the cast padding and should be applied in a similar manner. The first turn has 100% overlap, and each additional turn overlaps approximately 50%. To avoid transverse wrinkles, plaster rolls can be tucked (folded over) at the edges when redundancy occurs and smoothed with the palm of the hand (Fig. 187-12B and C). Avoid stretching and applying undue pressure with each turn. *Apply four to six layers* of plaster evenly, with extra reinforcement in areas under increased stress. Apply each roll in a consistent manner, either distal-to-proximal or proximal-to-distal, with the length of the area to be immobilized covered with each layer. Covering only a portion of the extremity with one roll and overlapping with the next roll may lead to inherent weakness and future difficulties with the cast. *Before placing the final layers, the ends of the stockinette should be folded over onto the initial layers*. Reinforcing strips or cast cushions, if used, should be added now (depending on the type of cast being applied; Fig. 187-12D).

9. Place the final layers of cast material and smooth the cast, using both hands. Make sure that it conforms to the contours of the local anatomy by using the palms to apply pressure to the cast (Fig. 187-12E). If the fingers are used to conform (or mold) the cast, subtle pressure areas under the cast may be created. After the cast is applied, plaster should never touch the patient's skin directly. Positioning of the injured area while casting is critical. The ankle joint should be at 90 degrees and the hand and wrist in a position of function (slightly extended, relaxed). This position should be closely rechecked before hardening of the cast. See Figure 187-2 for an example of the position of function used with short-arm casts. With certain fractures or tendon injuries, these positions may be altered to improve tissue healing. The provider should be aware of these needs before the application of the cast.

Application of *synthetic materials* follows a similar course, with a few noteworthy exceptions. Water used to activate the curing process should be kept no warmer than room temperature to avoid too rapid setting. Normally, setting occurs in 2 to 3 minutes. Because of the flexibility of the synthetic bandage rolls, tucking of edges is not necessary to avoid transverse creases. However, care must still be taken to avoid pulling the cast material too tight. Molding should occur between each layer, with most synthetic casts requiring only two to three layers of cast material, depending on the area immobilized (Fig. 187-13A to C). Strips of heavy-duty, reinforcing material are available and frequently applied (e.g., to the posterior aspect of a short-leg walking cast) to increase durability (Fig. 187-13D). After the final check of position, synthetic casts may require trimming of rough edges. If not trimmed, these edges may catch on clothing or injure the skin or soft tissue under the cast. Trimming can be done with a file, sandpaper, cast saw, or scissors, and it is done with less difficulty when the cast is still soft (Fig. 187-13E).

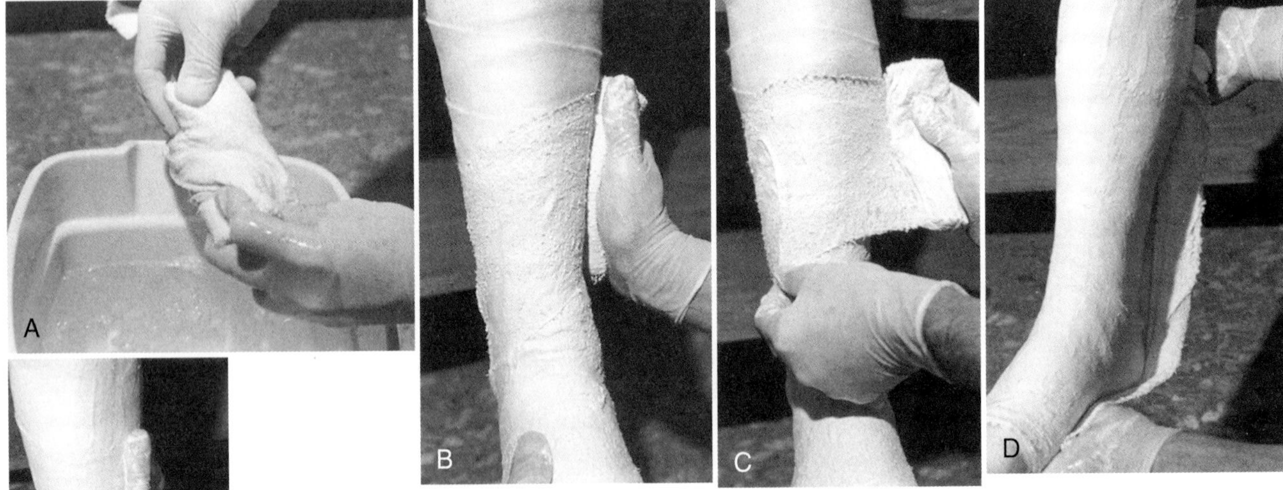

Figure 187-12 Application of plaster cast material. **A,** The plaster roll is removed from the water after the bubbles cease. The ends are pinched shut, and the roll is gently squeezed to expel excess water. Less water or excess wringing causes faster drying. **B,** Beginning at one end, the plaster is pushed onto the extremity by using gentle pressure from the thenar eminence against the middle of the roll. The roll should remain in contact with the limb and is usually not lifted from it. Additional rolls are started where the previous one ends. The roll is applied so that the opening side faces the operator and not the extremity. **C,** Tucks or pleats are taken as often as necessary to guide the roll and to accommodate any tapering of the limb. The stockinette is folded back and incorporated into the cast. **D,** Reinforcing splints five to ten layers thick applied to the sides or back add a great deal of strength without adding much weight. They are particularly useful at the ankle, where the cast is weakest and breakage is most common. **E,** The cast is molded with the flat surface of the hands, if necessary, and trimmed, especially at the small toe. (From Mercier LR: Practical Orthopedics, 5th ed. St Louis, Mosby, 2000.)

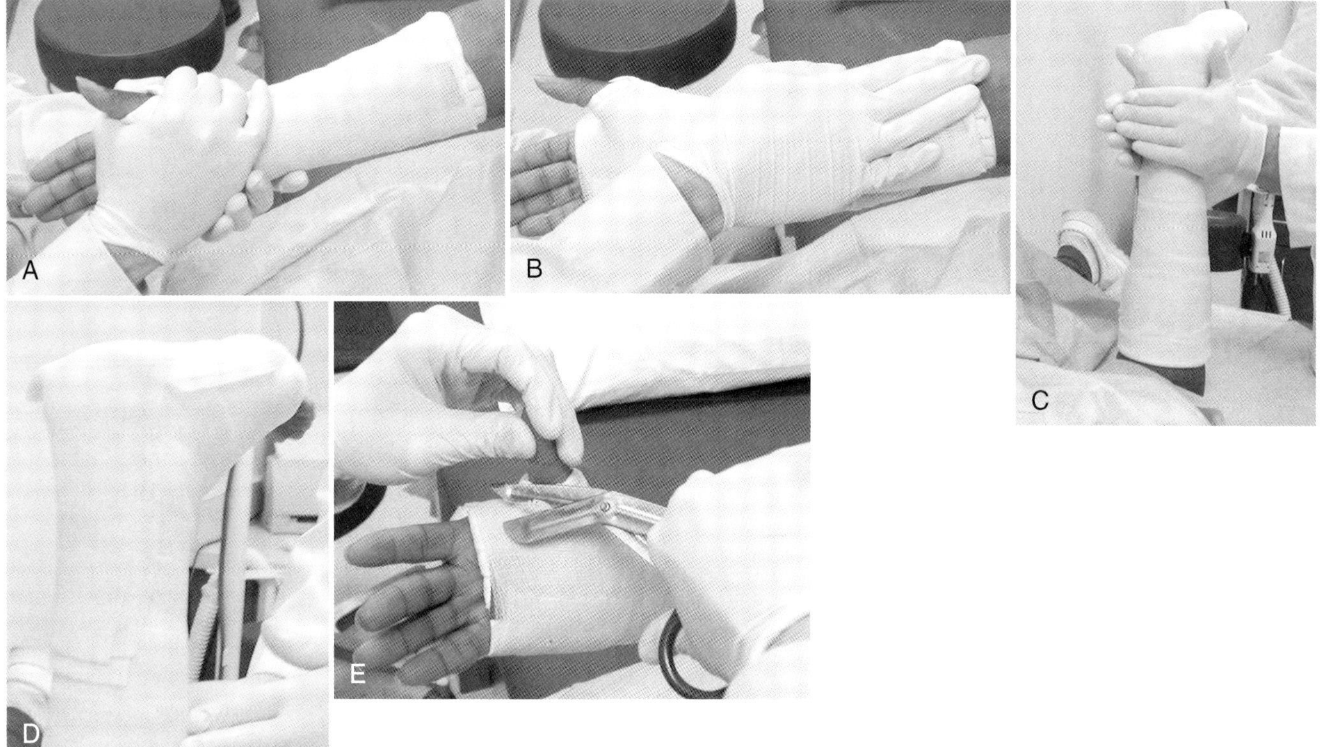

Figure 187-13 Application of synthetic materials. **A,** Molding short-arm cast at wrist. **B,** Molding short-arm cast at forearm. **C,** Molding short-leg walker at Achilles area. **D,** Position of posterior reinforcement strip for short-leg walker. **E,** Trimming excess cast material to avoid trauma to nearby skin.

Postprocedure Patient Education

After cast application, instruct the patient in proper cast care and advise of signs and symptoms that require immediate attention. For *plaster,* advise avoidance of unnecessary forces to the cast, such as weight bearing for at least the first 24 to 48 hours, as the material will still be in the curing process. *Synthetic* casts usually develop sufficient durability to bear increased forces after 12 to 24 hours. Depending on the acuity of injury, elevation for the initial 48 to 72 hours may be recommended to reduce swelling.

Crutch walking is necessary for lower-extremity injuries treated with casting until the cast has developed adequate strength to support weight bearing. Crutches that fit properly will be 1 to 1½ inches below the axilla when placed vertically between the arm and body. The handgrips should be adjusted to allow the patient to have slightly flexed elbows during use. It is also important to remind patients that crutches are not intended to support the weight in the axilla, since this can lead to paresthesias in the arm. The weight of the body should be supported in the hands and the unaffected lower extremity (using a three-point gait). Prior to discharging the patient, it is also helpful to observe his or her gait with the use of crutches and correct any problems that may occur.

Patients must take care to avoid getting the cast material wet and must be advised that submersion of even synthetic casts is unacceptable if routine stockinette and padding are used. If the cast should get wet, the patient may try drying it with an electric blow dryer on the cool setting, being careful not to overheat the cast material. Soaked plaster casts and synthetic casts (with traditional stockinette and padding) in which the underlying cast padding is saturated require attention by a clinician and possible replacement. If not evaluated, the patient may suffer loss of immobilization, or skin irritation or maceration from the moisture under the cast material.

The patient *must never introduce foreign objects (e.g., coat hangers) underneath the cast for any reason.* Strategies for the patient with pruritus under the cast include using cool air from an electric blow dryer or talc or baby powder applied under the cast.

Patients using waterproof cast liner and fiberglass cast material may allow their cast to get wet. Bathing with mild soap is permitted. In general, a synthetic cast will require 1 to 4 hours to dry after submersion. Common sense should dictate the avoidance of swimming in areas that might allow the introduction of foreign bodies beneath the cast (e.g., fish, debris).

Cast wearers should contact their clinician if they develop increased *pain* in the immobilized region; *numbness, tingling,* or *weakness* in the affected area; a *change in skin color* distal to the cast; or *persistent skin irritation.*

Cast Removal Equipment

- An electric, oscillating cast saw
- Cast spreaders
- Bandage/trauma scissors

Preprocedure Patient Preparation

Patient counseling before starting the procedure, especially in the pediatric population, is likely to be the most effective means of minimizing fear and apprehension. Some practitioners solve this potential problem by allowing ancillary staff (nurses or other clinicians) to perform this function. In either case, it is good practice to describe the technique to the patient and include descriptions of any sensations (e.g., warmth, vibration) likely to be experienced. Actually turning the cast saw on and applying it briefly to one's own skin to show that it will not cut is sometimes used to demonstrate the safety of the procedure. The fear related to the noise generated by the cast saw can be reduced with the use of hearing protection. This may be especially helpful in the pediatric population. Once the patient is prepared, actual removal of the cast is fairly easy.

TECHNIQUE

Removal techniques differ based on previous experience and training.

1. Stabilize the immobilized limb, with the patient in a comfortable position and with a drape covering any clothing likely to be exposed to cast saw dust. Some patients will also appreciate wearing a surgical mask to reduce the inhalation of cast dust.
2. Determine the cut line before starting. If possible, avoid potentially sensitive areas. If a protective strip was utilized, the cut line is between where it appears on the cuffs at each end.
3. Hold the cast saw in one hand and, using the thumb and a finger (usually the index) of the other hand, stabilize the saw against the cast (Fig. 187-14). This technique allows control of the depth of cut. Constantly changing the area of the blade in contact with the cast and avoiding prolonged cutting in a single area should decrease the heat generated and limit the potential for saw-induced burns. Another technique to reduce cast saw heat production is to cut in a manner similar to a sewing machine needle. With this method the depth of the cast saw is constantly changing and exposes different areas of the saw blade to cast material. Depending on the cast material and the type of cast, either one (univalve) or two (bivalve) cuts along the entire length of the cast will be required.
4. After full-thickness cuts have been made through the casting material, use the cast spreaders to expose the underlying padding and stockinette (Fig. 187-15), which can then be cut with bandage/trauma scissors. If a protective strip is in place, the cast spreaders should be used frequently to locate it and thereby maintain the cut line for the saw.
5. Once all material has been divided, remove the cast and allow the patient to cleanse the skin. Postprocedure cast care is injury specific and geared toward rehabilitation of the affected limb.

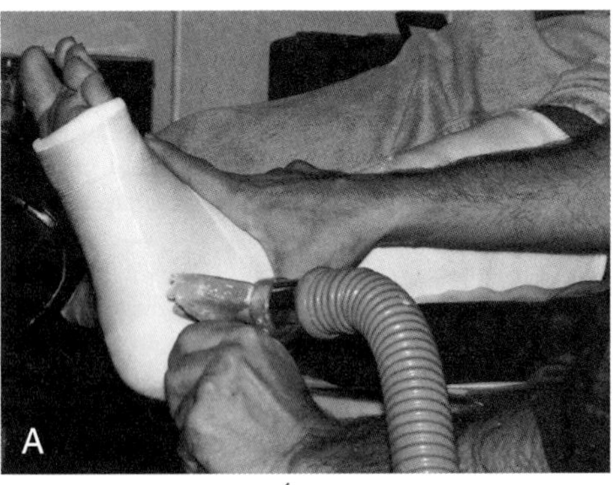

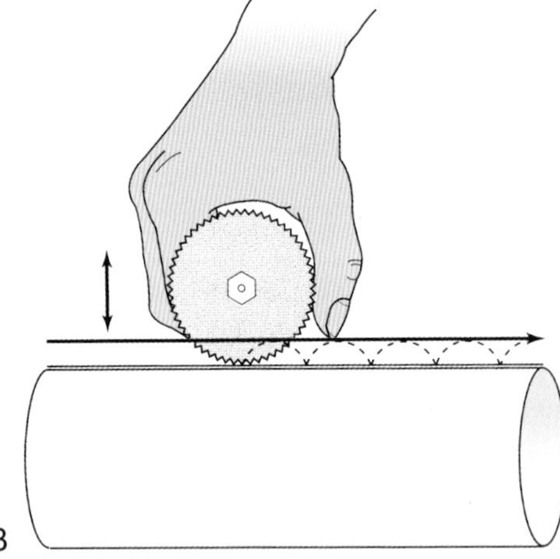

Figure 187-14 Cast removal. **A,** Hold the cast saw in one hand, and use the thumb and another finger (usually the index) to stabilize the saw against the cast, which prevents the blade from injuring the underlying skin. **B,** Cut down through both sides of the cast. Do not saw back and forth with the blade. Cut the cast at right angles to the material. (**B,** From Mercier LR: Practical Orthopedics, 5th ed. St Louis, Mosby, 2000.)

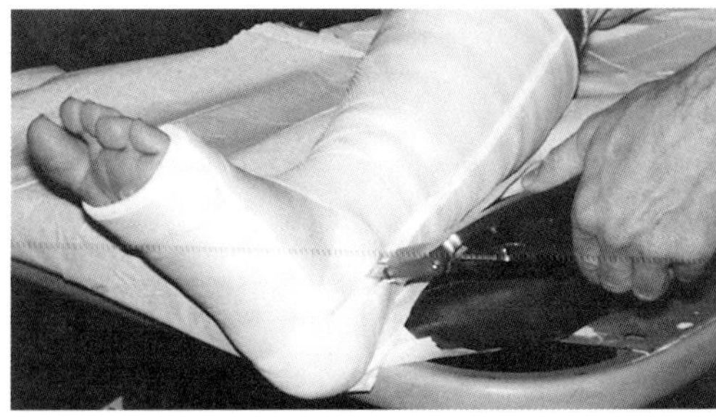

Figure 187-15 Cast spreader or pliers separate the upper and lower portions of the cast, which has been cut on both sides.

COMPLICATIONS

The most well-known and feared complication is the development of a compartment syndrome (see Chapter 188, Compartment Syndrome Evaluation). The process can occur with even a simple, benign-appearing injury. If a snug circumferential cast is applied and tissue swelling continues after the initial injury, conditions are set for compromise of the microcirculation to the immobilized tissue. This may lead to ischemia of the affected area, producing muscle necrosis and further edema. If this process continues untreated and compartmental pressures reach a critical level, irreversible damage to the involved tissues may ensue. Ultimately, ischemic contractures (e.g., Volkmann's) may occur with loss of limb function.

Signs and symptoms of compartment syndrome include *pain* that is out of proportion to the injury or is elicited with pressure over the affected compartment or with stretching of involved muscle groups. Additional indications of impending compartment syndrome include *paresthesias* in the corresponding dermatome, the *inability to generate a forceful muscle contraction*, and *normal pulses* in the affected limb. Pulselessness and pallor are not characteristics of compartment syndrome, because pressures will rarely rise high enough in a compartment to completely obstruct the major blood vessels in that area. *All patients who receive a cast as part of their therapy should be counseled regarding the signs and symptoms of compartment syndrome.* Should they occur, emphasis must be placed on the immediate need to contact the treating clinician or to seek care in an emergency department. *Delayed diagnosis and treatment can lead to irreversible muscle and nerve damage.*

Initial treatment in suspected cases of compartment syndrome is relief of the pressure generated by the cast, either through univalving, bivalving, or complete removal. Univalving results in a 30% drop in pressure while bivalving results in a 60% drop. Definitive diagnosis rests on characteristic signs, symptoms, and objective measurement of the compartmental pressure. Treatment of documented compartment syndrome may require surgical intervention in the form of fasciotomy.

Loss of reduction of the fracture is a possible complication. Therefore, every effort should be made to maintain the reduction as the extremity is being cast. Likewise, every effort should be made to maintain the integrity of the cast, especially as it is setting as well as afterward, when it is exposed to daily wear and the environment.

Various other skin conditions, nerve palsy, thermal injury, joint stiffness, disuse osteoporosis, and *thromboembolic events* may also complicate cast therapy. Of the skin conditions, *cast dermatitis* may be the most common, usually resulting in severe, bothersome pruritus from poor ventilation to the underlying skin. Use of absorbent powders (e.g., talc or baby powder) may help limit the incidence of this condition. Two problems may result if patients introduce objects under the cast to relieve intense itching. First, the object may become trapped under the cast, producing a pressure point that can cause severe ulceration. Second, such instruments as coat hangers can easily lacerate the skin if used too aggressively, forming a nidus for infection or even requiring suture repair. *Pressure necrosis or sores* may result from poorly fitting casts that are insufficiently padded over bony prominences or inadequately molded to local anatomic contours (Fig. 187-16). As mentioned, transverse wrinkles in stockinette or cast padding or ridges in the cast material can lead to pressure necrosis. Pressure sores can occur as soon as 2 hours after the application of a cast. The patient who complains of persistent skin irritation characterized by burning or pain should be seen for evaluation and for possible opening of a window over the symptomatic area to facilitate direct examination. Additional skin damage may occur during cast removal as a result of heat generated by the cast saw. These burns are preventable with use of good technique, and their frequency may be reduced with the use of protective strips under the cast (e.g., De-Flex Strip). The use of waterproof liner under the cast material *increases* the chance of burns during cast removal (this should be discussed with patients prior to cast application), and the use of a protective strip under the cast material is highly recommended. Many providers have patients sign a consent form prior to using waterproof liner because of increased risk of burns and because many insurance providers do not cover the additional cost of this material.

Any cast used to immobilize an anatomic region where superficial peripheral nerves lie in close proximity to underlying bone may lead to nerve *palsy*. Long-leg casts and those short-leg casts involving the head of the fibula can produce a common peroneal nerve palsy as the rigid cast compresses the nerve in its course over the fibular head (Fig. 187-17). Symptoms may include loss of sensation over the dorsolateral aspect of the involved foot, and "foot drop," or weakness in the ankle dorsiflexors. Other potential areas of involvement include the ulnar nerve as it passes through the cubital tunnel region, usually seen with long-arm casts, and the median nerve as it passes through the carpal tunnel (both short- and long-arm casts). These neurologic injuries can be complete or incomplete, reversible or irreversible, and should be recognized and treated in a timely fashion.

Risk of *thermal injury* can be minimized by avoiding water that is too warm (>24° C/75° F) when using plaster of Paris and by avoiding casting that is thicker than 10 ply. A nearly universal complaint following cast immobilization is *joint stiffness*, which is directly related to duration of immobilization. This fact should be discussed with the patient at the time of cast application and should be taken into consideration when determining length of treatment. Depending on the cause for initial treatment and response to therapy, the clinician can initiate fairly aggressive stretching exercises after cast removal to facilitate the return of normal joint function. Use of simple range-of-motion and other exercises involving nonimmobilized joints in the affected extremity (e.g., straight-leg raising, finger or toe flexion/extension) can minimize the effects of prolonged disuse. Casting in the position of function also seems to minimize the effects of disuse.

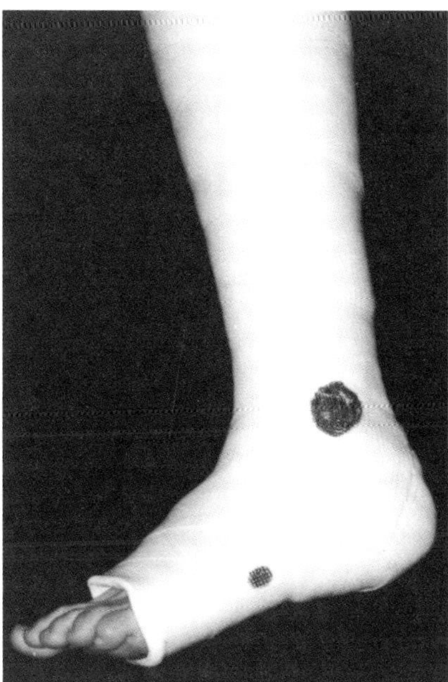

Figure 187-16 Common location for pressure sores (noted by ink on cast).

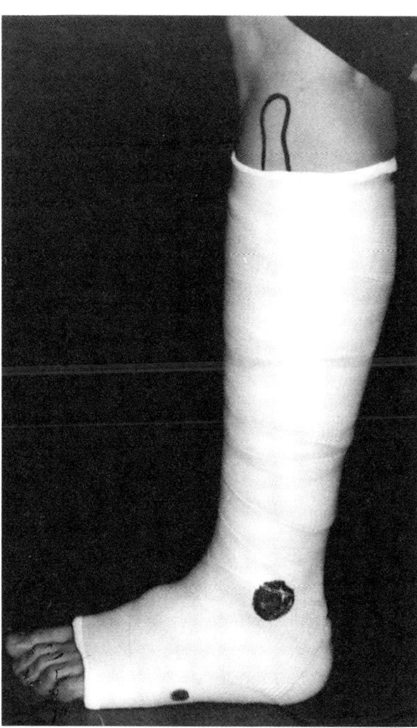

Figure 187-17 Outline on the skin denotes the fibular head and indicates where the peroneal nerve is located. Excess pressure in this area can lead to paralysis and foot drop.

Thromboembolic complications, such as deep venous thrombosis or pulmonary embolism, can occur with cast use (usually of the lower extremity) and must be considered when patients have suspicious symptoms. Diagnosis is difficult because of the presence of the original injury and limitations in examination. To exclude the diagnosis of venous thrombosis may require cast removal and ancillary testing (e.g., duplex ultrasound).

CPT/Billing Codes

The codes for fracture treatment include application of casts and splints. The clinician cannot use these codes for the *initial* application. Use the cast application codes listed here when any of the following occurs:

- Application of cast/splint is temporary and definitive treatment will be done later or by someone else (e.g., application performed in emergency room or office for patient comfort or to temporarily stabilize an injury).
- The cast must be replaced.
- The cast or splinting is performed as an initial service for treatment and no other procedure is planned (e.g., casting of a sprained ankle). Use a casting code in addition to an E/M code.

Casting and strapping codes include removal. Use removal codes only if the cast has been applied by another clinician.

If not listed here, see CPT codes 29000 to 29799 in the CPT code book.

Upper Extremity Casts

29065 Shoulder to hand (long arm)
29075 Elbow to finger (short arm)
29085 Hand and lower forearm (gauntlet)
29086 Finger (e.g., for contracture)

Upper Extremity Splints

29105 Application of long-arm splint (shoulder to hand)
29125 Application of short-arm splint (forearm to hand); static
29130 Application of finger splint; static

Lower Extremity Casts

29345 Application of long-leg cast (thigh to toes)
29355 Application of long-leg cast—walker or ambulatory type
29365 Application of cylinder cast (thigh to ankle)
29405 Application of short-leg cast (below knee to toes)
29425 Application of short-leg cast—walker or ambulatory type
29435 Application of patellar tendon bearing (PTB) cast
29440 Adding walker to previously applied cast
29445 Application of rigid total contact leg cast

Lower Extremity Splints

29505 Application of long-leg splint (thigh to ankle or toes)
29515 Application of short-leg splint (calf to foot)

Lower Extremity Strapping

29530 Strapping, knee
29540 Strapping, ankle
29550 Strapping, toes
29580 Unna boot

Removal or Repair

Codes for cast removal should be used only for casts applied by another clinician.

29700 Removal or bivalving, gauntlet, boot, or body cast
29705 Removal or bivalving, full-arm or full-leg cast
29730 Windowing of cast
29740 Wedging of cast (except clubfoot casts)
29799 Unlisted procedure, casting or strapping

Also see Chapter 190, Fracture Care, for appropriate ICD-9 codes.

Patient Education Guides

See the sample patient education handouts online at www.expertconsult.com.

ONLINE RESOURCE

University of Ottawa information and videos on casting: www.med.uottawa.ca/procedures/cast/.

BIBLIOGRAPHY

Anderson BC: Office Orthopedics for Primary Care: Diagnosis and Treatment, 2nd ed. Philadelphia, WB Saunders, 1999.

Black WS, Becker JA: Common forearm fractures in adults. Am Fam Physician 80:1096–1102, 2009.

Boyd AS, Benjamin HJ, Asplund C: Principles of casting and splinting. Am Fam Physician 79:16–24, 2009.

Bucholz RW, Heckman JD, Court-Brown C (eds): Rockwood and Green's Fractures in Adults, 6th ed. Philadelphia, Lippincott, Williams & Wilkins, 2006.

Eiff MP, Hatch RL, Calmbach WL: Fracture Management for Primary Care. Philadelphia, WB Saunders, 1998.

Huston AM, Rovinsky D: Casts and splints. In Reichman EF, Simon RR (eds): Emergency Medicine Procedures. New York, McGraw Hill, 2004.

Koval KJ, Zucherman JD: Handbook of Fractures, 3rd ed. Philadelphia, Lippincott, Williams & Wilkins, 2006.

Medley ES, Shirley SM, Brilliant HL: Fracture management by family physicians and guidelines for referral. J Fam Pract 8:701–710, 1979.

Wu K: Techniques in surgical casting and splinting. Philadelphia, Lea & Febiger, 1987.

CHAPTER 188

Compartment Syndrome Evaluation

Michelle E. Szczepanik • Francis G. O'Connor

Compartment syndrome occurs when the pressure inside the fascial compartment of an extremity is higher than the pressure of the blood in the vessels going into the compartment. This variance can be caused by bleeding into or edema in the area, which in turn can lead to compromise of the circulation to the soft tissues, especially the muscles and nerves, and cause tissue ischemia and eventual necrosis. If the compartment syndrome is present for 8 hours or more, irreversible tissue damage will likely occur and can lead to subsequent fibrosis and contracture of the muscles and compartment tendons. The flexor tendons are involved most often and are usually the earliest to be involved because they are in the deepest compartments of the calf and forearm. To merely monitor distal pulses for development of compartment syndrome is not adequate. An absent arterial pulse may indicate only damage to a single artery, congenital absence of an artery, or hypovolemia; conversely, normal pulses may be present despite dangerously elevated compartment pressures. Lack of pulse accompanied by pain and pallor are end-stage compartment syndrome signs and symptoms; if these are relied on to make the diagnosis, it will be too late for optimal treatment in most cases. Surgical release using an incision through the fascial compartments (fasciotomy) is required to relieve the excessive pressure.

Compartment syndrome can occur at any age but is much more common in adults than in children. Be aware that the swelling may not peak for 24 to 72 hours after an injury; therefore, the clinician needs to consider this diagnosis, perform a careful examination, and consider measuring compartment pressures up to 3 days after severe injuries.

Compartment pressures can be measured once (as a spot check), periodically, or continuously with a needle being left in place. This chapter discusses measurement of compartment pressures using a needle; wick or slit catheters can be used in a similar manner but are not covered here. Wick and slit catheters are generally used for more prolonged, in-hospital monitoring or research.

Conditions Associated with Compartment Syndrome

- Soft tissue injury only (without a fracture in forearm, calf, hand, or foot)
- Soft tissue injury with a fracture of forearm, calf, hand, or foot
- Supracondylar fracture of the elbow (Volkmann's ischemia)
- Crush injury to thigh
- Gluteal trauma
- Prolonged tourniquet application (>2 hours)
- Anticoagulated patient or patient with coagulopathy
- Electrical injury
- Burns
- Bites (e.g., dog, shark, snake) in susceptible areas
- Exercise-induced compartment syndrome

It is important to understand that compartment syndrome can occur as a result of many different types of insults. Although it is more common in the *calf* or the *forearm*, compartment syndrome can also occur in the hand, foot, thigh, or buttocks. The rule followed is the greater the amount of soft tissue trauma, the greater the chance of compartment syndrome. For this reason, any high-velocity injury should be treated with caution because the energy dissipated through the soft tissue can cause extreme swelling. Injuries commonly associated with compartment syndrome include automobile accidents and pedestrian trauma, especially bumper injuries to the buttocks, calf, or forearm.

Compartment syndrome is a common result of trauma or a fracture. "Volkmann's ischemia" is compartment syndrome in the forearm occurring after supracondylar fractures that cause a large amount of swelling around the elbow. Calcaneal fractures can also cause compartment syndrome, although this is rare. Compartment syndrome can occur in the thigh because of a severe crush injury. Gluteal compartment syndrome, which is frequently associated with an automobile accident or fall from a height, is due to the direct trauma and associated swelling of the muscle compartment. A patient with trauma, especially one with a coagulopathy or on anticoagulation, can develop bleeding into a muscle compartment, leading to increased pressure.

A chronic form of compartment syndrome can occur with exertion, usually increasing as a training program progresses. Also known as exercise-induced compartment syndrome, chronic exertional compartment syndrome presents as a gradual development of pain with activity followed by a gradual resolution of symptoms with cessation of the activity. It is more common in runners, usually involves the calf, and must be distinguished from other causes of chronic leg pain such as medial tibial stress syndrome, stress fracture, nerve or arterial entrapment, or muscle strain. A good history and postexercise examination are fundamental in differentiating between these different causes of chronic leg pain.

Finally, some less common but certainly notable causes of compartment syndrome include prolonged use of a tourniquet, large animal bites, snakebites, infection, electrical injuries, and burns. Prolonged application of a tourniquet (>2 hours) has been associated with development of compartment syndrome when the tourniquet is released and reperfusion causes swelling and increased pressure. Bites in an extremity from large animals such as sharks or dogs can cause crush injuries; snakebites are also associated with significant edema. Scratches, cuts, or bites from smaller animals or insects can result in infection that may cause a compartment syndrome or mask or restrict one. Patients who have electrical injuries, with or without a visible skin burn, can develop compartment syndrome. The mechanism is similar to that of a device available on the market to cook a hot dog, which is how the injury got its nickname "hot dogger." After a hot dog is punctured at both ends with a metal spike, an electrical current is delivered through the hot dog. This causes intense heat, thus cooking the hot dog. The same mechanism occurs with burn injuries with an entrance and exit point for the electrical energy. The "cooked" tissue inside swells, nearly to the point of bursting, but is restrained by the surrounding tissue. The extent of injury may not be visible on the patient's initial visit but can develop over the next 1 to 3 days. *A clinician should always consider compartment syndrome when evaluating burns of any source.*

Conditions That Can Create, Mask, or Worsen Compartment Syndrome

- Applying heat to injury
- Spinal cord injury or regional anesthetic block
- Intoxication, altered mental status, or changes in sensorium (e.g., head trauma, coma)
- Infection, burns, scarring, tight bandages, or being in a cast

An injury, with or without fracture, that is later subjected to warm water or any other intervention resulting in vasodilation will have increased swelling and an increased chance of compartment syndrome. Patients with a severe bruise from a fall who then soak it in a hot tub of water can develop compartment syndrome. It can also happen when expansion of the soft tissue envelope (skin) is constricted by a cast, scarring, or infection. If any patient has pain out of proportion to objective findings, especially after trauma to an extremity or placement of a cast, the cast and Webril should be removed entirely and the patient examined carefully for compartment syndrome. If removal of the cast and Webril does not bring immediate and complete relief of the intense pain, evaluation for compartment syndrome is indicated (with subsequent surgical treatment if present). Even without a cast, any feeling of tense, tight swelling in the forearm, hand, calf, or foot should lead to suspicion of compartment syndrome.

Another presentation for compartment syndrome is the intoxicated individual who falls and sustains an injury. Because of the intoxication (or any other reason for an altered sensorium), the pain is ignored. In addition, patients who have a spinal cord injury resulting from a motor vehicle accident will not have pain in the forearm or calf in spite of the swelling that may also occur as a result of the accident. Postoperative patients with a regional block may not have pain for the same reason. For the aforementioned reasons, immediate evaluation may be necessary and a fasciotomy considered in any such patient with a tense and swollen forearm, calf, hand, or foot.

Indications

A diagnosis of compartment syndrome made after loss of pulses and loss of capillary refill comes too late for optimal treatment. The most important and earliest symptom associated with compartment syndrome is *pain*. If pain after an injury is associated with swelling in an extremity and the pain is not relieved by medication (e.g., up to one or two Percocet tablets every 4 hours), compartment syndrome should be suspected, especially if the pain is progressive.

The earliest physical findings are (1) loss of fine touch and (2) pain with extension of the great toe or the thumb. Compartment syndrome most commonly occurs first in the volar/dorsal compartment of the forearm, where the long flexor tendon of the thumb travels, and in the calf, where the long flexor tendon for the great toe is located. By passively extending the thumb or great toe, the muscle tendon unit in this deep compartment is stretched. If the muscle is ischemic because of early compartment syndrome, pain will be present and increased by extension of the thumb or toe. Two-point discrimination is also impaired early.

For chronic exertional compartment syndrome, certain symptoms help distinguish it from other causes of chronic leg pain. Aching or cramping leg pain, gradual rather than immediate development of pain with activity, neurologic symptoms such as numbness or tingling, gradual resolution with cessation of activity, and shorter distances or intensities being required to produce the discomfort are all typical symptoms. Because routine physical examination is usually negative, a postexercise examination should be included to demonstrate tightness of the compartment involved, discomfort and tenderness with palpation, and involvement of the muscle mass rather than the muscle–tendon junction. The calf is most commonly involved, and about 80% of the time compartment syndrome occurs bilaterally.

Measurement of compartment pressures should be considered in any patient with a compatible history, a swollen and tense muscle group, and

- Pain (the earliest and most sensitive symptom)
- Pain out of proportion to objective findings, especially if progressive
- Increasing pain not relieved by usual narcotic pain medication
- Loss of fine touch or two-point discrimination
- Pain with passive motion of the affected muscles (e.g., extension of great toe or thumb of affected limb)
- Increased discomfort when muscle trapped in fascial compartment is moved (actively or passively), especially the flexor muscles
- Excessive constriction of the affected compartment
- Suspected chronic exertional compartment syndrome

Contraindications to Measurement

- When compartment syndrome is clinically obvious and measurement would delay definitive treatment
- Cellulitis directly over the area to be measured *(relative contraindication)*
- Anticoagulation *(relative contraindication)*

Preprocedure Patient Preparation

Indications, alternatives, risks, potential benefits, and expected results should be discussed with the patient or representative and signed informed consent should be obtained. The patient should expect some discomfort as needles are inserted. The procedure may need to be repeated at various locations and intermittently over time. Alternatively, a continuous monitor may be left in place (usually in a comatose patient). Let conscious patients know they will be warned before insertion of a needle. It will also be important for them to remain very still during certain portions of the procedure. If moderate (conscious) sedation is to be used, intravenous access should be obtained and the patient should be monitored with pulse oximetry.

Equipment

- Gloves and other necessary equipment for the clinician to follow universal blood and body fluid precautions
- Povidone–iodine (Betadine) or chlorhexidine (Hibiclens) antiseptic solution
- Sterile drapes and towels
- 4 × 4 gauze squares
- Band-Aids to cover needle insertion sites
- Local anesthetic (1% lidocaine), syringe, and needles *(optional)*

Stryker System

- Prefilled syringe with saline
- Side-port needle
- Diaphragm chamber
- Hand-held pressure monitor
- Stryker 295 quick-pressure monitor set (disposable pouch)

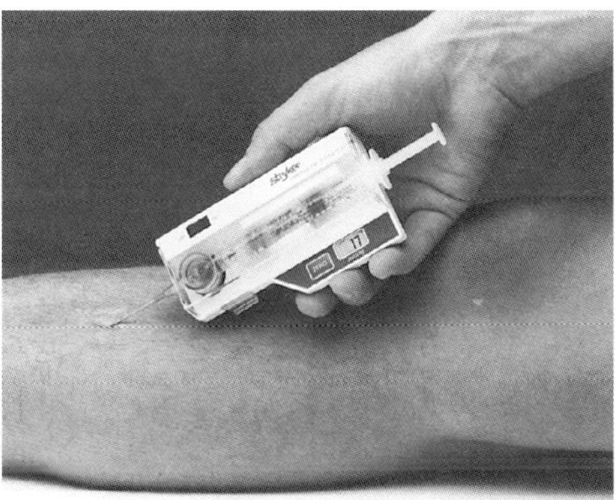

Figure 188-1 Stryker 295 intracompartmental pressure monitor system. (Courtesy of Stryker Instruments, Kalamazoo, Mich.)

Needle–Manometer or Arterial-Type Transducer System

- Two 18-gauge needles (18-gauge spinal needle may be needed for deep measurements such as thigh or gluteal compartments)
- Two sets of extension tubing
- 20-mL syringe
- Three-way stopcock
- Sterile normal saline solution
- Manometer or pressure transducer, cable, monitor, and adjustable transducer stand

Clinicians primarily use one of two pressure measurement systems, either the *Stryker 295 intracompartmental pressure monitor system*, which is a portable penlike compartment pressure device made by the Stryker Company, or a *needle–manometer or arterial-type transducer system*. The Stryker 295 (Fig. 188-1) is much like a tonometer for measuring glaucoma. All of these systems can also be converted to a continuous monitoring system.

Technique

Each body "compartment" can become compromised. Various compartments are shown in Figs. 188-2 to 188-13. Suggested sites for placement of the needle are noted in Table 188-1. Most experts recommend multiple measurements at multiple sites with at least one being at the site of maximal tightness as determined by the examining clinician. A study by Whitesides and Heckman (1996) suggests that with fractures, measurements should be performed at the level of the fracture as well as locations proximal and distal to the zone of the fracture. They used a distance of 5 cm proximal and distal to the fracture site.

General

1. Obtain informed consent.
2. The compartment to be measured should be at the level of the patient's heart and positioned so the needle can enter perpendicular to the compartment.
3. Avoid any external pressures to the area; the region tested may need to be slightly elevated off the bed by an assistant. The patient must be cooperative and not move or contract the muscle group.
4. Prepare skin with antiseptic solution. Sterile technique should be maintained when setting up the equipment and inserting the needles. Sterile drapes should be used if more than one measurement is to be obtained.
5. A *superficial* local anesthetic can be given.
6. When taking pressure measurements, squeeze the involved area to see if pressure increases (or have the patient contract the affected muscle), which confirms that the unit is functioning.
7. Consider measuring opposite-side pressures as a control and if there is any question about proper readings on affected side.
8. When the needle is pulled between measurements, flush it to be sure it has not become plugged with blood or tissue. After measurements are obtained, needle insertion sites should be covered properly (e.g., with a Band-Aid).

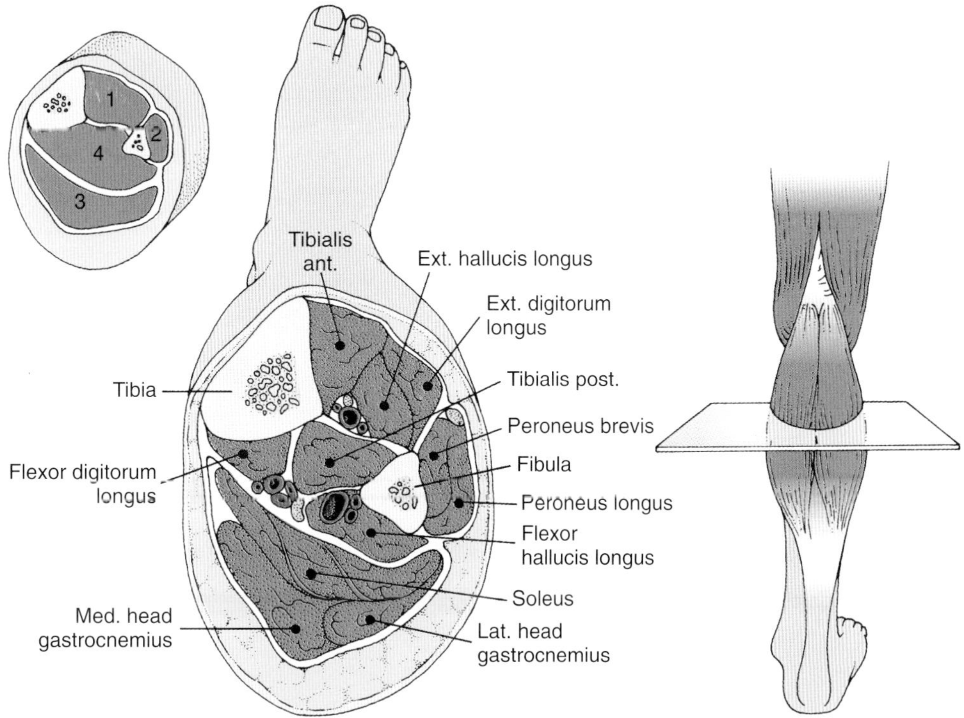

Figure 188-2 Fascial compartments of the lower leg with enclosed muscle groups: 1, anterior; 2, lateral; 3, superficial posterior; and 4, deep posterior compartments. (From Stack LB: Compartment syndrome evaluation. In Roberts JR, Hedges JR [eds]: Clinical Procedures in Emergency Medicine, 3rd ed. Philadelphia, WB Saunders, 1998.)

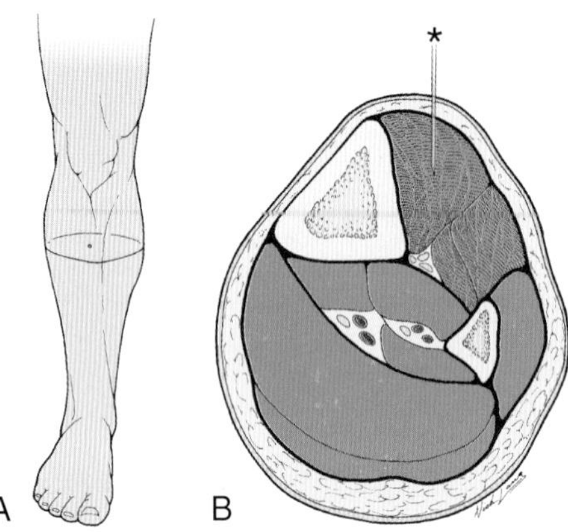

Figure 188-3 Anterior compartment syndrome of the lower leg. **A,** Suggested needle entry point is indicated by the small circle. **B,** The needle should be inserted (*) to a depth of 1 to 3 cm. (Modified from Matsen FA [ed]: Compartmental Syndromes. New York, Grune & Stratton, 1980. In Roberts JR, Hedges JR [eds]: Clinical Procedures in Emergency Medicine, 3rd ed. Philadelphia, WB Saunders, 1998.)

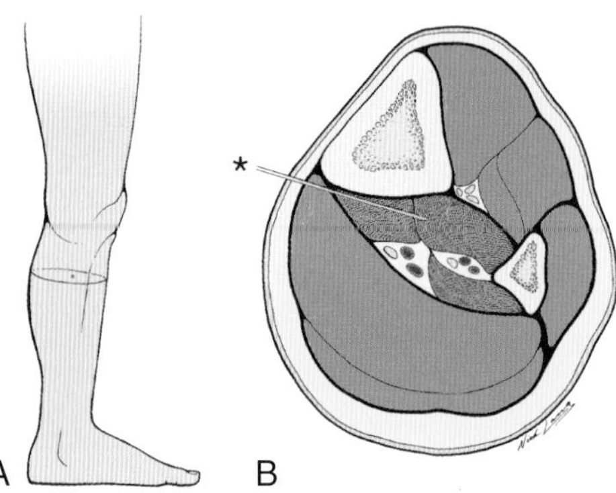

Figure 188-4 Deep posterior compartment syndrome of the lower leg. **A,** Suggested needle entry point indicated by the small circle. **B,** The needle should be inserted (*) to a depth of 2 to 4 cm. (Modified from Matsen FA [ed]: Compartmental Syndromes. New York, Grune & Stratton, 1980. In Roberts JR, Hedges JR [eds]: Clinical Procedures in Emergency Medicine, 3rd ed. Philadelphia, WB Saunders, 1998.)

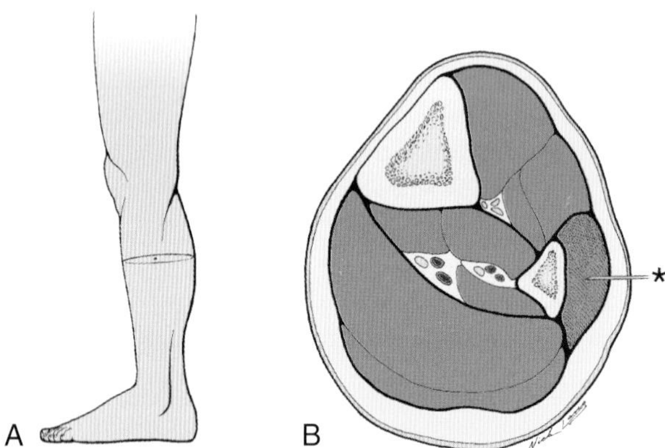

Figure 188-5 Lateral compartment syndrome of the lower leg. **A,** Suggested needle entry point indicated by the small circle. **B,** The needle should be inserted (*) to a depth of 1 to 1.5 cm. (Modified from Matsen FA [ed]: Compartmental Syndromes. New York, Grune & Stratton, 1980. In Roberts JR, Hedges JR [eds]: Clinical Procedures in Emergency Medicine, 3rd ed. Philadelphia, WB Saunders, 1998.)

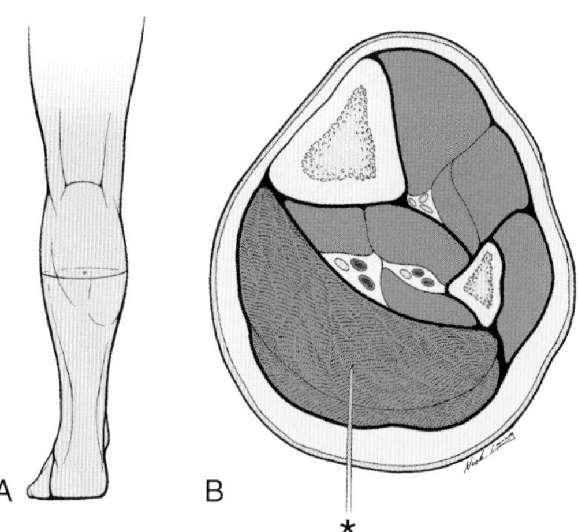

Figure 188-6 Superficial posterior compartment syndrome of the lower leg. **A,** Suggested needle entry point indicated by the small circle. **B,** The needle should be inserted (*) to a depth of 2 to 4 cm. (Modified from Matsen FA [ed]: Compartmental Syndromes. New York, Grune & Stratton, 1980. In Roberts JR, Hedges JR [eds]: Clinical Procedures in Emergency Medicine, 3rd ed. Philadelphia, WB Saunders, 1998.)

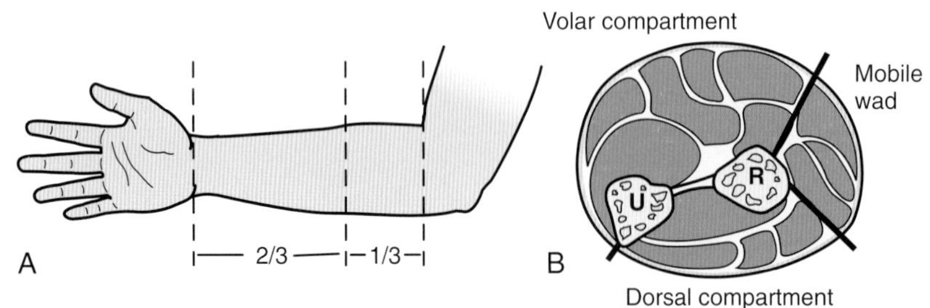

Figure 188-7 **A,** Level of needle insertion for the forearm. **B,** Cross-section through the upper third of the forearm demonstrating the three forearm compartments (volar, dorsal, mobile wad). R, radius; U, ulna. (From Green DP [ed]: Operative Hand Surgery. New York, Churchill Livingstone, 1982.)

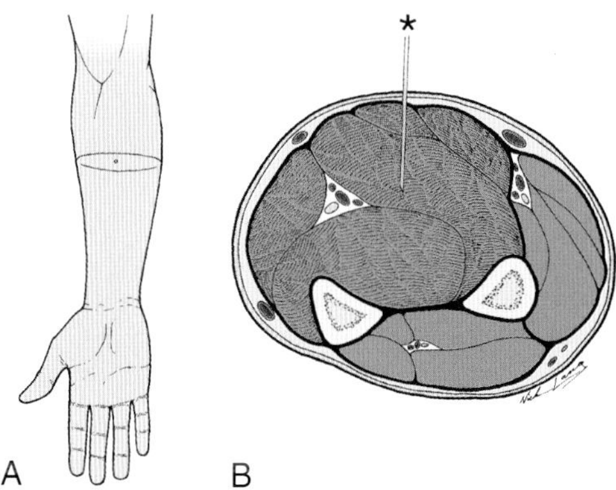

Figure 188-8 Volar compartment syndrome of the forearm. **A,** Suggested needle entry point indicated by the small circle. **B,** The needle should be inserted (*) to a depth of 1 to 2 cm. (Modified from Matsen FA [ed]: Compartmental Syndromes. New York, Grune & Stratton, 1980. In Roberts JR, Hedges JR [eds]: Clinical Procedures in Emergency Medicine, 3rd ed. Philadelphia, WB Saunders, 1998.)

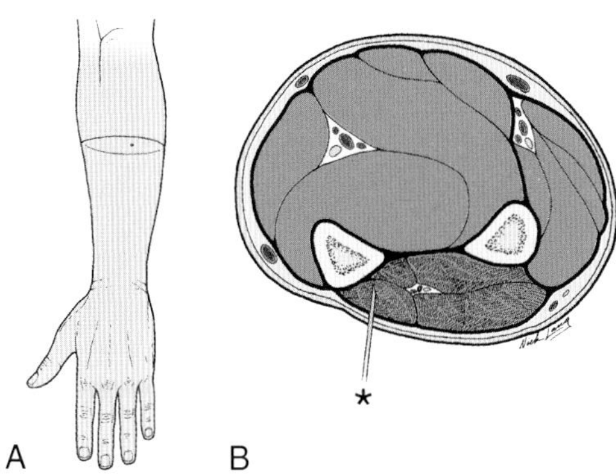

Figure 188-9 Dorsal compartment syndrome of the forearm. **A,** Suggested needle entry point indicated by the small circle. **B,** The needle should be inserted (*) to a depth of 1 to 2 cm. (Modified from Matsen FA [ed]: Compartmental Syndromes. New York, Grune & Stratton, 1980. In Roberts JR, Hedges JR [eds]: Clinical Procedures in Emergency Medicine, 3rd ed. Philadelphia, WB Saunders, 1998.)

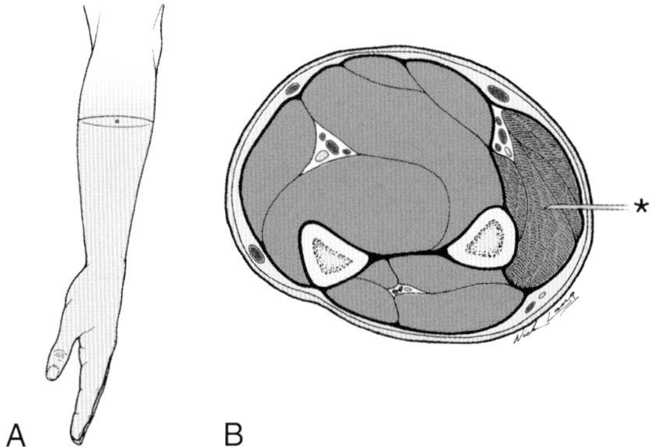

Figure 188-10 Mobile wad compartment syndrome of the forearm. **A,** Suggested needle entry point indicated by the small circle. **B,** The needle should be inserted (*) to a depth of 1 to 1.5 cm. (Modified from Matsen FA [ed]: Compartmental Syndromes. New York, Grune & Stratton, 1980. In Roberts JR, Hedges JR [eds]: Clinical Procedures in Emergency Medicine, 3rd ed. Philadelphia, WB Saunders, 1998.)

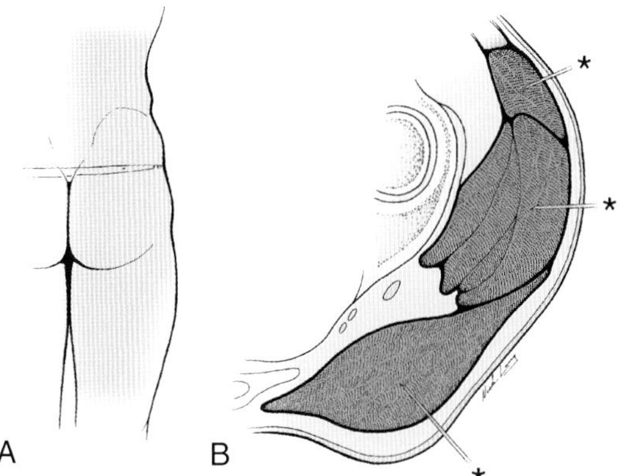

Figure 188-11 Gluteal compartment syndrome. **A,** Suggested needle entry point is indicated by the small circle. The needle should be inserted to a depth of 4 to 8 cm depending on which compartment is being measured. **B,** Needle tips (*) shown entering muscle compartments. (Modified from Owen CA, Moody PR, Mubarak SJ, Hargens AR: Gluteal compartment syndromes. Clin Orthop 132:57–60, 1978. In Roberts JR, Hedges JR [eds]: Clinical Procedures in Emergency Medicine, 3rd ed. Philadelphia, WB Saunders, 1998.)

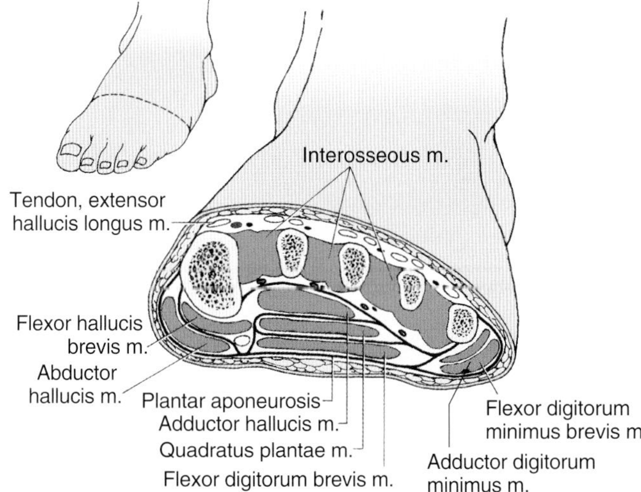

Figure 188-12 Compartments of the foot. (From Mubarak SJ, Hargens AR: Compartment Syndromes and Volkmann's Contracture. Philadelphia, WB Saunders, 1981.)

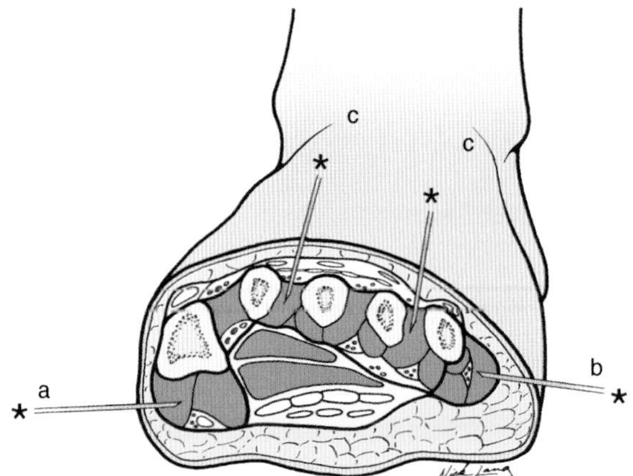

Figure 188-13 Compartment syndromes of the foot. Suggested needle pathways (*) to measure intracompartmental pressures are shown: Medial (a); lateral (b); and interosseous compartments (c). The central compartment is located between these compartments. (Modified from Myerson MS: Acute compartment syndromes of the foot. Bull Hosp Joint Dis Orthop Inst 47:251–261, 1987. In Roberts JR, Hedges JR [eds]: Clinical Procedures in Emergency Medicine, 3rd ed. Philadelphia, WB Saunders, 1998.)

TABLE 188-1 Landmarks for Suggested Needle Placement to Measure Compartment Pressures

Compartment	Position	Location	Insert Needle*	Depth (cm)	Confirm Proper Position by Pressure Variation
Lower Leg					
Anterior	Supine	Junction of proximal and middle thirds of tibia anteriorly	1 cm lateral to anterior tibia (see Fig. 188-3)	1–3	Compression proximal or distal Plantar flexion of foot Dorsiflexion of foot
Deep posterior	Supine	Junction of proximal and middle thirds of tibia anteriorly	Just posterior to medial border of tibia; direct at posterior border of fibula (see Fig. 188-4)	2–4	Toe extension Ankle inversion
Lateral	Supine	Junction of proximal and middle thirds, posterior border of fibula	Just anterior to posterior border of fibula; direct at fibula (see Fig. 188-5)	1–1.5	Compression inferior or superior to needle Inversion of foot and ankle
Superficial posterior	Prone	Junction of proximal and middle thirds of posterior leg	3–5 cm on either side of vertical line in middle of calf (see Fig. 188-6)	2–4	Compression inferior or superior to needle Foot dorsiflexion
Forearm					
Volar	Forearm in supination	Junction of proximal and middle thirds of forearm	Just medial to palmaris longus (midline of forearm); direct needle to palpated posterior border of ulna (see Fig. 188-7)	1–2	Compression proximal or distal to needle Extension of fingers or wrist
Dorsal	Forearm in supination	Junction of proximal and middle thirds of forearm, posterior aspect of ulna	1–2 cm lateral to posterior aspect of ulna (see Fig. 188-9)	1–2	Compression proximal or distal to needle Flex fingers or wrist
Mobile wad	Forearm in supination	Junction of proximal and middle thirds of forearm, most lateral portion of forearm	In muscle tissue lateral to radius	1–1.5	Compression proximal or distal to needle Ulnar deviation of wrist
Gluteal					
All three compartments	Prone	Point of maximal tenderness	Spinal needle	4–8	Compression of gluteal musculature
Foot					
Medial	Supine	Medial aspect of base of first metatarsal	Medial aspect of foot, inferior to base of first metatarsal into abductor hallucis	1–1.5	Compression of medial compartment
Central	Supine	Medial aspect of base of first metatarsal	Medial aspect foot inferior to base of first metatarsal, through abductor hallucis	3	Compression of central compartment
Lateral	Supine	Base of fifth metatarsal	Inferior to base of fifth metatarsal	1–1.5	Compression of lateral compartment
Interosseous	Supine	Dorsum, bases of second and fourth metatarsal	Dorsum of second and fourth web spaces	1	Compression of interosseous compartment

*Perpendicular to skin unless otherwise stated.

Stryker System

9. Open the disposable Stryker 295 quick-pressure monitor setup.
10. Assemble the equipment (Fig. 188-14).
11. Open the cover of the monitor and insert the chamber into the device well with the block surface down. Be sure it is firmly in place.
12. Snap the cover closed.
13. Remove the syringe cap and insert the plunger.
14. Purge the system of air. Tilt the end of the needle up 45 degrees and slowly fill the system with saline. *The saline must not roll back into the transducer well.*
15. Turn on the unit. Readings should be between 0 and 9 mm Hg.
16. Simulate the angle of insertion and press the "zero" button. If the monitor does not read "00," there is a problem. Review the instructions supplied with the kit if necessary. A reading of "00" must be displayed or readings will be inaccurate.
17. Insert needle into the tissue.
18. Inject up to 0.3 mL of saline.
19. Read the pressure once it stabilizes.
20. Repeat readings by turning the unit off and withdrawing the needle and repeating the previous steps.

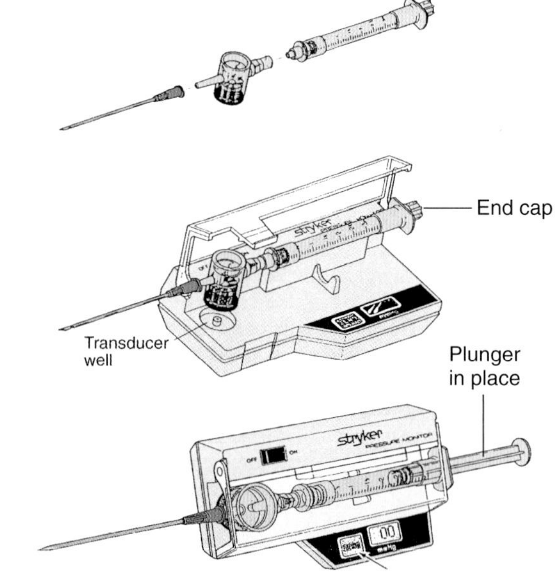

Figure 188-14 Stryker 295 intracompartmental pressure monitor system assembly. (Courtesy Stryker Instruments, Kalamazoo, Mich.)

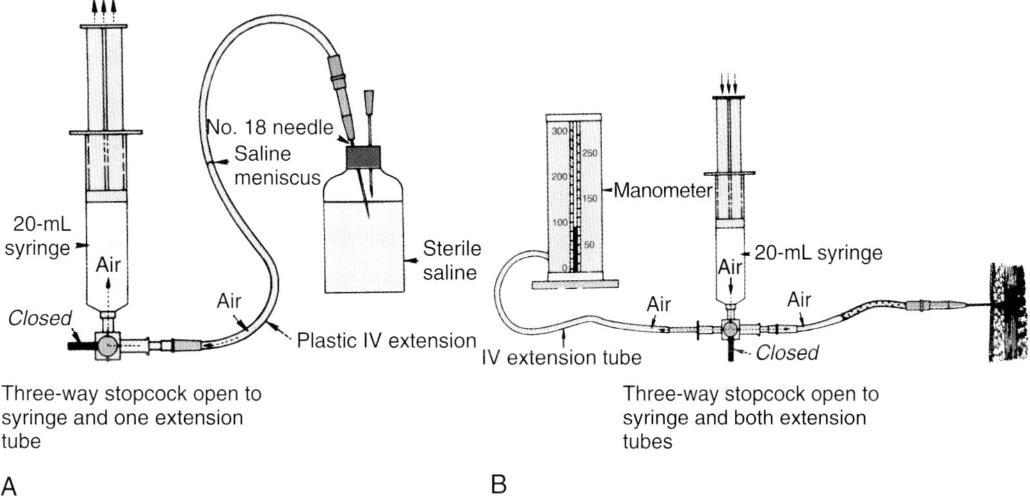

Figure 188-15 Needle–manometer technique for compartment pressure monitoring. **A,** Drawing up saline to partially fill tubing. **B,** Completed system setup with needle inserted into compartment. (From Whitesides TE Jr, Haney TC, Morimoto K, Harada K: Tissue pressure measurement as a determinant for the need of fasciotomy. Clin Orthop 113:43–51, 1975.)

Needle–Manometer System

Equipment for the needle–manometer technique is readily available and the least expensive but also the least accurate.

9. Prepare setup (Fig. 188-15A). Use one 18-gauge needle to ventilate the sterile saline solution (i.e., ventilate by inserting the needle, which opens the bag or bottle to atmospheric pressure and breaks the vacuum in the bottle or bag). This needle should be left in place, ventilating the saline, during the next step, while the extension tubing is being partially filled with saline.
10. Attach the 20-mL syringe to the stopcock. Attach one extension tubing (with the other 18-gauge needle attached) to another port on the stopcock.
11. Using the 20-mL syringe, draw enough saline into the extension tubing to fill it about halfway. Then close the stopcock to the extension tubing. Be sure there are no air bubbles in the saline in the extension tubing.
12. Remove the syringe from the stopcock and fill it about with about 15 mL of air. Reattach it to the stopcock.
13. Attach the other extension tubing to the stopcock. Attach the opposite end of this tubing to a manometer (Fig. 188-15B).
14. With the stopcock still closed to the extension tubing with the needle attached, pull the needle out of the saline. Insert the needle into the desired compartment for pressure measurement (see Table 188-1). For deep measurements (thigh or gluteal compartments), an 18-gauge spinal needle may be needed.
15. *Slowly* depress the syringe plunger. This gives the manometer time to move. Watch the meniscus on the column of saline in the extension tubing. When it flattens, right before the saline starts moving in the tubing, the pressure in the syringe has matched tissue pressure. Note the reading on the manometer, which is the compartment pressure.
16. Check a second recording by removing the needle and repeating as previously.

Arterial-Type Transducer System

Also see Chapter 208, Arterial Puncture and Percutaneous Arterial Line Placement.

Equipment for the arterial-type transducer system is also usually readily available. In the emergency department, the operating room, or the critical care unit, the nurse or respiratory therapist can often assist with flushing and hooking up the extension tubing, which is attached to a pressure transducer. The nurse or respiratory therapist also usually know how to assemble and calibrate the rest of the equipment.

9. Connect the cable to the monitor.
10. Assemble the equipment (Fig. 188-16). Using one 18-gauge needle, fill the 20-mL syringe with sterile saline. One extension tubing will be used to connect the stopcock to the transducer; the other will have the other 18-gauge needle attached.
11. Attach the 20-mL syringe to the stopcock and fill the transducer, both sets of extension tubing, and the attached 18-gauge needle with saline. Close the stopcock to the extension tubing attached to the 18-gauge needle.
12. Remove the 20-mL syringe and open the stopcock to air. Place the transducer at the level of the muscle compartment where pressures are being measured.
13. Calibrate to zero and close the stopcock.
14. Open the stopcock to the extension tubing with the 18-gauge needle attached (which will now be called the "arterial line" because the pressures will be measured and monitored like that of an artery) and insert the needle into the muscle

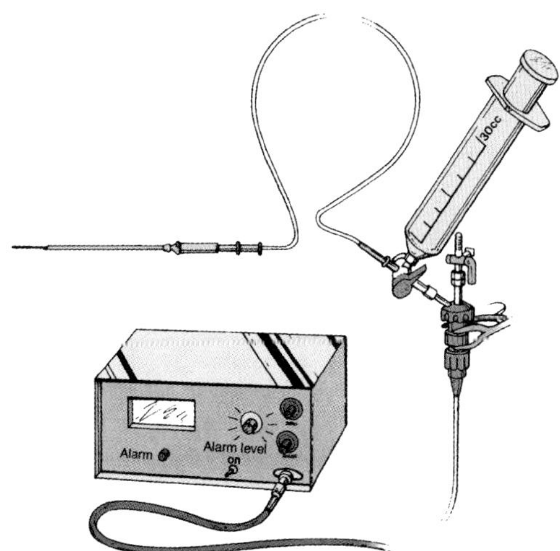

Figure 188-16 Arterial-type transducer system for compartment pressure measurement. (From Rorabeck CH: Compartment syndromes. In Browner BD, Jupiter JB, Levine AM, Trafton PG [eds]: Skeletal Trauma: Fractures, Dislocations, Ligamentous Injuries, vol 1, 2nd ed. Philadelphia, WB Saunders, 1992.)

compartment. Squeeze (or have the patient move) the muscles of the desired compartment. Pressures should elevate on the monitor. Allow the muscles to rest and measure the pressure.

15. Pull the needle and repeat the process for a second confirmatory measurement.

NOTE: Attempts should be made to minimize the injection of saline into the compartment being measured because it may elevate the pressure for subsequent measurements or worsen the compartment syndrome. Using a partially air-filled 20-mL syringe and a partially filled "arterial line" extension tubing, the technique described with the needle–manometer setup can also be used with the arterial-type transducer system. As the air-filled syringe is depressed, when the meniscus flattens and the saline starts moving toward the compartment, the measurement on the monitor will be equal to compartment pressure.

Criteria to Perform Fasciotomy

- Compartment pressure reading over 30 mm Hg
- High clinical suspicion despite normal pressure readings (symptoms of pain out of proportion to objective findings, decreased sensation and pain with passive extension of the thumb or great toe, a tense compartment with clinical signs of compartment syndrome)

Healthy compartment pressures range between 0 and 8 mm Hg. Readings in all compartments *should be 30 mm Hg or below*. Any reading above that level requires immediate consultation for possible surgical treatment of compartment syndrome. Compartment pressures 10 to 30 mm Hg below the patient's mean arterial pressure or the patient's diastolic pressure may also indicate need for a fasciotomy. If multiple measurements are taken, some experts recommend using the highest measured pressures to make the decision for further intervention.

Do not rely solely on pressures to make clinical decisions. Fasciotomy may be indicated if the compartment is tense to palpation, if there is pain out of proportion to objective findings, or if there is decreased sensation and pain with passive extension of the thumb or great toe. If any of these findings are present, even in the face of what appears to be normal compartment pressures, consultation should be obtained immediately. Compartment pressure measurements can give false-normal readings at times. Therefore, such measurements are of value only when combined with the other information on physical examination and pain level.

Criteria for Diagnosis of Chronic Exertional Compartment Syndrome

Once history and physical findings support the diagnosis, compartment pressures should be measured at rest followed by postexercise pressures after pain is reproduced. One of the following criteria must be met for the test to be positive:

- A pre-exercise compartment pressure greater than 15 mm Hg
- One-minute postexercise compartment pressure greater than 30 mm Hg
- Five-minute postexercise compartment pressure greater than 20 mm Hg

Complications

- Bleeding
- Infection
- Increased pressure from extra fluid injected
- Pain
- Inaccurate, falsely reassuring readings

Each of the first three (bleeding, infection, increased volume of fluid) could exacerbate a compartment syndrome.

Patient Education Guides

See the sample patient education form online at www.expertconsult.com.

CPT/Billing Code

29050 Monitoring of interstitial fluid pressure (includes insertion of device, e.g., wick catheter technique, needle–manometer technique) in detection of muscle compartment syndrome

ICD-9-CM Diagnostic Codes

729.71 Nontraumatic compartment syndrome of upper extremity
729.72 Nontraumatic compartment syndrome of lower extremity
729.73 Nontraumatic compartment syndrome of abdomen
729.79 Nontraumatic compartment syndrome of other sites
926.12 Crushing injury of buttock
927.03 Crushing injury of upper arm
927.10 Crushing injury of forearm
927.11 Crushing injury of elbow
928.00 Crushing injury of thigh
928.01 Crushing injury of hip
928.10 Crushing injury of lower leg
928.11 Crushing injury of knee
958.6 Volkmann's ischemic or post-traumatic muscle contracture
958.90 Compartment syndrome, unspecified
958.91 Traumatic compartment syndrome of upper extremity
958.92 Traumatic compartment syndrome of lower extremity
958.93 Traumatic compartment syndrome of abdomen
958.99 Traumatic compartment syndrome of other sites

Acknowledgment

The editors wish to recognize the many contributions by Robert L. Kalb, MD, to this chapter in a previous edition of this text.

Suppliers

(See contact information online at www.expertconsult.com.)

Miga Systems
Stryker Instruments

BIBLIOGRAPHY

d'Amato TA, Kaplan IB, Britt LD: High-voltage electrical injury: A role for mandatory exploration of deep muscle compartments. J Natl Med Assoc 86:535–537, 1994.

Dellaero DT, Levin LS: Compartment syndrome of the hand: Etiology, diagnosis, and treatment. Am J Orthop 25:404–408, 1996.

Gerow G, Matthews B, Jahn W, Gerow R: Compartment syndrome and shin splints of the lower leg. J Manipulative Physiol Ther 16:245–252, 1993.

Gourgiotis S, Villias C, Germanos S, et al: Acute limb compartment syndrome: A review. J Surg Educ 64:178–186, 2007.

Griffiths D, Jones DH: Spontaneous compartment syndrome in a patient on long-term anticoagulation. J Hand Surg Br 18:41–42, 1993.

Hutchinson MR, Ireland ML: Common compartment syndromes in athletes: Treatment and rehabilitation. Sports Med 17:200–208, 1994.

Hutson AM, Rovinsky D: Compartment pressure measurement. In Reichman EF, Simon RR (eds): Emergency Medicine Procedures. New York, McGraw-Hill, 2004, pp 541–550.

Myerson M, Manoli A: Compartment syndromes of the foot after calcaneal fractures. Clin Orthop 290:142–150, 1993.

Olson SA, Glasgow RR: Acute compartment syndrome in lower extremity musculoskeletal trauma. J Am Acad Orthop Surg 13:436–444, 2005.

Pedowitz RA, Hargens AR, Mubarak SJ, Gershuni DH: Modified criteria for the objective diagnosis of chronic compartment syndrome of the leg. Am J Sports Med 18:35–40, 1990.

Peters CL, Scott SM: Compartment syndrome in the forearm following fractures of the radial head or neck in children. J Bone Joint Surg Am 77:1070–1074, 1995.

Schnall SB, Holtom PD, Silva E: Compartment syndrome associated with infection of the upper extremity. Clin Orthop 306:128–131, 1994.

Seybold EA, Busconi BD: Anterior thigh compartment syndrome following prolonged tourniquet application and lateral positioning. Am J Orthop 25:493–496, 1996.

Simpson NS, Jupiter JB: Delayed onset of forearm compartment syndrome: A complication of distal radius fracture in young adults. J Orthop Trauma 9:411–418, 1995.

Stack LB: Compartment syndrome evaluation. In Roberts JR, Hedges JR: Clinical Procedures in Emergency Medicine, 3rd ed. Philadelphia, WB Saunders, 1998.

Vidal P, Sykes PJ, O'Shaughnessy M, Craddock K: Compartment syndrome after use of an automatic arterial pressure monitoring device. Br J Anaesth 71:902–904, 1993.

Whitesides TE, Heckman MH: Acute compartment syndrome: Update on diagnosis and treatment. J Am Acad Orthop Surg 4:209–218, 1996.

CHAPTER 189

EXTENSOR TENDON REPAIR

David T. Bortel

Acute extensor tendon injuries are common and for the most part may be addressed surgically as an outpatient procedure in an acute care setting with proper equipment. Extensor tendons are located superficially and are therefore very vulnerable to trauma. The specialized elastic fatty tissue that allows tendons to glide over the hand, forearm, or dorsum of the foot is called *paratenon*. This vascularized, filmy connective tissue envelops the extensor tendon and does not readily separate when lacerated. This makes these injuries more amenable to repair with less need for significant dissection compared with flexor tendons. However, the practitioner should not ignore the complexity of the extensor mechanism. In the hand, most clinicians consider the act of finger extension to be more intricate than finger flexion. The act of extension comprises two separate and neurologically independent (yet interdependent) systems: the extrinsic extensor system, originating from the forearm and innervated by the radial nerve, and the intrinsic extensor system, originating in the hand and innervated by the median and ulnar nerves (Fig. 189-1).

For years, extensor injuries have been classified by zones of injury (Kleinert zones; Fig. 189-2). Each zone has uniquely associated injury patterns and therefore different modes of treatment. Greater than 50% of extensor tendon injuries are accompanied by another injury (e.g., fracture, dislocation/ligamentous injury, capsular damage, or flexor tendon injury).

PRINCIPLES

Penetrating trauma to the dorsum of the hand needs to be examined carefully for any loss of the neurovascular status or motor/tendon function. The wound should be anesthetized and explored to *visualize the potentially involved tendon*; the wound should be extended, if necessary, to understand the personality of the specific injury (Fig. 189-3). When a tendon is completely transected, the cut ends can retract a considerable distance. Because a *partial tendon laceration* might appear to have full function on examination, the wound must be evaluated judiciously. Unrepaired partial tendon lacerations can result in delayed rupture 1 to several days after the initial injury. The entire tendon complex must be observed throughout the entire arc of motion at the injury location and function compared with that of the unaffected same finger on the opposite hand. Most practitioners believe *a repair is warranted if 50% or more cross-sectional damage has occurred*. After closure, a tendon repair must have healthy padded skin above it for viability, or tissue grafting will be necessary. Wounds older than 6 to 8 hours need aggressive cleansing with strong consideration toward leaving the wound open for a later staged irrigation or débridement with subsequent closure. During this interval, exposed bone, joint, and tendon tissue should be loosely covered with native tissue or a damp sterile gauze followed by a bulky dressing and an anterior-posterior splint,

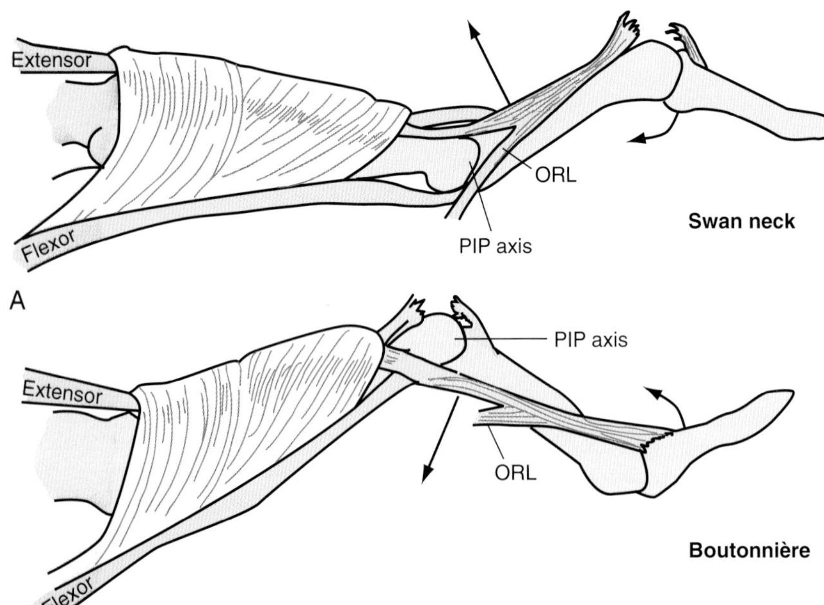

Figure 189-1 Note the intimate working relationship of the intrinsic and extrinsic extensor mechanisms. (Note that the flexor is not shown.) **A,** Mallet finger *(zone I injury)* that has resulted in a *swan-neck deformity* because the oblique retinacular ligament (ORL), also known as the conjoined lateral bands, has subluxated dorsal to the axis of rotation at the level of the proximal interphalangeal (PIP) joint. **B,** A *zone III injury* allows the ORL to subluxate volar to the axis of rotation at the PIP joint, resulting in a *boutonnière deformity.*

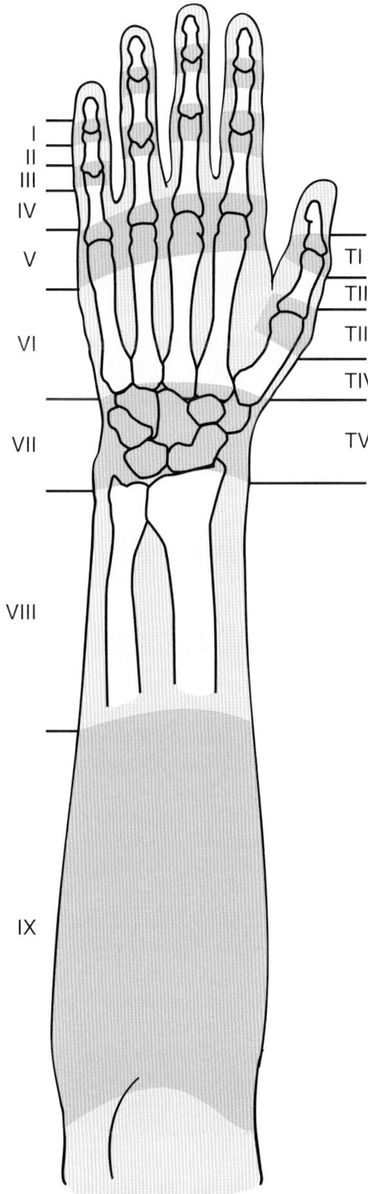

Figure 189-2 Zones of extensor injury (Kleinert zones). The extensor mechanism can be injured from the fingertip to the proximal forearm. Corresponding zones in the thumb are referred to as "T" plus the zone number.

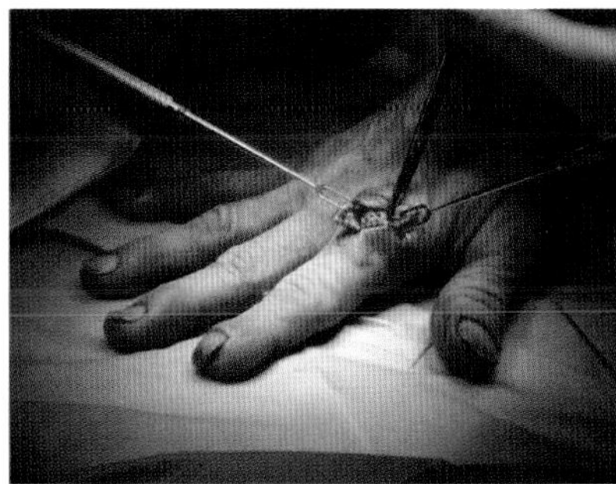

Figure 189-3 Exploration of an extensor tendon injury over the metacarpophalangeal joint with wound extension for appropriate visualization. (Courtesy of John Lubahn, MD.)

extending from fingertip to forearm. Tendon repair may be delayed up to 7 days.

A repaired tendon develops a fibroblastic bulbous connection during the first 2 weeks. Tendon collagen usually does not begin to form until the third week. At the end of the fourth week, swelling and vascularity will decrease. Once the junction becomes strong, the tendon can tolerate active gliding; therefore, physical therapy and rehabilitation can be initiated. Knowledge of appropriate splinting and necessary therapy is essential when caring for these injuries. Repaired tendons usually are immobilized to promote healing and to prevent tendon rupture. After hand extensor tendon repair, the splint typically can be placed on the dorsal surface from the forearm to the fingertips to protect and prevent active extension. The digits and wrist may be slightly flexed within the tolerances of the splint. These joints must be protected against flexion when changing dressings or splints. After a 3-week period of immobilization, depending on the particular circumstances, passive motion can generally be initiated under the guidance of a skilled hand therapist. Reasonable strength may return to this repaired tendon as early as 6 weeks after the injury, again depending on the patient's reliability and health status (e.g., neurologic status, tobacco use, metabolic and rheumatologic issues). Protected, nonloaded motion with a dynamic splint under the supervision of a hand therapist is increasingly chosen for postoperative care.

The vast majority of *flexor tendon* injuries should be treated by a clinician trained to repair these injuries in an appropriate surgical suite. In particular, flexor tendon injuries located in "no-man's land" (between the proximal palmar crease and the proximal interphalangeal joint) are significantly challenging. Results of tendon repair are consistently better when fixed primarily (within 7 days) rather than secondarily (after 7 days or delayed). Familiarity with the sources referenced is encouraged if managing tendon injuries (Baratz and colleagues, 2005; Hutson and Rovinsky, 2004; Thompson and Peimer, 2001; Wright, 2003).

Contraindications

- Less than 50% of the extensor tendon is lacerated and the finger functions as well as the same finger on the unaffected opposite hand.
- Clinician is unfamiliar with the anatomy of the hand or lacks the skills necessary for these repairs (in this situation, the wound should be loosely closed, the hand splinted, and the patient referred).
- There is an open joint space, a bony fracture, or inadequate soft tissue or skin to cover the defect or the subsequent repair (generally in this situation, the wound should be loosely closed, the hand splinted, and the patient referred).
- By zone (see Fig. 189-2)
  - Zone I open laceration: extensor tendon remnants are too short to repair.
  - Zone II (except in the thumb): extensor tendon remnants are too thin to repair.
  - Zones III and V: consider referral if tendon laceration has actual or potential joint or lateral band involvement.
  - Zone VII: consider referral if there is actual or potential extensor retinaculum involvement.
  - Zone VIII: consider referral if there is actual or potential need for tendon transfer. The wound should be loosely closed, the hand splinted, and the patient referred.

Equipment

- Surgical prep solution (e.g., povidone–iodine, chlorhexidine; from hand to elbow with particularly thorough cleansing of the contaminated tissues)
- Ruler marked in centimeters
- Irrigation device for contaminated wounds: 30-mL syringe with 18-gauge angiocatheter or commercially manufactured splash

shield device (see Chapter 22, Laceration and Incision Repair, Fig. 22-1) and sterile saline
- Appropriate anesthetic (see Chapter 4, Local Anesthesia, and Chapter 8, Peripheral Nerve Blocks and Field Blocks)
- 3- to 20-mL syringe
- 27-gauge, 1¼-inch needle (small-gauge needles are preferred to administer anesthesia)
- Additional 27-gauge, 1½-inch needles (useful to pierce and stabilize tendon end; *optional*)
- Sterile drapes; fenestrated drape applied over the lesion; appropriate larger barrier as indicated
- 4×4 gauze sponges; sterile cotton-tipped applicators are also useful
- Sterile pack containing 4½-inch needle holder; curved dissecting scissors; one or more mosquito hemostats; suture scissors; Adson forceps with and without teeth; skin hooks; small self-retaining retractor (e.g., Alm, Holzheimer, Weitlaner)
- Additional small (micro) instruments (may be helpful depending on the size of structures)
- No. 15 blade for excisions or wound lengthening with blade handle (or single disposable scalpel)
- Pack of folded sterile towels for patient arm positioning and clinician wrist support
- Appropriate suture: usually a 4-0 braided, nonabsorbable suture such as Tycron, Mersilene, or Ethibond for the tendon; a fine monofilament (e.g., 5-0 to 7-0 nylon) suture for closing the epitenon (see following text for specifics); also a monofilament (e.g., 4-0 to 5-0 nylon) suture for closing the skin (see Chapter 24, Laceration and Incision Repair: Suture Selection)
- Allis forceps for removal of deeper masses *(optional)*
- Skin-marking pen
- Electrocautery unit
- Specimen jar (if necessary)
- Sterile gloves
- Mask
- Protective glasses with shield
- Sterile gown
- Arm board
- Mayo or instrument holding stand draped in a sterile manner
- ¼-inch Penrose drain (to tag and protect critical structures)
- Appropriate finger or arm tourniquet (with routine use precautions; the maximum time for tourniquet application is generally 2 hours)
- Comfortable chair
- Operative microscope or magnifying loupes, particularly if considering neurovascular repair *(optional)*

Suture Material Considerations

Suture preferences can be quite variable among clinicians who perform tendon repairs. Currently, experienced clinicians usually choose nonabsorbable suture. (Absorbable materials such as Vicryl can precipitate an inflammatory response, which might lead to excessive tendon adhesion formation. Furthermore, an absorbable suture tends to break down while the tendon is very weakened and prone to failure.) If the tendon is of sufficient size with a transected pattern, most clinicians will place one or two "core sutures" using a braided, nonabsorbable material such as Tycron, Mersilene, or Ethibond (usually 4-0 is a good size for the repair, depending on the tendon size). If a running or interrupted epitenon repair is performed, ideally a fine monofilament material is implemented. This commonly will range from a 5-0 to a 7-0, with nylon being a frequently used material. Other suture material can be considered, depending on the clinician's preference and experience. Appropriate suture for the wound closure will also be needed (see Chapter 24, Laceration and Incision Repair: Suture Selection).

Preprocedure Patient Preparation

The risks, benefits, alternatives, and actual procedure should be explained to the patient. Informed consent should be obtained. If irrigation is necessary, this should be explained to the patient as well as the fact that he or she may feel some discomfort when the local anesthetic is being injected. Patients should understand the importance of remaining still during the procedure. They should be placed in a comfortable position, generally supine, in which they can remain still throughout the procedure.

Technique

Radiographic evaluation of the injured area is useful to rule out any residual foreign material in the soft tissues. Sometimes, depending on the mechanism, an unsuspected fracture might also be present. This information might influence the treatment plan. After verifying appropriate anesthesia (usually a digital or wrist block; see Chapter 8, Peripheral Nerve Blocks and Field Blocks) and completion of a thorough preparation and draping, the wound should be explored carefully to further delineate the injury. The clinician should follow universal blood and body fluid precautions. An additional irrigation and débridement might be necessary, depending on the nature of the injured tissues and if further foreign material is discovered. Any nonviable tissue must be removed. One should have little reluctance to extend the wound proximally and distally to understand the extent of the trauma, to satisfactorily visualize the damaged tissues, and to gain access to proximal and distal segments of the involved tendon(s). Electrocautery and a tourniquet are most useful to ensure appropriate hemostasis (although the maximal time for tourniquet application is generally 2 hours, most clinicians should not be performing a procedure that takes this long in the outpatient setting). Because these repairs can be quite tedious, most clinicians will perform them seated in a comfortable chair with the patient's arm positioned out to the side on an arm board. The primary surgeon will usually have his back facing the patient's head, allowing greater access to the extensor portion of the forearm and hand. With a large sterile field including the elbow through the hand and a sterile-gowned clinician, contamination is less likely when positioning the patient and providing stable wrist supports for the clinician performing these procedures.

Ragged tendon ends should be trimmed to allow a clean and direct reapproximation. It is imperative that the clinician be familiar with the associated anatomy for consideration of possible neurovascular injury. If a neurovascular injury is discovered, further referral to an experienced upper extremity surgeon is warranted. If critical structures are near the repair area, the clinician should take special precaution to protect these structures. Incomplete tendon lacerations can be repaired directly or débrided if considered an insignificant portion of the tendon. Occasionally, a tendon is lacerated in an oblique fashion, which is usually amenable to a direct repair with a fine nonabsorbable material. Most clinicians recommend a direct end-to-end (rather than side-to-side) repair of transverse extensor tendon lacerations. If a tendon has adequate substance, a "core" suture, particularly with a braided, nonabsorbable material is implemented. Typically one or two core sutures are placed. The stitch ideally has a buried knot (Fig. 189-4). A Kessler or Bunnell stitch or their modifications are commonly used, and these sutures redirect the force of the tendon perpendicular to the longitudinal axis to allow it to heal. Although no study has determined the optimal stitch for repair in each zone of injury, the modified Kessler and modified Bunnell stitches have been shown to produce the greatest strength for a core-type tendon repair. Although the literature supports the use of these modified core-type stitches, certain experts find them less useful in zones IV and VI because the tendons are so thin. These core-type stitches are most useful when repairing rounder, thicker tendons.

NOTE: If the tendon is not very thick, a loop of suture can be passed around the tendon (the solid vertical lines in Figs. 194-A, B, E, F and G). Granted this loop outside the tendon may later interfere with the tendon's ability to glide in its sheath, it may also be what is needed to best reapproximate the lacerated ends. If the tendon is

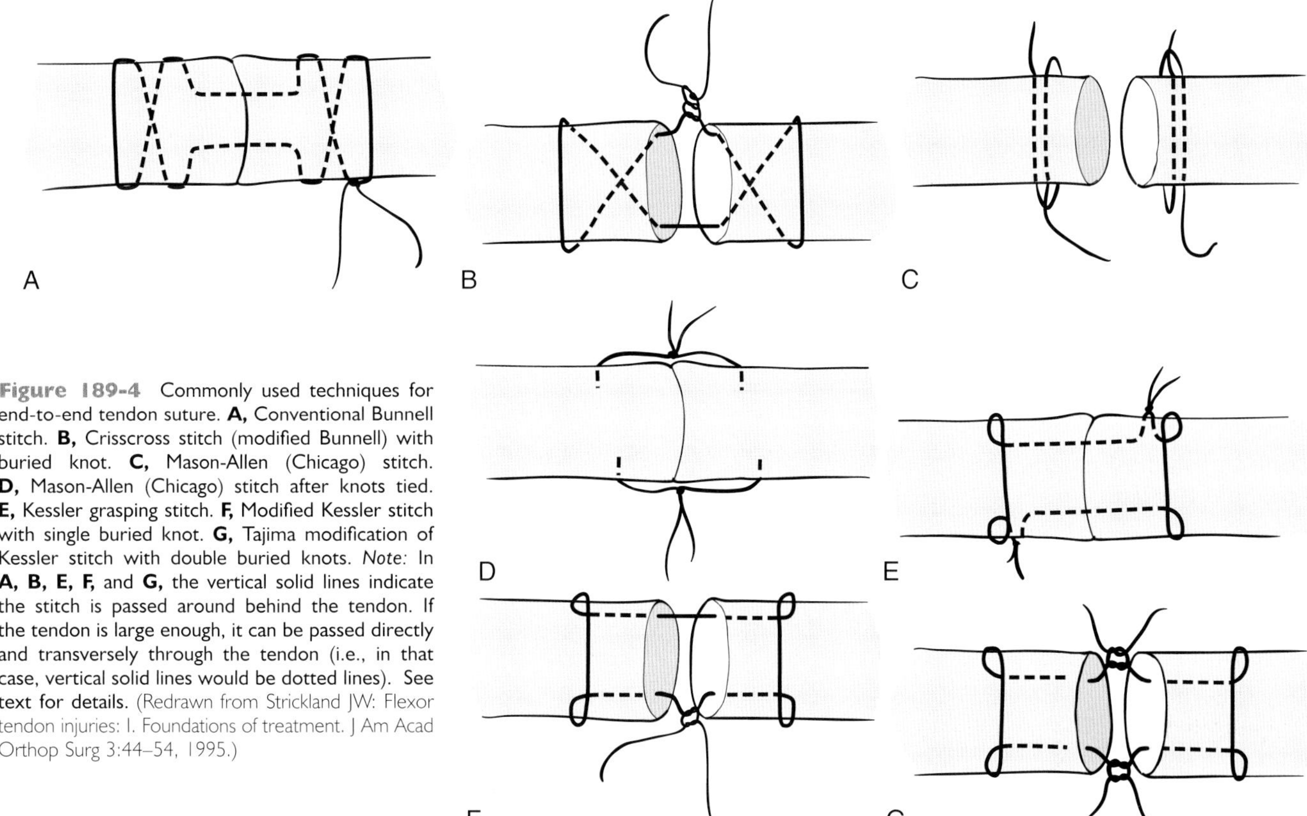

Figure 189-4 Commonly used techniques for end-to-end tendon suture. **A,** Conventional Bunnell stitch. **B,** Crisscross stitch (modified Bunnell) with buried knot. **C,** Mason-Allen (Chicago) stitch. **D,** Mason-Allen (Chicago) stitch after knots tied. **E,** Kessler grasping stitch. **F,** Modified Kessler stitch with single buried knot. **G,** Tajima modification of Kessler stitch with double buried knots. *Note:* In **A, B, E, F,** and **G,** the vertical solid lines indicate the stitch is passed around behind the tendon. If the tendon is large enough, it can be passed directly and transversely through the tendon (i.e., in that case, vertical solid lines would be dotted lines). See text for details. (Redrawn from Strickland JW: Flexor tendon injuries: I. Foundations of treatment. J Am Acad Orthop Surg 3:44–54, 1995.)

thick enough, the core suture can be passed directly and transversely through the tendon (in that case, the solid vertical lines in Figs. 194-A, B, E, F and G would be drawn as dotted vertical lines) which is how many experts have been suturing tendons for years.

Many clinicians use an epitenon running suture with or without a core stitch. The epitenon repair usually is with a fine, monofilament, nonabsorbable material that is appropriate for the size of the structures being repaired (Fig. 189-5). Simple interrupted sutures commonly fail by pulling through the tendon ends and fraying the tendon because of the fiber alignment. When the sutured tendon ends are brought together, a secured knot is present with minimal trauma to the tendon ends. During the repair, the tendon ends should be handled in an atraumatic technique with minimal tissue crushing. (Ideally, the tendon ends should be handled only by the clinician's fingers. Nontoothed forceps can also be quite helpful. A 27-gauge needle can be used to pierce the tendon perpendicularly and stabilize it, as can a single suture placed temporarily through the tendon. Traumatizing the tissue can result in disruption to the vascular and nutritional supplies and subsequent adhesions.) The approximated tendon ends should not buckle or be compressed excessively. A flat end repair promotes proper healing and return of the proper gliding action to the tendon. Particular considerations regarding the anatomic zones are detailed in the following sections.

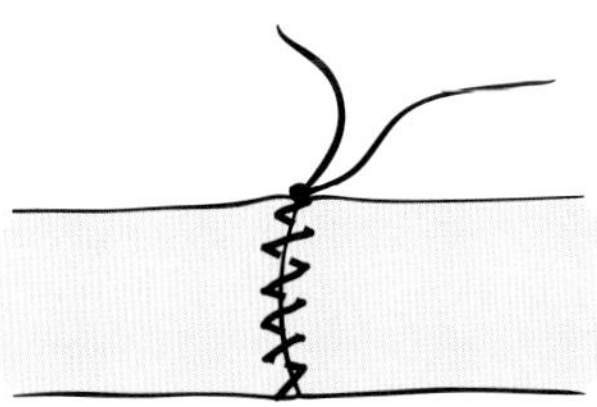

Figure 189-5 Simple running suture used for peripheral epitenon tendon repair. A locked running suture can also be used for greater strength.

By the Zones

Zone I: Distal Interphalangeal Joint

An extensor tendon disruption in this zone is by definition a "mallet finger" (flexion deformity at the distal interphalangeal [DIP] joint; see Fig. 189-1) unless the laceration is incomplete. These sometimes will progress to a "swan-neck" deformity as the conjoined lateral bands subluxate dorsally, resulting in proximal interphalangeal (PIP) joint hyperextension with the associated mallet deformity (see Fig. 189-1). Zone I injuries are commonly missed, especially when not associated with an open/laceration injury. These injuries usually occur when an athlete or manual laborer "jams" the fingertip. These frequently have a poor outcome, often needing a DIP fusion because the incomplete extensor mechanism at the unstable DIP joint interferes with dexterity and leads to subsequent arthritic changes at this joint.

Zone I injuries are classified into four subtypes:

- Type I: Closed or blunt trauma with loss of tendon continuity with or without a small avulsion fracture
- Type II: Laceration proximal to the DIP joint with loss of tendon continuity
- Type III: Deep abrasion with loss of skin, subcutaneous cover, and tendon substance
- Type IV: (1) Transepiphyseal plate fracture in children, (2) hyperflexion injury with fracture of 20% to 50% of the articular surface, (3) hyperextension injury with fracture of the articular

surface usually greater than 50% and with fairly early volar subluxation of the distal phalanx

A radiograph should be obtained with the lateral projection of the DIP joint being scrutinized. Fractures (typically interarticular) should be stabilized appropriately. Commonly, the fracture will need to be pinned.

Treatment

If not open, all zone I injuries should be splinted in extension or even hyperextension across the DIP joint (a digital block may be needed). Open lacerations can be repaired with care to avoid the vulnerable germinal nail matrix. These patients should be directed to a clinician who is skilled in treating these injuries. A temporary, retrograde, buried pin in full extension is often better tolerated than external splinting.

Zone II: Middle Phalanx and Thumb Proximal Phalanx

Zone II injuries typically can be treated similarly to zone I injuries. Many of these injuries are associated with a crush. The splint must be extended to include the PIP joint.

Zone III: Proximal Interphalangeal Joint

An injury at this location frequently will lead to a "boutonnière" deformity (see Fig. 189-1). A zone III deformity (and the previously noted mallet finger) are the most commonly missed closed injuries of the hand. The central slip is injured and the lateral bands can migrate in a volar direction past the axis of rotation at the PIP, resulting in a PIP flexion contracture with or without hyperextension at the DIP joint. Many patients have an associated collateral ligament or volar plate injury. If not recognized and treated early, no good salvage operation can restore normal function to these injuries.

Treatment

The PIP should be splinted in extension, possibly incorporating the DIP joint in extension. The patient should be referred to a clinician trained in these complex problems to have definitive care initiated within 7 days.

Zone IV: Proximal Phalanx

These injuries are normally easy to identify. The lateral band extension is rarely completely transected. A nonabsorbable suture repair, followed by protected motion while the PIP joint is splinted in extension, is typically used. Consider a bite wound (see next section, Zone V).

Zone V: Metacarpophalangeal Joint

Zone V injuries are *frequently* from a human tooth. Obtain a radiograph to rule out a fracture or foreign body. If there is *any* chance of a bite wound, it should be cleansed aggressively and *left open* with consideration of appropriate antibiotic coverage. Frequently, the metacarpophalangeal joint capsule is penetrated. Thus, these wounds should be opened, carefully explored in flexion and extension, and then normally left open (see Fig. 189-3). The hand should be splinted for later wound inspection and delayed tendon repair. An experienced practitioner can repair the wound primarily if it is considered *noncontaminated* and *not* associated with a bite wound.

NOTE: At this level of injury, disruption of the sagittal bands of the extensor hood may occur (e.g., dislocation of the extensor tendon) acutely or spontaneously. These injuries should be splinted and directed to a clinician skilled in managing hand and tendon injuries.

Zone VI: Metacarpal Level

A primary repair can be pursued routinely. Buried core sutures are the typical technique used. The practitioner must oversee a careful splinting and therapy program. Again, consider a bite wound.

Zone VII: Wrist Extensor Retinacular Area

Zone VII injuries may be repaired similarly to zone VI injuries, realizing that the extensor retinaculum is involved and may need repair or resection. Post-traumatic adhesions are not uncommon; hence many clinicians refer all zone VII injuries for retinaculum repair. These injuries should be managed with added diligence during hand therapy.

Zone VIII: Distal Forearm

Zone VIII injuries may be treated similarly to zone VI and VII injuries. At this level, adjacent structures can easily be injured, retracted, and difficult to appreciate. Sensory cutaneous nerves (radial branches and the antebrachial cutaneous nerve) should be protected carefully if in the field and repaired if observed to be lacerated.

Zone IX: Proximal Forearm

Zone IX injuries are frequently associated with neurovascular trauma. These injuries should be explored in an operating room by a clinician skilled in treating these problems.

If the practitioner has experience with extensor tendon injuries and is comfortable with splinting and therapy programs, repairs of zones IV through VI and maybe VIII can be addressed in an emergency department or an appropriately equipped office, if the inherent problems of each zone are understood. The remaining zones might be repaired in these settings relative to the clinician's experience and available equipment. The potential complications associated with these injuries and their repairs must be followed carefully. Complications can be quite significant, including primary failure of the repair, secondary later rupture of the tendon, stiffness, contractures with limited range of motion from resultant adhesions, residual pain, residual overlying tissue problems, infection, and problems related to other adjacent structures. The practitioner will never be faulted for leaving a wound open and splinted after an *aggressive* irrigation and débridement, especially over the metacarpophalangeal joint, and then referring. Ideally, tendon, bone, and joint tissues are kept moist in the wound with a damp sterile dressing to protect against desiccation of these vulnerable structures.

Extensor tendon lacerations to the feet occur less frequently than in the upper extremities because of activity patterns and the protection that shoes and pants can provide. However, when these injuries do occur, they commonly are associated with additional significant trauma to other tissues, including fractures. The clinician must be diligent to rule out other possible injuries by considering associated anatomic structures and obtaining appropriate radiographs. Isolated lower extremity extensor tendon injuries otherwise might be managed in a similar fashion to upper extremity injuries, taking into account the correlating anatomic zones (e.g., a tendon injury at the ankle under the retinacular tissues would correlate to a zone VII injury in the upper extremity). Foot flexor tendons should be addressed by a clinician skilled in these areas. (It is not uncommon for an isolated flexor tendon laceration to be relatively well tolerated without repair.)

Clinicians normally will give an appropriately dosed first- or second-generation cephalosporin for a clean open injury, which should provide satisfactory coverage for most gram-positive skin organisms. Consideration for gram-negative and anaerobic coverage should be entertained for contaminated wounds, especially if occurring at a farm. *Pseudomonas* coverage usually is wise for foot lacerations. Continued antibiotics are typically unnecessary unless there is gross contamination or a subsequent infection develops. It is safest to reevaluate these wounds and repairs 2 to 3 days later for possible early infection. Adjustment of antibiotic management might be necessary, especially when considering the patient's particular circumstances.

Patient Education Guides

See patient education and patient consent forms available online at www.expertconsult.com.

CPT/Billing Codes

25270 Repair, tendon or muscle, extensor, forearm and/or wrist; *primary*, single, *each* tendon or muscle
25272 Repair, tendon or muscle, extensor, forearm and/or wrist; *secondary*, single, *each* tendon or muscle
26410 Repair, extensor tendon, hand, primary or secondary; without free graft, each tendon
26418 Repair, extensor tendon, finger, primary or secondary; without free graft, each tendon
26432 Closed treatment of distal extensor tendon insertion, with or without percutaneous pinning (e.g., mallet finger)
28208 Repair, tendon, extensor, foot; primary or secondary, each tendon

ICD-9-CM Diagnostic Codes

727.63 Rupture of tendon, nontraumatic, extensor tendons of hand and wrist
727.68 Rupture of tendon, nontraumatic, other tendons of foot and ankle
736.1 Other acquired deformities of limbs, mallet finger
882.2 Open wound of hand except fingers(s) alone, with tendon involvement
883.2 Open wound of fingers(s) with tendon involvement
892.2 Open wound of foot except toe(s) alone with tendon involvement
893.2 Open wound of toe(s) with tendon involvement

Acknowledgment

Thanks for the many contributions of Thomas J. Zuber, MD, and John L. Pfenninger, MD, to this chapter in a previous edition of this text.

Bibliography

Baratz ME, Schmidt CC, Hughes TB: Extensor tendons injuries. In Green DP, Hotchkiss RN, Pederson WC, Wolfe SW (eds): Green's Operative Hand Surgery, 5th ed. New York, Churchill-Livingstone, 2005.

Carl HD, Forst R, Schaller P: Results of primary extensor tendon repair in relation to the zone of injury and the pre-operative outcome estimation. Arch Orthop Trauma Surg 127:115–119, 2007.

Dabezies EJ, Schutte JP: Fixation of metacarpal and phalangeal fractures with miniature plates and screws. J Hand Surg Am 11:283–288, 1986.

Hutson AM, Rovinsky D: Extensor tendon repair. In Reichman EF, Simon RR (eds): Emergency Medicine Procedures. New York, McGraw-Hill, 2004, pp 551–558.

Kleinert HE, Verdan C: Report of the Committee on Tendon Injuries (International Federation of Societies for Surgery of the Hand). J Hand Surg Am 8:794–798, 1983.

Newport ML, Blair WF, Steyers CM Jr: Long-term results of extensor tendon repair. J Hand Surg Am 15:961–966, 1990.

Rosenthal EA: Extensor surface injuries at the proximal interphalangeal joint. In Bowers WH (ed): The Interphalangeal Joints. New York, Churchill-Livingstone, 1987.

Thompson DS, Peimer CA: Extensor tendon injuries: Acute repair and late reconstruction. In Chapman MW (ed): Operative Orthopedics, 3rd ed. Philadelphia, Lippincott Williams & Wilkins, 2001.

Wright PE II: Flexor and extensor tendon injuries. In Canale ST (ed): Campbell's Operative Orthopaedics, 10th ed. St. Louis, Mosby, 2003, pp 3423–3482.

CHAPTER 190

FRACTURE CARE*

Robert L. Kalb • Grant C. Fowler

Primary care clinicians are able to manage a wide range of fractures with good outcomes. To do this optimally, however, it is important to have adequate orthopedic training (perhaps on a rotation in residency), as well as supportive orthopedic backup. In fact, primary care clinicians so equipped can manage more complicated fractures, including about a third of fractures requiring reduction. A patient with multiple fractures or open, displaced, intra-articular, or epiphyseal plate fractures should generally be referred to an orthopedic surgeon. Adverse outcomes can be avoided by carefully choosing which fractures primary care clinicians manage, based on their level of training or appropriate consultation. This chapter provides guidelines for the office, urgent care, and emergency center management of fractures by the primary care clinician.

Decisions regarding whether to manage a displaced fracture are often influenced by the state's malpractice climate, insurance carriers, and premiums. Managing fractures requiring reduction often necessitates a higher level of malpractice coverage and higher premiums. Those clinicians treating fractures, especially fractures that require reduction, must have a good working relationship with an orthopedic surgeon willing to provide informal advice on management and on specific cases. It is ideal to have a relationship with an orthopedist who is able occasionally to examine a patient and return the patient to the referring clinician for follow-up care.

All of the fractures discussed in this chapter can be treated by the primary care clinician, with or without local anesthesia. This chapter is intended to serve as a guide or a basic summary for primary care; it cannot possibly review the management of all fractures. Because the management of fractures in children often differs greatly from that of fractures in adults, children are considered separately.

With all fractures, healing starts when osteoclasts arrive at the fracture site, causing resorption of the dead, soon to be demineralized bone. This resorption results in the fracture line appearing larger in the follow-up radiograph (even in those fractures that are nondisplaced or initially have only hairline cracks). As the fracture heals further, callus forms and the pain and tenderness decrease. However, the radiograph will not show callus and healing until later, when it has mineralized. It is only when mineralization has occurred that the x-ray beam no longer easily penetrates the callus, which results in the image of healing observed on the radiograph.

Box 190-1 lists types of casts. Chapter 186, Ankle and Foot Splinting, Casting, and Taping, and Chapter 187, Cast Immobilization and Upper Extremity Splinting, contain more details on casts than are discussed in this chapter.

EQUIPMENT

See the discussions of equipment in Chapter 186, Ankle and Foot Splinting, Casting, and Taping, and Chapter 187, Cast Immobilization and Upper Extremity Splinting.

*Also see Chapter 231, Principles of X-Ray Interpretation.

TERMINOLOGY

Open fracture: This fracture communicates through a hole in the skin; therefore, by definition, an open fracture is contaminated and is more likely to become infected, especially if the hole is greater than 1 cm in diameter. Open fractures should almost always be referred to an orthopedic surgeon. (Previously, the term *compound fracture* was used to describe an open fracture.)

Closed fracture: This fracture is not openly communicating through a hole in the skin. The vast majority of fractures are closed, and the skin is unbroken.

Torus fracture: In this fracture only one of the cortices is buckled.

Greenstick fracture: A greenstick fracture is a level worse than a torus fracture. It involves an actual crack or disruption of one cortex and buckling of the opposite cortex. This fracture is so named because the bony deformation is much like that seen after cracking a green tree twig in springtime: the tension side of the bent twig cracks, whereas the compression side (i.e., the concave side) merely buckles.

Comminuted fracture: In this fracture the bone is in more than two pieces. Often an additional piece, which is small and shaped like a butterfly and therefore named a *butterfly fragment,* is found at the fracture site.

Fracture dislocation: A joint is dislocated and associated with a bony fracture on one or both sides of the joint.

Intra-articular fracture: This fracture extends into the joint or articular surface. If an intra-articular fracture is displaced, the patient should be referred to an orthopedic surgeon.

Delayed union: Delayed union occurs when a fracture is not healed after a time interval that is twice the normal healing time. For example, a fracture of the radius would be considered a delayed union if it has not healed in 4 months because it has an expected healing time of 2 months.

Nonunion: The bone has not united after three times the normal healing time. For example, a distal radius fracture is expected to heal completely in 2 months. If it has not healed in three times that amount, or 6 months, it is considered a nonunion fracture.

Atrophic nonunion: A bone end near the fracture becomes pointed like a partially consumed peppermint stick or icicle without any sign of new bone formation.

Hypertrophic nonunion: The bone end forms new bone even though it is not united.

Malunion: A fracture has united with unacceptable angulation, rotation, or shortening.

FRACTURES IN ADULTS

Cervical Spine Fracture

The possibility of a cervical spine fracture being unstable with associated spinal cord complications should always be considered (in fact, most are unstable). The exceptions would be a certain spinous process fracture (clay shoveler's fracture) or a simple anterior wedge fracture (defined as <25% loss of vertebral body height and no

Box 190-1. Types of Casts*

Long-arm cast (see Fig. 187-7): Always begins at the level of the proximal palmar crease and ends at the upper two thirds of the humerus. It always holds the elbow in 90 degrees of flexion. It begins as a short-arm cast and is then extended in a second stage.

Short-arm cast (see Fig. 187-4): Always begins at the proximal palmar crease and ends just below the elbow crease.

Short-leg cast (see Fig. 187-5): Always begins at the tips of the toes with the ankle in a neutral position and extends up to just behind the knee, allowing the patient to bend the knee at least 90 degrees without pinching from the cast.

Long-leg cast (see Fig. 187-7F): Always extends from the tips of the toes up to the proximal thigh. A long-leg cast is always a combination of first applying the short-leg cast and then extending it into a long-leg cast as the second stage, just as for a long-arm cast application.

If the knee is in approximately 30 degrees of flexion, crutch walking is easier because the foot is out of the way on the non–weight-bearing side. The 30 degrees of flexion helps control rotation of the tibia and ankle; it also prevents the patient from walking on the cast. Without 30 degrees of flexion, no rotational control is present.

*See Chapter 187, Cast Immobilization and Upper Extremity Splinting.

subluxation on dynamic flexion-extension radiographs of the cervical spine). The clay shoveler's fracture is an avulsion of the tip of the spinous process of C6 or C7 due to stress on the interspinous ligaments. These cervical fractures require nothing more than a soft cervical collar and symptomatic management.

All patients with a suspected cervical spine fracture should have a three-view series of cervical spine radiographs: cross-table lateral, anteroposterior (AP), and open-mouth odontoid views. In most cases, the lateral view should be taken first to rule out an occult fracture before the neck is moved. Overall, this view provides 90% of the information regarding the stability of the spine. The radiologist, neurosurgeon, or orthopedist can review the radiographs to exclude any associated problems. It should be noted that even minor fractures seen on plain radiographs may be associated with significant ligamentous injuries that render the cervical spine unstable; consultation with a neurosurgeon or orthopedist is helpful.

Thoracolumbar Spine Fractures

A thoracolumbar spine fracture can generally be treated with symptomatic management, brief (24 to 48 hours) bed rest with serial neurologic monitoring, followed by back support (thoracolumbosacral orthosis [TLSO]) and rehabilitative exercises. Exceptions include evidence of instability such as loss of greater than 50% of the anterior vertebral height (compared with posterior vertebral body height), presence of more than 20 degrees of angulation, an increased space between the spinous processes, and disruption of the facet joints; these patients should generally be referred. Burst fractures or fractures associated with any sign of neurologic injury should also be referred for orthopedic or neurosurgical consultation to rule out instability (which may require surgical stabilization). An exception to the use of a TLSO is a compression fracture occurring in an osteoporotic patient; in such cases, a TLSO is usually unnecessary and may impair return to function in the elderly.

Fractures of the upper thoracic spine (T1 to T9) tend to be more stable because of attachments of the rib cage, which in turn are further stabilized at the sternum. Fractures of L2 to L5 tend to be more stable because of the larger vertebral bodies; fractures of L5 and S1 tend to be unstable because of the high-energy forces required to cause injury at this level. Transverse process fractures, usually at L2, L3, or L4, and spinous process fractures are usually benign and do not affect spine stability. With a transverse or spinous process fracture in the general region of the kidneys, the possibility of a renal contusion should be considered.

For possible thoracolumbar spine fractures, radiographs should include AP, lateral, and oblique views of the entire thoracolumbar spine (patients often have fractures at more than one level). When managing a compression fracture, serial radiographs should be obtained at 3, 6, and 12 weeks to rule out a progressive kyphotic deformity (>20 degrees of angulation). Computed tomography (CT) scanning is particularly helpful in diagnosing multiple or occult fractures or bony impingement on the spinal canal. Magnetic resonance imaging (MRI) is useful for evaluating soft tissue injury. When managing these fractures, an accompanying ileus is fairly common. Always consider radiographs of the lumbar spine in a patient who has a calcaneal fracture because the axial loading associated with such an injury is often associated with a lumbar spine fracture.

Pelvic Fractures

Pelvic fractures managed by primary care clinicians tend to occur in osteoporotic older patients due to a fall. Otherwise, pelvic fractures are usually the result of significant trauma in a motor vehicle accident or a fall from a considerable height. Most fractures of the pelvis are diagnosed on the AP view. Additional views to assess the pelvis include inlet, outlet, and oblique views of the acetabulum. If there is concern for acetabular involvement, obturator (45 degrees of internal rotation) and iliac (45 degrees of external rotation) oblique views should be obtained; a radiologist or orthopedist will usually be able to determine from these views whether any question remains of acetabular involvement. If the acetabulum is involved, the patient should generally be referred to an orthopedist. If comminution is present, CT can be used for further delineation. Orthopedic referral should also be considered if the pelvic ring is unstable. However, there must be two breaks in the pelvic ring, either from two fractures or a fracture plus a joint dislocation (usually the sacroiliac joint), for a pelvic fracture to be unstable. Fractures external to the pelvic ring are generally considered stable (Fig. 190-1).

If the pelvic fracture is considered stable, the patient can be treated with bed rest, analgesics, walking as tolerated, or full weight bearing with a walker. The pubic and ischial rami function only as tie rods for the anterior portions of the pelvis; they are not weight bearing. The typical older woman who falls and breaks her pelvis has a pubic or ischial ramus fracture only (see Fig. 190-1) and does not require either surgical intervention or bed rest. Otherwise, the length of bed rest is variable, usually from 2 to 4 weeks; the patient may sit as tolerated. During bed rest, gentle range of motion exercises of the lower extremities should be performed, especially in the elderly. Although walking may be uncomfortable, explain to the patient that it is not dangerous or harmful.

If the pelvic fracture occurs in an individual younger than 50 years of age or one involved in a motor vehicle accident, be prepared to resuscitate the patient because hemorrhagic shock is the major cause of death. Consider the possibility of bladder, urethral, or external genitalia injury, especially with anterior pelvic fractures and especially in men. Always palpate the sacroiliac joint to ensure that it is nontender and therefore not involved in the injury.

Intertrochanteric Femur Fracture

The intertrochanteric femur fracture (Fig. 190-2) is the most common type of hip fracture. Occurring between the greater and lesser trochanter of the proximal femur, this fracture does not

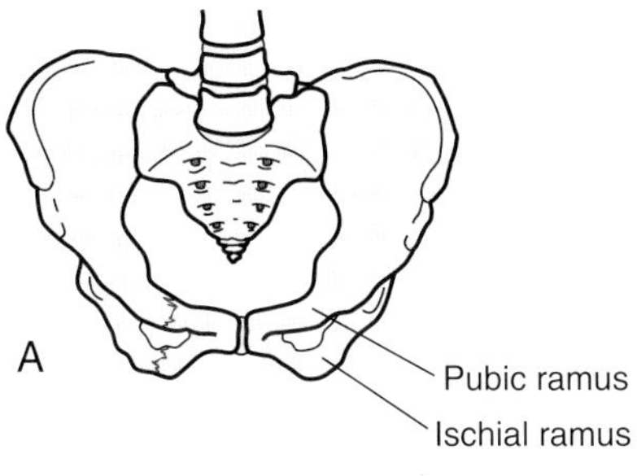

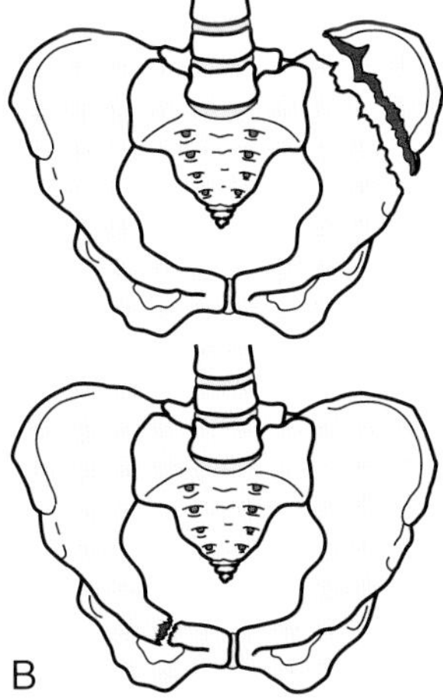

Figure 190-1 Stable pelvic fractures. **A,** Nondisplaced ramus fractures. **B,** Fracture of the pelvis not involving the ring (*top*). Stable, minimally displaced fracture of the ring (*bottom*).

involve the hip joint itself; it is an extra-articular, extracapsular fracture. The patient typically presents with a markedly shortened and externally rotated leg, painful with any movement of the hip. An intertrochanteric fracture usually results from the patient tripping over a carpet, pet, or step or slipping and falling; the force of the direct fall onto the intertrochanteric area causes the fracture. This scenario is entirely different from the femoral neck stress fracture discussed next. Repair of the intertrochanteric fracture requires hip pinning with a compression screw. It may require open reduction with use of a bone plate device to achieve near-anatomic alignment. Without repair, the intertrochanteric fracture, even if nondisplaced, is at high risk for displacement with such minor activities as rolling over or moving in bed. Therefore, if possible, these patients should be referred to an orthopedist for surgical repair. In the nonambulatory patient, such as the nursing home patient, nonoperative treatment may be a safer and less costly alternative. The patient should be managed symptomatically; Buck's traction can be used intermittently to reduce pain. The patient should be mobilized to a sitting position within 2 to 3 days. Nonoperative treatment for the ambulatory patient is a rare possibility; it is beyond the scope of this chapter.

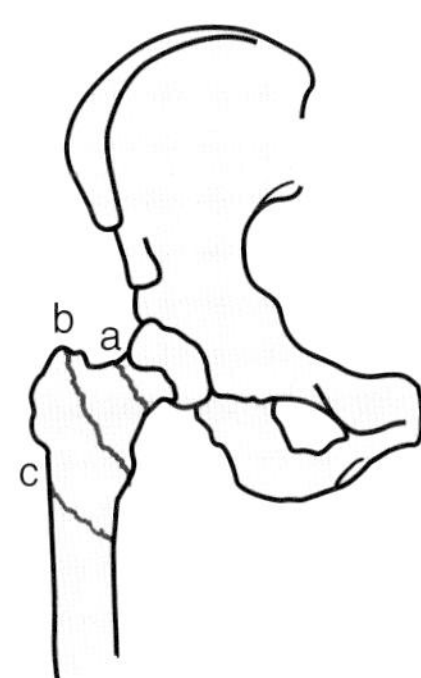

Figure 190-2 Fractures of the proximal femur: Neck (a); intertrochanteric (b); subtrochanteric (c).

Femoral Neck Fracture

Fracture of the femoral neck (see Fig. 190-2) is the second most common type of hip fracture. For a younger person to sustain a femoral neck fracture from trauma takes signficant force; therefore, most of these fractures occur in older osteoporotic patients, often while just walking in the home. The hip suddenly gives way, and the patient falls to the floor; no history of tripping over a carpet, pet, or step is usually reported and the patient does not know the reason for the fall. In most cases, an osteoporotic femoral neck fracture is actually a stress fracture, which ultimately becomes complete. As the fracture completes itself, it results in the instability that causes the patient to fall. Most of these fractures are displaced; therefore, appropriate treatment is prosthetic replacement (one half of a total hip). Occasionally, these fractures are nondisplaced and can be treated with pinning. Because the femoral neck (most of it) is intracapsular, the greater the displacement, the greater the risk of vascular compromise. Because of this tenuous blood supply, all femoral neck fractures should be monitored for the development of avascular necrosis, even if a prosthesis is placed.

If a patient does not have a history of falling but complains of pain in the groin aggravated by walking and weight bearing, rule out hip osteoarthritis with a weight-bearing radiograph. Always be certain to order a true lateral radiograph of the hip because it will often show a fracture not visible on the plain AP or "frog leg" AP view. If the hip joint is free of osteoarthritic findings, a diagnosis of impending stress fracture should be considered. In some patients, the fracture is not visible on the radiograph but can be observed on limited MRI. MRI is now considered the standard of care because it is more sensitive and specific than either a bone or CT scan for diagnosing femoral neck stress fractures. Nonathletes with nondisplaced stress fractures in progress demonstrated by bone scan or MRI can be treated with a walker and no weight bearing on the involved side. This treatment often allows the fracture to heal completely and prevents surgery.

Femoral neck stress fractures can also occur in athletes, and inguinal or anterior groin pain is the most frequent symptom. If the diagnosis is delayed, night pain can occur. On physical examination, discomfort is noted at the extremes of internal and external rotation, especially internal rotation. Compression-type stress fractures occur on the inferior medial border of the femoral neck and are considered more stable; tension-type stress fractures occur on the superior lateral border, are less stable, and are more prone to dislocate. Patients with an overt fracture line should be referred to an orthopedist. Conservative treatment consists of modified bed rest followed by assisted crutch-walking as tolerated until healing is seen (usually 6 weeks); cross-training with cycling or swimming will be helpful for maintaining fitness. Serial radiographs should be obtained every 1 to 2 weeks for the first month or at any time the patient stops improving; if sclerosis extends through both cortices or a crack develops, the patient should be referred. If the patient fails to heal with non-weight-bearing, he or she should be referred to an orthopedist. Otherwise, after 6 weeks, weight-bearing exercise can be resumed to preinjury levels over a span of 6 to 8 weeks; the patient should be able to walk a mile without pain before any running is allowed.

Femoral Shaft Fracture

Femoral shaft stress fractures can also occur in athletes. Lacking a history of trauma, the athlete often presents with vague thigh pain, diffuse tenderness, and a suspected quadriceps strain. These patients frequently wait 4 to 6 weeks following the onset of symptoms before seeking care; persistent, worsening symptoms finally bring them in. Fortunately, most femoral shaft stress fractures do not progress to complete fractures. Conservative care consists of relative rest with a switch to non-weight-bearing activities such as swimming or cycling for 6 to 8 weeks. Serial radiographs should be obtained and results managed as for a femoral neck stress fracture. Return to full activity can usually be anticipated after 3 to 4 months.

Other than stable stress fractures, femoral shaft fractures should always be referred for surgical stabilization. These fractures are at high risk for fat embolism and neurovascular problems. A distal femur fracture, which is often intra-articular (extending into the knee joint), should usually undergo surgery to stabilize the fracture, even if the fracture is nondisplaced.

Patellar Fractures

If the articular surface is smooth and the quadriceps mechanism intact, a nondisplaced patellar fracture (Fig. 190-3), whether comminuted or not, can be treated with a cylinder (from above malleoli to groin), full weight-bearing walking cast or with a knee immobilizer (in a reliable patient), crutches, and 10% partial weight-bearing activities. Consider referring severely comminuted fractures or fractures with more than 3 mm separation or more than 2 mm articular step-off to an orthopedist. Otherwise, a follow-up clinical examination is performed and AP and lateral radiographs assessed 3 weeks after initial treatment. If no displacement exists and tenderness with palpation is resolved, then gentle non-weight-bearing range of motion exercises can be started in an arc of 0 to 45 degrees. Another radiograph should be obtained 6 weeks after treatment; at this point, the fracture should be solidly healed and point tenderness over the patella resolved. Active and passive range of motion activities can now be initiated in therapy. During the healing phase, the patient should be encouraged to carry out quadriceps and hamstring isometric and straight-leg raising exercises to maintain muscle function and tone.

Marginal vertical fractures that are nondisplaced do not have to be immobilized. They can be treated with reduced activity for 4 to 6 weeks followed by progressive range of motion and strengthening exercises.

Tibial Plateau Fractures

The clinician should be certain that a tibial plateau fracture is not depressed or displaced, especially if it extends into the joint surface. Lateral, AP, and internal and external oblique radiographs should be obtained. A tunnel (notch) view is helpful for visualizing the intercondylar eminence. Tomograms are the only method to exclude displacement. CT will help delineate the extent of articular involvement and fracture displacement; MRI also provides this information and can detect ligamentous and meniscal injuries. If any depression or displacement has occurred, the patient must be referred; fractures associated with ligamentous or meniscal injury should also be referred. These referrals should generally occur within 24 to 48 hours.

If the fracture is extra-articularly displaced (intra-articularly nondisplaced), it can be treated with crutches, non-weight-bearing activities for 3 months, and gentle range of motion activities. Otherwise, the patient should remain non-weight-bearing for 4 to 6 weeks, until there is radiographic evidence of healing, and can then progress to partial weight bearing with crutches. Crutches should be used until solid union of the fracture is documented. These fractures need to be watched carefully with clinical examination and radiographs at 2-week intervals for the first month to be certain there is no displacement, which can occur with motion of the knee joint. Be certain to document the strength of the peroneal nerve.

Tibial Shaft Fractures

Tibial shaft fractures (Fig. 190-4) can be treated with a long-leg cast with the knee in 0 to 5 degrees of flexion and the ankle in neutral position (90 degrees). The patient can bear weight with this cast, and ambulation should be encouraged as soon as possible (as long as there is no risk for compartment syndrome [see Chapter 188, Compartment Syndrome Evaluation], which can occur at up to 10 days). As it turns out, most patients are not able to bear significant weight, due to discomfort, for 1 to 2 weeks.

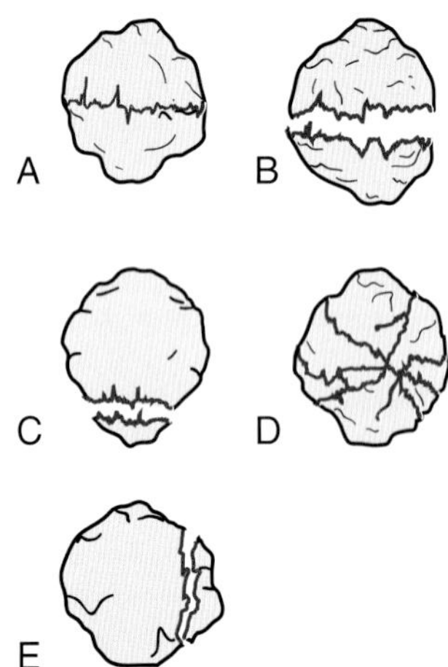

Figure 190-3 Classification of patellar fractures. **A,** Nondisplaced transverse. **B,** Displaced transverse. **C,** Upper or lower pole. **D,** Comminuted. **E,** Vertical.

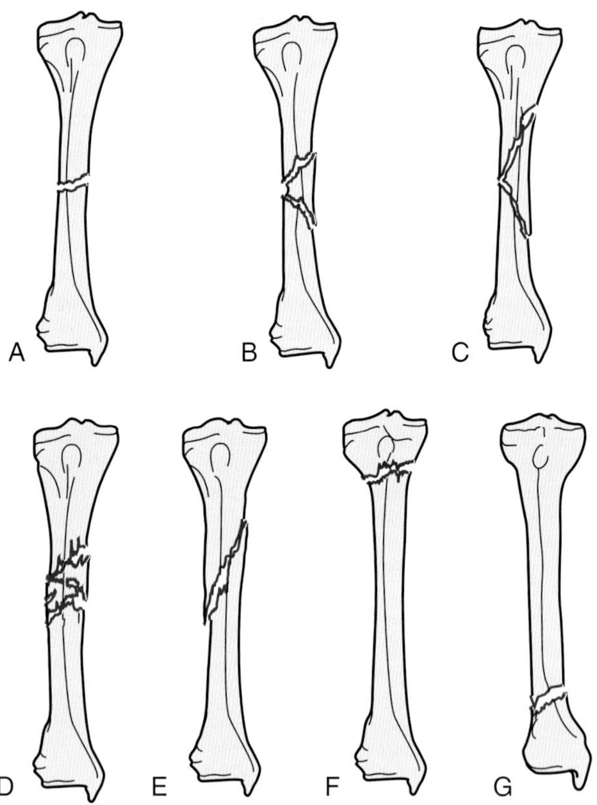

Figure 190-4 Tibial shaft fractures. **A,** Transverse or short oblique. **B,** Small butterfly fragment. **C,** Large butterfly fragment. **D,** Segmental comminution. **E,** Spiral. **F,** Proximal one fourth transverse or oblique. **G,** Distal one fourth transverse or oblique. The fracture in **A** is usually stable. The stability of the fractures shown in **B** and **C** is dependent on the size of the butterfly fragment. The fracture shown in **D** is usually unstable. The fractures shown in **E–G** are stable but difficult to control.

Proximal shaft fractures are often due to high-energy forces, but distal fractures are usually the result of low-energy injuries; this concept is important to consider during management. There should be less than 5 mm of *displacement* in both the AP and mediolateral planes; otherwise, the patient should be referred. If any *angulation* of the tibial shaft fracture has occurred, a *goniometer* must be used to assess the amount. Angulation up to 10 degrees in the AP radiograph and up to 5 degrees in the mediolateral plane is acceptable. Angulation greater than these amounts requires correction by wedging the cast; these patients should be referred.

If less than 50% bone surface contact between fracture fragments is observed in the AP or lateral views, then the patient should be referred to an orthopedic surgeon. Degree of *rotation* should be determined by the amount of discrepancy between transverse widths of the proximal and distal fragments; greater than 10 degrees of rotation should also be referred. *Shortening* greater than 2 cm is not acceptable and requires referral. If any doubt remains about the amount of overlap (which causes shortening), a bone length measurement radiograph can be obtained for the radiologist to compare the length of one tibia with the other.

For tibial fractures in which the fibula is not broken, very little chance exists of the tibia becoming unacceptably shortened because the fibula will splint the soft tissue at an appropriate length. *If the fibula is broken in addition to the tibia*, a higher incidence of shortening of the tibia exists as a result of unopposed muscle contraction. This is especially true in an oblique angle fracture; the oblique angle allows sliding of the fracture into a shortened position. If the fracture is transverse, then this sliding shortening cannot occur. Nevertheless, combined tibia–fibular fractures are frequently due to high-impact forces, are at high risk for compartment syndrome, and are rarely nondisplaced; these patients are frequently referred.

If the fracture is satisfactory in alignment and length, then a long-leg cast for a period of 4 to 6 weeks is appropriate. For the initial cast, plaster is usually easier to mold; fiberglass reinforcement can then be applied in a few days if this cast is left in place. The cast will usually need to be changed in 2 to 3 weeks because of loosening as the swelling decreases. After 4 to 6 weeks, the cast can be cut down to a short-leg walking cast or a walking cast brace for an additional 10 to 14 weeks, until clinically healed. To verify clinical healing, there should be minimal tenderness over the fracture site and no motion or pain with bending stress in any direction.

Tibial fractures are notorious for developing *compartment syndrome* (see Chapter 188, Compartment Syndrome Evaluation) when any significant soft tissue trauma has occurred. If the tibial fracture is the result of a fall from a height greater than 6 feet or the result of a high-velocity injury such as in an automobile accident, be very cautious about the possibility of compartment syndrome. Be certain that the patient elevates the leg at home so that the calf is 2 feet higher than the heart at all times, except when going to the bathroom, for 1 week. Explain to the patient that the heart is the pump, and that the fluid from the leg needs to drain toward the pump, which requires the fluid in the leg to be elevated higher than the pump. Seat cushions from the couch stacked three high under the calf can help achieve this elevation. The patient's chest must be flat, although pillows can be placed under the head to facilitate reading and eating. Sitting in a recliner, however, does not provide adequate elevation because the chest is only at the level of the calf.

Patients at risk for compartment syndrome may use their crutches to go to the bathroom, placing no weight on the injured side. They should return to the bed, couch, or floor, lie down, and resume elevation of the leg as soon as possible. If there is loss of fine-touch sensation or two-point discrimination, distention and swelling of the calf, pain with passive motion of muscle groups (especially extension of the great toe), progressive pain, or pain not relieved by oral pain medication such as narcotics, then emergent testing should be performed or referral made to rule out compartment syndrome (see Chapter 188, Compartment Syndrome Evaluation). *The peak time for compartment syndrome after a tibial fracture is on the third day after the injury.*

Tibial stress fractures are one of the most common stress fractures in young athletes and military recruits. They occur more commonly at the junction of the middle and distal thirds of the tibia in runners, in the middle third in ballet dancers, and in the proximal third in military recruits. Symptoms are usually insidious in onset, increase with physical activity, and may become severe enough to persist for hours after activity or even at night. There is usually pain with palpation but minimal swelling at the site of tenderness. However, pain can often be elicited at the site by applying a tuning fork or by percussing the tibia away from the site. Radiographs are frequently negative for 2 to 4 weeks after the onset of symptoms; a triple-phase bone scan can be helpful if a stress fracture is strongly suspected. Most tibial stress fractures are treated with elimination of impact activity for 4 to 6 weeks, cross-training, and crutches as needed for pain. Radiographs should be taken monthly to document healing.

Radiographs may demonstrate the "dreaded black line" fracture, which is an anterior midshaft tibial stress fracture associated with poor healing, a risk of nonunion, and risk of recurrence. These fractures typically take 6 to 12 months to heal; patients must refrain from impact loading activities until they are pain-free and there is complete radiographic healing.

Fibular Shaft Fractures

Fibular shaft fractures require no immobilization or restriction of weight-bearing activities, other than for pain management, because the fibula supports only 15% of the weight in the lower extremity. In fact, the fibula can be used elsewhere as a bone graft without a problem. *Fibular fractures, however, rarely occur alone*. Always check for associated injury around the ankle, over the medial and lateral collateral ligaments, and the tibiofibular distal joint. It is common for a severe ankle-twisting injury to result in a small fracture around the ankle and an associated fracture somewhere along the fibula, including the proximal fibula (Maisonneuve fracture). Isolated fibular fractures can occur from a direct blow to the side of the calf. Again, these fractures require no immobilization or restriction of weight-bearing activities and almost always heal uneventfully within 6 to 8 weeks. Use of a stirrup splint, a short-leg walking cast, or a cast boot for 3 to 4 weeks may help relieve moderate to severe pain.

Always evaluate the function of the peroneal nerve when treating a fibular fracture by documenting the strength of active foot flexion and extension at the ankle, as well as eversion. If the peroneal nerve is affected, document this and consider referral to an orthopedist. Also consider referral for severely displaced or comminuted fractures, ligament instability, or painful nonunion after treatment.

Ankle Fractures

Point tenderness over the lateral malleolus (distal fibula) or medial malleolus (distal tibia) often indicates an ankle fracture as opposed to a sprain. The area of the posterior malleolus (distal tibia, immediately behind the medial malleolus) should also be palpated for tenderness. If no point tenderness is felt over the malleoli, then an x-ray is rarely necessary. This decision is supported by the Ottawa Ankle Rules, which indicate a radiograph is most predictive of fracture if the patient has pain over the malleolus *and* tenderness over the malleolus *or* the patient was unable to bear weight immediately at the time of injury *and* at the initial clinician visit. Point tenderness over the anterior and lateral ligaments (anterior talofibular and lateral calcaneofibular ligament), but not the fibula, indicates an ankle sprain. A *first-degree ankle sprain* will have tenderness only over the anterior talofibular ligament, whereas a *second- or third-degree ankle sprain* has tenderness over the talofibular and calcaneofibular ligaments.

If ankle radiographs are indicated, obtain lateral, AP, and mortise (AP view with the foot in 15 degrees of adduction) views. The ankle mortise is the joint space between the top of the talus and the bottom of the tibia, as well as the medial and lateral malleoli. There should be symmetrical spacing throughout the mortise; in other words, there should be less than 1 mm of displacement of the talus in any direction greater than elsewhere in the mortise. A nondisplaced fracture of the ankle is frequently seen in only one radiographic view of the ankle.

Small avulsion fractures, nondisplaced single malleolar fractures, and stable bimalleolar fractures can be treated nonoperatively. Small, nondisplaced avulsion fractures are treated with early mobilization and weight bearing, as tolerated, similar to an ankle sprain. A functional stirrup splint worn in a shoe may be adequate; functional rehabilitation exercises can be started as soon as symptoms allow. Unstable fractures (e.g., malleolar fracture with ligament disruption on the opposite side), displaced single malleolar, large (>25% of articular surface) or displaced (>2 mm) posterior malleolar, or trimalleolar (bilateral plus posterior malleolar) fractures (or if clinician is unsure about the stability of the fracture) should be referred. Otherwise, medial and lateral malleolar fractures require a minimum of 4 weeks for clinical healing and possibly several months for radiographic healing. When following an ankle fracture with radiographs, the mortise view should always be examined for evidence of new instability or a shift.

If the patient smokes, the fracture healing time can be doubled; it can also be delayed in patients who are taking anti-inflammatory medications. Patients should be informed that the incidence of *reflex sympathetic dystrophy* (see Complications section) after any injury in this area, including a fracture, is much higher when they smoke.

NOTE: A cast boot should be prescribed for any patient wearing a short-leg splint or cast or a long-leg splint or cast. The cast boot protects the toes and cast and prevents material from slipping through the end of the cast and up underneath the foot.

Medial and Posterior Malleolar (Distal Tibia) Fractures

If an isolated medial or small (<25% of the articular surface) posterior malleolar fracture is shown to be nondisplaced in the lateral, AP, and mortise views of the ankle, treatment with a short-leg weight-bearing cast (or walking fracture boot in a trusted, compliant patient) is appropriate. (Suspect Maisonneuve fracture in isolated posterior malleolar fracture.) The ankle should be immobilized in the neutral (90 degrees) position to minimize Achilles tendon shortening. The patient should be seen again in 2 weeks to assess the condition of the cast (or compliance with the walking boot) and at 4 weeks to repeat radiographs. If the initial fracture line is below (distal to) the level of the ankle mortise, immediate full weight-bearing activities may be allowed, as tolerated. If the fracture is at or above the ankle mortise, and at 4 weeks is clinically healing (nontender over the fracture site and some evidence of radiographic healing such as callus formation), the patient may begin gradual weight bearing and ankle rehabilitation. If no radiographic evidence of healing is apparent at 4 weeks, the patient should remain in the cast another 2 weeks and return for repeat radiographs. At that point, if the patient is still not clinically healed, a fracture boot should be worn, and walking and ankle rehabilitation initiated.

Lateral Malleolar (Distal Fibula) Fractures

There are three types of fractures in the distal third of the fibula. Because these fractures can be associated with a medial ligament injury and subsequent instability, repeat radiographs should be obtained in 7 to 10 days to assess fracture alignment and the position of the mortise. A *Weber A* fracture occurs below the level of the ankle mortise and can be treated with an immediate weight-bearing short-leg cast or fracture boot for 6 weeks. A *Weber B* fracture occurs at the level of the ankle mortise. Again, if the lateral, AP, and mortise x-ray views show the fracture to be nondisplaced, it can be treated with a short-leg walking cast for 6 weeks. Because this fracture is at the level of the ankle mortise, weight bearing should not be allowed for the first 2 weeks. This restriction decreases stress at the ankle mortise, which could cause displacement at the fracture site. A *Weber C* distal fibular fracture occurs above the ankle mortise and has the greatest potential for displacement. This fracture disrupts a portion of the syndesmotic ligament area between the tibia and fibula distally, just above the ankle mortise. This fracture is also treated in a walking cast for 6 weeks with no weight bearing during the first 3 weeks.

Talar Fractures

Minor anterior and posterior avulsion fractures of the talus are occasionally seen in association with ankle injuries. Lateral avulsion fractures, just distal to the tip of the distal fibula, are occasionally seen in snowboarders (snowboarder's fracture) and can be large and comminuted. Small (<0.5 cm), nondisplaced, anterior and posterior avulsion fractures are treated with a short-leg walking cast for 1 month followed by range of motion, stretching, and strengthening rehabilitation exercises. Anterior avulsion fractures should be cast with the ankle in the neutral position (90 degrees); posterior avulsion fractures benefit from being cast in 15 degrees of equinus (plantar flexion), which allows tiptoe weight bearing. Small (<2 mm), nondisplaced, noncomminuted lateral avulsion fractures are probably best managed in a short-leg, non-weight-bearing cast for 4 weeks followed by 2 weeks of progressive weight bearing in a walking cast or cast boot. If displacement has occurred for an avulsion fracture, or the fragment is large or comminuted, the patient should be referred to an orthopedic surgeon.

Prolonged pain (several weeks to months) following an inversion injury of the ankle, often associated with point tenderness in the area, decreased range of motion, crepitus, and an effusion, should lead the clinician to suspect an osteochondral talar dome fracture. If plain films show no abnormality, a bone scan is highly effective for detecting these fractures. For positive bone scans, an MRI is effective at determining the exact location and stage. Symptomatic stage I (compressed, nondisplaced) and stage II (attached, nondisplaced) osteochondral talar dome fractures typically respond well to conservative treatment with immobilization for 6 to 8 weeks in a non-weight-bearing cast followed by rehabilitation; referral should be considered if symptoms persist after 4 to 6 months of conservative therapy. Stage III (detached, nondisplaced) and stage IV (displaced) talar dome fractures are best treated with early operative care (often just arthroscopy). Talar head fractures can be treated with a short-leg walking cast for 6 to 8 weeks followed by longitudinal arch support for several more weeks. Patients should be warned that this fracture may be complicated by persistent pain due to post-traumatic arthritis in the talonavicular joint.

The patient should be aware that despite perfect reduction, healing is often complicated by avascular necrosis in fractures of the talar neck and body. The nonunion rate may be as high as 50%, and there is an associated high incidence of osteoarthritis. Talar fractures are second only to scaphoid (navicular) fractures in the wrist as a site for chronic postfracture complications and pain. That said, nondisplaced talar neck fractures can be treated with a non-weight-bearing short-leg cast for 4 to 6 weeks followed by a short-leg walking cast for an additional 4 weeks. If there is no radiographic evidence of fracture union at 6 weeks, radiographs should be repeated every 2 to 3 weeks and the patient should remain in a walking cast until union is documented. CT scanning may be necessary to demonstrate fracture union. Nondisplaced talar body fractures should be immobilized in a short-leg non-weight-bearing cast for 6 to 8 weeks. All patients with a talar fracture should be instructed in range of motion, stretching, and strengthening rehabilitation exercises following cast removal. Patients should be seen 2 to 3 weeks into such a rehabilitation program and then followed until there is near-normal function.

Calcaneal Fractures

Obtain axial, lateral, and dorsoplantar radiographs of the calcaneus for suspected fractures. Comparison views of the opposite side may be helpful for diagnosing bilateral fractures (common) as well as for measuring anatomic angles. Oblique views may also be helpful. If any doubt remains about displacement, obtain a CT scan. A radiologist or orthopedist can offer suggestions about the need to obtain a CT scan after viewing the plain radiographs. Intra-articular (subtalar joint) fractures (approximately 70% of calcaneal fractures) or displaced extra-articular fractures should generally be referred to an orthopedist.

If the vertical forces were significant enough to cause a calcaneal fracture (e.g., a fall from a height), a radiograph of the thoracic and lumbar spine should also be obtained; there is a high incidence of associated axial fractures (e.g., thoracic and lumbar spine fractures). The clinician must also palpate the thoracic and lumbar spine for signs of tenderness in these patients.

For a nonarticular, nondisplaced fracture of the calcaneal body, pain management, treatment with a bulky compression soft wrap, and elevation are all that is needed. These fractures generally heal well regardless of treatment. Early, gentle, yet active range of motion exercises of the foot and ankle are appropriate to minimize the stiffness associated with these fractures. Maximal elevation is critical to minimize swelling and pain; swelling can be significant, even causing blisters or skin loss with subsequent infection. Elevation with the patient lying down and the hip and knee both flexed to 90 degrees with couch cushions under the calf is the best management for the first week. Patients may be up on crutches only to go to the bathroom; otherwise, they should be supine with the leg elevated.

AUTHOR'S NOTE: If the patient is not instructed to keep the hip and knee bent 90 degrees with elevation, he or she may complain of sciatica. When pillows or blankets are placed only underneath the heel, the knee remains straight and can result in the sciatic nerve being stretched.

For extra-articular fractures of the anterior, medial, or lateral calcaneal processes, the patient should be placed in a short-leg walking cast for 4 weeks. Fractures of the tuberosity or sustentaculum tali should be managed with a short-leg non-weight-bearing cast for 6 to 8 weeks. Tuberosity fractures should be cast in 5 to 10 degrees of equinus (plantar flexion) and repeat radiographs obtained at 1 week to check for alignment. The patient should be seen every 2 to 4 weeks for management of all of these fractures.

Midfoot Tarsal Bone (Cuneiforms, Cuboid, and Navicular) Fractures

Lateral, AP, and oblique radiographs should be obtained for suspected midfoot fractures. For nondisplaced fractures, apply a short-leg walking cast for weight-bearing activities as tolerated after the first week. For most, the cast should be in place for 4 to 6 weeks; fractures of the navicular body may benefit from casting for 8 weeks total. For nonunion of a navicular tuberosity fracture, 8 to 10 weeks of casting may be necessary. If fractures are displaced, severely comminuted, or there is nonunion of the navicular tuberosity after 10 weeks, or if there is a concomitant joint dislocation, refer the patient to an orthopedic surgeon.

Beware of a fracture or dislocation of the *Lisfranc joint,* which extends into the tarsometatarsal joint at the midfoot and occurs when an athlete falls forward on a plantar-flexed foot. To prevent future disability, it is critical to diagnose an unstable fracture of this area, so always obtain routine as well as weight-bearing lateral and AP radiographs for injuries to the bridge of the foot. Also suspect a Lis-franc injury when there is an avulsion "fleck" fracture of the lateral proximal first metatarsal or the medial proximal second metatarsal. The joint may appear nondislocated on the AP view; however, on the lateral view, anterior displacement may be observed. On the weight-bearing AP radiograph, widening may appear between the first and second metatarsals; on the weight-bearing lateral radiograph, a stepoff (evidence of joint disruption) between the tarsal and proximal metatarsal may appear. A CT scan can be used to confirm the diagnosis. If any questions remain about an injury to the midfoot or about the radiographic views, ask a radiologist or orthopedic surgeon to review the films. These fractures are rare because of the rigidity of the midfoot.

Metatarsal Fractures

The most common metatarsal fracture is at the base of the fifth metatarsal, and represents an avulsion fracture of the styloid where the peroneus brevis tendon inserts. With an inversion sprain-type injury to the forefoot and ankle, a small piece of bone can be pulled loose. The displacement is usually no greater than 3 mm; it is treated with a firm or wooden-soled fracture shoe with weight bearing as tolerated, and ice and elevation for comfort. The purpose of the wooden-soled shoe is to prevent flexion at the midfoot when the patient walks, thereby preventing stress at the fracture site. The wooden-soled shoe is worn for 3 weeks or longer until the patient is comfortable without it and can return to wearing a regular shoe. However, impact sports should be avoided for a minimum of 2 months.

A metatarsal avulsion fracture must be differentiated from a *Jones fracture,* which is much less common and treated entirely differently. A Jones fracture occurs in nearly the same location; however, it extends (if not initially, eventually) across the entire shaft just distal to the base of the fifth metatarsal and into the joint between the bases of the fourth and fifth metatarsals. If the fracture is displaced, the patient should be referred to an orthopedic surgeon. If nondisplaced, treatment includes a short-leg walking cast for 6 to 8 weeks with no weight bearing for the first 3 weeks. At this point, if neither clinical nor radiographic healing is apparent, a non-weight-bearing cast should be reapplied for 4 more weeks or the patient referred. This fracture is notorious for delayed union, especially in patients who smoke or take anti-inflammatory medications. No impact sports should be allowed after this injury for a minimum of 3 months.

A stress fracture of the fifth metatarsal can be confused with a Jones fracture, but it typically occurs in the proximal shaft. This fracture is also notoriously slow to heal. Although referral is not necessary in every case, referral should be considered because optimal conditions may require up to 20 weeks of immobilization and nonunion may still occur. With intramedullary screw fixation, the athlete may return to his or her sport much earlier. Stress fractures of the other metatarsal shafts are much more common and usually less severe. Symptoms may precede radiographic findings by 2 to 3 weeks. In most cases, these fractures can be managed without casting; merely eliminating impact (e.g., running, jumping) until clinical healing is documented is sufficient.

Nondisplaced fractures of metatarsal shafts can be treated with wooden-soled shoes. If there is significant pain (e.g., first metatarsal, multiple fractures), the patient can be in a short-leg walking cast for 4 to 7 weeks and minimize weight bearing for the first 2 to 3 weeks. Most displaced fractures of the first metatarsal should be referred. Patients with displaced fractures of multiple metatarsals, displaced fractures close to the metatarsal heads, and intra-articular fractures are probably best referred for pin fixation. Otherwise, fractures of the second through fourth metatarsals that are displaced only in the lateral or medial plane do not usually require reduction. Fractures of the second through fourth metatarsal shafts displaced more than 3 or 4 mm or angulated greater than 10 degrees in the dorsal or plantar plane should be reduced or referred. These fractures can often be reduced under local anesthesia hematoma block using Chinese finger (toe) traps and gravity or 2 to 5 lb of weight. After reduction, a short-leg walking cast can be used for 5 to 7 weeks with no weight bearing the first 2 to 3 weeks.

Although rare, clinicians must beware of *compartment syndrome* in the foot. This can occur with multiple fractures (e.g., three or more metatarsals) from a crushing-type injury, and resultant extreme swelling.

Toe Fractures

For the great toe, displaced intra-articular fractures and fractures that spontaneously become displaced when traction is released after reduction may benefit from internal fixation, so these patients should generally be referred. For the other toes, fracture dislocations and intra-articular fractures that involve more than 25% of the joint surface may benefit from referral. Otherwise, rarely is a surgical intervention required. Displaced fractures can be managed by reduction under digital block anesthesia followed by manual traction, pulling the toe into a corrected position. Many authorities recommend a short-leg walking cast with a toe platform for 2 to 3 weeks for fractures of the great toe followed by buddy taping and a wooden-soled shoe. For fractures of other toes, buddy taping to an adjacent toe for 3 to 6 weeks will stabilize the fracture. Use of wooden-soled shoes for 2 to 3 weeks, ice, and elevation may decrease pain. When taping digits together (fingers or toes), place dry cotton or gauze between them to prevent skin maceration from moisture. Patients can change this dressing after a shower and watch the alignment of the nail beds for development of a rotational deformity, which can be surgically repaired. Patients should be followed by the clinician every 2 to 4 weeks. Follow-up radiographs are generally not needed except for fractures of the great toe or intra-articular fractures.

Fractures in the distal phalanges of the fingers or toes sometimes involve injury to the nail bed or an open fracture caused by the bone pushing up through the nail bed. In these patients, the treatment should be digital block anesthesia followed by removal of the nail to irrigate the nail bed thoroughly at the site of the open fracture. The nail bed can be repaired with 5-0 absorbable suture, which will minimize nail deformity. Nail bed repair is usually more desirable for the fingers because many individuals will accept deformity of a nail plate in a toe but are concerned about a cosmetic deformity in a finger (see Chapter 27, Nail Bed Repair).

Clavicle Fractures

Because outcomes are basically the same, treatment for fractures of the clavicle is generally whatever best relieves the symptoms. Possibilities include a figure-eight brace or sling, both, or neither, depending on the patient's comfort level (see Fig. 190-8). Other considerations include whether the patient lives alone and can adjust a figure-eight; as opposed to a sling, use of a figure-eight also leaves the elbow and hand free for daily activities. If the fracture site produces pressure and tenting of the skin, refer the patient for possible surgery. Because nonunion of middle third (midshaft) fractures is rare (<1%), such fractures rarely require referral (usually only for symptomatic nonunion after 12 to 16 weeks). Inner third (proximal) clavicular fractures need be referred only if there is significant displacement or an associated sternoclavicular dislocation. Distal third (lateral) clavicular fractures should be referred if the coracoclavicular ligament is torn and the proximal fragment displaced (type IIB, Fig. 190-5). Because distal third fractures that extend into the acromioclavicular joint can lead to future degenerative changes in that joint, some primary care clinicians also refer these fractures (type III, see Fig. 190-5). Otherwise, symptomatic therapy is indicated for most clavicular fractures.

Clavicular fractures require a minimum of 2 months for solid union, and contact sports should be avoided for 8 to 10 weeks. (Do not be dismayed if the 1-month follow-up x-ray shows no sign of healing! In fact, this x-ray can be omitted if there are no new symptoms.) Patients should be seen every 2 to 3 weeks; radiographs are indicated only after clinical union (nontender locally and with full range of motion) has occurred or for late development of symptoms. Remember to adjust the figure-eight splint to ensure that it is tight enough to be supportive and keep the shoulders back ("position of attention"), yet loose enough to avoid tingling and numbness from

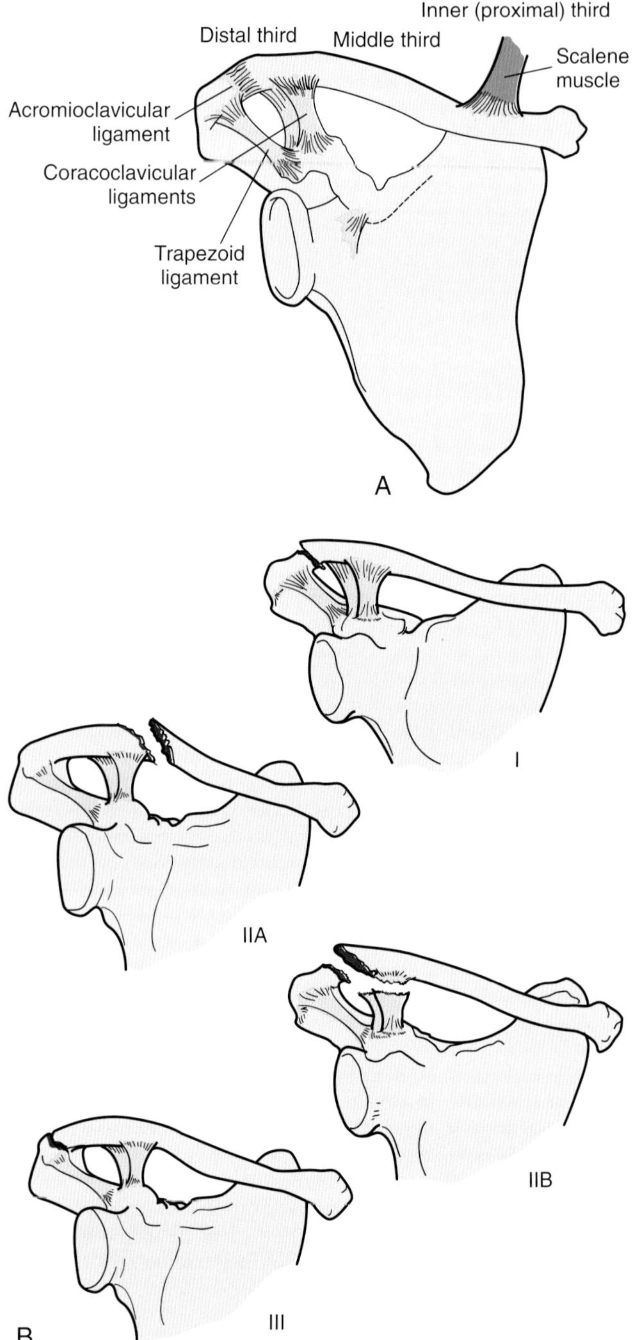

Figure 190-5 Clavicle fractures. **A,** Fractures of the clavicle are classified by location into the distal (15%), middle (80%), and inner (proximal) (5%) thirds. Clavicle fractures can be nondisplaced, displaced, angulated, or nonangulated. **B,** Classification of fractures of the distal third of the clavicle (Allman). Type I: minimal displacement with ligaments intact. Type IIA: proximal shaft is displaced with ligaments intact. Type IIB: clavicle displaced, coracoclavicular ligament ruptured but trapezoid ligament intact. Type III: fracture of the articular surface with no disruption of the ligaments.

pressure on the brachial plexus where the splint wraps around the armpit. Instruct the patient to loosen or tighten the brace for more support, if needed, or to reduce restriction if tingling and numbness occur. It should be worn until there is no more tenderness or crepitus at the fracture site.

For clavicular fractures, always listen to the chest to exclude a pneumothorax, especially for fractures due to motor vehicle accidents. A chest x-ray is also appropriate. Instruct the patient to report any shortness of breath immediately.

Scapular Fractures

The scapula is covered on all sides with muscle and has an excellent blood supply; therefore, fractures of the scapula (Fig. 190-6) heal extremely well, even when displaced. Most fractures of the scapula need only a sling or shoulder immobilizer for comfort for 2 weeks. Even these measures may not be needed for fractures of the scapular spine, body, or coracoid. For suspected scapular fractures, always obtain a true AP of the glenohumeral (shoulder) joint, an axillary view, and a true lateral scapular Y view. These views will help exclude any intra-articular extension into the glenoid shoulder socket. (A cephalic tilt view can help evaluate the coracoid process.) If any questions remain about a fracture being intra-articular or displaced at the glenoid, a CT scan should be obtained. Significantly displaced coracoid fractures, especially if combined with a complete acromioclavicular separation, displaced acromion fractures, displaced glenoid neck fractures associated with a clavicular fracture, and glenoid fractures involving more than 25% of the articular surface (or those with an associated subluxed humeral head) should be referred. For all others, early range of motion activities should be encouraged, as tolerated. Patients should be seen every 2 to 4 weeks to ensure adequate progress in their rehabilitation program. Evidence of radiographic healing should be present before resistance exercises are initiated.

Proximal Humerus Fractures

After obtaining true AP and lateral scapular Y or axillary views, fractures of the proximal humerus can be classified by the Neer system (Fig. 190-7) and are considered a one-part fracture if they are displaced less than 1 cm or angulated less than 45 degrees. Patients with fractures displaced more than 1 cm (the minority of fractures) or associated with joint instability or a dislocation should generally be referred. Fractures involving the bicipital groove may interfere with function and therefore also probably warrant referral. Angulation up to 45 degrees is tolerated amazingly well by most individuals, so referral is necessary only for greater angulation; however, athletic or very active individuals may warrant consultation when angulation approaches 20 degrees. Most fractures in older patients are immediately below the tubercles, in the area of the surgical neck, which generally has a good blood supply (as opposed to the anatomic neck, immediately beneath the humeral head). As long as there is at least 50% overlap of fracture segments on the AP and scapular Y views, treatment with a shoulder immobilizer for 2 weeks is appropriate, followed by gentle passive and active assistive range of motion exercises to minimize stiffness (Fig. 190-8). The shoulder immobilizer is worn 24 hours a day, except when performing physical therapy or exercise. The shoulder immobilizer prevents displacement of the fracture at night while sleeping. Remind the patient not to use the arm for heavy activity during the day. Protection of the shoulder for these fractures is appropriate for a total of 6 weeks before returning to regular activities.

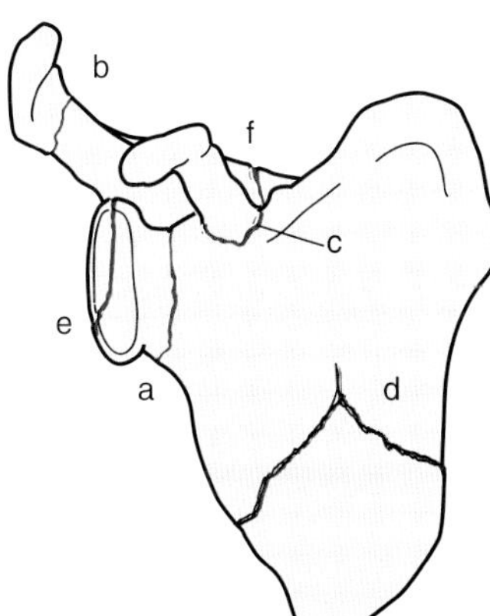

Figure 190-6 Scapular fractures (anterior view): neck (a); acromion process (b); coracoid process (c); body (d); glenoid rim or articular cartilage (e); spinous process (f), which is posterior and only partially seen here.

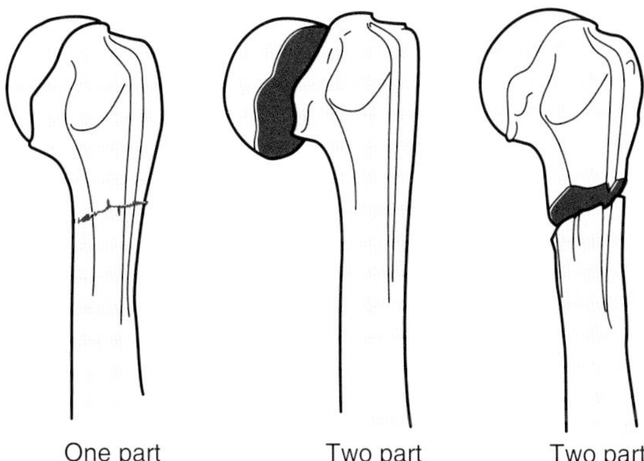

Figure 190-7 Neer classification of proximal humerus fractures. One-part or minimally displaced fracture is defined as no segments displaced more than 1.0 cm or angulated more than 45 degrees. A two-part fracture is defined as one segment displaced more than 1.0 cm or angulated more than 45 degrees.

In all fractures, palpation for resolution of point tenderness at the fracture site is a very reliable clinical index of solid fracture union. This finding combined with radiographic union determines when patients can return to full activity without restriction.

Humeral Shaft Fractures

Humeral shaft fractures are unique in the amount of angulation (of a long bone) that can be allowed; they are also unique in their excellent healing rate (low incidence of nonunion) for long bone shaft fractures. These distinctions are due to the excellent blood supply provided, in part, by a large amount of surrounding muscle tissue. This surrounding muscle tissue can also shelter significant angulation with little resultant cosmetic defect.

For these reasons, and because the shoulder and elbow have excellent motion, up to 30 degrees of mediolateral angulation, up to 20 degrees of anteroposterior angulation, and displacement of up to half the width of the humerus are acceptable when treating a humeral shaft fracture. Treatment consists of a hanging arm cast (see Fig. 190-8F) that extends from the humerus, around the elbow flexed at 90 degrees, and down to the wrist. This position is maintained until callus formation is detected and the fracture site is stable to manual stress, which can take from 8 to 14 weeks. Alternatively, if there is radiographic evidence of healing at 1 month and decreased tenderness at the fracture site, the hanging arm cast can be removed and a functional humerus cast brace (Fig. 190-9) applied.

Made from polyethylene, functional humerus cast braces are available "off the shelf" at local brace supply shops. They wrap around the midshaft of the humerus and provide circumferential compression of the muscle belly, resulting in some hydraulic stabilization at the fracture site. The patient may move the shoulder and elbow in the brace and begin using the arm with such light activities as eating, brushing the teeth, and reading a newspaper. When

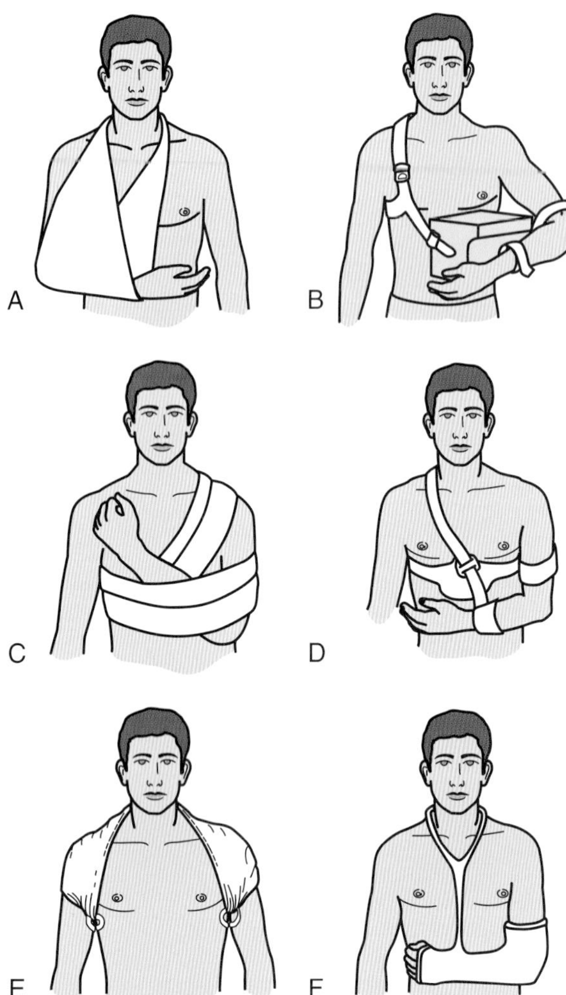

Figure 190-8 Possible methods of immobilization of the shoulder. **A,** Simple shoulder sling is used for humerus, clavicle, and radial head fractures. **B,** Abduction pillow shoulder immobilizer is used for rotator cuff tendon tear after surgery. **C,** Sling and swathe bandage is used for severe acromioclavicular separation and fractures of upper humerus. **D,** Shoulder immobilizer is used for humeral neck fractures. **E,** Figure-of-eight strap for fractures of the clavicle. **F,** The hanging arm cast is used for humeral neck and humeral shaft fractures. It provides weight and traction to align the fracture "pieces."

immobilized, even for a short period, the elbow is notorious for becoming stiff with possible permanent limitation of motion. For this reason, any time the elbow is immobilized for treatment of a humeral fracture at the shaft or shoulder, encourage the patient to adjust the brace and allow the elbow to hang straight in full extension for 15 minutes each day.

When managing these fractures, weekly radiographs are recommended for the first 4 to 6 weeks, until it is clear that the fracture fragments are not moving appreciably. At that point, the patient can be seen and radiographs repeated every 2 weeks until a satisfactory functional result is obtained.

At the time of the fracture, patients with neurovascular deficits should be referred emergently; surgical exploration may be necessary. Although radial nerve exploration is not always indicated when radial nerve function is absent or weak (e.g., weakness in finger or wrist extension), many primary care clinicians will refer in this situation. (As it turns out, radial nerve function almost always returns during the 6 months following an injury, but neither the clinician nor the patient may be willing to wait.) If the patient's radial nerve function is initially normal but becomes impaired after

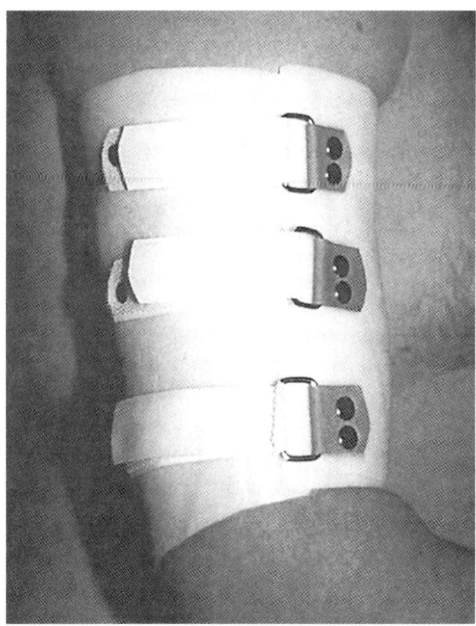

Figure 190-9 Functional humerus cast or fracture brace. (Courtesy of AliMed, Inc., Dedham, MA.)

splinting or casting, the splint or cast should be removed, a brace or shoulder immobilizer applied, and the patient referred to an orthopedist for evaluation and treatment. Other indications for referral at the time of the fracture include pathologic fractures, associated elbow injuries, and the presence of multiple injuries.

Supracondylar and Transcondylar Humeral Fractures

Nondisplaced or minimally displaced (<20 degrees apex anterior angulation on lateral x-ray) supracondylar and transcondylar fractures (Fig. 190-10) can be treated with a posterior long-arm, fiberglass, one-step prepadded splint. The elbow should be held at 90 degrees of flexion, and a shoulder immobilizer (see Fig. 190-8D) used. The distal pulses should be checked after splint application; if absent, the elbow should be extended until they return. True AP and lateral radiographs of the distal humerus should be obtained after immobilization to confirm that no displacement occurred during efforts to immobilize. During the first 7 to 10 days, frequent checks of neurovascular function are necessary. Follow-up radiographs should be reviewed weekly for the first 2 to 3 weeks, and then every 2 weeks until callus formation is seen. When significant tenderness is no longer felt at the fracture site, the splint can be removed to allow gentle range of motion activities (usually at 2 weeks). The patient should be instructed to avoid any passive motion at the elbow because it will predispose the elbow to ectopic bone formation and permanent stiffness. The splint is used for protection until adequate callus forms (usually 6 to 8 weeks), but is removed for showers, bathing, and gentle exercise, usually starting 2 weeks after the injury.

Intercondylar Fractures

Displaced intercondylar fractures (see Fig. 190-10A) are unstable and should be referred to an orthopedic surgeon. Nondisplaced fractures should be managed the same as nondisplaced supracondylar or transcondylar fractures; however, the risk of neurovascular compromise is less, so the patient does not need as many follow-up visits in the first 7 to 10 days.

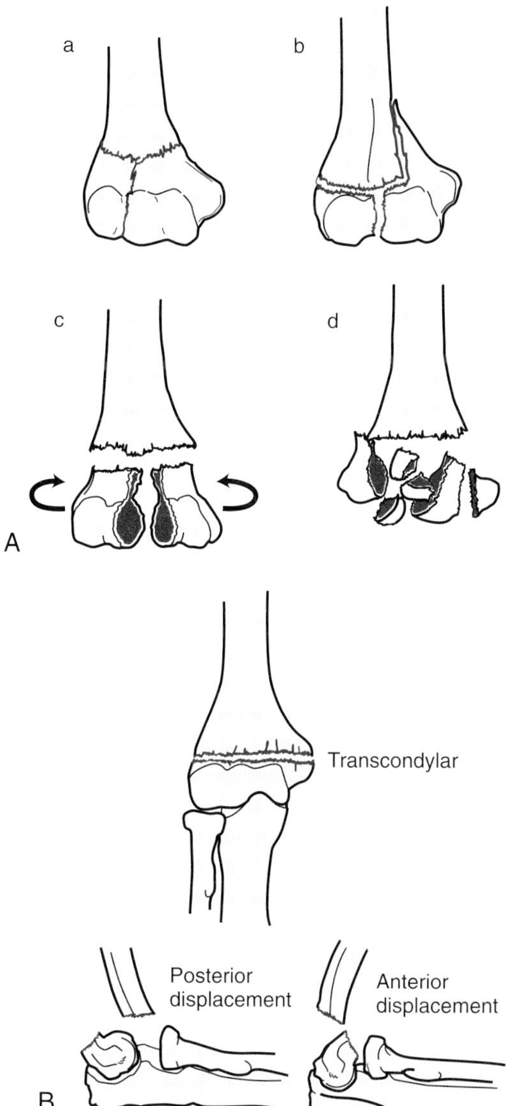

Figure 190-10 **A,** Intercondylar fractures of the humerus: No displacement of fragments (a); T-shaped fracture with the trochlear and capitellar fragments separated but not appreciably rotated in the frontal plane (b); T-shaped fracture with separation of the fragments and significant rotational deformity (c); T-shaped intercondylar fractures with severe comminution of the articular surface and wide separation of the humeral condyles (d). **B,** Transcondylar fractures of humerus, demonstrating significant posterior (*left*) and anterior (*right*) displacement.

Fractures of the Humeral Condyles

Type I fractures of the humeral (epi)condyles (Fig. 190-11) are treated with a splint in a manner similar to nondisplaced supracondylar and transcondylar fractures as previously discussed. The joint hemarthrosis should be aspirated and the elbow immobilized in a posterior splint with 90 degrees of flexion. For a medial condyle fracture, the forearm is placed in pronation and the wrist slightly flexed. For a lateral condyle fracture, the forearm is placed in supination and the wrist slightly extended. Radiographs should be obtained every 3 to 5 days for the first 2 weeks, then weekly thereafter to ensure no late displacement of the fragments. Patients with type II fractures of the humeral (epi)condyles should be referred to an orthopedic surgeon.

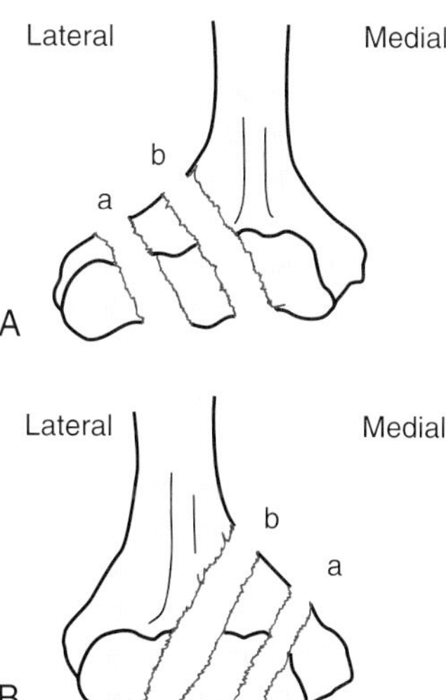

Figure 190-11 Fractures of the humeral (epi)condyles. **A,** Lateral humeral condyle: Type I, simple fracture of the lateral condyle with lateral wall of trochlea attached to main mass of the humerus (a); type II fracture with lateral wall of trochlea attached to fractured lateral condylar fragment (b). **B,** Medial humeral condyle: Type I, simple fracture of medial condyle with medial wall of trochlea attached to main mass of the humerus (a); type II fracture with medial wall of trochlea attached to fractured medial condylar fragment (b).

Elbow Fractures

All displaced (>2 mm) olecranon fractures (Fig. 190-12) should be referred to an orthopedic surgeon. If the patient is unable to actively extend the elbow (i.e., loss of triceps function), an orthopedic surgeon should be consulted. Otherwise, the patient should be immobilized in 60 to 90 degrees of flexion and seen in follow-up in 5 to 7 days. Radiographs should be evaluated in that visit to assure no displacement and at the 2- and 4-week visits. Range of motion activities should be started at 2 weeks with motion limited to 90 degrees of flexion until there is radiographic evidence of fracture healing.

Radial head fractures (Fig. 190-13) displaced more than 2 mm, involving more than a third of the articular surface, angulated more than 30 degrees, depressed more than 3 mm, severely comminuted, or with an associated dislocation should be referred to an orthopedic surgeon. Otherwise, treatment is range of motion activities such as pronation, supination, and elbow flexion and extension, as soon as pain permits, usually within 3 to 5 days. The patient should apply ice intermittently to the joint and keep it elevated for the first 48 hours. Significant pain relief can be provided by aspiration of blood from the joint followed by instillation of a local anesthetic. Immobilization is not required, but if the patient experiences too much pain without immobilization, a long-arm fiberglass one-step 90-degree splint and sling can be used. It should be removed as soon as possible to minimize stiffness. With radial head injuries, always check the wrist to ensure that there is no tenderness over the distal radius or ulna; associated injuries to the wrist often result in instability. If tenderness is present over the wrist, obtain true AP and lateral radiographs. For any displacement or dorsal subluxation of the ulna, with or without a fracture, the patient should be referred to an orthopedic surgeon.

Midforearm Fractures

An isolated fracture of the ulnar shaft (nightstick fracture) with no fracture or dislocation of the radius can be treated with a long-arm splint and sling with the elbow in 90 degrees of flexion. The splint remains in place for protection for 6 to 8 weeks. Weekly radiographs

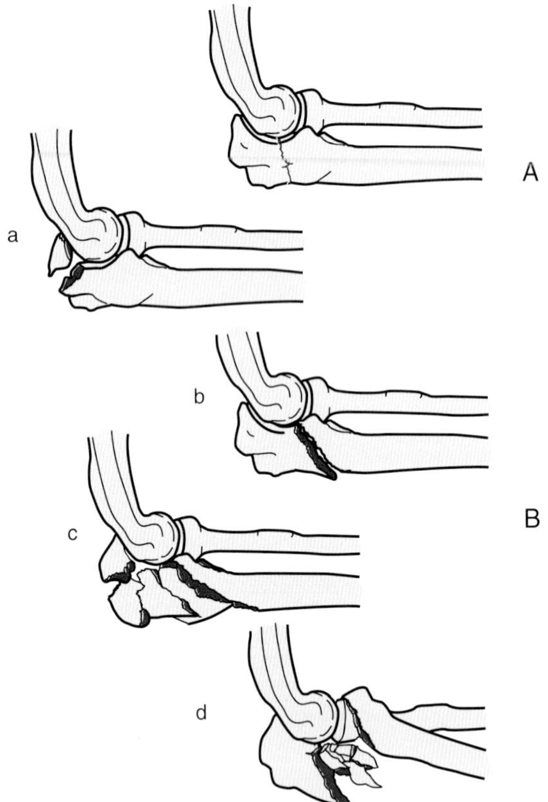

Figure 190-12 Olecranon fractures. **A,** Nondisplaced. **B,** Displaced fractures: Avulsion fracture (a); oblique and transverse fracture (b); comminuted fractures (c); fracture dislocations (d).

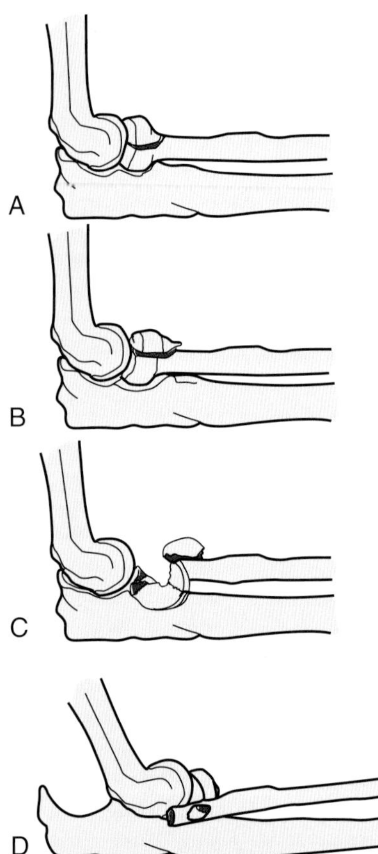

Figure 190-13 Radial head fractures (Mason classification with Johnston modification). **A,** Nondisplaced linear or transverse fractures. **B,** Fractures with minimal displacement (or comminuted fractures without displacement [not shown]). **C,** Comminuted fractures with marked displacement. **D,** Radial head fracture with associated elbow dislocation.

should be obtained for the first 3 weeks to detect any displacement and then at 6 to 8 weeks to document union. The fracture of the ulna will become sticky, stable, and less painful after 3 weeks, allowing removal of the splint for gentle range of motion activities of the elbow, including pronation and supination of the forearm twice a day for 15 minutes to minimize stiffness. Alternatively, a functional forearm brace can be applied after the intial swelling goes down in 7 to 10 days and remain in place until union is documented radiographically.

A fracture of the radial shaft (Galeazzi's fracture) requires surgery in all cases, so these patients should be referred to an orthopedic surgeon. Even if nondisplaced initially, the fracture will often become displaced, and the distal radioulnar joint is usually affected. Patients with both-bone shaft fractures (radial and ulnar shafts) should usually be referred to an orthopedic surgeon because these fractures usually require open reduction and internal fixation as a result of instability.

Distal Forearm Fractures

Colles' Fracture

A Colles' fracture involves the distal 2 cm of the radius, is angled dorsally (Fig. 190-14), and is the most common wrist fracture. If extra-articular and nondisplaced, it can be treated with a double sugar-tong splint (one splint from elbow to wrist, the other over initial splint and extending from elbow to axilla) for 3 to 5 days followed by a short-arm cast for 4 to 6 weeks. The fracture should be followed with radiographs at 1 (splint removed), 2, and 6 weeks to ensure no displacement and complete healing. At 6 weeks, the radiograph is taken after cast removal to assess fracture healing; if tenderness persists at the fracture site or there is incomplete union, an ulnar gutter splint should be applied. This splint can be removed to allow gentle range of motion activities, but should then be reapplied each time until all tenderness resolves and a solid fracture union is noted on the radiograph.

Colles' fractures require reduction if the lateral x-ray shows the distal radius articular surface to be tilted dorsally beyond the neutral position (determined by a line drawn straight through the distal radius, lunate, and capitate). After reduction, the distal articular surface should be perpendicular to the long axis of the forearm (neutral) or tilted volarly. If not reducible, unstable, comminuted, or intra-articular, these fractures are best treated by an orthopedic surgeon. Colles' fractures in the dominant wrist of the "high demand" (i.e., very active) patient are also more likely to require surgery for a satisfactory result.

On the AP view, if the radius is not equal to or longer than the length of the ulna, reduction is also indicated. Most patients have a radius that is longer than the ulna; this characteristic is referred to as negative ulnar variance as seen on the AP radiograph. (In a few patients, the radius and ulna are the same length; if any doubt remains, a comparison AP radiograph can be assessed). If there is displacement at the fracture site as defined by shortening of the radius on the AP view, reduction is indicated.

Reduction is simplified by injecting 10 mL of plain 1% lidocaine into the fracture site hematoma (hematoma block) for anesthesia. This injection should be performed slowly to minimize any pain associated with distention. The skin surface can be iced or sprayed with ethyl chloride to decrease the discomfort associated with the injection. Always clean the skin after applying the spray with an antiseptic preparation (e.g., povidone–iodine, chlorhexidine,

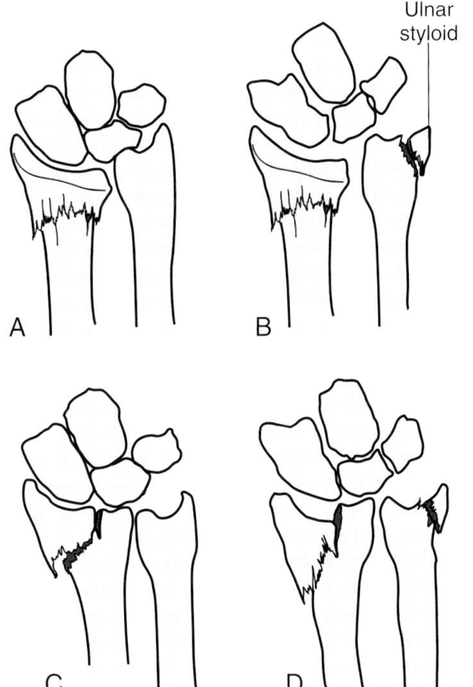

Figure 190-14 Distal radius fractures. **A,** Colles' fracture. **B,** Colles' fracture is commonly associated with fracture of ulnar styloid. **C,** Intra-articular fracture. **D,** Intra-articular fracture of radius with associated fracture of ulnar styloid.

alcohol) before injecting lidocaine. The patient should be supine during the entire procedure including the injection.

After the hematoma block has had time to take effect (10 minutes), hang the patient's hand in finger traps traction with the elbow flexed 90 degrees, and gradually add counterweights to a weight hanger, orthopedic felt sling, or stockinette draped over the humerus (Fig. 190-15). A weight of 5 to 10 lb is appropriate, and the patient should be in this suspended traction position for 15 to 20 minutes. At that point, reduction is usually achieved spontaneously by ligamentotaxis (the soft tissue attachments to the bone pull the bone into a reduced position in response to the traction). If any visible or palpable deformity remains after 15 to 20 minutes of traction, manual pressure can then be used to correct the deformity. Push from dorsal to volar over the distal radius, distal to the fracture site. Following reduction, with the arm still maintained in traction, as mentioned previously, the double sugar-tong splint should be applied. After 3 to 5 days, a long-arm, well-molded cast is applied (it is started as a short-arm cast and extended). Take great care to mold with your thenar cone at the base of the thumb, pressing into the patient's palm to prevent a gap in the volar portion of the cast

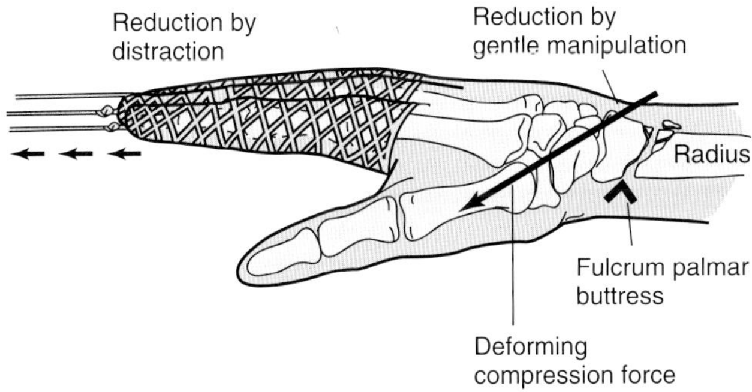

Figure 190-15 Treatment of Colles' fracture to effect reduction.

at the palm. After the cast is hard, trim it back to the proximal palmar crease to allow full flexion of the metacarpophalangeal (MP) joints to prevent joint stiffness.

After the cast is hard and three-point molding is applied (pushing volarly distal to the fracture site, dorsally just proximal to the fracture site, and volarly against the elbow), the cast is extended to the long-arm level, which is at least 5 inches more proximal, above the elbow. Be careful to pad the cast margins well, proximally and distally, and to stop application of plaster or fiberglass at least 1 inch before reaching the padding margin.

True AP and lateral postreduction radiographs should then be obtained. If the dorsal tilt of the distal radius articular surface or shortening of the radius in relation to the ulna persists, then the reduction is unacceptable and referral should be made for repeat reduction under general anesthetic and the possible application of skeletal external frame traction.

Ulnar styloid fractures indicate a larger force of injury and a higher chance of eventual loss of reduction. However, surgical treatment is never required for an isolated displaced ulnar styloid fracture. These fractures often remain nonunited on follow-up radiographs, but this has no clinical significance. Although patients may look at the radiograph and think they have a loose piece of bone floating around the wrist, they should be reminded that this bone is attached to soft tissue, does not float freely, and will not move.

Smith's Fracture

A *Smith's fracture* is similar to a Colles' fracture except that the angulation is volar (so it is sometimes called a reverse Colles'). After reduction, this fracture is treated the same as a Colles' fracture, with a double sugar-tong splint followed by a long-arm cast. If the fracture is intra-articular or the reduction is not anatomically correct, refer the patient to an orthopedic surgeon. This is an uncommon fracture and is often unstable; most should be referred.

Fractures of the Carpal Bones

Most chip and avulsion fractures of the carpal bones are treated with a gutter splint for comfort and protection for 4 to 6 weeks until symptoms resolve. The gutter splint can be removed for a shower. Hook of the hamate fractures should be referred to an orthopedist.

Scaphoid (Navicular) Fractures

When there is pain in the "snuffbox," always consider a scaphoid (navicular) injury (Fig. 190-16). Lateral, posteroanterior (PA), and motion (flexion-extension, radial deviation–ulnar deviation) views may be helpful. If a fracture is seen, a scaphoid magnification view

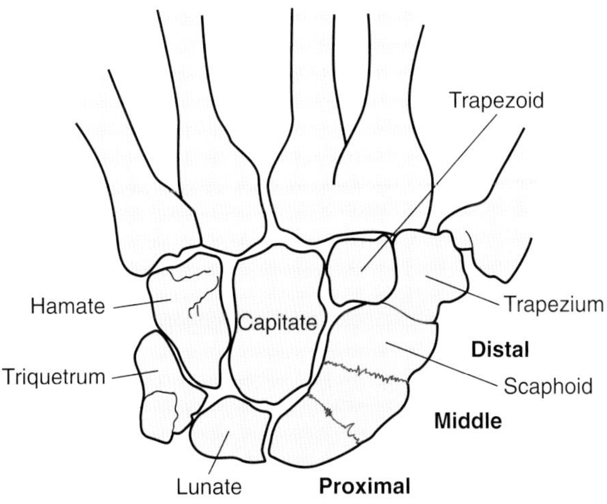

Figure 190-16 Scaphoid (navicular) fractures.

radiograph and consultation with a radiologist or orthopedist may help confirm that the fracture is, in fact, nondisplaced. A limited CT or MRI scan may also be helpful. Because the best blood supply (and highest likelihood of healing) is distal, nondisplaced distal third fractures (see Fig. 190-16) can be treated with a short-arm thumb spica cast for 4 to 6 weeks. Middle or proximal third fractures (see Fig. 190-16) need a longer cast and treatment; a long-arm thumb spica cast is applied for 6 weeks, followed by a short-arm thumb spica cast for another 6 weeks. Some clinicians continue the short-arm thumb spica cast for up to 14 more weeks for proximal third fractures.

A short-arm thumb spica cast is appropriate for any patient who has significant tenderness over the snuffbox (scaphoid), with follow-up radiograph and examination in 2 to 3 weeks without the cast. If at that time no tenderness is felt over the scaphoid and no fracture is visible, then there was no scaphoid fracture. Scaphoid fractures are notorious for being difficult to diagnose radiographically in the acute setting. For this reason, always err on the side of immobilization when a scaphoid fracture is suspected. If after 2 to 3 weeks the cast is removed and no fracture line is visible but persistent tenderness is noted over the fracture site, immobilization for an additional 2 to 3 weeks is appropriate, followed by repeat radiographs. At that point, if no fracture line is visible, then there was no scaphoid fracture and gentle range of motion exercises can be initiated. A bone scan may also help confirm a fracture.

Displaced scaphoid fractures should be referred to an orthopedic surgeon. Avascular necrosis, delayed union, nonunion, and arthritis are common complications of scaphoid fractures, even if managed appropriately; therefore, the patient needs to be made aware of these risks at the start.

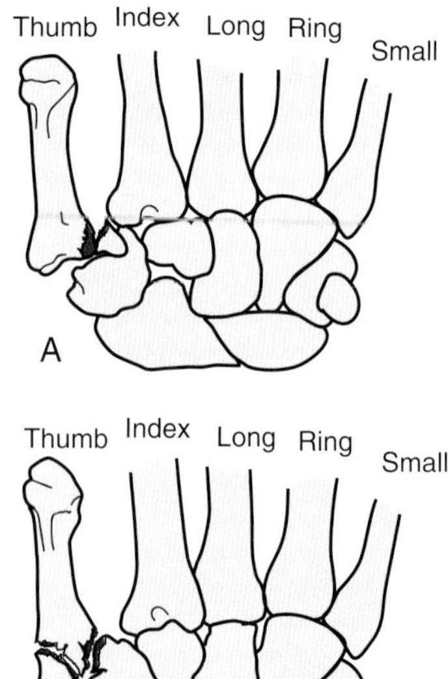

Figure 190-17 Displaced intra-articular fractures of the proximal thumb. **A,** Bennett fracture. **B,** Rolando fracture.

Metacarpal Fractures

Nondisplaced, noncomminuted metacarpal fractures, including those that are intra-articular (except thumb metacarpal), are treated with an ulnar or a radial gutter cast, depending on the fracture location. Nondisplaced, noncomminuted, nonarticular fractures of the thumb (first) metacarpal are treated with a thumb spica cast. An index (second) finger metacarpal fracture can be treated with a radial gutter cast with a hole cut out for the thumb to allow thumb function. Fractures of the middle (third), ring (fourth), and little (fifth) finger metacarpals are treated with an ulnar gutter splint. A gutter splint can be made using 6-inch wide one-step fiberglass prepadded splint material. Patients should be seen every 2 weeks.

Nondisplaced fractures of the metacarpal heads can be treated with a gutter splint for 2 to 3 weeks. Nondisplaced fractures of the second or third or mildly angulated fractures of the fourth (<30 degrees) or fifth metacarpal (<40 degrees) neck can be treated in the same manner for 3 to 4 weeks so long as there is no rotational deformity. If the fracture is in the midportion of the shaft, and there is no rotational deformity, mildly angulated second or third metacarpal (<10 degrees) or fourth or fifth metacarpal (<20 degrees) fractures can be managed with gutter splinting for 3 to 4 weeks. For angulation greater than these parameters, reduction can be attempted. If reduction is unsuccessful, or if there is a rotational deformity, the patient should be referred. Hematoma block reduction can be carried out with three-point pressure fixation in the splint, followed by postreduction radiographs. After 3 to 4 weeks, the gutter splint can be removed for range of motion exercises. When not performing range of motion movements, the metacarpal should remain protected in the splint for an additional 3 weeks.

Immobilize the metacarpals with 90-degree flexion at the MP joint and full extension of the interphalangeal (IP) and distal interphalangeal (DIP) joints of the fingers. Often referred to as the "intrinsic plus position," this position results in the MP joint lateral ligaments and those of the DIP and proximal interphalangeal (PIP) joints being in maximal stretch. This position prevents tightening during immobilization and secondary stiffness of the joint. The gutter cast should go from the tips of the fingers to the midforearm. Remember to place dry cotton ball padding between the fingers to prevent skin maceration from moisture accumulation.

Immobilizing all metacarpal fractures in an MP joint flexion 90-degree position minimizes the risk for future malrotation; the flexed finger at the MP joint serves to align the metacarpal in the correct direction with the adjacent metacarpals. This alignment acts as a reference angle because the protective fingers are also flexed 90 degrees.

Patients with displaced intra-articular fractures (Bennett and Rolando fractures) should be referred to an orthopedic surgeon, especially those who have intra-articular fractures at the base of the thumb (Fig. 190-17). Even nondisplaced intra-articular fractures of the base of the thumb should probably be referred. Nondisplaced fractures of the thumb shaft with more than 30 degrees of angulation should be reduced under a Bier or hematoma block and managed with a thumb spica cast for 4 weeks.

Boxer fractures occur at the fifth metacarpal neck. As mentioned previously, angulation up to 40 degrees is acceptable for this fracture. The clinician must be certain, however, not to confuse a boxer fracture (fifth metacarpal neck) with a fifth metacarpal shaft fracture (Fig. 190-18), because angulation of the shaft of the fifth metacarpal greater than 20 degrees is unacceptable. If the reduction is lost somewhat during healing of a fifth metacarpal neck, it will mainly

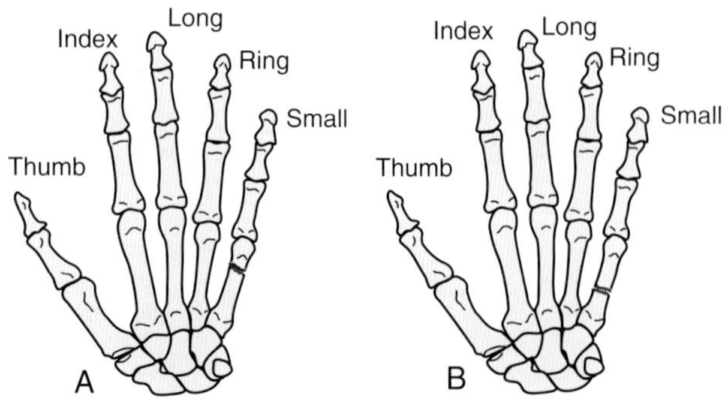

Figure 190-18 **A,** Boxer fracture. **B,** Metacarpal shaft fracture.

result in a cosmetic, as opposed to a functional, deformity. Also, explain to patients that with boxer fractures the bone will heal with abundant callus; consequently, they will have a bump over the dorsum of the hand because the callus is subcutaneous.

When treating boxer fractures, be cautious of any mark on the skin over the knuckle, which could suggest an open fracture or a human bite lesion that might become infected. If either is present, begin broad-spectrum antibiotics, possibly giving the first dose intravenously. The wound should be inspected again in 2 to 3 days to ensure no infection.

An isolated fracture involving one of the long or ring finger metacarpals can be treated without immobilization if the patient is comfortable and wishes to use the hand out of a cast. Approximately 3 to 5 mm of shortening of the finger may occur as the metacarpal overrides itself. However, no shortening will occur beyond this point because the fractured metacarpal is being suspended between the two intact metacarpals and associated interosseous ligaments that run between the metacarpals.

Phalangeal Fractures

Phalangeal fractures can be immobilized with aluminum foam splints, buddy taping, or stack splints (e.g., mallet finger fracture of distal phalanx). If there is any displacement of these fractures, closed reduction is unsuccessful, or reduction cannot be maintained, referral is appropriate. Volar plate avulsion fractures caused by hyperextension injuries at the PIP joint are best immobilized with a dorsal block splint holding the PIP joint in 45 degrees of flexion for 3 weeks.

Transverse or angulated fractures of the distal phalanx are often unstable and difficult to reduce because of interposition of soft tissue. Intra-articular fractures of one or more condyles of the middle or proximal phalanx at the level of the DIP or PIP joints, respectively, usually also need referral for internal fixation. Oblique or spiral proximal shaft fractures and large displaced avulsion fractures of the base of the proximal phalanx may also benefit from referral for operative repair. Conversely, mallet finger fractures should be treated with continuous slight hyperextension splinting for up to 8 weeks. Almost all other finger fractures can be treated with 3 or 4 weeks of buddy taping.

Always check the collateral ligaments by stress examination. Use a digital block if needed to perform the examination. If collateral ligaments are disrupted despite a negative x-ray, buddy taping is appropriate for protection for 1 month while allowing protected range of motion movement in the taped position.

In general, with metacarpal and phalangeal fractures, *malrotation* is the most common complication. To exclude malrotation with a metacarpal fracture, always hold the MP joints in 90 degrees of flexion to ensure perfect rotational alignment. For phalangeal fractures, always note the plane of the nail beds while looking at the fingers from the ends. Compare them with the opposite hand to ensure correct rotational alignment.

Any intra-articular fracture with displacement at the joint surface should be referred to an orthopedic surgeon for reduction and fixation. Proximal interphalangeal joint fractures involving more than 40% of joint surface should be referred for probable internal fixation. Extra-articular and intra-articular fractures without displacement at the joint surface can be treated without referral. If any doubt remains as to whether displacement in the joint surface is present, consult a radiologist or orthopedist.

Children's Fractures

Children's bone tissue is elastic, similar to a plastic flyswatter handle. For this reason, their bones can deform and bow without cracking the cortex. This elastic deformation commonly occurs in the shaft of the radius or ulna and is referred to as a bone bow fracture. If concerned about the alignment of the forearm, remember that the ulna is always straight and that a small 10- to 20-degree bow is normally present in the radius. Assessment of a *comparison film* can determine what is normal for the patient. When viewing comparison films, always make sure the views are taken in exactly the same projection so that a true comparison can be made. Comparison films in children are also beneficial because the growth plates ossify at different ages.

Comparison radiographs in children are especially important when treating any elbow injury, because numerous ossification centers develop at various ages (from 3 to 12 years). Because of these various centers of ossification, if any sign or question of fracture is present, a radiologist should be consulted or referral to an orthopedist considered to review the films. *Salter's classification* is commonly used for children's fractures involving the growth plate (Box 190-2 and Fig. 190-19).

Box 190-2. Salter's Classification of Fractures*

Salter type I fracture is diagnosed with a normal x-ray appearance and by point tenderness directly over the growth plate. No tenderness should be felt over the ligaments around the joint. This type of fracture is common in infants and young children. Treatment is always closed with cast immobilization.

Salter type II is a fracture through the growth plate and then through the metaphysis. This type of fracture is more common in older children. The prognosis for growth disturbance is very high when the fracture involves the distal femoral growth plate. Refer all patients with this type of fracture to an orthopedic surgeon if any displacement has occurred. Reduction is almost always performed with a general anesthetic to provide complete muscle relaxation. This relaxation allows the traction to decrease the force across the growth plate, which is required to set it. The less force required to set the fracture, the less recurrent injury to the growth plate itself (see Fig. 190-19).

Salter type III fracture involves the epiphysis extending into the epiphysial plate. If any displacement has occurred, the patient should be referred to an orthopedic surgeon. These fractures are most common in the distal tibia and can be associated with growth arrest. Anatomic reduction is always required, and surgery may be required.

Salter type IV fracture extends from the joint surface through the epiphysis and on through the epiphysial plate and out through the metaphysis. These fractures are often displaced and require open surgical treatment. This fracture most commonly occurs at the lateral humeral condyle at the elbow. These injuries extend into the joint. If the fracture appears nondisplaced and any question of displacement remains, it may be beneficial for a radiologist or an orthopedist to review the film and tomograms.

Salter type V injury is a crush injury of the epiphysial plate and is uncommon. When this fracture occurs, it is usually at the knee or ankle and associated with growth arrest. The x-ray appearance may be normal as for a Salter type I fracture. For this reason, parents (and the child) should be cautioned that growth arrest can occur if there is tenderness over the growth plate, whether it is a Salter I or Salter V fracture (and often this is difficult to determine) because it may have extended into the growth plate. Osteoarthritis can occur as a result of any fracture that extends into the joint itself, whether this occurs in an adult or a child.

*See Figure 190-19.

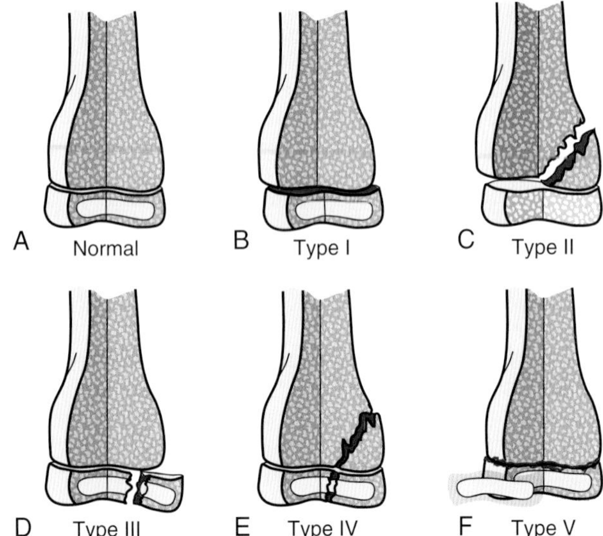

Figure 190-19 Illustrations of Salter's classification for fractures in children (also see Box 190-2). **A,** Normal. **B,** Type I. **C,** Type II. **D,** Type III. **E,** Type IV. **F,** Type V.

It is appropriate to refer all fractures in children involving the spine or knee because fractures around the spine and knee are at high risk for growth plate arrest or neurologic injury.

Upper Extremity Fractures

Clavicle fractures do not generally require referral, reduction, or intervention unless tenting of the skin is observed with whiteness over the skin as a result of loss of blood supply. Exceptions include a clavicular fracture near the acromioclavicular joint that is displaced or in the proximal third of the clavicle displaced posteriorly; these should be referred to an orthopedic surgeon. The vast majority of fractures, however, occur in the middle third of the clavicle or are nondisplaced and are treated with a figure-eight strap for immobilization and comfort. Remember, the figure-eight strap is applied only to increase comfort; children heal very rapidly (within weeks), and as soon as the child is comfortable without it, the strap is no longer required. In toddlers, a figure-eight strap is unnecessary because healing occurs so quickly. In older children, a sling may be more comfortable than a figure-eight strap. These straps and splints can be removed for bathing and then reapplied. To show patients how to put the straps back on and get the straps in the same position, instruct them to use a pen to make marks on the white straps at the level of the buckles. This "trick" will enable the patient to reapply the splint, sling, or brace in the same position with the same degree of tension as applied in the office.

Rib fractures, similar to those in adults, do not require treatment, immobilization, or bracing. Although patients may ask for any one of these treatments, remind them that splints or rib binders can cause atelectasis or pneumonia. Always auscultate the chest to exclude pneumothorax and respiratory compromise. Sometimes subcutaneous emphysema suggests lung puncture by a rib or clavicular fracture. This complication can be ruled out by palpating the skin around the area of the fracture to check for any crepitance.

Fractures around the shoulder usually involve only the surgical neck of the humerus. As long as there is 50% bone-on-bone contact and not too much angulation (<70 degrees before age 5, <40 degrees from age 5 to 16, <25 degrees after age 16), no reduction is necessary. As with adults, treatment is a hanging arm cast for 3 to 4 weeks until tenderness resolves on palpation and comfort is present. Humeral shaft fractures almost always heal well, and angulation up to 25 degrees on AP and lateral planes can be accepted. Always check for radial nerve dysfunction.

Distal humerus supracondylar fractures are best evaluated with comparison of true lateral radiographs. Remember that the distal humerus ordinarily has a tilt in an anterior direction. If the distal humerus is entirely straight, approximately 10 to 15 degrees of bending of the distal humerus has occurred in a posterior direction. This bending is acceptable, however, as long as the humerus is not bent backward beyond the straight position. As it turns out, most supracondylar fractures in children are displaced and require referral. Nondisplaced fractures with good alignment can be treated with a long-arm cast for 3 weeks with the elbow at 90 degrees and the forearm in neutral rotation.

A supracondylar fracture or radial head or neck fracture can be identified with a *posterior fat pad sign*. The posterior fat pad sign is the result of intra-articular bleeding in the elbow joint with any fracture that is intra-articular. The blood goes into the olecranon fossa in the distal humerus and causes the fat pad that resides there to float posteriorly; therefore, it is no longer hidden in the olecranon fossa. As it floats posteriorly, it is visible as a fat pad on the true lateral radiograph of the distal humerus. In the absence of any abnormality on the radiograph, a fat pad sign indicates bleeding into the joint and leads to a diagnosis of occult fracture most likely involving the radial head or neck. This involvement can be confirmed by point tenderness with palpation of the radial head and neck. Angulation up to 30 degrees and up to 4 mm translocation are acceptable in fractures of the radial head or neck; a child with greater angulation or translocation should be referred to an orthopedic surgeon for probable closed reduction.

Common fractures in the forearm include *torus fractures*. They are treated with a short-arm cast for 1 month until all tenderness resolves. *Greenstick fractures* are one level worse than torus fractures; these involve an actual crack or disruption of one cortex and often a buckling of the opposite cortex. These fractures are so named because they represent a deformation of the bone much like cracking a green twig on an apple tree in springtime. The tension side of the bent twig cracks, whereas the compression side (concave side) buckles and does not crack.

Any angulation in the radius greater than 10 degrees in children older than 8 (or >15 degrees in children younger than 8) requires reduction and should be referred. Significantly comminuted fractures or those associated with nerve injury should also be referred. With ulnar shaft fractures, angulation greater than 15 degrees should be reduced; if uncomfortable performing this reduction, the primary care clinician should refer the patient. For all other radial or ulnar shaft fractures (including both-bone fractures if nondisplaced or minimally displaced), a long-arm cast can be utilized for 6 to 8 weeks to prevent pronation and supination at the elbow. The cast is always applied with the elbow in at least 90 degrees of flexion, and the sling must always hold the arm in at least 90 degrees of flexion. If it does not do so or if the cast is applied in less than 90 degrees of flexion, the cast will continue to slip out of the sling.

Wrist and Hand Fractures

Fractures of the carpal bones are uncommon in children. Management of scaphoid fractures is very similar to that in adults. However, with a fall on the outstretched arm, the typical fracture is of the distal radius and ulna. These fractures can be reduced by hematoma block and finger traps traction, as in the adult. This technique should be reserved for the child who is 12 years or older and very cooperative and understanding. Younger children, who are uncooperative, anxious, or otherwise frightened of injections, should have a reduction under general anesthesia. This approach will provide a more comfortable, less frightening experience and allow maximum muscle relaxation for the least traumatic reduction potentially affecting later arm growth and length.

Metacarpal and phalangeal fractures that are nondisplaced are simply treated with ulnar or radial gutter splint immobilization. The position of immobilization and the angulation are the same as that used for treating adults. Remember, the fifth metacarpal neck can accept angulation up to 40 degrees, whereas the shaft angulation can be accepted only to 20 degrees. Phalangeal fractures, including mallet fingers, are treated the same for children and for adults.

The so-called *octave fracture* is common in children and occurs at the base of the proximal phalanx of the little finger (fifth digit), where it is angulated ulnarly. It is so named since playing the piano requires children to stretch their fingers into wide abduction. Reduction is required and is easily done using a finger digital block anesthetic, followed by placement of a pen or pencil between the fourth and fifth fingers. The pen acts as a fulcrum between the two fingers. The little finger is then pulled back into place with traction and radial deviation until it is perfectly straight using the pen or pencil deep against the web space as a bolster or fulcrum. This technique works extremely well, and should be followed by buddy taping and splint immobilization for a minimum of 3 weeks.

Again, a child with any displaced intra-articular fracture or displaced growth plate fracture should be referred to an orthopedic surgeon for reduction.

Lower Extremity Fractures

Fractures of the true pelvis are uncommon, except in automobile accidents or high-velocity trauma. Patients with these fractures should all be referred to rule out other associated injuries to the abdomen, genitourinary, and gynecologic systems. Apophyseal avulsion fractures are fairly common in young athletes. Those of the anterior inferior or superior iliac spine are usually minimally displaced; hamstring attachment avulsion fractures may result in a large displaced fragment. Conservative treatment consists of a brief period of rest followed by 2 to 3 weeks of crutch-assisted ambulation. Return to full function may take 6 to 12 weeks. Surgery is reserved for those with symptomatic nonunion.

Femur fractures are also uncommon and should be immediately referred to an orthopedic surgeon for further evaluation and treatment. Remember, a *slipped capital femoral epiphysis or avascular necrosis of the femoral head in children (Perthes disease)* can present with knee pain. The knee examination and radiograph may be entirely normal. The first clue to the diagnosis is limitation of hip internal rotation on the involved side. The *Trendelenburg test* often shows weakness in the gluteus medius on the involved side. *If a child under 17 years of age complains of knee pain and the knee examination and radiographs are negative, always examine and carry out radiographs of the pelvis and hips*. AP pelvic and true lateral radiographs of the hips are appropriate studies for this purpose.

Fractures of the distal femur that are nondisplaced and have normal radiographs are diagnosed by point tenderness over the distal femoral epiphysis, which is located 3 cm above the joint line. Treatment involves a cylinder cast for complete immobilization, crutches, and protective partial weight-bearing activities for 1 month. During the follow-up examination, a window can be placed in the cast through which the examiner's finger can palpate for tenderness. As long as tenderness is felt at the fracture site, the cast should remain in place. The tenderness should resolve within 8 weeks or sooner, depending on the child's age.

Patellar fractures are usually nondisplaced and are similarly treated with a knee immobilizer or cylinder cast. Immobilize the knee for 1 month until all tenderness resolves.

Beware of any *intra-articular avulsion fractures along the lateral tibial plateau*. This type of fracture indicates an anterior cruciate ligament avulsing a piece of bone. If there is any associated displacement, referral to an orthopedist should be carried out for surgical repair.

Proximal tibial fractures are treated the same as those of the distal femur and are diagnosed by point tenderness over the growth plate. Tibial shaft fractures can be treated in a long-leg cast without reduction if there is not more than 5 degrees angulation on the AP radiograph and not more than 10 degrees angulation on the lateral radiograph. If angulation exceeds these thresholds, referral to an orthopedic surgeon should be made for closed manipulation reduction.

Fibular fractures are of no concern and will heal uneventfully without treatment. However, if any angulation is present, an orthopedic surgeon should be consulted for probable closed manipulation reduction.

Foot and Ankle Fractures

Patients with any fracture around the ankle that is displaced should be referred to an orthopedist. Most fractures of the ankle should be managed by an orthopedist because most involve the growth plate. That said, fractures that are nondisplaced can be treated with a short-leg cast and no weight-bearing activity for 2 weeks, followed by advancing to weight-bearing activities for the remaining 3 to 4 weeks while in the cast.

Fracture of the talus, navicular, and cuneiform bones can be treated with a short-leg walking cast, provided there is no displacement. Fractures of the metatarsals are treated the same in children as for adults. Peroneus brevis avulsion fractures can be treated with a wooden-soled fracture shoe. Beware of the fracture of the proximal shaft of the fifth metatarsal (Jones fracture), which is different from a peroneus brevis avulsion fracture. For optimal healing, this type of fracture requires a short-leg fiberglass cast and no weight-bearing activities for 2 weeks, followed by weight-bearing activities for an additional 6 weeks.

Child Abuse

Any history or examination suspicious for child abuse should be assessed with long bone radiographs of the upper and lower extremities. This long bone study should be carefully reviewed for signs of fractures in various bones in different stages of healing, which would indicate a history of numerous injuries. A corner fracture is a typical radiographic finding, which is noted at the corner of the metaphysis of a long bone.

Complications (Adult and Pediatric)

Compartment syndrome (see Chapter 188, Compartment Syndrome Evaluation) is the most devastating complication in fracture treatment and is caused by swelling and a tight cast leading to neurovascular compromise. This syndrome most frequently occurs in the calf and forearm. Any patient who requires more than the average dose of oral pain medication for fractures of the forearm or tibia (or any other fracture, for that matter) should be evaluated emergently. If the patient feels the cast is too tight or if there is excess pain beyond what would be reasonably expected, or if any swelling in the digits occurs, then the cast and padding should be immediately split (bivalved). If pain relief does not occur, the entire cast should be removed and the extremity inspected for signs of tenseness of the skin. If the skin is not tense and the calf is involved, perform a Doppler study to rule out phlebitis. Treatment of the fracture and maintenance of reduction of the fracture are always a second priority to preserving the blood supply to the soft tissue and bone. If any question of compartment syndrome remains, compartmental pressure measurements must be obtained and a fasciotomy performed if pressures are elevated.

The higher the velocity of the injury, the more comminuted the fracture, the higher the energy of the force, the more soft tissue trauma, the higher the chance of swelling. For the upper extremity, always tell patients to carry the arm over the head in a "monkey-like" position for the first week. Children may go to school, but their arm should be propped up over the head or on a stack of books in front of them on their desk. At night, they should sleep with couch cushions elevating the arm. Parents should set their alarm clock for 3 AM and reposition the child's arm back up on the pillows because the child will have most likely wiggled the arm off the elevated position. Be certain that patients *do not* have slings to use for a long-arm cast for the first week. If they are given a sling, they will automatically carry the cast and arm down in front by their chest and it will be lower than the heart and promote swelling. The sling should not be used until after the first week.

Most *open fractures* should be referred to an orthopedist due to the increased risk of infection. The open fracture may be associated with only a small puncture wound in the skin, and this puncture may be located several inches from the fracture itself because of the forces of deformation at the time of the injury. Fractures of nail beds may become open fractures when the nail is removed; however, primary care clinicians can often repair these (see Chapter 27, Nail Bed Repair).

It is now known that *reflex sympathetic dystrophy* involves, in fact, a shutdown of the capillary circulation system and results in arterial blood being shunted in a bypass fashion from arterioles to venules without adequate capillary profusion. This phenomenon has been demonstrated by sampling the oxygen content of venous blood in the involved extremity compared with the uninvolved extremity. The oxygen content in the venous blood in an extremity with reflex sympathetic dystrophy is higher, which is due to the oxygen not being taken out by the tissues, as it would be if the blood were supplied normally to the capillary system.

The incidence of *postfracture stiffness* in a joint (especially at the elbow or where the fracture extends into the joint) is dramatically increased in patients who have diabetes and in those who smoke. Patients should understand that diabetes and smoking have similar effects on the capillary blood flow; they both diminish the flow.

Delayed union, nonunion, atrophic or hypertrophic union, and malunion are possible complications of fractures. Inadequate assessment of the initial radiographs, improper management of the fracture (including incomplete reduction), poor patient adherence and compliance, increased age, medications, and presence of osteopenia or osteoporosis are all possible causes of these complications. Smoking or taking anti-inflammatory medications delays the healing time and increases the risk for improper fracture healing, especially in weight-bearing bones (e.g., ankle, foot, calcaneus). If the patient smokes, the fracture healing time in the ankle is doubled compared to the nonsmoker. Colles' fracture healing may also be delayed in patients taking anti-inflammatory medications or smoking.

Among other factors, risk of *traumatic arthritis* is increased by the proximity of the fracture to a joint (especially if intra-articular), the forces causing the fracture (risk of damage to cartilage), repetitive fractures, and fracture healing.

CPT/Billing Codes

See Chapter 186, Ankle and Foot Splinting, Casting, and Taping, and Chapter 187, Cast Immobilization and Upper Extremity Splinting.

BIBLIOGRAPHY

Black WS, Becker JA: Common forearm fractures in adults. Am Fam Physician 80:1096–1102, 2009.

Boyd AS, Benjamin HJ, Asplund C: Principles of casting and splinting. Am Fam Physician 79:16–22, 23–24, 2009.

Bucholz RW, Heckman JD, Court-Brown C (eds): Rockwood and Green's Fractures in Adults, 6th ed. Philadelphia, Lippincott, Williams & Wilkins, 2006.

Eiff MP, Hatch RL, Calmbach WL: Fracture Management for Primary Care, 2nd ed. Philadelphia, Saunders, 2003.

Herring JA: Tachdjian's Pediatric Orthopedics from the Texas Scottish Rite Hospital for Children, 3rd ed. Philadelphia, WB Saunders, 2002.

Koval KJ, Zucherman JD: Handbook of Fractures, 3rd ed. Philadelphia, Lippincott, Williams & Wilkins, 2006.

Medley ES, Shirley SM, Brilliant HL: Fracture management by family physicians and guidelines for referral. J Fam Pract 8:701–710, 1979.

Rockwood CA, Wilkins KE, King RE (eds): Rockwood & Wilkins' Fractures in Children. New York, Lippincott, 2001.

Salter RB: Disorders and Injuries of the Musculoskeletal System. Baltimore, Williams & Wilkins, 1970.

Salter RB, Harris WR: Injuries involving epiphysial plate. J Bone Joint Surg 45A:587, 1963.

Spinner M: Monteggia fractures in children with nerve palsies. Clin Orthoped 58:141, 1968.

Stiell IG, McKnight RD, Greenberg GH, et al: Implementation of the Ottawa ankle rules. JAMA 271:827–832, 1994.

Usatine RP: The Color Atlas of Family Medicine. New York, McGraw-Hill, 2009.

Wilkins KE, Beaty JB, Kasser JR (eds): Rockwood & Wilkins' Fractures in Children. Philadelphia, Lippincott, 2001.

CHAPTER 191

GANGLION TREATMENT

David T. Bortel

The most common tumor of the hand or wrist is the ganglion, which has a propensity for women. A ganglion can occur at almost any location adjacent to a joint or tendon sheath. The most common site is the dorsal wrist (Fig. 191-1), accounting for about 65% of ganglions; for this location the scapholunate ligament and joint are usually the source or root of the pathology (Fig. 191-2). Volar cysts account for about 20% to 25% of ganglions and typically originate from the scaphotrapezial or trapeziometacarpal joints (Fig. 191-3). Another site of origin is the palmar fibro-osseous flexor tendon sheath, which accounts for about 10% of ganglions. A ganglion at this location normally presents as a hard, small or pea-sized, painful lesion at the proximal interphalangeal flexion crease (Fig. 191-4). Ganglion cysts can be seen at other body sites, with the foot and ankle being common locations (Figs. 191-5 and 191-6). Occasionally they can even be found intraosseously.

IDENTIFICATION AND CHARACTERISTICS

Patients usually present with an obvious mass and sometimes complain of pain and weakness. Ganglion cysts are usually easy to identify by their appearance. The most consistent characteristic is their location, as noted previously. The cyst is often rubbery, but it is sometimes firm. Occasionally a ganglion will allow fluid to be compressed from one septate area to another. The ganglion may transilluminate if it is of sufficient size. Seldom is it necessary to order additional studies to confirm the diagnosis; rather, confirmation is usually made by aspiration, which yields a viscous mucoid fluid (Fig. 191-7). A differential diagnosis includes extensor tenosynovitis, lipoma, sebaceous cyst, or other hand tumors.

The ganglion cyst is a fibrous-walled, mucin-filled structure typically connected to the joint capsule or tendon sheath by a tortuous stalk. In fact, it is basically a herniation of the synovial lining of tendons, ligaments, or joints. A "one-way valve" probably predicates the formation of these nonmalignant, yet frequently painful lesions. Use of the offending joint or tendon leads to increased production of the encapsulated mucin, thus magnifying the symptoms. The ganglion commonly is self-limiting (perhaps over several years) by rupture or resorption. These cysts *may reflect an underlying ligamentous pathology*.

NOTE: A close "cousin" of the ganglion cyst is the mucous (or mucinous) cyst. Both are nearly identical histologically, but the mucous cyst often involves a more ominous process. Mucous cysts arise from an arthritic distal interphalangeal (DIP) joint (i.e., the cyst is a direct drainage conduit to the DIP joint; Fig. 191-8). Unfortunately, as these cysts enlarge with time, they will commonly erode into the germinal nail matrix, causing discomfort and nail distortion. (Nail distortion is a hallmark of this type cyst.) Past treatments have included sclerosis, steroid injection, electrical or chemical cautery, cryotherapy, and simple incision and drainage. The thinned local subcutaneous tissue may rupture spontaneously, leading to a septic joint or osteomyelitis. These lesions are particularly difficult to manage, even by skilled hand surgeons. Aspiration or injection of mucous cysts can be attempted judiciously, but the risk of causing a septic joint must be appreciated. If such treatment is implemented, the patient needs to be aware of the signs of infection.

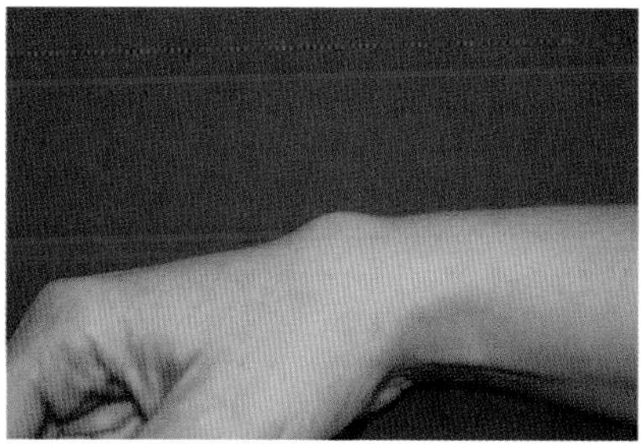

Figure 191-1 Dorsal wrist ganglion. (Courtesy of The Medical Procedures Center, Midland, Mich.)

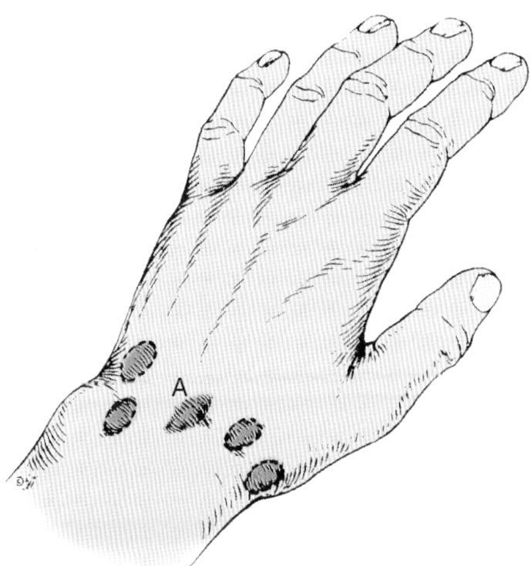

Figure 191-2 A few of the many possible locations of dorsal wrist ganglions. The most common site (A) is directly over the scapholunate ligament. The others are typically connected to the scapholunate ligament through an elongated pedicle. (Redrawn from Athanasian EA: Bone and soft tissue tumors. In Green DP, Hotchkiss RN, Pederson WC, Wolfe SW [eds]: Green's Operative Hand Surgery, 5th ed. Philadelphia, Churchill Livingstone, 2005, pp 2211–2264.)

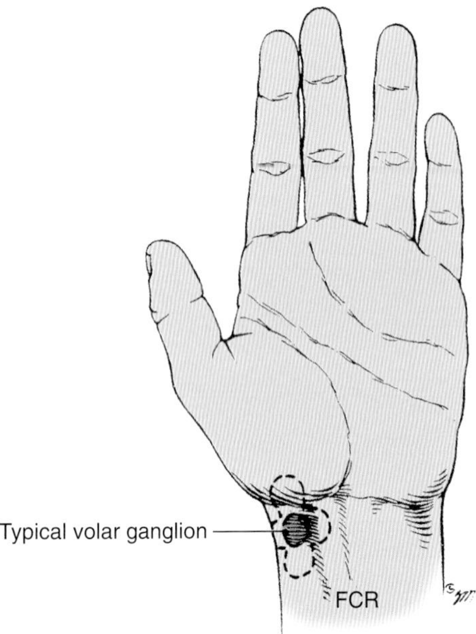

Figure 191-3 Typical location of a volar wrist ganglion. Possible subcutaneous extensions *(dotted lines)* are often palpable. FCR, flexor carpi radialis. (Redrawn from Athanasian EA: Bone and soft tissue tumors. In Green DP, Hotchkiss RN, Pederson WC, Wolfe SW [eds]: Green's Operative Hand Surgery, 5th ed. Philadelphia, Churchill Livingstone, 2005, pp 2211–2264.)

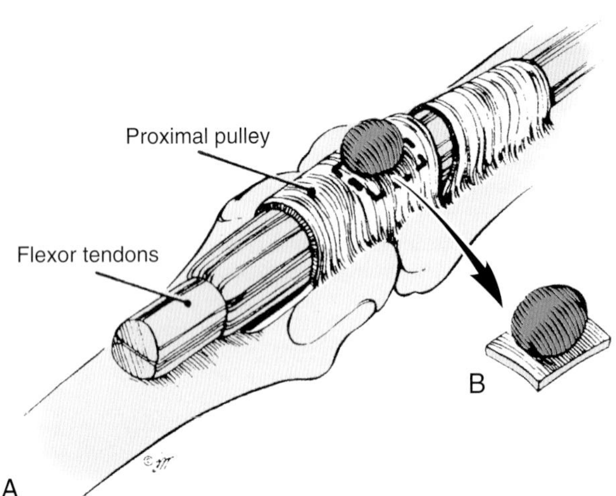

Figure 191-4 **A,** Volar retinacular ganglion in situ on the proximal annular ligament (A1 pulley) of the flexor tendon sheath. **B,** Excised specimen with a surrounding margin of tendon sheath. (Redrawn from Athanasian EA: Bone and soft tissue tumors. In Green DP, Hotchkiss RN, Pederson WC, Wolfe SW [eds]: Green's Operative Hand Surgery, 5th ed. Philadelphia, Churchill Livingstone, 2005, pp 2211–2264.)

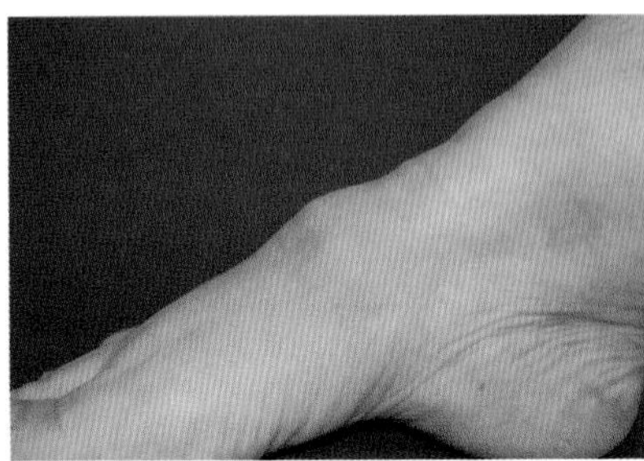

Figure 191-5 Dorsal foot ganglion (consider tarsal bossing).

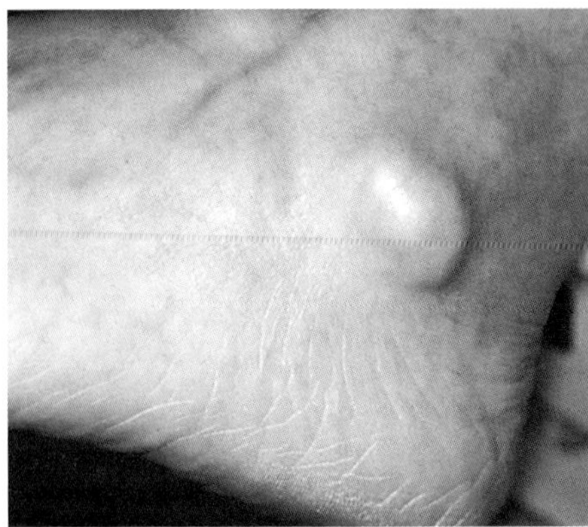

Figure 191-6 Ganglion inferior to malleolus of ankle. (Courtesy of The Medical Procedures Center, Midland, Mich.)

Preprocedure Patient Preparation

The patient should be informed that he or she will experience some discomfort similar to having a tooth numbed by a dentist. When the area is being anesthetized, a temporary burning sensation is felt. The local anesthetic typically lasts for 30 to 60 minutes. While anesthetized, the involved tissue could be prone to further unknown trauma until the anesthetic subsides. After the procedure, there will be a pressure-like sensation that may last for a few days. Typically a pressure dressing will be necessary for several days over the ganglion site. Any steroid placed may produce a local reaction, which can be as simple as skin irritation or as dramatic as dermal atrophy, significant hypopigmentation, or subsequent cutaneous slough. Fortunately, the dramatic reactions are rare. Similarly, systemic manifestations are rare because dosages and volumes for these lesions are usually very small.

Ganglion cysts of the volar wrist near the distal radius are near the radial artery (Fig. 191-9). In fact, excision of a cyst in this region often requires dissecting scar tissue off the radial artery. Theoretically, incision and drainage of a ganglion in this area might predispose the patient to an arteriovenous malformation; however, a cyst that spontaneously ruptures in this area or is surgically removed may also predispose the patient to such a lesion.

Ganglion Cyst Excision

The patient should be informed of the alternative to either simple observation or aspiration and injection, which is removal by a hand surgeon under regional or general anesthesia. Consequently, typical anesthetic risks should be discussed. The patient should be informed of additional risks of surgery of this nature, including infection, neurovascular injury, rarely a venous thromboembolic event (much more common in the lower extremities), or recurrence of the ganglion. If the ganglion has resulted from a capsular or ligamentous defect, additional problems such as underlying joint destabilization and stiffness may occur.

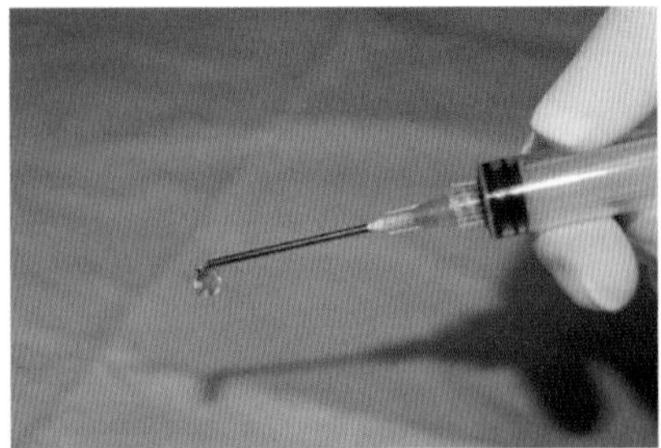

Figure 191-7 Typical thick, honey-like consistency of ganglion mucin. (Courtesy of The Medical Procedures Center, Midland, Mich.)

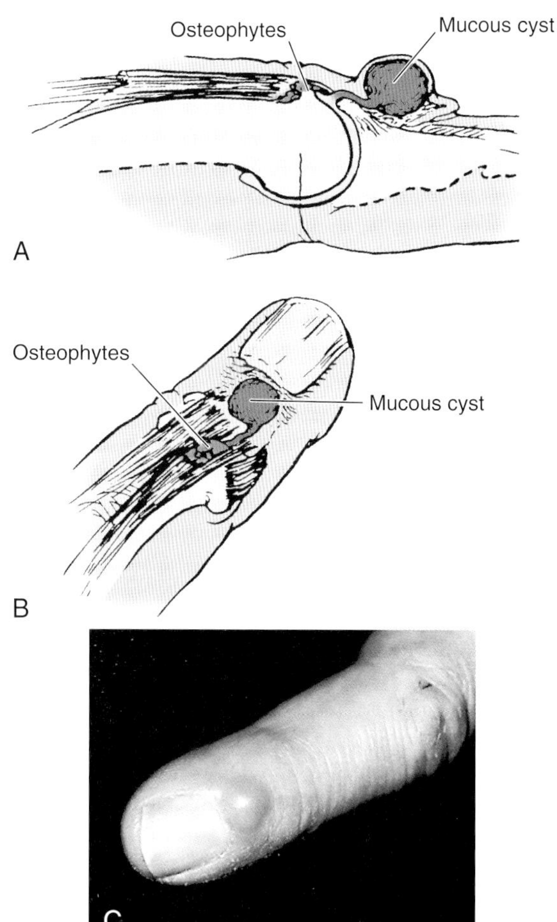

Figure 191-8 **A,** Relationship between mucous cyst and osteophyte of distal interphalangeal joint. Note that the cyst communicates with the joint. The osteophyte causes attrition of the extensor tendon, cyst formation, and decreased range of motion of the joint due to limited extension. **B,** As seen from above. **C,** Mucous cyst involving nailbed and distal interphalangeal joint. (A and B, Redrawn from Eaton RG, Dobranski AI, Littler JW: Marginal osteophyte excision in treatment of mucous cysts. J Bone Joint Surg Am 55:570–574, 1973. C, Courtesy of The Medical Procedures Center, Midland, Mich.)

Indications for Aspiration and Injection

- Symptomatic ganglion cyst (e.g., pain, paresthesias, motion limiting)
- Patient desires aspiration and/or injection (may be due to cosmetic deformity)

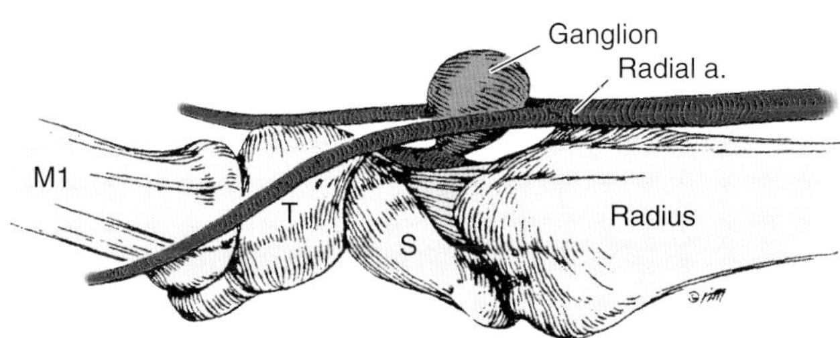

Figure 191-9 Usual relationship of the ganglion to the radial artery and volar joint capsule. M1, first metacarpal; S, scaphoid; T, trapezium. (Redrawn from Angelides AC: Ganglions of the hand and wrist. In Green DP, Hotchkiss RN, Pederson WC [eds]: Green's Operative Hand Surgery, 4th ed. New York, Churchill Livingstone, 1999, pp 2171–2183.)

- Diagnosis uncertain (although rare, malignant lesions can mimic ganglion cysts)

Contraindications to Aspiration and Injection

Be cautious and consider anatomic locations for critical neurovascular structures. The radial artery and dorsal sensory radial nerve are notable vulnerable structures, and as such should be avoided.

Equipment

- 25- or 27-gauge needle, 1 mL or less of lidocaine (1%), without epinephrine, in 1 or 3 mL syringe (if local anesthesia to be used)
- 18-gauge needle and 3- or 5-mL syringe for aspiration
- 1- or 3-mL syringe filled with steroid if injecting
- Small (2 to 4 inch) elastic bandage (e.g., Ace wrap) (*optional*)

Please refer to specified treatment techniques. Also see Chapter 192, Joint and Soft Tissue Aspiration and Injection (Arthrocentesis).

Treatment (Options)

1. *Observation*. Unless the ganglion is symptomatic (unsightly, painful, or limits motion), no treatment is necessary. Aspiration is indicated if there is uncertainty with the diagnosis.
2. *Digital pressure or rupture with a mallet, large book (e.g., the Bible), or blade*. These have all been tried historically with minimal success. Simple incision and drainage or rupturing with a needle are variants of this method.
3. *Aspiration and injection*. Aspiration followed by a steroid injection remains a commonly used technique. Although recurrence rates are high (up to 33%), some consider it the initial treatment of choice.
4. *Surgery*. Excision may be simple or quite complex. It is generally performed with a sterile environment. Even though recurrence rate is low with surgery, it can be as high as 20% if the surgeon cannot remove the entire stalk and a portion of the joint capsule.

Technique for Aspiration and Injection

Steroids

1. Using a 25- or 27-gauge needle, 1 mL or less of local lidocaine (1%) without epinephrine is deposited in a wheal over the most superficial portion of the ganglion. If the cyst is small, avoid this step because it may obscure (i.e., make it difficult to palpate) the underlying lesion.
2. The clinician first stabilizes and localizes the ganglion by grasping it (or the area around it) between the thumb and index finger of the nondominant hand. Using the clinician's dominant hand, an 18-gauge needle attached to a 3- to 5-mL syringe is inserted centrally into the ganglion while aspirating. Entry into the cyst is confirmed by a flash (it may be a small amount) of gelatinous fluid into the syringe. All of the thick, gelatinous fluid is then aspirated (Fig. 191-10). Applying pressure on the cyst by squeezing it between the thumb and index finger of the nondominant hand may be helpful. (If no fluid is aspirated, yet the clinician is certain that the needle has entered the cyst, the needle has probably become obstructed with a skin plug or very viscous fluid. Withdraw and detach the needle, fill the syringe with air, and attempt to flush this air back through the needle with the needle directed into a biohazard bin. This may remove an obstruction caused by either a skin plug or clotted, viscous fluid. Reinsert the needle into the ganglion.)
3. Secure this needle in place with a sterile hemostat (having verified that it is in the cyst) and remove the syringe filled with mucin.

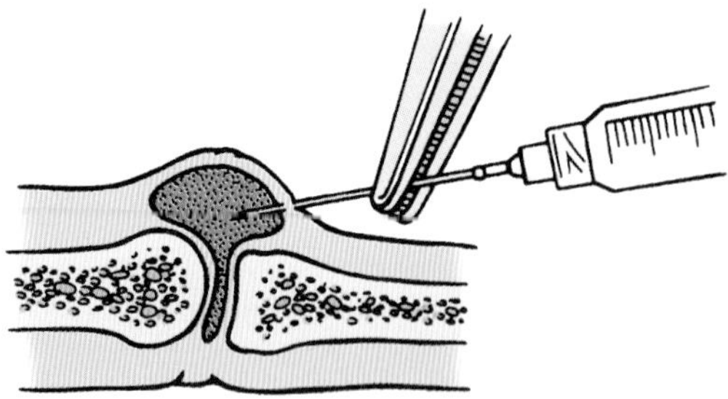

Figure 191-10 Use an 18-gauge needle and a 1- to 3-mL syringe to enter the ganglion and aspirate its contents. The contents are often thick, and there may be only minimal return of a gel-like material. Hold the needle in position with the hemostat and remove the syringe. Attach the steroid-containing syringe and inject the contents.

4. Attach another syringe (1 or 3 mL) filled with a 50/50 mixture of 1% lidocaine and steroid of choice (e.g., betamethasone; see Chapter 192, Joint and Soft Tissue Aspiration and Injection [Arthrocentesis]), and inject into the confines of the cyst. Variable amounts are used depending on the size of the cyst (0.1 to 1 mL). To reduce local steroid complications, consider starting with even smaller amounts of steroid. After injection, withdraw the needle.
5. Pressure is held over the needle track with a sterile gauze pad; then some clinicians wrap the area with a small elastic bandage (e.g., Ace wrap) to maintain occlusion of the cyst walls.
6. After successful aspiration, take all precautions to maintain the tip of the needle in the cyst until it is injected. After the cyst has been aspirated, if at all possible, *do not* withdraw the needle and then attempt a second insertion to inject (unless the needle becomes obstructed and has to be withdrawn to remove the obstruction).

Sclerosants

1. Technique is as noted for aspiration/injection. Instead of using steroids, substitute 1 mL of 3% sodium tetradecyl sulfate. This is the same solution used for sclerosing veins. Inject with approximately half the amount of the mucin withdrawn.

   NOTE: This technique reportedly has an 80% resolution rate.

2. Maintain compression continuously for 2 weeks.
3. After successful aspiration, take all precautions to maintain the tip of the needle in the cyst until it is injected. After the cyst has been aspirated, *do not* withdraw the needle and then attempt a second insertion to inject.

Postprocedure Patient Education

The patient should know to call the clinician's office or go to the emergency department for bleeding from the site, a significant increase in pain or fever, or signs or symptoms of infection. If a pressure dressing is applied, he or she should be instructed how to care for it and when it should be removed.

Complications

This procedure should *not* be taken lightly. Consideration of medical history and the location of the ganglion are of the utmost importance. The tissue overlying the ganglion commonly is thin with a poor blood supply and can slough because of bleeding, inadequate perfusion, or immune compromise. In addition, these cysts can be intertwined with neurovascular structures (see Fig. 191-9), and an intravascular or intraneural injection can have adverse results. Subcutaneous atrophy or depigmentation can occur if the steroid concentration is too high.

Operative Treatment

Surgical excision usually is 95% curative if the ganglion and stalk are removed with a small cuff of the adjacent joint capsule. The procedure should be approached with the same seriousness as any other hand surgery. A surgical suite with general or regional anesthesia is preferred. These operations should be performed by clinicians familiar with these lesions and the nearby anatomic structures. Even with surgical excision, the cysts can recur. The small, troublesome mucinous cyst on the dorsal DIP joint can actually require a fairly aggressive procedure to resolve.

CPT/Billing Codes

10160 Puncture aspiration of abscess, hematoma, bulla, or cyst
20600 Arthrocentesis, aspiration and/or injection, small joint or bursa (e.g., fingers, toes)
20605 Arthrocentesis, aspiration and/or injection, medium joint or bursa (e.g., wrist, elbow, ankle)
20612 Aspiration and/or injection of ganglion cyst(s) any location
25110 Excision, lesion of tendon sheath, forearm and/or wrist
25111 Excision of ganglion, wrist (dorsal or volar); primary

ICD-9-CM Diagnostic Codes

727.41 Ganglion; joint
727.42 Ganglion; tendon sheath

BIBLIOGRAPHY

Andrén L, Eiken O: Arthrographic studies of wrist ganglions. J Bone Joint Surg Am 53:299–302, 1971.
Athanasian EA: Bone and soft tissue tumors. In Green DP, Hotchkiss RN, Pederson WC, Wolfe SW (eds): Green's Operative Hand Surgery, 5th ed. New York, Churchill-Livingstone, 2005, pp 2211–2264.
Brown JS: Minor Surgery: A Text and Atlas, 4th ed. London, Oxford University Press, 2001.
Dias J, Buch K: Palmar wrist ganglion: Does intervention improve outcome? A prospective study of the natural history and patient-reported treatment outcomes. J Hand Surg Br 28:172–176, 2003.
Holm PCA, Pandey SD: Treatment of ganglia of the hand and wrist with aspiration and injection of hydrocortisone. Hand 5:63–68, 1973.
Jayson MIV, Dickson ASJ: Valvular mechanism in juxta-articular cysts. Ann Rheum Dis 29:415–420, 1970.
Kleinert HE, Kutz JE, Fishman JH, McCraw LH: Etiology and treatment of the so-called mucous cyst of the finger. J Bone Joint Surg Am 54:1455–1458, 1972.
Loder RT, Robinson JH, Jackson WT, Allen DJ: A surface ultrastructure study of ganglia and digital mucous cysts. J Hand Surg Am 13:758–762, 1988.
Nelson CL, Sawmiller S, Phalen GS: Ganglions of the wrist and hand. J Bone Joint Surg Am 54:1459–1464, 1972.
Peimer CA: Surgery of the hand and wrist. In Brunicardi FC, Andersen DK, Billiar TR, et al (eds): Schwartz's Principles of Surgery, 8th ed. New York, McGraw-Hill, 2005, pp 1721–1787.
Peimer CA, Thompson JS: Tumors of the hand. In Chapman MW (ed): Operative Orthopaedics, 3rd ed. Philadelphia, Lippincott Williams & Wilkins, 2001.
Richman JA, Gelberman RH, Engber WD, et al: Ganglions of the wrist and digits: Results of treatment by aspiration and cyst wall puncture. J Hand Surg Am 12:1041–1043, 1987.
Strenge KB, Mangan DB, Idusuyi OB: Postoperative toxic shock syndrome after excision of a ganglion cyst from the ankle. J Foot Ankle Surg 45:275–277, 2006.
Tallia AF, Cardone DA: Diagnostic and therapeutic injection of the wrist and hand region. Am Fam Physician 67:745–750, 2003.

CHAPTER 192

Joint and Soft Tissue Aspiration and Injection (Arthrocentesis)

Thad J. Barkdull • Francis G. O'Connor • John M. McShane

Joint and soft tissue aspiration and injection are both clinically rewarding and relatively simple office procedures. Steroid injection into joints fell into disfavor for many years because the procedure was overused and abused. When appropriate guidelines are followed, however, complications are extremely rare, and the injections can be very beneficial to the patient by reducing symptoms. The alternative to focal treatment with injection is usually systemic nonsteroidal anti-inflammatory drugs (NSAIDs), which have significant toxicity with prolonged use.

Primary care physicians should master the technique of aspiration and injection for many reasons. If the physician aspirates an inflamed joint, a diagnosis can be made immediately. If a joint is distended, pain can be relieved rapidly by aspirating the fluid. Injecting an anesthetic or steroid solution can give focal pain relief without the toxicity of the systemic medications and provide valuable information regarding diagnosis.

The clinician should not withhold the benefits of injection therapy because of incomplete familiarity with the precise anatomy involved. Knowledge of soft tissue and bony landmarks provides a reliable method for identification of needle insertion sites. The emerging role of musculoskeletal ultrasound in office-based practice additionally offers new opportunities to improve diagnostic and therapeutic techniques. The reader may want to refer to Chapter 191, Ganglion Treatment, for related information.

Indications

Diagnostic

- To evaluate synovial fluid and determine whether an effusion is from an infectious, rheumatic, traumatic, or crystal-induced origin
- To perform a therapeutic trial to differentiate between various conditions (e.g., costochondritis vs. coronary artery disease, trochanteric bursitis vs. deep hip disease, occipital trigger points vs. vertebral disease)
- To differentiate an intra-articular from extra-articular origin of pain symptoms

Therapeutic

- To remove exudative fluid from a septic joint
- To relieve pain in a grossly swollen joint (e.g., traumatic effusion)
- To reduce pain and inflammation by injecting lidocaine, with or without corticosteroids, or saline for trigger points (see Chapter 197, Trigger-Point Injection), noninfectious inflammatory arthritis, tendinitis, bursitis, or neuritis
- To stimulate the body's inflammatory cascade in order to promote healing (i.e., prolotherapy)

Indications for Corticosteroid Injections

Corticosteroids have a marked effect on inflammation. There are no good data to indicate that steroid injections decrease the long-term adverse effects of chronic degenerative osteoarthritis, but there is no doubt that they result in acute symptomatic improvement, especially over the first 1 to 4 weeks. The Cochrane Collaboration report on osteoarthritis supports the use of the intra-articular corticosteroids in the treatment of osteoarthritis (OA) of the knee.

Box 192-1 lists the conditions that are improved with local corticosteroid therapy. Localized pain that persists more than a few weeks after a trial of NSAIDs warrants an injection with steroids. Injections should be considered primarily when the potential toxicity or intolerance to NSAIDs outweighs the risk of local corticosteroids. Tramèr and colleagues noted in their meta-analysis that individuals chronically (≥2 months) using NSAIDs had a 1:1220 chance of dying from a gastrointestinal complication. In contrast, death occurring after intra-articular injections comes predominantly from septic arthritis, which occurs in anywhere from 1:3000 to 1:50,000 cases—with a mortality rate of about 15%. Morbidity risks associated with prolonged NSAID use are even greater.

Indications for Hyaluronic Acid Supplementation

Synovial fluid functions as a lubricant and a shock absorber in the joint. In OA, it retains very little of these intrinsic physical properties. At a critical load, normal synovial fluid changes its mechanical properties from viscous lubricant to elastic shock absorber. This change occurs between walking and running and is determined by the dynamic stress of both the frequency and the force of the load—a property which is diminished in OA. In addition, the concentration of hyaluronan in the synovial fluid in patients with OA is less than normal. Injected hylans and hyaluronans have properties similar to normal synovial fluid, and although they may only remain in the knee less than 2 weeks, the beneficial effects can persist up to a year (mean duration of 8.2 months). There is some evidence that they stimulate endogenous production of the synovial fluid. There is no evidence that viscosupplementation retards the progression of joint deterioration, but a recent Cochrane Review concluded that viscosupplementation showed beneficial effects on pain and patient function; this modality shows promise of postponing for years the need for total knee replacement. Studies are ongoing to assess its efficacy in other joints, because it is currently only Food and Drug Administration (FDA)–approved for use in the knee. The materials injected (hylans and hyaluronans) are

Box 192-1. Conditions Improved with Local Corticosteroid Injection

Articular Conditions

Coccydynia
Crystal-induced arthritis
  Gout
  Pseudogout
Ganglions
Osteoarthritis
Rheumatoid arthritis
Seronegative spondyloarthropathies
  Ankylosing spondylitis
  Arthritis associated with inflammatory bowel disease
  Psoriasis
  Reiter's syndrome

Nonarticular Conditions

Bursitis
  Anserine
  Olecranon
  Prepatellar
  Subacromial
  Trochanteric
Costochondritis
Fibrositis
  Localized (trigger points)
  Systemic
Morton's neuroma
Neuritis
  Carpal tunnel syndrome
  Cubital tunnel syndrome
  Tarsal tunnel syndrome
Periarthritis
  Adhesive capsulitis
Tenosynovitis/tendonitis
  Bicipital tendonitis
  de Quervain's disease
  Golfer's elbow (medial epicondylitis)
  Impingement syndrome
  Plantar fasciitis
  Rotator cuff
  Supraspinatus tendonitis
  Tennis elbow (lateral epicondylitis)
  Trigger finger
Tietze's syndrome

Adapted from Pfenninger JL: Injections of joints and soft tissue. Part I. General guidelines. Am Fam Physician 44:1196, 1991.

pharmacologically inert so the FDA classifies them as "devices," not "drugs."

- Approved for use in knee only
- May be used instead of, or after, intra-articular corticosteroid injections and before surgical intervention
- Effective in all stages of OA of the knee, although it wanes in the most advanced stages
- Is being studied for use in other joints

Indications for Prolotherapy

Prolotherapy is an alternative form of injection therapy, utilized by some clinicians to treat chronic musculoskeletal pain syndromes. *Prolo* is derived from proliferation, because the treatment causes the proliferation (growth and formation) of new connective tissue in areas that have become weak. The concept behind this technique is to stimulate the body's own inflammatory cascade in order to promote reabsorption of unhealthy tissue, such as degenerative fibroblasts in injured tendons, and the creation of new, healthy tissue. Inflammation-promoting agents (>10% dextrose solutions, phenol- or sodium-morrhuate–containing solutions, autologous blood, platelet rich plasma [PRP]) are injected into the area of injury, often with the aid of ultrasound to best localize the target.

Prolotherapy is most often described in use with tendinopathy, and there is some evidence to suggest that it is an effective therapy in treating the degenerative tissues identified. The treatment most likely achieves its maximal benefit when coupled with physical therapy focused on further stimulating growth of new tendinous tissue. As prolotherapy is an emerging technique that can be highly operator dependent, those interested in providing this service are encouraged to consult with a prolotherapist or complete a course of instruction prior to beginning prolotherapy injections in an office practice.

CONTRAINDICATIONS

- Cellulitis or broken skin over the intended entry site for the injection or aspiration
- Anticoagulant therapy that is not well controlled
- Severe primary coagulopathy
- Infected effusion of a bursa or a periarticular structure (for injection)
- More than three previous injections in a weight-bearing joint in the preceding 12-month period (*relative*—concern for theoretic joint destruction)
- Lack of response to two or three prior injections (*relative*)
- Suspected bacteremia (Unless the joint itself is suspected as the source of the bacteremia, it should not be tapped. Doing so could inoculate the joint space and *cause* infection.)
- Unstable joints (for steroid injection)
- Inaccessible joints (For many primary care physicians, this includes the hip joint, the sacroiliac joint, and the joints of the vertebral column.)
- Joint prostheses (If infection is suspected, consider a referral to the orthopedist that placed the prosthesis, if possible.)
- Pregnancy (*relative*)

EQUIPMENT

In the past, joint injections were frequently performed without gloves with only an alcohol wipe. In contrast, some physicians still use an extensive sterile draping procedure. Although the former is most likely inadequate, the latter is probably unnecessary unless the patient is immunosuppressed, diabetic, or at high risk of infection. Most injections are administered after an alcohol or povidone–iodine wipe. Gloves (sterile or nonsterile) should be used. When a culture is anticipated, sterile gloves are more customary. Masks are unnecessary.

Required equipment includes the following:

- Povidone–iodine wipes or alcohol wipes
- Sterile or nonsterile gloves
- Sterile drapes (*optional*)
- 22- to 27-gauge, 1½-inch needle for injections
- 18- to 21-gauge, 1½-inch needle for aspirations
- 30-gauge, ½-inch needle, if skin anesthesia is to be given (usually not needed)
- 1- to 10-mL syringe for injections (Luer-Lok is recommended.)
- 3- to 50-mL syringe for aspirations
- Single-dose vials of 1% lidocaine

NOTE: There are two reasons to use single-dose vials. First, no allergic reaction to lidocaine (an amide) has ever been reported. Although rare, reactions do occur to the preservative (parabens)

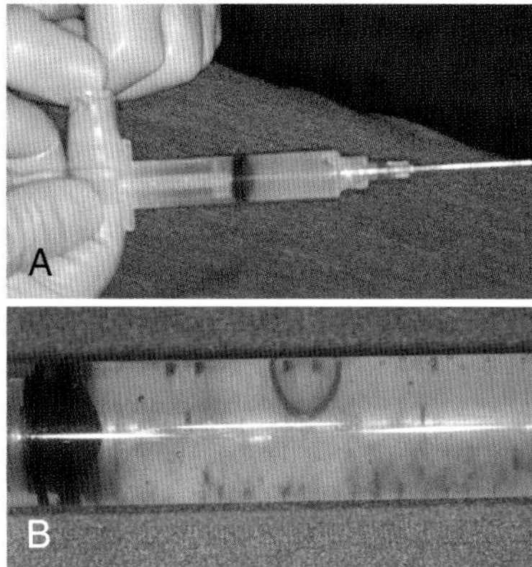

Figure 192-1 **A,** Example of precipitation of steroid (Celestone Soluspan) when mixed with lidocaine solution from a multidose vial. **B,** Steroid in solution (Celestone Soluspan) when mixed with lidocaine from a single-dose vial. It is preferable to have the steroid in solution rather than in precipitated form. (Courtesy of The Medical Procedures Center, PC, John L. Pfenninger, MD.)

TABLE 192-1 Relative Potency of Corticosteroids

Corticosteroid	Relative Anti-inflammatory Potency	Approximate Equivalent Dose (mg)
Short-acting Preparations		
Cortisone	0.8	25
Hydrocortisone	1	20
Intermediate-acting Preparations		
Prednisone	3.5	5
Prednisolone tebutate (Hydeltra-TBA)	4	5
Triamcinolone (Aristocort, Aristospan, Kenalog)	5	4
Methylprednisolone acetate (Depo-Medrol)	5	4
Long-acting Preparations		
Dexamethasone (Decadron-LA)	25	0.6
Betamethasone (Celestone Soluspan)	25	0.6

Adapted from Leversee JH: Aspiration of joints and soft tissue injections. Prim Care 13:572, 1986.

that is used in multidose vials. Local anesthetics with an ester base (e.g., procaine [Novocain]) can cause allergic reactions. So, using a single-dose vial of lidocaine makes it highly unlikely that there will be a reaction. Second, many steroids will precipitate when mixed with the parabens preservatives. This leads to uneven distribution in the syringe as well as the injection of small crystals into the site, and these crystals themselves could cause an inflammatory process (Fig. 192-1). Theoretically, a homogeneous solution would be more efficacious, although no studies have looked at the issue and many feel it is a moot point and of little concern. Certain manufacturers, however, do not recommend injecting precipitated steroids.

Many practitioners will use a longer-acting local anesthetic such as bupivacaine (Marcaine). Although this addition in most cases will not have any untoward effects, it should be noted that there have been instances of myotoxicity associated with bupivicaine, and given that it is only intended to provide short- to medium-term relief of symptoms, one might question its regular use.

- Hemostat (to be used if joint is to be aspirated then injected using different syringes but same needle)
- Tubes for culture or other laboratory studies (if aspiration is performed)
- Corticosteroid preparation (Tables 192-1 and 192-2)

A reasonable rule of thumb is that the greater the water solubility of the corticosteroid, the more rapid the onset of action, and the shorter the duration of effect. Thus, steroids with a lower degree of water solubility would in general be more effective in a chronic disease process, such as OA, whereas an acute inflammatory process might be more responsive to a shorter-acting preparation (Table 192-3).

NOTE: It is best to pick out one or two preparations and learn them well. It is not necessary to be familiar with all the drugs listed. There is no consensus in the literature as to the "best" drug or the optimal dosages. Table 192-2 offers our recommendations for appropriate dosing.

- Hyaluronic acid preparation (if used)—sodium hyaluronate (Hyalgan, Supartz, Euflexxa, Orthovisc) and hylan G-F 20 (Synvisc and Synvisc-one); dosages are as follows:
  - Hyalgan: five injections, 1 week apart ($691.60)
  - Supartz: five injections, 1 week apart ($709.72)
  - Euflexxa: three injections, 1 week apart ($599.15)
  - Orthovisc: three injections, 1 week apart ($801.57)
  - Synvisc: three injections, 1 week apart ($813.96)
  - Synvisc-one: one injection ($375.00)
- Adhesive bandage dressing
- Ultrasound (see later discussion for information regarding ultrasound-guided injections and Chapter 185, Musculoskeletal Ultrasonography)

Preprocedure Patient Preparation

Inform the patient of the risks, benefits, and possible complications of injection therapy. This information is especially important if steroids are used. Rarely is there ever a complication from the use of lidocaine alone. However, with steroids, and especially with repeated injections, there are some adverse consequences (see the "Complications" section and) Table 192-4. Inform the patient that there is always a possibility for *infection* with the injection, although this is extremely rare. *Bleeding* into a joint can occur, but this generally does not happen unless the patient has a coagulopathy. The injection may actually cause more *pain* during the first 24 to 36 hours. This reaction is called *steroid flare*. If the pain lasts for more than 72 hours, evaluate the patient for the possibility of a septic joint. Warn the patient of a possible *failure to obtain relief*, and that a second or even a third injection may be needed. Whether or not steroids have *significant adverse effects* on the cartilage and bone itself when steroids are injected into the joint space, and the degree of this reaction, is controversial. However, the effects would appear to be minimal, especially when used appropriately. *Allergic reactions* are very rare. *Tendon ruptures* should be avoidable if the injection is placed peritendinously instead of within the tendon itself. However, rupture is always a possibility. As a final precaution, warn the patient that a steroid placed too close to the surface of the skin occasionally causes *atrophy* (Fig. 192-2). This reaction may leave the patient with *depigmentation and a slight indentation* in the skin.

For diabetics, rapidly absorbed steroids can interfere with *glucose metabolism*. Therefore, glucose levels need to be followed more closely in the first 24 hours.

Pneumothorax has been reported after injection of trigger points and other conditions around the thorax. The following Technique section explains how to avoid this problem.

Technique

Before injection therapy, consider the differential diagnosis. If a tumor or fracture is possible, radiographs should be obtained. Many

TABLE 192-2 Common Corticosteroids and Recommended Dosages for Various Joint Injections

Corticosteroid	Concentration (mg/mL)	Large Joint* Dosage (mg)	Medium Joint† Dosage (mg)	Small Joint†‡ Dosage (mg)	Ganglia (mg)	Tendon Sheath (mg)	Bursa (mg)
Hydrocortisone acetate	25, 50	40–100	20–40	8–20	20–40	20–50	40–90
Prednisolone tebutate (Hydeltra-TBA)	20	20–30	10–20	8–10	10–20	4–10	20
Prednisolone sodium phosphate	20	10–20	5–10	4–5	5–10	3–8	20
Triamcinolone hexacetonide (Aristospan)	5, 20	20–30	10–20	8–10	10–20	4–10	20
Triamcinolone diacetate (Aristocrat)	25, 40	20–40	10–20	8–10	10–20	4–10	20
Triamcinolone acetonide (Kenalog)	10, 40	20–40	10–20	8–10	10–20	4–10	20
Methylprednisolone acetate (Depo-Medrol)	20, 40, 80	20–40	10–40	8–10	4–20	4–10	20
Dexamethasone sodium phosphate (Decadron)	4	2–4	1–3	0.8–1	1–2	0.4–1	2–3
Dexamethasone acetate (Decadron-LA)	8	2–4	1–3	0.8–1	1–2	0.4–1	2–3
Betamethasone acetate/phosphate (Celestine Soluspan)	6	6–12	3–6	1.5–3	1–3	1.5–2	3–6

*Such as knee, shoulder, ankle.
†Such as elbow, wrist.
‡Such as metacarpophalangeal, interphalangeal, acromioclavicular, temporomandibular.

times, especially with trigger-point injection (see Chapter 197, Trigger-Point Injection), x-rays are unnecessary. Other diagnoses may also be fairly straightforward and not require a prior radiographic examination either. If the diagnosis is in question or if the patient is at risk for bone metastases (e.g., a history of breast or prostate cancer), the condition should be clarified before injection therapy.

Generally, the clinician injects a combination of lidocaine with the steroid of choice. Single-dose vials of lidocaine should be used to avoid the preservative/precipitation problems (see earlier comments and the "Complications" section). Using a rather large volume of lidocaine may be beneficial. Not only does it disperse the steroid in a less concentrated solution, the volume itself may have a therapeutic effect. In some instances, only a minimal amount of lidocaine can be used (e.g., ganglion cysts, trigger fingers). In other sites, larger amounts are recommended (e.g., lidocaine 5 to 10 mL in a shoulder or knee mixed with 0.5 to 1 mL of selected steroid). A good rule of thumb is to use more, not less, when it comes to lidocaine.

The recommended dosages of medications (Table 192-5) and the specific techniques for various injection sites (Figs. 192-3 to 192-25) are included in this chapter.

General

The general approach is as follows:

1. *Identify the site of entry* and mark it with a thumbnail, ballpoint pen, or indelible marker. Making a circular indentation at the designated site with the retracted end of a ballpoint pen is an excellent way to avoid losing your landmarks when cleaning the area.
2. *Prep the area with an alcohol or povidone–iodine wipe.* (Note that alcohol often removes ink and skin marker solutions.)
3. *Draw up the proper amounts of steroid and anesthetic* into a single syringe and mix well by tipping the syringe backward and forward.
4. Note that although using smaller caliber needles may provide the patient with less pain, it is more difficult to determine whether the appropriate space for injection has been entered. In contrast, larger bore needles will be more painful. Based on the site of injection, and the constitution of the patient, you may decide to *inject a superficial anesthetic* (e.g., lidocaine) or use ethyl chloride spray on the skin prior to the intra-articular injection to allow for the use of a larger needle.
5. Using appropriate syringes and needles, either *aspirate* or *inject* the site as indicated. After insertion but before injection, pull back the plunger to be sure the needle is not in a blood vessel.
6. If aspiration of an effusion is to be followed by injection, there are two choices: (1) have two needle/syringe setups and enter the area twice, or (2) enter once, aspirate, grasp the needle with a hemostat (being careful not to change the position of the needle tip), remove the syringe with the aspirate, then replace it with the lidocaine/steroid syringe, and finally inject the contents.
7. If lidocaine or steroid is to be injected, it is often necessary to inject in two or three slightly different areas at the site of tenderness. This is not necessary when the joint space itself has been entered, although some practitioners advocate repositioning within bursal spaces because of the potential presence of

TABLE 192-3 Steroid Solubility

Steroid	Solubility (% wt/vol)
Triamcinolone hexacetonide	0.0002
Triamcinolone acetate	0.004
Prednisolone tebutate	0.001
Methylprednisolone acetate	0.001
Hydrocortisone acetate	0.002

TABLE 192-4 Adverse Effects of Local Corticosteroid Therapy

Complication	Estimated Prevalence
Postinjection flare	2%–5%
Steroid arthropathy	0.8%
Tendon rupture	<1%
Facial flushing	<1%
Skin atrophy, depigmentation	<1%
Iatrogenic infectious arthritis	0.01%
Transient paresis of injected extremity	Rare
Hypersensitivity reaction	Rare
Asymptomatic pericapsular calcification	43%
Acceleration of cartilage attrition	Unknown

From Gray RG, Gottlieb NL: Intra-articular corticosteroids: An updated assessment. Clin Orthop Relat Res 177:253, 1983.

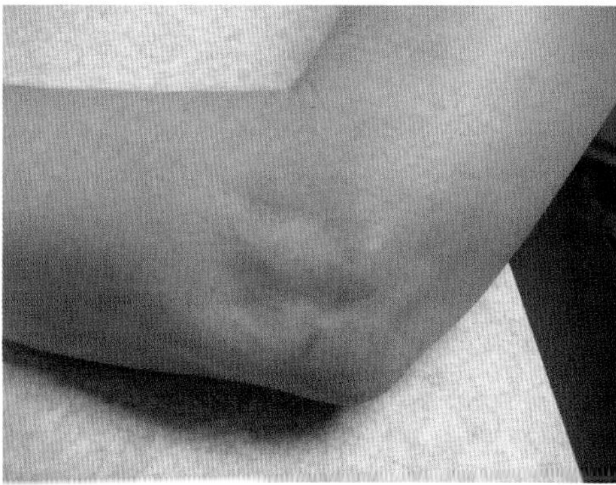

Figure 192-2 Fatty atrophy. This patient received a steroid injection for lateral epicondylosis approximately 11 months before this photo was taken, showing an example of steroid fatty atrophy and hypopigmentation. Such changes may take up to a year to resolve, and some can be permanent changes.

septations that may interfere with full dissolution within the desired area.

8. Although much has been written regarding *laboratory evaluation of joint fluid aspirates*, Schmerling and associates reported that the *white blood cell* (WBC) count and *polymorphonucleocyte percentage* (PMN) were the only helpful tests to determine the etiology of an exudate. Use lavender-topped Vacutainers for these studies. It is recommended that synovial fluid be examined within 1 hour after arthrocentesis. WBC counts of mildly inflammatory fluids can decrease to "noninflammatory range" within 5 to 6 hours. Glucose, protein, lactate dehydrogenase (LDH), complement fixation, electrolyte, uric acid levels, rheumatoid factor, and antinuclear antibodies were of little benefit. Fluids for chemistry testing if desired should be transported in green- or red-topped tubes and be analyzed within 4 hours.

If the exudate is cloudy, the WBC count is elevated, or a septic joint is strongly suspected, do not inject the area, and a *culture* is also indicated. For cultures, submit as much fluid as possible. "Swabbed samples" may not be adequate. Large-volume specimens (over 2 mL) support viability of most microorganisms for up to 24 hours at room temperature. Nevertheless, transport to the laboratory ASAP. *Do not refrigerate!* Large samples may be sent in the syringe used to aspirate them or in a sterile 5- or 10-mL container that has no additives (i.e., a red-topped glass tube). For volumes less than 2 mL, consider using bottles with culture media (e.g., Port-A-Cul) inside. Test tube containers with anticoagulant additives (i.e., lavender- or green-topped containers) should not be used.

If there is any suspicion of gouty arthritis, examine the fluid for crystals under polarized light.

A *peripheral smear* may be helpful when a bloody tap is obtained after trauma. The presence of fat cells indicates a fracture.

The Pfenninger articles listed in the bibliography contain many tables of other characteristics of synovial fluid for differential diagnosis, although the benefit of additional studies is unproved.

Technique of Injection for Hyaluronic Acid "Devices"

- Must be intra-articular.
- More demanding than steroid intra-articular injections because it must be placed within the synovial space, not the surrounding soft tissue.
- Some will use fluoroscopy or ultrasound to be certain of intra-articular injection.
- Do not mix with lidocaine or steroids.
- Drain all effusions before injection.
- Forced injections push material into the elasticity zone and then are very difficult to administer; slow injections must be given with a 22-gauge or larger needle (which again may necessitate the use of superficial anesthesia with lidocaine or ethyl chloride spray to allow for better tolerance by the patient).

TABLE 192-5 Needle Size and Drug Dosage for Injection Therapy

Anatomic Structure	Needle Gauge (Length)	Dose of 1% Lidocaine (mL)	Dose of Methylprednisolone Acetate (mg)
Abductor tendon of thumb (de Quervain's disease)	25 (1½ inch)	3–4	10–20
Acromioclavicular joint	22–25 (1–1½ inch)	2–4	4–10
Ankle	22 (1–1½ inch)	3–5	20–40
Anserine bursa	22–25 (1½ inch)	3–5	20–40
Biceps tendon	22 (1½ inch)	5–10	10–20
Calcaneal bursa	22 (1½ inch)	5	20–40
Carpal tunnel	25 (1½ inch)	1	20–40
Elbow	25 (1½ inch)	3–4	10–20
Radiohumeral joint	22 (1–1½ inch)	3–5	20–30
Lateral or medial epicondyle ("tennis elbow," "golfer's elbow")	22–25 (1–1½ inch)	3–5	10–30
Olecranon bursa	22 (1–1½ inch)	2–3	10–20
Finger and toe joints (interphalangeal)	25 (1 inch)	0.5–1.0	4–10
Flexor tendon sheath (trigger finger)	25 (1 inch)	0.25–0.5	4–10
Ganglion of wrist, other	18–20 (1–1½ inch)	0.25–0.5	4–10
Hip joint	20 (2½–3 inch)	5	40–80
Knee intra-articular space	20 (1½ inch)	5	20–80
Plantar fascia	22 (1½ inch)	2–4	15–30
Prepatellar bursa	20–22 (1–1½ inch)	3	20–40
Shoulder intra-articular space	20 (1½ inch)	5–7	20–40
Shoulder rotator cuff tendon	18–20 (1½ inch)	5	20–40
Shoulder subacromial bursa	22 (1½–2 inch)	5–7	30–40
Tarsal tunnel	25 (½–1 inch)	1–2	10–20
Temporomandibular joint	25 (½–1 inch)	1–2	5–20
Trigger point	25 (1½ inch)	3–5	10–30
Trochanteric bursa	22 (1½–2 inch)	5–10	20–40
Wrist joint	22–25 (1–1½ inch)	2–4	20–40

Modified from Pfenninger JL: Injections of joints and soft tissue. Part II. Guidelines for specific joints. Am Fam Physician 44:1690, 1991.

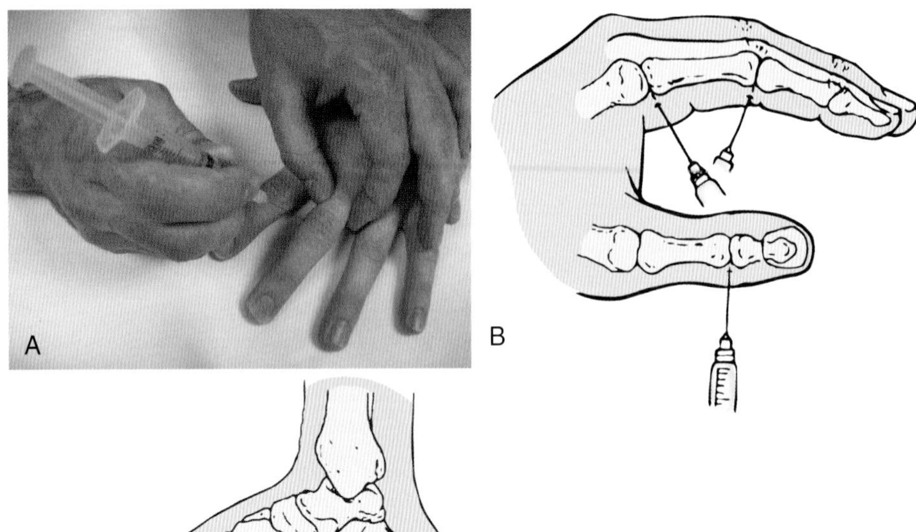

Figure 192-3 Injecting finger and toe joints. **A,** Appropriate technique for injecting a finger joint. Tendons run over the dorsum of the finger, whereas nerves and vessels run laterally. Open the joint slightly by flexing it and then inject between the ligaments and the vascular structures as noted. The needle enters at a 45-degree angle to the joint. Any of the finger (**B**) and toe (**C**) joints may be aspirated or injected in the lateral or medial aspect. Slightly flex the joint to open the joint space. Direct the needle to enter just medial or lateral to the extensor tendon, avoiding too lateral or medial an approach where the nerve and vascular structures run. Use a 25-gauge, 1-inch needle with 0.5 to 1.0 mL 1% lidocaine and 4 to 10 mg of methylprednisolone acetate or equivalent (see Tables 192-2 and 192-5).

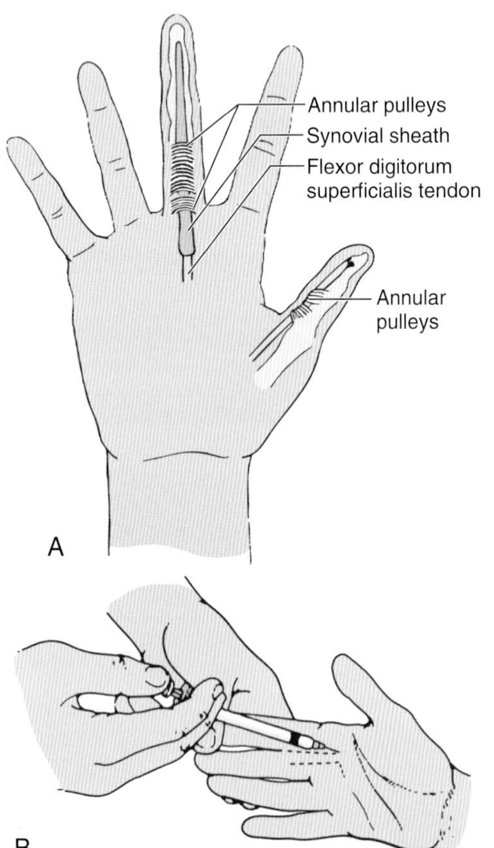

Figure 192-4 Trigger finger. **A,** The anatomy of a finger showing the annular pulleys, which maintain the flexor close to the bony structures. When the tendon becomes inflamed and enlarges, it catches on the pulleys, causing a snapping with extension or a "trigger finger." **B,** Identify the flexor tendon involved. Insert the needle at the distal palmar crease. Attempt to position it peritendinously. When the needle is in position, the syringe will move with flexion of the finger. Use a 25-gauge, 1-inch needle with 0.25 to 0.5 mL 1% lidocaine and 4 to 10 mg of methylprednisolone acetate or equivalent (see Tables 192-2 and 192-5).

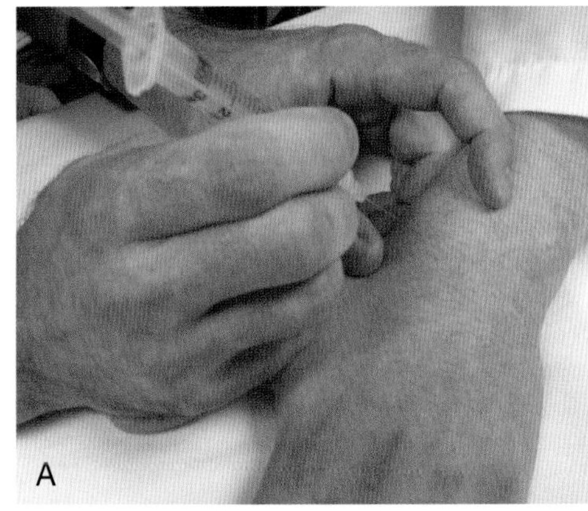

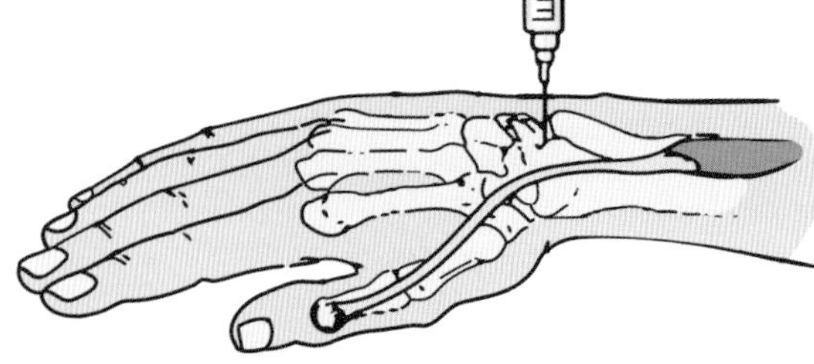

Figure 192-5 Wrist joint. **A,** Injection of the wrist joint. The hand is held in slight flexion, and the needle is inserted just distal to the radius in the "snuff box." **B,** Flex the joint 20 degrees to open the joint spaces. The dorsal approach is generally used. Position the needle perpendicular to the skin surface. Enter at a site distal to the radial head and lateral to the extensor pollicis longus tendon (just ulnar to the anatomic "snuff box"). If the needle can be easily inserted to 1 or 2 cm, it is correctly positioned in the joint space. The intercarpal joints have interconnecting synovial spaces, and the contents of one correctly placed injection will disperse into the entire joint complex. Use an 18- to 20-gauge, 1- to 1½-inch needle with 0.5 to 1.0 mL 1% lidocaine and 4 to 10 mg of methylprednisolone acetate or equivalent (see Tables 192-2 and 192-5).

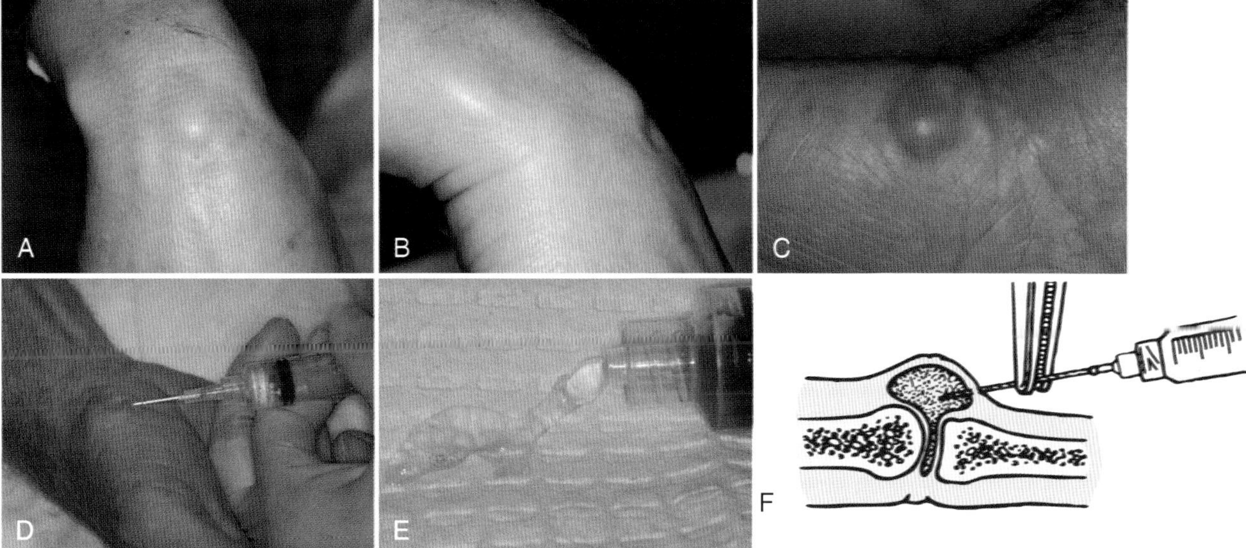

Figure 192-6 A ganglion is a manifestation of joint inflammation. **A,** Frontal view. **B,** Side view. **C,** Example of an unusual ganglion cyst on the thenar eminence. **D,** Aspiration of the cyst. Hold the needle in position with the hemostat and remove the syringe. Attach the steroid-containing syringe and inject the contents. (Some have used fibrin sealants, hypertonic saline, and other irritants for attempts to "scar down" the cyst.) **E,** The contents are often thick, and there may only be minimal return of a gel-like material. **F,** Use an 18- to 20-gauge, 1- to 1½-inch needle with 0.5 to 1.0 mL 1% lidocaine and 4 to 10 mg of methylprednisolone acetate or equivalent (see Tables 192-2 and 192-5). (**A–E,** Courtesy of The Medical Procedures Center, PC, John L. Pfenninger, MD.)

- Patient should avoid strenuous activity for 48 hours.
- Derived from chicken or rooster combs, so an allergy to eggs or feathers would dictate caution.

Technique of Injection for Prolotherapy

A complete course of instruction prior to beginning prolotherapy injections in an office practice is recommended.

- Typically used in areas of degenerative tissue (i.e., tendinoses).
- Because of common usage with tendinous tissues, care must be taken to inject into the peritendinous areas rather than into the body of the tendon itself.
- Ultrasound can be considered to confirm placement of agent into the desired area.
- Because an inflammatory response is the desired outcome, educating the patient regarding anticipated pain over the next 24 to 48 hours is strongly encouraged. Some practitioners even advocate the use of opioid analgesics for pain control in the immediate postinjection period.

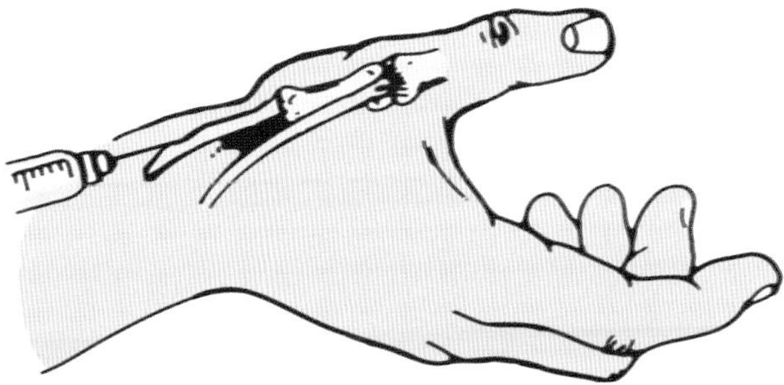

Figure 192-7 De Quervain's disease. Maximally abduct the thumb to accentuate and identify the tendon. Insert the needle parallel to (but not into) the tendon. Inject at the areas of greatest tenderness. Postinjection splinting may still be necessary. Use a 25-gauge, 1½-inch needle with 3 to 4 mL 1% lidocaine and 10 to 20 mg of methylprednisolone acetate or equivalent (see Tables 192-2 and 192-5).

- There are no current recommendations for the ideal proinflammatory agent; availability (i.e., dextrose solutions) or desire to utilize the patient's own fluids (i.e., autologous blood, platelet-rich plasma) are two of the considerations made in determining the appropriate agent.
- Lidocaine should be injected to provide local anesthesia prior to using the other agents.
- Volume of agent should be based on the size of the area involved most tendinous injections usually require no more than 5 mL of solution. Some areas will allow for a greater volume to be placed, but may cause more postinjection pain.
- Although there is no consensus as yet for the appropriate interval or total number of injections that should be administered, it is reasonable to wait at least 4 to 6 weeks between treatments. If more than five injections are necessary, consideration should be made for other therapies.

Ultrasound Guidance for Injections

Also see Chapter 185, Musculoskeletal Ultrasonography.

Ultrasound is an extremely valuable modality that can allow the physician to identify the structure to be injected and guide the needle to its precise location. This can be particularly beneficial in reducing the pain associated with "blind" localization of small joint spaces, making the patient more comfortable, and thus more compliant, during the procedure.

Ultrasound-guided injections also allow the clinician greater confidence in interpreting the results of an injection. For example, a missed injection into the acromioclavicular joint may suggest another etiology of a patient's shoulder pain, resulting in further erroneous testing and treatment regimens unless the error is identified on ultrasound. When the injection is performed with ultrasound, the physician has objective evidence of appropriate placement of the medication and can therefore derive more accurate conclusions regarding the efficacy of the medication.

In order to perform ultrasound-guided injections, the physician must have some training in the use of diagnostic ultrasound. The machine used should ideally have at least one multifrequency transducer, in order to allow for visualization of both superficial and

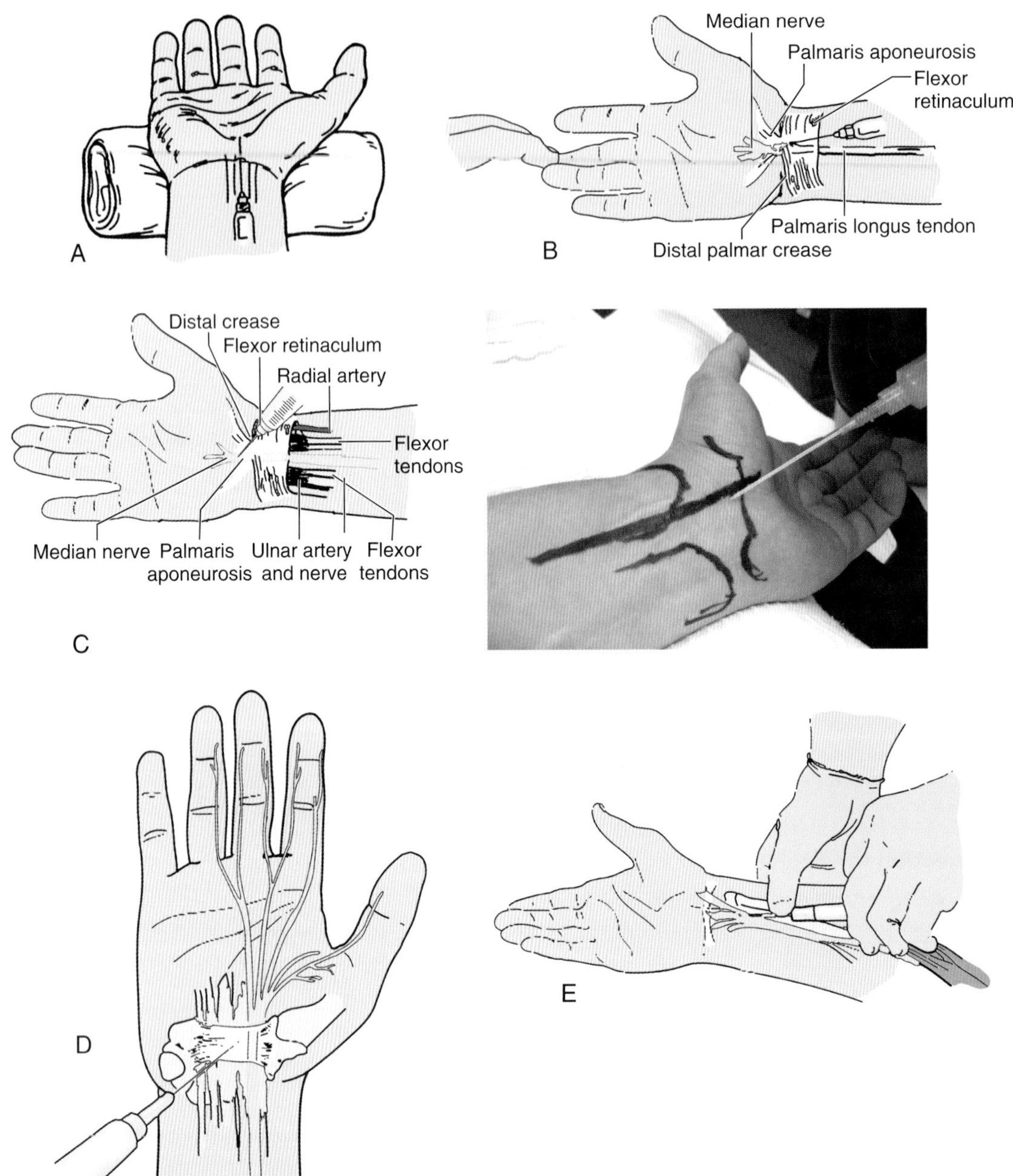

Figure 192-8 Carpal tunnel syndrome. Four approaches to injection: **A,** *Traditional method.* Dorsiflex the wrist 30 degrees and rest it on a rolled towel. Insert the needle at the distal crease of the wrist either lateral or medial to the palmaris longus tendon. **B,** Find the tendon by having the patient flex the middle finger against resistance or abduct the thumb and little finger together. Angle the needle downward at a 45-degree angle toward the tip of the middle finger. If there is any discomfort in the fingers, withdraw and reposition the needle. Advance 1 to 2 cm until there is *no* resistance, and then inject the medication. **C,** *Alternative method* (illustrated and pictured). Insertion of the needle directly over the carpal tunnel. Use a perpendicular approach going directly through the flexor retinaculum into the median nerve space. **D,** A *third method* of injecting the carpal tunnel. The needle is inserted just radial to the pisiform bone and directed toward the carpal tunnel just beneath the transverse carpal ligament. The needle goes dorsally and distally to terminate within the carpal tunnel just to the ulnar side and dorsal to the median nerve. **E,** A *more recent approach* is to inject on the volar aspect of the forearm 4 cm proximal to the wrist crease between the palmaris longus tendon (see previous description) and the radial flexor tendon. The needle is inserted in a distal direction with the syringe lifted 10 to 20 degrees up from the parallel. This approach supposedly minimizes chances of trauma to the nerve. In all cases (**A–E**), the injection should be given with minimal pressure, slowly. If there is resistance or if the patient feels "pins and needles" in the fingers, stop immediately. If an intraneural injection occurs, there will be significant pain after injection and surgical decompression may be needed. Use a 25-gauge, 1½-inch needle with 1 mL 1% lidocaine and 20 to 40 mg of methylprednisolone acetate or equivalent (see Tables 192-2 and 192-5).

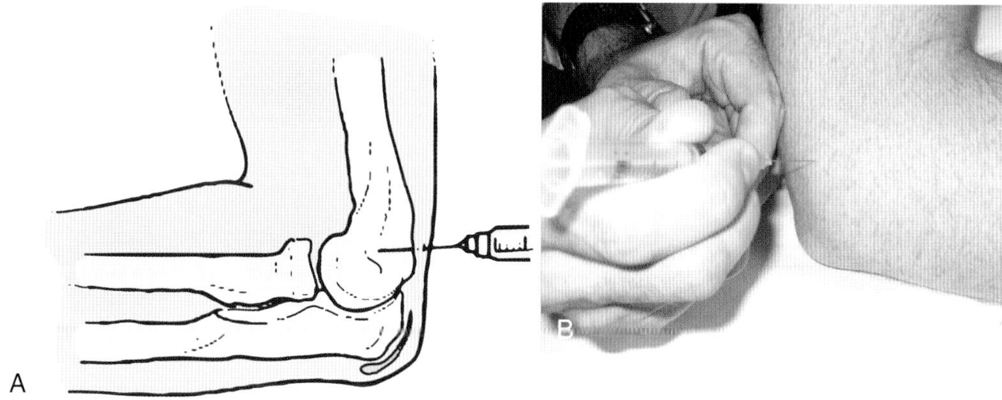

Figure 192-9 Lateral epicondylitis (tennis elbow). **A** and **B,** Find the area of greatest tenderness over the lateral epicondyle. Insert the needle perpendicularly until bone is felt. Withdraw the needle 1 to 2 mm and inject. It may be beneficial to fan out the injections in several directions into the extensor aponeurosis and the radial collateral ligament. Massage the injection site. If distal tenderness is still present after several minutes, another injection in a fanlike pattern may be necessary. Medial epicondylitis (golfer's elbow) is treated in a similar fashion. Use a 22- to 25-gauge, 1½-inch needle with 3 to 5 mL 1% lidocaine and 10 to 30 mg of methylprednisolone acetate or equivalent (see Tables 192-2 and 192-5).

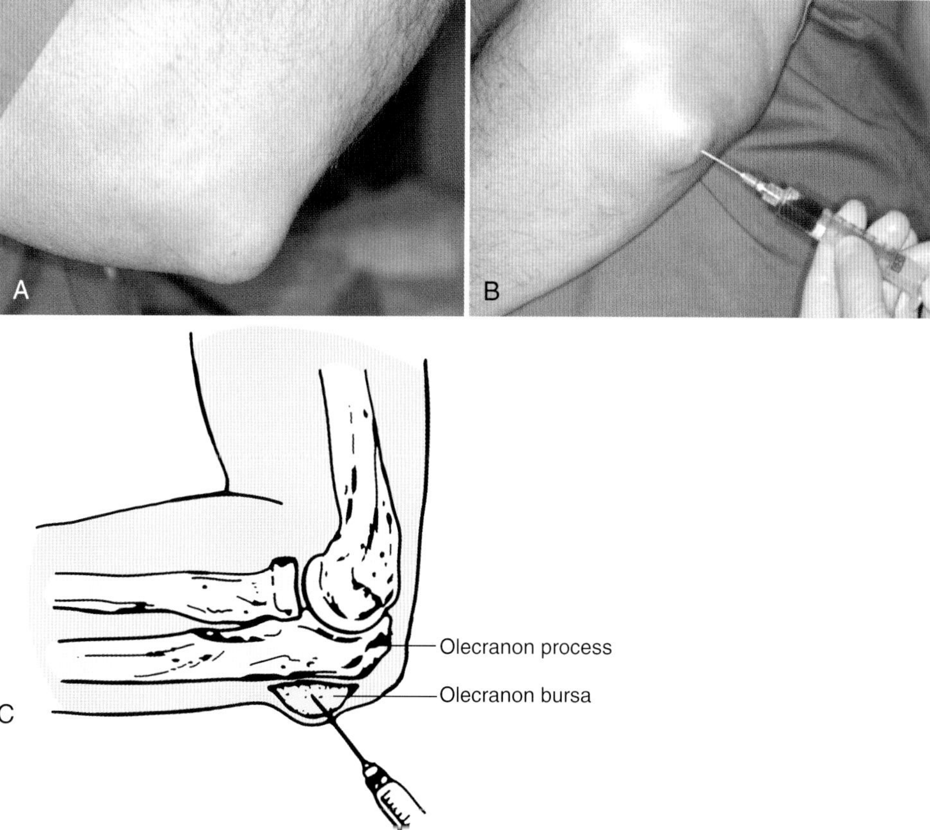

Figure 192-10 Olecranon bursa, aspiration and injection. **A,** An enlarged bursa secondary to bursitis. **B,** Aspirating the olecranon bursa. This bursa is easily identified and entered. **C,** Insert a large-bore needle directly into the bursa and aspirate until fluid is returned. Whether cloudy or not, the fluid should be submitted for culture and concurrent infection should be ruled out. Await the culture results before injecting with a steroid. It is next to impossible to tell whether the bursa is infected or not on a clinical basis. While waiting for the culture results, place the patient on nonsteroidal anti-inflammatory drugs (NSAIDs) and wrap the area tightly. If infection is suspected, start an antibiotic to cover gram-positive pathogens while waiting for culture results. Once infection is ruled out, steroids can be used. In a double-blind study comparing focal steroid injection into the olecranon bursa with systemic NSAIDs, the most rapid benefit and most lasting effect came from steroid injections. Use an 18- to 21-gauge needle for aspiration. Use a 22-gauge, 1- to 1½-inch needle with 2 to 3 mL 1% lidocaine and 10 to 20 mg of methylprednisolone acetate or equivalent for injection (see Tables 192-2 and 192-5). (Courtesy of The Medical Procedures Center, PC, John L. Pfenninger, MD.)

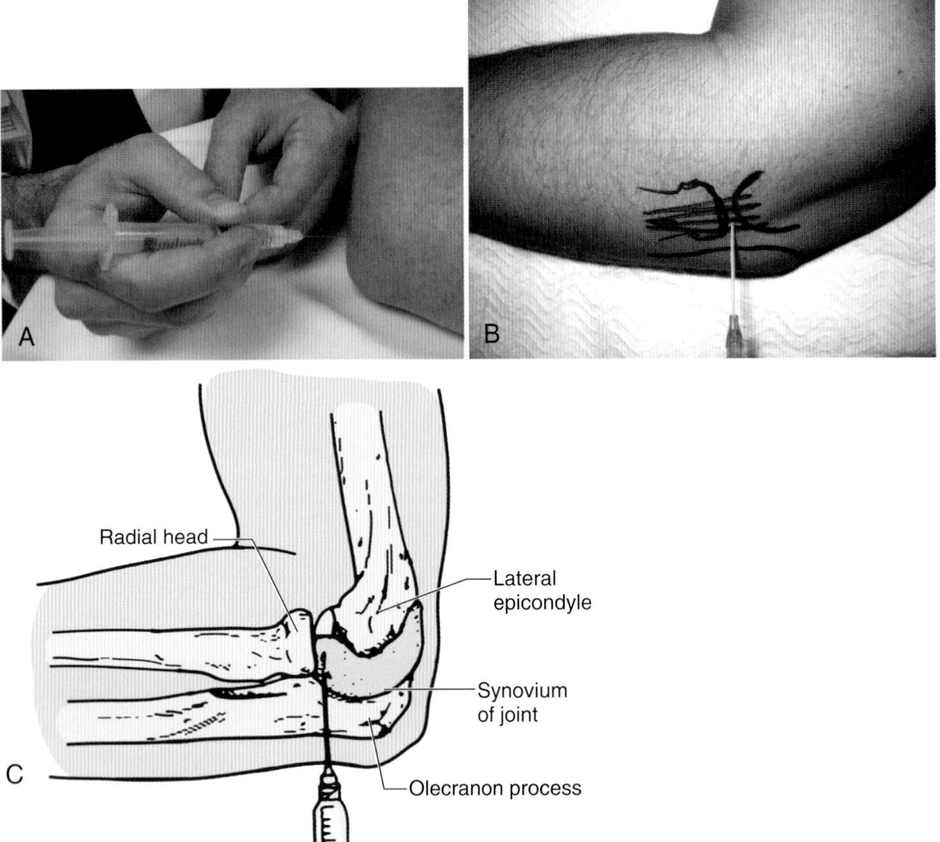

Figure 192-11 Elbow joint. **A,** Injection of the elbow joint. **B,** Flex the elbow 45 degrees. Identify the lateral epicondyle. Inject into the joint space just distal to the lateral epicondyle and superior to the olecranon process of the ulna. A slight concavity can be felt just inferior to the radial head and helps identify the proper point of insertion. **C,** Use a 22-gauge, 1- to 1½-inch needle with 3 to 5 mL 1% lidocaine and 20 to 30 mg of methylprednisolone acetate or equivalent (see Tables 192-2 and 192-5).

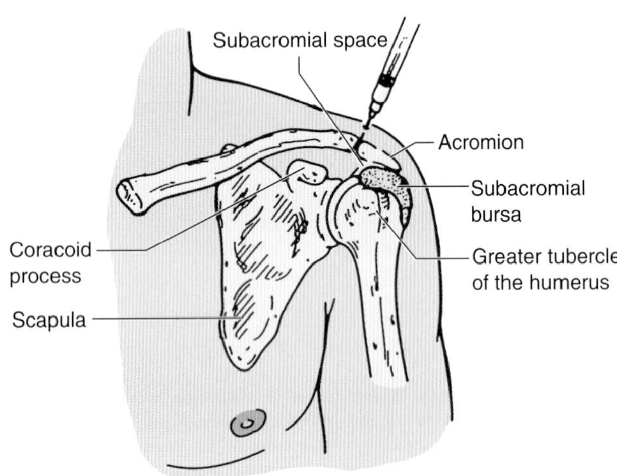

Figure 192-12 Acromioclavicular joint. With the patient seated and arm at the side, palpate the clavicle, moving laterally until a prominence is felt. This is the acromioclavicular joint. It is about 1.5 to 2 cm inward from the lateral edge to the acromion. Insert the needle from an anterior or superior position into the joint and angle it medially, then inject. Use a 22-gauge, 1- to 1½-inch needle with 5 to 7 mL 1% lidocaine and 30 to 40 mg of methylprednisolone acetate or equivalent (see Tables 192-2 and 192-5).

deeper structures. Power Doppler capability is also valuable because it allows the physician to avoid vasculature and to better observe the flow of the medication in the actual space intended.

When performing ultrasound-guided injections, the following supplies are needed:

- Ultrasound gel
- Antiseptic, such as alcohol or Betadine
- Gauze pads and adhesive bandages
- Ethyl chloride spray
- Syringes (It is important to ensure that all air has been cleared out of both the needle and the syringes to be used, because air bubbles obscure ultrasound images.)
- Needles of appropriate length to reach the target
- A pair of forceps or a needle holder

The standard technique for performing therapeutic injections under ultrasound guidance is as follows:

1. With the patient in a comfortable position, place some ultrasound gel over the area to be visualized and then use the ultrasound transducer to identify the structure to be injected.
2. Once the structure has been identified, place the transducer so that its long axis will be parallel to best line for the needle to take in order to reach its target (Fig. 192-26).
3. Use appropriate antiseptic solution to cleanse the skin at the end of the transducer where the needle will enter. Be sure not to move the transducer once the skin has been prepared.
4. Use the ethyl chloride spray to superficially anesthetize the skin that will be punctured by the needle.

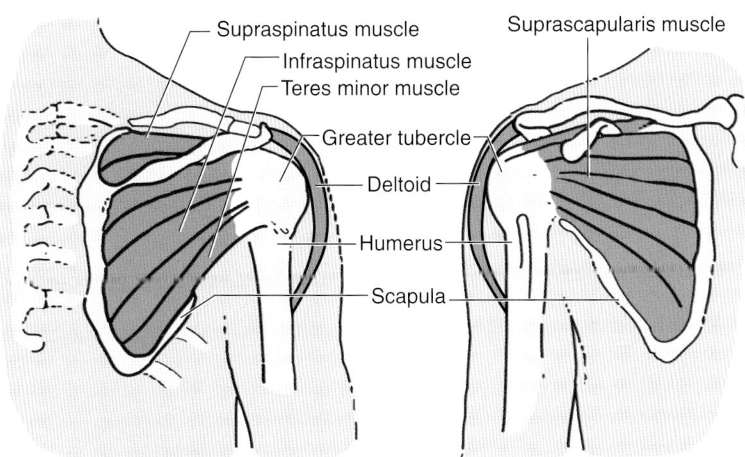

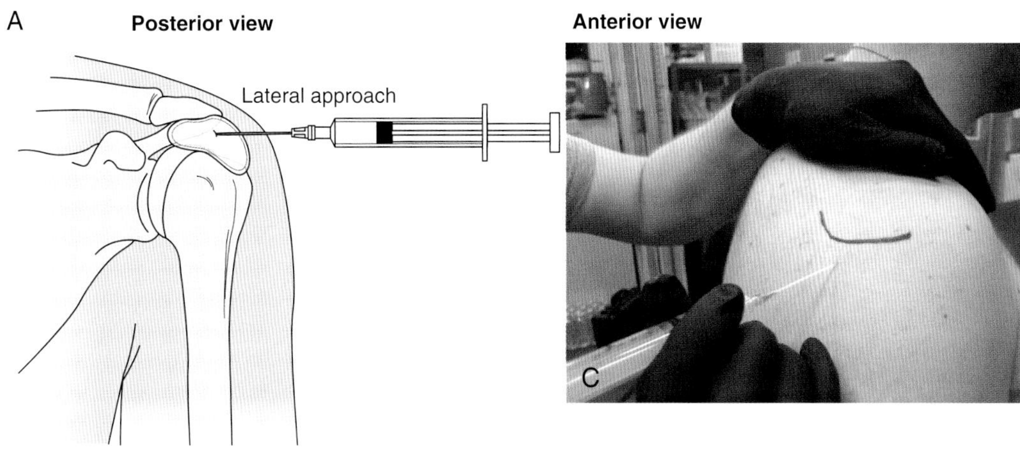

Figure 192-13 Shoulder: Subacromial bursa. Most injection procedures involving the shoulder will include an injection into the subacromial bursa. Palpate the superior surface of the shoulder, progressing laterally until there is a slight drop-off. This is the lateral edge of the acromion. The now palpable soft spot above the humeral head is the location of the subacromial bursa. Direct the needle perpendicular to the surface and insert the needle through the deltoid muscle into the bursa. The needle should be free floating, since it is within a space, not in a muscle or tendon. The tendon of the supraspinatus, the muscle most commonly involved in a rotator cuff syndrome, is directly medial to this bursa and can be entered by directing the needle deeper. If the tendon is calcified as it is entered, a gritty sensation may be felt. Inject within the bursa, not within the tendon. **A,** The muscles of the rotator cuff are demonstrated. They include the supraspinatus, the infraspinatus, teres minor, and the subscapularis. **B,** The technique of a subacromial bursa injection. **C,** Injecting the subacromial bursa. Use a 22-gauge, 1- to 1½-inch needle with 5 to 7 mL 1% lidocaine and 30 to 40 mg of methylprednisolone acetate or equivalent (see Tables 192-2 and 192-5). (**B,** Courtesy of Pharmacia Corp.)

5. Take the needle and syringe containing the local anesthetic and hold it parallel to the ultrasound transducer with the tip of the needle aimed at the skin that has been cleansed. Keeping the needle constantly parallel to the transducer, enter the skin and inject a small amount of anesthetic.
6. Using the ultrasound transducer, constantly keep the needle and the target to be injected in view. As the needle is advanced, repeatedly inject a small amount of anesthetic ahead of the tip. The fluid injected will be seen distending the tissue, and will help establish the location of the needle. If the needle is moved off target, slightly withdraw and redirect toward the target.
7. Once the structure to be injected is reached, turn on the power Doppler and center it over the tip of the needle. Inject some anesthetic into the targeted area and watch for flow on the Doppler. If the needle is placed accurately, it will be confirmed by seeing flow on the Doppler in the desired location.
8. Once the location of the needle is confirmed, the needle is held in place by the forceps/needle holder and the syringe is removed. The syringe containing the fluid to be injected is then attached to the needle and the fluid is then injected.
9. The needle is withdrawn, pressure is placed over the puncture site, and an adhesive bandage is placed.

COMPLICATIONS

Box 192-2 lists the possible complications of intra-articular or soft tissue injections. Also see Table 192-4.

Possible complications include the following:

- *Injection into a vein or artery* (This rarely causes a problem except that the therapeutic effect may not occur. Lidocaine and steroids are both given intravenously for other conditions.)

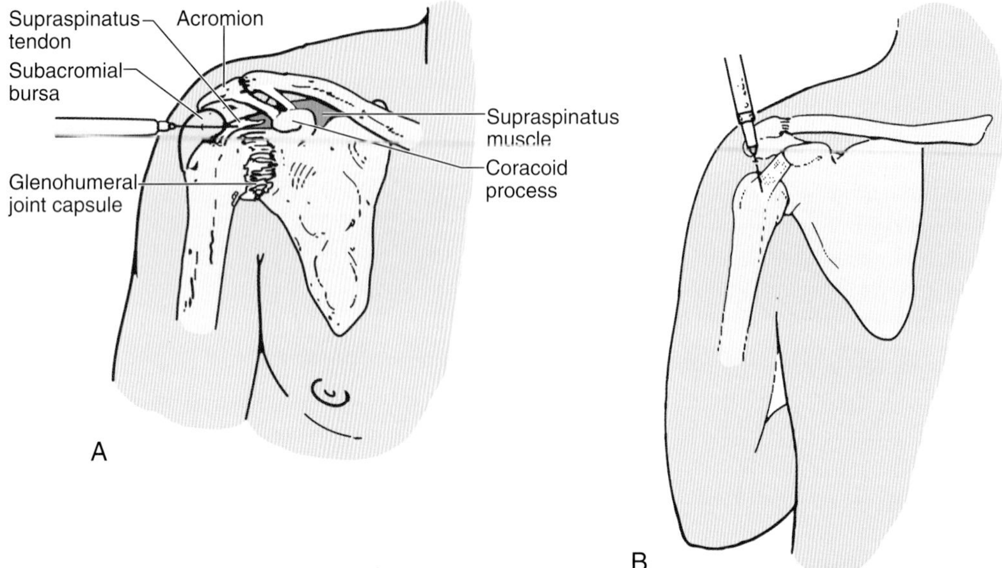

Figure 192-14 Shoulder: Rotator cuff (supraspinatus tendinitis). **A,** Use the same approach as that used for injecting the subacromial bursa (see Fig. 192-13). However, insert the needle deeper to reach the peritendinous area. **B,** Alternatively, have the patient rotate the flexed arm behind the back. Palpate the inferior edge of the acromion. The greater tuberosity of the humerus lies just below it. The tendon lies in the hollow between these two bones. Use an 18- to 20-gauge, 1½-inch needle with 5 mL 1% lidocaine and 20 to 40 mg of methylprednisolone acetate or equivalent (see Tables 192-2 and 192-5).

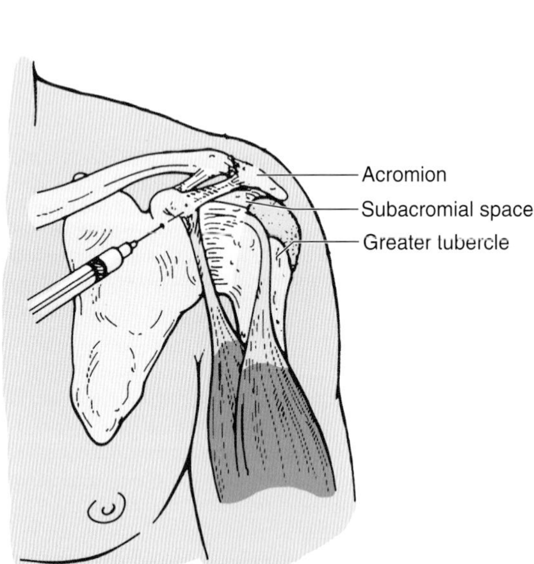

Figure 192-15 Shoulder: Short head of the biceps. The short head of the biceps attaches to the coracoid process. This is the palpable bony prominence located inferior to the clavicle and medial to the humerus over the anterior portion of the shoulder. Rarely does this area have to be injected, but should a patient have pain and discomfort over the coracoid process, insert a needle directly into the point of maximal tenderness until it reaches the bone. Withdraw the needle 1 or 2 mm and inject. Only a small volume of steroid is needed along with relatively larger amounts of lidocaine. Additional steroid may be injected parallel to the tendon distally (if it is palpable). Use a 22-gauge, 1½-inch needle with 5 to 10 mL 1% lidocaine and 10 to 20 mg of methylprednisolone acetate or equivalent (see Tables 192-2 and 192-5).

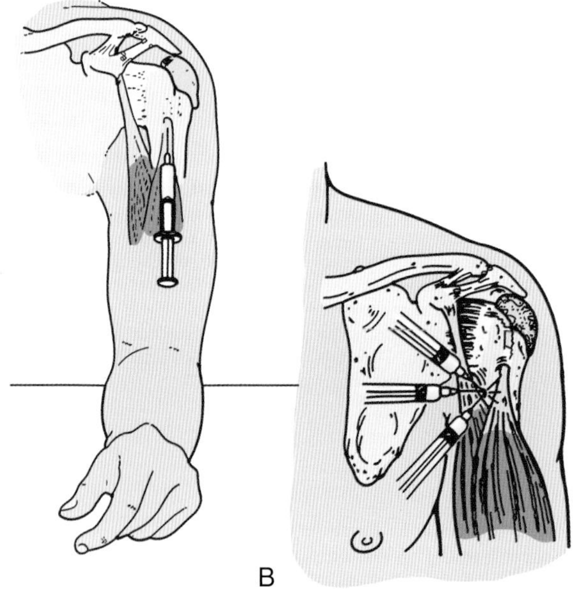

Figure 192-16 Shoulder: Bicipital tendinitis (injection of the long head of the biceps tendon). **A,** Have the patient seated with arm flexed 90 degrees. Identify the biceps tendon by placing your hand on the patient's shoulder with your fingers posteriorly and the thumb anteriorly over the proximal humerus. Internally and externally rotate the patient's arm. The bicipital groove is palpable anteriorly and the tendon "snap" can be felt under your thumb. Identify the most tender area of the tendon (usually in the bicipital groove on the humerus). Insert the needle into this groove and attempt to make a *peritendinous* injection of steroid and lidocaine. Often, a slip of the subacromial bursa surrounds the more proximal portion of the tendon. **B,** If pain persists on palpation after the injection, further injection in a fanlike *peritendinous* pattern may be needed more distally. Use a 22-gauge, 1½-inch needle with 5 to 10 mL 1% lidocaine and 10 to 20 mg of methylprednisolone acetate or equivalent (see Tables 192-2 and 192-5).

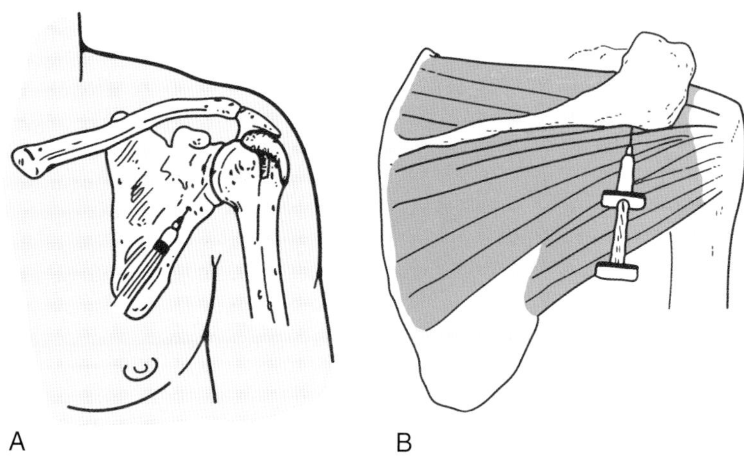

Figure 192-17 Shoulder: Intra-articular shoulder joint injection. A posterior or an anterior approach can be used to inject into the space of the shoulder joint (scapulohumeral or glenohumeral joint). **A,** In the anterior approach, externally rotate the shoulder. This movement opens the joint space. Identify the coracoid process. Insert the needle 1 cm inferior and 1 cm lateral to the coracoid process, and direct the needle perpendicularly, or slightly laterally, into the glenohumeral joint. The properly inserted needle should not contact bone. **B,** With the posterior approach, the patient is again seated with the arm internally rotated across the waist. Palpate the inferoposterior aspect of the acromion with the thumb. Place the index finger on the coracoid process. Insert the needle just below the acromion and aim toward the coracoid. Insert 2 to 3 cm deep. Use a 20-gauge, 1½-inch needle with 5 to 7 mL 1% lidocaine and 20 to 40 mg of methylprednisolone acetate or equivalent (see Tables 192-2 and 192-2).

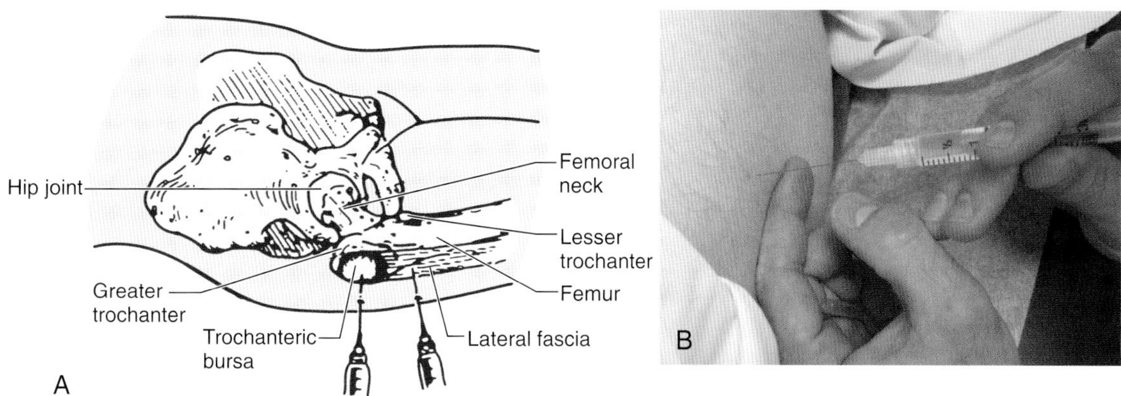

Figure 192-18 Trochanteric bursa. **A,** Trochanteric bursa is located at the most superior prominent portion of the femur. A bony prominence can be palpated. Tenderness in this area generally denotes trochanteric bursitis. Direct the needle perpendicular to the femur at the point of maximal tenderness, and insert until bone is felt. Withdraw the needle 2 to 3 mm and inject. Frequently the pain will radiate more distally (as it might with lateral epicondylitis in the arm) down the lateral portion of the femur along the fascia. If the patient is still experiencing discomfort 5 minutes after injection of the bursa and massage of the area, a more distal injection may be necessary at the areas of tenderness. **B,** Injecting for trochanteric bursitis. Use a 22-gauge, 1½- to 2-inch needle with 5 to 10 mL 1% lidocaine and 20 to 40 mg of methylprednisolone acetate or equivalent (see Tables 192-2 and 192-5).

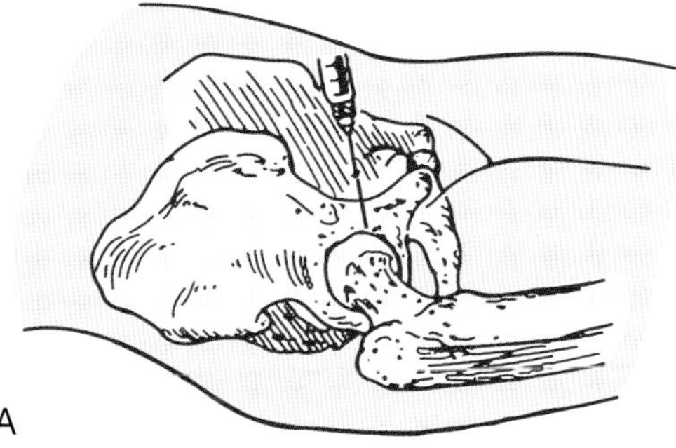

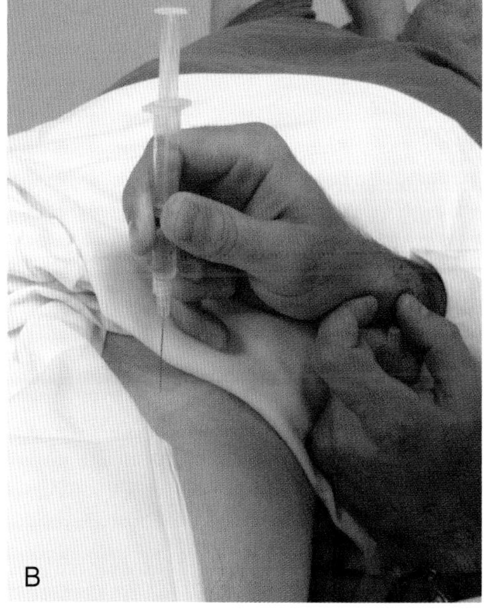

Figure 192-19 Hip joint proper. **A,** Experience is necessary to inject the hip joint itself. Even experienced practitioners often use fluoroscopy. An anterior or posterior approach can be taken. However, the anterior approach is most common. Great care must be taken to avoid entering any of the blood vessels or nerves coursing through the inguinal canal area. Position the hip so that the leg is maximally extended and internally rotated. Use a long needle to enter 2 to 3 cm below the anterior superior spine of the ilium and 2 to 3 cm lateral to the femoral pulse. The needle should point posteromedially at a 60-degree angle to the skin and then should course through the capsule ligaments until it reaches bone. Withdraw the needle slightly and aspirate for fluid. Injection may then be carried out, and there should be little resistance. **B,** Injecting the hip. Use a 20-gauge, 2½- to 3-inch needle with 5 mL 1% lidocaine and 40 to 80 mg of methylprednisolone acetate or equivalent (see Tables 192-2 and 192-5).

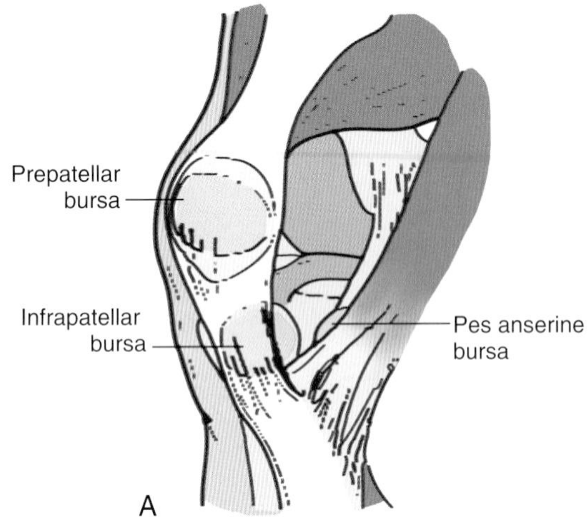

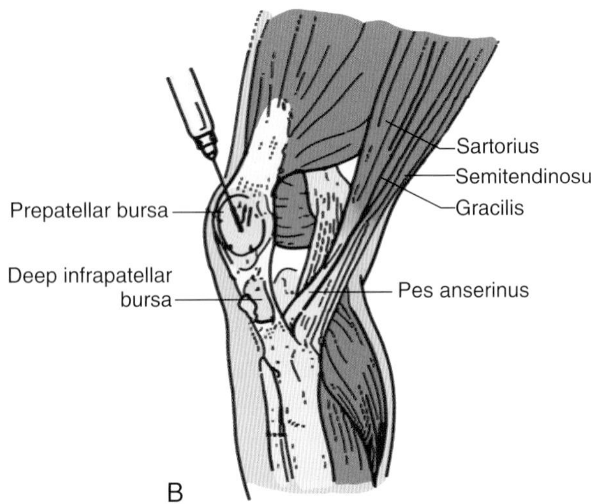

Figure 192-20 Prepatellar bursa. **A,** Identify the bursa, which is located between the skin and the patella. **B,** Insert the needle just above the patella and at the lateral portion of the bursa, and direct it to the center of swelling. Aspirate fluid (for culture), switch syringes, and then inject. (Although the data are not as documented as for olecranon bursitis, the protocol for injecting this bursa can be the same.) Use a 20- to 22-gauge, 1- to 1½-inch needle with 3 mL 1% lidocaine and 20 to 40 mg of methylprednisolone acetate or equivalent (see Tables 192-2 and 192-5).

- Introduction of *infection* (usually *Staphylococcus*) into joint space (18 infections per 250,000 injections [0.072%])
- *Trauma to articular cartilage*
- *Injury to nearby nerves* (e.g., median nerve in carpal tunnel injection)
- *Pneumothorax* (when injecting thoracic trigger points)
- *Subcutaneous fatty atrophy* (see Fig. 192-2)
- *Adverse drug reaction* (see Table 192-4)
- *Injection of steroid into a septic joint* (If there is any suspicion of infection, do not instill steroids until laboratory studies have ruled it out.)
- *Osteoporosis and cartilage damage* (This is rare; reported cases have usually occurred after 20 to 30 injections. For joints, especially weight-bearing joints, a limit of three steroid injections per year provides a wide margin of safety.)
- Inappropriate/missed diagnosis
- *Tendon rupture* (To reduce the possibility of tendon rupture, inject peritendinously instead of intratendinously. Ruptures usually occur after multiple injections and when the patient will not rest the area. Finger tendon ruptures have been reported after steroid injection. Gray and Gottlieb recommend setting a limit of five total injections per finger joint.)
- *Reactions to anesthetic agent* (True allergic reactions to lidocaine (an amide) itself have not been reported. Allergic reactions have been reported to the esters [e.g., procaine/Novocain]; when reactions to lidocaine are suspected, the lidocaine has usually been drawn up from a multidose vial. These vials contain parabens preservatives, which can cause a reaction. So, if suspicions of a "caine" allergy arise, single-dose vials of lidocaine should be used. Another reason to use single-dose vials is to avoid precipitation of the steroid; see earlier discussion.)
- *Steroid flare* (Steroid flares occur rarely but are very painful. The patient actually experiences more discomfort after the injection. The flare is not associated with fever, occurs within 12 to 24 hours of the injection, and resolves spontaneously within 72 hours. It may be controlled with ice and nonsteroidal drugs.)
- Problems with viscosupplementation injections
  - Injection site pain is more frequent.
  - Rash and itching, cramps, ankle edema, muscle pain, and tachyarrhythmia have been reported.
  - A local reaction can produce a massive effusion that resembles a septic joint; 69% with pain experience relief after effusion resolves.

Postprocedure Patient Care and Education

- An adhesive bandage dressing or other dressing should be left on for 8 to 12 hours.
- It is essential that the affected area be rested. Injection therapy is not a cure itself. It is used in conjunction with other modalities. Physical therapy, NSAIDs, and hot or cold compresses may all be indicated, depending on the specific problem. If a weight-bearing joint (such as the knee) is injected, rest is indicated for a longer period than that for a wrist ganglion cyst injection.
- The patient should report immediately if he or she develops fever, chills, or any sign of infection. If the discomfort from the injection does not resolve within 72 hours, the patient should be examined to rule out a septic joint.
- The patient may bathe normally.
- A short course of an NSAID is often beneficial at the time of injection; the two modalities combined may have a markedly beneficial effect.

Conclusion

A practitioner who is appropriately familiar with the indications and methods for joint and soft tissue injections and aspiration can better diagnosis and treat a number of conditions. The overall incidence of significant side effects is small when proper selection of the patient and technique are utilized.

Indications and techniques for injections are expanding, as are the medications incorporated. Growing interest has developed around the use of botulinum toxin in certain conditions, as well as consideration of NSAIDs intra-articularly to obviate the side effects that limit corticosteroid use. These modalities provide an opportunity for the primary care physician to either diagnose or treat debilitating conditions, and oftentimes to prolong the time to or alleviate the need for more invasive procedures.

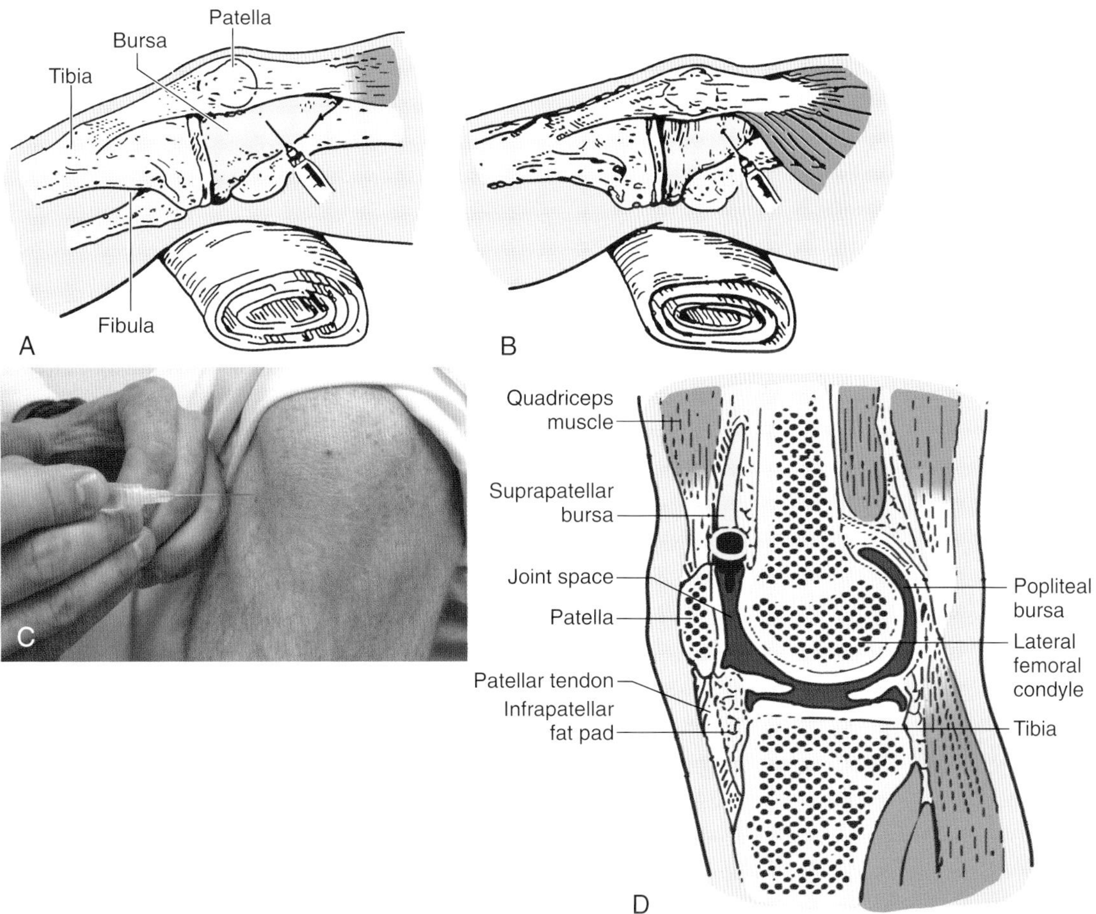

Figure 192-21 Knee joint. The knee is one of the easiest joints to enter and one of the most common joints to aspirate and inject. Slightly flex the knee using a towel in the popliteal space with the patient lying on an examination table. Either a lateral (**A**) or medial (**B**) approach may be used. For the lateral approach, palpate the superior lateral aspect of the patella and insert the needle 1 cm superior and 1 cm lateral to this point. Apply gentle pressure on the contralateral side of the knee to encourage the fluid to pool in the area of aspiration. Direct the needle under the patella at a 45-degree angle to the midjoint area. Aspirate all fluid before injection. There should be no resistance. **C,** Other approaches include entering medially or laterally directly above the joint line with the patient seated, or going directly through the patellar tendon just below the patella. **D,** The knee joint space is large and is readily entered from multiple approaches. Use a 20-gauge, 1- to 1½-inch needle with 5 mL 1% lidocaine and 20 to 80 mg of methylprednisolone acetate or equivalent (see Tables 192-2 and 192-5).

A Baker's cyst is a sac of synovial fluid that has leaked out of a hole in the posterior capsule of the knee. It generally indicates significant internal knee problems, and steroid injections are only a temporary relief frowned on by many clinicians. Insert the needle 3 cm medial to the midline and 3 cm below the popliteal crease. Take care to avoid the popliteal artery, vein, and nerve. Use a 20-gauge, 1 to 1½-inch needle with 5 mL 1% lidocaine and 20 to 80 mg of methylprednisolone acetate or equivalent (see Table 192-2).

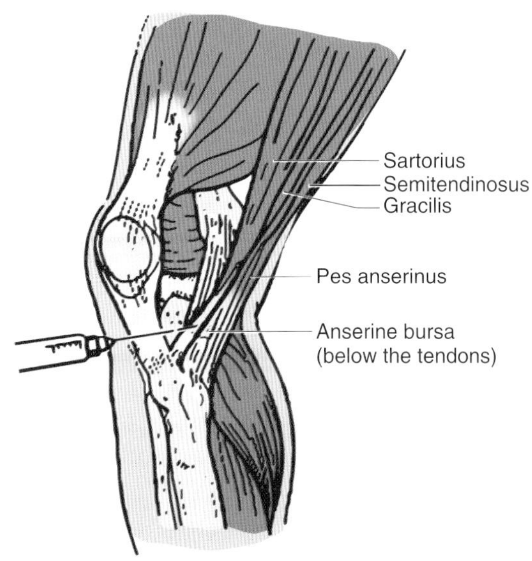

Figure 192-22 Anserine bursa. The anserine bursa is located on the upper medial portion of the tibia under the insertion of the sartorius, semitendinosus, and gracilis tendons. This bursa frequently becomes inflamed in elderly, somewhat obese women; the symptoms are aggravated by going up and down stairs. Palpate and find the point of maximal tenderness, and insert the needle perpendicular to the tibia. When bony resistance is encountered, withdraw the needle 2 or 3 mm and inject several areas in a fanlike fashion. Use a 22- to 25-gauge, 1½-inch needle with 3 to 5 mL 1% lidocaine and 20 to 40 mg of methylprednisolone acetate or equivalent (see Tables 192-2 and 192-5).

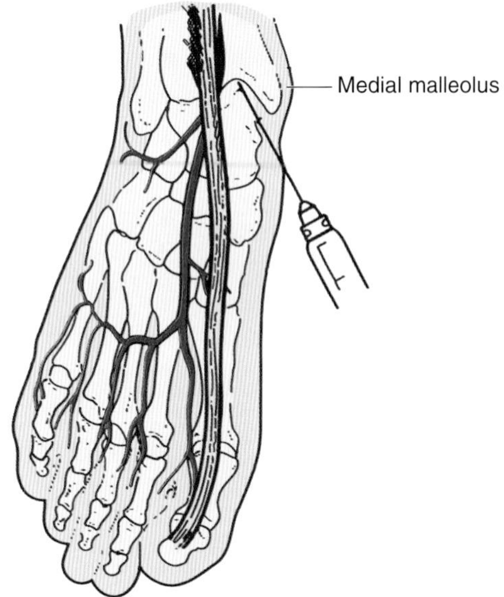

Figure 192-23 Ankle joint. Anteromedial approach is the easiest. Have the patient maximally dorsiflex the toe, accentuating the extensor tendon. Identify the hollow between the anterior medial malleolus and the long extensor tendon. This is the spot for injection. The needle must be inserted approximately 3 cm and directed slightly lateral. Use a 22-gauge, 1- to 1½-inch needle with 3 to 5 mL 1% lidocaine and 20 to 40 mg of methylprednisolone acetate or equivalent (see Tables 192-2 and 192-5).

CPT/Billing Codes

Healthcare Common Procedure Coding System (HCPCS) Codes*

20526 Injection: therapeutic (e.g., local anesthetic, corticosteroid), carpal tunnel
20550† Injection: tendon sheath, ligament, ganglion cyst
20551 Injection: therapeutic of tendon at its origin or insertion
20552 Injection: single or multiple trigger point(s), one or two muscle group(s)
20553 Injection: single or multiple trigger point(s), three or more muscle groups
20600 Arthrocentesis, aspiration, and injection; small joint, bursa, or ganglion cyst (e.g., fingers, toes)
20605† Arthrocentesis, aspiration, and injection, intermediate joint, bursa (e.g., temporomandibular, acromioclavicular, wrist, elbow, ankle, olecranon bursa)
20610† Arthrocentesis, aspiration, and injection, major joint or bursa (e.g., shoulder, hip, knee, subacromial bursa)
76942 Ultrasound guidance
M0076 Prolotherapy

*Can also charge for any injected medications using appropriate J code.
†Office visit can also be charged.

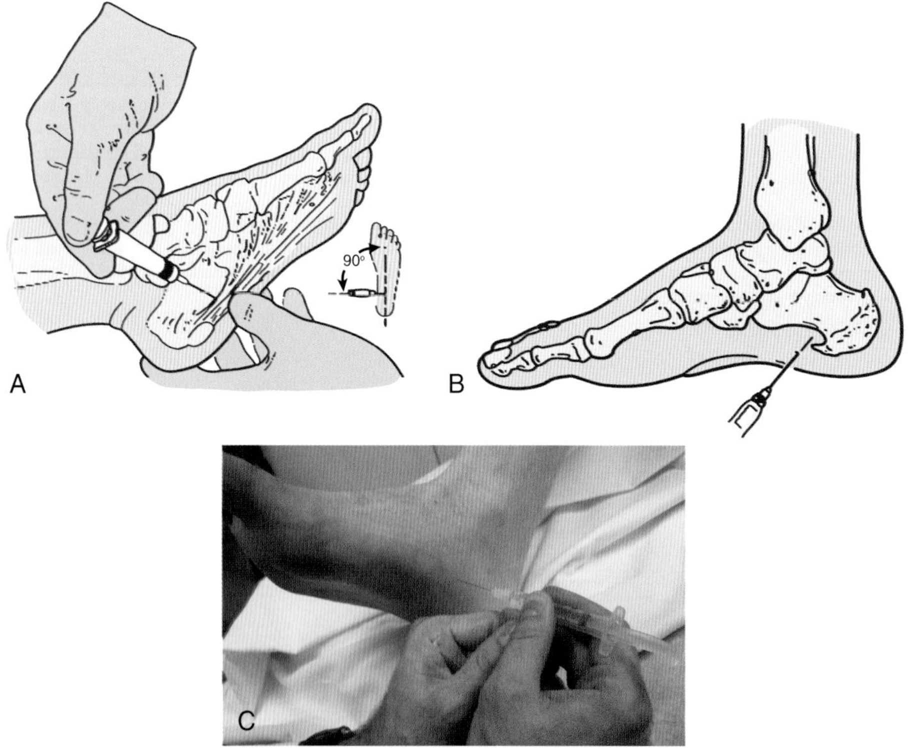

Figure 192-24 Calcaneal spur/plantar fasciitis. Two approaches can be used. Many physicians prefer to direct the needle from the lateral side of the foot (**A**) rather than from the inferior (plantar) side (**B**). The adipose tissue of the heel is uniquely segmented to provide cushion for the foot. If the plantar approach is used and steroid leaks out through the tract, atrophy could result, and thus the patient would have heel pain while walking. Nevertheless, many physicians approach directly from the plantar position to inject steroid right over a calcaneal spur. Using the lateral approach, the physician would direct the needle to enter just below the bony prominence of the calcaneus, and just anterior to the heel pad, and go to the midline until the point of maximal tenderness is reached (**C**). Use a 22-gauge, 1½-inch needle with 2 to 4 mL 1% lidocaine and 15 to 30 mg of methylprednisolone acetate or equivalent (see Tables 192-2 and 192-5).

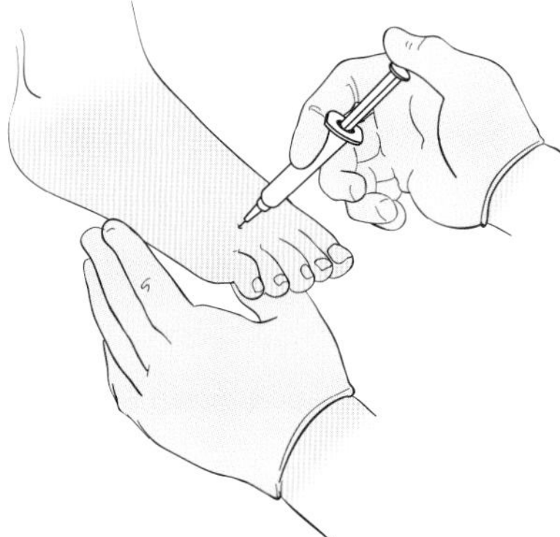

Figure 192-25 Morton's neuroma. Approach the foot from dorsal aspect. Insert needle 1 to 2 cm proximal to affected web space. Insert needle perpendicularly all the way to the plantar surface. Do not penetrate skin, but estimate depth by observing tenting of skin. Withdraw 1 cm and inject. Use a 25-gauge, 1½-inch needle with 3 to 5 mL 1% lidocaine and 10 to 30 mg of methylprednisolone acetate or equivalent (see Table 192-2).

Steroids

J0702 Betamethasone acetate (Celestone Soluspan)
J0810 Cortisone
J1021 Methylprednisolone acetate
J1040 Depo-Medrol
J1095 Dexamethasone acetate
J1100 Dexamethasone sodium phosphate (Decadron)
J1690 Prednisolone tebutate (Hydeltra-TBA)
J1700 Hydrocortisone acetate
J2640 Prednisolone sodium phosphate
J3301 Triamcinolone acetonide (Kenalog)
J3302 Triamcinolone diacetate (Aristocort)
J3303 Triamcinolone hexacetonide (Aristospan)
J7506 Prednisone

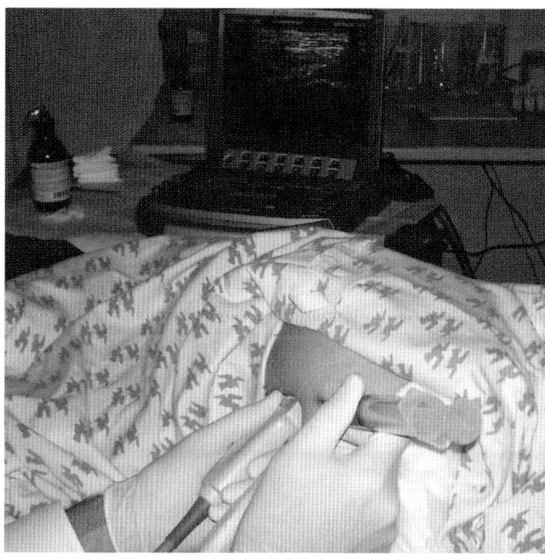

Figure 192-26 Ultrasound-guided injection. Physician demonstrates ultrasound guidance for injection of proximal hamstring tendinopathy. Note the needle is parallel to the longitudinal axis of the probe to facilitate visualization on the accompanying computer screen for identification. (Courtesy of John M. McShane, MD.)

Box 192-2. Possible Complications of Intra-articular or Soft Tissue Injections

Local Complications

Bleeding
Charcot-like arthropathy
Fat necrosis
Hemarthrosis
Iatrogenic infection; septic arthritis
Intra-articular calcification
Nerve damage from inadvertent injection
Osteonecrosis
Pain
Periarticular calcification
Pneumothorax (thoracic trigger points)
Postinjection flare
Skin depigmentation
Subcutaneous atrophy
Tendon rupture
Tenosynovitis

Systemic Complications

Acne
Adrenal suppression
Allergic reactions or anaphylaxis from local or preservatives in multidose vials
Avascular necrosis
Flushing of the face
Impaired glucose tolerance
Menstrual irregularity; uterine bleeding
Muscle wasting and myopathy
Osteoporosis
Pancreatitis
Posterior subcapsular cataracts
Psychological upset
Steroid arthropathy
Syncope

From McKeag D: Complication of joint aspiration/injection. Clin Atlas Office Proc 5:4, 2002.

Hyaluronic Acid Derivatives

Q4083 Sodium hyaluronate (Hyalgan)
Q4083 Sodium hyaluronate (Supartz)
Q4084 Hylan G-F 20 (Synvisc)
Q4085 Sodium hyaluronate (Euflexxa)
Q4086 Hyaluronan (Orthovisc)

ICD-9-CM Diagnostic Codes

274.0 Gouty arthropathy
354.0 Carpal tunnel syndrome
354.2 Cubital tunnel syndrome
355.5 Tarsal tunnel syndrome
355.6 Morton's neuroma
696.0 Psoriatic arthritis
714.0 Rheumatoid arthritis
715.11 Degenerative joint disease (DJD), shoulder
715.12 DJD, elbow
715.14 DJD, hand
715.16 DJD, knee
715.17 DJD, ankle
715.17 DJD, foot

719.41 Shoulder pain
719.42 Elbow pain
719.43 Wrist pain
719.44 Hand pain
719.45 Knee pain
719.46 Ankle pain
719.47 Foot pain
719.51 Shoulder stiffness
719.56 Knee stiffness
723.1 Neck pain
724.5 Back pain
724.3 Sciatica
724.79 Coccydynia
726.2 Impingement syndrome
726.5 Trochanteric bursitis
726.10 Bursitis, shoulder
726.10 Rotator cuff syndrome
726.11 Tendinitis shoulder
726.12 Bicipital tendinitis
726.31 Medial epicondylitis (golfer's elbow)
726.32 Lateral epicondylitis (tennis elbow)
726.33 Olecranon bursitis
726.61 Pes anserine bursitis
726.64 Patellar tendinitis
726.65 Prepatellar tendinitis
726.71 Achilles bursitis
726.73 Heel spur
727.03 Trigger finger
727.04 de Quervain's disease
727.05 Tendinitis, hand/wrist
727.06 Tendinitis, foot/ankle
727.3 Bursitis
727.41 Ganglion, joint
727.51 Baker's cyst
727.82 Calcific tendinitis
728.71 Plantar fasciitis
729.0 Fibrositis
729.4 Fasciitis
729.5 Arm pain
729.5 Leg pain
729.5 Toe pain

ACKNOWLEDGMENT

The editors wish to recognize the many contributions by John L. Pfenninger, MD, to this chapter in the previous edition of this text.

LEARNING RESOURCES

Alguire PC, Casey LM (eds): Arthrocentesis and Joint Injection, a videotape and slide presentation, 1999. American College of Physicians–American Society of Internal Medicine, 190 N. Independence Mall West, Philadelphia, PA, 19106-1572, 1-800-523-1546.

For courses on joint injection, contact The National Procedures Institute: www.npinstitute.com.

ONLINE RESOURCES

American Association of Orthopedic Medicine. http://www.aaomed.org/page.asp?id=88&name=Prolotherapy (accessed April 13, 2007).

Tuggy M, Garcia J: Procedures Consult. Available at www.proceduresconsult.com.

BIBLIOGRAPHY

Altman RD, Moskowitz R: Intraarticular sodium hyaluronate (Hyalgan) in the treatment of patients with osteoarthritis of the knee: A randomized clinical trial. J Rheumatol 25:2203, 1998.

Anderson B, Kaye S: Treatment of flexor tenosynovitis of the hand ("trigger finger") with corticosteroids: A prospective study of the response to local injection. Arch Intern Med 151:153, 1991.

Baker DG, Schumacher HR: Acute monarthritis. N Engl J Med 329:1013, 1993.

Bellamy N, Campbell J, Welch V, et al: Intraarticular corticosteroid for treatment of osteoarthritis of the knee. Cochrane Database Syst Rev Issue 2:CD005328, 2006.

Bellamy N, Campbell J, Welch V, et al: Viscosupplementation for the treatment of osteoarthritis of the knee. Cochrane Database Syst Rev Issue 2:CD005321, 2006.

Birrer RB: Aspiration and corticosteroid injection: Practical pointers for safety. Phys Sportsmed 20:57, 1992.

Blair B, Rokito AS, Cuomo F, et al: Efficacy of corticosteroids for subacromial impingement syndrome. J Bone Joint Surg 78-A:1685, 1996.

Cardone DA, Tallia AF: Joint and soft tissue injection. Am Fam Physician 66:283, 2002.

Carrabba M, Paresce E, Angelini M, et al: The safety and efficacy of different dose schedules of hyaluronic acid in the treatment of painful osteoarthritis of the knee with joint effusion. Eur J Rheumatol Inflamm 15:25, 1995.

Charalambous CP, Tryfonidis M, Sadiq S, et al: Septic arthritis following intra-articular steroid injection of the knee—A survey of current practice regarding antiseptic technique used during intra-articular steroid injection of the knee. Clin Rheumatol 22:386, 2003.

Chumacher HR, Chen LX: Injectable corticosteroids in treatment of arthritis of the knee. Am J Med 118:1208, 2005.

Dammers JW, Veering MM, Vermeulen M: Injection with methylprednisolone proximal to the carpal tunnel: Randomised double blind trial. BMJ 321:884, 2000.

Divine JG, Zazulak BT, Hewett TE: Viscosupplementation for knee osteoarthritis: A systematic review. Clin Orthop Relat Res 455:113, 2007.

Fadale PD, Wiggins ME: Corticosteroid injections: Their use and abuse. J Am Acad Orthop Surg 2:133, 1994.

Fitzgerald RH: Intrasynovial injection of steroids: Uses and abuses. Mayo Clin Proc 51:655, 1976.

Foster AH, Carlson BM: Myotoxicity of local anesthetics and regeneration of the damaged muscle fibers. Anesth Analg 59:727, 1980.

Gedda PO: Septic arthritis from cortisone. JAMA 155:597, 1954.

Genovese MC: Joint and soft tissue injection. Postgrad Med 103:125, 1998.

George E: Intra-articular hyaluronan treatment for osteoarthritis. Ann Rheum Dis 57:637, 1998.

Gowans JDC, Granieri PA. Septic arthritis: its relation to intra-articular injections of hydrocortisone acetate. N Engl J Med 261:502, 1959.

Gray RG, Gottlieb NL: Intra-articular corticosteroids: An updated assessment. Clin Orthop Relat Res 177:253, 1983.

Gray RG, Tenenbaum J, Gottlieb NL: Local corticosteroid injection therapy in rheumatic disorders. Semin Arthritis Rheum 10:231, 1981.

Hay EM, Paterson SM, Lewis M, et al: Pragmatic randomized controlled trial of local corticosteroid injection and naproxen for treatment of lateral epicondylitis of elbow in primary care. BMJ 319:964, 1999.

Hernandez-Diaz S, Garcia-Rodriguez LA: Epidemiologic assessment of the safety of conventional nonsteroidal anti-inflammatory drugs. Am J Med 110(Suppl 3A):20S, 2001.

Hollander JL: Intrasynovial corticosteroid therapy in arthritis. Maryland State Med J 19:62, 1970.

Jones A, Doherty M: Intra-articular corticosteroids are effective in osteoarthritis but there are no clinical predictors of response. Ann Rheum Dis 55:829, 1996.

Jones A, Regan M, Ledingham J, et al: Importance of placement of intra-articular steroid injections. BMJ 307:1329, 1993.

Kamm GL, Hagmeyer KO: Allergic-type reactions to corticosteroids, Ann Pharmacother 33:451, 1999.

Kendall H: Local corticosteroid injection therapy. Ann Phys Med 7:31, 1963.

Kim SR, Stitik TP, Foye PM, et al: Critical review of prolotherapy for osteoarthritis, low back pain, and other musculoskeletal conditions: A physiatric perspective. Am J Phys Med Rehabil 83:379, 2004.

Kotz R, Kolarz G: Intra-articular hyaluronic acid: Duration of effect and results of repeated treatment cycles. Am J Orthop 28:5, 1999.

Lavelle W: Intra-articular injections. Med Clin North Am 91: 241, 2007.

Leversee JH: Aspiration of joints and soft tissue injections. Prim Care 13:572, 1986.

McNabb JW: A Practical Guide to Joint and Soft Tissue Injection and Aspiration, 2nd ed. Philadelphia, Lippincott Williams & Wilkins, 2010.

Nelson KH, Briner W, Cummins J: Corticosteroid injection therapy for overuse injuries. Am Fam Physician 52:1811, 1995.

Nouette-Gaulain K, Sirvent P, Canal-Raffin M, et al: Effects of intermittent femoral nerve injections of bupivacaine, levobupivacaine, and ropivacaine on mitochondrial energy metabolism and intracellular calcium homeostasis in rat psoas muscle. Anesthesiology 106:1026, 2007.

Pfenninger JL: Injections of joints and soft tissue. Part I. General guidelines. Am Fam Physician 44:1196, 1991.

Pfenninger JL: Injections of joints and soft tissue. Part II. Guidelines for specific joints. Am Fam Physician 44:1690, 1991.

Pfenninger JL (ed): Joint injection techniques. Clin Atlas Office Proc 5:4, 2002.

Rifat SF, Moeller JL: Basics of joint injection. Postgrad Med 109:157, 2001.

Rifat SF, Moeller JL: Site-specific techniques of joint injection. Postgrad Med 109:123, 2001.

Rozental TD, Sculco TP: Intra-articular corticosteroids: An updated overview. Am J Orthop 29:18, 2000.

Ryan M, Wong A, Taunton J, Wong J: A pilot investigation on a new treatment for chronic plantar fasciitis: Ultrasound guided hyperosmolar dextrose injections. Clin J Sport Med 17:166, 2007.

Salzman KL, Lillegard WA, Butcher JD: Upper extremity bursitis. Am Fam Physician 56:1797, 1997.

Saunders S, Cameron G: Injection Techniques in Orthopaedic and Sports Medicine, 3rd ed. Philadelphia, WB Saunders, 2006.
EDITOR'S NOTE: This is an excellent manual.

Schmerling RH, Delbanco TL, Tosteson ANA, et al: Synovial fluid tests: What should be ordered? JAMA 264:1009, 1990.

Scott WA: Injection techniques and use in the treatment of sports injuries. Sports Med 22:406, 1996.

Sibbitt WL Jr, Peisajovich A, Michael AA, et al: Does sonographic needle guidance affect the clinical outcome of intraarticular injections? J Rheumatol 36:1892, 2009.

Slotkoff AT, Clauw DJ, Nashel DJ: Effects of soft tissue corticosteroid injection on glucose control in diabetics. Arthritis Rheum 37:S347, 1994.

Smith DL, McAfee JH, Lucas LM, et al: Treatment of nonseptic olecranon bursitis: A controlled, blinded prospective trial. Arch Intern Med 149:2527, 1989.

Stefanich RJ: Intra-articular corticosteroids in treatment of osteoarthritis. Orthop Rev 15:65, 1986.

Stitik TP, Kumar A, Foye PM: Corticosteroid injections for osteoarthritis. Am J Phys Med Rehabil 85(Suppl):S51, 2006.

Tramèr MR, Moore RA, Reynolds DJ, McQuay HJ: Quantitative estimation of rare adverse events which follow a biological progression: A new model applied to chronic NSAID use. Pain 91:401, 2001.

Troum OM: Office-based diagnostic needle arthroscopic lavage. In Pfenninger JL (ed): Joint injection techniques. Clin Atlas Office Proc 5:4, 2002.

Usatine RP: The Color Atlas of Family Medicine. New York, McGraw-Hill, 2009.

Uthman I, Raynauld JP, Haraoui B: Intra-articular therapy in osteoarthritis. Postgrad Med J 79:449, 2003.

Walker-Bone K, Javaid K, Arden N, et al: Medical management of osteoarthritis. BMJ 321:936, 2000.

Wen DY: Intra-articular hyaluronic acid injections for knee osteoarthritis. Am Fam Physician 62:565, 2000.

Wiggins ME, Fadale PD, Ehrlich MG, et al: Effects of corticosteroids on the healing of ligaments. J Bone Joint Surg 77-A:1682, 1995.

Wise CM: Arthrocentesis and injection of joints and soft tissue. In Firestein GS, Budd RS, Harris ED, et al (eds): Kelley's Textbook of Rheumatology, 8th ed. Philadelphia, Saunders, 2008, p 721.

Young CC, Rutherford DS, Neidfeldt MW: Treatment of plantar fasciitis. Am Fam Physician 63:467, 2001.

Zink W, Missler G, Sinner B, et al: Differential effects of bupivacaine and ropivacaine enantiomers on intracellular Ca^{2+} regulation in murine skeletal muscle fibers. Anesthesiology 102:793, 2005.

Zuckerman JD, Meislin RJ, Rothberg M: Injections for joint and soft tissue disorders; when and how to use them. Geriatrics 45:45, 1990.

CHAPTER 193

Knee Braces

Scott A. Paluska

The knee joint is the largest joint in the body, and traumatic, overuse, and degenerative knee injuries are common. Strength, flexibility, and technique modification have traditionally been essential components in the treatment of knee pain. Improved surgical techniques, arthroscopic advances, and smaller incisions have also enhanced therapy for knee disorders over the last few decades. More recently, knee braces have been used in an attempt to prevent or treat several knee conditions.

Knee braces typically fall into one of several broad categories:

- *Prophylactic:* Braces designed to reduce the occurrence or facilitate the recovery of injury to the knee's medial collateral ligament (MCL) or lateral collateral ligament (LCL).
- *Functional:* Braces designed to restore normal knee kinematics, minimize tibial rotation, and reduce translation for anterior cruciate ligament (ACL)–deficient or ACL-reconstructed knees.
- *Patellofemoral:* Braces designed to keep the patella centered in the femoral trochlea and improve patellofemoral joint alignment.
- *Postoperative:* Braces designed to immobilize the knee or limit motion after surgery or an injury.
- *Osteoarthritics:* Braces designed to diminish painful forces exerted on an affected knee's tibial-femoral compartment (medial or lateral) for unicompartmental knee osteoarthritis.

Despite their popularity, the appropriate indications and true benefits of many knee braces have not been clearly defined or validated by rigorous research. In addition, brace manufacturers market several different knee braces to address conditions that may be nonspecific and diverse. As a result, confusion often exists regarding when and if knee braces should be used for the prevention or treatment of various knee abnormalities. At this point, it can be said that some knee braces may minimize knee injuries, but the efficacy of most braces has not been confirmed by well-controlled studies. In general, most individuals using knee braces express subjective symptomatic improvements that exceed objective findings. Clinicians must assess the costs and potential risks of knee braces when deciding to use them for individuals. Although knee braces appear relatively safe when used appropriately, they should be used only in conjunction with appropriate education, muscular rehabilitation, technique enhancement, and activity modification.

Indications

Prophylactic Knee Braces

- MCL or LCL injury protection during significant valgus or varus knee forces
- MCL or LCL stabilization during recovery following an MCL or LCL sprain
- Athletes or individuals at high risk for MCL or LCL injuries

Functional Knee Braces

- Mild-to-moderate ACL instability
- ACL-deficient knees treated nonsurgically
- Postoperative support following ACL reconstruction
- Support for mild-to-moderate posterior cruciate ligament (PCL) or MCL instability

Patellofemoral Knee Braces

- Patellar subluxation or dislocation
- Anterior knee pain syndromes
- Patellar tendonitis
- Osgood-Schlatter disease
- Compression of a knee effusion

Postoperative Knee Braces

- Stabilization following an acute knee injury or ligament sprain
- Postoperative immobilization
- Customized range-of-motion limitations for various knee conditions
- Stabilization following a femoral or tibial fracture
- Graft protection following knee ligament reconstruction

Osteoarthritis Knee Braces

- Unicompartmental, symptomatic tibial-femoral knee osteoarthritis
- Neutral or varus knee alignment (for a valgus-force brace)
- Neutral or valgus alignment (for a varus-force brace)

Contraindications

In General

- Unstable knees requiring prompt surgical management
- Body contours that preclude effective brace positioning
- Regional compartment syndrome that may be exacerbated by brace tension
- Open wounds, cellulitis, or lacerations that will be occluded by the brace

Prophylactic Knee Braces

Prophylactic knee braces should not be used for control of tibial translation or rotation in ACL-deficient knees.

Functional Knee Braces

Functional knee braces should not be used for complex knee injuries, such as posterolateral corner injuries.

Patellofemoral Knee Braces

- Knee disorders unrelated to the patellofemoral joint
- Moderate-to-severe patellofemoral osteoarthritis

Osteoarthritis Knee Braces

- Multicompartmental knee osteoarthritis
- Moderate-to-severe patellofemoral osteoarthritis
- Knee arthritis related to other conditions such as inflammatory, infectious, or autoimmune

Equipment and Supplies

In General

- Tape measure
- Athletic tape (*optional*)
- Skin razor (*optional*)
- Prewrap on skin under brace to limit brace migration (*optional, not beneficial for patellofemoral braces*)
- Elastic wrap or brace cover (*optional*)

Prophylactic Knee Braces

- Custom or off-the-shelf (prefabricated) brace with unilateral or bilateral bars
- In addition to athletic tape, there may be manufacturer-supplied hook-and-pile fasteners

Functional Knee Braces

- Custom or off-the-shelf (prefabricated) brace
- In place of tape measure, there may be specific measuring device supplied by the brace manufacturer

Patellofemoral Knee Braces

- Custom or off-the-shelf (prefabricated) brace
- Counterbalancing straps (*optional*)
- Patellar buttresses (*optional*)
- Inflation device for inflatable air pocket (*optional*)

Postoperative Knee Braces

An off-the-shelf (prefabricated) universal-sized brace is used postoperatively.

Osteoarthritis Knee Braces

A custom or off-the-shelf (prefabricated) brace is used in cases of osteoarthritis.

Preprocedure Patient Education

The clinician should identify the appropriate indication for using a knee brace and explain that the brace may or may not be helpful for a given individual. An appropriately sized prefabricated brace is generally sufficient for most individuals. Although custom braces may distribute weight and fit better and be made of materials more worthwhile for high-level athletes or individuals with abnormal limb contours, they are more expensive. If the individual is a minor, consent should be obtained from the parent or guardian. (See the sample patient consent form online at www.expertconsult.com.) The initial fitting and brace application should be scheduled with adequate time allowed for correct sizing and an explanation of recommended brace care and usage. (See the sample patient education form online at www.expertconsult.com.)

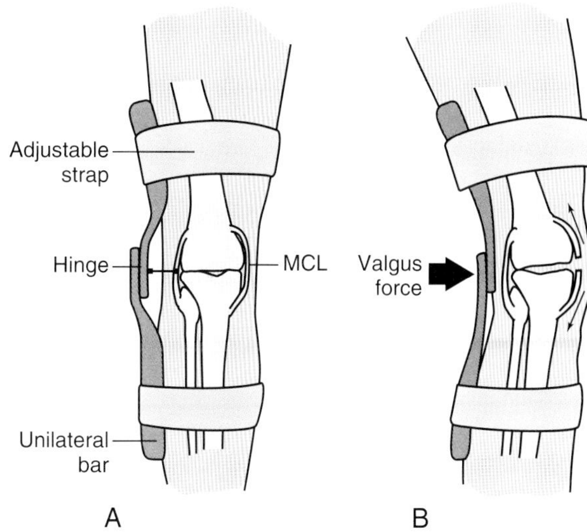

Figure 193-1 Representative prophylactic knee brace. **A,** Unilateral hinged bar prophylactic knee brace in a neutral position. **B,** Valgus-applied force causing increased medial collateral ligament (MCL) tension and potential ligament rupture. Use of the brace would hopefully prevent the MCL tear seen here.

Procedure

Prophylactic Knee Braces

Prophylactic knee braces are used to prevent injury to the MCL or LCL during contact sports or to provide stability during recovery after an MCL or LCL sprain (Fig. 193-1). Although the routine use prophylactic knee braces for collateral ligament injury prevention may be controversial, they do have a more well-defined role during MCL or LCL rehabilitation. Prophylactic knee braces are available as custom or off-the-shelf (prefabricated) models (Figs. 193-2 and 193-3). They have either a single lateral hinged support or bilateral supports with polycentric hinges that are connected by fabric and closures. Cost is greater for custom models, which appear to have greater efficacy during both knee flexion and extension. Although

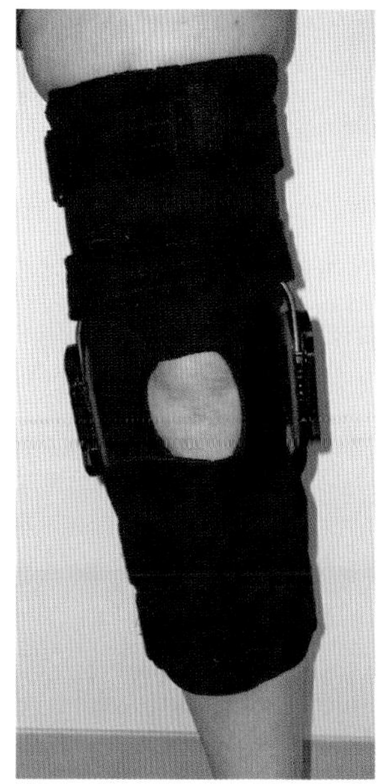

Figure 193-2 Representative prophylactic knee brace with bilateral hinged bars seen from the front.

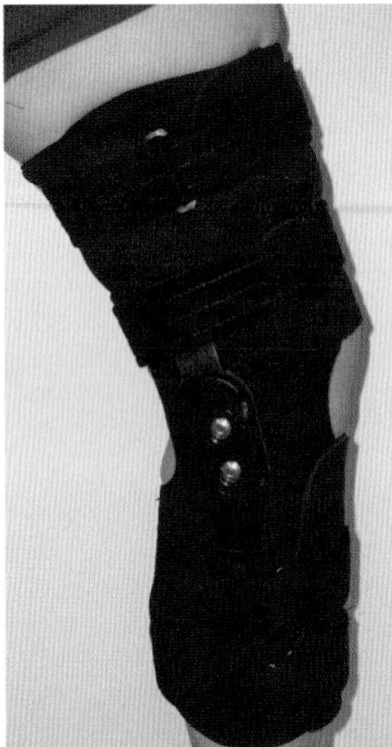

Figure 193-3 Representative prophylactic knee brace with bilateral hinged bars seen from the side.

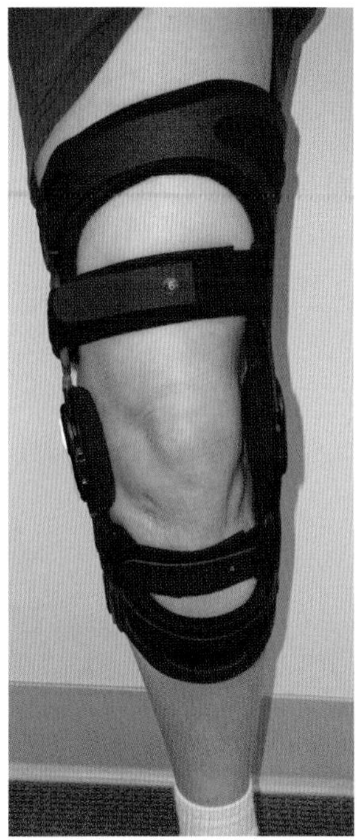

Figure 193-4 Representative functional knee brace seen from the front.

high-level athletes may profit from the weight distribution and fit characteristics of a custom brace, a prefabricated brace is sufficient for most individuals. At-risk athletes, such as football linemen, may particularly benefit from wearing well-fitting prophylactic knee braces on both knees during practices and games. However, it should be noted that prophylactic knee brace use may have a negative impact on an athlete's speed, agility, fatigability, and endurance.

1. Obtain the longest brace that the individual can wear comfortably (≥50 cm).
2. Select a brace with either unilateral or bilateral bars based on personal preference and cost. Bilateral bars may improve the brace's ability to transfer loads placed on the knee joint during impact.
3. Shave the skin under the brace, if desired, to maximize brace-to-skin contact.
4. Secure and adjust the athletic tape or brace enclosures to minimize brace movement.
5. Align the hinge(s) with the femoral condyles to minimize knee range-of-motion attenuation. Correct hinge placement relative to the knee joint is critical for optimal brace efficacy. The side bars may be bent if needed to accommodate the limb contours.
6. Cover the brace with the elastic wrap or brace cover, if desired, to minimize brace deterioration or injury to others during activities.
7. Tighten and adjust the brace regularly during prolonged athletic activities. It is common for the brace to migrate distally.
8. Hand wash and thoroughly dry the brace occasionally to prolong its life and reduce skin irritation.
9. Inspect the brace regularly for signs of deterioration or excessive wear.
10. Periodically apply a dry lubricant, such as Teflon spray, to the hinges.
11. Replace a broken or damaged brace.

Functional Knee Braces

The ACL is one of the knee's most important stabilizers for anterolateral motion, and an ACL tear can cause significant knee dysfunction. Functional braces are designed to limit instability in ACL-deficient knees or to stabilize the surgical graft for ACL-reconstructed knees. They are often antirotational. The braces may also enhance proprioception and muscle-timing during activity. Even though most individuals report subjective improvements with brace wear, the braces' ability to limit knee laxity during high-load, in vivo conditions is clearly less than what has been observed in laboratory models. Theoretically, functional braces may also provide protection for the ACL graft by limiting strain during the initial surgical recovery period. However, functional bracing has not been definitively shown in long-term studies to improve subjective or objective outcomes after ACL reconstruction. As such, functional bracing may be superfluous following uncomplicated ACL surgery.

Functional knee braces are available as custom or off-the-shelf (prefabricated) models (Figs. 193-4 and 193-5). They have similar designs and use either a "hinge-post-shell" or a "hinge-post-strap" design, which differ in the method of securing the brace around the user's thigh and calf. The "hinge-post-shell" braces provide better long-term durability and enhanced soft tissue contact. It is unclear whether the small mechanical and limb-contact advantages demonstrated in the laboratory for the more expensive custom models have clinically meaningful implications versus the less expensive off-the-shelf (prefabricated) knee braces. Custom braces may be more appropriate for individuals participating in high-level activities or

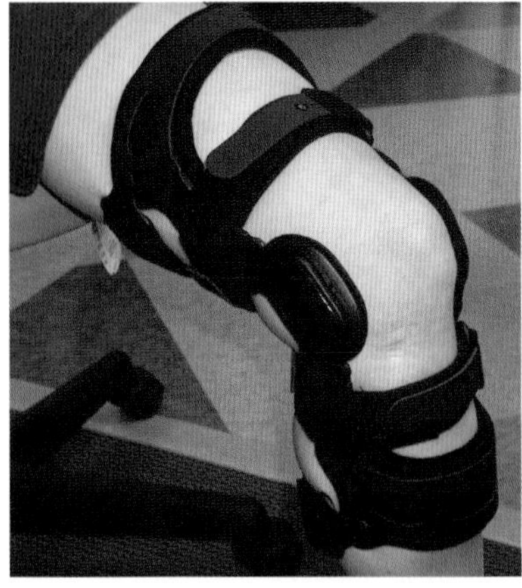

Figure 193-5 Representative functional knee brace seen from the side.

having abnormal limb contours. Prefabricated braces are usually sufficient for most individuals. It is more important that the brace be secured snugly and aligned correctly on the affected leg in order to maximize its efficacy.

1. Measure the thigh circumference 6 inches above the mid-patella if using a prefabricated brace and select the corresponding brace size according to the manufacturer's instructions.
2. Measure the thigh, knee, and calf dimensions with the manufacturer-specific instrument for custom braces. The submitted measurements will be used to fabricate a brace that closely meets the affected individual's leg.
3. Choose the longest length brace that the individual can comfortably wear, generally mid-thigh to mid-calf. Longer braces may be more uncomfortable, so balanced brace length and comfort is important to improve compliance.
4. Set the bilateral hinge extension stops at 10 to 20 degrees of flexion to minimize potentially harmful knee hyperextension.
5. Center the condylar hinge pads over the medial and lateral joint lines to allow the brace's flexion axis to conform to the knee joint.
6. Fasten the brace securely around the individual's leg using the brace closures or straps.
7. Cover the brace with the elastic wrap or brace cover, if desired, to minimize brace deterioration or injury to others during activities.
8. Tighten and adjust the brace regularly during prolonged athletic activities. It is common for the brace to migrate distally.
9. Hand wash and thoroughly dry the brace occasionally to prolong its life and reduce skin irritation.
10. Inspect the brace regularly for signs of deterioration or excessive wear.
11. Periodically apply a dry lubricant, such as Teflon spray, to the hinges.
12. Replace a broken or damaged brace.

Patellofemoral Knee Braces

Patellofemoral knee braces are designed to treat a variety of highly prevalent anterior knee symptoms that occur during activities such as ascending or descending stairs, prolonged sitting, or frequent squatting. Although their mechanism of action is uncertain, patellofemoral braces may diminish pain via improved patellar tracking, lessened lateral patellar tilt, augmented sensory feedback, reduced patellofemoral joint stress, and enhanced joint contact between the undersurface of the patella and the femoral trochlea. Generally, the subjectively reported benefits exceed the objectively measured findings for patellofemoral knee braces.

Patellofemoral knee braces are available in many different styles, but most use an elastic sleeve, a patellar cut-out, and padding around the patella (Figs. 193-6 and 193-7). Some braces also include adjustable straps or moveable buttresses. Most individuals can use a prefabricated brace without the need for customization. No patellofemoral brace type or materials appear to be superior.

1. Measure the extended and relaxed leg circumference 6 inches above and 6 inches below the knee joint line or around the mid-patella, depending on the manufacturer's instructions.
2. Obtain the corresponding brace size.
3. Pull the brace onto the individual's leg and center the patellar cut-out over the anterior knee.
4. Align the hinges, if present, with the medial and lateral femoral condyles.
5. Position the patellar buttress, if moveable, medial to the patella to apply laterally directed force (uncommon) or lateral to the patella to apply medially directed force (common).
6. Snugly secure the counterbalancing straps, if present, around the individual's thigh and calf. Moveable straps should be placed proximally to the patella for most individuals, except for those with patellar tendonitis who may benefit from a more distal placement.
7. Apply athletic tape to the top and bottom of the brace, if desired, to minimize brace migration during activities.
8. Hand wash and thoroughly dry the brace occasionally to prolong its life and reduce skin irritation.
9. Inspect the brace regularly for signs of deterioration or excessive wear.
10. Replace a broken or damaged brace.

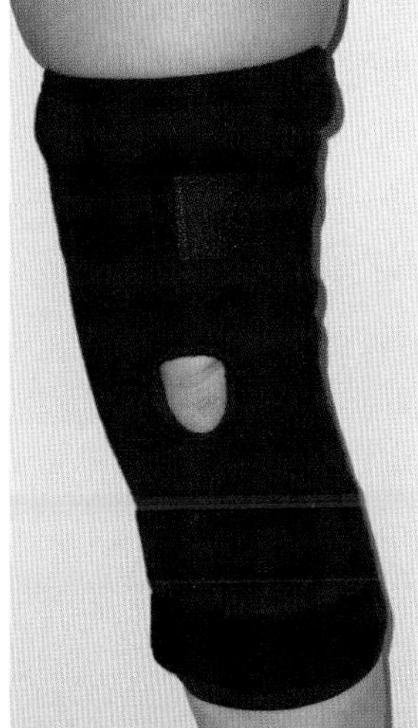

Figure 193-6 Representative patellofemoral knee brace seen from the front.

Postoperative Knee Braces

Postoperative knee braces are designed to provide immobilization and protected range of motion following a knee ligament injury, fracture, or surgical procedure. The braces may be used to keep the knee fully extended or limited within any desired range of motion. During the course of treatment or recovery, the allowable motion is typically advanced gradually. Postoperative knee braces are not designed to be worn during athletic endeavors but may be used during full or partial weight-bearing ambulation.

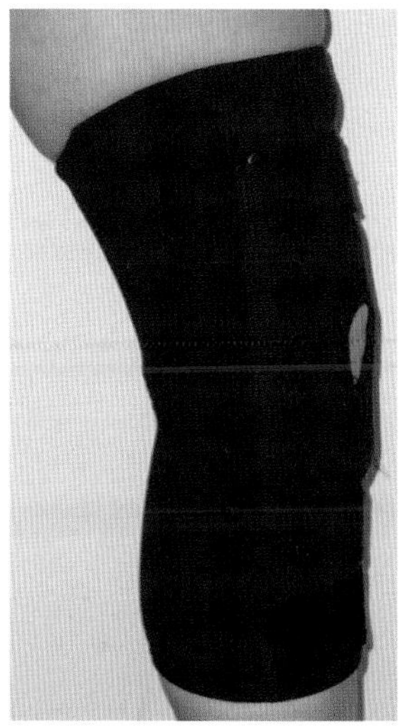

Figure 193-7 Representative patellofemoral knee brace seen from the side.

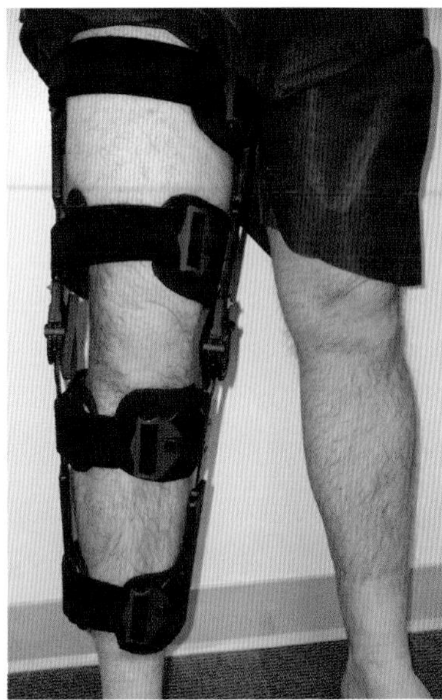

Figure 193-8 Representative postoperative knee brace seen from the front.

Postoperative knee braces are primarily prefabricated and universally sized (Figs. 193-8 and 193-9). Some individuals with abnormal limb contours may need a custom brace. It is essential that the brace be correctly positioned and securely attached on the affected leg in order to stabilize the knee adequately.

1. Unfasten all of the buckles and loosen the strap enclosures.
2. Pull the brace onto the individual's leg and center the patellar cut-out over the anterior knee.
3. Wrap the foam thigh and calf inserts securely around the leg and attach the free ends together. The foam may be trimmed if necessary.

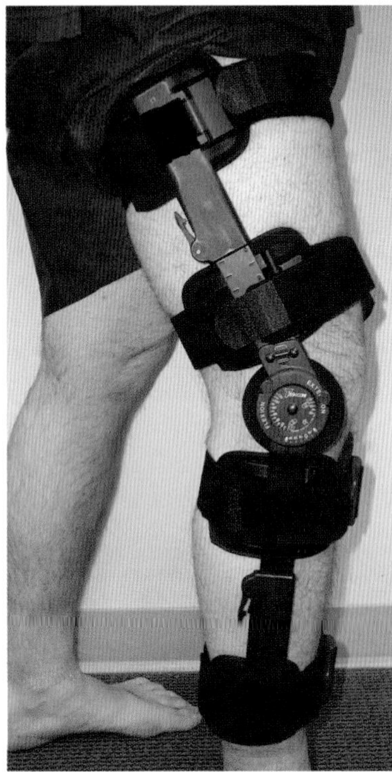

Figure 193-9 Representative postoperative knee brace seen from the side.

4. Adjust the brace length by pressing the medial and lateral release buttons, allowing the side bars to telescope to the desired length. If necessary, the bars may be fully extended from the upper thigh to the ankle. After finishing the adjustments, confirm that the release buttons have reengaged and that the side bars are equivalent in length.
5. Align the hinges with the patella and midline (anterior/posterior plane) of the affected leg. The lateral malleolus and greater trochanter may be used to verify midline placement. The hinge bars may be bent to fit varus or valgus knee alignments.
6. Confirm that the medial and lateral hinge heights are the same. Correct hinge placement is important for brace efficacy.
7. Adjust the brace's strap lengths and snap the buckles closed, starting with those closest to the patella.
8. Open the bilateral hinge covers and set the desired limitations of flexion and extension by moving the adjustment pins.
9. Tighten and adjust the brace regularly during prolonged wear. It is common for the brace to loosen slightly or migrate distally.
10. Hand wash and thoroughly dry the brace to prolong its life and reduce skin irritation.
11. Inspect the brace regularly for signs of deterioration or excessive wear.
12. Periodically apply a dry lubricant, such as Teflon spray, to the hinges.
13. Replace a broken or damaged brace.

Osteoarthritis Knee Braces

Knee osteoarthritis is a widespread disorder, and osteoarthritis knee braces have gained prominence as nonsurgical adjuncts in the treatment of unicompartmental degenerative changes. Many studies have confirmed the braces' subjective and objective benefits among symptomatic individuals. Osteoarthritis knee braces (Figs. 193-10 and 193-11) play an important role in addition to standard treatments of pharmacotherapy, intra-articular injections, heel wedges, regional muscle strengthening, and lifestyle modifications. The brace applies three-point forces periarticularly to reduce load on one side of the tibial-femoral knee joint. A varus (force is laterally directed) knee brace provides distracting pressure on the knee to

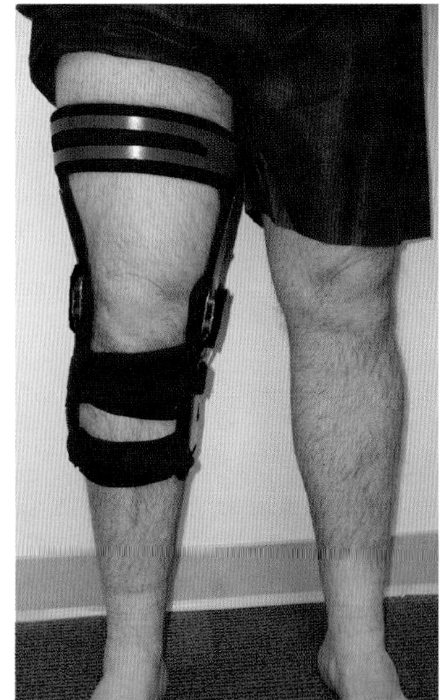

Figure 193-10 Representative osteoarthritis knee brace seen from the front.

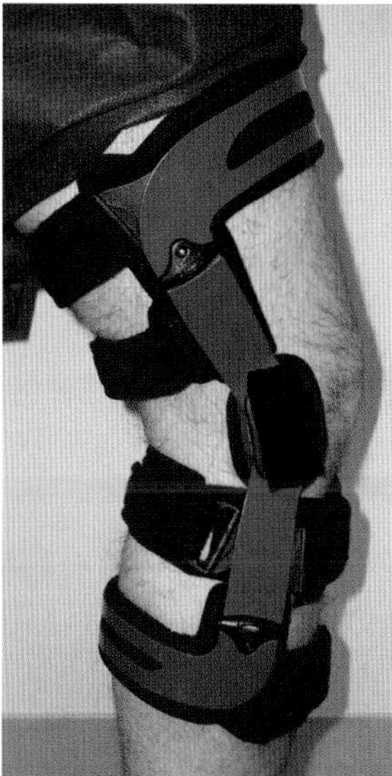

Figure 193-11 Representative osteoarthritis knee brace seen from the side.

off-load symptomatic lateral tibial-femoral osteoarthritis, and a valgus (force is medially directed) knee brace provides distracting pressure on the knee to off-load symptomatic medial tibial-femoral degenerative changes.

Most individuals can use a prefabricated brace without the need for more expensive customized osteoarthritis knee braces. No brace type or materials have been shown to be superior for improving pain or function. Obese individuals or those with abnormal limb contours typically have less success with the use of osteoarthritis knee braces. Moreover, some individuals are unable to tolerate the forces created by osteoarthritis knee braces very well during daily activities.

1. Measure the thigh circumference 6 inches above the mid-patella and select the corresponding brace size according to the manufacturer's instructions.
2. Some braces may also require measuring the calf circumference 6 inches below the mid-patella or the circumference of the knee at the joint line.
3. Loosely apply the brace to the leg without tightening the closure straps while the patient stands.
4. Adjust the varus and valgus alignment to fit the contours of the individual's leg. The side bars may be bent if needed.
5. Have the individual sit and flex the knee to 45 degrees. Position the side hinges 1 inch above the patella with the brace centered on the midline of the leg.
6. Secure the lower calf and the upper thigh straps snugly.
7. While the knee is still bent at 45 degrees, push both condylar hinges posteriorly to the midline of the leg. Hold the hinges in this position while securing the lower thigh strap.
8. While the knee is still bent at 45 degrees, pull both condylar hinges slightly forward but not anteriorly to the midline of the leg. Hold the hinges in place while securing the upper calf strap.
9. Confirm that both side hinges are centered just above the patella and slightly posterior to the leg's midline.
10. Tighten and adjust the straps after a few steps and then regularly during prolonged athletic activities. It is common for the brace to migrate distally or loosen slightly.
11. Trim the pads and straps as needed for comfort or to accommodate limb contours.
12. Cover the brace with the elastic wrap or a cover, if desired, to minimize brace deterioration or injury to others during activities.
13. Periodically apply a dry lubricant, such as Teflon spray, to the hinges.
14. Hand wash and thoroughly dry the brace occasionally to prolong its life and reduce skin irritation.
15. Inspect the brace regularly for signs of deterioration or excessive wear.
16. Periodically inspect and tighten the hinge screws as needed.
17. Replace a broken or damaged brace.

Common Errors and Complications

In general, knee braces are associated with few complications when selected and worn appropriately. Careful brace sizing and maintenance may limit unwanted side effects. However, the following may occur:

- Skin breakdown or irritation may occur from brace-to-skin contact over bony prominences. Regularly cleaning and air drying the brace may also help protect the skin's integrity.
- Athletes or highly active individuals may note diminished endurance, performance, speed, and range of motion.
- Brace wear may require increased energy expenditure during vigorous activities.
- Premature muscle fatigue resulting from regional muscle ischemia and lactic acid accumulation may limit activities.
- While wearing a knee brace, an individual may harbor a false sense of security or invincibility regarding the brace's efficacy and subsequently sustain a more significant knee injury.
- Some knee braces may interfere with an individual's knee proprioception.
- Brace-related contact injuries to others may occur.
- Excessive preloading of the knee ligaments by some braces may potentiate the severity of a knee injury.
- Some braces may cause symptomatic regional ipsilateral or contralateral lower extremity discomfort due to altered knee kinematics and gait.

Postprocedure Patient Education

Give the individual a copy of any materials provided by the brace manufacturer. It is also important to remind him or her of the following:

- Routinely inspect the brace for any signs of wear or deterioration. It is common for braces that are used for extended periods of time to need new pads, foam inserts, or enclosure straps.
- Knee braces are only one part of a comprehensive knee rehabilitation program. More important components of knee injury prevention and treatment include muscular strengthening, flexibility enhancement, and technique modification.
- The patient should report any of the following in regard to the knee brace: poor fit, mechanical dysfunction, skin breakdown or irritation, new-onset knee pain, or concerns regarding proper brace usage.

Suppliers

Full contact information is available online at www.expertconsult.com.

Functional Knee Braces

Bledsoe Ultimate CI (prefabricated)
Bledsoe, Inc.

Breg Fusion (prefabricated or custom)
Breg, Inc.

Donjoy Legend (prefabricated) or Defiance (custom)
dj Orthopedics

Össur C.Ti.2 (prefabricated or custom)
Össur

Townsend Design Rebel (prefabricated) or Premier (custom)
Townsend Design

Osteoarthritis Knee Braces

Bledsoe Thruster 3
Bledsoe, Inc.
Breg Fusion XT OA
Breg, Inc
DonJoy OA Adjuster
dj Orthopedics
Össur GII Unloader
Össur
Townsend Design Rebel Reliever
Townsend Design

Patellofemoral Knee Braces

BioSkin/Cropper Medical Q Lok
BioSkin/Cropper Medical
Breg Lateral J
Breg, Inc.
DonJoy Tru-Pull
dj Orthopedics
Hely Weber Shields Brace
Hely & Weber
Palumbo Patella Tracker
Palumbo Orthopedics

Postoperative Knee Braces

Bledsoe Merit OR
Bledsoe, Inc.
Breg T-Scope
Breg, Inc
Donjoy TROM
dj Orthopedics
Össur Innovator DLX
Össur
Townsend Adjusta-ROM
Townsend Design

Prophylactic Knee Braces

Bledsoe Sport Max (bilateral supports)
Bledsoe, Inc.
Breg RoadRunner (bilateral supports)
Breg, Inc.
DonJoy Playmaker (bilateral supports)
dj Orthopedics
Hely Weber Velocity (bilateral supports)
Hely & Weber
McDavid Protective Knee Guard (unilateral support) or Pro Stabilizer (bilateral supports)
McDavid Sports Medical Products

CPT/Billing Codes

For most fittings, E and M counseling codes will be used.

29530 Strapping, knee

HCPCS Brace Fitting and Application Codes

L1800 (Patella support) + L2795 (Patellar butress) billed together for patellofemoral brace
L1815 (Hinged knee support) + L2425 (Additional hinge) billed together for a unilateral support prophylactic brace or L1815 + L2425 (×2) for a bilateral support prophylactic brace
L1832: Postoperative hinged knee
L1845: Prefabricated functional or osteoarthritis brace
L1858: Custom functional or osteoarthritis brace

ICD-9-CM Diagnostic Codes

715.16 Osteoarthritis, lower leg
717.7 Chondromalacia of patella
717.83 Old disruption of ACL
719.06 Knee effusion
726.64 Patellar tendonitis
726.65 Prepatellar bursitis
726.69 Infrapatellar or subpatellar knee bursitis
823.00 Tibial plateau fracture
836.3 Dislocation of patella, closed
844.0 LCL sprain
844.1 MCL sprain
844.2 Cruciate ligament of knee sprain

Patient Education Guides

See the sample patient education and consent forms online at www.expertconsult.com.

BIBLIOGRAPHY

Dixit S, DiFiori JP, Burton M, Mines B: Management of patellofemoral pain syndrome. Am Fam Physician 75:194–202, 2007.
Lun VMY, Wiley JP, Meeuwisse WH, et al: Effectiveness of patellar bracing for treatment of patellofemoral pain syndrome. Clin J Sport Med 15: 235–240, 2005.
McDevitt ER, Taylor DC, Miller MD, et al: Functional bracing after anterior ligament reconstruction: A prospective, randomized, multicenter study. Am J Sports Med 32:1887–1892, 2004.
Najibi SH, Albright JP: The use of knee braces, part 1: Prophylactic knee braces in contact sports. Am J Sports Med 33:602–611, 2005.
Nadaud MC, Komistek RD, Mahfouz MR, et al: In vivo three-dimensional determination of the effectiveness of the osteoarthritic knee brace: A multiple brace analysis. J Bone Joint Surg Am 87A(Suppl 2):114–119, 2005.
Pollo FE, Jackson RW: Knee bracing for unicompartmental osteoarthritis. J Am Acad Orthop Surg 14:5–11, 2006.
Powers CM, Ward SR, Chan LD, et al: The effect of bracing on patella alignment and patellofemoral joint contact area. Med Sci Sports Exerc 36:1226–1232, 2004.
Soma CA, Cawley PW, Liu S, et al: Custom-fit versus premanufactured braces. Orthopedics 27:307–310, 2004.
Usatine RP: The Color Atlas of Family Medicine. New York, McGraw-Hill, 2009.
Wright RW, Fetzer GB: Bracing after ACL construction: A systematic review. Clin Orthop Relat Res 455:162–168, 2007.

CHAPTER 194

Nursemaid's Elbow: Radial Head Subluxation

Russell D. White • Christopher F. Adams

Nursemaid's elbow (radial head subluxation [RHS]) or "pulled elbow" is a common injury to children under 7 years old. The mechanism of injury is usually sudden axial traction of the outstretched, pronated forearm. It often occurs when a parent picks the child up and suspends the child's entire weight while holding only their hands. Alternatively, the child may have asked to be "swung around" while holding their hands. At times, the injury occurs unobserved by an adult. Regardless of mechanism, the child initially complains of pain and then refuses to use the arm. The concerned parents then take the child to seek medical attention.

The elbow consists of the articulation of the humerus, ulna, and radial head. The radius and ulna flex and extend against the humerus; the radial head can also rotate against the ulna and capitellum (humerus) to permit forearm pronation and supination. The radial head is held in place against the proximal ulna and capitellum by the annular ligament and joint capsule. In infants and young children, sudden traction on the distal forearm is sometimes more than the annular ligament can sustain; consequently, the radial head slides distally and partially dislocates or "subluxes." Presumably the annular ligament or synovial tissue becomes interposed between the radial head and capitellum, causing discomfort and preventing the radial head from spontaneous reduction.

Diagnosis

Often the history suggests the diagnosis. Typical scenarios for radial head subluxation include a caregiver pulling a child out of harm's way, a reluctant child being pulled along by the hand, a child suddenly dropping to the floor while being held, or a child being swung playfully by the arms. It is not uncommon for the subluxion to occur unwitnessed; in that case, the child may provide the history of having fallen or rolled over in bed. At presentation, the child expresses acute pain, refuses to move the affected extremity, and holds the elbow in a pronated and slightly flexed position (the nursemaid's position). Examination reveals no deformity and little if any swelling around the elbow. (Having the parent question the child and examine for areas of tenderness, with the clinician's guidance, may be less threatening than examination by the unknown clinician.) The child resists range of motion at the elbow, including further flexion or extension as well as supination and further pronation.

Some tenderness is noted over the radial head, but not the supracondylar regions. Neurovascular compromise is rare with this injury. Not infrequently, a child will have no known traction injury but holds the arm against the chest, refuses to use the arm, and has no significant deformity, swelling, or neurovascular compromise. The absence of a classic history of axial traction does not rule out the diagnosis of radial head subluxation. A small retrospective study found that a third of the 45 cases of nursemaid's elbow in the emergency department did not have a history of axial traction.

Radiographic Studies

The clinician should take standard elbow radiographs, including three views (anteroposterior, lateral, and oblique). Comparison radiographs of the contralateral elbow are essential in the young child because incomplete ossification increases the difficulty in evaluating the immature elbow structures and alignment. Radiographs of nursemaid's elbow are usually normal or reveal longitudinal misalignment of the radial head with the capitellum. The subluxation is occasionally reduced by the technician when taking the radiographs; the child is often distracted while being positioned for three radiographs and this may allow the elbow to be supinated and flexed. The child then returns to the clinical area using the affected extremity.

The clinician should evaluate the radiographs for the presence of a "fat pad sign" (joint effusion), location and alignment of epiphyseal growth centers, and the longitudinal alignment of the radial head with the capitellum. The fat pad sign is positive if a radiolucent stripe is visible at the posterior distal aspect of the humerus on the lateral view of the elbow and not visible on the comparison view. The periarticular fat is displaced posteriorly by an increase in intra-articular joint fluid, making it visible in the lateral view. This is a nonspecific finding. A positive fat pad sign associated with a history of trauma suggests a bloody joint effusion and intra-articular injury. In this case immediate orthopedic referral is recommended. A nursemaid's elbow can still be present despite the absence of a fat pad sign; in fact, that is generally the rule.

Misalignment of the ossification centers suggests a growth plate injury. Orthopedic referral is recommended for growth plate injury or other obvious fracture. Elbow fractures have a high complication rate.

We would never recommend manipulation of the patient, even with classic symptoms, before a radiographic study has been performed, although some clinicians do.

Indications

A child holding his or her arm in a pronated, partially flexed position, refusing to use it, often with a history of axial traction compatible with radial head subluxation (but not always), and negative radiographs indicates nursemaid's elbow.

Contraindications

- Edema or ecchymoses over the site
- Fracture (or suspicion of a fracture if no radiographs obtained)
- Mechanism of injury inconsistent with radial head subluxation (unless radiographs negative)
- Presence of distal neurologic or vascular compromise (orthopedic consultation recommended)

Preprocedure Patient Education

The procedure, as well as any risks and alternatives, should be explained to the patient and caregivers. Informed consent should be obtained. The patient can be sitting or supine on an examination table or sitting in a parent's lap. No preprocedure medications are generally required.

Technique

Supination and flexion of the forearm has been the usual method described in modern literature, including the first edition of this text, to reduce RHS. More recently, a method of hyperpronation with flexion has been evaluated as a safe and effective alternative technique for reduction of RHS, and has been shown in small studies to be a less painful method of reduction. The techniques differ in the direction the forearm is rotated.

Supination and Flexion Method

Figure 194-1 illustrates the supination and flexion method.

1. The elbow is held in one of the operator's hands (usually the nondominant hand) with either the thumb or second and third fingers exerting constant gentle pressure over the radial head in a medial direction.
2. While applying slight distal traction with the operator's other hand, the patient's wrist is supinated.
3. The patient's forearm is then rapidly raised toward the upper arm, flexing the elbow past 90 degrees. This should all be done in one smooth motion, and a click may be felt by the finger held over the radial head as it is reduced.
4. The forearm is moved so that the elbow is in 90 degrees of flexion and released.
5. The success of the manipulation is often tested by offering the child his or her favorite toy or a piece of candy on the side of the affected arm. If the child reaches with the affected arm, the manipulation was successful.
6. The child should be using the forearm normally within 30 minutes or else a repeat manipulation can be attempted. Using the alternative method of hyperpronating the forearm and rapid flexion has been successful even when repeat supination and flexion has failed.

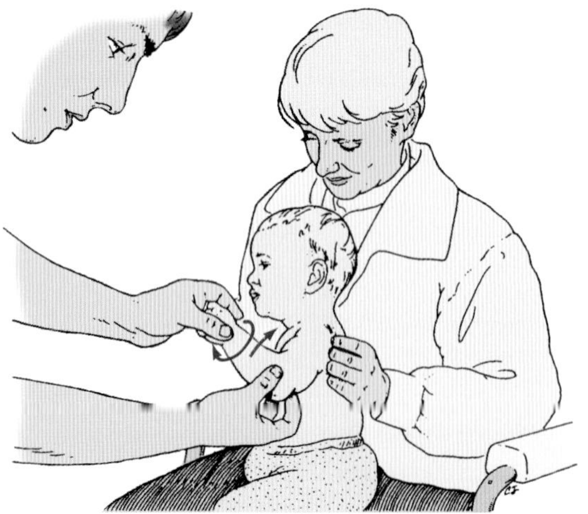

Figure 194-1 The reduction maneuver for a subluxed radial head (nursemaid's elbow) involves gentle supination of the forearm and flexion of the elbow. The examiner's thumb can be placed over the child's elbow to help palpate the radial head during the reduction process.

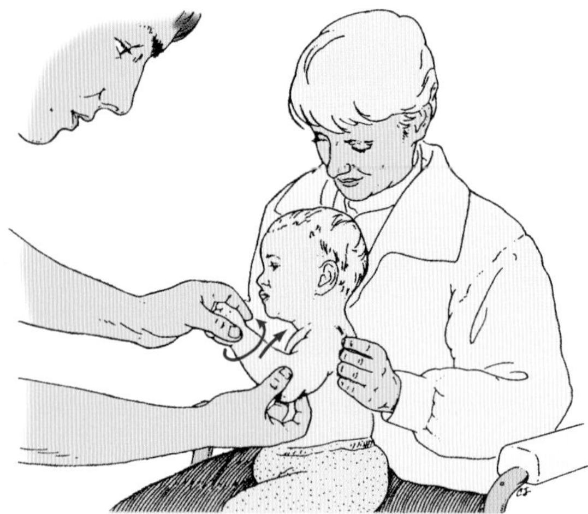

Figure 194-2 Pronation and flexion method.

Pronation and Flexion Method (Hyperpronation)

Figure 194-2 illustrates the pronation and flexion method.

1. The elbow is held with one of the operator's hands with the thumb or second and third fingers again exerting constant gentle medial pressure on the radial head.
2. While the operator applies slight distal traction, the patient's wrist is hyperpronated with the operator's other hand.
3. Rapid flexion at the elbow is performed; this should all be done in one smooth motion.
4. The elbow is extended to 90 degrees and released.
5. The success of manipulation is tested as noted previously.

Sometimes a click, snap, or satisfying clunk of the radial head may be felt, indicating reduction. Spontaneous reduction without manipulation may also occur before evaluation by the clinician. The caregivers generally need assurance that the child has suffered nothing serious.

Differential Diagnosis

If there is concern regarding the possibility of a growth plate injury, generally the best approach is to obtain an orthopedic consultation. Rarely, an arthrogram is needed to determine the extent of injury. Sedation or general anesthesia is often required to complete that study. The radiographic contrast material can help to outline articular surfaces and to give the examiner a better understanding of the nonossified anatomy.

Alternative diagnoses include osteomyelitis or clavicular, distal humeral, stress, or radial head fracture. Joint aspiration can be performed if there is concern regarding the possibility of more significant trauma or infection in the elbow (see Chapter 192, Joint and Soft Tissue Aspiration and Injection [Arthrocentesis]). Bloody fluid confirms the presence of a traumatic intracapsular injury, such as a fracture. Purulent material confirms the diagnosis of septic arthritis. Routine elbow aspiration is not recommended for a nursemaid's elbow; it is merely an adjunctive procedure that can be used in difficult diagnostic situations. Sedation or general anesthesia may be required. If any of the preceding diagnoses are being considered, an orthopedic surgeon should be consulted.

Postprocedure Patient Education

After successful reduction of a subluxed radial head, the provider should tell the child to rest the limb for several days and then reevaluate the child with follow-up clinical and possibly radiographic examination if symptoms do not totally resolve in 24 to 48 hours. If reduction is delayed more than 8 hours from the time of injury, it may take the full 24 to 48 hours to recover. A small percentage of patients will resublux the radial head within a few days of reduction, although the number and risk factors are not well defined. In a small randomized prospective study, immobilization in a flexed, supinated position with a posterior splint reduced the recurrence rate from 13% to zero ($p < .05$) at follow-up 2 days after manipulation (Taha, 2000). Children who remain reluctant to use their elbow in a normal fashion should be splinted from shoulder to hand. Follow-up evaluation in 2 or 3 days is recommended to determine normal joint function. If not normal at that point, orthopedic referral should be considered. Patients with splints should not remove the splint until the short-term follow-up examination.

Generally, children will let their symptoms be their guide in regard to activity level; once they are comfortable, they will resume their activities. It may take several days for them to do so. The long-term prognosis of nursemaid's elbow is generally favorable. Occasionally the child will have several episodes of subluxation, but the incidence drops off significantly after age 7. Caregivers should be educated regarding the mechanism of injury and how to avoid future subluxations. Long-term functional or growth problems are rare after appropriate treatment of this injury. Congenital radial head dislocation is a separate entity and is not related to the common pediatric problem of nursemaid's elbow.

CPT/Billing Codes

24640 Closed treatment of radial head subluxation in child, nursemaid elbow, with manipulation
29105 Splint, arm, long (shoulder to hand)

ICD-9-CM Diagnostic Code

755.59 Subluxation, joint, upper extremity

Acknowledgment

The editors wish to recognize the many contributions by Fred M. Hankin, MD, and James L. Telfer, MD, to this chapter in the previous two editions of this text.

BIBLIOGRAPHY

Green DA, Linares MYR, Garcia-Peña BM, et al: Randomized comparison of pain perception during radial head subluxation reduction using supination-flexion or forced pronation. Pediatr Emerg Care 22:235, 2006.
Kling MP, Reichman EF: Radial head subluxation ("nursemaid's elbow") reduction. In Reichman EF, Simon RR (eds): Emergency Medicine Procedures. New York, McGraw-Hill, 2004, pp 621–624.
Macias CG, Bothner J, Wiebe R: A comparison of supination/flexion to hyperpronation in the reduction of radial head subluxations. Pediatrics 102:e10, 1998.
McDonald J, Whitelaw C, Goldsmith LJ: Radial head subluxation: Comparing two methods of reduction. Acad Emerg Med 6:715, 1999.
Sacchetti A, Ramoska EE, Glascow C: Nonclassic history in children with radial head subluxations. J Emerg Med 8:151, 1990.
Taha AM: The treatment of pulled elbow: A prospective randomized study. Arch Orthop Trauma Surg 120:336, 2000.

CHAPTER 195

Podiatric Procedures

Gary L. Snyder • Grant C. Fowler

Orthotics

Orthotics are prescribed, in-shoe devices designed to protect and improve abnormal foot function. Orthotics are custom made and, as such, may differ in the materials from which they are manufactured. Each prescription may have various modifications and additions depending on the underlying diagnosis. The two most common types of orthotics are *functional* orthotics and *accommodative* orthotics. Both of these are made from precise casts, impressions, or scans of the patient's foot that has been placed in the position in which the practitioner wishes the foot to function. Although symptoms improve with conservative care in the vast majority of patients with plantar fasciitis in 3 to 6 months, no matter what the treatment, Cochrane evidence-based reviews found possible benefit with custom-made orthotics in patients with this disorder. Cochrane reviews also found possible benefit with custom orthotics in patients with painful pes cavus (high-arching foot), painful hallux valgus (bunion), rearfoot pain due to rheumatoid arthritis, and foot pain due to juvenile idiopathic arthritis (patients older than 5 years of age). Other reviews have found that 70% of patients improved with orthotics versus 30% with heel cups or injections. According to one study, after 1 year, most patients prefer custom orthotics to other devices (e.g., night splints) for preventing or managing foot pain.

EDITOR'S NOTE: Vendors with digital foot scanning systems have recently become much more common and offer custom orthotics. It should be noted that such orthotics will not be able to provide the frequently needed accommodative pads or customized balance support.

Most (70%) patients are heel strikers, and in these patients about 50% of the stress of weight bearing is borne or transferred through the calcaneus, whereas the other 50% is transferred to the first and fifth metatarsophalangeal (MTP) joints (about 35% to the first MTP). Although malalignment anywhere in the lower extremity can change this weight-bearing pattern, the normal pattern is therefore from the calcaneus, through the midfoot, and then off the first and fifth MTP joints. Orthotics can be useful for patients with abnormalities in their weight-bearing pattern. Corns and calluses may not only develop as a result of weight-bearing abnormalities, but their location may also help diagnose or confirm the abnormality. Exceptions to the normal weight-bearing pattern are patients with a very narrow heel and wide forefoot; they are likely forefoot strikers. Plantar warts, hammer (claw and mallet) toes, bunions, bunionettes, metatarsalgia, sesamoiditis, and hallux rigidus (stiff toe) can all be uncomfortable and have an impact on the weight-bearing pattern; significant relief is often provided by a simple podiatric adjustment or procedure.

Functional Orthotics

Functional orthotics are usually rigid or semirigid thermoplastic shells with built-in corrections or additions to change a foot's position or to control abnormal foot motion. Flexible deformities of the foot are most frequently treated with this type of orthotic.

Accommodative Orthotics

Accommodative orthotics are softer and more cushioned, designed to protect painful plantar lesions or bony deformities of the foot. A number of closed-cell and open-cell foam products—as well as cork, leather, rubber, and silicone—are used in the fabrication of accommodative orthotics. These designs are most frequently used with rigid foot deformities, arthritic foot changes, and certain diabetic conditions. In some cases, they may be useful early in a disease process that will later require surgery.

Indications (Rigid, Custom Orthotics)

- Plantar fasciitis (with or without heel spur syndrome)
- Pes cavus (Although people with this "high-arching foot" [defined as >3 cm height from ground measured at navicular bone] may never have a problem, they have a sixfold increased risk of injury with sports, largely because of an inflexible foot that does not adjust well to uneven surfaces; they also have a higher risk of plantar fasciitis.)
- Pes planus (flat foot)
- Excessive pronation (Fig. 195-1) resulting in problems (e.g., tibialis posterior dysfunction or medial tibial stress syndrome, metatarsalgia, tarsal tunnel syndrome)

  NOTE: Examination may reveal a long, narrow foot, usually resulting in the patient rolling the foot excessively (excessive pronation) with ambulation. Deviations from the normal leg–heel–forefoot alignment may also be noted. Direct observation or videotaping of training routines may also be necessary to diagnose biomechanical abnormalities that are not noticed on routine examination. Pes planus, tibia vara, tibial torsion, subtalar joint varus, and heel cord tightness are possible causes of malalignment.

- Painful corns and calluses (following treatment, to prevent recurrence)
- Hammer toes (flexible)
- Early bunion (hallux valgus) deformity
- Stiff toe (hallux rigidus)
- Morton's neuroma
- Chronic lateral ankle instability

Indications (Soft, Accomodative Custom Orthotics)

- Diabetic foot pathology such as Charcot changes or plantar ulcerations
- Patients with arthritis or arthrosis

Contraindications (Relative)

- Other than allergy to orthotic material, there are usually no contraindications.

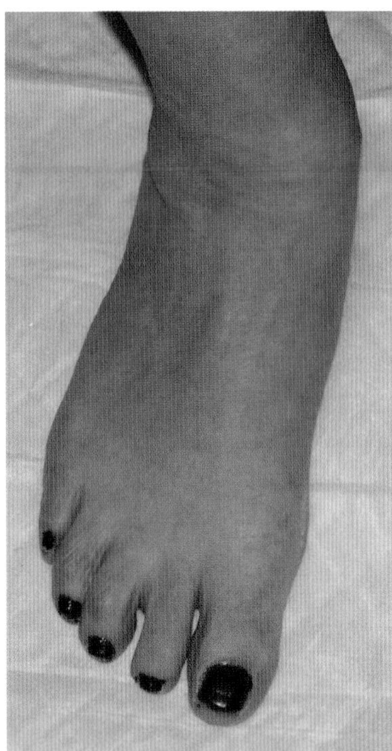

Figure 195-1 Excessive, unchecked pronation demonstrated with weight bearing.

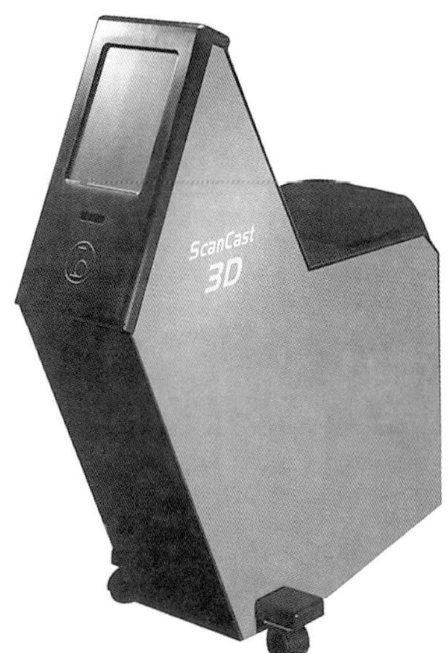

Figure 195-2 ScanCast 3D is a portable, self-contained unit. (Courtesy of Benefoot/Langer Biomechanics, Inc., Deer Park, NY.)

- Care must be taken with the neuropathic (e.g., diabetic) foot to ensure an exact fit.
- Some difficulty exists in fitting prescription orthotics for women's and men's dress shoes, although specialty laboratories do manufacture these devices.
- When anticipating a functional rigid or semirigid orthotic, the patient's range of ankle dorsiflexion must be greater than 10 degrees with the knee extended.

Equipment

More than 100 different prescription orthotic laboratories are accredited throughout the United States. The choice of laboratory is left to the discretion of the practitioner. Langer Biomechanics, Inc. (Deer Park, NY), is an example of an excellent facility and can be a very helpful resource.

Impressions taken in the office can be performed with the following techniques:

- Johnson & Johnson Extra-Fast Setting plaster casting tape (available from Moore Medical Corporation, New Britain, Conn)
- ScanCast Optical Scanner (Fig. 195-2; Benefoot/Langer)
- Biofoam Impression Kit (Smithers Bio-Medical Systems, Kent, Ohio)

Impression Techniques

Plaster Cast Technique

Four-inch-wide Johnson & Johnson Extra-Fast Setting casting splints can be used, usually two layers thick. The casting tape is wrapped around the foot to completely cover the heel, medial and lateral margins, plantar aspect, and toes (Fig. 195-3). The casting tape is then smoothed to ensure full contact with the foot, and the foot is immediately placed in the desired functional position. The procedure is repeated for the other foot. When the casting tape dries, the feet are easily released from these "slipper casts."

ScanCast Technique

Using ScanCast (Benefoot/Langer), the foot is placed in the desired functional position in front of the ScanCast screen (Fig. 195-4). Foot position is confirmed and visualized. The scan function is activated. Scanning takes approximately 1 second and is then repeated for the other foot. A digital image of the plantar surface of each foot is recorded. Orthotics are developed from these scans. (A positive model of each foot is constructed and the orthotic is molded onto this model.)

Biofoam Impression Technique

With one of the clinician's hands, the patient's ankle should be stabilized and held in a neutral position (preventing pronation) by supporting the talus. The patient's foot is then placed lightly over the foam in the impression kit, and the patient is instructed to avoid applying pressure. For additional stability, the clinician can quickly shift the stabilizing hand to the lateral aspect of the foot. Using the other hand, the clinician applies downward pressure on the patient's knee to make an impression of the foot in the foam. The foot should be pushed 1 to 1 ½ inches into the foam while simultaneous, stabilizing pressure is applied to the lateral aspect of the foot. Finish the

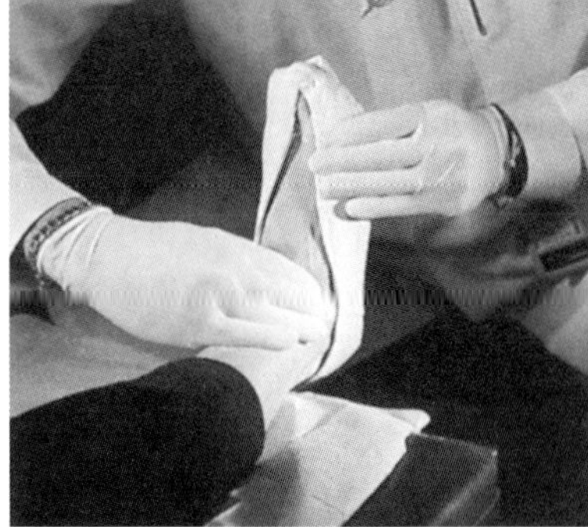

Figure 195-3 Casting tape applied to foot. (Courtesy of Benefoot/Langer Biomechanics, Inc., Deer Park, NY.)

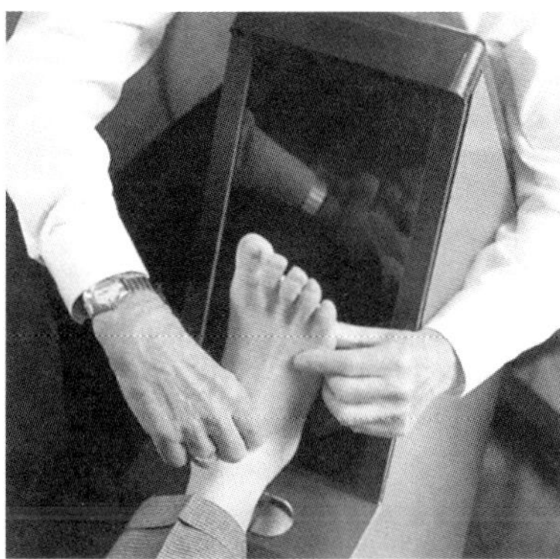

Figure 195-4 Using the ScanCast 3D to scan the foot. (Courtesy of Benefoot/Langer Biomechanics, Inc., Deer Park, NY.)

impression by using both hands to press the toes into the foam. In this manner, weight-bearing flow is simulated, from heel to midfoot to toes. Alternatively, with a good grasp on the lateral aspect of the foot, one hand can be used to both stabilize and push the foot into the foam and make the impression (Fig. 195-5A). Inspect each impression for defects, unevenness of the weight-bearing surface, or abnormal plantar contour (Fig. 195-5B). Repeat the procedure with the patient's other foot.

Foot Position

There are four basic positions that may be used to obtain a cast of the foot for an orthotic:

1. Subtalar neutral position, non-weight bearing
2. Subtalar neutral position, partial weight bearing
3. Rectus position
4. Full weight bearing

NOTE: One of the authors (GLS) suspects it is of little consequence which position is used to obtain the cast, scan, or impression as long as the mid-tarsal, subtalar, and ankle joints are in a neutral and "locked" position. His preference is to use the non–weight-bearing position for fitting custom orthotics and he reserves a weight-bearing position for obtaining certain radiographs.

Subtalar Neutral Position, Non-Weight Bearing

This technique is used most frequently and captures the "neutral" position of the foot. The patient may be sitting, supine, or prone with the feet hanging free over the end of the examination table. The ankle is kept at right angles to the leg. This technique can be used for the casting tape (see Fig. 195-3), ScanCast Optical Scanner (see Fig. 195-4), or Biofoam Impression (see Fig. 195-5). First, get a feel for what is the neutral position of the foot by inverting and everting, pronating and supinating it while palpating the medial and lateral aspects of the head of the talus with the thumb and index finger (at the talonavicular joint) of one hand. Next, stabilize the talonavicular joint in a neutral, congruous position, midway between inversion and eversion, pronation and supination. Then, with the other hand, grasp the foot on the dorsal and plantar aspects of the fifth metatarsal head (at the MTP joint) and maximally pronate the mid-tarsal joint (see Fig. 195-4). (One author [GLS] grasps the great toe and gently pulls down and lateral so that the foot is in approximately 15 degrees of external rotation.) The foot is held in this position until the casting tape dries (see Fig. 195-3) or the scanning is completed, or while a biofoam impression is made.

NOTE: Useful when maximum biomechanical control of forefoot and rearfoot deformities is required (e.g., flexible pes planus [flat foot] deformity, tibialis posterior dysfunction or medial tibialis stress syndrome, most pediatric deformities). Best for pes planus with greater than 10 degrees ankle dorsiflexion mobility. Most commonly used with sport orthotics.

Subtalar Neutral Position, Partial Weight Bearing

With this technique, the patient sits comfortably with the knee flexed at 90 degrees, the ankle at 90 degrees, and the center of the patella located directly over the second MTP joint. The foot is placed in the neutral position (Fig. 195-6), the position of function, and is then either wrapped in casting tape or placed over the Biofoam Impression Kit and carefully pressed into the foam (see Fig. 195-5). If casting tape is used, the patient is placed on a 2-inch-thick, plastic-wrapped foam pad until the casting tape dries. Care is taken to avoid inverting or everting the heel during the impression stage.

NOTE: This technique is indicated for most flexible foot deformities (e.g., pes cavus, pes planus, plantar fasciitis, heel spurs, bunions, painful corns, or calluses on the plantar aspect of the foot).

Rectus Position

This technique is similar to the non–weight-bearing neutral position, except that the forefoot is held parallel to the plantar aspect of the rearfoot during the time the plaster is drying or the foot is being scanned.

NOTE: This technique is indicated for childhood foot deformities (e.g., metatarsus adductus, pes cavus, pes planus, and calcaneal valgus).

Full Weight Bearing

The practitioner can choose plaster or a scanning system similar to the ScanCast Optical Scanner. The patient is instructed to stand in a normal angle and base-of-gait (with the foot held in the neutral

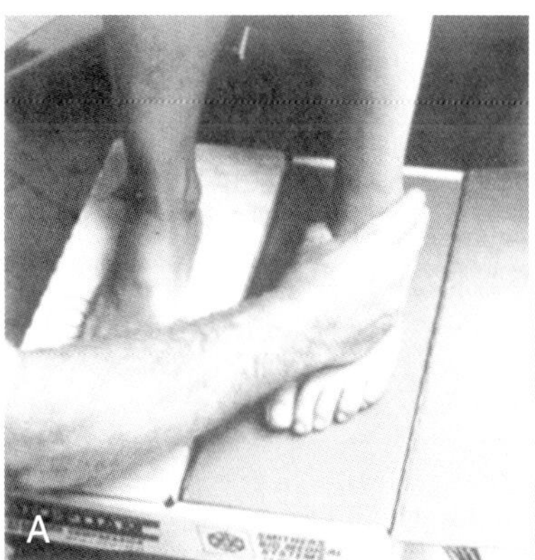

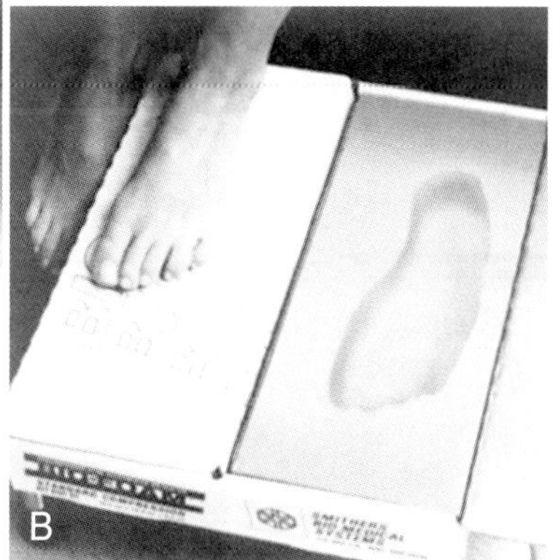

Figure 195-5 Taking foam impressions. **A,** Ankle should not be supinated or pronated. **B,** Inspect each impression for defects or unevenness of the weight-bearing surface, or abnormal plantar contour. (Courtesy of Smithers Bio-Medical Systems, Kent, Ohio.)

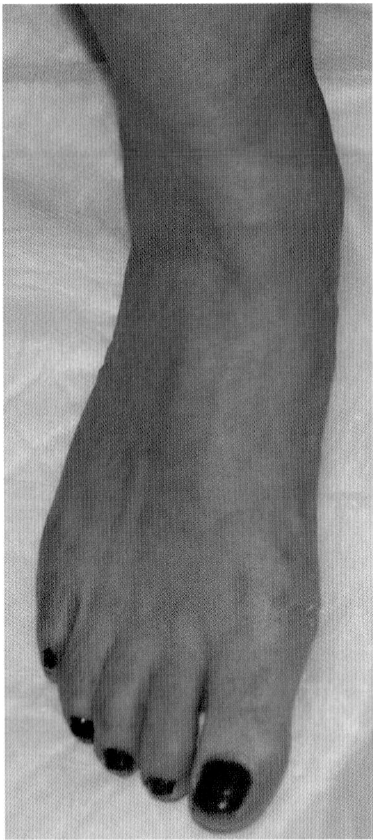

Figure 195-6 Partial weight-bearing, neutral functional position.

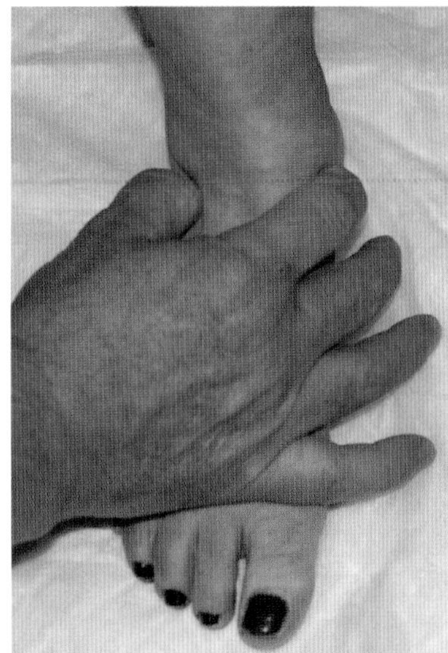

Figure 195-7 Weight-bearing, neutral position, demonstrated by palpating the talonavicular junction.

position by the clinician while palpating the talonavicular joint; Fig. 195-7) while plaster is drying or the foot is being scanned.

NOTE: Full weight-bearing impressions are useful for rigid and arthritic foot deformities, where accommodative padding under pressure points will be beneficial.

Complications

Reported adverse effects include additional foot pain, ankle instability, and skin irritation. Many adjustments can be performed in the office to minimize these or other adverse effects, usually relating to thickness, width, or position of accommodation. Shoe fitting can be difficult with some dress shoes.

Postprocedure Patient Education

Patients are instructed to initially wear an Oxford-style shoe, at least five eyelets per side, with a removable manufacturer's insole. They begin by wearing the orthotics approximately 1 hour per day; they can then increase the wearing time as tolerated. Average break-in period is between 4 and 12 weeks. If ankle equinus is present, the patient is instructed to continue with gastrocnemius-soleus–stretching exercises. It usually takes 12 weeks to obtain the maximum benefit from orthotics.

Corns (Helomas, Clavi), Calluses (Tylomas), and Plantar Keratomas

Corns are discrete, localized, well-circumscribed, round to oval hyperkeratotic lesions found on the toes, usually overlying bony prominences or digital deformities. They are usually painful and can be disabling. Corns involve the dermis and epidermis. *Soft corns* (heloma molle) are usually interdigital lesions resulting from abnormal pressure from deformed joints, bony prominences, or improper- or tight-fitting shoes (Fig. 195-8). Friction or structural deformities cause mechanical irritation between the toes. Soft corns are most commonly found between the fourth and fifth toes on the digital surface, but they can occur in any interdigital space or on the webspace. These lesions often become macerated (by absorbing moisture) and even secondarily infected. After paring or débridement, a small sinus tract can occasionally be identified and can be a source of underlying infection or inflammation. *Hard corns* (heloma durum) are usually found on the dorsum of an interphalangeal joint (second to fourth) or on the dorsolateral aspect of the fifth toe. These lesions result from structural deformities or bony prominences—pressure, shear forces, or friction from footgear over these prominences causes thickening and nucleation of the skin.

Corns are usually uniform in color and vary from whitish-gray to yellowish-gold. Subdermal hemorrhages can cause areas of discoloration that may appear dark red, brown, or black. Lesions are painful to direct and indirect pressure over the area. When débrided or pared down, a central, translucent, pearl-white core is usually found over the area of greatest pressure. Corns can be distinguished from warts by the lack of thrombosed tiny blood vessels on examination as well as the lack of punctate bleeding when débrided. Skin lines pass through corns but around warts (Box 195-1). These skin lines are often more apparent after alcohol is used to cleanse the area.

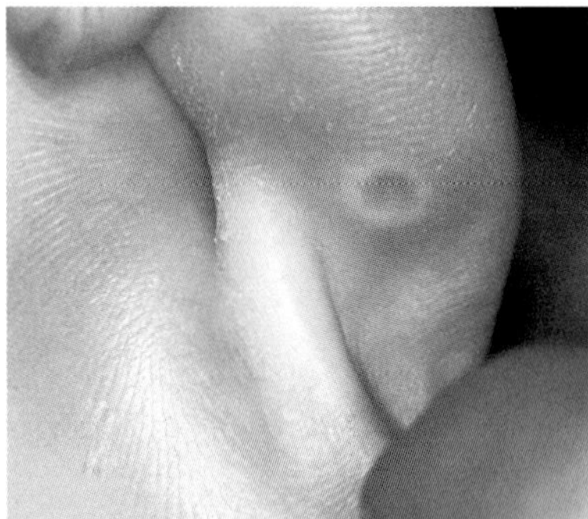

Figure 195-8 Soft corn on lateral aspect of the toe. (Courtesy of John L. Pfenninger, MD, The Medical Procedures Center, PC, Midland, Mich.)

Box 195-1. Distinguishing Features of Warts and Plantar Corns

Wart

- Relatively rapid onset
- May or may not be under bony prominences
- Skin lines pass around lesion
- Maximum pain on squeezing side to side
- End arteries visible as red or black dots on paring
- Rapid recurrence after shaving and padding

Plantar Corn

- Develops over months or years
- Located under bony prominences
- Skin lines pass through lesion
- Maximum pain with direct pressure
- No end arteries visible on paring
- Slower recurrence after shaving

From Singh D, Bentley G, Trevino SG: Callosities, corns, and calluses. BMJ 312:1403–1406, 1996.

Calluses are broad-based, poorly circumscribed, hyperkeratotic lesions commonly found on the plantar aspect of the foot at sites of friction or high pressure. They may be quite painful when located under the MTP joints. Calluses by definition involve primarily the epidermis and can occur diffusely around the heel or on the margins of the toes. Because most (70%) patients are heel strikers, and it is then normal to transfer weight through the midfoot and off the great (first) and fifth MTPs, calluses are common on the heels and under the first, second, and fifth MTP joints. (Calluses located between these areas often indicate abnormal foot structure or function.) A callus, differing from a corn, usually does not have a "nucleus" and instead consists of diffuse hyperkeratotic tissue (Fig. 195-9). The *intractable plantar keratoma* (Fig. 195-10) is a unique lesion consisting of an overlying callus with significant epidermal, dermal, and subdermal alterations, including fibrosis of the surrounding tissue. These are deep, nucleated plantar calluses found beneath an MTP joint and are often extremely painful with palpation and ambulation. They are usually circular, of smaller diameter than a tyloma, and exhibit a central "plug" or fibrous core on scalpel débridement. Intractable plantar keratomas are strong indicators of forefoot or rearfoot joint instability and therefore often benefit from rebalancing the weight-bearing surface with orthotics.

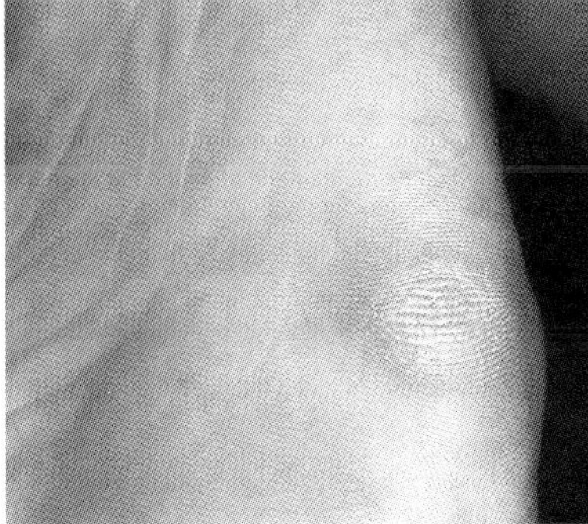

Figure 195-9 Callus on foot. The differential includes a plantar wart. (Courtesy of John L. Pfenninger, MD, The Medical Procedures Center, PC, Midland, Mich.)

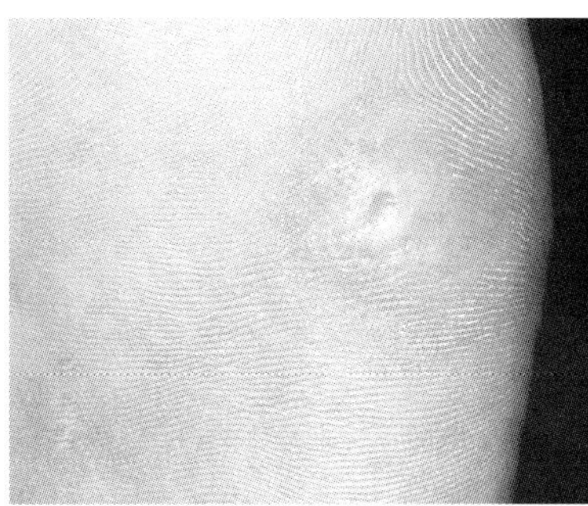

Figure 195-10 Intractable plantar keratoma showing solid, smooth, hard central core. There are no pinpoint bleeders characteristic of a wart. (Courtesy of John L. Pfenninger, MD, The Medical Procedures Center, PC, Midland, Mich.)

Etiology

Corns and calluses consist of multiple layers of flat sheets of α-keratin (β-keratin is found in reptile and fish scales), which has an underlying protein matrix consisting mostly of the amino acid cystine. Cystine, in turn, is formed by linking multiple molecules of the amino acid cysteine with disulfide bonds (Fig. 195-11). Clinicians are often familiar with the pungent sulfur odor released by these disulfide bonds when hair, skin, or a fingernail is cauterized or burned. Corns and calluses generally occur as a result of abnormally high pressure from a deformity, footgear, shear forces, or friction from ambulation. They can also be the result of permanently plantar flexed or hypermobile metatarsals as well as instability of the joints of the forefoot and rearfoot. Figure 195-12A shows normal metatarsal alignment; Figures 195-12B and C show how to test for permanently inflexible joints or hypermobile joints by moving the second and third metatarsal heads through their full range of motion.

Differential Diagnosis

- Verrucae
- Digital bursa
- Dermal and epidermal malignancies
- Porokeratosis plantaris discreta (caused by keratin-plugged sweat duct)

Techniques

Treatment should not only provide symptomatic relief, but attempt to lessen or alleviate the underlying biomechanical cause(s) inciting the problem. Use of shoes with a wider toe box or thicker socks may remove some of the pressure (see Postprocedure Patient Education for how to fit a shoe correctly using the Brannock device). Wearing a thin layer of cotton socks under a thicker layer of socks may reduce friction or shear forces on skin. Correcting or minimizing deformities with orthotics may prevent recurrence. Attempts should be made to correct bony angulation or flexibility defects with padding or orthotics, to see if they are beneficial, before performing corrective surgery.

Figure 195-11 Two molecules of cysteine are linked by disulfide bonds to form cystine, a major component of the underlying matrix in human keratin.

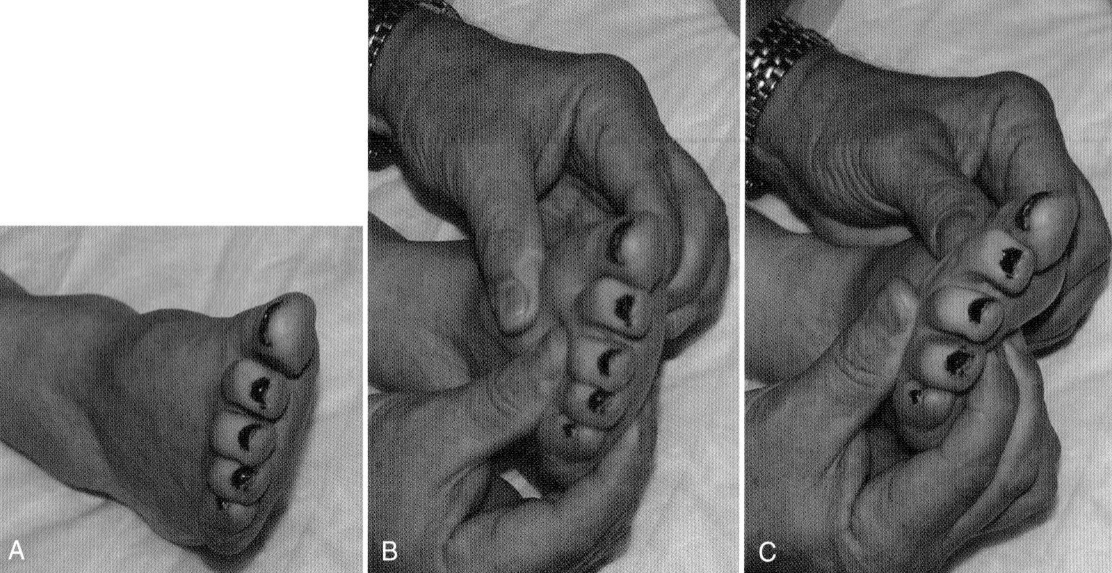

Figure 195-12 **A,** Normal metatarsal alignment. **B,** Testing metatarsal head flexibility with excessive pronation. **C,** Testing metatarsal head flexibility by hyperflexion.

Débridement

Débridement should be considered for hyperkeratotic lesions causing symptoms or showing signs of extreme dryness or intralesional cracking and fissuring. In the office, most clinicians use a no. 10 or no. 15 scalpel blade on a handle to remove hyperkeratotic tissue from corns or calluses. The scalpel is held parallel to the lesion and, using small, straight, or circular motions, the lesion is gradually shaved, débrided, or pared back. A thin layer is removed with each pass of the instrument. Because hyperkeratotic skin is devoid of innervation (has no sensation), the patient is usually able to tolerate débridement without a local anesthetic. To minimize discomfort, avoid placing pressure downward into the lesion; instead, pressure should be directed across the lesion with the scalpel. When most of the lesion has been removed, the clinician can usually visualize pink, viable skin just beneath it. This pink tissue has sensation, and as the clinician gets closer to shaving through it, the patient will usually sense or complain of some discomfort. This tissue also has a viable blood supply. In fact, the patient can guide and warn the clinician: as the sensation increases, the majority of the hyperkeratotic skin has been débrided and this is the point where bleeding is likely to start.

Débridement can also be accomplished with various razor blade–containing devices, a pumice stone, electric drill, or keratolytic agents such as weak salicylic acid plasters. It is easier to use a pumice stone if the area has been soaked and softened. Of course, débridement is only a temporary cure, and the lesion will recur unless the primary cause for the excessive pressure is corrected. Use of aperture pads (Fig. 195-13) may decrease the likelihood of recurrence by taking pressure off the original site. Shoes must be evaluated and modified if necessary.

NOTE: If the clinician is untrained or uncomfortable performing débridement, he or she may consider referral to a clinician comfortable performing it, especially for those patients with compromised circulation or diabetes; options include a competent podiatrist.

Combined Approaches

Therapy for these disorders can also include mechanical supportive orthotics (either functional or accommodative), nonsteroidal anti-inflammatory drugs (NSAIDs), accommodative footgear, digital or metatarsal pads, and accommodations made of moleskin, Cushlin (Dr. Scholl's/Schering-Plough Healthcare Products, Memphis, Tenn), or silicone (Silipos [New York] or Spenco [Waco, Tex]; all available through Moore Medical Corp.).

Surgical Treatment

Surgical removal of bone exostosis, correction of digital deformities, osteotomies for elevation of depressed metatarsals, arthrodesis of midfoot, hindfoot, or ankle joint, or various joint-limiting procedures may be recommended when conservative therapies fail to provide lasting relief.

Complications

Secondary infections can occur with untreated corns or calluses. Ulcerations are a serious complication with diabetic neuropathy. Bursitis can occur with untreated lesions.

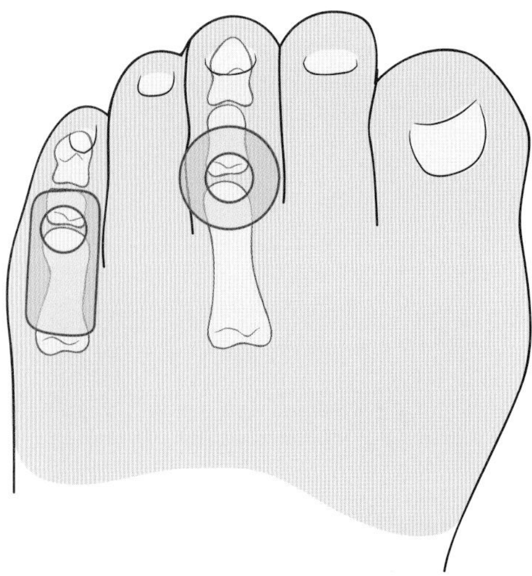

Figure 195-13 Self-adherent aperture pads, usually placed over previously pared area to relieve pressure, often overlying a bony prominence. (From Ehrlich M, Nemer JA: Management of select podiatric conditions. In Reichman EF, Simon RR [eds]: Emergency Medicine Procedures. New York, McGraw-Hill, 2004, p 1443.)

Warts (Verrucae Plantaris)

Verrucae plantaris ("plantar warts") are well-circumscribed, encapsulated, benign, tumorigenic, dermatotrophic lesions. The diagnosis is relatively simple, judging from appearance, the production of pain on lateral compression of the lesion, thrombosed tiny blood vessels, and pinpoint bleeding after débridement. Plantar verrucae appear different clinically from verrucae elsewhere because of being compressed and driven into the surrounding tissue.

Verrucae are encapsulated and well contained within the epidermis; the dermis is rarely involved. The lesion obliterates normal papillary skin lines. (This is an important diagnostic feature when treating warts. Often there is hyperkeratotic skin over the lesion. If this material is pared away after treatment and skin lines are then seen, the wart is considered resolved.) The appearance typically resembles grayish or brown papules with hypertrophic capillaries creating black or brown specks (end arteries, thrombosed capillaries) within the lesion. Plantar warts can occur singularly or in multiple clusters, which are referred to as *mosaic verrucae*. Smaller lesions surrounding the large centralized clusters are referred to as *satellite lesions*.

Etiology

Verrucae plantaris is caused by the human papillomavirus.

Differential Diagnosis

Warts are often confused with corns or deep calluses. Thrombosed tiny blood vessels and pinpoint bleeding after scalpel débridement are diagnostic hallmarks of verrucae plantaris. Other differential diagnoses include porokeratosis, epidermal malignancies (amelanotic melanoma), and various epidermal inflammatory conditions.

Treatment Options

There are a plethora of treatment methods, including chemical cautery with various acids, caustic chemotherapy such as 5-fluorouracil, cryotherapy, infrared coagulation, electrosurgery, immunotherapy (including imiquimod), injections (bleomycin, *Candida* antigen), CO_2 pulsed-dye laser, and surgical excision or curettage. Even duct tape has been reported to be beneficial, with an 85% cure rate! (Also see Chapter 42, Wart [Verruca] Treatment.)

Techniques

Chemocautery

Scalpel débridement of all hyperkeratotic tissue should be performed first. After débridement, the application of various acids, such as trichloracetic acid 85%, salicylic acid 60%, or pyrogallic acid 25%, can be used. Careful protection of the surrounding normal integument is paramount (some clinicians paint surrounding tissue with fingernail polish). The acids are usually followed by an occlusive, adhesive dressing. The patient is then instructed to keep the area dry and intact for approximately 2 to 7 days. This procedure is repeated until normal skin lines are visualized. Treatment response times vary greatly with individuals. If there is minimal improvement after a reasonable number of treatments, another form of treatment, such as cryotherapy or other options as mentioned, should be considered.

Other Techniques

Specifics of treatment using other modalities are noted in the specific chapter dealing with each technique. (See Chapter 12, Approach to Various Skin Lesions; Chapter 14, Cryosurgery; Chapter 30, Radiofrequency Surgery [Modern Electrosurgery]; and Chapter 42, Wart [Verruca] Treatment.)

Complications

Post-treatment pain can be controlled with ice, NSAIDs, and acetaminophen. Chemical burns can create a sterile abscess site; fortunately, these rarely become infected. Painful plantar scarring should be avoided because walking on scars can feel like stepping on a pebble.

Hammer (Claw and Mallet) Toes, Bunions (Hallux Varus and Valgus), and Bunionettes (Tailor's Bunion)

Hammer, claw, and mallet toes are usually due to atrophy of the intrinsic muscles of the interphalangeal joints with subsequent loss of their stabilizing effect on the interphalangeal joints. As a result, the extrinsic muscles overpower the joints and pull them into permanent flexion or extension. Atrophy of the intrinsic muscles may be due to biomechanical faults, arthrosis, or constant pressure from tight shoes, resulting in toes being held in a constantly flexed or bent position; atrophy may also be due to other causes such as neuropathy from diabetes, alcoholism, or normal aging.

Hammer toes, like most nonacute foot deformities, are progressive. They start as flexible deformities where biomechanical control may be all that is necessary to prevent progression and even allow regression. A severe hammer toe deformity can indicate that there has been enough atrophy of the plantar capsule of the MTP joint to allow the metatarsal head to drop through the degenerated, torn capsule. Often this metatarsal head can be palpated as a hard bump on the bottom of the foot. It will also often result in the affected toes being splayed, and this can even be seen radiographically. Usually affecting the second toe, which is often the longest toe, this results in a permanently extended, dorsiflexed MTP joint. Subsequent pressure on the dorsum of the toe combined with an imbalance of muscles results in permanent plantar flexion at the proximal interphalangeal (PIP) joint and the appearance of a hammer. This also often occurs in the third toe. If the distal interphalangeal (DIP) joint also becomes permanently plantar flexed, it results in a claw toe. Claw toes can affect all the toes with the exception of the great toe (which does not have a DIP joint). A mallet toe occurs when only the DIP joint is flexed, and although it can involve any of the toes, it frequently affects only the second toe because it is often the longest.

Such structural abnormalities and deformities often result in increased pressure on the overlying skin and development of hyperkeratotic lesions. The hammer toe frequently shows flexion of the PIP joint and extension of the DIP joint.

Bunions and bunionettes also result from the effects of biomechanical faults, footwear, osteoarthritis/osteoarthrosis, or various other anatomic, physiologic, and hereditary conditions. Just like the thumb, the MTP joint of the great toe is a common site for osteoarthritis. Bunions involve the first metatarsal head, resulting in lateral deviation of the great toe and medial deviation of the MTP joint (also known as hallux abducto valgus, the terms derived from movement related to the mid-sagittal plane of the foot); bunionettes affect the fifth metatarsal head, resulting in medial deviation of the fifth toe (adduction) and lateral deviation (abduction) of the fifth MTP joint (also known as *tailor's bunion*).

Differential Diagnosis

Trauma and infectious or other inflammatory diseases are possible causes for painful or deformed joints at all of these sites. Radiographs may be helpful not only for determining the magnitude of the problem but also for excluding other causes. Laboratory analysis may be helpful for ruling out infectious or inflammatory arthritis. The differential diagnosis of a bunion also includes bursitis of the first MTP joint; it can occur on the medial aspect of the joint.

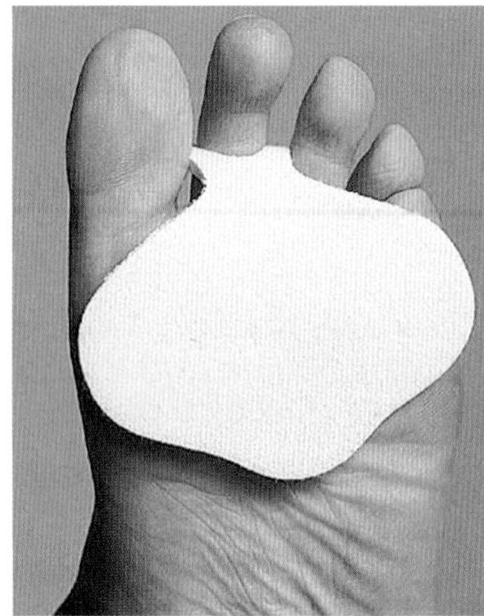

Figure 195-14 Commercially available metatarsal pad; a similar pad can be cut from self-adherent felt.

Techniques

The initial treatment of hammer, claw, and mallet toes and bunions or bunionettes is to consider changing footwear (see Postprocedure Patient Education for how to fit a shoe correctly using the Brannock device). Shoes with a roomier toe box or use of thicker socks should minimize pressure against the inflamed, affected areas and allow them to heal. Hyperkeratotic lesions should be débrided or pared down. Padding and accommodative shields may help disperse local pressure and change balance. Precut metatarsal pads (Fig. 195-14) or bars are available or may be cut from 1-cm-thick felt (see Suppliers section). For hammer or claw toes, decreasing the degree of plantar flexion of the MTP joint by using metatarsal pads (Fig. 195-15), placed just proximal to the metatarsal head, may decrease symptoms. This is partially accomplished by decreasing the pressure on the dorsum of the distal toe(s) from the inside top of the shoe. If a metatarsal pad is used early, it may even prevent the development of hammer or claw toes. Attempts should be made to correct bony angulation or flexibility defects with padding or orthotics, to see if they are beneficial, before performing corrective surgery.

Bunion shields (Fig. 195-16) are also available or may be cut from 1-cm felt. With a bunion shield in place, padding can be placed between the first and second toe to decrease the angle of lateral deviation of the bunion.

NSAIDs may help with pain and inflammation. The use of ice massage in the inflamed area after exercise may be helpful. An inflamed MTP bursa can be drained and reinjected with a steroid. Even if there is no bursitis, injection of corticosteroid into the area of inflammation may be helpful.

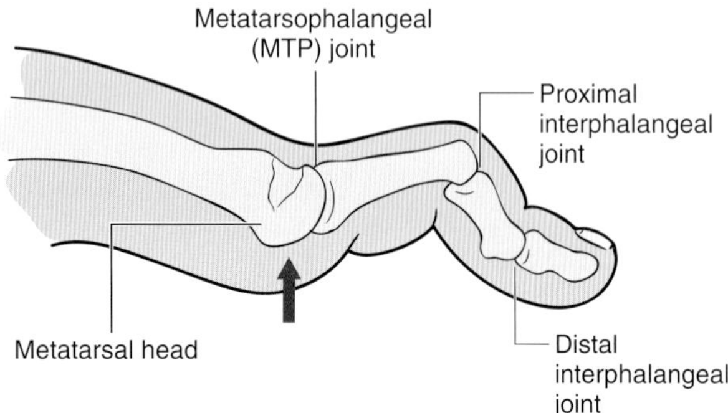

Figure 195-15 Adding padding such as a metatarsal bar may correct the angle of dorsiflexion of the MTP joint by putting pressure on the plantar aspect of the joint.

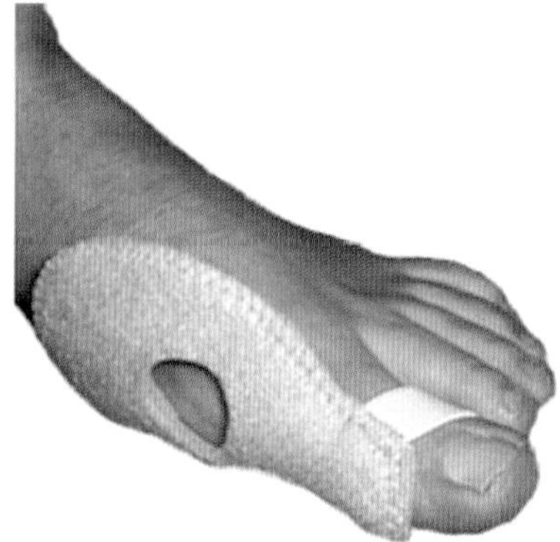

Figure 195-16 Bunion shields are commercially available or can be cut from self-adherent felt.

For those failing local care, surgical options include resection of the phalangeal head (arthroplasty), joint fusion (arthrodesis), removing tissue, or moving tendons in the toe joint. A fixed toe joint deformity usually requires surgery to relieve pain and correct the deformity.

METATARSALGIA, SESAMOIDITIS, AND STIFF TOE (HALLUX RIGIDUS)

Most commonly affecting the most distal portion of the metatarsal bone (i.e., the metatarsal head), metatarsalgia can affect the heads of any of the bones in the ball of the foot; however, it more commonly involves the second and third metatarsals. Frequently, a large callus is noted beneath the MTP joint. The ball of the foot is defined as the area between the arch of the foot and the toes.

Beneath the first metatarsal head are two sesamoid bones whose structure and function are similar to those of the patella. They may become painful as a result of overuse, a stress fracture, osteoarthritis, or chondromalacia. Because they are imbedded in the tendon, there is always an associated tendonitis. Plantar keratomas are frequently seen here, particularly with a plantar flexed first ray associated with high cavus foot deformity.

EDITOR'S NOTE: Anatomically, a "ray" is the digit plus the head and shaft of the respective metatarsal.

The great toe needs about 60 degrees of extension and 30 degrees of flexion for running and jumping sports; lack of flexibility causes discomfort. "Stiff toe," also known as *hallux rigidus*, is usually the result of a gradual process (over years) with a stiff, sore toe progressing to an inflexible first toe and pain even at rest. Although rheumatoid arthritis and gout can affect joint function, hallux rigidus is usually the result of a genetic predisposition combined with osteoarthritis. It can be a chronic, persistent cause of discomfort.

Differential Diagnosis

The location of hyperkeratotic lesions often helps differentiate between the possible causes of foot pain. Because of normal weight bearing, calluses are common under the first (and maybe second) and fifth MTPs; calluses between these locations may indicate other structural abnormalities of the foot or abnormal weight bearing, which may respond to orthotics or surgery.

The patient can often point to the most painful area. Pain beneath the second or third metatarsal heads usually indicates metatarsalgia. Pain beneath the first metatarsal head suggests sesamoiditis. Pain with sesamoiditis is usually gradual in onset; pain due to a stress fracture is usually immediate. A bursa can also form in this area, between the skin and usually the medial sesamoid bone, and result in bursitis. A torn ligament or arthritis of an individual joint can cause similar pain. A radiograph can help distinguish between metatarsalgia and a metatarsal stress fracture, or sesamoiditis and a sesamoid stress fracture. On radiographs, the lateral sesamoid is often bipartite with smooth edges as opposed to jagged edges seen with a fracture. Radiographs of the metatarsal or sesamoid bones may initially be negative; however, serial radiographs taken 2 to 4 weeks later may reveal a fracture.

Techniques

Hyperkeratotic lesions should be débrided or pared. Use of a metatarsal pad placed just proximal to the second or third metatarsal head, under the diaphysis, should alleviate some of the symptoms of metatarsalgia; alternatively, the pad can be placed beneath the first metatarsal to force it to bear more weight (i.e., change the balance). Sesamoiditis also often responds to the use of metatarsal pads or a donut pad (a felt pad cut in the shape of a donut) to change the balance. Orthotics may prevent excessive pronation and decrease strain in the area. For a stiff first toe, early use of a metatarsal pad beneath the MTP joint may take off some of the stress and increase the leverage and range of motion of the first toe, not only decreasing but also possibly slowing the progression of symptoms. Attaching a pad to an ordinary insole of a shoe (or custom orthotic with first ray support, also known as *first ray post*) under the first MTP may also change balance, increase range of motion, and decrease symptoms. NSAIDs may help with pain and inflammation in all of these disorders. The use of ice massage in the inflamed area after exercise may be helpful. Injection of corticosteroid into the area of inflammation or intracapsularly may also be helpful; caution should be observed in young athletes with such an injection to prevent fat pad atrophy and increased capsular laxity.

Postprocedure Patient Education

Care should be taken to fit shoes properly. As a general rule, a proper-fitting shoe is longer and narrower than what most people wear. A Brannock device (Fig. 195-17A) is the most common instrument used for measuring shoe size. It comes in three sizes: men's, women's, and children's. The measurement for the widest part of the shoe should be made just anterior to the first metatarsal head (Fig. 195-17B).

Shoes should also provide proper support, with steel shanks being preferable. It is simple to evaluate the effectiveness of any shank. Grasp the counter (heel) of the shoe with one hand and the toe box with the other hand (Fig. 195-18A), and attempt to twist the shoe. Observe the area of the shank, located between the center of the shoe and the heel; if that area deforms or twists (Fig. 195-18B), it will offer little support. A steel shank in a well-made shoe will result in little or no deformation with twisting.

Patient Education Guide

See the sample patient education handout online at www.expertconsult.com.

CPT/Billing Codes

Orthotics

A4580 Orthotic casting
L3030 Orthotics

Corns (Helomas)

L3030 Prescription orthotics
11055 Paring or cutting of benign hyperkeratotic lesion (e.g., corn or callus), single lesion
11056 Paring or cutting of benign hyperkeratotic lesions (e.g., corn or callus), two to four lesions
11057 Paring or cutting of benign hyperkeratotic lesions (e.g., corn or callus), more than four lesions

Warts (Verrucae Plantaris)

17000 Destruction (e.g., laser surgery, electrosurgery, cryosurgery, chemosurgery, surgical curettement), all benign or premalignant lesions, first lesion
17003 2 to 14 lesions (each)
17004 15 or more lesions (one set fee)

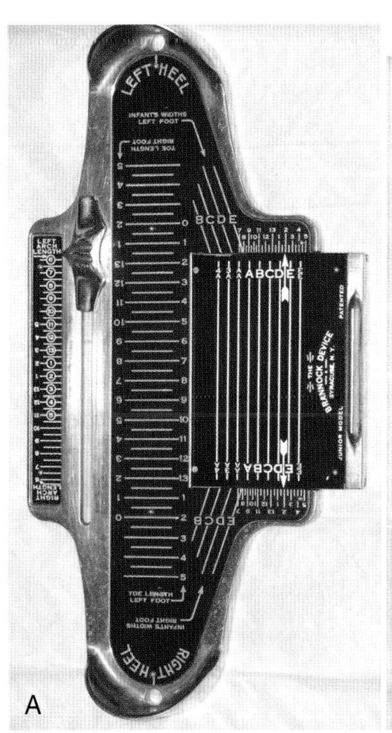

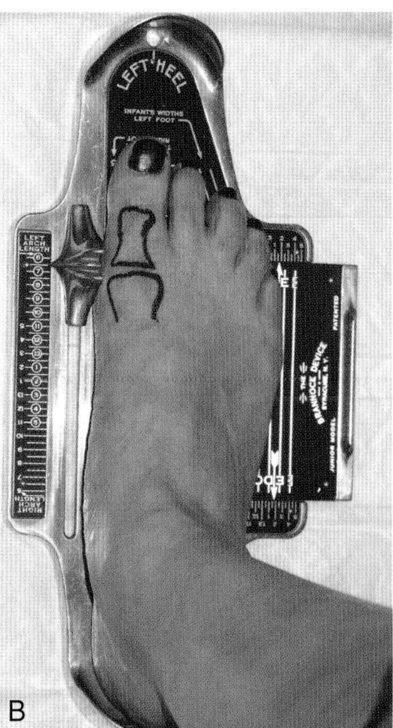

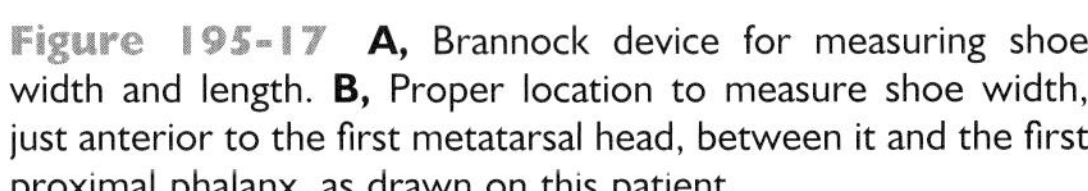
Figure 195-17 **A,** Brannock device for measuring shoe width and length. **B,** Proper location to measure shoe width, just anterior to the first metatarsal head, between it and the first proximal phalanx, as drawn on this patient.

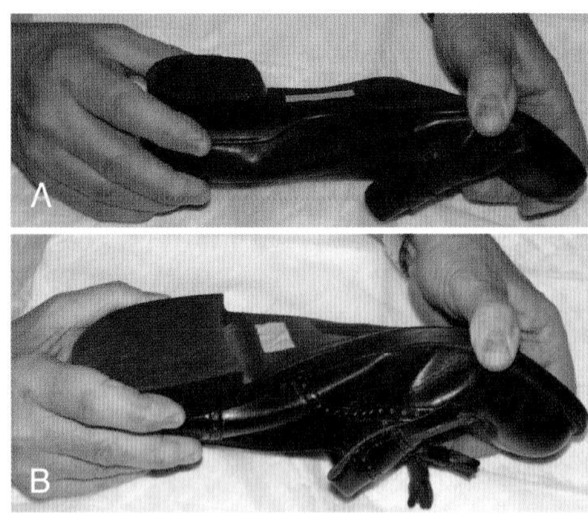

Figure 195-18 **A,** Determine shank stability by grasping counter (heel) and toe box and attempting to twist while observing the center of the shoe. **B,** Ability to twist the shank indicates it will not offer much support.

ICD-9-CM Diagnostic Codes

078.19 Verrucae (plana, plantaris or plantar warts)
355.6 Morton's neuroma
700 Corns and callosities (callus, heloma molle, heloma durum)
713.5 Charcot joint, neuropathic arthritis
715.17 Osteoarthrosis, localized, primary, ankle and foot
715.27 Osteoarthrosis, localized, secondary, ankle and foot
715.37 Osteoarthrosis, localized, not specified whether primary or secondary
716.17 Traumatic arthropathy, ankle and foot
719.47 Pain in joint, ankle and foot
726.73 Calcaneal (heel) spur
727.1 Bunion or bunionette
728.71 Plantar fasciitis
733.95 Stress fracture of other bone
733.99 Sesamoiditis
734 Pes planus (flat feet), acquired
735.0 Hallux valgus (similar to bunion)
735.1 Hallux varus
735.2 Hallux rigidus (inflexible or stiff big toe)
735.4 Hammer toes, acquired
736.73 Pes cavus
754.61 Pes planus, congenital (flat foot, rocker-bottom foot)

Acknowledgment

The editors wish to recognize the many contributions by Joseph Ellis, DPM, and David Snider, DPM, to this chapter in the previous two editions of this text.

Suppliers

(See contact information online at www.expertconsult.com.)

Corn, callus, hammer toe, and bunion supplies (also orthotics)
AliMed, Inc.
Feet Relief
Foot Smart
Moore Medical Corporation (subsidiary of McKesson Medical-Surgical, also supplies surgical instruments)
Myfootshop.com

Foam foot impression system
Smithers Bio-Medical Systems

Orthotics
Langer Biomechanics, Inc. (purchased Benefoot, Inc.)
Three Dimensional Systems, Inc.

ONLINE RESOURCES

American College of Foot and Ankle Surgeons: Offers patient information regarding most of the conditions described in this chapter. Available at www.footphysicians.com.

American Orthopaedic Foot & Ankle Society: Offers patient information regarding most of the conditions described in this chapter. Available at www.aofas.org.

BIBLIOGRAPHY

Banks AS, Downey MS, Martin DE, Miller SJ (eds): McGlamry's Comprehensive Textbook of Foot and Ankle Surgery, 3rd ed. Philadelphia, Lippincott Williams & Wilkins, 2001.

Bedinghaus JM, Niedfeldt MW: Over-the-counter foot remedies. Am Fam Physician 64:791–796, 2001.

Birrer RB, Dellacorte MP, Grisafi PJ: Common Foot Problems in Primary Care. Philadelphia, Hanley & Belfus, 1992.

Cole C, Seto C, Gazewood J: Plantar fasciitis: Evidence-based review of diagnosis and therapy. Am Fam Physician 72:2237–2242, 2005.

Ehrlich M, Nemer JA: Management of select podiatric conditions. In Reichman EF, Simon RR (eds): Emergency Medicine Procedures. New York, McGraw-Hill, 2004, p 1443.

Hawke F, Burns J, Radford JA, du Toit V: Custom-made foot orthoses for the treatment of foot pain. Cochrane Database Syst Rev 3:CD006801, 2008.

Jahss MH (ed): Disorders of the Foot and Ankle, 2nd ed. Philadelphia, WB Saunders, 1991.

Ringold S, Mendoza JA, Tarini BA, Sox C: Is duct tape occlusion therapy as effective as cryotherapy for the treatment of the common wart? Arch Pediatr Adolesc Med 156:975–977, 2002.

Samit MH, Dana AS: Cutaneous Lesions of the Lower Extremities. Philadelphia, JB Lippincott, 1971.

Singh D, Bentley G, Trevino SG: Callosities, corns, and calluses. BMJ 312:1403–1406, 1996.

Stadler TA, Johnson ED, Stephens MB: Clinical inquiries: What is the best treatment for plantar fasciitis? J Fam Pract 52:714–717, 2003.

CHAPTER 196

SHOULDER DISLOCATIONS

Jeffrey V. Smith

Dislocations of the shoulder are quite common. Approximately 50% of shoulder injuries in the emergency department are dislocations. Anterior dislocations are far more common than posterior dislocations. The four types of anterior dislocations account for 96% of all shoulder dislocations.

Of the four types of anterior dislocations, subcoracoid dislocations occur three times more frequently than all the others (subglenoid, subclavicular, and thoracic) combined. This chapter deals only with care of subcoracoid, anterior dislocations. All others should be treated with the assistance of an orthopedic surgeon.

The shoulder is the most flexible joint in the human body; consequently, it is the most unstable and most commonly dislocated joint. It is designed to enable a wide range of motion of the upper extremity, in all directions. To accomplish this feat, the actual bony articulation occupies only a very small part of the overall functional area of the joint. The glenohumeral joint surface and capsule are small sliding structures without significant fixed, ligamentous limitations. The tendons around the joint, making up the rotator cuff (Fig. 196-1), are the structures primarily responsible for the integrity of the joint and its complex function.

When the normal joint capsule and rotator cuff restraints are exceeded, the shoulder moves out of joint. Most frequently the clinician encounters a dislocation in which the humeral head has been pulled out of joint and is then held anteriorly and medially by spasm of the anterior chest wall muscles. This is the subcoracoid, anterior shoulder dislocation, usually occurring when an abducted, extended, and externally rotated upper extremity takes a major jolt. The resulting lever forces the proximal humerus anteriorly out of the glenoid socket. After the humeral head comes to rest under the coracoid process, the patient usually presents to the clinician in extreme pain with a nonfunctional arm. Dislocations may also occur during a seizure.

The patient will have a loss of the normal shoulder contour, with a step-off where the deltoid muscle used to be prominent. Instead, the acromion becomes very prominent. The contour of the humeral head may be noted in the anterior chest wall region. Clinically, a hollow can be appreciated beneath the acromion process, due to the missing humeral head. The arm will frequently be held in a slightly abducted, externally rotated posture. A neurologic deficit, most frequently involving the axillary nerve (provides innervation for shoulder abduction and sensation over the deltoid), may be noted on careful examination. Additional neurovascular compromise may be evident, but it is uncommon with subcoracoid, anterior dislocations.

Radiographs should be obtained; it is important to determine the presence (24% of anterior dislocations) or absence of a fracture before attempting to reduce the shoulder. Obtain standard radiographs of the shoulder. A single anteroposterior (AP) view of the shoulder will usually demonstrate the abnormal location of the humeral head. Another view at roughly 90 degrees will not only confirm the direction of humeral head movement, but help exclude a fracture or posterior dislocation. A lateral transcapular or a "Y"-type view will provide this information; an axillary view (Fig. 196-2) is preferred by some clinicians but it is often difficult to get the patient to move his or her arm into the necessary position. Alternatively, in some obese individuals, a computed tomography (CT) scan may be necessary to determine the direction of the shoulder dislocation and the presence of concomitant fractures.

INDICATIONS

A subcoracoid, anterior shoulder dislocation is the indication for treatment.

CONTRAINDICATIONS

The following findings or conditions should generate an immediate orthopedic consult:

- A shoulder dislocation, other than a subcoracoid, anterior dislocation
- Any fracture dislocation of the shoulder
- Dislocations that are more than a few days old (higher risk of vascular injury, especially in older patients)
- Other fractures of the shoulder, neck, ribs, or upper extremity
- Prior orthopedic surgery for chronic or recurrent shoulder dislocations
- Shoulder dislocations in children (if ossification centers are not fused, there is usually an associated Salter-Harris fracture)

EDITOR'S NOTE: A patient with neurovascular compromise (other than mild axillary nerve sensory defect) due to shoulder dislocation should undergo immediate reduction. Although it is beyond the scope of this book, even inferior or posterior shoulder dislocations should undergo immediate reduction if the distal pulse is compromised. Although immediate orthopedic assistance is optimal, it may not always be possible.

EQUIPMENT AND SUPPLIES

- Stretcher
- Washcloth or small towel
- Soft restraints such as sheets or blankets
- Cloth tape, gauze or elastic bandage, padded wrist restraint or commercially available device for hanging weights from wrist
- Weights (5 to 15 lbs) or bucket (½ to 1 gallon size and adequate tap water or intravenous [IV] fluid)
- Intra-articular anesthetic (10 to 20 mL of 50:50 mixture 1% or 2% lidocaine with sterile saline), antiseptic solution (e.g., chlorhexidine, povidone–iodine), 10- to 20-mL syringe, 25-gauge, 2½-inch needle
- Procedural sedation forms, consent, equipment (see Chapter 2, Procedural Sedation and Analgesia) and medications (e.g., analgesia, muscle relaxant, narcotics, benzodiazepines, reversal agents)
- Shoulder immobilizer or sling and swath

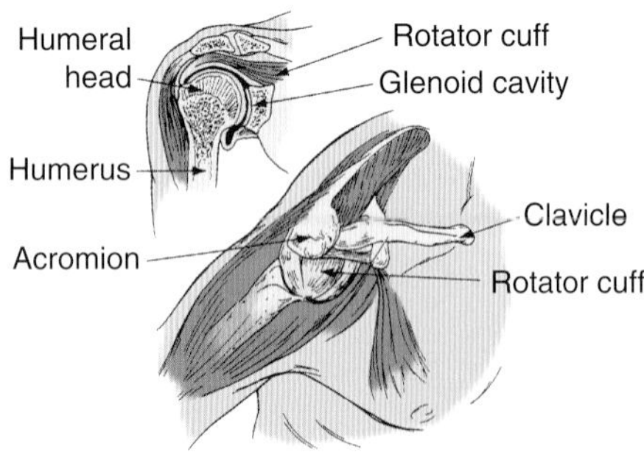

Figure 196-1 Anatomy of the shoulder joint and how the tendons of the muscles (supraspinatus, infraspinatus, subscapularis, and teres minor) form the rotator cuff. Also see Chapter 185, Musculoskeletal Ultrasonography, and Chapter 192, Joint and Soft Tissue Aspiration and Injection (Arthrocentesis).

Preprocedure Patient Preparation

Patients should be informed about the indications for shoulder reduction, as well as any alternatives and possible complications. They should know what to expect and try to relax as much as possible. If a local anesthetic injection will be used, the patient can be reassured that this should decrease the discomfort. Informed consent should be obtained appropriate for the procedure(s) to be performed.

Precautions

To be successful, this procedure takes some time and relaxation—on the part of both the patient and the clinician. The procedure is easy, but trying to rush it may result in an unsuccessful episode. One exception is the dislocation witnessed by the sports medicine clinician; if the dislocation is not associated with high-energy forces, some clinicians will reduce the shoulder immediately, fieldside, without radiographs and before the muscular spasm can occur.

Technique

There are a number of available techniques, all designed to apply gentle and persistent tension on the spasmodic chest wall muscles, to elongate them, and to reestablish the mobility of the humeral head. Once this is done, the humeral head will usually track or be gently manipulated back into the glenoid fossa. The patient is probably best served by the simplest technique, the one that minimizes both operator and patient stress. Typically, this is the Stimson technique, wherein weight loading and time can be used to gently stretch the muscles and reduce the joint. Certainly, this is the least traumatic technique for the shoulder and should help minimize the chances of a fracture developing related to the reduction process.

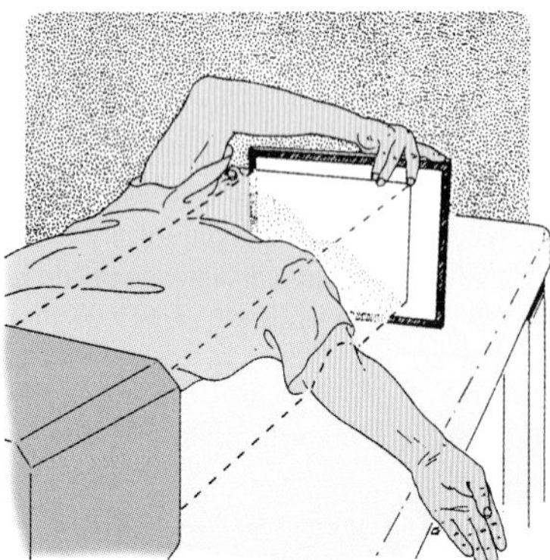

Figure 196-2 Radiographs should include a view at 90 degrees from the anteroposterior view, such as this axillary view. Such a projection helps document the direction (anterior vs. posterior) of the shoulder dislocation.

Other techniques may also be successful. Although many have been described in the literature, all of the listed techniques have been tested and are effective in a situation where the clinician is willing to take his or her time with the reduction. Experience suggests that the clinician should not attempt more than two reduction procedures. If the second attempt is unsuccessful, the resultant muscle spasm will likely prevent closed reduction in a safe manner. Call the orthopedic surgeon if the second attempt is unsuccessful.

Intra-articular Anesthetic

Some experts recommend the injection of intra-articular anesthetic with every shoulder reduction (see also Chapter 192, Joint and Soft Tissue Aspiration and Injection [Arthrocentesis]). It can also be used if procedural sedation is contraindicated.

1. Identify the hollow area where the humeral head used to be located, 2 cm (two fingerbreadths) directly inferior to the lateral border of the now prominent acromion process. Apply antiseptic solution to the skin over this area and allow to dry.
2. Using sterile technique, insert the 25-gauge, 2½-inch needle into this area, perpendicular to the skin, to a depth of 2 cm. Inject 10 to 20 mL of a 50:50 mixture of local anesthetic and sterile saline solution.

Stimson Technique

1. Using this technique, procedural sedation is often unnecessary; some experts use the injected local intra-articular anesthetic. Also, there are reports of a 96% success rate, and there is no need for an assistant. Conversely, the prone position may be impossible to use because of other injuries; procedural sedation is also not recommended because the prone position may interfere with respiration. Procedural sedation is even relatively contraindicated because of the prolonged nature of this technique.
2. The patient is placed in the prone position on a stretcher with the affected arm hanging over the side. A rolled-up washcloth or small towel can be placed beneath the coracoid process and pectoralis major muscle as needed for comfort. The clinician may want to wrap soft restraints (sheets or blankets) around the bed and the patient at the hips to prevent him or her from falling off the stretcher. A weight (usually from 5 to 15 lbs) is affixed to the wrist to provide longitudinal, sustained traction. Wrapping tape, a gauze or elastic bandage, or a padded wrist restraint around the wrist should provide secure fixation of the weight to the limb. Commercial devices are also available for securing and hanging a weight from the wrist. A bucket of water can be used if weights are not available; the disadvantage for the patient is having to hold the bucket for a considerable length of time. IV fluid can be used to gradually increase the traction as the bucket fills up (Fig. 196-3).
3. With time (usually 15 to 30 minutes) and relaxation, the shoulder will usually reduce itself. Occasionally (perhaps after 30 minutes), the clinician will need to facilitate the reduction by grasping the forearm and gently twisting it, externally first and then internally, while the arm is still under traction. Either the patient or clinician may feel a "clunk" as the joint is reduced, and there may be brief fasciculations of the deltoid muscle. However, the reduction may be more subtle; if the patient can touch his or her nose or the opposite shoulder with the index finger of the affected upper extremity, it usually indicates a successful reduction.
4. After the shoulder has been reduced, hold the limb in internal rotation against the abdomen and adduction (humerus against the lateral trunk) with a shoulder immobilizer or sling and swath

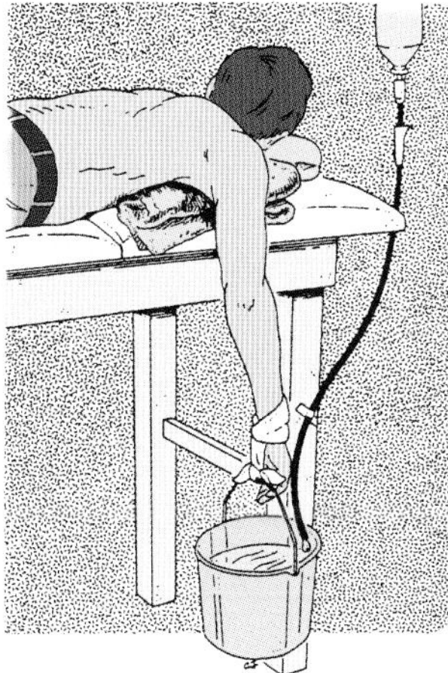

Figure 196-3 Gentle, sustained distal traction can provide an effective means for closed reduction of an anterior dislocation. As the intravenous fluid slowly empties into the bucket, the traction force gradually increases.

device. A careful postreduction neurovascular assessment is required.

5. While keeping the shoulder immobilized, obtain appropriate postreduction radiographs to determine whether adequate reduction of the joint surfaces has been achieved. A congruous-appearing joint without significant distraction (interposed tissue) between the glenoid and the humerus should be noted. Occasionally, comparison shoulder radiographs or a postreduction CT scan may be required. Some recent studies question the value of postreduction imaging, but in most communities it is still the standard of care.

Scapular Manipulation Technique

The patient may or may not require analgesia or injected anesthesia for this technique because there is somewhat less manipulation required (and less chance of injury) than with most other techniques. Using this technique, the glenoid fossa is repositioned rather than just the humeral head. Scapular manipulation may be performed with the patient prone, sitting, or supine. When the patient is prone or supine, traction is applied to the arm by an assistant (or by attached weights if the patient is prone). The shoulder is gently and gradually flexed by an assistant to a 90-degree position, and from 5 to 15 lbs of traction is required. The clinician then uses one hand to rotate the inferior aspect of the scapula upward and medially, and the other hand to rotate the superior aspect laterally (Fig. 196-4). When the patient is sitting, an assistant provides forward traction on the affected arm with countertraction against the head of the humerus to obtain the same 90 degrees of flexion. From behind the patient, the clinician manipulates the scapula as described previously. If reduction does not occur within 1 to 3 minutes, a small degree of dorsal displacement of the inferior scapular tip may be helpful. At this point, slight external rotation of the humerus by an assistant while traction is maintained on the humerus and the scapula is being manipulated may also be helpful. There have never been complications reported from using this technique; however, it is a cumbersome process. Reduction may also be very subtle when accomplished by this technique, without a perceived "clunk." This technique may be used when other injuries limit repositioning the patient.

Hennepin Technique

The Hennepin technique is named after the Hennepin County Emergency Medical Center (Minnesota), where the technique was

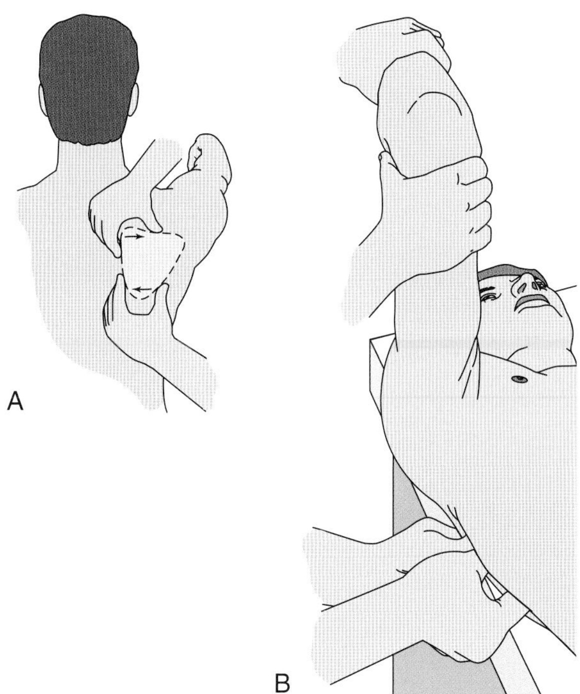

Figure 196-4 Scapular manipulation technique. **A,** An assistant flexes the patient's arm (or if the patient is prone, it can be flexed by gravity and weights, as with the Stimson technique). It must be slowly brought to a 90-degree position. The clinician then rotates the inferior scapular tip upward and medially, and the superior aspect laterally (clockwise on the right shoulder when viewed from back, counterclockwise on the left shoulder). **B,** The same technique with the patient in supine position. With the patient's shoulder and elbow both flexed 90 degrees, and the shoulder adducted, gentle upward pressure is maintained by an assistant while the scapula is manipulated as described.

first described. It is the technique preferred by some authors for anterior shoulder dislocations. There is less manipulation than with most other techniques, a lower probability of neurovascular or musculoskeletal damage, and little or no need for analgesia (although an injection of intra-articular anesthesia may be beneficial). The patient is seated upright, reclining at 45 degrees, or supine. With the clinician stabilizing the patient's elbow joint of the affected arm with one hand, the clinician's other hand is used to grasp the patient's wrist. Slowly (it can take up to 10 minutes to accomplish), the patient's forearm is externally rotated until there is 90 degrees of external rotation (Fig. 196-5). The procedure should be stopped if the patient experiences pain or discomfort, but do not release the arm or allow it to return to its original position. Usually, after allowing the musculature or spasm to relax, the procedure can be continued without analgesia. If pain or discomfort persists, the patient may require analgesia. The reduction usually occurs by the time the forearm has reached 90 degrees of external rotation; if it has not, the arm is slowly elevated. Occasionally, it will need to be elevated to the level that the patient can touch his or her contralateral ear (over the head). If reduction still does not occur, the humeral head is gently manipulated toward the glenoid until it reduces.

Modified Kocher Maneuver

The modified Kocher maneuver is similar to the Hennepin technique. The patient is placed supine with the arm of the affected shoulder over the edge of the gurney, and analgesia or injected anesthesia is provided if necessary. The patient's forearm, with the

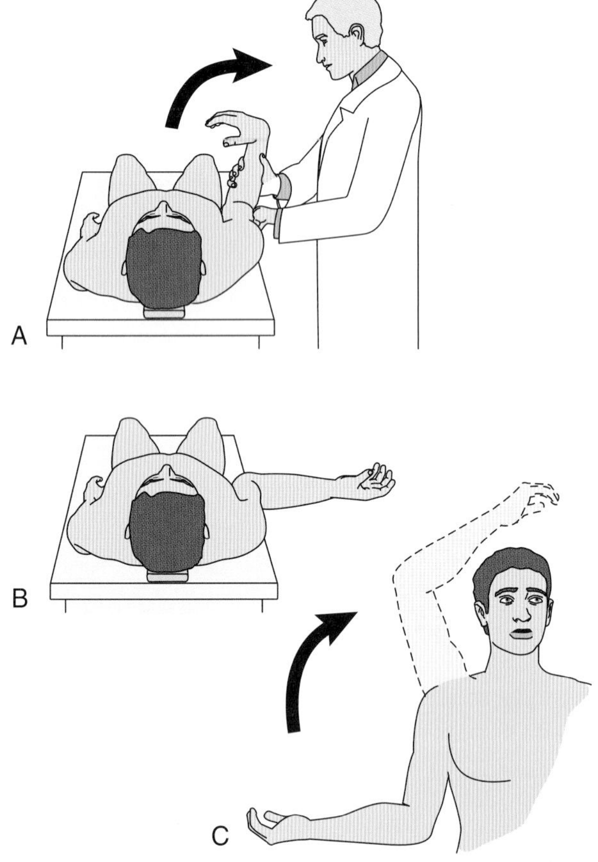

Figure 196-5 Hennepin and modified Kocher techniques. Both techniques start with the elbow flexed to 90 degrees (**A**), and then fully externally rotated (**B**). For the modified Kocher, the forearm is then returned to complete internal rotation while gentle shoulder joint pressure is applied. The Hennepin technique (**C**) is continued from (**B**), if necessary, with elevation of the arm and manipulation of the joint posteriorly until the arm is overhead and the dislocation is reduced.

elbow held at 90 degrees, is then rotated externally (abducting superiorly) over at least a 5-minute period (see Fig. 196-5), with simultaneous gentle downward pressure applied on the dislocation. After the arm reaches 120 degrees of rotation, the arm is brought back to internal rotation, at which time the reduction usually occurs.

Milch Technique

With the patient sitting or supine, the arm is moved to 10 to 20 degrees of forward flexion with slight abduction. One of the clinician's hands is then used to gently guide the patient's arm (grasping at the elbow) in this slightly abducted position and using slight traction, until it is directly overhead (Fig. 196-6). The patient may be able to move the arm without assistance to this position; however, there is usually too much pain and spasm. While this is occurring, the clinician's other hand is placed on the humeral head to prevent it from moving downward. When the arm is located directly overhead, the rotator cuff muscles are all in alignment, and all cross-stresses are eliminated. Using just his or her thumb, the clinician should be able to direct the humeral head superiorly over the rim of the glenoid and into the fossa. Otherwise, abduction of the arm and outward traction at the shoulder are increased and the arm brought through a full, lateral downward arc. Reduction is usually signified by an audible or palpable "clunk."

Fulcrum Technique

With the patient supine or sitting, a firmly rolled towel, sheet, or blanket, 6 to 8 inches in diameter, is placed as a fulcrum within the axilla of the affected shoulder. The distal humerus is used as a lever and is adducted gently, with simultaneous posterolateral manipulation of the humeral head. This technique increases the forces applied; therefore, the risk of complications is increased.

Boss-Holzach-Matter Technique

The patient sits against the maximally raised head of a gurney and wraps his or her forearms around the ipsilateral knee, which is flexed at 90 degrees. The head of the gurney is then lowered. The patient is asked to hyperextend the neck while leaning back and shrugging the shoulders anteriorly. This technique reportedly does not require analgesia.

Hippocratic Technique

Because the Hippocratic technique is no longer recommended, it is included only for historical interest. The clinician places his or her foot against the chest wall to provide countertraction and then manipulates the arm. This technique can cause serious neurovascular trauma.

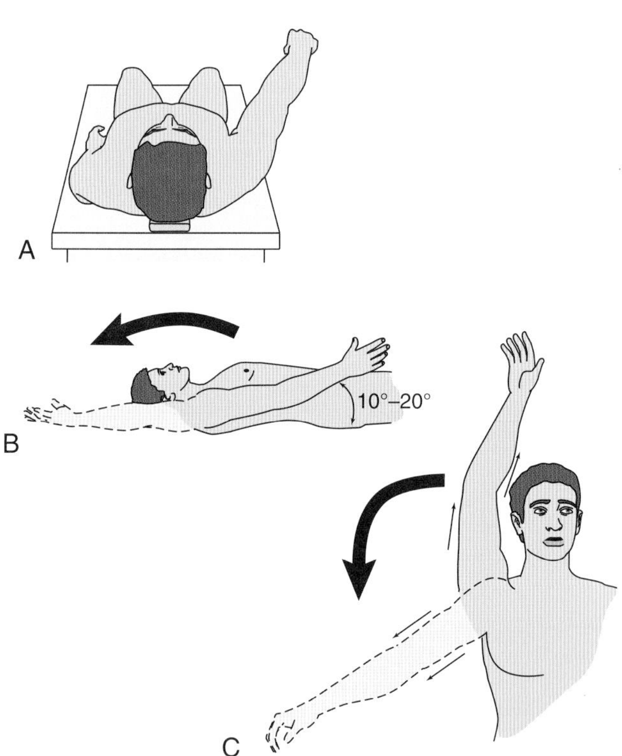

Figure 196-6 Milch technique. **A,** The arm is started at 10 to 20 degrees of flexion and slight abduction. **B,** Elevation continues slowly, with slight distal traction, until the arm is directly overhead. The patient may be able to raise the arm on his or her own. The head of humerus should be held immobile at this stage of maneuver. **C,** If no reduction occurs with gentle, direct manipulation of the head of the humerus, the arm is then slowly brought through a full, lateral downward arc, maintaining constant outward traction until reduction occurs. Note that this is the only step of the procedure in which outward traction is maintained.

COMPLICATIONS

If the shoulder dislocation proves *irreducible*, an orthopedic surgeon should be consulted and the use of general anesthesia considered. *Fracture* (due to the dislocation or reduction [iatrogenic]) and *neurovascular damage* are ever-present risks. Up to 50% of anterior dislocations have a Hill-Sachs deformity, an impaction fracture defect in the posterolateral portion of the humeral head. A Bankart lesion may also be noted, which is an avulsed fragment of the glenoid labrum with contiguous bone. Both lesions tend to get worse the longer the humeral head remains dislocated.

Many clinicians obtain postreduction radiographs to document reduction of the joint, any injury associated with the reduction, and any bony abnormalities such as the aforementioned lesions.

Another risk after a shoulder dislocation is *redislocation*. In patients followed for 10 years, age at initial dislocation was the only predictor of recurrence; duration of subsequent immobilization had no effect. *Rotator cuff tears* and *hemarthrosis* are more common with inferior dislocation and in patients older than 60 years of age. To avoid serious *complications of procedural sedation*, adequate respiratory support measures and monitoring should be present. Patients need to be observed after such sedation to ensure they are awake, alert, and oriented before discharge.

POSTPROCEDURE EDUCATION AND CARE

Patients may need oral analgesic medications, possibly even narcotics, for a few days. Those younger than 20 years of age should be immobilized for 3 weeks, patients aged 20 to 40 years should be immobilized for 1 to 2 weeks, and patients older than 60 years should have less than 1 week of immobilization. Appropriate clinical, neurologic, and radiographic follow-up examinations should be made throughout this time to confirm maintenance of the reduction. After the designated period of immobilization, assign a gentle strengthening program, with particular emphasis on the shoulder internal rotators. Unrestricted external rotation, abduction, and lifting activities are usually not permitted for a period of 3 months. Even combing the hair combines external rotation and abduction and should be avoided indefinitely on the side of dislocation. With recurrent dislocations, an arthrogram, CT arthrogram, magnetic resonance imaging, or arthroscopy might be warranted to help identify an anatomic variant that might make the patient more prone to redislocation. Patients with peripheral neuropathies, syringomyelia, and psychiatric histories may be more prone to dislocating their shoulders, and these underlying conditions should be considered in patients with repeated dislocations.

CPT/BILLING CODES

23650 Closed treatment of shoulder dislocation, with manipulation, without anesthesia
23655 Closed treatment of shoulder dislocation, with manipulation, requiring anesthesia

ICD-9-CM DIAGNOSTIC CODES

718.01 Articular cartilage disorder, shoulder region (old rupture of ligaments)
718.11 Loose body in joint, shoulder region
718.31 Recurrent dislocation of joint, shoulder region
831 Dislocation of shoulder
The following five-digit subclassification is for use with category 831:
- 0 Shoulder, unspecified (humerus NOS)
- 1 Anterior dislocation of humerus
- 2 Posterior dislocation of humerus
- 3 Inferior dislocation of humerus
- 4 Acromioclavicular (joint) (clavicle)
- 9 Other (scapula)

831.0 Closed dislocation
831.1 Open dislocation

ACKNOWLEDGMENT

The editors wish to recognize the many contributions by Fred M. Hankin, MD, and J. Mark Wiedemann, MD, MS, to this chapter in the previous two editions of this text.

BIBLIOGRAPHY

Doyle WL, Ragar T: Use of the scapular manipulation method to reduce an anterior shoulder dislocation in the supine position. Ann Emerg Med 27:92–94, 1996.

Eiff MP, Hatch RL, Calmbach WL: Fracture Management for Primary Care, 2nd ed. Philadelphia, Saunders, 2003.

Roberts JR, Hedges JR (eds): Clinical Procedures in Emergency Medicine, 4th ed. Philadelphia, Saunders, 2004.

Sineff SS, Reichman EF: Shoulder joint dislocation reduction. In Reichman EF, Simon RR (eds): Emergency Medicine Procedures. New York, McGraw-Hill, 2004, pp 593–613.

Stimson LA: An easy method of reducing dislocations of the shoulder and hip. Med Rec 57:356–357, 1900.

Tuggy M, Garcia J: Procedures Consult. Available at www.proceduresconsult.com, and as an application at www.apple.com/iTunes.

CHAPTER 197

Trigger-Point Injection

Ashley Christiani

Myofascial pain is among the most common complaints for which patients seek care. In many cases, there is a defined, reproducible site of tenderness in the affected muscle, called a *trigger point*, that can be targeted for relief of pain and spasm. Trigger points (TrPs) may be effectively treated in the office through the TrP injection technique described here. Understanding TrP pathology and treatment can aid the clinician in addressing one of the most common and debilitating acute complaints encountered in the outpatient setting.

The term *trigger point* was coined by Dr. Janet Travell in 1942 to describe the clinical finding of a painful nodule in an indurated cord or "taut band" of muscle (Fig. 197-1). According to the American College of Rheumatology, TrPs should be painful to palpation with 4 kg of pressure, approximately the point at which the examiner's fingernail would begin to blanch. The taut band of muscle fibers may respond during palpation or needle activation with a local twitch response (LTR). Although the LTR phenomenon is not always visible, when present this response predicts an effective response to TrP injection.

It is thought that any one of the over 600 striated muscles in the human body can develop TrPs, although not all can be accessed by direct palpation. Examples of the most common TrPs are shown in Figure 197-2. TrPs can form in response to an acute event such as a sudden strain placed on an already contracted muscle, or in the context of insidious, repetitive strain. TrPs are commonly classified as "active" or "latent." Active TrPs (Box 197-1) are symptomatic, causing pain, stiffness, decreased range of motion, and referred symptoms such as paresthesias or a disturbance in motor or autonomic function. The pain experienced by patients may be well localized or diffuse, ranging in character from a dull ache to sharp, burning, and debilitating. Motor dysfunction includes muscle weakness and easy fatigability as well as spasm of other muscles in the kinetic chain. Examples of autonomic dysfunction include abnormal sweating, lacrimation, and salivation, pilomotor disturbance, mild edema, imbalance, dizziness, and tinnitus. Palpation of active TrPs typically reproduces the patient's symptoms. Latent TrPs may also cause stiffness and restriction of motion but are generally not noted by the patient to be painful until directly palpated by the examiner or when "unmasked" during the treatment of active TrPs.

Approximately 20% of patients with active TrPs also have fibromyalgia; it is important to differentiate this subset (Table 197-1) because patients with fibromyalgia usually have diffuse pain that may be better managed with systemic regimens and physical therapy as opposed to localized TrP injections. Performing a TrP injection in patients with fibromyalgia may actually worsen the pain. It should be noted that TrPs are frequently located near a bony prominence, moving part, or where a muscle or tissue slides, whereas the tender points associated with fibromyalgia are often located in an area where the tissue is not subject to any local stress.

Trigger-point injection may be performed quickly and effectively in the office setting to treat myofascial pain, producing immediate and often long-term results, especially when combined with complementary therapies such as physical therapy, exercise, massage, "spray and stretch," or ergonomic retraining. TrP injection is thought to work by causing a temporary relaxation of the taut muscle, allowing for improved local perfusion, replenishment of the adenosine triphosphate (ATP) required to release actin–myosin chains, and clearance of noxious metabolites. In turn, this breaks the pain–tension cycle. Studies have demonstrated that it is the mechanical stimulation of the TrP by the needle that releases the muscle spasm, whereas the substance injected provides only adjuvant therapy. Response rates are similar regardless of the substance injected; whether it is saline, a steroid, a local anesthetic, or a paralytic agent such as botulinum toxin injected, none has proven to be more effective than "dry needling" alone. However, the latter two substances may produce longer-lasting results because of caustic damage to the muscle. Injection of local anesthetic offers the additional benefit of significantly reducing postprocedure pain compared with saline or dry needling, without adding undue risk to the procedure. Most authorities recommend the use of 0.25% to 1% lidocaine without epinephrine or 2% procaine diluted to 0.5% for TrP injections. We recommend against the use of steroids for TrP injection.

Indication

Focal tender area identifiable by palpation without other identifiable neurologic or musculoskeletal findings or pathology is the indication for treatment. The tender area should be accessible by needle without significant risk.

Contraindications

Absolute

- TrP not safely accessible by needle
- Cellulitis or other loss of skin integrity in area overlying TrP

Relative

- Poorly controlled psychiatric disorder
- Resuscitation equipment not available
- Poorly controlled systemic illness that may compromise healing or predispose to infection
- Bleeding disorder, including anticoagulant use
- Severe fibromyalgia or presence of numerous TrPs
- History of keloid formation
- Highly anxious or needle-phobic patient

Preprocedure Patient Preparation and Evaluation

History and Physical Examination

Screening should include any history of trauma, fibromyalgia, collagen vascular disease, inflammatory condition, bleeding disorder,

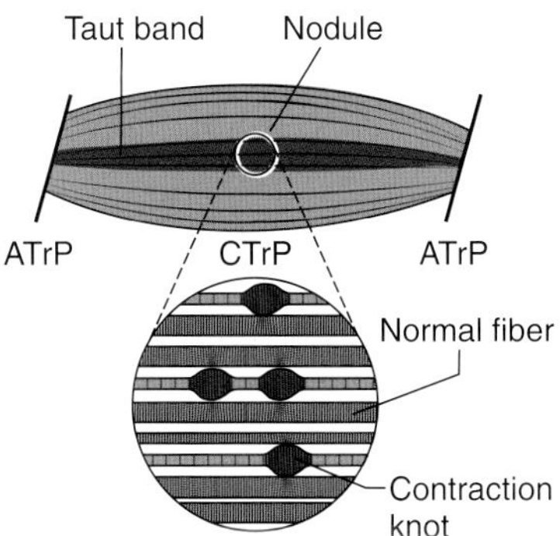

Figure 197-1 Trigger point complex in muscle. ATrP, attachment trigger point; CTrP, central trigger point. (From Simons DG, Travell JG, Simons LS: Travell & Simons' Myofascial Pain and Dysfunction: The Trigger Point Manual, 2nd ed. Philadelphia, Lippincott Williams & Wilkins, 1999.)

Box 197-1. Diagnostic Criteria for Active Trigger Points

- Pain recognition (patient identifies pain at the TrP as the pain he or she has been experiencing)
- Presence of an exquisitely tender nodule in a palpable taut band
- Referral of pain or symptoms in predictable pattern on palpation
- Painful limitation of range of motion

Helpful if Present

- Local twitch response observed when TrP is stimulated
- Associated autonomic responses triggered with palpation of TrP
- Electromyographic demonstration of spontaneous electrical activity in region of tender nodule in the taut band

TrP, trigger point.

hypothyroidism, diabetes, hepatitis C (often associated with generalized myalgia), and any other systemic diseases or chronic conditions. The physical examination should include evaluation of the affected musculature and any associated musculature innervated by the same spinal segment to identify active and latent TrPs and to assess for other potential causes of pain. Significant muscle atrophy or sensory deficit is not commonly seen in isolated TrP phenomena and should alert the clinician to other etiologies. Tender musculature should be palpated slowly and deliberately for taut bands and tender nodules with the muscle in a relaxed position. TrPs are commonly found in the mid-belly of the muscle where contraction is most acute, but the entire muscle from origin to insertion should be examined. Muscles that can be accessed in only one plane can be explored by flat palpation (Fig. 197-3), whereas those that can be partially enclosed in the fingers can be examined with the pincer grasp (Fig. 197-4). As discussed previously, palpation of an active TrP generally elicits wincing or involuntary guarding by the patient and may generate an LTR. The history and physical examination should also include investigation of mechanical etiologies and risk factors for development of recurrent TrPs such as leg length discrepancy, scoliosis, poor posture and body mechanics, or chronic trauma caused by carrying heavy items such as handbags, work equipment, or infants or young children. Behavior modification and physical therapy may help prevent further injury in these cases.

Informed Consent

Provide the patient with a detailed explanation about the procedure and its potential risks, benefits, and alternatives (specific to the condition being treated), and obtain informed consent. If multiple

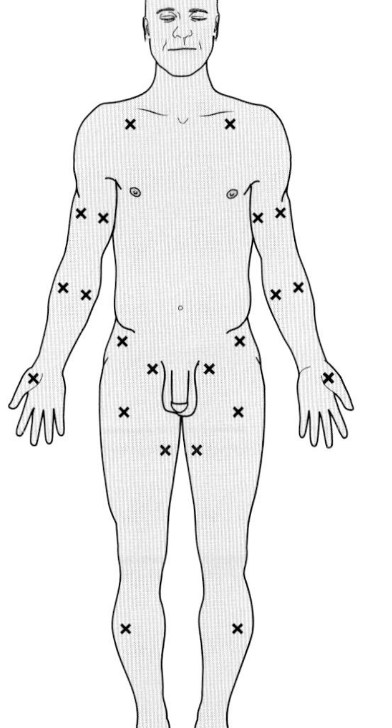
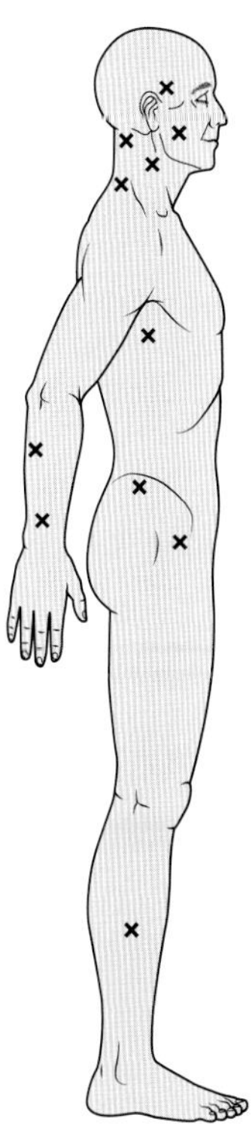
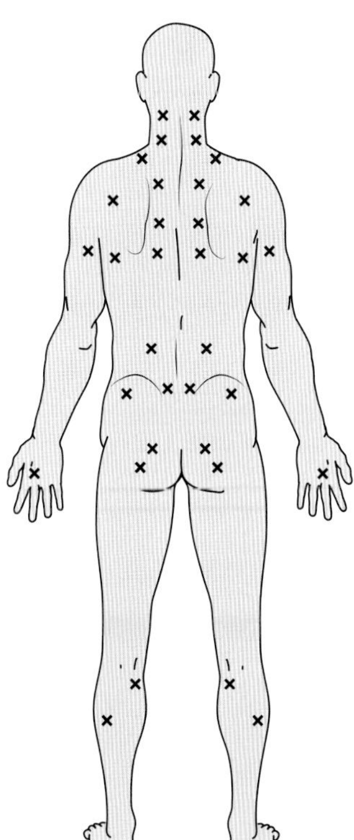

Figure 197-2 Anterior, lateral, and posterior views of common trigger points. (From Simons DG, Travell JG, Simons LS: Travell & Simons' Myofascial Pain and Dysfunction: The Trigger Point Manual, 2nd ed. Philadelphia, Lippincott Williams & Wilkins, 1999.)

TABLE 197-1 Myofascial Pain due to Trigger Points versus Fibromyalgia

Myofascial Pain Due to Trigger Points	Fibromyalgia
Male–female ratio 1 : 1	Male–female ratio ranges from 1 : 4 to 1 : 9
Local or regional pain and tenderness	Generalized or widespread pain* and tenderness
Taut muscle bands	Soft muscles
Muscle stiffness and decreased range of motion	Normal to hypermobile muscles and joints
"Trigger points"	Eleven of 18 "tender points"†
Immediate response to TrP injection	Poor or delayed response to TrP injection
Approximately 20% also have fibromyalgia	Approximately 70% also have active TrPs

TrP, trigger point.

*Widespread pain denotes pain that is bilateral and involving both the upper and lower body. Widespread pain must have been present for 3 months.

†Pain in at least 11 of the 18 specific tender points must be present. These tender points (bilateral) include the *occiput* (at suboccipital insertion), *lower cervical spine* (C5–C7 levels), *trapezius* (midpoint of upper border), *supraspinatus* (above scapular spine near medial border), *second rib* (at second costochondral junction), *lateral epicondyle* (2 cm distal to the epicondyle), *gluteus* (upper, outer quadrants of buttocks), *greater trochanter* (posterior to the trochanteric prominence), and *knee* (at the medial fat pad proximal to joint line).

Adapted from Simons DG, Travell JG, Simons LS: Travell & Simons' Myofascial Pain and Dysfunction: The Trigger Point Manual, 2nd ed. Philadelphia, Lippincott Williams & Wilkins, 1999.

TrPs are present on examination, they are generally best treated on the same visit unless they are too numerous (in which case other treatment modalities may be preferable). Explain to the patient that the relief resulting from the treatment can be followed by pain greater than the original pain either in the same location or as an "unmasking" effect with pain in other untreated muscle groups, and that follow-up injections may be appropriate.

Patient Preparation

If not medically contraindicated, it may be advisable to discontinue aspirin or other anticoagulants at least 3 days before the procedure to minimize bleeding. Patients who are anxious may benefit from pretreatment with a mild oral anxiolytic. In preparation for the procedure, the patient should generally be supine with pillows provided for rotational support, as needed, to minimize risk of vasovagal response.

EQUIPMENT

- Alcohol wipes.
- Gloves (nonsterile).
- Several gauze pads and Band-Aids.
- Ball-point pen (with retracted nib) or skin marker.
- Lidocaine (0.25% to 1% *without* epinephrine), procaine (2% diluted to 0.5%), or bupivacaine (0.125% to 0.25%).
- Sodium bicarbonate 5% to 8.4% solution, for injection, available in 50-mL bottles with 50 mEq/50 mL, may be added as a buffer to local anesthetic. Add 1 mL per 10 mL of anesthetic.
- 25- to 27-gauge needle, depending on site to be injected. A 27-gauge, 1½-inch needle is usually sufficient for the upper torso; a 25-gauge, 3½-inch spinal needle may be required for large back or leg muscles.

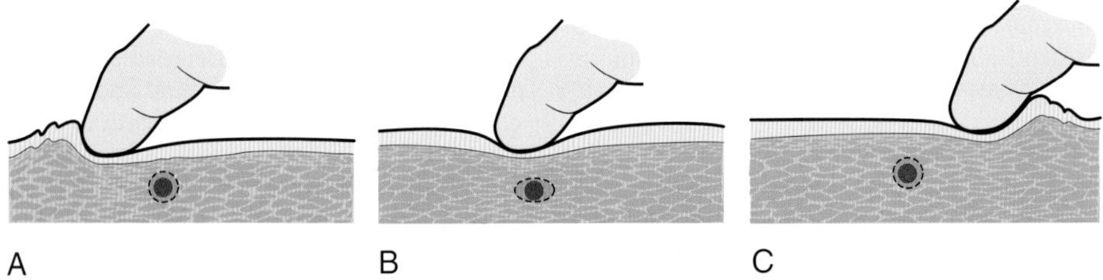

Figure 197-3 Flat palpation technique. **A,** Index finger pushes skin to one side. **B,** Fingertip sweeps across the muscle to feel the taut band rolling beneath. **C,** The skin is pushed to the other side, completing the movement. (From Simons DG, Travell JG, Simons LS: Travell & Simons' Myofascial Pain and Dysfunction: The Trigger Point Manual, 2nd ed. Philadelphia, Lippincott Williams & Wilkins, 1999.)

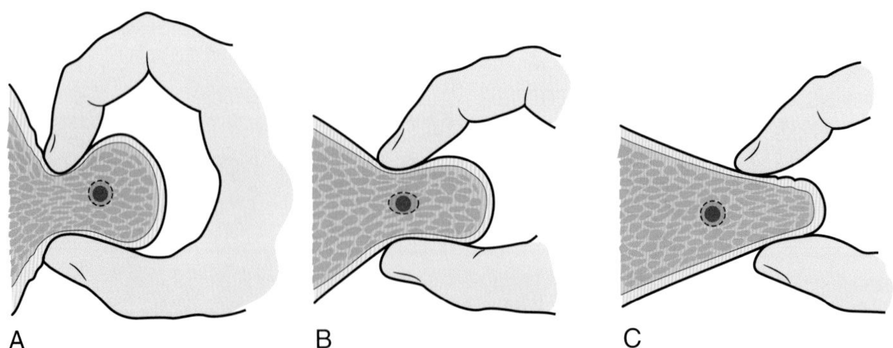

Figure 197-4 Pincer grasp technique. **A,** Muscles that are accessible from two sides may be gripped between the thumb and fingers. **B,** The taut band may be felt as it is rolled between the digits. **C,** The edge of the taut band is palpable as it rolls beneath the fingertips, often inciting a local twitch response. (From Simons DG, Travell JG, Simons LS: Travell & Simons' Myofascial Pain and Dysfunction: The Trigger Point Manual, 2nd ed. Philadelphia, Lippincott Williams & Wilkins, 1999.)

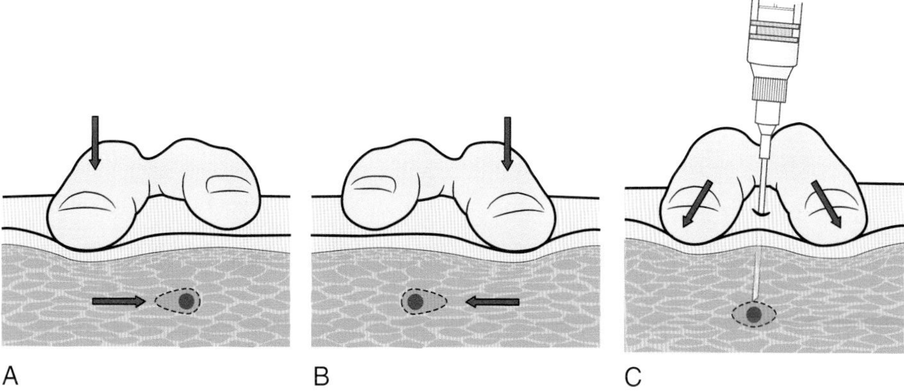

Figure 197-5 Localizing and securing a trigger point (TrP) for injection. **A** and **B,** The use of alternating pressure helps to precisely localize the TrP. **C,** The TrP is held in place with downward pressure and gentle traction to keep it from sliding away from the needle. (From Simons DG, Travell JG, Simons LS: Travell & Simons' Myofascial Pain and Dysfunction: The Trigger Point Manual, 2nd ed. Philadelphia, Lippincott Williams & Wilkins, 1999.)

- 3-, 5-, or 10-mL syringes.
- Resuscitation equipment (as with any injection).
- Pillows *(optional)*.
- Vapocoolant spray such as ethyl chloride for topical anesthesia *(optional)*.

Technique

1. Place the patient in a comfortable or recumbent position to protect the patient in the event of a vasovagal reaction.
2. Identify and mark the TrP.
3. Using an 18-gauge needle, draw up 5 to 10 mL of 1% lidocaine, 0.5% procaine, or 0.125% to 0.25% bupivacaine into the syringe. If desired, sodium bicarbonate solution may be added in a 1 : 10 ratio by volume.
4. Replace the needle with a 25- to 27-gauge needle as appropriate for TrP depth and muscle thickness.
5. Prepare the skin with an antiseptic solution or alcohol.
6. Reidentify the TrP with gloved hands, observing aseptic technique. The TrP should be stabilized between the fingers of the nondominant hand with downward pressure and slight tension on the skin surface (Fig. 197-5).
7. If superficial anesthesia is desired, 0.25 to 0.50 mL of local anesthetic may be injected into the skin to produce a wheal or a vapocoolant spray such as ethyl chloride may be applied to the site while maintaining stabilization of the TrP.
8. Slowly advance the needle perpendicular to the skin toward the TrP. Avoid infiltrating anesthetic until the needle is fully advanced into the target. A slight resistance should be felt on reaching the fascial plane of the muscle, at which point it is helpful to pause and inject 0.2 mL of solution. A gentle "pop" may be felt as the needle is advanced into the muscle itself. Once the needle is in the TrP site, observe for LTRs and aspirate to confirm a nonvascular position.
9. Inject 0.1 to 0.2 mL of solution once the TrP is located. Withdraw the needle slightly and reinject the site several times in a fanlike pattern, injecting as the needle is withdrawn (Fig. 197-6). No more than 2 mL should be injected into any particular muscle region. The patient will usually experience immediate relief if the injection is properly located.
10. Remove the needle and wipe the skin clean with a disinfectant.
11. After withdrawing the needle, massage the entire area to diffuse the anesthetic and check for pain relief. Put the affected muscle complex through full range of motion.

Complications

- Vasovagal symptoms or syncope.
- Skin infection.
- Injury to nerves, vasculature, or other nearby structures.
- Rebound pain.
- Reactions to the local anesthetic or steroid.
- Hematoma formation, bleeding, compartment syndrome.
- Pneumothorax *(rare)*. Special care should be observed when injecting muscles of the thorax. Use pincer grasp when possible. Carefully select appropriate needle length. Use a tangential (instead of vertical) vector for the needle. It may be helpful to have the patient hold his or her breath during injection.

Postprocedure Care

Active TrPs are generally treated with a series of injections over the course of days to weeks. Injections may be repeated as frequently as every 3 to 4 days. Temporary discomfort due to the injection itself may be treated with cold compresses or oral anti-inflammatory drugs. Patients should be instructed to report any redness, pus, streaking,

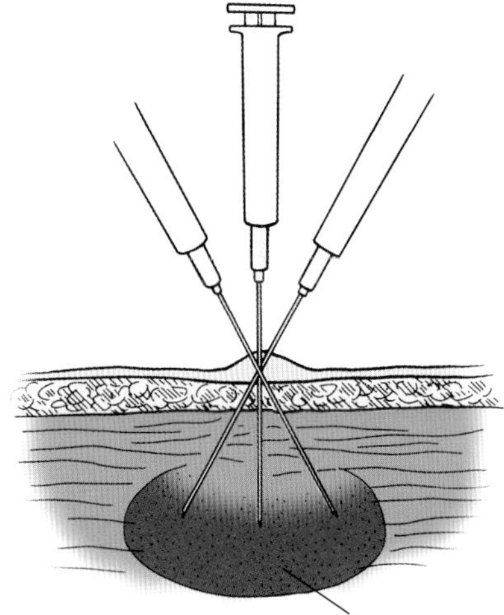

Figure 197-6 Injection of a trigger point.

increased pain, or other concerns. Activity modification and ergonomic retraining may help to avoid reinjury.

Patient Education Guide

See the sample patient consent form available online at www.expertconsult.com.

CPT/Billing Codes

20552 Injection; single or multiple trigger point(s), one or two muscle(s)

20553 Injection; single or multiple trigger point(s), three or more muscles

NOTE: These codes are per session not per injection.

ICD-9-CM Diagnostic Codes

723.1 Cervicalgia

723.9 Unspecified musculoskeletal disorders and symptoms referable to neck

724.1 Pain in thoracic spine

724.2 Lumbago

726.19 Other specified disorders (of rotator cuff syndrome of shoulder)

729.1 Myalgia and myositis, unspecified

Acknowledgment

The editors wish to recognize the contributions by Gary Ruoff, MD, to this chapter in the previous two editions of this text.

Bibliography

Christiani AK, Wallis D: Trigger point injection. In Pfenninger JL (ed): The Clinics Atlas of Office Procedures: Joint Injection Techniques. Philadelphia, Saunders, 2002.

Clauw DJ: Fibromyalgia. In Ruddy S, Harris ED, Sledge CB, et al (eds): Kelley's Textbook of Rheumatology, 6th ed. Philadelphia, WB Saunders, 2001, pp 417–428.

Hong CZ, Hsueh TC: Difference in pain relief after trigger point injections in myofascial pain patients with and without fibromyalgia. Arch Phys Med Rehabil 77:1161–1166, 1996.

Simons DG, Travell JG, Simons LS: Travell & Simons' Myofascial Pain and Dysfunction: The Trigger Point Manual, 2nd ed. Philadelphia, Lippincott Williams & Wilkins, 1999.

Sola AE: Trigger point therapy. In Roberts JR, Hedges JR (eds): Clinical Procedures in Emergency Medicine. Philadelphia, WB Saunders, 1985, pp 674–686.

Tough EA, White AR, Richards S, Campbell J: Variability of criteria used to diagnose myofascial trigger point pain syndrome: Evidence from a review of the literature. Clin J Pain 23:278–286, 2007.

Tuggy M, Garcia J: Procedures Consult. Available at www.proceduresconsult.com, and as an application at www.apple.com/iTunes.

SECTION 13

Hospitalist

Section Editor: JOE ESHERICK

CHAPTER 198

Intraosseous Vascular Access

Raymond F. Jarris, Jr. • Grant C. Fowler

One of the most frustrating and difficult challenges faced by a clinician is the establishment of vascular access in the critically ill patient. Establishment of peripheral intravenous (IV) access is often difficult in the patient who is in shock or cardiac arrest, and is notoriously difficult in the small pediatric patient. For children younger than 5 years of age, thin bones and a vascular marrow make intraosseous vascular access (IOVA) a fairly simple alternative. For years, plain hypodermic needles, spinal needles, or bone marrow aspiration needles (e.g., Jamshidi) were used for IOVA. Eventually, special IOVA needles with a handle and a screw tip were developed. Later models were developed with flanges to better secure them to the patient with tape after insertion. Recently, kits combining IOVA needles with either a small, portable, battery-powered drill or a spring-loaded disposable needle gun have increased the use of this technique in adults. In fact, many hospitalists now use IOVA in adults more often than in children. Using IOVA, after the needle traverses the cortex, the venous plexus in the marrow cavity (Fig. 198-1) functions as a rigid "vein" or conduit for fluid; it does not collapse with hypovolemia or even shock. This procedure is now so successful that many national and international organizations have recommended its use as the primary or secondary method of obtaining and maintaining vascular access in the critically ill patient. Use of IOVA is also increasingly common and accepted as an alternative to a central line for short-term infusions in nonemergent situations.

IOVA was originally described in the 1920s. However, with the introduction of plastic catheters and improved peripheral IV access skills, the need and interest for IOVA diminished. In the 1980s, IOVA saw a resurgence in use as a rapid method for vascular access in pediatric shock emergencies. It was also studied for use with regional anesthesia in Europe. IOVA has now been studied and proven to be a safe, reliable, and rapid temporary method for vascular access in adult shock emergencies, especially compared with percutaneous IV access. The American Heart Association, the American Academy of Pediatrics, and the American College of Surgeons recommend vascular access by IOVA in emergency situations when venous access is not immediately possible. Any medication or fluid that can be given IV can also be administered by IOVA. After a 5- to 10-mL flush with normal saline, medications are immediately absorbed into the systemic circulation; drug concentrations and onset of action match those given through a central venous line during cardiopulmonary resuscitation (CPR). In addition to serving as a route for fluid administration, the IOVA needle may be used for obtaining blood type, cross-matching, and blood chemistry determinations from the marrow cavity. Serum electrolyte, blood urea nitrogen, creatinine, glucose, and calcium levels are very similar to those in samples obtained from an IOVA aspirate.

One disadvantage of IOVA is the temporary nature of the procedure (it should not be used for more than 24 to 48 hours). Another, disadvantage is that infusion rates may be limited; however, rates can also reach more than 150 mL/min with a 16-gauge needle and a pressure infusor bag (blood pressure cuff inflated to 300 mm Hg around the IV fluid bag), an infusion pump, or with forceful manual pressure. The rate-limiting factor is usually the size of the marrow cavity. IOVA also is not universally successful; however, in the past, success rates were limited in older children and adults because needles often bent when attempting to penetrate thicker bones. Success rates have improved since the development of kits specially designed for this procedure.

One retrospective study of pediatric cardiopulmonary arrest patients revealed that, although the time to obtain peripheral IV was occasionally minimal, the average time was a disappointing 7.9 ± 4.2 minutes. The overall peripheral IV success rate was only 17%. Of all techniques used, the success rate was highest with IOVA (83%), next most successful was surgical cutdown (81%), and central venous line placement (CVP; 77%) came in third. The average time required to establish vascular access was 4.7 minutes for IOVA (using older equipment not specially designed for this procedure), followed by 8.4 minutes for CVP, in turn followed by 12.7 minutes for venous cutdown. Using newer kits specially designed for IOVA, the success rate has significantly improved over the prior 83%.

In the cardiopulmonary arrest situation, it is reasonable to use IOVA as the initial approach for vascular access because of the high success rate and the rapidity of the procedure. In fact, all providers of emergency care (including hospitalists) should be familiar with IOVA because in certain situations it may be the only available means of obtaining vascular access. It should be noted that since the last edition of this textbook was published (2003), this procedure has been moved from the Pediatrics section to the Hospitalist section; again, many hospitalists use IOVA in adults more often than in children. To learn the procedure or to maintain skills for IOVA, clinicians can practice on cadavers, raw chicken drumsticks, swine ribs, or piglet tibias. Mannequins are also available for practice from the manufacturers of the special IOVA kits.

The proximal tibia (Fig. 198-2), just below the growth plate, is the preferred site for IOVA for children younger than 5 years of age. At this level, the tibial tuberosity is a broad, flat surface close to the skin and there are few intervening muscles, nerves, and blood vessels; therefore, bony landmarks are easily recognized.

Recently, IOVA kits with either a battery-operated drill (EZ-IO; Vidacare, Dallas) or a spring-loaded needle gun (Bone Injection Gun [BIG]; WaisMed, Houston) have been demonstrated to be effective for use in the proximal humerus; having vascular access above the diaphragm during CPR is considered important by many clinicians. The distal tibia (Fig. 198-3), just above the medial malleolus, the lateral or medial malleolus, the distal radius, ulna, or femur (Fig. 198-4), the anterior-superior iliac spine, and the sternum are alternate sites for IOVA. Whereas the distal tibia is a good choice because the bone and tissues are thin, the distal femur is covered with muscles and fat, often making palpation of bony landmarks difficult. The distal femur should probably be reserved for those cases in which other sites cannot be used. The sternum and ilium are seldom used in children because the width of the marrow

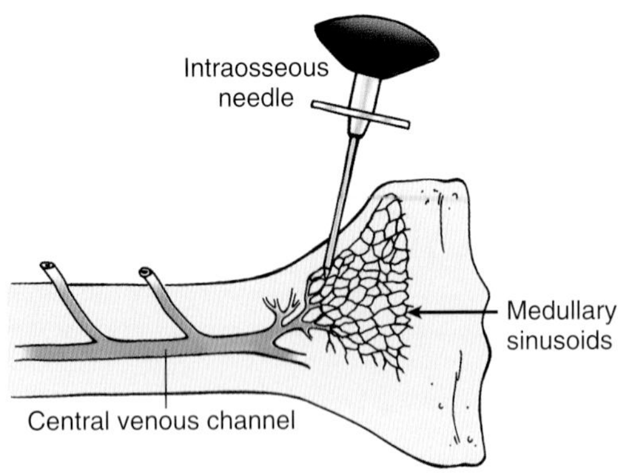

Figure 198-1 Intramedullary venous system. With intraosseous venous access, the marrow cavity functions as a "vein" that will not collapse.

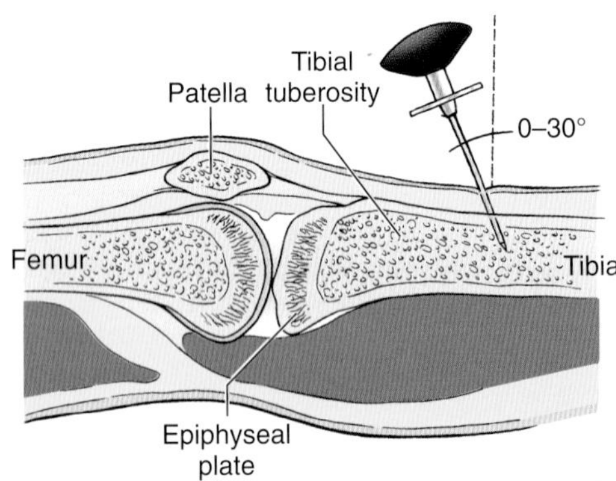

Figure 198-2 Proximal tibial needle insertion.

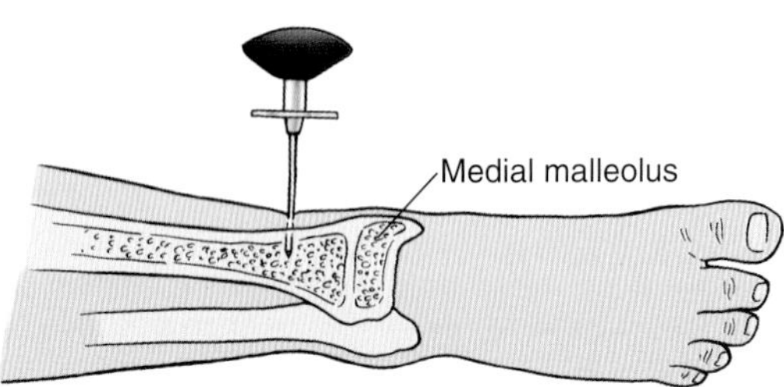

Figure 198-3 Distal tibial needle insertion.

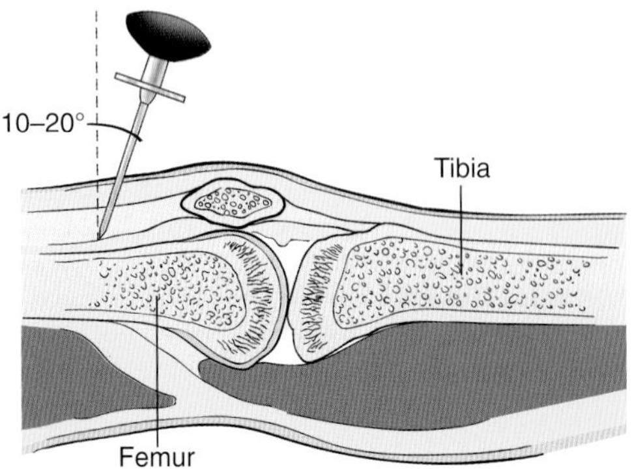

Figure 198-4 Distal femoral needle insertion.

space is inadequate if younger than 3 years of age, and insertion may be technically difficult and dangerous. In children and adults, the sternal site carries a risk of mediastinal puncture.

INDICATIONS

- As an alternative to a central line for short-term infusions
- Any emergency condition that requires immediate vascular access (IOVA can often be achieved in 30 to 60 seconds)
- When IV access cannot be achieved (e.g., small veins, venofibrosis, edema, obesity; also for regional anesthesia when the distal extremity is injured)

NOTE: When a large-volume infusion is needed very rapidly, bilateral IOVA may be necessary as well as the use of a pressure infusor bag, an infusion pump, a large syringe, or forceful manual pressure.

- IOVA is preferred over the endotracheal route for medication administration (certain fluids or medications can be given *only* by IV or IOVA route, and *not* through an endotracheal tube; e.g., blood, sodium bicarbonate, dextrose)

CONTRAINDICATIONS

Contraindications to IOVA are few and are all relative, especially because this is a very temporary, and occasionally a life-saving, procedure. However, the risks and benefits of the procedure should be considered.

- Ipsilateral fracture or crush injury of an extremity (increases the risk of subcutaneous extravasation, so another extremity should be used)
- Previous orthopedic procedure near the selected insertion site
- Previous IOVA attempts in the same bone (even if IOVA was obtained, fluid would leak out of the previously attempted site)
- Infection at the selected insertion site
- Inability to locate landmarks (e.g., excessive tissue over the insertion site)
- Brittle bones (e.g., osteogenesis imperfecta or anything increasing risk of fracture)

EQUIPMENT

- Disposable rigid needle, 16- to 20-gauge, preferably with stylet and designed as an intraosseous needle. Options include kits with a small, portable battery-powered drill, intraosseous needle, and integrated stylet that doubles as a drill bit (EZ-IO AD for patients ≥40 kg, EZ-IO PD for patients >6 kg, <40 kg; Fig. 198-5A) or a spring-loaded needle, disposable bone injection gun (BIG Adult or BIG Pedi; Fig. 198-5B), or a disposable needle with a built-in handle (Fig. 198-5C). If none of these is available, spinal needles (with a stylet) or bone marrow aspiration needles (e.g., Jamshidi) have been used to perform this procedure in children for years.
- Sterile latex gloves.
- Goggles.
- Sterile drapes.
- Antiseptic solution (povidone–iodine, chlorhexidine, or alcohol).
- Two 10-mL syringes for aspirating medullary contents and flushing with normal saline.
- 2 × 2 gauze pads.
- 4 × 4 gauze pads.
- Tape.
- IV solution (isotonic crystalloid or colloid), tubing, and pressure infusor bag (can use a blood pressure cuff) or infusion pump (large syringes can also be used for boluses).
- Extremity or torso restraints for the uncooperative patient.
- Plastic or Styrofoam cup.

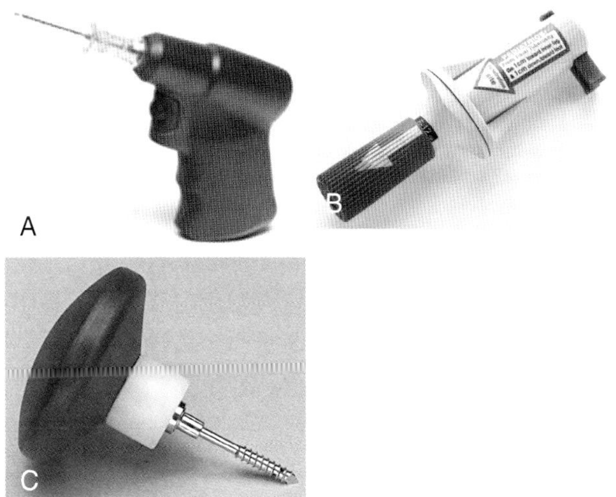

Figure 198-5 **A,** Intraosseous needle, drill bit stylet, battery-operated drill (EZ-IO). **B,** Spring-loaded needle gun (Bone Injection Gun [BIG]). **C,** Intraosseous vascular access needle with handle. (**A,** Courtesy of Vidacare, Dallas, TX. **B,** Courtesy of WaisMed, Houston, TX. **C,** Courtesy of Cook Critical Care, Bloomington, Ind.)

- In the alert patient, 2% lidocaine without preservatives (cardiac lidocaine) without epinephrine and a 10-mL syringe
- In the alert patient *(optional)*, 1% or 2% lidocaine for local anesthetic and a 3- or 5-mL syringe with a 25- or 27-gauge, ⅝-inch (1.6-cm) needle.

Preprocedure Patient Education

In most cases, IOVA is performed emergently. When time allows, the indications should be documented and explained to the parent or other relative, if present. If performed electively, the indications, alternatives, benefits, and risks should be explained to the patient or parent, and signed informed consent should be obtained.

Technique

NOTE: The following techniques and angles are for the standard IOVA needle. The battery-powered drill or bone injection gun is used most often at the proximal tibial site in adults and children and at the proximal humeral site in adults. The battery-powered drill is also used at the distal tibial site. The battery-powered drill and bone injection gun should be held perpendicular to the bone during insertion of the needle.

The operator should be familiar with the particular device available for IOVA and review the device specific protocol prior to use because the application of each device may vary slightly.

1. If an extremity is the chosen site, place a small sandbag beneath it. An assistant or restraint may be useful for an infant or a confused patient. *If an extremity is the desired site, everyone should avoid placing a hand behind the extremity in case of through-and-through bone penetration.*
2. Prepare the skin with antiseptic solution and drape the area. Follow universal blood and body fluid precautions.
3. Administer local anesthetic down to the periosteum (this is optional; it may not be necessary for patients with an altered mental status).
4. To avoid through-and-through bony penetration, hold your index finger approximately 1 cm from the needle tip and avoid pushing past this mark. This step is not necessary if using a kit with a battery-operated drill or spring-loaded bone injection gun.
5. Perform the procedure according to the selected insertion site:
   - Proximal tibia
     - Palpate the tibial tuberosity with your finger (it is the most prominent point on the tibia, noted immediately distal to the patella). In children, select a site approximately one or two fingerbreadths (1 to 2 cm) below the tibial tuberosity and one or two fingerbreadths medial to it. This should place the IOVA on the flat surface of the proximal, anteromedial tibia. In adults, the IOVA site can be found by first moving one or two fingerbreadths medial to the tibial tuberosity, and then moving one or two fingerbreadths above or below this location.
     - Grasp the medial aspect of the tibia with the thumb and fingers of your nondominant hand to secure it.
     - Using your dominant hand, with the stylet in place, insert the IOVA needle with a gentle, but firm, boring or screwing motion at an angle of 60 tp 80 degrees to the proximal skin (which is a 10- to 30-degree angle to verticle; see Fig. 198-2). *To avoid bending the needle, twist it rather than pushing it.* If the needle is threaded, it should be twisted clockwise to screw it into the bone. The needle should be pointed caudad, in the direction of the long axis of the bone, away from the epiphysis. The IOVA needle kits with either a battery-powered drill or bone injection gun can be used in the same location, but should be held perpendicular to the bone. Again, every effort should be made to avoid the epiphysis.
   - Head of humerus
     - Palpate the anterior aspect of the head of humerus.
     - Grasp the humerus in the nondominant hand to secure it. Make sure your nondominant hand is well below the insertion site in case there is through-and-through needle penetration of the bone.
     - Using your dominant hand, the IOVA needle kits with either a battery-powered drill or bone injection gun should be held perpendicular to the bone.
     - The needle should then be inserted. Care should be taken when disconnecting the needle from the drill or injection gun to avoid dislodging the needle.
   - Distal tibia
     - Insert the IOVA needle into the distal medial tibia at the broad, flat area proximal to the medial malleolus and posterior to the saphenous vein. It should be inserted at an angle perpendicular to the skin (see Fig. 198-3). Again, the IOVA needle kits with a battery-powered drill can be used at this location and directed at the same angle.
   - Distal femur (EZ-IO not indicated in this location)
     - Insert the needle 2 to 3 cm above the epicondyles in the anterior midline.
     - Direct the needle cephalad at an angle of 70 to 80 degrees to distal skin (10 to 20 degrees from the vertical; see Fig. 198-4).
6. Placement in the marrow space is confirmed by the following:
   - There is a decrease in resistance (it "gives") as the needle passes through the cortex into the softer medulla. The skin-to-cortex distance is rarely more than 1 cm in infants and children.
   - The needle should stand upright without support when the stylet is removed.
   - Marrow should be easily aspirated into a syringe, followed by blood (*note:* marrow or blood may not be aspirated in every case).
   - Fluids should infuse easily without extravasation.
7. Radiographs can be used to confirm needle position if time and the clinical situation permits *(optional)*.
8. Flush the needle with saline solution (heparin is optional). Check for swelling (extravasation of fluid) around the needle or behind the extremity. If the test injection is unsuccessful

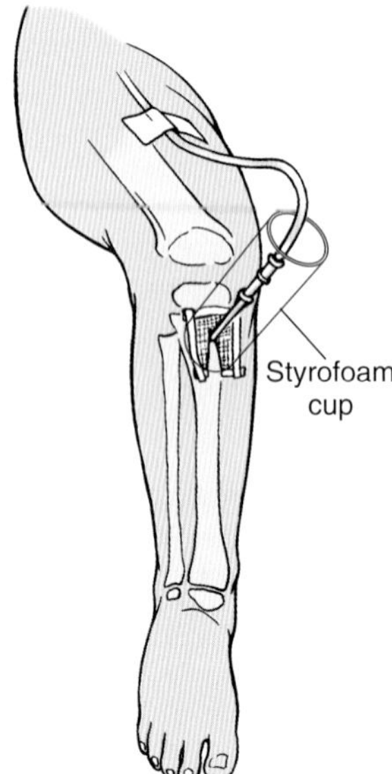

Figure 198-6 Completed intraosseous vascular access with cup protector.

(i.e., extravasation is noted), the IOVA should be removed and another site chosen. If an extremity is to be used, it should be another one. If the same extremity is used, fluid will leak through the prior hole in the cortex, possibly causing damage by extravasation.

NOTE: For the alert patient, 2% lidocaine without preservatives and without epinephrine (i.e., cardiac lidocaine, observing same contraindications and precautions as cardiac lidocaine; up to 5 mL in adults, less for children, adjusted for weight) can be infused very slowly (slow enough to prevent it being sent directly into the central circulation) to decrease the discomfort associated with later infusions. Lidocaine infused in this manner goes directly into the marrow to provide analgesia, prior to the saline flush.

9. If the IOVA has a flange, it should be taped down. A sterile 2 × 2 gauze pad cut to fit around the needle should also be taped down as a dressing. Next, place a cup (Styrofoam or plastic, with the bottom removed) over the IOVA site and firmly secure it with tape (Fig. 198-6).

   NOTE: The cup offers additional protection for the IOVA in the case of inadvertent extremity movement.

10. Attach the pressure bag infusor or an infusion pump to the IV bag, and tape the IV tubing in place. The tubing should be taped both to the patient (to avoid putting tension on the IOVA) and to the IV line (to avoid it being disconnected). Pressure bag infusors, infusion pumps, or forceful manual pressure can be used to administer large volumes. Large fluid boluses can also be given with a large syringe, either through a medication port in the IV line or through a saline lock attached to the IOVA. When giving large volumes under pressure, care should be taken to avoid air embolism.
11. Restrain the limb with soft restraints to avoid inadvertent movement.
12. Monitor the infusion site for evidence of needle displacement or extravasation. Needle displacement can result in severe complications from extravasation (e.g., compartment syndrome, tissue necrosis). Establish peripheral IV access within 24 to 48 hours after IOVA placement, and then remove the IOVA.

Removal

1. Rotate the needle slightly to loosen its seal. (If inserted by portable, battery-powered drill, rotate the needle clockwise.) Withdraw the needle with a firm, quick motion.
2. Place a sterile pressure pad over the puncture site; apply firm pressure for 5 minutes to prevent hematoma formation. Next, apply a sterile dressing to the extremity. Do not constrict the extremity with the dressing.

Postprocedure Management

After IOVA removal, the dressing must be changed daily. Dressings may be discontinued after 48 hours. The patient, his or her family, and the nursing staff should be taught to monitor for signs of infection and other possible complications.

Complications

- The most common complication is unsuccessful placement. This was previously due to the technical difficulty of the procedure; however, IOVA systems that include a battery-powered drill or spring-loaded needle gun have markedly increased the success rate. Technical failure is now most commonly due to a lack of familiarity with the equipment or the landmarks, or an improper technique.
- Clotting of marrow in the needle or displacement of the needle may lead to loss of vascular access.
- Subcutaneous, or occasionally subperiosteal, infiltration of fluid or leakage from the puncture site is common. This is especially common with use of pressure infusor bags, infusion pumps, or manual pressure, or with long-term use of intraosseous infusion. Extravasated crystalloid is usually not a problem, but solutions containing calcium chloride, epinephrine, or sodium bicarbonate (or other potentially cytotoxic agents) should be stopped or slowed to minimize extravasation. Muscle or tendon compartment syndromes from excessive fluid extravasation are a possibility.
- Slow infusion rates may be due to a small, fibrotic marrow cavity (rare). Initially, flow rates may be slow because the needle is plugged by marrow contents. Flushing the needle with 5 to 10 mL of saline often clears the needle.
- No lasting effects have been noted in bone, growth plate, or marrow elements after IOVA. The needle is directed away from the growth plate, or the insertion site is distal enough to avoid inadvertent injury to this structure. After successful placement, a small defect is created in the cortex that is visible as a small radiolucent area on radiographs. It should resolve in 30 to 40 days. In one case report, tibial fractures were seen after unsuccessful IOVA attempts, but these are very rare.
- Localized cellulitis or a subcutaneous abscess may be observed in less than 1% of cases. In most studies, the incidence of osteomyelitis was less than 1%. Infections were usually associated with prolonged catheter placement, placement in bacteremic patients, or use of hypertonic infusions.
- Hematomas are most likely caused by local trauma from needle insertion.
- Pain is possible with insertion and when intramedullary pressure is increased during infusion. It is generally not a problem with slow infusions or in the unconscious patient. Slowing the infusion rate in the conscious patient may relieve symptoms.
- A theoretical complication is creation of a bone embolus when a needle without a stylet is used. No documented cases of a bone embolism have been reported. A fat embolism has been reported from tibial infusion in adults but not in children, probably because the marrow in children is relatively fat free.
- Bone marrow elements (immature blood cells, including blasts) have been observed in venous blood sampled proximal to IOVA

infusion sites. Before more invasive diagnostic measures are undertaken, a repeat complete blood count with differential should be performed, preferably from the more permanent replacement IV site on another extremity.
- With sternal puncture, death has occurred from mediastinitis, hydrothorax, or injury to the heart or great vessels. This is avoidable if other sites are used rather than the sternum.
- Through-and-through placement of the needle can occur. Placing your index finger approximately 1 cm from the needle tip can prevent advancement of the needle through the opposite side of the bone. Your finger will prevent pushing too deep. (Some intraosseous needles have a preset depth indicator on the shaft.)

Patient Education Guides

See patient education and patient consent forms available online at www.expertconsult.com.

CPT/Billing Code

36680 Placement of needle for intraosseous infusion

ICD-9-CM Diagnostic Codes

276.51 Volume depletion, dehydration
345.11 Status epilepticus
427.5 Cardiorespiratory arrest
772.9 Hemorrhage, unspecified in newborn (NOS)
785.50 Shock (without trauma), unspecified
785.52 Shock, septic, endotoxic
785.59 Hypovolemic shock (NEC)
799.1 Respiratory arrest
958.4 Hemorrhagic shock or shock syndrome due to trauma
995.0 Shock, anaphylactic

Acknowledgment

The editors wish to recognize the contributions by Kelly T. Locke, MD, and Rafael F. Cruz, MD, to this chapter in the previous two editions of this text.

Thanks also to Dale Patterson, MD, for acting as the section editor for this chapter.

Suppliers

(See contact information online at www.expertconsult.com.)

Cook Medical: IOVA needles with handles, with or without flanges. Compact system, includes small, portable, battery-powered drill (EZ-IO AD for adults, EZ-IO PD for children). Training videos, equipment with which to practice, etc., are available.
Vidacare
WaisMed

BIBLIOGRAPHY

American Heart Association: Advanced Cardiac Life Support (ACLS) Provider Manual. Dallas, American Heart Association, 2006.

American Heart Association: Pediatric Advanced Life Support (PALS) Provider Manual. Dallas, American Heart Association, 2002.

Glaeser P, Hellmich T, Szewczuga D, et al: Five-year experience in prehospital intraosseous infusions in children and adults. Ann Emerg Med 22:1119–1124, 1993.

Hoffman ME, Ma OJ: Intraosseous infusion. In Reichman EF, Simon RR (eds): Emergency Medicine Procedures. New York, McGraw-Hill, 2004, pp 383–389.

Orlowski JP, Porembka DT, Gallagher JM, Van Lente F: The bone marrow as a source of laboratory studies. Ann Emerg Med 18:1348–1351, 1989.

Cricothyroid Catheter Insertion, Cricothyroidotomy, and Tracheostomy

David Roden

Establishing an airway is crucial to a patient's survival and is of paramount importance in an emergency. If endotracheal or nasotracheal intubation is impossible, several techniques can be used to establish a surgical airway. Cricothyroid catheter insertion (also known as percutaneous transtracheal jet ventilation) and cricothyroidotomy are usually performed in emergencies, whereas tracheostomy is usually performed under controlled conditions.

Cricothyroid catheter insertion is the least invasive procedure, requires the least surgical skill, does not require an assistant, and is the quickest technique. It also has the lowest risk of complications, such as bleeding, glottic stenosis, subglottic stenosis, or tracheal ulceration. This technique provides a temporary airway to preserve oxygenation until a larger airway can be established. (If used with intermittent jet of pressurized 100% oxygen at 50 pounds per square inch [psi], adequate ventilation is also provided; exhalation occurs passively due to secondary recoil of the lungs and chest wall.) Emergency personnel also use cricothyroidotomy as a lifesaving maneuver. One advantage of cricothyroid catheter insertion and cricothyroidotomy is the speed with which they can be performed. They also do not require a lot of equipment and result in less scarring than tracheosotomy. Because the airway is most superficial at the level of the cricothyroid membrane and anatomic landmarks are easily identifiable, this location is ideal for the clinician to create an airway. Serious bleeding and perforation of other structures can also usually be avoided at this site.

Tracheostomy is the most complicated surgical airway procedure and requires the most equipment. It is performed at a level two tracheal rings below the cricothyroid membrane. This site is farther away from the larynx, so the incidence of laryngeal injury is much lower, especially if the opening is maintained for a prolonged time. Dissection is more complicated because the trachea is located deeper than the cricothyroid membrane, so the clinician must be familiar with local anatomy to minimize risk. Tracheostomy is associated with two to five times the complication rate when performed as an emergency procedure; therefore, it is rarely performed except under controlled circumstances in the operating room. In addition, the complete procedure usually takes too long to be useful for emergency airway management and can be difficult for the untrained clinician to perform. The only situation in which emergency tracheostomy is preferred is when the specific location of the injury or disease (e.g., subglottic tumor, thyroid cartilage fracture) precludes alternatives.

Cricothyroid Catheter Insertion

Indications

- Temporary need for an airway
- Upper airway obstruction, usually resulting from foreign body, infection, neoplasm, edema, or trauma
- Preferred technique for establishing emergency airway in pediatric age group if endotracheal intubation fails

Contraindications

- There is an intact nonsurgical airway.
- Subglottic obstruction exists.
- Thyroid cartilage fracture or damage to larynx or cricoid cartilage: anterior neck trauma may be a contraindication if these structures are possibly damaged. In these situations, tracheostomy is preferred.
- Complete airway obstruction is a contraindication for jet ventilation (results in barotrauma or auto–positive end-expiratory pressure [auto-PEEP]; a patent airway is needed for outflow of gas with expiration).

Equipment

- Goggles or eye protection
- Mask, cap, gown, and sterile gloves
- 12-, 14- or 16-gauge, 2- to 3-inch over-the-needle catheter (angiocatheter)
- 5- or 10-mL syringe
- Lidocaine 1% with epinephrine in 10-mL syringe with 22-gauge, ⅝-inch needle
- Skin-sterilizing supplies such as povidine–iodine (if time allows)
- Adhesive tape
- Umbilical tape, 2-0 monofilament nylon suture and needle holder or commercially available endotracheal tube connecter
- High-pressure oxygen supply (30 to 60 psi) with a pressure gauge and a pressure-regulating valve (if high-pressure oxygen is not available, a 3-mL syringe barrel [without a plunger] can be attached to the catheter; a standard endotracheal tube connector can then be used to attach the catheter to a bag-mask-valve [Ambu bag] device)
- Hand-operated valve connected inline to tubing and catheter
- Alternate: an oxygen regulator and manual trigger

Preprocedure Patient Preparation

No patient education is needed in the emergency setting. Documentation should be made in the patient's chart that informed consent was obtained if time allows. If time does not allow, an explanation of the emergent need for this procedure should be documented.

Procedure

1. Position the patient in the supine position with the chin directly midline and maximally extended (if no cervical spine trauma). If a cervical fracture is suspected, the neck should remain immobilized in a neutral position.
2. Clean the neck with povidone–iodine or other antiseptic solution.
3. Observe universal blood and body fluid precautions. Observe sterile technique (cap, gloves, mask, gown, and drapes).
4. Use the nondominant hand to identify the cricothyroid membrane, which is located immediately caudal to the prominent thyroid cartilage (Adam's apple). It is the first small depression or indentation inferior to the hard thyroid cartilage, between the cricoid and thyroid cartilages. It should be easily palpable, even in obese individuals.
5. If the patient is awake, and time allows, infiltrate lidocaine as a wheal and then down to the membrane in the desired location using a 10-mL syringe with a 22-gauge needle.
6. With the nondominant hand, immobilize the thyroid cartilage and hold the skin taut over the cricothyroid membrane.
7. Direct the catheter-over-needle attached to the syringe downward in the midline and caudally at an angle of 45 degrees (Fig. 199-1). Inserting the catheter-over-needle in the inferior aspect of the cricothyroid membrane minimizes risk of injury to the cricothyroid arteries. Aspirate with the syringe during insertion. When air is obtained with aspiration, the needle has entered the trachea.
8. Advance the catheter over the needle, withdraw the needle and syringe, and attach the distal end of the high-pressure oxygen tubing to the catheter.
9. Open the hand-operated release valve to deliver pressurized oxygen to the trachea. As soon as the chest rises, assume that the patient has been oxygenated; the valve should then be closed. Open the valve, watch the chest rise, and close the valve—in a rhythmic pattern—to approximate actual breathing. Adjust the overall pressure level to allow adequate lung expansion.

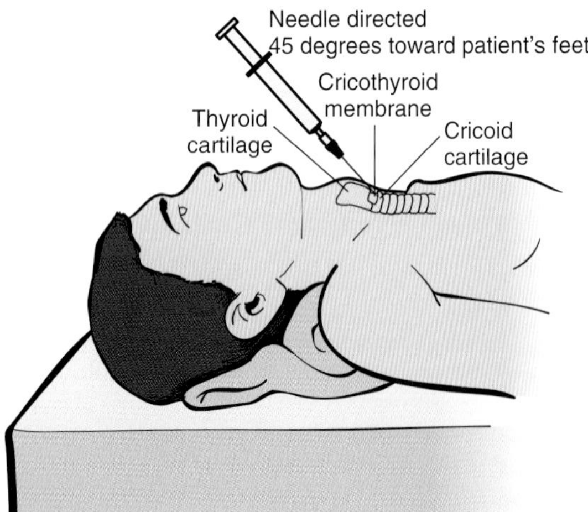

Figure 199-1 Over-the-needle catheter is inserted through cricothyroid membrane with syringe attached. The clinician should aspirate while inserting the needle.

10. Most upper airway obstructions are incomplete and allow some ventilation to occur with forced exhalations. (If the chest remains inflated during the exhalation phase, a complete proximal airway obstruction may be present. In this case, a second large-bore over-the-needle catheter can be inserted next to the original catheter. If the chest still remains distended, cricothyroidotomy should be performed.)
11. The oxygen line should be taped to the catheter. Next, secure the catheter and oxygen tubing by placing a stitch through the skin near the catheter (after infiltration of lidocaine in the conscious patient), wrapping one end of the suture around the catheter several times and tying it to the base of the other end of the suture near the skin. The other end of the suture can then be wrapped several times around the oxygen tubing and tied to the original end of the suture near the skin. Alternatively, a piece of umbilical tape or adhesive tape can be wrapped around the patient's neck, the catheter hub, and the oxygen tubing. Or a commercially available endotracheal tube holder can be wrapped around the patient's neck and connected to the oxygen tubing; the catheter will still have to be secured with suture or by being taped to the tubing and skin.
12. Obtain an arterial blood gas. Pulse oximetry, blood pressure, and telemetry should be monitored.

Complications

- Inadequate ventilation or hypoxia (often due to catheter kinking as it travels through the tissue; use of commercially available kink-resistant catheters minimizes this risk)
- Barotrauma (can cause pneumothorax, pneumomediastinum, or pneumopericardium; auto-PEEP can result in decreased mean arterial pressure)
- Subcutaneous emphysema
- Aspiration (pressurized airflow may minimize risk of aspiration; however, make sure to suction upper airway before discontinuing cricothyroid catheter)

NOTE: Cricothyroid catheter insertion through the cricothyroid membrane may maintain spontaneous respirations for a few minutes. This is the procedure of choice for children under 12 years old because the cricothyroid membrane is small. If this maneuver is inadequate, formal tracheostomy is indicated.

Cricothyroidotomy

Indications

- Upper airway obstruction, usually resulting from foreign body, infection, neoplasm, edema, or trauma
- When endotracheal or nasotracheal intubation has failed, is contraindicated, or is unavailable
- Patient with a cervical spine fracture who cannot extend neck for intubation
- Prior cricothyroidotomy catheter insertion complicated by carbon dioxide retention or air entrapment

Contraindications

- Intact nonsurgical airway
- Subglottic obstruction
- Thyroid cartilage fracture or damage to larynx or cricoid cartilage (anterior neck trauma may be contraindication if these structures are possibly damaged); in these situations, trachestomy preferred
- Patient younger than 8 years old (cricothyroid catheter insertion or needle cricothyroidotomy is the preferred procedure for this age group)
- *Relative contraindications*: a coagulopathy, massive neck swelling or hematoma, or previously prolonged endotracheal intubation (tracheostomy or conversion to tracheostomy may be preferred)

Equipment

- Goggles or eye protection
- No. 15 scalpel blade with handle
- Size 4 to 6 endotracheal tubes or size 4 to 6 Shiley cuffed tracheostomy tubes
- Adhesive tape
- Umbilical tape and 2-0 monofilament nylon suture and needle holder (if a tracheostomy tube is used)
- Sterile 4 × 4–inch gauze sponges
- Self-refilling bag-valve-mask unit (Ambu bag) with tubing and oxygen source
- Suction and suction catheters

If time allows

- Povidone–iodine (Betadine) or other antiseptic skin preparation
- Mask, cap, gown, and sterile gloves
- Sterile fenestrated drape
- Lidocaine 1% with epinephrine in 10-mL syringe with 22-gauge, ⅝-inch needle

If a tracheostomy tray is available:

- Hemostat clamps (2)
- Kelly clamps (2)
- Tracheal dilator (Trousseau)
- Curved scissors

Preprocedure Patient Preparation

No patient education is needed in the emergency setting. Documentation should be made in the patient's chart that informed consent was obtained, if time allows. If time does not allow, an explanation of the emergent need for this procedure should be documented.

Technique

NOTE: In extremely urgent situations, the goal is to save a life, so some concerns about sterile technique should be postponed.

1. Position the patient in the supine position with the chin directly midline and maximally extended (if no cervical spine trauma). If a cervical fracture is suspected, the neck should remain immobilized in a neutral position.
2. Clean the neck with povidone–iodine or other antiseptic solution.
3. Observe universal blood and body fluid precautions. Observe sterile technique (cap, gloves, gown, mask, and drapes).
4. Use the nondominant hand to identify the cricothyroid membrane, which is located immediately caudal to the prominent thyroid cartilage (Adam's apple). It is the first small depression or indentation inferior to the hard thyroid cartilage, between the cricoid and thyroid cartilages. It should be easily palpable, even in obese individuals.

   NOTE: The cricothyroid membrane averages 9 mm in the cephalad-caudad dimension and 30 mm in the left-to-right dimension in adults. It should be easily palpable and accessible.

5. If the patient is awake, and time allows, use the 10-mL syringe with the 22-gauge needle to infiltrate lidocaine in a large subcutaneous wheal encompassing the future vertical skin incision. Next, infuse lidocaine in a transverse line across the membrane.
6. With the nondominant hand, immobilize the thyroid cartilage and hold the skin taut over the cricothyroid membrane. Using the no. 15 blade, make a 3-cm vertical (longitudinal) skin incision centered over the cricothyroid membrane (Fig. 199-2).

   NOTE: Certain authorities recommend a transverse skin incision. Making a longitudinal incision slows down the procedure and requires repositioning after the skin incision; however, if the transverse skin incision is accidentally extended too far laterally (e.g., when the procedure is performed under duress), the anterior jugular veins may be injured. If a patient has a suspected laryngeal injury, the longitudinal incision is indicated in the event it needs to be extended inferiorly to perform an emergency high tracheostomy.

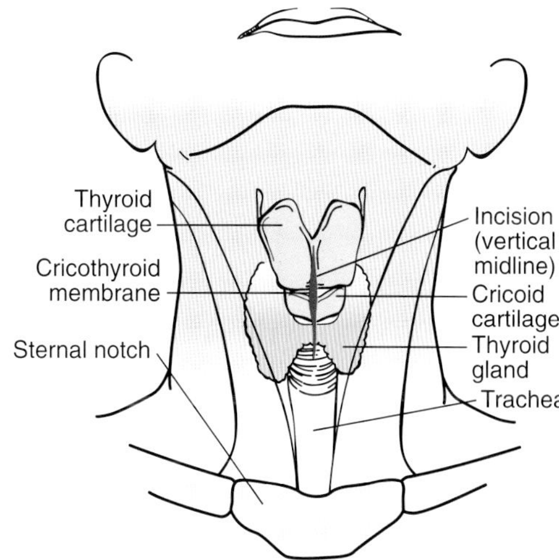

Figure 199-2 Neck extended, with cricothyroid membrane identified.

7. Use the finger and thumb of the nondominant hand to retract the incision edges laterally (Fig. 199-3).
8. Divide the neck fascia and strap muscles vertically in the midline with the scalpel until the thyroid and cricoid cartilages are encountered. In general, cartilage provides considerable resistance to the scalpel, so these structures are not easily injured.
9. Retracting soft tissue structures laterally, locate the cricothyroid membrane by palpation with the dominant hand and use the scalpel to create a 1- to 2-cm transverse incision centered in the midline, immediately above the cricoid cartilage. Be aware that at this point any respiratory effort by the patient will expel sputum, blood, and air into the wound. A low incision should avoid vocal cord injury and the cricothyroid arteries. The posterior aspect of the cricoid cartilage should be avoided, but even if the knife goes too deep, the cricoid cartilage should stop the progression of the knife.
10. Reverse the scalpel, placing the handle into the cricothyroidotomy incision horizontally. Rotate the handle 90 degrees to open the incision (Fig. 199-4).

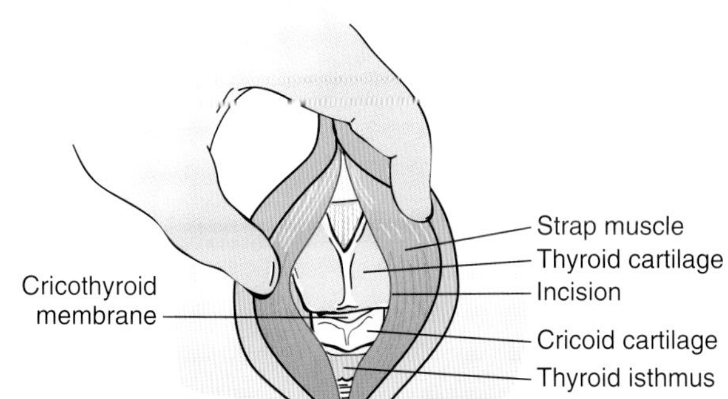

Figure 199-3 After a vertical skin incision, soft tissue structures are retracted laterally with the nondominant hand.

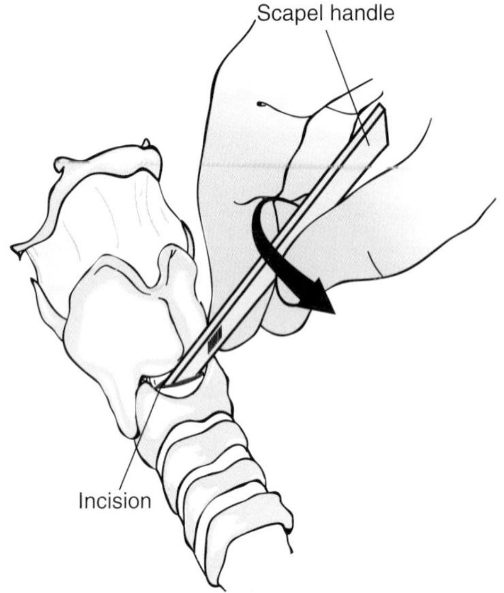

Figure 199-4 Scalpel handle inserted into incision and twisted vertically to open it.

If a tracheostomy tray is available, an alternative to Step 10 is as follows:

10. After using the scalpel to make a transverse midline incision in the cricothyroid membrane, insert a hemostat or Kelly clamp with the points downward into the trachea and spread laterally. A rush of air indicates patency of the airway. Alternatively, a tracheal dilator can extend the cricothyroid membrane incision laterally approximately 1 cm on each side of the midline. From here, continue with the remainder of the steps in the technique.
11. Use the nondominant hand to place the largest possible endotracheal tube or, preferably, tracheostomy tube into the incision. The scalpel handle can be used as both a retractor and a guide. Direct the tube tip toward the patient's feet and attempt to visualize its insertion into the trachea (Fig. 199-5). *Do not release the hold on the tracheostomy or endotracheal tube until it is secured.*
12. Connect the bag-valve-mask unit (Ambu bag) to the tube and ventilate with 100% oxygen. Check for bilateral breath sounds to ensure that the tube is properly placed above the carina.
13. Inflate the cuff with enough air to stop any audible air leaks.
14. Secure the tube and then apply a dressing. If an endotracheal tube is being used, secure the tube in place using tape. If a tracheostomy tube is being used, secure the tube with umbilical tape around the patient's neck. Place four interrupted sutures with 2-0 nylon through the tube's flange to secure it to the skin.

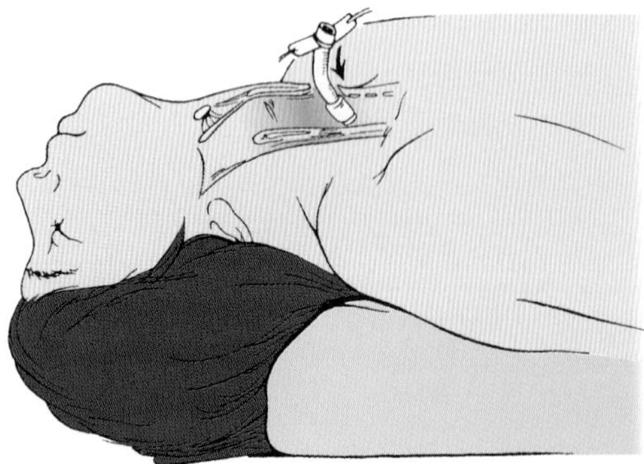

Figure 199-5 Tube is inserted into the incision. Scalpel handle is still in cricothyroid membrane (not shown for clarity).

15. Suction the trachea.
16. Obtain an arterial blood gas and a chest radiograph. The radiograph should demonstrate tube position above the carina and should ensure the absence of an iatrogenic pneumothorax.

Complications

- Intraoperative and postoperative bleeding (direct pressure will usually stop bleeding after the airway is established)
- Improper tube placement with asphyxia
- Tube displacement or obstruction with subsequent hypoxia or death
- Subcutaneous or mediastinal emphysema
- Laryngeal or vocal cord injury (especially if tracheostomy tube is larger than cricothyroid membrane)
- Voice changes (e.g., hoarseness)
- Infection
- Subglottic stenosis
- Perforated esophagus

To prevent subcutaneous or mediastinal emphysema or infection, the skin incision should not be closed around the tube. If the cricothyroidotomy is only necessary for 48 to 72 hours (e.g., resolving infection, angioedema of tongue), the patient can be decannulated without converting to a tracheostomy. If a longer period of intubation is required (see the "Tracheostomy" section for a discussion of the controversies of timing), the procedure should be revised to a tracheostomy to prevent subglottic stenosis.

Postprocedure Patient Education

If prolonged airway management is needed, convert the cricothyroidotomy to a tracheostomy and provide the appropriate patient education. If the cricothyroidotomy is able to be removed within 48 to 72 hours, give the patient instructions for the routine care of a skin laceration. The patient should be aware that the fistula will close spontaneously. He or she should have a follow-up appointment within a week and should call or go to the emergency room for signs of hemorrhage, infection, airway distress, or subcutaneous emphysema.

TRACHEOSTOMY

Indications

- Chronic ventilatory failure (most common indication)
- Upper airway obstruction usually resulting from infection, neoplasm, edema, or trauma; also obstructive sleep apnea and bilateral vocal cord paralysis
- Anticipated prolonged endotracheal intubation
- Facial, tracheal, or other head and neck trauma or surgery with compromised airway
- Fractured larynx or subglottic obstruction (cricothyroidotomy contraindicated)
- Chronic impaired pulmonary toilet
- Management of chronic aspiration
- Unstable cervical spine

NOTE: Management of bronchial secretions is much easier with a tracheostomy tube than with an endotracheal tube. Risk of endotracheal tube complications (e.g., tube displacement, sinusitis, tube kinking) is also reduced with conversion to a tracheostomy. However, the recommended timing for conversion has been debated extensively. Supporters for early conversion (7 days) suggest that laryngeal complication rates and patient comfort are improved with early conversion. Advocates for delayed placement of tracheostomy (14 to 21 days) state that unnecessary procedures will be avoided, reducing local wound and other surgical complications. Most experts have adopted an intermediate approach that is individualized to the patient. If the patient is expected to be intubated for considerably longer than 7 days, a tracheostomy is placed early. However, if the patient's course cannot be predicted, the conversion can be delayed until prolonged need becomes evident.

Contraindications

- Lack of familiarity with the procedure
- Known preexisting severe tracheal disease or trauma
- Uncontrolled coagulopathy

EDITOR'S NOTE: Cricothyroidotomy is the procedure of choice when an invasive approach to the airway is needed.

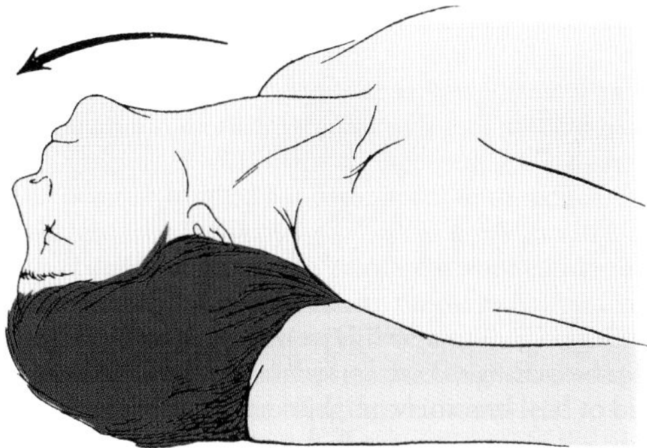

Figure 199-6 Patient is positioned for tracheostomy.

Equipment

- Povidone–iodine or other antiseptic solution
- 1 package of 4 × 4–inch sterile gauze sponges
- Sterile gown and gloves
- Sterile fenestrated drape
- Cap, mask, and eye protection
- Electrocautery machine
- 10- and 50-mL syringes
- 22- and 25-gauge, ⅝-inch needles
- No. 15 scalpel blade with handle
- Mosquito hemostats (4)
- Kelly clamps (2)
- Subcutaneous or Army-Navy retractors (2)
- Trousseau (tracheal) dilator
- Allis clamps (2)
- Tracheal hook
- Sizes 4, 6, and 8 cuffed Shiley tracheotomy tubes
- Needle holder
- Umbilical tape and 2-0 monofilament nylon suture
- Suction apparatus, tubing, and catheters
- Ventilation equipment: bag-valve-mask unit (Ambu bag) with tubing and 100% oxygen available
- 3-0 Dexon or chromic absorbable suture on a cutting needle

Preprocedure Patient Preparation

Education of the patient and family should include the indication for tracheostomy and possible complications. Benefits of the procedure, as well as the risks of not performing it, should be explained to the patient and family. If there are alternatives to this procedure, they should be explained. Informed consent should be obtained in nonemergent situations.

Technique

1. Tracheostomy can be performed under local anesthesia on a spontaneously breathing patient, or under general anesthesia on a previously intubated patient. Exercise caution in administering sedation to a nonintubated patient with a compromised airway.
2. Position the patient in the supine position with a roll under the shoulders and, if there is no cervical spine trauma, with the neck maximally extended (Fig. 199-6). Placement of an endotracheal tube before elective tracheostomy (or leaving an existing tube) allows for better airway control and minimizes complications, especially in children. The anesthetist should stand above the patient's head for better access to the endotracheal tube, if present.
3. Prep the neck with povidone–iodine or other antiseptic solution from sternum to chin, and laterally to the sternocleidomastoid muscles. Apply the fenestrated drape.
4. Check the tracheostomy tube cuff for leaks prior to making the incision. A second tube should be tested and available, if possible.
5. Palpate landmarks: the sternal notch, cricoid cartilage, and inferior border of the thyroid cartilage. Outline a horizontal incision two fingerbreadths above the sternal notch, centered in the midline over the trachea.
6. For conscious patients, inject lidocaine subcutaneously around the intended incision site. Lidocaine can then be injected down to the anterior tracheal wall beneath the incision.
7. Using the scalpel, make a horizontal incision through skin and subcutaneous tissue down to the strap muscles (Fig. 199-7). Alternatively, once the skin has been incised, electrocautery can be used to divide the subcutaneous tissue horizontally, deepening the incision until the strap muscles are encountered.
8. Clamp the subcutaneous tissue with Allis clamps and retract superiorly and inferiorly. Next, incise the fascia vertically in the midline, in the raphe between the strap muscles. Incise down to the pretracheal fascia (Fig. 199-8).

   NOTE: Often the strap muscles are fused in the midline and covered by a network of troublesome veins. Attempts should be made to cauterize or ligate these veins.
9. Place retractor(s) beneath the strap muscles and apply traction laterally. Incise the pretracheal fascia to expose the thyroid isthmus and tracheal rings (Fig. 199-9).
10. Retract the thyroid isthmus superiorly, if possible, to increase visibility. If exposure is inadequate, horizontally incise the fascia immediately caudal to the lower border of the cricoid cartilage but do not enter the trachea. Insert a hemostat through this

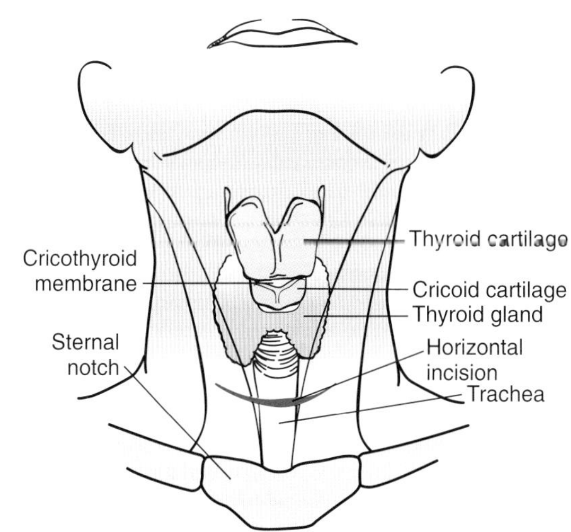

Figure 199-7 Horizontal incision is made through the skin.

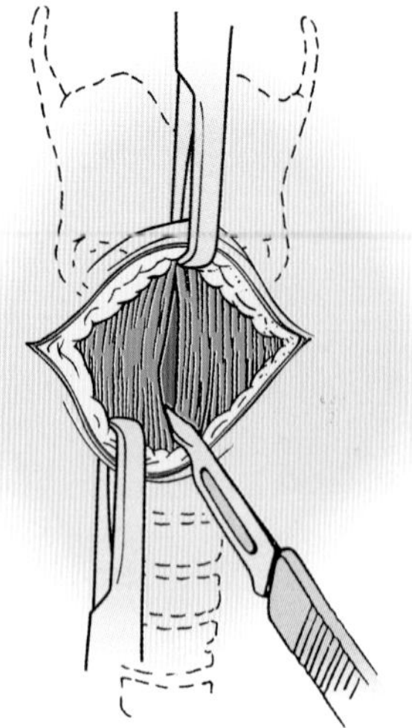

Figure 199-8 Fascia and strap muscles are divided in the midline.

incision pointed toward the patient's feet, parallel to the trachea. Bluntly dissect the thyroid isthmus off the anterior wall of the trachea. After an additional attempt at superior or inferior retraction, if visibility is still inadequate, it may be necessary to divide the thyroid isthmus with clamps and suture the ligated edges (Fig. 199-10). A 3-0 chromic suture is used to oversew each edge for hemostasis.

NOTE: It is important to remain in the midline with this procedure to minimize complications, especially in children.

11. If unsure that the object visualized is the trachea, aspirate for air with a small-bore needle to confirm before proceeding. Next, place a tracheal hook beneath the cricoid cartilage and elevate it toward the surgeon and toward the patient's head. If using local anesthesia, 1 to 2 mL should be injected beneath the second tracheal ring into the tracheal lumen. This should stimulate the nonanesthetized patient to cough.
12. Make a transverse incision between the second and third rings (Fig. 199-11). Be prepared for a spurt of blood, air, or sputum, and have suction ready. Do not use electrocautery to incise the trachea because there is a the risk of airway fire. Take care not to puncture the endotracheal tube cuff if present or the posterior wall of the trachea. (Alternatively, some clinicians make an inverted U-shaped incision. Others make a square "window" incision and remove the anterior portion of the second and third tracheal rings. A midline vertical incision through the second, third, and fourth tracheal rings is the incision of choice for an emergency tracheostomy.)

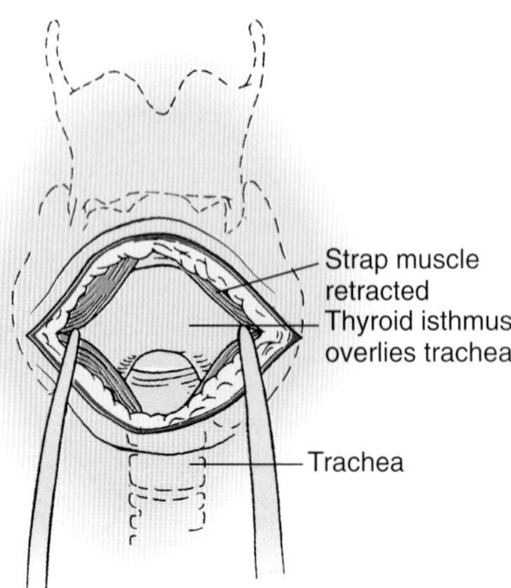

Figure 199-9 Strap muscles are retracted laterally to expose the thyroid isthmus.

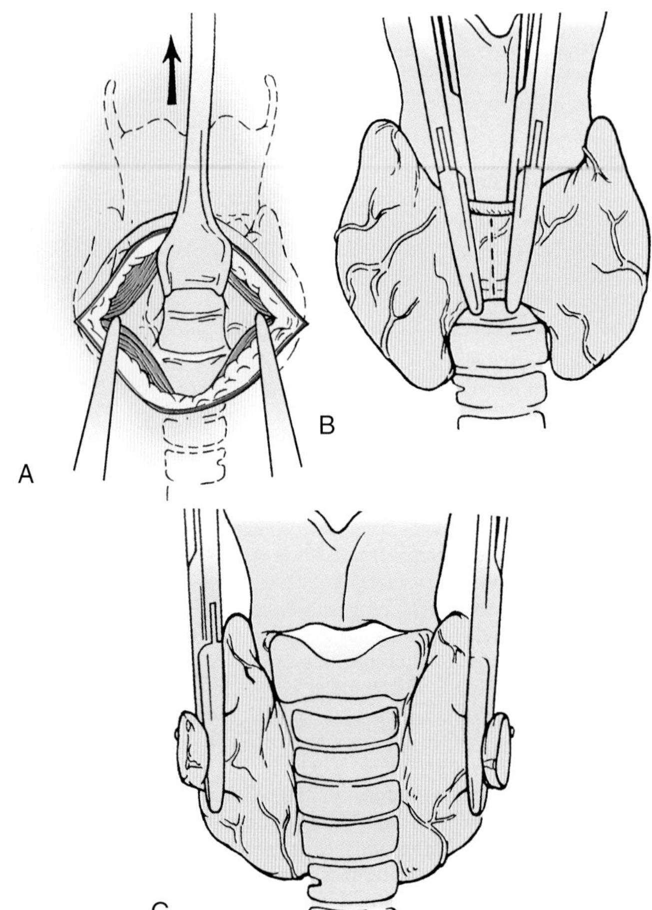

Figure 199-10 **A,** Thyroid isthmus is retracted. If exposure is inadequate, the thyroid isthmus should be clamped (**B**) and divided (**C**).

13. Insert a Trousseau dilator into the trachea and dilate laterally (Fig. 199-12).
14. Withdraw the endotracheal tube (if one is in place) until the tip is just above the tracheostomy. Under direct visualization, insert the appropriately sized tracheostomy tube through the dilated incision, with the tube tip directed downward (Fig. 199-13). Most adults will fit a size 8 Shiley tube. Inflate the tracheostomy tube cuff. Suction through the tube with a flexible suction catheter. Bronchoscopy can be performed at this point to confirm proper tracheostomy tube placement.
15. Attach the tube to the bag-valve-mask (Ambu bag) device and check for bilateral breath sounds with ventilation.
16. Remove the retractors and the cricoid hook when the tube is adequately positioned. Secure the tracheostomy tube around the neck with umbilical tape. Secure the flange to the patient's skin with four interrupted 2-0 nylon sutures.
17. Apply a sterile dressing around the tube.
18. A chest radiograph should be considered to assess tube placement above the carina and to ensure the absence of an iatrogenic pneumothorax.

To prevent infection, pneumomediastinum, or subcutaneous emphysema, do not close the skin incision around the tracheostomy tube. A tracheostomy tube provides access to the trachea for an unlimited amount of time. Once the indication for the tube has resolved, it is removed to allow the tracheocutaneous fistula to close spontaneously.

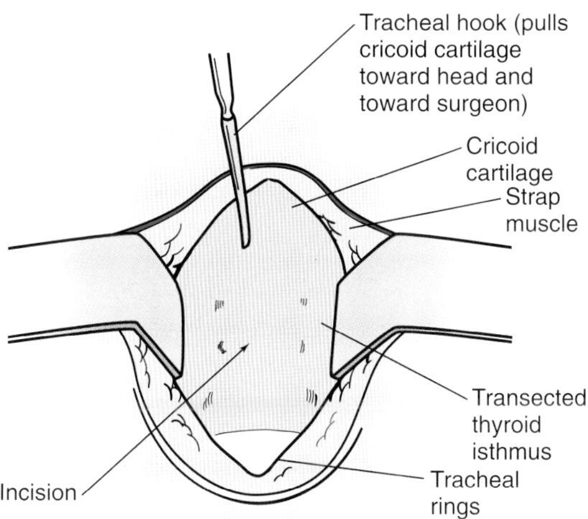

Figure 199-11 Tracheal hook is placed in the cricoid cartilage and elevated anteriorly. The incision is made between the second and third rings.

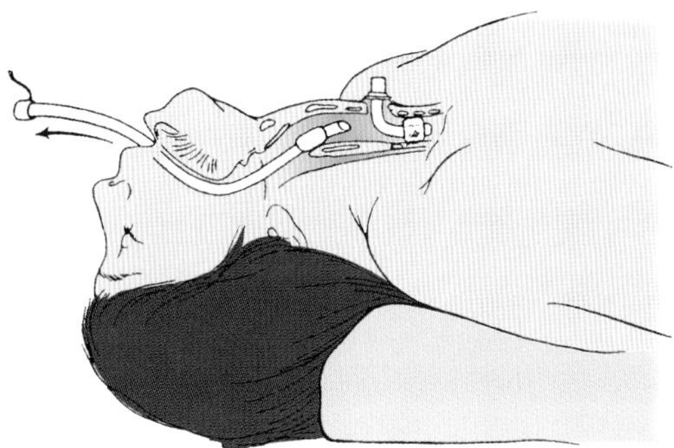

Figure 199-13 Remove the endotracheal tube after inserting the tracheostomy tube.

NOTE: Placement of tracheostomies can be technically difficult, especially in children, obese patients, and patients with deformed or fixed cervical spines. Complication rates are higher in children. For these individuals, tracheostomies should definitely be avoided in emergency situations and performed under controlled circumstances.

Complications

- Bleeding
- Subcutaneous emphysema
- Wound infection
- Pneumomediastinum
- Pneumothorax
- Tracheoesophageal fistula
- Tracheoinnominate artery fistula
- Recurrent laryngeal nerve damage
- Aspiration
- Tube obstruction
- Malpositioned or displaced tube with subsequent hypoxia or death
- Tracheal stenosis
- Dysphagia
- Sepsis

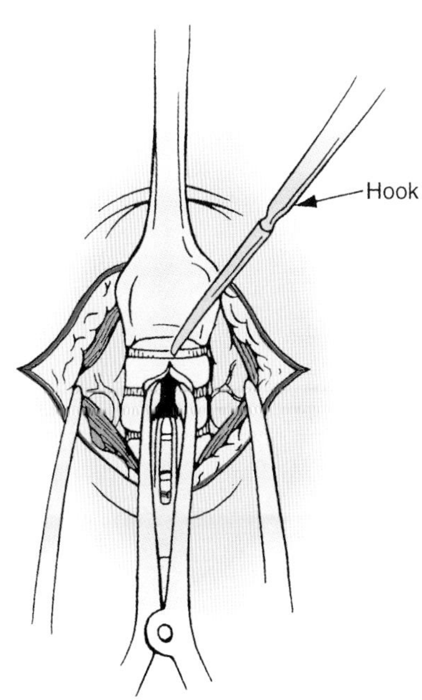

Figure 199-12 Insert the dilator into the trachea.

Postprocedure Patient Education

Initially, the patient will be cared for in the hospital. Postprocedure education includes cleaning of the appliance and suctioning. If the patient is discharged with a tracheostomy, caretakers will need to continue this care at home. Patients will not be able to speak if the tube balloon is inflated. If the balloon is deflated, patients can eat normally and can speak if the tube lumen is occluded with the patient's finger during exhalation. A speaking valve can also be fitted to passively close the lumen during exhalation.

CPT/Billing Codes

31600 Tracheostomy, planned (separate procedure)
31603 Tracheostomy, emergency procedure; transtracheal
31605 Tracheostomy, emergency procedure; cricothyroid membrane
31612 Tracheal puncture, percutaneous with transtracheal aspiration or injection

ICD-9-CM Diagnostic Codes

478.79 Unspecified diseases of larynx, not elsewhere classified (abscess, obstruction, necrosis)
518.5 Pulmonary insufficiency following trauma or surgery
518.81 Acute respiratory failure
518.83 Chronic respiratory failure
807.5 Fracture, larynx and trachea, closed

Patient Education Guides

See the sample patient education and consent forms online at www.expertconsult.com.

Suppliers

Full contact information is available online at www.expertconsult.com.

Percuteaneous transtracheal jet ventilation catheter
Life Medical Supplier
Shiley tracheostomy products
Bivona/Smith's Medical
Mallinckrodt/Covidien

BIBLIOGRAPHY

Boon JM, Abrahams PH, Meiring JH, Welch T: Cricothyroidotomy: A clinical anatomy review. Clin Anat 17:478–486, 2004.

Cabel JA: Percutaneous transtracheal jet ventilation. In Reichman EF, Simon RR (eds): Emergency Medicine Procedures. New York, McGraw-Hill, 2004.

Crosby KS: Tracheostomy. In Reichman EF, Simon RR (eds): Emergency Medicine Procedures. New York, McGraw-Hill, 2004.

Griffiths J, Barber VS, Morgan L, Young JD: Systematic review and meta-analysis of studies of the timing of tracheostomy in adult patients undergoing artificial ventilation. BMJ 330:1243, 2005.

Heffner JE: Tracheotomy application and timing. Clin Chest Med 24: 389–398, 2003.

Jackson C: Tracheotomy. Laryngoscope 19:285–290, 1909.

Nagy K: Cricothyroidotomy. In Reichman EF, Simon RR (eds): Emergency Medicine Procedures. New York, McGraw-Hill, 2004.

Rana S, Pendem S, Pogodzinski M, et al: Tracheostomy in critically ill patients. Mayo Clin Proc 80:1632–1638, 2005.

Weissler M: Tracheotomy and intubation. In Bailey B (ed): Head and Neck Surgery: Otolaryngology. Philadelphia, Lippincott Williams & Wilkins, 2006.

CHAPTER 200

Percutaneous Endoscopic Gastrostomy Placement and Replacement

Paul W. Davis

Percutaneous endoscopic gastrostomy (PEG) is the placement of a percutaneous gastrostomy tube with the aid of an endoscope. The PEG technique has largely replaced surgical gastrostomy as the procedure of choice for patients who require long-term enteral nutrition. It was first described in 1980 by Gauderer and colleagues for use in children but has since gained wide acceptance for use in patients of all ages. Along with other necessary supplies, commercial PEG tube kits usually contain the PEG tube, an internal bolster (to seal the gastric mucosa), and an external bolster (to stabilize and prevent migration of the tube). Choices for the internal bolster including a balloon, a soft dome, crossbars, a T-bar, a flange, a disk, a three-leaf retainer, and others; most are soft to avoid irritating the gastric mucosa.

The actual PEG placement procedure requires two trained individuals, one of whom must be skilled in esophagogastroduodenoscopy (EGD). Please see Chapter 101, Esophagogastroduodenoscopy, for a full discussion of EGD; this chapter will be limited to the application of EGD for PEG placement. The procedure can be performed in the operating room, the endoscopy suite, or at the bedside. Normally, the procedure can be performed under moderate sedation (see Chapter 2, Procedural Sedation and Analgesia, and Chapter 7, Pediatric Sedation and Analgesia), with a local anesthetic such as lidocaine also used at the cutaneous site (see Chapter 4, Local Anesthesia). However, if intravenous sedative agents are unlikely to be effective because of a history of prescribed or illicit controlled substance use, or if the patient is at risk of respiratory compromise secondary to oropharyngeal anatomy, risk of aspiration, or a history of obstructive sleep apnea, a third skilled provider will be needed to provide sedation and monitor the airway. Indeed, endotracheal intubation may be advisable because these patients often have underlying conditions that impair handling of secretions. In these circumstances, the assistance of an anesthesiologist, nurse anesthetist, or trained primary care colleague is advantageous.

After PEG placement, there is no reason for routine removal; however, occasionally they require replacement owing to accidental dislodgement or because they have become obstructed, worn out, kinked, or fractured. Although most of these problems can be avoided with diligent care, this chapter also briefly discusses PEG replacement.

Indications

Placement

The decision for PEG placement has to be made on a case-by-case basis, especially when rapidly progressive and incurable diseases are present. Certainly, this includes the various forms of severe dementia.

Most commonly, PEG tube placement is performed for patients who are unable or unwilling to ingest food orally. The usual conditions include major head and neck trauma, esophageal cancer, oropharyngeal cancers, cerebrovascular accidents, esophageal dysmotility, as well as other irreversible neurologic conditions such as amyotrophic lateral sclerosis. When used for provision of nutrients, the choice of PEG placement necessarily requires a functioning gastrointestinal tract and optimally involves a prior discussion with the patient or family concerning prognosis and underlying comorbid conditions. Other uses for the PEG procedure include treatment of gastric volvulus, decompression of patients with an intestinal obstruction or peritoneal carcinomatosis, administration of unpalatable medications to pediatric and mentally impaired patients, and enhanced enteral feeding of patients with hypercatabolic states, such as burn patients.

In brief, PEG tubes have two primary indications:

1. Enteral access for feeding or medication administration
2. Decompression of the gut

Replacement

- Accidental PEG dislodgement or removal
- PEG blockage or obstruction
- PEG damage (e.g., worn out, kinked, fractured)

Contraindications

Placement

Absolute

In general, any contraindication to endoscopy will apply to PEG insertion as well. In addition, the absence of one of three prerequisites for safe PEG placement is a good reason to abort the procedure. These prerequisites include ability to distend the stomach endoscopically with air, endoscopically visible finger invagination of the anterior gastric wall, and transillumination of the anterior abdominal incision site. Additional absolute contraindications include the following:

- Pharyngeal obstruction
- Esophageal obstruction
- Active coagulopathy
- Peritonitis
- Sepsis

- Recent myocardial infarction
- Hemodynamic instability

Relative

Either esophageal or oropharyngeal cancer is considered a relative contraindication because there is a theoretical potential for seeding of the gastrocutaneous tract with cancer cells. Although this hazard is rare, it is primarily seen with untreated oropharyngeal cancers, with an incidence of less than 1% in one reported series (Cruz and colleagues, 2005). Some have advocated use of the Russel or "poke" technique (see later), radiographically placed, or surgically placed gastrostomy tubes as more appropriate in this setting. With these techniques, the PEG tube is not drawn down the esophagus for placement.

The presence of gastroesophageal reflux with its attendant risk of aspiration has long been considered a contraindication to PEG. Historically, a surgically placed or, more recently, a radiologically placed jejunostomy tube has been preferred. However, jejunostomy does not prevent gastroesophageal reflux and it is now known that PEG placement may actually decrease reflux because the PEG effectively creates an anterior pseudogastropexy.

Other relative contraindications include the following:

- Portal hypertension
- Moderate or massive ascites
- Gastric varices
- Prior abdominal surgery
- Peritoneal dialysis
- Hepatomegaly or splenomegaly
- Large hiatal hernia
- Large ventral hernia
- Open abdominal wound
- Prior subtotal gastrectomy
- Morbid obesity
- Anorexia nervosa
- Infiltrative or malignant disorders of the stomach
- Limited life expectancy

Replacement

Absolute

- Immature PEG tract (e.g., <4 weeks after PEG placement)
- Existing PEG tube not removable with gentle, constant traction (endoscopic guidance necessary)
- Nonreplaceable catheter (e.g., needle jejunostomy with 5- to 7-Fr catheter)

Relative

- Jejunostomy (the tract can be stented with a replacement catheter, but more information should be obtained before resuming feedings)
- Witzel gastrostomy (these use a more circuitous tunnel and a smaller tube and may be difficult to maneuver)

Equipment and Materials

Placement

The equipment list in Chapter 101, Esophagogastroduodenoscopy, applies equally to the endoscopy needs of PEG placement. This includes topical benzocaine (e.g., Cetacaine, Hurricaine) spray, if desired. In addition, the following equipment and supplies are recommended (usually included in commercial PEG kits):

- Gloves and equipment necessary for clinician to follow universal blood and body fluid precautions
- Lidocaine 1% to 2% for local anesthesia of the skin and abdominal wall
- 22- and 25-gauge needles
- 50 or 10-mL syringe
- Antiseptic preparation solution such as povidone–iodine or chlorhexidine
- Scalpel with no. 11 blade
- 4 × 4 gauze sponges
- Fenestrated drape
- Introducer trocar
- Guidewire (standard or looped end, depending on technique used)
- Disposable snare for gastroscope
- Abdominal binder (for confused or impaired patients)
- PEG tube with external bolster
- Surgical jelly for PEG tube lubrication
- Large, 50- to 70-mL (e.g., Toomey) syringe to aspirate gastric contents
- Adapter to attach Foley catheter to feeding assembly or to cap it off
- Jejunal tube *(if warranted)*
- Low-profile device (Fig. 200-1)

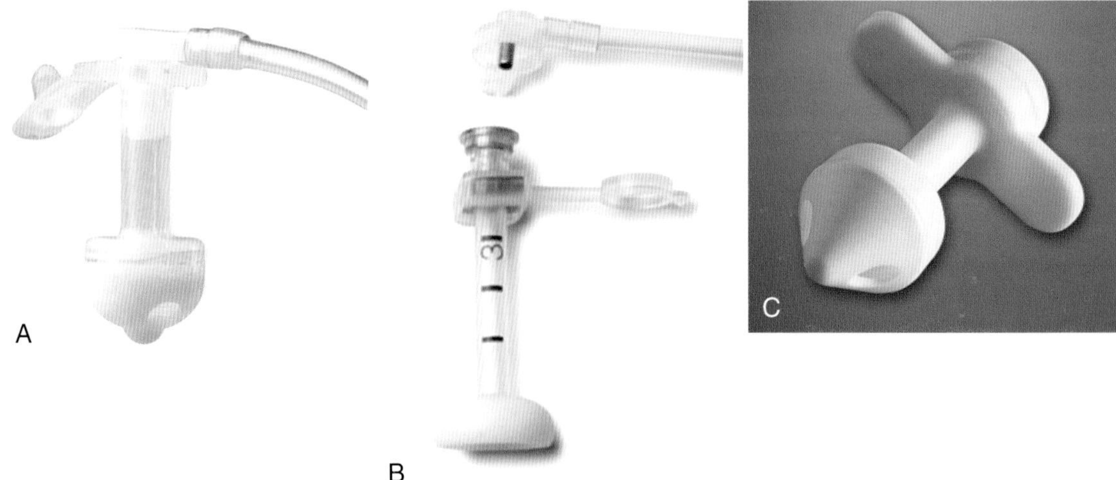

Figure 200-1 Low-profile devices (LPD). **A,** Bard Button. **B,** Bard Gauderer "Genie." **C,** Cook LPD.

Replacement

- Gloves and equipment necessary for clinician to follow universal blood and body fluid precautions
- Antiseptic preparation solution such as povidone–iodine or chlorhexidine
- 4 × 4 gauze sponges and adhesive tape
- Surgical jelly for PEG tube lubrication
- Foley catheter or commercial PEG replacement kit with PEG tube of similar diameter to the original PEG
- External bolster (Options include a retainer for a nasogastric tube, a short length [3 cm] of latex or Silicone tubing [cut from a Foley catheter or feeding tube] and a plastic cable tie or cut to form a T-bar, or a 0 or 2-0 silk suture. Commercial bolster kits are available; however, they are expensive, are not always available, and often do not properly fit the replacement PEG tube.)
- Large, 50- to 70-mL (e.g., Toomey) syringe to aspirate gastric contents
- Adapter to attach Foley catheter to feeding assembly or to cap it off
- Low-profile device (see Fig. 200-1)

Preprocedure Patient Preparation

The patient or legal guardian or family member who will be caring for the patient and assisting with tube feedings should be given a general description of EGD and the PEG placement or replacement procedure. Any available alternatives should be discussed. The possible risks and complications of these procedures need to be explained along with the symptoms and signs that might suggest late complications and problems. It is very important that caregivers be included in this conversation because patients requiring PEG frequently suffer from cognitive or neurologic impairments. Informed consent forms should be signed before EGD and PEG placement. It is prudent to provide a patient education handout and instructions to follow before the procedure(s). Diagrams and photographs are particularly useful for helping patients and families understand the anatomy and altered feeding pathway proposed with PEG placement.

Before PEG replacement, there may be an opportunity to explore with the patient or family whether PEG feeding is still the desired method of nutritional support. There may also need to be a discussion about PEG care to avoid the need for future replacement. The patient should experience minimal discomfort with PEG replacement; if there is more than minimal discomfort, the PEG should not be manipulated. Small children or anxious patients may benefit from mild sedation.

For PEG placement, it is essential to know if the patient is taking any anticoagulants or platelet-inhibiting medications and to withhold these for an appropriate interval before the procedure to minimize any risk of bleeding. The patient must have all solids and liquids withheld for at least 8 hours before the procedure to minimize risk of esophageal reflux and aspiration. Solids may need to be withheld for longer if diabetic gastroparesis or a similar neuropathic condition is present. The presence of a large phytobezoar in the gastric lumen may impair visualization of the gastric indentation by the assistant's finger as well as the sounding needle. Unless EGD is necessary, these precautions are not needed for PEG replacement.

Antibiotic Prophylaxis

Although antibiotic prophylaxis is neither necessary nor recommended for endoscopic procedures according to the most recent American Heart Association guidelines (see Chapter 221, Antibiotic Prophylaxis), preprocedure antibiotic administration is recommended before PEG insertion because of the risk of infection of the gastrocutaneous tract from oropharyngeal and cutaneous flora. It is important to recognize that PEG placement is a "clean" procedure, not a sterile procedure, and every effort should be made to make it as clean as possible. Usually, a cephalosporin or fluoroquinolone is satisfactory unless special considerations are present, such as methicillin-resistant *Staphylococcus aureus* (MRSA) or *Enterococcus* colonization of the skin or oropharyngeal cavity. Refer to recommendations later in the discussion of abscess and wound infection in the section on Postprocedure and Late Complications. If there is no sign of local irritation or infection and only minimal discomfort is experienced during the procedure, antibiotic prophylaxis is rarely necessary during PEG replacement.

Technique

Placement

Patient Positioning

1. The head of the patient's bed or gurney should be elevated 30 degrees to decrease the risk of aspiration of oral or gastric secretions.
2. The patient may be placed in either the left lateral decubitus or the supine position. Although the supine approach offers an added challenge for the endoscopist to identify the larynx and esophagus, this is more than compensated for by not having to rotate the patient after scope insertion.

Anesthetic Administration

3. At this point, conscious sedation can be achieved with appropriate intravenous medications. Depending on the endoscopist's preference, the posterior oropharynx and hypopharynx can be anesthetized with a topical anesthetic such as benzocaine spray.

Endoscope Insertion and Evaluation

4. Before introducing the gastroscope, it is essential to examine the oral cavity and oropharynx for food, debris, and retained secretions, which are quite common in patients undergoing this procedure. It is important to manually remove or suction this material to prevent aspiration during the procedure.
5. The gastroscope is then introduced and passed into the hypopharynx. Esophageal intubation can be difficult because of underlying pathology or the patient's inability to follow commands to swallow. One technique that can be helpful is to pass a snare catheter through the working channel of the scope and then into the proximal esophagus posterior to the arytenoid cartilages on either side of the visualized vocal cords. The gastroscope is then advanced over the closed snare catheter into the esophagus. The catheter is then retracted into the working channel before proceeding with the procedure.
6. It is prudent to perform a complete diagnostic examination of the esophagus, stomach, and duodenum before PEG placement. If a lesion is discovered that will require biopsy or some other therapy, this should be done after PEG placement.
7. Once the gastroscope is in the stomach, all residual fluid and food should be suctioned so that the stomach is completely empty. Occasionally, the standard-caliber endoscope cannot be passed beyond an esophageal stricture or tumor; use of a slim or ultrathin endoscope may be necessary. Rarely will esophageal dilation be required to advance the scope beyond an obstruction.

Identification of Percutaneous Endoscopic Gastrostomy Abdominal Insertion Site

8. Once the gastroscope is in the stomach, the second endoscopist (or trained assistant) can expose the anterior abdominal wall and carefully examine it for signs of transillumination. If necessary, the high light intensity feature on the light source can be used to help identify the insertion site. The assistant may also use a finger to palpate and indent the anterior abdominal wall; the endoscopist should then be able to visualize the

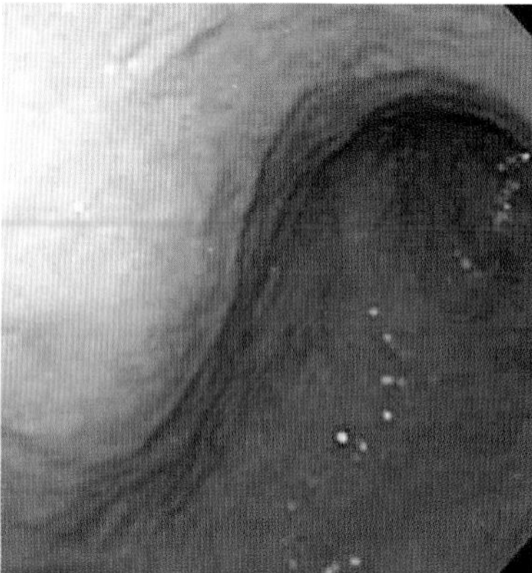

Figure 200-2 Endoscopic visualization of finger indentation.

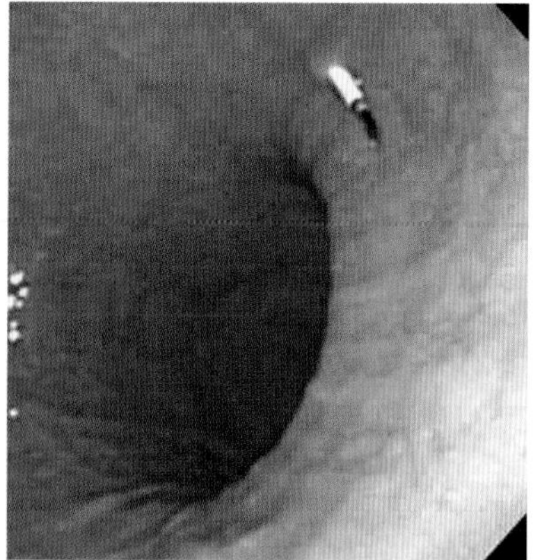

Figure 200-3 Introducer trocar visualized entering the gastric lumen.

corresponding indentation in the anterior wall of the stomach (Fig. 200-2).

NOTE: If a suitable site is not identifiable by either transillumination or finger palpation (preferably both), the procedure should be abandoned.

9. By convention, a PEG entry site is sought in the left upper quadrant of the abdomen, although a site to the right of midline is satisfactory as well. A site located a few centimeters below the costal margin will be more comfortable for the patient in the long run and will help prevent inadvertent laceration of the liver or spleen. Many endoscopists prefer a more distal site, in the anterior antrum. If the initial or subsequent plan is to convert the PEG to a jejunal enteral tube (PEG-J), an antral entry site will facilitate its advancement through the pylorus and beyond the ligament of Treitz, a measure found to minimize the risk of retrograde migration of the jejunostomy tube.
10. The assistant then prepares the anterior abdomen with an antiseptic solution, changes into sterile gloves, and covers the chosen site with a fenestrated sterile drape. Commercial PEG kits usually include a local anesthetic like lidocaine along with a syringe, a 22-gauge needle, and a 25-gauge needle. The anesthetic can be drawn up into the syringe using the 22-gauge needle and the smaller needle can be used to raise a skin wheal at the proposed entry site. The longer 22-gauge needle can then be reattached to the syringe.
11. As the assistant then passes the sounding needle through the abdominal wall into the stomach, the endoscopist watches for entry of the needle through the gastric wall. Some endoscopists recommend keeping slight negative pressure on the syringe plunger while the needle is advanced; if air enters the syringe before visualization of the needle in the gastric lumen, it can be presumed that the needle has entered another hollow viscus like the colon or a loop of small intestine. The needle is then withdrawn and another insertion site sought.

Percutaneous Endoscopic Gastrostomy Tube Placement

12. Once a suitable PEG insertion site has been identified, the assistant injects an additional 3 to 5 mL of anesthetic intradermally, and a no. 11 scalpel blade is used to make a horizontal or vertical skin incision.
13. While the assistant obtains the needle catheter from the PEG kit, the endoscopist can advance the snare catheter through the working channel of the gastroscope and into the gastric lumen.
14. The assistant then inserts the catheter rapidly through the skin incision and into the gastric lumen (Fig. 200-3), making certain that the catheter is directed at the same angle with respect to the skin as was just used with the sounding needle. This rapid "poke" should not be too slow or cautious; an assertive poke is necessary to ensure that the tip of the catheter successfully penetrates the tough gastric serosa instead of merely rebounding from the gastric wall.
15. As soon as the tip of the needle catheter enters the gastric lumen, the endoscopist snares it to hold it in place (Fig. 200-4). The assistant then withdraws the inner needle, leaving the outer plastic "introducer catheter" in place.

A. "PULL" TECHNIQUE. This is the most commonly used method of PEG placement, accounting for approximately 90% of PEGs.

16a. A looped guidewire is threaded through the catheter (Fig. 200-5) and this is grasped with the snare.
17a. The endoscope, along with snared guidewire, is withdrawn through the esophagus and out of the mouth under direct visualization.
18a. The looped guidewire is then released and looped to the wire guide for the gastrostomy tube included in the kit.
19a. The "skin" assistant pulls on the guidewire where it enters the abdominal wall to advance the gastrostomy tube through the esophagus and into the stomach.
20a. As the guidewire exits the abdominal incision, the tapered gastrostomy tip will follow. It should be advanced until the terminal bumper is snug against the anterior gastric wall.
21a. Finally, the assistant disconnects the looped guidewire from the gastrostomy tube assembly.

B. "PUSH" TECHNIQUE. Alternatively, the "push" (or Sacks-Vine) technique can be used.

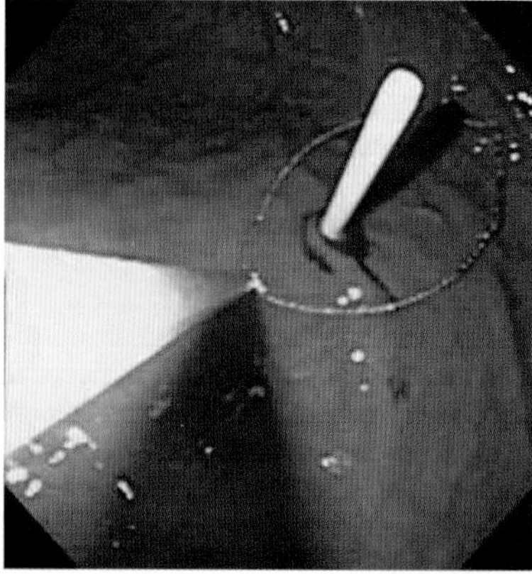

Figure 200-4 The snare is advanced through the working port of the gastroscope and here is seen looping around the introducer catheter.

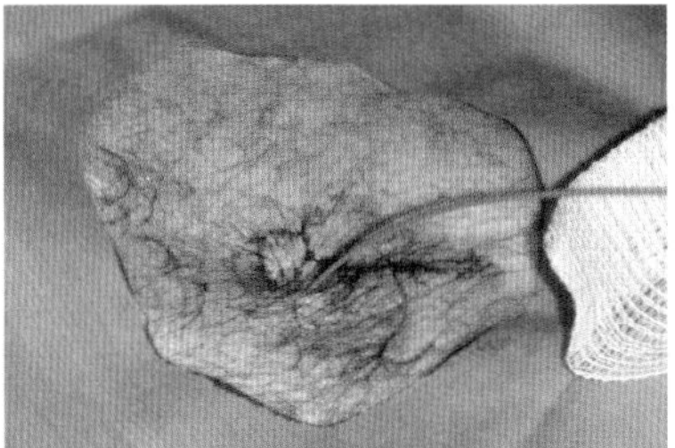

Figure 200-5 The guidewire is advanced through the introducer catheter and the catheter is subsequently removed.

16b. A standard (nonlooped) guidewire is threaded through the catheter (see Fig. 200-5) and grasped with the snare.
17b. The endoscope and snared guidewire assembly is withdrawn as a unit through the esophagus and out of the patient's mouth. Enough of the guidewire has to be threaded out of the mouth to enable the gastrostomy tube to be completely threaded over the guidewire (Fig. 200-6) so that it extends beyond the internal bolster on the proximal end.
18b. Both ends of the guidewire are then grasped in such a fashion as to create slight tension. The endoscopist maintains a firm grasp on this proximal end of the guidewire while the "skin" assistant maintains control of the abdominal end.
19b. The endoscopist then advances the gastrostomy tube over the taut guidewire, pushing the internal bolster into the patient's mouth until the dilating tip protrudes through the abdominal wall.
20b. The assistant then pulls the gastrostomy tube through the abdominal wall until the internal bolster is snug against the anterior gastric wall.
21b. Finally, the guidewire is removed from the abdominal end.

Postprocedure Endoscopy

22. The endoscope is reinserted after the gastrostomy has been pulled or pushed into place. This allows careful examination of the esophagus, stomach, and visible surrounding structures for any mucosal or other trauma caused during the procedure as well as confirmation of proper placement of the internal bolster adjacent to the anterior gastric wall (Fig. 200-7). A photograph is taken and any necessary biopsies are performed at this time.

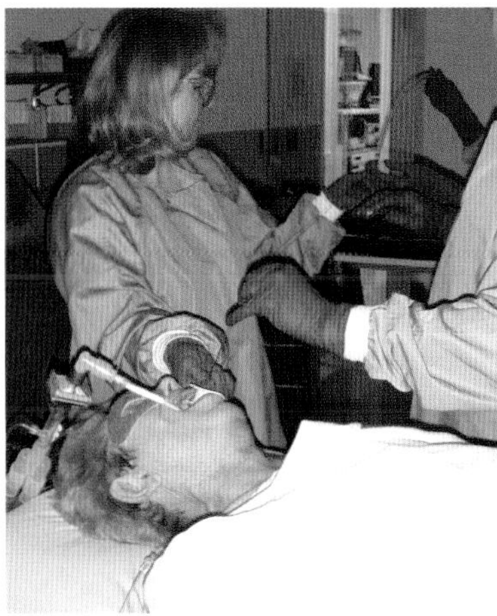

Figure 200-6 Threading the "push" percutaneous endoscopic gastrostomy tube over the guidewire.

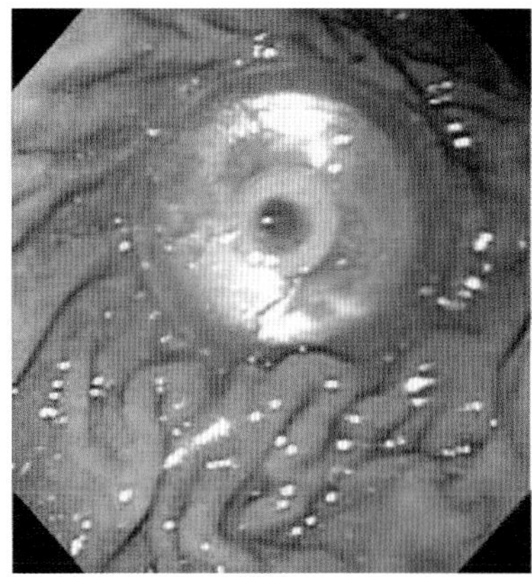

Figure 200-7 Endoscopic photograph of proper placement of internal bolster.

Post-Percutaneous Endoscopic Gastrostomy Placement

23. Once appropriate positioning of the internal bolster is confirmed, the endoscope is removed and an external bolster is slipped into place with the aid of some lubricant applied to the protruding gastrostomy tube.

    NOTE: Extra care must be taken when placing the external bolster to make sure it is not too tight. This will prevent such complications as PEG site infection, tissue necrosis, PEG entry site leakage, and "buried bumper syndrome" (see section on Postprocedure and Late Complications). Optimal external bumper placement allows the clinician's gloved index finger to slip easily between the abdominal entry site and the bumper.

24. If necessary, trim excess PEG tubing with scissors, leaving enough tubing to be looped around and taped to the skin of the abdomen, about 13 to 15 cm. This is also an ideal length to allow a jejunal tube to be inserted through the PEG and advanced beyond the ligament of Treitz, if necessary.
25. After a few minutes have passed, allowing the stomach to decompress from air introduced during the procedure, a feeding adapter is placed into the external end of the PEG tube.
26. The PEG site is then cleaned with soap and water and a split 4 × 4 gauze sponge placed around the PEG tube but *over* the external bolster. This dressing is not placed under the bolster because this will only cause more pressure on the healing wound. Dressings are changed daily and the wound is kept clean until complete healing has occurred. Dressings are changed as needed thereafter (Fig. 200-8).
27. Orders should be written to initiate tube feedings, medication administration, and tube irrigation 4 hours after placement.

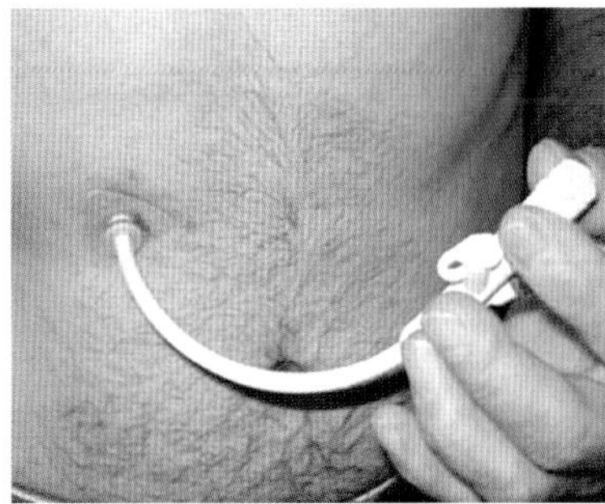

Figure 200-8 Final result with percutaneous endoscopic gastrostomy tube in place after tract has healed completely.

Special Considerations

Patients with unresected esophageal or oropharyngeal malignancies deserve special consideration; using either the "pull" or "push" technique raises the potential for seeding the abdominal wall with tumor cells. This is particularly true of oropharyngeal tumors. In many cases, long-term survival is not expected so the PEG can be placed in the usual fashion. If the PEG is to be placed for nutritional support before the planned tumor resection and there is a chance for long-term survival or cure, some endoscopists recommend the Russel or "introducer" method using a dilator with a peel-away sheath. This technique uses the Seldinger technique and fluoroscopy for placing an inflatable gastrostomy tube with a internal balloon bolster. The endoscope is used for direct visualization as well as to provide mucosal counterpressure during PEG insertion. The balloon tip is then inflated and an external bolster placed to secure the device. Advantages include the low risk of direct contamination of the tract with oral flora or malignant cells as well as a single passage of the gastroscope during the procedure and the avoidance of mucosal injury by the PEG tube during transesophageal passage (Vargo and Ponsky, 2000).

Obese patients present a special challenge. Transillumination of the abdominal wall may not be successful and the thickness of the subcutaneous layer may preclude successful sounding of the gastric lumen with the 1½-inch, 22-gauge needle. In this case, the PEG entry site can be identified by finger palpation alone, the skin and subcutaneous tissue anesthetized with lidocaine, and a transverse incision made with the scalpel down through the subcutaneous layer to the fascia. Transillumination should be possible at the base of the incision. Use of the high light intensity feature may be necessary and the stomach is then sounded with the 22-gauge needle, with additional local anesthetic provided for the patient's comfort.

Prior abdominal surgery is not an absolute contraindication to PEG placement but a PEG entry site should be found that is away from the surgical scar. Careful sounding can be performed using the technique described previously to identify an interposed air-filled viscus. If air enters the syringe before the sounding needle is seen in the gastric lumen by the endoscopist, the procedure should be aborted. Otherwise, a safe tract is confirmed by endoscopic visualization of the intragastric needle tip and concurrent aspiration of air from the syringe.

TECHNIQUE

Replacement

Perhaps more commonly than placing a PEG tube, primary care clinicians may be called on to replace one. This may be due to the PEG becoming dislodged (which is more common in confused or uncooperative patients) or nonfunctional (due to blockage or obstruction, fracture, or leaking). Techniques for attempting to clear blockage are discussed in a following section. Partial dislodgement presents a unique diagnostic challenge and can present as pain, buried bumper syndrome, or PEG tube blockage. Diagnostic approaches are also described for those complications in the section on Postprocedure and Late Complications. The management approach depends on the timing of dislodgement because the gastrocutaneous tract takes about 4 weeks to heal and mature. Therefore, as much information as possible should be gathered about the existing or prior PEG tube, especially regarding the procedure used to place the PEG, how long ago it was placed, and the type of PEG and internal bolster.

Dislodged Percutaneous Endoscopic Gastrostomy, Closed Mature Tract (≥4 Weeks after Placement)

Depending on the age, maturation, and diameter of the PEG, tracts begin to close as soon as the tube is removed; therefore, every effort should be made to replace a dislodged PEG tube as soon as possible. A lost tract may require a repeat procedure. Dilation of a closing PEG tract has been described using filiform catheters and followers adapted from urology (see Chapter 110, Bladder Catheterization [and Urethral Dilation]); however, consultation with a gastroenterologist or surgeon may be beneficial.

Dislodged Percutaneous Endoscopic Gastrostomy, Open Mature Tract (≥4 Weeks after Placement)

1. If the original PEG tube is in good condition, after the balloon is deflated it can simply be reinserted. Alternatively, a Foley catheter of similar diameter can be used. Either tube will act as a stent until a permanent replacement can be found.
2. Lubrication should be applied liberally to the tube being used for replacement, and it should then be gently inserted through the existing tract. This can be done without endoscopy.

   NOTE: Do not advance the tube against significant resistance; advancement against anything more than mild resistance can result in complications. Replacement should be painless and not require dissection or force. If these conditions occur, the procedure should be aborted.

3. Make sure that the balloon is well within the gastric lumen, and then slowly and carefully reinflate it with saline. Gentle external traction on the PEG tube should then be used to draw the balloon snugly against the anterior gastric wall. Plans for a permanent replacement PEG tube can then be made.

   NOTE: Inflation of the balloon within the gastrocutaneous tract can result in pain, hemorrhage, disruption of the tract, and even peritonitis.

4. Unless changes are deemed necessary, a permanent replacement PEG tube, often found in a commercial kit, should be similar in diameter and function to the original. Placement of a low-profile PEG tube (see Fig. 200-1) may prevent recurrence of dislodgement. Alternatively, a standard PEG tube can be used and an abdominal binder placed to prevent the patient from pulling the tube out again.
5. After any replacement, aspirate gastric contents with a large syringe or use gravity drainage of gastric contents to confirm placement. After the balloon is reinflated, pull the catheter snug to lodge the internal bolster against the anterior gastric wall, immediately behind the anterior abdominal wall. If there was any difficulty with replacement of the PEG tube, or if the return of gastric contents is equivocal, a water-soluble contrast study should be obtained before resuming feedings. This will also ensure proper positioning of the internal bolster. A small amount of water-soluble, radiopaque contrast material is injected through the PEG tube, and a flat plate radiograph of the abdomen obtained. It should show intraluminal distribution of the contrast material.

   NOTE: If the patient is known to have a jejunostomy tube, after stenting the tract with a replacement catheter, more information should be obtained before resuming feeding.

6. Perhaps more important than for the original PEG tube, unless a low-profile version is used (see Fig. 200-1), special attention should be paid to securing the external bolster for a replacement PEG. After bolstering, the catheter should be at approximately 90 degrees to the skin and anterior abdominal wall. It should be fixated to prevent internal migration of the catheter. Initially, 4 × 4 gauze sponges can be stacked several inches to create a pyramid-shaped dressing and taped to the skin and PEG catheter. Another temporary option is to use the same equipment provided to secure a nasogastric tube. However, temporary bolsters should usually be converted to a more permanent bolster. One option is to wrap a short (3-cm) segment of latex tubing (cut from another Foley catheter or nasogastric tube) around the base of the PEG tube and secure it with a plastic cable tie. This short segment should be wrapped perpendicularly around the PEG tube at the

skin level, and the resultant friction between the tubes should prevent PEG slippage or migration. Alternatively, a T-bar can be made from such a short segment by folding it in half and cutting small nicks from the two folded corners. After unfolding the segment, the tip of a hemostat can be inserted through the resulting two diamond-shaped holes, and across the short segment. The hemostat can then be used to grasp the distal end of the PEG tube and draw it through the T-bar. Make sure the diamond-shaped holes are large enough to avoid compressing the PEG tube lumen. The T-bar can then be drawn to the appropriate location on the PEG tube, approximately 0.5 to 1 cm from the skin surface, to act as a bolster. Placing a suture in a manner similar to that used to secure a chest tube may also be effective. Take a large bite of skin adjacent to the PEG exit site; tie a loose square knot at skin level, and then wrap the loose ends of the remaining suture several times in opposite directions around the PEG tube, finally securing the suture to the PEG tube in a snug fashion with another knot. The resultant tube fixation should be firm but allow some slack to prevent pressure necrosis if the patient changes position.

7. After placement is confirmed and the PEG tube is bolstered, the end of the tube should be clamped, capped, or fitted with the appropriate feeding adapter.

Dislodged Percutaneous Endoscopic Gastrostomy, Immature Tract (<4 Weeks after Placement)

Management of early dislodgement (<4 weeks) is different. The stomach may have separated from the anterior abdominal wall, resulting in free perforation with spillage of gastric contents, peritonitis, fever, or sepsis. In this event, broad-spectrum antibiotics should be administered, a nasogastric tube placed, and surgical consultation obtained. If the stomach has not separated from the anterior abdominal wall, a PEG tube can be replaced endoscopically, either through the same site or through a new one. Alternatively, the tract may be allowed to close spontaneously and a replacement PEG placed in 7 to 10 days if the patient remains stable.

Nonfunctioning Percutaneous Endoscopic Gastrostomy Needing Replacement

Again, as much information as possible should be gathered about the existing PEG tube, especially regarding the procedure used to place the PEG, how long ago it was placed, and the type of PEG and internal bolster.

1. If the PEG has a balloon for an internal bolster, deflation of the balloon should allow removal and replacement. If the balloon will not deflate, which is not unusual in long-standing PEG tubes, the inflation port may be clogged or damaged. Careful insertion of a guidewire into the balloon port may unclog it. If this attempt is unsuccessful, slightly further insertion of the guidewire may rupture the balloon. Alternatively, the balloon can be drawn close to the anterior abdominal wall by putting tension on the PEG tube. A needle inserted through the PEG tube can then be used to rupture the balloon. If these fail, endoscopic rupture of the balloon may be necessary. Another option is to cut the PEG tube close to the ports, which may allow the balloon to deflate on its own. After cutting, a firm external grip must be maintained with a clamp or hemostat on the portion of PEG tube remaining within the patient to prevent migration down the gastrointestinal tract; such migration may require endoscopic or surgical retrieval. If the PEG tube gets away and migrates, the majority of tubes will pass the gastrointestinal tract without incident and they can often be followed with plain radiographs every 48 hours, but there are reported cases of bowel obstruction and perforation. Endoscopic or surgical retrieval may be necessary for hardware that does not pass within 2 to 3 weeks or if the patient experiences obstructive symptoms. The risk of obstruction increases in children younger than 6 years of age or weighing less than 40 kg.
2. If the type of internal bolster cannot be determined or if it is thought to be soft or pliable, the application of constant, gentle external traction often results in PEG removal. Most PEGs can be removed in this manner.

NOTE: Never apply more than gentle traction when attempting to remove a PEG tube; either the internal bolster has become imbedded in the gastric wall or it was not intended to be removed externally and will likely need to be removed endoscopically.

COMPLICATIONS

Although deaths are not often directly attributable to the procedure, perioperative and postprocedure survival after PEG placement is exceedingly poor. In one study of 714 patients, 5.6% of patients died within 7 days of the procedure, whereas 22%, 31%, and 48% were dead at 30 days, 60 days, and 1 year from the procedure, respectively. The primary hospitalization mortality rate was 11%, with 50% of these patients dying within 1 week of PEG placement. Preprocedure predictors of mortality include older age, hemodialysis, mechanical ventilation, cancer, and coronary artery disease. Median survival for patients older than 70 years of age was less than 6 months, with length of survival decreasing rapidly with older age (Smith and colleagues, 2008).

It is important to emphasize to patients and caregivers that studies suggest PEG placement does not significantly alter survival. On retrospective review, many patients could have been fed or hydrated through a nasogastric tube until recovery or death. Thus, when obtaining informed consent, it is essential that the clinician emphasize both the direct technical risks of the PEG as well as the anticipated natural course of the patient's underlying medical condition(s). This being said, complications can be discussed in three categories: (1) complications of upper endoscopy, (2) direct complications of PEG placement, and (3) postprocedure complications.

Complications Associated with Endoscopy

The most common complications associated with endoscopy include aspiration, hypoxemia, hypotension, acute myocardial infarction, hemorrhage, and esophageal perforation. The cardiopulmonary complications are actually primarily related to conscious sedation. Refer to the respective chapters for a full discussion, including prevention, identification, and treatment. Reported mortality rates for upper endoscopy are exceedingly low, on the order of 0.005% to 0.01%, but these studies primarily include healthy patients, not the severely debilitated and poorly nourished patients requiring PEG feeding tubes. However, because the complications are serious, a careful and complete discussion with the patient or legal guardian before the procedure is essential.

Direct Complications of Percutaneous Endoscopic Gastrostomy Placement and Replacement (to a Lesser Degree)

- *Pneumoperitoneum:* This finding is very common (35% to 50% incidence) and usually follows a benign course. It results from air escaping from the stomach during the course of a prolonged EGD during PEG placement, possibly compounded by multiple abdominal needle punctures and excessive air insufflation. Conservative management is usually acceptable. If the patient develops signs of increasing intra-abdominal air, sepsis, peritonitis, a systemic inflammatory response, or air in the portal or mesenteric veins, surgical consultation will be necessary (Vargo and Ponsky, 2000).
- *Abdominal wall bleeding:* This is usually identified soon after PEG placement and is caused by nicking or puncturing an abdominal wall blood vessel. Risk can be minimized by avoiding a tract near the midline through the rectus abdominis muscle. Hemostasis can often be obtained by tightening the external bolster against the abdominal wall to provide compression. Care must be taken to

loosen the bolster again within 48 hours to prevent skin and mucosal maceration and ulceration. If bleeding is significant, standard resuscitative measures should be used. A standard "crash cart" should always be immediately available whenever an endoscopic procedure is performed.

- *Intraperitoneal and retroperitoneal bleeding:* Symptoms and signs that this has occurred include hypotension, decreasing hemoglobin or hematocrit, abdominal pain, a rigid abdomen, and an absence of blood seen endoscopically. It can occur from laceration of the liver, spleen, or a deep blood vessel. Diagnosis is confirmed by computed tomography (CT) imaging and treatment is by immediate surgery. Surgical consultation with possible evacuation of the hemoperitoneum, repair of any solid organ injury, control of bleeding, and revision of the gastrostomy is indicated.
- *Colon injury:* Prior abdominal surgery or anatomic variation may result in the transverse colon being displaced over the anterior gastric wall. Careful attention to the special instructions provided previously will minimize this complication. The usual presentation is peritonitis and the appropriate intervention is usually intravenous antibiotics and surgery. Occasionally, nonoperative management can be considered if the patient is hemodynamically stable and there are no signs of sepsis.
- *Hepatic injury:* This complication has been described only rarely and can be prevented by careful attention to the precautionary steps during placement. Close observation is often all that is necessary unless there is associated hemorrhage.
- *Splenic injury:* Splenic perforation or rupture has never been reported with PEG placement but has occurred rarely with other upper endoscopic procedures. It should be suspected if the patient develops hypotension or abdominal pain and resuscitation should immediately be initiated intravenously with crystalloid solution until blood is available. If the patient is hemodynamically stable, confirmation can be made by CT. Immediate surgical consultation with laparotomy and splenectomy is necessary if the patient becomes unstable.
- *Small bowel injury:* Small bowel perforation is often occult and difficult to diagnose early. Fortunately, this complication is rare because the small intestine is protected by the greater omentum, which prevents it from migrating into the upper abdomen. However, if the patient has postoperative adhesions or the omentum has been previously resected, this injury can occur. It becomes clinically significant if there is intra-abdominal leakage and consequent peritonitis or if an enterocutaneous fistula develops. Fistulas often come to light only after the PEG is manipulated or replaced.
- *Gastro-colo-cutaneous fistula:* This is a rare complication of PEG placement and occurs when the PEG is inserted directly through the lumen of the large bowel into the stomach, usually near the splenic flexure. The patient may have transient ileus or fever but often remains asymptomatic for months, the diagnosis being made only after gastrostomy tube replacement. In most cases, there is no evidence of stool leakage or fistula formation. If the replacement tube is inserted into the colon rather than the stomach, diarrhea becomes evident when feedings are restarted. This complication is prevented by careful attention to the details outlined in the Technique section. Good transillumination and finger palpation are paramount to avoidance. The diagnosis is made radiographically by introducing contrast through the PEG tube. Most can be managed nonsurgically by removing the PEG and allowing the fistula to close spontaneously. A surgeon can be consulted if an abscess forms or peritonitis develops.

Postprocedure and Late Complications Related to Percutaneous Endoscopic Gastrostomy Placement and Replacement

- *Pain at the PEG site:* This complication is also the primary presenting symptom of many of the complications listed in the following. Careful attention to proper technique during PEG placement and proper cleanliness and care after placement are essential to preventing pain and discomfort. An attentive and prudent diagnostic approach to uncover the cause of pain will usually be rewarded.
- *PEG tube blockage or obstruction:* This problem is extremely common, occurring in up to 45% of patients. Prevention is the key, with liberal PEG tube flushing using 30 to 60 mL of water every 4 hours with a large syringe. This should also be performed after feeding and medication administration, as well as after checking residual volumes. Saline solutions should be avoided because the salt tends to crystallize in the channel and gradually form a blockage. Liquid formulations of medication are preferred and bulking agents such as psyllium seed and resins like cholestyramine should be avoided. A variety of treatments are effective in unclogging PEG tubes. Plain warm water has been shown to be the best irrigant, with carbonated beverages also proving effective. Pancreatic enzymes mixed with bicarbonate have been effective for dissolving more resistant proteinaceous blockages, the solution being allowed to sit in the tube for several hours before flushing copiously with warm water. If these methods prove ineffective, commercially available plastic brushes can be used to manually clear the tube. Wires and metal brushes should be avoided because of risk of perforation. Endoscopic snares, biopsy forceps, or Fogarty catheters have been used successfully; however, consultation with a gastroenterologist or surgeon may be helpful. Before any of these maneuvers, make sure the tube is not kinked at the bolster; merely unkinking it may correct the blockage.

NOTE: Do not force irrigation fluid into the PEG tube because it may rupture and injure the patient.

- *Abscess and wound infection:* Peristomal wound infection is common in patients not receiving perioperative antibiotics. The incidence is 18% and can be reduced to about 3% with appropriate antibiotic prophylaxis. MRSA has emerged as a significant pathogen, and at least one study has shown that nasopharyngeal decontamination before planned PEG insertion can result in a significant reduction in the incidence of wound infections (Horiuchi and colleagues, 2006). If the patient has been hospitalized or institutionalized for a prolonged period or if there is any suspicion of colonization, a nasopharyngeal culture and sensitivity should be performed. A 10-day course of an appropriate antibiotic (trimethoprim/sulfamethoxazole, clindamycin, or vancomycin) is recommended before PEG placement. A confirmatory test to ensure MRSA eradication should be performed before the procedure.
- *Peristomal leakage:* This is a very common and significant problem that is often seen in patients with diabetes, immunodeficiency, and malnutrition. Other factors that have been implicated include wound infection, peristomal abscess, hypersecretory syndromes, traction on the PEG tube, and buried bumper syndrome. Treatment is aimed at correcting these underlying conditions as well as using barrier creams such as zinc oxide. If hypersecretion is thought to be a contributing factor, agents like hyoscyamine or glycopyrrolate can be administered. Replacing the PEG tube with a tube of larger diameter should be avoided because this frequently only exacerbates the problem. If all else fails, the PEG tube can be removed for a few days, any infection treated, and the tract allowed to heal, scar, and partially close before a new tube is placed. Alternatively, the PEG tube can be removed completely and a new PEG site chosen.
- *Diarrhea:* Diarrhea is common among patients receiving enteral feeding, occurring in 10% to 20% of patients. The possible causes are manifold, including infection, protein malnutrition, medications, and administration of hyperosmolar enteral solutions. Patients can also have other dietary contributors, including lactose intolerance, fat malabsorption, or celiac disease. Common pharmaceutical culprits include magnesium-containing antacids,

proton pump inhibitors (PPIs), antibiotics, prokinetic agents like metoclopramide, and hyperosmolar drug solutions. Management involves identifying the etiology and treating the patient accordingly. Protein malnutrition may require nutritional supplementation and delivery of isotonic feedings in the interim. Discontinuing unnecessary medications, using intravenous alternatives, and changing to a different brand or class of medication are all useful strategies. Antidiarrheals like loperamide are useful for some patients with medication-associated diarrhea. It is important to rule out pseudomembranous colitis and the rare cases of enterocutaneous fistula if diarrhea persists in spite of standard diagnostic and therapeutic measures.

- *Gastrointestinal bleeding and ulceration:* Gastrointestinal bleeding is a relatively infrequent late complication and occurs in about 2% of patients. It is caused by esophagitis, peptic ulcer disease, gastric pressure ulcers, and, rarely, erosion of the PEG tube into a gastric wall blood vessel. Once endoscopic diagnosis is determined, bleeding caused by a punctured gastroepiploic vessel in the stomach wall can be treated by tightening the external bolster against the abdominal wall, thus internally compressing the bleeding vessel. Care should be taken to loosen the bumper again within 48 hours to prevent pressure necrosis. Esophagitis and peptic ulcers can both be prevented and treated with PPIs; histamine type 2 receptor antagonists have not been noted to be very effective, especially in the former case. Gastric pressure ulcers are caused by the PEG tube and can occur either anteriorly, from direct pressure of the internal bolster, or posteriorly, caused by tall internal bolsters or protruding tips from Foley-type PEG tubes. Treatment is removal of the offending tube and replacement, which can often be done nearby (Fig. 200-9). Use of a low-profile device or a balloon-tipped device with a short (<3 mm) protruding tip for the replacement may minimize risk of recurrence. Use of a PPI alone will often be insufficient to heal these ulcers.
- *Ileus and gastroparesis:* Occasionally, postprocedure gastroparesis develops and can take longer than the usual 3 to 4 hours to resolve. Metoclopramide, erythromycin, or domperidone can be administered with good results in most cases. However, if persistent vomiting or abdominal distention occurs, the PEG should be unclamped to allow decompression and feedings should be discontinued for 24 to 48 hours. If abdominal distention and pain persist, an ileus should be suspected and perforation and peritonitis need to be ruled out. Often the cause is merely excessive pneumoperitoneum from the PEG procedure. Treatment often consists of nasogastric tube decompression, discontinuance of contributing medications, and clinical support. Intravenous broad-spectrum antibiotics and surgical consultation may be required if perforation is suspected.
- *Aspiration:* The risk of aspiration during the PEG procedure has already been discussed. The risk of aspiration, however, is much greater as a late complication and increases with supine positioning, use of sedative agents, advanced age, and neurologic impairment. Unfortunately, these are precisely the risk factors that predispose patients to need PEG placement. Again, prevention is superior to treating the sequelae of aspiration. The primary clinician is advised to avoid excessive use of sedative agents and the patient/caretaker is instructed to keep the head of the bed elevated for several hours after feedings.
- *Gastric outlet obstruction:* The presenting complaint is usually intermittent vomiting or upper abdominal cramping and the cause is generally distal migration of the PEG tube. It is much more common with Foley-type gastrostomy tubes with the balloon lodging in the pyloric channel or duodenum, creating an intermittent obstruction. In children, a displaced internal bolster can get wedged in the gastric outlet. Prevention is the best approach by ensuring proper placement of the external bolster. Diagnosis can be made by an upper gastrointestinal series or endoscopically. With the Foley-type tube, the balloon can be deflated and the tube repositioned and reinflated with proper external bolster positioning.
- *Buried bumper syndrome:* This is a rare (1% to 2%) but potentially serious complication that occurs late after PEG insertion, after an average of 4 months, but reported from 2 months to 7 years after PEG placement (Schrag and colleagues, 2007). The internal bumper retracts into the anterior gastric wall (Fig. 200-10) and becomes lodged at some point along the gastrocutaneous tract, resulting in either a partial or complete PEG obstruction. The gastric mucosa can completely reepithelialize the internal stoma, resulting in an inability to infuse feedings or medication. This is the usual presenting complaint, along with abdominal pain at the PEG site. Diagnosis can be made radiologically, endoscopically, by ultrasonography, or by endoscopic ultrasonography. The buried bumper should be removed regardless of whether the patient is symptomatic. Removal can be achieved surgically, endoscopically, or through a combination of approaches. Use of a needle knife through the biopsy port of the endoscope has been

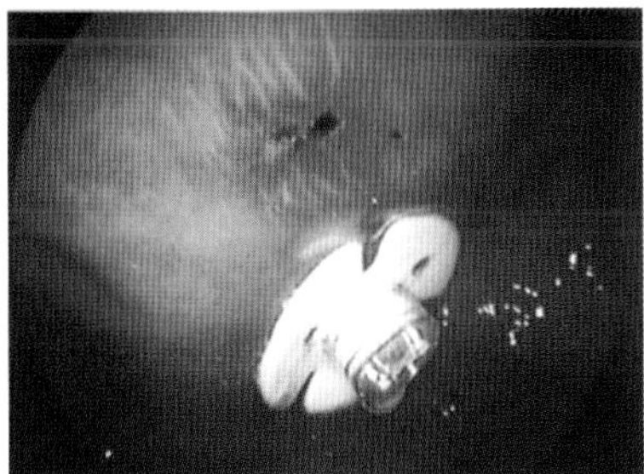

Figure 200-9 Healing pressure ulcer at previous percutaneous endoscopic gastrostomy (PEG) site with PEG tube placed at new site.

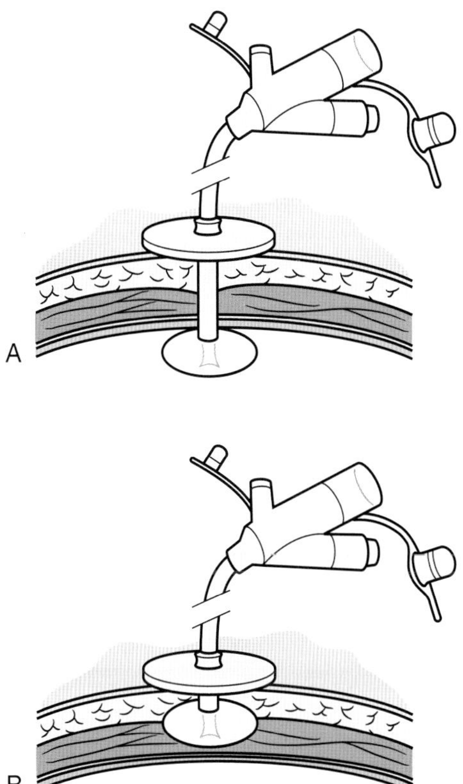

Figure 200-10 Buried bumper syndrome. **A,** Proper percutaneous endoscopic gastrostomy tube placement. **B,** Buried bumper with regrowth of gastric mucosa over gastrocutaneous tract.

found to be effective. A mucosal incision is made over the buried bumper to allow its mobilization and removal. A fresh PEG tube can then be inserted under endoscopic guidance. Occasionally, a more extensive surgical procedure is required.

- *Necrotizing fasciitis:* As noted earlier, pressure from the PEG tube and external bumper on the peristomal site can lead to this lethal complication. Patients who are diabetic, malnourished, or otherwise immunocompromised are predisposed and at increased risk, as are those with wound infections. Prevention is by proper placement and adequate spacing of the external bolster. There is good evidence that multiple aerobic and anaerobic organisms are synergistically responsible for necrotizing fasciitis. Treatment involves wide surgical débridement, broad-spectrum antibiotics, and planned operative reevaluation. Patients require transfer to the intensive care unit with extensive multisystem support.
- *PEG site herniation:* This complication has been reported only once in the literature and was a late sequela of deep ulceration. The diagnosis should be suspected whenever there is a peristomal bulge noted with Valsalva maneuver. It is confirmed by CT and repair, if indicated, is surgical.
- *Volvulus around PEG tube:* This rare complication is seen primarily in the pediatric population and can involve the small intestine, transverse colon, or stomach. It is more common if the PEG is introduced through the posterior wall of the stomach, which can lead to rotation of the gut and consequent volvulus. Prevention is by careful attention to placing the PEG through the anterior wall of the stomach with proper external bolster placement in order to achieve close apposition of the anterior gastric wall to the parietal peritoneum. Treatment requires surgical consultation with exploratory laparotomy, reduction of the volvulus, and repositioning of the gastrostomy. Gastropexy to the anterior abdominal wall may decrease the incidence of recurrence.
- *Tumor implantation in PEG tract:* As already mentioned, this late complication is extremely rare, occurring primarily in patients with oropharyngeal tumors and in less than 1% of this group. Direct seeding during the PEG placement is the accepted primary mechanism, although hematogenous or lymphatic spread is also thought to occur. This complication offers an exceedingly poor prognosis, with a 0% 1-year survival. Placement of the PEG after primary tumor resection or by using the Russell technique (nonendoscopic, using a peel-away catheter) is a reasonable approach to lowering the risk of seeding (Cruz and colleagues, 2005).
- *PEG tubes and pregnancy:* PEG tubes can be used successfully during pregnancy, although persistent emesis has been reported. Conversion of the PEG to a PEG-J may be attempted and has been reported to be successful in this condition (Wejda and colleagues, 2003).

Postprocedure Care

The external visible portion of the PEG tube can be cleaned with soap and water using a clean 4 × 4 sponge. Antibacterial ointment is not required and could result in inflammation caused by an allergy to one of the ingredients. A split 4 × 4 tracheostomy sponge is then placed *over* the external bolster—*not* between the bolster and the skin, which will cause excessive compression of the skin of the abdominal wall and possibly result in ostomy breakdown or buried bumper syndrome. The PEG tube is then looped back over the bolster and taped to the skin. If the patient is confused or unreliable, an abdominal binder can be placed to prevent manipulation and inadvertent removal of the tube. After 6 to 8 weeks, when the gastrocutaneous tract has healed and matured, the PEG can be removed and replaced with a low-profile device (see Fig. 200-1). This device is level with the skin with no permanent tubing extending from the abdominal wall, thus minimizing the opportunity for the patient to dislodge it.

Dressings over the PEG site are changed daily until there is no longer any drainage. The tube and ostomy site can be cleansed daily or as needed with soap and warm water, taking care to débride excessive granulation tissue and dried secretions. Tube feeding, medication administration, and water flushes can be initiated 4 hours after placement. An example of postprocedure orders is provided online at www.expertconsult.com.

Patient Education Guides

The following materials are available online at www.expertconsult.com:

- Sample post-PEG procedure instructions
- Sample patient consent form
- Also see the patient education handouts for Chapter 2, Sedation and Analgesia, and Chapter 101, Esophagogastroduodenoscopy.

CPT/Billing Codes

36000	Introduction of needle or intracatheter, vein
43234	Simple upper gastrointestinal endoscopy examination
43235	EGD, diagnostic, with or without brushings
43239	EGD, diagnostic, with biopsies
43246	EGD with directed placement of PEG tube
43760	Change of gastrostomy tube
94761	Noninvasive pulse oximetry for oxygen saturation; multiple determinations
96365	IV therapy, initial, up to 1 hour
96367	IV therapy each additional hour
96374	IV push, single or initial substance/drug
96376	IV push, each sequential new substance/drug

ICD-9-CM Diagnostic Codes

150.3	Ca, esophagus, upper third
150.4	Ca, esophagus, middle third
150.5	Ca, esophagus, lower third
260	Malignant malnutrition
263.9	Malnutrition, protein-calorie
520.3	Esophageal stricture
530.2	Esophageal ulcer
530.10	Esophagitis, unspecified
530.11	Esophagitis, reflux
530.12	Acute esophagitis
530.81	Esophageal reflux

Suppliers

(See contact information online at www.expertconsult.com.)

FASTRAC "Pull" Gastric Access Port Kit
Bard Access Systems, Inc.

Gastroscopes
Fujinon Corp.
Olympus Corp.
Pentax Corp.

Patient education materials
American Society for Gastrointestinal Endoscopy
Bard Access Systems, Inc.
Wilson-Cook Medical Inc.

Bibliography

Cosby KS: Gastrostomy tube replacement. In Reichman E, Simon R (eds): Emergency Medicine Procedures. New York, McGraw-Hill, 2004, pp 456–466.

Cruz I, Mamel JJ, Brady PG, Cass-Garcia M: Incidence of abdominal wall metastasis complicating PEG tube placement in untreated head and neck cancer. Gastrointest Endosc 62:708–711, 2005.

DeLegge MH: The experts corner: Percutaneous endoscopic gastrostomy. Am J Gastoenterol 102:2620–2623, 2007.

Dormann AJ, Huchzermeyer H: Endoscopic techniques for enteral nutrition: Standards and innovations. Dig Dis 20:145–153, 2002.

Gauderer MWL, Ponsky JL, Izant RJ Jr: Gastrostomy without laparotomy: A percutaneous endoscopic technique. J Pediatr Surg 15:872–875, 1980.

Horiuchi A, Nakayama Y, Kajiyama M, et al: Nasopharyngeal decolonization of methicillin-resistant *Staphylococcus aureus* can reduce PEG peristomal wound infection. Am J Gastroenterol 101:274–277, 2006.

Schrag SP, Sharma R, Jaik NP, et al: Complications related to percutaneous endoscopic gastrostomy (PEG) tubes: A comprehensive clinical review. J Gastrointest Liver Dis 16:407–418, 2007.

Smith BM, Perring P, Engoren M, Sferra JJ: Hospital and long-term outcome after percutaneous endoscopic gastrostomy. Surg Endosc 22:74–80, 2008.

Vargo JJ, Ponsky JL: Percutaneous endoscopic gastrostomy: Clinical applications. Medscape General Medicine 2(4), 2000. Available at www.medscape.com/viewarticle/407957.

Wejda BU, Soennichsen B, Huchzermeyer H, et al: Successful jejunal nutrition therapy in a pregnant patient with apallic syndrome. Clin Nutr 22:209–211, 2003.

CHAPTER 201

Abdominal Paracentesis

Eric Skye

Paracentesis, or an "abdominal tap," is an important clinical procedure for primary care clinicians. With the advent of new radiologic and minimally invasive techniques, diagnosis of intra-abdominal pathology has generally become less invasive. Nevertheless, paracentesis is the diagnostic test of choice in patients who have new-onset ascites, in patients with suspected malignant ascites, and to rule out infection in those with preexisting ascites. In addition, therapeutic large-volume paracentesis (>4 L) remains an important treatment option for many patients, particularly those with diuretic-resistant ascites. If ultrasonography is available for guidance, it simplifies this procedure and decreases the risk of complications (see Chapter 225, Emergency Department, Hospitalist, and Office Ultrasonography [Clinical Ultrasonography]).

Anatomy

Abdominal anatomy must be considered when performing paracentesis. Large volumes of ascitic fluid tend to float the air-filled bowel anteriorly and toward the midline when the patient is in the supine position. Other pelvic organs that must be considered include an overly distended bladder and a gravid uterus. In addition, the cecum is relatively fixed and less mobile than the sigmoid colon; thus, bowel perforation is more likely to occur in the right lower quadrant than in the left. Traditionally, the procedure has been performed through the linea alba using a midline insertion 2 cm below the umbilicus with the patient in a semiupright position (Fig. 201-1). Increasingly, a lateral approach has been advocated, with access 3 to 5 cm medial and cranial to the anterior superior iliac spine (Fig. 201-2). Using this approach, one must remain lateral to the rectus sheath to avoid the inferior epigastric artery. Paracentesis can be performed with the patient in the supine position or in the lateral decubitus position (or slight variants of these), which helps "float" the bowel away from the insertion site and can provide access to a deeper ascitic pool.

Indications

Diagnostic

- New-onset ascites
- Suspected malignant ascites
- Rule out infection (consider for all hospitalized patients with known ascites)

Therapeutic

- Temporary relief of tense ascites (causing gastrointestinal or cardiorespiratory symptoms such as pain or dyspnea)
- Symptom relief in patients with diuretic-resistant ascites

Contraindications

Absolute

- Acute abdomen requiring immediate surgery (and even in this situation, paracentesis may be performed by the surgeon at the time of surgery)
- Coagulopathy when there is evidence of disseminated intravascular coagulation (DIC) or fibrinolysis

Relative

- Current bowel obstruction or severe bowel distention (consider ultrasonographic guidance; see Chapter 225, Emergency Department, Hospitalist, and Office Ultrasonography [Clinical Ultrasonography])
- Previous abdominal surgery (bowel may be adherent to abdominal wall, so perform in an area away from prior incision or, even better, consider ultrasonographic guidance because pockets of fluid may have formed)
- Anticoagulated patient or patient with coagulopathy without evidence of DIC or fibrinolyis should have the process reversed before paracentesis (see Precautions section).
- Pregnancy (ultrasonography-guided paracentesis is recommended after the first trimester)
- Distended bladder that cannot be emptied with a urinary catheter (consider ultrasonographic guidance)
- Obvious infection at the intended site of needle insertion (cellulitis or abscess)

Equipment and Supplies

Commercially prepared kit or the following equipment:

- Skin cleansing solution (povidone–iodine or chlorhexidine)
- Sterile gloves and equipment necessary to follow universal blood and body fluid precautions
- Sterile marking pen (if area has not been marked indelibly before skin preparation)
- Sterile drapes
- 4 × 4 gauze squares
- 1% or 2% lidocaine with or without epinephrine
- 5-mL syringe for anesthetic
- 20-mL syringe for diagnostic paracentesis (also purple-topped blood collection tube for cell count, red-topped tubes for chemistries, blood culture bottles if infection suspected)
- 25- or 27-gauge, 1½-inch needle for local anesthesia
- 18-gauge, 1½- to 3-inch needle
  Alternative devices: 18- or 20-gauge spinal needle, 18- or 20-gauge, 1½- to 3-inch angiocatheter needle, 3¼-inch Caldwell needle (needle/cannula system designed for therapeutic large-volume

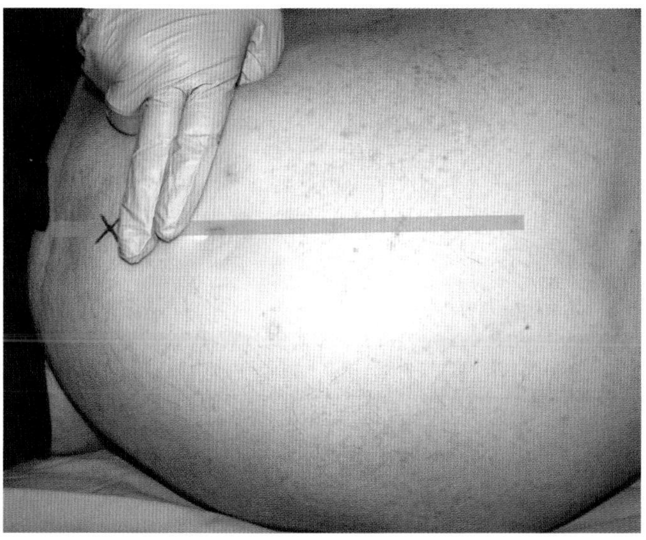

Figure 201-1 View of the midline approach with anatomic landmarks.

paracentesis; studies have suggested this is the most expedient technique), or catheter-over-wire system (Seldinger technique)

- No. 11 blade scalpel if large catheter to be inserted
- Sterile intravenous (IV) tubing
- 1-L vacuum bottles, a sufficient number if large-volume paracentesis is needed
- Foley catheter (if bladder decompression needed)
- Nasogastric tube (if gastric decompression needed)
- Three-way stopcock (for use with 50-mL syringe) *(optional)*
- 50-mL syringe, if using stopcock technique (*optional*)

Precautions

Careful attention to site selection as discussed in the section on Anatomy will minimize the risk of bleeding and injury to the bowel. In addition, entry near prior surgical scars should be avoided because there is a risk of adherent bowel loops near surgical scars. The *slow* introduction of the needle through the abdominal wall minimizes the risk of bowel injury because the needle can push mobile bowel away rather than injuring it. The application of intermittent negative pressure (aspiration) with the syringe while introducing the needle is generally preferred to constant negative pressure because the latter can quickly attract bowel or omentum on entry to the peritoneal cavity and occlude the needle. Needle occlusion can mask your entry into the peritoneal cavity and increase the risk of bowel injury as well as lead to a false sense of a "dry tap." Patients taking warfarin or who have any coagulopathy other than DIC or fibrinolysis should have the process reversed before paracentesis. If possible, antiplatelet medications should be held for 5 to 7 days. Warfarin can be held for 5 to 7 days (until the international normalized ratio [INR] normalizes) and the patient converted to low–molecular-weight heparin during this time, with the dose being held the day of the procedure. Alternatively, the INR can be reversed the day of the procedure with fresh-frozen plasma. Some experts suggest that patients with thrombocytopenia or an abnormal INR (for reasons other than taking warfarin) can be given platelets or the INR reversed with factor replacement; however, this process is considered controversial and there are no data to support it.

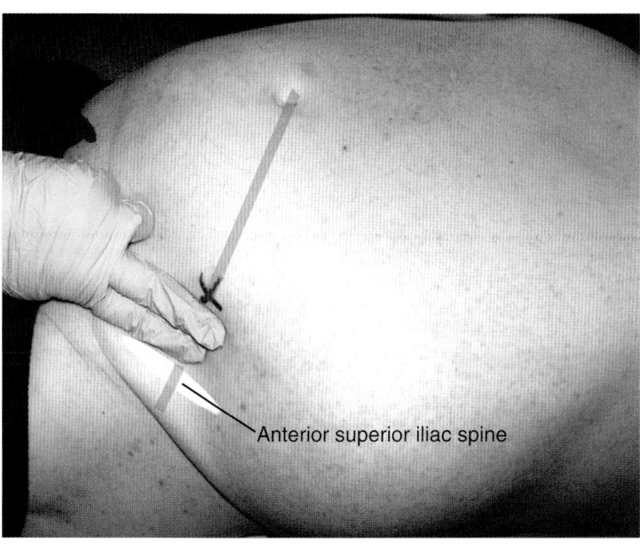

Figure 201-2 View of the lateral approach with anatomic landmarks.

Preprocedure Patient Education

Explain the procedure to the patient outlining the indications relevant to his or her medical situation and the anticipated benefits (diagnosis, ruling out infection, or decreased symptoms from therapeutic paracentesis). Risks of the procedure, as noted in the Complications section, should also be explained and informed consent obtained. Discuss anticipated patient positioning and ensure the patient is able to maintain the desired position. The patient should be aware that the local anesthetic may cause some discomfort, as well as the needle (or catheter) used to perform paracentesis.

Technique

1. Examine the abdomen, delineate areas of shifting dullness, and find landmarks. Mark if necessary. If clinical uncertainty exists about the presence of ascites, then ultrasonographic examination is recommended (see Chapter 225, Emergency Department, Hospitalist, and Office Ultrasonography [Clinical Ultrasonography]).
2. Assess for bowel and bladder distention and use a Foley catheter or nasogastric tube, if necessary, to decompress the bladder or stomach (see Chapter 110, Bladder Catheterization [and Urethral Dilation], and Chapter 203, Nasogastric and Nasoenteric Tube Insertion). Consider ultrasonographic guidance if needed.
3. Position the patient in the semiupright or lateral position, as tolerated, if the infraumbilical approach is used (see Fig. 201-1). Place the patient in the supine position if the lateral approach is taken (patient may be tilted slightly to the side of collection for improved fluid collection; see Fig. 201-2).
4. Prepare the abdominal skin at the puncture site with povidone–iodine or chlorhexidine solution.
5. Apply sterile drapes while confirming anatomic landmarks. The clinician should observe universal blood and body fluid precautions.
   - *Midline approach:* Insert the needle in the midline 2 to 3 cm below the umbilicus (two fingerbreadths). Patient is preferentially positioned in the semiupright or lateral position (see Fig. 201-1). Three "pops" will usually be felt as the needle penetrates the skin, the fascia, and the peritoneum.
   - *Lateral approach:* Enter 3 to 5 cm medial and cranial to the anterior superior iliac spine. Patient may be in the supine position or tilted slightly to the side of collection (see Fig. 201-2). At least two pops will be felt as the needle penetrates the skin and the peritoneum (fluid returns). One or two additional pops may be felt in between these two as the needle penetrates fascia before penetrating the peritoneum.
6. Infiltrate the skin, subcutaneous, and other tissues down to the peritoneum with lidocaine (with or without epinephrine). Attempt to locate the peritoneum and infiltrate a slight amount

of lidocaine across the peritoneum. Again, resistance is generally felt (a pop) as the needle perforates the peritoneum.

7. Direct the 18-gauge needle (or a catheter system) either perpendicular to the skin at the selected site or at a 45 degree angle to the skin and caudally. (A 20- or 22-gauge needle may be preferred for diagnostic paracentesis to minimize subsequent leakage of ascitic fluid.) A "Z-tract" technique should used (Fig. 201-3), especially if there is tense ascites. Two alternate Z-tract techniques are described: (a) the needle is inserted just through the skin, and the skin is then pulled taut from a cranial or caudal direction, moving the needle 1 or 2 cm, before the needle is advanced through deeper abdominal structures down to the peritoneum; or (b) the needle is inserted in a caudal direction at a 45-degree angle, just through skin and subcutaneous tissue. The skin is then pulled taut in a caudal direction, pulling the needle toward a more perpendicular position. It is then inserted down into the peritoneal cavity. The theoretical advantage of these techniques is the "self-sealing" of the needle tract when the tension on the skin is released after the procedure is completed, thus minimizing leaking of peritoneal fluid. With either method it is important to apply suction only intermittently as the needle is inserted through the deeper structures. Applying continuous suction after the needle has penetrated the peritoneum may attract bowel loops or omentum, occlude flow, and create the appearance of an unsuccessful tap, all of which increase the likelihood of bowel perforation. Insert the needle until fluid returns in the syringe. The needle can be rotated 180 degrees if peritoneal tenting is suspected because this helps enter the peritoneal cavity. If no fluid returns from an area of shifting dullness after rotating the needle, withdraw the needle to just below the skin and then redirect the needle in an area just inferior (midline approach) or just lateral (lateral approach) to the previous

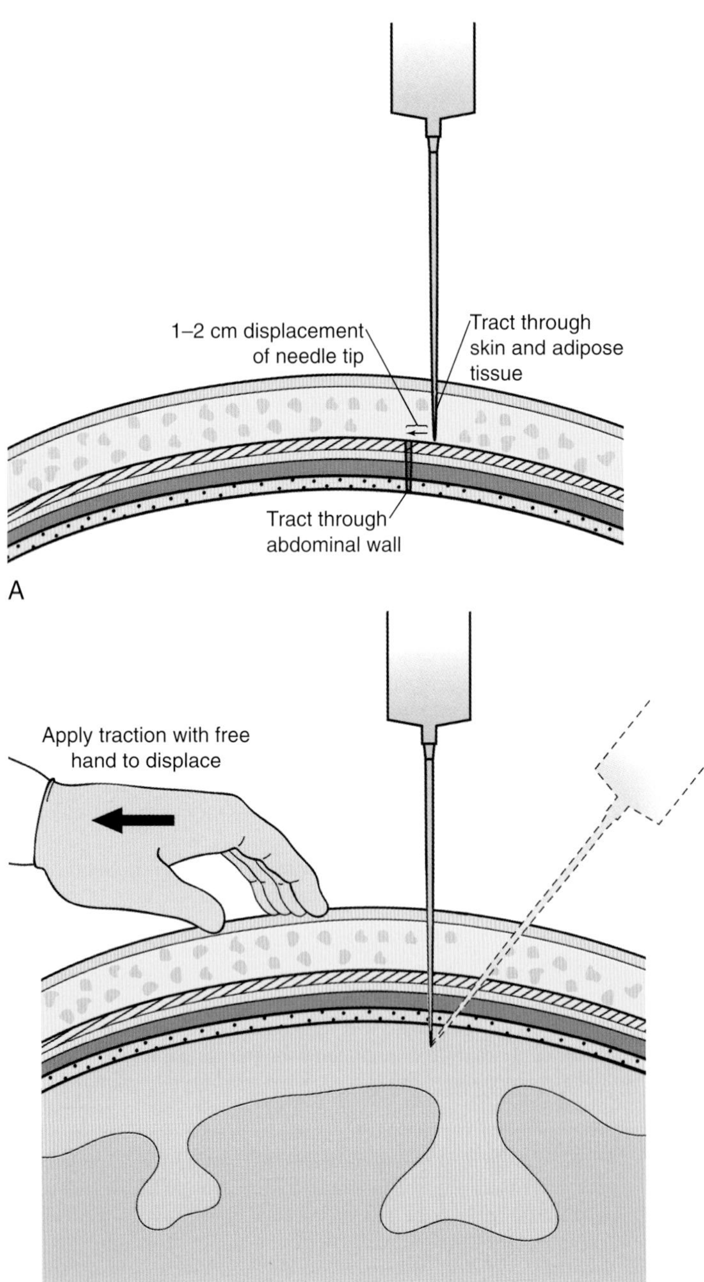

Figure 201-3 The Z-tract technique. **A,** Transverse view through the abdominal wall demonstrating the Z-tract. **B,** The needle is inserted perpendicular to the skin on the abdominal wall, which is then pulled taut or retracted a few centimeters caudad (or cephalad) by the non–needle-bearing hand *(arrow)*. The needle is then advanced through the subcutaneous and deeper structures until it pierces the peritoneum and fluid is obtained. (As an alternative, the needle can be inserted into just the skin and subcutaneous tissue at a 45-degree angle, directed caudally. When traction is placed on the skin or the skin is pulled taut in a caudal direction, the needle will be pulled more upright, toward a position more perpendicular to the skin. The needle is then advanced downward until fluid is obtained.) When the procedure is finished, the needle is withdrawn, traction is released, and the abdominal wall layers will shift back to their natural positions to facilitate closure of the needle tract.

attempt. If still no fluid returns, another attempt can be made using a different location. If the initial attempt was made in the midline, consider another attempt in the lateral location (if not contraindicated) or in the midline 1 cm below the prior attempt. If the initial attempt was in the lateral location, consider another attempt in the midline (if not contraindicated) or 1 cm lateral to the prior attempt. If these attempts are unsuccessful, ultrasonography should be used to guide the paracentesis. Ultrasonography can be used to quantify the amount of fluid expected (1 cm^3 of fluid equals 1 mL) as well as determine the direction necessary to obtain this fluid. It can also be used to make sure no vital organs are in the pathway chosen for aspiration (see Chapter 225, Emergency Department, Hospitalist, and Office Ultrasonography [Clinical Ultrasonography]).

If a catheter-over-needle system is used, advance the needle 1 to 2 mm after the flash of ascitic fluid is seen. Occlude the needle hub temporarily with a sterile gloved finger. Using the no. 11 blade scalpel, a small nick in the skin near the catheter (taking care not to cut the catheter) may facilitate passage of the catheter. Directing the needle toward a fluid-dependent position, advance the catheter over the needle, using a twisting motion, until the hub is against the skin. Gently withdraw the needle while holding the hub securely against the skin. Attach a syringe, if fluid is needed for diagnostic reasons, or the sterile IV tubing for therapeutic paracentesis.

For the Seldinger technique (catheter-over-wire system such as that used for central venous catheter insertion), advance the needle 1 to 2 mm after a flash of ascitic fluid is seen. (These are special needles tapered at the hub to facilitate advancement of the guidewire; standard hypodermics will generally not allow passage of a guidewire.) Occlude the needle hub temporarily with a sterile gloved finger, and then insert the guidewire through the hub. Insert the guidewire to the desired depth, always making sure at least several centimeters remains outside the beveled end of the hub. Holding the guidewire securely on the proximal end, remove the needle over the guidewire. After the needle tip has been removed from the skin, grasp the guidewire below the needle with sterile gloved fingers to prevent it from being pulled out of the peritoneal cavity. Using the no. 11 blade scalpel, a small nick in the skin near the guidewire (taking care not to cut the guidewire) may facilitate passage of the dilator/sheath unit through the skin. Place the dilator through the sheath to form a unit, and then advance the dilator/sheath unit over the guidewire, using a twisting motion, up to the hub. Holding the hub securely against the skin, remove the guidewire and dilator and attach a syringe to the hub, if fluid is needed for diagnostic reasons, or the sterile IV tubing for therapeutic paracentesis.

NOTE: When using a catheter-over-wire system, never let go completely of the proximal end of the wire. This precaution is to prevent loss of the wire into the peritoneal cavity.

8. After entry into the peritoneal cavity, fluid (usually 20 to 50 mL) should be withdrawn and collected for analysis (see Interpretation of Results section). Note the color and clarity of the fluid; normal ascitic fluid is clear and straw colored. If a therapeutic large-volume paracentesis is indicated, the needle may be attached to sterile IV tubing. This is then connected to vacuum bottles, if available, or a stopcock can be used with sequential aspiration using a 50-mL syringe. The needle may need to be repositioned to allow for continuous flow (omentum or a loop of bowel may have occluded the flow).

   NOTE: Never reposition the needle while the tip is within the peritoneal cavity; doing so may lacerate bowel, omentum, or a blood vessel. Instead, withdraw the needle into the subcutaneous tissue, redirect the needle, and then readvance it into the peritoneal cavity. Alternatively, the patient may need to be repositioned slightly or slight pressure applied to the abdomen.

   There is controversy regarding hypotension caused by a large-volume paracentesis (>4 L). Some clinicians give colloid replacement (e.g., albumin) as prophylaxis, especially in patients with cirrhosis and hypoalbuminemia; however, there is no evidence that this practice should be adopted universally and it is not recommended for procedures removing less than 6 L of ascitic fluid. After a large-volume paracentesis, there tends to be initial improvement in circulatory function; however, total paracentesis in patients with cirrhosis may cause delayed (>12 to 24 hours after the procedure) hypotension due to effective hypovolemia. Although the literature suggests this hypovolemia may be avoided by prophylactic colloid infusion, it is difficult to obtain albumin in the outpatient setting; therefore, these infusions typically have to be done in the hospital.
9. After the fluid is removed, gently remove the needle (or catheter), cover the entry site with 4 × 4 gauze pads, and apply pressure. If the wound is still leaking fluid after 5 minutes of direct pressure, consider suturing the puncture site using a mattress suture or apply a pressure dressing.

Complications

Complications are rare during paracentesis but include the risk of the following:

- Perforation of viscus organ (e.g., stomach, small bowel, colon; rare, and tend to be self-healing)
- Lacerations of major vessels with subsequent hemorrhage
- Abdominal wall hematoma
- Infection (local or intraperitoneal)
- Persistent ascitic fluid leak
- Hypotension (e.g., vasovagal reaction, hemorrhage, reaccumulation of fluid)
- Bladder perforation

Postprocedure Patient Management and Education

Complications of the procedure are rare and patients are usually able to return to their normal activities after this procedure. A brief observation period of 1 hour while monitoring vital signs is appropriate. Educate the patient about signs and symptoms of complications such as those listed (e.g., hypotension, bleeding, fever, abdominal pain or distention, nausea, vomiting), and instruct him or her to call or return to the clinician's office or the emergency department if these occur. If the site continues to ooze (e.g., tense ascites), the patient should be instructed in how to change the dressings regularly. When paracentesis is performed as an outpatient procedure, plans should be made to discuss with the patient the results of any tests performed.

Interpretation of Results

Although numerous tests are possible for ascitic fluid, the key questions of whether the fluid is infected and whether portal hypertension exists can usually be answered by obtaining the following:

- Cell count and differential (usually a purple-topped or EDTA tube)
- Bacterial culture (sensitivity and yield are increased by inoculating culture bottles at the bedside; the same bottles used for blood cultures may be used)
- Concurrent serum and ascitic fluid albumin and protein (usually a red-topped tube) to calculate serum–ascites albumin gradient (SAAG; see Table 201-1), which is approximately 97% accurate for diagnosing portal hypertension

To determine if preexisting ascites has become infected, some authors suggest using the cell count as the initial screen; if values are normal (<250/mm^3), the likelihood of infection is low. If the cell count is elevated, a confirmatory culture is required, but the patient should be admitted for empiric treatment with IV antibiotics (typically a third-generation cephalosporin, such as cefotaxime, which covers 98% of the causative agents for this disorder [*Escherichia coli* and streptococcal species; ampicillin should be added if *Enterococcus* is suspected]). It is also acceptable to culture all samples, but treat empirically only when cell counts are abnormal. For the evaluation of new-onset ascites, the initial evaluation often centers around whether the etiology is portal hypertension (often due to cirrhosis) or other factors. An increased red blood cell count can also be seen in malignancy, tuberculosis, endometriosis, mesenteric thrombosis, pancreatitis, abdominal trauma, and perforated viscus.

Additional studies on ascitic fluid to determine the etiology of new-onset ascites might include Gram stain (usually not helpful because bacterial concentrations are very low unless bowel is ruptured or perforated), triglyceride level (particularly if "milky" appearance, e.g., pancreatitis), smear for acid-fast bacteria (AFB), or assay for AFB by RNA polymerase chain reaction and AFB culture. (Suspect AFB in immunocompromised patients or those who have immigrated from areas where mycobacterial diseases are endemic; AFB culture has a sensitivity of about 50%.) Chemistries that might be obtained on both serum and ascitic fluid include glucose, lactate dehydrogenase, and amylase. Table 201-1 lists some common values to assist in laboratory interpretation.

Peritoneal carcinomatosis is possible in patients with a prior history of colon, breast, gastric, pancreatic, hepatobiliary, hepatocellular, ovarian, or other cancers. Ascitic fluid should be sent for cytologic study in these patients or anyone suspected of having a malignancy.

TABLE 201-1 Ascitic Fluid Analysis

Laboratory Test	Suggests Cirrhosis or Portal Hypertension*	Suggests Inflammatory Process†
White blood cell count (mm^3)	<250	>250 (often >500 with >50% polymorphonuclear leukocytes)
SAAG (g/dL)‡	≥1.1 suggests portal hypertension	<1.1
Protein (g/dL)	<3	>3
Lactate dehydrogenase (fluid/serum ratio)	<0.6	≥0.6

**Some causes of portal hypertension:* Cirrhosis, congestive heart failure (cardiac ascites), inferior vena caval obstruction or other veno-occlusive disease, Budd-Chiari syndrome (hepatic vein or inferior vena caval thrombosis), portal vein thrombosis, sarcoidosis, fulminant hepatic failure, alcoholic hepatitis, massive liver metastases, myxedema, mixed ascites.

†*Some causes of inflammatory processes:* Spontaneous bacterial peritonitis, malignancy, tuberculosis, pancreatitis, connective tissue disease. Nephrotic syndrome can cause ascites without an inflammatory process and SAAG < 1.1 g/dL.

‡Serum–ascites albumin gradient (SAAG) = [Serum albumin] − [Ascitic fluid albumin] alone is approximately 97% accurate in diagnosing portal hypertension. Increased red blood cell count can be seen in malignancy, tuberculosis, endometriosis, mesenteric thrombosis, pancreatitis, abdominal trauma, and perforated viscus.

CPT/Billing Codes

49080* Peritoneocentesis, abdominal paracentesis, or peritoneal lavage (therapeutic or diagnostic); initial
49081* Peritoneocentesis, abdominal paracentesis, or peritoneal lavage; subsequent
99070* Supplies and materials (except spectacles), provided by the physician over and above those usually included with the office visit or other services rendered (list drugs, trays, supplies, or materials provided)

ICD-9-CM Diagnostic Codes

014.0 Ascites, tuberculous
197.6 Ascites, malignant (secondary malignant neoplasm of respiratory and digestive system, retroperitoneum and peritoneum)
428.0 Ascites, cardiac
457.8 Ascites, chylous
567.23 Spontaneous bacterial peritonitis
571.2 Alcoholic cirrhosis of liver
789.50 Ascites, unspecified site
789.53 Ascites, right upper quadrant
789.57 Ascites, generalized

Acknowledgment

The editors wish to recognize the contributions by Michael Brown, MD, Brett White, MD, and Kenneth Hu, MD, to this chapter in the previous two editions of this text.

Supplier

(See contact information online at www.expertconsult.com.)

Abdominal paracentesis kit
Arrow International (Teleflex Medical)

ONLINE RESOURCE

Thompsen TW, Shaffer RW, White B, Setnik GS: Paracentesis. Videos in Clinical Medicine. N Engl J Med 355:e21, 2006, no. 19. Available at http://content.nejm.org/cgi/content/short/355/19/e21/.

BIBLIOGRAPHY

Marx JA: Peritoneal procedures. In Roberts JR, Hedges JR (eds): Clinical Procedures in Emergency Medicine, 4th ed. Philadelphia, Saunders, 2004, pp 841–856.
Ong JP: Paracentesis. Am J Gastroenterol 101:1954–1955, 2006.
Promes SB: Paracentesis. In Reichman EF, Simon RR (eds): Emergency Medicine Procedures. New York, McGraw-Hill, 2004, pp 467–477.
Runyon BA: Management of adult patients with ascites due to cirrhosis. Hepatology 39:841–856, 2004.
Runyon BA: Ascites and spontaneous bacterial peritonitis. In Feldman M, Friedman LS, Brandt LJ (eds): Sleisenger and Fordtran's Gastrointestinal and Liver Disease, 8th ed. Philadelphia, Saunders, 2006, pp 1935–1961.
Tuggy M, Garcia J: Procedures Consult. Available at www.proceduresconsult.com.

*Health Care Financing Administration (HCFA, for Medicare) allows additional payment for a tray for this procedure when performed in a physician's office.

CHAPTER 202

GASTROINTESTINAL DECONTAMINATION

Michael Zeringue • Grant C. Fowler

The overall mortality from acute poisoning is less than 1%; therefore, the challenge to clinicians is to determine which patients face serious complications from poisoning if not treated. If the decision is made to treat, activated charcoal has become the first-line treatment for most ingested toxins, especially for ingestion of a small or moderate amount. Multiple doses of charcoal are recommended by some experts, especially for toxins recycled in the enterohepatic circulation or those with long half-lives. Certain experts also add a laxative or cathartic to charcoal for more rapid elimination and to avoid constipation. Whole-bowel irrigation is a newer treatment; for most toxins, it is usually considered second-line treatment after activated charcoal. Rarely is gastric emptying (by lavage or induced emesis with substances like ipecac) recommended anymore, unless activated charcoal or whole-bowel irrigation is not available or gastric lavage or induced emesis can be performed very rapidly and will not delay administration of activated charcoal. It is rarely indicated for ingestion of corrosives or petroleum distillates because of risk of esophageal injury or aspiration. However, in certain cases, the potential benefit of removal of a highly toxic substance (e.g., benzene, pesticides) may outweigh the risk of complications. Consultation with a medical toxicologist or regional poison control center (1-800-222-1222) may help guide choice of intervention. For the sake of completeness, this chapter continues to cover techniques for gastric emptying.

MECHANISMS OF ACTION AND EVIDENCE

Charcoal is "activated" by the manufacturer by heating it to approximately 900° C and washing it in a stream of carbon dioxide gas or steam. This increases the surface area from 2 m^2/g to greater than 2000 m^2/g; consequently, a 50-g dose has the surface area of 10 football fields. When ingested, there is no modification of charcoal's structure by digestive enzymes as it passes through the stomach and intestines, nor is it absorbed across the intestinal wall. Activated charcoal binds with toxins and then passes through the gastrointestinal tract to be eliminated in the stool as a sticky black substance. As the charcoal absorbs the toxin in the intestine and passes distally, it creates a diffusion gradient. This in turn causes already absorbed toxins to diffuse back across the intestinal membrane and into the lumen; it somewhat dialyzes the intestinal blood. Thus, charcoal decreases systemic absorption of toxins by both its absorptive mechanism and its ability to form a diffusion gradient.

Charcoal has an excellent safety profile; it is even considered safe during pregnancy, in lactating women, and in the pediatric population. Although studies show a better safety profile and a more effective decrease in toxin absorption compared with lavage or ipecac-induced emesis, no significant decrease in mortality, length of hospital stay, or likelihood of clinical deterioration has been demonstrated with use of activated charcoal. In studies using a single dose of at least 50 g of activated charcoal, there was a 47% to 21% reduction in toxin absorption when administered 30 to 180 minutes after toxin ingestion, respectively. Although the clinical benefit of activated charcoal is less clear after 1 hour, "the potential for benefit ... cannot be excluded" (Position paper, 2005).

Similarly, although studies have shown statistical significance for multidose charcoal's effectiveness in removing toxins, it has not been shown to reduce morbidity or mortality. Therefore, multidosing is usually not recommended except for a select list of drugs (see Indications). Although there is no evidence supporting their use, cathartics are added to charcoal by some experts to hasten elimination. This may be especially helpful when large doses of charcoal have been administered, which can be constipating. If cathartics are used, it should be kept in mind that there are general, as well as specific, contraindications to certain agents. In the very young and elderly, cathartics can cause very large stools, dehydration, and electrolyte abnormalities such as hypernatremia. Sorbitol, which is used as a preservative and to decrease the grittiness of charcoal, also enhances the flavor of charcoal by making it slightly sweet. It is not absorbed and therefore encourages water secretion into the lumen, which in turn stimulates bowel peristalsis; however, it can cause severe cramping, hypotension, and vomiting and increase the risk of pulmonary aspiration. Sorbitol dosing in children is not clearly established and, therefore, if premixed with charcoal, may not be appropriate. Magnesium, another cathartic, is contraindicated in patients with hypermagnesemia, myasthenia gravis, renal insufficiency, or cardiac arrhythmias. Sodium-based cathartics should be avoided in patients with severe hypertension, renal failure, or congestive heart failure. Mineral oil– or other oil-based cathartics should not be used because of risk of aspiration.

Whole-bowel irrigation uses the infusion of polyethylene glycol (PEG) electrolyte solution (the same as used for preparation for colonoscopy) at a rate faster than normal for a bowel preparation. PEG infusion works by decreasing enteric transit time, thereby reducing toxin contact time with the intestinal wall and decreasing absorption. Whole-bowel irrigation has an advantage over cathartics in that it does not cause electrolyte disturbances because it does not create an osmotic differential across the intestinal membrane. Whole-bowel irrigation is especially useful for ingestions of toxins not absorbed by charcoal (e.g., iron, lithium, heavy metals), sustained-release or enteric-coated pills (if multidosing charcoal is not indicated), or illegal drug packets. Studies have found whole-bowel irrigation to decrease toxin bioavailability by up to two thirds.

Gastric lavage was at one time the chosen method to decontaminate the intestinal tract. However, in 1997, the American Academy of Clinical Toxicology/European Association of Poisons Centres and Toxicologists made the following statement: "Gastric lavage should not be considered unless a patient has ingested a potentially life-threatening amount of a poison and the procedure can be undertaken within 60 minutes of ingestion. Even then, clinical benefit has not been confirmed in controlled studies." Despite this knowledge, gastric lavage has not been completely abandoned. Some authorities believe that there are not enough data to direct decisions on all patients with potentially fatal ingestions. They believe that this lack of evidence should not lead to the discontinuance of gastric lavage, a logical, relatively safe, and inexpensive procedure. Gastric lavage can be considered when the substance ingested has high evidence of toxicity or risk of fatality or other supportive modalities are inadequate or unavailable. It is most effective for massive ingestions of solutions or small tablets, and is not as effective for large tablets or mushrooms, which may obstruct the orogastric tube when attempting to aspirate (see Indications and Contraindications). If performed within 5 minutes, 90% of ingestants are recovered, compared with 45% at 10 minutes, 30% at 19 minutes, and 8% at 60 minutes. Gastric lavage can also be used to evaluate gastric contents for poison or to administer charcoal. Specialized lavage (neutralizing) solutions may be indicated (after consultation with a toxicologist or poison control center) for ingested fluoride, formaldehyde, iodine, iron, or oxalic acid.

Syrup of ipecac has two pharmacologically active alkaloids, emetine and cephaeline, which stimulate both the gastric mucosal sensory receptors and the chemoreceptor trigger zone in the brain; given soon after toxin ingestion, ipecac can partially evacuate the gastric contents. However, there is no clear evidence for improved outcomes and its use is associated with the increased risks of pulmonary aspiration and delayed administration of activated charcoal. Therefore, like gastric lavage, induced emesis is no longer routinely recommended in poisoned patients. In fact, American poison centers recommended ipecac in only 0.6% of cases in 2002. That said, it may be considered in an alert patient who has ingested the toxin less than 60 minutes ago and for whom activated charcoal, whole-bowel irrigation, and gastric lavage are not indicated or available. Such may be the case at home or in the prehospital setting.

INDICATIONS

Activated Charcoal

- Most toxic substances
- Toxins metabolized by the liver and secreted into the bile
- Toxins that are recycled in the enterohepatic circulation and have long half-lives

Multidose Activated Charcoal

- Toxins that are recycled in the enterohepatic circulation and have long half-lives, including some sustained-release or enteric-coated preparations
- Amitriptyline
- Carbamazepine
- Dapsone
- Diazepam
- Digoxin
- Doxepin
- Phenobarbital
- Phenytoin
- Piroxicam
- Quinine
- Salicylates
- Tricyclic antidepressants
- Theophylline

Whole-Bowel Irrigation

- Life-threatening or serious ingestion not effectively removed by activated charcoal
- Medications with delayed absorption or sustained-release or enteric coatings
- Ingested packets of illicit drugs
- Iron (often seen on flat-plate radiograph)
- Lithium
- Heavy metals
- Activated charcoal not indicated or available

Gastric Lavage

Substances Able to Be Neutralized (after Consultation with Toxicologist or Poison Control Center)

- Fluoride
- Formaldehyde
- Iodine
- Iron
- Oxalic acid

Substances with High Risk of Morbidity or Mortality

- Beta blockers
- Calcium channel blockers
- Chloroquine
- Colchicine
- Cyanide
- Heavy metals
- Heterocyclic antidepressants
- Iron
- Paraquat
- Salicylates
- Selenious acid

Substances Poorly Absorbed by Activated Charcoal

- Iron
- Lithium
- Heavy metals
- Toxic levels of alcohol

Substances That Form Concretions

- Sustained-release or enteric-coated preparations
- Iron
- Phenothiazines
- Salicylates

Substances with Ineffective or No Antidotal Therapy Available

- Colchicine
- Paraquat
- Selenious acid

Induced Emesis (Syrup of Ipecac)

- Conscious, alert patient
- Potentially toxic dose of poison ingested within 60 minutes
- Activated charcoal, whole-bowel irrigation, gastric lavage are not indicated or available

CONTRAINDICATIONS

Activated Charcoal

- Unprotected airway
- Comatose or convulsing patient (unless the airway can be protected)
- Recent gastrointestinal surgery
- Ingestion of corrosive agent and endoscopy is planned
- Bowel obstruction or ileus
- Recent use of anticholinergic or antiperistaltic drugs
- Substances not absorbed by activated charcoal such as iron, lithium, lead, and other heavy metals, cyanide, acids, alkalis, alcohol, boric acid, petroleum distillates, pesticides

Use of Cathartic with Activated Charcoal

- Ingestion of a toxin that already causes diarrhea
- Electrolyte abnormality
- Debilitated or elderly patient who may not tolerate
- Children younger than 5 years of age
- Intestinal obstruction
- Severe dehydration
- Mineral oil– or other oil-based cathartics

Use of Sodium-Based Cathartics

- Severe hypertension
- Renal failure
- Congestive heart failure

Use of Magnesium-Based Cathartics

- Hypermagnesemia
- Myasthenia gravis
- Renal failure
- Abnormally slow heart rate

Whole-Bowel Irrigation

- Unprotected airway
- Abnormal gastrointestinal anatomy (e.g., strictures, anomaly) or recent gastrointestinal surgery
- Bowel perforation, obstruction, or ileus
- Ingestions of substances that cause an ileus (e.g., anticholinergics, antiperistaltics, opioids)
- Gastrointestinal bleed
- Vomiting
- Patient unable to remain sitting on toilet (*relative contraindication*)

Gastric Lavage

- Depressed mental status or inactive or diminished airway reflexes (unless airway can be protected)
- Active or substantial antecedent vomiting
- Abnormal pharyngeal or upper gastrointestinal anatomy
- Ingestion of corrosive agents
- Coagulopathy
- Large pills or particles (e.g., mushrooms)
- Large or sharp foreign body
- Nontoxic or minimally toxic ingestion
- Significant risk if aspirated (e.g., low-viscosity hydrocarbon or petroleum distillates)
- More than 60 minutes after ingestion
- Infants and neonates

Induced Emesis

- Depressed mental status
- Ingestion of corrosive agents
- Low-viscosity petroleum distillates or hydrocarbons (high risk of aspiration if vomiting occurs)
- Repeated vomiting would pose a health danger (e.g., recent gastrointestinal surgery, elderly or debilitated, third-trimester pregnancy, severe hypertension)

Equipment

- Equipment necessary for the clinician to follow universal blood and body fluid precautions (e.g., eye protection, mask, gloves, gown)
- Nasogastric tube (optional for administration of activated charcoal [i.e., for the patient who refuses to swallow charcoal], but use at least a 16-Fr diameter in adults for activated charcoal. A 10- to 12-Fr tube can be used for whole-bowel irrigation in anyone older than 1 year of age; infants can usually tolerate an 8-Fr tube.) An orogastric tube may be used instead for gastric lavage.
- 2% viscous lidocaine gel, or benzocaine; phenylephrine decongestant nasal spray for nasogastric tube insertion
- 50-mL tube syringe (Toomey)
- Towel or surgical Chux for covering patient's clothing
- Paper tissues
- Emesis basin
- Suction tube with vacuum generator
- Endotracheal tube with cuff for obtunded patients or those with an altered mental status or at risk of altered mental status or convulsions because of what they have ingested. Intubation should also be considered to protect the airway in patients who have ingested hydrocarbons.
- Intravenous (IV) antiemetics (e.g., promethazine); optional, but must avoid sedating dose

Activated Charcoal

Activated charcoal (1 g/kg): Flavored versions (e.g., cherry) are available. Preparations are also available containing sorbitol, which is an artificial sweetener and may make the charcoal slurry or solution seem less gritty and more palatable; however, sorbitol is also a laxative.

Whole-Bowel Irrigation

Use 4 to 8 L of balanced PEG electrolyte solution (e.g., Colyte, GoLYTELY, MoviPrep) at body temperature for whole-bowel irrigation.

Gastric Lavage

Use 3 L of normal saline at body temperature for gastric lavage.

Open-System Gastric Lavage

- Large-diameter gastric tube with extra holes cut near the tip (A 32- to 50-Fr orogastric tube is recommended for adults; a 16- to 32-Fr orogastric tube is recommended for children. Small children can generally accommodate a 24-Fr tube. Nasogastric tubes are discouraged (traumatize nasal mucosa and are too small for effective aspiration of gastric contents)
- Y-connector and clamp, with or without suction apparatus, and tubing

Closed-System Gastric Lavage

The EASI-LAV kit (Kimberly-Clark/Ballard Medical Products, Roswell, Ga) is an example of a closed system. It includes a fluid bag and tubing, a waste bag and tubing, a double-barrel syringe mechanism, a gastric tube, and a sample cup.

Induced Emesis

Use syrup of ipecac (2%), usually provided in 1-ounce bottle.

Preprocedure Patient Preparation

The patient or representative should know what to expect when activated charcoal is administered, especially if multiple doses will be needed or a cathartic will be used. The patient should be aware that if he or she is unwilling or refuses to swallow the charcoal, a nasogastric tube will be inserted. Likewise, a nasogastric tube will be inserted for whole-bowel irrigation, and a larger nasogastric or orogastric tube inserted for gastric lavage. The patient or representative should also know what to expect if whole-bowel irrigation, gastric lavage, or induced emesis will be performed. IV antiemetics may be used to minimize nausea when any of these procedures are performed (except, of course, induced emesis, unless vomiting is prolonged). Although administration of activated charcoal, whole-bowel irrigation, gastric lavage, or induced emesis is typically performed as an urgent or emergent procedure and most hospitals do not require written informed consent, the risks, benefits, indications, and any possible alternatives should be explained to the patient or representative.

Insertion of a nasogastric or orogastric tube can be very distressing for the conscious patient (see Preprocedure Patient Preparation section in Chapter 203, Nasogastric and Nasoenteric Tube Insertion, for additional information).

Airway protection with a cuffed endotracheal tube (see Preprocedure Patient Preparation section in Chapter 213, Tracheal Intubation) is very important for a patient whose level of consciousness is depressed, whose airway-protective reflexes are diminished, or who is otherwise in danger of aspiration (e.g., altered mental status, obtunded, unconscious, convulsing). For activated charcoal, whole-bowel irrigation, and induced emesis the patient should be upright or semiupright. For whole-bowel irrigation, the patient should optimally be capable of sitting on the toilet for a few hours. For gastric lavage, the patient should be positioned in the left lateral recumbent or decubitus position with the head lowered approximately 10 degrees (Trendelenburg position). These positions decrease the risk of aspiration should vomiting occur.

TECHNIQUE

Activated Charcoal

1. If the patient is unable, unwilling, or refuses to swallow the charcoal, place at least a 16-Fr nasogastric tube in adults and confirm its placement before administration of any fluids (see Chapter 203, Nasogastric and Nasoenteric Tube Insertion). Aspirated gastric contents can be saved or sent for analysis if the toxin is unknown. If the patient is unable to protect his or her airway, endotracheal intubation should be considered (see Chapter 213, Tracheal Intubation). (The absence of blinking after touching the eyelashes is strong evidence of inability to protect the airway from vomitus.) Intubation should also be considered in any patient who has ingested a central nervous system antidepressant or any substance that can cause altered mental status or seizures. The patient should not undergo endotracheal extubation until 4 hours after the last dose of charcoal is administered.
2. Charcoal can be ordered as capsules, tablets, powder, or oral suspension/solution. However, with an acute toxin ingestion, only powder mixed with water or a premixed oral suspension or solution, with or without a cathartic, is recommended. Older-style preparations or suspensions were gritty and, although they had no taste, were unpleasant to swallow. Newer-style preparations dissolve completely when added to water and form a solution. Flavored versions are also available.
3. Optimally, administration of charcoal should occur within the first hour of ingestion.
4. Powder comes in doses of 15 to 500 g. It should be mixed in water to achieve a slurry.
5. It has become standard practice to administer 50 to 100 g of charcoal for an adult and 1 g/kg (maximum 50 g) for a child.
6. An IV antiemetic can be administered to decrease vomiting/nausea. Avoid a sedating dose.
7. In adults, activated charcoal can be mixed with 70% sorbitol (1 g/kg) or 10% solution of magnesium citrate (typically given as 250 mL for adults).
8. For multidose charcoal treatment, follow the initial dose of 50 to 100 g with 25 to 50 g every 4 hours, possibly alternating with and without a cathartic. (A cathartic is not used with each dose to avoid side effects such as very large stools, dehydration, and electrolyte abnormalities.) Monitor the patient between doses to verify the presence of bowel sounds and to confirm the absence of distention or an ileus.
9. The nasogastric tube should be removed before extubation to avoid aspiration of charcoal as the nasogastric tube is being removed.

Whole-Bowel Irrigation

1. Place the nasogastric tube and confirm its placement before administration of any fluids (see Chapter 203, Nasogastric and Nasoenteric Tube Insertion). Consider endotracheal intubation in the patient who may become obtunded or sedated or may convulse. A 10- to 12-Fr tube can be used for whole-bowel irrigation in anyone older than 1 year of age; infants can usually tolerate an 8-Fr tube.
2. Introduce PEG electrolyte into the nasogastric tube at an initial rate at 25 mL/kg/hr. Increase the rate, depending on patient tolerance, while also trying to avoid vomiting and abdominal distention. Adults often tolerate greater than 3 L of PEG per hour.
3. Continue treatment until the patient passes the ingestant or clear rectal fluid.
4. The patient should be continually assessed for any signs of airway compromise, ileus, or abdominal distention. If significant abdominal distention occurs or there is a loss of bowel sounds, irrigation should be held for 30 to 90 minutes and the patient reassessed. If bowel sounds have returned, irrigation can be resumed at a reduced rate. If the patient tolerates irrigation at the reduced rate, and the clinical status improves, it can be continued at this rate or possibly increased gradually as tolerated.

Gastric Lavage

Lavage can be performed with either an open or a closed system. Open systems are generally more time-consuming and potentially messy, but they are also less expensive. Open systems use either an active or a passive process.

For passive lavage, once the intragastric tube is in place, it is merely used as a siphon. Active lavage uses a syringe to generate pressure as well as to aspirate and irrigate the stomach. A large syringe is used to inject and remove the fluid from the stomach through the gastric tube. This syringe must be disconnected from the tube to be filled and emptied after each lavage cycle. Alternatively, two tubes may be inserted, one in each nostril. One tube is used as the input port and the other as the output port.

Closed systems are available prepackaged in commercial kits, self-contained and easy to use. They generally provide more protection to the health care provider. Closed systems usually apply an active lavage process. A well-tested closed and active system, EASI-LAV, uses a double-barrel syringe with automatic two-way valves. The syringe remains attached to the gastric tube. Its stroke volume of 125 mL allows for rapid fluid movement and the creation of fluid turbulence, resulting in fast, easy removal of toxic substances or clots.

Again, specialized lavage solutions may be indicated (after consultation with a toxicologist or poison control center) if the ingested substance is fluoride, formaldehyde, iodine, iron, or oxalic acid.

1. Premeasure and mark the length of the tube needed by estimating the distance from the nose, around the ear, and down to the mid-epigastrium. To prepare the tube, larger holes may be cut in the end of the tube to accommodate larger pill or charcoal fragments.
2. In most cases, nasal intubation for gastric lavage is discouraged; it may cause injury to the mucosa and turbinates and severe hemorrhage, and the diameter is usually not large enough to aspirate particles effectively. However, if the tube is to be inserted nasally, spray both nostrils with the decongestant nasal spray and do not use larger than an 18-Fr tube. Lidocaine

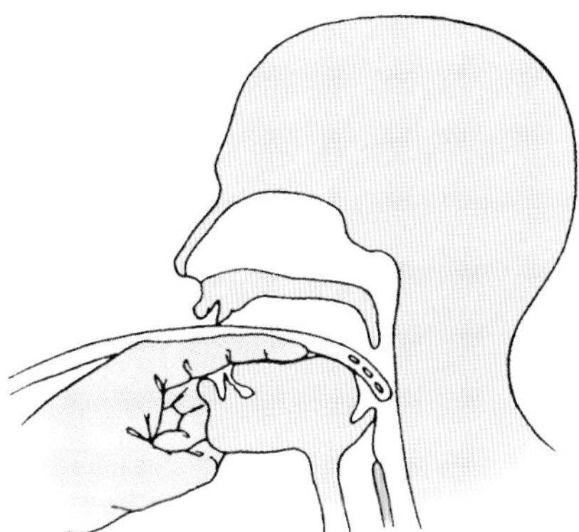

Figure 202-1 Orogastric tube insertion.

gel may be placed into the tube syringe and slowly instilled into one nostril. Ask the patient to "sniff and swallow," if he or she is able to do this. (See the procedure for nasogastric tube insertion in Chapter 203, Nasogastric and Nasoenteric Tube Insertion.) Consider endotracheal intubation in the patient who may become obtunded or sedated, or may convulse.

3. For orogastric tube insertion, if the patient is alert, spray the posterior pharynx with topical benzocaine or Cetacaine spray. Position the patient's head so that it is flexed as far forward as possible and, while ensuring against being bitten (i.e., bite block), insert your gloved index and middle fingers over the base of the patient's tongue. Guide the lubricated orogastric tube over the dorsum of your fingers as the patient swallows (Fig. 202-1). If the patient gags, advance the tube immediately after gagging. Advance the tube to the previously measured distance marked on the tube.
4. Confirm intragastric tube placement initially by auscultating the stomach while introducing air with the syringe. Verify the final placement by aspirating and confirming gastric contents. *It is critical to avoid infusion of fluids until tube placement is confirmed.* The aspirate may be sent for toxicologic analysis. Secure the tube with tape.

A. Open-System Procedure

See Figure 202-2.

5a. Introduce the normal saline at a rate of 1 to 2 mL/kg per cycle from an IV bag or large syringe attached to the tube with a Y-connector in the proximal circuit.

6a. During saline infusion, clamp the efferent drainage arm. After instilling approximately 150 to 200 mL (50 to 100 mL in children), clamp the afferent reservoir arm. Then open the drainage arm to allow gravity to siphon and evacuate the stomach contents. Intermittent suction may be applied to facilitate gastric emptying. Manual agitation of the stomach by gentle massage of the upper abdominal wall will enhance recovery of gastric contents.

7a. With an active system, use a syringe or vacuum suction equipment, instead of gravity, to irrigate and evacuate the gastric contents.

8a. Continue gastric irrigation until at least 3 L of lavage have been used and the return is clear on visual inspection.

9a. After gastric lavage has been completed, a slurry of activated charcoal can be used (see earlier sections for Indications and Contraindications for charcoal). It may be administered cleanly by adding 50 to 100 g (1 g/kg) of the powder through an opened upper corner of a partially full, hanging IV bag. Infuse this mixture through the orogastric circuit with the efferent arm clamped. Either the charcoal can be allowed to pass through the gastrointestinal tract, or additional saline lavages can be performed until the slurry is cleared of charcoal.

10a. When the procedure is completed, clamp or pinch the gastric tube during removal to prevent contaminating the lung with charcoal or gastric contents. If repeated doses of charcoal are deemed necessary, the large tube may be replaced with a standard, smaller nasogastric tube. In the obtunded, intubated patient, leave the endotracheal tube in place for at least 15 minutes after gastric tube removal to prevent aspiration. Confirm adequate spontaneous respirations and oxygenation by pulse oximetry before removing the endotracheal tube.

B. Closed-System Procedure

The procedure described here uses the EASI-LAV system (Fig. 202-3).

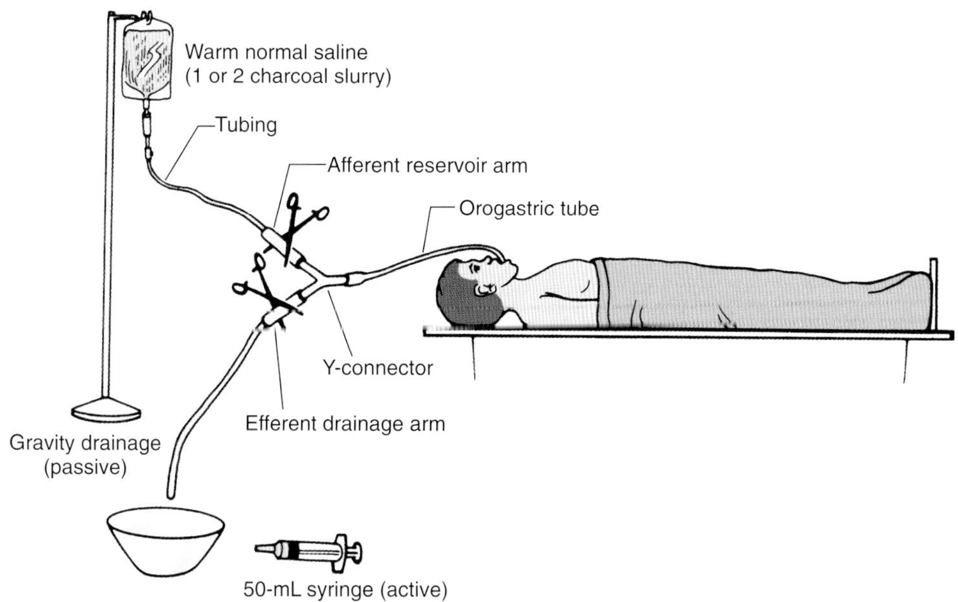

Figure 202-2 Open gastric lavage system assembly with components.

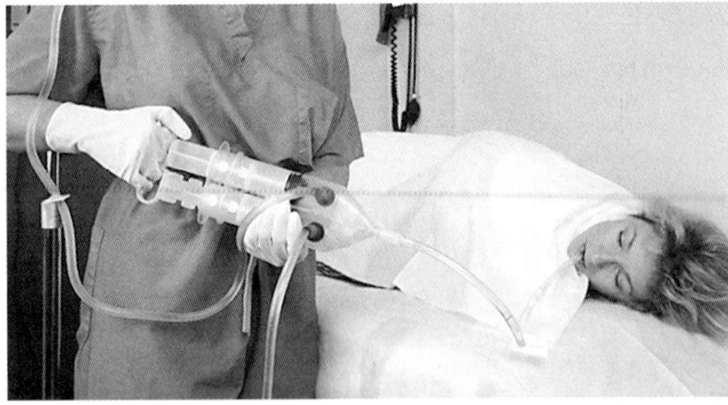

Figure 202-3 Performing gastric lavage with the closed double-barrel syringe system. (From Haynes JH: Gastric lavage for serious poisonings. Fam Pract Recert 14:45, 1992. Courtesy of Kimberly-Clark/Ballard Medical Products, Roswell, Ga.)

5b. Hang a waste bag from the bed. Close the sampling port clamp and cap. Close the fluid bag clamp and fill the fluid bag with normal saline solution. You can rest the fluid bag on the countertop when sealing it. Finally, hang the fluid bag from an IV pole.

6b. Next, evaluate the already inserted orogastric tube. Bending or kinking of the gastric tube may cause malfunction of the system. Ensure airway protection.

7b. Advance both syringe plungers to the fully forward position. Attach the syringe to the gastric lavage tube and pinch the retaining collar in place.

8b. Reconfirm proper tube placement, initially, by locking the red output plunger in the fully forward position and pumping the blue input plunger alone while listening for air bubbles in the stomach. Again verify correct placement finally by aspirating gastric fluid and confirming that it is indeed gastric fluid.

9b. Next, attach the blue tubing connection from the fluid bag to the blue input port on the syringe. Attach the red tubing connection from the waste bag to the red output port on the syringe. Ensure that both syringe plungers are in the fully forward position. Always leave the blue input plunger forward when not in use or fluid will flow into the patient's stomach. Open the clamp on the fluid bag.

10b. To empty the stomach, first confirm that the clamp on the waste bag line is opened. Next, pump the red output plunger alone until resistance is encountered or no return is obtained. To avoid mucosal injury, never pull the red plunger against stiff resistance.

11b. Lock the red output plunger in the forward position by pushing the plunger completely forward and rotating it clockwise 90 degrees. Prime the system by pumping the blue input plunger three times to partially fill the stomach.

12b. Unlock the red output plunger by rotating it 90 degrees counterclockwise. Perform the lavage as follows (see Fig. 202-3):
   a. Grasp both plunger handles, pull back, and then push forward. This will wash out and empty the stomach.
   b. Perform this lavage three times.
   c. With the blue input plunger fully forward, pump the red output plunger three times (or less, if resistance is met).

   Repeat steps 11b and 12b(a), 12b(b), and 12b(c) until the gastric return fluid is clear.

13b. To administer charcoal (see earlier sections for Indications and Contraindications), the following procedure is effective:
   a. Lock the red output plunger in the forward position by pushing it completely forward and rotating it clockwise 90 degrees.
   b. Pour charcoal into the fluid bag and reseal the bag.
   c. Lavage fluid (50 to 75 mL) may be added to thin the slurry and to speed up the administration.
   d. Pump the blue input plunger until all of the charcoal is in the stomach.

Induced Emesis

1. The patient should be in the upright or semiupright position as the ipecac is administered. The alert patient should be told that he or she may rapidly experience nausea and vomiting and that it will soon pass.
2. Adolescents or adults can be given 15 to 30 mL of syrup followed by 240 mL of water. Children 6 to 12 months of age should be given 5 to 10 mL of syrup of ipecac followed by 120 to 240 mL of water. Children 1 to 12 years of age should be given 15 mL of syrup followed by this same amount of water.
3. The dose may be repeated in all age groups if emesis does not occur in 20 to 30 minutes.

Complications

The main complications of activated charcoal administration are aspiration, intestinal obstruction, and electrolyte imbalances or dehydration from cathartic use. Aspiration is prevented by following the patient's alertness and gag reflexes as he or she is ingesting the activated charcoal, or by endotracheal intubation. Anticholinergic and antiperistaltic drugs should not be administered around the time of activated charcoal administration because they slow down gastrointestinal transit time and increase the risk of bezoar formation.

Caution should be taken when giving a cathartic with activated charcoal. Cathartics should be withheld in any patient who has ingested a toxin that may itself already cause diarrhea. Also, they should not be given to children younger than 5 years of age. Cathartic-induced hypernatremia is a serious side effect that has been reported in young children. Magnesium should not be administered in patients with hypermagnesemia, myasthenia gravis, an abnormally slow heart rate, intestinal obstruction, or kidney failure. Finally, cathartics are not recommended with every dose of multidose charcoal.

Pulmonary aspiration with subsequent chemical pneumonitis can be devastating complications of gastric lavage or induced emesis. In one study, the incidence of pneumonitis was found to be 56% with lavage, compared with 28% with induced emesis. It is less likely with whole-bowel irrigation. Such risk can be minimized by proper patient positioning and observing the patient closely. Laryngospasm and resultant hypoxia are possible complications of any aspiration. Risks versus benefits must be considered when performing any of these procedures.

Mucosal injury or perforation of the upper gastrointestinal tract is also a possible complication of nasogastric or orogastric intubation or gastric lavage. Up to 50% of patients will complain of nausea, gassiness, mild discomfort, or distention with whole-bowel irrigation; however, these symptoms do not mandate discontinuation of the procedure.

Fluid and electrolyte disturbances are possible with gastric lavage; these are more common when water is used instead of saline. Risk of hypothermia can be minimized by using body-temperature PEG or saline. Cardiac dysrhythmias, due to aspiration or otherwise, are possible complications of gastric lavage. Other possible complications are the same as for nasogastric tube insertion (see Chapter 203, Nasogastric and Nasoenteric Tube Insertion). The most common complications for induced emesis with ipecac syrup are diarrhea, lethargy/drowsiness, and prolonged (>1 hour) vomiting.

Patient Education Guides

See the sample patient education form available online at www.expertconsult.com.

CPT/Billing Code

91105 Gastric intubation, and aspiration or lavage for treatment (e.g., for ingested poisons)

ICD-9-CM Diagnostic Codes

NOTE: Most of these codes need a specific fourth digit.

960 Poisoning by antibiotics
961 Poisoning by other anti-infectives
962 Poisoning by hormones and synthetic substitutes
963 Poisoning by primarily systemic agents
964 Poisoning by agents primarily affecting blood constituents
965 Poisoning by analgesics, antipyretics, and antirheumatics
966 Poisoning by anticonvulsants and antiparkinsonian drugs
967 Poisoning by sedatives and hypnotics
968 Poisoning by other central nervous system depressants and anesthetics
969 Poisoning by psychotropic agents
970 Poisoning by central nervous system stimulants
971 Poisoning by drugs primarily affecting the autonomic nervous system
972 Poisoning by drugs primarily affecting the cardiovascular system
973 Poisoning by drugs primarily affecting the gastrointestinal system
974 Poisoning by water, mineral, and uric acid metabolism drugs
975 Poisoning by agents primarily acting on the smooth and skeletal muscles and respiratory system
980 Toxic effect of alcohol
981 Toxic effect of petroleum products
983 Toxic effect of corrosive aromatics, acids, and caustic alkalis
984 Toxic effect of lead and its compounds

Acknowledgment

The editors wish to recognize the contributions by John Harlan Haynes III, MD, and Andrew Thomas Haynes, MD, to this chapter in the previous two editions of this text.

Suppliers

(See contact information online at www.expertconsult.com)

Activated charcoal and syrup of ipecac
Paddock Laboratories
Gastric lavage: closed system
EASI-LAV and Char-Flo systems
Kimberly-Clark/Ballard Medical Products
TUM-E-VAC (available with activated charcoal systems)
Ethox Corp.
Gastric lavage open system: Argyle Edlich gastric lavage tray
Cardinal Health
The Kendall Company (Covidien)
Polyethylene glycol (PEG) solution
Braintree Laboratories

Bibliography

Bond G: The role of activated charcoal and gastric emptying in gastrointestinal decontamination: A state-of-the-art review. Ann Emerg Med 39:273–286, 2002.

Burns M, Schwartzstein R: Decontamination of poisoned adults. In Rose BD (ed): UpToDate. Waltham, Mass, UpToDate, 2005. Available at www.uptodate.com.

Haynes JH: Gastric lavage for serious poisonings. Fam Pract Recert 14:45, 1992.

Hoffman R: Importance of gastrointestinal decontamination. Internet J Med Toxicol [serial online] 2:5, 1999.

Gummin DD: Gastric lavage. In Reichman E., Simon R (eds): Emergency Medicine Procedures. New York, McGraw-Hill, 2004, pp 424–430

Gummin DD, Aks SE: Whole bowel irrigation. In Reichman E, Simon R (eds): Emergency Medicine Procedures. New York, McGraw-Hill, 2004, pp 431–435.

Leschke R, Bourn M: Activated charcoal administration. In Reichman E, Simon R (eds): Emergency Medicine Procedures. New York, McGraw-Hill, 2004, pp 420–423.

Marx JA, Hockberger RS, Walls RM (eds): Rosen's Emergency Medicine: Concepts and Clinical Practice, 5th ed. St. Louis, Mosby, 2001.

Olson KR: Poisoning. In McPhee SJ, Papadakis MA (eds): Current Medical Diagnosis and Treatment, 48th ed. New York, McGraw-Hill, 2009, pp 1388–1416.

Position paper: Cathartics. American Academy of Clinical Toxicology and European Association of Poisons Centres and Clinical Toxicologists. J Toxicol Clin Toxicol 42:243–253, 2004. Also available at www.clintox.org/documents/positionpapers/Cathartics.pdf. Last accessed May 11, 2010.

Position paper: Gastric lavage. American Academy of Clinical Toxicology and European Association of Poisons Centres and Clinical Toxicologists. J Toxicol Clin Toxicol 42:933–943, 2004. Also available at www.clintox.org/documents/positionpapers/GastricLavage.pdf. Last accessed May 11, 2010.

Position paper: Ipecac syrup. American Academy of Clinical Toxicology and European Association of Poisons Centres and Clinical Toxicologists. J Toxicol Clin Toxicol 42:133–143, 2004. Also available at www.clintox.org/documents/positionpapers/IpecacSyrup.pdf. Last accessed May 11, 2010.

Position paper: Single-dose activated charcoal in the treatment of acute poisoning. American Academy of Clinical Toxicology and European Association of Poisons Centres and Clinical Toxicologists. Clin Toxicol 43:61–87, 2005. Also available at www.clintox.org/documents/positionpapers/SingleDoseActivatedCharcoal.pdf. Last accessed May 11, 2010.

Position statement and practice guidelines on the use of multi-dose activated charcoal in the treatment of acute poisoning. American Academy of Clinical Toxicology and European Association of Poisons Centres and Clinical Toxicologists. J Toxicol Clin Toxicol 37:731–751, 1999. Also available at www.clintox.org/documents/positionpapers/MultipleDoseActivatedCharcoal.pdf. Last accessed May 11, 2010.

Reisdorff EJ, Roberts MR, Wiegenstein JG (eds): Pediatric Emergency Medicine. Philadelphia, WB Saunders, 1993.

Smith SW, Ling LJ, Halstenson CE: Whole bowel irrigation as a treatment for lithium overdose. Ann Emerg Med 20:536–539, 1991.

Tandberg D, Troutman WG: Gastric lavage in the poisoned patient. In Roberts JR, Hedges JR (eds): Clinical Procedures in Emergency Medicine, 2nd ed. Philadelphia, WB Saunders, 1991, pp 655–662.

Tenenbein M: Whole bowel irrigation. In Henretig FM, King C, Joffe MD, et al (eds): Textbook of Pediatric Emergency Procedures. Philadelphia, Lippincott Williams & Wilkins, 1997, pp 1309–1312.

Tintinalli JE, Kelen GD (eds): Emergency Medicine: A Comprehensive Study Guide. New York, McGraw-Hill, 2000.

CHAPTER 203

Nasogastric and Nasoenteric Tube Insertion

Yong Sik Kim

Nasogastric intubation (nasogastric tube insertion) is a common procedure performed in the hospital, emergency department, and office settings. The nasogastric tube was initially developed for gastric feeding in 1760. The indications were expanded to gastric lavage in the case of poisoning in the early 1800s. One current design, by Dr. Levin, became available in 1921 and soon became popular for preventing intraoperative and postoperative gastric distention. In the 1960s, improved technology allowed the manufacture of a double-lumen tube, which later developed into special soft tubes made of polyurethane and silicone. These tubes are also very thin and have a noncomplicated, smooth surface, useful characteristics for prolonged nasoenteric feeding.

A nasogastric tube can be used for either diagnostic or therapeutic purposes. The Levin nasogastric tube is a firm, straight, single-lumen tube with multiple distal side ports, and is used predominantly for diagnostic aspiration or to instill materials into the stomach. Unfortunately, even when low–flow-rate suction is applied to a Levin tube, or if it is applied for a very long time, the lumen frequently becomes occluded with gastric mucosa, and this can damage the gastric mucosa. In contrast, the Salem nasogastric sump tube is a double-lumen tube. The second lumen, or vent lumen, is smaller than the main suction lumen and runs alongside the larger lumen, providing a low level of continuous airflow to the stomach. This airflow prevents the main lumen from becoming occluded by gastric mucosa when suction is applied, thereby minimizing the risk of damage. The blue "pigtail" on the Salem sump is an extension of this vent lumen (Fig. 203-1). Similar to the Levin tube, the Salem sump has multiple distal side ports. Antireflux valves are available to prevent gastric contents from leaking out of the vent lumen and multiport adapters are available for the proximal end so that the same tube can be used for feeding, irrigating, suctioning, or medicating. Even though the Levin tube is still manufactured and available, hospitals predominantly stock the Salem sump tube because it can be used for most applications and is more effective and safer.

Salem sump tubes are usually clear, yet radiopaque, and made of polypropylene or Silicone, whereas Levin tubes are available in various versions, including red rubber and clear polypropylene. Levin tubes can be either radiopaque or radiolucent. Although both can be used for short-term (up to 4 weeks) gastric or nasoenteric feeding, most facilities now have the longer and smaller-diameter polyurethane tubes specially designed for this purpose. These softer tubes (especially softer at body temperatures) usually have a tungsten-weighted tip or balloon near the tip to facilitate passage beyond the pylorus. They may also have a stiffening wire or stylet available for use during insertion; many have also been designed to resist collapse when checking the gastric residual (Fig. 203-2). Other styles of tubes include those equipped with a large esophageal balloon that can be used to tamponade a bleeding esophageal lesion (e.g., esophageal varices). Larger gastric tubes are also available for gastric lavage (see Chapter 202, Gastrointestinal Decontamination).

Anatomy

The nasal cavity is lined by highly vascularized and innervated mucosa and continues posteriorly as the nasopharynx. Within the nasal cavity are the superior, inferior, and middle nasal conchae (turbinates), which divide the cavity into four passages (Fig. 203-3), the meatuses. Traditionally, the nasogastric tube is inserted blindly through middle and inferior meatuses. Beyond the nasal cavity, the pharynx extends from the base of the skull to the inferior border of the cricoid cartilage. It is divided into three parts: the nasopharynx, oropharynx, and laryngopharynx (hypopharynx). The nasopharynx gives rise to the oropharynx at the level of the soft palate, which then gives rise to the laryngopharynx (hypopharynx) at the superior border of the epiglottis (see Chapter 77, Nasolaryngoscopy, Fig. 77-6). The laryngopharynx becomes continuous with the esophagus at the inferior border of the cricoid cartilage. The posterior part of the upper nasopharynx is surrounded by the cribriform plate and the body of the ethmoid and sphenoid bones, which can easily be broken by a traumatic blow to the midface, resulting in a maxillofacial or basilar skull fracture. Such fractures can create a route into the cranial vault, which is a prerequisite for one of the most disastrous complications of inserting a nasogastric tube, intracranial intubation. This can result in brain damage or death. Therefore, placement of a nasogastric or nasoenteric tube in a patient with a possible skull or maxillofacial fracture should be avoided, if possible (an orogastric route may be a better option).

Beyond the laryngopharynx and the larynx, the trachea lies anterior to the esophagus at the level of the cricoid bone and is supported by fibrocartilaginous tracheal rings. The superior aperture is covered by the epiglottis of the larynx during swallowing.

The anatomy also confers the ability to estimate the length of tube that should be inserted. Because the median distance from the anterior aspect of the nasal septum to the cricopharyngeus muscle (tracheoesophageal junction) is about 8 inches, and the esophagus is on average about 10 inches long, and given that the tip of a nasogastric tube should lie 4 inches below the gastroesophageal junction when in place, the nasogastric tube should ideally be secured at the 20- to 24-inch mark at the nasal vestibule. Alternatively, the distance can be approximated by holding the tube up to the patient's ear and across to the nose, and then extending it to 6 inches below the xiphoid process (8 to 10 inches for a nasoenteric tube; this is described later in the Technique section).

The anatomy of children regarding the insertion of a nasogastric tube warrants a special note. Children have larger tonsils and adenoids, and their tongues are large compared to adults and may

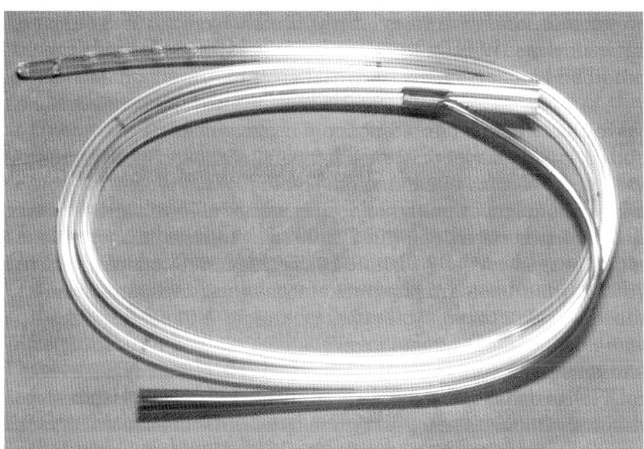

Figure 203-1 Sump suction (Salem) tube. (Argyle Salem Sump, courtesy of Tyco Healthcare, Gosport, United Kingdom.)

Figure 203-2 Feeding nasogastrostomy tube with weighted, radiopaque tip. (COMPAT Nasogastric Tube, courtesy of Nestlé Nutrition, Minnetonka, Minn.)

push into the oropharynx, all of which can hamper the insertion of a tube. At the same time, these tissues are soft and easily injured, thereby increasing the risk of bleeding with nasogastric intubation. Limiting the size of the tube to the smaller sizes of the nostrils and nasal cavity in children usually minimizes the difficulty with insertion, despite these anatomic differences.

Indications

Therapeutic

- Drainage of gastric contents/gastric decompression. *Examples:* small bowel or gastric outlet obstruction, paralytic ileus, upper gastrointestinal bleeding, refractory vomiting, severe pancreatitis with obstruction, gastric lavage (for drug overdose), prevention of aspiration, or before diagnostic peritoneal lavage or pericardiocentesis.
- Instillation of feedings or medications for patients unable to take by mouth. *Examples:* antacids, nutritional supplements, and activated charcoal for drug overdoses.

Diagnostic

- Sampling gastric contents. *Examples:* gastrointestinal bleeding and mycobacterial infection.
- Instillation of diagnostic agents. *Examples:* radiopaque contrast media for delineation of a transdiaphragmatic hernia or an abdominal radiologic procedure with air to assess for an intraperitoneal perforation.
- Radiologic procedure. *Example:* to visualize the stomach on chest radiography for assessment of a diaphragmatic hernia.

Contraindications

All the following contraindications are *relative.*

- Facial fractures, especially midface, or basilar skull fractures with possible cribriform plate injuries (may result in intracranial intubation; orogastric intubation may be a better option)
- Esophageal obstruction, strictures, or a history of alkali ingestion (increases the possibility of esophageal perforation)

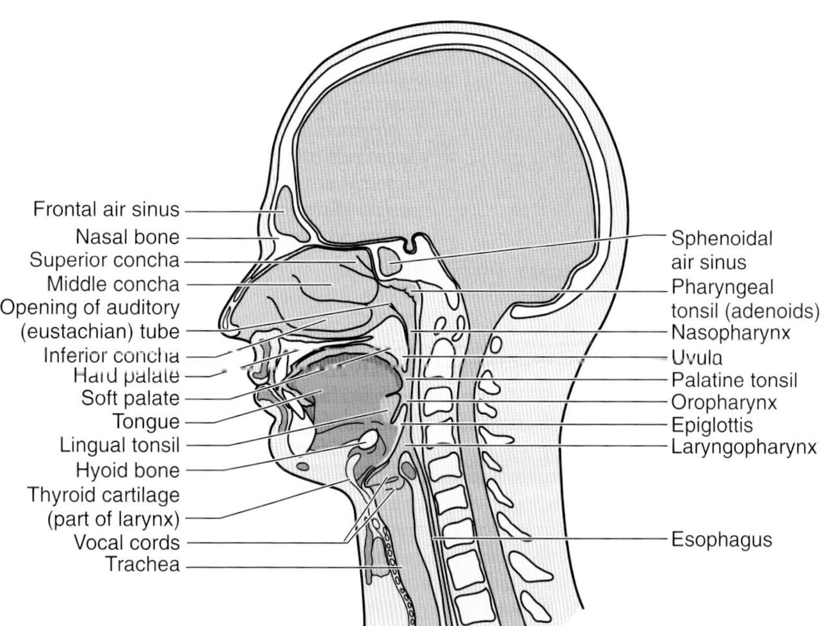

Figure 203-3 Pharyngeal anatomy: sagittal section of the head and neck. (From Thibodeau C, Patton KT: Structure and Function of the Body, 11th ed. St. Louis, Mosby, 2000.)

- Esophageal varices (may lead to rupture and uncontrollable hemorrhage)
- Comatose patients without protected airways (increases the risk of aspiration)
- Penetrating neck wounds in the awake trauma victim (gagging might stimulate increased bleeding from the wound)
- Choanal atresia
- Recent oropharyngeal, nasal, or gastric surgery
- Zenker's diverticulum
- Percutaneous endoscopic gastrostomy tube indicated (see Chapter 200, Percutaneous Endoscopic Gastrostomy Placement and Replacement).
- Severe coagulopathy (orogastric intubation may be a better option)
- Tube feeding in patients with advanced dementia (there is little evidence that the outcome will be improved)

Equipment and Supplies

- Gloves, mask, goggles, and an impervious gown
- Towel or surgical Chux for covering patient's clothing
- Paper tissues
- Emesis basin
- Nasogastric tube (For adults, use a 16- or 18-Fr Salem sump [with antireflux valve, if possible] or Levin tube. Use 10-Fr tube for children.) For nasoenteric feeding tubes (5 to 12 Fr), see Table 203-1. Larger tubes (12 Fr) should be used for shorter periods because they are less comfortable and more likely to become occluded than smaller tubes (5 to 8 Fr).
- Tincture of benzoin
- Hypoallergenic tape (e.g., Hy-Tape), NG Strip, or Tube Guard
- Stethoscope
- Large (60-mL) syringe with catheter tip (Toomey)
- Suction equipment
- Cup of water with drinking straw
- Decongestant such as phenylephrine (0.25% to 2%) spray (Neo-Synephrine, Vick's) or oxymetazoline hydrochloride 0.05% spray (Afrin, Neo-Synephrine 12 hour)
- Water-soluble lubricant gel (Surgilube) or 2% lidocaine gel (Xylocaine Jelly)
- Topical anesthetic spray such as benzocaine (Hurricaine) or tetracaine hydrochloride (Cetacaine), or both. Topical cocaine is an option, and it works as both a decongestant and anesthetic. However, its use may be a problem if the patient has to undergo drug testing. In addition, purchase and storage by clinician or hospital requires significant record-keeping, and may increase the risk of theft.
- Laryngoscope for difficult insertions
- pH indicator strips with 0.5 gradations or paper with a range of 0 to 6 or 1 to 11
- Soft nasal trumpet airway *(optional)*

Preprocedure Patient Preparation

Although the insertion of a nasogastric tube is a common and fairly simple procedure, serious complications can occur. The risk for complications can be minimized by taking a few precautions: obtaining the full cooperation of the patient, informing the patient carefully at each step of the process, using a decongestant and local anesthesia for the nasal and retropharyngeal mucosa, premeasuring and marking the length of the tube needed for insertion, using gentle technique during insertion, and carefully confirming that the tube is in the proper position before use.

Insertion of a nasogastric tube is considered by many patients to be one of the most uncomfortable and distressful procedures they have ever experienced. Although most hospitals do not require written informed consent, the risks, benefits, indications, and any possible alternatives should be explained to patients. Even with the use of decongestants and anesthetics, patients should be prepared for some discomfort. The unpleasant nature of the procedure should not be minimized.

Patients should know that their eyes may water and they may have some tearing. They may have an intense tickling sensation or an urge to sneeze. During insertion, they may experience a gagging sensation. Swallowing rapidly will minimize this response and shorten the total length of the procedure. At some point during the procedure, they will probably be asked to assist by sniffing or later by swallowing. To help them swallow, give them a glass of water and a straw. If they are not able to swallow, if they will mimic swallowing or make the sound "eeee" it may help. Patients should be reassured that after the tube has been placed, they will usually adapt to it very soon and no longer notice it.

Before nasogastric tube removal, the patient should be informed of the procedure and what to expect. Towels, surgical Chux, or other drapes should be placed around the patient's neck and chest. He or she should be handed an emesis basin and tissues.

Technique

Observe universal blood and body fluid precautions during the procedure. Wear gloves, goggles, a face mask, and an impervious gown.

1. Elevate the head of the bed into a high Fowler (sitting) position. Rest the back of the patient's head on a pillow or directly on the bed for support. The patient's clothing needs to be protected with a towel or surgical Chux. An emesis basin should be available on the patient's lap.
2. Check for a clear nasal passage. Various conditions may cause asymmetric nostril openings, for example, septal deviation, nasal polyps, septal spurs. So examine both nostrils to determine which is the largest and most open. You can also watch the patient inhaling through his or her nose to determine which nostril is more open.
3. Choose an optimal tube for the patient. A large-bore nasogastric tube (16 or 18 Fr), Salem sump (with antireflux valve, if available), or Levin tube should be used for adults. Select the largest tube possible for the patient's nostril size. The Salem sump tube has marks at 18, 22, 26, and 30 inches from the distal end. Measure the tube to fit the patient by holding the nasogastric tube above the patient, with the distal end 6 inches below the xiphoid process for a nasogastric tube and 8 to 10 inches for a nasoenteric tube; the proximal end extended to the nose. Loop the mid-portion over the patient's earlobe. Note the tube marks based on these measurements or mark the

TABLE 203-1 Enteral Alimentation Tubes

Trade Name	Material	Circumference (French)	Length (inches)	Feeding	Duration of Use
CORFLO (CORPAK MedSystems, Wheeling, Ill)	Polyurethane	5, 6, 8, 10, 12	15, 22, 36, 43, 55	Gastric or intestinal	Up to 6 weeks
COMPAT (Nestlé Nutrition, Minnetonka, Minn)	Polyurethane	8, 9, 10, 12, 14	42, 55	Gastric or intestinal	Up to 6 weeks
Dobhoff (Kendall/Covidien, Mansfield, Mass)	Polyurethane	3, 5	43, 55	Gastric or intestinal	Up to 6 weeks
Entriflex (Kendall/Covidien)	Polyurethane	5, 7	43, 55	Gastric or intestinal	Up to 6 weeks
Ross Nasoenteric (Abbott Laboratories, Abbott Park, Ill)	Polyurethane	8, 10, 12, 14	36, 45, 60	Gastric or intestinal	Up to 6 weeks

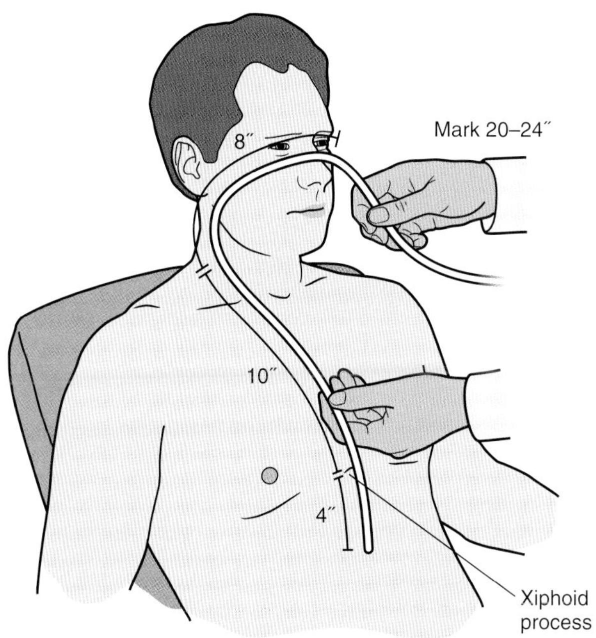

Figure 203-4 Measuring the length of nasogastric tube for placement into stomach.

tube with a piece of tape to avoid inserting the tube too far (Fig. 203-4). The nasogastric tube should generally be secured with the 20- to 24-inch mark at the nasal vestibule.

4. After application of a nasal decongestant such as phenylephrine or oxymetazoline, adding a topical anesthetic usually increases the patient's comfort. Although this procedure is usually brief, application of the decongestant before the anesthesia usually results in the anesthesia lasting longer. The decongestant may also may minimize damage to the nasal mucosa and decrease the incidence of epistaxis.

NOTE: A randomized, controlled trial (Singer and Konia, 1999) showed improved comfort when a decongestant/anesthetic was used, compared with plain lubrication for nasogastric tube insertion. In the study, topical anesthesia was applied (after the decongestant) by injecting 5 mL of 2% lidocaine gel (Xylocaine Jelly) into the nostril before insertion. The pharynx was then sprayed with both benzocaine (Hurricaine) and tetracaine hydrochloride (Cetacaine) spray to minimize the gag reflex. If possible, allow time for the decongestants and anesthetics to take effect before inserting the tube. Topical cocaine solution can also be used, but it often causes a strong burning sensation on application (see Equipment section for other warnings). Application of topical anesthesia should be considered the standard of care except in emergency situations where adequate lubrication alone may be acceptable.

5. An alternative option is to lubricate a soft nasal airway with 2% lidocaine gel and allow the patient to insert the lubricated airway into his or her nares. The nasogastric tube can then be inserted through the soft airway. As the patient swallows the gel, it will anesthetize the pharynx. A soft airway not only minimizes patient discomfort, it can also decrease the risk of severe epistaxis, intracranial intubation, and kinking of the nasogastric tube into the mouth.
6. Lubricate the tip of the tube with additional anesthetic jelly or a water-soluble lubricant. Curl the tube by rolling 18 to 20 inches of the distal tube clockwise onto the first three fingers of your nondominant hand.
7. Introduce the lubricated tube tip into the nostril, pointing straight to the back of the nasal cavity and toward the base of the skull (Fig. 203-5). Recalling the anatomy, it should be inserted horizontally, along the floor of the nasal passage, and directed straight back, not upward. Feed the tube slowly with the dominant hand into the nostril using continuous movement while unrolling the curled tube with the nondominant hand. The patient can sniff to assist the insertion. Never force a tube against resistance; however, spinning or twisting the tube slightly may help overcome resistance.
8. Have the patient flex his or her head slightly forward to narrow the pharyngeal airway. When the tip of the tube reaches the nasopharynx a slight increase in resistance will be noted (Fig. 203-6). Continue to advance the tube, and when the resistance decreases again, ask the patient to swallow or drink some water with a straw. Continue to push the tube with the same motion while asking the patient to continue swallowing. If the patient starts coughing or becomes distressed, or fog is seen in the tube, the tube has probably entered the trachea. The tube should be withdrawn a few inches, but not entirely, twisted slightly, and the process started again. If a patient cannot swallow, it is also helpful to mimic swallowing or to make the sound "eeee."
9. Continue to push the tube until the desired mark is reached if the patient is not coughing. In adults, this is slightly past the 22-inch mark—the second mark—on a Salem sump tube. The gastroesophageal junction is usually about 16 to 18 inches from the nose—the first mark—and the tube should be inserted about 4 inches beyond the gastroesophageal junction. If the stomach is full, an immediate return of fluid may occur. Use the emesis basin to collect this. If there is no return of fluid, open the patient's mouth to confirm that the tube is not curled in the mouth or pharynx.

NOTE: If significant resistance, respiratory distress, or a nasal hemorrhage occurs, or the patient suddenly becomes unable to speak, the tube should be withdrawn.

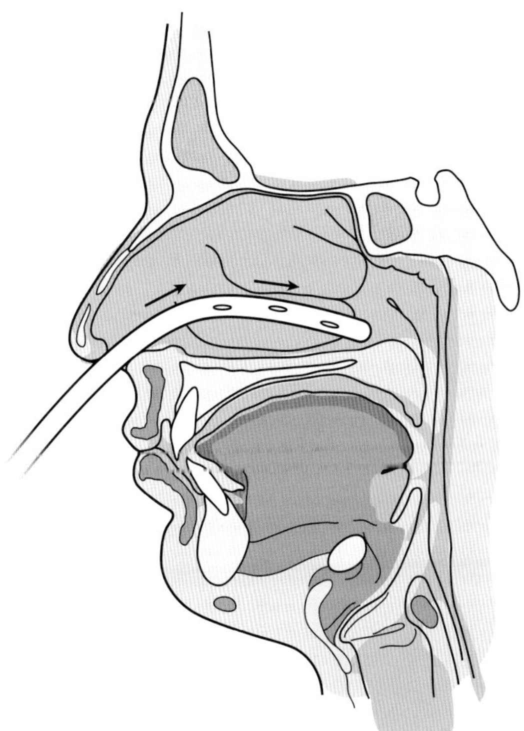

Figure 203-5 Horizontal insertion of nasogastric tube into nasopharynx.

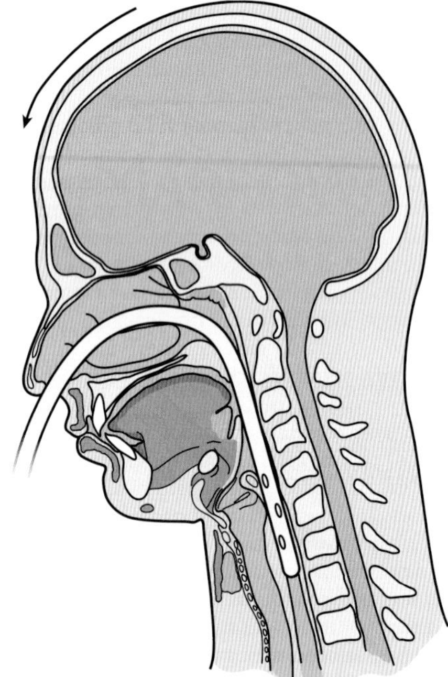

Figure 203-6 Have the patient flex his or her head. Next, gently advance the tube while asking the patient to swallow.

10a. Extra steps to facilitate placement of a *nasoenteric feeding tube* include the following:
- Having placed the tube into the stomach, leave some extra tubing or slack to facilitate passage of the tip into the duodenum.
- Place the patient in a right lateral decubitus (right side down) position.
- A 60-mL syringe (Toomey) can be used to inject 400 mL of air to distend the stomach. This may allow a feeding tube coiled in the fundus of the stomach to uncoil and pass more freely into the duodenum.
- In refractory cases, metoclopramide (Reglan) 10 mg may be given intravenously, with or without erythromycin 250 mg intravenously, to increase gastric motility.

10b. Extra steps to facilitate *any tube placement* include the following:
- If the tube persistently kinks or coils into the mouth, cooling the tube in ice chips or a refrigerator for 5 minutes may stiffen it to prevent coiling. A larger-bore tube is also less likely to coil.
- Applying external and medially directed pressure on the ipsilateral neck at the level of the thyrohyoid membrane may increase the success rate in difficult insertions. This maneuver collapses the piriform sinus and further clears the way for the nasogastric tube. If the tube passes to the level of the hypopharynx but then meets resistance, grasping the thyroid cartilage and lifting it anteriorly and upward may facilitate passage into the upper esophagus.
- Orotracheally intubated patients often present the most difficult challenge for inserting a nasogastric tube. If nasogastric insertion is deemed impossible, a second endotracheal tube may facilitate orogastric tube placement. Remove the respiratory adapter from the proximal end of the second endotracheal tube, lubricate it liberally, and insert it through the patient's mouth and into the esophagus. A well-lubricated nasogastric tube can then be inserted through the second endotracheal tube, which can then be removed over the proximal end of the nasogastric tube.
- Nasogastric placement may be facilitated manually through the oropharynx with three fingers, if necessary. However, unless the patient is unconscious or paralyzed, a bite block should be in place for this maneuver to prevent the clinician from being bitten.
- In difficult cases, a laryngoscope may be helpful for guiding or confirming proper placement.
- Fluoroscopic or endoscopic assistance may be necessary.

11. Confirm the location of the tip as soon as possible after the tube is passed. Ask the patient to speak after placement. If he or she is unable to speak, the tube is in the trachea and should be withdrawn. (Be aware that cases have been reported in which the patient could talk despite tracheal placement of a small-bore feeding tube.) Otherwise, the position of the tip should be confirmed by a chest radiograph. In addition, there are two traditional methods for confirming proper nasogastric placement: checking for absence of rhythmic airflow and auscultating for gastric bubbling when air is injected into the stomach. As it turns out, both of these techniques have been found to be inaccurate and therefore they are not recommended. Even if the tip of the tube is located in the esophagus, duodenum, jejunum, pleural space, or respiratory tract, a bubbling sound may be heard. If proper location is misdiagnosed, the instillation of feeds or air has been reported to result in a pneumonia or pneumothorax with a high chance of an adverse outcome. Fortunately, placement can also be confirmed by aspiration (to check for gastric contents) and by ultrasonography.

NOTE: If gastric juices are aspirated, correct placement has been demonstrated. Testing the pH of the aspirate will further verify placement. We recommend pH indicator strips with 0.5 gradations or paper with a range of 0 to 6 or 1 to 11. It is important that the resulting color change on any indicator strip or paper is easily distinguishable, particularly between the pH 5 to 6 range. The old type of litmus paper should not be used. Rakel and colleagues (1994) reviewed several studies regarding the significance of the pH value of the aspirate. They found that gastric fluid should have a pH of 0 to 4. If the patient is on antacids, histamine type 2 inhibitors, or proton pump inhibitors, the pH is between 0 and 6 approximately 70% to 80% of the time. Fluid aspirated from the duodenum averaged a pH of 6.5. Fluid aspirated from tracheobronchial secretions ranged from pH 6.74 to 8.79. In other words, suspect that fluid from the respiratory tract has been aspirated when the pH is greater than 6.

Neumann and colleagues (1995) concluded that when the pH of the nasogastric tube aspirate is less than 4.0, radiographs are not needed to confirm tube placement. In 2005, the National Patient Safety Agency in the United Kingdom recommended the use of a pH value of less than 5.5 for tube placement confirmation; they concluded a pH value of less than 4.0 (as recommended by Neumann and associates) is too low to evaluate patients practically. If the pH is greater than 5.5, a chest radiograph, still the gold standard, is required to confirm tube placement (Fig. 203-7). However, it chest radiography adds cost and prolongs waiting time before use (it can take up to 8 hours to receive notification from the radiologist). It also increases radiation exposure. There are also case reports of inaccurate confirmations by radiographs, with the tube being located in the midline after perforating the esophagus, subclavian vein, or atrium of the heart.

Recently, the bedside sonographic examination performed by experienced clinicians has been reported to be a sensitive method for confirming the position of nasogastric tubes. It is faster than conventional radiography and can easily be taught to nonradiologists. Confirmation must be done on all small-bore nasogastric or nasoenteric tubes used for feeding purposes before starting feeding to avoid massive aspiration. The distal

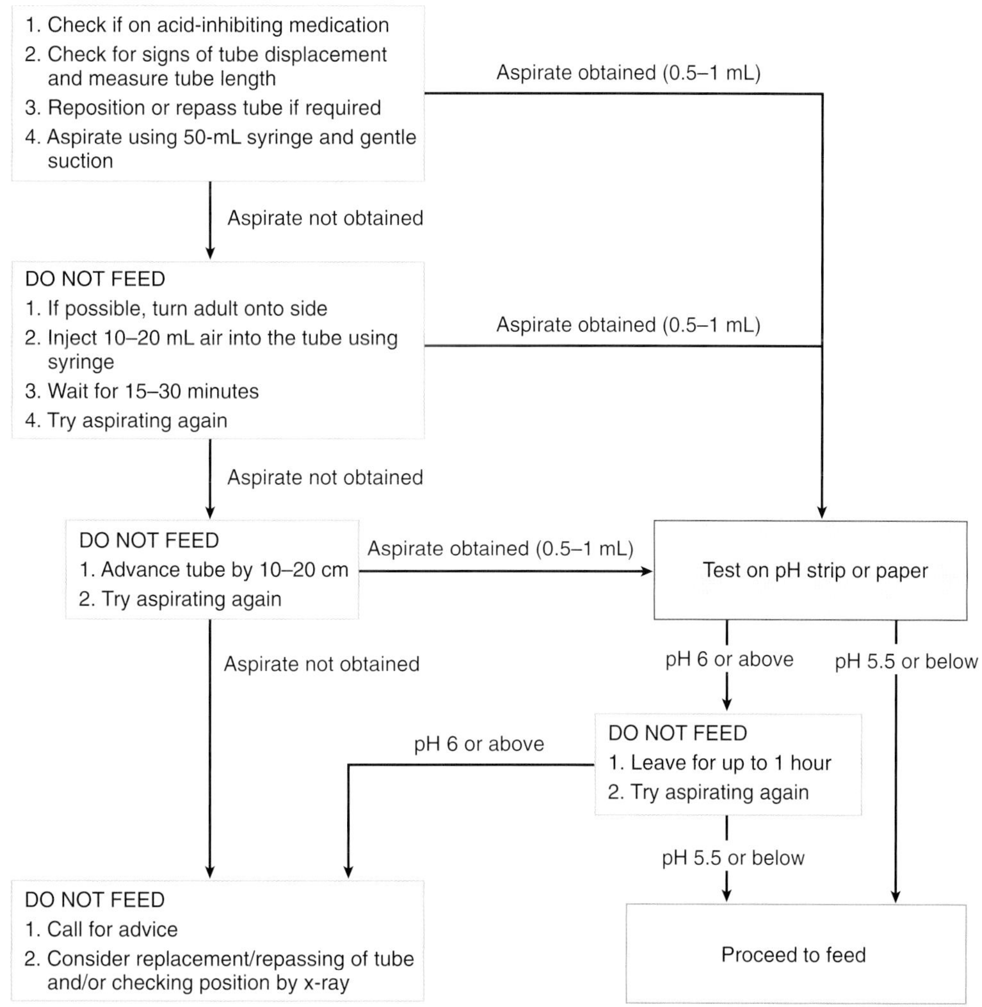
1. Check if on acid-inhibiting medication
2. Check for signs of tube displacement and measure tube length
3. Reposition or repass tube if required
4. Aspirate using 50-mL syringe and gentle suction
Aspirate obtained (0.5–1 mL)
Aspirate not obtained
DO NOT FEED
1. If possible, turn adult onto side
2. Inject 10–20 mL air into the tube using syringe
3. Wait for 15–30 minutes
4. Try aspirating again
Aspirate obtained (0.5–1 mL)
Aspirate not obtained
DO NOT FEED
1. Advance tube by 10–20 cm
2. Try aspirating again
Aspirate obtained (0.5–1 mL)
Test on pH strip or paper
Aspirate not obtained
pH 6 or above
pH 5.5 or below
pH 6 or above
DO NOT FEED
1. Leave for up to 1 hour
2. Try aspirating again
pH 5.5 or below
DO NOT FEED
1. Call for advice
2. Consider replacement/repassing of tube and/or checking position by x-ray
Proceed to feed
CAUTION: If there is ANY query about position and/or the clarity of the color change on the pH strip, particularly between ranges 5 and 6, then feeding should not commence.

Figure 203-7 Algorithm to confirm the correct position of nasogastric feeding tubes in adults. (From the National Patient Safety Agency [NPSA]: Reducing the harm caused by misplaced nasogastric feeding tubes: Interim advice for healthcare staff—February 2005; How to confirm the correct position of nasogastric feeding tubes in infants, children and adults. Available at www.nrls.npsa.nhs.uk/resources/?EntryId45=59794.)

tips of these tubes should be allowed to migrate to the duodenum before enteral feeding is initiated.

12. Secure the tube to the patient's nose after confirmation of proper placement. First, apply alcohol to the dorsum of the nose. If available, tincture of benzoin may then be applied after the alcohol dries. Next, obtain a 5-inch piece of 1-inch-wide hypoallergenic tape. Make a 3-inch cut lengthwise in the middle, thereby forming two narrow strips of tape at one end of the 5-inch piece (Fig. 203-8). The two narrow strips of tape should be applied in a spiral down and around the nasogastric tube, going away from the patient's nose. Attempt to tape the tube so that it will rest in the middle of the nostril to minimize direct contact of the tube with the skin of the nose and avoid pressure necrosis. Recently, several commercial products, NG Strip (Cardinal Health, Dublin, Ohio) and TubeGuard (Mormac TubeGuard, North Loup, Neb), have been developed for this special purpose.
13. Also secure the nasogastric tube to the patient's gown. Place a slipknot over the tube with a rubber band, and then pin it to the patient's gown. This should reduce the risk of the nasogastric tube being tugged out of position. The Salem sump tube vent, or blue pigtail, must remain above the patient's waistline at all times to prevent gravity from siphoning fluid. Inadvertent siphoning of gastric contents could block the sump vent. When suction is discontinued during ambulation, the pigtail should be attached to the connector of the main lumen to close the system and avoid the spillage of gastric fluids.
14. For removal, again place the patient in the sitting (Fowler) position and cover his or her neck and chest with towels, surgical Chux, or other drapes. Disconnect the nasogastric tube from the patient, from his or her nose, and from suction. Hand the patient an emesis basin and some tissues. Fold over the proximal end of the tube to prevent leakage and hold it tightly. Ask the patient to flex the neck, breath in, and hold his or her breath. Place a drape around the tube and withdraw the tube from the patient's nose through the drape. The patient can then resume breathing. Discard the tube and the drape.

Complications

The most common complication is discomfort of the patient. The traumatic insertion of a nasogastric tube can cause epistaxis, but this is often avoided by using careful technique and a decongestant.

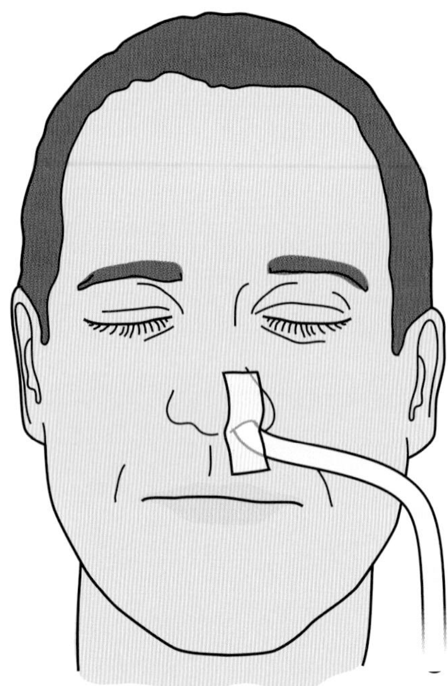

Figure 203-8 Secure the tube with a 5-inch piece of 1-inch-wide hypoallergenic tape, partially cut lengthwise. Apply to the dorsum of the nose and spiral the cut portions down the tube away from the nose.

Epistaxis can be massive and requires packing. It can even compromise the airway. Gagging can occur and induce vomiting with aspiration of gastric contents. This can cause an aspiration pneumonitis or pneumonia with a mortality rate as high as 30%. Patients with an altered mental status from severe trauma or other causes should have their airway secured with an endotracheal tube before placement of a nasogastric tube.

Another common complication is misplacement into the respiratory tree, which is estimated to occur in 15% of cases. This should be recognized rapidly in the conscious patient when it causes him or her to cough, choke, or develop respiratory distress or an inability to talk. The vocal cords may also be traumatized. In a patient with decreased consciousness, tracheal intubation can go undetected, creating multiple complications such as atelectasis, pulmonary edema, pneumonia, or lung abscess.

The "nasogastric tube syndrome" is a reported life-threatening complication with laryngeal and upper airway obstruction and vocal cord abduction paralysis. The nasogastric tube syndrome results from postcricoid ulceration and its effect on the posterior cricoarytenoid muscles. This can be prevented by early recognition and by checking the patient every day when making rounds. It is treated with emergent tracheostomy, immediate removal of the nasogastric tube, and administration of systemic antibiotics.

Penetration of a nasogastric tube into the pleural space is a rare but reported complication, with further possible complications including lung abscess, pneumothorax, isocalothorax, empyema, and sepsis. Intravascular penetration of the internal jugular and subclavian vessels has also been reported.

Perforation of the esophagus is a very serious reported complication that often results in mediastinitis, with a mortality rate of up to 30%. This may occur when the esophagus has been damaged by chemical burns, esophageal cancer, and multiple attempts, or if strictures are present, or with insertion after esophageal surgery. Prompt recognition of this complication, surgical repair, and parenteral antibiotics can significantly reduce the mortality rate. Bleeding from esophageal varices is not usually caused by nasogastric intubation. Duodenal perforation has also been reported. Tube knotting, coiling, kinking, obstruction, and rupture can occur.

With long-term use, sinusitis, erosion of nasal tissue, or even a tracheoesophageal fistula can occur. Tracheoesophageal fistulas are usually associated with simultaneous use of an endotracheal tube. Sinusitis can cause a fever of unknown origin in patients.

If the tube is forced against resistance, cribriform plate fracture may result, with subsequent intracranial intubation. Individuals with mid-facial or maxillofacial trauma or a basilar skull fracture have a significantly increased risk of inadvertent intracranial intubation. The risk of this complication can be reduced by using the orogastric route or by initially introducing a nasotracheal tube or a soft rubber nasal airway, through which a smaller-diameter nasogastric tube can then be passed. This technique decreases the danger of penetrating the cranium, reduces discomfort during insertion, decreases epistaxis, and decreases the frequency of the nasogastric tube kinking into the mouth. The long-term use of nasoenteric tube feeding may result in diarrhea, infection, electrolyte imbalance, and malnutrition.

Postprocedure Management

The nares should be assessed for skin irritation, erosion, or necrosis by health providers at regular intervals. The patient should be asked if he or she has any pain or pressure in the nose, throat, or sinuses. Any old or detached tape should be replaced after cleaning the skin of the nose with alcohol and applying tincture of benzoin. On a regular basis, the nursing team should record the patency of the tube, the level of graduated marks on the tube, any symptoms or patient complaints, the volume and nature of anything infused, and any residual volume. If it becomes difficult to aspirate from the tube, it should be flushed with 30 mL water. If patency is still uncertain, it should be repositioned by advancing 1 inch or withdrawing 1 inch. The same maneuver should then be tried again to confirm patency. Because the use of acidic substances for flushing can cause whole-protein formulas to coagulate and clog the tube, this practice should be discouraged. The tube should be flushed before and after each intermittent feeding, after medication administration, or every 4 to 6 hours in case of continuous infusion. When the volume of residual is higher than 300 to 400 mL or there is significant gastric distention, the clinician should be notified and any infusions held. Infusions should be held for several hours and the residual rechecked before restarting. For the infusion of medications, liquid forms should be used if possible. If pills are used they should be crushed to a fine powder and mixed with water. If the result is sticky or highly concentrated, dilute it further with water. When the tube is clogged, it can be irrigated with warm water or, if unsuccessful, a pancreatic enzyme solution injected. Reinsertion of a device, for example a stylet or guidewire, into a nasoenteric tube should never be tried because it can result in gastrointestinal tract injury. If there are unusual gastrointestinal symptoms like nausea, cramping, abdominal distention, or severe diarrhea, the infusion should be stopped and the clinician notified immediately. The clinician must assess the patient and the tube at this point.

When the nasogastric tube is used for gastric decompression or postoperative drainage, clinicians should understand the mechanics of nasogastric suction. Suction strength is inversely proportional to flow; therefore, the lower the flow rate through the suction lumen, the higher the suction strength. In addition, a suction force of more than 25 mm Hg causes tissue capillary fragility and may damage the gastric mucosa. One advantage of the double-lumen Salem sump tube over the Levin tube is that it allows constant airflow through the secondary lumen, keeping the necessary suction in the main lumen at a minimum. Therefore, the vent lumen must not be clamped or plugged. When the Levin tube is used, an intermittent suction pump should be connected to prevent injury of the gastrointestinal mucosa. The length of time the tube can be used depends on the patient's condition, feeding needs, and the tube design. With proper care and maintenance, most nasogastric tubes can be used for up to 30 days. For longer use, a percutaneous endoscopic gastrostomy tube should be considered (see Chapter 200, Percutaneous Endoscopic Gastrostomy Placement and Replacement).

CPT/Billing Codes

43219 Endoscopic guided insertion of plastic tube or stent
43752 Nasogastric or orogastric tube placement, necessitating physician's skill and fluoroscopic guidance
44500 Introduction of long gastrointestinal tube (e.g., Miller-Abbott)
74340 Introduction of long gastrointestinal tube (e.g., Miller-Abbott) with fluoroscopic guidance
89100 Duodenal intubation and aspiration; single specimen plus appropriate test procedure
89130 Gastric intubation and aspiration, diagnostic, each specimen, for chemical analysis or cytopathology
91105 Gastric intubation, and aspiration or lavage, for treatment (e.g., for ingested poisons)

ICD-9-CM Diagnostic Codes

014.82 Tuberculosis, gastrocolic, labs pending
261 Calorie deficiency, severe
263.9 Malnutrition, protein-calorie
536.2 Vomiting, persistent, nonpregnant
537.0 Gastric outlet obstruction, acquired or adult
560.1 Ileus, paralytic
561.81 Small intestine obstruction, due to adhesions
577.0 Pancreatitis, NOS or acute
577.1 Pancreatitis, chronic
578.0 Hematemesis or gastrointestinal hemorrhage
578.1 Hematochezia
578.9 Gastrointestinal bleeding, unspecified
787.01 Vomiting, NOS with nausea
787.03 Vomiting, NOS
977.9 Poisoning, unspecified drug or medicinal substances

Acknowledgment

The editors wish to recognize the contributions by Julie Graves Moy, MD, and Ramiro Sanchez, MD, to this chapter in the previous two editions of this text.

Suppliers

(See contact information online at www.expertconsult.com.)

Feeding tubes
Cook Incorporated (including percutaneous endoscopic gastrostomy tubes)
CORPAK MedSystems/VIASYS Healthcare/Cardinal Health

Latex-free, zinc oxide tape
Hy-Tape International

Levin, Salem sump, and feeding tubes
The Kendall Company (Covidien)

Nasogastric tube guard
Mormac TubeGuard
NG Strip (Cardinal Health)

pH indicator
pHion Nutrition

60-mL syringe with catheter tip (Toomey)
Becton, Dickinson and Co.

Topical anesthetic
Cetacaine
Cetylite Industries, Inc.
Xylocaine Jelly
AstraZeneca L.P.

Online Resources

National Patient Safety Agency (NPSA) UK: Reducing the harm caused by misplaced nasogastric feeding tubes: Interim advice for healthcare staff—February 2005. Available at www.npsa.nhs.uk/advice. Accessed May 15, 2010.

Thomsen TW, Shaffer RW, Setnik GS: Nasogastric intubation. Videos in Clinical Medicine. N Engl J Med 27 April, 2006. Available at http://content.nejm.org/cgi/video/354/17/e16/. Accessed May 15, 2010.

Bibliography

Fisman DN, Ward ME: Intrapleural placement of a nasogastric tube: An unusual complication of nasotracheal intubation. Can J Anaesth 43:1252–1256, 1996.

Leschke RR: Nasogastric intubation. In Reichman EF, Simon RR (eds): Emergency Medicine Procedures. New York, McGraw-Hill, 2004, pp 413–419.

Marcus EL, Caine Y, Hamdan K, et al: Nasogastric tube syndrome: A life-threatening laryngeal obstruction in a 72-year-old patient. Age Ageing 35:538–539, 2006.

Neumann MJ, Meyer CT, Dutton JL, et al: Hold that x-ray: Aspirate pH and auscultation prove enteral tube placement. J Clin Gastroenterol 20:293–295, 1995.

Pillai JB, Vegas A, Brister S: Thoracic complications of nasogastric tube: Review of safe practice. Interact Cardiovasc Thorac Surg 4:429–433, 2005.

Rakel BA, Titler M, Goode C, et al: Nasogastric and nasointestinal feeding tube placement: An integrative review of research. AACN Clin Issues Crit Care Nurs 5:194–206; quiz 218–219, 1994.

Singer AJ, Konia N: Comparison of topical anesthetics and vasoconstrictors vs lubricants prior to nasogastric intubation: A randomized, controlled trial. Acad Emerg Med 6:184–190, 1999.

Vigneau C, Baudel J-L, Guidet B, et al: Sonography as an alternative to radiography for nasogastric feeding tube location. Intensive Care Med 31:1570–1572, 2005.

CHAPTER 204

Diagnostic Peritoneal Lavage

Eric Skye

Diagnostic peritoneal lavage (DPL) is a procedure that consists of two components. The first part involves the attempt to aspirate any free blood that may be present in the peritoneal cavity. If this initial portion of the procedure reveals hemoperitoneum, the test is considered positive and the remainder of the procedure is aborted. Hemoperitoneum in this circumstance is highly predictive of intraperitoneal injury and warrants a laparotomy.

If no free blood is obtained during the initial aspiration, the second portion of the procedure is conducted. This involves the introduction of normal saline or lactated Ringer's into the peritoneal cavity. The instilled fluid is subsequently drained from the peritoneal cavity and analyzed; results may ultimately indicate the nature of the intra-abdominal pathology.

Physical examination can be misleading in up to 45% of patients with blunt abdominal trauma. Spiral (helical/real-time) abdominal computed tomography and focused abdominal sonography for trauma (FAST; often performed at the bedside; see Chapter 225, Emergency Department, Hospitalist, and Office Ultrasonography [Clinical Ultrasonography]) are generally considered the preferred initial diagnostic choices for evaluation of patients with blunt abdominal trauma that may necessitate surgical intervention. However, DPL continues to be an important diagnostic tool in patients with blunt abdominal trauma who are hemodynamically unstable and for whom bedside ultrasonography is not available or they cannot be transported safely from the emergency department for imaging studies. DPL also serves as an adjunct in the evaluation of the patient with penetrating trauma.

Anatomy

Diagnostic peritoneal lavage is traditionally performed in the midline, 1 to 2 cm below the umbilicus, which allows entry into the peritoneal cavity through the linea alba (the fibrous structure separating the rectus abdominis muscles). This fibrous band is relatively avascular and provides safe access for both the open and closed techniques. If DPL is performed above the umbilicus, the omentum frequently interferes with the catheter. When performed below the umbilicus, it is also usually easier to advance the catheter into a dependent location such as the pelvis.

Indications

- After blunt abdominal trauma in a patient who is either hemodynamically unstable or has an altered mental status or abnormal sensation (e.g., spinal cord injury) to assess for intraperitoneal hemorrhage or organ injury.
- After penetrating injuries (e.g., stab wound or gunshot wound) to the abdomen, flank, back, or lower chest to assess for intraperitoneal hemorrhage or organ injury. (Gunshot wounds that penetrate the peritoneum result in intraperitoneal injury in 98% of cases, so they warrant going straight to laparotomy; therefore, DPL should only be used for tangential gunshot wounds to the abdomen. Likewise, penetration into the peritoneum from a thoracoabdominal wound results in a diaphragmatic injury that, by definition, needs to be repaired, so such injuries warrant going straight to surgery. Penetration through the retroperitoneum from the back or flank will cause a significant injury in 73% of cases; DPL may help determine whether the retroperitoneum has been traversed. Only two thirds of stab wounds to the anterior abdomen will penetrate the peritoneum, and of these, only 50% will require repair. Use of DPL in these cases may reduce the laparotomy rate.)
- After penetrating injuries to the abdomen, flank, back, or lower chest or blunt abdominal trauma in a patient who has an unreliable physical examination or in whom serial physical examinations are not practical (e.g., patient under anesthesia for orthopedic or neurosurgical procedure or taking postoperative analgesics).
- For the patient in shock after trauma that has other potential sources of hemorrhage (e.g., thoracic, retroperitoneal) to determine whether intraperitoneal hemorrhage is contributing to shock.

Contraindications

Absolute

Acute abdomen requiring immediate surgery is the only absolute contraindication.

Relative

If DPL is performed, the open technique should be used.

- Previous abdominal surgery (bowel may be adherent to midline; although DPL may be performed in area away from scar, compartmentalization of abdomen may have occurred, preventing blood circulation and causing false-negative DPL result).
- Coagulopathy.
- Pregnancy (DPL should be performed above the level of the uterine fundus; possibly below umbilicus in early-stage pregnancy).
- Morbid obesity (the locator needle may not be long enough to pierce abdominal wall).
- Pelvic fracture (use open technique above the umbilicus; closed technique may result in penetration of a retroperitoneal hematoma, a false-positive result, and decompression of the hematoma).
- Inability to insert Foley catheter to decompress bladder (e.g., urethral injury or stricture).

Equipment

Commercially prepared kit or the following equipment:

- Skin-cleansing solution (povidone–iodine or chlorhexidine)
- Sterile gloves and mask

- Sterile marking pen (if area has not been marked indelibly before skin preparation)
- Sterile drapes
- 4 × 4 gauze squares
- 1% or 2% lidocaine with epinephrine
- Scalpel, no. 11 (and no. 15 blade for open technique)
- 9- to 18-Fr peritoneal catheter (kit equipped with catheter-over-wire system for closed or Seldinger technique)
- 10-mL syringe for anesthetic
- 10-mL syringe for diagnostic tap
- 50-mL syringe, if using stopcock technique
- 18-gauge, 1½- to 3-inch locator needle; alternatively, an 18- or 20-gauge, 1½- to 3-inch spinal needle may be substituted
- 25- or 27-gauge, 1½-inch needle
- Purple-topped blood collection tube
- Instruments for retractions such as hemostats or Army-Navy retractors
- Needle holder
- Nylon skin suture (4-0 or 5-0) on cutting needle
- Absorbable sutures (2-0 Vicryl) for peritoneum and fascia, if peritoneum is to be opened
- Sterile intravenous (IV) fluid (1 L warmed lactated Ringer's or normal saline, as opposed to fluid at room temperature, is preferred) and tubing
- Razor if open technique used
- Foley catheter
- Nasogastric tube
- Three-way stopcock (for use with 50-mL syringe) *(optional)*

PRECAUTIONS

- An open technique should be considered if the patient has a relative contraindication such as coagulopathy, pregnancy, previous abdominal surgery, pelvic fracture, or morbid obesity.
- A surgical assistant is recommended for an open DPL.
- DPL will not diagnose retroperitoneal hemorrhage.

PREPROCEDURE PATIENT PREPARATION

- Explain the procedure and its risks and benefits to the patient if possible (see the Complications section).
- Obtain verbal or written informed consent if possible.
- Place patient in the supine position.
- Use a Foley catheter and nasogastric tube for decompression of the bladder and stomach, respectively, if necessary.
- If necessary, use wrist restraints, especially for patients with altered mental status, to prevent contamination of the sterile field or self-injury.
- Consider procedural sedation (see Chapter 2, Procedural Sedation and Analgesia), especially if performing an open DPL.

EDITOR'S NOTE: Reviewing Chapter 201, Abdominal Paracentesis, may also be helpful.

TECHNIQUE

Procedural setup and fluid removal are identical for the open and closed techniques.

1. Decompress the stomach and bladder. (See Chapter 203, Nasogastric and Nasoenteric Tube Insertion, and Chapter 110, Bladder Catheterization [and Urethral Dilation].)
2. Prepare the abdominal skin at the puncture site with standard preparation solutions such as chlorhexidine or povidone–iodine, and apply sterile drapes as appropriate. The ideal site is immediately inferior to the umbilicus (Fig. 204-1). Again, the supraumbilical approach may be used in second- or third-trimester pregnant patients, patients with prior lower abdominal surgery, or patients with pelvic fractures.

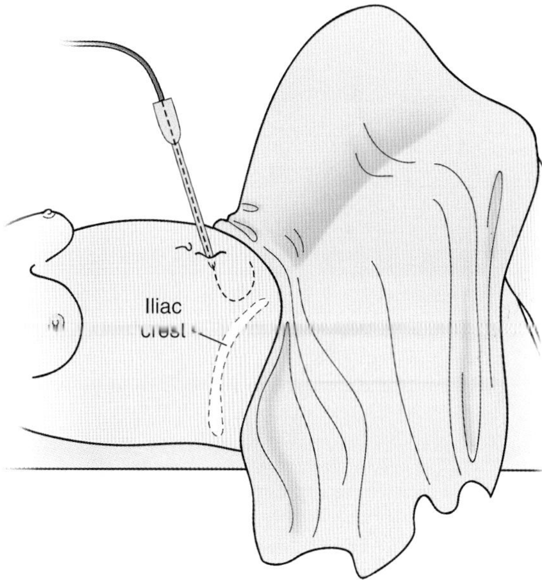

Figure 204-1 Insertion of the needle into the peritoneal cavity in the midline, immediately inferior to the umbilicus.

3. Infiltrate the skin, subcutaneous tissues, and fascia with lidocaine with epinephrine.

A. Closed (Seldinger) Technique

This is the preferred technique, if not contraindicated.

4a. Attach an 18-gauge locator needle to the syringe and insert it into the midline, 1 to 2 cm inferior to the umbilicus, directed at a 45-degree angle to the skin and toward the pelvis. Applying negative pressure on the syringe, insert the needle through the skin and directly into the peritoneal space. Three "pops" are felt as the needle penetrates the skin, the fascia, and the peritoneum. If blood is aspirated during this step, it is considered a positive result. If not, proceed to step 5.

5a. The guidewire is then introduced through the 18-gauge needle, until only 7 to 10 cm of the guidewire remains outside the needle. You may then safely remove the needle, although there must be continuous control of the wire to prevent migration and injury to peritoneal structures. If there is difficulty inserting the guidewire or the patient complains of pain, both the needle and guidewire should be removed as a unit. To avoid shearing it off, do not withdraw the guidewire through the needle.

6a. Slide the peritoneal catheter over the wire using gentle twisting motions. With the closed technique, it may be necessary to make a small skin nick at the entry site with the scalpel to allow for passage of the lavage catheter.

7a. Remove the wire after the catheter is in the peritoneum. Proceed to step 8.

B. Open Technique

4b. The skin should be shaved before preparation. Using the no.11 blade, create a 4- to 6-cm vertical skin incision in the midline.

5b. By blunt dissection, proceed down to the rectus fascia. Clamp and ligate any bleeders with absorbable suture before opening the fascia to prevent a false-positive test result. Open the rectus fascia using the no. 15 blade, and then proceed down to the peritoneum by sharp and blunt dissection.

6b. A 2- to 3-mm opening of the fascia is adequate for a semiopen technique. This technique provides room for the catheter to be inserted directly into the peritoneal space, even though visualization of the structures is not possible.

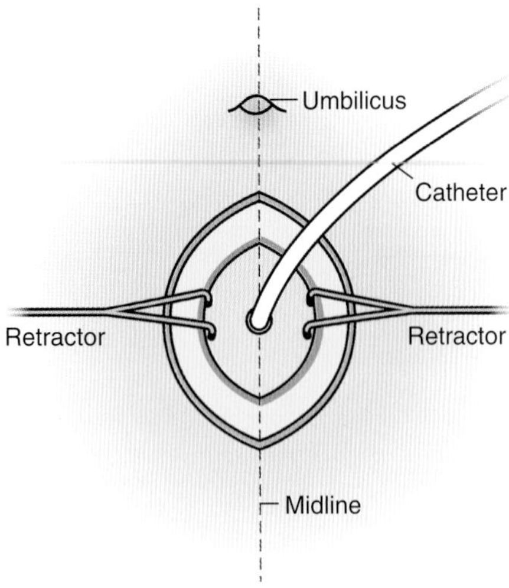

Figure 204-2 Open technique, view from above. Superficial layers have been opened and are retracted away from the field of view. Catheter is inserted through the opened peritoneum directly into the peritoneal space.

7b. A slightly longer incision of the fascia is required for the open technique. The longer incision allows for the peritoneal space to be opened and visualized. The catheter can then be inserted into the peritoneal space under direct visualization (Fig. 204-2). Proceed to step 8.

Both Techniques

8. Attach the syringe to the catheter and attempt to withdraw fluid. If more than 10 mL of blood is obtained, the patient should be prepared for emergent laparotomy. If the tap is dry, proceed to peritoneal lavage.
9. Connect the IV tubing and infuse lactated Ringer's solution or normal saline. The amount infused is 1 L for adults and 15 mL/kg for children.
10. The infused fluid is then removed by placing the IV bag on the floor and allowing the fluid to return by gravity. Alternatively, the IV tubing may be connected to a 1-L vacuum jar. The fluid should return at a steady rate of flow. If this flow is interrupted, it is probably due to omentum blocking the holes in the catheter. Placing pressure on the patient's abdomen may increase the flow; alternatively, the catheter may need to be withdrawn slightly and reinserted. If these maneuvers do not increase the return flow, a second liter of IV fluid may be infused.
11. At least 200 to 300 mL of lavage fluid should be returned for a valid test. After the maneuvers described previously have been performed, if less than 200 to 250 mL of return flow is obtained, a second catheter should be inserted. This should be inserted 1 cm below the first in the same manner as the first, in the midline. A second IV bag should then be attached and lowered to collect fluid via gravity drainage. After the fluid is removed, gently remove the catheter and apply pressure to the wound. When the open technique is used, close the peritoneum and rectus fascia with absorbable suture. The skin is then closed with nylon suture. If the closed technique was used, placement of a pressure dressing alone may suffice, although a single nylon skin suture may be necessary in some patients. A small amount of fluid should be transferred to the purple-topped tube for laboratory analysis.

Sample Operative Report

See the Sample Operative Report online at www.expertconsult.com.

Complications

Complication rates range from 0.6% to 2.3% of all DPLs. There is no difference in complication rates among the techniques discussed.

- Bladder perforation
- Bowel perforation
- Lacerations of major vessels
- Abdominal wall hematoma
- Abdominal wall dehiscence
- Infection (local, intraperitoneal, or systemic)
- False-positive result (vessel laceration during procedure) or false-negative result (poor catheter placement or loss of fluid into the thoracic cavity)

Postprocedure Patient Education

If the DPL result is positive, the patient should be informed of the need for emergent surgery. The patient with a negative DPL should be observed in the hospital for up to 24 hours. He or she should remain NPO during the initial observation period and receive analgesics as needed. Before discharge, it is useful to determine whether the patient can tolerate a regular diet. Also before discharge, educate the patient about the signs and symptoms of a complication such as bleeding, pain, vomiting, or infection. The patient should be given instructions regarding wound care.

Interpretation of Results

The aspiration of greater than 10 mL of gross blood on entering the peritoneal cavity or through the locator needle is considered a positive finding. If not grossly bloody, fluid aspirated through the catheter should be sent for a red blood cell (RBC) count, a white blood cell (WBC) count, and possibly to check for amylase. Findings of more than 100,000 RBCs/mm^3 are also considered positive (half these numbers if 2 L of fluid were infused). Findings of 20,000/mm^3 to 100,000/mm^3 RBCs should be considered equivocal. In these patients an observation period of 12 to 24 hours should be considered. Two situations provide exceptions to these general rules: (1) stab wounds to the low chest where diaphragmatic injury is suspected (the diaphragm does not bleed as readily as other abdominal organs); and (2) gunshot wounds. The threshold for a positive RBC count should be 5000 RBC/mm^3 in these situations. Always be mindful of the hemodynamic stability of the patient when interpreting these results.

A WBC count greater 500 cells/mm^3 is also considered a positive test and warrants laparotomy. Amylase may be elevated when there is injury to the gastrointestinal tract; however, a positive amylase test is neither sensitive nor specific. Confusion sometimes exists when a small amount of gross blood (<10 mL) is aspirated directly from the catheter (as opposed to the locator needle). This may have been the only blood located in a dependent portion of the abdomen and may not indicate the patient is unstable. The patient does not need a laparotomy if the subsequent lavage is negative.

CPT/Billing Codes

49080 Peritoneocentesis, abdominal paracentesis, or peritoneal lavage (diagnostic or therapeutic); initial
49081 Peritoneocentesis, abdominal paracentesis, or peritoneal lavage; subsequent

ICD-9-CM Diagnostic Codes

568.81 Hemoperitoneum (nontraumatic)
862.1 Injury, diaphragm, with open wound into cavity
863 Injury to gastrointestinal tract
864 Injury to liver
865 Injury to spleen

866 Injury to kidney
867 Injury to pelvic organs
868.00 Injury, other intra-abdominal organs, without mention of open wound into cavity
868.03 Injury, peritoneum, without mention of open wound into cavity

Acknowledgment

The editors wish to recognize the contributions by Michael Brown, MD, Brett White, MD, and Kenneth Hu, MD, to this chapter in the previous two editions of this text.

Supplier

(See contact information online at www.expertconsult.com.)

Peritoneal lavage kit
Arrow International (Teleflex Medical)

BIBLIOGRAPHY

Howell JM, Jolly BT, Lukens TW, et al: Clinical policy: Critical issues in the evaluation of adult patients presenting to the emergency department with acute blunt abdominal trauma. Ann Emerg Med 43:278–290, 2004.

Isenhour JL, Marx JA: Abdominal trauma. In Marx JA, Hockberger JS, Walls RM (eds): Rosen's Emergency Medicine: Concepts and Clinical Practice, 7th ed. Philadelphia, Mosby, 2010, pp 414–434.

Marx JA, Hockberger JS, Walls RM (eds): Rosen's Emergency Medicine: Concepts and Clinical Practice, 7th ed. Philadelphia, Mosby, 2010.

Nagy K: Diagnostic peritoneal lavage. In Reichman EF, Simon RR (eds): Emergency Medicine Procedures. New York, McGraw-Hill, 2004, pp 478–489.

Roberts JR, Hedges JR (eds): Clinical Procedures in Emergency Medicine, 3rd ed. Philadelphia, Saunders, 2004.

CHAPTER 205

Bone Marrow Aspiration and Biopsy

Beth A. Choby

Bone marrow examination is a useful adjunct in the evaluation of various diseases, both hematologic and nonhematologic in origin. Bone marrow aspiration and biopsy supply additional clinical information when peripheral blood smears or other routine laboratory tests are inconclusive. Certain patients require bone marrow sampling for cytogenetic analysis, molecular studies, flow cytometry, or microbiologic cultures. The two procedures are performed sequentially and supply complementary information. Bone marrow aspiration allows visualization of cell morphology and a count of marrow cellular elements, whereas bone marrow (trephine) biopsy evaluates marrow cellularity and detects focal lesions such as metastatic cancer, lymphoma, or granulomas.

Bone marrow aspiration and biopsy are performed through one skin incision but sample separate areas of bone about 5 mm apart. The aspirate is usually collected first. A drawback of this approach is aspiration artifact, the artifactual hypocellularity and contamination with sinusoidal blood seen on the subsequent marrow biopsy specimen. Although the bone marrow biopsy can be done first, thromboplastic substances are released, making it less likely to obtain an adequate aspirate.

Anatomy

Site selection for bone marrow aspiration depends on patient age and the clinician's experience. The posterior iliac crest is the most common site for bone marrow aspiration; bone marrow biopsy is nearly exclusively performed at this site (Fig. 205-1A). The sternum can be used for aspiration in adults, but it is never appropriate for biopsy (Fig. 205-1B; cardiac tamponade is a possibility if the posterior sternum were to be inadvertently penetrated). Figure 205-2 shows the Illinois needle, designed specifically for sternal bone marrow aspiration. The anterior iliac crest is an option for both bone marrow aspiration and biopsy, although the hard, thick cortical layer of bone makes this approach technically challenging. The anterior iliac crest is most often used when biopsy of the posterior iliac crest is contraindicated (e.g., significant obesity, physical disability, or presence of a cast). The anterior tibia is an option for marrow aspiration in infants younger than 18 months of age.

Aspiration and biopsy techniques for the posterior iliac crest are described in this chapter. Aspiration and biopsy at this site are both easily accessible and safe when performed properly.

Indications

- Evaluation of anemia or iron metabolism
- Thrombocytopenia
- Leukopenia or leukocytosis
- Pancytopenia
- Unexplained splenomegaly
- Work-up of fever of unknown origin
- Diagnosis and staging of leukemia and lymphoma
- Work-up for bone marrow transplantation
- Staging of nonhematologic cancers such as neuroblastoma
- Monitoring of chemotherapy- and radiation-induced damage from cancer treatment
- To obtain samples for chromosomal studies
- Work-up of dysproteinemia or lysosomal storage diseases
- Diagnosis of opportunistic infection in patients with human immunodeficiency virus infection/acquired immunodeficiency syndrome
- Unusual infections (e.g., tuberculosis, fungal infections)

Contraindications

Absolute

- Hemophilia and related bleeding disorders
- Uncooperative patient
- Skin infection or osteomyelitis at the proposed biopsy site

Relative

- Significant obesity
- Severe osteoporosis (risk of bone perforation and injury to underlying tissues)
- Previous radiation therapy at the biopsy site

NOTE: Isolated thrombocytopenia is *not* a contraindication to bone marrow aspiration or biopsy. When a patient requires anticoagulation therapy, it *does not* need to be reversed or held before the procedure. Patients taking anticoagulants should have an activated partial thromboplastin time (aPTT) and prothrombin time (PT)/international normalized ratio (INR) within the therapeutic range for heparin or warfarin before the procedure (i.e., not be excessively anticoagulated).

Equipment

Necessary equipment is available in sterile, disposable, prepackaged kits (Fig. 205-3).

- Antiseptic solution (e.g., povidone–iodine or chlorhexidine)
- Sterile fenestrated drape
- 1% lidocaine
- 5- and 10-mL syringes
- 22-gauge (1½-inch) and 25-gauge (⅝-inch) needles
- No. 11 scalpel
- Bone marrow aspiration needle (Fig. 205-4)
- 11-gauge Jamshidi bone marrow biopsy needle (Fig. 205-5)

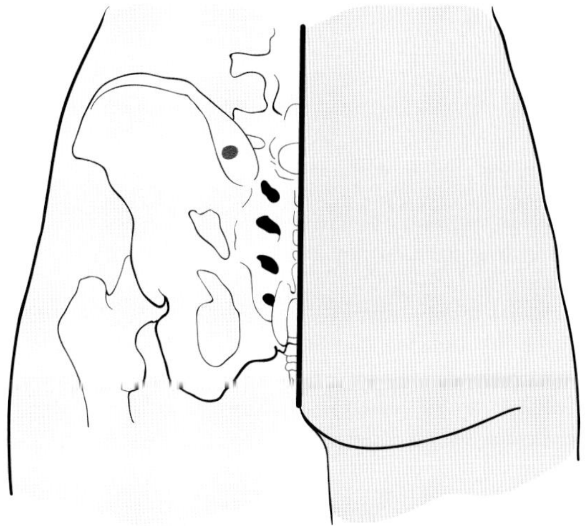

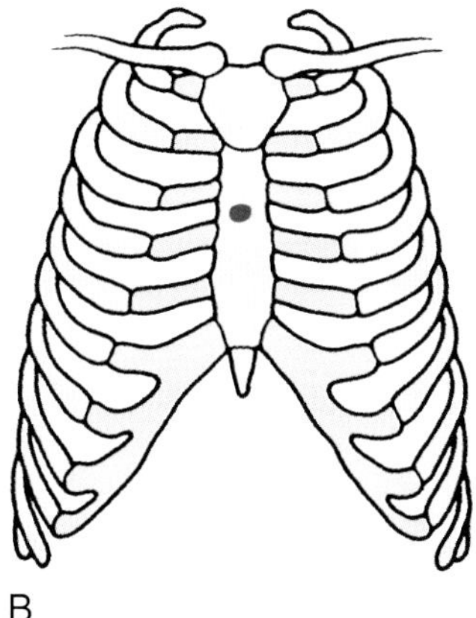

Figure 205-1 **A,** Posterior iliac sampling site. **B,** Sternal sampling site.

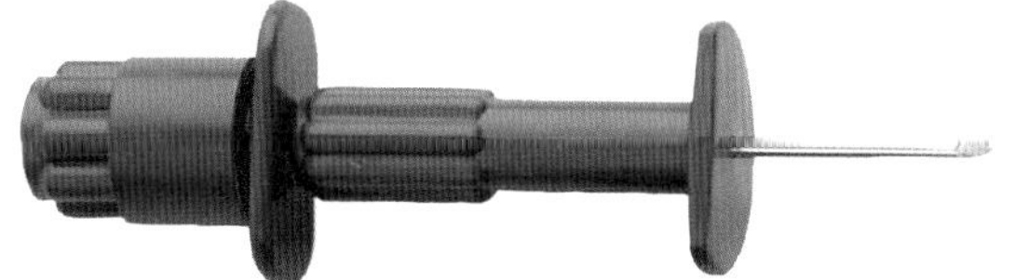

Figure 205-2 Illinois needle for sternal bone marrow aspiration. (Courtesy of Cardinal Health, Dublin, Ohio.)

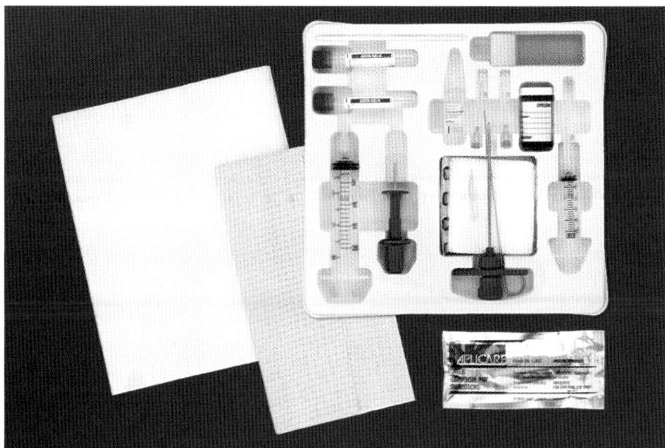

Figure 205-3 Prepackaged sterile Jamshidi bone marrow biopsy kit. (Courtesy of Cardinal Health, Dublin, Ohio.)

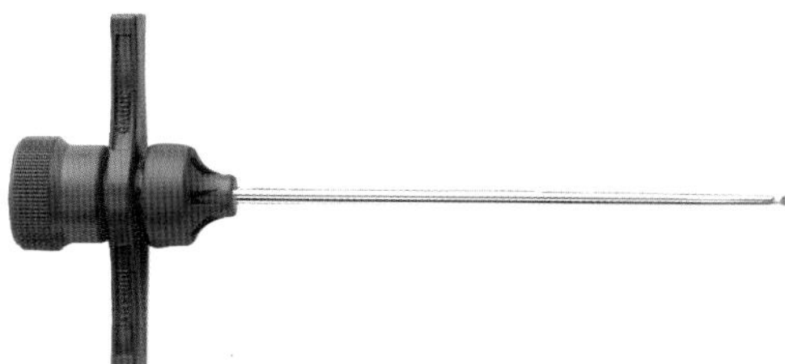

Figure 205-4 Bone marrow aspiration needle. (Courtesy of Cardinal Health, Dublin, Ohio.)

- 10-mL syringe rinsed with ethylenediamine tetra-acetic acid (EDTA)
- EDTA (purple-topped) tube
- Glass slides (10)
- Bottle or tube with fixative (formalin)
- 4 × 4 gauze
- Pressure dressing and tape

Precautions

Review the patient history and indications for bone marrow sampling. Question the patient about recent use of medications that might depress bone marrow function or stimulate blood formation (e.g., cytokines). Results of a complete blood count and peripheral blood smear should be reviewed before considering bone marrow aspiration and biopsy.

Preprocedure Patient Education

A cooperative patient is essential. Discuss indications for the procedure, as well as risks and benefits. Obtain a signed informed consent (see the sample patient consent form online at www.expertconsult.com). Inquire about any coagulation abnormalities or allergies (i.e., povidone–iodine or lidocaine). Explain that numbing the skin and periosteum, penetrating the iliac crest, and aspirating marrow is sometimes uncomfortable. Have the patient empty his or her bladder before the procedure. In overly apprehensive patients, premedication with a mild anxiolytic or analgesic is appropriate. Oral lorazepam (1 to 2 mg) and hydromorphone (1 to 2 mg) given 60 to 90 minutes before the biopsy lessen pain and induce varying degrees of amnesia.

Technique

Optimal bone marrow evaluation requires examination of both the marrow aspirate and a biopsy specimen (smear preparations and sections). Obtaining both samples simultaneously is better in terms of cost, patient comfort, and diagnostic information gleaned. The aspirate is usually performed first. The following instructions describe bone marrow aspiration and biopsy using the posterior iliac approach.

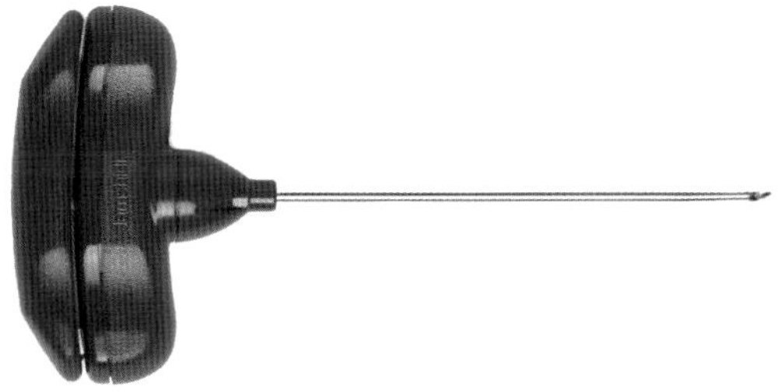

Figure 205-5 Jamshidi bone marrow biopsy needle. (Courtesy of Cardinal Health, Dublin, Ohio.)

Bone Marrow Aspiration

1. Have the patient lie either in the lateral decubitus position with knees flexed at the hip or in the prone position. Identify each iliac crest and follow it to its posterior superior spine (see Fig. 205-1). Mark this location using ink or pressure from a needle cap.
2. Put on sterile gloves and prepare the biopsy area with 10% povidone–iodine antiseptic in a circular pattern. Drape the site with the fenestrated sterile drape. Position the fenestration over the center of the intended biopsy site.
3. Using the 25-gauge needle and 5-mL syringe, make a skin wheal with 1% lidocaine. Switch to the 22-gauge needle/5-mL syringe to anesthetize deeper structures. Introduce the needle until the periosteum is encountered. Infiltrating the periosteum with 1 mL of lidocaine is important because most of the bone pain fibers are located here. Inject 2 to 3 mL of lidocaine along the outgoing tract as the needle is removed.
4. Make a 2- to 3-mm skin incision with the scalpel to enhance insertion of the aspiration needle.
5. Insert the aspiration needle perpendicularly to the bone; make sure the stylet is locked in place. Insert the needle until it rests against the anesthetized periosteum. Rotate the needle clockwise and counterclockwise using enough force to penetrate the bony cortex. "Give" is felt when the marrow cavity is entered. Stop pushing and check that the needle remains stationary without support.
6. Remove the stylet and attach a 10-mL EDTA-rinsed syringe. Warn the patient that he or she will experience pain as the marrow is aspirated. Pull the plunger and rapidly aspirate 0.2 to 2 mL of marrow for slide preparation (higher volumes dilute the specimen with blood). If more material is needed for other studies, an additional 5 mL of aspirate may be withdrawn.
7. Give the aspirated material to an assistant for slide preparation. Aspirate quality is assessed by the presence of grossly visible marrow spicules. Thin films should be prepared quickly with minimal specimen manipulation. Several drops of aspirate are placed on the edge of a glass slide while the edge of another slide is used to thinly spread the aspirate across the first slide. Four slides are prepared and allowed to air dry. Slides are stained with either Wright or May-Grünwald-Giemsa stain.
8. Place the remaining aspirate in a tube with EDTA, mix well, and allow it to clot for later fixation and processing by the histologist. If extra material is needed for flow cytometry, culture, cytogenetics, or other special studies, use another sterile syringe to withdraw more aspirate from the aspirate needle.
9. If a "dry tap" is encountered (no aspirate despite seemingly good needle placement), replace the stylet and advance the needle 1 to 2 mm. If still no aspirate is obtained, remove the needle and reinsert it at another part of anesthetized periosteum near the original site.
10. Once the aspirate sample is judged adequate, replace the stylet and remove the entire needle using a twisting motion.
11. Place dry gauze over the site and apply pressure until the bleeding stops. Cover the area with an adhesive bandage unless proceeding with a bone marrow biopsy.

Bone Marrow Biopsy

Bone marrow biopsy is performed immediately after aspiration. Once the bone marrow aspiration needle is removed, the following steps are taken:

1. Confirm that the stylet of the Jamshidi biopsy needle is locked into place with the cap secured (see Fig. 205-5). Place the capped end in the palm of your hand so that the shaft lies between the index and middle fingers. Introduce the needle into the skin incision and push past the soft tissue until the periosteum of the posterior iliac spine is reached. Position the needle at least 5 mm away from the periosteal entry point used for the aspirate collection (to avoid aspiration artifact). Using clockwise and counterclockwise rotation with considerable downward pressure, pierce the bony cortex and enter the marrow. The cortex is usually about 1 cm thick and entrance into the marrow cavity is detected by decreased resistance (Fig. 205-6).
2. Unlock the cap and remove the stylet.
3. Slowly and gently advance the needle millimeter by millimeter (1.5 to 2 cm) with an alternating clockwise-counterclockwise motion to obtain an adequate specimen.
4. Pull the needle back 2 to 3 mm and redirect the tip approximately 15 degrees. Advance the needle 2 to 3 mm forward in this new position to break off the specimen.

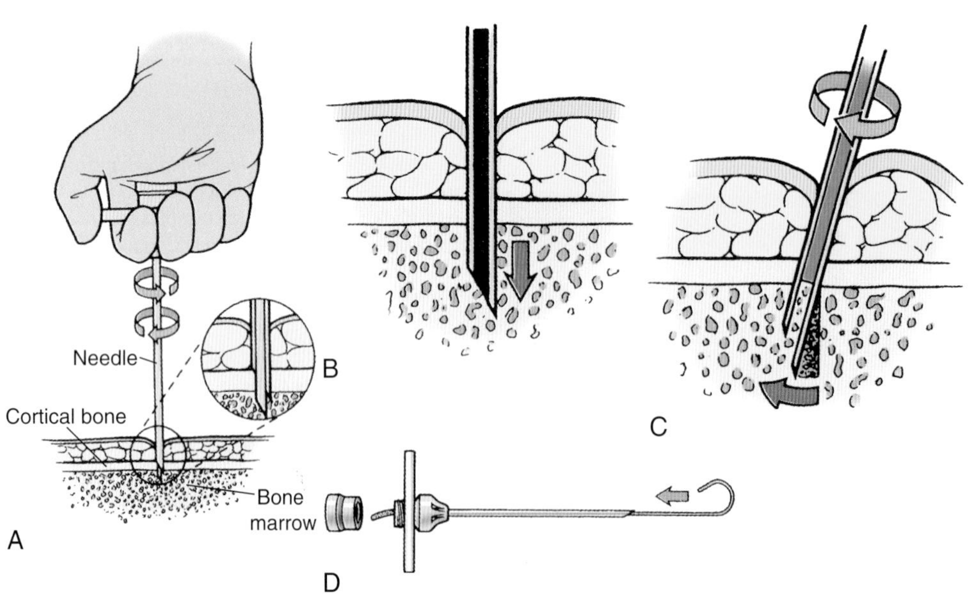

Figure 205-6 Technique for obtaining a bone marrow biopsy specimen. **A,** The needle is advanced through the cortical bone. **B,** The stylet is removed and the needle advanced an additional 1.5 to 2 cm using downward rotational force. **C,** The needle tip is redirected 15 degrees and rotated to break off the specimen. **D,** The probe is used to push the specimen onto gauze, threaded through the needle tip toward the biopsy needle handle.

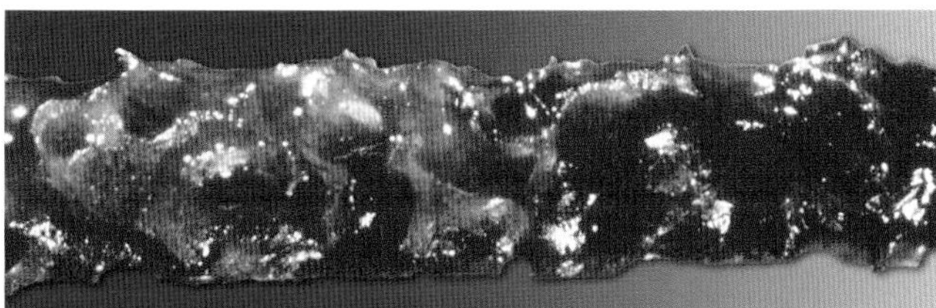

Figure 205-7 Biopsy specimen from bone marrow biopsy with Jamshidi needle. (Courtesy of Cardinal Health, Dublin, Ohio.)

5. Rotate the biopsy needle 360 degrees four times to the right and then four times to the left.
6. Remove the needle from the patient using rotational movements. The sample should stay in the Jamshidi needle.
7. Remove the biopsy specimen by inserting the blunt probe into the needle tip, pushing the specimen toward the hub/handle and out onto sterile gauze. Take care not to injure yourself on the sharp cutting edge (see Fig. 205-6D) of the needle tip.
8. Prepare the specimens or give the sample to the technician for preparation. Touch preparations (five) are made by gently pressing five glass slides against the biopsy specimen. The slides are usually stained with Wright or Giemsa stain. The remaining biopsy sample is placed into a container with formalin and sent for sectioning and staining (Fig. 205-7).
9. Cover the biopsy site with gauze and apply pressure until the bleeding stops. Cover the area with gauze and an adhesive bandage to form a pressure dressing. The patient should lie on the biopsy site for 60 minutes.

Sample Operative Report

See the Sample Operative Report online at www.expertconsult.com.

Common Errors

- *Failure to adequately anesthetize the periosteum.* Most of the bone pain fibers are located in this layer. The periosteum should be gently probed or tested with the sharp point of the 22-gauge needle before aspiration or biopsy. If the patient experiences sharp pain, an additional 1 to 2 mL of lidocaine should be injected.
- *Inadequate specimen length obtained on the bone marrow biopsy.* The ideal length of an adequate bone marrow biopsy is not well defined. Specimen lengths ranging from 1.6 to 3 cm have been recommended by various authorities. Because the core biopsy shrinks by up to 25% during processing, obtaining an adequate biopsy is important.
- *Dry tap.* A dry tap is the failure to aspirate fluid or find bone marrow particles during bone marrow aspiration. The most common cause is faulty positioning of the aspiration needle into the marrow cavity. The stylet can be replaced and the aspiration needle advanced to attempt a second aspirate. Dry taps occur in 4% to 7% of cases. A repeat dry tap is suggestive of myelofibrosis, hairy cell leukemia, aplastic anemia, myeloma, lymphoma, or leukemia. A bone marrow biopsy is then required to obtain touch imprints that "substitute" for the aspirate.
- *Preparation of low-quality aspirate smears.* Bone marrow clots quickly, so aspirate slides are usually prepared at the bedside by the provider or a trained technician. The simplest preparation is a wedge technique similar to that used for peripheral blood smears. A drop of marrow is placed at one end of a glass slide while a second slide held at a 30-degree angle is used to feather the aspirate across the first slide. Particle crush methods and coverslip preparations are more challenging to prepare.
- *Dilution by peripheral blood.* This happens when a large volume of bone marrow is aspirated.

Complications

Complications of bone marrow aspiration and biopsy are exceedingly rare. Major adverse events occur 0.2% of the time. Adverse outcomes include the following:

- Retroperitoneal hemorrhage or bowel damage from perforation of the iliac bone in osteoporotic patients
- Hemorrhage at the biopsy site
- Infection at the biopsy site (unusual if sterile technique is followed)
- Perforation of the lower sternal plate resulting in cardiac tamponade and sudden death
- Breakage of the bone marrow needle or handle separation during insertion into the bone (rare)
- Unilateral lower extremity weakness or numbness due to irritation of the sacral nerve plexus (rare and transient)
- Pain (usually resolves within a day)

Postprocedure Management

The patient lies on the bandaged biopsy site for 1 hour while being monitored. If the patient was thrombocytopenic before the procedure, a pressure bandage is applied and the site checked frequently for excessive bleeding.

Postprocedure Patient Education

Emergency contact numbers are provided and the patient instructed to call in case of bleeding, pain, fever, or erythema at the biopsy site. The pressure dressing is removed after 12 to 24 hours. Pain medication should be provided as needed.

Interpretation of Results

The bone marrow aspirate and biopsy specimens are examined by a trained histopathologist who interprets the results. A written report is generated and sent to the provider who performed the tests. Providing adequate clinical information aids the pathologist in reaching an accurate diagnosis.

Patient Education Guides

See patient education and patient consent forms available online at www.expertconsult.com.

CPT/Billing Codes

38220 Bone marrow aspiration
38221 Bone marrow biopsy
85060 Peripheral blood smear interpretation with written report
85097 Bone marrow smear with interpretation

ICD-9-CM Diagnostic Codes

018.90 Tuberculosis, disseminated, NOS
202.80 Lymphoma, NOS unspecified site
203.00 Multiple myeloma, without mention of remission
203.01 Multiple myeloma, in remission
208.00 Leukemia, acute, without mention of remission
208.10 Leukemia, chronic, without mention of remission
208.11 Leukemia, chronic, in remission
280.1 Anemia, iron deficiency, due to inadequate iron intake
284.1 Pancytopenia, acquired
287.5 Thrombocytopenia, NOS
288.50 Leukopenia, NOS

288.60 Leukocytosis
780.6 Fever of unknown origin
789.2 Splenomegaly, unspecified or unknown etiology

Acknowledgment

The editors wish to recognize the many contributions by John M. O'Brien, MD, to this chapter in the first edition of this text.

Suppliers

(See contact information online at www.expertconsult.com.)

Goldenberg Snarecoil bone marrow aspiration and biopsy tray
Illinois sternal/iliac bone marrow aspiration tray
Jamshidi bone marrow biopsy/aspiration needle
Allegiance Healthcare Corp. (a Cardinal Health company)
Jamshidi Economy bone marrow aspiration/biopsy tray

Online Resources

Maslak P: Atlas image set: Bone marrow aspiration slides. American Society of Hematology Image Bank. Available at http://ashimagebank.hematologylibrary.org/cgi/content/full/2002/0830/100430.

Riley RS, Ben-Ezra JM, Pavot DR, et al: An illustrated guide to performing the bone marrow aspiration and biopsy. Available at www.pathology.vcu.edu/education/lymph/How%20to%20Marrow.pdf.

Bibliography

Bain B: Bone marrow aspiration. J Clin Pathol 54:657–663, 2001.

Bain B: Bone marrow trephine biopsy. J Clin Pathol 54:737–742, 2001.

Islam A: Bone marrow aspiration before bone marrow core biopsy using the same bone marrow biopsy needle: A good or bad practice? J Clin Pathol 60:212–215, 2007.

Riley R, Hogan T, Pavot D, et al: A pathologist's perspective on bone marrow aspiration and biopsy: I. Performing a bone marrow examination. J Clin Lab Anal 18:70–90, 2004.

CHAPTER 206

Lumbar Puncture

Jeffrey A. German • John O'Brien

Lumbar puncture is performed to obtain cerebrospinal fluid (CSF) and is vital for making many neurologic diagnoses. In ordinary circumstances, the adult brain floats in about 150 mL of CSF and is capable of manufacturing about 500 mL/day. Examination of the CSF remains the most direct and accurate method of determining if there is a central nervous system infection. Lumbar puncture should be a routine procedure in febrile adults with an altered mental status and no source of fever and in febrile children who appear toxic, regardless of age. Whereas computed tomography (CT) and magnetic resonance imaging have somewhat superseded lumbar puncture for making various neurologic diagnoses, they have also increased the safety of performing a lumbar puncture. Although the sensitivity of CT for making the diagnosis of subarachnoid hemorrhage (SAH) can range from 92% to 98% when performed within 24 hours of the onset of symptoms, it decreases to 75% when performed 48 to 72 hours after the onset of symptoms. It is often negative in patients with a sentinel bleed, which occur in 20% to 50% of patients, hours, days, weeks, or months before a major SAH. Xanthochromia, when measured by spectrophotometry, has a sensitivity approaching 100% when performed between 12 hours and 2 weeks after SAH; therefore, a lumbar puncture must be performed if SAH is still suspected with a negative CT. If adequate time has elapsed (>2 hours), xanthochromia and red blood cells (RBCs) should be noted. If there has not been adequate time for RBCs to migrate to the lumbar spine area, a cerebral angiogram or repeat lumbar puncture in 12 to 18 hours should be performed. Although lumbar puncture is generally a diagnostic procedure, it can also have therapeutic applications (e.g., pseudotumor cerebri, elevated CSF pressure).

Indications

- Suspected central nervous system infection (e.g., meningitis, encephalitis)
- Suspected SAH (If available, a CT scan should be done first. It will exclude certain causes for increased intracranial pressure. However, CT has a false-negative rate of up to 25% for blood. With a bleed, xanthochromic color of CSF [visible >2 hours after the bleed] and an abnormal RBC count [>1000/mm^3] should be noted.)
- Pseudotumor cerebri (therapeutic) or normal-pressure hydrocephalus (diagnostic)
- Guillain-Barré syndrome (very high CSF protein level [>200 mg/dL])
- Multiple sclerosis (Usually the immunoglobulin G [IgG] level is elevated and oligoclonal banding is present on electrophoresis.)
- Spinal analgesia
- Lupus cerebritis (CSF may be normal, but some reports have noted elevated levels of anti-DNA antibodies, IgG, oligoclonal banding, immune complexes, interleukin-6, and the chemokine CXCL10.)
- Acute demyelinating disorders (e.g., encephalomyelitis, transverse myelitis)
- Dementia (if normal-pressure hydrocephalus, syphilis or other chronic infection, or vasculitis is suspected as a cause)
- Meningeal carcinomatosis
- Unexplained neurologic disorders if CT is negative (e.g., altered level of consciousness, polyneuropathy)
- Intrathecal antibiotics or chemotherapeutics
- Imaging procedures (e.g., myelography, cisternography)

Contraindications

- Local skin infection (*absolute* contraindication)
- Raised intracranial pressure (suggested by the presence of papilledema, suspected SAH, or clinical risk factor[s] for intracranial pathology [Box 206-1] unless the CT scan is negative)

  NOTE: The absence of papilledema is not always a reliable sign of normal intracranial pressure because it often takes more than 48 hours for papilledema to develop. Papilledema will be absent in up to 15% of adults and 50% of children with early increased intracranial pressure.

- Supratentorial mass lesions (should be evaluated by CT scan first)

  NOTE: Certain CT findings indicate a predisposition to herniation if a lumbar puncture is performed: (1) a midline shift, (2) a loss of the suprachiasmatic and basilar cisterns, or (3) any evidence of a posterior fossa mass or obliteration of the superior cerebellar cistern or the quadrigeminal plate cistern caudal to the midbrain.

Box 206-1. Clinical Findings Associated with Increased Risk of Intracranial Pathology

Abnormal language
Age 60 years or older
Altered level of consciousness
Arm drift
Facial palsy
Gaze palsy
History of central nervous system disease
Immunocompromised state
Inability to correctly answer two questions
Inability to follow two consecutive commands
Leg drift
Seizure within 1 week of presentation
Visual field abnormality

From Straus SE, Thorpe KE, Holroyd-Leduc J: How do I perform a lumbar puncture and analyze the results to diagnose bacterial meningitis? JAMA 296:2012–2022, 2006.

- Severe bleeding diathesis or coagulopathy (e.g., platelet count dropping rapidly or <20,000/mm^3 [platelets should be transfused]), or anticoagulated patient (international normalized ratio >1.4) *(relative contraindications; however, the most experienced clinician should perform the procedure using the smallest-gauge needle available)*
- Unstable patient (If patient has hypotension, shock, status asthmaticus, or unstable airway, lumbar puncture should be delayed until patient is stable.)

  NOTE: Meningitis itself can cause increased intracranial pressure. Consequently, patients with decorticate or decerebrate posturing, focal neurologic signs, or no response to pain should receive antibiotics without lumbar puncture even if the CT scan is negative.

- Uncooperative adult patient (Lumbar puncture should be delayed until patient is stable.)

Preprocedure Patient Preparation

Indications, alternatives, risks, potential benefits, and expected results should be discussed with the patient or representative, and he or she should sign an informed consent form (see the sample patient education and consent forms online at www.expertconsult.com). The patient should expect some discomfort with injection of the local anesthetic and as the spinal needle is inserted. It will be important for him or her to remain very still during certain portions of the procedure. If the patient is a child or minor, the parents or caregiver can be asked if they would like to be present during the procedure.

Equipment

Spinal tray (Fig. 206-1) containing the following:

- Povidone–iodine skin swabs
- Alcohol swab
- Fenestrated drape and sterile gloves
- Manometer, three-way stopcock
- 1% lidocaine
- 3-mL syringe with 20- to 23-gauge needle (for drawing up anesthetic)
- 25- to 27-gauge skin needle
- 20- to 22-gauge spinal needle plus a spare (traditional is Quincke spinal needle with sharp, beveled end)*
- Four numbered, capped test tubes
- Sterile dressing (Band-Aid)
- Pulse oximetry *(optional, may be especially helpful for children)*
- Lidocaine–prilocaine (eutectic mixture of local anesthetic or EMLA) cream *(optional; although shown to be more effective in adults than lidocaine infiltration alone, it must be applied 30 to 60 minutes before the procedure and local anesthetic should still be injected)*
- 1- mL syringe *(optional, but may be helpful if CSF not flowing)*
- 21- to 25-gauge butterfly needle *(optional)*

NOTE: Some experts advocate use of a butterfly needle in children; the tubing is then used to estimate opening pressure. However, epidermoid tumors due to implanted dermal cells are associated with use of a spinal needle without a stylet.

Technique

1. In patients with focal neurologic findings, altered mentation, immunocompromise, suspected SAH, or papilledema (see Box 206-1), consider CT scan first.

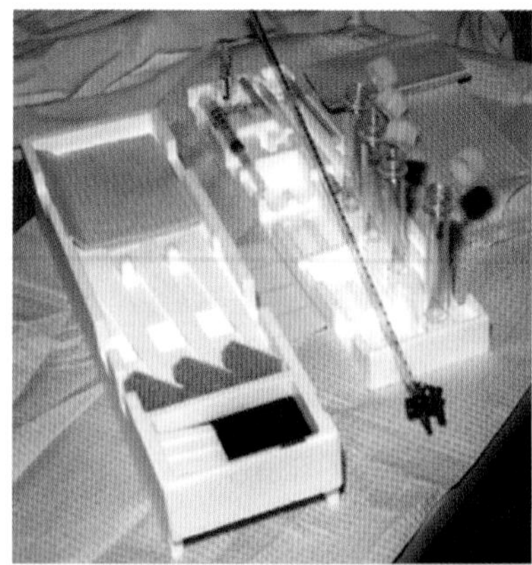

Figure 206-1 Lumbar puncture equipment tray.

   NOTE: If meningitis is suspected, the initiation of antibiotics should not be delayed while awaiting the CT scan results before performing the lumbar puncture.

2. Position the patient near the edge of the bed (or the examination table) in the lateral decubitus or sitting position. Slightly flex the neck anteriorly. If the patient is lying down, ask him or her to "roll up into a ball" with the knees drawn up to the abdomen (Fig. 206-2). The shoulders and pelvis should be aligned vertically without forward or backward tilt. If the patient is lying down, his or her shoulders, back, and hips should be exactly perpendicular to the bed. Identify the L3-L4 interspace (a line drawn between the superior aspect of the iliac crests intersects the body of L4). If necessary, the L2-L3 or L4-L5 interspaces can be used (Fig. 206-3). Some clinicians mark the site with a pen or make a small indention with the hub of a needle.

   NOTE: Although the lying position may be more comfortable for the patient, the sitting position is most commonly used in adults. With the patient sitting, it is usually easier to identify the midline and palpate the spinous processes, particularly when the patient is obese.

3. Open the spinal tray in a sterile manner. Put on sterile gloves and preassemble the manometer. It is usually in two pieces that slide together. Insert the manometer into the vertical port of the three-way stopcock and set this assembly to the side on the sterile field. Next, open the numbered test tubes. Place them upright, in order, in the slots provided in the plastic tray.
4. Prepare the skin at the selected interspace, plus the one above and below, with an antiseptic solution such as povidone–iodine. The prepared area is usually at least 10 cm in diameter; cover the area with a fenestrated drape. If lidocaine–prilocaine (EMLA) cream is used, it must be applied at least 30 to 60 minutes before beginning the procedure, and it only anesthetizes the skin and subcutaneous tissue, so a local anesthetic will still need to be injected.

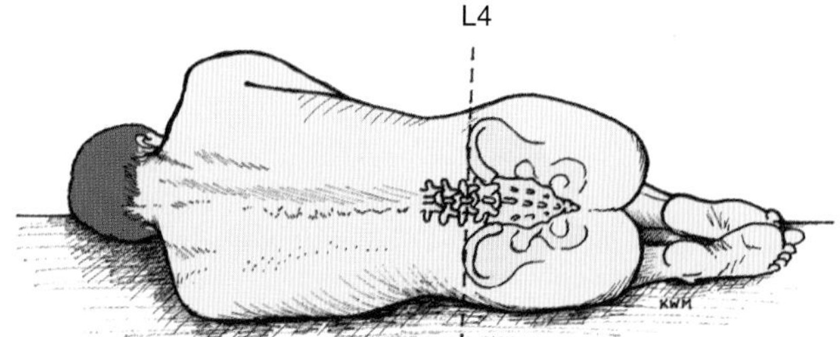

Figure 206-2 Location of anatomic landmarks.

*Atraumatic spinal needles have been shown to reduce the complication of spinal headache (i.e., less risk of a CSF leak).

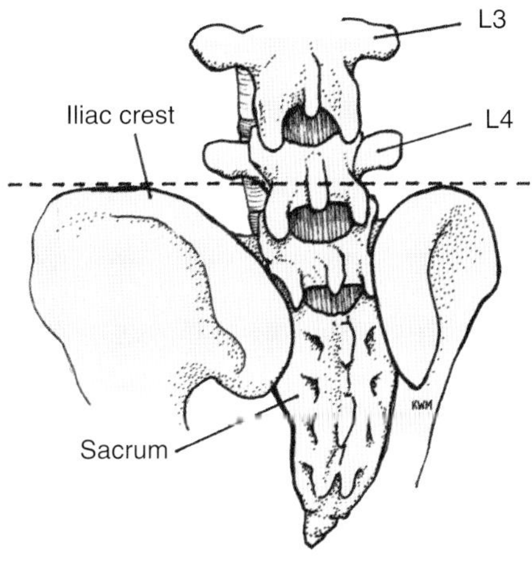

Figure 206-3 Line across the iliac crests intersects the body of L4.

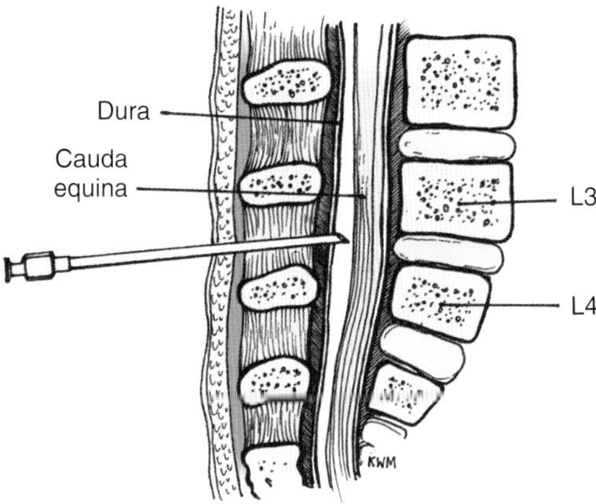

Figure 206-5 Drop in resistance will be felt as the needle penetrates the dura.

5. Draw 3 mL of 1% lidocaine into the syringe with the 20- to 23-gauge needle. Administer local anesthetic with the skin needle and raise a wheal over the L3-L4 interspace in the midline. Inject a small amount deeper into the posterior spinous region, in the direction that the spinal needle will follow. (Some experts perform a field block for anesthesia. Sensation to the interspinous ligaments and the periosteum is supplied by the recurrent spinal nerves, which branch off the nerve roots exiting the spinal canal at the same level. A field block is performed by first injecting a small amount of local anesthetic into the interspinous ligaments in the midline, and then above and below the intended location of the lumbar puncture. The block is completed by redirecting the needle laterally, to both sides of the intended lumbar puncture site, and injecting a small amount of anesthetic.)
6. Palpate the posterior spinous process. Using this and the umbilicus as landmarks, insert a 20- or 22-gauge spinal needle through the skin in the midline. The needle can be held with both index fingers and advanced with the thumb(s), or it can be guided with a thumb and forefinger near the puncture site while the other hand advances the needle by putting pressure on the hub. Angle the needle about 15 degrees cephalad, toward the umbilicus, keeping it level with the sagittal midplane of the body (Figs. 206-4 and 206-5). Keep the bevel of the needle parallel to the longitudinal axis of the spine (point turned upward or downward with the patient in the lateral decubitus position, or to one side if the patient is sitting) as the needle is advanced. If bone is encountered, withdraw the needle slightly and change its angle, usually more cephalad. Depending on the size of the patient, after the needle has advanced about 3 to 4 cm, stop, withdraw the stylus, and check the hub for fluid. If there is no fluid, replace the stylus and advance another fraction before repeating this again. Usually a slight "pop" is felt as the spinal needle penetrates the dura; however, this may not be felt using a Quincke needle. Advance the needle 1 to 2 mm farther and withdraw the stylus. Rotating the needle 90 to 180 degrees is sometimes helpful if no fluid returns. If the patient experiences pain radiating down one leg or the tap is "dry," remove the needle completely and make an attempt at a different interspace. A dry tap is more often due to a poorly positioned patient or an improperly placed needle than to an obliterated subarachnoid space; often the needle tip has migrated laterally out of the midline. For repeated dry taps, reposition the patient from lying to sitting, or vice versa, and attempt puncture again while making sure the needle is directed toward the midline. Approach from a lateral site can also be utilized as described later. CSF may fail to flow in certain low intracranial pressure situations (e.g., dehydrated patient), so gentle suction with a 1-mL syringe may be helpful.

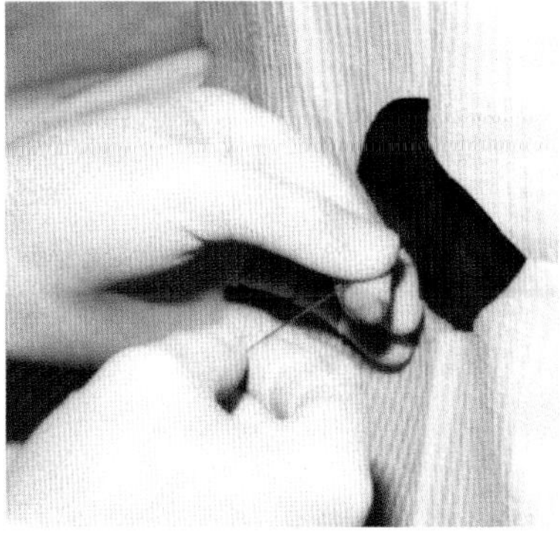

Figure 206-4 Proper angle for entering spinal canal (with patient seated). Needle is directed cephalad.

NOTE: For very large or obese patients, it may be impossible to palpate the spinous process for use as a landmark. Ultrasonography may help locate the bone in the spinous process (see Chapter 225, Emergency Department, Hospitalist, and Office Ultrasonography [Clinical Ultrasonography]).

7. Once fluid is obtained, the needle hub should be "anchored," or held firmly between the thumb and index finger of one hand that is braced against the patient's back, whenever anything is attached or removed from the needle using the other hand. Next, place the end of the stopcock with the attached manometer onto the hub of the needle. Have the patient straighten the legs and relax his or her position so that the opening pressure is not artificially elevated. The CSF should rise in the manometer to the level of the opening pressure. The pressure is accurate only if the patient is lying on his or her side in a relaxed position. If tubing is in between the needle and manometer, the base of the manometer should still be held at the level of the needle hub for accurate readings. Note the color of the fluid and the opening pressure. CSF pressure should oscillate slightly with respiration (and sometimes with the pulse).
8. In case the fluid is bloody and does not clear after the first few drops of fluid (bloody tap), replace the stylus and remove the spinal needle. Select an alternative lumbar interspace above or below the current level and reattempt lumbar puncture as described in steps 4 through 7.

NOTE: Bloody CSF due to SAH will *not* clot. Also, after spinning in a centrifuge, the supernatant is xanthochromic.

TABLE 206-1 Normal Cerebrospinal Fluid Values

Value	Term Infant	Child	Adult
Opening pressure (mm H_2O)	50–80	50–80	70–180
WBC count (WBC/mm^3)	8 (range, 0–22)	<7	<5
Neutrophils	61%	None	None
Glucose (ratio of blood/CSF glucose and CSF level [mg/dL])	44%–128% (34–119)	50% (40–80)	60%–70% (50–80)
Protein level (mg/dL)	20–170 (mean, 90)	5–40	15–45

CSF, cerebrospinal fluid; WBC, white blood cell.

9. Turn the stopcock to allow the CSF to flow into the test tubes. Keep track of the order in which they are filled. Fill at least three test tubes with 2 to 3 mL of CSF each (at least 2 mL is necessary for cytology or antigen testing). Label each tube in the order it was collected. A fourth tube can be filled and frozen in case further studies are needed. Table 206-1 shows normal CSF values, and Table 206-2 lists recommended CSF tests. Tube 1 is most likely to be contaminated with blood from the needle insertion; therefore, tube 3 should be tested for the cell count and differential. Minor blood contamination usually clears by the third tube.
10. Once you have obtained enough CSF, replace the stylus and withdraw the needle.
11. Cover the puncture site with a sterile dressing.
12. For a therapeutic lumbar puncture (i.e., for pseudotumor cerebri), remove enough CSF to reduce the closing pressure to 100 mm H_2O or less (usually 25 to 35 mL of CSF). For a diagnostic tap, removal of 35 to 50 mL may result in transient improvement in gait or cognition for suspected normal-pressure hydrocephalus.

Technique for Lateral Approach

The lateral approach technique may be preferred in elderly patients with calcified supraspinous and intraspinous ligaments. It may also be used if the midline approach has failed. The patient may be in either the sitting or the lateral decubitus position, and should be prepared and draped in the same interspaces as described previously. Anesthesia should be applied/injected in a location 1.5 to 2 cm lateral to the midline, on either side if the patient is in the sitting position or on the lower side if the patient is in the lateral decubitus position. Local anesthetic should be injected in the location and direction that the spinal needle will follow. The spinal needle should be directed approximately 15 degrees cephalad and 20 degrees to the midline (Fig. 206-6). From this location, the needle usually bypasses the supraspinous and infraspinous ligaments, and instead penetrates the erector spinae muscles and the paraspinous ligaments, and then the ligamantum flavum, dura, and subarachnoid space. If bone is encountered, the needle should be withdrawn slightly and redirected in the same angle toward the midline but slightly more cephalad. The remainder of the procedure is as described previously.

Technique for Pediatric Patients

The preferred position for infants (especially premature infants and neonates) is with the infant seated with the head only slightly flexed. Overflexion of the head can lead to hypoxia and respiratory arrest in young infants. Likewise, increased intra-abdominal pressure caused by flexing the knees into the abdomen may lead to compression of the diaphragm and hypoxia. Consequently, the child should be monitored visually and possibly with pulse oximetry during the procedure. Preoxygenation with 100% oxygen by face mask for 2 to 5 minutes before the procedure may prevent hypoxia. If the procedure is performed with the child lying, a modified lateral decubitus position should be used (i.e., hips flexed only to 90 degrees). Draping should be done conservatively to avoid interfering with any infant monitors. The skin can be anesthetized initially with a patch containing EMLA cream, if it is available, followed 30 to 60 minutes later by an injection with lidocaine. The spinal needle is directed slightly cephalad. In young infants a "pop" or change in resistance may not be felt as the needle penetrates the dura. Use a 20- to 22-gauge, 1½-inch needle for infants. A 3½-inch spinal needle can be used in children older than 12 years of age.

NOTE: Local anesthetic should be used in all children. There is evidence that pain perception is present even in premature neonates.

Complications

- *Post–lumbar (post–dural) puncture headache* occurs in 10% to 25% of patients and is usually self-limited. The headache usually lasts for only a few days, but may last longer than a week and can be debilitating. Ninety percent of spinal headaches occur within 48 hours after dural puncture, but it may occur up to 14 days later. It is exacerbated by sitting upright and is relieved by lying down. The incidence increases with repeat lumbar punctures in a patient. The incidence is reduced by using a higher-gauge (24- to 27-gauge) or atraumatic needle, but these smaller needles have a higher failure rate and take longer to obtain samples, and opening pressures cannot be measured; therefore, in practice, a 22-gauge needle is usually used. The incidence of headache is also reduced by keeping the bevel of the needle oriented parallel to the long axis of the patient's spine, thereby spreading rather than cutting

TABLE 206-2 Recommended Cerebrospinal Fluid Tests

Tube 1: Bacteriology	Tube 2: Biochemistry	Tube 3: Hematology	Tube 4: Optional
Gram stain	Glucose	Cell count	VDRL*
Acid-fast stain*	Protein	Differential	India ink*
Culture	Protein electrophoresis* (need concurrent serum study)		Cryptococcal antigen*
Bacteria			Cytology*
Fungal*			Oligoclonal bands*
Tuberculosis*			Myelin basic protein*
Viral*			Countercurrent immunoelectrophoresis*
			Serologic and genetic tests for other microorganisms*
			Anti-DNA antibodies, immune complexes, interleukin-6, chemokine, and CXCL10 levels*

*If clinically indicated.
CXCL10, chemokine (C-X-C motif) ligand 10; VDRL, Venereal Disease Research Laboratory.

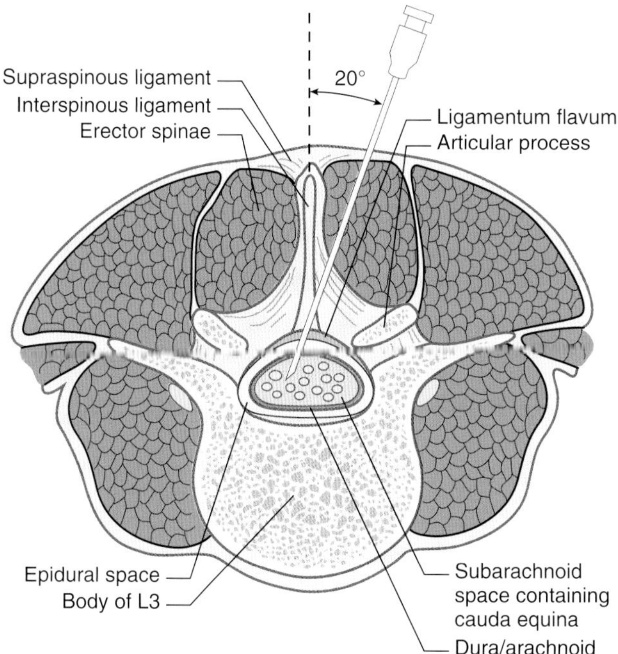

Figure 206-6 Using the lateral approach, the needle is inserted 1.5 to 2 cm lateral to the midline and is directed approximately 20 degrees toward the midline and 15 degrees cephalad. (From Fong B, VanBendegom JM: Lumbar puncture. In Reichman EF, Simon RR [eds]: Emergency Medicine Procedures. New York, McGraw-Hill, 2004, pp 859–880.)

the fibers of the ligamenta flava. Replacement of the stylet before removing the spinal needle has also been shown to decrease the risk of spinal headaches. Oral caffeine, 300 mg, or theophylline, 200 mg, if not contraindicated, may provide relief in adults. Intravenous caffeine benzoate, 500 mg given over a few minutes, can also be used to treat refractory spinal headaches in adults. A repeat dose can be given in 1 hour for an 85% chance of alleviation of symptoms. Twenty-four hours after lumbar puncture, if there has been no relief from caffeine, an epidural blood patch can be performed. This is performed by injecting 15 mL of autologous blood into the dural space. Although the mechanism of action is unclear, it usually provides immediate relief in up to 85% of patients. After a second patch is performed, if necessary, 98% of patients experience relief. Because the patient already has a spinal headache, the most experienced clinician available should probably perform the blood patch(es). Transient complications of the blood patch include back pain, paresthesias, radiculopathies, and weakness; rarely, spinal subdural hematoma has been reported.

- *Epidermoid tumors* have been associated with lumbar punctures performed in the neonatal period, especially when needles are used without a stylus.
- *Seizures* have been reported in a small percentage of patients with post–dural puncture headaches.
- A *traumatic or "bloody" tap* from inadvertent puncture of the spinal venous plexuses is possible. This is self-limiting in the majority of patients, but could lead to a spinal hematoma in patients with bleeding disorders. Some authorities recommend sending the first and fourth tubes for cell count (RBCs and WBCs with a differential) if a traumatic tap is suspected. The RBC count will decrease from tube 1 to tube 4 in the case of a traumatic tap. A correction can be made for CSF leukocytes and CSF protein if the tap is traumatic. For every 700 RBCs, CSF leukocytes increase by 1 and CSF protein rises 1 mg/dL.
- *Brain herniation* from a supratentorial mass or increased intracranial pressure is another complication. Always check the fundi for papilledema before performing lumbar puncture. If a tumor, intracranial bleed, intracranial pathology (see Box 206-1), or marked increased pressure is suspected, an emergency CT scan should be obtained before a lumbar puncture is done, to reduce the chance of herniation.
- *Intracranial subdural hematoma* is a rare complication, and is due to the same mechanism that causes post–lumbar puncture headache (especially with persistent CSF leakage) or brain herniation, that is, downward displacement of the brain. Such displacement can result in tearing of the bridging veins and lead to bilateral or unilateral subdural hematoma.
- *Spinal epidural or subdural hematoma* can present with paraplegia, lower extremity weakness, sensory deficits, or incontinence. Anticoagulated patients or those with a coagulopathy should be monitored closely for this complication.
- *Paresthesias* in the lower extremities are common and usually transient, but in rare cases can last for more than a year.
- *Local pain* in the back may be due to injury of the local tissue, the periosteum, or the spinal ligaments. Mild, transient pain is common.
- *Disk herniation* is a very rare complication and is caused by a needle passing through the entire subarachnoid space and into the annulus fibrosus. It can also result in diskitis or vertebral collapse.
- *Cranial nerve neuropathies* involving cranial nerves III, IV, V, VI, VII, and VIII have been reported. These are usually transient, present with visual and auditory symptoms, and are caused by traction on the nerve due to low intracranial pressure after lumbar puncture.
- *Nerve root aspiration* is a possible complication. Replacing the stylus before withdrawing the needle may prevent aspiration of nerve roots. Very rarely, nerve root diverticula can rupture as a result of lumbar puncture, causing a brief CSF leak and a spinal headache.
- *Meningitis* resulting from the procedure is a theoretical complication. Bacteremia is not a contraindication to lumbar puncture.

Patient Education Guides

See the sample patient education and consent forms available online at www.expertconsult.com. A video of ultrasonically directed lumbar puncture can be purchased at www.Sonosite.com.

CPT/Billing Codes

62270 Spinal puncture, lumbar, diagnostic
62272 Spinal puncture, therapeutic, for drainage of cerebrospinal fluid
62273 Injection, epidural, of blood or clot patch
62311 Injection, single, of diagnostic or therapeutic substances; (including anesthetic, antispasmotic, opioid, steroid, other solution), lumbar, sacral

ICD-9-CM Diagnostic Codes

239.7 Meningeal carcinoma or neoplasm
294.1 Dementia in conditions classified elsewhere
320.0 Meningitis due to *Hemophilus* meningitis
320.1 Pneumococcal meningitis
320.2 Streptococcal meningitis
320.3 Staphylococcal meningitis
320.9 Meningitis due to unspecified bacterium
322.0 Nonpyogenic meningitis
322.9 Meningitis, unspecified
323.9 Encephalitis, myelitis, and encephalomyelitis, unspecified cause

340 Multiple sclerosis
348.2 Pseudotumor cerebri
357.0 Guillain-Barré syndrome
430 Subarachnoid hemorrhage
710.0 Systemic lupus erythematosus
852.00 Subarachnoid hemorrhage after injury without open intracranial wound, unspecified state of consciousness

BIBLIOGRAPHY

Behrman RE, Kliegman RM, Jenson HB (eds): Nelson Textbook of Pediatrics, 17th ed. Philadelphia, Saunders, 2004.

Eng RH, Seligman SJ: Lumbar puncture-induced meningitis. JAMA 245:1456–1459, 1981.

Fong B, Van Bendegom JM: Lumbar puncture. In Reichman EF, Simon RR (eds): Emergency Medicine Procedures. New York, McGraw-Hill, 2004, pp 859–880.

Johnson KS, Sexton DJ: Lumbar puncture: Technique; indications; contraindications; and complications in adults. In Rose BD (ed): UpToDate. Waltham, Mass, UpToDate, 2005. Available at www.uptodate.com.

Siberry GK, Iannone R: The Harriet Lane Handbook, 17th ed. St. Louis, Mosby, 2005.

Straus SE, Thorpe KE, Holroyd-Leduc J: How do I perform a lumbar puncture and analyze the results to diagnose bacterial meningitis? JAMA 296:2012–2022, 2006.

Sun C, Lay CL: Post-lumbar puncture headache. In Rose BD (ed): UpToDate. Waltham, Mass, UpToDate, 2007. Available at www.uptodate.com.

Thomas SR, Jamieson DR, Muir KW: Randomized controlled trial of atraumatic versus standard needles for diagnostic lumbar puncture. BMJ 321:986–990, 2000.

Tuggy M, Garcia J: Procedures Consult. Available at www.proceduresconsult.com.

CHAPTER 207

MECHANICAL VENTILATION

Joe Esherick

Modern mechanical ventilation was developed out of necessity during the polio epidemic of the 1930s. The original machines were negative-pressure ventilators, known as "iron lungs." These devices soon became obsolete with the development of positive-pressure ventilators during the 1950s. The advent of positive-pressure ventilation ushered in the era of modern-day surgery, anesthesia, and critical care medicine.

Mechanical ventilators assist in the oxygenation and ventilation of patients. Ventilators improve pulmonary gas exchange and aim to reverse hypoxemia and acute respiratory acidosis. Mechanical ventilation also unloads the respiratory muscles and therefore significantly decreases the body's oxygen consumption in both shock and respiratory failure. Although positive-pressure ventilation can aid in pulmonary mechanics, it can also lead to ventilator-induced lung injury if improperly applied.

CLASSIFICATION OF MECHANICAL VENTILATION

All modern ventilators use positive-pressure ventilation. Positive-pressure ventilation can be administered noninvasively (e.g., bilevel positive airway pressure [BiPAP] or continuous positive airway pressure [CPAP] machines); however, this chapter focuses on positive-pressure ventilation delivered by an endotracheal or tracheostomy tube.

INDICATIONS

- Inability to protect one's airway
- Hypoxic respiratory failure
- Hypercapnic respiratory failure
- Cardiac arrest

CONTRAINDICATIONS

Advanced directives specifying no intubation or resuscitation are the contraindications for mechanical ventilation.

EQUIPMENT AND SUPPLIES

- Ventilator
- Ballard suction catheter
- Suction canister and suction tubing
- Yankauer suction tip
- Bite block or oral airway
- Heat and moisture exchanger
- Ventilator circuit tubing
- Metered-dose inhaler adapter
- Bag-valve-mask device

PRECAUTIONS

- Using inadequate sedation may lead to patient–ventilator dyssynchrony.
- High plateau pressures (>30 cm H_2O) lead to increased risk of barotrauma (e.g., pneumothorax, pneumomediastinum, pneumopericardium).
- Inadequate head elevation predisposes to ventilator-associated pneumonia.
- High positive end-expiratory pressure (PEEP) levels can decrease cardiac output, leading to hypotension, and can increase intracranial pressure.
- High tidal volume (VT > 10 mL/kg predicted body weight) ventilation may cause ventilator-induced lung injury and acute renal failure.
- Prolonged mechanical ventilation predisposes to
  - Stress gastric ulcers
  - Subglottic stenosis and tracheomalacia
  - Sinusitis
  - Decubitus pressure ulcers
  - Intensive care unit psychosis

TECHNIQUE

Modes of Ventilation

There are four main modes of ventilation: controlled mode, assist-control (AC) mode, synchronized intermittent mandatory ventilation (SIMV) mode, and support mode (Table 207-1). Each of these modes is subclassified into volume-cycled or pressure-cycled methods of ventilation.

Controlled Mode

Controlled ventilation (or intermittent mandatory ventilation) is restricted to use in heavily sedated or paralyzed patients. It is the principal mode of ventilation used for general anesthesia in the operating room. This mode will deliver a preset VT at a specified rate independent of patient effort. The advantage to its use is that the clinician controls with absolute certainty the patient's minute ventilation. However, the disadvantage is that heavy sedation is required to prevent the development of patient–ventilator dyssynchrony.

Assist-Control Mode

Assist-control ventilation is capable of both *assisted* ventilation and *controlled* ventilation. If patients are spontaneously breathing, the ventilator will synchronize with a patient-initiated breath and thereby assist ventilation. If the patient fails to initiate a breath within a given time (as determined by the preset ventilator rate), the machine will provide a controlled breath. AC mode can be volume-cycled (volume control), pressure-cycled, (pressure control), or a hybrid of the two (pressure-regulated volume control).

With volume control (VC) ventilation, each AC breath delivers a preset VT. In other words, both *assisted* breaths and *controlled* breaths receive a preset VT regardless of the pressure required. The machine ensures that the patient will receive a minimum number of breaths per minute, based on the set ventilator rate, even in the

TABLE 207-1 Modes of Ventilation

Controlled	Assist-Control	Synchronized Intermittent Mandatory Ventilation	Support
Pressure of volume preset	Pressure of volume preset	Usually volume preset	Usually pressure preset
Use in paralyzed patient	Use as an initial ventilatory mode	Use in spontaneously breathing patient	Use only in spontaneously breathing patient with adequate respiratory drive
Patient receives mandatory preset ventilator rate	Patient receives mandatory preset ventilator rate	Patient receives mandatory preset ventilator rate	Patient receives no mandatory preset ventilator rate
All breaths are ventilator initiated	All spontaneous breaths are ventilator assisted	Spontaneous breaths are not ventilator assisted	All spontaneous breaths are ventilator assisted
No spontaneous breathing problems		Can be used as a weaning mode	Can be used as a weaning mode

From Lapinsky SE, Slutsky AS: Ventilator management. In Wachter RM (ed): Hospital Medicine, 2nd ed. Philadelphia, Lippincott Williams & Wilkins, 2005, pp 173–182, Figure 23.1.

absence of patient effort. An advantage is that this mode requires less patient sedation. However, AC cannot limit the respiratory rate of patients who have a high spontaneous respiratory rate. Patients with obstructive lung disease (e.g., chronic obstructive pulmonary disease [COPD], status asthmaticus) and a rapid respiratory rate may develop air trapping. Air trapping can cause auto-PEEP and potentially barotrauma.

With pressure control (PC) ventilation, the ventilator delivers gas at a flow rate necessary to achieve a preset peak pressure. As in VC, the ventilator synchronizes with patient effort, when present, and ensures a minimum ventilatory rate. In PC ventilation the peak inspiratory pressure (PIP) remains constant, but its major disadvantage is that the VT varies from breath to breath depending on the dynamic lung compliance; therefore, the VT can fall to very low levels if the lungs are stiff, which can compromise the minute ventilation.

Pressure-regulated volume control (PRVC) is a hybrid between VC and PC. PRVC is essentially a volume-cycled mode of ventilation with gas flow characteristics similar to those of PC ventilation. The ventilator will deliver a preset tidal volume with each breath using a decelerating flow curve. PRVC allows the delivery of a preset VT at lower peak and mean airway pressures compared with VC.

The primary disadvantage for all modes of AC ventilation is the potential for developing auto-PEEP. At the same minute ventilation, auto-PEEP occurs with fairly equal frequency in VC, PC, and PRVC. See the discussion of auto-PEEP, later, for more details.

Synchronized Intermittent Mandatory Ventilation Mode

Synchronized intermittent mandatory ventilation is a mode of ventilation that ensures a preset minimum number of "machine breaths" while allowing spontaneous patient breaths in between. The ventilator waits for a preset time, allowing the patient to breathe spontaneously, and then delivers a "machine breath" synchronized with patient inspiratory effort. The main difference between the AC and SIMV modes is that every breath in the AC mode is ventilator assisted, whereas only a minimum number of breaths per minute are ventilator assisted in SIMV. SIMV can be administered in VC, PC, or PRVC mode; therefore, the ventilator mode can be set as SIMV/VC, SIMV/PC, or SIMV/PRVC. If necessary, pressure support (PS) or PEEP can be added to assist spontaneous breathing in the SIMV mode.

Pressure Support Mode

The PS mode is used solely for spontaneously breathing patients. All breaths in this mode are patient-initiated breaths and can be augmented by varying degrees of PS. The least amount of PS that should be added is 6 to 10 cm H_2O to overcome the resistance of the endotracheal or tracheostomy tube. Higher PS levels may be applied to aid respiratory mechanics and achieve an adequate VT.

Ventilator Settings and Terminology

- *Inspiratory time:* The inspiratory time (I_T) can be adjusted to change the inspiratory–expiratory (I:E) time ratio. The normal I:E ratio is 1:2. A decreased I_T is often helpful for conditions requiring a prolonged expiratory time, such as severe bronchospasm (e.g., COPD, asthma exacerbations). An increased I_T may be indicated for severe hypoxia refractory to high PEEP levels. A significantly prolonged I_T is usually very uncomfortable, typically requires heavy sedation, and may lead to auto-PEEP.
- *Triggering sensitivity:* The triggering sensitivity is the amount of negative pressure/flow needed to trigger a ventilator-assisted breath. This is set in all ventilator modes while watching patient effort. The aim is to achieve optimal patient comfort.
- *Positive end-expiratory pressure:* PEEP is applied by regulating the pressure in the expiratory limb of the ventilator circuit. The goal of PEEP is to keep the alveoli open after expiration to increase the surface area available for gas exchange. In addition, PEEP can recruit lung volume by opening closed alveoli; it also raises intrathoracic pressure, which can decrease cardiac preload. High levels of PEEP (>10 cm H_2O) can improve oxygenation so that lower levels of inspired oxygen (FIO_2) can be administered. Furthermore, a high level of PEEP is often needed during lung-protective ventilation in patients ventilated either for acute respiratory distress syndrome (ARDS) or for acute lung injury. PEEP must be used with extreme caution in shock states or if there is any evidence of increased intracranial pressure because high levels of PEEP can worsen both of these conditions.
- *Auto-PEEP:* Auto-PEEP occurs when there is inadequate time for expiration. It causes an increase in the functional residual capacity and raises intrathoracic pressure, increasing the risk of barotrauma. Volume-cycled AC modes have a higher risk of auto-PEEP compared with the SIMV modes of ventilation. Additional risk factors include severe bronchospasm, high respiratory rates, and a high I:E time ratio.
- *Tidal volume:* A preset VT is used for all volume-cycled modes of ventilation (VC or PRVC). The ventilator displays both an inspiratory VT and an expiratory VT, which should be the same unless the circuit is occluded or has a leak. VT should be monitored closely when ventilating in PS mode.
- *Peak inspiratory pressure:* The PIP is the maximal airway pressure experienced by the patient. The PIP is a measure of dynamic lung compliance and is a pressure preset in PC mode. The PIP levels vary in volume-cycled ventilation depending on the breath-to-breath changes in dynamic lung compliance. Causes of a high PIP are described later in the discussion of high airway pressures in the Ventilator Complications section.

- *Plateau pressure:* The plateau pressure (PPLAT) is the airway pressure measured after an end-inspiratory hold. This pressure reflects the static lung compliance and is a barometer for the risk of barotrauma. Every effort should be made to keep the PPLAT 30 cm H_2O or less. A patient with a high PPLAT may require a lower VT (if ARDS), increased sedation (if patient–ventilator dyssynchrony), loop diuretics (if congestive heart failure), or an investigation for abdominal compartment syndrome or pneumothorax.
- *Fraction of inspired oxygen:* The FIO_2 can vary from 0.21 (room air) to 1.0. The initial ventilator settings typically start with an FIO_2 between 0.8 and 1.0 until adequate oxygenation is ensured. Prolonged administration of an FIO_2 greater than 0.6 can lead to oxygen toxicity through formation of oxygen free radicals; therefore, every effort is made to wean the FIO_2 level down to at least 0.6 as quickly as possible.

Initiating Mechanical Ventilation

The steps involved in the initiation of mechanical ventilation and required monitoring are outlined in Box 207-1. The initial mode of ventilation is usually the AC mode.

Box 207-1. Initiating Mechanical Ventilation

1. Choose the mode of ventilation
   - AC if very limited patient effort or heavy sedation (VC or PRVC)
   - SIMV if some respiratory effort or patient–ventilator dyssynchrony on AC
2. Settings for oxygenation
   - Initial FIO_2 0.8 to 1.0, adjust according to SaO_2
   - Initial PEEP 5 cm H_2O, adjust according to FIO_2
   - Aim for SaO_2 ≥90%, PaO_2 ≥60 mm Hg
   - Aim to titrate FIO_2 ≤0.6
3. Settings for ventilation
   - Tidal volume: 6 to 10* mL/kg predicted body weight
   - Ventilator rate: 12 to 16/min, adjust based on $PaCO_2$ and pH (consider initial rate of 20 to 24 in ARDS)
   - Keep plateau pressure ≤30 cm H_2O
4. Additional ventilator settings
   - Triggering sensitivity: adjust to minimize patient effort
   - I:E ratio: initially 1:2, decrease inspiratory time for severe bronchospasm and can increase inspiratory time for refractory hypoxia
   - Pressure support: if SIMV mode, can adjust between 6 to 20 cm H_2O titrated to patient comfort
5. Monitoring
   - Continuous cardiopulmonary monitor
   - Ventilator: tidal volume, minute volume, airway pressures, serial arterial blood gases
   - $ETCO_2$ monitors desirable for ventilator weaning

AC, assist-control; ARDS, acute respiratory distress syndrome; $ETCO_2$, end-tidal carbon dioxide; FIO_2, fraction of inspired oxygen; I:E, inspiratory–expiratory time ratio; $PaCO_2$, partial pressure arterial carbon dioxide; PaO_2, partial pressure arterial oxygen; PEEP, positive end-expiratory pressure; SaO_2, arterial oxygen saturation; SIMV, synchronized intermittent mandatory ventilation; VC, volume control; PRVC, pressure-regulated volume control.
*Desire tidal volume 6 to 8 mL/kg predicted body weight.
Adapted from Lapinsky SE, Slutsky AS: Ventilator management. In Wachter RM (ed): Hospital Medicine, 2nd ed. Philadelphia, Lippincott Williams & Wilkins, 2005, pp 173–182, Figure 23.2.

Rules of Thumb for Mechanical Ventilation

- Adjust ventilation by changing minute volume, to modify the partial pressure of arterial carbon dioxide ($PaCO_2$) and pH:

$$\text{Minute volume} = \text{respiratory rate} \times \text{tidal volume (liters)}$$

- Methods to improve oxygenation are as follows:
  - Increase FIO_2 or PEEP first.
  - Increase the I_T for refractory hypoxia.
- Keep PPLAT no greater than 30 cm H_2O.
- Avoid ventilating with VT greater than 10 mL/kg (predicted body weight [PBW]).
  - Typical VT is 6 to 8 mL/kg (PBW).
  - PBW for men (kg) = 50 + (2.3 × [height in inches – 60]).
  - PBW for women (kg) = 45.5 + (2.3 × [height in inches – 60]).
- Avoid paralytics (if possible) because of concerns over critical illness polyneuropathy.
- Sedation during mechanical ventilation should include agents that provide anxiolysis, analgesia, and, ideally, amnesia. Sedation should be titrated to an accepted sedation scale (e.g., the Ramsey scale) and continuous sedation should be interrupted on a daily basis.
  - Opiate and benzodiazepine combination.
  - Opiate and propofol combination.
  - Ketamine and benzodiazepine combination.

Weaning from Mechanical Ventilation

Weaning from mechanical ventilation involves the transition from full ventilatory support to spontaneous breathing, and then to eventual extubation (Fig. 207-1). There have been numerous approaches to ventilator weaning, but none as successful as daily spontaneous breathing trials (SBT). Patients who pass an SBT can be successfully extubated 85% of the time.

Patients should be assessed on a daily basis as to whether they are ready for an SBT; in part, this consists of clinicians interrupting continuous sedation on a daily basis. Patients should meet the following criteria to be ready for an SBT: (1) awake, cooperative, and able to follow commands; (2) clinically stable and preferably off vasopressor medications; (3) the underlying disease leading to intubation has sufficiently resolved; (4) good gag reflex and a strong cough; (5) minimal pulmonary secretions, (6) spontaneous respirations with a PEEP less than 5 to 8 cm H_2O; (7) a partial pressure of arterial oxygen (PaO_2)/FIO_2 ratio of at least 150 to 200; (8) a pH of at least 7.25; and (9) a rapid shallow breathing index (RSBI) of less than 105. The RSBI is checked by placing the patient on CPAP of 5 cm H_2O with a PS of 0 cm H_2O for 3 minutes and determining the average respiratory rate divided by the VT (in liters). Patients who have an RSBI greater than 105 fail an SBT 95% of the time.

If the aforementioned criteria are met, an SBT should be performed daily. An SBT can be performed with the patient either on a CPAP level of 5 cm H_2O and PS of 6 to 8 cm H_2O or on a T-piece with an FIO_2 no greater than 0.4 to 0.5. Watch the patient for 30 to 120 minutes and terminate the SBT if the patient develops any of the following signs of intolerance: respiratory rate greater than 35/min, arterial oxygen saturation (SaO_2) less than 90%, PaO_2 less than 60 mm Hg, heart rate greater than 140/min, systolic blood pressure greater than 180 mm Hg or less than 90 mm Hg, agitation, diaphoresis, increased work of breathing, or a VT less than 325 mL (or less than 4 mL/kg PBW). After 30 to 120 minutes, an arterial blood gas can be drawn to ensure adequate oxygenation and ventilation. A $PaCO_2$ greater than 50 mm Hg (or a greater than 10 mm Hg increase) or a PaO_2 less than 55 mm Hg (on FIO_2 = 0.4) would be additional reasons to continue mechanical ventilation.

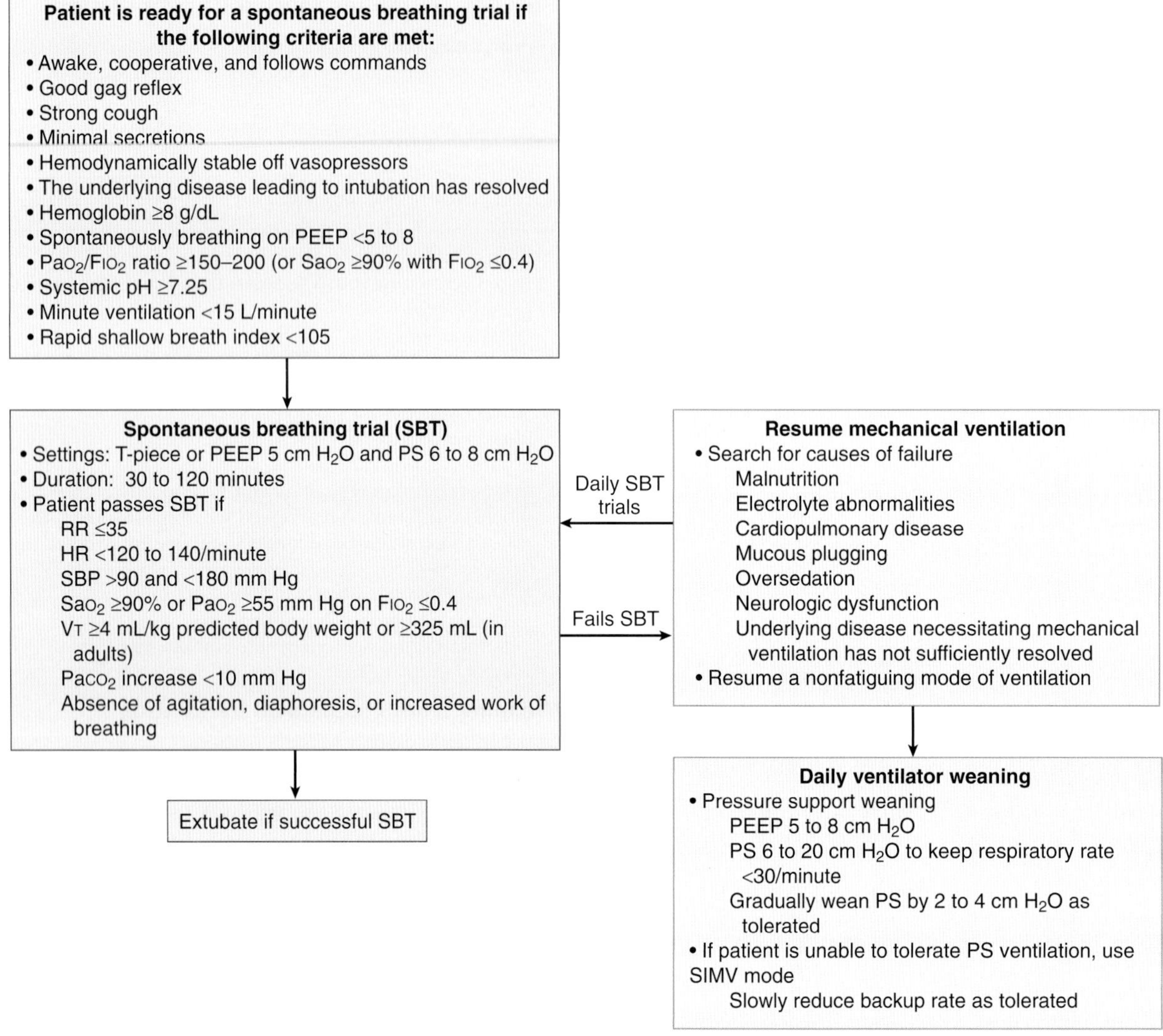

Patient is ready for a spontaneous breathing trial if the following criteria are met:
• Awake, cooperative, and follows commands
• Good gag reflex
• Strong cough
• Minimal secretions
• Hemodynamically stable off vasopressors
• The underlying disease leading to intubation has resolved
• Hemoglobin ≥8 g/dL
• Spontaneously breathing on PEEP <5 to 8
• Pa_{O_2}/F_{IO_2} ratio ≥150–200 (or Sa_{O_2} ≥90% with F_{IO_2} ≤0.4)
• Systemic pH ≥7.25
• Minute ventilation <15 L/minute
• Rapid shallow breath index <105
Spontaneous breathing trial (SBT)
• Settings: T-piece or PEEP 5 cm H_2O and PS 6 to 8 cm H_2O
• Duration: 30 to 120 minutes
• Patient passes SBT if
RR ≤35
HR <120 to 140/minute
SBP >90 and <180 mm Hg
Sa_{O_2} ≥90% or Pa_{O_2} ≥55 mm Hg on F_{IO_2} ≤0.4
V_T ≥4 mL/kg predicted body weight or ≥325 mL (in adults)
Pa_{CO_2} increase <10 mm Hg
Absence of agitation, diaphoresis, or increased work of breathing
Daily SBT trials
Fails SBT
Resume mechanical ventilation
• Search for causes of failure
Malnutrition
Electrolyte abnormalities
Cardiopulmonary disease
Mucous plugging
Oversedation
Neurologic dysfunction
Underlying disease necessitating mechanical ventilation has not sufficiently resolved
• Resume a nonfatiguing mode of ventilation
Extubate if successful SBT
Daily ventilator weaning
• Pressure support weaning
PEEP 5 to 8 cm H_2O
PS 6 to 20 cm H_2O to keep respiratory rate <30/minute
Gradually wean PS by 2 to 4 cm H_2O as tolerated
• If patient is unable to tolerate PS ventilation, use SIMV mode
Slowly reduce backup rate as tolerated

Figure 207-1 Weaning and liberation from mechanical ventilators. F_{IO_2}, fraction of inspired oxygen; HR, heart rate; Pa_{CO_2}, partial pressure of arterial carbon dioxide; Pa_{O_2}, partial pressure of arterial oxygen; PEEP, positive end-expiratory pressure; PS, pressure support; RR, respiratory rate; Sa_{O_2}, arterial oxygen saturation; SBP, systolic blood pressure; SIMV, synchronized intermittent mandatory ventilation; V_T, tidal volume. (Adapted from MacIntyre NR, Cook DJ, Ely EW Jr, et al: Evidence-based guidelines for weaning and discontinuing ventilatory support. Chest 120[6 Suppl]:375S–395S, 2001.)

Ventilator Complications

- *High airway pressures:* A high airway pressure can be divided into conditions associated with a high PIP or conditions associated with a high P_{PLAT}. The conditions associated with a high PIP, but an unchanged P_{PLAT}, include aspiration, bronchospasm, or endotracheal tube obstruction (kinking or secretions). Conditions that have an elevation in both the PIP and P_{PLAT} include "bucking the ventilator," pulmonary edema, pneumothorax, auto-PEEP, severe abdominal distention, ARDS, or chest wall noncompliance. "Bucking the ventilator" may be caused by inadequate sedation, paroxysms of coughing, or patient–ventilator dyssynchrony.
- *Barotrauma:* Barotrauma is defined as lung injury due to high mean airway pressures. It occurs when there is an alveolar leak causing one of the following clinical conditions: pneumomediastinum, pneumopericardium, pneumothorax, or subcutaneous emphysema. Those at highest risk for barotrauma have one of the following conditions: very stiff lungs (e.g., in ARDS); severe bronchospasm; P_{PLAT} greater than 30 cm H_2O; use of a high I_T; the development of auto-PEEP; and V_T greater than 10 mL/kg PBW.
- *Low airway pressures:* A low airway pressure usually means a leak in the ventilator circuit. This can be caused by the patient becoming disconnected from the ventilator, a loose tubing connection, or a large cuff leak.
- *Hypotension:* The causes of hypotension in a ventilated patient can be divided into ventilator-related causes, patient-related causes, and medication-induced hypotension. The ventilator-related causes include high PEEP levels, the development of auto-PEEP, or a tension pneumothorax. Patient-related causes include hypovolemia, a worsening shock state (e.g., septic, cardiogenic, anaphylactic), abdominal compartment syndrome, a massive pulmonary embolus, unstable arrhythmia, or a massive myocardial infarction. Finally, medication-induced hypotension may be caused by excessive sedation (e.g., opiates, propofol, benzodiazepines), medication hypersensitivity response, or the excessive use of antihypertensives.
- *Reversible causes of hypoxia:* The reversible causes of hypoxia in a ventilated patient can be remembered by the mnemonic CDSPIES (Box 207-2). Causes of *chronic* hypoxia are not included as etiologies. Splinting applies only to spontaneous breathing in a support mode when the V_T is limited by pain.

Box 207-2. Reversible Causes of Hypoxia in Ventilated Patients

C Congestive heart failure
D Drugs (oversedation leading to hypoventilation in spontaneously breathing patients)
S Secretions or splinting (leading to atelectasis in spontaneously breathing patients)
P Pneumothorax
I Infection (ventilator-associated pneumonia)
E Embolism (pulmonary embolism)
S Spasm (bronchospasm)

- *High respiratory rates:* The most common causes of a high respiratory rate in a ventilated patient are inadequate sedation, hypoxia, and anxiety. Other causes include a profound metabolic acidosis with a compensatory stimulus to hyperventilate, neurogenic hyperventilation, a pulmonary embolus, and toxic overdoses that stimulate the medullary respiratory center (e.g., salicylate overdose).
- *Apnea:* The most common cause of apnea in a ventilated patient is oversedation or the use of paralytics. Other potential causes include a central nervous system catastrophe or central sleep apnea.
- *Ventilator-induced lung injury:* Ventilator-induced lung injury results either from shear stress or from overdistention injury. Shear stress is caused by the repetitive opening and collapsing of alveoli. Overdistention injury results from the prolonged application of high-VT ventilation (VT >10 mL/kg PBW). Overdistention injury is especially common if there are areas of normal and diseased lung; the normal lung will be preferentially ventilated and therefore is at risk of overinflation. Conditions associated with poor lung compliance, like ARDS, are at highest risk for ventilator-induced lung injury, and therefore are indications for the use of lung-protective ventilation (Table 207-2).
- *Self-extubation:* Self-extubation can occur for several reasons. First, it can be the inadvertent consequence of moving the patient without adequate attention to the airway. It can also occur as a result of inadequate sedation or loose restraints in an agitated patient.
- *Decubitus pressure ulcers:* Patients who have been mechanically ventilated for a prolonged period are at risk for development of pressure ulcers of the occiput, sacrum, and heels. Frequent turning is imperative.
- *Venous thromboembolism:* Mechanical ventilation is a risk factor for venous thromboembolism. All ventilated patients should receive prophylactic heparin or sequential compression stockings to minimize the risk of a deep venous thrombosis.
- *Stress gastric ulcers:* Mechanical ventilation for longer than 48 hours places patients at risk for a stress ulcer. Therefore, histamine type 2 blockers or proton pump inhibitors should be administered as prophylaxis against the development of a stress gastric ulcer.
- *Ventilator-associated pneumonia:* Patients who have required mechanical ventilation for longer than 48 hours are at risk for a ventilator-associated pneumonia. The risk of ventilator-associated pneumonia can be decreased by performing the following interventions: raise the head of the bed to 45 degrees, avoid gastric overdistention, minimize ventilator circuit changes/manipulation, drain ventilator circuit condensate on a regular basis, use appropriate hand disinfection before patient care, consider kinetic bed therapy for prolonged mechanical ventilation, and administer twice-daily oral care with chlorhexidine rinses. Selective gut decontamination has a role in trauma patients. Other promising interventions include endotracheal tubes with either low-volume/high-compliance cuffs or those that allow for continuous subglottic suctioning.

Postprocedure Management

- Check a daily chest radiograph in all endotracheally intubated patients.
- Assess ventilator settings frequently and adjust accordingly.
- Ensure the patient is receiving interventions to prevent decubitus ulcers, gastric ulcers, a ventilator-associated pneumonia, or a deep venous thrombosis and assess daily for vent complications.
- Assess patients daily for potential to wean or discontinue ventilatory support.

CPT/Billing Codes

94002 Ventilation assist and management; hospital inpatient/observation, initial day
94003 Ventilation assist and management; hospital inpatient/observation, subsequent days

TABLE 207-2 Protocol for Lung-Protective Ventilation

1. Assist-control mode with FIO_2 = 100%
2. VT = 8 mL/kg predicted body weight (PBW)
   PBW for men (kg) = 50 + [2.3 × (height in inches − 60)]
   PBW for women (kg) = 45.5 + [2.3 × (height in inches − 60)]
   Decrease VT 1 mL/kg PBW every 1 to 2 hr until VT = 6 mL/kg PBW
3. Initial respiratory rate typically 12 to 16/min, but can increase up to 35/min
4. Initial PEEP 5 to 8 cm H_2O, and adjust based on PEEP-FIO_2 algorithm (see below)
5. Adjust PEEP and FIO2 to keep PaO_2 > 55 mm Hg or SaO_2 > 88%
6. Decrease VT as low as 4 mL/kg PBW if PPLAT >30 cm H_2O despite adequate suctioning and sedation
7. Allow permissive hypercapnia and may use sodium bicarbonate to keep pH > 7.15

PEEP-FIO_2 Algorithm for Lung-Protective Ventilation

FIO_2	0.3	0.4	0.4	0.5	0.5	0.6	0.7	0.7	0.7	0.8	0.9	0.9	0.9	1.0	1.0	1.0	1.0
PEEP*	5	5	8	8	10	10	10	12	14	14	14	16	18	18	20	22	24

FIO_2, fraction of inspired oxygen; PaO_2, partial pressure of arterial oxygen; PEEP, positive end-expiratory pressure; PPLAT, plateau pressure; SaO_2, arterial oxygen saturation; VT, tidal volume.
*PEEP measured in cm H_2O.
Adapted from Brower RG, Lanken PN, MacIntyre N, et al, for the ARDS Clinical Trials Network: Higher versus lower positive end-expiratory pressures in patients with the acute respiratory distress syndrome. N Engl J Med 351:327–336, 2004; and Brower RG, Matthay MA, Morris A, et al, for the ARDS Clinical Trials Network: Ventilation with lower tidal volumes as compared with traditional tidal volumes for acute lung injury and acute respiratory distress syndrome. N Engl J Med 342:1301–1308, 2000.

94004 Ventilation assist and management; nursing home, per day

(94002 to 94004 not to be reported with E/M services 99201–99499)

94005 Home ventilator management care plan oversight; in home or assisted living, within a calendar month, ≥30 minutes

(94005 code not to be reported with 99339–99340 or 99374–99378)

ICD-9-CM Diagnostic Codes

276.2 Acidosis
276.3 Alkalosis
276.4 Acid-base mixed disorder
427.5 Cardiac or cardiorespiratory arrest
428.1 Congestive heart failure, left-sided
491.20 Chronic obstructive bronchitis, without exacerbation
491.21 Chronic obstructive bronchitis, with or without emphysema, with acute exacerbation
492.8 Emphysema, NOS
493.01 Asthma, extrinsic with status asthmaticus
493.90 Asthma, unspecified with status asthmaticus
518.5 Pulmonary insufficiency following trauma and surgery
518.81 Acute respiratory failure, NOS
518.82 Respiratory distress, acute
518.83 Respiratory failure, chronic
780.01 Coma
785.50 Shock, unspecified, without mention of trauma
785.51 Shock, cardiogenic
785.52 Shock, septic
785.59 Shock, other (hypovolemic, anaphylactic)
786.09 Hypercapnia
799.02 Hypoxia
799.1 Respiratory arrest

Suppliers

(See contact information online at www.expertconsult.com.)

Maquet Critical Care AB
Puritan Bennett
Siemens

BIBLIOGRAPHY

Brower RG, Matthay MA, Morris A, et al, for the ARDS Clinical Trials Network: Ventilation with lower tidal volumes as compared with traditional tidal volumes for acute lung injury and acute respiratory distress syndrome. N Engl J Med 342:1301–1308, 2000.

Lapinsky SE, Slutsky AS: Ventilator management. In Wachter RM (ed): Hospital Medicine, 2nd ed. Philadelphia, Lippincott Williams & Wilkins, 2005, pp 173–182.

MacIntyre NR: Assist-control mechanical ventilation. In Fink MP, Abraham E, Vincent J-L, Kochanek P (eds): Textbook of Critical Care, 5th ed. Philadelphia, Saunders, 2005, pp 497–518.

MacIntyre NR, Cook DJ, Ely EW Jr, et al: Evidence-based guidelines for weaning and discontinuing ventilatory support. Chest 120(6 Suppl): 375S–395S, 2001.

Markowitz DH, Irwin RI: Mechanical ventilation: Initiation and discontinuation. In Irwin RI, Rippe JM (eds): Manual of Intensive Care Medicine, 4th ed. Philadelphia, Lippincott Williams & Wilkins, 2006, pp 301–311.

CHAPTER 208

ARTERIAL PUNCTURE AND PERCUTANEOUS ARTERIAL LINE PLACEMENT

Grant C. Fowler • Donna A. Landen

ARTERIAL PUNCTURE

An arterial puncture can be useful in certain urgent, acute, or chronic conditions, basically whenever an arterial blood sample is needed. If frequent sampling or (intra)arterial blood pressure monitoring is necessary, placement of an arterial line should be considered. With proper technique and equipment, an arterial puncture is a safe and simple procedure. However, advancements in technology for noninvasive monitoring may eventually make this procedure obsolete. Use of pulse oxymetry (arterial oxygen saturation) and end-tidal CO_2 ($ETCO_2$) monitoring has already markedly decreased the need for arterial puncture. In most cases, an arterial puncture is used now only to assess and confirm hypoxia or hypercapnia when indicated by pulse oxymetry or $ETCO_2$ monitoring. Although venous sampling may occasionally be used to monitor pH (e.g., diabetic ketoacidosis), venous blood pH is much less reliable as a surrogate marker for arterial pH in patients with shock and other critical illnesses; therefore, arterial puncture is still necessary in these patients.

Indications

- To confirm a clinically suspected acute problem with carbon dioxide or oxygen exchange, or with acid-base balance, such as patients with shock, asthma exacerbation, chronic obstructive pulmonary disease (COPD) exacerbation, pulmonary thromboembolism, diabetic ketoacidosis, or refractory cardiac dysrhythmias, or patients who are either newly comatose or have a depressed level of consciousness.
- To confirm the clinical status in a patient with a chronic condition that affects gas exchange or acid-base balance, such as chronic COPD. Long-term continuous oxygen therapy has proven beneficial (e.g., decreased mortality and hospitalizations) in patients with COPD with a partial pressure of arterial oxygen (PaO_2) less than 59 mm Hg (especially with comorbid disease, e.g., cor pulmonale, pulmonary hypertension), and even more if the PaO_2 is less than 55 mm Hg.
- To confirm hypoxia when pulse oximetry may not be reliable or is not available or obtainable (e.g., patient with severe hypoxia or severe hypotension).
- To confirm hypoxia, when pulse oximetry suggests this diagnosis.
- To confirm hypercapnia when $ETCO_2$ monitoring may underestimate (e.g., patient with large dead space ventilation or low cardiac output).
- To confirm the need for long-term continuous oxygen therapy. Medicare requires at least two blood gas determinations, while breathing room air for 20 minutes, with PaO_2 less than 59 mm Hg (with cor pulmonale, clinically diagnosed, or hematocrit ≥55%) or PaO_2 less than 55 mm Hg, to qualify for continuous oxygen therapy, or, alternatively, after 20 minutes of breathing room air and using pulse oximetry, two oxygen saturation readings ≤88%. The company providing the oxygen cannot be the same company that does the blood gas testing in the home.
- To obtain arterial blood for certain laboratory tests (lactate, ammonia, carboxyhemoglobin, methemoglobin, or carbon monoxide levels, although some laboratories can use venous blood).
- To obtain a blood sample in an emergent situation when phlebotomy cannot be performed or when there are no venous sites.

Contraindications

- When a functional arterial line is present
- Overlying skin compromised by trauma, burns, infection, severe dermatitis *(relative contraindication in life-threatening situation)*
- Known or suspected severe arterial disease of aneurysmal, atherosclerotic, inflammatory, or vasospastic nature *(relative contraindication in life-threatening situation)*
- Previous surgery in the area that may have caused scarring, thereby complicating the procedure *(relative contraindication, can always use hand-held Doppler technique)*
- Poor collateral perfusion from the ulnar or posterior tibial artery when the radial or dorsalis pedis artery, respectively, is the intended puncture site *(may be relative contraindication)*
- Inability to palpate arterial pulsation *(relative contraindication, can always use hand-held Doppler technique)*
- Synthetic vascular graft *(relative contraindication)*
- *Additional relative contraindications:* bleeding dyscrasias, anticoagulant therapy, or possible later thrombolytic or fibrinolytic therapy. These patients should be monitored carefully after arterial puncture to prevent complications.

NOTE: If drawing of frequent arterial specimens or continuous pressure monitoring is necessary, placement of an arterial line should be considered.

Equipment

- 3- to 5-mL sterile plastic or glass syringe with a freely movable plunger. (Kits are made in which the preheparinized syringe plunger should not be moved. A lyophilized heparin pellet may be in the syringe. These kits also contain the needle and rubber stopper or syringe plug.)
- 25-gauge, ⅝-inch (1.6-cm) needle for radial, brachial, dorsalis pedis, and femoral puncture. For femoral puncture in obese patients, a 22-gauge, 1½-inch (3.8-cm) needle may be helpful.

- 1 or 2 mL heparin (1000 U/mL)
- Plug for syringe or rubber stopper for end of needle
- Antiseptic skin preparation, such as povidone–iodine (Betadine) or 70% isopropyl alcohol
- Sterile 4 × 4 gauze pads
- Hypoallergenic adhesive tape
- Container with 2 to 3 inches of crushed ice for sample transport (e.g., plastic bag, emesis basin, cup)
- Sterile gloves
- Equipment for the clinician to observe universal blood and body fluid precautions
- In the alert patient *(optional)*, 1% or 2% lidocaine *without* epinephrine and a 1- or 3-mL syringe with 25- or 27-gauge, ⅝-inch (1.6-cm) needle
- Handheld Doppler or pulse oximeter *(optional)*

Arterial Site Selection

Each site for arterial puncture has its own risks and benefits. Because of its proximity to the skin surface, the radial artery in the patient's nondominant hand is the preferred site. It is an excellent location if there is adequate ulnar artery collateral circulation (see the following section) and if the clinical situation is stable. In severely hypotensive patients or during cardiopulmonary resuscitation, the femoral artery is usually the most readily palpable and most conveniently located artery, in spite of its higher risk of complications with puncture. Alternative sites, in decreasing order of preference, include the brachial, dorsalis pedis, and superficial temporal arteries. The brachial artery should be reserved for use when radial artery puncture cannot be performed or is contraindicated. Although the dorsalis pedis artery is absent, usually bilaterally, in 12% of the population, it is another option for puncture. Before dorsalis pedis artery puncture is performed, collateral flow should be demonstrated in a manner similar to the Allen test (see the following section). Superficial temporal artery puncture will not be discussed. Ultimately, clinician experience and local anatomy are the deciding factors in choice of site. If possible, the clinician should avoid an artery where the overlying cutaneous defenses are disrupted because of infection, burn, severe dermatitis, or other skin damage.

Assessment of Ulnar Collateral Circulation

Radial artery puncture can lead to thrombosis of the distal artery. Because 12% of hands have inadequate collateral flow because of an incomplete palmar arch (Fig. 208-1), to minimize the risk of permanent ischemic damage to the hand, many experts suggest confirming adequate collateral circulation before puncture. Even if there is excellent collateral flow, the nondominant hand should be used, if possible. However, other experts have questioned the value of testing for collateral circulation. At least one large case series of patients demonstrated the safety of radial artery cannulation without testing for collateral circulation with the modified Allen test in patients without major peripheral arterial disease (Slogoff and colleagues, 1983).

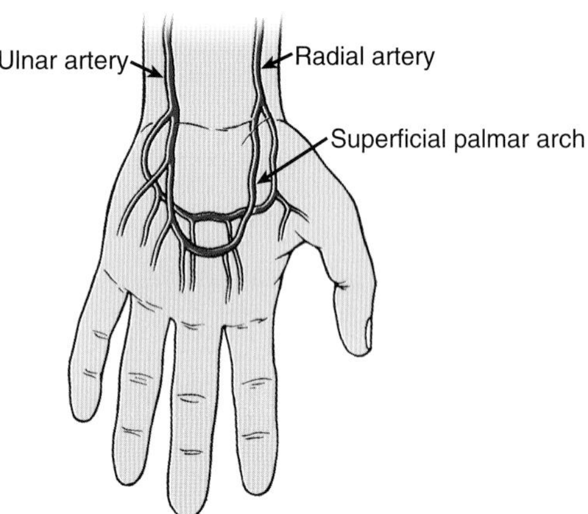

Figure 208-1 Anatomy of radial and ulnar arteries at wrist and superficial palmar arch.

MODIFIED ALLEN TEST. The Allen test, used to evaluate ulnar collateral flow, was first described in 1929. To minimize falsely abnormal results, the modified Allen test can be used:

1. The hand should be at least room temperature (>70° F). It can be warmed in water, if necessary. The patient should hold his or her arm above heart level, and then open and close the hand several times to exsanguinate it. Next, the patient should clench the fist tightly. The clinician then compresses both the radial and ulnar arteries (Fig. 208-2A). (In a comatose or anesthetized patient, the hand can be elevated and clenched passively by an assistant.)
2. After a minute is allowed for blood to drain from the hand, the fist should be lowered below the level of the heart, unclenched (Fig. 208-2B), and pressure on the ulnar artery (Fig. 208-2C) released. Care should be taken to avoid hyperextension of the wrist or fingers, which can lead to a falsely abnormal test result. When the pressure on the ulnar artery is released, the cadaveric color of the entire hand should return to its normal color within 6 seconds (Fig. 208-2D). Color usually returns to the palm first, and then to the entire hand. If any area of the hand does not rapidly (within 6 seconds) return to normal color, this is a positive modified Allen test. The thumb, index finger, and thenar eminence are the areas most commonly involved in a positive test. These areas often have inadequate collateral blood flow and may be entirely dependent on the radial artery for perfusion.

An abnormal or equivocal modified Allen test result, although it may not preclude arterial puncture or cannulation, should alert the clinician to potential complications, a need for caution when performing the procedure, and a need to monitor the patient closely postprocedure. Various types of noninvasive studies are also useful for further patient evaluation. Hand-held Doppler ultrasonography or pulse oximetry can be used to rapidly assess perfusion with techniques more sensitive and specific than the modified Allen test. If time allows, formal arterial Doppler ultrasonography, either portable or in the radiology department, can be used to further evaluate the collateral circulation or direct the puncture.

HAND-HELD DOPPLER EVALUATION

1. After placing the probe between the heads of the third and fourth metacarpals on the palm, angulate the probe and advance it proximally until maximal auditory signal is obtained (Fig. 208-3).
2. With the palmar arch identified and maximal signal obtained, compression of the radial artery should not cause a change of the signal if the palmar arch is complete and supplied by collateral ulnar circulation. A decrease in signal indicates poor collateral flow. This is a much more sensitive and specific test than the modified Allen test.

PULSE OXIMETRY EVALUATION. This is especially useful in the unconscious patient.

1. Place the sensor of a pulse oximeter with a visual pulse waveform display on the patient's thumb.
2. While examining the waveform on the monitor, occlude the radial artery. If the waveform remains unchanged after radial artery occlusion, the patient has adequate collateral circulation, probably from the ulnar artery.

Assessment of Dorsalis Pedis Collateral Circulation

To minimize the risk of permanent ischemic damage to the distal foot, some experts suggest confirming adequate collateral circulation before dorsalis pedis artery puncture is attempted.

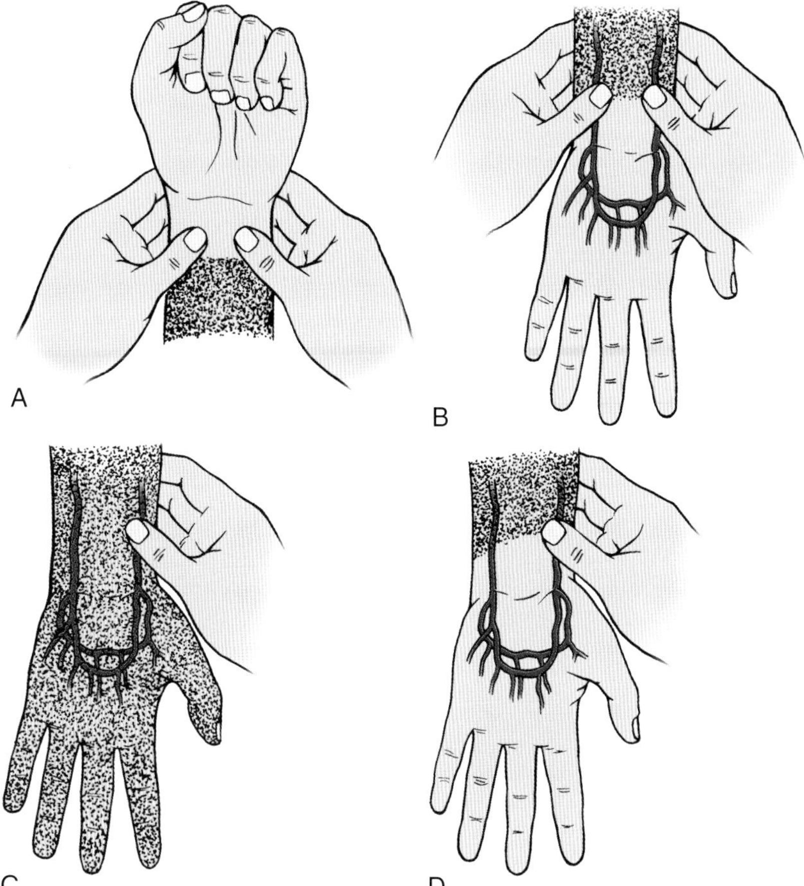

Figure 208-2 Modified Allen test. **A,** Hand is elevated and fist clenched while radial and ulnar arteries are occluded for 1 minute. **B,** Hand is lowered and fist is unclenched. Hand is cadaveric. **C,** Ulnar artery compression is released while radial artery compression is continued. In a negative test, the entire hand regains color within 6 seconds. **D,** Positive test. With inadequate collateral perfusion from the ulnar artery, the hand remains cadaveric as long as radial artery compression is maintained. When inadequate collateral perfusion is demonstrated, another puncture or cannulation site should be considered.

1. The foot should be at least room temperature (>70° F). It can be warmed in water, if necessary.
2. After locating and palpating the dorsalis pedis artery (Fig. 208-4), occlude it with compression.
3. Blanch the great toenail by compressing for several minutes.
4. Release pressure on the nail and observe for flushing. A rapid return of color indicates adequate collateral flow.

NOTE: In most persons, collateral circulation of the foot is provided by a branch of the posterior tibial artery. Hand-held Doppler ultrasonography can be used to assess collateral flow between the dorsalis pedis and posterior tibial arteries in a manner similar to that used in the palmar arch.

Preprocedure Patient Preparation

The clinician and patient should be in a comfortable position that can be maintained for 10 to 15 minutes. The procedure, its necessity, alternatives (if there are any), and possible complications should be explained to the alert patient. In nonemergent situations, informed consent should be obtained (see the sample patient consent form online at www.expertconsult.com). The patient should be prepared for some discomfort.

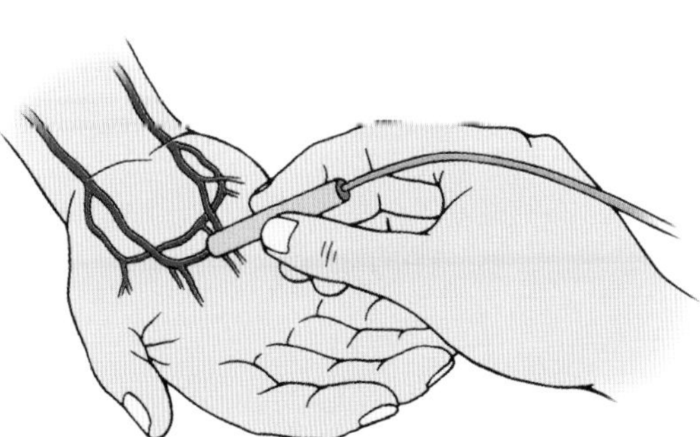

Figure 208-3 Assessment of the superficial palmar arch with hand-held Doppler ultrasonography.

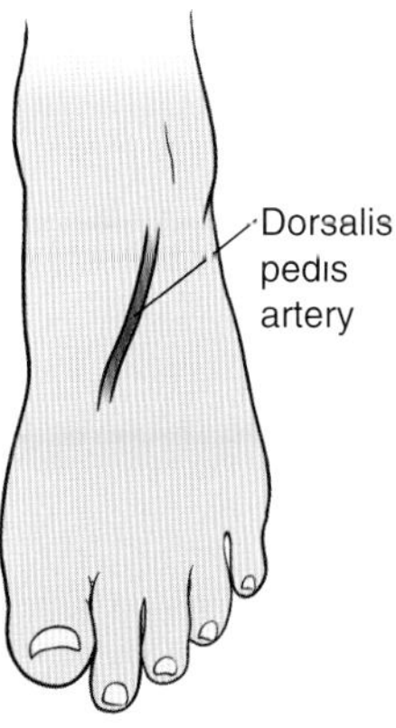

Figure 208-4 Location of the dorsalis pedis artery.

Technique

1. Rinse the syringe with a small amount (1 or 2 mL) of heparin and then empty it through the needle. For glass syringes, this step not only coats the syringe with heparin, it eliminates the dead space in the syringe and needle. Although heparin does not adhere to plastic syringes, performing this step with plastic syringes will displace any air and fill the dead space.

   NOTE: Certain kits contain syringes that are already heparinized (often containing a pellet of lyophilized heparin) and the plunger should not be moved.

2. Following universal blood and body fluid precautions, prepare the skin in an aseptic manner and put on sterile gloves.
3. The clinician should use his or her nondominant hand to palpate the selected artery with the balls of two or three fingers, and immobilize it with these fingers along its course.
4. *Optional:* Local anesthetic (lidocaine) can be injected for a particularly anxious patient to minimize hyperventilation artifact. However, use minimal amounts to avoid anatomic distortion, which could make it difficult to palpate and puncture the pulse.
5. Holding the barrel of the syringe like a pencil in the dominant hand, keep the needle bevel up.
6. Depending on the site selected, perform the puncture.
   - *Radial artery puncture:* Dorsiflex the supine wrist (about 30 degrees) of the patient's nondominant hand and rotate it outward (externally), slightly. The wrist should be supported by a firm surface, such as an assistant's hand, a rolled towel or washcloth, or a 500-mL intravenous (IV) fluid bag. Insert the needle where the pulse is most prominent—½ to 1 inch proximal to the wrist crease—at a 40- to 60-degree angle to the skin. Direct it slowly in the long axis of the artery toward the pulsation (Fig. 208-5).

   NOTE: Avoid "spearing" (going through) the artery. Osteomyelitis and large hematomas can result from "spearing" the artery.

   - *Brachial artery puncture:* Place the patient's elbow on a rolled towel or washcloth. Slightly hyperextend and supinate the arm (palm up) with the patient's wrist in the anatomic position but rotated slightly outward. The brachial artery pulsation should be palpable in the medial aspect of the antecubital fossa (Fig. 208-6), lateral to the medial epicondyle, but medial to the biceps tendon. Insert the needle at about a 45- to 60-degree angle, slightly above the elbow crease, in the antecubital fossa or slightly proximal to it. Aim along the long axis of the artery toward the pulsation.
   - *Femoral artery puncture* (Fig. 208-7): With the patient in a supine position and legs straight, rotated slightly outward, insert the needle 1 to 1½ inches distal to the inguinal ligament at about the inguinal crease. It should be at a 60- to 90- degree angle to the distal skin and aimed toward the pulsation (Fig. 208-8). Avoid puncturing lateral to the pulsation because the femoral nerve could be damaged.
   - *Dorsalis pedis artery puncture* (Fig. 208-9): With the patient in a supine position, insert the needle where the pulse is most prominent, at a 45- to 60- degree angle to the sole of the foot. Aim toward the pulsation.
7. Although penetration into the artery can occasionally be sensed, puncture is usually detected when blood enters the syringe. It should enter the syringe spontaneously without with-

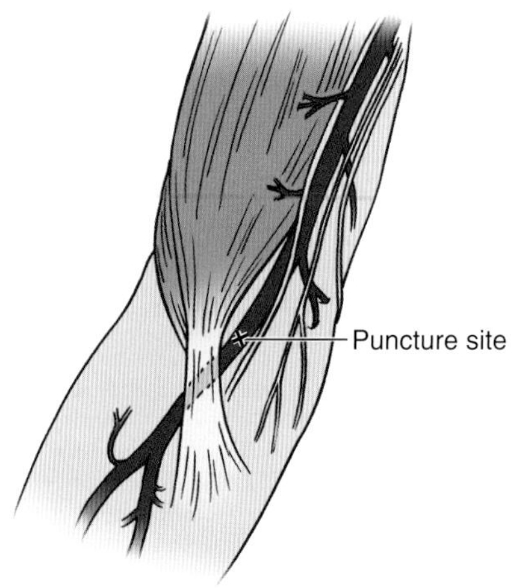

Figure 208-6 Right brachial artery and its branches, and the anatomic site for brachial artery puncture.

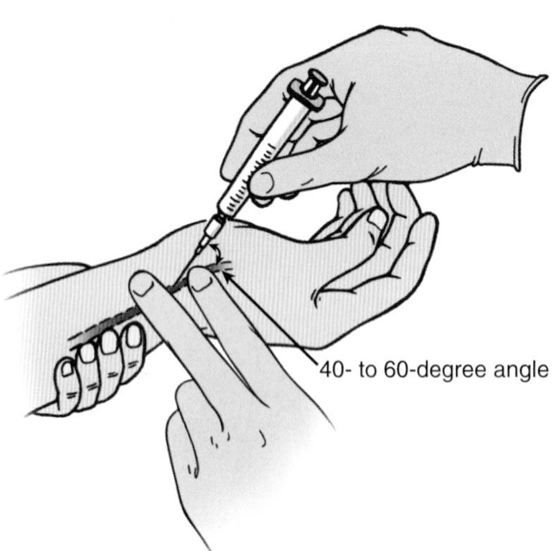

Figure 208-5 This patient is left-hand dominant. Palpate the patient's radial pulse with your left hand. While holding the heparinized syringe with your right hand (reverse hands if left-handed), puncture the skin at approximately a 60-degree angle to the skin, directing the needle toward the radial pulsation.

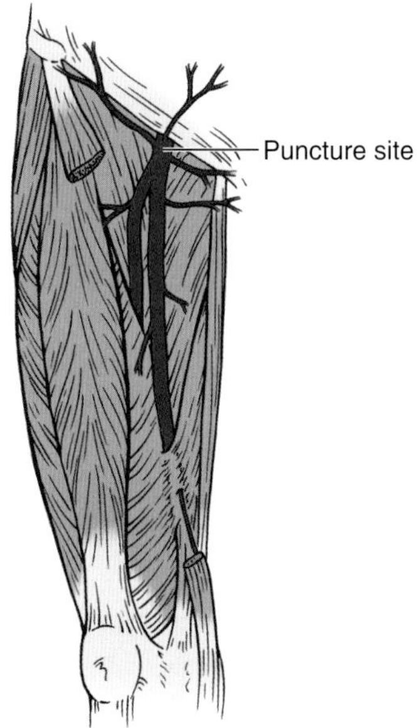

Figure 208-7 Right femoral artery and its branches, and the anatomic site for femoral artery puncture.

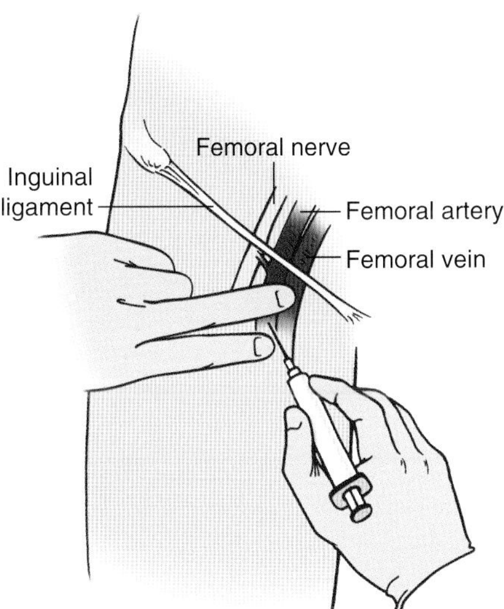

Figure 208-8 Technique of femoral artery puncture. The first two fingers of the free hand are used to palpate the femoral artery.

drawing the plunger if the syringe is specifically designed for arterial puncture. With plastic syringes or in severely hypotensive patients, slight aspiration may be necessary. Otherwise, attempt to avoid aspiration to decrease the chance of obtaining venous blood. If blood is not obtained during the insertion, slowly withdraw the needle and stop when blood appears.

8. If no blood appears, withdraw the needle completely and start again. For additional attempts, advance the needle without changing the angle of approach but with the needle directed ⅛ inch to either side of the previous attempt.
9. When blood appears, collect 3 mL of blood and remove the needle from the artery with a smooth, swift motion while applying pressure to the site. Steady pressure should be maintained for at least 5 minutes (longer in hypertensive patients and patients on anticoagulant therapy).
10. While applying pressure at the site with one hand, use the other hand to hold the syringe with the needle tip upright and expel any air bubbles. Tapping the syringe may help expel bubbles clinging to the sides.
11. Secure the needle tip by impaling it on a rubber stopper or remove the needle and cap the syringe securely. (Special rubber caps are available for this purpose.) Do not allow any room air to get into the syringe or any air bubbles to remain.

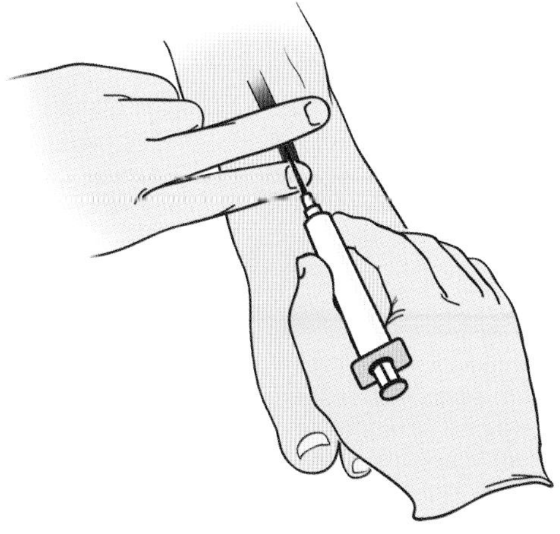

Figure 208-9 Technique of dorsalis pedis artery puncture.

12. Roll the syringe between the palms of the hands four or five times to mix the blood uniformly with the heparin.
13. Label the syringe appropriately with the patient's name and number(s), and place the syringe on ice. Immediately transport the syringe to the laboratory.
14. Return in 10 to 15 minutes and check the puncture site for hematoma formation and for adequate distal perfusion.

Complications

- Repeated punctures at the same site increase the risk of complications.
- Hemorrhage or hematoma is the most common complication. Risk can be minimized by prompt, continuous application (for 5 to 10 minutes) of pressure after the procedure, and by using a small-gauge (25-gauge) needle, if possible.
- Thrombosis is a possible complication of any arterial puncture. It more commonly results from puncture of the radial artery or any artery with occlusive disease. The risk increases with repeated punctures. For a diminished pulse after puncture, prompt vascular surgical consultation should be obtained. Ischemia and resulting gangrene are additional possible complications.
- Nerve damage can occur, either from direct needle insertion into the nerve or from the pressure of a resultant hematoma. This is more common with brachial and femoral artery punctures.
- Infection, including septic arthritis from a femoral artery puncture, is a possible complication. Try to avoid puncturing down to the bone with a femoral artery puncture (or any other puncture).
- Pseudoaneurysms have been reported, especially with femoral artery puncture. A pseudoaneurysm appears as a "pulsating tumor," anterior to the artery, often associated with a bruit. These occur more often after resolution of a large hematoma. Treatment is surgical removal of the pseudoaneurysm by a vascular surgeon.
- An arteriovenous fistula may form after femoral puncture. In part, this is why the radial artery is a preferred site because there is no accompanying large vein.
- Spurious laboratory results are most often the consequence of mixing venous blood with the arterial sample, but they can also be due to an excessive quantity of heparin in the syringe. Heparin has a very low pH; therefore, using too much can cause not only a falsely low partial pressure of arterial carbon dioxide ($PaCO_2$), but a low pH. Delay in analyzing the specimen or improper chilling can cause the blood to metabolize the oxygen, or the oxygen to dissociate from hemoglobin. This will falsely lower the oxygen and pH and falsely elevate the $PaCO_2$. Air in the syringe may markedly lower the $PaCO_2$ because room air contains little carbon dioxide. Depending on whether the initial partial pressure of arterial oxygen (PaO_2) was greater or less than room air, mixing the sample with air may either falsely lower or elevate the PaO_2. Vacutainers should not be used to draw arterial blood; even though they are filled with nitrogen, they contain measurable amounts of oxygen. Even this small amount of oxygen will significantly alter the PaO_2.

Postprocedure Patient Education

The patient should be instructed to avoid rubbing the site. He or she should report any bleeding, pain, swelling, numbness, or tingling after the arterial puncture. If the extremity turns cold or blue, the patient should inform the nurse or clinician. If the patient is awake and alert, he or she can help hold pressure on the site while the clinician is delivering the specimen to the laboratory.

Percutaneous Arterial Line Placement

Intra-arterial procedures are now common, with arterial dye studies and angioplasty even being performed by noncardiologists and nonsurgeons (e.g., interventional radiologists). The most common intra-arterial procedures performed are arterial puncture and arterial cannulation. If arterial cannulation is to be performed, support staff and facilities must be properly trained and prepared to deal with setup and possible complications, which can be more frequent and severe than with IV cannulation or arterial puncture. The site (radial, femoral, or dorsalis pedis artery) should be chosen according to the same risks and priorities established in the Arterial Puncture section. Benefits of arterial cannulation include accurate arterial pressure measurements, less discomfort and injury than with frequent arterial punctures, and the ability to obtain arterial samples without disturbing the steady state (e.g., pain induced with arterial puncture can cause hyperventilation, resulting in falsely low $PaCO_2$ measurements).

NOTE: For noninvasive monitoring of arterial pressure, Korotkoff sounds are commonly used. With increased wall tension (e.g., in vasoconstricted patients, such as those with increased systemic vascular resistance from shock), the ability of the arterial walls to produce the Korotkoff sounds may be altered. Therefore, in these patients, low cuff pressure does not necessarily indicate hypotension. Relying on Korotkoff sounds alone in such patients can result in dangerous errors in therapy. Stiff walls from atherosclerosis can also alter Korotkoff sounds.

Indications

- When there is difficulty obtaining or risk of inaccuracy of cuff blood pressure in a critically ill patient
- When continuous monitoring of arterial blood pressure is needed, especially in patients with shock, patients with resultant increased systemic vascular resistance, patients who have the potential to become hemodynamically unstable, and during major surgery or administration of parenteral vasopressor or dilator medications
- With labile or accelerated hypertension and evidence of progressive vascular damage (mean arterial pressure [MAP] is a much more consistent parameter for accelerated hypertension than the systolic or diastolic pressure alone)
- To monitor MAP in patients in whom it is necessary to maintain MAP at a certain level (e.g., to maintain cerebral perfusion pressure in a patient poststroke)
- When continuous access to arterial blood is needed (to avoid repeated arterial punctures)
- To measure cardiac output by the dye dilution method

Contraindications

Absolute

- Inadequate collateral blood flow distal to where the arterial line will be placed (e.g., abnormal modified Allen test or dorsalis pedis collateral flow test result, or hand-held Doppler ultrasonography or pulse oximetry reveals inadequate collateral arterial circulation; see the Arterial Puncture section)
- Patients with a significant injury to the same extremity, especially if it may compromise distal perfusion
- Hypercoagulable states

Relative

The following are relative contraindications; in life-threatening or certain other situations, the benefits of arterial cannulation may outweigh the risks. In some patients, arterial cannulation will decrease the risks of bleeding from multiple punctures.

- Severe atherosclerotic or vasospastic arterial disease
- Local skin compromise, such as with trauma, infection, burn, or severe dermatitis
- Anticoagulation from bleeding disorders, anticoagulant therapy, or potential future thrombolytic therapy
- Synthetic vascular graft

NOTE: Although certain experts no longer recommend cannulation of the brachial artery because of the increased potential for thrombosis and ischemia of the lower arm and hand, others prefer brachial artery cannulation to radial or dorsalis pedis artery cannulation in certain patients (e.g., the patient with anasarca). Brachial artery cannulation is also less likely to cause infection than femoral artery cannulation.

Equipment

- Sterile gloves, drapes, and 4 × 4 gauze sponges
- Equipment for the clinician to observe universal blood and body fluid precautions
- Antiseptic skin preparation, such as povidone–iodine or chlorhexidine solution
- In the alert patient *(optional)*, 1% or 2% lidocaine without epinephrine and a 3-mL syringe with 25- or 27-gauge, ⅝-inch (1.6-cm) needle
- Short arm board/wrist extensor splint and a rolled gauze, towel, or washcloth, about 3 inches in diameter, for radial artery cannulation; arm board and the same rolled gauze, towel, or washcloth for brachial artery cannulation
- For radial, dorsalis pedis, or brachial artery cannulation, a 20-gauge, 1¼- to 2-inch (3.2- to 5.1-cm) Teflon catheter-over-needle with a nontapered shaft
- For femoral artery cannulation, a 19- or 20-gauge or 4-Fr, 6-inch (15- to 16-cm) single-lumen cannula
- For the Seldinger or wire-guided technique, a flexible guidewire small enough to pass through the catheter and needle
- Fluid-filled connector tubing attached to sterile three-way stopcock and transducer (using a stiff, low-capacitance tubing will minimize the artifact; also, attempt to minimize the length of tubing); transducers are available with needleless sampling ports
- Antibiotic ointment, such as povidone–iodine ointment
- Nylon 3-0 or 4-0 suture, preferably on a skin needle
- Hypoallergenic adhesive tape
- Suture scissors
- Bag of sterile dextrose water (D_5W) IV fluid mixed with heparin to make a 1-U/mL solution for flushing (this should be in-line with the connector tubing)
- Scissors for clipping hair for femoral insertion
- Hand-held Doppler *(optional technique)*
- No. 11 or no. 15 blade scalpel, mosquito hemostat, and nylon 3-0 suture for cutdown *(optional technique)*

Preprocedure Patient Preparation

Explain the indications, complications, and necessity of the procedure to the patient if he or she is alert and awake. If the patient is unconscious, explain this to the next of kin. If there are alternatives available, discuss them as along with the benefits of this procedure. Discuss the importance of immobilization while the procedure is being performed, and warn the patient of the discomfort that will be felt with the insertion of the catheter. Inform the patient that this catheter is more dangerous than an IV catheter and that care must be taken with the catheter after insertion. Obtain written consent for the procedure or document implied consent in the chart if the patient is unconscious.

Technique

1. The clinician and the patient should be in a comfortable position that can be maintained as long as necessary to complete the procedure. When using nonclosed systems, observe universal blood and body fluid precautions.
2. The clinician should palpate the artery selected and immobilize it along its course with two or three fingers of his or her nondominant hand.

3. Prepare the skin in an aseptic manner. For femoral cannulation, use scissors to clip any long hairs in the area of the cannulation.
4. Local anesthetic (lidocaine) can be injected for a particularly anxious patient. It may also prevent arterial spasm when the artery is punctured. Use minimal amounts to prevent anatomic distortion, which may make it difficult to palpate the pulse. If the anatomy does get distorted from the anesthetic injection, attempt to massage it into the surrounding skin and soft tissue.
5. Drape the area with sterile towels.
6. Wearing sterile gloves, the clinician should hold the catheter needle hub like a pencil in his or her dominant hand with the needle bevel up.
7. Depending on the site selected, perform the cannulation.
   - *Radial artery cannulation:* On the patient's selected hand (preferably the nondominant hand), slightly dorsiflex (about 30 degrees), slightly rotate outward, and immobilize the wrist by taping a gauze roll between the supinated wrist and the dorsally applied arm board (Fig. 208-10A). The 3-inch roll should be between the arm and the board. Apply tape over the proximal interphalangeal joints (excluding the thumb) and around the arm board. Also apply tape more proximally, securing the forearm to the arm board. Insert the needle ½ to 1 inch proximal to the wrist crease, at about a 30-degree angle to the distal skin. Direct it slowly down the long axis of the artery toward the pulsation (Fig. 208-10B).
   - *Femoral artery cannulation:* With the patient in the supine position and legs straight, rotated slightly outward, insert the needle at a 45-degree angle to the skin and direct it toward the patient's head. Also, direct it toward the femoral artery pulsation, 2 to 5 cm distal to the inguinal ligament at the inguinal crease. After the flash of blood, the angle can be lowered to 20 or 30 degrees relative to the distal skin.

NOTE: Large hematomas are not uncommon in this area because of the amount of surrounding soft tissue. Femoral artery cannulation also carries the risk of more serious complications. Avoid puncturing proximal to the inguinal ligament, which could cause a retroperitoneal hematoma. The proximity of this location to the groin may increase the risk of infection. This location is also less popular for patients if they are awake; they should not ambulate with a femoral artery cannulation in place (see Fig. 208-7).

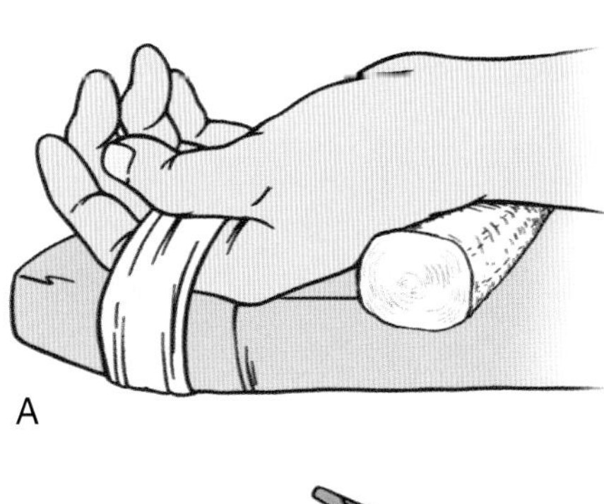

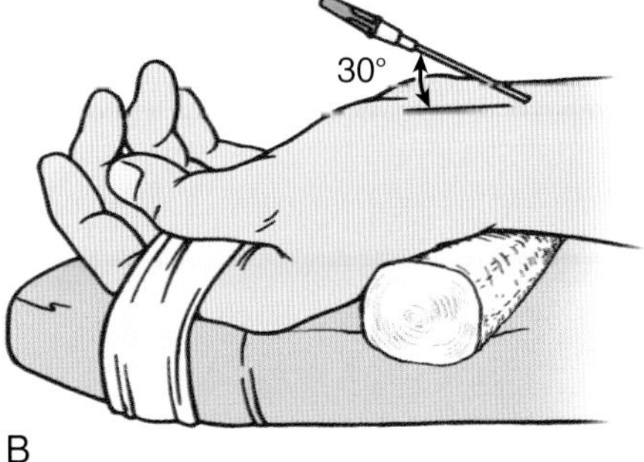

Figure 208-10 **A,** Position for radial artery cannulation. **B,** Catheter is directed along the long axis of the artery.

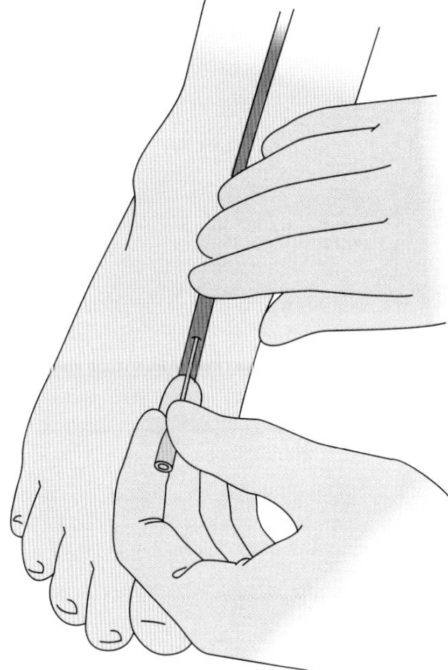

Figure 208-11 Dorsalis pedis artery cannulation. (Modified from American Heart Association: Textbook of Advanced Cardiac Life Support. Dallas, American Heart Association, 1997.)

   - *Dorsalis pedis artery cannulation:* With the patient in the supine position and the foot plantar flexed and stabilized on a firm surface, such as the bed, the dorsalis pedis artery should be palpated and stabilized using sterile technique (Fig. 208-11). Direct the needle tip and catheter slowly along the axis of the artery, aimed toward the arterial pulsation, at a 20- to 30-degree angle to the distal skin.

NOTE: Because collateral circulation in the foot is usually good, dorsalis pedis arterial cannulation should be considered when radial artery cannulation is not a good option. In patients with good cardiac output and palpable dorsalis pedis and posterior tibial pulses, dorsalis pedis arterial cannulation by experienced personnel has been demonstrated to have minimal risk of adverse events such as ischemia and thrombosis. It also allows the patient a little more mobility than with femoral artery cannulation.

   - *Brachial artery cannulation:* With the patient's elbow on a rolled towel or washcloth, slightly hyperextend and supinate the patient's nondominant arm so the patient's wrist lies in the anatomic position but rotated slightly outward. Immobilize the arm with tape and an arm board, preventing flexion at the elbow. The brachial artery lies lateral to the medial epicondyle but medial to the biceps tendon, and courses through the antecubital fossa. Palpate and stabilize the artery using sterile technique. Direct the needle tip and catheter slowly along the axis of the artery, aimed toward the arterial pulsation, at a 20- to 30- degree angle to the distal skin (Fig. 208-12).
8. Puncture is detected when blood appears in the needle hub. For radial, dorsalis pedis, and brachial artery cannulation, while holding the needle fixed, advance the catheter-over-needle into the artery (Fig. 208-13). For femoral artery cannulation, do the same unless the Seldinger technique is desired. With the Seldinger technique, insert the wire through the needle into the artery, remove the needle, insert the catheter over the wire, and

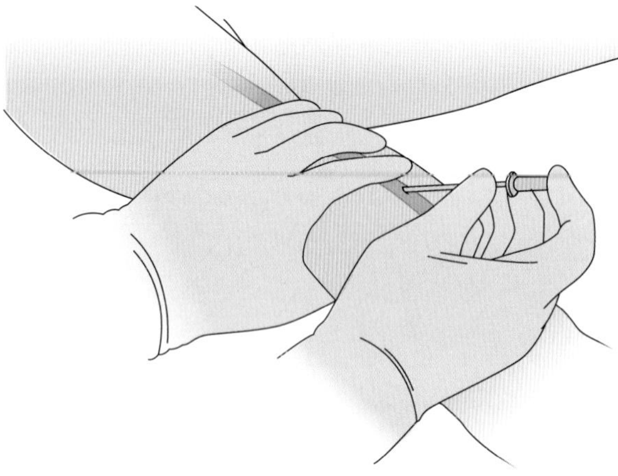

Figure 208-12 Brachial artery cannulation. (Modified from American Heart Association: Textbook of Advanced Cardiac Life Support. Dallas, American Heart Association, 1997.)

remove the wire. A modified Seldinger technique can be used for radial artery cannulation. Although the Seldinger technique is useful, an ordinary cannula is usually quicker and easier.

NOTE: The wire-guided technique may be more successful for arterial cannulation when the pulse is either weak or absent, especially in female patients.

9. If the artery cannot be cannulated after the flash of blood has appeared, the posterior artery wall has probably been penetrated. Remove the needle entirely, slowly withdraw the catheter until blood flows into it, and readvance the catheter.
10. For the Seldinger technique, to minimize the chance of intramural insertion or dissection, make sure the wire passes without *any* resistance.

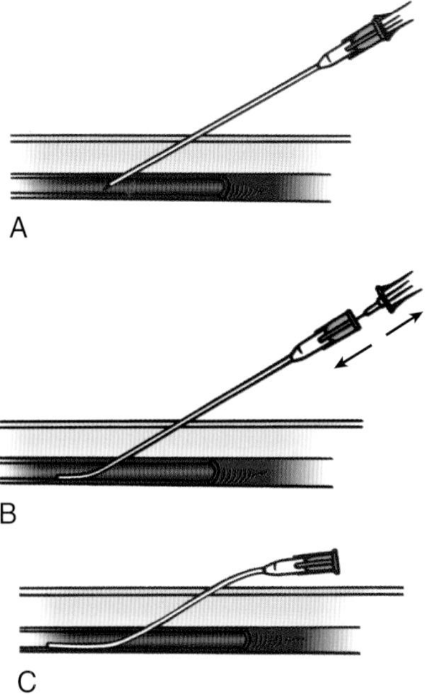

Figure 208-13 **A–C,** Technique for radial, dorsalis pedis, or brachial artery cannulation. Insert the angiocatheter through the skin and cannulate the artery.

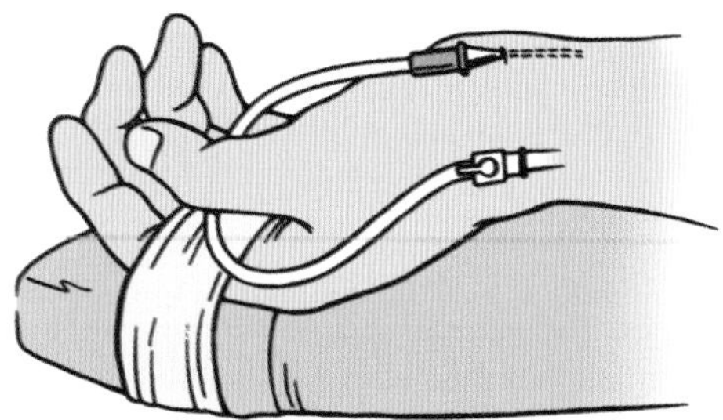

Figure 208-14 Attach connector tubing to the catheter and fix in position.

11. If after three attempts the artery has not been entered, discontinue the procedure on that side and attempt on the other side or at another site. Pressure should be applied to the unsuccessful site for at least 10 minutes, followed by a pressure dressing. A cutdown might also be considered, with the technique described in a later section being similar to that used for venous cutdown (see Chapter 209, Venous Cutdown).
12. After insertion, advance the catheter until the hub is in contact with the skin and attach it to the connector tubing (Fig. 208-14). Flush the catheter and zero the transducer system by opening the three-way stopcock to atmosphere and pushing the "zero" button on the pressure monitor. Return the three-way stopcock to the patient position and observe the arterial tracing. It should be sharp and clean. If it is not, reposition the catheter. If successful, stitch the catheter into position, apply antibiotic ointment, and cover with a sterile dressing. For radial or brachial artery cannulation, remove the 3-inch roll.
13. Staff should check the extremity every 4 hours for perfusion, and the site for signs of a hematoma or early cellulitis. The dressing should be changed daily along with regular flushing of the line as long as it remains cannulated. After catheter removal, observe the patient for bleeding, extremity pain, numbness, swelling, or discoloration.

NOTE: If the Seldinger technique is not used, the "liquid stylet" method may be useful. If a flash of blood is seen in the hub and the artery cannot be cannulated, fill a 10-mL syringe with 5 mL of sterile normal saline. Attach the syringe to the catheter hub and aspirate 1 to 2 mL of blood to verify intraluminal position. The blood should be very easy to aspirate. Slowly inject fluid from the syringe and advance the catheter behind the fluid wave.

Alternative Method for Artery Cannulation: Doppler Ultrasonography Guided

1. Position the extremity in the position previously described and prepare, anesthetize, and drape the area.
2. Using antiseptic ointment (e.g., povidone–iodine) as transmission gel, have an assistant align the hand-held Doppler with the artery, at a site slightly proximal to the puncture site. The assistant should pass it back and forth medial to lateral over the artery and determine the point of maximal flow. He or she should then hold the Doppler in place at the point of maximal volume.
3. Insert and advance the catheter-over-needle slowly and with constant pressure, at a 45-degree angle to the skin and directed toward the point of maximal flow (Fig. 208-15A and B).
4. Contact with the artery is discerned by a slight decrease in arterial flow sound.
5. As the needle compresses the artery before puncture, the flow sound may transiently decrease or cease (Fig. 208-15C and D).
6. The characteristic sound of arterial blood flow should resume as the artery is punctured and a flash of bright red blood is seen in the needle hub.

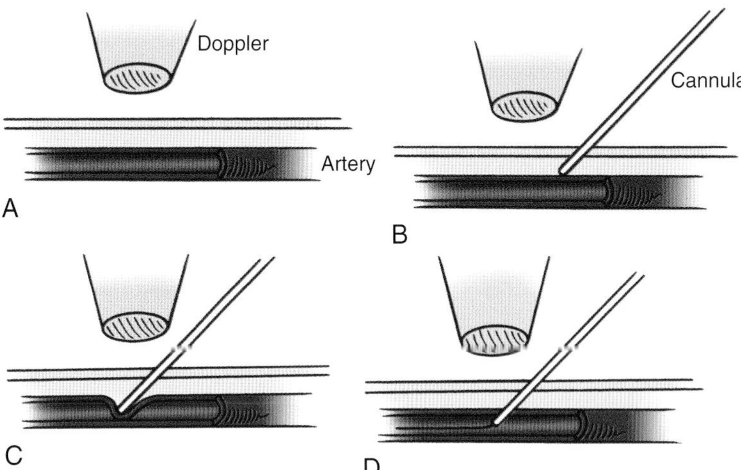

Figure 208-15 Radial artery cannulation guided by Doppler ultrasonography. **A** and **B,** Doppler locates the artery and helps in guiding the cannula. **C** and **D,** The catheter occludes the artery temporarily and then punctures the arterial wall (blood flashes in catheter), after which it is placed intraluminally.

7. Advance the cannula, and secure and calibrate it as described previously.

Alternative Method for Radial or Brachial Artery Cannulation: Cutdown

1. Position the wrist or arm in the previously described position and prepare, anesthetize, and drape the area.
2. Wearing sterile gloves and maintaining sterile technique, make a 1.5- to 2-cm transverse skin incision, perpendicular to the artery yet centered over it. Limit the depth of the incision to the skin; avoid cutting into the subcutaneous tissue to avoid damaging the nerve, artery, vein, lymphatics, tendons, or other nearby or deeper structures.
3. Using a mosquito hemostat, spread the subcutaneous tissue in a direction perpendicular to the incision, but along and above the artery. Expose approximately a 1-cm length of the artery.
4. Pass a nylon suture under the artery (internal suture), and prepare to elevate the artery to assist with cannulation.
5. Insert a catheter-over-needle through the skin, distal to the incision, and tunnel it under the skin and into the visible area of the incision.
6. While the clinician directly observes and controls the artery with two fingers of his or her nondominant hand or the suture, advance the catheter-over-needle into the artery. For the clinician to avoid being sprayed with arterial blood, the suture can be tied (lightly, without cutting the suture) proximal to where the catheter-over-needle will be inserted into the artery. After puncturing the artery with the catheter-over-needle, the knot in the suture can then be loosened (or released), as needed, to advance the catheter-over-needle further into the artery.
7. Advance the cannula, release the internal suture completely, and externally secure the arterial line and calibrate it as described previously. After the arterial line is secured externally and calibration confirmed, suture will also be needed to close the incision.

NOTE: Unlike venous cutdown (a procedure in which the internal suture is often tied, cut, and left within the incision), when an arterial cutdown is performed for arterial line insertion, the internal suture is only used temporarily to provide control while the artery is being cannulated.

Troubleshooting for a Variance between Cuff and Intra-arterial Pressure and Preventive Maintenance for Accurate Readings

A variance or disparity of 5 to 20 mm Hg between measured cuff (indirect) and intra-arterial (direct) pressures is normal and expected. If the intra-arterial pressure is higher than cuff pressure, possible causes include improper cuff size or placement and improper calibration or zeroing of the transducer.

If cuff pressure is recorded as higher than intra-arterial pressure, either improper cuff size, equipment malfunction, or technical error is likely. Damping of the arterial waveform suggests a problem with the intra-arterial measurement. Air bubbles or blood in the line or transducer dome, a clot at the catheter tip, mechanical occlusion of the catheter or tubing, and loose or open connections are all possibilities. If the arterial waveform is not dampened and the cuff size and placement are correct, other possible causes include failure to calibrate the sphygmomanometer or the transducer, or an error in electrically or mechanically zeroing the transducer.

The variance of 5 to 20 mm Hg may be physiologic because the arterial pulse wave is transformed as it travels peripherally. As a result, the systolic pressure may become higher and the diastolic pressure lower. MAP, however, is unchanged.

If the disparity is 20 to 30 mm Hg, severe vasoconstriction (e.g., patient with shock or hypothermia) may be the cause, and inevitably the auscultated cuff pressure is lower. With occlusive atherosclerotic peripheral disease, if the radial or dorsalis pedis artery has been cannulated, cuff pressures are frequently higher than the directly measured pressures because of the more distal location of cannulation.

If the disparity is greater than 30 mm Hg, the most common cause is resonance in the catheter system. This can be minimized by using stiff tubing that is kept as short as possible. Directly measured pressure may be significantly higher than cuff pressure when a single–end-hole catheter is used in a narrow artery with high flow. If the hole faces the flow, the direct blood pressure may be falsely elevated.

To minimize disparities and to maximize accurate readings, the following 10 preventive steps should be followed or considered:

1. Allow the transducer and the amplifier to warm up for at least 10 minutes before zeroing and calibrating the system.
2. Purge all air from the pressure system; always observe for bubbles in the line and attempt to remove them if seen.
3. Use stiff, noncompliant extension tubing of the shortest possible length. Avoid the use of more than one stopcock between the catheter and the transducer. Place the extension tube near the patient to prevent a pulsating line.
4. Electrically zero and calibrate the system with an accurate manometer or a water column.
5. Mechanically zero the transducer.
6. At least once a shift, staff should check all fittings for tightness, check the zero setting (both electrically and mechanically), and check the calibration.
7. Avoid draining blood samples from the full length of the plumbing system.

8. Maintain a continuous low-flow flushing system to avoid clotting.
9. When the level of the patient is changed, recheck the mechanical and electrical zero positions and recalibrate the system if necessary.
10. Avoid making adjustments to the amplifier except at the time of calibration.

Complications

- *Significant blood loss* can occur if the tubing becomes disconnected.
- *Arterial thrombosis* (risk minimized by reducing the duration of cannulation, by choosing larger arteries, and by flushing properly). The risk of thrombosis increases if the cannula is left in place for longer than 72 hours.
- *Embolism*, usually distal. Retrograde arterial embolism can also occur from retrograde flushing of the cannula, and may enter the cerebral circulation. This danger is greater with smaller patients. For all patients (and especially for smaller patients), make sure to either maintain a slow continuous flushing system or to use volumes of heparinized solution smaller than 3 mL to avoid dislodging thrombi.
- *Arterial occlusion.* With the Seldinger technique, it is possible to cause a small dissection and arterial occlusion by passing the guidewire between the intima and the media. With any technique, the result can be stenosis or permanent occlusion.
- *Ischemia or necrosis* distal to the site of arterial thrombosis, embolism, stenosis, or occlusion.
- *Hemorrhage or local hematoma.*
- *Aneurysm or pseudoaneurysm.* The patient will present with a pulsatile mass. Management is surgical removal.
- *Local infection or sepsis*, particularly after about 4 days.
- *Arteriovenous fistula.* This is more common with femoral artery cannulation because of the proximity of the large vein.
- *Neurologic complications*, same as with arterial puncture.
- *Vasovagal reactions.*

NOTE: A vascular surgeon should be consulted immediately if arterial flow is compromised in any way.

Postprocedure Patient Education

Explain to the alert patient and family the greater danger of a disconnected arterial line compared with a normal IV line. Instruct the patient not to rub or manipulate the site, line, or connectors. The patient should report any local pain, swelling, discoloration, or numbness at the site, or any bubbles in the line. He or she should also report any blood or dampness near the site. After catheter removal, the patient should report any bleeding, extremity pain, numbness, swelling, or discoloration.

Patient Education Guides

See patient education and consent forms online at www.expertconsult.com.

CPT/Billing Codes

Arterial Puncture

36600 Arterial puncture; withdrawal of blood for diagnosis

Percutaneous Arterial Line Placement

36620 Arterial catheterization or cannulation for sampling, monitoring, or transfusion (separate procedure); percutaneous
36625 Arterial cutdown

ICD-9-CM Diagnostic Codes

Arterial Puncture

250.1 Diabetic ketoacidosis, without mention of coma
276.2 Acidosis, lactic, metabolic or respiratory
276.3 Alkalosis, metabolic or respiratory
276.4 Acid-base mixed disorder
415.1 Pulmonary embolism and infarction
427.5 Cardiac or cardiorespiratory arrest
428.1 Left heart failure, with pulmonary edema or cardiac dyspnea (cardiac asthma)
491.20 Chronic obstructive bronchitis, with emphysema, without exacerbation
491.21 Chronic obstructive bronchitis (COPD), with acute exacerbation
492.8 Emphysema, NOS
493.00 Asthma, extrinsic, unspecified
493.01 Asthma, extrinsic with status asthmaticus
493.02 Asthma, extrinsic, with acute exacerbation
518.5 Pulmonary insufficiency following shock, trauma, or surgery
518.81 Respiratory failure, acute, NOS
518.82 Respiratory distress or other pulmonary insufficiency, acute, not elsewhere classified
518.83 Respiratory failure, chronic
518.84 Respiratory failure, acute and chronic
780.01 Coma
785.50 Shock, unspecified, without mention of trauma
785.51 Shock, cardiogenic
785.52 Shock, septic
785.59 Shock, other (hypovolemic, septic)
786.05 Shortness of breath
786.09 Respiratory distress or insufficiency, NOS
799.01 Asphyxia
799.02 Hypoxia
799.1 Respiratory arrest
986 Carbon monoxide, toxic effect

Percutaneous Arterial Line Placement

In addition to ICD-9-CM diagnostic codes used for arterial puncture, the following are commonly used for arterial lines:

V42 Organ or tissue replaced by transplant
V43 Organ or tissue replaced by other means
V45 Postprocedure states
V45.81 Postprocedure status, aortocoronary bypass
V46.1 Dependence on machines, respirator (ventilator)
401.0 Hypertension, accelerated, malignant
410.9 Myocardial infarction, acute, NOS or unspecified site
411.1 Angina, unstable
434.9 Cerebral artery occlusion, unspecified

Suppliers

(See contact information online at www.expertconsult.com.)

Arrow International (Teleflex Medical)
Becton, Dickinson and Co.
Cook Medical
Edwards Life Sciences Corp. (formerly a division of Baxter), closed needleless sampling systems

BIBLIOGRAPHY

Arterial Puncture

Allen EV: Thromboangiitis obliterans: Methods of diagnosis of chronic occlusive arterial lesions distal to the wrist with illustrative cases. Am J Med Sci 178:237–244, 1929.

Kamienski RW, Barnes RW: Critique of the Allen test for continuity of the palmar arch assessed by Doppler ultrasound. Surg Gynecol Obstet 142:861–864, 1976.

Lau J, Chew PW, Wang, C, White AC: Long term oxygen therapy for severe COPD. Rockville, Md, Agency for Health Care Research and Quality (AHRQ) Technology Assessment Program, U.S. Department of Health and Human Services, Public Health Services, June 11, 2004.

Slogoff S, Keats A, Arlund C: On the safety of radial artery cannulation. Anesthesiology 59:42–47, 1983.

Stroud S, Rodriguez R: Arterial puncture and cannulation. In Reichman EF, Simon RR (eds): Emergency Medicine Procedures. New York, McGraw-Hill, 2004, pp 398–412.

Percutaneous Arterial Line Placement

Gerber DR, Zeifman CW, Khouli HI, et al: Comparison of wire-guided and non-wire-guided radial artery catheters. Chest 109:761–764, 1996.

Maher JJ, Dougherty JM: Radial artery cannulation guided by Doppler ultrasound. Am J Emerg Med 7:260–262, 1989.

Mangar D, Thrush DN, Connell GR, Downs JB: Direct or modified Seldinger guide wire-directed technique for arterial catheter insertion. Anesth Analg 76:714–717, 1993.

Milzma D, Jaudan T: Arterial puncture and cannulation. In Roberts JR, Hedges JR (eds): Clinical Procedures in Emergency Medicine, 4th ed. Philadelphia, Saunders, 2004, pp 384–400.

Stroud S, Rodriguez R: Arterial puncture and cannulation. In Reichman EF, Simon RR (eds): Emergency Medicine Procedures. New York, McGraw-Hill, 2004, pp 398–412.

CHAPTER 209

VENOUS CUTDOWN

Wm. MacMillan Rodney • J.R. MacMillan Rodney

Obtaining vascular access is a life-saving procedure for critically ill patients in a variety of situations, but hypovolemic shock and cardiac arrest are the most common vascular access emergencies. Venous cutdowns were first described in World War II. With the advent of intensive care units in the 1960s, surgical cutdowns were frequently replaced by percutaneous approaches to the subclavian and internal jugular veins. In the 1970s, placement of these "central lines" became core curriculum in the newly established course known as Advanced Cardiac Life Support (ACLS). This course was usually taught by demonstration and did not require the traditional surgical skills of dissection and suture.

By 1980, the American College of Surgeons implemented the Advanced Trauma Life Support (ATLS) course, which required live tissue for the demonstration of vascular access techniques. These were "venous cutdowns," but percutaneous techniques have replaced most of the cutdowns. Plastic simulators do not realistically reproduce the in vivo experience. More recently, ultrasonography has dramatically improved the ability to visualize central and peripheral veins, often directing cannulation.

In situations where ongoing chest compressions, burns, or trauma make central line placement difficult, the intraosseous route (see Chapter 198, Intraosseous Vascular Access) is quickest and most reliable for clinicians with limited surgical experience. However, intraosseous needles and central line kits are not as universally available as scalpels, hemostats, and suture. In developing countries and most locations more than 1 mile from an academic medical center, venous cutdown is the most readily available method for rapid vascular access. Ironically, clinicians in these locations are often less likely to have any experience or training with venous cutdown.

This chapter describes cutdowns of the distal great saphenous vein near the ankle and the proximal great saphenous vein beneath the inguinal crease. Brachial or basilic vein cutdowns in the antecubital fossa are rarely a first choice because of the time required for dissection, but are also discussed. In cases where the patient is undergoing chest compressions, space around the patient can be limited, and choosing a more distal location is usually better.

INDICATIONS

- Multiple failed attempts at percutaneous insertion in a critically ill or injured patient
- Hypotensive shock
- Patient requiring immediate administration of intravenous (IV) fluids or drugs
- Cardiac or respiratory arrest
- Burns, trauma, or ongoing resuscitation preventing timely insertion of percutaneous central lines
- Intraosseous access contraindicated (see Chapter 198, Intraosseous Vascular Access) or equipment not available
- Surgical consultation not available (e.g., because of time or distance limitation)
- Lack of percutaneously accessible vein (e.g., obesity, unusually small or fragile veins [as in some adults and most infants], or venous sclerosis from aging, IV drug abuse, or previous multiple venipunctures)

CONTRAINDICATIONS

- When less invasive and adequate alternatives (e.g., intraosseous, percutaneous central or peripheral lines) are immediately available
- Long bone fracture present proximally in extremity
- Evidence of severe peripheral vascular disease such as thrombophlebitis, vascular insufficiency, history of vein stripping, history of vein sclerosis (clinician should consider different site)
- Lack of equipment
- Local infection, burns, or trauma in the area of the cutdown *(relative)*
- Prolonged use for administration of hypertonic fluids *(relative)*
- Inadequate local arterial supply (*relative*, arterial supply is important for postprocedural healing, so consider a different site)
- Bleeding disorder *(relative)*

EQUIPMENT

- Tourniquet and tape
- Sterile gloves, goggles, equipment to follow universal blood and body fluid precautions
- Sterile gauze sponges, gauze pads, and drapes
- Antiseptic skin preparation (if time permits), such as povidone–iodine or chlorhexidine soap or solution (alcohol is not preferred)
- A 3- to 5-mL syringe of local anesthetic (any kind of lidocaine; epinephrine is not necessary but is not harmful)
- Basic surgical equipment (e.g., scalpel [no. 10 or no. 15 blade for skin, no. 11 blade for minivenotomy), hemostats [large and mosquito, curved and straight], thumb forceps [pickups] with and without teeth, suture scissors, tissue dissection scissors [Metzenbaum], and a needle holder)
- Although silk ligatures (4-0) for the vein and nonabsorbable skin suture (4-0) have been recommended for the skin, this is an emergency and any suture will work. Generally, braided or monofilament absorbable sutures varying from 0 to 4-0 work fine. Concerns about infection risk with braided suture are more theoretical than real. Silk is the most reactive of all sutures in the skin and is not the first choice.
- IV fluids and setup. Cannulation is possible using a wide variety of tubes and catheters. Using the IV tubing itself (hub cut off) to cannulate permits the most rapid infusion but usually requires the proximal saphenous, and a backup IV catheter should be available. Ten- to 14-gauge plain peripheral IV catheters are almost as good for infusion of large amounts of fluid, but anything will work if cardioactive drugs are needed.
- High-frequency ultrasonography (5 to 10 MHz) and ultrasound gel to visualize or define the venous anatomy at the groin or antecubital fossa (*optional;* if time and the urgency of the situation allow)

Patient Preparation and General Considerations: Anatomy

1. The clinician should be familiar with the basic anatomy of the area (Fig. 209-1).
2. If the patient is alert, explain the need for IV access and the procedure. If time and the urgency of the situation allow, obtain informed consent.
3. For distal saphenous or basilic vein cutdowns, have an assistant apply a tourniquet proximal to the incision site and control it. This will enable the clinician to more easily visualize and palpate the vein. A tourniquet applied high on the thigh may help with locating the proximal saphenous vein. To minimize bleeding, tourniquets should be released at the time of venipuncture. Observe universal blood and body fluid precautions.
4. Cleanse the skin in the area around the vein and incision site thoroughly with antiseptic soap or solution.
5. To provide ample working space, if time and the urgency of the situation allow, extend a wide sterile field 8 to 10 cm proximally and distally and apply sterile drapes.
6. Regardless of which cutdown site is chosen, incisions can be made horizontally (i.e., laterally), which is also transversely. When subcutaneous fat protrudes from the incision, use blunt dissection and spread the tissue longitudinally along the axis of the vein. All of these veins are in superficial fat layers, so with a proximal saphenous or basilic vein cutdown, if the incision exposes muscle fascia, it is too deep.
7. The vein should appear pulseless and thin-walled, and it should blanch with the application of distal traction. If a vein is not readily identified, have an assistant tighten the tourniquet, which may make it more apparent or palpable.
8. With all cutdowns, the vein should be dissected free and isolated for 2 to 4 cm along its axis.

Cutdown

Distal Saphenous Vein (Ankle)

Advantages

- No interference or disruption of other resuscitative procedures (e.g., obtaining blood gases in same area, cardiopulmonary resuscitation [CPR], or endotracheal intubation)
- IV access on inferior side of diaphragm
- Minimal training needed and low risk of complications compared with central access
- No valves at this level of the vein because of the minimal volume and pressure
- Most consistent vein of the lower extremity, especially in its location anterior to the medial malleolus

Disadvantages

- Phlebitis and infection are common complications of the lower extremity cutdown
- Less than ideal route for cardiac drug administration (especially during CPR)
- Not good for hypertonic solutions (risk of sclerosis)
- May be absent if the patient has had vein stripping or harvest (e.g., used for a coronary artery bypass graft) or nonfunctional due to prior cutdown
- Older patients may have vein narrowing
- May not be useful in the patient with unstable pelvic fracture or major knee trauma because of iliofemoral venous interruption

Technique

1. With the tourniquet in place, palpate the distal saphenous vein just anterior to the medial malleolus (see Fig. 209-1B).

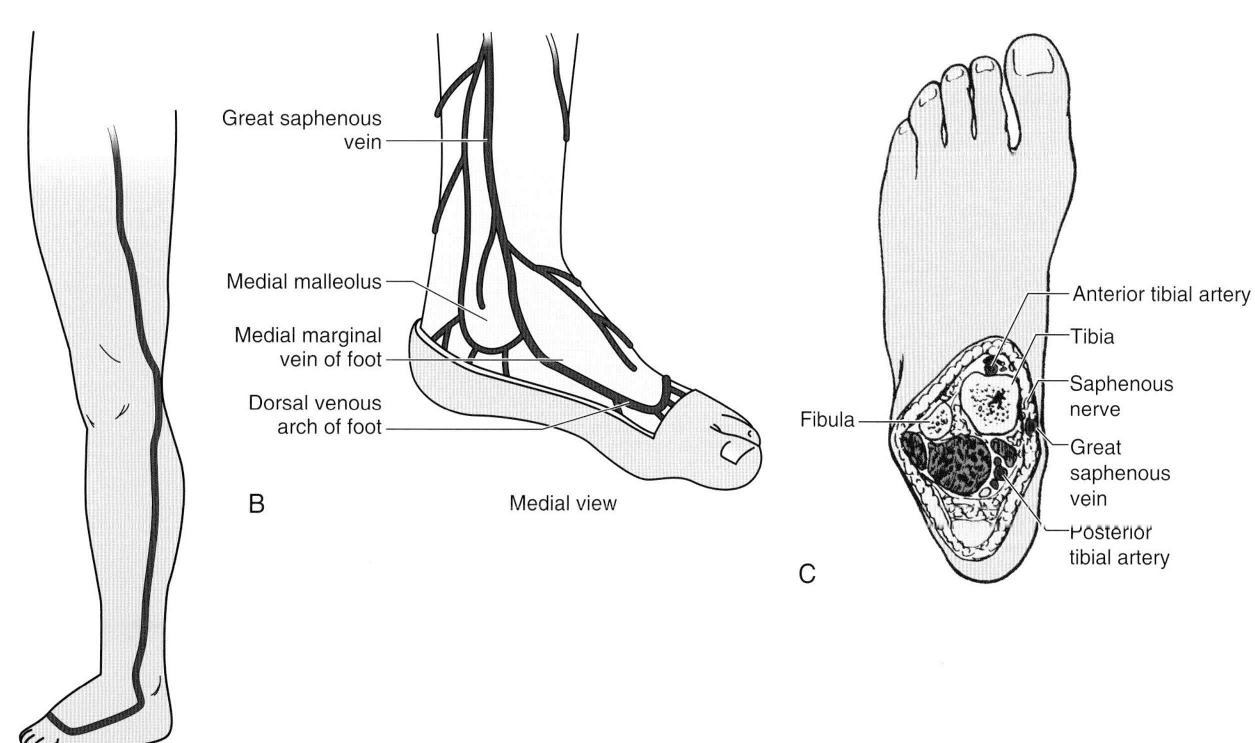

Figure 209-1 **A,** Anatomy of great saphenous vein of the lower extremity. **B,** Superficial veins of the leg and foot (great saphenous vein at the ankle). **C,** Cross-sectional view; the great saphenous vein may be isolated easily and safely at the ankle. Only the minor saphenous nerve lies nearby.

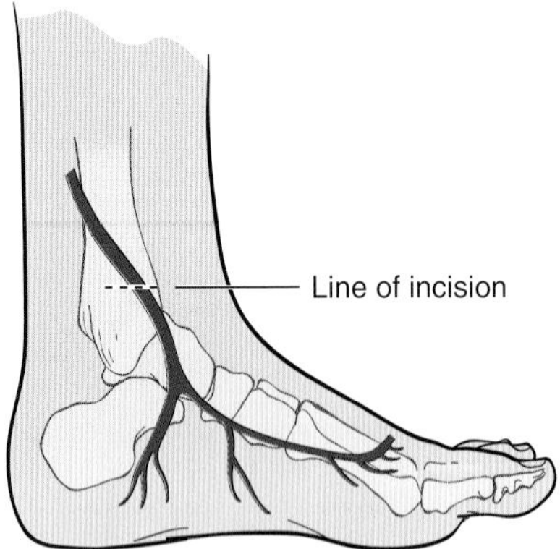

Figure 209-2 Anatomic relationship of the saphenous vein and the line of incision.

2. Incise skin above the medial malleolus starting at the proximal anterior border of the tibia and extending to the posterior border of the tibia (Fig. 209-2).
3. Using a closed, curved hemostat, with the point downward and adjacent to the tibia, advance the instrument in the line of the incision to lift the superficial tissue (Fig. 209-3).
4. Rotate the point upward, still holding the tissue. Spread to reveal the distal saphenous vein and nerve.
5. Proceed to cannulation as described in that section.
6. Apply dressing (Fig. 209-4).

Proximal Saphenous Vein (Groin)

Advantages

- IV access on inferior side of the diaphragm
- Minimal training and risk compared with central access
- Larger vein caliber facilitates cannulation and bolus infusion in profoundly hypovolemic patients

Disadvantages

- Phlebitis and infection are common complications in the groin
- Less than ideal route for cardiac drug administration (especially during CPR)
- Not good for hypertonic solutions (risk of sclerosis)
- Proximity of femoral neurovascular bundle and other structures may introduce greater risk for complications

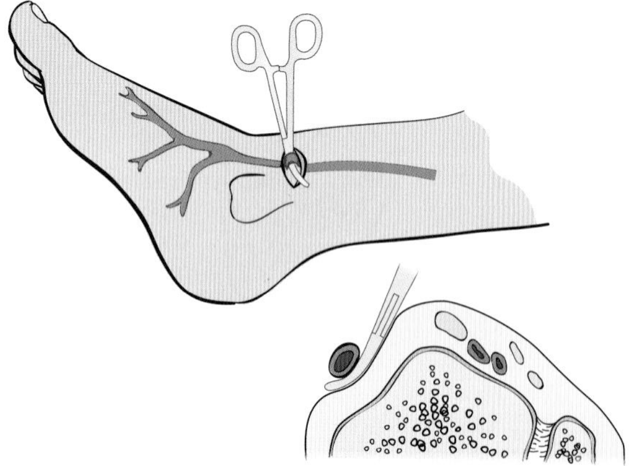

Figure 209-3 Curved mosquito clamp is inserted into the edge of the incision and the tip turned downward and placed adjacent to the tibia. It is then advanced under the saphenous vein and swept across the tibia. Then the clamp is turned over so that the tips are pointed upward. The tips are spread to reveal the saphenous vein and nerve.

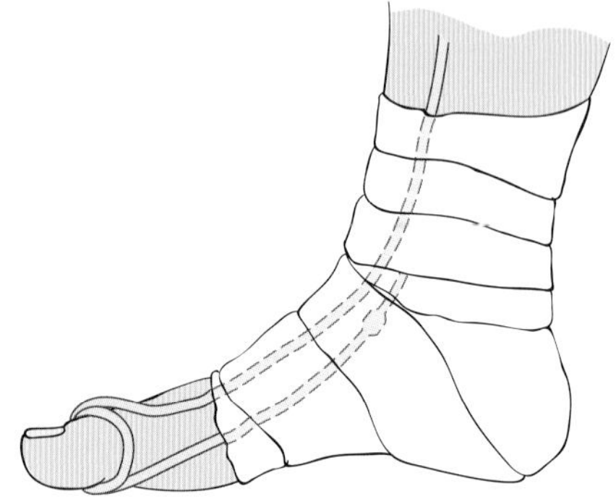

Figure 209-4 Dressing to prevent decannulation.

- May not be useful in patient with unstable pelvic fracture or major knee trauma because of iliofemoral venous interruption

Technique

1. If time and the urgency of the situation allow, identifying and visualizing the anatomy with a high-frequency (5 to 10 MHz) ultrasonography transducer is very helpful (Fig. 209-5). (Also see Chapter 225, Emergency Department, Hospitalist, and Office Ultrasonography [Clinical Ultrasonography].) The high-frequency probe (even the transvaginal probe is a high-frequency probe) can be applied directly to ultrasound jelly on the skin to obtain images.
2. Incise laterally starting at the junction of the scrotal/labial fold and the medial thigh (Fig. 209-6). Extend the incision to the outer portion of the mons pubis. Visible muscle fascia means the incision is too deep.
3. The proximal saphenous vein lies in the superficial fat layer where a vertical, imaginary line starting from the pubic tubercle crosses the incision (see Fig. 209-6). Cannulate as noted in that section.

Basilic Vein (Antecubital Fossa)

Advantages

- IV access on superior side of the diaphragm
- Minimal training and risk compared with central access
- Larger vein caliber facilitates cannulation and bolus infusion in profoundly hypovolemic patients

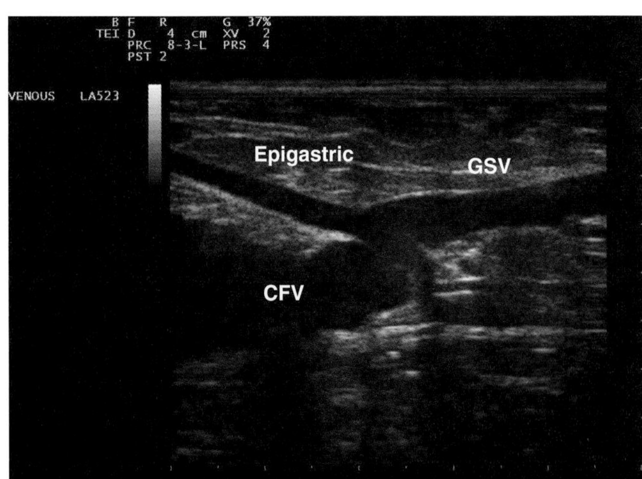

Figure 209-5 High-frequency (5 to 10 MHz) ultrasonogram of the groin, defining bifurcation of great saphenous vein (GSV) from common femoral vein (CFV).

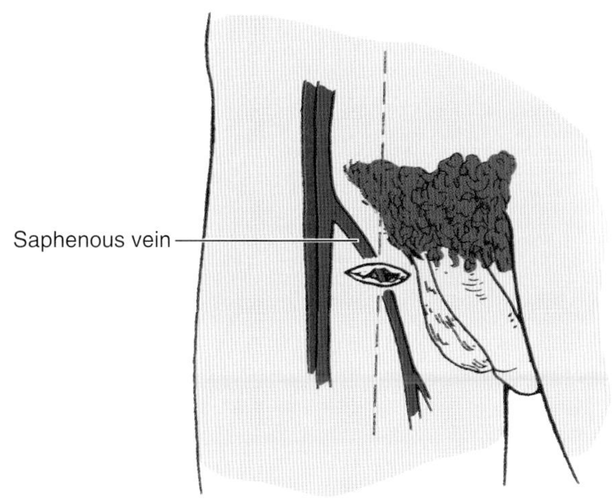

Figure 209-6 Cutdown location for great saphenous vein at the groin.

Disadvantages

- With ongoing CPR, percutaneous cannulation can be difficult at this site.
- Compared to the groin, the smaller diameter of the basilic vein theoretically limits rapid infusions of large volume. However, the cannulas are the same size in all sites; therefore, the basilica vein diameter is unlikely to be a negative factor.
- Deep dissection in the antecubital fossa can damage other structures.

Technique

1. Take the distance between the olecranon and the acromion and divide it into thirds. With the tourniquet applied proximally, palpate the vein on the medial aspect of the arm where it lies in the groove between the triceps and biceps muscles. On the medial arm, the vein follows a course slightly anterior and superficial to the brachial artery.
2. Make a horizontal, superficial incision from the biceps across the groove to the triceps (Fig. 209-7).
3. Locate the basilic vein by dissecting the superficial fat layer. Visible muscle fascia or the brachial artery means the incision is too deep.
4. If time and the urgency of the situation allow it, identifying and visualizing the anatomy with a high-frequency (10 MHz) ultrasonography transducer is very helpful (see Fig. 209-5; also see Chapter 225, Emergency Department, Hospitalist, and Office Ultrasonography [Clinical Ultrasonography]). The basilic vein will best be visualized with the tourniquet in place.
5. Proceed to cannulation.

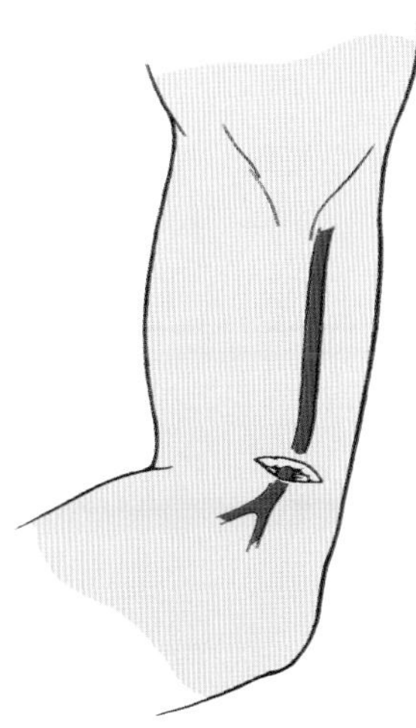

Figure 209-7 Incision is made between the biceps and triceps for basilic vein cutdown (right arm).

Cannulation

1. Isolate 3 to 4 cm of the chosen vein, dissecting aside loose adipose or adventitial tissue. The scissors can be spread longitudinally along the length of the vein to improve access and help visualize it.
2. Pass suture ties under the vein, both proximally and distally. Pass the distal suture as far distal as possible; use this as a retractor to bring the vein into the incision.
3. If the distal vein is to be sacrificed, the distal ligature should be tied and left long to help control and manipulate the vein. Clamp the ends of the ligature with a hemostat and use its weight to maintain tension on the ligature.
4. Place traction on the proximal suture to minimize rebleeding; it should not be tied at this point.
5. Loosen the tourniquet if one has been applied.
6. Select a site near the distal ligature for venotomy. If the vein is large enough, it can be catheterized directly. Otherwise, incise one third of the vein's diameter at a 45-degree angle to the skin in distal-to-proximal fashion (Fig. 209-8A). The result should be a V-shaped incision (Fig. 209-8B). While maintaining proximal ligature traction, expand the lumen with a mosquito hemostat (Fig. 209-8C).

   EDITOR'S NOTE: Avoid cutting the entire vein with the scissors or scalpel because it may result in retraction of the vein from the incision, thereby increasing the difficulty of the procedure.
7. Once the skin has been entered through a *separate* stab wound, introduce the cannula through the vein incision, maintaining the same 45-degree angle (Fig. 209-9). This is the most difficult portion of the procedure. Use caution in great saphenous vein cannulations, making sure not to occlude the femoral vein with the cannula (avoid advancing the cannula too far).
8. Aspirate air from the cannula; tie the proximal ligature around the cannula and vein wall.
9. Cut both ligatures and close the wound (Fig. 209-10).
10. Remove the tourniquet and observe for incision leakage of blood or fluid.
11. Secure the catheter hub to the skin with an additional stitch. Apply sterile dressing.

Minicutdown with Angiocatheter or Seldinger Wire

The minicutdown is the fastest technique when an angiocatheter needle (standard catheter-over-needle) of adequate size (16 to 18 gauge) or a Seldinger wire introducer or modified Seldinger wire kit is available. The vein is located and isolated surgically as previously described, but the incision can be much smaller ("mini," or just large enough to locate the vein). Then, the angiocatheter unit is placed through the skin approximately 1 cm distal to the incision. The angiocatheter is threaded into the vein in the same manner as with percutaneous catheterization. An optional suture through the skin proximal to the incision, around the catheter and vein, and then tied loosely can stabilize the catheter in the vein. However, inserting the angiocatheter through skin distally usually stabilizes it. Closure of the wound provides further stabilization. The hub should also be stabilized with an additional skin suture. In 1 to 2 days, after the patient is stable and has routine peripheral IV access, the hub (and optional catheter) sutures can be removed and the Teflon catheter withdrawn without reopening the incision.

To ease cannulation of the vein, a straight hemostat can be inserted beneath the vein and spread open. The scalpel can then be

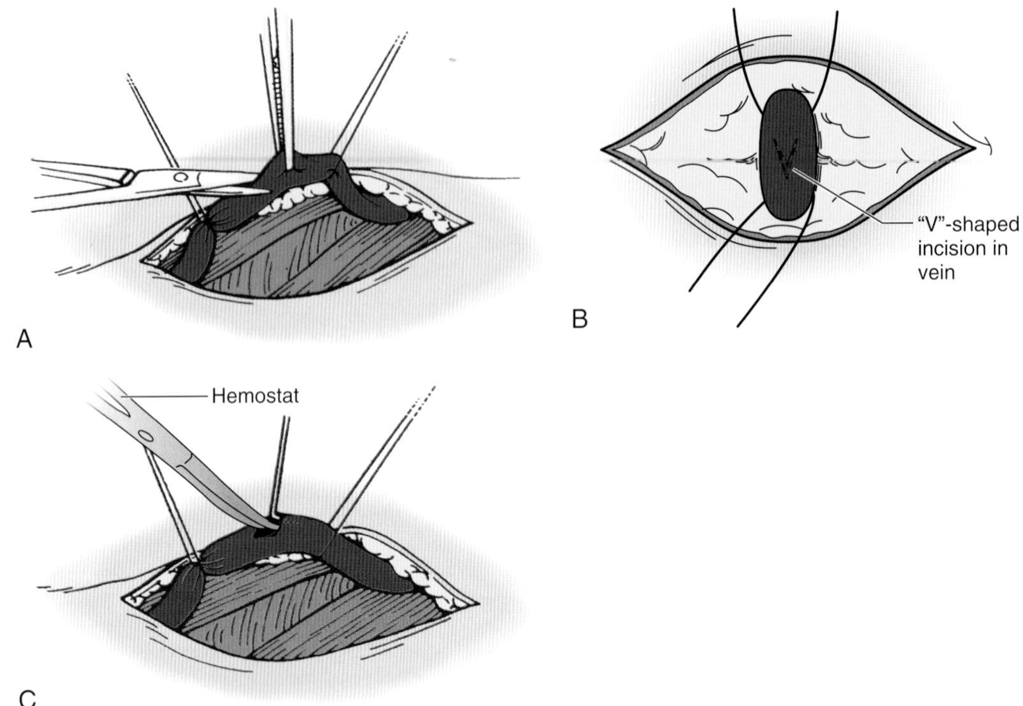

Figure 209-8 **A,** Angled wedge cut is made in the anterior wall of the vein. Traction should be maintained on the vein with proximal and distal ligatures. If sacrificed, the distal vein ligature can be tied. **B,** A V-shaped incision is made in vein. **C,** The vein is dilated with a hemostat.

used to make a 1- to 2-mm venotomy (Fig. 209-11) and the angiocatheter inserted through the venotomy.

The Seldinger technique for venous cutdown can also use a small, 1- to 2-mm, venotomy (see Fig. 209-11) and a Seldinger wire-guided catheter (found in prepackaged central line set). The Seldinger unit comes assembled with dilator and catheter. The catheter-over-needle is advanced though the skin 1 cm distal to the incision and then through the venotomy. The needle is removed and the wire advanced into the vein. The catheter is then removed while the guidewire stays in place. Next, place the dilator through the introducer sheath and thread the combined dilator–introducer sheath down the guidewire. Holding the free end of the guidewire to prevent it from advancing, and using a twisting motion, advance the dilator and introducer sheath further down the guidewire and into the venotomy. This effort also dilates the vein. Most of the time, this technique eliminates the need for tying off the distal vein. When the hub of the introducer sheath reaches the skin level, remove the guidewire and dilator as a unit, leaving the introducer sheath in place. Securing the introducer in the vein with a suture around them both is usually not necessary.

The modified Seldinger wire-guided technique for venous cutdown is even easier to learn and has been shown to be 22% faster than the classic technique. Assemble the unit (Fig. 209-12) by placing the dilator through the sheath and then inserting the guidewire through the dilator. The guidewire should protrude 3 to 4 mm beyond the tip of the dilator. This guidewire is then inserted through a 1- to 2-mm venotomy and advanced. With a twisting motion, the entire unit is then inserted over the guidewire, up to the hub.

The skin incision can then be closed with sutures and the catheter hub sutured in place. Even when pressure infusion techniques are used, additional sutures may not be necessary.

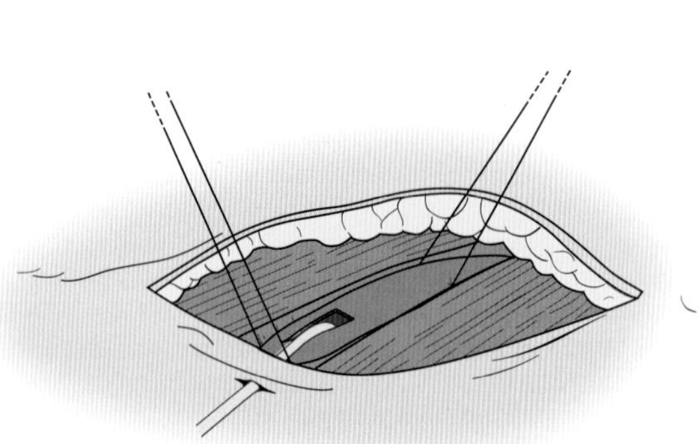

Figure 209-9 Catheter is threaded through a separate skin stab wound and then into vein.

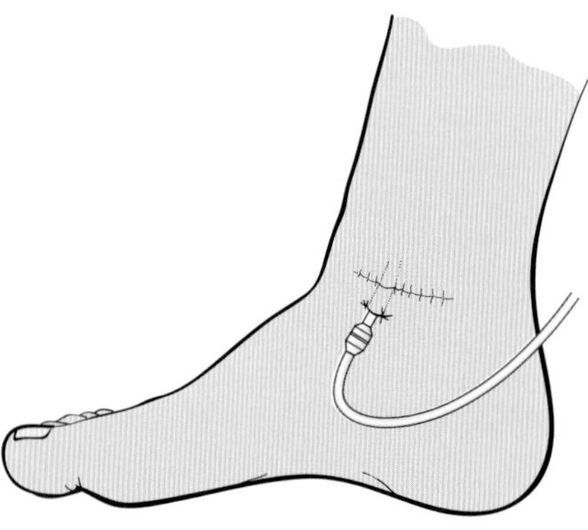

Figure 209-10 Incision is closed to minimize risk of infection and catheter is then sutured in place.

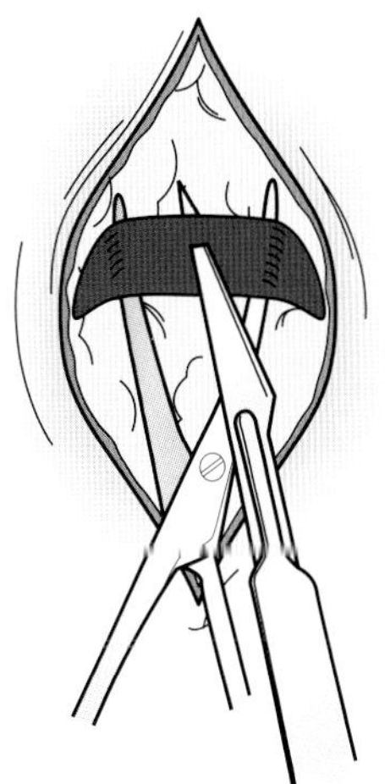

Figure 209-11 A spread straight hemostat and no. 11 blade used to make 2-mm minivenotomy incision. (From Klofas E: A quicker saphenous vein cutdown and a better way to teach it. J Trauma 43:985–987, 1997.)

Complications

Possible complications include hematoma, embolism, bacteremia, and sepsis. These are rare. There is always the possibility of injury to nearby structures, especially using the basilic vein technique, which is the most difficult approach. The second most difficult approach uses the proximal saphenous vein. The distal saphenous vein is least likely to result in damage to other structures. In the unstable emergency patient, there is the possibility of taking too much time during an attempt to perform venous cutdown, leading to a worsening of the clinical situation.

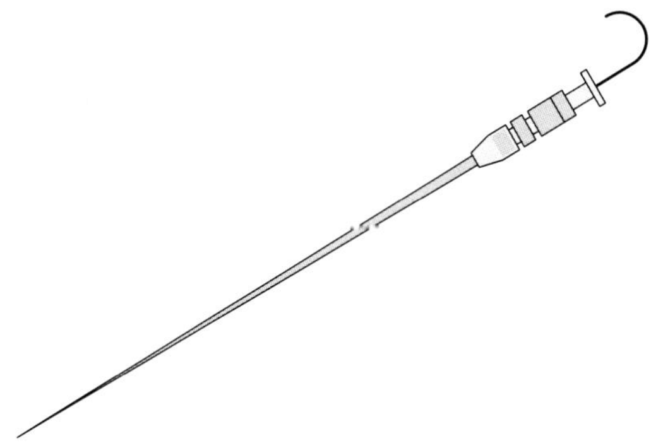

Figure 209-12 The wire-guided catheter, already mounted on the wire and dilator. (From Klofas E: A quicker saphenous vein cutdown and a better way to teach it. J Trauma 43:985–987, 1997.)

CPT/Billing Codes

36410 Venipuncture, child over 3 years or adult, necessitating physician's skill for diagnostic or therapeutic purposes (not to be used for routine venipuncture)
36425 Venipuncture, cutdown; aged 1 year or older
76937 Ultrasound guidance for vascular access

ICD-9-CM Diagnostic Codes

276.51 Volume depletion, dehydration
276.52 Volume depletion, hypovolemia
427.5 Cardiopulmonary arrest
459.0 Hemorrhage, nonspecific
459.89 Venofibrosis
772.9 Hemorrhage, unspecified in newborn (NOS)
785.50 Shock (without trauma), unspecified
785.52 Shock, septic or endotoxic
785.59 Hypovolemic shock (NEC)
799.1 Respiratory arrest
958.4 Hemorrhagic shock or shock syndrome due to trauma
995.0 Shock, anaphylactic

Acknowledgment

The editors wish to recognize the many contributions by Pauline Aham-Neze, MD, and Grant C. Fowler, MD, to this chapter in the previous two editions of this text

ONLINE RESOURCE

Blanchemaison P, Camponovo J, Greney P: Classical anatomy of the saphenous vein: Ultrasonographic anatomy. Phlebologia: Atlas of Anatomy of the Superficial Veins of the Lower Limbs. Available at www.phlebologia.com/en/anatomie_classique_04.asp.

Davies BW: Venous cutdown and intraosseous infusion. Update in Anaesthesia Issue 5, Article 3, 1995. Available at www.nda.ox.ac.uk/wfsa/html/u05/u05_004.htm.

BIBLIOGRAPHY

American College of Surgeons: Shock. In: Advanced Trauma Life Support Student Course Manual, 6th ed. Chicago, American College of Surgeons, 1997, pp 87–125.

Keenan SP: Use of ultrasound to place central lines. J Crit Care 17:126–137, 2002.

Klofas E: A quicker saphenous vein cutdown and a better way to teach it. J Trauma 39:985–987, 1997.

Nobay F: Peripheral venous cutdown. In Reichman EF, Simon RR (eds): Emergency Medicine Procedures. New York, McGraw-Hill, 2004, pp 367–382.

Shockley LW, Butzier DJ: A modified wire-guided technique for venous cutdown access. Ann Emerg Med 19:393–395, 1990.

CHAPTER 210

Electrical Cardioversion

Jeremy Fish

Transthoracic direct-current electrical shock, or electrical cardioversion, is a safe and effective procedure for terminating most sustained tachyarrhythmias. It is useful for converting acute arrhythmias that are causing clinical deterioration of the patient's condition, and for chronic arrhythmias that are symptomatic, carry a poor prognosis, or are unresponsive to drug therapy. Cardiac arrhythmias often can be converted to sinus rhythm with medications (chemical cardioversion), but electrical cardioversion refers to the direct application of electrical current.

Cardioversion versus Defibrillation

Cardioversion differs from defibrillation in that, with electrical cardioversion, the electrical discharge is synchronized with the R wave of ventricular depolarization to minimize the risk of triggering ventricular fibrillation. External paddles or patches are used to apply the electrical current, which causes total depolarization of the atria and ventricles. This depolarization frequently causes the instantaneous conversion of an arrhythmia to sinus rhythm.

Electrical defibrillation is a procedure in which nonsynchronized electrical current is applied to convert chaotic fibrillation, or pulseless ventricular tachycardia (VT), to a normal sinus rhythm. Defibrillation is warranted in an unconscious, pulseless, and apneic patient once ventricular fibrillation (VF) or pulseless VT is identified. Patients in VF or pulseless VT should receive immediate defibrillation at 360 joules (J) if using a monophasic device or 200 J if using a biphasic device. Defibrillation should be repeated at 360 J (monophasic energy) or 200 J (biphasic energy) if the rhythm does not convert. Defibrillation is an emergency procedure. One of the most generally accepted protocols for defibrillation is available through Advanced Cardiac Life Support (ACLS) courses given by many local hospitals and registered through the American Heart Association.

Indications

- Atrial fibrillation (AF)
- Atrial flutter
- Hemodynamically stable VT unresponsive to pharmacologic therapy
- Hemodynamically unstable VT with a pulse
- Hemodynamically unstable supraventricular tachycardic (SVT) arrhythmias
- Certain SVT arrhythmias unresponsive to pharmacologic therapy, including bypass tract SVT (e.g., Wolff-Parkinson-White syndrome)

Contraindications

Absolute

- Absent pulse (patient needs Basic Life Support measures or defibrillation)
- Severely unstable patient (patient needs resuscitation)
- Severe electrolyte disturbances
- Digitalis toxicity
- Left atrial or atrial appendage thrombus (for elective cardioversion)
- Left ventricular mural thrombus

Relative

- Large left atrial diameter (>4.5 cm) in patients with AF
- Sick sinus syndrome
- Ectopic or multifocal atrial tachycardia
- Junctional or sinus tachycardia
- Minimal hemodynamic or clinical improvement while in sinus rhythm
- AF duration greater than 6 months
- Inadequate anticoagulation and more than 48 hours' duration of AF (unless transesophageal echocardiography [TEE] negative)

A left atrial diameter greater than 4.5 cm or AF duration greater than 6 months is associated with a low likelihood of maintaining sinus rhythm. Patients with sick sinus syndrome or sinoatrial node block should not undergo cardioversion until a pacemaker has been placed. Ectopic or multifocal atrial, junctional, and sinus tachycardias do not normally respond to cardioversion. These rhythms have an automatic focus arising from cells that are depolarizing at a rapid rate; delivery of a shock may actually increase the rate of the tachyarrhythmia. Patients with a history of minimal hemodynamic or symptomatic improvement while in sinus rhythm should not undergo cardioversion because of an increased risk-to-benefit ratio. Inadequately anticoagulated patients with AF of longer than 48 hours' duration have an increased risk of thromboembolic stroke or arterial embolization (5% rate in the first 2 weeks after cardioversion).

Equipment

- Hand-held paddle electrodes, or 8- to 12-cm diameter, self-adherent pad electrodes or posterior paddle adapter
- Electrode gel or patches
- ACLS equipment
  - Oxygen source, nasal cannula or face mask
  - Pulse oximeter
  - Airway and intubation equipment
  - Ambu bag
  - Suction equipment, tubing, and catheter
  - Emergency drug kit, including IV drugs and lines
  - Medications needed to follow ACLS protocols
- Electrocardiography (ECG) electrodes and ECG monitoring capabilities
- Blood pressure monitoring equipment
- Direct-current defibrillator–cardioversion unit, with synchronization capabilities and optional "quick-look" paddles
- Sedatives for procedural sedation for elective cardioversion (see Chapter 2, Procedural Sedation and Analgesia)

Choice of Cardioversion Unit: Biphasic versus Monophasic

Biphasic waveform automated external defibrillators (AEDs) and cardioversion units were developed in the late 1990s and have been shown to provide superior atrial fibrillation conversion rates with lower-energy shocks compared with traditional monophasic units currently in use—86% of patients with AF returned to sinus rhythm after a single biphasic shock, versus 51% with the first monophasic shock. Most commercially available AEDs in the United States use biphasic waveforms, whereas most cardioversion units in hospitals and emergency departments continue to provide monophasic waveform shock. Cost and retraining of medical staff are likely barriers to wider use of biphasic cardioversion units.

Electrical versus Chemical Cardioversion

Given the procedural sedation (see Chapter 2, Procedural Sedation and Analgesia) required for nonemergent electrical cardioversion, much effort has been exerted to find an ideal antiarrhythmic medication for chemical cardioversion. The most effective agents, as recommended by the American College of Cardiology and American Heart Association (ACC/AHA), are the following:

- Ibutilide
- Dofetilide
- Propafenone
- Flecainide

Unfortunately, each of these agents has also been shown to be proarrhythmic—especially in the setting of decreased left ventricular ejection fraction (a relatively common finding in patients with AF). A less effective agent, amiodarone, has been shown to be safer in patients with a low ejection fraction, but it has delayed cardioversion effects in AF and is not currently approved for chemical cardioversion.

The advantage of chemical cardioversion is primarily related to the avoidance of procedural sedation in patients at high risk for airway compromise during procedural sedation (e.g., obstructive sleep apnea, known tracheal stenosis, prior tracheostomy, macroglossia). Like electrical cardioversion, chemical cardioversion in a nonurgent setting requires full anticoagulation for 3 weeks to avoid thromboembolic complications.

Rhythm Control versus Rate Control in Persistent Atrial Fibrillation

Five recent studies have demonstrated little difference in clinical outcome between rate and rhythm control strategies for patients with AF. In fact, rate control strategy is associated with fewer hospitalizations and less adverse drug effects when compared with rhythm control. Based on this evidence, some authors now recommend rate control and anticoagulation as primary therapy for persistent AF. The American Academy of Family Physicians and the American College of Physicians Joint Commission on Atrial Fibrillation recommends rate control with chronic anticoagulation for most patients with AF (Snow and colleagues, 2003). Drugs recommended for rate control are metoprolol, atenolol, diltiazem, and verapamil, with digoxin being moved into second-line therapy. The Joint Commission further recommends that most patients converted to sinus rhythm from AF not be placed on rhythm maintenance medications because of the risks outweighing any potential benefits. For patients who are unable to take warfarin, aspirin 325 mg orally daily or clopidogrel 75 mg may be used. These drugs have the advantage of not requiring monitoring of the international normalized ratio (INR), although aspirin and clopidogrel are clearly inferior to warfarin for preventing cardioembolic events. The role of oral direct thrombin inhibitors in place of warfarin remains controversial.

Preprocedure Patient Preparation

Urgent cardioversion is indicated when the patient is unstable. Examples include symptomatic hypotension with central nervous system changes or syncope resulting from decreased perfusion. If the patient is alert, briefly explain the procedure while connecting the equipment. Informed consent is unnecessary for a life-threatening situation. Document the indications and risks to the patient as time permits. The following preparation for elective cardioversion is not required for urgent cardioversion (i.e., if the clinical status of the patient is so tenuous that he or she would not survive).

Echocardiography

Transesophageal echocardiography is helpful before elective cardioversion to estimate left atrial diameter (see Chapter 90, Echocardiography). TEE can identify small atrial thrombi, especially in the left auricular appendage, that are not visible with transthoracic echocardiography in patients for whom anticoagulation with warfarin poses high risk.

Anticoagulation and Antiarrhythmics

All patients with AF for more than 48 hours should be anticoagulated adequately for 3 weeks before elective cardioversion because of the risk of embolizing intra-atrial thrombi when sinus rhythm (and atrial contractions) are reestablished. The incidence of emboli may be up to 5% for the first 2 weeks after cardioversion in nonanticoagulated patients. Recent trials indicate the benefits of anticoagulation in all patients with chronic AF. The INR for anticoagulation should be maintained between 2 and 3 for at least 3 weeks before and 4 weeks after the cardioversion. The routine use of anticoagulation in arrhythmias other than AF is controversial.

EDITOR'S NOTE: A TEE is much more sensitive than a transthoracic echocardiogram for detecting thrombi, especially in the atrial appendage. Although the absence of a detectable thrombus does not preclude thromboembolism after cardioversion, a TEE-guided strategy (Klein, 2000) for elective cardioversion of AF has resulted in outcomes comparable with those obtained using a conventional anticoagulation strategy.

There is some evidence suggesting that having the patient already on antiarrhythmic therapy before cardioversion may prevent recurrence. In the event the patient might chemically convert, he or she should have been adequately anticoagulated or have a TEE negative for thrombus before starting antiarrhythmics.

Fasting and Informed Consent

Instruct the patient to fast after midnight or for at least 4 to 6 hours before the procedure. Explain the indications for the procedure and the risk of complications. Explain that sedation will be used, but the patient may experience some achy discomfort in the arms and chest after the procedure. ECG monitoring for at least several hours will be necessary because of the risk of a recurrent or new arrhythmia. In addition, a minor skin irritation or burn may occur. Document the informed consent discussion and obtain the patient's signature on the consent form (see the sample patient consent form online at www.expertconsult.com).

Technical Considerations for Elective Cardioversion

Paddle and Electrode Selection and Placement

Apply the electrodes in either the standard paddle position (right upper parasternal [second or third interspace] and left apical [fourth

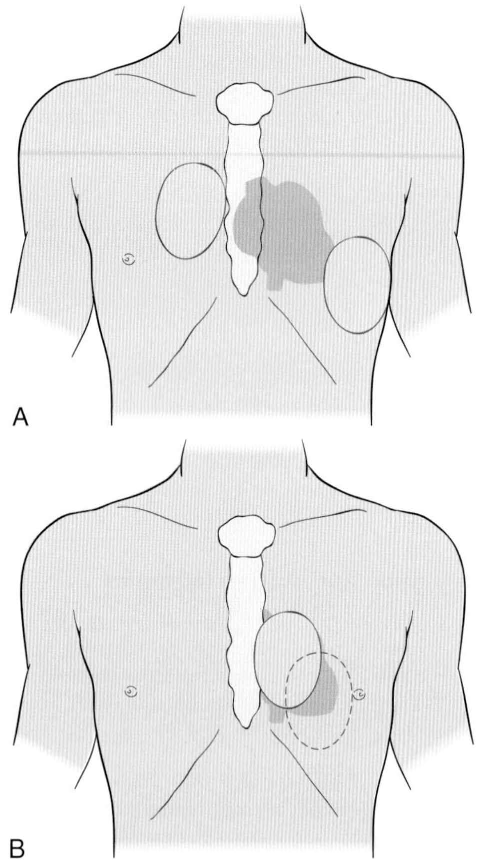

Figure 210-1 **A,** Standard electrode position. **B,** Alternative (anteroposterior) electrode position.

or fifth interspace, left mid-axillary line]; Fig. 210-1A) or the anteroposterior paddle position. For anteroposterior placement, the anterior electrode is centered over the sternum and the posterior electrode is placed between the scapulae, or both can be placed slightly to the patient's left, on the left side of the sternum and beneath the left scapula (Fig. 210-1B). Hand-held paddle electrodes or self-adherent pad electrodes 8 to 12 cm in diameter deliver adequate energy for cardioversion. To maximize the current flow to the heart, correct paddle or electrode placement is crucial. Either positioning technique is acceptable, but anteroposterior positioning may reduce energy requirements for cardioversion (through reduced electrical resistance) by up to 50%. In a large patient, this may increase cardioversion success. Anteroposterior placement is often used with disposable patches rather than paddles. Either paddles or electrodes must be positioned far enough apart so that electrical current travels through the heart. Gel or paste must be placed between the paddle or electrode and the chest wall to minimize resistance. However, avoid paste or gel smeared on the skin between electrodes, which might allow the current to travel along the external chest wall. Electrodes should also be placed far enough away from a pacemaker generator to prevent damage to its electrical components.

Electrocardiographic Monitoring

A set of ECG electrodes connected to the defibrillator should be placed on the patient so that the shock can be synchronized. An additional set of ECG electrodes can be connected to a telemetry monitor.

Synchronization

Synchronization refers to the delivery of electrical current to the myocardium during a nonrefractory period (e.g., not when repolarization of the entire myocardium is occurring). Shocking the myocardium during the relative refractory period (the T wave) can simulate the "R on T" phenomenon and induce VF. In synchronized mode, the energy is delivered at the peak of the QRS complex, the R wave. Synchronized administration reduces the energy requirements and complication rates of elective cardioversion.

Most defibrillators indicate when active synchronization is selected by highlighting the QRS peak (R wave). The practitioner can simply select and press the synchronization button for most cases of elective cardioversion. In cases with rapid ventricular response, the defibrillator in a synchronized mode may not be able to distinguish between the peak of the QRS complex and the peak of a T wave. As a safety feature, the defibrillator will not discharge if QRS complex and T waves cannot be distinguished. In this case, the provider should switch off the synchronization switch and perform unsynchronized defibrillation, realizing the increased risk of precipitating VT or VF. Alternatively, medications may be added to reduce the rapid ventricular response.

Energy Selection

Cardioversion is accomplished by passing an electrical current of sufficient magnitude through the heart to depolarize the myocardial tissues. Current flow is determined by the energy flow as measured in joules and by the resistance of the thoracic wall tissues as measured in ohms. The transthoracic resistance in an average adult is 70 to 80 ohms. If the transthoracic resistance is too high, the energy may fail to accomplish cardiac depolarization.

Some SVT arrhythmias are very sensitive to electrical current. Low energy settings may depolarize the myocardium in atrial flutter and allow the heart to resume a sinus rhythm. Recommended initial energy settings for cardioversion of various arrhythmias are listed in Table 210-1. For AF, the usual recommended initial energy setting is 100 J. However, recent evidence suggests that higher initial energy settings are more effective at achieving cardioversion, and some authors currently recommend an initial energy setting of 360 J.

Cardioversion energy for VT depends on the rate and morphologic features of the electrical activity. Monomorphic VT presents with a regular ECG form (wide-complex) and rate, and it is generally responsive to cardioversion beginning at energies of 100 J. Polymorphic VT has an irregular form and rate and is less responsive to electroshock therapy. Polymorphic VT behaves like VF, and the initial defibrillator shock energy should be 200 J (unsynchronized).

If the first shock fails to cardiovert any arrhythmia, repeated attempts should be undertaken with stepwise energy increases. The transthoracic resistance increases after each shock, so the energy must be increased to overcome that resistance. The standard sequence for synchronized cardioversion is 100, 200, 300, and 360 J; the energies used depend on the initial energy selected. For

TABLE 210-1 Recommended Initial Energy Settings for Electrical Cardioversion

	Initial Energy Settings (J)	
	Monophasic	**Biphasic**
Atrial flutter	50	50*
Atrial fibrillation	200	100*
Paroxysmal supraventricular tachycardia	50	50*
Monomorphic ventricular tachycardia	100	50*
Polymorphic ventricular tachycardia	200	100*

*Standards for biphasic cardioversion have not been established.

example, after starting with 200 J, the second attempt to convert polymorphic VT should be with an energy of 300 J. Patients with large thoraces, chest wall deformities, or large amounts of adipose tissue may require higher initial settings.

Energy levels differ between monophasic and biphasic cardioversion units. In general, the energy requirements for biphasic cardioversion units are about half those for monophasic units. For example, patients with chronic AF often require 200 to 360 J of monophasic countershock; however, only 100 to 150 J of biphasic countershock is usually required (see Table 210-1).

Environment and Personnel

Elective cardioversion should be performed in a prepared environment, usually in a cardiac care unit with telemetry capabilities. The ACC/AHA guidelines (Tracy and colleagues, 2000) review the cognitive and technical skills necessary to perform external direct-current cardioversion and suggest a minimum requirement of eight prior supervised electrical cardioversions. Sedation or anesthesia is typically used with elective cardioversion, requiring appropriate personnel and monitoring.

Choice of Sedation Agents

Many factors play into the decision for procedural sedation during elective cardioversion, including anticipated energy levels for cardioversion, patient factors (e.g., airway, obesity, hepatic and renal disorders), and desired length of sedation. In general, the extent of sedation needed depends on the amount of energy to be used:

- 50 to 100 J: mild sedation
- Over 100 to 150 J: moderate to deep sedation

Mild sedation usually requires only short-acting benzodiazepines, such as midazolam or lorazepam, and fentanyl, a narcotic with less hemodynamic effects than morphine.

Moderate to deep sedation agents often used for cardioversion include the following:

- Etomidate: advantage, little hemodynamic compromise; caution in liver disease
- Propofol: advantage, rapid on, rapid off; caution, may cause hypotension
- Barbiturates, primarily thiopental: losing favor because of long recovery

See Chapter 2, Procedural Sedation and Analgesia.

Technique

1. Review laboratory values and echocardiography results or obtain an echocardiogram (see Chapter 90, Echocardiography). Confirm adequate anticoagulation and normal electrolyte (particularly potassium and magnesium) and serum digoxin (if indicated) levels. If indicated, patients should already be on a therapeutic regimen of antiarrhythmic medication. Review echocardiogram findings, noting the absence of intra-atrial thrombi (if appropriate) and an atrial diameter less than 4.5 cm.
2. Ensure that the patient has fasted.
3. Obtain a resting 12-lead ECG and confirm the persistence of the rhythm disturbance.
4. Obtain informed consent (see the sample patient consent form, "Cardiac Procedure—Cardioversion," online at www.expertconsult.com).
5. Premedicate the patient with a sedative. Many experts recommend anesthesia standby if this service is available. Administration of a sedative (e.g., diazepam, midazolam) or a barbiturate can be combined with an analgesic (e.g., meperidine, fentanyl) to improve patient comfort.
6. The patient should be lying on a flat, dry surface.
7. Monitor the patient's ECG, pulse oximetry, and blood pressure throughout the procedure.
8. Initiate intravenous access. Apply supplemental oxygen.
9. Have suction, resuscitation equipment, and support staff immediately available.
10. Apply conductive material and electrodes. (If gel is applied directly to the paddles, the paddles can be rubbed together to coat the electrode surfaces completely.)
11. Turn on the cardioversion unit.
12. Select the appropriate energy level for the dysrhythmia, body habitus, and electrode positioning.
13. Turn on the synchronizer circuit. Look for markers on the R wave indicating synchronization mode. Adjust monitor gain, if necessary, until synchronization markers occur with each R wave.
14. Charge the capacitors to the preselected energy level.
15. Position the paddles or electrodes. Apply the pads firmly to the torso. (The paddles should be separated from each other by at least 2 to 3 cm to prevent arcing.)
16. Call "All clear!" to indicate all personnel should move away from the patient's bed to avoid receiving a shock. Double-check by visually confirming all personnel (including yourself) have moved back and have no physical contact with the patient or the bed.
17. Deliver electrical energy by depressing appropriate discharge buttons on both paddles. (There is often a brief delay. Keep buttons depressed until the shock is delivered.)
18. Assess the cardiac rhythm on the monitor.
19. Assess the patient and administer more sedation if needed.
20. If necessary, repeat cardioversion process (steps 12 through 17) at a higher energy setting.
21. Remember to reset the synchronization switch, if necessary. Some defibrillators reset the switch to the "off" position after a shock is delivered.
22. If cardioversion is unsuccessful after a shock at 360 J, abort the procedure and consider additional antiarrhythmic medications.

Complications

- Unsuccessful cardioversion
- Transient mild arrhythmias
- Conversion to VT or VF
- Bradycardia, heart block
- Elevated cardiac enzymes (up to three times normal values)
- Localized cutaneous burns
- Accidental shock to attending personnel because of contact with the patient or bed
- Damage to electrical equipment in contact with the patient or bed
- Thromboembolic events
- Recurrence of original arrhythmia

If the original arrhythmia persists after more than three shocks and up to 360 J, the cardioversion is considered unsuccessful. In this case, the procedure should be aborted. Allow the patient to waken. Explain that the cardioversion was unsuccessful despite maximal safe efforts, and list the various options available to the patient and anyone else present. Options include internal cardioversion, antiarrhythmic medications, devices such as pacemakers, and no further treatment. Catheter ablation techniques are also sometimes available. In a significant number of patients with unresponsive AF, internal cardioversion with intracardiac electrode catheters has been successful. In this case, anticoagulation needs to be withheld temporarily because of the risk of bleeding at the catheter site. Alternatively, additional, more specific antiarrhythmic medications could be considered. The cardioversion may be reattempted after therapeutic blood levels are achieved (usually a few days). The patient may decide that further attempts are not worth the perceived risks.

Other complications after cardioversion are uncommon in the absence of digitalis toxicity or hypokalemia and with a properly delivered shock. Bradycardia is sometimes noted immediately after cardioversion in patients with a history of inferior myocardial infarction. If the bradycardia is symptomatic, atropine may be used. Transient mild arrhythmias or creatine kinase elevations of less than three times normal may be noted, but they are generally inconsequential.

With any cardioversion, especially with rapid heart rates, there is a risk of producing a worse rhythm, such as VT or VF. Any attempted cardioversion that results in VF should be *defibrillated (synchronization off)* immediately, starting with 200 J of energy. On some defibrillators, the synchronization must be shut off manually to administer a nonsynchronized shock.

Application of adequate amounts of electrode paste to the paddles can minimize cutaneous burns. Electrical shock is a possibility for anyone in contact with the patient or the patient's bed. Any attached electrical equipment can be damaged. Systemic emboli may develop if the patient is not adequately anticoagulated, causing neurologic deficit or occlusion of a peripheral artery. The original arrhythmia may recur despite successful cardioversion.

Postprocedure Monitoring

Monitor the patient for 2 to 4 hours. An example of monitoring orders includes vital signs with neurologic checks every 15 minutes for 1 hour, then every hour for 2 hours. Provide continuous ECG telemetry during this time. Atrial or ventricular ectopy and bradycardia are not uncommon in the first 15 to 30 minutes after cardioversion.

CPT/Billing Codes

92950 Cardiopulmonary resuscitation
92960 Cardioversion, elective; electrical conversion of arrhythmia, external

Acknowledgment

The editors wish to recognize the many contributions by Thomas J. Zuber, MD, John L. Pfenninger, MD, Les B. Forgosh, MD, FACC, FACP, and David V. Power, MD, MPH, to this chapter in the previous two editions of this text.

Suppliers

Most hospitals have cardioversion equipment. Familiarize yourself with the equipment available in your particular setting.

BIBLIOGRAPHY

American Heart Association: Advanced Cardiovascular Life Support Provider Manual. Dallas, American Heart Association, 2006.

Boos CJ, Carlsson J, More RS: Rate or rhythm control in persistent atrial fibrillation? Q J Med 96:881–902, 2003.

Catherwood E, Fitzpatrick WD, Greenberg ML, et al: Cost-effectiveness of cardioversion and antiarrhythmic therapy in nonvalvular atrial fibrillation [see comments]. Ann Intern Med 130:625–636, 1999.

Joglar JA, Hamdan MH, Ramaswamy K, et al: Initial energy for elective external cardioversion of persistent atrial fibrillation. Am J Cardiol 86:348–350, 2000.

Klein EA: Assessment of cardioversion using transesophageal echocardiography (TEE) multicenter study (ACUTE I): Clinical outcomes at eight weeks. J Am Coll Cardiol 36:324, 2000.

Mathew TP, Moore A, McIntyre M, et al: Randomised comparison of electrode positions for cardioversion of atrial fibrillation. Heart 81:576–579, 1999.

Page RL, Kerber RE, Russell JK, et al, for the BiCard Investigators: Biphasic versus monophasic shock waveform for conversion of atrial fibrillation: The results of an international randomized, double-blind multicenter trial. J Am Coll Cardiol 39:1956–1963, 2002.

Sattar P: Cardioversion and defibrillation. In Reichman EF, Simon RR (eds): Emergency Medicine Procedures. New York, McGraw-Hill, 2004, pp 161–166.

Snow V, Weiss KB, LeFevre M, et al: Management of newly detected atrial fibrillation: A clinical practice guideline from the American Academy of Family Physicians and the American College of Physicians. Ann Intern Med 139:1009–1017, 2003.

Stroke Prevention in Atrial Fibrillation Investigators: Stroke Prevention in Atrial Fibrillation Study: Final results. Circulation 84:527–539, 1991.

Tracy CM, Akhtar M, DiMarco JP, et al: American College of Cardiology/American Heart Association clinical competence statement on invasive electrophysiology studies, catheter ablation, and cardioversion: A report of the American College of Cardiology/American Heart Association/American College of Physicians–American Society of Internal Medicine Task Force on Clinical Competence. J Am Coll Cardiol 36:1725–1736, 2000.

CHAPTER 211

Central Venous Catheter Insertion

David James

Over the past several decades, the use of central venous catheters has increased to keep pace with other medical and technological advances. Emergency resuscitation protocols, specialized cardiovascular monitoring techniques, transvenous pacer insertion, and total parenteral nutrition protocols all demand access to a large central vein.

Expeditious placement of a large central venous catheter presents a challenge to the clinician, because the central veins are neither readily visible to the eye nor distinctly palpable. If the patient is critically ill or hypovolemic, the challenge is magnified. Fortunately, the larger central veins have predictable and constant relationships to readily identifiable anatomic landmarks.

In recent years, increasing emphasis has been placed on using ultrasound to guide placement of central venous catheters (see Chapter 225, Emergency Department, Hospitalist, and Office Ultrasonography [Clinical Ultrasonography]). Although ultrasonic guidance was not considered the standard of care in a recent informal survey of hospitalists, recent Medicare guidelines suggest monitoring very closely for iatrogenic puncture wounds of vital organs in hospitalized patients.

NOTE: Remember that a short, large-diameter IV catheter (e.g., 14-, 16-, or 18-gauge peripheral catheter) *has less resistance to flow* than a long, skinny central catheter! Rapid, large-volume infusion is faster with a peripheral, large-bore catheter and is preferred in an emergent situation. Depending on local availability and expertise, newer kits are available to rapidly and dependably obtain intraosseous vascular access (IOVA; see Chapter 198, Intraosseous Vascular Access). In some facilities, this has become the preferred temporary backup or alternative to obtaining central or peripheral venous access, especially in children (see Chapter 182, Pediatric Arterial Puncture and Venous Minicutdown).

Indications

- Venous access in those patients who are either so obese or so debilitated that their peripheral veins are not accessible for intravenous (IV) cannulation
- Emergency venous access after a cardiac arrest
- Administration of cardiac medications during cardiopulmonary resuscitation (CPR)
- Large-volume parenteral fluid administration when peripheral IV cannulation is not readily obtainable
- Central venous pressure monitoring
- Administration of certain chemotherapeutic agents
- Administration of vasopressor medications
- Administration of hyperosmolar or other irritating solutions (e.g., total parenteral nutrition) that have the potential to cause thrombophlebitis or to cause soft tissue necrosis if extravasation occurs
- Patients with significant burns on peripheral areas that may prevent placement of a peripheral catheter
- Placement of a pulmonary artery (Swan-Ganz) catheter (see Chapter 215, Swan Ganz [Pulmonary Artery] Catheterization)
- Placement of a temporary transvenous pacemaker wire (see Chapter 216, Temporary Pacing)
- Performance of right cardiac catheterization and pulmonary angiography
- Performance of hemodialysis or plasmapheresis

Contraindications

Absolute

- Patient refusal
- Combative or agitated patient (may require procedural sedation, see Chapter 2, Procedural Sedation and Analgesia)
- Distortion of local anatomy or landmarks (e.g., prior surgery, trauma, radiation therapy, generalized obesity, orthopedic conditions, masses)
- Superior vena cava syndrome
- Bleeding diathesis or excessive anticoagulation and a noncompressible vessel
- Full-thickness burn or cellulitis over the proposed insertion site
- Pneumothorax or hemothorax on the contralateral side, or inability to tolerate a pneumothorax on the ipsilateral side (for subclavian and internal jugular locations)
- Prior injection of a sclerosing agent into the proposed vein
- Trauma to the proposed insertion site
- Venous thrombosis of the proposed vein
- Avoid internal jugular location if cervical spine fracture or penetrating neck injury
- Allergy to any component of the catheter such as latex
- Cardiac-paced patient (for Seldinger wire technique, whether pacer temporary, internal, or permanent)
- Highly unstable arrhythmias (for Seldinger wire technique, especially ventricular arrhythmias)
- Right-sided endocarditis or mural thrombus

Relative

- Suspected injury to proposed vein (may then use vein on contralateral side, if no associated hemothorax or pneumothorax, when using subclavian or internal jugular)
- Morbid obesity
- Marked cachexia
- Vasculitis that predisposes to sclerosis or thrombosis of veins
- Previous long-term central catheterization or recently discontinued central catheter in proposed vein
- Proposed mastectomy on same side of subclavian vein access

- Patients receiving ventilatory support with high end-expiratory pressures (if possible, for suclavian or internal jugular, ventilation should be briefly interrupted while central vein is cannulated with needle)
- Patients undergoing CPR (should use femoral or internal jugular vein locations)
- Children younger than 2 years old (for whom the internal jugular vein is preferred location)
- Severe hypovolemia (try large bore peripheral IV or IOVA first)
- Prosthetic right heart valve (Seldinger wire technique contraindicated)
- Avoid internal jugular or subclavian vein locations if patient unable to lie in the Trendelenburg position
- Left bundle branch block (use of Seldinger wire can cause complete heart block)
- Avoid internal jugular location if known severe carotid artery stenosis or atherosclerosis on the desired side (accidental artery puncture may result in plaque rupture and stroke)
- Personnel capable of handling complications not immediately available

Equipment

Many commercially prepared central venous catheter kits are available. Most institutions have a relationship with a hospital supplier that provides a catheter kit. These kits, often from a company such as Baxter or Cook, have all the components needed to insert a central venous catheter. These kits often utilize a Seldinger wire technique to place the catheter: a needle enters the vein, a guidewire is threaded through the needle into the vein lumen, and the cannulating needle is removed. A larger, flexible catheter is then passed over the guidewire into the vein, and the guidewire is removed.

- IV solution and connector tubing, flushed and ready
- Towel
- Pressure transducer and monitor, if monitoring central venous pressure
- Supplemental oxygen
- Continuous pulse oximetry and cardiac and blood pressure monitoring
- Fully stocked code cart and defibrillator nearby
- Surgeon's cap
- Sterile gloves and gown
- Sterile drapes
- Bio-occlusive dressing (e.g., Tegaderm, Opsite) to cover insertion site, especially useful if clear so the wound can be more easily inspected
- Goggles or eye protection

If a commercially prepared kit is unavailable, the following equipment list will supply what is needed:

- Sterile prep solution (chlorhexidine antisepsis preferred over povidone–iodine solution) and swabs
- Prep razor
- Sterile 4 × 4 inch gauze pads
- Lidocaine 1% to 2% with or without epinephrine for local anesthesia
- 3-mL syringe with 25-gauge needle for anesthetic injection
- 5-mL syringe with 22-gauge 1½- to 2½-inch seeker needle to find the vein
- 10-mL syringe with 2½-inch 18-gauge needle to introduce guidewire
- No. 11 scalpel blade and holder
- Guidewire or J-wire (flexible wire 45 cm long, 0.089 cm diameter, 3 mm radius of curvature)
- Central venous catheter
- 3-0 silk suture on straight needle to suture catheter into place
- Suture scissors
- Topical antimicrobial ointment
- Saline flushes

Preprocedure Patient Education

If the clinical situation permits, informed consent must be obtained prior to the procedure. Inform the patient (or family) of potential major complications and their management, which could require chest tube insertion, surgery, or cardioversion. To minimize patient anxiety during procedure, explain the major steps of the procedure, the possible necessity of remaining in a head down (Trendelenburg) position during placement, and the near impossibility of a completely painless procedure.

Techniques

Several distinct approaches are discussed for placement of a central venous catheter. These approaches include cannulation of the subclavian vein (using both the supra- and infraclavicular routes), the internal jugular vein, and the femoral vein.

Generally, the preferred veins are on the *right* side of the patient. This preference is because the right-sided veins have a more direct course to the right atrium, and thus can be utilized for placement of a pacemaker wire or Swan-Ganz catheter with greater ease than the left-sided veins. The left-sided veins tend to have a more tortuous course and are in closer proximity to the thoracic duct and dome of the lung pleura.

The internal jugular vein is accessible without terminating CPR, although chest compressions and the lack of a carotid pulse may make access more difficult. However, having an internal jugular line requires limited patient neck mobility, which can be uncomfortable, so the subclavian route may be preferable for long-term lines. Likewise, a femoral line limits ambulation, so the subclavian route may be preferable. Ongoing or impending thrombolytic or fibrinolytic therapy is a contraindication to internal jugular puncture. Femoral vein access may be the easiest to obtain and may be preferable in emergencies or during CPR. It may also be preferred for patients with respiratory distress and pulmonary edema because the patient should not be placed in the Trendelenburg position. Supplemental oxygen should be provided and the patient monitored continuously during this procedure. Passage of a guidewire into the right side of the heart can induce arrhythmias and complete heart block; the clinician should be prepared to treat these problems accordingly.

Subclavian Venipuncture

The subclavian vein begins as a continuation of the axillary vein at the lateral border of the first rib, and it joins the internal jugular vein to form the innominate vein (Fig. 211-1). As it crosses behind the first rib, the subclavian vein lies posterior to the medial third of the clavicle. It is only in this "middle region" that an intimate relationship exists between the subclavian vein and the clavicle. The subclavian vein contains no valves and is between 1 and 2 cm in diameter for most people. The subclavian artery is superior and posterior to the vein, and is separated from the vein by the anterior scalene muscle. Other important structures nearby include the phrenic nerve; the thoracic duct (left side); lymphatic duct (on the right side, it joins the subclavian vein near its merger with the internal jugular vein); and the dome of the pleura of the lung. The dome of the pleura may extend above the first rib on the left side but is rarely found this far cephalad on the right.

Patient Position

Proper positioning of the patient increases chances of a successful cannulation and reduces risk of complications of this procedure. Place the patient in Trendelenburg position at an angle of 15 to 20

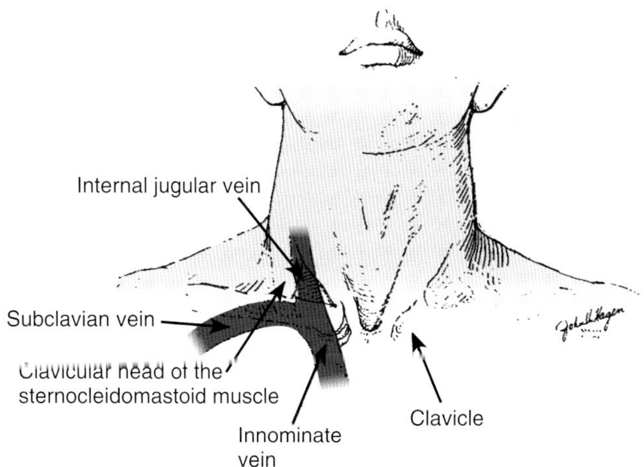

Figure 211-1 Relationship of great vessels in and about the right neck.

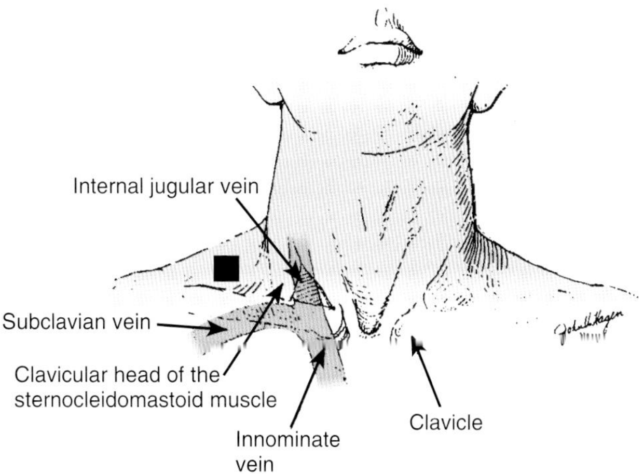

Figure 211-3 Supraclavicular approach: *black box* represents entry point 1 cm lateral to the clavicular head of the *sternocleidomastoid* muscle, and 1 cm above the superior border of the clavicle.

degrees (Fig. 211-2). This position fills these low-pressure great veins by gravity, thus making them swell in diameter and increasing your chances of finding them. It also reduces the risk of air embolism.

- Have the patient turn his or her head contralaterally. (Have an assistant turn the head if the patient is unable to do so.) This gives a wider field of operation.
- Consider placing a rolled-up towel vertically between the patient's shoulder blades. This may cause the shoulders to fall back from the clavicles, which could help to define the relevant anatomy and improve access the subclavian vein. However, it should be noted that certain experts avoid placing a towel between the shoulder blades because it can decrease the distance between the clavicle and first rib, thereby compressing the subclavian vein and making it more difficult to cannulate.

Supraclavicular Approach to the Subclavian Vein

This approach may sound complicated, but the author believes it to be the least complicated and most efficient technique. It is rapid, stays away from other vital structures, and is easily performed in patients undergoing CPR. Additionally, it is easily and reliably performed in an obese patient.

1. With the patient in the previously described position, locate the insertion area: *a spot 1 cm lateral to the lateral head of the sternocleidomastoid muscle and 1 cm superior to the clavicular border* (Fig. 211-3).
2. Review Figure 211-4 for an overview of the catheter-over-wire (Seldinger) technique described here.
3. Assemble equipment on a work surface of convenient height, and within your reach. Wash your hands and put on mask, cap, eye protection, sterile gown, and gloves. *Strict sterile technique should be observed from this point onward.* Cleanse the area with skin prep solution (some kits will have a chlorhexidine or povidone–iodine prep swab enclosed), and drape to define a sterile field. Optimally, the entire neck and clavicular area are prepped. That way, in case of unsuccessful cannulation, another site can be attempted without having to repeat the prep. Drape as large of an area as possible, including the majority of the patient and the bed. A three-quarter sheet works well for this purpose. Follow universal blood and body fluid precautions.
4. Draw up 2 mL of 1% lidocaine into the 3-mL syringe, and raise a skin wheal at the site of the proposed insertion; infiltrate the deeper tissues with the remainder of the lidocaine.
5. With the 22-gauge needle on a 5-mL syringe, seek the subclavian vein; insert the needle at the entry point diagrammed in Figure 211-3. *Aim just under the clavicle, angled toward the contralateral nipple*. Usually, in people of normal weight and habitus, the vein is quite shallowly located. In an obese patient, or those with chest hyperinflation from chronic obstructive pulmonary disease, the vein is deeper. Maintain suction on the syringe until *dark red blood* flows easily into the syringe.
6. Using the 18 gauge 2½-inch needle mounted on a 5- or 10-mL syringe, insert to parallel the seeker needle to enter the subclavian vein. The position of this needle should be identical to that of the seeker needle (i.e., the same direction, depth, and angle of penetration). Insert while aspirating with the syringe plunger. Placement within the vein is confirmed by easy return of *dark red blood*. Rotate the syringe/needle unit until the bevel of the needle faces caudally.
7. In many central line kits, a Raulerson syringe, which is an 18-gauge port that runs through the plunger and right out through the needle, is provided. This syringe allows guidewire insertion directly into the vein from the syringe plunger and allows the needle/syringe unit to be left in place where the subclavian vein was entered, thus minimizing the risk of unintentional movement of the needle out of the vein. If you do not have a kit with the plunger port, you will need to *remove the syringe from the 18-gauge 2½-inch needle hub, making sure the needle does not move from its position. Occlude the needle hub with your nondominant thumb*.

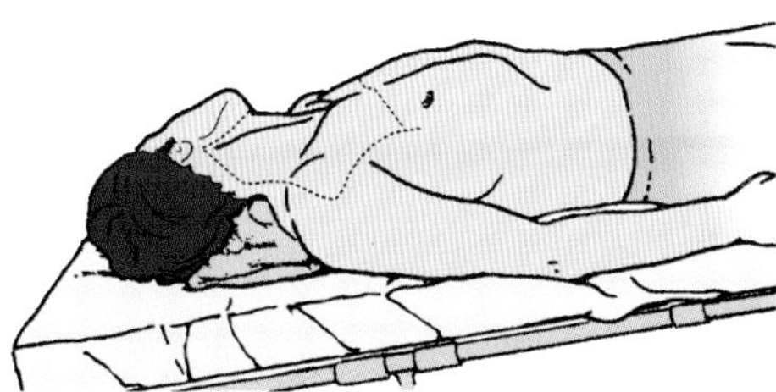

Figure 211-2 Moderate Trendelenburg position for subclavian central vein catheter insertion.

EDITOR'S NOTE: An intended benefit of use of a blue Raulerson syringe is the ability to differentiate arterial from venous blood by its color in the syringe. However, in patients with certain conditions (e.g., severe hypoxia, shock), arterial blood can be dark and mimic venous blood with adverse consequences. By disconnecting the introducer needle from the syringe, the clinician can determine whether the blood is pulsatile (arterial)

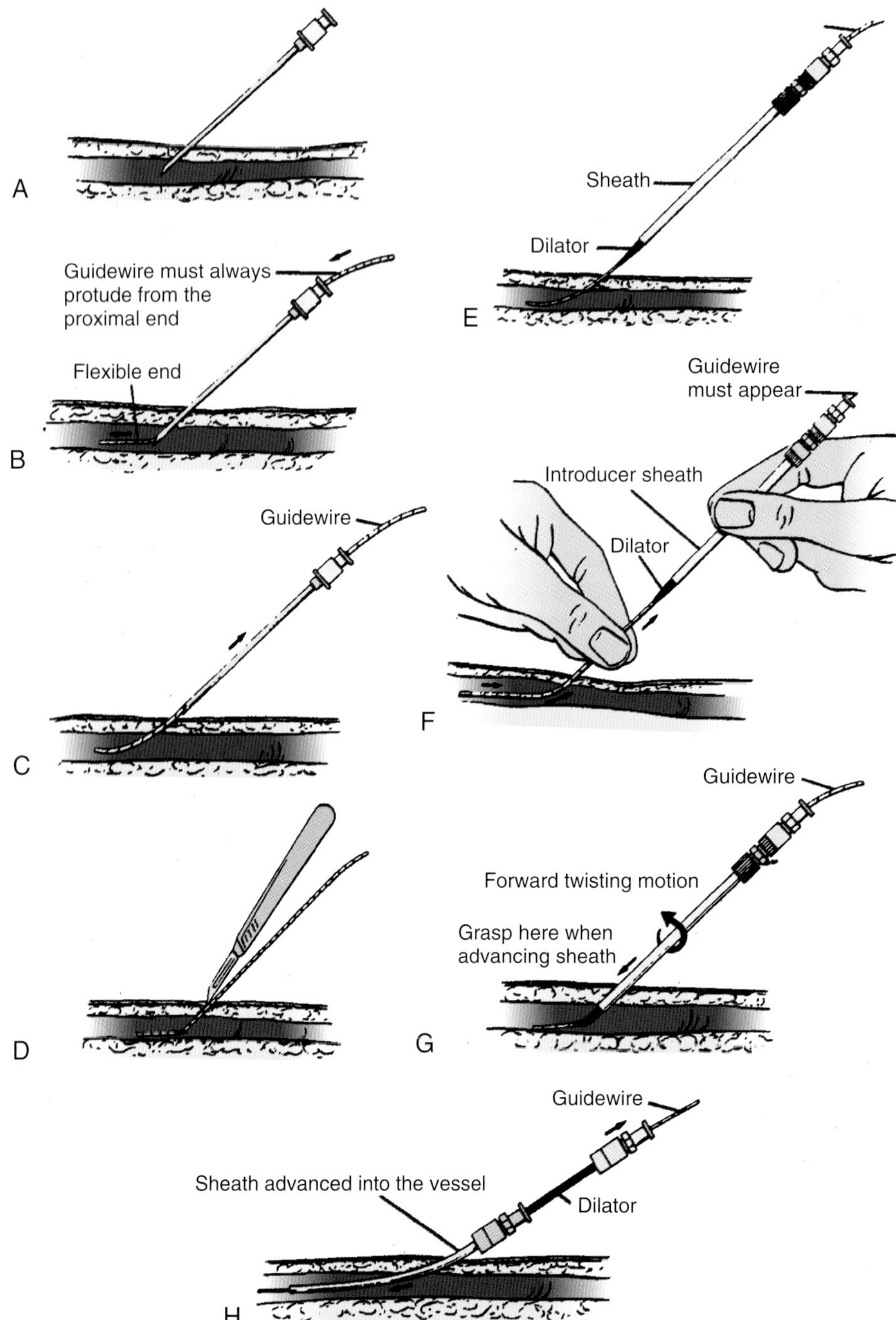

Figure 211-4 Placement of Seldinger-type guidewire and catheter. **A,** Introducing needle with tip in lumen. **B,** Advance guidewire into vein. **C,** Remove introducing needle over guidewire. **D,** Make small skin incision. **E,** Advance dilator and sheath until tip is near skin. **F,** If guidewire tip cannot be grasped, withdraw it slightly from the vein by grasping below the dilator tip. **G,** Advance dilator and sheath along guidewire and into vein. **H,** After sheath is fully advanced, slowly withdraw dilator and then guidewire. Immediately cover catheter hub with finger and attach to intravenous tubing. Also see text for details. (Modified from Roberts JR, Hedges JR [eds]: Clinical Procedures in Emergency Medicine, 3rd ed. Philadelphia, WB Saunders, 1998.)

or not. If there is any question, a sterile arterial blood gas syringe can be dropped into the field and a sample sent immediately for blood gas analysis. Make sure to cap the introducer needle hub while waiting for the result.

8. Insert the guidewire through the needle hub or plunger port. Most guidewires have a J loop at the end; straighten the loop by withdrawing the wire into its sheath. Then, once the straightened end of the wire is inserted into the needle, advance the guidewire approximately one half of its length into the subclavian vein.
9. Withdraw, over the wire, the introducer needle/syringe unit. Make sure the wire stays steady and does not advance inadvertently its entire length into the vein, where it could embolize.
10. Using the no. 11 scalpel blade, to make room for the dilator and introducer sheath, make a small nick in the skin where the guidewire enters; it is easiest just to slide the blade on top of the wire.
11. Slide the dilator over the wire, and insert/withdraw the dilator several times to dilate the entry site tissues. Using a twisting motion while inserting the dilator may facilitate its advance. Withdraw the dilator over the guidewire and set it aside.

12. If color-coded, remove the *brown hub* from the central venous catheter. In some kits, the catheter is stiff enough to be inserted alone, directly over the guidewire. Otherwise, insert the dilator into the catheter (or some kits have a smaller diameter introducer that fits into the catheter to stiffen it). Slide the catheter (and dilator/introducer if needed, as a unit) over the wire, and advance the guidewire *up into the catheter* until it just pokes out of the open port. Holding the end of the wire, slide the catheter (and dilator/introducer if needed) down over the wire to the desired depth of insertion. Using a twisting motion when advancing the catheter may facilitate its advance.
13. Remove the dilator/introducer over the guidewire and then remove the guidewire and set aside. This leaves the catheter in place.
14. Secure the catheter to the skin with a suture (most kits have a plastic hub that fits over the catheter and has preformed suture holes for securing to the skin). The insertion area and exposed catheter should be covered with a sterile dressing (a clear bio-occlusive dressing such as Tegaderm or Opsite provides added security).
15. Reattach the brown hub, or the required clave-type hub, to the catheter port, and aspirate each port to ensure easy blood return. Flush all ports with saline. You may hook up any IV tubing/fluids at this time.
16. Obtain a postinsertion chest radiograph to ensure that there is no iatrogenic pneumothorax and to check the catheter tip location.
17. If the catheter tip lies within the right atrium or ventricle, the catheter should be withdrawn so that the tip resides within the superior vena cava.

Infraclavicular Approach to the Subclavian Vein

This approach is very familiar because of the easily identified anatomic landmarks.

1. Position the patient in a moderate Trendelenburg position, as illustrated in Figure 211-2.
2. Orient yourself regarding landmarks, and establish an insertion site (Fig. 211-5). Place the thumb of your *nondominant* hand on the distal end of the clavicle and the middle finger of the same hand on the sternoclavicular joint. Let the index finger extend comfortably. The site for insertion will be immediately *under* the index finger, where it crosses the clavicle. Mark this site with your fingernail or a marker pen.
3. Open the central line catheter kit, wash your hands, don personal gear (mask, cap, eye protection, sterile gown, and gloves), and prep and drape the area in the usual fashion. Observe universal blood and body fluid precautions.
4. Using a 3-mL syringe with a 25-gauge needle attached, draw up 2 mL of 1% plain lidocaine and use this to anesthetize the insertion area. Infiltrate anesthesia into the deeper tissues under the clavicle as well.

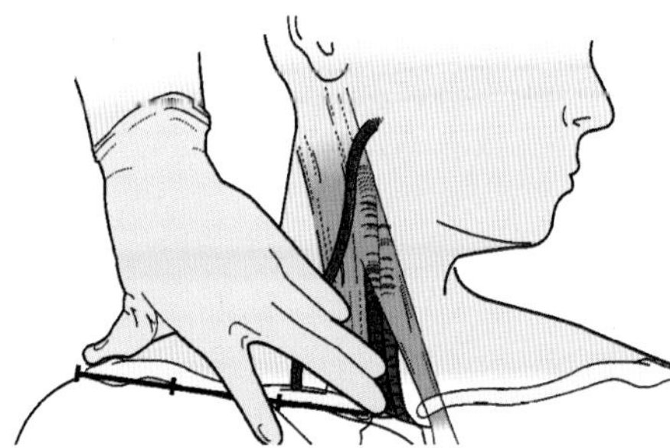

Figure 211-5 Orientation for subclavian catheter insertion, infraclavicular approach. Thumb of nondominant hand is on distal clavicle, middle finger on sternoclavicular joint.

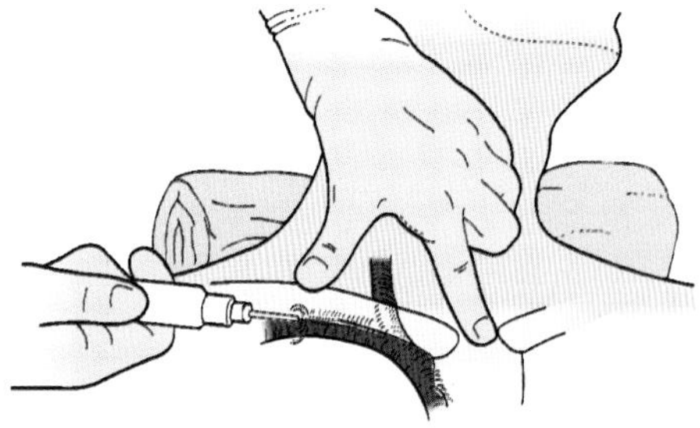

Figure 211-6 Inserting the seeker needle.

5. Have patient turn his or her head contralaterally, or have an assistant hold the head rotated contralaterally.
6. Use the 3-mL syringe with the 22-gauge needle as a "seeker" needle. Position the thumb of your nondominant hand over your mark and place the index finger of the same hand between the two clavicular heads in the suprasternal notch. Insert the seeker needle 1 to 2 cm *inferior* to the clavicle. Aim for the suprasternal notch (Fig. 211-6). Keep the shaft of the seeker needle in contact with the inferior border of the clavicle as you work it under the clavicle. Aspirate as you go; entry into the subclavian vein is confirmed by the easy return of dark venous blood into the syringe. If the first attempt is unsuccessful, withdraw the seeker needle, flush it, confirm landmarks, and reinsert it under the clavicle, directing the needle *somewhat cephalad and deeper*. At times, the 1½-inch "seeker" needle will be too short to enter the subclavian vein with the infraclavicular approach.
7. Once the subclavian vein has been located, remove the seeker needle. Using the 18-gauge 2½-inch needle on a 5-mL syringe, insert it along the track of the seeker needle (i.e., the same direction, angle, and depth of penetration) to enter the subclavian vein. Entry is confirmed by the easy return of dark red blood into the syringe. Once in the vein, roll the syringe, so that the bevel of the needle is directed inferiorly.
8. If the 5-mL syringe has a plunger entry port, insert the guidewire through the port and into the vein. Leave one third of the wire's length free, and maintain control of this end with your dominant hand. If the 5-mL syringe does not have a plunger entry port, remove the syringe from the needle hub, and occlude the needle hub with your nondominant thumb until you insert the guidewire. If you do not have to traverse the syringe's length, leave one half of the guidewire free and secured.
9. Using your nondominant hand, remove the syringe/needle assembly, gliding it along the guidewire. *Be sure to maintain the position of the guidewire in the superior vena cava.*
10. Nick the skin with the no. 11 scalpel blade by following the guidewire as it courses into the deeper tissues.
11. Slide the dilator over the guidewire, and run it along the guidewire into the subclavian vein up to the hub. Using a twisting motion while inserting the dilator may facilitate its advance. *Continue to maintain control of the guidewire*. Remove the dilator by sliding it out of the vein and off the guidewire.
12. Remove the central venous catheter from the kit, and if color coded, remove the *brown* port hub. In some kits, the catheter is stiff enough to be inserted alone, directly over the guidewire. Otherwise, insert the dilator into the catheter (or some kits have a smaller diameter introducer that fits into the catheter to stiffen it). Slide the catheter (and dilator/introducer if needed, as a unit) over the guidewire, and advance the guidewire *up into the catheter* until it just pokes out of the open port. Holding the end of the wire, slide the catheter and dilator/introducer down over the wire to the desired depth of insertion into the vein. Using a twisting motion when advancing the catheter may facilitate its advance. Leave 2 to 3 inches of the catheter free; otherwise the catheter will traverse too deeply into the heart. *Secure the position of the catheter with your nondominant hand.*

13. Remove the dilator/introducer over the guidewire and then remove the guidewire, pulling it free from the catheter. This leaves the catheter in place. Aspirate just to ensure that the catheter tip is in the superior vena cava; this is confirmed by the easy return of dark red blood into the syringe. Attach a flush syringe to the brown port, and flush with 5 to 10 mL of saline.
14. Remove the flush syringe, and hook up the IV line or clave-type connector.
15. Secure the catheter with a silk skin suture, and cover any exposed catheter with a sterile dressing.
16. Obtain an immediate chest radiograph to confirm position of catheter in the superior vena cava and to ensure that no pneumothorax was created during catheter insertion. You can always back the catheter out an inch or two if it is too deeply inserted into the right atrium. Ideally, the catheter tip should lie in the superior vena cava, just above the right atrium.

NOTE: Occasionally, the subclavian artery may be entered during placement of the catheter. This is marked by a rush of bright red arterial blood into the syringe or out of the needle hub. If this occurs, withdraw all needles, and place pressure over the site for 10 minutes. Obtain an urgent radiograph of the chest to check for pneumothorax/hemothorax, and check the distal arm pulse frequently. Recheck the hematocrit in 1 hour, and choose another site for venous access. If the catheter is seen to loop *up* the ipsilateral jugular vein, contralateral innominate vein, or contralateral subclavian vein on post-placement radiograph, the catheter will need repositioning. Because the sterile field has been removed, repositioning the catheter will involve a rewiring procedure. This procedure involves withdrawing the catheter until the tip lies just outside the ipsilateral jugular or innominate vein and then threading a sterile wire through the brown port of the preexisting catheter. The preexisting catheter is then removed leaving the wire in place and a new sterile catheter is introduced over wire using the Seldinger technique. Care must be taken to keep the wire sterile while discontinuing the "old" catheter.

Internal Jugular Vein Catheterization

Advantages of the internal jugular technique include the ability to cannulate the vessel during ongoing CPR and a relatively low iatrogenic complication rate. Bleeding complications are easily controlled by direct compression; hence this is the preferred approach for those patients who have a concurrent coagulopathy. Disadvantages include limited neck motion of the patient after insertion and injuries to the recurrent laryngeal nerve, phrenic nerve, and brachial plexus during insertion. A rare complication is ipsilateral pneumothorax. The central approach to internal jugular vein catheterization is described here:

1. Prepare the central catheter kit for use.
2. Position the patient as in Figure 211-2. Review the relevant anatomy, remembering that the internal jugular vein appears just under the triangular apex formed by the sternocleidomastoid muscle as it splits into sternal and clavicular heads. The vein then runs closely along the anterior border of the clavicular head of the sternocleidomastoid muscle and is lateral to the carotid artery.
3. Prep and drape the area to define a sterile field, and don mask, cap, eye protection, sterile gloves, and gown. Maintain strict sterile technique from here onward. Observe universal blood and body fluid precautions.
4. Anesthetize with 1% lidocaine a 1- to 2-cm diameter area just caudal to the apex of the sternocleidomastoid muscle. Attach the 22-gauge seeker needle to the 3-mL syringe.
5. The insertion site is located just at, or slightly caudal to, the apex of the sternocleidomastoid triangle, in the anesthetized field. Insert the seeker needle; aim toward the *ipsilateral nipple* at a 30-degree angle. Entry to the vein is marked by the easy return of dark red blood into the syringe. Figure 211-7 shows the needle's approach to the vein.

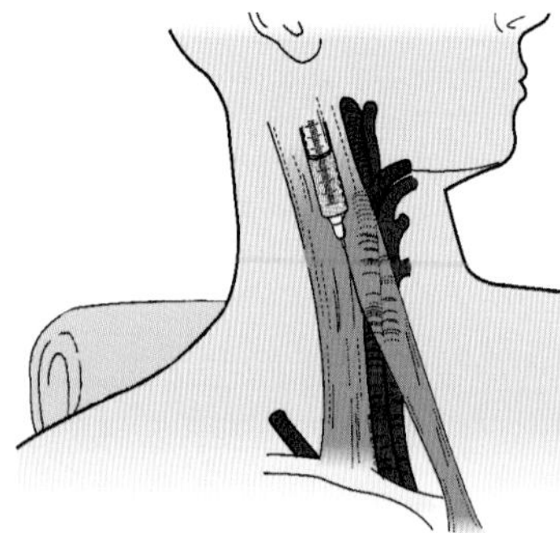

Figure 211-7 Needle approach to the internal jugular vein.

6. Once the internal jugular vein has been located, remove the seeker needle. Using the 18-gauge 2½-inch needle on a 5-mL syringe, insert it along the track of the seeker needle (i.e., the same direction, angle, and depth of penetration) to enter the internal jugular vein. Entry is confirmed by the easy return of dark red blood into the syringe.
7. If the 5-mL syringe has a plunger entry port, insert the guidewire through the port and into the vein. Leave one third of the wire's length free, and maintain control of this end with your dominant hand. If the 5-mL syringe does not have a plunger entry port, remove the syringe from the needle hub, and occlude the needle hub with your nondominant thumb until you insert the guidewire. If you do not have to traverse the syringe's length, leave one half of the guidewire free and secured.
8. Using your nondominant hand, remove the syringe/needle assembly, gliding it along the guidewire. *Be sure to maintain the position of the guidewire in the internal jugular vein.*
9. Nick the skin with the no. 11 scalpel blade by following the guidewire as it courses into the deeper tissues.
10. Slide the dilator over the guidewire, and run it along the guidewire into the internal jugular vein up to the hub. Using a twisting motion while inserting the dilator may facilitate its advance. *Continue to maintain control of the guidewire.* Remove the dilator by sliding it out of the body and off the guidewire.
11. Remove the central venous catheter from the kit, and if color coded, remove the *brown* port hub. In some kits, the catheter is stiff enough to be inserted alone, directly over the guidewire. Otherwise, insert the dilator into the catheter (some kits have a smaller diameter introducer that fits into the catheter to stiffen it). Slide the catheter (and dilator/introducer if needed, as a unit) over the guidewire, and advance the guidewire *up into the catheter* until it just pokes out of the open port. Holding the end of the wire, slide the catheter and dilator/introducer down over the wire to the desired depth of insertion into the vein. Using a twisting motion when advancing the catheter may facilitate its advance. Leave 2 to 3 inches of the catheter free; otherwise the catheter will traverse too deeply into the heart. *Secure the position of the catheter with your nondominant hand.*
12. Remove the dilator/introducer over the guidewire and then remove the guidewire, pulling it free from the catheter. This leaves the catheter in place. Aspirate to ensure position of the catheter tip in the vein; this is confirmed by easy return of dark red blood into the syringe. Attach a flush syringe to the brown port, and flush with 5 to 10 mL of saline.
13. Remove the flush syringe, and hook up the IV line or clave-type connector.
14. Secure catheter with a silk skin suture, and cover any exposed catheter with a plastic film dressing.
15. Obtain an immediate chest radiograph to confirm position of catheter in the superior vena cava, and to ensure that no pneu-

mothorax was created during catheter insertion. You can always withdraw the catheter an inch or two if it is too deeply inserted into the right atrium. Ideally, the catheter tip should lie in the superior vena cava just above the right atrium.

Femoral Vein Catheterization

Femoral vein catheterization is an alternative route to access the central venous system. Like the methods discussed previously, femoral vein catheterization may be used to deliver large volumes of fluid, chemotherapeutic agents, or total parenteral nutrition. By converting a femoral venous catheter to a percutaneous sheath introducer, a transvenous pacing wire or a Swan-Ganz catheter may be inserted. The femoral vein is easier to cannulate than the internal jugular or subclavian veins, and is readily accessible during CPR or other resuscitation. The few disadvantages to a femoral approach include the difficulty in sterilizing the groin insertion site, keeping it clean once the line is inserted, the increased risk of catheter-related venous thrombosis, and the fact that it limits patient mobility if the patient is ambulatory.

Contraindications to femoral line insertion include ipsilateral groin surgery or cellulitis over the proposed insertion site; a prosthetic vascular graft on the side of the proposed insertion; veno-occlusive diseases of the extremities or femoral venous thrombosis; and any uncontrolled bleeding diathesis. Because of the relatively superficial location of the femoral vein, direct pressure may be readily applied if required, and this author recommends this approach for those patients who are anticoagulated and require rapid central venous access.

Review the relevant anatomy in Figure 211-8. Note the neurovascular structures run in the following sequence from lateral to medial: nerve, artery, vein, "empty space," and lymphatics. The insertion site for femoral vein catheterization is just inferior to the femoral ligament, and 1 to 1.5 cm medial to the femoral artery, whose palpable pulse forms an important landmark for this procedure.

1. The patient should be flat in the supine position or in slight reverse Trendelenburg position. (The Trendelenburg position is contraindicated for this route of access due to the risk of venous air embolism.)
2. Set up the central venous catheter kit.
3. Wash hands and don mask, cap, eye protection, sterile gown, and gloves. Observe universal blood and body fluid precautions.
4. Prep and drape the groin area to obtain a sterile field. In obese persons, you may need an assistant to hold back any redundant pannus from the groin area in order to gain access to the femoral vein.
5. Locate the femoral pulse with fingers of your nondominant hand.
6. Using the 25-gauge needle on a 3-mL syringe, draw up 3 mL of lidocaine and anesthetize the area just medial to the femoral artery.

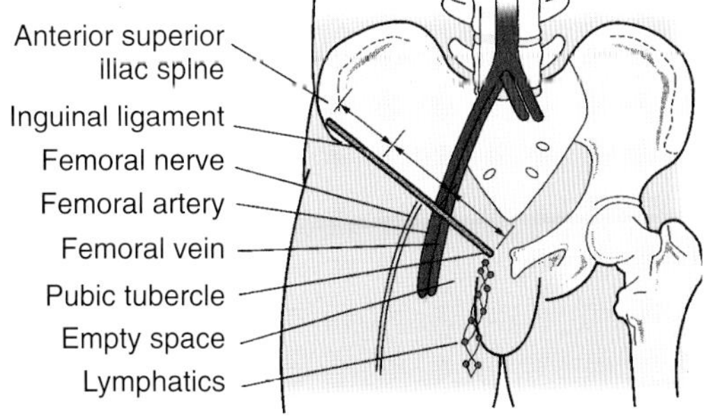

Figure 211-8 Relevant anatomy of groin showing relationship of femoral vein to surrounding structures.

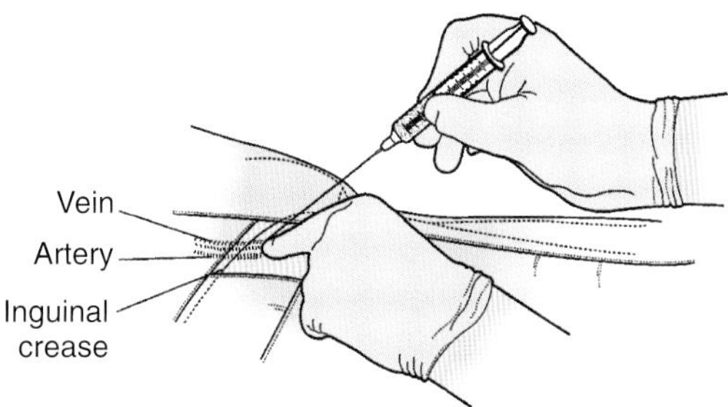

Figure 211-9 Approach to femoral vein cannulation.

7. You may use the 22-gauge needle on a 3-mL syringe as a seeker, or proceed directly with the 2½-inch 18-gauge needle on the 5-mL syringe with plunger port to find the femoral vein. Refer to Figure 211-9 for the approach to cannulation. With bevel down, angle the needle at 30 degrees to the skin, and aim at the ipsilateral nipple. Aspirate as you insert the needle. Entry into the femoral vein is marked by the easy return of dark red blood into the syringe. Once a free flow of blood is verified, *stop advancing the needle.*
8. Stabilize the 2½-inch needle and syringe assembly with your nondominant hand. If the syringe has a plunger port, pass the guidewire down this port, feeding approximately one half of the wire into the femoral vein. If there is no plunger port, carefully rotate the syringe off the needle hub, and advance the guidewire into the vein.
9. Maintain control of the distal end of the guidewire with your dominant hand, and remove the 2½-inch needle/syringe assembly over the wire with your nondominant hand.
10. Nick the skin at the entry site of the guidewire with the no. 11 scalpel blade. Thread the dilator over the guidewire, and run it into the groin several times to create a passage for the central venous catheter assembly. Maintain control of the distal end of the guidewire at all times.
11. Remove the dilator over the guidewire. If color coded, remove the *brown* hub from the central venous catheter. In some kits, the catheter is stiff enough to be inserted alone, directly over the guidewire. Otherwise, insert the dilator into the catheter (or some kits have a smaller diameter introducer that fits into the catheter to stiffen it). Slide the catheter and dilator/introducer as a unit over the wire, and advance the guidewire *up into the catheter* until it just pokes out of the open port. Holding the end of the wire, thread the catheter and dilator/introducer as a unit over the guidewire. Using a twisting motion when advancing the catheter may facilitate its advance. Advance the catheter over the wire until the catheter is fully within the femoral vein.
12. Remove the dilator/introducer over the guidewire and then remove the guidewire; this leaves the catheter in place. Stabilize the catheter with a free hand while the guidewire is pulled out.
13. Suture the catheter in place with a silk suture, and flush all catheter ports with saline; clave hubs may be attached at this time. Cover the insertion site with a sterile dressing.
14. Some practitioners may elect to perform an abdominal flat plate radiograph at this time to ensure placement of the catheter in the common iliac vein.
15. Lastly, some practitioners elect to give a dose of a broad-spectrum antibiotic at this time (although there is no evidence to support this practice).

COMPLICATIONS

- Thrombosis of the vein
- Hemorrhage or hematoma at the insertion site

- Local, systemic, or catheter-related infection (often from poor sterile technique, but not always)
- Hydrothorax from infusion of IV fluids into the chest cavity from erroneous placement of a catheter using subclavian or internal jugular approach
- Tracheal perforation
- Perforation of an endotracheal tube cuff
- Air embolus (usually with subclavian or internal jugular vein catheter insertion if patient was not placed in Trendelenburg position prior to vein cannulation)
- Guidewire fragment embolus (results from shear of guidewire when it is pulled back out of insertion needle)
- Lost guidewire
- Laceration of a lymphatic duct
- Arteriovenous fistula
- Superior vena caval obstruction
- Pericardial tamponade
- Injury to local nerve structures
- Catheter malposition (a catheter inserted into the subclavian or internal jugular vein may thread itself back up into the neck or the arm)
- Catheter kinking
- Cardiac dysrhythmias

CPT/Billing Codes

36010 Introduction of catheter into central vein
36011 Selective catheter placement, venous system, first order branch

ICD-9-CM Diagnostic Codes

See also ICD-9-CM codes for Chapter 215, Swan-Ganz (Pulmonary Artery) Catheterization, and Chapter 216, Temporary Pacing.

260 Protein calorie malnutrition
261 Severe calorie deficiency
276.51 Dehydration
276.52 Hypovolemia
276.6 Fluid overload or fluid retention
401.0 Accelerated or malignant essential hypertension
410.11 Myocardial infarction, initial episode, anterior wall (can include damage such as ruptured myocardium)
410.91 Myocardial infarction, acute, unspecified, initial episode (can include damage such as ruptured myocardium)
415.0 Cor pulmonale, acute
423.3 Cardiac tamponade
423.9 Pericardial effusion or unspecified disease of pericardium
427.1 Paroxysmal ventricular tachycardia
427.5 Cardiac or cardiorespiratory arrest
428.0 Right-sided heart failure, secondary to left or heart failure, congestive, unspecified
428.1 Pulmonary edema (left-sided heart failure)
584.9 Acute renal failure, unspecified
585.0 Chronic renal failure
669.1 Shock, obstetric
785.50 Shock, unspecified
785.51 Shock, cardiogenic
785.52 Shock, septic
785.59 Shock, other (hypovolemic)
958.4 Traumatic shock
995.4 Shock, anaphylactic
998.0 Surgical or postoperative shock

Acknowledgment

The editors wish to recognize the many contributions by John F. Donnelly, MD, John M. Passmore, Jr., MD, Thomas A. Bzoskie, MD, and Brian D. Madden, MD, to this chapter in the previous two editions of this text.

BIBLIOGRAPHY

Chen H, Sonnenday CJ: Manual of Common Bedside Surgical Procedures, 2nd ed. Philadelphia, Lippincott Williams & Wilkins, 2000, pp 35–55.
Custalow CB: Color Atlas of Emergency Department Procedures. Philadelphia, Elsevier, 2005, pp 15–18.
Feldman R: Central venous access. In Reichman EF, Simon RR (eds): Emergency Medicine Procedures. New York, McGraw-Hill, 2004.
James D (ed): Intravenous access techniques. In: A Field Guide to Urgent and Ambulatory Procedures. Philadelphia, Lippincott, 2001.
Roberts JR, Hedges JR (eds): Clinical Procedures in Emergency Medicine. Philadelphia, WB Saunders, 2002.

CHAPTER 212

Tube Thoracostomy and Emergency Needle Decompression of Tension Pneumothorax

Scott Savage

Tube thoracostomy, or chest tube insertion, is performed to evacuate air or fluid from the pleural space. A related procedure, emergency needle decompression, is performed to relieve a tension pneumothorax. Tension pneumothorax is a life-threatening condition. Air progressively accumulates in the pleural space, eventually compressing the lung and the mediastinum, causing decreased blood flow in the great vessels and subsequent death. Patients with tension pneumothorax present with dyspnea, tachycardia, and hypoxia. Jugular venous distention and midline tracheal shift are classically described but rarely present. Hypotension is an ominous sign that signifies obstructive shock.

The radiographic features of a tension pneumothorax are a 100% pneumothorax with a midline shift away from the collapsed lung. However, if clinically suspected, an emergency needle decompression should be performed; to wait for a confirming chest radiograph is unnecessary. A preprocedure chest radiograph should be obtained only in stable patients in whom the diagnosis is in question.

Diagnosing a tension pneumothorax in infants may be difficult because lobar emphysema can mimic a pneumothorax. Making the correct diagnosis is essential because chest tube insertion in the presence of lobar emphysema can make the infant worse. If the infant is hemodynamically stable, it is advisable to get three radiographic views of the chest—lateral, anteroposterior (AP), and lateral decubitus with the affected side inferior. A specialist in radiology, pediatrics, or pediatric emergency medicine should be consulted to help with film interpretation.

Emergency Needle Decompression

Indication

Tension pneumothorax indicates the need for emergency needle decompression.

Contraindication

Lobar emphysema in infants is a *relative* contraindication.

Equipment

- Antiseptic solution (e.g., povidone–iodine, chlorhexidine)
- Sterile hemostat
- 10-mL syringe half-filled with 2% lidocaine with epinephrine (or equivalent) attached to a large-bore (18-gauge or larger), 2-inch catheter-over-needle (angiocatheter)
- Supplemental oxygen, continuous cardiac and blood pressure monitoring

Technique

1. Place the patient in the semiupright position (head of bed elevated to 30 to 60 degrees).
2. Provide supplemental oxygen. If available, continuous cardiac and blood pressure monitoring is helpful.
3. Obtain rapid verbal consent with a witness present, if possible.
4. Apply antiseptic solution to a generous area of the second intercostal space where a line drawn laterally from the level of the sternomanubrial junction (Lewis's line) would intersect a line drawn down from the mid-clavicle (mid-clavicular line).
5. Locate the *upper border* of the rib at this intersection.
6. Insert the catheter-over-needle perpendicular to the skin just above the upper border of the rib (Fig. 212-1). (Remember that the neurovascular bundle runs below the ribs.) Once through the skin, infiltrate the tissue with half of the anesthetic solution.
7. Before proceeding further, attempt aspiration. If air is obtained, then the catheter-over-needle is not secured to the syringe tightly enough. Use the hemostat to tighten the catheter hub on the syringe before advancing the catheter-over-needle any farther.
8. After creating the skin wheal and testing the seal, advance the catheter-over-needle at a moderate rate with continuous aspiration until air is obtained—this will be noted by bubbles in the syringe and easy aspiration.
9. Advance the catheter-over-needle an additional half centimeter to prevent accidental dislodgement.
10. Using the hemostat, unscrew the syringe to allow free passage of air. *Do not* hook up the needle to suction. The air in the thoracic cavity is under pressure (under tension) and will exit the needle spontaneously; it should gush out. Intrathoracic pressure will equilibrate with room air, which is acceptable until tube thoracostomy is placed.

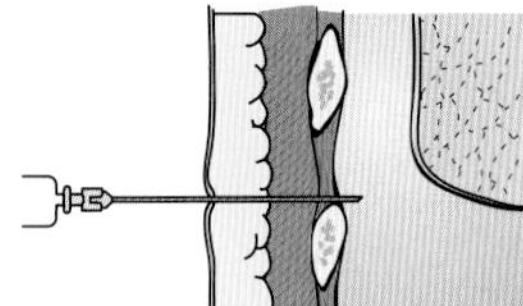

Figure 212-1 Placement of a catheter within a needle. Insert the needle slightly above the rib, and air should return or express itself through the needle.

11. *Do not* remove the needle at this point. In older texts, it was advised to remove the needle because the plastics in older catheters were much harder than the soft Silastic catheters now used. Unlike the older catheters, the new catheters are too soft to endure the tissue pressure of the intercostal muscles and will rapidly collapse, causing reaccumulation of the tension pneumothorax. Concerns that the re-expanding lung will be impaled on and lacerated by the needle (pulmonary laceration) are generally unfounded. There is a 100% pneumothorax present, and it is unlikely that lung tissue is near the needle tip so long as suction is not used. The purpose of this procedure is to relieve excessive intrathoracic pressure and allow blood circulation. Subsequent tube thoracostomy, hopefully performed very soon after emergency needle decompression, will provide full lung re-expansion. The time to remove the catheter-over-needle (angiocatheter) is just prior to applying suction to the chest tube.

EDITOR'S NOTE: In one ultrasound study (Ball and collegues, 2010), a 1¼-inch-long catheter-over-needle would fail to reach the pleural space in 65% of adults; however, a 1¾-inch catheter-over needle should reach the pleural space in 96% of adults.

TUBE THORACOSTOMY

Indications

- Pneumothorax
- After needle decompression of a tension pneumothorax
- Chylothorax
- Empyema
- Hemothorax
- Malignant pleural effusion
- Pleurodesis
- Recurrent pleural effusion
- Prevention of a hydrothorax after thoracotomy (cardiothoracic or lung resection surgery)

Contraindications

- No contraindications if the procedure is emergent.
- Bleeding dyscrasia.
- Severe thrombocytopenia (platelet count <50,000 cells/mL *relative contraindication*).
- Bullae (*relative contraindication*).
- Conditions causing pleural scarring in the area of planned insertion.
- Empyema with acid-fast organisms.
- History of pleurodesis.
- Use caution if loculated fluid collections are present.
- Pneumothorax of less than 20% that is stable for 6 hours (Fig. 212-2).
- Known or suspected mesothelioma.

There are many methods to determine whether or not a pneumothorax is greater than 20%. One method is to use the "1 cm and one third rule": if a pneumothorax creates no more than 1 cm distance between the pleural line and the inner chest wall and is also confined to the upper one third of the chest on an AP upright radiograph, then the pneumothorax is less than 20%. These may resolve without any intervention (see Fig. 212-2). Stability is gauged by comparing a chest radiograph taken initially to one obtained 6 hours later. Although it may require thoracostomy, a simple pneumothorax is the accumulation of air, not under pressure, within the pleural space.

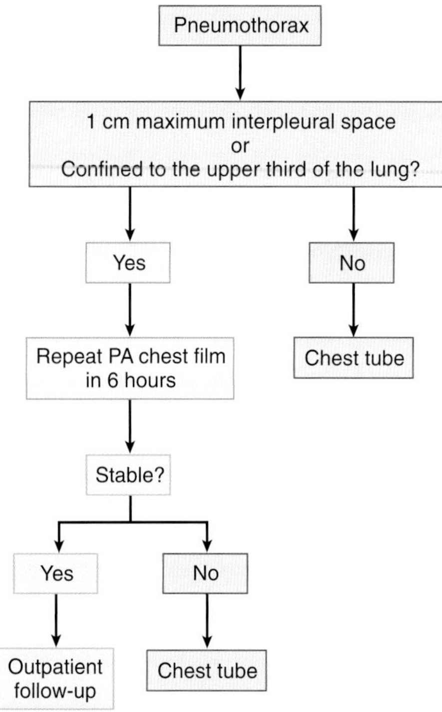

Figure 212-2 Algorithm used for deciding necessity of thoracostomy. PA, posteroanterior.

Results from some studies suggest that mere aspiration of a simple pneumothorax can be performed without placing a chest tube. However, this method is still controversial, because other studies indicate little better than a 50% success rate. The success rate may be higher in carefully selected patients.

Equipment

- Adhesive tape (Tensoplast or Elastoplast preferred)
- Antiseptic solution (e.g., povidone–iodine, chlorhexidine)
- Chest tube (alternatives are Seldinger guidewire kit or catheter-over-needle kit; Heimlich valve can be attached)
- Connector (5-in-1, also known as Christmas tree connector)
- Local anesthetic
- Petroleum impregnated gauze
- Sterile drapes
- Sterile gown and gloves
- Suction-drainage system (Fig. 212-3)
- Surgical mask, cap, and goggles
- Wall suction unit
- Supplemental oxygen, pulse oximetry, continuous cardiac and blood pressure monitoring
- Thoracostomy tray
  - 4 sterile towels
  - 1 package 4 × 4 inch sterile gauze pads
  - 4 towel clips (*optional*)
  - 1 large straight scissors
  - 1 large curved (Mayo) scissors
  - 2 large curved (Kelly) clamps
  - 2 medium-sized clamps
  - 1 needle holder
  - 1 package of 2-0 to 4-0 nonabsorbable suture
  - 1 no. 11 or no. 10 scalpel mounted onto a holder

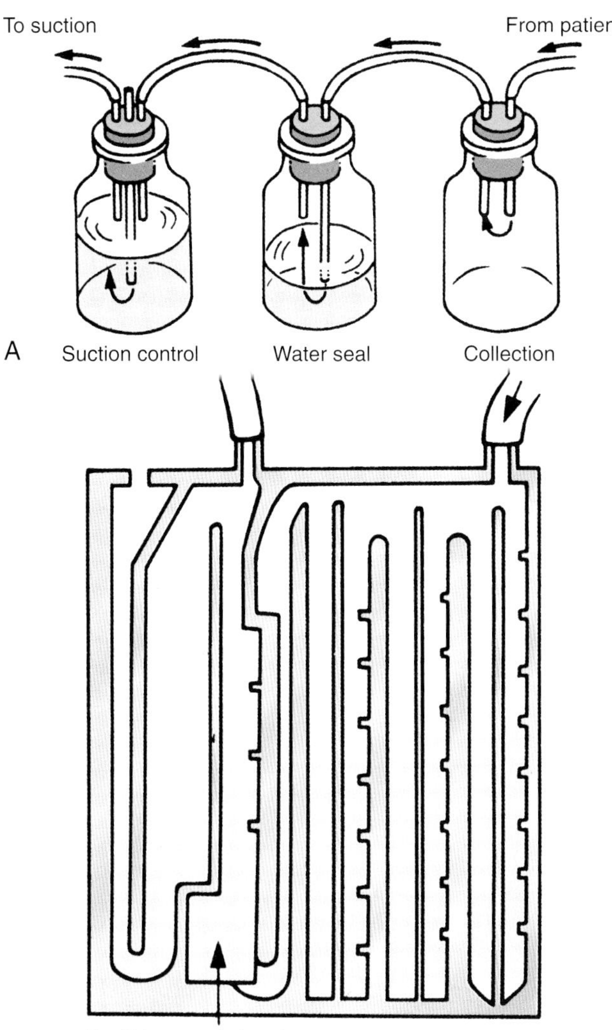

Figure 212-3 **A,** Three-bottle system: first bottle (*right*) is the collection chamber; second bottle (*center*) is the water seal; third bottle (*left*), closest to wall suction, is the suction control chamber. **B,** Disposable suction unit.

NOTE: Trocars have a high complication rate and should not be used.

Adult tube size selection

- Primary spontaneous pneumothorax: 7 F to 14 F
- Secondary spontaneous pneumothorax: 20 F to 28 F
- Trauma, mechanical ventilation, or detectable pleural fluid: 28 F to 40 F

Secondary spontaneous pneumothoraces are associated with underlying lung diseases such as chronic obstructive pulmonary disease (COPD), asthma, cystic fibrosis, infection, interstitial lung disease, neoplasms, connective tissue disease, pulmonary infarction, and endometriosis.

Procedures

Initial Preparation (for All Techniques)

1. Obtain written informed consent if possible. Patient should be aware of the indications, risks, and complications of the procedure, and whether any alternatives exist.
2. Because the procedure can be rather painful, the patient should be warned and prepared, even if a local anesthetic is used. Procedural sedation is recommended (see Chapter 2, Procedural Sedation and Analgesia). If time allows, obtain a partial thromboplastin time (PTT), international normalized ratio (INR), and platelet count.
3. Place the patient on 100% oxygen. (Use of oxygen increases the resorption rate of pneumothorax by fourfold.)
4. Monitor the patient with pulse oximetry and continuous cardiac and blood pressure monitoring.
5. An ultrasound (see Chapter 225, Emergency Department, Hospitalist, and Office Ultrasonography [Clinical Ultrasonography]) may be helpful for localizing the air or fluid levels and for possibly excluding any anatomic variants that could place the patient at risk.
6. Assemble the suction-drainage system according to the manufacturer's recommendations.
7. Connect the suction-drainage system to suction.
8. Create a sterile field for the equipment.
9. Measure the length of tube to be inserted: from the mid-axillary line at the fifth intercostal space to the inferior tip of the scapula. A piece of suture with the needle removed is often used to make this measurement.
10. In a sterile manner, open the package containing the tube and occlude the distal end at the properly measured distance with a large sterile clamp.
11. The distal end (usually beveled) of the tube can be cut so that it is "squared off," if needed to ensure a firm connection.
12. Place the patient in the semiupright position with the ipsilateral arm placed overhead and the wrist secured with a soft restraint. Use standard restraint monitoring.
13. Maintain sterile technique, including use of face mask, gown, and sterile gloves, and observe universal blood and body fluid precautions.
14. Mark the fifth intercostal space just slightly anterior to the mid-axillary line. In males, this is generally one space below the nipple line. In females, it is generally two fingerbreadths above the base (not the tip) of the xiphoid. Although an anterior approach was used in the past for pure pneumothoraces, it has fallen out of favor. (Studies have failed to demonstrate a significant clinical advantage and this approach leads to worse cosmetic results.) The posterior approach is generally reserved for thoracentesis.
15. Prepare the incision site area with antiseptic solution, and drape to create an adequate sterile field.
16. In a sterile fashion, infiltrate the skin with 2 to 4 mL of lidocaine 2% with epinephrine or equivalent local anesthesia at the *incision* site. Be careful to insert the needle just above the upper border of the rib. This avoids damage to the neurovascular bundle, which lies in a groove at the lower border of the ribs. Then use up to 6.5 mg/kg lidocaine with epinephrine (1 mL of 2% lidocaine contains 20 mg of lidocaine) to anesthetize the deeper structures along the tract that the chest tube will traverse and enter the pleural space (Fig. 212-4 shows a Z-tract technique).

Seldinger Guidewire Technique

1. Prepare as directed in "Initial Preparation" section.
2. The Seldinger guidewire technique requires use of a prepackaged kit, but it is generally preferred to the traditional open technique. For most operators, it is simpler, faster, and safer than the open technique. A Z-tract technique is unnecessary.
3. Open the kit and check the inventory to ensure all necessary materials are present and double check that the items listed on the package cover have been properly packaged. (Note that some kits do not include the ancillaries [cleaning swabs, tape, lidocaine for anesthetic].)
4. Using the locator needle, insert the tip just above the top of the rib in the anesthetized area, slowly advance the needle

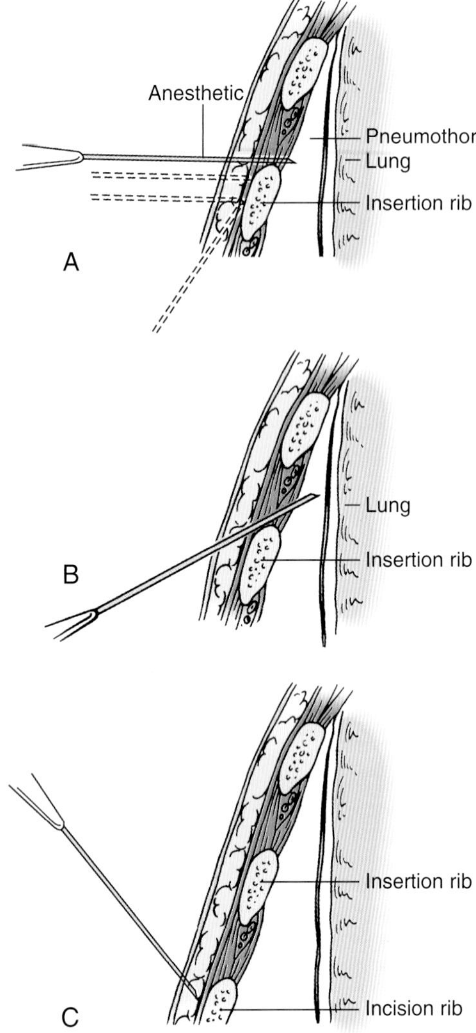

Figure 212-4 Infiltration of the skin, subcutaneous muscle, and periosteum of the rib (**A**); the pleura (**B**); and skin incision site (**C**) with local anesthetic.

perpendicular to the thorax, and enter the pleural cavity while aspirating for air, blood, or other fluid (similar to Fig. 212-1).

5. Once air, blood, or fluid is obtained, feed the guidewire posteriorly and superiorly toward the scapula in adults or anteriorly and superiorly toward the manubrium or sternal notch in small children.
6. Maintaining manual control of the guidewire at all times, remove the locator needle and nick the skin in a direction parallel to the rib with an 11-blade scalpel to about one third the depth of the scalpel.
7. Feed the smallest dilator over the guidewire with a twisting motion, and once through the skin, aim toward the tip of the scapula in adults and the sternal notch in small children.
8. If progressive dilators are available, use these to gradually widen the insertion track.
9. Remove the dilators and insert the chest tube over the guidewire to the premeasured length.
10. Remove the guidewire.
11. Attach the chest tube to the suction-drainage system. Be careful when removing the distal clamp, as blood or fluid may flow forcefully from the tube.
12. Have the patient cough, and check for bubbles in the water seal, which indicates good flow. (A Heimlich valve may then be used for a simple pneumothorax and no recurrent leaking.)
13. Secure the tube with tape (Tensoplast or Elastoplast tape is preferred; avoid taping the nipple), and obtain a chest radiograph. Suturing is not absolutely necessary, although it is recommended to ensure that the tube does not get dislodged. Likewise, petroleum gauze is not absolutely required unless an air leak is identified.
14. If no adjustment is needed, then tape the suction connector to the tube.
15. Consider use of prophylactic antibiotics.

Using Pneumothorax Evacuation Kits (Catheter-over-Needle, Heimlich Valve)

1. Special kits containing a single catheter-over-needle device, a connector, and a Heimlich valve are now available. They are used only in simple pneumothoraces but are very convenient and effective for that process.
2. Prepare as directed in the "Initial Preparation" section. Enter the interspace using the locator needle. Remove the needle.
3. Insert the catheter-over-needle tip just above the top of the rib in the anesthetized area, slowly advance the needle perpendicular to the thorax, and enter the pleural cavity while aspirating for air (similar to Fig. 212-1).
4. Once air is obtained, the catheter is advanced, the needle removed, and the Heimlich valve connected.
5. The Heimlich valve is taped to the anterior chest wall. This reduces the chance of the patient accidentally dislodging it with the elbow.
6. A postprocedure radiograph is required.
7. Although clinical judgment is required, it has been suggested that many patients receiving these types of devices may be discharged for next day follow-up.

Traditional (Open) Technique

1. Prepare as directed in "Initial Preparation" section.
2. At the fifth intercostal space in the mid-axillary line where the lower skin wheal was anesthetized, create a 2- to 4-cm skin incision (approximately two fingerbreadths) that follows the rib (Fig. 212-5).
3. Using a curved Kelly clamp, bluntly dissect until bone or muscle fascia is reached.
4. From this position, change the direction of the dissection superiorly, with the tips of the clamp directed upward, until the

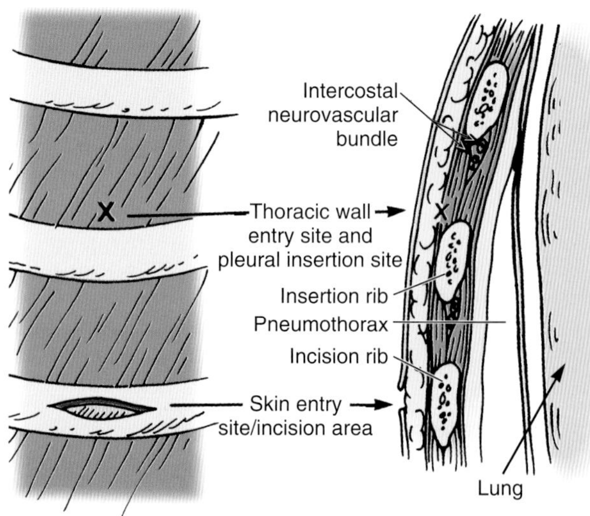

Figure 212-5 Skin incision is made one rib below the rib over which the tube will pass. Location of the intercostal neurovascular bundle is shown.

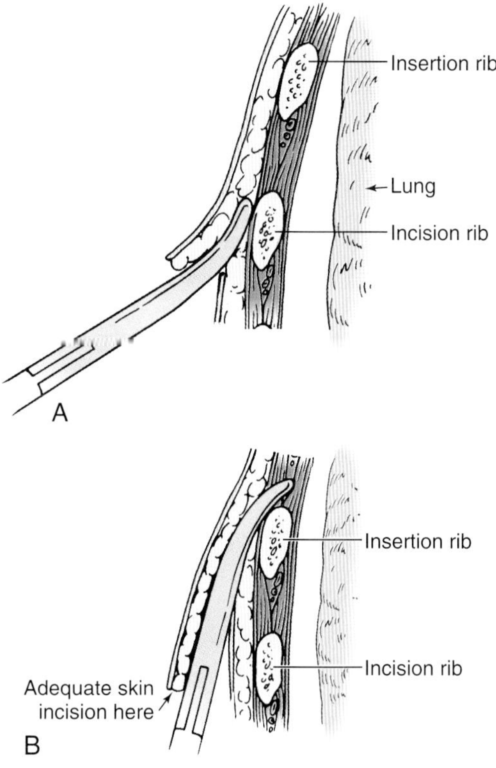

Figure 212-6 **A** and **B,** Tunneling procedure diagram that forms a Z-tract. (See text for details.)

upper border of the next rib is reached (Fig. 212-6). This should be at the level of the second anesthetic wheal.

5. From that position, rotate the tip of the curved clamp inward and use it to push through the intercostal muscle and parietal pleura. A popping sensation is often felt. (Do not push the clamp too far into the pleural space where it could cause damage to the great vessels, heart, diaphragm, or lungs.)
6. Once inside the pleural space, open the clamp and withdraw partially to widen the space. Be careful not to withdraw completely, as you may then lose the opening and therefore have to begin again.
7. Using the other hand, place a gloved finger in the pleural space (Fig. 212-7) as you withdraw the open curved clamp completely.

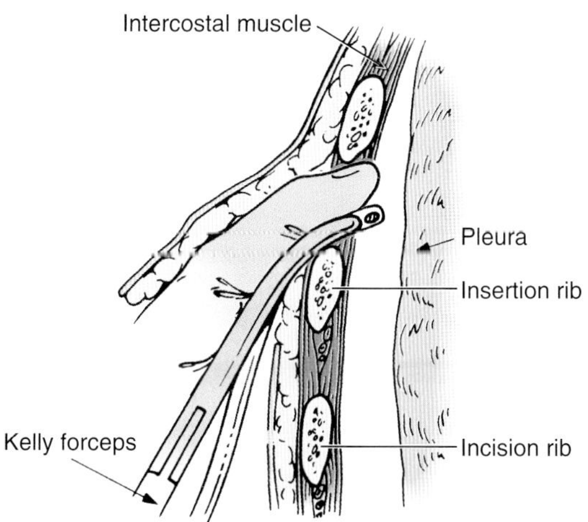

Figure 212-7 Tip placement in the pleural cavity, using the finger as a guide.

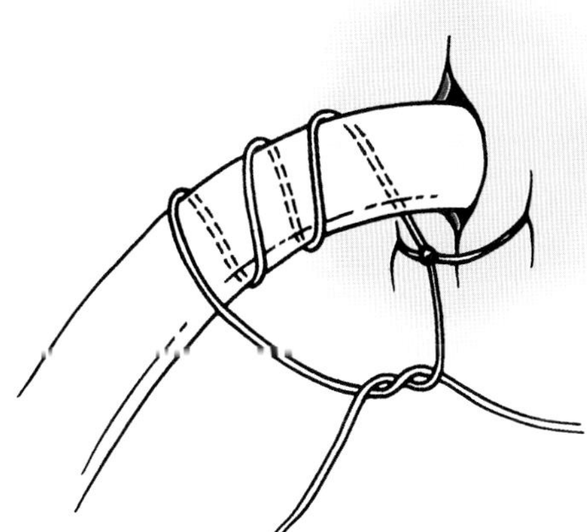

Figure 212-8 Chest tube is fastened with a stay suture.

The idea is to keep either the clamp or your finger in the hole at all times to prevent losing the opening.

8. Sweep the finger to confirm proper placement (you should not feel the diaphragm) and to detect any adhesions.
9. Using the curved clamp, grasp the proximal end of the tube (fenestrated end) and guide the tube into the pleural space, withdrawing your finger as you do so. Again, the idea is to keep either your finger or the tube in the hole at all times to prevent losing the opening.
10. Connect the tube to the suction-drainage system. Be careful when opening the distal clamp, as blood or fluid may flow forcefully from the tube.
11. Attach the suction-drainage system to suction.
12. Have the patient cough, and check for bubbles in the water seal, which indicates a patent system.
13. Suture the tube in place, taking care not to puncture the tubing. A variety of techniques are acceptable. A common one is to use a single horizontal mattress suture to close the incision around the tube. After tying a knot, and before cutting the suture ends, wind one around the tube several times and back to tie to the other end (Fig. 212-8). Alternatively, a second suture can be placed through the skin; it is then wound around the tube several times and secured with a knot.
14. Wrap the tube with petroleum gauze and secure the tube with tape (avoid taping the nipple).
15. Obtain a chest radiograph. Remove the chest tube and insert a new one if it is kinked, bent, in the fissure of the lung, or in the subcutaneous tissues.
16. If no adjustment is needed, then tape the suction connector to the tube, and the tube to the patient's side. (Tensoplast or Elastoplast tape is preferred.)
17. Consider the use of prophylactic antibiotics.

Management

After the chest tube is inserted, it should be connected to the suction-drainage system. Suction should be maintained until there is no air leak. Although many different protocols exist as to when to consider removing the tube, the most prudent method is to turn off the suction after the patient's lung re-expands and allow the patient to remain on water seal for 6 to 12 hours to detect occult air leaks. Chest tube dressings should be changed every 24 hours, or sooner if the dressing becomes saturated.

A chest radiograph taken 4 to 6 hours after chest tube insertion should show improvement in the pulmonary condition. If the patient's condition is not improved, check for persistent bubbling in the system. If bubbling is present, then check the connections between the chest tube, connectors, and hosing throughout the system. If the air leak continues, place cloth tape over all the connections. Examine a chest radiograph to confirm that all fenestrations are within the thoracic cavity. If not, replace the tube (advancing the current chest tube may track infectious material into the pleural cavity). If the air leak persists, check the tubing for holes or cracks, and replace any damaged tubing. If the air leak continues, place a second chest tube and prepare the patient for thoracoscopy, bronchoscopy, or esophagoscopy to diagnose the etiology of the leak.

Chest Tube Removal

Indications

- No air drainage for 24 hours
- Less than 150 mL fluid drainage in 24 hours

Contraindication

A persistent need for a chest tube contraindicates its removal.

Equipment

- Suture scissors
- Petroleum gauze
- Several sterile 4 × 4 inch gauze sponges
- Tape (Tensoplast or Elastoplast preferred)

Removal Technique

1. If sutures were used to secure the tube during placement, cut the sutures.
2. Disconnect the tube from the suction-drainage system.
3. If the patient is awake and cooperative, have the patient exhale and hold his or her breath. If the patient is nonalert and artificially ventilated, pause the ventilator in exhalation.
4. Swiftly and smoothly remove the tube.
5. Apply petroleum gauze covered by sterile 4 × 4 inch gauze sponges.
6. Apply a pressure dressing with tape (Tensoplast or Elastoplast preferred).
7. Repeat the chest radiograph in 6 to 12 hours.
8. Observe for complications.
9. After 48 hours, the dressing may be removed. The patient should follow routine wound care instructions.

Complications

- Injury to the heart, great vessels, lung, diaphragm, liver, spleen, or even the intestines
- Subdiaphragmatic placement of tube
- Open pneumothorax
- Tension pneumothorax
- Dislodgement of the tube
- Subcutaneous emphysema
- Re-expansion pulmonary edema
- Unexplained or persistent air leakage
- Hemorrhage from an injured intercostal artery
- Local or more generalized infection

CPT/Billing Codes

32002 Thoracentesis with insertion of tube with or without water seal (e.g., for pneumothorax)

32020 Tube thoracostomy with or without water seal (e.g., for abscess, hemothorax, empyema)

ICD-9-CM Diagnostic Codes

011.7 Pneumothorax, tuberculous

012.0 Empyema, tuberculous

197.2 Pleura malignant or pleural effusion, malignant

457.8 Chylous hydrothorax

510.9 Empyema, without mention of fistula (use additional code to identify infectious organism [041.0 to 041.9])

511.1 Pleurisy with effusion, bacterial, nontuberculous

511.8 Hemothorax or hemopneumothorax

511.9 Pleural effusion, unspecified

512.0 Pneumothorax, tension, spontaneous

512.1 Pneumothorax, due to operative injury of chest wall or lung

512.8 Pneumothorax, spontaneous

772.8 Hemothorax, newborn

860.0 Pneumothorax, traumatic, without mention of open wound into thorax

860.2 Hemothorax, traumatic, without mention of open wound into thorax

860.4 Pneumohemothorax, traumatic, without mention of open wound into thorax

Acknowledgment

The editors wish to recognize the many contributions by Nelly Otero, MD, and José Ramón García, MD, to this chapter in previous editions of this text.

Suppliers

(Full contact information is available online at www.expertconsult.com.)

Atrium Ocean Water Seal Chest Drain System and Thoracostomy Tubes
Atrium Medical Corporation

Emergency Pneumothorax Kits
Cook Medical, Inc.

Pleur-Evac Water Seal Chest Drain System and Thoracostomy Tubes
Teleflex Medical

Thoracentesis Tray with Catheter-over-Needle
Allegiance/Cardinal Healthcare Company

Water Seal Chest Drain Systems, Thoracostomy Tubes, Thoracentesis Trays, and Pneumothorax Tray with 8-F Catheter; Argyle Aqua-Seal Systems; Argyle Turkel Safety Thoracentesis and Pneumothorax Tray
The Kendall Company (Covidien)

Online Resources

www.icu-usa.com/tour/procedures/thoracostomy.htm (accessed April 23, 2010).

www.merck.com/mmpe/sec05/ch047/ch047i.html (accessed April 23, 2010).

www.proceduresconsult.com (accessed April 23, 2010).

Bibliography

Ball CG, Wyrzykowski AD, Kirkpatrick AW, et al: Thoracic needle decompression for tension pneumothorax: Clinical correlation with catheter length. Can J Surg 53:184–188, 2010.

Ma OJ, Cline DM (eds): Emergency Medicine: Just the Facts, 2nd ed. New York, McGraw-Hill, 2004.

Marx JA (ed): Rosen's Emergency Medicine, 6th ed. Philadelphia, Mosby, 2006.

Reichmann EF, Simon SR (eds): Emergency Medicine Procedures. New York, McGraw-Hill, 2004.

Tintinelli JE, Kelen GD, Stapczynski JS (eds): Emergency Medicine: A Comprehensive Study Guide, 6th ed. New York, McGraw-Hill, 2004.

CHAPTER 213

TRACHEAL INTUBATION

Scott Savage

Airway emergencies can be some of the most daunting situations a practitioner encounters. Radical advances in airway management have been made and are reviewed here.

INDICATIONS

- Hypoxia
- Respiratory distress
- Protection of the airway
- Cardiopulmonary arrest
- Need to maintain hyperventilation (e.g., with traumatic brain injury)

CONTRAINDICATIONS

- Cervical spine injury (may use video and optical laryngoscopes, fiberoptic laryngoscope, or digital [tactile] technique)
- Cervical spine severely immobilized due to arthritis (may use video and optical laryngoscopes, fiberoptic laryngoscope, or digital [tactile] technique)
- Expanding neck hematoma (relative, must use caution but may require surgical airway)
- Uncontrolled oropharyngeal hemorrhage (relative, may require surgical airway)
- Intact tracheostomy or stoma (replace tracheostomy tube)
- Combative patient (consider rapid-sequence intubation [RSI]—described in this chapter)
- Trismus (consider RSI or nasotracheal intubation)
- Severe facial or neck trauma (consider needle or surgical cricothyroidotomy; see Chapter 199, Cricothyroid Catheter Insertion, Cricothyroidotomy, and Tracheostomy)

EQUIPMENT

See Figure 213-1.

- Laryngoscope (and fresh batteries)
- Laryngoscope blades (at least two different types)
- Endotracheal tubes
  - Adult men sizes 7 to 9
  - Adult women sizes 6 to 8
  - Nasotracheal intubation sizes 5 to7
  - Pediatrics—consult Broselow tape or use the size equal to the width of the fingernail of the little finger. Use uncuffed tubes in infants and small children up to 8 years of age.
- Water-soluble lubricant
- 10-mL syringe
- Umbilical tape or endotracheal tube holding device
- Scissors
- Bag-valve-mask device (Ambu-bag) with 100% oxygen delivery system
- Pulse oximeter
- Capnograph, carbon dioxide detector, esophageal detector or other device to confirm tube placement
- Suction system with dental or Yankauer tip in children and adults, DeLee suction in neonates
- Stethoscope
- Cardiac monitor and defibrillator
- Blood pressure monitor
- Gloves
- Face mask, goggles or eye shield, and any other equipment necessary to follow universal blood and body fluid precautions
- Intravenous line (if possible)
- Ventilator
- Cricothyroidotomy kit
- Sedative medication to use for chemical restraint (e.g., propofol, benzodiazepines)

CRICOID PRESSURE (SELLICK MANEUVER)

Providing or performing cricoid pressure may help protect against regurgitation of gastric contents; it also increases visibility by moving the trachea into the visual field of the person intubating. To perform cricoid pressure (Sellick maneuver), first find the thyroid cartilage (Adam's apple), and then the small indentation beneath it (cricothyroid membrane). The cartilage beneath this small indentation is the cricoid bone. Cricoid pressure is performed by pinching the extended thumb, index, and middle finger together into a double "V," or tripod. This is then placed on the cricoid bone and pressed down with enough pressure to occlude the esophagus (Fig. 213-2). The pressure should be applied toward the patient's back and the head somewhat. Cricoid pressure should not be released until intubation is completed and confirmed and the cuff inflated.

NOTE: The effectiveness of the Sellick maneuver has been questioned. Because of the wide variation in pressure applied by operators, cricoid pressure should be removed if there is difficulty in visualizing the airway.

AIRWAY ASSESSMENT

Begin with the patient on 100% nonrebreather mask if spontaneously breathing. The jaw thrust maneuver can be used to keep the airway open (Fig. 213-3), or begin bag-valve-mask breathing with a second assistant providing cricoid pressure (Sellick maneuver). The practitioner should be familiar with the anatomic landmarks (Fig. 213-4). Many airway management failures can be traced to lack of airway assessment. Patients can be classified into three groups (shades) based on two criteria: anticipated difficulty in intubation and ability to maintain oxygen saturation greater than 90% by bag-valve-mask ventilation. Airway assessment is critical. An experienced person can assess an airway in less than 4 seconds, and an inexperienced person should be able to do so in less than 8 seconds.

The mnemonic for assessing difficulty in intubation is 332-NUTS:

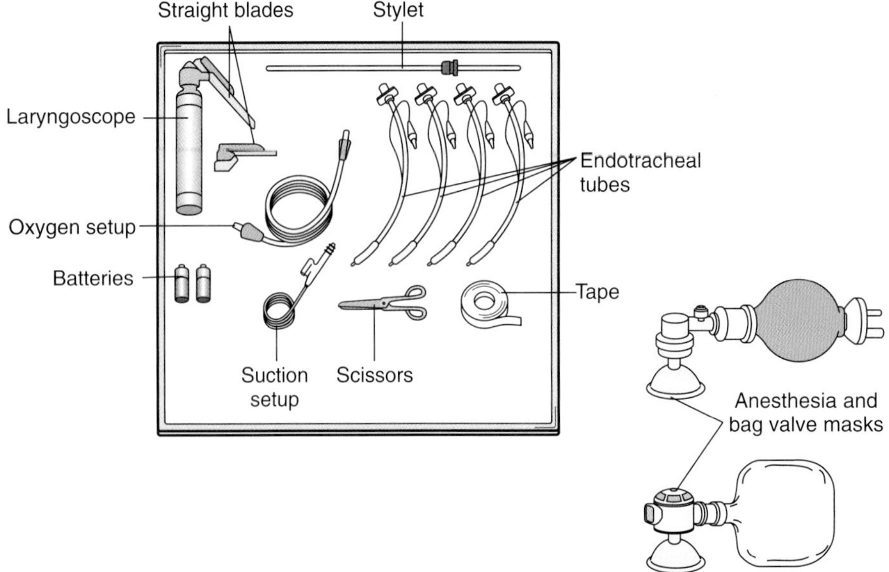

Figure 213-1 Suggested intubation equipment.

- 3—fingerbreadths, mouth opening
- 3—fingerbreadths, mentum (distance from the tip of the chin to the anterior soft tissue of the neck)
- 2—fingerbreadths, thyromental distance (distance from the top of the thyroid cartilage to the upper soft tissue angle of the neck)
- **N**—Normal neck flexion
- **U**—Uvula visible when opening the mouth
- **T**—no Tension pneumothorax
- **S**—no "Soup" (foreign body in the airway)

Meeting all these criteria indicates a low-risk intubation; conversely, the fewer the criteria present, the higher the risk. Although the last two categories, tension pneumothorax and "soup," do not strictly determine the anatomic difficulty of intubation, establishing their absence is a vital part of early airway assessment. The Mallampati system has previously been used to assess the uvular portion of the mnemonic; however, it is important to note that this classification was designed to assess a patient sitting upright with voluntary mouth opening—a condition rarely encountered in clinical practice outside anesthesiology. A simpler method is to open the mouth with the thumb while standing to either side of the patient's head. (Standing at the head of the patient changes the angle of view, and may produce a false result). If any portion of the uvula can be seen, then intubation will likely be unimpeded by this factor. The three risk groups (shades) are as follows:

- **Pink**—able to keep the oxygen saturation greater than 90%; anticipate easy intubation and use standard technique.
- **Purple**—able to keep the oxygen saturation greater than 90%, but anticipate difficult intubation. Attempt awake laryngoscopy. If successful, perform an assisted intubation with a gum elastic bougie, intubating or fiberoptic laryngoscope, lighted stylet, or similar device. If not, use an intermediate airway (laryngeal mask airway [LMA] or King LTS-D) if possible, and obtain expert assistance for further management.
- **Blue**—unable to keep the oxygen saturation greater than 90%. If possible, perform a single attempt at an intermediate airway (LMA or King LTS-D). If successful and easy intubation is anticipated, attempt assisted intubation as in the purple patient. If difficulty is anticipated, obtain expert assistance for further management if time permits. If not, needle or surgical cricothyroidotomy may be needed.

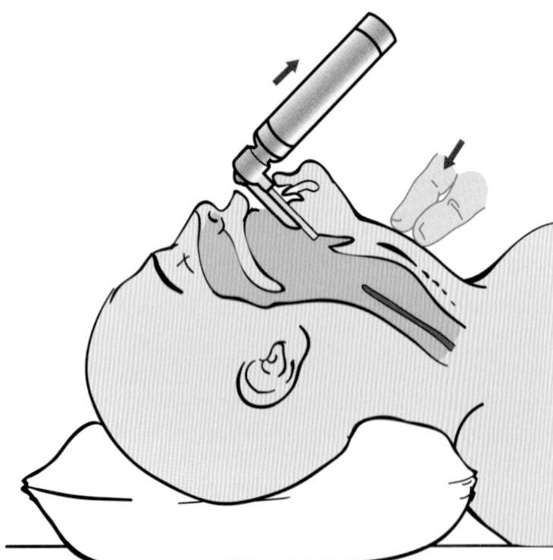

Figure 213-2 Sellick maneuver. Either the practitioner or assistant uses the thumb and index and middle fingers pinched into a double "V" or tripod. Posterior pressure is then applied to the cricoid to avoid aspiration and bring the larynx into view. Note the upward and forward direction of forces applied in a nonfulcrum manner by the laryngoscope.

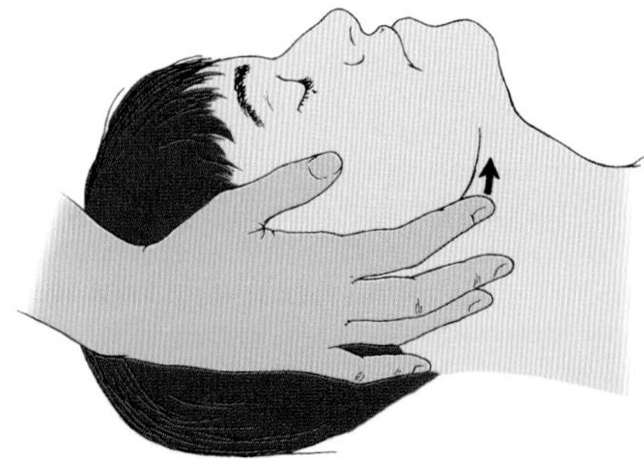

Figure 213-3 Jaw thrust. Rotate mandible forward with index fingers. *Arrow* indicates motion to bring soft tissues forward to relieve airway obstruction.

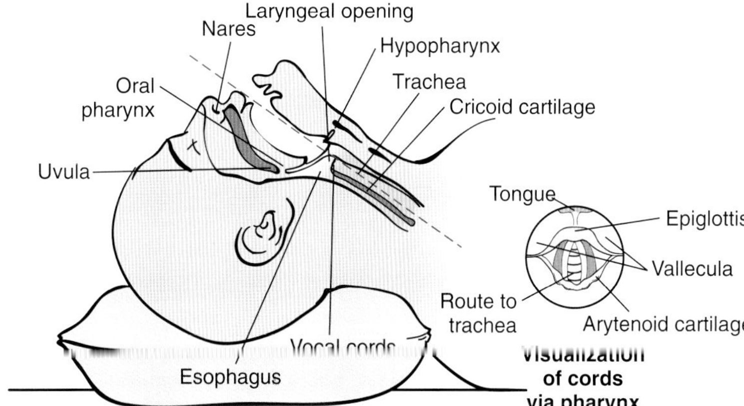

Figure 213-4 Anatomic landmarks of the head and neck.

STANDARD OROTRACHEAL INTUBATION

Preparation

Lack of proper preparation is another common reason for failure to intubate. If the airway risk is purple or blue, auxiliary techniques should be strongly considered. However, if the patient is classified in the pink group, attempt standard orotracheal intubation. Prepare for intubation using the mnemonic "airway START." The airway prefix distinguishes it from a similar mnemonic used for triage in mass disasters.

- S—Shade (classify the patient as pink, purple, or blue and select the proper technique)
- T—Technicians (respiratory technician and cricoid pressure technician)
- A—Assemble (ensure all the equipment and drugs are prepared)
- R—Respiration (preoxygenate with at least eight vital capacity breaths. If time permits, and the patient is breathing spontaneously, 5 minutes of preoxygenation provides 5 minutes of protection)
- T—Tilt (ensure both the patient and the practitioner are properly positioned)

Technique

The cricoid pressure technician should initiate cricoid pressure using the Sellick maneuver as soon as the respiratory therapist begins bagging. This will reduce stomach insufflation and the risk for vomiting. The cricoid pressure technician also watches the oxygen saturation of the patient and announces saturations below 90% to the practitioner. In addition, this technician holds the endotracheal tube and passes it to the practitioner so the practitioner can focus uninterrupted on the intubating view.

"Tilt" or position of the patient and the practitioner is often overlooked, but this is probably the most critical component of successful intubation. If the patient is not suspected of having neck problems that could be worsened by movement, place the patient in the "sniffing" position with the neck flexed and the head extended backward (Fig. 213-5). The neck may be flexed by raising the head several inches using a folded towel or firm pillow. It is important to remember that the padding should be placed under the head and not between the shoulders (see Fig. 213-4).

The position of the practitioner is even more important. The most common problem is having an angle of view that is too high to visualize the anatomy, which is caused by being both too close to and too high above the patient. Crowded conditions at the head of the bed in most care settings compound this problem. Unfortunately, the practitioner usually reacts by bending forward at the waist, which serves only to worsen the angle of view. Raise the bed and move it a full 2 feet or more forward if possible. If a lower angle of view is needed, the practitioner should bend at the knees and not at the waist.

Intubation

The paraglossal technique has supplanted older methods of intubation. It is easier to learn, has a higher success rate, and uses the same technique regardless of whether a curved or straight blade is used. I have nicknamed the method the "Diamond Technique," based on the four "Ds" of the steps used to intubate:

- **Dental**—Always hold the laryngoscope in the left hand. Place the flange of the blade against the right molars with no tongue intervening.
- **Deep**—Sweep the tongue centrally and insert the blade to the hilt or until resistance is met in the esophagus. If the patient is in the sniffing position, this is usually easy. If the patient cannot be moved safely into the sniffing position, follow the contour

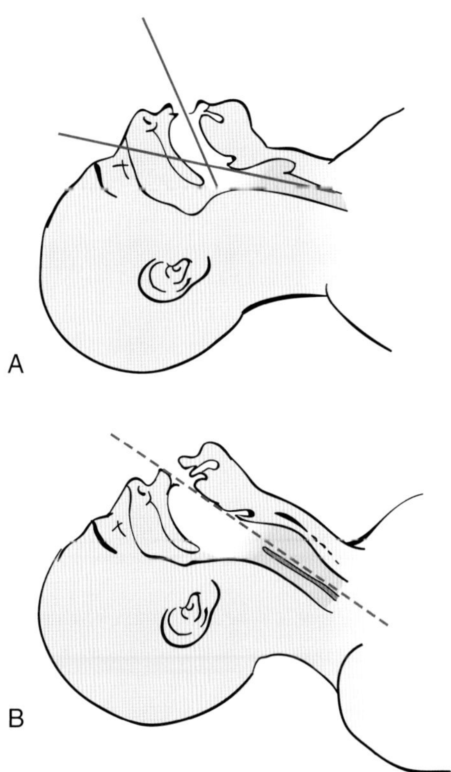

Figure 213-5 Proper head position is important for successful endotracheal intubation. Axes of the mouth, pharynx, and larynx need to be aligned. **A,** Divergent axes. **B,** Axes in line, or "sniffing position."

of the base of the tongue to reach the esophagus. Place the blade deeply and in the esophagus on purpose. In this position, the location of the tip of the blade is known and, more important, so is the location of the airway: shallow and superior to the blade tip.

- **Direct**—Once the blade is in the esophagus, lift the handle upward and forward (see Fig. 213-2), using the same technique as in the older methods of intubation.
- **Depart**—From this position, withdraw the blade while monitoring the view. Most of the time, there will be a slight sensation of "give" when the blade clears the esophagus, and a good intubating view is obtained.

From this position, the practitioner requests the tube from the cricoid pressure technician. Once received, the practitioner inserts it with the right hand guiding the tip down against the right buccal mucosa to avoid obstructing the intubating view (Fig. 213-6). A common mistake is to try to slide the tube straight down the center. This obstructs the view and increases the probability of accidental esophageal intubation. The endotracheal tube is advanced until the tip is at least 2 to 3 cm beyond the vocal cords.

Rarely, the tip of the epiglottis is encountered. If this is the case, lift the epiglottis with the blade tip. Using the right hand, after handing the tube back to the technician, replace the pressure on the cricoid cartilage that is being applied by the pressure technician. Manipulate the trachea to obtain a good view (commonly, the cricoid pressure technician will use too much pressure). When a good view is obtained, have the cricoid pressure technician replace the same amount of pressure to maintain a constant view. The technician then hands the endotracheal tube back to the practitioner, who intubates the trachea as described previously. The tube insertion depth can be approximated by the Chula formula: 4 cm + (patient height in inches/4). In most patients, this will be between 21 to 23 cm. Inflate the balloon according to manufacturer directions. Most balloons take 10 mL of air.

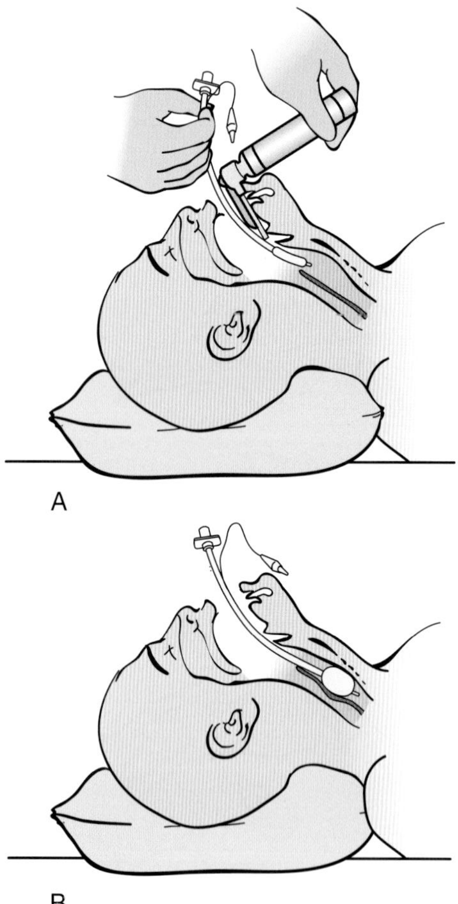

Figure 213-6 Insertion of tube with laryngoscope in place. **A,** Insert the tube with the tip initially against the right buccal mucosa so that a clear view of the vocal cords can be maintained at all times. As it advances, watch the tube pass through the cords. **B,** The tube is correctly placed when the tip is 2 to 3 cm beyond the vocal cords.

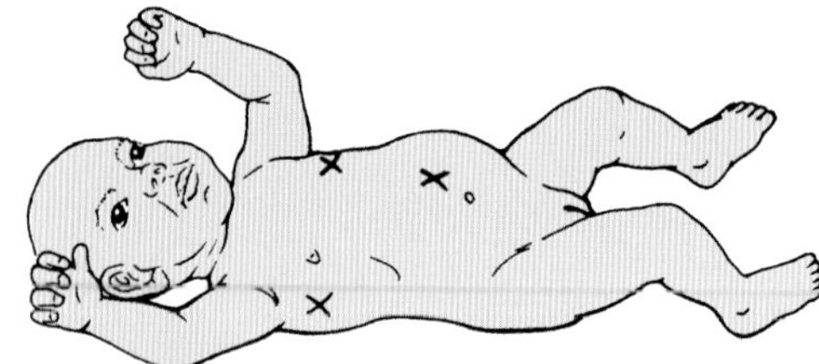

Figure 213-7 Auscultation points for confirmation of placement are over the stomach (should be lack of sound) and the axillae. The same locations should be used to auscultate in the adult.

Confirm Placement

Listen at the stomach to assess for an esophageal intubation, and then listen in each axilla to assess for equal breath sounds. Listening over the anterior chest is not as accurate as listening in the axillae for determining proper tube placement (Fig. 213-7). Asymmetric breath sounds suggests that the mainstem bronchus was intubated—typically, the right mainstem bronchus because it is more vertical than the left mainstem bronchus.

Next, use a secondary device to ensure proper placement. The devices available include bulb-type and syringe-type esophageal detector devices or carbon dioxide colorimetric devices. These devices are attached to the endotracheal tube after intubation. The bulb device is squeezed shut before being placed on the tube. If the bulb reinflates, the tube is in the proper location. One way to remember this is "reinflate means you're great." If a syringe device is used, aspiration of more than 30 mL of air indicates proper tube placement. Colorimetric devices, which change from yellow to purple with an elevated carbon dioxide level, are also useful. These end-tidal carbon dioxide detectors are placed between the tube and the bag-valve device after intubation: the detectors will change from purple to yellow if the tube is in the proper location. An easy way to remember the colors is "yellow, yellow in the bellow." Carbon dioxide capnographic devices should show adequate respiratory waveforms. These forms are characterized by three phases: baseline, rapid upstroke, and long alveolar plateau, similar to a small "r" written in longhand.

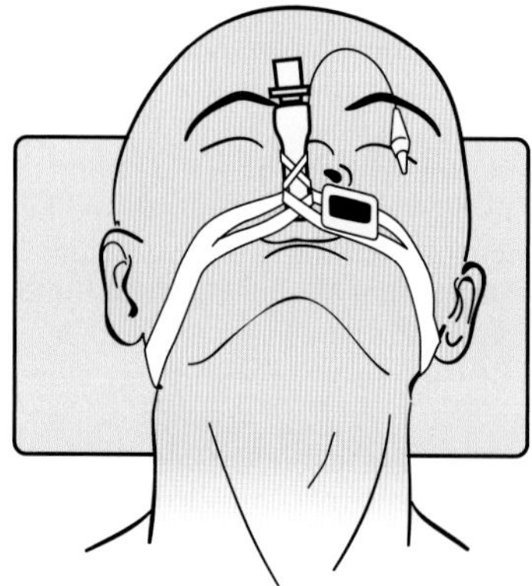

Figure 213-8 Secure the tube to minimize patient discomfort while maintaining correct positioning. Consider a bite block.

Secure

Secure the tube with umbilical tape or a commercial device made for that purpose (Fig. 213-8). Avoid using tape or tincture of benzoin on the face because facial irritation can cause at least temporary skin changes. Consider inserting a bite block if the patient might bite the tube. Insert a nasogastric or orogastric tube. Use chemical restraints with appropriate monitoring to prevent tube removal. Finally, take a chest radiograph to ensure proper depth and placement. The ideal location is to have the tube 2 to 3 cm above the carina.

Rapid-Sequence Intubation

Rapid-sequence intubation is an important technique to assist intubation in patients who are combative. It prevents laryngospasm and can have other therapeutic benefits. The prime candidate has been the "can't intubate, can't ventilate patient," but in actual practice this is rare. Airway assessment before the procedure should detect patients at risk for this problem, and often alternative methods can be used. Rarely, this may occur without warning, so an intermediate airway, such as a LMA or Combitube, as well as a cricothyroidotomy kit, needs to be readily available. There are many medications from which to choose and the topic can be complex. Here, only the most common technique is explained, and this will be suitable for patients without suspected bronchospasm or increased intracranial pressure.

- Choose the paralytic agent. Succinylcholine 1.5 mg/kg is the first choice unless contraindicated. Contraindications are conditions in which hyperkalemia may be worsened, where there is concern that increased intracranial pressure or intraocular pressure may worsen the patient's condition, or there is a risk of malignant hyperthermia such as the following:
  - End-stage renal disease with missed dialysis
  - Rhabdomyolysis (e.g., patients found down for a long time)
  - Muscular dystrophy of any type
  - History of spinal cord injuries
  - Open globe injury (of controversial significance)
  - Conditions under which there may be increased intracranial pressure
  - History of a recent cerebrovascular accident
  - Burns of greater than 10% body surface area more than 24 hours old but incompletely healed
  - Patients with crush injuries more than 24 hours old
  - Family history of an anesthetic reaction
- If succinylcholine is contraindicated, rocuronium 0.6 to 1 mg/kg is considered by many to be the best alternative. It has a rapid onset of action, but paralysis lasts an average of 50 minutes, placing it second to succinylcholine. However, if succinylcholine is indicated, then a standard dose is 2 mg/kg intravenously. It should not be given until other preparations are made.
- Choose the sedative agent. Etomidate (0.3 mg/kg intravenous perfusion) is the most common choice because of its lack of cardiovascular depression and versatility. Other agents include ketamine 1 to 2 mg/kg in bronchospasm, midazolam 0.2 mg/kg, or thiopental 3 mg/kg in increased intracranial pressure. Each has its benefits and drawbacks, which should be studied before use.
- Choose the adjuncts. Although not indicated in all cases, lidocaine 1.5 mg/kg is considered useful in patients with bronchospasm or concerns for increased intracranial pressure. Atropine should be administered to children younger than 10 years of age at 0.02 mg/kg (minimum 0.1 mg, maximum 1 mg) to inhibit reflex bradycardia before the use of succinylcholine. Atropine should be considered for any adult who is receiving either ketamine or a second dose of succinylcholine during the intubation or reintubation procedure to reduce complications.
- Three minutes before intubation, give adjuncts.
- Two minutes before intubation, give a priming dose (10% of the dose drawn up in the syringe) of succinylcholine (if this medication is to be used for paralysis).
- One minute before intubation, give the paralytic agent (succinylcholine or rocuronium), followed immediately by the sedative (etomidate, midazolam, or thiopental). Begin giving the patient eight vital capacity breaths.
- Assess for adequate paralysis by gently stroking the eyelashes. If there is no response, proceed with intubation as described in previous sections.

Nasotracheal Intubation

Nasotracheal intubation generally requires the patient to be breathing spontaneously, and has the complications of nasal bleeding and sinusitis. It is of limited usefulness except in cases where awake intubation is required. This technique is relatively contraindicated in the combative patient and in those patients with a coagulopathy or bleeding diathesis. It is important to examine the facial anatomy and nares for distortion, trauma, or other contraindications. If no contraindications are noted, use the side with the larger passage. If they are equal, use the right side because this helps reduce trauma from the tube bevel. Use a 6.5-mm tube or smaller, if anatomically indicated.

Preparation

Most nasotracheal intubation failures are the result of inadequate preparation.

- Get an assistant.
- Explain the procedure to the patient. This is the most important step.
- Place the patient in the standard "sniffing" position, as described previously.
- Determine if nasal vasoconstriction is safe. If the patient appears to be at risk for limited perfusion to the nasal area from either local or systemic disease, avoid the use of a vasoconstrictor.
- Prepare the nasopharyngeal path. Place 15 mL of 2% lidocaine with epinephrine (or plain lidocaine, if vasoconstriction is contraindicated) in a Toomey syringe.
- Have one assistant keep the syringe upright to prevent spillage, and connect the Toomey syringe to a small Foley catheter. A red Robinson catheter is preferred.
- While an assistant continues to hold the catheter upright, lubricate the distal catheter with a water-soluble lubricant.
- With the free hand, apply cricoid pressure. This facilitates entry of the catheter into the airway. Insert the catheter through the nose to the level of the vocal cords. This is approximately twice the distance from the front of the lips to the tragus of the ear. Ideally, the patient will cough, indicating vocal cord stimulation.
- Have the assistant turn the syringe upright and administer about 5 mL of the solution while the patient coughs, which helps disperse the solution.
- Withdraw the catheter, administering another 5 mL of the solution as the catheter is removed.
- Administer the last 5 mL at Kiesselbach's plexus in the anterior nasal passage of the septum. Allow the solution to work while lubricating the endotracheal tube and checking the balloon.

Two-Handed Nasotracheal Intubation Technique

- Standing at the side of the patient, insert the tube so the leading edge of the bevel is away from the septum. If the left nostril is used, the tube will be initially inserted with most of it positioned above the face and scalp, and then rotated 180 degrees once the turbinates are passed.
- Once the tube is about halfway in, apply cricoid pressure with the nondominant hand. Remember that unlike in training

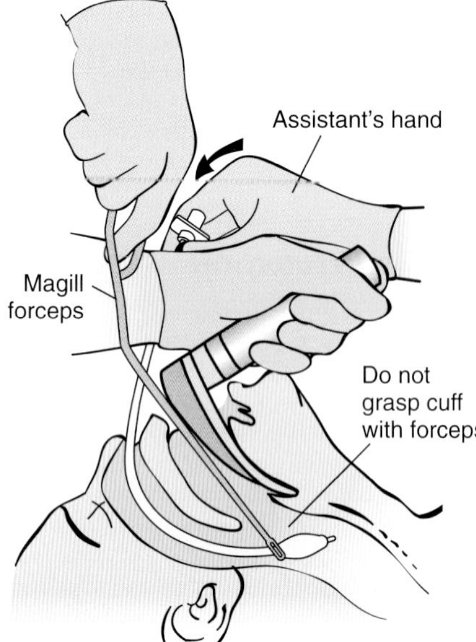

Figure 213-9 Nasotracheal intubation using a laryngoscope and Magill forceps. The forceps are not used to pull the tube; rather, they serve to guide the tip of the tube through the vocal cords while an assistant advances the tube. The cuff is frequently damaged if it is grasped. (Modified from Roberts JR, Hedges JR [eds]: Clinical Procedures in Emergency Medicine, 3rd ed. Philadelphia, WB Saunders, 1998.)

models, the trachea is a mobile structure. Use this advantage to move the trachea to assist placing the tube.

- Lean forward and listen for breath sounds through the end of the tube, adjusting both the tube and the trachea to create maximum breath sounds. Once resistance is felt at the vocal cord opening, await inspiration and then guide the tube past the vocal cords. This is often easily felt with the hand manipulating the trachea.
- Pass the tube 26 to 28 cm in an adult, depending on the size of the patient.
- Check and secure the tube in the standard fashion (see Fig. 213-8).
- Direct visualization can also be used for nasotracheal intubation. With the patient supine, use the laryngoscope in the same manner as for standard intubation. While visualizing the cords, use the Magill forceps to grasp the tube already inserted through the nasopharynx and pass it through the cords (Fig. 213-9). Avoid tearing the cuff when grasping the tube with forceps.

Postprocedure Patient Care

- Order daily chest radiographs to verify tube placement.
- The respiratory services department of the hospital usually supplies the ventilator, tape, and other equipment as well as providing care; however, the clinician is ultimately responsible.
- Check the patient and the respiratory setup frequently. Carbon dioxide detectors and whistles can be used to confirm expiratory efforts.

Complications

- Short-term laryngeal edema: Sore throat occurs in almost every patient after extubation (repeated attempts at intubation by unskilled personnel may cause enough edema to preclude intubation by highly skilled clinicians).
- Trauma
  - Broken teeth
  - Oral lacerations or ulcerations (lip, tongue, pharynx, esophagus, or trachea)
  - Bleeding, hematoma, or abscess formation as a result of trauma
  - Avulsion of arytenoid cartilage
- Hypoxia resulting from
  - Long duration of procedure
  - Esophageal intubation (most commonly results from not visualizing the vocal cords)
  - Intubation of a bronchus
  - Failure to recognize esophageal or bronchial intubation
  - Pneumothorax
  - Failure to secure the placement
  - Failure to recognize misplacement of the tube
  - Aspiration of vomited material, especially in unconscious or semiconscious patient
  - Laryngospasm
- Hypertension/hypotension
- Bradycardia
- Tachycardia with or without arrhythmias
- Sequelae of long-term endotracheal tube placement
  - Nosocomial infection
  - Pneumothorax
  - Corneal abrasions
  - Epistaxis
  - Sinusitis
  - Vocal cord damage or paralysis (left cord more frequently involved than right)
  - Tracheomalacia and stenosis (occur more frequently in men; are more common with older tubes that use higher cuff pressures)
  - Tracheoesophageal fistula
  - Innominate artery erosion by endotracheal cuff

NOTE: Rarely are teeth broken with nasotracheal intubation. However, acute epistaxis and nasal trauma can result. Pulmonary infection can also be caused by nasal flora introduced through the nasotracheal tube.

CPT/Billing Code

31500 Intubation, endotracheal; emergency procedure

ICD-9-CM Diagnostic Codes

276.2 Acidosis
276.3 Alkalosis
276.4 Acid-base mixed disorder
427.5 Cardiac or cardiorespiratory arrest
428.1 Pulmonary edema (left heart failure)
491.20 Chronic obstructive bronchitis, without exacerbation
491.21 Chronic obstructive bronchitis, with (acute) exacerbation
492.8 Emphysema, NOS
493.01 Asthma, extrinsic with status asthmaticus
493.91 Asthma, unspecified with status asthmaticus
518.5 Pulmonary insufficiency following trauma and surgery
518.81 Respiratory failure, NOS
518.82 Respiratory distress, insufficiency or syndrome; acute
518.83 Respiratory failure, chronic
780.01 Coma
785.50 Shock, unspecified
785.51 Shock, cardiogenic
785.52 Shock, septic
785.59 Shock, hypovolemic or other
786.09 Respiratory distress or insufficiency, other, including hypercapnia
799.02 Hypoxemia
799.1 Respiratory arrest or cardiorespiratory failure

Acknowledgment

The editors wish to recognize the many contributions by Len Scarpinato, DO, to this chapter in the previous two editions of this text.

Suppliers

(See contact information online at www.expertconsult.com.)

Cook Medical
Mallinckrodt, Inc.
Rusch
Sims Portex, Inc.

Bibliography

American Heart Association: Advanced Cardiovascular Life Support Provider Manual. Dallas, American Heart Association, 2006.

Butler J, Sen A: Best evidence topic report: Cricoid pressure in emergency rapid sequence intubation. Emerg Med J 22:815–816, 2005.

Ellis DY, Harris T, Zideman D: Cricoid pressure in emergency department rapid sequence tracheal intubations: A risk-benefit analysis. Ann Emerg Med 50:653–665, 2007.

Hagberg CA (ed): Manual of Difficult Airway Management. Philadelphia, Churchill Livingstone, 2000.

Kopman AF, Zhaku B, Lai KS: The "intubating dose" of succinylcholine: the effect of decreasing doses on recovery time. Anesthesiology 99:1050–1054, 2003.

Marx JA, Hockberger RS, Walls RM (eds): Rosen's Emergency Medicine: Concepts and Clinical Practice, 6th ed. Philadelphia, Mosby, 2006.

Naguib M, Samarkandi AH, El-Din ME, et al: The dose of succinylcholine required for excellent endotracheal intubating conditions. Anesth Analg 102:151–155, 2006.

Reichman EF, Simon RR (eds): Emergency Medicine Procedures. New York, McGraw-Hill, 2004.

Tintinalli, JE, Kelen GD, Stapczynski JS (eds): Emergency Medicine: A Comprehensive Study Guide, 6th ed. New York, McGraw-Hill, 2004.

Walls RM, Murphy MF, Luten RC, Schneider RE (eds): Manual of Emergency Airway Management, 2nd ed. Philadelphia, Lippincott Williams & Wilkins, 2004.

CHAPTER 214

Pericardiocentesis

David James

The normal pericardial space contains 10 to 30 mL of serous fluid, which serves to reduce friction between the surfaces of the visceral and parietal pericardium as the heart moves through the cardiac cycle. An increased amount of fluid in this space may result from a variety of disease processes or trauma. Because of the relatively nondistensible pericardial sac, an increased amount of pericardial fluid may exert pressure on the more compressible myocardium. This in turn may compromise cardiac performance and result in cardiac tamponade. Clinically, this is appreciated by markedly elevated jugular venous pressure (i.e., jugular venous distention), hypotension, and distant heart sounds. Although few patients will have all three of these clinical findings, almost all will have at least one unless they are hypovolemic. The patient may also exhibit restlessness, fatigue, and tachycardia; pulmonary edema may be present with corresponding tachypnea. Estimates of the volume of fluid required to accumulate acutely and produce tamponade range from 60 to 200 mL. A chest radiograph may show a dilated heart, classically in a "water-bottle" shape. Electrocardiographically, pericardial effusions are identified by low voltage in all leads or electrical alternans (i.e., the QRS amplitude or morphology changes on the electrocardiogram [ECG] as the heart swings to and fro within the pericardial fluid). However, electrocardiographic and radiographic signs of cardiac tamponade are often absent. If ultrasonography is available, a fluid echo will be present in the pericardial space. Further ultrasonographic confirmation includes collapse of the right and left ventricular chambers as a result of tamponade (see Chapter 225, Emergency Department, Hospitalist, and Office Ultrasonography [Clinical Ultrasonography]).

Additional findings on physical examination with tamponade include a paradoxical increase in jugular venous distention during inspiration and pulsus paradoxus (a drop in systolic pressure of >10 mm Hg during inspiration). To measure pulsus paradoxus, inflate the blood pressure cuff to greater than systolic pressure. Slowly release the cuff pressure until beats are heard only during expiration, and record this pressure. Keep deflating the cuff pressure until beats are heard continuously during expiration and inspiration, and record this pressure. The difference between these recorded pressures is pulsus paradoxus, as noted by Kussmaul, and is increased because the right ventricle and interventricular septum are forced into the left ventricle by tamponade.

Cardiac tamponade should always be considered as a cause of shock in a medical patient. This includes patients taking oral or parenteral anticoagulants or high-dose steroids, having known cancer or pericardial disease, suspected of having an aortic dissection, or having had a recent myocardial infarction (e.g., ruptured myocardium). In the trauma patient, cardiac tamponade is the most common presentation for a penetrating cardiac injury. It occurs in 80% to 90% of stab wounds and in 20% of gunshot wounds. Tamponade can also be due to iatrogenic causes such as central venous line placement, temporary pacing (transthoracic or transvenous), and cardiopulmonary resuscitation. The causes of effusions, in order of frequency from most to least, include cancer, idiopathic, infectious (including human immunodeficiency virus), postpericardiotomy, connective tissue disease, radiation therapy, trauma, and uremia.

Pericardial effusions may be asymptomatic or associated with life-threatening cardiac compromise. The aspiration of pericardial fluid (pericardiocentesis) has diagnostic and possibly therapeutic applications. Pericardiocentesis is an infrequently performed procedure that has the potential for significant patient morbidity and mortality. Optimally, the procedure should be performed in the cardiac catheterization laboratory or intensive care unit, where complete cardiac monitoring and trained support personnel are available. Ideally, the procedure should be performed under real-time ultrasonographic or fluoroscopic guidance to continuously visualize the pericardial fluid. With ultrasonographic or fluoroscopic experience, the clinician should be able to estimate the amount of fluid that can be aspirated and the depth and angle of penetration necessary for pericardiocentesis (see Chapter 225, Emergency Department, Hospitalist, and Office Ultrasonography [Clinical Ultrasonography]).

However, pericardiocentesis may be required under urgent or emergent conditions and in a suboptimal clinical setting if a patient presents with hemodynamic compromise from pericardial tamponade. Patients in whom urgent/emergent pericardiocentesis is contemplated should have intravenous (IV) access and continuous cardiac monitoring. Continuous oximetry, blood pressure monitoring, and supplemental oxygen may also be helpful. If the clinical situation permits, a 12-lead ECG and a chest radiograph should be obtained for review before the procedure (assess for mediastinal shift). Full resuscitation equipment should be readily available.

Before performing pericardiocentesis, the clinician should review the relevant anatomy of the heart, pericardium, and rib cage (Fig. 214-1). It may also be useful to insert a nasogastric tube to decompress the stomach (see Chapter 203, Nasogastric and Nasoenteric Tube Insertion). If time allows, efforts to stabilize the patient with cardiac tamponade include aggressive treatment with IV fluids and parenteral inotropic agents to increase ventricular filling pressures. Preload-reducing agents such as nitrates and diuretics may worsen the patient's condition or even be fatal.

Indications

Diagnostic

Determination of the etiology or confirmation of the presence of an effusion is the diagnostic indicator.

Therapeutic

The relief of cardiac tamponade (should be performed emergently only if diagnosis is consistent with known prior disease or mechanism of injury or in a resuscitation patient when other causes of electromechanical dissociation have been excluded [e.g., hypovolemia excluded by aggressive fluid replacement, tension pneumothorax excluded by needle thoracostomy]) is the therapeutic indication.

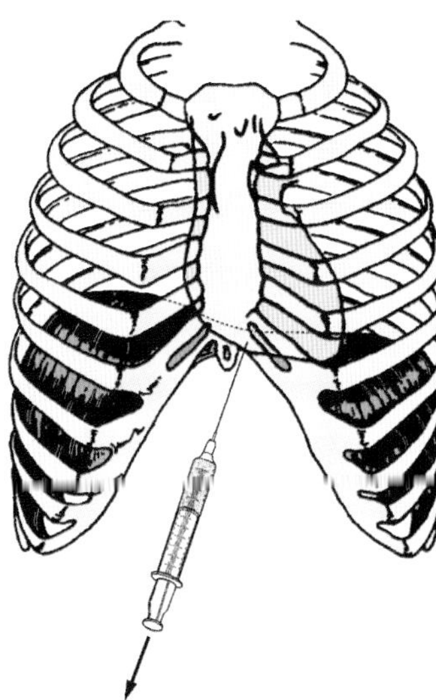

Figure 214-1 Anatomic relationships of the heart, pericardium, and rib cage. Note the inferior border of the pericardium in relation to the xiphoid process, and the angle the aspirating syringe takes as it enters under the rib cage.

Contraindications

- Anticoagulated patient or patient with uncontrolled coagulopathy (relative contraindication in life-threatening situation, absolute contraindication in stable patient).
- Because of the risk of complications, pericardiocentesis should not be performed if a safer alternative exists (e.g., medical management of an effusion).
- In stable patient, pericardiocentesis should not be performed without ultrasonographic or fluoroscopic demonstration of an effusion.
- In stable patient, diagnostic pericardiocentesis should be guided by ultrasonography or fluoroscopy in a cardiac catheterization laboratory or intensive care unit.
- In stable patient, pericardiocentesis should not be performed for small, loculated, or posteriorly located effusions.
- In trauma patients, some experts argue that prompt sternotomy should be performed instead of pericardiocentesis; in patients too unstable to make it to the operating room, they argue for an emergency thoracotomy.

Equipment

- Pericardiocentesis needle (18-gauge, 4-inch spinal needle with stylet)
- Two 10-mL syringes (Luer type), one with 25-gauge, 2-inch needle
- 50-mL syringe (Luer type)
- 10 mL local anesthetic (e.g., 1% lidocaine)
- ECG machine
- Wire connector with alligator clips (to connect pericardiocentesis needle to ECG lead)
- Basin
- Skin preparation solution (e.g., povidone–iodine, chlorhexidine)
- Sterile towels
- Mask, sterile gloves, eye protection, possibly sterile gown
- Kelly clamp
- Cardiac monitoring equipment, pulse oximetry, supplemental oxygen, automatic blood pressure cuff
- Nasogastric tube
- Access to chest radiography
- Bedside ultrasonography machine or fluoroscopy (in emergent situations, optional but desirable)
- Cook 8-Fr Fuhrman pericardiocentesis catheter kit (usually a soft, multihole catheter; in an emergency, a single-lumen, 6- to 10-Fr central venous catheter can be used), no. 11 blade scalpel, nylon suture (if inserting a catheter for continuous drainage)

Preprocedure Patient Education

If the clinical situation allows, describe the procedure to the patient or representative and obtain informed consent. Explain that there will be some discomfort involved, but that removal of even a small amount of pericardial fluid may make an enormous improvement in the patient's clinical status. The alert patient should attempt to remain as still as possible because the needle will be inserted near moving vital organs. If time allows, conscious sedation should be considered.

Technique

1. Assemble and connect supplemental oxygen and all cardiac, blood pressure, and oximetry monitoring equipment, and have IV access in place and resuscitation equipment nearby. Some clinicians insert an arterial line for monitoring.
2. Place patient in a semirecumbent position (Fig. 214-2) at about 30 to 45 degrees. This position allows the myocardium to "fall back" slightly within the pericardial sac and lessens the likelihood of puncturing the myocardium. The supine position is an acceptable alternative.
3. Hook up limb leads of ECG machine and attach one end of connector to lead V_1.
4. Prepare skin of epigastrium, xiphoid area, and lower chest. Drape with towels to define a sterile field. If time allows, consider using a sterile gown. The clinician should follow universal blood and body fluid precautions when performing this procedure.
5. If the patient is awake, anesthetize the subxiphoid area skin with 1% lidocaine solution. (Alternatively, the right or left sternocostal margin near the xiphoid can be used.) Anesthetize the deeper tissue with the 25-gauge, 2-inch needle. Direct the needle under the xiphoid or costal margin toward the left shoulder (alternatively, the suprasternal notch), aspirating continuously. If blood or pericardial fluid returns, withdraw the needle slightly.
6. Attach the pericardiocentesis needle to one of the 10-mL syringes and turn the ECG machine on.
7. Insert the pericardiocentesis needle through the subxiphoid skin, advancing toward the left shoulder (alternatively, the suprasternal notch), aspirating continuously. Remove the stylet, attach the other end of the ECG connector to the pericardiocentesis needle close to the hub, and then advance the needle 4 to 5 cm

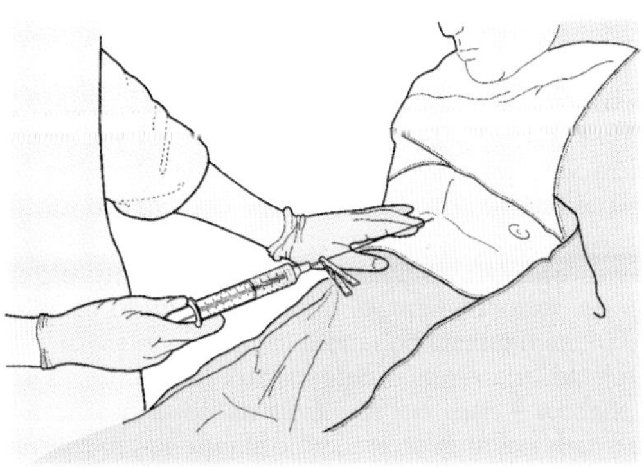

Figure 214-2 Patient lying in semirecumbent position.

while applying negative pressure to the syringe. *This may be guided by ultrasonography or fluoroscopy, if equipment is available*. Continue advancing the pericardiocentesis needle until blood or pericardial fluid is aspirated, cardiac pulsations are felt, or the ECG shows (a) increased P-wave amplitude, (b) ST segment elevation (i.e., current of injury), or (c) ectopic beats. All of these ECG findings are suggestive of penetration of the epicardium and require withdrawal of the needle slightly, in 1- to 2-mm increments, until the findings disappear.

NOTE: To minimize the risk of damaging vital organs, never rock or redirect the pericardiocentesis needle without withdrawing it almost completely (to just below the skin).

8. The clinician will often feel the needle give or a "pop" as it enters the pericardium. (The awake patient often complains of chest pain when the pericardium is entered.) Once blood or pericardial fluid begins to flow into the syringe, attach the Kelly clamp to the needle where it penetrates the skin. This will limit any further unwanted travel of the needle.
9. Remove the 10-mL syringe, attach the 50-mL syringe to the needle hub, and aspirate the desired amount of fluid. The fluid may be discarded into the basin or sterile containers if laboratory analysis is required. If the blood or pericardial fluid withdrawn clots, it is probably fresh blood from a cardiac chamber. Withdraw the needle slightly and aspirate again. Pericardial fluid may be bloody, but it should not clot.

Blind Insertion Technique

1. In an emergency, pericardiocentesis may have to be performed blindly (usually because connectors are not available to attach the ECG lead to the pericardiocentesis needle). In that situation, a 12-lead ECG machine should still be running continuously with the leads placed in the standard locations.
2. Follow previous steps 1 through 6, as much as possible. Next, insert the pericardiocentesis needle through the subxiphoid skin, advancing toward the left shoulder (alternatively, the suprasternal notch), aspirating continuously. Advance the spinal needle until blood or pericardial fluid is aspirated, cardiac pulsations are felt, or the 12-lead ECG shows (a) ST segment elevation (i.e., current of injury), or (b) ectopic beats. Again, these ECG findings are suggestive of penetration of the epicardium and require withdrawal of the needle slightly, in 1- to 2-mm increments, until the findings disappear.

Placing a Fuhrman Pericardial Drainage Catheter (Seldinger Technique)

Recurrence of an effusion is common; placing a pericardial catheter can minimize the risk of recurrence and decrease the risk of complications with repeat needlesticks.

1. Follow previous steps 1 through 8. Then, remove the 10-mL syringe from needle hub, grasp the needle firmly, and pass the guidewire through the needle into the pericardial space (Fig. 214-3). Advance the guidewire until approximately one third of its length is within the patient.
2. Stabilize the guidewire with one hand and remove the needle while leaving the guidewire in place. Nick the skin where the guidewire enters with a no. 11 blade.
3. Slide the dilator over the guidewire and dilate the skin tract. Several passes will be necessary. Slide the dilator off the guidewire and set it aside.

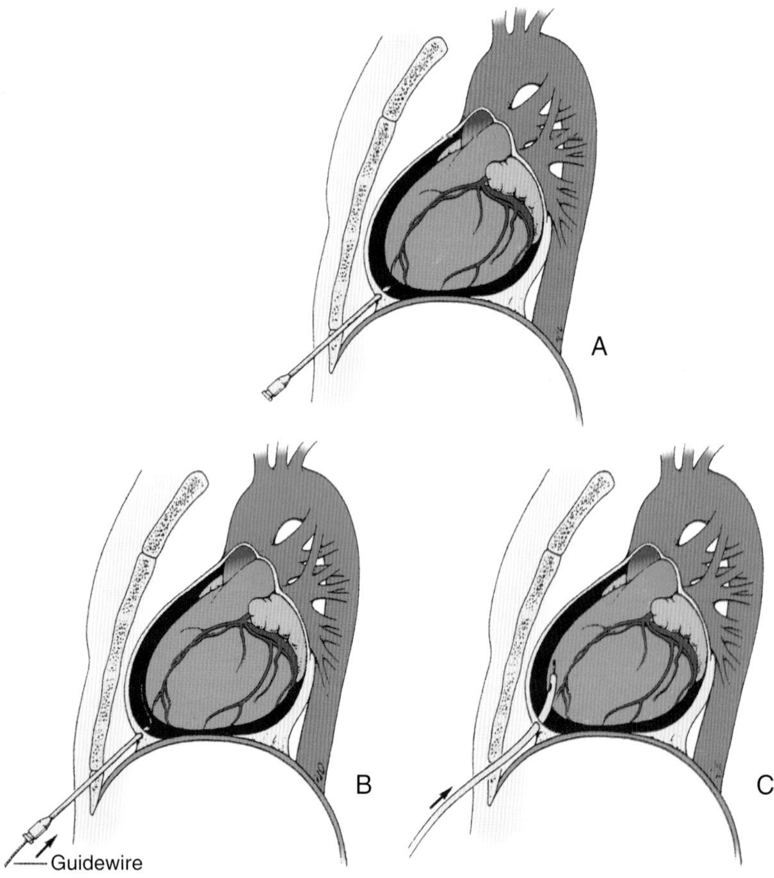

Figure 214-3 **A,** The needle is first advanced into the pericardial space. **B,** The syringe is then disconnected from the needle and the flexible guidewire advanced carefully into the pericardial space (best performed under fluoroscopic guidance). **C,** The needle is withdrawn over the guidewire, the needle tract dilated, and a multihole, soft pigtail catheter advanced into the pericardial space. (From Spodick DH: The technique of pericardiocentesis. J Crit Illn 2:91–96, 1987.)

NOTE: The clinician must obtain some assurance that the guidewire is not located in the myocardium; dilating a tract through the myocardium will result in cardiac tamponade or hemorrhage.

4. Again, stabilize the guidewire with one hand and with the other thread the 8-Fr pigtail (Fuhrman) catheter over the guidewire. Pass the catheter up through the dilated subcutaneous tract into the pericardium. Advance the entire catheter into the body except for the last 1 inch before the hub. Remove the guidewire and set it aside.
5. Suture the pigtail catheter onto the skin, wrapping suture around the catheter between the hub and where it enters the skin.
6. Attach and secure the suction device.

Postprocedure Patient Care

1. If just a simple aspiration was performed, remove the needle after aspiration is complete and dress the puncture site.
2. If a Fuhrman catheter is to be left in place, make sure *both* the catheter and drainage apparatus are secured. They tend to migrate out of the patient if they are not secured.
3. Obtain a postprocedure ECG to look for cardiac injury, and a chest radiograph, looking for pneumothorax. Repeat ultrasonography is also advisable to see if fluid remains. Repeat ultrasonography the next day may diagnose a reaccumulation.

Tamponade should be promptly relieved even with a small amount of fluid removed because of the steep pressure–volume relationship of the pericardium. False-negative aspiration rates as high as 80% have been reported with blind or ECG-directed pericardiocentesis. This false-negative aspiration result is often due to clotted blood in the pericardial space that cannot be aspirated or failure to transverse the pericardium. If fluid is removed and relief of tamponade with improvement in hemodynamic status does not occur, consider another diagnosis and arrange transfer of care to the appropriate consultant. Continue to monitor hemodynamic status in the meantime. Other diagnoses may include constrictive pericarditis, lung disease with left ventricular failure, right ventricular infarction, or biventricular failure. Consult a cardiothoracic surgeon if purulent material is expressed with pericardiocentesis.

After diagnostic pericardiocentesis, fluid should be sent for studies similar to those for pleural fluid (e.g., chemical, cytologic, microbiologic analyses). It can be sent for a cell count and differential, glucose, total protein (body fluid/serum ratio), lactate dehydrogenase, pH, appearance (e.g., clear, cloudy), Gram's stain and culture, acid-fast bacillus stain and culture, fungal culture, and cytology.

Complications

Complication rates vary from 4% to 40%, with potential complications including myocardial puncture with hemopericardium, laceration of the coronary vessels, bradyarrhythmias and tachyarrhythmias, pneumothorax, hemothorax, air embolism, liver laceration, hemorrhage, hypovolemic hypotension from removing large volumes of fluid (e.g., patients with >1 L pericardial effusions), infection, recurrence (up to 70% using blind technique; reduced to 25% if Fuhrman catheter placed), cardiac arrest, and even death. Death usually occurs as the result of recurrence or occurrence of tamponade, hemorrhage, or dysrhythmias. Few if any deaths have been associated with ultrasonography-guided pericardiocentesis. Overall, the complication rate of ultrasonography-guided pericardiocentesis has been reported to be less than 5%. A less serious complication is vasovagal reaction in the alert patient.

CPT/Billing Codes

33010 Pericardiocentesis, initial
33011 Pericardiocentesis, subsequent
33015 Tube pericardiostomy

ICD-9-CM Diagnostic Codes

017.9 Pericarditis, tuberculous
391.0 Acute rheumatic fever with pericarditis (can include effusion)
420.0 Acute pericarditis in diseases classified elsewhere (first, code the underlying disease; e.g., tuberculosis 017.9, chronic uremia 585.9, uremia NOS)
420.90 Acute pericarditis, unspecified
420.90 Effusion, pericardial (acute)
420.99 Pericarditis (acute), pneumococcal, purulent, staphylococcal, streptococcal, suppurative, or pyopericardium
423.0 Hemopericardium
423.3 Cardiac tamponade (first, code the underlying cause)
423.90 Effusion, pericardial

Bibliography

James D: Pericardiocentesis. In James D (ed): A Field Guide to Urgent and Ambulatory Procedures. Philadelphia, Lippincott Williams & Wilkins, 2001, pp 125–129.

Smith RF: Pericardiocentesis. In Reichman EF, Simon RR (eds): Emergency Medicine Procedures. New York, McGraw-Hill, 2004, pp 204–216.

CHAPTER 215

SWAN-GANZ (PULMONARY ARTERY) CATHETERIZATION

Stuart Forman

For over 30 years the use of the balloon-flotation, flow-directed pulmonary artery (PA) thermodilution (Swan-Ganz) catheter has symbolized modern care of the critically ill patient. However, in the past 10 years several studies have found that the PA catheter does not reduce morbidity or mortality. These studies are summarized in the Cochrane Collaborative paper that states "even though the trials measured numbers of deaths in each group at different points of time, all reported that there were no differences between patients who did and did not have a PA catheter inserted" (Harvey and colleagues, 2006). Another meta-analysis in the *Journal of the American Medical Association* similarly showed that "the use of PA catheter neither increased overall mortality in the hospital nor conferred benefit" (Shah and colleagues, 2005).

Alternatively, early goal-directed therapy (EGDT, which uses a regular central line and monitors central venous pressure [CVP] and central venous oxygen saturation [Scvo_2]) in patients with septic shock demonstrated impressive survival rates in a landmark study in 2001 (Rivers and colleagues, 2001). The standard therapy group had an in-hospital mortality rate of 46.5%, compared with 30.5% for those assigned to EGDT. Protocol patients were resuscitated to a CVP of 8 to 12 mm Hg and a mean arterial pressure of 65 mm Hg. If at this point their Scvo_2 was below 70%, packed red cells were transfused to a hematocrit of 30% and dobutamine added, if necessary, until their Scvo_2 normalized to 70%. If still not there, mean arterial pressure was titrated to 65 mm Hg with either norepinephrine or dopamine (Rivers and colleagues, 2001). Subsequent trials have validated these results with similar or better findings (Otero and colleagues, 2006). As a result, many intensive care units have moved away from the PA catheter and are using less invasive methods such as central lines for CVP monitoring and echocardiograms to evaluate cardiac function (see Chapter 90, Echocardiography, and Chapter 225, Emergency Department, Hospitalist, and Office Ultrasonography [Clinical Ultrasonography]). There is even exciting new technology available that provides continuous measurement of cardiac output using just a radial arterial line. That said, PA catheters still have a major role in critical care. Pinsky and Vincent (2005) proposed an algorithm for use of PA catheters (Fig. 215-1); their criteria for initiation of the protocol "would be ongoing circulatory shock despite initial fluid resuscitation efforts or, in the setting of normotension, persistent tachycardia, metabolic acidosis, lactic acidosis, altered mental status, or decreased urine output, since all these are signs or indirect markers of inadequate tissue perfusion." Further study is needed to compare PA catheter-derived outcomes with those using a mere central line. As of this writing, PA catheters still remain an important, although less frequently used, assessment tool in critical care.

This chapter was written for the primary care clinician preparing to insert a PA catheter. All PA catheters generate data such as cardiac output, pulmonary artery wedge pressure, systemic vascular resistance, and stroke work index; therefore, clinicians using PA catheters should be capable of interpreting and acting on these and other results. Many PA catheters are capable of continuously monitoring cardiac output and mixed venous oxygen saturation (Svo_2). Further specialized catheters often provide a port or built-in electrode for pacing, four lumens, or the ability to gather specific data regarding right ventricular function. These specialized catheters are beyond the scope of this chapter.

Although many clinicians are proficient with similar procedures and may have cross-over skills, beginners should first observe PA catheter placement several times. Attempts to place the first few catheters should be supervised by a trained, skilled, and experienced clinician. After the clinician gains mastery of the skill of insertion, further study and use of the catheter should increase his or her skills, interest, knowledge, and abilities in the maintenance of a PA catheter as well as in obtaining data. Attending courses devoted to the technology will further enhance proficiency, especially for the subtler applications.

INDICATIONS

- Refractory acute respiratory distress syndrome (ARDS) or pulmonary edema, especially in patients with renal failure
- Severe hypoxemia requiring high levels (>10 cm) of positive end-expiratory pressure (PEEP)
- Presence of hemodynamic deterioration due to a mechanical complication (e.g., differentiate between mitral regurgitation and acute ventricular septal defect)
- Evaluation of left ventricular function if echocardiogram not available
- Suspected right ventricular dysfunction or infarction
- Preoperative optimization of extremely high-risk surgical patients
- Oxygen delivery and consumption assessment
- The evaluation of and drug titration for severe pulmonary hypertension

Monitoring

- Titration of drugs or other interventions in a highly unstable patient (e.g., vasodilators, inotropes, pacemaker)
- Refractory heart failure
- Hemodynamically unstable patient unresponsive to conventional therapy
- Unstable myocardial infarction with severely decompensated heart failure
- Right-sided heart failure resulting from severe obstructive lung disease, ARDS, or pulmonary embolism
- Refractory sepsis

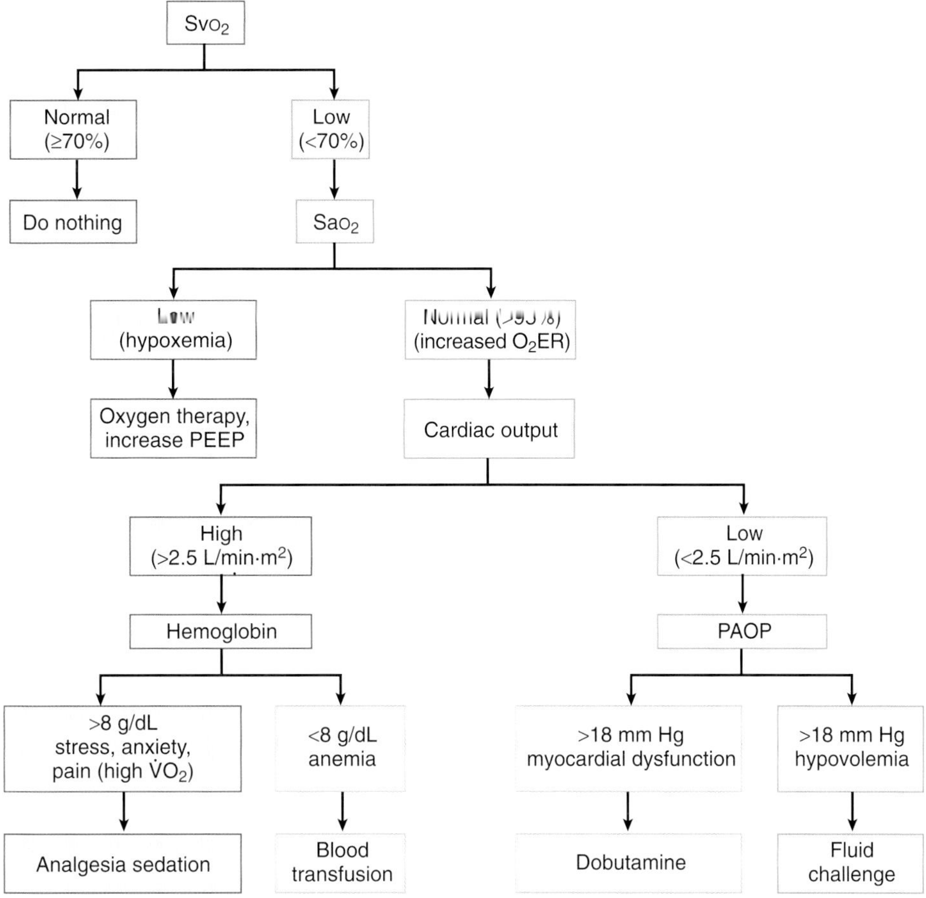

Figure 215-1 Diagnostic and therapeutic algorithm based on mixed venous oxygen saturation (SvO_2) measurements: therapeutic options to be considered are presented in the rectangles. SaO_2, arterial oxygen saturation; O_2ER, oxygen extraction ratio; PEEP, positive end-expiratory pressure; PAOP, pulmonary artery occlusion pressure; $\dot{V}O_2$, oxygen consumption. (From Pinsky MR, Vincent JL: Let us use the pulmonary artery catheter correctly and only when we need it. Crit Care Med 33:1119–1122, 2005.)

- Fluid management in certain complex situations (e.g., shock, postoperative state, ARDS, acute renal failure, intraoperative)

Therapeutic

- Pacing
- Aspiration of air emboli during seated neurosurgery

Contraindications

Contraindications are the same as those for central venous catheterization (see Chapter 211, Central Venous Catheter Insertion), plus the following *relative* contraindications:

- Diagnostic information could be provided by less invasive means (e.g., echocardiography, a therapeutic trial of fluid administration in the hypovolemic patient)
- Prosthetic right heart valve
- Cardiac-paced patient (temporary, internal, or permanent)*
- Severe hypotension
- Known pulmonary hypertension
- Highly unstable arrhythmias (especially ventricular)
- Right-sided endocarditis or mural thrombus
- Highly unstable respiratory status
- Lack of nursing staff or clinicians trained in use of PA catheters
- Lack of a compatible pressure monitoring apparatus
- Allergy to any component of the catheter (e.g., latex)

NOTE: If the underlying relative contraindication can be altered, catheterization may be worth the risk if there are no alternatives.

Equipment

- Central venous access with an 8.5-Fr percutaneous sheath introducer kit (see Chapter 211, Central Venous Catheter Insertion)
- Radiopaque PA catheter (7 to 7.5 Fr for adults; Fig. 215-2) with syringe for balloon inflation, occlusive caps for each port, and catheter protective shield

NOTE: Standard thermodilation catheters now usually have four lumens. The distal lumen at the tip measures PA and PA occlusion pressures, and is used for blood sampling. A more proximal

*Left bundle branch block (LBBB) was previously a contraindication because of the frequent occurrence of natural or induced right bundle branch block (RBBB) during passage of a PA catheter. This could cause complete heart block (i.e., RBBB + LBBB = complete heart block). A chronic indwelling catheter may also increase the risk of RBBB. Evidence suggests that the risk of complete bundle branch block is low; however, it may be prudent to use fluoroscopy when placing a PA catheter in a patient with an LBBB. A transvenous or transcutaneous pacer or a PA catheter with pacing capabilities should be available.

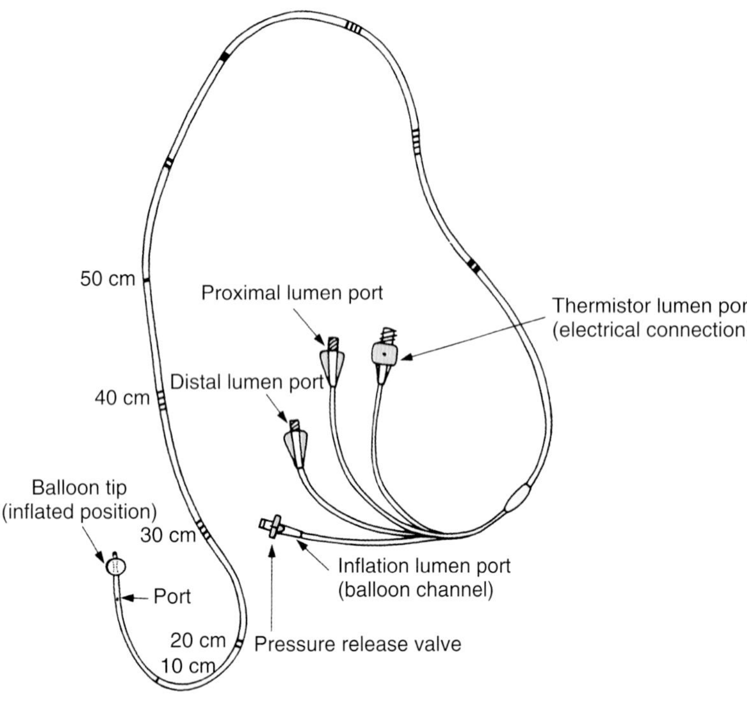

Figure 215-2 Balloon-tipped thermodilution catheter.

lumen (injectate) is used for injecting a thermal bolus for cardiac output measurement (if your Swan-Ganz catheter does not have continuous cardiac output capability). The third lumen is a proximal infusion port for medications; this port may also be used for a thermistor (electrical connection). A fourth lumen is used to inflate the balloon. There may be additional proximal lumens with ports. Catheters coated with chlorhexidine or heparin are also available to reduce the risk of infection and thrombosis, respectively.

- Pressure transducer and monitor (Fig. 215-3)
- High-pressure tubing, connectors, and two three-way stopcocks
- Heparinized saline flush system
- Povidone–iodine solution
- Sterile gowns, drapes, gloves, masks, and goggles
- Surgeon's cap
- Guidewire if changing central line to an introducer sheath (make sure it is the correct diameter and long enough to properly fit through both catheters)
- Suture and sterile dressing for site
- Supplemental oxygen
- Continuous pulse oximetry, cardiac, and blood pressure monitoring
- Fully stocked code cart and defibrillator nearby

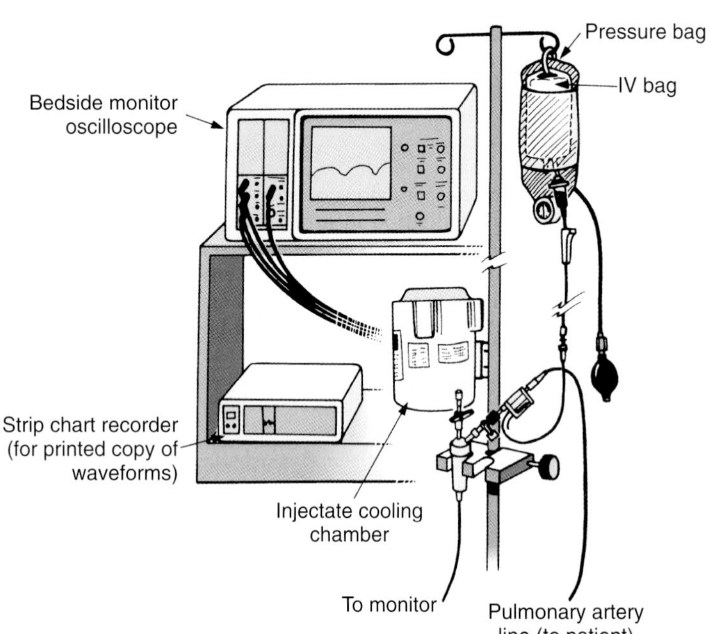

Figure 215-3 Pulmonary artery catheter setup.

Preprocedure Patient Preparation

Because PA catheterization is usually an emergency procedure, written informed consent cannot always be obtained. However, explain the indications, risks, benefits, and any available alternatives to the patient and the family, if possible. If the consent is implied, it should be documented. If time allows, the patient or family should sign for informed consent. Venous access may be established by the procedure outlined in Chapter 211, Central Venous Catheter Insertion. As delineated in Chapter 216, Temporary Pacing, catheterization of the right internal jugular vein provides the most direct access to the right atrium and ventricle, but its use may restrict patient mobility. The broad curve of the left subclavian vein may make it more difficult to traverse than the right internal jugular, but it is a reasonable second choice. The left internal jugular and right subclavian veins are acceptable alternatives. The femoral vein is another option, but it is infrequently used and often necessitates the use of fluoroscopy to properly advance the catheter. The external jugular, axillary, and basilic veins are additional options, but are also often difficult to traverse.

Technique

Before Insertion and General Guidelines

1. Supplemental oxygen should be supplied. If the patient is on a ventilator, the ventilatory settings and alarms should be checked. The endotracheal tube should be secured and suctioned.
2. Before the heart undergoes invasive monitoring or an area of the heart is traversed for any reason, record a baseline electrocardiogram (ECG).
3. A "time out" should be taken before this (and any) procedure to make sure you have the right procedure, site, and patient.
4. Because this procedure may induce arrhythmias, an additional, separate intravenous access site should be available. The introducer sheath has a separate intravenous access site if no other access is available.
5. To prevent the loss of a guidewire in a patient, *never* let go of the guidewire during catheter manipulation.
6. Observe strict sterile technique. Scrub after donning hair cover, goggles or eye protection, mask, and gown; wear sterile gloves and maintain sterile technique throughout the procedure. Optimally, the entire neck and clavicular area are prepared with povidone–iodine if the internal jugular or subclavian routes are to be used; a similarly sized area should be prepared if another route is to be used. Drape as large of an area as possible, including the majority of the patient and the bed. A three-quarter sheet works well for this purpose. Follow universal blood and body fluid precautions.

Conversion to a Sheath or an Introducer

If the venous catheter in place is a multilumen catheter or the single-lumen sheath is not large enough to accept the PA catheter, it must be converted. Use an 8.5-Fr introducer sheath for a 7- or 7.5-Fr PA catheter.

1. Insert a guidewire of proper diameter and sufficient length through the existing venous access line. Always maintain control of the guidewire. (Letting go could allow it to slip into the vein and embolize.) Carefully remove the existing venous access line (catheter or sheath) over the guidewire.
2. Leaving the guidewire in place, advance the dilator over the guidewire and into the vein to enlarge the lumen. A nick at the skin may be needed to advance the dilator; using a twisting motion when advancing may also be helpful.
3. Leaving the guidewire in place, remove the dilator.
4. Now place the dilator through the PA catheter introducer sheath and pass them both, as a unit, over the guidewire and into the patient's central circulation. Again, using a twisting motion while advancing the unit may facilitate this part of the procedure.
5. Remove the guidewire and the dilator, leaving the introducer sheath in place, and cap the sheath with the special cap that allows for PA catheter placement (usually a diaphragm on it).

Insertion of the Pulmonary Artery Catheter

1. Have an assistant set up, check, calibrate, and zero the electrical equipment. He or she should also level the transducer (see Fig. 215-3).
2. Remove the PA catheter from its sterile packaging. If used, thread the catheter protective sleeve (contamination shield) over the distal end of the catheter. Make sure that the docking mechanism is facing the correct direction. It should be able to be connected to the introducer sheath that was inserted earlier. Slide the protective sleeve up the PA catheter, far away from the tip, to keep it out of the way of the tip. Flush the catheter by injecting sterile heparinized saline into the three open ports of the catheter. Make sure that all ports are patent.
3. Next, test the balloon before insertion. Attach the smaller syringe to the balloon port and fill the balloon with air. A built-in safety mechanism in the syringe prevents overdistention of the balloon. Allow the balloon to deflate. (Never forcibly deflate the balloon.)
4. Hand the proximal end of the catheter to the assistant. Three-way stopcocks should be attached to the three lumens. Have the assistant connect the PA catheter to pressure tubing after internally flushing it with sterile saline.
5. Hook up the distal port to the PA transducer and jiggle the end of the catheter. You should see corresponding jiggling on the computer screen. If you do not, have your assistant check the connections.
6. Mark the patient's lateral midchest with an indelible ink spot so that the equipment can be lined up horizontally; this spot is considered the zero point. Record this height and the height of the bed mattress from the floor. The strict recording of heights is necessary because a change in height of 1 inch corresponds to a 1.8–mm Hg change in monitored pressure. An assistant or nurse will usually do this.
7. If using the right internal jugular approach, direct the catheter toward the superior vena cava. If using the right subclavian approach, aim the curve of the catheter so that it is pointing down clockwise toward the superior vena cava.

   EDITOR'S NOTE: The distance from the right internal jugular vein to the corresponding landmarks is about 5 cm more than when using the right subclavian vein approach.

8. ECG monitoring should be continuous throughout the procedure. Pass the deflated balloon-tipped catheter through diaphragm on the protective sleeve and then the sheath to the 20-cm mark; it is marked in 10-cm increments. Watch these distance markings carefully.
9. Watch the waveform monitor for a characteristic central venous tracing or a right atrial tracing. The normal range of pressure for the right atrium should be from 0 to 10 mm Hg and the monitor should show respiratory variation. An assistant should monitor the heart rhythm and record these pressures (Fig. 215-4). Three positive deflections can be seen if the scale is enlarged enough on the monitor: the a, c, and v waves.
10. Verify that the appropriate scale was picked on the monitor. If the patient is asked to cough, there should be an abrupt increase in the pressure tracing correlating with the abrupt increase in intrathoracic pressure.
11. After passing to 20 cm (out of the introducer sheath), rotate the entire catheter 180 degrees so the catheter tip is now pointing up (although you cannot see it) and counterclockwise,

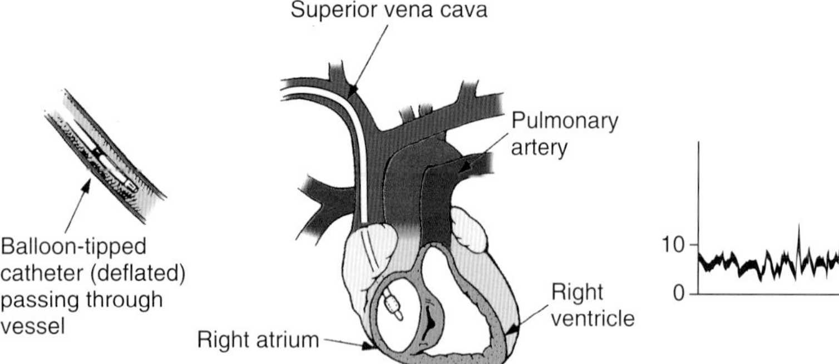

Figure 215-4 Balloon-tipped catheter passing through vessel to the 10- to 15-cm mark. If passed through internal jugular or subclavian vein, it enters right atrium at 15- to 20-cm mark. Note pressure.

matching the curve of the passage through the heart (see Fig. 215-4).

12. Using the syringe provided with the kit, inflate the balloon with air to the recommended full volume as indicated on the package or the syringe (0.8 to 1.5 mL of air). To avoid vessel damage, never advance the catheter beyond this point without an inflated balloon. The provided syringe is designed to prevent the entry of undesired air. As long as it is not overdistended, the balloon will typically provide a buffer around the distal hard tip of the catheter. Avoid overfilling the balloon! It can burst with dire consequences. Never force air into a PA catheter (Fig. 215-5).

   EDITOR'S NOTE: Once out of the introducer sheath, never advance the PA catheter without the balloon being inflated. Never withdraw the PA catheter without the balloon being deflated.

13. Pass the catheter to the 30- or 40-cm mark in a quick but not too rapid fashion. While passing the catheter, watch the pressure monitor for the characteristic right ventricular tracing. This tracing looks like a large square root sign without a dicrotic notch. A dramatic rise in the systolic pressure should occur during this manipulation (Fig. 215-6A). Record the right ventricular pressures. Also watch the ECG monitor for any ectopy at this stage.
14. After confirming its presence in the right ventricle, pass the catheter without delay to the 40- to 50-cm mark, into the PA. The PA will have the same systolic pressures as the right ventricle but the diastolic pressures will be higher. You will see a dicrotic notch on the downhill distal side of the triangles (Fig. 215-6B). Record the pressures. Normal PA pressures are 15 to 25 mm Hg systolic and 8 to 16 mm Hg diastolic, with a mean of 10 to 20 mm Hg.
15. Once in the PA, continue passing the catheter at a much slower pace, watching for the characteristic pulmonary capillary wedge pressure (PCWP) tracing at about the 50-cm mark on the catheter (Fig. 215-6C). With PCWP tracings, the systolic pressure is lost and you are left with the "wedge pressure." In fact, the PA diastolic pressure is a good estimate of the wedge pressure if for some reason you cannot get a wedge pressure. This is the place where the vessel has become occluded and the catheter no longer reads PA pressures; rather, it reads pressure reflected back from the left atrium through the capillaries. If the patient has a normal mitral valve, the PCWP approximates the left

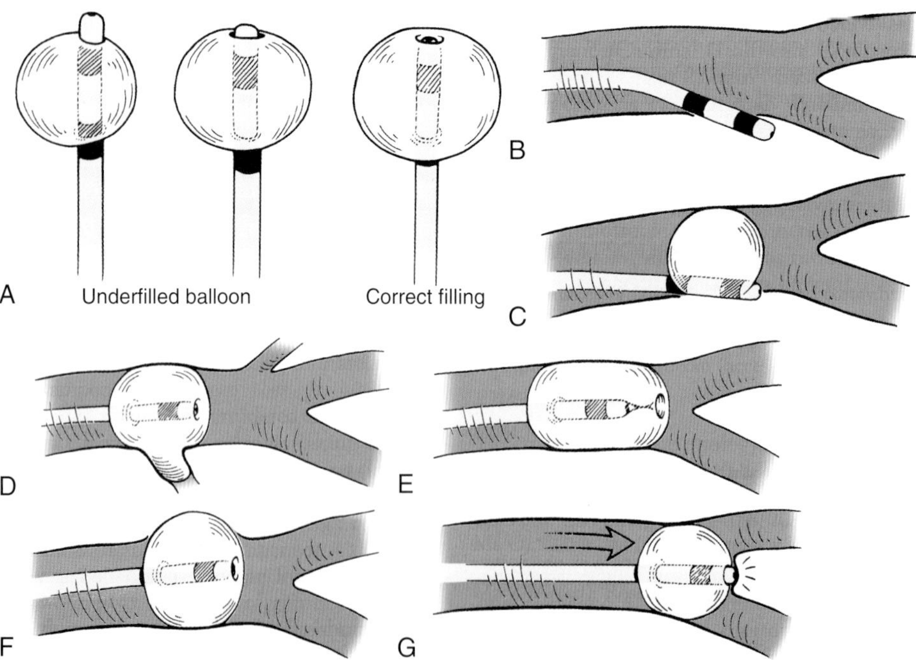

Figure 215-5 Correct filling of the balloon and possible complications. **A,** Underfilled and correct filling. **B,** Tip perforates wall of vessel when balloon is not inflated. **C,** Eccentric balloon (inaccurate wedge) with risk of wall rupture. **D,** Overfilled balloon inadvertently distending down side vessel. **E,** Inaccurate and overdistention of balloon can cause catheter tip occlusion. **F,** Overwedge (see Troubleshooting section). **G,** Underinflated catheter with protruding tip.

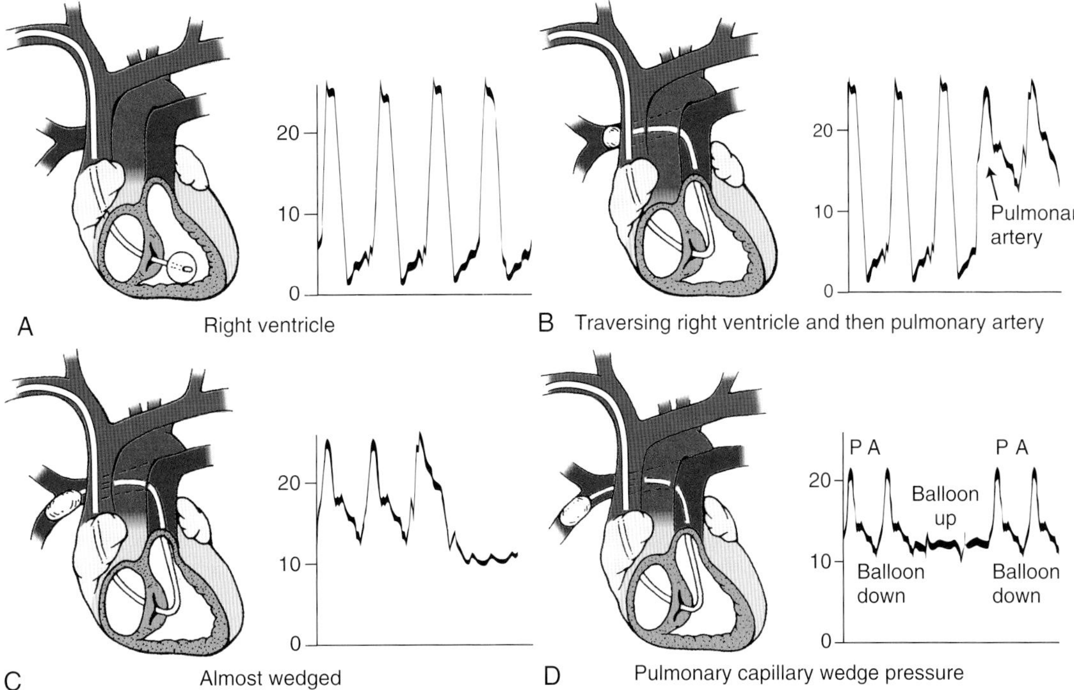

Figure 215-6 Tracings recorded through the catheter as it traverses the right ventricle and pulmonary artery and is wedged: the right ventricle (**A**), the pulmonary artery (**B**), almost wedged (**C**), and, finally, the wedged position (**D**).

ventricular diastolic pressure (Fig. 215-6D). In the absence of elevated end-expiratory pressures or obstruction of the pulmonary veins, PCWP approximates left atrial mean pressure to within 2 mm Hg. If desired, using the Starling pressure–volume relationships, left ventricular end-diastolic volume can also be estimated.

16. Once the balloon is wedged, allow it to passively deflate and watch for the phasic PA tracing. Do not aspirate to deflate the balloon; active deflation may cause rupture.
17. Inflate the balloon again and allow it to deflate to observe the two different tracings. If the syringe and balloon were designed to hold 1.5 mL, this should be the amount required to wedge the catheter safely. If any less accomplishes it, the catheter's location is too distal; withdraw it until 1.5 mL wedges it. If 1.5 mL does not wedge the balloon, pass the catheter further. Although the PCWP is called an occlusion pressure, the inflated balloon actually floats distally and *then* occludes the vessel. The vessel is not occluded from inflation at a fixed location. The catheter should be placed at the most proximal point where a wedge pressure is observed. If you deflate the balloon and do not see the PA pressures, either the balloon did not truly deflate, or you have a "permanent wedge." If the latter is the case, you must withdraw the catheter until you see PA pressures again and then refloat the catheter.
18. The wedge pressure should be read at end expiration and recorded.
19. Extend the catheter protective sleeve, if used, and attach it to the sheath with the docking mechanism.
20. Secure the entire assembly with suture and adequate tape. Apply a sterile dressing.
21. Order a chest radiograph and auscultate the chest bilaterally to exclude a pneumothorax.
22. Begin infusion of necessary fluids or medications.
23. If the patient was moved, the assistant should rezero the equipment.
24. Document the procedure in the chart, including the tracings, and record end-expiratory values. Additional documented values should include the PA pressure, the PCWP, and the cardiac output (performed by the assistant and not detailed here).

Confirmation of Proper Placement

1. Obstruction is excluded by the ability to flush the catheter before inflating the balloon.
2. When the balloon is inflated, the typical PA tracing disappears. It reappears promptly after the balloon deflates.
3. PCWP is lower than or equal to PA diastolic pressure.

TROUBLESHOOTING

It is common to get salvos of premature ventricular contractions as the catheter passes through the right ventricle. Usually this problem will resolve with passage of the catheter to the pulmonary artery. If the ectopy does not resolve, the balloon must be deflated and the catheter brought back to the superior vena cava. The catheter may also be coiling in the right ventricle. If further attempts to pass it are unsuccessful, administer an intravenous bolus of lidocaine (75 to 100 mg) and attempt passage under fluoroscopy.

If a PA or PCWP tracing cannot be obtained, keep the balloon deflated, pull the catheter back to 20 cm, and try inserting again. Consider inserting the catheter using a clockwise twisting action. If this fails, try counterclockwise reinsertion. Having the patient take some deep breaths may also help pass the catheter. Occasionally the tip of the PA catheter gets malpositioned in the chest. If the tip lies above the level of the left atrium (with the patient lying down, this would be anterior), the alveolar pressure may be greater than the pulmonary capillary pressures and you will get an errant reading. Again, fluoroscopy may be helpful here.

Some clinicians recommend injecting cold, sterile saline solution to enhance passage; this may stiffen the catheter, which may have softened because of the warmth of the body. Occasionally, a guidewire and fluoroscopy are necessary to advance the catheter. Repositioning the patient may help.

In patients with a very low ejection fraction, an inotrope may have to be administered to facilitate passage. It may also be difficult to pass a PA catheter in patients with tricuspid regurgitation or pulmonary hypertension. Again, having the patient take deep breaths may facilitate passage in all of these situations.

For a normal-sized adult, from the subclavian or internal jugular site, insertion beyond 50 cm (or 15 cm after entering the right ventricle) predisposes the catheter to coiling, which can lead to knotting.

When a catheter's location is too distal in the vessel, a tracing called an *overwedge* may be seen. This is likely to occur when the balloon is not filled with enough air. After allowing the balloon to deflate, withdraw the catheter and attempt to wedge it again, this time with the balloon fully inflated to its correct volume (see Fig. 215-5). Persistent underinflation of the balloon when wedging can damage the pulmonary vessels or the endocardium and may cause arrhythmias, especially if the catheter tip is exposed (see Fig. 215-5A and G). There are several possible mechanisms, such as overinflation or underinflation of the balloon (see Fig. 215-5B, C, F, and G), that could cause rupture of the PA; fortunately, these are unlikely.

When air is present in the catheter damping can occur, which has an opposite effect to that of overwedging. It appears like a regular tracing, but the variations are damped. Air bubbles should be removed from the connecting tubes by aspirating and flushing the catheter. If blood cannot be aspirated, yet the catheter flushes easily, suspect a ball-valve thrombus at the catheter tip. Inject 5000 U of heparin into the lumen and allow 15 to 30 minutes for it to take effect. Initiate a continuous drip of heparin (not to exceed 20,000 U for 24 hours). If still unsuccessful, withdraw the catheter gradually 5 cm at a time, watching for waveforms.

Lesions obstructing the mitral valve, such as mitral stenosis, can interfere with the accuracy of the PCWP as an estimate of left ventricular diastolic pressure. Respirations can also cause significant variations in the pressure readings for the PA catheter. Make calibrated strip chart recordings for all measurements derived from the catheter and then measure again at end expiration (Fig. 215-7). Finally, high PEEP settings on a ventilator can falsely elevate wedge pressures.

COMPLICATIONS

Possible complications are the same as for central venous catheterization (see Chapter 211, Central Venous Catheter Insertion), *plus* those discussed in the following sections.

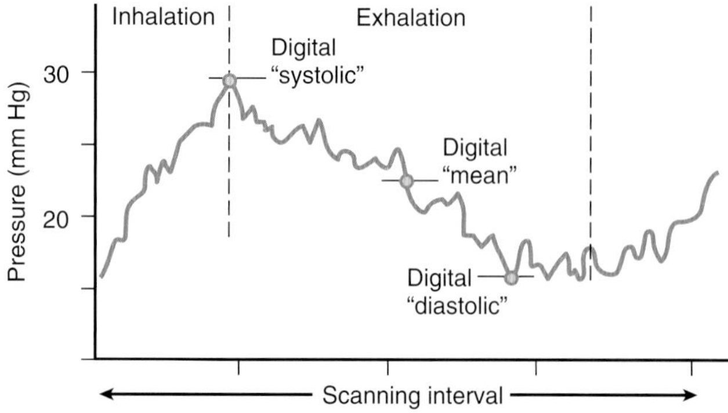

Figure 215-7 **Respiratory variation of the pulmonary artery catheter tracing.** (From Wiedemann HP, Matthay MA, Matthay RA: Cardiovascular-pulmonary monitoring in the intensive care unit: Part I. Chest 85:537–549, 1984.)

During Pulmonary Artery Catheter Placement

- *Pulmonary infarction:* Can result from leaving the balloon inflated too long.
- *Atrial and ventricular ectopy or conduction changes:* Advancement into the PA may decrease ectopy. However, withdrawal of the catheter may be necessary. Usually the ectopy is transitory, but if an unstable rhythm persists, medical treatment or electrical conversion may be necessary.
- *Knotting of the catheter* can occur inside or outside of the heart (more likely with smaller-bore catheters [e.g., 5 Fr]) and, rarely, cause injury to intracardiac structures. Inflating the balloon while in the subclavian vein or superior vena cava may minimize the risk of knotting. On the contrary, to avoid injury to the pulmonic or tricuspid valve, do not withdraw the catheter with the balloon inflated. Also, if resistance is noted with attempted withdrawal, obtain a chest radiograph to exclude the possibility of knotting or entanglement in the heart. The catheter rarely can get looped around the papillary muscle of the tricuspid valve so that removal is impossible.
- *Malposition:* The most common malposition occurs when the PA catheter turns up the internal jugular instead of down into the superior vena cava. If, while advancing, you feel resistance, deflate the balloon, do not advance any further, and get a radiograph. If the PA catheter is malpositioned, try to carefully reposition it or use fluoroscopy. Rarely, vessel wall puncture and insertion into undesirable places (e.g., subclavian artery, pleural space) may occur.
- *Cardiac perforation and tamponade* (extremely rare).

With Continued Presence of the Pulmonary Artery Catheter in the Central Circulation

- *Pulmonary infarction:* Leaving the balloon inflated too long or downstream displacement of the deflated balloon (causing "permanent wedge"—described earlier) can block an artery and cause infarction. Infarction can also result from thrombosis.
- *Pulmonary hemorrhage:* More common in the presence of pulmonary hypertension, possibly associated with the higher pressures forcing the tip through the vessel wall. Cautiously obtain PCWP in patients with pulmonary hypertension. Hemorrhage can also result from pulmonary infarction.
- *Mural (or elsewhere) thrombus formation:* Thrombosis may develop anywhere throughout the course of the catheter. It can occlude any of the veins through which the catheter has passed (or elsewhere).
- *Balloon rupture or catheter fracture:* If balloon rupture is suspected, aspirate into the syringe the same gas volume used for inflation, disconnect the syringe, and leave the stopcock open to vent the balloon. Remove the catheter immediately to prevent latex fragments from embolizing.
- *Endocarditis:* Aseptic vegetations are found on autopsy in approximately 30% of patients who have had a PA catheter. Both aseptic and septic vegetations may be more common in burn patients.
- *Sepsis:* Frequent manipulations of the catheter, as well as leaving the catheter in place more than 3 days, increase the risk of positive blood cultures. After 24 to 48 hours, if the catheter has become partially withdrawn, advancing the catheter may introduce bacteria from the skin insertion site or the catheter itself. No data show that aseptic protective sleeves prevent this from happening. PA catheters, like any other catheters, should be left in place only as long as necessary.
- *Hemoptysis:* Can be caused by flushing the catheter when it is in the wedged position.
- *Embolism* (air or thrombotic).
- *Pulmonary artery rupture.*

- *Pseudoaneurysm*.
- *Inaccurate diagnosis* because of malfunctioning or malpositioned catheter.

Postprocedure Catheter Care

- Flush the catheter with heparinized saline every 30 minutes.
- Inflate the balloon only when measuring the PCWP. To avoid pulmonary infarction, leave it inflated for a *maximum* of 60 seconds only. To exclude the possibility of catheter obstruction before inflation, flush the catheter each time before inflating the balloon. If the catheter is occluded, there is no point in inflating the balloon.
- For obstruction, attempt to reposition the catheter. If a thrombus is suspected, use the same technique as used for clearing a ball-valve thrombus.
- Adjust the position of the catheter as necessary. Otherwise, the catheter may soften and migrate to a more distal site, predisposing to distal or branch vessel occlusion. If the PA pressure tracing shows a loss in phasicity and begins to resemble the PCWP tracing (without balloon inflation), withdraw the catheter until the typical phasic PA tracing reappears. Always deflate when withdrawing to avoid damage to intracardiac structures.
- Remove, inspect, and replace the sterile dressing daily.
- Obtain daily chest radiographs to check for catheter migration and to exclude pulmonary infarction.

Patient Education Guides

See the sample patient education handout online at www.expertconsult.com.

CPT/Billing Code

93503 Insertion and placement of flow-directed catheter (e.g., Swan-Ganz) for monitoring purposes

ICD-9-CM Diagnostic Codes

401.0 Accelerated or malignant essential hypertension
410.11 Myocardial infarction, initial episode, anterior wall (can include damage such as ruptured myocardium)
410.91 Myocardial infarction, acute, unspecified, initial episode (can include damage such as ruptured myocardium)
411.1 Angina, unstable
415.0 Cor pulmonale, acute
415.11 Pulmonary embolism or infarct, postoperative or iatrogenic
415.19 Pulmonary embolism or infarct, unspecified
416.0 Pulmonary hypertension, chronic primary
416.8 Pulmonary hypertension, chronic secondary
423.0 Hemopericardium
423.3 Cardiac tamponade
423.9 Pericardial effusion or unspecified disease of pericardium
424.0 Mitral valve disorders
424.1 Aortic valve disorders
424.2 Tricuspid valve disorders
424.3 Pulmonic valve disorders
427.1 Paroxysmal ventricular tachycardia
427.5 Cardiac or cardiorespiratory arrest
428.0 Right heart failure, secondary to left
428.0 Heart failure, congestive, unspecified
428.1 Pulmonary edema (left heart failure)
518.5 Pulmonary insufficiency after trauma and surgery
785.50 Shock, unspecified
785.51 Shock, cardiogenic
785.52 Shock, septic
785.59 Shock, other (hypovolemic)

Acknowledgment

The editors wish to recognize the many contributions by Len Scarpinato, DO, to this chapter in the previous two editions of this text.

Suppliers

(See contact information online at www.expertconsult.com.)

Arrow International
Edwards Lifesciences Corp (formerly a division of Baxter)
Weslee Medical, Inc.

ONLINE RESOURCES

American College of Cardiology: Policy guidelines for cardiac catheterization, pulmonary artery catheterization, and the consensus statement on right heart catheterization. Available at www.acc.org.

American Society of Anesthesiologists: Practice guidelines for pulmonary artery catheterization: An updated report by the American Society of Anesthesiologists Task Force on Pulmonary Artery Catheterization. 2003. Available at www.asahq.org/publicationsAndServices/pulm_artery.pdf.

Manbit Technologies: PA catheter insertion simulators are available, and the online text describes the procedure. Available at www.manbit.com.

Pulmonary Artery Catheter Education Project: A free online resource that provides educational resources on how to use the pulmonary artery catheter. Available at www.pacep.org.

BIBLIOGRAPHY

American Heart Association: Textbook of Advanced Cardiac Life Support. Dallas, American Heart Association, 1997.

Bernard GR, Sopko G, Cerra F, et al: Pulmonary artery catheterization and clinical outcomes: National Heart, Lung, and Blood Institute and Food and Drug Administration Workshop Report Consensus Statement. JAMA 283:2568–2572, 2000.

Connors AF Jr, Speroff T, Dawson NV, et al: The effectiveness of right heart catheterization in the initial care of critically ill patients: SUPPORT investigators. JAMA 276:889–897, 1996.

Hall JB: Use of the pulmonary artery catheter in critically ill patients: Was invention the mother of necessity? JAMA 283:2577–2578, 2000.

Harvey S, Young D, Brampton W, et al: Pulmonary artery catheters for adult patients in intensive care [review]. Cochrane Database Syst Rev 3:CD003408, 2006.

Kelly RF, Franklin C: Pulmonary artery (Swan-Ganz) catheterization. In Reichman EF, Simon RR (eds): Emergency Medicine Procedures. New York, McGraw-Hill, 2004, pp 349–357.

Mueller HS, Chatterjee K, Davis KB, et al: ACC expert consensus document: Present use of bedside right heart catheterization in patients with cardiac disease. American College of Cardiology. J Am Coll Cardiol 32:840–864, 1998.

Otero RM, Nguyen HB, Huang DT, et al: Early goal-directed therapy in severe sepsis and septic shock revisited: Concepts, controversies, and contemporary findings. Chest 130:1579–1595, 2006.

Pinsky MR, Vincent JL: Let us use the pulmonary artery catheter correctly and only when we need it. Crit Care Med 33:1119–1122, 2005.

Rivers E, Nguyen B, Havstad S, et al: Early goal-directed therapy in the treatment of severe sepsis and septic shock. N Engl J Med 345:1368–1377, 2001.

Shah MR, Hasselblad V, Stevenson LW, et al: Impact of the pulmonary artery catheter in critically ill patients: Meta-analysis of randomized clinical trials. JAMA 294:1664–1670, 2005.

CHAPTER 216

Temporary Pacing

William Ellert

For various reasons, primary care clinicians may need to perform temporary cardiac pacing. Several types of pacing are available, with the primary purpose being to maintain circulatory stability until either the situation resolves or a permanent pacemaker can be installed. This chapter covers external (transcutaneous) and internal (transvenous) emergency ventricular pacing. Transesophageal pacing, usually limited to atrial pacing, and transmyocardial transthoracic pacing are beyond the scope of this chapter.

The basic uses for temporary cardiac pacing are as a standby should the patient become symptomatic or complete heart block occur and as a way to increase heart rate during periods of symptomatic bradycardia. In addition, overdrive pacing may be used to terminate arrhythmias (e.g., sustained supraventricular or ventricular tachycardia); atrioventricular (AV) sequential pacing may be used to prevent arrhythmias. "Medicinal" pacing (e.g., atropine, isoproterenol) is also available, with advanced cardiac life support (ACLS) guidelines being helpful to guide its use. Overall, the indications for temporary pacing can be divided into therapeutic, prophylactic, and diagnostic categories. For the purposes of this chapter, only therapeutic and prophylactic pacing are covered.

External (Transcutaneous) Pacing

Most defibrillator/cardioversion units are now capable of performing external transcutaneous pacing. Modern transcutaneous pacing units represent a major improvement over the units first developed in the 1950s. Those units frequently inflicted severe chest and back muscle stimulation and discomfort, and they often left burns on the skin. At least one suicide was recorded of a pacer-dependent patient who removed the leads from one of the older units to "end the pain." In the 1960s, transcutaneous pacing was largely replaced with the newly available transvenous pacing.

Subsequent discoveries rejuvenated transcutaneous pacing, especially since the 1980s. Researchers found that increasing the pulse duration from 2 to 20 milliseconds (msec) not only increased the safety of transcutaneous pacing (reduced the risk of ventricular fibrillation), but reduced the required current. Reduced current meant less pain and fewer burns. The development of electrodes with a larger surface area also decreased the pain and risk of tissue burn. Use of larger electrodes allows for a reduction in the current density, or the amount of current penetrating per square unit of skin. These developments have resulted in more frequent use of transcutaneous pacing, especially on a standby basis, and consequently decreased the use of transvenous pacing.

One of the shortfalls of external pacing, even with today's somewhat sophisticated equipment, is the difficulty of achieving capture in about one fifth of patients. Reasons for difficult or ineffective external pacing include increased intrathoracic air (such as barrel chests or chronic obstructive pulmonary disease), a large pericardial effusion or tamponade, recent thoracic surgery, obesity, and the improper placement of electrodes. Increased output for capture may be required in these individuals. Another shortfall is that it is rare for patients not to complain of some pectoral muscle stimulation. Although most patients rate the discomfort as mild or moderate and easily tolerable, approximately one third of patients rate the pain as severe or intolerable. Therefore, analgesics, narcotics, or sedatives should be considered when using the external pacer, especially if the required mean current for capture is 50 milliamperes (mA) or more (a common threshold).

Because the high voltages required for external pacing produce significant muscle twitching, conventional electrocardiographic (ECG) monitors and recorders are useless. To provide decent tracings despite the large pacer spikes and their aftermath, routine ECG monitors must be equipped with an *output adapter*. Fortunately, most external pacer units come equipped with a monitor capable of filtering the spikes. Without an adequate ECG monitor, treatable ventricular fibrillation could be masked by the large pacing spikes, with disastrous results. This is one of the grave risks of transcutaneous pacing.

Indications

- Short-term pacing until transvenous pacing can be initiated or underlying conditions requiring pacing are corrected (e.g., drug overdose, hyperkalemia)
- When medical therapy is not immediately available, or when significant bradyarrhythmias have not responded to medical therapy (e.g., atropine, isoproterenol)
- Symptomatic patients (e.g., syncope, presyncope, dizziness, fatigue) with type I or type II second-degree AV block, third-degree or complete AV block, asystolic pauses exceeding 3 seconds, or an escape pacemaker rate less than 40 beats per minute (bpm); also for patients who become symptomatic because of a bifascicular block or sinus node dysfunction
- As a standby or prophylaxis in conscious patients with hemodynamically stable bradycardia
- As a standby or prophylaxis before surgery in patients with a preexisting cardiac conduction block (anesthesia can exacerbate the block); also before cardiac diagnostic studies
- As a standby or prophylaxis in conscious patients with an expected bradyarrhythmia or a new type II second-degree, third-degree, or complete AV heart block in the setting of ischemia or infarction (frequently seen with acute anterior or inferior wall myocardial infarctions or digoxin overdose)

NOTE: Preliminary trial of pacing should be performed to ensure that capture is achievable and that pacing is tolerated by the patient.

- In children with primary bradycardia from congenital defects or after open-heart surgery
- To be considered when fluoroscopy (the preferred technique) is not available for transvenous pacer insertion

Contraindications

All of the contraindications are *relative*.

- Bradycardia in patient with significant hypothermia; as the core temperature drops, the ventricles become more irritable and prone to fibrillation that is resistant to defibrillation. In addition, bradycardia may be physiologic due to a decreased metabolic rate in these individuals.
- Bradycardia in children: usually due to hypoxia or hypoventilation, the best intervention is to provide an adequate airway as opposed to pacing (exceptions as mentioned in the Indications section).
- Overdrive pacing in tachyarrhythmias with rates greater than 180 bpm because that is the maximal rate of most external pacers.
- Bradyasystolic or asystolic arrest of more than 20 minutes' duration because of the well-documented poor resuscitation rates.
- Patient is unable to cooperate or tolerate the procedure (in life-threatening situation, provide sedation).
- Lack of therapeutic benefit because of advanced disease or terminal illness.

Equipment

- Two 8-cm electrodes. These are usually round or rectangular and packaged in pairs. The negative electrode may also be labeled "front," "apex," or "anterior"; the positive electrode may be labeled "back" or "posterior."
- Razor or scissors to remove body hair from the area of electrode placement.
- Pacing unit (contains pulse generator and monitor). The best units allow either fixed-rate or demand mode. Most allow a range from 30 to 180 bpm, with current output from 0 to 200 mA. Pulse durations vary from 20 to 40 msec and are not adjustable by the operator. To protect health care providers, some pacers shut off when an electrode falls off the chest.

NOTE: Most defibrillator/cardioversion units contain a transcutaneous pacing unit as an integral part of the system.

- ECG leads capable of monitoring during transcutaneous pacing. If not purchased as part of the pacing or defibrillator/cardioversion system, *an output adapter to a separate ECG monitor* is required to "blank" or neutralize the large electrical spikes from the pacer.

Preprocedure Patient Preparation

If time allows, explain the purpose and benefits of the procedure as well as the risks of not performing the procedure to the patient or representative. The patient should know what to expect, the sensations he or she may experience (e.g., muscle contractions, a slight tingling, burning or shocking sensation), and that although this may be uncomfortable, the majority of patients tolerate it well. Explain what will be done to minimize the discomfort (e.g., analgesic, sedation). A signed consent is not required to perform this procedure; however, implied consent should be documented in the medical record (e.g., "the risks and benefits have been explained to the patient, who agrees with having the procedure").

Any dirt or debris should be cleaned from the skin; however, avoid using any flammable liquids such as alcohol. Patients with significant body hair may need to be shaved (unconscious patients) or the hair clipped or trimmed (conscious) to ensure good skin–electrode contact. Shaving should be avoided, if possible, in the conscious patient because any nicks or lacerations can increase the discomfort and skin irritation during pacing.

Technique

1. Attach the exposed adhesive surfaces of two large electrode patches to the anterior and posterior chest walls (Fig. 216-1). The negative (anterior) electrode should be placed over the apex (at the point of maximal impulse) or the septum of the heart (the lead V_3 position), and the positive (posterior) electrode directly behind the anterior electrode, to the left of the thoracic spine, between the spine and the left scapula. Alternatively, the positive electrode can be placed on the right upper chest with the negative electrode over the apex of the heart.

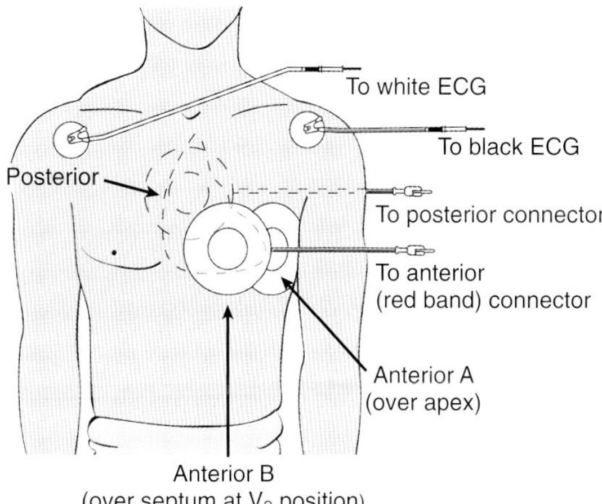

Figure 216-1 External (transcutaneous) pacing. The anterior electrode is placed at the apex (A), which is to the left of the sternum over the point of maximal impulse, or over the septum (B), which is the V_3 position. The posterior electrode is placed to the left of the spinal column on the back, directly behind the anterior electrode. (Adapted from Dahlberg ST, Benotti JR: Temporary cardiac pacing. In Rippe JM, Irwin RS, Alpert JS, Fink MP [eds]: Intensive Care Medicine, 2nd ed. Boston, Little, Brown, 1991.)

2. If time allows, prepare the patient with analgesia such as a narcotic or sedation with a benzodiazepine (especially helpful if the required mean current for capture is ≥50 mA).
3. Turn on the pacing unit. Set the heart rate (e.g., 80 bpm) to demand pacing. Set the current output and sensing thresholds at levels similar to those used for internal pacing; however, remember that larger outputs are necessary. Keep in mind that for demand pacing, external units often do not have sensing thresholds. The final current output setting is usually 1.25 times the initial capture threshold. Patients with conditions that cause difficult or ineffective pacing may require higher outputs for capture. At these higher outputs, the resultant muscle twitches may be so severe as to preclude external pacer use.
4. Apply the electrical stimulation to the electrodes. For conscious patients, slowly increase the output from the minimal setting, at 5- to 10-mA increments, until capture is achieved. Electrical capture is usually indicated by a widening of the QRS complex and especially by a broad T wave. The output required to obtain capture is defined as the pacing threshold. For asystolic or unconscious patients, begin at full output (200 mA) and decrease until capture is achieved, which defines the pacing threshold. The final current output should be set at the pacing threshold or 5 to 10 mA above it. When transcutaneous pacing is used as a standby technique, most clinicians document capture by initiating a brief period of pacing at a rate slightly higher than the patient's intrinsic rate. The pacing output threshold is then recorded and the pacing unit is returned to standby mode.
5. When successful pacing is achieved, prophylactic intravenous access (central venous [CV] catheter) through the right internal jugular vein may be helpful in case an internal pacer is needed urgently. Because external pacers have up to a 20% failure rate, having CV access available minimizes the risk of having to obtain it during a "code" situation.
6. Monitor continuously for capture and potential complications (e.g., treatable ventricular fibrillation, burns). The only sure sign of electrical capture is the presence of a consistent ST segment and T wave after each pacer spike. Palpation of the carotid to

confirm a pulse is not helpful because the muscle stimulation and contractions produced by the pacer simulate a carotid pulse.

NOTE: The increased use of external pacers has surely reduced the number of prophylactic internal pacers placed. However, in nontransient situations, external pacing is always a temporary measure until an internal pacer (probably transvenous, as described in the next section) can be placed.

Internal (Transvenous) Pacing

Clinicians who may need to insert a transvenous pacemaker should be familiar with the equipment and its use before needing it in an emergent situation. There are usually two lights, a sense indicator light, which is illuminated when a cardiac impulse is sensed, and a pace indicator light, which is illuminated whenever a pacing stimulus is generated. There is also usually a button to test the battery to ensure adequate voltage to operate the pacemaker generator. Although newer models have digital displays and more sophisticated pacing options, they function basically the same as older models.

Indications

Therapeutic

- Symptomatic, hemodynamically compromising or life-threatening bradyarrhythmias unresponsive to pharmacologic therapy (e.g., systolic blood pressure <80 mm Hg, change in mental status, angina, pulmonary edema), including sick sinus syndrome
- Bradycardia with ventricular escape rhythm, unresponsive to pharmacologic therapy

NOTE: For tachyarrhythmias of less than 150 bpm, neither immediate cardioversion nor an immediate pacer is necessary.

Prophylactic (in Setting of Acute Myocardial Infarction)

- Symptomatic sinus node dysfunction or Mobitz type I second-degree AV heart block that is not responsive to atropine therapy
- Second-degree Mobitz type II, third-degree, or complete AV heart block*
- Newly acquired bundle branch block with first-degree AV block
- Bilateral or alternating bundle branch blocks
- An old right bundle branch block with first-degree AV block and a new fascicular block

Contraindications

Contraindications include those listed in Chapter 211, Central Venous Catheter Insertion, and those listed previously for external pacing. Other contraindications include the following:

- A situation in which the bradycardia is well tolerated and the symptoms are intermittent, mild, or rare.*
- Bradycardia in patients with significant hypothermia; as the core temperature drops, the ventricles become more irritable and prone to fibrillation (especially if the pacing wire contacts the heart muscle) that is resistant to defibrillation. In addition, bradycardia may be physiologic because of a decreased metabolic rate in these individuals (*relative contraindication*).
- Digoxin toxicity and other drug ingestions that may increase the irritability of the myocardium (*relative contraindication* in life-threatening situation).
- Presence of a prosthetic tricuspid valve (*relative contraindication* in life-threatening situation).
- Depending on access site, planned neck or clavicle surgical procedures (*relative contraindication*, may affect choice of site).
- Distortion of local anatomy or landmarks; for insertion from subclavian, moderate to severe chest wall deformities that distort local anatomy (*relative contraindication*, may affect choice of site).
- Suspected injury to the superior vena cava (*relative contraindication*, may affect choice of site; e.g., superior vena cava syndrome, in which insertion from below the diaphragm is preferable).
- Bleeding diathesis, anticoagulation therapy, or concurrent thrombolysis or fibrinolysis (unless emergent pacing is required, and then antecubital venous cutdown access is preferred).
- Full-thickness burn, cellulitis, or other infection over the anticipated insertion site (*relative contraindication*, may affect choice of site).
- Pneumothorax or hemothorax on the contralateral side or inability to tolerate pneumothorax on the ipsilateral side (*relative contraindication* in life-threatening situation).
- The absence of informed consent (*relative contraindication* in life-threatening situation).
- Patient is unable to cooperate or tolerate the procedure (*relative contraindication* in life-threatening situation, provide sedation).
- Bradyasystolic and asystolic arrest of more than 20 minutes' duration because of the well-documented poor resuscitation rates (*relative contraindication*).
- Lack of therapeutic benefit because of advanced disease or terminal illness (*relative contraindication*).
- Suspected prior injury to the vein intended for insertion or vasculitis that predisposes to sclerosis or thrombosis of the veins (*relative contraindication* in life-threatening situation).
- Previous long-term catheterization, injection of hyperosmotic or irritant solution, or recently discontinued catheter in the same vein (*relative contraindication* in life-threatening situation).
- Contraindications specific to *internal jugular vein* access include significant carotid artery disease, distorted cervical anatomy, and recent, unsuccessful contralateral cannulation (to prevent bilateral neck hematomas, which could compromise the patient's airway).
- Subclavian insertion during cardiopulmonary resuscitation (CPR). (If CPR can be halted briefly, this may be beneficial; jugular access can usually be obtained without stopping CPR. Otherwise, peripheral access may be preferable.)
- Children (*relative contraindication* and rarely needed; better intervention is to treat the cause [e.g., hypoxia]. If pacing is needed, the internal jugular vein is the best access route.)
- Patients receiving ventilatory support with high end-expiratory pressures (e.g., positive end-expiratory pressure; *relative contraindication* in life-threatening situation; if possible, ventilation should be interrupted briefly while attempting to cannulate the vein for access).
- Patients with morbid obesity, marked cachexia, or severe hypovolemia may be better served by using common femoral or peripheral vein access.
- Severe hypovolemia (*relative contraindication* due to difficulty in insertion).

Equipment

- Bipolar transvenous pacing catheters (Fig. 216-2), 4 to 6 Fr, may be soft and pliable and made from extruded plastic or firm, relatively nonpliable, and made from woven Dacron. Some practitioners prefer soft, flexible, semifloating catheters; however, these are more difficult to maneuver and less stable once positioned. Flow-directed, flexible, balloon-tipped pacing catheters are also available. They are similar to balloon-tipped pulmonary artery catheters, but without an open lumen (see Fig. 216-2). Stiffer catheters are usually easier to maneuver than balloon-tipped

*In patients with an inferior myocardial infarction, relatively asymptomatic second- or third-degree heart block can occur. Pacing in such patients should be reserved for symptoms or the presence of a deteriorating bradycardia. If not paced, patients should be monitored closely with a pacer nearby or on standby. It should have been tested for capture and patient tolerance.

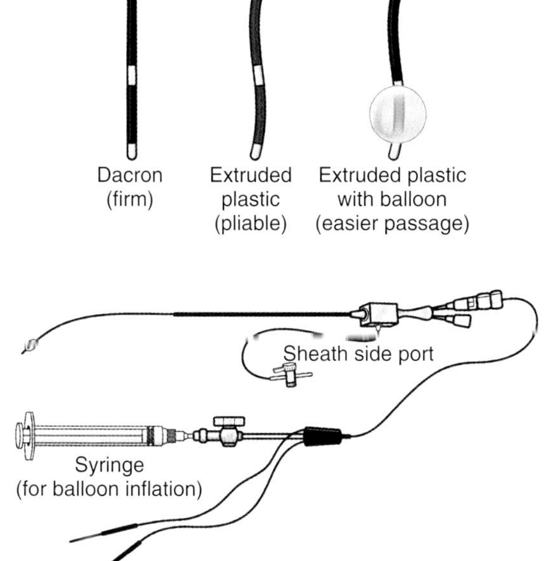

Figure 216-2 **A,** Distal tips of transvenous pacers. **B,** Transvenous balloon-tipped temporary pacer.

catheters; however, balloon-tipped catheters are easier to insert without fluoroscopy. There is also always the option of using a balloon-tipped, pacer-equipped pulmonary artery catheter (Swan-Ganz). One prospective, randomized trial (Ferguson and colleagues, 1997) demonstrated that balloon-flotation pacing wires are easier to insert, quicker to position, and more likely to be optimally positioned than semirigid electrode wires.

- Unipolar electrode catheters are available; however, unipolar catheters must rely on a second, external electrode to be placed on the skin. This electrode is very susceptible to any external electrical interference; therefore, bipolar catheters are preferred.
- A flexible "J"-shaped catheter is available specifically for temporary atrial pacing.
- Availability of fluoroscopy is ideal.
- Pacer pulse generator (Fig. 216-3) with a new or spare battery.
- Extension cable and alligator clips to connect pacer to catheter.
- ECG monitoring capability during insertion.
- Venous insertion site.
- Gauze squares.
- 3-0 nylon suture.
- Advanced cardiac life support equipment (defibrillator, airway management equipment, resuscitative drugs).

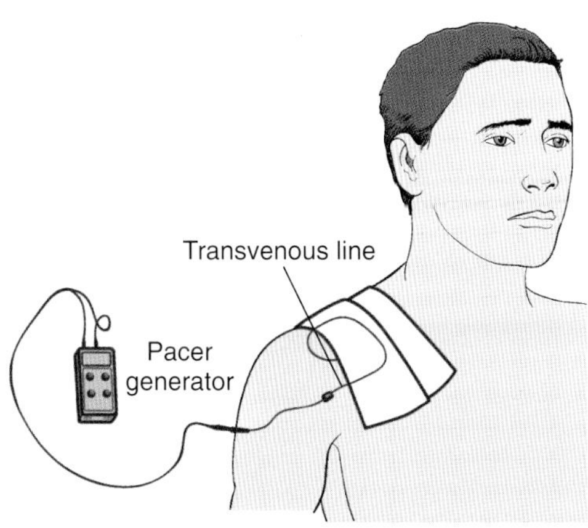

Figure 216-3 Transvenous line and pacer in place.

Preprocedure Patient Preparation

See Chapter 211, Central Venous Catheter Insertion.

If possible, obtain written informed consent. The conscious patient should know what to expect, the sensations he or she may experience (e.g., possibly being covered by a drape, needlesticks while obtaining central access), and that although this may be uncomfortable, everything possible will be done to minimize the discomfort (e.g., local anesthetic). In many cases, pacing is an emergency procedure and written informed consent cannot be obtained. However, after the patient is stabilized, the situation, risks, and benefits should be explained to the patient or representative. Implied consent should be documented in the medical record (e.g., in the conscious patient: "the risks and benefits have been explained to the patient, who agrees with having the procedure"). Always outline the complications of either performing or withholding the procedure.

Technique

All steps should be performed using aseptic technique and following universal blood and body fluid precautions. Venous access is established by the procedure outlined in Chapter 211, Central Venous Catheter Insertion. Inspect the leads on the pacing catheter for any breaks or manufacturing defects.

Access Route

The most direct route for internal pacemaker insertion is through a CV catheter in the right internal jugular (up to 8% failure rate). The subclavian vein (left preferred over right, and even then up to 17% failure rate) can also be used, especially for relatively long-term use, but this route of insertion may be more difficult because of the turns the electrode has to negotiate (Fig. 216-4). Brachial and femoral approaches are discouraged. The brachial approach has an increased risk of cardiac puncture and the femoral approach has an increased risk of deep venous thrombosis and infection.

Catheter Conversion

If necessary, insert a larger catheter into the established venous access site.

1. Place a guidewire down the CV access line.
2. Remove the catheter.
3. Use an obturator over the wire to enlarge the lumen.
4. Pass an introducer with catheter (e.g., Swan-Ganz or Cordis) assembly over the guidewire.
5. Remove the introducer.
6. Check for venous return.

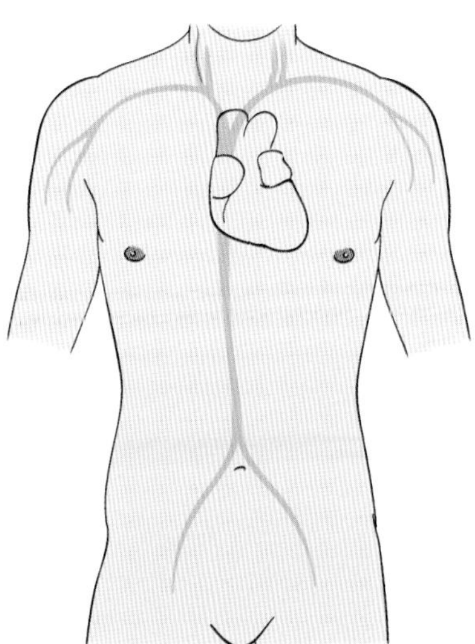

Figure 216-4 Temporary pacer in right internal jugular vein.

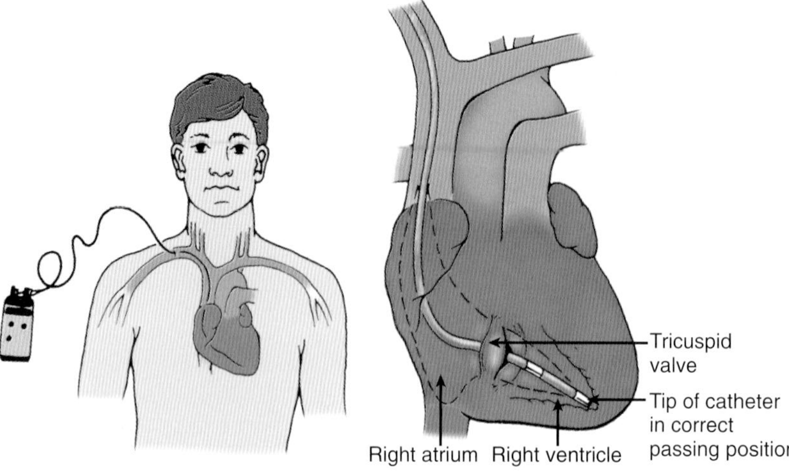

Figure 216-5 Correct positioning of pacer catheter. When the tip reaches the apex, it stops moving under fluoroscopy.

Pacer Placement

FLUOROSCOPY TECHNIQUE. By far, the best method of temporary pacer placement involves fluoroscopic guidance of the semifloating or balloon-tipped bipolar pacing leads. Many intensive care units and some emergency departments have beds that will accommodate C-arms for fluoroscopy. If C-arms cannot be accommodated, and if time and clinical conditions permit, the patient might also be moved to the radiology suite.

1. Pass the catheter through the rubber diaphragm of the introducer sheath and to the 10- to 12-cm mark (10-cm segments are marked on the catheter).
2. If the balloon is used, blow it up and advance the catheter; it should move easily into the right atrium (RA).
3. Pass the tip across the tricuspid valve and advance it to the apex of the right ventricle (RV). Ask the patient to take deep breaths or to cough; this will facilitate passage across the valve. Under fluoroscopy, once the radiopaque tip is at the apex, the last 2 to 3 cm of the lead should show minimal or no longitudinal motion if an attempt is made to advance the catheter farther. The remainder of the catheter may have horizontal and longitudinal motion (Fig. 216-5), but not the tip. If a balloon is used, deflate it as soon as it passes across the tricuspid valve and washes to the ventricular wall.

   If the catheter tip curls up against the atrial wall, advance it 1 to 2 cm to create a partial loop. Next, rotate it clockwise and watch it straighten as it enters the plane of the tricuspid valve.
4. The best final position for the catheter tip is at the right ventricular apex. Electrodes residing in the pulmonary outflow tract or along the free wall are less stable and more likely to cause perforation.
5. If a balloon is used, it must be deflated before withdrawal for repositioning.
6. Coiling the proximal electrode catheter around the insertion site and firmly suturing and taping it to the skin prevents inadvertent dislodgement of the distal electrode. Using the extension cable, connect the pacer electrodes to the pacer unit.

NONFLUOROSCOPY TECHNIQUE. A flexible, semiflotation or balloon-tipped catheter can be advanced and positioned much like a pulmonary artery catheter (see Chapter 215, Swan-Ganz [Pulmonary Artery] Catheterization), except that the distal negative catheter electrode is attached to an ECG machine (usually the V_1 lead, a unipolar lead) using a connector with alligator clips.

1. Connect the limb leads of an ECG machine to the patient.
2. Turn on the ECG machine and set it to the appropriate lead to monitor insertion (again, usually the V_1 lead). Use an alligator clip to attach the connector lead to the negative pacing catheter electrode. Next, touch the connector lead to the ECG monitor lead to confirm that the ECG is obtaining a signal. A large wave should be seen on the monitor when the connector lead touches the ECG lead.
3. Insert the pacemaker catheter through the rubber diaphragm of the introducer sheath and to the 10-cm mark. Using the other alligator clip, attach the connector lead to the ECG lead. If the balloon is used, inflate it and advance the catheter; it should move easily into the RA.
4. The change in the recorded QRS complex allows the practitioner to approximate the tip location (Fig. 216-6). Follow the same passage route: into the veins and then RA, across the tricuspid valve, and to the apex of the RV. In the internal jugular or subclavian vein, the P wave and the QRS complex are both small in amplitude and inverted. In the superior vena cava, the P wave increases in amplitude while the QRS complex is unchanged. As the electrode enters the RA, the P wave appears quite large but remains inverted until it reaches the lower RA, where it turns

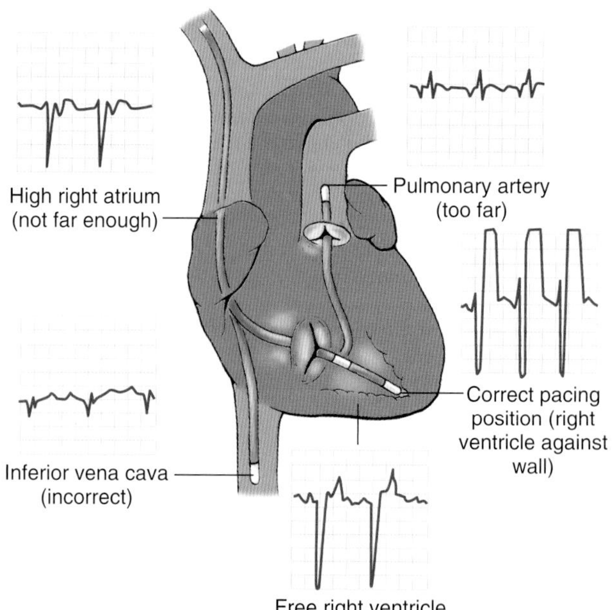

Figure 216-6 Pattern of recorded electrocardiogram from intracardiac pacemaker electrodes at various locations in the venous circulation.

upright. As it passes the tricuspid valve, the QRS amplitude increases. When the electrode is freely floating in the RV, the QRS amplitude appears large and normal (inverted in V_1 lead). The balloon should be deflated. Advance the catheter until a large, elevated ST segment is observed. This indicates the catheter is abutting the RV wall and is in the correct location.

5. If the catheter does not advance across the tricuspid valve, rotate it clockwise while advancing it 1 cm to flip the tip across the valve. If the catheter exits the RA and enters the inferior vena cava, the amplitudes of the P wave and QRS complex will decrease. Withdraw the catheter until the largest P wave is noted and then readvance the catheter. If the catheter exits the RA and enters the pulmonary artery, the P wave will become negative and the QRS will decrease. Withdraw the catheter until the normal right ventricular P wave and QRS complex are seen and then readvance the catheter.
6. Disconnect the negative pacemaker catheter lead from the connector and attach the positive and negative leads to the positive and negative terminals of the pacemaker generator, respectively.

EMERGENCY TECHNIQUE. Unfortunately, situations frequently require placement of a temporary pacer under emergent or extreme conditions, without fluoroscopic or ECG guidance, such as during a code with the patient lying in a hospital bed (often this is necessary because the alligator clips and connector are not available for ECG guidance).

1. A flexible catheter should be used, and it may be inserted blindly to about 12 cm. The catheter is then attached to the pacemaker and the pacemaker turned on.
2. Set the rate higher than the patient's highest native heart rate (usually 80 to 120 bpm), the amperage (ventricular output current) at 5 mA, and the mode at asynchronous (sensitivity off).
3. A surface or conventional ECG or rhythm strip should be running while the catheter is being passed. Capture is noted by an obviously paced rhythm seen on the surface ECG. Do not advance the catheter against resistance or more than 12 cm beyond the point at which the pacemaker was turned on. If capture does not occur at this point, withdraw the catheter and rotate it 90 degrees and readvance. Multiple attempts at passage may be necessary. When capture occurs, decrease the ventricular rate to 70 or 80 bpm.
4. Alternatively, the sensing indicator on the pacemaker can be used to guide placement. Advance the flexible catheter to about 12 cm, inflate the balloon, attach and turn on the pacemaker, and set it on demand mode with a rate twice the patient's highest native heart rate (again, usually 80 to 120 bpm) and the amperage at 1.5 to 2 mA. Advance the catheter, and when it enters the RV, the sensing indicator will illuminate with every other heart beat (because the pacemaker rate was set at twice the native heart rate). Deflate the balloon and increase the output to 5 mA. Slowly advance the catheter until ventricular capture occurs. Do not advance the catheter more than 10 cm beyond where the sensing indicator began to illuminate. If successful capture still has not occurred by this point, withdraw the catheter and rotate it 90 degrees. Readvance the catheter up to 10 cm. Continue to repeat the process until ventricular capture occurs and then decrease the ventricular rate to 70 or 80 bpm. Unfortunately, even experienced clinicians occasionally fail despite multiple attempts with either technique, underscoring the benefits of fluoroscopic guidance.

Parameter Settings

Determine the pacing parameters, and record each when it is set.

1. *Rate:* If the patient shows no intrinsic heart rate, set the pacing rate at 70 to 80 bpm to simulate the normal beating heart. If the patient is bradycardic, the same range can be used to raise the blood pressure and heart rate. Record the rate chosen after setting the machine.
2. *Ventricular output:* The sensitivity is the voltage used (set the sensitivity between 1.5 and 3 millivolts [mV]), whereas the ventricular output is the current generated by the pacer, adjustable from 0.1 to 20 mA. Depending on technique, start with 1.5 to 5 mA and increase until capture is seen on the monitor. After reaching the level of output necessary to capture the ventricle, large spikes are seen (Fig. 216-7) followed by bundle branch block pattern complexes (wide QRS complexes, ST-segment elevation, and T-wave inversion, depending on the lead). The bundle branch block pattern occurs because the complex originates in the ventricle. A pulse should also be palpable and it should generate a blood pressure. The ventricular output setting can then be reduced gradually, until capture is lost. The setting at which capture is lost is the pacing threshold, and this should be recorded. Resume pacing at 2 mA above this threshold. If capture occurs at less than 0.5 mA, the catheter may have become deeply embedded in the ventricular wall; be aware that withdrawal may cause perforation. If spikes are seen but no capture occurs, catheter manipulation is indicated. If levels of 5 to 6 mA or greater are required (which is common in fibrosis, but is usually a result of poor electrode positioning), attempt to reposition the electrode. If spikes and bundle branch block pattern are seen with no pulse, the possibility of pulseless electrical activity (electromechanical dissociation) must be considered. With electromechanical dissociation, the proper ACLS management protocol should be followed and there may be benefit of an emergent echocardiogram (see Chapter 225, Emergency Department, Hospitalist, and Office Ultrasonography [Clinical Ultrasonography]).

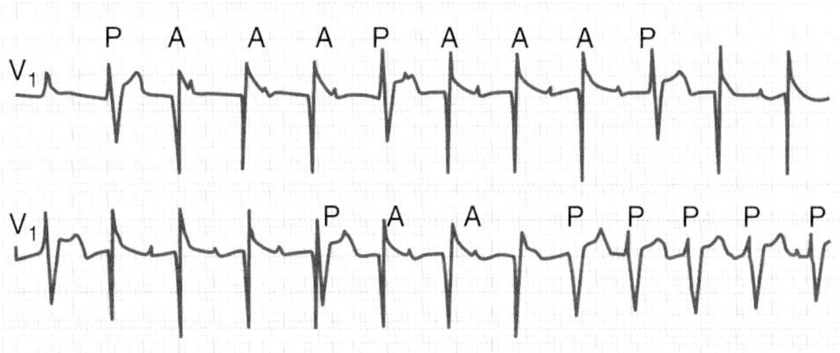

Figure 216-7 Pacing with intermittent capture. P indicates paced beats; A indicates pacer artifact without capture. (From Dahlberg ST, Benotti JR: Temporary cardiac pacing. In Rippe JM, Irwin RS, Alpert JS, Fink MP [eds]: Intensive Care Medicine, 2nd ed. Boston, Little, Brown, 1991.)

Demand Pacing

If the patient's intrinsic rhythm is inadequate, a sensing threshold must be determined with the sensitivity knob. Occasionally a sensing threshold cannot be determined when the patient has a very slow rhythm.

Sensitivity is the control on the pacer that detects the amplitude of the patient's intrinsic R wave. The most sensitive setting is 1 mV, corresponding to full clockwise rotation of the knob. In the least sensitive setting, called *asynchronous pacing*, the pacer does not "care" if there is a rhythm and functions oblivious to the intrinsic rate. The asynchronous setting should be avoided when there is an intrinsic rhythm because the additional electric spikes generated by the pacer can cause an arrhythmia.

To determine sensing threshold, first set the rate about 10 bpm below the patient's intrinsic rate. Gradually adjust the sensitivity control toward the highest sensitivity or entirely clockwise (to detect even the lowest-amplitude waves), which is known as the *full demand* setting. Pacer pulses should no longer be seen because all deflections are sensed and interpreted as QRS complexes. Every intrinsic or artifactual QRS complex should generate a flash of the sense indicator on the pacer. At this level the pacer senses almost all electrical activity and its firing is thus prevented. In fact, T waves, occasionally P waves (if the catheter is close to the atrium), chest muscle contractions, or even artifact may prevent the pacer from firing. This is called the *oversensing point*. This full demand setting is obviously too high for the pacer to function. The sensitivity control should then be turned counterclockwise, changing or decreasing the sensitivity toward higher numbers until ECG pacer spikes are seen that correspond to the patient's intrinsic rhythm, regardless of their capture. This level is the *sensing threshold* of the pacer. The pace indicator light (if the machine has one) should also flash. For *demand pacing* the sensing should be set at a level halfway between the oversensing point and the sensing threshold. This level should be recorded. Keep in mind that pacers can fail to sense when the sensitivity setting on the pacer is too low, when the lead is malpositioned, or when the intrinsic signal is of poor quality.

Once pacing is performing effectively, the length of wire that has been inserted transvenously should be recorded. Secure the electrode catheter to the skin with two sutures at two sites.

Confirmation of Lead Placement

1. A cross-table lateral and anteroposterior chest radiograph should be ordered. Pneumothorax should be ruled out. The tip of the catheter should be at the distal RV, in the apex, with no loops, kinks, or doublings. On the lateral view, the pacer should be to the left of the spine and slightly inferior and anterior, retrosternally.
2. A 12-lead ECG should demonstrate the expected left bundle branch block pattern because of the origination of electrical current in the RV (Fig. 216-8).
3. The pacer pulse generator should be secured to the bed, not the patient, for at least 24 hours. It should be covered to prevent inadvertent damage to the controls.

While a temporary pacer is in place, the patient's rhythm should be monitored and a hardwire or telemetry rhythm strip should be recorded frequently. Patients should be restricted to bed rest for at least 24 hours. Aseptic technique must be maintained when the catheter is handled, and appropriate skin care should be ordered. Sterile dressing changes should follow the intensive care unit's CV line protocol. Unnecessary catheter manipulations should be avoided. Pacemaker function should be checked daily with a 12-lead ECG. A change in the morphology of the paced QRS on the 12-lead ECG may be the first sign of electrode displacement. Daily physical examination for friction rubs (a clue to perforation) or clicking noises (muscle stimulation) must be documented. Pacing threshold should also be determined daily and documented.

Troubleshooting: Failure to Pace

Failure to pace can occur for a variety of reasons, including—but not limited to—a faulty battery, dislodged or malpositioned leads, a loose connection, a damaged or fractured wire, electronic interference, or a faulty pacer. Some cardiac conditions cause very high pacing thresholds or preclude intrinsic pacing, including myocardial fibrosis or ischemia, drug toxicity from cardiac agents, myocardial perforation, and ventricular refractoriness from a low-grade, unsensed, intrinsic QRS complex.

If the pacer fails to work after it had been functioning previously, several questions should be considered: Has the catheter become dislodged? Are the wires loose or disconnected? Are the pacemaker settings correct? Has the battery failed? Is there electrical interference? Has the ventricle been perforated as a result of synchronous diaphragmatic or intracostal muscle contractions?

In an emergency situation, consider increasing the stimulation or pacing threshold to regain capture. Occasionally the area in the heart near the electrode has become fibrotic, requiring a higher stimulation. Also, the catheter tip could have become partially dislodged. If the problem is oversensing, that threshold should be reset.

If all else fails, another emergency maneuver is to switch the polarity of the pacer lead connections. Occasionally this technique will regain pacing, although it has not been well documented in the medical literature.

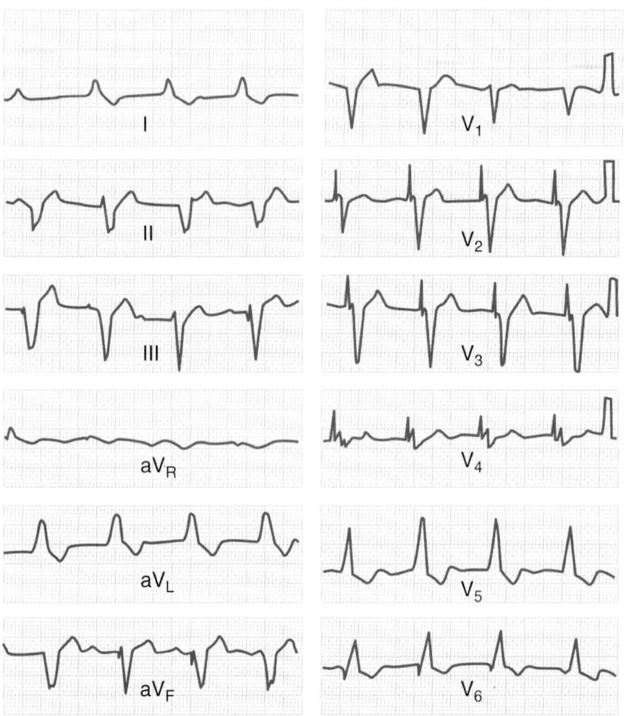

Figure 216-8 Finished product: 12-lead electrocardiogram with pacer in place. (From Morelli RL, Goldschlager N: Temporary transvenous pacing: Resolving postinsertion problems. J Crit Illness 2[3]:71, 1987.)

Postprocedure Patient Education

See the Postprocedure Patient Education section of Chapter 211, Central Venous Catheter Insertion. Also, if a patient will need a permanent pacemaker, see the Online Resources section of this chapter for patient education.

Complications

Most complications are infrequent and usually minor. Life-threatening complications are rare. Complications are seen more frequently as a result of pacing in an emergency, especially in a critically ill patient and when the operator is inexperienced.

- Pacing system dysfunction (18% to 43% of cases for transvenous), including failure to capture or sense the R wave properly. System malfunctions are usually due to problems with connections and lead placement or inappropriate setup of the device.
- Loss of pacing (failure of pacer, lead dislodgement, fracture of pacer wire).
- Failure to recognize that the pacer is not capturing or pacing.
- Pericardial friction rub, endocardial structural damage, myocardial damage, or infarction.
- Arrhythmia.
- Diaphragmatic stimulation; chest wall stimulation.

External (Transcutaneous)

- Failure to recognize the presence of underlying treatable ventricular fibrillation.

- Prolonged use is often associated with leads becoming dislodged; occasionally prolonged pacing is associated with a change in pacing threshold, requiring increased pacing current.
- Third-degree burns have been reported in children, even when large electrodes were used. The risk of a burn increases if the electrodes are placed improperly or if prolonged pacing is necessary.

Internal (Transvenous)

Complications include same as those for CV line insertion; see Chapter 211, Central Venous Catheter Insertion.

- Infection, including bacteremia and septicemia (up to 20% of patients developed microbiologically confirmed septicemia when the pacing wire was left in place >48 hours, and this increases risk of infection when a permanent pacemaker is placed).
- Interventricular septum or right ventricular perforation, with or without cardiac tamponade.
- Arterial or venous injury, including phlebitis and thrombosis (incidence is higher than expected).
- Pulmonary embolism.
- Air embolism.
- Electrical hazards (any extraneous currents, even microcurrents, can cause ventricular fibrillation if applied to a transvenous pacemaker catheter).

Patient Education Guides

See the sample patient education form available online at www.expertconsult.com.

CPT/Billing Codes

33210 Insertion or replacement of temporary transvenous single chamber cardiac electrode or pacemaker catheter
36556 Insertion of nontunneled centrally inserted central venous catheter, over age 5
92953 Temporary transcutaneous pacing

ICD-9-CM Diagnostic Codes

410.01 Acute myocardial infarction, initial episode of care, anterolateral wall, can include damage such as ruptured myocardium (ST elevation)
410.11 Acute myocardial infarction, initial episode of care, anterior, anteroapical, or anteroseptal wall, can include damage such as ruptured myocardium (ST elevation)
410.21 Acute myocardial infarction, initial episode of care, of inferolateral wall, can include damage such as ruptured myocardium (ST elevation)
410.41 Acute myocardial infarction, initial episode of care, other inferior wall, can include damage such as ruptured myocardium (ST elevation)
410.71 Acute myocardial infarction, initial episode of care, subendocardial or non-ST elevation infarction
410.91 Acute myocardial infarction, initial episode of care, unspecified site
426.0 Atrioventricular block, complete or third-degree heart block
426.2 Left bundle branch hemiblock
426.3 Left bundle branch block, complete
426.4 Right bundle branch block
426.11 First-degree atrioventricular block
426.12 Mobitz type II block
426.13 Other second-degree atrioventricular block, including Mobitz type I (Wenckebach's)
426.53 Bifascicular or bilateral bundle branch block
427.5 Cardiac arrest or asystole
427.81 Sinoatrial node dysfunction or sinus bradycardia, persistent, severe, or sick sinus syndrome

Acknowledgment

The editors wish to recognize the many contributions by Len Scarpinato, DO, to this chapter in the two previous editions of this text.

Suppliers

(See contact information online at www.expertconsult.com.)

See suppliers of pulmonary artery (Swan-Ganz) catheters, as well as the following:

Biosense Webster
Medtronic
St. Jude Medical

Online Resources

American Heart Association: Information regarding pacemakers, temporary and permanent. Available at www.heart.org.

Levine MD, Brown DFM: Heart block, third degree. eMedicine. Updated April 13, 2009. Available at www.emedicine.com/EMERG/topic235.htm.

For patient information from the manufacturers regarding permanent pacemakers: www.guidant.com (Guidant); www.medtronic.com (Medtronic); www.biotronik.com (Biotronic; available in German, English, Italian, and French); www.sjm.com (St. Jude Medical).

Bibliography

American Heart Association: Advanced Cardiovascular Life Support Provider Manual. Dallas, American Heart Association, 2006.

Dahlberg ST, Mooradd MG: Temporary cardiac pacing. In Irwin RS, Cerra FB, Rippe JM (eds): Irwin and Rippe's Intensive Care Medicine, 4th ed. Philadelphia, Lippincott Williams & Wilkins, 1999, pp 71–77.

Davis WR: Temporary cardiac pacemakers. In Civetta JM, Taylor RW, Kirby RR (eds): Critical Care, 3rd ed. Philadelphia, Lippincott Raven, 1997.

Doukky R, Rajanahally, RS: Transcutaneous cardiac pacing. In Reichman EF, Simon RR (eds): Emergency Medicine Procedures. New York, McGraw-Hill, 2004, pp 167–172.

Ferguson JD, Banning AP, Bashir Y: Randomised trial of temporary cardiac pacing with semirigid and balloon-flotation electrode catheters. Lancet 349:1883, 1997.

Francis GC, Williams SV, Achord JL, et al: Clinical competence in insertion of a temporary transvenous ventricular pacemaker: A statement for physicians from the ACP/ACC/AHA Task Force on Clinical Privileges in Cardiology. Circulation 89:1913, 1994. http://www.ncbi.nlm.nih.gov/pubmed/8149566.

James DM: Temporary pacing techniques: External and transvenous. In James DM (ed): Field Guide to Urgent and Ambulatory Care Procedures. Philadelphia, Lippincott Williams & Wilkins, 2001, pp 136–141.

Olshansky B: Temporary cardiac pacing. In Rose BD (ed): UpToDate. Waltham, Mass, UpToDate, 2007. Available at www.uptodate.com.

Wilson DD, Reichman EF: Transvenous cardiac pacing. In Reichman EF, Simon RR (eds): Emergency Medicine Procedures. New York, McGraw-Hill, 2004, pp 178–185.

CHAPTER 217

Drawing Blood Cultures

Theodore O'Connell

Bacteremia and septicemia are potentially life-threatening conditions caused by a variety of microorganisms. The successful isolation of microorganisms from blood requires an understanding of the intermittent nature of most bacteremias, the low order of magnitude of most bacteremias, and the great variety of organisms capable of causing septicemia.

Consideration must first be given to the patient's clinical status. Indications for obtaining blood cultures are outlined later. Note that 25% of patients with documented bacteremia have periods without fever. In the elderly population, the proportion is even higher, with 50% of bacteremic patients older than 65 years of age being afebrile.

Because most bacteremias are intermittent, blood collections for culture ideally should be made intermittently during a 24-hour period. Two separate blood culture sets should be collected within a 24-hour period. However, if urgent administration of antibiotics is clinically indicated, two sets of cultures from two different sites should be obtained, separated by 20 to 30 minutes if possible. Cultures should also be obtained through any vascular access devices that have been in place at least 48 hours. Each set of culture bottles has one aerobic and one anaerobic bottle.

Most bacteremias are of a very low magnitude, so an adequate volume of blood should be collected for each set of cultures. Small children usually have higher numbers (concentrations) of bacteria in the blood than adults, which means that smaller quantities of blood may be obtained from children. Appropriate volumes are noted in Table 217-1.

Indications

- Fever and unexplained alterations in mental status, functional status, or autonomic status in a previously healthy patient
- Fever and no source of infection, especially in a patient younger than 2 years of age or older than 65 years of age
- Fever of unknown origin
- Immunocompromised status with a fever and no source
- All febrile infants younger than 3 months of age
- Persistent rigors, with or without fever
- Fever, or no fever in a patient with a toxic or "septic" appearance (including unexplained hypotension, altered mental status, or shock)
- Possible infectious endocarditis (hematuria and elevated sedimentation rate)
- Serious focal infections such as meningitis, septic arthritis, and osteomyelitis
- Patients with pneumonia or pyelonephritis and need for hospitalization or with signs of toxicity

Contraindications

There are essentially no contraindications to drawing blood cultures. As with any patient, blood should not be drawn through infected skin sites.

Equipment

- Alcohol pads.
- 2% tincture of iodine in 70% alcohol (alternatively, 2% iodine solution or 10% povidone–iodine [Betadine] may be used).
- Chlorhexidine (Hibiclens) may be used in the iodine-allergic patient.
- Tourniquet.
- Gloves and any equipment needed to follow universal blood and body fluid precautions.
- 21-gauge needle.
- 30-mL syringe.
- Set of blood culture bottles, aerobic and anaerobic, with labels.

Preprocedure Patient Preparation

Drawing blood for culture does not entail any more risk than drawing blood for any other purpose. Patients should be warned about the needlestick and the potential for bleeding, bruising, and infection. Written consent for this procedure is not necessary.

Technique

1. Fill in the laboratory request form and explain the procedure to the patient.
2. Apply the tourniquet and determine the location of the vein to be used for venipuncture (Fig. 217-1A).
3. Cleanse the skin with alcohol swabs three times or until pads are free of surface dirt.
4. Allow the skin to dry.
5. Apply iodine three times in centrifugal circles from the anticipated site of venipuncture.
6. After the third swab, allow to dry at least 60 seconds.
7. Remove the protective cap and cleanse the top of the culture bottles with alcohol swabs.
8. Wipe off dry iodine at the venipuncture site with alcohol swabs. Do not palpate the vein or the area where the needle will be inserted after disinfecting the site. Clinicians should follow universal blood and body fluid precautions.
9. Obtain the required volume of blood (see Table 217-1 for recommended blood volumes by patient size).
10. Immediately apply pressure to the puncture site (after removing the needle) with a clean cotton sponge.
11. Place up to 10 mL of blood in each culture bottle. (These two bottles constitute one blood culture "set.")
12. Inoculate both bottles without changing needles.
13. Repeat at different sites or different times for the requisite number of blood culture sets.
14. Transport the blood cultures as soon as possible to start the incubating process.
15. Specimens need to be held for an extended duration when culturing blood for fungi or fastidious bacteria.

TABLE 217-1 Optimal Specimen Volumes to Be Drawn per Blood Culture Set

Age Group	Ideal Volume per Set (mL)
Neonates	1–2
Infants 5–10 kg	2–4
Children 7–20 kg	3–8
Children 20–40 kg	10
Children >40 kg	20–30
Adults	20–30

Complications

- Bleeding
- Bruising
- Infection

Interpretation of Results

In the case of a positive blood culture, the offending organism(s) are identified. If sensitivities have been ordered, the antibiotic susceptibility or resistance is reported.

One of the more challenging aspects of interpreting blood culture results is determining which positive blood cultures are actually false-positive results. Features of false-positive blood cultures are outlined as follows:

- Coagulase-negative staphylococci (*Staphylococcus epidermidis)* and *Streptococcus viridans* in a single bottle in patients not suspected of having infectious endocarditis and without chronic indwelling intravenous catheters are usually contaminants.
- *Corynebacterium*, *Propionibacterium acnes*, and *Bacillus* species are usually contaminants, but they can be pathogens in immunocompromised hosts.
- Multiple organisms growing from the same bottle suggests contamination.
- Species that grow out after a prolonged culture have a greater likelihood of being contaminants.
- The patient's symptoms have resolved or are inconsistent with sepsis. However, special consideration must be given to infectious endocarditis, which can have an indolent course.
- A primary infected source, such as urine, yields a different pathogenic isolate.

CPT/Billing Codes

If cultures are grown in the office and organisms identified, laboratory codes are as follows:

87040 Culture, bacterial; blood, aerobic, with isolation and presumptive identification of isolates (includes anaerobic culture, if appropriate)

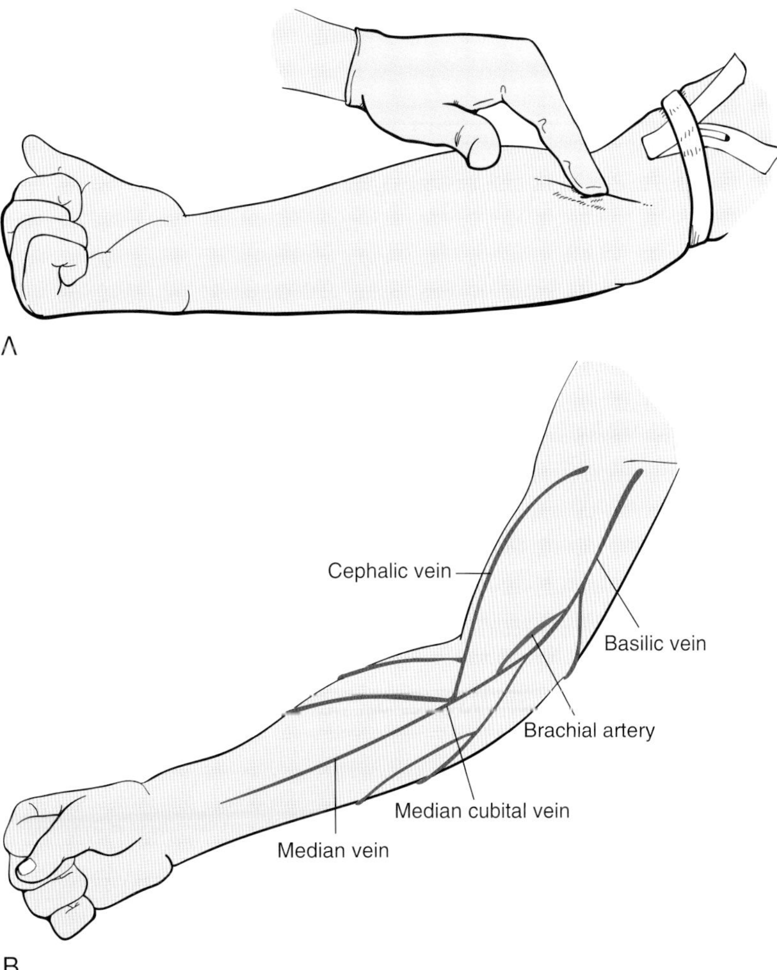

Figure 217-1 Venipuncture. **A,** After the tourniquet is applied, the vein is located. **B,** Veins in arm.

87103 Culture, fungi (mold or yeast) isolation, with presumptive identification of isolates, blood

There is no specific code for drawing blood. Add laboratory handling fee (99000) to office visit.

ICD-9-CM Diagnostic Codes

038.0 Septicemia, streptococcal
038.2 Septicemia, pneumococcal
038.3 Septicemia, anaerobic
038.9 Septicemia, unspecified
771.83 Bacteremia, newborn
790.7 Bacteremia

Supplier

(See contact information online at www.expertconsult.com.)

BacT/Alert blood culture bottles
Organon Teknika Corp.

Bibliography

Larosa S, Opal SM: Sepsis. In Dale DC (ed): Infectious Diseases: The Clinician's Guide to Diagnosis, Treatment, and Prevention. New York, WebMD Professional Publishing, 2007.

Little JR, Murray PR, Traynor PS, Spitznagel E: A randomized trial of povidone–iodine compared with iodine tincture for venipuncture site disinfection: Effects on rates of blood culture contamination. Am J Med 107:119–125, 1999.

Madell GL, Bennett JE, Dolin R (eds): Principles and Practice of Infectious Diseases, 5th ed. New York, Churchill Livingstone, 2000.

Mimoz O, Karim A, Mercat A: Chlorhexidine compared with povidone-iodine as skin preparation before blood culture: A randomized, controlled trial. Ann Intern Med 131:834–837, 1999.

SECTION 14

Miscellaneous

Section Editor: MIKE PETRIZZI

CHAPTER 218

ACUPUNCTURE

Victor S. Sierpina

The insertion of fine needles into the body at specific points, or "channels of energy flow," called *meridians* has been used in the treatment of human and animal disease for thousands of years. The oldest reference to this traditional East Asian medical procedure dates to 2600 BC, when fine, sharpened stone or bamboo needles were reported to be used in the treatment and prevention of illness.

Contemporary use of acupuncture has become increasingly popular. It is offered not only by traditionally trained doctors of Oriental medicine, but by allopathic and osteopathic physicians and clinicians. Patient interest and acceptance of acupuncture in the United States have resulted in its investigation and recognition by such bodies as the National Institutes of Health's (NIH) Office of Alternative Medicine. Their advisory panel recently released a consensus statement supporting the efficacy of acupuncture and acknowledging the potential benefit of acupuncture in a number of acute and chronic conditions (NIH, 2005). Furthermore, they recommended that the insurance industry consider wider coverage for this safe and effective technique. These statements have begun changing the perceptions of this ancient medical art from that of a curiosity or an "experimental treatment" to that of an acceptable procedure within medical science.

Although the exact mechanism of its action is not known, acupuncture is the most widely studied alternative therapy, and a wide variety of theories attempt to explain its effects. After use for many centuries, the traditional concept used by the Chinese and others to explain acupuncture is that it is a method of balancing *qi* (or *chi*), an invisible yet essential, ceaselessly flowing life energy that circulates silently and invisibly in the body. Because no scientist has ever measured or seen *qi*, only its effects can be observed. These effects are best demonstrated when the body is performing normally, an amalgamation of all the physiologic, immunologic, and homeostatic functions of a living organism. The blockage of the flow of *qi*, an inadequate or waning supply of it, or an excess amount of *qi* can all lead to conditions of pain, disease, and loss of homeostasis.

This quasi-mystical explanation is not always satisfying to the medical scientist's theorizing mind. Thus, attempts have been made over the years to derive a more robust explanation, one that is understandable in terms of Western scientific tradition and terminology. The work of Pomeranz and others showed that some of the effects of acupuncture are achieved by activating the endorphin neuropeptide system and can be blocked by the opiate receptor antagonist naloxone. Others have looked into the quantum physics realm and found parallels there in nonlocal effects, standing wave theory, and other quantum principles now used by physicists. Certain hybrid models apply Western medical and physiologic terminology to explain the effect of needling. These models discuss the ionic and electrical milieu of cells and tissues as well as the foreign body effect and the pattern of injury currents induced by needling. Additional theories explain acupuncture results as being due to a "neurogate blocking phenomenon," various neural or endocrinologic events, effects on cytokine and prostaglandin inflammatory pathways, or electromagnetic field realignment. Given the sheer range and diversity of these explanations, it is likely that acupuncture works through a number of mechanisms and perhaps is not yet fully explicable with our current science. However, its effects on humans and animals, its longevity as a healing art, and its resurgence in the Western medical community are all inductive evidence of the value of acupuncture, whatever its mechanism of action.

Although there is considerable variability among training approaches for physicians, the annual 300-hour course called Medical Acupuncture for Physicians offered by the Helms Medical Institute (1-510-649-8488; www.hmieducation.com) and Stanford University (http://cme.stanford.edu/courses) is widely acknowledged as a benchmark minimum for those wanting to practice acupuncture. Classes are offered over several months, including distance learning by DVD and video, and are designed to give practical knowledge without requiring too much time away from a medical practice. The longer, 3- to 4-year courses offered at Asian medical colleges are not usually required by states for licensure for physicians and are often impractical for the practicing clinician to complete.

Laws governing physician acupuncture are listed on the American Academy of Medical Acupuncture's website, www.medicalacupuncture.org.

Blending this ancient medical art into a medical practice can be a source of satisfaction to both professionals and their patients. It can serve as a practice builder and provide new opportunities to attract patients. With the NIH consensus panel's opinion on record, health care professionals have reason to anticipate better insurance coverage for acupuncture and a resulting increase in demand. In fact, some HMOs already reimburse for alternative therapies, including acupuncture.

INDICATIONS

Although acupuncture has been used to treat every imaginable human condition, to treat animals, and to prevent disease, most clinicians performing acupuncture find its greatest usefulness in the following conditions:

- Arthritis
- Asthma
- Back pain
- Carpal tunnel syndrome
- Dizziness
- Dysmenorrhea
- Gastrointestinal disorders
- Gynecologic problems
- Headache
- Irritable bowel syndrome
- Mental and mood disturbances
- Musculoskeletal pain
- Neuralgia
- Sciatica
- Sinusitis
- Skin disorders
- Substance addiction

- Tendonitis
- Tennis elbow
- Upper respiratory infections
- Urologic disease

Contraindications

- Septic or extremely weakened patient.
- Local skin infection or loss of skin integrity (e.g., burns, cellulitis).
- Uncooperative patients or patients with delusions, hallucinations, or paranoia.
- Electroacupuncture should not be applied across the brain or heart.
- During pregnancy, a number of points are to be avoided (see acupuncture references for details) because some of these points may stimulate labor.
- The umbilicus, the nipple, points over major vessels and nerves, and an infant's fontanelle are points forbidden by both classic and contemporary practitioners.
- During menses (*relative contraindication*).
- Patient unable to lie down (*relative contraindication*; sitting or standing treatments should usually be avoided, especially for first treatment).

Equipment

A variety of needles are available, ranging from very fine, 34- or 36-gauge needles, to 18-gauge needles used for veterinary acupuncture. The most commonly used needles are those from 0.5 to 3 inches in length and in the 30- to 34-gauge size. Acupuncture needles usually have solid stainless steel shafts and a copper, silver, or wound-steel-wire handle. The longer needles are used in thicker muscle groups, such as the back, buttocks, and legs, whereas the shorter, more delicate needles are used in the hands, face, and ears.

In addition to the needles, acupuncturists both in the United States and abroad, including China, now commonly use electrostimulation units (Fig. 218-1). These are small, hand-held, battery-operated units, similar in design to transcutaneous electrical stimulation (TENS) units used for pain control. Instead of the electrode pad that is used with the TENS unit, a small alligator clip is placed on the shaft of an acupuncture needle to deliver the electrical current.

Other materials that may be used by an acupuncturist include embedded ear needles; metallic or magnetic beads; the herb moxa (*Artemisia vulgaris*), which is burned to heat the skin, needle, or acupuncture points; glass or bamboo cups used for a corollary procedure called *cupping*; small hammers with several needles on the tip (plum blossom or seven-star needles); and electrical point locators, probes, or stimulators.

In general, four sizes of needles and a few electrostimulator devices are all that is necessary for most medical acupuncture applications. The cost of these supplies varies, but a reasonable, complete set of equipment will usually cost less than $1000 (see the list of Suppliers).

Preprocedure Patient Preparation

Although acupuncture is among the safest of invasive medical therapies, some precautions are needed. A thorough standard examination and diagnostic evaluation by a clinician are needed before acupuncture. Interestingly, performing these procedures often prepares the patient for acupuncture by giving him or her confidence through a known, established medical ritual—the routine physical. If the patient has never had acupuncture, the clinician should first show him or her the needles and stimulation devices. It is essential to assure the patient that the needles are sterile and disposed of after every treatment to allay fears of disease transmission. It is helpful to explain the risk of a needle reaction and the occasional endorphin rush, or "high," that follows some treatments.

Like any other medical treatment or procedure, it is wise to discuss the pros and cons of treatment, any conventional therapy options that may not have been tried, the likelihood of success with acupuncture, its possible costs, and the expected number and length of treatments. Most conditions amenable to acupuncture will show a positive response in 4 to 10 treatments. With initial treatments, the patient may experience no response, a temporary worsening of the condition, or a gradual (or even sudden) improvement. For most chronic conditions, such as low back pain, a series of 4 to 10 treatments at $50 to $100 per treatment is often worth the investment for the patient seeking relief.

The topics just mentioned should be discussed with every patient before initiating a course of acupuncture treatments. The initial

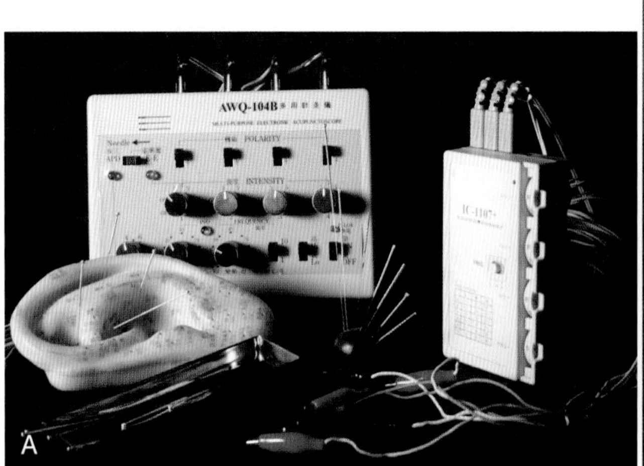

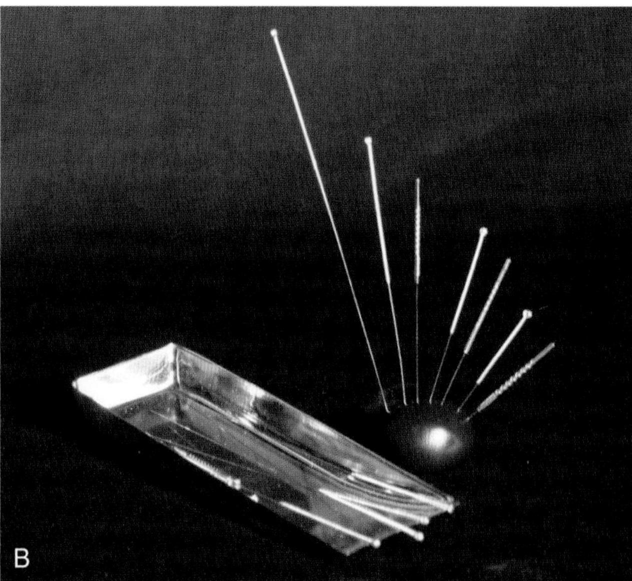

Figure 218-1 Examples of an electroacupuncture stimulator (**A**) and acupuncture needles of various sizes (**B**).

evaluation, review of records, discussion of options, and development of care plan usually occupy the entire first visit. Needle treatment is often deferred until the second visit. Usually no informed consent forms or releases are used in acupuncture therapy, although they may be useful in certain practice situations.

Technique

Although the choice and location of points and the details of acupuncture therapeutics are beyond the scope of this chapter, the following text should give a general idea of how to interact with the patient, and how a treatment session is staged and integrated into a medical practice.

1. After the patient and acupuncturist agree that a trial of acupuncture is appropriate and mutually acceptable, the patient is draped or gowned. Special efforts should be made to ensure patient comfort on the treatment table, using supports such as pillows, towels, and bolsters, because the patient will be lying down for a session lasting 15 to 30 minutes or more. As noted earlier, sitting or standing treatments are avoided unless the patient is known to have tolerated them previously.
2. Acupuncture points are palpated on the body, extremities, ears, face, or scalp, and the needle is inserted deftly with a slight twirling motion (Figs. 218-2 to 218-4). A sufficient depth of insertion has been reached when the patient feels a slight aching sensation, indicating that the *qi* has been reached (*de qi* sensation). Needle insertion should be painless other than the mild *de qi* sensation and a tiny prick the patient may feel as the needle penetrates the skin. Although some acupuncturists wipe the area of insertion with an alcohol swab, this is not necessary. However, cleansing before needling may be prudent in certain cases (e.g., patients who have an immune deficiency or diabetes or those who are concerned or worried).
3. A typical treatment may require 15 to 30 needles. After all of the needles are in place, electroacupuncture electrodes are usually attached to several, but not all, of the needles. The electrostimulator is turned on and the current is gradually increased until the patient can feel a pulsing sensation. The current is then increased to the patient's maximal tolerance level and then backed off slightly (Fig. 218-5).
4. A timer is set, and a health care professional should remain within hailing distance to assist the patient if needed. The patient may be given a bell to ring if assistance is needed (e.g., if a needle falls out, the patient becomes uncomfortable or for some other reason needs the presence of another person).
5. At the end of the session, a nurse or medical assistant removes the wires and clips from the needles, removes the needles and disposes of them in a sharps container, and allows the patient to dress. The clinician or acupuncturist may return to evaluate the treatment or the patient may be discharged without further attention until the next visit. Usually the clinician is seeing or managing other patients while an acupuncture session is in progress. He or she may start another or even two more acupuncture sessions while the first is occurring, or the clinician may attend to other standard medical cases.
6. Follow-up treatments are done at intervals of up to 2 weeks. During return visits, the acupuncturist interviews, examines, and reevaluates the patient and his or her progress. Treatment and needle location may be altered based on the patient's response, or the same or a similar pattern may be used. As the patient starts to improve, treatment intervals are spaced farther apart. Whereas some patients obtain permanent relief from acupuncture, others may require periodic "tune-up" treatments to sustain their improvement.
7. The patient's diagnosis, his or her vital signs, type of treatment, and needle application points used should be dictated into the medical record.

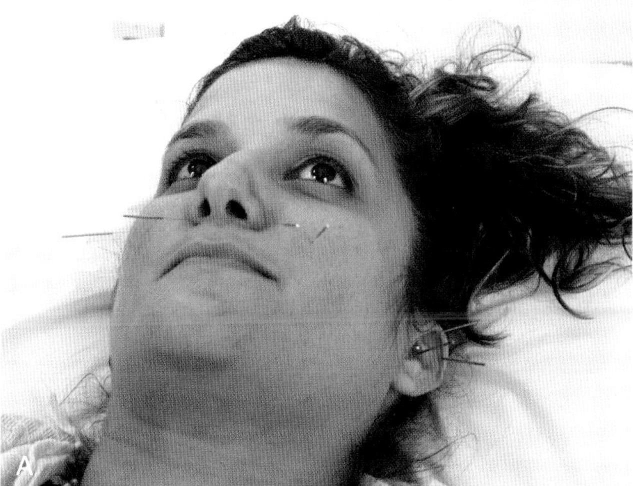

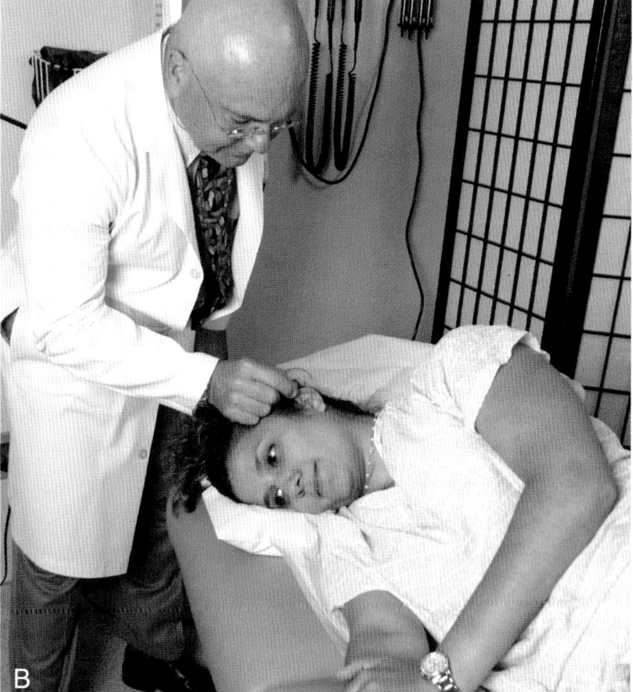

Figure 218-2 **A,** Example of treatment of facial and ear points. **B,** Ear acupuncture.

Complications

Complications are rare in acupuncture, but of those reported, the most common are local pain; swelling; hematoma formation; organ puncture; pneumothorax; metal allergy; needle reaction (fainting); a post-treatment period of euphoria; and local infections, such as perichondritis, or even more serious infections, such as endocarditis. Systemic infections, such as hepatitis and acquired immunodeficiency syndrome, have been reported as transmitted by acupuncture needle. However, poorly qualified practitioners who reused needles and did not use sterile technique were the cause of these infections.

Postprocedure Patient Education

Depending on the type of treatment, no special instructions are usually necessary. Band-Aids are not needed. Some patients,

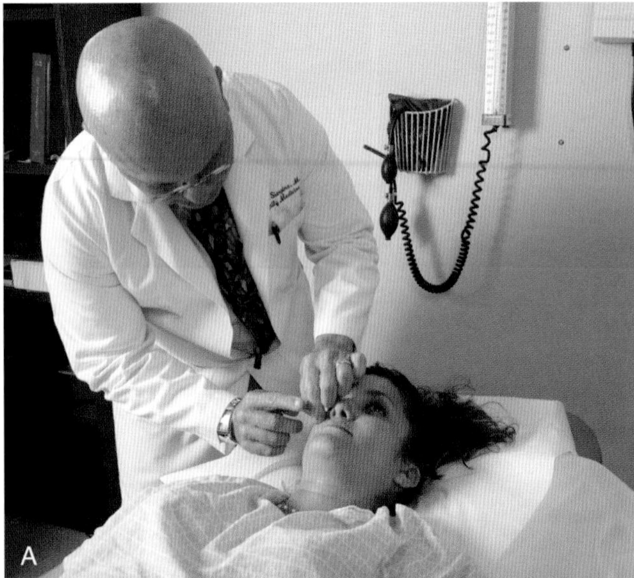

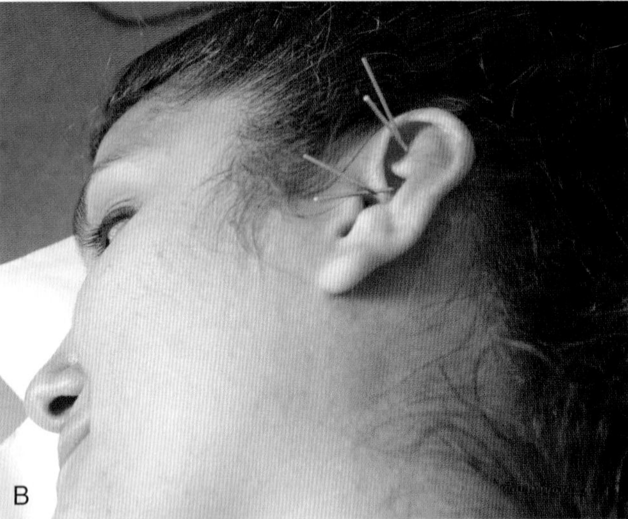

Figure 218-3 **A,** Facial points used for sinus problems. **B,** Auricular points used for an addiction.

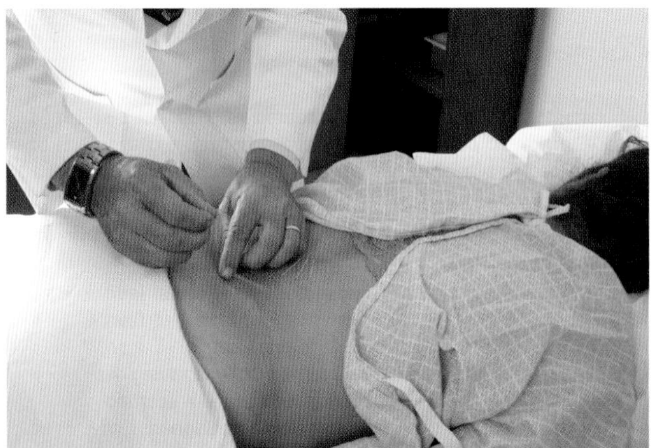

Figure 218-4 Needle insertion in abdomen.

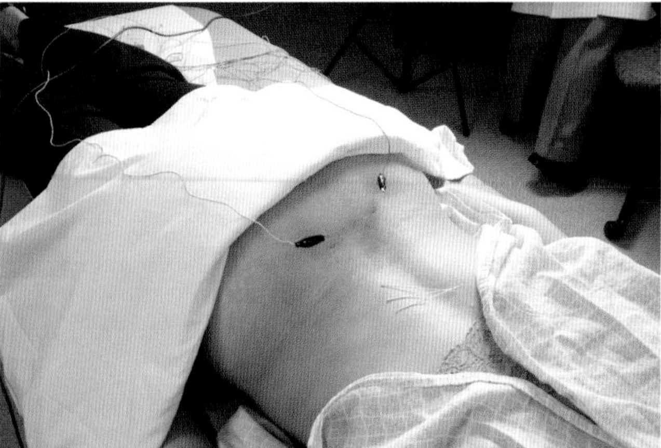

Figure 218-5 Adjusting treatment settings (after checking pulse).

particularly at their first treatment, experience a euphoric spell thought to be related to endorphin release. The practitioner may instruct patients to drive carefully after a treatment or to have someone drive them home.

Some treatments are designed to increase general energy and vigor, especially in chronically weakened patients. Advice should be given to these patients to avoid heavy meals, alcoholic beverages, sexual relations, and intense exercise for about 8 hours after the treatment. This should enhance treatment benefits.

Referral Process

If you choose not to learn to use acupuncture in your practice, the clinical algorithm shown in Figure 218-6 can be very useful in selecting proper cases for referral, assessing evidence, and managing follow-up for patients who are seen by an acupuncturist outside of your practice.

Patient Education Guides

See the sample patient education form available online at www.expertconsult.com.

CPT/Billing Codes

97810 Acupuncture, one or more needles; *without* electrical stimulation, initial 15 minutes of personal one-on-one contact with the patient

97811 Each additional 15 minutes of personal one-on-one contact with the patient, with reinsertion of needles(s) *without* electrical stimulation

97813 Acupuncture, one or more needles; *with* electrical stimulation, initial 15 minutes of personal one-on-one contact with the patient

97814 Each additional 15 minutes of personal one-on-one contact with the patient, with reinsertion of needles(s) *with* electrical stimulation

New codes are based on 15-minute increments, and time must be documented in the chart for billing purposes. Most patients pay out of pocket, however, thus minimizing billing procedures.

Standardized fees depend on the client population, geography, and, increasingly, the rate of insurance reimbursement. However, treatments are billed in the range of $50 to $100 in most cases and locations.

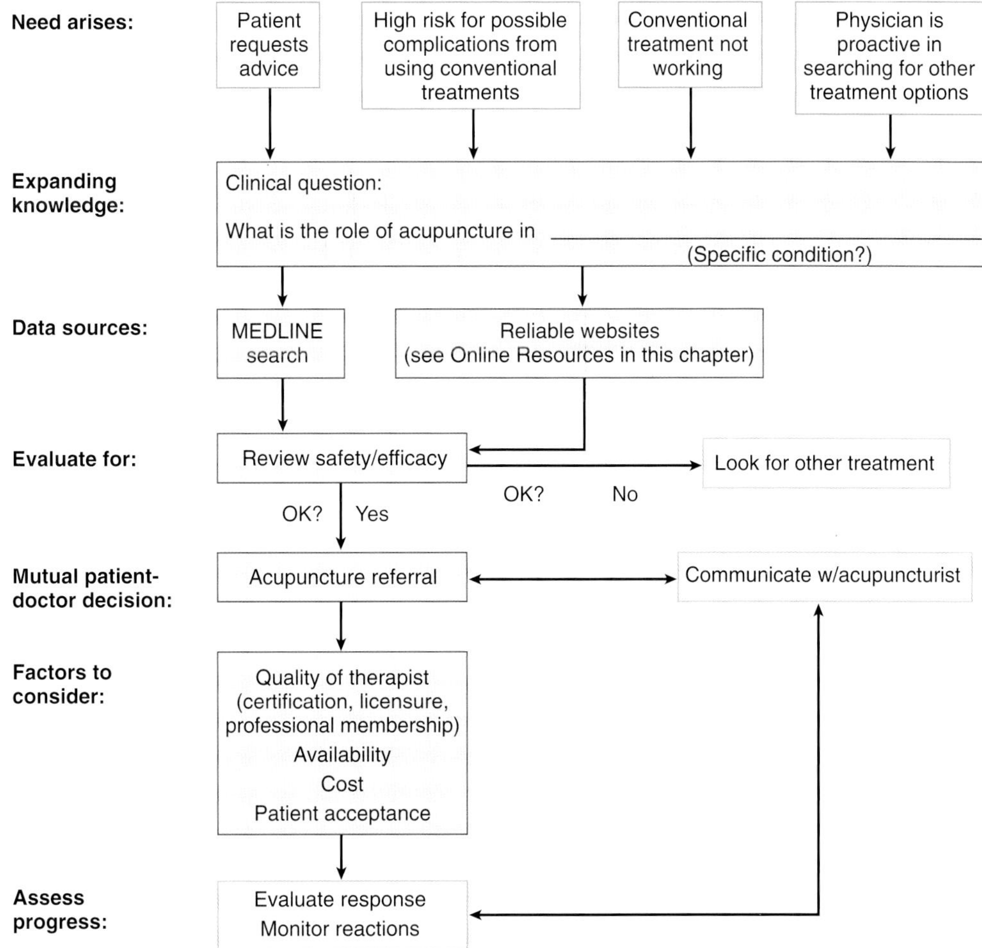

Figure 218-6 Algorithm for integrating acupuncture into medical practice.

ICD-9-CM Diagnostic Codes

300.0 Anxiety
303.90 Alcohol dependence syndrome, chronic, unspecified
304.00 Drug dependence, opioid, unspecified
304.10 Drug dependence, barbiturate, unspecified
304.20 Drug dependence, cocaine, unspecified
304.40 Drug dependence, amphetamine, unspecified
307.81 Headache, tension
309.0 Depressive reaction, brief
309.1 Depressive reaction, prolonged
311 Depressive disorder not otherwise classified
346.00 Headache, classical migraine, not intractable
346.10 Headache, common migraine, not intractable
346.20 Headache, cluster, without intractable migraine
354.0 Carpal tunnel syndrome
473.9 Sinusitis, chronic
493.0 Asthma, without mention of status asthmaticus
519.8 Upper respiratory infection, chronic
564.1 Irritable bowel syndrome
595.1 Cystitis, chronic interstitial
617 Endometriosis
625.3 Dysmenorrhea
625.9 Pelvic pain
691.8 Dermatitis, atopic (eczema)
696.1 Psoriasis
714.0 Arthritis, rheumatoid, adult
715.0 Arthrosis, osteoarthrosis, site unspecified or generalized
722.10 Sciatica, discogenic
724.2 Back pain, low, or low back syndrome
726.32 Lateral epicondylitis
726.90 Tendonitis, site not otherwise specified
729.2 Neuralgia, unspecified
729.89 Musculoskeletal pain, limbs
780.4 Dizziness
789.00 Abdominal pain, unspecified site

Suppliers

(See contact information online at ww.expertconsult.com.)

Acupuncture needles and other equipment
Lhasa Medical, Inc.
OMS Medical Supplies

Books and references on acupuncture
Redwing Book Company

ONLINE RESOURCES

A large number of websites can be found on the Internet by searching under the keyword acupuncture.

American Academy of Medical Acupuncture: A physician-oriented site supported by the Medical Acupuncture Research Foundation to make available online the most comprehensive database of references on acupuncture in the English language. Available at www.medicalacupuncture.org/aama_marf/marf.html.

Helms Medical Institute: Medical Acupuncture for Physicians. Courses and physician education in acupuncture. Available at www.hmieducation.com.

MedlinePlus: Acupuncture. A number of reliable links. Available at www.nlm.nih.gov/medlineplus/acupuncture.html.

World Health Organization: Acupuncture Research. List of common conditions treatable by Chinese medicine and acupuncture. Available at http://tcm.health-info.org/WHO-treatment-list.htm.

BIBLIOGRAPHY

Allen JJ, Schnyer RN, Chambers AS, et al: Acupuncture for depression: A randomized controlled trial. J Clin Psychiatry 67:1665–1673, 2006.

Berman BM, Ezzo J, Hadhazy V, et al: Is acupuncture effective in the treatment of fibromyalgia? J Fam Pract 48:213–218, 1999.

Berman BM, Lao L, Langenberg P, et al: Effectiveness of acupuncture as adjunctive therapy in osteoarthritis of the knee: A randomized, controlled trial. Ann Intern Med 141:901–910, 2004.

Burke A, Upchurch D, Dye C, Chyu L: Acupuncture use in the United States: Findings from the National Health Interview Survey. J Altern Complement Med 12:639–648, 2006.

Ernst E: Acupuncture: A critical analysis. J Intern Med 259:125–137, 2006.

Ezzo J, Hadhazy V, Birch S, et al: Acupuncture for osteoarthritis of the knee. Arthritis Rheum 44:819–825, 2001.

Filshie J, White A: Medical Acupuncture: A Western Scientific Approach. New York, Churchill Livingstone, 1998.

Helms J: Acupuncture Energetics. Berkeley, Calif, Medical Acupuncture Publishers, 1996.

Helms J: An overview of medical acupuncture. Altern Ther Health Med 4:35–45, 1998.

MacPherson H, Hammerschlag R, Lewith G, Schnyer R: Acupuncture Research: Strategies for Establishing an Evidence Base. London, Churchill Livingstone, 2007.

Melchart D, Thormaehlen J, Hager S, et al: Acupuncture versus placebo versus sumatriptan for early treatment of migraine attacks: A randomized controlled trial. J Intern Med 253:181–188, 2003.

National Institutes of Health: Acupuncture. NIH Consensus Statement 15(5), November 3–5, 1997. Available at http://consensus.nih.gov/1997/1997Acupuncture107pdf.pdf.

Pomeranz B, Chiu D: Naloxone blockade of acupuncture analgesia: Endorphin implicated. Life Sci 19:1757–1762, 1976.

Richardson M, Freedman J: A model for acupuncture training in primary care. Acupunct Med 23:135–136, 2005.

Rubik B: Can Western science provide a foundation for acupuncture? Altern Ther Health Med 1:41–47, 1995.

Sierpina V, Frenkel M: Acupuncture: A clinical review. South Med J 98:330–337, 2005.

Stux G, Pomeranz G: Scientific Basis of Acupuncture: Acupuncture Textbook and Atlas. New York, Springer-Verlag, 1987.

White A, Tough E, Cummings M: A review of acupuncture clinical trials indexed during 2005. Acupunct Med 24:39–49, 2006.

CHAPTER 219

Allergy Testing and Immunotherapy

Harold H. Hedges III

The primary methods of allergy skin testing are (1) *single skin prick tests* (SPT; pricking the skin at a 45-degree angle through previously placed allergens); (2) *skin puncture tests* (puncturing the skin at a 90-degree angle through previously placed allergens); and (3) using *preloaded multiple-allergen testing devices* that apply multiple allergens simultaneously. All three of these tests are confined to the epidermis. Multiple-allergen applicators have gained in popularity because of their safety, ease of use, and test reproducibility and readability. The three that are commercially available are the Multi-Test II (Lincoln Diagnostics, Decatur, Ill; Fig. 219-1), Quintest (Hollister-Stier Laboratories, Spokane, Wash; Fig. 219-2), and Omni (Greer Laboratories, Lenoir, NC).

Although considered an SPT, Multi-Test II is comparable with an *intradermal* (ID) test using a 1 : 1000 dilution of allergen. Several studies have shown that a positive ID skin test (1 : 100 dilution) after a negative SPT (using 1 : 20 concentrates) has little or no clinical significance; thus it is not recommended (see later discussion).

As opposed to the prick and puncture tests, the ID test goes deeper, into the dermis.

Older *scratch testing* methods are not as reproducible or reliable as SPT and are not recommended.

In vitro blood tests (e.g., radioallergosorbent test [RAST]) are performed by a reference laboratory. No "kits" are available for office testing because this procedure involves just the drawing and testing of a blood sample. It is the test of choice for patients exhibiting dermographism, hyporeactive skin, poorly controlled asthma, eczema, or any skin condition limiting the placement of skin tests.

The identification of allergens helps direct patient avoidance measures and medical therapy; it also provides the basis for immunotherapy. As Nelson and colleagues (1996) state, "Immunotherapy provides the only potentially curative treatment available because of its unique ability to change the natural history of allergic respiratory disease and Hymenoptera sensitivity. Many suggest that starting immunotherapy is a reasonable option that can provide safe and cost effective management for a substantial number of patients." Starting immunotherapy earlier in allergic conditions may prevent (rather than just reduce) the inflammatory response, prevent the development of asthma in children with rhinitis, and allow treatment to begin at lower levels of patient sensitivity. It may be the only safe modality for patients whose jobs require alertness and who cannot tolerate antihistamines (e.g., pilots, truck drivers). *It is accepted that a positive SPT or in vitro test does not necessarily mean clinical sensitivity, so correlation with the clinical history is essential if immunotherapy is to be successful.*

Indications

Perennial or seasonal rhinitis, rhinosinusitis, rhinoconjunctivitis, rhinitis with otitis media, and anaphylaxis from Hymenoptera stings are the major indications for allergy testing. Patients should be tested for tree, grass, and weed pollens; mold sensitivity; and appropriate insects or animal danders. Limited food testing may be performed. There is increased risk when testing asthmatic patients and when placing them on immunotherapy, so the risk–benefit ratio must be considered carefully. Many people with asthma have concomitant allergic rhinitis, which, when treated, aids in asthma control.

Contraindications

- Any condition that compromises the patient's ability to withstand the rare anaphylactic reaction (e.g., patients with uncontrolled hypertension or significant unstable cardiovascular disease).
- Although most allergic patients can be safely tested and treated by the primary care physician, an allergist should be consulted for the evaluation and treatment of patients with history of anaphylactic reactions (particularly to stinging insects), reactions to anesthetics, and difficult-to-control, moderate to severe, persistent asthma. Great caution must be exercised.
- Immunotherapy usually is not initiated during pregnancy. Allergic patients on maintenance therapy who become pregnant may continue the desensitization process through the pregnancy.
- Patients taking beta blockers should have alternative medications prescribed before they are tested and placed on immunotherapy because beta blockers interfere with the response to epinephrine, which is needed to treat anaphylaxis should it occur.
- Those with dermographism (which makes skin testing unreliable), those with chronic skin diseases that limit access to normal skin, and those (physically or psychologically) unable to communicate symptoms should be tested by in vitro testing.
- There is no specific age limit (young or old) for allergy testing to check for suspected inhaled allergens, but usually it is not done before the age of 3 years. Allergic food reactions can be detected by limited food testing (SPT or RAST). Other (nonallergic) adverse food reactions require single or multiple food elimination diets.
- Antihistamines and steroids may blunt the response to skin testing and should be eliminated before testing. Older, short-acting antihistamines should be stopped 48 hours before testing. Longer-acting antihistamines require a drug-free period of 7 to 10 days. Steroids may need to be withheld for 2 to 4 weeks. Positive and negative controls are essential, especially when these medications have been used, and help to validate skin test results. The positive control (histamine) usually responds with a 7- to 10-mm wheal (and is always read as a 3+ reaction). If the response is less, it is still being blunted by the antihistamine or other medication. In vitro tests (e.g., RAST) are not affected by any

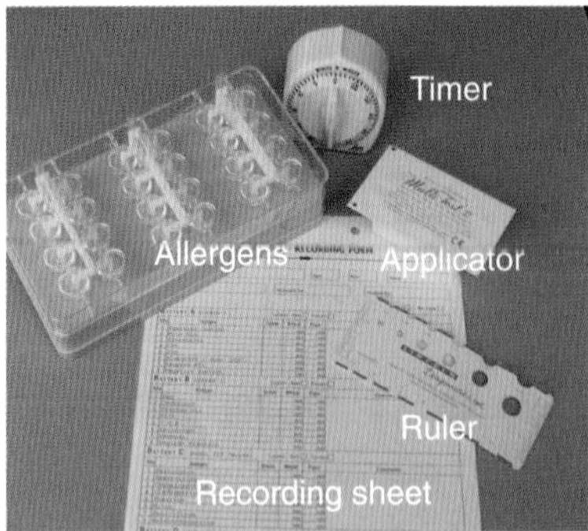

Figure 219-1 Lincoln Diagnostics Multi-Test. (Courtesy of Lincoln Diagnostics, Decatur, Ill.)

antihistamines, steroids, or other medication and thus can be used at any time.

Screening for Allergies

It is appropriate and cost effective to *screen* patients for allergies with a limited set of 6 to 10 allergens before applying a complete geographic panel of allergens (Fig. 219-3). A typical screen consists of a positive (histamine) and negative (glycerol-saline) control; house dust mite mix; cat; and the most tree, grass, weed, and mold allergens of the geographic area. Physicians and patients reluctant to rely on only six allergens for *screening* may use a second panel of eight allergens consisting of dog; cockroach; feathers; silk; and secondary tree, grass, weed, and mold preparations.

Always check the positive and negative control sites before interpreting the response to the allergens. When all screening test sites are negative (excluding the positive control; see Fig. 219-13), the probability of allergy is less than 3%. Approximately 50% of patients with rhinitis tested by Multi-Test or an in vitro test will have negative findings. These patients have *nonallergic rhinitis*. Identification of nonallergic triggers is critical for medical care. Decongestants (not antihistamines), nasal steroids, and nasal astemizole are the appropriate medications indicated for nonallergic rhinitis. However, roughly 50% of patients with rhinitis have an allergic basis to their symptoms. Many patients have mixed rhinitis, meaning they have both allergic and nonallergic rhinitis simultaneously.

As noted, allergy screening can be performed using either SPT or in vitro methods. Phadiatop (Pharmacia & Upjohn Diagnostics, Uppsala, Sweden) and the Multiple Inhalant Allergy screen (MIA; LabCorp, Burlington, NC) are two RAST screens using 10 allergens. In vitro screens usually have ±10 of the most common allergens, including tree, grass, weed, and molds from a geographic area; house dust mite; and cat. In vitro screens are performed by the various laboratories. A blood sample is sent to the company for testing. There is no office "kit."

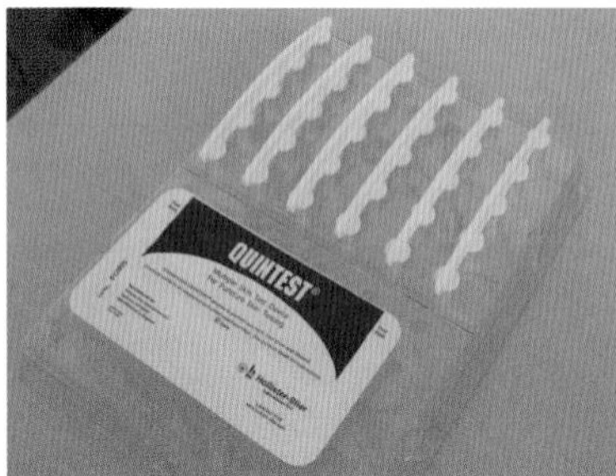

Figure 219-2 Hollister-Stier Quintest. (Courtesy of Hollister-Stier Laboratories, Spokane, Wash.)

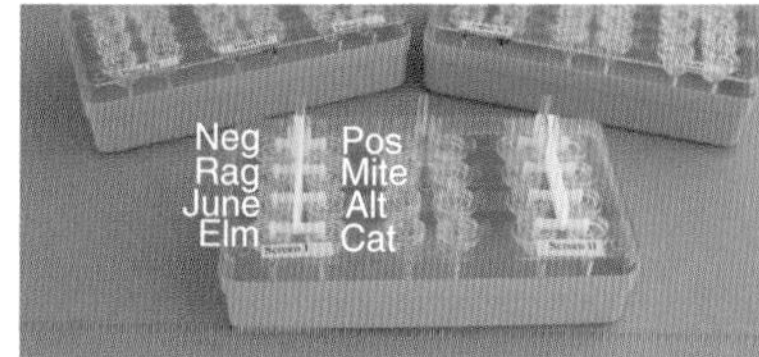

Figure 219-3 A typical screening panel with six allergens.

When the aforementioned screening tests are negative, no further testing is needed. Screening is very cost effective in selecting out the nonallergic patient. (The Blue Cross/Blue Shield usual and customary reimbursement for SPTs is currently $7.00 per allergen. The negative and positive controls are not reimbursed, hence the $42 payment. The $15 to $25 fee for in vitro testing varies from company to company.)

A history of symptoms in early *spring* generally correlates with positive skin tests to tree allergens. *Summer* symptoms correlate with grass sensitivity, and *fall* symptoms correlate with weed sensitivity. In the warmer climates there is much overlap. *Year-round (perennial) symptoms* correlate with house dust mite, mold, or insect or animal sensitivity. Perennial symptoms with seasonal exacerbations frequently occur in the same patient.

Preprocedure Patient Preparation

- *Establish the history* compatible with rhinitis or asthma.
- *Explore hereditary factors, allergic and nonallergic triggers*, previous and present medications, severity and duration of symptoms, secondary infections, and quality-of-life limitations caused by the symptoms.
- *Perform a physical examination* to evaluate for signs of atopic disease: rhinorrhea (especially if clear and combined with nasal congestion and pale blue, swollen turbinates), allergic "shiners" under the eyes, conjunctivitis, and evidence of reversible airway disease.
- *Spirometry or peak expiratory flow rates* are helpful to identify and follow associated asthma (see Chapter 91, Pulmonary Function Testing). Patients with poorly controlled asthma (forced expiratory volume in 1 second [FEV_1] <70% of their *personal best effort*) should *not* be skin tested or receive immunotherapy until treated and stable. In vitro testing, however, is safe and recommended in this situation.
- Inform patients about the nature of testing, the risk of possible reactions, the types of reactions encountered (local and systemic), and the treatment available should a reaction occur. Patients or parents of minors should sign an informed consent. (Refer to Lockey and colleagues, 2004.)
- Instruct patients to avoid older, short-acting antihistamines 48 hours before skin testing. *Longer-acting antihistamines should be avoided 7 to 14 days before testing.* Remember, the positive histamine control must produce a 7- to 10-mm wheal to validate skin testing.
- Explain the frequency and duration of immunotherapy (weekly or biweekly injections for 3 to 5 years), the expected response, and the criteria for discontinuation (symptom-free control with little or no medication and no increase in symptoms with increasing intervals between injections).

Equipment

For Skin Testing

- Multiple allergen applicators and loading docks (Multi-Test II, Quintest, Greer)
- Individual applicators for the occasional testing of one or two allergens (Duotip [Lincoln Diagnostics], Morrow Brown Needle

[Alkaline Corporation, Oakhurst, NJ]); or a tip from a multiple-allergen applicator can be broken off and used separately
- Alcohol sponges to clean the testing site
- 30 to 50 standardized or 1:20 weight/volume [w/v] allergen concentrates identified for the specific geographic locale by published data or suggested by providers of allergy diagnostics (house dust mite comes only as a 1:100 dilution as the concentrate)
- Histamine phosphate (2.75 mg/mL) for the positive control and saline for the negative control
- Recording form (Fig. 219-4)
- Black skin-marking pen
- Timer capable of timing at least 20 minutes
- Millimeter ruler
- EpiPen, Ana Kit, or epinephrine, and albuterol
- Resuscitation equipment in the rare event of anaphylactic reaction (the same as that for giving any injections in the office; see Chapter 220, Anaphylaxis)
- Disposable tuberculin syringes fitted with a 26- or 27-gauge needle for the "vial test" (see the section on Intradermal Testing and the Vial Test)

For Radioallergosorbent Testing or Other in Vitro Tests

- Equipment for drawing blood
- Mailing packages or instructions provided by the RAST laboratory

TECHNIQUE

Skin Prick and Puncture Tests

Skin *prick* tests are performed by placing a drop of allergen concentrate (usually 1:20 w/v) on the arm or back, then pressing a needle through the drop into the epidermis at a 45-degree angle. The tip of the needle is then lifted up, producing the pricking sensation. If performed correctly, no bleeding should occur (Figs. 219-5 and 219-6A). The skin *puncture* test is similar, but the skin is punctured at a 90-degree angle (Fig. 219-6B). Several *skin testing devices* were listed previously. The use of Multi-Test II is described in detail here because it has been found to be safe, easily learned, reproducible, and reliable. A videotape of the procedure is available from Lincoln Diagnostics.

Multi-Test Applicator Method

Multi-Test II is a sterile, disposable, multiple-test applicator used to apply eight allergens simultaneously. Although considered an SPT, its reliability is comparable to ID techniques using a 1:1000 dilution of allergen. Laboratories that supply the allergen concentrates will help determine the most relevant allergens for the patient's geographic area based on established patterns. The system consists of plastic applicators and the Dipwell tray (Fig. 219-7).

Loading the Dipwell Tray

1. Establish a master list of allergen panels (each containing eight allergens) to be tested and enter them on the recording form. It is crucial to load each allergen in the same test well each time. Make copies of this list for recording test results and refer to it when replenishing allergens.
2. Label (number) each panel A, B, C, D, etc.
3. Allergen panels are made by adding 1 mL (enough for 100 applications) of each allergen concentrate (1:20 w/v in 50% glycerin or standardized extract) to each well numbered 1 through 8. Applicator heads are numbered 1 through 8 also and correspond to the numbered wells. Each Dipwell tray accommodates three allergen panels, each with eight testing heads (see Fig. 219-7).
4. Panel A (*screening* panel) contains the positive control in well A1 and the negative control in well A8. A2 through A7 contain the most common tree, grass, weed, and mold allergens from a geographic area, plus house dust mite mix and cat.

   NOTE: *This panel will identify over 95% of those in the allergic population. A negative (except for the positive control) screen indicates a nonallergic cause of rhinitis or asthma. No further allergy testing is indicated.* This reduces the cost of total allergy testing. When the screen is positive, additional allergens of the geographic area are tested (usually 30 to 40). An additional panel can also be used to check for allergies to common foods (e.g., milk, corn, wheat, egg, soy, sugar, baker's yeast, and pork).
5. Trays are stored in the refrigerator and stack easily.

Application of Multi-Test

1. Place the Dipwell tray, which has been filled as noted previously, on a flat surface with the "cradle" for the "T" handle facing away from you.
2. Remove the sterile applicator from the package (held with the blue dot at the top) by pulling the label at the blue dot. This positions the "T" handle away from you for correct placement in the Dipwell tray (Fig. 219-8).
3. Place the applicator in the loaded Dipwell tray (see Fig. 219-7). The applicator now has the allergen on the respective tips.
4. Cleanse the skin with an alcohol wipe and allow it to dry.
5. Mark (number) the test sites on the skin corresponding to the placement of the applicators (A, B, C, D, etc.) with a black skin-marking pen.
6. Apply panel A (screening panel) to the volar surface of the forearm (supported with a pillow to keep the arm flat) with the "T" handle toward the patient's head (Fig. 219-9). Apply with a rocking motion, to and fro and side to side. When applied with correct pressure, a footprint of each testing head will be visible. No bleeding should occur; if it does, reduce the amount of pressure applied. The correct amount of pressure will be realized after several applications.
7. A positive reaction to any one of the tree, grass, weed, or mold allergen(s) is followed by testing all remaining significant allergens of the area suggested by history. Total number is variable from area to area, usually 20 to 40. These are placed on the patient's back with the patient lying face down and can be applied at this visit (Fig. 219-10). Sites must be kept flat to prevent allergens from running and contaminating other sites. Hairy sites should be avoided because this interferes with readability.

Interpretation of Results

See Box 219-1. Positive responses are noted by wheals. Erythema may be present but is not used in scoring.

- The wheal is the white or gray raised area at the test site. This wheal may be surrounded by an area of erythema called the *flare*. The size and shape of the *wheal* only are used in scoring reactions (see Box 219-1) and are noted on the recording form in rhe corresponding position.
- The wheal produced at the positive (histamine) control site (Fig. 219-11), usually 7 to 10 mm in an adult and 6 mm in a child, is read and recorded as a 3+ reaction. Should the reaction at the positive control site be less than 7 mm or more than 10 mm, it should always be scored as a 3+ reaction, and should be read and recorded at 10 minutes because it will begin to fade. Other sites should be read at 20 minutes.
- Reactions comparable with those at the negative control site (saline or glycerol-saline) are negative. It is not unusual to see a small wheal (1 to 3 mm) at the negative control site (Fig. 219-12). 2+ reactions are generally 3 to 5 mm in size, and 3+ reactions 5 to 7 mm. Reactions read as 4+ are greater than the

Multi-Test Recording Form

Patient Name: ____________________________ Age: _____ Sex: _____ Date: __________________

Patient ID: ______________________ Ordered by: _________________ Tested by: ______________

❒ Initial Test ❒ Re-test

Battery A Screen I		Location: ❒ Back ❒ Forearm			
Site	Antigen	Grade	Wheal	Flare	Comments
1	Positive control		mm	mm	
2	Mite mix		mm	mm	
3	Alternaria		mm	mm	
4	Cat		mm	mm	
5	Elm		mm	mm	
6	Bluegrass/June (std.)		mm	mm	
7	Ragweed mix		mm	mm	
8	Negative control		mm	mm	

Battery B Screen II		Location: ❒ Back ❒ Forearm			
Site	Antigen	Grade	Wheal	Flare	Comments
1	Dog		mm	mm	
2	Cockroach		mm	mm	
3	Feather mix		mm	mm	
4	Silk		mm	mm	
5	T.O.E.		mm	mm	
6	Epicoccum		mm	mm	
7	Bermuda		mm	mm	
8	English Plantain		mm	mm	

Battery C Panel III (molds)		Location: ❒ Back ❒ Forearm			
Site	Antigen	Grade	Wheal	Flare	Comments
1	Pullularia		mm	mm	
2	Aspergillus		mm	mm	
3	Cephalosporium		mm	mm	
4	Cladosporium		mm	mm	
5	Fusarium		mm	mm	
6	Mucor		mm	mm	
7	Penicillium		mm	mm	
8	Helminthosporium		mm	mm	

Battery D Panel IV (trees)		Location: ❒ Back ❒ Forearm			
Site	Antigen	Grade	Wheal	Flare	Comments
1	Alder		mm	mm	
2	Birch		mm	mm	
3	E. Cottonwood		mm	mm	
4	Hackberry		mm	mm	
5	Maple/Box Elder		mm	mm	
6	Pine		mm	mm	
7	Sweet Gum		mm	mm	
8	Sycamore		mm	mm	

Figure 219-4 Sample recording form. (Courtesy of Lincoln Diagnostics, Decatur, Ill.)

Battery E Panel V (grass)		Location: ❐ Back		❐ Forearm	
Site	Antigen	Grade	Wheal	Flare	Comments
1	Oak		mm	mm	
2	Hickory/Pecan		mm	mm	
3	Mtn. Cedar		mm	mm	
4	Timothy (std.)		mm	mm	
5	Grass Smuts		mm	mm	
6	Bermuda (std.)		mm	mm	
7	Johnson		mm	mm	
8	Bahia		mm	mm	

Battery F Panel VI (weeds)		Location: ❐ Back		❐ Forearm	
Site	Antigen	Grade	Wheal	Flare	Comments
1	Cocklebur		mm	mm	
2	Dock		mm	mm	
3	Lambsquarter		mm	mm	
4	Nettle		mm	mm	
5	Pigweed/Careless		mm	mm	
6	Marshelder, R.		mm	mm	
7	Russian Thistle		mm	mm	
8	W. Water Hemp		mm	mm	

Battery G Foods		Location: ❐ Back		❐ Forearm	
Site	Antigen	Grade	Wheal	Flare	Comments
1	Beef		mm	mm	
2	Corn		mm	mm	
3	Egg		mm	mm	
4	Milk		mm	mm	
5	Pork		mm	mm	
6	Soybean		mm	mm	
7	Wheat		mm	mm	
8	Baker's Yeast		mm	mm	

Battery H		Location: ❐ Back		❐ Forearm	
Site	Antigen	Grade	Wheal	Flare	Comments

Figure 219-4, cont.

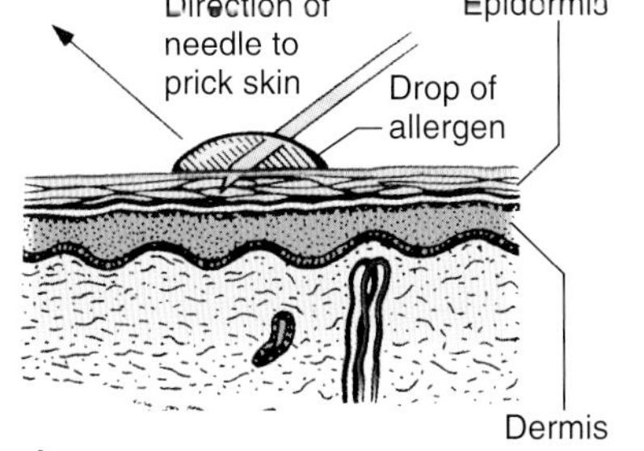

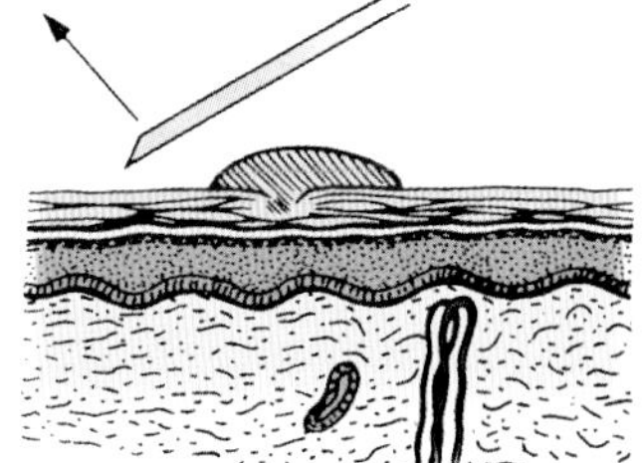

Figure 219-5 Method for percutaneous skin prick testing. **A,** The drop of allergen is placed on the skin and a 27-gauge needle (bevel up) is placed through the allergen drop into the superficial epidermis. **B,** The needle pricks the skin at a 45-degree angle, allowing allergen to come in contact with sensitized mast cells located in the epidermis, and then is lifted up. The dermis is not violated and bleeding at the site is nonexistent or minimal.

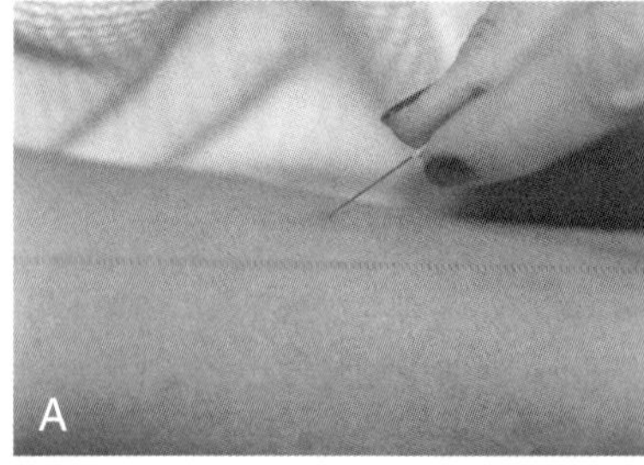

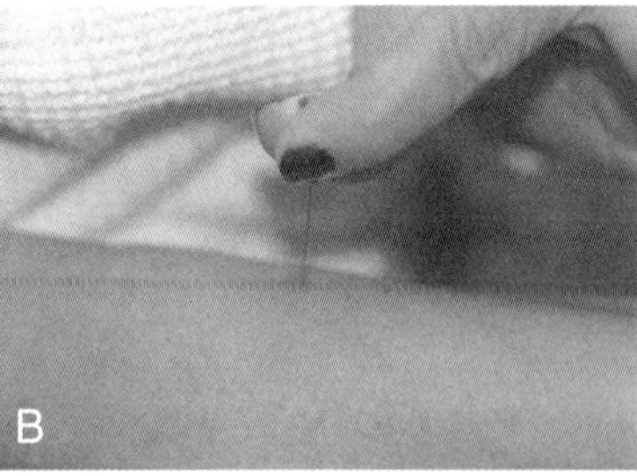

Figure 219-6 **A,** Skin prick test (45-degree angle). **B,** Skin puncture test (90-degree angle). In both methods, only the epidermis is penetrated.

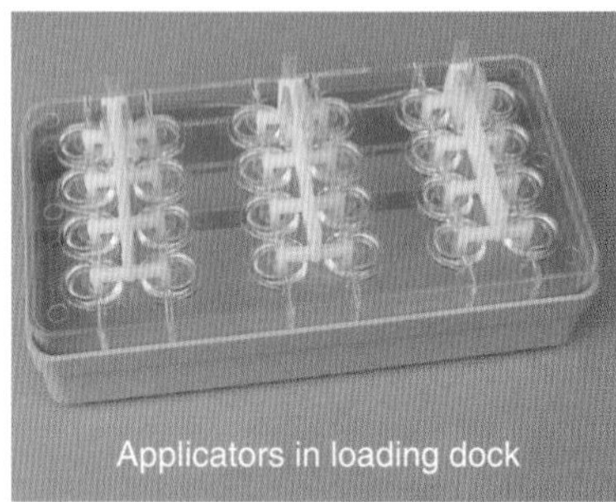

Figure 219-7 Plastic applicators in the Dipwell tray.

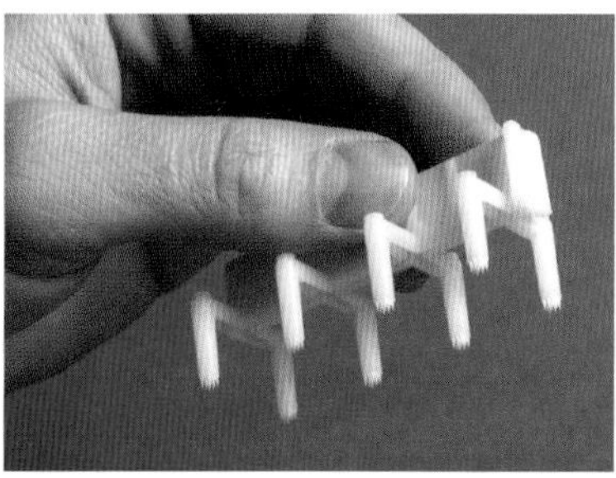

Figure 219-8 Disposable plastic applicator for Multi-Test II.

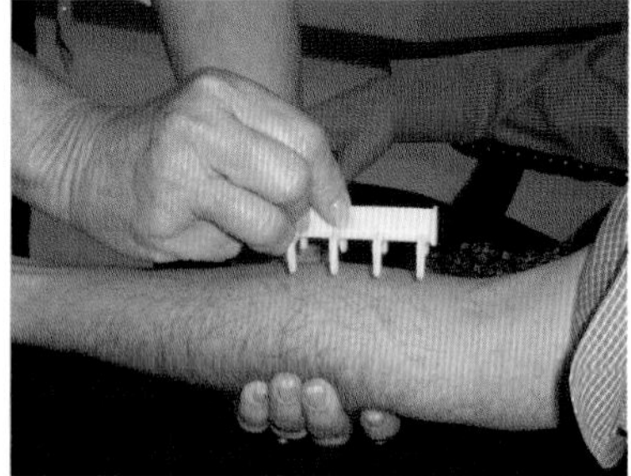

Figure 219-9 Applying loaded applicator.

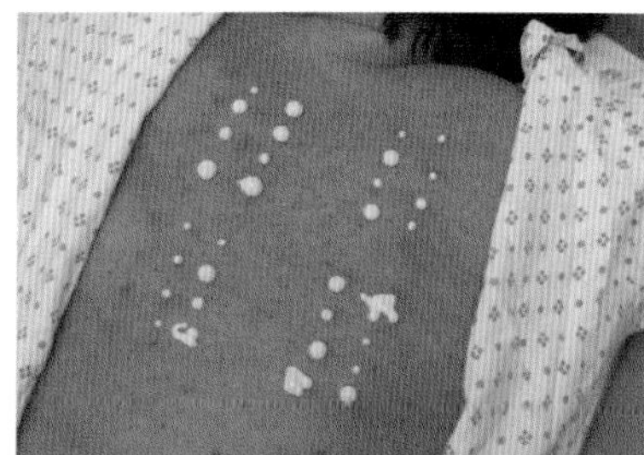

Figure 219-10 Additional panels on patient's back.

Box 219-1. Scoring of Multi-Test (Used in Fivefold Dilution Systems)

Multi-Test is scored by comparing the reaction of allergens to the negative (glycerol–saline) and positive (histamine 1 mg/mL) controls applied at the same time and in the same general location.

- 0 No reaction or a wheal up to 3 mm in size may occur at the negative control site
- 1+ Wheal larger than the negative control, usually 3–4 mm
- 2+ Wheal 5–7 mm
- 3+ Wheal 7–10 mm (size of the positive control)
- 4+ Any reaction with a wheal larger than the positive control without pseudopods
- 5+ Any reaction larger than the positive control with pseudopods

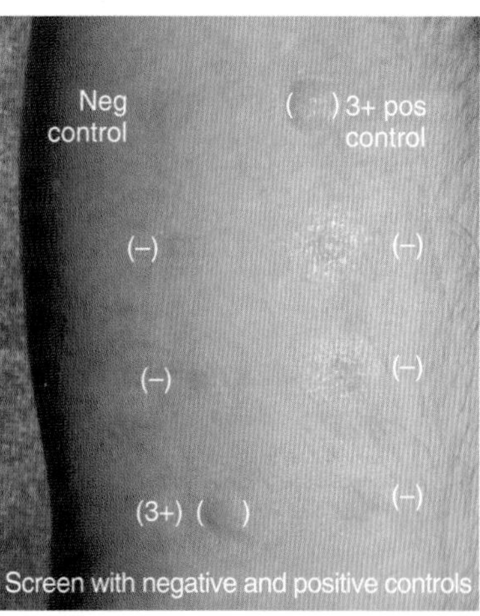

Figure 219-11 Example of a positive allergy screen (3+ reaction). A positive reaction at the tree, grass, weed, or mold site dicatates completing local allergy panels.

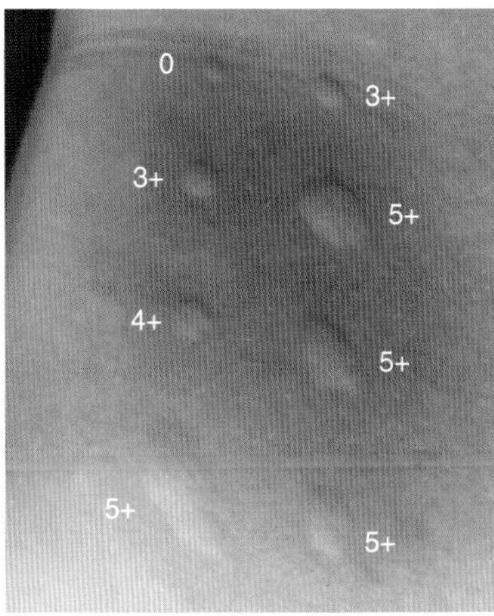

Figure 219-12 Scoring results. See text for explanation. The negative control in the left upper corner shows a 1+ reaction.

reaction at the positive control site but retain their circular form. Reactions read as 5+ are larger than the positive control site with spreading pseudopods.

- Reactions equal to or greater than the positive (histamine) control site generally correlate the best with history of exposure to allergic triggers. 2+ reactions correlate less, and 1+ reactions even less. Correlation of all test responses to history is important in compounding immunotherapy sets.
- When the positive control is positive and all other tests are negative (Fig. 219-13), nonallergic rhinitis or asthma is present. This result occurs 50% of the time.
- Dermographism (Fig. 219-14) should be suspected when *all* tests are positive, including the negative control. Such patients must be tested by RAST.
- When reactions at all test sites are negative (Fig. 219-15), including the positive control site, suspect antihistamine or other medication, which may decrease the skin response.
- Results of tests are recorded (see Fig. 219-4), and a signed copy is the prescription sent to the laboratory for compounding immunotherapy (see later discussion).
- When house dust mite (Fig. 219-16), cat (Fig. 219-17), or both, are the only positive reactions, *no further testing need be done at this time.* Avoidance measures *and immunotherapy* are instituted for either or both of these allergens. *House dust mite avoidance* includes covering pillows and mattresses, dusting regularly, and removing stuffed animals, carpets, and overstuffed furniture. Bedding should be washed weekly with water at 130° F. Lowering humidity to below 50% is helpful. HEPA filtration helps remove small particulate matter. Ideally, cats should be eliminated from

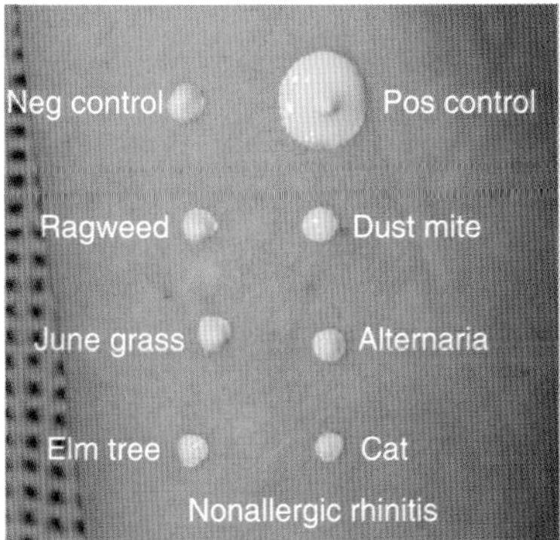

Figure 219-13 Nonallergic allergy screen. Positive and negative controls are appropriate; all other test sites are negative. The diagnosis is nonallergic rhinitis or asthma.

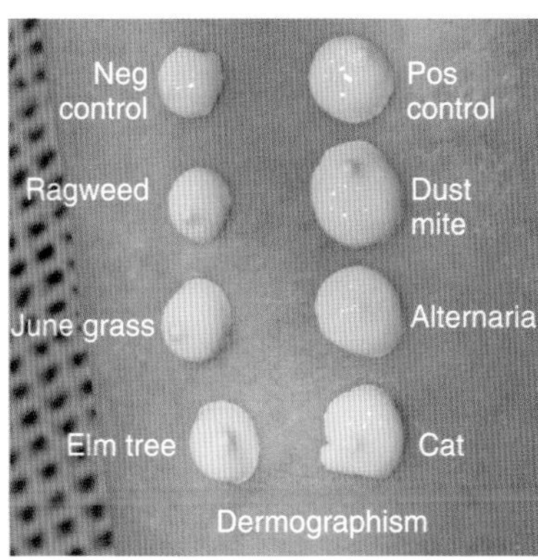

Figure 219-14 Dermographism. Negative control is positive and all other test sites are positive.

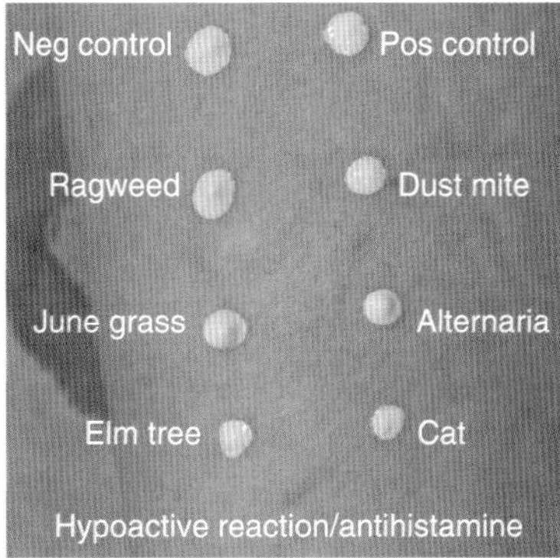

Figure 219-15 Positive (histamine) control is nonreactive, which invalidates skin response at other test sites. Suspect antihistamine or other medications.

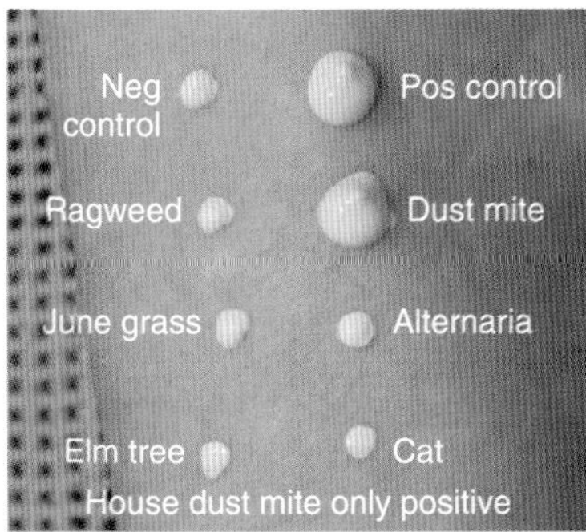

Figure 219-16 House dust mite is the only positive.

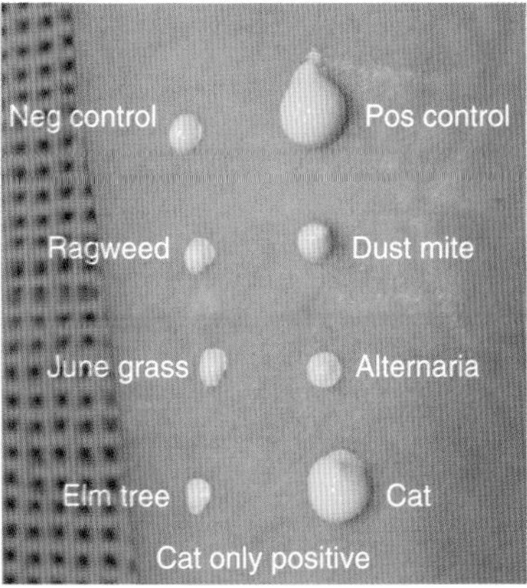

Figure 219-17 Cat is the only positive.

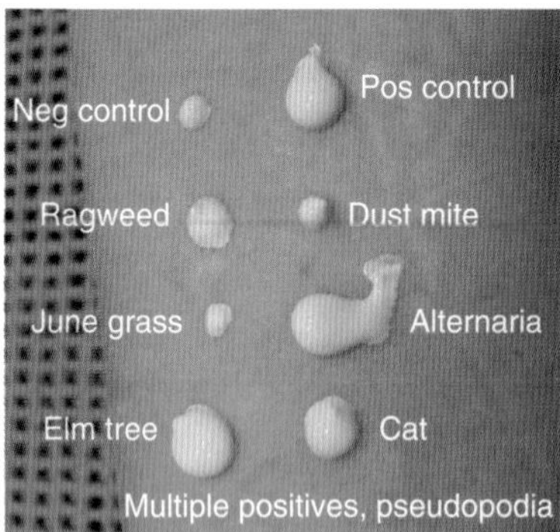

Figure 219-18 Allergic rhinitis. Pseudopod is best seen with the *Alternaria* allergen.

the home, but it has been shown that less than 25% of patients or families comply. (At the very least, cats should be kept out of the bedroom and off the bed.) Weekly *washing of the cat* will decrease the allergen load. *Later, additional allergy testing can be done if symptoms do not improve.*

- Pseudopods (Fig. 219-18) occur frequently and are recorded as 4+ or 5+ reactions.
- Testing for other nonpollen allergens, such as dog, cockroach, feathers, and laboratory and farm animals, may be suggested by history.

Complications

- *Itching* at the positive test sites is expected. Highly allergic patients may have rapid and large skin responses and will begin to show whealing, erythema, and itching within minutes. These individual reactions should be wiped clean with alcohol, being careful not to contaminate a nearby test site. These will proceed to react despite wiping and can be treated with oral antihistamines or steroid creams if necessary. The reaction will usually resolve in 30 minutes to 1 hour.
- Rarely, *systemic symptoms* occur that may include hives, urticaria, itching of the roof of the mouth, a sensation of throat closure, shortness of breath, an increase in presenting symptoms (sneezing, rhinorrhea, or wheezing), and anxiety. All allergens should be removed with alcohol. Give 50 to 100 mg of diphenhydramine (Benadryl) orally or intramuscularly and observe closely, monitoring vital signs. Epinephrine, 0.3 mL (1 : 1000 dilution) for adults and 0.1 to 0.15 mL for children, should be nearby and used as needed if symptoms proceed to anaphylaxis. This occurrence is very rare. In addition to epinephrine, maintenance of the airway, correction of hypotension, and other general measures are used for treatment. Bronchodilation per inhaled albuterol should be given if asthma is precipitated. Monitor the patient's general condition, including blood pressure and respiration using peak flow measurement or spirometry, for several hours as needed. Transfer to an emergency department for more intensive help may be indicated (see Chapter 220, Anaphylaxis).
- *False-negative results.*
- When there is *no reaction whatsoever at the positive control site*, hypoactive skin due to antihistamines, steroids, or other medications should be suspected. The clinician should retest after an appropriate time off medication or consider an in vitro test, which is not affected by any medication.
- *Delayed reactions* (usually at mold sites) may occur up to hours after testing and last for 2 to 7 days. This reaction is an inflammatory response rather than immunoglobulin E (IgE) mediated, and it does not respond to immunotherapy. Local steroids may be helpful.

Intradermal Testing and the Vial Test

Historically, ID testing has followed negative or equivocal SPT results when the history strongly indicates a particular allergen. Studies have questioned the presence of clinically significant sensitivity if the SPT is negative but the ID test is positive. The use of positive ID tests after negative SPTs may not be an appropriate basis for selecting patients for immunotherapy. An ID test is used for the "vial test" before starting immunotherapy. The vial test affirms the safety of the immunotherapy set. It is needed only with the initial vial. The clinician should create a 4-mm ID wheal (Fig. 219-19) by injecting about 0.03 mL of the weakest vial (1 : 100,000 dilution) on the upper outer arm, using an allergy syringe and a 26- or 27-gauge needle. The test is read in 15 minutes. Growth of the ID wheal beyond 15 mm indicates increased sensitivity, and a further 10-fold (1 : 1,000,000) or 5-fold dilution of the vial is necessary. The clinician should take 0.5 mL of the allergen vial and add it to 4.5 mL of phenolated saline (diluting fluid) and repeat the vial test. Rarely, the vial test may cause reproduction of presenting symptoms (e.g., sneezing, rhinorrhea, congestion, or asthma). This recurrence indicates increased exposure to an allergen(s) in the mix that may have pollinated since testing and initiation of immunotherapy. Further dilution of the immunotherapy may be indicated.

Radioallergosorbent Blood Test

A reference laboratory processes in vitro tests. The same principles of *screening* apply as for SPT, and most laboratories will provide a geographic screening panel before completing an extensive specific regional in vitro panel; if not, one can be designed based the allergens in the clinician's local area. A negative in vitro screen requires no further testing. In vitro testing is not affected by any medication. Box 219-2 shows indications for in vitro testing.

In in vitro testing, an allergen is coupled to a paper disk or placed in a cellulose suspension to which the patient's serum is added. An antigen–antibody complex is formed that, when tagged with radioactive anti-IgE, forms an antigen–antibody–anti-IgE complex scored by a gamma counter. A grading system provides quantifying levels of IgE antibody on which immunotherapy is based. In vitro–based immunotherapy uses either 5-fold or 10-fold dilutions. In vitro laboratories usually provide immunotherapy sets or will suggest an immunotherapy-compounding laboratory. In vitro testing is efficacious. As with skin testing, results must be interpreted in light of the clinical history.

In vitro testing is an accepted method of testing for specific allergies and can be used by physicians who do not want to perform skin testing.

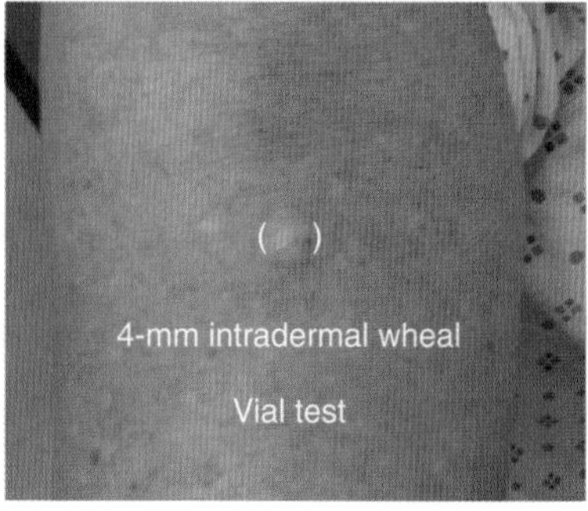

Figure 219-19 A 4-mm intradermal wheal for the vial test.

Box 219-2. Indications for Radioallergosorbent Testing

Atrophic or very young skin
Dermographism
Extensive eczema or other dermatoses
History of anaphylaxis
Immunodeficiency disorders
Long-acting antihistamines, steroids
Presence of beta blockers
Unstable cardiac condition
Unstable or severe asthma

ADVANTAGES OF SKIN TESTING

- The patient can be tested and results known within minutes, whereas in vitro results may not be available for a week or longer, depending on the laboratory.
- The patient sees and experiences the reaction, which reinforces the need for avoidance. This is especially helpful in house dust mite avoidance and cat or dog allergy.
- There is much less difficulty with insurance companies over payment for skin allergy testing. A significant number of HMOs and other insurance carriers will deny payment for in vitro testing.
- In vitro testing is more expensive than SPT ($3 to $4 per skin test versus $8 to $15 per RAST).

POSTPROCEDURE PATIENT EDUCATION

Avoidance procedures and medications are prescribed where appropriate. Brochures describing general allergen avoidance and specific house dust mite and animal dander measures are readily available. Immunotherapy is considered an adjunct to treatment.

IMMUNOTHERAPY

Immunotherapy is indicated based on the demonstration of immediate hypersensitivity by SPT, Multi-Test, or any in vitro test that correlates with the patient's history and physical findings. This correlation is imperative for success. When beginning therapy on a patient for the first time, perform an ID test (the vial test) as noted previously. Increasing amounts of allergen are given subcutaneously until the highest tolerated dose is reached.

Conventional immunotherapy is based on a 10-fold dilution system and is started at 0.1 mL of 1 : 100,000 dilution of each allergen. Injections are graduated (0.1, 0.2, 0.3, 0.4, 0.5 mL) weekly through dilutions of 1 : 100,000, 1 : 10,000, 1 : 1000, and 1 : 100 until maintenance is reached. Some laboratories use a fivefold dilution system (1 : 325,000, 1 : 62,500, 1 : 12,5000, 1 : 2500, 1 : 500, 1 : 100) for immunotherapy. *The maintenance dose in either system is the highest tolerated dose that can be attained without causing a significant local (painful knot or erythema lasting more than 24 hours) or systemic reaction.* Some patients may not be able to tolerate injections in the 1 : 100 dilutions because of local or systemic reactions, but immunotherapy at lower dilutions usually will be effective for them. Using the fivefold dilution system, Multi-Test and in vitro testing allow the starting dose to be tailored based on the degree of sensitivity to the allergen. The higher the sensitivity, the more dilute the starting dose; the lower the sensitivity, the more concentrated the starting dose. Immunotherapy is usually started at a level 5 to 25 times weaker than the test scores, and then graduated until maintenance is reached.

Based on testing, an allergy laboratory will compound an immunotherapy set consisting of four vials each containing increasing concentrations of all the relevant allergens. If more than 12 allergens are to be included, 2 sets are needed. As a clinician's allergy practice grows, compounding immunotherapy in the office can be considered. This requires additional space and personnel. By law, immunotherapy sets made by commercial laboratories are "quarantined" for 2 weeks to ensure sterility. This does not apply in office compounding. Phenolated saline with glycerin or glycerinated saline is used as the diluent in mixing, providing ample sterility and stability.

Escalation of immunotherapy (Box 219-3) proceeds on a weekly schedule with doses adjusted as needed because of local or systemic reactions. Increasing symptoms and skin responses that occur during a pollinating season may require slowing or holding of escalation until pollination ceases. As the season passes, escalation can then proceed with no further problem. Local swelling, whealing, or "knot" formation greater that 2 cm lasting more than 24 hours is considered significant. The subsequent dose should be reduced to one not causing a reaction and escalated at a slower rate for patient comfort. Doses for smaller local reactions of swelling and redness

Box 219-3. Example of Escalation Schedule for Weekly Immunotherapy*

Vial D

1 : 100,000 w/v	**Green vial**
Dose no. 1	0.05 mL
2	0.10
3	0.20
4	0.30
5	0.40
6	0.50

Vial C

1 : 10,000 w/v	**Blue vial**
Dose no. 7	0.05 mL
8	0.10
9	0.20
10	0.30
11	0.40
12	0.50

Vial B

1 : 1000 w/v	**Gold vial**
Dose no. 13	0.10 mL
14	0.20
15	0.30
16	0.40
17	0.50

Vial A

1 : 100 w/v	**Red vial**
Dose no. 18	0.05 mL
19	0.10
20	0.15
21	0.20
22	0.25
23	0.30
24	0.35
25	0.40
26	0.45
27	0.50

Maintain for 1 year, then go to every 2 weeks for 3 to 5 years, then try to discontinue.

*The same antigen mixture is used in vials A through D, but with varying concentrations.

Box 219-4. Reasons for Allergy Treatment Failures

Development of new allergens
Erratic dosage schedule
Inaccurate diagnoses
Inadequate dose of immunotherapy
Incomplete diagnoses (allergic and nonallergic factors)
Immunotherapy dose beyond the optimal dose
Lack of appropriate patient education
Nonallergic food and chemical sensitivities
Noncompliance with avoidance
Noncompliance with medication
Rhinitis medicamentosa

should be repeated or reduced as tolerated. *Immunotherapy should be omitted or delayed* (1) when a febrile illness is present, (2) when the patient is extremely fatigued, (3) after acute exacerbation of allergic symptoms during a pollinating season, (4) or during or after an asthma attack. The peak expiratory flow rate should be above 70% of the patient's personal best effort. Asthmatic patients should be free of wheezing, cough, or shortness of breath before being tested or receiving an allergy injection. Asthmatic patients should monitor their own status with a peak flow meter.

Actions *to prevent untoward reactions and anaphylaxis* during immunotherapy include the following:

- Evaluate the patient's condition before injection.
- Minimize the chance of errors in dosing and administration by checking and rechecking the patient's dosing schedule and reactions to previous injections.
- Have the patient identify the vial to be used by name and birthday on the vial.
- Use more dilute allergen in highly sensitive patients (by history or testing).
- Observe patients in the office for 20 to 30 minutes after injection.
- Check the patient and injection site before allowing the patient to leave.
- Reduce the first dose of newly prepared extracts by half.
- Reduce the dose when local or systemic reactions occur.
- Avoid shots to asthmatic patients whose peak flow is less than 70% of their personal best effort.
- Avoid immunotherapy in the presence of a febrile illness.
- Avoid giving immunotherapy to patients on beta blockers.

About 80% of allergic patients respond to immunotherapy, whereas some 20% show little or no response (Box 219-4). Maintenance doses should be continued for 3 to 5 years, and the time between doses increased to 2 weeks after the first year, then 2 to 4 weeks after the second year, with symptom return used as the guide. The patient may miss doses in the buildup and maintenance phases of immunotherapy. Guidelines for treatment after missed doses are found in Boxes 219-5 and 219-6.

Box 219-5. Resuming Immunotherapy after Missed Doses during Escalation

3–10 days	Continue escalation
10–14 days	Repeat last dose
14–21 days	Reduce dose 0.1 mL
Over 21 days	Reduce dose by half and gradually re-escalate

Box 219-6. Resuming Immunotherapy after Missed Doses during Maintenance

1–4 weeks	Continue maintenance dose
4–12 weeks	½ maintenance dose, rebuild to maintenance
3–6 months	Drop dilution by full 10-fold (i.e., if maintenance is 0.5 mL of vial A [1 : 100 dilution], drop back to 0.5 mL of vial B [1 : 1000 dilution])

Attempts to discontinue immunotherapy can be made after 3 to 5 years if the patient is symptom free. The interval between injections can be lengthened from every 2 weeks to 3 or 4 weeks. If there is no exacerbation of symptoms after 6 months to 1 year, immunotherapy may be discontinued. Approximately one third of patients will return within 2 years to restart their immunotherapy program.

On completion and discontinuance of a program after 5 years of therapy, one third of patients may return to restart immunotherapy because of return of symptoms. Reasons for allergy treatment failures are given in Box 219-4.

Sublingual Immunotherapy

Sublingual immunotherapy (SLIT), first described in 1934 in the United States, is being increasingly recognized by U.S. physicians as an alternative to allergy shots. It is a common practice in European countries, especially in Italy and France. The safety and efficacy of SLIT are well documented in peer reviewed journals in the United States and abroad. SLIT is an evidence-based practice and recommended by the World Health Organization and the Cochrane Review. There has never been a death or serious anaphylactic reaction reported in patients using SLIT. A Joint Task Force of the American Academy of Allergy, Asthma, and Immunology (AAAAI) states, "Despite clear evidence that SLIT is an effective treatment, many questions remain unanswered, including effective dose, treatment schedules, and duration of treatment. SLIT does appear to be associated with few serious side effects" (Cox and colleagues, 2006).

At present, SLIT is an off-label use of immunotherapy. Allergens used for compounding SLIT are the same as those used for subcutaneous administration and are approved by the U.S. Food and Drug Administration (FDA). Low-dose and high-dose treatments have been shown to be effective. Efficacious weekly doses are nearly identical to those used in subcutaneous immunotherapy (SCIT). SLIT is used for 3 to 5 years before discontinuing it, similar to SCIT. The route of administration is the only significant difference.

In addition to its efficacy and safety profile, *advantages of SLIT* include the following:

- Sublingual drops can be given at home daily.
- The cost of preparation of sublingual drops is similar to that of injections.
- The cost of allergen administration decreases because no injection is necessary.
- There is no loss of time or income or inconvenience incurred in driving to and from an office to obtain an allergy injection, wait for the injection, wait after the injection, and return to work.
- There is no loss of time from school or missing after-school activities to get an allergy shot.
- There is no needle fear, as seen in children (and some adults).
- There is no erythema or painful local reaction at the injection site.
- SLIT can be used in children 3 years of age and older.

Studies are ongoing to gain FDA approval for SLIT. When SLIT is approved and covered by insurance, many more patients will be able to benefit from immunotherapy.

The disadvantages of SLIT are few:

- Doses have to be given on a daily basis rather than weekly.
- It may be difficult to get children to hold a sublingual dose in the mouth for 30 seconds or longer.
- The immune response may be somewhat slower than with SCIT.

Labeling and Storage of Extracts

- Each vial of extract should be labeled with the patient's name, chart number, birth date, expiration date, and dilution strength.
- Vials are stored in the refrigerator overnight but may be kept out and readily accessible for daily use.
- Dilutions *should be discarded and remade after* 6 *months* if not used. Glycerin is added to ensure stability.
- 2.5-mL vials are used in sets for escalation of doses (five doses will be used in 5 weeks [0.1, 0.2, 0.3, 0.4, 0.5 mL = 1.5 mL]). The remainder may be used to repeat doses if necessary, or simply discarded.
- Ten dose vials (number of milliliters [usually 5 mL] will vary depending on the maintenance dose) are formulated for maintenance therapy.

Summary

Studies have shown beneficial effects on acute allergic disease as well as long-lasting symptom control after a successful course of immunotherapy. The measurable anti-inflammatory influences of immunotherapy do not occur with antihistamines and steroids, suggesting that immunotherapy should be used earlier and more often in the treatment of allergic rhinitis and asthma.

Educational Guide

Lincoln Diagnostics provides a videotape describing the Multi-Test II.

CPT/Billing Codes

Testing and Immunotherapy

86003 RAST per test
86005 RAST multiallergen disk (screen)
95004 Multiple puncture test, SPT, per test
95024 Intradermal test, per test; vial test (intradermal)

Allergy Injections

95115 Allergy injection, single (injection only)
95117 Allergy injection, multiple (injection only)
95120 Allergy injection, single antigen (plus antigen if provided)
95125 Allergy injection, multiple antigen (plus antigen if provided)
95165 Allergy extract (specify number of doses) (vial of antigen)

Other Services

99002 Mail out charge
99071 Educational supplies
99080 Medical reports

ICD-9-CM Diagnostic Codes

346.20 Allergic headache
372.14 Allergic conjunctivitis
381.04 Allergic otitis media
477.8 Allergic rhinitis
477.9 Allergic sinusitis
493.00 Asthma
558.9 Allergic gastroenteritis
691.8 Eczema dermatitis
708.0 Allergic urticaria/hives
786.2 Chronic cough
995.0 Anaphylaxis
995.1 Angioedema

Suppliers

(See contact information online at www.expertconsult.com.)

Allergen extracts, immunotherapy sets, supplies
Allergy Laboratories
ALK-Abello Laboratory
Antigen Lab, Inc.
Center Laboratories
Greer Laboratories, Inc.

Devices for skin testing (multiple-allergen applicators)
Greer Laboratories, Inc.
Hollister-Stiert Laboratories LLC
Lincoln Diagnostics

Laboratories providing RAST services
Antigen Laboratories
Commonwealth Medical Laboratories
LabCorp
MRT Laboratories
Serolab
SmithKline Beecham Clinical Laboratories

Miles Allergy Products
Hollister-Stier Laboratories LLC

Bibliography

Ahlstedt S, Murray CS: In vitro diagnosis of allergy: How to interpret IgE antibody results in clinical practice. Prim Care Respir J 15:228–236, 2006.

Altman CA, Becker WB, Williams PV (eds): Allergy in Primary Care. Philadelphia, WB Saunders, 2000.

American Academy of Allergy, Asthma, and Immunology: The Allergy Report (Volume I: Overview of Allergic Diseases; Volume II: Diseases of the Atopic Diathesis; Volume III: Conditions That May Have an Allergic Component). St. Louis, Mosby, 2001.

Bierman CW, Pearlman DS, Shapiro GG, Busse WW (eds): Allergy, Asthma, and Immunology from Infancy to Adulthood, 3rd ed. Philadelphia, WB Saunders, 1996.

Bousquet J, van Cauwenberge P, Khaltaev N: Allergic rhinitis and its impact on asthma. In collaboration with the World Health Organization: Executive summary of the workshop report, 7–10 December 1999, Geneva, Switzerland. Allergy 57:841–855, 2002.

Canonica GW, Bousquet J, Casale T, et al: Sub-lingual immunotherapy: World Allergy Organization Position Paper 2009. Allergy 64(suppl 91): 1–59, 2009.

Cox LS, Linnemann DL, Nolte H, et al: Sublingual immunotherapy: A comprehensive review. J Allergy Clin Immunol 117:1021–1035, 2006.

Craig T, Sawyer AM, Fornadley JA: Use of immunotherapy in a primary care office. Am Fam Physician 57:1888–1894, 1998.

Emanuel I: In-vitro testing for allergy diagnosis. Otolaryngol Clin North Am 36:879–893, 2003.

Hedges H, Squillace S: Asthma, Allergic Rhinitis, and Immunotherapy. AAFP Home Study Monograph 235. Kansas City, Mo, American Academy of Family Physicians, 1998.

Joint Task Force on Practice Parameters: Allergen immunotherapy: A practice parameter. American Academy of Allergy, Asthma and Immunology, and American College of Allergy, Asthma and Immunology. Ann Allergy Asthma Immunol 90(1 Suppl 1):1–40, 2003.

Kaliner MA: Current Review of Allergic Diseases. Philadelphia, Current Medicine, 2000.
Kaplan AP (ed): Allergy, 2nd ed. Philadelphia, WB Saunders, 1997.
Kniker WT: Multi-Test skin testing in allergy: A review of published findings. Ann Allergy 71:485–491, 1993.
Krouse JH, Sadrazodi K, Kerswill K: Sensitivity and specificity of prick and intradermal testing in predicting response to nasal provocation with timothy grass antigen. Otolaryngol Head Neck Surg 131:215–219, 2004.
Li JT: Allergy testing. Am Fam Physician 66:621–624, 2002.
Lockey RA, Buckantz S, Bousquet J (eds): Allergens and Allergen Immunotherapy, 3rd ed. New York, Marcel Dekker, 2004.
Middleton E Jr, Reed CE, Ellis EF, et al. (eds): Allergy: Principles and Practice, 5th ed. St. Louis, Mosby, 2003.
Nelson HS, Lahr J, Buchmeier A, McCormick D: Evaluation of devices for skin prick testing. J Allergy Clin Immunol 101:153–156, 1998.
Nelson HS, Oppenheimer J, Buchmeier A, et al: An assessment of the role of intradermal skin testing in the diagnosis of clinically relevant allergy to timothy grass. J Allergy Clin Immunol 97:1193–1201, 1996.
Schwindt CD, Dykewicz MS, Hutcheson GA, et al: Role of intradermal skin tests in the evaluation of clinically relevant respiratory allergy assessed using patient history and nasal challenge. Ann Allergy Asthma Immunol 94:627–633, 2005.
Titus K: Lab-based allergy testing on the march. College of American Pathologists. CAP Today April 2002.
Wilson D, Torres-Lima M, Durham S: Sublingual immunotherapy for allergic rhinitis. Cochrane Database Syst Rev 2003(2):CD002893.

CHAPTER 220

Anaphylaxis

Daniel J. Derksen

Anaphylaxis is an acute and serious allergic reaction in response to antigen exposure in a previously sensitized patient. It can be encountered after administration of intramuscular (IM) antibiotics; vaccines; contrast material, such as intravenous pyelography or computed tomography contrast; local anesthetics; allergy injection in the office setting; or exposure to latex. Patients may also report to the physician's office with a clinical picture of anaphylaxis after being bitten by an insect (Fig. 220-1) or snake or exposed to some other allergen (e.g., pollen, latex, certain food products). The source of the allergic reaction may be unknown to the patient.

Medical procedures frequently require injections or use of foreign materials. The clinician must be prepared to treat the rare but serious complication of anaphylaxis.

Diagnosis

Depending on the severity of reaction, patients may have a variety of symptoms, including swelling, rash, urticaria, pruritus, dyspnea, abdominal pain, vomiting, and decreased blood pressure from baseline (Figs. 220-2 and 220-3). As the anaphylaxis proceeds, respiratory compromise may occur with laryngeal edema, bronchospasm, and hypoxia. The patient may progress into shock as manifested by hypotension, bradycardia, peripheral vasodilation, and mental status changes. If the physician does not take immediate steps to reverse the anaphylactoid reaction in the final stages, vascular collapse and death can occur within minutes.

Vasovagal reactions (e.g., fainting and seizure-like activity) and injection of intravascular anesthetic that can cause lightheadedness and ringing in the ears may be confused with an anaphylactic response.

Equipment

Physicians and practitioners should be prepared to treat anaphylaxis in the office, especially if any injections are given. A collection of medications and equipment, the "crash cart," can be gathered and placed in one area. Alternatively, a fishing tackle box or medical emergency kit can be made. The simplest and best-organized method is to use commercially available Banyan kits (Fig. 220-4). These kits, similar to suitcases, are stocked with various medications. They vary in size, contents, and cost ($800 to $1000). The Banyan Stat Kit 900 is essentially a portable crash cart, lacking only a defibrillator. The specifics on medications and equipment needed are too extensive to detail in this chapter. The Banyan Corporation provides check sheets that can be reviewed regularly to reorder out-of-date stock (see the Suppliers section).

Whether the commercially available kits are used or a do-it-yourself collection is assembled, the entire office staff must know where the kit is stored. One person must be in charge of keeping the medications current. Drugs cannot be borrowed from this kit for other purposes.

The physician in charge of office procedures must be prepared for emergencies. Assembling a crash cart or obtaining a Banyan kit may appear expensive, but it is a good practice to have one available and is an inexpensive form of malpractice coverage in the event of an emergency.

Technique

Patients who exhibit signs and symptoms of anaphylaxis should be treated immediately. In the earliest stages, anxiety, swelling, urticaria, pruritus, and mild dyspnea respond quickly to *epinephrine*. The dose can be *0.3 to 0.5 mL of a 1 : 1000 solution, given subcutaneously every 20 to 30 minutes* as needed (to a maximum of three doses). In the milder reactions, antihistamines such as *diphenhydramine hydrochloride (Benadryl), 25 to 50 mg by the intravenous (IV), IM, or oral (PO) route every 6 hours*, can be given. Some suggest using both histamine type 1 and type receptor antagonists (H_1 and H_2 blockers), such as 50 mg of diphenhydramine and 50 mg of ranitidine, may be more effective than diphenhydramine alone. Systemic *steroids* can be given as a prednisone taper, beginning with 30 to 60 mg the first day and gradually tapering to nothing over a 2-week period.

In truly emergent situations, give 100 mg methylprednisolone (Solu-Medrol) IV. For life-threatening reactions, 5 mL of a *1 : 10,000* solution of epinephrine should be given IV over 10 minutes and repeated every 5 minutes as needed. In addition, consider summoning an ambulance. *Patients on beta blockers* may exhibit more severe anaphylactic symptoms and be refractory to epinephrine. Administration of *glucagon* (1-mg ampule), *atropine* (1 mg IV), or *isoproterenol* (0.1 mg/kg initially) may be necessary to stabilize patients on beta blockers who do not respond to epinephrine.

Physicians should consider basic life support (BLS) and advanced cardiac life support (ACLS) training and certification as appropriate if administering medications or therapies that might cause anaphylactic reactions. If the patient responds rapidly to epinephrine and has no further symptoms, a shorter monitoring period may be possible. For those patients refractory to treatment, or those requiring multiple doses, it may be necessary to be more aggressive, including summoning an ambulance to an emergency department, while following BLS and ACLS protocols until the patient is safely transported.

Patients with anaphylaxis or anaphylactoid reactions must be observed for an appropriate period of time after treatment of a reaction to ensure that there is no recurrence.

NOTE: A quick way to administer epinephrine is to have a preloaded syringe system of epinephrine (e.g., *EpiPen Epinephrine 0.3 mg Auto-Injector* for those weighing more than 30 kg [66 lbs], *EpiPen Jr. 0.15 mg Auto-Injector* for those weighing 15 to 30 kg [33 to 66 lbs], and *Ana-Kit Anaphylaxis Emergency Treatment Kit* 1-mL syringe) available in the office. This system eliminates the delay involved in drawing up epinephrine in a syringe before administration. Appropriate examination and treatment rooms should have one of these injection systems taped to a cabinet door for easy accessibility.

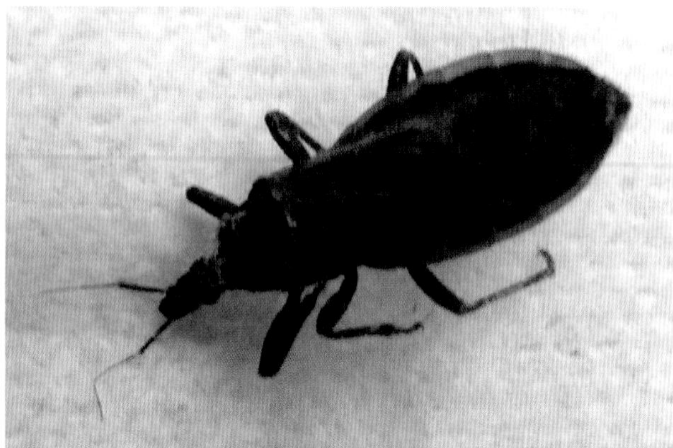

Figure 220-1 Insect bites, such as those caused by kissing bugs (Reduviidae kissing bugs), can cause anaphylactic reactions in a small percentage of the population. The reaction may start as urticaria (hives) at the site of the bite.

Prevention with Previous History

Some patients may require tests that necessitate the use of known allergens. For example, patients may require a computed tomography scan with *contrast material that previously caused urticaria, dyspnea, or other signs of early anaphylaxis.* If an alternative contrast agent cannot be used and the test is critical to the diagnostic work-up, the patient can be counseled about the risks, asked to sign an informed consent form, and premedicated with Benadryl and steroids to minimize the risk of an anaphylactic reaction. This premedication can be done with 50 to 100 mg of Benadryl orally and 100 mg of hydrocortisone or 50 mg of methylprednisolone (Solu-Medrol) intravenously; both the oral and intravenous forms of premedication are given 1 hour before the procedure. The patient should be observed carefully for at least 6 hours after the procedure.

For patients with a *history of allergies to local anesthetics*, a few simple steps need to be followed. Allergies have been reported to ester drugs (e.g., procaine [Novocain]) but not to amide derivatives (e.g., lidocaine [Xylocaine]). If someone is suspected of having an allergy to a local anesthetic, the clinician should use an amide drug from a *single-dose vial*. Single-dose vials do not contain any preservatives (parabens), which can also be the source of allergy. To date, *there have been no reported allergic reactions to amide local anesthetics from single-dose vials*. It is still judicious, however, to observe the reaction to a small wheal of injected solution (0.05 mL) for 10 to 15 minutes before injecting a larger volume.

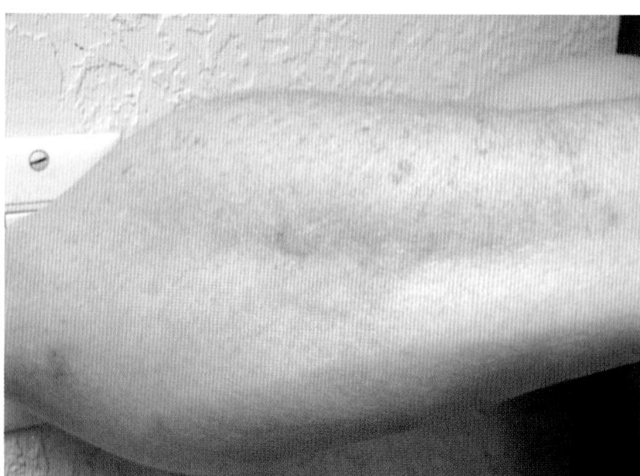

Figure 220-2 Urticaria. Without prompt treatment, urticaria can quickly progress to angioedema.

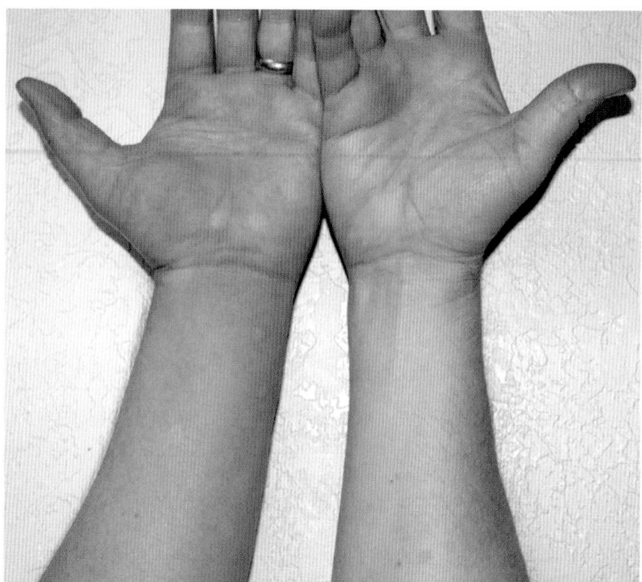

Figure 220-3 Angioedema of the left arm and generalized anaphylaxis.

Precautions

Procedures and medications that could result in anaphylaxis should not be administered unless the office is equipped to deal with this complication. At a minimum, the office should be able to administer subcutaneous epinephrine, supply supplemental oxygen, and provide ventilation to the patient until emergency services can arrive. In general, procedures and medications that carry a high risk of anaphylaxis should be followed by an appropriate observation period after the procedure to watch for signs and symptoms.

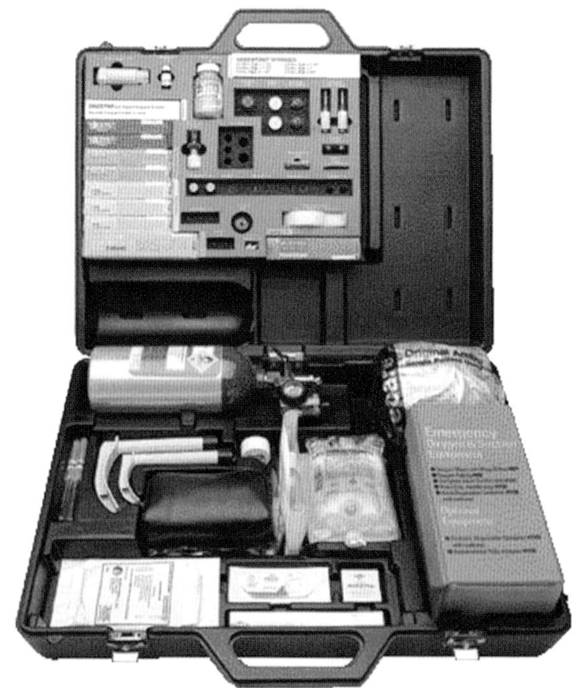

Figure 220-4 Banyan kit. (Courtesy of Banyan International Corporation, Abilene, Tex.)

Postprocedure Patient Education

Sensitized patients should receive detailed patient education. Such patients should be encouraged to wear a medical identification bracelet that identifies the agent that could cause anaphylaxis (e.g., penicillin, bee sting, intravenous pyelography contrast). Some patients with recurrent, severe anaphylactoid reactions should carry a kit with them (containing 1 : 1000 epinephrine that can be injected) so that initial treatment can begin without delay. For example, a beekeeper with a known sensitivity to bee stings and who refuses to explore a new profession should be encouraged to carry a kit. Patients with previous anaphylaxis should be instructed to seek prompt medical attention for the following symptoms:

- Shortness of breath
- Swelling of eyes, legs, or hands
- Dizziness
- Sensation of swelling in the throat
- Raised, red rashes (urticaria)
- Change in mental status

ICD-9-CM Diagnostic Codes

Purpura	287.0
Overdose or wrong substance given or taken	977.9
Following sting(s)	989.5
Anaphylactic shock or reaction (correct substance properly administered)	995.0
Due to food	995.60
Peanuts	995.61
Crustaceans	995.62
Fruits; vegetables	995.63
Nuts (including tree nuts); seeds	995.64
Fish	995.65
Additives	995.66
Milk products	995.67
Eggs	995.68
Specified NEC	995.69
Immunization; serum	999.4
Specified drug (see Table of Drugs and Chemicals)	

Suppliers

(See contact information online at www.expertconsult.com.)

Ana-Kit anaphylaxis emergency treatment kit
Bayer Corporation

Banyan kits
Banyan International Corporation

EpiPen
Dey, LP

BIBLIOGRAPHY

deShazo RD, Kemp SF: Allergic reactions to drugs and biologic agents. JAMA 178:1895–1906, 1997.

Ewan PW: ABC of allergies: Anaphylaxis. BMJ 316:1442–1445, 1998.

Fader DJ, Johnson TM: Medical issues and emergencies in the dermatology office. J Am Acad Dermatol 36:1–16, 1997.

Hash RB: Intravascular radiographic contrast media: Issues for family physicians. J Am Board Fam Pract 12:32–42, 1999.

Joint Task Force on Practice Parameters; American Academy of Allergy, Asthma, and Immunology; American College of Allergy, Asthma, and Immunology; Joint Council of Allergy, Asthma, and Immunology: The diagnosis and management of anaphylaxis: An updated practice parameter. J Allergy Clin Immunol 115(suppl 2):S483–S523, 2005. Full text available at http://www.guideline.gov/summary/summary.aspx?ss=15&doc_id=6887&nbr=4211.

Kemp SF, Lockey RF, Simons FE: Epinephrine: The drug of choice for anaphlaxis. A statement of the World Allergy Organization. Allergy 63:1061–1070, 2008.

Kemp SF, Lockey RF, Wolf BL, Lieberman P: Anaphylaxis: A review of 266 cases. Arch Intern Med 155:1749–1754, 1995.

Lieberman P: Epidemiology of anaphylaxis. Curr Opin Allergy Clin Immunol 8:316–320, 2008.

Lin RY, Curry A, Pesola GR, et al: Improved outcomes in patients with acute allergic syndromes who are treated with combined H_1 and H_2 antagonists. Ann Emerg Med 36:462–468, 2000.

Sampson HA, Munoz-Furlong A, Campbell RL, et al: Second symposium on the definition and management of anaphylaxis: Summary report—Second National Institute of Allergy and Infectious Disease/Food Allergy and Anaphylaxis Network Symposium. Ann Emerg Med 47:373–380, 2006.

Wyatt R: Anaphylaxis: How to recognize, treat, and prevent potentially fatal attacks. Postgrad Med 100:87–99, 1996.

CHAPTER 221

ANTIBIOTIC PROPHYLAXIS

Coral D. Matus • Scott F. Ross

ANTIBIOTIC PROPHYLAXIS FOR INFECTIVE ENDOCARDITIS

The publication of new American Heart Association guidelines for the prevention of infective endocarditis by Wilson and associates (2007) in *Circulation* represents a major change. The American Heart Association originally published guidelines for infective endocarditis prevention in 1955. Before the 2007 update, the last changes were in 1997. Since that time, the efficacy of antimicrobial prophylaxis to prevent infective endocarditis in patients undergoing dental, gastrointestinal, and genitourinary procedures has been questioned by many groups. Those seeking further discussion beyond that presented here are referred to the American Heart Association guideline.

Major changes in the guidelines include the following:

- Emphasizes that most cases of infective endocarditis are caused by random bacteremia related to daily exposures, such as chewing, tooth brushing, flossing, and use of toothpicks.
- Review of the literature shows that prophylaxis prevents a very small number of cases of infective endocarditis.
- The risk of antibiotic-associated adverse events appears to exceed the benefit of prophylactic antibiotic therapy, which seems to be very small.
- Current recommendations are based on consideration of those conditions that are most likely to have an adverse outcome from infective endocarditis, not necessarily those with the highest lifetime risk of acquiring infective endocarditis.
- Although the committee acknowledges that there is no convincing evidence that prophylaxis is effective, prophylaxis is considered reasonable for those with the highest risk of adverse outcomes from infective endocarditis.
- Mitral valve prolapse, which is the most common underlying condition that might predispose to infective endocarditis, is not on the list of recommended conditions for prophylactic antibiotic use because the absolute incidence of infective endocarditis in this population is very low, and poor outcomes are extremely uncommon.

Box 221-1 lists the *conditions that are at highest* risk for poor outcomes with infective endocarditis and should therefore be considered for prophylaxis with antibiotics for some procedures. No other cardiac conditions should be considered for prophylaxis for any dental, gastrointestinal, or genitourinary procedures.

Prior recommendations separated *dental procedures* into those for which prophylaxis was or was not recommended, based on risk of bacteremia and subsequent development of infective endocarditis. The updated recommendations indicate prophylaxis for any dental procedure that might involve manipulation of the gingival tissues or apical region of the teeth or perforation of the oral mucosa, including teeth cleaning, only for those at high risk (see Box 221-1). Box 221-2 lists dental procedures for which antibiotic prophylaxis is *not* recommended for anyone.

For those undergoing incision or biopsy of the *respiratory mucosa*, such as tonsillectomy or adenoidectomy, prophylaxis for infective endocarditis with antibiotics is recommended for those with the cardiac conditions at highest risk for poor outcomes (see Box 221-1). This recommendation is in spite of a lack of conclusive data linking respiratory tract procedures to infective endocarditis.

In contrast to prior American Heart Association guidelines, prophylaxis for infective endocarditis is *not recommended for gastrointestinal or genitourinary procedures*, including diagnostic esophagogastroduodenoscopy or colonoscopy with or without biopsy. The only exception to this guideline is for those patients with cardiac conditions at highest risk for poor outcomes who have an enterococcal urinary tract infection or colonization at the time of a genitourinary procedure. The new guidelines reaffirm that vaginal hysterectomy, vaginal delivery, cesarean section, dilation and curettage, therapeutic abortion, insertion of an intrauterine device, and sterilization procedures do not need prophylactic antibiotics in anyone.

Antibiotic prophylaxis for infective endocarditis for *routine skin procedures* is not recommended. For surgical procedures involving *infected* skin, skin structures, or musculoskeletal tissue, antibiotic choice should be active against staphylococci and beta-hemolytic streptococci but again, only for those patients listed in Box 221-1.

Box 221-1. Cardiac Conditions with High Risk of Adverse Outcome

Prosthetic cardiac valve
Previous infectious endocarditis
Congenital heart disease including only the following:
- Unrepaired cyanotic congenital heart disease
- Palliative shunts and conduits
- Completely repaired congenital heart defect with prosthetic material or device (placed surgically or by catheter) during first 6 months after procedure (until endothelialization of prosthetic material occurs)
- Repaired congenital heart disease with residual defects at site of prosthetic patch or device (because endothelialization may be inhibited)

Cardiac transplant recipients with cardiac valvulopathy

Adapted from Wilson W, Taubert KA, Gewitz M, et al: Prevention of infective endocarditis: Guidelines from the American Heart Association. A guideline from the American Heart Association Rheumatic Fever, Endocarditis, and Kawasaki Disease Committee, Council on Cardiovascular Disease in the Young, and the Council on Clinical Cardiology, Council on Cardiovascular Surgery and Anesthesia, and the Quality of Care and Outcomes Research Interdisciplinary Working Group. Circulation 116:1736–1754, 2007.

Box 221-2. Dental Procedures for Which Antibiotic Prophylaxis Is Not Recommended

Adjustment of orthodontic appliances
Bleeding from trauma to the lips or oral mucosa
Dental radiographs
Placement of orthodontic brackets
Placement of removable prosthodontic or orthodontic appliances
Routine anesthetic injection through noninfected tissue
Shedding of deciduous teeth

Adapted from Wilson W, Taubert KA, Gewitz M, et al: Prevention of infective endocarditis: Guidelines from the American Heart Association. A guideline from the American Heart Association Rheumatic Fever, Endocarditis, and Kawasaki Disease Committee, Council on Cardiovascular Disease in the Young, and the Council on Clinical Cardiology, Council on Cardiovascular Surgery and Anesthesia, and the Quality of Care and Outcomes Research Interdisciplinary Working Group. Circulation 116:1736–1754, 2007.

The new American Heart Association guidelines not only simplify the decision-making process for physicians regarding who should or should not receive antibiotic prophylaxis for infective endocarditis, they shift the emphasis to improved dental care and oral health to decrease routine exposure to bacteremia from oral microflora related to daily activities, which likely cause the vast majority of cases of infective endocarditis.

Figure 221-1 illustrates an approach to appropriate antibiotic selection for those high-risk individuals undergoing a procedure for which prophylaxis for infective endocarditis is indicated. Table 221-1 indicates appropriate doses for adults and children of selected antibiotics used for prophylaxis.

WOUND PROPHYLAXIS

Also see Chapter 222, Prevention and Treatment of Wound Infections.

Although antibiotic prophylaxis can reduce wound infection, the benefits must be weighed against the risks of toxic and allergic reactions, selecting for resistant bacteria, drug interactions, and possibly unnecessarily increasing the costs of health care. Prophylaxis is generally recommended only when prosthetic materials are involved, for patients in whom infection can have serious consequence, and in major surgeries. The 2006 reference from *The Medical Letter* reviews current recommendations for prophylaxis.

Patients with *prosthetic joints* generally do not require antimicrobial prophylaxis even for dental, gastrointestinal (GI), or genitourinary (GU) procedures.

For most elective *dermatologic and plastic surgeries*, antibiotic prophylaxis for wound infection is not routinely indicated unless the procedure is expected to last more than 3 hours or the patient is at high risk for wound infection. Patients at *high risk include those with diabetes mellitus, significant obesity, immunosuppression, vascular insufficiency, malnutrition, chronic steroid use, and lymphedema, as well as older patients*, among others. It is best to give the antibiotic 1 hour before surgery, but there are benefits to administration even up to 4 hours later. There is no benefit to extending prophylactic therapy beyond 24 to 48 hours. For most procedures, cefazolin, which is effective against streptococci and staphylococci, is an effective and narrow-spectrum choice. However, any antibiotic effective against streptococci and staphylococci, such as erythromycin, may be used. For office surgeries in which prophylaxis is desired, also consider cephalexin and drugs effective against methicillin-resistant *Staphylococcus*.

Wound care is an important part of a busy outpatient and office practice. For dirty, traumatic wounds, copious irrigation is the most important means of decreasing the incidence of wound infection. Smaller, low-risk wounds and those in more vascular areas usually require less volume, but in most cases the best approach is to follow the dictum: "The solution to pollution is dilution." Irrigation with

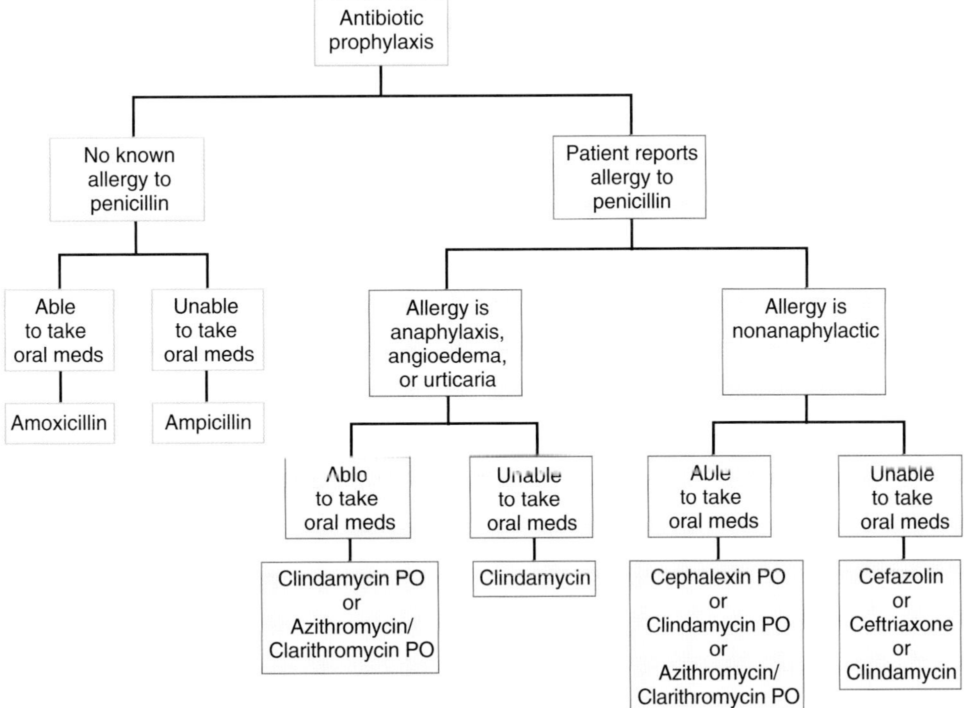

Figure 221-1 Appropriate antibiotic selection for high-risk individuals undergoing a procedure for which prophylaxis for infective endocarditis is indicated. PO, orally.

TABLE 221-1 Antibiotic Doses for Prophylaxis of Infective Endocarditis

Antibiotic	Adult Oral Dose	Pediatric Oral Dose	Adult IV/IM* Dose	Pediatric IV/IM* Dose
Amoxicillin	2 g	50 mg/kg	N/A	N/A
Ampicillin	N/A	N/A	2 g	50 mg/kg
Cefazolin	N/A	N/A	1 g	50 mg/kg
Ceftriaxone	N/A	N/A	1 g	50 mg/kg
Cephalexin	2 g	50 mg/kg	N/A	N/A
Clindamycin	600 mg	20 mg/kg	600 mg	20 mg/kg
Azithromycin or clarithromycin	500 mg	15 mg/kg	N/A	N/A

IM, intramuscular; IV, intravenous; N/A, not applicable.
*Avoid IM doses in patients who are anticoagulated.
Adapted from Wilson W, Taubert KA, Gewitz M, et al: Prevention of infective endocarditis: Guidelines from the American Heart Association. A guideline from the American Heart Association Rheumatic Fever, Endocarditis, and Kawasaki Disease Committee, Council on Cardiovascular Disease in the Young, and the Council on Clinical Cardiology, Council on Cardiovascular Surgery and Anesthesia, and the Quality of Care and Outcomes Research Interdisciplinary Working Group. Circulation 116:1736–1754, 2007.

normal saline is recommended (and warmed saline offers the additional benefit of increased patient comfort over room-temperature solution), but tap water may be an acceptable alternative in nonbite wounds. Povidone–iodine (Betadine) surgical scrub solution, and other antiseptic solutions such as hydrogen peroxide, may be toxic to wound tissue and therefore impede healing. A dilute Betadine solution (1 : 10), however, may be useful for contaminated wounds. Débridement of the wound plays an equally important role in preventing infection because permanently devitalized tissue impairs the wound's ability to resist infection. In situations in which foreign bodies such as particulate matter or bone fragments may be present, exploration with a metal probe and use of radiographs are indicated. Opening the wound further to permit adequate visualization may be necessary in some cases.

The most common bacteria causing wound infections are *Staphylococcus aureus*, group A streptococci, and *Clostridium* species. If significant injury exists, consider cefazolin, if available, 1 to 2 g intravenous (IV) every 8 hours for one to three doses. For less extensive injuries, oral antibiotics that cover these organisms are also acceptable.

For *bite wounds* in which likely pathogens may also include oral anaerobes, such as *Eikenella corrodens* (human) or *Pasteurella multocida* (dog and cat), amoxicillin with clavulanic acid (Augmentin) or ampicillin sulbactam (Unasyn) is recommended. A 7- to 10-day course may be advisable.

A *human bite* wound over the metacarpophalangeal joints in the hand, commonly caused by fist fighting, can be very serious. If it is suspected that the joint capsule has been entered, IV or intramuscular antibiotics may be indicated. Close follow-up is essential.

For other high-risk wounds, such as those obtained in a barnyard, sewer, or meat packing plant, antibiotics are required for 7 to 14 days. Gentamicin and clindamycin IV may be initially needed.

Clean, sterile technique is mandatory in the excision and repair of any wound in the skin. The 11 most common causes of a wound infection may truly be the naso-oral area and the 10 fingers of the operating physician!

Also, see the discussion on wound prophylaxis in Chapter 22, Laceration and Incision Repair. Chapter 145, Intrauterine Device Insertion, discusses the use of antibiotics at the time of device insertion to prevent endomyometritis and pelvic inflammatory disease. Routine use is not recommended.

BIBLIOGRAPHY

American College of Obstetricians and Gynecologists: Antibiotic prophylaxis for gynecologic procedures. ACOG Practice Bulletin no. 104. Washington DC, ACOG, 2009.

Antibacterial prophylaxis for dental, GI, and GU procedures. Med Lett Drugs Ther 47:59–60, 2005.

Antimicrobial prophylaxis for surgery. Treat Guidelines Med Lett 4:83–88, 2006.

Bonow RO, Carabello BA, Chatterjee K, et al: ACC/AHA 2006 guidelines for the management of patients with valvular heart disease. A report of the American College of Cardiology/American Heart Association Task Force on Practice Guidelines. J Am Coll Cardiol 48:e1–e148, 2006.

Dajani AS, Taubert KA, Wilson W, et al: Prevention of bacterial endocarditis: Recommendations by the American Heart Association. JAMA 277:1794–1801, 1997.

Ernst AA, Gershoff L, Miller P, et al: Warmed versus room temperature saline for laceration irrigation: A randomized clinical trial. South Med J 96:436–439, 2003.

Graham L: AHA releases updated guidelines on prevention of infective endocarditis. Am Fam Physician 77:538–545, 2008.

Haas AF: Antibiotics. In Robinson JK, Hanke CW, Sengelmann RD, Siegel DM (eds): Surgery of the Skin: Procedural Dermatology. Philadelphia, Mosby, 2005, pp 137–146.

Hollander JE: Laceration management. Ann Emerg Med 34:356–367, 1999.

Lammers RL: Principles of wound management. In Roberts JR, Hedges JR (eds): Clinical Procedures in Emergency Medicine, 4th ed. Philadelphia, Saunders, 2004, pp 623–654.

Taubert K: Endocarditis prophylaxis: An evolution of change. Am Fam Physician 77:421–422, 2008.

Wilson W, Taubert KA, Gewitz M, et al: Prevention of infective endocarditis: Guidelines from the American Heart Association. A guideline from the American Heart Association Rheumatic Fever, Endocarditis, and Kawasaki Disease Committee, Council on Cardiovascular Disease in the Young, and the Council on Clinical Cardiology, Council on Cardiovascular Surgery and Anesthesia, and the Quality of Care and Outcomes Research Interdisciplinary Working Group. Circulation 116:1736–1754, 2007.

CHAPTER 222

Prevention and Treatment of Wound Infections

Madelyn Pollock • Farin W. Smith

Infection is one of the possible adverse outcomes of many procedures. Generally, infection rates in the controlled environment of an office procedure are low and prophylactic antibiotic use is usually *not* indicated. The rate of infection in traumatic wounds is somewhat higher. Physicians must decide whether to use prophylactic antibiotics in managing surgical or traumatic wounds. Making the right choice involves evaluating the wound, the patient, and the risk–benefit balance. Much of the information available in making that choice is based on opinion, with little being evidence based.

Initial Wound Management

After ensuring that the patient is medically stable, treatment of any wound should begin with hemostasis and a thorough physical examination, with particular attention to motor, sensory, and vascular components. The wound should be anesthetized and copiously irrigated, and any devitalized tissue should be débrided. Use a 30-mL syringe with a large-bore needle (16 to 18 gauge), with a steady, firm force. For large wounds, use at least 500 mL of fluid. A quick method is to hook up a three-way stopcock to a bag of saline. Clean wounds do not need irrigation. However, if there is significant manipulation of a wound (e.g., difficult removal of a deep lesion) or if a cyst has been ruptured during removal, irrigation will help remove small pieces of adipose or cystic contents. In the Cochrane Review "Water for Wound Cleansing" (Fernandez and Griffiths, 2008), tap water is determined to be as safe as sterile water or saline for this irrigation. If the possibility of a retained foreign body exists, a radiograph should be considered (see Chapter 22, Laceration and Incision Repair, for more details). Most wounds can be closed for up to 12 hours from the time of injury. The American College of Emergency Physicians (ACEP) guidelines recommend no more than 8 to 10 hours from injury to closure and less time (6 hours or less is optimal) for wounds of the hands and feet; however, clinical judgment may allow the time in the lowest-risk wounds to extend up to 20 hours. Clean superficial wounds on the head and neck can be safely closed for up to 12 hours or longer in healthy patients. Grossly contaminated wounds and most wounds older than 12 hours should be allowed to heal by secondary intention or undergo delayed closure in 4 to 5 days. Puncture wounds should not be closed. Buried absorbable subcutaneous sutures increase the infection rate in irrigated contaminated wounds and should be avoided. Shaving of wound sites should be avoided if possible because it increases the likelihood of infection.

Patient Factors

Certain patient or wound characteristics are associated with a possible increase in wound infection. When these higher-risk situations apply, there is little evidence to guide the practitioner's decision to use or not use prophylaxis. Conditions to consider are listed in Box 222-1. All of these conditions or characteristics can increase the risk of infection. The use of the antibiotic itself carries the risk of allergic reactions, development of resistant organisms, antibiotic-associated colitis, fungal superinfections, and increased costs to the medical system. A careful assessment of risk and potential benefit should be made before making the choice.

Box 222-1. When to Consider Antibiotic Prophylaxis for Surgical and Traumatic Wounds

Comorbid Conditions

- Diabetes mellitus
- Peripheral vascular disease (if wound on extremity involved)
- Elderly
- Immunocompromised
- History of radiation to site of wound
- Malnutrition (e.g., alcoholic, chemotherapy, chronic debility)
- History of previous wound infection or slow healing
- Chronic steroid use
- Obesity
- Pedal edema with leg wounds
- History of poor healing
- Collagen vascular diseases

Wound Locations and Characteristics

- Increased bacteria—axilla, inguinal fold, mouth, anogenital area
- Over joint spaces where invasion of space possible (finger and toe joints in particular)
- Residual devitalized tissue (should be rare)
- Penetrating injury, particularly if mucous membrane perforation possible
- Stellate wounds
- Wounds deeper than the subcutaneous tissue

Contamination

- Dirty wounds, particularly if contaminated with feces, meat, seawater
- Break in sterile technique
- Deep puncture wounds
- Bites (human and cat; <5% of dog bites result in infection)
- Presence of residual foreign body

WOUND FACTORS

Prophylaxis in Clean Surgical Wounds

The use of prophylactic antimicrobials is *not* indicated in the vast majority of dermatologic procedures. In certain patient types and in some wound locations, antimicrobial prophylaxis may be indicated (see Box 222-1). If an antibiotic is indicated, the most common regimen for adults is a first-generation cephalosporin in a dose of 1 g given orally. Clindamycin 300 mg orally is the alternative for allergic patients. The dose should be given at least 30 minutes but not longer than 1 hour before the incision in clean, scheduled cases. This timing is important. Efficacy decreases with doses given earlier or later.

Topical application of antibiotic ointment has been shown to decrease wound infections better than petrolatum alone. Mupirocin applied after clean procedures was not more effective than commonly available triple-antibiotic ointment in preventing infection and is much more expensive. A generic mupirocin ointment (not cream) has become available and is somewhat less expensive. Because of risk of hypersensitivity, topical neomycin should be avoided if possible. Neomycin is present in most generic triple-antibiotic formulations and in Neosporin; it is not present in Polysporin or Bacitracin. If a patient complains of redness and itching, and is using a neomycin product (or some other topical antibiotic), the clinician should suspect allergy, rather than a resistant organism and infection.

Prophylaxis in Traumatic Wounds

Prophylactic antimicrobials in traumatic wounds are those used within 24 hours of the event and before there is evidence of infection. Their use is not indicated in the vast majority of traumatic wounds in healthy patients. Copious and thorough wound irrigation is the most important intervention to prevent infection. When risks are particularly high, either because of patient factors or wound characteristics, prophylactic antibiotics may be used. First-generation cephalosporins are the drugs of choice. Injuries associated with contamination from saliva, blood, feces, meat, and seawater are more likely to become infected. However, there is no clear indication for antibiotics versus copious irrigation and early treatment for signs of infection (Table 222-1).

Rabies Prophylaxis in Animal Bites

The Cochrane Database (Medeiros and Saconato, 2001) reports that there is good evidence to support routine use of prophylactic antibiotics in wounds from *cat and human* bites because these are likely to get infected even when copiously irrigated (see Table 222-1). Blunt trauma resulting from contact with the human mouth (e.g., a punch to the face) should be treated as a *human bite* if the skin is broken. Dog bites tend to become infected less than 5% of the time. Ampicillin–clavulanate is the recommended antibiotic for prophylaxis in bite wounds. Rabies should always be a consideration when treating patients with animal bites. The animal's location and rabies vaccination status should be assessed and the local public health department should be contacted. Decisions regarding post-exposure rabies prophylaxis are complex and depend on the animal involved, the degree of contact, local epidemiology, and the results of testing, when available. In most states a period of observation is required and rabies prophylaxis can be delayed unless and until the offending animal exhibits clinical signs of infection.

TREATMENT OF WOUND INFECTIONS

Patients should always be educated about the signs and symptoms of wound infection after a procedure and asked to return for early evaluation should the classic signs of redness, swelling, warmth, increased pain, or purulent drainage occur. An early postoperative evaluation of the wound at 48 to 72 hours might be useful in patients at high risk of infection. If infection is detected, extraction of some or all suture material with irrigation and exploration of the wound may be indicated if there is no marked improvement in 24 hours with antibiotics. Devitalized or obviously infected tissue should be débrided. A Gram stain and culture of the wound should guide the choice of antibiotic therapy.

The most common organisms present are staphylococci or streptococci. More often in recent years, methicillin-resistant *Staphylococcus aureus* is the culprit. Therefore, trimethoprim/sulfamethoxazole preparations are now recommended as first-line therapy, replacing cephalexin or other first-generation cephalosporins. It is important to be guided by resistance profiles in your area. Clindamycin is recommended for allergic patients. In the specific setting of bite wounds, ampicillin–clavulanate is recommended as first-line therapy if *not* used as a prophylactic antibiotic. For cat bites, the most common cause of infection is *Pasteurella multocida*, which has a high rate of resistance to dicloxacillin and cephalexin; therefore, these should not be used. As an alternative to systemic antibiotics, topical mupirocin has been shown to perform as well as systemic cephalosporins in treating uncomplicated surgical skin infections. In wounds close to bony structures, osteomyelitis should be considered when the response is not prompt, and consideration given to ciprofloxacin.

TABLE 222-1 Choice of Antibiotic Prophylaxis when Indicated

Setting	Recommendation	Comments
Adult bites (or child >40 kg) with wound from human mouth contact (bite or punch)	Ampicillin–clavulanate 875/125 mg PO every 12 hr for 3–5 days	Even small skin breaks should receive prophylaxis because infection rates are high. Hand wounds are especially worrisome if over joint spaces.
Child bites (>3 mo and <40 kg) with hand wound from human mouth contact (bite or punch)	First dose parenteral: ampicillin–sulbactam 50 mg/kg of ampicillin to max. 3 g; then 45 mg/kg/day divided every 12 hr for 3–5 days	Alternative is clindamycin 5–10 mg/kg IV to max. of 600 mg, then PO clindamycin 10–30 mg/kg/day PO divided every 6–8 hr, *plus* trimethoprim/sulfamethoxazole 8–10 mg/kg/day of trimethoprim divided every 12 hr for 3–5 days.
Dog bites, low risk	No antibiotics in healthy patients	Infection rate <5% if wound well irrigated.
Dog bites, high risk, and cat bites	Same as above for human bite	High-risk dog bites include hand bites, deep punctures.
Wounds sustained in seawater or in wet/dirty environments (e.g., plumber)	Tetracycline	*Vibrio* species often the organism; treat based on culture when possible.
Intraoral wounds, full thickness or "through-and-through" in adults	Penicillin VK 500 mg every 6 hr for 5 days *or* Clindamycin 150–450 mg PO every 6 hr for 5 days	Increased rate of infection if sutures used.
Most surgical wounds, clean		Copious irrigation recommended for most traumatic wounds.
Surgical wounds when risk factors present (see Box 222-1)	First-generation cephalosporin 1 g PO 30–60 min before procedure	If allergic, clindamycin 300 mg PO.

IV, intravenous; PO, oral.

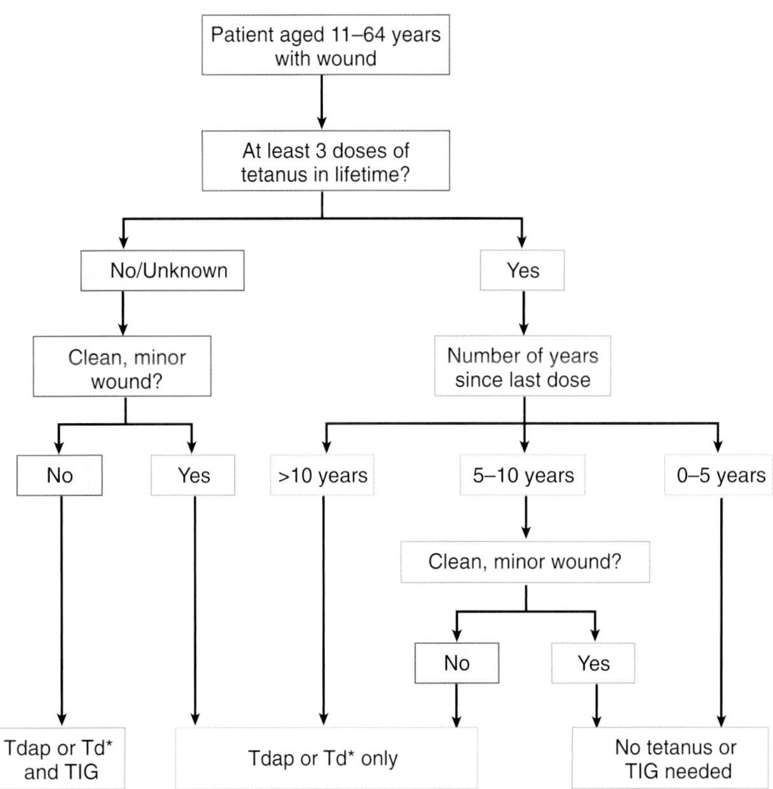

Figure 222-1 Tetanus prophylaxis decision tree. A wound does not qualify as a "clean, minor wound" if it is contaminated with dirt, feces, soil, or saliva; is a puncture wound or avulsion; or is a wound resulting from missiles, crushing, burns, or frostbite. Td, tetanus and diphtheria toxoids vaccine; Tdap, tetanus toxoid, reduced diphtheria toxoid, and acellular pertussis vaccine; TIG, tetanus immunoglobulin; TT, tetanus toxoid, *Tdap is preferred to Td for adults or adolescents who have never received Tdap. Td is preferred to TT for adults/adolescents who received Tdap previously or when Tdap is not available. If TT and TIG are both used, Tetanus Toxoid Adsorbed rather than tetanus toxoid for booster use only (fluid vaccine) should be used. (From Broder KR, Cortese MM, Iskander JK, et al: Preventing tetanus, diphtheria, and pertussis among adolescents: Use of tetanus toxoid, reduced diphtheria toxoid and acellular pertussis vaccines. Recommendations of the Advisory Committee on Immunization Practices [ACIP]. MMWR Recomm Rep 55[RR-3]:1–34, 2006; and Kretsinger K, Broder KR, Cortese MM, et al: Preventing tetanus, diphtheria, and pertussis among adults: Use of tetanus toxoid, reduced diphtheria toxoid and acellular pertussis vaccine. Recommendations of the Advisory Committee on Immunization Practices [ACIP] and recommendation of ACIP, supported by the Healthcare Infection Control Practices Advisory Committee [HICPAC], for use of Tdap among health-care personnel. MMWR Recomm Rep 55[RR-17]:1–33, 2006.)

Seawater Wounds

For the special circumstances of wounds associated with exposure to seawater, and the possibility of infection with *Vibrio* species, tetracycline has been shown to be the drug of choice, but many other choices are effective. Treatment should be based on culture when possible.

Tetanus Prophylaxis

An important, and too often overlooked, aspect of wound management is tetanus prophylaxis. It is easy to overlook in atypical wounds, such as foreign bodies in the eye or superficial burns. All wounds that penetrate the superficial skin should be considered for tetanus prophylaxis based on immunization history and type of wound (Fig. 222-1). The recent release of the tetanus toxoid, reduced diphtheria toxoid, and acellular pertussis (Tdap) vaccines Boostrix and Adacel has changed the Centers for Disease Control and Prevention (CDC) recommendations for use of tetanus in adults and adolescents (Table 222-2). Of note, for individuals with an unknown number or less than three tetanus-containing immunizations before the injury, the CDC recommends use of tetanus immunoglobulin (TIG) for all but "clean, small" wounds. These guidelines do not use age of wound, mechanism of injury, or presence of devitalized tissue to distinguish between wounds that might be an indication for TIG and those that are not.

TABLE 222-2 Guide to Tetanus Prophylaxis in Routine Wound Management among Adults and Adolescents Aged 11 to 64 Years

History of Tetanus Doses	Clean, Minor Wound		All Other Wounds*	
	Tdap or Td[†]	TIG	Tdap or Td[†]	TIG
Unknown or <3	Yes	No	Yes	Yes
≥3	No[‡]	No	No[§]	No

Tdap, tetanus toxoid, reduced diphtheria toxoid, and acellular pertussis vaccine; Td, tetanus and diphtheria toxoids vaccine; TIG, tetanus immunoglobulin; TT, tetanus toxoid.

*Such as, but not limited to, wounds contaminated with dirt, feces, soil, and saliva; puncture wounds; avulsions; and wounds resulting from missiles, crushing, burns, and frostbite.

[†]Tdap is preferred to Td for adults or adolescents who have never received Tdap. Td is preferred to TT for adults or adolescents who received Tdap previously or when Tdap is not available. If TT and TIG are both used, Tetanus Toxoid Adsorbed rather than tetanus toxoid for booster use only (fluid vaccine) should be used.

[‡]Yes, if ≥10 years since the last tetanus toxoid–containing vaccine dose.

[§]Yes, if ≥5 years since the last tetanus toxoid–containing vaccine dose.

From Broder KR, Cortese MM, Iskander JK, et al: Preventing tetanus, diphtheria, and pertussis among adolescents: Use of tetanus toxiod, reduced diphtheria toxoid and acellular pertussis vaccines. Recommendations of the Advisory Committee on Immunization Practices (ACIP). MMWR Recomm Rep 55(RR-3):1–34, 2006; and Kretsinger K, Broder KR, Cortese MM, et al: Preventing tetanus, diphtheria, and pertussis among adults: Use of tetanus toxoid, reduced diphtheria toxoid and acellular pertussis vaccine. Recommendations of the Advisory Committee on Immunization Practices (ACIP) and recommendation of ACIP, supported by the Healthcare Infection Control Practices Advisory Committee (HICPAC), for use of Tdap among health-care personnel. MMWR Recomm Rep 55(RR-17):1–33, 2006.

CPT/Billing Codes

The postoperative management of wound infections usually will be included in the initial charge for the wound management or operative procedure if it occurs within 10 days ("10-day global period"). If the treatment of the infection is complex, the following code can be used:

10180 Incision and drainage of complex postoperative wound infection

Other codes that may be useful in certain situations include the following:

12020 Treatment of superficial wound dehiscence, simple closure
12021 Treatment of superficial wound dehiscence with packing
13160 Secondary closure of surgical wound or dehiscence, extensive or complicated

ICD-9-CM Diagnostic Codes

NOTE: Always include date of injury and measurement of wound.

027.2 Infection by *Pasteurella multocida* including septic infection (cat or dog bite)
958.3 Post-traumatic wound infection, not elsewhere classified
Excludes: infected open wounds—code to complicated open wound of site

998.3 Disruption, dehiscence, or rupture of operation wound
998.5 Postoperative infection
Excludes: infection due to implanted device or postoperative obstetric wound

BIBLIOGRAPHY

Antimicrobial prophylaxis for surgery. Treat Guidelines Med Lett 4:83–88, 2006.

DeBoard RH, Rondeau DF: Principles of basic wound evaluation and management in the emergency department. Emerg Med Clin North Am 25:23–39, 2007.

Fernandez R, Griffiths R: Water for wound cleansing. Cochrane Database Syst Rev 1:CD003861, 2008.

Gilbert DN, Moellering RC, Eliopoulos GM, Sande MA: The Sanford Guide to Antimicrobial Therapy, 37th ed. Sperryville, Va, Antimicrobial Therapy, 2007.

Mcmanus J, Wedmore I, Schwartz RB (eds): Emergency Department Wound Management. Emerg Med Clin North Am 25:1–248, 2007.

Medeiros I, Saconato H: Antibiotic prophylaxis for mammalian bites. Cochrane Database Syst Rev 2:CD001738, 2001.

Mehta PH, Dunn KA, Bradfield JF, Austin PE: Contaminated wounds: Infection rates with subcutaneous sutures. Ann Emerg Med 27:43–48, 1996.

Rupprecht CE, Gibbons RV: Prophylaxis against rabies. N Engl J Med 351:2626–2635, 2004.

Usatine RP, Moy RL, Tobinick EL, Siegel DM (eds): Skin Surgery: A Practical Guide. St. Louis, Mosby, 1998.

CHAPTER 223

Body Fat Analysis

Russell D. White • Darrin Ashbrooks

Body fat analysis is a quantitative method for assessing obesity and lean body mass. Several methods of body fat analysis are listed in Table 223-1, and each has advantages and disadvantages. Body fat analysis is more accurate than using body mass index (BMI) for evaluation.

Traditional methods such as densitometry and skin-fold measurements are based on the two-compartment model (fat and fat-free mass). Densitometry (underwater weighing) is cumbersome and not readily available. Alternative methods include dual energy x-ray absorptiometry (DEXA) and total-body electrical conductivity (TOBEC), which distinguish four compartments (water, protein, fat, and bone). Imaging techniques such as computed tomography (CT) scanning and magnetic resonance imaging (MRI) also can give estimates of subcutaneous and visceral fat. Although some of these methods are impractical and require expensive and bulky instruments, several methods can be performed quickly and easily in the office setting. These include skin-fold measurements, bioelectrical impedance, and infrared interactance.

Indications

- Assessment of conditioning or fitness level
- Assessment of nutritional status
- Obesity
- Risk stratification for disease states (e.g., hypertension, diabetes, coronary artery disease)

Contraindications

- Patient refusal
- For MRI, patients with pacemakers, implantable defibrillators, spinal cord stimulators, or implantable pain pumps
- For bioelectrical impedance, caution in patients with implantable defibrillators or pacemakers

Skin-Fold Measurements

In the outpatient setting the most widely used method is the measurement of skin-fold thickness in various predetermined sites.

Equipment

- Marking pen *(optional)*
- Measuring tape *(optional)*
- Skin-fold calipers (Fig. 223-1)

Technique

1. Although it matters little on which side of the body measurements are taken, by convention, measurements are taken on the right side.
2. Measure the exact same sites for serial comparisons.
3. Be familiar with the skin-fold site to be measured, and pull the skin fold once or twice before the actual measurement.
4. Grasp the skin fold with the index finger and thumb of one hand and pull a fold away from the body with the sides approximately parallel. Asking the patient to contract the underlying muscle will help in grasping only skin and fat.
5. Place the caliper heads approximately 0.5 cm away from the fingers holding the skin fold. Place the caliper heads perpendicular to the skin fold and measure 4 to 5 seconds after releasing the lever arm of the calipers.
6. Maintain constant pressure with the thumb and index finger throughout the measurement.
7. Take a minimum of two measurements 15 seconds apart at each site until consecutive measurements vary by no more than 1 mm, to ensure consistency.
8. Measuring obese subjects may require both hands to pull a skin fold away with parallel sides. In this case, an assistant is needed to place the caliper heads on the skin fold.
9. Take measurements when the skin is dry and when the subject is not overheated (e.g., after exercise). Vasodilation of the skin in these conditions will inflate normal skin-fold size.
10. Proficiency and accuracy require practice.

Measurements at seven common sites are described as follows:

1. *Chest:* Pick up the pectoral skin fold at the anterior axillary line with the long axis directed to the nipple. Place the skin-fold calipers approximately 2 cm anterior to the anterior axillary line (Fig. 223-2).
2. *Subscapular:* Lift a diagonal fold parallel to the medial border of the scapula at a point just below the inferior angle of the scapula (Fig. 223-3).
3. *Triceps:* Pick up a vertical fold on the posterior arm 1 cm above the midway point between the lateral edge of the acromion and

TABLE 223-1 Comparative Analysis of Methods for Body Fat Analysis*

Method	Cost	Difficulty	Accuracy
Skinfold measurements	1	2	3†
Bioelectrical impedance	3	1	3‡
Near-infrared interactance (NIR)	3	1	3‡
Underwater weighing (hydrostatic)	3	4	5
BOD POD (air displacement)	4	2	5
Magnetic resonance imaging	5	3	5
Computerized tomography	4	3	5
Dual-energy x-ray absorptiometry (DEXA)	5	2	5
Total-body electrical conductivity test	5	2	5

*Range: 1 is low; 5 is high.
†Accuracy depends on quality of instrument and skills of the technician.
‡Accuracy diminishes in very lean or very obese subjects.

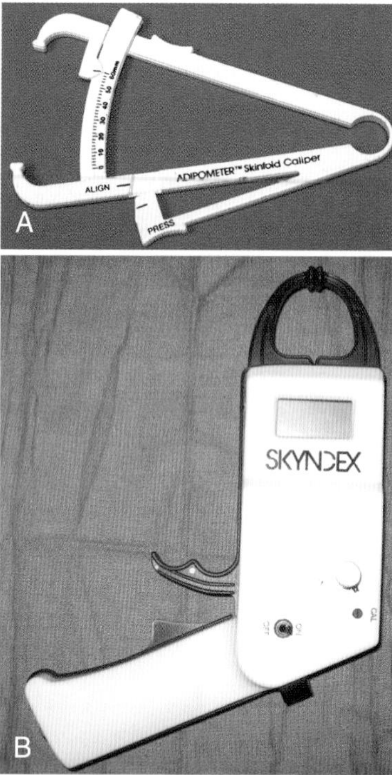

Figure 223-1 **A** and **B,** Skin-fold calipers.

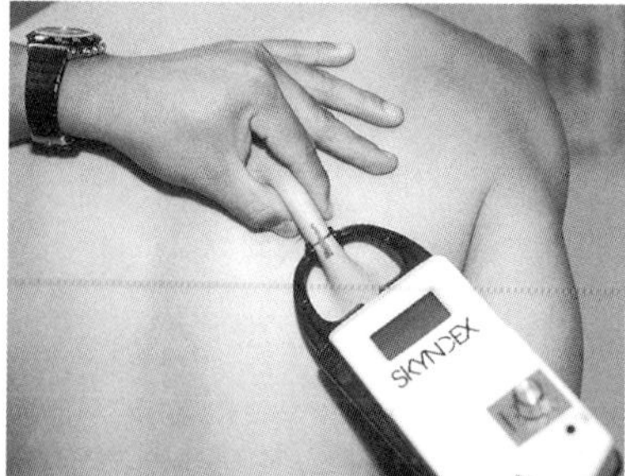

Figure 223-3 Measurement of the subscapular skin fold.

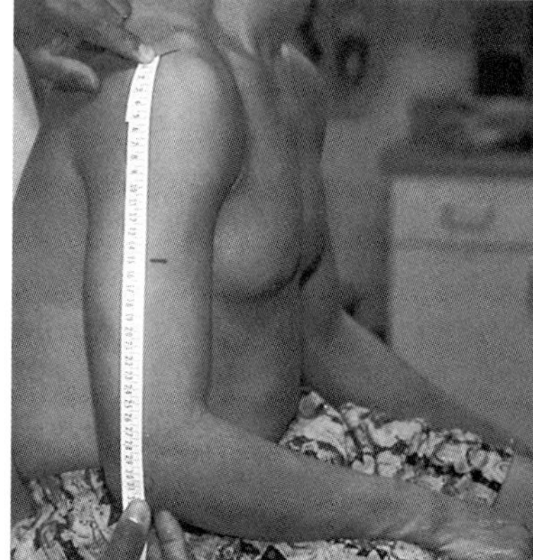

Figure 223-4 Determining the midpoint between the lateral edge of the acromion and the inferior border of the olecranon.

the inferior border of the olecranon. A measuring tape may be helpful in determining the midpoint (Fig. 223-4). Measurements are taken with the arm hanging loosely at the side and with the caliper heads placed precisely at the midpoint (Fig. 223-5).

4. *Abdomen:* Pick up a horizontal fold 3 cm lateral to and 1 cm below the navel (Fig. 223-6).
5. *Suprailiac:* Pick up a diagonal fold along Langer's lines above the iliac crest just posterior to the mid-axillary line, with the calipers placed approximately 1 cm anterior to the grasping fingers. The arm should hang naturally to the side but can be moved slightly to improve access (Fig. 223-7).
6. *Thigh:* Measure a vertical fold midway between the inguinal crease and the superior border of the patella. It may be helpful to use a measuring tape to determine the midpoint of the anterior thigh (Fig. 223-8). Pick up the skin fold 1 cm above this point. The subject should have his or her body weight shifted to the opposite side, with the measured leg in slight knee flexion and the foot flat on the floor (Fig. 223-9).
7. *Medial calf:* Measure a vertical fold at the level of the maximum calf circumference on the medial side of the calf. The measured leg should not bear weight and can be measured with the patient in either the standing or the seated position (Fig. 223-10).

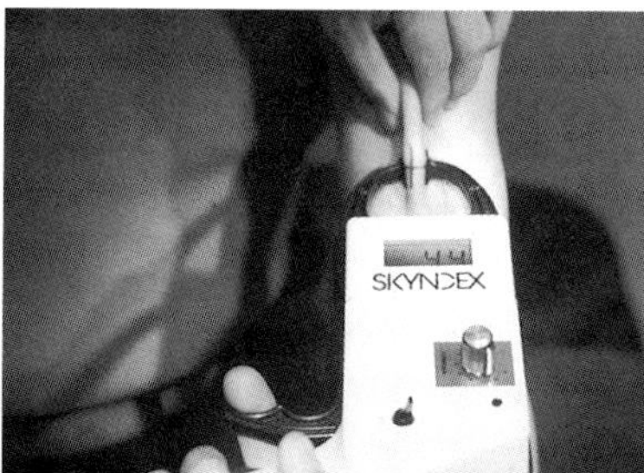

Figure 223-5 Measurement of the triceps skin fold.

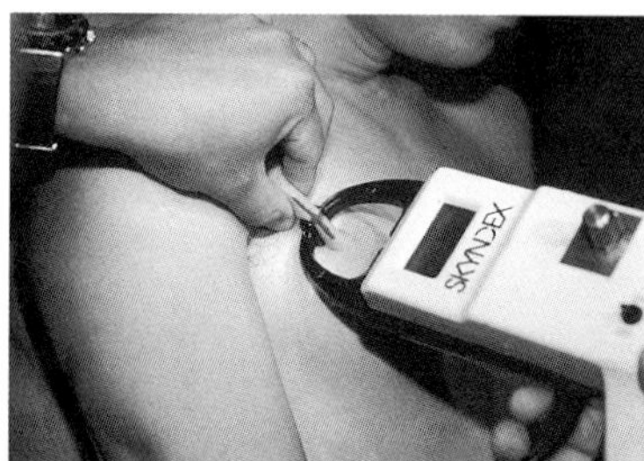

Figure 223-2 Measurement of the chest or pectoral skin fold.

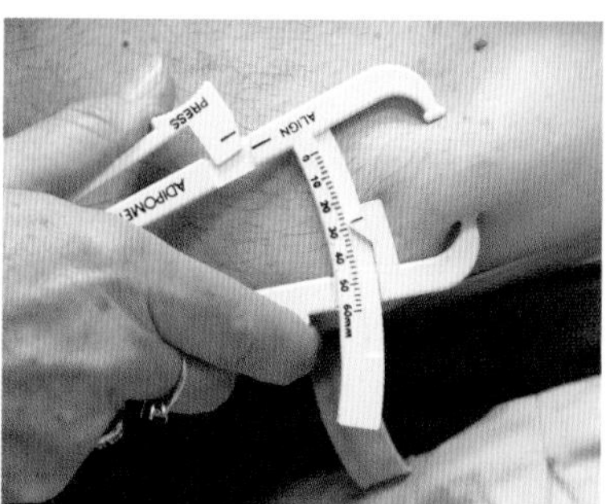

Figure 223-6 Measurement of the abdominal skin fold.

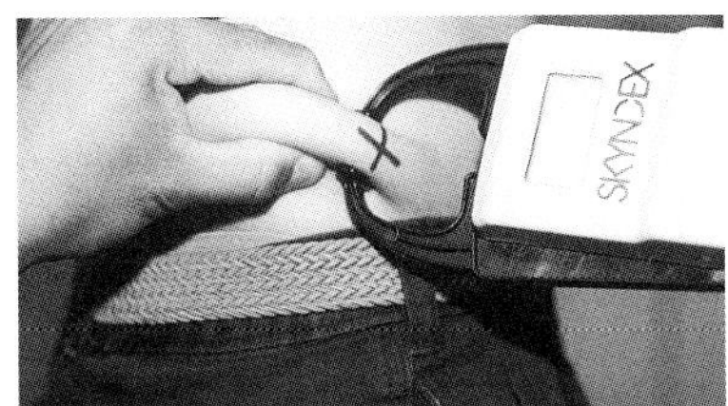

Figure 223-7 Measurement of the suprailiac skin fold.

Calculations

Numerous regression equations with various anthropometric measurements have been used to calculate body fat percentage. However, the following equations by the American Alliance for Health, Physical Education, Recreation, and Dance (AAHPERD), used in children and youth (6 to 17 years of age), and those developed by Jackson and Pollock for adults are among the most widely used and accepted.

- For children and youth, a *two-site* skin-fold test is done, using the triceps and medial calf sites:
  - *Boys 6 to 17 years:* % body fat = (0.735 × Sum of skin folds in mm) + 1.0
  - *Girls 6 to 17 years:* % body fat = (0.610 × Sum of skin folds in mm) + 5.0
- For adults, the *three-site* equations developed by Jackson and Pollock are as follows:
  - *Men:* Body density = 1.1093800 − 0.0008267(x) + 0.0000016$(x)^2$ − 0.0002574(Age)

    where x = sum of chest, abdomen, and thigh skin folds in mm

    % body fat = (495/Body density) − 450

    or

    % body fat = 0.39287(x) − 0.00105$(x)^2$ + 0.15772(Age) − 5.18845

    where x = sum of abdomen, suprailiac, and triceps skin folds in mm
  - *Women:* Body density = 1.0994921 − 0.0009929(x) + 0.0000023$(x)^2$ − 0.0001392(Age)

    where x = sum of triceps, suprailiac, and thigh skin folds in mm

    % body fat = (495/Body density) − 450

    or

    % body fat = 0.41563(x) − 0.00112$(x)^2$ + 0.03661(Age) + 4.03653

    where x = sum of triceps, abdomen, and suprailiac skin folds in mm

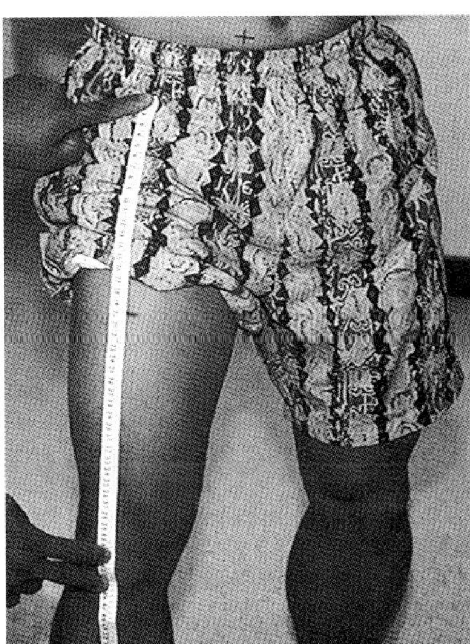

Figure 223-8 Determining the midpoint of the anterior thigh between the inguinal crease and the superior border of the patella.

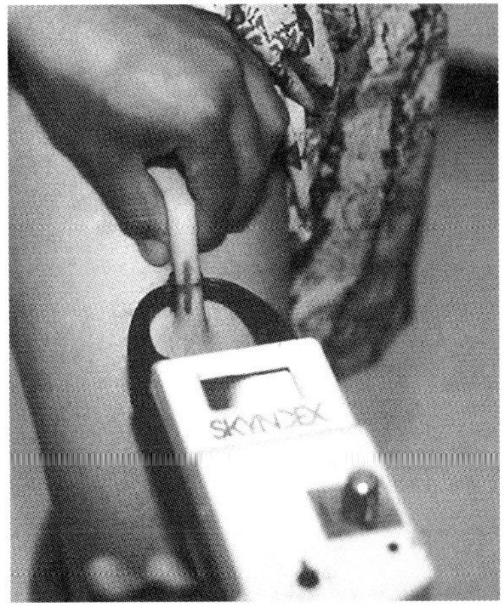

Figure 223-9 Measurement of the thigh skin fold.

Other formulas have been used, such as those developed by Durnin and Womersley. Also, many clinicians have found the nomogram from AAHPERD useful for determining body fat percentage (Fig. 223-11). Table 223-2 shows weight classifications for men and women.

Bioelectrical Impedance

Bioelectrical impedance is based on differences in electrical conductivity through tissue depending on the amount of fat-free mass. A greater percentage of fat-free mass increases electrical conductivity, which decreases impedance. Mass is measured by applying an electrode to one leg and one arm or by standing on the foot plate of a special scale. A variety of formulas have been developed to convert the impedance, which measures body water, into an estimate of body fat.

Equipment

- Bioelectrical impedance measuring device (Fig. 223-12A)
- Foot plate of special scale (Fig. 223-12B)

Technique A

See Figure 223-12C and D.

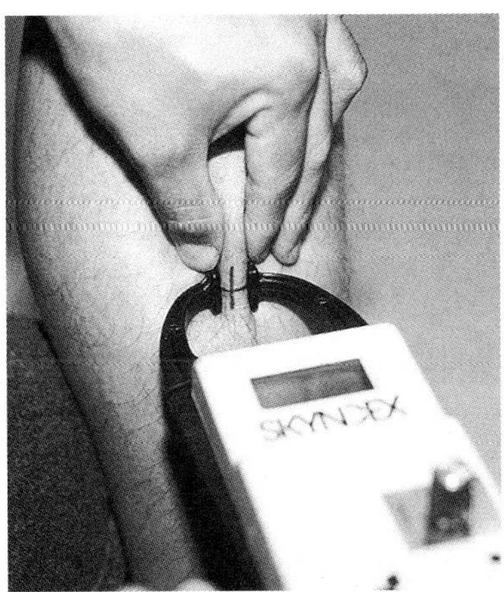

Figure 223-10 Measurement of the medial calf skin fold.

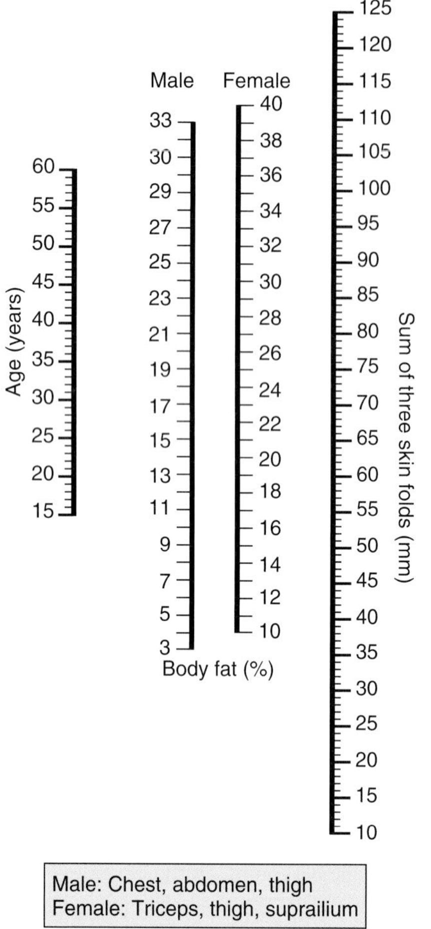

Figure 223-11 Nomogram for estimating body fat percentage by using the sum of three skin folds and age. (From Baun WB, Baun MR, Raven PB: A nomogram for the estimate of percent body fat from generalized equations. Res Q Exerc Sport 52:380–384, 1981.)

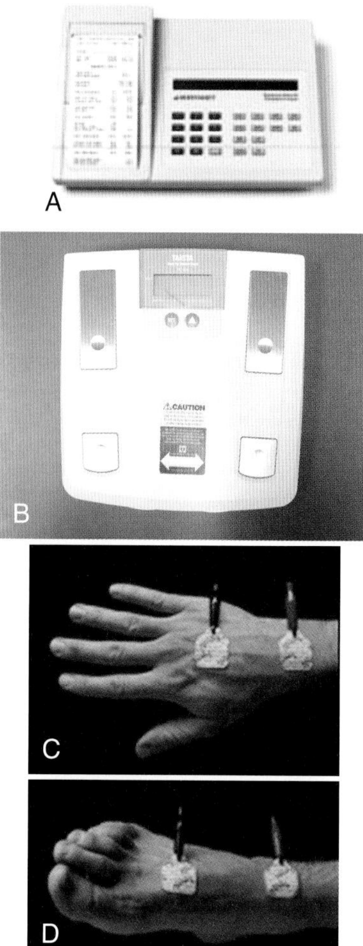

Figure 223-12 **A,** Bioelectrical impedance measuring device. **B,** Foot plate of special scale. **C** and **D,** Electrodes are placed on the right hand and right foot. (Courtesy of Biodynamics Corp., Seattle, Wash.)

1. Subject should
   - Be in a fasting state for at least 4 hours.
   - Void completely before testing.
   - Avoid alcohol ingestion within 4 hours of test.
   - Avoid diuretics within 24 hours of test.
   - Avoid exercising for 12 hours before test.
2. Have the subject lie flat on a table with the limbs not touching the body.
3. Electrodes are placed on the right hand and right foot. A harmless, 50-kHz current at 800 μA is generated and passed through the subject.
4. Electrical conductance (or impedance) is measured and percentage lean body mass is subsequently automatically calculated by the machine.

Technique B

1. Have the subject follow the guidelines given in step 1 of technique A.
2. Have the subject stand in limited clothing on the foot plate of a special scale (see Fig. 223-12B).
3. Electrical conductance (or impedance) is measured and percentage lean body mass is subsequently automatically calculated by the instrument.

Complications

Bioelectrical impedance should not be used in patients with implantable defibrillators or pacemakers.

TABLE 223-2 Weight Classification (General Body Fat Percentage Categories)

Classification	Women (% of Fat)	Men (% of Fat)
Essential fat	10%–13%	1%–3%
Athletes	14%–20%	6%–13%
Fitness	21%–24%	14%–17%
Acceptable	25%–31%	18%–30%
Obese	32+%	31+%

From American Council of Exercise: http://www.acefitness.org/blog/112/what-are-the-guidelines-for-percentage-of-body-fat/

Near-Infrared Interactance

Near-infrared interactance (NIR) is based on the principles of light absorption and reflection and uses near-infrared spectroscopy. The degree of infrared energy absorption is related to the composition of the substance through which the energy is passing and the particular wavelength of the energy. Hence, lean body mass and fat can be distinguished from each other and a percentage calculated.

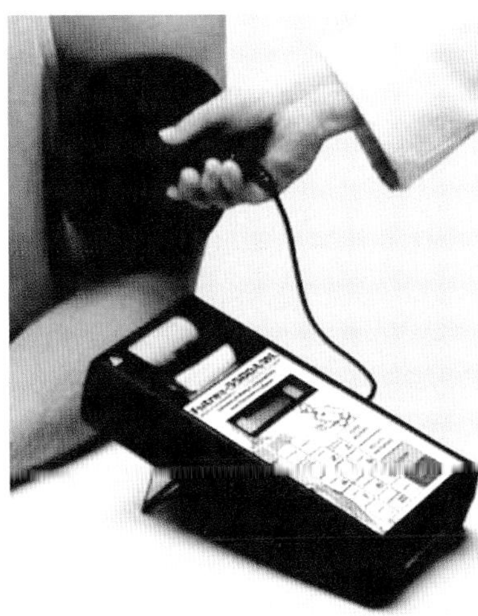

Figure 223-13 Measurement using computerized, near-infrared spectrophotometer with fiberoptic probe. (Courtesy of Futrex, Inc., Gaithersburg, Md.)

Equipment

A computerized, near-infrared spectrophotometer with fiberoptic probe, practical for office use (Fig. 223-13), is necessary.

Technique

The fiberoptic probe commonly is placed over the belly of the biceps muscle to gather the near-infrared data. Specific requirements, including anatomic location for probe placement, may differ depending on the individual spectrophotometer (see Fig. 223-13).

Complications

There are no complications associated with NIR.

Dual-Energy X-Ray Absorptiometry

Densitometry has been the gold standard for determining body fat. However, this technique has now been replaced by dual energy x-ray absorptiometry (DEXA) because of its ease of use.

NOTE: There have been questions regarding DEXA's accuracy in child and adolescent models. Compared with other methods, DEXA overestimated body fatness at lower values. It has been recommended that this method not be used for calibration of field methods in the pediatric population.

DEXA estimates lean mass, body fat, and bone mineral density by using the differential absorption of photon beams of two levels of intensity. DEXA relies on the principle that the intensity of a photon beam is altered by the thickness, density, and chemical composition of an object in its path. In children, the scan takes approximately 10 minutes. The average radiation dose is barely higher than normal background radiation, and well below that of a chest radiograph.

Equipment

A DEXA scanner is required.

Complications

Although it is minimal, there is radiation exposure. DEXA is contraindicated in the first trimester of pregnancy and relatively contraindicated in the second and third trimesters.

Magnetic Resonance Imaging and Computed Tomography Scans

Regional body fat distribution can be determined reliably by either CT or MRI scan. CT uses x-radiation and computer analysis to determine the structure of internal organs. It is possible to obtain an accuracy within less than a 1% margin of error for body fat using a series of scans. With MRI the patient is placed in an electromagnetic field that creates tissue (body) images. Hydrogenated (^{1}H) atoms possess an unpaired proton and exhibit a spin that results in a magnet moment. ^{1}H atoms react to an external magnetic field when radiowaves are pulsed to a patient at a specific frequency and are absorbed by the nuclei. Fatty tissue is high signal on T1-weighted images, while fluid (water) is high signal on T2-weighted images. In addition, fat suppression techniques that cause fat to lose signal or become dark while fluid stays bright or high signal are available. The ratio of whole body fat/nonfat tissue can be determined because the human body is primarily fat and water. MRI takes longer to perform than CT and is considerably more expensive.

Equipment

An MRI or CT scanner is necessary.

Technique

These scans are used mainly for analysis of body fat in a certain region, most commonly the abdomen. There are different methods of CT scanning, but the most common is to take a single cut through the L4-5 position and compute the regional body fat percentage from this cut. This method minimizes the patient's exposure to radiation. Likewise, MRI methods usually consist of scanning a region such as the abdomen and computing data from this region.

Complications

There is moderate radiation exposure with CT scans and they are relatively contraindicated in pregnancy. MRI is contraindicated in patients with pacemakers, implantable defibrillators, and intracranial metal clips (until 8 weeks after CNS surgery) or following documentation of material utilized in the procedure. After implantation, patients are issued a medical card indicating whether MRI is acceptable. Since 1995, new materials have been used for pacers and defibrillators, and many are now acceptable.

BOD POD

BOD POD (Air Displacement) is based on the same principle as underwater weighing and uses computerized sensors to measure how much air is displaced while a person sits for 20 seconds in a capsule. The BOD POD determines body mass and volume and from these two variables computes body density. From this calculation body fat is determined. The equipment is very expensive and limited in availability. Studies have shown that it is comparable with underwater weighing. There has been some variance in outcomes (−3.0% to 1.7%) when air displacement is compared with other methods, such as DEXA scanning. These differences are likely due in part to differences in laboratory equipment, study design, and subject characteristics, and in some cases to failure to follow the manufacturer's recommended protocol.

Equipment

The BOD POD capsule and associated computerized equipment are required.

Technique

1. The subject should avoid eating or exercising for at least 2 hours before testing.

2. The subject removes clothing, jewelry, and eyeglasses and should wear form-fitting clothing (e.g., Spandex or Lycra swimsuit).
3. A swim cap is worn to compress air pockets from the hair.
4. The subject avoids moving, talking, or laughing.
5. During the test, slight pressure changes occur, similar to what is experienced in a moving elevator.

CPT/Billing Codes

6028T DEXA
93701 Bioelectrical impedance
99213 Infrared interactance
99214 Skin-fold measurement

ICD-9-CM Diagnostic Codes

278.00 Obesity (BMI ≥30.0)
278.01 Obesity, morbid (BMI ≥40.0)
278.02 Overweight (BMI = 25.0–29.9)

Acknowledgment

The editors wish to recognize the contributions of Arnold M. Ramirez, MD, to this chapter in the previous edition of this text.

Suppliers

(See contact information online at www.expertconsult.com.)

Bioelectric impedance measuring device (approximate cost: $1500 to $2200)
Biodynamics Corporation
Near-infrared spectrophotometer (approximate cost: $3000 to $4000)
Futrex Inc.
Skin-fold calipers (approximate cost: $250 to $500)
Medco Supply Company
Micro Bio-Medics

Bibliography

Baun WB, Baun MR, Raven PB: A nomogram for the estimate of percent body fat from generalized equations. Res Q Exerc Sport 52:380–384, 1981.

Boneva-Asiova Z, Boyanov MA: Body composition analysis by leg-to-leg bioelectrical impedance and dual-energy x-ray absorptiometry in non-obese and obese individuals. Diabetes Obes Metab 11:1012–1018, 2008.

Brodie DA: Techniques of measurement of body composition: Part I. Sports Med 5:11–40, 1988.

Brodie DA: Techniques of measurement of body composition: Part II. Sports Med 5:74–98, 1988.

Durnin JV, Wormersley J: Body fat assessment from total body density and its estimation from skinfold thickness: Measurements on 481 men and women aged 16–72 years. Br J Nutr 32:77, 1974.

Fields DA, Goran MI, McCrory MA: Body-composition assessment via air-displacement plethysmography in adults and children: A review. Am J Clin Nutr 75:453–467, 2002.

Goodpasture BH: Measuring body fat distribution and content in humans. Curr Opin Clin Nutr Metab Care 5:481–487, 2002.

Helba M, Blinkovitz LA: Pediatric body absorption analysis with dual-energy X-ray absorptiometry. Pediatr Radiol 39:647–656, 2009.

Heymsfield SB, Wang ZM, Baumgartner RN, et al: Human body composition: Advances in models and methods. Annu Rev Nutr 17:527–558, 1997.

Horie LM, Barbosa-Silva MC, Torrinhas RS, et al: New body fat prediction equations for severely obese patients. Clin Nutr 27:350–356, 2008.

Jackson AS, Pollock ML: Practical assessment of body composition: Traditional and new. Phys Sports Med 13:76, 1986.

Kyle UG, Piccoli A, Pichard C: Body composition measurements: Interpretation finally made easy for clinical use. Curr Opin Clin Nutr Metab Care 6:387–393, 2003.

Lazzer S, Bedogni G, Agosti F, et al: Comparison of dual-energy x-ray absorptiometry, air displacement plethysmography and bioelectrical impedance analysis for the assessment of body composition in severely obese Caucasian children and adolescents. Br J Nutr 100:918–924, 2008.

Lee SY, Gallagher D: Assessment methods in human body composition. Curr Opin Clin Nutr Metab Care 11:566–572, 2008.

Lukaski HC: Methods for the assessment of human body composition: Traditional and new. Am J Clin Nutr 46:537–556, 1987.

Mattsson S, Thomas BJ: Development of methods for body composition studies. Phys Med Biol 51:R203–R228, 2006.

Pietrobelli A, Tato L: Body composition measurements: From the past to the future. Acta Paediatr Suppl 94:8–13, 2005.

Reilly JJ, Gerasimidis K, Paparacleous N, et al: Validation of dual-energy x-ray absorptiometry and foot-foot impedance against deuterium dilution measures of fatness in children. Int J Pediatric Obes 5:111–1115, 2010.

Ritz P, Salle A, Audran M: Comparison of different methods to assess body composition of weight loss in obese and diabetic patients. Diabetes Res Clin Pract 77:405–411, 2007.

Van der Kooy K, Seidell JC: Techniques for the measurement of visceral fat: A practical guide. Int J Obes 17:187–196, 1993.

Vescovi JD, Zimmerman SL, Miller WC, et al: Evaluation of the BOD POD for estimating percentage body fat in a heterogeneous group of adult humans. Eur J Appl Physiol 85:326–332, 2001.

Volgyi E, Tylavsky FA, Lyytikainen A, et al: Assessing body composition with DXA and bioimpedance: Effects of obesity, physical activity, and age. Obesity 16:700–705, 2008.

Wagner DR, Heywrd VH: Techniques of body composition assessment: A review of laboratory and field methods. Res Q Exerc Sport 70:135–149, 1999.

Wells JC, Haroun D, Williams JE, et al: Evaluation of DXA against the four-component model of body composition in obese children and adolescents aged 5–21 years. Int J Obes 34:649–655, 2010.

CHAPTER 224

NC-stat Nerve Conduction Testing

Thomas A. Kintanar

The NC-stat System (NeuroMetrix, Inc., Waltham, Mass) is designed to perform standard noninvasive nerve conduction studies. The system has three components that work together to accurately and rapidly evaluate peripheral nerve function. This enables physicians to manage patient care more effectively and efficiently—all within the office or clinic setting. This diagnostic tool has the capability of approximating the results of more invasive electromyographic (EMG) testing, but with the purported advantage of patient comfort without sacrificing diagnostic accuracy. The neural waveform analysis provided is parallel to traditional EMG analysis without the pain conferred by traditional EMG. The unit, connectors, and biosensors are all available from NeuroMetrix.

The NC-stat system is termed an *automated system*, which clearly delineates it from a standard EMG system, which is a manual system. There are some advantages, but also disadvantages, conferred by an automated system. The *advantages* include standardized methods and reference ranges; technical setup can be performed by staff with basic training; the process is rapid and consistent; support systems can aid the clinician with reports to assist in diagnosis; and the procedure is completely automated. The *disadvantages* of this system in deference to traditional needle EMG are that it is limited to nerves for which the system was specifically designed; is less flexible than other systems; is not suitable for children; and may not work well in anatomically challenged patients (e.g., amputees).

Anatomy

Neurons serve as the primary functional unit of the nervous system. The basis of the evaluation is centered around the basic components of a *neuron*. The components consist of a *cell body* that contains a nucleus and axon (nerve fiber) and creates an electrochemical action potential to stimulate communication with other neurons or muscle fibers; a *dendrite* that receives input from other neurons and transmits the signal to the cell body for interpretation; and the *synapse*, which is the connecting point between a neuron and muscle fiber or two neurons.

Peripheral nerves are a collection of thousands of nerve fibers whose cell bodies are located in either the dorsal root ganglia *(sensory neurons)* or the anterior horn *(motor neurons)* of the spinal cord. Nerve fibers can be characterized by the amount of myelin surrounding each axon. Myelin is an insulator that enhances the speed of action potential propagation. Thus, axons can be *thinly myelinated* (A-delta pain fibers), *unmyelinated* (temperature and pin prick), or *thickly myelinated* (motor or sensory fibers that carry vibration, light touch, and proprioception). Thin myelination is considered to be less than 0.5 mm, whereas thick myelination is greater than 1 mm.

Indications

Indications for NC-stat testing include the EMG diagnosis of the following:

- Polyneuropathies: diabetes, chronic inflammatory demyelinating polyneuropathy (toxic, metabolic, drug-induced polyneuropathy), acute demyelinating polyneuropathy (i.e., Guillain-Barré syndrome)
- Upper extremity neuropathies: carpal tunnel syndrome, cubital tunnel syndrome
- Spine and lower extremity disorders: tarsal tunnel syndrome, spinal stenosis, lumbosacral radiculopathy
- Generalized disorders: myopathy, motor neuron disease, disorders of neuromuscular transmission (e.g., myasthenia gravis)

Contraindications

Relative

- Anticoagulation (for the needle examination).
- Check for medication administration (e.g., if patient has myasthenia gravis, medication may alter the validity of the examination).

Absolute

Other than placing a needle through an infected area, there are no absolute contraindications.

Equipment and Supplies

NC-stat Biosensors

A biosensor is a preconfigured standard array of electrodes, eliminating the need for placement of multiple needles in very precise locations; multiple sites can be studied instead (Figs. 224-1 to 224-6). The NC-stat biosensor integrates flexible circuitry and a proprietary electrochemical gel with stimulus and sensing electrodes. An embedded chip monitors skin surface temperature, an important covariant for nerve conduction studies. A unique serial number is also embedded in the chip to conveniently link patients to their test results. Currently, biosensors are available for the median, ulnar, cubital, peroneal, sural, and tibial nerves.

NC-stat Monitor

The NC-stat monitor houses sophisticated proprietary technology for conducting accurate nerve conduction studies. The monitor

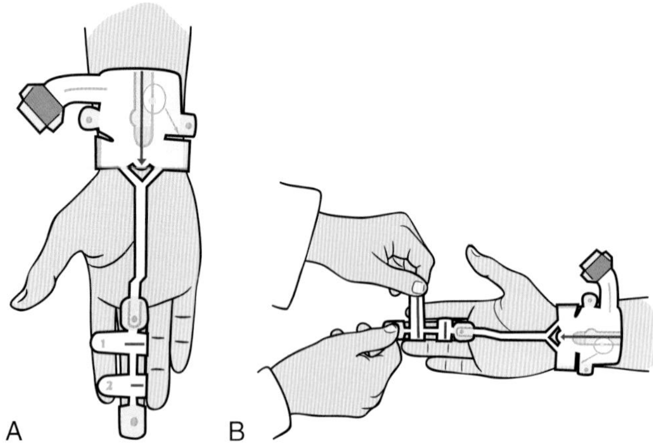

Figure 224-1 **A** and **B,** Median nerve biosensor.

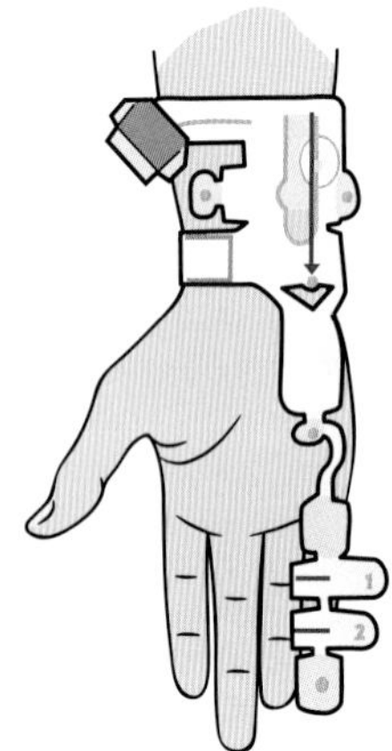

Figure 224-2 Ulnar nerve biosensor.

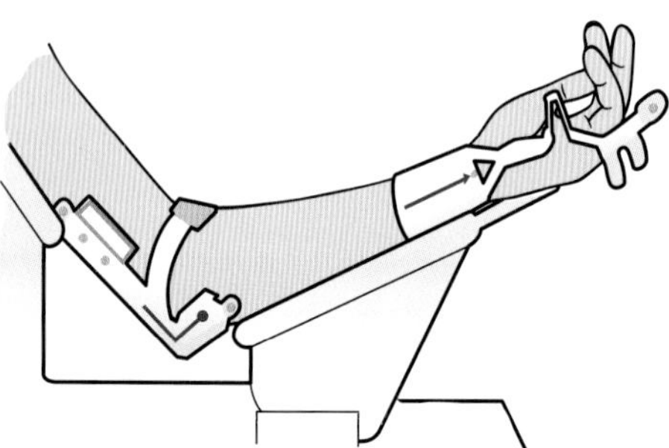

Figure 224-3 Cubital nerve biosensor.

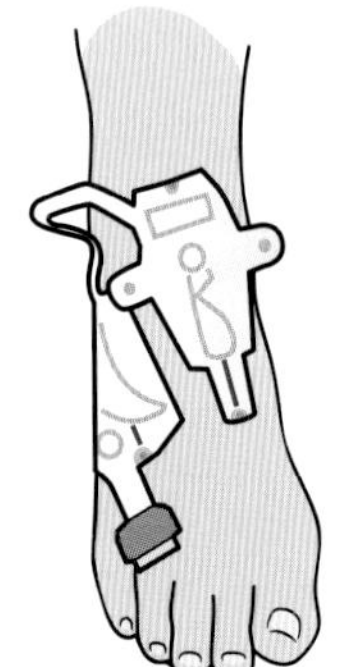

Figure 224-4 Peroneal nerve biosensor.

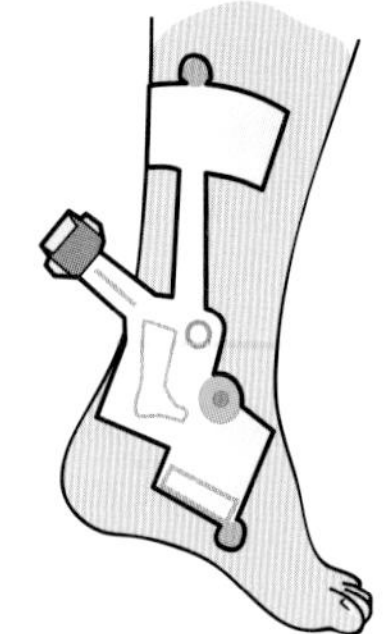

Figure 224-5 Sural nerve biosensor.

measures standard nerve conduction parameters—amplitude, latency, and conduction velocity—of the motor and sensory nerves. The NC-stat can record the smallest signals for early detection of disease.

A nerve conduction study is initiated with the press of a button. The monitor automatically stimulates the nerve, acquires all the response waveforms, and displays response parameters in real time on the liquid crystal display screen. Using advanced signal processing and control algorithms, the monitor determines stimulation intensity, waveform validity, real-time response parameters, noise artifacts, and appropriate NC-stat biosensor contact.

NC-stat Docking Station

This component receives nerve conduction data and waveforms from the monitor and, at the physician's direction, can automatically transmit the data to the On-Call Information System at NeuroMetrix through any available analog telephone line (such as those used by facsimile machines) in minutes. The monitor can also be remotely upgraded by the docking station, thus ensuring that the system is always up to date with the latest software (Fig. 224-7).

On-Call Information System

This component at NeuroMetrix receives data from the docking station and automatically generates a report in real time that is returned to the physician within minutes by facsimile or e-mail. The report includes nerve conduction data originally displayed by the monitor, response waveforms, comparison with reference data, and summary data. Nerve conduction data are archived for sequential testing and trending. Suggested interpretation and diagnostic considerations are provided.

PRECAUTIONS

No general precautions are needed, except to remind the patient not to use lotions or oils, which may alter the quality of the signals evaluated. Alcohol wipes are sufficient to remove oils from contact points.

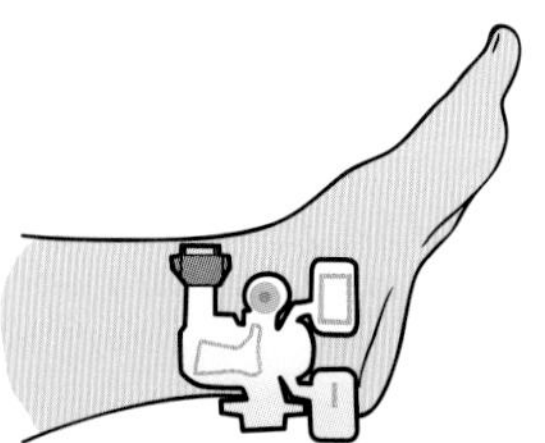

Figure 224-6 Tibial nerve biosensor.

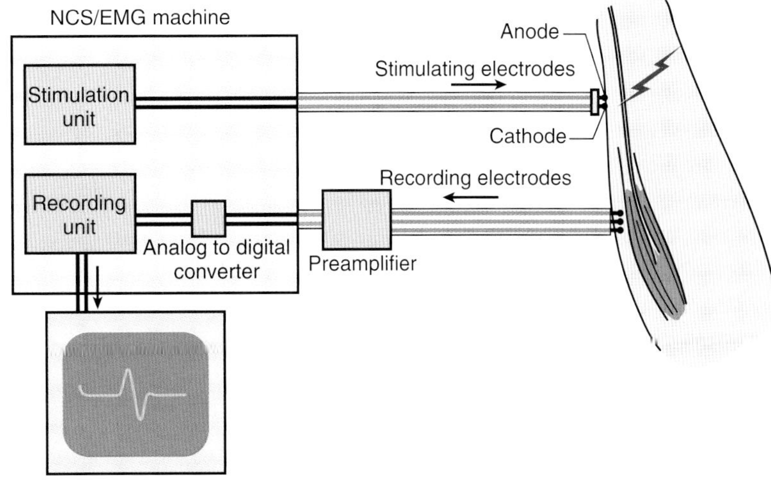

Figure 224-7 The basic unit of operation in obtaining the recorded data.

PREPROCEDURE PATIENT EDUCATION AND FORMS

Patient education forms and insurance/Medicare/Medicaid waiver forms are available online at www.neurometrix.com.

PROCEDURE

The bulk of this procedure is performed by ancillary staff. The biosensors are placed by staff who are trained in the proper technique or by the physician/clinician. Proper placement of the biosensors is essential for accurate interpretation of the submitted data (see Figs. 224-1 to 224-6). Instructions for the accurate placement of the leads and operation of the NC-stat module are found online at www.neurometrix.com. Proficiency in the use of the NC-stat system is easily attained. However, it is important to highlight the basic elements of interpretation of the traditional EMG, which correlate with the NC-stat system interpretation. *The two major evaluative points of EMG or nerve conduction include (1) evaluation of spontaneous muscle activity performed while the muscle is at rest, and (2) evaluation of voluntary activity performed when the patient is requested to contract the muscle.* The oscilloscope findings may demonstrate the muscle electrical potential tracings shown in Figures 224-8 to 224-10.

SAMPLE OPERATIVE REPORT

A sample operative report is available online at www.neurometrix.com. The clinician uses the initial interpretation along with his or her cognitive knowledge of neural wave patterns and the clinical presentation of the patient to agree with or supplement the initial interpretation, or to synthesize another interpretation germane to the patient.

COMPLICATIONS

- For needle EMG: infection, bleeding, pain
- For NC-stat: none apparent except surface allergies to the biosensors

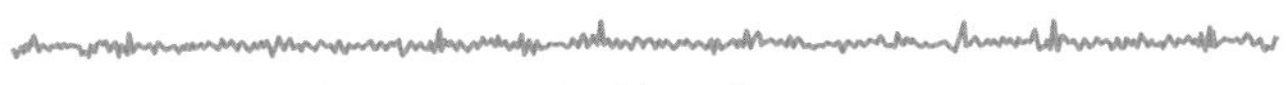

Figure 224-8 Normal wave pattern.

POSTPROCEDURE PATIENT EDUCATION

An appointment should be scheduled to review the results with the patient.

INTERPRETATION OF RESULTS

The basic electrophysiologic assessment of peripheral nerve conduction depends on the response of nerves to electrical stimulation. The study is objective and independent of patient input. It is also quantitative, providing numeric values that can be compared rigorously against reference ranges. The results of a nerve conduction study are reproducible and assess peripheral sensory neurons, motor neurons, and the neuromuscular junction. Nerve conduction studies also document the presence, nature, distribution, and severity of peripheral nerve impairment and have high diagnostic sensitivity and specificity for most types of peripheral nerve disorders.

There are no standard or normative reference ranges used for conduction studies. Each laboratory usually has it own reference range or uses published parameters determined using rigorous clinical study design. Reference values may depend on height, age, and sex. Only reference data that are demographically matched should be used for determining an abnormality. Obviating this detail may lead to poor sensitivity and specificity of resultant data. The basic components of a sensory nerve conduction study starting with baseline at 0 milliseconds are shown in Figure 224-11.

When stimulating the nerve, the stimulus should be strong enough to stimulate all axons in the nerve, which is termed *supramaximal*. A *submaximal* stimulus may lead to inaccurate data being recorded. This potential problem is minimized by the NC-stat technology.

Under the usual needle protocol, a strong, appropriate stimulus is achieved by slowly and gradually increasing the intensity and duration of the stimulus until maximal stimulus is achieved. The NC-stat technology performs this function through its biosensor units. In *motor conduction studies*, the nerve is stimulated at two or more points along its course while the electrical response of one of the muscles supplied is recorded. The muscle response is recorded by surface (biosensors) or subcutaneous needle electrodes, with the

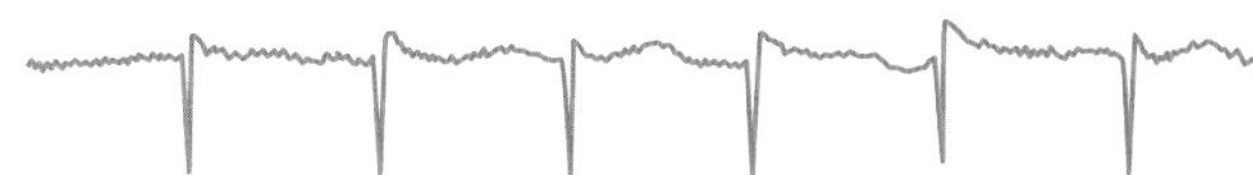

Figure 224-9 Abnormal wave pattern demonstrating positive sharp wave.

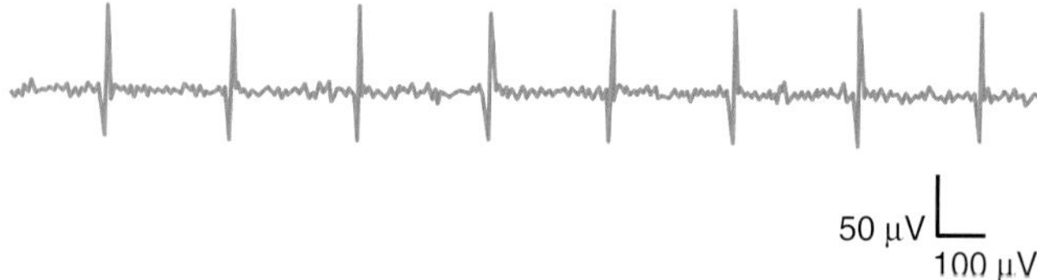

Figure 224-10 Abnormal wave pattern demonstrating fibrillation potential.

active electrode being placed over the end-plate region and the reference electrode over the muscle tendon. The response recorded is called the *compound muscle action potential* (CMAP), or M *wave*, and it represents the sum of the electrical activity of all the activated muscle fibers within the pickup region of the recording electrode. The shape, size, and latency of the response obtained by stimulating the nerve at different sites are measured. The conduction velocity can then be determined by measuring the distance between stimulation sites and the time it takes to measure a response. This measurement can determine the fastest conducting fibers along the intervening segments of the nerve. *The normal range of maximal motor conduction velocity is between 50 and 70 m/sec in the arms, and between 40 and 60 m/sec in the legs.*

Sensory nerve conduction studies involve stimulating a sensory nerve and recording the response at another point along the course of the same nerve. Responses can also be recorded from a purely sensory nerve after stimulation of the parent nerve trunk from which it originates, or vice versa. This response is called the *sensory nerve action potential.*

Nerve Conduction Study Components

The parameters for interpretation of the EMG/NC-stat are (1) the standard sensory nerve conduction study, (2) the standard motor nerve conduction study, and (3) an F-wave study.

Sensory Nerve Conduction Study

The components to evaluate this part of an EMG/NC-stat evaluation are as described earlier. The sensory response is termed the *sensory nerve action potential (SNAP)*.

Standard Motor Nerve Conduction Study

The components to evaluate this part of an EMG/NC-stat include recording, reference, and stimulating electrodes, as noted previously. This portion of the study creates a characteristic waveform. The calculation for motor velocity conduction occurs at proximal and distal sites along the nerve and is called the CMAP (Figs. 224-12 and 224-13).

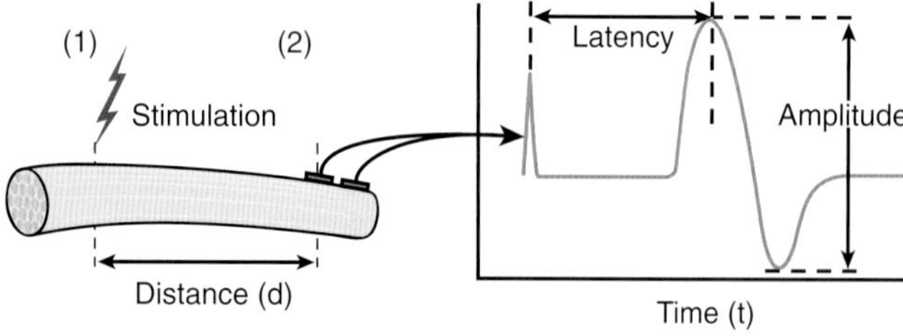

Figure 224-11 The testing sequence. Components of a sensory nerve conduction study are defined as follows: *Latency* is the time it takes the impulse to travel the distance (d) between the stimulator (1) and the detector (2), usually measured in milliseconds. *Conduction velocity* is the speed with which the impulse propagates, calculated as d/t, usually measured in meters per second. *Amplitude* is the height of the response, and can be measured from the baseline to the peak or from peak to peak for sensory responses.

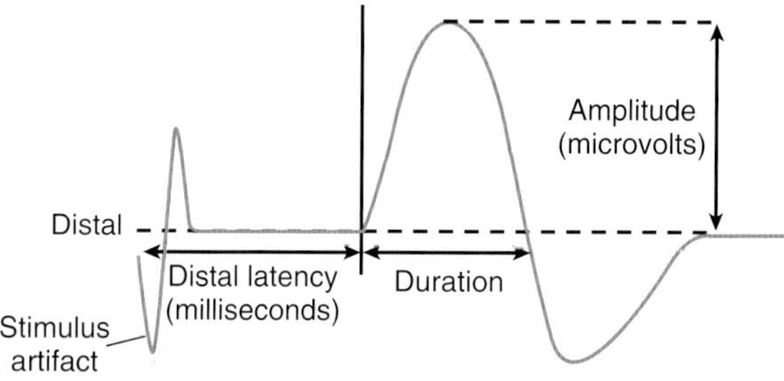

Figure 224-12 Compound motor action potential.

Differentiating CMAP (Motor) and SNAP (Sensory) Responses

Several parameters differentiate CMAP and SNAP. The size of the signal involved is larger with CMAP. The signal is measured in millivolts rather than microvolts for SNAP. Although muscle can amplify the signal in CMAP, noise and other small artifacts can alter the quality of the reading with SNAP. CMAP can detect pathology in nerve and muscle, whereas SNAP can identify nerve changes only. The SNAP response is not affected by radiculopathies, whereas CMAP can be. The sensitivity of amplitude decrement to axonal loss is very high in SNAP because of the proportional relationship of amplitude to the number of axons in this study. This sensitivity is hard to overcome in CMAP because of vigorous muscle fiber reinnervation until advanced axonal loss occurs. As mentioned earlier, CMAP requires stimulation at two locations to evaluate conduction velocity, whereas SNAP requires only one stimulation site.

The F Wave

The F wave provides information on the integrity of the entire nerve, from the root to the muscle. Because its measurement requires evaluating signals from every nerve traversing the entire spine, its latency is considerably longer than the CMAP's. The *minimum latency* is the most frequently reported parameter in most traditional studies. Its limitation lies in its having the lowest sensitivity because a single normal nerve fiber can read as a normal minimum latency. Measurement of these parameters is the function of the biosensor system of NC-stat (Fig. 224-14).

There are several F-wave response parameters that help to generate optimal sensitivity and specificity. These include *minimum F wave*, which is the earliest latency among the ensemble of recorded F waves; *chronodispersion*, which is the time between the earliest and latest responses in the ensemble; and *persistence*, which is the per-

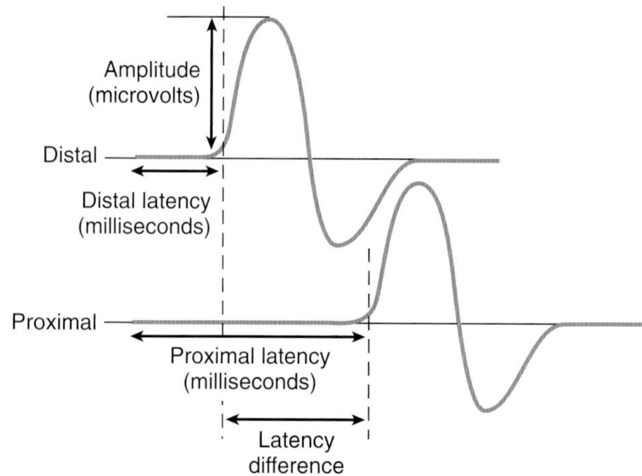

Figure 224-13 Comparison of proximal and distal compound motor action potential responses.

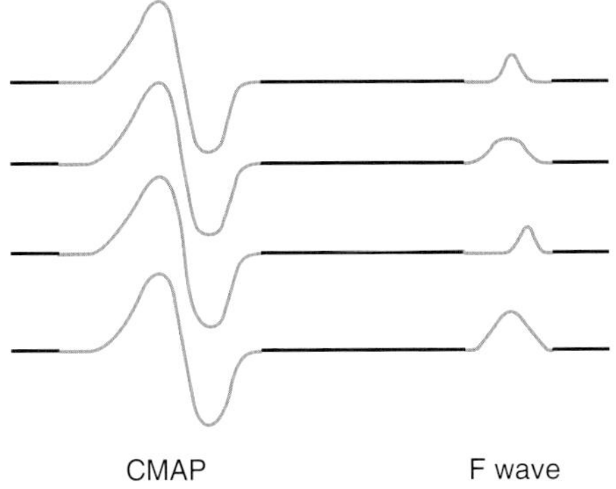

Figure 224-14 Illustration of a compound motor action potential (CMAP) and F wave.

centage of stimuli that lead to a recordable F wave. Other factors that affect interpretation are the age, height, and temperature of the patient as well as appropriate stimulation and placement of electrodes or biosensors. The sum of all of these parameters, collectively, provide data to assist the clinician in coming to a meaningful clinical conclusion. By evaluating the nerve conduction data in their entirety, the clinician can assess how severe a nerve problem happens to be, the duration of the problem, and whether a nerve injury or muscle anomaly is generalized or involves specific nerves and muscles.

It is *highly recommended* that a clinician who wants to perform nerve conduction/EMG studies participate in a dedicated course in EMG waveform interpretation to understand the nuances of EMG interpretation. Suggested courses are found on the NeuroMetrix website. There is, however, a distinct advantage conferred with the NC-stat system in that the real-time automatic reports generated include very detailed waveform analysis and explanations that assist the clinician to correlate clinical findings with the most likely diagnosis without the patient experiencing the pain or discomfort of a needle prick. The report includes not only the waveforms and data but a preliminary diagnostic impression, which the clinician can confirm, refute, or include as additional commentary in the final diagnosis.

Billing and Coding

CPT/Billing Codes

95900 Nerve conduction, amplitude and latency/velocity study, each nerve; motor, without F-wave study

95903 Nerve conduction, amplitude and latency/velocity study, each nerve; motor, with F-wave study

95904 Nerve conduction, amplitude and latency/velocity study, each nerve; sensory

95999 Select Medicare carriers require the use of 95999, unlisted neurologic or neuromuscular code

Coding Multiple Nerves

Units are used to indicate the number of nerves tested when coding nerve conduction studies. When performed with the NC-stat, a motor study with F wave of two separate nerves might be described as two units of 95903. Some payers have specific requirements for modifiers. For example, certain payers will require a specific local modifier to indicate billing for multiple nerves and, if not used, will reimburse for one nerve/unit of the procedure. Although nerve conduction CPT codes are designed to be billed per nerve by definition (no modifier needed), payers might not recognize this and reject this usage on a regular basis. A CMS 2000 OCI edit update suggested that the "-59" modifier be used with CPT code to indicate it is a "distinct procedural service" being performed on a different area of the body (different nerve). It is good practice to regularly cross-reference units billed with reimbursement received.

Coding Components

Nerve conduction studies consist of a professional component, the amount paid for the physician's interpretation of the results of the study and associated overhead, and a technical component (TC), the amount paid for all other services (including technician and equipment costs). The global charge describes both the professional and technical components. Most payers will process and reimburse for the global (entire) procedure when nerve conduction studies are billed without modifiers indicating the separate components (TC or -26 modifier). Note that some payers have specific requirements for modifiers. For example, certain payers require a local modifier to indicate billing for the entire procedure and, if not used, will reimburse for one component of the procedure.

In essence, the real-time interpretation provided by NeuroMetrix is subject to the confirmation of the clinician providing direct service to the patient. Thus, the eligible charges are credited to the primary provider of the service. NeuroMetrix is able to sustain its support to the medical community by the sale of its biosensors. An example of characteristic payment for the procedure is given in Table 224-1.

Nerve Conduction Policy

Medicare and other payers reimburse for medically appropriate nerve conduction studies. Most Medicare carriers have established lists of pertinent ICD-9 codes that indicate medical necessity for nerve conduction studies. Studies submitted with other diagnoses are considered not medically necessary and denied. Additional details for billing nerve conduction studies can be found in Medicare carrier Local Coverage Decisions (LCDs). The LCDs provide detailed conditions of coverage for nerve conduction procedures that address the following: type of procedures covered, number of nerves allowed, patients who are eligible to receive the procedure, requirements for providers of the procedure, the allowed testing frequency, and coding instruction.

Frequency of Testing

Electrodiagnostic testing frequency guidelines have been established according to the American Association of Neuromuscular and Electrodiagnostic Medicine (AANEM). Repeat electrodiagnostic testing should not be necessary in a 12-month period in most cases. Tests refer here to any area tested with a group or region of nerve distribution, not the number of nerves. These guidelines have been incorporated into many Medicare and other payer policies. These limits should not apply if the patient requires evaluation by more than one electrodiagnostic consultant (i.e., a second opinion or an expert opinion at a tertiary care center) in a given year or if the patient requires evaluation for a second diagnosis in a given year. Additional tests may be required or appropriate over and above these guidelines. In such situations, the reason for the repeat test should be included in the body of the report or in the patient's chart. Comparison with the previous test results should be documented.

TABLE 224-1 Sample Reimbursement Rates for Nerve Conduction Studies

CPT Code	Global	-26 Modifier	TC Modifier
95900	$90.88	$32.38	$57.98
95903	$96.63	$46.48	$50.14
95904	$77.30	$26.64	$50.66

TC, technical component.

Reimbursement

Medicare, workers' compensation carriers, and other payers reimburse medical providers for nerve conduction studies. Payment amounts and coverage policies for specific procedures vary by geographic location. To confirm reimbursement rates, consult with your local carrier or fiscal intermediary for specific procedure code reimbursement rates.

Location

Nerve conduction studies are reimbursed in hospital and office settings. The Medicare Diagnostic Related Group (DRG) covers the technical component of Medicare services for inpatients. When submitting bills to Medicare, the physician may submit and be reimbursed for only the professional component of these studies. Although the physician cannot bill the carrier for the technical component under the DRG system, he or she may either bill the institution or establish a separate contract to receive the appropriate reimbursement. This rule also applies to non-Medicare payers using DRG payment methods.

Technical Specifications

The NC-stat nerve conduction system meets or exceeds all the technical requirements for standard electrodiagnostic equipment. A detailed chart demonstrating each specification is available from NeuroMetrix on request.

Caveats

- Because this technology is relatively new, a number of insurers consider this automated methodology "experimental" and will not pay for the procedures performed. New CPT codes that should specifically reflect this procedure with commensurate charges are scheduled to be released in 2010.
- The biosensors are expensive, but their accuracy is impressive. Always make sure that lead placement is accurate and contact points are clean. If there seems to be a malfunctioning unit, always recheck electrical contact points to ensure power is adequate.
- In the unlikely event reports are not timely, one can usually contact NeuroMetrix for support.
- Do your due diligence to evaluate the payment policy in your practice arena. One size does not fit all. Take advantage of some of the patient handouts supplied by NeuroMetrix. These remind the patient this is *not* a needle procedure.

SUPPLIER

(See contact information online at www.expertconsult.com.)

NeuroMetrix, Inc.

BIBLIOGRAPHY

Gozani SN, Fisher MA, Kong X, et al: Electrodiagnostic automation: Principles and practice. Phys Med Rehabil Clin N Am 16:1015–1032, 2005.

Jabre JF, Salzsieder BT, Gnemi KE: Criterion validity of the NC-stat automated nerve conduction measurement instrument. Physiol Meas 28:95–104, 2007.

Kong X, Gozani SN, Hayes MT, Weinberg DH: NC-stat sensory nerve conduction studies in the median and ulnar nerves of symptomatic patients. Clin Neurophysiol 117:405–413, 2006.

Megerian JT, Kong X, Gozani SG: Utility of nerve conduction studies for carpal tunnel syndrome by family medicine, primary care, and internal medicine physicians. J Am Board Fam Med 20:60–64, 2007.

Morse J: Technology assessment: NC-stat System, NeuroMetrix, Inc. Olympia, Wash, Office of the Medical Director, Washington State Department of Labor and Industries, June 8, 2006.

Emergency Department, Hospitalist, and Office Ultrasonography (Clinical Ultrasonography)

Grant C. Fowler

For many reasons—including improvements in image quality, portability, and affordability, high-quality research about applications, and more widely available educational programs—real-time sonography has become a valuable tool for the primary care clinician. In many settings, patient care quality has been improved and lives have been saved because of immediately available information from real-time ultrasonographic scanning. Studies continue to demonstrate the safety and efficacy of sonography in the hands of nonradiologists, as well as to clarify its indications. As a result, the American College of Emergency Physicians (ACEP) has recognized the need for emergency ultrasonography imaging on a 24-hour basis and states that emergency physicians should perform such examinations. Such policy has been endorsed by the Society for Academic Emergency Medicine (SAEM), and since SAEM began encouraging residency programs to offer ultrasonography training, nearly all now provide it. ACEP considers focused, bedside ultrasonographic imaging to be within the scope of practicing emergency clinicians in the following areas: cardiac, pelvis, aorta, biliary, renal, trauma, venous thrombosis, and ultrasonography-guided procedures (an excellent reference is the ACEP Emergency Ultrasound Imaging Criteria Compendium, 2006). The American College of Surgeons now also offers courses and a CD-ROM on ultrasonography.

Although many of the applications in emergency medicine are useful for hospitalists and in the offices of primary care clinicians, ultrasonography in those settings has not been studied as extensively. However, when the principles of sonography are understood and the equipment is available, certain diagnostic and procedural applications can be learned during or after residency. Ultrasonography may improve not only the accuracy of making diagnoses and the performance of procedures, but how rapidly these are made and performed.

Because ultrasonography enhances physical examination skills, its use is also anticipated to enhance periodic health evaluations (PHEs). In so doing, cancer, carotid atherosclerosis, urinary retention, hydronephrosis, abdominal aortic aneurysms (AAAs), and other disease processes might be diagnosed earlier. One study (Siepel and colleagues, 2000) of ultrasonography-enhanced PHE in the elderly found a new diagnosis in 31% of patients who had already undergone a conventional physical examination. Seven percent of the patients required prompt treatment for a serious, unsuspected condition. Musculoskeletal ultrasonography has also evolved as an adjunct to the history and physical examination and to guide procedures for primary care clinicians providing musculoskeletal care, especially those skilled in sports medicine (see Chapter 185, Musculoskeletal Ultrasonography). Both screening for atherosclerosis with ultrasonography and musculoskeletal ultrasonography have been endorsed by the American Institute for Ultrasound in Medicine (AIUM), and guidelines and videos have been developed. Ultrasonography has also been used by primary care clinicians to direct prostate biopsy (see Chapter 121, Prostate and Seminal Vesicle Ultrasonography and Biopsy).

Primary care clinicians already performing obstetric ultrasonography (see Chapter 172, Obstetric Ultrasonography) are often comfortable with the principles of sonography and capable of extending its use beyond obstetrics with little additional training. Primary care clinicians who use sonography when covering emergency departments or urgent care centers often extend its use into their hospital and office practices. Even primary care clinicians not comfortable using ultrasonography for diagnostic purposes may find it useful for procedures (e.g., insertion of central lines; guiding aspiration of bladder, breast or thyroid cysts, abscesses, or pericardial, pleural, peritoneal, or joint fluid), especially invasive procedures. Such use may help identify relative anatomy and pathology to minimize the number of attempts necessary when performing a procedure, thereby increasing patient safety. Having ultrasonography available may also increase clinician confidence when performing procedures. Gastroenterologists and nephrologists now use ultrasonography to direct liver and renal biopsies. The subspecialty of interventional radiology has grown very rapidly, and clinicians in this field frequently use ultrasonography to guide procedures formerly performed "blindly" by primary care clinicians. Surely, clinicians who have been performing these procedures "blindly" in the past should be able to enhance their skills with ultrasonography.

When first getting started, it is important to ask what clinical question(s) can be answered while scanning. Perhaps the answer in the emergency department can be provided with a *limited* scan rather than a *standard* or complete ultrasonographic survey. Sonographers and radiologists are trained for formal, complete ultrasonographic surveys. Applications for sonography in the emergency department are also defined as either *primary*, which have been evaluated and defined in the medical literature, or *extended*, which generally require more training or experience. Primary scans are often brief and goal oriented to answer specific questions raised by the clinical presentation. If a definitive clinical answer cannot be obtained with portable scanning, a formal study can then be ordered or consultation obtained.

Clinical ultrasonography is used as a component of the overall clinical evaluation of the patient. It is used in conjunction with historical, physical, and laboratory information and provides additional data for decision making and guiding procedures. It usually answers specific questions about a particular patient's condition or anatomy. Although other tests may provide more information in more detail, have greater anatomic specificity, or identify alternative diagnoses, clinical ultrasonography is noninvasive and rapidly deployed, and does not require the patient to visit another unit or facility. Furthermore, use of clinical ultrasonography avoids or minimizes the delays, costs, use of specialized technical personnel, and administration of contrast agents or exposure to biohazards (e.g., radiation). These advantages make clinical ultrasonography a valuable addition to available diagnostic and procedural resources. It is particular useful in time-sensitive or emergent situations.

Principles of Ultrasonography

Similar to sonar used by submarines and fishing boats, ultrasonographic technology analyzes echoes from pulsed sound waves to generate images. Real-time sonography provides continuously updated or "live" images while the patient is being scanned. Live images often allow the clinician to immediately exclude certain diagnoses and to redirect clinical suspicions elsewhere. Live images may also improve the clinician's understanding of a particular patient's underlying anatomy. In addition, the best images are often obtained when scanning "live" because the clinician can immediately reposition the patient, if needed.

One general principle of ultrasonography is that the higher the frequency, the sharper the resolution of the image. However, the higher the frequency, the less depth of penetration there is into tissue (Fig. 225-1). With these principles in mind, the clinician chooses the probe, or *transducer*, that best matches his or her needs. Although recently developed probes can actually change between frequencies, most probes are dedicated to one frequency range—a *high-* (7.5 to 10 megahertz [MHz]), an *intermediate-* (5 to 7.5 MHz), or a *low-* (3.5 to 5 MHz) frequency probe. High-frequency probes are useful for scanning tissue close to the skin surface, such as breast or thyroid lumps, testicles, arteries, veins, or foreign bodies in the skin. Low-frequency probes are useful for scanning deep internal structures such as those of the abdomen, pelvis, and chest. (Even lower-frequency probes [2 to 2.25 MHz] are being used to scan obese patients.) Intermediate-frequency probes may be useful for scanning children. *Linear* probes are elongated and use parallel sound waves to produce a square or rectangular image (Fig. 225-2A). They require more surface contact, basically throughout the length of the probe, than *sector* probes. With sector probes, sound waves originate from one point source and are directed through a field to produce a pie-shaped image (Fig. 225-2B). *Curvilinear* probes are basically linear probes with a curved surface, also requiring less surface contact (Fig. 225-2C) and making it easier to scan areas where it is difficult to maintain good surface contact with a linear probe (e.g., between ribs).

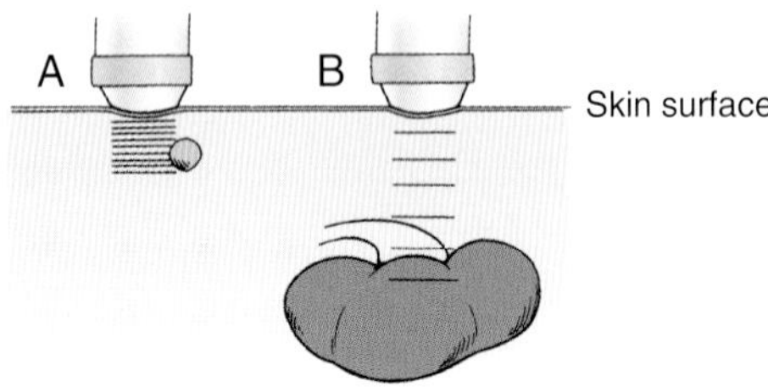

Figure 225-1 **A,** High-frequency probe (7.5 to 10 MHz) provides higher-resolution images but cannot be used to scan deep organs. This probe is especially useful for organs or structures near the skin surface such as breast or thyroid tissue, veins, or arteries. **B,** Low-frequency probe (3.5 to 5 MHz) for deeper tissue such as abdominal or pelvic organs.

Another principle of ultrasonography is that sound waves travel more readily and rapidly through solids and liquids than through air. Consequently, organs that are predominantly air filled (e.g., lungs, bowel), or any organs posterior to or surrounded by air-filled organs, may be difficult to image with sonography. In contrast, the liver, spleen, heart, bladder, and uterus (during pregnancy) are predominantly fluid filled and therefore provide their own excellent "windows" for imaging. They also provide windows to view surrounding organs or structures. A "window" is an area or organ near the body surface through which sound waves can easily be transmitted to obtain images. For tissue very close to the skin surface, such as thyroid, breast, and femoral veins, there is little tissue to be used for a window. In other words, there is little fluid between the probe and the organ. As a result, high-frequency probes often have their own built-in windows. Because ultrasound is best transmitted through solids and liquids, ample acoustic gel must also be applied between the body surface and any probe to form a good interface. Nevertheless, even with ample gel applied and excellent equipment, there will sometimes be difficulty obtaining images of certain organs for various reasons (e.g., inadequate window, organ obscured by bowel gas, body habitus, local trauma). In that situation, the reasons for being unable to scan an area or an organ should be documented and other imaging modalities considered.

NOTE: An after-market standoff or water path can usually be purchased and attached to a low-frequency probe so that, in addition to scanning deep organs, the same probe can be used for scanning near the body surface. If the clinician is not concerned about seeing bubbles, a bag of intravenous (IV) fluid can be used in the same manner, even if it is sometimes awkward to scan through it. Although a higher-frequency probe would certainly produce better images in this situation, for beginners, using a standoff with a low-frequency probe can save the cost of a high-frequency probe. This allows the primary care clinician to become very proficient with his or her "workhorse" or primary probe, usually a low-frequency 3.5-MHz probe.

Fluid such as amniotic fluid, urine, pus, or blood in the aorta or inferior vena cava appears dark by convention on an ultrasonographic image and is *sonolucent* (sound waves pass through it). Predominantly fluid-filled organs such as the liver, spleen, or renal cortex appear dark or gray on the screen with intermittent bright echoes within their structure. Solid objects such as polyps, bones, or gallstones are white or *echogenic* (i.e., produce a lot of echoes). If a solid object (calcified or hardened such as a gallstone) is larger than 3 mm, it should cast a well-defined shadow. This type of well-demarcated or "sharp" shadow can be differentiated from shadows cast by air, such as air in the gut. Artifact and shadows produced by air are often diffuse or "soft" and change considerably with changes in the placement, angle, or pressure of the probe or with peristalsis.

From a sonographic perspective, a cyst is any fluid-filled structure with smooth walls. Examples include cysts in the ovary, liver, or kidney, but also a full gallbladder, uterus during pregnancy, or full urinary bladder. In some ways, the inferior vena cava and abdominal aorta demonstrate cystic properties, such as the following:

- Cysts have smooth walls.
- No echoes or shadows are normally found in simple cysts.
- There is enhanced visualization of structures or tissue posterior to cysts.
- Cysts demonstrate a penumbra effect.

Because of the third property, cystic structures often serve as excellent windows for tissue being scanned behind or around them. The fourth property manifests as "semishadows," or what appear to

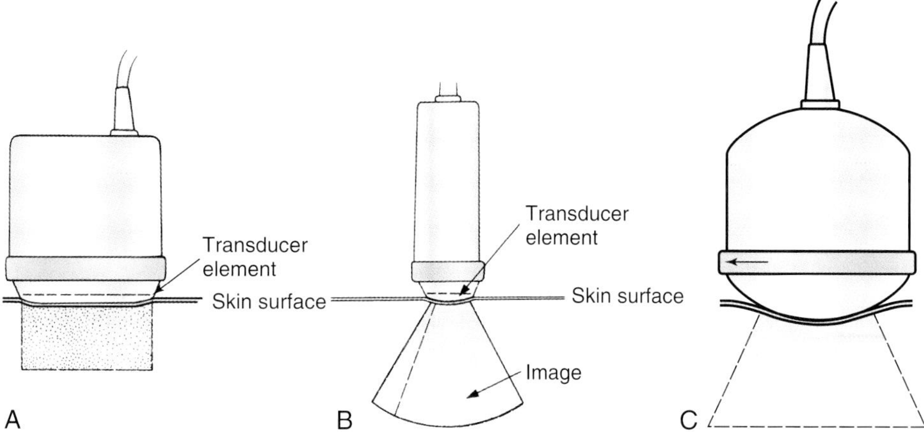

Figure 225-2 **A,** Linear probe produces a rectangular image and works especially well for obstetric scans. **B,** Wedge-shaped image produced by sector scanning probe may be adequate for most applications, depending on width of image. **C,** Curvilinear probe may be easier to maneuver between ribs. Note wedge-shaped image with curved anterior edge.

be shadows, often seen below both sides of a cyst and spreading outward (i.e., the penumbra effect). Combined, the appearance of all four acoustic properties may help confirm that whatever is being scanned is a cystic structure. These phenomena may be important after localizing a palpable mass, especially when trying to determine whether it is truly a cyst and might benefit from draining, or whether it is an adenoma.

QUALITY ASSURANCE

For diagnostic purposes, to maximize accuracy and to minimize liability—especially for emergency scans—again, perhaps only limited, goal-directed scans should be performed. If the patient is possibly unstable, there may be time only for a limited study. Limited or focused studies can be used to answer a particular clinical question, to improve patient care, or as a follow-up to streamline patient care. Similar to interpreting plain radiographs, the clinician at the bedside knows exactly where the patient is experiencing pain. This information is helpful when interpreting limited scans, especially when there are abnormalities. In complex cases or in cases in which portable ultrasonography is inconclusive, if the patient is stable, referral for a formal study can be considered. If the clinical question cannot be answered with certainty, referral or consultation should be considered, especially if it might change the management. If these principles are followed, perhaps the rare yet most dreaded error of failure to diagnose can be avoided.

A quality assurance program should be implemented. This could consist of some method of tracking outcomes or comparing results. One method of comparing outcomes while the clinician is learning is to not charge for "beginner" or "learner" scans and to follow up every scan with a formal scan in the radiology department. Log sheets should be created and used to compare results with formal scans. Results should continue to be compared until an acceptable level of clinical accuracy is achieved. Although formal interpretations may differ slightly from "beginner" or "learner" interpretations, the evaluation standard is whether the formal interpretation will lead to a change in clinical management. Having a radiologist over-read every scan is another method of ensuring quality; standard images could be obtained with each scan and then reviewed by a radiologist. Internet over-reading services by a radiologist are now continuously available (see the Suppliers section). With either method of quality assurance, proof of high-quality clinical data can be maintained and liability minimized, especially the liability of failure to diagnose. With these methods of quality assurance, the process of verifying and documenting clinician competence can be customized for each individual clinician.

For procedural purposes, there has been speculation that national hospital accrediting organizations will someday require many emergency department and hospital procedures to be ultrasonography guided. At the time of this publication, the author informally surveyed hospitalists and emergency medicine experts and found that none saw the need for such guidelines. Although there is individual variation, the literature suggests that the vast majority (>80%) of hospital and emergency medicine procedures are not currently ultrasonography guided. The majority of clinicians use ultrasonographic guidance only in those patients with a challenging body habitus or when there has been difficulty performing a procedure.

As with many procedures in primary care, beginners should develop a relationship with a consultant, either a radiologist or a clinician competent with ultrasonography (sonologist). Ultrasonography technicians (sonographers) often have extensive skill in multiple areas of ultrasonography and can be helpful consultants, especially in rural areas. As the clinician begins performing ultrasonography, cases should be discussed and consultation or supervision should be available.

CREDENTIALING

For departments implementing ultrasonography as a procedure, in addition to quality assurance, policies should be in place regarding credentialing. Such policies should identify eligible providers, specify training or experience requirements, and specify the ultrasonography privileges. For certain clinicians, ultrasonography can seem quite simplistic, and it can even be seductive; operators may become overconfident. Without credentialing, the liability of failing to diagnose may increase with potentially catastrophic outcomes, especially in urgent care centers or emergency departments. The author knows of cases in which watchful waiting (e.g., leaking abdominal aortic aneurysm, ectopic pregnancy) was inappropriate management. These near-catastrophes could have been avoided with appropriate departmental policies, credentialing, or a supervision process.

Reasonable guidelines for credentialing nonradiologists in an emergency department require a minimum of 150 recorded scans for general emergency ultrasonography privileges or 25 scans per primary indication. For procedural ultrasonography, the clinician should demonstrate competence in the use of basic ultrasonography by being credentialed for at least one primary indication. ACEP (and the literature) supports these numbers and notes that the range needed to document proficiency is between 25 to 50 scans per primary indication. These scans should be followed up with formal scans, over-reading, or by tracking clinical outcomes to document and demonstrate accuracy. At least 50% of the scans should show an abnormality. When competence for primary scans has been documented, scanning for other diagnoses (extended scans) can be managed on a case-by-case basis. Although there is much more to ultrasonography than can be learned by performing a certain number of scans, using these numbers as guidelines is helpful when attempting to decide whether a clinician is ready to demonstrate competence. There is also a process by which clinicians can be certified as registered diagnostic medical sonographers (RDMSs) after passing certain examinations and being supervised with scanning. It should be noted that the American Academy of Family Physicians does not endorse using a particular number of procedures performed (or documented) to credential for this or most other procedures.

Liability

When deciding whether using ultrasonography will raise a clinician's liability, the risk of not having ultrasonography immediately available should be weighed against making an incorrect diagnosis using ultrasound as a nonradiologist. For example, if certain diagnoses are not made urgently (e.g., pericardial tamponade, ectopic pregnancy, leaking aortic aneurysm, hemoperitoneum), patients may be endangered and liability may increase. In fact, failure to diagnose ectopic pregnancy is the second leading cause (in total dollar amounts) of malpractice awards against emergency physicians; ultrasonography is the initial procedure of choice to exclude ectopic pregnancy. For these and many other reasons, emergency clinicians now perform ultrasonography in most large emergency departments. Since ultrasonography training became routine for residents in emergency medicine, the standard of care also changed to that of a prudent emergency department physician, not a radiologist. Unfortunately, the standards of care for hospitalists and other primary care clinicians are not as well defined; therefore, documentation of competence, absolute certainty of interpretation, and overreading may be important.

Documentation

In many cases, ultrasonographic images are interpreted by the primary care clinician as they are being obtained. These interpretations often guide contemporaneous clinical decisions; however, a report needs to be placed on the patient's chart. It can be a handwritten, dictated, or templated note and should include the indication for the ultrasonography (e.g., preliminary diagnosis), what organs or structures were imaged, a copy of recorded images, appropriate measurements, and the final interpretation. If bowel gas or other technical factors prevent a thorough scan, these limitations should be identified and documented. Whenever feasible, images should be stored as part of the medical record and done so in accordance with facility policy requirements. Documentation is especially important if the clinician will be billing for ultrasonography; however, given the possible emergent use of ultrasonography by primary care clinicians, the timely delivery of care should not be delayed to archive images.

Equipment

- Acoustic gel.
- For cardiac and abdominal scanning, a 2.5- to 5-MHz sector or curvilinear transducer and scanner is needed. These scanners, or a linear scanner of the same frequency, can also be used for transabdominal obstetric–gynecologic scanning.
- For transvaginal scanning, a 3.5-, 5-, or 7.5-MHz sector, linear, or curvilinear transducer can be used. Special transvaginal probes are manufactured at those frequencies. Again, the higher the frequency, the higher the resolution and the sharper the image. However, the depth of scanning is decreased with a high-frequency probe, so the transvaginal probe must be applied directly to the cervix. For transvaginal scanning, a probe cover, plain-tipped condom, or examination glove is necessary to place over the probe.
- For pediatric or vascular scans, a 5- to 10-MHz sector, curvilinear, or linear scanner can be used.
- For scanning tissue close to the body surface (e.g., thyroid, testicular, breast)—also known as "small-parts scanning"—a high-frequency, 7.5- to 10-MHz sector, curvilinear, or linear scanner can be used (Box 225-1).

Box 225-1. Probe Frequencies and Potential Applications (from Low to High Frequency)

3.5 MHz

Abdominal
Cardiac
Lumbar puncture in morbidly obese
Pelvic and obstetric
Pleural effusion

5 MHz

Pediatric, including bladder
Transvaginal

7.5–10 MHz

Breast mass or cyst
Carotid arteries
Pediatric bladder
Testicular mass
Thyroid mass or cyst
Transvaginal
Venous vessels in neck and extremities

Beginner Scanning

Most clinicians learn human anatomy in three dimensions by dissection. Interpreting ultrasonographic images requires an ability to translate that knowledge into two dimensions. For proper probe placement and angulations, beginners should know that the best image is generated when the probe is perpendicular to the tissue being studied (Fig. 225-3). It may be helpful for beginners to minimize the planes of anatomy they have to learn by limiting their scanning to transverse and longitudinal planes. In other words, beginners should consider placing the transducer marker dot only toward the patient's right side (transverse) or head (longitudinal), while holding the probe perpendicular to the organ or tissue being scanned. If the probe can be held perpendicular to the skin surface, it is also usually easier to scan. Even for experienced sonographers, using these techniques may be helpful when getting oriented to a patient's anatomy at the beginning of any scan.

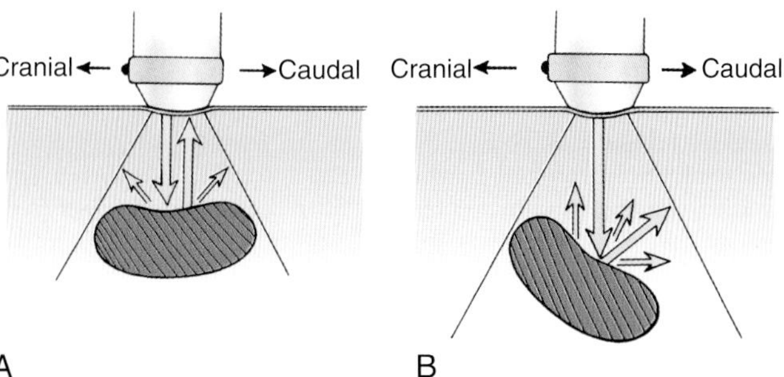

Figure 225-3 **A,** Best image is produced when the ultrasound beam is perpendicular to the organ interface. **B,** When the ultrasound beam is not perpendicular to the organ interface, scatter is seen, which may cause artifacts.

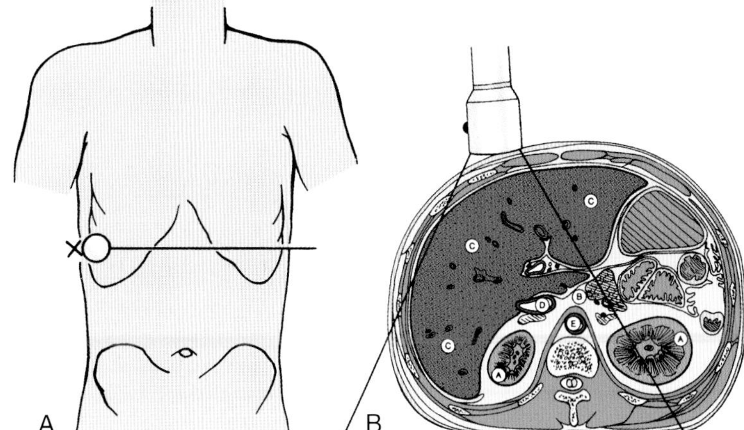

Figure 225-4 **A,** Marker dot toward the patient's right side produces a transverse image of the abdomen. **B,** Transverse image: kidneys (A), pancreas (B), liver (C), inferior vena cava (D), and aorta (E).

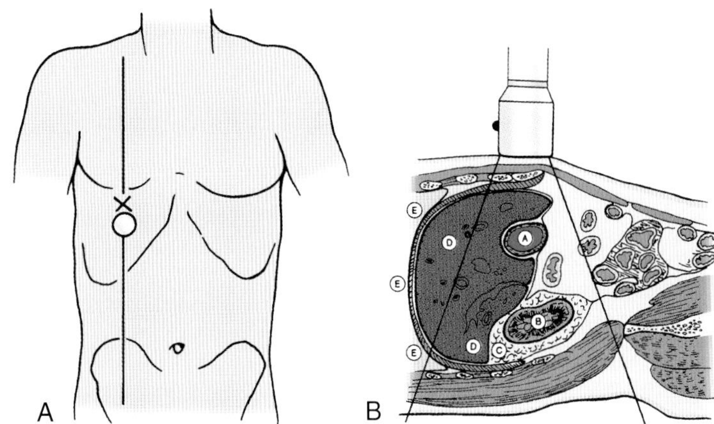

Figure 225-5 **A,** Marker dot toward the patient's head produces a longitudinal image of the abdomen. **B,** Longitudinal image: gallbladder (A), right kidney (B), perirenal fat (C), liver (D), and diaphragm (E).

By convention, when the marker dot is to the patient's right side, it produces a transverse image similar to computed tomography (CT) orientation (Fig. 225-4). The patient's right side will be to the left of the image on the screen. With the marker dot toward the patient's head, the image is what the clinician would see if the patient were dissected longitudinally and viewed looking into the body from the right side with the patient's head to the left of the screen (Fig. 225-5). A good impression of all of the anatomy and images of most organs can be obtained with longitudinal scanning, alone, at first.

NOTE: Some European manufacturers reverse the orientation so that the marker dot is found on the right side of the image.

INDICATIONS

Diagnostic Ultrasonography

Cardiac Indications

- Electromechanical dissociation (EMD): narrow electrical complexes on electrocardiogram (ECG) without measurable blood pressure or clinical evidence of perfusion*
- Evaluation of gross cardiac activity in setting of cardiopulmonary resuscitation*
- Suspected pericardial effusion (enlarged cardiac silhouette on chest x-ray, electrical alternans or decreased voltage on ECG)*
- Suspected pericardial tamponade (unexplained hypotension, prominent jugular venous distention, pulsus paradoxus, or EMD)*
- Penetrating wounds to the chest (to exclude hemopericardium*; see also the discussion of the focused assessment with sonography for trauma [FAST] examination, in the section on Trauma)
- Evaluation of global left ventricular function*
- Gross estimation of intravascular volume status and cardiac preload
- Identification of acute right ventricular dysfunction or acute pulmonary hypertension in the setting of acute or unexplained chest pain, dyspnea, or hemodynamic instability
- Identification of proximal aortic dissection or thoracic aortic aneurysm

Obstetric–Gynecologic Indications

- First-trimester vaginal bleeding*
- Suspected ectopic pregnancy*
- Threatened abortion*
- Evaluation of fetal viability (e.g., maternal demise, maternal trauma, or inability to auscultate fetal heart tones by Doppler)*
- Misplaced intrauterine device
- Suspected ovarian cyst, tubo-ovarian abscess, or adnexal/ovarian torsion
- Uterine fibroid

*These indications have been evaluated and defined in the medical literature and are considered primary applications in emergency medicine. The remaining indications listed for scanning by nonradiologists have also been published, and in many cases studied extensively.

Abdominal Indications

- Right upper quadrant (RUQ) pain*
- Symptoms suggestive of biliary tract disease*
- Suspected acute cholecystitis*
- Obstructive uropathy and renal colic*
- Hematuria
- Suspected renal abscess
- Pulsatile abdominal mass or suspected AAA*

Trauma

- Suspected hemoperitoneum or hemopericardium (e.g., FAST examination),* especially when real-time spiral (helical) CT is not available or the patient is not stable enough for CT (hemoperitoneum and hemopericardium need to be excluded in a patient with a history of blunt or penetrating trauma to the chest or abdomen or with an altered mental status and an acute abdomen)

Miscellaneous Indications

- Rib fracture
- Pneumothorax
- Suspected proximal deep venous thrombosis*
- Ultrasonographic evaluation of the bladder before suprapubic aspiration (SPA) or cannulation in infants or adults, or for documentation of postvoid residual (PVR)
- Subcutaneous foreign body
- Testicular pain or mass

Combined Diagnostic–Procedural Ultrasonography

- Insertion of central lines*
- Arterial puncture and cannulation
- Lumbar puncture or other spinal procedures in a morbidly obese individual (increasingly used by anesthesiologists, at least for localization of puncture site; see Chapter 206, Lumbar Puncture)
- Thyroid or breast mass or cyst, diagnosis or aspiration
- Pericardial effusion and ultrasonography-guided pericardiocentesis (see Chapter 214, Pericardiocentesis)
- Pleural effusion and ultrasonography-guided thoracentesis (see Chapter 95, Thoracentesis)
- Ascites and ultrasonography-guided paracentesis (see Chapter 201, Abdominal Paracentesis)
- Soft tissue abscess and ultrasonography-guided drainage (see Chapter 185, Musculoskeletal Ultrasonography)
- Joint effusion and arthrocentesis (see Chapter 185, Musculoskeletal Ultrasonography)
- Fracture, long bone, and fracture reduction (see Chapter 185, Musculoskeletal Ultrasonography)
- Endotracheal tube placement confirmation (see Chapter 213, Tracheal Intubation)
- Transvenous and transthoracic pacemaker placement (for localization of insertion site and when having difficulty with capture; see Chapter 216, Temporary Pacing)

CARDIAC ULTRASONOGRAPHY

In the unstable hypotensive patient or the patient in shock, if there are narrow QRS complexes on the ECG, the diagnosis is EMD. The differential includes anything that could cause abrupt cessation of venous return to the heart (including massive pulmonary embolism, tension pneumothorax, cardiac tamponade), acute malfunction of a prosthetic valve, and exsanguination. During resuscitative measures, exclusion of reversible causes is imperative, especially tamponade. Cardiac ultrasonography (echocardiography) is the diagnostic procedure of choice for excluding reversible causes of EMD.

A patient with a large pericardial effusion can be completely asymptomatic, deteriorate rapidly as a result of tamponade, or be in between. Several scenarios may lead the clinician to suspect a pericardial effusion (e.g., an enlarged cardiac silhouette on the chest radiograph, electrical alternans or decreased voltage on an ECG), especially in a patient at risk of an effusion. Pericardial tamponade may also result from a penetrating wound to the chest or be the cause of unexplained hypotension, prominent jugular venous distention, or a pulsus paradoxus on physical examination. Echocardiography is also the diagnostic procedure of choice for identifying and quantifying a pericardial effusion. Because rapid intervention is often a necessity in tamponade, ultrasonically directed aspiration of a hemodynamically significant effusion has become the treatment of choice.

Many emergency department clinicians, hospitalists, and cardiologists now also include a quick portable ultrasound of the heart when evaluating patients with chest pain. (See also Chapter 90, Echocardiography.) With this evaluation, gross cardiac activity can be assessed, including left ventricular function. Wall motion abnormalities (suggesting ischemia or scar) or severe valvular dysfunction may be noted, often early in the evaluation. Intravascular volume status can often be estimated, and right ventricular dysfunction or acute pulmonary hypertension identified (possibly indicating a pulmonary embolism). In the setting of chest pain, occasionally the diagnosis of proximal aortic dissection or a thoracic aortic aneurysm can be made.

Preprocedure Patient Preparation

Indications for the study and possible findings should be explained to the patient. The patient should be prepared to change positions, if possible, during scanning. He or she may experience some pressure from the probe as images are being obtained. Adequate gel should be applied to the parasternal, apical, and possibly subxiphoid areas of the chest wall. The patient should be in the supine or left lateral decubitus position when scanning is initiated.

Technique

While viewing the front of the chest—if the 12 o'clock position is considered cephalic and the 6 o'clock direction caudal—note that the axis of the heart is directed toward the 4 o'clock position. Placing the marker dot of the transducer at about the 4 o'clock position produces the long-axis view of the heart, especially if the probe is located parasternally. The long-axis view is essentially the longitudinal view of the heart, if described in the conventional terminology of ultrasonography for the remainder of the body. Rotating the marker dot almost 90 degrees to the 8 o'clock position produces the short-axis view of the heart, which is actually a transverse view of the heart (Fig. 225-6). For unresponsive patients, those who cannot be moved, or patients with pulmonary hyperinflation (e.g., chronic obstructive pulmonary disease, intubated), a subxiphoid view may be useful. However, a subxiphoid view may not be possible in patients with abdominal distention or pain, so the clinician should be comfortable using several cardiac windows.

1. With the patient in the supine position, place the low-frequency transducer in the parasternal (third to fourth or fifth intercostal space) or apical (inferolateral to the left nipple at the point of palpated maximal cardiac impulse) location. These are the same two traditional locations used for auscultation with a stethoscope.

*These indications have been evaluated and defined in the medical literature and are considered primary applications in emergency medicine. The remaining indications listed for scanning by nonradiologists have also been published, and in many cases studied extensively.

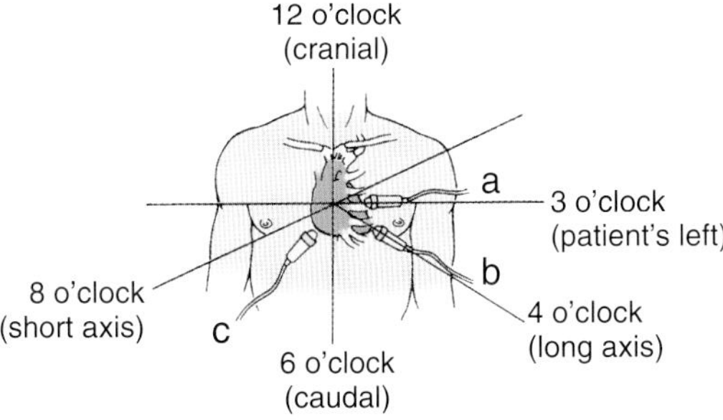

Figure 225-6 Typical probe positions (placement) for emergency department echocardiography: a, parasternal position of probe; b, apical position of probe; and c, probe in subxiphoid position.

2. In the parasternal space, the probe or marker dot will be rotated to either the 4 o'clock (long axis) or 8 o'clock (short axis) position.
3. The short-axis view at the level of the mitral valve is often used to assess the adequacy of the window because the mitral valve is usually prominent and easy to locate. In this view, with the probe directed almost straight posteriorly, nearly perpendicular to the bed, the mitral valve produces the characteristic "fish-mouth" image (Fig. 225-7), especially if there is any degree of stenosis. This is basically a transverse view of the mitral valve. After this transverse view is obtained, if the probe is directed or angled superiorly, toward the patient's right scapula, the aortic valve can often be seen in cross-section. (This is more of an extended scan, so see also Chapter 90, Echocardiography, and Fig. 90-4.) Conversely, from the transverse view of the mitral valve, if the probe is directed or angled inferiorly, toward the patient's left hip, the papillary muscles of the mitral valve can be seen in cross-section (see Chapter 90, Echocardiography, Fig. 90-5). They are echogenic (bright white) structures, surrounded by fluid in the heart (dark), which in turn is enclosed by the echogenic left ventricular walls seen in cross-section.

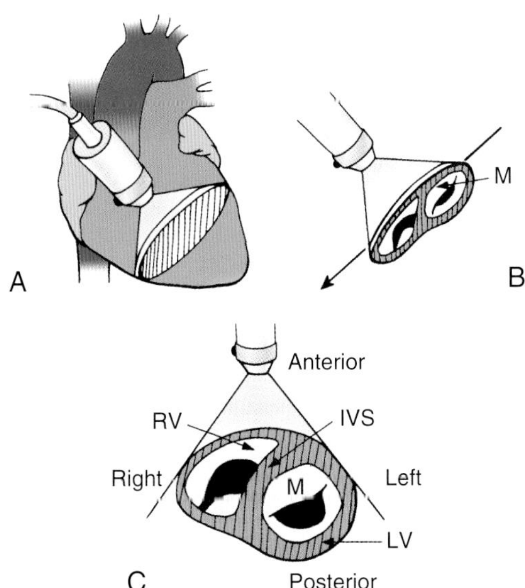

Figure 225-7 Short-axis view at mitral valve level. Probe is in parasternal position with marker dot at the 8 o'clock position. **A,** Ultrasonographic plane transects the short axis of the heart at the level of the mitral valve. **B,** Actual endocardiac structures viewed with probe in this position. M, mitral valve. **C,** Short-axis view as it appears on the ultrasonography screen. The image is displayed as if it is being viewed from the apex of the heart looking up toward the base. Note "fish mouth" appearance of mitral valve (M) as seen from this view. IVS, interventricular septum; LV, left ventricle; RV, right ventricle.

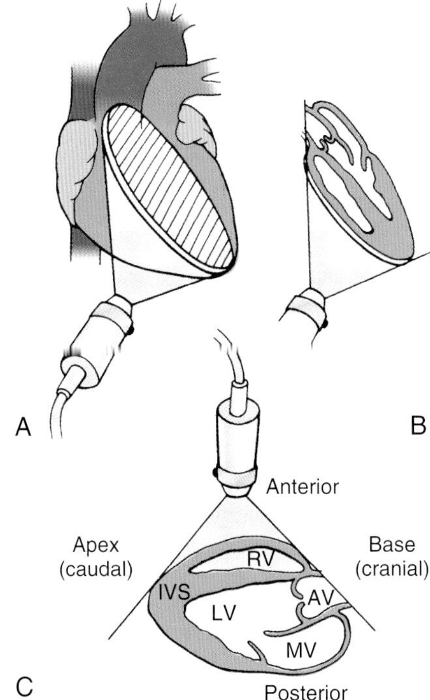

Figure 225-8 Parasternal long-axis view of the heart. Probe is in parasternal position with the marker dot at the 4 o'clock position. **A,** Ultrasonographic plane transects heart through the long axis. **B,** Actual endocardiac structures viewed. **C,** Image as it appears on ultrasonography screen. AV, aortic valve; IVS, interventricular septum; LV, left ventricle; MV, mitral valve; RV, right ventricle.

4. Directing the probe straight posteriorly, again perpendicular to the bed, the parasternal long-axis view can be obtained from the short-axis view by simply rotating the probe about 90 degrees counterclockwise (i.e., marker dot directed toward the 4 o'clock position; Fig. 225-8A and B). This is basically a longitudinal view of the mitral valve, with the echogenic ventricular septum located above the mitral valve on the image and the posterior wall located below it. The dark, fluid-filled right ventricle is located above the septum, and the left ventricle below it (Fig. 225-8C). To the right side of the image will be the aortic root, located to the right of the aortic valve and above the left atrium (see Fig. 225-8C). The left atrium in this view is located to the right of the mitral valve. The aortic valve cusps will also be seen opening and closing in a longitudinal view.
5. If the patient's position can be changed easily, place the patient on his or her left side. This allows the lingula of the lung to fall away from the heart and often provides a better window for all cardiac imaging.

   NOTE: Some ultrasound equipment places the marker dot 180 degrees away from this standard orientation (i.e., the 6 o'clock position for some is the 12 o'clock position for others). To allow the user to determine the orientation of the probe, the marker on the image should be found. It corresponds with the marker dot on the probe.

6. In the apical location (again, a more extended scan, so see also Chapter 90, Echocardiography), the majority of scanning can be performed with the marker dot rotated toward the patient's right side or at the 8 o'clock position. The probe is then directed toward the patient's right shoulder. The apex of the heart will be in the center at the top of the image, with the septum also in

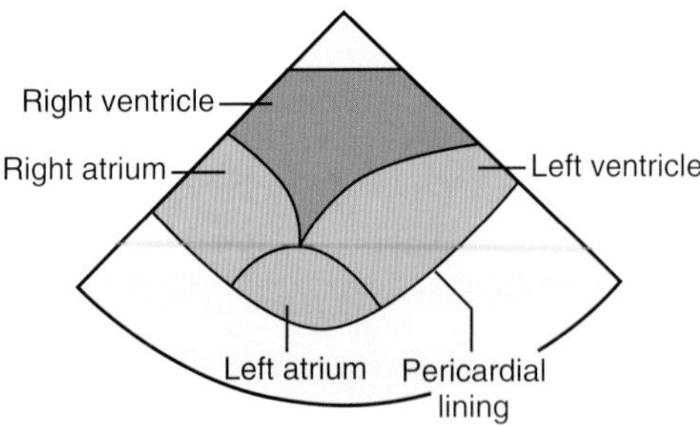

Figure 225-9 Subxiphoid (subcostal) view of heart.

the center and coursing vertically downward. The left ventricle and atrium will be on the right side of the image, and the right ventricle and atrium on the left, so it is called the *apical four-chamber view* (see Chapter 90, Echocardiography, Fig. 90-7).

7. A subxiphoid view may be needed to obtain a good window. Place the transducer directly below the xiphoid with the marker dot toward the patient's right side and angle it toward the patient's left scapula or even higher on the back. In fact, because the heart lies immediately beneath the sternum, the angle or plane of the probe will be almost horizontal or parallel to the patient's bed. A portion of liver will typically be seen at the top of the image (Fig. 225-9). Firm downward pressure may need to be applied with the probe, especially if the patient has a protuberant abdomen. Cardiac structures from this window will appear similar, but in a mirror image (rotated 180 degrees), to the parasternal long-axis view.
8. Search for fluid posterior to the heart. If present, it will usually appear at the bottom of the image. If found, quantify the amount of fluid (see Fig. 225-10). For various reasons (including body habitus) up to 10% of patients cannot be scanned adequately for a complete echocardiogram with portable equipment, even under optimal conditions. However, almost all patients with a clinically significant effusion can be diagnosed, so scan patiently and methodically. With a significant effusion, almost any view is acceptable. If an effusion is not readily apparent, vary the probe angles and amount of pressure applied on the probe for 5 to 10 minutes, if necessary, to find a window. Changing the patient's position may be helpful. All of these maneuvers may be necessary when there is a challenging body habitus or too much air in the lungs obscuring the image. If a good window is found with the parasternal short-axis view, many experts suggest using the parasternal long-axis view to exclude an effusion (see Fig. 225-8) because it provides a lengthwise image of the gravity-dependent portion of the heart (the posterior wall) when the patient is lying down. This is where a nonloculated effusion is most likely to settle.

NOTE: Even large effusions may develop gradually and not cause EMD or tamponade.

Interpretation

Electromechanical Dissociation

For patients undergoing cardiopulmonary resuscitation or with EMD, a subjective estimate of the organized cardiac activity can be made. Terminal cardiac dysfunction typically progresses from global ventricular hypokinesis with incomplete valve closure, to absence of ventricular wall and valve motion, to eventual cardiac standstill. This information, combined with the clinical scenario, may be helpful for determining futility during resuscitative efforts. Patients with poorly organized or absent cardiac activity on ultrasonography have a prognosis similar to that of patients with the ECG pattern of asystole (very poor). Patients with no obtainable blood pressure yet good cardiac contractility appear to carry a better prognosis, so an aggressive search for reversible causes of EMD should be pursued. If the EMD is due to pericardial tamponade, at least one chamber of the heart should collapse during diastole, and there will usually be a moderate to large pericardial effusion. However, even without identified collapse of a chamber, hemodynamic instability associated with a moderate to large pericardial effusion is suspect for tamponade. The cardiac activity is often well organized, with the rhythm regular and the rate tachycardic. Pericardiocentesis may be lifesaving. After the patient has been stabilized the findings should be recorded, including the size of the effusion.

Effusions

A small amount of pericardial fluid may be physiologic. If an effusion is diagnosed, it should be quantified (small, moderate, large, or very large) and recorded (Fig. 225-10). Any hemodynamic compromise should also be noted.

- *Small:* With the patient in the supine position, pericardial fluid is confined posteriorly without anterior, lateral, or apical spread. It will be less than 10 mm width in diastole.
- *Moderate:* Effusion more evenly distributed anteriorly, laterally, and apically, no part greater than 10 mm width in diastole.
- *Large:* Effusion extends entirely around the heart, 10 to 20 mm width in diastole.
- *Very large:* Greater than 20 mm width as well as evidence of tamponade.

Epicardial fat pads can occasionally be mistaken for a pericardial effusion. However, epicardial fat pads usually have some internal echoes and are not distributed evenly around the heart. The descending aorta can also be mistaken for a pericardial effusion, but rotating the probe into a transverse plane will often help distinguish that structure. See Chapter 214, Pericardiocentesis, for treatment of a pericardial effusion.

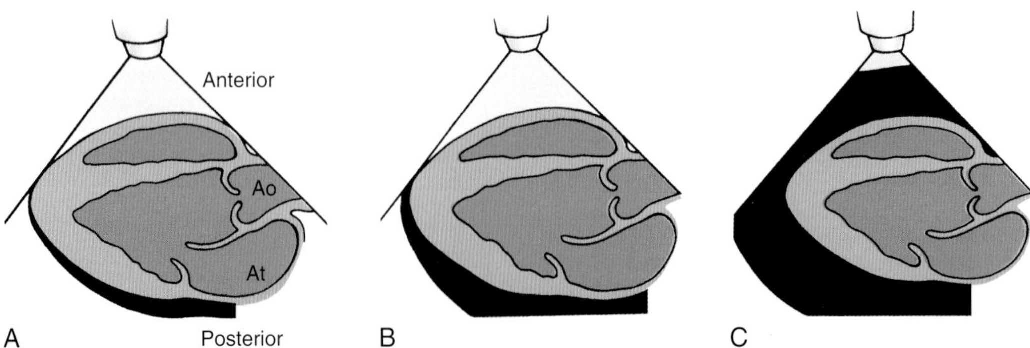

Figure 225-10 Effusions using a parasternal long-axis view. **A,** Small (may be physiologic). Ao, aortic root; At, left atrium. **B,** Moderate. **C,** Large.

Global Left Ventricular Systolic Function

Published reports indicate clinicians can accurately estimate left ventricular ejection fraction (EF) as normal (EF >50%), moderately impaired (EF 30% to 50%), or severely impaired (EF <30%) with little training and experience.

Dilated Left Atrium or Aortic Root

The diameter of the left atrium should be approximately the same as that of the aortic root on the parasternal long-axis view (see Fig. 225-10), and normal for both is about 2 cm. Disparities may suggest the need for a formal echocardiogram. A dilated aortic root may be suggestive of a thoracic aortic aneurysm, whereas an enlarged atrium increases the risk for atrial fibrillation and may indicate valvular or left ventricular dysfunction.

Right Ventricular Function, Intravascular Volume, and Preload Assessment

Using the subxiphoid view (or during abdominal scanning), the inferior vena cava can be located. Comparing the maximal diameter of the inferior vena cava during exhalation with the minimal diameter during inhalation may provide a quantitative estimate of preload. Collapse of 50% to 99% is normal, complete collapse may indicate volume depletion, and less than 50% collapse may indicate volume overload, pericardial tamponade, or right ventricular strain or failure. However, it can also indicate acute right ventricular infarct, pulmonic stenosis, and chronic pulmonary hypertension. An estimate of preload can also be made by measuring the height of the meniscus sonographically in the internal jugular from the sternal notch and adding 5 cm.

NOTE: Lack of right ventricular strain on ultrasonography does not exclude pulmonary embolism.

Mitral Valve Function

The parasternal long-axis view (because it cuts the mitral valve lengthwise) can be used to assess the mitral valve quantitatively (M-mode) and qualitavely. The anterior leaflet is seen on the superior aspect of the image, and the posterior leaflet is located inferiorly (see Fig. 225-8). With real-time scanning, leaflets can be observed opening and closing. In systole, the leaflets should close to about a 90-degree angle from the septal and posterior walls and lie flat against the plane of the annulus. If the leaflets close and then billow beyond the 90-degree angle or the plane of the annulus, they are prolapsing, and a formal echocardiogram may be helpful to confirm the diagnosis. Severe prolapse can be the result of papillary muscle dysfunction or disruption due to an acute myocardial infarction. The apical four-chamber view (see Chapter 90, Echocardiography, Fig. 90-7) is also helpful for assessing mitral valve function.

Obstetric–Gynecologic Ultrasonography

With the advent of transvaginal probes, an alternative to transabdominal scanning became available for evaluating the female pelvis. Advantages of transvaginal over transabdominal scanning include the use of a higher-frequency probe with higher resolution, fewer tissue layers through which to scan (nine layers on transabdominal), resulting in less artifact, and less patient preparation required, especially regarding the bladder. These advantages allow an intrauterine pregnancy to be diagnosed by about 5 weeks after the first day of the patient's last menstrual period. Fetal cardiac activity can frequently be seen by 6 weeks. With transvaginal scanning, there is also a greater likelihood of visualizing an ectopic pregnancy in a tube or the adnexa. Disadvantages to transvaginal scanning include the necessities of an extra probe, a sheath, and additional training. Interpretation is slightly more confusing and the field of imaging is slightly narrower. Despite the fact that patients are becoming more familiar with and accepting of this technology, transvaginal scanning is also slightly more invasive.

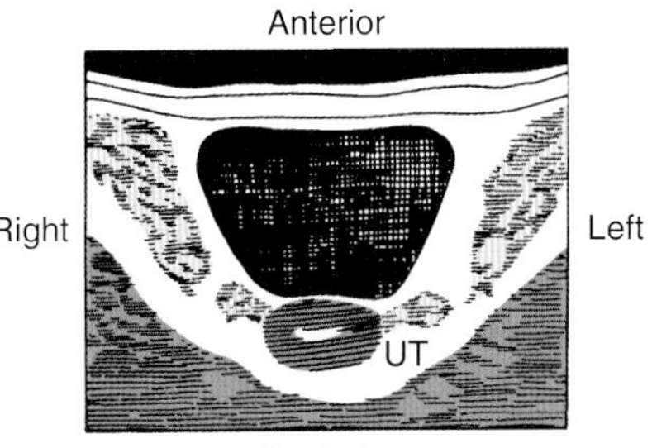

Figure 225-11 Transverse view of the bladder. Note uterus (UT), viewed transversely, is found posterior to the bladder.

Transabdominal Scanning

Preprocedure Patient Preparation

The patient is scanned in the supine position. For an adequate window, the patient's bladder must be full, occasionally to the point of discomfort. For best scanning, the bladder should be so full that the dome extends 1 or 2 cm above the fundus. If scanning above the pubis does not immediately provide an adequate view, the patient's clinical stability should be evaluated. If she is stable, either a Foley catheter infusion of fluid (300 to 500 mL) or oral or IV hydration can be used to fill the bladder. If a Foley catheter is used to infuse fluid, the clinician should try to avoid instilling air bubbles into the bladder, which can cause echoes and produce a confusing image.

Technique

1. Scanning the bladder first with a low-frequency probe and the marker dot at the patient's right side may help determine the shape and orientation of the uterus behind the bladder (Fig. 225-11). Because the bladder is rarely full of floating debris, the gain should be lowered until a minimal number of echoes are demonstrated in the bladder. This will decrease artifact. Confirm that the bladder, as opposed to a large ovarian cyst, is being used as a window. A large ovarian cyst is usually irregularly shaped, is oval or round, and often contains complex or echogenic contents. The bladder is basically square in a transverse view.
2. Turn the marker dot cephalad for a longitudinal view (Fig. 225-12). Often the uterus is not quite in the midline, as will have been demonstrated on the transverse view, so the probe may need to be rotated slightly out of the midline for a longitudinal image of the uterus. An echogenic line in the midline of the uterus is normal and represents the interface between the anterior and posterior endometria. A pair of dark fluid lines anterior and posterior to the central echogenic line represents endometrium during the proliferative phase. During the secretory phase, the

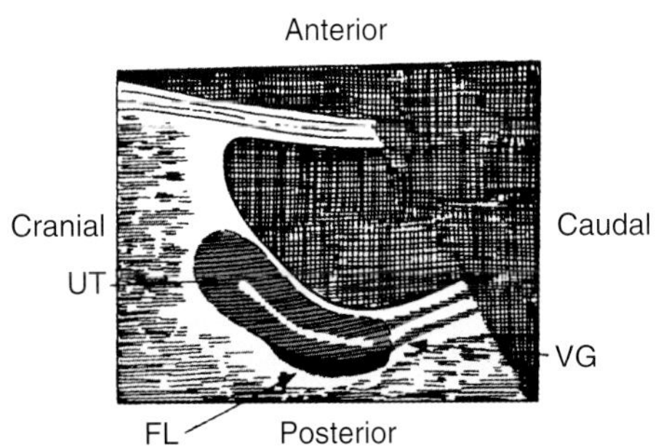

Figure 225-12 Longitudinal view of the bladder. Note uterus (UT), viewed longitudinally, behind the bladder. Fluid in the cul de sac (FL) is found posterior to the uterus. VG, vagina.

endometrium becomes progressively thicker and echogenic. Scan the uterus from fundus to cervix. Occasionally an echogenic line known as the *vaginal stripe* may be visualized in the vagina, distal to the cervix. It represents another interface.

3. Photograph and document any object or fluid accumulation within the uterus or posterior to it in the cul de sac (pouch of Douglas).
4. Scan the adnexa and note any fluid accumulations or abnormalities. Adnexa are usually located by first finding the midline of the uterus and then rotating the probe slightly. More specifically, with the probe producing a longitudinal view of the uterus, rotate it slightly clockwise (left adnexa) or counterclockwise (right adnexa) so that the marker dot is somewhat oblique to the uterus. If the adnexa cannot be located with this maneuver, move the probe laterally off of the midline and, while maintaining a longitudinal orientation, scan across and through the bladder to the opposite adnexa. In other words, angle the probe about 15 degrees off of the vertical to scan from the patient's left paramedian position. Scan across the midline through the bladder to visualize the patient's right adnexa, and vice versa for the left. The ovary often indents the wall of the bladder. Ovaries are oval structures of medium echogenicity and lie immediately anterior and medial to the internal iliac arteries, which are pulsatile and have echogenic walls. The iliac veins are also nearby. In women of reproductive age, demonstration of internal follicles often distinguishes ovaries from surrounding structures. Normal ovaries are 2.5 to 5 cm long, 1.5 to 3 cm wide, and 0.6 to 1.5 cm thick. Evidence of peristalsis on the patient's left side confirms that the colon is being scanned instead of the ovary.

Transvaginal Scanning

Preprocedure Patient Preparation

The patient is scanned in the supine or lithotomy position. Transvaginal scanning is usually preceded by transabdominal scanning with a full bladder, perhaps allowing the clinician to make the diagnosis and, if not, to assess the overall anatomy. The bladder can then be emptied; however, some residual urine can serve as a useful marker for locating the bladder.

Technique

1. Prepare the probe by covering it with a probe sheath, a plain-ended latex condom, or an examination glove. Adequate gel should be placed on the tip of the transducer before covering it. Any bubbles between the cover and transducer should be smoothed out before scanning.
2. Perform a preliminary pelvic examination to relax the vagina as well as to evaluate for palpable masses. Determine the size, shape, and position of the uterus and define any areas of tenderness. Any tampons should be removed. Counsel the patient about the transvaginal ultrasonographic examination and obtain verbal consent.
3. While continuing to wear examination gloves, apply more gel to the transducer cover and gently insert the probe with posterior vaginal pressure to a position anterior to the cervix.
4. Scanning starts as soon as the transducer is inserted; avoid inserting the transducer too far, which can cause the clinician to miss the cervix and lower uterine segment. With the marker dot anterior, locate the midline of the uterus in the image.
5. Obtain both longitudinal and coronal scans of the uterus and adnexa by turning the marker dot anterior to the patient or toward her right side. For longitudinal scanning, the image orientation changes slightly (Fig. 225-13) compared with transabdominal scanning. Because the marker dot is pointed toward the anterior abdominal wall of the patient, the left side of the resultant image is actually anterior instead of cranial. Transverse orientation also changes slightly because true anteroposterior (AP) images of the uterus cannot be obtained by scanning from below. However, various coronal images are obtained that are similar to transverse images. The patient's right side remains on the left side of the image because the marker dot is turned to the patient's right side (Fig. 225-14).
6. Scan the uterus by performing a series of longitudinal, coronal, and oblique scans with the transducer at varying depths of penetration. Oblique views are obtained by rotating the probe with the marker dot in the longitudinal position to either the right or left side of the patient. Oblique views are used to scan the adnexa.
7. Note any evidence of a fetus or fluid accumulations. Any areas of tenderness should be documented, along with any other important findings.

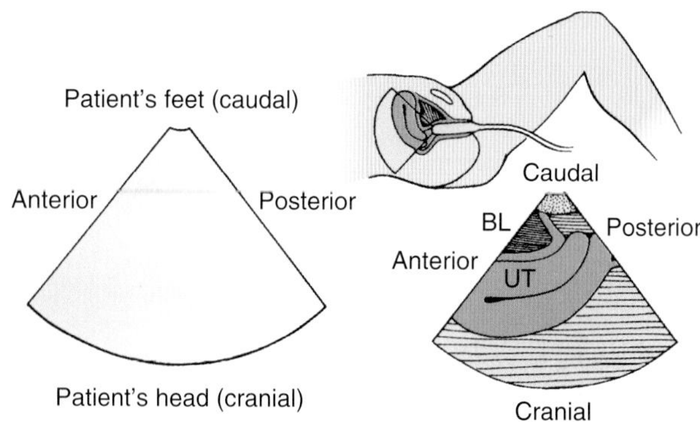

Figure 225-13 Longitudinal orientation with transvaginal scanning. BL, bladder; UT, uterus.

First-Trimester Vaginal Bleeding

Approximately 25% of all pregnancies experience bleeding during the first half (see Chapter 172, Obstetric Ultrasonography, for differential). Abdominal pain is also common during pregnancy. Ultrasonography is recommended as the first test in patients experiencing bleeding or pain beyond 5 to 7 weeks after their last menstrual period. Two frequent causes of first-trimester vaginal bleeding are ectopic pregnancy and threatened abortion.

NOTE: If a fetal heart beat is demonstrated by the less expensive hand-held Doppler, pregnancy loss has effectively been ruled out and ectopic pregnancy is much less likely. Doppler heart beats are not heard until 9 or 10 weeks, and most ectopic pregnancies become symptomatic before that time. With a threatened abortion, demonstration of fetal heart beats decreases the likelihood of miscarriage to less than 10%. If the Doppler is used during a bimanual pelvic

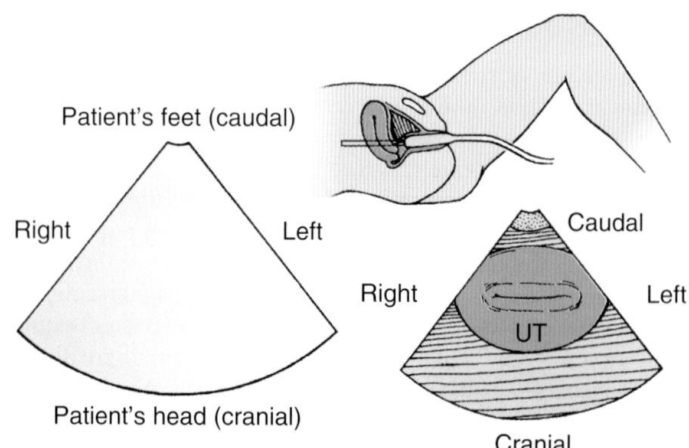

Figure 225-14 Transverse orientation with transvaginal scanning. UT, uterus.

examination and aimed directly at the uterine fundus as it is elevated by the examiner's hand, the likelihood of hearing fetal heart beats is much improved.

Suspected Ectopic Pregnancy

Ectopic pregnancies vary in prevalence from 1 in 28 to 1 in 200 pregnancies. They account for the majority of first-trimester maternal deaths. The incidence has quadrupled since 1970, and there has been a sevenfold increase in maternal mortality. More than 40% of ectopic pregnancies are misdiagnosed on first presentation to the health care provider.

Clinical ultrasonography coupled with immediately available sensitive radioimmunoassay for human chorionic gonadotropin (hCG) has decreased the morbidity and mortality of ectopic pregnancies. It is important to correlate quantitative hCG levels in your laboratory with the type of equipment available to determine at what level of hCG an intrauterine pregnancy should be visible by sonography. This will vary depending on whether transabdominal or transvaginal scanning is performed.

RISK FACTORS FOR ECTOPIC PREGNANCY (IN DESCENDING ORDER OF SIGNIFICANCE) AND SYMPTOMS

- Intrauterine device currently in place or recently used
- Previous tubal, abdominal, or pelvic surgery
- Prior ectopic pregnancy
- Prior sexually transmitted infection, especially pelvic inflammatory disease
- Infertility
- Recent therapeutic abortion

In several large studies, pain (97% to 100% of patients) and amenorrhea (74% to 84%) were more common complaints than vaginal bleeding, although bleeding occurred in the majority of ectopic pregnancies.

INTERPRETATION: TRANSABDOMINAL SCANNING. One technique for excluding or *ruling out* an ectopic pregnancy is to confirm or *rule in* an intrauterine pregnancy. With transabdominal scanning, to diagnose an ectopic pregnancy by actually visualizing the fetus in a tube or the adnexa is rare (<10% of ectopic pregnancies). Even with higher-resolution transvaginal scanning, only occasionally will the ectopic pregnancy be visualized (<25% of ectopic pregnancies).

To confirm an intrauterine pregnancy, a gestational sac with a fetus or fetal pole should be noted. A gestational sac appears as an anechoic (dark) structure within the uterus with highly echogenic borders. The first small echogenic structure seen in the gestational sac is the yolk sac at about 5½ weeks. About a week later, a small collection of echoes may be seen; they constitute the fetal pole. The presence of a gestational sac *with* a fetal pole in the uterus reduces the chance of an ectopic pregnancy to about 1 in 30,000 cases. This figure represents the likelihood of a concomitant ectopic during an intrauterine pregnancy, the so-called combination pregnancy. Exceptions to this statistic are found in patients undergoing assisted reproduction in which the risk of combination pregnancy may be as high as 1 in 7000, or in patients taking ovulation-stimulating fertility drugs (e.g., clomiphene), in which the incidence may be as high as 1 in 100. If no fetal pole is seen within what appears to be a gestational sac, the clinician must consider that 10% to 20% of ectopic pregnancies produce pseudogestational sacs in the uterus and that the possibility of an ectopic pregnancy cannot be completely dismissed.The gold standard for diagnosing an intrauterine pregnancy is the visualization of embryonic cardiac activity. This may be seen as early as 7 weeks after the first day of the patient's last menstrual period or when the mean sac diameter is 12 to 16 mm, depending on the resolution of the equipment and the skill of the examiner. *Mean sac diameter* is determined by measuring a single diameter if the sac is round. It is the average of the three largest diameters (transverse, longitudinal, and AP) if the sac is oval. If a fetus is seen, gestational age can also be determined from what else is visualized (Table 225-1). When a gestational sac with a mean diameter greater than 25 mm (17 mm for transvaginal scanning) lacks an embryo or when the gestational sac is grossly distorted, abnormal pregnancy is almost certain. Using these criteria, 76% of abnormal pregnancies and 93% of normal pregnancies will be correctly classified by only one ultrasonographic scan. The most accurate estimate of gestational age is at 9 to 11 weeks, using the crown–rump length.

TABLE 225-1 Dates from Last Menstrual Period Correlated to Findings by Transabdominal Imaging*

Finding	Weeks
Gestational sac	5–6
Yolk sac	5–6
Fetal pole	6–7
Cardiac activity	7–8
Placenta	8–9
Somatic activity	9–10

*Transvaginal imaging can usually locate the same finding 1 week earlier.

If the patient is obese or her bladder is empty, transabdominal ultrasonographic findings may be limited; transvaginal scanning may be the only option. In all cases, failure to define an intrauterine pregnancy is interpreted in the proper clinical setting as an ectopic pregnancy until proven otherwise. Eight options exist when an intrauterine pregnancy is not demonstrated by ultrasonography (Table 225-2). Correlation with hCG titers may be necessary to complete the interpretation. With a healthy intrauterine pregnancy, hCG values rise predictably, doubling every 2 to 3 days for the first 8 weeks. In contrast, the hCG titer tends to rise at a slower rate in a patient with an ectopic pregnancy.

Evaluation of the medical literature for quantitative hCG titers correlated with sonographic findings often leads to confusion regarding the standards being used (for a crude conversion, the Second International Standard equals about 50% of the International Reference Preparation [IRP]). Most hospital laboratories are currently using the Second International Standard, whereas much of the early research used IRP. If the IRP standard of hCG quantities is used, transabdominal ultrasonography should detect an intrauterine pregnancy in 94% of cases when the quantitative hCG reaches 6000 to 6500 mIU/mL (3000 to 3250 mIU/mL for the Second Standard). This correlates with about 42 days' gestation.

Even if an ectopic pregnancy is not demonstrated by ultrasonography, there are associated sonographic findings (Table 225-3) that, if seen, significantly increase the likelihood of ectopic pregnancy. In the case of a ruptured ectopic, scanning the upper abdomen may reveal free fluid representing intra-abdominal hemorrhage. Although a moderate to large amount of fluid is highly correlated with an ectopic pregnancy, any free fluid is significant in the proper clinical situation. A demonstrated echogenic pelvic mass also significantly increases the likelihood of ectopic pregnancy.

If a normal intrauterine pregnancy is demonstrated, the search for other causes of the patient's symptoms might be facilitated with ultrasonography. The clinician should scan for evidence of urolithiasis, intact or ruptured ovarian or corpus luteum cyst, adnexal/ovarian torsion, tubo-ovarian abscess (dilated fallopian tubes/hydrosalpinx, usually bilateral, indicate pelvic inflammatory disease), or appendiceal abscess (appendicitis). Although a thorough description of the ultrasonographic findings for most of these situations is beyond the scope of this chapter, a ruptured ovarian cyst frequently is noted as an irregular adnexal mass, accompanied by fluid in the cul de sac, and evidence of clotting blood seen as an echogenic mass difficult to separate from the uterus. The appearance will be the same with a ruptured corpus luteum cyst; however, the ovary will be noted in the middle of the irregular adnexal mass. If color Doppler

TABLE 225-2 Possible Diagnoses If an Intrauterine Pregnancy Is Not Demonstrated by Transabdominal Ultrasonography

Diagnosis	Finding	Management
Confirmed ectopic pregnancy	Empty uterus and ectopic fetal heart activity	Surgery or emergent consultation
Highly likely ectopic pregnancy	Empty uterus and echogenic pelvic mass or free pelvic fluid or hemoperitoneum	Surgery, culdocentesis or emergent consultation
Very early normal pregnancy	Serum quantitative hCG <6000 mIU/mL IRP (3000–3250 mIU/mL Second Standard)	Repeat quantitative hCG in 48–72 hr
Occult unruptured ectopic pregnancy	Empty uterus or may see pseudogestational sac in uterus (seen in 10%–20% of ectopic pregnancies)	Surgery, consultation, or repeat quantitative hCG in 48–72 hr if stable
Complete or incomplete spontaneous abortion	Empty uterus or atypical echogenic or sonolucent findings in uterus such as a misshapen sac, located low in the uterus, or debris in the sac	D&C to treat or confirm, consultation, or repeat quantitative hCG; emergency treatment necessary if cannot exclude ectopic pregnancy, if patient is unstable, or for heavy bleeding
Dead embryo	Crown–rump length >5 mm and no cardiac motion after continuous observation	Serial quantitative hCGs or repeat ultrasonography in a few days; emergency treatment necessary only for heavy bleeding
Embryonic resorption/blighted ovum	Mean sac diameter of >2.5 cm and no fetal pole or >2.0 cm and no yolk sac (see text for calculating mean sac diameter); also, a misshapen empty sac, located low in uterus, or debris in the sac	Emergency treatment necessary only for heavy bleeding
Hydatidiform mole or trophoblastic disease	Snowstorm appearance of uterine contents	Consultation or D&C

D&C, Dilation and curettage; hCG, human chorionic gonadotropin; IRP, International Reference Preparation.

is available, it may diagnose probable adnexal/ovarian torsion by demonstrating an enlarged ovary with absent blood flow compared with the opposite adnexa. However, two arterial sources supply the ovary, the ovarian and the uterine arteries, so normal blood flow does not exclude ovarian torsion. A torsioned cyst is often associated with a torsioned ovary, and may have a fluid–fluid level and a thickened rim of tissue, and be tender with palpation with the transvaginal probe. Urolithiasis is discussed in a separate section of this chapter.

INTERPRETATION: TRANSVAGINAL SCANNING. The interpretation for transvaginal scanning is the same as for transabdominal scanning, except that with a fetus everything is visualized approximately 1 week earlier than with transabdominal scanning. The correlations with hCG must also be corrected (see Table 225-1). Transvaginal scanning can usually detect an intrauterine gestational sac at 2000 mIU/mL IRP (1000 mIU/mL Second Standard) or about 35 days' gestation. For a patient with a quantitative hCG above this level and no intrauterine pregnancy visualized, ectopic pregnancy must be considered. If there is no vaginal bleeding, ectopic pregnancy becomes almost certain.

Threatened Abortion

Management of a threatened abortion consists of ruling out possible causes (or treating them), assessing the amount of bleeding, and predicting the prognosis for the pregnancy. If bleeding is minimal and no specific cause is identified, such as infection (e.g., urinary tract or cervix) or anemia, the patient is discharged in most cases with instructions for bed rest, to minimize stress, and to increase hydration. If the evaluation can be completed entirely in the emergency department or the office, treatment goals are more readily accomplished than if the patient must undergo a stressful evaluation in another department. Using specific sonographic criteria, the clinician may determine which patients need additional ultrasonographic studies as well as reasonably estimate the prognosis of the early pregnancy. Without ultrasonography, the only prediction the clinician can make is that 50% of threatened abortions will progress to miscarriage.

TABLE 225-3 Using Transabdominal Ultrasonography to Determine Risk of Ectopic Pregnancy in Patients with Positive Human Chorionic Gonadotropin and Empty Uterus

Ancillary Findings	Risk of Ectopic Pregnancy (%)
Any free fluid	20
Echogenic mass	71
Moderate to large amount of fluid	95
Echogenic mass with fluid	100
No ancillary findings	20

INTERPRETATION. Frequently, the diagnosis of threatened abortion is made after ruling out ectopic pregnancy. Presence of fetal cardiac activity is an encouraging finding in an early pregnancy because the risk of spontaneous abortion is less than 2% to 4% if fetal cardiac activity is seen after 12 weeks. The risk of miscarriage is less than 16% if cardiac activity is noted at less than 8 postmenstrual weeks, which is much lower than the 50% predicted if ultrasonography is not available or performed.

With earlier pregnancies (even before the embryo is visible), major and minor criteria are available for evaluating gestational sacs (see Chapter 172, Obstetric Ultrasonography). Again, patients with gestational sacs meeting most or all of these criteria by ultrasonography are much less likely to miscarry than the 50% rate predicted if the patients are evaluated by clinical means alone.

Failure to meet at least one major criterion is 100% specific in predicting spontaneous abortion. Fifty-three percent of abnormal pregnancies are identified by the same criteria. If there is a question about an abnormal sac, the patient should be scanned 7 to 10 days later. As an additional criterion during that time, the mean sac diameter in normal pregnancies should increase by about 1 mm per day.

Examples of abnormalities include low-lying gestational sacs (sacs in the cervical region) and abnormally shaped sacs. Both of these are worrisome findings and should be followed with a scan 1 week later. Frequently, low-lying sacs lead to spontaneous abortions, whereas abnormally shaped sacs lead to abnormal pregnancies. Worrisome findings also include failure of the sac to gain 1 cm in mean diameter in 1 week or the inability to visualize an embryo when the sac reaches 2.5 cm in mean sac diameter. These findings may assist the clinician in preparing the patient for the possibility of an abnormal pregnancy, such as one resulting in a spontaneous miscarriage.

Fibroids are present in 40% of women older than 40 years of age, have an echogenicity similar to the uterus (although the tissue is frequently organized in whorls), and can calcify. They are an overgrowth of uterine tissue and may be intracavitary, submucosal, intramural, subserosal, or pedunculated. Intracavitary fibroids almost always cause cramping and bleeding. Subserosal fibroids lie on the edge of the uterus and may indent the bladder, submucosal fibroids border on the endometrial lining, and intramural fibroids lie entirely within the myometrium. Pedunculated fibroids are connected by a neck to the body of the uterus and may be confused with adnexal masses.

Evaluation of Fetal Viability

Detection of fetal heart activity by the second and third trimester of pregnancy should be reliable by transabdominal scanning (see Chapter 172, Obstetric Ultrasonography). Earlier detection may require transvaginal scanning.

Interpretation

Absence of fetal movement after scanning for a 5-minute interval in a pregnancy of more than 20 weeks' gestation is said to be 100% reliable for diagnosing a fetal demise. For a first-trimester pregnancy, if uncertainty exists about fetal heart activity, rescanning should be performed in 1 to 2 weeks.

Secondary criteria for fetal demise using ultrasonography include fetal anomalies such as hydrops, ascites, and pleural or pericardial effusions. Echogenic gas in the fetal heart and vessels may be early findings. Late findings include morphologic changes such as skeletal anomalies and unusual fetal positioning.

Reaction to external stimulation or uterine manipulation should cause brisk reflexes in viable fetuses as opposed to the passive motions seen with a fetal demise. Avoid misinterpreting the passive motions from uterine contractions around a dead fetus as fetal activity.

Because abruptio placentae cannot always be diagnosed with ultrasonography (i.e., it is a clinical diagnosis), ultrasonographic studies should be used in conjunction with maternal–fetal monitoring in the pregnant patient with significant abdominal trauma. A 4-hour monitoring period should be sufficient to identify fetal distress.

Misplaced Intrauterine Device

Intrauterine contraceptive devices (IUDs) are approved for 5 to 10 years of continuous use. This length of time offers many opportunities to lose the string. When a string is not palpable on an IUD, possible causes include a properly positioned IUD in the uterus that has lost its string, an extruded IUD, or an IUD that has perforated the uterus and may even be lying in the abdomen. IUD users who have not lost the string also warrant further evaluation if they are experiencing cramping, pain, or abnormal bleeding. A flat-plate radiograph may document the presence of the IUD, but it will not help determine whether the IUD is in the uterus. Gynecologic instrumentation is another option, but instrumentation places the patient at risk of infection. In most cases, it should be reserved for removal of the IUD after the location is documented. Ultrasonography is usually the diagnostic procedure of choice to determine the location of an IUD. However, the diameter of most IUDs is less than 3 mm; therefore, scanning for IUDs in some cases is more difficult than expected.

Interpretation

An IUD on ultrasonography produces a very straight, sharp-edged, echogenic image. Document the location of the IUD in both longitudinal (Fig. 225-15A) and transverse or coronal views (Fig. 225-15B). It may be accompanied by a small "ball" of echoes in the cervix—the string coiled up, which can often be retrieved with a cervical brush used for Papanicolaou (Pap) smears (see Chapter 146, Intrauterine Device Removal). If an IUD is not demonstrated and the posterior wall of the uterus is not easily identified, formal scanning may be necessary. IUDs may be difficult to locate when the uterus is retroverted.

Decidual reaction may mimic an IUD. To differentiate, an IUD should produce shadowing in at least one plane. Echoes from an IUD are typically straighter and sharper-edged than those from a decidual reaction.

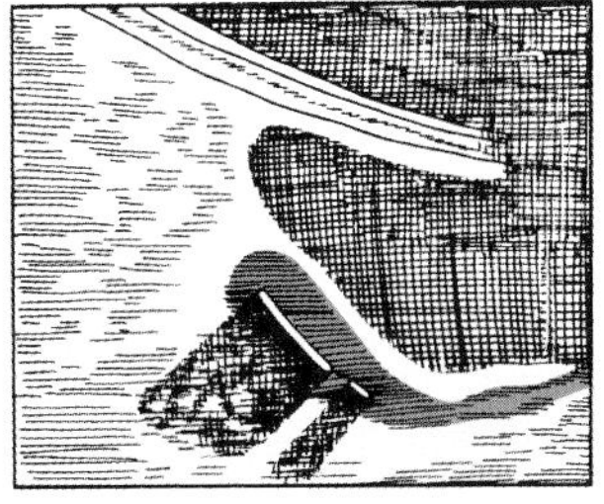

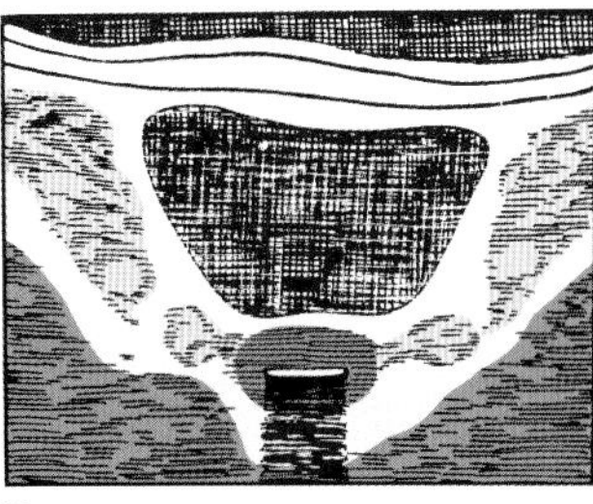

Figure 225-15 Intrauterine device in longitudinal (**A**) and transverse (**B**) views.

A perforation should be recorded as either complete or incomplete. For an incomplete perforation, a portion of the IUD can be demonstrated within the uterine wall. A flat-plate x-ray film may be necessary to document a complete perforation if it is not visible by ultrasonography.

Abdominal Ultrasonography

Various tests can be used when deciding whether conditions are good enough to perform a complete abdominal survey, especially if using portable equipment. The gain can also be set when performing these tests. First, if the bladder is full, an attempt should be made to scan it; if a full bladder cannot be scanned, the body habitus or conditions are probably not conducive for obtaining a complete abdominal survey. If the bladder can be scanned, the gain on the machine should be set low enough to eliminate echoes from a normally nonechogenic organ. Next, the clinician should attempt to scan the aorta lengthwise. Repositioning may be required, and the liver may be needed as a window. If the aorta is located, the gain should be set to minimize internal echoes because this organ normally has no echoes. (This gain setting can then generally be used to scan the majority of the abdomen.) If the clinician is unable to locate the aorta after several attempts and several minutes of scanning, body habitus or conditions may preclude a complete abdominal survey or scan. The clinician may be restricted to a focused or limited scan. The pelvis with a full bladder and the liver, right kidney, and RUQ structures will probably be easiest to scan. A referral may be necessary for a formal, complete scan for other abdominal structures.

Biliary Tract Disease

Acute cholecystitis in the ambulatory setting in the United States results from obstruction of the cystic duct by gallstones in approximately 95% of cases. Unfortunately, the diagnosis of acute cholecystitis by purely clinical means (without ultrasonography) has an accuracy of only 50%, even with a positive Murphy's sign (pain over the gallbladder with palpation during inspiration). Therefore, real-time ultrasonography is the preferred diagnostic test for acute cholecystitis. A "sonographic Murphy's sign" combined with the presence of gallstones increases the diagnostic accuracy for acute cholecystitis to more than 90%. A sonographic Murphy's sign is described as pain elicited with probe compression over the gallbladder. Because early surgical management is now the treatment of choice for acute cholecystitis, early diagnosis is also important. Bedside ultrasonography is useful in diagnosing most cases of cholelithiasis and acute cholecystitis; however, obscure cases may require additional studies.

Preprocedure Patient Preparation

If possible, the patient should have been in the fasting state for at least 8 hours; this ensures that the gallbladder is fully distended. Early-morning scanning may minimize bowel gas interference.

Technique

1. Scan the patient in the supine position, longitudinally, with a low-frequency probe until you locate the gallbladder. It is usually located in about the mid-clavicular line, just above the inferior edge of the liver; however, it can be located anywhere between the midline and the anterior axillary line. A combination of subcostal and intercostal windows may be needed. Sustained inspiration by the patient may move the liver below the ribs and improve the subcostal window. The normal gallbladder is a cystic structure; when distended, it demonstrates the sonographic properties of cysts elsewhere in the body. The walls are smooth, usually no echogenic matter exists between them, and tissue behind the posterior wall is more clearly defined.

   Other cystic structures located nearby that can be confused with the gallbladder include hepatic cysts, hepatic veins, the portal vein, renal cysts, the duodenum, the inferior vena cava, and the abdominal aorta. Hepatic cysts have very thin walls and are usually located much deeper in the hepatic parenchyma than the gallbladder. Hepatic veins usually run vertically within the liver when the patient is supine. They also have very thin walls that are compressible with probe pressure. Veins also collapse with inspiration and expand with a Valsalva maneuver. If followed posteriorly, the location just below the diaphragm where the hepatic veins empty into the inferior vena cava can usually be seen. Although the portal vein has echogenic sidewalls similar to the gallbladder, it can usually be viewed coursing horizontally through the liver. Often, tributaries to the portal vein, such as the splenic vein, can be traced from their origin to where they join to form the portal vein near the liver. Renal cysts can usually be demonstrated as very thin walled and contiguous with renal tissue (Fig. 225-16). They are located much further lateral and posterior than the gallbladder. Although the abdominal aorta has echogenic walls, it demonstrates pulsations and can be followed distally. Pulsations transmitted from the aorta may also be noted in the inferior vena cava. Having the patient take in a large breath should collapse the vena cava; a Valsalva maneuver should cause significant dilation. The duodenum can usually be distinguished from the gallbladder because peristalsis is observed. Having the patient drink water can also stimulate and demonstrate peristalsis in the duodenum. Air in the duodenum usually casts confusing, irregular shadows as opposed to the sharp shadows of gallstones.
2. Compared with other abdominal organs, the gallbladder usually has a rather superficial location on the inferior edge of the liver. After locating the gallbladder with the probe in the longitudinal position, obtain a long-axis view by rotating the probe out of the longitudinal plane of the body until the maximal length of the gallbladder is visualized and an image recorded. The maximal transverse diameter of the gallbladder should also be measured and recorded.
3. Obtain additional views of the gallbladder by moving the patient into one other position: the decubitus (right side up) position or the erect position. Repositioning the patient helps to avoid missing stones that may have rolled into a dependent position out of view.
4. Attempt to identify the source of any local tenderness and scan that area. The porta hepatis, which consists of the common bile duct, the hepatic artery, and the portal vein, can often be located by following the portal vein from the confluence of the splenic vein and the superior mesenteric vein. Conversely, the portal vessels in the liver can be followed horizontally until they coalesce as the portal vein at the hepatic hilum. The porta hepatis also can be located by tracking the hepatic artery from the celiac axis. Color Doppler can help distinguish the common bile duct from the hepatic artery.

Interpretation

An echogenic structure within the gallbladder is a gallstone if it shows prominent posterior shadowing, has circumferential bile visible in at least one view, and has demonstrated mobility when the patient is placed in various positions (Fig. 225-17). When

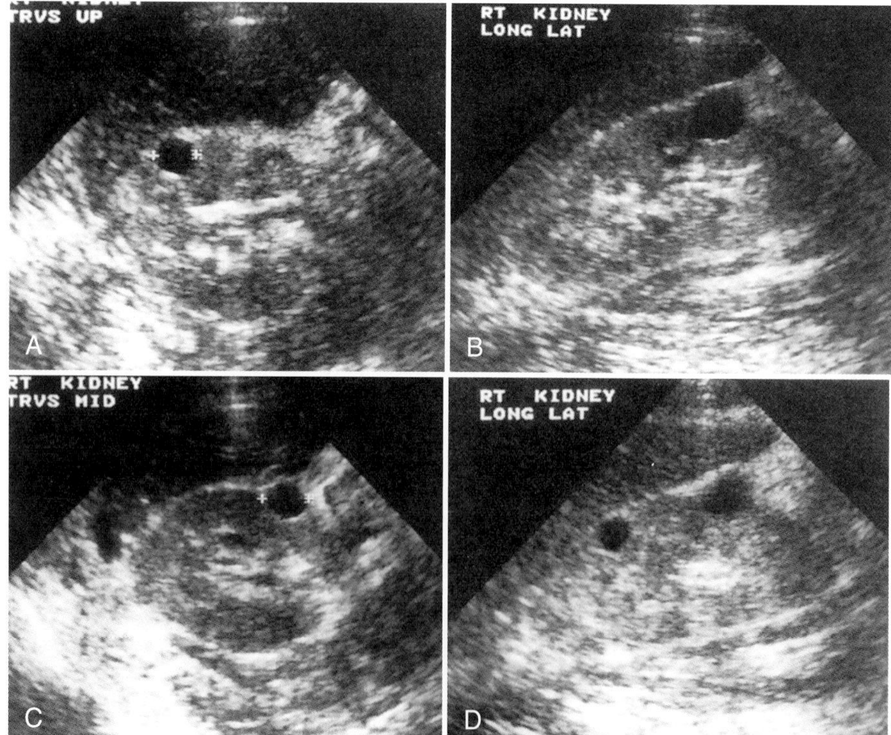

Figure 225-16 Transverse (**A** and **C**) and longitudinal (**B** and **D**) scans of two small renal cysts along the lateral wall of the kidney. Borders are smooth and well defined. No echoes are present. (From Hagen-Ansert SL [ed]: Textbook of Diagnostic Ultrasonography, 4th ed. St. Louis, Mosby, 1995.)

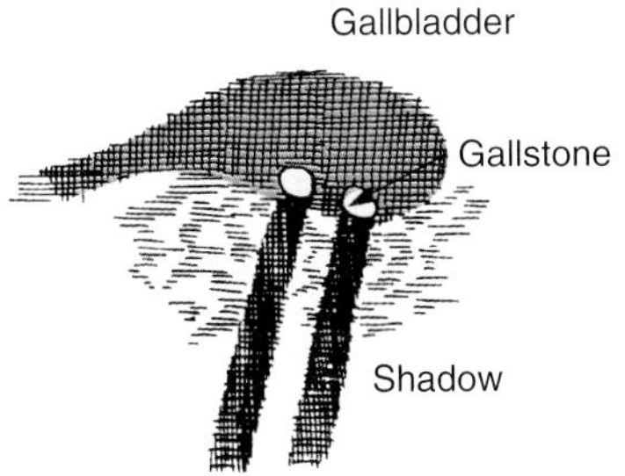

Figure 225-17 Acoustic shadowing behind two gallstones. Note the "sharpness" of the shadow.

coupled with a positive sonographic Murphy's sign, this is diagnostic of acute cholecystitis. Otherwise, gallstones can have several variations when viewed sonographically:

- *Nonshadowing:* Gallstones less than 2 to 3 mm in size often do not cast a shadow. In that situation the differential also includes echogenic structures such as polyps or folds in the gallbladder. In fact, echogenic structures in the gallbladder that are nonshadowing are calculi in only 50% of cases. If, however, an echogenic structure is noted to have gravity-dependent motion, it is usually a stone (Fig. 225-18).
- *Intermittent shadowing:* Multiple small stones may form an irregular layer in the most dependent portion of the gallbladder. They may also cast a variable or intermittent shadow. This may be highly suspect for cholelithiasis, but further studies are necessary if there is no well-defined shadowing.
- *Filled gallbladder:* If the gallbladder is entirely filled with stones, bile may not be noted circumferentially around any one stone. Shadowing may be less prominent or hazy. Because a gas-filled duodenum can have the same appearance, it must be carefully eliminated from the differential by studying for other characteristics (e.g., peristalsis).
- *Adherent stones:* These can appear as echogenic structures that are not gravity dependent. If no shadowing is seen, further studies may be necessary to exclude a polyp, tumor, or fold, which can also be echogenic.
- *Floating stones:* Either one stone or a collection of stones may float and appear as an echogenic structure or a line of echoes in a nondependent portion of the gallbladder. If they do not cast a shadow, further studies may be necessary.
- *Absent gallbladder:* This sonographic finding (absence) may also be noted in a nonfasting patient or in one with chronic cholecystitis and severe scarring preventing expansion of the gallbladder. A patient with a completely stone-filled gallbladder, with a previous cholecystectomy, or with congenital absence of a gallbladder may also have a nonvisible gallbladder. If the gallbladder is not readily imaged and the patient is clinically stable, additional scanning should be performed several hours later with the patient fasting.

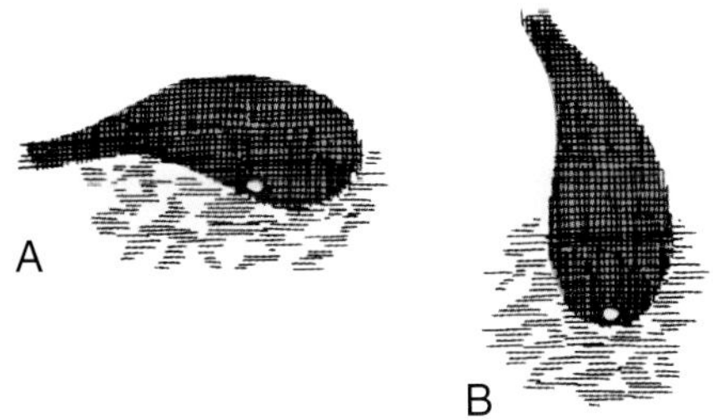

Figure 225-18 **A,** Gallstone is small and shadowing is not seen. **B,** However, it moves when the patient is repositioned.

Additional echogenic structures that can be noted in the gallbladder include folds and septations (very common) or polyps (less common). These are immobile and do not cast shadows. Other possible findings within and around the gallbladder include the following:

- *Increased diameter:* A gallbladder diameter greater than 5 cm may be evidence of cholecystitis.
- *Sludge:* Low-level to mixed echogenic material that is slow to layer out after the patient changes positions may be gallbladder sludge. It most commonly represents biliary stasis and may occur in various conditions (e.g., obstructive jaundice, liver disease, sepsis) or in patients receiving hyperalimentation or certain other medications. It may also precede the formation of gallstones by a few years.
- *Edema:* A thin, dark line of fluid around the gallbladder wall may represent gallbladder edema, which can be found in acute cholecystitis or other conditions such as hypoalbuminemia, hepatitis, and ascites. In the situation where the patient has a sonographic Murphy's sign, discrete pockets of fluid may represent small abscesses. These abscesses are often near the fundus and are definitive evidence of acute cholecystitis.
- *Thickening:* Wall thickening is not specific for acute cholecystitis. The anterior wall is usually the easiest to measure. A rim of diffuse echogenicity greater than 3 mm thick may represent contraction after a recent meal, hepatic dysfunction, congestive heart failure, renal disease, ascites, sepsis, or neoplasms elsewhere (decreased osmotic pressure or elevated portal venous pressure). Patients with acquired immunodeficiency syndrome may also have diffuse thickening. Irregular wall thickening is also common with both acute and chronic cholecystitis. If no stone is present, yet the patient has a positive sonographic Murphy's sign, acalculous cholecystitis is a possibility.
- *Dilated common bile duct:* The normal common bile duct is less than 3 mm in diameter, but it can increase with age by 1 mm per decade without indicating a pathologic process.

Other entities, including hepatic tumors and abnormalities of the pancreas or portal system, would not usually be identified by a limited or focused examination. However, hepatic cysts are common (although not as common as renal cysts), are usually smooth walled, and demonstrate properties of cysts elsewhere. Hepatic malignancies usually demonstrate a variation in density from the normal surrounding tissue, but this can be very subtle.

Obstructive Uropathy, Renal Colic, Hematuria, Renal Abscess

Obstruction of the collecting ducts of the kidney may be acute or chronic and unilateral or bilateral. Renal failure due to obstruction may be relatively asymptomatic, so an ultrasonographic study may be helpful, especially in those at risk (e.g., older man with benign prostatic hyperplasia). As much as 15% of American men will experience an episode of renal colic severe enough to require emergent medical attention. With flank pain and hematuria being the hallmark signs and symptoms for a stone, if a small stone is identified and the patient responds to analgesics, expectant management may be adequate. If available, real-time spiral CT scanning using a stone protocol has somewhat become the diagnostic procedure of choice for identifying stones. If a spiral CT is not available, studies have found that plain radiographs (KUB: kidney, ureter, and bladder) rarely change the clinician's management of renal colic. Intravenous pyelograms (IVPs) can be used when direct imaging of the urinary tract is necessary. Studies comparing sensitivity of ultrasonography and IVP have found them to be relatively comparable. However, most studies have found IVP to be somewhat more specific. Nonetheless, in certain situations, ultrasonography may be preferred over IVP (Box 225-2). Even if ultrasonography does not reveal the

Box 225-2. Conditions in Which Ultrasonography May Be Preferable to Intravenous Pyelography

- Dehydration
- Contrast allergy
- Diabetes mellitus
- Differential diagnosis includes dissecting aortic aneurysm or acute cholecystitis
- Inadequate abdominal preparation for intravenous pyelography
- Poor venous access
- Pregnancy
- Renal failure or proteinuria
- Time constraints

diagnosis, at least it is noninvasive and certainly can be followed up with an IVP.

Evaluation of hematuria in the asymptomatic person probably warrants cystoscopy (see Chapter 111, Diagnostic Cystourethroscopy); however, it may warrant an ultrasonographic scan, even though evaluating all of the possible sources requires considerable ultrasonographic experience. The patient with a possible renal abscess (e.g., fever from pyelonephritis defervesced on IV antibiotics for a few days and then spiked again) may also benefit from ultrasonography, especially in the area of the original flank pain. Scanning the patient for possible renal trauma is discussed with the FAST examination.

NOTE: A leaking or dissecting AAA may produce signs and symptoms similar to left-sided renal colic, including hematuria. In fact, left-sided renal colic is the most common misdiagnosis in elderly patients with a symptomatic AAA. In patients older than 55 years of age with left-sided renal colic, CT or ultrasonography should be considered to exclude this potentially fatal diagnosis that may be missed with an IVP.

Preprocedure Patient Preparation

Under optimal conditions, the patient should have been in the fasting state for at least 8 hours to minimize bowel gas. Early-morning scanning may be preferable; bowel gas is usually minimal. Understanding that patients do not always come to the hospital or the office under these conditions, the clinician may need to hydrate the patient to increase hydronephrosis and enhance the acoustic window. Therefore, administering IV fluids may be not only therapeutic but helpful for making the diagnosis.

Technique

1. Scan the patient in the supine position, longitudinally, with a low-frequency probe until the kidney is located. Kidneys are football shaped with a white stripe (echogenic renal sinus) down the middle. The renal sinus is surrounded by the echolucent renal cortex, which in turn is surrounded by the echogenic renal capsule (Fig. 225-19A). Compared with other abdominal organs, the kidneys are very posterior and lateral organs. On the right, the kidney is located at the posterior inferior edge of the liver, far lateral to the mid-clavicular line. Prolonged deep inspiration by the patient should bring the liver edge down from under the subcostal margin to improve the window and facilitate locating the kidney. Scanning between the ribs may also be necessary to obtain a good window through the liver.
2. The left kidney is located slightly higher than the right. On the left, the same maneuvers may enhance the use of the spleen as an acoustic window. Having the patient turn completely onto his or her right side to facilitate scanning in the coronal and transverse planes may also be helpful. Even scanning between

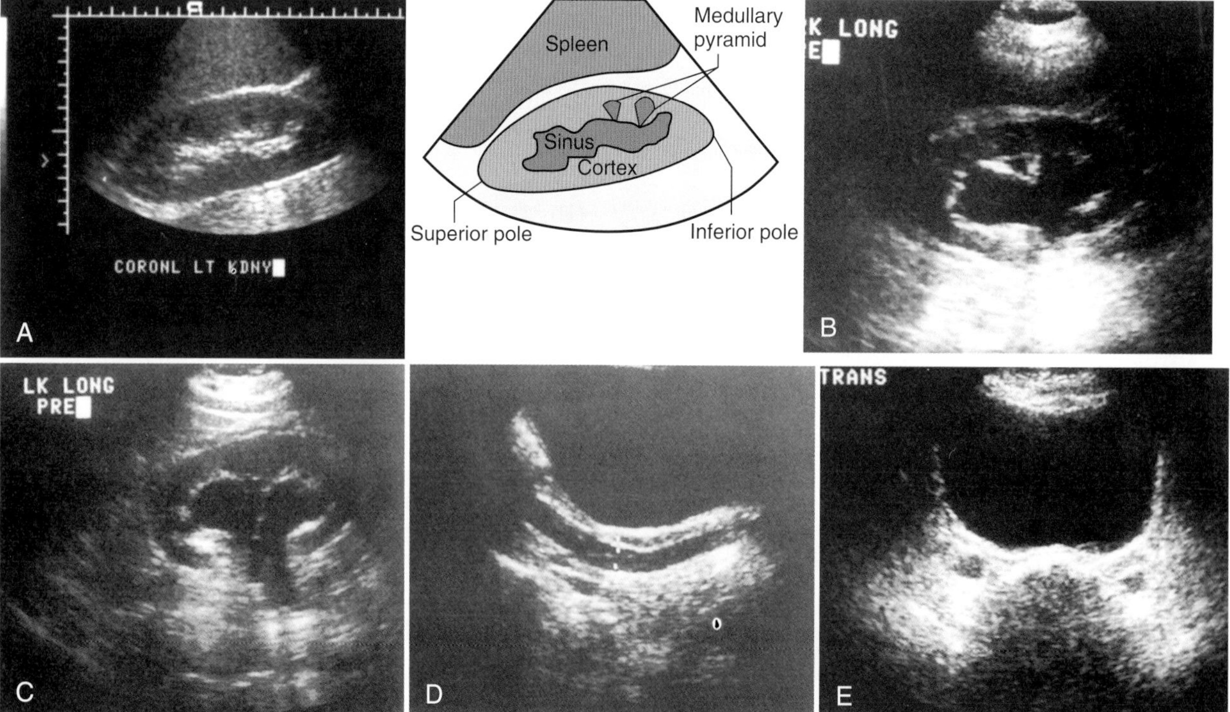

Figure 225-19 Longitudinal view of the left kidney (**A**), including inferior and superior poles. Pseudohydronephrosis of both kidneys (**B** and **C**) and ureters (**D**) associated with a full bladder (**E**). (**A,** From Simon BC, Snoey ER [eds]: Ultrasound in Emergency and Ambulatory Medicine. St. Louis, Mosby, 1997. **B,** From Hagen-Ansert SL [ed]: Textbook of Diagnostic Ultrasonography, 4th ed. St. Louis, Mosby, 1995.)

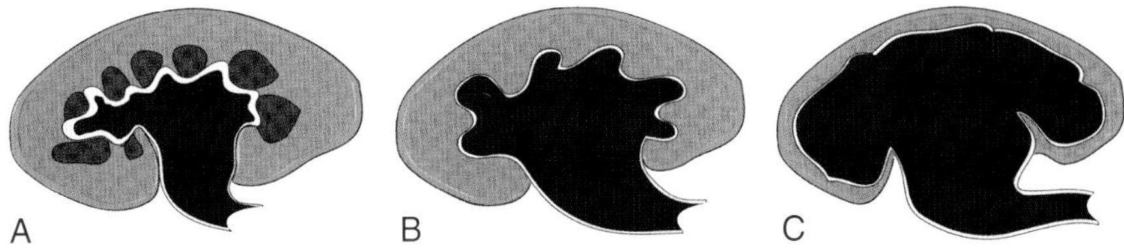

Figure 225-20 **A,** Mild hydronephrosis. Note hydroureters. **B,** Moderate hydronephrosis. **C,** Severe hydronephrosis.

the ribs from the back may be useful. Occasionally, having the patient sit in the erect position will bring the kidney into view. If no kidney is found on the left side, attempt to locate the kidney by scanning the pelvis for a pelvic kidney or the midline for a horseshoe kidney.

3. After locating each kidney, with the probe in the longitudinal position, obtain a long-axis view. Rotate the probe out of the longitudinal plane of the body until the maximal length of the organ is visualized.
4. Attempt to assess for the presence or absence of hydronephrosis or hydroureter in both kidneys. Also attempt to locate any other intrarenal or extrarenal fluid collections, masses, or calcifications. The bladder should be scanned (see the section on Ultrasonographic Evaluation of the Bladder), especially if there is hydronephrosis or hydroureter.

Interpretation

Because most episodes of renal colic are caused by small stones (2 to 4 mm), it is uncommon to actually visualize the stone. The confirmation of renal colic is usually made by demonstrating hydronephrosis or hydroureter in the correct clinical setting (flank pain, hematuria). Associated intrarenal calcifications further support the diagnosis. However, absence of hydronephrosis does not exclude the possibility of a stone; it may be small or have already passed.

The normal ureter is rarely visualized with the bedside ultrasonographic examination, so demonstration of a dark, fluid-filled ureter (hydroureter) is usually abnormal. With accumulation of additional fluid, as seen in hydronephrosis, the normal echogenic renal sinus stripe may actually be split by fluid, appearing as an intervening dark stripe. Along with this intervening stripe, the full appearance of hydronephrosis is characterized by increased fluid throughout the kidney, often contiguous with the hydroureter. Make sure the patient has voided before the sonographic examination because a very full or overdistended bladder can cause pseudohydronephrosis, which appears identical to mild or moderate hydronephrosis (Fig. 225-19B and C). Dehydration may also mask hydronephrosis, so IV hydration may be necessary before the scan.

When hydronephrosis is noted, an attempt should be made to follow the hydroureter(s) distally to the source of the obstruction. When associated with hydronephrosis, an echogenic structure found as the source of an obstruction, with or without prominent posterior shadowing, is diagnostic of urolithiasis. A stone larger than 3 mm should be highly echogenic and cast a well-defined shadow. With a good acoustic window and minimal bowel gas, the ureterovesical junction may be visualized and is a common place to find stones; stones commonly lodge at this level. Occasionally a stone will have passed this junction and be found in the bladder. Even if a stone cannot be located distally, scanning the kidney may reveal intrarenal calcifications. As mentioned previously, intrarenal calcifications associated with hydroureter support the diagnosis of renal colic due to a stone.

With moderate chronic hydronephrosis there is thinning of the renal medulla (Fig. 225-20A). With severe, long-standing, chronic hydronephrosis, there may also be thinning of the renal cortex (Fig. 225-20B and C). If bilateral obstructions are found, they are more likely due to an obstruction at the bladder outlet. In this situation, the bladder will be distended, should be easily scanned, and should be scanned carefully for the source of obstruction. One system grades hydronephrosis as mild or grade I (any hydronephrosis up to grade II), moderate/grade II (renal sinus is split and confluent with calyces), or severe/grade III (causing effacement of renal parenchyma).

Hydronephrosis can be a normal finding in pregnancy, especially on the right side. Renal cysts may also mimic hydronephrosis. With ultrasonography, simple renal cysts appear like cysts elsewhere in the body. They have smooth borders and no echogenic material within them. Renal cysts are common, occurring in 50% of individuals older than 50 years of age. As opposed to hydronephrosis, renal cysts are well circumscribed and do not communicate with fluid outside the kidney (see Fig. 225-17). Renal cell carcinoma, which may appear as an echogenic mass in the kidney, can also cause hematuria. Transitional cell carcinoma can be seen as a mass anywhere along the length of a ureter or in the bladder. Fluid around the capsule, which appears as a dark stripe and can be irregular, may represent a perinephric abscess or, in the trauma patient, hemoperitoneum or a hematoma; hence, clinical correlation will be important.

Suspected Abdominal Aortic Aneurysm

Unlike coronary artery disease and cerebrovascular disease, the incidence and associated mortality rate of AAAs continue to increase. Men are affected three to four times more frequently than women. The prevalence of AAA has climbed to 10% in people older than 65 years of age, and ruptured AAA has also become the 10th leading cause of death in men older than the age of 55 years.

The natural history of an AAA is to expand at a rate of 0.21 to 0.4 cm/year. Over 5 years, a 4-cm AAA has a 10% chance of rupture, a 5-cm aneurysm an 18% chance, and a 6-cm aneurysm a 30% or greater likelihood of rupturing. Controlling blood pressure and cessation of smoking may diminish the risk of rupture. At all comparable sizes, women may have a higher risk of rupture. Elective repair in most large centers has a mortality risk of less than 5%, compared with up to 80% in those patients who live long enough to reach the operating room after rupture. Therefore, elective resection is indicated for low- to moderate-risk patients with aneurysms that measure more than 5 cm in diameter.

Risk Factors

- Male sex.
- 50 years of age or older.
- Use of tobacco.
- Hypertension.
- Family history of AAA.*
- Other atherosclerotic risk factors may also be AAA risk factors.

The classic triad of ruptured AAA is pulsatile abdominal mass; low back, flank, or abdominal pain; and hypotension. Less than 50% of victims, however, possess this triad, and less than 25% are hypotensive on admission. Unfortunately, low back, flank, or abdominal pain is a frequent complaint for patients in the age group at risk for AAA. Patients with a leaking AAA may have many other signs and symptoms as well, including chest pain, ecchymoses, or a scrotal

*Family history is most significant when a female relative has been diagnosed. Elastinolytic enzymes, decreased type III collagen, decreased elastin, and other biochemical variants are being studied to determine what is probably a multifactorially inherited etiology.

mass. The most common incorrect diagnosis in an elderly patient with a symptomatic AAA is left-sided renal colic. A leaking AAA may even be associated with hematuria; therefore any elderly patient with left-sided renal colic should be considered to have an AAA until proven otherwise.

Most aortic aneurysms are found in the mid-abdomen, just above the iliac bifurcation (about the level of the umbilicus). Physical examination is extremely inaccurate for diagnosing AAA. Aortography may underestimate the size of an aneurysm if it is filled with thrombus or is dissecting, and lateral radiographs overestimate the possibility and size. Ultrasonography has been shown to be accurate in identifying both aneurysmal and normal aortas, especially infrarenally. For screening, ultrasonography is comparable with CT scanning, which is the gold standard for both diagnosis and estimation of size. However, ultrasonography may be a difficult study if there is a large amount of bowel gas, retained barium, or marked obesity. In addition, CT scanning is better than ultrasonography for identifying a leaking aneurysm, although ultrasonography may be useful when there is not enough time to perform a CT scan (emergent situation).

Preprocedure Patient Preparation

Under optimal conditions, the patient should have fasted for at least 8 hours to minimize bowel gas. Early-morning scanning may also be preferable because bowel gas is usually minimal. Patients do not always present to the primary care clinician under these conditions; however, if a pulsatile mass is palpable through the anterior abdominal wall, it should be readily scannable. The patient should be informed of possible diagnoses and the indication for scanning.

Technique

1. With a low-frequency probe and the patient in the supine position, attempt to define the general outline of the aorta with longitudinal scanning (Fig. 225-21). It is thick walled and pulsating. The inferior vena cava runs parallel and may be transmitting pulsations, but will be thin walled and will collapse with inspiration and distend with a Valsalva maneuver. If a pulsatile mass is palpated, it should not be difficult to determine whether it is contiguous with the abdominal aorta. If the aorta cannot be identified with longitudinal scanning, rotate the probe for a transverse scan and the aorta will often be revealed slightly anterior and to the left of the patient's vertebral body. A transverse view of the inferior vena cava will be noted to the patient's right (to the left of the image).
2. After defining the general outline, measurements should be taken of the largest AP diameter on transverse scanning at 1 to 2 cm increments from immediately below the diaphragm (at level of xiphoid) to a level 3 cm below the umbilicus. Measurements are taken from the outside wall to the opposite outside wall. Be aware that the transverse diameter of the aorta on a transverse scan may be exaggerated if the aorta is tangentially imaged when it makes a lateral turn. In addition, avoid applying too much probe pressure, which can also distort AP measurements. That being said, both AP and lateral transverse diameters should be measured because the lateral diameter of an AAA is often larger than the AP diameter. The lateral diameter may be slightly more difficult to obtain because the AP walls and diameter are usually more sharply demarcated.
3. If there is considerable truncal obesity or overlying bowel gas, increased surface pressure with the probe may enhance visualization. Immediately below the xiphoid, the liver can often be used as a window, especially if the patient suspends breathing briefly after a deep inspiration. Despite these maneuvers, bowel gas frequently obscures a 4- or 5-cm segment between the xiphoid and umbilicus. Using a rocking motion with the probe and scanning from above and below this segment may allow for a complete, systematic evaluation of the entire abdominal aorta. Turning the patient to the right or left lateral decubitus position may enhance scanning the aorta in the area of the kidneys, although the iliac bifurcation may not be visible unless the liver or spleen is enlarged. With the patient in the left lateral decubitus position (left side down), scanning intercostally from the right mid-axillary line may reveal the aorta lying "deep" to the inferior vena cava. Alternatively, placing the probe in the left paraumbilical region may allow evaluation of the distal aorta.

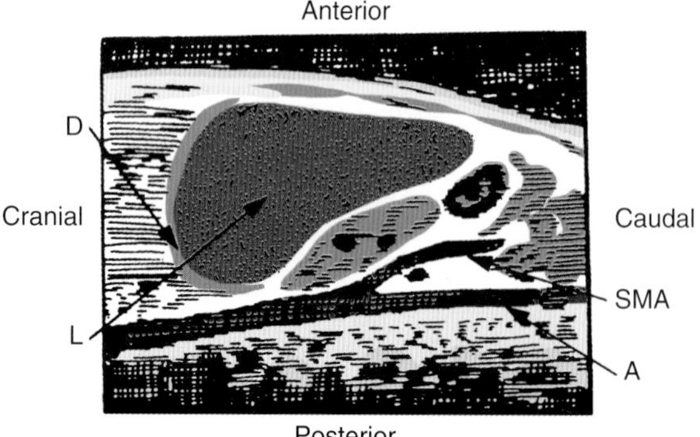

Figure 225-21 Longitudinal scan slightly to the left of the midline showing normal structures and orientation. A, aorta; D, diaphragm; L, liver; SMA, superior mesenteric artery.

Interpretation

With normal anatomy, mean abdominal aortic diameters are approximately equal in males and females during the second decade of life: 12.2 mm and 12.3 mm, respectively. By the eighth decade, the mean diameter increases to 22.8 mm in men and 16.9 mm in women. An AAA is defined by an aortic diameter of greater than 3 cm in a man and greater than 2.5 cm in a woman, or an enlargement of greater than 0.5 cm throughout the length of the aorta (the normal aorta tapers and decreases in diameter as it descends to its bifurcation). Surgery should be considered for any patient with symptoms compatible with an acute AAA and meeting these definitions because he or she is at risk for rupture.

If an AAA is found (Fig. 225-22) and the patient is hemodynamically stable, the clinician should attempt to determine whether branching vessels are involved and whether there is free intraperitoneal (in the manner of the FAST examination; see the section on Trauma) or retroperitoneal fluid (although ultrasonography is not always reliable for diagnosing retroperitoneal hemorrhage). Usually located along the left side of the spine or anterior to a kidney, the presence of fluid may indicate a ruptured or leaking aneurysm; surgical consultation should be obtained immediately. It should be noted that the lack of free intraperitoneal fluid does not rule out an acute AAA because the majority of acute AAAs present without free intraperitoneal fluid. If no fluid is visualized and the patient is hemodynamically stable, a CT scan may be useful to check for retroperitoneal hemorrhage. CT angiography and magnetic resonance angiography are best for delineating whether other arteries are involved. Again, surgery should be considered in any patient with persistent abdominal pain and a known AAA. At the same time, because AAAs are common in older patients, just because a patient has a new or known AAA does not guarantee it is the source of symptoms. Stents are now offered as an alternative (and probably safer choice) for patients with asymptomatic AAAs, especially those greater than 5 cm.

Most AAAs are fusiform and extend over a segment of the aorta; however, saccular aneurysms are often confined to a short segment. Therefore, to avoid overlooking an AAA, all segments of the aorta should be scanned methodically and systematically.

Echogenic material in the lumen may represent a thrombus or dissection. Alternatively, the clinician should check the gain setting elsewhere on the aorta to make sure it is not artifact. Large para-

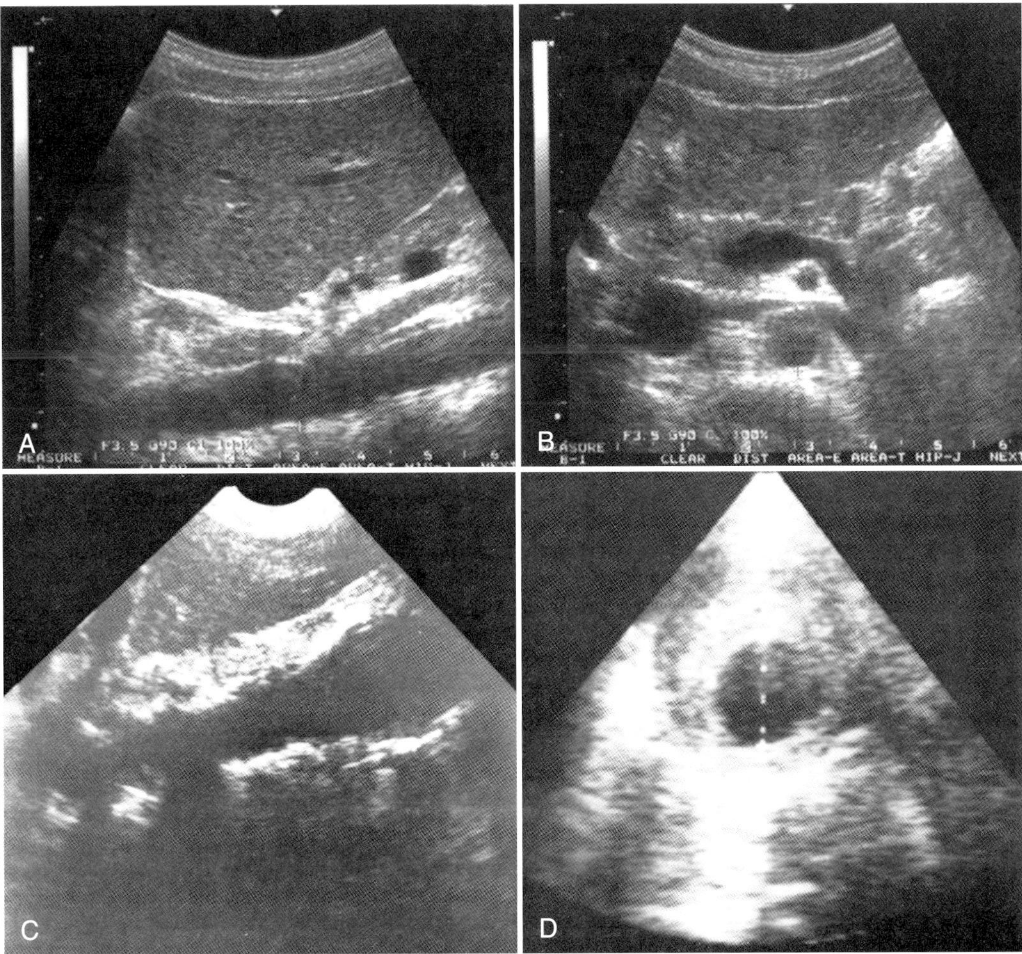

Figure 225-22 **A,** Longitudinal view of an abdominal aortic aneurysm (AAA). **B,** Transverse view of an AAA. **C,** Longitudinal view of intrarenal AAA. **D,** Transverse view of a rupturing AAA with thrombus. (**A** and **B,** From Simon BC, Snoey ER [eds]: Ultrasound in Emergency and Ambulatory Medicine. St. Louis, Mosby, 1997. **C** and **D,** From Heller M, Jehle D [eds]: Ultrasound in Emergency Medicine. Philadelphia, WB Saunders, 1995.)

aortic lymph nodes (usually anterior, but may be posterior and even displace the aorta away from the vertebrae) may be confused with the aorta or an AAA. However, compared with the aorta, nodes are usually irregular and nodular; color Doppler will demonstrate an absence of blood flow.

Trauma

Studies indicate that physical examination fails to reveal significant injuries in 25% to 40% of trauma patients. Although a spiral CT scan may detect damage to abdominal organs, free fluid released from injured organs has long been used as a marker for significant injury. Over these years in the United States, diagnosis of intraperitoneal blood was made almost exclusively with diagnostic peritoneal lavage (DPL; see Chapter 204, Diagnostic Peritoneal Lavage). However, after dozens of prospective, controlled studies demonstrated the accuracy of ultrasonography for detection of hemoperitoneum, diagnostic techniques changed, first in Europe and Japan, and then in the United States. Investigators demonstrated that in the hands of capable, properly trained personnel, the sensitivity of ultrasonography for diagnosing hemoperitoneum was at least as great as that of DPL. In recent years, the FAST (focused assessment with sonography for trauma) examination was developed, which also includes a quick scan of the heart and pleural space. (See also the Miscellaneous section for a brief discussion of scanning for rib fractures or pneumothorax.) The indications for the FAST examination include but are not limited to traumatic injury to the torso. Not only is such rapidly available diagnostic information very valuable in the emergency department, it may be very useful for triage in the setting of mass casualties or on the battlefield. There are no absolute contraindications to the FAST examination, and the only relative contraindications include morbid obesity, massive subcutaneous emphysema, and extensive abdominal or chest wall trauma because these patients may be difficult to scan. Patients with intra-abdominal fluid due to ascites, peritoneal dialysis, a ventriculoperitoneal shunt, a prior DPL, a ruptured ovarian cyst, or other pelvic inflammatory processes may also be difficult to evaluate. It may also be difficult to detect free fluid in some children and patients with isolated penetrating injury to the torso. The emergent need for laparotomy may be a relative contraindication; however, it may be important to make the diagnosis of pericardial tamponade or hematothorax with the FAST examination before taking such a patient to surgery.

NOTE: Unfortunately, individuals who already have free fluid in the abdomen (e.g., ascites due to alcoholic cirrhosis) are often prone to abdominal trauma, and yet they frequently are not the best candidates for DPL or surgery. Serial ultrasonographic scans can be used in such patients to document rapidly increasing fluid; the decision can then be made whether this is likely due to bleeding and thereby justifies surgery.

Preprocedure Patient Preparation

If the patient is hemodynamically compromised, attempts should be made to stabilize him or her before scanning. A full bladder may enhance scanning. The patient may experience some discomfort when scanning is performed over a contusion. The patient may also be asked to change positions.

Technique

1. If the bladder is about to be emptied, consider proceeding to step 5. The location of initial scanning may also be determined by a history of or evidence of trauma over a particular area. Otherwise, most clinicians scan the RUQ first. This is the most important and easiest region to visualize and is usually the earliest and most accurate for detecting blood. Factors that may affect the sensitivity include the positioning of the patient and a history of prior abdominal surgery or intra-abdominal adhesions. If no fluid is seen in the supine position, Trendelenburg positioning may increase the sensitivity. Scan the patient's RUQ longitudinally with a low-frequency probe until you locate the right kidney. It is quite lateral and behind the organ used as a window, the liver. If the kidney is not immediately visible and the patient is conscious, have him or her inspire and briefly suspend breathing to bring the liver down. This often provides a better window and pushes bowel gas out of the way. If not, it may be necessary to scan between the ribs. The probe may need to be turned counterclockwise out of the longitudinal orientation to scan between the ribs. The probe may also need to be moved as far posterior as the posterior axillary line if bowel gas is interfering. The potential space located between the liver and the kidney is Morison's pouch (Fig. 225-23), also known as the *hepatorenal space*. This area, as well as the other spaces, should be scanned meticulously and in at least two perpendicular planes to rule out even a small collection of fluid.
2. If no fluid is seen in Morison's pouch, three additional potential spaces should be scanned in the RUQ. By angling the probe cephalad and using a gentle rocking motion, the pleural space above the echogenic diaphragm can usually be seen. The diaphragm will be moving with inspiration and expiration. Fluid above the diaphragm indicates either a hemothorax or a preexisting fluid collection (e.g., pleural effusion, empyema); fluid below it, in the subphrenic space, indicates intra-abdominal fluid. The potential space immediately below the kidney should also be scanned; it is actually an extension of Morison's pouch from above and the right paracolic gutter below.
3. Next, with the marker dot turned to the patient's right side, the probe should be moved to the midline and angled upward for a subxiphoid (subcostal) view of the heart and pericardium. The probe should be angled toward the patient's left scapula or even higher on the back, almost horizontal or parallel to the patient's bed. Again, the liver is usually used as a window. The area around the heart should be searched for fluid (usually located posteriorly, and possibly extending laterally) or evidence of tamponade. Avoid confusing a dark stripe due to pericardial fat pads, a pericardial cyst, or the descending thoracic aorta with a pericardial effusion. Scanning in more than one plane will usually help define the aorta. (See the section on Cardiac Ultrasonography for a discussion of subxiphoid scanning as well as alternative windows to use, such as the parasternal and apical windows, in case the subxiphoid view cannot be used owing to local trauma or body habitus.) Also, if pericardial fluid is noted, an attempt should be made to determine whether the patient has a diagnosis that could be associated with a preexisting effusion.
4. The probe should then be moved to the left upper quadrant (LUQ). Scan it longitudinally and survey the same four potential spaces that were scanned around the right kidney. The area should be scanned meticulously and the probe rotated to scan in at least two perpendicular planes to rule out small pockets of fluid. Scan the areas around the left kidney and spleen, the space between the kidney and spleen (splenorenal space), the pleural space above the diaphragm, the subphrenic space, and the space below the left kidney. The splenorenal ligament on the left side may prevent accumulation of fluid in the splenorenal space, so scanning the other areas around the spleen becomes more important. Similar to the right side, the space below the left kidney is an extension of the splenorenal space from above and the paracolic gutter below. Realizing that the spleen is smaller than the liver and often more difficult to locate, use modest inspiration to bring it down to facilitate a window. If subcostal scanning does not provide an adequate window, intercostal scanning may be necessary. Rotate the probe counterclockwise to fit between the ribs. Because it is even more likely that bowel gas will interfere when scanning the LUQ, the clinician needs to be very patient when scanning, rocking the probe gently. The probe may need to be moved even more laterally than on the patient's right side, beyond the posterior axillary line to the flank or the back.

   NOTE: Scanning the paracolic gutters requires considerable sonographic experience. When scanning immediately beneath the kidneys, windows from above are usually available; however, when attempting to scan inferiorly, windows next to the iliac crests may be more difficult to locate. Large amounts of fluid surrounding the bowel may facilitate scanning; however, it usually requires more experience to be comfortable with declaring an absence of fluid. Although studies indicate that scanning this area only minimally improves the sensitivity, such scanning significantly increases the time required. Clinicians should also be aware that scanning these areas increases the number of false-positive findings because of confusion of soft tissue for fluid.

5. If the preceding scans are negative and the patient remains stable, the region of the pelvic cul de sac can be scanned after placing the patient in the reverse Trendelenburg or sitting position. Scan transversely by placing the probe immediately above the suprapubic bone, turning the marker dot toward the patient's right side, and angling the probe downward into the pelvis. Rock it gently and scan meticulously all planes of tissue from the dome of the bladder to the inferior aspect of the cul de sac. The marker dot can then be turned cephalad for a longitudinal scan, which sometimes allows a better appreciation of the pelvic anatomy. If time allows, a full bladder increases the sensitivity of scanning in this area; however, adequate views can often be obtained with a partly full bladder, especially if there are large amounts of blood. Conversely, if the bladder is empty, small amounts of blood in the cul de sac may be missed. In women, transvaginal scanning replaces the need for a full bladder and is exquisitely sensitive for free fluid (capable of visualizing as little as 5 mL).
6. If the patient remains stable, serial scans may be helpful for detection of newly accumulating fluid. Conversely, if the patient suddenly becomes unstable, another scan may locate the cause.

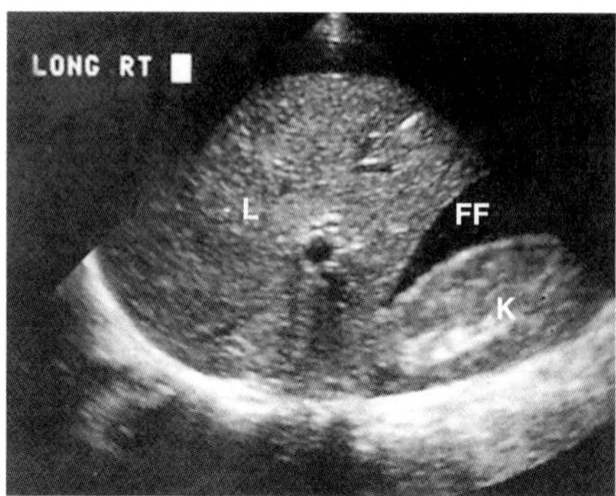

Figure 225-23 Fluid in Morison's pouch or hemoperitoneum. FF, free fluid; K, right kidney; L, liver. (From Simon BC, Snoey ER [eds]: Ultrasound in Emergency and Ambulatory Medicine. St. Louis, Mosby, 1997.)

Interpretation

The entire examination can be performed very rapidly, with all four areas being scanned in less than 5 minutes. Intraperitoneal blood in small amounts usually first accumulates lateral to the right kidney. Fresh, unclotted blood has the same appearance as any free fluid in the abdomen. In the setting of a patient with a possible hemoperitoneum, the appearance of free fluid as a "dark stripe" is diagnostic (Fig. 225-24, and see Fig. 225-23) or a positive examination. As little as 10 mL has been diagnosed in the upper abdomen with transabdominal scanning; however, studies indicate the usual threshold for diagnosing hemoperitoneum is 500 mL. Therefore, a negative FAST examination does not preclude early or slowly bleeding injuries. A 1-cm fluid stripe roughly corresponds to 1 L of intra-abdominal fluid. Again, Morison's pouch in the RUQ is one of the most sensitive areas to find fluid.

In the setting of trauma, the spleen is the most commonly injured abdominal organ. In the LUQ, fluid does not always accumulate between the spleen and the kidney; it can be located between the spleen and the abdominal wall. Conversely, it may completely surround the spleen (Fig. 225-24). Spontaneous rupture of the spleen occurs occasionally, such as in teenagers or individuals in their early twenties after an Epstein-Barr virus infection (mononucleosis). In that situation, fluid will usually be found surrounding the spleen.

Free fluid in the abdomen may also be due to urine or bile and denote injury to the urinary or biliary tract, respectively. With large amounts of blood, fluid may be visible from almost anywhere in the abdomen or pelvis. It may accumulate as fluid in the cul de sac (see Fig. 225-12). As soon as the clotting process begins, blood may produce variable echoes as the fibrin and degenerating cells become more prominent. As clotting progresses further, which can occur rapidly, the fluid may develop the sonographic qualities of soft tissue; however, such an accumulation of soft tissue is unusual in dependent areas such as the cul de sac.

Avoid confusing fluid in the stomach or bowels as free fluid; search for the peristalsis associated with this fluid. Likewise, avoid confusing a dark stripe due to perinephric fat with free fluid. Obese patients may have a significant amount of such hypoechoic perinephric fat. However, fat tends to accumulate along the upper and lateral aspect of the kidney, whereas fluid often completely surrounds the kidney. Comparison with the opposite kidney may demonstrate a similar accumulation of fat, confirming the false-positive result. Patients with multiple abdominal surgical scars and adhesions may accumulate fluid in different patterns and locations because the normal flow of fluid in the abdomen (Fig. 225-25) is disrupted.

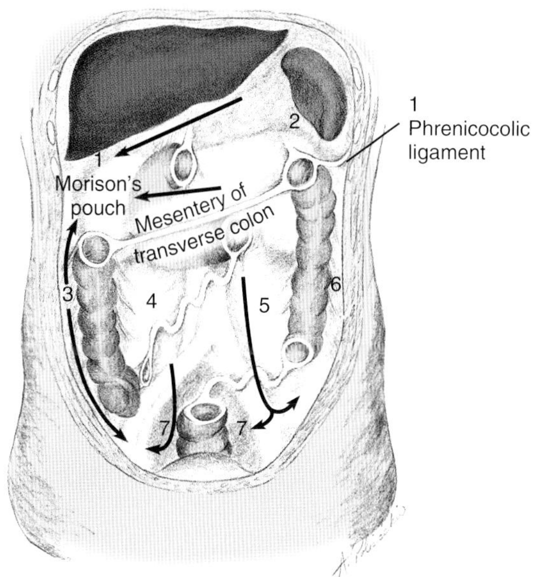

Figure 225-25 Posterior peritoneum and reflections, indicating potential sites of intra-abdominal fluid localization and spread. 1 and 2, Right and left supramesocolic regions—above the transverse mesocolon and separated by the ridge of the lumbar spine; 3, right paracolic gutter; 4, right inframesocolic gutter; 5, left inframesocolic gutter; 6, left paracolic gutter; 7, pelvic cul de sac. *Arrows* indicate movement of free fluid (hemorrhage). (From Simon BC, Snoey ER [eds]: Ultrasound in Emergency and Ambulatory Medicine. St. Louis, Mosby, 1997.)

Likewise, adhesions in the chest may result in fluid accumulating in areas other than a dependent location.

After examining all four areas for free fluid, the liver, spleen, and kidney capsules and the parenchyma should be reexamined for disruption or hematoma. After a recent hepatic, renal, or splenic contusion, if an intracapsular hematoma accumulates it will usually appear cystic with irregular borders. A renal or splenic contusion with a ruptured capsule often appears as fluid surrounding either the kidney or spleen. Keep in mind it is more difficult to evaluate the spleen for such injuries because the spleen is normally hypoechoic in texture. Consequently, large intraparenchymal and subcapsular splenic injuries can be missed. To avoid missing clinically significant splenic injuries, the ultrasound, along with a hematocrit, should be repeated in 2 to 3 hours or if there is a change in vital signs. As it turns out, a negative FAST examination does not exclude most solid organ, mesenteric vascular, hollow viscus, or diaphragmatic injuries. Major disruptions of the capsules of all of these organs can be missed by ultrasonography; spiral CT scanning is more likely to diagnose such injuries.

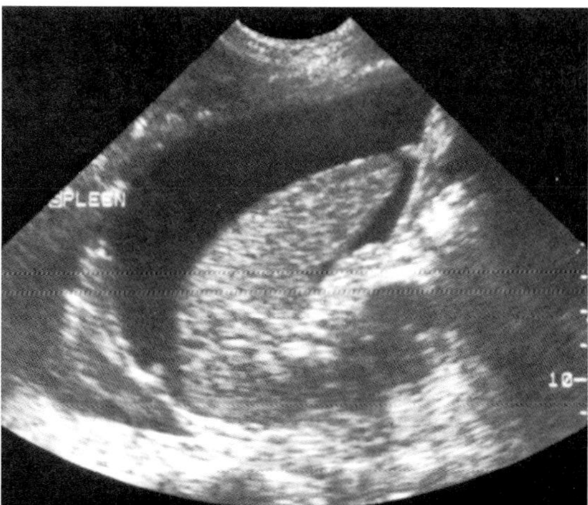

Figure 225-24 Free fluid in the left upper quadrant. (From Heller M, Jehle D [eds]: Ultrasound in Emergency Medicine. Philadelphia, WB Saunders, 1995.)

MISCELLANEOUS

There are many applications being used and further studied for ultrasonography in the emergency department, hospitalist, and office settings. For example, one published study found that rib fractures can be accurately diagnosed with ultrasonography. The entire outline of the affected ribs was scanned with high-frequency ultrasonography, searching for breaks in the normal smooth cortex. Accuracy, in certain situations, was better than that found with radiographs. Use of ultrasonography also spared the patient from radiation exposure. A pneumothorax may also be detected by scanning the rib interspaces anteriorly and longitudinally in the midclavicular line using a high-frequency probe. In the normal lung, pleural sliding should be noted in the somewhat superficial visceral–parietal pleural interface during respiration. Absence of normal pleural sliding suggests separation of the visceral and parietal pleura due to pneumothorax. Although the following section is certainly not all-inclusive, it lists some of the indications in the emergency department, hospital, or office for which an ultrasonographic application has been either studied or published.

Suspected Deep Venous Thrombosis

See Chapter 88, Noninvasive Venous and Arterial Studies of the Lower Extremities. Even when duplex equipment is available, compression ultrasonographic scanning using the high-frequency probe should be the initial study performed in most cases.

Ultrasonographic Evaluation of the Bladder

Up to 8% of infants younger than 8 weeks of age in the emergency department with a temperature of 100.6° F or higher have a urinary tract infection (UTI). As much as 5% of infants younger than 2 years of age with unexplained fever have UTIs. The rate is 8% in girls and uncircumcised boys but less than 1% in circumcised boys. White girls have a much higher rate (up to 15%) than black girls. Boys are at the highest risk during the first 3 to 6 months of life.

Using an evidence-based approach, in those infants or children sufficiently ill to warrant immediate antibiotic therapy, the practice parameter of the American Academy of Pediatrics (AAP) recommends either SPA or transurethral catheterization to obtain a urine specimen. In those not sufficiently ill to require immediate antibiotics, the same diagnostic approach can be used; however, another option is available. If a urinalysis obtained by the most convenient means indicates a UTI, a sterile urine specimen should then be obtained in the same manner as listed earlier. These recommendations are based on a summary of the evidence and good clinical judgment; however, although a negative culture from a bagged specimen effectively rules out UTI, culture results are not available immediately. Bagged specimen cultures are also rarely negative, and unfortunately culture results cannot be predicted from urinalysis in most cases. Therefore, many clinicians opt for SPA or catheterization.

Although catheterization is less invasive than SPA, the process of catheterization may actually cause a UTI. SPA is inherently invasive, yet few serious complications have been reported, and numerous studies have demonstrated the superiority of SPA over alternative techniques. Limiting SPA to patients with proven full bladders further minimizes the risk to the infant (see Chapter 183, Pediatric Suprapubic Bladder Aspiration).

In adults, there are indications in the emergency department, hospital, and the office for SPA or suprapubic cannulation (SPC). SPA can be useful for obtaining a urine culture whenever a urethral catheter cannot be placed (or is contraindicated) or may be particularly useful in critically ill, potentially septic, or unresponsive adults. SPC is indicated whenever a urethral catheter is indicated yet cannot or should not be placed (e.g., trauma patients who have serious injury to the urethra, patients who recently underwent bladder or gynecologic surgery, or when a sufficiently wide catheter is unable to be passed through the urethra for diagnostic cystometry; see also Chapter 113, Suprapubic Catheter Insertion and/or Change, and Chapter 114, Suprapubic Tap or Aspiration).

Ultrasonography may also be used in adults to estimate PVR to evaluate the significance or status of urethral obstruction (e.g., significant prostatic hyperplasia) or a neurogenic bladder. PVR can be measured more precisely, albeit more invasively, by inserting a catheter; however, ultrasonography provides reasonable estimates of PVR in a much more comfortable manner with less risk of inducing an infection. Given the fact that recent studies have failed to document an exact level of PVR that would benefit from transurethral resection of the prostate (TURP) as opposed to watchful waiting, PVR estimates from ultrasonography may be more than adequate in that situation (considering TURP).

Preprocedure Patient Preparation

The patient (or his or her parents or caregiver) should be informed about the indication for the study. If a suprapubic tap or cannulation is to be performed, counseling should be given for informed consent.

Technique

1. Infants should be placed in the supine, frog-leg position; adults should be supine. Perform the scanning in a transverse manner with a high-frequency transducer in infants. The marker dot should be directed toward the infant's right side, with the transducer placed slightly above the symphysis pubis. The transducer should be directed posteriorly or slightly caudad to locate the bladder. In adults, a low-frequency probe is used with the transducer and marker dot in the same location. The transducer should be angled in more of a caudal direction.

   NOTE: In infants younger than 2 years of age, the bladder is an abdominal organ. As the pelvis grows, the bladder moves into the pelvis; therefore the transducer should be angled more caudad.

2. Move and angle the probe to locate the maximal transverse diameter of the bladder. In infants, this is the probe location and angle to take measurements for determining whether the bladder is full. Take measurements in both the AP and transverse diameters.
3. For aspiration or cannulation, note the angulation of the probe necessary to locate the maximal transverse diameter of the bladder. Note the depth necessary to penetrate the bladder. The same angulation and depth should be used when directing the aspiration needle or trocar.
4. To estimate bladder volume in an adult, including PVR, three diameters should be determined. First, measure and record the greatest transverse measurement (*w* in Fig. 225-26A). Next, turn the marker dot cephalad and find the longest longitudinal plane. Measure and record the maximal superoinferior measurement (*h* in Fig. 225-26B) in this plane. In the same plane, with that same image, measure and record the maximal AP measurement (Fig. 225-27; see *d* in Fig. 225-26B).

Interpretation and Results

In infants, a pocket of fluid larger than 2 × 2 cm in the retropubic area measured in the AP and maximal transverse diameters defines a "full" bladder (see Fig. 225-27). In adults, the pocket should be much larger in order to reach it with a needle or trocar. Again, SPA

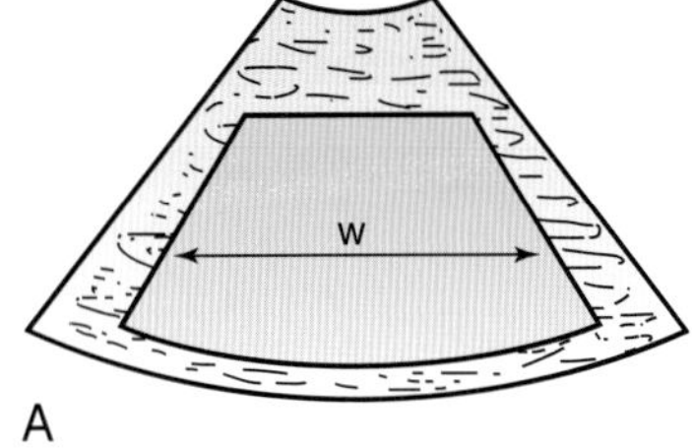

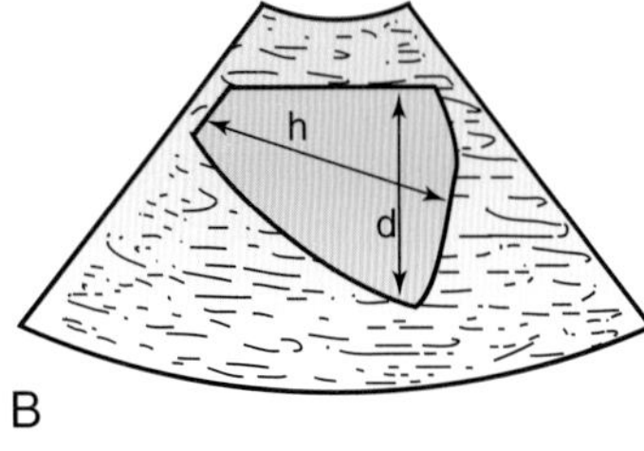

Figure 225-26 **A,** Greatest transverse diameter of bladder is shown by *w*. **B,** Maximal superoinferior measurement is shown by *h*; the maximal anteroposterior measurement is shown by *d*.

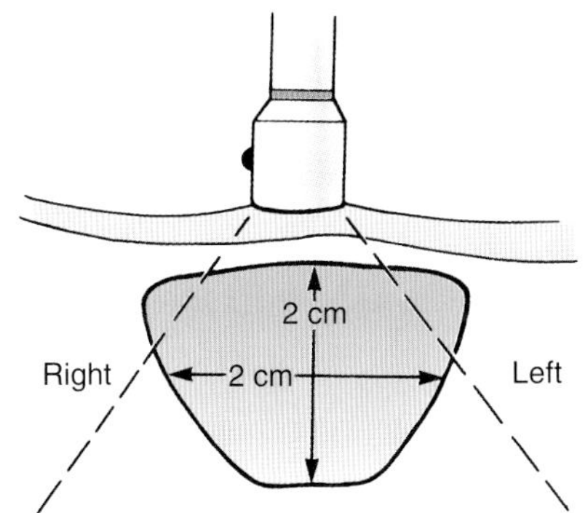

Figure 225-27 Transverse view of a full infant bladder.

or SPC should be attempted at the same angle with which the maximal transverse bladder diameter was measured (Fig. 225-28). One study resulted in obtaining urine in 79% of children meeting these criteria and undergoing aspiration. If the bladder is found to be empty and the patient is clinically stable, repeat scanning to search for a full bladder should be performed 30 minutes to 1 hour after the initial scan. If a full bladder cannot be found on the repeat scan, bladder catheterization should be considered.

In adults, bladder volume can be calculated with this formula:

$$0.7 \times h \times d \times w$$

This yields a standard error of approximately 21%. Although 21% may seem like a large error, as mentioned earlier, it is now known that no certain PVR threshold exists where surgery (TURP) ensures success and avoids future morbidity. For that reason, this crude measurement may be more than adequate. If more precise volumes are needed, more sophisticated formulas are available. In addition, software packages are available for more precise estimates using large machines that can take more precise measurements. Portable ultrasonographic equipment is also available that is used solely for making urologic measurements. Such equipment has been studied extensively and its accuracy has been documented.

Subcutaneous Foreign Bodies

Missed foreign bodies are the second most frequent cause of lawsuits against emergency medicine clinicians. Objects composed of wood, plastic, glass, and vegetable material may not be radiopaque or visible with standard x-ray examinations. Modern military armor is also an example. Most is now fiberglass or cloth and therefore shrapnel is not often visible on routine radiographs. Although fine needles and splinters may be missed, high-frequency ultrasonography is usually helpful not only for confirming the presence of a foreign body but for localization before removal. (See also Chapter 18, Foreign Body Removal from Skin and Soft Tissue, and Chapter 185, Musculoskeletal Ultrasonography.)

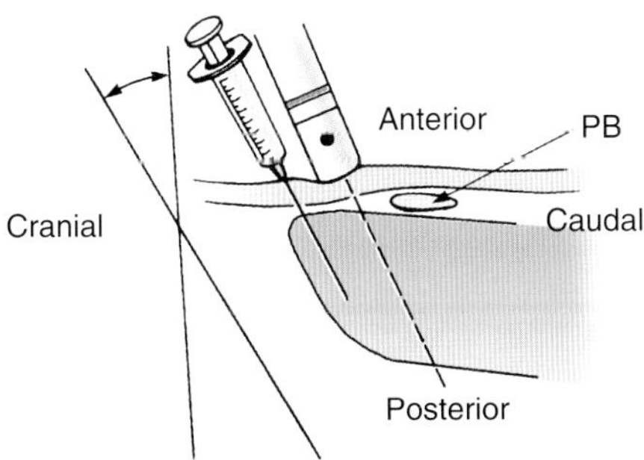

Figure 225-28 Needle should be inserted next to the probe and parallel to whatever angle demonstrated the greatest diameter of the bladder. PB, pubic bone.

Preprocedure Patient Preparation

The patient should be informed about the indication for the study and should understand that not all foreign bodies are visible with either ultrasonography or standard x-ray examinations. If a foreign body is located, the patient should decide whether he or she wants it removed. The patient needs an understanding of the possible complications of removing the object as opposed to not removing the object. (See Chapter 18, Foreign Body Removal from Skin and Soft Tissue.)

Technique

1. In most cases, a high-frequency probe is preferred. For objects very near the skin surface, a standoff pad may be needed to raise the probe several millimeters off the skin. Such a device can either be purchased commercially or created using a latex glove filled with water or acoustic gel. Place the glove or pad on the skin and scan through it with the transducer.
2. Understanding that layers of normal subcutaneous tissue are not always uniform, scan in the area of the possible foreign body. Scan the contralateral "normal" side if unsure of the finding. Scan both longitudinally and transversely, and attempt to clarify the largest dimensions when located.

Interpretation and Results

Foreign bodies may appear as hyperechoic in contrast to the surrounding tissue. If the resolution of the probe is great enough and the foreign body thick enough, an acoustic shadow may also be seen. Metal and glass are more echoic than plastic or wood. Foreign bodies may also be surrounded by a hypoechoic halo representing fluid or inflammation. The exact location of the foreign body should be marked; if it is not round, the predominant direction in which it is lying should be noted. The depth of the object, especially if it is to be removed, should also be noted.

Testicular Mass or Possible Torsion

High-frequency ultrasonography is helpful in diagnosing testicular cancer as well as for differentiating the four most common causes for a scrotal mass: spermatocele, hydrocele, varicocele, and tumor. Transillumination with a bright penlight can often differentiate a spermatocele or hydrocele from other possible causes of a scrotal mass. When there is still a question after transillumination, ultrasonography is the procedure of choice.

Although radioisotope scans have been the procedure of choice for diagnosing a torsioned testicle, they often take hours to obtain, and time is of the essence when making this diagnosis. Because it can be performed fairly rapidly, color Doppler ultrasonography is becoming the diagnostic procedure of choice for testicular torsion.

Preprocedure Patient Preparation

The patient should be informed about the indication for the study. Using a towel, the patient can retract the penis. The testicle and the scrotum are supported by the clinician's hand or by a towel under the scrotum. Either a very cooperative patient or an assistant may be needed to allow the clinician to use both hands for the ultrasonographic equipment.

Technique

1. Using the same orientation as for the rest of the body, first turn the marker dot toward the patient's head for a longitudinal scan. Parallel longitudinal scans should be made with the high-frequency probe about every 5 mm.
2. Next, turn the marker dot toward the patient's right side for a transverse scan. Transverse scans should also be made approximately every 5 mm.

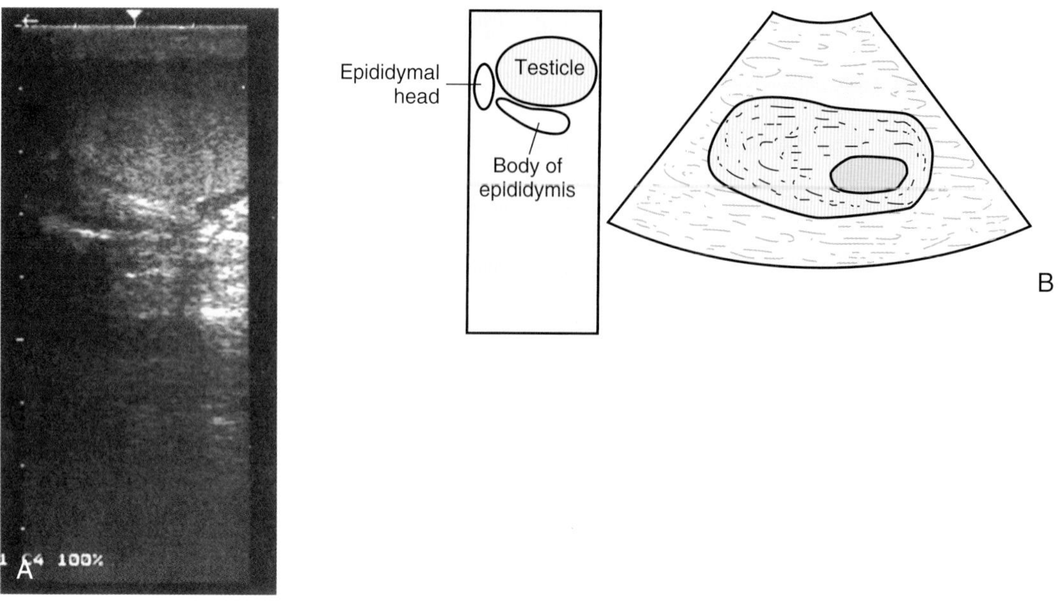

Figure 225-29 **A,** Normal testicular tissue with mediastinum testis. **B,** Testicular mass suspect for cancer. (**A,** From Simon BC, Snoey ER [eds]: Ultrasound in Emergency and Ambulatory Medicine. St. Louis, Mosby, 1997.)

3. The opposite testicle should be scanned, if indicated, or for a comparison for questionable areas. Any palpable abnormalities should be scanned.

Interpretation and Results

Testicles are normally symmetric in size. A small amount of fluid in the scrotal sac is normal. A normal sonographic finding known as the *mediastinum testis* is seen as an echogenic longitudinal central line within the testicle (Fig. 225-29A). The epididymis usually appears as a slightly sonolucent structure posterior to the testes.

A small mass within the testicle is cancer until proven otherwise, especially in a patient younger than 40 years of age (Fig. 225-29B). A seminoma, the most common testicular tumor, usually appears as a hypoechoic mass within the testicle. Teratomas and embryonal cell cancers are usually irregularly echogenic.

Hydroceles, spermatoceles, and varicoceles should all be extratesticular. Spermatoceles are usually found superior to the testicle and attached to the vas deferens. Hydroceles may surround the testicle and are predominantly fluid filled. Varicoceles are usually found in the region of the epididymis, extending superiorly. They will often increase considerably in size with a Valsalva maneuver.

A torsioned testicle often appears enlarged, less dense, and less echogenic compared with the normal testicle (Fig. 225-30A and B). The texture of the ischemic testicle is often blurry, and even sharp intratesticular markings (mediastinum testis) may be diminished. If available, color Doppler (especially spectral Doppler) usually reveals decreased blood flow on the torsioned side. However, flow cannot always be established by certainty with Doppler; if flow cannot be demonstrated in the opposite testicle, a radioisotope scan may be necessary to exclude torsion. If bilateral blood flow is documented and symmetric, the intratesticular markings are sharp and symmetric, and there is a difference in appearance between epididymides, epididymitis on the tender side is the likely diagnosis.

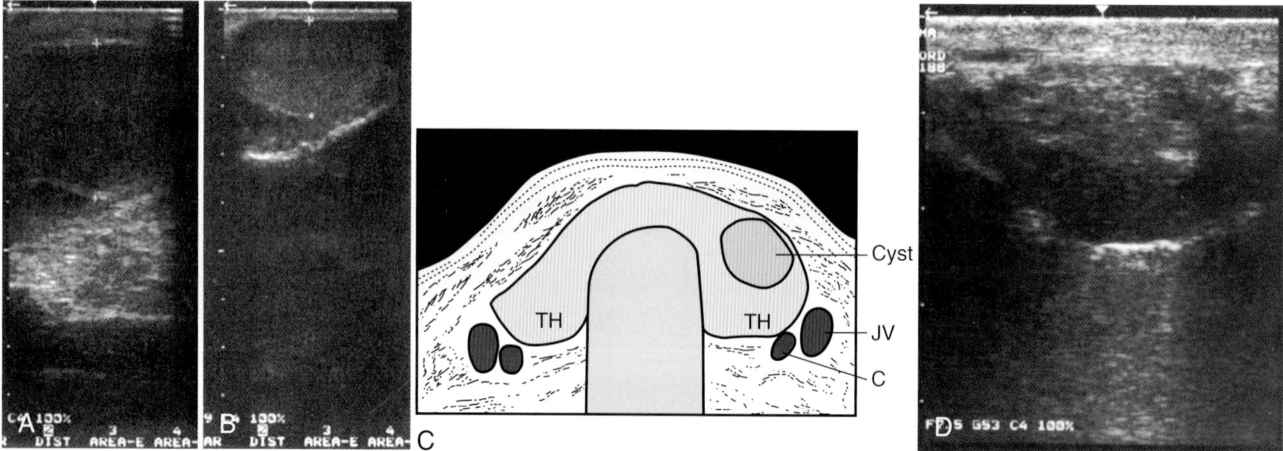

Figure 225-30 **A,** Torsion of right testicle demonstrated by an enlarged, hypoechoic testicle. **B,** Normal left testicle. **C,** Thyroid cyst. C, carotid artery; JV, internal jugular vein; TH, thyroid. **D,** Thyroid mass (adenoma). (**A, B,** and **D,** From Simon BC, Snoey ER [eds]: Ultrasound in Emergency and Ambulatory Medicine. St. Louis, Mosby, 1997.)

Combined Diagnostic–Procedural Ultrasonography

Procedures can be guided either statically with ultrasonography or in real time. For the static technique, anatomic structures, the insertion site, and the angle and depth of insertion are first identified with ultrasonography, and then the probe is laid aside. If a fluid collection is to be aspirated, the amount can also be estimated (e.g., 1 cm^3 equates to approximately 1 mL of fluid). The key portions of the procedure are then performed without ultrasonographic imaging. For the real-time technique, a sterile probe cover is used and the key components of the procedure are performed with simultaneous ultrasonographic imaging. A needle guide for the probe is helpful for real-time guidance; either a one-person or two-person technique can be used.

Insertion of Central Lines

Several studies indicate that the use of ultrasonography as an adjunct for inserting central venous catheters not only decreases the failure rate, it decreases the overall incidence of complications as well as the number of attempts necessary. Consequently, the Institute of Medicine, the Agency for Healthcare Research and Quality, and the National Institute for Health and Clinical Excellence now recommend this technique. Patient satisfaction should also be improved. A real-time, two-person technique for internal jugular cannulation is described here. Similar techniques can be used for other sites (e.g., external jugular, subclavian, femoral). With the advent of tunneled catheters, such techniques can also be used to cannulate the brachial and cephalic veins for central venous access. Equipment is now available in many large intensive care units and other areas of the hospital that is portable and dedicated to the insertion of central lines. Such equipment may facilitate a one-person technique. It also frequently has a needle guide that attaches to or is built into the probe.

Preprocedure Patient Preparation

See Chapter 211, Central Venous Catheter Insertion.

Technique

1. For internal jugular cannulation, the patient is positioned supine, in 15 degrees of Trendelenburg, with the head turned slightly to the opposite side. (See Chapter 211, Central Venous Catheter Insertion, for techniques in locations other than the internal jugular.)
2. Perform a preliminary transverse scan with the high-frequency probe just above the clavicle near the insertion of the two heads of the sternocleidomastoid muscle. The pulsatile internal carotid artery should appear in cross-sectional view beside and medial to the larger internal jugular vein. With a Valsalva maneuver, the internal jugular will increase in diameter, significantly. Avoid applying too much pressure with the probe initially, which may temporarily collapse the vein and make it hard to locate. After it is identified, apply pressure to demonstrate that it is indeed collapsible as opposed to the noncollapsible carotid artery.
3. Cover the probe with a sterile cover (e.g., a sterile glove). A ribbon of acoustic gel should have been placed on the probe before covering; pay special attention to eliminating all bubbles between the cover and the head of the transducer. Prepare and drape the patient in the usual sterile fashion.
4. A small amount of sterile acoustic gel is placed over the site to be scanned. The sterilely gowned and gloved ultrasonography operator should be located next to the clinician (similarly gowned and gloved) performing the cannulation. The ultrasonographic probe should be operated beneath the drape to avoid interfering with the cannulation.
5. Position the probe so that the internal jugular vein is centered under the probe, which also means centered in the monitor screen. The person performing the cannulation should aim the needle toward the center of the probe. Unless there is a needle guide, the needle will not always be visualized; if it is, it will appear as a linear, echogenic structure with shadowing. The needle will typically cause slight tenting of the vessel as it enters. The flash of blood in the syringe is often anticipated by the sonographer when he or she sees tenting of the vein immediately before the needle enters. After the flash of blood and confirmation of needle placement, if a guidewire is used it can often be visualized as it passes into the vein.

Arterial Puncture and Cannulation

Techniques are described using a hand-held Doppler to assess collateral flow before arterial puncture and to facilitate arterial cannulation in Chapter 208, Arterial Puncture and Percutaneous Arterial Line Placement. The technique just described for ultrasonography-guided central venous catheter insertion can also be used to localize the vessel and then for arterial puncture and cannulation.

Lumbar Puncture in the Morbidly Obese Individual

In morbidly obese individuals, lumber puncture is often complicated by the inability to palpate the spinous processes. The goal of ultrasonography is to locate the midline of the spine. (Ultrasonographic localization of the spine is also helpful for performing other spinal procedures and is being used more frequently by anesthesiologists.)

Preprocedure Patient Preparation

See Chapter 206, Lumbar Puncture.

Technique

1. Ultrasonography can be performed either under nonsterile conditions, to mark the midline, or under sterile conditions for ultrasonographic guidance of the needle. A low-frequency probe is usually preferred.
2. With the patient in either the lateral recumbent or sitting position, apply adequate acoustic gel over the midline of the spine. Scan initially in transverse dimensions to locate a vertebra. The L4 spinous process should be noted below a line drawn between the iliac crests. When this vertebra is noted, maneuver the transducer so that the spinous process is centered on the monitor. Next, rotate the probe 90 degrees to scan longitudinally and locate several spinous processes. Mark the location and note the angle necessary to penetrate between the L3 and L4 spinous processes. After local anesthetic is given, insert the spinal needle and follow the remaining technique as described in Chapter 206, Lumbar Puncture.
3. To perform the scan under sterile conditions, cover the probe with a sterile barrier (sterile glove) as noted previously for central line insertion. When performing the lumbar puncture, use the same technique as for central line insertion and observe the needle passing over the L4 spinous process.

Interpretation and Results

The spinous process should appear hyperechoic in contrast to surrounding tissue. The vertebral bodies should also be hyperechoic and cast shadows. Spinal fluid is rarely imaged between the spinous processes in adults, but the angles and depths to the vertebral bodes can usually be more clearly defined.

Thyroid Mass

Palpable thyroid nodules occur in 3% to 4% of the population. One important goal when scanning a thyroid nodule is to determine whether there is more than one nodule. If multiple nodules are present (40% possibility), the risk of malignancy is very low (1% to

6%), with the exception of those who underwent low-dose irradiation. In the past, this was usually done for children with croup or acne; however, these treatments were stopped so many years ago that patients have likely outlived their risk (i.e., they would have already developed their malignancies). More recently, patients exposed to nuclear accidents such as Chernobyl or those exposed in the future to a terrorist "dirty bomb" may be at risk. These patients have a 30% to 40% lifetime risk of malignancy.

The next goal of scanning a thyroid nodule is to determine whether it is cystic (Fig. 225-30C), solid (Fig. 225-30D), or both (complex). Cold nodules on nuclear studies can be cystic with low risk of malignancy (20%), malignant (20%), or benign (60%).

If the nodule is cystic, aspiration may be an option and the fluid may be sent for cytologic analysis. Fine-needle aspiration is also an option for solid lesions.

Preprocedure Patient Preparation

The patient should be informed about the indication for the study. If an aspiration is to be performed, the patient should be counseled for informed consent.

Technique

1. With the patient in the supine position and the neck slightly hyperextended, apply an adequate amount of acoustic gel. Using a high frequency probe, scan transversely (marker dot to the patient's right side) in a lateral-to-medial fashion on one side. Next, scan the opposite side at the same level from lateral to medial. Apply minimal pressure at the midline to avoid obscuring the texture of the isthmus. Proceed in 5-mm increments throughout the entire gland.
2. Next, scan with longitudinal planes at 5-mm intervals. Observe each plane and then move medially from the carotid artery. Good surface contact is usually obtained at a 10- or 20-degree angle from the vertical. Scan the opposite side in the same manner.
3. For aspiration, see the next section, Breast Mass. If aspiration is to be attempted, mark the location. Note the angle and depth of any nearby structures that need to be avoided.

Interpretation and Results

Carcinomas of the thyroid are usually single nodules with irregular borders, and most are hypoechoic. They can be cystic, solid, or both (complex), and they are frequently accompanied by adenopathy. However, there is no pathognomonic feature of cancer of the thyroid. If unsure, the clinician should consider fine-needle aspiration or surgical removal, especially for solitary nodules.

The most common thyroid masses are adenomas. Adenomas almost invariably occur as multiple lesions. They can appear with a halo of hypoechoic tissue surrounding a more echogenic mass, as a solid homogeneous mass with few internal echoes, or as a densely echogenic mass. Goiters appear as a diffuse, asymmetric expansion of the thyroid with a coarse texture. Multiple nodules are often present. Thyroiditis usually appears as a diffuse enlargement of the thyroid with multiple nodules. Parathyroid glands are rarely seen and usually appear on the posterior aspect of the thyroid near the carotid artery. They are relatively sonolucent; if larger than 5 mm, they are abnormal.

Breast Mass

Ultrasonography is very helpful for evaluating breast masses, whether confirming the presence of a palpable mass or locating a nonpalpable mass seen on mammography, evaluating young fibroglandular breasts where mammography is less helpful, or differentiating solid from cystic lesions.

Preprocedure Patient Preparation

The patient should be informed about the indication for the study. The patient should be aware that this procedure is being used only to evaluate palpable lesions (or lesions noted on mammograms), to localize them, or to determine whether they are cystic or solid. It is not being used solely to exclude cancer. Portable ultrasonography may also be used to assist with aspiration of a breast cyst or with fine-needle aspiration of a suspected adenoma. Informed consent should be obtained if aspiration will be attempted.

Technique

1. Place the patient in the supine position. After application of acoustic gel, scan palpable lesions with a high-frequency probe. To locate nonpalpable lesions noted on a mammogram, scan longitudinally in 5-mm parallel increments in the appropriate quadrant. If the lesion is not located, scan in transverse increments through the same quadrant.
2. For cyst aspiration, either a one- or two-person technique can be used. The one-person technique may be adequate for large cysts, especially if they are readily palpable. The ultrasonography can be performed under nonsterile conditions. The goal of the ultrasonographic study is to locate the cyst, note the surrounding structures (especially those that should be avoided), determine the necessary depth for puncture, and mark the puncture site. The transducer can then be set aside and the procedure performed under sterile conditions as noted elsewhere (e.g., suprapubic aspiration, thoracentesis).
3. For smaller or deeper cysts that are difficult to localize, use the two-person technique. Just as with insertion of central lines, one person localizes the cyst with a high-frequency probe and keeps it in the center of the image while maintaining sterile conditions. The second clinician then punctures the cyst, also under aseptic conditions. Occasionally the needle can be visualized on the screen as it enters the cyst. The needle usually indents the cyst wall before it punctures.
4. After aspiration, the contents should be sent for cytology. A sample can also be prepared as a smear between two microscope slides that are then pulled apart, sprayed with the same fixative used for Pap smears, allowed to air dry, and sent for cytology.

Interpretation and Results

Breast cysts have the sonographic appearance of cysts elsewhere in the body and are the most common breast masses in women between 35 and 50 years of age. They normally have smooth walls and an absence of internal echoes; therefore they are uniformly hypoechoic. Tissue behind the posterior wall of the cyst is usually more sharply defined than tissue anterior to the cyst. The penumbra effect may be seen.

The cyst should be measured in three dimensions: AP, longitudinal, and transverse. If aspiration is to be attempted, the depth necessary for penetration should be recorded. Nearby structures should also be noted.

Adenomas are usually ovoid, with lateral diameters larger than AP diameters. They usually have uniform and regular borders. If the gain is set improperly (too low) and no internal echoes are noted, adenomas may also appear cystic.

In contrast, ductal carcinomas usually have irregular borders and may be dense enough to cast acoustic shadows. Their AP diameter may be as great or greater than the lateral diameter. If they are blocking ducts, the ducts can often be traced to the site of the mass. Medullary carcinoma may be difficult to differentiate from adenomas, with the only differences being a more irregular border and more internal echoes. For this reason, solid solitary breast lesions should undergo either fine-needle aspiration or surgical removal.

Papillary carcinoma is fairly rare, but it can appear as finger-like projections protruding from a cyst wall. After cyst aspiration, if any tissue remains palpable, it should probably be surgically removed to exclude the possibility of papillary carcinoma. Also after aspiration, air can be reinjected into the cyst and a repeat mammogram performed. The location of the cyst will be marked by the air when the mammogram is repeated. In this manner a mammogram can be used to help exclude papillary carcinoma.

Pericardial Effusion and Ultrasonography-Guided Pericardiocentesis

See Chapter 214, Pericardiocentesis. Even when duplex equipment is available, plain ultrasonographic scanning using the low-frequency probe should be the initial study performed in most cases.

Pleural Effusion and Ultrasonography-Guided Thoracentesis

Ultrasonography is an alternative to the use of decubitus x-ray films for confirmation of an effusion (e.g., patient with blunting of costovertebral angles on radiography). Once the effusion is confirmed, not only can the amount of fluid be quantified, but the best angle and the depth necessary for inserting the needle can be determined. In patients with a small amount of pleural fluid or a loculated effusion, routine thoracentesis is often unsuccessful and possibly dangerous. Ultrasonography-directed thoracentesis should minimize the danger while maximizing the results.

Preprocedure Patient Preparation

The patient should be informed about the indications for the procedure as well as the risks and possible complications. The usual risks of pneumothorax, solid organ puncture, and procedural failure are reduced when thoracentesis is ultrasonography guided. Signed, informal consent should be obtained for thoracentesis. (See Chapter 95, Thoracentesis.)

Technique

1. With the patient in the proper position (usually sitting and leaning forward, but can be supine or lateral decubitus), use a low-frequency probe to scan the back intercostally on the appropriate side, just above the liver or spleen. It may be helpful to actually scan the liver or spleen first, and to then move the probe in a cranial direction to locate the effusion. With the patient in the sitting position and the marker dot located cephalad, scan the entire thorax in longitudinal planes. After scanning near the midline, move the transducer laterally and map the dimensions of the effusion from superior to inferior, medial to lateral. Then turn the marker dot counterclockwise to fit between the ribs, and again scan to note the lateral dimensions of the effusion.
2. Mark the location of the largest collection of effusion that is safely accessible with the needle. The diaphragm will appear echogenic and moving with respiration; also note the location of the spleen or liver, and avoid inserting the needle in those locations. If the procedure will be performed with the patient in the supine or lateral decubitus position, be sure to demarcate the extent of the effusion relative to the hemithorax that will be accessible.

   Effusions may move with respiration, so note where to direct the needle relative to each phase of respiration. Plan to perform the insertion during the optimal phase. Note the depth necessary to reach fluid, especially for large or obese patients; an extra-long needle may be necessary for these patients. A needle stop, set to the appropriate depth, may be helpful for preventing penetration of lung tissue and causing a pneumothorax.
3. For smaller or loculated effusions, the thoracentesis is best performed with ultrasonographic guidance. Cover the probe with a sterile barrier (e.g., sterile glove) as noted previously for central line insertion. This procedure may also require two persons: one to hold the transducer while the other performs the aspiration. When performing ultrasonography-guided thoracentesis, use the same technique as for central line insertion. With the probe held scanning longitudinally, the top of the rib over which the thoracentesis is to be performed should be highlighted by the transducer. If a curvilinear or sector scanner is being used, the transducer should be held at the same optimal angle as that needed to reach the effusion. The thoracentesis needle should then be advanced to the appropriate depth at the same angle as the transducer. Again, a properly set needle stop may prevent penetrating lung tissue and causing a pneumothorax. Occasionally the echogenic needle will be observed passing over the rib. Once fluid is obtained, complete the procedure in the same manner as if it were not ultrasonography guided.

Interpretation and Results

Pleural effusions that are predominantly fluid appear dark or hypoechoic on ultrasonography. They are located above the echogenic diaphragm, which moves with respiration (Fig. 225-31). An empyema may demonstrate echogenic objects in the fluid. Loculations and the diaphragm appear as echogenic borders to the fluid. Fluid located below the diaphragm (and not within an organ) is ascites.

Ascites and Ultrasonography-Guided Paracentesis

As discussed in the Trauma section, the presence of abdominal fluid is not always obvious on physical examination. Ultrasonography can be used to confirm the presence of ascites and to determine the best location for diagnostic paracentesis. Although routine paracentesis may be contraindicated in certain situations (e.g., in patients with adhesions from prior abdominal surgery), paracentesis directed by ultrasonography may remain an option for those patients. Similar to the FAST examination, ascites is usually diagnosed earliest (even small amounts) in Morison's (hepatorenal) pouch.

Preprocedure Patient Preparation

The patient should be informed about the indications for the procedure as well as the risks and possible complications. The usual risks for paracentesis of solid organ perforation, vascular injury,

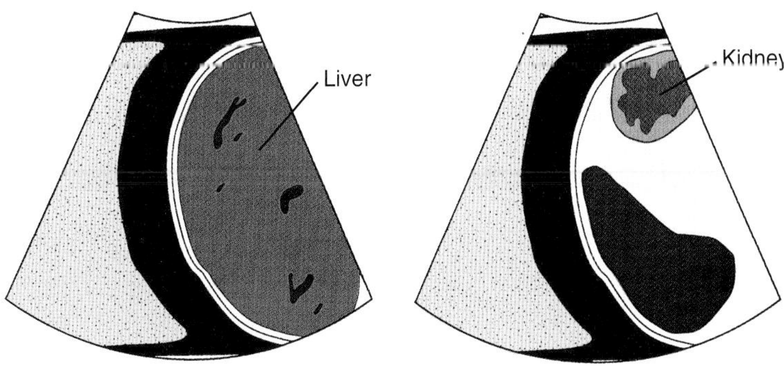

Figure 225-31 Pleural effusion. Note the fluid is above the diaphragm.

bowel perforation, and procedural failure are decreased when ultrasonographic guidance is used. If there is a relative contraindication, the patient should be informed of the increased risk. (See Chapter 201, Abdominal Paracentesis.)

Technique

1. With the patient in the supine or sitting upright position, use a low-frequency probe to scan the usual location for performing paracentesis (in the midline, approximately one-third the distance from the umbilicus to the pubic symphysis, or in a lower quadrant [left usually preferred] about one-third the distance from the umbilicus to the anterior iliac crest). Note the location of any solid organs to avoid. Next, locate the largest, safest collection of fluid for a successful paracentesis. Also, confirm absence of bowel (would be floating in fluid; air in bowel usually causes scatter artifact) and whether the bladder has been emptied adequately. If these conditions are met, perform the procedure in the usual manner.
2. For small amounts of fluid, or if there is need for stereotactic paracentesis, perform it under ultrasonographic guidance. Cover the probe with a sterile barrier (e.g., sterile glove) as noted previously for central line insertion. When performing the paracentesis, use the same technique for ultrasonographic guidance as for central line insertion or thoracentesis. In some cases, the echogenic needle may be observed passing into the fluid.

Interpretation and Results

Peritoneal fluid appears dark or hypoechoic on ultrasonography. Bowel or bladder wall is relatively echogenic. With peritonitis, echogenic objects will occasionally be seen floating in the fluid.

Over-Reading Services

Over-reading services are available through the following websites, among others: www.nighthawkradiologyservices.net and www.radisphere.net.

NOTE: These require T1 internet access; DSL is not compliant with the Health Insurance Portability and Accountability Act (HIPAA) Privacy Rule.

Patient Education Guide

See the sample patient consent form available online at www.expertconsult.com.

CPT/Billing Codes

NOTE: Only one limited scan can be billed per patient encounter.

Cardiac

93307 Echocardiography, transthoracic, real time with image documentation (2D) with or without M-mode recording; complete
93308 Echocardiography, follow-up or limited study

Obstetric–Gynecologic

See also Chapter 172, Obstetric Ultrasonography.

76801 Ultrasound, pregnant uterus, real-time with image documentation, <14 weeks, transabdominal, single or first gestation
76802 Ultrasound, pregnant uterus, transabdominal, each additional gestation
76805 Ultrasound, pregnant uterus, >14 weeks, transabdominal, single or first gestation
76810 Ultrasound, pregnant uterus, >14 weeks, transabdominal, each additional gestation
76815 Ultrasound, pregnant uterus, real-time with image documentation, limited (e.g., fetal heart beat, placental location, fetal position and/or qualitative amniotic fluid volume), one or more fetuses
76816 Ultrasound, pregnant uterus, real-time with image documentation, follow-up (e.g., reevaluation of fetal size, reevaluation of organ system[s] suspected or documented to be abnormal on previous scan), transabdominal approach
76817 Ultrasound, pregnant uterus, real-time with image documentation, transvaginal

Gynecologic

76830 Ultrasound, transvaginal
76856 Ultrasound, pelvic (nonobstetric), real-time with image documentation; complete
76857 Ultrasound, pelvic (nonobstetric), limited or follow-up study (e.g., for follicles)

Abdominal and Trauma

76700 Ultrasound, abdominal, real-time with image documentation; complete
76705 Ultrasound, abdominal, limited (e.g., single organ, quadrant, follow-up)
76770 Ultrasound, retroperitoneal (e.g., renal, aorta, nodes), real-time with image documentation; complete
76775 Ultrasound, retroperitoneal, limited study

Miscellaneous

See also Chapter 88, Noninvasive Venous and Arterial Studies of the Lower Extremities.

76604 Ultrasound, chest (includes mediastinum), real-time with image documentation
76870 Ultrasound, scrotum and contents

Combined Diagnostic–Procedural

76536 Ultrasound, soft tissue of head and neck (e.g., thyroid, parathyroid, parotid), real-time with image documentation
76645 Ultrasound, breast(s) (unilateral or bilateral), real-time with image documentation
76930 Ultrasonic guidance for pericardiocentesis, imaging supervision and interpretation
76937 Ultrasonic guidance for vascular access requiring ultrasound evaluation of potential access sites, documentation of selected vessel patency, concurrent real-time ultrasound visualization of vascular needle entry, with permanent recording and reporting (list separately in addition to code for primary procedure)
76942 Ultrasonic guidance for needle placement (e.g., biopsy, aspiration, injection, localization device), imaging, supervision and interpretation

ICD-9-CM Diagnostic Codes

Cardiac

420.90 Pericardial effusion, acute
420.91 Pericarditis, acute, idiopathic
420.99 Pericarditis, acute purulent
423.3 Cardiac tamponade

423.9 Pericardial effusion (chronic), or unspecified disease of pericardium
427.5 Asystole

Obstetric–Gynecologic

See also Chapter 172, Obstetric Ultrasonography, for additional coding on gravid uterus.

V25.42 Intrauterine device, checking, reinsertion, or removal
218.9 Uterine fibroid, unspecified
614.2 Tubo-ovarian, ovarian, or fallopian tube abscess, salpingitis, or oophoritis, acute or chronic
620.1 Ovarian cyst, corpus luteum
620.2 Ovarian cyst, unspecified
620.5 Torsioned ovary, ovarian pedicle or fallopian tube
623.8 Vaginal bleeding
630 Hydatidiform mole
631 Blighted ovum
632 Missed abortion
633.0 Abdominal pregnancy
633.1 Tubal pregnancy
633.9 Ectopic pregnancy, unspecified
634.91 Abortion or miscarriage, incomplete, without any complications
634.92 Abortion or miscarriage, complete, without complication
640.03 Threatened abortion, antepartum
655.73 Decreased fetal movements, antepartum
656.43 Intrauterine fetal death, late (after 22 weeks' gestation)

Abdominal

441.02 Abdominal aortic aneurysm, dissecting
441.3 Abdominal aortic aneurysm, ruptured
441.4 Abdominal aortic aneurysm, without mention of rupture
574.20 Cholelithiasis, without obstruction, without mention of cholecystitis
574.21 Cholelithiasis, with obstruction, without mention of cholecystitis
574.60 Calculus of gallbladder and bile duct with acute cholecystitis, without mention of obstruction
575.2 Obstruction of gallbladder
575.9 Pain, gallbladder
575.10 Cholecystitis, unspecified
575.11 Cholecystitis, chronic
575.12 Cholecystitis, acute and chronic
576.8 Cholestasis
576.9 Pain, bile duct
590.2 Renal abscess
591 Hydronephrosis
592.0 Calculus of kidney
592.1 Calculus of ureter
593.5 Hydroureter
594.1 Urinary bladder stone
599.7 Hematuria
788.0 Renal colic
789.01 Pain, abdominal, right upper quadrant
789.3 Abdominal mass

Trauma

See also Chapter 204, Diagnostic Peritoneal Lavage, and Chapter 214, Pericardiocentesis.

423.0 Hemopericardium
459.0 Hemorrhage, unspecified
568.81 Hemoperitoneum
573.8 Hematoma, traumatic liver, subcapsular
861.0 Injury to heart, without mention of open wound into thorax
861.1 Injury to heart, with open wound into thorax
861.2 Injury to lung, without mention of open wound into thorax
861.3 Injury to lung, with open wound into thorax
862.29 Traumatic pleural effusion
864.01 Injury to liver, without mention of open wound, hematoma without rupture of capsule
865.01 Injury to spleen, without mention of open wound, hematoma without rupture of capsule
866.01 Injury to kidney, without mention of open wound, hematoma without rupture of capsule

Miscellaneous

See also Chapter 18, Foreign Body Removal from Skin and Soft Tissue, Chapter 88, Noninvasive Venous and Arterial Studies of the Lower Extremities, Chapter 114, Suprapubic Tap or Aspiration, and Chapter 183, Pediatric Suprapubic Bladder Aspiration.

186.9 Primary neoplasm of testicle
512.8 Pneumothorax, spontaneous, acute or chronic
595.0 Cystitis, acute
599.0 Urinary tract infection, site not specified
608.89 Testicular mass
788.20 Urinary retention, NEC
788.21 Urinary retention, bladder incomplete emptying
729.6 Residual foreign body in soft tissue
807.00 Rib fracture, closed, unspecified number of ribs
807.01 Rib facture, closed, one rib

Combined Diagnostic–Procedural

See also Chapter 185, Musculoskeletal Ultrasonography, Chapter 206, Lumbar Puncture, and Chapter 211, Central Venous Catheter Insertion.

012.0 Tuberculous pleurisy, pleural effusion, empyema, or hydrothorax
047.9 Unspecified viral meningitis, or abacterial or aseptic meningitis
174.8 Primary breast neoplasm, upper or lower
193 Malignant neoplasm of thyroid gland
197.2 Pleural effusion, malignant
226 Benign neoplasm of thyroid
241.1 Nontoxic multinodular goiter
242.2 Toxic multinodular goiter
246.2 Cyst of thyroid
320.9 Meningitis due to unspecified bacterium
511.1 Bacterial, nontuberculous pleural effusion
511.9 Pleural effusion
567.2 Suppurative peritonitis
610.0 Solitary cyst of breast
610.1 (Fibro) Cystic breast
611.72 Lump or mass in breast
682.9 Other cellulitis and abscess, unspecified site
789.5 Ascites
998.7 Chemical peritonitis

SUPPLIERS

See Suppliers sections in Chapter 172, Obstetric Ultrasonography, and Chapter 185, Musculoskeletal Ultrasonography.

ONLINE RESOURCES

American College of Surgeons: Educational CD-ROM. Available at www.facs.org.

American Institute of Ultrasound in Medicine (AIUM): Short guidelines and DVDs available for many areas of scanning (e.g., abdominal aorta, abdominal/retroperitoneal scanning, FAST exam, musculoskeletal system, pelvis). Available at www.aium.org.

Challenger Fundamentals: EM Ultrasound: CD-ROM–based course designed to teach the basic techniques of emergency ultrasonography. The course contains a combination of still and video segments, as well as diagrams, three-dimensional animations, and interactive multimedia that describe the key concepts of ultrasonography. Available at www.chall.com/emus.htm.

Society for Academic Emergency Medicine: Online teaching and narrated slides, including ultrasound images, for various emergency medicine topics. Available at www.saem.org.

Sonosite: Several video series for learning ultrasound, from bedside invasive procedures, to emergency medicine, critical care medicine, and anesthesiology procedures. Available at www.sonosite.com.

BIBLIOGRAPHY

American College of Emergency Physicians: ACEP emergency ultrasound guidelines—2001. Ann Emerg Med 38:470–481, 2001.

American College of Emergency Physicians: Clinical policy: Critical issues in the evaluation of adult patients presenting to the emergency department with acute blunt abdominal trauma. Ann Emerg Med 43:278–290, 2004.

American College of Emergency Physicians: ACEP policy statement: Emergency ultrasound imaging criteria compendium. Ann Emerg Med 48:487–510, 2006.

American Institute of Ultrasound in Medicine: AIUM practice guideline for the performance of the focused assessment with sonography for trauma (FAST) examination. October 1, 2007. Available at www.aium.org/publications/guidelines/fast.pdf.

American Institute of Ultrasound in Medicine: AIUM practice guideline for the performance of scrotal ultrasound examinations. October 1, 2006. Available at www.aium.org/publications/guidelines/scrotal.pdf.

Deutchman M: The problematic first-trimester pregnancy. Am Fam Physician 39:185–198, 1989.

Gochman RF, Karasic RB, Heller MB: Use of portable ultrasound to assist urine collection by suprapubic aspiration. Ann Emerg Med 20:631–635, 1991.

Heller M, Jehle D (eds): Ultrasound in Emergency Medicine. Philadelphia, WB Saunders, 1995.

Jehle D, Davis E, Evans T, et al: Emergency department sonography by emergency physicians. Am J Emerg Med 7:605–611, 1989.

Mahoney BS, Filly RA, Nyberg DA, Callen PW: Sonographic evaluation of ectopic pregnancy. J Ultrasound Med 4:221–228, 1985.

Mortality results for randomized controlled trial of early elective surgery or ultrasonographic surveillance for small abdominal aortic aneurysms: The UK Small Aneurysm Trial Participants. Lancet 352:1649–1655, 1998.

Roberts KB: The AAP practice parameter on urinary tract infections in febrile infants and young children. Am Fam Physician 62:1815–1822, 2000.

Sanders RC, Winter TC (eds): Clinical Sonography: A Practical Guide, 4th ed. Philadelphia, Lippincott Williams & Wilkins, 2007.

Schlager D, Lazzareschi G, Whitten D, et al: A prospective study of ultrasonography in the ED by emergency physicians. Am J Emerg Med 12:185–189, 1994.

Siepel T, Clifford DS, James PA, Cowan TM: The ultrasound-assisted physical examination in the periodic health evaluation of the elderly. J Fam Pract 49:628–632, 2000.

Simon B, Snoey E (eds): Ultrasound in Emergency and Ambulatory Medicine. St. Louis, Mosby, 1997.

CHAPTER 226

Fine-Needle Aspiration Cytology and Biopsy

Lee A. Green

Fine-needle aspiration (FNA) and biopsy is a rapid, safe, relatively painless method of sampling solid and cystic masses in a variety of anatomic sites for cytologic examination. Both benign and suspected malignant conditions can be diagnosed with FNA.

Although the procedure is successfully used to sample lesions of the prostate, salivary glands, and intra-abdominal and intrathoracic organs, as well as for culturing cellulitis, the primary care physician will find FNA most useful for masses in the *breast* and *thyroid*, and for *lymph nodes* (especially solitary supraclavicular nodes). For tumors of these sites, positive and negative predictive values for malignancy are typically in the 92% to 98% range, with overall diagnostic accuracy of greater than 70%. However, these rates are highly dependent on the skill of the clinician. It is clear from the literature that FNA should be performed by clinicians who are skilled at technical procedures and well trained in FNA in order to obtain adequate diagnostic accuracy. The availability of a cytopathologist skilled in reading FNA specimens is crucial. Liquid-based cytology (e.g., CytoLyt; Cytec Corporation, Marlborough, Mass) is now standard, obviating the potentially error-prone step of direct slide smear preparation at the time of aspiration.

As implied by the overall diagnostic accuracy rate, as much as one fourth of specimens will return with nondiagnostic results, necessitating repeat aspiration or open biopsy. However, FNA will provide diagnosis in most cases with a procedure that is safer, more comfortable, less invasive, and less costly than open biopsy. These same advantages allow FNA to be used with less hesitation than would open biopsy. For example, many samples can be drawn over time from breast lesions in a patient with fibrocystic disease, whereas repeated open biopsy with subsequent scarring would be unacceptable.

Although false-negative results are generally more common than false-positive results with FNA, the reverse is true for breast aspirations among young women; more than half of all "suspect" FNAs of palpable breast masses among women younger than 30 years of age prove to be benign on excisional biopsy. Fibroadenomas can show cellular atypia, nuclear overlapping, hyperchromasia, and epithelial clustering, and are thus easily overinterpreted.

Some authors advocate use of FNA of breast lesions as one component of a *triple test*, comprising clinical examination, mammography or ultrasonography, and FNA. When all three elements are concordant for malignancy or nonmalignancy, the negative predictive value of the triple test approaches 100%. The majority of the predictive value of the triple test is the FNA result, but attention to a discordance—suspect abnormal clinical and imaging findings with a negative or nonspecific FNA—may help the clinician identify potential false-negative FNAs for further work-up. In the breast, *any palpable mass that is new and clinically suspect must be removed if fluid cannot be aspirated, regardless of other test findings*.

In all breast complaints, FNA provides significant information. If a mass is palpable, FNA is carried out. If nonbloody cystic fluid is retrieved and the mass is gone, the woman can be reassured of the extremely low likelihood of cancer if the mass does not recur within 6 to 8 weeks. If it does recur, repeat aspiration should be performed. If it recurs a third time, it should be excised. Mammograms are usually done for baseline or confirmation a week after the aspiration.

FNA is widely used for evaluation of thyroid masses, where it has similar predictive values. Nondiagnostic thyroid FNAs prove malignant in approximately 7% of cases. Malignancy is more likely in younger and in male patients, those with high-normal thyroid-stimulating hormone (TSH) levels, and in solitary lesions. Solitary hyperfunctioning nodules with low-normal TSH or patients with more than two nodules are less likely to harbor malignancy. Two successive nondiagnostic FNAs of a thyroid mass should prompt suspicion. More than two FNAs are not generally useful.

Indications

- Presence of a palpable, suspect mass in the breast
- Thyroid nodule
- Clinically suspect lymph node or group of nodes
- Any palpable, superficial, nonpulsatile mass

The primary care physician ordinarily does not perform plain radiography– or computed tomography–guided FNA of nonpalpable lesions, but if an office ultrasonography machine is available it can readily be used to guide FNA. FNA is the procedure of first choice, even over imaging studies, for evaluating thyroid nodules and detecting the rare parathyroid tumor.

Contraindications

- Unskilled clinician *(relative)*
- Absence of a cytopathologist capable of proper interpretation of the resulting slides
- Sites of active pyogenic infection, although suspected granulomatous infection (fungal or mycobacterial) of a node does not contraindicate FNA, and FNA can be used (with sensitivity of roughly 20% to 30%) to obtain culture material from cellulitis
- Nonpalpable lesion (unless readily visualized on ultrasonography and office ultrasonography is available)

FNA may be performed safely in the anticoagulated patient if studies are in the therapeutic range, with proper attention to compression of the site afterward to avoid hematoma. It may be performed in all but the most severely immunocompromised patients.

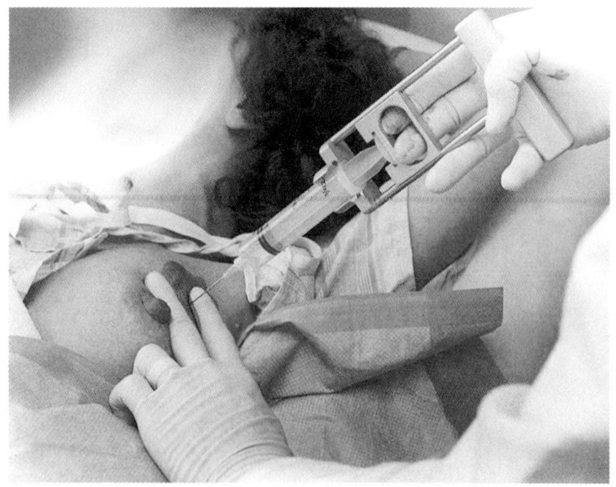

Figure 226-1 Breast fine-needle aspiration using Cameco syringe holder.

EQUIPMENT

- *One* of the following syringe or needle systems:
  - The syringe pistol shown in Figure 226-1 is available in various sizes from Belpro (Anjou, Quebec).
  - A spring-loaded device called the Tao Aspirator, designed to allow a pencil-type grip on the syringe, is available from Tao & Tao Technology (Camano Island, Wash; Fig. 226-2).
  - Milex Products (Chicago) supplies a breast aspiration biopsy needle (Fig. 226-3), which is unique because of its separate cutting port near the tip.
  - A 21- or 23-gauge butterfly needle can be connected to a syringe. The assistant aspirates the syringe while the clinician manipulates the needle.
  - A 21- or 23-gauge needle can be used on the end of a regular 3-, 5-, or 10-mL syringe.
- Two sterile, plain (nonanticoagulant), evacuated blood tubes.
- 21-, 22-, or 23-gauge needle.
- Syringe of appropriate size.
- 120-mL specimen containers containing 30 mL CytoLyt solution each.
- 4 × 4 gauze pads.
- Sterile gloves.
- Isopropyl alcohol pads or povidone–iodine swabs.
- 1-mL syringe with 30-gauge ½-inch needle (or insulin syringe and needle) and 1% plain lidocaine for anesthesia of skin *(optional)*.

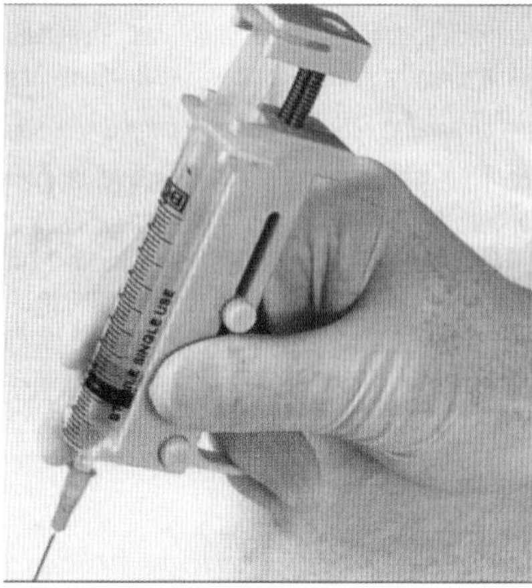

Figure 226-2 Tao Aspirator. (Courtesy of Tao & Tao Technology, Camano Island, Wash.)

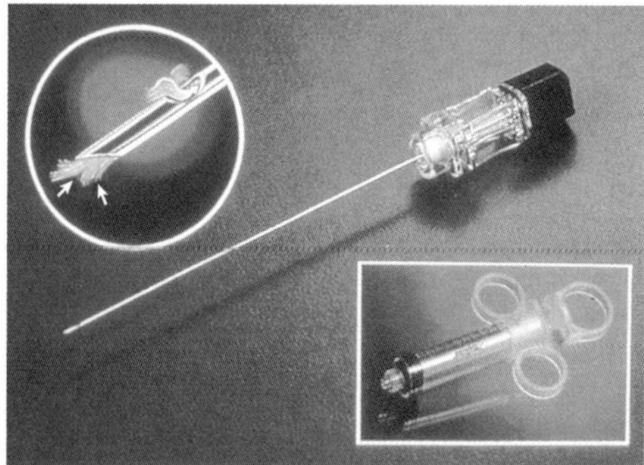

Figure 226-3 Milex needle used for needle biopsy. Note the special extra side port to sample more tissue. (Courtesy of Milex Products, Chicago.)

PREPROCEDURE PATIENT PREPARATION

Advise patients of the risks and benefits of the procedure, the indications, the alternatives, and the comparative risks and benefits of the alternatives. (See the sample patient education and consent forms online at www.expertconsult.com.)

Significant complications of FNA are rare. A small hematoma or ecchymosis for a few days (especially from thyroid FNA) and some mild soreness are to be expected. The patient must understand that nondiagnostic results occur commonly and may require repeat FNA or open biopsy, and that false-negative and false-positive results are possible. Patients undergoing FNA of breast lesions should wear a supportive brassiere.

TECHNIQUE

Setup and Preparation

1. Prophylaxis for bacterial endocarditis is not required.
2. Prepare the skin with 70% isopropyl alcohol. Povidone–iodine preparation may be used but is not required for FNA. Sterile draping is not required, although neither the needle nor the skin entry site should be touched except with a sterile glove after the skin is prepared.
3. Figure 226-4 illustrates the typical equipment setup for FNA. The sterile tray contains both a 5-mL syringe for free-hand aspiration and a 20-mL syringe for use with the aspirator handle; ordinarily one or the other is used, not both. Both 21- and 23-gauge needles are illustrated; either size may be used, although 23-gauge may be preferred in the thyroid and 21-gauge for dense masses and the breast. The 1-mL syringe with a 30-gauge, ½-inch needle may be used for skin anesthesia, if desired. The specimen containers use the same CytoLyt fluid used for ThinPrep-method Papanicolaou (Pap) smears, but it is best to use a container distinct from that used for Pap smears because the laboratory may mistakenly process the FNA specimen as a

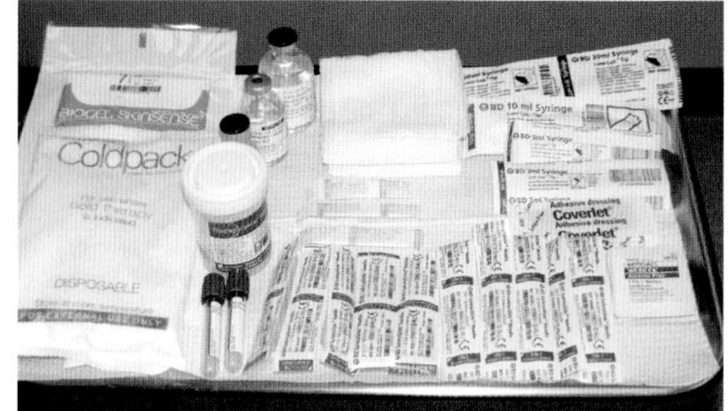

Figure 226-4 Setup tray for fine-needle aspiration.

Pap, destroying it. The sterile plain (nonanticoagulant) blood specimen tubes are for cyst fluid, if obtained. Alternatively, the fluid can just be placed in the CytoLyt. If breast fluid is nonbloody (urine colored or green), it does *not* need to be sent to pathology (for cell block, cytology, or anything else) and should be discarded.

4. Skin anesthesia is often not necessary for FNA because the needles are small and not painful. If desired, however, excellent anesthesia can be obtained with 1% lidocaine (plain or with epinephrine) by using a 30-gauge needle on a 1-mL syringe. If the lidocaine is injected slowly and in small volume (approximately 0.5 mL) into the subcutaneous tissues without raising a skin wheal, and then allowed to remain for 5 minutes, anesthesia can be achieved painlessly and without obscuring the lesion to be aspirated. Buffering the lidocaine to near-neutral pH just before injection by mixing it in a 9:1 ratio with 1 mEq/mL sodium bicarbonate solution can further reduce injection discomfort.

Sampling

Pneumothorax has been reported with needle aspiration and needle biopsy of the breast. To prevent this, aspirate with the mass positioned over a rib, or keep the needle at a tangential angle as opposed to perpendicular to the body. If the person is thin or the lesion is deep, it may be prudent to have the patient hold her breath while sampling.

Figure 226-5 illustrates the aspiration of a thyroid nodule using one-handed manual withdrawal of the syringe plunger to create vacuum. The fingers hold the plunger while the thumb exerts pressure on the syringe top flange. Figure 226-1 illustrates aspiration of a breast cyst using the syringe holder to withdraw the plunger. Whatever technique is used, the fingers of the nondominant hand stabilize the lesion to be aspirated and provide tactile feedback when the needle has been placed in the lesion.

Before the puncture is made, draw air into the syringe, filling approximately one fifth of its volume. The purpose of this is to have the air to flush out the needle and its contents onto a slide. Without the air, there is no good way to empty the needle. (*Do not* aspirate air after withdrawing the needle from the mass because this will spread the sparse contents all over the inside of the syringe, making it hard to retrieve.) Carefully note the position of the plunger against the syringe markings, and then introduce the needle into the lesion. The standard technique is to then withdraw the plunger to create vacuum and sample the lesion, but recent research suggests that suctionless fine-needle sampling may be equally effective.

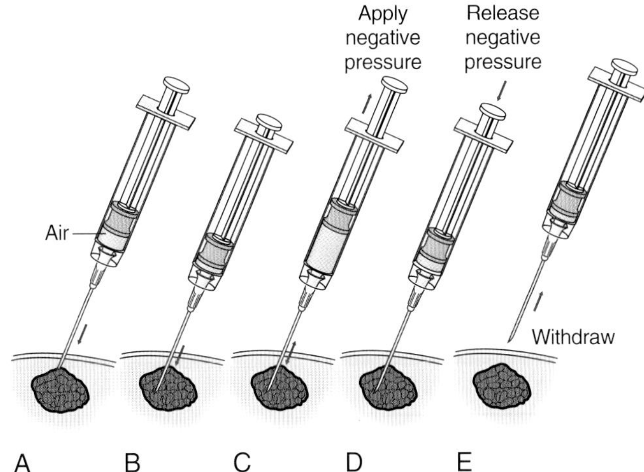

Figure 226-6 Fine-needle aspiration technique of a solid lesion or cyst (a palpable breast mass, in this case) that remains palpable after fluid has been drained. **A,** Aspirate 1 to 2 mL of air into syringe before inserting needle. **B,** Insert the needle into the mass and aspirate. If cystic fluid is not obtained or the mass does not resolve, the mass is solid. **C,** Maintain negative pressure in the syringe and move the needle back and forth through the tissue 15 to 20 times to collect cells for analysis (see Fig. 226-7). **D,** Release the plunger. **E,** Withdraw needle and spread contents on a slide, which is immediately fixed.

Figure 226-6 illustrates the technique of sampling a solid lesion or a cyst that remains palpable after fluid has been drained. Make several (10 to 20) passes into the lesion, filling the needle with cells and sampling all areas of the lesion (Fig. 226-7). Return the plunger to its previously noted resting position *before withdrawing the needle from the mass* to avoid aspirating the cells into the syringe when the needle is withdrawn. Withdraw the needle from the lesion and skin and use the air that was in the syringe to express the sample from the needle into the specimen container. Aspirate 1 to 2 mL of the liquid cytology solution into the syringe, agitate it gently, and express it gently back into the container. Repeat the procedure if necessary.

If a lesion is cystic and fluid is obtained, draw as much as possible into the syringe. Withdraw the needle and empty the syringe, then perform another aspiration if more fluid remains. Alternatively, detach the needle from the syringe and leave the needle in place, empty the syringe and reattach it, and withdraw more fluid. As

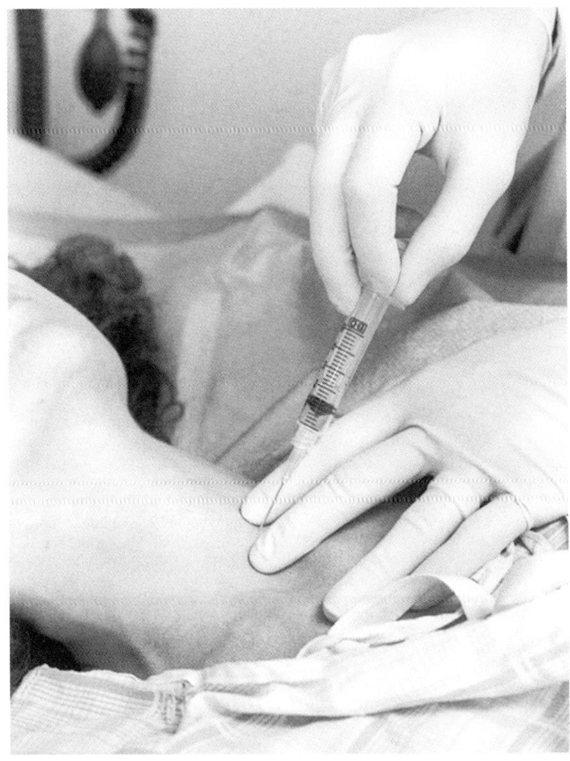

Figure 226-5 Thyroid fine-needle aspiration using ordinary syringe.

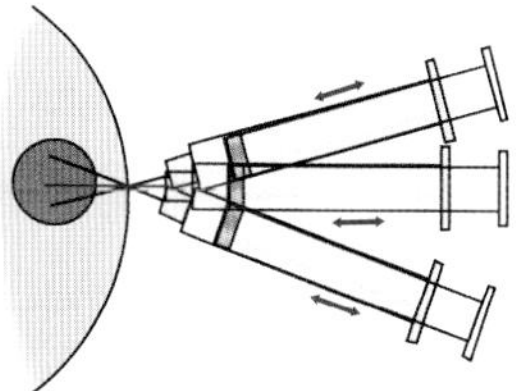

Figure 226-7 Depiction of how to carry out step **C** in Figure 226-6. The needle is passed multiple times into the mass to obtain adequate sampling.

noted, for nonbloody cystic masses of the breast, the fluid can be discarded and there is no need to send it to pathology.

Fluid obtained from cysts can be placed in liquid cytology solution or submitted in bulk in a sterile tube. (Standard evacuated blood tubes are sterile; those without anticoagulant should be used.) When a breast cyst is aspirated, the fluid should be submitted for pathologic evaluation only if tinged with blood. Yellow or green fluid is diagnostic of benign cysts, and cytology is unnecessary. A sterile tube can also be used to submit semisolid material such as that obtained from a lymph node for culture. If infection is suspected, fluid and solid specimens can be submitted in transport media as well.

Postprocedure Care

Compression of the site with a gauze pad for 5 to 15 minutes will minimize bruising, especially of the highly vascular thyroid area. A compression dressing of folded gauze pads under Elastoplast tape can be applied on suitable sites. In breast biopsies, placement of a stack of folded gauze pads under a snug brassiere forms an effective compression dressing that may be left in place for several hours to prevent hematoma formation. Some physicians apply a small ice pack to the FNA site for 15 to 60 minutes after the procedure.

Complications

Complications of FNA are limited primarily to *diagnostic failure* or to false-negative and false-positive results. The incidence of failure is strongly dependent on the operator. *Minor hematoma* formation is a frequent occurrence but is seldom of clinical significance. *Pneumothorax* has been reported in rare instances. Before the widespread use of FNA, concern was often expressed about the possibility of seeding the needle track with malignant cells or releasing malignant cells to spread through lymphatics. Neither of these theoretical complications has been documented to occur, and they should not be considered complications of FNA. *Damage to local anatomic structures* (e.g., recurrent laryngeal nerve injury with thyroid FNA) is possible but occurs rarely; most large case series have not reported such injuries. The lack of complications is probably due to the small diameter of the needles used for FNA, in contrast to cutting-needle biopsies, which do cause injury with some frequency.

Patient Education Guides

See the sample patient education and consent forms online at www.expertconsult.com.

CPT/Billing Codes

10021 Fine-needle biopsy w/o imaging
19000 Aspiration drainage of a breast cyst; one cyst
19001 Aspiration drainage of a breast cyst; additional cyst
19100 Core needle biopsy breast
20206 Muscle biopsy, needle
38505 Lymph node biopsy, needle
60001 Aspiration and/or injection, thyroid cyst
60100 Biopsy thyroid, percutaneous, core needle

ICD-9-CM Diagnostic Codes

174.0 Cancer, breast, areola
174.1 Cancer, breast, central
174.2 Cancer, breast, upper inner quadrant
174.3 Cancer, breast, lower inner quadrant
174.4 Cancer, breast, upper outer quadrant
174.5 Cancer, breast, lower outer quadrant
174.6 Cancer, breast, axillary tail
193 Malignant neoplasm of thyroid
217 Benign lesion breast
226 Benign neoplasm of thyroid
610.0 Solitary cyst of breast
610.1 Fibrocystic breast disease
610.2 Fibroadenosis of breast
611.72 Breast lump
785.6 Enlarged lymph node

Suppliers

(See contact information online at www.expertconsult.com.)

Cameco syringe
Belpro Medical, Inc.
CytoLyt solution
Cytyc Corp.
Special syringe
Milex Products, Inc.
Tao Aspirator
Tao & Tao Technology, Inc.

Online Resources

Papanicolaou Society of Cytopathology: Available at www.papsociety.org/fna.html.

Tuggy M, Garcia J: Procedures Consult. Available at www.proceduresconsult.com, and as an application at www.apple.com/iTunes.

Bibliography

Abati A, Simsir A: Breast fine needle aspiration biopsy: Prevailing recommendations and contemporary practices. Clin Lab Med 25:631–654, 2005.

Baloch ZW, LiVolsi VA: Fine-needle aspiration of thyroid nodules: Past, present, and future. Endocr Pract 10:234–241, 2004.

Cady B, Steele GD Jr, Morrow M, et al: Evaluation of common breast problems: Guidance for primary care providers. CA Cancer J Clin 48:49–63, 1998.

Caruso DR, Mazzaferri EL: Practical evaluation of thyroid nodules. Hosp Med 28:46, 1992.

Conry C: Evaluation of a breast complaint: Is it cancer? Am Fam Physician 49:445–450, 1994.

Donnegan WL: Evaluation of a palpable breast mass. N Engl J Med 327:937–942, 1992.

Florentine BD, Staymates B, Rabadi M, et al, Cancer Committee of the Henry Mayo Newhall Memorial Hospital: The reliability of fine-needle aspiration biopsy as the initial diagnostic procedure for palpable masses: A 4-year experience of 730 patients from a community hospital-based outpatient aspiration biopsy clinic. Cancer 107:406–416, 2006.

Gupta RK, Naran S, Lallu S, Fauck R: The diagnostic value of fine needle aspiration cytology (FNAC) in the assessment of palpable supraclavicular lymph nodes: A study of 218 cases. Cytopathology 14:201–207, 2003.

Hammond S, Keyhani-Rofagha S, O'Toole RV: Statistical analysis of fine-needle aspiration cytology of the breast. Acta Cytol 3:276–280, 1987.

Handa U, Mohan H, Bal A: Role of fine needle aspiration cytology in evaluation of paediatric lymphadenopathy. Cytopathology 14:66–69, 2003.

Kopicki MT: Management of the palpable breast mass. Female Patient 23:45, 1998.

Layfield LJ, Chrischilles EA, Cohen MB, Bottles K: The palpable breast nodule: A cost-effectiveness analysis of alternate diagnostic approaches. Cancer 72:1642–1651, 1993.

Layfield LJ, Cibas ES, Gharib H, Mandel SJ: Thyroid aspiration cytology: Current status. CA Cancer J Clin 59:99–110, 2009.

Lau SK, McKee GT, Weir MM, et al: The negative predicative value of breast fine-needle aspiration biopsy: The Massachusetts General Hospital experience. Breast J 10:487–491, 2004.

Ogilvie JB, Piatigorsky EJ, Clark OH: Current status of fine needle aspiration for thyroid nodules. Adv Surg 40:223–238, 2006.

Perez-Reyes N, Mulford DK, Rutkowski MA, et al: Breast fine-needle aspiration: A comparison of thin-layer and conventional preparation. Am J Clin Pathol 102:349–353, 1994.

Pothier DD, Narula AA: Should we apply suction during fine needle cytology of thyroid lesions? A systematic review and meta-analysis. Ann R Coll Surg Engl 88:643–645, 2006.

CHAPTER 227

HEIMLICH MANEUVER

Raymond F. Jarris, Jr.

Each year in the United States, 3000 people die from swallowing or aspirating objects. When a patient displays the distress signal for choking (i.e., clutching the neck) or becomes cyanotic, unconscious, or unable to cough or breathe effectively (suggesting complete obstruction), efforts to clear the obstruction are warranted. The Heimlich maneuver (abdominal thrusts) causes a sudden increase in intrathoracic pressure, forcing an obstructing object from the glottis (Fig. 227-1).

NOTE: In the event of partial foreign body aspiration, *if the patient is able to move air or speak*, the Heimlich maneuver and probing of the oropharynx should be avoided and the patient should be transported to a source of emergency medical care.

INDICATION

Asphyxiation from a foreign body obstruction of the upper airway indicates treatment. If forceful coughing is occurring, do not interfere with the coughing. However, the Heimlich maneuver is indicated if the cough becomes silent, respiratory difficulty increases and is accompanied by stridor, or the victim becomes unresponsive. In the unresponsive patient, a "finger sweep" of the posterior oropharynx should only be used when the provider can see solid material obstructing the airway.

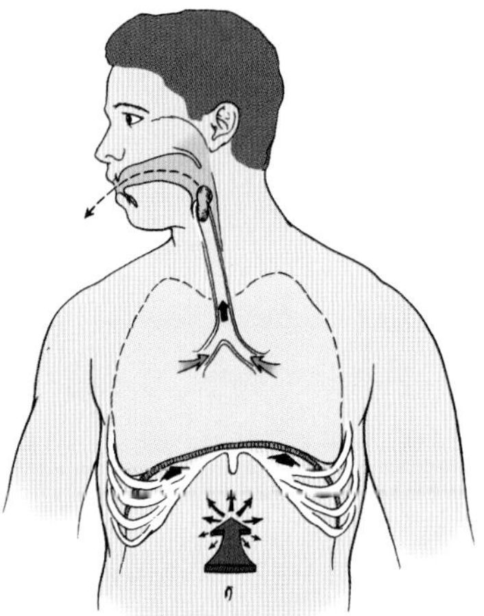

Figure 227-1 The Heimlich maneuver causes a sudden increase in intrathoracic pressure, forcing an obstructing object from the glottis. If the patient is sitting or standing, the clinician should stand behind the patient and wrap his or her arms around the patient's waist. The clinician's fist should be placed with the thumb side against the patient's abdomen, above the umbilicus but below the rib cage.

CONTRAINDICATIONS

The Heimlich maneuver is contraindicated in infants, small children, and pregnant women (abdominal thrusts inappropriate). It may also be difficult to accomplish in obese patients if the clinician is unable to encircle the victim's abdomen. In obese patients and in pregnant women, chest thrusts may be appropriate.

TECHNIQUE

Adults and Children Older Than 1 Year of Age

Sitting or Standing

Apply three to five abdominal or chest thrusts (Fig. 227-2A). These thrusts lift the diaphragm and force enough air from the lungs to create an artificial cough to move and expel an obstructing foreign body in an airway.

Lying

1. Place the patient in the supine position.
2. Place one hand on top of the other, with the heel of the bottom hand positioned in the midline of the patient, between the umbilicus and xiphoid.
3. Lean forward with shoulders over the patient's abdomen and quickly press inward and upward three to five times (Fig. 227-2B).
4. In pregnant or obese patients, use chest thrusts delivered in the same fashion as step 3, but place hands over the sternum.
5. Clear visible material from the oropharynx with a finger sweep or Magill forceps.

Infants to 1 Year of Age

1. Place the child face down on your arm with head directed downward, supporting head and neck with knee and one hand (Fig. 227-3).
2. Deliver three to five gentle back blows between the scapulae with the palm of the hand.
3. If obstruction is still present, roll the child over, lower his or her head, and deliver chest thrusts gently with two to three fingers as in cardiopulmonary resuscitation.
4. Repeat steps 2 and 3 until the object is cleared or surgical intervention is required (see Chapter 199, Cricothyroid Catheter Insertion, Crycothyroidotomy, and Tracheostomy).

COMPLICATIONS

- Abdominal aortic aneurysm thrombosis
- Internal carotid artery dissection
- Esophageal rupture
- Gastric rupture
- Jejunal rupture
- Liver, spleen, or pancreas injury

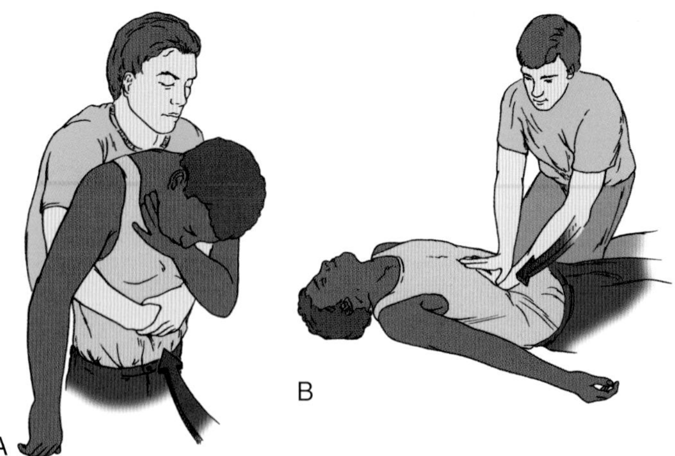

Figure 227-2 Abdominal thrusts. **A,** If the patient is sitting or standing, the clinician should stand behind the patient, wrap his or her arms around the patient's waist, grasp the fist or wrist of one hand with the other, place the hands against the patient's abdomen between the navel and rib cage, and press the fist into the patient's abdomen with a quick thrust upward. This should be repeated up to three to five times. **B,** If the patient has collapsed or is unable to be lifted, he or she should be placed in the supine position and the clinician should kneel beside the patient's abdomen or straddle it. The clinician should place one hand on top of the other, with the heel of the bottom hand in the midline between the patient's navel and rib cage. He or she should lean forward so that the shoulders are over the patient's abdomen and press toward the diaphragm with a quick thrust, inward and upward. The clinician should not press to the right or left of the midline. This should be repeated up to three to five times if necessary.

- Pneumomediastinum
- Regurgitation
- Rib fracture

The Heimlich maneuver is usually performed outside of medical facilities. Although complications are rare, most of the complications are severe and can be life-threatening. For example, gastric rupture has a high mortality rate. A physician should evaluate all persons who have been subjected to the Heimlich maneuver. Focused evaluation by the physician should include history and physical examination of the respiratory and gastrointestinal system. Early intervention may reduce the morbidity and mortality associated with these complications.

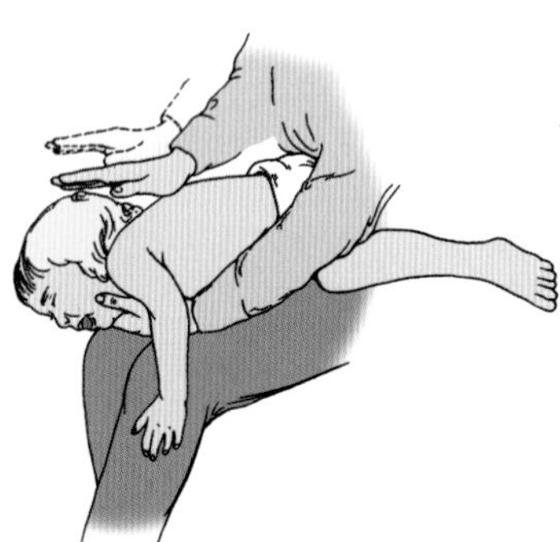

Figure 227-3 Back blows for infants and small children. See text for details.

ACKNOWLEDGMENT

The editors wish to recognize the many contributions of Timothy J. Downs, MD, to this chapter in the previous edition of this text.

BIBLIOGRAPHY

American Heart Association Guidelines for Cardiopulmonary Resuscitation and Emergency Cardiovascular Care: Part 4: Adult Basic Life Support. Circulation 112:IV-19–IV-34, 2005. Also available online at http://circ.ahajournals.org/content/vol112/24_suppl/. Accessed August 8, 2010.

Bintz M, Cogbill TH: Gastric rupture after the Heimlich maneuver. J Trauma 40:159–160, 1996.

Haynes DE, Haynes BE, Yong YV: Esophageal rupture complicating Heimlich maneuver. Am J Emerg Med 2:507–509, 1984.

Kirschner RL, Green RM: Acute thrombosis of abdominal aortic aneurysm subsequent to Heimlich maneuver: A case report. J Vasc Surg 2:594–596, 1985.

Majumdar A, Sedman PC: Gastric rupture secondary to successful Heimlich maneuver. Postgrad Med J 74:609–610, 1998.

Otero Palleiro MM, Barbagelata López C, Fernández Pretel MC, Salgado Fernández J: Hepatic rupture after Heimlich maneuver. Ann Emerg Med 49:825–826, 2007.

Razaboni RM, Brathwaite CE, Dwyer WA Jr: Ruptured jejunum following Heimlich maneuver. J Emerg Med 4:95–98, 1986.

CHAPTER 228

Muscle Biopsy

James R. Shepich

Many disorders of the motor unit can be identified by clinical presentation, but occasionally a muscle biopsy is necessary for diagnosis. Muscle biopsy is a relatively straightforward procedure that may be performed under local anesthesia. However, many authorities contend that a better-quality specimen can be obtained under general anesthesia because injudicious local infiltration can affect the histology. The site of biopsy and the type of biopsy (open vs. core needle) vary with the patient and disease.

The *muscle of choice* should show the effects of the disease process. However, the most severely affected muscles *should be avoided* because the muscle mass may be replaced by scar tissue or fat, and an adequate pathologic diagnosis may not be possible. Muscles with recent trauma, including recent electromyography (EMG) or infection, should not be sampled. Muscle in areas of tendinous transition should be avoided because the increased connective tissue may be mistaken for fibrosis during pathologic assessment. Some commonly sampled muscles include the lateral aspect of quadriceps femoris, deltoid, biceps brachii, tibialis anterior, and gastrocnemius.

The *biopsy method* depends on clinical judgment. *Core needle biopsy* is less invasive and causes less pain and scarring than open biopsy. It is easier to perform, especially in children, and allows repeat biopsy of the same muscle if necessary. *Open biopsy* allows a larger specimen to be taken, which increases the chance of definitive diagnosis and allows multiple modalities of pathologic preparation of the specimen if needed, including electron microscopy. Open biopsy is also ideal if disease of the motor end plate is suspected. With either approach the muscle to be sampled should be placed in an extended, relaxed position.

Indications

A muscle biopsy is performed to identify syndromes of muscle weakness that do not present with classic findings. Several diseases, such as Duchenne's muscular dystrophy, Werdnig-Hoffmann disease, and myasthenia gravis, have classic presentations and muscle biopsy is not necessary. Muscle biopsy can be used to distinguish between neurogenic and myopathic processes, identify congenital myopathies, and diagnose connective tissue disorders and muscle infections, such as trichinosis and toxoplasmosis. Metabolic disorders of the muscle may also be found by biopsy. Biopsy is also indicated in the identification and indexing of hereditary disorders.

Contraindications

- Anticoagulation and bleeding disorders
- Recent trauma of the muscle, including EMG
- Clinical appearance of Duchenne's muscular dystrophy (biopsy can cause scarring and contracture of muscle)
- Infection in region of proposed biopsy

Equipment

Open Biopsy

- Sterile drapes
- Povidone–iodine
- Local anesthesia (1% lidocaine without epinephrine)
- Scalpel with no. 11 or no. 15 blade
- Forceps, iris scissors, suture scissors
- 3-0 Vicryl or Monocryl sutures
- 4-0 Vicryl or Monocryl sutures
- Electrocautery or diathermy (not to be used until after biopsy sample is procured)
- 4 × 4 gauze sponges
- Tongue blade, cut into 6- to 7-cm lengths, with V-groove in ends, or 22-gauge needles to pin specimen
- 3-0 nylon or Prolene suture
- Steri-Strips, Tegaderm, Op-Site, or dressing of choice

Core Needle Biopsy

- Sterile drape
- Povidone–iodine
- Local anesthesia
- Tru-Cut, Biopty, Conchotome, or equivalent needle
- Band-Aid

Preprocedure Patient Preparation

The patient should be informed that the procedure is relatively painless, but that the biopsy site may be sore for several days. Many patients experience a sensation of muscle bruising and occasionally a pulling sensation. The patient does not need to restrict food and fluids before the procedure, but he or she should be instructed to wear loose-fitting clothes that readily allow access to the intended biopsy site. Little postprocedural disability or recovery time is expected and the patient may return to usual activity immediately. Analgesic medication is rarely needed, and when it is necessary, it is usually only for 24 to 48 hours. Risks, benefits, and potential complications should be discussed with the patient before the procedure (see the sample patient education handout online at www.expertconsult.com).

Technique

Open Biopsy

The patient should be prepared and draped, with the muscle in an extended, relaxed position. To prevent a vasovagal episode, the patient should be lying down. The *skin* overlying the muscle to be

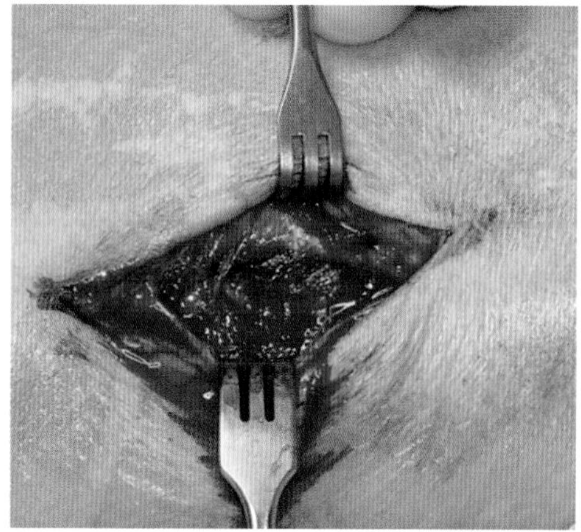

Figure 228-1 Incision for biopsy of rectus femoris muscle.

sampled is infiltrated with local anesthesia. Care should be taken to avoid infiltration of the muscle itself. A 3- to 4-cm incision is made over the muscle belly, in an axial orientation to the muscle (Fig. 228-1). The skin and subcutaneous tissue are retracted and the fascia exposed. The fascia is opened sharply in a longitudinal fashion, and the muscle is exposed. Care should be taken to avoid injuring cutaneous nerve branches, which often lie on the fascia. A portion of muscle approximately 3 to 4 cm in length and 5 mm in diameter is excised after a nonabsorbable suture is placed at each end. The excisional sites are "outside" of the sutures. The specimen is maintained in an extended state and transferred to the tongue depressor, where the suture can be placed in a V-groove on either end or pinned to the surface with 22-gauge needles (Fig. 228-2). Hemostasis is achieved with diathermy or electrocautery.

Many pathologists require two specimens for a muscle biopsy. The first is a piece of muscle measuring 0.5 to 1 cm, and the second is an additional fascicle 2 to 3 cm in length and 5 mm in diameter that is tied to a splinter of tongue blade in situ, before it is excised (Figs. 228-3 to 228-5).

The fascia is then closed with 3-0 Vicryl sutures to prevent muscle herniation. The skin is closed with a running subcuticular stitch. Steri-Strips and a sterile dressing are applied. Dermabond or other skin adhesive may also be used.

Core Needle Biopsy

The patient is prepared, draped, and anesthetized as previously described for an open biopsy. A small nick is made in the skin with a no. 11 blade, and the bioptome is introduced. Care should be taken that the throw of the needle does not carry it into vital structures or bone. The bioptome is then activated. Multiple passes may be taken through the muscle in different areas, and usually three cores

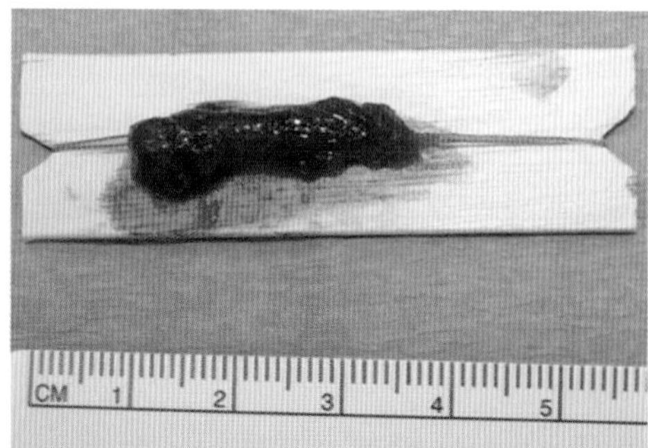

Figure 228-2 Muscle portion approximately 1 × 1 × 2 cm stretched on a tongue blade.

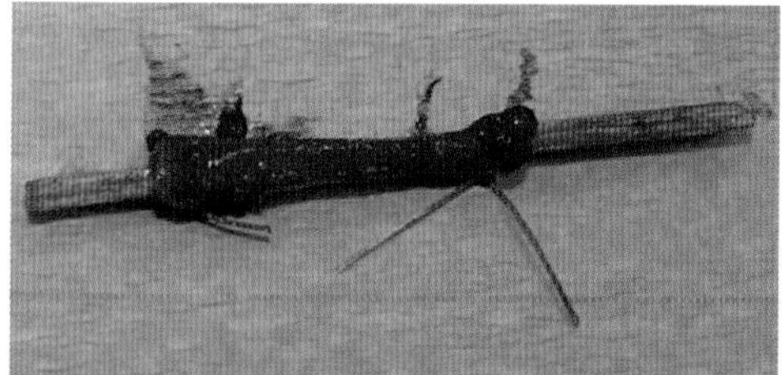

Figure 228-3 Muscle fascicle tied in situ to splinter of tongue blade.

of tissue are obtained. Pressure is held at the site for 2 to 3 minutes, and a Band-Aid is then applied.

Complications

Potential complications include bleeding, hematoma, or bruising at site of biopsy. The wound may become infected or be slow to heal, especially in patients with connective tissue disorders who have been on steroids. In some conditions biopsy may lead to fibrosis and contracture of the muscle. Mild postprocedural discomfort is usual, and prolonged paresthesia can be experienced if a sensory nerve is injured. Also, the biopsy may be nondiagnostic, requiring a repeat biopsy.

Handling of Tissue and Interpretation of Results

Note the muscle sampled for the pathologist. (The deltoid muscle has an unusual connective tissue pattern that may be misinterpreted.) Other information supplied to the pathologist should include a clinical summary of symptoms and their distribution and duration. The results of EMG, nerve conduction velocity, and pertinent laboratory studies should also be included. Muscle biopsy should be performed in coordination with a pathologist because the specimen should *never be placed in a fixative* and should be processed within 30 minutes of its removal. A longer interval will cause specimen desiccation and architectural distortion. Standard pathologic assessment includes sectioning after cryostat freezing of the specimen, electron microscopy, and immunohistochemical analysis. The pathologic diagnosis is based on the architecture of the muscle group, the characteristics of the individual fibers, and the presence of increased connective tissue or inflammatory cells. Electron microscopy will reveal abnormalities of the mitochondria and other cellular infrastructure. Special staining for oxidative, glycolytic, and hydrolytic enzymes will add information about enzyme deficiency, inflammation, and mitochondrial and lysosomal abnormalities. Stains with periodic acid-Schiff reagent and Oil Red O will help diagnose glycogen and lipid storage disorders. Immunohistochemical assay will add information regarding dystrophin, major histocompatibility complex receptors, and autoimmune disorders.

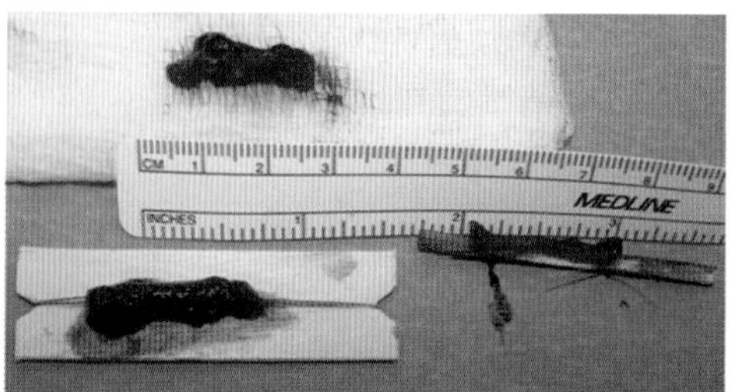

Figure 228-4 Three specimens for histology, immunochemistry, and electron microscopy.

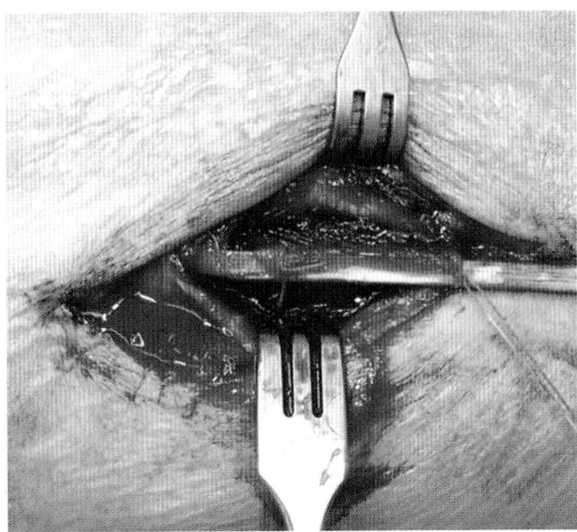

Figure 228-5 Technique for in situ harvest of muscle fascicle.

Postprocedure Patient Education

The patient should be instructed to monitor the area of biopsy for signs or symptoms of infection, excessive bleeding, or hematoma formation. A small amount of serosanguineous fluid may accumulate beneath the dressing. The outer dressing should be maintained for at least 48 hours and then removed. The Steri-Strips may be removed between the fifth and seventh days after the biopsy (see the sample patient education handout online at www.expertconsult.com).

Patient Education Guides

See the sample patient education and consent forms online at www.expertconsult.com.

CPT/Billing Codes

20200 Muscle biopsy, superficial
20205 Muscle biopsy, deep
20206 Muscle biopsy, needle

ICD-9-CM Diagnostic Codes

335.0 Werdnig-Hoffmann syndrome (muscular atrophy)
359.9 Myopathy
359.89 Myopathy, primary
710.3 Dermatomyositis
710.4 Polymyositis
728.2 Muscular atrophy (NOS or idiopathy)
728.9 Muscle weakness

Also, see numerous specific conditions.

Online Resources

Neuromuscular: Muscle biopsy. Available at www.neuro.wustl.edu/neuromuscular/lab/mbiopsy.htm.

University of Iowa, Department of Pathology, Laboratory Services Handbook: Muscle biopsy: General instructions. Available at www.medicine.uiowa.edu/path_handbook/Appendix/Anatomicpath/ex_muscle_biopsy.html.

Bibliography

DuBowitz V, Sewry C: Muscle Biopsy: A Practical Approach, 3rd ed. Philadelphia, Saunders, 2006.

Rubin E, Farber J (eds): Pathology. Philadelphia, JB Lippincott, 1988.

CHAPTER 229

Transcutaneous Electrical Nerve Stimulation, Phonophoresis, and Iontophoresis

Russell D. White • Mary Beth Brown

The procedures described in this chapter—transcutaneous electrical nerve stimulation (TENS), phonophoresis, and iontophoresis—can be performed either by primary care clinicians in their office or by physical therapists when ordered by a clinician. The procedures are often used with other physical therapy modalities such as manual therapy or therapeutic exercise. The choice of procedure depends on the size (localized vs. diffuse) and depth (superficial vs. deep) of the proposed treatment area as well as the specific pathologic process.

Equipment

- Scissors to trim hair
- Isopropyl alcohol 70% to cleanse skin
- For *TENS*: TENS unit with either disposable or reusable electrodes and gel
- For *phonophoresis*: therapeutic ultrasound unit, appropriate medication, and coupling gel
- For *iontophoresis*: direct-current generator with constant current output (calibrated in milliamperes), electrodes, and appropriate medications

Preprocedure Patient Preparation

After discussing the patient's diagnosis, the risks and benefits of the selected treatment should be explained, along with any treatment options. Oral or written consent should be obtained from the patient. Patients should be aware that their skin will be cleansed and that their hair may be trimmed. The anticipated treatment plan and total number of treatments should also be discussed.

Transcutaneous Electrical Nerve Stimulation

Transcutaneous electrical nerve stimulation therapy uses low-voltage electrical pulses to stimulate the nervous system and is used for the treatment of pain syndromes. Skin surface electrodes are used to pass the electricity into the affected area. TENS units are Class II, U.S. Food and Drug Administration–approved devices and are *typically selected for larger, generalized areas of pain, for chronic joint pains, or for persistent myalgias*. This procedure can be performed in the clinician's office and is reimbursable if performed by the clinician. However, TENS therapy is usually prescribed by a clinician and performed by the physical therapist. When prescribed for home use, the patient must be competent in operating a TENS unit.

TENS therapy is based on the *gate theory of pain*. According to this theory, nociperception (injury information) is transmitted through T cells that convey information to the higher brain centers. This information is presynaptically inhibited by interneurons in the substantia gelatinosa. TENS therapy bombards these interneurons, attempting to modulate or decrease the pain transmission by effectively blocking transmission of pain sensation. Other theories suggest that TENS therapy achieves its result by an acupuncture effect, by release of natural opiates, or by direct local vasodilation, which may reduce relative ischemia.

The goal of TENS therapy is to reduce or relieve pain and discomfort. This result may be either short lived or prolonged. TENS therapy may slowly break the *pain–spasm–pain cycle* and reduce perceived discomfort. Unfortunately, TENS therapy is not effective for pain of central origin (e.g., headache).

Treatment parameters are chosen based on several factors:

- *Intensity:* Small unmyelinated fibers require more current than large myelinated fibers. (Intensity is set according to patient comfort [strong but not painful] and can vary widely by body part undergoing treatment, by device used, and by individual sensation and tolerance.)
- *Pulse rate:* Small unmyelinated fibers respond better to a low-frequency rate (<100 Hz), whereas large myelinated fibers respond better to a high-frequency rate (>100 Hz).
- *Wave characteristics:* These characteristics are either monophasic (positive rectangular pattern) or biphasic (negative spike pattern).
- *Pulse width:* Small unmyelinated fibers respond to a long pulse (200 milliseconds [msec]), whereas large myelinated fibers respond to a short pulse (50 msec).
- *Modulation:* Modulation allows gradual variation of the frequency or pulse width and retards accommodation of the nervous tissue.

Indications

- Chronic pain
- Acute pain
- Musculoskeletal pain
- Neurologic pain (e.g., herpes zoster)
- Phantom limb pain

- Before another procedure to elevate the pain threshold and to decrease patient discomfort after the procedure
- Postoperative pain
- Obstetric pain (after the first trimester)

Contraindications

- Patients with demand-type pacemakers (Newer pacemakers with improved shielding are not affected by TENS units. Check with a cardiologist or the manufacturer.)
- Patients in first-trimester pregnancy
- Patients with known cardiac dysrhythmias
- Mentally incompetent patients, uncooperative patients, those with paranoid disorders, or pediatric patients without adult supervision
- Undiagnosed pain syndromes without established etiology
- TENS therapy is also contraindicated over the following areas:
  - Carotid sinuses
  - Chest areas in patients with a cardiac history
  - Head or neck area of patients with an epileptic history
  - Laryngeal or pharyngeal muscles
  - Local areas of skin irritation or loss of skin integrity
  - Mucosal surfaces
  - Eyes

Technique

1. Before initiating therapy, organize the necessary materials (Fig. 229-1) and prepare the skin area to which the electrodes will be attached. Trimming hair and cleansing the skin with 70% isopropyl alcohol will promote the adhesion and conductivity of the electrodes.
2. Select the proper electrodes. For 24 hours or more of use, select either a carbon-impregnated rubber electrode with gel or a carbon-filled silicone electrode.
3. Attach electrodes to the selected treatment site, whether isolated trigger points, individual dermatomes or myotomes, or in the distribution of a specific nerve. Position the electrodes so that a paresthesia will be felt in the area of pain or dysfunction (Fig. 229-2). If the electrodes are secured poorly to the skin, they may cause a burning sensation instead of a paresthesia. In addition, electrodes should be placed at least 2 inches apart. Placing electrodes closer together can cause a burning sensation. The electrodes should also be placed so that the perimeter of the painful area is entirely surrounded by the electrodes.

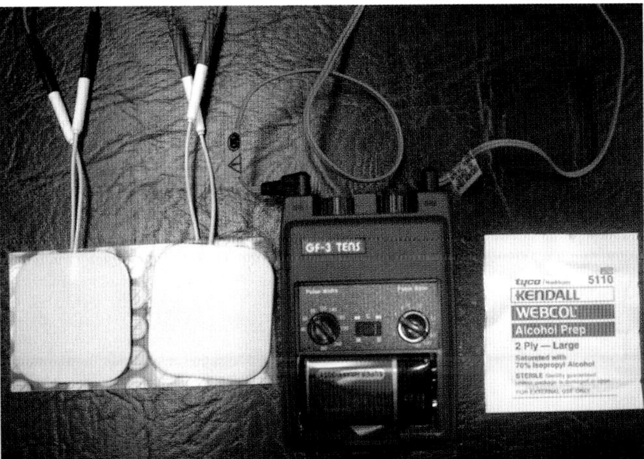

Figure 229-1 Transcutaneous electrical nerve stimulation (TENS) unit (generator) with supplies for skin preparation, electrodes, and electrode wires.

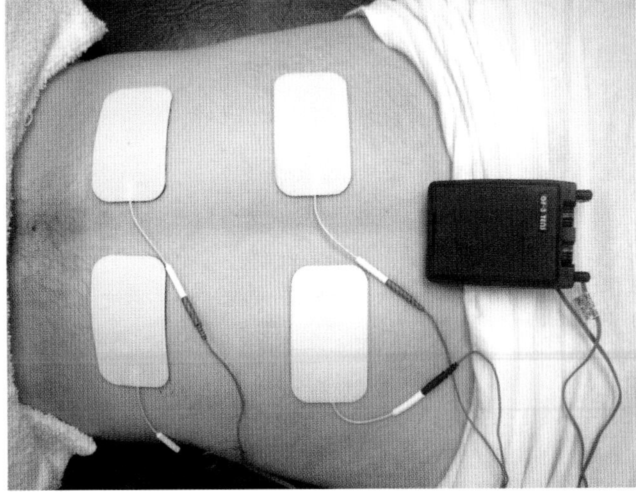

Figure 229-2 TENS treatment.

4. Select the treatment parameters. Conventional settings use a high-frequency rate with a narrow pulse width. The intensity level is *less than* that which results in muscle stimulation.
5. With the amplitude control in the *off* position, attach wires to the TENS unit. Turn on the generator unit and increase the amplitude slowly, up to the patient's comfort level. Again, paresthesia should be felt by the patient before the threshold for motor stimulation.
6. If desired results (paresthesia with control of pain) are not achieved, change the stimulation sites or adjust the treatment settings.
7. Typically, patients are treated once or twice daily for a duration of 30 to 60 minutes. Some patients may benefit from more frequent treatments and may require a home unit for therapy.
8. When the treatment is completed, turn off the unit, return the settings to zero, and remove the electrodes.

Complications

- Skin irritation from electrode placement
- Contact dermatitis resulting from electrode gels
- Pacemaker malfunction (typically an older pacemaker)
- Twitch response secondary to stimulation of a motor nerve or end plate in the treatment area by inappropriate current

PHONOPHORESIS

Phonophoresis uses therapeutic ultrasound to enhance the diffusion of medications across the skin and into body tissues. Commonly used medications include dexamethasone, hydrocortisone, and lidocaine. Although phonophoresis is usually performed by the physical therapist, some clinicians provide this modality in the office setting. Clinicians can be reimbursed for phonophoresis, even if not performed by a physical therapist.

The dual action of phonophoresis—thermal and mechanical—counteracts the inflammatory response by a process called *acoustic streaming*, which increases cell membrane permeability. This effect also facilitates the passage of medications into body tissue. With *acute* inflammation, using pulse-mode ultrasound avoids an increase in tissue temperature. In addition to the alteration of tissue permeability, beneficial effects are obtained through nonthermal changes (e.g., stimulation of fibroblasts). With *chronic* inflammation, using continuous or nonpulsed ultrasound can produce thermal changes that counteract or prevent the chronic changes of scarring and tissue edema.

Ultrasound dose is measured in intensity (intensity = W/cm^2), which is the acoustic energy delivered through the surface area of the head of the transducer. Areas of inflammation are usually treated with 1 to 2 W/cm^2 for 5 to 10 minutes. Results are measured by the improvement (either immediate or gradual) in pain or function of the treated area.

Indications

- Superficial periarticular disorders: bursitis, tendinitis, ligament sprains
- Contracture of joint capsules or adhesive scars
- Neuromas
- Reflex sympathetic dystrophy
- Plantar warts
- Muscular strains, fibrosis, spasm, myositis (limited evidence)

Contraindications

- Allergy to medications being used
- Tumors
- Thrombophlebitis
- Pregnancy (*therapeutic* ultrasound is contraindicated over the abdomen and pelvis)
- Hemorrhagic or infected areas
- Cardiac disease (*therapeutic* ultrasound over the cervical ganglia, cardiac area, or an implanted pacemaker may produce a detrimental cardiac reflex)
- Unhealed fracture sites
- Phonophoresis should also be avoided over the following areas:
  - Epiphyseal plate in growing bones
  - Spinal cord
  - Area of previous radiation therapy (wait 6 months before applying ultrasound)
  - Eyes

Technique

1. A clinician's prescription is required for the medications when phonophoresis is administered by a physical therapist.
2. Select an area of inflammation for treatment that is no greater than twice the surface area of the sound head.
3. Select the proper ultrasound equipment (Figs. 229-3 and 229-4).
4. Cleanse the general area to be treated. Inspect the skin for excessive dryness and trim excess hair. Skin areas may be pretreated with moist heat packs to facilitate drug absorption by dilating the hair follicles.
5. Because the chosen agent can affect ultrasound transmission, select only topical agents that transmit ultrasound. (Hydrocortisone 10% or ketoprofen 2.5 % in an aqueous base are commonly used medications for phonophoresis.) Apply the medication followed by the coupling gel or use coupling gels impregnated with medication.
6. Apply phonophoresis through the sound head in a moving pattern of overlapping strokes or circles (Fig. 229-5).
7. Recommended *intensities* of 1 to 2 W/cm^2 usually provide effective results. Use *frequencies* of 3 MHz for superficial tissues and 1 MHz for deeper tissues. Apply for 5 to 10 minutes. Treatment

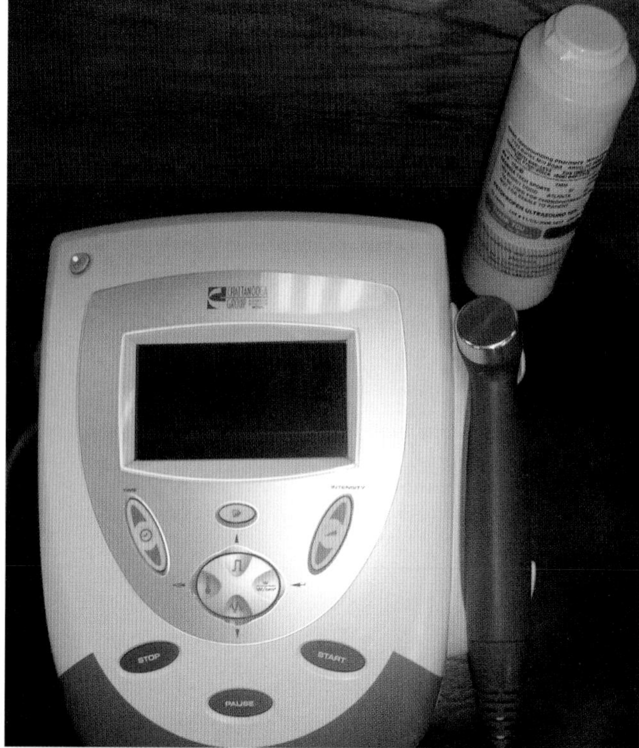

Figure 229-4 Ultrasound unit.

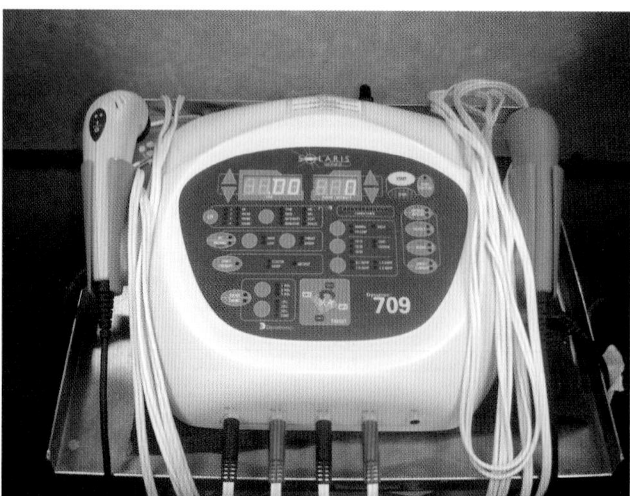

Figure 229-3 Ultrasound–electrical stimulation combination unit used for phonophoresis and TENS.

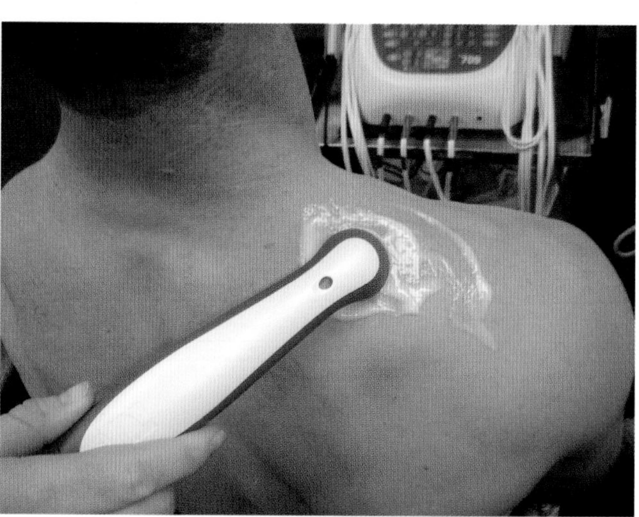

Figure 229-5 Phonophoresis treatment.

for greater than 10 minutes increases the risk of a negative effect (e.g., periosteal burn).

8. When finished, wipe away coupling gel but do not cleanse skin; there is some evidence that an occlusive dressing may further promote continued medication absorption.

Complications

- Previously unknown allergy or sensitivity to medication
- Systemic side effects from excessive absorption of applied medication
- Damage to susceptible areas (listed in Contraindications section)

IONTOPHORESIS

Iontophoresis uses direct electrical current to enhance the diffusion and absorption of charged medications across the skin and mucous membranes. With this technique, medicinal ions can penetrate tissue for 0.2 to 1.5 cm, depending on the drug used and the characteristics of the local tissue. This technique is based on repulsion of similarly charged ions; charged ions in solution are driven away from like-charged electrodes.

Iontophoresis works best when the pathologic process is superficial and localized. This treatment is usually performed in an outpatient rehabilitation setting or in the clinician's office. Primary care clinicians can be reimbursed for the procedure, even if it is not performed by a physical therapist.

The most common *medications* used are dexamethasone or lidocaine and the amount depends on the size of the treatment area. The amount used also depends on the electrode size and the volume it takes to fill it. Electrode size varies from 1.5 to 3.5 cm^3. Dexamethasone is the primary agent indicated for inflammatory lesions. Lidocaine is the agent typically used for preoperative topical anesthesia.

The *electrical* dose for administration is expressed in milliampere minutes (mA minutes) and is the product of the *intensity* (milliamperes) and *duration* (minutes). Most treatments last 10 to 20 minutes each and are repeated three to eight times (depending on patient response).

Indications

- Same indications as for a superficial injection of a therapeutic agent (superficial, because the medications *penetrate* only up to 1.5 cm with iontophoresis)
- Inflammation
  - Bursitis
  - Tendinitis
  - Fasciitis
  - Sprain
  - Strain
  - Trigger points
  - Carpal tunnel syndrome
  - de Quervain's disease
- Analgesia
  - Neuritis
  - Local anesthesia for invasive procedures, such as dermatologic procedures
- Other (limited case reports; Table 229-1)
  - Ganglion
  - Hyperhidrosis of feet or palms
  - Ischemic ulcer
  - Neuroma
  - Post-traumatic edema
  - Scar tissue
  - Tinea pedis
  - Turf toe
  - Warts
  - Wound healing

TABLE 229-1 Indications and Dosages for Common Iontophoresis Agents

Ion (Dose)	Polarity	Therapeutic Use
Acetic acid (3–4 mA × 10–20 min)	Negative	Calcified tendinitis, calcium deposit
Chloride, sodium (4 mA × 20–45 min)	Negative	Keloids, scar tissue
Copper sulfate (4 mA × 20–30 min)	Positive	Fungal infection
Dexamethasone (1–4 mA × 15–20 min)	Negative	Tendinitis, tenosynovitis, bursitis, arthritis
Hyaluronidase (1–2 mA × 20–40 min)	Positive	Edema, lymphedema, scleroderma
Iodine (2 mA × 1 min; then 4 mA × 5 min)	Negative	Fibrosis, scar tissue, trigger finger
Lidocaine 4% (4 mA × 20–30 min)	Positive	Skin anesthesia
Methylprednisolone (1–4 mA × 15–20 min)	Negative	Postherpetic neuralgia
Salicylate (4 mA × 45 min)	Negative	Analgesia, myalgia, plantar warts
Zinc (4 mA × 15 min)	Positive	Wound healing, ulcers

Contraindications

- Allergy or sensitivity to therapeutic agent
- Patients with pacemakers because electric current could interfere with sensitive implanted devices
- Iontophoresis should also be avoided over the following areas:
  - Areas of abnormal skin sensation (patients must be able to give feedback so that the intensity can be set correctly)
  - Superficial abrasions, cuts, and bruises
  - Areas of recent bleeding
  - Areas surrounding or superficial to an implanted or embedded wire, screws, staples, or other metallic objects
  - Recent scars or skin graft
  - Area over heart
  - Area over carotid sinus

Areas of abnormal sensation or a loss of skin integrity have decreased skin resistance; this raises the risk that an increased current dose may be given. Such a dose may lead to undesired skin reactions. Areas of increased vascularity or those near metal objects can also be subjected to enhanced current dosage.

Technique

1. A clinician's prescription is required for the medications administered by a physical therapist using iontophoresis.
2. Position the patient to obtain good exposure for the area to be treated. Inspect the skin of the treatment area for any recent injury or any contraindications previously listed.
3. Clip excessive hair but do not shave. Clean the skin treatment area with 70% isopropyl alcohol to remove surface oils and skin cells.
4. Before initiating therapy, the clinician should organize the equipment and select a direct-current generator (Fig. 229-6). Next, inject the premeasured medication into the electrode reservoir according to the manufacturer's recommendations. (Properly filling electrodes to specified volumes decreases skin irritation.)
5. The *active* electrode *(drug containment electrode)* should be attached over the treatment area. It should have the same polarity as the medication to be used. Attach the larger *dispersive* electrode *(indifferent electrode)* over an area that is at least 3 inches distant (Fig. 229-7) from the active electrode.
6. Connect the electrode leads to the current generator. Current settings should range from 0.1 to 4 mA.

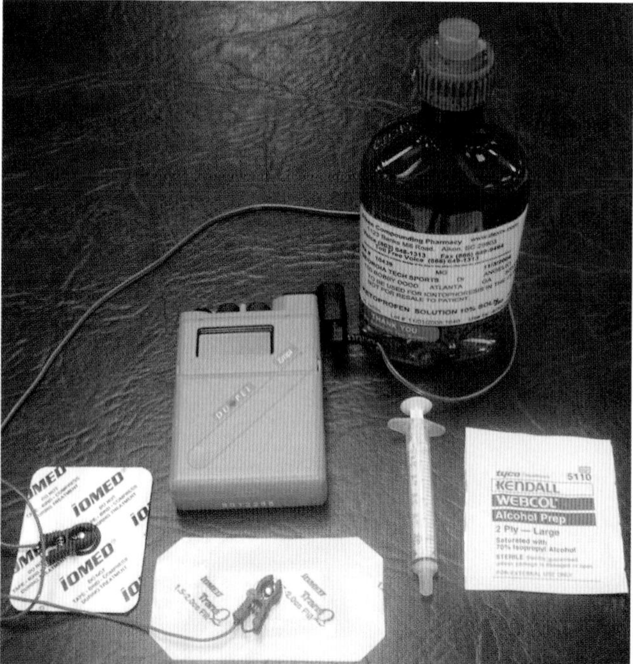

Figure 229-6 Iontophoresis current generator with iontophoresis agent, measuring syringe, alcohol wipe for skin preparation, electrodes, and electrode leads.

7. Determine the current dosage on the basis of the diagnosis and treatment. The recommended dosage for dexamethasone or lidocaine is listed in Table 229-1 and measured in mA × min. (milliamperes [current] × minutes [time] = mA × min [dosage]).
8. *Gradually* increase the current until the patient barely feels it. Any *sudden* change in current may produce burning, stinging, or a twitch response. With most units, the treatment time is automatically set by the device once the intensity (current) and dosage are determined and entered.
9. During and after the procedure, ask the patient every 2 to 4 minutes if he or she is experiencing any adverse effects.
10. When the procedure is completed, remove the attached electrodes. Instruct the patient to report any delayed adverse effects. (Post-treatment erythema is common, resulting from either changes in skin pH or a histamine reaction.)
11. An alternative, recently developed technique is the use of a wearable, battery-powered iontophoresis patch. The patch is filled with medication by a physician or a physical therapist in the clinic and applied directly to prepared skin. Medication is iontophoretically delivered using a constant 0.06- to 0.45-mA current over 3 to 24 hours (varies by manufacturer) with automatic current shut-off when desired dosage is reached.

Complications

- Previously unknown drug allergy or sensitivity to medications
- Galvanic rash: hypersensitivity reaction to the direct current that develops within 5 minutes of initiating the electrical stimulation
- Twitch response secondary to stimulation of a nerve in the treatment area by inappropriate current
- "Negative electrode burn": skin burn resulting from a decrease in skin resistance and an alkaline reaction when the negative electrode (cathode) is the active electrode (newer electrodes stabilize the pH better and cause less skin irritation)
- Local immunologic inhibition from the steroid (dexamethasone is not detected in the bloodstream after treatment)

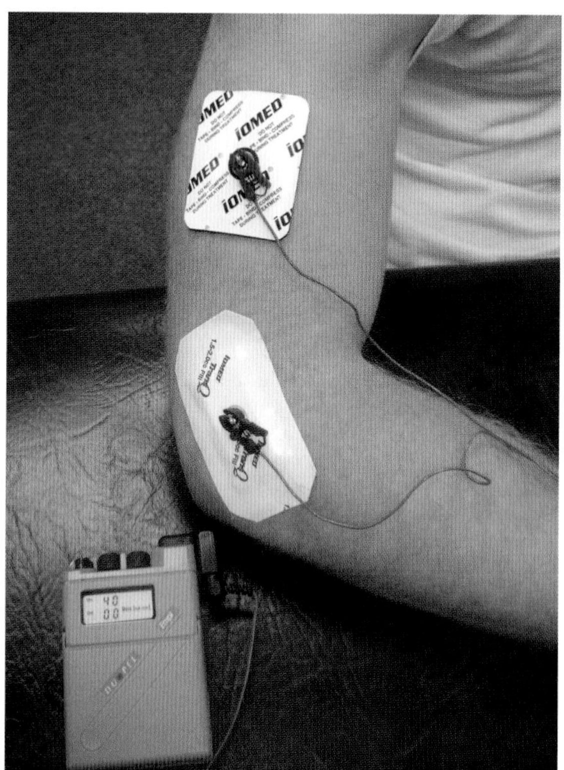

Figure 229-7 Iontophoresis treatment.

Postprocedure Patient Care and Education

The patient's results are evaluated by determining the decrease in pain or inflammation after treatment(s). Treatment(s) can be terminated when the patient has reached the desired clinical goal. The number or frequency of treatments can be increased to improve the results, as long as no adverse effects have been noted. On the contrary, after five treatments with any of these modalities, if there are no results, another type of therapy should be considered.

The patient should know to report any delayed adverse reactions to the clinician. He or she should also know when to make a follow-up appointment.

Patient Education Guides

See the patient education form available online at www.expertconsult.com.

CPT/Billing Codes

NOTE: Healthcare Common Procedure Coding System (HCPCS) codes are used for procedures and supplies when there is no CPT code. They are the alphanumeric codes listed here, and reimbursement is variable.

TENS

64550 Application of surface transcutaneous neurostimulator (TENS)

TENS Unit

E0720 TENS, two lead localized stimulation*
E0730 TENS, four lead, larger/multiple nerve stimulation*

Phonophoresis

97035 Ultrasound therapy
A4558 Conductive paste or gel supplies

Iontophoresis

97033 Iontophoresis, each 15 minutes or application of each wearable patch

Medication and Supplies

A4556 Electrodes, per pair
J1100 Dexamethasone sodium phosphate, 4 mg/mL
J1020 Methylprednisolone acetate, 20 mg
J1030 Methylprednisolone acetate, 40 mg
J1040 Methylprednisolone acetate, 80 mg

ICD-9-CM Diagnostic Codes

053.9 Postherpetic neuralgia
078.19 Plantar warts
110.4 Tinea pedis
337.20 Reflex sympathetic dystrophy
350.1 Trigeminal neuralgia
353.6 Phantom limb pain
354.0 Carpal tunnel syndrome
355.0 Piriformis syndrome
355.6 Neuroma, Morton's
457.1 Lymphedema
524.60 Temporomandibular syndrome
625.9 Pain, obstetric (by site)
701.4 Keloids
707.1 Ulcer, lower limbs
709.2 Scar tissue
715.0 Osteoarthrosis, general
715.00 Osteoarthrosis, unspecified
715.01 Osteoarthrosis, shoulder
715.02 Osteoarthrosis, upper arm
715.03 Osteoarthrosis, forearm
715.04 Osteoarthrosis, hand
715.06 Osteoarthrosis, lower leg
715.07 Osteoarthrosis, ankle/foot
715.08 Osteoarthrosis, specified sites
715.9 Arthritis, unspecified
715.16 Osteoarthrosis, lower leg
715.17 Osteoarthrosis, ankle and foot
724.2 Low back pain
726.0 Adhesive capsulitis of shoulder
726.0 Tendinitis, shoulder
726.5 Tendinitis or bursitis, hip
726.10 Bursitis, shoulder
726.31 Medial epicondylitis
726.32 Lateral epicondylitis
726.60 Enthesopathy or bursitis, knee
726.61 Enthesopat, pes anserinus
726.64 Tendonitis, patellar
726.65 Bursitis, prepatellar
726.71 Tendinitis, Achilles
726.90 Capsulitis, periarthritis, or tendinitis, NOS
727.00 Tenosynovitis and synovitis, unspecified
727.03 Trigger finger
727.04 de Quervain's disease
727.41 Ganglion of joint
727.42 Ganglion, tendon sheath
727.82 Calcific tendonitis
728.2 Muscle wasting/fibrosis
728.12 Myositis ossificans, traumatic
728.71 Fasciitis, plantar
728.85 Muscle spasm
729.1 Myalgias and myositis, unspecified
729.2 Neuritis
780.8 Hyperhidrosis
782.0 Dermal pain
782.3 Edema
845.0 Ankle, sprains/strains
845.01 Deltoid ligament
845.02 Calcaneofibular ligament
845.03 Tibiofibular ligament
845.09 Achilles tendon
845.1 Foot, sprains/strains
845.12 Turf toe
848.9 Sprains/strains, unspecified site

NOTE: 900 series need date of injury.

923.00 Contusion, shoulder
923.03 Contusion, upper arm
923.10 Contusion, forearm
924.00 Contusion, hip
924.01 Contusion, thigh
924.10 Contusion, lower leg
924.11 Contusion, knee
959.1 Injury, trunk
959.2 Injury, shoulder and upper arm
959.7 Injury, knee, leg, ankle, and foot

Suppliers

(See contact information online at www.expertconsult.com.)

Iontophoresis
EMPI, Inc
IOMED, Inc.
Smith & Nephew
Stoetling
Travanti Pharma, Inc. (formerly Birch Point Medical, Inc.) for IontoPatch

Phonophoresis
AliMed, Inc.
Chattanooga Group, Inc.
Dynatronics
DynaWave Corporation

TENS units
AliMed, Inc.
Electro-Med Health Industries
EMPI, Inc.
RS Medical
Thera-Tronics, Inc.

BIBLIOGRAPHY

Abram SE: Advances in chronic pain management since gate control. Reg Anesth 18:66–81, 1993.
Anderson CR, Morris RL, Boeh SD, et al: Effects of iontophoresis current magnitude and duration on dexamethasone deposition and localized drug retention. Phys Ther 83:161–170, 2003.

*Prior authorization is required by Medicare for this item.

Bolin DJ: Transdermal approaches to pain in sports medicine management. Curr Sports Med Rep 2:303–309, 2003.

Byl NN: The use of ultrasound as an enhancer for transcutaneous drug delivery: Phonophoresis. Phys Ther 75:539–553, 1995.

Cagnie B, Vinck E, Rimbaut S, Vanderstraeten G: Phonophoresis versus topical application of ketoprofen: Comparison between tissue and plasma levels. Phys Ther 83:707–712, 2003.

Costello CT, Jeske AH: Iontophoresis: Applications in transdermal medication delivery. Phys Ther 75:554–563, 1995.

DeSantana JM, Walsh DM, Vance C, et al: Effectiveness of transcutaneous electrical nerve stimulation for treatment of hyperalgesia and pain. Curr Rheumatol Rep 10:492–499, 2008.

Deyo RA, Walsh NE, Martin DC, et al: A controlled trial of transcutaneous electrical nerve stimulation (TENS) and exercise for low back pain. N Engl J Med 322:1627–1634, 1990.

Gudeman SC, Eisele SA, Heidt RS Jr, et al: Treatment of plantar fasciitis by iontophoresis of 0.4% dexamethasone: A randomized, double-blind, placebo-controlled study. Am J Sports Med 25:312–316, 1997.

Guy RH, Kalia YN, Delgado-Charro MB, et al: Iontophoresis: Repulsion and electroosmosis. J Control Release 64:129–132, 2000.

Klaiman MD, Shrader JA, Danoff JV, et al: Phonophoresis versus ultrasound in the treatment of common musculoskeletal conditions. Med Sci Sports Exerc 30:1349–1355, 1998.

Kuntz AR, Griffiths CM, Rankin JM, et al: Cortisol concentrations in human skeletal muscle tissue after phonophoresis with 10% hydrocortisone gel. J Athl Train 41:321–324, 2006.

Mehreteab TA: Iontophoresis. In Hecox B, Mehreteab TA, Weisberg J (eds): Physical Agents: A Comprehensive Text for Physical Therapists. East Norwalk, Conn, Appleton & Lange, 1994, pp 295–298.

Moll MJ: A new approach to pain: Lidocaine and Decadron with ultrasound. USAF Med Serv Dig 30:8–11, 1979.

Nnoaham KE, Kumbang J: Transcutaneous electrical nerve stimulation (TENS) for chronic pain. Cochrane Database Syst Rev 3:CD003222, 2008.

Robinson AJ: Transcutaneous electrical nerve stimulation for the control of pain in musculoskeletal disorders. J Orthop Sports Phys Ther 24:208–226, 1996.

Rose JB, Galinkin JL, Jantzen EC, Chiavacci RM: A study of lidocaine iontophoresis for pediatric venipuncture. Anesth Analg 94:867–871, 2002.

Semalty A, Semalty M, Singh R, et al: Iontophoretic drug delivery system: A review. Technol Health Care 15:237–245, 2007.

Spielholz NI, Nolan MF: Conventional TENS and the phenomena of accommodation, adaptation, habituation, and electrode polarization. J Clin Electrophysiol 7:16–19, 1995.

Sweitzer RW: Ultrasound. In Hecox B, Mehreteab TA, Weisberg J (eds): Physical Agents: A Comprehensive Text for Physical Therapists. East Norwalk, Conn, Appleton & Lange, 1994, pp 163–192.

Wang Y, Thakur R, Fan Q, Michniak B: Transdermal iontophoresis: Combination strategies to improve transdermal iontophoretic drug delivery. Eur J Pharm Biopharm 60:179–191, 2005.

Zempsky WT, Sullivan J, Paulson DM, Hoath SB: Evaluation of a low-dose lidocaine iontophoresis system for topical anesthesia in adults and children: A randomized, controlled trial. Clin Ther 26:1110–1119, 2004.

CHAPTER 230

Preoperative Evaluation*

Maury J. Greenberg

The preoperative medical consultation may be one of the most misunderstood services provided by primary care clinicians. Often incorrectly referred to as a "clearance," it is more properly a consultation provided by the patient's primary clinician, at the request of the operating surgeon. The goal of this consultation is to assess the patient's medical condition to minimize risks of untoward events related to the proposed surgical intervention.

In some instances, the operating surgeon is also the primary care clinician, in which case the preoperative evaluation may be conducted as part of the overall decision-making process surrounding the need for an office- or hospital-based diagnostic or therapeutic procedure. In others, the consultation may be performed before surgery by another clinician. In either case, it provides an opportunity for the primary care clinician to review the patient's overall health status and bring up to date a variety of issues such as recommended screening tests, medication adjustments, and lifestyle modifications. It may also afford an opportunity to review previously offered recommendations the patient has failed to pursue, such as screening colonoscopy, smoking cessation, weight loss, vaccination, or, in the case of children, developmental assessments.

As a consultation, the results must be reported to the requesting surgeon in a timely fashion and in a usable format, and must include clear, concise, and specific recommendations related to the proposed surgical procedure.

It should also be noted that, particularly in the case of procedures performed in hospitals, the preoperative evaluation will become a part of the patient's medical record. As such, should complications arise or unexpected events occur, this evaluation may provide the only comprehensive medical history immediately available.

Finally, it must be recognized that "standards" change. Ongoing research and evidence results in changes to our understanding of what is best for optimizing a patient's condition and to limit risks. For example, changes to American Heart Association guidelines for prevention of bacterial endocarditis (www.americanheart.org) have altered the use of preoperative antibiotic prophylaxis in many patients. It is important, therefore, for every clinician to maintain access to current guidelines and to seek expert consultation when indicated.

Surgical Risk

Determining the relative risk of a given procedure must take into account the patient's underlying condition, the specific risks of the procedure itself, the risks of anesthesia, and the possibility of postoperative complications. In most cases, "risk" refers to the possibility of cardiovascular complications in adults or respiratory complications in children. However, in the face of underlying conditions such as bleeding disorders, asthma, steroid dependence, or renal insufficiency, an otherwise simple procedure can present risks that require careful preoperative preparation. The timing of an elective procedure can also modify the risk, particularly during the postpartum period, or in a patient with a recent myocardial event such as an infarction.

Risk from Procedures

- *High-risk procedures* (often >5% risk) include cardiac procedures, aortic and other major vessel vascular procedures, and peripheral arterial procedures.
- *Intermediate-risk procedures* (1% to 5% risk) include intraperitoneal, intrathoracic, carotid or aortic stent, carotid endarterectomy, orthopedic, head and neck, and prostate procedures. Although each of these types of surgery may entail specific risks such as anticipated blood loss, risk of airway compromise, or risk of intraoperative or postoperative neurologic complications, they are not unanticipated and are addressed by the operating surgeon together with the anesthesiologist as part of the operative plan.
- *Low-risk procedures* (<1% risk) include cataract surgery, most endoscopic procedures, and breast, superficial skin, and ambulatory noncardiac surgeries.

Most office-based procedures such as skin biopsy, colposcopy, vasectomy, and others that require no anesthesia or only topical or local anesthesia do not increase the risk of cardiac or pulmonary events in otherwise healthy individuals and are considered low risk. Such procedures, including dental procedures performed with self-administered 50% nitrous oxide and other diagnostic or therapeutic procedures performed without sedation or analgesia, do not usually require a separate or specific preoperative consultation, especially if the procedure is performed by the patient's primary care clinician, who is familiar with the individual's medical history.

Patient Risk Factors

Risk is further determined by considering the patient's medical conditions, including that which resulted in the need for surgery. Clinical predictors of increased risk of cardiac complications associated with surgery include uncontrolled coronary occlusive disease including unstable angina, uncontrolled congestive heart failure, significant valvular disease (especially aortic or mitral stenosis), recent (<30 days) myocardial infarction, and cardiac dysrhythmias associated with hemodynamic instability.

Concurrent medical conditions, including uncontrolled hypertension, diabetes, obstructive pulmonary disease (asthma or emphysema), poor nutritional status, bleeding disorders, hypercoagulable states, ischemic cerebrovascular disease, liver disease, kidney disease, or immune deficiency, will also require assessment and specific interventions to reduce risk, if possible.

In some cases, the decision may need to be made that an elective procedure should be deferred until risk factors have been fully evaluated and appropriate interventions performed.

*The opinions contained in this chapter are solely those of the author and do not represent the official policy or doctrine of the Department of Defense, the U.S. Public Health Service, or the Uniformed Services University of the Health Sciences.

Although it may be intuitive to assign greater risk of a given procedure to patients of advanced age, there is no evidence for age as an independent variable correlating with increased incidence of poor outcomes. The perception of increasing age resulting in increased risk is more likely associated with increased incidence of comorbid conditions. Simply put, healthy old people will have the same risks of surgery as healthy young people. This may be a good incentive for younger patients to maintain healthy lifestyles and physical fitness in anticipation of the increased likelihood that they may require surgery when they are older.

Risk from Anesthesia

Selection of type of anesthesia may also affect the overall risk of surgery, but the notion that local, regional, or spinal anesthesia is automatically safer than general anesthesia is not valid. The availability of a tracheal tube in a patient under general anesthesia allows optimal airway control and protection, which may offset the risks of such anesthesia in some patients. The use of "sedation analgesia," also known as *conscious sedation*, for some procedures allows the performance of certain procedures while the patient is still able to respond to commands and maintain his or her own airway (see Chapter 2, Procedural Sedation and Analgesia).

The selection of this technique, however, mandates strict adherence to monitoring and the availability of resuscitative equipment. Clinicians who use conscious sedation for procedures performed in office settings make considerable investments in training, equipment, and personnel in order to provide essentially the same level of care as is provided in a hospital setting.

For procedures performed in hospitals or ambulatory facilities that provide anesthesia team services, in the absence of compelling issues, it is usually best to leave selection of specific anesthetic modalities to the anesthesiologist. Specific concerns should of course be discussed with the surgeon and anesthesia team when indicated. It is helpful, however, for all clinicians to have an understanding of the risk classification system used by anesthesiologists (Box 230-1).

Box 230-1. Shortcuts to Determine Indicators for Noninvasive Testing before Noncardiac Surgery

No testing is necessary if the answer is "Yes" to any of the following four questions:

1. Is this low-risk surgery (e.g., endoscopic, superficial, cataract, breast, ambulatory surgery)?
2. Does the patient have fair functional/exercise capacity (≥4 METs) and no symptoms?
3. Has the patient undergone revascularization (coronary artery bypass grafting or percutaneous coronary intervention) within last 5 years without a change in symptoms indicating ischemia?
4. Has the patient had a thorough cardiac evaluation within last 2 years without a change in symptoms indicating ischemia?

Conversely, if vascular surgery is planned and the patient has three or more clinical risk factors (CAD, CHF, ASCVD, diabetes, or renal insufficiency), noninvasive testing is reasonable if the results will change the management.

Also, if the answer is "Yes" to both of the following two questions, noninvasive testing is reasonable:

1. Does the patient have poor functional/exercise capacity by questionnaire or specific questioning (<4 METs, or inability to climb one flight of stairs)?
2. Is a clinical risk factor present (CAD, CHF, ASCVD, diabetes, or renal insufficiency)?

ASCVD, arteriosclerotic cardiovascular disease; CAD, coronary artery disease; CHF, congestive heart failure; METs, metabolic equivalents.

From Fleisher LA, Beckman JA, Brown KA, et al: ACC/AHA 2007 Guidelines on perioperative cardiovascular evaluation and care for noncardiac surgery: Executive summary. A report of the American College of Cardiology/American Heart Association Task Force on Practice Guidelines (Writing Committee to Revise the 2002 Guidelines on Perioperative Cardiovascular Evaluation for Noncardiac Surgery). Circulation 116:1971–1996, 2007; originally published online September 27, 2007.

Preoperative History and Physical Examination

History

It has been noted that the history provides 90% of the information needed to tender good medical care, the physical examination provides 10%, and laboratory testing only confuses the matter. Although this may be a slight exaggeration, it is true that a careful and complete history is critical to good care and the ability of the consultant to provide appropriate recommendations.

The *reasons for the planned procedure* should be noted and should include the laterality of the affected organ or body part if appropriate. Events leading up to the procedure, especially those associated with trauma, should be reviewed for possible indicators of medical causes. For example, a fractured hip may be secondary to a fall, but the fall may be secondary to syncope related to intermittent complete heart block, which in turn may be secondary to Lyme disease.

The *past surgical history*, including any reactions to anesthesia as well as family history of such reactions, must be noted and investigated, and any allergies to medications as well as sensitivity to latex must be prominently included in the report forwarded to the surgeon.

A complete *list of medications* being taken by the patient, including dose, route, and frequency, should include not only prescribed medications but vitamins, supplements, and herbal treatments. The common use of aspirin is an obvious concern, but other products such as nonsteroidal anti-inflammatory drugs (NSAIDs), omega-3 fatty acids, ginkgo biloba, or high-dose vitamin E can also affect bleeding. St. John's wort interacts with many medications.

Aspirin, which irreversibly interferes with *platelet function* by inhibiting cyclooxygenase, has effects that last the entire 10-day lifespan of platelets, and must therefore be discontinued 10 to 14 days before surgery that has a risk for bleeding. The exception to this is for patients with known coronary or cardiovascular disease. Neither aspirin nor any other antiplatelet medications should be discontinued before dermatologic or dental procedures. Other NSAIDs such as ibuprofen also affect cyclooxygenase, but in a reversible fashion that lasts until the drug has effectively been cleared, usually after approximately five half-lives (10 hours for ibuprofen, which has an elimination half-life of 2 hours, but 3 days for naproxen, which has an elimination half-life of about 15 hours).

Patients should be questioned about history of angina, myocardial infarction, and symptoms suggestive of congestive heart failure such as dyspnea, orthopnea, or edema, as well as any recent cardiac testing such as stress tests or echocardiograms, the availability of which might obviate the need for repeat studies.

History of respiratory or cardiac conditions that might suggest the need for preoperative testing, or interventions such as bronchodilator treatments, should be noted and appropriate recommendations made. Factors such as obesity, likelihood of immobility, or altered coagulation and immunologic states should also prompt appropriate suggestions for both preoperative and postoperative care. Risk of postoperative deep venous thrombosis with secondary pulmonary embolism is increased by immobility and should prompt suggestions for prevention, which may include early ambulation if possible, use of sequential leg compression devices, or postoperative anticoagulation with heparin, enoxaparin, or warfarin. In some cases it may be prudent to discontinue medications that have prothrombotic properties, such as estrogen or oral contraceptives that contain estrogen.

Family history of deep venous thrombosis, early stroke, or other events that might suggest the possibility of an inherited tendency to hypercoagulability might prompt testing for such issues as factor V Leyden mutation, prothrombin mutation, or abnormalities of protein S or protein C, among others.

The history includes an *assessment of functional cardiac capacity* based on questions of tolerance of physical activity. The inability of the adult patient with more than minimal risk predictors to perform activity equaling at least 4 metabolic equivalents (METs) usually suggests the need for additional preoperative cardiac evaluation. Examples of activities that correspond to 4 METs include playing doubles tennis, climbing a flight of stairs, walking on level ground at 4 miles per hour, running a short distance, or doing moderately heavy housework such as scrubbing floors or moving heavy furniture.

For children, the history should include the birth history, any prenatal or perinatal complications, growth and developmental milestones, immunization status, and any recent illness, particularly respiratory infections.

The *last menstrual period* for women must be noted, as well as methods of birth control, menstrual history, and date of last Papanicolaou (Pap) test and mammogram. For patients with planned gynecologic surgery a pregnancy history should be taken, including types of delivery, obstetric anesthesia, and birth outcomes.

A *history of nutritional deficiency* for adults as well as children may have profound implications for wound healing and postoperative morbidity, and must be mentioned. It should prompt specific recommendations for preoperative nutritional evaluation and possibly the need for preoperative or postoperative nutritional support.

Smoking status must be reviewed and noted. Discontinuation of smoking 6 to 8 weeks before surgery is clearly beneficial in terms of reduced risk of cardiac and respiratory complications, as well as long-term health if the patient does not resume smoking. There is debate, however, about the effects of more proximate smoking cessation, especially if the patient discontinues cigarette use only a few days before surgery, which may lead to increased mucus mobilization as well as nicotine withdrawal symptoms. *Alcohol consumption* and nonmedical drug use are also important factors that should be considered in order to avoid unexpected withdrawal.

Elements of the patient's history will affect recommendations for antibiotic prophylaxis, including recent prosthetic joint surgery or other implanted devices, the need for endocarditis prophylaxis, or the need for other specific pharmacologic pretreatment such as stress doses of cortisone for dependent patients (e.g., patients with steroid-dependent asthma or Addison's disease).

Physical Examination

The physical examination starts with an accurate recording of the patient's vital signs, including temperature, pulse, respiratory rate, and blood pressure. Document height, weight, body mass index, and head circumference for children younger than 2 years of age. Orthostatic testing should be performed if there is risk or suspicion of hemodynamic compromise. The temptation simply to ask a patient his or her weight must be avoided, and only values and measurements actually obtained at the time of the consultation should be considered valid.

A full examination is performed with emphasis on the patient's known medical conditions and the type of surgery anticipated, remembering that the patient's care may not be ultimately limited to the procedures, interventions, and types of anesthesia initially planned.

The report of the physical examination should mention pupil equality and reactivity, especially if the patient exhibits anisocoria (unequal pupils) at baseline. The condition of his or her dentition and the presence of braces, dentures, or other removable dental appliances should be noted, as should the absence of teeth, which should be identified by tooth number.

The presence of previously uninvestigated carotid bruits indicates the need for further work-up.

Recalling that the most serious surgical risk is associated with cardiovascular and pulmonary complications, careful attention should be paid to the examination of the heart and lungs, being alert for murmurs, gallops, wheezes, rales, crackles, or other signs of valvular disease, respiratory conditions, or congestive heart failure. The abdominal examination should include palpation for pulsatile abdominal findings that might prompt an assessment for aortic aneurism, and for renal bruits. The presence of ascites or a previously undocumented enlarged liver or spleen will prompt additional evaluation.

Assessment of extremity function, including motor strength, is important in patients undergoing joint surgery, but evaluation of peripheral vascular competency, including distal pulses and capillary refill, is essential in all patients because peripheral vascular disease is an important predictor of postoperative cardiac complications.

The neurologic examination should at minimum include a mental status evaluation that will serve as a baseline against which postoperative neurologic compromise will be measured. In some cases it may also be important in establishing the patient's ability to give informed consent.

As mentioned previously, the preoperative medical evaluation may be the patient's only opportunity for a complete medical assessment, and it may be appropriate to include an examination of the prostate, a breast and pelvic examination, or performance of a Pap test, even if they are not directly related to the planned procedure.

Laboratory and Radiographic Testing

Preoperative laboratory testing should be based on the individual patient's underlying conditions, the potential for surgically related problems that relate to laboratory findings, or the potential that baseline or preoperative laboratory results might be helpful, should complications arise perioperatively. Most laboratory and diagnostic tests are *unnecessary* in healthy patients undergoing low- or intermediate-risk procedures, and in fact may lead to additional unnecessary testing if insignificant abnormalities are identified.

A *baseline electrocardiogram* should be obtained in patients with a history of diabetes, coronary artery disease, congestive heart failure, or poor functional capacity (<4 METs), or with evidence of peripheral vascular disease, cerebrovascular disease, or renal insufficiency. It is also probably reasonable in anyone undergoing vascular surgery.

Loss of physiologic variability in heart rate normally seen with respiration suggests possible autonomic dysfunction, which increases the risk of coronary artery disease in diabetic patients.

The patient with chest pain, new symptoms of congestive heart failure, or arrhythmias including ectopic beats should also be considered for noninvasive cardiac testing (e.g., exercise electrocardiography testing, nuclear stress testing, stress echocardiography). An echocardiogram with Doppler flow studies may also be helpful in assessing risk in patients with murmurs, physical findings suggestive of cardiomegaly, or symptoms that indicate decreased ventricular function. Results of recent testing may obviate the need for repeat studies if the patient's symptoms are chronic and unchanged in the past year or two.

The emergence of medications for treatment of erectile dysfunction has improved awareness of this condition as a marker for peripheral vascular disease and possible concomitant coronary artery disease. Patients taking these medications who have not previously been evaluated might benefit from preoperative noninvasive cardiac testing.

Hemoglobin should be measured in patients with history of anemia, bleeding disorders, diabetes, renal disease, hepatic disorders, human immunodeficiency virus infection, hypertension, or cardiovascular disease, or with planned surgery in which significant blood loss is anticipated. The optimal hemoglobin level is related more to the patient's baseline and functional capacity than to a specific value. Although the traditional lower limit of 10 to 11 g/dL hemoglobin is a good approximation, the risks of transfusion must also be considered, especially in patients who normally function without difficulty at somewhat lower levels.

Preoperative supplementation of iron, vitamin C, and, when documented deficiency exists, folic acid or vitamin B_{12}, may help to optimize hemoglobin levels. The use of erythropoietin should be avoided in the absence of documented deficiency, usually related to renal or neoplastic disease. Serum creatinine and potassium should also be documented in such patients, along with serum glucose for patients with diabetes. Liver function tests (aspartate and alanine aminotransferases, gamma-glutamyltransferase, alkaline phosphatase, serum bilirubin) should be checked in patients with liver disease.

Use of diuretics or digoxin indicates the need for measuring potassium and magnesium serum levels as part of the preoperative evaluation.

On a practical basis, it is often simpler and frequently cost effective to obtain these tests as part of automated panels (complete blood count [CBC], basic metabolic panel, or comprehensive metabolic panel).

Patients on warfarin therapy will need to have the international normalized ratio (INR) checked before surgery, to ensure return to normal if treatment was stopped or to ensure therapeutic values if treatment is to continue uninterrupted. Patients at high risk of a cardiovascular event if warfarin therapy is discontinued should obtain "bridging" therapy with low-molecular-weight heparin or heparin.

A history or suspicion of cardiovascular or pulmonary disease will prompt the performance of a *preoperative chest radiograph.* They are otherwise generally not indicated unless related to the planned procedure, particularly if the patient has had a negative chest film in the past year.

Assessment of nutritional status can be very helpful in planning the need for nutritional support, especially in patients with signs of malnutrition. Measurement of *serum albumin below 3.2 g/dL* or prealbumin below 15 mg/dL suggests the need for nutritional evaluation and possible supplementation before and after surgery. In some cases it may be prudent to postpone nonemergent surgery in nutritionally depleted individuals until this issue has been addressed.

Other preoperative laboratory evaluation should be specific to the patient's comorbid conditions or the specific nature and risks of the planned procedure. This may include a pregnancy test for women of childbearing age. Diabetic patients will benefit from urine protein screening and possibly measurement of creatinine clearance to assess for diabetic kidney disease.

PATIENTS WITH CARDIAC AND PULMONARY DISEASE

Patients with past history of cardiac disease or at high risk of cardiac disease should be evaluated and managed preoperatively (Fig. 230-1). Such patients include those with recent myocardial infarction, unstable angina, significant valvular disease, hemodynamically significant dysrhythmias, or uncompensated heart failure, and those with poor functional capacity. Comorbid conditions such as pulmonary disease, diabetes (especially insulin requiring), kidney disease, and uncontrolled hypertension (diastolic blood pressure >100 mm Hg) require careful consideration for preoperative evaluation and management.

Cardiac Risk Factors

Individuals with controlled angina, moderate symptoms of heart failure, or mild valve disease and those with borderline functional capacity should be considered for preoperative cardiac testing, especially if the planned procedure is high risk, because perioperative stresses may unmask or exacerbate previously controlled or compensated disease. Patients whose history and clinical presentation suggest the need for a cardiac evaluation independent of the planned surgery should have such evaluation regardless of their risk factors or the calculated risk of the specific procedure.

Patients who have had a recent coronary evaluation (within 2 years) or a revascularization procedure (within 5 years), and who are free of angina, ectopy, and clinical signs of heart failure, are at lower risk for perioperative complications, especially those with a fair exercise capacity (>4 METs). In the absence of such recent testing or interventions, the performance of preoperative testing for patients with significant cardiac risk factors should be considered. Exercise electrocardiography testing (see Chapter 93, Exercise Electrocardiography [Stress] Testing), stress echocardiography (see Chapter 94, Stress Echocardiography), or nuclear cardiac stress testing may be appropriate, and patients who are unable to perform treadmill testing should be evaluated with pharmacologic stress testing using dipyridamole, adenosine, dobutamine, or arbutamine. Table 230-1 provides shortcuts for determining whether a patient needs noninvasive testing. For intermediate- or high-risk surgery with only one or two clinical risk factors present, there is insufficient evidence to determine the best management, beta blockade therapy versus noninvasive testing.

Recent coronary stent placement (<10 weeks) presents specific issues related to the risk of early stent thrombosis. Long-term aspirin therapy for nearly all patients with coronary artery disease is supplemented with long-term clopidogrel in patients who have received coronary stents to prevent early stent occlusion until epithelialization has occurred. The use of drug-eluting stents has reduced the risk of early stent closure but presents the need for longer, perhaps lifelong antiplatelet therapy, with the risk of late stent thrombosis if such therapy is discontinued. Decisions regarding the risk of bleeding in a particular procedure weighed against the risk of stent closure must be made, as well as the timing of discontinuation and reinstitution of aspirin alone, or both aspirin and clopidogrel.

When considering the value of various cardiac tests as part of a preoperative medical consultation, the clinician must consider the individual patient's risk of progressive disease as well as the risk of the test itself compared with the risks of the surgery. Local expertise is also a consideration. The concerns of the patient, the anesthesiologist, and the surgeon who will be performing the procedure must be factored into the decision-making process. It is therefore important to maintain an open dialogue with patients, surgeons, and anesthesiologists to achieve trust and confidence among all involved.

Anticoagulation

Long-term anticoagulation with warfarin is common among patients with atrial fibrillation, artificial heart valves, history of recurrent thrombosis, and other conditions.

The safety of discontinuing warfarin before surgery depends on the underlying condition, and in some cases the patient may require heparin therapy while warfarin is discontinued, and again after surgery until a therapeutic INR is achieved. Such patients include those with mechanical heart valves or with a history of recurrent deep venous thrombosis associated with hypercoagulable states. The use of low-molecular-weight heparin such as enoxaparin on a short-term basis may be acceptable in some of these patients, but has been less studied than the use of intravenous heparin.

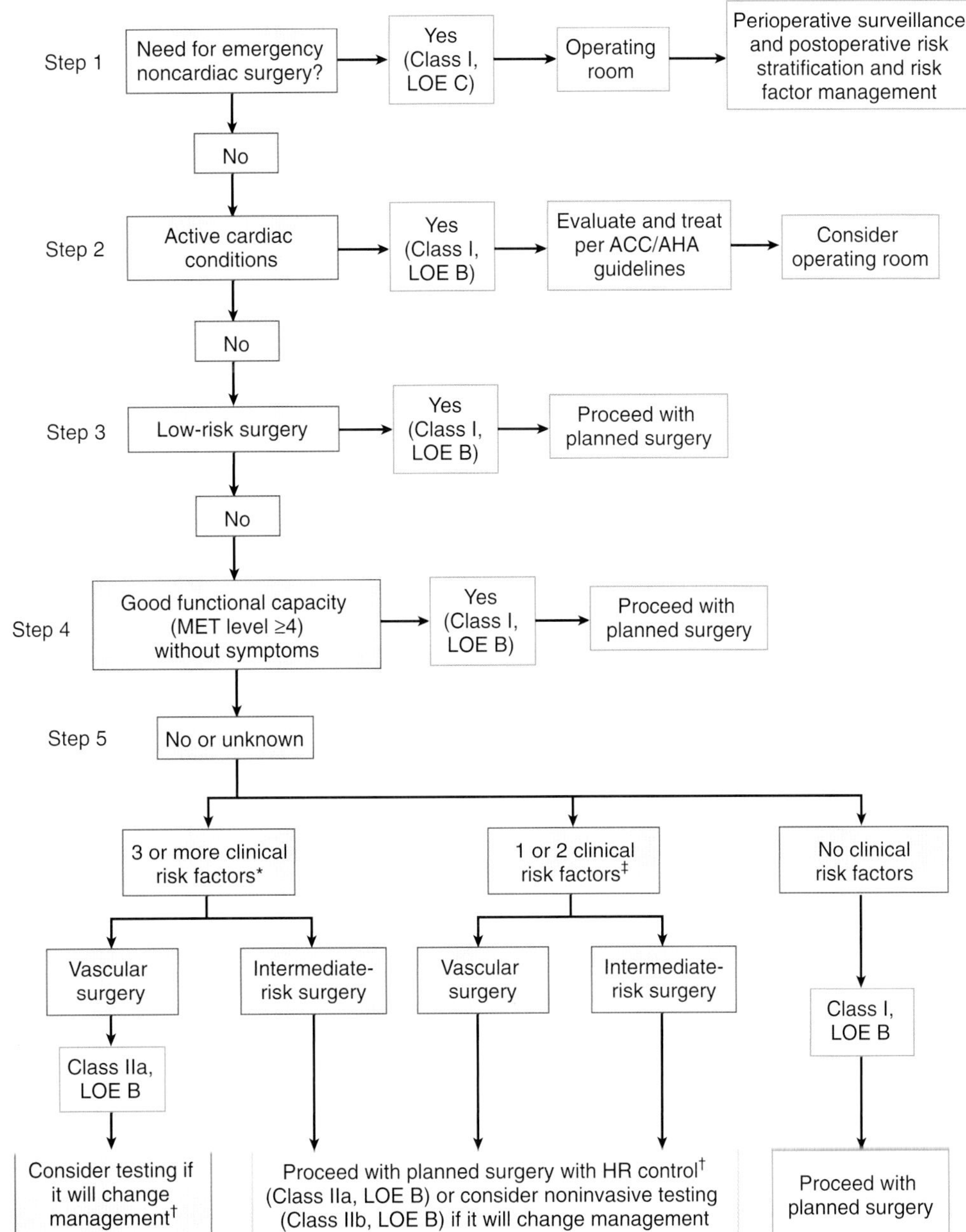

Figure 230-1 Cardiac evaluation and care algorithm for noncardiac surgery based on active clinical conditions, known cardiovascular disease, or cardiac risk factors for patients 50 years of age or older. *Clinical risk factors include ischemic heart disease, compensated or prior heart failure, diabetes mellitus, renal insufficiency, and cerebrovascular disease. †Consider perioperative beta blockade for populations in which this has been shown to reduce cardiac morbidity/mortality. ACC/AHA, American College of Cardiology/American Heart Association; HR, heart rate; LOE, level of evidence; MET, metabolic equivalent. (From Fleisher LA, Beckman JA, Brown KA, et al: ACC/AHA 2007 Guidelines on perioperative cardiovascular evaluation and care for noncardiac surgery: Executive summary. A report of the American College of Cardiology/American Heart Association Task Force on Practice Guidelines [Writing Committee to Revise the 2002 Guidelines on Perioperative Cardiovascular Evaluation for Noncardiac Surgery]. Circulation 116:1971–1996, 2007; originally published online September 27, 2007.)

For patients taking warfarin because of atrial fibrillation or ischemic cerebrovascular disease (recurrent transient ischemic attacks), the drug can usually be discontinued 3 days before surgery and restarted at the usual dose on the first postoperative day if the surgeon deems the risk of postoperative bleeding to be low. This would allow the patient's INR to slowly return to normal around the time of surgery, and slowly return to a therapeutic level after surgery without leaving the patient fully untreated for more than 72 hours. Such a regimen is frequently used for outpatient dental procedures, although many dentists and oral surgeons will allow patients to continue warfarin therapy uninterrupted. Bridging therapy with low-molecular-weight heparin or heparin may be considered in patients with atrial fibrillation and at high risk for thromboembolism.

Patients with protein S or C deficiency, factor V Leyden mutation, or other inherited causes of hypercoagulability may require heparin therapy while warfarin treatment is restarted to avoid thrombosis if loading doses of warfarin are used.

Close communication with the operating clinician, surgeon, or dentist is important to avoid conflicting and confusing instructions to the patient.

TABLE 230-1 American Society of Anesthesiologists Physical Status Classification System

Class	Description
1	A healthy patient with no significant medical problems
2	A patient with mild systemic disease
3	A patient with severe systemic disease that is not incapacitating
4	A patient with severe systemic disease that is a constant threat to life
5	A moribund patient, not expected to live 24 hours regardless of treatment
6	A brain-dead patient who is an organ donor
E	The "E" suffix is added to any class to indicate that the surgery is emergent.

Other Medications

Beta blockers should be continued in most patients already taking them, and initiation of such treatment before surgery should be considered in patients with high cardiac risk (ischemia on preoperative testing) who are scheduled for vascular surgery and other procedures that present increased risk of cardiac stress. These patients may be at high risk of perioperative cardiac events and expert consultation may be of benefit in determining appropriate therapy. Several authors have suggested withholding angiotensin-converting enzyme inhibitors and angiotensin receptor blockers the day of surgery and only restarting them postoperatively after euvolemia has been established in order to decrease the risk of perioperative renal dysfunction. A meta-analysis of 11 studies with 1007 patients (Mukherjee and Eagle, 2003) suggested that calcium channel blockers significantly reduced ischemia and risk of supraventricular tachyarrhythmias and were associated with trends toward reduced perioperative death and myocardial infarction. α_2-Adrenergic agonists have been shown to reduce mortality and myocardial infarction in patients undergoing vascular surgery. More specifically, clonidine has been studied prospectively and found to cause minimal hemodynamic effects and reduce postoperative mortality for up to 2 years.

Statins, widely used for long-term control of serum cholesterol, are also known to have beneficial effects in stabilizing atherosclerotic plaques. Their use preoperatively in patients with known coronary artery and ischemic cerebrovascular disease should be considered.

Pulmonary Disease

Preoperative evaluation of patients with pulmonary disease, including asthma, emphysema, or conditions that may affect oxygen diffusion such as lupus or sarcoidosis, may benefit from pulmonary function testing and baseline measurement of oxygen saturation as well as diffusing capacity. Optimization of therapy with inhaled beta agonists, inhaled steroids, and oral steroids may help reduce postoperative complications such as atelectasis, pneumonia, and exacerbations of obstruction. Intravenous stress doses of steroids (e.g., hydrocortisone sodium succinate [Solu-Cortef] 100 mg) might also be considered in patients who are steroid dependent. This may need to be balanced against considerations of steroid effects on wound healing and fluid balance. A preoperative nebulizer treatment with albuterol or another beta-active medication is often helpful. Patients with increased risk of postoperative atelectasis, including those with planned thoracic or abdominal surgery, may also benefit from preoperative teaching in the use of an incentive spirometer.

Sleep apnea, most common in adult men, should be noted in previously diagnosed individuals and considered in patients with typical body habitus (obese, short neck) and history of snoring, fatigue, and observed apneic episodes while sleeping. Sleep studies may be appropriate and the use of postoperative continuous positive airway pressure (CPAP) might be considered.

Patients with Diabetes

Control of blood glucose levels, as well as recognition of conditions that frequently are associated with diabetes, are important concerns in the preoperative evaluation of diabetic patients. If sufficient time is available before surgery, an attempt should be made to bring the patient under good glycemic control through adjustment in their usual oral medications or insulin dosages, or initiation of insulin therapy if necessary. Attempting to maintain normal blood sugars postoperatively, especially after major surgeries, has been proven beneficial for diabetic patients. In addition, undiagnosed patients at risk for metabolic disease, including diabetes, would benefit from screening before surgery.

The stress response to surgery can result in hyperglycemia, and this should be considered in the planning of diabetic therapy. Perioperative dehydration may also result in elevated blood glucose, ketosis, and potential acidosis, especially in patients with type 1 diabetes.

Non–insulin-requiring patients with diabetes with planned minor surgical procedures, who are expected to be able to resume normal diets soon after surgery, may be able to continue their oral medications up to the morning of surgery. Patients with type 2 diabetes who are scheduled for such procedures, and who will be NPO for more than 4 to 6 hours, may be instructed to discontinue short-acting insulin on the evening before surgery and take half their usual intermediate- or long-acting insulin dose on the morning of surgery.

Patients taking glargine (Lantus) may be instructed to take half of their usual dose the evening before surgery and to discontinue oral medication at that time. Normal insulin and oral regimens may be resumed when the patient returns to a normal diet.

Longer procedures that entail more extensive periods of NPO status require a more detailed approach to preoperative glycemic control. This may include discontinuation of oral medications 48 to 72 hours before surgery and institution of intermediate-acting insulin (NPH, Novolin) with preprandial blood glucose measurements and sliding scale administration of short-acting insulin (Humalog, Regular, NovoLog). Type 1 and some type 2 insulin-requiring diabetic patients may require continuous insulin infusion preoperatively along with a separate intravenous glucose infusion. The use of subcutaneous doses of short-acting insulin may yield unpredictable responses in patients with altered peripheral perfusion, and these patients may also benefit from continuous intravenous insulin infusion that can be monitored and adjusted with greater accuracy. Careful attention to fluid balance and serum electrolytes, especially potassium, is also critical to avoiding complications.

Patients with diabetes are at risk for silent ischemia as well as ventricular dysfunction and may benefit from preoperative cardiac evaluation if not recently performed. Renal status should also be confirmed, understanding that a normal preoperative serum creatinine level, although somewhat comforting, may not reflect the patient's reserve capacity and response to surgical stress.

Communication with the surgeon, anesthesia team, and postoperative nursing staff is important in the management of diabetic patients, and may best be done directly rather than through written means if concerns about the patient's perioperative management exist. The trend toward ambulatory surgery and early discharge also requires careful instructions to the patient about postoperative management and may warrant specific preadmission teaching.

Patients with Liver or Kidney Disease

Liver Disease

The presence of known liver disease, including cirrhosis, hepatitis, or obstructive biliary disease, may predispose patients to nutritional deficiency as well as coagulation disorders. Preoperative evaluation should include studies to identify such disorders, including serum albumin or prealbumin, clotting time, prothrombin time (INR), and CBC to assess hemoglobin and platelets. Some patients may require perioperative administration of fresh frozen plasma or other blood products, supplementation of vitamin K to correct elevated INR, or specific clotting factors. Platelet infusions have very brief benefit and should be used only if counts are critically low. Most patients with platelet counts above 60,000 do not exhibit abnormal bleeding on the basis of thrombocytopenia.

Antibiotics that are cleared through the liver should be avoided or dosages adjusted appropriately, and sedatives with hepatic metabolism must be used with caution. Amide anesthetics (lidocaine, bupivacaine, mepivacaine) commonly used for local and regional anesthesia are cleared through the liver and must be used with caution in patients with known liver disease, as well as elderly patients whose hepatic function may be naturally reduced.

Kidney Disease

Patients with kidney disease may have stable mild chronic renal insufficiency, which, if their reserve is minimal, may progress to acute renal failure perioperatively.

Others may already be on dialysis, and others may be categorized as somewhere between these two extremes.

Chronic renal disease predisposes patients to anemia, platelet dysfunction, metabolic acidosis, hyperkalemia, and uremia. They also have higher incidences of peripheral vascular disease, coronary artery disease, and ischemic cerebrovascular disease. Preoperative evaluation therefore must identify individuals at risk of electrolyte imbalance and fluid status abnormalities and increased risk of worsening renal impairment, as well as of cardiac and respiratory disease.

Preoperative testing should include measurement of serum electrolytes, bicarbonate, creatinine, blood urea nitrogen, calcium, CBC with platelet count, coagulation studies (prothrombin time/INR, bleeding time), urinalysis, and arterial blood gas if bicarbonate is decreased (<16 to 18 mEq/L). The electrocardiogram and chest radiograph should be reviewed and repeated if not recent. Unless the patient is undergoing dialysis, results of recent measurement of renal function, including creatinine clearance, should be reviewed.

Timing of dialysis in enrolled patients should be discussed with the nephrology or dialysis team, and is usually performed on the day before surgery to optimize fluid status and reduce uremic bleeding complications. Serum potassium levels should be checked within 3 to 6 hours before surgery and corrected to less than 5 to 5.5 mEq/L using bicarbonate/dextrose/insulin infusion, unless the patient has responded well to previous use of binding resins. Anemia as low as 7 to 8 g/dL hemoglobin may be well tolerated in patients with chronic renal failure; however, if functional capacity, coronary ischemia, respiratory compromise, or likelihood of significant surgical blood loss are a concern, the patient may benefit from judicious transfusion of packed red cells. If time permits, erythropoietin therapy may be considered.

Bariatric Surgery

The growth of the availability and variety of surgical procedures aimed at treating obesity has offered hope for many patients who have struggled with weight loss. In many cases these procedures offer life-changing remedies, and the results of surgery are often encouraging to patients, their families, and their clinicians. In many cases, however, the results are transient because behaviors and extrinsic factors return the patient to an obese state, now with an altered alimentary tract. The true nature and helpfulness of bariatric surgery will require ongoing research, and the perioperative risks remain underestimated and poorly understood.

The immediate concern for many primary care clinicians whose patients undergo evaluation for bariatric surgery is the preoperative surgical protocol followed by many, if not most, bariatric surgeons. This protocol mandates a standard list of subspecialty consultations, usually including cardiology, pulmonary, endocrinology, gastroenterology, and frequently psychiatry, in addition to dietary and nutritional counseling. The patient is also usually told to see his or her primary care clinician, for "clearance."

The question in the mind of the primary care clinician may then be, what additional service or advice can he or she offer that has not already been offered by the myriad of medical professionals already consulted? Or, what is the motivation of the surgeon in asking for a "clearance" from the patient's primary care clinician, when the decision has apparently already been made that expertise beyond the scope of the primary care clinician is required?

Although many primary care clinicians enthusiastically advocate for the role of "patient manager," others see this situation as a result of proactive medicolegal defensiveness on the part of the surgeon. These primary care clinicians understand the risks, both known and unknown, of these particular planned procedures, and understand the perception of the surgeon about how many consultations should be on the patient's chart and of what variety.

It has consequently become the usual and customary practice of many primary care clinicians to withhold an opinion as to the fitness of their patients for bariatric surgery, to limit their consultative reports to an accounting of the patient's medical history, including that of their obesity and attempts at weight loss, and to leave recommendations about preoperative optimization to the other specialists involved.

Pregnant Patients

Nonobstetric surgery may be required during the course of nearly 2% of otherwise normal pregnancies. Appendectomy, cholecystectomy, orthopedic procedures after trauma, or other emergent procedures must not be delayed because of concurrent pregnancy. Surgery that is nonobstetric but related to pregnancy, such as urologic interventions or ovarian surgery, may also be required. In these cases, the axiom that *a pregnant patient is treated in the same fashion as a nonpregnant patient* applies. The safety and well-being of the fetus depend in the greatest degree on the health of the mother.

When possible, elective surgical procedures should be performed during the second trimester, when organogenesis is less affected and the risk of preterm labor is decreased. Advanced pregnancy may affect diaphragmatic excursion and predispose the patient to atelectasis and postoperative risk of pneumonia; therefore, pulmonary function should be evaluated and the use of incentive spirometry considered. Antibiotic selection should avoid drugs with known fetal adversities, such as tetracycline in early pregnancy or NSAIDs near term.

Preoperative medical evaluation of the pregnant patient centers on the same considerations of operative and anesthesia risk, patient risk factors, and the need for perioperative care as with a nonpregnant patient.

Communicating Recommendations

The results and report of the preoperative consultation should be forwarded to the requesting surgeon (or dentist, clinician) promptly. Inpatient consultations will be posted to the patient's chart and reviewed by the surgeon and anesthesia team. Although local protocols may request that reports of outpatient medical evaluations be sent directly to the hospital or ambulatory surgical center, it is the responsibility of the consultant (the primary care provider in this case) to ensure that findings and recommendations are in fact received by the surgeon. For this reason, many clinicians forward the preoperative evaluation to the surgeon and directly communicate the need for him or her to provide the results to the hospital or other surgical facility. The establishment of good communication and relationships helps to guarantee effective information sharing for the benefit of the patient.

Many formats, forms, and designs for both printed and electronic transmittal of preoperative medical evaluations are available, but the standard dictated letter that includes the patient history, physical examination, laboratory, and diagnostic findings and recommendations may be most useful and, as noted at the beginning of this chapter, may constitute the only comprehensive document containing this information in the patient's chart. It should include a statement of the patient's condition relative to his or her fitness for the planned procedure, indicating that no "current medical contraindications" exist, or, if they do exist, what specific steps need to be taken to reduce the risks compared with the urgency of the surgery.

CPT/Billing Codes

99241–99245 Office consultations
99251–99255 Inpatient consultations

NOTE: Determining the level of complexity for consultations is similar to determining use for other office- and hospital-based evaluation and management (E&M) services.

ICD-9-CM Diagnostic Codes

V72.81 Preoperative cardiovascular examination
V72.82 Preoperative respiratory examination
V72.84 Preoperative examination, unspecified

NOTE: V72.84 can be used in addition to the specific diagnosis code for the underlying condition.

BIBLIOGRAPHY

Ebell MH: Preoperative evaluation for noncardiac surgery. Am Fam Physician 69:1977–1980, 2004.

Fleisher LA, Beckman JA, Brown KA, et al: ACC/AHA 2007 guidelines on perioperative cardiovascular evaluation and care for noncardiac surgery: Executive summary. A report of the American College of Cardiology/American Heart Association Task Force on Practice Guidelines (Writing Committee to Revise the 2002 Guidelines on Perioperative Cardiovascular Evaluation for Noncardiac Surgery). Circulation 116:1971–1996, 2007. Also available online at circ.ahajournals.org/cgi/content/full/116/17/1971. Accessed March 11, 2009.

Flood C, Fleishe LA: Preparation of the cardiac patient for noncardiac surgery. Am Fam Physician 75:656–665, 2007.

Institute for Clinical Systems Improvement (ICSI): Preoperative evaluation. Bloomington, Minn, ISCI, 2006.

Katz RI, Cimino L, Vitkun SA: Preoperative medical consultations: Impact on perioperative management and surgical outcome. Can J Anaesth 52:697–702, 2005.

King MS: Preoperative evaluation. Am Fam Physician 62:387–396, 2000.

Marks JB: Perioperative management of diabetes. Am Fam Physician 67: 93–100, 2003.

Mukherjee D, Eagle K: Perioperative cardiac assessment for noncardiac surgery: Eight steps to the best possible outcome. Circulation 107: 2771–2774, 2003.

CHAPTER 231

PRINCIPLES OF X-RAY INTERPRETATION

Wm. MacMillan Rodney • J.R. MacMillan Rodney • K.M.R. Arnold

INTRODUCTION

Studies on imaging outcomes have documented quality of care for interpretation of radiographs by nonradiologists in family medicine and emergency medicine. This chapter provides a "how-to-do-it" guideline on the interpretation of the most common adult x-ray studies needed in primary care: common fractures of the long bones and the chest radiograph (posteroanterior and lateral). (For the treatment of fractures and further discussion, see Chapter 190, Fracture Care.) There will also be an overview of the purchase, maintenance, and staffing of equipment in the office. This includes the decision to have all or selected images interpreted by outside consultation. Published data suggest that consultation significantly changes management in less than 2% of cases if the physician has basic interpretation skills.

Who Reads the Film and Who Collects the Fee?

Practicing medicine in today's world entails medicolegal risk. It cannot be eliminated, but it can be lessened by timely application of procedural skills such as interpretation of radiologic images at the point of service. The advantages of bedside correlation and subsequent follow-up cannot be overemphasized.

Primary care residency training is adequate to train clinicians to interpret images or to seek consultation when needed. Levels of comfort vary from physician to physician. There is no legal requirement to have images interpreted by a radiologist. Physicians are entitled to reimbursement for the technical component (TC) and the professional component of the CPT-4 charges for the image if they own the equipment, and create the formal report for the medical record. Only the physician signing the final report is entitled to bill for the professional component of the fee.

Buying the Equipment

Digital radiography offers lower-cost and more reliable technology in the office. From a storage perspective, the space that developers, darkrooms, and films (both exposed and unexposed) occupy can be more efficiently used for patient care. Digital technology also promotes safety by eliminating developer chemicals that must be stored and disposed. Also, by decreasing the number of retakes, radiation to patients and office staff is reduced. Finally, images are easily stored and can be shared more quickly and efficiently, which prevents unnecessary repeated studies and minimizes expense and radiation exposure.

Computed radiography (CR) is less expensive and equally accurate as the picture archiving and communication systems purchased by hospitals. CR refers to the use of phosphor films that function in the cassettes of traditional x-ray equipment. The image is taken; the plate is transferred to a developer; and then the image is loaded digitally to the computer. Installation of a new digital CR system costs less than $60,000. Digital images can be inserted directly into most electronic medical record systems.

State Certification, Licensing Laws, and Insurances Vary

A lead-lined room is necessary to obtain state certification. This can be done for less than $10,000. Physicians do not require additional licensing to provide radiographs, but unlicensed staff must usually take a 6- to 10-day course and pass a state test for licensing. Hiring a dedicated radiology technician is an expensive option that may be beyond the budget of an office taking fewer than 25 images a day. Data suggest that offices order 3 to 8 radiographs per 100 patients per day. Geriatric and urgent care–open access practices have higher demand.

Planning and cost–benefit analyses must be completed before the purchase of equipment and staff training (see Appendix L: Buying Major Office Equipment). Some HMO contracts forbid reimbursement to office-based physicians, but some emergency departments are charging over $200 per chest film. An average Medicaid reimbursement may be less than $40 per image. Local reimbursement rates, insurance rules, governmental policies, and patient mix must be reviewed before purchasing an x-ray unit.

CHEST RADIOGRAPHY

One example of documentation that helps ensure that all aspects of the radiograph are reviewed is shown in Figure 231-1. This documentation form helps maintain quality of care. Obtaining a second opinion (over-reading by a second physician) is suggested until the reader becomes comfortable with the many variations of normal versus abnormal.

Interpretation Guidelines for the Adult Posteroanterior and Lateral Chest Radiograph

Clinical Context

The clinician who performs the history and bedside examination has a tremendous advantage compared with a radiologist remote in time and space. The immediacy of clinical data differentiates imaging as a diagnostic procedure for the patient in real time versus a radiologic consultation, which usually occurs after the patient has left the office. The bedside examination at the point of service minimizes errors of interpretation.

Validity

Images must be labeled and dated and there must be a system in place to ensure this is done.

INTERPRETATION OF THE CHEST X-RAY

Please fill this form out completely.

I. CLINICAL CONTEXT

Patient ID#/Name____________________________Age:______ Sex:_____ Date: _________

Are old films available for comparison? Yes No

REVIEW OF SYSTEMS (circle those that apply)

Cough Dyspnea Pleuritic Pain Chest pain Hemoptysis HTN

Other illnesses, signs, or symptoms ____________________________

DURATION OF PROBLEM in days, weeks, or months ______________________

Circle the techniques used PA Lateral AP Portable Decubitus

Is this film significantly rotated? Yes No

Is there an adequate inspiration? Yes No

Is the amount of penetration[exposure]within normal limits? Yes No

II. VALIDITY—Does the image need to be repeated? Yes No

III. Check the lateral—Are there abnormalities of the spine, diaphragms, anterior clear space or the posterior cardiac space? Yes No

IV. Bones and soft tissues. See any significant abnormalities? Yes No

V. Mediastinum. Is it normal? Yes No

VI. Cardiac silhouette. Is it normal? Yes No

VII. Diaphragms. Are there any significant abnormalities? Yes No

VIII. Lungs

A. Are there any significant abnormalities on the left or right hilum? Yes No

B. Any significant abnormalities to the lung parenchyma? Yes No

C. Any significant abnormalities of the lung pleurae? Yes No

IX. My interpretation is[circle one]:

A. Within normal limits.

B. Normal, but I want to comment on some findings which are probably insignificant. Consultation not required.

____

C. Questionable findings exist and consultation will be requested.

D. Abnormal findings:

____

X. PLAN

XI. SIGNATURES

Student/Resident:____________________Attending Physician: ____________________CC:_______ Date:_________

Figure 231-1 Interpretation of the chest x-ray report form.

Posteroanterior (PA) and *lateral* views are the standard views for the cooperative adult. "PA" simply means the beam travels in the direction from the back to the chest (vs. "AP" [anteroposterior], from chest to back). The patient stands and takes a deep breath. Views are standardized as noted later. Cardiomegaly definitions are different on PA versus AP views, so it is important that radiographs be taken appropriately. Without a lateral view, lesions in the retrocardiac and poststernal (anterior clear space) space can be missed. Other potential views are not covered here.

"Perfect views" are not necessary to gain useful information, but a disclaimer describing any technique limitations must be inserted with every film. For chest films, the acronym *RIP* describes the characteristics of *rotation, inspiration, and penetration* (i.e., exposure). These validity checks must be addressed before any interpretation of findings.

POSTEROANTERIOR VIEW

- *Is this film rotated?* In the PA film, measure the distance from the spinous processes of the vertebral bodies to the medial heads of each of the clavicles. These are easily identifiable bony landmarks. Commonly, there is a 2- to 3-mm difference because of slight rotation, which does not invalidate the film, but in general, the distances on the right and the left should be approximately the same.
- *Is there an adequate inspiration?* Inadequate inspiration is a cause of decreased specificity (increased opacity) for lung parenchyma. The "best" method for measuring inspiration is by counting *posterior* ribs as they join the spine. A minimally adequate inspiration uncovers nine ribs. Avoid counting anterior ribs, which are less predictable.
- *Is the amount of penetration within normal limits?* Penetration describes the amount of radiation exposure applied to the tissue. A practical rule of thumb for evaluating overpenetration and underpenetration is the anatomic point at which the vertebral interspaces are no longer visible. An *overpenetrated* PA chest image will create a "spine film" with all elements of the vertebral bodies visible down into the abdomen. An *underpenetrated* film will be too "white." When *penetration technique is ideal*, intervertebral spaces disappear somewhere in the cardiac shadow and do not appear beneath the diaphragm.

Overexposure "burns out" the ability to see the lung parenchyma and vessels, that is, turns the lung fields black. The vessels normally start to disappear as they approach within 3 to 4 mm of the chest wall. Overexposure increases the probability of false-negative interpretation.

Physicians should comment on limitations of interpretation caused by suboptimal technique. The physician should request additional views or insert a disclaimer about technique if necessary. This includes the need for a lateral image in the ambulatory adult and older child.

These validity checks, and the following system for reviewing the film, establish guidelines for quality assurance.

Check the Lateral Image

Review the spine, diaphragms, anterior clear space, and the retrocardiac space. The majority of diagnoses will come from the PA view.

Does a Survey of the Bones and Soft Tissues Reveal Any Significant Abnormalities?

This area is of limited value when the radiograph has been ordered to investigate dyspnea, cough, hypertension, and other routine cardiovascular issues. However, a systematic sweep of the bones and soft tissues is mandatory.

Is the Appearance of the Mediastinum within Normal Limits?

The physician cannot miss a shifted or widened mediastinum, which is associated with aortic dissections, pericardial tamponade, tumors of the thymus and thyroid, lymphoma, and germ cell teratomas. A quoted dimension for "wide" is 8 cm in the average adult. Another method measures the mediastinal width at the level of the carina. If it is more than 25% of the thoracic diameter, it is considered "wide." A "thin" mediastinum has no significance. However, aortic dissections have occurred in mediastina measuring less than 8 cm. Normal children younger than 5 years of age frequently have a "wide" mediastinum and large cardiac silhouette.

Does a Review of the Cardiac Silhouette Reveal Any Significant Abnormalities on the Posteroanterior View?

Cardiomegaly exists if the transverse diameter of the heart on a PA view is greater than 50% of the transthoracic diameter measured at the same level. The *thoracic diameter* is measured from one side of the rib cage to the other at the level of the middle of the heart. An *enlarged pulmonary artery segment* can be seen as an extra hump on the left side of the PA heart. *On the lateral, left ventricular enlargement* can cause a shadow more than 2 cm posterior to the shadow of the inferior vena cava. *Pneumopericardium* creates a black line around the border of the heart. The *thin heart* of deep inspiration, such as in chronic obstructive pulmonary disease, is not indicative of cardiac disease.

Does a Review of the Diaphragms Reveal Any Significant Abnormalities (Posteroanterior View)?

Air beneath the diaphragms is a surgical emergency until proven otherwise (it documents a bowel perforation). Normally the right diaphragm is higher than the left by 2 to 20 mm. Abnormal elevation occurs from lung atelectasis, paralysis, effusion, lobectomy, and other causes.

Lungs

Now the lung tissue itself is evaluated.

1. *Are there any significant abnormalities on the left or right hilum?* In 70% of normal patients, the left hilum is higher than the right, and at equal elevations in 30%. The right hilum in not normally higher than the left. *Abnormal hilar adenopathy indicates serious infection, sarcoid, or malignancy in most cases.*
2. *Are there any significant abnormalities to the lung parenchyma?* A rapid visual "ping-pong" comparison of the left and right lung fields should detect flagrant asymmetries caused by pathologic processes such as *hemothorax, metastatic nodules, sarcoid, primary tuberculosis, and pneumonias*. Failure to detect an obvious abnormality in the face of a seriously ill patient may require consultation or hospitalization.

Poor inspirations and AP views cause false-positive "fluffiness" similar to congestive heart failure (CHF) patterns. Normally on the PA film, the vascular markings stop short of the lung wall by 3 to 5 mm. Gravity causes subtle tapering of the vessels as they go toward the head (cephalad). "Cephalization of flow" is jargon for the phenomenon of enlarged lung vessels in the upper lung fields secondary to CHF.

The *silhouette sign* helps the clinician to localize the lesion. In the chest, there are anatomic structures that exist in fixed air–soft tissue relationships. Given proper rotation and penetration, the heart borders, the ascending and descending aorta, the aortic knob, and the diaphragms are visible (Figs. 231-2 and 231-3). The silhouette sign describes the situation where parenchymal pathology masks the silhouette of a common anatomic landmark. The heart and diaphragm are most commonly affected. For example, when anterior left upper lobe pneumonia obscures the border of the left heart, it is called a silhouette sign. When pleural effusion obscures the contour of the diaphragm, it is a silhouette sign.

Nodules are classified by their diameter of 5 to 30 mm. Above 30 mm, these lesions are classified as *masses*. Small lesions (2 to 10 mm) are common. Most of these are *calcified granulomas*, and vessels on end. They are small and innocent, and do not grow over time. They can be followed by serial radiographs and clinical history. Positron emission tomography scans can differentiate

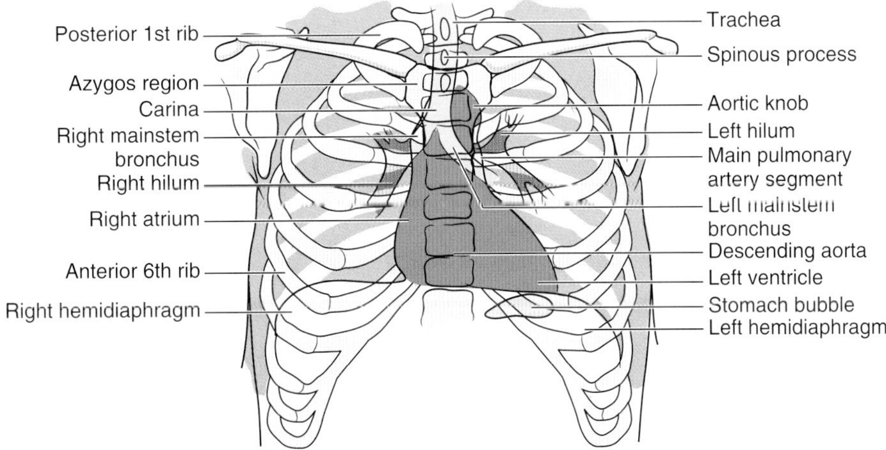

Figure 231-2 Schematic anatomy of posteroanterior chest images.

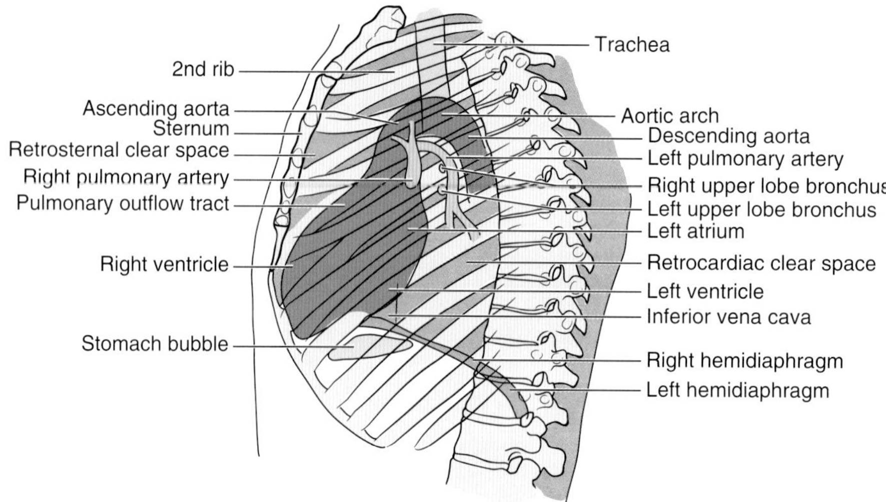

Figure 231-3 Landmarks of the lateral chest film.

metabolically active lesions (malignant, infectious) from those that are metabolically quiescent (benign).

3. *Are there any significant abnormalities of the lung pleurae?* The absence of pulmonary vasculature extending out to the bony inner edge of the thorax indicates a *pneumothorax* until proven otherwise. The *visceral pleura* is the outer lining of the lung, and the *parietal pleura* is the inner lining of the chest cavity up against the bones and muscles. The area between the two, the *pleural space*, under normal conditions, is a potential space. *Pleural effusions* are caused by primary disease processes such as infection, neoplasm, and inflammation. Specific diseases such as subphrenic abscess, hepatitis, and pancreatitis can cause effusions. Cardiac failure, renal failure, or any disease that alters the osmolar and hydrostatic equilibrium among the body compartments can cause effusions. Untreated chronic pleural effusions can cause loculations and adhesions.

Interpretation

1. *Within normal limits.*
2. *Normal, but I want to comment* on some findings which are probably insignificant. *Consultation not required,* but … (perhaps the penetration was not ideal or the entire right shoulder was not seen, etc.).
3. *Questionable findings exist and consultation will be requested.* This could include a computed tomography scan of the chest, which is the most commonly ordered test for ambiguous findings on the plain radiograph. Consultation reports can be ambiguous or wrong. CHF can appear to be pneumonia, and vice versa.
4. *Abnormalities include the following:* Naming the disease is not necessary. Stating that the entire right lung is "whited out," or that "multiple 2- to 3-cm nodules are present in both lungs," will lead to dramatic changes in management that will be mentioned in the plan.

Plan

By offering an interpretation or a "preliminary interpretation" in the office at the point of service, quality is improved. Clearly indicate in the report any intention of further diagnostic studies or follow-up, which can then be immediately explained to the patient. Poorly worded or ambiguous interpretations that arrive hours or days after the patient has left the office decrease the quality of care.

Consultant reports can be lost or misplaced. The beauty of imaging in the office is the high predictive value of a positive finding. Specificity is high when lesions are obvious, and delay of management pending formal interpretation is often not wise. The risk of a false-negative result (low sensitivity) is always present. Multiple studies have documented, however, that the rate of failure to diagnose a lesion of significance is less than 1% to 2%.

Top 10 "Normal" Tips

1. You are at the bedside. Integrate the history with the physical findings and be sure they correlate.
2. The clavicular heads are equidistant from the spinous processes.
3. There are at least nine ribs visible on a normal inspiratory PA view.
4. The intervertebral spaces should not be visible beneath the diaphragm.
5. Before 5 years of age, a normal thymus can make a large-appearing mediastinum.
6. In adults, the mediastinum should not measure more than 8 cm.
7. The left hilum is higher than the right hilum.
8. The right diaphragm is higher than the left.
9. The exact boundary distinguishing a granuloma from a nodule may not be as important as the clinical context, which includes a history for risk and the rate of growth. Lesions greater than 10 mm in diameter may benefit from a second opinion.
10. There is no exact formula for hilar enlargement and subtle parenchymal change. Chance favors the prepared mind. Read or perish.

Sample Chest Radiograph Presentations

Make copies of the report form (see Fig. 231-1) and fill it out for each of the following images. Check your findings against the information given in the figure legends.

Figure 231-4: This is a 43-year-old African-American woman with a 3-month history of increasing fatigue and shortness of breath. Other than being overweight, her past medical history is noncontributory. Her lungs were clear to auscultation and vital signs were normal.

Figure 231-5: A 59-year-old white man with a long history of chronic obstructive pulmonary disease reports a mild cough, a mild increase in dyspnea, and a fever last night. He has dropped out from care in the cardiology and pulmonary clinics. Many years ago he was told he needed a heart operation, but he has refused. He is demanding an antibiotic shot because his "pneumonias" start like this. His lungs are clear and his heart sounds are distant. His vital signs are normal, including a respiratory rate of 16 per minute.

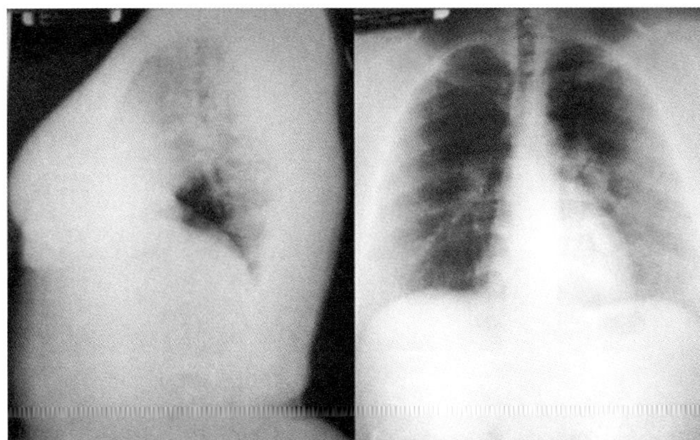

Figure 231-4 On the posteroanterior (PA) film *(right)*, there is clinically insignificant rotation with an adequate inspiratory effort. The left costophrenic angle is partially cut off. Penetration (exposure) is somewhat strong but not clinically significant. The bones are normal, but soft tissue breast shadows are causing transparent opacity over the lower outer lung fields bilaterally. The mediastinum and cardiac shape are normal. The right hemidiaphragm is slightly higher than the left, and the left hilum is slightly higher than the right. Both hilar areas are enlarged and there is paratracheal node enlargement on the right in the area of the clavicle. There are parenchymal streaks extending down and outward from the hilar areas, but they do not constitute infiltrates.

Although the lateral film *(left)* does not record an optimal inspiration, it does not change the findings on the PA film. Taken together, the films are adequate for an interpretation of "abnormal chest." Rather than repeating the films, the patient was sent for computed tomography of the chest. The differential diagnosis includes sarcoidosis, lymphoma, and tuberculosis, among others. This was biopsy-proven sarcoidosis.

Figure 231-6: This patient complains of acute chest pain radiating to the back. A 33-year-old Latino man with an unremarkable past medical history walked away from a motor vehicle accident last night. He reports that he was hit in the chest very hard. He is in moderate distress, with a pulse of 110 beats per minute and blood pressure of 100/70.

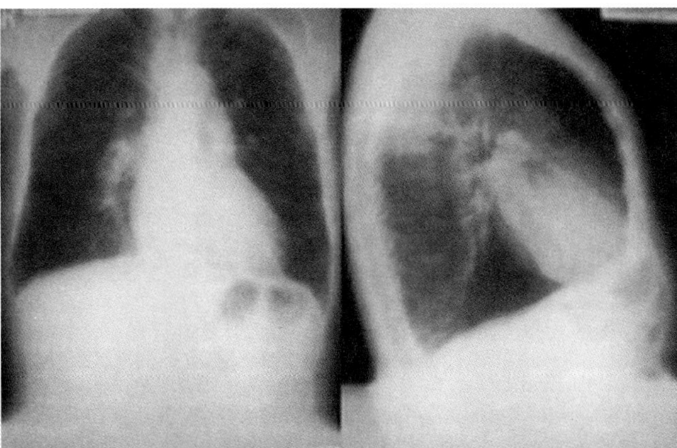

Figure 231-5 The initial impression is overexposure with blackening of the lung fields, but the vertebral interspaces are not obvious. Clearly, there is an adequate inspiration without rotation. Bones and soft tissues are unremarkable, but the mediastinal and cardiac contours look abnormal. The diaphragms are flattened, as is common with patients with chronic obstructive pulmonary disease, suggesting a hyperaeration common with these patients. The opacities on the right do not constitute a mass or an infiltrate of significance. The lateral view *(right)* reveals flattened diaphragms and a barrel chest. This accentuates the anterior clear space in front of the heart and the retrocardiac space, which do not contain any abnormal findings. The extra hump on the left side of the heart is significant enlargement of the pulmonary artery segment, and it is likely that the patient has a compensated congenital heart defect.

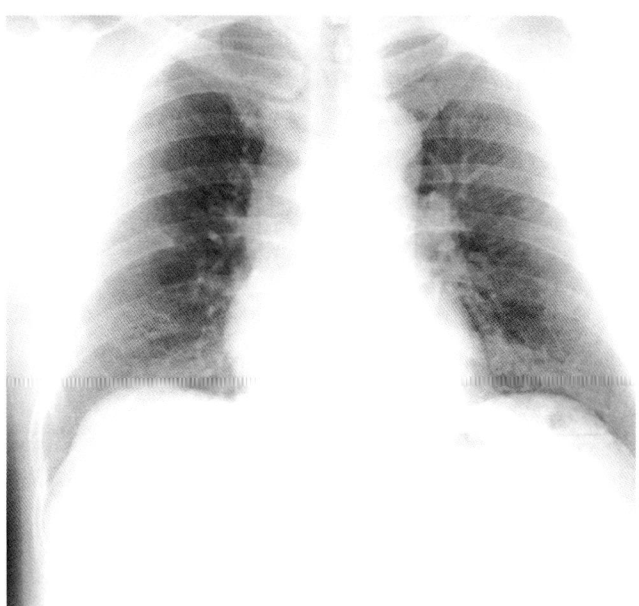

Figure 231-6 The mediastinum is widened, and the diagnosis is traumatic aortic dissection. Overall, the film is insignificantly rotated with an adequate inspiration. Nine posterior ribs are showing, but the film is mildly underpenetrated–underexposed. Minor imperfections in technique are the rule, not the exception. The mediastinal findings are sufficient to send the patient to the hospital.

The bones and soft tissues are inconsequential. The left hilum is higher than the right, and the right hemidiaphragm is higher than the left. The underexposure makes the parenchymal markings more prominent, but they do not represent infiltrates. As with all previous images, there is no air under the diaphragms.

Figure 231-7: A 23-year-old Latina woman presents with cough and fevers for 1 month. Past medical history is noncontributory.

Figure 231-8: A 68-year-old white woman with a history of uncontrolled hypertension and dyspnea, worsening today. Vital signs are pulse 105, blood pressure 190/115, temperature 98° F, and respiratory rate 24 per minute. She is in mild distress.

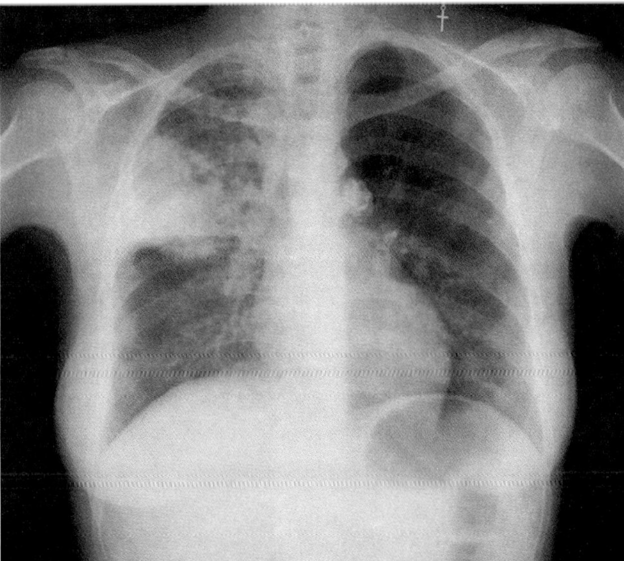

Figure 231-7 Example of infiltrate on right, calcified hilar node on left, visible sequestration in minor fissure on left—and more. Lateral image did not add to the information seen here. The diagnosis is tuberculosis.

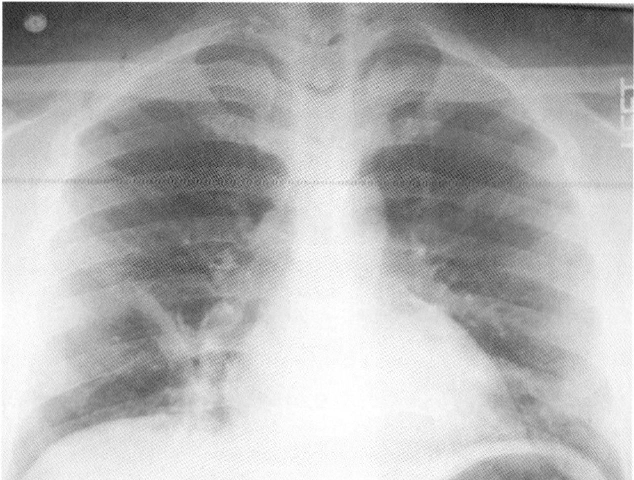

Figure 231-8 Good example of cardiomegaly and "cephalization" of flow. Inspiration is adequate, with nine visible posterior ribs. The heart measures greater than 50% of the transthoracic distance. Blood vessels at a level superior to the tracheal bifurcation appear larger than those at the level of the midheart. This is the reverse of what would normally be seen. *Cephalization* is another term for the "reversal of flow" seen in congestive heart failure. This is a good view demonstrating the clavicular heads as equidistant from the spinous processes of the spinal column. In this case, the lateral image did not change the management.

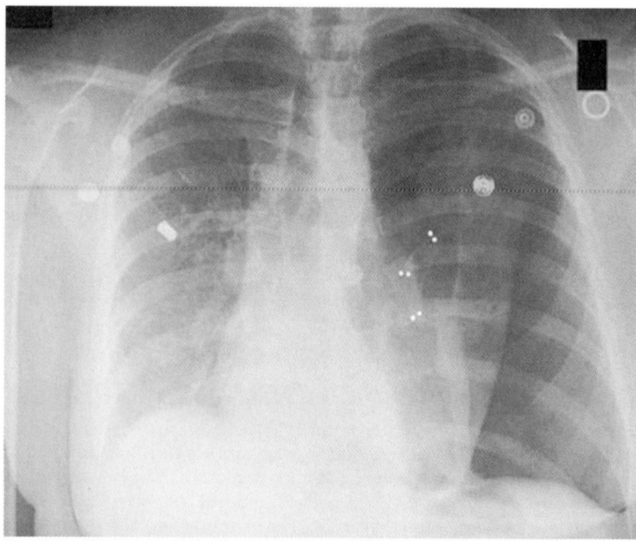

Figure 231-10 Because the patient is unable to raise his arms, the scapulae are in the lung fields, but interpretation of the most significant event is reasonable. There is a bullet in the right side and buckshot in the left. The heart is shifted to the right and the radiograph confirms the need for chest tube insertion. The entire left lung is collapsed. Note the absence of vascular markings on the left. Although a lateral image would localize the depth of the bullet and buckshot, the emphasis should be on stabilizing these critical injuries.

Figure 231-9: A 55-year-old smoker coughed up blood this morning and presents with cough, fever, and purulent sputum. Lateral view does not change management.

Figure 231-10: This patient is a 27-year-old man with reported gunshot wounds to chest and pneumothorax. The patient is unable to stand and is tachycardic and clammy. The image was obtained using portable technique, AP view.

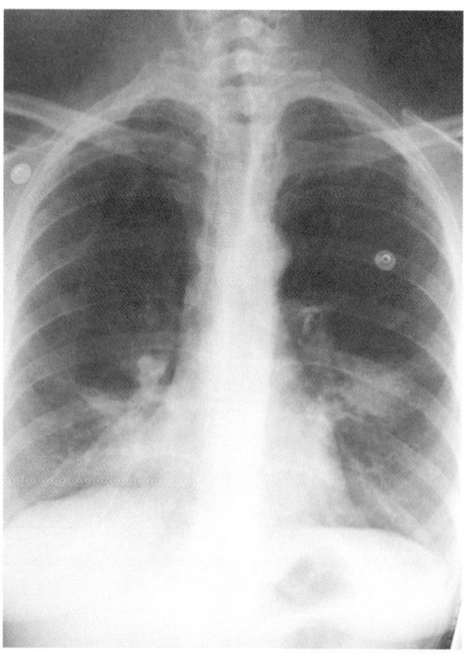

Figure 231-9 Bilateral acute pneumonia. Note abnormalities of cardiac border on the left and right. This is a good example of the silhouette sign with the right heart border obscured by an inflammatory process. This man was sent for computed tomography, which led to tissue diagnosis of lung cancer.

Long Bone Fracture Radiographs

Tips for Reading Long Bone Fractures

- Study the terminology of fractures as given in Chapter 190, Fracture Care, and in a reprint of *Musculoskeletal Medicine/Office Orthopedics* by Wm. Rodney, MD (available online at www.psot.com [see under rural family medicine, predoctoral section, ortho 101, assigned reading]).
- Use comparison images of the injured with the noninjured bone in children with growth plates.
- Study the Salter system for fractures in children. Prognosis worsens as the Salter number increases. Salter 1 and 2 fractures can be managed conservatively.
- When any radiographic image is indicated, take the time to view each one in detail, looking at the bones too. This is what develops one's sense of "normal."

Finding fractures is guided by the location of the point tenderness. The clinician then requests two or three views to determine stability features such as displacement, angulation, and involvement of a joint. Positioning is an art, not a science. Make sure that you follow the cortex (edge of the bone) for any breaks in the line. These small defects are fractures, especially when they are associated with point tenderness.

Fracture detection is made more difficult by technique that is overpenetrated (too black). Nondigital films may be clarified by the use of a hot lamp technique in which the film is placed directly over a bright light. Digital films can be electronically corrected in several ways. Underpenetrated films (too white) may lead to false-negative findings. Without digital software, these images need to be retaken. Digital manipulations can correct some of the underpenetration errors in technique.

There are specific soft tissue clues that increase the probability of a fracture even when one is not immediately visible. The best known is the *fat pad sign* associated with occult fractures of the bones surrounding the elbow. This sign is defined by a hypolucent (i.e., dark) space immediately adjacent to the injured bone. It usually represents blood released by the acute injury. A *posterior fat pad sign* is clearly abnormal, whereas an anterior fat pad may normally be visible for 1 to 2 mm. Larger than that is abnormal.

Primary bone tumors are rare, but appear as hyperopaque (osteoblastic) or hypo-opaque (osteoclastic) lesions, with occasional detection by the spontaneous occurrence of pathologic fractures. Metastatic bone cancers, for example, from the prostate or breast, are more common. Fractures may be the first sign of an undiagnosed malignancy.

Those taking and reading their own radiographs should be reassured by the fact that most orthopedists depend on their own interpretations. The opportunity for clinical correlation is a tremendous help in achieving optimal management for the patient. The importance of examining the cortex with specific attention to the area of point tenderness cannot be overemphasized. Digital films allow magnification for subtle lesions. In the extremities, particularly in children, comparison views of the noninjured limb may lead to a more accurate diagnosis.

General Guidelines for Fracture Care

See Chapter 190, Fracture Care, for more detail.

- Even after the bones heal, many fractures have minor, but residual discomfort and possible minor changes in function for up to 1 year later. Physical therapy will not remove this.
- Open (compound) fractures require immediate antibiotics.
- Stability governs prognosis as well as the possible need for consultation.
- Fractures that are nondisplaced, nonangulated, transverse/oblique, and without involvement of the joint space are more stable.
- Fractures that are comminuted, spiral, and involving the joint space are less stable.
- Review the patient context and factor in comorbidity. For example, fractures in the elderly heal more slowly and are at higher risk of sustained discomfort. Patients with mental illness or sociopathic behavior require additional care.
- If providing care for a fracture, see the patient on days 2, 7, and 14 postinjury. If the pain is not resolving, consultation should be considered.
- Healing times and follow-up protocols vary. For nonoperative fractures, young people heal more rapidly than seniors.

Common Fractures

Make copies of the report form (Fig. 231-11) and fill it out for each of the following images. Check your findings against the information given in the figure legends.

X-RAYS FOR SPORTS, TRAUMA, AND WORKPLACE INJURIES

Medicos para la Familia; www.psot.com
Method of Wm. MacMillan Rodney, MD, FAAFP, FACEP
Original 1992; Updated June 3, 2008

Please fill this form out completely

I. CLINICAL CONTEXT
Patient Name/MRN #:________________________Age:_____Sex:____Date:________

REVIEW OF SYSTEMS (briefly describe PMH, mechanism of injury, signs, and/or significant symptoms)
____
____

DURATION OF PROBLEM in days/wks/m/yrs________________________________
Old Films Available for Comparison? Yes No

II. LOCATION-ANATOMICAL AREA: Please circle areas of imaging interest
Shoulder Arm Forearm Wrist Hand Fingers
Pelvis Thigh Knee Leg Ankle Foot Toes
CSpine Lspine Sinus Skull

III. VIEWS
Views requested AP/PA Lateral Oblique Other-specify
Number of views 1 2 other

IV. VALIDITY
Is the amount of penetration acceptable to allow interpretation? Yes No
Is the film labeled correctly Yes No

V. FINDINGS
A. Are there any significant abnormalities to the bones? Yes No
B. Any significant abnormalities to the soft tissue? Yes No
C. Any significant abnormalities to the joint? Yes No

VI. My Interpretation Is:
A. Within normal limits.
Normal, but I want to comment on some findings which are probably insignificant. Consultation not required.
____
Questionable findings exist and consultation will be requested.
Abnormalities include the following: ____________________________________

VII. PLAN: ____

VIII. SIGNATURES:
Student/Resident: ____________________Attending MD/DO:__________________Date:__________

Figure 231-11 X-rays for sports, trauma, and workplace injuries report form.

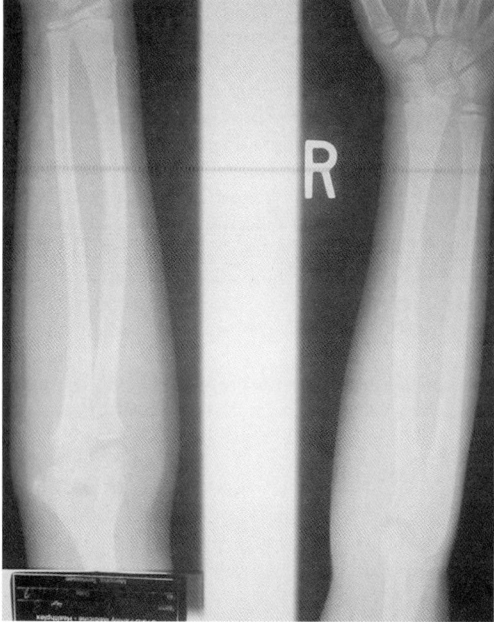

Figure 231-12 A "bump" is visible on the radius proximal to normal epiphyses (growth plates). This is a torus fracture where the cortex of the bone has buckled. Although classified as a fracture, there is no displacement, angulation, joint involvement, or visible fracture line. Conservative management with simple protective devices will lead to a good result.

Figure 231-12: A 10-year-old girl fell on her arm 2 hours ago while playing outside. There is point tenderness over the left distal radius, but otherwise she has no significant physical findings.

Figure 231-13: A 19–year-old man "broke his arm 3 months ago and the cast was removed 4 weeks ago." He fell again today and wants to know if he refractured the forearm.

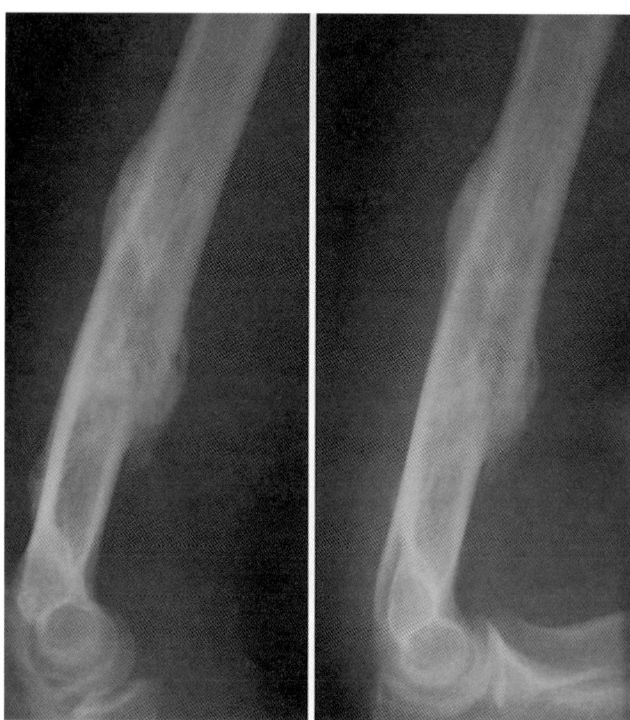

Figure 231-13 Lateral views demonstrating normal callus formation with no evidence of a new fracture. Patient and family can be reassured. No additional casting is necessary.

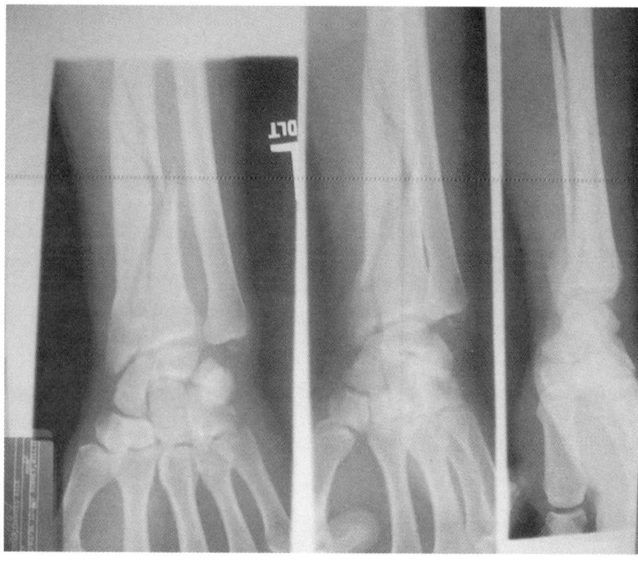

Figure 231-14 Lateral, posteroanterior, and oblique views are the recommended views. Physicians should consider characteristics that affect fracture management. In this fracture, the joint space is involved and this is associated with instability and a higher risk of subsequent arthritic pain. Instead of being transverse or oblique, this fracture has a spiral nature, but it is not distinctly comminuted (i.e., more than two pieces). It is a classic example of a complicated fracture destined for orthopedic surgery.

Figure 231-14: A 27-year-old man fell on his arm yesterday, and he could not sleep last night. The arm is swollen and extremely painful to the touch. His neurovascular examination is negative, but there is limited range of motion secondary to pain.

Figure 231-15: A 10–year-old boy experienced a collision on the soccer field this afternoon. He continued to play briefly, but states that he does not wish to move his arm.

Figure 231-16: A 23-year-old man tripped playing touch football. He was unable to walk.

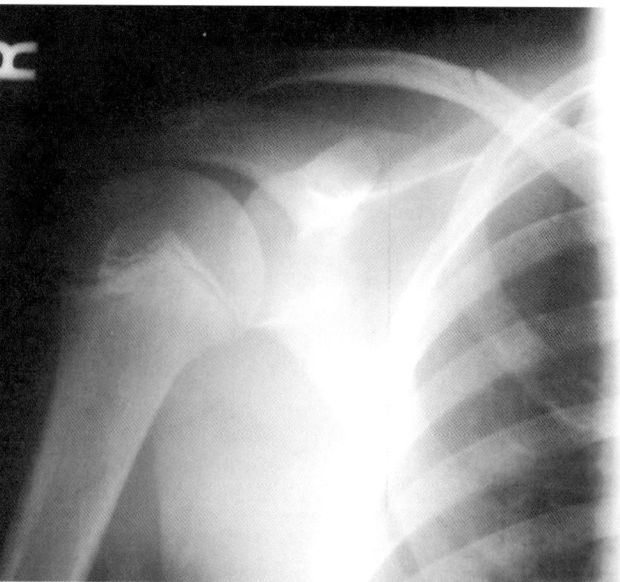

Figure 231-15 The focal point of this image is the shoulder and its growth plate, which is normal. However, there is a nondisplaced, nonangulated fracture of the clavicle. We treated this with a sling and range-of-motion exercises three times a day.

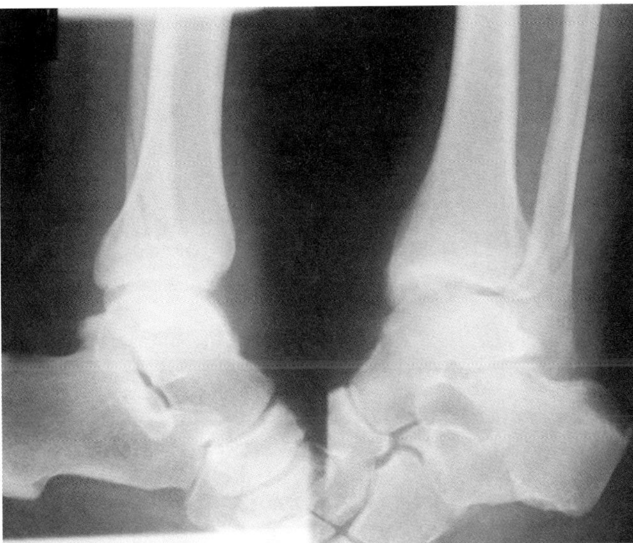

Figure 231-16 Lateral *(left)* and oblique *(right)* views reveal a fracture of the distal fibula, which is simple, oblique, nonangulated, and nondisplaced, and does not involve an articular surface. It was immobilized with a cast for 6 weeks. No orthopedic consult was obtained.

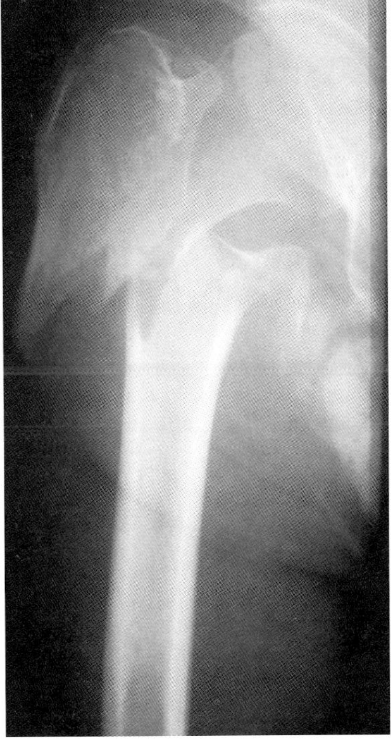

Figure 231-18 This is a nonangulated but seriously displaced fracture of the proximal femur. It is probably intertrochanteric and transverse. It is not comminuted, but a request for surgical consultation should be noted in the medical record. The patient refused surgery and left with his walker. He died of pneumonia 9 months later (at home).

Figure 231-17: A 38-year-old jogger hit a pothole and inverted his ankle. There was an audible "pop," and exquisite pain was immediate. The neurovascular examination is negative.

Figure 231-18: A 79-year-old farmer was brought by his daughter, who insisted that he be evaluated after a fall from a dumpster the preceding day. He is ambulating with a walker, and insisting that he "only needs a tetanus shot."

Figure 231-19: A 23-year-old basketball fan hit the wall with his fist yesterday. The pain is great and he would like an evaluation. His

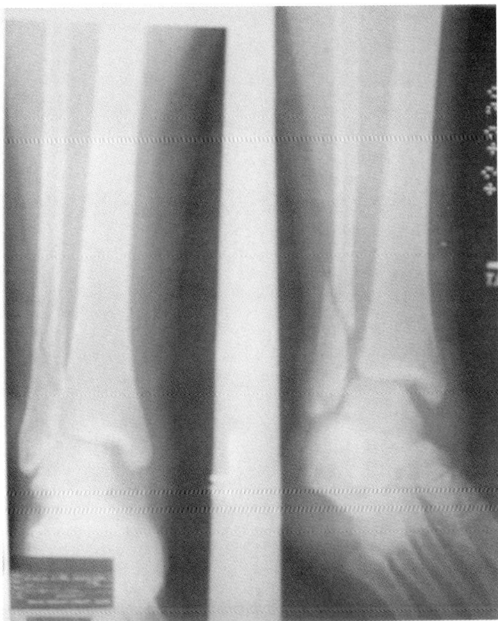

Figure 231-17 This is a noncomminuted, nonangulated, nondisplaced, oblique fracture of the distal third of the fibula. There is no involvement of an articular surface. There is a spiral component to the fracture on the posteroanterior view *(left)*. Worse yet, there is displacement of the tibia on the talus. Note the abnormally large distance from the medial malleolus to the talus. This indicates separation of the interosseous membrane. This is a highly unstable fracture that received orthopedic surgery.

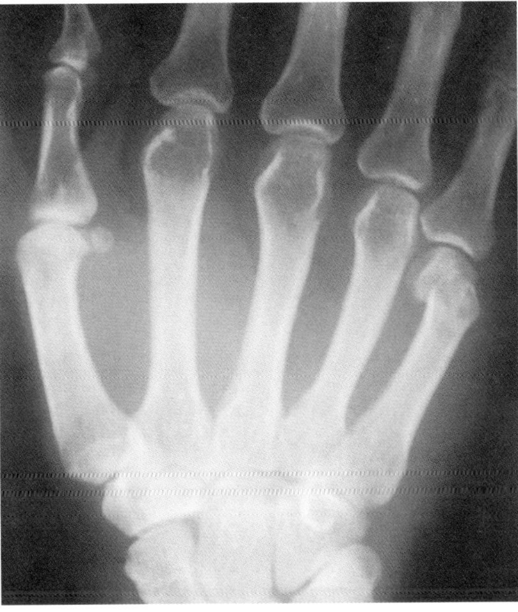

Figure 231-19 In contrast to "compound" fractures, simple fractures are those in which the skin is unbroken and the bone is not "sticking out." This was the case here. There is a fracture at the distal fifth metacarpal bone, but it does not involve the articular surface of the joint. There is 45 degrees of angulation, but no displacement. This is the classic "Boxer's fracture." Attempts at reduction are unlikely to affect the end result, which is good function and minor cosmetic deformity.

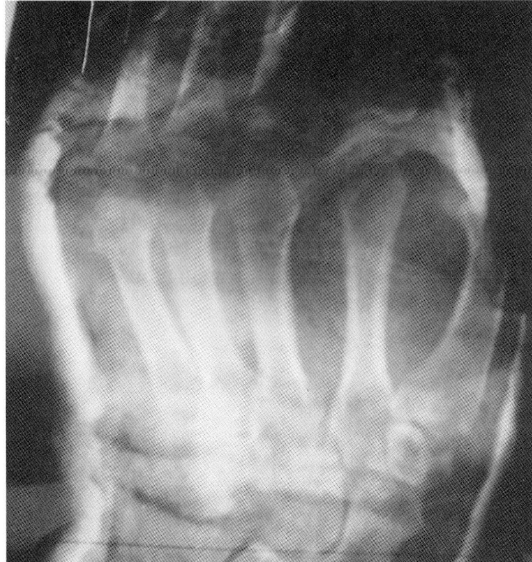

Figure 231-20 A cast has been placed on the hand after a reduction maneuver. The radiograph has been taken with the cast on. It is tempting to deduce that the bone fragments are in better alignment, but at least two views would be necessary to make this judgment. Complete immobilization would require encasing the entire hand in concrete. This is not possible, and these fractures almost always return to their original position.

neurovascular examination is negative, but pain limits his ability to flex and extend the fourth and fifth digits.

Figure 231-20: What has happened to the preceding case?

Figure 231-21: A 14-year-old boy's hand was stepped on during his first football game. It is painful and swollen, but the worst pain occurs in the area of the third metacarpophalangeal joint. Is there a fracture?

Figure 231-22: A 17-year-old female basketball player was trying to perform a dunk and landed on her outstretched hand with immediate pain, but little swelling. Neurovascular examination is negative, but there is a loss of range in motion at the wrist secondary to pain. Pain localizes to the area between the first metacarpal and distal radius.

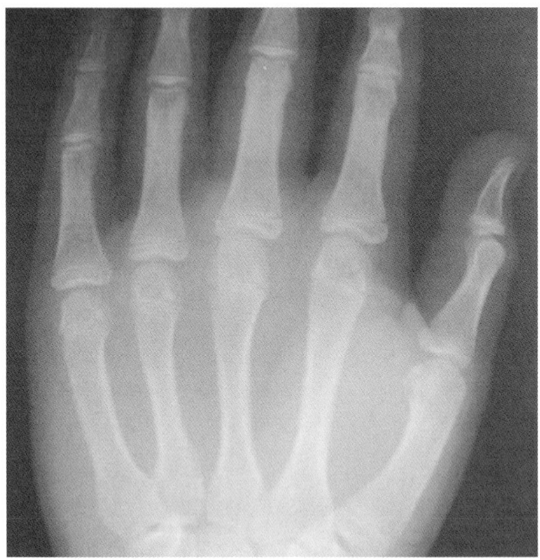

Figure 231-21 A Canadian family physician, Robert Salter, created the Salter classification of pediatric fractures. This is a Salter 3 fracture with a fracture on the ulnar side of the epiphysis of the proximal third digit. It involves the joint space, but the size of the fracture is so small that it was treated conservatively.

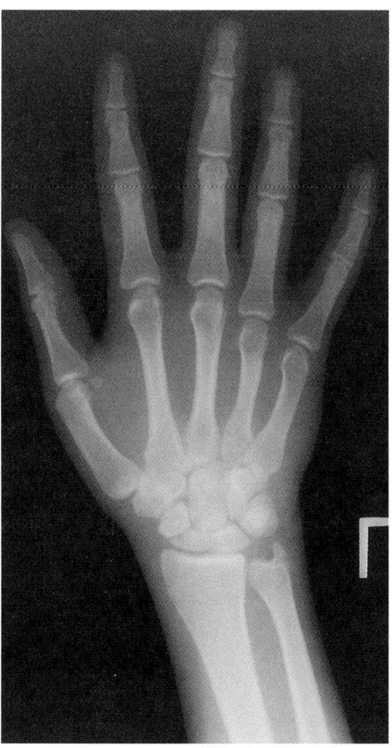

Figure 231-22 This is a simple, noncomminuted, nondisplaced, nonangulated fracture of the scaphoid bone. A thumb spica cast should be applied for 6 to 8 weeks, and the patient should be warned about the possibility of nonunion.

ONLINE RESOURCES

LearningRadiology: Available at www.learningradiology.com.

Rodney W (senior ed): Procedural Skills and Office Technology. Available at www.psot.com.

BIBLIOGRAPHY

Ballinger PW, Frank EV (eds): Merrill's Atlas of Radiographic Positions and Radiographic Procedures. St. Louis, Mosby, 2003.

Black WS, Becker JA: Common forearm fractures in adults. Am Fam Physician 80:1107–1114, 2009.

Connolly JF: Fractures and Dislocations: Closed Management. Philadelphia, WB Saunders, 1995.

Griffin L (ed): Essentials of Musculoskeletal Care, 3rd ed. Rosemont, Ill, American Academy of Orthopaedic Surgeons, 2005.

Halvorsen JG, Kunian A, Gjerdingen D, et al: The interpretation of office radiographs by family physicians. J Fam Pract 28:426–432, 1989.

Hatch RL, Rosenbaum CI: Fracture care by family physicians: A review of 295 cases. J Fam Pract 38:238–244, 1994.

Muller NL, Silva CIS (eds): Imaging of the Chest. Philadelphia, Saunders, 2008.

Simon HK, Khan NS, Nordenberg DF, Wright JA: Pediatric emergency physician interpretation of plain radiographs: Is routine review by a radiologist necessary and cost-effective? Ann Emerg Med 27:295–298, 1996.

Smith P, Temte J, Beasley J, Mundt M: Radiographs in the office: Is a second reading always needed? J Am Board Fam Pract 17:256–263, 2004.

Warren JS, Lara K, Hahn RG: Correlation of emergency department radiographs: Results of a quality assurance review in an urban community hospital. J Am Board Fam Pract 6:255–259, 1993.

CHAPTER 232

Special Considerations in Geriatric Patients

Gerald A. Amundsen • Kalyanakrishnan Ramakrishnan • Robert Salinas

Patients in the geriatric age group often have multiple chronic illnesses associated with functional decline of major organ systems. In addition, there are normal physiologic changes associated with aging that are universal to all. These diseases and changes, along with the medications used to treat them, may complicate outcomes of office procedures and influence physician decisions regarding timing, technique, aftercare, and whether or not to perform the procedure at all.

Currently, people 65 years of age and older account for approximately 12% of the U.S. population, a number expected to approach 20% by the year 2030. This group consumes approximately one third of health care provided, and a higher percentage of office surgical procedures. The physician performing office procedures must understand the underlying physiologic changes associated with aging and approach them with caution to achieve the common goals of diagnostic accuracy and relief from symptoms, while maintaining functional independence, and improving quality of life.

The subclinical losses in organ function with advancing age, although rarely the cause of substantial illness or disability, impede optimal recovery and increase susceptibility to complications (Table 232-1).

Influence of Comorbidities

The elderly are more likely to have poorly controlled chronic diseases such as coronary artery disease, diabetes mellitus, hypertension, peripheral vascular disease, or chronic obstructive pulmonary disease. In the absence of significant functional reserves, exposure to sustained physiologic stress may result in acute decompensation and organ failure.

Heart disease affects over half the population 65 years of age and older. Orthopnea associated with congestive heart failure (CHF) influences patient positioning, frequently dictating the need to avoid Trendelenburg and flat supine positions, which may cause dyspnea. Electrolyte imbalance caused by diuretics may induce arrhythmias during procedures. Valvular heart lesions may dictate the need for endocarditis prophylaxis. In the presence of coronary artery disease, sublingual nitroglycerin should be available during surgery, and perioperative use of epinephrine should be minimized or avoided.

Hypertension is associated with perioperative bleeding and cardiovascular complications, as well as postoperative hematoma formation. Achieving normotension before even minor, elective surgery minimizes bleeding. Hypertensive responses to pain, hypoxia, hypercarbia, and hypothermia during surgery may be avoided through judicious use of analgesics, respiratory support, and maintaining ambient room temperature. Procedures may be performed while taking precautions to minimize stimuli elevating blood pressure and ensuring perioperative cardiovascular stability.

Patients with *diabetes mellitus* have defects in immune function, vasculopathy, and neuropathy, which increase risk for infection and poor healing. Efforts should be made to tighten blood sugar control before any significant procedure. Prophylactic antibiotics should be a strong consideration.

Hypoxemia and hypercapnia associated with *chronic obstructive pulmonary disease* can be associated with respiratory decompensation as well as right-sided CHF, tissue edema, and impaired mental status. These patients may also be steroid dependent. Hypoxia, coexisting CHF, and steroid use delay wound healing. Once again, consider antibiotic prophylaxis for any surgical procedure. Oxygen, nebulized bronchodilators, and positioning options should be available for potential respiratory decompensation.

Peripheral vascular disease is chronic, progressive, and debilitating and adversely affects the patient's ability to perform daily activities. Ischemia and tissue hypoxemia associated with peripheral vascular disease delays wound healing. Postoperative infection may precipitate gangrene in areas already affected by critical ischemia. Prophylactic antibiotics may help prevent this.

Bleeding diathesis due to anticoagulants or diseases such as myeloproliferative disorders may result in intraoperative bleeding and postoperative hematomas. These risks should be detected and corrected to minimize surgical complications.

Stroke victims more commonly have associated cardiac arrhythmias or coronary artery disease, so extra precaution needs to be taken in this population. In addition, commonly used antiplatelet agents or anticoagulants place this group at higher risk for wound hematoma and subsequent infection. Neurologic deficits may hinder recovery and postoperative care and may also present difficulties in obtaining informed consent.

Hypothyroidism may have protean manifestations (e.g., musculoskeletal or mobility disorders, depression and dementia, slowing of speech and thought processes, cerebellar dysfunction, neuropathy, and macrocytic anemia with or without pernicious anemia). Patients with mild to severe hypothyroidism may also have exaggerated responses to local anesthetics.

Neuropsychiatric manifestations of *vitamin B_{12} deficiency* may include fatigue, weakness, memory loss, and depression. Peripheral or sensory neuropathy may result in urinary or fecal incontinence, ataxia, spasticity, and abnormal gait. Hematologic features include pancytopenia and hepatic dysfunction. These manifestations may influence the informed consent process, as well as anesthetic and surgical techniques.

Hyperviscosity syndrome due to multiple myeloma, other plasma cell dyscrasias, leukemias, or polycythemia is generally not diagnosed until the seventh decade of life. Associated fatigue, weakness, skin and mucosal bleeding, and neurologic manifestations such as paresthesias and ataxia impede healing. Features of the illness and treatment measures (antimitotic agents and plasmapheresis) delay

TABLE 232-1 Senescent Changes with Aging

Organ	Changes and Effect
Skin	• Loss of subcutaneous fat, thinning of epidermis and dermis • Decreased sensory perception • Decrease in collagen, mast cells, fibroblasts, vascularity • Greater susceptibility to injury, delay in wound healing, slowed reepithelization
Cardiovascular system	• Thickening of LV, delayed LV relaxation, reduced LV filling • Diminished cardiac output and vessel compliance • Coronary atherosclerosis • Decreased baroreceptor reflex sensitivity • Cardiac decompensation and postural hypotension
Respiratory system	• Weakness of pharyngeal muscles and diaphragm, intercostal muscle atrophy • Diminished protective reflexes (cough, swallow), chest wall compliance • Senile emphysema • Diminished ventilatory response to congestive heart failure, chronic obstructive pulmonary disease, pneumonia
Central nervous system	• Decrease in cognitive ability, increase in emotional lability • Weakness, ataxia, instability
Kidney	• Decreased glomerular filtration rate, renal blood flow, creatinine clearance*, impaired excretion of acid load, impaired concentrating/diluting capacity and ability to excrete/conserve elements • Increased risk of renal failure in response to various stresses • Reduced renal clearance of drugs; doses of medications need to be adjusted
Gastrointestinal tract	• Delayed relaxation of lower esophageal sphincter and stomach emptying, diminished pepsin secretion, diminished strength and contractility of the colon
Liver	• Diminished hepatic metabolism
Immune system	• Decrease in T-cell–mediated immunity, decrease in delayed hypersensitivity • Enhanced risk of infection
General	• Loss in height and weight, increased fat to lean body mass, and increase in total body water • Effect on drug distribution, binding

LV, left ventricle.
*Serum creatinine is not an accurate reflection of creatinine clearance in the elderly.

wound healing, increase risk of infection, and influence the impact of any procedure.

Pedal edema not only can make lower extremity surgery more difficult, it increases the likelihood of slow healing and infection. Whether the edema is from CHF, venous insufficiency, or other causes, any surgical intervention on the area should be accompanied by leg elevation, prophylactic antibiotics, and delayed removal of sutures.

Approximately 10% of elderly patients have some form of *cognitive impairment*, increasing to 47% among those institutionalized. Cognitive impairment may limit ability to give informed consent, follow instructions regarding aftercare, or comply with medication requirements. These patients are not excluded from office procedures, but there is an increased need to assess the level of functional independence and address the potential need to involve a surrogate caregiver.

Preoperative Assessment

It may be best to schedule the assessment weeks before the procedure so that a focused history, examination, and relevant tests can be carried out. This also allows for optimizing treatment of comorbidities, identification of barriers to obtaining informed consent, and mobilization of support systems. Most elderly patients depend on numerous family and social systems to maintain their independence, and these caregivers should be informed as to the treatment plan and details of postoperative care. Modifications to medications, antibiotic prophylaxis, and bowel preparation should also be addressed at the initial visit. In patients with multiple comorbidities, it may be beneficial to consult with other physician colleagues to minimize risks and optimize outcomes.

The approach to the patient must be geriatric oriented. In addition to the history and physical, elements of functional assessment should be evaluated. The extent of assessment should be determined by the level and potential impact of the procedure on the patient. Psychosocial assessment should address cognitive, affective, functional, environmental, and economic issues.

Most, if not all, *office procedures* are "low risk" and there is insufficient evidence either to advocate routinely performing any given test on the basis of age or to clearly define preoperative tests that are of value. Morbidity after office procedures is not affected by commonly ordered preoperative tests, so *laboratory tests should be ordered only when the history or an examination finding indicates a need.* A chest radiograph and electrocardiogram do not reduce adverse postoperative outcomes and are not usually required.

Medication Issues

A detailed list of medications, including those available over-the-counter (OTC) and herbal preparations, is important in assessing risks associated with office procedures. Medications can influence perioperative and postoperative outcomes by their effect on wound healing and hemostasis, and through drug interactions. Classes of *drugs affecting surgery include antiplatelet agents, anticoagulants, corticosteroids, nicotine, antineoplastic drugs, antihypertensives, antidepressants, and herbal medications.* Most older Americans (80%) take at least one prescription medication and three OTC drugs every day, and there is a linear relationship between the number of drugs taken and the potential for complications. Although it usually is unnecessary to alter or withhold medications, the risks and benefits of discontinuing medications must be carefully weighed with particular emphasis on potential complications, always with the goal of minimizing complications.

Aspirin, antiplatelet agents, selective serotonin reuptake inhibitors, and nonsteroidal anti-inflammatory drugs (NSAIDs) may cause perioperative bleeding by inhibiting platelet aggregation. Traditionally, aspirin has been discontinued for 2 weeks and most NSAIDs 2 days before elective surgery. Nonaspirin, non-NSAID pain relievers are recommended postoperatively. Warfarin, a potent inhibitor of vitamin K–dependent factors, also increases bleeding risk. Recent publications have encouraged continuing both NSAIDs and other anticoagulants during *cutaneous* surgical procedures by demonstrating that complications are not reduced by their brief perioperative discontinuation. If it is necessary to stop oral anticoagulant therapy before performing the office procedure, warfarin can be replaced with *bridge therapy* using low-molecular-weight heparin (enoxaparin). Warfarin is usually stopped 5 days before the procedure and recommenced the day after. Enoxaparin is dosed at 1 mg/kg every 12 hours or 1.5 mg/kg daily in the interim. Both the low-molecular-weight heparin and warfarin are given for 2 to 3 days after the procedure to ensure anticoagulation while the warfarin takes effect. With any of these agents, meticulous hemostasis during office procedures must be ensured.

Unwanted *drug interactions* are typically avoidable with careful preoperative assessment. *Electrolyte levels* should be monitored if indicated based on comorbid illness or medication use, and imbalances corrected before surgery. The use of epinephrine in the presence of hypokalemia can induce cardiac arrhythmia. *Propranolol,* when used with epinephrine, has been known to cause malignant hypertension and reflex bradycardia. However, rebound hypertension and worsening angina may follow abrupt discontinuation of

TABLE 232-2 Medications Interfering with Wound Healing

Agent	Mechanism
Aspirin, ticlopidine, dipyridamole, clopidogrel (Plavix)	• Wound hematoma • Disturbance of fibrin matrix
Corticosteroids	• Decrease fibroblast and epidermal proliferation, formation of granulation tissue, protein and collagen production • Decreased inflammatory response • Increase wound infection rates
Nicotine	• Vasoconstriction
Antineoplastic agents	• Decreases immune response to infection, increased infection rates • Interference with cell division
Colchicine, penicillamine, phenytoin	• Interference with cellular turnover

propranolol or other beta blockers. Abrupt withdrawal of *benzodiazepines* and *antipsychotics* may lead to significant hypertension and mental status changes; their use should therefore be continued. *Monoamine oxidase inhibitors* may interact with epinephrine, phenylephrine, and meperidine, leading to serotonin syndrome (hypertensive crises, mental status changes, fever, muscle cramps, seizures, and coma). *Tricyclic antidepressants* or *selective serotonin reuptake inhibitors* administered for chronic depression need not be discontinued before surgery because this may worsen anxiety, agitation, and depressed mood. It has been suggested that tricyclic antidepressants be stopped 1 to 2 weeks before surgery if use of epinephrine is anticipated, because of the potential arrhythmogenic effect; with the minimal doses used in the office setting, however, this is rarely, if ever, a significant factor. Potential complications of *herbal supplements* include coronary ischemia, stroke, bleeding, and interactions with anesthetic agents. Vitamin E, ginkgo biloba, ginseng, and garlic all inhibit platelet aggregation and increase risk of bleeding and hematoma.

Several agents commonly used in the elderly population delay wound healing (Table 232-2).

Assistive Devices

Many older patients may have eyeglasses, hearing aids, and dentures that are essential to their independence, nutrition, and social interaction. Other assistive devices to be considered include *pacemakers, prosthetic joints or extremities, and assistive mobility devices such as wheelchairs, canes, and walkers*. Procedures should be modified to minimize intraoperative problems associated with these devices and minimally affect their postoperative use. In *pacemaker-dependent patients*, electrosurgery near the heart or pacemaker site should be avoided. If such surgery is contemplated, the indifferent (ground) electrode is placed far away from the pacemaker site and short bursts of current lasting less than 5 seconds should be used. The cutting currents have a higher likelihood of interfering with the pacer.

Competence and Informed Consent

Physical competence specifically refers to the patient's physical ability to participate in the preoperative, intraoperative, and postoperative phases of office procedures. Mental capacity, on the other hand, is defined as the patient's ability to understand the nature and risk of the procedure, along with postoperative care instructions. The elements required to give informed consent include the ability to understand and remember treatment options, risks, and benefits, and the capacity to make decisions consistent with personal values and goals. Sensory and cognitive impairment are associated with impaired understanding and difficulties in communication. Several effective methods have been used to improve understanding in these patients before obtaining consent, including simplified instructions, videos, instructions printed in large font, and use of health educators, patient quizzes, and multiple office visits to alleviate potential confusion. These strategies should be considered in designing materials, forms, policies, and procedures for obtaining informed consent. When the patient is deemed unable to fully understand the information and instructions, the next-of-kin or a legally appointed caregiver should participate in the process.

Antibiotic Prophylaxis

See Chapter 221, Antibiotic Prophylaxis, and Chapter 222, Prevention and Treatment of Wound Infections.

The goals of prophylactic antibiotics are (1) to prevent wound infection and (2) to avoid endocarditis. Antibiotics to prevent wound infection are probably indicated even in clean wounds in the oral cavity, axilla, and perineum, or when there are minor breaks in aseptic technique, where the infection rate is less than 10%. Contaminated wounds (post-traumatic wounds, major breaks in sterile technique, wounds compounded by inflammation) have a 20% to 30% risk of infection and require antibiotics for 3 to 7 days. Wounds grossly contaminated with foreign bodies or with devitalized tissue have a 30% to 40% risk of infection and require more prolonged antibiotic treatment (7 to 14 days). There are no reliable studies confirming the effectiveness of this approach and the optimal duration of antibiotics in these classes of wounds.

In addition, for the office practice, wound prophylaxis should be strongly considered in the very old, those with suspected poor nutrition, those who are immunosuppressed for any reason or have diabetes, and for large wounds and for surgery on the lower extremities in the presence of edema or peripheral vascular disease.

Topical antibiotics facilitate wound healing by keeping the wound moist, increasing the removal of debris, and reducing the surface bacterial count. They may both promote and retard the rate of reepithelialization of wounds, and may also cause allergic reactions. Sterile petrolatum is an inexpensive and effective alternative that is less likely to cause an allergic dermatitis or promote bacterial resistance. Although "moist healing" is the standard in the elderly, the moist environment may lead to maceration and skin breakdown. After the first few days, wounds may do better being left open to "dry" for a good portion of the day.

A significant proportion of reported cases of *infective endocarditis* have no known predisposing source, and most cases are not due to invasive procedures. Although antibiotic prophylaxis against endocarditis had been recommended in the past for dermatologic procedures in patients with valvular heart disease and prosthetic valves, more recent recommendations by the American Heart Association have not mandated this because of the low risk of endocarditis after these procedures. Office procedures associated with development of endocarditis include oral hygiene and dental procedures, especially in the presence of gum disease, nasal cautery for epistaxis, fiberoptic endoscopy of the gastrointestinal tract, barium enema, and genitourinary procedures such as urethral catheterization. Patients at high risk of development of endocarditis include those with cardiac prosthetic valves and those with previous episodes of endocarditis. Indwelling pacemakers pose a low risk of development of endocarditis. Most evaluations have also found routine prophylaxis for patients with prosthetic joints unnecessary.

Aftercare and Follow-up

In the absence of any significant physical or cognitive limitations, most patients recover well after office procedures. Patients should be encouraged to resume activities of daily living as early as possible. Medication changes should be reviewed carefully. Written and verbal postprocedure instructions for wound care, pharmacotherapy, and follow-up should be given to the patient or caregiver.

If significant pain is anticipated after the procedure, analgesics should be continued, making allowances for temporary functional limitations they may impose. If narcotic analgesics are used, they should be accompanied by a gentle bowel stimulant such as senna to prevent constipation and fecal impaction. Symptoms suggesting complications (e.g., wound infection, sepsis, deep venous thrombosis if immobilization is anticipated, bleeding and bowel perforation after endoscopy) should be explained to both patient and caregiver to maximize opportunities for early intervention. In cognitively impaired or homebound patients, a home health care agency or skilled nursing services may be useful in assisting with postprocedure monitoring and ensuring optimal recovery.

CONCLUSION

The turn of the century has brought with it a large group of older people in need of health care and support. When contemplating office procedures, it is mandatory that physicians familiarize themselves with the additional demands that aging, illness, polypharmacy, and the presence of assistive devices place on these patients.

BIBLIOGRAPHY

American Society of Health-System Pharmacists: Snapshot of medication use in the U.S. ASHP Research Report, December, 2000. Available at http://www.ashp.org/s_ashp/docs/files/PR_snapshot.pdf. Accessed June 17, 2010.

Fleisher LA: Routine laboratory testing in the elderly: Is it indicated? Anesth Analg 93:249–250, 2001.

Haas AF, Grekin RC: Antibiotic prophylaxis in dermatologic surgery. J Am Acad Dermatol 32:155–176, 1995.

Khazan M, Scheuering S, Adamson R, Mathis AS: Prescribing patterns and outcomes of enoxaparin for anticoagulation of atrial fibrillation. Pharmacotherapy 23:651–658, 2003.

Otley CC, Fewkes JL, Frank W, et al: Complications of cutaneous surgery in patients who are taking warfarin, aspirin, or non-steroidal anti-inflammatory drugs. Arch Dermatol 132:161–166, 1996.

Perron VD, Robinson BE: The aging process and functional assessment. Arch Am Acad Orthop Surg 2:1–8, 1998.

Smack DP, Harrington AC, Dunn C, et al: Infection and allergy incidence in ambulatory surgery patients using white petrolatum vs bacitracin ointment: A randomized controlled trial. JAMA 276:972–977, 1996.

Winton G: Anesthesia for dermatologic surgery. J Dermatol Surg Oncol 14:41–54, 1988.

CHAPTER 233

Body Piercing

Peter Valenzuela

Modification of the body in the form of piercing and skin art has been demonstrated in virtually every culture dating back to at least 2000 BC. Egyptian pharaohs pierced their navels, and Roman soldiers pierced their nipples. Perhaps better known are the piercings and body art of African and Native American communities. In the United States, female ear piercing has long been accepted, but in the last 25 years male ear piercing and the piercing of other body areas have become widespread. Today, navel piercing is one of the most fashionable piercings. More extreme piercings of the eyebrows, nipples, lips, tongue, and genitals have also become common. With this in mind, primary care physicians may decide to offer body piercing to their patients.

Physicians have the advantage of being trained in anatomy, physiology, and aseptic technique, which are vital to performing safe piercings. In addition, physicians can recognize potential complications and have the capacity to therapeutically intervene early and effectively. Even if physicians choose not to perform body piercing, they need to be familiar with the techniques and complications that are unique to body piercing.

Anatomy

Commonly pierced areas of the body include the ears, eyebrows, tongue, nose (i.e., ala, septum, and bridge), umbilicus, nipples, lips, and genitals. Each site carries unique risks. The physician needs to be cognizant of these risks when evaluating whether to pierce a specific location, and needs to counsel the patient accordingly.

Indications

- Cosmetic procedure
- No traditional medical indications
- The clitoral hood piercing may improve the sexual experience for women who have lost sensitivity

Contraindications

- *Skin and systemic disorders:* Medical contraindications to body piercing are related to external factors involving the skin and to systemic conditions. Local skin infection, a cyst, severe eczema, or any other significant skin disorder at the site is a contraindication to piercing. A history of keloid formation, not necessarily hypertrophic scarring, is also a condition that warns against piercing.
- *Steroid use and coagulation disorders:* Chronic steroid use or a coagulation disorder also precludes the procedure.
- *Immunodeficiency syndromes:* Patients with an immunodeficiency disorder, such as acquired immunodeficiency syndrome (AIDS), present unique difficulties. For many of these patients, body modification is an important part of life, and the piercing would benefit their overall sense of well-being. Although, theoretically, AIDS might be considered a contraindication to piercing, realistically, unless the patient's T-cell levels are significantly compromised, piercing can be successfully accomplished in the patient with AIDS.
- *Pregnancy:* Clinicians should discuss pregnancy intentions with women seeking nipple or navel piercings because healing can take 2 to 4 months. Controversy exists regarding whether a nipple piercing affects lactation. There are 15 to 20 milk ducts in the nipple. Although scar tissue may occlude some ducts, a properly placed piercing with appropriate jewelry should not adversely affect breast function. Excessive scarring may lead to duct occlusion, which could cause decreased or absent milk expression, persistent breast engorgement, and increased risk of infection or abscess formation during lactation. Women interested in nipple piercings should be aware of the unknown and potentially adverse effects on the ability to breast-feed. Also, because the infant may aspirate the jewelry or develop metal allergies, the jewelry is removed during actual breast-feeding.

  Navel piercings can take 6 to 10 months to heal. This should also be taken into consideration if a pregnancy is being considered. Navel piercings also tend to migrate. Tissue distortion that occurs during pregnancy can exacerbate this problem, and it may be necessary to remove the jewelry as gestation progresses.

Equipment

Jewelry

It is important to use the proper jewelry to avoid complications. Patients should wear only jewelry made of surgical-grade stainless steel (316 L [low carbon], 316 LVM [low carbon, volume melt]), titanium, niobium, platinum, solid white or yellow gold (14K or 18K), or Tygon. Gold-plated jewelry contains reactive metals such as nickel and can cause allergic reactions. Silver will tarnish in the moist environment of a new piercing or in contact with any mucosal surface.

The most common types of jewelry are bead ring, captive bead ring, straight barbell, circular barbell, and curved barbell (Fig. 233-1). Size is defined in terms of gauge and either diameter or length. If the jewelry is not provided by the physician's office, patients should be advised to purchase the jewelry that is appropriate for the piercing they desire and bring it with them. Table 233-1 summarizes the initial jewelry commonly used for each location.

The bead ring and captive bead ring are opened and closed either by hand or with specialized ring-opening, ring-closing pliers. The use of other pliers may distort the shape of the ring. It is important to maintain the integrity and shape when opening and closing the ring.

Piercing Equipment

- Appropriate jewelry: sterilize in an autoclave.
- Antiseptic cleanser: use povidone iodine (Betadine), Techni-Care, or ethyl alcohol.

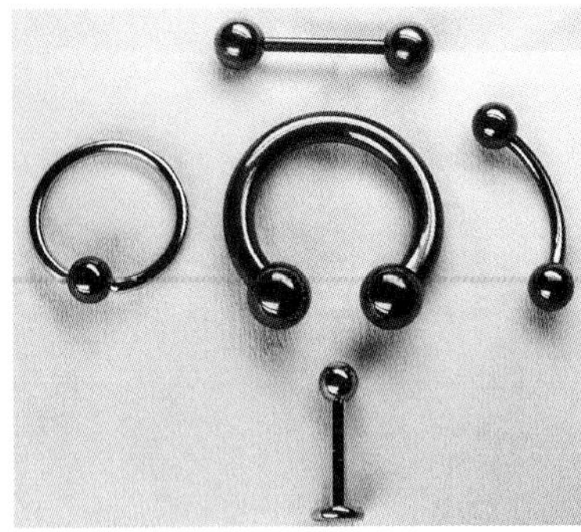

Figure 233-1 Jewelry styles: straight barbell *(top)*, captive ring *(left)*, circular barbell *(center)*, curved barbell *(right)*, and labret stud *(bottom)*.

- Ring-closing pliers: use with captive or bead rings; usually not needed if jewelry is annealed. (The annealing process allows jewelry to be manipulated more easily, particularly by hand.)
- Piercing needles: have various sizes available, including 10, 12, 14, 16, and 18 gauge. (For most piercings, the needle size should match the gauge of the jewelry being inserted [Fig. 233-2].)
- Needle-receiving tube: use for piercings involving the nostril, septum, penis, clitoral hood, and some parts of the ear cartilage (Fig. 233-3).
- Rubber bands: use to provide tension for piercing clamps.
- Insertion taper: a solid metal rod that is larger at one end and gradually becomes smaller at the other end; gauge measurement is based on size of larger end; use to help transfer jewelry or for stretching; in a fresh piercing the taper's gauge will be the same as the jewelry gauge. *Transfer* means to place the tip of the jewelry into the needle or taper and pass it into place in the hole previously made by the needle.
- Needle pusher/acrylic needle holder: helps pass the needle through skin.
- Tissue forceps: use Pennington, mini-Pennington, or ring forceps; slotted style is optional. (The forceps is tensioned with two rubber bands; this helps avoid clamping skin too tightly.)
- Surgical marking pen: use very fine point. (Sharpie Fine Point pens can be used.)
- Gentian violet: to mark tongue and oral cavity piercings.
- Toothpicks: to apply gentian violet.
- Cotton applicators: use to adjust the size or site of insertion marks at the piercing site; erase or fine-tune the marks with alcohol-soaked applicators.

Figure 233-2 Piercing needle. This is a hollow, tribeveled needle. Jewelry is held against the nonpointed end of the needle for passage through the skin. After passage, a cork can be placed on the needle tip to prevent needlestick injuries.

- Gauze: to cleanse the site after piercing.
- Gauge wheel: confirm gauge of needle or jewelry.
- Caliper: confirm size of jewelry.
- Sterile barrier field: cover instrument tray.
- Cork: cover needle tip after insertion. (Protects against needle injury.)
- Ethyl alcohol (70%): can use as a skin cleanser. (Removes excess ink marks.)

Sterilization

Most piercing equipment can be sterilized in an autoclave (270° F under high-pressure steam for at least 10 minutes). Items that are reusable should be cleansed in an ultrasonic cleaner before sterilization. Those items that are heat sensitive can be cleansed with a broad-spectrum, environmentally safe germicidal that kills such organisms as human immunodeficiency virus (HIV), hepatitis (particularly B), and tuberculosis. When possible, piercing guns should be avoided because most cannot be properly sterilized. Those patients choosing to have a body piercing done at a piercing salon should be advised to search for members of the Association of Professional Piercers. In addition, the piercer should possess certifications for basic life support/cardiopulmonary resuscitation and blood-borne pathogens training.

Preprocedure Patient Education and Forms

Inform the patient of all possible complications of piercing in general and those specific to the location requested. Thorough documentation of the informed consent is mandatory. All patients younger than 18 years of age need legal guardian consent. Patients should anticipate the average healing time depending on the loca-

TABLE 233-1 Jewelry Selection

Location	Type and Size	Gauges*	Comments
Ear lobe	BR, CBR, or LB; 3/8–1/2 inch	18–10 gauge	Avoid ear studs; occlusive and difficult to clean
Ear cartilage (outer)	BR, CBR, or LB; 5/16–7/16 inch	18–14 gauge	Choose jewelry least likely to be uncomfortable during sleep
Ear cartilage (tragus)	BR, CBR, or BB; 5/16–3/8 inch	18 or 16 gauge	Choose jewelry least likely to be uncomfortable during sleep
Eyebrow	BR, CBR, BB, or LB; 3/8–7/16 inch	18 or 16 gauge	Risk of tearing with smaller gauges; risk of migration with larger gauges
Nostril	Nostril screw; BR, CBR; 5/16–7/16 inch	20 gauge; 18 gauge	Nostril screw has small loop at right angle to hold it in place
Nasal septum	BR, CBR, BB or CB; 3/8–1/2 inch	16–10 gauge	Use a needle-receiving tube
Tongue	BB; 3/4–1 inch	14–10 gauge	Length accounts for initial edema; downsize jewelry in 2–3 weeks; minimum ball size is 6 mm
Labret	Labret stud; 3/8–1/2 inch	14 gauge	Minimum ball size is 5 mm; can downsize later
Nipple (female)	BR, CBR, BB, or CB; 5/8–3/4 inch	14–10 gauge	Consider future breast-feeding plans; postpone piercing if pregnancy is in the near future
Nipple (male)	BR, CBR, BB, or CB; 9/16 inch	14 or 12 gauge	
Navel	BR, CBR, or LB; 7/16–5/8 inch	14 or 12 gauge	Pierce navel fold; avoid small jewelry that can constrict skin
Clitoral hood (vertical)	BR, CBR, or LB; 7/16–9/16 inch	14 or 12 gauge	Position jewelry so that ball rests on the clitoris
Penis (Prince Albert)	BR, CBR, LB, or CB; 9/16–1 inch	12 or 10 gauge	Use a needle-receiving tube

BB, straight barbell; BR, bead ring; CB, circular barbell; CBR, captive bead ring; LB, curved barbell.
*When using gauge readings, the size actually decreases as the gauge number gets larger.

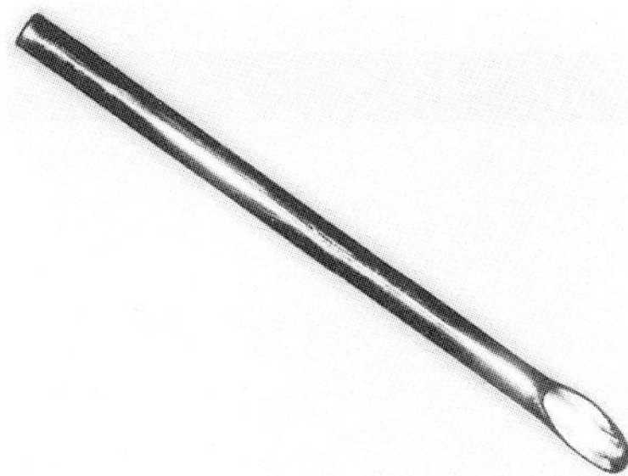

Figure 233-3 Needle-receiving tube. This is a hollow tube that is used in ear cartilage, nostril, and genital piercings. The needle is passed through the area being pierced into the tube. The tube protects adjacent structures from inadvertent injury.

tion of the piercing (Table 233-2). (See the sample patient education and consent forms online at www.expertconsult.com.)

Technique

Universal precautions should always be followed. Instruments and jewelry need to be appropriately sterilized. In rare circumstances, certain jewelry will need to be soaked in an antiseptic solution for 30 minutes. This solution is removed with alcohol before insertion. Anesthesia is usually not indicated for these procedures. However, for sensitive areas such as the genitals and mucosa, topical anesthetics like topical lidocaine (EMLA cream) or benzocaine (Hurricaine) can be applied before the procedures.

Navel Piercing

1. Prepare the sterile instrument tray (Fig. 233-4).
2. Clean the navel and the surrounding abdominal wall with an antiseptic solution (sterile preparation).
3. Mark entry and exit points with the surgical marker (Fig. 233-5). Confirm acceptability of location with the patient before proceeding. Use the crest of the navel fold as a guide. On the abdominal wall, mark the entrance site at a distance half the length of the curved barbell or the diameter of the ring from the edge of the skin fold. On the undersurface of the navel skin fold, mark the exit site at the same distance from the edge of the fold as the entrance site. This is above the deep, flat base of the umbilicus. Have the patient lie, sit, stand, protrude, and retract the abdomen to evaluate placement of the markings as they vary with each position. Make adjustments in the markings if needed. If an umbilical hernia or other anatomic variants are present, a navel piercing should be avoided.

TABLE 233-2 Average Healing Times for Piercing Locations

Location	Healing Times
Ear lobe	4–6 wk
Ear cartilage	2–3 mo
Eyebrow	6–8 wk
Nostril	2–3 mo
Nasal septum	4–6 wk
Tongue	4–6 wk
Labret	6–8 wk
Nipple (female)	2–3 mo
Nipple (male)	2–3 mo
Navel	6–10 mo
Clitoral hood	4–6 wk
Penis (Prince Albert)	4–6 wk

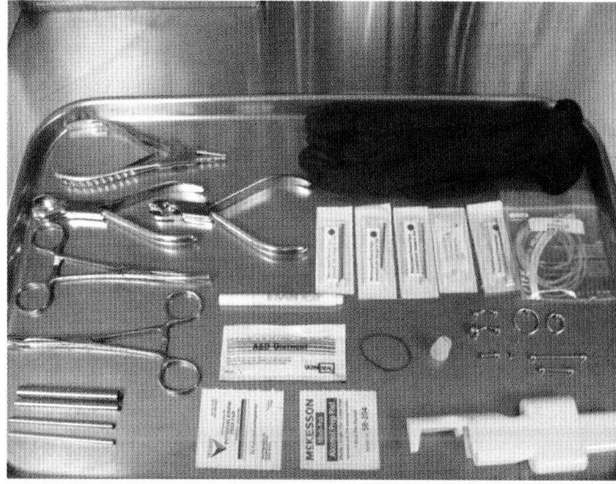

Figure 233-4 Instrument tray. Items shown: gloves, marking pen, cotton applicators, calipers, gauze, captive bead ring, piercing needle, insertion taper, Pennington forceps, and rubber bands. All items are appropriately sterilized. (Courtesy of Armando Escajeda, Jr.)

NOTE: Our preferred method is to start with the patient in a supine position and mark the exit hole within the fold of skin over the navel. Have the patient stand, and evaluate tissue above the navel fold for a natural indentation. Mark this site as the entrance hole. Choose the appropriate jewelry size ($\frac{7}{16}$, $\frac{1}{2}$, $\frac{9}{16}$, or $\frac{5}{8}$) to match the navel's anatomy as determined by the placement of the markings.

4. Place rubber bands on the forceps and adjust the tension. Grasp and tent the skin with traction. Avoid actually clamping the forceps because this will crush the skin (Fig. 233-6).
5. Position the piercing needle perpendicular to the tented skin and parallel to the floor and the markings (Fig. 233-7).
6. Pass the needle through the skin. Remove the forceps. Attach the jewelry to the nonpointed end (see Fig. 233-2) of the needle, then pass the jewelry into the piercing. For a captive ring, the ring needs to be twisted back and forth to allow easy transfer (Fig. 233-8). After the ring is in place, straighten the ring and insert the ball (Fig. 233-9).
7. Remove the antiseptic cleansing agent with sterile saline.

Other Piercings

Ear Lobe

1. Cleanse the front and back of the lobe.
2. Mark the front and back in the center of the lobe.
3. Use the Pennington forceps to stabilize the lobe when passing the needle. Do not ratchet down the forceps. (Disposable ear piercing kits are also available.)
4. Pierce perpendicular to the plane of the lobe.

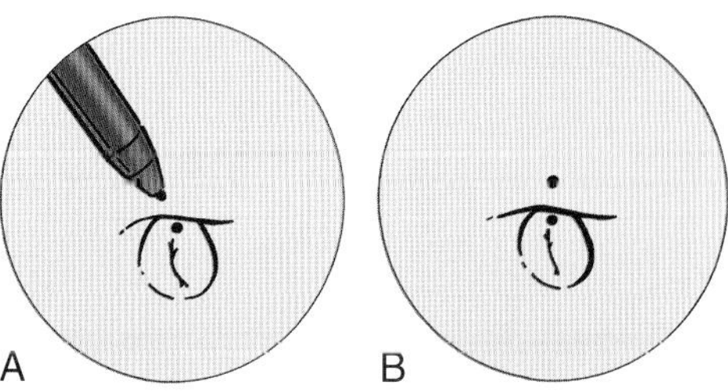

Figure 233-5 **A** and **B,** Schematic representation of the skin markings for umbilical piercing. The longitudinal line in the circular area represents the base of the umbilicus. The transverse line represents the navel skin fold. The area between the longitudinal and transverse lines represents the undersurface of the skin fold. The markings are usually equidistant from the edge of the fold.

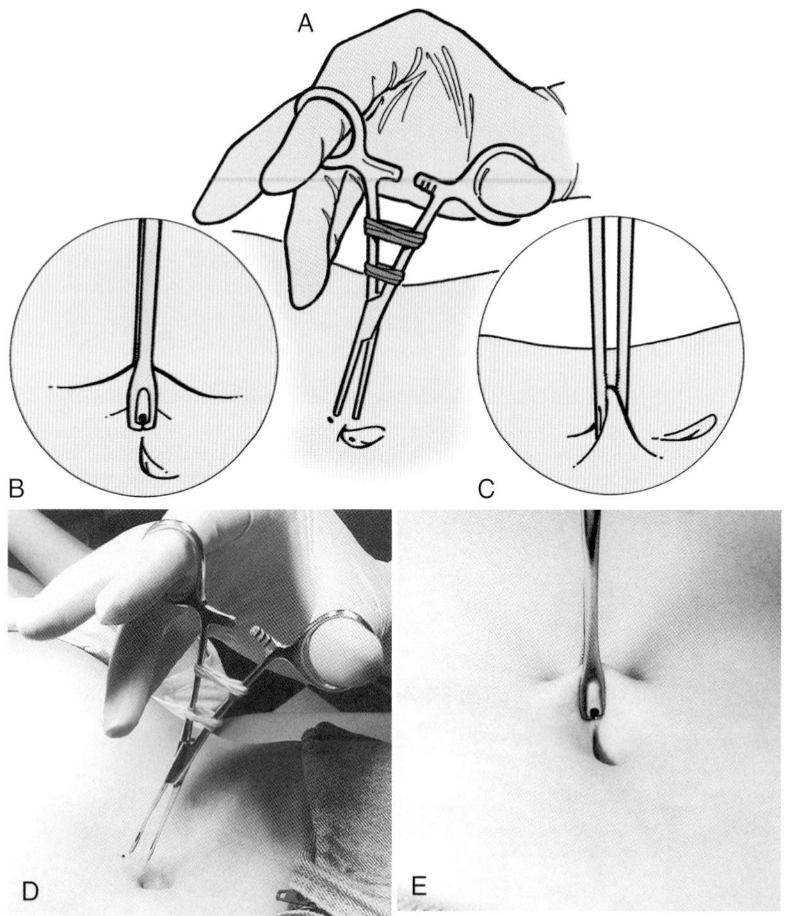

Figure 233-6 Schematic representation of forceps application for umbilical piercing. The patient is supine. **A,** The navel skin fold has been marked (*center*). (Note markings above and below the marked skin fold.) The forceps have two rubber bands in place for tensioning. The skin fold will be gently held by the forceps. **B,** The markings are positioned at the edge of the clamp opening. The skin fold is then gently tented and held perpendicular to the floor. It is important not to engage the clamp's ratchets. **C,** Forceps application. The skin fold is gently tented and held perpendicular to the floor. Note the deep aspect of the umbilicus is not involved in the piercing. **D,** Photograph of step A. **E,** Photograph of step B.

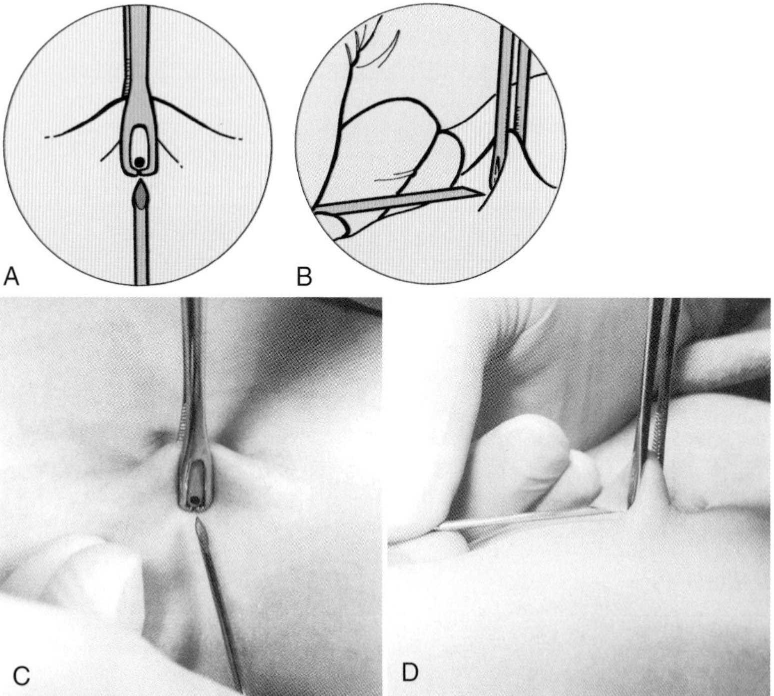

Figure 233-7 Schematic representation of the needle position for umbilical piercing. **A,** With the skin gently tented, the needle is positioned perpendicular to the skin and parallel to the floor. The direction of the piercing is cranial to caudal (i.e., the needle is pointing toward the foot). **B,** The needle is positioned perpendicular to the skin fold and parallel to the floor. The needle is aligned with the markings and is pointing cranial to caudal (i.e., toward the foot). **C,** Photograph of step A. **D,** Photograph of step B.

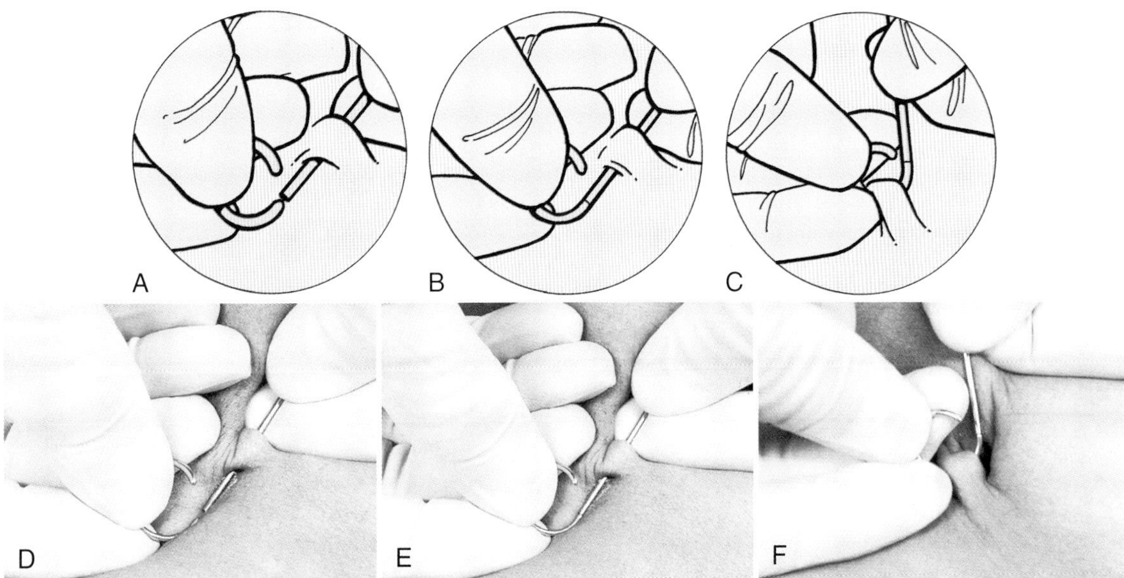

Figure 233-8 Schematic representation of jewelry transfer for umbilical piercing. **A,** The sharp end of the needle is held with the fingers of one hand. The point can be protected with a cork. **B,** The jewelry is positioned against the nonpointed end. **C,** The skin fold is stabilized against the finger during transfer. The jewelry is gently twisted to help clear the skin fold. **D,** Photograph of step A, showing jewelry positioning. The sharp end of the jewelry is held with the fingers of one hand. The jewelry is being placed on the nonpointed end of the needle. The jewelry is gently twisted to help clear the skin fold. **E,** Photograph of step B. The jewelry abuts the nonpointed end of the needle. The skin fold is stabilized against the finger holding the sharp end. **F,** Photograph of step **C** showing jewelry transfer. The jewelry has been transferred through the skin fold. During the transfer, the jewelry is held against the nonpointed end of the needle. The jewelry is gently twisted to help clear the skin fold.

Ear Cartilage

1. Clamping is not recommended for cartilage because of potential crushing and increased risk of complication.
2. Use a free-hand technique or a needle-receiving tube.
3. Pierce perpendicular to the plane of the cartilage.

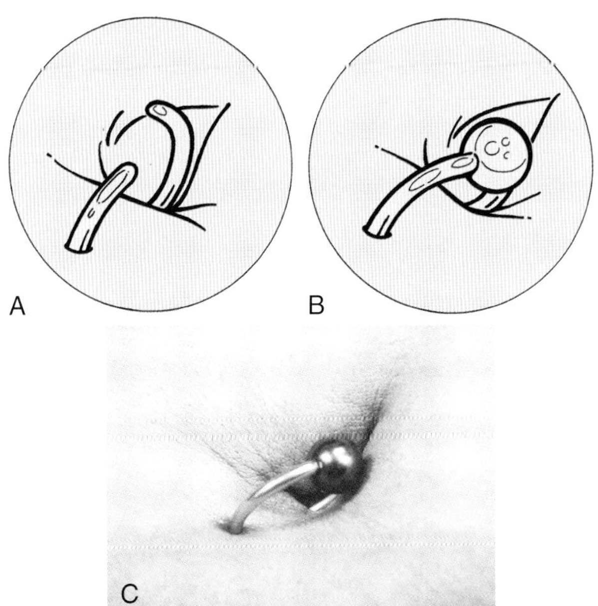

Figure 233-9 Schematic representation of jewelry for umbilical piercing. **A,** The ring has a gentle twist and must be untwisted for bead placement. **B,** The bead has indentations, and these are positioned between the ends of the ring. **C,** The captive bead ring is positioned in the navel's skin fold.

Eyebrow

1. Can be performed similar to the navel technique.
2. The piercing is placed over the lateral third of the eyebrow to avoid the supraorbital nerve.
3. Slant the piercing toward the nose with the lower mark made medial to the upper mark.
4. Avoid a shallow piercing because this can lead to migration.

Nostril

1. The entrance point is at the natural indentation of the alar fold; the direction of the piercing is external to internal.
2. Use a needle-receiving tube placed inside the nostril to avoid tissue damage.
3. Avoid using a clamp on the ala because this will crush the cartilage.

Nasal Septum

1. Piercing is done through the soft membrane inferior to the nasal cartilage.
2. The piercing is located $\frac{3}{4}$ inch from the external tip of the nose and $\frac{1}{8}$ inch below the cartilaginous edge.
3. Use a needle-receiving tube to stabilize the septum.

Labret or Lip

1. These are unique piercings because they involve two different tissue surfaces, facial skin and the mucosa of the oral cavity.
2. The piercing site in the skin is usually placed below the vermillion border of the lip.
3. On the mucosal surface, the site is positioned so the jewelry does not rest on the gums.
4. Appropriate jewelry for these piercings are rings or labret studs (see Fig. 233-1). Jewelry size is $\frac{3}{8}$ to $\frac{1}{2}$ inch.

Cheek

1. Before the piercing, use a penlight to identify vascular structures, particularly the branches of the facial artery and vein. This will help avoid the branches of the facial nerve.

2. Pierce through the facial skin anterior to the laugh line into the oral cavity.
3. Inside the oral cavity, the hole should avoid the parotid duct.

Tongue

1. Choose a central and midline location in the natural bend of the tongue. Have the patient cup the tongue to find this indentation.
2. The exit site is anterior to the frenulum. Avoid the veins that are easily visualized on the underside of the tongue.
3. Use gentian violet to mark the entrance and exit sites. With the tongue in an extended position, the entrance and exit sites should be perpendicular. This allows for a slightly angulated position when the tongue is retracted.
4. During the piercing, hold the tongue in an extended position with gauze or a sponge forceps.

Nipple

1. The horizontal axis is preferred for women, but they may prefer the piercing to be vertical. The horizontal or vertical axis can be used for men.
2. For women, the piercing is placed through the base of the nipple at or just below the midline. In men, placement is at the junction of the nipple with the areola at or just above the midline.

Clitoral Hood

Actual clitoral piercings are rare, and they depend on the size of the clitoris. Damage to the neural tissue can occur. Most patients who request a clitoral piercing actually desire the clitoral hood piercing.

VERTICAL PIERCING

1. Find the apex of the hood at the base of the clitoris.
2. Mark the outer skin of the hood at this site.
3. Measure the distance to the edge of the hood and to the head of the clitoris. Choose a jewelry size that allows the ball to rest on the head. Typically the jewelry will be a ½-inch curved barbell.
4. Insert the jewelry; the preferred jewelry is a curved barbell.

HORIZONTAL PIERCING

1. Pierce through the clitoral hood tissue at a similar distance from the clitoris as in the vertical piercing.
2. Avoid the veins that pass down the hood; use a penlight to identify the veins.
3. Use lightweight jewelry because the weight of the jewelry can pull the hood beyond the clitoris, and the desired effect will be lost.

Penis (Prince Albert)

1. This is the most commonly requested penile piercing.
2. Place the piercing in the thin, soft, triangular skin on the ventral side of the penis just below the corona of the glans at the frenulum.
3. Evaluate the penis in both a flaccid and an erect state to locate the entrance site that accommodates an erection.
4. Choose the jewelry size based on the erect state of the penis; the jewelry is generally ⅝ to ¾ inch long.
5. Mark the entrance site at the frenulum.
6. Place a needle-receiving tube through the meatus into the urethra. Position the end of the tube (which is now inside the urethra) at the entrance site.
7. Pass the needle through the skin into the receiving tube.
8. Remove the tube and protect the sharp end of the needle with a cork.
9. Position the jewelry on the needle and transfer.

NOTE: The Prince Albert has a tendency to bleed for several days after the piercing.

COMPLICATIONS

General

Some complications are inherent in all piercing procedures.

- The most common complication is infection from staphylococcal or streptococcal species. Bacterial infections can occur because of improper piercing technique or poor hygiene. Local infections can be cared for using warm compresses, antibacterial soap, and topical mupirocin. In severe skin infections, oral antibiotics such as the first-generation cephalosporins (i.e., cephalexin, cefadroxil, dicloxacillin) may be indicated and are appropriate treatment options for more serious wound infections. If *Pseudomonas* is suspected, use ciprofloxacin. If methicillin-resistant *Staphylococcus aureus* is suspected, consider oral trimethoprim/sulfamethoxazole (Bactrim).
- Other infection: Tuberculosis, tetanus, hepatitis, HIV infection, and toxic shock syndrome have been attributed to contamination at the time of piercing. Genital piercings increase the risk of hepatitis and HIV infections from sexual contact because of the open wounds and associated trauma.
- Pain.
- Bleeding.
- Hypertrophic scarring.
- Keloid formation.
- Granuloma or cyst formation.
- Migration or expulsion of jewelry.
- Contact dermatitis or other skin reaction.
- Possible social stigma.

Specific Complications by Location

Navel

- Migration
- Frictional irritation
- Scar formation

Ear Cartilage

- Associated with poor healing and more serious infection because of the avascular nature of auricular cartilage
- Auricular perichondritis and perichondrial abscess (typically occur in the first month after piercing, especially during warm-weather months)
- Infection from *Lactobacillus*, *Pseudomonas* more common
- Toxic shock syndrome (very rare)
- In one study, 34% of ear piercings experienced complications such as mild infection, pain, and allergic reaction

Ear Lobe

- Keloids, especially in black individuals
- Enlargement of the opening and traumatic lacerations tearing through the lobe
- Lack of symmetry between the two sides

Eyebrow

- Periorbital infection
- Damage to supraorbital nerve

Nostril

- Damage to cartilage
- Infection (staphylococcal)

Nasal Septum

- Pressure necrosis of cartilaginous border and alae

Tongue

- Damage to dentition and gums
- Loss of bone supporting the teeth
- Lingual nerve damage
- Hematoma
- Aspiration of jewelry

Labret and Lips

- Damage to dentition and gums

Cheek

- Damage to parotid duct branches of the facial artery, vein, and nerve
- Uncontrolled drooling

Nipple

- Interference with lactation
- Mastitis and abscess formation

Postprocedure Patient Education

Advise the following:

- Always wash hands thoroughly before touching the piercing.
- Avoid tight clothing that can cause increased friction at the piercing site.
- Expect serosanguineous fluid to ooze and crust around the entrance and exit sites. This crusting will last until the piercing has completely healed. Only when the crusting has stopped can jewelry exchange or a stretching procedure be considered. The crusted material harbors bacteria and needs to be removed. Soak the piercing site with a warm sea salt solution (¼ teaspoon of sea salt in 8 oz of distilled water) using a soft cloth, gauze, or an inverted glass for 5 to 10 minutes. Then remove the crusted material with a clean, damp cloth or cotton-tipped applicators before carefully twisting the jewelry in the moistened area to ensure it is not trapped.
- Use a mild antibacterial soap that does not contain fragrances. We prefer Provon (GOJO Laboratories, Akron, Ohio) and Septicare (Sage Laboratories, Hudson, NH). If using soap, lather the area and the jewelry, then rinse well with water. Allow to air dry. If using Septicare, allow it to dry without rinsing.
- If redness and swelling develop, use warm compresses four times a day for 24 hours. If the redness and swelling do not go away or if a purulent discharge (pus) develops, see a physician.
- For tongue piercings, use an antibacterial mouthwash that does not contain alcohol or a saline solution after meals and smoking. Gargle for 30 to 60 seconds. It is preferable to avoid smoking. Use a new toothbrush and change it every 30 days. Brush the jewelry with the toothbrush to remove plaque.
- Do not use antibacterial ointments such as polymyxin B sulfate, neomycin sulfate, and bacitracin (Neosporin); bacitracin; or polymyxin B sulfate and bacitracin zinc (Polysporin). These ointments are petroleum based and can occlude the piercing. Occlusion will trap serosanguineous fluid and dead cells, delay healing, and promote possible infections. Prolonged use of antibacterial ointments can also irritate the skin. If necessary, prescribe mupirocin (Bactroban) ointment for the first 24 to 48 hours if mild redness or swelling develops. Rub the ointment gently on the jewelry and the surrounding skin until a thin, invisible layer is present.
- Avoid using alcohol, which can dry the skin and the cells involved in healing the piercing.
- Avoid using hydrogen peroxide and povidone–iodine, which are toxic to healing tissues.

Conclusion

Body piercing is an elective procedure that patients may be surprised to learn a physician understands and can perform. Anatomic evaluation, aseptic technique, appropriate aftercare, and proper selection of jewelry to fit the location are keys to a successful piercing procedure. Understanding the patient who requests a piercing is necessary to obtain an excellent result.

Patient Education Guides

See the sample patient education and consent forms online at www.expertconsult.com.

The following brochures are available from the Association of Professional Piercers (APP) (www.safepiercing.org). The APP has also written the *APP Procedural Manual*.

- Picking Your Piercer
- Aftercare Guidelines for Facial and Body Piercings
- Aftercare Guidelines for Oral Piercings
- Body Piercing Troubleshooting: For You and Your Healthcare Professional

Billing and Coding

Because this is a cosmetic procedure, providers need to collect payment directly from the patient. However, there is an ICD-9 code for ear piercing (V50.3).

Suppliers

(See contact information online at www.expertconsult.com.)

Anatometal
Body Circle Designs
Body Vision
Custom Steel
Industrial Strength
Unimax Supply Company

Online Resources

Answers.com: Body piercing. Available at www.answers.com/topic/body-piercing.
Association of Professional Piercers: Available at www.safepiercing.org.
Atomic Tattoos and Body Piercing: Available at www.atomictattoos.com.
Body Jewellery Shop: Available at www.bodyjewelleryshop.com.
Body Work Productions: Available at www.bodyworkprod.com.
Piercinglinks.com: An aggregator website with a very complete listing of body piercing links. Available at www.piercinglinks.com.
Tribalectic Body Piercing Community: Available at www.tribalectic.com.
Yahoo! Body Art: Yahoo! Directory links to body piercing websites. Available at dir.yahoo.com/Arts/Visual_Arts/Body_Art/.

Bibliography

American Academy of Dermatology: Tattoos, body piercings, and other skin adornments. Available at www.aad.org/public/Publications/pamphlets/tattoo.htm. Accessed April 1, 2007.
Angel E: The worst piercing story. The Point 23:15, 2002.
Campbell A, Moore A, Williams E, et al: Tongue piercing: Impact of time and barbell stem length on lingual gingival recession and tooth chipping. J Periodontol 73:289–287, 2002.
Er N, Ozkavaf A, Berberoglu A, Yamalik N: An unusual cause of gingival recession: Oral piercing. J Periodontol 71:1767–1769, 2000.
Gawkrodger DJ: Nickel dermatitis: How much nickel is safe? Contact Dermatitis 35:267–271, 1996.
Landeck A, Newman N, Breadon J, Zahner S: A simple technique for ear piercing. J Am Acad Dermatol 39:795–796, 1998.

Liden C, Menne T, Burrows D: Nickel-containing alloys and platings and their ability to cause dermatitis. Br J Dermatol 134:193–198, 1996.

Meltzer D: Complications of body piercing. Am Fam Physician 72: 2029–2034, 2005.

Meyer D: Body piercing: Old traditions creating new challenges. J Emerg Nurs 26:612–614, 2000.

More DR, Seidel JS, Bryan PA: Ear-piercing techniques as a cause of auricular chondritis. Pediatr Emerg Care 15:189–192, 1999.

Samantha S, Tweeten M, Rickman LS: Infectious complications of body piercing. Clin Infect Dis 26:735–740, 1998.

Staley R, Fitzgibbon JJ, Anderson C: Auricular infections caused by high ear piercing in adolescents. Pediatrics 99:610–611, 1997.

CHAPTER 234

INTERVENTIONAL PROCEDURES FOR HEADACHES: ACUTE AND PREVENTATIVE

Duren Michael Ready

Headaches are an almost universal condition. They are as old as humankind. Headache management evolved beyond "taking two aspirins" with the development of the ergots and migraine-specific triptan medications. Physicians frequently still encounter patients who have broken through their prophylaxis, failed acute treatments, and are in need of rescue therapies.

The introduction of sumatriptan and the subsequent development of additional triptans have proven to be a great enhancement for the acute and rescue treatment of migraine and cluster headaches. Triptans are still considered to be underused medications. However, even they have their limits. They work best when used at the onset of mild pain and are of very limited utility 24 hours after onset of the headache. Unfortunately, when we encounter many of these difficult patients, it is too late to use them.

Several of the procedures discussed here are older (greater and lesser occipital nerve blocks and sphenopalatine nerve blocks) and well established in the medical literature. However, newer techniques (botulinum toxin and paracervical intramuscular spinal blocks) are under increasing study and use.

There are multiple benefits to incorporating injection procedures into the management of headaches. They can provide some of the fastest relief (occipital nerve blocks, paracervical intramuscular spinal blocks), are the most comfortable (sphenopalatine ganglion blocks), and the most beneficial to patients with refractory headache (botulinum toxin). They are relatively simple, easy to learn, and provide a great deal of patient satisfaction.

An additional benefit to using injection procedures for acute or rescue management of headaches is to stem the use of narcotics. A recent study surveyed Canadian emergency department acute headache treatments and reported that over half of patients had their first exposure to narcotics in the emergency department as a rescue therapy. There has been a growing consensus among physicians treating headaches that narcotics should be used, if at all, only as a last resort. This is because of their almost universal tendency to sensitize the central nervous system and ultimately make the headaches refractory to treatment.

A history and physical examination are essential before initiating treatment to rule out any "red flags" for secondary headaches that are caused by treatable conditions. Usually the history will reveal a primary headache disorder that allows for a satisfactory treatment plan. But it is also important to discover potential contraindications to these procedures, such as prior cranial surgery. The physical primarily identifies secondary causes of headaches. In primary headache disorders such as migraine or tension-type headache, the physical examination is usually unrevealing (Table 234-1).

Most patients have sought help only after they have failed their usual prophylaxis and available acute treatments. Although pharmacologic interventions are still an option, procedural treatments for the most part are simple and safe, and they can be a beneficial asset for the treatment and prevention of many headache disorders. In this chapter, we discuss lower cervical intramuscular blocks, occipital nerve blocks, sphenopalatine ganglion blocks, and botulinum toxin injections.

Also, see Chapter 8, Peripheral Nerve Blocks and Field Blocks, Chapter 9, Oral and Facial Anesthesia, and Chapter 56, Botulinum Toxin.

LOWER CERVICAL INTRAMUSCULAR INJECTIONS

In 2006, Mellick and colleagues reported a 1-year retrospective review of lower cervical intramuscular injections in over 400 emergency department patients treated for headaches. The results were impressive: 65.1% had resolution within 15 minutes and an additional 20.4% had partial relief within 20 minutes. When patients who were not pain free 20 minutes after treatment were reinjected, additional improvement was seen in 59.5% of the patients. The study did not attempt to differentiate between headache subtypes, so the procedure can be tried with most headaches.

Anatomy

Landmarks to identify include the spinous processes of T1, C6, and C7. The injections are placed 2 to 3 cm lateral to the midline either at the level of C6 or C7, so there is some latitude as to their placement. Although there are no major arteries in the area it is always a good practice to aspirate before injections.

Indications

Although indications have not been well established, generally this procedure is beneficial for *migraine, tension-type, post-traumatic, and cervicogenic headaches.*

Relative and Absolute Contraindications

Secondary headache disorders are a relative contraindication (see Table 234-1).Treatment of the headache should not interfere with treatment of the underlying condition. Allergy to the local anesthetics is also a contraindication.

TABLE 234-1 Red Flags for Acute Secondary Headache Disorders

Red Flag	Differential Diagnosis	Possible Work-up
Headache beginning after 50 years of age	Temporal arteritis, mass lesion	Erythrocyte sedimentation rate, neuroimaging
Sudden onset of headache	Subarachnoid hemorrhage, pituitary apoplexy, hemorrhage into a mass lesion or vascular malformation, mass lesion (especially posterior mass)	Neuroimaging; lumbar puncture if neuroimaging is negative*
Headaches increasing in frequency and severity	Mass lesion, subdural hematoma, medication overuse	Neuroimaging, drug screen
New-onset headache in a patient with risk factors for human immunodeficiency virus infection or cancer	Meningitis (chronic or carcinomatous), brain abscess (including toxoplasmosis), metastasis	Neuroimaging; lumbar puncture if neuroimaging is negative*
Headache with signs of systemic illness (fever, stiff neck, rash)	Meningitis, encephalitis, Lyme disease, systemic infection, collagen vascular disease	Neuroimaging, lumbar puncture,† serology
Focal neurologic signs or symptoms of disease (other than typical aura)	Mass lesion, vascular malformation, stroke, collagen vascular disease	Neuroimaging, collagen vascular disease evaluation (including anti-phospholipid antibodies)
Papilledema	Mass lesion, pseudotumor cerebri, meningitis	Neuroimaging, lumbar puncture†
Headache subsequent to head trauma	Intracranial hemorrhage, subdural hematoma, epidural hematoma, post-traumatic headache	Neuroimaging of brain, skull, and, possibly, cervical spine

*Lumbar puncture may follow a negative neuroimaging procedure if suspicion of hemorrhage, infection, or malignancy remains high.
†Suspicion of specific central nervous system infections (e.g., Lyme disease, syphilis) or intracranial hypertension (pseudotumor cerebri) warrants lumbar puncture with cerebrospinal fluid analysis and pressure measurement.
From Newman LC, Lipton RB: Emergency department evaluation of headache. Neurol Clin 16:285–303, 1998.

Equipment and Supplies

- Bupivacaine 0.5% 3 mL (1.5 mL injected bilaterally)
- Syringe with 25-gauge, 1½-inch needle
- Gebauer's ethyl chloride (optional vapocoolant spray to minimize injection discomfort)

Precautions

As with all injections, sterile technique is essential. Inject slowly to minimize risk of a vasovagal reaction.

Technique

See Figure 234-1.

1. Have the patient seated with the neck flexed, chin toward chest. The forehead can rest on crossed forearms.
2. Identify the T1 spinous process by finding the superiormost rib. Walk your fingertips medially to the spinous process and move up one or two levels to the C6 or C7 level. Identify the areas for injection bilaterally, 2 to 3 cm lateral to the selected spinous process (two fingerbreadths approximates 3 cm for many people).
3. Insert the needle to the hub perpendicular to the cervical spine, toward the anterior neck.
4. Once fully inserted to the needle's hub, aspirate, and if there is no return, inject all of the bupivacaine slowly in one spot. After all of the bupivacaine is injected, withdraw the needle and apply an adhesive strip (Band-Aid) at the site of the injection.
5. Repeat the injection on other side.
6. The injection may be repeated once in 20 to 30 minutes if the headache has not resolved.

It is not known whether relief is a function of resolution of muscle tension, reflex arc to the spinal trigeminal nucleus, a combination of the two, or some other mechanism of action.

Common Errors

The procedure itself is very simple and does not lend itself to many errors.

Complications

Adverse events are uncommon and limited, but have been reported as muscle soreness at injection sites, transient weakness of posterior neck muscles, and vasovagal reactions.

Postprocedure Management

Typically, placement of a bandage is all that is required after an injection; however, if any complications develop they should be managed before patient discharge.

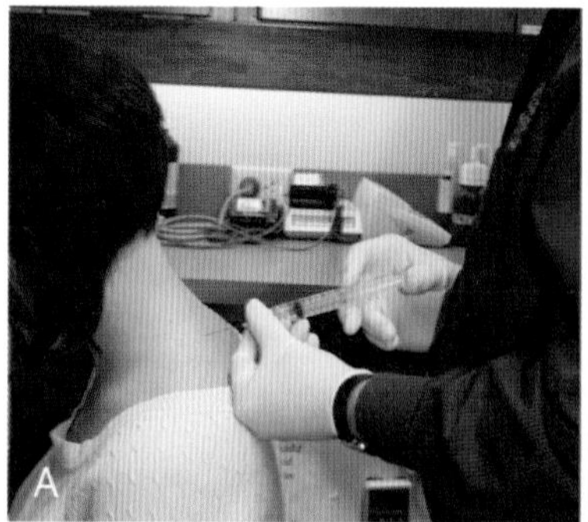

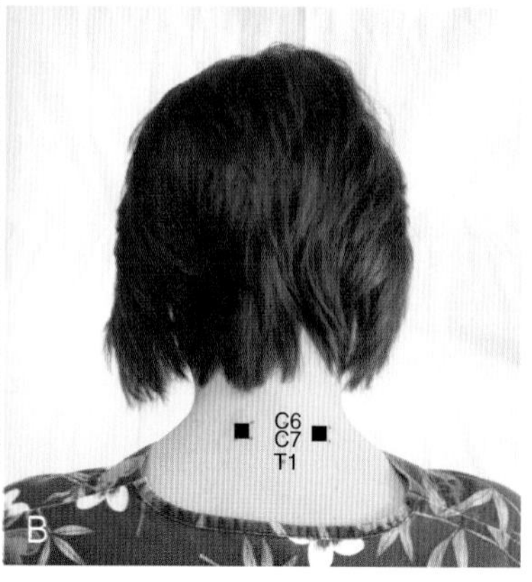

Figure 234-1 Lower cervical intramuscular injection. **A,** A 25-gauge, 1½-inch needle attached to a 10-mL syringe filled with 3 mL of 0.5% bupivacaine is inserted up to the hub into the paraspinous muscles, 2 to 3 cm lateral to the midline at a level between the C6 and C7 spinous processes and at an angle perpendicular to the cervical spine. The bupivacaine is injected slowly to minimize patient discomfort. After 1.5 mL of the bupivacaine has been injected, the needle is withdrawn, the injection site is bandaged, and the procedure is repeated on the other side. **B,** Lower cervical intermuscular injection. The injections are placed perpendicular to the cervical spine, 2 to 3 cm lateral to the area between the C6 and C7 spinous processes.

CPT/Billing Code

20552 Injection(s); single or multiple trigger point(s), one or two muscles

This is a common code for cervicalgia, which is frequently associated with headaches.

Greater and Lesser Occipital Nerve Blocks

The greater and lesser occipital nerve blocks are additional beneficial procedures that are well established and relatively simple to learn. In a study by Ashkenazi and Young (2005), 89.5% of patients with episodic or transformed migraines responded to greater occipital nerve blocks (GONB). The GONB has been used as an acute and a preventative treatment for *migraine, cluster, and tension-type headaches*. This block is a popular treatment for individuals who need quick relief without sedation, although it is slightly more uncomfortable than the lower cervical intramuscular injection. Patients who describe their headaches as "exploding" typically find the greatest relief. The recent discovery of transcranial sensory nerves connecting the scalp and the dura offers an interesting possibility for a mechanism of action, although the exact mechanism has yet to be defined.

Anatomy

The greater occipital nerve (GON) rises out of the dorsal primary rami of cervical spinal nerves 2 and 3. It provides cutaneous sensation to the medial posterior portion of the scalp. The lesser occipital nerve (LON) represents the ventral branches of C2 and C3. These origins suggest a possible mechanism of action: a reflex signal transmitted to the spinal trigeminal nucleus through the C2 nerve.

The GON and LON emerge from underneath the muscles at the level of the nuchal ridge. The GON lies about 2 to 3 cm lateral to the greater occipital protuberance and adjacent to the greater occipital artery. Attempt to palpate the greater occipital artery to approximate the GON. The GON is frequently tender to palpation during acute headaches.

Indications

The GONB is indicated for prevention and treatment of *primary headache conditions and other cephalgias in the back of the neck*. In earlier clinical trials steroids have not been shown to significantly enhance the effectiveness of an ONB, with the noted exception of cluster headaches. When corticosteroids are used, their frequency should be moderated to typically no greater than one every 3 months, with a continuing assessment of individual risks and benefits. If no steroids are used, the risks and benefits of repeated injections of local anesthetic should guide decisions about frequency.

Relative and Absolute Contraindications

Occipital nerve block is relatively contraindicated in the presence of a bony defect. Patients with a prior occipital or mastoid craniotomy should be injected only by a skilled clinician familiar with the patient to avoid any risk of spinal anesthesia. Caution should also be used in patients with impaired glucose tolerance or diabetes because the steroids may worsen hyperglycemia. In these instances the blocks may be performed with local anesthetic alone.

Equipment and Supplies

Amounts listed here are for *unilateral* injections. They will need to be doubled for bilateral injections.

- Steroid: typically no more than 1 mL per side.
  - Intermediate-acting, moderate-potency: triamcinolone acetonide 20 to 40 mg (Kenalog 40 mg/mL).
  - Long-acting, high-potency: dexamethasone 4 mg (Decadron 4 mg/mL)
- Local anesthetic: 0.5% bupivacaine 3 mL.
- Local anesthetic: 1% lidocaine with or without epinephrine (*optional*). If lidocaine is used, the patient may report onset of the anesthetic effects of the block while it is still being administered, thereby making the block more tolerable.
- 10-mL syringe with a 25-gauge needle
- The desired quantity of steroid is drawn up into the syringe using a 20-gauge needle and sterile technique, followed by the desired quantities of the bupivacaine or lidocaine. The total volume should be 3 to 4 mL of solution for a unilateral block and 6 to 8 mL of solution for a bilateral block.

Precautions

Always confirm a patient's allergies to medications before any procedure.

Procedure

Many techniques have been reported in the literature, but this is no comparison study of the merits of one injection technique over another. It appears best to block the GON and LON by inserting the needle between them and advancing it toward the respective nerves (always aspirating before injection), thereby providing a block that is complete over the superior nuchal ridge. Other clinicians have reported success with blocking the GON and LON using two separate injections.

Greater and Lesser Occipital Nerve Block with One Injection Site

See Figure 234-2.

1. Have the patient lean forward with the chin flexed forward toward the chest and the head resting on the forearms.
2. Identify the superior nuchal ridge from the medial greater occipital protuberance to the lateral mastoid process. Attempt to palpate the greater occipital artery.
3. Introduce the needle between the approximated GON and LON and advance to the skull, withdraw the needle slightly, and administer a small bolus of the solution.
4. Advance the needle medially toward the GON (staying above the nuchal line), aspirate, and inject approximately 2 mL of solution.
5. Withdraw the needle and redirect toward the mastoid process, aspirate, and inject the remaining solution.
6. Repeat the procedure on contralateral side if the headache is bilateral.

Greater and Lesser Occipital Nerve Blocks as Individual Injections

In this variation of the GONB, the GON and LON are blocked by two separate injections placed medial and lateral to the anatomic position of the GON and LON.

1. Have the patient lean forward with the chin flexed forward toward the chest and the head resting on the forearms.
2. Identify the greater occipital protuberance at the midline.
3. Inject approximately 2.5 cm lateral to the greater occipital protuberance, just medial to the palpable greater occipital artery. Advance the needle at a slight angle toward the vertex until it strikes the skull. Now withdraw the needle slightly, aspirate, and inject around the target (medially and laterally by approximately 0.5 mm).

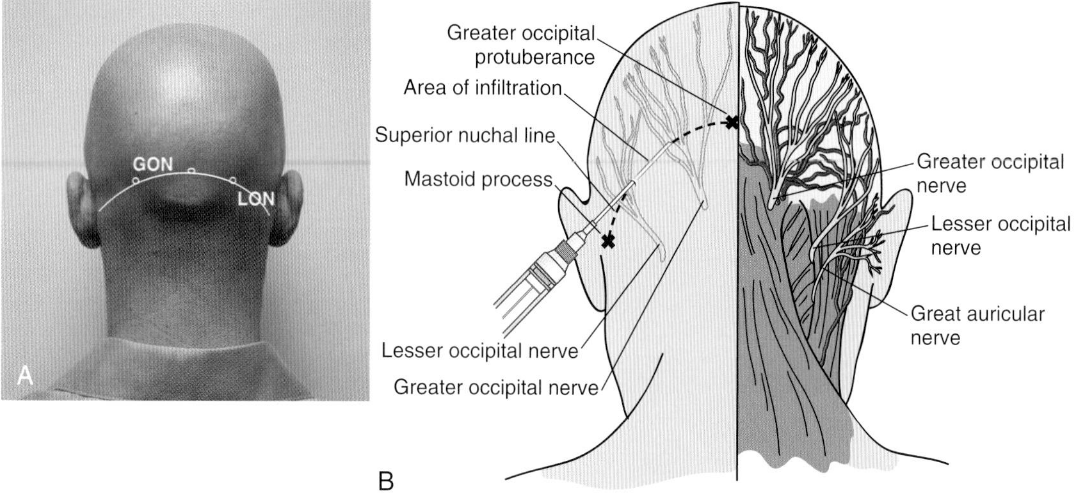

Figure 234-2 **A,** Occipital nerve block. An imaginary curvilinear line is drawn over the superior nuchal line between the greater occipital protuberance and the mastoid process. The line is then divided into thirds. The medial division represents the approximate position of the greater occipital nerve (GON). The lateral division represents the position of the lesser occipital nerve (LON). Injections may be placed over the GON and LON (*circles* [i.e., nerve sites]) or the injection maybe placed between the nerves at the superior nuchal line and directed toward the GON and LON. **B,** Occipital nerve block. An imaginary curvilinear line is drawn over the superior nuchal line between then greater occipital protuberance and the mastoid process. The line is then divided into thirds. The medial division represents the approximate position of the GON. The lateral division represents the position of the LON. Injections may be placed over the GON and LON (their approximate position [i.e., nerve sites] as labeled on the imaginary curvilinear line), or the injections may be placed between the nerves (marked by the Xs) at the superior nuchal line and directed medially toward the GON and then redirected laterally toward the LON. (**B,** From Cousins MJ, Carr DB, Horlocker TT, Bridenbough P [eds]: Cousins and Bridenbough's Neural Blockade in Clinical Anesthesia and Pain, 4th ed. Philadelphia, Lippincott Williams & Wilkins, 2008, p 421.)

4. Place the second injection an additional 2.5 cm lateral to the previous site, approximately two thirds of the distance along a line drawn from the greater occipital protuberance to the mastoid process. As before, the needle is directed in a slight angle toward the vertex, advanced until contact is made with the skull, and withdrawn slightly; then aspirate and inject in a trigger-point manner.
5. Repeat on contralateral side if needed.

Common Errors

Intra-arterial injection of local anesthetic can usually be prevented by aspirating before injection.

Complications

In addition to the complications reported for lower cervical intramuscular injections, the following may arise:

- As with any repeated steroid injection, it has been suggested that the patient may develop Cushing's syndrome or *fatty atrophy* at the injection site (see Chapter 192, Joint and Soft Tissue Aspiration and Injection [Arthrocentesis]).
- It has been suggested that a *seizure* may result from intra-arterial injection of the local anesthesia; aspiration before injection will prevent this adverse event.
- *Spinal anesthesia* has been reported with ONB in a patient with a history of prior cranial surgery. In such patients, it would be best not to perform these procedures unless absolutely necessary, and then only with great caution and appropriate resources. If spinal anesthesia does occur, support the patient until the condition resolves (until the local anesthesia has worn off). The patient may need to be transported to an emergency department or hospital until recovery occurs. The reported cases of spinal anesthesia all occurred in individuals who have bony anomalies or prior craniotomies, and all recovered once the effects of the local anesthesia had resolved.

Postprocedure Management

Postprocedure management is primarily limited to observation of the patient to see if the headache has resolved and to offer additional treatment if needed. If the patient had a vasovagal response, a brief period of observation is appropriate.

CPT/Billing Code

64405 Greater occipital nerve blocks

No specific code exists for lesser occipital nerve blocks. Consider using 64450: Injection, anesthetic agent, other peripheral nerve or branch. You can also charge for the steroid using J-Codes (see Chapter 192, Joint and Soft Tissue Aspiration and Injection [Arthrocentesis]).

Some insurance companies may consider ONBs investigational or experimental, so it will be important to document the need for the injection in the patient's chart. These reasons could include failure to respond to more conservative therapies, prior positive response, or the acute need for the procedure. Injections with steroids should be limited to no more than four times a year, typically waiting at least 2 months between injections at the earliest. The Michigan Head Pain and Neurological Institute has reported a patient who was self-administering GONBs about four times a day, so any treatment has the potential for abuse. It is hoped that if any clinician encounters these situations, he or she will consult appropriately.

Sphenopalatine Ganglion Nerve Block

The sphenopalatine ganglion (SPG) block was first described over 100 years ago by Greenfield Sluder as a treatment for a variety of headaches and facial pain syndromes. The block originally used a cocaine solution. As the medical applications of cocaine came under increasing scrutiny, the procedure became more uncommon. Another likely explanation for the SPG block's fall from favor as a preferred treatment for headaches was the development of ergotamine derivatives, which provided an easier treatment. In the early 1980s, interest in the procedure returned as headache specialists started to report success treating difficult and refractory cephalalgias. Because the SPG represents a "crossroad" of neurons involved in pain processing, clinicians using SPG blocks have reported its effectiveness in a variety of central pain syndromes, from complex regional pain syndrome to fibromyalgia. A common thread through many of the modern articles about SPG blocks is the question, why is this procedure underused? There are also multiple reports of patients being successfully taught this procedure for self-administration. Although this is a realistic option for some patients, they should be selected carefully on a case-by-case basis.

Anatomy

The SPG (also known as the pterygopalatine or Meckel's ganglion) is the largest collection of neuronal cell bodies outside the central nervous system. It is located in the pterygopalatine fossa behind the mid-nasal fossa and in front of the pterygoid canal. Physiologically, there are three major roots: motor, sensory, and sympathetic. It connects the trigeminal and facial nerves and communicates directly with the cervical sympathetic ganglia by the deep petrosal nerve. An SPG block potentially blocks three types of nerve fibers: sensory, sympathetic, and parasympathetic. The zygomatic arch can be an important external landmark because it corresponds to the level of the medial turbinate in the nasopharynx (see also Chapter 9, Oral and Facial Anesthesia).

Indications

The SPG block is indicated for *acute migraine, cluster headaches, and facial neuralgias*. It may be useful for *status migrainosus and chronic cluster headaches*. There are reports of varying response to the SPG block for a variety of central pain processes, and given its simplicity and lack of significant adverse events, it is not unreasonable to offer it as a treatment. For central pain conditions (e.g., fibromyalgia, complex regional pain syndrome), it is common to perform several blocks over the space of 1 to 2 weeks.

Relative and Absolute Contraindications

Contraindications are as described for the previously discussed blocks. In addition, a history of nasopharyngeal neoplasms might allow the local anesthetic to cross to the dura and produce spinal anesthesia. History of epistaxis should signal the examiner to proceed with caution; however, this risk is minimized with the use of topical nasal decongestants. Anatomic anomalies in the nasopharynx (e.g., deviated septum, nasal polyps) may also complicate the procedure.

Equipment and Supplies

- Topical, over-the-counter nasal decongestant spray (e.g., Afrin, Neo-Synephrine)
- Sterile cotton swabs (solid wood or hollow plastic)
- 2-inch intravenous catheter (if using the intravenous [IV] catheter technique)
- Local anesthetic: viscous lidocaine 2%, or lidocaine 4% compounded with 1% phenylephrine

Precautions

Nasopharyngeal cancers that communicate with the dura might lead to a spinal block. There has been a single reported case of respiratory arrest due to spinal anesthesia. The patient had a complete recovery after the local anesthesia had worn off.

Procedure

The goal is to apply topical anesthesia to the inferior branch of the SPG unilaterally, or bilaterally if needed. Two techniques are commonly described. The traditional technique involves sterile cotton swabs (either wood or hollow plastic—both have advantages that will be discussed). The more recent involves a flexible 1- to 2-inch IV catheter attached to a syringe. A positive response typically occurs in 5 to 10 minutes, although most clinicians keep the applicators in place for 20 to 30 minutes and repeat when necessary.

Sphenopalatine Ganglion Block with Cotton-Tipped Applicators

See Figure 234-3A and B.

1. With the patient sitting, spray nasal decongestant bilaterally.
2. Apply local anesthetic (viscous lidocaine or lidocaine with phenylephrine) topically to the mucosa of the nasal vestibule and antrum to minimize patient discomfort.
3. Have the patient lie down with a pillow or a towel roll under the shoulders to extend the neck and point the nose toward the ceiling. Allow several minutes for the nasal decongestant and local anesthesia to take effect.
4. Identify the zygomatic arch and use it as a landmark for the middle turbinate.
5. Pass a lidocaine-saturated cotton-tipped applicator into the nasal antrum. Do not force the swab. If you encounter resistance, wait a moment to allow for greater topical anesthesia to occur and then continue advancing the swab gently. Slowly twisting the swab between your fingers as you progress will also ease passage. Continue advancing the swab posteriorly until contact is made with the posterior pharyngeal wall, and then withdraw slightly. At this point, the swab has been inserted to a depth of about 4 inches (10 cm).
6. You may place a second swab unilaterally, posteriorly and superiorly.
7. Repeat insertion if needed on the contralateral side.
8. Leave the swabs in place for 20 to 30 minutes and then withdraw them slowly while rotating them to increase exposure of the ganglion to the topical anesthetic.

PEARLS: Greater exposure to the nasal antrum can be achieved by elevating the nasal apex, thereby opening the nares. Some clinicians have reported additional benefits to rotating the swabs once they are in place, thereby exposing additional anesthetic to the SPG. Some patients are more comfortable having the applicators placed while sitting instead of lying down. One advantage that the hollow plastic swab may have is that once it is in place, small amounts of local anesthesia can be reinstilled through the swab. However, much the same can be accomplished with the wooden swabs by slowly dripping the local anesthetic down the side of the swab. When introducing the additional anesthetic, proceed slowly, using only small amounts to minimize the chance of the patient swallowing the medication. Continued anesthesia can also be accomplished by withdrawing the swabs and replacing them with new ones. Any patient discomfort during the second insertion is greatly diminished because of the preceding anesthesia.

Sphenopalatine Ganglion Block with Flexible Intravenous Catheter

This technique is primarily for unilateral headaches, so treat the affected side (Fig. 234-3C and D).

1. Instill 4 mL of 2% viscous lidocaine in a 10-mL syringe, then attach a 2-inch flexible IV catheter from which the needle has been removed.
2. Insert the catheter through the nares toward the posterior nasopharynx, through the middle turbinate.
3. Have the patient turn the head to the side of his or her pain.

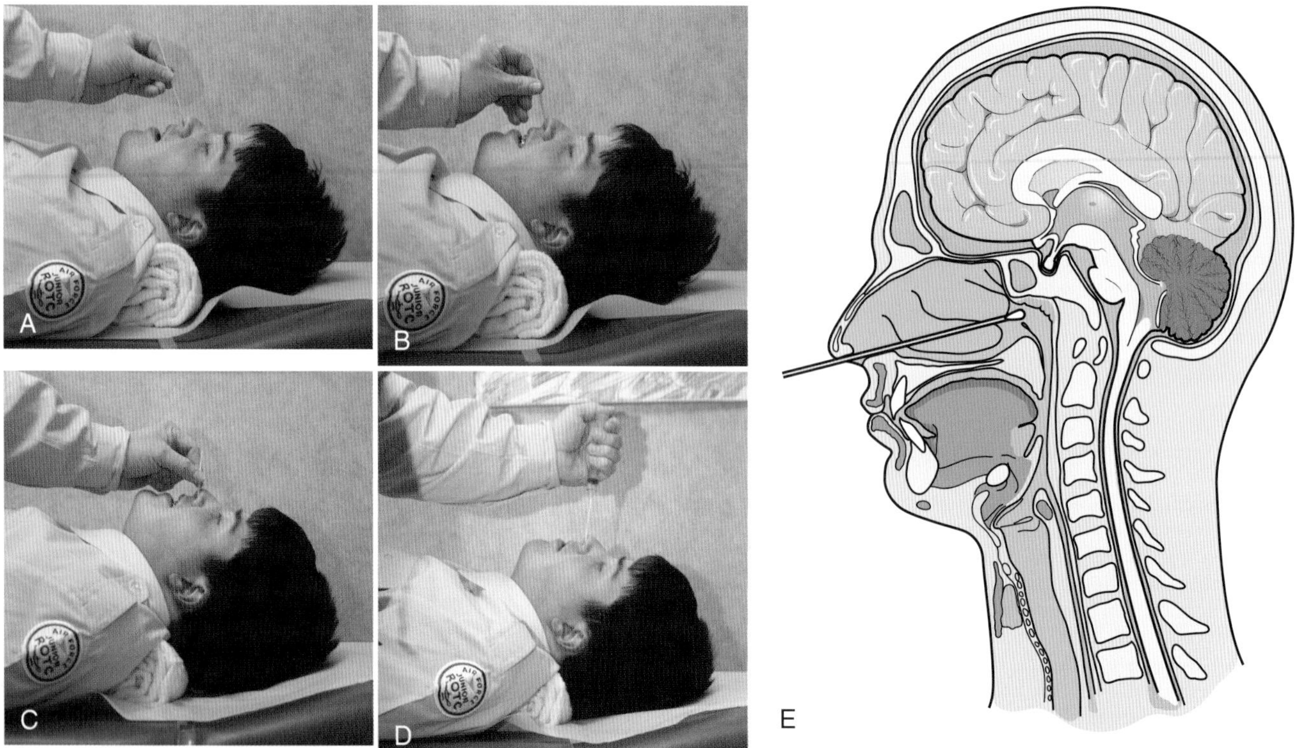

Figure 234-3 Sphenopalatine ganglion (SPG) block. **A,** Step 1: The patient is placed face up with a towel roll under the neck to extend the neck. After applying topical anesthetic to the nasal antrum, the cotton-tipped applicator is introduced into the nostril (targeting the level of the zygomatic arch—the level of the SPG between the first and second turbinates). **B,** Step 2: The cotton-tipped applicator is gently advanced, never forced. A twisting motion of the swab between the fingers may ease passage. **C,** Step 3: The cotton-tipped applicator is advanced until it touches the posterior pharyngeal wall. It is then withdrawn about 1 cm. It is left in place 15 to 20 minutes and replaced if needed. **D,** Step 4: After placement of the applicator, the process may be repeated or additional anesthetic may be applied slowly down the shaft. It will drain down to the cotton tip and replenish the absorbed anesthetic. If a plastic applicator is used, the local anesthetic may be placed inside the hollow shaft. **E,** Diagram demonstrating placement of cotton-tipped applicator in the nasopharynx.

4. Slowly administer 2 mL of the viscous lidocaine while having the patient refrain from swallowing or moving the head. Instill the remaining 2 mL after 10 minutes. If the patient is unable to refrain from swallowing, use the cotton swab applicators.

Common Errors

- Incorrect placement of the swab not producing adequate blockade; withdraw and replace the swab or try the IV catheter technique

Complications

- Epistaxis can occur. It is managed in the usual manner.
- Rarely, toxic effects of the local anesthetic might occur as a result of resorption into a very well-vascularized tumor.
- It has also been suggested that in patients who self-administer the SPG block, mucosal erosions might develop, and that this might lead to some spinal resorption of the local anesthetic. This can be prevented by using a nasal rinse such as the Sinus Rinse (NeilMed Pharmaceuticals, Inc., Santa Rosa, Calif) after removal of the cotton-tipped applicator.

Postprocedure Patient Education

- If posterior pharyngeal numbness develops, the patient should not eat or drink until it resolves, typically within 1 hour.

CPT/Billing Code

64505 Injection, anesthetic agent; sphenopalatine ganglion

Botulinum Toxin Type A

EDITOR'S NOTE: The reader should become totally familiar with the information included in Chapter 56, Botulinum Toxin, as well as the information in this chapter before injecting Botox for the treatment of headaches.

In the early 1980s, Alan Scott was the first physician to use onabotulinumtoxinA (also known as botulinum toxin type A [BTX-A] or Botox) to treat strabismus in humans. To date, BTX-A is the most widely used and studied form of botulinum toxin. It was during clinical trials using BTX-A for treating brow lines that William Binder, an otolaryngologist, discovered that migraineurs receiving Botox injections for wrinkles experienced fewer headaches. Many of these patients reported fewer migraines or total elimination of migraine pain.

When injected locally, BTX-A binds to acceptor sites on motor or sympathetic nerve terminals and inhibits acetylcholine release by cleaving the SNAP-25 component of the SNARE complex responsible for docking and fusion of the acetylcholine vesicles. BTX-A has also been shown to inhibit release of glutamate, substance P, and calcitonin gene–related peptide from nociceptive neurons, thereby providing a secondary mechanism of action different from neuromuscular junction blockade. The effect is temporary (although it should last several months) and is overcome by regeneration of proximal axons and neuromuscular junctions.

At the International Headache Congress at Philadelphia in 2009, David Doddick from the Mayo Clinic reported that the "pooled analyses from the PREEMPT 1 and 2 trials demonstrate that treatment with onabotulinumtoxin A resulted in a highly significant improvements in onabotulinumtoxin A treated patients versus placebo-treated patients in frequency of headache days in patients suffering from chronic migraine" (www.neurologyreviews.com/09oct/c1botox.html).

Although the PREEMPT 1 and 2 trials have shown promising results for certain refractory headache populations, the use of BTX-A for treatment of headaches remains an off-label use, so there are no standardized protocols for the injection of BTX-A for headaches. Consequently, several different methodologies have been developed.

BTX-A can be used as a treatment for patients with *recurrent headache, primarily migraines*. Because the goal of headache treatment is to reduce their frequency, severity, and associated disability, and improve the patient's quality of life by reducing headache-related distress and symptoms, it is essential to start with an accurate history and diagnosis. As with the previously discussed treatments, it is mandatory to rule out secondary headache disorders.

More importantly than for any of the other headache procedures, informed consent with a discussion of costs and expectations must be obtained. Because the level of coverage can vary significantly from one insurance carrier to another, it is essential to determine if the patient can afford the treatment course before starting. BTX-A is very expensive and a treatment can average around $500 or more. Documenting prior treatment failure or adverse events to prior therapies can increase the chance of insurance coverage. Improvement may not be noticed for 1 to 2 weeks after injections; in general, improvements are typically seen in 80% of patients.

BTX-A (Botox), manufactured by Allergan, Inc. (Irvine, Calif), is supplied in single-use vials containing 100 or 200 U of vacuum-dried *Clostridium botulinum* type A neurotoxin complex, 0.5 mg of human albumin, and 0.9 mg of sodium chloride in a sterile, vacuum-dried, preservative-free form. See Chapter 56, Botulinum Toxin, for a description of its use and injection techniques.

Indications

Ninan Mathew, Director of the Houston Headache Clinic, has suggested that the indications for BTX-A include a *lack of improvement with preventive pharmacotherapy; severe and intolerable adverse events from preventive therapy; and patient refusal or inability to use daily medications*. Contraindications include *acute migraine therapy or an elderly patient with chronic migraine*. In 2007, Roger Cady and Curtis Schreiber of the Headache Care Center in Springfield, Missouri, suggested BTX-A as an ideal prophylactic agent for patients with frequent disabling headache who have been poorly controlled with previous preventatives secondary to compliance, adherence, or inability to use conventional preventive therapies as a result of adverse events. In a small study of 63 migraineurs, Jakubowski and colleagues (2006) found that 74% of BTX-A responders described their headaches as a pressure from the outside, imploding, or as an "eye-popping" sensation. Conversely, 92% of the nonresponders described their headaches as "exploding," with pressure building up from the inside.

Relative and Absolute Contraindications

- Infection at the injection site.
- Known hypersensitivity to any ingredient in the formulation.
- Presence of a neuromuscular disorder (e.g., myasthenia gravis, Eaton-Lambert syndrome).
- BTX-A is labeled category C in pregnancy, and its safety in nursing mothers is unknown.

Equipment and Supplies

- Botulinum toxin type A
- 1-mL tuberculin syringe

Other gauge needles can be used, but it is generally believed that smaller-gauge needles are less painful.

Precautions

Because the U.S. Food and Drug Administration has not approved BTX-A for the treatment any headache disorder, it may be prudent to limit the amount of BTX-A to 60 U per session until the patient's response to therapy is known.

Preprocedure Patient Education and Forms

- Insurance preauthorization forms. Allergan offers physician and patient assistance through their Botox Reimbursement Solutions website (www.botoxreimbursement.us/Home.apx).
- Checklist visit/encounter form (go to www.expertconsult.com).
- Consent forms.

Botulinum Toxin for Headache Prevention

Three injection paradigms have been used in clinical trials for patients with chronic daily headache and chronic migraine: *fixed-site, fixed-dose; follow the pain; or a combination of the two*. A study published in *Headache* demonstrated a positive response with single bilateral injections of 25 U of BTX-A (Behmand and colleagues, 2003).

Basic Tenets

1. Preplan the injections using an anatomic drawing for injection sites and units used (see Chapter 56, Botulinum Toxin, for areas of caution).
2. Use a 25-, 27-, 30-, or 31-gauge needle affixed to a tuberculin syringe. Some research has suggested that using a smaller-gauge and slightly longer needle, such as the 31-gauge, 13-mm SteriJect needle, minimizes discomfort and allows for injection of the deeper muscles of the head and neck.
3. Inject intramuscularly in a manner that will allow for greater infiltration, avoiding intradermal or periosteal injections.
4. In cosmetically sensitive areas, inject in a symmetric fashion.
5. Injecting at multiple sites in the targeted muscle group allows for a more even dispersal of toxin through the target region.
6. Visualization and avoidance of facial vessels minimizes any subsequent bruising.

Preparation

See Chapter 56, Botulinum Toxin.

1. Reconstitute the BTX-A and draw up into two syringes (one syringe for each side). Dilution with 2 mL of preservative-free normal saline will yield 50 U/syringe, or 5 U/0.01 mL.
2. Return any unused BTX-A to the refrigerator for storage.
3. BTX-A must be used within 24 hours of being reconstituted.

Fixed-Site Protocol

See Figure 234-4.

- *Glabellar region* (the area around the smooth prominence between the eyebrows).
  - Smaller fluid volumes minimize spread to adjacent muscles.
  - Inject *procerus* (small muscle that originates at the nasal bone and inserts upward between the eyebrows): Treat as one region, injecting with 2.5 to 4 U.
  - Inject *corrugators*: Inject two sites bilaterally, totaling four sites, 1.5 to 3 cm apart. The corrugators are identified by having the patient frown. Apply pressure at the supraorbital ridge to reduce the potential for inferior extravasation. Grasping the mid-lateral portion of the corrugators between two fingers while injecting the toxin diminishes risk of eyelid ptosis. See the Precautions section in Chapter 56, Botulinum Toxin.
- *Forehead*.
  - Inject the *frontalis* (forehead muscle, anterior aspect of the occipitofrontalis) with a larger volume (20 to 30 U) over a

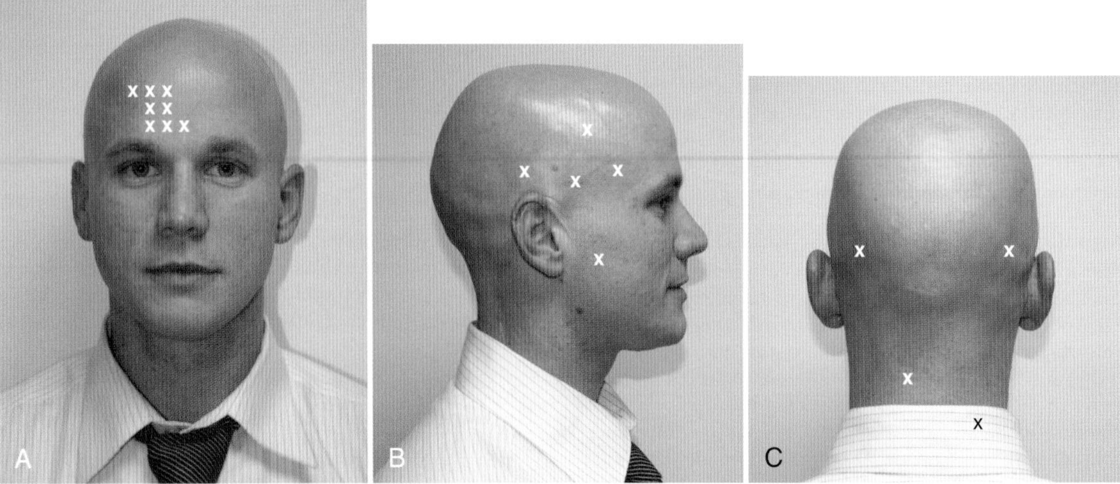

Figure 234-4 Approximate site of botulinum toxin injections over the face (**A**), temple and jaw (**B**), and occiput and neck (**C**).

greater area, typically 8 to 12 sites. Have the patient elevate the eyebrows before injection. Remember to inject symmetrically.
  - If the inferolateral frontalis is not painful, do not inject over the lateral third; this will decrease the risk of brow ptosis.
- *Lateral injections*.
  - If painful, inject the temporalis (large muscle over the temporal fossa). The temporalis is identified by having the patient clench his or her teeth. Injections are given bilaterally, posterior, superior, and inferior, using 0.2 mL per site in four sites, for a total of 20 U.
  - If there is a history of temporomandibular joint syndrome, inject the masseters (large muscle originating from the zygomatic arch and process and inserting into the mandibular ramus and gonial angle) with 5 to 15 U per side.
- *Posterior neck muscles*.
  - Inject the *trapezius* (bilateral large triangular muscle of the upper back that originates at the occipital bone, ligamentum nuchae, and the spinous processes of C7–T12 and inserts into the distal clavicle, acromion, and scapular spine).
  - If the trapezius is involved or suspected as a pain generator, inject bilaterally at one to three sites with 5 to 15 U total.
  - If posterior neck pain is present, evaluate occipital/cervical paraspinal muscles. Inject one or two sites on each side. The doses varies from 5 to 15 U per side.

"Follow the Pain" Protocol (Most Commonly Treats Tension-Type Headaches)

1. Have the patient identify the areas of origination and radiation of the pain.
2. Inject areas associated with pain and tenderness on palpation.
3. Inject the identified areas with 4 to 12 U, 1.5 to 3 cm apart.

Common sites of injection include glabellar and frontal regions, temporalis muscle, occipitalis muscle, and cervical paraspinal region. Inject in similar fashion to the fixed-site injections.

Bilateral Single-Site Protocol

See Figure 234-5. Significant improvement has been reported with single bilateral injections into the corrugator supercilii muscles with 25 U of BTX-A using a 1-inch, 30-gauge needle. Patients were asked to frown to identify the most lateral attachment of the corrugator supercilii muscle. The needle was then inserted at this most lateral attachment and advanced medially toward the root of the nose. BTX-A was then infiltrated evenly across this path as the needle was withdrawn. Be sure to avoid areas where major nerve branches are present, such as the supraorbital nerve; if injected, significant paralysis may result (see Chapter 56, Botulinum Toxin).

Common Errors

To avoid a ptosis, avoid injecting lateral to the pupil in an area 1 cm superior to the supraorbital rim, out to the lateral eyebrow. Only time will correct this error; typically, ptosis may take upward of 3 months to resolve.

Complications

- Most commonly involve bruising and swelling.
- Some patients develop a transient headache that usually resolves within 24 to 48 hours.
- Occasional flulike symptoms may develop and resolve within a day or two.
- A transient ptosis may develop that will resolve over 3 months. This is best avoided by not injecting over the lateral supraorbital muscles. However, if this is an area of pain, this complication may be unavoidable, but it will be essential to warn the patient that a ptosis may result.
- Muscle paralysis at site of injection may occur (although this is a desired effect for the most part).
- There have been reports of antibody formation in patients treated with BTX-A for cervical dystonia or torticollis. These procedures used an older, "less clean" formulation of BTX-A in much higher doses than those used for treating migraines. To prevent antibody formation, current recommendations are to limit BTX-A administration to a minimum of 3-month intervals between injections, with an annual load of 300 to 600 U/year.

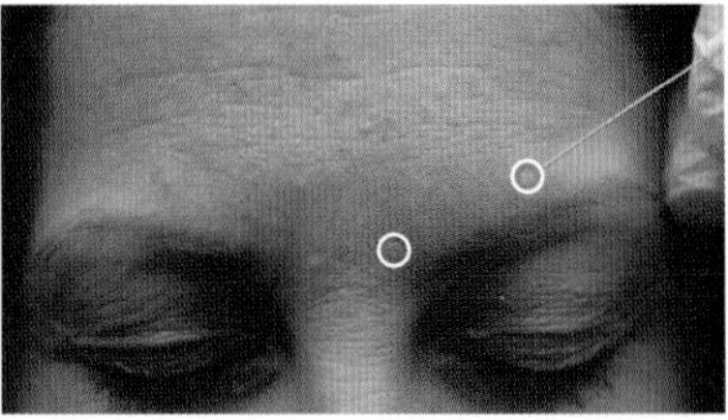

Figure 234-5 Single-site botulinum toxin type A (BTX-A) injection. Insert the needle at the designated site over the medial brow and advance toward the target on the medial aspect of the procerus. Slowly infiltrate the 25 U of BTX-A while withdrawing the needle to evenly dispense the drug.

Postprocedure Management

Remind patients that improvement is gradual and mostly cumulative over several sessions.

Suppliers

See contact information online at www.expertconsult.com.

Botulinum toxin type A
Allergan, Inc.
Tuberculin syringe 1 mL
Air-Tite Products Company

POSTPROCEDURE PATIENT EDUCATION FOR ANY TREATMENT

It will be important to maintain a headache diary to provide objective measures for determining effectiveness of treatment and direction for future treatments. The goal of most preventive treatments for headache is a 50% reduction in the frequency and severity of the headaches. In the absence of headache diaries, this is very difficult to quantify. If any postinjection wheals or blebs develop, inform the patient that they usually resolve within 2 hours. There may be a reduction in hyperfunctional lines of the face. This should be expected and is not considered an adverse event. It may take several weeks for headache relief, and the greatest benefit is seen with repeated treatments.

ONLINE RESOURCES

Allergan: Allergan's Botox Reimbursement Solutions website. Allergan will help your office preauthorize patients and this is their portal to offer assistance for those patients without insurance who are in need. Available at www.botoxreimbursement.us/.
American Headache Society: Professional Resources: Headache Journal toolbox. Available at www.americanheadachesociety.org/professionalresources/headacheresources/Toolbox.asp.
Binder WJ: Beverly Hills Botox treatment. Available at www.doctorbinder.com/proc_botoxmigraines.asp.
Edderai JJ: Sphenopalatine ganglion block. Available at www.drjjedderai.com/headaches.php.
http://drmiltonreder.com.
The Johns Hopkins Headache Center: Available at www.hopkinsneuro.org/headache/procedure_nerveblock.cfm.
www.centenoschulz.com/uploads/Ocipital_Nerve_Block.pdf.

BIBLIOGRAPHY

Ashkenazi A, Young WB: The effects of greater occipital nerve block and trigger point injection on brush allodynia and pain in migraine. Headache 45:350–354, 2005.
Behmand RA, Tucker T, Guyron B: Single-site botulinum toxin type A injection for elimination of migraine trigger points. Headache 43: 1085–1089, 2003.
Blumenfeld AM, Binder W, Silberstein S, Blitzer A: Procedures for administering botulinum toxin type A for migraine and tension-type headache. Headache 43:884–891, 2003.
Botox is safe and effective as preventative treatment for chronic migraine. Clinical Trends and Reviews in Neurology 17(10), 2009. Available at http://www.neurologyreviews.com/09oct/c1botox.html.
Cady, R, Schreiber, C: Botulinum toxin type A as migraine preventive treatment in patients previously failing oral prophylactic treatment due to compliance issues. Headache 48:900–913, 2008.
Jakubowski M, McAllister PJ, Bajwa ZH, et al: Exploding vs. imploding headache in migraine prophylaxis with botulinum toxin A. Pain 125: 286–295, 2006.
Jankovic D, Wells C: Nasal block of the pterygopalatine ganglion. In Regional Nerve Blocks: Textbook and Color Atlas, 2nd ed. Berlin, Blackwell, 2001, pp 29–30.
Jankovic D, Wells C: Occipital nerve blocks. In Regional Nerve Blocks: Textbook and Color Atlas, 2nd ed. Berlin, Blackwell, 2001, pp 14–16.
Krusz JC: Aggressive interventional treatment of intractable headaches in the clinic setting. Clin Fam Pract 7:545–565, 2005.
Lavin PJ, Workman R: Cushing syndrome induced by serial occipital nerve blocks containing corticosteroid. Headache 41:902–904, 2001.
Lebovits AH, Lefkowitiz M: Sphenopalatine ganglion block: Clinical use in the pain management clinic. Clin J Pain 6:131–136, 1990.
Mellick LB, McIlrath ST, Mellick GA: Treatment of headaches in the ED with lower cervical intramuscular bupivacaine injections: A 1-year retrospective review of 417 patients. Headache 46:1441–1449, 2006.
Quevedo JP, Purgavie K, Platt H, Strax TE: Complex regional pain syndrome involving the lower extremity: A report of 2 cases of sphenopalatine block as a treatment option. Arch Phys Med Rehabil 86:335–337, 2005.
Racz, GB, Morton AB, Diede JH: Sphenopalatine ganglion block. In Waldman SD, Winnie AP (eds): Interventional Pain Management. Philadelphia, WB Saunders, 1996, pp 223–225.
Smith, KC, Alum P: Botulinum toxin for pain relief and treatment of headache. In Carruthers A, Carruthers J (eds): Procedures in Cosmetic Dermatology Series: Botulinum Toxin, 2nd ed. Oxford, Elsevier, 2007, pp 101–111.
Tobin J, Flitman S: Occipital nerve blocks: When and what to inject? Headache 49:1521–1533, 2009.
Winner P: Botulinum toxins in the treatment of migraine and tension-type headaches. Phys Med Rehabil Clin N Am 14:885–899, 2003.
Yarnitsky D, Goor-Aryeh I, Bajwa ZH, et al: 2003 Wolff Award: Possible parasympathetic contributions to peripheral and central sensitization during migraine. Headache 43:704–714, 2003.

APPENDIX A

Commonly Used Instruments and Equipment*

John L. Pfenninger

Listed here are the most commonly used instruments in a primary care physician's office. This list provides a basic beginning for ordering equipment for the office. A physician can alter the equipment depending on the procedures performed.

Anoscope

- Every primary care office must have an anoscope to evaluate anal complaints. The Ive's slotted anoscope is recommended, although others are acceptable (see Chapter 98, Anoscopy).

Biopsy instruments (skin, cervix, endometrial, colon, breast)

- *Skin*: 2-, 3-, 4-, 5-mm disposable punches are inexpensive and stay sharp. They are preferable to the reusable Keyes punches (noted next). (See Chapter 32, Skin Biopsy.)
- *Skin*: A set of Keyes reusable punches is also an option for doing skin biopsies (Fig. A-1). However, they become dull quickly. Considering the time it takes to sterilize them and the sharpening costs, it may be advisable to consider the disposable punches.
- *Cervical*: Mini-Townsend, Baby Tischler, Kevorkian instruments are preferred (see Chapter 137, Colposcopic Examination, Fig. 137-6).
- *Endometrial*: Reusable Novak and disposable Endocell (Wallach), PipetCuret (Milex), and Pipelle (Unimar, CooperSurgical) instruments are useful (see Chapter 143, Endometrial Biopsy).
- *Colon/rectum*: For flexible sigmoidoscopy, colonoscopy, and esophagogastroduodenoscopy (EGD) procedures, see Chapter 103, Flexible Sigmoidoscopy, Fig. 103-6. The small flexible biopsy forceps used for flexible sigmoidoscopy can be inserted through an anoscope to obtain adequate biopsies without causing excess bleeding. These can also be readily used for the high-resolution anoscopy procedure (see Chapter 99, High-Resolution Anoscopy).
- *Breast*: Milex breast biopsy needle and Comeco syringe are optional (see Figs. 226-1 and 226-3).

Dermal curettes

- Fox type (3-, 4-, 5-, 6-mm reusable; 2-, 3-, 4-, 5-mm disposable) (Fig. A-2): Reusables work well for soft or necrotic tissue such as basal cell carcinomas. However, unless sharpened regularly, they perform poorly for more fibrotic tissue such as with warts. On the other hand, the disposables are so sharp that they readily cut through any tissue so, if used for curetting out a basal cell, they may actually cut into normal tissue. It is advisable, then, to have both types of curettes.

  A disadvantage of using the disposables for larger very fibrotic lesions is that they bend. An excellent addition is the Curetteblade. The curette is disposable so it stays sharp, and it fits on a scalpel handle. It is stronger and does not bend under pressure (see Chapter 32, Skin Biopsy, Fig. 32-2C).

Forceps

- Adson forceps with and without teeth, 4¼ inches (Fig. A-3)
- Splinter (Fig. A-4)
- Allis (Fig. A-5)
- Uterine packing (look like long, large hemostats)
- Ring (sponge)

Ring forceps can grasp tissue or clot during gynecologic procedures, and are useful for holding gauze or cotton to apply solutions (such as antiseptics or acetic acid to the cervix during colposcopy) or to stop bleeding in the vagina or rectum (Fig. A-6).

Hemostats and clamps

- Mosquito: 5-inch straight, 5-inch curved (for fine application) (Fig. A-7)
- Kelly: 5½-inch straight, 5½-inch curved (for larger application) (Fig. A-8)
- Towel clips (Fig. A-9)

Scissors

- Suture removal (Spencer 3½-inch) (Fig. A-10)
- Suture cutting (William 4½-inch) (Fig. A-11)
- Tissue
  - Mayo 6¾-inch (Fig. A-12)
  - Curved Metzenbaum 5-inch, 7-inch (Fig. A-13)
  - Fine tissue (iris) 4⅛-inch (Fig. A-14)
- Bandage 5½-inch (Fig. A-15)

Needle driver 5-inch (9-inch for vaginal/uterine procedures)

- Webster serrated jaws

NOTE: This is not the place to save a few pennies. Buy the best needle holders (Fig. A-16). They are often designated as the ones used for plastic surgery repairs. They are well worth it. Do not become frustrated by using the types provided in the disposable sets.

Minor surgery pack

- Scalpel handle with metric ruler inscribed on it (Fig. A-17)
- Fine hemostats (2), curved and straight
- 5-inch curved Metzenbaum scissors
- Pick-ups with teeth
- Pick-ups without teeth
- Suture scissors
- Stainless steel basin
- 4 × 4 gauze pads (8–10)
- Glass jar for specimen
- Needle driver
- Also have available: sterile fenestrated drapes, appropriate suture, skin marking pens, alcohol wipes, betadine solution, dressings for the wound

*For a full list of supplier information, see Appendix D.

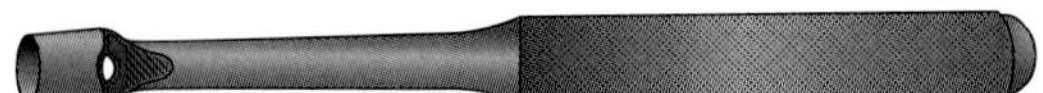

Figure A-1 Keyes cutaneous punch, 4 mm.

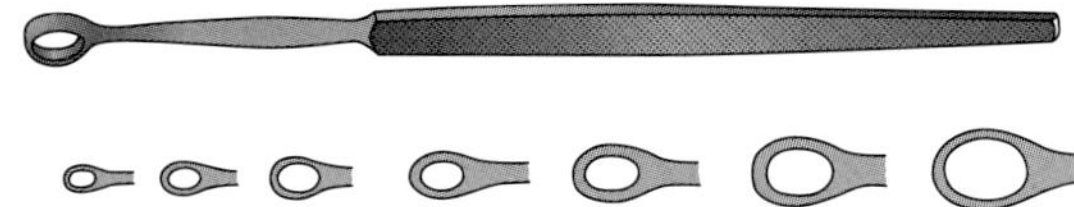

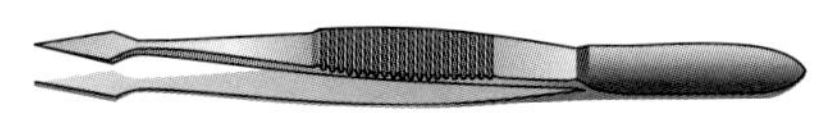

Figure A-2 Fox dermal curette.

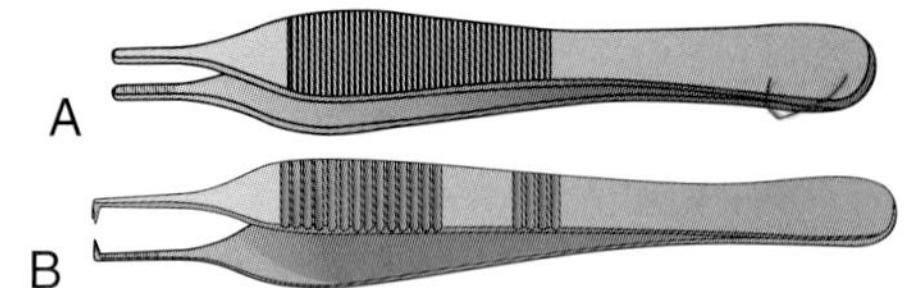

Figure A-3 Adson forceps. **A,** Serrated jaws. **B,** With teeth.

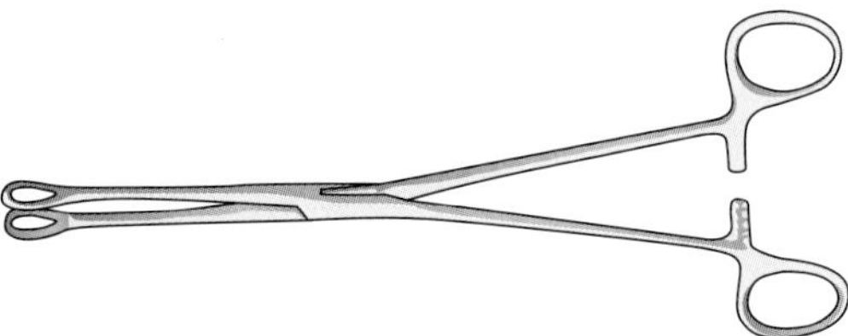

Figure A-4 Carmalt splinter.

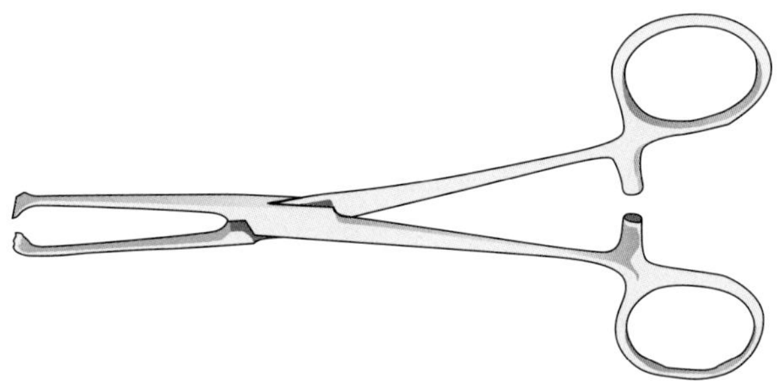

Figure A-5 Allis tissue forceps.

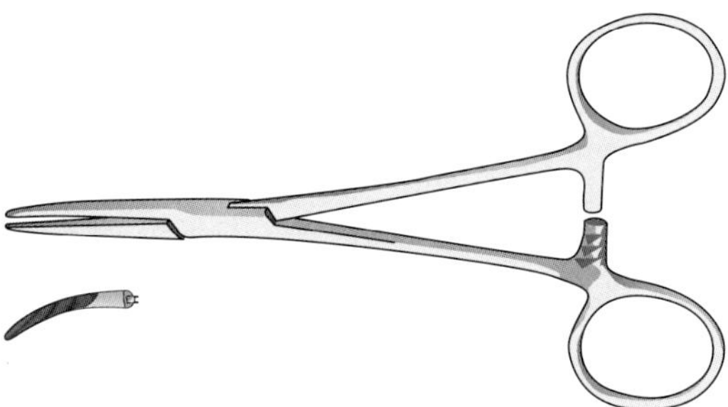

Figure A-6 Foerster sponge/ring forceps.

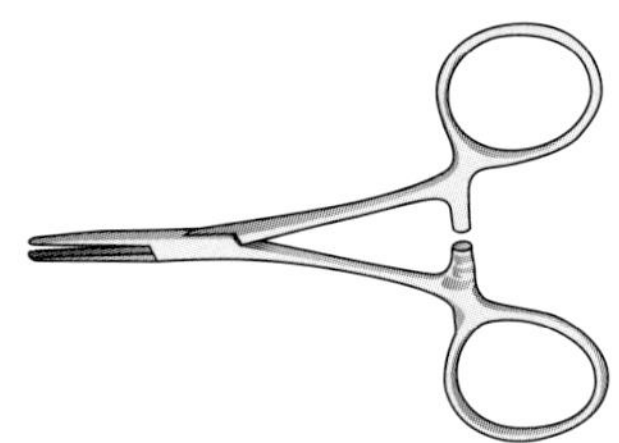

Figure A-7 Pedifine Hartman mosquito hemostats.

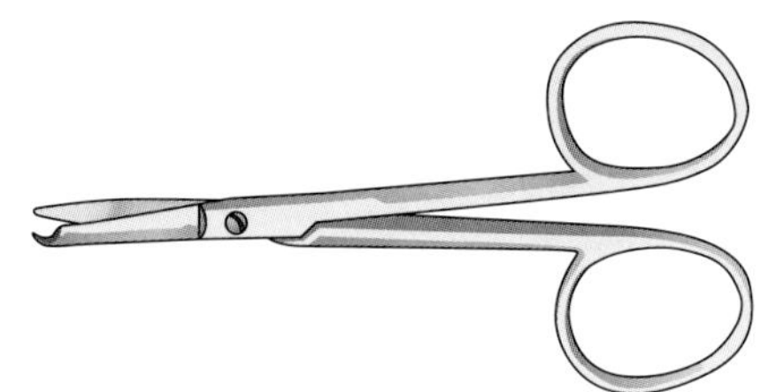

Figure A-8 Kelly straight and curved (*inset*) hemostats.

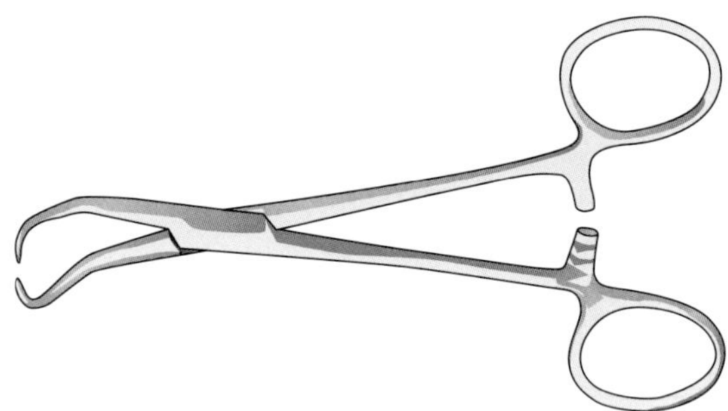

Figure A-9 Backhaus towel clamps.

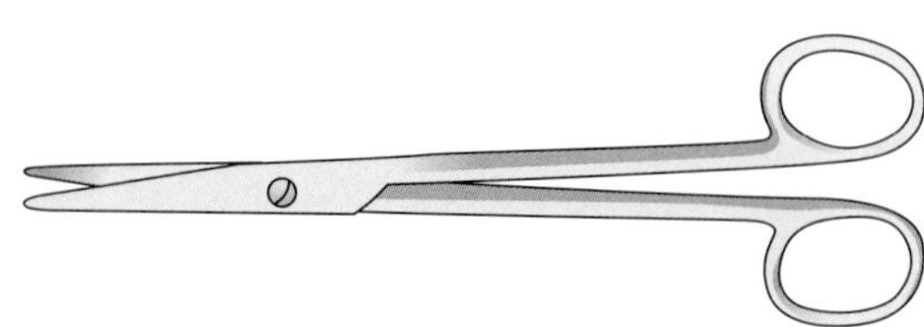

Figure A-10 Spencer 3½-inch suture removal scissors.

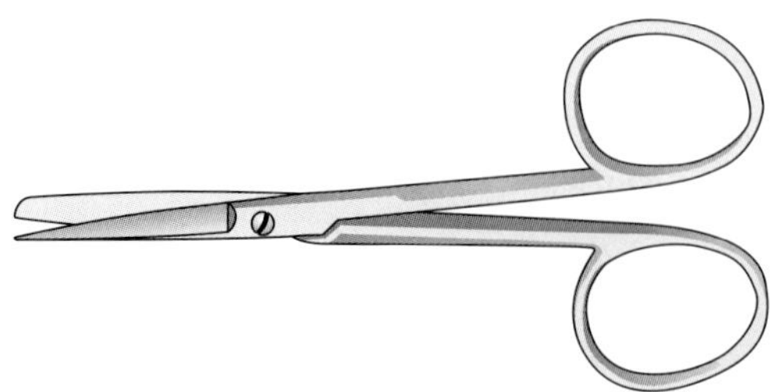

Figure A-11 William 4½-inch suture cutting scissors.

Figure A-12 Mayo 6¾-inch operating scissors.

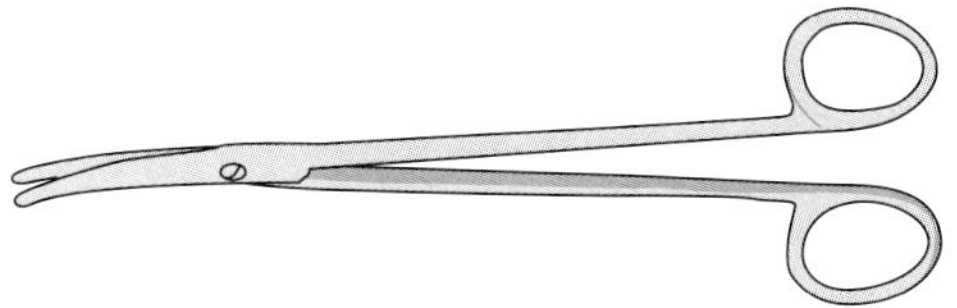

Figure A-13 Curved Metzenbaum 5- and 7-inch operating scissors.

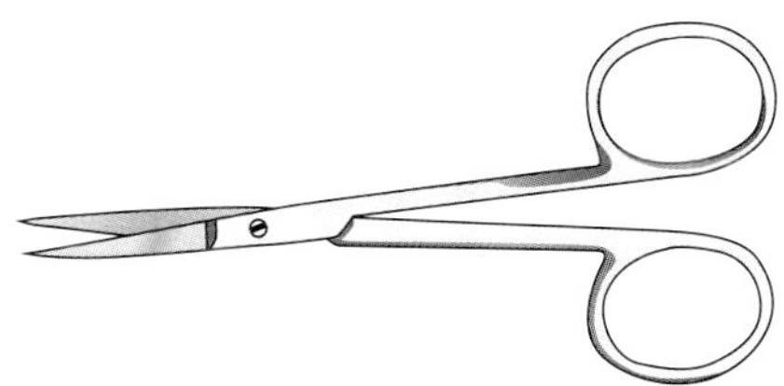

Figure A-14 Fine tissue (iris) 4⅛-inch scissors.

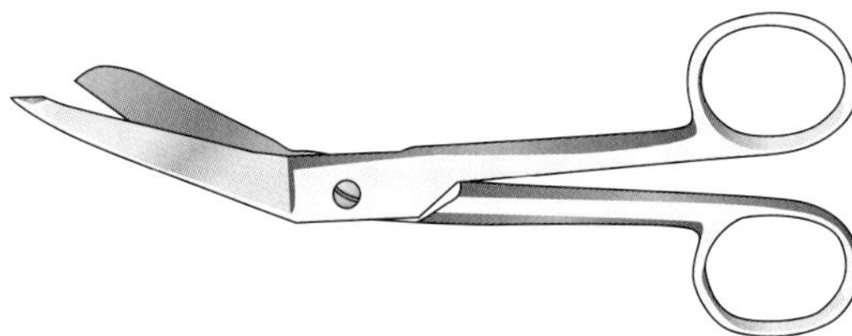

Figure A-15 Bandage removal scissors.

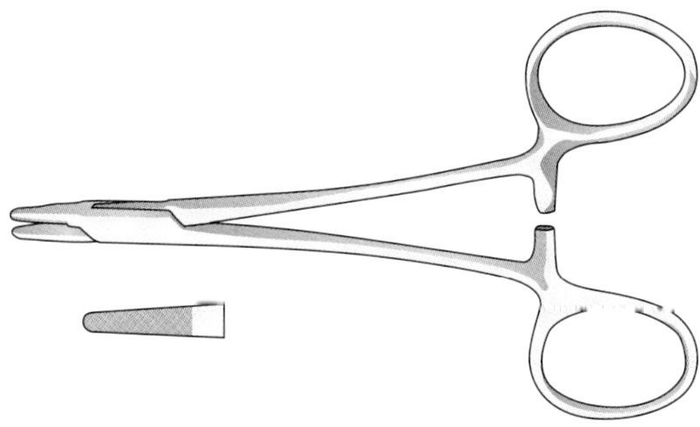

Figure A-16 Webster serrated jaw needle holder.

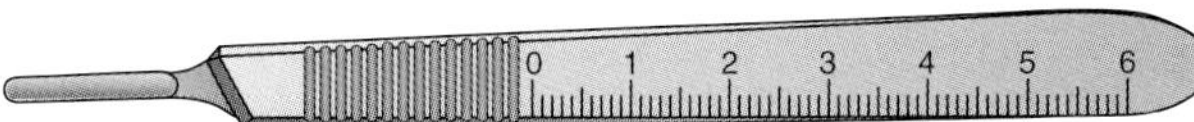

Figure A-17 Scalpel handle with metric rule.

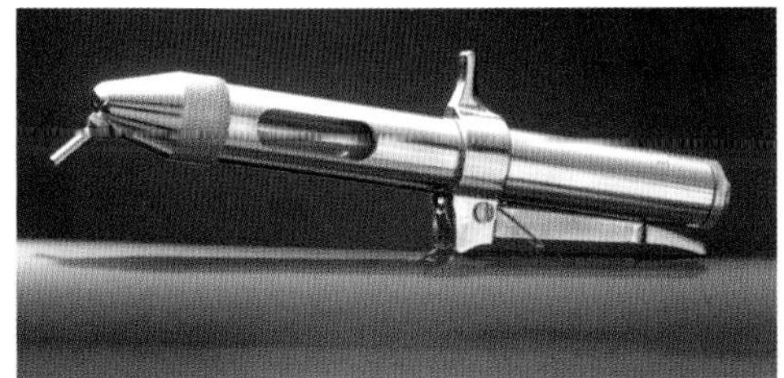

Figure A-18 Madajet SL anesthetic injector. (Courtesy of Mada Medical, Carlstadt, NJ.)

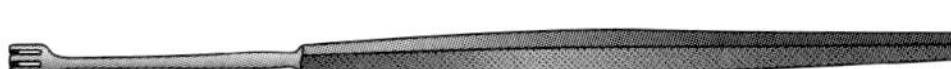

Figure A-19 Seltzer skin hook.

Vasectomy setup (no-scalpel)

- Small curved hemostats (2)
- Hemoclip applicator (medium) and clips (or suture)
- Vas dissecting forceps
- Vas clamp (Wilson or Li)
- Sharp tissue scissors
- Battery-powered cautery unit
- Medicine cup
- 4 × 4 gauze pads, large pack
- For the no-needle method, will also need the Madajet anesthetic injector (urology version) (Fig. A-18) (see Chapter 126, Vasectomy)

Skin hooks

- Useful for nontraumatic skin or wound edge retraction (Fig. A-19)

Staple applicator

- See Chapter 34, Skin Stapling.

Staple remover

- Removes surgical stainless steel skin staples. Removers are sold as disposable, and many patients have staples, especially after being treated in the emergency room. Staple removers may be reused, however, with appropriate sterilization (Fig. A-20).

Syringes

- Clinicians need mostly 1-mL syringes for skin procedures (e.g., biopsies), as well as some 3-mL, a few 5-mL, and even fewer 10-mL (for excisions) syringes. Two 25-mL syringes may also come in handy for thoracenteses, knee aspirations, irrigations, and so forth.

Needles (for injection)

NOTE: *The larger the number, the smaller the needle!* Clinicians need mostly 1½-inch, 25-gauge and ½-inch, 30-gauge needles for skin local anesthesia. The larger 21-gauge and 18-gauge needles are used to aspirate viscous fluid (e.g., ganglions, 18G) or large amounts of fluid (e.g., knee aspiration). Eighteen-gauge needles are also used to draw up anesthetic; it goes much more quickly than with needles that are smaller.

5-inch needle extender

- After twisting the extender on a syringe, the practitioner then locks the needle to this "extender." It is reusable and can be used to reach deep areas like the cervix, posterior pharynx, anus, etc. (See Chapter 149, Loop Electrosurgical Excision Procedure for Treating Cervical Intraepithelial Neoplasia, Fig, 149-4.)

Madajet

- A unique instrument for injecting solutions without a needle and with virtually no pain is the Madajet. Each application provides 0.1 mL of liquid for the intended site. It can be used to anesthetize for a simple skin biopsy or used in combination with steroids to treat hypertrophic and keloid scars. It is especially helpful in dense tissue where injecting with a needle is difficult. The instrument is cocked and then activated by pushing a button. This is the same basic unit that has been

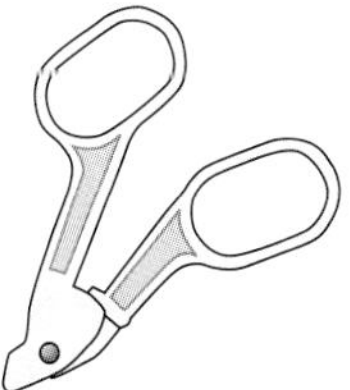

Figure A-20 Davis & Geck staple remover.

adapted for the no-needle vasectomy. (Be sure to order the correct device depending on whether it will be used for dermal applications or for vasectomies.) By using small volumes it also prevents distortion of tissue. Extenda Tips are available in varying lengths to reach tissue in the back of the mouth, the rectum, and other areas. It is easily cleaned between patients. Possible indications as listed by the manufacturer include anesthesia for digital block or prior to treating verrucae; steroids for keloids, lichen planus, lichen chronicus simplex, erythema nodosum, and lichen planus; injecting fasciitis, Morton's neuralgia, and more.

Suture
- Use cutting needles for the majority of patients:
  Skin: 3-0, 4-0, 5-0, and 6-0 nylon (for most interrupted skin closures)
  4-0 and 5-0 Prolene (for subcuticular procedures)
  Deep inverted: 3-0, 4-0, and 5-0 Vicryl
- See Chapter 24, Laceration and Incision Repair: Suture Selection.

Sterile drapes, fenestrated and nonfenestrated
- Both polyurethane and paper drapes are available in solid and fenestrated versions. The area around the fenestration has an adhesive backing to keep it in place. The paper is cheaper but doesn't lie in place as well and can become soiled with blood.

Mayo stand with tray to hold instruments

Magnification loupes
- Welch Allyn: 2.5× to 3×; has light with battery pack

Comedone extractor
- Saalfield or Unna types (Fig. A-21)

Ear irrigation setup
- A variety of units are available. One of the least expensive (approximately $40), most effective, and easiest to use is the Elephant Ear Wash System (Fig. A-22).

Ear loop curette
- For cerumen removal: Sklar #67-2513. These are available in both reusable metal and disposable, softer plastic. The latter are less traumatic and reduce the discomfort of removing cerumen.

For ingrown toenails
- Locke periosteal nail elevator (Fig. A-23)
- Nail splitter (Fig. A-24)

Chalazion clamp (small) with curette (Figs. A-25 and A-26)

Vaginal speculum
- Small, medium, large Graves'
- Nonconductive, vented for loop electrosurgical excision procedure (LEEP)
- Extra long (Snowman by CooperSurgical) for obese patients; very helpful for difficult cases

Endocervical curette (Kevorkian, without a basket)

Endocervical speculum (small, large)
- For colposcopy and removal of cervical polyps (see Chapter 137, Colposcopic Examination)

Cervical dilators (including silver probe)
- For endometrial biopsy, cervical stenosis, and dilation and curettage (D&C) (see appropriate chapters)

Dilateria (thin, medium thick, thick)
- For cervical stenosis
- Used to dilate a cervix atraumatically
- See Chapter 136, Cervical Stenosis and Cervial Dilation

Word Bartholin cyst catheter

Uterine sound
- Malleable rod is used to determine the depth of the uterus (from external os to back wall). Such information decreases the likelihood of uterine perforation during procedures.

Vaginal sidewall retractors
- Use for cryotherapy of cervix, LEEP (see Chapter 149, Loop Electrosurgical Excision Procedure for Treating Cervical Intraepithelial Neoplasia)

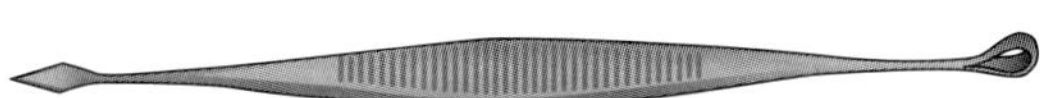

Figure A-21 Saalfield comedone extractor.

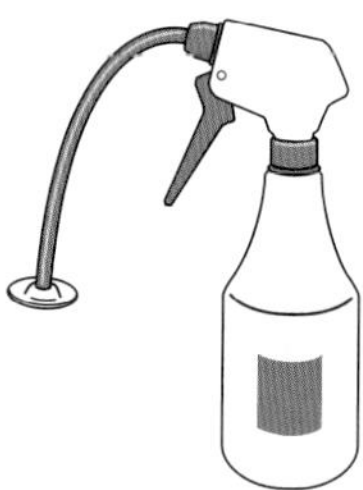

Figure A-22 Elephant ear washer system.

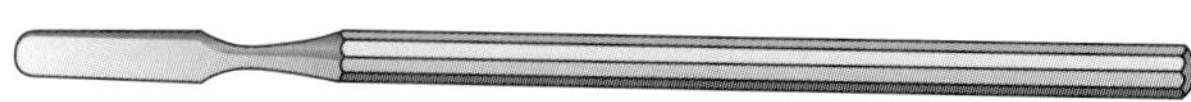

Figure A-23 Locke elevator.

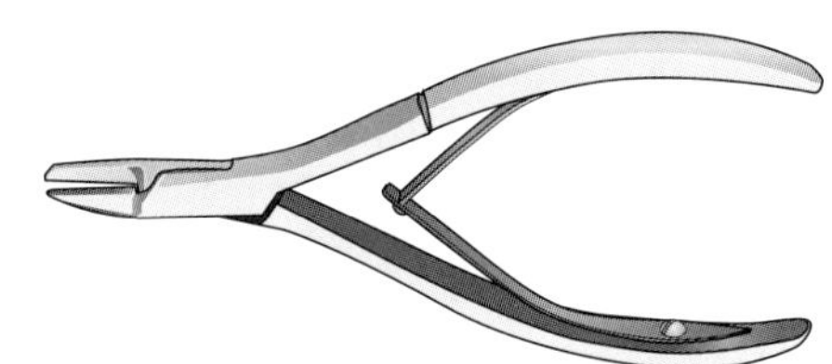

Figure A-24 Nail splitter.

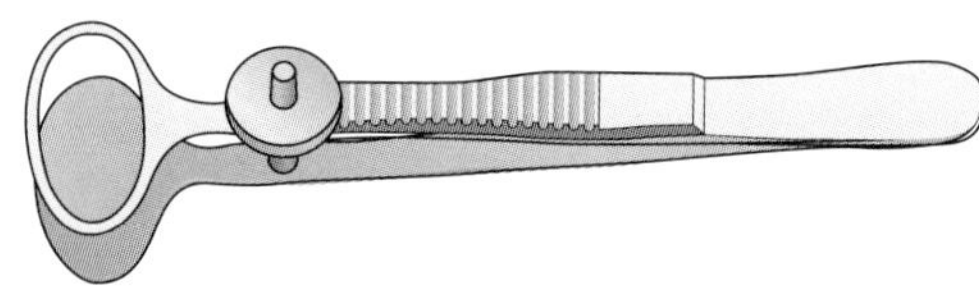

Figure A-25 Desmarres chalazion clamp.

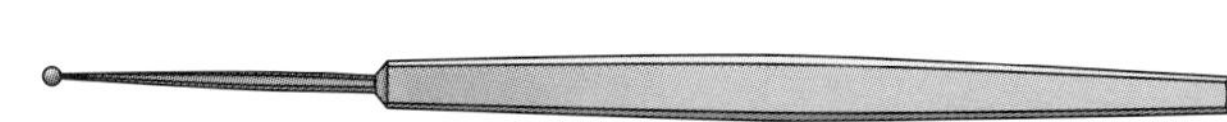

Figure A-26 Skeele chalazion curette.

Single-tooth tenaculum for cervix
- Used to stabilize the cervix for intrauterine device (IUD) placement, endometrial biopsy, laminaria insertion, or dilation, or to perform colpocentesis (see Chapter 127, Pregnancy Termination: First-Trimester Suction Aspiration)

IUD remover
- See Chapter 146, Intrauterine Device Removal

Anoscope
- Ive's slotted (see Chapter 98, Anoscopy; Fig. 98-1D)
- Plastic, disposable
- Pediatric

McGivney hemorrhoid ligator
- See Chapter 106, Office Treatment of Hemorrhoids; Fig. 106-4

Infrared coagulator (Redfield)
- See Chapter 106, Office Treatment of Hemorrhoids; Fig. 106-7
- Used for hemorrhoids, warts, tattoos, nasal turbinates, and bleeders

Silver probe
- This small malleable metal probe is basically a thickened wire with slightly bulbous ends. It is used to probe suspected fistulae

around the anus and to probe for the cervical canal when the os is stenotic (see Chapter 96, Anal Fissure and Lateral Sphincterotomy and Anal Fistula).

Liquid nitrogen cryogun and Dewar (Brymill, Wallach) for skin
- See Chapter 14, Cryosurgery

Casting supplies
- See Chapter 186, Ankle and Foot Splinting, Casting, and Taping and Chapter 187, Cast Immobilization and Upper Extremity Splinting

Wall blood pressure cuff with stethoscope
Glucose monitor
Oxygen tank on mobile cart
Electrocardiography machine
Pulse oximeter and vital signs monitor (Welch Allyn)
Defibrillator
Banyon Emergency Kit
- See Chapter 220, Anaphylaxis

Electrosurgical coagulation unit (ESU)
- See Chapter 30, Radiofrequency Surgery (Modern Electrosurgery) and Fig. 30-1
- Spend a little more and purchase a high-frequency unit for cutting (Ellman, Wallach, CooperSurgical)

Smoke evacuator for electrosurgical application
- See Chapter 30, Radiofrequency Surgery, Fig. 30-1

Cart for ESU unit and smoke evacuator
- See Chapter 30, Radiofrequency Surgery (Modern Electrosurgery).

Otoscope and ophthalmoscope
Sharps containers
Safety goggles
Examination tables, powered
- A matter of an inch or two makes a big difference. (Twenty-four inches is the ideal height when the table is as low as it can go. It cannot be higher.)

Examination stools
Refrigerator for medications
- Must be separate unit from the one used to store lunches!

Autoclave
Portable DVD player(s) for patient education
Binocular microscope

Optional Equipment to Consider

Air purifier
Colonoscope
- See Chapter 100, Colonoscopy

Colposcope
- See Chapter 137, Colposcopic Examination, Fig. 137-8

Flexible sigmoidoscope with suction pump and light source, cart
- See Chapter 103, Flexible Sigmoidoscopy

Gastroscope
- See Chapter 101, Esophagogastroduodenoscopy
- Consider the new thin-diameter versions that do not require sedation.

Halogen flexible floor light or mobile high-intensity ceiling surgical light
Intravenous pole
Nasopharyngoscope
- See Chapter 77, Nasolaryngoscopy

Nitrous oxide cryotherapy unit
- See Chapter 138, Cryotherapy of the Cervix, Fig. 138-1
- Tips: 19- and 25-mm flat and slight conical for *cervix*
- Slanted end tips for *skin*
- Hemorrhoid tip (multifunctional for *skin* lesions; virtually never used for hemorrhoids!)

Stress electrocardiography unit
- See Chapter 93, Exercise (Stress) Testing

VE-11 Handzfree anesthetic bottle holder
- See Chapter 4, Local Anesthesia, Fig. 4-1
- Saves time; holds multidose vials of anesthetic; inexpensive

APPENDIX B

INFORMED CONSENT

*Patrick J. Haddad**

Before a physician or other health care provider performs any procedure or offers other treatment, the *patient and the physician must discuss the reasons for it; the available alternatives; the possible material complications from the procedure or treatment, as well as those from forgoing it; and the patient must consent.* Consent is often considered to be simply a form which the patient needs to sign before a procedure or treatment begins, rather than being a process that results in the patient deciding, on an informed basis, whether to accept or reject treatment. Many physicians mistakenly believe or hope that a signed consent form, by itself, will prevent a professional liability lawsuit. However, a consent form alone is not legally sufficient to protect a physician from litigation or from liability if a suit is filed.

LEGAL CONSENT

A patient's consent to treatment is important to physicians for various reasons, including liability exposure. *Physicians have a legal liability exposure to claims for battery and the failure to obtain informed consent.* A physician commits battery by treating a patient without consent. Battery is an intentional tort that does not require proof of negligence or of the intent to do harm. Generally, a person commits battery by intentionally touching another individual without consent. The individual may be permitted to recover monetary damages absent bodily injury, although the damages awarded in such circumstances may be nominal. For medical care, consent may be express or implied by the patient seeking treatment or otherwise manifesting consent, or consent may be implied by law, such as in an emergency. If consent is given or implied, however, it is not limitless. A physician remains exposed to liability for battery if the treatment furnished exceeds the boundaries of the consent given or implied.

A patient's consent may be sufficient for a physician to successfully defend a battery claim. However, if the consent, or the patient's refusal of treatment, was not preceded by disclosure of the material benefits, risks, and alternatives, the physician may continue to have a liability exposure, even if the procedure or treatment itself was furnished in a competent manner without technical error or if the procedure was declined. *In order for there to be liability for lack of informed consent, the patient generally must show that the physician was negligent, the patient was injured and sustained damages, and the negligence was a proximate cause of the injury and damages.* Lack of informed consent is a claim based on professional negligence (i.e., malpractice). Unlike battery, which requires proof of an intentional touching without consent, a negligence claim requires proof of the applicable standard of care and that the physician failed to furnish care in conformity with that standard, in addition to proof of injury, damages, and causation. The standard of care, and whether the standard has been satisfied or breached, is typically established through the testimony of expert witnesses.

Across the United States, there are generally two alternative ways by which the standard of care is measured when lack of informed consent is alleged. One way is from *the perspective of physicians—the reasonable physician standard.* Under this standard, timely information must be given to the patient and in accordance with accepted standards of practice among physicians with similar training and experience in the community, or nationally for care furnished by a specialist. This view is followed by a slight majority of jurisdictions in the United States. The alternative view, adopted by slightly less than one half of the jurisdictions in the United States, is from *the perspective of patients—the reasonable person standard,* under which the patient must be informed of the risks and alternatives that a reasonable person in the patient's position would consider material in deciding whether to accept or to reject the proposed treatment.

Both standards are measured objectively, rather than by the subjective intent of the physician and the patient who are parties to a malpractice suit. Under either standard, risks that are not serious or are remote, or which are already known by the patient or which patients typically know, are generally not considered material.

Adults who are not competent to make decisions about their own health may not give or withold consent, or if they purport to do so, their consent will not be effective legally. Similarly, minor children typically may not consent to medical treatment, although some states have enacted exceptions by statute. For incompetent adults and minors, consent must be obtained from a legal guardian or parent. In emergencies, it is usually permissible to perform procedures or furnish treatment necessary to save the patient's life without consent when it cannot be obtained in a timely fashion.

Some jurisdictions may excuse the obtaining of informed consent when the information might have a detrimental effect on the patient's physical or psychological well-being. The availability and scope of this so-called "therapeutic privilege" can vary among jurisdictions, and physicians should use caution—and consult with legal counsel or with their liability carrier's risk management—before relying on it.

Additionally, physicians need to consider the ethical issues raised by postponing the disclosure of information to patients. Ethically, it may be appropriate in special circumstances to postpone or delay disclosure of certain information if early communication is clearly contraindicated. However, withholding medical information from patients without their knowledge is not ethically permissible. Although all information need not be communicated to the patient immediately or all at once, physicians should assess the amount of information a patient is capable of receiving at a given time.

Some states have codified by statute certain informed consent procedures. Texas, for example, has established panels of physicians and lawyers who together write rules for informed consent for many surgical procedures, including the use of consent forms (Fig. B-1).

*Mr. Haddad is a member of Kerr, Russell and Weber, PLC, Detroit, Mich. Mr. Haddad is co-chair of the firm's healthcare law practice and is a member of the State Bar of Michigan Healthcare Law Section, the American Bar Association Health Law Section, and the American Health Lawyers Association. This chapter is presented for informational purposes only and does not constitute legal advice by Kerr, Russell and Weber, PLC, or Mr. Haddad. Physicians should consult with legal counsel knowledgeable in the laws of the jurisdictions in which they practice medicine.

State of Texas: 25 TAC §601.4(a)(1)

DISCLOSURE AND CONSENT

Medical and Surgical Procedures

TO THE PATIENT: You have the right, as a patient, to be informed about your condition and the recommended surgical, medical, or diagnostic procedure to be used so that you may make the decision whether or not to undergo the procedure after knowing the risks and hazards involved. This disclosure is not meant to scare or alarm you; it is simply an effort to make you better informed so you may give or withhold your consent to the procedure.

I (we) voluntarily request Dr. ____________________ as my physician, and such associates, technical assistants, and other health care providers as they may deem necessary, to treat my condition which has been explained to me (us) as:

____

____

____.

I (we) understand that the following surgical, medical, and/or diagnostic procedures are planned for me and I (we) voluntarily consent and authorize these procedures:

____

____

____.

I (we) understand that my physician may discover other or different conditions which require additional or different procedures than those planned. I (we) authorize my physician, and such associates, technical assistants, and other health care providers, to perform such other procedures which are advisable in their professional judgment.

I (we) (do) (do not) consent to the use of blood and blood products as deemed necessary.

I (we) understand that no warranty or guarantee has been made to me (us) as to result or cure.

Just as there may be risks and hazards in continuing my present condition without treatment, there are also risks and hazards related to the performance of the surgical, medical, and/or diagnostic procedures planned for me. I (we) realize that common to surgical, medical, and/or diagnostic procedures is the potential for infection, blood clots in veins and lungs, hemorrhage, allergic reactions, and even death. I (we) also realize that the following risks and hazards may occur in connection with this particular procedure:

____

____

____.

I (we) understand that anesthesia involves additional risks and hazards but I (we) request the use of anesthetics for the relief and protection from pain during the planned and additional procedures. I (we) realize the anesthesia may have to be changed, possibly without explanation to me (us).

I (we) understand that certain complications may result from the use of any anesthetic including respiratory problems, drug reaction, paralysis, brain damage, or even death. Other risks and hazards which may result from the use of general anesthetics range from minor discomfort to injury to vocal cords, teeth, or eyes. I (we) understand that other risks and hazards resulting from spinal or epidural anesthetics include headache and chronic pain.

I (we) have been given an opportunity to ask questions about my condition, alternative forms of anesthesia and treatment, risks of nontreatment, the procedures to be used, and the risks and hazards involved, and I (we) believe that I (we) have sufficient information to give this informed consent.

I (we) certify this form has been fully explained to me (us), that I (we) have read it or have had it read to me (us), that the blank spaces have been filled in, and that I (we) understand its contents.

Figure B-1 State of Texas Disclosure and Consent Form for Medical and Surgical Procedures. (Courtesy of Texas Medical Board, http://www.tmb.state.tx.us/.)

Figure continues on following page.

PATIENT/OTHER LEGALLY RESPONSIBLE PERSON (signature required)

____

DATE:________________ TIME:________________ AM/PM

WITNESS:

____

Signature

____

Name (Print)

____

Address (Street or PO Box)

____

City, State, Zip Code

Figure B-1, cont.

Also, Michigan mandates that all women receive a state-approved booklet before mastectomy for breast cancer.

Physicians should be aware of the law in their respective states, both legislative and judicial. Physicians often have many resources available on consent issues, such as state and specialty medical societies. Additionally, liability insurers will often furnish guidance to their insured physicians on consent issues and may have available model consent forms.

In cases in which a legally mandated consent form is not required, a general consent form that identifies the patient, the procedure, the indications, and the risks can be used to document the physician's disclosures and discussion with the patient, and the patient's consent (Fig. B-2). Some states may require a witness to sign the consent form. Many physicians in office practices may ask nurses or other office staff to witness. Because of potential conflict-of-interest issues that may be raised in litigation, physicians may consider having a family member or friend of the patient also witness the consent process, in addition to the physician's staff, if possible.

Patient Consent Form

I came to the office of Dr. ________ on ________ (date) for evaluation and treatment of the following condition:

____

(description of diagnosis, etiology, and different diagnosis)

We discussed the different treatments possible, and discussed the risks of not treating the condition. Based on the advice given by Dr. ________ and my own judgment, I agree to undergo the following procedure:

____

(description of anesthetic, procedure, and dressing)

We discussed the different outcomes that could occur, and most of the possible complications. I am aware that other complications could occur that we could not foresee. I agree to follow the instructions for self-care after the procedure, and to return for follow-up care on: ________. I will call the office or answering service if any problems arise before the scheduled follow-up visit.

________________	________________
Patient's signature	Date/time
Witness's signature	Physician's signature

One copy for chart, one copy for patient.

Figure B-2 Sample of patient consent form.

Models of Medical Decision Making

The courts have been criticized for setting standards that do not actually reflect medical practice and may interfere with the doctor-patient relationship. The problem may lie in the implementation, not in the actual concept. The ethical concept of informed consent includes the legal concept of consent, but it goes further: *the patient must be a partner in the decision-making process* (Box B-1). Just as the laws have evolved in clarifying informed consent, the transition toward involving the patient more in the process has also changed.

There are essentially four models of medical decision making:

1. *Traditional model*: The physician decides whether to perform a procedure and which procedure to perform; the patient's trust and confidence in the doctor replace the need for consent.
2. *Traditional informed consent*: The physician decides whether to perform a procedure and which procedure to perform with the patient's informed consent.
3. *Collaboration*: The physician and the patient work together to make a joint decision about the procedure.
4. *Patient choice*: The patient decides with the physician's counsel.

If given a choice, some patients will choose the traditional model, and a few will choose the fourth model. Most patients and physicians are more comfortable with either traditional informed consent or collaboration, and physicians should learn how to use both of these models as well as how to determine which model to use for a specific patient.

Notwithstanding the model of medical decision making utilized, a physician will be held, for liability purposes, to the standard of informed consent adopted by the jurisdiction in which he or she practices. This means that for liability purposes, the physician must ensure that the necessary disclosures to the patient have been made and documented in the medical record and in any consent form used.

Box B-1. Elements of Informed Consent

- Disclosure of information
- Competency (the patient is not a minor, unconscious, intoxicated, or incapable of participating in the process)
- Understanding
- Voluntarism
- Decision making
- Patient participation

Consent Is a Process

With the possible exception of treatment needed in emergencies, there is rarely an exception to the rule that all procedures or other treatment—whether office or facility based—should be preceded by disclosure of the material risks and benefits and discussion that allows the patient to participate in and to decide whether to have the procedure or other treatment. In many instances, it may be permissible to obtain and to rely on the patient's oral consent, which should be documented explicitly by the physician in the medical record summarizing all the essential points (risks, benefits, possible complications, alternatives, etc.). In other instances, particularly those involving surgical procedures, the patient should sign a consent form that documents the process utilized. Some states have laws that specify certain language on consent forms for certain procedures.

The process of discussing the procedure with the patient or guardian and providing education about the procedure itself, the possible complications, and aftercare responsibilities of the patient should all be considered part of the consent process. The consent form can be used as a patient education tool, with a copy containing the patient's signature to be given to the patient for reference. Patients can be educated during the consent process about the legal requirements for the signed form and the fact that results of medical procedures are not guaranteed. However, bringing the form out at the last minute for signature can produce some patient anxiety and suspicion. A better approach may be to start the process by giving the patient the consent form to read, then using the form to guide the discussion. For certain procedures, such as vasectomy, the form can be sent out before the consultation visit or given at the time of the consultation. The patient can read it, think about it, then return it before surgery. The consent form can include postprocedure instructions as well as instructions for contacting the physician or an associate if complications occur after hours.

Many liability insurance companies advise that patients view videotapes discussing the proposed procedure. This ensures that the patient has an opportunity to consider all the pertinent information and serves as a record for defense of a lawsuit. However, a videotape is not a substitute for discussion between physician and patient.

The process of informed consent can be summarized as follows:

1. Establish responsibility:
   - The doctor's role
   - The patient's role
2. Establish expected duration of responsibility.
3. Define the problem with the patient.
4. Set goals for treatment and establish whether cure is a reasonable expectation.
5. Select an approach to treatment; during this step the informed consent form is signed.
6. Perform extended treatment and follow-up.

Complications Happen and the Consent Process Will Be Scrutinized

Surgical and other complications are at the core of many malpractice suits. Physicians should not rely solely on a signed consent form for protection in a malpractice suit. Rather, they should rely on the process that resulted in the patient's consent, including the patient's participation in that process. In malpractice litigation, that process will be viewed through the lens of hindsight. A physician who brings out a highly technical consent form to be signed by the patient at the last minute is not likely to be viewed favorably. By itself, such a form may not necessarily be evidence that the patient's consent was informed. A consent form is only one piece of evidence, and in lawsuits other evidence, such as the patient's testimony, is examined as well. *A consent form itself cannot—and is not intended to—substitute for a candid discussion* with the patient about the procedure and the inclusion of the patient in the decision-making process, or for documentation in the medical record of the discussion before the patient signs the form. For some patients, particularly uninformed or anxious patients, knowledge of the risk may dissuade them from undergoing an otherwise needed procedure.

Many consent forms use language that is too technical; the forms are often too long to read and interpret during an office visit. Consent forms are often handed to patients during hospital registration by nonprofessional personnel, and some patients are unable to comprehend the procedure even after explanation. The consent form should be meaningful to the patient. *Likewise, in order to provide the additional type of documentation that is also useful in a court case, the physician should include in the patient's chart a narrative of the discussion between doctor and patient during the decision-making process, in addition to the actual consent form.*

Clinicians should always *be careful not to "overpromise" what* a procedure can do. Honesty is best. "Never say never and never say always!" There are always exceptions. If someone asks about a rare complication, the clinician should not say it *won't* happen! It could. An example should be given instead. If the patient plays the lotto, the clinician should ask if he or she is likely to win. The answer is usually "No." But could the patient win? Is it possible? The answer is usually "Yes." So it goes with complications. Will it happen? "Most likely not. But, in rare instances, it could."

It goes without saying that *no consent form will protect a physician from true malpractice*. Competence and keeping up to date educationally are essential. Seeking expert advice and second opinions is encouraged, and knowing one's limits is essential. Especially in primary care, clinicians must be sure to inform the patient of their training and background; they should not pretend to be an orthopedist, or obstetrician, or plastic surgeon. The patient should seek another opinion if he or she is at all uncomfortable.

As many have said before, the best way to minimize the risk of a lawsuit is to have an excellent physician-patient relationship with both the patient and the family. Each patient is different. Some have a lot of questions that need to be addressed and answered. Some have been let down by the medical system in the past and are fearful. Some have extreme anxiety and no amount of reassurance helps them. Some want absolute assurances that are impossible.

Ultimately, it is the patient's decision whether to accept or reject treatment. As a matter of practicality, sometimes personalities just aren't compatible. When "the vibes are bad" between the patient and the caretaker, clinicians should learn to sense this and not try to "force" things. Providers should recognize that they can't always be all things to all people and that referring a patient to "other experts" is often best for the relationship and to reduce liability exposure.

Complications occur, even though the physician has furnished good quality care with technical perfection. Unfortunately, mistakes can and do happen. Physicians are typically advised by their hospitals, insurers, and legal counsel—and maybe are ordered by their employers—to refrain from expressing sympathy or compassion to the patient or family in these circumstances. The reason is that such statements can be construed as an admission of malpractice and used as evidence against the physician in litigation. Expressions of sympathy also have been seen as inviting malpractice suits. Nevertheless, some institutions have enacted policies of transparency and accountability by admitting errors and volunteering fair settlements. Anecdotal reports suggest that this practice may reduce the number of malpractice suits, the dollar amount of settlements, and defense costs, although there is some debate as to whether the quantity of claims is affected. Approximately 35 states have enacted laws—referred to as "I'm sorry" laws—which provide that expressions of sympathy and compassion by physicians are inadmissible as an admission of liability in malpractice litigation. The scope of these laws varies among jurisdictions, but typically are narrowly drawn and normally will not shield statements that admit—or can be construed as admitting—fault. Consequently, physicians, when caught up in the moment, could unwittingly express sympathy or compassion in such a way as to unfairly implicate himself or herself before a jury.

BILLING ISSUES

Evaluation and management codes are used to bill for surgical consultation, evaluation, and management services furnished by a physician in the office. The informed consent process is included in the evaluation and management codes and is not a separately reimbursable service. The range of available evaluation and management codes varies according to the degree of the examination performed, the history taken, the complexity of the medical decision making, and the time spent with the patient and family. When extended counseling with the patient or family is necessary, the physician should consult with his or her billing advisor to ensure that the appropriate evaluation and management codes are reimbursable and billed.

ACKNOWLEDGMENT

The editors wish to recognize the many contributions by Julie Graves Moy, MD, to this chapter in the previous edition of this text.

ONLINE RESOURCES

College of Registered Nurses of British Columbia statement on informed consent: http://www.crnbc.ca/downloads/359.pdf.
State of Texas Medical Board: http://www.tmb.state.tx.us/.

BIBLIOGRAPHY

American Medical Association, Ethics Opinions E-8.082 (Informed Consent) and E-8.122 (Withholding Information from Patients).
Caterine JM, Miller B: Informed consent: Procedure specific. Iowa Med 79:231, 1989.
Green JA: Minimizing malpractice risk by role clarification: The confusing transition from tort to contract. Ann Intern Med 109:234, 1988.
Hansson MO: Balancing the quality of consent. J Med Ethics 24:182, 1998.
Kaibara PD: 8 ways to improve the informed consent process. J Fam Pract 59:373, 2010.
King JS, Moulton BW: Rethinking conformed consent: The case for shared medical decision-making. Am J Law Med 32:429, 2006.
Lidz CW, Appelbaum PS, Meisel A: Two models of implementing informed consent. Ann Intern Med 148:1385, 1988.
Loewy EH: Textbook of Healthcare Ethics. New York, Plenum Press, 1996.
Mazur DJ: What should patients be told prior to a medical procedure? Ethical and legal perspectives on medical informed consent. Am J Med 81:1051, 1986.
Peters SK, Finberg J, Kroll JD: The Law of Medical Practice in Michigan. Ann Arbor, Mich., Institute of Continuing Legal Education, 1981.
Savulescu J, Momeyer RW: Should informed consent be based on rational beliefs? J Med Ethics 23:282, 1997.
Sprung CL, Winick BJ: Informed consent in theory and practice: Legal and medical perspectives on the informed consent doctrine and a proposed reconceptualization. Crit Care Med 17:1346, 1989.
Walter P: The doctrine of informed consent: A tale of two cultures and two legal traditions. Issues Law Med 14:357, 1999.

APPENDIX C

LATEX ALLERGY GUIDELINES

Sumana Reddy

Sensitivity to natural rubber latex (NRL) has gained increasing prominence over the last three decades. Latex is now likely the second most important cause of intraoperative anaphylaxis, behind muscle relaxants. Although NRL has been in widespread use for over a century, multiple factors, including a dramatic increase in use and changes in production time and production quality, have led to now well-established reports of severe reactions. In 1997, the National Institute for Occupational Safety and Health (NIOSH) issued an advisory recommending that latex gloves be used only by those workers exposed to blood or body fluids, and not by food handlers, hobbyists, and those performing many housekeeping activities. NIOSH also recommends that if NRL gloves are to be used, they should be *low protein and powder free*. Increasingly, hospitals are making the decision to be latex-free in terms of glove purchases. It is a reasonable decision, given the prevalence of latex allergy, to do all procedures with nonlatex gloves. Although there are a variety of alternatives to latex, not all have the tensile strength, flexibility, and impermeability of NRL. The solution may be to use different glove materials for examination versus surgery and procedural use.

SYMPTOMS OF LATEX ALLERGY

Reactions to NRL are type I, immediate hypersensitivity reactions. They can cause local or systemic urticaria, symptoms of rhinoconjunctivitis or bronchospasm, and anaphylaxis. The proteins of NRL have been described as unique in that an unpredictable course may occur in the progression from no or mild symptoms to anaphylaxis. The sensitization begins and is perpetuated both as a contact allergen and as an inhalant. The *greatest degree of sensitization* occurs in areas where powdered latex gloves with a high NRL protein content are used. In these situations, the cornstarch powder particles appear to adsorb latex to the surface. These latex-cornstarch *powder particles* have been demonstrated to aerosolize, especially when gloves are removed. Prolonged exposure through the lungs appears to cause high rates of sensitization. Those who are sensitized may cross-react to certain foods such as banana, kiwi, chestnut, or avocado. NRL gloves may also cause an irritant contact dermatitis from occlusion and frequent handwashing, or a delayed hypersensitivity reaction from chemicals used in processing. These are not reactions to latex itself (Box C-1).

RISK GROUPS

Those at greatest risk of sensitization are all those groups with cumulatively prolonged exposure to latex. The greatest prevalence appears to be in those who have undergone repeated surgeries, especially children with spina bifida or urogenital abnormalities. Others at risk include workers in the latex manufacturing industry and health care workers. Studies indicate 10% to 17% of health care workers have already become sensitized, and over 2% have occupational asthma as a result of latex exposure. In addition, over 50% of persons who are sensitive to latex have a history of atopic illness, or hay fever (Box C-2).

NONLATEX MATERIALS

The establishment of universal precautions in 1985 has led to an increased use of latex gloves through the spectrum of health services from phlebotomy to nursing home care. This use is now being reevaluated in light of our growing understanding of the process of sensitization. As recommended by NIOSH, all health care providers should make purchasing decisions avoiding the use of powdered, high-protein latex gloves, in favor of powder-free, low-protein gloves. Where possible, nonlatex gloves should be used. As mentioned, in the last decade this has become an increasingly popular solution. These measures have led to a probable drop in the incidence of latex allergy, and certainly a deceleration in the rate of newly sensitized individuals.

There is a range of surgical and nonsurgical gloves available in nonlatex materials. These have been ASTM (American Society for Testing and Materials) tested for barrier integrity and are expected to provide protection against viral particles such as human immunodeficiency virus (HIV) when used as recommended. Vinyl gloves are not as effective as other materials against viral penetration.

Box C-1. Symptoms and Signs Associated with Latex Glove Use

Irritant Contact Dermatitis (Nonimmune)

Gradual onset, over days, caused by handwashing, occlusion, antiseptics, and glove chemicals
Redness
Cracks, fissures
Scaling

Allergic Contact Dermatitis, or Type IV (Delayed Hypersensitivity)

Onset 6 to 48 hours after contact, caused by chemicals
Erythema
Vesicles
Papules
Pruritus
Blisters
Crusting

Immediate Hypersensitivity, or Type I

Local and generalized urticaria onset within minutes, very rarely longer than 2 hours; caused by latex
Feeling of faintness
Feeling of impending doom
Angioedema
Nausea, vomiting, abdominal cramps
Rhinoconjunctivitis
Bronchospasm
Anaphylactic shock

Box C-2. Risk Groups for Latex Allergy

Occupational latex exposure
- Health care workers
- Rubber industry workers

Medical patient exposure
- Spina bifida
- Urogenital abnormalities
- Other repeated or prolonged surgeries or mucous membrane exposure to latex devices, especially early in life

Atopic history or food allergy (especially bananas, avocados, kiwis, and chestnuts) (cross-reacting protein epitopes)

Low risk: no identifiable risk factors

DIAGNOSIS

In performing procedures, there are issues of identifying the patient who may be latex allergic, and avoiding exposure through inadvertent use of a product containing latex. Use of a standardized questionnaire is recommended where any suspicion may exist (Box C-3). It is also important to prevent the development of latex sensitization in the health care workers performing and assisting in the procedure. The use of nonlatex gloves and supplies can streamline processes, and has become more of an option as these gloves become competitively priced.

The diagnosis of latex sensitivity is not straightforward. It is made through a combination of thorough medical history and immunologic testing. Because symptoms can be generalized and nonspecific, the sensitized individual often remains unaware of the condition. Standardized extracts for prick testing are not available in the United States. Therefore, such skin testing should be carried out only by centers with experience in preparing extracts and may cause a high incidence of anaphylaxis. Food and Drug Administration (FDA)–approved in vitro tests to measure latex-specific IgE are available (Pharmacia CAP, Pharmacia-UpJohn Diagnostics Inc.; AlaSTAT, Diagnostic Products Corp.; and HYTEC, HYCOR Biomedical). The low specificity of these tests, with at least 20% false-negative results and unclear positive predictive value, gives them limitations. Negative serologic testing with a strongly positive history would suggest the value of skin prick testing in experienced hands to confirm the diagnosis. Because individuals with no risk factors or prior symptoms have had anaphylactic reactions, those who are asymptomatic with positive tests should be advised to exercise caution.

If in doubt at the time of performing a procedure, it is best to avoid use of latex-containing medical devices and products. Especially prone to cause reactions are gloves and urinary catheters placed in direct contact with mucosal surfaces (e.g., during pelvic examinations).

The task of identifying latex-containing medical devices has been simplified by FDA requirements indicating on packaging whether latex is contained in a product. Lists of latex-containing

Box C-3. Screening Questionnaire for Latex Sensitivity

I. Allergies
- Have you had a history of hay fever, asthma, eczema, allergies, or problems with rashes?
- Are you allergic (rash, oral itching, swelling, or wheezing) to any foods, especially bananas, avocados, kiwi, or chestnuts?

II. Job-Related Symptoms
- Does your work involve any exposure to latex products, including latex gloves? Have you ever had allergic reactions to something in your work environment?
- If you have had a rash on your hands after wearing latex gloves, how long after putting on the gloves did the rash develop? What did it look like?

III. Hidden Reactions to Latex
- Have you ever had swelling, itching, hives, shortness of breath, cough, or other allergic symptoms during or after blowing up a balloon, undergoing a dental procedure, using condoms or diaphragms, or following a vaginal or rectal examination?
- Have you ever had an allergic reaction of unknown cause, especially during a medical or dental procedure?

IV. Surgical History
- Have you ever had surgery, and if so, what type?
- Do you have spina bifida or any urinary tract problem requiring surgery or catheterization?

Box C-4. Sources of Possible Latex Exposure

Medical Devices with Potential Latex Content

Adhesive tape
Ambu-bags
Bandages
Bulb syringes
Dental devices
Electrode pads
Face masks
Gloves
Injection ports
Mattresses on stretchers
PCA syringes
Rubber syringe stoppers and medication vial stoppers
Stethoscope and BP cuff tubing
Tourniquets
Urinary catheters
Wound drains

Household Items with Potential Latex Content

Balloons
Buttons on electronic equipment
Carpet backing
Clothing, including elastic on underwear
Computer mouse pads
Condoms and diaphragms
Diapers
Erasers
Feeding nipples and pacifiers
Food handled with powdered latex gloves
Handles on racquets, tools
Many toys
Rubber bands
Sanitary and incontinence pads
Shoe soles
Sports equipment

BP, blood pressure; PCA, patient-controlled analgesia.
A more detailed and periodically updated list of latex-containing products and nonlatex substitutes by brand name is available from the Spina Bifida Association of America (1-800-621-3141 or http://www.sbaa.org).

Box C-5. Latex Allergy Management Guidelines for the Hospital Setting

- Ask all patients about latex sensitivity, using a screening questionnaire if relevant.
- Place latex allergy identification bracelet on patient in admitting area.
- Label room as latex-safe and enter in all relevant areas of signage, notes, and databases.
- Disseminate latex allergy protocol and lists of nonlatex substitutes for latex-containing materials that may contact the patient.
- Remove all latex products that would contact the patient and remove all latex gloves. Use PVC tubing or wrap cotton gauze over the extremity if using latex cuffs and tubing or tourniquets.
- Ensure that adhesives and tapes, including ECG electrodes and dressing supplies, are checked for latex content.
- Have a latex-free crash cart available to follow the patient through his or her stay.
- Notify Pharmacy and Central Supply that the patient is latex-sensitive so that latex contact can be eliminated in preparation of materials or drugs for the patient.
- Notify Dietary of relevant food allergies and avoid handling food with powdered latex gloves (NIOSH recommended and mandated by many states).

ECG, electrocardiogram; NIOSH, National Institute of Occupational Safety and Health; PVC, polyvinyl chloride.

and latex-free devices may be obtained both directly from individual manufacturers and from the Spina Bifida Association of America. As Box C-4 shows, many medical and household items contain latex. To a sensitized person, all of these may be problematic. To an unsensitized person, the thin stretchy rubber of gloves, condoms, and balloons provides the greatest source of rubber particles leaching from the surface. Solid, molded rubber objects are less likely to leach proteins from their surfaces.

Management

A history of type 1 immediate hypersensitivity reactions necessitates a latex-safe environment. Patient records should be identified clearly for latex allergy, and at no time in treatment should latex gloves, tourniquets, catheters, or other materials come in direct contact with the patient. If blood pressure cuffs and tubing are made of latex, the patient's extremities should be wrapped to prevent contact. Although rubber medication vial and syringe stoppers are listed, to date there have been only rare reactions to medication in contact with latex. For the most part, then, extreme measures (e.g., only using medication from glass ampules or glass syringes) are not recommended. The hospital guidelines provided may be adapted as applicable for an outpatient setting (Box C-5).

Premedication with antihistamines or steroids is not helpful. It may only mask symptoms leading to anaphylaxis without preventing anaphylactic reactions. Persons with latex hypersensitivity should carry an epinephrine autoinjection kit and wear MedicAlert identification. In the medical office it is always advisable to have available sterile nonlatex gloves for use.

Suppliers

See Table C-1 for a list of suppliers of hypoallergenic nonlatex gloves.

Conclusion

For those who have been sensitized, avoidance is the cornerstone of management. In all settings where gloves are heavily used, avoiding sensitization through purchase of powder-free gloves is recommended. Almost all hospitals have gone toward powder-free and low-protein gloves, and increasing numbers are opting to convert to entirely nonlatex products. This choice has already begun to have a positive impact on the patient with latex allergy and to prevent sensitization in the health care worker. Ironically, with this condition, it is the health care worker who is often the patient.

ICD-9-CM Diagnostic Code

989.82 Latex allergy

TABLE C-1 Suppliers of Nonlatex Gloves*

Name of Glove	Material	Company/Phone Number/Website
Dermaprene	Neoprene (polychloroprene polymer)	Ansell (1-800-321-9752), www.ansellpro.com
Sensicare	Polyisoprene	Medline (1-800-346-8849), www.medline.com
Elastyfree and Elastylite	Polyisoprene (no accelerators and nonchlorinated)	ECI Medical Technologies (1-800-668-5289), www.ecimedical.com
Neotech Biogel	Neoprene (polychloroprene polymer)	Regent Medical (1-800-843-8497)
Pure Advantage and Ultra Preserve	Butadiene-acrylonitrile (nitrile) and polychloroprene	Tillotson (1-800-445-6830), www.thcnet.com
Elastylite and QualiTouch	Styrene butadiene co-polymer and butadiene-acrylonitrile (nitrile)	Smartpractice (1-800-522-0595)
Safeskin	Butadiene-acrylonitrile (nitrile), polyvinyl chloride	Kimberly Clark (1 800-524-3577), www.kchealthcare.com Ammex (1-800-274-7354), www.ammex.com
FreeForm, Supreno, NeoproEC	Nitrile† (butadiene co-polymer), polyvinyl chloride and polychloroprene	Microflex (1-800-876-6866), www.microflex.com
Nitrastretch, Synthatech	Nitrile† (butadiene co-polymer), polyvinyl chloride	Top Quality Manufacturing (1-800-483-8559), www.topqualitygloves.com
Allerderm	Polyvinyl chloride and nitrile	Allerderm (1-800-365-6868), www.allerderm.com
Duraprene and Esteem	Duraprene and polyisoprene	CardinalHealth (1-800-964-5227), www.cardinal.com
Allergard	Styrene butadiene block polymer	Allergard (1-800-255-2500)
N-DEX	Nitrile* (butadiene co-polymer)	Best Glove/Best (1-800-241-0323)

*Kits containing everything needed for one latex-safe surgical procedure are obtainable from DeRoyal Surgical (1-800-251-9864), www.deroyal.com.
†Gloves made from nitrile are produced with the same accelerator (mercaptobenzathiazole) as some latex gloves. Those with suspected irritant or allergic contact dermatitis to latex gloves may also react to nitrile.

ONLINE RESOURCES

Patient education and additional information are available through the following groups:

American Latex Allergy Association: http://www.latexallergyresources.org/ or 1-888-972-5378.

Latex allergy links: http://latexallergylinks.tripod.com/.

Spina Bifida Association of America website: www.sbaa.org.

BIBLIOGRAPHY

Ahmed S, Aw T-C, Adisesh A: Toxicological and immunological aspects of occupational latex allergy. Toxicol Rev 23:123–134, 2004.

Arellano R, Bradley J, Sussman G: Prevalence of latex sensitization among hospital physicians occupationally exposed to latex gloves. Anesthesiology 77:905, 1992.

Beezhold DH, Beck WC: Surgical glove powders bind latex antigens. Arch Surg 127:1354, 1992.

Condemi J: Allergic reactions to natural rubber latex at home, to rubber products and to cross-reacting foods. J Allergy Clin Immunol 110:2, 2002.

Food and Drug Administration: Latex-containing devices: User labeling. Fed Register 61:32618–32620, 1996.

Kwittken PL, Becker J, Oyefara B, et al: Latex hypersensitivity reactions despite prophylaxis. Allergy Proc 13:123, 1992.

Lieberman P: Anaphylactic reactions during surgical and medical procedures. J Allergy Clin Immunol 110(2 Suppl):S64–S69, 2002.

U.S. Department of Health and Human Services, Public Health Service, Centers for Disease Control and Prevention, National Institute for Occupational Safety and Health: Preventing allergic reactions to natural rubber latex in the workplace. NIOSH Pub. No. 97-135. Cincinnati, Government Printing Office, 1997.

APPENDIX D

SUPPLIER INFORMATION

Accutome
263 Great Valley Parkway
Malvern, PA 19355
Phone: 1-800-979-2020
www.accutome.com

Accutron, Inc.
Phone: 1-800-531-2221
www.accutron-inc.com

ACMI Circon
136 Turnpike Rd.
Southborough, MA 01772-2104
Phone: 1-508-804-2600
www.circoncorp.com

Acuderm
5370 NW 35 Terrace
Ft. Lauderdale, FL 33309
Phone: 1-800-327-0015
www.acuderm.com

Acuson (owned by Siemens)
1220 Charleston Rd.
P.O. Box 7393
Mountain View, CA 94039-7393
Phone: 1-800-422-8766
www.acuson.com or www.medical.siemens.com

Advanced BioSensor, Inc.
400 Arbor Lake Dr., Suite B450
Columbia, SC 29223
Phone: 1-800-443-3816
www.advancedbiosensor.com

Advanced Laser Centers
1900 E. Golf Rd.
Schaumburg, IL 60173
Phone: 1-888-525-2737
www.dermaglide.com

Advanced Meditech International, Inc. (AMI)
86-38 53rd Ave.
Flushing, NY 11373
Phone: 1-800-635-2452
www.ameditech.com

Advanced Surgi-Pharm, Inc.
850 Halpern Ave.
Dorval, Quebec
H9P 1G6 Canada
Phone: 1-800-661-5432
www.surgmed.com

Aesculap
3773 Corporate Parkway
Center Valley, PA 18034
Phone: 1-800-282-9000
www.aesculapusa.com

Aesthetic Lasers, Inc.
530 College Parkway
#D
Annapolis, MD 21401
Phone: 1-800-925-5022
www.powerpeel.com

Aesthetic Solutions
651 Canyon Rd.
Novato, CA 94947
Phone: 1-888-345-4569
www.dermaglow.com

Aesthetic Technologies, Inc.
2150 W. Sixth Ave.
Bloomfield, CO 80020
Phone: 1-800-262-4412
www.parisianpeel.com

Ageless Aesthetics
6500 S. Quebec St.
#270
Denver, CO 80122
Phone: 1-877-721-7975
www.agelessaesthetics.com

Agilent Technology (formerly Hewlett-Packard)
5301 Stevens Creek Blvd.
Santa Clara, CA 95051
Phone: 1-405-345-8886
www.home.agilent.com

Aircast, Inc. ([and DonJoy] now owned by DJO)
1430 Decision St.
Vista, CA 92081
Phone: 1-800-336-6569
www.aircast.com or www.djoglobal.com

Air-Tite Products Company
565 Central Dr.
Virginia Beach, VA 23455
Phone: 1-800-231-7762
www.air-tite.shop.com

Akorn Pharmaceuticals
1925 W. Field Ct.
Suite 300
Lake Forest, IL 60045
Phone: 1-800-932-5676
www.akorn.com

Alderm
17951 Sky Park Circle
Suite G
Irvine, CA 92614
Phone: 1-949-250-8955 or 1-800-254-8505
Fax: 1-949-250-8821
www.aldermna.com

AliMed, Inc.
297 High St.
Dedham, MA 02026
Phone: 1-800-225-2610
www.alimed.com

ALK Laboratory
1700 Royston Lane
Round Rock, TX 78664
Phone: 1-800-252-9778

Alkaline Corporation
Allergy Diagnostics Division
714 West Park Ave
P.O. Box 306
Oakhurst, NJ 07755-0306
Phone: 1-800-686-6483

Allegiance Healthcare Corp. (a Cardinal Health company)
7000 Cardinal Pl.
Dublin, OH 43017
Phone: 1-614-757-5000 or 1-800-234-8701
www.cardinal.com

Allergan, Inc.
2525 Dupont Dr.
P.O. Box 19534
Irvine, CA 92623-9534
Phone: 1-800-433-8871 or 1-800-44BOTOX
www.allergan.com
www.botoxcosmetic.com (physician and consumer information)
www.aestheticenhance.org (CME accredited website; injection techniques)

Allergy Laboratories
P.O. Box 26492
Oklahoma City, OK 73126
Phone: 1-405-235-1451

Allermed Laboratories
7203 Convoy Court
San Diego, CA 92111
Phone: 1-800-221-2748
www.allermed.com

Allied Biomedical Corp.
3850 Ramada Dr., C-2
Paso Robles, CA 93446
Phone: 1-800-276-1322
www.alliedbiomedical.com

Allied Healthcare Products, Inc.
1720 Sublette Ave.
St. Louis, MO 63110
Phone: 1-800-444-3940
www.alliedhpi.com

Alma Lasers
485 Half Day Rd.
#100
Buffalo Grove, IL 60089
Phone: 1-866-414-2562
Fax: 1-224-377-2050
www.almalasers.com

Aloka
10 Fairfield Blvd.
Wallingford, CT 06492
Phone: 1-203-269-5088
www.aloka.com

Altair Instruments
321 Aviador St.
Suite 113
Camarillo, CA 93010
Phone: 1-805-388-8503
www.diamondtome.com

American Academy of Dermatology Association
930 North Meacham Rd.
P.O. Box 4014
Schaumburg, IL 60168-4014
Phone: 1-847-330-0230
www.aadassociation.com

American Academy of Family Physicians
11400 Tomahawk Creek Parkway
Leawood, KS 66211-2672
Phone: 1-800-274-2237
www.aafp.org

American Academy of Pediatrics
Division of Publications
141 Northwest Point Blvd.
Elk Grove Village, IL 60007-1098
Phone: 1-847-434-4000
www.aap.org

American College of Obstetricians and Gynecologists
409 12th St., S.W.
P.O. Box 96920
Washington, D.C. 20090-6920
Phone: 1-202-638-5577
www.acog.org

American Medical Systems
10700 Bren Rd. West
Minnetonka, MN 55343
Phone: 1-800-328-3881
www.heroption.com
www.americanmedicalsystems.com

American Social Health Association
P.O. Box 13827
Research Triangle Park, NC 27709
Phone: 1-919-361-8400
www.ashastd.org

American Society for Colposcopy and Cervical Pathology (ASCCP)
152 West Washington St.
Hagerstown, MD 21740
Phone: 1-800-787-7227 or 1-301-733-3640
www.asccp.org

American Society for Gastrointestinal Endoscopy
13 Elm St.
Manchester, MA 01944
Phone: 1-508-526-8330
www.asge.org

American Urological Association
1120 North Charles St.
Baltimore, MD 21201
Phone: 1-800-908-9414
www.auanet.com

Anatometal
411 Ingalls St.
Santa Cruz, CA 95060
Phone: 1-888-262-8663
www.anatometal.com

Angiodynamics
14 Plaza Dr.
Latham, NY 12110
Phone: 1-518-795-1400
Fax: 1-518-795-1401
www.auanet.org

Antigen Laboratories, Inc.
P.O. Box 123
Liberty, MO 64069
Phone: 1-800-821-7013
www.antigenlab.com

APEX Radiology, Inc.
1999 University Dr., Suite 204
Coral Springs, FL 33071
Phone: 1-954-345-1161
Fax: 1-954-345-2262
24-hr. contact: 888-557-3617
info@apexrad.com
www.apexrad.com

Arrow International Inc.
2400 Bernville Rd
Reading, PA 19605
Phone: 1-800-523-8446
www.arrowintl.com

ArthroCare ENT
7500 Rialto Blvd.
Building Two
Suite 100
Austin, TX 78735
Phone: 1-800-797-6520
www.arthrocareent.com

Association for Primary Care Endoscopy
11400 Tomahawk Creek Parkway
Leawood, KS 66211-2672
Phone: 1-913-906-6000, ext: 6706
Fax: 1-913-906-6092
www.aapce.org

Astra Tech Inc.
Urology Division
21535 Hawthorne Blvd.
Suite 525
Torrence, CA 90503
Phone: 1-877-456-3742
www.astratech.us

AstraZeneca L.P.
725 Chesterbrook Blvd.
Wayne, PA 19087
Phone: 1-610-695-1000
www.astrazeneca.com

Atrium Medical Corp.
5 Wentworth Dr.
Hudson, NH 03051
Phone: 1-800-528-7486
www.atriummed.com

Augusta Medical Systems
1027 Broad St.
Augusta, GA 30903
Phone: 1-877-827-8382
www.augustams.com

B. Braun Medical, Inc.
824 12th Ave.
Bethlehem, PA 18018
Phone: 1-800-854-6851
www.bbraunusa.com

B-Met Endoscopic, Inc.
Rte. 5
Box 156
Dallas, PA
Phone: 1-570-255-1288

Banyan International Corp.
P.O. Box 1779
Abilene, TX 79604-1779
Phone: 1-888-STAT-KIT (1-888-782-8548)
www.statkit.com

Bard Access Systems, Inc.
Salt Lake City, UT 84116
Phone: 1-800-545-0890 or 1-801-595-0700
Technical and clinical support: 1-866-893-2691
www.bardaccess.com
medical.services@crbard.com

Bard Medical
8195 Industrial Blvd.
Covington, GA 30014
Phone: 1-800-526-4455
www.bardmedical.com

Barr Pharmaceuticals
223 Quaker Rd.
Pomona, NY 10970
Phone: 1-800-222-4043
www.tevapharm.com

Bartor Pharmacal Co.
70 High St.
Rye, NY 10580
Phone: 1-914-967-4219

Bausch and Lomb
7 Giralda Farms
Suite 1001
Madison, NJ 07940
Phone: 1-877-442-6925 or 1-800-338-2020

Baxter Healthcare Corp.
95 Spring St.
New Providence, NJ 07974
Phone: 1-800-667-0959
www.baxter.com

Bayer Corp.
100 Bayer Road
Pittsburgh, PA 15205-9741
Phone: 1-412-777-2000
http://pharma.bayer.com/

BD Diagnostics
780 Plantation Dr.
Burlington, NC 27215
Phone: 1-336-222-9707 or 1-800-426-2176
Fax: 1-336-222-8819
www.bd.com

Becton, Dickinson and Co.
1 Becton Dr.
Franklin Lakes, NJ 07417
Phone: 1-888-237-2762

Beiersdorf
P.O. Box 5529
Norwalk, CT 06856-5529
Phone: 1-203-853-8008
www.beiersdorf.org

Bella Products, Inc.
27136 Burbank
Foothill Ranch, CA 92610
Phone: 1-877-550-5655
www.bellaproducts.com

Belpro Medical, Inc.
9915 Place York
Anjou, Quebec
Canada H1J 1Z3
Phone: 1-888-230-1010
Fax: 1-514-355-5554
www.belpro.ca

Benson Medical Instruments
310 Fourth Ave. South
Suite 5000
Minneapolis, MN 55415
Phone: 1-612-827-2222
Fax: 1-612-827-2277
www.bensonmedical.com

Bergen Brunswig Medical Corp.
5301 Peoria
Unit B
Denver, CO 80239
Phone: 1-800-411-9022

Berkeley Medevices
1330 South 51st St.
Richmond, CA 94804-4628
Phone: 1-800-227-2388
Fax: 1-510-231-9880
www.berkeleymedevices.com/

Beutlich LP Pharmaceuticals
1541 Shields Dr.
Waukegan, IL 60085
Phone: 1-800-238-8542
www.beutlich.com

Bio-Therapeutic
4822 California Ave., SW
Seattle, WA 98116
Phone: 1-800-976-2544
www.bio-therapeutic.com

BIOCAM GmbH
Friedenstrasse 30
D-93053 Regensburg
Germany
Phone: +49 (0)941-78-53-98-0
www.finde24.de

Biodermis
3078 East Sunset Rd.
Suite 1
Las Vegas, NV 89120
Phone: 1-800-322-3729
www.biodermis.com

Biodynamics Corp.
3511 NE 45th St.
#2
Seattle, WA 98105
Phone: 1-800-869-6987
www.biodyncorp.com

BioForm Medical
1875 South Grant St.
Suite 200
San Mateo, CA 94402
Phone: 1-650-286-4000
Fax: 1-650-286-4090
www.bioform.com

Biolitec
515 Shaker Rd.
East Longmeadow, MA 01028
Phone: 1-800-934-2377
Fax: 1-413-525-0611
www.biolitec.com

BioMedic
4602 East Hammond Lane
Phoenix, AZ 85034
Phone: 1-800-736-5155
www.biomedic.com

BioMedix
4205 White Bear Parkway
St. Paul, MN 55110
Phone: 1-877-854-0012
www.biomedix.com

Bionix Corp.
757 Warehouse Rd.
Toledo, OH 43615
Phone: 1-800-551-7096
www.bionix.com

Biosense Webster
3333 Diamond Canyon Rd.
Diamond Bar, CA 91765
Phone: 1-800-729-9010
www.biosensewebster.com

BioSkin/Cropper Medical
240 E. Hersey St.
Suite 2
Ashland, OR 07520-5201
Phone: 1-800-541-2455
www.bioskin.com

Biosound Esaote, Inc.
8000 Castleway Dr.
Indianapolis, IN 46250
Phone: 1-800-428-4374
www.biosound.com

BioTherapeutics, Education and Research (BTER) Foundation
36 Urey Court
Irvine, CA 92612
Phone: 1-949-509-0989
Fax: 1-949-509-7040

Birtcher Medical Systems, Inc.
1435 Henry Brennan Dr.
#J
El Paso, TX 79936
Phone: 1-915-858-1895

Bivona Medical Technologies
5700 West 23rd Ave.
Gary, IN 46406

Bledsoe, Inc.
2601 Pinewood Dr.
Grand Prairie, TX 75051
Phone: 1-888-253-3763
www.bledsoebrace.com

Body Circle Designs
P.O. Box 68249
Seattle, WA 98168
Phone: 1-800-244-8430
www.bodycircle.com

Body Vision
220 West Fifth St.
Suite 802
Los Angeles, CA 90013
Phone: 1-888-991-2639
www.bodyvision.net

Boston Medical Products
117 Flanders Rd.
Westborough, MA 10581
Phone: 1-508-898-9300
www.bosmed.com

Boston Scientific
One Boston Scientific Place
Natick, MA 01760-1537
Phone: 1-508-650-8000
www.bostonscientific.com

Bovie Medical Corporation
7100 30th Ave.
N. St. Petersburg, FL 33710
Phone: 1-800-537-2790
www.boviemedical.com

Braintree Laboratories
60 W. Columbian St.
Braintree, MA 02185
Phone: 1-800-874-6756
www.braintreelabs.com

Breg, Inc.
2611 Commerce Way
Vista, CA 92081
Phone: 1-800-897-2734
www.breg.com

Briggs Corporation (Hollister Global)
P.O. Box 1698
Des Moines, IA 50306-1698
Phone: 1-877-307-1744
www.briggscorp.com/Hollister

Brymill Cryogenic Systems
105 Windmere Ave.
Ellington, CT 06029
Phone: 1-860-875-2460
www.brymill.com

BSN-Jobst Institute, Inc.
Rutherford College
100 Beiersdorf Dr.
P.O. Box 390
Rutherford College, NC 28671
Phone: 1-828-879-5100
www.jobst.com

Burton Medical Products
21100 Lassen St.
Chatsworth, CA 91311
Phone: 1-800-444-9909
Fax: 1-800-765-1770
www.burtonmedical.com

Byron Medical
602 West Rillito
Tucson, AZ 85705
Phone: 1-800-777-3434
www.mentorcorp.com

Candela Corp./Candela Lasers
530 Boston Post Rd.
Wayland, MA 01778
Phone: 1-508-358-7637 or 1-800-733-8550
Fax: 1-508-358-5602
www.clzr.com
www.candelalaser.com

Cardiac Science (from merger of Burdick and Quinton Instrument Co.)
3303 Monte Villa Parkway
Bothell, WA 98021
Phone: 1-800-426-0337
www.cardiacscience.com

Cardinal Health
7000 Cardinal Place
Dublin, OH 43017
Phone: 1-800-964-5227
www.cardinal.com

CareFusion
3750 Torrey View Court
San Diego, CA 92130
Phone: 1-858-617-2000 or 1-888-876-4287
Fax: 1-858-617-2900
www.carefusion.com

Carl Zeiss Surgical, Inc.
5160 Hacienda Dr.
Dublin, CA 94568
Phone: 1-925-557-4100
www.zeiss.com

Carolon Health Care Products
601 Forum Parkway
Rural Hall, NC 27045
Phone: 1-800-334-0414
Contact: Info@carolon.com
www.carolon.com

Castle Group
Scarborough Business Park
Salter Road
Scarborough
North Yorkshire YO11 3UZ
United Kingdom
Phone: +44 (0)1723 584250
Fax: +44 (0)1723 583728
Contact: enquiries@castlegroup.co.uk
www.castlegroup.co.uk

Center Laboratories
35 Channel Dr.
Port Washington, NY 11050-2216
Phone: 1-800-223-6837

Cetylite Industries, Inc.
9051 River Rd.
Pennsauken, NJ 08110
Phone: 1-800-257-7740
www.cetylite.com

Dr. Charles Wilson
The Vasectomy Clinic
5402 47th Ave. NE
Seattle, WA 98105
Phone: 1-206-525-4090
www.thevasectomyclinic.com

Chattanooga Group, Inc.
4717 Adams Rd.
Hixson, TN 37343
Phone: 1-800-592-7329
www.chattgroup.com

Cheshire Medical Specialties, Inc.
P.O. Box 894
Cheshire, CT 06410
Phone: 1-800-243-3020 or 1-203-272-1364
Fax: 1-203-250-0557
Contact: chesmed@cheshire-medical.com
www.cheshire-medical.com

Claflin Medical Equipment
1206 Jefferson Blvd.
Warwick, RI 02886
1-800-338-2372
1-401-732-9150
www.claflinequip.com

Clarion Medical
125 Fleming Dr.
Cambridge, Ontario
Canada N1T 2B8
Phone: 1-519-620-3900 or 1-800-668-5236
Fax: 1-519-621-0313 or 1-866-320-7287 (orders)
www.clarionmedical.com

Clinical Innovations, Inc.
747 W. 4170 South
Murray, UT 84123
Phone: 1-888-268-6222 (main) or 1-801-268-8200
clinicalinnovations.com

CNexGen Lasers, Inc.
112 Commerce Park Dr.
Units D & E
Barrie, Ontario
Canada L4N 8W8
Phone: 1-888-527-3711
Fax: 1-705-719-1658
www.nexgenlasers.com

Colin Medical (Omron)
5859 Farinon Dr.
San Antonio, TX 78249
Phone: 1-800-829-6427
www.colinmedical.com/

College Pharmacy
3505 Austin Bluffs Parkway
Colorado Springs, CO 80907
Phone: 1-800-888-9358
www.collegepharmacy.com

Coloplast Corporation (formerly Mentor Corporation)
200 South 6th St.
Suite 900
Minneapolis, MN 55402
www.coloplast.com
Phone: 1-800-533-0464

Commonwealth Medical Laboratories
11150 Main St.
Suite 550
Fairfax, VA 22030
Phone: 1-800-222-5775
www.allergytest.com

Conceptus, Inc.
331 E. Evelyn Ave.
Mountain View, CA 94041
Phone: 1-650-962-4000 (main) or 1-877-377-8732 (orders/training/support)
Fax: 1-650-962-5200
www.essuremd.com

ConMed
525 French Rd.
Utica, NY 13402
Phone: 1-800-448-6505
www.conmed.com

Contemporary Health Communications
16714 Benton Taylor Dr.
Chesterfield, MO 63005
Phone: 1-800-234-1742

Convatec (division of Bristol-Myers Squibb)
P.O. Box 5254
Princeton, NJ 08543-5254
Phone: 1-800-422-8811
www.convatec.com

Cook, Inc.
925 South Curry Pike
P.O. Box 489
Bloomington, IN 47402-0489
Phone: 1-800-457-4500
www.cookcriticalcare.com

Cook Medical
P.O. Box 4195
Bloomington, IN 47402
Phone: 1-800-457-4500
www.cookmedical.com

Cook Women's Health
1100 West Morgan St.
P.O. Box 271
Spencer, IN 47460
Phone: 1-800-541-5591
Fax: 1-812-829-2022
www.cookmedical.com

Cooley and Cooley
8550 Westland West Blvd.
Houston, TX 77041
Phone: 1-800-215-4487
www.copalite.com

CoolTouch
Roseville, CA
www.cooltouch.com

CooperSurgical
95 Corporate Dr.
Trumball, CT 06611
Phone: 1-800-243-2974
www.coopersurgical.com

Corpak MedSystems/VIASYS Healthcare/Cardinal Healthcare
100 Chaddick Dr.
Wheeling, IL 60090
Phone: 1-800-323-6305
www.viasyshealthcare.com

Corthel, Inc.
2107 Emmorton Park Rd.
Suite 105
Edgewood, MD 21040
Phone: 1-410-612-9440
www.corthel.com

Cosmetic R & D
4125 Pine Crest Ct.
Rocklin, CA 95677
Phone: 1-916-632-9134
www.dermasweep.com

Cosmos Medical Technology, Inc.
42230 Zevo Dr.
Temecula, CA 92590
Phone: 1-800-634-7921

Covidien
6135 Gunbarrel Ave.
Boulder, CO 80301
Phone: 1-800-NELLCOR
respiratorysolutions.covidien.com

Creative Health Communications
4675 South Portsmouth Rd.
Bridgeport, MI 48722
Phone: 1-989-777-8485
www.creativehealthcommunications.com

CryoPen LLC
800 North Shoreline
Suite 900
Corpus Christi, TX 78401
Phone: 1-361-888-7708
www.cryopen.com

CryoSurgery, Inc.
5829 Old Harding Rd.
Nashville, TN 37205
Phone: 1-800-729-1624
www.cryosurgeryinc.com

Curetteblade, Inc.
194 Mayfair Dr.
Pittsburgh, PA 15228-1145
Phone: 1-866-curette (287-3883) or 1-412-563-4121
Fax: 1-412-563-4520
info@curetteblade.com

Custom Scripts Pharmacy
4600 North Habana Ave.
Tampa, FL 33614
Phone: 1-800-226-7094
www.custom-rx.com; rx@custom-rx.com

Custom Steel
13 Custom Steel Dr.
Paguate, NM 87040
Phone: 1-800-877-5855
www.customsteel.com

Cutera
3240 Bayshore Blvd.
Brisbane, CA 94005
Phone: 1-888-4-CUTERA or 1-415-657-5500
Fax: 1-415-330-2444
www.cutera.com

Cynosure Inc.
5 Carlisle Rd.
Westford, MA 01886
Phone: 1-978-256-4200
www.cynosure.com

CYTYC Corp.
250 Campus Dr.
Marlborough, MA 01752
Phone: 1-800-442-9892
Fax: 1-508-229-2860
www.hologic.com

Davol, Inc.
100 Sockanossett Crossroad
P.O. Box 8500
Cranston, RI 02920
Phone: 1-401-463-7000
www.davol.com

Delasco Dermatologic Lab and Supply Co.
608 13th Ave.
Council Bluffs, IA 57501-6401
Phone: 1-800-831-6273
www.delasco.com

Dentsply International
Susquehanna Commerce Center
221 W. Philadelphia St.
York, PA 17405
Phone: 1-800-877-0020
www.dentsply.com

DermaMed, Inc.
394 Parkmount Rd.
P.O. Box 198
Lenni, PA 19052-0198
Phone: 1-877-789-MEGA
www.megapeel.com

Dermatology Lab & Supply, Inc. (Delasco)
608 13th Ave.
Council Bluffs, IA 51501-6401
Phone: 1-800-831-6273 or 1-712-323-3269
Fax: 1-800-320-9612 or 1-712-323-1156
Contact: questions@delasco.com
www.delasco.com

Dey, LP
2751 Napa Valley Corporate Dr.
Napa, CA 94558
Phone: 1-707-224-3200
http://www.epipen.com/

Diamond Medical Aesthetics
One Madison St.
Bldg. C
East Rutherford, NJ 07073
Phone: 1-877-754-6749

Diomed
1 Dundee Park Dr.
Ste. 4
Andover, MA 01810
Phone: 1-978-475-1089
venacure-evlt.com

dj Orthopedics
1430 Decision St.
Vista, CA 92081
Phone: 1-800-321-9549
www.donjoy.com

Duramed Pharmaceuticals, Inc.
223 Quaker Rd.
Pomona, NY 10970
Phone: 1-800-222-0190
www.paragardiud.com

Dusa Pharmaceuticals Inc.
25 Upton Dr.
Wilmington, MA 01887
Phone: 1-877-533- DUSA (3872)
www.dusapharma.com

Dynatronics
7030 Park Centre Dr.
Salt Lake City, UT 84121
Phone: 1-800-874-6251
www.dynatronics.com

DynaWave Corporation
2520 Kaneville Ct.
Geneva, IL 60134
Phone: 1-630-232-4945
my.inil.com/~dynawave/

Eclipse, Ltd.
16850 Dallas Parkway
Dallas, TX 75248
Phone: 1-972-380-2911 or 1-800-759-6876
Fax: 1-972-380-2953
Contact: sales@eclipsemed.com
www.eclipsemed.com

Edge Systems
2277 Redondo Ave.
Signal Hill, CA 90755
Phone: 1-800-603-4996
www.edgesystem.net

Edwards Life Sciences Corp (formerly a division of Baxter; closed needle-less sampling systems)
One Edwards Way
Irvine, CA 92614
Phone: 1-800-424-3278
www.edwards.com

Electro-Med Health Industries
11601 Biscayne Blvd.
Suite 200-A
North Miami, FL 33181
Phone: 1-800-232-3644

Ellman International
3333 Royal Ave.
Oceanside, NY 11572
Phone: 1-800-835-5355
www.ellman.com

EMPI, Inc.
599 Cardigan Rd.
St. Paul, MN 55126-4099
Phone: 1-888-FOR-EMPI
www.empi.com

Endoscopy Support Services, Inc.
3 Fallsview Lane
Brewster, NY 10509
Phone: 1-800-349-3636
www.endoscopy.com

EngenderHealth
440 Ninth Ave.
New York, NY 10001
Phone: 1-212-561-8000
www.engenderhealth.org

Envy Medical, Inc. (formerly Emed, Inc.)
31340 Via Colinas
Suite 101
Westlake Village, CA 91362
Phone: 1-888-848-3633
www.silkpeel.com

ERBE USA, Inc.
2225 Northwest Parkway
Marietta, GA 30067
Phone: 1-800-778-3723

Ethicon, Inc.
Hwy. 22
P.O. Box 151
Somerville, NJ 08876-0151
Phone: 1-800-438-4426 or 1-908-218-0707
www.ethiconinc.com

Ethicon Endo-Surgery, Inc. (Johnson and Johnson)
4545 Creek Rd.
Cincinnati, OH 45242
Phone: 1-800-USE-ENDO
www.jnjgateway.com (video available)

Ethox Corp.
251 Seneca St.
Buffalo, NY 14204
Phone: 1-800-521-1022
www.ethoxcorp.com

Everything Birth, Inc.
P.O. Box 66781
Falmouth, ME 04105
Phone: 1-800-370-1683
www.midwifesupplies.com

Feet Relief
1032 Irving St.
PMB 507
San Francisco, CA 94122-2200
Phone: 1-888-671-8027
www.feetrelief.com

Fem Cap
14058 Mira Montana Dr.
Del Mar, CA 92014
Phone: 858-922-7673
Fax: 858-792-2624
contact@femcap.com
www.femcap.com

Female Health Company
919 N. Michigan Ave.
Suite 2208
Chicago, IL 60611
Phone: 1-312-280-2201
Fax: 1-312-280-9360
www.femalehealth.com

FLA Orthopedics
2881 Corporate Way
Miramar, FL 33025
Phone: 1-800-327-4110
www.flaorthopedics.com

Focus Medical, LLC
23 Francis J. Clark Cir.
Bethel, CT 06801
Phone: 1-866-633-5273
www.focusmedical.com

Foot Smart
5250 Triangle Parkway
Suite 200
Norcross, GA 30092
Phone: 1-800-707-9928
www.footsmart.com

Fredericks–Jobst Institute Inc.
P.O. Box 653
Toledo, OH 43697-0653

Fujinon Medical
10 High Point Dr.
Wayne, NJ 07470
Phone: 1-800-490-0661
www.fujinon.com

Futrex Inc.
6 Montgomery Village Ave.
#620
Gaithersburg, MD 20879
Phone: 1-800-255-4206
www.futrex.com

GC America, Inc.
3737 W. 127th
Alsip, IL 60803
Phone: 1-800-323-7063

GE Healthcare
3000 N. Grandview
Waukesha, WI 53188
www.gehealthcare.com/usen/cardiology/diagnostic_ecg/products/amb_centerpg.html

General Electric Medical Systems and General Electric Healthcare
800 Centennial Ave.
P.O. Box 1327
Piscataway, NJ 08855-1327
Phone: 1-800-526-3593
www.gemedicalsystems.com
www.gehealthcare.com

Genesis Biosystems
1500 Eagle Ct.
Lewisville, TX 75057
Phone: 1-888-577-7335
www.dermagenesis.com

Genzyme Biosurgery
64 Sidney St.
Cambridge, MA 02142
Phone: 1-800-232-7546
www.genzyme.com/business/biosurgery/burn/burn_home.asp

George Tiemann and Co.
25 Plant Ave.
Hauppauge, NY 11788-3804
Phone: 1-800-843-6266
www.georgetiemann.com

Gieserlab Equipment and Supply
P.O. Box 659
Chestertown, MD 21620
Phone: 1-888-778-7829
www.gieserlab.com

Gill Podiatry Supply and Equipment
22400 Acoa Ct.
Strongsville, OH 44149-4766
Phone: 1-800-432-9445
www.gillpodiatry.com

Gordon Stowe
Phone: 1-800-323-4371
www.gordonstowe.com

GPT Glendale, Inc.
5300 Region Ct.
Lakeland, FL 33815
Phone: 1-800-500-4739

Graham-Field, Inc.
400 Rabro Dr.
East Hauppauge, NY 11788
Phone: 1-516-582-5900

Grason-Stadler, Inc.
7625 Golden Triangle Dr.
Suite F
Eden Prairie, MN 55344
Phone: 1-800-700 2282 (U.S.) or +1 952-278 4402 (international)
Fax: +1 952-278 4401
Contact: info@grason-stadler.com
www.grasonstadler.com

Greer Laboratories, Inc.
P.O. Box 800
639 Nuway Cir.
Lenoir, NC 28645-0088
Phone: 1-800-438-0088

Gulden Ophthalmics
225 Cadwalader Ave.
Elkins Park, PA 19027
Phone: 1-800-659-2250
www.guldenophthalmics.com

Gynecare, Inc. (Division of Ethicon, Inc.)
P.O. Box 151
Somerville, NJ 08876-0151
Phone: 1-888-496-3227
www.gynecare.com
Instructional: www.interact3d.com/modules/

Gyne-Tech Instrument Corp.
2819 Burton St.
Burbank, CA 91504
Phone: 1-818-842-0933

Gynex
2789 152nd Ave. NE
Redmond, WA 98052
Phone: 1-888-486-4644 or 1-800-220-5988
Fax: 1-425-895-0115
service@gynex.com

Gyrus ACMI Corporation (Olympus)
136 Turnpike Rd.
Southborough, MA 01772
Phone: 1-800-852-9361
www.circoncorp.com

Haag-Streit
3535 Kings Mills Rd.
Mason, OH 45040
Phone: 1-866-417-3802
www.haag-streit-usa.com

Hardwood Products Co.
P.O. Box 149
Guilford, ME 04443
Phone: 1-800-321-2313
www.hwppuritan.com

Hardy Diagnostics
1430 West McCoy Ln.
Santa Maria, CA 93455
Phone: 1-805-346-2766 or 1-800-266-2222
Fax: 1-805-346-2760
www.HardyDiagnostics.com

Health Sciences Center for Educational Resources University of Washington
P.O. Box 357161
T-252 Health Sciences Bldg.
Seattle, WA 98195-7161
Phone: 1-206-685-1158
www.hscer.washington.edu/hscer

Heine USA
1 Washington St.
Suite 555
Dover, NH 03820-3851
Phone: 1-800-367-4872
www.heine.com

Hely & Weber
P.O. Box 832
Santa Paula, CA 93061-0832
Phone: 1-800-654-3241
www.hely-weber.com

HemCon Medical Technologies, Inc.
10575 SW Cascade Ave.
Suite 130
Portland, OR 97223-4363
Phone: 1-503-245-0459
Fax: 1-503-245-1326
www.hemcon.com

Henry Schein Dental
135 Duryea Rd.
Melville, NY 11747
Phone: 1-631-843-5500 or 1-800-372-4346
www.henryscheindental.com

Hitachi Medical Corp.
1959 Summit Commerce Park
Twinsburg, OH 44087
Phone: 1-800-800-3106
www.hitachiultrasound.com

Hollister-Stier Labs
3525 North Regal
Spokane, WA 99220-3145

HOYA Conbio
http://www.conbio.com

HPSRx Enterprises, Inc. (Ipas distributor)
3229 Brandon Ave.
Suite 2
Roanoke, VA 24018
Phone: 1-800-850-1657
Fax: 1-800-361-6984
www.hpsrx.com

Hull Anesthesia, Inc.
7521 Talbert Ave.
Huntington Beach, CA 92648
Phone: 1-800-400-4484
Fax: 1-714-375-2658
www.hullanesthesia.com

Huot Instruments LLC (Wittenberg VisiPunch and ElliptiPunch)
N50 W13740 Overview Dr.
Suite A
Menomonee Falls, WI 53051
Phone: 1-262-373-1700 or 1-866-212-8466
Fax: 1-262-373-1800
info@huotinstruments.com or Cust.Service@HuotInstruments.com
www.huotinstruments.com/

Hy-Tape International
P.O. Box 540
Patterson, NY 12563-0540
Phone: 1-800-248-0101
www.hytape.com

ImageDerm
3032 Dolores St.
Los Angeles, CA 90065
Phone: 1-818-500-9034
imagederm.com

Industrial Strength
1945 Martin Luther King, Jr. Way
Berkeley, CA 94704
Phone: 1-510-644-0968
www.isbodyjewelry.com

Inhealth Industries
1110 Mark Ave.
Carpinteria, CA 93013-2918
Phone: 1-800-477-5968
www.inhealth.com

Innovative Med, Inc.
4 Autry
Suite B
Irvine, CA 92618
Phone: 1-877-779-9492
www.imibeauty.com

Instromedix
6779 Mesa Ridge Rd.
Suite 200
San Diego, CA 92121
1-800-633-3361
www.lifewatch.com

Instrument Specialists, Inc.
32390 IH-10
West Boerne, TX 78006-9214
Phone: 1-800-537-1945
www.isisurgery.com/

Integra LifeSciences Corp.
311 Enterprise Dr.
Plainsboro, NJ 08538
Phone: 1-877-444-1122 or 1-609-275-9004
www.integraskin.com

Integrated Medical Systems, Inc.
1823 27th Ave. South
Birmingham, AL 35209
Phone: 1-800-783-9251
www.imsready.com

Interstitial Cystitis Association (ICA) National
100 Park Ave.
Suite 108A
Rockville, MD 20850
Phone: 800-HELP-ICA (1-800-435-7422)
Fax: 1-301-610-5308
ICAmail@ichelp.org
www.ichelp.org

Interstitial Cystitis Network (ICN) National (A Division of J.H. Osborne, Inc.)
P.O. Box 2159
Healdsburg, CA 95448
Phone: 1-707-433-0413 (orders) or 1-707-538-9442 (patient assistance)
www.ic-network.com

IOMED, Inc.
Phone: 1-800-621-3347
www.seeiomed.com

Ipas
300 Market St.
Suite 200
Chapel Hill, NC 27516
Phone: 1-919-960-6453
Fax: 1-919-929-7687
www.ipas.org
customerservice@ipas.org

IQDr. Inc.
34 Sandra Ln.
Manitou Springs, CO 80829
Phone: 1-800-747-3184
www.iqdr.com

Iridex
1212 Terra Bella Ave.
Mountain View, CA 94043
Phone: 1-650-940-4700
Fax: 1-650-940-4710
www.iridex.com

Jobst/BSN Medical
5825 Carnegie Blvd.
Charlotte, NC 28209
Phone: 1-800-552-1157
www.bsnmedical.com

Johnson & Johnson Professional, Inc. (extra-fast-setting casting splints available)
325 Paramount Dr.
Raynham, MA 02767-0350
Phone: 1-800-526-2459
www.jandj.com/connect

Juzo (Julius Zorn), Inc.
3690 Zorn Dr.
P.O. Box 1088
Cuyahoga Falls, OH 44223
Phone: 1-800-222-4999
www.juzo.com

Karl Storz Endoscopy-America, Inc.
600 Corporate Pointe
Culver City, CA 90230-7600
Phone: 1-800-421-0837
www.karlstorz.com

Kendall Healthcare Products
15 Hampshire St.
Mansfield, MA 02048
Phone: 1-800-962-9888
www.kendallhq.com

Keystone Pharmacy (Compounding Pharmacy)
4021 Cascade Rd. SE
Grand Rapids, MI 49546
Phone: 1-616-974-9792
www.keystonerx.com

Kimberly-Clark/Ballard Medical Products
12050 Lone Peak Parkway
Draper, UT 84020
Phone: 1-800-528-5591
www.kchealthcare.com

Krames Communications
1100 Grundy Ln.
San Bruno, CA 94066
Phone: 1-800-333-3032
www.krames.com

LabCorp
358 South Main St.
Burlington, NC 27215
Phone: 1-336-584-5171
www.labcorp.com

Laborie Medical Technologies
400 Avenue D
Suite 10
Williston, VT 05495
Phone: 1-800-522-6743
www.laborie.com

Langer Biomechanics (purchased Benefoot Inc.)
450 Commack Rd.
Deer Park, NY 11729
Phone: 1-800-645-5520
www.langerbiomechanics.com

LASERING USA
2246 Camino Ramon
San Ramon, CA 94583
Phone: 1-866-471-0469
Contact: info@laseringusa.com
www.laseringusa.com

Levin, Salem (sump and feeding tubes; Bard Medical Division)
8195 Industrial Blvd.
Covington, GA 30014
Phone: 1-800-526-4455
www.bardmedical.com

Lhasa Medical, Inc.
539 Accord Station
Accord, MA 02018-0539
Phone: 1-800-722-8775
www.lhasamedical.com

LifeCell Corporation
One Millennium Way
Branchburg, NJ 08876-3876
Phone: 1-908-947-1100
www.lifecell.com

Lifesource Medical (A & D Medical)
1756 Automation Parkway
San Jose, CA 95131
Phone: 1-888-726-9966
www.lifesource.com

Life-Tech, Inc.
4235 Greenbriar Dr.
Stafford, TX 77477-3995
Phone: 1-281-491-6600
www.life-tech.com

Lincoln Diagnostics
P.O. Box 1128
Decatur, IL 62525
Phone: 1-800-537-1336
www.lincolndiagnostics.com

LPG
10800 Biscayne Blvd.
Suite 850
Miami, FL 33131
Phone: 1-305-892-4588
Fax: 1-305-892-4589
www.endermologie.com

Lumenis (formerly ESC Medical Systems)
100 Morse St.
Norwood, MA 02062
Phone: 1-800-562-5916
www.lumenis.com

Lutronic
51 Everett Dr.
Unit A-50
Princeton Junction, NJ 08550
Phone: 1-888-588-7644
Fax: 1-609-275-3800
Contact: officeusa@lutronic.com
www.lutronic.com

Luxtec
99 Hartwell St.
West Boylston, MA 01583
Phone: 1-800-325-8966
www.luxtec.com

MADA Medical Products
625 Washington Ave.
Carlstadt, NJ 07072
Phone: 1-800-526-6370
www.madamedical.com

Madsen (product)
GN Otometrics A/S
Dybendalsvænget 2
DK-2630 Taastrup
Denmark
Phone: +45 45 75 55 55 or 1-800-777-4130 (U.S.)
Fax: +45 45 75 55 59
Contact: info@gnotometrics.dk
www.otometrics.com

Maico Diagnostics
2545 Chicago Ave.
Minneapolis, MN
Phone: 1-888-941-4201 or 1-952-941-4200
www.maico-diagnostics.com

Mallinckrodt
675 McDonnell Blvd.
Hazelwood, MO 63042
Phone: 1-800-635-5267
www.mallinckrodt.com/respiratory/resp/index.html

Maquet Critical Care AB
SE-171 95 SOLNA
Sweden
Phone: +46-8-730-73-00
www.maquet.com/criticalcare

Marina Medical
955 Shotgun Rd.
Sunrise, FL 33326
Phone: 1-954-924-4418 or 1-800-697-1119
Fax: 1-954-924-4419 or 1-800-748-2089

Matlock Endoscopic
2969 Armory Dr.
Suite 400
Nashville, TN 37204
Phone: 1-800-394-9822
www.matlockendo.com

Mattioli Engineering
4200 Wilson Blvd.
Suite 750
Arlington, VA 22203
Phone: 1-877-628-8364
www.mattiolienginering.com

McDavid Sports Medical Products
10305 Argonne Dr.
Woodridge, IL 60517
Phone: 1-800-237-8254
www.mcdavidinc.com or www.mcdavidusa.com

Med-Aesthetic Solutions
2033 San Elijo Ave.
Suite 200
Cardiff-by-the-Sea, CA 92007
Phone: 1-760-942-8815
www.medaestheticsolutions.com

MedaSonics (CooperSurgical)
95 Corporate Dr.
Trumbull, CT 06611
Phone: 1-800-243-2974
www.coopersurgical.com

Medco Supply Company
500 Fillmore Ave.
Tonawanda, NY 14150
Phone: 1-800-556-3326
www.medco-athletics.com

MedGyn
328 N. Eisenhower Ln.
Lombard, IL 60148
Phone: 1-630-627-4105
Toll-free: 1-800-451-9667
Fax: 1-630-627-0127
www.medgyn.com
medgyn@medgyn.com

Medical Graphics
350 Oak Grove Parkway
St. Paul, MN 55127
Phone: 1-800-950-5597
www.medgraph.com

Medical Optics
559 Sawgrass Corporate Parkway
Sunrise, FL 33325
Phone: 1-800-286-9542
www.medicaloptics.com

Medical Replacement Parts LLC
6302 Manatee Ave. West
Suite F1
Bradenton, FL 34209
Phone: 1-800-363-6726
www.endoscopepartsplus.com

Medicis Aesthetics Inc.
7720 North Dobson Rd.
Scottsdale, AZ 85256
Phone: 1-866-222-1480
www.dysportusa.com

Medison America, Inc.
11075 Knott Ave.
Suite C
Cypress, CA 90630
Phone: 1-800-829-7666
www.medisonusa.com

MediUSA
6481 Franz Warner Parkway
Whitsett, NC 27377
Phone: 1-800-633-6334
www.mediusa.com

MedSurge Advances, Inc.
14850 Quorum Dr.
Suite 120
Dallas, TX 75254
Phone: 1-972-720-0425
www.medsurgeadvances.com

MedTech International
P.O. Box 162992
Altamonte Springs, FL 32716-2992
Phone: 1-800-447-0014

Medtronic
710 Medtronic Parkway NE
Minneapolis, MN 55432-5604
Phone: 1-800-633-8766 or 1-800-505-4636 (bradyarrhythmia products)
www.medtronic.com

Medtronic Functional Diagnostics
3850 Victoria St. North
MS V215
Shoreview, MN 55126-2978
Phone: 1-612-514-1700
www.medtronic.com

Medtronic Xomed Surgical Products, Inc.
6743 Southpoint Dr. North
Jacksonville, FL 32216-0980
Phone: 1-800-874-5797
www.medtronic.com

Merz Pharmaceuticals
4215 Tudor Ln.
Greensboro, NC 27410
Phone: 1-888-925-8989
www.mederma.com

Micro Audiometrics
655 Keller Road
Murphy, NC 28906
Phone (toll-free): 1-866-EARSCAN (327-7226) or 1-800-729-9509
Phone: 1-828-644-0771
Fax: 1-866-683-4447
www.microaudiometrics.com

Micro Bio-Medics
846 Pelham Parkway
Pelham Manor, NY 10803
Phone: 1-800-431-2743
www.microbiomedics.com

Micro-Imaging Solutions, Inc.
6400 S. Fiddlers Green Circle
Suite 1840
Englewood, CO 80111
Phone: 303-221-3677, ext. 2
www.micro-imaging.us

Microsulis
Parklands Business Park
Denmead, Hampshire
United Kingdom P07 6XP
Phone: +44(0)-2392-240011
www.microsulis.com

Miga Systems
3500 N. Holly Ln.
Suite 40
Plymouth, MN 55447
Phone: 1-800-913-6442
www.miga.com

Miles Inc. (Pharmaceutical Division)
1127 Myrtle St.
Elkhart, IN 46514
Phone: 1-800-800-4793

Milex Products, Inc.
4311 N. Normandy
Chicago, IL 60634
Phone: 1-800-621-1278
Fax: 1-800-972-0696
www.milexproducts.com

Miltex, Inc.
700 Hicksville Rd.
Bethpage, NY 11714-3490
Phone: 1-800-645-8000
www.miltex.com

Mindray DP-6600
8650 154th Ave. NE
Redmond, WA 98052
Phone: 1-888-816-8188
www.mindray.com

Minogue Medical
180 W. Dundas St.
Toronto, Ontario
Canada M5G 1Z8

MJD Patient Communications
4641 Montgomery Ave.
Suite 350
Bethesda, MD 20814
Phone: 1-301-657-8010
www.mjdpc.com

Mobile Instrument Service
333 Water Ave.
Bellefontaine, OH 43311
Phone: 1-800-722-3675
www.mobileinstrument.com

Mogen Instrument Co.
437 Crown St.
Brooklyn, NY 11225
Phone: 1-718-604-8833

Monarch Labs
17875 Sky Park Cr.
Suite K
Irvine, CA 92614
Phone: 1-949-679-3000
Fax: 1-949-679-3001

Moore Medical Corp
1690 New Britain Ave.
P.O. Box 4067
Farmington, CT 06032-4067
Phone: 1-800-234-1464
www.mooremedical.com

Mormac TubeGuard
P.O. Box 40
North Loup, NE 68859-0040
Phone: 1-800-445-2868
Fax: 1-308-496-4786

Mortara
7865 N. 86th St.
Milwaukee, WI 53224
Phone: 1-800-231-7437
www.mortara.com

M-Pact (now owned by Jobst/BSN Medical)
5825 Carnegie Blvd.
Charlotte, NC 28209
Phone: 1-800-537-1063
www.m-pactmed.com or www.jobst.com

MRT Laboratories
50 Johnson Ave.
Hackensack, NJ 07601
Phone: 1-800-631-1379
www.mrtlabs.com

Myfootshop.com
1159 Cherry Valley Rd.
Newark, OH 43055
Phone: 1-888-859-8901
www.myfootshop.com

Nasostat Gottschalk
Los Angeles, CA 90049
Phone: 1-310-207-1445
www.nasostat.com

The National Procedures Institute (NPI)
12012 Technology Blvd.
Suite 200
Austin, TX 78727
Phone: 1-866-NIP-CME1 or 1-512-870-8051
Fax: 1-512-329-0442
Contact: Info@npinstitute.com
www.npinstitute.com

Natus Medical, Inc.
Corporate Headquarters
1501 Industrial Rd.
San Carlos, CA 94070
Phone: 1-800-255-3901
www.natus.com

Nellcor (product)
Covidien
6135 Gunbarrel Ave.
Boulder, CO 80301
Phone: 1-800-NELLCOR
respiratorysolutions.covidien.com

NEUROMetrix, Inc.
62 Fourth Ave.
Waltham, MA 02451
Phone (general assistance): 1-781-890-9989
Toll-free (customer service): 1-888-786-7287
www.neurometrix.com

Newport Cosmeceuticals, Inc.
Newport Beach, CA 92660
Phone: 1-949-955-DERM (3376)
Fax: 1-949-955-0977
www.nciskincare.com

NG Strip (Cardinal Health)
7000 Cardinal Place
Dublin, OH 43017
Phone: 1-800-323-9088
www.cardinal.com

Nighthawk Radiology Services
601 Front Ave.
Suite 502
Coeur d'Alene, ID 83814
Phone: 1-866-400-4295
Fax: 1-208-664-2720
www.nighthawkrad.net

Norscam
Phone: 1-800-376-3541
www.laminaria.net

Northern Optotronics, Inc
151 Savage Dr.
Unit 2
Cambridge, Ontario
Canada N1T 1S4
Phone: 1-519-621-2666
dcraig@noi.ca
www.noi.ca

Nova Medical Systems Corp.
4101 Southwest 47th Ave.
Suite 105
Ft. Lauderdale, FL 33314
Phone: 1-954-581-3616
www.medicalsystems.com

Nuell, Inc.
P.O. Box 55
Warsaw, IN 46581-0055
Phone: 1-800-829-7694
www.nuell.com

OBP Medical, Inc.
360 Merrimack St.
Lawrence, MA 01843
Phone: 1-888-257-9253
www.obpmedical.com

Olympic Medical Corp. (Natus)
5900 First Ave. South
Seattle, WA 98108
Phone: 1-800-426-0353
www.natus.com

Olympus America Inc.
3500 Corporate Parkway
P.O. Box 610
Center Valley, PA 11747
Phone: 1-800-848-9024
Medical Instrument Division
8370 Dow Circle
Strongsville, OH 44136
Phone: 1-800-627-6264
www.olympusamerica.com

OMS Medical Supplies
1950 Washington St.
Braintree, MA 02184
Phone: 1-800-323-1839
www.omsmedical.com

OraSure Technologies
220 E. First St.
Bethlehem, PA 18015
Phone: 1-800-869-3538
www.orasure.com

Organon Teknika Corp.
100 Rodolphe St.
Durham, NC 27712
Phone: 1-800-682-2666
www.biomerieux-usa.com

Ortho-McNeil Janssen Scientific Affairs, LLC/Ortho-McNeil Janssen Pharmaceuticals
Customer Communications Center
1125 Trenton-Harbourton Rd.
P.O. Box 200
Titusville, NJ 08560-200
Phone: 1-800-526-7736
www.ortho-mcneil.com
www.thepill.com

Össur
2741 Aliso Viejo Parkway
Aliso Viejo, CA 92656
Phone: 1-800-233-6263
www.ossur.com

Otometrics
Phone: 1-800-289-2150
www.otometrics.com

Overread
Pleasanton, CA
Phone: 1-925-426-3111

Paddock Laboratories
3940 Quebec Ave.
Minneapolis, MN 55427
Phone: 1-800-328-5113
www.paddocklabs.com

Padgett Instruments, Inc.
1520 Grand St.
Kansas City, MO 64108-1404
Phone: 1-800-842-1029

Palomar Medical Technologies, Inc.
82 Cambridge St.
Burlington, MA 01803
Phone: 1-781-993-2300
Toll-free: 1-800-PALOMAR (725-6627)
Fax: 1-781-993-2330
www.palomarmedical.com

Palumbo Orthopedics
8206 Leesburg Pike
Suite 402
Vienna, VA 22182
Phone: 1-800-292-7223
www.palumbobraces.com

Parks Medical Electronics
19460 SW Shaw
Aloha, OR 97006
Phone: 1-800-547-6427
www.parksmed.com

Path Scientific, LLC
P. O. Box 102
Carlisle, MA 01741
Fax: 1-978-369-7325
info@pathscientific.com

Pedicraft
4134 Saint Augustine Rd.
Jacksonville, FL 32247
Phone: 1-800-223-7649
www.pedicraft.com

Pentax Medical Company
102 Chestnut Ridge Rd.
Montvale, NJ 07645
Phone: 1-201-571-2300
www.pentax.com

Pentax Precision Instruments Corp.
30 Ramland Rd.
Orangeburg, NY 10962-2699
Phone: 1-800-431-5880
www.pentaxmedical.com

Pharmacia and Upjohn Company (A Division of Pfizer)
235 East 42nd St.
New York, NY 10017
Phone: 1-212-733-2323
www.pfizer.com

Pharmacy Specialists (Sam Pratt, RPh)
650 Maitland Ave.
Altemonte Springs, FL 32701
Phone: 1-800-224-7711

Philips Medical Systems
Heartstream Operation
2401 4th Ave.
Suite 500
Seattle, WA 98121-1436
Phone: 1-800-263-3342

pHion Nutrition
14201 North Hayden Rd.
Suite A4
Scottsdale, AZ 85260
Phone: 1-888-744-8589
www.ph-ion.com/

Phlebology and Aesthetic Concepts
3725 S US Hwy
Ste 1
Edgewater, FL 32141

Photo Therapeutics, Inc.
2335 Camino Vida Roble
Suite A
Carlsbad, CA 92011
Phone (main): 1-760-607-0488 or 1-800-743-8150
Fax: 1-760-607-0288
Contact: salesinfo@phototherapeutics.com
www.phototherapeutics.com

Precordial Stethoscopes
Sedation Resource, Inc.
Phone: 1-800-753-6376
www.sedationresource.com

Premier Medical Products
1710 Romano Dr.
P.O. Box 4500
Plymouth Meeting, PA 19462
Phone: 1-888-670-6100
www.premusa.com

Procter & Gamble Pharmaceuticals
1 Procter & Gamble Plaza
Cincinnati, OH 45201
Phone: 1-513-983-1100
www.wcrx.com

Pulpdent Corp.
80 Oakland St.
Watertown, MA 02471
Phone: 1-800-343-4342
www.pulpdent.com

Puritan Bennett (product)
Covidien
6135 Gunbarrel Ave.
Boulder, CO 80301
Phone: 1-800-NELLCOR
www.respiratorysolutions.covidien.com

QIAGEN Inc.
27220 Turnberry Ln.
Valencia, CA 91355
Phone (orders): 1-800-426-8157
Fax: 1-800-718-2056
Technical assistance: 1-800-DNA-PREP (800-362-7737)
www.thehpvtest.com

QuickMedical
Phone: 1-425-222-5963, ext. 1010 or 1-888-345-4858
Fax: 1-425-222-6030
www.quickmedical.com

Raja Medical
801 South Olive Ave.
Suite 124
West Palm Beach, FL 33401
Phone: 1-561-868-4600
www.rajamedical.com

Redfield Corp.
210 Summit Ave.
Montvale, NJ 07645
Phone: 1-800-678-4472

Redwing Book Company
44 Linden St.
Brookline, MA 02445
Phone: 1-800-873-3946
www.redwingbooks.com

Refine USA, LLC
340 S. 3rd Ave.
Jacksonville Beach, FL 32250
Phone: 1- 866-491-7546
www.refineusa.com

Reichert
3362 Walden Ave.
Depew, NY 14043
Phone: 1-888-849-8955
www.reichert.com

Rejuveness, LLC
28 Clinton St.
Suite 6
Saratoga Springs, NY 12866
Phone: 1-800-588-7455 or 1-518-584-5017
Fax: 1-518-584-3618
www.rejuveness.com

Reliant Technologies
464 Ellis St.
Mountain View, CA 94043
Phone: 1-888-437-2935
Fax: 1-650-473-0119

Richard Wolf Medical Instruments
353 Corporate Woods Parkway
Vernon Hills, IL 60061-3110
Phone: 1-800-829-7694
www.richard-wolf.com

RS Medical
14001 SE 1st St.
Vancouver, WA 98684
Phone: 1-800-935-7763

Rusch, Inc.
2450 Meadowbrook Parkway
Duluth, GA 30096
Phone: 1-800-553-5214
www.ruschinc.com

Sam Wagner
P.O. Box 431
202 Dodd St.
Middlebourne, WV 26149
Phone: 1-304-758-2370

Sandstone Medical Technologies
105 Citation Ct.
Homewood, AL 35209
Phone: 1205-290-8251
Fax: 1-205-290-4269
www.sandstonemedicaltechnologies.com

Saratoga Diagnostics
12619 Paseo Olivos
Saratoga, CA 95070
Phone: 1-800-998-1555
www.saratogadiagnostics.com

Save-A-Tooth System
18 South Roland St.
Pottsdown, PA 19464
Phone: 1-888-788-6684
www.save-a-tooth.com

ScarHeal Inc.
352 150th Ave.
Bldg. G
Madeira Beach, FL 33708-2008
Phone: 1-888-722-7432 or 1-727-397-7227
Fax: 1-877-722-7329
www.scarheal.com

Schering-Plough Corporation
2000 Galloping Hill Rd.
Kenilworth, NJ 07033-0530
Phone: 1-908-298-4000
www.IMPLANON-USA.com

Science Innovative Aesthetics
30 Montgomery St.
Suite 660
Jersey City, NJ 07302
Phone: 1-201-332-4100
www.scienceaesthetics.com

Sciton
925 Commercial St.
Palo Alto, CA 94303
Phone: 1-888-646-6999
Fax: 1-650-493-9146
www.sciton.com

The Scope Exchange
4210 Tudor Ln.
Greensboro, NC 27410
Phone: 1-888-252-1542
www.sterilmed.com

Scripts Pharmacy
4059 Hollywood Rd.
St. Joseph, MI 49085
Phone: 1-269-428-2500
Fax: 1-269-428-2555.

SDI Diagnostics, Inc.
10 Hampden Dr.
Easton, MA 02375
Phone: 1-800-678-5782
www.sdidiagnostics.com

Seiler Colposcope
3433 Tree Court Industrial Blvd.
St. Louis, MO 63122
Phone: 1-314-968-2282 or 1-800-489-2282
www.seilmicro.com

Serolab
P.O. Box 3307
Waco, TX 76707-3307
Phone: 1-800-460-4867

Shippert Medical Technologies
6248 S. Troy Circle
Suite A
Centennial, CO 80111
Phone: 1-800-888-8663
www.shippertmedical.com

Siemens/Acuson
1220 Charleston Rd.
P.O. Box 7393
Mountain View, CA 94039-7393
Phone: 1-800-422-8766
www.medical.siemens.com

Sigvaris
P.O. Box 570
Branford, CT 06405
Phone: 1-800-322-7744
www.sigvaris.com

Silhouet-Tone USA
7 Champlain Commons
St. Albans, VT 05478
Phone: 1-800-552-0418
www.silhouettone.com

Sims Portex, Inc.
10 Bowman Dr.
Keene, NH 03431
Phone: 1-800-258-5361
www.portexusa.com

Sirchie Fingerprint Laboratories, Inc.
100 Hunter Pl.
Youngsville, NC 27596
Phone: 1-800-356-7311
www.sirchie.com

SkinMedica, Inc.
5909 Sea Lion Pl.
Suite H
Carlsbad, CA 90210
Phone: 1-877-944-1412
www.SkinMedica.com

SkinRx Distribution Inc.
Phone: 1-905-640-9113 or 1-416-450-5663 (cell)
Fax: 1-905-640-0747
Contact: Chantal.ward@sympatico.ca
www.isolaz.com

Slate Pharmaceuticals
318 Blackwell St.
Suite 240
Durham, NC 27701
Phone: 1-866-SLATE-50 (1-866-752-8350)
Fax: 1-866-596-8350
www.testopel.com

Smart Practice
3400 E. McDowell Rd.
Phoenix, AZ 85008-7899
Phone: 1-602-225-0595 or 1-800-522-0800
Fax: 800.522.8329
www.smartpractice.com

Smith & Nephew, Inc.
11775 Starkey Rd.
Largo, FL 33773
Phone: 1-727-392-1261
Call for local distributor: 1-800-876-1261

Smithers Bio-Medical Systems
P.O. Box 790
Kent, OH 44240
Phone: 1-800-321-8286
www.biofoamimpression.com

SmithKline Beecham Clinical Laboratories
11636 Administration Dr.
St. Louis, MO 63146
Phone: 1-800-669-8077

Smiths Medical USA
1265 Grey Fox Rd.
St. Paul, MN 55112
Phone: 1-800-258-5361
www.smiths-medical.com

Solta Medical, Inc.
25881 Industrial Blvd.
Hayward, CA 94545
Phone: 1-877-782-2286
Fax: 1-510-782-2287
www.solta.com

Sonoscape USA
6160 Peachtree Dunwoody Rd.
Suite B-201
Atlanta, GA 30328
Phone: 1-800-797-4546

SonoSite
21919 30th Dr. SE
Bothell, WA 98021-3904
Phone: 1-888-482-9449
www.sonosite.com

SOS Medical
740 East Arrow Highway
Covina, CA 91722
Phone: 1-888-592-5550
www.sos-medical.com

SoundSkin Corp.
429 S. Main St.
Oswego, IL 60543
Phone: 1-888-596-5277
www.soundskin.com

SpaceLabs Healthcare
5150 220th Ave. SE
Issaquah, WA 98029
Phone: 1-800-522-7025
www.spacelabshealthcare.com

SSR Surgical Instruments
5 Shore Ave.
P.O. Box 537
Oyster Bay, NY 11771
Phone: 1-800-932-7364
www.ssrsurgical.com

STD Pharmaceutical
Fields Yard, Plough Ln.
Hereford, UK HR4 0EL
Phone: +44-(0)1432-353684
www.stdpharm.co.uk

SterilMed
11400 N. 73rd Ave.
Maple Grove, MN
Phone: 1-888-856-4870
www.sterilmed.com/

St. Jude Medical
One Lillehei Plaza
St. Paul, MN 55117-9983
Phone: 1-800-328-9634
www.sjm.com

Stoetling
620 Wheat Ln.
Wood Dale, IL 60191
Phone: 1-800-860-9775 or 1-630-860-9700
Fax: 1-630-860-9775
Contact: Info@StoeltingCo.com
www.stoetlingco.com

Storz (Bausch and Lomb)
180 Villa Verde Dr.
San Dimas, CA 91773
Phone: 1-800-338-2020
www.storz.com

Stryker Instruments
1410 Lakeside Parkway
Flower Mound, TX 75028
Phone: 1-866-726-3705
www.stryker.com

SunTech Medical
507 Airport Blvd.
Suite 117
Morrisville, NC 27560
Phone: 1-800-421-8626
www.suntechmed.com

Surgical Optics LLC
1900 Wyatt Dr.
Suite 7
Santa Clara, CA 95054
Phone: 1-888-884-6887
www.surgical-optics.com

Surgical Repair Technologies
930 Blue Gentian Rd.
Suite 1400
Eagan, MN 55121
Phone: 1-800-495-0297
www.sohniks.com

Surgical Specialties Corporation
100 Denis Dr.
Reading, PA 19606

Surgical Supply Service
500 Fillmore Ave.
Tonawanda, NY 14150
Phone: 1-800-523-0706 (U.S.) or 1-716-743-1529 (worldwide)
Fax (24-hour): 1-800-222-1934
Contact: customersupport@SurgicalSupplyService.com
www.surgicalsupplyservice.com

Swede-O, Inc.
611 Ash St.
P.O. Box 610
North Branch, MN 55056
Phone: 1-800-525-9339
www.swedeo.com

Sybaritic
9220 S. James Ave.
Bloomington, MN 55431
Phone: 1-800-445-8418
www.sybaritic.com

Syneron Inc.
28 Fulton Way
Unit 8
Richmond Hill, Ontario
Canada L4B 1L5
Phone: 1-905-886-9235 or 1-866-259-6661
Fax: 1-905-886-7046
www.syneron.com

SYNOVA Healthcare Inc.
1400 N. Providence Rd.
Suite 6010
Media, PA 19063
Phone: 1-610-565-7080
www.todaysponge.com

Tao & Tao Technology, Inc.
886 Sands Ln.
Camano Island, WA 98282
Phone: 1-360-387-6186
Fax: 1-360-387-6269
info@taoaspirator.com
www.taoaspirator.com

Teleflex Medical
2917 Weck Dr.
Research Triangle Park, NC 27709
Phone: 1-866-246-6990
www.teleflexmedical.com/pleurevac/pe.html

Terarecon
2955 Campus Dr.
#325
San Mateo, CA 94403
Phone: 1-650-372-1100
Fax: 1-650-372-1101
Contact: info@terarecon.com
www.terarecon.com

Terason Ultrasound (Division of Teratech Corporation)
77 Terrace Hall Ave.
Burlington, MA 01803
Phone: 1-866-837-2766 (U.S. only) or 1-781-270-4143
Fax: 1-781-270-4145
www.terason.com

Terumo Medical Corp.
2101 Cottontail Ln.
Somerset, NJ 08873
www.terumotmp.com

Theraplex Company
3380 Peasson Rd.
Memphis, TN 38118
Phone: 1-888-437-2753
www.theraplex.com

Thera-Tronics, Inc.
623 Mamaroneck Ave.
Mamaroneck, NY 10543
Phone: 1-914-698-9802
www.theratronicsinc.com

Thermage, Inc.
25881 Industrial Blvd.
Hayward, CA 94545-2991
www.thermage.com

ThermoTek Inc.
1200 Lakeside Parkway
Suite 200 (Building 2)
Flower Mound, TX 75028
Phone: 1-972-874-4949 or 1-877-242-3232
Fax: 1-972-874-4945
Contact: info@thermotekusa.com
www.thermotekusa.com

Thomas Medical, Inc.
4100-C Nine McFarland Dr.
Alpharetta, GA 30004
Phone: 1-800-556-0349

Three Dimensional Systems, Inc.
210 W. Kensinger Dr.
Suite 400
Cranberry Twp., PA 16066
Phone: 1-888-529-3734
www.lazerfit.com

3Gen, LLC
31521 Rancho Viejo Rd.
Suite 104
San Juan Capistrano, CA 92675
Phone: 1-949-481-6384
Fax: 1-949-240-7492
Contact: info@3GenLLC.com
www.dermlite.com/

3M Health Care
3M Center
Bldg. 275-4E-01
St. Paul, MN 55144-1000
Phone: 1-800-228-3957
www.3m.com

TIMM Medical Technologies
6585 City West Parkway
Eden Prairie, MN 55344
Phone: 1-800-344-9688
www.timmmedical.com

Topix Pharmaceuticals
155 Knickerbocker Ave.
Bohemia, NY 11716
174 Rte. 109
West Babylon, NY 11704
Phone: 1-800-445-2595
www.topixpharm.com

Toshiba America
2441 Michelle Dr.
Tustin, CA 92780
Phone: 1-800-421-1968
www.medical.toshiba.com

Townsend Design
4615 Shepard St.
Bakersfield, CA 93313
Phone: 1-800-432-3466
www.townsenddesign.com

Travanti Pharma, Inc. (formerly Birch Point Medical, Inc.; for Ionto-Patch)
Phone: 1-866-467-2824
www.iontopatch.com

Ultradent Products Inc.
555 W. 10200
South Jordan, UT 84095
Phone: 1-800-552-5512
www.ultradent.com

Unimax Supply Company
365 Canal St.
New York, NY 10013
Phone: 1-800-986-4629
www.unimaxsupply.com

United Endoscopy
10405 San Sevaine Way
Suite B
Mira Lorma, CA 91752-1150
Phone: 1-800-899-4847
www.endoscope.com

United Medical
832 Jury Ct.
San Jose CA, 95112
Phone: 1-408-278-9300 or 1-877-490-7036
Fax: 1-408-278-9797
www.umiultrasound.com

Universal Endoscopic Services
6861 SW 196th Ave.
Suite 402
Pembroke Pines, FL 33332
Phone: 1-800-266-1464
www.ues1.com

University Compounding Pharmacy
1875 Third Ave.
San Diego, CA 92101
Phone: 1-800-985-8065
www.ucprx.com

Used Medical Equipment and Devices Medline
278 S. Lincoln St.
Minster, OH 45865
Phone: 1-419-628-2548

USSDG Sutures (Now Syneture after U.S. Surgical acquiring Davis & Geck, a subsidiary of TYCO Healthcare)
150 Glover Ave.
Norwalk, CT 06856
Phone: 1-800-544-8772
www.syneture.com

Utah Medical Products, Inc. (Europe)
Athlone Business and Research Park
Dublin Rd.
Athlone, County Westmeath
Republic of Ireland
Phone: 353-90-647-3932
www.utahmed.com

Utah Medical Products, Inc. (United States)
7043 South 300 West
Midvale, UT 84047-1048
Phone: 1-866-754-9789 (main, toll-free) or 1-800-533-4984 (customer support)

Valiant Pharmaceuticals
3300 Hyland Dr.
Costa Mesa, CA 92626
Phone: 1-800-556-1937

Valleylab, Inc.
5920 Longbow Dr.
Boulder, CO 80301-3299
Phone: 1-800-255-8522
www.valleylab.com

VBM Medical, Inc.
15013 Herriman Blvd.
Noblesville, IN 46060
Phone: 1-800-580-7117
www.vbm-medical.de

Venosan
300 Industrial Park Ave.
P.O. Box 1067
Asheboro, NC 27204-1067
Phone: 1-800-432-5347
www.venosanusa.com

Vibraderm Inc.
2100 N. Hwy. 360
Suite 1502
Grand Prairie, TX 75050
Phone: 1-800-494-7181

Vidacare
722 Isom Rd.
San Antonio, TX 78216
Phone: 1-866-479-8500
www.vidacare.com

Viora, Inc.
30 Montgomery St.
Suite 660
Jersey City, NJ 07302
Phone: 1-201-332-4100
www.vioramed.com

Vision Sciences
40 S. Ramland Rd.
Orangeburg, NY 10962
Phone: 1-845-365-0600 or 1-800-431-5420
Fax: 1-835-365-0620
info@visionsciences.com
www.visionsciences.com

Visual Changes Skin Care
Phone: 1-800-400-8901
customerservice@visualchanges.com
www.visualchanges.com/

Vita Medical Technologies
1286 University Ave.
#264
San Diego, CA 92103
Phone: 1-619-795-7953
www.vitamedtech.com

Vitalograph
8347 Quivira
Lenexa, KS 66215
Phone: 1-800-255-6626
www.vitalograph.com

VNUS Medical
5799 Fontanoso Way
San Jose, CA 95138
Phone: 1-408-360-7200 or 1-888-797-8346
Fax: 1-408-365-8480
Contact: info@vnus.com
www.vnus.com

WaisMed
3050 Post Oak Blvd.
Houston, TX 77056
Phone: 1-866-924-7633
www.waismed.com

Wallach Surgical Devices, Inc.
235 Edison Rd.
Orange, CT 06477
Phone: 1-203-799-2002 or 1-800-243-2463
www.wallachsurgical.com
wallach@wallachsurgical.com

Walls Precision Instruments
38800 Deer Creek Rd.
Baker City, OR 97814
Phone: 1-888-445-6534
www.tympanocentesis.com

Weck Closure Systems (product)
Teleflex Medical
2917 Weck Dr.
Research Triangle Park, NC 27709
Phone: 1-866-246-6990
www.teleflexmedical.com

Welch Allyn Corporation
4341 State Street Rd.
P.O. Box 220
Skaneateles Falls, NY 13153-0220
Phone: 1-800-535-6663
www.welchallyn.com

Weslee Medical, Inc.
1187 Wilmette Ave.
PMB 149
Wilmette, IL 60091-2719
Phone: 1-877-624-6681

Westone
2235 Executive Cr.
Colorado Springs, CO 80906
Telephone: 1-800-525-5071
www.westone.com

Wilson-Cook Medical, Inc.
4900 Behania Station Rd.
Winston-Salem, NC 27105
Phone: 1-336-744-0157
Fax: 1-336-744-1147

Wilson Ophthalmic Corp.
932 W. State Hwy. 152
Mustang, OK 73064
Phone: 1-405-376-9114
www.hilco.com

Xomed (Medtronics)
Medtronic ENT
6743 N. Southpoint Dr.
Jacksonville, FL 32216
Phone: 1-800-874-5797
www.medtronic.com

Yama, Inc.
650 Liberty Ave.
Union, NJ 07083
Phone: 1-800-699-8130
Fax: 1-908-206-8725
info@leasshield.com

Z-Medica Corp.
4 Fairfield Blvd.
Wallingford, CT 06492
Phone: 1-203-294-0000
Fax: 1-203-294-0688
www.z-medica.com

Zeiss
One Zeiss Dr.
Thornwood, NY 10594
Phone: 1-914-747-1800
www.meditec.zeiss.com

Zerowet
P.O. Box 4375
Palos Verdes Peninsula, CA 90274
Phone: 1-800-438-0938

Zimmer, Inc.
727 N. Detroit St.
Warsaw, IN 46580
Phone: 1-800-613-6131
www.zimmer.com

Zimmer Medizin Systems
25 Mauchly
Suite 300
Irvine, CA 92618
Phone (office): 1-800-327-3576
Fax: 1-949-727-2154
info@zimmerusa.com
zimmerusa.com

APPENDIX E

RESOURCES FOR LEARNING AND TEACHING PROCEDURES

Stephen J. Wetmore • Steven E. Roskos

The well-rounded primary care physician performs a variety of medical and surgical procedures in his or her practice. The skill in performing such procedures and resultant success will depend strongly on the training that one has received in performing those procedures. Advancing technology and changing practice patterns lead primary care physicians to add new procedures to their practices and to update their skills in procedures that they already perform. Regardless of whether the clinician is learning a procedure for the first time or wishing to update skills, it is helpful to have a good understanding of the resources that are available to facilitate learning.

This appendix provides information about the variety of resources available for learning procedures and how these can be accessed. A new section in this appendix includes some tips for teaching and learning procedures in family medicine. This is also of considerable interest to teachers of procedural skills. It is not possible to include every resource, but each section will have examples and provide ideas about where to search for other similar resources.

COURSES IN PROCEDURES FOR PRIMARY CARE PHYSICIANS

In both Canada and the United States, national medical associations such as the College of Family Physicians of Canada and the American Academy of Family Physicians provide opportunities to learn and update procedure skills. National and state or provincial meetings of these bodies often have seminars or workshops on common procedures in primary care. Seminars and workshops are excellent starting points for physicians hoping to learn procedures because they will include the pertinent background knowledge for each procedure, including indications, contraindications, technical details, and complications. Many of these workshops also include opportunities for "hands-on" experience, which allows physicians to become familiar with equipment and techniques. These sessions are suitable as updates for physicians already familiar with the procedures but often do not provide enough practical experience in some procedures for new learners to commence performing them right away. They are, nevertheless, good starting points.

The National Procedures Institute (Texas) is a joint venture of The Texas Academy of Family Physicians, The American Academy of Family Physicians, and The Society of Teachers of Family Medicine. A variety of courses in procedure skills can be found on its website (www.npinstitute.com). The range of procedures covered in these courses is extensive, and readers are referred to the course outlines on the website for details.

The following are examples of nationally recognized programs with standards and hands-on practical training that must be met to receive credit:

Advanced Cardiac Life Support (ACLS)
Advanced Life Support in Obstetrics (ALSO)
Advanced Trauma Life Support (ATLS)
American College of Sports Medicine (www.acsm.org)
Basic Life Support (BLS)
Canadian Academy of Sports Medicine (www.casm-acsm.org)
MORE^{OB} program (http://moreob.com)
Neonatal Resuscitation Program (NRP)
Pediatric Advanced Life Support (PALS) (www.americanheart.org)

TEACHING PROCEDURES

Physicians find themselves teaching procedures in various settings, both formal and informal. You may give a workshop to family medicine residents on a certain procedure. You may teach a procedure to a medical student spending time in your office. The principles of effective instruction remain the same, though their application to these different situations may vary.

Which procedures should be taught and learned? Each practice situation will require different procedural skills, so no list will be universal. Some good starting points include the core list of procedures for family physicians developed by the Working Group on Procedure Skills of the College of Family Physicians of Canada or the list of core procedures for family medicine developed by the Society of Teachers of Family Medicine (STFM) Group on Hospital Medicine and Procedural Training.

Several other papers in the medical literature provide valuable information about procedure skills training in American and Canadian family medicine training programs. What should the content of teaching and learning procedures include? Although the first component that comes to mind is the technical skill, there is much more to learn about a medical procedure. The Working Group on the Certification Process of the College of Family Physicians of Canada has defined the key features that must be included for each procedure. These features are discussed in the following section.

KEY FEATURES OF PROCEDURAL SKILLS

1. In order to decide whether or not you are going to perform a procedure, consider the following:
   - The indications and contraindications to the procedure
   - Your own skills and readiness to do the procedure (e.g., your level of fatigue and any personal distracters)
   - The context of the procedure, including the patient involved, the complexity of the task, the time needed, the need for assistance, and location.

2. Before deciding to go ahead with the procedure, consider the following:
   - Discuss the procedure with the patient, including a description of the procedure and possible outcomes, both positive and negative, as part of obtaining consent.
   - Prepare for the procedure by ensuring appropriate equipment is ready.
   - Mentally rehearse the following:
     - The anatomic landmarks necessary to perform the procedure
     - The technical steps necessary in sequential fashion, including any preliminary examination
     - The potential complications and their management
4. During performance of the procedure
   - Keep the patient informed to reduce anxiety.
   - Ensure patient comfort and safety always.
5. When the procedure is not going as expected, stop, reevaluate the situation, and seek assistance as required.
6. Develop a plan with your patient for aftercare and follow-up after completion of a procedure.

Good working understanding of these key features is prerequisite to performing any procedure and needs to be taught and learned in addition to the technical skill itself. The goal of teaching a procedure is that the learner be able to perform the procedure in the real world on a real patient. When teaching medical procedures, it is best to treat them as a relatively "closed" skill, in other words, with specific steps that the learner should not deviate from. Once the procedure is mastered, variations can be introduced to address different anatomy or other variations in the clinical situation.

The OOMPA ED WASDM PF SIOMT acronym explained in the following sections can help you remember to incorporate all the steps to effective instruction.

Introduction

O—**O**bjective. To perform a given procedure on real patients in the real world.

O—**O**verview. Provide a quick summary of the steps involved.

M—**M**otivation. Why should the learner gain proficiency in this procedure? Provide information on how often this procedure is required, what the benefits are, and the consequences of not acquiring skill in this procedure.

P—**P**rerequisites. Before learning the technical skills required to perform a procedure, the learner needs to know the indications, risks, anatomy, and so forth. This is a good opportunity to refer the learner to a chapter in this text. The best way to assure that the learner knows the prerequisite information is to ask questions: "What are the indications for this procedure?" "What are the risks?" "What complications would you keep your eye out for?" Role playing works as well: "Pretend I am the patient and obtain informed consent for this procedure from me." Pictures and models are also very helpful in cementing this information in the learner's mind.

A—**A**genda. Describe what the learner can expect. If you are giving a formal lesson or workshop, describe what it will contain. If this is informal teaching in the office, explain that you will list and explain the steps, demonstrate them in some way, and ask the learner to demonstrate them as well.

Core Material

ED—**E**xplanation and **d**emonstration. This portion of the instruction is key. Even if the learner has performed this procedure several times, it is helpful to review the steps and then have the learner repeat them, and even have the learner demonstrate the procedure in some way before beginning the actual procedure on a patient.

The explanation and demonstration phase can be outlined by the WASDM acronym:

W—"You **w**ill perform this procedure."

A—"**A**ttend to these steps as I show you how to do them."

SD—**S**ay each step before **d**oing it.

M—Ask the learner to **m**emorize the steps and recall them before the practice.

Sometimes dividing the procedure into discrete steps can be difficult and it is easy to leave a step out. Use this text as a starting point to list all the steps for a procedure. If the instruction is for a formal setting, ask others who are familiar with the procedure to review the steps. Then, ask someone who is unfamiliar with the procedure, perhaps someone who is nonmedical, to try to learn the procedure using this method. This person can often point out missing steps or incomplete instruction. If the situation is informal, add steps as you go if you realize that you have left some out. When teaching complex procedures, it may be best to divide them into segments, and teach the segments separately, combining them later. For example, when teaching laceration repair, local anesthesia may be separated from suturing.

You may demonstrate a procedure in several ways. The best way is on a real patient. However, if you want the learner to perform a procedure on that patient, the patient probably doesn't need two procedures. On the other hand, if the patient needs both knees injected or two moles removed, this is the perfect opportunity to demonstrate and then have the learner perform the procedure, a classic case of "see one, do one." If several procedures are being performed in succession, for example, several colonoscopies are scheduled in the endoscopy laboratory, you can demonstrate on the first one and let the learner try the second one. It is very important to follow the WASDM acronym when demonstrating so that the learner gains maximum benefit from the demonstration.

If a real patient is unavailable for demonstration, mock demonstration using capped needles or covered scalpels is useful. Video demonstration is an excellent alternative and there are many resources available for video demonstration (see Table E-2).

PF—Following demonstration, **p**ractice with **f**eedback is very important. The learner can practice on a real or simulated patient. The learner should state the steps as they do them ("**s**ay, then **d**o"). It is important that the practice be in an environment that is encouraging and pleasant. If there really isn't time to teach the procedure, it is better to wait for another opportunity. A stressful and high-pressure setting is not conducive to learning and may discourage the learner from future attempts at learning a procedure. Do your best to be encouraging and positive during the practice. If the learner is forgetting a step or not performing it properly, ask them to stop and think "What step are you missing?" or "That's not quite right. How should you perform this step?" Specific feedback is very important. Rather than saying "good job," try pointing out specific things that were done well, for example, "you really kept that site sterile throughout the procedure" or "your conversation with the patient put him at ease."

Conclusion

Whether in a formal or informal instructional situation, it is important to review and summarize (SIOMT):

S—**S**ummary. Review the steps.

I—**I**ntegration. Explain how this procedure might fit in with other treatments for the same condition or other procedures that are related.

O—**O**bjective. Review the objective (to perform the procedure on a real patient in the real world).

M—**M**otivation. Review the motivation.

T—**T**est. If you need to assess competency, have the learner perform the procedure while you observe. The best situation is performing the procedure on a real patient. If this is not possible, then performing the procedure in some simulated fashion may suffice.

Teaching procedures is challenging and rewarding. Seeing a learner achieve competence and independence in performing procedures is one of the greatest rewards of the physician–educator. Following these tips can help you do so effectively and efficiently.

Gaining Practical Experience in Procedures

Although formal courses or workshops are suitable for learning information about procedures, equipment, and techniques, it may not be possible for the clinician to gain enough experience in this way to begin performing the procedure. Supervised practice is necessary to gain confidence in many procedures. In most cases there is no consensus on how many supervised procedures are necessary to achieve competence. The number of supervised procedures necessary to achieve competence for any given procedure depends on the complexity of the procedure, and the confidence and physical dexterity of the operator, among other things. For example, a learner may need to perform 25 to 30 supervised flexible sigmoidoscopies to achieve competence but only 10 to 15 supervised no-scalpel vasectomies. Clinicians should consider performing procedures under the supervision of an experienced colleague until both are comfortable with the learner's competence. Supportive colleagues can be a major resource toward getting started in procedures and providing backup and support when difficulties arise.

Books on Procedures in Primary Care

With the rise in technology and increasing use of CD-ROMs, computer animations, and virtual reality, there is less emphasis on books for many of the things we do in practice. Nevertheless, textbooks remain a readily available source of practical information. One or two texts on procedural skills are an essential part of the primary care physician's library. This book, *Pfenninger and Fowler's Procedures for Primary Care,* 3rd ed., is one example of an ideal resource book because of its comprehensive nature, inclusion of background material, patient education, description of technique, helpful illustrations, company names and addresses for obtaining equipment, and billing and coding information. Many common primary care procedures are covered in *The Essential Guide to Primary Care Procedures,* by E.J. Mayeaux, Jr. (2009), and there is access to a companion website with patient education handouts and videos (Lippincott Williams & Wilkins). Another excellent resource for dermatology procedures is Habif's *Clinical Dermatology: A Color Guide to Diagnosis and Therapy,* 4th ed. (WB Saunders, 2004) and its associated website www.clinderm.com. Usatine's text *Dermatologic and Cosmetic Procedures in Office Practice* (Elsevier, 2011) is a comprehensive review of dermatologic procedures.

The following are examples of other important texts; they are but a few of the "must have" texts for any library:

Apgar's Colposcopy: Principles and Practice, 2nd ed. (Saunders, 2008)
Diagnosis and Office Orthopedics for Primary Care, by B.C. Anderson (WB Saunders, 2006)
Emergency Medicine Procedures, by E.F. Reichman and R.R. Simon (McGraw-Hill, 2004)
Essentials of Musculoskeletal Care, 3rd ed., by L.Y. Griffin, comes with a DVD (American Academy of Orthopedic Surgeons, 2005)
Essential Orthopedics, by M. Miller (Elsevier, 2009), comes with a DVD (videos on how to perform 29 joint injections, 7 common physical examinations, and 6 splinting and casting procedures) and full-text online access
A Practical Guide to Joint and Soft Tissue Injection and Aspiration: An Illustrated Text for Primary Care Providers, by James W. McNabb (Lippincott Williams & Wilkins, 2009)
Surgery of the Skin, by J.K. Robinson, et al. (Mosby, 2005)

A more complete list of other available texts can be found in Table E-1.

CD-ROM/DVD Resources for Procedures in Primary Care

CD-ROMs and DVDs are useful resources for learning procedures because the technology allows the integration of text with voice, pictures, computer animation, and videotape. These can be searched easily to focus on specific details of any given procedure. Like textbooks, CD-ROMs can provide all the relevant background information necessary to perform the procedure. Texts now often contain a DVD and online access (see Miller's *Essential Orthopedics*, cited previously). One strength of this technology is the capacity to incorporate video footage; the visual presentation of the technique is a powerful learning aid. CD-ROMs are portable and can be used in a variety of settings, including the office, clinic, or even the home. As an example is a DVD, *Multimedia Primary Care Procedures* by Tuggy, Garcia, and Newkirk. The quality of the DVD and visualization of the techniques are excellent. This DVD includes patient guides, voice or text instruction for each procedure, and access to ICD-9/CPT codes for each procedure. The purchase of *Multimedia Primary Care Procedures* also provides access to the website (www.primarycareprocedures.com), which is regularly updated, and video footage of additional procedures is available. This works well for teaching many students and residents in a lecture format as well as small groups. Box E-1. lists the contents of this DVD.

Deutchman has produced two excellent DVDs: *Emergency and Trauma Ultrasound* and *Cesarean Delivery*. Links to these products can be found at http://www.chall.com/emus.htm and http://www.chall.com/cesarean.htm, respectively. Descriptions and contents can be found in Box E-2.

The National Procedures Institute produces a series of learning DVDs that are listed in Box E-3.

MeisterMed recently launched its *Procedures: Hospital Collection* for iPhone and iPod touch (www.meistermed.com/procedures). It includes videos, images, and step-by-step details for 15 key inpatient procedures.

The American College of Physicians-American Society of Internal Medicine has two products: *Arthrocentesis and Joint Injection* (Alguire PC, Casey LM, eds., 1999) and *Common Skin Biopsy Techniques* (Alquire PC, Casey LM, eds., 1999) that include videotapes of the procedures.

Websites

First Consult (www.firstconsult.com) is an informative website that is constantly being updated. Many procedural topics are outlined and each includes a short video clip of the procedure as well the indications, contraindications, techniques, outcomes, and resources. Subscription is required but the value of the resource is worth it.

Another good resource for teaching is The Family Medicine Digital Resources Library (FMDRL), produced by the Society of Teachers in Family Medicine (STFM), available at www.fmdrl.org. This website contains user-posted conference presentations and handouts, and shared curricular materials such as PowerPoint lectures, learning modules, syllabi, digital images, video and audio recordings, and recommended websites. All of the content has been peer reviewed and anyone can search the database and download materials. Registration is required but free if you want to upload material to share with others. One example is a PowerPoint presentation entitled "Procedure World: A New Paradigm for Teaching Procedural Skills" by Ellen Johnson which illustrates one teaching program for procedural skills.

The American Academy of Family Physicians website now includes a self-study program on clinical procedures designed for physicians to review and build confidence in procedural skills. Most of the programs (e.g., Joint Injection and Aspiration, No Scalpel

TABLE E-1 Procedures Books	
Book Title	**Authors and Publishing Data**
Ambulatory Gynaecological Surgery	PJ O'Donnovan, N. Amso Publisher: Bailliere Tindall 2005
Atlas of Primary Care Procedures, for PDA	Thomas J. Zuber, EJ Mayeux Publisher: Lippincott Williams & Wilkins, 2004
Basic Soft-Tissue Surgery: An Illustrated Guide for the Family Physician	Thomas J. Zuber, Donald E. Dewitt Publisher: American Academy of Family Physicians, 2004
Blueprints Clinical Procedures	Laurie L. Marbas, Erin Case Publisher: Blackwell, 2004
Clinical Procedures for Medical Assistants	Kathy Bonewit-West Publisher: Saunders, 2004
Clinical Procedures for Ocular Examination	Nancy B. Carlson, Daniel Kurtz Publisher: McGraw-Hill Medical Publishers, 2004
Clinical Procedures in Emergency Medicine	James R. Roberts, Jerris R. Hedges, Arjun S. Chanmugam, MD Consult LLC, et al. Publisher: Mosby, 2004
Clinical Procedures in Primary Eye Care	David B. Elliott Publisher: Butterworth-Heinemann, 2003
Clinical Skills for the Ophthalmic Examination: Basic Procedures	Lindy DuBois Publisher: SLACK Inc., 2006
Clinician's Pocket Reference	Leonard G. Gomella, Steven A. Haist, University of Kentucky College of Medicine Publisher: McGraw-Hill, 2007
Color Atlas of Emergency Department Procedures	Catherine B. Custalow Publisher: Saunders, 2005
Current Procedures—Pediatrics	Denise M. Goodman, NetLibrary, Inc., et al. Publisher: McGraw-Hill, 2007
Emergency Medicine Procedures	Eric Reichman, Robert R. Simon Publisher: McGraw-Hill Medical Publishing, 2004
Emergency Procedures and Techniques	Robert R. Simon, Barry E. Brenner Publisher: Lippincott Williams & Wilkins, 2002
Essential Clinical Procedures	Richard W. Dehn, David P. Asprey Publisher: Saunders, 2007
Essential Emergency Procedures	Kaushal Shah, Chilembwe Mason Publisher: Wolters Kluwer Health/Lippincott Williams & Wilkins, 2008
The Essential Guide to Primary Care Procedures	EJ Mayeaux Publisher: Lippincott Williams & Wilkins, 2009
Handbook of Emergency Department Procedures	John B. Bache, Carolyn R. Armitt, Cathy Gadd Publisher: Mosby, 2003
Handbook of Primary Care Procedures	No author listed Publisher: Lippincott Williams & Wilkins, 2002
Medicine for the Outdoors: The Essential Guide to Emergency Medical Procedures and First Aid	Paul S. Auerbach Publisher: Lyons Press, 2003
Merrill's Atlas of Radiographic Positioning & Procedures	Eugene D. Frank, Bruce W. Long, Barbara J. Smith, et al. Publisher: Mosby, 2007
Murtagh's Practice Tips	John Murtagh Publisher: McGraw-Hill, 2008
Office Procedures	Robert S. Wigton, Thomas G. Tape Publisher: Mosby, 2004
Office Surgery	Gerald Amundsen, Brian Coleman, Kalyanakrishnan Ramakrishnan, Rhonda Sparks, American Academy of Family Physicians Publisher: American Academy of Family Physicians, 2003
On Call Procedures	Gregg A. Adams, Stephen D. Bresnick Publisher: Saunders, 2006
Ophthalmic Office Procedures: A Step-by-Step Approach	Kenneth C. Chern, Eliot Foley, Ashok Reddy Publisher: McGraw-Hill Medical Publishing (New York); McGraw-Hill (London), 2004
Orthopedics for Primary Care Physicians	Rene Cailliet Publisher: AMA Press, 2003
Pfenninger and Fowler's Procedures for Primary Care	John L. Pfenninger, Grant C. Fowler Publisher: Mosby, 2003
Pfenninger and Fowler's Procedures for Primary Care, 2nd ed. + Multimedia Primary Care Procedures DVD, Online, and Pocket Procedures Manual	John L. Pfenninger, Michael Tuggy, Grant C. Fowler, Jorge Garcia Publisher: Saunders, 2005
Pocket Guide to Orthopedic and Sports Medicine Procedures: 111 Commonly Performed Procedures for the Health Care Professional	J. Konin Publisher: SLACK, 2009
Primary Care Procedures in Women's Health	CB Heath, SM Sulik Publisher: Springer, 2009
Procedures for Primary Care Practitioners	Marilyn W. Edmunds, Maren Stewart Mayhew Publisher: Mosby, 2003
Roenigk's Dermatologic Surgery: Current Techniques in Procedural Dermatology	Randall K. Roenigk, John L. Ratz, Henry H. Roenigk Publisher: Informa Healthcare, 2007
Text and Atlas of Emergency Medicine Procedures	E. Reichman Publisher: McGraw-Hill, 2003
Textbook of Pediatric Emergency Procedures	Christopher King, Fred M. Henretig, John Loiselle, Richard M. Ruddy Publisher: Wolters Kluwer Health/Lippincott Williams & Wilkins, 2008
Ultrasound-Guided Procedures in Emergency Medicine	Daniel Price, Jerris R. Hedges Publisher: Hanley & Belfus (Philadelphia); Elsevier Health Sciences (London), 2003

Box E-1. Procedures Included in *Multimedia Primary Care Procedures*

Abdominal paracentesis
Amniotomy
Anoscopy
Arthrocentesis—knee aspiration
Banding of internal hemorrhoids
Barrier contraceptives (diaphragm)
Bartholin's gland—marsupialization
Bartholin's gland—Word catheter placement
Bladder catheterization—female
Bladder catheterization—male
Burn débridement
Cerumen impaction removal
Cervical polyp removal
Cervical sampling (wet smear with KOH preparation)
Cesarean section
Colposcopy
Complete nail removal
Curettage and cautery—basal cell carcinoma
Digital block
Endometrial biopsy
Episiotomy—laceration repair
Excisional skin biopsy
Flexible sigmoidoscopy
Ganglion injection/aspiration
Incision and drainage of abscesses
Incision and drainage of thrombosed hemorrhoids
Inverted subcuticular stitches
IUD insertion
IUD removal
Joint injection—knee
Joint injection—shoulder
Lipoma removal
Lipoma removal by extrusion
Local anesthesia
Loop electrosurgical excision procedure (LEEP)
Lumbar puncture
Mattress stitches
Nasogastric intubation
Nasopharyngoscopy
Needle aspiration of breast cysts
Neonatal circumcision
No-scalpel vasectomy
Obstetric ultrasound
Optimal circumcision anesthesia
Pap smear (and wet prep Pap smear with HPV sampling)
Paracervical block
Performing an instrument tie
Pilonidal cyst excision
Placing an Unna boot
Punch biopsy
Radiofrequency mole excision/shave biopsy
Radiofrequency spider vein ablation
Removal of ingrown toenail
Ring removal
Scalp cyst excision
Shave biopsy
Skin tag removal
Subacromial shoulder injection
Subclavian line placement
Subcuticular running stitches
Subrapubic taps or aspirations
Thoracentesis
Thyroid fine needle aspiration
Tissue adhesives—use of tissue glues
Topical anesthesia
Topical hemostasis
Trigger point injection
Tubal ligation
Vaginal delivery
Vulvar biopsy
V-Y flap closure
Wart treatment (peripheral and plantar)

HPV, human papillomavirus; KOH, potassium hydroxide; IUD, intrauterine device; Pap, Papanicolaou.
From www.primarycareprocedures.com (Tuggy M, Garcia J: Procedures Consult. Philadelphia, Elsevier, 2009; also available at www.proceduresconsult.com).

Vasectomy, and Soft Tissue Surgery) include a DVD and syllabus, which can be purchased online by both AAFP members and nonmembers. The website www.proceduresconsult.com is paired with this text. Models are animated in three-dimensional (3-D) imagery.

The site www.primarycareprocedures.com is paired with Tuggy's *Multimedia Primary Care Procedures* (Elsevier) and is accessible when the DVDs are purchased.

Ethicon has several resources online. Not only is there a catalog of sutures, but a full 229-page comprehensive wound closure manual can be found at http:www.pilonidal.org/pdfs/wound_closure.pdf.

More and more video clips of procedures and other resources are becoming available on the Internet. A more complete list is found in Table E-2.

ARTIFICIAL MODELS AND LEARNING PROCEDURES

Lack of opportunities for enough practice is a common obstacle to learning procedures in primary care. Models and simulations provide an opportunity to practice skills when patients requiring the procedure are not available. Many physicians who have taken such courses as Advanced Cardiac Life Support (ACLS), Advanced Trauma Life Support (ATLS), Advanced Life Support in Obstetrics (ALSO), and the Neonatal Resuscitation Program (NRP) can appreciate the value of practicing and learning with models. Similar models are widely used in courses for teaching procedures. Research has shown that artificial models can be effective for learning and retaining technical skills. They can also be helpful in the clinical setting to rehearse a procedure before performing it on a patient. Companies such as Medisim Corp. (www.medisim.ca), Sawbones (www.sawbones.com), 3-Dmed Surgical Training Aids (www.3-Dmed.com), and Limbs & Things Ltd. (www.limbsandthings.com) offer highly realistic models for learning and practicing medical and surgical procedures. You will find a full listing of available models and costs at their websites.

Figure E-1 shows a realistic pelvic model developed by Medisim Corp. in cooperation with Ontario College of Family Physicians as part of the Benign Uterine Conditions Project. The soft tissue component of this model was developed from a casting of a human model. Its highly realistic features allow for practicing pelvic examination, endometrial biopsy, intrauterine device insertion, and pessary fitting. This model has proved itself in teaching skills to family physicians and family medicine residents as part of the skills transfer workshop associated with the Benign Uterine Conditions Initiative (www.machealth.ca/programs/buc).

Box E-2. Contents of Deutchman's Emergency and Trauma Ultrasound Examination and Cesarean Delivery DVDs

Emergency and Trauma Ultrasound Examination

This CD-ROM–based course is designed to teach the basic technique of emergency ultrasound examination. The course contains a combination of still and video segments as well as diagrams, three-dimensional animation, and interactive multimedia that describe the key concepts of ultrasonography.

Chapters include the following:

Introduction
Physics and orientation
Trauma ultrasound examination
Cardiac examination
Right upper quadrant examination
Abdominal aorta examination
Renal examination
OB/GYN examination
Lower extremity venous examination (DVT)
Sonographic guidance of procedures

20 hours of AMA Category 1 CME credit
Link to product: http://www.chall.com/emus.htm

Cesarean Delivery

This DVD contains 50+ minutes of high-quality surgical video demonstrating all aspects and multiple variations of cesarean surgical technique and tubal ligation technique, as well as assisting at surgery. Although the procedure must ultimately be taught in the operating room, viewing high-quality DVD video of the standard technique and its variation is helpful both to new learners and to more experienced physicians interested in improving their skills.

These techniques are included:

Patient positioning and preparation
Abdominal incisions: vertical and transverse
Opening the uterus
Delivery of the infant from cephalic and breech presentations
Use of vacuum extractor
Delivery of the placenta
Closure of the uterus
Tubal ligation technique
Closure of the abdomen and skin

6 hours of AMA Category I CME credit
Link to product: http://www.chall.com/emus.htm
AMA, American Medical Association; CME, continuing medical education; DVT, deep vein thrombosis; OB/GYN, obstetrics/gynecology.
Courtesy of Mark Deutchman, Aurora, CO.

Figure E-2 shows the artificial breast model developed by Medisim. The texture and feel of the skin and breast tissue are highly lifelike. With this model a breast cyst can be palpated and aspirated. The cyst will actually disappear when aspirated properly in a very realistic simulation of a clinical situation.

Figure E-3 shows the simulated skin model produced by Limbs & Things Ltd. Once again the skin is very lifelike when handled with instruments. Modifications of this model can be used to practice cyst or lipoma excision in a realistic fashion. The skin simulator can be adapted for different features, as is illustrated in Figure E-4, which shows how the model can be used to simulate excision of a sebaceous cyst.

Box E-3. DVDs Available from the National Procedures Institute

The Basics of Cardiac Stress Testing
The Basics of Radiofrequency Surgery
Billing and Coding for Dermatologic Procedures
Common Office Dermatologic Procedures: Patient Cases
Excisions and Common Wound Repairs: Patient Cases
Hospitalist Procedures: Collection 1
Hospitalist Procedures: Collection 2
How to Perform Skin Biopsies
Learning No-Scalpel Vasectomy: A Guide for Clinicians—From Counseling Through Procedure
Learning to Work with Botox (Botulinum Toxin A): A Guide for Clinicians
No-Scalpel Vasectomy: 6 Patient Cases
Removal of Condyloma with Radiofrequency/Electrosurgery
Suturing and Excision Techniques: Exercises on Pigs' Feet
Working with Collagen and Newer Tissue Fillers: A Guide for Clinicians

Figure E-5 shows the Face with Lesions, produced by Limbs & Things. Some of these lesions can be excised, creating a realistic simulation of skin surgery of the face, where scar orientation, lines of tension, and similar issues have to be considered.

Figure E-6 shows the NPI Down's Cervical Model, which can be biopsied, frozen, and used for performing an endocervical curettage.

Figure E-7 shows the very realistic NPI vasectomy model.

Figure E-8 shows the use of an orange to practice shave biopsy.

3-Dmed Surgical Training Aids provides multiple models and simulators (www.3-Dmed.com). These items include portable endoscopic/laparoscopic trainers, open procedure surgical trainers (episiotomy repair, suturing pads, coordination models, etc.), computer interface equipment, and more.

The cost of commercially available models for practicing procedure skills can be considerable. There is always the possibility of using less expensive, less realistic models for learning procedures. In fact many of these have been developed and described in various articles. Some of the models have been used in studies and shown success in improving a trainee's knowledge and confidence in procedure performance. In Table E-3 a variety of such models is listed. Some are quite traditional; some are very innovative. Nearly all are low cost, easily available, or reproducible. Appropriate references are provided in the table.

Computer Simulation and Virtual Reality in Learning Procedures

Simulation as a teaching technique has played a significant role in the training of pilots. The advent of virtual reality means that there is now the capability to combine 3-D visual imagery with the ability to interact. This can create very realistic simulations, which are

TABLE E-2 Procedural Skills Videos on the Web

Title/Author	Address/Description
Canadian Family Physician Video Series	http://www.cfp.ca/cgi/search?tocsectionid=Video%20Series Collections > Video Series ~10 procedures including: cryotherapy, toenail resection, pilar cyst removal, skin tag removal, elliptical excision, punch biopsy, and more. Free.
Casting and Splinting Videos. University of Ottawa Dept. of Emergency Medicine	http://intermed.med.uottawa.ca/procedures/cast/ Free.
Clinical Skills Online. St. George's e-Learning Unit, University of London	http://www.elu.sgul.ac.uk/cso/index.htm A project aimed at providing online videos demonstrating core clinical skills common to a wide range of medical and health-based courses. Free.
The Common Currency Project. Dalhousie University	http://currency.medicine.dal.ca/video.htm A project to develop general guidelines and concrete examples for the creation of a standard format, or "common currency," for shareable multimedia medical education materials. Free.
Google Video	http://video.google.com Type "medicine procedural skills" or name of specific skill. As with all resources, consider the source in evaluating usefulness.
Multimedia Primary Care Procedures: DVD, Online, and Pocket Procedures Manual. Tuggy M, et al.	http://www.elsevier.com/wps/find/bookdescription.cws_home/705622/description#description ISBN-13: 978-1-4160-0091-4, ISBN-10: 1-4160-0091-7 Saunders, 2006. $110.00
NEJM Videos in Clinical Medicine	http://content.nejm.org/ > Recent NEJM Video and More procedure videos (lower right-hand panel) Free, registration required.
Papanicolaou Society of Cytopathology	http://www.papsociety.org/fna.html Fine Needle Aspiration video tutorials
PocketSnips Procedural Skills Project. PocketSnips.org	http://normedsps.lakeheadu.ca/pocketsnips/default.aspx Free.
Procedures Consult. Elsevier	http://www.proceduresconsult.com/medical-procedures/ An online multimedia resource to with learning, performing, and testing of knowledge of the most frequent medical procedures. ~140 procedures. Annual subscription.
Procedural Skills Resources. University of Iowa Libraries	http://guides.lib.uiowa.edu/content.php?pid=5859&sid=36906 Lists resources under specific procedures; for example, Abscess Incision and Drainage, Casting & Splinting
Root Atlas	http://www.rootatlas.com/ Ophthalmology videos showing how to use the slit lamp and manage foreign bodies. Free.
The Thorndale Lion's Medical Center	http://www.ingrowntoenails.ca/ Informational site on ingrown toenails, including speaking engagements
Vidéos sur la petite chirurgie La Fédération des médecins omnipraticiens du Québec (FMOQ)	http://www.fmoq.org/Accueil/Accueil/Index.aspx > Formation professionnelle > Outils de formation > Boîte à outils Free.
Webmed. University of Alberta	http://www.webmedtechnology.com/physician/video.html Procedures ranging from lumbar puncture to managing psychotic patients. ~15 procedures. Free.
YouTube	http://ca.youtube.com/ Type "medicine procedural skills" or name of specific skill. As with all resources, consider the source in evaluating usefulness.

Compiled by The Library Service of The College of Family Physicians of Canada, Room 106K, Natural Sciences Centre, UWO, London, Ontario, Canada N6A 5B7. Phone: 519-661-3170. Fax: 519-661-3880. clfm@uwo.ca or www.cpfc.ca/clfm, 2009.

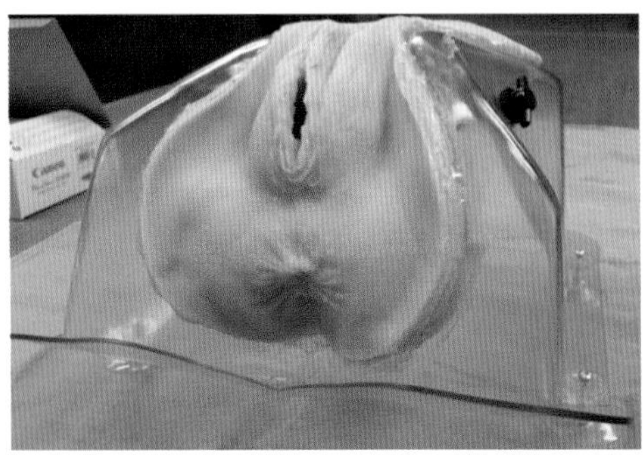

Figure E-1 Artificial pelvis model. This model can be used to teach and learn pelvic examination, endometrial biopsy, intrauterine device insertion, and pessary fitting. (Courtesy of Medisim Corp., Ontario, Canada.)

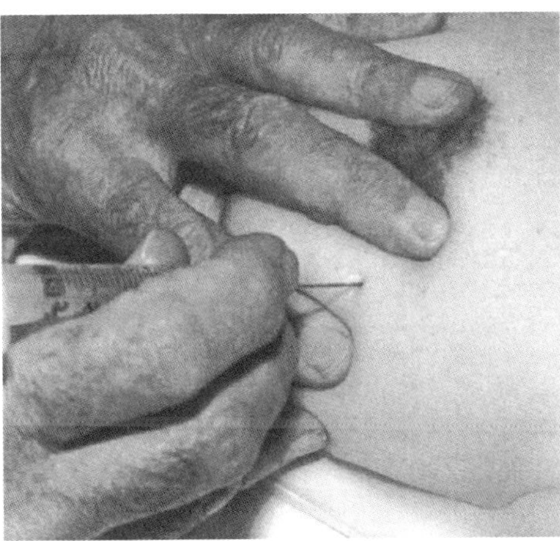

Figure E-2 Artificial breast model. This lifelike model contains a cyst that can be aspirated as shown to simulate aspiration in a real clinical situation. (Courtesy of Medisim Corp., Ontario, Canada.)

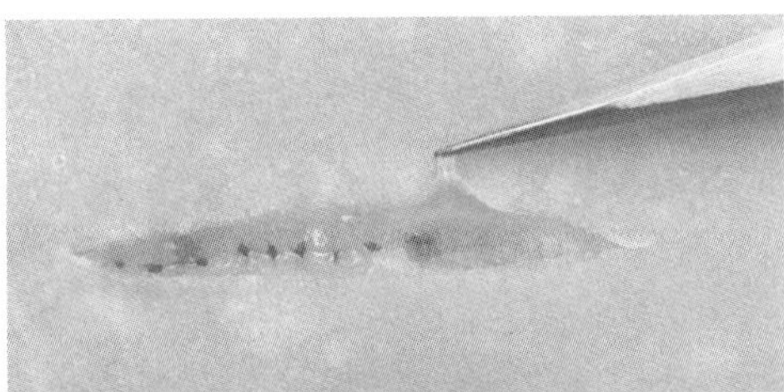

Figure E-3 Skin simulator model. The artificial skin is very lifelike and feels realistic when using a scalpel or other instruments. It can be used to practice incisions and suture techniques. (Courtesy of Limbs & Things Ltd., United Kingdom.)

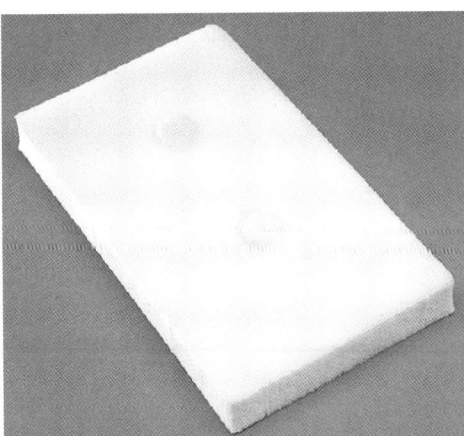

Figure E-4 Adaptation of the skin simulator model, showing a sebaceous cyst that can be excised by the operator. The texture of the artificial skin and cyst is very lifelike and produces a realistic cyst excision procedure. (Courtesy of Limbs & Things Ltd., United Kingdom.)

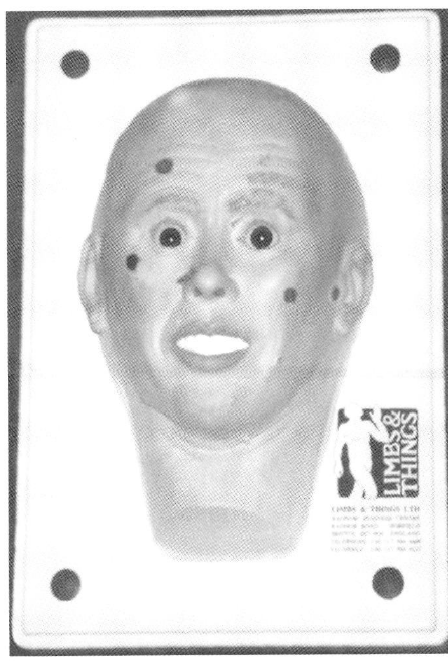

Figure E-5 The Face with Lesions model has realistic skin lesions for diagnosis. Some lesions can be excised and the skin repaired to practice the fine surgical techniques necessary for the face. (Courtesy of Limbs & Things Ltd., United Kingdom.)

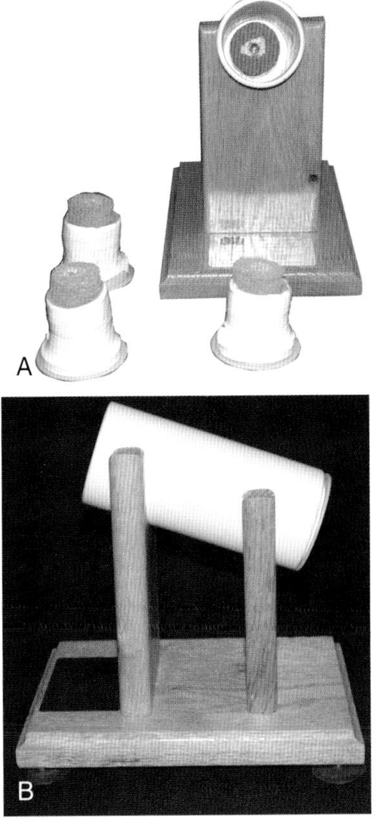

Figure E-6 NPI Down's cervical model. This cervical model is unique because biopsies can be performed, endocervical curettage (ECC) can be practiced, and it can be frozen. **A,** With replaceable inserts. **B,** Side view. (Courtesy of The National Procedures Institute, Midland, Mich.)

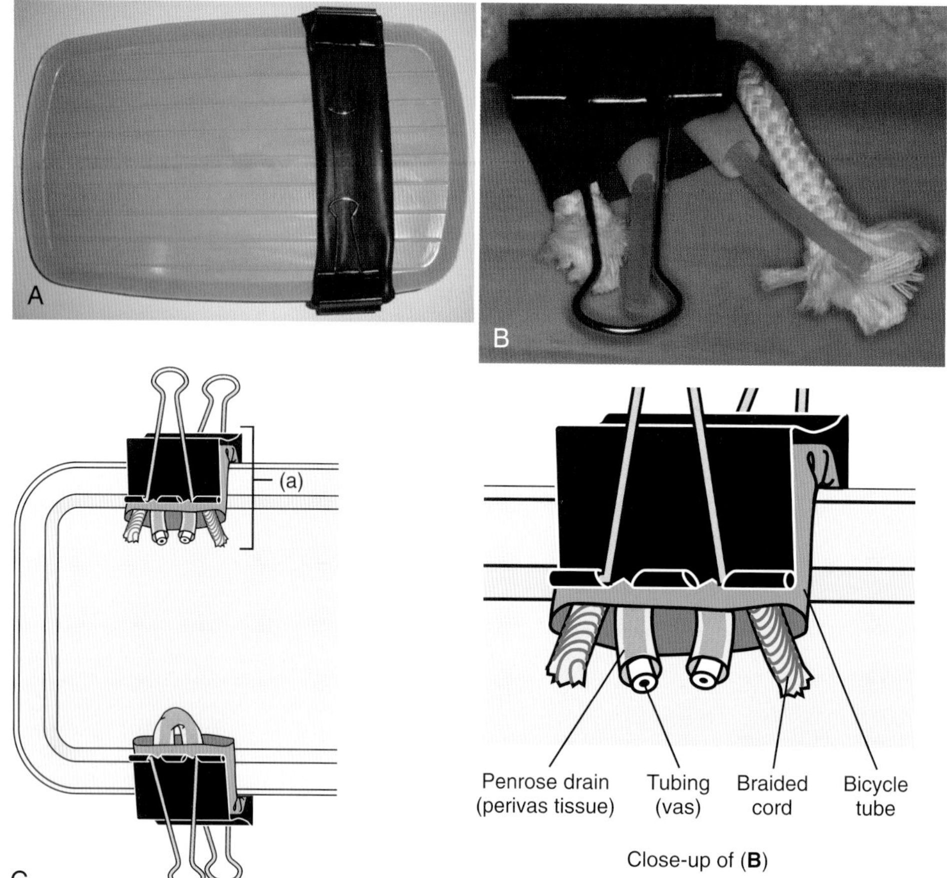

Figure E-7 NPI vasectomy model. **A,** Model. **B,** An "underside view" of the components of the NPI vasectomy model. See diagram for explanation. **C,** Illustration detailing the makeup of the model (underside) and what each material represents. The model is very realistic and provides a lifelike experience. (Courtesy of The National Procedures Institute, Midland, Mich.)

useful for training surgeons. The use of simulation has been demonstrated for laparoscopic and neurosurgical procedures and will be valuable for such techniques as sigmoidoscopy, colonoscopy, and hysteroscopy, among others. These simulations have proved very valuable for training in the various endoscopic techniques and ultrasound. While much of the attention has been given to invasive or minimally invasive surgical procedures, such devices will be helpful for training in suturing, line placement, biopsy, lumbar puncture, and many other procedures in emergency medicine. It should be pointed out that a systematic review of simulation methods currently used for surgical training has not shown them to be any better than other forms of training but, as there are such rapid advances in technology being made, there has to be continuous research in this area. In general, the more lifelike the simulations, the better the learning. Issenberg and associates have shown that high-fidelity medical simulations are educationally effective and complement usual medical training. Their value lies in the ability to receive feedback and experience repetitive practice. Application of such sophisticated training to the more common family medicine and emergency medicine procedures would be welcome. Although such virtual simulations are very expensive to develop, they can be reused indefinitely without deterioration and may be available, in part or in total, for long-distance learning over the Internet. There is currently an excellent computer simulator available from Immersion Medical (www.immersion.com) and (www.cae.com/en/healthcare/surgical.solutions.asp) to teach upper and lower gastrointestinal endoscopy. Although expensive, this unit comes as close to the real-life experience as possible.

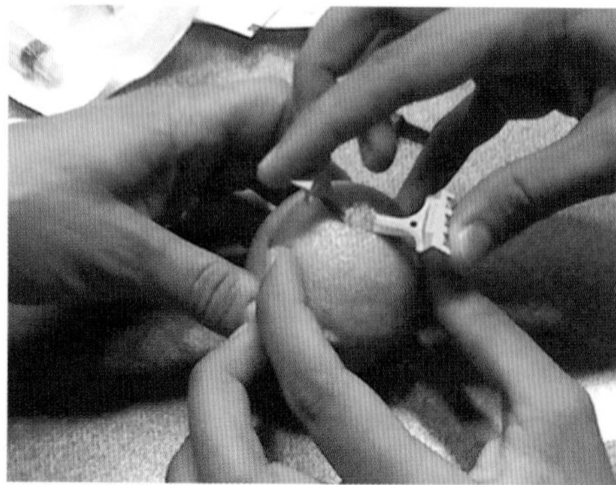

Figure E-8 Using an orange to practice shave biopsy. (Courtesy of Linda Prine, MD.)

Many medical schools now have simulation centers, where models and computer simulations are used to train students and residents. You may wish to contact the nearest medical school to see if they have such a center and if it would be available to you for practice or teaching.

PROCEDURE-ORIENTED ASSOCIATIONS

In addition to the general societies, those interested should be made aware of The American Association for Primary Care Endoscopy (AAPACE, www.aapace.org) and The American Society for Colposcopy and Cervical Pathology (ASCCP, www.asccp.org),

TABLE E-3 Models to Simulate and Practice Procedures

Model Type/Materials	Practice Use	Comments	Reference
Pig's feet	Suturing Minor skin surgery Laceration repair	Readily available from butchers and abbatoirs	Snell GF: A method for teaching techniques of office surgery. J Fam Pract 7:987–990, 1978.
Pig abdominal skin	Suturing Minor skin surgery	Tough	
Chicken breast	Cryosurgery		
Beefsteak	Electrosurgery		
Chicken legs	Tendon repair		
Breast cyst aspiration model (balloons, flour, Vitamin E capsules, or bath beads for cysts)	Breast cyst aspiration	Easy to prepare Teaches importance of release of suction before withdrawal	Delva D, Tomatly L, Payne P: Practice tips: Fine needle aspiration of breast lumps. Can Fam Physician 48:1055–1056, 2002.
Neonatal circumcision (cocktail wiener and surgical glove)	Neonatal circumcision		Brill JR, Wallace B: Neonatal circumcision model and competency evaluation for family medicine residents. Fam Med 39:241–243, 2007.
Surgical towel/Face cloth model	Perineal laceration or episiotomy repair	Low cost Practice anywhere	Cain JJ, Shirar E: A new method for teaching the repair of perineal trauma of birth. Fam Med 2:107–110, 1996.
Sponge perineum	Fourth-degree perineal laceration repair	Low cost	Sparks RA, Beesley AD, Jones AD: The Sponge Perineum: An innovative method of teaching fourth-degree obstetrical perineal laceration repair to family medicine residents. Fam Med 38:542–544, 2006. (more info available at www.fmdrl.org)
Papaya fruit	Uterine aspiration		Paul M, Nobel K: Papaya: A simulation model for training in uterine aspiration. Fam Med 37:242–244, 2005.
Kiwi fruit	Endometrial aspiration, IUD insertion		
Bovine cervix	Cervical surgery		Ferris DG, Waxman AG, Miller MD: Colposcopy and cervical biopsy educational training models. Fam Med 26:30, 1994.
Beefsteak	Electrosurgical loop excision		
Bovine colon	Sigmoidoscopy, colonoscopy		Sedlack RE, Baron TH, Downing SM, Schwartz AJ: Validation of a colonoscopy simulation for skills assessment. Am J Gastroenterol 102:64–74, 2007.
Hollowed-out fruit	Sigmoidoscopy	String fruit together	Empkie TM: Another exciting use for the cantaloupe. Fam Med 19:430, 1987.
Liver, beef or kidney (in surgical glove)	Fine needle aspiration of lumps		
Cow's eye	Corneal foreign body removal		
Peach	Musculoskeletal injections	Use a ripe peach and cut one side off flat for stability	
Sequential teaching model (surgical gloves and foam)	Perineal laceration repair		Montiel T. Rosenthal, MD Assistant Clinical Professor and Director of Maternity Services Department of Family Medicine University of Cincinnati The Christ Hospital/University of Cincinnati Family Medicine Residency Program 2123 Auburn Ave. Suite 340 Cincinnati, OH 45219 513-721-2221, ext. 12
Butternut pumpkin	Hysteroscopy		Kingston A, Abbott J, Lenart M, Vancaillie T: Hysteroscopic training: The butternut pumpkin model. J Am Assoc Gynecol Laparosc 11:256–261, 2004.
Orange	Shave biopsy	See Fig. E-8	Photo courtesy of Linda Prine, lindaprine@earthlink.net

which provide detailed learning in special interest areas. The Society of Teachers of Family Medicine (STFM) Group on Hospital Medicine and Procedural Training is focused on all aspects of teaching procedural skills.

Conclusion

In conclusion, the resources available for learning procedures range from courses at medical association meetings, books, CD-ROMs, DVDs, artificial models, and simulations all the way to virtual reality.

Clinicians can learn the background for each procedure, indications, contraindications, complications, and techniques from books, CD-ROMs, and DVDs. However, the ability to practice psychomotor skills is crucial to gaining confidence. Suitable practice can be achieved by using appropriate artificial models, biologic models, and other simulations. Such practice will facilitate learning in the clinical setting and skill maintenance.

Primary care physicians should remember that their primary care colleagues and specialist consultants are valuable resources for learning procedures through their teaching, encouragement, and support during skill learning.

The listing of resources provided in this chapter should be helpful for teachers and learners in developing the skills and the support necessary to provide our patients with quality care in primary care procedures.

BIBLIOGRAPHY

Anastakis DJ, Regehr G, Reznick R, et al: Assessment of technical skills transfer from the bench training model to the human model. Am J Surg 177:167–170, 1999.

Harper MB, Mayeaux EJ, Pope JB, Goel R: Procedural training in family practice residencies: Current status and impact on resident recruitment. J Am Board Fam Pract 8:189–194, 1995.

Issenberg SB, McGaghie WC, Petrusa ER, et al: Features and uses of high-fidelity medical simulations that lead to effective learning: A BEME systematic review. Med Teach 27:10–28, 2005.

Kelly BF, Sicilia JM, Forman S, et al: Advanced procedural training in family medicine: A group consensus statement. Fam Med 41:398–404, 2009.

Norris TE, Felmar E, Tolleson G: Which procedures should be taught in family practice residency programs? Fam Med 29:99–104, 1997.

Nothnagle M, Sicilia JM, Forman D, et al: Required procedural training in family medicine residency: A consensus statement. Fam Med 40:248–252, 2008.

Rodney WM, Hahn RC: Impact of the limited generalist (no hospital, no procedures) model on the viability of family practice training. J Am Board Fam Pract 15:191–200, 2002.

Sierpina VS, Volk RJ: Teaching outpatient procedures: Most common settings, evaluation methods, and training barriers in family practice residencies. Fam Med 30:421–423, 1998.

Sutherland LM, Middleton PF, Anthony A, et al: Surgical simulation: A systematic review. Ann Surg 243:291–300, 2006.

Sweet RM, McDougall EM: Simulation and computer-assisted devices: The new minimally invasive skills training paradigm. Urol Clin North Am 35:519–531, 2008.

van der Goes T, Grzybowski SC, Thommasen H: Procedural skills training. Canadian family practice residency programs. Can Fam Physician 45:78–85, 1999.

Wetmore S, Allen T, Brailovsky C, et al (The Working Group on the Certification Process, The College of Family Physicians of Canada): The General Key Features of Procedure Skills (personal communication).

Wetmore S, Rivet C, Tepper J, et al (The Working Group on Procedure Skills): Defining core procedure skills for Canadian family medicine training. Can Fam Physician 51:1364–1365, 2005.

Yelon S: Powerful Principles of Instruction. New York, Addison Wesley/Longman, 1996.

UNIVERSAL PRECAUTIONS

Madelyn Pollock

In discussion of universal precautions, it is important to understand the terminology used by the entities that promulgate the guidelines: primarily the Centers for Disease Control and Prevention (CDC) and the Occupational Safety and Health Administration (OSHA). Before 1983, the recommendations of public health agencies in handling blood and body fluids centered on special precautions taken with individuals known or suspected of being infected with bloodborne pathogens. These guidelines were known in the health care industry as "Blood and Body Fluid Precautions." With the increasing prevalence of human immunodeficiency virus (HIV) and hepatitis B virus (HBV) infections and the possibility that these diseases could be undiagnosed in patients, the CDC published "universal precautions" in 1983, recommending that blood and body fluids from *all patients* be considered potentially infectious and that rigorous infection control precautions be taken to minimize the risk of exposure to health care workers.

In 1996, the CDC modified its recommendations for infection control in the hospital setting, introducing the terminology "standard precautions." To quote the CDC in *Guideline for Isolation Precautions in Hospitals*, "Standard Precautions synthesize the major features of Universal (Blood and Body Fluid) Precautions (designed to reduce the risk of transmission of bloodborne pathogens) and Body Substance Isolation (designed to reduce the risk of transmission of pathogens from moist body substances). Standard Precautions apply to (1) blood; (2) all body fluids, secretions, and excretions except sweat, regardless of whether or not they contain visible blood; (3) nonintact skin; and, (4) mucous membranes."

In 1991, OSHA, a federal agency within the Department of Labor, issued a separate standard. OSHA's Bloodborne Pathogen Standards is based on the concept of universal precautions. It is intended to protect employees who might be exposed to blood or body fluids on the job. (See Online Resources for citation of the complete statute.)

A physician or other administrator managing a health care facility must attend to both the practical matters of reducing risk to people as well as satisfying regulatory agencies through appropriate documentation and follow-through. This appendix focuses on the procedures, policies, and equipment recommended for reducing risk to health care workers (HCWs) and patients, as well as meeting statutory regulations, especially as they apply to office procedures. It also outlines the requirements of an "Exposure Control Plan" as required for all health care employers by OSHA. Be aware that OSHA focuses only on employee protection.

INFECTION PREVENTION STRATEGY: WORKERS

Recommended guidelines for prevention of infections in HCWs encompass four domains: (1) formulation and implementation of site-specific policies in infection control (an "Exposure Control Plan"), (2) HCW screening and education at time of employment, (3) HCW immunization at the time of entry into an employment situation with risk, and (4) HCW use of barrier protection at time of risk of exposure. *All aspects of the prevention strategy require regular reevaluation and updating* as well as ongoing education of all workers.

The elements of an OSHA-compliant "Exposure Control Plan" are detailed in the statute and must be adapted to each individual site. Twenty-four states have adopted their own occupational safety guidelines and enforcement policies. They are usually identical to the federal guidelines, but you should check specifics for your state. In general, your plan must include common policies (Table F-1) as well as documentation of orientation and ongoing training of personnel. It must also delineate policies for record keeping (employee health screen information, records of training, records of any incidents or injuries, and so forth). The plan must be in written form and available to all employees. There should be evidence of periodic review of the plan for currency and accuracy. Proprietary agencies, including some medical supply marketers, sell "kits" for preparation of a site's "Exposure Control Plan" that include templates customizable to a site. Federal regulations require that all HCWs be evaluated initially with a health inventory. This should include determination of suitability for a position at risk for infectious exposure as well as determination of the worker's immune status for vaccine-preventable illnesses (OSHA's only *required* immunization policy is for hepatitis B virus vaccine). These health screens must be recorded in written form, and workers must be reevaluated periodically. Each employee in the facility should have a health record available and updated with the necessary information. This health record should be maintained separately from the employee's other employment record and must be maintained for 30 years by OSHA regulations. At this initial evaluation, a determination of the need for additional vaccination should be made. Current CDC recommendations are listed in Table F-2.

After initial assessment, infection control in HCWs continues with education. Simple hand washing is the most important activity in reducing transmission of infections in the workplace. Education about policies such as sharps disposal, no recapping of needles, and prompt reporting of injury is crucial. Health care facilities should take steps to ensure initial orientation to infection control policies for all employees and periodic reinstruction of all established personnel. Policies should be written clearly and include supporting information so that employees can understand the rationale for the policies. Employees should be evaluated for the specific risk associated with their particular job and special education for risk reduction implemented and documented.

An often overlooked aspect of an infection control strategy is the immunization of HCWs who are at risk for vaccine-preventable diseases. Appropriate use of vaccines in susceptible individuals can not only help prevent nosocomial infections in HCWs but also reduce loss of workdays because of isolation following potential exposures. In addition, prevention of infection through optimal use of vaccinations and laboratory determination of immune status is much more cost effective than case management following an exposure in a nonimmunized HCW. Immune status of all health care

TABLE F-1 Infection Control Policies for a Typical Physician's Office

Area	Specific Details to Include
Handwashing	Rules for areas with and without running water; handwashing before and *after* eating, drinking, smoking, applying cosmetics, handling contact lenses, or using the restroom as well as between patients
Contaminated sharps	Both disposable and reusable sharps; no recapping of needles or using one-handed recapping technique; disposal of filled sharps containers
Areas for eating, drinking, smoking, and applying cosmetics	Application of lip balm
Contaminated equipment	Manufacturers' guidelines for disinfection
Personal protection equipment (PPE)	Use of gloves, gowns, masks, goggles, and impervious aprons
Cleaning/disposal of PPE	Method of documentation of cleaning
Contaminated spills	Choice of cleaning agent
Contaminated laundry	Bagging in room of use; use of closed bags for transport
Employee hepatitis B virus vaccination	Hepatitis B vaccine declination form (OSHA Regulation, see Fig. F-1)
Postexposure evaluation and follow-up	Procedure to document details of injury; testing of both employee and source individual; document counseling; procedure for administration of antiretroviral agents
Employee training	Initial and ongoing training schedule
Specimen handling	Separation of food items and specimens; use of gloves when handling specimens
Triage of patients	Carefully screen patients for communicable diseases at check-in so that susceptible workers can avoid contact, and infectious patients can be removed promptly from contact with other waiting patients

facility personnel should be recorded at initiation of employment, and the hepatitis B vaccination series should be made available to all susceptible employees (OSHA Regulation, 2001). An employee who declines the vaccine should sign the Hepatitis B Vaccine Declination Form (Fig. F-1). Barrier protection using personal protection equipment (PPE) is the last line of prevention for HCW exposure to potentially infectious material. All HCWs must use appropriate PPE for the task at hand. In summary

- Gloves should be worn when contact with any blood, body fluids, mucous membranes, or broken skin is anticipated or possible; this exposure includes contact with soiled items or surfaces and performing venipuncture.
- Masks and eye shields should be worn when splashes of blood or body fluids are possible or during procedures in which blood, body fluids, or tissue could be aerosolized.
- Gowns or impervious aprons should be worn in situations in which blood or body fluids could contaminate the HCW's clothing.
- Gowns, aprons, and gloves must be changed and discarded between patients.
- Mouth-to-mouth ventilation should be performed using a "mouth-to-mask" ventilation device with no direct contact between the patient's mouth and the HCW's.

See Table F-1 for an example of an office guideline, and consult the OSHA statute for a detailed discussion of the regulations.

Environmental Considerations

Environmental considerations for prevention of infection from the HCW to the patient (or between patients) can be defined in three areas: (1) surface disinfection, (2) instrument sterilization/disinfection, and (3) policies regarding function of actively infected HCWs in the health care facility.

A full discussion of all the issues in the choice and use of agents for disinfection of surfaces and instruments is beyond of the scope of this appendix. The Association for Professionals in Infection Control and Epidemiology, Inc. (APIC) has published a comprehensive guideline that can serve as a reference for further details. In general, it is important to know some of the history of this area in order to understand some of the terminology. A classification developed in the 1960s by E. H. Spaulding is still used today to determine appropriate levels of decontamination of medical surfaces and equipment.

In general, Spaulding divided devices into three levels of decontamination. The first level is *critical*, meaning that the device enters sterile tissue or the vascular system. These devices must be *sterilized*, that is, devoid of microbial life, including spores. This can be accomplished by heat, ethylene oxide gas, and a number of immersion techniques. For many physicians' offices, a small autoclave accomplishes the task of rendering reusable devices and instruments sterile between patients. For critical instruments that cannot be subjected to heat or for facilities in which use of heat or ethylene oxide sterilization is not available, several immersion fluids are available.

TABLE F-2 Summary of Advisory Committee on Immunization Practices Recommendations for Health Care Workers, Including Special Conditions

Worker Status	Hepatitis B Recombinant Vaccine	Influenza Vaccine	Measles/Mumps/Rubella Live-Virus Vaccine	Varicella Zoster Live-Virus Vaccine
Healthy, nonpregnant	R	R	R	R
Pregnant	R	R	C	C
HIV-positive	R	R	R*	C
Severe immunosuppression	R	R	C	C
Asplenia	R	R	R	R
Renal failure	R	R	R	R
Diabetes	R	R	R	R
Alcoholism and cirrhosis	R	R	R	R

C, Contraindicated; HIV, human immunodeficiency virus; R, recommended.
*Contraindicated in persons with HIV infection and severe immunosuppression.
Adapted from Centers for Disease Control and Prevention. Immunization of Health-Care Workers: Recommendations of the Advisory Committee on Immunization Practices (ACIP) and the Hospital Infection Control Practices Advisory Committee (HICPAC). MMWR 46(No. RR-18):36, 1997. Available at http://www.cdc.gov/mmwr/preview/mmwrhtml/00050577.htm.

Hepatitis B Vaccine Declination Form

I understand that due to my occupational exposure to blood or other potentially infectious materials I may be at risk of acquiring hepatitis B virus (HBV) infection. I have been given the opportunity to be vaccinated with hepatitis B vaccine, at no charge to myself. However, I decline hepatitis B vaccination at this time. I understand that by declining this vaccine, I continue to be at risk of acquiring hepatitis B, a serious disease. If in the future I continue to have occupational exposure to blood or other potentially infectious materials and I want to be vaccinated with hepatitis B vaccine, I can receive the vaccination series at no charge to me.

________________________ __________
Signature of employee Date

Figure F-1 Hepatitis B Vaccine Declination (Mandatory) form. (From OSHA [Occupational Safety and Health Administration] Regulations [Standards, 29 CFR Part 1910.1030] [56 Fed. Reg. 64,004, Dec. 6, 1991, as amended at 57 Fed. Reg. 12,717, April 13, 1992; 57 Fed. Reg. 29,206, July 1, 1992; 61 Fed. Reg. 5507, Feb. 1996].)

Manufacturers' recommendations for use of these solutions, with special attention to treatment time, should be followed closely.

The second level is *semi-critical* and applies to devices that touch mucous membranes. These instruments include endoscopes, endotracheal tubes, and laryngoscopes as well as thermometers. These devices must be subjected to *high-level disinfection*. Because many of these instruments cannot be subjected to heat, special cleaning devices and fluids must be used for their disinfection. It is important to follow manufacturers' recommendations completely to avoid incomplete disinfection as well as damage to the instruments. Again, thorough cleaning of instruments prior to disinfection is important. Routine changing of fluids and cleaning tools is an important part of an effective routine.

The third level of decontamination according to Spaulding is *noncritical* and includes stethoscopes, examination room surfaces, and bedpans. These items should be cleansed appropriately with agents that are known to kill most surface microbes without significant corrosion of the items or without being excessively toxic to the HCW. Typical agents in this category include alcohols (ethyl and isopropyl), household bleach (5.2% sodium hypochlorite), phenols, iodophors, and quaternary ammonium compounds. These agents are commonly sold by medical supply companies for use on surfaces. Manufacturers' guidelines must be understood and followed. Be aware of the corrosive nature of some of these products on certain surfaces, and follow instructions for protection of HCWs from any potentially toxic fumes.

An important concept in the handling of reusable instruments is the direction of workflow. It is important that "clean" and "soiled" areas are separated and policies are established so that item flow does not risk contamination of "clean" items. There should be clearly defined areas for the receipt of contaminated items with physical barriers preventing accidental contamination. Policies for maintaining these processing standards should be clear to all workers.

Use and maintenance of autoclaves in an office should be governed by policies and routine, reflecting good infection control practices. The first step in sterilization of instruments is thorough cleaning (removal of surface debris) of all instruments to be sterilized. Biologic and chemical indicators for use in heat sterilizers should be used and checked consistently. Temperature and pressure and results of indicators should be recorded in a log form. Remember, biologic indicators require use of a manufacturer-recommended incubator for proper use.

Regarding transmission of disease from the ill or potentially ill HCW to the patient, the health care facility's administration is responsible for development and implementation of policies to address this issue. At times, such policies may result in restriction of HCWs from patient contact; therefore, it is important that policies be designed to encourage reporting of exposures and illnesses protecting wages, benefits, and job status if possible. The policies should reflect exclusions resulting from both acute infection and known exposure. The policies should be clear regarding who in the facility is responsible for making isolation exclusions.

The decision making falls into two broad categories that require quite different management and follow-through. For chronic bloodborne communicable diseases such as HIV and HBV, the CDC recommends the HCW "...not perform exposure-prone, invasive procedures until counsel from an expert review panel has been sought, which will determine under what circumstances the worker may or may not perform exposure-prone, invasive procedures." Exposure-prone invasive procedures include those that involve manipulating a needle inside the body or placing the fingers and a needle or other sharp instrument in a poorly visualized or highly confined anatomic site. The CDC recommends no restrictions for workers with chronic hepatitis B if hepatitis B e antigen becomes negative and currently recommends no restriction regarding workers with hepatitis C. Each facility should develop its own policy regarding HIV and hepatitis B- and C-infected workers.

For more acute disease entities, the CDC has developed guidelines that can be adapted for most facilities (Table F-3). The guidelines summarize recommended work restrictions including duration. These guidelines apply to both exposure and infection with the disease. They should always be compared with any local or state guidelines that may apply in your area. Consideration of your facility's patient population and the worker's level of patient exposure is important. In jobs in which close contact with patients is unlikely, a worker might be able to remain on the job but could use certain precautions (such as wearing a mask) and still not jeopardize patients or coworkers.

CONCLUSION

It is important that the leadership of every health care facility, regardless of size, become familiar with the standards and regulations regarding infection control in the workplace. The facility must formulate and implement policies to protect health care workers as well as patients from communicable diseases. These policies should reflect current guidelines from the CDC and comply with regulations promulgated by OSHA. In addition to this appendix, the infection control officer of your local hospital should be considered as an ally and information source in development or review of policies and procedures for your particular site.

GENERAL RESOURCES

Association for Professionals in Infection Control and Epidemiology, Inc.
1275 K Street, NW, Suite 1000
Washington, DC 20005-4006
Phone: 1-202-789-1890
Website: www.apic.org

Centers for Disease Control and Prevention
1600 Clifton Road, NE
Atlanta, GA 30333
Phone: 1-404-639-3311
Division of AIDS/HIV Prevention: 1-800-843-6356
Website: www.cdc.gov

U.S. Department of Labor
Occupational Safety and Health Administration
200 Constitution Avenue, NW
Washington, DC 20210
Website: www.osha.gov

TABLE F-3 Summary of Suggested Work Restrictions for Health Care Workers Exposed to or Infected with the Most Common Acute Communicable Diseases of Importance in the Ambulatory Setting

Disease/Problem	Work Restriction	Duration
Conjunctivitis	Restrict from patient contact and contact with the patient's environment	Until discharge ceases
CMV infection	No restriction	
Diarrheal diseases		
Acute stage	Restrict from patient contact, contact with the patient's environment, and food handling	Until symptoms resolve
Convalescent stage (*Salmonella* spp.)	Restrict from care of high-risk patients	Until symptoms resolve; consult with local health agencies regarding need for negative cultures
Enteroviral infections	Restrict from care of infants, neonates, and immunocompromised patients and their environments	Until symptoms resolve
Hepatitis A	Restrict from patient contact, contact with the patient's environment, and food handling	Until 7 days after onset of jaundice
Herpes simplex		
Genital	No restriction	
Hands (Whitlow)	Restrict from patient contact and contact with the patient's environment	Until lesions heal
Orofacial	Evaluate for need to restrict from care of high-risk patients	
Measles		
Active	Exclude from duty	Until 7 days after rash appears
Postexposure (susceptible)	Exclude from duty	From 5th day after first exposure through 21st day after last exposure or 4 days after rash appears
Meningococcal infection	Exclude from duty	Until 24 hours after start of effective therapy
Mumps		
Active	Exclude from duty	Until 9 days after onset of parotitis
Postexposure (susceptible)	Exclude from duty	From 12th day after first exposure through 26th day after last exposure or until 9 days after onset of parotitis
Pediculosis	Restrict from patient contact	Until treated and observed to be free of adult and immature lice
Rubella		
Active	Exclude from duty	Until 5 days after rash appears
Postexposure (susceptible)	Exclude from duty	From 7th day after first exposure through the 21st day after last exposure
Scabies	Restrict from patient contact	Until cleared by medical evaluation
Staphylococcus aureus infection		
Active, still draining lesions	Restrict from patient contact, contact with patient's environment, and food handling	Until lesions have resolved
Carrier state	No restriction unless personnel are epidemiologically linked to transmission of the organisms	
Streptococcus, group A infection	Restrict from patient contact, contact with patient's environment, and food handling	Until 24 hr after adequate treatment started
Tuberculosis		
Active disease	Exclude from duty	Until proved noninfectious
PPD converter	No restriction	
Varicella		
Active	Exclude from duty	Until all lesions dry and crusted
Postexposure (susceptible)	Exclude from duty	From 10th day after first exposure through the 21st day (28th day if VZIG given) after last exposure
Zoster		
Localized in healthy person	Cover lesions, restrict from care of high-risk patients	Until all lesions dry and crusted
Generalized or localized in the immunocompromised person	Restrict from patient contact	Until all lesions dry and crusted
Postexposure (susceptible)	Restrict from patient contact	From 10th day after first exposure through the 21st day (28th day if VZIG given) after last exposure, or if varicella occurs, until all lesions dry and crusted
Viral URI, acute febrile	Consider excluding from the care of high-risk patients or contact with their environment during community outbreak of RSV and influenza	Until acute symptoms resolve

CMV, cytomegalovirus; PPO, purified protein derivative; RSV, respiratory syncytial virus; URI, upper respiratory infection; VZIG, varicella zoster immunoglobulin.
From Current Postexposure Prophylaxis Recommendations. MMWR Recomm Rep 47(RR-7):1, 1998. Available at http://www.cdc.gov/ncidod/dhqp/gl_occupational.html.

ONLINE RESOURCES

Centers for Disease Control and Prevention: "Sharps Injury Prevention Workbook." For use in establishing a sharps policy, can be downloaded at http://www.cdc.gov/sharpssafety/resources.html.

Centers for Disease Control and Prevention: Updated U.S. Public Health Service Guidelines for the Management of Occupational Exposures to HBV, HCV, and HIV and Recommendations for Postexposure Prophylaxis. MMWR 2001;50(No. RR-11) Available at http://www.cdc.gov/ncidod/dhqp/gl_occupational.html.

OSHA Regulation: Exposure Control Plan. Occupational Safety and Health Administration, Department of Labor. 29 CFR Part 1910.1030, Occupational exposure to bloodborne pathogens; final rule. Revised 2001. Available at http://www.osha.gov/SLTC/bloodbornepathogens/index.html.

BIBLIOGRAPHY

Bolyard EA, Tablan OC, Williams WW, et al: The Hospital Infection Control Practices Advisory Committee: Special article: Guideline for infection control in healthcare personnel, 1998. Am J Infect Control 26:289, 1998.

Garner JS, and the Hospital Infection Control Practices Advisory Committee: Guidelines for isolation precautions in hospitals. CDC Guidelines published Jan. 1, 1996.

Rutala WA: APIC guideline for selection and use of disinfectants: 1994, 1995, and 1996 APIC Guidelines Committee: Association for Professionals in Infection Control and Epidemiology. Am J Infect Control 24:313, 1996.

APPENDIX G

NEOPLASMS OF THE SKIN: ICD-9 DIAGNOSTIC CODES

John L. Pfenninger

- For excision and repair CPT codes, see Chapter 22, Laceration and Incision Repair. Understand that "shave excisions" and "biopsies" have their own CPT codes.
- The following ICD-9 codes are *only for neoplasms originating in the skin*. Other, subcutaneous tumors have their own codes (see the section on Selected Tumor Codes).

	Malignant					
Site	**Primary**	**Secondary**	**Carcinoma in situ**	**Benign**	**Uncertain Behavior**	**Unspecified**
Skin NEC	173.9	198.2	232.9	216.9	238.2	239.2
Abdominal wall	173.5	198.2	232.5	216.5	238.2	239.2
Ala nasi	173.3	198.2	232.3	216.3	238.2	239.2
Ankle	173.7	198.2	232.7	216.7	238.2	239.2
Antecubital space	173.6	198.2	232.6	216.6	238.2	239.2
Anus*	173.5	198.2	232.5	216.5	238.2	239.2
Arm	173.6	198.2	232.6	216.6	238.2	239.2
Auditory canal (external)	173.2	198.2	232.2	216.2	238.2	239.2
Auricle (ear)	173.2	198.2	232.2	216.2	238.2	239.2
Auricular canal (external)	173.2	198.2	232.2	216.2	238.2	239.2
Axilla, axillary fold	173.5	198.2	232.5	216.5	238.2	239.2
Back	173.5	198.2	232.5	216.5	216.5	239.2
Breast	173.5	198.2	232.5	216.5	238.2	239.2
Brow	173.3	198.2	232.3	216.3	238.2	239.2
Buttock	173.5	198.2	232.5	216.5	238.2	239.2
Calf	173.7	198.2	232.7	216.7	238.2	239.2
Canthus (eye) (inner) (outer)	173.1	198.2	232.1	216.1	238.2	239.2
Cervical region	173.4	198.2	232.4	216.4	238.2	239.2
Cheek (external)	173.3	198.2	232.3	216.3	238.2	239.2
Chest (wall)	173.5	198.2	232.5	216.5	238.2	239.2
Chin	173.3	198.2	232.3	216.3	238.2	239.2
Clavicular area	173.5	198.2	232.5	216.5	238.2	239.2
Clitoris	184.3	198.82	232.3	221.2	236.3	239.5
Columnella	173.3	198.2	232.3	216.3	238.2	239.2
Concha	173.2	198.2	232.2	216.2	238.2	239.2
Contiguous sites	173.8					
Ear (external)	173.2	198.2	232.2	216.2	238.2	239.2
Elbow	173.6	198.2	232.6	216.6	238.2	239.2
Eyebrow	173.3	198.2	232.3	216.3	238.2	239.2
Eyelid	173.1	198.2	232.1	216.1	238.2	239.2
Face NEC	173.3	198.2	232.3	216.3	238.2	239.2
Female genital organs (external)	184.4	198.82	233.3	221.2	236.3	239.5
Clitoris	184.3	198.82	233.3	221.2	236.2	239.5
Labium NEC	184.4	198.82	233.3	221.2	236.3	239.5
Majus	184.1	198.82	233.3	221.2	236.3	239.5
Minus	184.2	198.82	233.3	221.2	236.3	239.5
Pudendum	184.4	198.82	233.3	221.2	236.3	239.5
Vulva	184.4	198.82	233.3	221.2	236.3	239.5
Finger	173.6	198.2	232.6	216.6	238.2	239.2
Flank	173.5	198.2	232.5	216.5	238.2	239.2
Foot	173.7	198.2	232.7	216.7	238.2	239.2
Forearm	173.6	198.2	232.6	216.6	238.2	239.2
Forehead	173.3	198.1	232.3	216.3	238.2	239.2

Site	Malignant			Benign	Uncertain Behavior	Unspecified
	Primary	Secondary	Carcinoma in situ			
Glabella	173.3	198.2	232.3	216.3	238.2	239.2
Gluteal region	173.5	198.2	232.5	216.5	238.2	239.2
Groin	173.5	198.2	232.5	216.5	238.2	239.2
Hand	173.6	198.2	232.6	216.6	238.2	239.2
Head NEC	173.4	198.2	232.4	216.4	238.2	239.2
Heel	173.7	198.2	232.7	216.7	238.2	239.2
Helix	173.2	198.2	232.2	216.2	238.2	239.2
Hip	173.7	198.2	232.7	216.7	238.2	239.2
Infraclavicular region	173.5	198.2	232.5	216.5	238.2	239.2
Inguinal region	173.5	198.2	232.5	216.5	238.2	239.2
Jaw	173.3	198.2	232.3	216.3	238.2	239.2
Knee	173.7	198.2	232.7	216.7	238.2	239.2
Labia						
Majora	184.1	198.82	233.3	221.2	236.3	239.5
Minora	184.2	198.82	233.3	221.2	236.3	239.5
Leg	173.7	198.2	232.7	216.7	238.2	239.2
Lid (lower or upper)	173.1	198.2	232.1	216.1	238.2	239.2
Limb NEC	173.9	198.2	232.9	216.9	238.2	239.2
Lower	173.7	198.2	232.7	216.7	238.2	239.2
Upper	173.6	198.2	232.6	216.6	238.2	239.2
Lip (upper or lower)	173.0	198.2	232.0	216.0	238.2	239.2
Male genital organs	187.9	198.82	232.6	222.9	236.6	239.5
Penis	187.4	198.82	232.5	222.1	236.6	239.5
Prepuce	187.1	198.82	232.5	222.1	236.6	239.5
Scrotum	187.7	198.82	232.6	222.4	236.6	239.5
Mastectomy site	173.5	198.2				
Specified as breast tissue	174.8	198.81				
Meatus, acoustic (external)	173.2	198.2	232.2	216.2	238.2	239.2
Melanoma[†]						
Nates	173.5	198.2	232.5	216.5	238.2	239.0
Neck	173.4	198.2	232.4	216.4	238.2	239.2
Nose (external)	173.3	198.2	232.3	216.3	238.2	239.2
Palm	173.6	198.2	232.6	216.6	238.2	239.2
Palpebra	173.1	198.2	232.1	216.1	238.2	239.2
Penis NEC	187.4	198.82	233.5	222.1	236.6	239.5
Perianal	173.5	198.2	232.5	216.5	238.2	239.2
Perineum	173.5	198.2	232.5	216.5	238.2	239.2
Pinna	173.2	198.2	232.2	216.2	238.2	239.2
Plantar	173.7	198.2	232.7	216.7	238.2	239.2
Popliteal fossa or space	173.7	198.2	232.7	216.7	238.2	239.2
Prepuce	187.1	198.82	233.5	222.1	236.6	239.5
Pubes	173.5	198.2	232.5	216.5	238.2	239.2
Sacrococcygeal region	173.5	198.2	232.5	216.5	238.2	239.2
Scalp	173.4	198.2	232.4	216.4	238.2	239.2
Scapular region	173.5	198.2	232.5	216.5	238.2	239.2
Scrotum	187.7	198.82	233.6	222.4	236.6	239.5
Shoulder	173.6	198.2	232.6	216.6	238.2	239.2
Sole (foot)	173.7	198.2	232.7	216.7	238.2	239.2
Specified sites NEC	173.8	198.2	232.8	216.8	232.8	239.2
Submammary fold	173.5	198.2	232.5	216.5	238.2	239.2
Supraclavicular region	173.4	198.2	232.4	216.4	238.2	239.2
Temple	173.3	198.2	232.3	216.3	238.2	239.2
Thigh	173.7	198.2	232.7	216.7	238.2	239.2
Thoracic wall	173.5	198.2	232.5	216.5	238.2	239.2
Thumb	173.6	198.2	232.6	216.6	238.2	239.2
Toe	173.7	198.2	232.7	216.7	238.2	239.2
Tragus	173.2	198.2	232.2	216.2	238.2	239.2
Trunk	173.5	198.2	232.5	216.5	238.2	239.2
Umbilicus	173.5	198.2	232.5	216.5	238.2	239.2
Vulva	184.4	198.8	233.3	221.2	236.3	239.5
Wrist	173.6	198.2	232.6	216.6	238.2	239.2

NEC, neuroendocrine carcinoma.

*Intra-anal lesions have separate codes.

[†]Melanoma skin sites use the 172.X codes, where "X" notes the site on the skin. See the ICD-9 code book. Acceptable, but less accurate, coding would be to use the generic "primary, malignant" category by site.

From International Classification of Diseases, rev 9: ICD-9-CM 2003, 6th ed. Ingenix/St. Anthony Publishing, 2003.

Selected Tumor Codes

Lesions below the skin have their own ICD-9 diagnostic codes depending on the location. They are divided into similar categories including the following:

- Malignant
  - Primary
  - Secondary
- Benign
- Uncertain behavior
- Unspecified

Each lesion must be looked up individually. Some examples of benign tumors:

215.0 Neoplasm of the face
215.2 Neoplasm of the shoulder
215.7 Neoplasm of the trunk

Another way of coding some of these lesions would be more specific:

214.0 Lipoma, face, subcutaneous (SQ)
214.1 Lipoma, other, SQ

Some examples of malignant tumors:

171.0 Malignant tumor of the face
171.2 Malignant tumor of the shoulder
171.7 Malignant tumor of the back

It is important to recognize that skin neoplasms are coded distinctly differently than tumors below the skin. For excision of these tumors, a separate set of CPT codes is used, based on the size (usually <3 cm or >3 cm) and whether they were subcutaneous or subfascial, or whether a radical removal/excision was required. See Chapter 22, Laceration and Incision Repair.

Using the "unspecified" codes for either skin neoplasms or for subcutaneous tumors is likely to generate rejections from insurance carriers or requests for further information.

PEARLS OF PRACTICE

John L. Pfenninger • Grant C. Fowler

"I don't think I'm unique. Anybody can do quite a lot by refusing to give in to limitations."

Christopher Reeves

1. When repairing or removing *scalp lesions*, remember that patients do not like to have their hair shaved unless it is absolutely necessary. *Remove minor lesions without shaving*. To keep the hair from continually falling into the operative field, use antibiotic ointment to flatten it down. Apply the ointment after performing the usual preparation.
2. The majority of *skin lesion removals* are performed either with a shave technique or with curettement and cautery. *Moist healing* is the key to an excellent long-term outcome with *minimal scarring*. Eschars (scabs) impair the normal healing process. Healing tissue is much like a new lawn: It needs to be kept moist. Unless under clothes, wounds should remain without a dressing, except for ointment, when possible. If under clothes, wounds will obviously need to be covered with an adhesive strip or other dressing. Likewise, facial areas will need to be covered at night. Basically, the patient just gently washes the area three to four times a day with mild soap and water and applies an ointment afterward. It does not necessarily have to be an antibacterial ointment; even petrolatum (Vaseline) will do. Avoid neomycin, hydrogen peroxide, or povidine–iodine (Betadine). The deeper the open wound, the longer it will be necessary to keep the area moist (generally 7 to 14 days).

   With sutured wounds, have the patient gently wash the area within 12 hours and apply antibiotic ointment three or four times a day (unless tissue glue or Steri-Strips have been applied). Cover with other dressings only as noted previously. An easier method for the patient that causes less inflammation is to use a moist healing occlusive dressing such as Tegaderm. This is applied immediately after excision (or laceration repair) and left in place until the sutures are removed, unless blood accumulates and then it can be changed.

   See the sample patient education handout online at www.expertconsult.com.
3. *There is no need to stop warfarin (Coumadin), clopidogrel (Plavix), or aspirin for routine dermatologic procedures*. Several articles have been published documenting that embolic events occur during the period of stopping and restarting the medications. Meticulous attention must be paid to hemostasis. Clotting parameters should be checked before significant excisional surgery. However, for shaves, curettements, and most excisions, it is unnecessary to stop any of these medications or to check laboratory results (see Alcalay 2001; Schanbacher and Bennett 2000).
4. *Bridge therapy is for patients on chronic anticoagulation* who need elective surgery. It is defined as protected periprocedural discontinuation of warfarin (Coumadin) 3 to 4 days before performing procedures in patients at high risk for thromboembolism. The first step is initiation of low-molecular-weight heparin (LMWH) at full therapeutic dose on the day after warfarin is stopped (e.g., no warfarin Monday, begin LMWH on Tuesday morning). The patient receives the last dose of LMWH the morning of the day before the procedure. Then the invasive procedure or surgery occurs. Warfarin and LMWH are reintroduced later that day if deemed safe and hemostasis has been achieved. Subsequently, LMWH is discontinued after discharge once the international normalized ratio (INR) has been therapeutic for 3 or 4 days.

   Bridge therapy is used for patients with a high risk of atrial fibrillation (i.e., for cerebrovascular accident [CVA] prevention), prosthetic valves, a recent (last 3 months) thromboembolic event, indications for prolonged warfarin therapy, or a history of a hypercoagulable state.

   This therapy avoids prolonged hospitalization, changing of anticoagulation while preparing for surgery, vitamin K administration, and a prolonged period without anticoagulation with the attendant risk for thromboembolism.

   The disadvantages are cost of LMWH, self-injection, and a relative lack of reversibility. (From James Lile, pharmacist, MidMichigan Medical Center, Midland, Mich.)
5. For those who want to *diminish the pain of anesthetic injections*, add a little bicarbonate to the anesthetic (1 part bicarbonate to 9 parts of anesthetic). Anesthetics sting with injection because of a low pH; this supposedly inhibits bacterial growth but at the same time is uncomfortable. The bicarbonate takes the "sting" out of the injection. Also, use a small needle (27 or 30 gauge), use warm solutions, and inject slowly. Injecting deeper into the dermis will cause less pain, but it takes longer for the anesthetic to work. Injecting more superficially will hurt a little more, but the anesthetic will work faster. Do not add sodium bicarbonate to bupivicaine (Marcaine) because it will precipitate in a neutral pH.
6. When *injecting lidocaine* into an area that needs to be palpable later (e.g., to feel a foreign body, find a vas during vasectomy), you can massage the lidocaine into the skin so that it does not obstruct your fine touch. Alternatively, perform a nerve block or a field block, thus eliminating any anesthetic in the area.
7. Melman and Siegel (1999) have shown that it is perfectly okay *to draw up anesthetic solutions in syringes up to 7 days before use*. There is no increased bacterial contamination or growth, and the anesthetic still functions. We used to pull up our syringes at the beginning of the day and then discard them at the end of the day, but there was no need. We now fill numerous 1-mL syringes, date them, and continue to use them throughout the week. It is much more efficient for the nurse to pull up multiple syringes than to do just one at a time. It is inefficient for the physician to spend time pulling up anesthetic!
8. Consider using the *MadaJet for local injections*. It is a small handheld "gun" that "injects" medications without a needle. It is only for superficial injections but can be used to treat keloids and hypertrophic scars with steroids, etc. It has also been adapted for the no-needle vasectomy (Wilson 2001). It is available from Delasco at 1-800-831-6273 (website: www.delasco.

com) and Advanced Meditech International (1-800-635-2452 or www.ameditech.com).

9. When someone complains of an *allergy to local anesthetics* (including Novocain), he or she has usually received an *ester*. To date, there have been no reported allergic reactions to the *amides* such as lidocaine (Xylocaine). Some patients still report that they have had a reaction to lidocaine or to "all local anesthetics." In these instances, they have usually had medication drawn from a multidose vial, which has preservatives (parabens) in it. If someone does complain of having a history of local anesthetic reaction, use single-dose vials of lidoocaine and he or she will be able to tolerate it without incident. It is inexpensive and helpful to have around. (Also see pearl 43.)
10. Advanced Meditech International (AMI) has designed *a small anesthetic bottle holder that mounts on the wall* (VE-11 Handzfree anesthetic bottle holder). The cost is only around $40, and in our office it is indispensable. It holds the anesthetic where it is readily available and makes filling syringes an easy task. It also allows the entire staff to see how much anesthetic is left in the bottle. There is nothing more frustrating than pulling out the drawer with the anesthetic solution and finding that the bottle is empty! Contact AMI at 1-800-635-2452 (website: www.ameditech.com).
11. Physicians must *maximize their time in the office*. Inefficiency has to be eliminated. I (JLP) literally try to find *30 seconds to save on every patient*. Having the syringes prefilled (see pearl 7) saves time! When I discuss this at our courses, initially there are chuckles about "the 30 seconds." Then I do the math. I am usually able to see 20 to 25 patients in a day. If I save 30 seconds on each one, this is 10 to 12 minutes per day, which actually allows an extra office visit or procedure in a day. If you work 4 days a week, that is four extra visits a week. Working 45 weeks out of the year, this amounts to 180 visits. If you average $100 per visit, that is an extra $18,000 per year. At $150 per visit, that is an extra $27,000 a year—just for saving 30 seconds per patient! If you see more than 20 to 25 patients per day, even more can be earned. *Efficiency is essential*.
12. OSHA has numerous requirements for a safe office practice. One of them is the use of *fluid-resistant coats* when performing procedures. My (JLP's) staff ordered these coats for me. They made an error and selected the coats with the *knit cuff sleeves*—how fortuitous! As residents rotate through the office, they frequently have the large sleeves that look like the old nuns' habits! The ends of the sleeves hang down 8 to 10 inches from the wrist. Subsequently when they reach for an instrument, the sleeve often drags across the sterile field. Knit cuffs help protect a sterile field and I highly recommend them. The fluid-resistant coats are also beneficial in that any fluid that gets on them is easily wiped off, and the coats last a long time. And remember, not using them could make you liable for a $25,000 OSHA fine!
13. I (JLP) have found that a *good way to explain the risk of complications* to patients is to use the example of a lottery. In medicine, you "never say 'never' and never say 'always'". And yet, the likelihood of some things happening is almost "never." So I ask the patients if they play the lotto. Most of them do sometimes. I then ask them if they will ever win. Most of them say, "No." I then reply, "But you could, right?" and they say, "Yes." I then explain that many complications are just like that. It is not going to happen, but if you play "the lotto," it could. This example really helps them understand the risk of complications. (So one day, a patient called up and said that he had won the lotto. A resident who was working with me got excited. I had to tell him that that wasn't good!)
14. I (JLP) have always liked to explain to patients how the particular surgery or procedure went. I try to be very honest. I will often say, "Technically, things went well," or "Technically, this case was quite difficult and we had a few problems." *Patients appreciate honesty*. They know things cannot go perfectly all the time. I never tell patients that it was "an easy case"; should complications arise, they think you have done something wrong. If you tell them, however, that the case was difficult, you are not looked on so negatively if complications do arise. Also, if there are no complications with tough cases, they think you have done a better job. The point of this tip: *Never overstate how well something went*. Just say that technically things went well, but complications can still occur.
15. I (JLP) have done perhaps 125 or 130 medicolegal cases as an expert witness. *A brief tip to avoid litigation:* When a patient comes in to the office, always review the last note to see what the complaint was. Ask the patient if the problem has resolved. Just jot a little note (e.g., "breast mass resolved" with the date, or "rectal bleeding gone" with the date, or perhaps "cough cleared"). Many times patients come into the office for a new complaint and the physician forgets about a significant old complaint, but the patient thinks the physician remembers. Just looking back at the record and asking that simple question could have cleared many physicians from later malpractice suits. You would also be amazed how many problems persist that the patients don't complain about and physicians subsequently overlook.
16. The *height of your examination table* is extremely important. When I (JLP) opened a new office, I purchased a table that was only 2 inches higher than my current one. I found that older patients had a difficult time getting up on the table. The lowest height can be no more than 24 inches for these patients. *A power table is essential* if you are going to be doing procedures.
17. There are really few *medical emergencies* in a physician's office. However, one of them can be *anaphylaxis* (see Chapter 220). In addition to the *Banyan kit* ("a crash cart in a suitcase") that is mentioned there, I keep an *EpiPen* taped to one of our cupboard doors. Right beside it is a vial of *atropine* and some *ammonia salts*. I have only had occasion to use the EpiPen once after an injection with *Candida*. However, people were not rushing around looking for the proper dose of epinephrine, or the syringe, or even trying to find the Epi! We just opened the cupboard door where it was taped, and gave the injection. Consider having these three medications readily available in your office, especially if you perform a significant number of procedures or injections. The Banyan Kit is the most cost efficient, safe, and practical way to maintain resuscitation capabilities in your office.
18. I (JLP) have developed a simple method for *determining whether or not a patient is likely to faint during a procedure*. I think vasovagal symptoms have occurred more with vasectomy than with any other procedure I do. Subsequently, I ask the patient how well they tolerate pain. The options are "well," "okay," and "poorly." I also ask them if they have a tendency to faint or if they faint when they see blood. If the answer is that they tolerate pain well, I just use a local anesthetic. If they tolerate pain "okay," I'll offer them 10 mg of diazepam an hour before significant procedures (e.g., vasectomy). If they tolerate pain poorly or if they say they have a tendency to faint, in addition to the 10 mg of diazepam orally, I'll give 0.5 of atropine intramuscularly on arrival to the office. (I'll often listen to the partner's answers, too, in addition to the man's response!) Since using this approach, I haven't had a single patient have a vasovagal episode while on the table during a vasectomy or any other procedure.
19. In the past it was felt that *epinephrine should not be used in fingers, nose, penis, and toes*. These are end-arterial and it was thought that the vessels could go into spasm leading to necrosis. As with many past "teachings," this was an empirical one. Studies have not found this to be true and "epi," in the doses used in local anesthetics, appears to be safe. By reducing blood flow, it may improve visualization of the anatomy and aid in closure. See the references in Chapter 4, Local Anesthesia. Interestingly,

these very same areas (in addition to the anal and vulvar regions) are very sensitive. Warn patients that injections are very uncomfortable.

20. Now that I (JLP) receive numerous referrals from primary care physicians, I think the *single largest error that I see involves anal complaints*. Frequently patients are sent to me for "hemorrhoids" and I have found fissures, fistulas, cancers, polyps, warts, and solitary anal ulcers. It seems that for both physicians and patients, when there is any rectal bleeding, it is automatically assumed to be "hemorrhoids." My only plea would be to look. Many times just spreading the glutei will give you the diagnosis. If nothing else, *perform a digital examination and a good anoscopy*. In my opinion, the only anoscope to use is the *Ive's slotted anoscope*. The long cylindrical scopes just do not allow adequate visualization for anorectal complaints. If you as a clinician do not feel comfortable evaluating anorectal complaints, then don't treat them; but don't make a diagnosis for the patient. Just send them to a clinician who is willing to evaluate them.
21. It always amazes me (JLP) that when patients have anal complaints, one of the first things they are treated with is *hydrocortisone cream for presumed hemorrhoids*. I ask at many of my courses how many physicians treat varicosities of the lower extremities with steroids. Not surprisingly, no one does. Then why does everyone treat "hemorrhoids," which are engorged veins, with steroids? It is an appropriate thing to do if the hemorrhoids are inflamed, but probably less than 10% of those with rectal bleeding truly have inflammation. Again, the rule should be to *examine the patient first before making the diagnosis of hemorrhoids* and to use hydrocortisone preparations only if inflammation is present.
22. A study was performed that looked at *absorbable vs. nonabsorbable sutures after a punch biopsy*. The study found that the cosmetic results 3 months later were equal.
23. When performing a *punch biopsy of the skin, routinely use a 3-mm punch*. The advantage is that it provides enough tissue for diagnosis but will not need suture closure. A 4-mm punch often requires a suture, and a 5-mm punch definitely does. However, when you close a circular lesion that is 5 mm with suture, you will end up with dog ears on each side. A 2-mm punch may not be adequate for diagnosis. The tissue is often macerated and it is difficult to give the pathologist a good specimen. If a 3-mm punch defect is not closed, there will usually be no visible scar remaining. At the very worst, the patient may end up with a small acne pockmark-like lesion.
24. Performing a *needle biopsy does not spread malignant cells* in the needle track. It is safe even with nodes that contain metastatic melanoma. Similarly, shaving a nevus does not lead to malignant transformation.
25. *The work-up for abnormal uterine bleeding* is now generally managed with an endometrial biopsy (see Chapter 143). In the past, when dilation and curettage (D&C) procedures were performed, a "fractional" D&C was recommended. This meant that an endocervical curettage preceded the D&C. When the studies confirmed that endometrial biopsies alone were an adequate method of evaluating abnormal uterine bleeding, many dropped the endocervical curettage (ECC). However, an ACOG Bulletin recommends that the *evaluation for abnormal uterine bleeding includes an ECC along with the endometrial biopsy*. If these studies are negative and symptoms resolve, no further work-up is necessary. Although many of us have jumped to performing *vaginal ultrasounds* to evaluate abnormal uterine bleeding, there is an *ethnic variance*. Although the safe cut-off quoted is 5 mm of endometrial stripe, cancers have been found with only 3 mm of stripe in Japanese patients. Endometrial biopsy with ECC is still, in my (JLP's) estimation, the best way to evaluate abnormal uterine bleeding. The caveat is to be sure that the bleeding is "uterine" and that other potential causes are not overlooked.
26. Unless extensive stitching is to be done, *sterile gloves are not needed for routine biopsies and most skin procedures*.
27. A potential *pitfall in interpreting Papanicolaou (Pap) smear results* is to confuse atypical squamous cells of uncertain significance (ASC-US) with atypical glandular cells (AGC) and ASC-H (atypical squamous cells, high-grade lesion cannot be ruled out). Should a Pap smear come back with either AGC or ASC-H, it is imperative that the patient undergo a complete work-up, beginning with colposcopy. A consensus of studies shows that approximately 10% of patients with atypical glandular cells will have a cancer somewhere in the genital tract if indeed the cells are glandular and atypical. Another 10% to 15% will have high-grade dysplastic lesions. *Be careful not to confuse atypical squamous cells with atypical glandular cells*.
28. I (JLP) have found that using the *medium titanium hemoclips for performing vasectomies for fascial occlusion* has been a timesaver, reduces the amount of bleeding present during the procedure, and is cost-effective. When introduced to the clips, I was resistant because I was going to have to incur another cost for the applicators. However, when suture material is used to perform the purse string around the fascia, the suture material also adds to the cost. In addition, bleeding often occurs with the insertion of the needle and it takes more time. Now, if there is bleeding in the fascial tissues around the vas, the titanium clip will readily and quickly control it. Patients often ask if the clips set off metal detectors. Since they are nonmagnetic, they do not. After a vas there will often be a slight palpable nodule, but by 3 months, patients are unable to detect any sign of the clip. If the patient continues to be worried, I just tell him to think about all the men who have fought in various battles during wars and who have shrapnel remaining in their bodies that does not cause them problems. This example usually eases the patient's mind.
29. In regard to billing, consider billing a *handling fee (99000)* when any labs are sent out to the hospital or other laboratory. Although many health maintenance organizations (HMOs), Medicare, and Medicaid may not reimburse it, a good portion of private insurance companies do. This covers your costs for documenting that the labs were sent out, for receiving the labs back, and for calling the patient. Even if only a small percentage of these fees is paid, it is still worthwhile charging for them.
30. *"Insurance only" statements on your bills may get you into trouble*. If you write "insurance only," it negates the insurance company's obligation to pay you. Treating certain patients, such as physicians and friends, for free is a medical tradition, but be careful. The changes in the law have made it a bad idea. The courts ruled in 1991 that physicians cannot charge insurance companies if they make this statement! (Don't you just love how everyone else tells us what to do? My suggestion: Be creative and be the doctor you want to be. You can figure out a way around this bureaucratic hassle.)
31. *If you write off the patient portion of a Medicare bill*, document well why it is a hardship case. Otherwise, Medicare can sue you and reclaim many of the fees they have paid you.
32. *For Medicare, you cannot bill for treating your own family*, which includes husband, wife, parents (even if you are adopted), children, siblings, step-relatives, grandparents, and domestic employees. It is okay for your partner to treat them, but not for insurance only. See pearl 30.
33. For those of you who are audited and your CPT coding is questioned, see King and Lipsky, 2000. They found that giving the same procedure to various coding experts resulted in various methods of coding out the procedure. Their conclusion was that CPT coding is not objective. This finding may help you in court!
34. I (GCF) suggest that you spend some quality time on coding and that you *buy a good book on coding*. While writing the foreign body removal chapter, I found that "10120" is the

routine code for general removal of a subcutaneous foreign body. However, if the foreign body is located in the area of the shoulder, and is subcutaneous, the code is 23330 and the relative value units (RVUs) for this code are almost three times that for 10120! Knowing your coding and billing can markedly increase reimbursement. Consider the National Procedure Institute's *Reimbursement Manual,* which is updated annually (Phone: 1-866-NPI-CME1; website: www.npinstitute.com).

35. It is difficult for us to know exactly *what to charge for each procedure*. I (JLP) commonly refer to three books, which are updated annually: Yale Wasserman DMD Medical Publishers Ltd., *Physicians Fee Reference*; The Health Care Consultants of America, Inc., *Physicians Fee & Coding Guide;* and the *Ingenix National Fee Analyzer.* Over the past 16 years, The National Procedures Institute has published a 53-page manual that is especially helpful for office practices. It lists all the common procedures normally performed by primary care physicians. For each CPT code, the RVUs and National Medicare, Michigan Medicaid, Michigan Blue Cross/Blue Shield, and the 50th percentile of the fees *charged* for each are listed. The three preceding references list fees based on national surveys of what physicians charge. The 50th percentile from each book is averaged together to come up with the 50th percentile charge. This would give at least a starting point to determine what to charge patients. For instance, what is reasonable for removing an ingrown toenail? A vasectomy? Sclerotherapy? Incision of a thrombosed hemorrhoid? Many physicians are undercharging. This manual, which is updated annually, does a lot of the work for you and is available from The National Procedures Institute (www.npinstitute.com).
36. Medicare did have a list of procedures in which they would reimburse a surgical tray. However, as of 2003, a *surgical tray fee* is not allowed. They claim to have incorporated the cost of the tray into the reimbursement for the procedure (in other words, a nice way to cut reimbursement without admitting that they've done it!). However, a surgical tray can still be charged to other insurances with the procedures that require more medical supplies (e.g., loop electrosurgical excision procedure [LEEP]). A surgical tray should never be charged for routine laceration repair or lesion removal, because it is indeed incorporated into the usual reimbursement fee.
37. With *coding and billing multiple procedures* performed on the same day, always have the biller code out the highest reimbursed procedure first. The procedures listed second, third, fourth, and fifth will be reduced by 50%. Those listed after that will be reduced to only 25% of the routine allowable charge. *When seeing a new patient,* it is essential to obtain a past medical history and evaluate the patient for other medical problems before performing the procedure. Proper coding and billing (current procedural terminology [CPT]) allows for payment of an initial office visit along with the procedure that same day. However, if the patient has been seen *in the practice* within the last 3 years, only the procedure can be charged. If the procedure is performed and another separate identifiable service has been provided (e.g., treatment for diabetes), a *modifier 25* is used to receive reimbursement for both the procedure and the visit.
38. Some patients are sensitive to *nonsteroidal anti-inflammatory drugs* (NSAIDs) and will have *increased bleeding* when using them. A simple way to check for this sensitivity is just to obtain a bleeding time on and off the drug. If the bleeding time is prolonged while on the drug, patients are indeed sensitive.
39. It is amazing to us that more physicians are not *incorporating ultrasound into the office practice*. The newer units are cheaper, smaller, often can use a PC for the screen, and the definition has really been improved. Ultrasound is the modern stethoscope. If the stethoscope were developed today, we would call the HMO and get approval before we listen to someone's lungs to rule out pneumonia or congestive heart failure. Of course, approval for this procedure ("auscultation of the lungs") would probably cost $24.99! Physicians should be embracing ultrasound technology as a means to enhance diagnostic capabilities, reduce delay in diagnosis, and actually bring down health care costs. It is reimbursed better than colonoscopy. After a 6-year review, one academic family medicine department found that a complete abdominal ultrasound was the best reimbursed procedure for the amount of time it took to perform it.
40. It concerns me (JLP) that so many physicians are jumping to the *LEEP procedure* to treat every dysplastic lesion on the cervix. *Cryotherapy has worked* for 30 years, and the documentation is excellent on efficacy and lack of complications. Cryotherapy fails only when there is a large extensive lesion or if the lesion goes into the os. It treats small CIN III lesions as well as conization (whether it be by laser, cold knife, or the LEEP procedure). Appropriate treatment with cryotherapy removes approximately 3 to 4 mm of cervix. Treatment with LEEP not only costs four to six times more (don't forget about the pathology fee to interpret the sample), but removes a minimum of 8 mm of cervix, and often 15 mm. Every study that has been done shows that in properly selected patients, cryotherapy of the cervix has the same cure rate as the LEEP procedure. (See, for example, Mitchell MF and colleagues, 1998; Pfenninger, 1999.). Some OB/GYN residency programs do not even teach cryotherapy anymore! I have a difficult time understanding the lack of science in medicine. Studies have documented that one in 17 women who have had a LEEP will experience a complication of pregnancy. See Chapter 149 on the LEEP procedure and Appendix K for further information.
41. A fantastic *buying resource for dermatologic equipment* is Delasco (available at 1-800-831-6273 or www.delasco.com).
42. Now do you want to read something really interesting? See Harris and colleagues, 1999, and Cha and colleagues, 2001. When treating patients, always try to emphasize treating the "whole" patient. We need to include surgery, medicines, x-rays, faith, and the person him- or herself in the healing process. The second reference is fascinating. Women attending an infertility clinic in South Korea were placed in the study to evaluate the effects of prayer. Half of the group was prayed for in the United States; the other half was treated routinely. The average fertility rate for the clinic was 27% for the previous 2 years. For the control group, the average rate of pregnancy was 28%. For the group that was prayed for, the average pregnancy rate was 56%! And the rest of the story: None of these patients or their doctors even knew that they were enrolled in a study, let alone that they were being prayed for in the United States (while they were in South Korea)! I don't think we understand extrasensory perception, clairvoyance, or the power of prayer. But just because we don't understand it doesn't mean we shouldn't use it!
43. When *injecting steroids* into joints, many of the steroids will precipitate when mixed with multidose vials of anesthetic. (See Chapter 192, Joint and Soft Tissue Aspiration and Injection [Arthrocentesis].) When the steroids precipitate, small crystals are then injected into the joint space. Some have postulated that this may be one of the causes for the *postinjection flare* some people experience. To avoid this complication, use single-dose vials of the anesthetics that lack parabens, and the steroid will remain in solution. It is the reaction with the parabens that causes the precipitation.
44. For those who have to treat *umbilical stump granulomas*, an article by Lotan and colleagues (2002) suggests using two ligatures rather than silver nitrate or other methods. The first ligature is tied to hold the stump and pull it up while a deeper ligature is placed to necrose the entire stump. It will fall off in 7 to 14 days and apparently has a better outcome than using silver nitrate.

45. Many people think that *taking photographs of pathology* (e.g., colposcopic findings) is beneficial and will help in a lawsuit situation. However, if you illustrate the findings, you are "the expert." In a photograph, a plaintiff's expert can contest what you identified. Drawing your findings may be more protective than photographing them.
46. *Hypnotherapy* can be a remarkable aid for controlling pain. Even if full hypnosis is not used, several relaxation techniques can be employed. Use a low monotone voice during painful or uncomfortable procedures. Avoid noisy interruptions by the staff or too much noise in the hallways and around the room. Soft, soothing music helps. Engaging the patient to help relax is important.
47. *Compounding pharmacists* are now making a comeback. They can make lollipops with lidocaine for anesthesia for oral procedures for children and with nicotine for those trying to stop smoking. "Rectal rockets" can make treatment of inflamed hemorrhoids easier. It is beneficial to learn what a compounding pharmacist can do.
48. Consider using a *skin hook* for vasectomies if you do not have the no-scalpel vasectomy instruments. It not only helps stabilize the vas, it is also reassuring that the vas is isolated, because fascia will flatten out or tear with pressure or tension. The skin hook can also be used for the minimally invasive sebaceous cyst removal. It can fixate the cyst sac, making it easier to invert and remove the sac itself.
49. *Aesthetic procedures* are really "hot" at this time. Not only are patients demanding them, but reimbursement is reasonable! A 15- or 30-minute therapy may reimburse as much as 3 hours in the intensive care unit working on someone with diabetic ketoacidosis or cardiogenic shock.

    CAUTION: Many of the new instruments being offered are very expensive. Be sure to do your homework and determine what the maintenance fees will be per year. They can often run to $10,000! Also, check on costs for supplies. Be cautious about the sale's pitch that "everyone will be running to your office." Many of us have been caught with equipment that generates cash—not for the doctor, but for the salesperson and the manufacturer!

50. The *correct suture removal scissors* can make a tough job much easier. Fine, tightly spaced sutures are often difficult to remove. It is worth the money to obtain Shortbent Stitch Scissors (3½ inch), curved, delicate (Miltex no. 9-101).
51. *Good 2.5× to 3× optical loops* do help to evaluate lesions, treat telangiectasias, and remove foreign bodies and sutures. Consider the Welch Allyn LumiView portable binocular microscope or flat surface magnifier (Welch Allyn, Inc., 4341 State Street Rd., Skaneateles Falls, NY 13153-0220; phone: 1-800-535-6663; website: www.welchallyn.com) or Keeler Loupes (Keeler, Clewer Hill Road, Windsor, Berkshire, SL4 4AA; phone: +44 (0)1753 857177; website: www.keeler.co.uk).
52. If you are having difficulty *passing the sigmoidoscope or colonoscope* at 25 cm, roll the patient all the way onto his or her back. This opens up the rectosigmoid junction and allows the scope to pass more easily (GCF).
53. Pay critical attention to proper patient positioning for the *slit-lamp examination*, because this will greatly facilitate obtaining a good examination. Most ocular pathology can be visualized appropriately under low magnification. Use of high magnification causes many users to miss the forests for the trees (From Christopher J. Bigelow, Midland, Mich.).
54. The extensor tendons have a significant excursion over the metacarpophalangeal joints. When lacerations occur in this area, carefully explore the underlying joint capsule for penetration throughout the entire arc of motion. *Unrecognized open joint injuries* can lead to significant infection if not treated appropriately. Bites or tooth lacerations (usually resulting from fistfights) are especially bad. Use a low index of suspicion to start broad-spectrum antibiotics.

    A sizeable *ganglion will typically transilluminate*, thereby providing affirmation of the diagnosis (From David T. Bortel, Midland, Mich.).
55. Take a lot of time to establish rapport with a young female patient. The pelvic–genital examination itself takes no more than 5 minutes if the fearful patient trusts you long enough to be cooperative.

    Don't expect the *child* who has just received *nasal midazolam* to sleep through your procedure. However, he or she will be cooperative.

    Do not be tempted to use *DeLee suctioning* to clear the airway of particulate meconium in a newborn. Use an appropriately sized endotracheal tube (From David B. Bosscher, Knoxville, Tenn.).
56. Because fewer elective vaginal breech deliveries are being attempted, *external cephalic version* often provides the only option in attempting to avoid a cesarean section for breech presentation. If the initial attempt is unsuccessful, it is safe and cost effective to repeat the procedure in 1 week (From Andrew Coco, Hershey, Penn.).
57. Practice is the key to master *laceration and incision repair*. Begin with easy procedures and work up to larger excisions and skin flaps. Remember, it is okay to cut a suture that is incorrect and replace it (From William Jackson Epperson, Murrells Inlet, SC).
58. Consider *event monitoring rather than Holter monitoring* if the patient's symptoms are infrequent (From Dave Feller, Gainesville, Fla.).
59. *Infarction q waves* can be normal in limb leads III, AVL, and precordial lead V_1. *ST segment elevation* can be normal in healthy people but is ominous in the patient with chest pain (From Victor F. Froelicher, Stanford, Calif.).
60. The *cesarean section* is a lifesaving procedure that can be performed competently by family physicians with adequate training. Hospital privileges should be granted on the basis of experience with the operation and expertise of the surgeon.

    The evaluation and selection of the patient for cesarean section is the most important step in the procedure. Knowledge of risk factors and indications for cesarean section is essential to proper patient care (From Rebecca H. Gladu, Houston, Tex.).
61. *Allergy screening* with only six to ten allergens can separate your allergic patient from nonallergic patients in a cost-effective way.

    Immunotherapy is the patient's only "cure" for allergic rhinitis (From Harold Hedges, Little Rock, Ark.).
62. Every *spider vein*, no matter how small, comes from venous incompetence that can be traced back to a perforator. Always try to inject the vein that is closest to the source of this incompetence.

    The longer *postinjection compression* (≤3weeks) is used, the better the result (From Stanley A. Hirsch, Pittsburgh, Penn.).
63. Many *paracentesis* kits have a 16- or 18-gauge needle for the paracentesis. This size is generally too large. A smaller needle can limit the amount of "leakage" of ascitic fluid from the entry site after the procedure is completed (From Kenneth Hu, Santa Monica, Calif.).
64. *Knee braces* should be used only in conjunction with a rehabilitation program incorporating strength training, flexibility, activity modification, and technique refinement (From Scott A. Paluska, Seattle, Wash.).
65. A tissue diagnosis is required for any *dominant breast mass*, even if the mammogram and ultrasound are negative.

    Plan incisions carefully to achieve optimal cosmesis while preserving future surgical options if the lesion proves unexpectedly malignant (From Helen A. Pass, Royal Oak, Mich.).

66. *Electrical cardioversion,* unlike defibrillation, is the administration of DC current synchronized with the R wave of the QRS complex.

    Adequate anticoagulation of 3 weeks' duration and performance of an echocardiogram to evaluate left atrial diameter are generally considered necessary before *cardioversion of atrial fibrillation* of longer than 48 hours' duration (From David V. Power, Minneapolis, Minn.).
67. Send *thoracocentesis* fluid for protein, pH, and lactate dehydrogenase (LDH). Do not order other tests unless the fluid is an exudate (From Terry S. Ruhl, Altoona, Penn.).
68. When injecting a *trigger point,* inject directly into the area and then fan the needle to each side along the lines of the skin for best results. Trigger points are usually not round, but are oblong and amenable to fanning (From Gary E. Ruoff, East Lansing, Mich.).
69. To best visualize the sides and top of the bladder, the *cystoscope* should be rotated around the long axis of the scope rather than levered from side to side. This minimizes patient discomfort (From Andrew C. Steele, Travis AFB, Calif.).
70. *Endometrial ablation* significantly improves PMS, moodiness, and dysmenorrhea.

    Postmenopausal bleeding resulting from hormone replacement therapy can be controlled completely by *endometrial ablation* (From Duane E. Townsend, Park City, UT).
71. *When performing a punch biopsy, it is not necessary to obtain normal skin.* The only time normal tissue is needed is with vesicular and bullous disease. For these entities, perform the biopsy on a new, fresh lesion right at the edge where it lifts up off the dermis. This location will afford the pathologist a better chance of making the correct diagnosis.
72. When using *plastic endometrial aspirators* for endometrial biopsy, it may be difficult to insert the unit into the os because of the flexibility of the tube. The aspirator can be "stiffened" by placing it in a freezer for a few minutes. When cold, it may easily enter the os. A full bladder often pushes the fundus posteriorly, opening the internal os if traction with a tenaculum has not succeeded in doing the same thing. Alternatively, a metal cervical dilator can be used.
73. The Centers for Disease Control and Prevention and other organizations have made the recommendation that, rather than frequent handwashing with soap and water, medical caretakers should use an *antimicrobial hand gel.* Various brands are available. In our office (JLP), we use *Prevacare* (Johnson & Johnson). It's hypoallergenic and has moisturizers. Several of my staff have eczema, and frequent handwashing was really exacerbating symptoms. Using the new gels without any water improved their symptoms while producing a better compliance and efficacy rate than soap and water. We get the hand pump container and feel it's well worth the cost.
74. Some patients are *allergic to iodine,* even in topical preparations (e.g., Betadine). Consider Techni-Care surgical scrub (Care-Tech Laboratories, Inc., St. Louis, MO [phone: 1-800-325-9681]) with such cases. It's a broad-spectrum topical antiseptic microbicide with a 99.99% bacterial reduction in 30 seconds of contact. There is minimal to no dermal irritation. It's nonstinging and also safe on mucous membranes. The only difficulty is its tendency to foam up.
75. Children undergoing surgery develop more postsurgical scarring than adults. This is probably due to increased elasticity of the skin as well as an inability to get the children to limit activity. A report in the *Family Practice News* gives several pearls to limit the scarring:
    - Use more subcutaneous sutures and place them deeper. The report suggests that if you normally would use four sutures, then use eight for children! If the wound is fairly deep, consider using clear nylon for buried sutures, which will give permanent strength to the wound.
    - Leave in nondissolving running subcuticular stitches. If not visible, they won't hurt anything. If the stitch begins to work out, remove it later.
    - Place bulky dressings over the wound. This will inhibit some movement and help the child remember that surgery has occurred.
    - Immobilize the joints if there are any incisions over them.
    - Provide written instructions and emphasize the necessity of limiting activity.

BIBLIOGRAPHY

Alcalay J: Cutaneous surgery in patients receiving warfarin therapy. Dermatol Surg 27:756, 2001.

Cha KY, Wirth DP, Lobo RA: Does prayer influence the success of in vitro fertilization-embryo transfer? Report of a masked, randomized trial. J Reprod Med 46:9, 2001.

Family Practice News: Sept. 15, 2002, p. 30.

Gabel EA, Jimenez GP, Eaglestein WH, et al: Performance comparison of nylon and an absorbable suture material (Polyglactin 910) in the closure of punch biopsy sites. Dermatol Surg 26:750, 2000.

Harris WS, Gowda M, Kolb JW, et al: A randomized, controlled trial of the effects of remote, intercessory prayer on outcomes in patients admitted to the coronary care unit. Arch Intern Med 159:2273, 1999.

King MS, Lipsky MS, Sharp L: Current procedural terminology coding: Do the experts agree? J Am Board Fam Pract 13:144, 2000.

Lotan G, Klin B, Efrati Y: Double-ligature: A treatment for pedunculated umbilical granulomas in children. Am Fam Physician 65:2067, 2002.

Melman D, Siegel DM: Dermatol Surg 25:492, 1999.

Mitchell MF, Tortolero-Luna G, Cook E, et al: A randomized clinical trial of cryotherapy, laser vaporization, and loop electrosurgical excision for treatment of squamous intraepithelial lesions of the cervix. Obstet Gynecol 92:737, 1998.

Pfenninger JL: Good things still come in old packages: Cryosurgery vs LEEP (Loop electrosurgical excision procedure). J Am Board Fam Pract 12:416, 1999.

Schanbacher CF, Bennett RG: Dermatol Surg 26:785, 2000.

Wilson CL: No-needle anesthetic for no-scalpel vasectomy. Am Fam Physician 63:1295, 2001.

UNIVERSAL PROCEDURAL TRAINING IN FAMILY MEDICINE

Julie M. Sicilia • Stuart Forman

Box I-1. Procedure Categories

A: All family medicine residency programs must provide training in each of these procedures.
- A0: Residents will have the ability to perform these basic procedures either upon graduation from medical school or through normal residency experience. These procedures do not require specific documentation of training or numbers performed.
- A1: All residents must be able to perform these procedures independently by graduation.
- A2: All residents must have exposure to these procedures and be given the opportunity to be trained to perform them independently by graduation.

B: These procedures are within the scope of family medicine and require focused training for residents to be able to perform independently by graduation.

C: These procedures are within the scope of family medicine and may require additional training beyond the usual 3 years of training for family physicians to perform independently.

There has been a great deal of controversy over the fact that there are no universal standards defining which procedures are taught in family medicine residencies. In addition, there is a huge variance in regional and local areas. The inconsistent standardization of procedural training in family medicine residencies is the source of much consternation for patients, credentialing bodies, insurance companies, regulatory organizations, and other medical specialists, all of whom struggle to understand the scope of practice of family physicians, and which procedures family physicians are trained to perform.

The Society of Teachers of Family Medicine (STFM) Group on Hospital Medicine and Procedural Training met as a Task Force in 2007 and again in 2008 to propose a standard procedural training curriculum. The group consisted of 17 family physician educators (15 faculty members, 2 in private practice) from rural, suburban, and urban areas. Ten states were represented. During the first Task Force meeting, multiple procedures were considered and classified into different categories based on the need to be included in the curriculum (Box I-1). A paper was published in *Family Medicine* that outlined the agreed-upon core procedures. Recommendations were sent to the American Academy of Family Physicians (AAFP) Commission on Education for potential consideration by the Residency Review Committee (RRC). The group met again in 2008 and revised and updated the core procedures, which are printed as Table I-1. Advanced procedures were also discussed (Table I-2), and a summary was published in 2009 in *Family Medicine*.

TABLE I-1 Core Procedures in Family Medicine

	Category		
Area of Care	**A0***	**A1†**	**A2‡**
Skin	Remove corn/callous Drain subungual hematoma Skin staples Fungal studies (KOH) Laceration repair with tissue glues	Biopsies: punch, excisional, incisional Cryosurgery Remove warts, fingernail, toenail, foreign body Incision and drainage of abscess Simple laceration repair with sutures	Electrosurgery
Maternity care		Spontaneous vaginal delivery, including Fetal monitoring Fetal scalp electrode IUPC and amnioinfusion Amniotomy Labor induction/augmentation First- and second-degree laceration repair Vacuum-assisted vaginal delivery	Third- and fourth-degree laceration repair Manual extraction of placenta
Women's health	Wet mount, KOH Diaphragm fitting	Pap smear Vulvar biopsy Bartholin's cyst management Remove cervical polyp Endometrial biopsy IUD insertion/removal FNA of breast	Pessary fitting Paracervical block Cervical dilation Colposcopy Cervical cryotherapy Uterine aspiration/D&C

Table continues on following page.

TABLE I-1 Core Procedures in Family Medicine—cont.

Area of Care	Category		
	A0*	A1†	A2‡
Life support courses	Electrocardiography performance and interpretation	ACLS, NRP, PALS, ALSO, ATLS, or equivalent programs	
Musculoskeletal		Initial management of simple fractures Closed reduction Upper and lower extremity splints Injection/aspiration: large joint, bursa, ganglion cyst, trigger point Reduction of nursemaid's elbow	Upper and lower extremity casts Reduction of shoulder dislocation
Pulmonary	Hand-held spirometry		
ultrasound		Basic OB ultrasound: AFI, fetal presentation, placental location U/S guidance for central vascular access, paracentesis, thoracentesis	Advanced OB ultrasound: dating, anatomic survey
Urgent care and hospital	Foreign body removal: ear, nose Ring removal Fish hook removal Phlebotomy Peripheral venous access	Eye procedures Fluorescein examination Foreign body removal Anterior nasal packing for epistaxis Lumbar puncture FNA of mass or cyst	Frenlotomy Slit lamp exam Endotracheal intubation Ventilator management Thoracentesis Paracentesis Arterial line Central venous catheter Venous cutdown Pediatric vascular access: peripheral, intraosseus, umbilical vein
Gastrointestinal and colorectal	Nasogastric tube, enteral feeding tube Fecal disimpaction Digital rectal exam	Anoscopy Excision of thrombosed hemorrhoid Incision and drainage of perirectal abscess Remove perianal skin tags	Flexible sigmoidoscopy or colonoscopy
Genitourinary	Urine microscopy Bladder catheterization	Newborn circumcision	Vasectomy Suprapubic tap
Anesthesia		Topical anesthesia Local anesthesia/Field block Digital block	Peripheral nerve block Conscious sedation

ACLS, advanced cardiac life support; AFI, amniotic fluid index; ALSO, advanced life support in obstetrics; ATLS, advanced trauma life support; D&C, dilation and curettage; FNA, fine needle aspiration; IUD, interuterine device; IUPC, intrauterine pressure catheterization; KOH, potassium hydroxide; NRP, neonatal resuscitation program; OB, obstetrics; PALS, pediatric advanced life support; Pap, Papanicolaou.
*All residents must be able to perform, but documentation not required.
†All residents must be able to perform independently by graduation.
‡All residents must be exposed to and have the opportunity to train to independent performance.

TABLE I-2 Advanced Procedures Within the Scope of Family Medicine

Area of Care	Category	
	B*	C†
Skin	Allergy testing Botulinum toxin injection Nonsurgical cosmetic aesthetics Skin flap advanced closures	
Maternity care	Amniocentesis Cesarean delivery Dilation and evacuation External cephalic version Forceps-assisted delivery	Cervical cerclage Vaginal twin delivery
Women's health	Contraceptive implant insertion and removal Loop electrosurgical excision procedure (LEEP) Non-FNA breast biopsy Tubal ligation	Hysteroscopy Laparoscopy
Musculoskeletal		Acupuncture

TABLE I-2 Advanced Procedures Within the Scope of Family Medicine—cont.

	Category	
Area of Care	**B***	**C†**
Urgent care and hospital	Bone marrow biopsy Cardioversion Chest tube insertion, management, and removal Exercise stress test Nasorhinolaryngoscopy Peritonsillar abscess incision and drainage Swan-Ganz catheter insertion and management Tooth extraction	Bronchoscopy Myringotomy (PE) tubes Sleep study: perform and interpret Tonsillectomy
Gastrointestinal and colorectal	Endoscopic gastroduodenoscopy (EGD)	Appendectomy Anal fissure treatment including sphinctotomy and Botox injection
Genitourinary	Emergency dorsal slit procedure	Non-neonatal circumcision
Anesthesia	Intrathecal anesthesia	Epidural anesthesia

FNA, fine needle aspiration.
*Require focused training in residency.
†May require additional training beyond residency or fellowship.

This information is included here to provide a ready reference for those who need it. It is not meant to be all inclusive, or exclusive of any procedure.

BIBLIOGRAPHY

Harper MB, Mayeaux EJ, Pope JB, Goel R: Procedural training in family practice residencies: Current status and impact on resident recruitment. J Am Board Fam Pract 8:189–194, 1995.

Kelly BF, Sicilia JM, Forman S, et al: Advanced procedural training in family medicine: A group consensus statement. Fam Med 41:398–404, 2009.

Norris TE, Felmar E, Tolleson G: Which procedures should be taught in family practice residency programs? Fam Med 29:99–104, 1997.

Nothnagle M, Sicilia JM, Forman S, et al: Required procedural training in family medicine residency: A consensus statement. Fam Med 40:248–252, 2008.

Rodney WM, Hahn RC: Impact of the limited generalist (no hospital, no procedures) model on the viability of family practice training. J Am Board Fam Pract 15:191–200, 2002.

Tenore JL, Sharp LK, Lipsky MS: A national survey of procedural skill requirements in family practice residency programs. Fam Med 33:28–38, 2001.

APPENDIX J

OUTLINE FOR A COMPREHENSIVE OPERATIVE NOTE

John L. Pfenninger

Procedure(s) performed:
(1)
(2)
Surgeon:
Assistant:
Indications:
Preoperative diagnosis:
Postoperative diagnosis:
Findings:
Anesthesia:
Estimated blood loss:
Complications:
Pathology specimen sent?
Disposition:
Describe the patient's condition on the completion of the procedure and whether the patient was sent home, returned to the recovery room, and so on. If postoperative monitoring occurred, record that too.
Procedure:
Describe the surgical technique. Include the position of the patient; preparation; measurements; anesthetic administration; draping; details of the procedure itself, on the findings, any specifics; if tissue was removed, and if it was sent to the pathology department; methods of controlling bleeding, if applicable; closure (including types of sutures used, if applicable); dressing; and any other necessary pertinent information.

Management Guidelines for Abnormal Cervical Cancer Screening Tests and Histologic Findings

Gary R. Newkirk

In September 2006 a group of 146 experts representing 29 organizations and professional societies met in Bethesda, Maryland, to develop revised evidence-based consensus guidelines for the management of women with abnormal cervical cancer screening tests. The process of revising these guidelines, which were originally published in their first version in 2001, was started in 2005 by the American Society for Colposcopy and Cervical Pathology (ASCCP) in collaboration with its partner professional societies and federal and international organizations. This effort culminated with the adoption and publication of two new consensus guidelines and a series of 12 management algorithms that provide suggested clinical responses to a variety of situations for both abnormal cervical screening testing and cervical histologic biopsy results (Figs. K-1 through K-3).

These guidelines are based on evidence whenever possible. However, for certain clinical situations, there is limited high-quality evidence, and in these situations the guidelines have, by necessity, been based on consensus expert opinion. The terms "recommended," "preferred," "acceptable," and "unacceptable" are used in these guidelines to describe various interventions. Table K-1 explains this terminology.

Several introductory caveats are provided with these guidelines and include the following: (1) clinical judgment should always be used when applying a guideline to an individual patient and (2) these guidelines should never substitute for clinical judgment. The expansion of these guidelines included management recommendations for special populations such as adolescent (younger than age 21 years) and pregnant women. Furthermore, given the potentially aggressive and increasingly prevalent nature of adenomatous or glandular precancerous and cancerous cervical disease, special guidelines provide specific management strategies for women with either cytologic or histologic glandular changes.

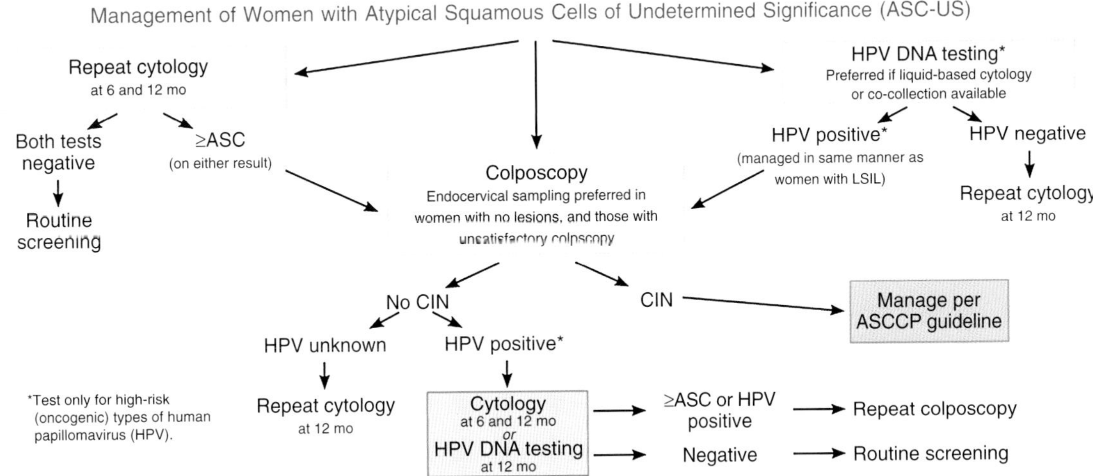

Figure K-1 **A–J,** Cytologic consensus guidelines for the management of women with abnormal cervical cancer screening tests.

Figure continues on following page.

Management of Adolescent Women with Either Atypical Squamous Cells of Undetermined Significance (ASC-US) or Low-Grade Squamous Intraepithelial Lesion (LSIL)

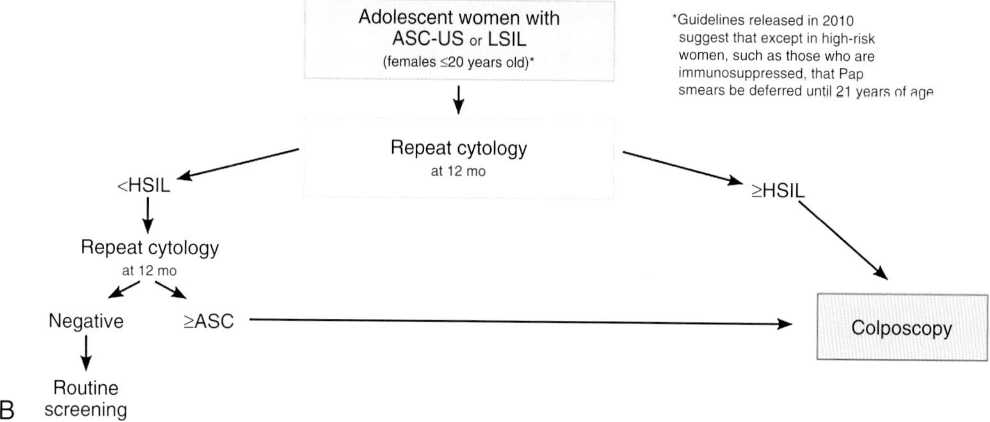

Management of Women with Atypical Squamous Cells: Cannot Exclude High-Grade Squamous Intraepithelial Lesion (ASC-H)

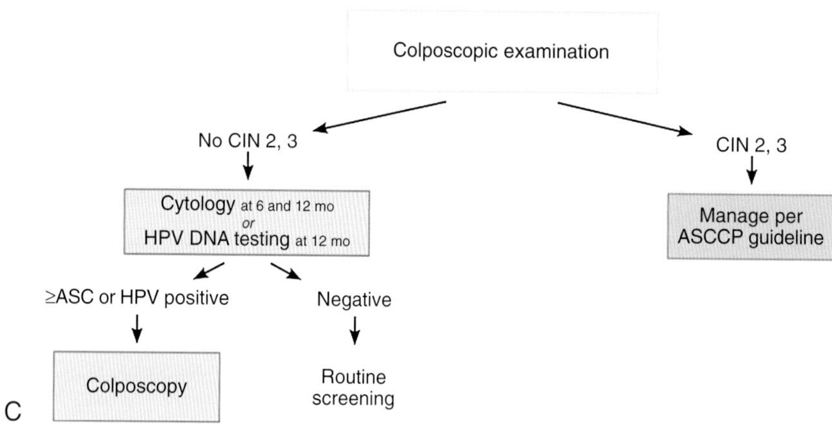

Management of Women with Low-Grade Squamous Intraepithelial Lesion (LSIL)

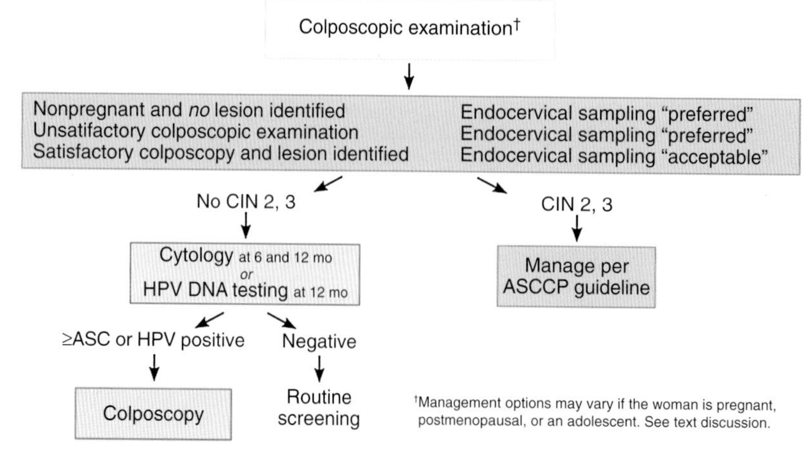

Figure K-1, cont.

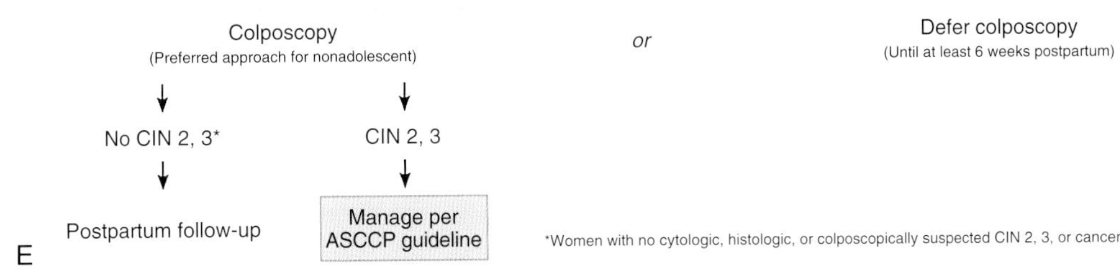

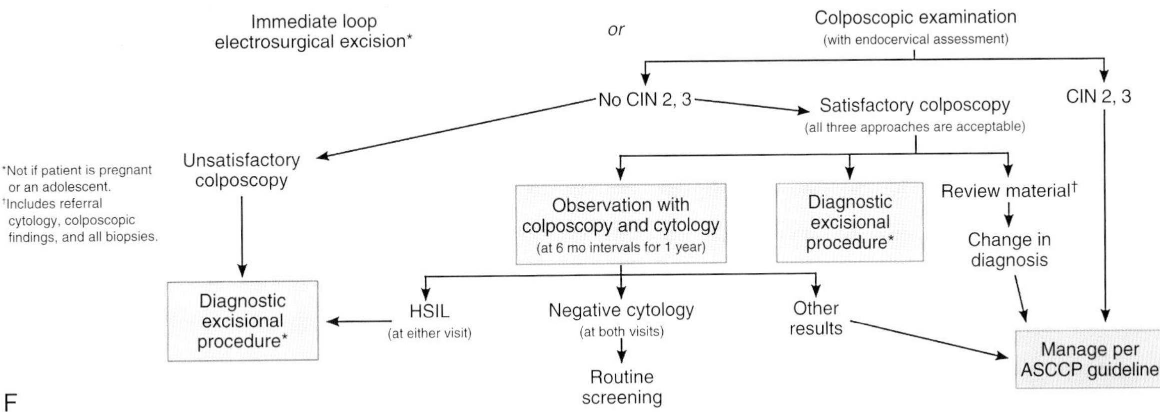

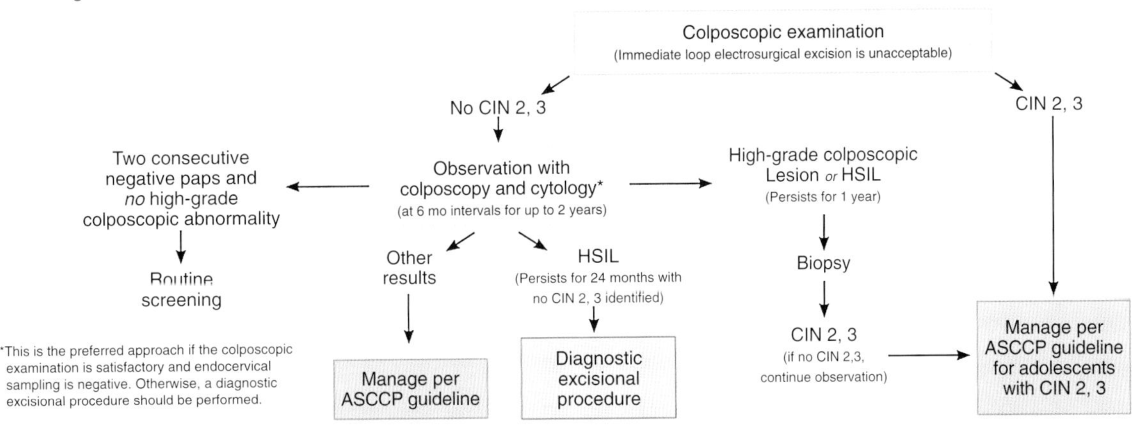

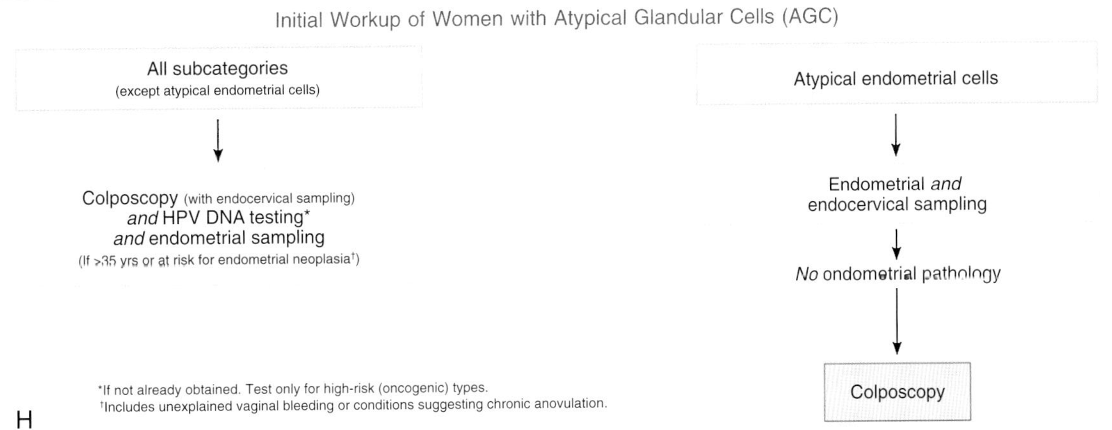

Figure K-1, cont.

Figure continues on following page.

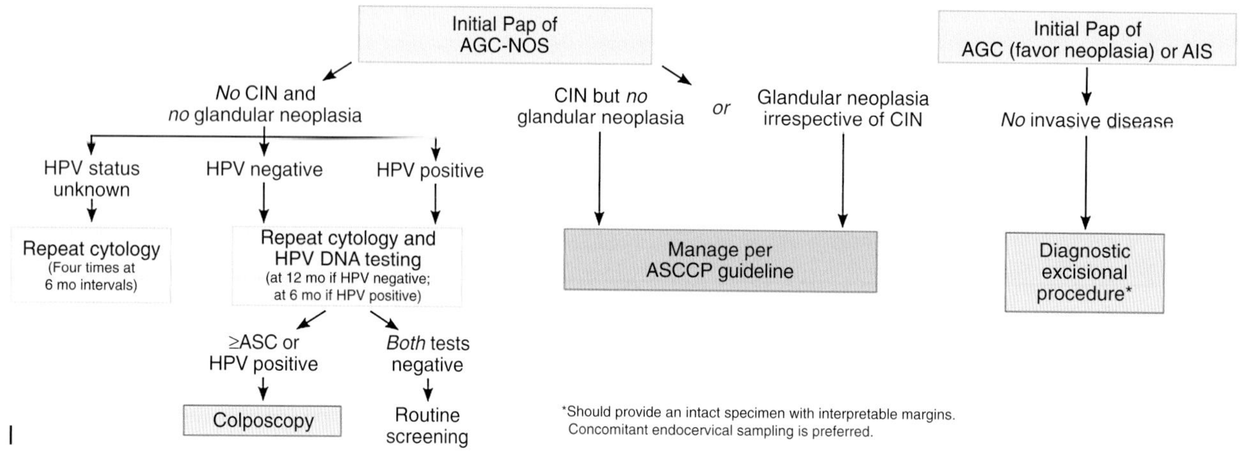

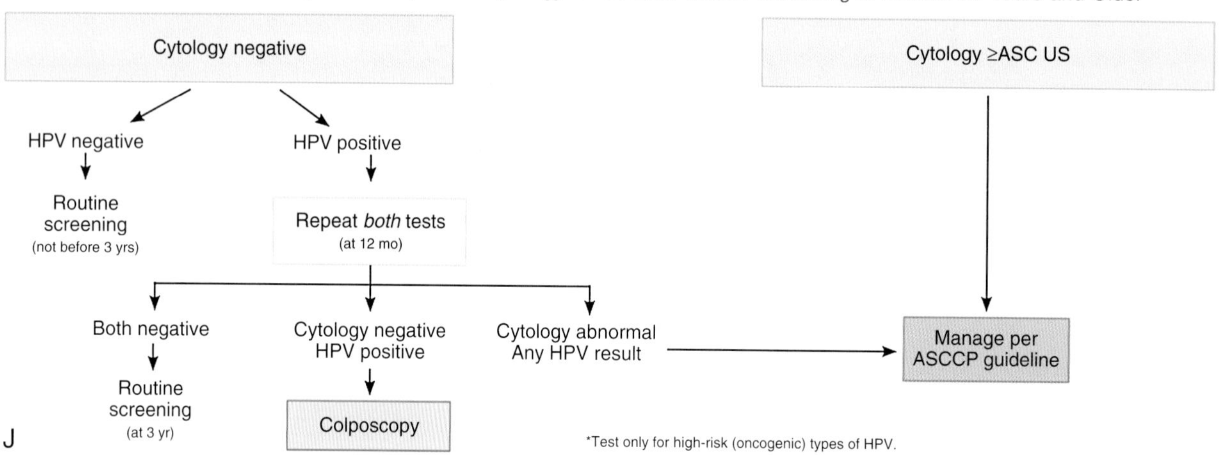

Figure K-1, cont. (**A–J,** Copyright 2006, 2007 American Society for Colposcopy and Cervical Pathology. All rights reserved. Available at http://www.asccp.org/pdfs/consensus.)

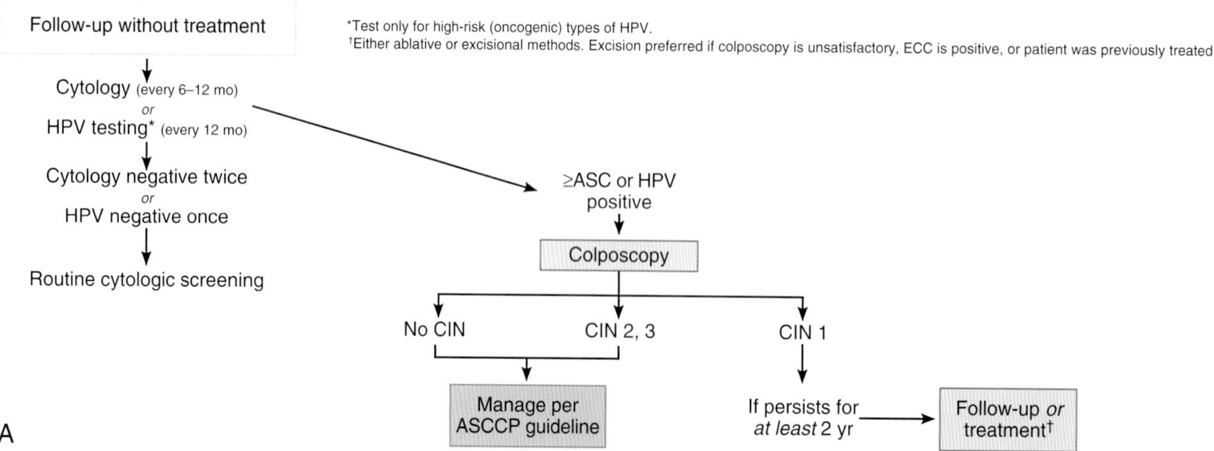

Figure K-2 **A–E,** Histologic consensus guidelines for the management of women with abnormal cervical cancer screening tests.

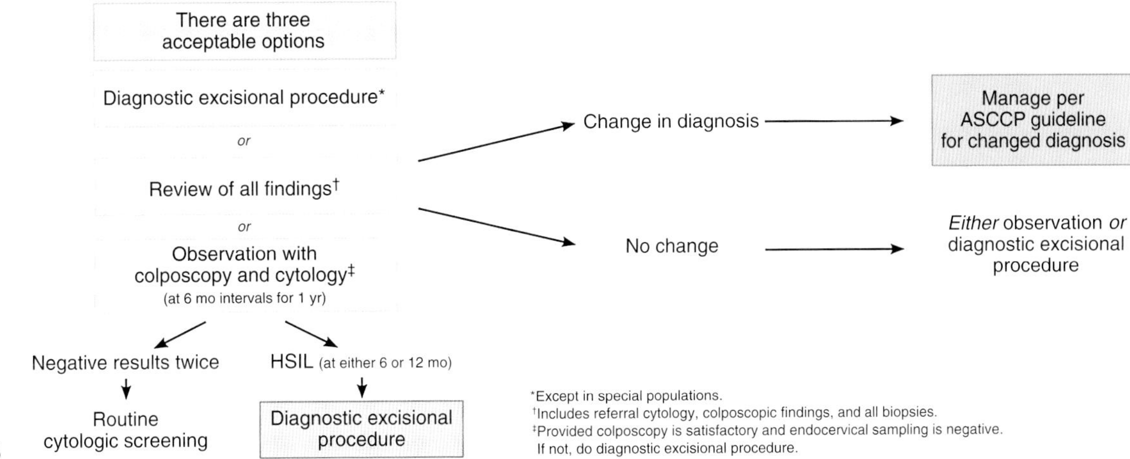

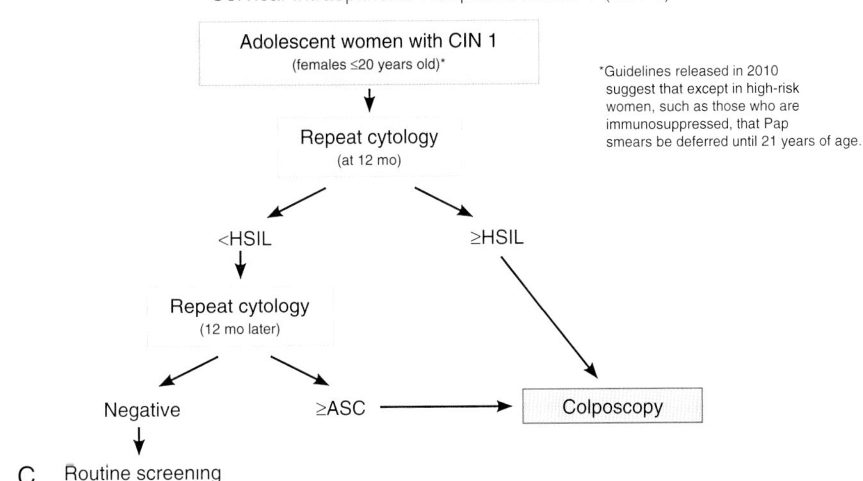

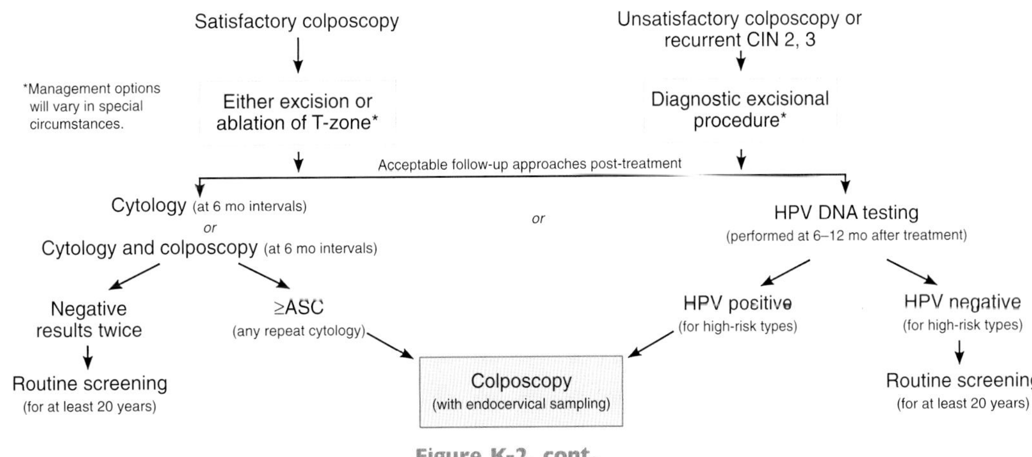

Figure K-2, cont.

Figure continues on following page.

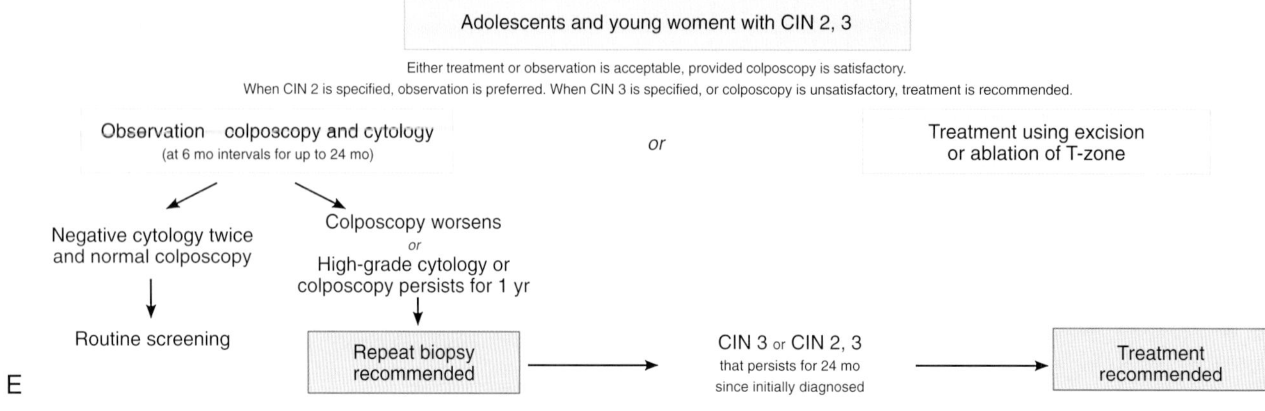

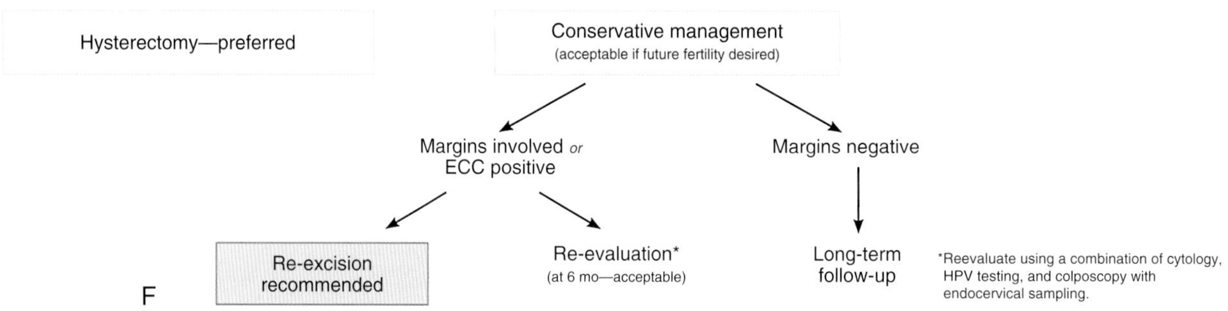

Figure K-2, cont. (**A–F,** Copyright 2006, 2007 American Society for Colposcopy and Cervical Pathology. All rights reserved. Available at http://www.asccp.org/pdfs/consensusf.)

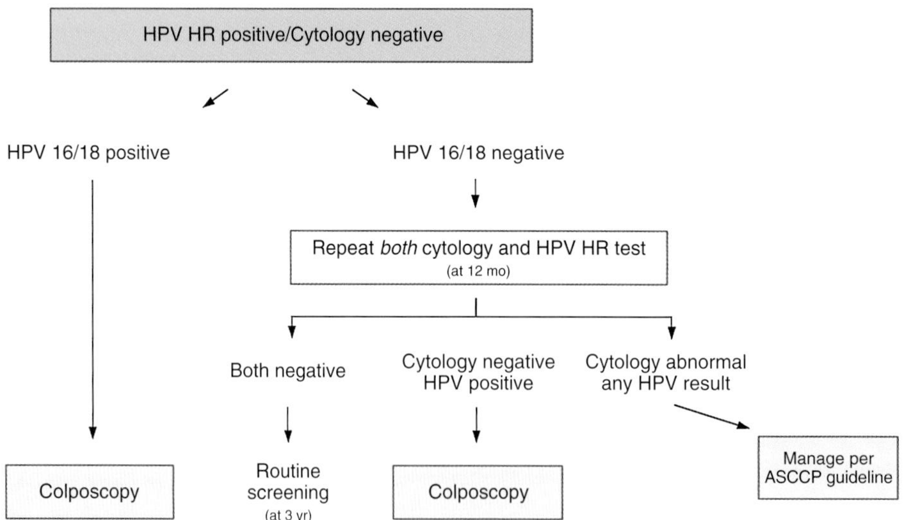

Figure K-3 Based on the data available at the time, the 2006 Consensus Guidelines included a recommendation that in cytology-negative women 30 years of age and older who are HPV DNA positive (for any of the 13 or 14 high-risk types of HPV detected by the high-risk HPV assays), molecular genotyping assays that detect HPV 16 and 18 would be clinically useful for determining which women should be referred for immediate colposcopy, and which could be followed up with repeat cytologic and high-risk HPV testing in 12 months. Because an FDA-approved HPV genotyping assay was not available in 2006, this recommendation was made contingent on approval of a HPV genotyping assay by the FDA. The first HPV genotyping assay was approved in March 2009. HPV, human papillomavirus; HR, high risk. (Copyright 2004, 2009 American Society for Colposcopy and Cervical Pathology. All rights reserved. Available at http://www.asccp.org/pdfs/consensus/hpv_genotyping_20090320.pdf; accessed 5/3/10.)

TABLE K-1 Terminology Used to Describe Interventions

Guideline Terminology	Interpretation
Recommended	Good data to support use when only one option is available
Preferred	Option is the best (or one of the best) when there are multiple other options
Acceptable	One of multiple options when there are either data indicating that another approach is superior or when there are no data to favor any single options
Unacceptable	Good data against use

The published algorithms for the 2006 Consensus Guidelines are presented as a valuable resource to clinicians who provide screening, diagnostic, and therapeutic management of cervical cancer precursors in women across the reproductive years and into the postmenopausal period. Appreciation is expressed to the ASCCP for granting inclusion of these guidelines. The complete guidelines are available at the ASCCP website and as cited in the references to this appendix.

These guidelines are cited throughout applicable areas of the text. Please see the following chapters:

- Chapter 134, Cervical Conization
- Chapter 137, Coloscopic Examination
- Chapter 138, Cryotherapy of the Cervix
- Chapter 142, Human Papillomavirus DNA Typing
- Chapter 149, Loop Electrosurgical Excision Procedure for Treating Cervical Intraepithelial Neoplasia
- Chapter 151, Pap Smear and Related Techniques for Cervical Cancer Screening

BIBLIOGRAPHY

American Society of Colposcopy and Cervical Pathology (ASCCP) website: www.asccp.org.

Wright TC, Massad LS, Dunton CJ, et al: 2006 consensus guidelines for the management of women with abnormal cervical cancer screening tests. Am J Obstet Gynecol 197:346–355, 2007.

Wright TC, Massad LS, Dunton CJ, et al: 2006 consensus guidelines for the management of women with cervical intraepithelial neoplasia or adenocarcinoma in situ. Am J Obstet Gynecol 197:340–345, 2007.

APPENDIX L

BUYING MAJOR OFFICE EQUIPMENT

Mark Needham • Bernard Katz

Throughout their careers, family physicians will be confronted with financial decisions that involve the investment of money with the hope for a profitable return. Buying a major piece of office equipment for a new diagnostic or therapeutic service is one example. Certain decisions, such as paying for office maintenance, are relatively straightforward. If the office isn't maintained properly or the roof leaks, the practice obviously will do poorly. However, buying some office equipment is optional and requires investing money in a piece of equipment now with hopes of earning profit in the future. Certain financial tools, in particular the *calculation of the net present value*, can greatly increase the ability to determine whether to invest in the office equipment and how much to pay for it. This appendix explains how to estimate the value of a piece of office equipment over time so that you can make the right buying decisions.

If a physician has a very strong desire to offer a certain procedure for personal or career goals, and is not strictly motivated by the financial result, the financial analysis that drives the purchase decision may be less important. However, for the most part, physicians should base their decisions on sound financial principles. In so doing they should receive the best possible financial return for their investment.

Wise use of the tools of financial analysis increases the likelihood of making the correct decision so that the value of future dollars will exceed the value of the dollars invested today.

Presented here is a step-by-step approach that will increase the chances that the purchase will turn out to be financially successful. It is based on a simple Excel spreadsheet that includes all the financial information necessary for you to make an informed decision. To help understand how this is acheived, we will use an example of a practice that is considering whether to buy a bone densitometer (Fig. L-1). Make the following entries as shown in the sample in Figure L-1.

ESTIMATE THE LIFETIME OF THE PROJECT

All equipment has a finite useful life. Equipment wears out; technology becomes obsolete; spare parts become unavailable; and so on. Estimate how long the equipment under consideration will last and enter those years across the top of your spreadsheet. For the example of buying a bone densitometer (a DEXA unit) we have estimated a useful life of 10 years.

FORECAST THE ANNUAL REVENUE

Estimate the number of procedures that will be performed on a daily basis and then scale that up to an annual number of procedures. Base your estimate on what you think will happen during the first year of operation. Later you will estimate what the growth rate in the number of procedures will be. Try to be conservative when you make an estimate. If your project exceeds your forecasts, you will only be pleased, but if your forecast is overly optimistic, the result may be a significant financial loss if time, money, and effort will have been expended on a losing project. In the example it is estimated that during the first year 220 densitometry procedures will be performed.

FORECAST THE ANNUAL EXPENSE

Forecasting the annual expense is more complicated than forecasting revenue but equally important. Take a look at a recent income statement from your practice in order to ascertain all the categories of expense that need to be included and to assist with estimates in each category. There are generally two categories of expenses; those associated with *startup* and those that are *recurring annual expenses*. The recurrent expenses comprise both *fixed* and *variable* expenses. Fixed expenses will be incurred regardless of the number of procedures performed, and variable expenses will be dependent on the number of procedures done during the year.

Startup expenses include installation fees, delivery fees, remodeling or construction that may have to be done to ready the premises, licensing, staff training, and any other one-time expenses associated with getting the machine ready to go. Typical recurring annual expenses will include supplies and materials required to operate the machine, staff labor and benefit expense, repair and maintenance, marketing and advertising if required, travel for training, rent, telephone, data lines, insurance, and any other recurring expense associated with the annual operation of the machine.

CONSIDER THE OPPORTUNITY COST

It may not be easy to place a value on the *opportunity cost* but it should be considered. In the example of the densitometry machine you need to know whether it is going to be placed into a vacant/unused area in the office, will displace some existing program, or requires new construction. Vacant and unused office space offers the best upside opportunity because the space is not currently generating any revenue for the practice. In that case the financial analysis simply compares the financial return from one project against the other. If a new piece of equipment is going to displace an existing program, then one has to consider the revenue lost in displacing that program as part of the ongoing annual expense of the new project. It is important to factor in the lost revenue as an expense to the new project to properly decide if buying the new piece of equipment makes financial sense. If new office space has to be acquired or constructed to make room for the new equipment, then the cost of the new construction has to be included in the annual expense, but one can safely allocate that expense over a long time period and then apportion the expense only during the time period under consideration for this project. In the example of densitometry, the assumption is that the machine will be going into unused space in the office so the opportunity cost is stated as zero dollars.

One must also factor in the opportunity cost of the *physician's time* related to the equipment under consideration. Adding laser or colonoscopy equipment to the practice will ultimately require that the physician spend time performing the procedure. That means when he or she is doing colonoscopy or laser procedures, the

Example: Should I buy a DEXA machine?
Excel spreadsheet example

Name of project under consideration	Bone Densitometry									
Estimated lifetime of project 10 years										
Year of project	**1**	**2**	**3**	**4**	**5**	**6**	**7**	**8**	**9**	**10**
Estimated number of units of service per year	220	227	233	240	248	255	263	271	279	287
Estimated annual growth rate of units provided per year	3.00%									
Estimated revenue per unit of service	$ 110	$ 111	$ 112	$ 113	$ 114	$ 116	$ 117	$ 118	$ 119	$ 120
Estimated annual growth rate of revenue per unit	1%									
Forecasted annual revenue	$ 24,200	$ 25,175	$ 26,190	$ 27,245	$ 28,343	$ 29,485	$ 30,674	$ 31,910	$ 33,196	$ 34,534
Expense categories										
One-time expenses										
Installation	$ 1,000									
Delivery	$ 300									
Remodel/Construction	$ 5,000									
License	$ -									
Training	$ 2,500									
Other One-time expense	$ -									
Other One-time expense	$ -									
Total One-time expense	$ 8,800									
Recurrent expenses										
Materials and supplies	$ 1,000									
Labor	$ 10,000									
Benefits	$ 1,000									
Repair and maintenance	$ 1,800									
Marketing and advertising	$ 500									
Travel	$ -									
Rent	$ -									
Telephone	$ -									
Utilities	$ 300									
Insurance	$ 300									
Taxes	$ 250									
Opportunity cost/Expense	$ -									
Physician expense	$ -									
Other recurring expense	$ -									
Other recurring expense	$ -									
Other recurring expense	$ -									
Total recurring expense	$ 15,150	$ 15,908	$ 16,703	$ 17,538	$ 18,415	$ 19,336	$ 20,302	$ 21,318	$ 22,383	$ 23,503
Interest on loans	$ -	$ -	$ -	$ -	$ -	$ -	$ -	$ -	$ -	$ -
Total annual expenses	$ 23,950	$ 15,908	$ 16,703	$ 17,538	$ 18,415	$ 19,336	$ 20,302	$ 21,318	$ 22,383	$ 23,503
Estimated annual growth rate in recurring expenses	5.00%									
Forecasted annual expense	$ 23,950	$ 15,908	$ 16,703	$ 17,538	$ 18,415	$ 19,336	$ 20,302	$ 21,318	$ 22,383	$ 23,503
Forecasted annual net income	$ 250	$ 9,268	$ 9,487	$ 9,707	$ 9,928	$ 10,150	$ 10,371	$ 10,592	$ 10,812	$ 11,031

Net present value (NPV) calculation

This estimates the present value of the future annual net income stream
Calculation is based on your selected discount rate

Selected discount rate	15.00%
Net present value	$ 41,499
Initial cost of project (price of equipment)	$ 40,000

Sensitivity analysis

This shows the reduction in net present value if revenue forecasts fall short of the original estimate

90% of forecasted revenue NPV	$ 27,534
80% of forecasted revenue NPV	$ 13,569
70% of forecasted revenue NPV	$ (396)

Figure L-1 Example of a spreadsheet that can help determine if purchasing equipment makes fiscal sense for a practice.

physician can't also be seeing patients in the office or otherwise generating revenue. For physician-intense equipment, such as colonoscopes and lasers, you must factor in the physician time expense into the annual expenses. Other office-based procedures, such as densitometry, are performed by a technician and require very little time for the physician to interpret the results. Adding a procedure or service that does not require much time input from the physician, although modest in revenue, may ultimately prove to be a better investment for the practice than adding a procedure that requires a lot of physician labor, even though that procedure may produce more revenue. An exception might be a situation such as a laser procedure in which a technician administers the treatment under supervision of the physician. Under those circumstances physician time must be considered at least for the initial consultation, and the technician cost must be included in the expenses.

It is a good exercise for any practice to determine what the average hourly net income is for each physician in the practice. Once that number is determined you can estimate the average hourly net income for an examination room in the office. It is not a good idea to place machinery in an examination room that ultimately produces net income less than that produced by usual patient care, unless the examination room is underutilized anyway. Similarly, it is not a good idea to have physicians switch to doing procedures that result in an hourly net income that is lower than what they produce through usual patient care. Therefore, certain strategic and career decisions may significantly affect this sort of decision. Just be aware that, because of limited resources, a decision to do one thing will typically result in an inability to do another thing.

Forecast the Annual Growth Rate for Revenue and Expense

Revenue growth depends on the *expected increase in number of procedures* performed as well as the *change in reimbursement per procedure*. In the densitometry example it is forecasted that there will be a 3% annual growth rate in number of procedures performed and a 1% growth rate in revenue per procedure performed. If you don't think the growth will be a simple percentage annual increase, but instead might increase rapidly over the first few years and then taper off, then go ahead and manually enter the annual number of procedures forecast to be performed each year.

At the minimum, you should estimate that expenses will increase at a typical inflation rate, maybe 3% to 4%. However, for various reasons, medical expense growth seems to have outpaced inflation in recent years. For the densitometry example we have forecasted an annual growth in expenses of 5%.

Estimate the Terminal Value

Most medical equipment wears out, becomes obsolete, or for some reason has to be replaced after some finite period of time. You may be able to sell the equipment to a used machinery vendor or get some trade-in value if buying a replacement, but often the equipment has minimal value at the end of its useful life. It may be that you will be building some sort of business or revenue stream that might have value to a third party. If you can estimate what the resale value of the equipment or the sale value of the business would be at the end of the term under consideration, then you can add that value to the revenue received during the final year of the project. There are other ways to handle the so-called "terminal value," but for our purposes this method will work well.

Estimate the Risk of the Project

If you have gotten this far in your financial analysis then you should have a series of net annual income numbers along the bottom of your spreadsheet. That is what would be called the *annual cash flow for the project*. The Excel spreadsheet program has an extremely useful function called *net present value (NPV)* that indicates what the value of those cash flows is right now. When we compute the NPV of those cash flows we can then easily compare the value of the cash flows over time, the NPV, to the cost or purchase price of the piece of equipment under consideration. If the NPV exceeds the purchase price, then the project is likely to be profitable. If the NPV does not meet the purchase price, then the project is a loser. When comparing two possible projects for likelihood of success, the project with the greatest NPV will likely be more financially successful. In calculating the value of the cash flows in today's dollars, the NPV calculation is easily able to compare projects of different duration, projects that may or may not have any residual value at the end of their expected lifetime, and projects with cash flows that vary over time.

In order to compute the NPV in Excel you will need the annual cash flows. To use Excel correctly, create and label a cell called NPV below your annual cash flow line. Next, insert the function called NPV. A dialogue box will appear that asks for "Rate," which will be described next, and "Value 1." Click on the "Value 1" box and then drag the cursor across the annual cash flow line from the beginning to the end of the project. That will enter the annual cash flows into the formula. Ignore "Value 2."

You will also need to insert a number in your spreadsheet called the *discount rate*. When you open the dialogue box for the NPV function in Excel it is called "Rate." The discount rate is a numerical estimate of the risk of the project. Think of the discount rate as the interest rate you would have to pay an outside investor to invest money in your project. If you were selling Treasury bonds backed by the U.S. government, an investor would not require much of a premium beyond the bonds' interest rate to buy Treasury bonds from you because the payment of the interest and principle is virtually a sure thing. However, if you were buying a piece of office equipment to start a medical service in which you had little experience and there was a great deal of competition in your area providing the same service, then an outside investor might ask for a high interest rate, say 20%, because your chance of success and the investor's chance of being repaid is much less than if Treasury bills were the investment. The riskier the project, the higher the interest rate an investor will require because the failure rate increases and the risk of not being fully repaid increases. Investors require higher potential returns for assuming more risk.

Choosing a high discount rate, reflecting a high-risk venture, will cause the NPV of the future cash flows to be lower, whereas a low discount rate will increase the NPV. There is no ideal or perfect way to choose a discount rate. Using 15% is a reasonable discount rate to start with, adding 5 percentage points if you think the project is high risk, and reducing by 5 percentage points if you think the project is rock solid. By varying the discount rate you can see the rate at which the project breaks even; that is, it returns over time the initial investment in the purchase or startup price of the project. If a discount rate less than 10% is required just to break even, you don't have much room for error on your project. Conversely, if a 30% discount rate still yields a NPV above your startup cost, then you have a project with a greater chance of profitability.

You can find the NPV function on the Excel spreadsheet by going to the menu across the top of the worksheet and finding "Insert." Pull down to "Function" and you will be given a list of possibilities. Choose NPV, or Net Present Value, and you will be shown a dialog box where you enter your chosen discount rate and your estimated annual cash flows. Enter the annual cash flows in the box called "Value 1," and enter your chosen discount rate in the box called "Rate." Percentage is entered as a decimal; for example, a chosen rate of 15% is entered in the "Rate" box as .15. Excel will then return the NPV for you to consider when you click "OK." You can ignore the box called "Value 2."

Perform a Sensitivity Analysis

The next step is to challenge some of your forecasts. In performing a sensitivity analysis, you are going to make your forecasts for growth in annual revenue less optimistic, and your forecasts for expense growth more pessimistic. In making these changes in your forecast observe the effect the changes have on the NPV. The greater the amount that the NPV (i.e., the worth of the project over time) exceeds the cost of doing the project, the more likely that the project will be a financial success for you. Similarly, if the NPV exceeds the cost of doing the project, even when your sensitivity analysis subjects your revenue forecasts to only 60% or 70% of the originally forecasted net income, the more likely that your project will be a financial success. Conversely, if the NPV barely exceeds the cost of the project or the NPV actually drops below the cost of the project with minimal reduction in the net income forecasted, then it becomes more likely that the project will be a financial failure, especially when you factor in any "lost" opportunity cost.

It may be true that certain projects have "value" beyond the NPV. Adding a service line through purchase of new equipment may prevent a competitor from doing the same. By adding a procedure to your practice, you may learn a new skill that will allow you to do something else later that has financial benefits. The addition of a service line or procedure may simply make your practice more interesting and enjoyable. However, although these "intangibles" may have bearing on the final decision, just as the opportunity cost may, the most useful and reliable analytic tool that you can bring to the decision-making table is the NPV. Learning to make a forecast of cash flows for your project, estimating risk, calculating the NPV, and relying on this result to guide your decision to buy office equipment will greatly increase your chance of making the right decision.

Take a look at the dexitometry example. The NPV of the cash flows over the 10 years of the project using a 15% discount rate is $41,499. That barely exceeds the asking price of the machine, which is $40,000. Effectively, that means that 10 years of densitometry will result in a profit of $1,499. That is a paltry return on a $40,000 investment. You'd be better off buying Treasury bonds and leaving that examination room empty or using it for storage until you find something better to do with it. However, let's say you went back to the salesperson and offered $28,000 for the machine and the offer was accepted. The expected profit would then increase to $13,499, which is around a 3% annual return on the $40,000, still not a great return but beginning to look more reasonable. You can see how knowing the NPV gives you a much firmer foundation to negotiate. A price of $40,000 would simply be unacceptable for the machine under these circumstances.

Establishing your demand price and walk-away price for purposes of negotiation is a great use of the NPV. You will be much less likely to overpay for equipment, office space, or any capital asset if you have a good sense of the current value (NPV) of your proposed project. The NPV is also useful when two or more potential projects might be competing in your mind for the same space, financial resources, or staff resources. If you use the same rigorous approach to developing the annual cash flows for each project, and appropriately assign a discount rate to each project based upon a fair estimate of the inherent risk of each project, then you will arrive at two NPVs that can be easily compared. Obviously, forecasts are subjective and subject to bias, but if you are even-handed in preparing your financial analysis, and then subject each project to a sensitivity analysis, you can create a best case, expected case, and worst case scenario for each project and then compare them side by side. This method requires less of a "gut" reaction or "seat of the pants" decision, but you will be far more competent at making financial decisions.

Conclusion

Just as you might practice suturing on pig's foot, you have to practice NPV estimates by making a spreadsheet and "tinkering" around with the revenue forecasts, the expense forecasts, and the discount rate. In so doing you will get a better understanding of what drives the value in a project, just as you might learn how different suture techniques affect the final appearance of a wound closure. Although your goal in a wound closure is an aesthetically appealing result for your patient, your goal in learning how to calculate the NPV is to win the negotiation with your vendor, your landlord, your banker, your broker, or anybody otherwise trying to take advantage of you in a sale. This may not be what you went to medical school for, but it is a handy skill if you want your practice to be more successful.

Bibliography

Buford GA, House S: Beauty and the Business. Garden City, NY, Morgan James, 2010.

ONLINE ASSETS

The following forms are available at www.expertconsult.com.

PATIENT EDUCATION HANDOUTS

ActiveFX Laser Fractional Skin Resurfacing Patient Education Handout
ActiveFX Laser Fractional Skin Resurfacing (Postprocedure) Patient Education Handout
ActiveFX Laser Fractional Skin Resurfacing (Preprocedure) Patient Education Handout
Acupuncture Patient Education Handout
Adult Circumcision Patient Education Handout
Ambulatory Blood Pressure Monitoring Patient Education Handout
Amniocentesis (Postprocedure) Patient Education Handout
Anal Fissures Patient Education Handout
Androscopy Patient Education Handout
Anesthesia for Upper Endoscopy Patient Education Handout
Arterial Puncture Patient Education Handout
Bifid Earlobe Repair Patient Education Handout
Body Piercing Patient Education Handout
Bone Marrow Aspiration/Biopsy Patient Education Handout
Botox Injections: Treatment for Skin Wrinkles, Excessive Sweating, and Headaches Patient Education Handout
Bowel Preparation for Sigmoidoscopy Patient Education Handout
Breast Biopsy Patient Education Handout
Cast Care Patient Education Handout
Casts and Splint Care Patient Education Handout
Cervical Polyps/Polypectomy Patient Education Handout
Cervical Stenosis and Cervical Dilation Patient Education Handout
Chemical Peels Patient Education Handout
Cold-Knife Conization of the Cervix (Cone Biopsy) Patient Education Handout
Colonoscopy: GoLYTELY Preparation Patient Education Handout
Colonoscopy Patient Education Handout
Colonoscopy (Preprocedure) Patient Education Handout
Colposcopy Patient Education Handout
Colposcopy and Biopsy (Postprocedure) Patient Education Handout
Contraction Stress Test Patient Education Handout
Corns and Calluses of the Feet Patient Education Handout
Crutch Use Patient Education Handout
Cryotherapy (Freezing) Patient Education Handout
Cryotherapy of the Cervix Patient Education Handout
Cryotherapy of the Cervix (Postprocedure) Patient Education Handout
Dilation and Curettage (D&C) Patient Education Handout
Dorsal Slit for Phimosis Patient Education Handout
Emergency Contraception Patient Education Handout
Endometrial Ablation Patient Education Handout
Endometrial Biopsy Patient Education Handout
Endovenous Radiofrequency/Laser Treatment for Varicose Veins (Postprocedure)
Endovenous Radiofrequency/Laser Treatment for Varicose Veins (Preprocedure)
Epidural Anesthesia Patient Education Handout
Epilation of Isolated Hairs (Postprocedure) Patient Education Handout
Epistaxis (Nosebleed) Patient Education Handout
Esophagogastroduodenoscopy (EGD) Patient Education Handout
Esophagogastroduodenoscopy (EGD) (Postprocedure) Patient Education Handout
Esophagogastroduodenoscopy (EGD) (Preprocedure) Patient Education Handout
External Cephalic Version (ECV) Patient Education Handout
Fetal Movement Counting Patient Education Handout
Fine-Needle Aspiration (FNA) Patient Education Handout
Flexible Sigmoidoscopy Patient Education Handout
Foreign Body Removal from Nose or Ear Patient Education Handout
Gastric Lavage Patient Education Handout
Hemorrhoids Patient Education Handout
Hemorrhoids (Postprocedure) Patient Education Handout
Home Wound Care Patient Education Handout
How to Insert and Use a Diaphragm Patient Education Handout
How to Use Condoms for Contraception and Disease Prevention Patient Education Handout
HPV and Genital Warts Patient Education Handout
Ingrown Toenails Patient Education Handout
Intense Pulsed Light and Nd:YAG Laser Patient Education Handout
Intraosseous Venous Access (IOVA) Patient Education Handout
Intrathecal Analgesia for Labor Patient Education Handout
Knee Braces Patient Education Handout
Laser Hair Removal Patient Education Handout
Loop Electrosurgical Excision Procedure (LEEP) Patient Education Handout
Lumbar Puncture Patient Education Handout
MDT (Maggot Débridement Therapy) Patient Education Handout
Microdermabrasion Patient Education Handout
Moist Healing after Skin Surgery Patient Education Handout
Mucocele Treatment Patient Education Handout
Muscle Biopsy Patient Education Handout
Nail Biopsy Patient Education Handout
Newborn Circumcision Patient Education Handout
Nonstress Test Patient Education Handout
Obstetric Ultrasound Patient Education Handout
Office Electrocardiograms (ECG) Patient Education Handout
Pap Smear Patient Education Handout
Paracervical Block Patient Education Handout
Pediatric Sedation Patient Education Handout
Peripheral Nerve Blocks and Field Blocks Patient Education Handout
Permanent Female Sterilization (Tubal Ligation) Patient Education Handout
Pessary Patient Education Handout
Photodynamic Therapy Procedure Patient Education Handout
Photoepilation/Laser Hair Removal Patient Education Handout
Postpartum Tubal Ligation Patient Education Handout
Procedural Sedation Patient Education Handout
Prostate Ultrasound and Biopsy Patient Education Handout
Pulmonary Artery Catheterization Patient Education Handout
Radiage Patient Education Handout
Radiofrequency Hair Removal Patient Education Handout
Repair of Extensor Tendon(s) Injury Patient Education Handout
Saddle Block Anesthesia Patient Education Handout
Sclerotherapy (Postprocedure) Patient Education Handout
Sclerotherapy (Vein Injection) Patient Education Handout
Self-Injection Therapy for Impotence Patient Education Handout
Sexual Abuse Patient Education Handout
Sexual Assault Patient Education Handout
SilkPeel Dermalinfusion System Patient Education Handout
Skin Graft (Postprocedure) Patient Education Handout
Skin Peels Patient Education Handout
Subungual Hematoma Evacuation Patient Education Handout
Suture Care Patient Education Handout
Tattoo Removal (Post-Laser) Patient Education Handout
Temporary Pacing Patient Education Handout
Thoracentesis Patient Education Handout
Thoracentesis (Postprocedure) Patient Education Handout
Tick-borne Diseases: What You Should Know Patient Education Handout
Tick Removal and Prevention of Infection Patient Education Handout
Tonometry Patient Education Handout
Tonsillectomy and/or Adenoidectomy Patient Education Handout
Tracheostomy Patient Education Handout
Transcervical Amnioinfusion Patient Education Handout
Transcutaneous Electrical Nerve Stimulation (TENS), Phonophoresis, and Iontophoresis Patient Education Handout

Trauma to Extremities and Avoidance of Compartment Syndrome Patient Education Handout
Tubal Ligation (Postprocedure) Patient Education Handout
Tympanocentesis/Myringotomy Postprocedure Patient Education Handout
Urinary Catheter Care Patient Education Handout
Urodynamic Testing Patient Education Handout
Uterine Aspiration (Postprocedure) Patient Education Handout
Vacuum Devices for Erectile Dysfunction Patient Education Handout
Vaginal Delivery Aftercare Patient Education Handout
Vasectomy Patient Education Worksheet
Vasectomy (Postprocedure) Patient Education Handout
Vulvar Biopsy Patient Education Handout
Wart Removal Patient Education Handout
Wart (Verruca) Treatment Patient Education Handout
Wound Care after Cryosurgery Patient Education Handout
Wound Care after Treatment with Topical Skin Adhesive (Tissue Glue) Patient Education Handout

PATIENT CONSENT FORMS

ActiveFX Laser Fractional Skin Resurfacing Patient Consent Form
ALA Photodynamic Therapy Procedure Patient Consent Form
Ambulatory Phlebectomy Patient Consent Form
Amniocentesis Patient Consent Form
Amniotomy Patient Consent Form
Arterial Puncture Patient Consent Form
Body Piercing Patient Consent Form
Bone Marrow Aspiration/Biopsy Patient Consent Form
Botox Cosmetic Patient Consent Form
Botox Injections Patient Consent Form
Breast Biopsy Patient Consent Form
Breast Mass Aspiration/Thyroid Mass Aspiration Patient Consent Form
Cardiac Exercise Testing Patient Consent Form
Cardiac Procedure: Cardioversion Patient Consent Form
Cervical Conization Patient Consent Form
Cervical Polypectomy Patient Consent Form
Cervical Stenosis and Cervical Dilation Patient Consent Form
Chalazion Excision Patient Consent Form
Circumcision/Dorsal Penile Nerve Block Patient Consent Form
Colonoscopy, Biopsy, and Polypectomy Patient Consent Form
Contraction Stress Test Patient Consent Form
Dilation and Curettage (D&C) Request Patient Consent Form
Dorsal Slit for Phimosis Patient Consent Form
Endometrial Biopsy Patient Consent Form
Endovenous Laser Treatment for Varicose Veins Patient Consent Form
Epistaxis (Nosebleed) Patient Consent Form
Esophagogastroduodenoscopy (EGD) Patient Consent Form
External Cephalic Version (ECV) Patient Consent Form
Fetal Movement Counting Patient Consent Form
Fine-Needle Aspiration (FNA) Patient Consent Form
Flexible Sigmoidoscopy Patient Consent Form
Foreign Body Removal from Nose or Ear Patient Consent Form
Forensic Evaluation Patient Consent Form
Hysteroscopic Sterilization (Essure) Procedure Patient Consent Form
Implanon (Etonogestrel Implant) Patient Consent Form
Intraosseous Venous Access (IOVA) Patient Consent Form
Intrathecal Analgesia in Labor Patient Consent Form
Knee Braces Patient Consent Form
Laser Hair Removal Patient Consent Form
Laser Surgery for Spider Veins Patient Consent Form
Lumbar Puncture Patient Consent Form
McDonald's Cerclage Patient Consent Form
Microdermabrasion Patient Consent Form
Mifepristone/Misoprostol Abortion Patient Consent Form
Muscle Biopsy Patient Consent Form
Nail Biopsy Patient Consent Form
Nonstress Test Patient Consent Form
Obstetric Ultrasound Patient Consent Form
Occipital Nerve Block Patient Consent Form
Paracervical Block Patient Consent Form
Peripheral Nerve Blocks and Field Blocks Patient Consent Form
Photoepilation/Laser Hair Removal Patient Consent Form
Procedural Sedation Patient Consent Form
Radiofrequency Hair Removal Patient Consent Form
Repair of Extensor Tendon(s) Injury Patient Consent Form
Sclerotherapy Patient Consent Form
SilkPeel Dermalinfusion System Patient Consent Form
Skin Lesion Excision (Elective) Patient Consent Form
Skin Surgery Patient Consent Form
Subungual Hematoma Evacuation Patient Consent Form
Tattoo Removal Patient Consent Form
Thoracentesis Patient Consent Form
Tonometry Patient Consent Form
Tracheostomy Patient Consent Form
Transcervical Amnioinfusion Patient Consent Form
Transrectal Ultrasound of the Prostate with or without Biopsy Patient Consent Form
Trigger-Point Injection Patient Consent Form
Tympanocentesis/Myringotomy Patient Consent Form
Uterine Aspiration Patient Consent Form
Vacuum Devices for Erectile Dysfunction Patient Consent Form
Vaginal Delivery Patient Consent Form
Vasectomy Patient Consent Form
Vitalize Peel Treatment Patient Consent Form
Vulvar Biopsy Patient Consent Form

MISCELLANEOUS

ActiveFX Laser Fractional Skin Resurfacing Patient Encounter Form
Aesthetic Dermafiller Treatment Record
Aesthetic Services Patient Profile: Burn Treatment
Ambulatory Phlebectomy Sample Operative Report
American Academy of Family Physicians' Position Paper on Endoscopy
Amniotomy Sample Operative Report
Androscopy Patient Encounter Form
Androscopy Procedure Follow-up Form
Blepharoplasty Sample Operative Report
Bone Marrow Aspiration/Biopsy Sample Operative Report
Botox (OnabotulinumtoxinA) Injection Record
Breast Biopsy Sample Operative Report
BTX-A Headache Treatment Record
Cervical Polyps Sample Operative Report
Cesarean Section Sample Operative Report
Chalazion Excision Sample Operative Report
Chemical Peels Progress Note
Colon Cancer Screening Options Vary (Editorial)
Colposcopy Patient Encounter Form
Cryotherapy of the Cervix Sample Operative Report
Diagnostic Peritoneal Lavage Sample Operative Report
Diagnostic Ultrasonography Checklist
Dorsal Slit Technique Sample Operative Report
Endometrial Biopsy Patient Encounter Form
Endovenous Laser Vein Closure Treatment Form
Epilation of Isolated Hairs Sample Operative Report
Essure Confirmation Test Checklist
Essure Confirmation Test Overview
External Cephalic Version (ECV) Sample Operative Report
Hemorrhoids Initial Encounter Form
Hemorrhoid Treatment Summary
Implanon Insertion/Removal Patient Encounter Form
Intrathecal Analgesia Sample Operative Report
Intrauterine Pressure Catheter Insertion Sample Operative Report
Nail Biopsy Patient Encounter Form
NC-stat System for Office EMGs Sample Operative Report
Occipital Nerve Block Patient Encounter Form
Office Testing and Treatment Options for Interstitial Cystitis: Permeability Study
Office Testing and Treatment Options for Interstitial Cystitis: PORIS Form
Pediatric Arterial Puncture Sample Operative Report
Pediatric Venous Minicutdown Sample Operative Report
Peritonsillar Abscess Drainage Sample Operative Report
Preprocedure Sedation Assessment Flowsheet
Radiofrequency Hair Removal Patient Encounter Form
Sclerotherapy Billing Procedures Physician Handout
Thoracentesis Sample Operative Report
Tongue-Tie Snipping (Frenotomy) for Ankyloglossia Sample Operative Report
Ultrasonography-guided Preprocedure Checklist
Vasectomy Patient Encounter Form
Vasectomy Questionnaire

INDEX

Page numbers followed by f refer to figures; page numbers followed by t refer to tables; page numbers followed by b refer to boxes.

A

B

E

O

S

T

V

W